Cardiology

Section Editors

Gerard P. Aurigemma MD
Professor of Medicine and Radiology
University of Massachusetts Medical School
Director of Noninvasive Cardiology
Director, Cardiology Fellowship Training Program
UMass Memorial Medical Center
Worcester, Massachusetts

George L. Bakris MD
Professor of Medicine
University of Chicago Pritzker School of Medicine
Director, Hypertensive Diseases Unit
Section of Endocrinology, Diabetes and Metabolism
University of Chicago Medical Center
Chicago, Illinois

Helmut Drexler MD
Professor of Medicine
Chief, Division of Cardiology
Medical University of Hannover
Hannover, Germany

Erling Falk MD, PhD
Professor of Cardiovascular Pathology
Institute of Clinical Medicine
Aarhus University Hospital Skejby
Aarhus, Denmark

Michael A. Gatzoulis MD, PhD, FACC, FESC
Professor of Cardiology
National Heart and Lung Institute
Imperial College London
Head, Adult Congenital Heart Centre and
Centre for Pulmonary Hypertension
Royal Brompton Hospital
London, United Kingdom

George J. Klein MD, FRCPC, FACC
Professor, Department of Medicine
University of Western Ontario
London, Ontario, Canada

William J. Kostuk MD, FRCPC
Emeritus Professor of Medicine
Schulich School of Medicine & Dentistry
University of Western Ontario
Consultant, Cardiology Division
University Hospital
London, Ontario, Canada

Gregory Y H Lip MD, FRCP, DFM, FESC, FACC
Professor of Cardiovascular Medicine
University Department of Medicine
City Hospital
Birmingham, United Kingdom

Barry M. Massie MD
Professor of Medicine
UCSF School of Medicine
Chief, Cardiology Division
San Francisco VA Medical Center
San Francisco, California

David J. Sahn MD, MACC, FAHA
Professor of Pediatrics (Cardiology),
Diagnostic Radiology, Obstetrics and
Gynecology, and Biomedical Engineering
Oregon Health & Science University
Portland, Oregon

Prediman K. Shah MD, FACC, FACP, FCCP
Shapell and Webb Chair and Director
Division of Cardiology
Oppenheimer Atherosclerosis Research Center
Cedars Sinai Medical Center
Professor of Medicine
David Geffen School of Medicine at UCLA
Los Angeles, California

David Waters MD
Emeritus Professor
Department of Medicine
UCSF School of Medicine
San Francisco, California

Cardiology

Third Edition

Michael H. Crawford MD
Professor of Medicine
Lucie Stern Chair in Cardiology
University of California, San Francisco
Interim Chief of Cardiology
UCSF Medical Center
San Francisco, California

John P. DiMarco MD, PhD
Julian R. Beckwith Professor of Medicine
University of Virginia School of Medicine
Director, Cardiac Electrophysiology Laboratory
Cardiovascular Division
University of Virginia Health System
Charlottesville, Virginia

Walter J. Paulus MD, PhD, FESC
Professor of Cardiac Pathophysiology
Department of Physiology
Faculty of Medicine
Free University Amsterdam
Associate Director
Cardiovascular Center
VU University Medical Center
Amsterdam, The Netherlands

MOSBY

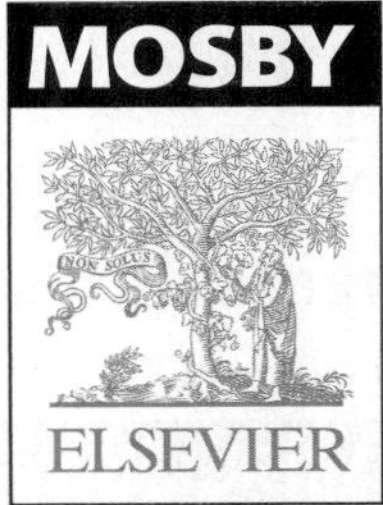

ELSEVIER

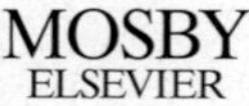

1600 John F. Kennedy Blvd.
Ste 1800
Philadelphia, PA 19103-2899

CARDIOLOGY ISBN: 978-0-7234-3485-6

Notice

Knowledge and best practice in this field are constantly changing. As new research and experience broaden our knowledge, changes in practice, treatment, and drug therapy may become necessary or appropriate. Readers are advised to check the most current information provided (i) on procedures featured or (ii) by the manufacturer of each product to be administered, to verify the recommended dose or formula, the method and duration of administration, and contraindications. It is the responsibility of the practitioner, relying on his or her experience and knowledge of the patient, to make diagnoses, to determine dosages and the best treatment for each individual patient, and to take all appropriate safety precautions. To the fullest extent of the law, neither the Publisher nor the Editors assume any liability for any injury and/or damage to persons or property arising out of or related to any use of the material contained in this book.

The Publisher

Library of Congress Cataloging-in-Publication Data
Cardiology / [edited by] Michael H. Crawford . . . [et al.]. — 3rd ed.
p. ; cm.
Includes bibliographical references and index.
ISBN 978-0-7234-3485-6
1. Cardiology. I. Crawford, Michael H., 1943–
[DNLM: 1. Heart Diseases—diagnosis. 2. Heart Diseases—etiology. 3. Heart Diseases—therapy.
WG 100 C2655 2010]
RC667.C377 2010
616.1′2—dc22 2009018142

Acquisitions Editor: Natasha Andjelkovic
Developmental Editor: Pamela Hetherington
Publishing Services Manager: Linda Van Pelt
Project Manager: Frank Morales
Design Direction: Lou Forgione

Printed in China

Last digit is the print number: 9 8 7 6 5 4 3 2 1

Contributors

Nicola Abate, MD
Professor, Chief Division of Endocrinology, University of Texas Medical Branch, Galveston, Texas, USA

Ahmed Tageldien Abdellah, MD
Professor of Cardiology, Hull York Medical School, University of Hull, Castle Hill Hospital, Kingston upon Hull, United Kingdom

Jonathan Abrams, MD
Professor of Medicine, Division of Cardiology, Department of Internal Medicine, University of New Mexico School of Medicine, Albuquerque, New Mexico, USA

Christophe Acar, MD
Professor of Cardiac Surgery, Université Pierre et Marie Curie–Paris VI, Staff Surgeon, CHU Pitié-Salpêtrière Hospital, Paris, France

Jean Acar, MD
Professor Emeritus of Cardiology, Université Pierre et Marie Curie–Paris VI, Former Chief, Department of Cardiology, CHU Tenon Hospital, Paris, France

Harry Acquatella, MD, FACC, FAHA
Professor of Medicine, Faculty of Medicine, Universidad Central de Venezuela, Centro Medico, Caracas, Venezuela

M. Jacob Adams, MD, MPH
Assistant Professor of Community and Preventive Medicine, Division of Epidemiology, University of Rochester School of Medicine and Dentistry, Rochester, New York, USA

Teiji Akagi, MD, PhD, FACC, FAHA
Associate Professor, Department of Cardiovascular Surgery, Okayama University Graduate School of Medicine and Dentistry, Attending, Cardiac Intensive Care Unit, Okayama University Hospital, Okayama, Japan

Inder S. Anand, MD, FRCP, DPhil (Oxon)
Professor of Medicine, University of Minnesota Medical School, Director, Heart Failure Program, Minneapolis VA Medical Center, Minneapolis, Minnesota, USA

David E. Anderson, PhD
Senior Investigator, Cancer research Branch, National Institute on Aging, Baltimore, Maryland, USA

Henning Rud Andersen, MD, DMSc
Associate Professor of Cardiology, University of Aarhus Faculty of Health Sciences, Cardiac Electrophysiologist, Aarhus University Hospital Skejby, Aarhus, Denmark

Mark E. Anderson, MD, PhD
Professor of Internal Medicine, University of Iowa Carver College of Medicine, Director, Division of Cardiovascular Medicine, University of Iowa Hospitals and Clinics, Iowa City, Iowa, USA

Christiane E. Angermann, MD
Professor of Medicine and Cardiology, University of Würzburg Faculty of Medicine, Head, Division of Cardiology (Polyclinic), Department of Medicine I, University Hospital Würzburg, Würzburg, Germany

Stefan D. Anker, MD, PhD
Professor of Cardiology and Cachexia Research, Division of Applied Cachexia Research, Department of Cardiology, Charité University Medical School, Campus Virchow-Klinikum, Berlin, Germany

Ramon Arroyo-Espliguero, MD
Associate Professor of Cardiology, University of Guadalajara Faculty of Medicine, Consultant Cardiologist, Hospital General Universitario, Guadalajara, Spain

Gerard P. Aurigemma, MD
Professor of Medicine and Radiology, University of Massachusetts Medical School, Director of Noninvasive Cardiology, Director, Cardiology Fellowship Training Program, UMass Memorial Medical Center, Worcester, Massachusetts, USA

Sonya V. Babu-Narayan, MBBS, BSc, MRCP
Honorary Clinical Research Fellow, National Heart and Lung Institute, Imperial College London, Specialist Registrar, Adult Congenital Heart Disease, Royal Brompton Hospital, London, United Kingdom

George L. Bakris, MD
Professor of Medicine, University of Chicago Pritzker School of Medicine, Director, Hypertensive Diseases Unit, Section of Endocrinology, Diabetes and Metabolism University of Chicago Medical Center, Chicago, Illinois, USA

Malcolm Barlow, MBBS, FRACP, FCANZCS
Conjoint Senior Lecturer, School of Medicine and Public Health, Faculty of Health, University of Newcastle, Newcastle, Senior Staff Specialist, John Hunter Hospital, New Lambton, New South Wales, Australia

Margot M. Bartelings, MD, PhD
Assistant Professor of Cardiac Pathophysiology, Department of Anatomy and Embryology, Leiden University Medical Center, Leiden, The Netherlands

George A. Beller, MD
Ruth C. Heede Professor of Cardiology and Internal Medicine, University of Virginia School of Medicine, Charlottesville, Virginia, USA

Lisa J. Bergerson, MD
Assistant Professor in Pediatrics, Harvard Medical School, Associate in Cardiology, Children's Hospital Boston, Boston, Massachusetts, USA

Sandro Betocchi, MD, FACC, FESC
Professor of Cardiology, Department of Clinical Medicine–Cardiovascular and Immunological Sciences, University of Naples Federico II School of Medicine and Surgery, Chief, Cardiology Consultant Service, Federico II University Hospital, Naples, Italy

Ami B. Bhatt, MD
Fellow in Cardiology, Brigham and Women's Hospital, Boston, Massachusetts, USA

Kalkidan G. Bishu, MD
Resident, Department of Medicine, Minneapolis VA Medical Center, Minneapolis, Minnesota, USA

Reidar Bjørnerheim, MD, PhD, FESC
Head, Department of Cardiology, Oslo University Hospital, Ulleval, Oslo, Norway

Hans Erik Bøtker, MD, PhD, DMSc
Professor of Cardiology, University of Aarhus Faculty of Health Sciences, Consultant Interventional Cardiologist, Aarhus University Hospital Skejby, Aarhus, Denmark

Harm Jan Bosaard, MD, PhD
Assistant Professor of Medicine, Department of Internal Medicine, Virginia Commonwealth University School of Medicine, Victoria W. Johnson Center for Obstructive Lung Disease Research, VCU Health System, Richmond, Virginia, USA

Jamieson Bourque, MD, MHS (ClinRes)
Fellow in Advanced Imaging and Cardiovascular Disease, University of Virginia Health System, Charlottesville, Virginia, USA

Craig Broberg, MD, FACC
Assistant Professor of Medicine, Oregon Health & Science University School of Medicine, Director, Adult Congenital Heart Disease Program, OHSU Hospital, Portland, Oregon, USA

Fiona Brodie, MBBS, MRCP(UK)
Stroke Research Fellow, University of Leicester College of Medicine, Biological and Psychological Science, Leicester, United Kingdom

W. Virgil Brown, MD
Charles Howard Candler Professor of Medicine, Emory University School of Medicine, Chief of Medicine, Atlanta VA Medical Center, Atlanta, Georgia, USA

David A. Calhoun, MD
Professor of Medicine, Vascular Biology and Hypertension Program, University of Alabama at Birmingham School of Medicine, Birmingham, Alabama, USA

Francesco P. Cappuccio, MBBS, MD, MSc, FRCP, FFPH, FAHA
Professor and Cephalon Chair of Cardiovascular Medicine & Epidemiology, University of Warwick Medical School/ Clinical Sciences Research Institute, Consultant Cardiovascular Physician, University Hospitals Coventry & Warwickshire NHS Trust, Coventry, United Kingdom

Blase A. Carabello, MD, FACC
Professor of Medicine, Baylor College of Medicine, Chief of Medicine, Michael E. DeBakey VA Medical Center, Houston, Texas, USA

John G. Carr, MD
Assistant Professor of Medicine, Boston University School of Medicine, Cardiac Electrophysiologist, Boston Medical Center, Boston, Massachusetts, USA

John D. Carroll, MD
Professor of Medicine, University of Colorado Denver School of Medicine, Director, Section of Interventional Cardiology, University of Colorado Hospital, Aurora, Colorado, USA

Filip P. Casselman, MD, PhD, FETCS
Staff Surgeon, Department of Cardiovascular and Thoracic Surgery, Atrial Fibrillation Clinic, Onze Lieve Vrouw (OLV) Hospital, Aalst, Belgium

David Celermajer, MBBS, PhD, DSc, FRACP
Scandrett Professor of Cardiology, University of Sydney Faculty of Medicine, Clinical Academic Cardiologist, Director, Adult Congenital Heart Disease, Royal Prince Albert Hospital, Sydney, New South Wales, Australia

Bojan Cercek, MD, PhD
Professor of Medicine, David Geffen School of Medicine at UCLA, Director, Coronary Care Units, Co-Director, Atherosclerosis Research Center at Cedars-Sinai Medical Center, Los Angeles, California, USA

Philippe Charron, MD, PhD
Associate Professor, Université Pierre et Marie Curie–Paris VI, Department of Genetics, CHU Pitié-Salpêtrière Hospital, Paris, France

Shi-Ann Chen, MD
Professor of Medicine, Department of Medicine, Division of Cardiology, National Yang-Ming University School of Medicine, Attending Cardiologist, Taipei Veterans General Hospital, Taipei, Taiwan

Alice Yuk-Yan Cheng, MD, FRCPC
Assistant Professor (Adjunct), Department of Medicine, University of Toronto Faculty of Medicine, Staff Endocrinologist, St. Michael's Hospital, Toronto, Staff Endocrinologist, Credit Valley Hospital, Mississauga, Ontario, Canada

Margaret A. Chesney, PhD
Professor of Medicine, University of Maryland School of Medicine, Baltimore, Maryland, USA

Bernard Cheung, PhD, FRCP
Professor of Clinical Pharmacology and Therapeutics, College of Medical and Dental Sciences, University of Birmingham, Honorary Consultant, University Hospital Birmingham, Birmingham, United Kingdom

Massimo Chiarello, MD
Professor of Cardiology, Department of Clinical Medicine–Cardiovascular and Immunological Sciences, University of Naples Federico II School of Medicine and Surgery, Chief, Cardiology, Federico II University Hospital, Naples, Italy

Dave C.Y. Chua, MD, MS
Cardiologist, Dreyer Medical Clinic, Auroa, Illinois, USA

Natali A.Y. Chung, MD, MRCP
Specialist Registrar, Adult Congenital Heart Disease, Royal Brompton Hospital, London, United Kingdom

David Churchill, MBChB, MD, FRCOG
Consultant Obstetrician, Clinical Director of Governance, The Royal Wolverhampton Hospitals NHS Trust, New Cross Hospital, Wolverhampton, United Kingdom

John G.F. Cleland, MD
Professor of Cardiology, Hull York Medical School, University of Hull, Castle Hill Hospital, Kingston upon Hull, United Kingdom

Peter Clemmensen, MD, PhD
Associate Professor of Medicine, University of Copenhagen Faculty of Health Sciences, Director, CAO Services, Department of Cardiology, Rigshospitalet, Copenhagen University Hospital, Copenhagen, Denmark

Laura J. Collins, MD, FACC, FAHA
Associate Professor of Medicine, Division of Cardiology, University of Texas Southwestern Medical School, Staff Cardiologist, Dallas VA Medical Center, Parkland Memorial Hospital, and University Hospital St. Paul, Dallas, Texas, USA

Louis S. Constine, MD, FASTRO
Professor of Radiation Oncology and Pediatrics, University of Rochester School of Medicine and Dentistry, Vice Chair and Director, Fellowship Program, Department of Radiation Oncology, James P. Wilmot Cancer Center, University of Rochester Medical Center, Rochester, New York, USA

Michael H. Crawford, MD
Professor of Medicine, Lucie Stern Chair in Cardiology, University of California, San Francisco, Interim Chief of Cardiology, UCSF Medical Center, San Francisco, California, USA

Alain Cribier, MD
Professor of Medicine, University of Rouen Medical School, Chief, Department of Cardiology, Charles Nicolle Hospital, Rouen, France

Laura Cupper, BSW
Vocational Counselor, Minto Prevention and Rehabilitation Centre, University of Ottawa Heart Institute, Ottawa, Ontario, Canada

William A. Dafoe, MD, FRCPC
Associate Professor of Medicine, Division of Cardiology, University of Alberta Faculty of Medicine & Dentistry, Regional Director, Cardiac Rehabilitation, Walter Mackenzie Centre/University of Alberta Hospitals, Edmonton, Alberta, Canada

Jayanta Das, MD
Fellow in Cardiovascular Medicine, Cedars-Sinai Medical Center, Los Angeles, California, USA

Warren Davis, MD

Professor of Medicine (retired), Emory University School of Medicine, Atlanta, Georgia, USA

G. William Dec, MD

Roman DeSanctis Professor of Medicine, Harvard Medical School, Chief, Cardiology Division, Massachusetts General Hospital, Boston, Massachusetts, USA

Prakash Deedwania, MD, FACC, FACP, FAHA

Professor of Medicine, University of California, San Francisco, School of Medicine, San Francisco, Chief, Cardiology Section, VA Medical Center Fresno, Director, Cardiovascular Research, VACCHCS/UCSF Program, Fresno, California, USA

Livio Dei Cas, MD

Divisions of Cardiac Surgery and Cardiology, University of Brescia Medical School, Brescia, Italy

Pim J. de Feyter, MD

Professor of Cardiac Imaging, Department of Cardiology, Erasmus University Medical Center, Rotterdam, The Netherlands

Gilles de Keulenaer, MD, PhD

Professor of Physiology, Department of Pharmaceutical Sciences, University of Antwerp Faculty of Medicine, Director, Laboratory of Physiology, University Hospital of Antwerp, Cardiologist and Specialist in Cardiac Rehabilitation, Middelheim Hospital, Antwerp, Belgium

Marco C. DeRuiter, PhD

Associate Professor of Anatomy and Embryology, Leiden University Medical Center, Leiden, The Netherlands

Richard B. Devereux, MD

Professor of Medicine, Weill Cornell Medical College, Attending Physician, NewYork–Presbyterian Hospital, New York, New York, USA

Abhay J. Dhond, MD, MPH, FACP

Associate Professor of Medicine, Drexel University College of Medicine, Attending, Hahnemann University Hospital, Philadelphia, Pennsylvania, USA

John P. DiMarco, MD, PhD

Julian R. Beckwith Professor of Medicine, University of Virginia School of Medicine, Director, Cardiac Electrophysiology Laboratory, Cardiovascular Division, University of Virginia Health System, Charlottesville, Virginia, USA

Konstantinos Dimopoulos, MD, MSc, PhD

Senior Fellow, National Heart and Lung Institute, Imperial College London, Associate Specialist, Royal Brompton Hospital, London, United Kingdom

Annie Dore, MD

Associate Professor of Medicine, University of Montreal Faculty of Medicine, Cardiologist, Adult Congenital Heart Center, Montreal Heart Institute, Montreal, Quebec, Canada

Paul Dorian, MD, MSc, FRCPC

Professor of Medicine, Director, Cardiology Division, University of Toronto Faculty of Medicine, Cardiac Electrophysiologist, St. Michael's Hospital, Toronto, Ontario, Canada

Pamela S. Douglas, MD, FACC

Ursula Geller Professor of Research in Cardiovascular Diseases, Professor of Medicine, Division of Neurology, Duke University School of Medicine, Head, Cardiovascular Medicine Section, Duke Clinical Research Institute, Durham, North Carolina, USA

Helmut Drexler, MD

Professor of Medicine, Chief, Division of Cardiology, Medical University of Hannover, Hannover, Germany

Jean G. Dumesnil, MD, FRCPC, FACC

Professor of Medicine, Laval University Faculty of Medicine, Cardiologist, Quebec Lung and Heart Institute, Quebec City, Quebec, Canada

Amgad El Sherif, MD

Clinical Instructor in Cardiothoracic Surgery, UPMC Presbyterian, Pittsburgh, Pennsylvania, USA

Uri Elkayam, MD

Professor of Medicine, Division of Cardiovascular Medicine, Keck School of Medicine of USC, University of Southern California, Los Angeles, California, USA

Perry M. Elliott, MD

Reader in Inherited Cardiovascular Disease, University College London Medical School, Consultant Cardiologist, University College London Hospital, London, United Kingdom

William J. Elliott, MD, PhD

Professor of Preventive Medicine, Internal Medicine, and Pharmacology, Rush Medical College, Attending Physician, Rush University Medical Center, Chicago, Illinois, USA

Alexander Ellis, MD, MSc, FAAP

Assistant Professor of Internal Medicine and Pediatrics, Eastern Virginia Medical School, Pediatric and Adult Congenital Cardiologist, Children's Hospital of the King's Daughters, Norfolk, Virginia, USA

Hélène Eltchaninoff, MD

Professor of Medicine, University of Rouen Medical School, Head, Cardiac Catheterization Unit, Department of Cardiology, Charles Nicolle Hospital, Rouen, France

Jeanette Erdmann, PhD

Professor of Genetics, Faculty of Medicine, University of Lübeck, Head, Molecular Genetics Laboratory, Lübeck University Hospital, Lübeck, Germany

Mohammed Rafique Essop, MBBCh, MRCP(UK), FCP(SA), FRCP(Lond), FACC

Associate Professor of Medicine–Cardiology, Faculty of Health Sciences, University of the Witwatersrand, Head, Division of Cardiology, Baragwanath Hospital, Johannesburg, South Africa

Michael D. Ezekowitz, MD, PhD

Vice President, Lankenau Institute for Medical Research, Wynnewood, Pennsylvania, USA

Bengt Fagrell, MD, PhD

Professor Emeritus, Department of Internal Medicine, Karolinska Institute, Stockholm, Sweden

Erling Falk, MD, PhD

Professor of Cardiovascular Pathology, University of Aarhus Faculty of Health Sciences, Cardiovascular Pathologist, Department of Cardiology, Aarhus University Hospital Skejby, Aarhus, Denmark

William F. Fearon, MD

Assistant Professor of Medicine, Stanford University School of Medicine, Associate Director, Interventional Cardiology, Stanford University Medical Center, Stanford, California, USA

Eric O. Feigl, MD

Professor, Department of Physiology and Biophysics, University of Washington School of Medicine, Seattle, Washington, USA

Craig E. Fleishman, MD

Director, Noninvasive Cardiology, Congenital Heart Institute at Miami Children's Hospital, Miami, Arnold Palmer Hospital for Children, Orlando, Florida, USA

Gerald F. Fletcher, MD

Professor of Medicine, Mayo College of Medicine, Cardiologist, Mayo Clinic Jacksonville, Jacksonville, Florida, USA

Andrew S. Flett, MBBS, BSc

Clinical Fellow, University College London, London, United Kingdom

Thomas R. Flipse, MD

Assistant Professor of Medicine, Mayo College of Medicine, Jacksonville, Florida, USA

Gregory P. Fontana, MD

Vice Chairman, Department of Surgery, Cedars-Sinai Medical Center, Los Angeles, California, USA

Thomas Force, MD
James C. Wilson Professor of Medicine, Jefferson Medical College of Thomas Jefferson University, Clinical Director, Center for Translational Medicine, Thomas Jefferson University Hospitals, Philadelphia, Pennsylvania, USA

Anne Fournier, MD
Associate Professor, Department of Pediatrics, University of Montreal Faculty of Medicine, Director, Electrophysiology Section, Ste. Justine Hospital, Montreal, Quebec, Canada

Gary S. Francis, MD, FACC
Professor of Medicine, University of Minnesota Medical School, Minneapolis, Minnesota, USA

Ian J. Franklin, MS, FRCS(GenSurg)
Honorary Clinical Senior Lecturer, Imperial College London School of Medicine, Consultant Vascular Surgeon, Charing Cross Hospital, Imperial College Healthcare NHS Trust, London, United Kingdom

William H. Gaasch, MD
Professor of Medicine, University of Massachusetts Medical School, Worcester, Tufts University School of Medicine, Boston, Senior Consultant in Cardiology, Lahey Clinic, Burlington, Massachusetts, USA

Michael A. Gatzoulis, MD, PhD, FACC, FESC
Professor of Cardiology, National Heart and Lung Institute, Imperial College London, Head, Adult Congenital Heart Centre and Centre for Pulmonary Hypertension, Royal Brompton Hospital, London, United Kingdom

Peter Geelen, MD, PhD
Head, Arrhythmia Unit and Atrial Fibrillation Clinic, Cardiovascular Center, Onze Lieve Vrouw (OLV) Hospital, Aalst, Belgium

Tal Geva, MD
Professor of Pediatrics, Harvard Medical School, Chief, Division of Noninvasive Imaging, Senior Associate in Cardiology, Children's Hospital Boston, Boston, Massachusetts, USA

Marc Gewillig, MD, PhD
Professor of Pediatric Cardiology, University of Leuven Faculty of Medicine, Head, Pediatric Cardiology, University Hospital Leuven, Leuven, Belgium

Aziz Ghaly, MD
Fellow in Cardiothoracic Surgery, Cedars-Sinai Medical Center, Los Angeles, California, USA

Adrianna C. Gittenberger-de Groot, PhD
Professor and Chair, Department of Anatomy and Embryology, Leiden University Medical Center, Leiden, The Netherlands

James A. Goldstein, MD
Medical Director, Cardiovascular Research & Education, William Beaumont Hospital, Royal Oak, Michigan, USA

Eric M. Graham, MD
Assistant Professor of Pediatric Cardiology, Medical University of South Carolina College of Medicine, Charleston, South Carolina, USA

Peer Grande, MD, PhD
Associate Professor of Medicine, University of Copenhagen Faculty of Health Sciences, Chief, Acute Coronary Care Service, Rigshospitalet Heart Center, Copenhagen University Hospital, Copenhagen, Denmark

Paul A. Grayburn, MD
Paul J. Thomas Professor of Medicine, Baylor College of Medicine, Director, Cardiology Research, Baylor University Medical Center, Dallas, Texas, USA

Ehud Grossman, MD
Professor of Medicine, Sackler Faculty of Medicine, Tel-Aviv University, Tel-Aviv, Head, Internal Medicine D and Hypertension Unit, Chaim Sheba Medical Center, Tel-Hashomer, Israel

Scott M. Grundy, MD, PhD
Director of the Center for Human Nutrition, Chairman of the Department of Clinical Nutrition, University of Texas Southwestern Medical School, Chief of the Metabolic Unit, Veterans Affairs Medical Center, Dallas, Texas, USA

Colette Guiraudon, MD, FRCPC, FACP
Emeritus Professor of Pathology, Schulich School of Medicine & Dentistry, University of Western Ontario, Consultant, Department of Pathology, University Hospital, London Health Sciences Centre, London, Ontario, Canada

Lorne J. Gula, MD
Assistant Professor of Medicine, Division of Cardiology, Schulich School of Medicine & Dentistry, University of Western Ontario, Cardiologist, University Hospital, London Health Sciences Centre, London, Ontario, Canada

Donald J. Hagler, MD
Professor of Pediatrics, Mayo Clinic College of Medicine, Consultant, Pediatric Cardiology–Cardiovascular Diseases, Consultant, Circulatory System Devices Panel, Medical Devices Advisory Committee, Mayo Clinic, Rochester, Minnesota, USA

David E. Haines, MD
Chief, Department of Cardiovascular Medicine, Beaumont Hospitals, Royal Oak, Michigan, USA

Sharif A. Halim, MD
Resident and House Officer, Department of Internal Medicine, Duke University Medical Center, Durham, North Carolina, USA

Afshan Hameed, MD, FACC
Assistant Professor of Cardiology and Maternal Fetal Medicine, University of California, Irvine, School of Medicine, Orange, California, USA

Frank L. Hanley, MD
Professor of Cardiothoracic Surgery, Stanford University School of Medicine, Director, Children's Heart Center, Lucile Packard Children's Hospital, Stanford, California, USA

Göran K. Hansson, MD, PhD
Professor, Center for Molecular Medicine, Department of Medicine, Karolinska Institute, Stockholm, Sweden

Peter D. Hart, MD, FACP
Associate Professor of Medicine, Rush Medical College, Chair, Division of Nephrology, Stroger Hospital of Cook County, Chicago, Illinois, USA

Gerd Hasenfuss, MD, FAHA
Professor of Medicine, Department of Cardiology and Pulmonary Medicine, Faculty of Medicine, Georg August University of Göttingen, Göttingen, Germany

Emily Hass, MD
Cardiology Fellow, University of North Carolina at Chapel Hill School of Medicine/North Carolina Memorial Hospital, Chapel Hill, North Carolina, USA

Harvey S. Hecht, MD
Director of Cardiovascular Computed Tomography, Lenox Hill Heart & Vascular Institute, New York, New York, USA

Otto M. Hess, MD, FESC, FAHA
Professor of Cardiology, Faculty of Medicine, University of Bern, Bern, University of Zurich, Zurich, Switzerland, Faculty of Medicine and Surgery, University of Bari, Bari, University of Verona, Verona, Italy, Chair, Department of Cardiology, Swiss Cardiovascular Center, Bern University Hospital, Bern, Switzerland

Li-Wei Ho, MD
Lecturer in Medicine, Department of Medicine, Division of Cardiology, National Yang-Ming University School of Medicine, Attending Cardiologist, Taipei Veterans General Hospital, Taipei, Taiwan

Richard Hobbs, MBChB, FRCGP, FRCP, FESC, FMedSci
Professor and Head, Primary Care Clinical Sciences, School of Medicine, University of Birmingham, Birmingham, United Kingdom

Neil Hobson, MD
Consultant Cardiologist, Castle Hill Hospital, Kingston upon Hull, United Kingdom

Steven Hollenberg, MD
Professor of Medicine, UMDNJ–Robert Wood Johnson Medical School, Director, Coronary Care Unit, Cooper University Hospital, Camden, New Jersey, USA

Babak Hooshmand, MD
Aging Research Center, Karolinska Institute, Stockholm, Sweden

Priscilla Y. Hsue, MD
Assistant Professor of Medicine, University of California, San Francisco, School of Medicine, Attending, Division of Cardiology, San Francisco General Hospital, San Francisco, California, USA

Judy Hung, MD
Assistant Professor of Pathology, Harvard Medical School, Associate Director, Echocardiography, Cardiology Division, Massachusetts General Hospital, Boston, Massachusetts, USA

Stuart J. Hutchison, MD
Clinical Professor of Medicine, University of Calgary, Foothills Medical Center, Calgary, Alberta, Canada

Michael Dilou Jacobsen, MD
Senior Resident, Department of Cardiology, Rigshospitalet, Copenhagen University Hospital, Copenhagen, Denmark

Jose A. Joglar, MD
Associate Professor of Internal Medicine, Elizabeth Thaxton Page and Ellis Batten Page Professorship in Cardiac Electrophysiology Research, University of Texas Southwestern Medical School, Director, Clinical Cardiac Electrophysiology, University of Texas Southwestern Medical Center, Dallas, Texas, USA

Monique R.M. Jongbloed, MD, PhD
Assistant Professor of Anatomy and Embryology, Leiden University Medical Center, Leiden, The Netherlands

Priya Kansal, MD
Fellow, Division of Cardiology, Northwestern University Feinberg School of Medicine, Chicago, Illinois, USA

Juan Carlos Kaski, MD, DSc, FRCP, FESC, FACC
Professor of Cardiovascular Science, Director, Cardiovascular Research Centre, St. George's University of London, Consultant Cardiologist, Deputy Head, Division of Cardiac and Vascular Sciences, St. George's Hospital NHS Trust, London, United Kingdom

Wolfgang Kasper, MD
Professor of Cardiology, Faculty of Medicine, Albert Ludwigs University of Freiburg, Medical Clinic III, University Medical Center Freiburg, Freiburg, Chief of Cardiology, St. Josef's Hospital, Wiesbaden, Germany

Hirohisa Kato, MD, PhD, FACC
Professor Emeritus of Pediatrics, Kurume University School of Medicine, Honorary President, Cardiovascular Research Institute, Kurume, Japan

Sanjay Kaul, MD
Director, Cardiology Training Fellowship Program, Division of Cardiology, Cedars-Sinai Heart Institute, Director, Vascular Physiology and Thrombosis Research Laboratory, Burns and Allen Research Institute, Cedars-Sinai Medical Center, Los Angeles, California, USA

Gautam Kedia, MD
Fellow in Cardiology, Cedars-Sinai Medical Center, Los Angeles, California, USA

John A. Kern, MD
Associate Professor of Surgery, Department of Surgery, University of Virginia School of Medicine, Medical Director, Non-Invasive Vascular Laboratory, University of Virginia Hospital, Charlottesville, Virginia, USA

Paul Khairy, MD, PhD
Associate Professor of Medicine, University of Montreal Faculty of Medicine, Canada Research Chair, Electrophysiology and Adult Congenital Heart Disease, Director, Adult Congenital Heart Center, Montreal Heart Institute, Montreal, Quebec, Canada, Research Director, Boston Adult Congenital Heart Service, Boston, Massachusetts, USA

Apurv Khanna, MD
Assistant Professor of Medicine, University of Connecticut School of Medicine, Attending Physician, John Dempsey Hospital, Farmington, Connecticut, USA

Michael S. Kim, MD
Chief Fellow, Cardiovascular Diseases, Clinical Fellow, Section of Interventional Cardiology, University of Colorado Denver School of Medicine/University of Colorado Hospital, Aurora, Colorado, USA

Thomas R. Kimball, MD
Professor of Pediatrics, University of Cincinnati College of Medicine, Director, Cardiac Ultrasound, Director, Cardiovascular Imaging Core Research Laboratory, Cincinnati Children's Hospital, Cincinnati, Ohio, USA

Miia Kivipelto, MD, PhD
Associate Professor, Department of Neuroscience and Neurology, Faculty of Medicine, University of Kuopio, Kuopio, Finland, Aging Research Center, Department of Neurobiology, Karolinska Institute, Stockholm, Sweden

George J. Klein, MD, FRCPC
Professor of Medicine, Division of Cardiology, Schulich School of Medicine & Dentistry, University of Western Ontario, Cardiologist, University Hospital, London Health Sciences Centre, London, Ontario, Canada

Michel Komajda, MD, PhD
Professor of Cardiology, Université Pierre et Marie Curie–Paris VI, Head, Department of Cardiology, CHU Pitié-Salpêtrière Hospital, INSERM UMR 621, Paris, France

Marvin A. Konstam, MD
Professor of Medicine, Tufts University School of Medicine, Chief Physician Executive, The Cardiovascular Center, Tufts Medical Center, Boston, Massachusetts, USA

Stavros Konstantinides, MD
Professor of Medicine, Department of Cardiology and Pulmonary Medicine, Faculty of Medicine, Georg August University of Göttingen, Göttingen, Germany

Alexander Kopelnik, MD
Fellow in Cardiology, University of California, San Diego, School of Medicine/ UCSD Medical Center, San Diego, California, USA

William J. Kostuk, MD, FRCPC, FACC, FACP, FAHA
Emeritus Professor of Medicine (Cardiology), Schulich School of Medicine & Dentistry, University of Western Ontario, Cardiologist, University Hospital, London Health Sciences Centre, London, Ontario, Canada

Andrew D. Krahn, MD
Professor of Medicine, Division of Cardiology, Schulich School of Medicine & Dentistry, University of Western Ontario, Cardiologist, University Hospital, London Health Sciences Centre, London, Ontario, Canada

Richard Krasuski, MD
Assistant Professor of Medicine, Cleveland Clinic Lerner College of Medicine of Case Western Reserve University, Director, Adult Congenital Heart Disease Services, Cleveland Clinic, Cleveland, Ohio, USA

Jacqueline Kreutzer, MD, FACC, FSCAI
Associate Professor of Medicine, University of Pittsburgh School of Medicine, Director, Cardiac Catheterization Laboratory, Children's Hospital of Pittsburgh of UPMC, Pittsburgh, Pennsylvania, USA

Henry Krum, MBBS, PhD, FRACP
Professor of Medicine, Chair of Medical Therapeutics, Monash University Faculty of Medicine, Nursing and Health Sciences, Head, Clinical Pharmacology, Physician, Heart Centre, Alfred Hospital, Melbourne, Victoria, Australia

Uwe Kühl, MD, PhD
Department of Cardiology and Pneumonology, Medical Clinic II, Charité University Medicine Berlin, Campus Benjamin Franklin, Berlin, Germany

Michael J. Landzberg, MD
Assistant Professor of Medicine, Harvard Medical School, Director, Boston Adult Congenital Heart (BACH) and Pulmonary Hypertension Service, Department of Cardiology, Children's Hospital Boston/ Brigham and Women's Hospital, Boston, Massachusetts, USA

Chim C. Lang, MD, FRCP(Lond, Edinb)
Professor of Cardiology, Division of Medical Sciences, College of Medicine, Dentistry and Nursing, University of Dundee, Honorary Consultant Cardiologist, Ninewells Hospital and Medical School, Dundee, United Kingdom

Mark Langsfeld, MD
Professor of Surgery, University of New Mexico School of Medicine, Albuquerque, New Mexico, USA

Guido Lastra, MD
Endocrinology Fellow, University of Missouri–Columbia School of Medicine/ Harry S. Truman Memorial Veterans' Hospital, Columbia, Missouri, USA

Decebal-Gabriel Latcu, MD
Assistant Specialist, Cardiology Service, Princess Grace Hospital Center, Monaco (Principality)

Chu-Pak Lau, MD
Honorary Clinical Assistant Professor, Department of Medicine, Li Ka Shing Faculty of Medicine/Queen Mary Hospital, University of Hong Kong, Director, Institute of Cardiovascular Science & Medicine, Hong Kong, China

Wendy Lau, MBBS, MD
Honorary Physician to the Pacemaker Clinic, The Royal Melbourne Hospital, Melbourne, Victoria, Australia

Agnes Y.Y. Lee, MD, MSc, FRCPC
Associate Professor of Medicine, University of British Columbia Faculty of Medicine, Medical Director of Thrombosis, Vancouver General Hospital, Vancouver, British Columbia, Canada

Kathy L. Lee, MBBS, MRCP, FRCP, FHKCP, FHKAM, FACC
Honorary Clinical Assistant Professor, Li Ka Shing Faculty of Medicine, University of Hong Kong, Senior Medical Officer, Queen Mary Hospital, Hong Kong, China

James Leitch, MBBS, FRACP, FCANZCS
Conjoint Senior Lecturer, School of Medicine and Public Health, Faculty of Health, University of Newcastle, Newcastle, Senior Staff Specialist, John Hunter Hospital, New Lambton, New South Wales, Australia

Paul LeLorier, MD
Assistant Professor of Medicine, Boston University School of Medicine, Director, Electrophysiology Training Program, Boston Medical Center, Boston, Massachusetts, USA

Oren Lev-Ran, MD
Department of Cardiothoracic Surgery, Onze Lieve Vrouw Gasthuis (OLVG) Hospital, Amsterdam, The Netherlands

Martin M. LeWinter, MD
Professor of Medicine and Molecular Physiology and Biophysics, University of Vermont College of Medicine, Attending Physician and Director, Heart Failure and Cardiomyopathy Program, Fletcher Allen Health Care, Burlington, Vermont, USA

Bertil Lindal, MD, PhD
Associate Professor of Cardiology, Department of Medical Sciences, Uppsala University Faculty of Medicine, Co-Director, Uppsala Clinical Research Centre, Uppsala University Hospital, Uppsala, Sweden

Gregory Y.H. Lip, MD, FRCP, DFM, FESC, FACC
Professor of Cardiovascular Medicine, School of Medicine, University of Birmingham, Consultant Cardiologist, Director, Haemostasis, Thrombosis and Vascular Biology Unit, University Department of Medicine, City Hospital, Birmingham, United Kingdom

Steven E. Lipshultz, MD
George E. Batchelor Professor and Chairman, Department of Pediatrics, Associate Executive Dean for Child Health, Professor of Epidemiology and Public Health, Professor of Medicine (Oncology), University of Miami Leonard M. Miller School of Medicine, Chief-of-Staff, Holtz Children's Hospital, Director, Batchelor Children's Research Center, Associate Director, Mailman Center for Child Development, Member, Sylvester Comprehensive Cancer Center, University of Miami–Jackson Memorial Medical Center, Miami, Florida, USA

Li-Wei Lo, MD
Professor of Medicine, Department of Medicine, Division of Cardiology, National Yang-Ming University School of Medicine, Attending Cardiologist, Taipei Veterans General Hospital, Institute of Clinical Medicine, Taipei, Taiwan

Maria-Angela Losi, MD
Assistant Professor of Cardiology, Department of Clinical Medicine–Cardiovascular Sciences, University of Naples Federico II School of Medicine and Surgery, Chief, Echocardiography Laboratory, Federico II University Hospital, Naples, Italy

Nidal Maarouf, MD
Consultant Cardiologist, Castle Hill Hospital, Kingston upon Hull, United Kingdom

Malcolm J. MacDonald, MD
Clinical Assistant Professor, Department of Cardiothoracic Surgery, Division of Pediatric Cardiac Surgery, Stanford University School of Medicine, Stanford, Attending Surgeon, Pediatric Cardiac Surgery, Children's Hospital of Central California, Madera, California, USA

Yasuki Maeno, MD
Associate Professor of Pediatrics, Department of Pediatrics and Child Health, Kurume University School of Medicine, Staff Neonatologist, Maternal and Perinatal Medical Center, Kurume University Hospital, Kurume, Fukuoka, Japan

Binu Malhotra, MD
Clinical Associate of Medicine, Rittenhouse Hospitalist Associates, University of Pennsylvania Health System, Philadelphia, Pennsylvania, USA

Efstathios Manios, MD
Research Fellow, Department of Cardiovascular Sciences, University of Leicester College of Medicine, Biological and Psychological Science/University Hospitals of Leicester NHS Trust, Leicester, United Kingdom, Consultant, Department of Clinical Therapeutics, University of Athens School of Medicine/Alexandra Hospital, Athens, Greece

Calin V. Maniu, MD
Cardiologist, Cardiovascular Specialists, Inc., Portsmouth, Virginia, USA

Barry J. Maron, MD
Director, Hypertrophic Cardiomyopathy Center, Minneapolis Heart Institute Foundation, Minneapolis, Minnesota, Professor of Medicine, Tufts University School of Medicine, Boston, Massachusetts, USA

David Martins, MD, MS
Assistant Professor of Medicine, College of Medicine, Charles Drew University of Medicine and Science, Los Angeles, California, USA

Thomas H. Marwick, MBBS, PhD
Professor of Medicine, School of Medicine, University of Queensland, Director of Echocardiography, Princess Alexandra Hospital, Brisbane, Queensland, Australia

Gerald R. Marx, MD
Associate Professor of Pediatrics, Harvard Medical School, Senior Associate in Cardiology, Children's Hospital Boston, Boston, Massachusetts, USA

Yasmin Masood, MD
Assistant Professor of Medicine, Penn State University College of Medicine, Heart and Vascular Institute, Hershey, Pennsylvania, USA

Barry M. Massie, MD
Professor of Medicine, University of California, San Francisco, School of Medicine, Chief, Cardiology Division, San Francisco VA Medical Center, San Francisco, California, USA

Henry Masur, MD
Chief, Critical Care Medicine, National Institutes of Health Clinical Center, Bethesda, Maryland, USA

David McCarty, MBBCh
Research Fellow, Harvard Medical School, Clinical and Research Fellow, Cardiology Division, Massachusetts General Hospital, Boston, Massachusetts, USA

Samy I. McFarlane, MD, MPH
Professor of Medicine–Endocrinology, Medical Director of Clinical Research, SUNY Downstate School of Medicine, Chief, Division of Endocrinology, Department of Medicine, SUNY Downstate Medical Center, Attending, University Hospital of Brooklyn and Kings County Hospital, Brooklyn, New York, USA

William J. McKenna, MD, DSc, FRCP, FESC, FACC
Professor of Cardiology, Institute of Cardiovascular Science, University College London Medical School, Clinical Director, The Heart Hospital, University College London Hospitals, NHS Foundation Trust, London, United Kingdom

Alison Knauth Meadows, MD, PhD
Assistant Professor of Radiology and Pediatric Cardiology, University of California, San Francisco, School of Medicine, San Francisco, California, USA

Lise-Andreé Mercier, MD
Associate Professor of Medicine, University of Montreal Faculty of Medicine, Cardiologist, Adult Congenital Heart Center, Montreal Heart Institute, Montreal, Quebec, Canada

Luc Mertens, MD, PhD
Associate Professor of Pediatrics, University of Toronto Faculty of Medicine, Section Head, Echocardiography, Hospital for Sick Children, Toronto, Ontario, Canada, Associate Professor of Pediatrics, University of Leuven Faculty of Medicine, Pediatric Cardiologist, University Hospital Leuven, Leuven, Belgium

Marco Metra, MD
Institute of Cardiology, Department of Experimental and Applied Medicine, University of Brescia, Brescia, Italy

Bret Mettler, MD
Fellow in Cardiac Surgery, University of Virginia School of Medicine/Medical Center, Charlottesville, Virginia, USA

Theo E. Meyer, MD, DPhil
Professor of Medicine, University of Massachusetts Medical School, Chief of Clinical Cardiology, Director, Advanced Heart Failure Program and Heart Failure Wellness Center, UMass Memorial Medical Center, Worcester, Massachusetts, USA

Pierre-Louis Michel, MD
Professor of Cardiology, Université Pierre et Marie Curie–Paris VI, Chief, Division of Cardiology, CHU Tenon Hospital, Paris, France

John M. Miller, MD
Professor of Medicine, Indiana University School of Medicine, Director, Clinical Cardiac Electrophysiology, Clarian Health System, Indianapolis, Indiana, USA

Mary Minette, MD
Assistant Professor, Oregon Health & Science University, Director, Pediatric Echocardiography Laboratory, Doernbecher Children's Hospital, Portland, Oregon, USA

Michelle C. Montpetit, MD
Private Practitioner, Kane Cardiology, Geneva, Illinois, USA

Carlos A. Morillo, MD, FRCPC, FACC, FHRS, FESC
Professor of Medicine, McMaster University Faculty of Medicine, Director, Arrhythmia and Pacing Service, Hamilton Health Sciences, Hamilton, Ontario, Canada

Cynthia D. Morris, PhD, MPH
Professor of Medical Informatics and Clinical Epidemiology; Medicine (Research), Division of Cardiology; and Public Health and Preventive Medicine, Oregon Health & Science University School of Medicine, Portland, Oregon, USA

Lori Mosca, MD, MPH, PhD
Professor of Medicine, Columbia University College of Physicians and Surgeons, Director, Preventive Cardiology, NewYork–Presbyterian Hospital, New York, New York

Barbara J.M. Mulder, MD, PhD
Professor of Cardiology, Academic Medical Center, University of Amsterdam, Amsterdam, The Netherlands

Francis D. Murgatroyd, MD, FRCP, FACC
Director of Cardiac Electrophysiology, King's College Hospital, London, United Kingdom

Daniel J. Murphy, Jr., MD
Associate Professor of Pediatrics (Cardiology), Stanford University School of Medicine, Director, Congenital Cardiac Clinic, Stanford Hospital & Clinics, Stanford, Associate Chief, Pediatric Cardiology, Lucile Packard Children's Hospital, Palo Alto, California, USA

Katherine T. Murray, MD
Associate Professor, Departments of Medicine and Pharmacology, Vanderbilt University School of Medicine, Nashville, Tennessee, USA

M.L. Myers, MD, FRCSC
Associate Professor, Schulich School of Medicine & Dentistry, University of Western Ontario, Cardiac Surgeon, University Hospital, London Health Sciences Centre, London, Ontario, Canada

Rangadham Nagarakanti, MD
Lead Clinical Research Physician, Lankenau Institute for Medical Research, Wynnewood, Pennsylvania, USA

Shawna D. Nesbitt, MD
Associate Professor of Internal Medicine, Division of Hypertension, University of Texas Southwestern Medical School, Dallas, Texas, USA

Pavlo I. Netrebko, MD
Electrophysiology Fellow, Geisenger Medical Center, Danville, Pennsylvania, USA

L. Kristin Newby, MD, MHS
Associate Professor of Medicine, Division of Cardiovascular Medicine, Duke University School of Medicine, Co-Director, Cardiac Care Unit, Duke University Hospital, Durham, North Carolina, USA

David Newman, MD
Associate Professor of Medicine, University of Toronto Faculty of Medicine, Staff Physician, Division of Cardiology, St. Michael's Hospital, Toronto, Ontario, Canada

Jens Cosedis Nielsen, MD, PhD, DMSc
Associate Professor of Cardiology, University of Aarhus Faculty of Health Sciences, Chief Cardiac Electrophysiologist, Department of Cardiology B, Aarhus University Hospital Skejby, Aarhus, Denmark

Jan Nilsson, MD, PhD
Professor of Experimental Cardiovascular Research, Department of Clinical Sciences, Lund University Faculty of Medicine, Malmö, Sweden

Sigurd Nitter-Hauge, MD, PhD
Professor Emeritus, Department of Cardiology, University of Oslo Faculty of Medicine, Head, Medical Department B, Rikshospitalet, Oslo, Norway

Keith C. Norris, MD
Professor of Medicine, Department of Internal Medicine, Executive VP for Research and Health Affairs, Charles Drew University of Medicine and Science, Los Angeles, California, USA

John B. O'Connell, MD
Executive Director, Heart Failure Program, Heart and Vascular Institute, St. Joseph's Hospital, Atlanta, Georgia, USA

E. Magnus Ohman, MD
Professor of Medicine, Duke University School of Medicine, Associate Director, Duke Heart Center–Ambulatory Care, Director, Program for Advanced Coronary Disease, Duke University Medical Center, Durham, North Carolina, USA

Tanvier Omar, MBBCh, FRPath(SA)
Lecturer in Anatomical Pathology, School of Pathology, Faculty of Health Sciences, University of the Witwatersrand, Principal Pathologist and Head, Division of Cytopathology, Department of Anatomical Pathology, National Health Laboratory Service, Johannesburg, South Africa

Suzanne Oparil, PhD, MD
Professor of Medicine, Physiology, and Biophysics, Director, Vascular Biology and Hypertension Program, University of Alabama at Birmingham School of Medicine, Birmingham, Alabama, USA

Kristina Orth-Gomér, MD, PhD
Professor of Community Medicine, Department of Public Health Sciences, Karolinska Institute, Stockholm, Sweden, Charité University Medicine Berlin, Berlin, Germany

Catherine M. Otto, MD
J. Ward Kennedy-Hamilton Endowed Professor of Cardiology, Director, Cardiology Fellowship Programs, Department of Medicine, Division of Cardiology, University of Washington School of Medicine, Associate Director, Echocardiography, University of Washington Medical Center, Seattle, Washington, USA

Richard L. Page, MD
Professor and Head, Division of Cardiology, Robert A. Bruce Endowed Chair in Cardiovascular Research, Department of Medicine, University of Washington School of Medicine, Seattle, Washington, USA

Joseph E. Parrillo, MD
Professor of Medicine, UMDNJ–Robert Wood Johnson Medical School, Chief and Edward D. Viner Chair, Department of Medicine, Director, Cooper Heart Institute, Cooper University Hospital, Camden, New Jersey, USA

Ayan R. Patel, MD
Associate Professor of Medicine, Tufts University School of Medicine, Director, Cardiovascular Imaging and Hemodynamic Laboratory, Tufts Medical Center, Boston, Massachusetts, USA

J. Norman Patton, MD
Assistant Professor of Medicine, Mayo College of Medicine, Chair, Department of Cardiovascular Disease, Mayo Clinic Jacksonville, Jacksonville, Florida

Walter J. Paulus, MD, PhD, FESC
Professor of Cardiac Pathophysiology, Department of Physiology, Faculty of Medicine, Free University, Amsterdam, Associate Director, Cardiovascular Center, VU University Medical Center, Amsterdam, The Netherlands

Naveen Pereira, MD
Assistant Professor of Medicine, Mayo Clinic College of Medicine, Consultant, Cardiovascular Diseases and Internal Medicine, Mayo Clinic, Rochester, Minnesota, USA

Phillippe Pibarot, DVM, PhD, FACC, FAHA
Professor of Medicine, Laval University Faculty of Medicine, Director, Research Group in Valvular Heart Diseases, Quebec Lung and Heart Institute, Quebec City, Quebec, Canada

Eduardo Pimenta, MD
Hypertension Unit, Princess Alexandra Hospital, Brisbane, Queensland, Australia

Arnold Pinter, MD, FRCPC
Assistant Professor of Medicine, University of Toronto Faculty of Medicine, Cardiac Electrophysiologist, St. Michael's Hospital, Toronto, Ontario, Canada

Robert E. Poelmann, PhD
Professor of Anatomy and Embryology, Leiden University Medical Center, Leiden, The Netherlands

Piotr Ponikowski, MD
Cardiology Department, Military Hospital, Wroclaw, Poland

Shakeel Ahmed Qureshi, MBChB, FRCP
Honorary Senior Lecturer, Guy's, King's and St. Thomas' School of Medicine, University of London, Consultant Paediatric Cardiologist, Evelina Children's Hospital, Guy's & St. Thomas Hospital Foundation Trust, London, United Kingdom

Michael Ragosta, MD
Professor of Medicine, University of Virginia School of Medicine, Director, Cardiac Catheterization Laboratories, Director, Interventional Cardiology, University of Virginia Health System, Charlottesville, Virginia, USA

P. Syamasundar Rao, MD
Professor of Pediatrics and Medicine, University of Texas Houston Medical School, Director, Division of Pediatric Cardiology, Children's Memorial Hermann Hospital, Houston, Texas, USA

Rajni Rao, MD
Asistant Professor of Medicine, University of California, San Francisco, School of Medicine, San Francisco, California, USA

Michael W. Rich, MD
Professor of Medicine, Washington University in St. Louis School of Medicine, Director, Cardiac Rapid Evaluation Unit, Barnes-Jewish Hospital, St. Louis, Missouri, USA

Kurt C. Roberts-Thomson, MBBS, PhD, FRACP
Electrophysiology Postdoctoral Fellow, School of Medicine, University of Adelaide Faculty of Medicine, Electrophysiology Fellow, Royal Adelaide Hospital, Adelaide, South Australia, Australia

Thompson Robinson, BMedSci, MD, FRCP
Professor of Stroke Medicine, University of Leicester College of Medicine, Biological and Psychological Science, Honorary Consultant Physician, Department of Aging and Stroke Medicine, Leicester General Hospital, University Hospitals of Leicester NHS Trust, Leicester, United Kingdom

Dan M. Roden, MD
Professor of Medicine and Pharmacology, Director, Oates Institute for Experimental Therapeutics, Assistant Vice-Chancellor for Personalized Medicine, Vanderbilt University School of Medicine, Nashville, Tennesseee, USA

Carlos A. Roldan, MD, FACC, FASE
Professor of Medicine, University of New Mexcio School of Medicine, Staff Cardiologist, University of New Mexico Health Sciences Center, Director, Echocardiography Laboratory, Raymond G. Murphy VA Medical Center, Albuquerque, New Mexico, USA

Jolien Roos-Hesselink, MD, PhD
Associate Professor, Erasmus University Rotterdam, Cardiologist, Director, Adult Congenital Heart Disease Program, Thoraxcenter, Erasmus Medical Center, Rotterdam, The Netherlands

Prashanthan Sanders, MBBS(Hons), PhD, FRACP, FESC
Knapman-NHF Chair of Cardiology Research, University of Adelaide, Director of Cardiac Electrophysiology, Royal Adelaide Hospital, Adelaide, South Australia

Nadir Saoudi, MD, PhD
Professor and Chief, Cardiology Service, Princess Grace Hospital Center, Monaco (Principality)

Wolfgang Schaper, MD, PhD
Professor of Physiology, Justus-Liebig University Giessen, Giessen, Director Emeritus, Division of Thoracic and Cardiovascular Surgery, Max Planck Institute, Bad Neuheim, Germany

Heinz-Peter Schultheiss, MD
Clinical Director, Department of Cardiology and Pneumology, Medical Clinic II, Charité University Medicine Berlin, Campus Benjamin Franklin, Berlin, Germany

Heribert Schunkert, MD
Professor of Medicine, Faculty of Medicine, University of Lübeck, Head of Cardiology, Clinic for Internal Medicine II, Schleswig-Holstein University Hospital, Lübeck, Germany

Prediman K. Shah, MD
Professor of Medicine, David Geffen School of Medicine at UCLA, Director, Division of Cardiology, and Oppenheimer Atherosclerosis Research Center, Shapell and Webb Family Endowed Chair in Cardiology, Cedars-Sinai Heart Institute, Ceadrs-Sinai Medical Center, Los Angeles, California, USA

Joseph Shalhoub, BSc(Hons), MBBS (Hons), AICSM, MRCS(Eng)
Clinical Research Fellow and Honorary Clinical Lecturer, Department of Vascular Surgery, Imperial College London School of Medicine, Honorary Registrar in Vascular Surgery, Charing Cross Hospital, Imperial College Healthcare NHS Trust, London, United Kingdom

Robin D. Shaughnessy, MD
Attending Pediatric Cardiologist Doernbecher Children's Hospital Oregon Health & Science University Portland, Oregon

David M. Shavelle, MD, FACC, FSCAI
Assistant Clinical Professor of Medicine, David Geffen School of Medicine at UCLA, Director, Interventional Cardiology Fellowship, Los Angeles County–Harbor UCLA Medical Center, Los Angeles, California, USA

Girish S. Shirali, MBBS
Assistant Professor of Pediatric Cardiology and OB/GYN, Medical University of South Carolina College of Medicine, Director, Pediatric Echocardiography, Children's Heart Program, Charleston, South Carolina, USA

Darryl F. Shore, MD, FRCS
Director, Heart Division, Consultant Cardiac Surgeon, Department of Cardiac Surgery, Royal Brompton and Harefield NHS Trust, London, United Kingdom

Alfonso Siani, MD
Head, Unit of Epidemiology and Population Genetics, Institute of Food Sciences, CNR, Avellino, Italy

Domenic Sica, MD
Professor of Medicine and Pharmacology, Virginia Commonwealth University School of Medicine, Chairman, Clinical Pharmacology and Hypertension, Virginia Commonwealth University Health System, Richmond, Virginia, USA

Agneta Siebahn, MD, PhD
Professor of Coagulation Sciences, Department of Medical Sciences, Uppsala University Faculty of Medicine, Head, Coagulation Laboratory and UCR Laboratory, Department of Clinical Chemistry, Uppsala Clinical Research Centre, Uppsala University Hospital, Uppsala, Sweden

Henrik Sillesen, MD, DMSc
Associate Professor of Medicine, University of Copenhagen Faculty of Health Sciences, Chief of Vascular Surgery, Department of Cardiology, Rigshospitalet, Gentofte Hospital, Copenhagen University Hospital, Copenhagen, Denmark

David K. Singh, MD
Chief Cardiology Fellow, Cedars-Sinai Medical Center, Los Angeles, California, USA

Gautam K. Singh, MD, MRCP, FACC
Associate Professor of Pediatrics, Division of Cardiology, Washington University in St. Louis School of Medicine, Attending Pediatric Cardiologist, Director of Noninvasive Imaging Research, Co-Director, Echocardiography Laboratory, St. Louis Children's Hospital, St. Louis, Missouri, USA

Allan C. Skanes, MD
Associate Professor of Medicine, Division of Cardiology, Schulich School of Medicine & Dentistry, University of Western Ontario, Cardiologist, University Hospital, London Health Sciences Centre, London, Ontario, Canada

Otto A. Smiseth, MD, PhD
Professor of Medicine, Department of Cardiology, University of Oslo Faculty of Medicine, Head, Division of Cardiovascular and Respiratory Medicine and Surgery, Rikshospitalet, Oslo University Hospital, Oslo, Norway

Frank C. Smith, MD
Clinical Professor of Pediatrics, SUNY Upstate Medical University College of Medicine, Syracuse, New York, USA

Sidney C. Smith, Jr., MD
Professor of Medicine, University of North Carolina at Chapel Hill School of Medicine, Director, Center for Cardiovascular Science and Medicine, Chapel Hill, North Carolina, USA

Alina Solomon, MD
Researcher, Department of Neurology, Faculty of Medicine, University of Kuopio, Kuopio, Finland, Aging Research Center, Karolinska Institute, Stockholm, Sweden

James R. Sowers, MD
Professor of Medicine, Pharmacology, and Physiology, University of Missouri–Columbia School of Medicine, Columbia, Missouri, USA

George S. Stergiou, MD
Associate Professor of Medicine, University of Athens School of Medicine, Hypertension Center, Third Department of Medicine, University of Athens Sotiria Hospital, Athens, Greece

Martin K. Stiles, MBcHB, PhD, FRACP
Postdoctoral Fellow, University of Adelaide, Electrophysiology Fellow, Royal Adelaide Hospital, Adelaide, South Australia, Australia

Joshua M. Stolker, MD
Resident, Department of Cardiology, Mid-America Heart Institute, Saint Luke's Hospital, Kansas City, Missouri, USA

Saverio Stranges, MD, PhD
Associate Professor of Cardiovascular Epidemiology, Clinical Sciences Research Institute, University of Warwick Medical School, Coventry, United Kingdom

Mary Ellen Sweeney, MD
Associate Professor of Medicine, Endocrinology, Diabetes and Lipid Metabolism, Emory University School of Medicine, Director, Lipid and Hypertension Clinics, Atlanta VA Medical Center, Atlanta, Georgia, USA

W.H. Wilson Tang, MD
Assistant Professor of Medicine, Cleveland Clinic Lerner College of Medicine of Case Western Reserve University, Staff Cardiologist and Director of Research, Section of Heart Failure and Cardiac Transplantation Medicine, Heart and Vascular Institute, Cleveland Clinic, Cleveland, Ohio, USA

Allen Taylor, MD
Professor of Medicine, Uniformed Services University of the Health Sciences F. Edward Hébert School of Medicine, Chief of Cardiology, Walter Reed Army Medical Center, Washington, DC, USA

Christian Juhl Terkelsen, MD, PhD
Department of Cardiology B, Aarhus University Hospital Skejby, Aarhus, Denmark

Udho Thadani, MD
Professor Emeritus of Medicine, University of Oklahoma College of Medicine, Consultant Cardiologist, Oklahoma City VA Medical Center, Oklahoma City, Oklahoma, USA

Pierre Theodore, MD
Van Auken Endowed Chair in Thoracic Oncology, Assistant Professor of Surgery, University of California, San Francisco, School of Medicine, Thoracic Oncology Program, UCSF Comprehensive Cancer Center, Medical Center Heart and Lung Transplantation Program, UCSF Medical Center, San Francisco, California, USA

John Thomson, BM, BS, MD, FRCP
Senior Lecturer, School of Medicine, University of Leeds, Consultant Paediatric Cardiologist, Leeds General Infirmary, Leeds, United Kingdom

Dennis A. Tighe, MD
Professor of Medicine, University of Massachusetts Medical School, Director, Ambulatory Cardiology, Associate Director, Non-invasive Cardiology, UMass Memorial Medical Center, Worcester, Massachusetts, USA

Christophe Tron, MD
Head of ICU, Department of Cardiology, Charles Nicolle Hospital, Rouen, France

Hung Fat Tse, MBBS, MD, PhD
William M.W. Mong Professor in Cardiology, Academic Chief, Li Ka Shing Faculty of Medicine, University of Hong Kong, Consultant Cardiologist, Queen Mary Hospital, Hong Kong, China

Anuradha Tunuguntla, MD
Fellow in Cardiology, Louisiana State University School of Medicine/Health Sciences Center, Shreveport, Louisiana, USA

Hideki Uemura, MD, FRCS
Consultant Cardiac Surgeon, Brompton Hospital, London, United Kingdom

Hirotsugu Ueshima, MD
Professor, Department of Health Science, Shiga University of Medical Science, Otsu, Shiga, Japan

Peter van der Meer, MD, PhD
Fellow in Cardiology, Department of Cardiology, University Medical Center Groningen, Groningen, The Netherlands

Frank Van Praet, MD
Staff Surgeon, Department of Cardiovascular and Thoracic Surgery, Onze Lieve Vrouw (OLV) Hospital, Aalst, Belgium

Dirk J. van Veldhuisen, MD, PhD
Professor of Cardiology, University of Groningen Faculty of Medical Sciences, Chief, Department of Cardiology, University Medical Center Groningen, Groningen, The Netherlands

Hugo Vanerman, MD
Head, Department of Cardiovascular and Thoracic Surgery, Onze Lieve Vrouw (OLV) Hospital, Aalst, Belgium

Victoria L. Vetter, MD
Professor of Pediatrics, University of Pennsylvania School of Medicine, Director of Electrophysiology, Medical Director, Youth Heart Watch (an affiliate of Project ADAM), The Children's Hospital of Philadelphia, Philadelphia, Pennsylvania, USA

Ronald G. Victor, MD
Professor of Internal Medicine, University of Texas Southwestern Medical School, Norman and Audrey Kaplan Chair in Hypertension, Dallas Heart Ball Chair in Hypertension and Heart Disease, Director, Florence A. and Houston J. Doswell Center for the Development of New Approaches in the Treatment of Hypertension, Chief, Hypertension Division, University of Texas Southwestern Medical Center, Dallas, Texas, USA

Renu Virmani, MD
Medical Director, CV Path, International Registry of Pathology, Gaithersburg, Maryland, USA

Norbert F. Voelkel, MD
Professor of Medicine, E. Raymond Fenton, M.D., Chair in Pulmonary Disease, Department of Internal Medicine, Virginia Commonwealth University School of Medicine, Director, Victoria W. Johnson Center for Obstructive Lung Disease Research, VCU Health System, Richmond, Virginia, USA

Wanpen Vongpatanasin, MD
Associate Professor, Department of Internal Medicine, Division of Hypertension, University of Texas Southwestern Medical School, Dallas, Texas, USA

Anton Vonk-Noordegraaf, MD, PhD
Associate Professor of Medicine, Department of Pulmonology, Faculty of Medicine, Vrije Universiteit, Amsterdam, VU University Medical Center, Amsterdam, The Netherlands

J. Deane Waldman, MD, MBA
Professor of Pediatrics and Pathology, University of New Mexico School of Medicine, Professor of Healthcare Strategy, Robert O. Anderson Graduate Schools of Management, University of New Mexico, Albuquerque, New Mexico, USA

Bruce D. Walker, MBBS, PhD
Cardiologist, St. Vincent's Hospital, Darlinghurst, New South Wales, Australia

Lars Wallentin, MD, PhD
Professor of Cardiology, Department of Medical Sciences, Uppsala University Faculty of Medicine, Consultant, Department of Cardiology, Co-Director, Uppsala Clinical Research Center, Uppsala University Hospital, Uppsala, Sweden

David D. Waters, MD
Emeritus Professor, Department of Medicine, University of California, San Francisco, School of Medicine, San Francisco, California, USA

Gary Webb, MDCM
Professor of Medicine, University of Pennsylvania School of Medicine, Director, Philadelphia Adult Congenital Heart Center, Hospital of the University of Pennsylvania and The Children's Hospital of Philadelphia, Philadelphia, Pennsylvania, USA

Gerdi Weidner, PhD
Professor of Biology, San Francisco State University, Tiburon, California, USA, Professor of Psychology, Johannes Gutenberg University, Mainz, Germany

Peter Wenaweser, MD
Assistant Professor of Cardiology, Faculty of Medicine, University of Bern, Attending Physician, Interventional Cardiology, Swiss Cardiovascular Center, Bern University Hospital, Bern, Switzerland

Jorge Wernly, MD
W. Sterling Edwards Professor of Surgery, University of New Mexico School of Medicine, Chief, Division of Cardiothoracic Surgery, University of New Mexico Health Sciences Center, Albuquerque, New Mexico, USA

William B. White, MD, FACP, FAHA
Professor of Medicine, University of Connecticut School of Medicine, Chief, Division of Hypertension and Clinical Pharmacology, Calhoun Cardiology Center, Lead Physician, Hypertension and Vascular Diseases Associates, Medical Director, Clinical Trials Unit, University of Connecticut Health Center/John Dempsey Hospital, Farmington, Connecticut, USA

William Williams, BSc, MDCM

Co-Chair, Undergraduate Cardiology Teaching, University of Ottawa, Staff Cardiologist, University of Ottawa Heart Institute, Ottawa, Ontario, Canada

Stephan Windecker, MD

Professor of Medicine, Faculty of Medicine, University of Bern, Director, Invasive Cardiology, Bern University Hospital, Bern, Switzerland

Kai C. Wollert

Professor of Medicine–Cardiology, Department of Cardiology and Angiology, Hannover Medical School, Hannover, Germany

Mark A. Wood, MD

Professor of Medicine, Virginia Commonwealth University School of Medicine, Richmond, Virginia, USA

Fred M. Wu, MD

Instructor in Pediatrics, Harvard Medical School, Assistant in Cardiology, Children's Hospital Boston, Brigham and Women's Hospital, Boston, Massachusetts, USA

Raymond Yee, MD

Professor of Medicine, Division of Cardiology, Schulich School of Medicine & Dentistry, University of Western Ontario, Cardiologist, University Hospital, London Health Sciences Centre, London, Ontario, Canada

Glenn D. Young, MBBS, FRACP

Senior Lecturer, School of Medicine, University of Adelaide Faculty of Medicine, Cardiac Electrophysiologist, Royal Adelaide Hospital, Adelaide, South Australia, Australia

James B. Young, MD

Executive Dean and Professor of Medicine, Cleveland Clinic Lerner College of Medicine of Case Western Reserve University, Chairman, Endocrinology and Metabolism Institute, Cleveland Clinic, Celeveland, Ohio, USA

Alan Zajarias, MD

Assistant Professor of Medicine, Cardiovascular Division, Washington University in St. Louis School of Medicine, St. Louis, Missouri, USA

Jonathan G. Zaroff, MD

Adjunct Investigator, Kaiser Northern California Division of Research, Oakland, Staff Cardiologist, Kaiser San Francisco Medical Center, San Francisco, California, USA

Kenton J. Zehr, MD

Professor of Surgery and Chief, Division of Cardiac Surgery, University of Pittsburgh School of Medicine, Pittsburgh, Pennsylvania, USA

Michael R. Zile, MD

Professor of Cardiology, Medical University of South Carolina College of Medicine, Charleston, South Carolina, USA

Preface

The primary goals of *Cardiology* were to (1) provide a global perspective on cardiovascular disease, rather than one focused almost exclusively on the USA; (2) provide a clinical focus with practical advice on prevention, diagnosis and treatment of heart disease supported by an expert's summary of relevant scientific advances; (3) take advantage of advances in publishing technology to provide high-quality color illustrations and a web site for downloading the figures; (4) tightly organize the book for minimal redundancy, and employ color coding to aid navigation; and (5) create case-based special problems to cover issues that fall through cracks of most textbooks. We hoped to provide practicing cardiologists, cardiology trainees, and other physicians with an up-to-date clinical reference they could use in their everyday practice and an instructional resource they could use for teaching.

That we largely succeeded is evidenced by the very positive reviews the first edition received; accolades such as Medical Book of the Year for 2002 by the British Medical Association; enough demand for a full-translation Spanish edition; and worldwide sales that considerably exceeded the publisher's expectations. This success led to a second edition and now a third edition.

For this new edition, Michael Gatzoulis has joined the Section Editors. He is a recognized expert in congenital heart disease.

A few chapters have been eliminated or merged into others as a result of changes in our understanding of certain diseases. Several new chapters have been added in areas where knowledge is rapidly expanding. In addition, many of the Special Problems have been eliminated or updated, or are new. Finally, all chapters have been extensively revised and the references updated.

The Third Edition now includes access to a dedicated Expert Consult website, where the entire contents of the book and index can be searched and perused independently. We believe the changes outlined above have strengthened this successful textbook and have added to the quality, practical utility, and easy navigability of the first edition.

Michael H. Crawford, MD
John P. DiMarco, MD, PhD
Walter J. Paulus, MD, PhD
2009

Contents

SECTION 1

ATHEROSCLEROSIS AND ITS PREVENTION

SECTION 2

ISCHEMIC HEART DISEASE

Stable Coronary Syndromes

Acute Coronary Syndromes

Nonpharmacologic Treatment of Ischemic Heart Disease

SECTION 3

HYPERTENSIVE HEART DISEASE

SECTION 4

CARDIAC ARRHYTHMIAS

Bradyarrhythmias

Supraventricular Arrhythmias

SECTION 5
HEART FAILURE AND CARDIOMYOPATHY

Aortic Valve Diseases

Right-Sided Heart Valve Disease and Endocarditis

Surgical Treatment of Valvular Heart Disease

SECTION 7
CONGENITAL HEART DISEASE

Cardiac Defects

Vascular Abnormalities

SECTION 8

SECONDARY HEART DISEASE

Systemic Diseases and the Heart

Cardiac Responses to Physiologic Stress

Cardiac Responses to Environmental Stress

Consult Issues

ATHEROSCLEROSIS AND ITS PREVENTION

SECTION

1

chapter 1

Pathogenesis of Atherosclerosis

Göran K. Hansson and Jan Nilsson

Definition

- Atherosclerosis is a focal disease of the inner layer of large and medium-sized arteries.

Key Features

- Atherosclerosis is an inflammatory and fibrotic disease of the arterial intima.
- The basic lesion of atherosclerosis is a raised, focal, fibrofatty plaque or atheroma.
- Atheromas contain a core of lipid, largely cholesterol, surrounded by a fibrous cap.
- The development of atherosclerotic lesions is aggravated by risk factors including hypercholesterolemia, hypertension, smoking, and diabetes.
- Inflow and accumulation of low-density lipoprotein and monocyte-derived macrophages in the arterial intima result in a fatty streak.
- Cytokines and growth factors released from inflammatory cells promote the development of a fibrofatty plaque, which contains a cap of smooth muscle cells and collagen.
- Clinical syndromes are usually caused by plaque activation.
- This process appears to be precipitated by inflammatory activation and protease secretion in the plaque, which leads to fissuring and endothelial defects that elicit thrombosis.
- The role of specific antigens, cytokines, and growth factors remains controversial, as does the possible role of microorganisms.

Clinical Implications

- Atherosclerosis is the underlying cause of approximately 90% of all myocardial infarction and a large proportion of strokes and ischemic gangrenes.
- Atherosclerotic lesions can cause ischemic symptoms, such as angina pectoris, but do not usually lead to ischemic necrosis of the end organs unless thrombi form on their surfaces.
- In addition to management of classic cardiovascular risk factors, treatment of atherosclerosis in patients with established coronary heart disease should focus on plaque stabilization.
- Atherosclerosis is an inflammatory and fibrotic disease of the arterial intima.
- The basic lesion of atherosclerosis is a raised, focal, fibrofatty plaque or atheroma.
- Atheromas contain a core of lipid, largely cholesterol, surrounded by a fibrous cap.

Atherosclerosis is the most common cause of death and serious morbidity in the Western world. The World Health Organization has predicted that in the near future, it will also become the number one cause of mortality in the entire world.[1] Atherosclerosis is a disease of elastic arteries (i.e., aorta, carotid, and iliac arteries) and large and medium-sized muscular arteries (i.e., coronary and popliteal arteries), whereas smaller arteries rarely become affected. It is part of a family of arterial disorders characterized by thickening and loss of elasticity of the vascular wall. The common term used for these diseases is *arteriosclerosis*, which literally means "hardening of the arteries." The other diseases of this group include arteriolosclerosis, which is marked by proliferation and hyaline thickening of the walls of small arteries and arterioles, and Mönckeberg's medial calcific sclerosis, which is characterized by calcification of the media of muscular arteries. Atherosclerosis is by far the most common and important form of arteriosclerosis, and the terms are sometimes used synonymously.

The disease process of atherosclerosis is primarily restricted to the intimal layer of the artery wall, which becomes infiltrated by lipids and inflammatory cells and develops various degrees of fibrosis. This observation has led to the belief that atherosclerosis is caused, at least in part, by activation of vascular repair responses. Arterial trauma initiates a healing reaction that involves phenotypic modulation of medial smooth muscle cells into fibroblast-like repair cells that migrate into the intima, where they proliferate and produce extracellular matrix. The accumulation of lipoprotein-derived lipids, including oxidatively and enzymatically modified components of low-density lipoprotein (LDL), is believed to damage the artery, to induce local inflammation, and to activate the repair process.[2] This leads to formation of intimal lesions that may progress into atheroma.

Although the atherosclerotic process is so strikingly located in the intima, other layers of the artery wall are not unaffected by the disease. The media behind plaques frequently shows atrophy, with loss of smooth muscle cells. This may be caused by a decreased supply of nutrients to the medial cells and by the fact that many of the medial smooth muscle cells have migrated into the intima. As a result of the medial atrophy, the artery dilates. However, even before this final phase, remodeling of the media occurs, tending to enlarge the vessel to accommodate the plaque and thus to preserve the dimensions of the lumen (Fig. 1.1).[3] As a result, the artery may appear quite normal at an angiographic evaluation even though it is severely affected by atherosclerosis. This represents a serious problem in angiographic

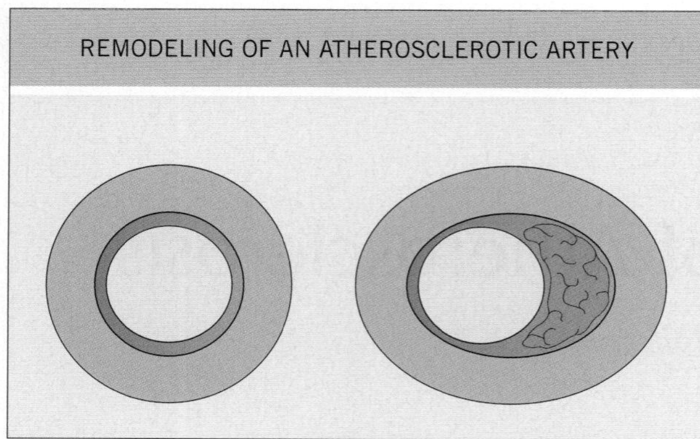

Figure 1.1 Remodeling of an atherosclerotic artery. During the initial stages of plaque growth, the artery may compensate for the increased intimal thickness by remodeling of the extracellular matrix in the media and the adventitia, leading to a more oval shape of the vessel.

evaluation of atherosclerosis. In general, it can be assumed that once a plaque becomes visible at angiography, it is not a new plaque but rather the "tip of an iceberg." Novel methods that visualize actual plaques rather than the lumen are being developed and are being used in clinical research. They include ultrasound imaging (particularly intravascular ultrasonography), computed tomography, and magnetic resonance imaging. By tagging of molecules that accumulate in lesions or certain types or areas of lesions, such structures can be visualized (e.g., by positron emission tomography or magnetic resonance imaging). For future studies, such molecular imaging is a promising approach.

Atherosclerosis does not affect arteries uniformly; it is a focal disease. This is highlighted by the term *plaque,* which was used by the first pathologists who at autopsy described dotted lesions covering the aortic surface. The focal nature of the disease is in apparent contrast to the fact that most risk factors for development of atherosclerosis, such as hyperlipidemia, hypertension, smoking, and diabetes, are systemic and are likely to affect all parts of the arterial system similarly. This clearly shows that the systemic risk factors must act in concert with local factors. One such factor is the local shear stress exerted by the blood flow. Atherosclerotic plaques do not develop randomly in the arterial system. They are preferentially located close to branching sites in areas of low shear stress, where the time of interaction between blood-borne particles (such as LDL) and the lumen surface is increased. This is associated with increased transendothelial passage of lipoproteins and, when hyperlipidemia is present, increased accumulation of lipid in the subendothelial matrix.[2] For reasons that remain to be fully understood, low shear stress is also associated with a local activation of proinflammatory genes that further contributes to the risk for lesion development at these sites.[4]

More recently, attention has focused on the role of microorganisms in atherosclerosis. Several epidemiologic studies have demonstrated an association between *Chlamydia pneumoniae* infection and cardiovascular disease.[5] *Chlamydia,* cytomegalovirus, and other pathogens have been found in vascular specimens removed at surgery, but it remains unclear whether they contribute to disease development or are "passengers" trapped in the lesions. Cell culture studies support a pathogenic role for some of these pathogens. However, the observation from several randomized clinical trials that long-term treatment with antibiotics does not reduce coronary event rates has questioned the validity of the concept that bacterial pathogens contribute to atherosclerosis.[6]

It has become increasingly evident that the clinical symptoms of atherosclerosis are related not so much to plaque development and growth but rather to the degeneration and rupture of established plaques. Plaque growth by lipid accumulation and fibrosis rarely gives rise to lesions large enough to significantly limit blood flow (i.e., more than 75% lumen reduction). Even so, when plaques occur in the coronary arteries, the slow growth of a plaque gives ample time for small collateral vessels to develop. In the case of acute myocardial infarction and unstable angina, they can almost invariably be attributed to thrombus formation on ruptured lesions. Also, the rapid plaque growth that can sometimes be observed on sequential angiographic evaluations is probably caused by plaque rupture followed by fissure healing and encapsulation of the thrombus and other blood cells. Accordingly, it is likely that the treatment of atherosclerosis in patients with established coronary heart disease should primarily focus on achieving plaque stabilization. Experience from intervention trials using lipid-lowering agents (statins) also suggests that plaque stabilization may be a major factor responsible for the reduction in cardiovascular events.

In this chapter, we first provide a brief overview of the anatomy of the normal arterial wall, the substrate for the disease. The cellular components of the artery as well as the inflammatory cells that infiltrate the arterial intima during atherosclerosis are discussed. The different histopathologic stages of atherosclerosis are described, and we finally discuss the pathogenesis of the disease and some of its complications. More detailed insights into the epidemiology of atherosclerosis and the biology of risk factors for the disease are provided in other sections of this volume.

ANATOMY AND CELL BIOLOGY OF THE ARTERIAL WALL

Histologic Organization

The normal artery has a very simple anatomy. It consists of three layers: the tunica intima, which forms a barrier between the artery wall and the circulating blood; the thick muscle layer, the tunica media; and a connective tissue layer, the tunica adventitia, which fuses with connective tissue of the surrounding organs (Fig. 1.2).

The tunica media is the largest layer of the artery wall. It is composed of one single cell type, the vascular smooth muscle cell, which provides the bulk of the cell mass of the artery and also produces the extracellular matrix components of the media. The smooth muscle cells are elongated, spindle-shaped cells that adhere to each other through junctional complexes. The cells are organized into circular layers that surround the arterial lumen in concentric circles. They produce large amounts of elastic fibers, which form lamellae between the layers of muscle cells. The media therefore has a multilayered organization: two elastic lamellae surround a layer of smooth muscle cells and form a lamellar unit. In elastic arteries such as the aorta, 20 to 50 such lamellar units build up the tunica media. In the smaller muscular

Figure 1.2 Histologic organization of the normal artery wall. This schematic drawing shows a cross section through the wall of a medium-sized muscular artery.

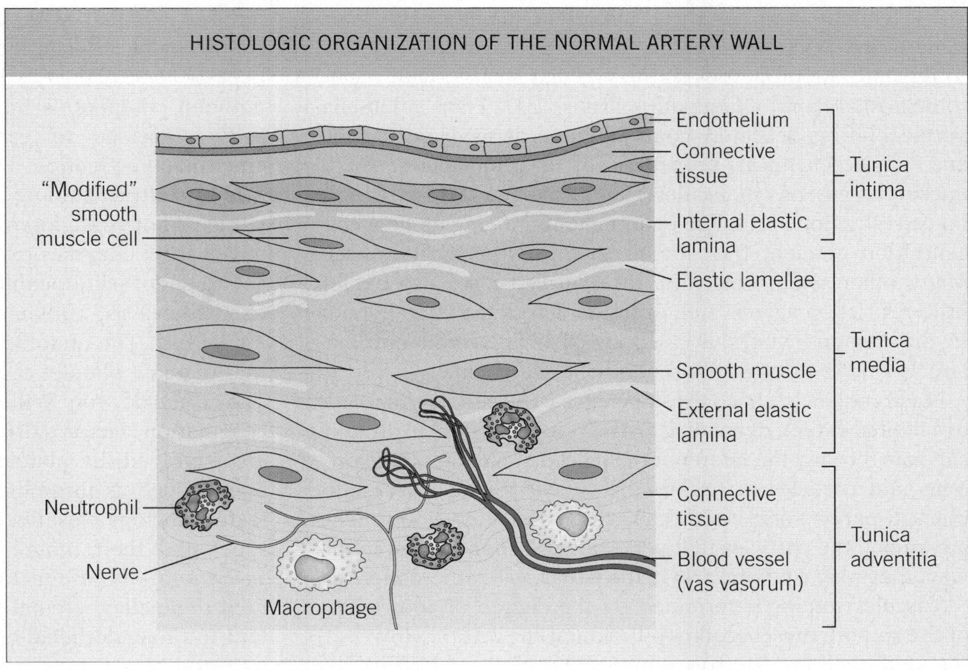

arteries, the organization is less developed, although layers of smooth muscle and elastic fibers can be discerned.

The outermost elastic lamellae form a thick elastic membrane, the lamina elastica externa, which demarcates the border between the media and the adventitia. Similarly, the innermost elastic lamella, the lamina elastica interna, is thickened and constitutes the border between media and intima.

The adventitia is a connective tissue structure that continues into the surrounding connective tissue stroma. Its inner part is fibrous and dominated by collagen and elastin, but this gradually gives way to loose connective tissue with increasing distance from the media. In addition to fibers, the adventitia contains fibroblasts, mast cells, adipocytes, and sympathetic nerve endings. It also carries blood and lymph vessels that penetrate into the outer third of the media. In the normal artery, the inner part of the media and the entire intima are avascular. However, during pathologic conditions such as atherosclerosis, angiogenic factors stimulate neovascularization that extends as far as the intima.

The intima consists of a continuous, single-cell layer, the endothelium, and its basement membrane and a connective tissue layer with occasional primitive mesenchymal cells. In the newborn, this layer extends for only a few micrometers. However, it undergoes a progressive intimal thickening during life and can be several hundred micrometers thick in the adult aorta. This is caused by a continued accumulation of connective tissue fibers, proteoglycans, and mesenchymal cells. The mesenchymal cells appear to be "modified" smooth muscle cells that have lost contractile capacity and function as fibroblasts (i.e., by producing connective tissue elements).

"Cushions" of increased intimal size and arterial disorganization are found at branching points in the arterial tree. Here, the endothelium exhibits increased permeability and has a higher proliferation rate. The intima is thickened, the lamellar organization of the media is disturbed, and the smooth muscle cells proliferate at an increased rate. These sites are hot spots for cell division and tissue renewal and might contain vascular stem cells.[7] It is also possible, however, that they represent a tissue response to increased hemodynamic strain because they are often found at sites of disturbed flow. It is striking that the anatomic distribution of atherosclerotic lesions overlaps with that of intimal cushions. It remains unclear whether the cushions are substrata for lesion formation or whether the same factors (e.g., hemodynamic strain) that induce cushion formation also promote atherosclerosis.[8]

CELLS OF THE ARTERY WALL

Endothelial Cells

The endothelial cell is a thin, elongated epithelial cell that is specialized to constitute a barrier and to control the blood-artery permeability. Its cytoplasm is filled with pinocytotic vesicles, which may form chains that penetrate through the cell, whereas the borders between adjacent endothelial cells are developed into junctional complexes with specialized structures that increase mechanical strength and control macromolecular permeability. Endothelial cells of arteries and veins, and those of most capillaries, form a continuous monolayer of polygonal cells that are tightly fitted to each other through such junctions. They develop embryonally from hemangiopoietic stem cells, which form blood islands as well as primitive endothelial sacks and tubes. The primitive endothelium penetrates all organs of the embryo, forming a continuous vasculature and recruiting local mesenchymal cells to develop into smooth muscle cells that surround the endothelial tubes. In adults, endothelial cells may also originate from bone marrow–derived stem cells, so-called endothelial progenitor cells. Whether treatment with such endothelial progenitor cells may improve myocardial function after an infarct is presently the subject of intense investigations.

The endothelium has three important functions: to determine blood-tissue permeability, to control vascular tone, and to regulate the properties of the vascular surface with regard to hemostasis and inflammation (Table 1.1). Transendothelial permeability is delicately controlled and depends on the size and physicochemical properties of the molecules. Small uncharged gaseous molecules such as oxygen diffuse without much restriction across the endothelium, moving along a concentration gradient from blood to the extravascular space. Many other small molecules, including glucose, also exhibit little restriction against free diffusion across the endothelium. In arteries and veins, the supply of oxygen and nutrients largely occurs through transendothelial diffusion.

Macromolecules, in contrast, penetrate the endothelium only to a limited extent, depending on their size. Thus, small proteins can pass through the interendothelial clefts, whereas large proteins and particles can reach the subendothelial space only through endocytotic vesicles. As discussed later, lipoproteins are among the particles that penetrate the endothelium in this way; they play a pivotal role in the initiation of atherosclerosis.

Vascular tone is determined by the degree of contraction of the smooth muscle cell population of the artery. However, the endothelium controls smooth muscle contractility by releasing paracrine vasoactive mediators (see Table 1.1). Nitric oxide is an inorganic gas that is produced from L-arginine by an endothelial enzyme, nitric oxide synthase. This production occurs constitutively but is increased when the intracellular calcium level is raised in the endothelial cell as a result of the action of acetylcholine, bradykinin, and some other circulating mediators. Nitric oxide diffuses through the endothelial plasma membrane, passes the extracellular space, and activates an enzymatic cascade in the smooth muscle cell. This leads to smooth muscle relaxation and reduced vascular tone. Other vasoactive endothelial factors counterbalance this effect. They include the vasoconstrictive peptide endothelin 1, which is expressed as a large preproendothelin polypeptide by the endothelial cell and proteolytically processed to generate active endothelin-1 during endothelial activation. Like endothelin-1, angiotensin-II also acts to contract smooth muscle cells. It is present as a circulating proform, angiotensinogen, which is processed to angiotensin II by enzymes expressed by endothelial cells.

The endothelium exhibits active functions that are related to hemostasis, inflammation, and vascular tone (see Table 1.1). The endothelial surface contains a set of factors that regulate platelet adhesion, coagulation, and fibrinolysis. They include von Willebrand factor (a component of the coagulation factor VIII complex), surface molecules that are involved in platelet adhesion, coagulation-regulating factors such as thrombomodulin, and fibrinolysis-regulating factors such as plasminogen activators (tissue and urokinase type) and their inhibitor (plasminogen activator inhibitor 1). Several of these factors are stored in specialized intracellular organelles, Weibel-Palade bodies, that empty their content to the endothelial cell surface when the cell is activated by thrombin or some other mediators. Similarly, endothelial cells control the inflammatory properties of the vascular surface by expressing leukocyte adhesion molecules, such as E-selectin and the intercellular adhesion molecule-1; chemokines that promote the recruitment of leukocytes, such as monocyte chemotactic protein-1 and interleukin-8; and cytokines that can activate immune cells, such as interleukin-1.

Prostacyclin (PGI_2) is a bioactive lipid produced by the endothelium. It is a powerful inhibitor of platelet aggregation and also promotes vascular relaxation. Counterbalancing its effect, thromboxane A_2 (TXA_2) produced by platelets stimulates platelet aggregation. The balance between PGI_2 and TXA_2 determines whether platelet microthrombi are permitted to form on the endothelium. Under normal conditions, PGI_2 dominates and prevents thrombus formation. Aspirin inhibits TXA_2 formation to a greater extent than PGI_2 formation and therefore prevents thrombosis, whereas cyclooxygenase-2 inhibitors (coxibs) reduce PGI_2 production, which may lead to thrombosis.

FUNCTIONS OF THE VASCULAR ENDOTHELIUM		
Permeability regulator (filter function)	Large molecules	Vesicular transport Passage through intercellular junctions
	Small molecules	Vesicles, junctions, and through the cytoplasm
Regulator of vascular tone (regulation of smooth muscle contractility)	Smooth muscle relaxation	Nitric oxide, others
	Smooth muscle contraction	Endothelin, angiotensin II
Regulator of hemostasis and inflammation	Platelet adhesion and activation	von Willebrand factor, P-selectin, E-selectin, platelet-activating factor, PGI_2
	Coagulation	Thrombomodulin, heparan sulfate, others
	Fibrinolysis	t-PA, u-PA, PAI-1

PAI-1, plasminogen activator inhibitor; t-PA, tissue plasminogen activator; u-PA, urokinase-type plasminogen activator.

Table 1.1 Functions of the vascular endothelium.

Smooth Muscle Cells

The smooth muscle cell is by far the most prevalent cell type in the artery, where it constitutes more than 95% of all cells. Smooth muscle cells contain myosin and actin filaments but have a less advanced contractile apparatus than the striated muscle cells of the heart and skeletal muscle. The vascular smooth muscle cell is particularly primitive and combines a capacity to change its tone with a fibroblast-like role as producer of the large extracellular matrix of the vessel wall. Smooth muscle cells are recruited from the local mesenchyme during embryonal development. This is probably initiated by a molecular signal from the embryonal endothelium, which induces mesenchymal cells to form a circular layer around the endothelial tube.

In the adult artery, almost all smooth muscle cells are present in the medial layer. They are fitted to each other by junctional complexes that include tight and gap junctions. This not only increases the tensile strength of the smooth muscle layer but also permits rapid transfer of signaling molecules between cells throughout the arterial smooth muscle population. The contractile apparatus of smooth muscle cells is dominated by actin filaments that are mainly composed of a unique actin isoform, α-smooth muscle cell actin. Although the contractile filaments are associated with each other and form specialized structures termed dense bodies, they are not at all as well developed as in striated muscle, and no sarcomeres can be discerned. This reduces the contractile capacity of the smooth muscle cell compared with the striated one. In most of the arterial tree, the contractile repertoire of the smooth muscle cell is limited to changes in vascular tone. However, this not only permits fluctuations in blood pressure but also regulates perfusion of different organs and tissues.

Smooth muscle tone is regulated by several mechanisms. Local regulation by the endothelium is of key importance, as mentioned before. In addition, metabolites produced by the surrounding tissue, autonomous nerve control from sympathetic nerve endings, and circulating mediators control smooth muscle tone. Together, all of these stimuli orchestrate a fine-tuned regulation of vascular tone, blood pressure, and local perfusion.

The matrix produced by the smooth muscle is composed of two major types of fiber, elastic and collagen fibers, together with a ground substance containing a loose proteoglycan network. The elastic fibers are particularly important for the mechanical properties of the vessel media, whereas collagen is a major secretory product of smooth muscle cells in the intima.

Smooth muscle cells as well as endothelial cells are normally quiescent cells that do not divide. However, vascular injury elicits a proliferative response in which medial smooth muscle cells divide, migrate into the intima, and then divide repeatedly to form an intimal thickening. This process, which resembles the restenosis observed after angioplasty and vascular surgery, is controlled by growth factors.[9] Thus, the first round of replication in the media is initiated by the basic isoform of fibroblast growth factor, which is released from extracellular stores in the tissue. The subsequent migration and continued proliferation depend on stimulation by the platelet-derived growth factor (PDGF), which is released from adherent, activated platelets on the vascular surface, from infiltrating monocytes, and, at certain stages, from vascular endothelial and smooth muscle cells themselves. It has also been proposed that some intimal smooth muscle cells are derived from bone marrow–derived stem cells.[7]

Infiltrating Leukocytes and Other Nonvascular Cells

Macrophages form a small but significant component of the cell population in the normal artery. They are derived from blood monocytes, enter by interacting with leukocyte adhesion molecules on the endothelium (probably both the luminal endothelium and that of the vasa vasorum), and settle in the intima and the adventitia.

Lymphocytes are also found in the artery, although not as frequently as macrophages. T cells are present in the intima and the adventitia, whereas B cells are largely confined to the adventitia. Periarterial lymph nodes are normally present along the aorta and its major branches. They permit immune activation by circulating antigens that penetrate into the arterial wall, from which they are transported to the local lymph nodes by lymph vessels of the arterial wall.

Mast cells, which are derived from hematopoietic stem cells and present throughout the connective tissue, are also found in the arterial wall, particularly in the adventitia.

Adipocytes, finally, are common in the adventitia and a major cell type in the loose connective tissue that surrounds the artery. They are derived from local fibroblasts, and their size and number obviously depend on the nutritional state.

HISTOPATHOLOGY OF ATHEROSCLEROSIS

On the basis of morphologic studies performed by pathologists during many years, three types of atherosclerotic plaque have been described:

- fatty streaks;
- fibrous plaques; and
- complicated lesions.

Fatty streaks consist of intimal accumulations of macrophages filled with numerous lipid droplets (foam cells). The lipid droplets consist of cholesterol esters derived from oxidized or aggregated LDL that is taken up by a specific family of scavenger receptors. On gross examination, they are visible as yellow streaks that follow the direction of the blood flow. Fatty streaks do not affect the blood flow.

In fibrous plaques, lipids are present both in macrophage foam cells and in the extracellular matrix. The intima is thickened because of accumulation of smooth muscle cells and extracellular matrix. Lipids and macrophages are usually most frequent in the core region, which also contains T lymphocytes and occasional B cells and mast cells. Smooth muscle cells and the extracellular matrix are more abundant in the subendothelial region, often forming a fibrous cap covering the lipid and inflammatory cells in the deeper part of the plaque (Fig. 1.3). In coronary arteries, fibrous plaques are often eccentric, covering only a part of the vessel. Even if fibrous plaques grow to significantly reduce the lumen of the vessel, they are not believed to be a major cause of clinical symptoms as long as they remain intact. However, fibrous plaques are heterogeneous in their nature, mainly depending on the balance between the amount of lipids and inflammatory cells on one hand and the amount of fibrous tissue on the other. Plaques with a thin fibrous cap and a large core of lipids and inflammatory cells have a high risk of rupture and are sometimes referred to as thin cap atheromas or vulnerable plaques. This risk does not appear to be dependent on the size of the plaque.

Complicated lesions are plaques that in addition to lipids, inflammatory cells, and fibrous tissue also contain a hematoma or hemorrhage and thrombotic deposits. Complicated lesions predominantly develop as a result of a rupture of a fibrous plaque. Another possible cause may be bleeding from capillaries entering the plaque from the adventitial vasa vasorum. Bleeding from intraplaque capillaries may cause rapid plaque growth, and much of the cholesterol in such lesions is derived from erythrocyte membranes rather than lipoproteins. Fissures, erosions, and ulcerations in the fibrous cap and luminal surface are other frequent characteristics. The morbidity and mortality from coronary atherosclerosis derive mainly from these lesions; it is estimated that of all acute thrombotic events, about two thirds are caused by

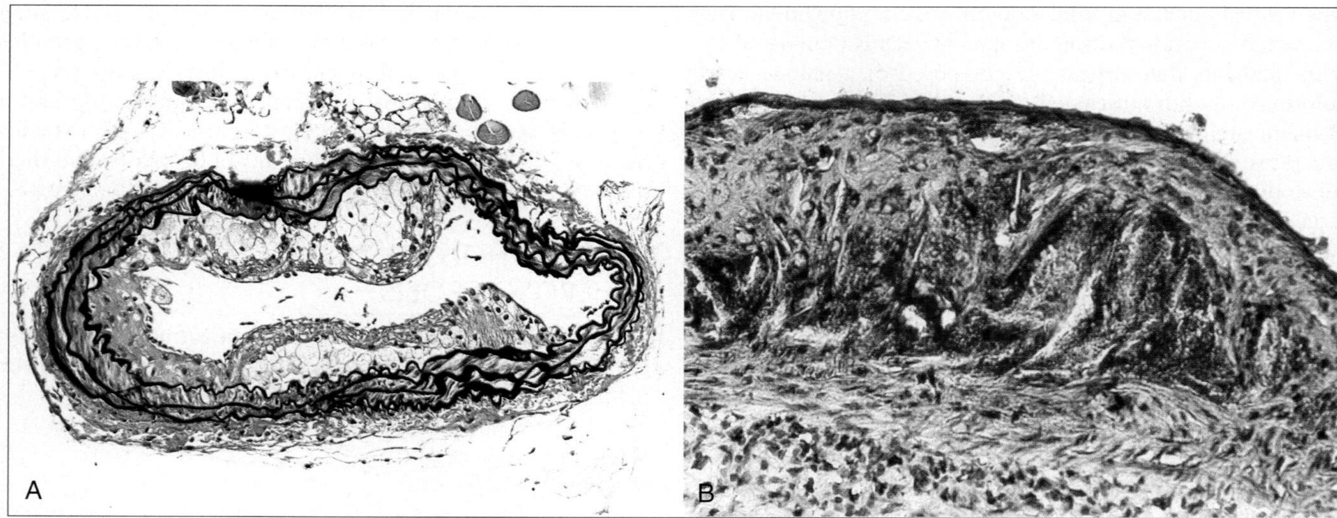

Figure 1.3 Early stages of plaque growth in apoE$^{-/-}$ mice. A, Early stage of a fibrous plaque consisting of a cap of smooth muscle cells and collagen covering a core of lipid-rich macrophages. **B,** A more advanced plaque with massive accumulation of macrophages (brown) in the core of the lesion.

plaque ruptures, whereas one third are due to thrombus formation on an eroded endothelial surface with an intact fibrous cap. At older ages, these lesions often contain calcium deposits. The pathophysiologic relevance of these calcium deposits is not clear, but they may make the plaques more brittle and likely to rupture in response to tensile stress.

Again, it may be useful to look on these different types of lesion from the perspective of healing reactions in response to injury. From this point of view, intimal lipid accumulation appears to play a key role as a cause of the vascular injury. The fact that macrophages are initially recruited to the intima suggests the presence of minor injuries caused by toxic effects of lipid accumulations in the extracellular matrix. The removal of extracellular lipids through macrophage uptake represents an effective early defense mechanism in response to this injury. The failure of this defense would then lead to formation of fibrous plaques. If macrophages were unable to remove toxic lipid products, resulting tissue injury would activate a repair process involving recruitment of smooth muscle cells from the media. A successful repair process would keep the intimal layer intact. However, if the repair process fails to fulfill its function, the fibrous component of the plaque will become too weak to resist the tensile forces of the blood flow and rupture.

On the basis of their morphologic characteristics as well as experience from different animal models of atherosclerosis, it has been assumed that the three plaque types represent different stages of atherosclerosis and develop in a chronologic order from fatty streaks into fibrous plaques and finally into complicated lesions. However, as our knowledge about the atherosclerotic process has increased, it has become clear that this view does not sufficiently describe the complex nature of the disease. Only a certain population of fatty streaks appears to be at risk of progressing into more advanced lesions. The rapid changes in plaque characteristics in response to rupture have important clinical implications that need to be taken into account. A new classification has been proposed by the American Heart Association Committee on Vascular Lesions, categorizing the process of lesion progression into eight different phases (Fig. 1.4).[10] Although the terminology initially appears complicated, it has the advantage of integrating morphologic changes and clinical consequences in a way that is meaningful for both investigators and clinicians. It also takes into account the role of what

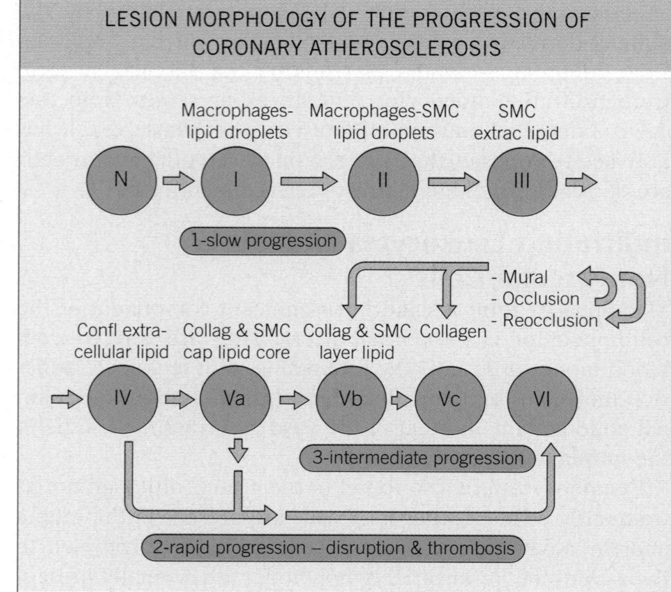

Figure 1.4 Lesion morphology of the progression of coronary atherosclerosis according to the histopathologic findings. Collag, collagen; Confl, confluent; Extrac, extracellular; N, normal; SMC, smooth muscle cells.

are considered physiologic changes in the vascular wall, such as adaptive intimal thickening.

Human arteries normally have both thin and thick segments. These differences are already present at birth and reflect physiologic variations in shear and tensile forces. The thicker intima segments are found near branches and are called adaptive intimal thickening. They are self-limited in growth and never obstruct the blood flow. In cross section, an adaptive thickening is seen as an eccentric, crescent-shaped increase of the outer wall of the bifurcation. The adaptive intimal thickening consists of a subendothelial layer of proteoglycan-rich extracellular matrix containing sparse smooth muscle cells covering a deeper layer of tissue with abundant elastic fibers, collagen, and smooth muscle cells. These intimal thickenings result from normal physiologic adaptation and are not regarded as part of the atherosclerotic process. However, at the same time, intimal adaptive thickenings appear to be particularly susceptible to the development of atherosclerotic lesions.

The type I lesion is the earliest lesion and is characterized by minor lipid depositions and sparse macrophage foam cells. In the coronary arteries, type I lesions are usually colocalized with adaptive intimal thickenings, suggesting that the same shear stress factors that give rise to these changes also are involved in the formation of atherosclerotic plaques. Immediately after birth, 45% of infants have type I lesions. They become less frequent during the first years of childhood but begin to increase again around the age of 10 years.

In type II lesions, macrophage foam cells are more numerous and organized in what is classically recognized as fatty streaks. Type II lesions also contain occasional T cells, mast cells, and lipid-filled smooth muscle cells. They are usually present at certain lesion-prone locations, and segments with adaptive intimal thickening are at greatest risk in this respect.

The type III lesion is the first stage to be recognized by classic pathology as an atherosclerotic plaque or atheroma. The most important distinction versus type II lesions is the presence of small extracellular lipid deposits. This lipid accumulates in the deepest regions of the lesion below the macrophages and the T cells. The lipid deposits expand the extracellular matrix compartment and disrupt the cellular organization of the intima. The presence of type III lesions is believed to be predictive of future clinical disease.

In type IV lesions, the amount of extracellular lipid has increased to form a continuous cell-free pool of cholesterol deposits. The lipid may be derived both from degenerating foam cells and from direct deposition of lipoprotein lipids. According to the old classification, the disease has now reached the stage of an advanced lesion. The lipid core is surrounded by inflammatory cells and covered by a thin layer of smooth muscle cells and connective tissue. Capillaries, originating from the adventitial vasa vasorum, start to grow into the deeper parts of the plaque. In accordance with the earlier lesions, type IV lesions initially develop at the same sites as adaptive intimal thickenings. Type IV lesions are generally crescent shaped and increase the thickness of the artery wall opposite the flow divider of a bifurcation. At this stage, the artery remodels to maintain its original lumen volume. The outer contour of the vessel becomes oval, and as a consequence, these lesions are difficult to visualize by angiography (see Fig. 1.1). Although type IV lesions are generally clinically silent, their recognition by intravascular ultrasonography, magnetic resonance imaging, or radiolabeled ligands with high affinity for vascular lesions will become important as they have the potential to rapidly develop symptom-producing ruptures. Thrombus formation on ruptured type IV lesions is the most likely explanation when occlusions or significant stenoses develop in a section of a coronary artery that on recent angiographic evaluation has appeared normal.

Type V lesions are characterized by an increase in the fibrous tissue that covers the lipid core in type IV lesions. This fibrosis is caused by smooth muscle cells that proliferate and secrete extracellular matrix proteins such as collagen and proteoglycans. Animal experiments suggest that these smooth muscle cells are recruited from the media, where some cells undergo a phenotypic modulation into fibroblast-like repair cells. In contrast to the contractile smooth muscle cells, these "synthetic" smooth muscle cells contain abundant rough endoplasmic reticulum but no filament bundles. The human arterial intima, in contrast to that of most animals, normally contains some smooth muscle cells. It remains to be finally determined whether the cells that form the fibrous tissue in type V lesions in humans originate from the media or from preexisting intimal cells. Collagen often becomes the predominant feature of type V lesions and may account for most of the volume of the plaque. The ingrowth of capillaries is also more prominent than in type IV lesions. Type V lesions are often too large for the artery to compensate by remodeling, resulting in a narrowing of the lumen. The contour of these narrowings remains smooth, but they are usually detectable by angiography.

Although type V lesions have more fibrous tissue than type IV, most ruptures still take place in this lesion type. Rupture-prone type V lesions typically have a thin layer of fibrous tissue at the border region between the plaque and the surrounding normal intima. This region is characterized by increased smooth muscle cell death and degradation of extracellular matrix by infiltrating inflammatory cells. Because type V lesions often invade the lumen and disturb the laminar blood flow, they are also more exposed to tensile forces.

Type VI lesions are plaques that contain thrombotic deposits or hemorrhage. The major cause of development of type VI lesions is plaque rupture, and fissures, erosions, and ulcerations of the subendothelial fibrous tissue are frequently observed. It is also possible that development of type VI lesions may be a result of bleeding from the capillaries that reaches into the plaque from the vasa vasorum. The occurrence of clinical events, such as acute myocardial infarction and unstable angina, is with few exceptions dependent on a type VI lesion.

However, development of type VI lesions can also take place in the absence of clinical symptoms. Autopsy studies in subjects who had coronary atherosclerosis but who died of noncardiac causes showed presence of recent intraplaque thrombus in 16% of those with hypertension and diabetes and in 8% of those without these factors. In another study of a population aged 30 to 59 years, 38% of those with advanced lesions in the aorta had thrombi on the surface of the lesions. Much of the thrombus that forms on top of a ruptured plaque is likely to be removed by the fibrinolytic system, but some of the material can also be incorporated into the plaque, which reseals. This process is responsible for most cases of rapid plaque progression that can be seen with angiography. The thrombotic material gradually becomes colonized by smooth muscle cells, which convert it back to fibrous tissue. As a result of this healing process, the lesion returns to a type V morphology.

Type VII and type VIII lesions are advanced plaques that have no or only minor amounts of lipids but contain masses of calcium deposits (type VII lesions) or predominantly consist of collagen (type VIII lesions). These lesions are believed to represent the end stage of the disease. Calcification is an age-related phenomenon and is widely present in the coronary arteries of subjects older than 70 years. Because calcification takes place in preexisting tissue, it does not generally contribute to plaque growth. The clinical importance of plaque calcification is unclear, but it is likely to make lesions less elastic and more sensitive to tensile forces. Type VIII lesions are more stable than type V and VI lesions. From a clinical point of view, much would be gained if type V and VI lesions could be converted into type VIII lesions. Lipid-lowering intervention trials using angiographic endpoints have shown that the beneficial effect on cardiovascular events is much greater than can be expected from the modest effect on plaque size. This observation suggests that the effect of lipid-lowering treatment is plaque stabilization rather than plaque regression. This notion is also supported by studies demonstrating that statins decrease plaque lipids and inflammation and increase the plaque collagen content.[11]

PATHOGENESIS OF ATHEROSCLEROSIS

Historical Background

The mechanisms by which atherosclerotic lesions form and expand have puzzled scientists for 150 years. The brilliant German pathologist Rudolf Virchow proposed in 1856 that atherosclerosis is caused when plasma components (including lipids) elicit an inflammatory response in the arterial wall. Another pathologist, von Rokitansky, suggested that the atherosclerotic lesion is formed by organization of thrombi on the surface of the arteries. In the first years of the last century, a major piece was added to the puzzle when Anitschkov in St. Petersburg observed the large lipid deposits in atherosclerotic plaques, speculated that cholesterol might cause atherosclerosis, and tested this idea by feeding rabbits cholesterol. This led to atherosclerotic lesions similar to those in humans. A few years later, two other Russian investigators, Starokadomskij and Sobolev, showed that mechanical injury to the aorta leads to intimal lesions resembling atherosclerosis. This fitted in with Virchow's hypothesis because injury would increase the infiltration of plasma components into the artery. In the 1950s, Florey and coworkers tied some of these observations together by showing that a de-endothelializing injury increases the accumulation of lipids and macrophages in the artery.[12]

With the advent of molecular medicine, it became possible to formulate more specific hypotheses for the pathogenesis of atherosclerosis. Ross and colleagues[13] in 1974 proposed that arterial injury causes local release of PDGF from adherent platelets or other cells. This would initiate a proliferative response in the smooth muscle population that could lead to atherosclerosis. An alternative hypothesis advocated by Benditt[14] stated that atherosclerosis is due to uncontrolled smooth muscle cell proliferation similar to that in a benign tumor.

The discovery by Brown and Goldstein[15] of LDL receptors and the mechanisms of cholesterol metabolism permitted testing of the "cholesterol hypothesis" with efficient pharmacologic and genetic tools. It clearly showed, in humans as well as in experimental models, a direct correlation between serum cholesterol (in particular LDL-cholesterol) and the extent of atherosclerosis. With these findings, it became obvious that any hypothesis concerning the pathogenesis of atherosclerosis must attempt to explain the role of cholesterol in this disease. New genetic disease models based on disturbances in lipid metabolism in gene knockout mice have permitted a detailed dissection of pathogenetic steps and have advanced our understanding of atherosclerosis significantly during the last 10 years.[16]

ATHEROSCLEROSIS: A CURRENT HYPOTHESIS

Studies of human lesions have identified molecules and cells that participate in the disease process. The recent development of genetic mouse models has made it possible to test the role of such specific factors in the formation and progression of atherosclerotic lesions. However, certain factors that may be of great importance in atherogenesis (e.g., several growth factors and adhesion molecules) cannot be studied by this approach because defects in the genes that encode these factors are not compatible with life. New technical achievements in knockout technology permit the induction of gene defects at a certain time point or in a certain tissue; the use of such methods has improved our understanding even further. A unifying hypothesis can now be proposed on the basis of these studies.[2] It is presented here and outlined in Figure 1.5.

Low-Density Lipoprotein Accumulation and Modification

The first detectable changes in an experimental animal subjected to proatherogenic stimuli, such as hypercholesterolemia, are an appearance of blood-derived lipids in the subendothelial intima and the expression of leukocyte adhesion molecules on the endothelial surface. When LDL levels rise in plasma, increasing amounts pass across the endothelium and into the intima. This process is enhanced at sites of increased transendothelial permeability, which are found at branches of the arterial tree.

The elimination of LDL from the intima is limited because of the lack of a microvasculature in this region. The capacity to eliminate LDL is therefore quickly exceeded, and LDL is trapped in the extracellular matrix. Proteoglycans of the matrix have an affinity for LDL, which leads to binding of LDL to the matrix and the buildup of an LDL pool.[17] In the intima, LDL undergoes a series of modifications that include aggregation, oxidation, and degradation of LDL components. They can be explained by an oxidative attack on the LDL particle, possibly by oxygen radicals generated

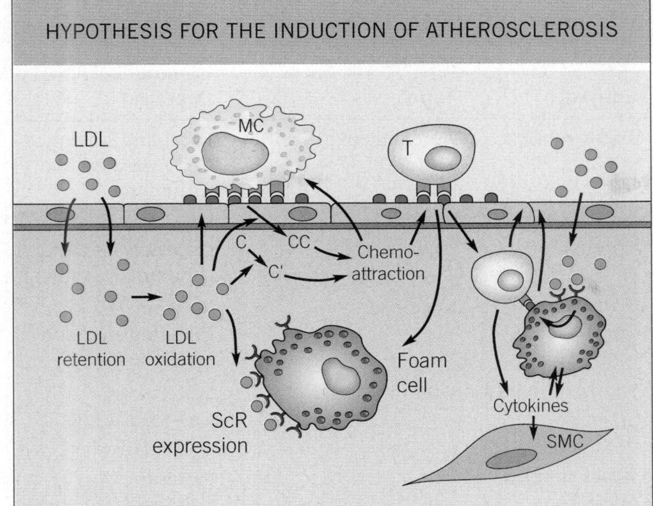

Figure 1.5 Hypothesis for the induction of atherosclerosis. Low-density lipoprotein (LDL) enters the arterial intima through an intact endothelium. In hypercholesterolemia, the influx of LDL exceeds the eliminating capacity, and an extracellular pool of LDL is formed. This is enhanced by association of LDL with proteoglycans of the extracellular matrix. Intimal LDL is oxidized through the action of free oxygen radicals formed by enzymatic or nonenzymatic reactions. This generates proinflammatory lipids that induce endothelial expression of the adhesion molecule vascular cell adhesion molecule 1, activate complement (C′), and stimulate chemokine (CC) secretion. All of these factors cause adhesion and entry of mononuclear leukocytes, particularly monocytes (MC) and T lymphocytes (T). Monocytes differentiate into macrophages, a process that is promoted by local macrophage colony-stimulating factor secretion in the forming lesion. Macrophages up-regulate scavenger receptors (ScR), which internalize oxidized LDL and transform into foam cells. Macrophage uptake of oxidized LDL also leads to presentation of fragments of it to antigen-specific T cells. This induces an autoimmune reaction that leads to production of proinflammatory cytokines. Such cytokines include interferon-γ, tumor necrosis factor-α, and interleukin-1, which act on endothelial cells to stimulate expression of adhesion molecules and procoagulant activity; on macrophages to activate proteases, endocytosis, nitric oxide, and cytokines; and on smooth muscle cells (SMCs) to induce nitric oxide production and to inhibit growth, collagen, and actin expression.

in tissue macrophages.[18] However, it is unclear why the antioxidants that protect LDL from oxidation in the blood cannot prevent the same process in the intima. Oxidation of LDL is described in more detail in other sections of this volume.

Recruitment of Inflammatory Cells

Oxidation of LDL leads to the release of modified lipids such as lysophosphatidylcholine. Several of these lipid species can act as signaling molecules that activate endothelial and smooth muscle cells.[19,20] This leads to expression of the leukocyte adhesion molecule vascular cell adhesion molecule-1 (VCAM-1), which is a receptor for monocytes and T lymphocytes.[21] Such cells express a "counterreceptor," very late activation antigen-4, which can ligate VCAM-1 as well as certain matrix molecules on the vascular surface. In concert with other adhesion molecule interactions, VCAM-1 ligation leads to sticking of monocytes and T cells on the endothelial surface at sites of lipid accumulation and modification.

Chemokines (i.e., chemotactic cytokines) are produced by macrophages, endothelial cells, and smooth muscle cells.[22] Their induction appears to be related to lipid accumulation and oxidation,[23] although the precise mechanisms are not fully clarified. In addition, aggregates of oxidized cholesterol induce complement activation, which also generates chemotactic signals.[24] Both these stimuli can promote the migration of mononuclear cells from the endothelial surface, through intercellular clefts of the endothelial layer, and into the subendothelial intima.

It is possible that other stimuli apart from lipids activate the endothelium and initiate leukocyte recruitment to the intima. In particular, heat shock proteins expressed during cell injury have been shown to activate the endothelium and to promote entry of monocytes and T cells.[25] Interestingly, immunization with such heat shock proteins substantially aggravates atherosclerosis.

Once present in the intima, monocytes differentiate into macrophages. This process is promoted by the cytokine monocyte colony-stimulating factor (M-CSF), which is produced by activated vascular cells. Because the monocyte is a relatively inert proform of the active macrophage, the differentiation process is of critical importance for pathology. This is illustrated by the observation that M-CSF–deficient mice do not develop atherosclerosis even if they are exposed to hypercholesterolemia or bred with atherosclerosis-prone mice.[26]

Foam Cell Formation

The macrophage plays a pivotal role in the forming atherosclerotic lesion. By virtue of its capacity to internalize oxidized lipoproteins, it accumulates cholesterol and transforms into a lipid-laden foam cell, which is the prototypic cell of atherosclerosis. Brown and Goldstein, who received the Nobel Prize for their discoveries concerning lipoprotein receptors and cholesterol metabolism, observed that macrophages do not take up significant amounts of normal, native LDL. However, they can internalize huge amounts of oxidized LDL through a set of scavenger receptors.[15,27] These cell surface receptors recognize "macromolecular patterns" containing clustered negative charges; such patterns are present on oxidized LDL but also on bacterial endotoxins and several other macromolecules.[28] Such ligands are bound to scavenger receptors, internalized, and degraded in the lysosomes. Cholesterol esters that are present in oxidized LDL are hydrolyzed, and free cholesterol escapes into the cytoplasm. It is re-esterified by cytosolic enzymes, and a pool of cholesterol esters start to form intracellular droplets in the macrophage. With continued uptake of oxidized LDL, such lipid droplets pile up in the cytoplasm until the macrophage is transformed into a lipid-laden foam cell. The fatty streak is essentially an accumulation of foam cells together with some T cells and extracellular cholesterol (largely lipoproteins) under an intact endothelium.

The scavenger receptor family, which includes the receptors SR-A, SR-B1, MARCO, CD36, and others, might have developed during evolution to protect us from endotoxinemia rather than to handle oxidized LDL,[29] and the number of scavenger receptors on the surface of the macrophage is not controlled by the intracellular cholesterol content. Therefore, the macrophage will continue to internalize oxidized LDL until its cytoplasm is overloaded with cholesterol ester. Scavenger receptors are regulated, however, by cytokines of the immune system and by metabolic factors other than cholesterol. In general, inflammatory cytokines tend to reduce receptor levels, whereas those cytokines that stimulate macrophage growth and differentiation up-regulate them. This focuses our attention on the inflammatory and immune aspects of the fatty streak.

The Toll-like receptors (TLRs) are another family of pattern recognition receptors involved in atherosclerosis. The TLRs are an important part of the innate immune system and mediate a rapid inflammatory response to a number of different structures exclusively expressed by viral and bacterial pathogens. These receptors are abundantly expressed in human atherosclerotic lesions.[30] Hypercholesterolemic mice lacking the TLR signal protein MyD88 develop less atherosclerosis, suggesting that hypercholesterolemia results in formation of endogenous ligands that react with TLRs and contribute to the formation of atherosclerotic plaques.[31]

IMMUNE INTERACTIONS IN THE FORMING LESION

Antigens and Immune Activation

T cells, like macrophages, enter the arterial intima after binding to an activated endothelium. Almost all the T cells are of the memory-effector type (i.e., they have been primed by a previous encounter with their respective antigen in lymphoid organs).[32] Once in the forming lesion, the T cells can be reactivated, provided their cognate antigens are present. In addition, there is a need for antigen-presenting cells because T cells, in contrast to B cells, cannot recognize free, soluble antigens. Instead, they require antigen to be "presented" in fragmented form and bound to major histocompatibility complex (MHC) molecules. In the plaque, antigen presentation appears to occur largely after uptake of antigen by macrophages, which present antigen fragments bound to MHC class II molecules (in humans, HLA-DR, DQ, and DP). Such antigen-MHC complexes are recognized by $CD4^+$ T cells, which are the predominating T-cell type in the plaque. Recognition leads to activation, which is a chain reaction of intracellular signals. It causes production of autocrine growth factors, DNA synthesis, T-cell division, secretion of cytokines, and, in some cases, development of cytotoxic properties. As discussed later, the cytokines serve to transduce antigen recognition into effector mechanisms.

Isolation and cloning of T cells from human plaques have revealed that a significant proportion of them recognize components of oxidized LDL.[33] Therefore, LDL can be viewed as an endogenous particle that is transformed into an autoantigen by oxidation. Antibodies to oxidized LDL are present in high titers in patients with atherosclerosis as well as in experimental models of the disease. However, it remains unclear whether antibody titers actually predict extent of disease progression.[34]

In addition to oxidized LDL, several other candidate antigens have been proposed for atherosclerosis.[35] They are listed in Table 1.2. Several of them, including heat shock protein 60, *Chlamydia pneumoniae* proteins, and oxidized LDL, not only function as T cell–dependent antigens but also act directly on macrophages to promote inflammation. This dual action of "atheroantigens" may be important for the progression of the disease.

CANDIDATE ANTIGENS IN ATHEROSCLEROSIS

Antigen	Type	Immune Responses Detected
Oxidized LDL	Autoantigen	Local and systemic Cell-mediated and humoral
Heat shock protein 60	Autoantigen, cross-reacts with microbial antigens	Local and systemic Cell-mediated and humoral
Chlamydia pneumoniae	Microbial	Systemic Cell-mediated and humoral
Cytomegalovirus	Viral	Systemic Cell-mediated and humoral
Herpes simplex type I	Viral	Systemic Cell-mediated and humoral

Table 1.2 Candidate antigens in atherosclerosis.

Immune Cytokines and Effector Mechanisms

T-cell cytokines produced after activation include proinflammatory cytokines that activate macrophages, endothelial cells, and smooth muscle cells but also cytokines that can inhibit inflammation and promote fibrosis. Different T-cell subtypes produce discrete sets of cytokines, which leads to different functional responses (Table 1.3). In the human plaque, most T cells are of the T_H1 type, which causes macrophage activation and inflammation.[36] Another proinflammatory T-cell subset, T_H17, plays a major role in some other inflammatory diseases, but its role in atherosclerosis is still unclear. The most important T_H1 cytokine is interferon-γ, which has profound vascular activities. It activates endothelial cells to express adhesion molecules and procoagulant activity, inhibits smooth muscle cells from making actins and collagens, and modulates cell division in the vessel wall. In addition, and most important, interferon-γ is a major macrophage-activating cytokine. It stimulates the macrophage to increase phagocytosis, to secrete inflammatory cytokines such as tumor necrosis factor-α (TNF-α) and interleukin-1, to release proteolytic enzymes, and to produce large amounts of toxic oxygen and nitric oxide radicals. In addition, TNF-α inhibits lipolytic enzymes, induces procoagulant activity, and changes the balance between fibrinolytic and antifibrinolytic factors on the endothelial surface.[22] All of these effects act to promote atherosclerosis, and interferon-γ appears to be the major cytokine causing the special form of arteriosclerosis that develops in transplanted organs.

The proinflammatory T_H1 effector activity is counterbalanced by regulatory T cells. These cells protect against autoimmunity and release anti-inflammatory cytokines such as interleukin-10 and transforming growth factor-β. They can also inhibit the activity of T_H1 cells by direct cell-to-cell

SOME CYTOKINES EXPRESSED IN ATHEROSCLEROTIC LESIONS			
Immune-regulating cytokines	Interferon-γ	T cells (T_H1-type $CD4^+$; $CD8^+$); NK cells	MØ activation, inflammation, EC and SMC activation, nitric oxide production, growth inhibition, reduced matrix formation, ScR regulation
	IL-2	T cells	T-cell proliferation
	IL-4	T cells (T_H2)	Allergic responses, B-cell activation, T-cell proliferation
	IL-12	MØ, EC, SMC	Induces T_H1 responses
	IL-10	MØ, T cells Treg	T_H2 stimulation, T_H1 inhibition
Proinflammatory cytokines	TNF-α	MØ, T_H1 cells	Adhesion molecules, growth factors, prostaglandins, nitric oxide, proteases, procoagulant
	IL-1	MØ, EC, SMC	Similar to TNF; promotes T-cell activation
	IL-6	MØ, T cells, EC, SMC	Acute-phase proteins; B-cell activation
Chemokines	MCP-1	MØ, EC, SMC	Attracts MC and T cells
	IL-8	MØ, T cells, EC, SMC	Attracts granulocytes
Growth factors	PDGF	Platelets, MØ, EC, SMC	SMC proliferation
	bFGF	SMC, EC	SMC and EC proliferation
	VEGF	MØ, SMC	EC proliferation
	TGF-β	MØ, EC, SMC, Treg platelets	Growth regulation; fibrogenic; anti-inflammatory
	M-CSF	MØ, T cells, EC	Stimulates MØ differentiation and ScR expression
	GM-CSF	MØ, T cells, EC	Differentiation of MC and granulocytes

bFGF, basic fibroblast growth factor; EC, endothelial cell; GM-CSF, granulocyte-macrophage colony-stimulating factor; IL, interleukin; MC, monocyte; M-CSF, macrophage colony-stimulating factor; MCP-1, monocyte chemoattractant protein 1; MØ, macrophage; PDGF, platelet-derived growth factor; ScR, scavenger receptor; SMC, smooth muscle cell; TNF, tumor necrosis factor; TGF, transforming growth factor; Treg, regulatory cells; VEGF, vascular endothelial growth factor.

Table 1.3 Some cytokines expressed in atherosclerotic lesions.

contact. Several lines of evidence have shown that regulatory T cells protect against atherosclerosis in hypercholesterolemic animals.[37,38] The balance between the different subsets varies between organs, with time during the course of an inflammatory disease, and also with the metabolic state of the host. This appears to depend on the levels of antigen, the conditions under which antigens are presented, and the presence or absence of immune-regulatory cytokines such as interleukin-10 and interleukin-12. The latter has also been detected in atherosclerotic plaques, where it may promote proinflammatory immune responses.[39]

Although cytokines are soluble, hormone-like substances, some cell surface factors may also be important in cell-cell signaling during atherogenesis. CD40 is a cell surface receptor on macrophages, B cells, and vascular cells. It binds to CD40 ligand, another surface protein that is present on T cells (but under some conditions expressed also by vascular cells). Their interaction leads to immune activation. When it occurs in the forming atherosclerotic lesion, it is an important driving force for disease progression and appears to act in a manner similar to the proinflammatory cytokines.[40] CD40 ligand and several other cell surface proteins display structural similarities to TNF-α, hence the name the TNF superfamily. Other family members such as lymphotoxin, OX40 ligand, LIGHT, RANK ligand, and CD137 have also been associated with atherosclerosis on the basis of genetic association, presence in lesions, and functional properties.[2,22,41]

Certain immune responses may be protective rather than proatherogenic. Thus, immunization with oxidized LDL inhibits atherosclerosis in several animal models.[42,43] Similarly, transfer of B cells from atherosclerotic to disease-prone mice protects them from severe disease.[44] This seemingly paradoxical effect may be caused by production of protective antibodies or anti-inflammatory or otherwise vasculoprotective cytokines.

Several therapeutic approaches that modulate immune activity have been used successfully to inhibit atherosclerosis in animal models. They include the use of polyclonal immunoglobulins[45] and anti-CD40L antibodies,[40] immunization with oxidized LDL,[46] peptide fragments of apolipoprotein B,[47] and anti–MDA-apoB peptide antibodies.[48] We are now awaiting clinical studies of these approaches.

PROGRESSION FROM FATTY STREAK TO ATHEROSCLEROTIC PLAQUE

The fatty streak is of no clinical significance. In fact, many of them disappear spontaneously. However, certain fatty streaks progress into true atherosclerotic, fibrofatty plaques. This characteristically occurs at sites of hemodynamic strain. Smooth muscle cells migrate to the subendothelial space, divide, and synthesize extracellular matrix. The result is a fibrous cap that separates the lipid-filled core of the lesion from the endothelial surface. It consists of fibrocyte-like, elongated smooth muscle cells surrounded by thick layers of their own matrix.

The stimuli that induce fibrous cap formation probably act by inducing smooth muscle activation.[2] Cell migration and proliferation will ensue, together with the synthesis by the cells of collagen and proteoglycans. In view of the focal localization of plaques, it is likely that local factors of the artery wall activate the smooth muscle cells. Most interest has been focused on growth factors, and data from vascular injury models show that basic fibroblast growth factor (bFGF) and PDGF can induce proliferation of quiescent arterial smooth muscle cells in vivo. In addition, PDGF acts as a chemotactic factor for smooth muscle cells. Whereas bFGF is deposited in the arterial extracellular matrix and can be released on injury, PDGF expression by endothelial cells can be up-regulated by flow changes.[49]

Hematopoietic cells can also release PDGF, and in particular, platelets and macrophages may be important sources of this growth factor. Interestingly, endothelial damage with defects covered by platelet microthrombi is observed in this phase of the disease in experimental models. A plausible scenario for the transition from fatty streak to fibrous plaque is therefore that hemodynamic stress or inflammatory activation causes growth factor release from platelets or macrophages. This stimulates smooth muscle cells to migrate, divide, and form the fibrous cap. The lipid core has been physically separated from the endothelial surface, and the plaque is stabilized. The price for this is obviously an encroachment on the lumen of the artery.

PLAQUE ACTIVATION AND THE PRECIPITATION OF CLINICAL SYNDROMES

The progressive reduction in luminal size can lead to clinical syndromes such as effort angina and intermittent claudication, but it is remarkable that even very large plaques may be completely asymptomatic. The development of acute clinical complications usually requires an additional pathogenetic event to occur, which is the formation of a thrombus on the plaque.[50] When this takes place, acute coronary syndromes such as myocardial infarction are observed. In other vascular beds, transitory cerebral ischemic attacks, brain infarction, and acute ischemic gangrene are caused by plaque thrombosis.

Several lines of research have established the role of thrombosis in the precipitation of acute ischemia. Injection of radioactive fibrinogen into patients with acute coronary syndromes has revealed incorporation into fresh coronary thrombi, and histopathologic analysis of coronary arteries has made it possible to identify mural thrombi on "culprit lesions." Interestingly, such lesions almost always show evidence of surface damage; approximately 80% of them exhibit small fissures through the endothelium and down into the plaque, whereas the remaining 20% appear to have areas of endothelial desquamation.[51,52] Such surface defects lead to exposure of prothrombotic subendothelial material and will rapidly result in thrombosis.

The superficial fissures found in most culprit lesions have been taken as evidence of plaque rupture. This term does not imply a crack through the entire endothelial wall; rather, the intimal plaque structure or part of it fissures. A plaque fissure usually extends from the endothelial surface through the fibrous cap and down into the lipid core of the plaque.

Why do plaques rupture? An important clue came from the observation that activated macrophages, T cells, and mast cells abound in the vicinity of the rupture.[53,54] This points to an inflammatory mechanism as the inducer of rupture. Such an interpretation is supported by the finding of circulating cytokines and activated T cells in patients with acute coronary syndromes such as unstable angina.[55] Subsequent immunohistochemical, biochemical, and cell biological studies have made it possible to propose a scenario for plaque activation and rupture.[2,56]

According to this hypothesis (Fig. 1.6), inflammatory cells of the plaque are activated by proinflammatory lipids, cytokines, antigens, or microbes. The ensuing immune or inflammatory activation results in macrophage activation. As part of it, the macrophage releases matrix metalloproteinases, which are enzymes that digest the collagen of the fibrous cap. Proinflammatory cytokines present in the inflammatory area prevent rebuilding of the collagen fibers by inhibiting collagen gene expression. Such cytokines (in particular, interferon-γ and TNF-α) also inhibit smooth muscle proliferation and actin gene expression, which eliminates the mechanisms for repair of the fibrous cap. Cytotoxic oxygen and nitric oxide radicals released by the macrophages contribute to the process by causing apoptotic cell death. All of these events reduce the tensile strength of the fibrous cap to such an extent that it succumbs to the mechanical stress exerted by the pulsating blood flow.

Advanced plaques contain cells that produce prostaglandin-like molecules called leukotrienes.[57,58] They are bioactive lipids with proinflammatory and vasoconstrictive effects. Molecular epidemiologic studies identify genes controlling

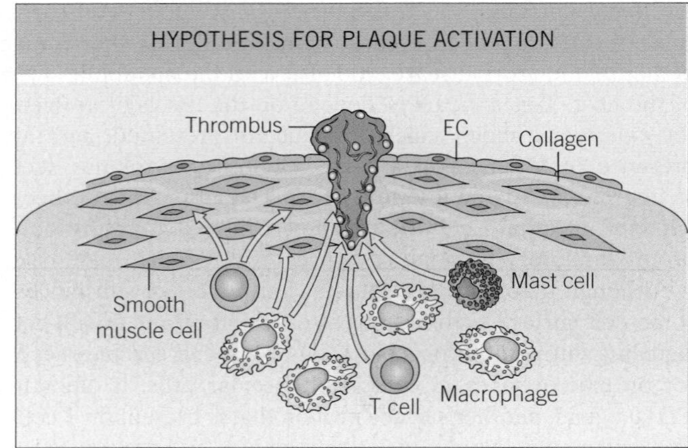

Figure 1.6 Hypothesis for plaque activation. Inflammatory activation in coronary plaques may be induced by lipids, cytokines, antigens, or microorganisms. Activated macrophages release matrix metalloproteinases, which digest collagen fibers of the plaque cap. Activated T cells produce cytokines, which inhibit proliferation and collagen secretion by cap smooth muscle cells. Activated mast cells release proteases such as chymase, which can also degrade cap structures. All of these factors weaken the fibrous cap, which eventually leads to the formation of fissures in the surface of the plaque. Such fissures serve as sites for thrombus formation by exposing subendothelial adhesive and procoagulant structures and also because inflammation can induce tissue factor expression by plaque cells. Thrombi may build up to eventually occlude the lumen; this precipitates myocardial infarction. EC, endothelial cell.

leukotriene biosynthesis as risk factors for cardiovascular disease,[59] and experimental studies show important, proatherogenic effects of leukotrienes on vascular endothelial and smooth muscle cells.[60]

When blood components are exposed to the subendothelium, platelets are immediately activated. They adhere to the surface and start to aggregate. A set of surface receptors mediate attachment between the platelet and the tissue; they include glycoprotein IIb/IIIa, which binds fibrinogen, and glycoprotein Ib, which binds the von Willebrand factor. Adenosine diphosphate and other factors released by the adhering platelet induce activation of other platelets, and the exposure of platelet membrane structures promotes activation of the humoral coagulation cascade. This is initiated when the protein tissue factor (thromboplastin) is exposed on the surface. It can be induced on macrophages, endothelial cells, and smooth muscle cells by proinflammatory cytokines and the CD40 system. Thus, inflammatory and immune activation promotes thrombosis in two ways: by causing plaque rupture and by inducing tissue factor expression.[2,56] In addition to tissue factor, cofactors such as membrane phospholipids and the von Willebrand–factor VIII complex are also important for humoral coagulation. The end result is the formation of a fibrin clot that surrounds and stabilizes the platelet thrombus.

With the formation of a solid thrombus, an acute coronary syndrome is often precipitated. However, defense mechanisms intrinsic to the blood and vessel wall may counteract thrombosis and prevent or eliminate complete obstruction. The most important of these defense mechanisms is the fibrinolytic system. It is a proteolytic cascade that is activated by plasminogen activators (tissue plasminogen activator and urokinase-type plasminogen activator), both of which can be expressed by endothelial cells. An inhibitor of fibrinolysis, the plasminogen activator inhibitor 1 (PAI-1), is also expressed by endothelial cells, and the balance between fibrinolysis and antifibrinolysis is therefore pivotal for the control of thrombus formation. By modulating the expression of plasminogen activator and PAI-1 genes, proinflammatory cytokines are important regulatory factors of this balance.

Research into the pathogenetic mechanisms that lead from silent atherosclerosis to myocardial infarction have been hampered by lack of suitable models. However, new mouse models may be useful for dissecting the pathogenetic sequence of acute coronary syndromes.[61,62]

SUMMARY

Is atherosclerosis a metabolic, inflammatory, infectious, or hemodynamic disease? In the past, scientists have debated whether atherosclerosis should be considered a disturbance of cholesterol metabolism, an inflammatory and fibrotic disease of the vessel wall, or a dysregulation of hemodynamic homeostasis. As evident from this chapter, all of these factors participate in the formation and activation of atherosclerotic plaques. Without hypercholesterolemia, it is unlikely that LDL would accumulate in the intima. Therefore, the chain of events that leads to atherosclerosis would never start. This view is confirmed by the success of lipid-lowering therapy against cardiovascular disease.

It could equally well be claimed that atherosclerosis would not occur if inflammatory cells did not enter the vessel wall. A large body of evidence shows that the disease can be prevented if leukocyte adhesion or macrophage differentiation cannot take place. Similarly, disease progression is retarded dramatically when immune activation is prevented.

The acceleration of disease in hypertension and the success of antihypertensive therapy show that a disturbed blood flow should be considered an important aggravating factor for atherosclerosis. Similarly, hemostatic factors, including those regulating platelet adhesion, humoral coagulation, and fibrinolysis, are involved in plaque activation. Blocking of platelet adhesion is an important therapeutic strategy against complications of angioplasty and vascular surgery and, together with anticoagulant therapy, also in acute coronary syndromes and cerebral and peripheral ischemia.

Our limited understanding of the roles of diabetes and smoking in the pathogenesis of atherosclerosis is in striking contrast to our knowledge of the effects of hypercholesterolemia and hypertension. Diabetes may act by perturbing the local carbohydrate metabolism in the vessel wall, but it could also affect the regulation of cellular functions by affecting growth regulation through insulin-like growth factors. Furthermore, hyperglycemia, which is usually present in diabetes, may result in nonenzymatic glycation of extracellular proteins, which is followed by uptake through specific receptors, resulting in both intracellular accumulation and signaling pathways that may affect hemostasis, angiogenesis, and cellular activation. Finally, non–insulin-dependent diabetes mellitus is often part of a metabolic syndrome that also includes hypertriglyceridemia and abdominal obesity. Abnormal triglyceride metabolism, which is part of this syndrome, may modulate vascular gene expression through specific transcriptional mechanisms (in particular through so-called peroxisome proliferator-activated receptors) and also cause release of proinflammatory cytokines from adipose tissue. Intense research into these aspects of diabetes and the metabolic syndrome may lead to new concepts of these risk factors for atherosclerosis within the next few years.

Information concerning smoking as a pathogenic factor in atherosclerosis is even more limited than information about diabetes. Epidemiologic studies show that the proatherogenic effect is not due to nicotine. Scientists have therefore proposed that complex biomolecular components of tar and cigarette smoke may damage endothelial cells or activate immune mechanisms. However, no definitive evidence links any of these factors to atherosclerotic disease.

It is apparent from this brief summary that several factors are epidemiologically linked to atherosclerosis, and at least three of them—hypercholesterolemia, inflammation, and hypertension—can be placed in a pathogenetic scheme. Our final conclusion must therefore be that atherosclerosis is a true multifactorial disease. The formation, progression, and activation of atherosclerotic plaques require an interaction between metabolic, inflammatory, hemodynamic, and hemostatic factors. All of them may turn out to be important targets for therapy, and all of these pathways are worth exploring in trying to develop new therapies against this major lethal disease of the Western world.

chapter

2 Genetics of Atherosclerosis

Heribert Schunkert and Jeanette Erdmann

- Myocardial infarction in a first-degree relative (man < 55 years, woman < 65 years) is an established cardiovascular risk factor.
- Positive family history increases the risk of myocardial infarction 1.5- to 2.0-fold.
- Twin and family studies revealed an estimate for heritability (h^2) of up to 60% for myocardial infarction.
- Some features of coronary disease, including calcification, left main disease, and proximal location of lesions, carry a high heritability.
- In rare cases (<1%), myocardial infarction displays a mendelian pattern of inheritance, mostly autosomal dominant.
- Major cardiovascular risk factors including hypercholesterolemia, hypertension, and diabetes mellitus are also in part genetically determined.
- Several genomic variants increase the risk of hypertension, hypercholesterolemia, and diabetes mellitus and—as a consequence of mendelian randomization to a risk factor—contribute to the genetic risk of myocardial infarction.
- Genome-wide association studies identified further common risk alleles that contribute to the manifestation of coronary artery disease, many by as yet unknown mechanisms.

Atherosclerosis is a complex disease caused by multiple genetic and environmental factors. Likewise, a multifactorial etiology applies to many of the underlying cardiovascular risk factors, including hypercholesterolemia, hypertension, diabetes mellitus, and smoking addiction. Thus, endogenous (genetic) and exogenous (e.g., nutrition, physical activity, therapy) mechanisms may affect the manifestation of atherosclerotic lesions either directly in the arterial wall or indirectly by modulation of traditional risk factors. On a cellular level, atherosclerosis is also complex, characterized by endothelial dysfunction, lipid and matrix accumulation, smooth muscle cell proliferation and migration, calcification, inflammation, and, finally, thrombus formation. In this scenario, the potential involvement of genetically modulated mechanisms may occur at multiple stages of the disease.

Evaluation of the family history long served as a guide to approach a patient's genetic risk for coronary events. Beyond the information conferred by a positive family history, identification of the underlying gene defects is thought to improve risk prediction and the knowledge of pathogenetic mechanisms.

Consequently, during the past 3 decades, a great deal of research has focused on defining such genetic components of myocardial infarction and of atherosclerosis and its risk factors. The hope for the future is that knowledge of the genes and gene variants will lead to improvements in the diagnosis and treatment of coronary disease. Indeed, emerging data suggest that some of the gene variants identified in recent years allow improved genetic risk prediction with sufficient reproducibility for the clinical setting.

This research initially focused on candidate genes that hypothetically might affect known traits involved in the atherosclerotic process, including the renin-angiotensin system, lipoprotein metabolism, inflammation, and coagulation. Many of these attempts failed replication in consecutive studies. Another difficulty in this research is that unlike mendelian traits, genetic studies of complex cardiovascular disorders are complicated by variable cosegregation between the risk allele and the disease. In fact, many genetic variants subsequently associated with the disorders were found to be relatively common in the overall population and thus—albeit to a variable degree—prevalent in both healthy and affected individuals.

In the beginning of this decade, genome-wide linkage analysis searched without a priori hypothesis for chromosomal regions shared in family members with myocardial infarction. Whereas this approach allowed identification of several chromosomal regions harboring myocardial infarction genes, it proved to be difficult to precisely define these. However, success came with genome-wide association studies that most recently identified multiple gene variants reproducibly associated with coronary heart disease, hypercholesterolemia, or diabetes mellitus. Surprisingly, most of the genes identified thus far are not expected to play a role in the development of atherosclerosis. Thus, an important task for the immediate future is to understand the fundamental pathophysiologic mechanisms affected by these genes in the development of atherosclerosis. Accordingly, functional information on these genetic factors and related gene expression as well as protein expression patterns is very much in need. Subsequently, genetic research may enhance diagnostic testing and development of new treatment targets.

DIAGNOSTIC CRITERIA

Assessment of Family History

For the time being, the assessment of family history is fundamental for approaching the genetic components in the complex disease processes leading to myocardial infarction. Particularly, a familial predisposition is assumed when myocardial infarction is diagnosed before the 55th year of life in a male first-degree relative or before the 65th year in a female first-degree relative. The Framingham Heart Study revealed that such positive family history for premature myocardial infarction increases the risk by a slightly different extent, depending on parental premature coronary artery disease (1.45-fold) or sibling coronary artery disease (1.99-fold). Moreover, the familial risk was found to be greater the lower the age of first manifestation of disease in the affected family.[1-3] To a lesser degree, genetic effects regarding myocardial infarction risk can be traced in an affected second-degree relative.[4] Interestingly, the excess risk related to a positive family history was found to be largely independent of the traditional risk factors tested.[5]

In families with several affected family members, traditional cardiovascular risk factors are often found with increased frequency.[6] Furthermore, lifestyle habits associated with a raised incidence of myocardial infarction (e.g., smoking) are more frequently shared in affected family members. Interestingly, the Northwick Park Heart Study as well as the Reykjavik Cohort Study revealed that the increase in risk in terms of a positive family history remains highly significant (odds ratio [OR], 1.5-1.8), even after adjustment for traditional risk factors.[7,8]

Furthermore, a high risk for recurrence of myocardial infarction was found in identical twins of myocardial infarction patients. Such form of a positive family history was related to an eightfold increased probability to die of myocardial infarction before the age of 55 years when the twin was affected at an early age as well (Fig. 2.1).[9] The highest risk related to family history, however, is found in rare families with an autosomal dominant pattern of inheritance for myocardial infarction.[10,11] In such families, up to 50% of individuals may be affected before the age of 70 years.

Heritability of Myocardial Infarction

The classic measure of the genetic component for a phenotype (trait), termed heritability, is defined as the percentage of the total variance of the trait that is explained by inheritance. By examining the increased similarity of trait values

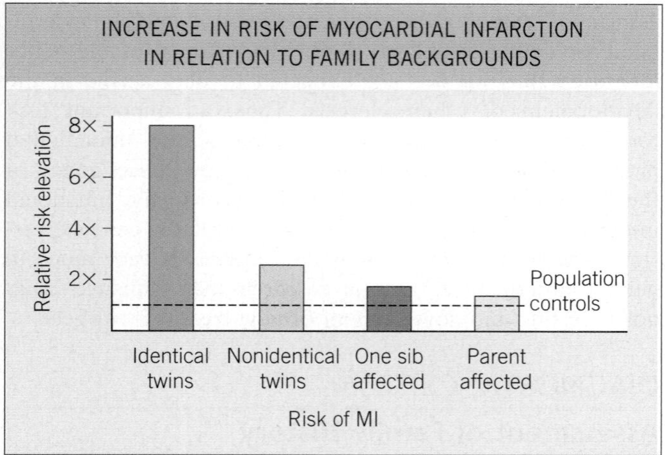

Figure 2.1 The relative increase in risk of myocardial infarction (MI) and coronary artery disease is shown in relation to different familial backgrounds. The risk for identical and nonidentical twins is based on the hypothesis that the partner twin had died of myocardial infarction at an age of ≤ 55 years.

HERITABILITY ESTIMATES FOR MYOCARDIAL INFARCTION AND VARIOUS RISK FACTORS

Trait	Heritability Estimate (%)*
Myocardial infarction	25-60
Total cholesterol level	40-60
High-density lipoprotein cholesterol level	45-75
Total triglyceride level	40-80
Body mass index	25-60
Systolic blood pressure	50-70
Diastolic blood pressure	50-65
Lipoprotein(a) level	90
Homocysteine level	45
Type 2 diabetes	40-80
Fibrinogen level	20-50

*Heritability estimates, in most cases based on multiple studies, are taken from Jee et al.,[12] King et al.,[13] and Lusis et al.[14]

Table 2.1 Heritability estimates for myocardial infarction and various risk factors.

in related individuals compared with unrelated or less-related individuals, one can estimate the heritability. The simplest conceptual study design is the comparison of monozygotic and dizygotic twins. Thus, monozygotic twins share 100% of their genes, whereas dizygotic twins share, on average, 50% of their genes. If a trait has a genetic component, monozygotic twins are likely to resemble each other to a greater extent than dizygotic twins do. Table 2.1 lists heritability estimates for myocardial infarction and various risk factors.[12–14] Because of assumptions that are required for estimates of heritability, the calculated heritabilities must be considered approximate.

Heritability of Coronary Anatomy and Disease

The heritability estimates of coronary artery disease have been demonstrated to depend in part on the pattern of coronary morphology.[16] Particularly, left main disease and proximal coronary artery stenoses displayed high recurrence rates in affected siblings. The heritability estimate for ostial and proximal coronary stenoses was found to be $h^2 = 0.32$, indicating that about one third of the variability of this phenotype is explained by genetic factors ($P = .008$). Likewise, a highly significant heritability was found for the ectatic form of coronary atherosclerosis and extraluminal calcification of the coronary arteries as well as the abdominal aorta.[15] Thus, in addition to family history, knowledge of the coronary disease in an affected family member may enhance risk prediction in first-degree relatives of this patient.

Molecular Genetic Testing

In addition to the assessment of family history, molecular genetic testing may be reasonable to estimate the predisposition for coronary artery disease or the presumed pharmacodynamic or pharmacokinetic effects of drugs.

To become a useful tool in the clinical setting, a molecular genetic test should be characterized by high analytical and clinical validity as well as a reasonable clinical utility.[17] Whereas the precision of molecular genetic testing (analytical validity) is generally high, the degree to which the test predicts the risks of health or disease (clinical validity) remains to be established for most genetic variants associated with myocardial infarction. In addition, it is currently unclear to what extent clinical decision making (clinical utility) can be improved by molecular genetic testing for myocardial infarction risk. Particularly, with the background of currently validated tools for risk prediction (e.g., Framingham risk score, PROCAM score, ESC score), novel molecular, genetically based tests have to demonstrate how the diagnostic precision of such scores can be improved.[18] This challenge is particularly true for a molecular-based risk score that ultimately may consider the interaction of multiple risk alleles for disease prediction.[19-21] Irrespective of such uncertainties, molecular diagnostic testing is being commercially offered. It is questionable, however, whether the information gathered by such testing is meaningful, particularly when no genetic counseling accompanies such analysis.

Prevalence of Genetic Risk Markers

Atherosclerotic heart disease involving the coronary arteries (coronary heart disease) is the most common cause of death in Europe and the United States, accounting for one third of all deaths. In the setting of large epidemiologic surveys, 35% of all patients with coronary artery disease were found to fulfill the criteria for a positive family history. This high prevalence of familial recurrence underscores the quantitative significance of genetically mediated risk factors.[8]

Sizeable differences can be observed with respect to the prevalence of alleles conferring a risk for myocardial infarction. The spectrum reaches from private mutations found only in a single family or a few families to common risk alleles prevalent in more than 50% of individuals in a given population. Examples for such alleles are presented in Table 2.2. Given the large number of genes affecting the risk of myocardial infarction and the high prevalence of some of the risk-conferring variants, it is obvious that almost every person in a population carries some alleles associated with myocardial infarction risk. However, many of the common risk variants confer only a small relative risk increase, that is, an odds ratio of 1.2 to 1.5 per allele. Given that the absolute risk for myocardial infarction per year is small in most individuals (e.g., the annual risk for an unselected man at the age of 50 years in a mid-European population is 0.25%), a small risk increase mediated by a single genetic variant may be clinically irrelevant. In fact, given that the individuals used as a reference for this comparison are also carrying the average number of risk alleles found in the respective population, genotypic information of a single variant is unlikely to improve risk prediction in the clinical setting.

It is currently unclear whether certain patterns of risk alleles or the mere additive effect of such variants will ultimately precipitate the clinical event. In the case that several genetic variants jointly confer risk of myocardial infarction, it has been estimated that knowledge of 40 to 80 risk alleles may allow clinically meaningful risk prediction (population attributable risk). In this regard, it is important to distinguish between common sequence variants with a small effect (low odds ratio) and rare sequence variants with a large effect. Particularly those variants with a high prevalence and a strong effect may confer a profound effect at the population level. In the case of the chromosome 9p21.3 locus, the population attributable risk is about 21%. This reaches the same

GENES AND GENE LOCI IDENTIFIED IN CORONARY ARTERY DISEASE–MYOCARDIAL INFARCTION*

Genes and Gene Loci	Function	References
I. Beyond controversy		
More than three large independent replication studies (>10,000 cases and 10,000 controls), no negative study, positive association results in different ethnicities		
9p21.3	Unknown	18, 37-44
II. Beyond controversy (at least in one ethnicity)		
More than two large independent replication studies (>1000 cases and 1000 controls) in the same ethnicity, negative association results in different ethnicities, positive meta-analysis		
LP(a)	Lipoprotein	45
ApoE4	Lipoprotein handling	46
LPL	Lipoprotein lipase	40
CETP	Lipoprotein handling	47
PCSK9	Lipoprotein handling	48
LDLR	Lipoprotein handling	70
LTA	Inflammation	49
Galectin 2	Inflammation	50
ALOX5AP	Inflammation	51
LTA4H	Inflammation	52
III. Still controversy		
More than three small independent replication studies (<500 cases and 500 controls), plus negative association studies in different ethnicities		
MHC2TA	Inflammation	53
Kalirin	Inflammation	54
IV. Involvement in pathophysiologic process beyond controversy, impact on common forms of coronary artery disease–myocardial infarction still doubtful		
Mutations in mendelian forms of coronary artery disease–myocardial infarction, plus positive and negative association studies in different ethnicities		
MEF2A	Endothelial integrity	10, 36
LRP6	Lipoprotein	11

*Listed are some genes and gene loci identified in coronary artery disease–myocardial infarction. The genes and gene loci are prioritized (I to IV) according to the current evidence for association with coronary artery disease–myocardial infarction on the basis of independent replication studies in different ethnicities.

Table 2.2 Genes and gene loci identified in coronary artery disease–myocardial infarction*.

magnitude as many of the traditional risk factors (e.g., diabetes mellitus) that carry a relatively high risk but occurs at a much lower frequency in the population.

Genetic Risk Factors

Molecular Genetics of Coronary Artery Disease and Myocardial Infarction

Genes that are associated with complex human diseases like coronary artery disease and myocardial infarction can be classified into two categories: disease-causing genes and susceptibility genes.

Disease-causing genes are those genes that are directly responsible for the pathogenesis of disease when they are mutated. For example, mutations in β-myosin heavy chain gene (*MYH7*) cause hypertrophic cardiomyopathy,[22,23] and mutations in Titin gene (*TTN*) cause dilated cardiomyopathy.[24] Such disease-causing genes have great predictive values and can be used directly for genetic testing.[17]

Susceptibility genes are those that increase or decrease the risk for development of a specific disease. However, these variants may or may not cause the disease in the context of other genetic and environmental factors. Risk-predicting variants of these genes are present in both normal and diseased individuals of a given population, but the frequencies differ in the two groups. For a single individual, susceptibility genes have less predictive value for the development and prognosis of the disease.

Disease-Causing Genes for Coronary Artery Disease and Myocardial Infarction

Among the best-established genetic risk factors for coronary artery disease and myocardial infarction are single-gene disorders affecting plasma levels of low-density lipoprotein (LDL) cholesterol and high-density lipoprotein (HDL) cholesterol. In fact, genes responsible for familial hypercholesterolemia (FH) and Tangier disease are the prototypic examples of causal genes for coronary artery disease and myocardial infarction.

Familial Hypercholesterolemia

The heterozygous state of this autosomal dominant condition, present in around 1 in 500 to 1000 of most Western populations, is associated with elevated cholesterol levels and premature coronary heart disease. The homozygous state leads to accelerated vascular disease, and without treatment, survival into the teenage years is unusual. The ranges of LDL-cholesterol levels are 200 to 400 mg/dL in heterozygotes and more than 450 mg/dL in homozygous carriers of FH mutations compared with 75 to 175 mg/dL in healthy individuals. As a consequence, progressive coronary artery disease and myocardial infarction may occur in the fourth or fifth decade in heterozygotes and already in the first decade of life in homozygote mutation carriers.

In most families, the underlying defect can be identified in the LDL receptor gene (*LDLR*) located on chromosome 19p13.2. The LDL receptor is responsible for the majority of uptake of circulating LDL by the liver. Besides rare mutations, studies have identified common genetic variants affecting the variability of LDL-cholesterol levels and thus the risk of coronary artery disease.

Other disease-causing genes for coronary artery disease–myocardial infarction that act through markedly altered LDL-cholesterol levels are *APOB* (chromosome 2q24) and *PCSK9* (chromosome 1p34.1-p32).[25]

Familial Defective Apolipoprotein B-100

Apolipoprotein B (apoB) is the primary apolipoprotein of LDL that is responsible for carrying cholesterol to tissues. Although it is unclear exactly what functional role apoB plays in LDL, it is the primary apolipoprotein component and is absolutely required for its formation. The most important molecular defect responsible for familial defective apoB-100 is a single mutation (R3500Q) in *APOB* gene.[26]

PCSK9

In FH families with no mutation in the *LDLR* gene and lack of the APOB3500 variant, a new FH locus was identified recently on chromosome 1p34.1-32. Subsequent sequencing analysis identified missense mutations in the proprotein convertase subtilisin/kexin 9 (PCSK9) gene. *PCSK9* was found to play a major role in the LDL-LDLR pathway, even if the exact mechanism of its influence remains incompletely understood (see also later).[27-29]

Tangier Disease

Tangier disease is a very rare autosomal recessive condition characterized by low levels of HDL-cholesterol in the blood, accumulation of cholesterol in many organs of the body, and an increased risk of arteriosclerosis. This disease is due to mutations in *ABCA1* gene.[30] *ABCA1* gene encodes a protein that regulates the cellular efflux of cholesterol and phospholipids to an apolipoprotein transporter. Until now, several mutations responsible for Tangier disease have been identified, all of which result in a complete or partial loss of function that leads to an accumulation of cellular cholesterol, low plasma HDL levels, and increased risk of coronary artery disease.

Apolipoprotein A-I (APOA1) (Milano, Arg173Cys)

Franceschini and colleagues[31] identified a family with hypertriglyceridemia and a marked decrease of HDL levels. Further studies revealed an arginine-to-cysteine exchange at position 173 of the amino acid sequence of apolipoprotein A-I resulting in an anomalous protein designated APOA-I (Milano). Gualandri and associates[32] traced the origin of this variant to Limone sul Garda, a small community of about 1000 persons in northern Italy. In a study of the entire population, 33 living carriers were found, ranging in age from 2 to 81 years. The genealogy showed origin of all cases from a single couple living in the 18th century. Despite low HDL-cholesterol levels and increased mean level of triglycerides, no evidence of increased atherosclerosis was found. Shah and colleagues[33] formulated recombinant APOA-I (Milano) in a complex with naturally occurring phospholipids. Studies in mice and rabbits with experimental atherosclerosis demonstrated that such complexes rapidly mobilized cholesterol and thereby reduced atherosclerotic plaque burden. The anti-atherosclerotic effects occurred in animals as rapidly as 48 hours after a single infusion.[33] In humans, Nissen and coworkers[34] found that this complex, administered intravenously for five doses at weekly intervals, produced significant regression of coronary atherosclerosis as measured by consecutive intravascular ultrasound studies.

Autosomal Dominant Coronary Artery Disease–Myocardial Infarction Families

Some families present with an extremely raised prevalence of coronary artery disease–myocardial infarction in multiple members in subsequent generations. With the exception of two large families studied by Wang and coworkers[10] and Mani and associates[11] (see next paragraphs), many such families could not be systematically analyzed genetically because of the high lethality of the disease. In the German Myocardial Infarction Family Study, we specifically looked for myocardial infarction in large families with at least four surviving affected individuals. We systematically interviewed and investigated members of 19 such families.[35,36] On the basis of family pedigree analysis and statistical simulations, the presence of an autosomal dominant inheritance pattern was probable in all cases. The family pedigrees will, it is hoped, extend the knowledge of genes involved in myocardial infarction in the near future (Fig. 2.2). However, the prevalence of such families with a mendelian pattern of coronary artery disease is low and estimated to account for approximately 1% of all myocardial infarction cases.[35]

MEF2A

Wang and coworkers[10] recently succeeded in identifying a mutation in the gene of the transcription factor myocyte enhancer factor 2A (MEF2A) in a family with an autosomal dominant form of myocardial infarction. For the first time, a familial genetic defect was shown to give rise to myocardial infarction in humans. A 21-bp deletion in the gene appeared to result in alterations of the coronary walls, thus favoring plaque deposition, which ultimately may lead to myocardial infarction. Interestingly, the same pathway is crucial in preventing apoptosis in endothelial cells and death due to vascular obstruction in mice. However, at present, the significance of this gene with respect to the heritability in humans is still unclear given several studies showing no association between single nucleotide polymorphisms (SNPs) in the *MEF2A* gene and coronary artery disease and myocardial infarction in other families or large case-control studies.[36]

LRP6

In 2007, Mani and associates[11] described a large Iranian family segregating autosomal dominant coronary artery disease with hyperlipidemia, hypertension, type 2 diabetes, and osteoporosis. They identified a C-to-T transition in exon 9 of the *LRP6* gene, resulting in an arginine-to-cysteine substitution at codon 611 (R611C). The index case in this family was found to be homozygous for this mutation, whereas all other affected family members were heterozygous. However, even heterozygous subjects manifested early coronary artery disease and metabolic syndrome. Expression of *LRP6* containing this mutation in NIH3T3 cells showed a 49% reduction of Wnt signaling compared with that of wild-type *LRP6*. The addition of low doses of Wnt3a also demonstrated markedly reduced signaling of *LRP6* carrying the R611C mutation.

Candidate Genes for Coronary Artery Disease and Myocardial Infarction

Hundreds of association studies and dozens of genome scans have been conducted to identify genes contributing to common forms of coronary artery disease–myocardial infarction and its risk factors. For the majority of studies, it proved to be difficult to reproduce originally reported associations. The most likely cause is a false-positive finding in relatively small study populations with an elevated possibility of spurious association. Moreover, ethnic variation (differences in genetic structure, namely, differences in SNP linkage

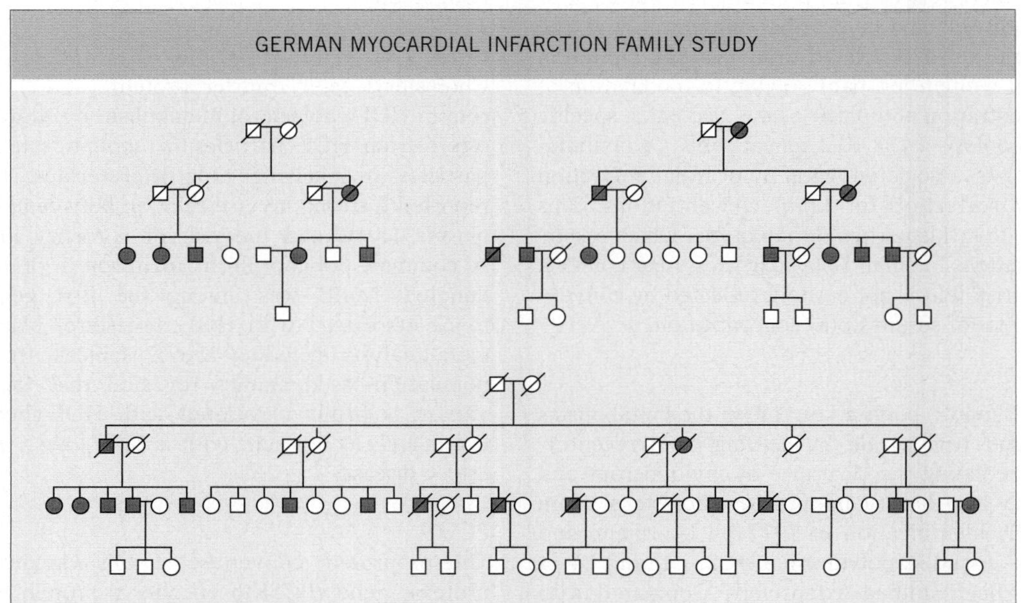

Figure 2.2 Examples of multiplex families with myocardial infarction presenting an autosomal dominant inheritance pattern from the German Myocardial Infarction Family Study. Men are encoded with squares, women with circles. Affected individuals are designated in black, unaffected individuals are bordered, and deceased persons are crossed out.

disequilibrium and haplotype structure) must be taken into consideration in the appraisal of divergent results. Finally, the functional relevance of most polymorphisms still needs demonstration; alternatively, these variants may display association with disease only because of their close neighborhood or linkage disequilibrium with responsible mutations.

Despite these problems, a number of genes have exhibited consistent evidence of linkage or association with coronary artery disease–myocardial infarction or its risk factors or have exhibited similar effects when studied in animal models. Some examples of these genes contributing to atherosclerosis or its risk factors are described in the next paragraphs and in Table 2-2.[37-54]

However, none of these genes allows risk prediction with sufficient reproducibility for the conditions in the clinical setting. Both positive and negative associations were found for all of these variants.

Lipoprotein(a)

Lipoprotein(a) serum levels have been repeatedly associated with coronary artery disease or myocardial infarction in large observational studies.[55,56] The interindividual variability of Lp(a) levels is very high and is largely determined by the polymorphic apolipoprotein(a) gene on chromosome 6q27.[45,57] Besides several polymorphisms located in the promoter region of the gene, the apolipoprotein(a) kringle IV (KIV) repeat polymorphism (38 known alleles) that generates apolipoprotein(a) molecules ranging from 250 to 800 kDa appears to determine about half of the variability of Lp(a) serum levels, with an inverse relationship between the number of KIV repeats and Lp(a) serum concentration. In addition, a pentanucleotide repeat polymorphism (seven known alleles) at position −1373 from the ATG site may be of particular interest because a consistent association with Lp(a) levels was found in small populations. A study by Holmer and colleagues[45] suggests that at least three factors affect the association between lipoprotein(a) and the risk of coronary artery disease and myocardial infarction. First, the kringle IV polymorphism is related to myocardial infarction in both men and women, probably owing to modulation of both Lp(a) concentration and particle size. Second, a specific and frequent haplotype (≤22 KIV repeats and ≤8 pentanucleotide repeats) is associated with myocardial infarction in women after correction for Lp(a) concentrations. This finding indicates that this particular haplotype, which results in high concentrations of small Lp(a) particles, may confer a specifically high risk that is not entirely reflected by conventional measurement of serum Lp(a) concentration.

Apolipoprotein E

Apolipoprotein E (apoE) plays a key role in the metabolisms of cholesterol and triglyceride by serving as a receptor-binding ligand mediating the clearance of chylomicrons and remnants of very-low-density lipoprotein cholesterol from plasma. Since the identification in 1977 by Utermann and colleagues,[58] the common polymorphism ε2, ε3, and ε4 of *APOE* gene has been studied extensively. Compared with ε3 homozygotes, carriers of the ε2 allele, which has defective receptor-binding ability, have lower circulating cholesterol levels and higher triglyceride levels, whereas carriers of the ε4 allele appear to have higher plasma levels of total cholesterol and LDL-cholesterol.[59] A meta-analysis of 48 studies including 15,492 cases and 32,965 controls revealed that carriers of the apoE ε4 allele had a 42% higher risk for coronary artery disease than did persons with the ε3/3 genotype (OR, 1.42; 95% confidence interval [CI], 1.26-1.61) (for review, see reference 46).

Lipoprotein Lipase

Lipoprotein lipase (LPL) hydrolyzes triglycerides contained in the core of both chylomicrons and very-low-density lipoproteins, thus causing these particles to be transformed into chylomicron remnants and intermediate-density or low-density lipoproteins, respectively. Genetic defects of LPL are responsible for the reduced triglyceride-rich lipoprotein clearance, and mutations in the *LPL* gene have been shown to play a central role in the development of hypertriglyceridemia in the general population. Approximately 143 different variants have been identified to date in the human *LPL* gene, 90% of which occur in the coding regions and affect LPL functions through catalytic activity, dimerization, secretion, and heparin binding.[60] Moreover, several common variants like the S447X polymorphism located in exon 9 of the human *LPL* gene have been identified and associated with decreased levels of blood triglycerides and an increase in LPL activity. Associations between LPL genetic variation and coronary artery disease have been contradictory, but a recent candidate gene analysis based on genome-wide association data for coronary artery disease and myocardial infarction in more than 2500 cases and 4500 controls confirmed the association between *LPL* gene variants and disease risk. Although several SNPs in different candidate genes showed significant association with coronary artery disease in the Wellcome Trust Case Control Consortium study or with myocardial infarction in the German study, only two linked SNPs (rs17489268 and rs17411031) tagging the Ser447X variant in the *LPL* gene showed a significant association in both studies.[40]

CETP

Cholesteryl ester transfer protein (CETP) plays a central role in HDL-cholesterol metabolism by shuttling cholesteryl esters from HDL particles to apolipoprotein B–containing particles in exchange for triglycerides. Several studies reported a strong inverse relation between HDL-cholesterol plasma levels and the risk of coronary artery disease.[61] A common polymorphism in intron 1 of the *CETP* gene denoted *Taq*IB was among the first genetic variations to be associated with HDL-cholesterol plasma levels.[62] A meta-analysis including 13,677 subjects from seven large, population-based studies revealed that the *CETP Taq*IB variant is firmly associated with HDL-cholesterol plasma levels and, as a result, with a 20% lower risk of coronary artery disease.[47]

PCSK9

The proprotein convertase subtilisin/kexin type 9 serine protease gene *(PCSK9)* encodes a protein that is involved in the regulation of the number of LDL receptors on the cell surface and was first identified by Seidah and coworkers.[27] Genetic variation at *PCSK9* has been reported to significantly affect LDL-cholesterol levels in the plasma,

LDL-cholesterol–lowering response to statins, and risk for premature coronary artery disease.[48] By resequencing of the *PCSK9* gene, a broad spectrum of sequence variations was found with a wide range of frequency (0.2% to 34%) and magnitude of LDL-cholesterol–lowering effects (from a 3% increase to a 49% decrease).[63] The clinical impact of functional variants (like the Y142X, C679X, or R46L) was studied in a large epidemiologic cohort known as the Atherosclerosis Risk in Communities (ARIC) study, which had 15-year follow-up of about 13,000 individuals. Variants in *PCSK9* causing a decrease in LDL-cholesterol were associated with a marked reduction of coronary events, consisting of coronary artery disease–related death, myocardial infarction, or need for a revascularization procedure. These findings strongly point out the protective effect of having low LDL levels from birth, which is quite disparate from the way LDL reduction is achieved clinically with statins beginning in the fifth or sixth decade of life.[64]

LDLR

Whereas FH is perhaps the most prominent example of a genetic disorder associated with coronary artery disease, missense mutations in *LDLR* resulting in FH have a frequency of only 0.01% to 0.02% in populations of European descent. Much less is known about common genetic variation in the *LDLR* gene associated with LDL-cholesterol levels and risk of coronary artery disease. Two studies have identified a common polymorphism located in exon 12 of *LDLR* (rs688) that decreases splicing efficiency of the *LDLR* mRNA and is associated with increased LDL-cholesterol levels.[65,66] More recently, three reports of genome-wide association studies on serum lipoprotein levels have identified two variants in strong linkage disequilibrium (rs2228671 and rs6511720) that affect LDL-cholesterol levels across multiple populations.[67-69] The minor allele (frequency 11%) of SNP rs2228671 results in a lifelong LDL lowering of 16 mg/dL, and this reduction in LDL-cholesterol translates into a decreased risk of coronary artery disease across multiple case-control studies.[70]

Lymphotoxin α (LTA)

In a stepwise genome-wide association study, Ozaki and colleagues[49] identified in 2002 a susceptibility locus for myocardial infarction on chromosome 6p21 in a Japanese population. Five SNPs within a 50-kb genomic locus region comprising *BAT1* (encoding HLA-B–associated transcript 1), *NFKBIL1* (encoding nuclear factor of κ light chain gene enhancer in B cells inhibitor-like 1), and *LTA* (encoding lymphotoxin α) were in high linkage disequilibrium and significantly associated with myocardial infarction (*LTA* exon 1 G10A; OR, 1.78; 95% CI, 1.39-2.27; $P = .0000033$; recessive model). Functional data as well as involvement of the gene product in the inflammatory pathways further supported their hypothesis.

Galectin 2 (LGALS2)

In another study, the same authors identified an SNP (rs7291467) in the galectin 2 (*LGALS2*) gene associated significantly with susceptibility to myocardial infarction (OR, 1.57; 95% CI, 1.30-1.90; $P = .0000026$ for recessive model of inheritance), which in vitro affected the transcriptional level of the galectin 2 protein.[50] The authors demonstrated binding of LTA protein to galectin 2 and speculated that altered biologic availability of the LTA protein might affect disease pathogenesis.

Nevertheless, for both genes, controversial results were obtained in subsequent replication studies. Whereas two groups were able to replicate the original findings in the *LTA* and *LGALS2* genomic region, others failed to provide additional evidence for the association of *LTA* with myocardial infarction.[71]

ALOX5AP

In two studies, Helgadottir and colleagues[51,52] reported a strong genetic association between the *ALOX5AP* gene and risk of myocardial infarction and stroke in the Icelandic population.

ALOX5AP encodes arachidonate 5-lipoxygenase–activating protein (FLAP), which plays a key role in the biosynthesis of proinflammatory leukotriene B mediators, providing a potential link between inflammation and cardiovascular disease. In a genome-wide scan of Icelandic families with myocardial infarction, suggestive linkage led to the identification of the *ALOX5AP* gene as a strong candidate gene for myocardial infarction. Within the *ALOX5AP* gene, the authors identified a four-SNP haplotype (haplotype A) conferring a twofold risk for myocardial infarction. In functional studies using isolated neutrophils from carriers of haplotype A, an increased production of the proinflammatory leukotriene B was demonstrated.[51]

In a subsequent report, the same authors who first reported the association of haplotype A with myocardial infarction in the Icelandic population were unable to confirm this association in a cohort of British patients. However, the authors identified another four-SNP haplotype of the *ALOX5AP* gene, termed haplotype B, that conferred significant risk of both myocardial infarction and stroke.[72] Similarly, an angiography-based study from Italy has detected an increased risk of angiographically proven coronary artery disease for carriers of haplotype B but not for carriers of haplotype A.[73] In analogy to these two studies, Linsel-Nitschke and colleagues[74] detected an increased risk of myocardial infarction for carriers of haplotype B of the *ALOX5AP* gene in a large German study. In contrast to the aforementioned European studies, no association of either haplotype A or haplotype B of the *ALOX5AP* gene with myocardial infarction was detected in further studies from the United States and Japan.

LTA4H

The *LTA4H* gene encodes leukotriene A_4 hydrolase, a protein in the same biochemical pathway as FLAP, the gene product of *ALOX5AP*. Helgadottir and colleagues[52] reported a moderately increased risk of myocardial infarction for carriers of a haplotype in the *LTA4H* gene (haplotype K). In a similar fashion as previously demonstrated for *ALOX5AP*, the authors were again able to show an increased production of proinflammatory leukotriene B associated with haplotype K of the *LTA4H* gene. In the same report, the authors replicated the association of haplotype K with myocardial infarction and stroke in pooled populations from three North American cities comprising 1591 myocardial infarction cases with European ancestry and 197 myocardial infarction cases with African American ancestry. The increased chance conferred by haplotype K was markedly higher in African Americans and for subjects with myocardial infarction and concomitant cerebrovascular disease. This association was not replicated in a large German population.[74]

Susceptibility Genes and Gene Regions for Coronary Artery Disease–Myocardial Infarction From Genome-Wide Association Studies

Completion of the human genome reference sequence in 2004, the systematic cataloguing of sequence variation by the SNP Consortium and the HapMap Project in 2005, and novel high-throughput technologies for SNP typing now enable interrogation of the genome with approximately 80% coverage currently using 500,000 to 1,000,000 SNPs simultaneously. These technologic advances opened a new era of the exploration of common diseases like coronary artery disease and myocardial infarction. Indeed, in the past months, four independent genome-wide association studies were completed on coronary artery disease.[37,39-41] Most excitingly, all studies revealed uniformly that a single chromosomal locus (9p21.3) confers the strongest association with coronary artery disease and myocardial infarction (Table 2.3 and Fig. 2.3). Six additional loci were identified by Samani and coworkers[40] on chromosome 1 (1p13.3 and 1q41), chromosome 2 (2q36.3), chromosome 6 (6q25.1), chromosome 10 (10q11.21), and chromosome 15 (15q22.33). To date, for chromosome 9p21.3, large studies showing subsequent replication of the original association signal in different populations are published.[18,38,42-44,75] Moreover, a locus at chromosome 1p13.3 displayed strong association

COMPILATION OF STUDIES SHOWING THE ASSOCIATION OF GENETIC VARIANTS AT CHROMOSOME 9p21.3 AND DIFFERENT CARDIOVASCULAR PHENOTYPES

Cohort	No. of Cases	No. of Controls	Phenotype	*P* value	Reference
Ottawa Heart Study-1	322	312	CAD	3.7×10^{-6} (rs10757274)	37
Ottawa Heart Study-2	311	326	CAD	.0009 (rs10757274)	
Atherosclerosis Risk in Communities	1347	9054	CAD	.004 (rs10757274)	
Copenhagen City Heart Study	1525	9053	CAD	.0004 (rs10757274)	
Dallas Heart Study	154	527	CAD	.025 (rs10757274)	
Ottawa Heart Study-3	647	847	CAD	.0003 (rs10757274)	
Iceland	2274	10,260	CAD	1.9×10^{-7} (rs10757278)	39
United States	2315	2508	CAD-MI	1.5×10^{-10} (rs10757278)	
British Family Heart Study and Global Registry of Acute Coronary Events	1926	2938	CAD-MI	1.80×10^{-14} (rs1333049)	41
German Myocardial Infarction Family Study	875	1644	MI	6.70×10^{-5} (rs1333049)	40
PROCARDIS	4251	4443	CAD-MI	6×10^{-13} (rs2891168)	44
Iceland, Belgium, Canada, United States, Netherlands, New Zealand, United Kingdom	2836	14,259 2476	AAA	1.2×10^{-12} (rs10757278)	38
Iceland, Netherlands, Finland	1134	1222	IA	2.5×10^{-6} (rs10757278)	
Iceland, Italy, Sweden, New Zealand	2599	787	PAD	6.1×10^{-5} (rs10757278)	
Iceland, Sweden	705	734	LAA	.015 (rs10757278)	
South Korea	611	294	CAD	.024 (rs10757274)	42
Italy	416	308	CAD	.007 (rs10757274)	43
Northwick Park Heart Study II	270	2472	Incident CAD	.01 (rs10757274)	18
German Myocardial Infarction Family Study II	701	911	MI	.0028 (rs1333049)	75
U.K. Myocardial Infarction Study	772	734	MI	.0102 (rs1333049)	
AtheroGene	392	355	CAD	.0175 (rs1333049)	
Left Main Disease Study	483	480	Left main disease	.0024 (rs1333049)	
MONICA/KORA Study	589	1056	MI	8.79×10^{-5} (rs1333049)	
PopGen	1085	1021	CAD	2.38×10^{-6} (rs1333049)	
PRIME	617	620	CAD	.0081 (rs1333049)	
Total numbers	29,157	69,641			

AAA, abdominal aortic aneurysm; CAD, coronary artery disease; IA, intracranial aneurysm; LAA, large artery atherosclerosis–cardiogenic stroke; MI, myocardial infarction; PAD, peripheral arterial disease.

Table 2.3 Compilation of studies showing the association of genetic variants at chromosome 9p21.3 and different cardiovascular phenotypes.

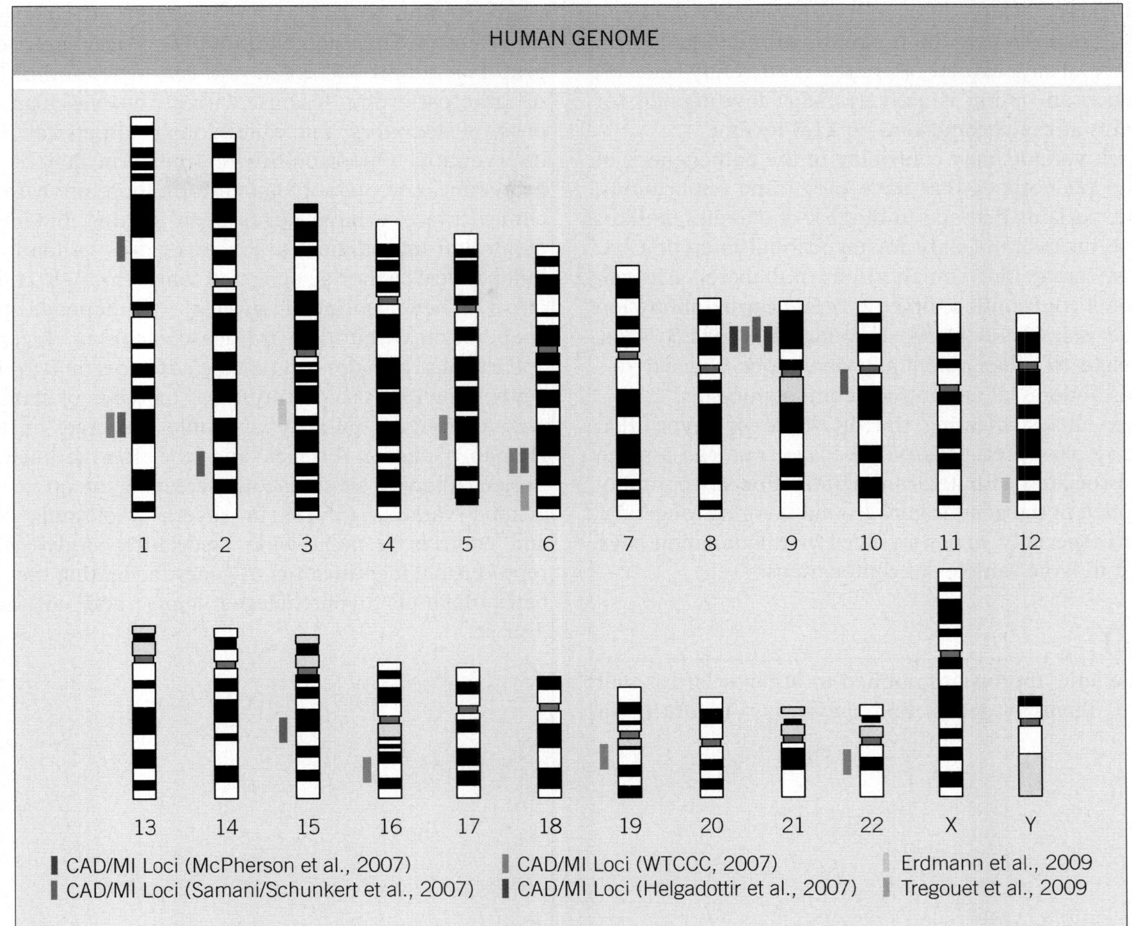

Figure 2.3 Schematic representation of the human genome. Chromosomal coronary artery disease–myocardial infarction gene regions (red) and myocardial infarction genes (green) identified so far by genome-wide association analyses.

with LDL levels in several genome-wide association studies and subsequent replication studies.[68,69]

Chromosome 9p21.3

Initially, the locus on chromosome 9p21.3 was reported to be associated with type 2 diabetes in three of five genome-wide association studies for type 2 diabetes.[76-78] McPherson and colleagues,[37] Helgadottir and coworkers,[39] and Samani and coworkers[40] were the first to report strong evidence for association between SNPs at the same chromosomal region and coronary artery disease–myocardial infarction. It is interesting that the same chromosomal region on chromosome 9p21.3 but not the same SNPs are repeatedly associated with type 2 diabetes (a risk factor for coronary artery disease) and coronary artery disease–myocardial infarction. A simultaneous test of coronary artery disease and diabetes susceptibility with coronary artery disease and type 2 diabetes–associated SNPs indicated that these associations were independent of each other.[44]

Helgadottir and colleagues[38] provided further data showing that this locus not only affects coronary artery disease–myocardial infarction risk but also affects the risk of abdominal aortic aneurysm, intracranial aneurysm, peripheral arterial disease, and large artery atherosclerosis–cardiogenic stroke in many populations. These findings may extend our knowledge about the role of sequence variants within the chromosome 9p21.3 region and show that it is not restricted to atherosclerotic diseases.

In parallel, Broadbent and associates[44] reported that a large antisense noncoding RNA gene *(ANRIL)* colocates with the high-risk haplotype at chromosome 9p21.3. This gene is expressed in tissues and cell types that are affected by atherosclerosis and is therefore a prime candidate gene for the chromosome 9p21.3 coronary artery disease–myocardial infarction locus.

At present, a total of 29,157 patients with cardiovascular diseases and 69,641 controls are genotyped for SNPs at this locus, making this gene region the most often replicated coronary artery disease–myocardial infarction region ever studied (see Table 2.3).

PROGNOSIS

Little work has been done to study the prognostic implications of genetic variants affecting the risk of myocardial infarction. Theoretically, multiple mechanisms may be of relevance in this respect. First, such variants may impair the prognosis of patients with known coronary artery disease. This certainly applies to some of the rare mutations causing familial hypercholesterolemia or other autosomal dominant forms of coronary artery disease.[10,11,35] Whether common risk alleles likewise impair the prognosis of individuals with known history of myocardial infarction is currently unclear. However, such an option is actively being investigated for the risk alleles at the chromosome 9p21.3 locus.

Second, risk variants may contribute to the pathogenesis of other disease phenotypes that have prognostic implications. For example, variants that add to the risk of diabetes mellitus may increase the risk not only for myocardial infarction but also for other threatening complications of diabetes. Alternatively, variants contributing directly to myocardial infarction risk, like the risk alleles at the chromosome 9p21.3 locus, may also relate to other potentially dangerous vascular diseases such as abdominal and intracerebral aneurysms.[38]

Third, risk alleles affecting the incidence of myocardial infarction may also affect longevity because one can assume that alleles associated with myocardial infarction susceptibility are not included in the genetic background favoring longevity. In this regard especially, genes involved in inflammation have been studied in large samples of centenarians.[79]

SUMMARY

Molecular genetic approaches applied to atherosclerosis will continue to identify genes and pathways involved in predisposition to and pathophysiologic mechanisms of this often life-threatening condition. Moreover, gene expression profiling studies will refine the understanding of the nature of atherosclerotic lesions within the vascular wall and promise discovery and validation of targets for therapeutic intervention. Opportunities to transform genetic, genomic, proteomic, and metabolomic information into cardiovascular clinical practice have never been greater, but their implementation into clinical practice requires validation in large independent cohorts, achieved only through collaborative effort. Their continued success will depend on ongoing cooperation within the cardiovascular research community.

Particularly, major technologic advances in high-throughput genotyping (SNP chip arrays) and methods of statistical analysis as well as publicly available resources including the Human Genome Project and the International HapMap Project allowed simultaneous screening of up to 1,000,000 genetic variants (SNPs) in several thousands of patients and controls (genome-wide association study) with highly reproducible identification of genes facilitating the risk of diabetes mellitus, hypercholesterolemia, and coronary artery disease.

chapter 3

Risk Factors for Cardiovascular Disease

David D. Waters

Issue

- Cardiovascular events are the leading cause of mortality in industrialized countries and are rapidly increasing in prevalence in developing countries.

Key Features

- For the main, important cardiovascular risk factors, clinical trials have demonstrated that controlling or eliminating the risk factor reduces the risk of an event.
- The underlying causative factors of the metabolic syndrome are universally recognized to be excess calorie intake and inadequate physical activity, leading to truncal obesity.
- Risk calculators, such as those derived from Framingham, PROCAM, and SCORE, are useful, but the concept of lifetime risk is important for the assessment of risk in younger individuals.

Clinical Implications

- Traditional risk factors (smoking diabetes, hypertension, obesity, and lipids) account for nearly all of the population attributable risk for coronary heart disease. Acccurate risk assessment improves the appropriateness of risk factor treament.

The accurate assessment of cardiovascular risk is important because overtreatment of low-risk individuals is wasteful and undertreatment of intermediate- or high-risk individuals leads to preventable cardiovascular events. Treatment of each of the major cardiovascular risk factors—low-density lipoprotein (LDL) cholesterol, hypertension, diabetes, and smoking—has been shown in clinical trials to reduce events. Cardiovascular events are the leading cause of mortality in industrialized countries and are rapidly increasing in prevalence in developing countries.

This chapter discusses the concept of a risk factor and how it relates to cardiovascular events. Methods of assessing risk are covered, and the concept of lifetime risk is compared with 10-year risk calculations. The chapter discusses additional tests available to refine risk assessment and the effect of appropriate treatment of risk factors on the level of risk.

WHAT IS A RISK FACTOR?

A cardiovascular risk factor can be broadly defined as a variable that is statistically associated with cardiovascular events. To be useful, the statistical association should be strong and independent of other variables. Furthermore, the risk factor should play a significant role in the pathogenesis of atherosclerosis. Ideally, a risk factor should be modifiable. For the main, important cardiovascular risk factors, clinical trials have demonstrated that controlling or eliminating the risk factor reduces the risk of an event.

The main cardiovascular risk factors are listed in Table 3.1 Several important predictors of cardiovascular events are not included in this list. For example, educational level and socioeconomic status are strong predictors of cardiovascular events in most populations. However, these variables exert their effects partly through some of the listed risk factors as well as through incompletely defined mechanisms, and these variables are not good targets for intervention to reduce risk in an individual patient. Poor diet is also not listed; it increases cardiovascular risk through multiple pathways, such as increased salt intake, increased calorie intake, and *trans* fats.

The importance of individual risk factors varies across cultural and ethnic groups. Hypertension is more important in African American and East Asian populations, whereas diabetes and low levels of high-density lipoprotein (HDL) cholesterol are stronger risk factors in South Asians.[1] As a consequence of improving economic conditions in many parts of the world, LDL-cholesterol levels and smoking rates are increasing rapidly. In the United States, smoking rates and cholesterol levels have declined, but the prevalence of obesity has increased dramatically.

Important linkages exist among the major risk factors. The prevalence of hypertension and diabetes increases with age. Obesity is an important risk factor for glucose intolerance and diabetes. Cigarette smokers have lower HDL-cholesterol and higher C-reactive protein levels. Risk factors tend to cluster, and the most important cluster has been termed the metabolic syndrome.

THE METABOLIC SYNDROME

The features of the metabolic syndrome and the criteria for diagnosis according to the National Cholesterol Education Program Adult Treatment Panel III guidelines[2] are listed in Table 3.2. The World Health Organization and the American Association of Clinical Endocrinologists have proposed different criteria that emphasize the central role of insulin resistance and diabetes.[3,4] The underlying causative factors of the metabolic syndrome are universally recognized to be excess calorie intake and inadequate physical activity, leading to truncal obesity. Obesity contributes to hypertension and diabetes. Excess adipose tissue releases several products that lead to increased cardiovascular risk: nonesterified fatty acids overload liver and muscle with lipids, enhancing insulin

MAIN CARDIOVASCULAR RISK FACTORS
Nonmodifiable
Age
Gender
Family history
Modifiable
Hypertension
Lipid abnormalities
High LDL-cholesterol
Low HDL-cholesterol
Hypertriglyceridemia
Cigarette smoking
Glucose intolerance and diabetes
Obesity
Physical inactivity
Cocaine
Depression
Laboratory abnormalities
Left ventricular hypertrophy
Fibrinogen
Lipoprotein(a)
C-reactive protein

Table 3.1 Main cardiovascular risk factors.

METABOLIC SYNDROME
Features
Abdominal obesity: increased waist circumference
Atherogenic dyslipidemia: low HDL-cholesterol, high triglycerides, increased remnant lipoproteins, small LDL and HDL particle size
Elevated blood pressure
Insulin resistance → glucose intolerance → type 2 diabetes
Proinflammatory state: increased C-reactive protein
Prothrombotic state: increased fibrinogen and plasminogen activator inhibitor 1
Criteria for diagnosis according to Adult Treatment Panel III
Three of five required for diagnosis, but each additional factor increases risk: 1. waist circumference >40 inches for men or >35 inches for women 2. triglycerides ≥150 mg/dL 3. HDL-cholesterol <40 mg/dL for men or <50 mg/dL for women 4. blood pressure ≥130/≥85 mm Hg 5. fasting glucose concentration ≥110 mg/dL

Table 3.2 Metabolic syndrome.

resistance; cytokines promote higher C-reactive protein levels, denoting a proinflammatory state; and high plasminogen activator inhibitor 1 levels and fibrinogen are markers of a prothrombotic milieu.[3]

ETHNIC-SPECIFIC VALUES FOR WAIST CIRCUMFERENCE

Central obesity is most easily measured by waist circumference with use of these guidelines that are gender and ethnic group (not country of residence) specific.

Country or Ethnic Group	Waist Circumference: Males	Waist Circumference: Females
Europids	≥94 cm	≥80 cm
United States (Adult Treatment Panel III cutpoints)	≥102 cm	≥88 cm
South Asians (based on a Chinese, Malay, and Asian Indian population)	≥90 cm	≥80 cm
Chinese	≥90 cm	≥80 cm
Japanese	≥90 cm	≥80 cm
Ethnic South and Central Americans, use South Asian recommendations until more specific data are available.		
Sub-Saharan Africans, Eastern Mediterranean and Middle East (Arab) populations, use Europid recommendations until more specific data are available.		

Modified from International Diabetes Foundation. The IDF consensus worldwide definition of the metabolic syndrome. Available at http://www.idf.org. Accessed March 13, 2008.

Table 3.3 Ethnic-specific values for waist circumference.

The age-adjusted prevalence of the metabolic syndrome was 24% among adults in the United States and nearly 10% among children 12 years of age or older at the time of the Third National Health and Nutritional Survey, between 1988 and 1994.[5,6] Higher rates were present in Mexican Americans and in African American women compared with men. The prevalence of obesity has increased considerably in the United States since these data were collected, and it is likely that the prevalence of the metabolic syndrome has increased as well.

As shown in Table 3.3, different cutpoints for waist circumference have been proposed in different populations to define abdominal obesity. Asians are at risk for diabetes and cardiovascular disease at lower waist circumferences and body mass indices compared with white individuals.[7] The prevalence of the metabolic syndrome is increasing in many Asian countries as they become more prosperous.

In both European and American populations, the metabolic syndrome increases the risk of a cardiovascular event by approximately twofold.[8,9] The metabolic syndrome is also associated with an increased risk of cardiovascular events in survivors of myocardial infarction.[10] The metabolic syndrome does not appear to increase risk beyond what would be expected for the individual risk factors taken together.[3] As shown in the Framingham cohort, most of the risk associated with the metabolic syndrome is captured by age, blood pressure, total cholesterol level, diabetes, and HDL-cholesterol level.[3]

CONTRIBUTION OF RISK FACTORS

It used to be thought that conventional risk factors accounted for approximately half of coronary disease and that as yet undiscovered risk factors would turn out to play an important role. However, more recent studies with more stringent definitions of risk factors indicate that this is not so. For example, in a study of more than 120,000 patients with coronary events, no risk factors were identified in only 15% of women and less than 20% of men.[11] Diabetes, hypertension, smoking, elevated lipids, or more than one of these factors were present in the remainder.

The INTERHEART study examined the relative contribution of various risk factors in approximately 15,000 cases with acute myocardial infarction and 15,000 controls in 52 countries.[12] Current smoking, raised apoB/apoA1 ratio, history of hypertension, diabetes, abdominal obesity, psychosocial factors, lack of daily consumption of fruits and vegetables, regular alcohol consumption, and regular physical activity were all related to myocardial infarction ($P < .0001$ for all risk factors and $P = .03$ for alcohol). These associations were present in both men and women and in all regions of the world. These nine risk factors collectively accounted for 90% of the population attributable risk (PAR) in men and 94% in women.[12]

The odds ratio associated with each risk factor and the PAR for each are listed in Table 3-4. PAR is a useful concept because it combines both the prevalence of a risk factor and its relative strength. A potent risk factor that is uncommon in a group will have a lower PAR than a slightly weaker risk factor with a much higher prevalence. Considerable overlap of the PAR exists for the major traditional risk factors.

As shown in Figure 3.1, risk increases dramatically in patients with clusters of risk factors. The odds ratio for each of the four standard risk factors—diabetes, hypertension, smoking, and lipid abnormality—ranges from 1.9 to 3.3; however, when all four are present, the odds ratio jumps to 42.3.

The graded relationship between exposure to a risk factor and level of risk was also clearly seen in INTERHEART. Smoking one to five cigarettes/day was associated with an odds ratio of myocardial infarction compared with never smoked of 1.38; this increased to 3.83 for 16 to 20 cigarettes/day and to an odds ratio of 9.16 for those who smoked more than 40 cigarettes/day. Similarly, risk increases as the ratio of apoB/apoA1 increases. The severity and duration of both hypertension and diabetes have been shown in other studies to increase risk compared with milder levels or shorter duration of these risk factors.

The PAR of each risk factor varies somewhat by geographic area, depending mainly on its prevalence. For example, in INTERHEART, obesity accounted for only 5.5% of the PAR in China compared with 35.8% for smoking. On the other hand, in western Europe, obesity accounted for 63.4% of the PAR and smoking 29.3%.

The importance of lifestyle is emphasized by the INTERHEART data: nonsmokers who get regular exercise, use alcohol, and eat fruits and vegetables regularly have an odds ratio of only 0.20 for myocardial infarction. Similar data have been reported in other populations. In a study of five cohorts from the United States,[13] the absence of five risk factors (abnormal electrocardiographic recording, diabetes, smoking, cholesterol level, and blood pressure) was associated with an 80% to 90% lower risk of coronary disease. In an analysis from Göteborg, Sweden, subjects with low blood pressure and low cholesterol level who did not smoke had a relative risk of 0.09 for a coronary event.[14]

RISK FACTORS FOR MYOCARDIAL INFARCTION IN THE INTERHEART STUDY

Risk Factor	Prevalence: Controls (%)	Prevalence: Cases (%)	Odds Ratio (99% CI), Adjusted for Other Risk Factors	Population Attributable Risk (%)
Current smoking	26.7	45.2	2.87 (2.58-3.19)	—
Current and former smoking	48.1	65.2	2.04 (1.86-2.25)	35.7
Diabetes	7.5	18.5	2.37 (2.07-2.71)	9.9
Hypertension	21.9	39.0	1.91 (1.74-2.10)	17.9
Abdominal obesity (3 vs 1*)	33.3	46.3	1.62 (1.45-1.80)	20.1
All psychosocial†	—	—	2.67 (2.21-3.22)	32.5
Vegetables and fruit daily	42.4	35.8	0.70 (0.62-0.79)	13.7
Exercise	19.3	14.3	0.86 (0.76-0.97)	12.2
Alcohol intake	24.5	24.0	0.91 (0.82-1.02)	6.7
ApoB/apoA1 ratio (2 vs 1*)	20.0	14.3	1.42 (1.22-1.65)	—
ApoB/apoA1 ratio (3 vs 1*)	20.0	18.1	1.84 (1.58-2.13)	—
ApoB/apoA1 ratio (4 vs 1*)	20.0	24.2	2.41 (2.09-2.79)	—
ApoB/apoA1 ratio (5 vs 1*)	20.0	33.5	3.25 (2.81-3.76)	49.2
All risk factors combined	—	—	129.2 (90.2-185.0)	90.4

*Comparison of tertiles or quintiles.

†A model-dependent index combining positive exposure to depression, perceived stress at home or work (general stress), low locus of control, and major life events, all referenced against nonexposure for all five factors.

Modified from Yusuf S, Hawken S, Ounpuu S, et al. Effect of potentially modifiable risk factors associated with myocardial infarction in 52 countries (the INTERHEART study): case-controlled study. Lancet 2004;364:937-952.

Table 3-4 Risk factors for myocardial infarction in the INTERHEART study.

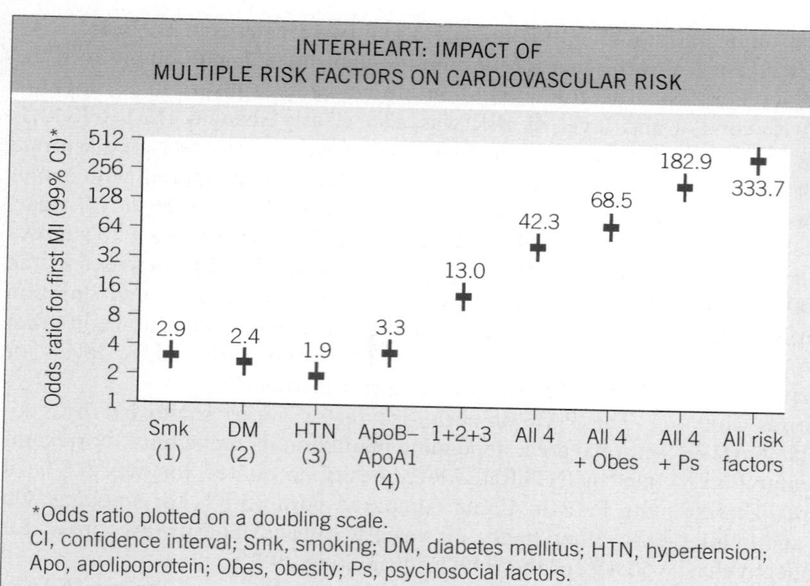

Figure 3.1 Impact of single and multiple risk factors from INTERHEART. The odds ratio for a first myocardial infarction (MI) increase dramatically when multiple risk factors are present. (From Yusuf S, Hawken S, Ounpuu S, et al. Effect of potentially modifiable risk factors associated with myocardial infarction in 52 countries [the INTERHEART study]: case-controlled study. Lancet 2004;364:937-952.)

FAMILY HISTORY AND GENETIC RISK FACTORS

A family history of coronary disease is useful clinically, particularly as a screening tool in younger populations. In INTERHEART, a family history of premature coronary heart disease was associated with an odds ratio of 1.55 (99% CI, 1.44-1.67), adjusted for age, sex, smoking, and geographic region.[12] The PAR for family history was 12%. However, family history is largely expressed through other risk factors; when family history is added to the other nine risk factors in INTERHEART, PAR increased from 90.4% to only 91.4%. For this reason, family history is not usually used as a risk factor in risk assessment algorithms.

The mechanisms whereby genes lead to the development of myocardial infarction are complex and incompletely defined.[15] Four distinct pathways have been identified. The first of these is alterations in lipoprotein handling, an example of which is polymorphisms of the apolipoprotein E (apoE) gene. Of the three variants of apoE (apoE2, apoE3, and apoE4), apoE4 has been associated with an increased risk of myocardial infarction as documented in a recent meta-analysis of 48 studies.[16] Although the functional genomics of this polymorphism are not well understood, affected individuals have a predisposition to increased LDL-cholesterol levels.

Other mutations associated with variations in LDL-cholesterol levels have also recently been described. Variants in the *PCSK9* (proprotein convertase subtilisin/kexin type 9) gene have been associated with both high and low LDL-cholesterol levels.[17] A mutation of the *LRP6* gene leads to hyperlipidemia and early onset of coronary disease.[18]

The second pathway leading to an increased risk of myocardial infarction is through disruption of endothelial integrity. A doubling of the risk of myocardial infarction has been reported and confirmed in subjects with a variant of the thrombospondin family of matrix proteins.[15,19] These patients exhibit a reduction in the capacity for endothelial proliferation and repair.

The third pathway is through genetic variants that increase the risk of myocardial infarction through inflammatory mechanisms. At least eight genes have been identified that act through inflammation, as recently summarized by Demani and Topol.[15] Two genes in the inflammatory pathway of leukotriene production, 5-lipoxygenase–activating protein (FLAP) and leukotriene A_4 hydrolase *(LTA4H)*, have haplotype variants associated with an increased risk of myocardial infarction.[20,21] The fourth pathway is through genes that influence thrombosis and clot formation; four have been identified, including plasminogen activator inhibitor 1, factor V, and prothrombin.[15]

Should we use genetic screening to help identify patients at high risk for coronary disease? The benefit of such a strategy is currently unclear because the incremental benefit of genetic information beyond clinical risk factors has not been defined and is likely to be small at present.

CALCULATION OF RISK

A large number of Internet sites and charts are available for the calculation of cardiovascular risk. Risk calculators can also be downloaded to hand-held devices. However, these risk calculators are based on a much smaller number of studied populations, the oldest and most widely used of which is the Framingham Study.[22] The original Framingham risk factors were age, sex, blood pressure, total cholesterol, LDL-cholesterol, HDL-cholesterol, smoking, diabetes, and electrocardiographic left ventricular hypertrophy. Left ventricular hypertrophy correlates strongly with high blood pressure and was not included in the main updated publication of the Framingham risk tables.[23] An electronic calculator with these variables is available.[24] The risk calculator of the National Cholesterol Education Program,[25] and many other Framingham-based risk calculators, omit LDL-cholesterol, diastolic blood pressure, and left ventricular hypertrophy.

The Framingham risk score has undergone revisions to overcome some of its limitations. A workshop sponsored by the National Heart, Lung, and Blood Institute in 2001 was devoted to the applicability of Framingham data to minority populations.[26] The prediction models have been updated to include more recently collected Framingham data.[27]

The Framingham equations predict risk quite well in white and African American men and women in the United States who are between the ages of 30 and 65 years but predict risk less well in other groups: U.S. ethnic groups such as Japanese men, Hispanic men, and Native American women; men and women outside the 30- to 65-year age range; and diabetics.[28] Framingham risk covers only cardiovascular death and myocardial infarction, thus neglecting the risk of stroke, unstable angina, and coronary revascularization. Adding to the Framingham risk assessment additional important risk factors, such as blood glucose level or hemoglobin A_{1c}, triglycerides, weight or body mass index, and some measure of physical activity, might improve the accuracy of prediction, but this has not been well studied.

Besides Framingham, other populations are available for use in risk assessment. The Prospective Cardiovascular Münster (PROCAM) study included 5389 middle-aged men without evidence of heart disease at the time of recruitment.[29] The risk factors included in the PROCAM model in order of importance are age, LDL-cholesterol, smoking, HDL-cholesterol, systolic blood pressure, family history of premature myocardial infarction, diabetes, and triglycerides. The PROCAM calculator is available on-line at the Web site of the International Task Force for Prevention of Coronary Heart Disease.[30] PROCAM is slightly more accurate in western European men, in whom Framingham tends to overestimate risk. A major limitation of the original PROCAM risk calculator is that it includes no women, no minorities, and no subjects older than 65 years at the time of recruitment. In a more recent report from PROCAM,[31] women and older subjects are included, and endpoint events include stroke and transient ischemic attack as well as coronary events. PROCAM is probably superior to Framingham for risk assessment in European populations.

The SCORE (Systematic Coronary Risk Evaluation) project developed a risk scoring system for use in clinical practice in Europe.[32] Datasets were pooled from 12 European cohort studies covering high- and low-risk regions of Europe. The risk factors that were included are age, sex, smoking, systolic blood pressure, and either total cholesterol or total cholesterol/HDL-cholesterol ratio. The main advantage of SCORE is its broad geographic coverage within Europe. Among its limitations are the exclusion of diabetes and its emphasis on cardiovascular mortality as opposed to a broader endpoint.

The Joint British Societies have produced coronary risk prediction charts, as illustrated in Figure 3.2.[33,34] These are based on Framingham data and thus use the same risk factor variables as Framingham does.

A risk engine for new cardiovascular events has been developed from the United Kingdom Prospective Diabetes Study.[35] This model is specific to patients with diabetes. It includes age, sex, ethnic group, smoking, time since the diagnosis of diabetes, hemoglobin A_{1c}, systolic blood pressure, and total cholesterol/HDL-cholesterol ratio.

Is risk assessment with use of any of these tools of any clinical value? Do physicians use any of these methods of risk assessment widely in practice? Do risk assessment tools lead to favorable behavioral modifications from patients or to changes in prescribing patterns in physicians? Answers to the last of these questions are incomplete and somewhat contradictory[36,37] but provide some reason for optimism.

THE CONCEPT OF LIFETIME RISK

A limitation of current risk assessment calculators is that they usually cover a 10-year time frame. As a consequence, calculated risk in almost all young subjects will be quite low, even when multiple risk factors are present. Aggressive treatment may thus be deferred. For example, with use of the National Cholesterol Education Program Adult Treatment Panel III on-line risk estimator, a 45-year-old obese, nonsmoking, nondiabetic man with a total cholesterol concentration of 200 mg/dL, an HDL-cholesterol concentration of 40 mg/dL, and an untreated systolic blood pressure of 135 mm Hg has an estimated 10-year risk of a hard coronary event of 3%.[38] Yet his lifetime risk for cardiovascular disease is 50%, and his predicted mean survival is more than 10 years shorter than that of a man at the same age with optimal risk factors.

The concept of lifetime risk has been promoted by Lloyd-Jones and colleagues[38-40] based on long-term follow-up data from the Chicago Heart Association Detection Project in Industry and from the Framingham Study. In Framingham, among 3564 men and 4362 women free of cardiovascular disease at the age of 50 years, 1757 died of cardiovascular disease and 1641 died free of cardiovascular disease during long-term follow-up.[39] The lifetime risk at age 50 years for a cardiovascular event was 51.7% in men and 39.2% in women. As illustrated in Figure 3.3, risk factors had a major influence on outcome: lifetime risk with two or more risk factors was 68.9% in men and 50.2% in women. Lifetime risk with optimal risk factors, a circumstance present in less than 5% of subjects, was 5.2% in men and 8.2% in women.

The concept of lifetime risk logically leads to more aggressive treatment of younger subjects with multiple risk factors. Atherosclerosis is known to be a gradual, insidious process, beginning in childhood and developing without symptoms for decades. Earlier control of risk factors should be expected to produce more benefit than treatment of later onset. This concept, although highly plausible, remains unproven.

NEWER BIOCHEMICAL MARKERS OF RISK

An inflammatory component to atherosclerosis has become increasingly recognized in recent years.[41] The inflammatory marker high-sensitivity C-reactive protein (hs-CRP) has been extensively studied in large datasets and has been shown to be predictive of future cardiovascular events in diverse populations.[42] A limitation of hs-CRP measurements in the risk classification of individual patients is a high level of intertest variability.[43] However, as illustrated in Figure 3.4,

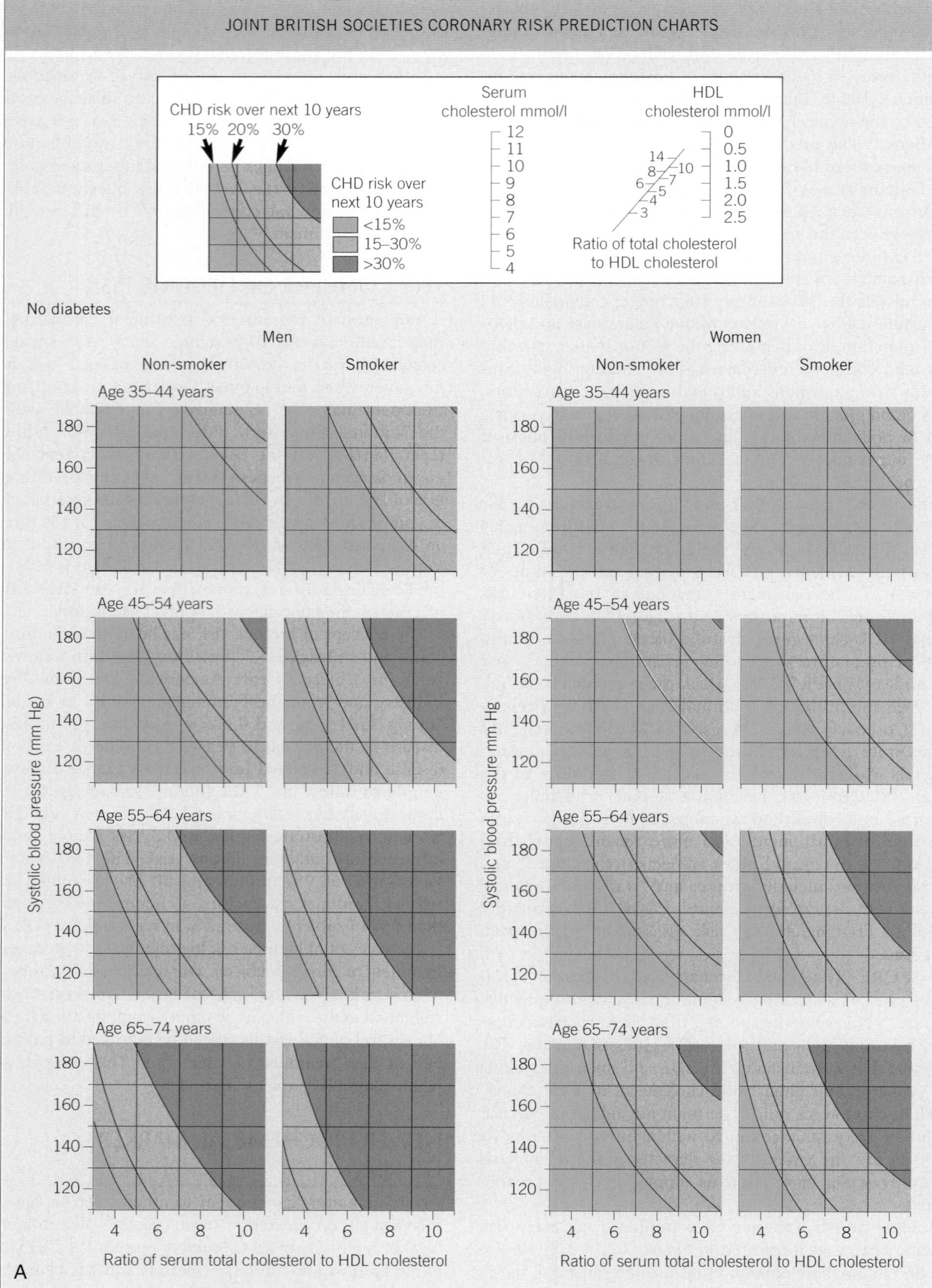

Figure 3.2 Joint British Societies coronary risk prediction charts. A, No diabetes. **B,** Diabetes. (From British Cardiac Society, British Hyperlipidaemia Association, British Hypertension Society, British Diabetic Association. Joint British recommendations on prevention of coronary heart disease in clinical practice: summary. BMJ 2000;320:705-708.)

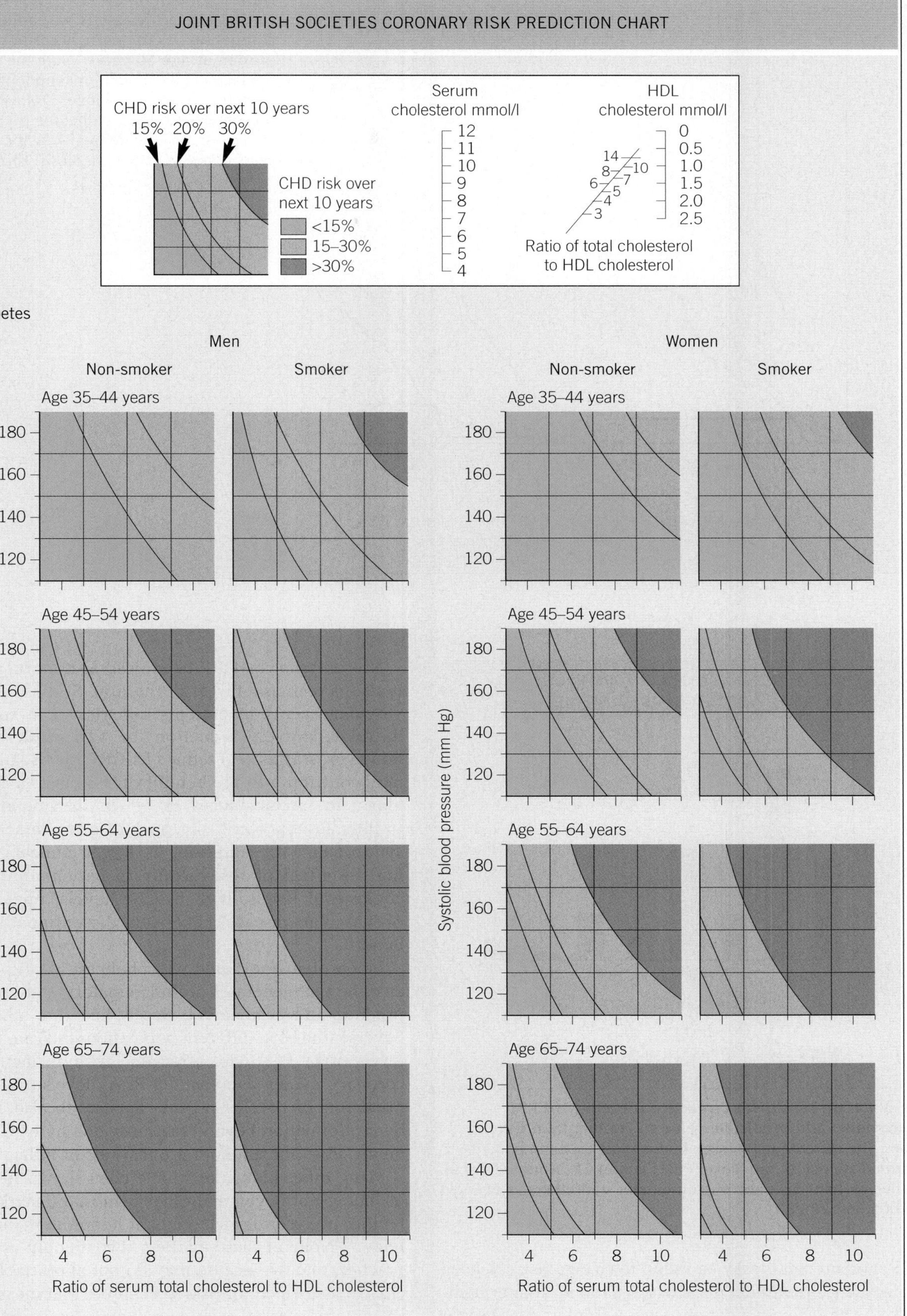

Figure 3.2—cont'd.

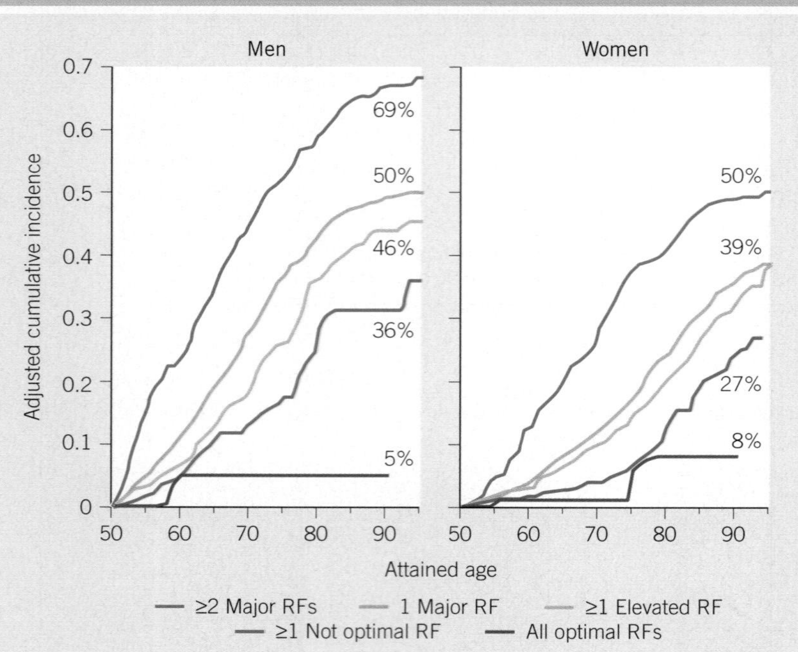

Figure 3.3 Cumulative incidence of cardiovascular disease (CVD) adjusted for competing risk of death, according to risk factor burden at age 50 years. Note the importance of risk factors (RFs) in determining long-term outcome. (From Lloyd-Jones DM, Leip EP, Larson MG, et al. Prediction of lifetime risk for cardiovascular disease by risk factor burden at 50 years of age. Circulation 2006;113:791-798.)

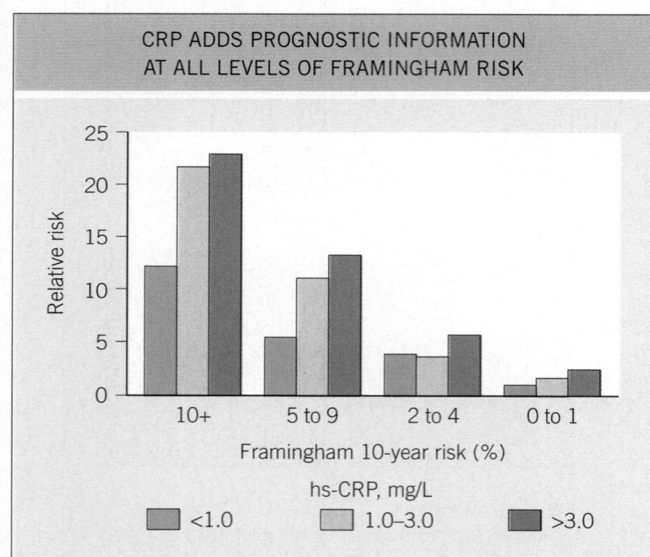

Figure 3.4 High-sensitivity C-reactive protein (hs-CRP) measurements add predictive value to Framingham risk in women. The incremental information is most useful in patients at intermediate risk. (From Ridker PM, Cannon CP, Morrow D, et al. C-reactive protein levels and outcomes after statin therapy. N Engl J Med 2005;352:20-28.)

hs-CRP measurements may be useful to change risk category and to influence treatment decisions in patients at intermediate risk.[44] The recommendations from a Centers for Disease Control and Prevention and American Heart Association workshop for use of hs-CRP measurements in clinical practice are listed in Table 3-5.[45]

Not only has hs-CRP been used as a marker of risk, but it also is seen as a target of therapy. Statins reduce cardiovascular events in patients and risk. The risk reduction is related to a reduction in LDL-cholesterol levels; however, statins also reduce hs-CRP levels, and this action may contribute to the benefit of this class of drugs, particularly in circumstances in which inflammation appears to play an important role, such as after an acute coronary syndrome.[46] In addition, a large clinical trial assessing the effect of rosuvastatin in patients with low LDL-cholesterol levels, high hs-CRP levels, and no evidence of vascular disease has been discontinued because of benefit.[47]

Lipoprotein-associated phospholipase A_2 (Lp-PLA_2) is an enzyme that generates proinflammatory and proatherogenic products and thus may be closely linked to atherogenesis.[48] Several studies in different populations indicate that elevated levels of Lp-PLA_2 are associated with an increased risk of coronary events and that Lp-PLA_2 levels are independent predictors of risk.[49] Lp-PLA_2 appears to also add independent information beyond that provided by hs-CRP measurements, even though both are markers of inflammation.

Many other biomarkers have been shown to predict risk, including fibrinogen and other hemostatic markers, lipoprotein(a), triglyceride-rich remnant lipoproteins, and homocysteine.[50] None of these markers is commonly used in clinical practice, mainly because they do not appreciably add to the clinical assessment of risk. Techniques that measure subclinical atherosclerosis, such as scanning for coronary calcium, carotid intima-media thickness measurement, and ankle-brachial index, are useful to classify risk but are beyond the topic of this chapter.

RECOMMENDATIONS FOR THE USE OF hs-CRP MEASUREMENTS IN CLINICAL PRACTICE
1. High-sensitivity C-reactive protein (hs-CRP) is an independent marker of risk that may be used at the discretion of the physician in patients judged by global risk assessment to be at intermediate risk (10% to 20% risk of coronary heart disease [CHD] per 10 years) for cardiovascular disease (CVD). hs-CRP may help direct further evaluation and therapy in the primary prevention of CVD. The benefits of such therapy based on this strategy remain uncertain. (Class IIa, Level of Evidence: B)
2. hs-CRP is an independent marker of risk and may be used at the discretion of the physician as part of a global coronary risk assessment in adults without known CVD. The benefits of this strategy remain uncertain. (Class IIb, Level of Evidence: C)
3. hs-CRP levels may be useful in motivating patients to improve their lifestyle behaviors. The benefits of this strategy remain uncertain. (Class IIb, Level of Evidence: C)
4. Patients with persistently unexplained marked elevation of hs-CRP ($\geq$10 mg/L) after repeated testing should be evaluated for noncardiovascular causes. (Class IIa, Level of Evidence: B)
5. Inflammatory markers (cytokines, other acute-phase reactants) other than hs-CRP should not be measured for the determination of coronary risk. (Class III, Level of Evidence: C)
6. hs-CRP measurement in patients with stable coronary disease or acute coronary syndromes (ACS) may be useful as an independent marker of prognosis for recurrent events, including death, myocardial infarction, and restenosis after percutaneous coronary intervention (PCI). The benefits of therapy based on this strategy remain uncertain. (Class IIa, Level of Evidence: B)
7. Application of secondary prevention measures should not depend on hs-CRP determination. (Class III, Level of Evidence: A)
8. Application of management guidelines for ACS should not depend on hs-CRP levels. (Class III, Level of Evidence: A)
9. Serial testing of hs-CRP should not be used to monitor the effects of treatment. (Class III, Level of Evidence: C)
From Smith SC Jr, Anderson JL, Cannon RO III, et al. CDC/AHA workshop on markers of inflammation and cardiovascular disease. Application to clinical and public health practice: report from the clinical practice discussion group. Circulation 2004;110:e550-e553.

Table 3-5 Recommendations for the use of hs-CRP measurements in clinical practice

chapter 4

Assessment of Cardiovascular Risk

F. D. Richard Hobbs

Summary

- Cardiovascular disease is the most important cause of mortality in the world and by 2020 will be the most common global cause of death and disability.
- The evidence base on what causes cardiovascular disease and which interventions reduce cardiovascular risks is one of the largest in medicine.
- Because cardiovascular disease is multifactorial, the risk factors coexist in many patients, and these risk factors are variably additive in their influence on overall risk, identification of people at highest risk is clinically difficult.
- Identification of people with established cardiovascular disease is an essential component of good clinical practice and requires the accurate recording of established disease, such as angina or peripheral arterial disease. Such patients warrant immediate interventions. Increasingly, guidelines advocate similar action in patients with diabetes.
- Identification of people at risk of cardiovascular disease, but without current disease, is more difficult and requires the routine monitoring of blood pressure in adults, occasional assessment of serum lipid levels, and calculation of overall cardiovascular disease risk.
- The use of cardiovascular disease risk scores, based on the observed cardiovascular disease event rates among well-phenotyped population cohorts followed up for years and expressing absolute risk during a defined period, is the most practical method for determining which people without established cardiovascular disease have most to gain from interventions.

Cardiovascular disease is the world's major cause of death, responsible for one third of total global deaths in 2001. The World Health Organization predicts that by 2020, with the rise in cardiovascular disease incidence, coronary heart disease and stroke will become the most important global causes of death and disability (Table 4.1).[1] In 2001, 80% of all cardiovascular deaths occurred in developing, low- and middle-income countries, whereas these countries accounted for 86% of the total global burden of cardiovascular disease. The number of people at risk of cardiovascular disease is rising as average life expectancy increases and social change leading to increases in vascular risk factors continues, notably the rapid rise in obesity in children and adolescents[2] due to increased calorie intake coupled with increasingly sedentary lifestyle. Perversely, increased survival and better secondary prevention in patients suffering cardiovascular events are further increasing overall prevalence of cardiovascular disease.

Long-term follow-up of well-phenotyped population cohorts provides the best data on the occurrence of cardiovascular disease and development of cardiovascular risk factors over time. The most widely cited of these cohorts (Table 4.2)[3-10] is the Framingham Heart Study.[11] These cohorts also provide data on which of the risk factors are most strongly correlated with observed cardiovascular outcomes. The widely agreed methods for assessing future cardiovascular risk are based on these historical observed risk and event correlations.

Risk factors for cardiovascular disease may be present in childhood or early adulthood, but it may be decades before clinical disease is manifested. Therefore, cardiovascular disease prevention strategies must encompass early identification of patients with individual risk factors coupled with formal cardiovascular risk assessment to determine the extent of optimal risk management needed.

RISK FACTORS FOR CARDIOVASCULAR DISEASE

Risk factors for cardiovascular disease are well established (Table 4.3). Major nonmodifiable risk factors include family history of premature cardiovascular disease, age, gender, and ethnicity. Modifiable risk factors include dyslipidemia—high levels of low-density lipoprotein (LDL) cholesterol and triglycerides and low levels of high-density lipoprotein (HDL) cholesterol (Fig. 4.1); hypertension, especially systolic elevations (Fig. 4.2); cigarette smoking; and diabetes.[11-14]

The pivotal data on risk factors came from the Framingham Heart Study,[11] initiated in 1948 to identify and evaluate factors influencing the development of cardiovascular disease in men and women free of these conditions at the outset. In 1971, the Framingham Offspring Study was initiated in children and spouses of the original cohort to study family patterns of cardiovascular disease and risk factors. In 2002, the Third Generation Study began enrolling grandchildren of the original enrollees. Another important cohort of healthy men aged 40 to 59 years, the Seven Countries Study,[4] showed that cardiovascular risk is strongly related to both serum cholesterol and the proportion of saturated fatty acids in the diet. More recently, the INTERHEART study[10] confirmed that nine potentially modifiable risk factors (Fig. 4.3) remain strongly associated with the

TEN LEADING CAUSES OF DEATH AND DISABILITY IN THE WORLD					
1990			2020		
Rank	Cause	%	Rank	Cause	%
1	Lower respiratory infections	8.2	1	Ischemic heart disease	5.9
2	Diarrheal diseases	7.2	2	Major depression	5.7
3	Perinatal conditions	6.7	3	Road traffic accidents	5.1
4	Major depression	3.7	4	Cerebrovascular disease	4.4
5	Ischemic heart disease	3.4	5	Chronic obstructive pulmonary disease	4.2
6	Cerebrovascular disease	2.8	6	Lower respiratory infections	3.1
7	Tuberculosis	2.8	7	Tuberculosis	3.0
8	Measles	2.7	8	War	3.0
9	Road traffic accidents	2.5	9	Diarrheal diseases	2.7
10	Congenital abnormalities	2.4	10	Human immunodeficiency virus infection	2.6

From the Global Burden of Disease Project, World Health Organization, 1996.

Table 4.1 Ten leading causes of death and disability in the world.

MAJOR POPULATION-BASED COHORT STUDIES THAT PROVIDE DATA ON THE OCCURRENCE AND DETERMINANTS OF CARDIOVASCULAR DISEASE						
Study	Countries	Numbers	Ethnicity	Diabetes	Age (yr)	Period
Framingham Heart Study[3,11]	United States	2590 men 2983 women	Mostly white	337	30-74	1948-present
SCORE[38]	11 European countries	88,080 men 117,098 women	European, mostly white	NA	19-80	2003-present
Seven Countries Study[4]	Italy, Finland, Greece, Japan, Netherlands, United States, Yugoslavia	11,579 men	Mostly white	NA	40-59	1957-present
United Kingdom Prospective Diabetes Study[27,34]	United Kingdom	2643 men 1897 women	U.K., mostly white	All	25-85	NA
Study of men born in 1913[5]	Sweden	792 men	Swedish, mostly white	NA	54	1963-present
Whitehall Study	England	17,530 men	British, mostly white	NA	20-64	1967-1977
PROCAM[6]	Germany	10,856 men	German, mostly white	1205 impaired fasting glucose 406 diabetes	36-65	1978-present
MONICA[7]	Worldwide	10 million men and women	Multiethnic	NA	25-64	1980-1995
Cardiovascular Health Study[8]	United States	5888 men and women	Mostly white	NA	65+	1989-1999
Rotterdam Study[9]	Netherlands	10,994 men and women	Mostly white	NA	55+	1990-1999
INTERHEART[10,50]	Worldwide	15,152 cases 14,820 controls Men and women	Multiethnic	NA	No age restriction, but no ranges	1999-2002

Table 4.2 Major population-based cohort studies that provide data on the occurrence and determinants of cardiovascular disease.

development of a first myocardial infarction by comparing patients with a first myocardial infarction with asymptomatic individuals from 52 countries. These risk factors, including smoking, hypertension, diabetes, dyslipidemia, and obesity, were associated with 90% of the population risk of myocardial infarction in all ethnic groups and across all geographic regions.

These risks factors are additive but to variable degrees (Fig. 4.4) and also cluster in individuals; 80% to 90% of cardiovascular disease patients have at least one of these

CARDIOVASCULAR RISK FACTORS		
Major Risk Factors		
Nonmodifiable	**Modifiable**	**Emerging Risk Factors[a]**
Established cardiovascular disease[b] Age Male gender Family history of premature coronary heart disease	Cigarette smoking High saturated fat diet Body mass index[c]/waist circumference Physical activity Systolic and diastolic blood pressure LDL-cholesterol HDL-cholesterol Triglycerides Diabetes/blood glucose Socioeconomic status Left ventricular mass	Homocysteine C-reactive protein Albuminuria Coagulation factors (e.g., fibrinogen) Other lipid factors (e.g., apolipoproteins) Ankle-brachial index Carotid artery intima-media thickness (ultrasonography) Calcifications in the aorta or coronaries (computed tomographic scanning or other imaging techniques)

*Does not imply direct causality.
[a]Value in addition to the major risk factors; clinical practice for assessing absolute cardiovascular risk remains to be established.
[b]Includes angina, myocardial infarction, angioplasty, coronary artery bypass grafting, transient ischemic attack, ischemic stroke, or peripheral arterial disease.
[c]Body mass index = weight (kg) per length (m)^2.

Table 4.3 Cardiovascular risk factors.

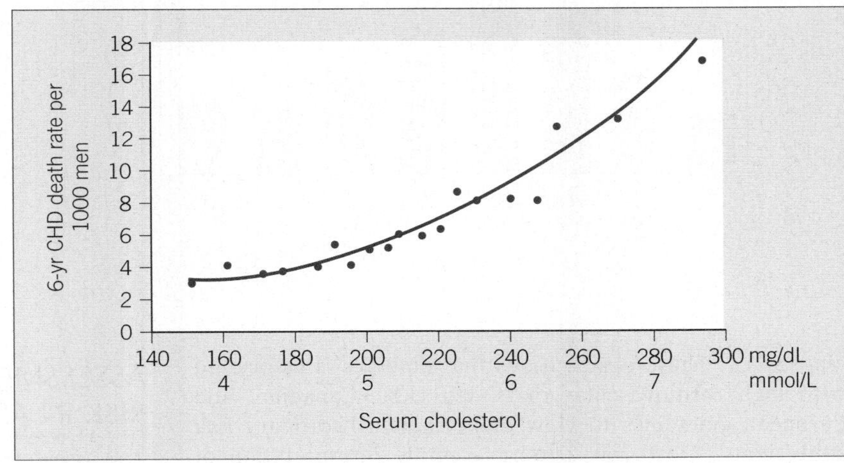

Figure 4.1 Age-adjusted coronary heart disease (CHD) death rate and serum cholesterol in 361,662 U.S. men. (From Martin MJ, Hulley SB, Browner WS, Kuller LH, Wentworth D. Serum cholesterol, blood pressure, and mortality: implications from a cohort of 361,662 men. Lancet 1986;2:933-936.)

four risk factors (Fig. 4.5),[15,16] and each risk factor has a continuous, dose-dependent impact on cardiovascular disease risk.[17] Treatment of these cardiovascular risk factors reduces subsequent cardiovascular events, whether coronary heart disease or stroke.[18-23]

ASSESSMENT OF CARDIOVASCULAR RISK IN PEOPLE WITH ESTABLISHED CARDIOVASCULAR DISEASE

Based on the major epidemiologic studies and intervention trials, the level of continued risk in people with established cardiovascular disease (acute coronary syndromes, myocardial infarction, prior revascularization, angina, peripheral arterial disease, stroke, transient ischemic attack) is sufficiently high to warrant immediate access to the full range of multiple lifestyle and therapeutic interventions to modify continued risk. The main challenge to clinicians is the accurate and early recognition of people presenting with symptoms or signs suggestive of cardiovascular disease. This requires the formal investigation of symptomatic disease, such as suspected angina (by assessments such as exercise electrocardiographic testing and cardiac imaging) and peripheral vascular disease (ankle–brachial plexus index), and the validation of events, such as myocardial infarction or stroke.

Once cardiovascular disease in an individual is established, there is no need to assess future risk. Immediate prevention strategies are warranted to control blood pressure, lipids, and weight to guideline targets, to cease smoking, and to maintain recommended levels of exercise.

ASSESSMENT OF CARDIOVASCULAR RISK IN PEOPLE WITH DIABETES

Prospective studies show that cardiovascular risk is two to five times higher in patients with diabetes than in the population at large, but the magnitude of this increased risk depends on diabetes-related factors, notably the time since

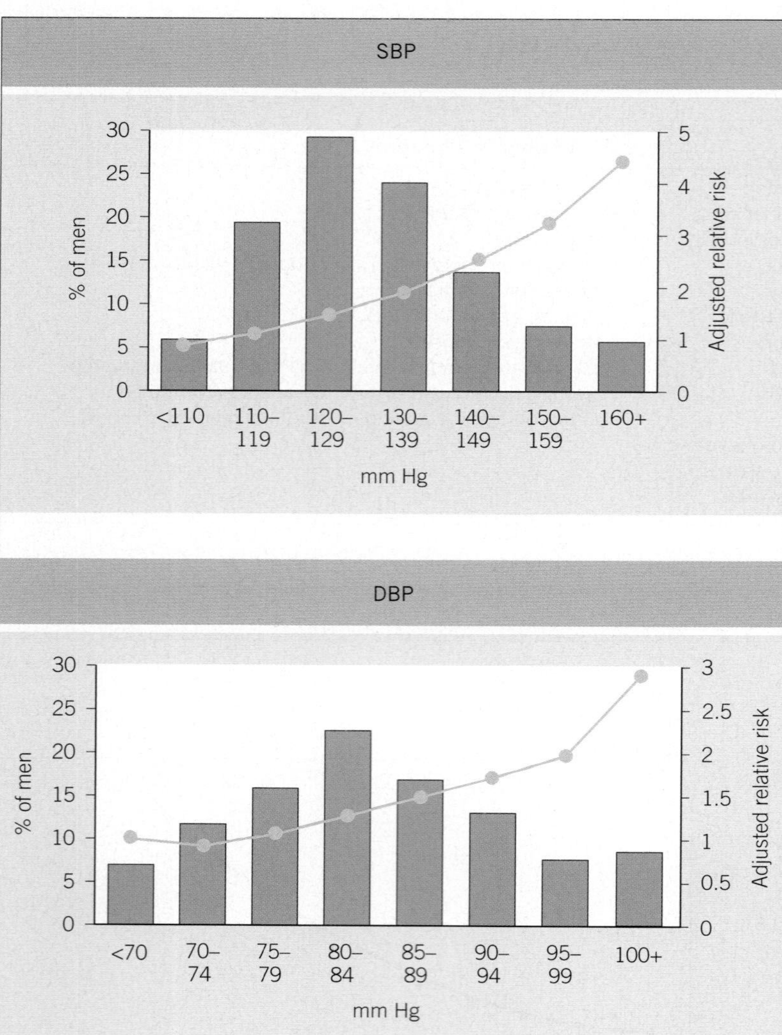

Figure 4.2 Adjusted relative risk of cardiovascular mortality by systolic blood pressure (SBP) and diastolic blood pressure (DBP) in men screened for the Multiple Risk Factor Intervention Trial. (From the National High Blood Pressure Education Program Working Group report on primary prevention of hypertension. Arch Intern Med 1993;153:186.)

diagnosis.[24] These observations that diabetes is associated with high cardiovascular risk[25] led U.S., Canadian, and European guidelines to view diabetes as a "coronary risk equivalent." However, a more accurate interpretation of the evidence is that in people who have suffered diabetes for some time (perhaps a decade in established diabetic populations or those with a delay in diagnosis) and in those with additional cardiovascular risk factors, diabetes represents a coronary risk equivalent. There is therefore no need to assess future cardiovascular disease risk formally, and patients are eligible for secondary prevention strategies automatically.

There are good pragmatic arguments for supporting this viewpoint. Diabetes is much more common,[26] so secondary risks are an increasing issue, and crucially, if a cardiovascular event occurs in a patient with diabetes, it will likely be a more serious event, whether a stroke or myocardial infarction, than among nondiabetics. However, when this simple policy is not supported, cardiovascular disease risk scores can be used to estimate risk but will underestimate future risk of events in most patients with established diabetes, unless adjustment is made or an algorithm incorporating glycemic levels is used, such as from the United Kingdom Prospective Diabetes Study (UKPDS).[27]

ASSESSMENT OF CARDIOVASCULAR RISK IN ASYMPTOMATIC INDIVIDUALS

The assessment of cardiovascular risk in the general population is more of a problem because people will not have presented themselves to clinicians with symptoms or with events. Cardiovascular risk estimation tools help identify those at greatest absolute risk of disease to prioritize management of those with most to gain. Many countries advocate that the threshold for considering initiation of pharmacologic intervention should be set, at most, at a 10-year risk of major cardiovascular events of 20% (or coronary heart disease of 15%) or equivalent. Cardiovascular risk estimation tools are based on a variety of biometric measures in adults, including age, gender, smoking status, blood pressure, and lipid ratio estimation (in all risk scores), and sometimes family history of cardiovascular disease, glycemia levels, and socioeconomic status (in some risk scores). The health system challenge is to develop strategies to collect the requisite information for all adults, commencing at a certain age and repeating at appropriate intervals. Unfortunately, there are no reliable data to determine the most cost-effective strategy as to when to start and how to deliver this function. Methods therefore vary across countries, although a number of steps are uniform.

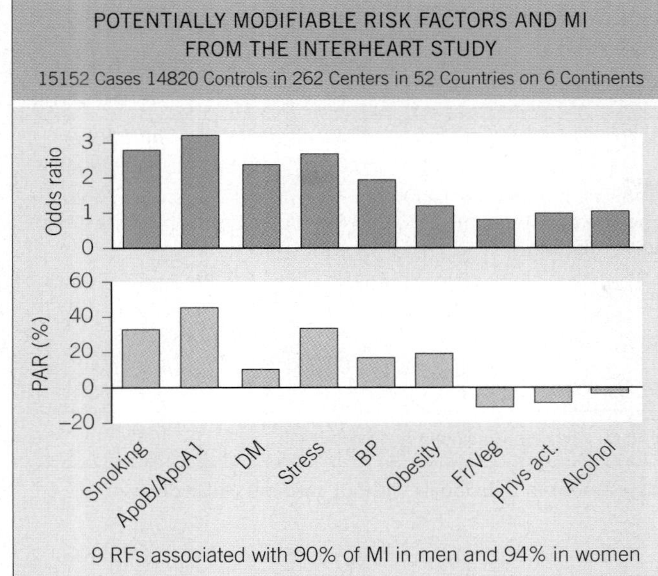

Figure 4.3 Main risk factors associated with cardiovascular disease in INTERHEART. BP, blood pressure; DM, diabetes mellitus; MI, myocardial infarction; PAR, population attributable risk; RFs, risk factors. (From Yusuf S, Hawken S, Ounpuu S, on behalf of the INTERHEART Study Investigators. Effect of potentially modifiable risk factors associated with myocardial infarction in 52 countries [the INTERHEART study]: case-control study. Lancet 2004;364:937-952.)

Selecting People for Cardiovascular Risk Assessment

Total population screening is advocated in the U.S. National Cholesterol Education Program, Adult Treatment Panel III guidelines,[28] which recommend screening for raised blood pressure and lipids in all adults without cardiovascular disease every 5 years and with cardiovascular disease every 2 to 3 years. Certain population groups are more likely than others to be at increased risk, such as older people (especially older than 65 years), certain ethnic groups (especially South Asians), and people with a family history of premature cardiovascular disease. Many of the different country guideline recommendations prioritize these groups for assessment (Table 4.4). For example, Canadian guidelines recommend screening of all

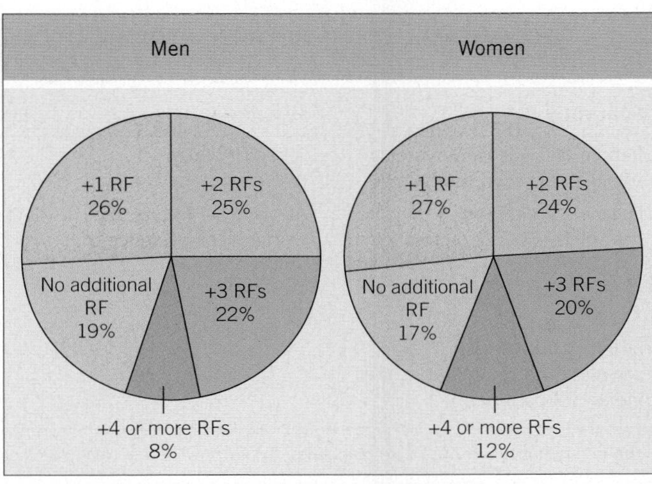

Figure 4.5 Presence of additional risk factors (RFs) in hypertensive patients in the Framingham cohort. (From Kannel WB. Risk stratification in hypertension: new insights from the Framingham Study. Am J Hypertens 2000;13:3S-10S.)

men older than 40 years and all women older than 50 years.[29] The New Zealand guidelines recommend screening of Maori, Pacific peoples, and people from the Indian subcontinent 10 years earlier than other population groups.[30] The evidence underlying most of these recommendations is poor, and their cost-effectiveness has not been evaluated.

A less ambitious alternative is opportunistic case finding of those at higher cardiovascular risk through formal risk estimation only in all those who have the detected presence of any single cardiovascular disease risk factor, however so detected. The European[31] and U.K.[32] guidelines emphasize such opportunistic cardiovascular risk assessment in patients with any cardiovascular risk factor but also stress the need to screen close relatives of patients with early cardiovascular disease (men < 55 years, women < 65 years) and families with inherited dyslipidemia.

Measuring Cardiovascular Risk Factors

Once a patient has been identified for assessment, a comprehensive risk assessment should be carried out, involving

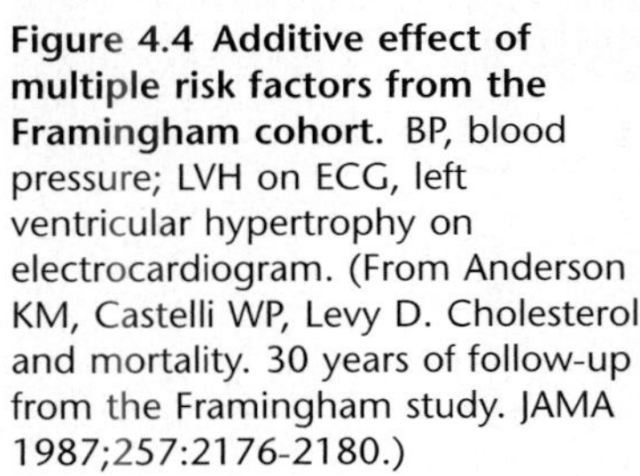
Figure 4.4 Additive effect of multiple risk factors from the Framingham cohort. BP, blood pressure; LVH on ECG, left ventricular hypertrophy on electrocardiogram. (From Anderson KM, Castelli WP, Levy D. Cholesterol and mortality. 30 years of follow-up from the Framingham study. JAMA 1987;257:2176-2180.)

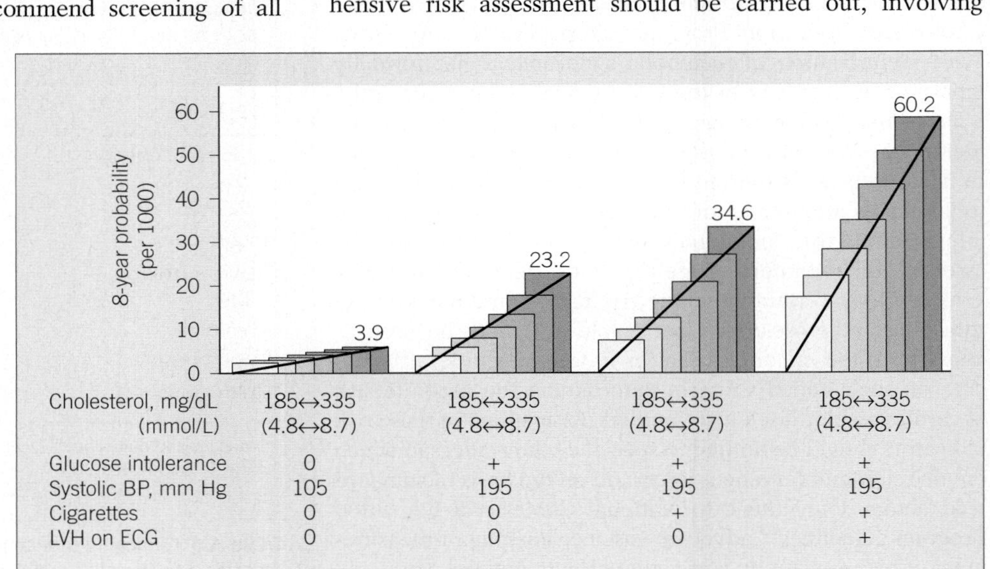

RECOMMENDED GUIDELINE CRITERIA FOR USE OF CARDIOVASCULAR RISK ASSESSMENT IN INDIVIDUALS WITHOUT CARDIOVASCULAR DISEASE				
Subgroup	**Canada**	**Europe**	**New Zealand**	**United States**
People without cardiovascular disease or known risk factors	All >40/>50 yr (men/women)	—	All >45/>55 yr (men/women)	All >20 yr (men/women)
People with known cardiovascular risk factors	All with 1+ risk factor, diabetes, or evidence of atherosclerosis	All with diabetes, multiple risk factors, or family history of premature cardiovascular disease	All >35/>45 yr (men/women) with known risk factors or a high risk of diabetes	All >20 yr (men/women)
Ethnic groups Maori, Pacific peoples, and people from the Indian subcontinent	—	—	All >35/>45 yr (men/women)	—

The International and Australian guidelines do not provide any clearly defined guidance on selecting people for risk assessment.

Table 4.4 Recommended guideline criteria for use of cardiovascular risk assessment in individuals without cardiovascular disease.

measurement of all major risk indicators (Table 4.5), because the magnitude of cardiovascular risk is determined by the synergistic effect of the combined risk factors.

The assessment of people with diabetes differs between the guidelines. For example, diabetes is not listed in the calculations of the American National Cholesterol Education Program and the Canadian guidelines, as people with diabetes are categorized as coronary heart disease equivalents.[33] Most other guidelines consider diabetes a risk factor and include it in the risk assessment. The New Zealand guidelines, for example, make a 5% 5-year cardiovascular risk adjustment to patients with diabetes diagnosed more than 10 years, in addition to the weighting given to diabetes in the Framingham-based risk score.[30] Only the UKPDS risk score[34] requires measurement of blood glucose concentration for inclusion in the algorithm.

Most guidelines now recognize the "metabolic syndrome," in which clustering of cardiovascular risk indicators is associated with increased risk of a cardiovascular event.[35] Three or more of the five risk factors (all continuous variables that have been arbitrarily dichotomized) are required for a diagnosis of metabolic syndrome according to the U.S. National Cholesterol Education Program criteria (Table 4.6). However, identification of metabolic syndrome is not formally incorporated into any of the risk calculators, and currently, none of the guidelines suggest automatic adjustment for the metabolic syndrome in the calculated cardiovascular risk. Its measurement is therefore mainly as a guide to clinicians to intensify attainment of treatment goals or to consider intervention for individuals who would otherwise be assessed to have intermediate risk (most likely the young).

In addition, certain emerging risk factors and measures of subclinical atherosclerosis (see Table 4.3) may be used as adjuncts to the major risk factors in assessing risk, although data on their added value in determining the absolute risk of cardiovascular disease are limited. Assessment of these risk indicators should be limited to special circumstances in which the decision to intervene is uncertain on the basis of standard risk factors. Only the U.S. National Cholesterol Education Program guidelines[33] advocate vascular imaging or measurement of high-sensitivity C-reactive protein in these cases.

RISK INDICATORS TYPICALLY MEASURED AND RECORDED IN ASSESSING CARDIOVASCULAR RISK
Age
Gender
Ethnicity*
Smoking history
Lipid profile (note: fasting is unnecessary for total cholesterol or HDL-cholesterol level)
Fasting plasma glucose concentration/diabetes
Blood pressure
Family history of premature cardiovascular disease
Body mass index/waist circumference
Presence of left ventricular hypertrophy

*Not all guidelines take ethnicity into account in assessing risk.

Table 4.5 Risk indicators typically measured and recorded in assessing cardiovascular risk.

CLINICAL IDENTIFICATION OF THE METABOLIC SYNDROME, ACCORDING TO THE NATIONAL CHOLESTEROL EDUCATION PROGRAM	
Risk Factor	**Defining Level**
Abdominal obesity	Waist circumference
Men	≥102 cm*
Women	≥88 cm*
Triglycerides	≥1.7 mmol/L
HDL-cholesterol	
Men	<1.0 mmol/L
Women	<1.3 mmol/L
Blood pressure	≥130/85 mm Hg
Fasting glucose	≥6.1 mmol/L†

*New Zealand guidelines[30] recommend levels of 100 cm and 90 cm for men and women, respectively.
†Canadian guidelines[29] recommend levels of 6.2-7.0 mmol/L.

Table 4.6 Clinical identification of the metabolic syndrome, according to the National Cholesterol Education Program.

Assessment of Cardiovascular Risk Level by Use of Risk Calculators

Because cardiovascular risk assessment in individual patients is complicated by the interaction of multiple risk factors, a number of risk calculators have been developed (Table 4.7) and are recommended in guidelines. Although there is some variation between the different calculators,[36,37] the majority are based on logistic regression (or similar) equations based on the observed associations between risk factors and events in the various population cohorts. The calculators estimate an individual's risk of experiencing a cardiovascular event during a given time, usually 10 or 5 years. This time period as well as the specific outcome (either fatal or the combination of fatal and nonfatal coronary heart disease or cardiovascular disease) varies between calculators. In most guidelines, the risk determined is categorized as high, intermediate, and low risk (Table 4.8). Higher risk demands more intensive intervention and stricter treatment goals.

Cardiovascular risk estimation can be performed with use of any of the risk calculator tools that are based on observational outcome data from large population cohorts, of which the most widely used are based on the Framingham Heart Study (see Table 4.1), although it may overestimate risk in some populations. The European Systematic Coronary Risk Evaluation (SCORE) charts[38] were created to address the perceived limitations of the Framingham Heart Study.[39] SCORE is based on asymptomatic individuals from 12 European cohort studies with no evidence of preexisting cardiovascular disease. Studies across multiple countries enabled charts to be drawn up for high- and low-risk countries, and because atherosclerotic cardiovascular disease mortality was the endpoint, these charts may provide more accurate estimates of overall cardiovascular risk.

However, major differences in risk estimation are observed when populations are assessed by use of different risk calculators,[40-42] hence the trend for more risk-scoring algorithms using data from the population in which the algorithm will be used, as is the case for SCORE,[38] ASSIGN,[43] the Italian Risk Charts,[44] PROCAM,[45,46] and QRISK.[47] Some of these more recent algorithms may benefit from the inclusion of additional risk factors into the equation. For example, the Scottish Intercollegiate Guidelines Network (SIGN) developed its own risk-scoring tool (ASSIGN)[43] to address two risks omitted in most risk-scoring algorithms—social deprivation and family history. Social deprivation refers to low-income populations who may have limited access to health care and health education and whose cardiovascular disease risk is underestimated by the Framingham Heart Study.[48,49] In ASSIGN, social deprivation is estimated by region with use of the Scottish Index of Multiple Deprivation. QRISK also accounts for social deprivation,[47] developed from a cohort of 1.28 million patients in the United Kingdom between the ages of 35 and 74 years and who were free of diabetes or cardiovascular disease at the time of enrollment. Data on the first diagnosis of cardiovascular disease, including myocardial infarction, coronary heart disease, stroke, and transient ischemic attack, were available for 8.2 million person-years of observation. QRISK shares many common parameters with other risk-scoring algorithms, including age, total cholesterol/HDL-cholesterol ratio, systolic blood pressure, body mass index, family history of early-onset cardiovascular disease, and smoking status, but includes the Townsend score, a surrogate measure of social deprivation that is based on geographic region. Cardiovascular risk calculators are available as risk charts (Figs. 4.6 to 4.9) and downloadable computer-assisted algorithms (Table 4.9) to assist office-based assessment of patients.

LIST OF RISK CALCULATORS INCORPORATED INTO CARDIOVASCULAR GUIDELINES	
Framingham	
Australia	National Heart Foundation of Australia and the Cardiac Society of Australia and New Zealand: Lipid Management Guidelines
Canada	Working Group on Hypercholesterolemia and Other Dyslipidemias
New Zealand	The New Zealand Guidelines Group, the National Heart Foundation of New Zealand, and the Stroke Foundation of New Zealand
United States	Third Report of the National Cholesterol Education Program
International	International Atherosclerosis Society
SCORE	
Europe	Third Joint European Task Force
PROCAM	
International	International Atherosclerosis Society

Table 4.7 List of risk calculators incorporated into cardiovascular guidelines.

RISK CATEGORIES ACCORDING TO DIFFERENT GUIDELINES				
		Risk Per Year (%)		
Guideline	**Outcomes***	**High**	**Moderate-Intermediate**	**Low**
Australia	Fatal and nonfatal CVD risk	>3		
Canada	Fatal and nonfatal CHD risk	>2	1-2	<1
Europe	Fatal CVD risk	≥0.5		<0.5
New Zealand	Fatal and nonfatal CVD risk	>3	2-3	<2
United States	Fatal and nonfatal CHD risk	>2	1-2	<1
International	Fatal and nonfatal CHD risk	>2	1-2	<1

*Fatal or the combination of fatal and nonfatal coronary heart disease (CHD) or cardiovascular disease (CVD).

Table 4.8 Risk categories according to different guidelines.

ATP III: FRAMINGHAM POINT SCORES ESTIMATE OF 10-YEAR RISK FOR MEN

1

Age	Points
20–34	–9
35–39	–4
40–44	0
45–49	3
50–54	6
55–59	8
60–64	10
65–69	11
70–74	12
75–79	13

2

TC	Age 20–39	Age 40–49	Age 50–59	Age 60–69	Age 70–79
<160	0	0	0	0	0
160–199	4	3	2	1	0
200–239	7	5	3	1	0
240–279	9	6	4	2	1
≥280	11	8	5	3	1

3

SBP mm Hg	If untreated	If treated
<120	0	0
120–129	0	1
130–139	1	2
140–159	1	2
≥160	2	3

4

HDL mg/dL	Points
≥60	–1
50–59	0
40–49	1
<40	2

5

	Age 20–39	Age 40–49	Age 50–59	Age 60–69	Age 70–79
Nonsmoker	0	0	0	0	0
Smoker	8	5	3	1	1

6

Point total	10-year risk, %
<0	<1
0	1
1	1
2	1
3	1
4	1
5	2
6	2
7	3
8	4
9	5
10	6
11	8
12	10
13	12
14	16
15	20
16	25
≥17	≥30

HDL = high-density lipoprotein
Expert panel on detection, evaluation, and treatment of high blood cholesterol in adults. *JAMA.* 2001;285:2486–2497.

Age (Low-risk level)*	30–34 (2%)	35–39 (3%)	40–44 (3%)	45–49 (4%)	50–54 (5%)	55–59 (7%)	60–64 (8%)	65–69 (10%)	70–74 (13%)	Absolute risk‡ Total CHD‡	Absolute risk‡ Total CHD¶
Points†											
0	1.0									2%	2%
1	1.5	1.0	1.0							3%	2%
2	2.0	1.3	1.3	1.0						4%	3%
3	2.5	1.7	1.7	1.3	1.0					5%	4%
4	3.5	2.3	2.3	1.8	1.4	1.0				7%	5%
5	4.0	2.6	2.6	2.0	1.6	1.1	1.0			8%	6%
6	5.0	3.3	3.3	2.5	2.0	1.4	1.3	1.0		10%	7%
7	6.5	4.3	4.3	3.3	2.6	1.9	1.6	1.3	1.0	13%	9%
8	8.0	5.3	5.3	4.0	3.2	2.3	2.0	1.6	1.2	16%	13%
9	10.0	6.7	6.7	5.0	4.0	2.9	2.5	2.0	1.5	20%	16%
10	12.5	8.3	8.3	6.3	5.0	3.6	3.1	2.5	1.9	25%	20%
11	15.5	10.3	10.3	7.8	6.1	4.4	3.9	3.1	2.3	31%	25%
12	18.5	12.3	12.3	9.3	7.4	5.2	4.6	3.7	2.8	37%	30%
13	22.5	15.0	15.0	11.3	9.0	6.4	5.6	4.5	3.5	45%	35%
> 14	26.5	> 17.7	> 17.7	> 13.3	> 10.6	> 7.6	> 6.6	> 5.3	> 4.1	> 53%	> 45%

Color key for relative risk	
Green	Below average risk
Blue	Average risk
Yellow	Moderately above average risk
Red	High risk

* Low absolute risk level = 10-year risk for total CHD endpoints for a person the same age, BP <120/<80 mm Hg, TC 160–199 mg/dL, HDL cholesterol ≥45 mg/dL, nonsmoker, no diabetes. Percentages show 10-year absolute risk for total CHD endpoints.
† Framingham points.
‡ 10-year absolute risk for total CHD endpoints estimated from Framingham data corresponding to Framingham points.
¶ 10-year absolute risk for hard CHD endpoints approximated from Framingham data corresponding to Framingham points.

Figure 4.6 U.S. National Cholesterol Education Program Adult Treatment Panel III (ATP III) algorithm to estimate 10-year coronary heart disease risk. CHD, coronary heart disease; SBP, systolic blood pressure; TC, total cholesterol. (From Expert Panel on Detection, Evaluation, and Treatment of High Blood Cholesterol in Adults. Executive Summary of the Third Report of the National Cholesterol Education Program [NCEP] Expert Panel on Detection, Evaluation, and Treatment of High Blood Cholesterol in Adults [Adult Treatment Panel III]. JAMA 2001;285:2486-2497; and Grundy SM, Pasternak R, Greenland P, Smith S Jr, Fuster V. Assessment of cardiovascular risk by use of multiple-risk-factor assessment equations: a statement for healthcare professionals from the American Heart Association and the American College of Cardiology. Circulation 1999;100:1481-1492.)

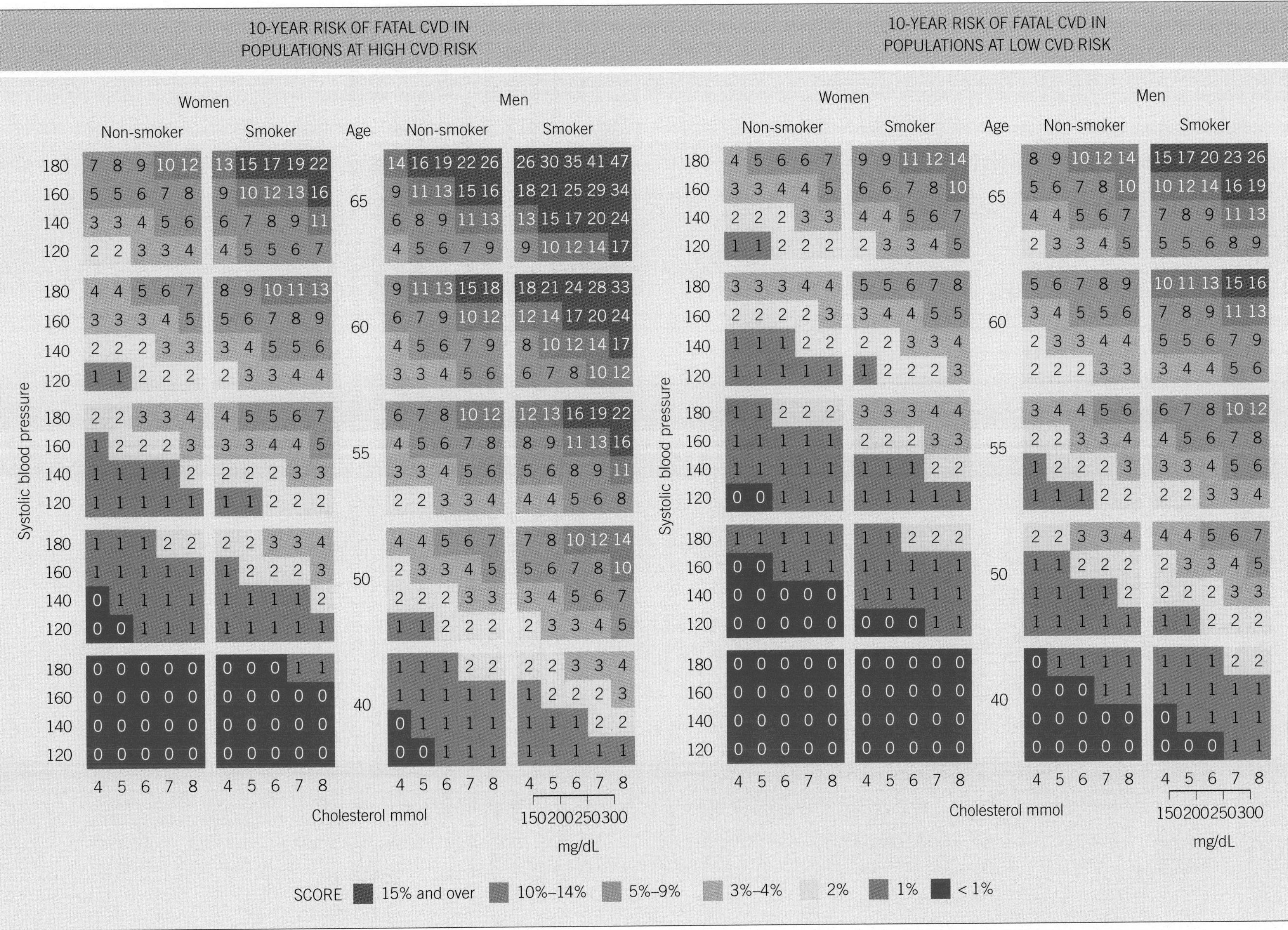

10-YEAR RISK OF FATAL CVD IN POPULATIONS AT HIGH CVD RISK

Age	Systolic blood pressure	Women Non-smoker 4	5	6	7	8	Women Smoker 4	5	6	7	8	Men Non-smoker 4	5	6	7	8	Men Smoker 4	5	6	7	8
65	180	7	8	9	10	12	13	15	17	19	22	14	16	19	22	26	26	30	35	41	47
	160	5	5	6	7	8	9	10	12	13	16	9	11	13	15	16	18	21	25	29	34
	140	3	3	4	5	6	6	7	8	9	11	6	8	9	11	13	13	15	17	20	24
	120	2	2	3	3	4	4	5	5	6	7	4	5	6	7	9	9	10	12	14	17
60	180	4	4	5	6	7	8	9	10	11	13	9	11	13	15	18	18	21	24	28	33
	160	3	3	3	4	5	5	6	7	8	9	6	7	9	10	12	12	14	17	20	24
	140	2	2	2	3	3	3	4	5	5	6	4	5	6	7	9	8	10	12	14	17
	120	1	1	2	2	2	2	3	3	4	4	3	3	4	5	6	6	7	8	10	12
55	180	2	2	3	3	4	4	5	5	6	7	6	7	8	10	12	12	13	16	19	22
	160	1	2	2	2	3	3	3	4	4	5	4	5	6	7	8	8	9	11	13	16
	140	1	1	1	1	2	2	2	2	3	3	3	3	4	5	6	5	6	8	9	11
	120	1	1	1	1	1	1	1	2	2	2	2	2	3	3	4	4	4	5	6	8
50	180	1	1	1	2	2	2	2	3	3	4	4	4	5	6	7	7	8	10	12	14
	160	1	1	1	1	1	1	2	2	2	3	2	3	3	4	5	5	6	7	8	10
	140	0	1	1	1	1	1	1	1	1	2	2	2	2	3	3	3	4	5	6	7
	120	0	0	1	1	1	1	1	1	1	1	1	1	2	2	2	2	3	3	4	5
40	180	0	0	0	0	0	0	0	0	1	1	1	1	1	2	2	2	2	3	3	4
	160	0	0	0	0	0	0	0	0	0	0	1	1	1	1	1	1	2	2	2	3
	140	0	0	0	0	0	0	0	0	0	0	0	1	1	1	1	1	1	1	2	2
	120	0	0	0	0	0	0	0	0	0	0	0	0	1	1	1	1	1	1	1	1

10-YEAR RISK OF FATAL CVD IN POPULATIONS AT LOW CVD RISK

Age	Systolic blood pressure	Women Non-smoker 4	5	6	7	8	Women Smoker 4	5	6	7	8	Men Non-smoker 4	5	6	7	8	Men Smoker 4	5	6	7	8
65	180	4	5	6	6	7	9	9	11	12	14	8	9	10	12	14	15	17	20	23	26
	160	3	3	4	4	5	6	6	7	8	10	5	6	7	8	10	10	12	14	16	19
	140	2	2	2	3	3	4	4	5	6	7	4	4	5	6	7	7	8	9	11	13
	120	1	1	2	2	2	2	3	3	4	5	2	3	3	4	5	5	5	6	8	9
60	180	3	3	3	4	4	5	5	6	7	8	5	6	7	8	9	10	11	13	15	16
	160	2	2	2	2	3	3	4	4	5	5	3	4	5	5	6	7	8	9	11	13
	140	1	1	1	2	2	2	2	3	3	4	2	3	3	4	4	5	5	6	7	9
	120	1	1	1	1	1	1	2	2	2	3	2	2	2	3	3	3	4	4	5	6
55	180	1	1	2	2	2	3	3	3	4	4	3	4	4	5	6	6	7	8	10	12
	160	1	1	1	1	1	2	2	2	3	3	2	2	3	3	4	4	5	6	7	8
	140	1	1	1	1	1	1	1	1	2	2	1	2	2	2	3	3	3	4	5	6
	120	0	0	1	1	1	1	1	1	1	1	1	1	1	2	2	2	2	3	3	4
50	180	1	1	1	1	1	1	1	2	2	2	2	2	3	3	4	4	4	5	6	7
	160	0	0	1	1	1	1	1	1	1	1	1	1	2	2	2	2	3	3	4	5
	140	0	0	0	0	0	1	1	1	1	1	1	1	1	1	2	2	2	2	3	3
	120	0	0	0	0	0	0	0	0	1	1	1	1	1	1	1	1	1	2	2	2
40	180	0	0	0	0	0	0	0	0	0	0	0	1	1	1	1	1	1	1	2	2
	160	0	0	0	0	0	0	0	0	0	0	0	0	0	1	1	1	1	1	1	1
	140	0	0	0	0	0	0	0	0	0	0	0	0	0	0	0	0	1	1	1	1
	120	0	0	0	0	0	0	0	0	0	0	0	0	0	0	0	0	0	0	1	1

Figure 4.7 SCORE risk charts in high-risk and low-risk regions based on total cholesterol. CVD, cardiovascular disease. (From Conroy RM, Pyorala K, Fitzgerald AP, et al. Estimation of ten-year risk of fatal cardiovascular disease in Europe: the SCORE project. Eur Heart J 2003;24:987-1003.)

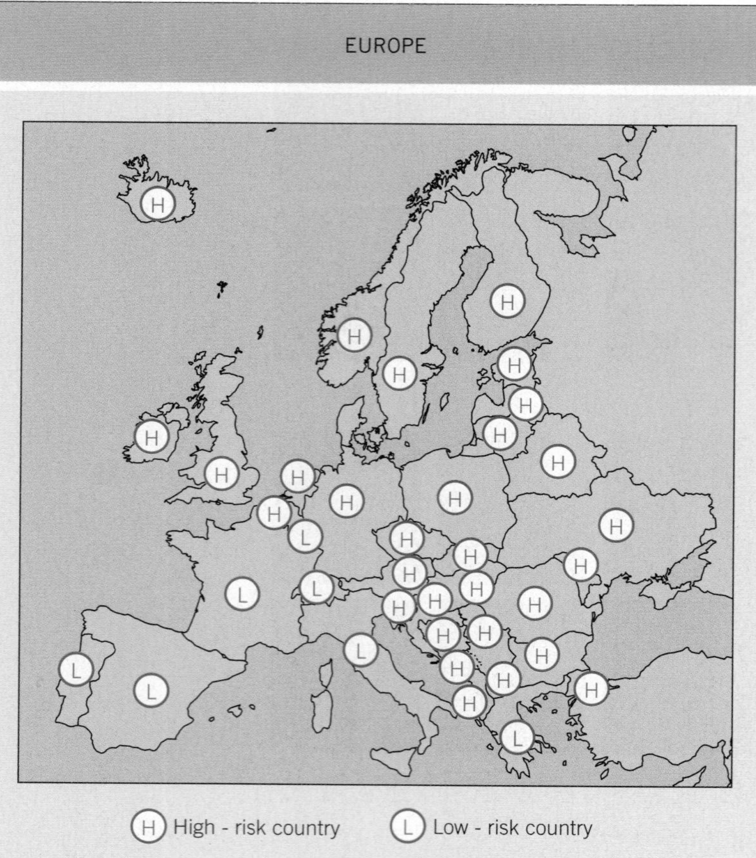

Figure 4.8 Regions of Europe with low and high cardiovascular disease risk.

Whatever the limitations of scores in terms of precision, there is strong trial evidence that patients derive significant vascular gains from treatment of coronary heart disease 10-year risk levels down to as low as 6%. Therefore, even if scores overestimate risk, a threshold for intervention set at 20% 10-year risk remains well above the levels for which evidence of benefit is established.

SUMMARY

Cardiovascular disease is the most important cause of death and disability in the world but encompasses the strongest evidence base on which health professionals can base their interventions to modify risk. It is therefore essential that clinicians determine those who have most to gain from intervention, which requires the early and accurate recognition of those with established disease, for secondary prevention, and the assessment of cardiovascular risk in those without apparent disease, for primary prevention. However, for primary prevention of cardiovascular disease, although there is considerable evidence on what to do, in terms of which risk factors are important and how to reduce their impact, the major limitation is how to efficiently identify those individuals who are at most risk.

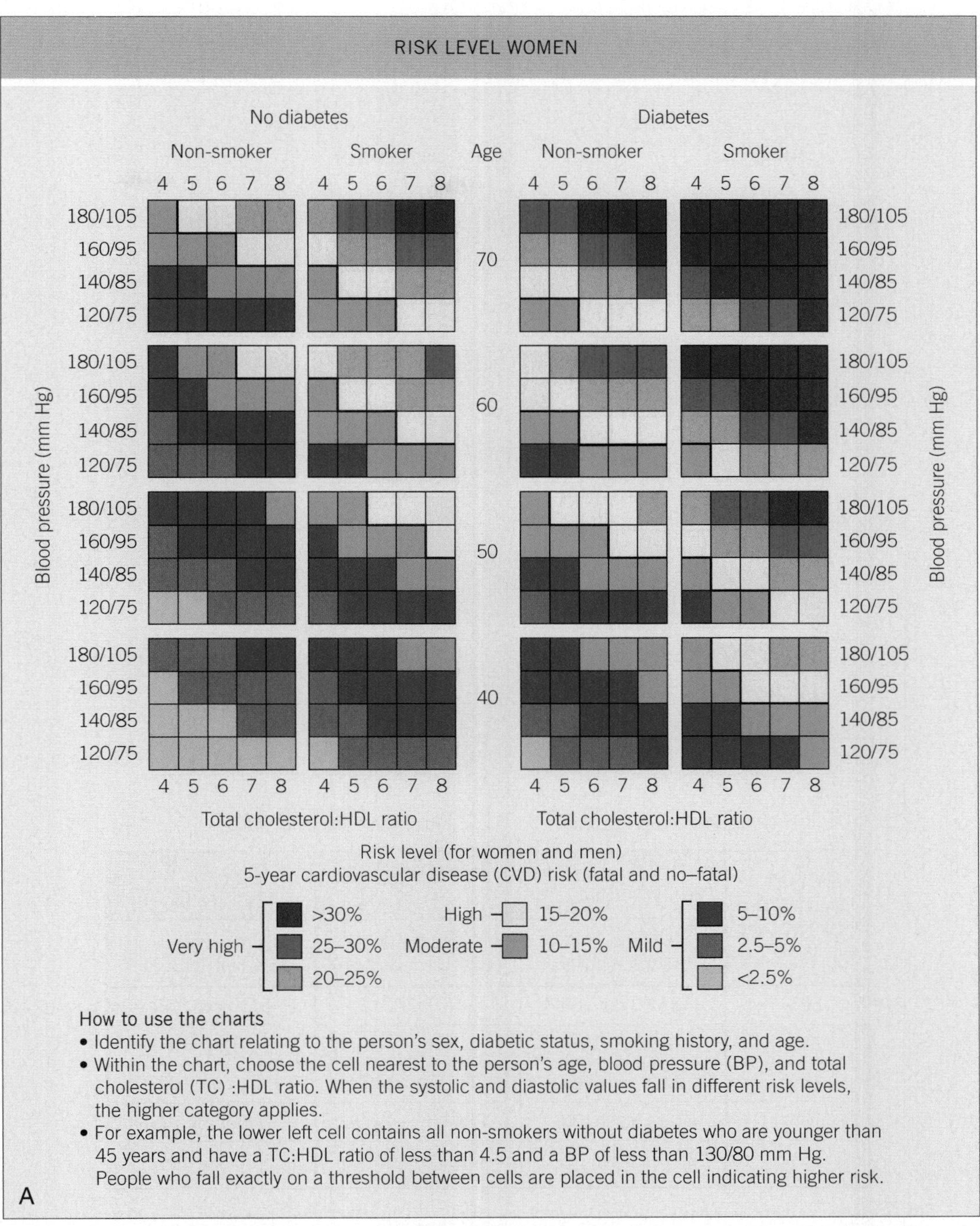

Figure 4.9 Risk assessment charts from the New Zealand guidelines, based on the Framingham algorithm. A, Risk level in women. **B,** Risk level in men. (From Assessment and Management of Cardiovascular Risk. Available at: http://www.nzgg.org.nz/index.cfm?fuseaction=fuseaction_10&fusesubaction=docs&documentid=22. Accessed December 2007.)

(*Continued*)

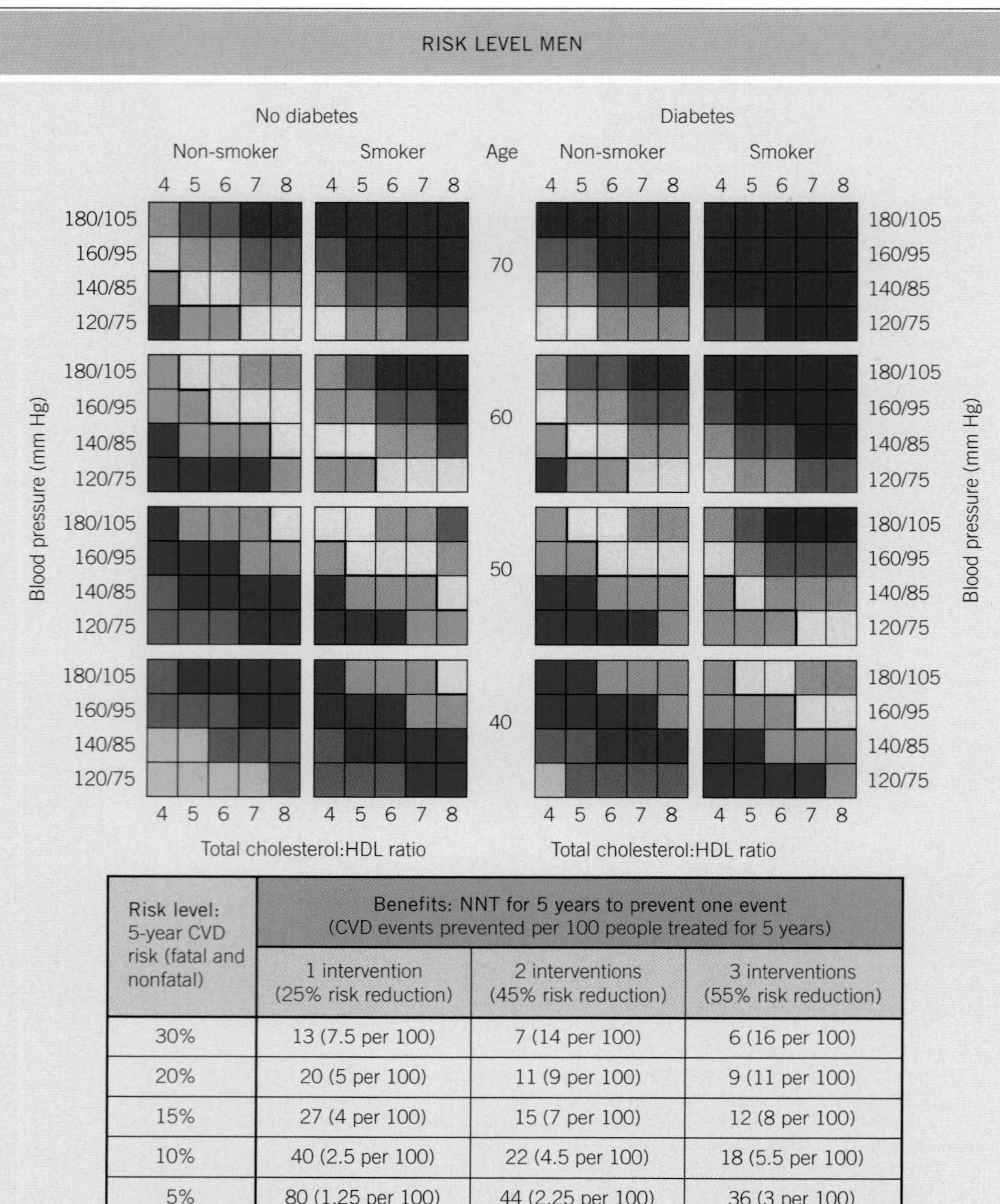

Risk level: 5-year CVD risk (fatal and nonfatal)	Benefits: NNT for 5 years to prevent one event (CVD events prevented per 100 people treated for 5 years)		
	1 intervention (25% risk reduction)	2 interventions (45% risk reduction)	3 interventions (55% risk reduction)
30%	13 (7.5 per 100)	7 (14 per 100)	6 (16 per 100)
20%	20 (5 per 100)	11 (9 per 100)	9 (11 per 100)
15%	27 (4 per 100)	15 (7 per 100)	12 (8 per 100)
10%	40 (2.5 per 100)	22 (4.5 per 100)	18 (5.5 per 100)
5%	80 (1.25 per 100)	44 (2.25 per 100)	36 (3 per 100)

Based on the conservative estimate that each intervention — aspirin, BP treatment (lowering systolic BP by 10 mm Hg), or lipid modification (lowering LDL-C by 20%) — reduces cardiovascular risk by about 25% over 5 years.

Note: Cardiovascular events are defined as myocardial infarction, new angina, ischemic stroke, transient ischemic attack (TIA), peripheral vascular disease, congestive heart failure, and cardiovascular-related death.

NNT = Number needed to treat

B

Figure 4.9—cont'd

CARDIOVASCULAR RISK CALCULATORS AVAILABLE ON-LINE
Framingham
Adapted by National Cholesterol Education Program, Adult Treatment Panel III ■ Risk calculator: http://hin.nhlbi.nih.gov/atpiii/calculator.asp?usertype=prof (on-line version) ■ Risk calculator: http://hin.nhlbi.nih.gov/atpiii/riskcalc.htm (downloadable version) ■ Risk calculator spreadsheet: http://www.nhlbi.nih.gov/guidelines/cholesterol/risk_tbl.htm Adapted by New Zealand Guidelines Group ■ Risk tables: http://www.nzgg.org.nz/guidelines/0035/CARDIOVASCULAR DISEASE_Risk_Chart.pdf
SCORE
■ SCORE risk charts: http://www.escardio.org/initiatives/prevention/SCORE+Risk+Charts.htm ■ HeartScore: http://www.escardio.org/knowledge/decision_tools/heartscore/Program+Download.htm
PROCAM
■ Risk calculator: http://chdrisk.uni-muenster.de/calculator.php?iSprache=1&iVersion=1&iSiVersion=0 ■ Risk score: http://chdrisk.uni-muenster.de/risk.php?iSprache=1&iVersion=1&iSiVersion=0 ■ PROCAM Neuronal Network Analysis: http://chdrisk.uni-muenster.de/n_network.php?iSprache=1&iVersion=1&iSiVersion=0
United Kingdom Prospective Diabetes Study
■ UKPDS Risk Engine: http://www.dtu.ox.ac.uk/index.html?maindoc=/ukpds/

Table 4.9 Cardiovascular risk calculators available on-line.

chapter 5

Special Problems in the Prevention of Cardiovascular Disease

a. Diabetes Mellitus Type 2

Warren W. Davis and W. Virgil Brown

DEFINITION OF PROBLEM

Diabetes significantly increases the risk for atherosclerotic disease. Patients with type 2 diabetes (non–insulin dependent) in their fourth to seventh decades of life without known heart or vascular disease have been found to have an incidence of myocardial infarction and cardiac death equal to that of nondiabetic patients with manifest arteriosclerotic cardiovascular disease (Fig. 5A.1). The reasons for this increased risk are only partially understood. The common coincidence of high blood pressure and obesity plays a role. Plasma levels of cholesterol and triglycerides can be normal in the presence of diabetes; however, elevated triglycerides and reduced high-density lipoprotein (HDL) cholesterol are common. These risk factors are not sufficient to explain the magnitude of the risk in diabetics. Hyperglycemia and insulin resistance are probably direct culprits at the cellular level as well. When control of blood glucose concentration is suboptimal, these abnormalities will be exacerbated. The reduction of risk involves (1) reduction of low-density lipoprotein (LDL) cholesterol, (2) reduction of non–HDL-cholesterol when triglyceride levels are above 200 mg/dL, (3) reduction of blood pressure, and (4) control of blood glucose concentration.

TYPICAL CASE

A 55-year-old postmenopausal woman was diagnosed with type 2 diabetes 5 years ago. Initially, her blood glucose concentration fell with diet and weight loss of 10 pounds. However, she regained her weight after 1 year, and the fasting plasma glucose concentration at home rose to values above 200 mg/dL. The addition of glyburide, 5 mg daily, improved control, with fasting plasma glucose concentration ranging between 130 and 160 mg/dL. Her blood pressure has ranged from 135 to 150 mm Hg systolic and 80 to 95 mm Hg diastolic without medication. She has had no signs or symptoms of coronary, cerebral, or peripheral vascular disease. There is no history of smoking, and she is unaware of a cholesterol elevation in the past. On physical examination, she weighs 196 pounds (89 kg) and is 5 feet 6 inches (168 cm) tall, giving a body mass index of 32. Her waist size is 40 inches. Blood pressure is 145/90 mm Hg, and pulse rate is 82 and regular. There is no evidence of retinopathy or neuropathy, and the cardiovascular examination findings are within normal limits. The electrocardiogram reveals nonspecific ST- and T-wave abnormalities. The total cholesterol level is 236 mg/dL, with triglycerides of 380 mg/dL, HDL-cholesterol of 28 mg/dL, and calculated LDL-cholesterol of 130 mg/dL. The retinas have a few microaneurysms. The neurologic examination reveals no sensory loss. Urinalysis reveals an albumin/creatinine ratio of 60. Hemoglobin A_{1c} is 9%, and the fasting glucose concentration is 230 mg/dL.

DIFFERENTIAL DIAGNOSIS

This patient currently has no symptoms and no objective findings of atherosclerotic cardiovascular disease. However, she does have findings of microvascular involvement. According to the U.S. National Cholesterol Education Program Adult Treatment Panel III guidelines, this patient is considered to have coronary equivalency in terms of cardiovascular risk because of diabetes. The retinal findings and small amount of proteinuria are a major warning of ongoing vascular damage in major arteries as well. Furthermore, the low HDL-cholesterol level and high blood pressure are major warnings that must be considered in the planning of her treatment.

Although the obesity is a fundamental cause of the metabolic derangement, it is not classified as an independent risk factor because most of the effects are expressed through other risk factors. Genetic insulin resistance becomes manifested much earlier in persons with excess adipose tissue, particularly intra-abdominal fat. The triglyceride elevation may also have independent genetic determinants, but the final value is greatly influenced by the failure of adequate insulin action in both adipose tissue and liver. Rising triglyceride levels reduce the HDL-cholesterol level and appear to compromise the reverse cholesterol transport for peripheral tissues to liver. Furthermore, the higher triglyceride values are a reflection of inadequate clearance of partially digested very-low-density lipoprotein and chylomicrons. These "remnants" of triglyceride-rich lipoproteins are atherogenic.

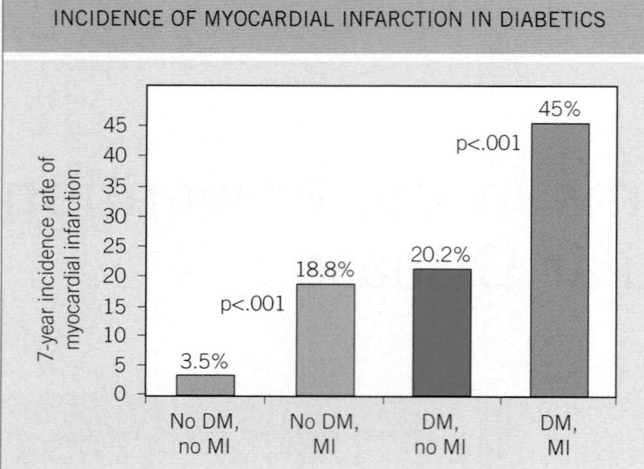

Figure 5A.1 Incidence of myocardial infarction in diabetes. In Finland, the incidence of fatal and nonfatal myocardial infarction (MI) was 45% in diabetics known to have a previous MI. Middle-aged adults without diabetes (DM) but with a history of MI experienced a 20.2% incidence of a second MI (fatal or nonfatal). Diabetics had a similar risk (18.8%) without evidence of previous MI. The diabetics with nonclinical vascular disease experienced almost sixfold more myocardial infarctions. (From Haffner S, Lehto S, Ronnemaa T, Pyorala K, Lakso M. Mortality from coronary heart disease in subjects with type II diabetes and in nondiabetic subjects with and without prior myocardial infarction. N Engl J Med 1998;339:229-234.)

According to U.S. National Cholesterol Education Program guidelines, the goal of therapy is to reduce LDL-cholesterol to below 100 mg/dL and non–HDL-cholesterol to less than 130 mg/dL when the triglyceride level is above 200 mg/dL. Therefore, optimal control of risk factors might be defined as the following:

- hemoglobin A_{1c} <7%
- LDL-cholesterol <100 mg/dL
- non–HDL-cholesterol <130 mg/dL
- blood pressure ≤135/85 mm Hg
- weight of 70 kg
- disappearance of proteinuria

HDL-cholesterol may rise to more desirable levels when these goals are achieved. A direct attack on the low HDL otherwise is not documented to be beneficial by controlled clinical trials.

Before treatment is begun to achieve these goals, it is important to document normal thyroid, liver, and other aspects of renal function.

TREATMENT OPTIONS

The most effective treatment for this woman would be weight loss. With current modes of therapy, attaining her optimal body mass index of 25 is highly improbable. However, 10% to 15% loss of body weight as adipose tissue would be expected to markedly improve diabetic control, to reduce the blood pressure and triglycerides, and to raise the HDL-cholesterol. A moderate reduction in calories with a regular exercise program is the most suitable approach and the one that is most likely to achieve the long-term effects that are necessary to reduce cardiovascular disease. Reducing the cholesterol and saturated fat in the diet may also reduce the LDL-cholesterol level. Monitoring of those parameters for which goals have been set is essential for success. The patient's testing of her glucose before breakfast, before dinner, and at bedtime on at least 2 days of each week should demonstrate a rapid improvement in diabetic control as the body weight falls. Office visits at 6- to 8-week intervals to measure the hemoglobin A_{1c}, blood pressure, and lipoproteins as well as the body weight provide important feedback and motivation for the patient. Discontinuation of the oral hypoglycemic agent may be possible at an early stage of this treatment.

There may be no need to add new medications in this patient if the weight loss is achieved; however, the frequent story is that a new lower weight is achieved, but this does not produce optimal control of risk. If the hemoglobin A_{1c} remains at levels above 7%, adding metformin to the regimen may provide improved glucose control as well as aid in weight loss. In the United Kingdom Prospective Diabetes Study, metformin, among all hypoglycemic agents used, was associated with the most significant reduction in vascular events and the greatest weight loss. Recently, pioglitazone has been shown not only to improve diabetic control but to have a beneficial effect on coronary and carotid lesions and to reduce coronary events. Another choice is the addition of long-acting insulin (glargine insulin). A bedtime dose of insulin at about half of the estimated daily requirements may markedly improve the hemoglobin A_{1c} concentration without hypoglycemia as a common occurrence.

If the LDL-cholesterol level persists above 100 mg/dL, this patient should be treated with a statin. This class of drugs has been demonstrated to reduce risk markedly in diabetics with a wide range of cholesterol values (Fig. 5A.2). The Collaborative Atorvastatin Diabetes Study (CARDS) trial comparing statin therapy with placebo in type 2 diabetic patients was stopped early because of the dramatic reduction in cardiovascular endpoints. The 6000 patients with diabetes in the Heart Protection Study showed significant reductions in cardiac events at all levels of initial LDL-cholesterol value. Because of this clinical trial, consideration of statin use in most if not all diabetics may be warranted. Once optimal LDL levels are achieved, the non–HDL-cholesterol level should be below 130 mg/dL. Fibric acid derivatives or niacin can be used to lower the triglyceride and non–HDL-cholesterol levels in combination with the statin. This may also raise the HDL-cholesterol level. The side effect of flushing has been a major impediment to niacin use. Preparations of extended-release niacin have reduced the frequency and severity of this problem. In one recent trial, only 7% of subjects discontinued the drug. Niacin will occasionally raise blood glucose concentration or aggravate gout or hyperuricemia. However, these effects do not appear to reduce the beneficial effects on vascular disease incidence but require monitoring. If the initial triglycerides rise to values above 300 mg/dL, a fibric acid derivative might be used as initial therapy and a statin added later to achieve the desirable LDL-cholesterol level. Fenofibrate has been shown to reduce

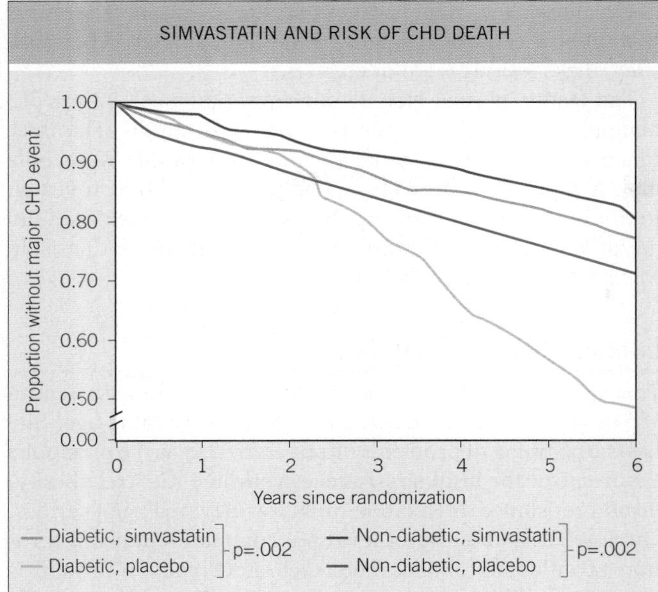

Figure 5A.2 Simvastatin and risk of coronary heart disease (CHD) death. Treatment with simvastatin in the 4S study greatly reduced the risk of CHD death or nonfatal myocardial infarction in those with diabetes. The benefit was statistically significant in both nondiabetics and diabetics considered separately. The risk for treated diabetes was similar to that of the nondiabetic treated group. The much greater risk for diabetics is clear with comparison of the two groups treated with placebo. (From Pyorala K, Pedersen TR, Kjekshus J, Faergeman O, Olsson AG, Thorgeirsson G. Cholesterol lowering with simvastatin improves prognosis of diabetic patients with coronary heart disease: a subgroup analysis of the Scandinavian Simvastatin Survival Study [4S]. Diabetes Care 1997;20:614-620.)

progression of microvascular disease as well. Fibrate data on macrovascular disease prevention have been difficult to interpret. Gemfibrozil was documented to reduce events in middle-aged men with elevated non–HDL-cholesterol without evidence of preexisting vascular disease in the Helsinki Heart Study as well as in men with cardiovascular disease and low HDL-cholesterol in the Veterans Affairs HDL Intervention Trial (VA-HIT). Both trials contained a minority of diabetic patients. Fenofibrate has been tested in the Fenofibrate Intervention and Event Lowering in Diabetes (FIELD) study that contained 10,000 patients with type 2 diabetes. Unfortunately, this was an open trial, and the groups receiving placebo with higher risk status were selectively treated by the physicians with other drugs, primarily statins. This reduced the differential in lipid reduction between the groups with coronary heart disease and may have resulted in the lack of a demonstrable benefit. Those diabetics without preexisting vascular disease in the FIELD study had a 25% reduction in myocardial infarction or coronary death. Unfortunately, no trial has selectively studied diabetics with elevated triglycerides, and we are therefore without demonstration of the preventive effects of either fibrates or niacin in the group of patients who are usually chosen for therapy with these drugs, that is, those with hypertriglyceridemia and low HDL-cholesterol levels.

At this point, borderline elevations in blood pressure might be treated with an angiotensin-converting enzyme inhibitor, an angiotensin receptor blocker, or a calcium channel blocker. Low doses of hydrochlorothiazide ($\leq$25 mg/day) may add significant further reduction of blood pressure as a second-line drug if needed. Such low doses have been found to have minimal effect on glucose control.

This patient has a set of problems seen frequently by every busy practitioner. Making the diagnosis and deciding what needs to be done provide no challenge to the physician. It is in the doing that our best efforts seem to meet with failure. Reducing the progression of arteriosclerosis and microvascular disease should remain the focus. At present, the best approach is a systematic evaluation, setting of goals in collaboration with the patient, and following through with a plan of monitoring and appropriate adjustments of therapy. In theory, optimal diet therapy should provide the most effective treatment, and therefore it deserves a sustained effort in this patient. The patient's compliance with planned goals and management strategy should significantly reduce the insulin resistance that is typical of type 2 diabetes, achieve goal levels of triglyceride and LDL-cholesterol, and reduce the progression of the atherosclerotic process and the risk of major clinical events.

b. Menopausal Women

W. Virgil Brown and Warren W. Davis

DEFINITION OF PROBLEM

Women in the United States and other Western populations have a significant rise in the mean low-density lipoprotein (LDL) cholesterol and triglyceride concentrations beginning with the end of the fifth decade of life. During this period, which coincides with ovarian failure, one can also detect acceleration in the incidence of coronary heart disease. Ultimately, almost as many women as men die of coronary heart disease, and more die of stroke (Fig. 5B-1). Clinical trial evidence confirms that hormone replacement therapy with estrogen and progestin does not reduce the risk of coronary events in women either with or without known coronary disease. (Women with high concentrations of lipoprotein(a) are an exception to this rule.) However, the diagnosis and treatment of hypercholesterolemia and other cardiovascular risk factors in menopausal women have been shown to improve their outcome. Hypertriglyceridemia and diabetes mellitus are particularly powerful causative risk factors in women, and these deserve monitoring and adequate treatment. Such treatment remains underused.

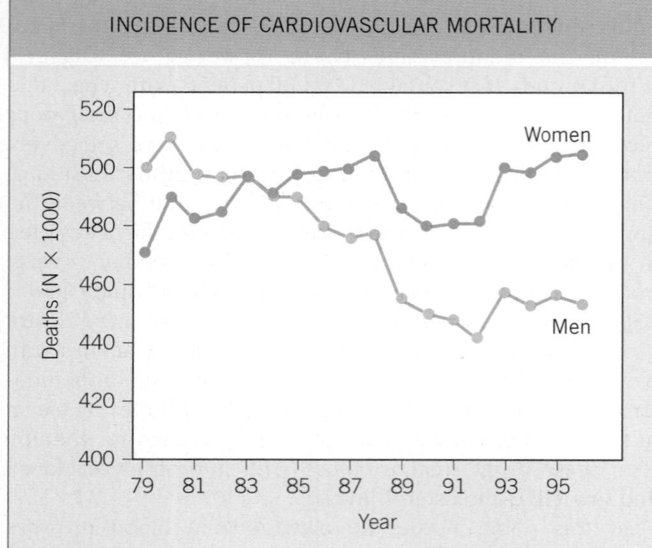

Figure 5B.1 The decline in the incidence of cardiovascular mortality is evident only with age adjustment. In the aging population of the United States, disease appears later. The total mortality attributable to this cause has declined modestly in men but has not changed in women in recent years. (From American Heart Association. 1999 Heart and Stroke Statistical Update. Dallas, Texas, American Heart Association.)

TYPICAL CASE

A 58-year-old woman with a myocardial infarction 3 months earlier is seen as an outpatient. On the morning after admission to the hospital, the blood pressure had been 170/105 mm Hg. A fasting plasma glucose concentration was 153 mg/dL; the total cholesterol level was 315 mg/dL, with triglycerides of 420 mg/dL and high-density lipoprotein (HDL) cholesterol of 32 mg/dL. She made an uneventful recovery and was discharged after 1 week; she was prescribed atenolol (100 mg/day) and oral equine estrogen (0.625 mg/day). She had immediately terminated her habit of smoking one package of cigarettes per day.

Previously, the patient was thought to be in good health. She was unaware of high blood pressure or elevated blood cholesterol or glucose concentration. She underwent a total abdominal hysterectomy at the age of 51 years after developing menometrorrhagia. Subsequently, she had taken equine estrogens for 3 months but stopped because of breast tenderness. Since the age of 40 years, the patient had gained some 35 pounds (16 kg); her current weight is 170 pounds (77.3 kg) at 5 feet 6 inches (168 cm) in height. She noted that she had gained an additional 5 pounds since discharge from the hospital after the myocardial infarction. Her blood pressure is 145/90 mm Hg, and the pulse rate is 64/minute. The excess adiposity is most evident in the abdominal and chest areas (waist circumference of 38 inches). The optic fundi revealed pale pink vessels, and it was difficult to tell arteries from veins by color. The neck, chest, cardiac, and abdominal examination findings were within normal limits. There was no peripheral edema and no tendon xanthomas. The skin over the lateral aspects of the upper arms, buttocks, and lateral upper legs demonstrated scattered raised red lesions with yellow centers averaging 3 mm in diameter. At certain sites, these lesions were in clusters.

The fasting plasma glucose concentration was 122 mg/dL; hemoglobin A_{1c}, 7.4%; and uric acid, 8.9 mg/dL. The liver function, thyroid, and renal function test results were normal. A repeated fasting plasma lipoprotein analysis revealed total cholesterol of 520 mg/dL, with triglycerides of 3750 mg/dL and HDL-cholesterol of 18 mg/dL. It was not possible to calculate the LDL-cholesterol level.

DIFFERENTIAL DIAGNOSIS

This woman has multiple risk factors that combined to cause active coronary heart disease at a relatively young age. She has the complex of problems often referred to as the metabolic syndrome or the insulin resistance syndrome. Central obesity, insulin resistance, high blood pressure, elevated triglycerides, and low HDL-cholesterol level are common features. Elevation of inflammatory markers such as C-reactive protein is common, and high uric acid concentration is also occasionally observed. This patient also had a lipoprotein disorder, which was probably separately inherited. The most likely diagnosis is familial combined hyperlipidemia, a common problem of overproduction of very-low-density lipoprotein (VLDL), which also leads to overproduction of LDL as well—therefore the combined elevation of triglycerides (VLDL) and cholesterol (LDL).

THERAPY

These patients tend to respond to change in diet with reduction in calories, saturated fat, and cholesterol, particularly if a decrease in body weight is achieved. Screening of first-degree relatives and documentation of autosomal dominant inheritance would be required to apply this diagnosis with certainty. Cigarette smoking was an accelerant for vascular disease. Although stopping was totally appropriate, this probably set the stage for further weight gain in the absence of a diet and exercise program. The addition of atenolol may have increased the triglycerides modestly, but a major stimulus to overproduction of VLDL can come from the use of oral estrogens. Oral estrogens are now considered of no benefit as indicated in the early period after an acute vascular event from the results of the Heart and Estrogen/Progestin Replacement Study (HERS) trial. In this study, women with a history of myocardial infarction had more serious coronary artery disease–related events during the first year of treatment compared with placebo.

Estrogen was discontinued, and a diet low in saturated fat and cholesterol and restricted in calories was prescribed. She also began an angiotensin-converting enzyme inhibitor, and atenolol was continued. The patient began a walking program and during the next 8 weeks lost some 10 pounds. On return, her blood pressure was 130/84 mm Hg; blood chemistries were as follows: fasting plasma glucose concentration, 103 mg/dL; uric acid, 8.8 mg/dL; cholesterol, 285 mg/dL; triglycerides, 290 mg/dL; HDL-cholesterol, 38 mg/dL; LDL-cholesterol, 189 mg/dL; and lipoprotein(a), 22 mg/dL. Further weight loss may improve lipoproteins over time, but it is unlikely that the LDL-cholesterol will be brought to the goal of less than 100 mg/dL as defined by the current National Cholesterol Education Program Adult Treatment Panel III guidelines. An LDL-cholesterol–reducing medication was thus indicated. Choosing a drug that would lower LDL-cholesterol and the elevated triglycerides while further raising the low HDL-cholesterol level would be ideal. Niacin is the most effective at accomplishing all these tasks. However, niacin would not be a good first choice in a patient with hyperuricemia and marked insulin resistance, although niacin can be used successfully in patients with insulin resistance with an occasional adjustment in blood glucose therapy. Instead, we chose one of the more potent statin drugs, such as simvastatin, atorvastatin, or rosuvastatin, because we needed to reduce the LDL-cholesterol level approximately 50% to achieve the stated goal (Fig. 5B-2). If the triglycerides remain above 200 mg/dL and the LDL-cholesterol has achieved the target level, one should assess the non–HDL-cholesterol level. This represents all the cholesterol in the atherogenic lipoprotein, including very-low-density, intermediate-density, and low-density lipoproteins. If the target LDL-cholesterol level is below 100 mg/dL, then the target level for non-HDL cholesterol is less than 130 mg/dL. Additional reduction may be achieved by adding a fibric acid derivative, such as gemfibrozil or fenofibrate, to the statin treatment. The dose of statins must remain at or near the lower end of the approved range if gemfibrozil is chosen because this drug tends to interfere with the metabolism of statins (except fluvastatin). Fenofibrate does not have this limitation, and the wider range of statin dosing is permitted. One must sequentially monitor the liver function measures (alanine and aspartate aminotransferases) during the first 3 months after a change in the dosage of these medications. It is also important to carefully avoid other drugs that might inhibit the metabolism of the statin, particularly when the combination with a fibrate is being used.

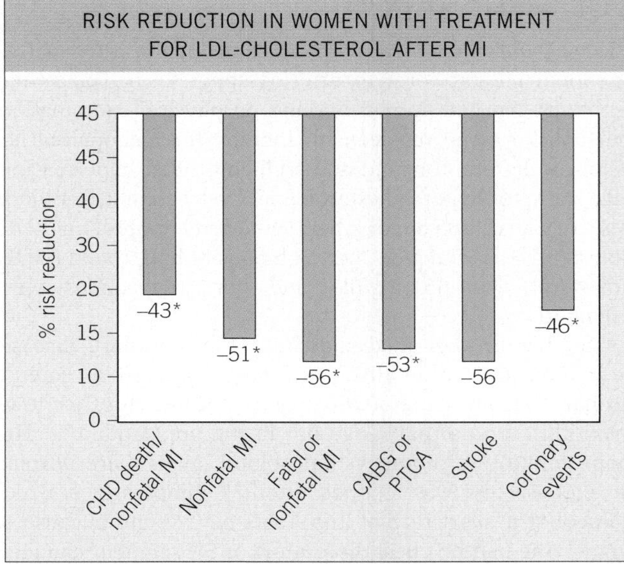

Figure 5B.2 Risk reduction in women with treatment for LDL-cholesterol after myocardial infarction (MI). Women have experienced significant risk reduction with treatment for LDL-cholesterol after myocardial infarction. In the Cholesterol and Recurrent Events (CARE) study, 14% of the participants were women. Half took pravastatin (40 mg/day) and half placebo by random assignment. After 5 years, the relative number of cardiovascular events was reduced as shown. CABG, coronary artery bypass graft; CHD, coronary heart disease; PTCA, percutaneous transluminal coronary angioplasty.

SUMMARY

Women with insulin resistance syndrome may be particularly subject to other risk factors and develop coronary artery disease as early in life as men do. The entry into menopause should cause the physician to evaluate all risk factors and to begin the planning process for risk management. Control of the other risk factors, such as cigarette smoking, high blood pressure, insulin resistance, and hyperlipidemia, is documented to be effective in reducing vascular events. After the event, as in this patient, reduction of LDL-cholesterol becomes the top priority, but aggressive blood pressure control and management of the insulin resistance are clearly indicated.

c. Nontraditional Risk Factors for Coronary Disease

David D. Waters

DEFINITION OF PROBLEM

Diabetes, hypertension, hyperlipidemia, and smoking are the main traditional risk factors for coronary disease. They are important because they are common and because it has been shown that successful treatment of them improves outcome. Physical inactivity and obesity should be corrected as well, but these two risk factors exert part of their detrimental effect through the four major risk factors listed. Other risk factors, such as age and a positive family history, cannot be modified.

In the past decade, new risk factors have been widely publicized, specifically, high blood levels of lipoprotein(a), homocysteine, and markers of inflammation, most commonly C-reactive protein (CRP). The data that link these factors to an increased risk of coronary events are strong. However, it has not been shown that treatment to lower the blood levels of these markers reduces risk.

In addition, noninvasive tests that detect and quantify aspects of the underlying atherosclerotic process have become popular, namely, electron beam computed tomography (EBCT) and B-mode ultrasonography to assess carotid atherosclerosis. EBCT detects coronary calcification and scores its severity. The risk of a coronary event increases with increasing scores, and the coronary artery calcification score adds useful prognostic information to the Framingham risk calculation in some subsets of patients.

CASE PRESENTATION

A 55-year-old woman requested a second opinion as to whether she should undergo coronary arteriography. She had no cardiac symptoms and had normal findings on physical examination. She took hormone replacement therapy for menopausal hot flashes, a diuretic for mild and well-controlled hypertension, and a statin for hypercholesterolemia. On treatment, her blood pressure was 125/85 mm Hg, her low-density lipoprotein (LDL) cholesterol was 95 mg/dL, her high-density lipoprotein (HDL) cholesterol was 65 mg/dL, and her triglycerides were 170 mg/dL.

After her brother died suddenly from coronary disease, the patient underwent EBCT scanning. This test revealed a coronary calcium score of 300 angstrom units. Her CRP level was within the normal range but in the upper quintile. Her lipoprotein(a) and homocysteine blood levels were normal. An exercise test was stopped after 11 minutes of a Bruce protocol at a heart rate of 165 beats per minute because of fatigue. She had no chest discomfort or ST-segment changes, and the nuclear perfusion component of the test was normal.

The patient asked whether coronary arteriography might reveal advanced coronary disease that could be amenable to revascularization, thus prolonging her life.

DIFFERENTIAL DIAGNOSIS

According to the Framingham risk calculation included in the National Cholesterol Education Program Adult Treatment Panel III guidelines, this woman's risk of experiencing cardiac death or myocardial infarction within the next 10 years is 1%. However, the Framingham risk calculation is based on traditional risk factors only. In a middle-aged woman without known coronary disease, a CRP level in the upper quintile of the normal range confers a threefold increased risk of a coronary event during the next 5 years. Unfortunately, considerable variability has been shown to exist in the measurement of CRP, so that a repeated measurement often leads to a reclassification of risk.

Similarly, a high calcium score increases the risk for future coronary events. The presence of coronary calcium indicates that coronary atherosclerosis is present; however, some degree of atherosclerosis is ubiquitous in middle-aged adults in affluent countries, and the underlying atherosclerotic process may not be encroaching on the lumen. On the other hand, advanced atherosclerosis may be present without calcification. In a recent, large registry with a mean follow-up of 6.8 years, the risk of all-cause mortality increased from 2.2-fold for a calcium score between 11 and 100 to 12.5-fold for a score above 1000, compared with a score of zero. The American College of Cardiology Foundation/American Heart Association 2007 clinical expert consensus document on coronary artery calcification scoring suggests that the test might be most useful in patients judged to be at intermediate risk, when a high score would indicate the need for much more aggressive risk factor treatment.

High blood levels of homocysteine have been associated with an increased risk of cardiovascular disease in epidemiologic studies. The magnitude of the incremental risk is similar in some studies to that associated with smoking or hypertension. Some subjects with high homocysteine levels are homozygotes for a variant of the methylenetetrahydrofolate reductase *(MTHFR)* enzyme, but curiously, an increased risk for myocardial infarction was not present in the Physicians' Health Study in this subgroup. High homocysteine levels probably cause cardiovascular disease through prothrombotic effects and impairment of endothelial function.

Homocysteine is a sulfur-containing amino acid that is formed during the metabolism of methionine, an essential amino acid derived from dietary protein. Methionine metabolism and homocysteine levels are dependent on the availability of folate, vitamin B_6, and vitamin B_{12}.

Treatment of hyperhomocysteinemia is inexpensive and effective in reducing blood homocysteine levels, but whether this reduces the risk of future coronary events is still being debated. Clinical trials have generally not shown benefit; for example, in the Heart Outcomes Prevention Evaluation-2 (HOPE-2) trial, vitamin treatment did not reduce the primary endpoint composed of cardiovascular death, myocardial infarction, and stroke. A significant reduction in stroke was seen, but also a significant increase in hospitalizations for unstable angina. Since 1998, federally mandated folic acid fortification of all enriched grain products in the United States has decreased the prevalence of high homocysteine levels by approximately half.

Lipoprotein(a) is structurally similar to plasminogen and thus is prothrombotic. It binds fibrin and fibrinogen competitively with plasminogen and inhibits fibrinolysis. In most prospective studies, high lipoprotein(a) levels were linked to an increased risk of subsequent coronary events. In the Framingham population, the risk of an elevated lipoprotein(a) level was approximately equal in both men and women to the risk of an elevated total cholesterol or a low HDL-cholesterol level.

CRP is a nonspecific marker of inflammation, and atherosclerosis is a low-grade inflammatory process. Epidemiologic studies clearly indicate that both men and women with higher CRP levels, although still within the normal range, are at increased risk for myocardial infarction for at least 5 years. Most of these studies use a high-sensitivity assay that is now widely available. Higher levels of CRP and other inflammatory markers (interleukin 6, serum amyloid A, tumor necrosis factor α) are associated with a worse prognosis in patients with acute coronary syndromes. Estrogen increases CRP levels, as does diabetes, obesity (particularly central adiposity), and smoking.

Although not as extensively studied, lipoprotein-associated phospholipase A_2 may prove to be a better marker of risk than CRP because it is more reproducible. CRP measurements often vary within an individual enough to change risk category.

TREATMENT OPTIONS

If coronary arteriography revealed severe coronary narrowings in this woman, she would likely undergo coronary revascularization if she were being treated in the United States. However, in the absence of symptoms, inducible myocardial ischemia, or left ventricular dysfunction, there is no evidence that she would derive benefit from either bypass surgery or angioplasty.

Homocysteine levels can be reduced by folic acid doses of 400 μg/day, but the usual dose is 1 mg/day or even higher.

Some physicians prescribe vitamins B_6 and B_{12} with folic acid, but this does not appear to be necessary. Fortification of enriched grain with folic acid was begun in the United States in 1997 by a Food and Drug Administration regulation. As a result, serum folate levels have risen and homocysteine levels have decreased in the general population. The available evidence from clinical trials suggests that this treatment would not reduce coronary risk.

The commonly used cholesterol-lowering drugs do not alter lipoprotein(a) levels. Benzafibrate (but not clofibrate or gemfibrozil), high-dose niacin, estrogen, and combined estrogen and progesterone therapy reduce lipoprotein(a) levels. Women with high lipoprotein(a) levels appeared to respond better to hormone replacement therapy than did women with low levels in a post hoc analysis of the Heart and Estrogen/Progestin Replacement Study (HERS). However, there is no other evidence that lowering of lipoprotein(a) blood levels reduces cardiovascular risk.

CRP levels are usually not measured clinically and are not treated directly. Aspirin reduces risk in coronary patients, particularly those with high CRP levels, but aspirin does not reduce CRP levels. Statins reduce CRP levels within weeks, but whether this effect is related to the event reduction associated with statins is not known. In one secondary prevention trial, patients with higher levels of inflammatory markers not only had a higher risk but also obtained the most benefit from a statin. In a recent primary prevention trial (JUPITER), a statin reduced events in patients with high CRP levels but without elevated LDL-cholesterol levels.

Measurement of high-sensitivity CRP might thus be useful in deciding whether to treat some patients more aggressively, such as with a statin. Smoking cessation, weight loss, and exercise each reduce CRP levels.

SUMMARY

The addition of newer risk factors to the traditional ones increases the accuracy of risk assessment and thus may alter treatment for specific patients, usually those considered to be at intermediate risk. The measurement of high-sensitivity CRP and calcium score as measured by EBCT are now used for this purpose in clinical practice. Specifically, treatment of lipoprotein(a) or homocysteine has not been shown to reduce the risk of future coronary events. Such evidence is available for the traditional risk factors of smoking, hypertension, hypercholesterolemia, and diabetes.

chapter 6

Therapeutic Approaches to the Diabetic Patient

Mary Ellen Sweeney

Definition and Description

- Diabetes mellitus is diagnosed when one of the following is present: (1) symptoms of diabetes and a casual (random) plasma glucose concentration above 200 mg/dL (11.1 mmol/L); or (2) the fasting plasma glucose concentration is above 126 mg/dL (7.0 mmol/L); or (3) the 2-hour post–glucose load value is above 200 mg/dL (11.1 mmol/L), confirmed on repeated testing.
- "Prediabetes" encompasses impaired fasting glucose concentration and impaired glucose tolerance. Impaired fasting glucose concentration is defined as fasting plasma glucose level between 100 and 125 mg/dL (5.6-6.9 mmol/L). Impaired glucose tolerance is defined as a 2-hour post–glucose load value above 140 mg/dL (7.8 mmol/L) and below 200 mg/dL (11.1 mmol/L).
- In the absence of unequivocal hyperglycemia, these criteria should be confirmed by repeated testing on a different day. The oral glucose tolerance test is not recommended for routine clinical use but may be required in the evaluation of patients with impaired fasting glucose concentration (see text) or when diabetes is still suspected despite a normal fasting plasma glucose concentration, as with the postpartum evaluation of women with gestational diabetes.

Key Features

- Type 2 diabetes confers a twofold to fourfold increased risk of coronary heart disease (CHD); in those with type 1 diabetes, the risk may be increased more than 10-fold.
- Specific changes in the lipoprotein profiles associated with insulin resistance contribute to the increased risk in type 2 diabetes. Hyperlipidemia and hypertension predominate as risk factors in type 1 and type 2 diabetes.
- Data on the role of glycemic control as a risk factor for CHD in diabetes are building, but its role as a primary determinant of microvascular complications and of cardiovascular risk factors mandates reasonable (and possibly rigorous) attention.

Clinical Implications

- The screening of high-risk diabetic subjects for CHD is recommended, given the increased prevalence and case fatality of CHD as well as the more frequent silent ischemia in diabetes. Similarly, screening for diabetes is recommended in patients with CHD.
- Vigorous control of blood pressure (goal, 130/80 mm Hg) and dyslipidemia prevents cardiovascular events in diabetes.

Diabetes mellitus has reached epidemic proportions in the United States, affecting in excess of 20 million individuals. In addition, 26% have impaired fasting glucose concentration.[1] Both type 1 (caused by autoimmune beta-cell destruction) and the more common type 2 (related to obesity and insulin resistance) are associated with dramatically increased rates of coronary heart disease (CHD). The risk is usually increased twofold to fourfold in type 2 diabetes and as high as 10-fold in type 1 diabetes, reflecting the younger age at onset in these subjects. These increased CHD rates are seen not only for incidence (i.e., the number of new cases per year) but also for case fatality (i.e., reduced survival after a cardiovascular event). This means that it is important to pursue both primary and secondary prevention. Another important epidemiologic observation is that at least for CHD mortality, the usual female protection is greatly diminished, which means that the diabetic woman is an extremely high-risk CHD patient. Approximately 6% of the middle-aged population (those aged 45 to 74 years) in the United States have diabetes, and twice as many as this have prediabetes. Patients with impaired fasting glucose concentration and impaired glucose tolerance are now categorized as having prediabetes, which refers to their increased risk for development of both diabetes and cardiovascular disease (CVD). Thus, from a primary community-wide viewpoint, diabetes should be a major target for preventive cardiology. Of further note for the practicing cardiologist is the observation that approximately one quarter of hospital admissions for myocardial infarction are in patients who have diabetes; a similar proportion of patients who undergo revascularization are known to have diabetes.[2]

Given the potential vascular and cardiovascular consequences of diabetes, it is imperative that it be recognized early. It is thus incumbent on cardiologists to look for diabetes in all of their patients who have CHD and on all internists, general practitioners, and diabetologists to look for heart disease in their diabetes patients. This point is particularly important given the increased prevalence of silent ischemia in diabetes. Therefore, this chapter addresses screening in both the primary and secondary prevention settings.

The major focus, however, is on the management of the diabetes and of CVD risk factors. Major questions remain unanswered in terms of glucose control, and the trial evidence to date is inconclusive, as discussed later.[3-6] Nonetheless, certain conclusions can be drawn and appropriate guidelines developed. In terms of the standard cardiovascular risk factors, which are still operative in diabetes[7,8] but do not fully explain the excessive cardiovascular risk, evidence from clinical trials is mounting and exists for both primary prevention by blood pressure control[9-12] and secondary prevention with cholesterol lowering.[13,14]

DESCRIPTION OF TECHNIQUE AND PROCEDURE

Screening for Diabetes Mellitus

To manage cardiovascular risk in diabetes effectively, it is imperative to know the cardiac status of all diabetic patients and the diabetes status of all cardiac patients. In terms of the latter, cardiologists and internists should question every patient as to their diabetes status. Patients should be screened by determination of fasting blood glucose concentration every 3 years if they are older than 45 years or if they are younger than 45 years and overweight (body mass index above 25 kg/m^2). Testing should also be considered in other circumstances (Table 6.1).

If there is any doubt or if it has not been checked during the past 3 years at the maximum (1 year at the minimum), a fasting plasma glucose test should be ordered (Fig. 6.1). Indeed, this should be considered to be as important as the fasting lipid profile and, similarly, should be repeated annually. If the result is 126 mg/dL (7.0 mmol/L) or more, the test should be repeated on a second occasion, and if this level is then confirmed, the patient is diagnosed with diabetes type 1 and thus requires a specialized approach to both management and secondary prevention. Alternatively, diabetes may be diagnosed by two criteria: (1) a casual plasma glucose concentration above 200 mg/dL (11.1 mmol/L) accompanied by symptoms of hyperglycemia, such as polyuria, polydipsia, and unexplained weight loss; or (2) a 2-hour plasma glucose concentration above 200 mg/dL after a 75-g oral glucose load (oral glucose tolerance test). With both the fasting glucose determination and the oral glucose tolerance test, a lesser state of glucose intolerance or prediabetes is diagnosed. Prediabetes is defined as either impaired fasting glucose concentration or impaired glucose tolerance. Impaired fasting glucose concentration is defined as a fasting plasma glucose concentration of 100 mg/dL (5.6 mmol/L) to 125 mg/dL (6.9 mmol/L). Impaired glucose tolerance is diagnosed by plasma glucose concentration of 140 mg/dL (7.8 mmol/L) to 199 mg/dL (11.0 mmol/L) after an oral glucose tolerance test. Data are accumulating that patients with prediabetes may be at a similarly increased cardiovascular risk as those who have diabetes.[15] Subjects who have either impaired fasting glucose concentration or impaired glucose tolerance should be treated aggressively as they have an increased risk of CHD and of diabetes. The risk for development of diabetes for those with impaired glucose tolerance is approximately 5% or more per year. These subjects are also more likely to have metabolic syndrome.[16] Metabolic syndrome is diagnosed when a patient is found to meet three or more of the criteria (Table 6.2). Together, these features may enhance thrombotic tendencies as well as atherosclerosis.[17] Although not every patient who has impaired fasting glucose concentration or impaired glucose tolerance has all of the risk factors associated with insulin resistance

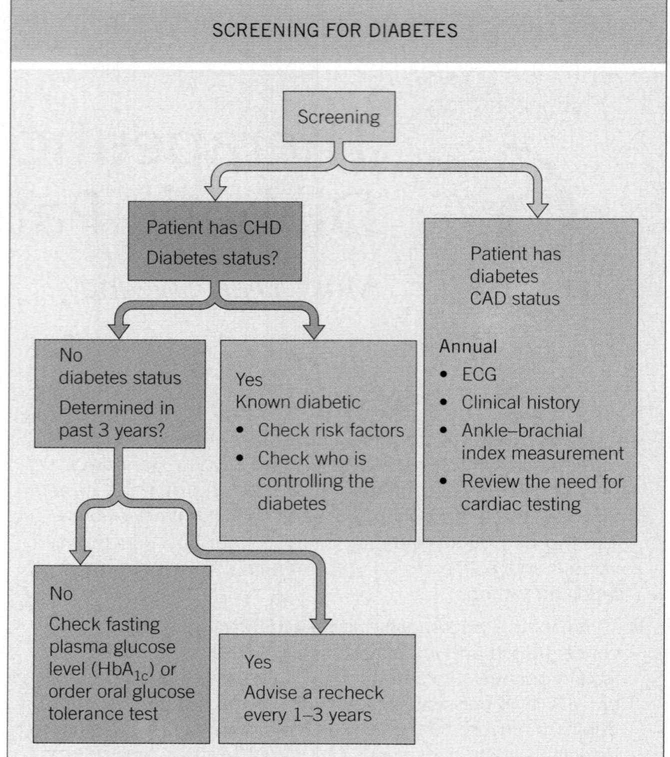

Figure 6.1 Screening for diabetes. The fasting plasma glucose concentration recommended by the American Diabetes Association and the World Health Organization (WHO) as being diagnostic but needing to be confirmed is above 126 mg/dL (7.0 mmol/L). The plasma glucose concentration by the oral glucose tolerance test recommended by the WHO as being diagnostic but needing to be confirmed is 200 mg/dL (11.1 mmol/L) at 2 hours after a glucose load of 75 g. (CAD, coronary artery disease; CHD, coronary heart disease; ECG, electrocardiography.)

WHO SHOULD BE TESTED FOR DIABETES?

Testing for diabetes should be considered in all individuals at age 45 years and older, particularly in those with a body mass index $\geq$ 25 kg/m^2; if the result is normal, the test should be repeated at 3-year intervals.

Testing should be considered at a younger age or be carried out more frequently in individuals who are overweight (body mass index $\geq$ 25 kg/m^2) and have additional risk factors:

- are habitually physically inactive
- have a first-degree relative with diabetes
- are members of a high-risk ethnic population (e.g., African American, Latino, Native American, Asian American, Pacific Islander)
- have delivered a baby weighing more than 9 pounds or have been diagnosed with gestational diabetes mellitus
- are hypertensive ($\geq$140/90 mm Hg)
- have an HDL-cholesterol level <35 mg/dL (0.90 mmol/L) or a triglyceride level >250 mg/dL (2.82 mmol/L)
- have polycystic ovary syndrome
- on previous testing, had impaired glucose tolerance or impaired fasting glucose concentration
- have other clinical conditions associated with insulin resistance (e.g., polycystic ovary syndrome or acanthosis nigricans)
- have a history of vascular disease

From the American Diabetes Association. Standards for medical care for patients with diabetes mellitus. Diabetes Care 2008;31:S12-S49.

Table 6.1 Who should be tested for diabetes?

DIAGNOSTIC CRITERIA FOR THE METABOLIC SYNDROME BASED ON NCEP ATP III GUIDELINES*
Fasting blood glucose concentration ≥100 mg/dL (5.6 mmol/L)
Hypertension (blood pressure ≥130 mm Hg systolic or ≥85 mm Hg diastolic or taking antihypertensive medication)
HDL-cholesterol <40 mg/dL (1.04 mmol/L) for men or <50 mg/dL (1.29 mmol/L) for women
Triglycerides ≥150 mg/dL (1.69 mmol/L)
Waist circumference >102 cm (40 inches) for men or >88 cm (35 inches) for women

*The presence of three of the five criteria confirms the diagnosis.

From Executive Summary of the Third Report of the National Cholesterol Education Program (NCEP) Expert Panel on Detection, Evaluation, and Treatment of High Blood Cholesterol in Adults (Adult Treatment Panel III). JAMA 2001;285:2486-2497.

Table 6.2 Diagnostic criteria for the metabolic syndrome based on AHA/NHLBI scientific statement.[17]

syndrome (indeed, some statistical analyses have suggested different "subtypes" with specific risk factor disturbances), recognition of these subjects is helpful because it focuses attention on the underlying mechanism of risk (insulin resistance) and the fundamental therapy (diet for weight loss and exercise). The level of glycated hemoglobin (HbA_{1c}) is used for long-term monitoring of glucose control. However, neither the American Diabetes Association (ADA) nor the World Health Organization has endorsed this test for diagnostic purposes because of the great variability in assay methodologies and normal ranges. Any patient with CHD who is found to have diabetes by any of these methods should also be carefully assessed for risk factors and diabetes control (Table 6.3). Most important, it must be determined who will take responsibility for future management of CVD risk factors and diabetes in such patients. The cardiologist should be instrumental in making sure these aspects of the management of patients with both CHD and diabetes are addressed.

PREVENTION CHECKLIST FOR ALL DIABETIC PATIENTS WHO HAVE CORONARY HEART DISEASE
Who is looking after the diabetes?
If no one is, assume responsibility personally or make referral.
Is blood pressure less than 130/80 mm Hg?
If not, instigate or modify treatment or contact the primary care provider.
Is LDL-cholesterol less than 100 mg/dL (or <70 mg/dL if very high risk)?
If not, instigate or modify treatment or contact the primary care provider.
Is hemoglobin A_{1c} concentration above 7.0%?
If so, instigate or modify treatment or contact the primary care provider or diabetologist.
Is patient a current smoker?
If so, instigate or modify cessation strategy or contact the primary care provider.

Table 6.3 Prevention checklist for all diabetic patients who have coronary heart disease.

Screening for Heart Disease

Screening for heart disease in known diabetic patients is a more complex and controversial area than screening for diabetes mellitus. Because the risk is so high, periodic screening for CHD is recommended. Indeed, as Haffner and colleagues[18] have demonstrated, the heart disease mortality risk of diabetic subjects who do not have known heart disease is equivalent to that of nondiabetic subjects who do have known heart disease. It could thus be argued that all patients who have type 2 diabetes should be treated as if they have CHD; for patients who have both diabetes and CHD, an even more intensive intervention should be mounted. Jaffe and coworkers[19] categorized the 10-year cardiovascular risk among U.S. adults with diabetes as a percentage per year estimated by the Third National Health and Nutrition Examination Survey using the U.K. Prospective Diabetes Study outcomes model. In that model, 42.7% of diabetics fell within the lowest risk group (>0% to 1% per year), 23.3% in the moderate-risk group (>1% to 2% per year), 27.0% in the high-risk group (>2% to 4% per year), and 7.0% in the highest risk group (>4% per year). Therefore, the majority of patients with type 2 diabetes have a moderate to high risk for development of coronary artery disease (CAD), and a small percentage have a very high risk.

Another justification for screening for heart disease in diabetes is the higher prevalence of silent ischemia that is seen in many studies (but not all). This silent ischemia is related to vagal denervation, which results from autonomic neuropathy, a condition that itself has been associated with excess cardiovascular mortality. Although much of this excess mortality is related to concurrent CVD risk factor disturbances and renal disease, detection of those who have significant silent ischemia is important because it enables more intensive risk factor modification to be focused on these patients. A 2007 ADA consensus statement on screening for CAD in diabetic patients specifically defined certain clinical features that help identify those patients who are at increased risk of myocardial infarction or cardiac death (Table 6.4).[20] For risk stratification of new patients with diabetes who are seen

CLINICAL FEATURES IN DIABETIC PATIENTS INDICATING AN INCREASED RISK FOR CARDIOVASCULAR OUTCOMES
Other atherosclerotic vascular disease (peripheral, cerebral, renal, or mesenteric)
Microalbuminuria and chronic kidney disease
Abnormal resting electrocardiogram
Autonomic neuropathy
Retinopathy
Chronic undertreated hyperglycemia
Age older than 65 years
Male sex
Unexplained dyspnea
Multiple cardiac risk factors*

*Hypertension, dyslipidemia, inactivity, smoking, and abdominal obesity.

Table 6.4 Clinical features in diabetic patients indicating an increased risk for cardiovascular outcomes.

in the cardiologist's office, certain baseline studies should be done. These include routine medical history with focus on duration of diabetes and level of control; history of smoking; functional status; symptoms of autonomic neuropathy, including delayed gastric emptying and orthostatic hypotension; and past medical history of hypertension, kidney disease, stroke, claudication, or vascular procedures. Laboratory evaluation should include fasting plasma glucose concentration, creatinine concentration, urine microalbumin test, and fasting lipid level. A routine annual resting electrocardiogram is inexpensive and should be done on every patient. An ankle-brachial index measurement should also be obtained annually (as recommended by a joint ADA and American Heart Association workshop).[21] The ankle-brachial index is an inexpensive quick measure of subclinical atherosclerosis that is predictive of future CVD. The index is the ratio of the systolic blood pressure in either of the two ankle arteries (posterior tibial artery or dorsalis pedis) in either leg to the systolic pressure in the arm. If the result is positive (i.e., a ratio of less than 0.9), intensive risk factor management is advised and possible consideration of further cardiac testing is warranted. Referral to a peripheral vascular specialist is indicated if the ratio is less than 0.5.

The type of testing to be undertaken in the asymptomatic diabetic patient varies according to the circumstances. For instance, if the patient has a high probability of CHD (e.g., Q waves on the electrocardiogram), stress perfusion imaging or stress echocardiography may be appropriate; for patients who have a lesser risk (e.g., two or more risk factors), a plain exercise stress test is recommended as the initial test.

Electron beam computed tomography (also known as ultrafast computed tomography) is a new modality that can detect coronary atherosclerosis by identifying coronary calcium. Testing in asymptomatic patients may be valuable in identifying patients with a high likelihood of inducible myocardial ischemia, but it is not as valuable in low-risk patients. However, asymptomatic diabetic patients who have a high calcium score may represent a higher risk group. Anand and colleagues[22] demonstrated that 46.3% of asymptomatic patients with type 2 diabetes had a significant coronary artery calcification score on testing.[22]

The action that should be prompted by a positive result to the initial screening test depends on the individual circumstances of the patient and the local cardiology facilities and practices. Clearly, markedly positive results should lead to evaluation by a cardiologist and possible catheterization. Detection of left main coronary artery disease or multivessel disease would normally lead to consideration for revascularization, and some patients with lesser disease may be candidates for "early" revascularization. However, analysis of patients in the COURAGE trial did not show benefit for percutaneous coronary intervention over medical management in diabetic patients with CAD.[23] At the very least, all patients with positive findings are candidates for close follow-up and intensive risk factor intervention.

Not only is the presence of diabetes an indicator of increased cardiovascular risk and a risk equivalent, but it has been recently shown that myocardial infarction may be considered a prediabetes risk equivalent. Mozaffarian and colleagues[24] studied 8291 Italian patients with myocardial infarction within the past 3 months. In those patients free of any glucose abnormalities in the peri-infarct period, one third developed new diabetes or impaired fasting glucose concentration within 3.5 years, and this number increased to two thirds when the lower limit of 100 mg/dL (5.6 mmol/L) was used as the cutoff.

INDICATIONS, CONTRAINDICATIONS, AND OBJECTIVES

Diabetes Management and Glucose Control

One of the fundamental questions that faces the cardiologist who is treating a diabetic patient is how involved he or she should become in the patient's diabetes management. The answer to this question depends partly on the extent and nature of the patient's other health care and the insurance plan. However, the cardiologist should, at a minimum, ask about the patient's diabetes management plan and ensure that at least twice-yearly HbA_{1c} levels are measured in all patients (the frequency of HbA_{1c} testing should be quarterly for those who do not meet treatment goals) and reviewed by the appropriate health care professional. If the HbA_{1c} level is noted to be above 7.0% by an assay that has an upper limit of normal of 6.0% (or if it is equivalently elevated in other assays), the cardiologist should ensure that whoever is managing the diabetes is aware of the result because the ADA recommends a change or intensification of therapy in such cases. The goal of management should be HbA_{1c} level of less than 7% according to the ADA 2008 clinical guidelines.[1] The relative benefit of achieving this goal is documented in controlled clinical trials with relative risk reductions of 15% to 30% per 1% absolute reduction in HbA_{1c}.[1] The major limitations include hypoglycemia, weight gain, and other adverse effects.

Controversy about whether blood glucose levels are themselves related to CVD has existed for many years in both epidemiologic and clinical trial arenas, both in diabetic and in nondiabetic populations. Jarrett and Shipley,[25] using data from the Whitehall study, showed no difference in the risk of heart disease between those who were newly diagnosed with diabetes and those who were diagnosed for 7 years or more. The alternative that they proposed is that diabetes and CVD share a common (possibly genetic) antecedent. The lack of a simple relationship between blood glucose level and CVD received further support from a pooling of prospective studies, which showed little association in the nondiabetic population between blood glucose level and CVD, although the two largest such studies did show a threshold relationship such that the highest blood glucose levels in the nondiabetic range predicted increased risk. Subsequent studies have provided evidence in both directions, but no clear consensus has arisen, although it seems likely that the lack of relationship between duration of diabetes and CHD may reflect an increased CVD risk that is also seen in early type 2 diabetes owing to antecedent insulin resistance. This may thus obscure a diabetes effect as such, which may become apparent only after a longer duration of diabetes. For example, in the Nurses' Health Study, a duration effect was seen only after 10 years or longer.[8] It is thus likely that hyperglycemia in the high-normal and low diabetic range reflects hyperinsulinemia, which may explain the association of impaired glucose tolerance with CVD. In type 1 diabetes, cross-sectional and prospective studies also cast doubt on a clear and strong relationship between blood glucose concentration and CHD risk.[26] However, the most recent report does suggest that in women who have type 1 diabetes, HbA_{1c} is indeed a predictor of CHD mortality but not of CHD morbidity.[27]

For younger patients (those younger than 50 years) who have type 1 diabetes, however, a goal closer to 6.0% (i.e., normal) should be considered, given the results of the Diabetes Control and Complications Trial (DCCT)[6] and the fact that such a reduction confers considerable benefit in terms of microvascular complications, one of which (nephropathy) is also a major cardiovascular risk factor. Exceptions to this goal for type 1 patients are those with recurrent difficulties with hypoglycemia and those with advanced microvascular disease (e.g., visual loss and renal failure). The main reason that a normal glycemic level is given great prominence in the younger type 1 diabetic patient is that younger patients have a life expectancy that allows a reasonable probability for development of the advanced, symptomatic microvascular complications. It has been estimated that patients who have an HbA_{1c} level that is constantly more than 2 percentage points above normal would take, on average, 42 years to develop the major complications; if the HbA_{1c} is 5 percentage points above normal, major complications will develop after only 18 years. The other reason for the lower goal in type 1 diabetes is that the DCCT, which is the definitive trial, was carried out in young adult and adolescent patients with type 1 diabetes and provided nonsignificant but suggestive evidence of benefits from intensive therapy for the prevention of macrovascular (largely peripheral arterial) disease.[28] The DCCT trial involved young patients with type 1 diabetes who were within 5 years of diagnosis (primary cohort) or 15 years of diagnosis (secondary cohort) and whose mean age at randomization into intensive therapy (goal HbA_{1c} in the normal range) or conventional therapy was 27 years. This volunteer population agreed to be randomized to either regimen for 6 years or longer and thus possibly to be committed to multiple insulin injections (three or more times daily) and glucose testing (four times daily and once weekly in the middle of night). Therefore, the patients were a highly motivated group. They also represented a relatively low CVD risk group because significant hyperlipidemia and any hypertension were exclusion criteria.

The Epidemiology of Diabetes Interventions and Complications (EDIC) study, an observational follow-up of the DCCT type 1 diabetes cohort, has reported[28] that DCCT intensive therapy significantly reduced the long-term risk of clinical CVD by 42%; however, the cumulative incidence of such events remains low. More recently, the DCCT/EDIC diabetes cohort was assessed by coronary artery calcification (CAC), an index of atherosclerosis, with computed tomography. The 1205 EDIC patients were assessed at about 7 to 9 years after the end of the DCCT. The investigators therefore examined the influence of the 6.5 years of prior conventional versus intensive diabetes treatment during the DCCT as well as the effects of CVD risk factors on CAC. The prevalences of CAC >0 and >200 Agatston units were 31.0% and 8.5%, respectively. Compared with the conventional treatment group, the intensive group had significantly lower geometric mean CAC scores and a lower prevalence of CAC >0 in the primary retinopathy prevention cohort, but not in the secondary intervention cohort, and a lower prevalence of CAC >200 in the combined cohorts.[29] These findings were consistent with those of the Pittsburgh Epidemiology of Diabetes Complications (EDC) study, which showed a positive relationship between HbA_{1c} and CAD.[30]

The decision as to whether the goal HbA_{1c} in type 2 diabetics should be slightly less than, equal to, or slightly greater than 7.0% largely rests on a balance between the physician's interpretation of the risks accompanying the treatment and the benefits in terms of cardiovascular morbidity and mortality based on available trial evidence. There have been few long-term clinical trial data available on the risk versus benefit of more intensive treatment of type 2 diabetes until the past 15 years. The selection and achievement of an intensive glucose target vary considerably (Table 6.5), with achieved goals in published studies ranging from 8.0% to 6.4%. The Kumamoto Study in Japan, a study of normal-weight patients with type 2 diabetes, provides useful confirmatory data for the value of intensive glycemic therapy on microvascular outcomes, but it included only five macrovascular events, an insufficient number to permit any conclusions.[31] The 20-year U.K. Prospective Diabetes Study Group (UKPDS) has been the landmark trial in type 2 diabetes.[5] This trial of newly diagnosed type 2 diabetic patients, despite some 27,000 patient-years of intensive glycemic therapy (goal fasting plasma glucose concentration <108 mg/dL [6.0 mmol/L]), failed to show a significant benefit compared with conventional therapy (diet, fasting plasma glucose levels <270 mg/dL [15 mmol/L]) in terms of cardiovascular events (e.g., fatal or nonfatal myocardial infarction, fatal and sudden cardiac death), although the results were borderline (16% reduction; $P = .052$). Again, a low risk of CVD may partly be responsible for these results. Early epidemiologic data from the study showed a weaker relationship between glycemia and CVD than was apparent for microvascular complications.[32] Indeed, this study, which compared three different intensive therapies (sulfonylurea, insulin therapy, and, in a subgroup of obese subjects, metformin) showed an overall significant benefit for all diabetes-related events ($P = .02$) but did not show a clear benefit for the other major outcomes and diabetes-related deaths ($P = .34$) and all-cause mortality ($P = .44$). However, in the subgroup of obese subjects who were randomized to metformin, there were significant reductions in myocardial events (39%; $P = .01$) as well as in the primary endpoints described before (e.g., any diabetes-related endpoint [32%; $P = .002$]) and total mortality (36%; $P = .01$).[33] In both the intensive and the conventional groups, stable degrees of glucose control could not be achieved during the entire study period, and the mean in both groups drifted upward from 6.6% to 8.1% and from 7.4% to 8.7% in the intervention and conventional groups, respectively. Because of considerable crossover of therapy in the UKPDS, it is difficult to interpret whether any specific therapy carries greater benefit than any other. However, from these data, metformin alone for obese subjects may be a wise initial approach.

The decision, therefore, as to how much farther one would drive the HbA_{1c} below 7.0% in those who have type

INTENSIVE VERSUS STANDARD DIABETES CONTROL					
			HbA_{1c} at Study End (%)		
Study	N	Mean Follow-up (yr)	Intensive	Control	Difference (%)
Type 1					
DCCT primary prevention	726	6.5	7.1	9.0	−1.9
DCCT secondary prevention	715	6.5	7.1	9.0	−1.9
Type 2					
Veterans Affairs	153	2.3	7.1	9.2	−2.1
UKPDS normal weight	2022	10.3	7.5	8.3	−0.8
UKPDS overweight	1845	9.7	8.0	8.3	−0.3
UKPDS metformin	753	10.7	8.0	8.3	−0.03
Kumamoto primary prevention	55	8.0	7.2	8.4	−2.2
Kumamoto secondary prevention	55	8.0	7.2	9.4	−2.2
ACCORD*	10,251	5+	6.4	7.5	−1.1
ADVANCE*	11,140	5+	6.4	7.0	−0.6

*Preliminary data. These trials will be completed in 2008 and 2009.

Table 6.5 Intensive versus standard diabetes control.

2 diabetes largely rests on a balance between the physician's interpretation of the risks for CVD (which accounts for more than two thirds of the mortality in type 2 diabetes). In February of 2008, the National Heart, Lung, and Blood Institute announced the early termination of the intensive glycemia arm in the ACCORD (Action to Control Cardiovascular Risk in Diabetes) trial.[34] ACCORD is an ongoing trial of 10,251 men and women with type 2 diabetes who have either preexisting CHD or significant CAD risk factors.[35] Patients were randomized to either standard glycemia control with a target HbA_{1c} of 7.5% (achieved goal = 7.5%; range, 7.0% to 7.9%) or intensive control with HbA_{1c} below 6.0% (achieved goal = 6.4%). Patients were then further randomized to either a lipid or blood pressure intervention. At baseline, the average age was 62 years and the duration of diabetes was 10 years. After approximately 5 years, there was a 20% increase in total mortality noted in the intensive group produced predominantly through cardiovascular events. This translated to 14 deaths per 1000 persons/year in the intensive group versus 11 deaths per 1000 persons/year in the standard group. The expected death rate in this group of high-risk diabetics would be 50 deaths per 1000 persons/year. Therefore, one could also interpret the finding as glycemic control, either standard or intensive, improves outcomes over usual care. The initial HbA_{1c} at entrance into the study was 8.4%. There was a 10% improvement in the primary outcome of nonfatal myocardial infarction, nonfatal stroke, and CVD death, but this was not statistically significant. Because of the mortality finding, the Data and Safety Monitoring Board and the National Heart, Lung, and Blood Institute recommended that all patients in the intensive glycemia arm be transitioned to the standard glycemia arm. They will continue until the study ends in June 2009. In response to this finding, the investigators of the ADVANCE trial, a similar trial in 11,140 high-risk type 2 diabetics conducted in Australia and other non-U.S. countries, undertook an interim analysis that provided no evidence of increased mortality risk in the intensive glucose control arm, which had also achieved a similar HbA_{1c} of 6.4%.[36] The results of this trial and of the Veterans Affairs diabetes trial showed no differences in mortality with glycemic control.[36a,36b]

Another recently published trial addressed cardiovascular mortality in type 2 diabetics. Gaede and associates[37] published a follow-up study to the Steno-2 trial. In this trial, 160 Danish patients with type 2 diabetes and microalbuminuria were randomized to intensive versus standard risk factor control. The intensive arm included a target HbA_{1c} of 6.5%, along with lipid and blood pressure goals. Patients were observed for a mean of 13.3 years (7.8 years of intervention and an additional 5.5 years of follow-up). There was a 20% absolute risk reduction for death from any cause and a 29% reduction in cardiovascular events in the intensive arm. The rate of death among patients in the conventional group during the entire follow-up period was 50%, which underscores the need for aggressive intervention when multiple risk factors are present.

Management of Hyperglycemia

The choice of agents for glycemia control should be predicated on their efficacy in lowering blood glucose concentration and their effects on other comorbid conditions commonly seen in the diabetic patient (Table 6.6). Lifestyle interventions that improve diet, lower body weight, and increase activity level should be tried as initial therapy in all patients with type 2 diabetes. The Look AHEAD trial demonstrated that significant weight loss and improvement in cardiovascular risk factors and diabetes control are achievable with intensive lifestyle changes.[38] In this study, 5145 overweight patients with type 2 diabetes were randomized to standard diabetes education versus a combination of calorie restriction and physical activity. Patients assigned to the intensive group lost 8.6% of their initial weight versus 0.7% in the standard diabetes education group after 1 year ($P < .001$). They also had significantly greater improvement

GLUCOSE LOWERING AND CARDIOVASCULAR RISK IN DIABETES		
Study	**Intervention**	**Result**
UGDP[3]	Tolbutamide	Possible increased cardiovascular risk
	Phenformin	Increased lactic acidosis
	Insulin variable	No benefit
	Insulin standard	No benefit
DCCT[28]	Intensive (insulin) and EDIC[29] glycemic therapy in type 1 diabetes	Possible decrease in macrovascular events (largely lower extremity arterial disease). No effect on carotid intima–medial wall thickness or ankle-brachial index
VACSDM[4]	Intensive (insulin and sulfonylurea) therapy in type 2 diabetes	Borderline increased cardiovascular risk
UKPDS[5]	Intensive (insulin and sulfonylurea) therapy	Borderline reduction in risk of myocardial infarction ($P = .052$)
	Metformin in obese subjects	Significant reduction in risk of myocardial infarction ($P = .01$)
ACCORD[35]	Intensive glucose lowering, all drug classes, type 2 diabetes	Increase in total mortality ($P < .04$)

Table 6.6 Glucose lowering and cardiovascular risk in diabetes.

in blood pressure, lipid profiles, and HbA_{1c}. Referral to a nutritionist or, in the case of cardiac patients, participation in a cardiac rehabilitation program should be recommended in all sedentary or overweight patients.

The next step in control of hyperglycemia is the addition of medications. Naturally, the lead should come from the patient's diabetologist or internist (if there is one). The effectiveness of the current therapies rests not only on the intrinsic characteristics of the drugs but on the level of hyperglycemia, the degree of insulin resistance, the duration of diabetes, and other factors. The mainstay of oral therapy is the biguanide metformin. A suggested flow diagram for treatment options appears in Figure 6-2. On the basis of the UKPDS, it would seem that monotherapy with the hepatic insulin sensitizer metformin in the obese patient in whom diet and exercise are failing to maintain control would be the best approach. Metformin has the advantage of a favorable lowering of triglycerides and of causing less weight gain than the sulfonylureas (indeed, many patients may lose a small amount of weight). For the nonobese patient who has type 2 diabetes, sulfonylurea therapy may be appropriate first-line therapy.[5] Sulfonylureas act by enhancing insulin secretion and may lower HbA_{1c} by up to 1.5%. The glinides repaglinide and nateglinide are another class of oral hypoglycemic agents that also enhance insulin secretion but bind to a different insulin receptor and have a much shorter circulating half-life. They are given immediately before meals and are ideal in patients with an erratic daily routine. In general, they produce less hypoglycemia. Sulfonylurea or glinide plus metformin combinations may also be used when the monotherapy approach fails. The α-glucosidase inhibitors acarbose and miglitol inhibit the enzyme α-glucosidase at the intestinal brush border and inhibit carbohydrate breakdown. They may also be added to further lower glycemic levels; however, the gastrointestinal side effects may limit their use in many patients.

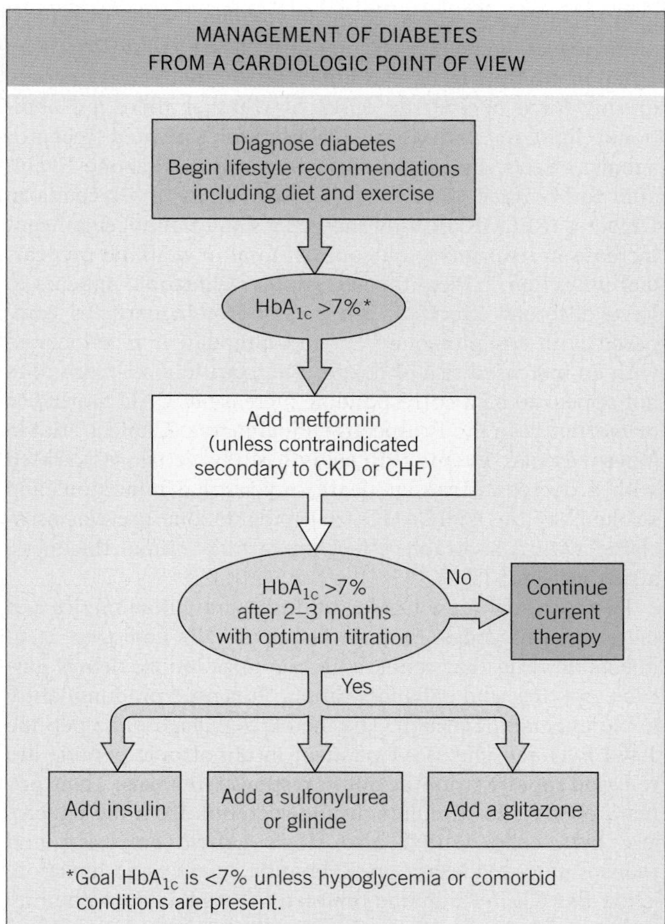

Figure 6.2 Management of type 2 diabetes from a cardiologic viewpoint. CHF, congestive heart failure; CKD, chronic kidney disease.

Another insulin sensitizer group is the thiazolidinedione or glitazone class. The first drug produced in this class has been removed from the market secondary to problems with hepatotoxicity. However, drugs in the subsequent generation including rosiglitazone and pioglitazone are available and appear to have a low risk of hepatotoxicity. These agents activate the nuclear receptor peroxisome proliferator-activated receptor γ, increasing peripheral insulin sensitivity, and they also improve hepatic insulin sensitivity without increasing insulin levels. In addition to their insulin-sensitizing effects, glitazones may have protective affects on the beta cell, reduce free fatty acid levels, raise high-density lipoprotein levels, and possess anti-inflammatory and antioxidant properties.[39] Although there is a low risk of hypoglycemia, both drugs can cause significant edema and weight gain and may exacerbate congestive heart failure.

In a controversial meta-analysis of rosiglitazone studies published in the *New England Journal of Medicine*, Nissen and Wolski[40] concluded that the use of rosiglitazone may lead to an increased risk of cardiovascular events. Although an increased incidence of congestive heart failure has been noted in multiple trials, it is not clear whether this is the only driving force behind the effect or whether there are additional lipid or peroxisome proliferator-activated receptor agonist effects. Interim analysis of the Rosiglitazone Evaluated for Cardiac Outcomes and Regulation of Glycemia in Diabetes (RECORD) study showed a slight but not significant increase in its primary outcome of fatal or nonfatal myocardial infarction.[41] Pioglitazone, another glitazone, appears to have different effects on serum lipoprotein particles compared with rosiglitazone,[42,43] and although it is associated with an increased risk of congestive heart failure, there does not appear to be a corresponding increase in CAD morbidity or mortality. In the Prospective Pioglitazone Clinical Trial in Macrovascular Events (PROactive) study, it was associated with a decreased risk of death, myocardial infarction, and stroke.[44] In the CHICAGO trial, pioglitazone use was associated with a favorable effect on carotid intimal thickness, a surrogate for CVD.[45]

There are two new classes of drugs, amylinomimetics and incretin-based drugs. Pramlintide, an amylin analogue, is an injectable drug that reduces glucagon secretion, delays gastric emptying, and enhances satiety. It is used predominantly in patients taking insulin. The incretins glucagon-like peptide 1 (GLP-1) and glucose-dependent insulinotropic peptide are released rapidly from the gut in response to meals. Their primary effect is to stimulate insulin secretion from the pancreatic beta cells. GLP-1 also slows gastric emptying and reduces glucagon secretion. Exenatide, given as an injection, is the first GLP-1 mimetic that can be used as monotherapy or in combination with metformin or a glitazone. It reduces HbA_{1c} about 1% but also has an added benefit of producing significant weight loss. Sitaglipitin is an oral inhibitor of dipeptidyl peptidase 4. This widely expressed enzyme metabolizes incretins. Inhibition of this enzyme increases circulating levels of both GLP-1 and glucose-dependent insulinotropic peptide, reducing postprandial glucose levels.

If all of these oral approaches fail to yield adequate control, insulin therapy should be instigated. Many endocrinologists will begin with bedtime insulin, either intermediate-acting NPH or one of the longer acting basal insulins, glargine or detemir, and continue the oral agents. If glucose control is still inadequate, multiple insulin injections may be required.

Inpatient Hyperglycemia

Inpatient hyperglycemia has gradually come to the forefront as the number of patients with diabetes as a discharge diagnosis has increased dramatically. The treatment of hyperglycemia in the acute care setting has remained haphazard for a number of reasons, the most prominent being the perception that hypoglycemia should be avoided at all costs. Not only are patients with diabetes at risk, but the common phenomenon of stress hyperglycemia is often overlooked in nondiabetic patients admitted to the hospital. A Swedish study showed that 31% of patients admitted for acute myocardial infarction had hyperglycemia at the time of discharge.[46] Hyperglycemia contributes to overall morbidity and mortality in the hospitalized patient regardless of the initial diagnosis. A meta-analysis of 15 studies of patients with and without diabetes hospitalized for acute myocardial infarction reported that glucose levels above 110 mg/dL were associated with increases in both in-hospital mortality and congestive heart failure.[47] In addition, elevated glucose levels have been associated with larger infarct size in patients without a prior history of diabetes who were being treated with perfusion therapy for ST-segment elevation myocardial infarction.[48] In the first DIGAMI (Diabetes and Insulin-Glucose Infusion in Acute Myocardial Infarction) study,[49] patients with acute myocardial infarction received intravenous insulin therapy for 24 hours, followed by multiple daily injections of insulin for 3 months or more, and had a 29% reduction in mortality at 1 year and a 28% reduction at 3.4 years in comparison with the control group. The DIGAMI 2 study[50] was designed to compare three treatment strategies in patients with acute myocardial infarction: group 1 received acute insulin-glucose infusion followed by insulin-based long-term glucose control; group 2 received insulin-glucose infusion followed by standard glucose control; and group 3 received routine metabolic management in accordance with local practice. Unfortunately, this study did not reach recruitment goals and showed no treatment differences. Moreover, the primary treatment target of a fasting blood glucose level of 90 to 126 mg/dL for those in group 1 was never achieved. Mean fasting blood glucose levels (149 mg/dL) and HbA_{1c} (6.8%) were similar among the three study groups. Thus, if glycemia is predictive of outcomes, no differences would have been expected, and no differences were observed. In a landmark study by Van den Berghe and colleagues,[51] intensive care unit mortality rates were reduced from 8.0% to 4.6% in surgical patients and 10.9% to 7.2% in nonsurgical patients by targeting glucose to a level of 80 to 110 mg/dL through intensive insulin treatment. The American Heart Association in a consensus statement on hyperglycemia and acute coronary syndromes recommends the following[52]:

1. Glucose levels should be a part of the initial laboratory evaluation in all patients with suspected or confirmed acute coronary syndrome.
2. In patients with significant hyperglycemia (>180 mg/dL), intensive insulin therapy should be considered to treat to a goal of 90 to 140 mg/dL with care to avoid hypoglycemia.
3. In non–intensive care patients, glucose levels should be maintained below 180 mg/dL through the use of subcutaneous insulin regimens.

Cardiologists treating patients admitted to the hospital, whether as a consultant or the admitting physician, should be cognizant of these glycemia goals. In patients with documented hyperglycemia either with or without a prior diagnosis of diabetes, consultation with an endocrinologist should be considered early in their hospitalization to institute appropriate insulin regimens.

Lipid Management

Many data, ranging from early data of the Framingham study[53] to more recent data of follow-up studies of men (the Multiple Risk Factor Intervention Trial[7]) and women (the Nurses' Health Study[8]), have demonstrated the predictive power of cholesterol levels, both low-density lipoprotein (LDL) cholesterol (positively) and high-density lipoprotein

(HDL) cholesterol (negatively), for CVD in type 2 diabetes. Also apparent in diabetes is a greater predictive power of triglycerides,[54,55] which probably reflects an association with overproduction and impaired clearance of very-low-density lipoprotein (VLDL) particles and remnants.[56] These features are linked to insulin resistance, the key metabolic abnormality seen in type 2 diabetes. Also associated with decreased VLDL catabolism is a reduction in HDL-cholesterol level. However, total cholesterol and LDL-cholesterol concentrations are not usually greatly altered in moderately well controlled type 2 diabetes. Thus, triglyceride levels are characteristically elevated and HDL-cholesterol levels are characteristically depressed, and these findings form the hallmark of traditional diabetic dyslipidemia. Another characteristic lipid abnormality seen in type 2 diabetes and insulin resistance is a shift in density of the LDL particle to the more dense (type B) particle.[57] This change is thought to enhance the atherogenicity of LDL[34] and is correlated with triglyceride levels and with postmenopausal status in women. It is thus difficult, both statistically and pathophysiologically, to distinguish which of these disturbances (VLDL remnants, triglycerides, HDL-cholesterol, and LDL phenotype B) are the key players.

Our knowledge of lipid-CVD relationships in type 1 diabetes is even more limited, although in general terms, similar relationships to the general population appear to be present from the Pittsburgh EDC, DCCT/EDIC, and EURODIAB studies, with, as in type 2 diabetes, a suggestion that triglycerides may play a greater role than in the general population.[58,59] Interestingly, in moderately well controlled type 1 diabetes, absolute lipid concentrations are not greatly disturbed. Lipoprotein concentration may therefore account for little of the excess CVD risk seen in type 1 diabetes. This has led to an increased focus on lipoprotein composition, and a number of differences have been identified, including triglyceride enrichment of LDL and HDL particles and disturbed reverse cholesterol transport, LDL oxidation and immune complex formation may be particularly important risk factors.[60] Further study is needed to determine whether interventions directed at improving these compositional changes or oxidative properties will result in a reduction in CVD events.

Until recently, most of the large lipid intervention trials had either ignored or excluded patients with diabetes. This means that we have not had evidence on which to base cholesterol-lowering (or other lipid modulation) therapy in diabetes, despite the fact that the lipid-CVD connection is just as strong in diabetes as it is in the general population, if not stronger (see earlier).[56] Fortunately, a number of trials have recently reported data that involve diabetic subjects; this has helped to address some of these issues, but others are left unanswered.

The Third National Cholesterol Education Program (NCEP) Expert Panel[16] acknowledged what many practitioners have accepted as standard of care, that diabetes mellitus is considered a CAD risk equivalent (i.e., that patients with diabetes should have the same LDL-cholesterol goals as patients with existing CAD).

In 2004, Grundy and colleagues[61] published an NCEP report, endorsed by the American College of Cardiology, the American Heart Association, and the National Heart, Lung, and Blood Institute, which addressed the implications of five major clinical statin trials that had been published since NCEP III. They confirmed the benefit of therapeutic lifestyle intervention and the NCEP III LDL-cholesterol goal of less than 100 mg/dL (2.6 mmol/L) for diabetics and patients and non–HDL-cholesterol goal of less than 130 mg/dL. In addition, they introduced the term *very high risk*, which identifies patients with CAD who have one or more additional risk factors that confer a very high risk of near future events. For these patients, the suggested treatment goal is less than 70 mg/dL (1.8 mmol/L), even if the baseline LDL level is already below 100 mg/dL (2.6 mmol/L). For moderately high risk patients (2+ risk factors and a 10-year risk of 10% to 20%), the recommended LDL-cholesterol goal is less than 100 mg/dL (2.6 mmol/L) but with the therapeutic option of less than 70 mg/dL. It is also suggested that when a patient at high or very high risk also has a high triglyceride level or low HDL-cholesterol concentration that consideration be given to the addition of a fibric acid or niacin (Table 6.7).

The ADA[1] also recommends an LDL-cholesterol goal of less than 100 mg/dL (2.6 mmol/L) and further recommends lowering of triglycerides to less than 150 mg/dL (1.7 mmol/L) and raising of HDL-cholesterol to above 45 mg/dL (1.15 mmol/L) in men and above 55 mg/dL (1.40 mmol/L) in women with diabetes. The addition of HDL-cholesterol–raising and triglyceride-lowering strategies to the LDL-cholesterol recommendation is due in part to results obtained from studies with fibric acid derivatives, such as the Veterans Affairs High-Density Lipoprotein Cholesterol Intervention Trial (VA-HIT).[62] In addition, the American Heart Association has also made recommendations for women.[63]

With respect to primary prevention in diabetics, the evidence for lipid-lowering therapy comes from two major trials. The Heart Protection Study included a subset of 5963 patients with diabetes who were randomized to simvastatin or placebo.[63] Simvastatin treatment was associated with a 27% reduction in CAD events after 5 years, and the benefit was independent of the degree of LDL lowering. In the Collaborative Atorvastatin Diabetes Study (CARDS), 2838 patients with type 2 diabetes were randomized to atorvastatin or placebo.[64] CVD events were reduced by 36% and overall death rate by 27% in the treatment group. On the basis of these studies, all patients with type 2 diabetes should be considered for statin treatment.

The first study to report on secondary prevention was the Scandinavian Simvastatin Survival Study (4S),[65] which was also the first of the new generation of trials that used statins. This trial involved 4444 men and women who had stable angina or previous myocardial infarction and moderately high cholesterol levels (213 to 309 mg/dL [5.5-8.0 mmol/L]) and triglyceride levels below 221 mg/dL (2.5 mmol/L). This latter restriction, plus the exclusion of conditions likely to reduce life expectancy, probably explains why only 202 (4.5%) of the trial population had diabetes, almost certainly type 2 in the majority of cases. Overall, the trial reported three highly significant findings:

- a 35% fall in LDL-cholesterol accompanied by a 30% fall in total mortality (the primary outcome);
- a 42% fall in CHD mortality; and
- a 34% fall in major CHD events.

GOALS AND INTERVENTION LEVELS FOR LOW-DENSITY LIPOPROTEIN CHOLESTEROL				
Risk Category	**Risk Factors***	**LDL-Cholesterol Goal**	**Initiate TLC**	**Consider Drug Therapy**
Low risk	0-1	<160 mg/dL	≥160 mg/dL	≥190 mg/dL (160-189 mg/dL): LDL-lowering drug optional
Moderate risk	2+ (10-year risk <10%)	<130 mg/dL	≥130 mg/dL	≥160 mg/dL
Moderately high risk	2+ (10-year risk 10%-20%)	<130 mg/dL	≥130 mg/dL	≥130 mg/dL (100-129 mg/dL): consider drug options
High risk	CHD† or CHD risk equivalents‡	<100 mg/dL (optional goal: <70 mg/dL)	≥100 mg/dL	≥100 mg/dL
Very high risk	CHD + other risk factor (10-year risk >20%)	<70 mg/dL		>70 mg/dL: consider drug options

*Risk factors include cigarette smoking, hypertension (blood pressure, 140/90 mm Hg) or taking antihypertension medications, low HDL-cholesterol, family history of premature CHD (first-degree male relative < 55 years; female relative < 65 years).

†Coronary heart disease (CHD) includes a history of myocardial infarction, unstable angina, coronary artery procedures, or evidence of significant myocardial ischemia.

‡CHD risk equivalents include clinical manifestations of noncoronary forms of atherosclerotic disease (peripheral artery disease, abdominal aortic aneurysm, and carotid artery disease), diabetes, and 2+ risk factors with a 10-year risk for hard CHD of more than 20%.

TLC, therapeutic lifestyle change.

Table 6.7 Goals and intervention levels for low-density lipoprotein cholesterol.

In the 202 diabetic subjects, a 36% fall in LDL-cholesterol was seen, along with a Cox regression–adjusted 43% fall in total mortality ($P = .09$), a 36% fall in CHD mortality ($P = .24$), and a 55% fall in major CHD events ($P = .002$). It thus seems that the diabetic subgroup parallels the main study population, and indeed for major CHD events, it had a greater overall benefit. The medication was well tolerated and had no apparent effect on fasting blood glucose levels. This is very encouraging, particularly in conjunction with the Helsinki study, but both of these studies need to be seen in the context that they are post hoc subgroup analyses of nonrepresentative diabetic subjects, most of whom would have relatively mild glucose disturbances. Of the diabetic subjects in 4S, 50% were diet controlled, as were 71% of the Helsinki study participants; however, the degree of control of their diabetes is unknown.

The second trial of statins to report data about diabetes was the Cholesterol and Recurrent Event (CARE) study.[14] This study involved a more representative group of 588 diabetic subjects (who made up 14% of all subjects). Although subjects who had severe hyperglycemia (fasting glucose levels >220 mg/dL [12.2 mmol/L]), severe hypertriglyceridemia (>350 mg/dL [3.9 mmol/L]), or heart failure were still excluded, the diabetic patients were, in the main, treated (only 10% were untreated and 30% were treated with diet alone). The CARE study focused on subjects with modest, not severe, cholesterol elevation (total cholesterol levels, <240 mg/dL [6.2 mmol/L]; LDL-cholesterol levels, 115-174 mg/dL [3.0-4.5 mmol/L]; and triglyceride levels, <350 mg/dL [3.9 mmol/L]). Thus, the diabetic dyslipidemic patient group in the CARE study was somewhat more typical than the one in the 4S study in that the patients had lower LDL-cholesterol levels (138 versus 187 mg/dL [3.5 versus 4.8 mmol/L]), which reflected the different selection criteria and higher triglyceride levels (164 versus 152 mg/dL [1.8 versus 1.72 mmol/L]). Importantly, although the CARE diabetic subjects also had lower LDL-cholesterol levels and higher triglyceride levels than the CARE nondiabetic subjects (whose LDL-cholesterol level was 139 mg/dL [3.59 mmol/L] and whose triglyceride level was 154 mg/dL [1.74 mmol/L]), they experienced LDL-cholesterol lowering almost identical to that of the nondiabetic subjects (27% versus 28%). The reduction in the primary endpoint (CHD death plus nonfatal myocardial infarction) was, however, only about half of that seen in the nondiabetic group (13% versus 26%). Nonetheless, the reduction (25%) in the expanded endpoint (which also included revascularization) was similar to that seen in the nondiabetic group. This different effect reflects a lack of reduction of CHD mortality in the diabetic group. A significant reduction ($P = .04$) in revascularization alone was also seen in those diabetic subjects treated with pravastatin. There is no obvious explanation for why pravastatin had only a weak effect on CHD mortality in the CARE study in the diabetic group, but it is encouraging that overall CHD events are reduced in a similar manner to that seen in the nondiabetic population. It is possible that the more severe patient population studied in CARE was a contributory factor to the lack of effect in CHD mortality. Finally, CARE included postmenopausal women and therefore further extends the results from the all-male 4S study, although only 20% of the subjects were women. As in 4S, diabetes in CARE was not a primary stratification variable before randomization, nor was it a prespecified subgroup; therefore, the results have to be treated as being post hoc.

The Long-Term Intervention with Pravastatin in Ischaemic Disease (LIPID) study was an Australian-based study of 9014 patients with a past history of myocardial infarction or hospitalized unstable angina.[13] Somewhat broader ranges of total cholesterol levels (155-271 mg/dL [4.0-7.0 mmol/L]) and fasting triglyceride levels (<445 mg/dL [5.0 mmol/L]) were allowed than in the CARE or 4S, and the primary outcome was CHD death. Of the cohort, 9% had diabetes, which is a somewhat lower than expected frequency of diabetes in such a CHD-based population. The relative risk reduction was 15.8% (crude) or 19% (Cox model adjusted), which was not significant (95% CI, −10 to +41) but was comparable to the 25% reduction seen in the nondiabetic population. The Heart Protection Study[63] was both a primary and secondary prevention study of simvastatin (40 mg/day) and a combination antioxidant therapy. Of the 5963 participants with diabetes, 1981 had had a previous CAD event. There was a highly significant 13% reduction in all-cause mortality because of an 18% reduction in coronary death. In the diabetic group, there was a 12% reduction in the incidence of first major vascular event. Antioxidant vitamin therapy failed to show any effect. The ALLHAT (Antihypertensive and Lipid-Lowering Treatment in the Prevention of Heart Attack Trial) study was a large multicenter, primarily community-based trial that had both a lipid and a hypertension component. Fourteen percent of the patients had CAD, and 35% had type 2 diabetes. In the lipid arm, patients were randomized to pravastatin or placebo and observed for 4.8 years.[66] All-cause mortality was not different between groups, although LDL-cholesterol was reduced by 28% and 11% in the treatment and usual care group, respectively. The lack of a significant difference between groups was thought to be partially associated with the fact that about a third of the usual care patients both with and without CAD began taking lipid-lowering medications at some point during the trial. The ASPEN (Atorvastatin Study for the Prevention of Coronary Heart Disease Endpoints in Non–Insulin Dependent Diabetes Mellitus) study was a double-blinded 4-year study of 2410 patients with type 2 diabetes randomized to receive 10 mg of atorvastatin or placebo.[67] The mean reduction in LDL-cholesterol was 29%. There was no difference in the composite endpoint of cardiovascular death, nonfatal myocardial infarction, nonfatal stroke, recanalization, coronary artery bypass grafting, resuscitated cardiac arrest, or worsening or unstable angina. There was, however, a nonsignificant 27% reduction in fatal and nonfatal myocardial infarction. At the end of the study, the reported HbA_{1c} level was about the same in both groups (7.8% ± 1.4% in the atorvastatin group and 7.7% ± 1.4% in the placebo group), thus eliminating degree of diabetes control as a confounder.

More recent studies have addressed the question of a lower threshold of risk reduction. In other words, how low can we drive down the LDL and still reduce CAD risk? The Treating to New Targets (TNT) trial was a multicenter, double-blinded, randomized clinical trial that compared the effects of 10 mg versus 80 mg of atorvastatin in 10,001 patients observed for 4.9 years.[68] The diabetes substudy involved 1501 patients with CAD and type 2 diabetes. The primary outcome was death from CHD, nonfatal myocardial infarction, resuscitated cardiac arrest, or fatal or nonfatal stroke. High-dose atorvastatin reduced the rate of cardiovascular events by 25%. The time to a cerebrovascular or CVD event was significantly prolonged with more aggressive LDL lowering. Objective evidence of the benefit of aggressive LDL lowering was provided by the ASTEROID trial (A Study to Evaluate the Effect of Rosuvastatin on Intravascular Ultrasound-derived Coronary Atheroma Burden) using intravascular ultrasonography to assess the change in atheroma volume.[69] Patients were treated with rosuvastatin (40 mg) for 2 years. LDL-cholesterol decreased to 60.8 mg/dL (1.6 mmol/L), and HDL-cholesterol increased to 49.0 mg/dL (1.3 mmol/L). Of the 349 patients who completed the trial, 46 had a previous diagnosis of diabetes. Total atheroma volume decreased by 6.8%. The authors concluded that high-intensity statin therapy can regress atherosclerosis in CAD patients.

Fibric acid derivatives have also been shown to produce beneficial effects not only in the treatment of diabetic dyslipidemia by lowering triglycerides and raising HDL but also in reducing CAD events. The Helsinki Heart Study[69] did include a small group of type 2 diabetic patients. This trial remains one of two fully described studies of lipid modulation in diabetes by drugs in the primary prevention setting (i.e., in patients without known CAD). In general, this study, using a fibric acid (whose principal action is to enhance VLDL catabolism through stimulation of lipoprotein lipase), was remarkably successful, yielding a 34% fall in the primary endpoint of CHD death or myocardial infarction. The trial was initially conceived as a trial to raise HDL-cholesterol, but it was later reformatted so that the entry criterion was a non–HDL-cholesterol level of more than 200 mg/dL (5.2 mmol/L). The mean LDL-cholesterol level (200 mg/dL [5.2 mmol/L]) was a little lower ($P = .03$) and the mean triglyceride level was a little higher (239 mg/dL [2.7 mmol/L]) in the 135 type 2 subjects compared with the 3946 nondiabetic subjects (205 mg/dL [5.3 mmol/L] and 177 mg/dL [2.0 mmol/L], respectively). HDL-cholesterol was also lower in the type 2 diabetic subjects (45.7mg/dL [1.18 mmol/L] versus 48.8 mg/dL [1.26 mmol/L]; $P = .001$). Gemfibrozil had similar lipid-altering effects in the diabetic subjects compared with nondiabetic subjects, although each effect was slightly less than that seen overall (exact reductions were not reported). Although gemfibrozil was associated with a 68% relative reduction in the incidence of CHD death or myocardial infarction (7.1% absolute reduction), because only 10 subjects with type 2 diabetes had the endpoint, this was not significant, despite the risk reduction being greater than in the main trial. This result helped to reestablish the use of fibric acids in CHD prevention, which had been dealt a severe blow by the World Health Organization clofibrate trial. Of particular importance and relevance to diabetes is the subsequent demonstration that the bulk of the benefit in the Helsinki Heart Study was seen in subjects with a mixed dyslipidemia (i.e., LDL-cholesterol levels above 175 mg/dL [4.5 mmol/L], triglyceride levels above 200 mg/dL [2.2 mmol/L], and HDL-cholesterol levels below 35 mg/dL [0.9 mmol/L], the so-called triopathy). Because gemfibrozil is predominantly a triglyceride-lowering agent (it may even raise LDL-cholesterol in some subjects), this finding is not surprising and should be remembered before the drug is prescribed. It is clearly a useful agent for patients who have increased levels of triglyceride and decreased levels of HDL-cholesterol, but it is not useful for patients who have isolated LDL-cholesterol elevation. A lack of effect on blood glucose levels is also encouraging. Whether the diabetic subgroup in this study is representative is also questionable because not only were subjects with type 1 diabetes excluded, but the 135 subjects with type 2 diabetes represented less than 3.5% of the population, far less than the

14% or more that would be expected. Furthermore, the Helsinki study involved only men.

The VA-HIT[62] addressed the importance of HDL raising and triglyceride lowering in CAD risk. In this trial, men with CAD, low HDL-cholesterol level, and average LDL-cholesterol level (110 mg/dL [2.86 mmol/L]) were treated with gemfibrozil for a 5-year period. There was a 22% reduction in new events in the treatment group, without a significant change in LDL-cholesterol concentration. About 25% (627 patients) in the trial had diabetes. In this subgroup, there was a similar reduction in event rates even though the diabetic placebo group event rates were nearly twice those of the nondiabetic placebo group. One could hypothesize that part of this higher risk may be associated with LDL-cholesterol levels that were still above the ADA and NCEP III goal of 100 mg/dL (2.86 mmol/L). It may be that combined therapy is necessary in diabetics to reduce CAD risk.

The clinical management of dyslipidemia in patients who have diabetes is basically the same as in the general population with one major exception—glycemic control must go hand-in-hand with lipid control. This cannot be overemphasized, and its failure underlies the failure of lipid control in most cases. The enhanced VLDL production and decreased catabolism are central to the classic disturbances of raised triglyceride levels and depressed HDL-cholesterol levels (see earlier). Other relatively minor differences in the management of dyslipidemia between patients who have diabetes and the general population are the potential side effects of the medication (Table 6.8). The bile acid sequestrants (cholestyramine, colesevelam, and colestipol) are effective, but the gastrointestinal side effects may be particularly troublesome in those who have autonomic neuropathy. In patients with combined hyperlipidemia, these drugs may further elevate triglycerides. The statins are well tolerated and are probably the first choice for most patients who do not have severe hypertriglyceridemia, for whom the fibric acids should be considered. Both fibric acid derivatives gemfibrozil and fenofibrate lower triglycerides. Caution must be used in combining gemfibrozil with a statin as gemfibrozil interferes with statin glucuronidation, leading to dramatically elevated levels of the statin, increasing the risk for myopathy and myositis. Fenofibrate does not cause this reaction and can therefore be used with higher dose statins. The dose of fenofibrate should be reduced in renal disease. Ezetimibe inhibits cholesterol absorption through the Niemann-Pick C1-like 1 receptor in the intestine. It lowers LDL-cholesterol an average 15% when it is used as monotherapy and may be used in combination with other drugs, particularly statins. Niacin in its various forms has been thought to be contraindicated in diabetes as it can increase insulin resistance and worsen glycemic control. Newer niacin formulations, especially the extended-release form, have been shown to have minimal effects on glucose and HbA_{1c} levels. Perhaps the one group of patients in whom it should be avoided is those who have impaired glucose tolerance or early diabetes but who do not yet require oral therapy because niacin may make such patients frankly diabetic with a need for hypoglycemic therapy. Niacin lowers total cholesterol and LDL-cholesterol levels and raises HDL-cholesterol level. It is also a potent reducer of lipoprotein(a).

LIPID-MODULATING AGENTS AND DIABETES	
Drug Class	**Comments**
Bile acid resins	Effective, but constipating side effects may be exacerbated by gastrointestinal autonomic neuropathy Indicated for elevated LDL; may increase triglycerides
Statins	Effective and well tolerated Indicated for elevated LDL; has mild HDL-raising and triglyceride-lowering effects
Fibric acids	Effective and generally well tolerated Indicated for elevated VLDL-cholesterol and triglycerides and low HDL
Niacin	Effective but may worsen glucose tolerance Avoid in those bordering on the need for oral hypoglycemic therapy Indicated for elevated LDL, VLDL, and triglycerides and low HDL; also lowers lipoprotein(a)
Ezetimibe	Effective and well tolerated; synergistic effect with statins; indicated for elevated LDL

Table 6.8 Lipid-modulating agents and diabetes.

Blood Pressure Management

Hypertension is as major a risk factor for vascular disease in the diabetic population as it is in the general population. Indeed, studies have repeatedly demonstrated a similar risk gradient, from the Framingham study[53] to the recent Multiple Risk Factor Intervention Trial[7] and Nurses' Health Study[8] reports. As with blood cholesterol level, the absolute risk at any given level is considerably higher for those who have diabetes. The recommendations of the Seventh Joint National Committee on Prevention, Detection, Evaluation, and Treatment of High Blood Pressure[70] are consistent with guidelines from the American Diabetes Association, which has also recommended a goal blood pressure in diabetics to be 130/80 mm Hg or lower (Table 6.9). Most patients will require two or more medications for blood pressure control, and clinical trials with diuretics, angiotensin-converting enzyme (ACE) inhibitors, beta blockers, angiotensin receptor blockers, and calcium antagonists have demonstrated benefit in the treatment of hypertension in both type 1 and type 2 diabetics.

CHANGES BETWEEN JNC 6 AND JNC 7		
JNC 6	**Blood Pressure (mm Hg)**	**JNC 7**
Optimal	<120/80	Normal
Normal	120-129/80-84	Prehypertension
Borderline	130-139/84-89	Prehypertension
Hypertension	≥140/90	Hypertension
Stage 1	140-159/90-99	Stage 1
Stage 2	160-179/100-109	Stage 2
Stage 3	≥180/110	Stage 2

JNC, Joint National Committee on Prevention, Detection, Evaluation, and Treatment of High Blood Pressure.

Table 6.9 Changes between JNC 6 and JNC 7.

Although these recommendations mainly concern type 2 diabetes, blood pressure elevation is just as important in type 1 diabetes. In the Pittsburgh EDC cohort, hypertension was a strong consistent prospective predictor of CHD and largely explained the "renal" prediction in multivariate Cox modeling.[30] Hypertension is strongly related to the progression of renal disease[71] and also explains the renal link with proliferative retinopathy.[72] Furthermore, hypertension is also a major risk factor for neuropathy.[73] The importance, therefore, of good blood pressure control in diabetes cannot be overstated.

The evidence that blood pressure lowering delays the progression of proteinuria and nephropathy is well established, and blood pressure lowering is recommended in type 1 and type 2 diabetes,[74] as is the apparent specific additional benefit of ACE inhibition beyond blood pressure lowering.[75] This specific additional benefit is particularly apparent when mean arterial pressure is above 100 mm Hg. However, for macrovascular disease, the evidence is less extensive because, again, those who have diabetes were largely excluded from the early major blood pressure–lowering trials.

The Hypertension Detection and Follow-up Program (HDFP)[76] did not, however, exclude those with a history of diabetes, who appeared to experience little benefit in terms of overall mortality from the enhanced stepped care provided in the intervention group to that seen in the referred care group (Table 6.10). However, those who were initially untreated and had mild hypertension (90-104 mm Hg diastolic) experienced a marginally greater benefit if they had diabetes (26.5%) than did those who did not have diabetes (20.9%). Regrettably, however, this trial was not a placebo-controlled trial, and little can be concluded about blood pressure lowering per se.

The first clear data from a large trial were reported by the Systolic Hypertension in the Elderly Program (SHEP),[9] which, as its name implies, was limited to those with isolated systolic hypertension, defined as a systolic blood pressure above 160 mm Hg and a diastolic blood pressure below 90 mm Hg. Twelve percent (n = 583) of those studied had type 2 diabetes. An important exclusion, however, was treatment with insulin. Consequently, the diabetic subjects included in SHEP had milder diabetes in terms of metabolic disturbance. The SHEP results suggest that for the primary endpoint (all stroke), the adjusted relative risk (0.78) of events in the treated group was not as substantially (or significantly) reduced as it was for nondiabetic subjects (0.62); whereas for all CVD events, identical relative risks were seen (0.66). Importantly, for CHD events (myocardial infarction and CHD death), the relative risk was substantially lower in those who had diabetes (0.46) than in those who did not (0.81). A somewhat greater benefit (RR = 0.74) was also seen for total mortality compared with those who did not have diabetes (RR = 0.85). These findings are thus in contrast to those of HDFP, in which mortality was reduced only in those who had previously untreated mild hypertension. Drug choice may be a concern, and the SHEP data are reassuring in terms of chlorthalidone-atenolol, despite earlier reports from observational studies that diuretics are associated with increased mortality in diabetes.[77] Biochemical changes (e.g., blood glucose) were relatively minor in SHEP participants receiving diuretic and beta-blocker therapy and not sufficient to deter the use of chlorthalidone-atenolol in those who have diabetes and isolated systolic hypertension. The Syst-Eur Study[12] also focused on isolated systolic hypertension and reported a reduction of 55% (P = .06) in total mortality in the treatment group (nitrendipine plus enalapril-hydrochlorothiazide) compared with placebo in the diabetic subgroup. Substantial reductions were also seen for stroke (73%; P = .13) and CAD (63%; P = .12).

None of the other trials in Tables 6.10 and 6.11 was placebo controlled; however, all of these trials provide some relevant data. Perhaps the most important is the recent UKPDS study.[78] The blood pressure intervention in this study (which was described earlier in connection with its major objective of assessing the effect of intensive glycemic control) involved 1148 subjects who were recruited in the latter part of the study (and are not therefore truly comparable with the whole study population). Two treatments were tested: an ACE inhibitor (captopril) and a beta blocker (atenolol). Both of these drugs were used to achieve a goal blood pressure of less than 150/85 mm Hg and were compared with a control group that were not given ACE inhibitors and beta blockers and had a goal blood pressure of less than 180/105 mm Hg. A meaningful difference in blood pressure was maintained (10 mm Hg systolic and 5 mm Hg diastolic) between the two groups, and 43% of the person-year experience of the control group was without blood pressure medication. Significant reductions in all diabetes-related endpoints and in diabetes-related mortality were seen (primary endpoint); significant reductions were also seen in stroke and microvascular disease (secondary endpoints). Although reductions were also seen in all-cause mortality (18%), myocardial infarction (21%), and peripheral vascular disease (49%), these were not significant (P = .13-.17), largely because of the small number of events. In contrast to the glycemic control component of the trial in terms of macrovascular events, these results are clear and consistent and should encourage treatment to reduce blood pressure to at least 150/85 mm Hg. No major differences were noted when captopril was compared with atenolol.[78]

Even lower goal diastolic pressures are suggested by the Hypertension Optimal Treatment (HOT) trial. This study,[11] which included subjects who had diabetes and subjects who did not, examined three "target" diastolic pressures (<90 mm Hg, <85 mm Hg, and <80 mm Hg). In contrast to the overall results, in which a trend for increasing benefit with lower blood pressure goals was seen only for myocardial infarction, in those with diabetes, a greater benefit of a goal diastolic blood pressure of less than 80 mm Hg was evident for each of the seven macrovascular endpoints studied. This pattern was most marked for cardiovascular mortality and least marked for myocardial infarction when silent myocardial infarctions were included. The interpretation of these results, therefore, is that in diabetes, a goal diastolic blood pressure of less than 80 mm Hg is probably justified, although the mean diastolic blood pressure achieved in the lowest target group was 82 mm Hg. Two other studies suggest that calcium channel blockers may be less appropriate than ACE inhibitors for those who have diabetes. In the first trial, Appropriate Blood Pressure Control in Diabetes (ABCD), a fivefold higher rate of myocardial infarction was

BLOOD PRESSURE–LOWERING TRIALS THAT INCLUDED DIABETIC SUBJECTS (PART 1)

Study	Year	Diabetic Subjects (n)	Intervention	Primary Secondary Prevention	Entry Criteria	Duration of Study (yr)	Endpoint	Treatment Crude Incidence (%)	Control Crude Incidence (%)	Crude Risk Reduction (%; Increase Shown as ↑) [Absoulte Risk Reduction (%)]	Reported Adusted Risk Reduction (%; Increases Shown as ↑) (*P*; 95% CI)
HDFP Group Research	1985	256 (fasting PG >140 mg/dL)	Stepped care versus referred care	—	Diastolic blood pressure >90 mm Hg and age 30-69 years	5	Mortality	12.1	11.2	↑3.5 (↑0.9)	↑3.2*
		1378 (1-hour PG > 205 mg/dL						6.0	7.5	13.4 (0.9)	17.9†
		772 (history of diabetes)						11.0	12.5	5.3 (1.5)	4.9*
Curb et al.[9] (SHEP)	1996	583	Chlorthalidone 12.5-25 mg/day plus atenolol 25-50 mg/day or reserpine 0.05-0.10 mg/day	Primary and secondary	Systolic blood pressure >160 mm Hg and diastolic blood pressure >90 mm Hg	5	Primary: stroke (fatal or nonfatal)	8.8	12.0	26.7 (3.2)	22 (34-55)
							Secondary: CHD death or myocardial infarction	6.4	11.3	43.6 (4.9)	54 (12-76)
							All cardiovascular events**	20.1	27.7	27.3 (7.6)	34 (6-54)
Estacio et al.[79] (ABCD)	1998 (study continues for a second normotensive cohort)	470	Intensive antihypertensive treatment	Primary and secondary	Diastolic blood pressure >80 mm Hg	5	Primary: 24-hour creatine clearance	Not reported			

			Diastolic blood pressure 75 mm Hg vs 80-85 mm Hg		Diabetes (Subjects with end-stage renal disease, severe congestive heart failure, or a recent history of cardiovascular disease excluded)	5	Secondary: myocardial infarction (fatal or nonfatal)***)	10.6	2.1 (rates and risk reduction reflect increased risk of nisoldipine compared with enalapril)	↑405 (85)	↑700 (230-2140)
			Nisoldipine vs enalapril								
Califf and Granger [80] (FACET)	1998	380	Fosinapril 20 mg/day vs amlodipine 10 mg/day	Primary	Type 2 diabetes Systolic blood pressure >160 mm/Hg or diastolic blood pressure >90 mm/Hg	3.5	Primary: lipids and BP Secondary: major vascular events	7.4	14.1	47.1 (6.7)	51(.03; 5-74)

*P values not available; ** includes myocardial infarction, CHD death, cardiac revascularization, stroke, transient ischemic attacks, aneurysm, and endarterectomy; *** includes any cardiovascular death, myocardial infarction, stroke, hospitalized heart failure, and pulmonary infarction.

†Test of homogeneity suggests no difference from overall results, which showed 16.9% reduction by stepped care.

BP, blood pressure; CHD, coronary heart disease; PG, plasma glucose.

Table 6.10 Blood pressure–lowering trials that included diabetic subjects (Part 1).

BLOOD PRESSURE–LOWERING TRIALS THAT INCLUDED DIABETIC SUBJECTS (PART 2)

Study	Year	Diabetic Subjects (n)	Intervention	Primary or Secondary Prevention	Entry Criteria	Duration of Study (yr)	Endpoint	Treatment Crude Incidence (%)	Control Crude Incidence (%)	Crude Risk Reduction (%) [Absolute Risk Reduction (%)]	Reported Adjusted Risk Reduction (95% CI)
U.K. Prospective Diabetes Study Group[5]	1998	1148	ACE inhibitor or beta blocker; goal blood pressure <150/85 mm Hg vs 180/105 mm Hg (if treatment needed, ACE inhibitor or beta blocker avoided)	Primary and secondary	Newly diagnosed type 2 diabetes	8.4	Diabetes-related events	34.0	47.2	28.0 (13.2)	24% (8-38; $P = .005$)
							Diabetes-related death	10.8	15.9	32.0 (5.1)	32% (6-51); $P = .019$
							All-cause mortality	17.6	21.2	17.4 (3.7)	18% (increased 8-37); $P = .17$
Hansson et al.[11] (HOT)	1998	1501	Felodipine with three diastolic blood pressure goals: <90, <85, <80 mm Hg Aspirin 75 mg/day vs placebo	—	Age 50-80 years and diastolic blood pressure 100-115 mm Hg	3.8	Major cardiovascular events (all myocardial infarction, stroke, and cardiovascular deaths) Total mortality	Cardiovascular events per 1000 patient-years ($P = .005$) <90 24.4 <85 18.6 <80 11.9		Mortality per 1000 patient-years ($P = .068$) <90 15.9 <85 15.5 <80 9.0	Cardiovascular disease 90 vs 80: 51% reduction RR 90 vs 80: 2.06 (1.24-3.41) Mortality 90 vs 80: 43% reduction RR 90 vs 80: 1.77 (0.48-3.21)

Tuomilehto et al.[12] (Syst-Eur)	1999	492	Nitrendipine plus enalapril-hydrochlorothiazide vs placebo	—	Age older than 60 years and systolic blood pressure 160-219 mm Hg and diastolic blood pressure <95 mm Hg	2		Events per 1000 patient-years		
							Total mortality	6.4	10.8	41.2 (4.4) 55%; $P = .04$
							Cerebrovascular events	2.0	6.3	68.3 (4.3) 73% $P = .13$
							Coronary artery disease-related events	2.8	6.3	56.0 (3.5) 63% $P = .12$
Hansson et al.[82] (CAPPP)	1999	572	Captopril vs diuretics plus beta blockers	Primary and secondary	Aged 25-66 years and diastolic blood pressure >100 mm Hg	5	Primary: fatal cardiovascular disease plus nonfatal myocardial infarction or stroke	—	—	41% (9-62;) $P = .019$
							Secondary: all stroke	—	—	2% (increased 88-45); $P = .95$
							Secondary: all myocardial infarction	—	—	76% (33-85); $P = .002$

ACE, angiotensin-converting enzyme; RR, relative risk.

Table 6.11 Blood pressure–lowering trials that included diabetic subjects (Part 2).

seen in those patients with type 2 diabetes who were treated with nisoldipine compared with those who were treated with enalapril; this difference caused the safety committee to terminate nisoldipine therapy early.[79] In the second trial, the Fosinopril versus Amlodipine Cardiovascular Events Trial (FACET), another comparison of an ACE inhibitor and a calcium channel blocker was made.[80] In this trial, the primary objective was to compare lipid and glycemic control in type 2 diabetic subjects who were receiving, as primary therapy, fosinopril (an ACE inhibitor) with those who were receiving amlodipine (a calcium channel blocker). The two drugs were comparable in their blood pressure–lowering effects and in their effects on lipid and glucose levels. However, fosinopril subjects had a significantly lower risk of major vascular events. The Multicenter Isradipine Diuretic Atherosclerosis Study (MIDAS) compared isradipine with hydrochlorothiazide in patients aged 40 years or older who had ultrasonographically demonstrated carotid atherosclerosis and a diastolic blood pressure above 90 mm Hg. Although this study excluded subjects who had frank diabetes, it demonstrated that the adverse cardiovascular risk shown in the overall trial was concentrated in "prediabetic" subjects who had high HbA_{1c}; this provided further evidence that calcium channel blockers may not be advisable for those with glucose intolerance.[81] The Captopril Prevention Project (CAPPP) is a large study that compared captopril with diuretics plus beta blockers in 572 diabetic subjects. It showed essentially better results for captopril, with a greater reduction in all CVD events and myocardial infarction, whereas in the 10,413 nondiabetic subjects, little difference between the interventions was noted.[56,82] The ALLHAT trial assessed more than 40,000 patients with hypertension and CAD risk factors including a large number of patients with diabetes.[83] In the prespecified diabetic subgroup of ALLHAT, therapy that began with chlorthalidone reduced the primary endpoint of fatal CHD and myocardial infarction to the same degree as therapy based on lisinopril or amlodipine. The incidences of hyperglycemia and hypoglycemia were not significant between groups. Of potential concern is the tendency for thiazide-type diuretics to worsen hyperglycemia, but this effect tended to be small and did not produce more cardiovascular events compared with the other drug classes.

The ADA has recommended ACE inhibitors for diabetic patients older than 55 years at high risk for CVD and beta blockers for those with known CAD.[84] In the MICRO-HOPE subanalysis of the Heart Outcomes Prevention Evaluation (HOPE) Study, which included both hypertensive and normotensive individuals,[85] high-risk diabetic patients treated with ACE inhibition added to conventional therapy showed a reduction in combined myocardial infarction, stroke, and CVD death of about 25% and reduction in stroke of about 33% compared with placebo plus conventional therapy. With respect to microvascular complications, the ADA has recommended both ACE inhibitors and angiotensin receptor blockers for use in type 2 diabetic patients with chronic kidney disease because these agents delay the deterioration in glomerular filtration rate and the worsening of albuminuria. With calcium channel blocker therapy in the diabetic cohort of ALLHAT, amlodipine was as effective as chlorthalidone in all categories except heart failure, in which it was significantly inferior.[83] The ABCD study in diabetics was stopped prematurely when it was found that the dihydropyridine-nitrendipine was inferior to lisinopril in reducing the incidence of ischemic cardiac events.[79] More recent data concerning early hypertension come from the Strong Heart Study, in which 2629 participants free of CAD and hypertension at baseline were followed up for 12 years to observe the development of CVD. The investigators found that prehypertension was more prevalent in diabetic than in nondiabetic patients (59.4% versus 48.2%; $P < .001$, adjusted for age). Compared with nondiabetics, the hazard ratios for CAD were 3.70 (95% CI: 2.66, 5.15) for those with both prehypertension and diabetes, 1.80 (1.28, 2.54) for those with prehypertension alone, and 2.90 (2.03, 4.16) for those with diabetes alone.[86] Impaired fasting glucose and glucose intolerance also increased the risk of CVD in those with prehypertension.

In conclusion, from a macrovascular viewpoint, vigorous blood pressure control is appropriate for those with diabetes, both with and without clinical CAD. Diuretics,[9] ACE inhibitors,[79,80,82] and beta blockers[78] would all seem appropriate primary drugs, whereas calcium channel blockers[79-81] would seem less appropriate.

Smoking

Although there is no randomized clinical trial evidence that stopping smoking is of benefit, stopping smoking is strongly recommended, given the evidence that smoking is still a risk factor for CVD in type 2 diabetes[7,8]; furthermore, although it is not a clear risk factor in type 1 diabetes for CAD,[26] it does appear to be a risk factor for the progression of nephropathy,[87] which is in turn a major risk factor for CAD. Various antismoking programs have been tried in diabetes, and cardiologists are urged to refer diabetic patients to appropriate sources of help.

Beta Blockers and Angiotensin-Converting Enzyme Inhibitors

Because of perceived contraindications, the use of beta blockers and ACE inhibitors after myocardial infarction has been lower in diabetic patients than in the general population. This is most unfortunate because both of these drug classes are effective in diabetic patients, who because of their poorer post–myocardial infarction survival have a special need for this additional protection. Although much of the excess case mortality in diabetes is probably related to cardiac failure,[88] beta blockers may be even more effective in those with diabetes. For example, in a review of beta blockers and sudden cardiac death, Kendall and associates[89] reported that early post–myocardial infarction treatment with beta blockers reduces mortality by 13% overall and by 37% in those who have diabetes. Furthermore, although long-term use was associated with a 33% reduction in mortality in all patients, in those with diabetes, the reduction was 45%. The feared worsening of glycemic control and masking of (and diminished response to) hypoglycemia are not serious problems when cardioselective beta blockers are used. Tse and Kendall[90] have reported a useful review of the use of beta blockers in diabetes. ACE inhibition appears to be particularly beneficial in diabetes, according to the GISSI-3 data.[91] Indeed, in this study, the combined use of a beta blocker and lisinopril reduced the rates of mortality or severe left ventricular dysfunction from 12.6 to 5.5, which suggests that the full beta-blocker effect is not evident without ACE inhibition.[91]

Aspirin

Although aspirin was not shown to prevent proliferative eye disease in the Early Treatment Diabetic Retinopathy Study,[92] it did seem to provide some protection against CAD, as was seen in a secondary prevention setting in the Antiplatelet Trialists' Collaboration.[63,93] It has been suggested that diabetic subjects may require higher doses to affect thromboxane A_2 synthesis, which may explain the lack of effect in the Second International Study of Infarct Survival (ISIS-2).[64,94] Further evidence of benefit from aspirin use comes from the HOT study.[11] In this trial, apart from the blood pressure arm, subjects were randomized to 75 mg of aspirin per day or to placebo. Those with diabetes are reported to have a similar benefit (i.e., reduction of myocardial infarction by 35% [$P = .002$] or by 15% [$P = .13$] if silent myocardial infarctions are included) to the benefit that was seen overall. The rates of stroke, CVD, and total mortality were not, however, reduced. Also, although fatal bleeds were not increased, all bleeds were twice as common in the aspirin group. These results suggest that aspirin can be used with benefit even in hypertensive subjects who were previously thought to have a relative contraindication.

Bypass Surgery Versus Angioplasty

In a significant report, the Bypass Angioplasty Revascularization Investigation (BARI) investigators reported that unlike in the general population, in which no difference in outcome was noted between bypass grafting and angioplasty, 5-year survival was dramatically lower (65.5% versus 80.6%; $P = .003$) in diabetics who had angioplasty compared with those who had bypass surgery.[95] This finding led to a clinical alert and a general understanding that in diabetes, bypass surgery is the preferable means of revascularization. This benefit, on subsequent analyses, was limited to those who had a left internal mammary artery graft.[96] The underlying mechanism is unclear, although the enhanced endothelial disturbance of angioplasty may be particularly damaging in the atherogenic milieu of diabetes, or it may simply be that the provision of a new arterial supply in a high-risk group enables the myocardium to cope better with future insults. Although these data preceded the use of stents and were not confirmed in the BARI registry of revascularization procedures,[97] it would seem at present that bypass grafting is preferable for diabetic patients who need revascularization.

SUMMARY

Diabetes is without doubt a major contributor to the morbidity and mortality of CVD, in both primary and secondary settings. Although there are many gaps in our knowledge, and a lack of trial evidence in many areas, certain preventive actions are currently warranted. These include the constant surveillance of all CHD patients for diabetes and the repeated screening of all diabetic patients for CHD.

Vigorous risk factor management (blood pressure <130/80 mm Hg, LDL-cholesterol levels <100 mg/dL [2.6 mmol/L], cholesterol levels <100 mg/dL [2.6 mmol/L]) is indicated for the majority of diabetic subjects, as is adequate glycemic control (HbA_{1c} <7.0%). Beta blockers, ACE inhibitors, and aspirin should also be used as vigorously as they are in the general population. Of fundamental importance, however, is the assumption of responsibility for these aspects of care, and the cardiologist must ensure that these preventive measures are fully addressed.

chapter 7 Physical Activity and the Cardiovascular System

Calin V. Maniu, Thomas R. Flipse, J. Norman Patton, and Gerald Fletcher

Definitions

- Isotonic exercise: contraction of large skeletal muscle groups resulting in limb movement.
- Isometric exercise: contraction of smaller skeletal muscle groups without limb movement.
- Resistance exercise: a combination of isotonic and isometric exercise.

Key Features

- Neural and chemical factors during exercise increase cardiac output and redistribute flow to meet metabolic demands.
- Prolonged exercise training will lead to anatomic and physiologic changes in the cardiovascular system.
- Cessation of exercise training leads to a rapid reversal of these changes.

Clinical Implications

- Normal adaptations to exercise (athlete's heart) must be distinguished from disease.
- Exercise is beneficial for primary and secondary prevention of ischemic cardiovascular disease.
- An exercise prescription is required to avoid the risks of exercise in patients with cardiovascular disease.

The primary function of the cardiovascular system is to deliver components needed for tissue metabolism and growth and to remove the products of metabolism. During physical exercise, energy expenditure increases, requiring appropriate adjustments in blood flow. These changes are the result of a combination and integration of neural, chemical, and other physiologic factors.

The higher areas of the brain provide a coordinated and rapid response of the cardiovascular system to optimize tissue perfusion and to maintain central blood pressure in relation to motor cortex activity. They are also involved in the pre-exercise anticipatory period. The central command explains the significant influence of emotional state on the cardiovascular responses.

The cardiovascular control center is believed to be in the ventrolateral medulla and receives inputs that modulate its activity. These include mechanoreceptors found in muscles, joints, and vascular system; chemoreceptors from the muscles and vascular system; and vascular baroreceptors. The control center regulates the output of blood from the heart and its preferential distribution to tissues.

CIRCULATORY ADJUSTMENTS WITH EXERCISE

Integrated Response in Exercise

The circulatory response to exercise involves a complex series of adjustments that result in an increased cardiac output, proportional to the augmented metabolic demands. These changes ensure that the metabolic needs of the exercising muscles are met, that hyperthermia does not occur, and that blood flow to essential organs is protected. Two major effects occur during exercise: an increase in cardiac output and a redistribution of blood flow.

Cardiac output is defined as the product of stroke volume and heart rate. The average cardiac output at rest is about 5 L/min for men. In women, the value is usually 25% lower.

Resting cardiac output increases immediately before the onset of physical exercise as a result of anticipatory changes in the autonomic nervous system, resulting in tachycardia and increased venous return. The cardiac output then increases rapidly until steady-state exercise is reached. This is followed by a gradual rise until a plateau is achieved. The magnitude of hemodynamic response during physical activity depends on the intensity of exercise and the muscle mass involved. In sedentary individuals, the cardiac output during maximal exercise increases approximately four times, whereas in elite-class athletes, it may rise eightfold.

Heart Rate Response to Exercise

At the transition from rest to strenuous exercise, the heart rate increases rapidly to values of 160 to 180 beats per minute. During short bouts of maximal exercise, even higher heart rates have been recorded. The initial rapid increase is believed to be the result of central command influences or a rapid reflex from muscle mechanoreceptors. The almost instant acceleration in heart rate is mainly due to vagal withdrawal. Later increases result from reflex activation of the pulmonary stretch receptors, which trigger increased sympathetic tone and further parasympathetic withdrawal. The increased circulating catecholamines play a role as well. During exercise, the heart rate increase accounts for a greater percentage of the increase in cardiac output than does the increase in stroke volume. The stroke volume normally reaches its maximum when the cardiac output has increased by only half of its maximum. Any further increase in cardiac output occurs by increasing the heart rate.

Stroke Volume Changes with Exercise

Two physiologic mechanisms influence the stroke volume. The first one is intrinsic to heart muscle and involves enhanced cardiac filling in diastole secondary to increased venous return. The second mechanism involves normal ventricular filling followed by a more forceful contraction secondary to neurohormonal influences.

Greater ventricular filling during diastole, or preload, is caused by slower heart rate and increased venous return. The relationship between contractile force and resting length of the myocardial fibers represents the Frank-Starling law. As muscle fibers stretch, there is a more optimal arrangement of the sarcomere's myofilaments, resulting in enhanced contractility. This mechanism is responsible for the increased stroke volume during transition from rest to exercise or from the upright to the supine position. Cardiac output is highest in the supine position. Stroke volume is nearly maximal at rest and increases only slightly during exercise. In the upright position, at rest, the venous return to the heart is diminished, resulting in a smaller stroke volume and cardiac output. During upright exercise, however, stroke volume can increase to the point at which it approaches the maximum stroke volume observed in the recumbent position. In the upright position, in the early phase of exercise, cardiac output rises as a result of a simultaneous increase in stroke volume and heart rate. In the later phases of exercise, the increase in heart rate is primarily responsible for the further increase in cardiac output.

Distribution of Cardiac Output During Exercise

Blood flow to different tissues is generally proportional to their metabolic activity; but in certain organs, blood flow varies secondary to the metabolic demands of the exercising muscle. At rest, about 20% of the cardiac output is distributed to the skeletal muscle. The majority (up to 85%) of the increased cardiac output during exercise is diverted to the working muscles (Fig. 7.1). Within active muscle, blood flow is highly regulated, so that the greatest amount is delivered to the oxidative portions of the muscle at the expense of the tissue with high glycolytic capacity. Local metabolic conditions and neural and hormonal vascular regulation control the shunting of blood from nonmuscular tissues to the active muscles. The local response is due primarily to the buildup of vasodilatory metabolites in the exercising muscle.

During exertion, parasympathetic activity is withdrawn and sympathetic discharge is maximal. Plasma epinephrine levels are also increased. As a result, the majority of the vascular beds of the body are constricted, except those in exercising muscles and in the coronary and cerebral circulations. Blood flow to the skin increases during light and moderate exercise, favoring body cooling. Further increases in workload cause a progressive decrease in skin flow as the rising cutaneous sympathetic vascular tone overcomes the thermoregulatory vasodilatory response. At rest, the kidneys and splanchnic tissues use only 10% to 25% of the oxygen available in the blood supply. Consequently, considerable reductions in blood flow to these tissues can be tolerated because of increased extraction of oxygen from the available blood supply. In contrast, at rest, the heart extracts about 75% of the oxygen in the coronary blood flow. Because of a limited margin of reserve, the increased myocardial demands during exercise are met mainly by a fourfold increase in coronary blood flow. Cerebral blood flow also increases during exercise by approximately 25% to 30%. During maximal exercise, however, cerebral flow may also decrease in association with hyperventilation and respiratory alkalosis. The systolic and mean arterial pressure, pulse pressure, skeletal muscle blood flow, and oxygen extraction increase. The total peripheral resistance decreases, whereas the diastolic blood pressure is unchanged or may increase or decrease. Venous tone also increases with exercise.

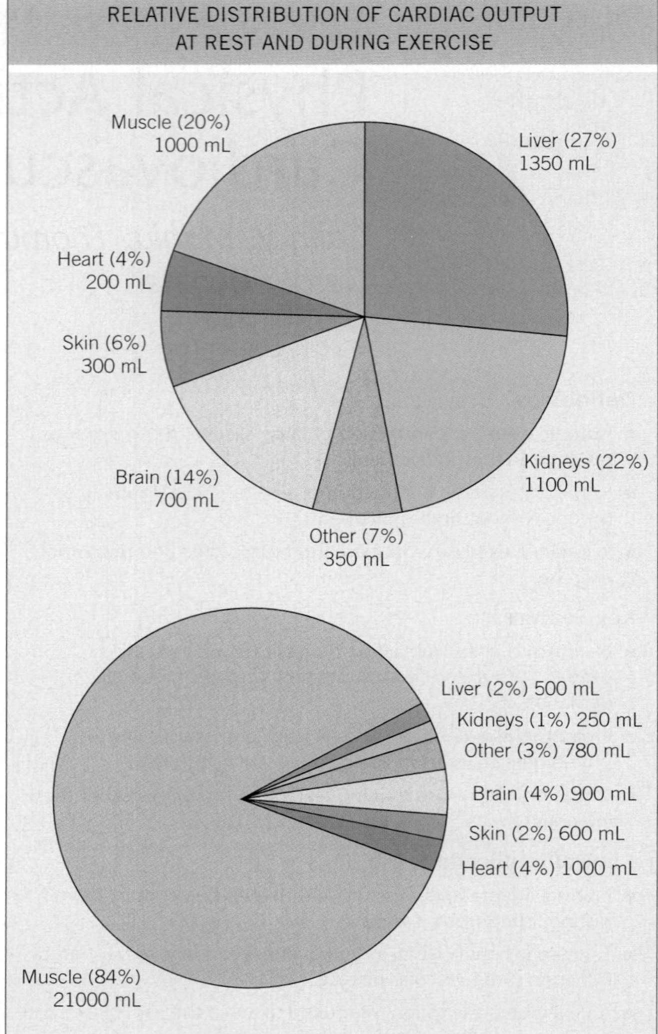

Figure 7.1 Relative distribution of cardiac output at rest *(top)* and during exercise *(bottom)*. From McArdle WD, Katch FI, Katch VL. Exercise Physiology, 4th ed. Baltimore, Md, Williams & Wilkins, 1996.

When exercise stops, there is an abrupt decrease in heart rate and cardiac output secondary to removal of the sympathetic drive and reactivation of vagal activity. In contrast, systemic vascular resistance remains lower for some time because of persistent vasodilatation in the muscles. As a result, arterial pressure falls, often below pre-exercise levels, for periods up to 12 hours into recovery. Blood pressure is then stabilized at normal levels by the baroreceptor reflexes.

EXERCISE TYPE AND CARDIOVASCULAR RESPONSE

Different types of exercise impose various loads on the cardiovascular system. Isotonic (dynamic) exercise is defined as muscle contraction of large muscle groups resulting in movement. Isometric (static) exercise is defined as a constant muscle contraction of smaller muscle groups without movement. A third type of exercise is resistance exercise. This is a combination of isometric and isotonic exercise by use of muscle contraction with movement. Most activities usually combine all types of exercise.

Isotonic (Dynamic) Exercise

During acute isotonic exercise, the total peripheral vascular resistance falls as a result of the marked vasodilatation of the vessels in exercising muscles, which overcomes the vasoconstriction of the splanchnic and renal vessels. As a result, afterload decreases and the increased cardiac output is redistributed, mainly to the active muscles. These changes develop through local autoregulation and are mediated by local factors related to the level of tissue metabolism (hypoxia, acidic pH, increased local temperature), the stimulation of sympathetic vasodilatory nerve endings, and the effects of circulating catecholamines.

During prolonged dynamic exercise, skeletal muscle metabolism is primarily aerobic and requires a significant increase in oxygen supply. In normal sedentary individuals, the oxygen consumption typically increases 10-fold from rest to maximal exertion, and in world-class athletes, the increase can be even greater. Maximal oxygen consumption is considered to be an indicator of the degree of training. The increased oxygen requirements are fulfilled by an augmentation of the local blood flow and improved oxygen extraction.

Isometric (Static) Exercise

The oxygen requirements necessary to sustain the contraction of a smaller muscle group without performing external work are lower. These are maintained with a smaller increase in cardiac output. An increase in regional blood flow is limited because local vasodilatation is impeded by the mechanical compression of the blood vessels during the sustained muscle contraction. To maintain regional perfusion, a pressor response is evoked, which is thought to be, at least in part, mediated locally by reflexes that originate in the muscles. The amplitude of the increase in blood pressure is proportional both to relative muscle tension and to the mass of the muscle groups involved. Significant increases in mean arterial pressure have, however, been recorded during sustained isometric contraction of relatively small muscle groups. As a result of the increase in blood pressure and in the absence of an increased venous return, stroke volume usually declines. To maintain the higher cardiac output, the heart rate must increase, often out of proportion to the metabolic needs of the active muscle groups.

Resistance (Resistive) Exercise

The acute cardiovascular response to resistance exercise is determined by the extent of the isotonic and isometric components. Repetitive weightlifting is considered to be the prototype resistance exercise. It is usually considered to have a high isometric component. Weight-training exercises have been shown to cause an acute increase in blood pressure. The heart rate response during maximal upper body resistance exercise is lower than that seen during maximal isotonic exercise.

Previous concerns about safety have been rebutted by several reports that showed that moderate resistance training programs are safe even in subjects with cardiac disease.[1] At this time, it is believed that resistance training is useful for promoting muscle strength and flexibility but probably contributes less significantly to cardiovascular health.

CHRONIC ADAPTATIONS TO EXERCISE

Physical conditioning or exercise training improves work performance, and the cardiovascular system increases its capacity to deliver oxygen to the active muscle. Physical training also improves the ability of the muscles to use oxygen. Through conditioning induced by repetitive bouts of dynamic exercise, the maximal oxygen consumption may increase twofold to threefold. About half of this increase is due to an increased cardiac output and about half is induced by the peripheral adaptations that improve oxygen extraction. Through physical training, an individual is able to increase maximal exercise intensity and duration and to achieve submaximal workloads with less cardiovascular effort.

At rest, cardiac output is similar for both trained and untrained individuals. Endurance training induces an increase in resting parasympathetic tone, associated with a concomitant reduction in resting sympathetic activity. The effect is bradycardia, with heart rates averaging about 50 beats per minute, although values below 30 beats per minute have been recorded for healthy athletes. The cardiac output is maintained by an increase in stroke volume, although the underlying physiologic mechanisms are not fully understood.

During exercise, trained individuals achieve a larger maximal cardiac output than do sedentary persons. In the untrained person, there is only a small increase in stroke volume during the transition from rest to exercise, and the major augmentation in cardiac output is induced by tachycardia. The improved cardiac performance after conditioning involves both the Frank-Starling mechanism and augmented myocardial contraction and relaxation. It has been shown that in previously sedentary individuals, 8 weeks of aerobic training will increase stroke volume. After cessation of training, these changes largely regress within 3 weeks.[2]

Several factors are likely to contribute to the chronic adaptations seen with training. An increased parasympathetic tone induces bradycardia, which prolongs diastolic filling time, resulting in ventricular dilatation. The plasma volume expands in response to aerobic training. Some studies have revealed that endurance training brings about increased compliance of the left ventricle.[3] This is probably caused by enhanced early diastolic filling and increased peak myocardial lengthening during exercise. These physiologic changes are accompanied by biochemical and ultrastructural alterations of the myocardial fibers, which have been demonstrated in the hearts of physically conditioned animals. There is an increase in lactic dehydrogenase and pyruvate kinase activity, which enhances the respiratory capacity of the cardiac myocytes. The size of the myocardial cells as well as the number of mitochondria and myofibrils in every fiber increases. In addition, changes in sarcolemma and sarcoplasmic reticulum have been noted.

The cross-sectional area of the epicardial coronary arteries increases in response to exercise. Alterations in the microcirculation have been identified in animal studies, revealing an increased capillary density and a decrease in the diffusion distance between the capillaries and the myocytes. Some data suggest that conditioning promotes coronary collateral formation to a potentially ischemic vascular bed.[4] The functional significance of these changes is unknown. These adaptations may enable the heart to better tolerate and to recover from transient episodes of ischemia and to function at a lower percentage of its total oxidative capacity during exercise. It is therefore likely that training-induced myocardial adaptations provide protection from myocardial ischemia.

Skeletal muscle also undergoes adaptations with training that favor an enhanced oxygen extraction. With long-term training, capillary density and the capillary-to-fiber ratio in skeletal muscles increase. The number of mitochondria increases, as do the oxidative enzymes in the mitochondria. Other cellular adaptations include increases in myoglobin, enzymes involved in lipid metabolism, and ATPase activity.

THE ATHLETE'S HEART

The structural characteristics of the hearts of apparently healthy, highly trained athletes differ considerably from those of normal individuals. Regardless of age, exercise training is followed by an increase in heart size, and this cardiac hypertrophy is viewed as a biologic reaction to an increased workload.

The duration of training affects cardiac size and structure. Short-term training is not associated with changes in cardiac dimensions, even though there is an improvement in maximal oxygen consumption and submaximal heart response. Prolonged endurance training is followed by left ventricular enlargement, which returns to pretraining levels after cessation of the exercise program.

Isotonically trained athletes undergo an eccentric hypertrophy characterized by a slight increase in wall thickness, an enlarged end-diastolic volume with a normal ratio of volume to thickness. In contrast, athletes involved in isometric training develop a concentric hypertrophy defined by symmetrically thickened ventricular walls and little difference in end-diastolic volume compared with sedentary persons. The wall thickness-to-volume ratio is increased.

The implications of these changes for myocardial blood flow and long-term cardiovascular health are unknown. The functional hypertrophy that occurs in response to exercise training is different from the pathologic hypertrophy secondary to chronic disease states. Even though the hearts of elite athletes are larger than the hearts of sedentary controls, the size is usually within the upper range of normal limits in relation to body size or to the increased end-diastolic volume. There is no compelling scientific evidence that specific forms of exercise training can harm a normal heart. On the contrary, the cardiac functional capacity of the athlete's heart is much greater, in terms of stroke volume and maximal cardiac output, than that of the hearts of healthy sedentary individuals.

The cardiovascular examination of an athlete has distinctive features. There is resting bradycardia with pulse rates as low as 30 to 40 beats per minute and an exaggerated normal respiratory variation in heart rate. Blood pressure and jugular venous pulsations are normal. The apical impulse may be slightly displaced because of left ventricular enlargement, but wide displacements suggest concurrent cardiac disease. The first and second heart sounds are normal. Both S_3 and S_4 gallop sounds are not uncommonly encountered in athletes, especially in the supine position, but are considered normal. Short systolic murmurs are also relatively common, reflecting a larger stroke volume or functional regurgitation caused by enlarged annuli of the atrioventricular valves. Diastolic murmurs or thrills, however, need to be further investigated.

The clinician's role is to recognize physiologic adaptations to the conditioned state and to distinguish them from pathologic cardiac conditions, which occur in athletes with the same frequency as in the general population.

GENDER DIFFERENCES

Few studies have assessed the physiologic responses of women to exercise. There are some quantitative differences, although the qualitative aspects of these responses are similar to those seen in men. Teenage women have a 5% to 10% larger cardiac output at any level of submaximal oxygen uptake than that of men. This is explained by the 10% lower hemoglobin concentration in women than in men.

The maximal aerobic capacity in women is lower than that in men. If adjusted to lean body mass, the difference is reduced to about 10% to 15%, which probably represents a true gender-specific difference. The explanation reflects the lower hemoglobin concentration and smaller blood volume of women, although differences in level of conditioning could play a role as well. The capacity to perform isotonic exercise is greater in women, a fact observed also during dynamic endurance competitions. A possible explanation might be the effect of estrogen, which induces the use of fatty acids as preferential energy substrate during exercise while relatively sparing the glycogen stores.

In men, during acute dynamic exercise, there is an increase in ejection fraction with little or no increase in end-diastolic volume. In contrast, women have been reported to increase end-diastolic volume without a significant increase in ejection fraction.[5] Therefore, the lesser rise in ejection fraction during exercise stress testing in a woman may be a normal manifestation and not an abnormal finding.

AGE-ASSOCIATED CHANGES IN CARDIOVASCULAR RESPONSE TO EXERCISE

Aging results in changes in cardiovascular structure and function that vary significantly among individuals. An increased frequency of acquired heart disease occurs with age, and there needs to be a strict differentiation between normal aging and the interplay of aging and disease.

The aortic wall stiffens with age as a result of alterations in the vascular media. These alterations consist of a reduction in the amount of elastic tissue and its fragmentation and degeneration and an increased amount of collagen. Because the left ventricle is ejecting blood into a "stiffer" central aorta, the systolic blood pressure tends to be higher in older individuals, even in the absence of disease. The diastolic blood pressure changes less and may actually decrease, resulting in a widened arterial pulse pressure.

Because of the age-associated rise in blood pressure, mild to moderate left ventricle hypertrophy occurs without overall cardiac size change, even in subjects without heart disease. This appears to be a physiologic adaptation. It is associated with an increase in myocyte size despite a reduction in the number of myocytes. There are also increased degenerative changes in myocardial collagen, lipids, and lipofuscin. The response to stimulation of β-sympathetic receptors in cardiac myocytes is significantly less in the elderly. The responsible mechanism is probably related to a defect in signal recognition or transduction. This decrease in β-sympathetic response results in decreased chronotropic and inotropic response of cardiac muscle and reduced arterial vasodilating response. Cardiac function in young individuals in the presence of beta blockade appears similar to that in older persons not receiving beta blockade, suggesting that the decreased β-sympathetic response is a major factor contributing to aging-related changes in the cardiovascular system. Left ventricular hypertrophy and prolongation of the isovolumic relaxation period cause a decrease in early left ventricle diastolic compliance. As a result, left ventricular end-diastolic volume does not decrease with age, but the end-diastolic pressure is often higher in older subjects. The rest ejection fraction remains stable in healthy subjects with aging, whereas the resting cardiac output decreases or remains unchanged.

It has been noted that with aging, exercise capacity and maximal oxygen consumption decrease. When it is adjusted for lean body mass, however, the age difference in maximal oxygen consumption is minimized. Measurements of cardiac output during exercise have failed to unequivocally substantiate claims that a failure of cardiac output to increase limits peak oxygen consumption or work capacity in older subjects. To date, there is no clear explanation for these phenomena. There are, however, several mechanisms that have been postulated: skeletal muscle fatigue or sense of fatigue; increased work of breathing or overall decrease in pulmonary function; differences in muscle mass; reduced blood flow to skeletal muscle; decreased oxygen extraction; and psychological factors. These age-related changes can be, at least partially, overcome through physical conditioning. Potential mechanisms for this improvement include an improved β-adrenergic sensitivity and a decrease in afterload.

There are significant changes in the effect of exercise on the cardiovascular system in the elderly. There is a lower maximal heart rate response during exercise at any workload. This could be explained by a decreased sympathetic response. The end-systolic volume also fails to decrease with exercise. This is thought to represent a diminished cardiac inotropy and the increased impedance to ejection mentioned before. These alterations are not attributable to decreased circulating catecholamines, as these are actually higher during exercise in the elderly. There is a greater increase in end-diastolic volume. These changes result in a similar cardiac output in elderly and younger individuals at any specific exercise load. However, the underlying mechanisms differ markedly. Whereas in young individuals this is produced by use of adrenergically mediated responses (increased heart rate, decreased end-systolic volume, and decreased impedance to left ventricle ejection), the elderly rely mainly on the effective use of the Frank-Starling mechanism. Ejection fraction at rest is unchanged with age and increases during exercise in elderly healthy subjects. This increase is less in older individuals, however, because of a lesser decrease in end-systolic volume.

EXERCISE AND PRIMARY PREVENTION OF CARDIOVASCULAR DISEASE

Epidemiologic studies published during the past half-century have documented the link between physical activity and decreased incidence of myocardial infarction and sudden death in the more physically active individuals.[6]

More studies have examined cardiac event rates between physically active and inactive individuals categorized by energy expenditure during leisure-time activities assessed from activity questionnaires. In the Harvard alumni study,[7] those who were more physically active at baseline showed reductions in myocardial infarctions and sudden death rates compared with more sedentary counterparts. The Multiple Risk Factor Intervention Trial[8] revealed that even low-intensity activity resulted in significant reduction in manifestations of coronary disease. For a more objective assessment of physical conditioning, several studies used exercise performance during an exercise treadmill test. They revealed that the least exercise-conditioned individuals have a higher rate of cardiovascular disease compared with the best-conditioned individuals. An analysis of previous exercise trials revealed that a physically inactive lifestyle was associated with twice the risk for development of coronary disease, a risk similar to that of other modifiable risk factors.[9] Studies indicate that those at highest risk might benefit most from vigorous physical activity. It is estimated that approximately 12% of the total mortality in the United States, 250,000 deaths per year, is attributable to physical inactivity.[10]

The majority of the population studies reveal that active people develop coronary artery disease less frequently. This association implies but does not guarantee that intervention through increased physical activity will reduce the incidence of coronary artery diseases. Self-selection and confounding variables can never be eliminated from this type of study.

A dose-response relationship between physical inactivity and development of coronary artery disease has been noted. Some suggest that the risk reduction might depend on a threshold effect or reaching of peak load rather than a composite or average exertion level. In recent years, this view has been questioned as there appears to be benefit with only moderate physical activity that does not need to be strenuous or prolonged and includes daily leisure activities readily attainable by large sections of the population.[11]

The American Heart Association classifies physical inactivity as a major risk factor. The extent to which physical inactivity raises coronary risk independent of the major risk factors is uncertain.[12] Some authors consider it a predisposing risk factor that contributes to the major, causal risk factors.[13]

An important observation is that the habitual level of physical activity in middle life has been associated with a low risk of cardiovascular morbidity and mortality. Men who were physically active initially and subsequently became inactive had the same risk of death as did men who were constantly inactive. Men who were inactive at baseline but later took up moderately vigorous activity had a lower risk of mortality compared with constantly inactive men.[7]

A randomized, controlled study to prove that regular exercise as primary prevention decreases the cardiovascular event rate has never been performed. Cost, methodologic and logistic problems, and the difficulty of ensuring long-term compliance by treatment groups greatly limit the ability to conduct such a trial.

The data available at this time support the concept that physical activity may lower cardiovascular risk and is not simply a marker of favorable genetic predisposition. The potential benefits of physical exercise outweigh the risks. The large number of sedentary persons predisposed to coronary artery disease makes the impact of more active lifestyles comparable with intervention of other risk factors. It has been estimated that conversion from a sedentary to an active lifestyle could eliminate 33% of coronary artery disease risk.

The majority of studies that examined the effect of exercise on cardiovascular risk have included predominantly young and middle-aged men. There has been a concern that the results might not be readily translated to other population subgroups. In addressing another population, the National Children and Youth Fitness Studies found that approximately 60% of U.S. schoolchildren engage in appropriate physical activity.[14] Physical activity levels in children peak in the early teenage years and then drastically decline so that by early adulthood, only 10% of the population is regularly active. More recent reports raise the concern that a large percentage of young Americans are less physically active than is desirable. Cardiovascular endpoints are extremely rare in children, so the importance of studying physical activity in childhood is related to its ability to predict physical activity in adulthood and its impact on other coronary risk factors.

The number of women who took part in studies examining the effect of risk factors on cardiovascular disease has been very small. The available evidence, although limited, suggests that cardiorespiratory fitness has the same effect on cardiovascular endpoints in women as in men.[15]

Elderly individuals are the fastest-growing segment of the U.S. population. Studies that enrolled only elderly patients revealed that regular exercise was associated with a significant decrease in risk of death.[16] Persons older than 65 years appear to benefit from exercise training at least as much as younger adults do, and maintaining a physically active lifestyle can reduce the risk of coronary heart disease and extend the active life span.[17]

ROLE OF PHYSICAL ACTIVITY IN SECONDARY PREVENTION OF CARDIOVASCULAR DISEASE

In the United States, approximately 6 million people are estimated to be living with diagnosed coronary artery disease, and a larger number are believed to be living with significant, yet undiagnosed, silent myocardial ischemia. Several studies have evaluated the cardioprotective effect of exercise training in the setting of cardiac rehabilitation programs for survivors of myocardial infarctions. A review of these trials reported that cardiovascular rehabilitation programs led to improved functional capacity and cardiovascular efficiency as well as enhanced physiologic well-being.[18] The evidence, however, fell short of indicating that exercise conditioning programs could independently reduce recurrence of fatal or nonfatal coronary events. The largest trial performed in the United States was the National Exercise and Heart Disease Project, in which the favorable trends seen in both overall mortality and cardiovascular mortality after 3 years in the exercise group failed to reach statistical significance.[19]

The most recent and comprehensive review of cardiovascular rehabilitation included 51 randomized controlled trials of exercise-based cardiovascular rehabilitation and added about 4000 patients to the prior widely quoted meta-analyses.[20,21] It confirms that exercise-based cardiac rehabilitation results in a 27% reduction in overall mortality and a 31% reduction in cardiac mortality but not in a reduction of the risk of recurrent myocardial infarctions. The reason for the lack of effect on recurrent nonfatal myocardial infarctions remains unclear.[22]

Changes in cardiac function and coronary blood flow consequent to exercise might be possible in humans, as suggested by improved thallium exercise scans and ejection fractions in some patients.[4] Beneficial changes in work capacity and hemodynamics could also be a result of noncardiac adaptations in the skeletal muscles, catecholamine levels, sympathetic tone, and peripheral circulation.

Exercise training is the mainstay of cardiac rehabilitation and can be used with impressive benefits for many cardiac patients. Studies have shown significant regression or lack of progression of coronary lesions in patients who performed high-intensity exercise and were also on a low-fat diet.[23] High-intensity exercise training has been shown to result in higher left ventricular ejection fractions in men with coronary artery disease compared with low-intensity exercise.[24] Other studies report that exercise training programs have significant beneficial effects on ventricular function and "remodeling" in subjects with coronary artery disease.[25] The available studies do suggest that cardiac rehabilitation, in which exercise is a major component, is cost-effective for enhancing quality-adjusted life-year gains[26] and is associated with lower cardiac rehospitalization rates and hospital charges. The benefits of cardiac rehabilitation extend to the elderly patients.[27]

EFFECT OF PHYSICAL ACTIVITY ON ATHEROSCLEROTIC RISK FACTORS

The level of physical activity predicts future development of other risk factors. The direct impact of exercise on a given risk factor is frequently confounded by changes in other physiologic variables that result from exercise training. It has been observed that physically inactive subjects more often have other coronary risk factors as well. Physical activity appears to influence favorably a number of coronary risk factors, as shown in Table 7.1. After adjustment for other

RISK FACTORS FAVORABLY AFFECTED BY PHYSICAL ACTIVITY	
Blood lipids	High-density lipoproteins and triglycerides
Hypertension	
Obesity	
Diabetes	Weight control and decreased insulin resistance
Other risk factors	Fibrinolytic system Platelet aggregation Hypercoagulant states Circulatory catecholamines Psychological (i.e., depression and some type A behavior)

Table 7.1 Risk factors favorably affected by physical activity.

risk factors, the significance of exercise is reduced. However, the benefit of exercise on risk factors is suggestive of protection until a definite causal relationship is proved.

Although some long-term studies have demonstrated a benefit of physical activity on the lipid profile, others have not. The contribution of weight loss after exercise toward changes in lipid profile is controversial. Exercise training has been shown to have a favorable effect on the lipid profile, including a reduction in triglycerides and increases in high-density lipoprotein.[28] It has been suggested that exercise training needs to be of long enough duration and of a certain intensity to induce changes in the lipid profile.

A sedentary lifestyle may be associated with hypertension, and physical inactivity predicts the future development of hypertension. Exercise training adds an independent blood pressure–lowering effect in both normotensive and hypertensive individuals.[29] Studies suggest that obese hypertensive patients benefit most significantly and that the benefit of exercise is limited to the period of exercise training.

Obesity has been associated with increased coronary risk. In population studies, active individuals have better controlled weights. Because the calorie expenditure of exercise is small, exercise alone results in little weight loss, but physical activity is an important adjunct to diet in achieving and maintaining weight loss.[30] Maintaining the reduced weight depends on adherence to an exercise program.

Currently, there is no conclusive evidence that exercise training has a positive effect on smoking cessation.[31] Some studies suggest a favorable effect in patients involved in cardiac rehabilitation programs, but psychological counseling and nicotine replacement were used in addition to physical exercise. Nonetheless, exercise training is often incorporated as part of smoking cessation programs. Preliminary evidence suggests that physical activity facilitates long-term smoking cessation by increasing the initial quit rate.[32]

Exercise improves insulin resistance and glycemic control.[33] Physical activity has a positive role in preventing the development of type 2 (non–insulin-dependent) diabetes mellitus.[34] There seems to be an intensity and duration threshold for exercise that needs to be reached to obtain the beneficial effects. Exercise conditioning has a favorable effect on blood clotting by stimulation of the fibrinolytic system, reduction of hypercoagulable states,[35] inhibition of platelet aggregation, and reduction of circulating catecholamines.

Several studies suggested that physical activity had psychological benefits, but the intervention groups often received counseling in addition to exercise training. However, active individuals were reported to be at lower risk for depression, and in individuals with depression, physical exercise was shown to reduce the severity of depression.[36] Regular exercise promotes a sense of well-being, is “anxiolytic,” and modifies some type A personality behaviors.

IMPLEMENTATION OF PHYSICAL EXERCISE PROGRAMS

The type of activity and its frequency, duration, intensity, and progression are important variables that influence the benefit obtained from different types of physical activity. Published recommendations are available for the quantity and quality of exercise for achieving substantial health benefits over and above the routine light-intensity activities of daily living.[37] Thirty minutes of moderate-intensity physical activity 5 days or more per week or 20 minutes of vigorous-intensity physical activity on 3 days per week, or a combination of moderate- and vigorous-intensity activity in the range of 450 to 750 metabolic equivalent value minutes per week, is the minimal amount of activity recommended to achieve these benefits. This activity can be accumulated in at least 10-minutes bouts. Suggested activities are those that use large muscle groups, can be maintained continuously, and are rhythmic and aerobic in nature (walking, jogging, biking, swimming). Larger amounts of physical activity, including more activity at higher intensities, provide additional benefits. Resistance training at least twice per week provides a safe and effective method for improving muscle strength and endurance and represents a complement to rather than a replacement for aerobic exercise.[1] At present, less than half of the U.S. adults meet the 1995 Centers for Disease Control and Prevention and American College of Sports Medicine physical activity recommendation of “30 minutes or more of moderate-intensity physical activity on most, preferably all, days of the week.”[38] It is suggested that sedentary people begin with levels of activity that are comfortable and then gradually work up to the preset goals. Resistance exercise can be added to the activity program to increase muscle strength, and the physical activity should be preceded by a warm-up period and followed by a cool-down period.

Improvement in physical conditioning is an important consideration in designing exercise programs for the elderly, but for many elderly persons, enhancing the ability to perform daily activities and improving and maintaining the quality of life will be the most important goals. In general, many of the basic guidelines of exercise prescription that have been developed for the younger and middle-aged populations are appropriate for the elderly. These individuals are, however, more susceptible to fatigue, musculoskeletal injury, and potential cardiovascular problems. Thus, the exercise prescription for the elderly should include activities of low impact, performed at a more moderate intensity and implemented more gradually. Muscle-strengthening activity is particularly important in older adults, given its role in preventing age-related loss of muscle mass and bone and the beneficial effects on functional limitations.[17]

An exercise prescription should be individualized and updated periodically for each individual and should include the following information: types of exercise, desired intensity, duration of exercise sessions, anticipated rate of progression, specific warm-up and cool-down activities, and warning symptoms necessitating the termination of the exercise session. Before starting an exercise program, patients with cardiovascular disease should undergo an exercise test, which provides initial levels of working capacity, specific precautions, and heart rates used to prescribe activity.

COMPLICATIONS OF EXERCISE

Physical activity has been demonstrated to decrease cardiovascular disease risks, yet there is still a risk of sudden death associated with physical exercise. Table 7.2 lists causes of sudden cardiac death during exercise.

There are different estimates of the risk of exercise. In high-school and college athletes, the absolute exercise-related death rate was 1 per 133,000 men per year and 1 per 769,000 women per year,[39] and these estimates included all sports-related nontraumatic deaths. Another study estimated that approximately 1 in 200,000 athletes is at risk of sudden cardiac death and that male athletes have a higher risk.[40] In Seattle, Washington, the annual incidence of exercise-related cardiac arrests among previously healthy adults was 1 for every 18,000.[41]

Age is an important variable in predicting the cause of sudden cardiac deaths. The leading cause of sudden death for athletes older than 35 years is coronary atherosclerosis. The majority of younger athletes die of structural nonatherosclerotic heart disease. Hypertrophic cardiomyopathy is the predominant cause of death in young athletes, occurring in up to a third of cases in some series.[42] Ventricular dysrhythmias and dynamic obstruction to left ventricular outflow are the most likely mechanisms of sudden death in this group of patients. Some of the other more common structural abnormalities responsible for sudden death in the young athlete are anomalous coronary arteries, idiopathic left ventricular hypertrophy, and myocarditis. Up to 2% of athletes who die suddenly have no structural abnormalities at necropsy. Ion channel disorders such as long QT syndrome and Brugada syndrome, Wolff-Parkinson-White syndrome, and coronary vasospasm are some of the disorders in this category.[43] Commotio cordis is increasingly recognized as a cause of sudden death during athletic competition. A blow to the chest, most commonly by a projectile, during a vulnerable period in the cardiac cycle can result in ventricular fibrillation. Overall survival is poor, and successful resuscitation depends on early defibrillation.[44] Gender and racial differences exist in the frequency and cause of sudden death during exercise. The risk of sudden death for women is considerably less than that for men, probably a result of gender differences in athletic participation.[45] In the United States, the majority of athletes dying of hypertrophic cardiomyopathy during exercise are African American, illustrating the need for improved preparticipation screening to recognize this condition.[46]

In athletes older than 35 years, coronary artery disease is responsible for about 80% of sudden deaths, with 50% having prodromal symptoms or known coronary artery disease. Other causes of sudden death in the older athlete include hypertrophic cardiomyopathy, right ventricular dysplasia, coronary artery anomalies, and aortic dissection.

Despite the low absolute risk of exercise in previously healthy men, the death rate per hour of exercise is increased.[41] The heart rate profile during exercise and recovery may predict risk for sudden death in those being affected by the alteration in autonomic influence on cardiac function.[47] Paradoxically, the risk of experiencing a myocardial infarction during exercise is higher in sedentary than in habitually active individuals.[48] There are no established strategies to decrease that risk in this population of patients, but it would appear that maintaining physical fitness through regular physical activity may help decrease sudden death events.[49] Exertion-related myocardial infarction is more common in men who smoke and have hypercholesterolemia.[48] They are more likely to have ventricular fibrillation, heart failure, single-vessel disease, and a large thrombus burden in the infarct artery than are patients with myocardial infarction not related to effort.[48] It is noteworthy that among previously healthy men with hypercholesterolemia, there were more myocardial infarctions during exercise than sudden cardiac deaths.[50] In contrast, among cardiac rehabilitation participants with coronary artery disease, the ratio of myocardial infarctions to sudden cardiac deaths during exercise is reversed, probably as a result of myocardial scarring that increases the risk of ventricular fibrillation.[51]

Several hypotheses have been postulated to explain how exercise might provoke acute coronary events. Usually, exercise dilates normal coronary arteries, but it can induce spasm in diseased segments.[52] Plaque rupture could occur through

CAUSES OF SUDDEN CARDIAC DEATH DURING EXERCISE	
Older than 35 years	Coronary artery disease
Younger than 35 years	Hypertrophic cardiomyopathy Commotio cordis Coronary artery anomalies Idiopathic left ventricular hypertrophy Myocarditis
Less common causes (<5% of sudden cardiac death)	Arrhythmogenic right ventricular cardiomyopathy Idiopathic dilated cardiomyopathy Aortic stenosis Ruptured aortic aneurysm (Marfan's syndrome) Mitral valve prolapse Drug abuse (primarily cocaine) Kawasaki's disease Sarcoidosis Coronary artery vasospasm Wolff-Parkinson-White syndrome Long QT syndrome Brugada syndrome Catecholaminergic polymorphic tachycardia Conduction system abnormalities
Modified from Maron.[42,43]	

Table 7.2 Causes of sudden cardiac death during exercise.

contraction of a noncompliant atherosclerotic plaque. Physical exertion increases systolic blood pressure through the coronary arteries, thereby increasing shear forces and possibly inducing plaque rupture. The "twisting" of the epicardial coronary arteries brought about by the exaggerated changes in cardiac dimensions during exercise might contribute to plaque rupture as well, and the increased level of catecholamines may increase thrombosis by favoring platelet aggregation.

In older athletes, exercise testing is thought by some to be of benefit in identifying subjects at increased risk for sudden death. The American College of Sports Medicine recommends routine use of exercise testing to screen high-risk individuals before vigorous exercise.[53] However, exercise testing in asymptomatic individuals has a limited sensitivity for acute coronary events. This is explained by the fact that a truly positive test result requires a hemodynamically significant lesion, whereas acute coronary events often occur at the site of previous nonobstructive atherosclerotic plaque. The American Heart Association does not recommend the nonselective use of exercise testing for screening of apparently healthy individuals. The test may be considered helpful for motivational purposes and for designating exercise on prescription.[54] Radionuclide or echocardiographic imaging, in conjunction with exercise testing, will reduce the incidence of false-positive electrocardiographic recordings, but it is probably not justified to identify asymptomatic individuals who are at risk for exercise-related cardiac events.

Another approach is to restrict routine preparticipation exercise testing to high-risk subjects. One study[50] addressed this issue and found that the positive predictive value for an acute exercise-related event was only 4%, in part because such events are rare even in a high-risk group. Thus, the value of routine exercise testing to prevent acute exercise-related cardiac events is limited even in high-risk individuals.

Several attempts have been made to identify high-risk athletes in the hope of preventing sudden cardiac death. In several studies, screening echocardiography has been used, but no cases of hypertrophic cardiomyopathy were detected. Mitral valve prolapse is the most common valvular disorder, and clinical judgment dictates that athletic participation should not be prohibited solely because of its presence. It is therefore recommended that echocardiographic screening not be done routinely in young athletes. In Italy, a nationwide preparticipation screening program has proved effective at decreasing the incidence of sudden death during athletic training and competition. This was most dramatic in the Veneto region, where arrhythmogenic right ventricular cardiomyopathy is prevalent—the annual incidence of sudden death in athletes declined by 89% with their screening program.[55] In Italy, the use of the history, physical examination, and 12-lead electrocardiography proved efficient in identifying athletes with hypertrophic cardiomyopathy, leading to timely disqualification from competitive sports.[56]

Therefore, it is recommended that all athletes undergo a brief cardiovascular examination in conjunction with an adequate history. Cardiac auscultation should be performed with subjects sitting or standing to minimize the chance of producing innocent flow murmurs and to increase the chance of detecting the murmur of hypertrophic cardiomyopathy. Athletes with abnormalities should be referred for further evaluation. It is important to educate the athletes about prodromal cardiac symptoms, and new symptoms of exercise intolerance should be carefully evaluated.

SUMMARY

During exercise, the increased metabolic demands of the body are met by alterations in the cardiovascular system induced by a combination of neural and chemical factors. The main adjustments are increase in cardiac output and redistribution of blood flow. These changes are a result of the interplay between neurohormonal and intrinsic cardiac factors.

There are three types of physical activity that impose different loads on the cardiovascular system: isotonic, isometric, and resistance exercise. Chronic repetition of physical exercise, especially isotonic, results in physical conditioning, which improves the work performance of the cardiovascular and skeletal muscle systems.

The heart of an athlete undergoes anatomic and physiologic changes as an adaptation to the increased workload. Prolonged training is required for these changes to occur. After cessation of exercise, the modifications gradually disappear.

Despite some quantitative differences, the qualitative aspects of physical responses and adaptation to exercise are similar in men and women. Aging brings about changes in the cardiovascular structure and function that need to be strictly differentiated from the pathologic alterations induced by disease.

Although a randomized, controlled study to prove the beneficial effects of physical exercise on cardiovascular disease has never been performed in humans, the data available at this time strongly support that regular physical activity lowers cardiovascular risk. This conclusion applies to primary as well as to secondary prevention of cardiovascular disease. Physical activity appears to influence several coronary risk factors favorably.

Implementation of physical exercise programs is dependent on different variables. There are general recommendations for the quantity and quality of exercise that need to be adjusted for each participant.

Despite the fact that physical activity decreases cardiovascular disease risk overall, there are certain risks associated with physical exercise that should be considered.

chapter 8

Cholesterol-Lowering Therapy

Lori Mosca and David D. Waters

Definitions

- Plasma lipoproteins are complexes of lipids (cholesterol and triglycerides) and proteins that are classified according to their density, electrophoretic mobility, and apolipoprotein content.

Key Features

- High levels of low-density lipoprotein (LDL) and triglycerides or low levels of high-density lipoprotein (HDL) increase the risk of coronary heart disease.
- Decreasing LDL-cholesterol has been shown to reduce cardiovascular events across a wide range of at-risk patients.
- Recent evidence suggests that aggressive LDL-cholesterol lowering yields an incremental reduction in events compared with less aggressive treatment.

Clinical Implications

- The goal of lipid-altering therapy is to reduce the incidence and recurrence of cardiovascular events while minimizing side effects and costs of therapy.
- Secondary causes of dyslipidemia should be identified and target lipid levels established, depending on the presence of cardiac disease and risk factor status, before therapy is initiated.

Compelling laboratory, epidemiologic, and clinical trial evidence supports a central role of lipids in the genesis of atherosclerosis. Cholesterol, triglycerides, free fatty acids, and phospholipids are major lipids and, because of their insolubility in plasma, circulate as lipoprotein complexes. Lipoproteins are spherical particles that contain a nonpolar core of esterified cholesterol and triglyceride and have a polar surface layer made up of apolipoproteins, phospholipids, and free cholesterol (Fig. 8.1).[1] Lipoproteins vary in the amount of core cholesteryl ester and triglyceride that they contain and are classified according to their density and electrophoretic mobility (Table 8.1). The large, more buoyant particles have a triglyceride-rich core, whereas the smaller, denser particles have more cholesteryl ester. Specific apoproteins associate with lipoproteins and mediate important steps in lipid metabolism.

Concentrations of lipids and lipoproteins are highly correlated with the incidence of coronary heart disease (CHD) globally. There is an increased recognition that atherogenesis is not simply a manifestation of cholesterol burden. The number, density, size, apoprotein and lipid content, and oxidation status of lipoproteins appear to play an important role in the risk of cardiovascular events. Low-density lipoprotein (LDL) cholesterol is causally related to atherosclerotic risk, but other major lipoproteins are also important markers of and contributors to cardiovascular disease (CVD). Some studies suggest that increased levels of C-reactive protein, lipoprotein(a), homocysteine, and other factors may also be associated with increased risk of CVD, but data showing altering their levels improves clinical outcomes is lacking.

Surrogate endpoints have been used in clinical trials to demonstrate benefit from lipid-lowering therapies. In more than a dozen studies using coronary angiographic measurements, treatment (usually statins, but also diet and lifestyle interventions and even ileal bypass surgery) reduced progression of coronary disease, increased regression, and was associated with less new lesion development.[2] These beneficial angiographic findings have been shown to be predictive of subsequent improvement in clinical outcomes. Carotid intima-media thickness as assessed by B-mode ultrasonography increases over time and is predictive of both coronary and cerebrovascular events. Lipid-lowering therapy, mainly with statins, has been shown to slow or to halt this progression.[3] Intracoronary ultrasonography has demonstrated that lipid lowering slows the progression of atherosclerosis within the arterial wall and favors regression[4]; however, the clinical significance of these changes has not been documented.

Lipid lowering has been associated with a reduction in CHD mortality, nonfatal myocardial infarction (MI), hospitalization for unstable angina, need for coronary revascularization, and stroke. The reduction in clinical cardiovascular events that has been observed with lipid-lowering therapy has been ascribed to numerous mechanisms, including a reduced tendency for plaque disruption and thrombosis and beneficial effects on vasomotor tone.[5] Increased plaque lipid core, lipid concentrations, and lipid peroxidation are associated with impaired endothelial function, which predisposes to vasoconstriction, thrombosis, and inflammatory cell recruitment. Numerous clinical trials have demonstrated improvements in endothelial function and vascular reactivity with cholesterol lowering. Other pathophysiologic mechanisms of potential benefit include modulation of immune function, effects on hemostatic and rheologic parameters, reduced macrophage density within plaque, and increased matrix synthesis.

More than 100,000 patients have been randomized into lipid-lowering trials with hard clinical endpoints. The results of these trials support the recommendations of the National Cholesterol Education Program Adult Treatment Panel III (NCEP ATP III) guidelines, which emphasize primary prevention in people with multiple risk factors and recommend more intensive LDL-lowering therapy in high-risk groups.[6]

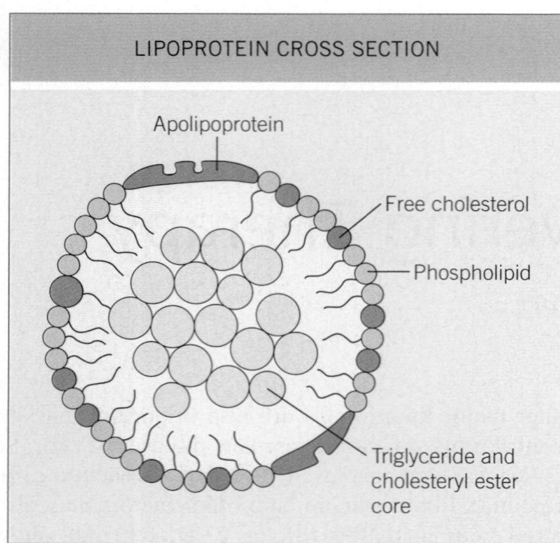

Figure 8.1 Lipoprotein cross section. (From Miller M, Vogel RA. The Practice of Coronary Disease Prevention. Baltimore, Md, Williams & Wilkins, 1996.)

EVIDENCE FROM MAJOR CLINICAL ENDPOINT LIPID-LOWERING TRIALS

Trials with Drugs Other than Statins

One of the first randomized, double-blind studies to establish that lowering of cholesterol reduced the incidence of CHD was the landmark Lipid Research Clinics Coronary Primary Prevention Trial[7] (1984). The study randomized 3806 men aged 35 to 59 years without symptomatic CHD and with an average LDL-cholesterol concentration of 204 mg/dL to diet plus cholestyramine or diet plus placebo. After an average of 7.4 years, the active drug treatment was associated with a 12% reduction in LDL-cholesterol and a 19% reduced risk of nonfatal MI or CHD death compared with the diet-only group (one-tailed $P < .05$).

Four major trials with clinical endpoints have been completed within the past 2 decades using fibrates. The Helsinki Heart Study (1987) randomized 4081 asymptomatic men aged 40 to 55 years with a mean LDL-cholesterol concentration of 188 mg/dL to diet plus gemfibrozil or diet plus placebo.[8] During the 5-year follow-up, gemfibrozil was associated with 34% fewer cardiac deaths and nonfatal MIs. The trial was not designed to assess all-cause mortality; however, concern was raised about more deaths from accidents and suicide in the treatment group. Before this study, the World Health Organization Clofibrate Trial[9] (1978) also raised concerns about nonspecific excess in mortality associated with clofibrate treatment, despite a 20% reduction in the coronary event rate. This adverse finding has not been borne out in more contemporary studies using gemfibrozil.

The first secondary prevention trial of gemfibrozil, the Veterans Affairs High-Density Lipoprotein Cholesterol Intervention Trial (VA-HIT) (1999), demonstrated that treatment was associated with a significant 24% reduction in risk of nonfatal MI, stroke, and CHD death in 2531 men with CHD whose primary lipid abnormality was a low high-density lipoprotein (HDL) cholesterol level.[10] At 1 year, the mean HDL-cholesterol level was 6% higher and the mean triglyceride level was 31% lower in the gemfibrozil group compared with placebo. This trial provided important evidence that raising HDL-cholesterol levels and lowering triglyceride levels without altering LDL-cholesterol levels reduced major cardiovascular events in men with CHD.

In contrast to these two gemfibrozil trials with positive results, two trials with other fibrates have yielded disappointing results. In the Bezafibrate Infarction Prevention (BIP) study[11] (2000), 3090 men with documented CHD were randomized to bezafibrate (400 mg/day) or placebo. Mean HDL-cholesterol level was 35 mg/dL, and mean LDL-cholesterol level was 149 mg/dL. In the active treatment group, LDL-cholesterol decreased by 7%, HDL-cholesterol increased by 18%, and triglycerides fell by 21%; however, the primary endpoint, MI or sudden death, was not significantly reduced during 6.2 years of follow-up (13.6% versus 15.0%; $P = .26$).

The Fenofibrate Intervention and Event Lowering in Diabetes (FIELD) study (2006) randomized 9795 patients with type 2 diabetes to fenofibrate (200 mg/day) or to placebo and observed them for 5 years.[12] The primary endpoint, CHD

CLASSIFICATION AND PROPERTIES OF PLASMA LIPOPROTEINS				
Lipoprotein Class	**Major Lipid Components**	**Apolipoproteins**	**Density (g/mL)**	**Electrophoretic Mobility**
Chylomicron	TG	A-I, A-II, A-IV, Cs, B-48, E	<0.95	Origin
Chylomicron remnant	CE, TG	B-48, E	<1.006	Origin
VLDL	TG	B-100, Cs, E	<1.006	Pre-beta
IDL	CE	B-100, Cs, E	1.006-1.019	Broad beta
LDL*	CE	B-100	1.019-1.063	Beta
HDL				
HDL2	CE, PL	A-I, A-II†	1.063-1.125	Alpha
HDL3	PL	A-I, A-II†	1.125-1.210	Alpha

*A usually minor but variable fraction of LDL is complexed to apolipoprotein(a) and constitutes a lipoprotein subclass termed lipoprotein(a).
†Minor apolipoproteins of HDL are C-I, C-II, C-III, A-IV, and D.
CE, cholesteryl ester; HDL, high-density lipoprotein; IDL, intermediate-density lipoprotein; LDL, low-density lipoprotein; PL, phospholipid; TG, triglyceride; VLDL, very-low-density lipoprotein.
From Gotto AM Jr, Pownall H. Manual of Lipid Disorders: Reducing the Risk for Coronary Heart Disease. Baltimore, Md, Williams & Wilkins, 1999.

Table 8.1 Classification and properties of plasma lipoproteins.

death or nonfatal MI, occurred in 5.2% of fenofibrate patients and 5.9% of placebo patients, a nonsignificant difference. A significant 24% reduction in nonfatal MI was counterbalanced by a nonsignificant 19% increase in CHD mortality.

Statin Trials: Primary Prevention

The effect of statin therapy on cardiovascular events has now been studied in numerous major randomized controlled trials, as summarized in Table 8.2. These trials cover a broad spectrum of patient populations. Six involved populations with no clinically evident CHD: the West of Scotland Coronary Prevention Study (WOSCOPS)[13] in hypercholesterolemic men, the Air Force/Texas Coronary Atherosclerosis Prevention Study (AFCAPS/TexCAPS)[14] in men and women with low HDL-cholesterol levels, the Anglo-Scandinavian Cardiac Outcomes Trial–Lipid Lowering Arm (ASCOT-LLA)[15] and the Antihypertensive and Lipid-Lowering Treatment to Prevent Heart Attack Trial (ALLHAT)[16] in subjects with hypertension, the Collaborative Atorvastatin Diabetes Study (CARDS)[17] in diabetics, and the Prospective Study of Pravastatin in the Elderly at Risk (PROSPER) study.[18]

Recently, results from the Justification for the Use of Statins in Prevention: an Intervention Trial Evaluating Rosuvastatin (JUPITER) demonstrated significant benefit with statin therapy in a population of 17,802 healthy individuals with low to moderate levels of LDL-cholesterol (≤130 mg/dL C-reactive protein and elevated (CRP, >2 mg/L).[18a] The trial included 38% women, and it compared the effects of 20 mg rosuvastatin vs. placebo on a combined primary end point of MI, hospitalization for unstable angina, and cardiovascular death. After a median follow-up of 1.9 years, the trial was stopped due to early evidence of efficacy. The treatment group demonstrated a 50% reduction in LDL-cholesterol and the mean level was near 50 mg/dL. This translated into a relative 44% reduction in the primary end point, 54% reduction in the risk for MI, 48% reduction in the risk for stroke, 47% reduction for revascularization or unstable angina, and 20% reduction for all-cause mortality. Benefit was consistent across all subgroups. The results from JUPITER suggest statins may be beneficial in the primary prevention in men over 50 years and women over 60 years that are at-risk.

In all but one of these primary prevention trials, the primary endpoint was significantly lower in the statin group compared with the placebo group. The one exception, ALLHAT, was impacted by a high crossover rate of placebo patients to unblinded statin therapy so that the difference in LDL-cholesterol levels between the pravastatin and placebo groups was only 17%. On the other hand, both the ASCOT-LLA and the CARDS trials were stopped early because of a statistically significant benefit in the atorvastatin groups compared with the placebo groups. In PROSPER, nearly half of the patients had a history of vascular disease at baseline. Although pravastatin significantly reduced events in the entire study population, the benefit was not statistically significant among patients with no history of vascular disease.

Although variation exists from one trial to another, in general, statin-treated patients were at lower risk not only for MI and cardiac death but also for other cardiovascular events, including unstable angina, coronary revascularization, and stroke. One of the early criticisms of cholesterol-lowering therapy was that it had no effect on total mortality. Even though total mortality tends to be quite low in primary prevention trials, it was significantly reduced the JUPITER trial.

The Heart Protection Study (2002) recruited 20,536 men and women at high risk because of either a history of CHD (secondary prevention) or risk factors (primary prevention).[19] Patients had to be 40 to 80 years old and to have a baseline total cholesterol level of only 135 mg/dL or greater. Patients were randomly assigned to placebo or simvastatin (40 mg/day) and were observed for 5 years. Compared with placebo, treatment with simvastatin was associated with significant reductions in all-cause mortality (13%), cardiovascular death (17%), stroke (25%), and major cardiovascular events (24% relative reduction, 5.4% absolute reduction). Importantly, the reduction in events was uniform across all patient groups, including women and patients up to the age of 80 years, and was not related to baseline LDL-cholesterol levels. Even among the 3421 patients whose baseline LDL-cholesterol level was less than 100 mg/dL, simvastatin reduced events, with a rate of 16.4% compared with 21.0% in the placebo group ($P = .0006$).

This result from the Heart Protection Study has shifted the target for statin therapy. Patients should be treated if they are at high risk, irrespective of their cholesterol level. Lowering of LDL-cholesterol, even when it is already within the average range, reduces events in patients at high risk. This approach was confirmed in ASCOT and CARDS, in which hypertensives and diabetics, respectively, experienced benefit irrespective of baseline cholesterol level.

Statin Trials: Stable Coronary Heart Disease

Five large randomized trials of statins have been completed in patients with stable CHD, as summarized in Table 8.2. The first of these (1994), the Scandinavian Simvastatin Survival Study (4S),[20] included 4444 patients with angina pectoris or previous MI and with total cholesterol levels between 212 and 309 mg/dL and triglycerides less than 220 mg/dL. Participants were randomized to simvastatin (20 or 40 mg/day) or placebo and observed for a median of 5.4 years. LDL-cholesterol was reduced by 35%. The primary endpoint, all-cause mortality, was reduced by 30% ($P = .0003$), major coronary events were reduced by 34%, and the need for revascularization was lowered by 37% with simvastatin relative to placebo.

In the CARE trial (1996), 4159 post-MI patients with average total and LDL-cholesterol levels of 209 mg/dL and 139 mg/dL, respectively, were randomized to pravastatin (40 mg/day) or to placebo.[21] During 5 years of follow-up, LDL-cholesterol levels were 28% lower in the pravastatin group, and the primary endpoint, nonfatal MI and CHD death, was reduced by 24% ($P = .003$). The Long-Term Intervention with Pravastatin in Ischaemic Disease (LIPID) trial[22] (1998) randomized 9014 men and women with CHD to pravastatin (40 mg/day) or to placebo and observed them for 6.1 years. Pravastatin reduced CHD mortality by 24%, overall mortality by 22%, MI by 29%, coronary revascularization by 20%, and stroke by 19%, with all of the differences being statistically significant.

In the Treating to New Targets (TNT) trial (2005), 10,001 patients with stable CHD were randomized to 10 or 80 mg/day of atorvastatin and observed for 4.9 years.[23] The study was designed so that patients receiving 10 mg would have a mean LDL-cholesterol level of 100 mg/dL and those

RANDOMIZED CONTROLLED TRIALS OF STATINS WITH CLINICAL ENDPOINTS

					LDL-Cholesterol						
Trial	**Year**	**Drug and Dose**	**Control**	**Patients**	**Follow-up (yr)**	**Therapy (mg/dL)**	**Control (mg/dL)**	**Difference (%)**	**Primary Endpoint**	**Event Rates (%), Therapy vs Control**	**HR (95% CI) *P* Value**
Primary prevention											
WOSCOPS (high LDL-C)	1995	Pravastatin, 40 mg	Placebo	6595 men	4.9	142	192	26	CHD death + MI	5.5 vs 7.9	0.69 (0.57-0.83) $P < .001$
AFCAPS/TexCAPS (low HDL-C)	1998	Lovastatin, 20-40 mg	Placebo	6605	5.2	115	156	26	CHD death, MI, or UA	6.8 vs 10.9	0.63 (0.50-0.79) $P < .001$
ASCOT-LLA (↑BP)	2003	Atorvastatin, 10 mg	Placebo	10,305	3.3	87	133	35	CHD death or MI	6.0 vs 9.4	0.64 (0.50-0.83) $P = .0005$
ALLHAT-LLT (↑BP)	2002	Pravastatin, 40 mg	Placebo	10,355	4.8	111	135	17	All-cause mortality	12.2 vs 12.4	0.99 (0.89-1.11) $P = .88$
CARDS (diabetes)	2004	Atorvastatin, 10 mg	Placebo	2838	3.9	72	120	40	CHD death, MI, UA, cardiac arrest, CABG, PCI, or stroke	5.8 vs 9.0	0.63 (0.48-0.83) $P < .001$
PROSPER (elderly)	2002	Pravastatin, 40 mg	Placebo	5804	3.2	107	147	27	CHD death, MI, or stroke	14.1 vs 16.2	0.85 (0.74-0.97 $P = .014$
JUPITER (hscRP72)	2003	Rosuvastatin	Placebo	17,802	1.9	55	110		MI, stroke revascularization VA, CVD death	0.77/100 person-y vs 1.36/100 person-y	0.56 (0.46-0.69) $P < .00001$
Stable CAD											
4S	1994	Simvastatin, 20-40 mg	Placebo	4444	5.4	122	188	36	Total mortality	8.2 vs 11.5	0.70 (0.58-0.85) $P = .0003$
CARE	1996	Pravastatin, 40 mg	Placebo	4159	5.0	97	125	28	CHD death or MI	10.2 vs 13.2	0.76 (0.64-0.91) $P = .003$
LIPID	1998	Pravastatin, 40 mg	Placebo	9014	6.1	113	150	25	CHD death	6.4 vs 8.3	0.76 (0.65-0.88) $P < .001$

TNT	2005	Atorvastatin, 80 mg	Atorvastatin, 10 mg	10,001	4.9	77	101	24	CHD death, MI, stroke, or cardiac arrest	8.7 vs 10.9	0.78 (0.69-0.89) $P = .0002$
IDEAL	2005	Atorvastatin, 80 mg	Simvastatin, 20 mg	8888	4.8	81	104	22	CHD death, MI, or cardiac arrest	9.3 vs 10.4	0.89 (0.78-1.01) $P = .07$
Post-ACS											
MIRACL	2001	Atorvastatin, 80 mg	Placebo	3086	16 weeks	72	135	40	Death, MI, cardiac arrest, UA → hospitalization	14.8 vs 17.4	0.84 (0.70-1.0) $P = .048$
PROVE-IT	2004	Atorvastatin, 80 mg	Pravastatin, 40 mg	4162	2.0	62	95	35	Death, MI, UA, PCI, CABG, or stroke	22.4 vs 26.3	0.84 (0.74-0.95)
A to Z	2004	High-dose simvastatin	Placebo → low dose	4497	2.0	Varied	Varied	Variable	CHD death, MI, ACS, or stroke	14.4 vs 16.7	0.89 (0.76-1.04) $P = .14$
Special populations											
Heart Protection Study (high risk)	2002	Simvastatin, 40 mg	Placebo	20,536	5.0	89	127	29	All-cause mortality	12.9 vs 14.7	0.82 (0.77-0.87) $P = .0003$
4D (diabetes + ESRD)	2005	Atorvastatin, 20 mg	Placebo	1255	4.0	72	120	41	All-cause mortality, MI, or stroke	37 vs 38	0.92 (0.77-1.10) $P = .37$
SPARCL (stroke)	2006	Atorvastatin, 80 mg	Placebo	4731	4.9	73	129	43	Stroke	11.2 vs 13.1	0.84 (0.71-0.99) $P = .03$
CORONA (heart failure)	2007	Rosuvastatin, 10 mg	Placebo	5011	2.7	76	136	45	All-cause mortality, MI, or stroke	11.4 vs 12.3	0.92 (0.83-1.02) $P = .12$

ACS, acute coronary syndrome; BP, blood pressure; CABG, coronary artery bypass grafting; CAD, coronary artery disease; CHD, coronary heart disease; ESRD, end-stage renal disease; HDL-C, high-density lipoprotein cholesterol; HR, hazard rate; LDL-C, low-density lipoprotein cholesterol; MI, myocardial infarction; PCI, percutaneous coronary intervention; UA, unstable angina.

Table 8.2 Randomized controlled trials of statins with clinical endpoints.

receiving 80 mg would have LDL-cholesterol in the range of 75 to 80 mg/dL. The primary endpoint, CHD death, MI, resuscitated cardiac arrest, or stroke, occurred in 8.7% of the group receiving 80 mg and 10.9% of the group receiving 10 mg, a relative risk reduction of 22% ($P < .001$).

The Incremental Decrease in End Points Through Aggressive Lipid Lowering (IDEAL) study (2005) randomized 8888 CHD patients to atorvastatin (80 mg) or to simvastatin (20 to 40 mg/day) and observed them for 4.8 years.[24] Mean LDL-cholesterol levels were 81 mg/dL in the atorvastatin group and 104 mg/dL in the simvastatin group. The primary endpoint, CHD death, MI, or resuscitated cardiac arrest, occurred in 9.3% of atorvastatin patients and 10.4% of simvastatin patients ($P = .07$). MI ($P = .02$), coronary revascularization ($P < .001$), and any CHD event ($P < .001$) were reduced in the atorvastatin group.[25]

The results of TNT and IDEAL indicate that in patients with stable CHD, lower LDL-cholesterol levels on treatment are associated with lower event rates, even below the LDL-cholesterol target of 100 mg/dL. In a post hoc analysis from TNT, patients were divided into quintiles according to LDL-cholesterol level on treatment.[26] Coronary events decreased with decreasing LDL-cholesterol quintiles, with the lowest rate in the lowest quintile, in which mean LDL-cholesterol level was 54 mg/dL, similar to the mean level achieved in the JUPITER trial.

Statin Trials: Acute Coronary Syndromes

The use of a statin in the period immediately after an acute coronary episode was evaluated in three large trials. The Myocardial Ischemia Reduction with Aggressive Cholesterol Lowering (MIRACL) study[26] (2001) randomly assigned 3086 patients to receive 16 weeks of treatment with atorvastatin (80 mg/day) or placebo starting 24 to 96 hours after hospital admission for unstable angina or non–Q wave acute MI. LDL-cholesterol levels at the end of the treatment period were 125 mg/dL in the placebo group and 72 mg/dL in the atorvastatin group. The composite primary endpoint (death, MI, resuscitated cardiac arrest, and worsening angina with new objective evidence of ischemia requiring hospitalization) occurred in 17.4% of the placebo group and 14.8% of the atorvastatin group ($P = .048$).

The Pravastatin or Atorvastatin Evaluation and Infection Therapy (PROVE-IT) trial (2004) randomized 4162 patients hospitalized with an acute coronary syndrome within 10 days to pravastatin (40 mg) or atorvastatin (80 mg/day).[27] LDL-cholesterol averaged 95 mg/dL in the pravastatin group and 62 mg/dL in the atorvastatin group. During a mean follow-up of 24 months, the primary composite endpoint (death, MI, stroke, unstable angina requiring hospitalization, and coronary revascularization) occurred in 26.3% of the pravastatin group and 22.4% of the atorvastatin group ($P = .005$).

In the Aggrastat to Zocor (A to Z) trial[28] (2004), 4497 patients stabilized after an acute coronary syndrome were randomized to simvastatin (40 mg increasing to 80 mg/day after 1 month) or to placebo for 4 months followed by simvastatin (20 mg/day). At 1 month, LDL-cholesterol levels were 68 mg/dL in the aggressively treated group compared with 122 mg/dL in the placebo group. The primary endpoint (cardiovascular death, MI, stroke, or readmission for an acute coronary syndrome) was reduced by 11% during the 2 years of follow-up, but the difference was not statistically significant ($P = .14$).

Other Statin Trials

As listed in Table 8.2, the utility of statins has also been assessed in special populations. The German Diabetes and Dialysis Study (4D) investigators (2005) randomized 1255 patients with diabetes and end-stage renal disease undergoing hemodialysis to atorvastatin (20 mg/day) or placebo and observed them for 4 years.[29] LDL-cholesterol levels were reduced by 42% in atorvastatin-treated patients, to a mean of 72 mg/dL. However, the primary composite endpoint (cardiac death, MI, or stroke) occurred in 37% of atorvastatin patients and 38% of placebo patients, a nonsignificant difference. All cardiac events combined were reduced by 18% in the atorvastatin group ($P = .03$), and there was a trend toward a lower all-cause mortality (20% versus 23%; $P = .08$).

The Stroke Prevention by Aggressive Reduction in Cholesterol Levels (SPARCL) trial (2006) included 4731 patients without known coronary disease but with a stroke or transient ischemic attack within 6 months, randomized to atorvastatin (80 mg/day) or to placebo.[30] LDL-cholesterol decreased by an average of 53% to 61 mg/dL in the atorvastatin group. During 4.9 years of follow-up, the primary endpoint, fatal or nonfatal stroke, occurred in 11.2% of patients in the atorvastatin group compared with 13.1% in the placebo group (adjusted $P = .03$), a 16% relative risk reduction. Despite the reduction in overall stroke, hemorrhagic stroke, although rare, occurred more frequently in the atorvastatin group. Major coronary events were reduced by 35% ($P = .003$). Thus, statins are indicated for secondary prevention of ischemic stroke, just as they are indicated for secondary prevention of coronary disease.

Patients with heart failure were either excluded or underrepresented in most of the major statin trials; yet experimental evidence from a variety of sources suggests that these drugs might be beneficial for this condition. The Controlled Rosuvastatin Multinational Trial in Heart Failure (CORONA)[31] (2007) included 5011 patients at least 60 years of age with systolic heart failure and coronary disease. They were randomized to rosuvastatin (10 mg/day) or to placebo and observed for a mean of nearly 3 years. The primary outcome (cardiovascular death, MI, or stroke) occurred in 11.4% of rosuvastatin patients and 12.3% of placebo patients, a nonsignificant reduction ($P = .12$). Total hospitalizations and hospitalizations for heart failure were significantly reduced in the rosuvastatin group.

Taken together, the results of the major statin trials provide conclusive evidence for cholesterol lowering in the prevention of clinical CVD in diverse populations, including patients at risk with average LDL-cholesterol levels. Overall, the statins were well tolerated. Although the absolute risk reduction is greater in the highest risk patients (e.g., 4S), statins have been shown to be cost-effective for both primary and secondary prevention.

GENERAL MANAGEMENT STRATEGIES

A key initial step in determining the appropriate therapy for hyperlipidemia is a comprehensive clinical evaluation to identify the lipid phenotype, to rule out secondary causes of dyslipidemia, and to assess overall CVD risk.

The screening examination should begin with a detailed medical history that documents any existing CVD, diabetes mellitus, or symptoms suggestive of ischemia. A thorough search for secondary causes of dyslipidemia, including lifestyle factors, is an important part of the evaluation of hyperlipidemia (Table 8.3). Numerous medications may have lipid-altering effects; therefore, information about prescription and nonprescription medications should be sought. A careful family history that focuses on family patterns of dyslipidemia and premature CVD is essential to establishing a diagnosis of primary hyperlipidemia.

The physical examination is an important element of the evaluation of hyperlipidemia. Assessment of cardiovascular status, including documentation of peripheral pulses, presence of bruits, blood pressure, height, weight, and abdominal girth, is a standard component of a targeted clinical evaluation. In addition, clinical manifestations of hyperlipidemia, especially the presence of xanthomas (commonly found in patients with familial hypercholesterolemia), can help establish a primary diagnosis. The examination should include an evaluation of conditions, such as thyroid abnormalities and other endocrine disorders, that predispose to dyslipidemia (see Table 8.3).

The laboratory evaluation should include an assessment of liver and thyroid function, a fasting blood glucose determination, estrogen status in women, and urinalysis to help rule out secondary causes of dyslipidemia. NCEP ATP III guidelines recommend obtaining a complete fasting lipoprotein profile once every 5 years for all adults 20 years or older, rather than screening for total cholesterol and HDL-cholesterol alone. (NCEP ATP III guidelines are available on-line at *http://www.nhlbi.nih.gov/guidelines/cholesterol/index.htm*). Included in the profile are total cholesterol, LDL-cholesterol, HDL-cholesterol, and triglycerides. LDL-cholesterol is the primary atherogenic lipoprotein and the most important measure for estimating lipoprotein-related risks for CVD. LDL-cholesterol levels are closely correlated with CHD risk from low to very high. According to the NCEP ATP III guidelines,[6] an LDL-cholesterol level below 100 mg/dL is optimal and levels of 160 mg/dL and above are high; LDL-cholesterol of 130 to 159 mg/dL is classified as borderline high. An update to the ATP III guidelines recommends an optional target LDL-cholesterol level of 70 mg/dL in the highest risk patients.[32] Triglycerides, which are also associated with increased CHD risk, are considered borderline high at levels of 150 to 199 mg/dL and high at levels of 200 mg/dL and above. Although a high HDL-cholesterol level (>60 mg/dL) is considered to be a negative risk factor that is protective against CHD, low HDL-cholesterol (<40 mg/dL) is also a CHD risk factor.[6]

The most recent European guidelines[33] were developed independently but are similar to the NCEP guidelines. They can be accessed at *http://www.guideline.gov/summary/summary.aspx?doc_id=4766*. They recommend that the 10-year risk of fatal CVD be assessed by the Systematic Coronary Risk Evaluation (SCORE) system, which is based on European epidemiologic data. Lifestyle changes are recommended for risk levels of 5% or greater, followed by drug therapy if risk remains at this level.

Studies and NCEP ATP III guidelines have suggested an additional measure, non–HDL-cholesterol, defined as the difference between total cholesterol and HDL-cholesterol levels. Unlike LDL-cholesterol, non–HDL-cholesterol reflects all atherogenic lipoproteins, including LDL, lipoprotein(a), intermediate-density lipoprotein, and very-low-density lipoprotein (VLDL) remnants. Preliminary research suggests that non–HDL-cholesterol level may be a somewhat better predictor of CVD mortality than the LDL-cholesterol level is.[34] The NCEP ATP III guidelines consider non–HDL-cholesterol to be a secondary target of therapy (after the primary target, LDL-cholesterol) in patients with elevated triglyceride levels (≥200 mg/dL).[6] Other emerging risk factors, such as total apolipoprotein B, lipoprotein(a), homocysteine, fibrinogen, and C-reactive protein, may also help guide risk-reduction therapy in certain patients.

Results of the fasting lipoprotein analysis may also be used to determine the lipid phenotype according to the Fredrickson classification (Table 8.4). This system is based on the patient's triglyceride and lipoprotein patterns, exclusive of HDL-cholesterol. Each lipid phenotype is associated with multiple genetic and secondary causes of dyslipidemia. The Fredrickson classification is useful to guide therapeutic decisions but does not establish a diagnosis of a specific lipid disorder.

Determination of a primary genetic lipid disorder may be useful for family counseling. Common primary lipid disorders encountered in clinical practice include polygenic

SELECTED CAUSES OF SECONDARY HYPERLIPIDEMIA	
Related to hypercholesterolemia	
Hypothyroidism	Dysglobulinemia
Nephrotic syndrome	Cushing's syndrome
Chronic liver disease (mainly primary biliary cirrhosis)	Hyperparathyroidism
Acute intermittent porphyria	
Related to hypertriglyceridemia	
Alcoholism	Hypothyroidism
Diabetes mellitus	Pancreatitis
Obesity	Dysglobulinemia
Estrogen use	Glycogen storage disease
Chronic renal failure	Lipodystrophy
Cushing's syndrome	Acute intermittent porphyria
Glucocorticoid use	Pregnancy
Beta-blocker use	Stress
Diuretic use	Uremia
Hypopituitarism	

From Gotto AM Jr. Lipid and lipoprotein disorders. In Pearson TA, ed. Primer in Preventive Cardiology. Dallas, Texas, American Heart Association, 1994:107-129.

Table 8.3 Selected causes of secondary hyperlipidemia.

FREDRICKSON CLASSIFICATION OF THE HYPERLIPIDEMIAS					
Phenotype	Lipoproteins Elevated	Result	Atherogenicity	Associated with Genetic Disorders	Selected Conditions Associated with Secondary Hyperlipidemia
I	Chylomicrons	Very high TG	?	Familial chylomicronemia (familial LPL deficiency, apoC-II deficiency)	Dysglobulinemia, pancreatitis, poorly controlled diabetes mellitus
IIa	LDL	Elevated cholesterol	+++	FH, FCH, polygenic hypercholesterolemia, familial defective apoB	Hypothyroidism, acute intermittent porphyria, nephrosis, idiopathic globulinemia, anorexia nervosa
IIb	LDL and VLDL	Elevated cholesterol and TG	+++	FH, FCH	Hypothyroidism, acute intermittent porphyria, nephrosis, idiopathic globulinemia, anorexia nervosa
III	IDL	Elevated cholesterol and TG	+++	Familial dysbetalipoproteinemia	Diabetes mellitus, hypothyroidism, dysglobulinemia
IV	VLDL	Elevated TG and normal to slightly elevated cholesterol	+	Familial endogenous hypertriglyceridemia, FCH	Glycogen storage disease, hypothyroidism, disseminated lupus erythematosus, diabetes mellitus, nephrotic syndrome, renal failure, ethanol abuse
V	VLDL and chylomicrons	Very high TG and normal to slightly elevated cholesterol	+	Familial mixed hypertriglyceridemia	Poorly controlled diabetes mellitus, glycogen storage disease, hypothyroidism, nephrotic syndrome, dysglobulinemia, pregnancy

apo, apolipoprotein; FCH, familial combined hyperlipidemia; FH, familial hypercholesterolemia; IDL, intermediate-density lipoprotein; LDL, low-density lipoprotein; LPL, lipoprotein lipase; TG, triglycerides; VLDL, very-low-density lipoprotein.
From Gotto AM Jr, Pownall H. Manual of Lipid Disorders: Reducing the Risk for Coronary Heart Disease. Baltimore, Md, Williams & Wilkins, 1999.

Table 8.4 Fredrickson classification of the hyperlipidemias.

hypercholesterolemia, familial hypercholesterolemia, familial combined hyperlipidemia, familial hypertriglyceridemia, type III hyperlipidemia (dysbetalipoproteinemia), and primary hypoalphalipoproteinemia (HDL-cholesterol ranges from 20 to 35 mg/dL). Not all low HDL-cholesterol syndromes resulting from genetic mutations are associated with an increased risk of premature CVD. For example, lecithin–cholesterol acyltransferase (LCAT) deficiency, fish eye disease (a rare form of LCAT deficiency), Tangier disease, and apoA1 variants seem to involve preserved functional reverse cholesterol transport and to confer no significant increase in CHD risk.

The approach to the patient with a secondary cause of dyslipidemia is to treat the underlying disorder or to remove the offending agent if possible. Examples of the latter are changing a patient with CHD from a nonselective beta blocker, which may decrease HDL-cholesterol by 10% to 20% and increase triglycerides by 15% to 30%, to a beta blocker with intrinsic sympathomimetic activity and less adverse effects on lipids and discontinuation of oral contraceptives in a woman presenting with severe hypertriglyceridemia.

Many people exhibit a cluster of metabolic risk factors and lifestyle factors that constitute a condition called the metabolic syndrome. Characteristic features are abdominal obesity, atherogenic dyslipidemia (elevated triglycerides, small LDL particles, low HDL-cholesterol), elevated blood pressure, insulin resistance (with or without glucose intolerance), and prothrombotic and proinflammatory states (Table 8.5).[35]

CLINICAL IDENTIFICATION OF THE METABOLIC SYNDROME	
Risk Factor	Defining Level
Abdominal obesity*	Waist circumference†
Men	>102 cm (>40 inches)
Women	>88 cm (>35 inches)
Triglycerides	≥150 mg/dL
High-density lipoprotein cholesterol	
Men	<40 mg/dL
Women	<50 mg/dL
Blood pressure	≥130/≥85 mm Hg
Fasting glucose	≥110 mg/dL

*Overweight and obesity are associated with insulin resistance and the metabolic syndrome. However, the presence of abdominal obesity is more highly correlated with the metabolic risk factors than is an elevated body mass index. Therefore, the simple measure of waist circumference is recommended to identify the body weight component of the metabolic syndrome.
†Some male patients can develop multiple metabolic risk factors when the waist circumference is only marginally increased, for example, 94 to 102 cm (37 to 40 inches). Such patients may have strong genetic contribution to insulin resistance, and they should benefit from changes in life habits, similar to men with categorical increases in waist circumference.
From Executive Summary of the Third Report of the National Cholesterol Education Program (NCEP) Expert Panel on Detection, Evaluation, and Treatment of High Blood Cholesterol in Adults (Adult Treatment Panel III). JAMA 2001;285:2486-2497.

Table 8.5 Clinical identification of the metabolic syndrome.

The presence of three or more of these cardiovascular risk factors is necessary for the diagnosis of the metabolic syndrome, according to current NCEP guidelines.[6] Nutrition and lifestyle approaches (weight reduction, increased physical activity) are the first-line therapy. However, drug treatment of dyslipidemia and hypertension is often necessary.[35] Most other secondary causes of dyslipidemia are also related to unhealthy lifestyle, which should be addressed in practice. All patients with dyslipidemia should be counseled on appropriate lifestyle interventions as described in the next section.

At present, there is increasing focus on primary prevention through the assessment of absolute risk—the estimated probability that a person with a certain set of characteristics will develop any particular disease within a fixed period.[6] Absolute global risk assessment reflects the synergistic effect of multiple risk factors and allows better prediction than a single factor. The NCEP ATP III guidelines use Framingham risk scores, developed for the Framingham Heart Study, to determine 10-year CHD risk. Risk factors included in the Framingham calculation are age, total cholesterol, HDL-cholesterol, systolic blood pressure, and cigarette smoking. The same risk factors, with the exception of HDL-cholesterol, are used in the European SCORE system. Treatment decisions may then be based on whether a patient is at low risk, moderate risk, or highest risk for CHD. However, the Framingham calculations exclude certain relevant factors, such as obesity, physical inactivity, evidence of subclinical disease (e.g., carotid artery stenosis on ultrasound examination), and family history of premature MI. These additional factors should be noted in the initial screening examination.

The NCEP ATP III has developed specific algorithms for initiation of diet and drug treatment, based primarily on the level of LDL-cholesterol and the number of other CVD risk factors that are present (Table 8.6). For patients with high triglycerides, non–HDL-cholesterol becomes a target of therapy. The goal for non–HDL-cholesterol in patients with hypertriglyceridemia in all three risk categories is 30 mg/dL higher than the corresponding goals for LDL-cholesterol.[6] In the United States, some persons at 10% to 20% risk are considered candidates for drug treatment if an adequate trial of diet and lifestyle therapy does not lower LDL-cholesterol to target levels. Individuals with established CVD and LDL-cholesterol levels exceeding 130 mg/dL may be started on drug therapy immediately. For patients with atherosclerotic disease and LDL-cholesterol levels in a more moderate range (100 to 130 mg/dL), a short trial (6 weeks) of lifestyle therapy may be reasonable.

Target LDL levels are based on the presence of CVD and the number of risk factors present. Diabetes is considered a CHD risk equivalent, according to the NCEP ATP III guidelines.[6] An LDL goal of less than 100 mg/dL may be appropriate in this population as well as in persons with CHD or other clinical forms of atherosclerotic disease, such as peripheral arterial disease. More recent clinical trial data have stimulated the NCEP to suggest the optional LDL-cholesterol target of 70 mg/dL in the highest risk patients with known atherosclerosis.[32] An LDL-cholesterol level below which further lowering does not produce additional risk reduction has not yet been identified.

LIFESTYLE APPROACHES TO HYPERLIPIDEMIA

Nutritional Therapy

Several dietary factors have been linked to the incidence of CHD, either through promotion of atherosclerosis or thrombosis or by protective mechanisms. This section is concerned with dietary factors that may influence the concentration, composition, or function of atherogenic lipids and lipoproteins. Following a description of specific nutritional factors and their role in lipid management, a summary of recommendations for other lifestyle interventions for lipid management is provided.

Total Fat and Saturated Fatty Acids

Consumption of total fat in populations is correlated with rates of mortality from CHD (Fig. 8.2).[36] Dietary therapy for hypercholesterolemia should focus on a reduction in fat intake, primarily saturated fat intake. The Seven Countries Study published more than 30 years ago by Keys[37] correlated population death rates from CVD with saturated fat intake. Since then, a wealth of epidemiologic and experimental data

NCEP ATP III LDL-CHOLESTEROL GOALS AND CUTPOINTS FOR THERAPEUTIC LIFESTYLE CHANGES AND DRUG THERAPY IN DIFFERENT RISK CATEGORIES

Risk Category	LDL-C Goal	LDL-C Level at Which to Initiate TLC	LDL-C Level at Which to Consider Drug Therapy
CHD or CHD risk equivalents (10-year risk >20%)	<100 mg/dL	≥100 mg/dL	≥130 mg/dL (100-129 mg/dL, drug optional*)
2+ risk factors (10-year risk ≤20%)	<130 mg/dL	≥130 mg/dL	10-year risk 10%-20%: ≥130 10-year risk <10%: ≥160
0-1 risk factor†	<160 mg/dL	≥160 mg/dL	≥190 mg/dL (160-189 mg/dL, drug optional)

*Some authorities recommend use of LDL-lowering drugs in this category if an LDL-cholesterol level below 100 mg/dL cannot be achieved by therapeutic lifestyle changes. Others prefer use of drugs that primarily modify triglycerides and high-density lipoprotein (e.g., nicotinic acid or a fibrate). Clinical judgment also may call for deferral of drug therapy in this subcategory.

†Almost all people with 0-1 risk factor have a 10-year risk of less than 10%; thus, 10-year risk assessment in people with 0-1 risk factor is not necessary.

CHD, coronary heart disease; LDL-C, low-density lipoprotein cholesterol; TLC, therapeutic lifestyle change.

From Executive Summary of the Third Report of the National Cholesterol Education Program (NCEP) Expert Panel on Detection, Evaluation, and Treatment of High Blood Cholesterol in Adults (Adult Treatment Panel III). JAMA 2001;285:2486-2497.

Table 8.6 NCEP ATP III LDL-cholesterol goals and cutpoints for therapeutic lifestyle changes and drug therapy in different risk categories.

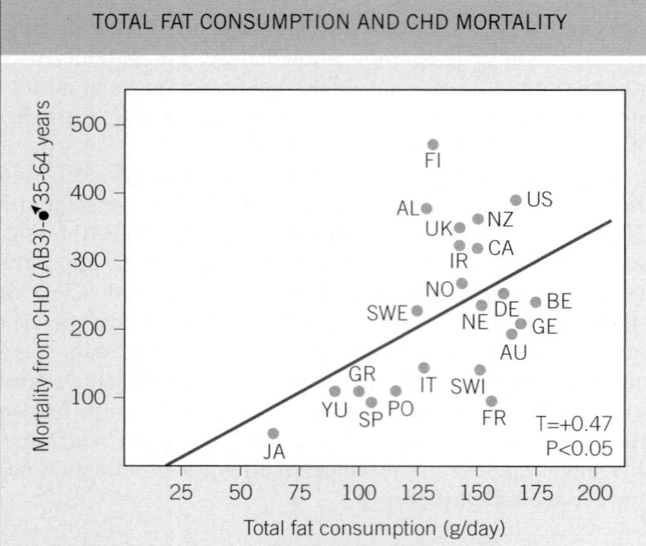

Figure 8.2 Correlation between total fat consumption and mortality from coronary heart disease (CHD). AL, Australia; AU, Austria; BE, Belgium; CA, Canada; DE, Denmark; FI, Finland; FR, France; GE, Germany (West); GR, Greece; IR, Ireland; IT, Italy; JA, Japan; NE, The Netherlands; NO, Norway; NZ, New Zealand; PO, Portugal; SP, Spain; SWE, Sweden; SWI, Switzerland; UK, United Kingdom; US, United States; YU, Yugoslavia. (From Turpeinen O. Effect of cholesterol-lowering diet on mortality from coronary heart disease and other causes. Circulation 1979;59:1-7.)

have shown that diets high in saturated fat are associated with elevated serum cholesterol levels, which in turn elevate coronary risk. Classic migration studies, such as the Ni-Hon-San study,[38] showed that Japanese living in the continental United States had a higher intake of fat than did Japanese living in Hawaii, whose fat intake was higher than that of those living in Japan. The gradient in fat intake corresponded with increased cholesterol levels and incidence of coronary disease. In countries in which fat intake has recently increased, such as Japan and Taiwan, there has been a corresponding increase in cholesterol levels.[39,40] Cardiovascular mortality rates may not necessarily correspond to shifts in dietary fat and population cholesterol levels because of advances in the treatment of CVD and the increased use of preventive therapies.

Dietary fat consists mainly of triglycerides, which are composed of three fatty acid molecules esterified to a glycerol backbone. The three basic types of fatty acid are saturated, monounsaturated, and polyunsaturated, with several subspecies, each having unique effects on lipid metabolism, depending on the number of carbon atoms and double bonds (Table 8.7).

The proportion of calories derived from saturated fat is a major determinant of serum cholesterol levels. For every 1% of calories consumed as saturated fat, there is an approximate 2.7 mg/dL increase in total cholesterol. Although it is generally agreed that saturated fat is the most significant dietary risk factor for CHD, not all saturated fatty acids in the diet have similar effects on cholesterol (see Table 8.7). Fatty acids range in chain length from 8 to 18 carbon atoms, with the longer chain fatty acids lauric acid (12:0), myristic acid (14:0), and palmitic acid (16:0) being associated with increased serum cholesterol levels. In contrast, those with 8 and 10 carbon atoms (medium-chain fatty acids) do not raise cholesterol. Stearic acid (18 carbons) also does not raise cholesterol levels, which explains why beef fat (high in stearic acid content) does not raise cholesterol levels to the same degree as butter fat (rich in myristic and palmitic acids).

INFLUENCE OF SPECIFIC NUTRIENTS ON SERUM LIPID AND LIPOPROTEIN LEVELS

	Serum Lipids and Lipoproteins			
Specific Nutrient	**Total Cholesterol**	**Triglycerides**	**LDL**	**HDL**
Dietary cholesterol	↑	–	↑↑	↑
Saturated fatty acids				
Palmitic acid	↑↑↑	–	↑↑↑	↑
Myristic acid	↑↑↑↑	–	↑↑↑↑	–
Lauric acid	↑↑	–	↑↑	–
Medium-chain fatty acids	↑	↑	↑	–
Stearic acid	–	–	–	–
Monounsaturated fatty acids				
Oleic acid	–	–	–	–
Trans fatty acids	↑↑	–	↑↑	↓
Polyunsaturated fatty acids				
Omega-6 (linolenic acid)	↓	↓	↓	↓
Omega-3 (EPA, DHA)	↓	↓↓↓	–	–
Carbohydrates	–	↑↑	–	↓↓

↑ increase (number of arrows indicates relative increase); ↓ decrease; – no change.
DHA, docosahexaenoic acid; EPA, eicosapentaenoic acid; HDL, high-density lipoprotein; LDL, low-density lipoprotein.
From Grundy M. Lipids, nutrition, and coronary heart disease. In Fuster V, Ross R, Topol EJ, eds. Atherosclerosis and Coronary Artery Disease. Philadelphia, Lippincott-Raven, 1996:45-68.

Table 8.7 Influence of specific nutrients on serum lipid and lipoprotein levels.

Mechanisms by which saturated fatty acids may raise cholesterol include suppression of the activity of LDL receptors and possibly enhanced secretion of apoB-containing lipoproteins.

Numerous studies have shown that a reduction in dietary saturated fatty acids is associated with lowering of plasma total cholesterol and LDL-cholesterol. The DELTA-1 study, a randomized crossover trial in 103 healthy adults, compared the impact of a typical American diet (34.3% kcal fat and 15% kcal saturated fat) with an American Heart Association (AHA) Step I diet (28.6% kcal fat and 9% kcal saturated fat) and a low–saturated fat diet (25.3% kcal fat and 6.1% kcal saturated fat) on plasma lipids and lipoproteins.[41] Plasma total cholesterol fell by 5% in the Step I diet group and by 9% in the low–saturated fat diet group compared with the typical American diet. Plasma LDL-cholesterol also fell 7% and 11% with the Step I diet and low–saturated fat diet, respectively. Stepwise reductions in cholesterol were similar for all subgroups, including men and premenopausal and postmenopausal women.

The Women's Health Initiative Randomized Controlled Dietary Trial was an attempt to demonstrate that dietary intervention could reduce the risk of CHD and stroke.[42] A total of 48,835 postmenopausal women aged 50 to 79 years were randomized to the intervention or control groups and observed for a mean of 8.1 years. The goal of intervention was to reduce fat intake to 20% of calories and to increase intakes of vegetables, fruit, and grain. By year 6, fat intake was reduced by 8.2% of energy intake in the intervention group compared with controls, and LDL-cholesterol levels and diastolic blood pressure were slightly lower as well. The diet had no significant effect on the incidence of CHD or stroke, although a trend toward less invasive breast cancer was seen in the low-fat group.[43] Although disappointing, this trial suggests that longer or more intensive interventions are required to reduce the incidence of CHD with a low-fat diet.

Very-low-fat diets (15% to 20% of calories from fat) may produce reductions in LDL-cholesterol by 10% to 20% over higher fat diets (35% to 40% of calories from fat). Whether these diets are associated with additional long-term cardiovascular benefits is not established.[44] The Lifestyle Heart Trial showed that among patients with established coronary disease, a 10% fat diet was associated with more coronary regression, fewer cardiovascular events, and a 72% reduction in angina after 5 years compared with a control group. However, the results were based on a small number of participants, and the intervention included other intensive lifestyle changes.[45] Concern has been raised about the nutritional adequacy of very-low-fat diets among vulnerable populations, such as pregnant women, children, and the elderly.[44] In clinical practice, very-low-fat diets may be a reasonable intervention in motivated patients, but they should be monitored closely.

There is significant individual variation in the response of total cholesterol and LDL-cholesterol levels to a reduction in saturated fat intake. The apoE4 allele has been associated with hyperresponsiveness; other predictors include baseline concentrations of apoB and triglycerides, plasma cholesteryl transferase activity, and polygenic factors.[46] Variation in dietary responsiveness is an important observation because many patients in clinical practice may have a much greater response to dietary intervention than what might be expected on the basis of the mean response observed in clinical trials.

Reduction in saturated fat intake is often associated with a decline in HDL-cholesterol levels. This occurs regardless of what nutrient replaces the saturated fat, although the greatest decline is associated with increased carbohydrate intake.[47] In the DELTA-1 trial described before, HDL-cholesterol fell by 7% when saturated fat intake was reduced from 15% to 9% of calories and by an additional 4% when intake was further reduced.[48] The reduction in HDL-cholesterol is associated with increased fractional clearance and decreased secretion of apoA1. Although low HDL-cholesterol in observational studies is predictive of coronary events, the clinical relevance of reduced HDL-cholesterol in response to a low-fat diet is not known. Consumption of a low-fat diet has been associated with increased lipoprotein-(a) levels, but the significance of this finding is also not known.[48] On the basis of the well-documented association between lower fat intake and lower LDL-cholesterol levels, it is prudent to recommend reduced saturated fat intake for all individuals, not just for patients with hypercholesterolemia. NCEP ATP III guidelines recommend that total fat intake should be restricted to 25% to 35% of total calories, with a reduction in intake of saturated fats to less than 7% of total calories and a reduction of cholesterol intake to less than 200 mg/day, in conjunction with weight reduction, increased physical activity, and other lifestyle changes. In addition, the latest AHA Dietary Guidelines emphasize consumption of a variety of foods, including fruits, vegetables, grains, fat-free and low-fat dairy products, fish, legumes, poultry, and lean meats, while limiting alcohol and foods high in saturated fat and cholesterol.[49]

Monounsaturated Fatty Acids

Unsaturated fatty acids include monounsaturated fatty acids and polyunsaturated fatty acids. The major monounsaturated fatty acid that occurs in the diet is oleic acid (omega-9, *cis*-18:1). Olive oil and canola oil are concentrated sources of monounsaturated fatty acids also found in other vegetable and animal products. Substitution of polyunsaturated or monounsaturated fatty acids for saturated fatty acids in the diet is associated with an LDL-cholesterol–lowering effect.[50] Studies that have compared the relative benefits of substituting either polyunsaturated or monounsaturated fatty acids for saturated fatty acids have yielded inconsistent results. One meta-analysis examined whether oils high in monounsaturated fatty acids versus polyunsaturated fatty acids had a differential effect on serum lipid levels and found that LDL-cholesterol and HDL-cholesterol levels were not different when oils were exchanged in the diet.[51] The DELTA study showed that HDL-cholesterol levels were reduced to a lesser degree with a high (22%) monounsaturated fatty acid diet than with an AHA Step I diet (15% monounsaturated fatty acids).[43] Lipoproteins derived from a monounsaturated fat diet may be less susceptible to oxidation, but the clinical relevance of this is not established. The Mediterranean diet, rich in monounsaturated fatty acids, has been associated with a lower risk of death and recurrent MI among survivors of first MI than in control subjects

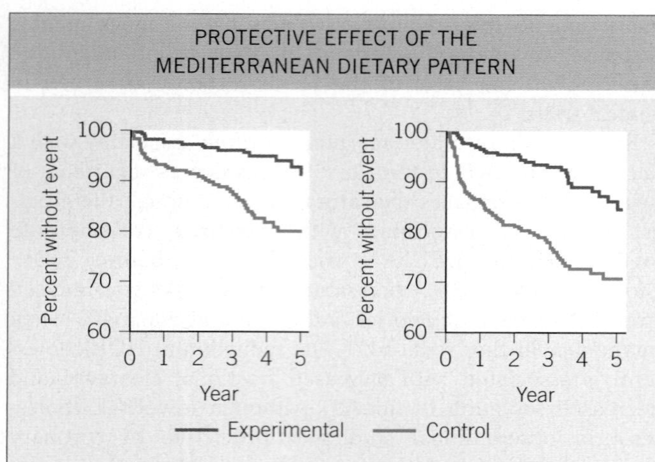

Figure 8.3 Protective effect of the Mediterranean dietary pattern on long-term survival after a first myocardial infarction. Cumulative survival without nonfatal myocardial infarction *(graph on left)* and without either nonfatal infarction or major secondary endpoints *(graph on right)* among experimental (Mediterranean diet) and control (prudent Western diet) subjects. (From de Lorgeril M, Salen P, Martin JL, Monjaud I, Delaye J, Mamelle N. Mediterranean diet, traditional risk factors, and the rate of cardiovascular complications after myocardial infarction: final report of the Lyon Diet Heart Study. Circulation 1999;99:779-785.)

consuming North American or northern European diets (Fig. 8.3).[52] Despite this, concerns have been raised that recommendations for higher fat monounsaturated fatty acid diets may contribute to obesity.

Trans *Fatty Acids*

Another type of monounsaturated fatty acid derived from the hydrogenation of polyunsaturated fats to produce margarine and shortenings is *trans* fatty acid. Oils rich in *cis* double bonds are generally liquid at room temperature because of a bent carbon chain interfering with packing of molecules and lowering the temperature at which crystallization occurs. Higher temperatures are required for crystallization; therefore, *trans* fatty acids are solid at room temperature, making them popular for use in prepared foods such as cookies, crackers, and commercially prepared fried foods.[49] Relative to oleic acid, *trans* monounsaturates raise LDL-cholesterol levels. They may also produce small increases in triglycerides and lipoprotein(a) and lower HDL levels and thus may be considered atherogenic. Epidemiologic studies have demonstrated a correlation between intake of *trans* fatty acids and increased risk of CHD.[53] Therefore, it may be prudent to limit the use of solid vegetable shortening and margarine until more definitive data are available.

Polyunsaturated Fatty Acids

The two major types of polyunsaturates are omega-6 and omega-3 acids. Linoleic acid (18:2) is the major type of omega-6 fatty acid. When linoleic acid replaces carbohydrate in the diet, total cholesterol will decrease approximately 1.4 mg/dL for each 1% decrease in calories from fat.[54] Linoleic acid is associated with increased oxidation, tumor promotion, and gallstones if it is consumed in large amounts, so intake should be limited to less than 10% of total calories.[40,54] α-Linolenic acid (18:3), found in soybean, flaxseed, rapeseed, and linseed oils and tofu, is the predominant omega-3 fatty acid. The Lyon Diet Heart Study reported that a Mediterranean diet rich in α-linolenic acid, in the setting of secondary prevention, was associated with a 70% reduction in all-cause mortality. The benefit was due to a reduction in CHD mortality and comparable reductions in nonfatal MI after 27 months of follow-up.[52] The protective effect of the diet was maintained for 4 years with remarkable adherence, suggesting that a Mediterranean-type diet is a feasible long-term intervention.

Fish oils contain the longer chain omega-3 fatty acids eicosapentaenoic acid and docosahexaenoic acid. Both eicosapentaenoic acid and docosahexaenoic acid can be synthesized from α-linolenic acid. The major lipid effect of fish oils is to decrease triglycerides by reducing secretion of VLDL (as much as 35%). Very high doses of fish oil may lower LDL-cholesterol, but to a lesser degree than triglycerides. Most epidemiologic studies have supported an association between fish oil intake and risk of CHD. The Diet and Reinfarction Trial (DART) demonstrated a 29% reduction in overall mortality among men with CVD who ate fatty fish twice a week.[55] The Gruppo Italiano per lo Studio della Sopravvivenza nell'Infarto Miocardico (GISSI)–Prevenzione study showed that supplementation with omega-3 polyunsaturated fatty acid, at a dose of 1 g/day, reduced the risk of death, nonfatal MI, and nonfatal stroke by 15% compared with placebo.[56] Potential cardioprotective mechanisms include antithrombotic and antiarrhythmic effects as well as reduced VLDL and triglycerides.

Dietary Cholesterol

The LDL-raising effect of dietary cholesterol is less than that of saturated fatty acids but is significant. Increases of dietary cholesterol of 100 mg/1000 kcal will raise the serum total cholesterol an average of 6 to 10 mg/dL; however, individual responses vary. Dietary cholesterol may increase the risk of CVD independently of its effect on lipids.[50] The AHA Step I and Step II diets recommend intakes of less than 300 and 200 mg/day, respectively. Egg yolks and organ meats are especially high in dietary cholesterol; therefore, limiting their intake can help reduce dietary cholesterol.

Carbohydrates and Fiber

Carbohydrates are either absorbable or nondigestible (fiber). Absorbable forms include simple sugars (monoglycerides and diglycerides) and complex carbohydrates (polysaccharides or starches). The influence of carbohydrate on lipid metabolism is not fully understood. Digestible carbohydrates have neutral effects on LDL-cholesterol. High-carbohydrate, low-fat diets are associated with reductions in both LDL and HDL levels. Increased consumption of sugars appears to increase triglyceride and to depress HDL levels, although the response is not always consistent. Physiologic mechanisms are not completely defined, but elevations in triglycerides appear to be independent of reductions in HDL-cholesterol. The clinical impact of diet-induced triglyceride and HDL changes is not known, but it may be advantageous to avoid high intake of simple carbohydrates.

Indigestible fiber has been shown to lower cholesterol levels, and the effect appears to be greater for soluble fiber than for insoluble fiber.[40] Soluble fiber includes gums, pectin, psyllium, guar gum, and oat bran. Food sources include fruits, vegetables, legumes, oats, and barley. Two or more servings of soluble fiber added to a Step I or Step II diet may lower LDL-cholesterol and total cholesterol levels by an additional 2% to 3%, with little effect on HDL-cholesterol.[50] Alternatively, adding 3 g of soluble fiber per day lowers cholesterol by approximately 5 to 6 mg/dL. Epidemiologic studies have demonstrated an inverse relation between fiber intake and risk of CHD. In one study, men in the highest quintile of dietary fiber intake (median, 28.9 g/day) had nearly a 40% reduced risk of CHD compared with men in the lowest quintile (12.4 g/day).[57] In addition to beneficial lipid effects, high fiber intake is associated with reduced blood pressure, increased insulin sensitivity, decreased factor VIIc, and enhanced weight control.[54] Some studies have shown that fiber supplements are associated with lower LDL levels; however, no long-term trials have demonstrated a relationship between use of fiber supplements and reduced CVD. Although AHA guidelines do not recommend fiber supplements for decreasing the risk of heart disease,[49] the newest NCEP ATP III guidelines recommend consumption of 10 to 25 g/day of soluble fiber.[6]

Soy and Phytochemicals

Soy protein is associated with a reduction in cholesterol when it is substituted for animal protein. Soy products are a major source of dietary protein for the Japanese, who have low rates of heart disease compared with those of cultures that consume higher amounts of animal protein. A meta-analysis of clinical trials of soy intake revealed that serum cholesterol was significantly lowered with intakes of 31 to 47 g of soy protein per day.[58] In general, the higher the level of cholesterol at baseline, the greater the reduction observed with soy. Among men and women with type II hypercholesterolemia, a textured soybean preparation reduced plasma cholesterol by 23% and 25%, respectively.[59] Recent double-blind, placebo-controlled trials showed that 20 to 50 g of soy protein daily significantly reduced LDL-cholesterol in mildly hypercholesterolemic persons.[60] Consumption of 25 g of soy protein per day can be expected to reduce serum cholesterol by approximately 9 mg/dL. The mechanisms responsible for lipid lowering are not established but may be related to bile acid or cholesterol absorption, glucagon or insulin levels, or hepatic cholesterol synthesis.[54]

Phytochemicals, such as the isoflavones genistein and daidzein found in soy, have weak estrogenic activity, which may help lower cholesterol.[50,61] The risk for CVD may be lowered by soy phytoestrogens through antioxidant properties and antiplatelet effects as well as lipid-lowering effects. In normal postmenopausal women, consumption of whole soy foods containing 60 mg/day of isoflavones significantly reduced total cholesterol/HDL-cholesterol ratios and other clinical risk factors for CVD and for osteoporosis.[62] Flaxseed, the richest food source of lignans, a major group of phytoestrogens, has also been shown to significantly lower both serum total cholesterol and non–HDL-cholesterol in postmenopausal women.[63] Garlic contains another phytosterol, tocotrienol, and is associated with improved cholesterol levels. Intermediate endpoint studies for soy and phytochemicals are promising, but long-term clinical endpoint data are not available.

Plant Sterols and Stanols

Plant sterols, including sitosterol, stigmasterol, and campesterol, have a structural resemblance to cholesterol and may inhibit absorption of both dietary and biliary cholesterol from the small intestine. Sitostanol is the saturated form of sitosterol and more effectively reduces serum cholesterol. In patients with mild hypercholesterolemia, intake of sitostanol ester margarine (1.8 g or 2.6 g of sitostanol per day) was associated with a 10.2% reduction in serum cholesterol, compared with a 0.1% increase in a control group after 1 year.[64] Because sitostanol is not absorbable, it is believed to be a safe, well-tolerated lipid-lowering agent and is available without a prescription in margarines. Additional, clinically significant reductions in serum cholesterol levels above what is obtained with a Step II diet alone have been demonstrated in hypercholesterolemic subjects using a low-fat, stanol ester–containing margarine.[65] In a randomized, double-blind, placebo-controlled clinical trial of men and women with elevated LDL-cholesterol and triglycerides on a stable regimen of statin therapy, consumption of a spread that provided 5.1 g/day of plant stanol esters significantly reduced elevated total and LDL-cholesterol levels.[66] The long-term impact of plant stanols and sterols on clinical CVD is not established; however, the NCEP ATP III guidelines recommend consumption of 2 g/day of plant stanols or sterols to enhance LDL lowering.[6]

Chinese Yeast

Consumption of red yeast rice, a dietary staple in many Asian countries that contains the statin-like substance monacolin K, has been shown to reduce cholesterol concentrations by approximately 20% in patients with hyperlipidemia in China.[67] In an American population consuming a Step I diet, total cholesterol and LDL levels were also significantly reduced by a red yeast rice supplement (2.4 g/day) compared with placebo after 8 weeks of treatment.[68] The long-term safety and efficacy of red yeast rice are not established, but it may be a reasonable adjunct and food-based approach to the patient with hypercholesterolemia.

Antioxidants

The oxidative modification of LDL is believed to be a key step in the pathogenesis of atherosclerosis.[69] Oxidized LDL is rapidly internalized by macrophages, leading to the formation of foam cells. Although many epidemiologic studies have shown an inverse correlation of CVD with intake of antioxidant nutrients, randomized clinical trials have been disappointing. In fact, a recent meta-analysis of 68 randomized trials involving 232,606 subjects suggested that beta-carotene, vitamin A, and vitamin E may actually increase overall mortality, with no benefit on cardiovascular endpoints.[70] Although the mechanism for this effect is not understood, it may be prudent to encourage intake of antioxidants from food sources rather than from supplements until further data are available. Diets that are rich in fruits and vegetables and therefore rich in antioxidant nutrients have been consistently associated with a reduced risk of CVD.

Alcohol

Moderate alcohol intake is associated with a reduced risk of CHD that is partly attributable to an HDL-raising effect.[71]

A J-shaped curve has been documented, with a protective effect observed for one or two drinks per day but an excess of CVD risk at three or more glasses per day. The adverse effects of heavier drinking that are observed at the population level may occur at more moderate levels of consumption in some individuals, particularly among women. Although epidemiologic studies support an association between alcohol intake and lower risk, these results are confounded by lifestyle, diet, and other cultural factors. The rate of CVD in France is significantly lower than that in many other countries in which lower quantities of fat are consumed, and this paradox may be due to increased intake of wine, especially red wine, among the French.

Nearly 80 experimental studies have evaluated the impact of alcohol on intermediate cardiovascular risk factors, including lipoproteins. Most prospective cohort studies do not support an association between type of alcoholic beverage, such as red wine, and lower cardiovascular risk. In epidemiologic studies, 45% to 55% of the protective effect of alcohol appears to be mediated through increased levels of HDL. The protective effect of alcohol that is not related to HDL-cholesterol is probably caused by its effects of decreasing fibrinogen, inhibiting platelet aggregation, and increasing tissue plasminogen activator secretion. The nonethanol effects of wine (e.g., polyphenol substances as antioxidants) that might provide additional benefit are theoretical; they are supported by canine models but are not definitively proved in humans. Because alcohol is an addictive substance, recommendations for its use to increase HDL levels and possibly to lower CHD risk should be weighed against the known adverse consequences of drinking. AHA guidelines do not recommend alcohol (or wine specifically) as a cardioprotective strategy.[72]

Exercise Therapy

Persons who engage in regular physical activity have lower rates of CHD, which may be mediated in part by the beneficial effects of exercise on lipoproteins. Physical activity is associated with increased levels of HDL-cholesterol, reduced concentrations of triglycerides and VLDL-cholesterol, and, in some patients, lowering of LDL-cholesterol.[73] The weight loss that may accompany increased exercise is probably a significant contributor to improved lipid profiles. Reductions in postprandial chylomicrons and triglycerides may result from an increase in lipoprotein lipase associated with exercise. The amount of exercise needed to improve lipoproteins is not firmly established, but it appears that high-intensity exercise is not necessary. The time frame and magnitude of change in HDL-cholesterol levels with physical activity vary by the baseline level of HDL and the age of the population studied. Physical activity has been shown to prevent the lowering of HDL-cholesterol that may result from a low-fat diet.[74] In a clinical trial of 180 postmenopausal women and 197 men with hypercholesterolemia, the combination of a Step II diet and an aerobic exercise program significantly reduced LDL-cholesterol by 14.5% in women and 20% in men, with no significant lipid changes observed with either diet or exercise alone.[75] These findings highlight the synergy between physical activity and nutritional approaches to management of hyperlipidemia.

Smoking Cessation Therapy

The adverse effects of smoking on cardiovascular health are well established. A dose-response relationship exists between the amount of smoking and increased concentrations of total cholesterol, LDL-cholesterol, VLDL-cholesterol, and triglycerides (Fig. 8.4). In addition, HDL-cholesterol and apoA1 levels are inversely related to cigarette consumption. Smoking increases small, dense LDL particles and may render them more susceptible to oxidation. Smoking may increase lipolysis by increasing circulating catecholamines, leading to increased concentrations of free fatty acids and enhanced VLDL secretion.

Smoking is a major preventable cause of CHD and dyslipidemia. Cessation of smoking is associated with a rapid reversal of its deleterious effects and should be a top priority in clinical practice. The role of the physician is critical in helping patients to quit. Complete cessation should be the primary goal; however, a reduction in intake is beneficial as a step toward that goal. At each visit, patients and family members should be counseled to stop smoking, or nonsmoking status should be reinforced. Smokers should be offered a formal cessation program that includes behavioral therapy in conjunction with nicotine replacement therapy or other pharmacotherapy as indicated.

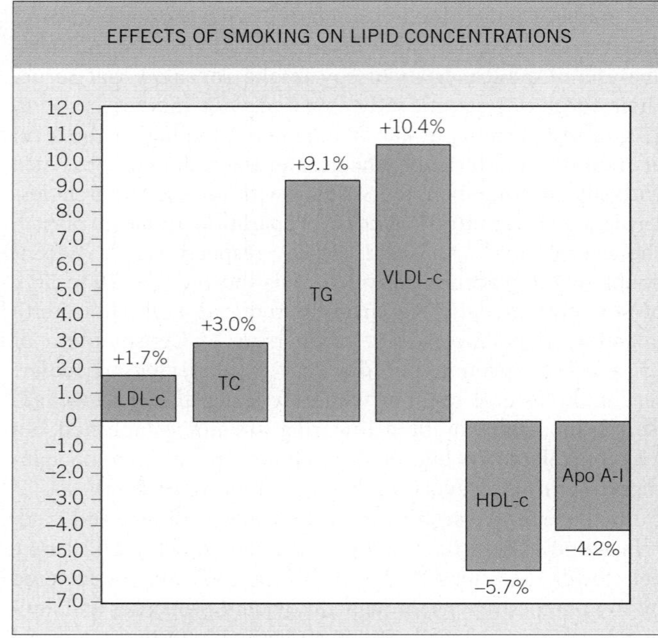

Figure 8.4 Effects of smoking on lipid concentrations, from a pooled analysis of 54 published studies. Effects in heavy smokers only were total cholesterol (TC), +4.5%; low-density lipoprotein cholesterol (LDL-c), +18.0%; very-low-density lipoprotein cholesterol (VLDL-c), +39.0%; high-density lipoprotein cholesterol (HDL-c), −8.9%; and apolipoprotein (apo) A-I, −5.7%. Increased triglycerides (TG) and decreased HDL-c are aspects of the insulin resistance syndrome, a syndrome that may play an important role in the high risk for death from cardiovascular disease among smokers. All values are $P < .001$ versus nonsmokers. (From Gotto AM Jr, Pownall H. Manual of Lipid Disorders: Reducing the Risk for Coronary Heart Disease. Baltimore, Md, Williams & Wilkins, 1999.)

PHARMACOTHERAPY FOR HYPERLIPIDEMIA

There are five classes of drug that are available to treat lipid disorders as an adjunct to lifestyle interventions (Table 8.8). These are

- statins (HMG-CoA reductase inhibitors);
- bile acid sequestrants (resins);
- fibric acid derivatives (fibrates);
- niacin (nicotinic acid); and
- cholesterol absorption inhibitors.

The decision about which class of agent to use depends on the lipid phenotype and the target lipid levels that need to be achieved in the patient. Drugs should be used when they not only ameliorate lipid levels but also have been shown to reduce events in clinical trials. Mechanisms of action, complications, and indications for each major antilipidemic drug class are described here.

Statins

The lipid-lowering effects of statins were discovered serendipitously by Endo and colleagues[76] in 1976. They were introduced into clinical practice in the late 1980s. As discussed earlier in this chapter, they have been shown to reduce coronary events and stroke in both primary and secondary prevention settings.

Mechanisms of Action

The primary action of statins is to lower the level of LDL-cholesterol. This hypolipidemic effect of statins is due to suppression of the biosynthesis of cholesterol. Hepatic cholesterol synthesis involves successive condensations of acetyl coenzyme A leading to the formation of 3-hydroxy-3-methylglutaryl coenzyme A (HMG-CoA), which is then reduced to mevalonate. The conversion to mevalonate is catalyzed by the enzyme HMG-CoA reductase and is a major rate-limiting step in cholesterol synthesis. Statins competitively inhibit HMG-CoA reductase and therefore reduce hepatic cholesterol synthesis. As a consequence, LDL receptor activity in the liver is up-regulated. This leads to lower LDL-cholesterol levels by promoting the direct uptake of LDL by the liver. Enhanced hepatic uptake of the precursors of LDL (VLDL and VLDL remnants) may also lower LDL levels by reducing the conversion of VLDL to LDL. Decreased hepatic production of VLDL and increased catabolism of VLDL remnants contribute to the triglyceride-lowering effect of statins.

Statins lower total and LDL-cholesterol in a dose-dependent manner (Table 8.9). A daily dose of 2.5 mg of rosuvastatin, 5 mg of atorvastatin, 10 mg of simvastatin, 20 mg of pravastatin or lovastatin, or 40 mg of fluvastatin is associated with an approximately 22% reduction in total cholesterol and a 27% lowering of LDL-cholesterol. (These doses of rosuvastatin and atorvastatin are below recommended starting doses.)

MECHANISMS OF ACTION AND LIPID-REGULATING EFFECTS OF THE FIVE AVAILABLE CLASSES OF LIPID-ALTERING DRUGS

Lipid-Regulating Agents	Mechanisms	Effects on Lipids
Bile acid sequestrants Cholestyramine Colestipol Colesevelam	↓Intrahepatic cholesterol by nonspecific binding of bile acids ↑Activity of LDL receptors	LDL-C ↓15%-30% HDL-C ↑3%-5% TG No change or ↑
Nicotinic acid	↓Production of VLDL ↓Mobilization of free fatty acids from peripheral adipocytes	LDL-C ↓5%-25% HDL-C ↑15%-35% TG ↓20%-50%
HMG-CoA reductase inhibitors Atorvastatin Fluvastatin Lovastatin Pravastatin Rosuvastatin Simvastatin	↓Cholesterol synthesis caused by partial inhibition of HMG-CoA reductase	LDL-C ↓18%-60% HDL-C ↑5%-15% TG ↓7%-37%
Fibric acid derivatives Bezafibrate Ciprofibrate Clofibrate Fenofibrate Gemfibrozil	↑Activity of lipoprotein lipase ↓Release of free fatty acids from peripheral adipose tissue	LDL-C ↓5%-20% with high LDL-C; may ↑ with high TG HDL-C ↑10%-20% TG ↓20%-50%
Cholesterol absorption inhibitors Ezetimibe	↓Intestinal absorption of cholesterol	LDL-C ↓18% HDL-C ↑1% TG ↓8%

HDL-C, high-density lipoprotein cholesterol; LDL, low-density lipoprotein; LDL-C, low-density lipoprotein cholesterol; TG, triglyceride; VLDL, very-low-density lipoprotein.

From Jones P, Gotto A. Special issues in the management of dyslipidemias. In Robinson K, ed. Preventive Cardiology: A Guide for Clinical Practice. Armonk, NY, Futura, 1998:142. Modified with data from Executive Summary of the Third Report of the National Cholesterol Education Program (NCEP) Expert Panel on Detection, Evaluation, and Treatment of High Blood Cholesterol in Adults (Adult Treatment Panel III). JAMA 2001;285:2486-2497; and Physicians' Desk Reference. Montvale, NJ, Thomson Medical Economics Company, 2002.

Table 8.8 Mechanisms of action and lipid-regulating effects of the five available classes of lipid-altering drugs.

COMPARATIVE EFFICACY OF FIVE STATIN DRUGS								
Statin Drug (mg)					Cholesterol Levels			
Atorvastatin	Simvastatin	Lovastatin	Pravastatin	Fluvastatin	Total	LDL	HDL	LE↑ >3× ULN
5*	10	20	20	40	22%↓	27%↓	↑	0.25%
10	20	40	40	80	27%↓	34%↓		0.50%
20	40	80			32%↓	41%↓	7%↑	1%
40	80				37%↓	48%↓		2%
80	160*				42%↓	55%↓	↓	2%

*Not an approved dose.
LE↑ >3× ULN, liver enzyme increase to more than three times the upper limit of normal. HDL, high-density lipoprotein; LDL, low-density lipoprotein.
From Roberts W. The rule of 5 and the rule of 7 in lipid-lowering by statin drugs. Am J Cardiol 1997;49:106-107.

Table 8.9 Comparative efficacy of the five currently available statin drugs.

Each doubling of the statin dose results in an additional 5% reduction in total cholesterol and 7% reduction in LDL-cholesterol. This pattern is referred to as the rule of 5 and rule of 7 in lipid lowering by statin drugs.[77] At higher doses of rosuvastatin (40 mg), atorvastatin (80 mg), and simvastatin (80 mg), reductions in LDL-cholesterol of up to 60% have been observed.[78,79] Reductions in LDL are accompanied by reductions in apolipoproteins B, C-II, C-III, and E.

Statins increase HDL-cholesterol levels by 5% to 15% and reduce triglyceride levels by 7% to 37% in patients without hypertriglyceridemia, but responses are variable.[6,78,79] Differential effects on HDL-cholesterol have been observed, but it is not known whether these translate to different effects on clinical outcomes. In patients with severe hypertriglyceridemia, the triglyceride-lowering effect of statins is magnified and can be in the range of 50% with a high dose of a potent statin. Comparisons of lipid-lowering effects among the statins are not always standardized because of differences in the populations studied, the doses of drugs used, and variations in the baseline levels of lipids.

The beneficial effect of statins on cardiovascular events have been attributed to several mechanisms other than lipid lowering (Table 8.10).[80] Statins may prevent thrombosis, inhibit platelet adhesion and activation, and improve the rheologic profile. They have been shown to reverse endothelial dysfunction, most probably through direct effects on endothelial vasoactive factors, endothelin 1, and nitric oxide. Moreover, statins may inhibit the production of inflammatory cytokines involved in monocyte adhesion, chemotaxis, and metalloproteinase secretion. An alternative explanation is that these beneficial effects are a consequence of cholesterol lowering.

The statins are generally most effective when they are given in the evening because the rate of endogenous cholesterol synthesis is highest at night. Atorvastatin and pravastatin, however, can be taken any time of day without affecting efficacy. Food has little effect on the absorption of statins, except for pravastatin, which should be taken on an empty stomach, and lovastatin, which is better absorbed when it is taken with meals. Pregnant women should not take statins because of possible teratogenic effects. Women of childbearing age should use reliable methods of contraception if they are prescribed statins. Persons with hepatic disease should avoid statins or be given lower than standard doses.

Complications

Clinical trial data and postmarketing surveillance data for statins support an excellent safety record. Adverse effects may range from mild gastrointestinal complaints to rare cases of rhabdomyolysis. Approximately 1% of persons taking HMG-CoA reductase inhibitors experience an elevation in serum hepatic transaminases to more than three times the upper limit of normal. These changes are usually transient, even when the drug is continued, and are rarely associated with clinical consequences. Symptoms of hepatitis may rarely occur and resemble those of an influenza-like syndrome. A clinical indication that such an adverse effect has occurred is that the levels of LDL-cholesterol and HDL-cholesterol may be much lower than expected with treatment. Symptoms tend to resolve, and increases in hepatic enzymes tend to return to normal on removal of the drug. Mild elevations in aminotransferases (less than twice normal) do not usually require cessation of drug therapy. Liver enzymes may rise in the setting of alcohol abuse, and statins should be used with caution in this situation. Liver function tests should be performed before initiation of therapy, at 2 to 12 weeks after the start of therapy, and after increases in dosage. Liver enzymes almost never increase after the first few months of therapy unless the drug dose has been increased or a concomitant condition has arisen.

The spectrum of myopathic syndromes that may occur with statin therapy includes myalgia (muscle aches and tenderness), myositis (pain and muscle weakness with malaise or fever and elevated creatine kinase), and rhabdomyolysis (severe myositis that may lead to acute renal failure).[81] An increased risk of myopathy is associated with concomitant use of fibrates, nicotinic acid, erythromycin, protease inhibitors, and cyclosporine.[82] Simvastatin is more myopathic than other available statins at higher doses, and it is contraindicated at the 40- and 80-mg dose in combination with a fibrate. Cerivastatin was withdrawn from the market in August 2001 because of its myotoxicity after 52 deaths from rhabdomyolysis had been recorded worldwide.[83] A U.S. Food and Drug Administration review showed that many deaths occurred in patients who received very high doses or who also received gemfibrozil, a combination that had been contraindicated. The rate of fatal rhabdomyolysis associated with

MECHANISMS OF ACTION OF STATINS OTHER THAN LIPID LOWERING

Antiatherosclerotic Properties of Statins

Statin	Endothelial Dilatation	LDL Oxidation Resistance	VSMC Proliferation	VSMC Apoptosis
Lovastatin	↑	↑	↓	↑
Pravastatin	↑	↑	Neutral	Neutral
Simvastatin	↑, neutral	↑	↓	↑
Fluvastatin		NA	↓	↑
Atorvastatin	NA	NA	↓	↑

Anti-inflammatory Properties of Statins

	Mononuclear Cell Functions			Proinflammatory Cytokine Production				
Statin	**Endothelial Adhesion**	**Chemotaxis**	**Metalloproteinase Secretion**	**TNF-α**	**IL-1β**	**IL-6**	**IL-8**	**MCP-1**
Lovastatin	↓	↓	NA	↑	↑	NA	↑	↑,⁻
Pravastatin	NA	NA	Neutral	↓, neutral	Neutral	↓	Neutral	Neutral
Simvastatin	↓	NA	↓	↑	↑	NA	↑	↑
Fluvastatin	NA	NA	↓	NA	NA	NA	NA	NA
Atorvastatin	↓	↓	NA	↑	↑	NA	↑	↑

Antithrombotic Properties of Statins

				Fibrinolysis			
Statin	**TF**	**TFPI**	**Platelet Aggregation**	**Fibrinogen**	**Plasma Viscosity**	**PAI-1**	**Lp(a)**
Lovastatin	NA	NA	↑	↑, neutral	↓, neutral	↓, Neutral	↑
Pravastatin	Neutral	Neutral	↓	↓, neutral	↓	↓	↑
Simvastatin	↓	↑	Neutral	Neutral	Neutral	↑	↑
Fluvastatin	↓	↑	NA	Neutral	NA	NA	↑
Atorvastatin	NA	NA	NA	↑	NA	NA	↑

↑ increase; ↓ decrease; IL, interleukin; LDL, low-density lipoprotein; Lp(a), lipoprotein(a); MCP-1, monocyte chemoattractant protein 1; NA, not available; PAI-1, plasminogen activator inhibitor 1; TF, tissue factor; TFPI, tissue factor pathway inhibitor; TNF-α, tumor necrosis factor α; VSMC, vascular smooth muscle cell.
From Rosenson R. Non–lipid-lowering effects of statins on atherosclerosis. Curr Cardiol Rep 1999;1:225-232. © Current Science Inc.

Table 8.10 Mechanisms of action of statins other than lipid lowering.

cerivastatin therapy was 10 to 50 times higher than the rates associated with the other statins, which reaffirms that current statin therapy is very safe.[84]

Indications

The HMG-CoA reductase inhibitors are indicated to treat several types of hyperlipidemia, including types IIa, IIb, and III (dysbetalipoproteinemia), in conjunction with a lifestyle program. They are the agents of choice in patients with heterozygous familial hypercholesterolemia and other forms of primary hypercholesterolemia, such as familial combined hyperlipidemia and polygenic hypercholesterolemia. Statins are effective therapy in patients with mild to moderate hypercholesterolemia who have other risk factors for CVD. They are also indicated in patients with mixed hyperlipidemia, diabetic dyslipidemia, remnant removal disease (familial dysbetalipoproteinemia), and the nephrotic syndrome.

The demonstration in recent clinical trials that statins decrease risk irrespective of baseline LDL-cholesterol levels has made this class of drugs a treatment for elevated risk, not just elevated cholesterol levels. Thus, statins are indicated for patients with atherosclerosis without a contraindication as well as for patients at equivalent risk, such as diabetics. As the safety of long-term statin use becomes better established, and as the cost of statin therapy decreases with increased availability of generic statins, the indications for statin treatment are likely to continue to broaden.

Bile Acid Sequestrants

Three bile acid sequestrants, cholestyramine, colestipol, and colesevelam, are available for clinical use. Cholestyramine (4 to 8 g) is mixed with a suspension of juice or water and taken before meals two or three times a day up to a maximum of 24 g. It may also be mixed with puréed fruit. Colestipol (5 to 10 mg) may be taken in a similar manner or as a 1-mg tablet. Colesevelam, a polymeric, high-potency, water-absorbing hydrogel, is formulated as a tablet and so does not need to be mixed with liquid.[85] The recommended dosing is

6 tablets once daily or 3 tablets twice a day (total daily dose, 1.95 g). Bile acid sequestrants are often used as an adjunct to statin therapy or as a second-line agent in individuals who do not tolerate statins. Both cholestyramine and colestipol reduce the absorption of vitamin D and other fat-soluble vitamins. They bind polar compounds such as digoxin, warfarin, thiazide diuretics, beta blockers, thyroid preparations, and statins. Because of this, other medications should be taken at least 1 hour before or 4 hours after the bile acid sequestrants are taken.

Mechanism of Action

Normally, almost 98% of bile acids that enter the small intestine are reabsorbed in the ileum and return to the liver through the portal vein to be cleared in their first pass through the liver. They are resecreted into bile to complete the enterohepatic circulation. Resins bind to bile acids in the small intestine and prevent their absorption. Thus, they interrupt the enterohepatic circulation of bile acids, which increases the conversion of cholesterol into bile acids in the liver as a result of loss of feedback inhibition. The hypocholesterolemic effect of resin therapy is due to enhanced LDL receptor activity on the surface of the liver. This leads to increased clearance of LDL from plasma and promotes the clearance of VLDL and VLDL remnants, which decreases the conversion of VLDL to LDL. However, reduced cholesterol content of hepatic cells stimulates a compensatory increase in cholesterol synthesis. This in turn increases the secretion of VLDL into the circulation and explains why resin therapy may be associated with increased concentrations of triglycerides. A marked increase in triglycerides may occur in patients with a tendency toward hypertriglyceridemia; in severe cases, resins should be avoided.

Typical responses to monotherapy with bile acid sequestrants are reductions in LDL-cholesterol in the range of 15% to 30%, no change or slight increases in triglycerides (10% to 15%), and increases in HDL-cholesterol of 3% to 5%. The mechanism for the increase in HDL levels is not established.

Complications

Bile acid sequestrants are not absorbed systemically; therefore, their side effects are generally limited to the gastrointestinal tract. The advantage of nonabsorption makes bile acid sequestrants a good option for women with moderate hypercholesterolemia who are in their childbearing years. Constipation, fullness, and gas are most frequently associated with use, occurring in 30% of patients. Symptoms are worse at higher doses and can often be avoided by gradually increasing the dose of resin. If constipation persists, it can be treated by increasing the daily intake of water and foods with wheat fiber or by adding psyllium or prune juice to the diet. Dosage reduction may be indicated if symptoms do not resolve. Studies suggest that colesevelam lacks the constipating effect seen with the other bile acid sequestrants; however, it appears to reduce intestinal absorption of beta-carotene.[85] As previously mentioned, resins may interfere with the absorption of other drugs, and levels of some medications may need to be monitored. Prothrombin times may be altered in patients receiving anticoagulant therapy.

Indications

The primary indication for resin therapy is for use in combination with statin therapy to reduce LDL-cholesterol levels. For example, in one study of 94 hypercholesterolemic men and women, coadministered colesevelam and atorvastatin produced additive LDL-cholesterol reductions comparable to those observed with maximum atorvastatin dosage, and notably, triglyceride levels were not negatively affected by colesevelam alone or in combination.[86] Bile acid sequestrants may be first-line therapy in patients with mild hypercholesterolemia who are not able to tolerate statin therapy or for patients who desire a nonsystemic agent, such as women of childbearing potential. They are less effective in the setting of mixed hyperlipidemia.

Fibric Acid Derivatives

Several fibrates are available for clinical use, including gemfibrozil, bezafibrate, ciprofibrate, and fenofibrate. Gemfibrozil is widely used in combination with a lifestyle approach to lower levels of triglycerides. It is typically given as one 600-mg tablet twice daily, 30 minutes before the morning and evening meals. In contrast, fenofibrate should be given with meals. It is commonly dosed at 160 mg/day in patients with primary hypercholesterolemia or mixed hyperlipidemia and at 54 to 160 mg/day in patients with hypertriglyceridemia. In addition to their primary action of reducing serum triglycerides, fibrates increase serum HDL-cholesterol and, to a lesser extent, lower LDL-cholesterol.

Mechanism of Action

Several different mechanisms are postulated for the lipid-altering effects of fibrates. They appear to enhance the oxidation of fatty acids in liver and muscle, increase the activity of lipoprotein lipase, enhance the catabolism of LDL-cholesterol, and reduce the rate of VLDL synthesis. These effects result in reductions in LDL-cholesterol and serum triglyceride levels. The extent of reduction in total and LDL-cholesterol levels in response to fibrate therapy depends on initial levels but is in the range of 5% to 20%. Triglycerides may be lowered by between 20% and 50%. Fibric acid derivatives also raise HDL-cholesterol levels by 10% to 20%, but the precise mechanism for this effect is not completely understood. Concentrations of the major apolipoproteins (A-I and A-II) found in HDL have been shown to increase in response to gemfibrozil treatment. Fibrates have been shown to increase the buoyancy of LDL particles, but the clinical significance of this effect is not established.

Complications

The fibrates are generally well tolerated. The major side effects reported with their use are gastrointestinal complaints (nausea, abdominal and epigastric pain). Because fibrates increase biliary cholesterol concentrations, they may be associated with an increased incidence of gallstones. Their use is contraindicated in persons with severe renal or hepatic disease.[6] Other adverse effects that have been reported include erectile dysfunction in men using clofibrate, increased serum transaminases, and myositis in patients with impaired renal dysfunction. A reduction in the dose of warfarin by as much as 30% may be necessary because fibrates displace it from albumin-binding sites. As previously mentioned, the use of statins, particularly simvastatin, in conjunction with fibric acid derivatives may increase the risk of myositis and rhabdomyolysis.

Indications

Fibrates are clearly indicated in patients with type V hyperlipoproteinemia and triglyceride levels above 1000 mg/dL to prevent acute pancreatitis. They are also used in patients with type IV and IIb mixed hyperlipidemia. Less commonly, they may be given to patients with type IIa hyperlipidemia when other agents are not tolerated. They are also used in patients with hypoalphalipoproteinemia who are at increased risk of CVD because of other lipid abnormalities or concomitant risk factors.

Niacin (Nicotinic Acid)

Niacin (nicotinic acid) is a water-soluble B vitamin that has beneficial effects on several lipid parameters when it is given in pharmacologic doses (1 to 6 g/day). It is the most effective agent to increase levels of HDL-cholesterol. Niacin is available in a crystalline form or as timed-release formulations (e.g., Niaspan). The slow-release formulations are associated with a lower incidence of cutaneous flushing and itching, a frequent side effect of niacin, but they may have a greater incidence of hepatotoxicity. Studies indicate that immediate-release, intermediate-release, and extended-release, once-a-day prescription forms of niacin are essentially equivalent in their efficacy in reducing triglycerides and increasing HDL-cholesterol.[87] Niacin is taken with a large glass of water at mealtimes while avoiding hot beverages to help avoid flushing. It is suggested that prolonged exposure to the sun be avoided and that sun protection be used in conjunction with niacin.

Mechanism of Action

Niacin inhibits the mobilization of free fatty acids from peripheral tissues to the liver, an effect that reduces hepatic synthesis of triglycerides and secretion of VLDL. Reductions in triglycerides observed with niacin are similar to those obtained with fibric acid derivatives (20% to 50%) and partly depend on the formulation (Fig. 8.5). The conversion of VLDL to LDL is also inhibited by niacin, thereby lowering LDL-cholesterol levels by 5% to 25%. The amount of total and LDL-cholesterol lowering depends on initial serum triglyceride levels, with smaller decreases observed for patients with the highest initial levels of triglycerides. Reduction in LDL-cholesterol may also result from increased clearance of VLDL remnants and decreased synthesis of LDL-cholesterol. Levels of HDL-cholesterol may be increased up to 35% with niacin and may be secondary to a decrease in VLDL triglyceride concentrations. In addition, niacin has been shown to lower levels of lipoprotein(a) and may cause a shift in LDL particle size from small, dense particles to the less atherogenic large, buoyant type.

Complications

Cutaneous flushing mediated by prostaglandins is a common side effect of niacin that can be prevented by administration of aspirin (325 mg) 30 to 60 minutes before each dose during the initial week of therapy. Tolerance to flushing generally develops after several days. This side effect may also be minimized by gradually increasing the dose of niacin during several weeks to months.

Other dermatologic side effects include itching, rash, and acanthosis nigricans. In addition to hepatotoxicity, adverse gastrointestinal effects associated with niacin use are epigastric distress and activation of peptic ulcer disease and chronic bowel disease. Glucose intolerance is reported with niacin; therefore, the drug should be avoided or used with caution in patients with diabetes. In addition, hyperuricemia, cardiac arrhythmias, and toxic amblyopia have been reported with niacin.

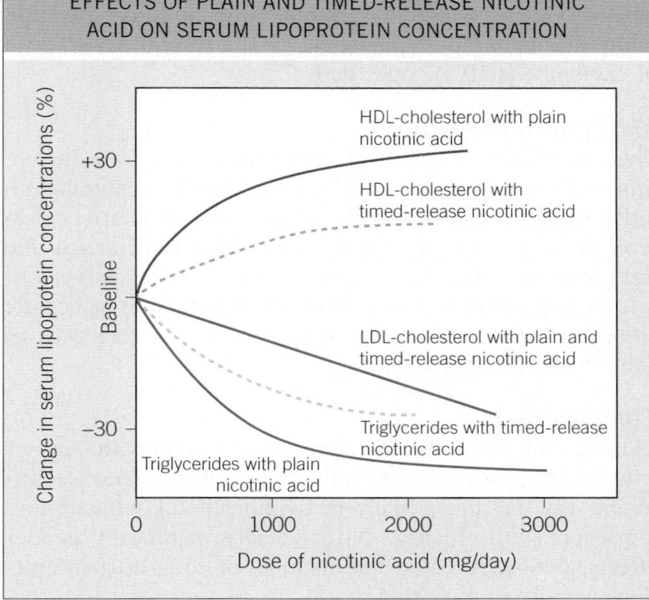

Figure 8.5 Effects of plain and timed-release nicotinic acid on serum lipoprotein concentration. HDL, high-density lipoprotein; LDL, low-density lipoprotein. (From Knopp RH. Drug treatment of lipid disorders. N Engl J Med 1999;341:498-511. © Massachusetts Medical Society.)

Indications

Niacin is indicated for patients with mixed lipid disorders, often in conjunction with a statin. It may be used in patients with primary hypercholesterolemia; however, high doses (>3000 mg/day) are often necessary to achieve a significant LDL-lowering effect. Niacin is also an option in patients with modest elevations in LDL and in those with non-LDL lipid disorders. Although niacin may raise HDL levels in patients with primary hypoalphalipoproteinemia, the clinical significance of raising an isolated low HDL-cholesterol concentration remains unknown. The effect of niacin on cardiovascular events is currently being evaluated in two large randomized clinical trials.

Cholesterol Absorption Inhibitors

A new category of agents, the selective cholesterol absorption inhibitors, directly block the absorption of cholesterol by the small intestine. Ezetimibe is the first such agent to be approved for clinical use. Ezetimibe has shown clinical benefits when it is used as monotherapy and in combination with other lipid-modifying agents.[88] The recommended dose of ezetimibe is 10 mg once daily.[88]

Mechanism of Action

The mechanism of action of ezetimibe differs from that of other classes of cholesterol-lowering drugs. Ezetimibe inhibits the intestinal absorption of dietary and biliary cholesterol by impeding the transport of cholesterol across the intestinal wall. This leads to a decrease in the delivery of intestinal cholesterol to the liver and a reduction of hepatic cholesterol stores, resulting in an increase in clearance of cholesterol from the blood.

Complications

Clinical trials of ezetimibe (administered as monotherapy or with a statin) showed that ezetimibe was well tolerated. Ezetimibe can be taken with or without food without any impairment in efficacy. No clinically significant gender effects, P450 3A4 drug interactions, or drug-drug interactions have been identified.[88]

Indications

Ezetimibe is indicated as adjunctive therapy to diet for the reduction of elevated total cholesterol, LDL-cholesterol, and apoB in patients with primary (heterozygous familial and nonfamilial) hypercholesterolemia. Ezetimibe, administered in combination with a statin, is indicated as adjunctive therapy to diet for the reduction of elevated total cholesterol, LDL-cholesterol, and apoB in patients with primary (heterozygous familial and nonfamilial) hypercholesterolemia.[88]

Concerns have recently been raised about ezetimibe, both with respect to efficacy and safety. The addition of ezetimibe to simvastatin failed to have a beneficial effect on carotid intima-media thickness change in a clinical trial of patients with familial hypercholesterolemia.[89] In another trial,[90] cancer and cancer-related mortality were significantly increased in patients in the ezetimibe treatment group.[91]

Estrogen and Selective Estrogen Receptor Modulators

Despite some beneficial effects on lipid levels, combination hormone replacement therapy (i.e., estrogen given in combination with a progestin) does not appear to be a viable option for CVD prevention. Data from the Heart and Estrogen/Progestin Replacement Study Follow-up (HERS II), a randomized, blinded, placebo-controlled clinical trial of estrogen combined with medroxyprogesterone acetate, found that long-term (6.8 years) use of hormone replacement therapy did not reduce the risk of cardiovascular events in postmenopausal women with CHD.[92] Furthermore, the Women's Health Initiative, a randomized trial of conjugated equine estrogen and medroxyprogesterone acetate in 16,000 healthy postmenopausal women, revealed a higher risk of CHD, stroke, pulmonary embolism, and invasive breast cancer in the active treatment group.[93] The estrogen-only arm of the trial showed no cardiovascular benefit but an increased risk of stroke.[94]

Selective estrogen receptor modulators (SERMs) are a potential alternative to estrogen therapy in postmenopausal women. SERMs bind to estrogen receptors and produce beneficial estrogen-like effects on bone and on lipoprotein metabolism. However, like estrogen, SERMS are associated with increased risk of deep venous thrombosis, and they increase the incidence of hot flushes.[95] The Raloxifene Use for the Heart (RUTH) study randomized 10,101 postmenopausal women at high risk for CHD to raloxifene or placebo and observed them for a median of 5.6 years.[96] Raloxifene had no significant effect on coronary events, the co-primary endpoint, but invasive breast cancers and vertebral fractures were reduced, at the cost of an increase in venous thromboembolism and fatal stroke.

Indications

On the basis of findings from the HERS and the Women's Health Initiative studies, the initiation or continuation of hormone therapy for the purpose of prevention of CHD is not recommended, despite its beneficial effects on lipids.[97] Based on the results of the RUTH study, raloxifene is also not recommended for CHD prevention.

THERAPY FOR REFRACTORY HYPERLIPIDEMIA

In patients with refractory hyperlipidemia, LDL plasmapheresis can be an effective therapeutic modality. Patients with CHD who have LDL-cholesterol levels above 200 mg/dL (or above 300 mg/dL if there is no CHD) despite maximal lifestyle and drug therapy may be considered candidates for plasmapheresis. Several systems that remove apoB-containing lipoproteins from the blood, including heparin precipitation and models that use immunoabsorption or dextran sulfate cellulose columns, are available. A single treatment may reduce LDL-cholesterol by up to 150 mg/dL and lipoprotein(a) levels by 50%. Side effects associated with therapy include hypotension, nausea and vomiting, and flushing. Major limitations to the use of LDL apheresis include cost and inconvenience. Ex vivo gene therapy has reportedly been successful in a small number of patients with familial hypercholesterolemia.

SUMMARY

Therapy for hyperlipidemia has been shown to reduce all-cause mortality and major cardiovascular events. It is associated with few adverse effects and is cost-effective. Appropriate management of lipids begins with a clinical assessment to identify any underlying causes of dyslipidemia. Once a diagnosis is established, lifestyle therapy should be prescribed for all patients. Pharmacotherapy is an increasingly important adjunct to dietary approaches to hyperlipidemia for both primary and secondary prevention of cardiovascular events. Statins have been proved to reduce events for high-risk patients even with average or low LDL-cholesterol levels. The initiation of drug therapy and aggressiveness of treatment depend on the presence of CVD or risk factors for CHD. Selection of a specific drug therapy depends on the lipid phenotype and the need to minimize side effects and costs. Underuse of lipid-altering therapy in high-risk patients has been documented worldwide.

chapter 9 Special Problems in Hyperlipidemia Therapy

a. Child with Hypercholesterolemia

Warren W. Davis and W. Virgil Brown

DEFINITION OF PROBLEM

Children with two defective genes for the low-density lipoprotein (LDL) receptor develop severe familial hypercholesterolemia with LDL-cholesterol concentrations in plasma between 500 and 1000 mg/dL. In these children, severe arteriosclerotic lesions are evident histologically, causing coronary events in the first decade of life. Raised complex lesions appear in the second and early third decades in children with heterozygous familial hypercholesterolemia; the LDL-cholesterol level is usually between 200 and 300 mg/dL. In very young adults with only moderately elevated LDL-cholesterol (130 to 200 mg/dL) and other risk factors such as smoking and low concentration of high-density lipoprotein (HDL) cholesterol, lesions may be obvious in the late teens and 20s. These pathologic studies have made it clear that risk factors are operative early in life. The severity of the lesions correlates with these risk factors, and these findings raise important questions about the current lack of more systematic programs to evaluate and to prevent vascular disease in children (Figs. 9A.1 and 9A.2). Most of these questions are only being formulated and need more studies to demonstrate benefit. What we do know is that vascular disease begins early in life and is accelerated by the classic risk factors.

CASE PRESENTATION

During the preschool physical for a healthy-appearing 12-year-old girl, the pediatrician notes small nodules in her calcaneal tendons consistent with tendon xanthomas. All other physical findings are within normal limits. There is a family history of myocardial infarction in the maternal grandfather at age 48 years and sudden death at age 51 years. He did not smoke cigarettes and was not diabetic. As a result, the pediatrician requests determination of plasma cholesterol and HDL-cholesterol concentrations, which return as 352 mg/dL and 54 mg/dL, respectively. The child, a younger brother, and both parents return after a 12-hour fast for a complete lipoprotein analysis. The father and brother are within normal limits. The mother's LDL-cholesterol is 290 mg/dL. The patient's total plasma cholesterol level is now 344 mg/dL; triglycerides are 90 mg/dL, HDL-cholesterol is 55 mg/dL, and LDL-cholesterol is 271 mg/dL. There is no evidence of endocrine, renal, or liver dysfunction.

DIFFERENTIAL DIAGNOSIS

The findings in this child and the family are typical of heterozygous familial hypercholesterolemia. The maternal grandfather almost certainly had elevated LDL-cholesterol in the same range as now seen in the patient and her mother. It is not totally clear as to the impact of other risk factors because the family is not aware of his blood pressure or HDL-cholesterol level.

His clinical event at age 48 years is a clear warning to the 37-year-old mother, who was previously unaware of her hypercholesterolemia. It is important to plan dietary change for this family that is effective for both mother and daughter and that respects the lifestyle choices of the father and brother. This requires some thought and planning best done in collaboration with a registered dietitian. The reduction of the daily intake of cholesterol to less than 100 mg and of the saturated fat to less than 7% of calories is feasible. This may require the child to become vegetarian at home, leaving the cholesterol and saturated fat intake for meals outside the home to make socialization easier for this 12-year-old. The mother would need to adopt a similar approach to her daily habits. Because the mother is probably 15 years away from entering a high-risk period for acute coronary events, monitoring the effect of these lifestyle changes on lipoprotein concentrations for several months is useful. Some patients are remarkably dietary responsive; others are resistant. The patient may show a significant fall in LDL-cholesterol of 20% to 40% with dietary change. Children usually are more diet responsive than adults are. The experiment should be done thoroughly before medications are considered because the period of treatment will be long, and the true benefit of any drug regimen should be judged against a background of the most effective diet. Avoidance of other risk is imperative. Cigarette smoking should be avoided absolutely. The body weight should be controlled. An annual physical examination with careful monitoring of blood pressure should be part of the plan.

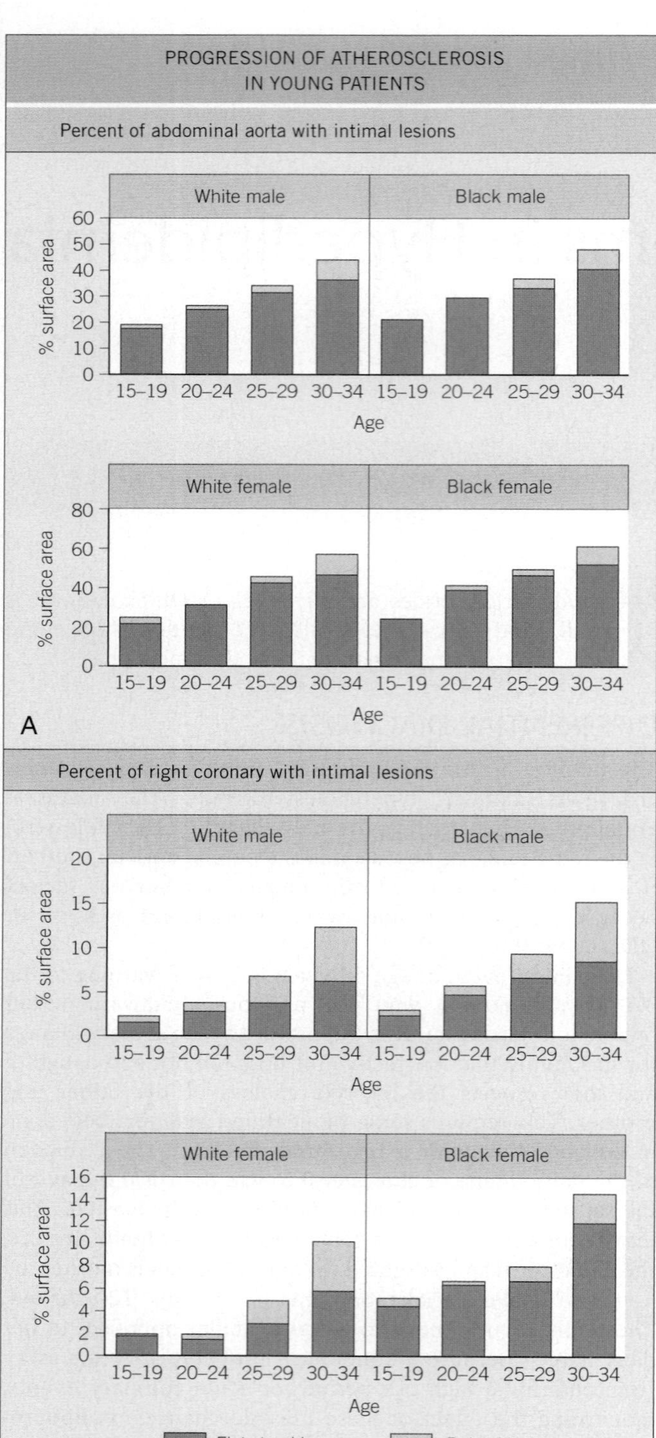

Figure 9A.1 **Progression of atherosclerosis in young patients.** The Pathobiological Determinants of Atherosclerosis in Youth (PDAY) study demonstrated that young persons in the United States have demonstrable vascular disease that increases with age. Blood vessels analyzed from postmortem specimens provide data on the distribution of fatty streaks as well as raised and more complicated arteriosclerotic lesions. **A,** The percentage of the aortic surface involved with intimal lesions was seen to increase with each 5-year interval. **B,** A similar increase was seen in the coronary arteries. (From Strong JP, Malcom GT, McMahan CA, et al. Prevalence and extent of atherosclerosis in adolescents and young adults: implications for prevention from the Pathobiological Determinants of Atherosclerosis in Youth Study. JAMA 1999;281:727-735.)

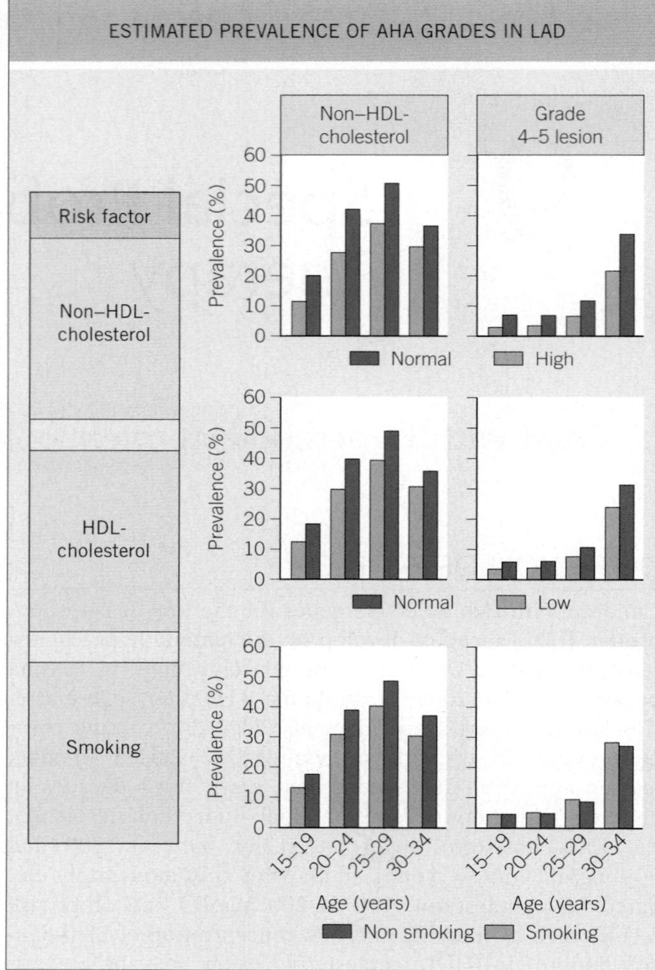

Figure 9A.2 Estimated prevalence of American Heart Association (AHA) grades in left anterior descending coronary artery (LAD). Estimated prevalence of AHA grades in LAD by high versus normal non–HDL-cholesterol concentration *(top);* low versus normal HDL-cholesterol concentration *(middle);* smoking versus nonsmoking status *(bottom);* and 5-year age group, adjusted for race, sex, and other risk factors. (From McGill HC Jr, McMahan CA, Zieske AW, et al. Association of coronary heart disease risk factors with microscopic qualities of coronary atherosclerosis in youth. Circulation 2000;102:374-379.)

The goal for the mother is to reduce her LDL-cholesterol to well below 160 mg/dL if no other risk factors are evident. At the time of her menopause, this goal can be reconsidered with new evidence from clinical trials accruing during this 10- to 15-year period and with consideration of new drugs available at that time. In the interval, statin or bile acid resin therapy would be indicated to achieve and to maintain the LDL-cholesterol goal.

The patient's risk will be affected positively by the dietary change, and if no other risk factors are added, it is unlikely that coronary artery disease will appear for several decades. However, moderate reduction for many years is far better than marked reduction after vascular disease is manifested. The opportunities for definitive treatment will certainly expand during this interval. If the LDL-cholesterol remains above 190 mg/dL on diet, adding small doses of bile acid sequestrants (cholestyramine or colestipol) before dinner often provides a 20% reduction or more. Some children are motivated and will sustain this regimen for years. Use of the encapsulated resin (1 g/tablet) may prove easier for many children. Taking three to five of these before the major meal at home is effective. Constipation is minimal at this dose. Because both cholestyramine and colestipol can bind other drugs, preventing their absorption, any needed medications should be taken at least 1 hour before or 4 hours after the resin dose. The use of colesevelam as the bile acid sequestrant may also improve compliance. Statins have been used clinically for more than 20 years, and multiple studies in children indicate that they are safe. They do not affect growth, and adverse effects do not appear any more frequent than in adult populations. Pravastatin has been given the indication for treatment in children by the Food and Drug Administration. Therefore, patients with elevations of LDL-cholesterol or with other risk factors, including a family history of very early clinical events, can be treated with pravastatin. For the severely involved child with LDL-cholesterol above 300 mg/dL, other statins or more than one drug may be needed. Cholesterol absorption may be reduced with the drug ezetimibe. In view of the minimal systemic absorption and minimal side effects that have been noted to date, this should be considered because it will provide a 20% further reduction when it is combined with a statin.

SUMMARY

This case illustrates the astute pediatrician's recognizing clues as to the existence of hypercholesterolemia in a family on the basis of both physical findings and family history. The first and most important result is the identification of an adult woman (mother of the patient) who is in clear need of medical management to reduce the risk of cardiovascular disease. Furthermore, the environment is altered, which can possibly alter the child's long-term risk at relatively little cost. Of most importance to the child is the awareness and development of a sensible lifestyle that involves monitoring for risk factors as she grows into adulthood and, it is hoped, into a long and healthful life with the benefits of current drugs and of future knowledge. For these children with severe hypercholesterolemia, management in a specialized lipid clinic is advised.

b. Transplant Patient

Warren W. Davis and W. Virgil Brown

DEFINITION OF PROBLEM

The probability of clinical events related to arteriosclerosis is significantly higher in post-transplantation patients compared with those with similar risk factors but no transplanted organs. Although not all reasons for this accelerated vascular disease are known, high blood pressure and diabetes contribute, and many patients undergoing organ transplantation will develop hyperlipidemia. The drugs that are used to suppress the immune system have significant effects on these risk factors, including lipid metabolism, and make management of the hyperlipidemia difficult. Furthermore, the potential for serious drug interactions between the immunosuppressive drugs and the drugs used to lower lipids increases the difficulty. Treatment objectives include prevention of coronary, cerebral, and peripheral arteriosclerosis as well as vascular disease in the transplanted organ. The prolonged survival after organ transplantation in many patients has made this objective of the utmost importance. Furthermore, the vascular changes in the transplanted organ that have been associated with chronic rejection have many of the characteristics of arteriosclerosis, such as lipid deposition and foam cells. Infiltration of the artery wall with T cells and the other manifestations of an inflammatory process, including the release of cytokines, may be part of the rejection process. Significant clinical disease in the transplanted organ can be evident as soon as 1 year after transplantation. Elevated lipoproteins may play a role in this accelerated disease, and lipid-lowering drugs have reduced the incidence of this problem.

TYPICAL CASE

A 42-year-old man presents 6 months after renal transplantation. He currently has no evidence of organ rejection, and the renal function is good with a blood urea nitrogen concentration of 18 mg/dL and creatinine concentration of 1.4 mg/dL. He was discovered to have albuminuria in his teens, diagnosed as chronic glomerulonephritis. During the subsequent years, the urinary protein concentration had been measured at 2 to 4 g/day, the serum albumin concentration was between 2.5 and 3.0 g/dL, and the cholesterol and triglyceride levels had remained between 250 and 300 mg/dL. This nephrotic syndrome was treated by diet only. Elevated blood pressure had been controlled by lisinopril. End-stage renal disease required hemodialysis at the age of 39 years. His current medications are lisinopril, 10 mg; azathioprine, 100 mg daily; cyclosporine, 400 mg daily; and prednisone, 10 mg daily.

A lipoprotein analysis immediately before the current visit revealed total cholesterol, 280 mg/dL; triglycerides, 325 mg/dL; high-density lipoprotein (HDL) cholesterol, 31 mg/dL; low-density lipoprotein (LDL) cholesterol, 184 mg/dL; and lipoprotein(a), 78 mg/dL.

DIFFERENTIAL DIAGNOSIS

After full recovery from surgery, all risk factors should be evaluated. This includes measurements of total cholesterol, HDL-cholesterol, LDL-cholesterol, triglycerides, and lipoprotein(a). Secondary causes of elevated lipids, such as liver disease, nephrotic syndrome, and hypothyroidism, need to be eliminated. Inadequate control of diabetes can also be a factor. The presence of hyperlipidemia related to the renal disease before the transplantation will be common, but genetic causes of lipid elevations may also be operative. The use of cyclosporine or tacrolimus (FK 506) is associated with the significant abnormalities in lipids, including elevated cholesterol and triglycerides. In addition, higher doses of steroids are also a factor in aggravating the elevation of triglycerides and cholesterol. Lipoprotein(a) tends to rise significantly in some patients and may confer additional risk.

TREATMENT OPTIONS

Treatment should include evaluation of diet and exercise patterns and prescription of important changes. Loss of excess adipose tissue can have profound effects on triglyceride concentrations and to a lesser extent on LDL-cholesterol. One may also achieve a rise in HDL and a drop in blood pressure. An American Heart Association Step II diet is recommended. Additional saturated fat and cholesterol restriction may be possible with the help of a dietitian. High blood pressure needs to be treated and in this patient may have been aggravated by immunosuppressive therapy.

Many patients will still have unacceptable levels of cholesterol and triglycerides after these interventions. The LDL-cholesterol goal of less than 130 mg/dL should be set and appropriate drug therapy prescribed after dietary effects have been evaluated for 8 to 12 weeks. Triglycerides should be reduced below 200 mg/dL. If hypercholesterolemia is the main abnormality, treatment with a statin drug can be started. Tacrolimus causes less severe alterations in lipid values than cyclosporine does, and the use of tacrolimus can be considered when lipid changes are prominent. Pravastatin in doses of 20 to 80 mg has a theoretical advantage because its metabolism does not involve the cytochrome P450 system (Fig. 9B.1). Cyclosporine and many other drugs are powerful competitive inhibitors of this system (specifically the 3A4 enzyme) and may cause accumulation of several members of the statin class of drugs. In addition, reduced rejection and improved survival have been demonstrated with pravastatin in heart transplant patients compared with those given no statin therapy (Figs. 9B.2 and 9B.3). Other statins may prove effective but low doses should be used, and careful monitoring of aspartate transaminase and alanine transaminase is recommended to guard against liver and muscle dysfunction. Theoretically, full doses of fluvastatin or rosuvastatin could be used because they are not metabolized by the 3A4 isoenzyme of the P450 system. However, the clearance of rosuvastatin by the liver is inhibited by cyclosporine, which interferes with uptake of this drug from the plasma space. Bile acid

EFFECT OF PRAVASTATIN ON CHOLESTEROL IN HEART TRANSPLANT PATIENTS

Figure 9B.1 Effect of pravastatin on cholesterol in heart transplant patients. Heart transplant patients assigned randomly to pravastatin (40 mg/day) maintained much lower mean cholesterol levels than did those treated with placebo during 12 months. (From Kobashigawa JA, Kasiske BL. Hyperlipidemia in solid organ transplantation. Transplantation 1997;63:331-338.)

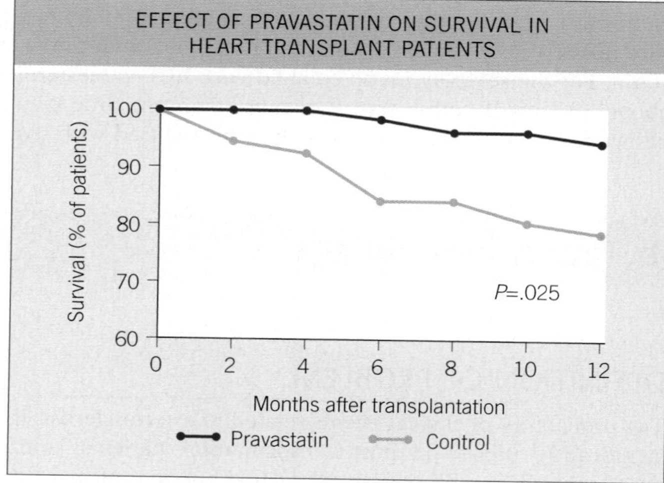

Figure 9B.2 Effect of pravastatin on survival in heart transplant patients. The pravastatin-treated patients experienced a significant improvement in survival. (From Kobashigawa JA, Kasiske BL. Hyperlipidemia in solid organ transplantation. Transplantation 1997;63:331-338.)

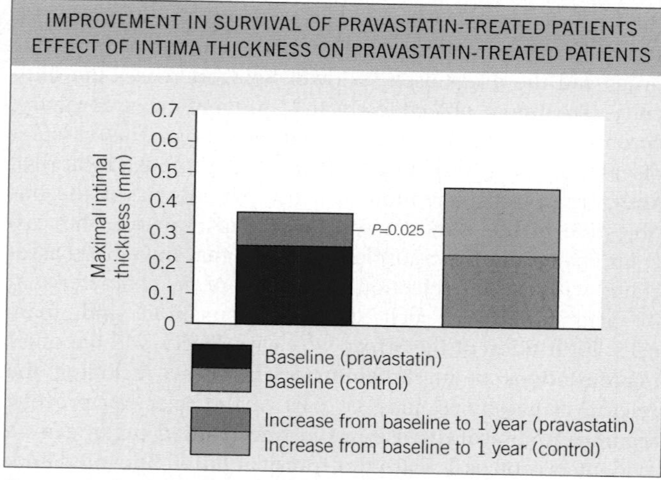

Figure 9B.3 Effect of pravastatin on intimal thickness. The major difference in survival of pravastatin-treated patients (see Fig. 9B.2) appeared to be secondary to reduced proliferative change in the intima of their coronary arteries. (From Kobashigawa JA, Kasiske BL. Hyperlipidemia in solid organ transplantation. Transplantation 1997;63:331-338.)

sequestrants or the cholesterol absorption inhibitor ezetimibe can also be combined with a statin to achieve further reduction in LDL-cholesterol. Timing of the dose of bile acid sequestrants is critical to prevent inhibition of absorption of other drugs that are critical in management of the transplant patient.

Fibric acid derivatives might also be used when triglyceride levels remain high. Pravastatin or fluvastatin might be combined with these agents in severely hyperlipidemic patients. Education of the patient and monitoring are doubly necessary in these patients because drug combinations may increase the incidence of rhabdomyolysis or liver dysfunction.

SUMMARY

Transplant patients have higher than expected risk of atherosclerotic events related to abnormalities in HDL-cholesterol, LDL-cholesterol, and triglycerides. Patients with organ transplantation can have prolonged survival if they are properly managed. Benefits are demonstrated in clinical trials, and therefore drug therapy for lipid abnormalities should be undertaken. It is mandatory that appropriate attention be given to drug interactions if significant adverse reactions are to be avoided.

c. Hypercholesterolemia in the Elderly

Warren W. Davis and W. Virgil Brown

DEFINITION OF PROBLEM

Elevated cholesterol is often found in patients older than 75 years with no history of cardiovascular disease. On occasion, this is due to elevated high-density lipoprotein (HDL) cholesterol, but low-density lipoprotein (LDL) cholesterol above 160 mg/dL (>4.2 mmol/L) is a more common finding. When evaluation of renal, liver, and endocrine status is within normal limits, it might be assumed that this elevated plasma cholesterol is relatively benign because the patient has lived a long life without apparent consequences. However, population studies tell us that myocardial infarction and stroke are most frequent in this age group and that elevated LDL-cholesterol and reduced HDL-cholesterol continue to be risk factors. Expensive hospitalization, disability, and long-term nursing care are the result in many of these patients. We have powerful drugs for reducing cholesterol, and benefit in those older than 70 years has now been proved. The absolute benefit in a population of the elderly is actually greater than in middle-aged patients because the incidence of disease is so great in this age group.

TYPICAL CASE

A 78-year-old retired physician is seen as a new patient. He notes remarkably good health over the years, having been hospitalized only once—tonsillectomy at age 11 years. He plays golf at least once weekly, takes care of his small garden without help, and travels frequently with his wife. There have been no symptoms suggesting angina, claudication, or dyspnea on exertion, and his activity level has been relatively stable. His blood pressure was found to be 165/100 mm Hg approximately 5 years ago and has been treated with hydrochlorothiazide. His cholesterol level has always been approximately 250 mg/dL, but the HDL level was 48 to 50 mg/dL (1.2 mmol/L). This was treated with dietary advice, but he has never taken lipid-lowering medications. He reports eating little dairy fat and meat only once daily. This is often fish or chicken with no skin. He has never smoked, and his blood glucose concentration has always been less than 100 mg/dL. His brother, who smoked, died of a myocardial infarction at 68 years. He is unaware of hypercholesterolemia in the family. His two sons, aged 46 and 50 years, are thought to be healthy and with cholesterol concentrations below 200 mg/dL.

On physical examination, he weighs 175 pounds (79.5 kg) at 5 feet 11 inches (180 cm). His blood pressure is 155/92 mm Hg. There is a moderate corneal arcus bilaterally. There is a soft bruit over the left subclavian artery. The chest and cardiac examination findings are otherwise normal. The abdominal examination reveals a murmur over the right inguinal area. There are no tendon or cutaneous xanthomas, and the pulses are easily palpable. The ankle-brachial blood pressure ratio is 1.0. The neurologic examination is within normal limits.

Laboratory analyses confirm normal renal, liver, and thyroid status. The fasting plasma glucose concentration is 88 mg/dL. A fasting lipoprotein analysis reveals a total cholesterol level of 265 mg/dL (6.88 mmol/L), triglycerides of 280 mg/dL (3.18 mmol/L), HDL-cholesterol of 42 mg/dL (1.1 mmol/L), and calculated LDL-cholesterol of 167 mg/dL (4.34 mmol/L).

DIFFERENTIAL DIAGNOSIS

This is an active man continuing to enjoy life and making contributions to his community and family. The bruit suggests but does not prove that some arteriosclerotic lesions already exist. These may be due to stable lesions that will never cause a clinical event; however, unstable plaque in his aorta and coronary or cerebral arteries may lead to a life-damaging or life-destroying episode. The probability of this is increased by his age and his elevated blood pressure as well as by his elevated LDL-cholesterol. The blood pressure may be due in part to his large-vessel disease with some segmental renal compromise. The elevated LDL-cholesterol is probably polygenic in origin because the family history does not suggest a major genetic defect, his diet is consistent with guidelines, and there are no other metabolic abnormalities evident.

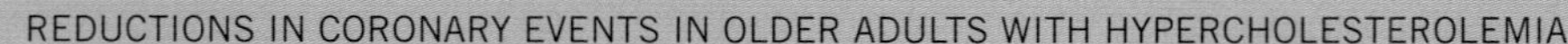

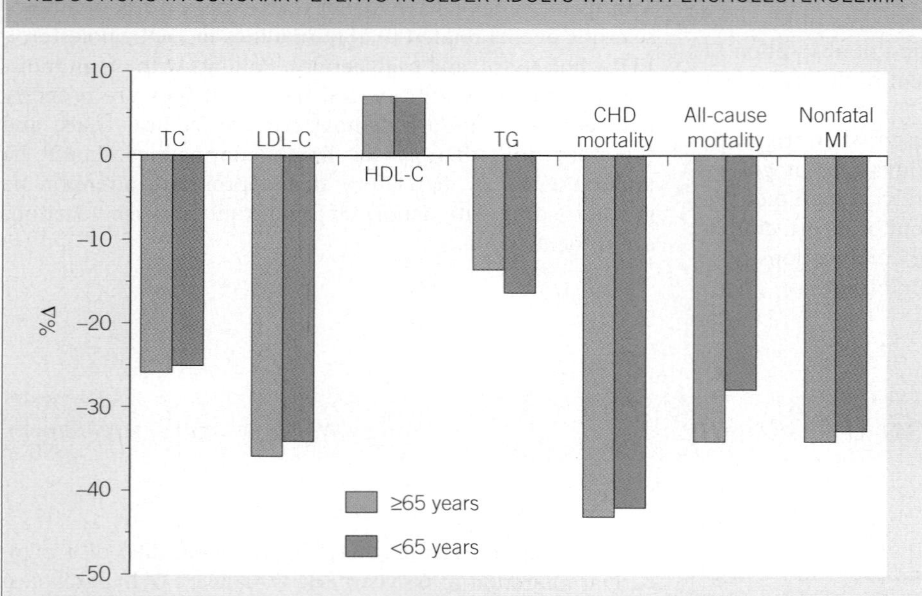

Figure 9C.1 Reductions in coronary events in older adults with hypercholesterolemia. The response to statin therapy has been observed to be similar in middle-aged and elderly persons. The Scandinavian Simvastatin Survival Study (4S) found no difference in the sustained response of lipoprotein concentrations to simvastatin in those older than 65 years. CHD, coronary heart disease; HDL-C, high-density lipoprotein cholesterol; LDL-C, low-density lipoprotein cholesterol; MI, myocardial infarction; TC, total cholesterol; TG, triglycerides. (From Miettinen TA, Pyörälä K, Olsson AG, et al. Cholesterol-lowering therapy in women and elderly patients with myocardial infarction or angina pectoris: findings from the Scandinavian Simvastatin Survival Study [4S]. Circulation 1997;96:4211-4218.)

By current National Cholesterol Education Program Adult Treatment Panel III (NCEP ATP III) guidelines, this patient has two risk factors, age and blood pressure. His 10-year risk by use of the ATP III model is above 30%; this is a coronary disease equivalent, and his LDL-cholesterol goal is below 100 mg/dL.

TREATMENT OPTIONS

A review of this patient's diet revealed that he had essentially eliminated egg yolks, dairy fat, and coconut oil. He had reduced the size of meat and poultry portions and limited them to once daily. He was unwilling to make further changes.

The current medications included hydrochlorothiazide, 25 mg/day, and a daily multivitamin tablet containing folate at 400 mg. Additional medication, such as low-dose angiotensin-converting enzyme inhibition, might reduce the blood pressure another 10 to 15 mm Hg with predicted benefit in stroke and perhaps coronary disease risk. The debatable question is whether to add a drug to specifically reduce the LDL-cholesterol. Although LDL-cholesterol is relatively weaker as a risk predictor in those older than 65 years, the prevalence of disease is greater in this age group. In fact, more than 80% of cardiovascular death occurs in this age group. His 10-year risk is in the coronary equivalent category by NCEP guidelines. Furthermore, the large clinical trials have shown benefit in cardiovascular event reduction that in those aged 65 to 75 years is comparable to that in those younger than 65 years (Figs. 9C.1 and 9C.2). The Heart Protection Study that observed slightly more than 20,000 patients 40 to 80 years old during 5 years found the same or a greater reduction in vascular events in subjects older than 75 years as in those younger. Stroke reduction has averaged 30% in those with known preexisting vascular disease treated with statins in these trials. Certainly, stroke prevention would be a major goal for treatment in this patient. Therefore, the use of a statin as well as more aggressive blood pressure reduction should be initiated in this patient. This patient should enjoy a reduction of 40% or more in the LDL-cholesterol with customary doses of several of the statin drugs, and this would reduce this value to less that 100 mg/dL as called for in the NCEP guidelines.

SUMMARY

Prevention of vascular disease is a key element in a therapeutic plan to reduce morbidity in the elderly. All the usual independent risk factors should be considered and treated in appropriate fashion. The benefits of LDL-cholesterol reduction are evident in those between 65 and 75 years in many studies as well as in one study conducted exclusively in more than 6000 individuals older than 70 years (PROSPER). Although other factors regarding functionality may be important considerations, the current guidelines in North America and in Europe should apply without regard to age in management of lipoprotein disorders.

Figure 9C.2 Survival without major coronary events: older versus younger adults. Patients older than 65 years enjoyed similar risk reduction during the Scandinavian Simvastatin Survival Study (4S). CHD, coronary heart disease. (From Miettinen TA, Pyörälä K, Olsson AG, et al. Cholesterol-lowering therapy in women and elderly patients with myocardial infarction or angina pectoris: findings from the Scandinavian Simvastatin Survival Study [4S]. Circulation 1997;96:4211-4218.)

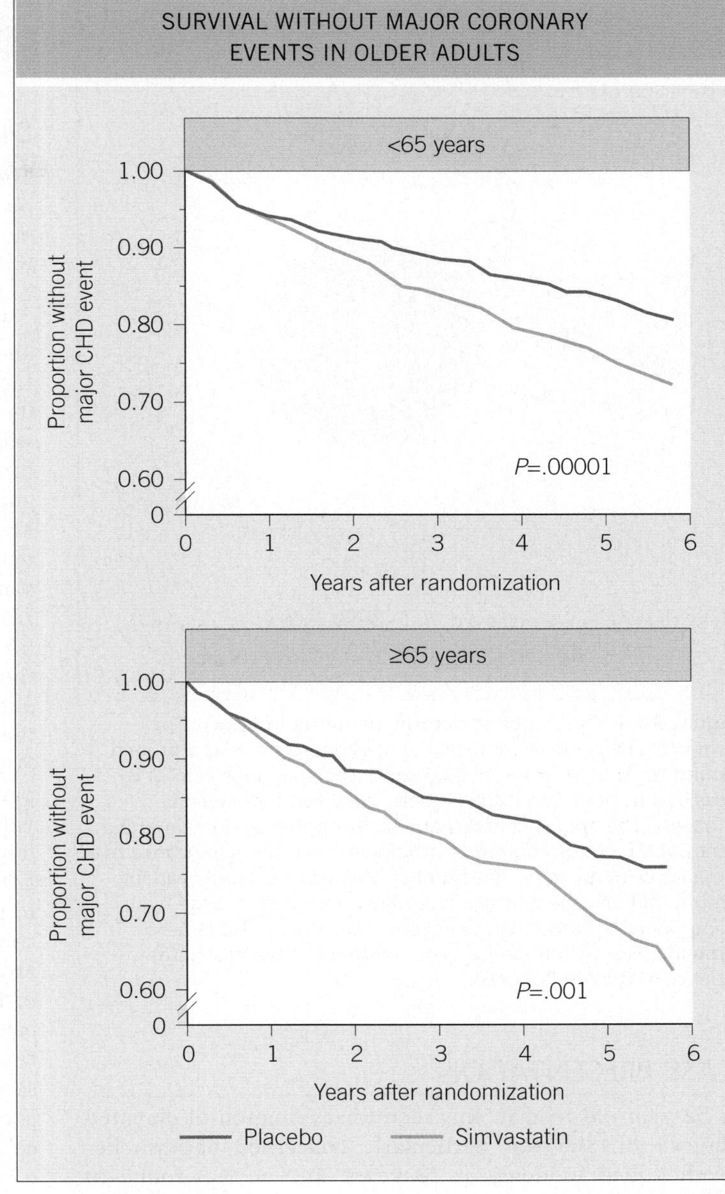

d. Elevated Lipoprotein(a)

W. Virgil Brown and Warren W. Davis

DEFINITION OF PROBLEM

An increase in levels of lipoprotein(a), or Lp(a), has been associated with increased risk for cardiovascular disease. Lp(a) is a combination of low-density lipoprotein (LDL) and a glycoprotein ("little a") linked by a sulfhydryl bridge with apolipoprotein B, the major protein of LDL (Fig. 9D.1). Many but not all population studies have shown an increase in the risk for cardiovascular disease with elevations in this lipoprotein. The plasma levels in any given individual are determined genetically, with diet and lifestyle having little impact. Very high levels are seen in certain families, and some of these demonstrate strong linkage between those affected with cardiovascular disease and the early onset of vascular disease. The "little a" protein is highly variable in its structure, with molecular weights ranging from 300,000 to more than 800,000. There are more than 30 isoforms defined, and only some of these seem to confer increased risk. Plasma levels of Lp(a) are not routinely measured with standard lipid profiles because these families are uncommon.

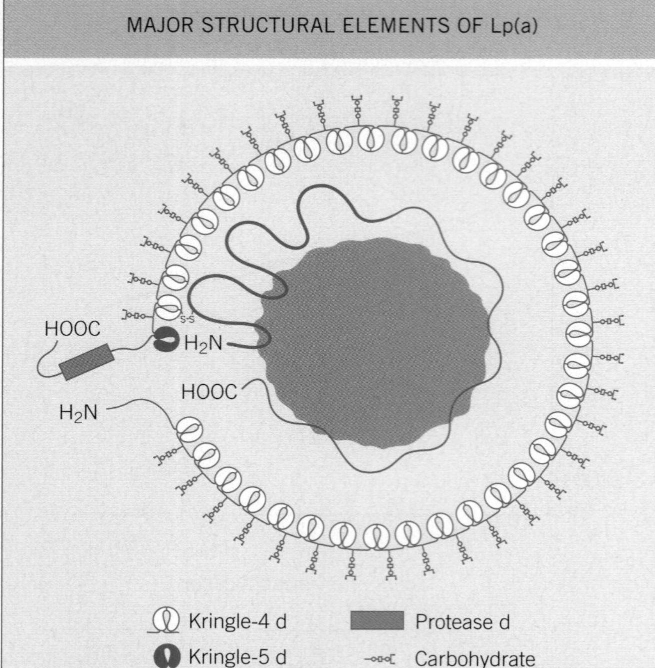

Figure 9D.1 The major structural elements of Lp(a). The spherical LDL particle contains the apolipoprotein B as a protein bound to its outer phospholipid shell. The apolipoprotein(a) is attached through the disulfide bond between two cysteine moieties. The apo(a) contains an inactive protease domain and a series of structures referred to as kringles after the appearance of a popular Danish pastry. The number of kringles is highly variable among different genetically determined isoforms. A large component of carbohydrate increases the size of this large protein. (From Utermann G. The mysteries of lipoprotein(a). Science 1989;246:904-910.)

CASE PRESENTATION

A 52-year-old woman was seen for evaluation of elevated cholesterol. She was particularly concerned because her brother died suddenly at 28 years, and he was found to have extensive arteriosclerosis on postmortem examination. His cholesterol values were not known. Recently, her total cholesterol concentration was found to be 310 mg/dL, with high-density lipoprotein cholesterol of 65 mg/dL and triglycerides of 210 mg/dL. During the past several months, rapid walking, particularly uphill, caused a pressure sensation over the back of her neck. There had been no leg pain with exercise and no pain on rest. She denied cigarette smoking, high blood pressure, or elevated blood glucose concentration. She had regular menses. Her only medication was a multivitamin taken once daily. She also reported that her son, aged 20 years, was found to have a total plasma cholesterol concentration of about 300 mg/dL but otherwise was believed to be healthy.

The physical examination revealed a faint corneal arcus but no cutaneous or tendon xanthomas. The blood pressure was 122/78 mm Hg, and the cardiovascular examination was within normal limits.

The patient underwent an exercise electrocardiographic examination that was markedly positive, and a subsequent cardiac catheterization demonstrated lesions in both the right and circumflex coronary arteries producing stenoses of 70% to 80%. These were treated with angioplasty.

DIFFERENTIAL DIAGNOSIS

The early appearance of coronary artery disease in a premenopausal woman with no major risk factors other than elevated LDL-cholesterol and a strong family history should raise the question of additional inheritable factors. Elevated Lp(a) and homocysteine fall into this category.

Fasting blood samples were obtained for both the patient and her son. The homocysteine values were 7 and 9 μmol/L in each, respectively, values considered within normal limits (<14 μmol/L). However, the patient's Lp(a) concentration was 159 mg/dL, and the son's was 175 mg/dL. The mean Lp-(a) value in white populations is approximately 10 mg/dL, and above 30 mg/dL is considered to confer increased risk. The elevated LDL-cholesterol was also confirmed with values of 235 mg/dL in the patient and 247 mg/dL in the son. The Lp(a) cholesterol is measured as part of the total LDL-cholesterol; however, the amount contributed by Lp-(a) does not explain the elevations in LDL-cholesterol in these patients. The reported values for Lp(a) include the entire mass of the molecule, including the proteins and all the lipid components. The cholesterol may be only 15% to 20% of this mass, and accordingly, the levels in these patients could add only 25 to 35 mg to the LDL-cholesterol value. Thus, a second genetic abnormality, such as familial hypercholesterolemia, must be present to explain the high LDL-cholesterol level. Elevations of both these lipoproteins in the same patient are probably a chance occurrence. Their coincidence markedly increases the risk and requires therapy. The family history is the clue to the unusual features of this case. In fact, the Framingham risk for this patient is calculated to be only 2% (Fig. 9D.2). Therefore, standard risk factors underestimate the risk in this patient. The reasons for increased vascular risk related to elevated LDL-cholesterol are consistent with the increased delivery to the cells of the intima. The mechanism for the higher incidence of disease with Lp(a) has been attributed to its apparent rapid uptake by macrophages, its susceptibility to oxidative damage, and the inhibition of plasminogen conversion to plasmin by binding to fibrinogen activation sites.

Lowering of LDL-cholesterol appears to lower the atherosclerotic risk in these patients in the absence of changes in Lp(a) levels. On the other hand, no studies have selectively lowered Lp(a) and demonstrated an associated risk reduction. Therefore, the emphasis in these patients should be on optimal reduction of LDL-cholesterol. The goal should be to achieve a long-term value for LDL-cholesterol well below 100 mg/dL. Reducing the saturated fat and cholesterol in the diet may help reduce the LDL-cholesterol but would be expected to produce no change in Lp(a). Drugs, which can produce a 50% reduction in LDL-cholesterol, will be needed. These include statins alone or perhaps in combination with another agent. In choosing that second agent, consideration of one that might lower Lp(a) would seem appropriate. Elevations of Lp(a) do not respond to treatment with statin drugs or fibric acid derivatives. Niacin lowers Lp-(a) concentrations by approximately 30% at doses of 2 to

FRAMINGHAM RISK ASSESSMENT–WOMEN

Age	Points
20–34	–7
35–39	–3
40–44	0
45–49	3
50–54	6
55–59	8
60–64	10
65–69	12
70–74	14
75–79	16

Total cholesterol	Points				
	Age 20-39	Age 40-49	Age 50-59	Age 60-69	Age 70-79
<160	0	0	0	0	0
160–199	4	3	2	1	1
200–239	8	6	4	2	1
240–279	11	8	5	3	2
≥280	13	10	7	4	2
Nonsmoker	0	0	0	0	0
Smoker	9	7	4	2	1

Point total	10-year risk (%)
< 9	< 1
9	1
10	1
11	1
12	1
13	2
14	2
15	3
16	4
17	5
18	6
19	8
20	11
21	14
22	17
23	22
24	27
≥ 25	≥ 30

Systolic BP (mm Hg)	If untreated	If treated
<120	0	0
120–129	1	3
130–139	2	4
140–159	3	5
≥160	4	6

HDL (mg/dL)	Points
≥60	–1
50–59	0
40–49	1
<40	2

Score = 13
Risk = 2
LDL-C goal: <130 mg/dL

Figure 9D.2 Framingham risk assessment in women. Framingham risk assessment in this patient according to the Adult Treatment Panel III model. The patient's values are highlighted. (From Executive Summary of the Third Report of the National Cholesterol Education Program [NCEP] Expert Panel on Detection, Evaluation, and Treatment of High Blood Cholesterol in Adults [Adult Treatment Panel III]. JAMA 2001;285:2486-2497.)

3 g/day. Additional reduction of LDL-cholesterol may also be achieved. The only other drug that reduces Lp(a) to a comparable degree is estrogen, and Lp(a) values often rise with ovarian failure. The patient's son should also be treated. This is emphasized by the death of his uncle at age 28 years of coronary artery disease, and it must be assumed that this risk factor was a major causative element. Statin therapy would be the first choice, and a reduction of LDL-cholesterol well below 100 mg/dL would seem justified. This may require other lipid-lowering drugs, and niacin would be a logical choice for a second drug because it not only lowers LDL-cholesterol but also reduces Lp(a) by 20% to 40%. Ezetimibe or bile acid sequestrants could also be considered if the response to statins is less than expected. The results of liver function tests should be followed 6 to 8 weeks after each dose change and up to 3 months with stable doses of the combination.

No formal test of reducing Lp(a) as a means of reducing vascular events has been completed with niacin; small studies using combinations of drugs with niacin have shown impressive reductions in growth of vascular lesions and clinical events. The patients with Lp(a) above the mean benefited more than those below the mean values at baseline. Estrogen also reduces Lp(a), and in the Heart and Estrogen/Progestin Replacement Study (HERS), the subgroup of women who had Lp(a) concentrations above the 75th percentile (>27 mg/dL) and received hormone replacement therapy had a significant reduction in recurrent coronary events. Women with high Lp(a) may be particularly benefited by estrogen replacement therapy as they enter the menopause. This hypothesis needs clinical testing.

SUMMARY

Lp(a) elevations represent a significant risk for atherosclerotic events in the presence of high-normal or elevated LDL-cholesterol. A very strong family history or earlier onset of vascular disease than seems compatible with a given risk factor profile should prompt the measurement of Lp(a) in the patient and in all first-degree relatives. These patients, once identified, should be treated aggressively to lower their LDL-cholesterol. The only specific treatments that might be considered for reducing Lp(a) are niacin and perhaps hormone replacement therapy in postmenopausal women.

chapter 10

Arterial Diseases of the Limbs

Bengt Fagrell

Definition

- Peripheral arterial diseases can be divided into obliterative arterial diseases, vasospastic disorders, and inflammatory diseases.

Key Features

- Peripheral arterial occlusive disease is a manifestation of atherosclerosis.
- Buerger's disease is an inflammatory process related to tobacco smoking.
- Vasospastic diseases and erythromelalgia are caused by a disturbed regulation of the reactivity of the macrovessels and microvessels in the skin and sometimes also in other tissues.

Peripheral arterial disease is a major cause of morbidity in Western countries today. The main reason for the arterial insufficiency is atherosclerosis, which has reached epidemic proportions in many countries. One of the most common symptoms of peripheral arterial occlusive disease (PAOD) is intermittent claudication, and the prevalence of this symptom is 1% to 2% in the adult population. The number of people who have asymptomatic disease is about three or four times higher than this. There is no major difference between men and women in this regard.[1]

The most severe symptom in patients with PAOD is critical leg ischemia, and the incidence is estimated to be about 500 to 1000 patients per million of the population per year. The fate of patients who have this serious symptom is very poor. One year after first presentation, 25% of patients require a major amputation. After 5 years, only half of them are still alive and with two legs, and 20% are dead.[1,2]

There are also other disorders in the peripheral arterial system that disable patients. In countries with cold climate, vasospastic disorders are common, and about 20% of the healthy population of women in Sweden have symptoms of peripheral vasospasm or so-called Raynaud's phenomenon in the hands and feet.[3,4] Another serious peripheral vascular disorder is thromboangiitis obliterans or Buerger's disease.[3,5]

ANATOMY AND PATHOLOGY

Anatomy

The anatomy of peripheral arteries of the lower leg is illustrated in Figure 10.1. The distal part of the abdominal aorta is divided into the common iliac arteries, each of which after about 5 to 8 cm gives off the internal iliac artery and continues as the external iliac artery. The internal iliac artery is divided into several small branches that give blood to the pelvic organs and that, through collaterals, support the thigh with blood. The external iliac artery continues below the inguinal ligament into the femoral artery down to the popliteal artery at the knee region. About 5 to 10 cm below the inguinal ligament, the femoral artery gives off the profunda femoris artery, which mainly provides the thigh muscles with blood. Below the knee region, the popliteal artery divides into three branches, the anterior tibial artery, the posterior tibial artery, and the peroneal artery. The anterior tibial artery later changes its name to the dorsal artery of the foot.

Pathology

Atherosclerosis and Thrombosis

The main pathologic finding in PAOD is atherosclerosis, the pathogenesis of which is described in Chapter 1.

In the peripheral leg arteries, the atherosclerotic process is spread in most parts of the vessels. It is seldom that atherosclerotic obstruction gives rise to any clinical symptoms when it is located in the aorta because of the large diameter of the aorta, but sometimes thrombotic material can add to the atherosclerotic process and be responsible for a final occlusion. Occlusion of the aorta most often occurs where it branches off into the iliac arteries, which sometimes results in an acute and severe ischemia in one or both legs, the so-called Leriche syndrome.[6]

Symptomatic stenoses are also found in the iliac and femoral arteries but most often in the arteries of the lower leg. About 20% of the obstructions are located in the iliac arteries, about 40% in the femoral arteries, and 20% in the lower leg arteries. In about 20% of the patients, the atherosclerotic process is found at all levels of the leg arteries. The most prominent places for atherosclerotic lesions are at the sites of arterial bifurcations and in Hunter's canal in the lower third of the thigh.

Macroembolism

Acute occlusions of the arteries of the legs are usually caused by embolism, thrombosis, or trauma. Embolism is the most common cause and represents about 75% to 80% of the events. The true incidence of arterial macroembolism is difficult to establish because it is possible to determine with any degree of certainty whether there is an embolus or a thrombus only in patients who are operated on. Data from a nationwide vascular register in Sweden have shown that the annual incidence of embolic events varies from 0.04%

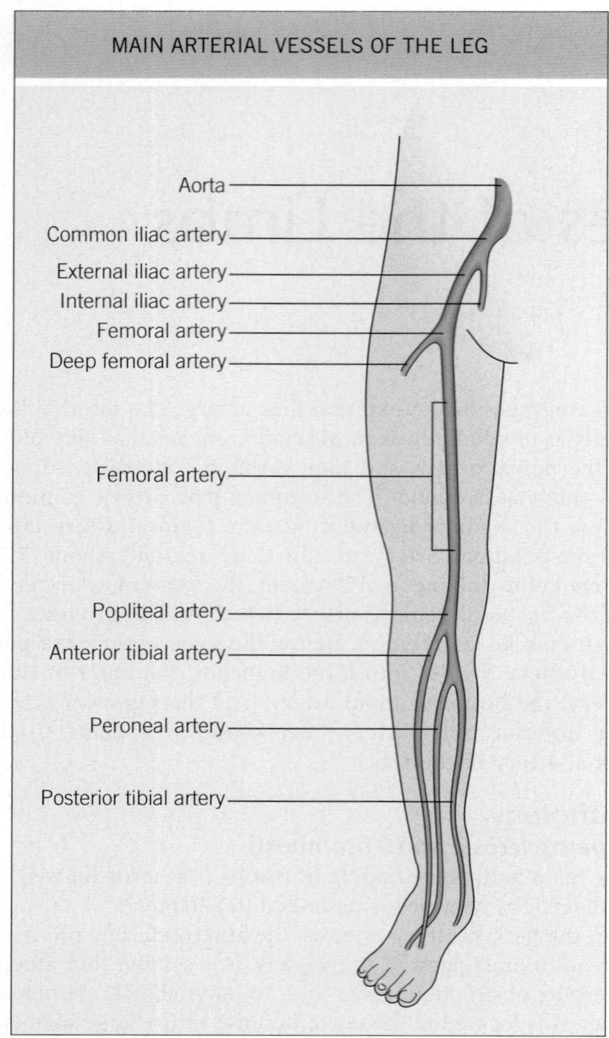

Figure 10.1 Main arterial vessels of the leg.

in people aged 20 to 30 years up to 8% in those older than 90 years.[7] Most often the origin of the embolus is thrombotic material in an atherosclerotic heart with arterial fibrillation (70%),[8] but some may also come from thrombotic material in the aorta or other main arteries.

Microembolism

Microembolism is uncommon in the lower extremities and is often clinically silent. There are mainly two types, cholesterol emboli and thrombotic emboli.[9] Both types are often generated from ulcerated atherosclerotic plaques located proximally in the arterial system. They may sometimes give rise to local severe ischemia in the most distal parts of the digits. The clinical presentation of microembolism is often discoloration of one or several toes, and the syndrome is therefore often called the blue toe syndrome. Other organs, such as the kidney, are sometimes involved, and the clinical manifestation can range from a cyanotic toe to diffuse multiorgan disease, which may present as serious systemic illness.[10]

Buerger's Disease

Buerger's disease (thromboangiitis obliterans) does not have an atherosclerotic pathology, but it is important to know about its existence because of the serious symptoms and the relatively low age of the patients. In 1908, Leo Buerger published details of the first series of patients with the typical features of the disease, and he was also the first to call it thromboangiitis obliterans.[11] He later presented about 500 patients with the disease.[12] During the 1950s and 1960s, it was strongly questioned by several authorities whether Buerger's disease was a true entity or simply an early variant of atherosclerosis. However, it is now well established that the cause of the disease is not atherosclerosis but a specific inflammatory process both in the arteries and in the veins.[5,13]

PATHOPHYSIOLOGY

Peripheral Arterial Occlusive Disease

Atherosclerotic lesions in the peripheral arteries do not give any symptoms as long as the blood flow through the vessel is sufficient to support the tissues with oxygen and nutrients. On occasion, an artery can be occluded without the patient's having any symptoms because of a good collateral circulation in the region. However, when a stenotic artery becomes severely occluded, symptoms often occur. Such thrombotic occlusions are common in the leg arteries. If stenoses or occlusions occur in the arteries above the knee region, intermittent claudication is often the result. If the obstruction affects the lower leg arteries, rest pain and skin ulcers or gangrene may be the final outcome.

Buerger's Disease

The etiology of Buerger's disease is still unknown, but it is well established that it is an inflammatory process in which smoking plays a crucial role.[14] The combination of smoke and other factors that leads to the development of the syndrome is obscure. It has been suggested that the disease is caused by an immunologic disorder (Table 10.1).[14] Most probably, it is caused by a combination of different factors that lead to the development of the symptoms.[5] However, the fact that smoking plays a major role in the development and prognosis of the disease has been proved.[12,14]

EVIDENCE FOR AN IMMUNOLOGIC BASIS OF BUERGER'S DISEASE	
Inflammatory disease of medium to small-sized vessels	Increased incidence of HLA antigens (DR4, A9, B5, and B8) Increased complement Sensitivity to human collagen types I and III Anticollagen antibodies
Arteries or veins are affected focally	Cellular infiltration in the whole vessel wall Endothelial and fibroblast proliferation (often giant cells) Often thrombus formation with similar changes Angiogenesis in the vessel wall
Mainly peripheral vessels are affected, but inner organ vessels may also be involved.	

Table 10.1 Evidence for an immunologic basis of Buerger's disease.

Vasospastic Disorders

In 1862, Maurice Raynaud described episodic digital ischemia provoked by cold and emotion, and this phenomenon has since been called Raynaud's syndrome. It is defined as episodic pathologic attacks of white or blue fingers produced by cold provocation or emotional stress or both. A higher frequency of vasospastic symptoms in other organs, such as migraine and variant angina, indicates that the syndrome has a more general manifestation.[4] The patients are usually divided into two groups, depending on the etiology. The most common form of the disorder is primary Raynaud's phenomenon (Raynaud's disease). This form is called primary because no underlying disease has been found and etiology is, so far, unknown. The other form is secondary Raynaud's phenomenon, in which the etiology and underlying disease in most cases are thought to be known. Today we know that a large number of different causes can produce the phenomenon (Table 10.2).[3,4,15]

CAUSES OF RAYNAUD'S PHENOMENON
Primary Raynaud's phenomenon (also known as Raynaud's disease or idiopathic episodic vasospasm)
Secondary Raynaud's phenomenon
Autoimmune diseases
Scleroderma or CREST syndrome (calcinosis cutis, Raynaud's phenomenon, esophageal involvement, sclerodactyly, and telangiectasia)
Systemic lupus erythematosus
Mixed connective tissue disease
Vasculitis
Polyarteritis nodosa
Polymyositis
Thromboangütis obliterans
Temporal arteritis
Polymyalgia rheumatica
Drug induced
Beta blockers
Ergotamine
Clonidine
Bleomycin
Lithium
Rheologic changes
Macroglobulinemia
Polycythemia
Cryoglobulinemia
Cryofibrinogenemia
Cold agglutinins
Other causes
Macrothrombosis and microthrombosis or embolism
Atherosclerosis
Smoking
Allergy
External causes
Vibration (from vibrating tools)
Digital trauma (piano players)
Nerve lesion or compression

Table 10.2 Causes of Raynaud's phenomenon.

CLINICAL PRESENTATIONS

The symptoms of patients who have PAOD are

- intermittent claudication, and
- symptoms due to chronic critical leg ischemia (i.e., rest pain and ischemic ulcerations or gangrene).

Intermittent Claudication

The major symptom of intermittent claudication is pain in the muscles of the buttocks or lower limb during walking. The pain starts after a certain walking distance, depending on the location and severity of the obstruction (Fig. 10.2). When the obstruction is located in the pelvic arteries, the pain is often localized to the buttock or thigh region; and when it is localized in the femoral or popliteal arteries, the pain occurs in the calf muscle.

Medical History

The symptoms are most often typical, with a muscle pain that increases gradually during walking and disappears rather quickly, often within a few minutes, after stopping. When the patient starts walking again, the pain successively comes back after a constant distance. The symptoms are usually so typical that the diagnosis can be made almost solely by the medical history.

Clinical Examination

The physical examination includes palpation of arterial pulses at different locations of the leg and auscultation over the femoral and iliac vessels. The pulses are weak or absent distal to a stenosis or occlusion. However, normal pulsations can sometimes be found in patients who have typical symptoms of claudication. These patients usually have a short but narrow stenosis in the iliac artery that during rest does not have a high enough resistance to reduce the pulse wave. However, during walking, the blood flow may be significantly reduced, leading to typical symptoms of claudication. In these patients, auscultation over the iliac and femoral arteries is imperative. An easy and clear way of presenting the results of pulse palpation and auscultation is in the form of a graph.

Ankle Pressure Measurements

Most patients who have claudication are elderly and retired, and a medical history and a thorough clinical investigation are usually enough to reach a diagnosis. However, ankle pressure measurements should be performed. This test is usually the only laboratory investigation required because conservative treatment is most often the treatment of choice in this patient group. In younger patients, who may be handicapped at work, further investigation should be performed to find out whether angioplasty or surgical intervention is possible. This applies also to a few elderly patients who are socially handicapped in such a way that they have difficulty living a normal daily life, and angioplasty or surgical intervention should be considered in these patients. The technique of distal blood pressure measurements is described in more detail later.

Chronic Critical Leg Ischemia

Chronic critical leg ischemia (CCLI) is the most severe condition in patients who have PAOD. Several attempts

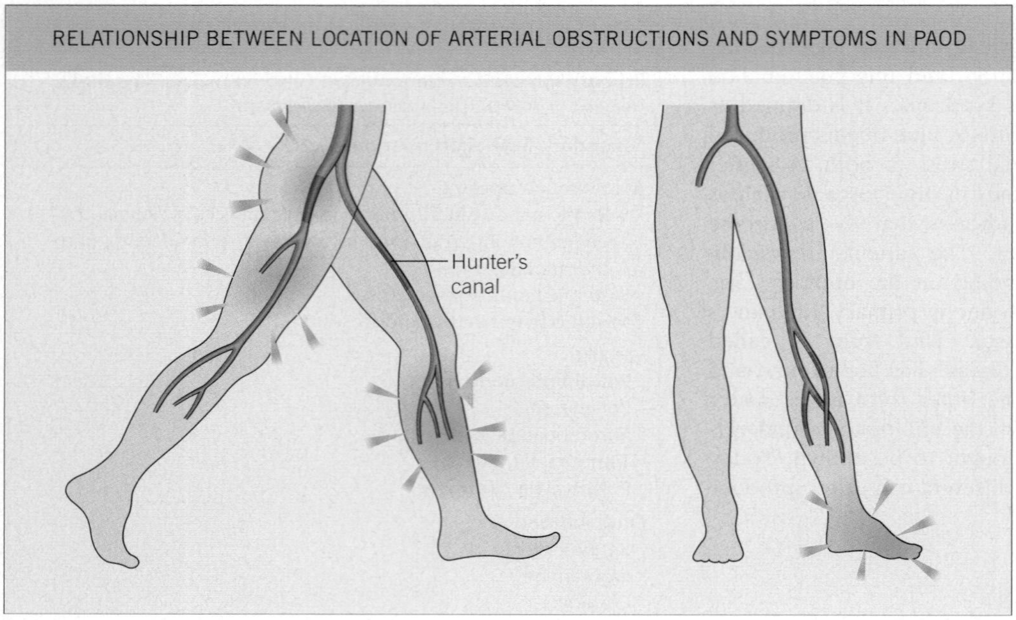

RELATIONSHIP BETWEEN LOCATION OF ARTERIAL OBSTRUCTIONS AND SYMPTOMS IN PAOD

Hunter's canal

Figure 10.2 Relationship between location of arterial obstructions and symptoms in peripheral arterial occlusive disease (PAOD). Obstructions in the iliac artery give rise to pain in the buttock and thigh, femoral stenosis gives rise to pain in the calf muscles, and obstructions of the lower leg arteries most often give rise to rest pain and skin necrosis.

have been made to define it. One of the latest and most thorough ones was made in a consensus process at the beginning of the 1990s in which CCLI was defined as follows[16,17]:

- persistently occurring rest pain that requires regular analgesia for longer than 2 weeks, with an ankle systolic blood pressure of 50 mm Hg or less or a toe systolic blood pressure of 30 mm Hg or less (or both); and
- ulceration or gangrene of the foot or toes, with an ankle systolic blood pressure of 50 mm Hg or less or a toe systolic blood pressure of 30 mm Hg or less (or both).

These definitions were later challenged, and other pressure levels and criteria have been suggested.[17] Regardless of the criteria agreed on, it is crucial to have strict criteria for classifying CCLI patients to be able to evaluate, for example, the results of different treatments.

One of the earliest symptoms in patients with CCLI is rest pain. This is predominantly localized to the most distal parts of the leg (i.e., the foot and toes). The pain usually appears first in the supine position (e.g., in bed at night). How early in the disease process the pain appears depends on the severity and location of the arterial obstruction. The patient most often experiences relief if the lower leg is moved out of bed into a hanging position. This increases the hydrostatic pressure and improves the blood filling of the nutritional vessels in the ischemic region, resulting in pain relief. In severe cases, the patient has to sit, stand up, or walk around to be relieved of pain. If the obstructions are marked, the pain will also be present in the sitting and standing position, and it is then often intolerable in the supine position.

The most severe signs of CCLI are ischemic ulcers and gangrene, localized in the most distal parts of the leg (i.e., the toes) and predominantly in the first, fourth, and fifth toes.[18,19] The heel is sometimes also involved. The reason for these locations is almost certainly that these regions are most frequently exposed to trauma from shoes (Fig. 10.3). In patients who have severely compromised blood supply

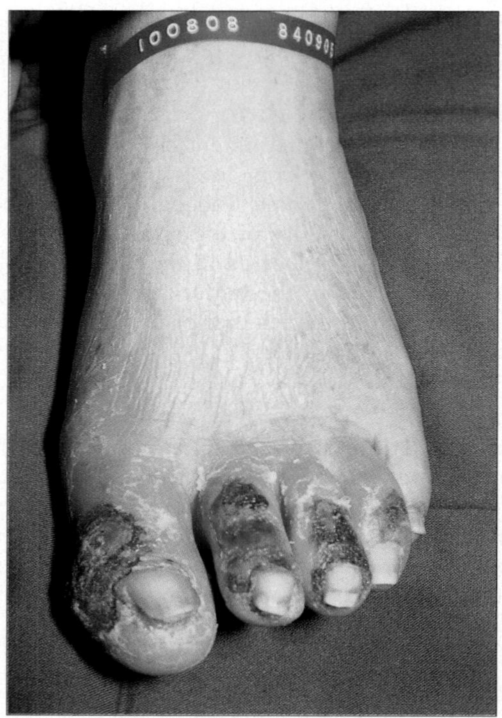

Figure 10.3 Ischemic skin ulcer induced by trauma from shoes. This patient with peripheral arterial occlusive disease suffered severe superficial skin necrosis of several toes because of shoes that were too tight.

to the foot, even a slight pressure from a shoe may lead to abolition of skin microcirculation in the area, resulting in tissue necrosis.[19] Consequently, it is of the utmost importance that patients be told to wear large enough shoes so that no pressure is applied to ischemic regions.

The primary reason for the development of ischemic skin ulcers in patients who have CCLI is, of course, obstructions in the main arteries of the leg. However, necrosis of the skin does not occur until the blood flow in the nutritional capillaries of the ischemic region decreases below the minimal demand of oxygen and nutrients to the tissue.[18-21] This is clearly demonstrated by the fact that only about half of the patients who have CCLI will develop skin necrosis in the ischemic foot during a 3-month observation period.[21] Consequently, microcirculatory methods must be used to predict the risk of skin necrosis in CCLI patients.

Clinical Examination

The examination of a patient who has CCLI is largely the same as for a patient who has claudication (i.e., palpation of leg pulses and auscultation over the femoral and iliac vessels). Inspection of the skin of distal parts of the extremity often gives valuable information about the severity of the reduction in blood flow in the region.

By evaluating the skin color during changes in leg position, it is possible to determine the degree of reduction of arterial circulation in the leg. When the leg is elevated, the ischemic leg becomes pale. The patient should be in a horizontal position with the leg elevated at 45 degrees. To strengthen the outcome of the test, the patient should then be asked to move his or her feet back and forth, which will empty the veins of the leg. If significant obstructions are present in the leg arteries, little or no blood will enter the foot vessels, resulting in blanching of the foot.

After this procedure, the patient should sit up quickly, and the length of time for color to return to the foot is recorded. This is mainly a test of the time of venous filling. In patients who have marked reduction of the arterial blood supply, the filling will be delayed for one or several minutes, after which the ischemic foot most often takes on a red-blue color (Fig. 10.4). The reason for this is that the vessels are paralyzed and the normal microvascular reactivity of the skin is abolished, resulting in a passive filling of the skin microvascular vessels.

The blood filling of the nutritional skin capillaries cannot be estimated by the color of the skin. The reason for this is that the amount of blood in the nutritional skin capillaries represents only about 1% to 3% of the total skin microvascular blood volume,[22] and consequently the contribution of this amount to skin color is totally insignificant. From this it follows that it is impossible to determine whether blood enters the nutritional skin capillaries of ischemic areas in patients who have CCLI by looking at the skin color. Objective microcirculatory methods have to be used (see later).

In patients who have CCLI, the structure of the skin often deteriorates, and all hair on the dorsal side of the foot disappears. Marked decrease in the growth of nails is also a distinctive sign of severe reduction of the nutritional circulation of an ischemic foot. In patients with claudication, skin changes are seldom seen.

Patients who have CCLI usually have a low skin temperature in the supine position because of the reduced perfusion pressure and blood flow. However, in the sitting or standing position, when the foot is in a dependent position, the skin temperature is often increased, and it may become several degrees warmer than the nonischemic foot, especially in diabetic patients (see Fig. 10.4). As mentioned previously, this is due to large amounts of blood entering the paralyzed, dilated subpapillary, thermoregulatory vascular beds of the ischemic region because of the hydrostatic pressure. Nevertheless, no blood may enter the nutritional vessels, with skin necrosis as a consequence.[18-21]

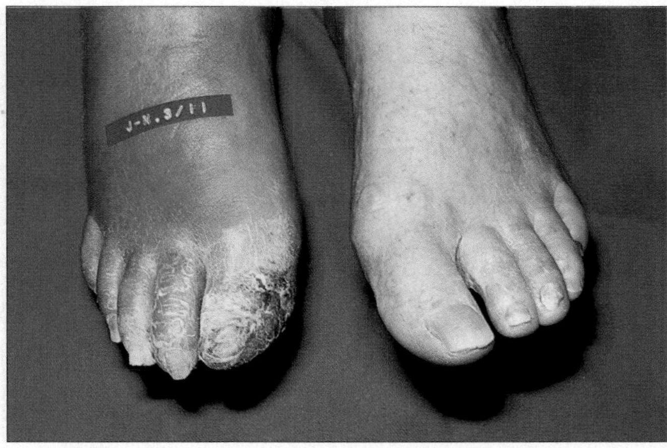

Figure 10.4 Red and warm ischemic foot in dependent position. In patients who have severe chronic critical leg ischemia, the skin is often red and the temperature is increased in the sitting or standing position. The skin temperature of this patient was 5.4°F (3°C) higher at the dorsum of the ischemic right foot than at the same area of the left nonischemic foot.

Vasospastic Disorders

Primary Raynaud's Phenomenon

Medical History

The majority of patients with Raynaud's phenomenon have so-called primary Raynaud's phenomenon or Raynaud's disease. It is about 9 or 10 times more common in women than in men, and in northern countries, about 20% of young women have Raynaud-like symptoms.[4,23]

From the medical history, it is usually possible to determine whether a patient has primary or secondary Raynaud's phenomenon. If the symptoms start at or around puberty, it is most likely that it is a primary Raynaud's phenomenon. The patient will clearly describe how one or several digits have cold-induced blanching, with subsequent hyperemia when the patient comes into a warm environment. Emotional stress can also provoke attacks, as can tobacco smoke, hormones, and trauma. The thumb is seldom involved in patients with primary Raynaud's phenomenon.

Clinical Examination

In young women, the patient group in whom primary Raynaud's phenomenon is most common, medical history and clinical investigation are often sufficient to establish the diagnosis. It is, in routine clinical practice, unnecessary to perform various cold provocation tests in patients who clearly describe the symptoms.

Secondary Raynaud's Phenomenon

The clinical features of secondary Raynaud's phenomenon are

- older age at onset than that for primary Raynaud's phenomenon;
- often marked ischemia, sometimes with necrosis of the tip of the digits (Fig. 10.5);

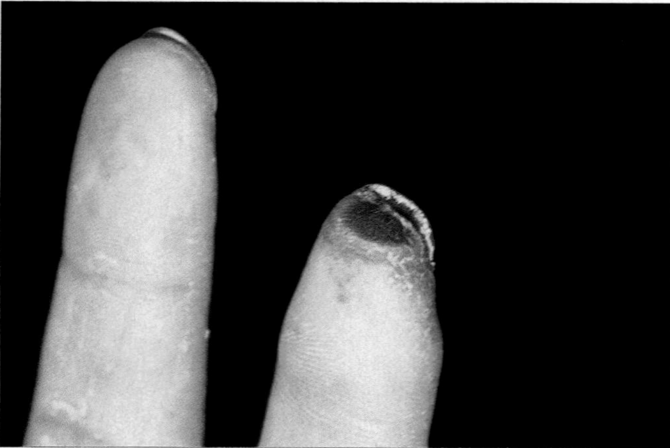

Figure 10.5 Finger necrosis in secondary Raynaud's phenomenon. The second and third fingers of a 42-year-old woman with scleroderma. A typical sclerosis of the skin often leads to a cuff-like strangulation of the microcirculation, with concomitant fingertip necrosis.

- vasospasm, most often throughout the year;
- asymmetric attacks; and
- involvement of the thumb.

In patients in whom there is a suspicion of secondary Raynaud's phenomenon, further investigations should include a complete clinical evaluation of the heart and vascular system.

Laboratory Investigations

Several different techniques can be used to evaluate the digital macrocirculation and microcirculation in patients who have Raynaud's phenomenon. The main principle of all these techniques is to determine whether vasospasm occurs during local digital cooling or general body cooling.

Several different techniques for measuring digital blood pressure have been described. Small miniature pressure cuffs are applied around the base of the digits, and the systolic blood pressure is recorded before, during, and after local or systemic cold provocation. The reduction in digital blood pressure is recorded and gives an estimate of the degree of vasospasm.[24]

Laser Doppler fluxmetry measures the blood flow in the total skin microcirculation. It can be used to determine whether blood flow decreases during cold exposure.[25]

Capillary microscopy has been shown to be useful in differentiating between primary and secondary Raynaud's phenomenon.[26] The nail fold capillaries of the affected digits are investigated with an ordinary light microscope and a magnification factor of between 10 and 50.[27] In normal subjects, the capillaries are long and slender and have a hairpin shape. In patients who have primary Raynaud's phenomenon, the nail fold capillaries usually look ordinary (Fig. 10.6). On occasion, they may be somewhat dilated, especially if they are investigated in the hyperemic phase, but the morphologic appearance is normal. In patients who have secondary Raynaud's phenomenon, especially in those patients who have scleroderma or CREST syndrome (calcinosis cutis, Raynaud's phenomenon, esophageal hypomobility, sclerodactyly, telangiectasia), marked morphologic changes of the capillaries can be seen (see Fig. 10.6). A proposed classification of nail fold microvascular changes[28] is shown in Table 10.3. The morphologic changes in the capillaries very often precede other symptoms of the disease, and therefore this method is often a useful tool to determine whether a primary or secondary Raynaud's phenomenon is present and also to monitor the progression or improvement of the vascular component in patients with secondary Raynaud's phenomenon.

Blood Tests

As a rule, patients who have primary Raynaud's phenomenon have completely normal laboratory test results. However, some laboratory tests may help in the diagnosis of secondary Raynaud's phenomenon:

- erythrocyte sedimentation rate;
- detection of antibodies;
- von Willebrand factor antigen;
- radiography to determine whether a cervical rib is present;
- antinuclear antibody screening; and
- cryoglobulin, cryofibrinogen, and cold agglutinin titers (these blood samples must be taken in a warm room at temperatures above 95°F [35°C]).

Erythromelalgia

Erythromelalgia is characterized by skin redness, increased skin temperature, and burning pain, predominantly localized to the feet. Excellent, condensed reviews have been published.[29,30]

Buerger's Disease

Medical History

The diagnosis of Buerger's disease or thromboangiitis obliterans is primarily set from the medical history and clinical presentation.[4,5,13,14] The following clinical criteria have been noted:

- It occurs in young patients, usually younger than 40 years.
- It is more common in men than in women.
- It occurs almost exclusively in smokers or ex-smokers.
- Inflammatory activity is most often in both arteries and veins, and there is sometimes migrating thrombophlebitis.
- Ischemia is most often present in the digits of both upper and lower limbs.

As the disease is more common in certain populations (e.g., in the eastern part of the Mediterranean and in Asia), information on ethnic origin should be obtained.

Smoking Habits

Because almost all patients who have Buerger's disease are or have been heavy smokers, a detailed medical history on this point is essential. There are only anecdotal cases described in the literature of patients in whom smoking has not been a major factor in Buerger's disease, but it cannot be excluded that such patients have been exposed to passive smoking.

Clinical Examination

The first sign of the disease is often thrombophlebitis in the legs or arms. The vessel feels hard, and a strong inflammatory

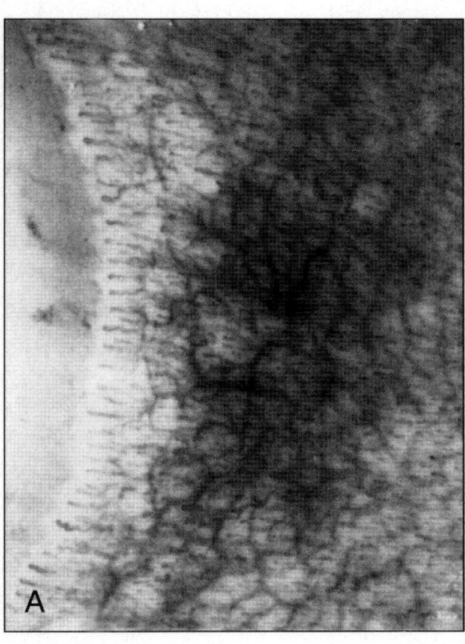

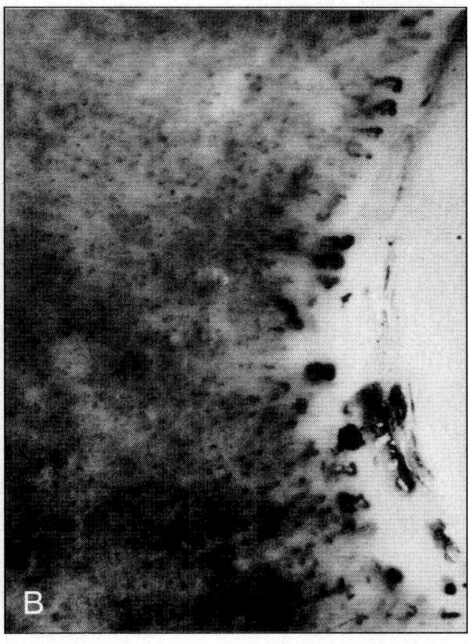

Figure 10.6 Nail fold capillaroscopy in patients with Raynaud's phenomenon. A, Microscopic image from a finger nail fold of a patient with primary Raynaud's phenomenon. The capillaries are normal, but the subpapillary venous plexuses are more prominent. **B,** Finger nail fold capillaroscopy from a patient with secondary Raynaud's phenomenon (scleroderma). Note the clear reduction in the number of capillaries. Several giant and deformed capillaries are also seen, with avascular areas in between. (Courtesy of Professor H. Maricq, Charleston, South Carolina.)

CLASSIFICATION OF NAIL FOLD VASCULAR CHANGES
Capillary morphology
Normal capillaries
Enlarged, dilated capillaries
Giant capillaries (diameter >50 μm)
Loss of capillaries
No obvious avascular areas
Small avascular areas
Moderate avascular areas
Extensive avascular areas
Microvascular changes in other skin areas

Table 10.3 Classification of nail fold vascular changes.

reaction is often noted. The patient may also sometimes have changes in inner organ vessels, such as the coronary arteries, but this is not common.

Angiography

Angiography (Fig. 10.7) often reveals the following:

- segmental lesions in otherwise normal, nonatherosclerotic arteries;
- involvement of small and medium-sized vessels;
- more severe changes distally;
- corkscrew-like collateral vessels; and
- larger vessels (e.g., the aorta and the iliac arteries) usually unaffected.

Laboratory Tests

Laboratory findings include

- increased incidence of HLA antigens DR4, A9, B5, and B8;
- increased complement activity;
- sensitivity to human collagens type I and type III; and
- anticollagen antibodies.

One or several of these test results are usually pathologic, but they may, in occasional patients, be completely normal.

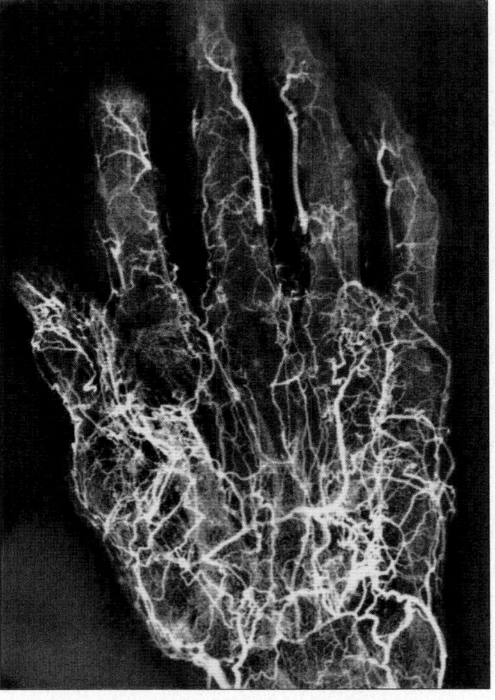

Figure 10.7 Angiographic findings in the hand of a patient with Buerger's disease. Several of the digital arteries are occluded, with acral skin necrosis as a result. (Courtesy of Professor Bollinger, Zurich, Switzerland.)

DIAGNOSTIC TECHNIQUES

A number of tests can be performed to evaluate the peripheral arterial circulation of the extremities. Angiography is one of the most common techniques to visualize the abdominal and leg arteries. However, as it is invasive, and serious complications (bleeding, local trauma on the vessel wall) occurs in 1% to 3%, it should be performed only in patients for whom an operative procedure (percutaneous transluminal angioplasty or surgery) is planned.

Magnetic resonance angiography is a noninvasive technique for computerized imaging of the vascular system. A gadolinium contrast medium is injected intravenously to improve the images and to reduce disturbances.

During the past few decades, noninvasive techniques have been improved and successfully applied in clinical practice.

Local Blood Pressure Measurements

The simplest test for evaluating the arterial circulation of the lower extremity is to measure the ankle systolic blood pressure. This can be performed in any consultation room. The equipment consists of an ordinary blood pressure cuff and some kind of detector for recording blood flow, which should be placed distally to the cuff. Simple, hand-held Doppler ultrasound velocity detectors are most often used. However, other types of recording devices can also be used (e.g., photoplethysmographs or strain-gauge plethysmographs).

Measuring Procedure

The pressure in the cuff is elevated to suprasystolic values, after which the cuff is slowly deflated. The pressure is then measured when blood flow returns, as detected by the recording device. This pressure is equal to the systolic blood pressure at the point in the vessel that is located under the cuff. The pressure can be measured at different levels of the extremity. When the pressure is measured at the level of the ankle, the pressure in both the dorsal pedal artery and the posterior tibial artery should be recorded. The brachial blood pressure should be measured simultaneously. An ankle-brachial pressure index can then be obtained. In normal subjects, this index ranges from 0.9 to 1. Values below 0.9 indicate a significant arterial stenosis in any of the vessels proximal to the ankle region, with moderate reduction of blood flow. Patients who have ischemic rest pain or ulcerations usually have an index of less than 0.5. The measurements may also be performed after a treadmill exercise test, in which case the time until the ankle blood pressure has resumed its pre-exercise value is recorded.[31]

The ankle-brachial index is of importance only for evaluating the degree of obstruction. The local arterial systolic pressure in itself gives a more direct indication of the severity of the reduction in arterial perfusion down to the region distal from the cuff. For example, if a patient has an ankle pressure of 100 mm Hg and a systolic brachial pressure of 200 mm Hg, the index is 0.5, whereas another patient may have an ankle pressure of 50 mm Hg and a brachial pressure of 100 mm Hg, which will give the same index of 0.5. However, it is obvious that this last patient is much worse off than the former patient, who had an ankle pressure of 100 mm Hg. Consequently, both the ankle pressure itself and the ankle-brachial index should be recorded.

Segmental Blood Pressure Measurements

The blood pressure can be measured at different levels of the leg.[31] The most frequently used levels are the proximal and distal thigh level, below the knee, and at the ankle. Pressure measurements can also be performed in the big toe by applying a miniature cuff around the base of the toe. In this region, Doppler ultrasonography cannot be used for determining when blood flow starts distally to the cuff, and strain-gauge plethysmography or photoplethysmography is usually used as a detecting device.

Pressure measurements may be hazardous in some patients with PAOD, especially in those who also have diabetes. On occasion, the arteries may be so stiff from calcification that they can hardly be compressed, and consequently the recorded pressure values will be falsely high. In diabetic patients, this is most often due to the media sclerosis of the leg arteries. In patients in whom a falsely high pressure is suspected, toe blood pressure can be measured instead, as marked calcification of digital arteries is rare.

Venous Occlusion Plethysmography

Several techniques have been used over the years to assess limb blood flow by plethysmography. The most common methods for detecting the volume changes are air plethysmography, photoplethysmography, and strain-gauge plethysmography.

Pulse Volume Recording

Pulse volume recording systems have been used for decades in the evaluation of peripheral arterial disease. Various kinds of transducers for recording the pulse waves are available. These are primarily air cuffs and strain gauges, but photoplethysmography has also been used. Different kinds of calculations can be performed from the recorded pulse waves, including the amplitude of the wave, the time to the peak of the pulse wave, and the inclination time.

Since the introduction of Doppler ultrasound techniques, the importance of pulse volume analyses has been markedly reduced. However, analyses of the most distal pulse wave (i.e., those in the toes) still give valuable information on the degree of reduction in arterial blood flow to the most distal parts of the extremity.

Vascular Ultrasound Techniques

Several different ultrasound principles and types of investigations are available for the evaluation of peripheral arteries:

- Doppler ultrasonography, which can be continuous or pulsed; and
- echo ultrasonography.

Three different types of recording devices are used:

- A (amplitude) mode;
- B (brightness) mode; and
- M (motion) mode, also known as colored Duplex ultrasonography.

The A-mode technique primarily gives information about whether flow is present in the vessel, and the B mode also images the lumen of the vessel. The M-mode technique is a combination of the two other methods and gives both flow information and an actual image of the vessel. This technique can also be color coded to facilitate the localization and type of vessel and the atherosclerotic obstruction. Through directional imaging, arterial blood flow is represented by one color and venous blood flow by another.

Microvascular Techniques

During the past decades, it has clearly been shown that the microcirculation is of major importance for the symptoms in CCLI,[18,27] and various methods for studying blood flow in different parts of the microvascular bed have been developed.[27,32] The final event that produces symptoms in CCLI is a markedly reduced or abolished nutritional circulation in the region, and it is therefore necessary to use microcirculatory methods for evaluation of the nutritional status of local tissue.[18,20,21,27]

Vital Capillaroscopy

Vital capillaroscopy is a technique in use in clinical practice that evaluates, directly and noninvasively, the blood filling and morphologic features of the nutritional skin.[27] Because ulcers are most often localized to limited areas, such as a toe, it is necessary to use a technique that can map the microcirculation in all parts of the foot. This can be performed by capillaroscopy. It has been shown that if a normal structure and blood filling of the capillaries are seen in the skin (stage A in Fig. 10.8), the risk for development of necrosis is less than 10% during an observation period of 3 months, regardless of the macrocirculatory status. However, if marked destruction of the capillary bed is present (stage B in Fig. 10.8) or if no blood enters the nutritional capillaries (stage C in Fig. 10.8) in the sitting position, there is an almost 100% risk for development of skin necrosis during the same period.[21,27] The technique has been shown to be valuable for predicting the risk of skin ulcers in patients who have CCLI and also for evaluating the prognosis of ischemic foot ulcers.[21,27]

A more sophisticated technique is dynamic capillaroscopy, with which blood flow in single skin capillaries can be directly and noninvasively studied.[26,32] With this technique, blood flow in single nutritional skin capillaries can be measured directly in the ischemic regions of patients with peripheral vascular disorders. However, this technique is not useful in clinical practice.

Laser Doppler Fluxmetry

This method, which mainly evaluates the blood circulation through the non-nutritional, thermoregulatory vascular bed of the skin, may also be used to give a crude estimation of the total microcirculation in ischemic areas.[27] However, the technique does not seem to be useful for predicting the risk of skin necrosis, probably because it measures only the total skin microcirculation and does not give any information about whether blood reaches the nutritional capillaries.[27,33,34]

Transcutaneous Oxygen Pressure Measurement

Transcutaneous oxygen pressure measurement has also been used for evaluating the reduction in skin circulation. The method does not seem to be useful for predicting the risk of skin necrosis, but if it is combined with inhalation of oxygen, it has been shown to be a good predictor of the prognosis for a severely ischemic leg.[32] Provocation tests or a combination of methods seem to be necessary to classify the degree of arterial insufficiency in patients who have PAOD.[32,35,36]

Blood Tests

The prognosis for the ischemic leg has been shown to be strongly influenced by several components in the blood. Therefore, a laboratory chemistry analysis, including erythrocyte sedimentation rate, plasma viscosity, prothrombin time, and fibrinogen, should be performed. A number of studies have shown that the hemoglobin value, the fibrinogen level, and the platelet and leukocyte counts are strong predictors of the fate of the ischemic leg, for instance, after vascular reconstructive surgery.[16,17]

Additional, Optional Investigations

As noted, it is of great importance to assess the whole cardiovascular system for optimizing the central circulation. Exercise electrocardiography may be useful for evaluating the status of the coronary arteries, possibly supplemented by coronary angiography. Patients who have CCLI are seldom able to perform a bicycle or walking test, but these patients may do an arm exercise test instead.

MANAGEMENT

The management of patients who have PAOD differs markedly according to the symptoms, and therefore the management of intermittent claudication and of CCLI is discussed separately. Patients who have asymptomatic atherosclerosis in the leg arteries should be investigated for possible risk factors (see Chapter 3). A summary of the management of PAOD is presented in Figure 10.9.

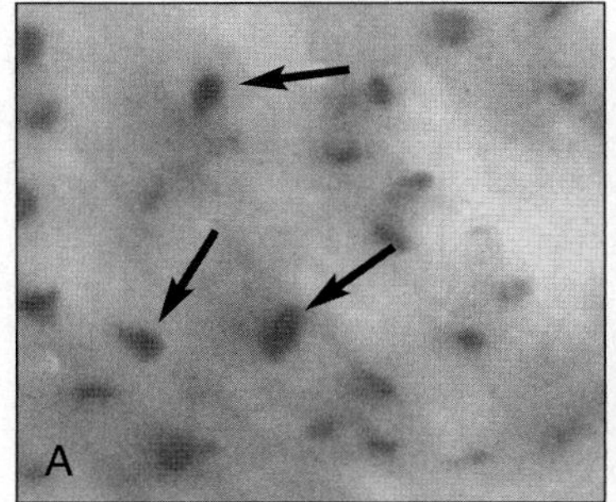

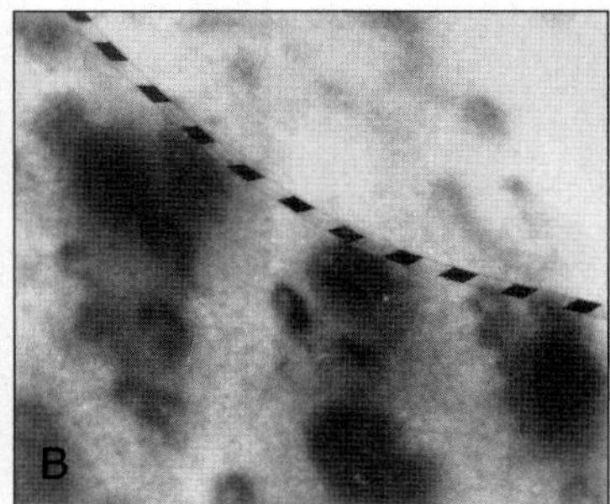

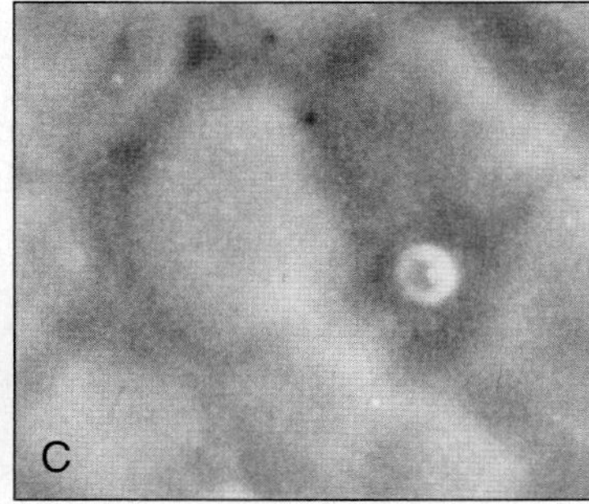

Figure 10.8 Capillary changes in a patient with chronic critical leg ischemia. Note the changes in capillary morphology and blood filling. The investigation was performed in the sitting position. There are marked differences between skin areas in the same foot. **A,** Stage A is normal, with dot- or comma-shaped capillaries that are well filled with blood *(arrows)*. **B,** Stage B shows indistinct capillaries, caused by edema and capillary hemorrhages. **C,** In stage C, only a few or no blood-filled capillaries can be seen.

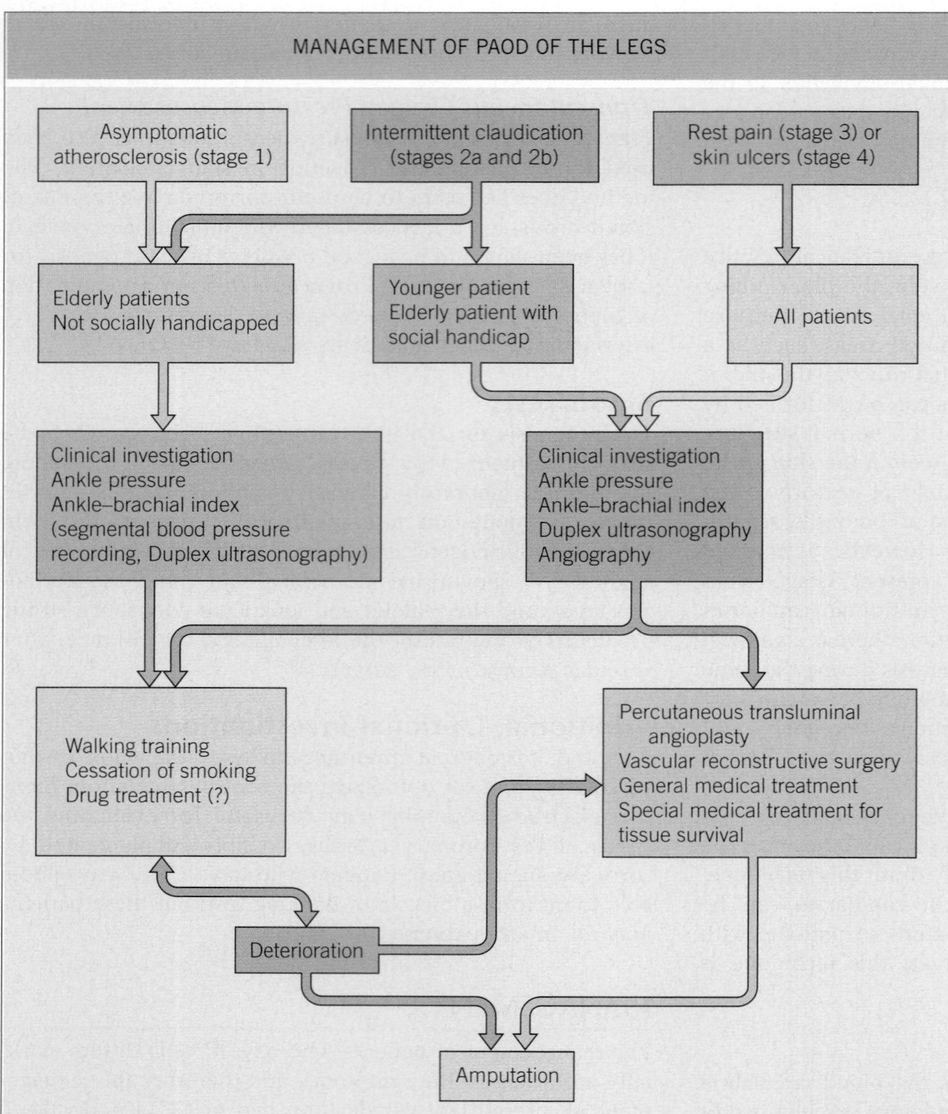

Figure 10.9 Management of peripheral arterial occlusive disease (PAOD) of the legs. The stages referred to are according to Fontaine's classification: stage 1, asymptomatic disease; stage 2, intermittent claudication; stage 3, rest pain; stage 4, skin ulcers or gangrene.

Intermittent Claudication

The optimal treatment of patients who have intermittent claudication has been a matter of long-standing debate. Substantial evidence has accumulated to show that basic treatment of these patients should be conservative, and in several recent reviews, it has been stated that exercise training is the treatment of choice.[37-41]

Natural History of Intermittent Claudication

Patients who have PAOD have a high incidence of symptomatic atherosclerotic disease in many other organs of the body (Table 10.4).[17,42,43]

Annual mortality is around 5% in this group of patients, and life table analyses show that about 50% of the patients either have developed critical ischemia or are dead within 5 years.[17,43] It has also been shown that smoking habits have a major adverse influence on the natural course of the disease.[17,43]

PREVALENCE OF ATHEROSCLEROTIC DISEASE IN PATIENTS WITH PERIPHERAL ARTERIAL OCCLUSIVE DISEASE (PAOD)

Disease	Prevalence (%)
Coronary atheroasclerosis	30-50
Cerebrovascular disease	5-10
Diabetes	5-30
Hypertension	30-55
Hyperlipidemia	30-50

Data from Coffman.[42]

Table 10.4 Prevalence of atherosclerotic disease in patients with peripheral arterial occlusive disease (PAOD).

Conservative Treatment

All patients with claudication should be strongly advised to stop smoking. If they are able to do so, the prognosis, both for the local symptoms of the ischemic leg and for the risk of other cardiovascular complications, will be reduced.[43,44]

The beneficial effect of exercise training in patients who have intermittent claudication is now well proved.[37-41] The improvement in walking distance has been reported to be between 30% and 200%.[45] Several factors are involved in the positive effects:

- muscle adaptation to exercise;
- improved walking technique that will reduce the metabolic demand of the muscle;
- increased tolerance to the pain; and
- insight that the pain is not harmful.

There are no definite data showing that there is increased redistribution of blood or collateralization triggered by the exercise itself. A specific exercise program gives a more marked improvement than if the patient tries to exercise on his or her own.[37,44] The greatest improvement in walking distance until pain develops seems to occur with an exercise duration of longer than 30 minutes per session and a frequency of at least three sessions per week. Walking should be used as the mode of exercise, and it should be performed at nearly maximum pain. The program should last at least 6 months.

Thus, intermittent walking to nearly maximum pain during a special supervised program for at least 6 months gives the best results in terms of walking distance. However, for several reasons, this is not easy to implement in all patients because of cost, transportation difficulties, and successively decreased power of endurance of the patients. Therefore, it is crucial always to encourage the individual patient to walk as often as possible to nearly maximum pain and to do so on a regular basis.

Angioplasty

Dilatation of stenotic or occluded arteries has been the treatment of choice for PAOD since the late 1960s, but it was not until around 1980 that the method came into use in routine treatment of PAOD.[46] Catheter opening procedures now have an established place in the treatment of PAOD, but they are indicated more for patients who have critical limb ischemia.[44]

A few randomized trials have concluded that approximately 10% of claudicants have lesions that are suitable for percutaneous transluminal angioplasty (PTA).[41] The effects of PTA in these patients seem to be a short-term improvement in walking distance and quality of life. Two years after PTA, patients have less extensive vascular disease than medically treated patients, but it does not seem to translate into improved walking ability or better quality of life. The procedure should be considered in younger patients who have limited working capacity because of claudication. With catheter procedures, local thrombolysis may also be applied in combination with balloon dilatation (Fig. 10.10). If a longer occlusion is present, it is also possible to perform a thrombectomy through the catheter, and large amounts of thrombotic material may be extracted. The risk of complications must also be considered after PTA. In the nationwide Swedevasc Registry for vascular procedures in Sweden, the 30-day mortality after PTA for claudication was 0.2%, amputation rates were 0.9%, and about 5% of the patients needed open surgery within 30 days.[7] These figures must be compared with the beneficial effects of conservative treatment.

Reconstructive Vascular Surgery

The place for reconstructive vascular surgery in intermittent claudication is limited. In the iliac vessel, there is rarely an indication for surgery in patients who have claudication. In these patients, the treatment of choice is walking exercise or PTA, or both. In femoropopliteal obstructions, bypass surgery is usually restricted to patients in whom the disease still severely impairs social life after at least 6 months of

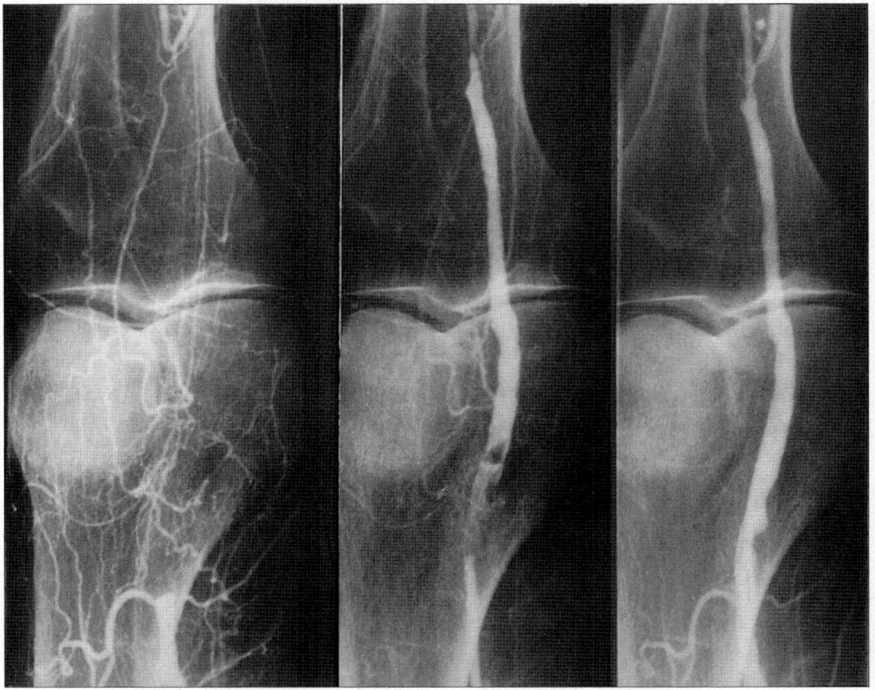

Figure 10.10 Result of thrombolysis and percutaneous transluminal angioplasty (PTA) of a popliteal occlusion. Thrombolysis of a subacute thromboembolus in the popliteal artery. The procedure was followed by conventional PTA. (Courtesy of Professor Bollinger, Zurich, Switzerland.)

conservative treatment. This surgery should be performed only in centers with extensive experience of the procedure (see Chapter 16).[44]

Pharmacotherapy

Several vasoactive drugs have been tried in intermittent claudication, but few have shown convincing positive effects on walking distance. Pentoxifylline affects the rheologic properties of blood and has been tried in several studies. A meta-analysis of the controlled studies of this drug has shown positive effects on walking distance, but the patients usually did not experience any subjective improvement. Naftidrofuryl, a 5-hydroxytryptamine type 2 serotonergic receptor inhibitor, has been shown to exert some beneficial effects on pain-free walking distance in patients who have claudication. However, the marginal increase in walking distance produced by drugs is limited compared with the increase produced by exercise training alone.[44]

Aspirin is now an accepted treatment of patients who have generalized atherosclerosis, and it should therefore be used also in patients who have PAOD, although convincing data on its direct effect on walking distance are limited. Other antiplatelet drugs (ticlopidine and clopidogrel) have shown improvement of walking distance in patients who have claudication. Like aspirin, these drugs also seem to reduce the risk of other vascular events in patients who have PAOD.[47] Oral anticoagulants seem to reduce the incidence of thromboembolic episodes in patients who have atherosclerosis.

Chronic Critical Limb Ischemia

General Management[44]

When rest pain and ulcers are present in the foot, the patient should be advised to avoid extensive walking because this may harm the vulnerable ischemic tissue and cause deterioration. As rest pain and ulcers are signs of severely impaired circulation in the nutritional skin capillaries, great efforts should be made to improve blood flow in these vessels.[27] To improve the pressure gradient across the vessel wall in the ischemic area, it is recommended that the ischemic foot be kept in the lowest possible position without inducing edema. The patient should be instructed to contract the calf muscle repeatedly to improve blood reflow from the leg.

Most patients with CCLI have other concomitant diseases, especially in the cardiovascular and renal systems. Lung diseases, such as chronic bronchitis and bronchial carcinoma, also often occur owing to the high proportion of smokers. It is therefore compulsory to inform patients strongly of the necessity to stop smoking. Several studies have shown that both the macrocirculation and microcirculation of ischemic areas may be improved by smoking cessation. The reason for this is that the rheologic properties of the blood, the oxygen transport by red blood cells, and the blood viscosity improve, resulting in enhanced nutritional skin circulation.[48]

Foot Care

Ulcers and necrosis in CCLI are most frequently observed in the first, fourth, and fifth toes. Occlusions of the precapillary arterioles (30 to 50 μm) and empty nutritional capillaries have also been found in increased frequencies in these toes in patients who have CCLI.[18,19] Even the slightest pressure from a shoe may damage ischemic skin tissue and completely block blood from entering the nutritional skin capillaries, resulting in an ischemic ulcer (see Figs. 10.3 and 10.4). Patients are instructed to wear shoes that are large enough to minimize local pressure. Thick foam rubber inner soles may be used to distribute the pressure of the ischemic foot more evenly during walking.

Cardiac Disease

Coronary heart disease is present in the majority of patients who have CCLI. The possible need for coronary bypass surgery should be evaluated before any intervention of the peripheral leg arteries is performed. Other severe cardiac symptoms, such as heart failure, should be treated optimally. This is necessary regardless of what kind of treatment procedures will be used for the ischemic limb. An improved cardiac function is also of great importance for the surgical outcome in patients who have CCLI.

Edema

Edema in the ischemic area compromises the nutritional skin circulation and must be intensively treated. It has been shown that edema, especially in diabetic patients, may totally compress the nutritional skin capillaries in ischemic areas so that they become completely void of blood.[18,21] By reducing the edema in such areas, blood may enter the capillaries with a concomitant improvement and even healing of the ischemic ulcer. However, treatment with diuretics may reduce the systemic blood pressure, and this can be deleterious for the nutritional circulation in the ischemic region. Consequently, systolic blood pressure must be carefully monitored during treatment of edema.

Hypertension

Blood pressure should as a rule be controlled to normal levels in patients who have PAOD. However, in patients who have CCLI, an elevated blood pressure may be necessary to improve the perfusion of the ischemic region, and in the European Consensus Document, it was agreed that blood pressure up to 180/100 mm Hg could be accepted for a limited period to optimize the nutritional circulation.[16] Patients who are taking antihypertensive drugs and have a low or normal blood pressure may sometimes benefit dramatically if the systemic and local blood pressure is increased by 10 to 20 mm Hg. Consequently, temporary cessation of the antihypertensive treatment should always be considered in these patients. If antihypertensive drugs must be given, beta blockers should be avoided because these drugs may have a deleterious effect on the skin microcirculation in ischemic areas. Diuretics, angiotensin-converting enzyme inhibitors, calcium channel blockers, or other vasodilating substances should be considered instead.

Infection

One of the most serious threats to patients who have CCLI is bacterial infection in the ischemic region.[16] To minimize the spread of infection, the area should be kept dry. If the skin around the ulcer can be kept dry, the risk of bacterial infiltration of the ischemic tissue is minimized. Wet bandages may macerate the skin with a markedly increased risk of spreading the infection. Infection can spread rapidly in ischemic tissue, and antibiotics should therefore be instituted immediately at first signs of infection. Before antibiotic therapy is started, bacterial cultures should be taken for determination of drug resistance.

Revascularization Procedures

Most patients with CCLI have stenotic or occluding lesions of the leg arteries in a multilevel fashion, and stenotic changes can be successfully treated with angioplasty in almost all patients who have iliac or femoral obstructions.[46] This is the first-choice procedure, provided a specialized interventional vascular radiologist or angiologist is available.[16,46] Limb salvage rates of more than 80% after 2 years have been achieved with this procedure.[49] Intra-arterial stents can be used in combination with PTA and may improve the patency rate after PTA.

Thrombolytic therapy, for example, with the use of streptokinase, urokinase, or tissue plasminogen activator, is now used routinely (see Fig. 10.10).[50,51] The lysis can be performed in a systemic form, but intra-arterial thrombolysis has emerged as the primary method. The procedure is most often combined with PTA of the underlying stenosis. The different treatment regimens have been discussed and presented by an international consensus panel.[51]

PTA can also be combined with removal of embolic and thrombotic material.

Pharmacologic Treatment

The main purpose of all treatment procedures in patients with CCLI is to improve the nutritional blood flow in the ischemic tissue. As the ischemic symptoms in these patients are primarily due to macrovascular obstructions, opening procedures should be performed if possible.

If this cannot be done, conservative treatment must be implemented. The possibility of improving the nutritional blood flow in severe ischemic skin areas with pharmacologic agents is limited because of the marked reduction in total blood flow to the region. Another reason very few drug trials have shown any statistically significant improvement in CCLI is that it is difficult to collect a homogeneous group of patients if only macrocirculatory parameters are used to classify the patients. As noted before, microcirculatory methods must be used to determine the nutritional status in an ischemic skin area,[21] and very few such studies have been performed. Nevertheless, remarkable positive effects of different vasoactive drugs can sometimes be demonstrated in single patients (Fig. 10.11).

The only drug therapy that has convincingly been shown to have a positive effect on rest pain and skin necrosis is intravenous infusion of prostanoids. The first studies were reported in the 1970s with prostaglandin E_1 and prostaglandin I_2, but the results were inconclusive. More recently, stable prostacyclin analogues have been tested, and there is now good scientific evidence that these compounds have a positive effect on reducing rest pain and healing ulcers.[52]

Antiplatelet drugs may be used for long-term treatment to reduce progression of atherothrombosis in leg arteries. It has been shown that these agents may also reduce vascular events such as stroke and myocardial infarction in about 25% of patients who have atherosclerotic disease.[47]

Anticoagulant treatment may also be considered in patients who have CCLI to reduce the risk of microthromboembolism or macrothromboembolism in stenotic, atherosclerotic vessels.

No vasoactive drug except prostanoids has, as yet, shown scientifically convincing positive effects on the symptoms of patients who have CCLI. Hyperbaric oxygen therapy and hemodilution have been tried, but there is no scientific support for these interventions. However, advances in molecular biology may generate new principles for the treatment of patients who have PAOD. For instance, in pilot studies, vascular endothelial growth factor seemed to promote angiogenesis in selected patients who have CCLI.[53]

Spinal Cord Stimulation

A few studies have been performed in which electrical spinal cord stimulation has been tried in CCLI. Although promising results have been reported in pilot studies, the treatment is costly and the effect does not seem to be very long lasting.[54]

Amputation

Amputation may be the ultimate but also the best treatment of some patients who have CCLI when all other treatments have failed. Major amputations must be considered in all patients who have CCLI if the probability of successful treatment with other procedures has been ruled out. However, it was agreed in the European consensus process that "reopening procedures should be tried if there is a 25% chance, based on local audited past experience, of saving a useful limb for the patient for at least 1 year."[16] Patients who have a severe ischemia that makes amputation necessary also face an extremely poor long-term prognosis regardless of treatment. Only about half of these patients will be alive after 2 to 3 years.[55]

Buerger's Disease

There is no specific treatment for Buerger's disease as yet. The main treatment of these patients is to avoid tobacco smoke completely (Fig. 10.12). The patient should be informed that some substance in the smoke triggers the inflammatory process. Patients who stop smoking will most often improve spontaneously and dramatically. The stenotic lesions that have developed will not disappear, but they may diminish and symptoms will improve. If the patient does not start to smoke again, new lesions or attacks can be prevented. However, in some patients, passive contact with smoke may be enough to trigger a new attack, with deleterious results.

In the acute stage of Buerger's disease, it may be necessary to try to improve the nutritional circulation of the ischemic areas as fast as possible. Anti-inflammatory drugs such as aspirin, cortisone, and immunosuppressive agents have been tried with limited success. The best treatment so far seems to be prostaglandins, but the effect on ulcer healing is still limited.[56]

Vasospastic Disorders

In patients who have primary Raynaud's phenomenon, the most important approach is to inform them that the disease has a benign course. The patient should also be advised to avoid smoking, to avoid cold exposure, and to not wear rings on the fingers.

Smoking Cessation

Patients who smoke should be told to stop. Cigarette smoking has a long-lasting negative effect on the microcirculation in patients who have Raynaud's phenomenon, and cessation of smoking can result in marked improvement of the symptoms.

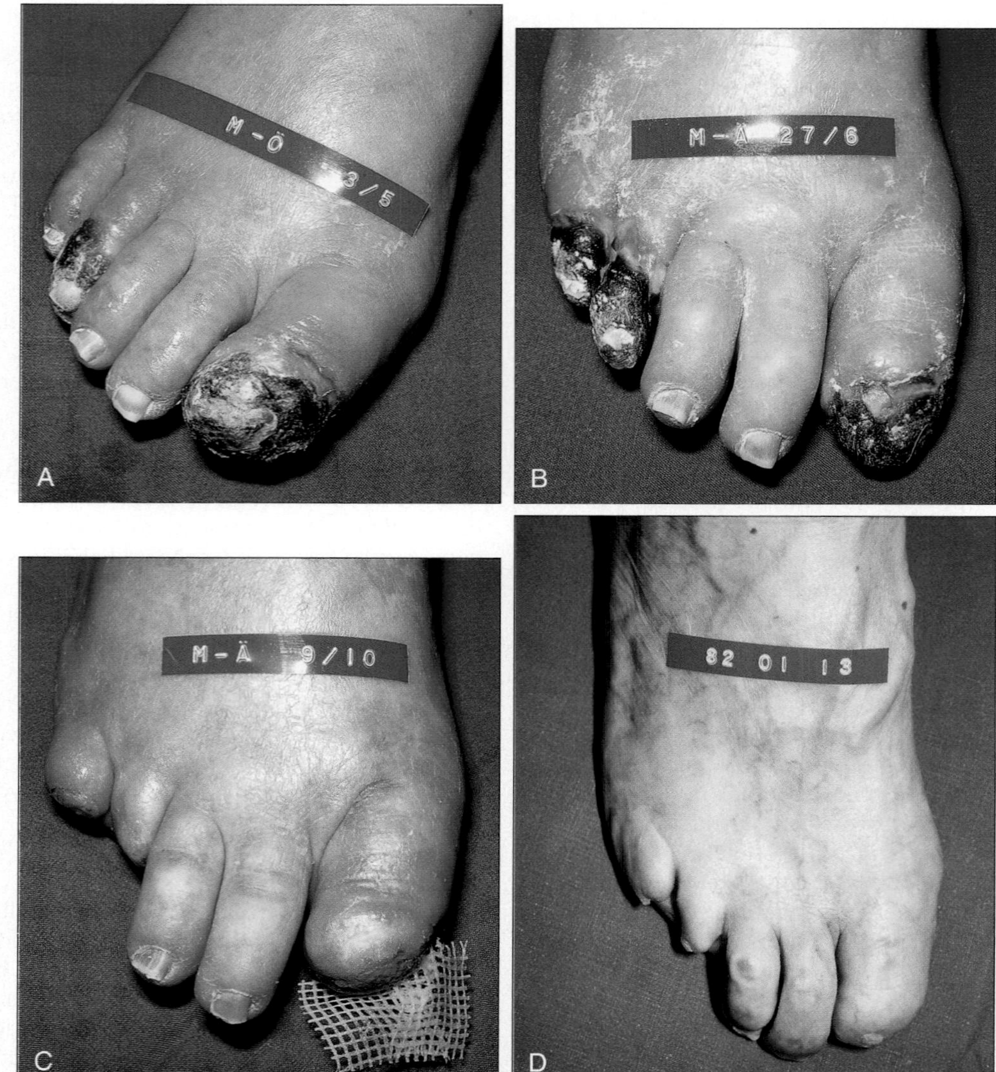

Figure 10.11 Successful result of medical treatment in a patient with severe leg ischemia. A 62-year-old woman with diabetes and marked peripheral arterial occlusive disease in the lower leg arteries had a right great toe blood pressure of 10 mm Hg. A lower leg amputation was planned but she refused and entered a 4-month randomized, placebo-controlled study with buflomedil. **A,** Before treatment, no blood-filled capillaries were visible on the fourth and fifth toes or at the rim of the ulcer at the great toe. The second and third toes had normal capillaries filled with blood. **B,** After 8 weeks of placebo treatment, extensive gangrene of fourth and fifth toes and increased necrosis on the great toe were noted. **C,** After 8 weeks of buflomedil treatment, all patients previously taking placebo received buflomedil for the next 8 weeks, and this is the picture after this period. The capillary bed surrounding the ischemic ulcers became filled with blood after 2 weeks, with concomitant disappearance of rest pain and the start of ulcer healing. The toe blood pressure was still 10 mm Hg. **D,** Six years after buflomedil treatment was ended, the patient had no ischemic symptoms in the foot, except a slight rest pain in the supine position. The toe blood pressure was still only 20 mm Hg.

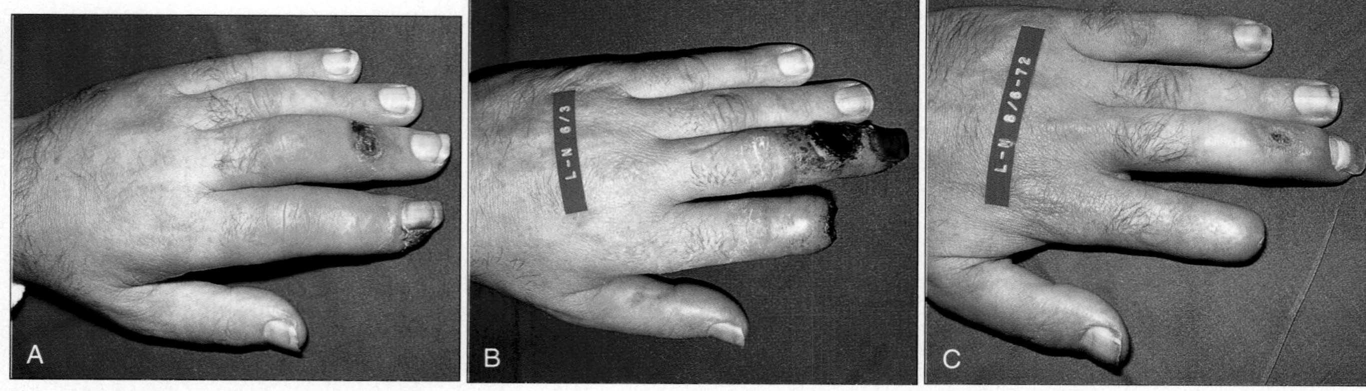

Figure 10.12 Buerger's disease. A 42-year-old man with typical criteria for Buerger's disease.Two toes on the left foot were amputated 5 years ago, after which the patient stopped smoking. **A** and **B,** Three weeks before these photographs were taken, he started smoking again and developed severe ischemia in several fingers. **C,** Four weeks after cessation of smoking, healing of the ulcers was complete.

Avoidance of Cold Exposure

Patients should avoid cold exposure of the peripheral parts of the extremities and should dress carefully. In severe cases, electrically heated gloves and socks are often a very great help in reducing the frequency and severity of attacks.

Avoidance of Rings on the Fingers

The patients should be informed not to wear rings on the fingers. There are a number of Raynaud's patients who have lost a finger because of too tight a ring. The reason for this serious complication is the hyperemia that is induced when patients with Raynaud's disease enter warm surroundings after an ischemic attack. The spasm in the arteries ceases, and a marked vasodilatation follows. A tight ring can then induce venous stasis, and if the ring is not removed immediately, venous gangrene leading to amputation may be the end result.

Drug Treatment

Many studies have been performed with different kinds of vasoactive drugs in patients who have Raynaud's phenomenon. Local nitroglycerin ointment is a simple and often good solution for many of the patients, especially those who have primary Raynaud's phenomenon. This should be applied on the affected digits in a 1% ointment about 20 minutes before exposure to cold, and it will often reduce or prevent the vasospastic attacks.

Some calcium channel blockers (nifedipine and isradipine) have shown positive effects on the vasospastic symptoms.[15] However, because these substances must be given systemically, they sometimes have unpleasant side effects, including flushing, headache, and ankle swelling, which limits their use, especially in younger patients.

In very severe cases, prostaglandin infusions may be helpful, especially in patients who have secondary Raynaud's phenomenon, but it is not yet licensed for this indication in many countries. Moreover, because of its intravenous administration, it is not feasible to use this treatment for longer periods.

SUMMARY

The importance of peripheral arterial diseases is obvious because vascular diseases have a great impact on morbidity and mortality in westernized countries today. This has become more obvious during recent decades with the aging of the population. Several other factors have also renewed interest in peripheral vascular diseases. One of the main reasons for this is the increasing knowledge of vascular biology and pathology, which has opened up a new field in research and clinical practice. New sophisticated methods of investigation have also improved the possibility of making a more precise diagnosis at both the macrovascular and microvascular levels. New treatment modalities, such as intra-arterial thrombolysis, antiplatelet drugs, and possibly also gene therapy, have further increased the interest for patients with various vascular diseases.

chapter 11

Cardiovascular Disease, Stroke, and Dementia

Miia Kivipelto, Babak Hooshmand, and Alina Solomon

The brain is entirely dependent on a properly functioning vascular system. During the past decade, the approach to cerebrovascular disease has been undergoing major changes. It is no longer enough to pay attention only to clinically obvious strokes, and it has become unrealistic to regard vascular disease in the brain as completely separated from neurodegenerative disease. Stroke, dementia (both vascular and Alzheimer's), and cardiovascular disease, all common major health problems, share several risk factors and often occur simultaneously, interacting with one another and warranting a transdisciplinary approach.

According to World Health Organization Statistics 2008, ischemic heart disease and stroke are predicted to remain the leading causes of death in the world even in 2030.[1] Moreover, obvious stroke is only the tip of the "cerebrovascular iceberg" because "silent" (subclinical) strokes are the most common stroke type, occurring five times as often as clinical stroke.[2] Silent events thus place a heavy burden on public health because of the substantially larger number of affected persons. One subclinical stroke is associated with an increased chance of having others and of experiencing clinical stroke or dementia.[3] Subclinical strokes may seem silent because of the habit of leaving out cognition from most stroke studies and "vascular" clinical practice, but persons with so-called silent infarcts have subtle cognitive deficits due to cumulative brain damage.

Just like clinical stroke, dementia is an extreme condition. According to the 2003 World Health Report, the disability weight for dementia was higher than for almost any other health condition, apart from spinal cord injury and terminal cancer.[4] However, milder forms of cognitive impairment are far more common than full-blown dementia, and they often develop insidiously over time, creating a window of opportunity for primary or secondary prevention. Alzheimer's disease (AD), the most common cause of dementia, is a progressive neurodegenerative disease with a long preclinical phase. Although AD has traditionally been separated from vascular dementias, evidence has accumulated during recent years that there is significant overlap between AD and vascular dementia in terms of risk factors, clinical features, and pathologic changes. "Pure" AD and "pure" vascular dementia can be considered the opposite ends of a dementia etiology continuum; most cases are "in between" and have combinations of AD-type and vascular changes in different degrees.[5]

The very concept of "vascular dementia" has been heavily criticized as focusing only on the late stages of cognitive impairment, when it is already too late to intervene effectively. Vascular dementia is currently being replaced with "vascular cognitive impairment," defined as cognitive impairment caused by or associated with vascular factors. Vascular cognitive impairment can occur either alone or in association with AD, and individuals having both pathologic processes frequently show greater cognitive impairment than do those having either pathologic process alone.[6]

Recent results from the Framingham study indicate that the lifetime risk of stroke in middle-aged adults is substantial, at one in six or higher. This risk is higher in women (one in five) compared with men, largely because of the greater life expectancy in women. Moreover, the lifetime risk of stroke either equals or is greater than the lifetime risk of AD. The combined lifetime risk for development of either stroke or dementia is less than 30% in men but nearly 40% in women (exceeding their lifetime risk for development of symptomatic coronary artery disease).[7]

STROKE

EPIDEMIOLOGY

Although the average age-adjusted stroke mortality for developed countries is about 50 to 100 per 100,000 people per year, there are wide differences between countries, suggesting differences in the prevalence of risk factors, genetic factors, and differences in stroke management. Several East European countries have high and increasing stroke mortality rates, whereas low and decreasing rates are reported from most West European countries.[8] According to WHO-MONICA findings, the changes in mortality are principally explained by changes in case fatality (rather than by changes in event rates). Whether this is due to changes in stroke management or disease severity remains to be determined.[9]

Stroke in developing countries accounts for about 70% of global stroke deaths, and 40% of stroke deaths in developing countries were in China. The Sino-MONICA-Beijing Project has recently reported a decreased proportion of deaths of cerebrovascular disease and an increased proportion of ischemic heart disease in China.[10] This study also found a significant increase in the incidence rate of ischemic stroke, declining incidence rates of hemorrhagic stroke, and reduced case fatality rates. However, the total stroke burden was significantly increased.

Projections to the year 2025 suggest that even with stable stroke incidence rates, there will be a marked increase in the number of stroke patients in the next decades.[11] One important contributing factor is the aging of the population. Apart from increasing total stroke burden, demographic changes may also cause a shift of stroke subtype, with a more marked increase in ischemic strokes. The incidence of hemorrhagic stroke reaches a peak around the age of 55 to 65 years and begins to decrease slightly thereafter, whereas the incidence of ischemic stroke increases continuously with age.[12]

CLASSIFICATIONS

Strokes are either ischemic or hemorrhagic, and the different types of stroke have specific courses requiring special treatment and rehabilitation. There are currently two main classification systems, the TOAST (Trial of ORG 10172 in Acute Stroke Treatment) criteria and the OCSP (Oxfordshire Community Stroke Project) classification.[8] The TOAST criteria identify the most probable pathophysiologic mechanism on the basis of clinical findings and results of investigations:

- large-artery atherosclerosis (embolus or thrombosis);
- cardioembolism;
- small-vessel occlusion (lacune);
- stroke of other determined cause; and
- stroke of undetermined cause (two or more causes identified or negative evaluation or incomplete evaluation).

The OCSP classification relies exclusively on clinical findings and is therefore broadly applicable in settings with restricted access to investigations:

- ischemic stroke;
- transient ischemic attack (TIA);
- intracerebral hemorrhage; and
- subarachnoid hemorrhage.

Classification based on the OCSP system can be done in the emergency department and gives important prognostic information. The TOAST criteria help identify the mechanism, which is needed to decide both acute treatments and secondary prevention measures.

CAUSES OF CEREBRAL ISCHEMIA

About 80% of all strokes are ischemic.[8] The description of acute ischemic stroke as a "heart attack" of the brain emphasizes the similarities with myocardial infarction and especially the time-sensitiveness of evaluation and emergency management. However, the causes of acute ischemic stroke are much more heterogeneous than for acute myocardial infarction, implying different prognosis, therapy, and secondary prevention. About 25% of cases are due to large-artery atherosclerosis, 25% to small-vessel disease, 25% to cardioembolism, and 5% to less common mechanisms (such as arterial dissection, vasculitis, hypercoagulability); in about 20% of cases, the etiology remains uncertain despite advanced diagnostic techniques.[13]

Large artery–related acute ischemic stroke has two main similarities to myocardial infarction with respect to underlying pathophysiologic processes: the buildup and destabilization of atherosclerotic plaques in the internal carotid artery or vertebral-basilar arteries; and the development of acute thrombosis on superimposed arterial plaques. However, the clot formed on a ruptured arterial plaque is more likely to cause an ischemic event in the brain by embolizing distally into the intracranial vasculature (artery-to-artery embolization) than by locally compromising vascular patency with secondary distal hypoperfusion. Isolated stenosis of intracranial vessels with associated in situ thrombosis is uncommon in white populations but much more common in Asian populations.[13]

Lacunar infarcts are deep, small infarcts with a diameter of less than 1.5 cm. The main etiology in small vessel–related stroke is the formation of microatheroma in deep, small, penetrating arteries that supply vital structures (i.e., internal capsule, basis pontis). Whether obstruction is predominantly caused by destabilization of microatheromas or as a consequence of superimposed small thrombi is unclear. In a small percentage of cases, small-vessel lacunar strokes may be related to embolization of thrombi from large, more proximal vessels, such as the internal carotid artery, to small penetrating arteries; an even smaller percentage could theoretically be related to cardiac emboli. In patients with lacunar stroke and with evidence of significant ipsilateral carotid artery disease or a cardiac source for emboli, these potential stroke sources are usually considered incidental findings unrelated to the development of the acute lacunar stroke.

An enhanced ability to detect potential sources of cardiac and pericardiac emboli has led to an increased recognition of cardioembolism in the etiology of acute ischemic stroke (Table 11.1). Ischemic heart disorders, such as acute myocardial infarction with a dyskinetic ventricular segment, ventricular aneurysm, and ischemic cardiomyopathy, are recognized sources for emboli to the brain. The existence of a potential source of cardiac emboli does not necessarily imply that the

CARDIOEMBOLIC SOURCES AND EMBOLIC RISK

High Risk	Low or Uncertain Risk
Atrial	**Atrial**
Atrial fibrillation Sustained atrial flutter Sick sinus syndrome Left atrial thrombus Left atrial appendage thrombus Left atrial myxoma	Patent foramen ovale Atrial septal aneurysm Atrial autocontrast
Valvular	**Valvular**
Mitral stenosis Prosthetic valve Infective endocarditis Nonbacterial thrombotic endocarditis	Mitral annulus calcification Mitral valve prolapse Calcified aortic stenosis Fibroelastoma Giant Lambl's excrescences Aortic atheroma Mitral valve strands
Ventricular	**Ventricular**
Left ventricular thrombus Left ventricular myxoma Recent myocardial infarct Left ventricular aneurysm Dilated cardiomyopathy	Akinetic or dyskinetic ventricular segment Hypertrophic cardiomyopathy Congestive heart failure

Modified from Ferro JM. Cardioembolic stroke: an update. Lancet Neurol 2003;2:177-188.

Table 11.1 Cardioembolic sources and embolic risk.

stroke was directly related to the cardiac disorder. For a lacunar stroke, intracranial small-vessel disease is the more likely etiology; for ischemic stroke in a large-vessel territory in patients with coexistent large-artery atherosclerosis, vascular compromise may have been the cause.[13]

DEFINITION OF CEREBRAL INFARCTION

An interesting parallel can be drawn between defining myocardial infarction or unstable angina and defining stroke or TIA. Establishment of the boundary for myocardial infarction also defines unstable angina, and cardiologists have reformulated the definition of myocardial infarction over time on the basis of a tissue criterion. Similarly, establishment of the boundary for TIA also defines cerebral infarction, but the complexity of the brain has long limited neurologists to use of an arbitrary time criterion to distinguish them. The time-based definition of TIA implied that transient clinical symptoms disappeared completely because no permanent brain injury had occurred. Advances in neuroimaging (paralleling advances in serum biomarkers in cardiology) allowed better identification of injury and showed that no single threshold for clinical symptom duration could distinguish patients with and without brain infarction with high sensitivity and specificity.[14] In 2002, the TIA Working Group proposed the following, more tissue-oriented, definition: "a brief episode of neurological dysfunction caused by focal brain or retinal ischemia, with clinical symptoms typically lasting less than one hour, and without evidence of acute infarction." The corollary to the proposed TIA definition is that "persistent clinical signs or characteristic imaging abnormalities define infarction—that is, stroke."[14] However, the current tissue definitions of cerebral infarction are still nonuniform and not operationalizable.

A "universal definition" of myocardial infarction, demarcating any ischemia-related myocyte loss as myocardial infarction, has recently been formulated.[15] A similar trend toward a universal definition exists in vascular neurology, with proposals for defining cerebral infarction as "brain or retinal cell death due to prolonged ischemia."[14] Both "complete" neuropathologic infarcts (regions of complete pannecrosis with tissue collapse) and "incomplete" ones (regions of neuronal dropout with preservation of some supportive tissue) would thus become cerebral infarcts.

The main advantage of a broad tissue definition of cerebral infarcts is that it would include both symptomatic and silent events.[14] TIA must be symptomatic, but cerebral infarcts will not necessarily have to be. Subclinical strokes are actually far more common than clinically obvious ones, and little strokes mean big trouble if they are not detected and treated in time.

Also, the list of stroke symptoms is traditionally focused on motor and sensory deficits, aphasia, and dysphagia. From a practical point of view, it has become important to recognize that some of the symptoms that patients (especially the elderly) manifest, such as changes in cognitive abilities, personality changes, and depression, may be associated with subclinical strokes.[16]

HEMORRHAGIC STROKE

The most common mechanism of intracerebral hemorrhage is hypertensive small-vessel disease, which causes small lipohyalinotic aneurysms that subsequently rupture. Other contributing factors, such as hemorrhage into a previous infarction, may also be important. About two thirds of patients with primary cerebral hemorrhage have either preexisting or newly diagnosed hypertension.[8] The remaining patients may have intracranial vascular malformations (cavernous angiomas or arteriovenous malformations), cerebral amyloid angiopathy, or infarcts into which secondary hemorrhage has occurred.

Subarachnoid hemorrhage accounts for about 5% of all strokes.[8] The main cause is rupture of saccular aneurysms within the subarachnoid space. There is a hereditary propensity for aneurysms, and they sometimes occur together with other pathologic processes, such as polycystic kidney disease and aortic aneurysms. Another cause is represented by arteriovenous malformations.

DIAGNOSIS OF STROKE

The first aim is to confirm that the patient's symptoms are due to a stroke rather than to other medical disorders. Easily recognized symptoms of stroke are

- sudden numbness or weakness of face, arm, or leg;
- sudden deterioration of vision of one or both eyes;
- sudden difficulty in walking, dizziness, and loss of balance or coordination;
- impaired consciousness or difficulty in speaking or understanding; and
- sudden, severe headache with no known cause.

The onset of stroke symptoms is usually sudden, but a gradual progression of neurologic deficits is occasionally elicited in the history. The accuracy of clinical examination by an emergency physician is good (sensitivity, 85%; specificity, 99%). Less often recognized are the "silent" strokes and the cognitive impairment they lead to. The common mimics of stroke are listed in Table 11.2.

Medical history and examination should focus on identification of risk factors for atherosclerotic and cardiac disease, including hypertension, diabetes mellitus, tobacco use, high cholesterol concentration, and history or signs of coronary artery disease, coronary artery bypass, or atrial fibrillation. In younger patients, elicit a history of recent trauma, coagulopathies, illicit drug use (especially cocaine), migraines, or use of oral contraceptives. In alcoholics and elderly people with confusion, it is wise to think of subdural hemorrhage—look for a recent head trauma. The ability to swallow should be tested in all patients to avoid later problems with aspiration.

Laboratory Chemistry

All patients arriving in an emergency department with a possible stroke should have some acute blood tests. Time is crucial.

- Serum glucose: Hypoglycemia is a common cause of stroke-like symptoms. It is easily corrected, and correction leads to rapid resolution of symptoms. Blood glucose testing can also help identify previously unknown diabetes.
- Complete blood count provides information on hemoglobin, hematocrit, and platelet count (important in fibrinolytic candidates). In addition, sickle cell disease, polycythemia, and thrombocytosis increase the risk for stroke.

COMMON MIMICS OF STROKE
Neurologic
Seizure, postictal state Complicated or hemiplegic migraine Subdural hematoma Abscess Tumor, malignant neoplasm, or metastatic brain tumors Hypertensive encephalopathy Multiple sclerosis or other demyelinating process Vertigo Cranial and peripheral neuropathies Spinal cord or disk disease Transient global amnesia Bell's palsy Encephalitis
Metabolic
Hypoglycemia Hyperglycemia Hyponatremia Hepatic encephalopathy Drug overdose
Psychiatric
Conversion disorder Malingering
Other
Syncope
Modified from Khaja AM, Grotta JC. Established treatments for acute ischemic stroke. Lancet 2007;369:319-330.

Table 11.2 Common mimics of stroke.

- Coagulation studies: Prothrombin time, activated partial thromboplastin time, and international normalized ratio (INR) tests need to be done because many patients with acute stroke are receiving anticoagulants; thrombolytic treatment decisions are based on coagulation status.
- Cardiac enzymes and electrocardiography: Not infrequently, patients with acute stroke also have acute myocardial ischemia. In addition to electrocardiographic findings, increased cardiac enzymes may suggest concomitant cardiac injury. Electrocardiography may also demonstrate cardiac arrhythmias, such as atrial fibrillation. At a later phase, transthoracic echocardiography and transesophageal echocardiography are useful tools in evaluating patients with possible cardiogenic sources of their stroke.
- Additional laboratory tests that should be considered for all patients include serum electrolyte determinations, renal function tests, and oxygen saturation.[17]
- Other measures are tailored to the individual patient: hepatic function tests, blood alcohol level, toxicology screen, pregnancy test, arterial blood gas analysis. Measurement of fasting lipid profile, homocysteine concentration, antinuclear antibody, and rheumatoid factor may also be considered. Moreover, in patients with possible hypercoagulable states, certain blood markers, such as antithrombotic proteins (e.g., protein C, protein S, antithrombin III) and antiphospholipid antibodies (e.g., anticardiolipin antibody, lupus anticoagulants), and factor V Leiden testing may be required.
- A lumbar puncture may be required to rule out meningitis or subarachnoid hemorrhage when the computed tomographic scan is normal but the clinical suspicion remains high. Electroencephalography is performed if seizures are suspected. Chest radiography is performed if lung disease is suspected.

Neurologic Examination

A neurologic examination seems to be a powerful tool for prediction of prognosis. Based on the U.S. National Institutes of Health Stroke Scale (NIHSS), which is the most widely used stroke scale in the United States, ischemic stroke patients with an NIHSS score of less than 10 have a 60% to 70% chance of favorable outcome at 1 year compared with only 4% to 16% chance if the score is more than 20.[18] The scale includes 11 items (levels of consciousness, gaze, visual fields, facial movement, motor function for arm and leg, limb ataxia, sensory, language, articulation, and inattention) that are scored. In addition, to facilitate communication between health care professionals, these scores also help quantify the degree of neurologic deficit, identify the possible location of vessel occlusion, and help identify the patient's eligibility for various interventions and the potential for complications.[17]

Imaging Studies

Computed tomography (CT) is the most commonly used form of neuroimaging in the acute evaluation of patients with stroke and in most cases provides the information that is needed to make decisions about emergency management. Non–contrast-enhanced CT is very sensitive in detecting intracerebral and subarachnoid hemorrhage as well as subdural hematomas (Fig. 11.1). Treatment strategies are decided according to the presence or absence of intracranial blood (recanalization strategies for ischemic stroke require the absence of intracranial hemorrhage). CT is not very sensitive for early ischemia (<6 hours), but some findings (i.e., loss of the gray-white matter interface, loss of sulci, loss of the insular ribbon) can suggest relatively early ischemic changes. CT is not ideal in detecting small infarcts and changes in the brainstem area. CT may show other causes of the patient's symptoms, such as tumor, hemorrhagic stroke, and hydrocephalus. A multimodal CT approach, such as CT angiography (may demonstrate the location of vascular occlusion) and perfusion CT (may provide measure of blood volume or flow), may become more available and used in the acute evaluation of stroke patients.[17]

Magnetic resonance imaging (MRI) is an important advance in the neuroimaging of stroke, providing great structural detail (Fig. 11.2). A major limitation of MRI is its availability and the skills required to interpret the images. Diffusion-weighted MRI can detect areas of ischemic brain injury earlier in the evolution of ischemia than can standard T1- or T2-weighted MRI images or CT scan by detecting changes in water molecule mobility. Diffusion-weighted MRI can also better visualize small subcortical lesions and brainstem and cerebellar lesions. Perfusion-weighted MRI uses injected contrast material to show areas of delayed perfusion. A combination of these sequences can yield areas of "diffusion-perfusion mismatch," theoretically identifying

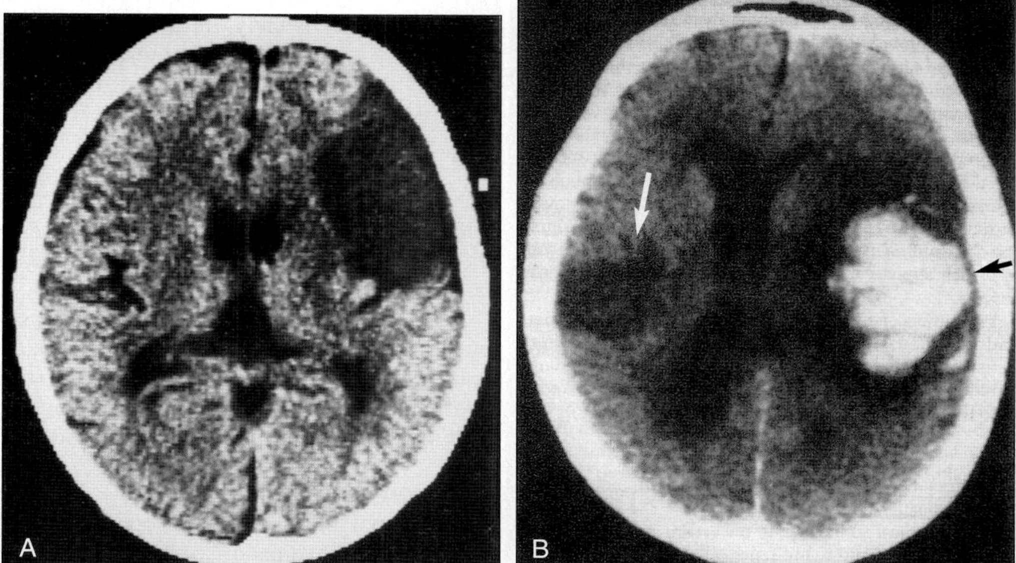

Figure 11.1 Embolic stroke. A, CT scan showing a large cortical infarct in the middle cerebral artery in a patient with atrial fibrillation. **B,** Embolic brain infarct in the right hemisphere *(white arrow)* treated with heparin, which has caused an intracerebral hemorrhage in the contralateral hemisphere *(black arrow).*

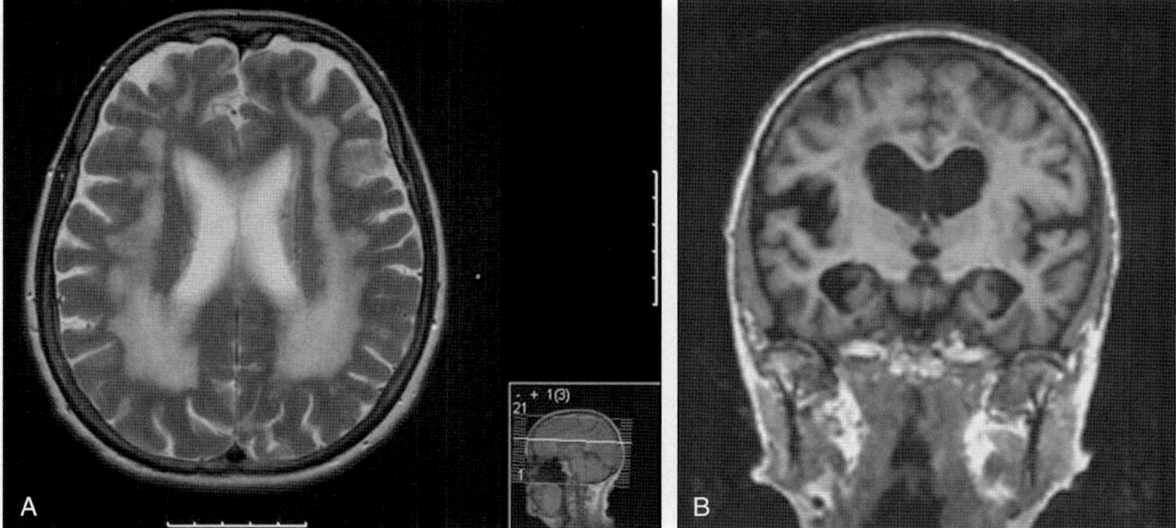

Figure 11.2 MRI of white matter lesions and brain atrophy. MRI brain scan provides valuable information for early diagnosis of cerebrovascular and dementing disorders. White matter lesions **(A)** are commonly seen on MRI scans, especially in elderly persons, and may impair cognitive functions. The picture shows severe white matter lesions commonly seen in vascular dementia. Medial temporal lobe and central atrophy **(B)** are typical structural brain changes in Alzheimer's disease. (**A,** From Dr. Maria Kristoffersen Wiberg, Department of Radiology, Karolinska University Hospital, Huddinge, Sweden; **B,** From Professor Lars-Olof Wahlund, Department of Clinical Geriatrics, Karolinska University Hospital, Huddinge, Sweden).

potentially salvageable tissues (ischemic penumbra; Fig. 11.3). Magnetic resonance angiography, a noninvasive technique, demonstrates cerebral vasculature and occlusive disease.[17]

Digital subtraction angiography is considered the definitive method for demonstrating vascular lesions, including occlusions, stenoses, dissections, and aneurysms. Cerebrovascular angiography not only provides useful information on the extracranial and intracranial vasculature but also allows intra-arterial therapies, both intra-arterial thrombolytics and investigational catheter devices. Angiography requires special facilities and a skilled operator.

Magnetic resonance spectroscopy is an experimental technique that may have potential for distinguishing areas of salvageable neurons from those that are injured irreversibly.

Carotid duplex scanning is one of the most useful tests in evaluating patients with stroke. Increasingly, it is being performed earlier in the evaluation, not only to define the cause of the stroke but also to stratify patients for either medical management or carotid intervention if they have carotid stenoses. Patients with symptomatic critical stenoses on carotid duplex scanning may require anticoagulation before intervention is performed.

Transcranial Doppler ultrasonography can assess the location and degree of arterial occlusions in the extracranial carotid and large intracranial vessels, including the middle cerebral and vertebrobasilar arteries. It can also be used to detect restoration of flow after thrombolytic therapy, and the recent Combined Lysis of Thrombus in Brain Ischemia

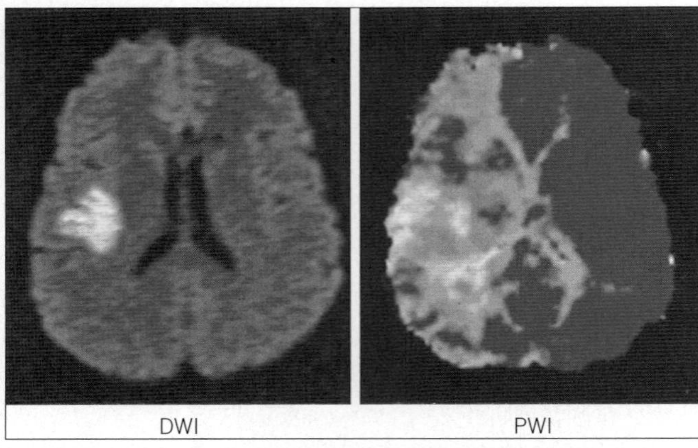

Figure 11.3 MRI of the ischemic penumbra. Mismatch between large perfusion deficit seen on perfusion-weighted image (PWI) and infarct core seen on small diffusion-weighted image (DWI) represents penumbral target for therapy. The mismatch between the diffusion-weighted and perfusion-weighted images is increasingly being used to identify patients who are most likely to benefit from new interventions in acute ischemic stroke. (From Donnan GA, Fisher M, Macleod M, Davis SM. Stroke. Lancet 2008;371:1612-1623.)

Using Transcranial Ultrasound and Systemic TPA (CLOTBUST) study has suggested that transcranial Doppler ultrasonography may even facilitate recanalization.

Single-photon emission computed tomography in stroke is still relatively experimental and available only at select institutions; it can define areas of altered regional blood flow.[17]

STROKE MANAGEMENT

Without doubt, the most substantial advance in stroke has been the routine management of patients in stroke care units, which is effective and appropriate for all stroke subtypes and provides a focus for professionals in stroke care.[8] There is a clear reduction in the proportion with poor outcome when patients treated in a stroke unit early after stroke are compared with patients treated in general wards. Management of patients within a stroke care unit has been shown to reduce mortality by about 20% and to improve functional outcome by about the same amount.[8] In a community-based epidemiologic study, in which all patients eligible for possible acute stroke interventions were considered, stroke care unit management had the potential to prevent death or disability for around 50 patients for every 1000 strokes, compared with 6 per 1000 with tissue plasminogen activator (t-PA) and 4 per 1000 with aspirin.[19]

Acute Ischemic Stroke

Intravenous Thrombolysis

Intravenous thrombolytic therapy for acute stroke is now generally accepted.[17] The use of recombinant tissue plasminogen activator (rt-PA) is associated with improved outcomes for a broad spectrum of patients who can be treated within 3 hours of stroke onset. Earlier treatment (i.e., within 90 minutes) may be more likely to result in a favorable outcome. Later treatment, at 90 to 180 minutes, also is beneficial. Patients with major strokes have a very poor prognosis, but some positive treatment effect with rt-PA has been documented.[17] However, the eligibility to receive rt-PA must be carefully determined on the basis of special criteria[17] because of the risk of hemorrhage. In many trials, there were an excess number of symptomatic intracerebral hemorrhages (about 6% to 7% of cases).[8] The risk increases with age, high blood pressure, very severe neurologic deficits, and severe hyperglycemia and possibly with early ischemic changes on CT.[8] Moreover, this risk has been shown to increase with delay of onset of symptoms to start of treatment and size of the ischemic area. Besides bleeding complications, physicians should also be aware of the potential side effect of angioedema that may cause partial airway obstruction.[17]

The intravenous administration of streptokinase for treatment of stroke is not recommended. Also, the intravenous administration of ancrod, tenecteplase, reteplase, desmoteplase, urokinase, or other thrombolytic agents outside the setting of a clinical trial is not recommended.[17]

Intra-arterial Thrombolysis

Intra-arterial thrombolysis is an option for treatment of selected patients who have major stroke of less than 6 hours' duration due to occlusions of the middle cerebral artery and who are not otherwise candidates for intravenous rt-PA. It is mostly reasonable in those who have contraindications for intravenous thrombolysis, such as a recent surgery. An experienced stroke center with immediate access to cerebral angiography and qualified interventionalists is required for this kind of treatment.[17]

Anticoagulants

For more than 50 years, anticoagulants have been used to treat acute ischemic stroke and continue to be commonly prescribed.[20] However, the usefulness of emergency anticoagulation is debatable.[17,18] Urgent anticoagulation with the goal of preventing early recurrent stroke, halting neurologic worsening, or improving outcomes after ischemic stroke is not recommended.[17] However, this may change if additional data demonstrate the usefulness of very early intravenous administration of anticoagulants for treatment of patients with infarctions secondary to large-artery thrombosis or cardioembolism. Urgent anticoagulation should not be used instead of intravenous thrombolysis for treatment of otherwise eligible patients (and anticoagulant therapy should not be initiated within 24 hours of intravenous rt-PA treatment). In addition, because of an increased risk of serious intracranial hemorrhage, urgent anticoagulation is not recommended in patients with moderate to severe strokes.[17]

Antiplatelet Agents

Oral administration of aspirin (initial dose, 325 mg) is recommended for most patients within 24 to 48 hours after stroke onset. However, aspirin is not a substitute for other acute stroke interventions, including the intravenous administration of rt-PA. Ongoing research is testing the usefulness of intravenously administered antiplatelet agents such as abciximab (a glycoprotein IIb/IIIa receptor inhibitor), given alone or in combination with other interventions.[17]

Hemodilution

Hemodilution is achieved by administration of plasma volume expanders (dextran, hydroxyethyl starch, albumin) or by the combination of plasma expanders and bloodletting. The goal is to improve cerebral blood flow to hyperperfuse potentially viable brain tissue supplied by leptomeningeal collaterals in an attempt to perfuse the ischemic penumbra. However, present data indicate that hemodilution does not reduce case fatality or improve functional outcome in survivors. It is thus not recommended for treatment of acute ischemic stroke (with the exception of stroke patients with severe polycythemia).[17]

Neuroprotection

Potential therapeutic strategies that may limit the cellular effects of acute ischemia or reperfusion include curbing the effects of excitatory amino acids such as glutamate, transmembrane fluxes of calcium, intracellular activation of proteases, apoptosis, free radical damage, inflammatory responses, and membrane repair. Although numerous interventions were promising in experimental studies, most clinical trials produced disappointing results. Several steps to improve research have been recommended, and it is hoped that ongoing studies will demonstrate safety and efficacy.[17]

Intracerebral Hemorrhage

Initial stabilization, prevention of hematoma growth, treatment of complications, and identification of the underlying cause are considered the basic principles of intracerebral hemorrhage management.[21] Management usually depends on the size and location of the lesion. The mass effect of a cerebral hematoma is far greater than in a large cerebral infarction in the acute phase, and it poses greater risk for herniation and death. On the other hand, hemorrhagic patients have a much better prognosis for recovery in the chronic phase than ischemic stroke patients do. Therefore, reducing mass effect is usually the key for treatment of acute hemorrhage.[21,22] Surgical decompression should be considered urgently in patients with cerebellar hemorrhage of more than 3 cm who are deteriorating neurologically or who have brainstem compression or hydrocephalus from ventricular obstruction.[23]

Recombinant factor VII (for attenuating hematoma expansion) and minimally invasive clot evacuation with a variety of mechanical devices or endoscopy are approaches in need of further testing in clinical trials.[8,21,23,24]

Subarachnoid Hemorrhage

Careful management of blood pressure and fluid and electrolyte balance with prevention of hypovolemia is the basis of treatment of all patients with subarachnoid hemorrhage. Rebleeding, delayed brain ischemia, and hydrocephalus are the three main neurologic complications of a ruptured intracranial aneurysm in patients who survive the initial hours after the hemorrhage.[25]

The risk of rebleeding in patients who survive the first day is evenly distributed during the next 4 weeks, with a cumulative risk of 40% without intervention. Rebleeding makes prognosis poor. During the past decade and in specialized centers, endovascular occlusion by means of detachable coils (coiling) of aneurysms has largely replaced surgical occlusion as the intervention of choice for rebleeding prevention.[25] Surgical clipping for occlusion of the aneurysm (usually within 3 days of the initial bleed and if possible within 24 hours) has become the second choice for most patients. Antifibrinolytic drugs (i.e., tranexamic acid) can also prevent bleeding after aneurysmal rupture, but because they increase the risk of cerebral ischemia, they have no useful effect on overall outcome.[25]

Intracerebral extension of the hemorrhage occurs in at least a third of patients, with poor prognosis. Patients with a large hematoma and depressed consciousness might require immediate evacuation, preferably preceded by occlusion of the aneurysm, or extensive hemicraniectomy that allows external expansion of the brain.[25]

Unlike thromboembolic stroke, cerebral ischemia after subarachnoid hemorrhage has a gradual onset, with hemispheric focal deficits or reduction in the level of consciousness evolving during several hours. The peak frequency is 5 to 14 days after subarachnoid hemorrhage. Calcium channel blockers have been shown to improve outcome and to reduce the risk of secondary ischemia after aneurysmal subarachnoid hemorrhage. Oral nimodipine is currently indicated on the basis of several studies.[25,26] Tirilazad, a scavenger of free radicals, may also improve the outcome in subarachnoid hemorrhage in men (but not in women). It may be used in combination with nimodipine.

A gradual reduction in consciousness in the next few hours in a previously alert patient is a typical presentation of acute hydrocephalus.[25] Repeated CT scanning is needed to diagnose or to exclude hydrocephalus. External drainage of the cerebrospinal fluid by a catheter inserted through a burr hole is the usual method for treatment of acute hydrocephalus. Ventriculitis is a common complication, especially if drainage is continued for more than 3 days.[25]

MANAGEMENT OF ACUTE COMPLICATIONS

Brain Edema

Brain edema is a leading cause of death after a major ischemic stroke and represents a pressing issue. At present, evidence is still needed to establish the effectiveness of medical and surgical interventions in controlling brain edema, preventing the neurologic consequences of increased intracranial pressure or herniation, or improving outcomes after stroke. Corticosteroids are not recommended for treatment of cerebral edema because of the lack of evidence for efficacy and the potential to increase the risk of infectious complications.[17] Hyperventilation, furosemide, mannitol, and glycerol are traditionally used, but these measures are still unproven. Decompressive surgery for malignant edema of the cerebral hemisphere may be lifesaving, but the impact on morbidity is unknown. It appears that earlier interventions may be associated with better clinical outcomes than waiting for the patient to have signs of profound neurologic dysfunction, such as herniation.[17]

Elevated Blood Pressure

About 70% of ischemic stroke patients have high blood pressure at onset.[8] For every increase of 10 mm Hg above 180 mm Hg, the risk of neurologic deterioration was shown to increase by 40% and the risk of poor outcome by 23%. Blood pressure elevation may be secondary to the stress of the cerebrovascular event, a full bladder, nausea, pain, preexisting hypertension, a physiologic response to hypoxia, or a response to increased intracranial pressure. Blood pressure decline may occur within the first hours after stroke even without any specific medical treatment.[17] However, urgent antihypertensive therapy may be needed in patients who also have hypertensive encephalopathy, aortic dissection, acute renal failure, acute pulmonary edema, or acute myocardial infarction.

Uncertainty exists about how to manage high blood pressure in the early stages of stroke. By consensus, medications should be withheld unless the systolic blood pressure is above 220 mm Hg or the diastolic blood pressure is above 120 mm Hg.[17] Evidence from one clinical trial indicates that initiation of antihypertensive therapy within 24 hours of stroke is relatively safe, and it is generally agreed that it should be restarted at about 24 hours for patients who have preexisting hypertension and are neurologically stable unless there is an identified contraindication to restarting treatment.[17]

In patients otherwise eligible for rt-PA treatment, blood pressure should be lowered to maintain systolic blood pressure of 185 mm Hg or lower and diastolic blood pressure of 110 mm Hg or lower before lytic therapy is started. Because there is a short maximum interval from stroke onset until rt-PA treatment, many patients with sustained hypertension above recommended levels cannot be treated with intravenous rt-PA.[17]

Overall, suggested guidelines for treatment of elevated blood pressure in spontaneous intracerebral hemorrhage state that aggressive reduction of blood pressure with continuous intravenous infusion should be considered if systolic blood pressure is above 200 mm Hg or mean arterial pressure is above 150 mm Hg, with blood pressure monitoring every 5 minutes.[23] If systolic blood pressure is above 180 mm Hg or mean arterial pressure is above 130 mm Hg and there is evidence or suspicion of elevated intracranial pressure, then monitoring of intracranial pressure and reduction of blood pressure to keep cerebral perfusion above 60 to 80 mm Hg may be considered.[23] For systolic blood pressure above 180 mm Hg or mean arterial pressure above 130 mm Hg without evidence or suspicion of elevated intracranial pressure, a modest blood pressure reduction (e.g., mean arterial pressure of 110 mm Hg or target blood pressure of 160/90 mm Hg) may be considered, and patients should be reexamined every 15 minutes. Some of the intravenous medications to be considered for blood pressure control in intracerebral hemorrhage are labetalol, nicardipine, esmolol, enalapril, hydralazine, nitroprusside, and nitroglycerin.[23]

Deep Venous Thrombosis and Pulmonary Embolism

Approximately 10% of deaths after ischemic stroke are due to pulmonary embolism.[17] Pulmonary emboli generally arise from venous thrombi developed in a paralyzed lower extremity or pelvis. Early mobilization, antithrombotic agents, and the use of external compression devices may reduce risk. In immobilized patients, subcutaneous anticoagulants are recommended for prevention of deep venous thrombosis. Aspirin can also prevent deep venous thrombosis but is less effective than anticoagulants. Intermittent external compression devices can be used in patients who cannot receive anticoagulants.[17]

Patients with acute primary intracerebral hemorrhage and hemiparesis or hemiplegia should have intermittent pneumatic compression for prevention of venous thromboembolism.[23] After cessation of bleeding, low-dose subcutaneous low-molecular-weight heparin or unfractionated heparin may be considered in patients with hemiplegia. Intracerebral hemorrhage patients who develop acute proximal venous thrombosis, particularly those with clinical or subclinical pulmonary emboli, may be considered for acute placement of a vena cava filter.[23]

Fever

Elevated body temperature after stroke is associated with poor neurologic outcome.[17,23] This is possibly secondary to increased metabolic demands, enhanced neurotransmitter release, and increased free radical production. The source of any fever should be identified (i.e., a cause of stroke, like infective endocarditis; a complication, such as pneumonia). It is generally agreed that sources of fever should be treated and antipyretics should be administered to lower temperature.[17,23]

Hyperglycemia

Hyperglycemia is present in as many as one third of patients with stroke. It may be secondary to the stress of the acute cerebrovascular event.[17] Persistent hyperglycemia (>140 mg/dL) during the first 24 hours after stroke is associated with poor outcomes; it is generally agreed that treatment is needed.[17,23] The detrimental effects of hyperglycemia are not clearly understood, but they include increasing tissue acidosis secondary to anaerobic glycolysis, lactic acidosis, and free radical production. It may also affect the blood-brain barrier and the development of brain edema and may be associated with an increased risk of hemorrhagic transformation of the infarction. Close monitoring of glucose concentration with adjustment of insulin doses to avoid hypoglycemia is recommended. Simultaneous administration of glucose and potassium also may be appropriate.[17]

Seizures

Seizures commonly occur after intracerebral hemorrhage and may be nonconvulsive.[23] In ischemic stroke, however, seizures are more likely to occur within the first 24 hours and are usually partial, with or without secondary generalization. Recurrent seizures may occur as well, but status epilepticus is uncommon. Recurrent seizures after stroke require treatment, but prophylactic administration of anticonvulsants to stroke patients without seizures is not recommended.[17]

Acute Confusion

Some degree of acute confusion (delirium) is present in as many as 40% to 50% of patients at some time during the acute phase of stroke.[27] The confusion is often caused by the brain lesion itself, but it may also be drug induced (anticholinergic agents, in particular) or associated with complications like pneumonia, urinary retention, pulmonary emboli, myocardial infarction, or sleep apnea. If drug therapy is required to alleviate the delirium, short-acting sedatives without anticholinergic action are preferred. Most confusional states are transient, but they may predict later development of dementia.

Neuropsychiatric Complications

Depression is the most frequently occurring psychiatric disorder after stroke. The reported prevalence varies from 20% to 50% within the first year, with an apparent peak within the first 6 months of onset event.[28] Post-stroke depression has been consistently associated with poor cognitive status and functional outcome. Despite high prevalence and serious sequels, post-stroke depression most often remains undetected and untreated. Because stroke patients are sensitive to cardiovascular and other adverse effects of tricyclics, serotonin reuptake inhibitors are preferred.[29]

Other conditions such as post-stroke anxiety disorder, catastrophic reaction (emotional outbursts, usually short-lived and related to trigger stressors such as performance of a cognitive task), anosognosia, pathologic affect (uncontrollable episodes of laughter or crying, discordant or disproportionate to the situation), psychosis, and apathy can also be observed in stroke patients.[30]

REHABILITATION AFTER STROKE

- The effects of stroke units are well documented; very early start of reactivation and rehabilitation is a key feature of stroke unit care.
- In constraint-induced training, the affected limb is immobilized and the affected side is trained intensively, for many hours a day. This strategy has been reported to be very effective also in the late phase after stroke.[31]
- There is no good scientific proof that any of the other physiotherapeutic techniques applied in stroke patients is superior (if the therapies are conducted with the same intensity).
- Documented beneficial long-term effects of systematic training of perception deficits and cognitive dysfunction are lacking.
- In patients with aphasia or dysphasia, it is still controversial whether specific speech therapy provided by professionals is superior to unspecific training of speech, for example, by family members or stroke club volunteers.

Brain plasticity is a much-unexplored area of research, and it may well be that in the near future, there will be major scientific breakthroughs to the benefit of stroke patients in their rehabilitation. Drugs that facilitate rehabilitation are an area of great interest.

STROKE PROGNOSIS

The prognosis is better for ischemic stroke compared with hemorrhagic stroke (for which 1-month mortality is about 50%).[8] Early mortality is usually due to neurologic deterioration and other causes, such as infections secondary to aspiration (if not managed aggressively). Later mortality is commonly caused by cardiac disease or complications of stroke. In the OCSP classification, the 1-year mortality for patients with stroke affecting the entire anterior circulation supplying one side of the brain (total anterior circulation syndromes) is about 60%, substantially higher than for those with partial anterior circulation and posterior circulation syndromes (about 15% to 20%), which in turn is higher than that for patients with lacunar syndromes (10%).[8]

The best predictors of stroke recovery at 3 months are the initial neurologic deficit and age; other factors include high blood glucose concentrations, body temperature, and previous stroke. After TIA or minor stroke, the risk of further stroke is substantially higher than previously thought, reaching as high as 30% within the first month in some subgroups.[8] Patients at very high risk (>30%) of recurrence within 7 days can be identified on the basis of simple scores (Table 11.3). Neuroimaging findings (e.g., diffusion-weighted image lesions on MRI or occluded vessels on magnetic resonance angiography) can also identify patients at increased risk of recurrence.

ABCD PROGNOSTIC SCORE FOR EARLY RISK OF STROKE AFTER TRANSIENT ISCHEMIC ATTACK

Feature	Points
Age 60 years or older	1
Blood pressure elevation on first assessment (≥140 mm Hg systolic, ≥90 mm Hg diastolic)	1
Clinical features of transient ischemic stroke	
Unilateral weakness	2
Speech impairment without weakness	1
Duration of transient ischemic attack	
≥60 minutes	2
10–59 minutes	1
Diabetes	1

A score of ≥4 might justify admission to the hospital or urgent evaluation, treatment, and observation because 30-day stroke risk is on the order of 5% to 15%.

Modified from Donnan GA, Fisher M, Macleod M, Davis SM. Stroke. Lancet 2008;371:1612-1623.

Table 11.3 ABCD prognostic score for early risk of stroke after transient ischemic attack.

SECONDARY STROKE PREVENTION

In the past 30 years, recurrent stroke prevention has been one of the major therapeutic advances in stroke management. There was no proven secondary prevention strategy for stroke in 1977. Aspirin and aspirin plus dipyridamole were introduced in 1978 and 1987, respectively; warfarin for patients with atrial fibrillation, in 1993; carotid endarterectomy for symptomatic carotid artery stenosis of greater than 70%, in 1991; clopidogrel, in 1996; blood pressure reduction with perindopril and indapamide or ramipril, in 2001; and cholesterol reduction with atorvastatin, in 2006. Hence, a formidable array of secondary prevention strategies is now available, with most patients qualifying for at least one and many for up to three or more interventions at hospital discharge.[8] The current recommended strategies usually include monitoring and treatment of vascular risk factors, use of low-dose aspirin and dipyridamole in patients with ischemic stroke of arterial origin, oral anticoagulation in patients with cardiac embolism, and carotid endarterectomy in patients with substantial ipsilateral carotid stenosis.[32]

RISK FACTOR CONTROL IN PATIENTS WITH TRANSIENT ISCHEMIC ATTACK OR ISCHEMIC STROKE

Hypertension

Antihypertensive treatment is recommended for all ischemic stroke or TIA patients beyond the hyperacute period, even for patients with no hypertensive history. An absolute target blood pressure level and the amount of reduction are still uncertain, but a reduction of about 10/5 mm Hg has been proved to be beneficial, and normal blood pressure has been defined as below 120/80 mm Hg by the Seventh Report of the Joint National Committee on Prevention, Detection, Evaluation, and Treatment of High Blood Pressure (JNC-7). It is still undetermined whether a particular class of antihypertensive drugs or a particular drug within a given class can offer a particular advantage for patients after ischemic stroke. Much discussion has been focused on the role of angiotensin-converting enzyme inhibitors.[33] The Heart Outcomes Prevention Evaluation (HOPE) study, comparing ramipril and placebo, found a 24% risk reduction for stroke, myocardial infarction, or vascular death among high-risk patients with a history of stroke or TIA.[34] The Perindopril Protection Against Recurrent Stroke Study (PROGRESS), a large multinational trial, showed that combination therapy (perindopril plus the diuretic indapamide) can result in a 43% reduction in the risk of the recurrent stroke, with the effects present in both hypertensive and normotensive groups. Interestingly, there was no significant benefit when the angiotensin-converting enzyme inhibitor was given alone.[35] Therefore, whereas the blood pressure targets and specific drug choices should be individualized, available data give support for the use of diuretics and the combination of diuretics and an angiotensin-converting enzyme inhibitor.[33]

Diabetes

In patients with TIA or ischemic stroke, maintenance of nearly normal levels of glucose is recommended (hemoglobin A_{1c} level $\leq 7\%$) to reduce microvascular and macrovascular complications.[33] However, if glucose control is excessively tight, hypoglycemia may increase the risk of mortality.[36] Moreover, strict control of lipid levels and blood pressure is recommended for diabetic patients. In addition, most patients will require more than one agent to control their blood pressure. Angiotensin-converting enzyme inhibitors and angiotensin receptor blockers are recommended as first-line antihypertensives as they can reduce the progression of renal disease.[33]

Lipids

Although the relationship between lipid levels and ischemic stroke has not been as clearly established as the relationship between lipids and cardiac disease, evidence supports lowering of lipid levels to reduce the risks of initial and recurrent stroke.[36] For ischemic stroke and TIA patients with elevated cholesterol, comorbid coronary heart disease, or evidence of atherosclerotic origin, it is recommended that clinicians follow National Cholesterol Education Program Adult Treatment Panel III guidelines for lifestyle modification, dietary guidelines, and medications.[33] Statin therapy is recommended with the goal of low-density lipoprotein cholesterol level below 100 mg/dL in those with coronary heart disease or symptomatic atherosclerotic disease and below 70 mg/dL in very high risk patients with multiple risk factors.[33] On the basis of the SPARCL (Stroke Prevention by Aggressive Reduction in Cholesterol Levels) trial, statin therapy with intensive lipid-lowering effects is recommended for all patients with atherosclerotic ischemic stroke or TIA, even for those without any known coronary heart disease, to reduce the risk of stroke and cardiovascular events.[37,38] Mechanisms other than cholesterol lowering, so-called pleiotropic effects of statins (e.g., anti-inflammatory, improved fibrinolytic activity, increased cerebral blood flow), also may be involved.[39] Moreover, management with niacin or gemfibrozil can be considered for ischemic stroke or TIA patients with low levels of high-density lipoprotein cholesterol.[37]

Lifestyle-Related Modifications

Avoidance of smoking (even passive smoking) should be recommended to all patients with ischemic stroke or TIA. Counseling and nicotine products can help facilitate cessation.[33] It is recommended that heavy drinkers with prior ischemic stroke or TIA eliminate or reduce their alcohol consumption. However, light to moderate levels ($\leq$2 alcohol drinks/day for men and $\leq$1 drink/day for nonpregnant women) may be permitted.[33] To maintain a goal of a normal body mass index (18.5 to 25 kg/m^2) and a waist circumference of less than 35 inches for women and less than 40 inches for men, weight management through an appropriate balance of calorie intake, physical activity, and behavioral counseling is encouraged for all overweight ischemic stroke or TIA patients. In addition, 30 minutes or more of moderate-intensity physical activity on most days is recommended in ischemic stroke or TIA patients who are able to engage in physical activity. A supervised therapeutic exercise regimen is recommended for those with disability after ischemic stroke.[33]

Anticoagulation for Patients with Cardiogenic Embolism

Patients with cardiac disease and cerebral infarction face a high risk of recurrent stroke. Because it is often difficult to determine the exact mechanism, the choice of a platelet inhibitor or anticoagulant drug may be difficult. Patients with a high-risk source of cardiogenic embolism and ischemic stroke should generally be treated with anticoagulants to prevent recurrence.

- Atrial fibrillation: Both persistent atrial fibrillation and paroxysmal atrial fibrillation are potent predictors of first and recurrent stroke, and therefore long-term oral anticoagulant treatment should be initiated within 2 weeks of the stroke. Warfarin targeted to an INR of 2.5 (range, 2.0 to 3.0) is recommended. Aspirin (325 mg/day) may be considered for patients unable to take oral anticoagulants.[33]
- Acute myocardial infarction: In cases of ischemic stroke or TIA due to myocardial infarction and cardiac imaging shows a left ventricular mural thrombus, treatment with oral anticoagulants for 3 months to 1 year is reasonable (target INR, 2.0 to 3.0). In addition, concurrent use of aspirin for ischemic coronary artery disease with doses up to 162 mg/day during oral anticoagulant therapy may be considered.
- Cardiomyopathy: Warfarin (INR, 2.0 to 3.0) or antiplatelet therapy may be recommended for prevention of recurrent events in ischemic stroke or TIA patients.[33]
- Valvular heart diseases: Long-term warfarin therapy with a target INR of 2.5 (range, 2.0 to 3.0) is recommended in patients with ischemic stroke or TIA who have rheumatic mitral valve disease, whether or not atrial fibrillation is present. To avoid additional bleeding risk, antiplatelet

agents should not be routinely added to warfarin. However, in cases of embolism recurrence while warfarin is being taken, the addition of aspirin (81 mg/day) may be suggested whether or not atrial fibrillation is present.[33]

In mitral valve prolapse, long-term antiplatelet therapy has been suggested for ischemic stroke and TIA patients. Antiplatelet therapy may also be considered in patients with aortic valve disease who do not have atrial fibrillation.[33] Finally, in patients with modern mechanical prosthetic heart valves, oral anticoagulants targeted to an INR of 3.0 (range, 2.5 to 3.5) have been recommended. However, if ischemic stroke or systemic embolism occurs while oral anticoagulant therapy is adequate, addition of 75 to 100 mg/day of aspirin and maintenance of the INR at a target of 3.0 (range, 2.5 to 3.5) are reasonable. On the other hand, for ischemic stroke and TIA patients with bioprosthetic heart valves and no other source of thromboembolism, warfarin, targeted to an INR of 2.0 to 3.0, may be considered.[33]

Antithrombotic Therapy for Noncardioembolic Stroke or Transient Ischemic Attack

For all noncardioembolic ischemic stroke and TIA patients (specifically atherosclerosis, lacunar infarcts, or cryptogenic infarcts), antiplatelet agents rather than oral anticoagulation are recommended to reduce the risk of recurrent stroke and other cardiovascular events.[33,37] The selection of an antiplatelet agent should be individualized on the basis of patient risk factor profiles, tolerance, and other clinical characteristics. Acceptable options for initial therapy are aspirin (50 to 325 mg/day) monotherapy, the combination of aspirin and extended-release dipyridamole, and clopidogrel monotherapy.[37]

However, the new American Heart Association/American Stroke Association guideline recommends the use of the combination of aspirin and extended-release dipyridamole over aspirin alone. For patients who experienced an ischemic stroke event while using aspirin, there is no evidence that increasing the dose of aspirin provides additional benefits.[37] On the basis of direct-comparison trials, clopidogrel may be considered over aspirin alone. This drug is also advised for patients allergic to aspirin. The addition of aspirin to clopidogrel increases the risk of hemorrhage, and this combination therapy is not routinely recommended for ischemic stroke or TIA patients unless they have a specific indication for this therapy, like coronary stent or acute coronary syndrome.[37]

Interventional Approaches for the Patient with Large-Artery Atherosclerosis

Carotid endarterectomy is recommended for patients who had ischemic stroke or TIA in the previous 6 months and severe ipsilateral (70% to 99%) carotid artery stenosis. In case of moderate ipsilateral carotid stenosis (50% to 69%), carotid endarterectomy may be recommended, depending on patient-specific factors such as age, gender, comorbidities, and severity of initial symptoms. There is no indication for carotid endarterectomy when the degree of stenosis is less than 50%. Surgery within 2 weeks rather than delayed surgery is recommended when carotid endarterectomy is indicated.[33]

If stenosis is severe (>70%) and symptomatic and is difficult to access surgically or is radiation induced, if it results after a prior endarterectomy, or if comorbid conditions make surgery a high-risk procedure, carotid artery balloon angioplasty and stenting should be considered.[33]

In cases of symptomatic extracranial vertebral artery stenosis, endovascular therapy (e.g., angioplasty, stenting) may be considered when patients are having symptoms despite treatment with antithrombotics, statins, and other medical therapies.[33,36]

DEMENTIA

A useful comparison for understanding dementia would be a "heart failure" of the brain. Both heart failure and dementia are major and growing health problems, and they are both primarily conditions of the elderly. Just as heart failure can result from several cardiac disorders, dementia is a complex clinical syndrome with several possible causes, the most frequent of which are Alzheimer's disease (AD) and cerebrovascular disease. For dementia, cognitive, behavioral, and psychiatric symptoms correspond to the three cardinal heart failure manifestations (dyspnea, fatigue, fluid retention). These categories of symptoms do not necessarily dominate the clinical picture at the same time, and they can vary over time. A parallel can also be drawn between acute and chronic heart failure and delirium and dementia. Delirium (acute confusional state) can be either the beginning of a dementia syndrome or a transient result of various medical conditions (in the brain or elsewhere in the body). The management, however, is different from dementia management.

The dementia syndrome caused by AD is typically dominated by memory impairment and continuous progression, whereas the typical vascular dementia syndrome is dominated by impairment of executive functioning (involved in processes such as planning, cognitive flexibility, abstract thinking, initiation of appropriate actions and inhibition of inappropriate actions, selection of relevant sensory information) and focal neurologic signs. The progression can be stepwise; but in small-vessel disease or vascular dementia due to small lacunar infarcts, the progression is often continuous. There is no single diagnostic test for dementia or for heart failure; they are largely clinical diagnoses based on careful history and examination. Neuroimaging (preferably MRI; see Fig. 11.3), cerebrospinal fluid analyses, and careful neuropsychological examination give valuable information for early diagnosis of dementing disorders. Full-blown heart failure, just like full-blown dementia, represents the end stage of the underlying disease. Thus, the best approach implies not only early diagnosis and treatment but especially prevention.

The American College of Cardiology/American Heart Association classification of heart failure,[40] which emphasizes both the development and progression of disease, has some similarities with the current trends in the dementia field (Fig. 11.4). Stage A corresponds to the "brain at risk" stage, when risk factors for AD and stroke are present but without structural brain changes or symptoms. Interestingly, cardiovascular disease, stroke, AD, and vascular dementia have many risk factors in common (Table 11.4), warranting

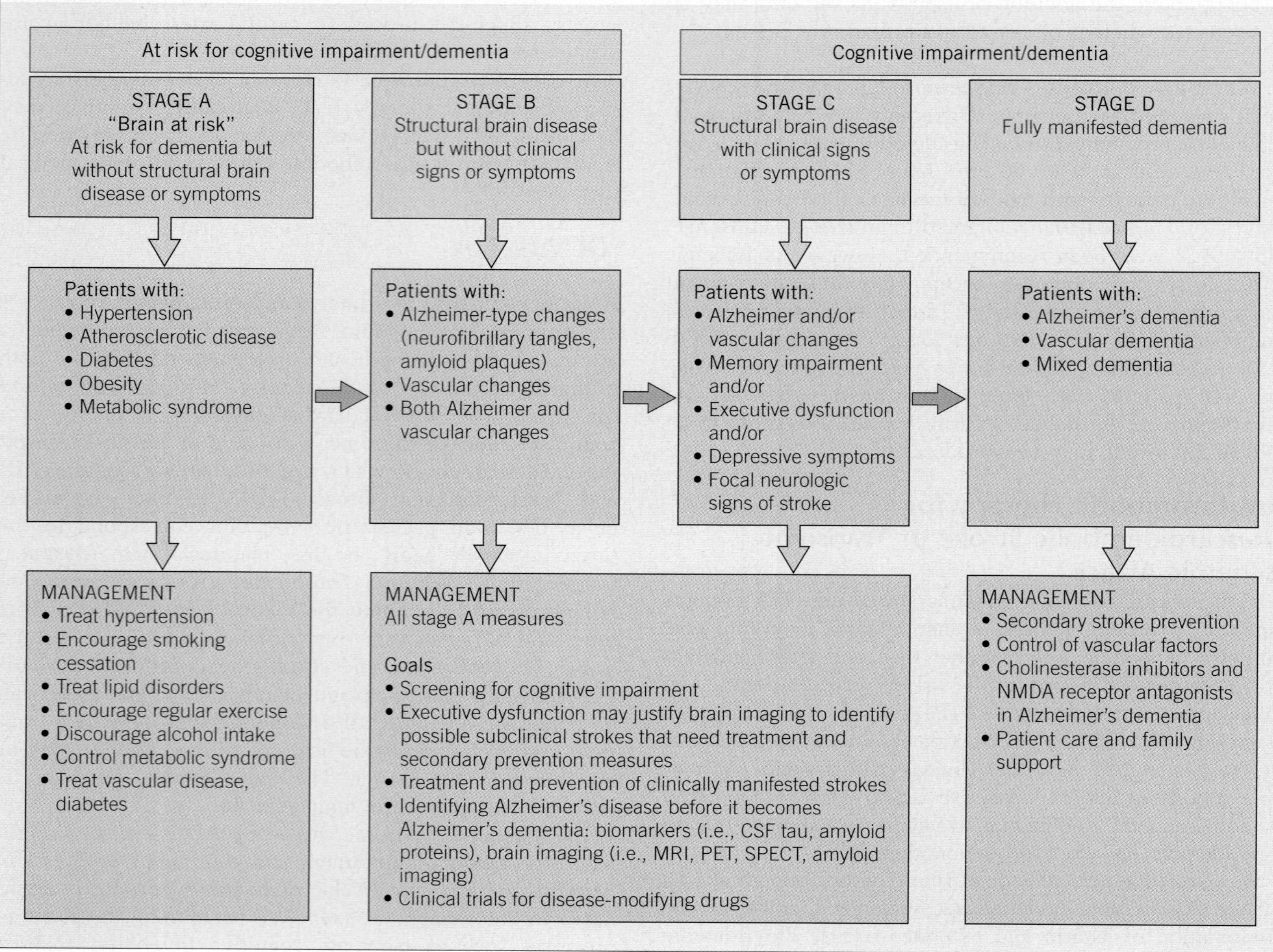

Figure 11.4 Stages leading to dementia development.

a transdisciplinary approach to prevention. Stage B is the equivalent of structural brain changes without clinical signs or symptoms. AD has a long, clinically silent stage characterized by progressive neuropathologic changes (neurofibrillary tangles and amyloid plaques). Similarly, cerebrovascular changes may be asymptomatic. Moreover, neurodegenerative and vascular pathologic processes can occur together and interact in many cases. Stage C is characterized by the onset of clinical manifestations. The concepts of mild cognitive impairment and vascular cognitive impairment have been formulated to shift the focus from fully developed dementia to earlier disease stages, when treatment or secondary prevention may have better effects. Efforts are being made to formulate standardized diagnostic criteria for Alzheimer's disease (instead of Alzheimer's dementia) and for vascular cognitive impairment. Stage D is a late-stage, full-blown dementia, with already advanced brain lesions. It has been shown that individuals can carry a heavy load of typical AD changes without having cognitive impairment as long as they do not have, in addition, cerebrovascular lesions. Cerebrovascular lesions thus have the potential to tip the balance so that persons with AD pathology express a dementia syndrome. For the same degree of dementia severity, AD patients with cerebrovascular lesions can present a lower burden of degenerative lesions than in "pure" AD cases. Also, in many individuals, especially the elderly, a combination of minor AD-type and vascular pathologic changes may cause dementia, when these minor pathologic changes would not have done so individually, which indicates their synergistic effect.

RISK FACTORS AND PRIMARY PREVENTION IN STROKE AND DEMENTIA

Age, Sex, and Genetic Predisposition

Age is the overriding risk factor for both stroke and dementia, with an exponential increase with increasing age. After adjustment for age, men have, on average, a 40% higher risk

RISK FACTORS FOR STROKE AND DEMENTIA			
Risk factor	**Association with stroke**	**Association with dementia**	**Effect of intervention/Risk reduction with treatment**
Hypertension	The most important risk factor; the relationship is continuous, consistent, and independent of other risk factors.	High BP at midlife is associated with increased risk of subsequent dementia/AD. At late-life (75+), more complex association; high SBP but also low DBP are associated with increased dementia risk.	Compelling evidence for more than 30 years that controlling high BP contributes to stroke prevention. Epidemiological evidence and RCTs indicate that antihypertensive drugs may protect against dementia.
Smoking	Doubles ischemic stroke risk and is associated with 2-4 fold increased risk for hemorrhagic stroke.	Current smoking is associated with a moderately increased risk of dementia (AD and VaD)	Smoking cessation reduces stroke risk: 50% within 1 year, baseline after 5 years. Effects on dementia: to be investigated.
Diabetes	Has an independent effect on ischemic stroke, with a 1.8-6 fold increase in relative risk.	Associated with both VaD and AD, but methods and results vary between studies.	Reduction of stroke risk in hypertensive diabetic patients with blood pressure control. Reduction of stroke risk with statins. Rosiglitazone and insulin have been associated with better cognitive outcomes in small studies. Larger studies ongoing.
Atrial Fibrillation (AF)	Associated with a 3-4 fold increase in stroke risk. About one quarter of strokes in very elderly (>80 years old) are due to AF.	Associated with cognitive impairment and dementia (both AD and VaD) in some studies; the link needs further investigation.	RCTs have firmly established the value of antithrombotic therapies for reducing the risk of stroke in patients with AF. Risk is reduced by 60% with warfarin and 20% with aspirin. Effects on dementia: to be investigated.
Other cardiac conditions	Incidence of stroke is inversely proportional to cardiac ejection fraction.	Only recently investigated in relation to dementia/AD; increased risk.	Considering practice guidelines which recommend strategies to reduce the risk of stroke in patients with cardiac conditions can reduce the risk in these patients.
High total cholesterol	About 25% increase in ischemic stroke rates for every 1-mmol (38.7 mg/dl) increase in total cholesterol. Relative risk is about 2.0 for persons younger than 55 years.	High total cholesterol at midlife is a risk factor for subsequent dementia (AD and VaD). More complex association in late-life.	Near 30% risk reduction by treatment with statins in high risk patients with coronary heart diseases, hypertension, or diabetes. Unclear effects of statins in dementia prevention or treatment. No safety concerns or cognitive side effects related to statin treatment in AD patients.
Low HDL cholesterol	Relative risk for ischemic stroke 1.5-2.5 in men. More data needed to verify the effect in women.	Related to poorer memory performance in some studies.	Unknown
Diet and nutrition	Fruits and vegetables are considered as protective factors. High sodium intake increases and high potassium reduces stroke risk.	Saturated fat and cholesterol may increase dementia/AD risk; polyunsaturated fatty acids, fish and 'Mediterranean diet' may be protective	One serving/day increment in fruit and vegetable intake may reduce stroke risk by 6%. Reduced sodium and increased potassium intake are recommended to lower blood pressure. Dietary fat recommendations for heart disease may reduce dementia risk.
Physical inactivity	A sedentary lifestyle is associated with an increased risk of stroke.	A sedentary lifestyle is associated with an increased risk of dementia/AD.	CDC and NIH guidelines recommend moderate exercise for at least 30 minutes on most days of the week. Effects size in stroke and dementia to be investigated in RCTs.

(Continued)

Risk factor	Association with stroke	Association with dementia	Effect of intervention/Risk reduction with treatment
Obesity and body fat distribution	Increased weight associated with increased stroke risk in a dose-response fashion. Abdominal obesity stronger predictor of stroke risk than high BMI.	High BMI and abdominal obesity increase dementia risk.	Weight reduction influences several cardiovascular risk factors for stroke and dementia. Effects on stroke and dementia to be evaluated in RCTs.
Carotid stenosis	Relative risk 2 for increasing the risk of stroke.	Have been associated with worse cognitive functioning in some studies.	~ 50% reduction in stroke risk with endarterectomy. Aggressive management of other identifiable vascular risk factors
Metablic Syndrome (MetS)	Individual components of MetS have been associated with an increased risk of ischemic stroke and should be treated as appropriate. The specific risk of stroke in persons with MetS is uncertain.	MetS and individual components of MetS have been associated with cognitive impairment and an increased risk of dementia (AD and VaD). The added values of MetS beyond its components on dementia risk is uncertain.	The impact of treatment of the combined syndrome is uncertain. However, management of the individual components of the MetS is endorsed. It is not known whether agents that ameliorate aspects of the insulin resistance syndrome are useful for reducing stroke or dementia risk
Alcohol Abuse	Strong evidence suggests that alcoholism and heavy drinking are risk factors for all stroke subtypes.	Alcohol abuse increases dementia risk but moderate consumption has been suggested to be protective	Effect size to be evaluated. Possible beneficial effects need to be investigated.
Oral Contraceptive Use (women age 25-44 y)	The association is still conflicting, but certain women, particularly those who have had a prior thrombotic event, may be at somewhat higher risk.	Unknown	None (and may increase risk for stroke)
Postmenopausal hormone therapy	The risk of stroke is increased with active treatment by tested forms of hormone therapy (RR=1.4). Data for other forms of hormone therapy are lacking.	Epidemiological evidence indicate protective roll but RTCs risk increase for dementia. There may be critical time window for putative protective roll.	None (and may increase risk)
Hyperhomocysteinemia	Several studies have shown that baseline total homocysteine levels were an independent risk factor for incident stroke in the elderly.	Homocysteine has been associated with an increased dementia risk in some studies.	No RCTs have been conducted showing that lowering elevated homocysteine levels reduces the risk of a first stroke or dementia.
Inflammation	Elevated CRP levels have been associated with cerebrovascular events in several studies (RR 2-3)	Elevated CRP levels have been associated with dementia and cognitive decline in some studies	Unknown

Table 11.4 Risk factors for stroke and dementia.

for stroke than women do, at least up to the age of 80 years. Nevertheless, because there are more women than men in stroke-prone ages, the total numbers of male and female stroke victims are about the same in most populations. No clear differences in the severity, subtype, location, and size of the infarct between men and women have been reported.[41] Dementia is more common among women due to the fact that women have greater longevity, but other factors (e.g., hormonal) may also be involved.

The causation of stroke and dementia is multifactorial (a combination of environmental and genetic risk factors), and the genetic part is very complex (polygenic, multiple genes play a role). Many common risk factors for stroke (i.e., hypertension, diabetes) are partly inherited, so many genetic loci contribute more or less to the stroke phenotype. The relation between genotype and phenotype in sporadic stroke is thus complicated. For instance, a family history of myocardial infarction may be more common than a family history of stroke in probands with a TIA.[42] Also, there is a strong association between having both a history of hypertension and a family history of stroke or myocardial infarction.[42] So, even in seemingly sporadic stroke in the elderly, careful taking of family history of cardiovascular risk factors should be considered important. There is also familial aggregation for dementia that may be mediated through genetic factors or shared environmental factors.

A large number of reports have linked stroke and dementia to specific genetic polymorphisms, but most of these findings have not been replicated by independent investigators. There are, however, some polymorphisms showing more consistent associations. The gene encoding apolipoprotein E (apoE) has a central role in lipid metabolism, and the apoE $\varepsilon 4$ allele is associated with increased cholesterol levels, atherosclerosis, and coronary heart disease, but its role in ischemic stroke remains more controversial. Both apoE2 and apoE4 alleles have been associated with increased risk of intracerebral hemorrhage[43]; apoE4 is associated with worse outcome after stroke. Other polymorphisms located in the genes for fibrinogen, platelet glycoprotein receptors, and angiotensin-converting enzyme have been linked with stroke.[42]

To date, the apoE ε4 allele is the only genetic risk factor for AD of established general significance. The apoE ε4 allele is a susceptibility gene for AD, being neither necessary nor sufficient for AD development. The risk of AD increases and the age at onset decreases with the number of the ε4 alleles, in a dose-dependent manner. The very mechanisms relating apoE ε4 allele to AD are not completely understood, but the effect for AD seems to be at least partly independent of the effects on peripheral vascular factors.[44] ApoE4 has been linked to all the major features in AD pathogenesis including β-amyloid generation and clearance, neurofibrillary tangle formation, oxidative stress, apoptosis, dysfunction in lipid transport and homeostasis, modulation of intracellular signaling, and synaptic plasticity.[43,45] Epidemiologic studies have also suggested that apoE ε4 carriers may be more vulnerable to a variety of environmental factors (e.g., physical inactivity, saturated fat intake, alcohol drinking, diabetes, high blood pressure).[46] Interestingly, many of the other suggested candidate genes for AD are vascular related, such as CYP46 (cholesterol 24-hydroxylase), insulin-degrading enzyme, angiotensin-converting enzyme, peroxisome proliferator-activated receptor γ, and interleukin 1.

Very rarely, stroke and dementia may result from a monogenic familial disorder. A syndrome of cerebral autosomal dominant arteriopathy with subcortical infarcts and leukoencephalopathy (CADASIL) has been described and a genetic locus has been identified in the Notch3 gene on chromosome 19. A syndrome of mitochondrial encephalopathy with lactate acidosis and stroke-like episodes (MELAS) is caused by a number of different point mutations within the tRNA-Leu gene. Familial forms of AD (representing about 1% to 2% of all AD cases) can be caused by mutations on chromosome 21 (*APP* gene), 14 (*PSEN1* gene), or 1 (*PSEN2* gene).

Modifiable Risk Factors

Evidence has been accumulating during recent years that stroke and dementia share many modifiable vascular and lifestyle-related risk factors (see Table 11.4).

Hypertension

Hypertension is the most important risk factor for stroke. The relationship is continuous, consistent, and independent of other risk factors, that is, the higher the blood pressure, the greater the stroke risk.[47] There is compelling evidence for more than 30 years that control of high blood pressure contributes to the prevention of stroke. Antihypertensive therapy is associated with a 35% to 44% reduction in the incidence of stroke (38%).[47] The risk is also reduced when isolated systolic hypertension is treated. However, lack of diagnosis and inadequate treatment still represent important problems, particularly in minority populations and in the elderly.[47]

High blood pressure (especially systolic blood pressure) has been constantly associated with a higher risk of dementia and AD. Long-term population-based follow-up studies have shown that high blood pressure, especially at midlife, is associated with an increased AD risk later in life.[44,48] High blood pressure even later in life[49] and closer to dementia onset has also been linked with a higher AD risk, but results have been more inconsistent. Hypertension has been related to increased brain atrophy and AD lesions at autopsy, suggesting that hypertension may be linked with neurodegenerative changes besides its known contributions as a risk factor for cerebrovascular lesions.

Blood pressure values often fall during aging, before the manifestation of dementia and during the course of AD. AD is a catabolic disorder and, besides blood pressure, cholesterol values and body weight often decline during the disease course. Decline in blood pressure may be at least partly related to neurodegenerative processes and brain lesions (e.g., several brain regions affected in AD are involved in blood pressure regulation) and thus be secondary to the AD process, but other factors may also be involved. Whether low blood pressure accelerates the AD process is still a matter of debate.

Some observational studies indicated that antihypertensive medication, especially long-term treatment, may reduce the risk of dementia, including AD.[50] In the Systolic Hypertension in Europe (Syst-Eur) trial, active treatment of isolated systolic hypertension with nitrendipine, a calcium channel blocker, was found to halve the incidence of AD. Antihypertensive drugs affecting the renin-angiotensin system have also been associated with preservation of cognitive function.[51]

Hypercholesterolemia

Plasma lipids and lipoproteins affect the risk of ischemic stroke, but the exact relationships still need to be clarified. There is a nearly 25% increase in ischemic stroke rates for every 1-mmol (38.7 mg/dL) increase in total cholesterol concentration.[47] The relative risk is about 2.0 for persons younger than 55 years. Low concentration of high-density lipoprotein seems to be a risk factor for ischemic stroke in men (relative risk, 1.5 to 2.5), but more data are needed to verify its effect in women. There is about a 30% risk reduction by treatment with statins in high-risk patients with coronary heart diseases, hypertension, or diabetes.[47] It is recommended that management of patients with known coronary artery disease and high-risk hypertensive patients even with normal low-density lipoprotein concentration include lifestyle-related changes and a statin.[47]

High midlife total cholesterol level also increases the risk of late-life dementia.[44,52] Midlife total cholesterol level has been related to AD-type brain changes in autopsy studies.[53,54] The significance of high cholesterol level later in life and closer to dementia onset is more complex; cholesterol values seem to decrease after midlife, especially in persons who go on to develop dementia. Results from studies suggest a bidirectional relationship: high cholesterol is a risk factor for subsequent AD, but decreasing cholesterol after midlife may reflect ongoing disease processes and may represent a risk marker for late-life dementia.[55,56] A decrease over time in blood pressure and body mass index has also been described.

As serum and brain cholesterol concentrations are two separate pools, studies measuring serum cholesterol concentration can only observe the tip of the iceberg. The brain is the most cholesterol-rich organ in the body, and disturbances in brain cholesterol metabolism have been linked with all the main neuropathologic changes in AD. The links between serum and brain cholesterol concentrations are not fully known, but one link is represented by oxysterols, monooxygenated derivates of cholesterol with a unique ability to pass the blood-brain barrier. This may be important for neurodegeneration and may be one of the links between hypercholesterolemia and AD.[57]

Some (but not all) observational studies have suggested that statins may be beneficial in prevention of AD.[58] Cognitive arms were added to the Heart Protection Study and PROSPER study, but no significant influence of statins on cognition or dementia incidence was found. However, the add-on design and the possible lack of power question the results. Two small studies indicated that statins might be effective in delaying the progression of cognitive decline in persons with AD.[59,60] In two larger studies (LEADe and CLASP)[61] of patients with mild to moderate AD with normal cholesterol values and receiving background therapy of a cholinesterase inhibitor (established treatment for AD), statins had no additional benefits on cognition and global function during 18 months (main results presented during the International Conference of Alzheimer Disease 2008). Importantly, there were no safety concerns.

Obesity

General obesity (increased body mass index) and abdominal obesity (increased waist-to-hip ratio) have been reported as independent risk factors for stroke (even after controlling for hypertension, diabetes, and cholesterol levels). Abdominal obesity seems to be a stronger predictor of stroke risk than is general obesity.[47] No clinical trials have so far tested the effects of weight reduction on stroke outcomes; however, weight reduction is associated with a lowering in blood pressure and may thereby contribute to a reduced stroke risk.[47]

The association between obesity and dementia or AD risk has been less studied. Weight loss seems to occur during the preclinical phases of dementia, and in some persons, low body mass index may be an early dementia sign. Long-term population-based studies have shown that high body mass index or abdominal obesity at midlife or high body mass index at late life 9 to 18 years before dementia is associated with increased AD risk.[62]

Obesity is related to vascular disorders, which could be the link to dementia and AD. For example, obesity is an essential feature in metabolic syndrome. Metabolic syndrome has been related to an increased risk of both stroke and dementia.[63,64] Higher body mass index and waist-to-hip ratio were related to white matter lesions in some studies, and higher body mass index was associated with greater temporal lobe atrophy and greater brain atrophy rate.[62] Insulin resistance is one possible factor related to AD pathogenesis.[65] Furthermore, adipose tissue is an important endocrine organ and secretes hormones and several other bioactive compounds (e.g., sex hormones, leptin, interleukins, growth factors) that may be involved.

Atrial Fibrillation

Atrial fibrillation represents a major risk factor for stroke, increasing the risk three to four times after adjustment for other risk factors. For those without prior TIA or stroke, 2% to 4% per year have an ischemic stroke.[47] About one quarter of strokes in the very elderly (>80 years) are due to atrial fibrillation. Strokes associated with atrial fibrillation are especially large and disabling.

Randomized controlled trials have firmly established the value of antithrombotic therapies for reducing the risk of stroke in patients with atrial fibrillation.[47] The risk is reduced by 60% with warfarin and by 20% with aspirin. Warfarin (INR, 2.0 to 3.0) is recommended for atrial fibrillation patients with high risk (>0.4% annual risk of stroke) and for most patients with moderate risk (according to an assessment of bleeding risk) who have no clinically significant contraindications to oral anticoagulants.[47] The optimal target level of anticoagulation in those at risk of increased bleeding is still debated. Unfortunately, this results in many atrial fibrillation patients, particularly those older than 75 years, not receiving anticoagulation treatment.[47]

Atrial fibrillation has also been associated with cognitive dysfunction and dementia (both Alzheimer's and vascular). Impaired cognition and vascular dementia may be the result of multiple episodes of cerebral ischemia (clinically manifested or silent) caused by atrial fibrillation. Patients with atrial fibrillation show activation of the plasmatic and cellular clotting system, and in addition to thromboembolic events, there is cardiac beat-to-beat variability inducing cerebral hypoperfusion.[66] However, several studies have shown that the association between atrial fibrillation and cognitive impairment is independent of stroke and other cardiovascular risk factors, so other mechanisms may exist as well. Interestingly, atrial fibrillation was identified as a risk factor for AD and has been associated with memory impairment and hippocampal atrophy in stroke-free patients.[66] Amyloid fibrils occur in AD as well as in subgroups of patients with atrial fibrillation, although the fibril proteins are different. It remains to be determined if these diseases share a common pathophysiologic basis with regard to amyloidogenesis. Another issue to be investigated is whether the occurrence of atrial fibrillation is followed by cerebral alterations or whether atrial fibrillation may be secondarily due to autonomic dysbalance induced by localized brain atrophy.[66]

It is possible that atrial fibrillation treatment may be important not only in stroke prevention but in dementia prevention as well. Because atrial fibrillation seems to contribute to cognitive decline independently of stroke, future interventional studies and possible treatment guidelines need to consider cognition as an outcome parameter.

Vascular Diseases

Other cardiac conditions, such as dilated cardiomyopathy, valvular heart diseases (mitral valve prolapse, endocarditis, prosthetic cardiac valves), and intracardiac congenital defects (patent foramen ovale, atrial septal defect, atrial septal aneurysms), can increase stroke risk. The incidence of stroke is inversely proportional to cardiac ejection fraction. Myocardial infarction patients who have an ejection fraction below 29% have a relative risk of stroke of 1.86, compared with patients who have an ejection fraction of more than 35% (an 18% increase in stroke risk for every 5% decline in ejection fraction).[47]

Until recently, clinical vascular diseases (which can be considered consequences of elevated blood pressure, cholesterol, and obesity) have quite seldom been studied in relation to AD. Because of the diagnostic criteria for AD, patients with clinical vascular diseases are less likely to be diagnosed with AD. However, studies have reported an association between various vascular disorders like myocardial infarction, atrial fibrillation, and heart failure and AD. In addition, coronary artery disease at autopsy has been linked with an increase in cortical senile plaques. Generalized atherosclerosis also seems to be associated with AD.[67]

Diabetes and Metabolic Syndrome

Diabetes has an independent effect on ischemic stroke, with a 1.8- to 6-fold increased relative risk.[47] Reduction of stroke risk with blood pressure control has been shown in hypertensive diabetic patients.[47] Tight glycemic control does not seem to have a significant direct effect on stroke risk reduction, but there is a demonstrated reduction in other complications. Statin treatment and aggressive management of other identifiable vascular risk factors in patients with diabetes also reduce stroke risk.[47]

Diabetes has been associated with an increased risk of AD and dementia in several cohort studies.[68] In the elderly, the true prevalence of diabetes mellitus is above 30%, and more than half of them are asymptomatic and undiagnosed. In addition, more than 30% have impaired glucose tolerance, which makes more than half of elderly people affected with hyperglycemia. The potential biologic mechanisms underlying the diabetes-AD association are many. These associations may reflect the direct effects on the brain of hyperglycemia and advanced glycation end products or the effects of diabetes-associated comorbidities (hypertension, dyslipidemia, or hyperinsulinemia). Diabetes is associated with changes in cerebral microvessels and the blood-brain barrier. Some studies have indicated that higher insulin levels are associated with the risk of dementia or AD. Insulin resistance may be important in AD pathogenesis by influencing β-amyloid regulation, cerebral glucose metabolism, and inflammatory processes. Insulin-degrading enzyme has received a lot of interest recently as a potential link between hyperinsulinemia and AD; the enzyme degrades insulin, amylin, and β-amyloid, and hyperinsulinemia may elevate β-amyloid through insulin's competition with β-amyloid for insulin-degrading enzyme.[65] Recent trials with the insulin-sensitizing drug rosiglitazone have suggested benefits in cognition in AD patients, but larger trials are under way to verify the results.[69]

Dietary Factors

Diet (especially fat intake) has a well-known association with coronary heart disease. The relationship with stroke or dementia is less clear, however. There is a lack of well-designed epidemiologic studies addressing the role of dietary fats in different stroke subtypes.[70] A proper outcome definition in such studies is crucial, as atherosclerotic changes may have different causes in different types of cerebral arteries. Atherosclerosis may be involved in large-artery infarction, but other factors (e.g., blood pressure) may have more important roles in other types of ischemic stroke (lacunar and cardioembolic infarction).

Fruits and vegetables are considered protective factors for stroke. For each increment of one serving per day in fruit and vegetable intake, the risk of stroke may be reduced by 6%.[47] A reduced intake of sodium (<2.3 g/day) and increased intake of potassium (<4.7 g/day) are recommended to lower blood pressure, which may thereby reduce the risk of stroke.[47]

The pattern for fat intake and dementia or AD seems to follow that for coronary heart disease. Intake of unsaturated fats and fish may be protective, whereas moderate intake of saturated fats may increase AD risk.[71] A high saturated fat intake is linked to vascular factors and oxidative stress. Unsaturated fatty acids may confer protection through their anti-inflammatory properties. Fatty acids may be important in the synthesis and fluidity of nerve cell membranes, for synaptic plasticity and neuronal degeneration.

Oxidative stress is important in both stroke and dementia or AD, and some studies (but not all) suggested that a diet rich in antioxidants might be protective.[72,73] Low vitamin B_{12} and folate levels and their marker high homocysteine have been linked with an increased risk of both stroke and dementia or AD.[73]

The "Mediterranean diet" seems to protect against dementia and AD, even after controlling for several vascular factors.[74] A similar association was found for stroke.[73]

Physical Exercise and Active Lifestyle

A sedentary lifestyle is associated with an increased risk of stroke (relative risk, 2.7). Clinical trials documenting a reduction in the risk of a first stroke with regular exercise have not been done; however, exercise has beneficial effects on other cardiovascular risk factors and is associated with a reduction in stroke risk in epidemiologic studies. The Centers for Disease Control and Prevention and National Institutes of Health guidelines recommend that people exercise moderately for at least 30 minutes on most (preferably all) days of the week.[47] For stroke, the benefits are apparent even for light to moderate activities, such as walking, and the data support additional benefit from increasing the level and duration of physical activity.[47]

Regular leisure-time physical activity at midlife seems to protect against dementia and AD later in life. A risk reduction of 50% for dementia and 60% for AD was reported, even after controlling for several vascular and lifestyle-related factors.[75] This association was more pronounced among apoE4 carriers. However, not all studies have shown such an effect.[76]

Physical activity is important in promoting general and vascular health, but it may confer its effects through other mechanisms as well: promoting brain plasticity[77] and affecting several gene transcripts and neurotrophic factors relevant for maintenance of cognitive functions.[78] Social and mental activities have also been suggested to protect against dementia and AD.[76] Generally active lifestyle may increase cognitive reserve, reduce stress, and protect against development or expression of dementia also through these mechanisms.

Smoking and Alcohol Drinking

Smoking doubles ischemic stroke risk and has also been clearly associated with a twofold to fourfold increased risk for hemorrhagic stroke. Smoking may also potentiate the effects of other stroke risk factors (e.g., oral contraceptive pills).[47] Several studies suggest that environmental tobacco smoke is also a substantial risk factor for stroke.[47] Smoking cessation is associated with a rapid reduction in the risk of stroke: 50% within 1 year, baseline after 5 years.[47] Current smoking has also been related to a moderately increased risk of AD and vascular

SIMILARITIES OF PREDICTORS IN RISK SCORES FOR CORONARY HEART DISEASE AND STROKE (FRAMINGHAM STUDY)			
Coronary Heart Disease			Stroke
2-year Risk	10-year Risk	Hard CHD* 10-year Risk	10-year Risk
Age High-density lipoprotein and total cholesterol levels Diabetes Systolic blood pressure Hypertension treatment Smoking status	Age Low-density lipoprotein or total cholesterol level High-density lipoprotein level Blood pressure Diabetes Smoking status	Age Total cholesterol level High-density lipoprotein level Systolic blood pressure Hypertension treatment Smoking status	Age Systolic blood pressure Diabetes Smoking status Prior cardiovascular disease Atrial fibrillation Left ventricular hypertrophy Hypertension treatment

*Hard coronary heart disease (myocardial infarction or coronary death).

Table 11.5 Similarities of predictors in risk scores for coronary heart disease and stroke (Framingham study).

dementia, partly because of the association with cardiovascular diseases and also with oxidative stress.

Strong evidence suggests that alcoholism and heavy drinking are risk factors for all stroke subtypes.[47] Many studies have suggested a J-shaped relationship between alcohol consumption and ischemic stroke risk, with a protective effect in light or moderate drinkers and an elevated risk with heavy alcohol consumption.[47] The pattern of association seems to be similar for dementia. Moderate alcohol drinking has also been associated with fewer brain infarcts, and a U-shaped relationship with white matter lesions has been described.[79] On the other hand, excessive alcohol drinking has clear detrimental effects on the brain (even relatively light drinking levels have been related to increased brain atrophy)[80] and can lead to hypertension, hypercoagulability, and increased likelihood of atrial fibrillation.[47]

Alcohol may also have beneficial effects on several cardiovascular risk factors, including lipid and lipoprotein levels and inflammatory and hemostatic factors, and moderate alcohol drinking has been related to a reduced risk of cardiovascular diseases. The protective effect of alcohol may also be due to the effect of specific antioxidant substances in wine.

Risk Prediction Models

Primary prevention can be categorized into long-term and short-term prevention. Long-term prevention aims to reduce the risk for heart disease, stroke, and dementia over a lifetime (to prevent the initiation and progression of underlying causal disease). Short-term prevention is directed toward persons who in all probability already have such disease and who are at risk of acute coronary syndromes or stroke during the next few years (e.g., $\leq$10 years). There are two main approaches in primary prevention, the counting of risk factors and the integrated, global risk assessment. Whereas it is important to keep track of and to manage all risk factors, estimation of absolute risks can provide a quantitative overview of the patient's situation and help both physicians and patients (on a clinical level) and the general population (on a public health level) set goals and make decisions about necessary lifestyle-related changes and pharmacologic treatment.

Practical tools are already available for predicting the risk of cardiovascular outcomes or stroke (e.g., the Framingham scores). There is a striking resemblance between these tools (Table 11.5). Recently, similar tools were developed within the dementia field. The CAIDE Dementia Risk Score includes easily measurable variables at midlife and predicts dementia risk 2 decades later (Table 11.6). Developed in a Finnish population,[81] the CAIDE Dementia Risk Score has been validated in a large, diverse population of members of a health care delivery system in the United States (Kaiser Permanente).[82] The risk score provides a quantitative estimation of the probability of becoming demented, but it cannot definitely state whether someone will develop dementia.

CAIDE DEMENTIA RISK SCORE: PROBABILITY OF DEMENTIA IN LATE LIFE ACCORDING TO THE RISK SCORE CATEGORIES IN MIDDLE AGE		
Risk Factor		Points
Age	<47 years	0
	47-53 years	3
	>53 years	4
Education	>10 years	0
	7–9 years	2
	<9 years	3
Sex	Female	0
	Male	1
Blood pressure	<140 mm Hg	0
	>140 mm Hg	2
Body mass index	<30 kg/m^2	0
	>30 kg/m^2	2
Total cholesterol	<6.5 mmol/L	0
	>6.5 mmol/L	2
Physical activity	Yes	0
	No	1
Total Score		**Dementia Risk**
0-5		1.0%
6-7		1.9%
8-9		4.2%
10-11		7.4%
12-15		16.4%

Table 11.6 CAIDE Dementia Risk Score: Probability of dementia in late life according to the risk score categories in middle age.

It should therefore be used mainly to target preventive measures to those most at risk and not to place labels on individuals. This first version will be further developed (e.g., by adding new variables) to increase its predictive value, but it can already be used as an educational tool to demonstrate the role of modifiable factors in dementia, together with cardiovascular disease or stroke. Shorter term predictive models for dementia development (i.e., in persons who are older at the time of risk factor assessment) are currently being formulated.

SUMMARY

In the aging population, stroke and dementia are increasing public health challenges and leading causes of death and disability worldwide. Both stroke and dementia are late events (clinical endpoints) and present only the tip of the "cerebrovascular iceberg." It is now known that silent stroke and milder forms of cognitive impairments are much more common than clinical stroke and full-blown dementia, and these "silent" events place a heavy burden on public health. Thus, one of the main changes in approaching cerebrovascular diseases is the shift from clinically obvious strokes and dementia to prevention and identification of "brain at risk" stages.

Acute stroke management has developed during recent years, and here without doubt, management in a stroke care unit has been the most substantial advantage. Intravenous thrombolysis within 3 hours or aspirin within 48 hours of stroke onset and decompressive surgery for supratentorial malignant cerebral infarction are interventions of proven benefit. Several other interventions are being assessed. Neuroprotective agents have been beneficial in reducing the size of brain infarcts in animal models but not so far in clinical settings; new studies are ongoing. New and sensitive neuroimaging techniques have quickly developed (e.g., diffusion-weighted MRI) and improved early detection of cerebrovascular lesions.

Secondary prevention of stroke has developed, and the current recommended strategies usually include monitoring and treatment of vascular risk factors (including cholesterol reduction), use of low-dose aspirin and dipyridamole in patients with ischemic stroke of arterial origin, oral anticoagulation in patients with cardiac embolism, and carotid endarterectomy in patients with substantial ipsilateral carotid stenosis.

Stroke and dementia (both vascular and Alzheimer's) share several cardiovascular risk factors, highlighting the importance of integrated interventions and transdisciplinary approaches. Evidence has been accumulating that minding heart health may prevent dementia as well, which may add motivation for patients to better control vascular risk factors. Stroke and dementia risk scores have been developed and can be used to target interventions for those most at risk.

chapter 12

Thoracic Aorta Disease

Jorge A. Wernly

Definitions

- Aortic dissection is a sudden event in which blood penetrates the aortic wall through an intimal tear and creates a false channel by dissection of the media.
- Aortic aneurysm is abnormal dilatation of the aorta with a tendency to expand.

Key Features

- Middle-aged or elderly hypertensive men with atherosclerosis and young patients with Marfan's syndrome or other connective tissue disorders are affected.
- Acute aortic dissection presents with chest pain, hemodynamic instability, absent or unequal peripheral pulses, various neurologic complications, and aortic regurgitation.
- Widened mediastinum on chest radiography may indicate dissection or aneurysm formation.

Therapy

- Ascending aortic dissection should lead to emergency surgery. Stable dissection limited to the descending aorta can, in general, be treated medically.
- Aortic aneurysms often require surgery or stent-grafts, depending on their size and location.

Acute dissection, the most frequent catastrophic disorder involving the aorta, occurs in an estimated 10 to 20 cases per million people per year. Acute aortic dissection is at least twice as common as ruptured abdominal aneurysm. More than three quarters of patients are older than 40 years. Acute aortic dissection occurs two to three times more frequently in men between the ages of 50 and 70 years than in women of the same age. It is rare in young patients, except for those with familial predisposition, Marfan's syndrome, other connective tissue disorders, or congenital lesions such as bicuspid aortic valve or coarctation of the aorta. Before the age of 40 years, there is a nearly equal male-to-female distribution; half of the dissections in women occur during pregnancy.

Two variants of acute aortic disease different from classic aortic dissection have been identified with the introduction of high-resolution imaging of the aorta by computed tomography, magnetic resonance imaging, and transesophageal echocardiography. Penetrating aortic ulcer and intramural aortic hematoma were virtually unknown in the era when angiography was the diagnostic standard for aortic disease. Not only are these two conditions distinct radiographic lesions, but it appears that they are also distinct clinical entities. Even though the exact pathologic mechanism of these two conditions is still being debated and although, in some cases, penetrating aortic ulcer leads to the development of a hematoma, there is enough evidence to support the concept that "spontaneous" or "primary" intramural aortic hematoma is different from penetrating aortic ulcer.[1,2] Intramural aortic hematoma is discussed as a variant of aortic dissection, and penetrating aortic ulcer is discussed along with other manifestations of atherosclerotic disease.

Aortic aneurysm is an abnormal dilatation of the aorta to at least 50% larger than normal. The incidence of thoracic aortic aneurysms appears to have increased significantly in the last 2 decades. Thoracic aneurysms are now estimated to affect 10 of every 100,000 patients per year.

Of all thoracic aortic aneurysms, the ascending aorta is affected in approximately 50% of the cases, the aortic arch in 10%, and the descending aorta in 40%. The mean age at diagnosis is 59 to 69 years. Men predominate over women with a ratio of 2:1. Peripheral vascular disease, including abdominal aortic aneurysm, stroke, and distal arterial occlusive disease, is also common in this population of patients.[3]

ACUTE AORTIC DISSECTION

ANATOMY AND PATHOLOGY

The natural history of the aortic dissection depends almost exclusively on whether the ascending aorta is involved. The Stanford clinical classification system is based solely on whether the ascending aorta is involved, irrespective of the site of the primary intimal tear and the extent of the dissection. All dissections that involve the ascending aorta, regardless of the site of entry, are defined as type A. All dissections that do not include the ascending aorta are defined as type B. This includes all dissections of the descending thoracic aorta and the aortic arch (Fig. 12.1).

Aortic dissection has often been related to structural changes in the media. Histopathologic changes such as medionecrosis, cystic medial necrosis, fibrosis, and fragmentation of elastin fibers have been considered to be specific for this disease. Studies of undissected aortas indicate that these changes are not specific and occur as part of the aging process. The terms *cystic medial necrosis* and *medionecrosis* are probably also misleading because there are no true cystic lesions in cystic medial necrosis and actual necrosis is rare in both.

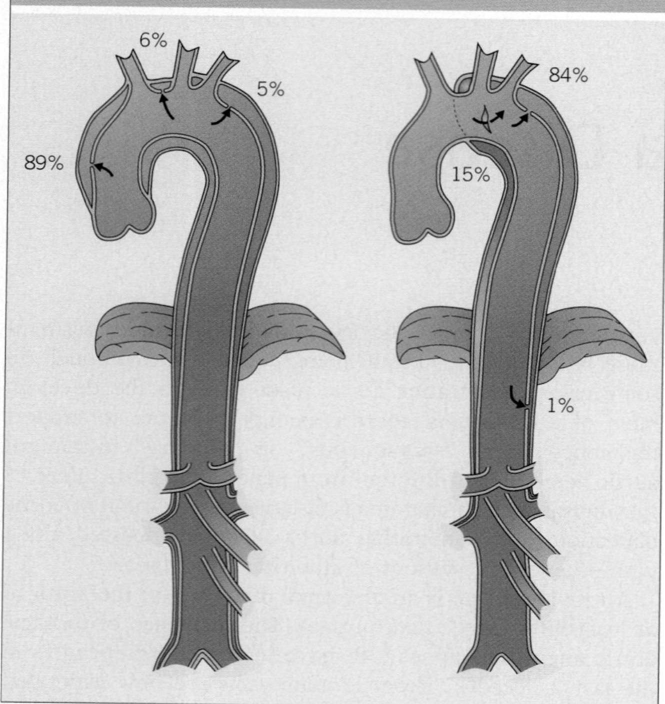

Figure 12.1 Aortic dissection classification system. Type A is defined by the involvement of the ascending aorta irrespective of the location of the tear. In type B, the dissection does not extend into the ascending aorta. Note the distribution of the location of the entry point for each type.

Histologic changes secondary to aging are more pronounced in the ascending aorta and the aortic arch than in the descending aorta and the abdominal aorta. Several investigators have postulated that these changes represent an injury repair process secondary to the long-standing trauma to the media caused by the pulse wave. Lesions that involve elastin and collagen have been found predominantly in people younger than 40 years and in patients with Marfan's syndrome and other connective tissue disorders. These defects in the extracellular matrix cause a severe loss of integrity of the vessel wall, and dissection often develops in the absence of hypertension. Degenerative changes in the smooth muscle cells have been found more commonly in older patients. Without associated defects in the extracellular matrix, these cause a less marked loss of aortal integrity than do the collagen and elastin lesions; hypertension has been identified as a major predisposing factor in these patients.

Patients with bicuspid aortic valves have a risk nine times greater for development of acute dissection than that of patients with normal aortic valves. Studies suggest that there may be associated congenital anomalies of the aortic wall. Aortic coarctation has also been associated with an increased incidence of aortic dissection. This is most probably caused by proximal arterial hypertension and the frequent association with a congenital bicuspid aortic valve and not directly related to the coarctation. The association of aortic dissection with pregnancy is poorly understood; the event may be partially related to the increase in blood volume and systemic blood pressure observed late in pregnancy. The other causes of dissection include trauma, cardiac catheterization, intra-aortic balloon valvuloplasty, cannulation for cardiopulmonary bypass, and other surgical manipulations of the ascending aorta.

In spontaneous aortic dissections, the primary tears are located in the ascending aorta in two thirds of cases; in half of these cases, the tears are located in the first few centimeters of the aortic root. The second most common location of entry tears (20%) is the descending aorta next to the isthmus of the aorta. The tear is located in the aortic arch in 8% to 10% of the cases and rarely (>2%) in the abdominal aorta.

PATHOPHYSIOLOGY

The process of dissection involves an initial phase during which the intimal tear occurs and a second phase in which the dissection propagates. Several hemodynamic factors as well as intrinsic properties of the aortic wall determine the propensity for development of primary tears. The pulsatile load—as determined by the contractility of the heart, the stroke volume, the arterial wall compliance, and the blood pressure—appears to be greatest in the ascending aorta, hence the increased incidence of tears in this location.

The false channel develops and propagates rapidly, usually involving one half to two thirds of the circumference. Experimental evidence suggests that propagation of the dissection is directly related to the rate of rise in blood pressure (dP/dt). The walls of the branches of the aorta may be involved by the dissection or may be sheared off from the true lumen. The avulsed branches may stay open, connected only to the false channel, or may be closed by the dissection. The extent of the involvement of the aortic branches determines the symptoms and signs found on presentation.

The dissection is initially contained by the thin outer layer of the media and the adventitia of the aorta. Blood can re-enter the true lumen anywhere along its length through re-entry points. The false channel can rupture into the pericardium or the left pleural space. Before the rupture, blood can extravasate and form large mediastinal hematomas. Spontaneous thrombosis of the false lumen is rare. In most of the patients who survive the acute dissection, the false lumen enlarges and reaches aneurysmal proportions; late rupture may eventually occur. Partial thrombosis of the false lumen does not protect from late rupture.

CLINICAL PRESENTATIONS

The dissection is considered acute if the time from clinical onset of the dissection is less than 2 weeks and chronic if this period exceeds 2 weeks. Patients with type A dissection tend to be younger (an average age of 49 years versus 60 years for those with type B) and are less likely to have a history of hypertension (30% versus 71% with type B).[4] Patients with type A dissection are also more likely to have associated congenital defects that predispose to dissection, such as bicuspid aortic valve, Marfan's syndrome, or other connective tissue disorders.

In most cases, no specific activity precedes the dissection. Contrary to common opinion, only a small group of patients have reported strenuous physical exertion before the onset of dissection. Acute dissections that have been reported in weightlifters are probably secondary to the acute hypertension produced by the isometric exercise. Acute aortic dissection has been reported in patients who have recently smoked crack cocaine.[5] The peak incidence of aortic dissection is in the morning hours and the winter months.[6]

The clinical presentations of aortic dissection include shock, hypertension, various neurologic symptoms, and sudden death (within 15 minutes of the onset of dissection). Sudden death may be caused by free rupture or by sudden occlusion of a coronary artery. A significant number of the patients who present with aortic dissection are in shock. This can be classic hypovolemic shock from blood loss in the channel and soft pericardial tissues or cardiogenic shock from acute aortic valve regurgitation, myocardial infarction, or cardiac tamponade. Many patients who are sweaty and clammy and appear to be in shock are actually hypertensive, as are more than half of the patients who reach the hospital.

Although the acute dissection produces no significant symptoms in a few patients, pain is the most frequent symptom. Interestingly, in patients with type B dissection, the absence of pain on presentation is a powerful predictor of death. The onset of pain is sudden and unremitting. Obvious discomfort and the fear of death are common. Localization of the pain varies. Because the entire aorta is frequently involved, a spectrum of presentations is seen. Although the localization of the pain does not indicate the site of the intimal tear, it occasionally suggests the extent of the process. For example, pain in the flank usually indicates involvement of the renal arteries.

Pulses may be diminished or absent in one or more extremities (usually the left leg). Oliguria or anuria suggests involvement of the renal arteries. New cardiac murmurs can also be heard. A diastolic murmur of aortic regurgitation, suggesting involvement of the ascending aorta, is present in more than 50% of cases of type A dissection. Systolic bruits may be heard over narrowed arteries. A pericardial rub is infrequent but an ominous sign when it is present because it indicates leakage of blood into the pericardial space.

In approximately 40% of patients, there are diverse neurologic findings ranging from Horner's syndrome to syncope, paraplegia, and stroke. Symptoms of neurologic origin may be temporary and related to the location of the dissection. The reappearance of pulses and wandering paralysis usually indicate either re-entry of the false channel or intermittent occlusion of the vessel by an intimal flap.[7]

DIAGNOSTIC TECHNIQUES

The nonspecific nature of the presenting symptoms of aortic dissection and its dismal prognosis if it is left untreated require immediate confirmatory diagnosis to allow institution of appropriate therapy.

Electrocardiography

Changes of chronic left ventricular hypertrophy from longstanding hypertension are often present. Acute ischemic changes can occur when the dissection involves the coronary arteries. Because the dissection most commonly involves the right coronary artery, ischemic changes in the inferior leads are more common.

Chest Radiography

Plain films of the chest may show several changes that are suggestive of dissection: widening of the superior mediastinum, double shadow of the aortic wall, and disparity in size of the ascending and descending aortas. Cardiomegaly secondary to pericardial effusion or signs of pleural effusion, particularly on the left side of the chest, are sometimes present. However, in many patients, there is no visible mediastinal enlargement in the early phases of acute dissection.

Imaging Techniques

Retrograde aortography was considered the "gold standard" in aortic dissection, and for many years it was the only accurate diagnostic procedure. Newer imaging techniques have revealed that aortography is not as sensitive as previously thought. Aortographic findings in aortic dissection include visualization of the false lumen in 80% to 90% of cases, the intimal flap in 70%, and the site of entry in approximately 50%. Overall sensitivity is 80% to 90%, with a specificity of 90% to 100% and a positive predictive value of about 95%. False-negative studies can occur in several situations: equal opacification of both lumens, flap not tangential to the x-ray beam, or tears proximal to the tip of the catheter. Retrograde aortography has a number of disadvantages. It requires the administration of contrast material and has the usual risks of any invasive procedure. Also, laboratory preparation and patient transport often prolong the time necessary to perform the study. In addition, it is more expensive than other imaging procedures.

Computed tomography (CT) equipment is readily available in most hospitals, and the procedure is rapid and noninvasive. Spiral CT allows complete imaging of the thoracic aorta after a single injection of contrast material in less than 1 minute. Imaging is performed with optimal contrast enhancement, giving a better definition of intimal flaps, entry points, and proximal coronary arteries (Fig. 12.2). The two lumens with a visible intimal flap are visualized by CT in more than 70%

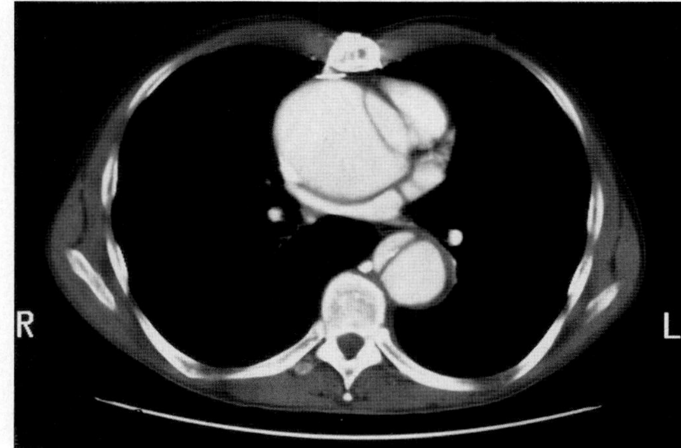

Figure 12.2 Spiral CT in acute type A dissection extending into the descending aorta. The ascending aorta is dilated. The intimal flap is clearly seen in both the ascending and descending aorta. (Courtesy of Dr. Loren Ketai, University of New Mexico, Albuquerque.)

of cases. The high density of a fresh intramural hematoma also can readily be identified. In addition, CT is helpful in identifying other causes of aortic widening, such as periaortic hematomas, abnormal mediastinal fat, and adjacent tumor. Although CT scanning in the diagnosis of dissection shows a sensitivity of 79% to 93% and a specificity of 86% to 100%, it cannot reliably identify aortic regurgitation, detect the entry site or the involvement of branch vessels, or delineate distal coronary arteries.

Magnetic resonance imaging (MRI) has emerged as one of the most accurate techniques for detecting aortic dissection in hemodynamically stable patients. It provides high-quality images in multiple planes (transverse, coronal, sagittal, and oblique) and better definition of the location and extent of the dissection. Moreover, no intravenous contrast material is required. Dissection is best seen when there is flow in both the true and false lumens (Fig. 12.3). Slow flow can sometimes resemble thrombosis. In such cases, it may be difficult to distinguish the dissection from an aortic aneurysm with mural thrombosis. Characteristic flow signals can identify communications between the true and false lumens and thrombus formation. Cine and gradient MRI supplies images that simulate real-time cardiac imaging. It can detect valvular regurgitation by identifying areas of turbulent flow. Acute intramural hematomas are well seen on T2 images because of the high signal intensity of blood. Older hemorrhages (1 to 5 days) have a higher signal intensity on T1 spin-echo images.[1] Studies of MRI efficacy in diagnosis of aortic dissection show sensitivity and specificity of almost 100%. Identification of the entry site was also high (sensitivity, 85%; specificity, 100%). The presence of aortic regurgitation was assessed with cine MRI with 85% sensitivity and 100% specificity.

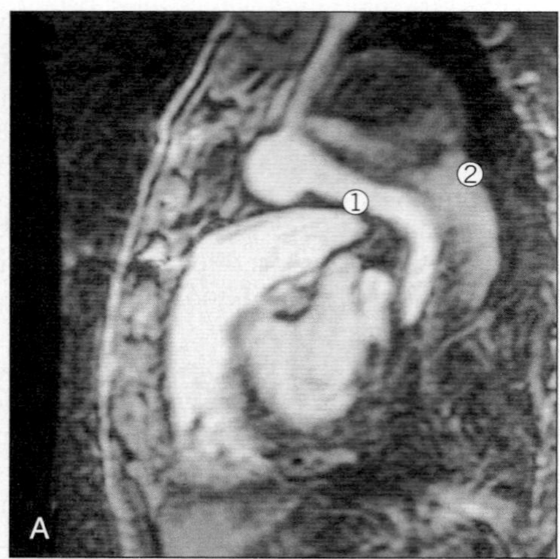

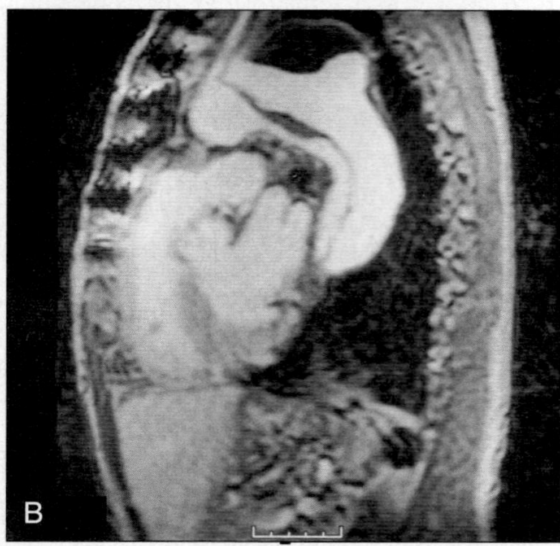

Figure 12.3 Longitudinal MRI in a chronic type B dissection extending into the arch. A, Early phase showing (1) the entry point and (2) a faint visualization of the outline of the aneurysm. **B,** Late phase demonstrating partial opacification of the aneurysm and the extension of the dissection along the subclavian artery. (Courtesy of Dr. Loren Ketai, University of New Mexico, Albuquerque.)

Although MRI is an accurate method of diagnosing aortic dissection, several disadvantages limit its use in unstable patients. The time necessary to perform the test (significantly longer than that of a CT scan and echocardiography) and the relatively limited access to the patient during imaging make MRI less than ideal for these patients, who are frequently intubated and receiving vasoactive drugs intravenously and are therefore in need of close monitoring. In addition, in many hospitals, MRI scanners are located in decentralized special facilities that complicate the issues of patient transport. Patients with implanted metal objects, such as pacemakers and defibrillators, or with claustrophobia cannot undergo MRI.

Echocardiography is an excellent test for patients with suspected aortic dissection because it is widely available and easily performed at the bedside. Transthoracic echocardiography can detect proximal ascending thoracic aorta dissections; but in adults, the aortic arch and descending thoracic aorta are not visualized well enough to identify aortic dissections reliably. Transesophageal echocardiography (TEE) is the preferred technique because the echo probe lies in the esophagus close to the descending thoracic aorta and provides excellent images of the entire thoracic aorta. Excellent visualization is possible because of the multiple planes that can be scanned as the probe is advanced and rotated. The procedure is quick, requiring only 5 to 18 minutes; it can be rapidly and safely performed in the emergency department, intensive care unit, and other clinical environments such as the operating room. TEE is playing an increasingly important role in the evaluation of aortic disease and has several advantages in the diagnosis of acute aortic dissection. It requires minimal preparation of the patient, avoids the contrast material and x-ray exposure associated with CT and angiography, and eliminates the delays and practical difficulties of MRI. In the majority of cases, the esophagus can be intubated with minimal distress by use of conscious sedation. The incidence of complications during TEE is less than 1%.

The diagnostic features sought are identification of intimal flaps, false lumens, intramural hematoma, ulcerated plaques, and blood flow between the true and false lumens (entry site). A number of studies examining the clinical value of TEE in diagnosis of aortic dissection have demonstrated a sensitivity of 92% to 100%, a specificity of 82% to 95%, a positive predictive value of 79% to 96%, and a negative predictive value of 97% to 100%. False-positive test results are usually due to reverberations from sclerotic or calcific ascending aortic disease and tortuous descending aortas.

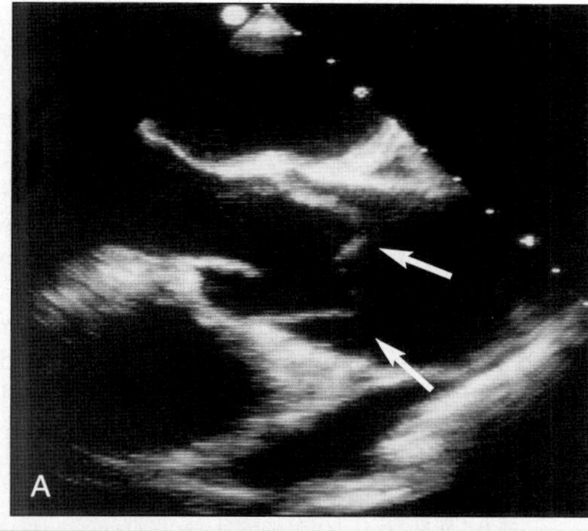

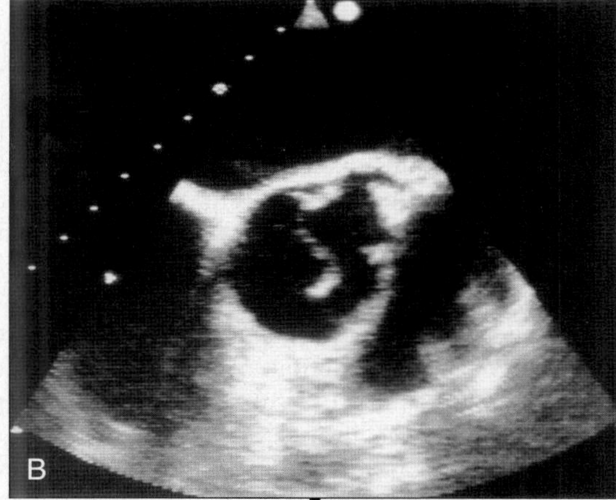

Figure 12.4 Visualization of the intimal flap. A, TEE long-axis view of the aortic valve and ascending thoracic aorta showing a circumferential intimal flap at the junction of the sinuses of Valsalva and the ascending aorta *(arrows)*. **B,** Cross-sectional view of the flap.

Imaging artifacts, which are often linear and parallel to the aortic wall, can arise from several factors, including variable contact with the esophageal wall and atherosclerotic disease. To minimize the possibility of false-positive examination findings, the intimal flap should be visualized in more than one plane (Fig. 12.4). False-negative test results are usually aortic arch dissections because the aortic arch is occasionally difficult to visualize completely on TEE.

Color-flow Doppler is extremely valuable for identifying the main channel of aortic flow (usually the true lumen) and other channels (Fig. 12.5). Color-flow imaging can help distinguish true intimal flaps and false channels from artifacts by observing different flow patterns on either side of the structure in question. Color-flow imaging can also detect the entry and exit points into the false lumen (Fig. 12.6).

Important precursors of aortic dissection and rupture, such as ulcerated plaques and intramural hematoma, can also be detected by TEE.[1] The diagnosis of intramural hematoma relies on the visualization of localized increases in aortic wall thickness caused by blood. Differentiation from severe atherosclerosis can be difficult, but in contrast to aortic plaque, intramural hematoma is a homogeneous, moderately echodense expansion of the aortic wall. Aortic plaque is nonhomogeneous, more echo dense, and more prominent on the

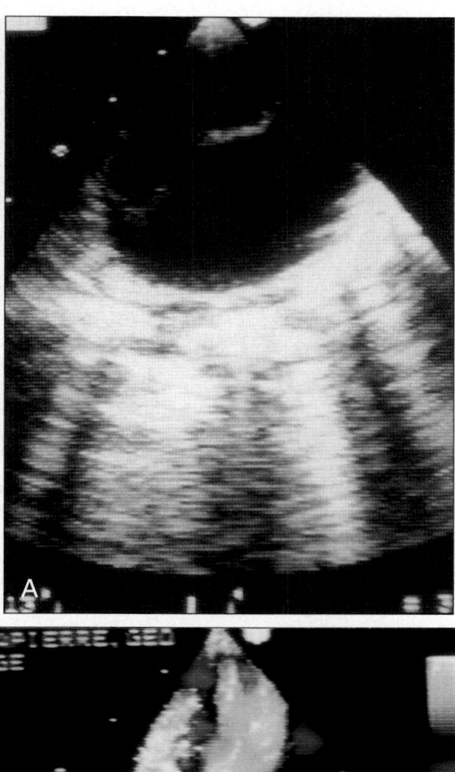

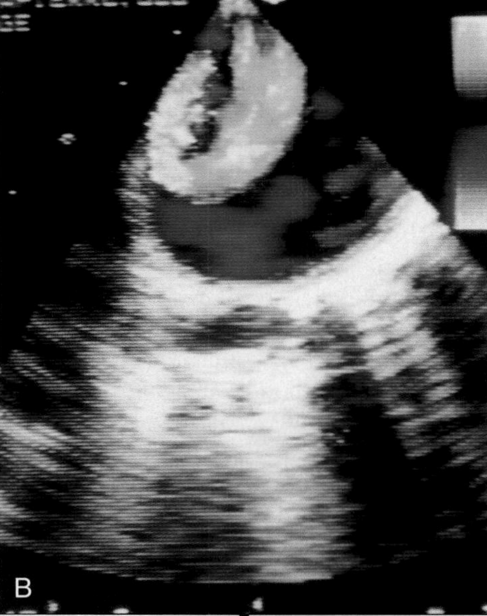

Figure 12.5 Identification of the main channel of aortic flow by color Doppler imaging. A, Possible intimal flap and false channel in a cross-sectional TEE view of the descending thoracic aorta. **B,** Color-flow Doppler imaging shows high-velocity flow in the smaller true lumen *(top)* and slow flow in the false channel *(bottom)*.

luminal surface of the aorta, often protruding into the lumen. Severe aortic atherosclerotic disease may result in mobile masses attached to the aortic wall, which could resemble intimal flaps, but usually they are thicker, are more echo dense, and arise from a markedly plaqued aortic wall.

TEE can readily identify complications of aortic dissection, such as aortic regurgitation and pericardial effusion, as well as rupture. TEE also provides detailed morphologic information about involvement of the proximal coronary arteries; false-negative results are unusual. This compares favorably with aortography in diagnosis of proximal dissection of the coronary arteries. Assessment of distal coronary arteriosclerosis, however, requires coronary angiography. In addition,

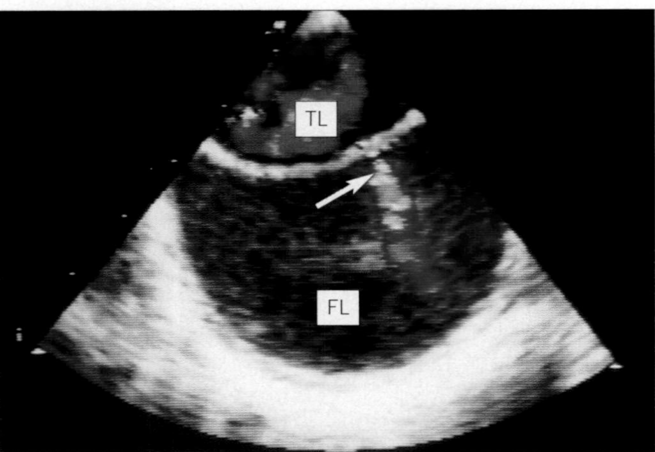

Figure 12.6 Cross-sectional TEE view of the descending thoracic aorta showing on color-flow imaging an entry point from the true lumen to the false lumen *(arrow).* FL, false lumen; TL, true lumen.

TEE can often assess aortic branch vessel involvement. Another advantage of TEE is that imaging can be easily performed in the operating room without affecting the performance of the operation. Intraoperative imaging by TEE can eliminate any uncertainty as to which structures are involved in the dissection and can provide critical information for the surgeon's management of the operation.

Selection of the Imaging Method

Each of the aortic imaging methods has advantages and disadvantages in the diagnosis of aortic dissection. Proper understanding of the accuracy, limitations, and relative merits of each of the diagnostic procedures is paramount. In selecting the best method of imaging for each individual patient, the physician must consider several factors. The ideal test should rapidly and safely confirm or exclude the diagnosis of dissection, determine whether the dissection involves the ascending aorta, and identify the anatomic features of the dissection, such as the presence of pericardial effusion, sites of entry and re-entry, extension of the dissection, and severity of aortic regurgitation. The accuracy of the information must be considered. A false-negative diagnosis might lead to death; a false-positive diagnosis can result in unnecessary surgery, carrying a significant risk. The physician must carefully assess the clinical condition of the patient, which will, of course, influence the selection of the imaging method. The availability of the equipment and personnel, the need for transportation, the length of time necessary to perform the procedure, and overall safety must also be considered (Table 12.1).

In most hospitals, TEE and spiral CT scanning have become the preferred diagnostic strategy for the initial evaluation of patients with suspected acute aortic disease. The use of MRI has been limited by the restricted availability of the magnets and by considerations of the patient's safety while undergoing the study. Aortography is seldom indicated, and coronary angiography is not recommended. Each institution should develop a strategy based on availability and areas of greatest local expertise. A low threshold for repeated imaging of the same or complementary type is critical to achieve a good outcome.[1]

Differential Diagnosis

Acute aortic dissection is the great clinical masquerader, and it can be misdiagnosed like almost any other acute medical or surgical illness. A high clinical index of suspicion is therefore imperative. Acute dissection should be considered whenever there is simultaneous acute involvement of multiple diverse organ systems without an obvious common explanation.

Careful evaluation of the presenting symptoms and signs permits an accurate differential diagnosis, including diseases as varied as myocardial infarction, cerebrovascular accident, pulmonary embolus, and acute surgical abdomen. Of paramount importance is the proper distinction between cases of aortic dissection and those of myocardial infarction because the administration of thrombolytic agents to patients with acute dissection can be catastrophic.

MANAGEMENT

Prevention

Many cases of acute dissection may be prevented in the general population by proper treatment of systemic hypertension. Hypertension control is not enough to prevent dissection in patients with Marfan's syndrome, other connective tissue disorders, and bicuspid aortic valve because they can develop acute dissection, with or without hypertension. These patients must be observed carefully for changes in aortic size. Several general recommendations that have emerged from the follow-up of patients with Marfan's syndrome are probably applicable to all patients with connective tissue disorders. Because the risk for development of

COMPARISON OF DIAGNOSTIC STUDIES				
Advantage	Aortography	CT	MRI	TEE
Readily available	Fairly	Quite	Fairly	Very
Rapid	Fairly	Quite	Fairly	Very
Performed at patient's bedside	No	No	No	Yes
Intravenous administration of iodinated contrast material	Yes	Yes	No	No
Cost	High	Reasonable	Moderate	Reasonable

CT, computed tomography; MRI, magnetic resonance imaging; TEE, transesophageal echocardiography.

Table 12.1 Comparison of diagnostic studies.

acute dissection is three times higher in patients with a hereditary history of dissection and a dilated aortic root, Marfan's patients should undergo a cardiologic evaluation, including transthoracic echocardiography, at least annually. When the aortic root diameter reaches a ratio of 1.3 above normal dimension, the evaluation interval should be shortened to 6 months. Patients with a ratio between 1.3 and 1.5 should be considered for elective surgical repair because of the high risk of dissection. The relationship between dilatation of the aortic root and the potential for dissection should be extrapolated to all patients undergoing cardiac surgical procedures for other indications. For instance, the risk of aortic dissection after aortic valve replacement is several times higher if the ascending aorta is dilated.[8] In such cases, the surgeon should consider replacing the ascending aorta at the time of valve replacement. With current improvements in surgical techniques and myocardial protection, elective replacement of the aorta does not add a significant risk to the heart operation.

Treatment

Optimal treatment of patients with aortic dissection requires that the diagnosis and the extent of the process be identified as soon as possible. Advances in treatment during the past few decades have produced a remarkable improvement in the prognosis of patients affected by this highly lethal disease. Although the mortality rate of untreated aortic dissection during the first 48 hours is as high as 1% per hour, the rapid initiation of medical therapy followed by prompt surgical therapy when indicated is associated with a significant improvement in survival. Most if not all patients with type A dissection require urgent surgical repair, whereas those with uncomplicated type B dissection can usually be treated successfully with medical therapy alone.

Acute Management

All patients suspected of having aortic dissection should be evaluated and treated as a real emergency. Regardless of the location of the dissection, all patients should receive anti-impulse pharmacologic therapy as soon as possible. The initial goal is to stabilize the propagation of the dissection to prevent rupture. Patients who present at a hospital without appropriate facilities should be transferred to a tertiary hospital with a cardiac surgery service as expeditiously as possible. In our opinion, transfer should not be delayed for confirmatory diagnosis. Patients suspected of having aortic dissection should be directly admitted to an intensive care unit for continuation of medical therapy, appropriate monitoring, and confirmatory imaging studies. Patients suspected of having type A dissections with pericardial effusion should probably be moved directly to the operating room where, if necessary, the diagnosis can be confirmed by TEE.

Acute reduction in arterial pressure is effectively accomplished by the administration of intravenous sodium nitroprusside (2 to 10 mcg/kg per minute). The dose is titrated against the blood pressure response. Blood pressure is reduced to the lowest level compatible with normal cerebral, renal, and cardiac function. Because nitroprusside alone can increase dP/dt, adequate simultaneous β-adrenergic blockade is routinely used. Intravenous esmolol or metoprolol is administered to maintain heart rate in the range of 65 to 70 beats per minute. Alternatively, labetalol (20 to 40 mg intravenously every 10 minutes) can be used. Other agents to reduce blood pressure and to decrease dP/dt include trimetaphan and reserpine. While the medical treatment is instituted, preparations should be made for aortic imaging and consultation with a cardiovascular surgeon.

Medical Treatment as Primary Therapy

Medical treatment is generally considered the primary treatment of dissection that involves the descending aorta as well as of most patients with aortic arch involvement (type B). In rare circumstances, medical therapy is the only treatment of patients with ascending aortic dissection who have serious associated medical conditions that contraindicate surgery.[9]

It is always advisable to restrict patients to intravenous nutrition for the first 48 hours after medical treatment, in case surgery becomes necessary. Many patients have an ileus, and a nasogastric tube may be required. When the condition of the patient stabilizes after 2 to 3 days of treatment, oral feeding may be started. Antihypertensive medications are gradually switched to the oral route by the third day. Patients without complications can be moved out of the intensive care area, and ambulation can begin. Approximately 85% to 90% of patients with medically treated uncomplicated type B dissection can be discharged from the hospital in 7 to 10 days. Patients who develop complications usually have a prolonged course of treatment that often requires endotracheal intubation, dialysis, and other therapies. Acute renal failure, other organ dysfunction, and neurologic deficits are common. Few patients with multiple complications survive.

Surgical Treatment

The goal of surgical treatment is to prevent death from aortic rupture and to reestablish blood flow to arteries occluded by the dissection. In cases of ascending aortic dissection, a secondary goal is to correct aortic regurgitation. With the exception of a few patients with very localized dissections, the operation does not remove the entire false channel. Only areas of actual or impending rupture are excised. The indications and surgical procedures used for the treatment of type A and B dissection are quite different and are reviewed.

The development of endovascular stent-grafts and their relatively recent application for the treatment of type B dissection probably represent the most remarkable advance in the management of this disease. The implantation of endovascular stent-grafts permits the coverage of the primary tear with redirection of flow into the true lumen, which appears to reduce the risk of rupture, to increase the likelihood of false lumen thrombosis, and to eliminate the propensity for late aneurysmal dilatation of the false lumen.

Indications

Acute Type A Dissection

Emergency surgical intervention is the treatment of choice in essentially all patients who have acute type A dissection; exceptions, which should be based on individual judgment, include the very old (>80 years), those with an irreversible stroke, and those with other severe, chronic, life-threatening illnesses. Serial aortic imaging and close clinical follow-up are mandatory if patients are not operated on immediately.[9] Patients with hemiplegia or paraplegia should not be denied emergency operation. In a recent report, most patients presenting with a stroke experienced partial or complete neurologic recovery after repair. On the other hand, in patients with paraplegia, chances of spinal cord deficit recovery are low. No worsening of the neurologic condition after repair was observed.[10]

Acute Type B Dissection

The optimal management of patients with acute type B dissection is controversial. In most centers, patients with type B dissections are treated medically. The recommendation for medical treatment of patients with type B dissections is based on the relatively high operative mortality rates for these patients and the observation that medical management can generally prevent death during the acute phase.

Surgery is reserved for patients with complications such as rupture, compromise of distal organs, persistence or recurrence of intractable pain, uncontrollable hypertension, or progression of dissection during medical treatment.[11] Several other conditions should prompt strong considerations for surgery but have not yet been accepted universally: Marfan's syndrome, a large localized aneurysm in the descending thoracic aorta, diffuse enlargement of the aorta (>5 cm), and, in very carefully selected patients, involvement of the aortic arch.

When medical treatment fails and complications develop, the course is usually catastrophic. It is paradoxical but not surprising that the indications for operation are those same factors that increase the surgical risk. The prognosis in such cases is dismal even if an emergency operation is performed. Early operative intervention for selected patients at low surgical risk with uncomplicated acute type B dissection may reduce the incidence of late death secondary to rupture of distal false aneurysm and redissection. In some centers, urgent surgery is the treatment of choice for carefully selected patients with acute type B dissections, even if they are uncomplicated. With this approach, current surgical mortality rates of patients with uncomplicated type B dissection have improved significantly during the past 10 years and may now be lower than 10%.[12] On the other hand, elderly patients and those with uncomplicated acute type B dissections who have severe pulmonary, cardiac, renal, or central nervous system disease, however, have a better prognosis if they are treated medically.

Endovascular repairs have been used in selected patients with acute type B dissection with satisfactory results. Whereas the indications are not yet clear, endovascular repairs are now a new viable treatment option. At this time, indications include patients who develop complications, particularly the elderly, who are not suitable for open repair. Further studies are necessary to compare endovascular stent-graft placement with medical treatment in patients with uncomplicated dissections. Given the relatively low mortality for uncomplicated type B dissections, the benefit of stent-grafting may be difficult to prove. The indication for endografts in chronic dissections is less clear. Given the stiffness and the multiple fenestrations of the chronically dissected septum and the fact that the circulation of distal organs and limbs is frequently dependent on the patency of the false lumen, it seems unlikely that stent-graft insertion could repair the consequences of the dissection.

Surgical Procedure for Type A Dissection

Current surgical management for acute type A dissection recommends a local and expeditious operation consisting of a supracoronary graft replacement of the ascending aorta redirecting forward flow into the true lumen and correction of aortic regurgitation. The native aortic valve should be preserved whenever possible. Valve reconstruction can be performed in approximately 75% of patients with acute type A dissection and in 50% of patients with chronic dissection with aortic insufficiency.[13] This approach prevents most deaths and is associated with the lowest operative risk. Although it is debatable, this conservative surgical approach should not be used in patients with Marfan's syndrome, Ehlers-Danlos syndrome, or other connective tissue disorders because of the questions about limited durability of aortic valve reconstruction. The most radical replacement of the ascending aorta and the aortic valve with a composite graft-valve prosthesis and the complex valve-sparing replacement of the aorta with coronary reimplantation are reserved for patients with severe involvement of the sinuses and proximal coronaries.

Given the negative impact of a patent false lumen on aortic expansion and late survival, every effort should be made to avoid the persistence of the false lumen. This includes avoidance of aortic clamping, open distal anastomosis, resection of the entry point and adjacent friable aorta, and use of perfusion strategies that direct flow into the true lumen. One of the most important controversies in the surgical treatment of acute dissection with entry sites in the aortic arch is whether the entire arch should be included in the repair (Fig. 12.7). Many authors agree that if the tear can be visualized in the proximal arch through the open aorta, it should be included in the repair (hemiarch repair). On the other hand, if the primary intimal tear cannot be exposed and resected safely (e.g., type A dissection with a tear in the distal aortic arch or the descending thoracic aorta), it should not be included in the resection because the operative risk for a complete arch replacement is extremely high. Early and late survivals are not affected adversely with this approach, but the subsequent reoperation rate is higher. The exception to this recommendation is selected low-risk younger patients, in whom it may be prudent to use profound hypothermic circulatory arrest and to include the aortic arch in the repair. The risk of the arch operation in this situation approaches 10% to 15%. If the arch has ruptured, concomitant arch replacement is mandatory, but the operative risk is substantially higher (25% to 50%).

Surgical Procedure for Type B Dissection

The repair involves resection of the intimal tear and placement of an interposition graft to obliterate the distal false lumen by approximating the layers of the aortic wall. Distal perfusion should be maintained during the procedure to prevent spinal cord and visceral ischemia. The risk of paraplegia is greater in patients with acute dissection than with atherosclerotic aneurysm, probably because there is no collateral flow. Visceral malperfusion usually improves with restoration of flow into the true lumen. Major aortic branches involved by the dissection may need to be stented or directly revascularized to restore flow. In other cases, as a last resort, a distal fenestration procedure between the true and false

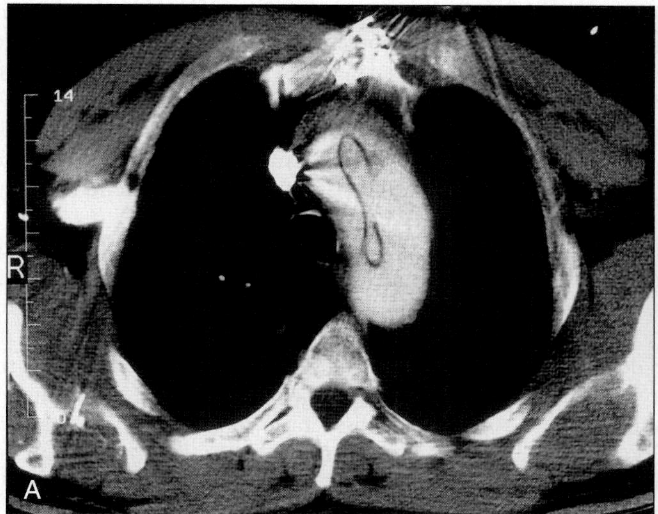

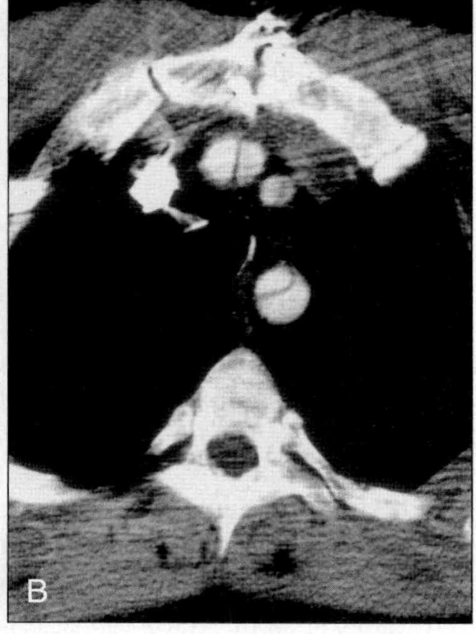

Figure 12.7 Surgical repair of dissection of the aortic arch. A, Chronic dissection of the aortic arch 6 months after ascending aortic repair of a type A dissection. The true lumen is completely detached from the adventitia. A large intimal tear is clearly seen. **B,** Dissection extending distally into the brachiocephalic vessels. (Courtesy of Dr. Loren Ketai, University of New Mexico, Albuquerque.)

lumens can be performed percutaneously in an attempt to improve perfusion of organs or limbs that communicated only with the false lumen.

Endovascular Stent-Graft Techniques

A primary goal of the procedure is the exclusion of the primary tear to redirect blood flow into the true lumen. This may increase the likelihood of false lumen thrombosis and may eliminate the risk for late aneurysmal dilatation. In addition, the implantation of endovascular stent-grafts inside of the true lumen permits the internal coverage of friable, enlarging, or even ruptured areas of the aorta, decreasing the risk of acute rupture. A limitation of this technique is the need to anchor the graft in a relatively normal segment of the aorta both proximally and distally. Critical aortic branches originating from the anchoring segments may be occluded. Additional revascularization procedures to ensure flow to these vessels are necessary in one third of the patients. The most common of these is a left carotid–subclavian bypass when the origin of the subclavian is covered by the stent-graft. Selected cases of retrograde dissection from a distal tear around the arch into the ascending aorta have been treated successfully by limited endograft coverage of the entry point. Endovascular stent-grafts have also been used for the treatment of acute dissection involving the arch in combination with open revascularization of the neck vessels before graft deployment. The use of uncovered stents in branch vessels and the creation of controlled re-entry tears in dissection flaps with use of balloon catheters can improve visceral malperfusion syndromes secondary to acute dissections.[14]

Surgical Results

The current operative mortality rate for patients with acute type A dissection remains between 10% and 25%[13]; for uncomplicated acute type B dissection, it is 13% ± 12%.[14] Selected centers have reported even lower operative mortality for uncomplicated cases.[12] The mortality rate has been much higher (25% to 60%) for type B patients with complications. Most deaths that occur shortly after operations for acute dissection are secondary to hemorrhage, heart failure, brain damage, or respiratory failure.[7,11]

Independent determinants of operative risk for type A dissections are age older than 70 years, shock at presentation, neurologic deficits, tamponade, myocardial ischemia or infarction, renal failure, and renal or visceral ischemia. Concomitant total arch replacement or coronary artery bypass is a risk factor for early death. For type B dissections, the determinants of risk include an older age, rupture, renal or visceral ischemia, and infarction. The incidence and types of postoperative complications appear to be similar for both type A and type B dissections. The most significant exception to this is the development of new paraplegia after repair of descending thoracic aortic dissection; this is quite rare after type A dissection but can occur in approximately 4% of patients after type B dissection repair.

Results of Endovascular Grafting for Type B Dissection

Despite the improvements in device technology and growing clinical experience, the use of stent-grafts for the treatment of aortic dissection is still in a developmental phase.[15] Several single-center reports have demonstrated that endovascular repair is technically successful in most cases and that procedure-related risks appear to compare favorably with those of surgery, particularly in patients with complications.[14] A recently published meta-analysis[16] of 39 studies that included 609 patients showed that overall mortality was 5.3% and major complications occurred in 14% of the patients (21% for acute and 9% for chronic dissection). The incidence of neurologic complications was low (3%); however, in contrast to open repair, stroke was twice more common than paraplegia. Despite those encouraging early results, some concern exists about mid- and long-term outcomes. Thrombosis of the false lumen in the stented segment was achieved in more than 80% of the cases, but occlusion of the false lumen in the distal thoracic and abdominal aorta was observed in only 10%. Late complications occurred in a third of the patients, including endoleaks, device migration, and distal aortic enlargement, with a 10% risk of aortic rupture at 2 years. In addition, retrograde type A dissection developed in 4% of the patients.[16] Strict follow-up with aortic imaging is necessary to detect and to manage these complications.

Long-term Management

All patients who survive acute dissection should be followed up medically for life. The late mortality rate related to aortic complications accounts for one third of late deaths. In many postoperative patients and almost all medically treated patients, the false channel persists, leading to the development of complications and death.[17] Progressive expansion of the dissected segment of the aorta is common and occurs in 25% to 40% of patients. Effective control of blood pressure and dP/dt should be continued after the initial episode, even if the patient is normotensive. Maximal blood pressure response to exercise should be assessed with treadmill testing. In one study, aneurysms developed in 45% of patients without good blood pressure control, compared with only 17% of patients with satisfactory control. The ideal drug should have a negative inotropic as well as a hypotensive effect (e.g., beta blockers).[18] Pure vasodilator drugs such as hydralazine and minoxidil increase dP/dt and should be used only in the presence of adequate beta-blocker therapy. Calcium channel blockers and angiotensin-converting enzyme inhibitors are potentially beneficial for the long-term management of aortic dissection (as a supplement to the traditional beta-blocker agents).

Accurate information of the extent of the dissection at the time of discharge is mandatory for proper follow-up. The aortic size and the status of the false lumen should be monitored periodically. Aortic imaging should be performed on a regular basis to evaluate the involved and uninvolved aorta after treatment and to detect extension of the dissection or enlargement of distal false aneurysms before rupture can occur.[7]

Recommendations for follow-up after discharge of patients with aortic dissection include regular examinations and chest radiography every 3 months during the first year and every 6 months thereafter. Aortic imaging should initially be performed at 3 months and then at 6 months. For patients with significantly dilated aortas, the intervals should remain at 3 months. If the aorta is not significantly dilated and no clinical or anatomic changes develop between imaging studies, the initial studies can be done at 6-month intervals. Studies can be performed annually after that period; it is probably not safe to exceed 1 year between examinations. Early recognition of aortic disease permits both prevention of aortic rupture and timely reoperation. Unfortunately, late death from aortic rupture can be reduced but not completely eliminated with this policy.[17]

PROGNOSIS

Natural History of Untreated Patients

The risk of death during the initial phase of acute dissection is very high. It is generally believed that approximately 10% to 15% of patients die suddenly in the first 15 minutes. Approximately 50% of patients are alive 48 hours later, and only 10% of patients are alive after 3 months. These statistics, however, ignore the clear difference in prognosis between acute dissections involving the ascending aorta and those involving only the descending aorta. Without treatment, only 8% of patients with ascending dissection survive for more than a month, whereas almost 75% may survive after dissection of the descending thoracic aorta.

Long-term Prognosis after Treatment

The prognosis of patients with acute aortic dissection in general has improved significantly as a result of earlier and more accurate diagnosis, more effective medical therapy, better surgical techniques, and improved perioperative management. During the past 2 decades, the annual mortality rate for aortic dissection in the United States has declined steadily by more than 50%.

There is scant information about the long-term survival of acute type A dissection treated medically. As mentioned before, a clear difference in early prognosis exists between patients with acute dissections that involve the ascending aorta and those that involve only the descending thoracic aorta. In a series of medically treated patients, only 43% of patients with type A dissection were alive 1 month after the dissection, compared with 91% of patients with type B dissection. Interestingly, for survivors of the acute episode, the difference in prognosis disappears after the first month. The 5-year survival rate for patients who survived an acute dissection followed by medical treatment alone was not different between type A and type B dissections. Several factors adversely affect the long-term prognosis of medically treated patients; these include age, presence of serious early complications before therapy was instituted, and large diameter of the descending aorta (>5 cm).

Even though patients who survive the acute dissection continue to be at a significantly greater risk of death than the general population, their long-term survival after surgical treatment shows a relatively satisfactory prognosis. Published results for long-term survival after repair of acute dissection are between 70% and 85% at 5 years and between 54% and 66% at 10 years.[17] The actuarial survival rate of patients with acute type A dissection showed a slightly (yet significantly) lower life expectancy at 10 years than that of the general U.S. population, matched for age and sex. For patients with acute type B dissection, the actuarial survival rate was 48% at 5 years and 29% at 10 years, not significantly different from that of a matched population.

A report focusing on the long-term outcome of all types of dissections showed that 18% of late deaths were caused by rupture of another region of the aorta, 38% were cardiovascular in nature, and 28% were sudden and not defined. Even considering that many patients had cardiovascular disease, some (if not many) of these sudden deaths may have been due to aortic rupture. These results underscore the importance of indefinite clinical follow-up. The surgical nature of the late sequelae suggests that surveillance should ideally be performed by the surgeon (who is the one who must decide when to reoperate).[7]

Reoperations are common in patients with treated aortic dissections. In the Stanford experience, the incidence of reoperation was 13% ± 4% at 5 years and 23% ± 6% at 10 years (linearized rate, 3.1% per patient-year). The type of dissection has no significant influence on the probability of reoperation, which is more likely in younger patients and in those with Marfan's syndrome (31% versus 8%).[17]

INTRAMURAL AORTIC HEMATOMA

The term *intramural hematoma* (IMH) was introduced to describe a localized aortic dissection without intimal disruption. It is thought to begin with the rupture of the vasa vasorum of the aortic wall. This results in a collection of blood oriented circumferentially around the lumen of the aorta. In the early stages, the blood extravasated in the media or in the subadventitial space does not communicate with the aortic lumen; therefore, it does not show enhancement with the administration of contrast material, nor does it show blood flow into the space on TEE.[2] The absence of an intimal tear has been confirmed in several surgical and autopsy cases. Even though IMH can develop in any location of the aorta, two thirds of the patients have involvement of the descending aorta.

Echocardiographic findings that are suggestive of the diagnosis of IMH include the following (Fig. 12.8):

- the typical reflection pattern of loculated blood with formation of a thrombus between the adventitia and the media;
- eccentric aortic lumen;
- displaced intimal calcium; and
- areas of echolucency within the aortic wall.

Because the echocardiographic criteria for IMH may not be confirmatory, a second imaging modality is frequently necessary after TEE to secure its diagnosis. On CT images, the IMH is recognized as a nonenhancing circular or crescent-shaped thickening of the aortic wall without evidence of an intimal flap. A fresh hematoma is evidenced by a high-density signal compared with that of the aortic layers (Fig. 12.9). Thrombosis is identified by a multilayered pattern.[8] On MRI, acute IMH is demonstrated as a circular or crescent-shaped thickening of the aortic wall without evidence of a classic intimal flap and absence of blood flow in the false lumen. Fresh bleeding is isodense on T1-weighted images but has a high signal intensity on T2-weighted images. Subacute IMH, on the other hand, has a high signal intensity on both T1- and T2-weighted images because of the formation of methemoglobin.

Spontaneous IMH affects patients with long-standing hypertension. They present with severe chest or back pain similar to that of aortic dissection, but the signs and symptoms of arterial branch involvement are lacking. Aortic regurgitation can occur in some cases of ascending aortic IMH. Pericardial and pleural effusions are common and

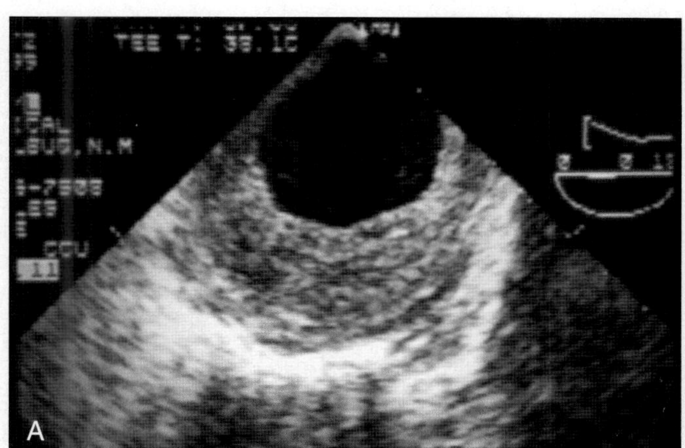

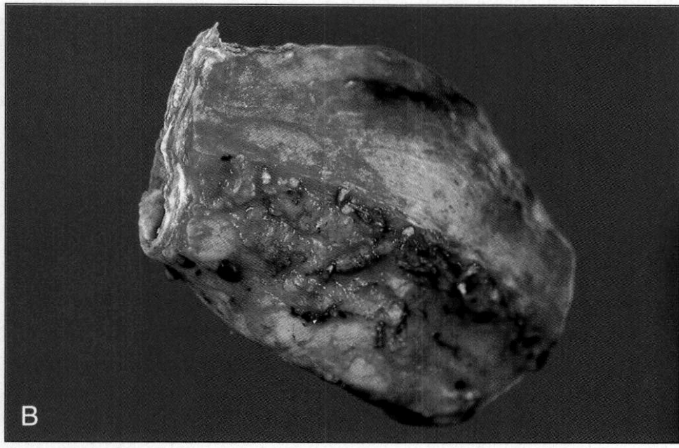

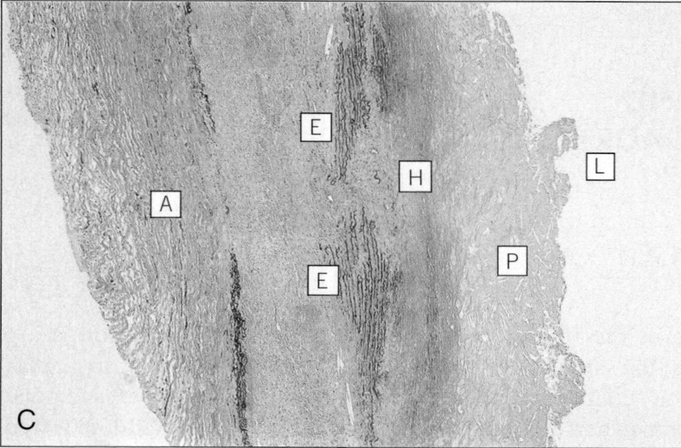

Figure 12.8 Intramural hematoma. A, Cross-sectional transesophageal echocardiogram of the descending thoracic aorta showing a large intramural hematoma *(bottom)*. **B,** Gross surgical specimen of the excised section of aorta. **C,** Histologic section of the affected aortic wall with a Verhoeff–van Gieson stain for elastin showing penetration of the luminal plaque through the elastic media, with the resultant hematoma separating the elastic layers. A, adventitia; E, elastin fibers; H, hematoma; L, lumen; P, plaque.

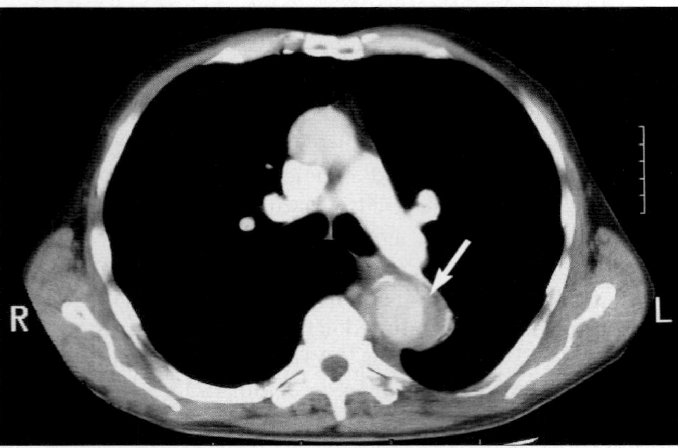

Figure 12.9 Transverse CT image at the level of the pulmonary trunk. The arrow marks a discrete localized wall thickening of high density. This is considered strong evidence of fresh hematoma.

represent impending external rupture. Spontaneous progression of IMH to classic dissection may occur regardless of the location of the hematoma and characterizes IMH as a precursor of dissection.

From collective experience, it appears that IMH of the ascending aorta has a worse prognosis with medical treatment than with early surgery.[2] These patients should be managed like those with classic ascending aortic dissection. Patients with descending aortic IMH can probably initially be treated medically. However, several series have also demonstrated the potential for poor outcome in patients with descending aortic IMH treated medically. Thus, follow-up imaging to rule out progression should be carried out in 2 to 4 days. If the findings demonstrate progression, surgery should be performed preemptively to prevent rupture. If patients tolerate medical management without deterioration, they may continue to be treated conservatively. Several patients have shown involution of the lesions over time. These recommendations should be adjusted to the individual condition of the patient. IMH is a lesion of the elderly, frequently with major associated comorbidities. Many patients may not be appropriate candidates for the aggressive surgical approach described.

CHRONIC THORACIC AND THORACOABDOMINAL AORTIC ANEURYSMS

ANATOMY AND PATHOLOGY

Annuloaortic Ectasia

Annuloaortic ectasia is a disease of the fibrous component of the aortic annulus in which the annulus is primarily enlarged. In its progression, the dilatation includes the sinuses of Valsalva and the proximal part of the ascending aorta. Because the dilatation occurs almost exclusively on the right side of the aortic root, which is not muscular, the noncoronary sinus is the first one to become dilated. As the process advances, the right and left aortic sinuses also dilate. Patients with annuloaortic ectasia frequently have enlarged mitral valves, which may or may not be abnormal. Annuloaortic ectasia is often associated with Marfan's syndrome and other connective tissue disorders. It is also common in patients with bicuspid aortic valve. Dilatation of the aortic root due to annuloaortic ectasia frequently leads to aortic valve insufficiency, acute aortic dissection, or a combination of these problems.

Arteriosclerotic or Degenerative Aneurysms

Arteriosclerosis or nonspecific degenerative disease is the most common cause of descending thoracic and thoracoabdominal aneurysms. More than half of the aneurysms reported in surgical series are in this category. Although atheromatous changes have long been recognized in these aneurysms, the causative role of atherosclerosis in their development is not clearly established. Several deficiencies of collagen, elastin, and smooth cells have been described in these aneurysms.

Chronic Aortic Dissection

When the false lumen persists after an acute aortic dissection, the thin outer wall has a strong tendency to enlarge gradually. Chronic aortic dissection with a persistent false channel is the second most common cause for the development of chronic thoracic aneurysms. They have a propensity to enlarge and rupture.

Chronic Traumatic Aortic Transection

Untreated, acute traumatic transection leads to the extravasation of blood into the periaortic area. If the patient survives, the periaortic hematoma remains in communication with the aorta and forms a false aneurysm that is contained only by the aortic adventitia or mediastinal tissues. The false aneurysm has a tendency to enlarge and rupture. Less than 10% of descending aortic aneurysms have a traumatic origin.

Aortitis

Infection is an uncommon cause of thoracic aortic aneurysm and represents a small percentage of cases in modern series. Granulomatous aortitis is an uncommon condition in which the microscopic appearance suggests an infectious etiology, but bacteriologic studies are negative. Granulomatous aortitis may produce simultaneous aortic and pulmonary aneurysms. Secondary syphilis was a common cause of ascending aortic aneurysm in the past. It causes the destruction of the elastic fibers in the aortic media, leading to progressive expansion and rupture.

PATHOPHYSIOLOGY

Aneurysm formation is a progressive and self-perpetuating phenomenon due to Laplace's law. As the radius increases, wall stress increases exponentially, leading to further expansion. Aortic dilatation is frequently associated with deposition of laminated thrombus along the walls of the aneurysm. Thrombus formation does not protect against expansion and potential rupture. Eventually, most aneurysms will rupture. The natural history may depend in part on the etiology of the aneurysm. In patients whose aneurysm is related to a previous dissection, the prognosis is worse than for the degenerative ones. Hypertension is an important factor in the development of dilatation.[19]

Aneurysms of the ascending aorta are frequently associated with aortic valve regurgitation. Aortic regurgitation results from the dilatation of the sinotubular junction. This causes passive stretching of the otherwise normal leaflets, which are pulled away by the displacement of the commissures. Dilatation of the aorta at the level of the sinotubular junction is the most common cause of isolated aortic valvular regurgitation, frequently in the presence of a normal valve and, in many instances, a normal-sized annulus. In typical ascending aortic aneurysms, the aortic annulus often dilates much less than the sinuses and the sinotubular junction. As described before, this is not the case, however, in annuloaortic ectasia, in which annular dilatation is the first pathologic development, followed later by the dilatation of the sinotubular junction.

Progressive dilatation and increase in the wall tension of the aneurysm can lead to the development of acute dissection. The relationship between aortic size and risk of dissection is better described in Marfan's syndrome than in other pathologic processes. However, several findings suggest that the risk of complications is also related to the size of the aorta in other diseases. For instance, in most aortic dissection series, the diameter of the aortic root at the time of presentation is clearly enlarged in the majority of patients, suggesting the presence of preexisting abnormal dilatation. The incidence of postoperative dissection after aortic valve replacement is also significantly higher if the aorta is 5 cm or larger at the time of the operation. In all contemporary natural history studies, the probability of rupture increases significantly beyond an aortic diameter of 6 cm, and the risk increases as the aneurysm increases even further.[16]

After size, other risk factors associated with aneurysm growth identified by multivariate regression analysis include chronic dissection, Marfan's syndrome, aneurysm location, age, smoking, hypertension, and sex. Descending thoracoabdominal aneurysms expand faster than ascending or aortic arch aneurysms do. The presence of chronic obstructive pulmonary disease is also a powerful predictor of rupture,[20] independent of smoking.

Clinical Presentations

Many patients are asymptomatic at the time of presentation; the diagnosis is often made during evaluation for other medical conditions, such as aortic regurgitation, hypertension, or atypical chest pain. When symptoms are present, they are often of recent onset and coincide with a change in the rate of expansion of the aneurysm. In other cases, pain may be chronic and of several months' duration. Location of the pain may be precordial in the case of ascending aorta, or it may radiate to the neck and jaw when arch involvement exists. Aneurysms of the descending thoracic aorta tend to produce back pain. Of great clinical significance is the fact that in most of the patients who present with sudden rupture, the diagnosis of aneurysm was not known before the development of the complication. A constellation of symptoms may result from the aneurysm's compressing adjacent structures. This may include superior vena cava obstruction, stretching of the left recurring laryngeal or phrenic nerve, airway compression, dysphagia, and hemoptysis. Evidence of atherosclerotic disease is frequently present in patients with thoracic aortic aneurysms. This includes coronary artery disease, peripheral vascular disease, and cerebral vascular disease. About 10% of the patients have an associated aortic abdominal aneurysm.

DIAGNOSTIC TECHNIQUES

The plain chest radiograph can readily identify dilatation and aneurysms because of the natural contrast between the thoracic aorta and the surrounding lung. Conventional CT scanning can identify aneurysms well but provides only axial images and requires contrast material. Three-dimensional reconstructions permit an excellent evaluation of the size and extent of the aneurysm.

MRI is a useful technique because it can identify and characterize aortic aneurysms and assess their physiologic consequences. The ability to image the entire aorta in sagittal planes allows assessment of the location and extent of aneurysms. The use of oblique planes permits accurate measurements of aneurysm diameter and the relation of the aneurysm to branch vessels. In addition, coronal plane images can identify ascending aortic aneurysms, and with spin-echo or phase mapping techniques, associated aortic regurgitation and hemopericardium can be assessed.

Echocardiography is used to further define the morphologic character of the aorta as well as to evaluate cardiac function. Transthoracic echocardiography can visualize the proximal ascending aorta adequately, permitting the diagnosis of annuloaortic ectasia or postaortic stenosis dilatation. It can also identify thoracic aortic aneurysms, but only MRI and intravascular ultrasonography can also interrogate the abdominal aorta. Aortic angiography, until recently the gold standard, is not generally necessary.

MANAGEMENT

The size of the aorta remains the most important factor in the decision-making process to recommend treatment for asymptomatic aortic aneurysms. Because of the significant operative risks associated with the repair, operation is not advised for an asymptomatic patient before the aorta reaches a size associated with a risk of rupture that is greater than the surgical risk. The decision to operate is not simple, and there is a great deal of discussion about the current recommendations for elective resection of aortic aneurysms.[20,21]

Most recommendations are based on absolute measurements of the aorta that ignore the relationship between aortic size, age, and body surface area. Furthermore, these recommendations are based on the observation that the mean diameter of the aorta at the time of the development of dissection or rupture is around 6 cm for the ascending aorta and 7 cm for the descending aorta. If operation is delayed until this point, it means that half of the patients would have experienced a complication by the time that treatment is recommended. This policy, which may have been justified in an era when the surgical morbidity and mortality were relatively high, is undoubtedly too conservative.

Nomograms that permit accurate assessment of the degree of aortic dilatation in relation to the expected size of the aorta based on body surface area, age, and sex have been developed. Decisions should be based on the determination of aortic diameter to expected diameter ratios for each individual patient. Current guidelines for elective aortic replacement in patients at low surgical risk recommend operation when the aortic ratio is 1.3 or greater. For higher risk patients, surgery is recommended for a ratio of 1.5 or greater for ascending aortic lesions and 2.0 or greater for descending aortic lesions. For patients who are under observation, operative repair is recommended if the aneurysm expands by more than 0.3 cm per year. Mandatory indications for replacement of the aorta include development of symptoms, acute dissection, intramural hematoma, and rupture. Severe atherosclerosis with mobile plaque is also an emerging indication for operation.

Techniques of Operation

Several operative techniques are available for surgical treatment of a dilated ascending aorta. They include the separate replacement of the aortic valve and ascending aorta, a valve-sparing root replacement procedure, and the traditional composite root replacement with a valved conduit. Options for a valved conduit replacement include a synthetic graft, a homograft, and a pulmonary autograft. Choosing of the technique appropriate for the individual patient and the specific pathologic process requires careful consideration of several important factors. Among these factors are

- age and expected survival;
- underlying pathologic changes;
- anatomic condition of the aortic valve, sinuses, and sinotubular junction;
- risk of anticoagulation; and
- presence of active infection.

The goals of surgical treatment for descending aortic aneurysm are to resect the diseased segment and to reestablish continuity with an in situ graft. The procedure varies, depending on the location and size of the aneurysm. On occasion, in long aneurysms involving several aortic segments, the operation is staged. Temporary cross-clamping of the aorta produces an increase in cardiac afterload and temporary ischemia of visceral organs, including the spinal cord. Numerous methods have been recommended to minimize the consequences of aortic cross-clamping during the repair. Temporary shunts, partial or total cardiopulmonary bypass, and hypothermic circulatory arrest are recommended for different situations. The choice depends largely on the surgeon's preference. Interruption of critical intercostal vessels is avoided as much as possible.

Techniques for the placement of endovascular stent-grafts have recently been developed. This procedure offers a promising alternative for the treatment of patients with aneurysms. The need for a 2-cm neck proximal and distal to permit a stable seal remains a major limitation to its use, as does the necessity for a large introducer sheath, usually inserted through a femoral cutdown. Initially reserved for patients at very high risk who were not considered candidates for conventional surgical repair, endovascular stent-grafts are proving to be an effective means of treatment in a significant number of patients with favorable anatomic features.[22]

PROGNOSIS

Appropriate choice of surgical procedure for the aortic root and the ascending aorta yields excellent immediate and long-term results. Hospital mortality after elective operation ranges between 4% and 12%, whereas the mortality of emergency operation is still very high. Late survival after operation is approximately 65% at 5 years and 55% at 7 years. The occurrence of dissection severely affects long-term prognosis. Expected mortality for patients undergoing elective resection of descending thoracic aneurysms is higher, in the range of 5% to 15%. Morbidity includes the risk of paraplegia, renal dysfunction, low cardiac output, and bleeding. The incidence of paraplegia for elective procedures ranges between 0% and 20% and averages 4%. The operative morbidity and mortality for emergency procedures are increased several-fold over that for elective repair. Late survival after operation is 70% at 5 years and 40% at 10 years. Interestingly, endovascular stent-grafts have been associated with a low incidence of development of paraplegia, even when all the intercostal vessels between T8 and L1 have been covered. Paraplegia has occurred only when an abdominal aortic aneurysm repair was performed simultaneously with the thoracic endografting.[22]

PENETRATING AORTIC ULCERS

The penetrating aortic ulcer, a unique pathologic event with special prognostic and therapeutic implications, is quite different from the simple superficial ulceration of an arteriosclerotic lesion. Penetrating aortic ulcers are atheromatous plaques that ulcerate and disrupt the internal elastic lamina, burrowing deeply into the aortic media and beyond. Microscopic findings demonstrate intimal degeneration and cholesterol infiltration mimicking clefts that penetrate through the media. Depending on the depth of penetration, blood is found at varying levels of the aortic wall.[21]

Depending on the degree of local inflammation and fibrosis, the plaque may precipitate a localized hematoma within the aortic wall. The hematoma may break through into the adventitia to form a pseudoaneurysm or may rupture freely into the mediastinum. Penetrating ulcers are frequently misdiagnosed as dissection because they are much less common than classic dissection.[23]

The clinical presentation is similar to that of classic aortic dissection. However, the symptoms and signs secondary to peripheral arterial compromise, which are so typical of dissection, are lacking. Accurate recognition and differentiation of penetrating ulcers from classic aortic dissection are critical for optimal management because their prognosis may be more serious than with classic dissection.

The mean age at presentation is significantly older than that of patients with type A or type B dissection. Close to half the patients have a concomitant abdominal aortic aneurysm.[23] The incidence of acute rupture at the time of presentation of the penetrating aortic ulcer has been reported to be higher than that of type A or type B dissection.

The diagnosis of penetrating aortic ulcer can be made by most imaging techniques with the demonstration of a contrast material–filled outpouching in the aorta in the absence

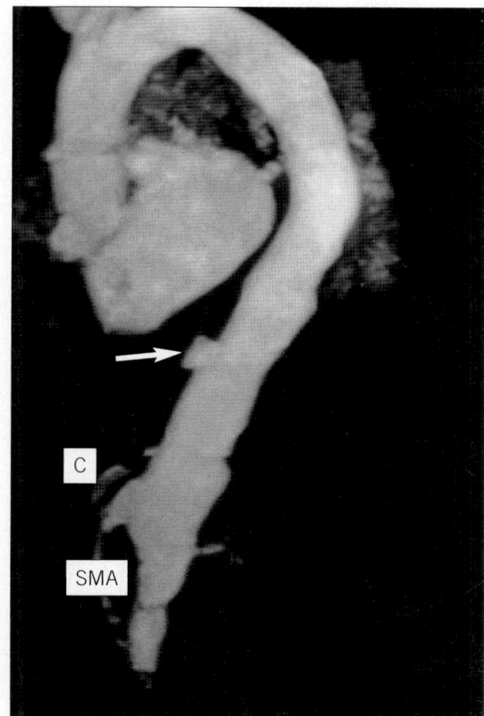

Figure 12.10 MRI clearly demonstrating a penetrating ulcer *(arrow)* and diffuse atherosclerotic disease. The celiac axis (C) and the superior mesenteric artery (SMA) are seen. Both are severely atherosclerotic.

of a dissection flap or false lumen. TEE demonstrates a crater-like ulcer with jagged edges in the presence of extensive aortic atheroma but in the absence of an intimal flap or false lumen. On CT scans, the diagnosis is confirmed with the demonstration of an outpouching of the aorta in the absence of a dissection flap or false lumen. On MRI, penetrating ulcer is identified by visualization of a distinct ulcer crater in the absence of a dissection (Fig. 12.10). On angiography, penetrating ulcers are recognized as a characteristic localized contrast-filled outpouching. Cobblestoning in the region of the ulcer signifies the presence of severe atherosclerosis. Complicated penetrating ulcers can be accompanied by localized intramural hematoma surrounding hemorrhage and pleural effusion.[24]

Regardless of the location of a penetrating aortic ulcer, patients should undergo immediate medical treatment to control pain and to prevent rupture. Persistent pain, hemodynamic instability, and radiographic expansion are indications for surgical treatment. On the basis of several reports that have shown that penetrating aortic ulcers of the ascending aorta are prone to rupture, patients with ascending penetrating aortic ulcer should undergo immediate operation.[24] Uncomplicated ulcers in the descending aorta may initially be managed medically with a high index of suspicion for potential expansion or rupture. Surgical treatment becomes necessary in the case of clinical or radiologic deterioration. Patients who tolerate medical management without clinical signs of expansion should undergo follow-up imaging studies at 3 to 5 days to confirm the safety of this approach. Although the preferred operation is resection and graft interposition of the affected area of the aorta, there are special situations in which patch repair and external wrapping of the aorta can be lifesaving in patients who are moribund. Endovascular stent-grafts play a significant role in the treatment of these challenging patients and are gradually becoming the first approach to treatment. Endovascular stent-grafting is a less invasive alternative to conventional operations. Unfortunately, in many cases, the severity of the atherosclerotic disease and the size of the aorta limit its application.

Penetrating aortic ulcer can be a life-threatening condition that may not be recognized unless the treating physician is aware of this entity.[2] In one series, 40% of patients with penetrating aortic ulcer of the descending aorta suffered rupture during observation in the intensive care unit while being treated for what was thought to be type B dissection. Medically treated patients should be followed up indefinitely with periodic imaging studies. Surgical results depend on several factors, such as age, diffuse aortic atherosclerotic involvement, associated medical conditions, and the frequently nonelective nature of the operation. Best results are seen in nondelayed operations in hemodynamically stable patients. Emergency operation for rupture is associated with a very high morbidity and mortality. As is the case with repair of aneurysm disease, operations in the aortic arch and descending thoracic aorta carry a higher mortality than those in the ascending aorta.

SUMMARY

Aortic dissection is a catastrophic event, and urgent diagnosis and aggressive medical treatment are vital. Regardless of the location of the initial tear, surgical intervention is mandatory when the ascending aorta is involved. Descending aortic dissections are initially managed medically, but operative repair is indicated as complications develop. Long-term medical management with periodic imaging evaluation of all patients is of paramount importance because of the high incidence of late complications from the dissection. Potential improvements in overall survival of patients in the future will most probably be obtained by earlier and more accurate diagnosis, earlier initiation of pharmacologic management, and, when indicated, more expeditious operation.

chapter 13

Abdominal Aortic Aneurysms

Joseph Shalhoub and Ian J. Franklin

Definition

- Abdominal aortic aneurysm (AAA) is defined as dilatation of the abdominal aorta to more than 3 cm in diameter.
- These can be infrarenal, juxtarenal, or suprarenal, according to the relationship to the renal arteries.

Key Features

- AAA is common; 5% of men older than 65 years have a degree of aortic dilatation.
- AAA is a common cause of sudden death, annually more than 100 per million in Western countries.
- Most AAAs are asymptomatic until they rupture.
- Ruptured AAA has a high mortality; most patients die before reaching the hospital. Emergency surgery saves around 60% of those who survive to the operating theater.
- AAA size remains the best indicator of risk of rupture.

Therapy

- There is no proven survival advantage in intervening for AAAs of less than 5.5 cm in diameter; surveillance by ultrasonography is safe.
- There are two treatments of aortic aneurysm: open surgical repair and endovascular repair. Open surgical repair was once considered the "gold standard" treatment of AAAs and is a relatively safe and durable procedure.
- Endovascular repair is now supported by a strong body of evidence, with a lower morbidity and a faster return to work compared with open surgery, particularly in fit patients. However, follow-up is required, and there is a significant reintervention rate to maintain stent-graft function.
- There is currently no proven pharmacotherapy to limit aneurysm development, but greater understanding of the pathogenesis of AAA may allow the introduction of drugs to limit aneurysm growth.

The first successful repair of an abdominal aortic aneurysm was performed by Pierre Dubost in Paris on March 29, 1951. He used a cadaveric homograft, and the patient, then aged 51 years, survived another 8 years before dying suddenly at home, probably of a heart attack. Until the early 20th century, syphilis was the most common cause of aortic aneurysms, mainly affecting the aortic arch. Of the first 10 abdominal aortic aneurysm repairs performed by Eastcott in London in 1954-1955, four were tuberculous or syphilitic. Such thoracic aneurysms are now rare, and the most common in current clinical practice are aneurysms of the infrarenal abdominal aorta (Fig. 13.1). This, along with evidence we present later, shows that there has been an etiologic and diagnostic shift in the story of aortic aneurysms in general.

There is no clear-cut definition of abdominal aortic aneurysm. Various attempts have been made to relate aortic diameter to height, sex, weight, and the diameter of the suprarenal aorta; but for most practical purposes, the infrarenal aorta is considered aneurysmal when the diameter exceeds 3 cm, implying a 50% increase. This chapter uses the term *aneurysm* to mean abdominal aortic aneurysm (AAA) unless otherwise stated.

Aneurysm is a disease of later life, with the incidence rising progressively with age. Men are eight times more likely to develop an aneurysm than are women. Around 5% of men older than 65 years have an aneurysm, and as more people live longer, the incidence is rising. In one study, aneurysms were detected in 11.4% of men 60 years of age and older undergoing abdominal ultrasound examination for reasons other than a suspected aneurysm.[1] Autopsy-based studies indicate that the incidence of ruptured aneurysm is 8.4 per 100,000 of the population for men and 3.0 per 100,000 for women.[2] Around 7500 deaths per year in the United Kingdom are caused by ruptured AAA, similar to the number dying of upper gastrointestinal tract malignant disease. Although aneurysms are less common in women, female gender confers a threefold increased risk of aneurysm rupture.[3]

ANATOMY AND PATHOLOGY

Normal aortic wall comprises tunica intima, media, and adventitia. In health, the intima and adventitia are thin, and the tensile strength of the wall is derived from the media. The tunica media consists of vascular smooth muscle cells in a well-organized matrix of concentric lamellae. The smooth muscle cells provide tensile strength and secrete the bulk of the matrix proteins. The two main extracellular proteins are elastin and collagen. Elastin is extensile and can extend to double its resting length yet return to its normal size. This property allows the aorta to expand during systole, thus storing the energy of the cardiac impulse and driving the blood into the tissues as the aorta contracts during diastole.

Fibrillar collagen (types I and III) is the main provider of tensile strength in the aortic wall. Collagen is inelastic, but in the aorta, it is wound in a coiled form that allows expansion without altering the length of each fiber. As the aorta is distended, the initial load is taken by elastin. As further expansion occurs, the coiled collagen fibers become taut, and further expansion is prevented.[4]

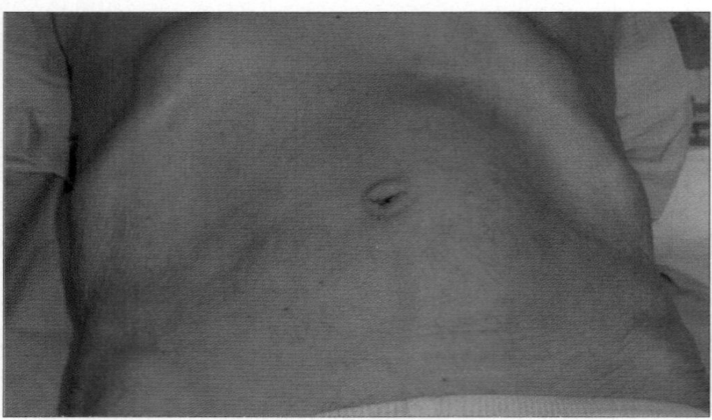

Figure 13.1 In thin individuals, an aortic aneurysm may be seen as a pulsating swelling in the upper abdomen. (Courtesy of Mr. S. Ray.)

On histologic examination, there are striking differences between normal and aneurysmal aorta. Aneurysm wall is usually thicker, but the structure is disorganized and weaker. AAA wall frequently has atherosclerotic lesions on the luminal surface. The normal lamellar structure of the tunica media is disrupted, and the media is thin with marked loss of smooth muscle cells. Elastin is conspicuous by its absence, but there is a relative increase in collagen. The adventitia is thick and inflamed, with infiltrating lymphocytes and macrophages especially around the vasa vasorum.

In the past, aortic aneurysms were considered to be a complication of atherosclerosis, and most aneurysms that were not obviously inflammatory or infective were referred to, almost without question, as atherosclerotic aneurysms. It is now evident that earlier models of aneurysm development were overly simplistic and that aneurysms do not simply result from an artery wall somehow weakened by atheroma.

Three crucial processes have emerged as being central to the vascular remodeling that results in aortic aneurysms. These are

- inflammation;
- loss of vascular smooth muscle; and
- excessive proteolysis.

The pathogenesis of AAAs involves progressive cycles of proteolysis and inflammation, the product of proteolysis driving subsequent inflammation. Little is yet known about the initiating events, and uncertainty of a "chicken and egg" nature exists over which is the primary abnormality. Chronic inflammation in the aneurysm wall leads to an imbalance of proteolytic enzyme activity, causing degradation of the matrix proteins.[3] The inflammation also causes depletion of smooth muscle cells.[5] These changes result in weakening, dilatation, and eventually rupture of the aorta.

There are large gaps in this model. The influence of genetic factors is far from clear. The mechanisms by which risk factors (such as male sex, smoking, hypertension, and atherosclerosis) contribute to aneurysm development have not been firmly established. The trigger for aneurysm formation might even be infective, and several organisms have been implicated, most prominently *Chlamydia pneumoniae* (see later). Nonetheless, the interactions between inflammatory pathways, smooth muscle cell function, and extracellular matrix turnover are being discovered, revealing potential strategies for drugs designed to prevent aneurysm growth.

PATHOPHYSIOLOGY

Mechanical Considerations

Blood Pressure

Several mechanical factors are pertinent to aortic aneurysms. Blood pressure exerts an effect on the incidence, the rate of dilatation, and the risk of rupture. Hypertension, both systolic and diastolic, is a weak risk factor for aneurysm formation. The incidence of AAA in patients with uncomplicated hypertension has been reported to be as low as 3%, rising to 18% in patients with coexisting advanced vascular disease.[6,7]

Modulation of blood pressure may influence dilatation. A randomized controlled trial of β-adrenergic blockade in Marfan's syndrome conducted with 70 patients during 10 years demonstrated that propranolol protects against development of aneurysms of the aortic root, a characteristic complication of the condition.[8] The rate of aortic dilatation was around one quarter that in the untreated control patients. This was associated with a reduction in systolic and diastolic blood pressure, and the rate of rise of pressure during systole was also diminished. In one nonrandomized study of 121 infrarenal AAAs, those patients with large aneurysms ($\geq$5 cm) receiving beta blockers had a significantly reduced mean expansion rate compared with those without β-adrenergic blockade.[9]

Whereas hypertension is only a weak factor for aneurysm incidence, mean blood pressure is significantly and independently associated with increased risk of aneurysm rupture.[3] It is therefore likely that control of blood pressure is important in reducing rupture rates of aortic aneurysms. It is intuitive that elevated blood pressure increases the strain on the aorta, but studies in experimentally induced aneurysms in rats suggest that hypertension also exacerbates inflammation in the aneurysm wall, indicating that hemodynamic load may affect aneurysm development in more than one way.

Aortic Shape

As the shape and diameter of the aorta change with aneurysm formation, the stresses within the vessel wall alter. A consequence of Laplace's law is that for a given intraluminal pressure, the tension in the wall is proportional to the diameter. Thus, as an aneurysm dilates, the tension in the wall increases, leading to further expansion and ultimately rupture. The wall thickening seen as the aneurysm dilates may be a compensatory mechanism to withstand increasing strain because Laplace's law predicts that the tension in the vessel wall is inversely proportional to the wall thickness. The change in shape toward that of a sphere may also confer some protection against rupture because the tension in the wall of a sphere is half that of a cylinder of the same radius, pressure, and wall thickness.[4]

Hemodynamic factors have been postulated to account for the localization of the majority of aortic aneurysms to the infrarenal aorta. The pulse pressure increases as the pressure wave progresses distally from the aortic root, although the mean arterial pressure does not increase. The aortic bifurcation has been reported to be a source of pressure wave reflections, but direct measurements of intraluminal pressure have failed to detect regions of unexpectedly high pressure.[10]

Despite wide-ranging investigations into the physical aspects of aneurysm development, few useful facts have found their way into practical management of aneurysm patients. These are that hypertension should be controlled and that aneurysm diameter is the best indicator of risk of rupture. Other risk factors affecting aneurysm formation, growth, and rupture are discussed later.

Inflammation

Inflammatory and Atherosclerotic Aneurysms: Two Ends of the Same Spectrum?

Surgeons commonly speak of aortic aneurysms as being of one of two types: atherosclerotic or inflammatory. Inflammatory aneurysms are easily recognized by their thick white wall, densely adherent to surrounding structures. Dissection is more difficult, increasing the risk of inadvertent damage to surrounding structures, such as the ureters and duodenum. Fortunately, such aneurysms are less common than the "ordinary" atherosclerotic variety. However, there is now a substantial body of evidence to suggest that inflammation plays a key part in the formation of so-called atherosclerotic aneurysms, even that inflammatory aneurysms may simply represent one end of a broad spectrum (see also Chapter 1).

Characteristics of the Inflammatory Infiltrate in Abdominal Aortic Aneurysm

The clear distinction observed macroscopically between inflammatory and ordinary aneurysms is not apparent under the microscope. The typical histologic appearance of an AAA is shown in Figure 13.2. When analyzed histologically, more than 80% of aneurysms exhibit a variable degree of inflammation.[11] Heavily inflamed aneurysms are more likely to be symptomatic,[12] and there is a positive correlation between degree of inflammation and aneurysm diameter.[13]

Whereas inflammatory changes can be detected in aortas affected by stenosing arterial disease, the nature of the infiltrate seen in aortic aneurysms is different. The appearances are those of a chronic inflammatory response with a high proportion of lymphocytes and macrophages but few neutrophils. In contrast to occlusive atherosclerotic disease, which is mainly a disorder of the tunica intima, the infiltrate is concentrated in the outer layers of the vessel wall, in the adventitia and media. The infiltrate frequently surrounds vasa vasorum.

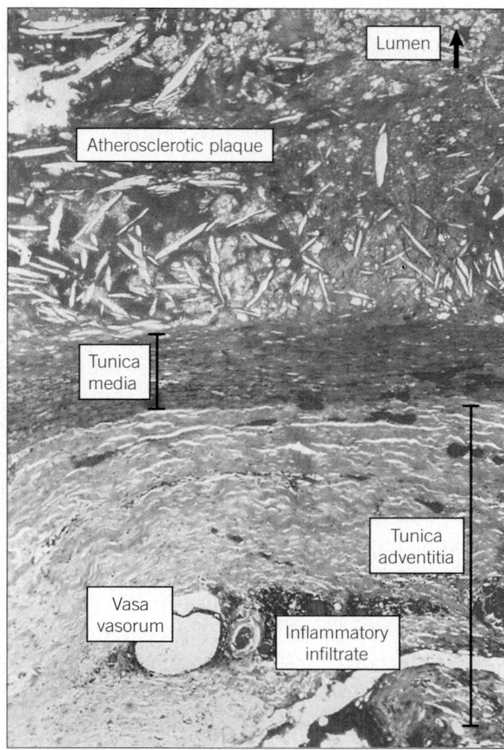

Figure 13.2 Histologic section through the wall of a typical abdominal aortic aneurysm. There is an atherosclerotic plaque on the luminal surface. The tunica media, which in normal aorta comprises a thick layer of smooth muscle and elastin, is thin and exhibits marked loss of smooth muscle cells. The tunica adventitia is thick, disorganized, and inflamed. The inflammatory infiltrate is particularly prominent around the vasa vasorum.

Immunoglobulins and Complement

Elevated immunoglobulin content (IgG) is a feature of tissues affected by an autoimmune process, including disorders such as rheumatoid arthritis and glomerulonephritis. IgG secretion and complement activation are associated with tissue destruction. Increased concentrations of all four subclasses of IgG together with complement degradation products are present, suggesting that the complement cascade is activated in aneurysm wall.[14]

Inflammatory Mediators, Cytokines, and Prostaglandin E_2

Numerous studies have confirmed high cytokine levels in aneurysm wall. Compared with normal or occlusive aorta, elevated amounts have been detected of tumor necrosis factor α, interleukin (IL)–1β, IL-6, IL-8, monocyte chemoattractant protein 1, and interferon γ.[15] These cytokines have the ability to promote production of proteolytic enzymes by macrophages and to induce apoptosis in vascular smooth muscle,[16] processes strongly implicated in aneurysm development.

Aneurysm biopsy specimens in explant culture produce large quantities of prostaglandin E_2 (PGE_2) compared with normal aorta, which produces very little.[17] PGE_2 is synthesized by the enzyme cyclooxygenase (COX), of which there are two isoenzymes, COX-1 and COX-2. COX-2 has been identified and localized to macrophages in the inflammatory infiltrate in AAA wall by immunohistochemistry and in situ hybridization.[17] Because the action of matrix metalloproteinases has been shown to be PGE_2 dependent, these findings raise the possibility that PGE_2 is an important mediator of aneurysm formation and that its synthesis results from COX-2 expression in adventitial macrophages. Moreover, PGE_2 appears to depress replication of aortic smooth muscle cells,[18] which could account for the loss of smooth muscle seen in the tunica media of AAAs.

All explant models of aortic aneurysm have limitations. Human explant specimens represent only late-stage disease, and animal models may differ greatly from the human condition.

The inflammatory processes seen in AAA are not confined to the aortic wall. Aortic aneurysms are associated with increased levels of several circulating cytokines.[19] There is some evidence that the concentration of interferon γ is linked to aneurysm growth rate.[20] Aneurysms also seem to be an important source of circulating IL-6, and the IL-6 genotype is prognostic of cardiovascular mortality,[21] an important finding indicating that aneurysms may affect pathologic processes distant from the aorta.

Is Infection of the Vessel Wall the Cause of the Inflammation?

It has been recognized for centuries that syphilis causes aneurysms of the aortic arch. Tuberculosis is known to cause inflammatory aneurysms of the abdominal aorta.[22] The notion that stenosing atherosclerotic disease might be caused by infection was first proposed by Sir William Osler in 1908.[23] This concept received little attention until 1988, when a Finnish study demonstrated that acute myocardial infarction was associated with raised antibodies to part of the newly identified organism *Chlamydia pneumoniae*. In the subsequent decade, more than 1000 papers have been published exploring the possible role of this organism in the pathogenesis of vascular disease. *C. pneumoniae* has now been identified in every large artery in the body, including coronary, carotid, iliac, and lower limb arteries. *C. pneumoniae* has been identified in the walls of aortic aneurysms; the incidence varies according to the technique used[24] and ranges between 0% and 100%; most studies find evidence of the presence of *C. pneumoniae* in around 35% to 45% of cases.

The detection of chlamydial DNA by polymerase chain reaction does not demonstrate the presence of active infection. Indeed, viable *C. pneumoniae* has been cultured only once from vascular tissue, from the coronary artery of one patient. It seems likely that infection of the vessel wall may leave remnants of chlamydial DNA and membrane components long after active infection has terminated.

C. pneumoniae infection of endothelial cells induces procoagulant activity[25] and stimulates expression of adhesion molecules essential for leukocyte migration, including intercellular adhesion molecule 1 and vascular cell adhesion molecule 1.[26] Moreover, chlamydial infections are frequently chronic, and in the case of the closely related organism *Chlamydia trachomatis,* the tissue damage may be delayed by several years. In an experimental aneurysm model in rabbits, *C. pneumoniae* appears to contribute to aortic dilatation by specific activation of macrophages.[27]

Despite extensive literature that *C. pneumoniae* is associated with atherosclerosis and plausible circumstantial evidence that it could contribute to the inflammation seen in aneurysm formation, there is no proof that the presence of this organism is anything other than coincidental. Interestingly, one group could not find evidence of *C. pneumoniae* in the majority of analyzed AAA walls; however, all samples showed a strong cross-reaction between chlamydial antibodies and human immunoglobulin.[28] This raises the hypothesis that AAA is an autoimmune disease, perhaps triggered by an initial *C. pneumoniae* infection.

Although bacteria have received the most attention in searching for triggers for vascular disease, viruses, especially herpes viruses, have also been implicated. One study reported finding cytomegalovirus DNA in 86% of inflammatory aneurysms, 65% of so-called atherosclerotic aneurysms, and 31% of normal aortas.[29] The herpes simplex virus has also been detected in inflammatory and atherosclerotic aneurysms: 29% of inflammatory aneurysms and 27% of atherosclerotic aneurysms compared with 6% of normal aortas.[29] As with *C. pneumoniae,* the presence of the infectious agent does not constitute proof of a role in the pathogenesis of aneurysms but merely demonstrates an association between the two.

Summary: Inflammation in Abdominal Aortic Aneurysms

Studies in humans showing an abundance of inflammatory cells in aneurysm wall, high circulating inflammatory markers, and high localized production of cytokines together with IgG secretion and complement activation suggest that inflammation is intricately involved with aneurysm development. Further corroborative evidence is provided by the experimental aneurysms in animals. The initial stimuli that provoke the reaction are not identified, although infectious agents have been implicated; nor is it clear whether the inflammation is a consequence or a cause of aortic dilatation. Nonetheless, this growing body of evidence points to the concept that the excessive proteolysis seen in aneurysm wall is driven by chronic inflammation.

Proteolysis

Structure of Aortic Wall: Elastin and Collagen

The transformation of normal aorta into aneurysm involves profound changes in the cellular composition and extracellular matrix of the vessel wall. Lack of elastin is a striking histologic feature of aortic aneurysm wall, and the normal lamellar pattern of concentric rings of smooth muscle and elastin is absent. Loss of elastin appears to be a critical component of aneurysm formation, occurring early in the process. The proportion of elastin in normal aorta progressively decreases from the root to the bifurcation, making the infrarenal segment the most inelastic part and the most vulnerable to further depletion of elastin.[30]

Elastin is normally a stable component of the extracellular matrix, showing very little turnover in adult aorta or other tissues. Elastin depletion is due to destruction rather than to diminished production. As elastin is destroyed, the hemodynamic load is taken up by the remaining collagen, and whether the aorta goes on to dilate and to rupture depends on the collagen metabolism in the individual concerned. Collagen turnover is greatly increased in aneurysm wall, with large amounts synthesized in the adventitia, leading to the characteristic thick outer layer. The new collagen is not laid down in a lamellar pattern, and although thicker, the wall is less strong than normal aorta.

Matrix Metalloproteinases

Matrix metalloproteinases (MMPs) are a family of enzymes responsible for degradation of extracellular matrix components, including elastin and collagen.

Studies in experimental aneurysms support the hypothesis that proteolytic activity is important in aneurysm expansion. Perfusion of rat aortas with elastase rapidly generates aneurysmal dilatation. In the same model, treatment with doxycycline, an MMP inhibitor, reduces aneurysm development, and this is associated with depression of MMP-9 activity.[31]

Several different laboratories using different methodologies have provided convincing evidence that the principal cell type secreting MMPs in AAA wall is the macrophage.[32] MMP-2 and MMP-9 in particular have been localized to macrophages at the adventitial-medial junction.[33]

Numerous studies have demonstrated abnormal proteolytic activity in human aortic aneurysm wall compared with normal or atherosclerotic aorta.[34] Aneurysm tissue contains high concentrations of a range of matrix-degrading enzymes, including serine proteases and MMPs. MMPs appear to play the dominant role in disrupting the aortic wall.[35] MMPs 2, 3, and 9 have been identified in high amounts. Studies have shown MMP-2 to be the dominant enzyme in small aneurysms (4 to 5.5 cm); MMP-9 predominates for aneurysms in the 5- to 7-cm range.[13,36] MMP-9 concentration actually declines in large (>7 cm) aneurysms, implying that as aneurysms enlarge, hemodynamic rather than biochemical factors may dominate the rate of expansion. Distribution of MMP within aneurysm wall is not homogeneous, and it has been suggested that localized pockets of very high MMP-9 activity could predispose toward aneurysm rupture.

Summary: Proteolysis in Aortic Aneurysm Wall

On histologic examination, elastolysis is one of the earliest observable events in aneurysm genesis. Aneurysm tissue, compared with normal and athero-occlusive aorta, contains high levels of proteases, particularly MMPs, the main source of which is infiltrating macrophages. These enzymes degrade the extracellular components of the aortic wall, in particular elastin and collagen. Inhibition of MMP activity in experimental aneurysms attenuates aneurysm growth. These observations support the concept of excessive proteolytic activity in aortic wall that causes destruction of the extracellular matrix, leading to weakening, dilatation, and eventually rupture of the aorta.

Smooth Muscle Cell Loss

In addition to the changes in the extracellular matrix, aortic aneurysms exhibit marked changes in cellular structure of the vessel wall. The infiltration of the aortic wall with inflammatory cells has been discussed. In the normal aorta, the predominant cell type is the vascular smooth muscle cell (SMC), arranged in concentric elastic lamellae in the tunica media. The SMCs both contribute to the tone of the vessel wall and synthesize the bulk of the matrix proteins and are therefore important in maintaining structural integrity. In addition, SMCs influence extracellular matrix turnover by expression of MMPs and tissue inhibitors of metalloproteinases. In the aneurysm wall, therefore, there is an apparent conflict between synthesis of connective tissue proteins by aortic SMCs and matrix degradation by infiltrating inflammatory cells. This suggests that SMC function might be a pivotal factor in the formation of aortic aneurysms. Any diminution in SMC numbers would deplete a population of cells capable of synthesizing components of the vessel wall and could contribute to weakening and dilatation of the aorta.

There is a notable reduction in the number of SMCs in the media of aortic aneurysms relative to normal and atherosclerotic aortas as measured by immunohistochemistry for α–SMC actin and a reduction in SMC density of 74%.[37] The decrease in the SMC population of aneurysm wall coincides with chemical and ultrastructural evidence of SMC apoptosis.[38] Intact SMCs remaining within the aneurysm wall display loss of cell volume, cytoplasmic contracture, dissolution of cytoskeletal actin fragments, and distortion of intracellular organelles. The nuclei show clumping and fragmentation of chromatin, changes consistent with apoptosis.

These morphologic and histochemical findings are supported by molecular studies. The protein p53 has been implicated in the induction of physiologic cell death in a range of tissues including vascular SMCs[39] and is used as a marker for apoptosis. By use of a combination of immunohistochemistry and reverse transcriptase–polymerase chain reaction, p53 and p53 mRNA were localized to the cytoplasm and nuclei of SMCs and detected in greater quantities in aneurysm tissue (by nearly fourfold) compared with normal and atherosclerotic occlusive aorta.

These findings taken together suggest that the SMC population in aortic aneurysms is depleted by apoptosis and that this process may occur, at least in part, through mechanisms involving increased expression of p53. The stimuli leading to induction of physiologic cell death remain to be defined, although a number of different mechanisms have been proposed.

Atherosclerotic lesions produce high concentrations of oxidants such as nitric oxide, oxygen free radicals, and oxidized low-density lipoproteins. These substances have been reported to induce apoptosis of vascular SMCs in vitro.[40] The proximity of SMCs in aneurysm wall to intimal plaque may allow diffusion of these oxidants into the media, resulting in cytotoxic effects on SMCs. This concept alone could not account for SMC depletion in aneurysms or one would expect to see aneurysmal dilatation wherever there is atheroma; clearly, this is not the case.

The paucity of vasa vasorum in the infrarenal aorta has been implicated in the development of aortic aneurysms.[41] Healthy infrarenal aorta has far fewer vasa vasorum than the proximal aorta or other mammalian aorta of similar size, and the cells of the media are more dependent on diffusion from the lumen for delivery of oxygen and nutrients. Development of atherosclerosis and intimal thickening may exacerbate the situation, resulting in a chronic insufficiency of oxygen and nutrients in the aortic media. Both hypoxia and serum deprivation induce apoptosis of vascular SMCs in vitro, so it is reasonable to speculate that the same effects might occur in aneurysm wall.

The chronic inflammation seen in the media and adventitia of aneurysms may have deleterious effects on SMCs. Many of the cytokines produced by inflammatory cells, for example, IL-1β, tumor necrosis factor α, and interferon γ, are known to induce apoptosis in vascular SMCs in vitro,[42] and these mediators are present in high concentrations in aneurysmal wall. PGE_2 in particular, originating in adventitial macrophages, is present in very high levels[43] and has a concentration-dependent deleterious effect on aortic SMC proliferation.[5] PGE_2 may also increase SMC apoptosis.[5]

There are therefore several mechanisms that could account for the diminution of SMCs seen in AAA.

The Role of Risk Factors in Aneurysm Development and Rupture

Gender: Abdominal Aortic Aneurysms Are Less Common but More Dangerous in Women

Since the publication of the U.K. Small Aneurysm Trial results, it has become necessary to make a distinction between the risk factors predisposing to aneurysm development and those leading to rupture. The trial yielded a cohort of 2257 patients, of whom 103 suffered AAA rupture during the 7-year period of follow-up. This permitted analysis of the factors that influence aneurysm rupture.[3] The study confirmed that even quite small aneurysms may rupture, but such events are rare. Five factors, each of which was associated with an increased risk of rupture, were identified: female gender, mean arterial blood pressure, active smoking, reduced FEV_1 (forced expiratory volume in 1 second), and aneurysm diameter.

Screening studies have shown that the prevalence of AAA is much lower in women than in men.[44] Consequently, advocates of screening usually suggest that such programs be aimed at the male population. The striking finding from the U.K. Small Aneurysm Trial was that female sex conferred a threefold greater risk of rupture, even after adjustment for age, initial aneurysm diameter, body mass index, and height. Moreover, the mean AAA diameter preceding rupture was smaller in women (5.0 ± 0.8 cm) than in men (6.0 ± 1.4 cm). This study therefore demonstrated that although aneurysms are less common in women, those female patients who do develop aneurysms are at substantially higher risk of rupture than their male counterparts are. This suggests that the diameter at which repair of an AAA is indicated is smaller in women than in men.

Smoking

Cigarette smoking is strongly associated with the development of aortic aneurysms[6] and appears to be the strongest risk factor after age. In the North American Aneurysm Detection and Management (ADAM) study,[45] smoking was the strongest risk factor for aortic aneurysms, with an odds ratio of 5.57. Aneurysm risk increased with the number of years of smoking and decreased with number of years since stopping smoking. Cigarette smoking has been found to be much more common in young patients (<50 years) presenting with aortic aneurysms and is associated with more proximal (i.e., juxtarenal and suprarenal) aneurysms in older patients.[46] Smoking appeared to have a direct effect on aneurysm risk that is independent of atherosclerosis. Number of cigarettes smoked and depth of inhalation are both associated with increased risk of aortic aneurysm, but not tar content or nicotine yield.

Smoking is associated with increased growth rates of small aneurysms.[47] MacSweeney and colleagues[48] observed 43 patients with small aortic aneurysms for 3 years. Aneurysm diameter increased significantly faster in smokers (0.16 cm per year) compared with nonsmokers (0.09 cm per year), and this was strongly associated with elevated serum cotinine (a nicotine metabolite). Smoking is associated not only with increased aneurysm growth rates but also with greater risk of rupture.[3]

The mechanisms through which smoking influences aneurysm development and expansion are not established. Two mechanisms that have been suggested include direct elastin disruption by the nitrite ion[49] and potentiation of neutrophil elastase activity.[50]

Smoking therefore is a risk factor for development and expansion of aortic aneurysms and appears to have effects independent of promoting atherosclerosis, perhaps by potentiating elastin degeneration. Although smoking is associated with increased aneurysm growth rates, it has not yet been demonstrated that stopping smoking slows aneurysm expansion. Most patients find it difficult to stop smoking, and it is problematic to randomize patients to a "stopping smoking" arm of a trial.

Hypertension

The role of blood pressure in aneurysm development was discussed earlier (see the section on pathophysiology, mechanical considerations). Hypertension has been shown to be associated with aneurysm rupture,[3] an important finding because hypertension is treatable and control of blood pressure may reduce the likelihood of rupture.

Aneurysm Diameter

The changes in mechanical stresses that occur in aneurysm wall in the course of dilatation were discussed earlier (see the section on pathophysiology, mechanical considerations). The alterations in tension within an aneurysm wall are predictable according to Laplace's law and go some way toward explaining the observation in practice that risk of rupture increases as an aneurysm enlarges. Measurement of aneurysm diameter is the best-known indicator of rupture risk but unfortunately has serious limitations. Small aneurysms can and do rupture (especially in women), although the risk is low. The risk escalates sharply for aneurysms of more than 6 cm in diameter.[3]

Atherosclerosis

The concept that atherosclerosis causes aortic aneurysms is well ingrained in surgical thinking and goes unchallenged in many textbooks. This view is based on the almost universal finding of atheromatous plaque on the luminal surface of aortic aneurysms and the fact that certain of the risk factors for atherosclerosis and aneurysmal disease are shared.[51] The conventional wisdom is that atherosclerosis somehow weakens the aortic wall, leading to dilatation and eventually rupture. Zarins and colleagues[51a] reported induction of aortic aneurysms in a small number of monkeys fed a high-fat diet to generate atheroma, then transferred to a low-fat regimen to cause the plaque to regress. They suggested that atheroma weakens the vessel wall but the rigidity of the plaque prevents dilatation; on regression of the atheroma, aneurysms resulted. In humans, however, there has been no sign of aneurysms occurring in individuals undergoing dietary manipulations or taking lipid-lowering agents, nor does this reasoning explain the characteristic distribution of aneurysms and their absence in many areas of the vascular system where atheroma is common.

A substantial body of evidence has accumulated that aortic aneurysms are genetically and biochemically different from aortas with athero-occlusive disease. Patients with stenosing peripheral vascular disease have serum lipid and lipoprotein profiles different from those of patients with dilating vascular disease.[52] The pattern of inheritance of aneurysmal disease is distinct from atherosclerosis, and patients with aneurysms are more likely to be male and less likely to be diabetic than are individuals affected by athero-occlusive disease.[45] On histologic examination, atherosclerosis affects primarily the tunica intima, whereas aneurysm development characteristically shows marked changes in the media and adventitia.

As understanding of aneurysm pathogenesis has advanced, it has become clear that although atherosclerosis and aortic aneurysm share certain risk factors and frequently coexist, there are important differences, and the latter is not simply a complication of the former. Otherwise, one would expect to find aortic dilatation wherever atherosclerosis is present. Clearly, this is not so; therefore, whereas atherosclerosis is frequently almost a prerequisite, additional explanation is sought for the dilatation process.

Genetic Factors

The first report of a familial clustering of aortic aneurysms in an otherwise healthy family was in 1977 and described three siblings with ruptured aneurysms.[53] Many reports since published have suggested a strong genetic basis for aortic aneurysm, but there is disagreement on the patterns of inheritance. There is a clear distinction in genetics between the aneurysms seen in association with a defined connective tissue disorder and the more common "standard" aneurysm. A mutation in the fibrillin gene gives rise to aneurysms of the ascending aorta in Marfan's syndrome,[54] and several defects in the type III collagen gene result in arterial dilatation as part of the Ehlers-Danlos syndrome.[55] As expected in single-gene disorders, these conditions display clear-cut mendelian patterns of inheritance; however, neither condition gives rise to AAA.

Genetic abnormalities in the elastin gene have never been detected in patients with aneurysms. There are rare examples of AAAs occurring in conjunction with mutations in genes coding for collagen.[56] It seems that although specific genetic defects in connective tissue proteins may lead to aortic aneurysm formation, the great majority of aneurysms are not caused by such abnormalities.

Aside from abnormalities in genes coding for connective tissue proteins, there are other mechanisms by which genetic defects might precipitate aneurysms. MMP regulation is complex and involves several different enzymes and cytokines. Aberrant expression of a crucial control mediator could give rise to unbalanced proteolysis and matrix destruction. α_1-Antitrypsin has been suggested as such a candidate.[57] Faulty expression of genes coding for tissue inhibitors of metalloproteinases has also been considered a possible mechanism for a genetic predisposition for aortic aneurysm, but DNA sequencing studies have not identified any increased incidence of mutations or polymorphisms in these genes in aneurysm patients.

These diverse results support the concept of a strong genetic element in the pathogenesis of aortic aneurysms, but the mode of inheritance and the precise mechanisms involved are obscure.

Diabetes Mellitus

Aneurysms seem to occur less frequently in diabetics. The reasons for this are unknown, but one possibility is that glycosylation of collagen confers some resistance to degradation by collagenases. Diabetes is found in approximately 1% of patients with aneurysmal disease, 10% of patients with intermittent claudication, and 20% of patients with critical limb ischemia. It would seem that the diabetic process is associated with a more distal small-vessel disease.

CLINICAL PRESENTATIONS

Asymptomatic Aneurysms and Screening

AAA is frequently detected as an incidental finding during clinical examination or investigation for a different problem. In particular, there is a significant coexistence of AAA with intra-abdominal malignant disease, including colorectal carcinoma, posing a therapeutic dilemma in the order of management. Some patients notice their aneurysm as a pulsatile mass when in bed or in the bath, but most aortic aneurysms are asymptomatic and go undetected unless they rupture.

Two major U.K. studies have demonstrated that screening for aneurysms reduces aneurysm-related mortality. A major randomized trial, the Multicentre Aneurysm Screening Study (MASS), was conducted across four U.K. centers. In a population-based sample, 67,770 men aged between 65 and 74 years were observed for 7 years.[58] Aneurysm-related mortality in the screened group approached half that of the unscreened group. Screening had no significant effect on all-cause mortality. With regard to cost-effectiveness, AAA-related mortality cost $19,500 per life-year gained. On this basis, if a health service provider were willing to pay $40,000 per life-year gained, the probability that AAA screening would be cost-effective is 98%. It is thought that in the MASS trial, the treatment effect has been underestimated by including rupture of aneurysms from unspecified sites, such as thoracoabdominal aneurysms. Similarly, the Gloucestershire Aneurysm Screening Programme reported a 66% reduction in AAA deaths in men aged 65 to 73 years.[59]

Painful or Tender Nonruptured Aortic Aneurysm

Some nonruptured aneurysms may give rise to pain, experienced typically as an ache in the abdomen, back, or flanks. The discomfort may persist for days or even weeks and is sometimes difficult to distinguish from musculoskeletal back pain. There may be associated aneurysm tenderness. The mechanism of the pain is not known, but possibilities include stretching of the periaortic tissue due to rapid aneurysm expansion and pain due to the inflammation in the aorta and periaortic tissue. Most vascular surgeons consider a painful or tender aneurysm to be at high risk of imminent rupture regardless of its size and advise urgent repair in all but the least fit patients. There is, however, no high-quality evidence for this policy, and it is clear from observation of patients who are unfit for surgery that a painful aneurysm considered at risk of imminent rupture may settle and become painless again. This is especially so in patients with painful inflammatory aneurysms who may benefit from a period of treatment with steroids. It is always difficult to proclaim an aneurysm to be "symptomatic," and even "tenderness" is variable according to the examining fingers.

Abdominal Aortic Aneurysm Rupture

This is the third most common cause of sudden death according to British autopsy statistics. Approximately 75% die before reaching the hospital.[3] The presentation of a ruptured aortic aneurysm is variable, depending on the size and site of the rupture. This commonly leads to diagnostic confusion. Misdiagnoses, such as ureteric colic and pancreatitis, are recorded with monotonous regularity, leading to delayed diagnosis with disastrous results.

A large leak, especially one that ruptures into the peritoneal cavity, causes a swift death. Other patients have a contained retroperitoneal bleed causing pain of sudden onset, which is severe and continuous in the central abdomen and radiates to the back. The site of pain may be variable and may be felt only in the back or one or other flank. The signs of acute hemorrhage, tachycardia, hypotension, peripheral vasoconstriction, and depressed conscious level, depend on the size of leak. In many patients, the initial rupture is contained and tamponaded by the periaortic tissue and posterior peritoneum to the extent that no hemodynamic disturbance occurs; indeed, the patient may even be hypertensive during this early stage. A pulsatile, expansile mass in the epigastrium is sought, but this is not always found in larger patients. Moreover, retroperitoneal hematoma surrounding the aorta may mask the aortic pulsation and be evident simply as a large, tender mass. For these reasons, the abdominal signs of aortic aneurysm rupture are not as clear-cut as might be expected.

Embolization

AAAs are usually lined to a variable extent by mural thrombus. Pieces of this may dislodge and embolize, causing ischemia of one or both lower limbs. This may occur suddenly, causing acute ischemia, or insidiously with multiple small emboli for a long time, causing no symptoms until the patient presents with intermittent claudication, ulceration, or rest pain due to occlusion of the distal vessels (trash foot).

Fistula Formation

Aortoenteric fistula is a rare cause of upper gastrointestinal hemorrhage. Most aortoenteric fistulas are into the fourth part of the duodenum and occur after previous aortic surgery. It is very rare but not unknown for an unoperated aorta to fistulate into the gastrointestinal tract—primary aortoenteric fistula.

Fistulization into the vena cava is a very rare cause of high-output cardiac failure. Aortocaval fistula may occur during contained aneurysm rupture; it is manifested as massive venous bleeding when the aneurysm is opened during emergency aneurysm repair. A leak into the vena cava is another "lucky site" for the patient, provided the condition is recognized before or early during surgery.

DIAGNOSTIC TECHNIQUES

Clinical examination is an unreliable method of diagnosing and estimating the position and diameter of AAAs. In obese patients, quite large aneurysms may not be palpable, and even in thinner individuals, estimation of aneurysm size by palpation is highly inaccurate.[60] It is thought that being able to palpate normal-caliber abdominal aorta proximally suggests the AAA is infrarenal.

The simplest diagnostic test for aortic aneurysm is ultrasonography. This has a high sensitivity and specificity for aortic aneurysms and allows measurement of aneurysm diameter (Fig. 13.3). The presence of mural thrombus is readily detected. Duplex ultrasonography allows detailed assessment of the iliac arteries, which are also commonly aneurysmal. Whereas ultrasonography is invaluable to diagnose AAA and to assess diameter, aneurysm rupture is frequently not confirmed by this technique. Another disadvantage is that the proximal limit of the aneurysm and the relationship to the renal arteries are poorly visualized with ultrasound examination.

Computed tomography (CT) scanning offers few advantages over ultrasonography for simple diagnostic purposes but is invaluable in assessing the painful aneurysm to confirm or to exclude the presence of rupture (Fig. 13.4). The great advantage of CT scanning is the excellent visualization of the proximal limit of the aneurysm and the relationship to the renal arteries. The iliac arteries are also well demonstrated by CT; such preoperative knowledge of the anatomy makes surgery easier, especially in an emergency.

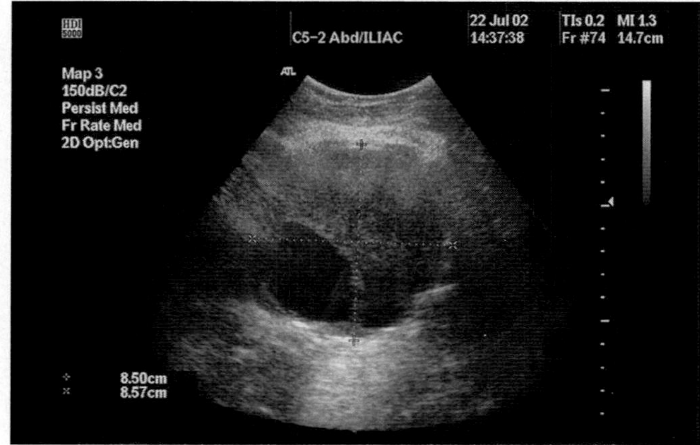

Figure 13.3 Ultrasound appearance of an abdominal aortic aneurysm, seen in cross section. Sonography is highly accurate in diagnosis and measurement of infrarenal aortic aneurysms. (Courtesy of M. Ellis.)

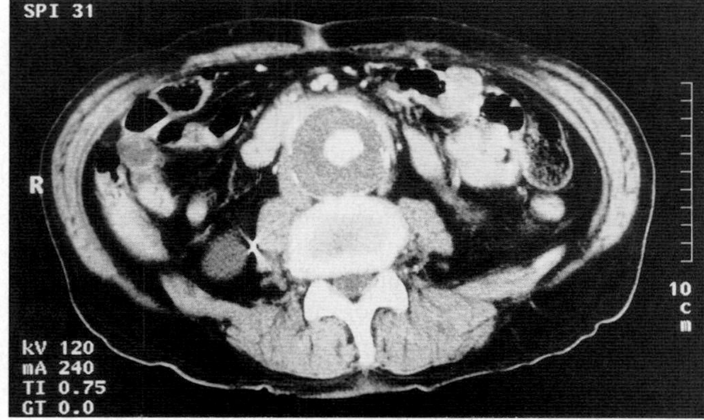

Figure 13.4 CT scan of an abdominal aortic aneurysm. Contrast material in the lumen of the vessel, a thick layer of mural thrombus, and calcification in the aneurysm wall are shown.

Angiography is not a useful investigation to image aortic aneurysms. It can be misleading because mural thrombus in the aneurysm sac mimics the true wall of the vessel, giving an underestimate of aortic diameter. CT workstation analysis has replaced calibrated catheter angiography.

Endovascular treatment has altered the preoperative assessment of aneurysms. Although a CT scan is desirable before conventional open surgery, mainly to determine that the aneurysm is not juxtarenal or suprarenal, many surgeons without access to CT facilities perform perfectly adequate surgery with only a preoperative abdominal ultrasound examination, tailoring the operative procedure according to the findings at surgery. In contrast, accurate measurements of aortoiliac anatomy are crucial for the planning of successful endoluminal repair; such accuracy, particularly relating to the superior aortic neck, is not attainable by duplex ultrasonography or plain axial CT scanning. Contrast-enhanced spiral CT scanning allows computer-generated reconstructions in different planes, permitting excellent visualization of complex and tortuous aneurysm.

Preoperative planning has become more complicated since the advent of fenestrated and branched endovascular grafts (discussed later), which necessitate a high level of accuracy in establishing the dimensions for the manufacturing of these grafts.[61]

MANAGEMENT

The management of the asymptomatic patient with an aortic aneurysm poses a number of problems. Elective repair even in the best hands carries significant risk, but aneurysm rupture is usually catastrophic. Aneurysm patients are usually elderly with significant comorbidity. The difficulty lies in balancing the potential increased life expectancy of a successful operation against the early operative risk.

Central to this dilemma is the uncertainty of predicting the risk of rupture of a particular aneurysm. The risk of rupture increases with aneurysm diameter, and those larger than 6 cm have a high risk. However, some small aneurysms do leak with disastrous results, and others grow to alarming dimensions without causing problems. If it were possible precisely to distinguish those aneurysms threatening imminent rupture from those that could be safely observed, surgery could be targeted to those patients at highest risk. This would reduce unnecessary operations without increasing the incidence of rupture.

A rate of expansion of more than 1.0 cm during a 12-month period is thought to be of greater risk regardless of initial size, although there are no published data to support this belief. Clearly, such estimates of expansion rate require a number of measurements during the period, with all the attendant difficulties of reproducibility and interobserver variation. Aneurysm wall is stiffer and less compliant than normal aorta, which is attributable in part to decreased elastin content.[62] Aortic compliance can be assessed noninvasively, but such measurements do not appear to relate to risk of rupture.[63]

In principle, it would be useful to risk stratify aneurysms by use of circulating markers that are associated with elevated expansion rate.[19,20] High circulating levels of the cytokine interferon γ seem to be associated with increased AAA expansion, and such estimations might potentially be used to identify the more dangerous aneurysms. Whereas no single parameter reliably predicts risk of rupture, it is possible that combining the results of different measurements (e.g., diameter, compliance, and circulating markers) might allow the development of a scoring system to assist in estimating rupture risk. Unfortunately, at present, aneurysm diameter remains the best available indicator of risk of rupture for asymptomatic AAAs, with the use of serum markers yet to materialize in the clinical arena.

Aneurysms of Less than 5.5 cm in Diameter

Until 1998, there was great uncertainty as to how to treat aneurysms in the range of 4 to 5.5 cm in diameter. Few surgeons advised surgery for aneurysms smaller than 4.0 cm, whereas most recommended repair for aneurysms larger than 5.5 cm in all but very elderly or unfit individuals. The range between these sizes constituted a gray area, with widely divergent practices between different surgeons. The U.K. Small Aneurysm Trial was a prospective, randomized, controlled trial designed to address this question.[64] A total of 1090 patients were randomized to either ultrasound surveillance or operation within 3 months. Mean duration of follow-up was 8 years. Surgery was performed for patients randomized to the observation arm of the trial if the aneurysm diameter reached 5.5 cm, if the aneurysm became painful or tender, or if the aneurysm grew more than 1.0 cm per year.

The trial was set up to show that early surgery within 3 months in a younger patient with small aneurysm would clearly do better than waiting. A 2% rupture rate per year for the observation arm and 2% 30-day mortality for the early surgery arm was predicted. In the event, early surgery patients had a 5.8% 30-day mortality, and rupture rate during follow-up was only 1% per year. In addition, a majority of the surveillance patients came to surgery. Early surgery was more costly and no better in terms of all-cause mortality. These findings are in close agreement with the ADAM trial in North America, which also showed no survival benefit for patients with small aneurysms offered early prophylactic surgery.[65]

Aneurysms of More than 5.5 cm in Diameter

Preoperative Assessment

Elective aortic aneurysm repair is a prophylactic operation for an asymptomatic condition, so it is essential to identify coexistent conditions that might threaten life expectancy or a successful operative outcome. Patients of any age with advanced cancer or degenerative neurologic disease are clearly not candidates for surgery. Operative mortality is approximately double for patients older than 80 years compared with those younger than 80 years.[66] This applies to operations for both ruptured and nonruptured aneurysms. Successful aneurysm repair can be achieved in patients older than 80 years; when to attempt it is a matter for individual judgment.

The main concerns for the majority of patients are impaired respiratory, cardiac, and renal function. As with stenosing atherosclerotic disease, most individuals with aneurysms are or have been smokers. Standard spirometric respiratory function tests are normally adequate to assess the extent of respiratory impairment. Chronic obstructive airways disease and impaired respiratory function are important risk factors for increased postoperative complications.[67]

There is great debate concerning the most accurate method of assessing cardiac risk in aneurysm surgery, in particular how best to quantify the risk attributable to asymptomatic coronary artery disease. Routine 12-lead electrocardiography is essential, but many abnormalities will become apparent only on stress testing or during 24-hour monitoring. Echocardiography is performed in many centers to determine ejection fraction. Isotope scanning may reveal asymptomatic areas of poor myocardial perfusion. Coronary angiography may be indicated in patients found to have significantly impaired myocardial perfusion to determine whether correction of coronary artery stenosis is required before aneurysm repair. Determination of the priority of treatment in such patients is difficult and requires close cooperation between the cardiologist and the vascular and cardiac surgeons.

Cardiopulmonary exercise testing noninvasively measures how efficiently subjects meet increased metabolic demand, and combined with simple comorbidity scoring, it has been shown to identify elective AAA open repair patients unlikely to survive in the mid term and those likely to suffer complications.[68] Cardiopulmonary exercise is particularly useful in the preoperative risk stratification and in predicting postoperative outcomes of older patients undergoing major abdominal surgery.

Impaired renal function confers higher operative risk. This is particularly so for patients undergoing endovascular repair, in which administration of a significant volume of contrast medium is required. Interestingly, the excess mortality in these patients is due to septic complications rather than to renal failure.

A number of scoring systems, with the aim of predicting outcome for patients after aneurysm surgery, have been devised, implemented, and scrutinized. These include the POSSUM, VBHOM, and APACHE models; a statistical comparison of these concluded that the last is the most accurate in risk stratification owing to its facility to account for hospital-related "effect" and the patient case mix.[69]

Open Repair (Fig. 13.5)

Dubost performed the first successful repair of an AAA in 1951 using a cadaveric human aorta.[70] Knitted Dacron is now the standard graft material and was introduced by Michael DeBakey. A midline abdominal incision is used for most repairs, although some surgeons prefer a transverse incision. The retroperitoneal approach is indicated when access to the aorta through the abdomen is impeded, for example, by a horseshoe kidney, adhesions from previous surgery, or a colostomy. A minimal dissection technique is used to expose the aorta above the aneurysm and the iliac arteries below. After administration of heparin, the iliac arteries and aorta are clamped, the aneurysm is opened, and mural thrombus is removed. Backbleeding from lumbar arteries and the inferior mesenteric arteries is controlled by oversewing. The Dacron graft is sutured to the neck of the aneurysm by an inlay technique; the distal anastomosis is formed in the same way. The aneurysm wall is then closed over the graft to reduce the risk of aortoenteric fistula. Tube grafts are suitable for most patients. When the iliac arteries are aneurysmal, a bifurcation "trouser" graft is used.

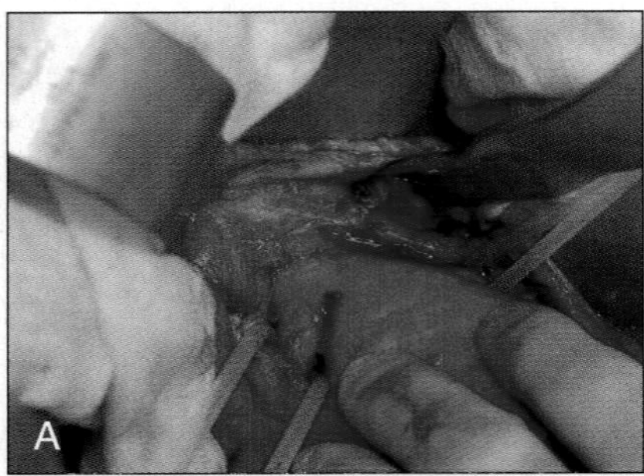

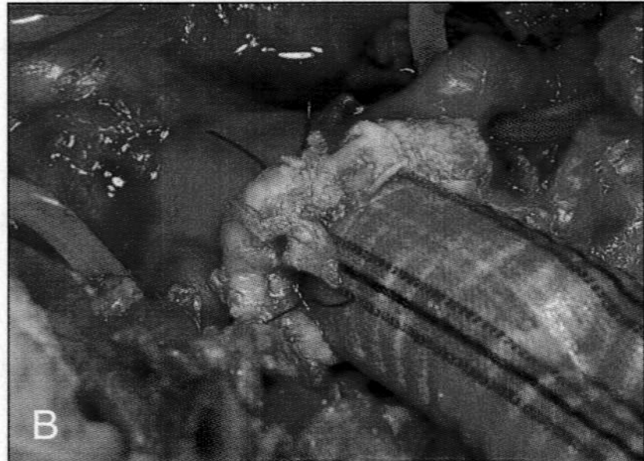

Figure 13.5 Operative repair of a juxtarenal abdominal aortic aneurysm. In **A,** the proximity of the top end of the aneurysm to the renal arteries (controlled with Silastic slings) is evident. In **B,** the aneurysm has been replaced by a bifurcated Dacron graft. (Courtesy of Mr. S. Ray.)

A number of studies and analyses have been completed that demonstrate improved outcomes for patients when elective and urgent open repairs of AAAs are performed in centers where a high volume of such procedures are undertaken annually.[71] A recent systematic review and meta-analysis identified thresholds of 43 and 15 aneurysm repairs per annum for elective and ruptured AAAs, respectively. It was above these numbers that high-volume institutions reported improved outcomes.[72] In another contemporary systematic review and meta-analysis of six randomized controlled trials, significant relationships between higher surgeon caseload and lower mortality were demonstrated in 12 of 14 studies. A critical volume threshold was identified as 13 cases per annum for individual surgeons.[73] Such evidence supports the principle that management of AAA should be centralized to specialist vascular centers.

Endovascular Repair

The technique of endovascular aortic aneurysm repair (EVAR) was introduced by Parodi and colleagues[74] in 1991. This method permits the stent-graft to be introduced and secured inside the aneurysm through the femoral arteries under fluoroscopic control (Figs. 13.6 to 13.8). The advantages are obvious; EVAR is carried out usually under local or regional anesthesia, through two small groin incisions, with less blood loss, reduced duration of hospital stay, and more rapid convalescence.

There are two main disadvantages. The first relates to anatomic suitability of patients for endovascular repair. Successful deployment of a stent-graft relies on achieving a good seal between graft and aortic wall at each end. This requires

ENDOVASCULAR REPAIR OF AAA

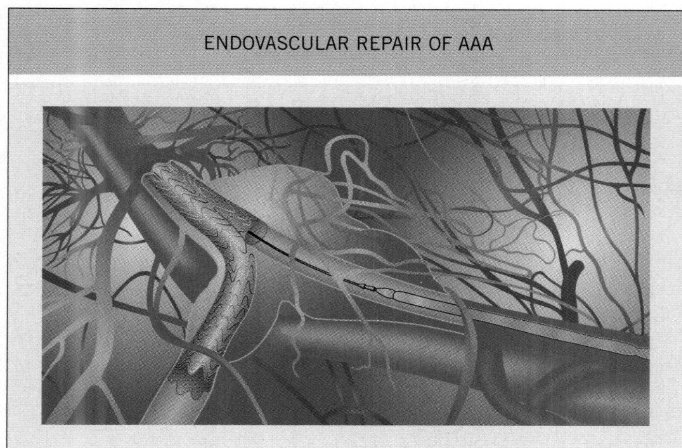

Figure 13.6 Stylized depiction of endovascular deployment of a two-part bifurcation stent-graft. (With permission from W. L. Gore and Associates.)

a length of ideally more than 1 cm of normal-caliber aorta between the renal arteries and the top of the aneurysm without excessive mural thrombus or irregular atherosclerotic plaque. In addition, the iliac arteries must be of adequate diameter to allow passage of the delivery system. Although graft technology is improving rapidly, especially the development of uncovered suprarenal stents, the anatomy of a number of patients is such that there is inadequate length of normal vessel above and below the aneurysm to permit secure fixation of the graft.

The second main concern regarding EVAR relates to the durability of the technique. Despite widespread initial enthusiasm, longer term follow-up data indicate a significant incidence of problems after endovascular repair. After endovascular treatment, the morphologic character of the aneurysm continues to change, which may cause the stent-graft to migrate and sometimes to disintegrate. The resulting endoleaks fall into five broad groups, some of which cause the aneurysm to repressurize and so necessitate reintervention to prevent potential aneurysm rupture (Table 13.1).

The EVAR 1 trial compared open repair with endovascular repair in patients who were fit for conventional open aortic surgery and anatomically suitable for EVAR.[75] Between 1999 and 2003, 1082 patients were randomized across U.K. centers. The 30-day mortality was 1.7% for EVAR versus 4.7% for open repair (hazard ratio [HR], 0.35; $P = .009$). At 4 years of follow-up, all-cause mortality was similar at approximately 28% (HR, 0.9). AAA-related mortality was 4% in the EVAR group, being 7% with open surgery (HR, 0.55; $P = .04$). Complications of EVAR totaled 41%, most of these being minor, compared with only 9% in the open group (HR, 4.9. $P < .0001$). Similarly, the reintervention rate for EVAR was as high as 20%, versus 6% with open repair (HR, 2.7; $P < .0001$). At 12 months, there was a negligible difference with respect to health-related quality of life, but EVAR was more than £3,000 more expensive.

TECHNIQUES OF ENDOVASCULAR AORTIC ANEURYSM REPAIR

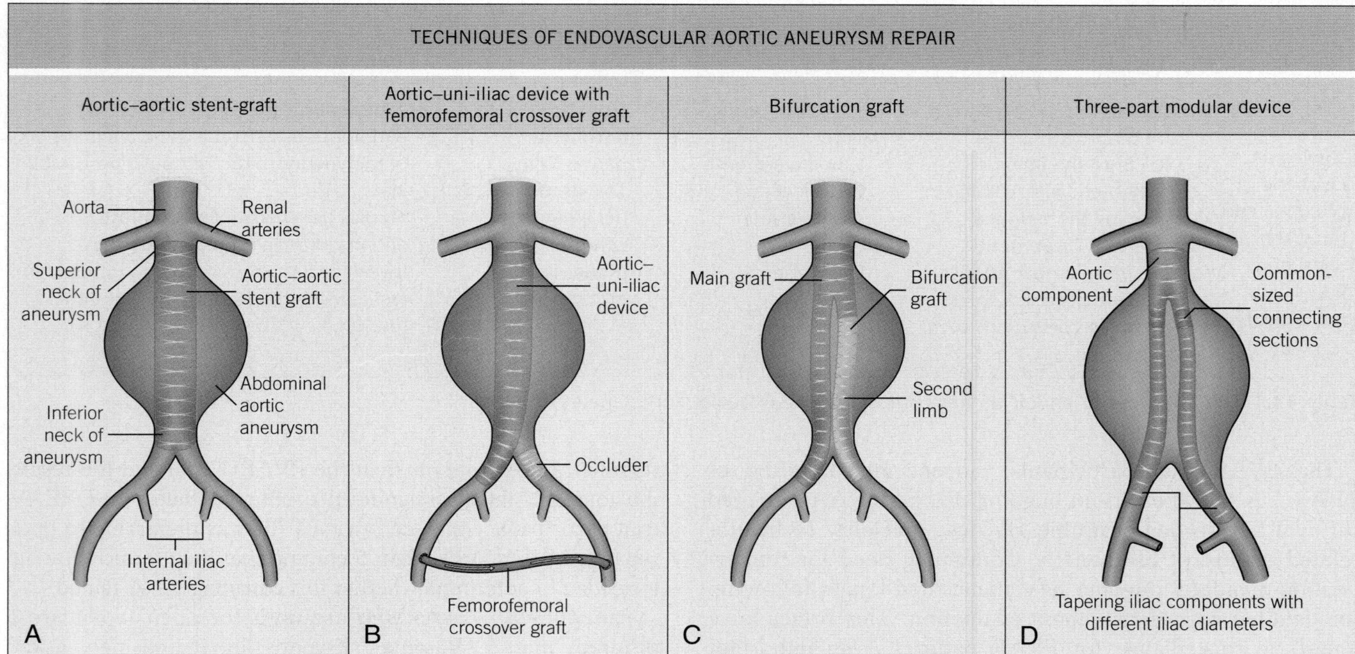

Figure 13.7 Techniques of endovascular aortic aneurysm repair. The aortic-aortic stent-graft **(A)** was the configuration of the early aneurysm stent-graft systems. In practice, the inferior aneurysm neck is not usually of adequate length to achieve a seal, and aortic-aortic tube grafts are now rarely used. The aortic–uni-iliac device with femorofemoral crossover graft **(B)** appears inelegant at first glance, but aortic–uni-iliac grafts, particularly the custom-made devices, permit great flexibility in anatomic dimensions and so enable patients whose aneurysms are not suitable for other graft configurations to receive endovascular treatment. The bifurcation graft **(C)** is the configuration of choice for most patients. Most bifurcation grafts are modular devices **(D)** in which the main graft resembles a pair of long trousers with one leg cut short. This is deployed in the aneurysm, with the upper neck placed below the renal arteries and the long limb secured in the common iliac artery. The second "trouser leg" is then deployed through the contralateral groin to join the short limb of the main graft to the opposite common iliac artery. The early endovascular bifurcation grafts were complicated to use and required thick delivery systems; improvements in technology have simplified use and slimmed down delivery catheters to allow percutaneous deployment in some cases.

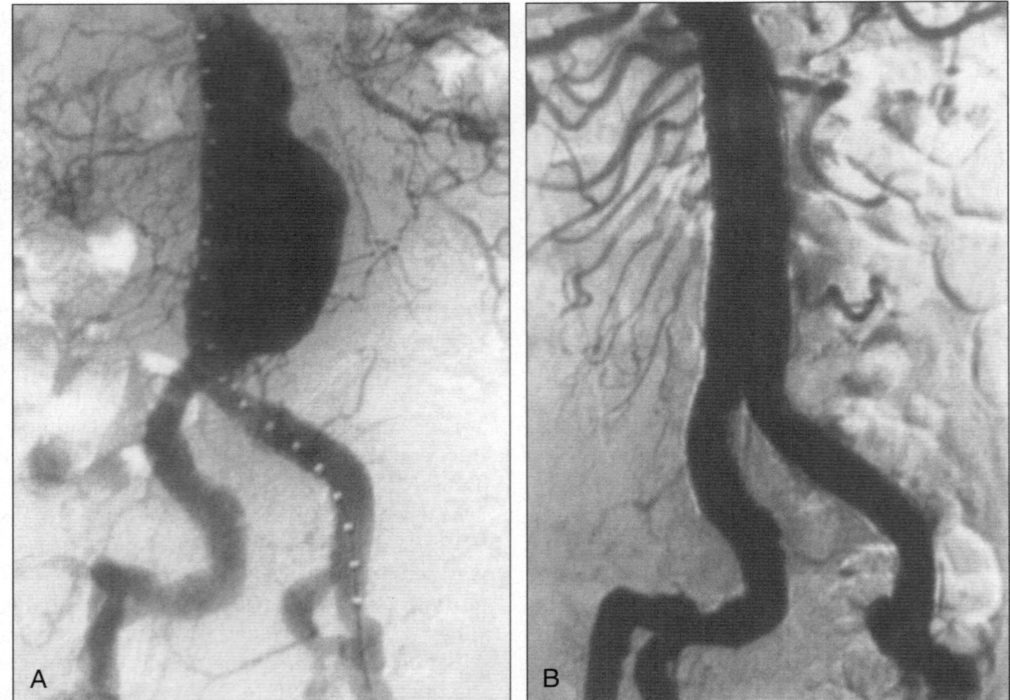

Figure 13.8 Endovascular aneurysm repair angiography. Angiograms taken before **(A)** and after **(B)** deployment of a modular bifurcation stent-graft. In **A,** the calibrated catheter is seen passing up the left iliac system into the aorta; the dilated aneurysm lumen is well demonstrated. In **B,** the aneurysm cavity has been excluded. (With permission from W. L. Gore and Associates.)

THE FIVE TYPES OF ENDOLEAK THAT COMPLICATE ENDOVASCULAR AORTIC ANEURYSM REPAIR				
Type I	**Type II**	**Type III**	**Type IV**	**Type V**
Occur at an end of a stent-graft Ia: at the proximal end Ib: at the distal end Require reintervention	Due to retrograde flow from aortic branches IIa: from the inferior mesenteric artery being filled by the marginal artery of Drummond IIb: from lumbar arteries Need treatment if follow-up reveals aneurysm sac expansion	Secondary to graft failure Fabric tears, limb disconnection, graft disintegration Require reintervention	From graft wall porosity or permeability This group is becoming less common with modern stent-grafts.	Attributed to the phenomenon of endotension, whereby there is expansion of the aneurysm sac without a detectable leak Studies using advanced contrast-enhanced imaging techniques have revealed that a proportion of these are in fact low-flow leaks of one of the other four types.

Table 13.1 The five types of endoleak that complicate endovascular aortic aneurysm repair.

The EVAR trial participants' current interpretation of EVAR 1 is that there is an ongoing 3% better AAA-related survival but no demonstrable all-cause mortality or health-related quality of life benefit. Continuing need for reintervention mandates ongoing surveillance and longer follow-up for detailed cost-effectiveness evaluation. This principle of long-term surveillance for EVAR patients is an important consideration before embarking on such intervention.

Similarly, the Dutch Randomized Endovascular Aneurysm Management (DREAM) trial also assessed EVAR in patients who were deemed fit for open aortic repair.[76] A total of 345 aneurysms were randomized to EVAR or open surgery. The operative mortality was reported as 1.2% in the EVAR arm versus 4.6% in the open group ($P = .10$). Operative mortality plus severe complications were 4.7% for EVAR compared with 9.8% for surgical repair ($P = .10$). The DREAM trial recruited fewer patients than the EVAR 1 trial and the results did not reach statistical significance, but nonetheless the DREAM trial participants concluded that EVAR was preferable to open repair in AAAs larger than 5 cm and that long-term follow-up is needed to determine whether this advantage is sustained.

Patients with AAAs who are unfit for open repair are a different matter. Vascular surgeons are increasingly asked to treat elderly, frail patients with severe comorbidities. In the U.K. Small Aneurysm Trial, 50% of patients unfit for surgery were dead within 2 years. The pressing issue is whether EVAR can alter this morbidity. The EVAR 2 trial compared endovascular therapy against best medical treatment for patients who are unfit for open surgery.[77] A total of 338 patients were randomized to EVAR plus best medical therapy or best medical therapy alone. The 30-day mortality was 9% in the EVAR arm, with no difference in all-cause or

AAA-related mortality. There was no significant difference in health-related quality of life, but EVAR was more than £8,600 more expensive.

There have been a number of criticisms of the EVAR 2 trial, including that there was a significant number of patients crossing over from the best medical therapy arm to the EVAR arm. The methods used to assess fitness were controversial, and during follow-up, a proportion of patients categorized as unfit had subsequently undergone and survived open aneurysm repair. In addition, there was no stratification for aneurysm size.

The current interpretation of EVAR 2 by the EVAR trial investigators is that EVAR had a considerable 30-day mortality in patients already unfit for open repair. There was no improvement in long-term survival, with associated need for continued surveillance and reintervention, at substantially increased cost. In these sick patients, emphasis has shifted toward improving the patient's fitness.

In a study that applied a validated fitness score to patients in the EVAR 1 and 2 trials to determine whether fitter patients with large aneurysms benefited from having open rather than endovascular repair, only in the fitter group did 30-day mortality convincingly favor endovascular repair.[78] Consequently, there is continuing argument with regard to the role of EVAR in the unfit patient.

There are a number of ongoing trials comparing endovascular and open techniques for aortic aneurysm that will further contribute to the decision-making process in our patients. The French ACE trial and the Open Versus Endovascular Repair (OVER) study from the United States are two such examples. The Positive Impact of Endovascular Options for Treating Aneurysms Early (PIVOTAL) and Comparison of surveillance vs Aortic Endografting for Small Aneurysm Repair (CAESAR)[79] studies are investigating the potential benefit of endovascular intervention on small aneurysms by comparing EVAR with surveillance for aneurysms between 4 and 5.5 cm in diameter.

The importance of these studies is highlighted by research reporting that preoperative aneurysm size is an important determinant of long-term outcome after endovascular repair, raising the question of whether suitability for EVAR decreases with increasing aneurysm size. This work may represent a paradigm shift and raises the question of whether surveillance could mean missed opportunities for optimal intervention on smaller aneurysms with less complex anatomy.[80] One group has shown that patients with small AAAs (<5.0 cm) are more favorable candidates for EVAR and have the best long-term outcomes.[81]

The natural history of aortic aneurysms of less than 5.5 cm is a rupture rate of 1% per annum.[3] As such, to improve on this, EVAR for small aneurysms would have to have outstanding results.

More than 10,000 patients undergoing EVAR were entered into the EUROSTAR registry database in the 10 years between 1996 and 2006. At 6 years of follow-up, this cohort of patients suffered a rupture rate of 12%. Multivariate analysis of the risk factors for rupture showed that device-related aspects predominate, commonly migration or other device failure, highlighting the need to focus on device durability as key to the long-term success of EVAR. Endovascular devices are made by a variety of manufacturers with many different fixation mechanisms. The EUROSTAR analysis revealed that endograft performance varied, with some having higher rates of graft failure than others.[82] Later generation devices, such as those analyzed by the EVAR trial collaborators, tend to have more stable fixation, with broadly similar medium-term outcomes.[83]

The 12% graft failure rate reported by the EUROSTAR group is alarmingly high, but this seems to have improved as the EVAR learning curve has been negotiated.[84] There is a reintervention rate of around 7% per year, and each procedure carries significant complication risk. Moreover, revision of an endovascular repair to an open reconstruction carries a substantially higher risk than a primary open repair. These long-term difficulties must be weighed against the early advantages of EVAR over open surgery.

Significant design modifications have been made to stent-grafts, such as to broaden the indications for endovascular aortic repair. Devices with a scalloped proximal end to accommodate the renal arteries allow higher deployment (Fig. 13.9). This maximizes the aneurysm neck, against which the endoprosthesis must form a tight seal to prevent graft failure by way of a proximal endoleak. Fenestrated and branched endovascular devices have been developed, have been shown to be feasible, and are being used to include aneurysms with short necks and that involve branches, such as the renal and internal iliac arteries. A fundamental worry with regard to renal branched grafts is that they involve the stenting of otherwise normal renal arteries, with the knowledge that all stents carry a risk of stenosis and occlusion. Controversy surrounding iliac branched devices is very much in relation to the indications for their use. The vascular world is divided, with some groups preserving, by way of stent branches, both internal iliac arteries, others preserving one, with the remainder happy to sacrifice both

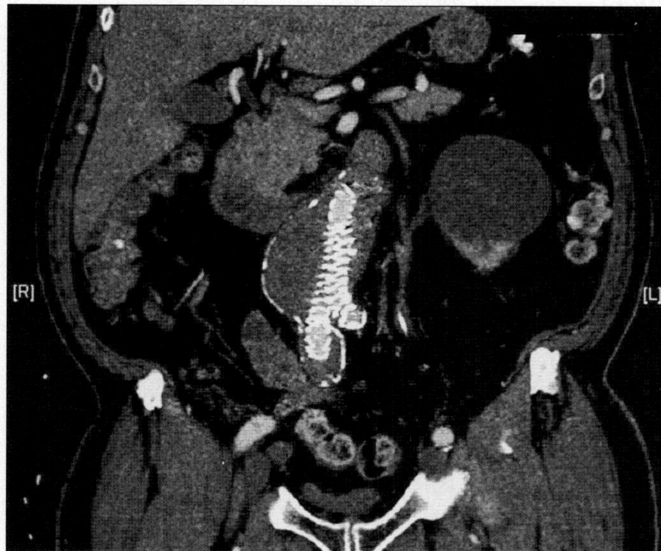

Figure 13.9 Coronal reconstruction of a CT scan showing an endovascular stent-graft within an abdominal aortic aneurysm, thereby excluding the aneurysm sac from the circulation. This particular endovascular device has a scalloped proximal end to accommodate the renal arteries, thereby allowing higher deployment and maximizing the aneurysm neck, against which the endoprosthesis must form a tight seal to prevent graft failure by way of a type Ia endoleak.

with the expectation that the patient will experience some postprocedure buttock claudication and impotence (Leriche syndrome). There is ongoing debate and study, with long-term outcomes yet to be determined.

Emergency Repair of Ruptured Abdominal Aortic Aneurysm

Hemorrhage from a leaking aortic aneurysm is reduced by reflex contraction of the abdominal wall musculature to generate a high intra-abdominal pressure. This protective mechanism is lost the moment anesthesia is induced and muscle relaxants are administered, causing rapid collapse of blood pressure. It is therefore vital that all preparations for operation, including insertion of venous and arterial lines, skin preparation, and draping, are completed on the operating table (not in the anesthetic room) before induction of anesthesia. On entering of the abdomen, proximal control is obtained by rapidly exposing and clamping the supraceliac aorta through the lesser omentum. This reduces blood loss during the more difficult dissection of the aorta below the renal arteries, which may be obscured by hematoma. As soon as the infrarenal aorta is controlled, the proximal clamp is released. The remainder of the operation proceeds along the same lines as for elective repair.

Emergency EVAR has great potential to reduce the mortality of surgery for ruptured aneurysms (Fig. 13.10). Of the patients who survive long enough to reach the operating theater, only around half will be discharged from the hospital alive after emergency open repair. There is, therefore, huge scope for improvement. Endovascular repair has been used to treat contained aneurysm ruptures[85] with limited success to date. We have recently used an aorto–uni-iliac endovascular stent-graft, in conjunction with a femorofemoral crossover graft, to successfully manage a contained aortic aneurysm rupture in a Jehovah's witness who was refusing blood transfusion (Fig. 13.11).

Pharmacologic Treatment of Abdominal Aortic Aneurysm

Pharmacologic treatment for abdominal aneurysms is eagerly sought to treat the large number of small aneurysms being diagnosed by screening programs.[86] This is a rapidly evolving field and one in which translation from experimental research to clinical practice is anticipated. Although there is currently no effective nonsurgical treatment to limit aneurysm growth, developments in the understanding of the pathogenesis of AAA formation are hoped to revolutionize treatment of the condition in coming years.

Cessation of smoking and control of blood pressure delay aneurysm development and reduce risk of rupture. As alluded to earlier, there is a potential role for β-adrenergic blockade in the control of the rate of expansion of larger aneurysms,[87] but this benefit needs to be balanced against the potential drug side effects. Losartan, an angiotensin II type 1 receptor blocker, prevents aortic aneurysm in a mouse model of Marfan's syndrome[88]; the same group published their recommendation for, rationale of, and design of a randomized clinical trial of beta-blocker therapy, with atenolol, versus angiotensin II receptor blockade, with losartan, in individuals with Marfan's syndrome.[89] With this in mind, Marfan's syndrome tends to affect the proximal aorta first.

Although there is circumstantial evidence to link aortic aneurysms and atherosclerosis with *C. pneumoniae,* no causative link has been established.

The inflammatory and proteolytic processes occurring in AAA wall are attractive targets for pharmacotherapy aimed at limiting aneurysm growth. The MMP-mediated degradation of elastin and collagen could potentially be attenuated by an MMP inhibitor that achieves adequate concentration in the aortic wall. Low-molecular-weight heparin has been shown to lower plasma MMP-9 levels in AAA patients[90]; however, most attention has focused on the tetracycline family of antibiotics and its derivatives, which include direct MMP inhibition among their several biologic activities.[91] These compounds have been shown to prevent the collagen destruction due to excessive MMP activity in periodontitis; a similar rationale is suggested to treat aneurysms. Doxycycline has been shown to reduce the growth of experimental aneurysms in rats, and this is associated with depressed activity of MMP-9. Tetracycline has both anti-MMP and anti-inflammatory activity on human AAA tissue in vitro, but high concentrations are required; such concentrations are not readily achieved in AAA wall in vivo.[92]

In one study, prolonged administration of doxycycline was shown to be safe and well tolerated by patients with small asymptomatic AAAs and was associated with a gradual reduction in plasma MMP-9 levels.[93] Baxter and coworkers concluded that further studies are needed to evaluate the long-term effects of doxycycline on the rate and extent of aneurysm growth and the potential use of plasma MMP-9 levels as a biomarker of aneurysm disease progression. Tetracycline derivatives offer a number of distinct advantages as MMP inhibitors for patients with small AAAs, but drug therapy for AAA based on MMP inhibition will require the development of agents with equivalent potency teamed with greater penetration of aneurysm wall.

Statins have been shown to significantly reduce MMP-9 (by up to 40%) and other protease activity in the wall of AAAs of patients who were receiving statins preoperatively compared with those who were not on a lipid-lowering pharmacologic regimen.[94] In a cohort of patients whose AAAs were under surveillance, statin users had a 1.16 mm

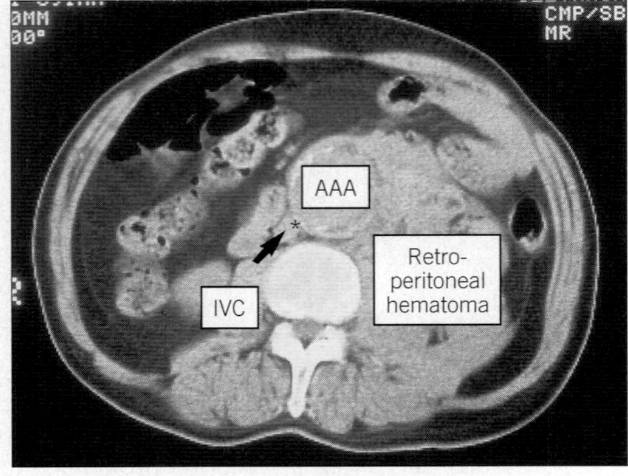

Figure 13.10 CT scan of an abdominal aortic aneurysm. A large retroperitoneal hematoma to the left of the aneurysm is shown. AAA, abdominal aortic aneurysm; IVC, inferior vena cava. (Courtesy of Mr. S. Selvakumar.)

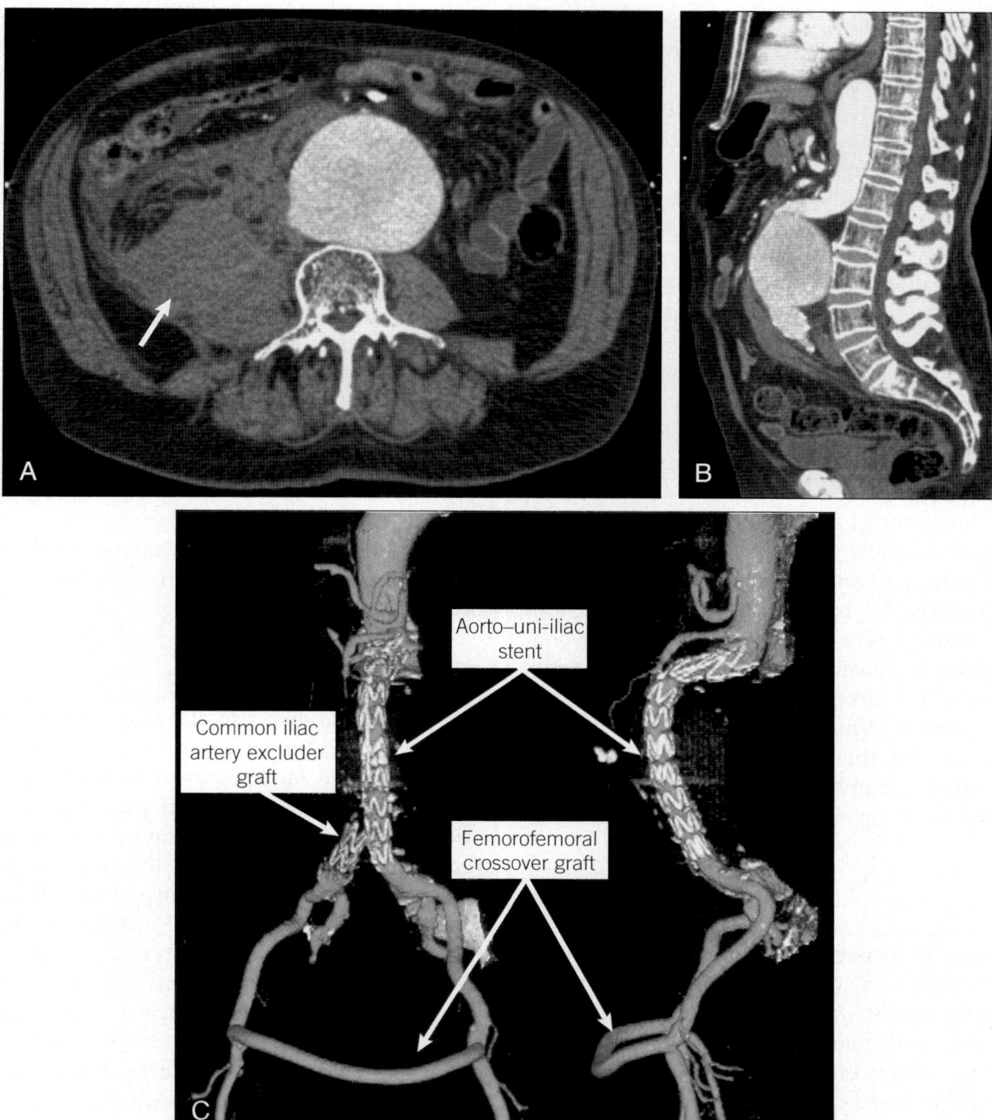

Figure 13.11 Images relating to a Jehovah's witness who presented acutely with an abdominal aortic aneurysm rupture. He refused all forms of transfusion of blood products, including autotransfusion. A, Axial slice of a CT scan showing an abdominal aortic aneurysm and a right retroperitoneal hematoma *(arrow)* due to contained rupture of the aneurysm. **B,** Sagittal reconstruction of the CT scan showing the angulated neck of this aneurysm. **C,** CT angiogram three-dimensional reconstruction to show how this ruptured aneurysm was successfully managed by endovascular techniques. An aorto–uni-iliac stent-graft was sited. The contralateral (right) common iliac artery was occluded with an excluder graft. Perfusion to the right lower limb was restored by way of a left-to-right femorofemoral crossover graft. (Courtesy of Mr. Farokh Pakzad.)

per year lower AAA growth rate compared with that of nonusers.[95] The use of nonsteroidal anti-inflammatory drugs in this study was not independently associated with AAA growth, with the conclusion that statins appear to be associated with attenuation of AAA growth, irrespective of other known factors influencing aneurysm growth.

The chronic inflammation in the aneurysm wall that appears to underlie and to drive the excessive proteolysis is also a tempting target for drugs. Some authorities advocate corticosteroid treatment for so-called inflammatory aneurysms. Of the inflammatory mediators and cytokines present in AAA wall, PGE_2 is of particular interest. It is produced in very high concentrations, mainly by adventitial macrophages, and apart from potentiating the action of other inflammatory mediators and MMPs, it appears to depress smooth muscle cell replication.[5] Treatment with indomethacin readily abolishes PGE_2 secretion by AAA tissue in vitro and also suppresses production of the cytokines IL-1β and IL-6.[96] The nonselective cyclooxygenase inhibitor indomethacin and the selective COX-2 inhibitor MF-tricyclic have both been shown to attenuate the growth of experimental aneurysms in rats.[97,98] One small case-control study has suggested that AAA may expand more slowly in patients who happen to be taking nonsteroidal anti-inflammatory drugs for joint problems; however, this has not been reproduced in larger studies.[5,99]

In a murine aneurysm model,[100] the selective inducible nitric oxide synthase activity inhibitor 1400 W significantly decreased aneurysm size and preserved aortic elastin without altering MMP-9 levels, suggesting an MMP-9–independent mechanism. Indomethacin significantly decreased MMP-9 expression, but to an extent insufficient to limit aneurysm size. In the same study, rofecoxib, another selective COX-2 inhibitor, did not significantly decrease MMP-9 expression or aneurysm size. Such observations centered on inhibition of the cyclooxygenase pathway have yielded mixed and disappointing results in both the preclinical and clinical arenas, and further work is necessary to determine whether anti-inflammatory drugs have a role in the pharmacotherapy of AAAs.

Gene therapy has yet to find widespread application even for clear-cut single-gene disorders. The genetic element contributing to AAA pathogenesis is far from understood and certainly involves a number of genes. For example, cystatin C, an inhibitor of proteolytic enzymes, is expressed in arterial smooth muscle cells, and an imbalance in cystatin C has been implicated in AAAs.[101] In a study of more than 400 small aneurysms, there was a weak association between cystatin C gene polymorphism and AAA growth. Aortic aneurysms are, however, unlikely candidates for gene therapy for the foreseeable future. Similarly, therapeutic options such as stem cell therapy, the use of medicinal foods, and vaccination require considerable study and development before they can approach clinical relevance in AAA.[102]

PROGNOSIS

There is no evidence of benefit to operate on nontender aneurysms smaller than 5.5 cm in diameter; for these patients, early surgery confers no survival advantage. However, 54% of patients with aneurysms in the 4- to 5.5-cm range may expect to require elective repair within 5 years of diagnosis as the aneurysm expands.

Elective open surgical repair of an AAA with a Dacron graft is a safe, standard, and durable procedure. Dacron is inert and outlives the patient, provided no infection occurs at operation. The 30-day mortality rate across Britain for open elective surgical repair is around 6%. The 30-day mortality for elective repair in the U.K. Small Aneurysm Trial was 5.8%. In this study, all deaths that occurred within 2 weeks of surgery were attributed to the operation. Repair of symptomatic, nonruptured aneurysms seems to carry a higher risk. In the Charing Cross series, 30-day mortality for asymptomatic aneurysm repair was 1.4% compared with 9.2% for tender and painful aneurysms.[103]

The perioperative mortality for EVAR in fit patients is less than 2%, at least half that of open repair.[75,76] At 4 years of follow-up, all-cause mortality is approximately 28%, similar to that of patients who have open surgery. Aneurysm-related mortality in fit patients is 4% after EVAR and 7% after open surgery. Surveillance after EVAR is necessary, and reintervention rates are significant.

The outcome for patients whose aneurysms rupture is dismal. Around three quarters die before reaching the hospital. Of those who make the operating theater, half do not survive the operation. For the remainder, a 30-day mortality of 42% is fairly typical.[103]

SUMMARY

AAA is a common cause of sudden death. AAA size remains the best indicator of future rupture, with elective repair being indicated for aneurysms larger than 5.5 cm in diameter, those growing faster than 1 cm per year, and symptomatic aneurysms by way of pain or tenderness. Open surgical repair, previously considered the gold standard in treatment, is a safe and durable procedure in fit patients. Endovascular repair is an evidence-based method of treatment, with a lower morbidity and a faster return to work compared with open surgery. Fit patients have been shown to do particularly well after endovascular repair, with an ongoing argument regarding the role of endovascular repair in the unfit. The pathogenesis of aortic aneurysm development is complex. Inflammation, proteolysis, and smooth muscle cell loss in the aortic wall are key elements of aneurysmal dilatation. Drugs to treat aneurysm are being developed; none has yet proved effective.

chapter

14 Venous Disease

Agnes Y. Y. Lee

Definition

- Abnormal conditions of the veins are due to thrombotic or inflammatory processes that impair the function of the vessels in returning blood to the heart and may result in thromboembolic events to the cardiorespiratory vasculature.

Key Features

- The most common venous disease is acute venous thromboembolism involving deep veins of the legs, with or without pulmonary embolism.
- Classic clinical features are swelling and pain of the involved extremity, but significant disease can be clinically silent.
- Diagnosis requires objective investigations because clinical features are nonspecific.
- Venous thrombosis can be associated with significant short- and long-term morbidity and, potentially, mortality.

Therapy

- Systemic anticoagulant therapy is highly effective and remains the mainstay of treatment for acute venous thromboembolism.
- Duration of therapy depends on balancing the risks of recurrence and anticoagulant-related bleeding.
- Indications for second-line therapy, such as thrombolytic treatment and vena cava filter insertion, remain poorly established.

Although venous disease has generally received less attention than arterial disease, acute and chronic conditions can be associated with significant morbidity and, potentially, mortality. Approximately 1 per 1000 persons is affected by venous thrombosis annually.[1] The most common condition is acute venous thromboembolism involving the deep veins of the legs, with or without pulmonary embolism. Rarely, thrombus can form in the venae cavae as well as in the veins of the liver and the kidneys and in the mesenteric, portal, or central nervous system. A good understanding of the anatomy and pathophysiology is helpful in making an accurate diagnosis, but objective testing is essential because the clinical features of venous thrombosis are nonspecific. Although highly effective treatment is available, serious short- and long-term sequelae can still result from the disease process, underlying comorbid conditions, and treatment-related complications.

ANATOMY AND PHYSIOLOGY

The veins are vessels that convey blood back to the heart. The smallest veins are called venules. These arise from capillaries, and they unite to form larger veins or tributaries and venous plexuses. Large veins from the lower limbs and torso form the inferior vena cava; veins draining the upper extremities, head, and neck join to form the superior vena cava. The venae cavae lead into the right atrium and complete the circulatory system. Compared with arteries, the veins are distensible, high-capacitance vessels that can accommodate 60% to 75% of the blood volume of the body. Because the walls of veins contain less elastic tissue and smooth muscle than the arterial walls do, the competency of veins in directing blood back to the heart is highly dependent on bicuspid valves, which normally allow only unidirectional blood flow.[2]

Veins of the Lower Extremities

The venous system of the lower extremities is composed of three sets of veins: the deep veins, the superficial veins, and the communicating veins.

The deep veins, unlike the superficial and communicating veins, accompany the major arteries. The proximal veins include the common femoral, deep femoral, superficial femoral, and popliteal veins (Fig. 14.1). A single vein usually accompanies the corresponding artery, although duplication of the superficial femoral vein and popliteal vein is not uncommon. The deep veins of the calf are usually paired when they accompany the corresponding artery. These include the anterior tibial, posterior tibial, and peroneal veins.

The superficial venous network includes veins in the thigh, calf, and foot. These vessels course close to the skin and are sometimes visible. The most significant superficial veins are the greater and lesser saphenous veins. The greater saphenous vein begins at the medial malleolus of the ankle and courses medially up the entire length of the calf and thigh to enter into the common femoral vein in the groin. The lesser saphenous vein arises from the lateral part of the foot and ascends behind the lateral malleolus. It courses along the posterolateral aspect of the calf and ends in the popliteal vein at the lower part of the popliteal fossa.

The communicating veins connect the superficial veins with the deep veins. The two types are the perforating veins, which course through the deeper fascial layers outside the muscles, and the intramuscular sinusoids, which course through the muscles of the lower extremity.

Veins of the Upper Extremities

The deep veins parallel the corresponding upper extremity arteries. These are the subclavian, axillary, and brachial veins in the upper arm and the radial and ulnar veins in the forearm. The largest superficial veins are the basilic and

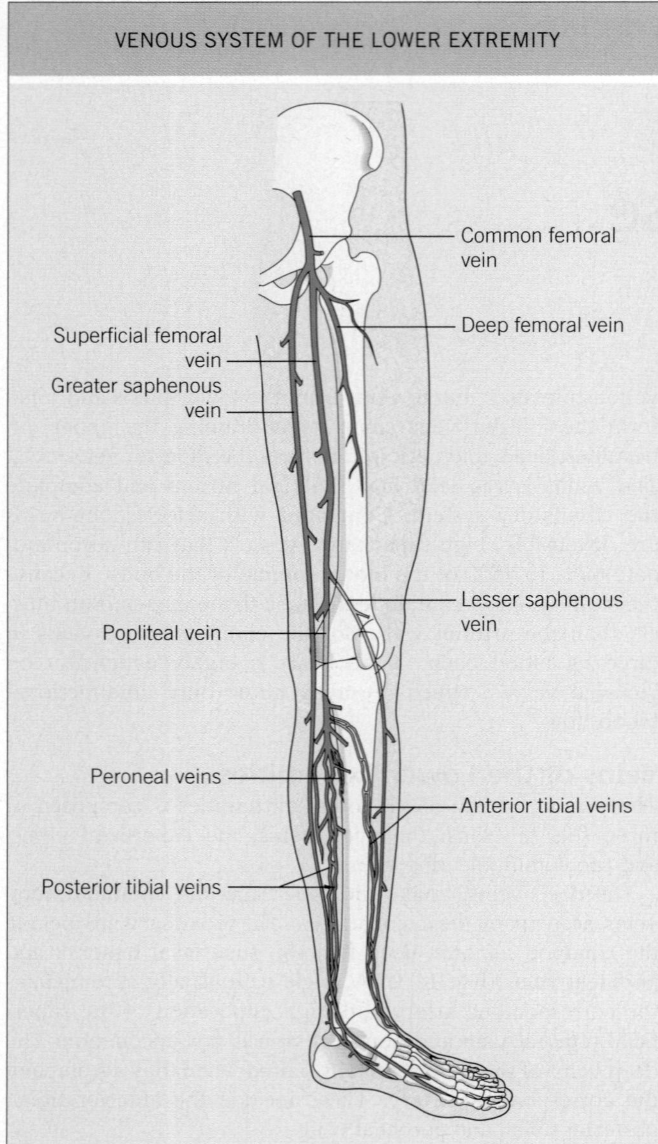

Figure 14.1 Venous system of the lower extremity.

cephalic veins in the upper arm, which join the deep venous system in the region of the shoulder (Fig. 14.2).

The subclavian vein traverses the relatively narrow space between the first rib and the clavicle to enter the thorax. The subclavius and scalene muscle tendons and other ligaments can encroach on this space, occasionally leading to venous obstruction. Cervical ribs can also compress the neurovascular bundle at the junction of the arm with the thorax, usually leading to nerve, arterial, and venous compression.

Central Veins

The major veins emptying into the right atrium are the superior vena cava and the inferior vena cava (Fig. 14.3). The superior vena cava is formed on the right side of the mediastinum by the joining of the right and left brachiocephalic (innominate) veins, which receive venous tributaries from the upper torso, including the arms, the head, the neck, and the overlying soft tissues of the thorax. The subclavian veins and the internal jugular veins, which carry blood from the

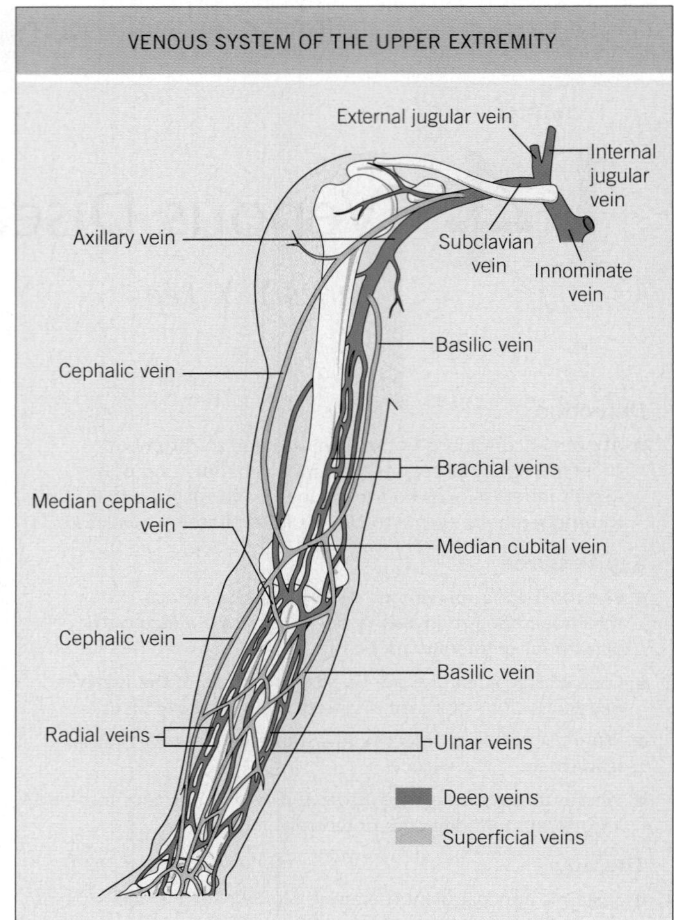

Figure 14.2 Venous system of the upper extremity.

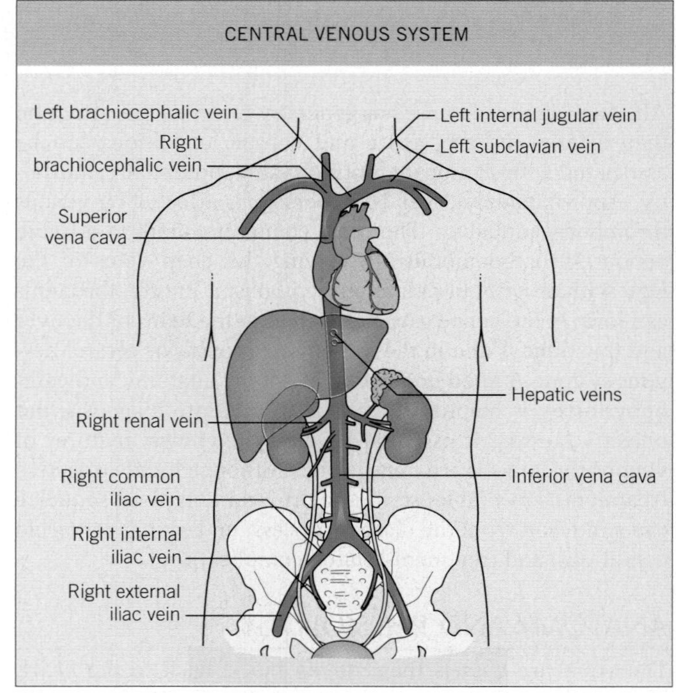

Figure 14.3 Central venous system. Only major vessels are included.

head and neck, join to form the right and left brachiocephalic veins.

The inferior vena cava is formed by the right and left common iliac veins in the pelvis and receives tributaries from the pelvic and abdominal viscera as well as from the overlying soft tissues of the lower torso. The common iliac veins are formed by the external iliac veins, which carry blood predominantly from the legs, and the internal iliac veins, which carry blood from the pelvic viscera. The inferior vena cava also receives venous tributaries from the abdominal viscera, most notably the liver and the kidneys. The hepatic veins and renal veins empty directly into the inferior vena cava; the venous drainage from most of the gut, the pancreas, and the spleen passes through the portal vein into the hepatic sinusoids and then through the hepatic veins into the inferior vena cava.

PATHOPHYSIOLOGY

Venous disease primarily arises from pathologic processes that lead to thrombosis of the circulating blood. This is often accompanied by an inflammatory response of the vessel walls, which can further propagate the thrombotic process. Thrombus formation is dependent on thrombin generation, which is promoted through the activation of the coagulation pathways (Fig. 14.4). The interruption of normal blood flow by the thrombus produces venous hypertension, which results in the clinical manifestations of deep venous thrombosis. Damage to the venous valves, either secondary to previous thrombosis or from inherent structural defects, leads to chronic venous reflux, formation of varicose veins, and skin changes.

Mechanisms

Virchow's triad describes the three basic mechanisms that can lead to thrombus formation: venous stasis, vessel wall damage, and hypercoagulability.[3] In many clinical situations, all three mechanisms may play a role. Venous stasis is usually caused by extrinsic compression of the vessel by tumor masses, adenopathy, fibrosis, or anatomic strictures. Conditions resulting in prolonged immobility, such as paralysis or casting of a lower limb, can also predispose to venous stasis and thrombosis. Thrombi within the deep veins are thought to arise most commonly at the valves within the soleal sinusoids in the calf and to propagate into the deep calf veins (Fig. 14.5).[4] Vessel wall or endothelial damage leads to exposure of the subendothelium, whereby exposure of membrane-bound tissue factor results in activation of the extrinsic coagulation pathway.

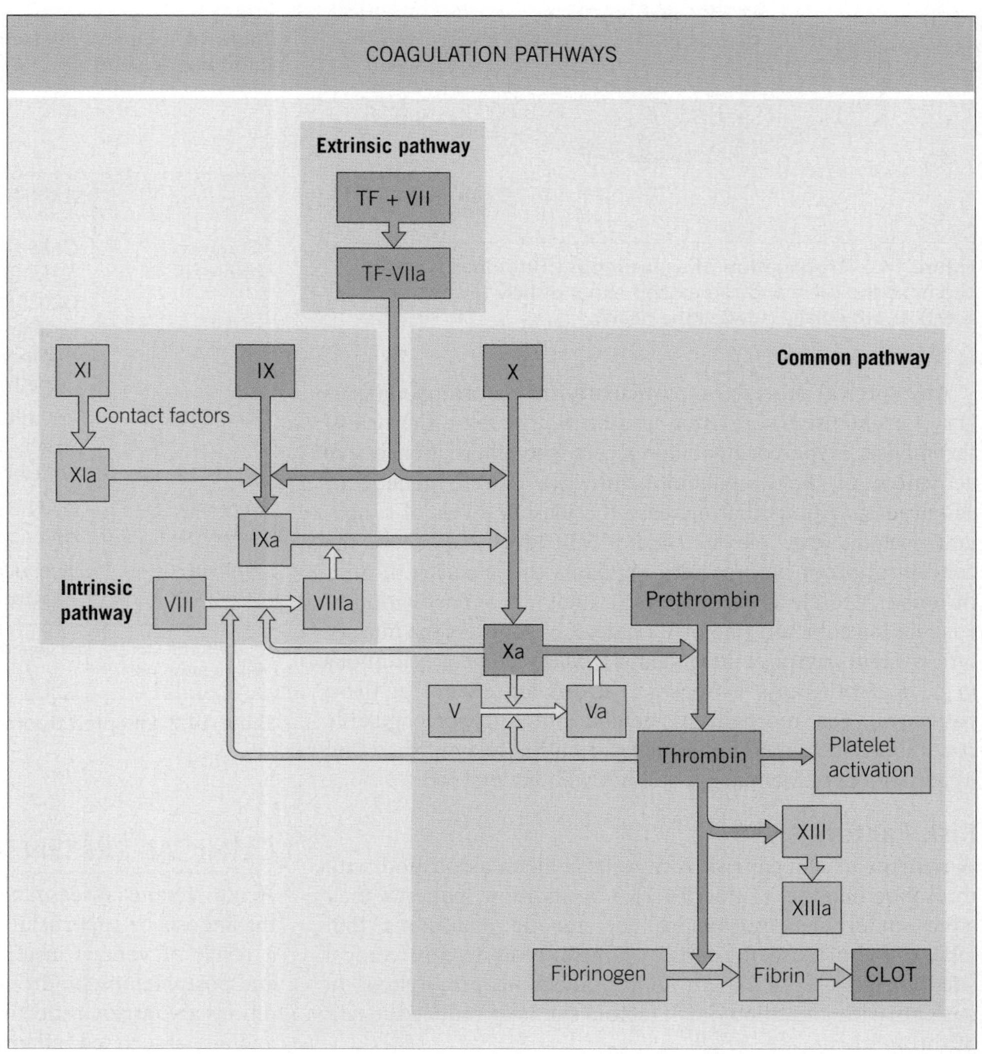

Figure 14.4 Coagulation pathways. A simplified schematic of the extrinsic, intrinsic, and common pathways of the coagulation cascade. TF, tissue factor.

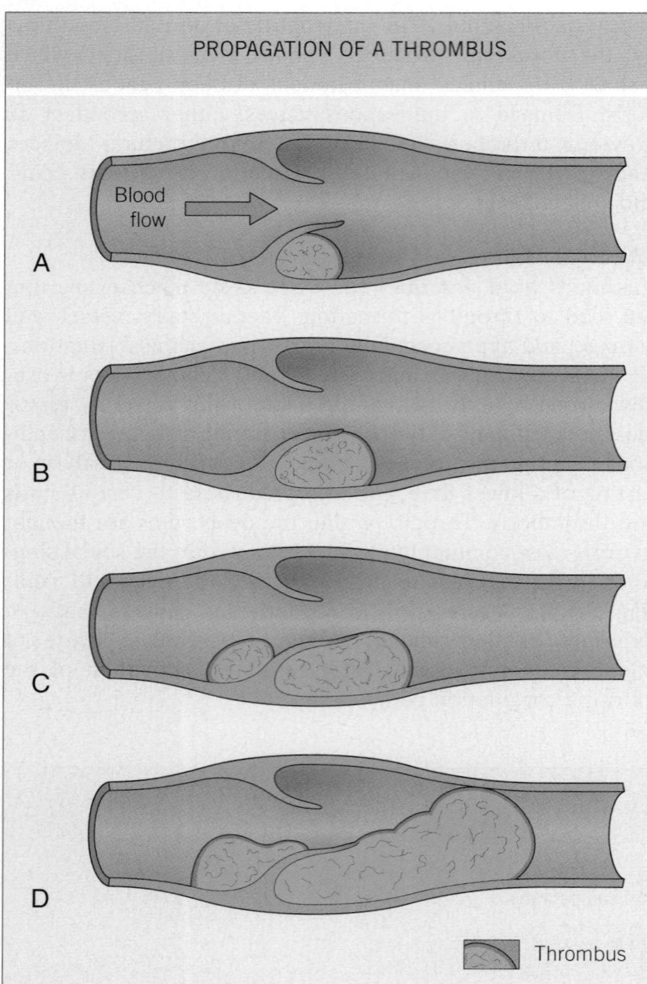

Figure 14.5 Propagation of a thrombus. Thrombus typically begins at the valve and can extend either distally (away from the heart) or proximally (toward the heart).

Any surgical procedure, particularly major orthopedic surgery, or extensive soft tissue trauma will increase the risk of thrombosis. Hypercoagulability occurs when there is excessive activation of the coagulation pathways due to genetic or acquired conditions that increase the plasma levels of coagulant proteins (e.g., elevated factor VIII levels), decrease the concentration of natural anticoagulants (deficiencies of antithrombin, protein C, or protein S), inhibit the inactivation of coagulation cofactors (factor V Leiden), or suppress the fibrinolytic system (dysplasminogenemia). Many clinical conditions (e.g., chemotherapy, estrogens) can impair several of these pathways. The mechanisms behind other hypercoagulable conditions, such as antiphospholipid antibody syndrome and hyperhomocysteinemia, are still not well understood.

Risk Factors

A number of clinical risk factors have been associated with thromboembolism (Table 14.1).[5] In addition, patients may have underlying biochemical or genetic conditions that inherently increase their risk of thrombosis in any clinical situation (Table 14.2).[6] Providing adequate prophylaxis in patients with identifiable risk factors can help reduce the risk of thrombosis.

CLINICAL RISK FACTORS ASSOCIATED WITH VENOUS THROMBOEMBOLISM

Physiologic conditions	Advanced age Obesity Postpartum Pregnancy
Surgery or trauma	Major trauma Major surgery Pelvic or hip fracture Paralysis or stroke Spinal cord injury Prolonged immobilization
Medical conditions	Cancer Acute myocardial infarction Congestive heart failure Chronic respiratory failure Inflammatory bowel disease Hematologic disorders Nephrotic syndrome Inherited thrombophilia
Medications	Anticancer therapy Oral contraceptives Hormone replacement therapy
Other	History of venous thromboembolism Central venous catheter

Table 14.1 Clinical risk factors associated with venous thromboembolism.

INHERITED THROMBOPHILIA

Common disorders	G1691A mutation in the factor V gene (factor V Leiden) G20210A mutation in the prothrombin (factor II) gene Homozygous C677T mutation in the methylenetetrahydrofolate reductase gene
Rare disorders	Antithrombin deficiency Protein C deficiency Protein S deficiency
Very rare disorders	Dysfibrinogenemia Homozygous homocystinuria
Probably inherited	Increased levels of factor VIII, factor IX, factor XI, or fibrinogen*

*Levels of factor VIII and fibrinogen may also increase as part of the acute-phase response.

Table 14.2 Inherited thrombophilia.

CLINICAL PRESENTATIONS

Acute venous disease may be manifested as deep venous thrombosis or superficial phlebitis. Chronic venous disease is a result of venous insufficiency and includes varicose veins and postphlebitic syndrome. The clinical features in these conditions are largely reflective of the resultant venous congestion and any associated inflammation of the involved vessel walls.

Veins of the Lower Extremities

Deep Venous Thrombosis

The majority of patients presenting with deep venous thrombosis complain of pain or swelling of the involved leg. The pain is often nonspecific, and it is usually described as a dull, aching sensation in the calf or entire leg. With more extensive thrombosis, some patients experience a heavy or "charley horse" sensation of the leg. Pain that is described as sharp, pinpointed in a specific location, or isolated to the anterior aspect of the lower leg is almost never associated with deep venous thrombosis. Swelling is also a frequent symptom that prompts the patient to seek medical attention. The swelling is usually unilateral, beginning in the lower leg or ankle, and it gradually advances proximally. Because bilateral deep venous thrombosis is uncommon, patients presenting with bilateral leg edema are less likely to have deep venous thrombosis than are those with swelling in one leg. On occasion, the patient will notice erythema and may describe having a bluish hue of the involved leg after prolonged standing or sitting.

Physical examination may demonstrate pitting edema, discoloration, and tenderness to palpation along the deep venous distribution of the leg (calf, popliteal fossa, and medial thigh). The involved calf may feel heavier, and its circumference at 10 cm below the tibial tuberosity will often show enlargement compared with the unaffected calf. The classic Homans sign of pain elicited on dorsiflexion of the foot is uncommon and nonspecific for deep venous thrombosis. A palpable cord underneath the skin is not characteristic of deep venous thrombosis unless there is accompanying superficial thrombophlebitis. When there is extensive thrombosis with complete obstruction of the deep venous system, severe venous congestion can result in tissue ischemia. This condition (phlegmasia cerulea dolens) is relatively rare and is manifested as severe pain of the lower extremity accompanied by cyanosis and swelling.

Many other leg pathologic processes (e.g., ruptured Baker's cyst, cellulitis, musculoskeletal conditions) can mimic the presentation of deep venous thrombosis. Patients may occasionally present with signs and symptoms from pulmonary emboli as the first manifestation of clinically silent lower extremity deep venous thrombosis (see Chapter 85).

Superficial Thrombophlebitis

Superficial thrombophlebitis is common in the elderly and is usually a benign condition. It usually is manifested as redness and pain in the thrombosed vein and is more common in the lower extremities. Physical examination will reveal a tender, red, warm cord beneath the skin that follows the course of a superficial vein. Swelling of the involved leg is not a typical feature of isolated superficial thrombophlebitis, and its presence suggests that there may be underlying deep venous thrombosis. Approximately 10% to 20% of cases are associated with deep venous thrombosis.

Chronic Venous Insufficiency

Chronic venous insufficiency is a common clinical problem. Varicose veins are dilatations of the superficial veins secondary to venous reflux and are considered the hallmark of venous insufficiency. However, patients with venous insufficiency do not always have varicosities and may be asymptomatic. Some will present with patches of reticular superficial venules or chronic skin changes, including hyperpigmentation (stasis dermatitis) and ulcerations. Up to half of patients with deep venous thrombosis of the legs may go on to develop postphlebitic syndrome.[7] This is characterized by fluctuating but chronic discomfort and swelling of the involved leg. These symptoms are exacerbated by prolonged sitting or standing and vigorous exercise. Severe cases may develop venous ulcerations of the skin, which typically occur over the medial aspect of the lower leg near the ankle. The severity of chronic venous disease can be classified according to the grading system recommended by the American Venous Forum (Table 14.3).[8]

CLASSIFICATION OF CHRONIC VENOUS INSUFFICIENCY

Class	Description
0	No signs of venous disease
1	Telangiectases or reticular veins
2	Varicose veins
3	Edema
4	Skin changes ascribed to venous disease
5	Skin changes with healed ulceration
6	Skin changes with active ulceration

Table 14.3 Classification of chronic venous insufficiency.

Veins of the Upper Extremities

Deep Venous Thrombosis

Upper extremity deep venous thrombosis may occur spontaneously or secondary to vessel trauma from instrumentation or catheterization. Spontaneous or primary thrombosis of the subclavian or axillary vein is known as the Paget-Schroetter syndrome.[9] This is also referred to as effort-related thrombosis because repetitive or strenuous upper extremity exercise is occasionally reported in association with the thrombotic event. This typically occurs in young patients in the second or third decade, with a slightly higher prevalence in men. About 60% of cases occur in the dominant arm. Patients usually complain of dull, aching pain in the shoulder or axilla and swelling of the arm. Symptoms worsen with vigorous use of the arm and improve with rest and elevation. Physical examination usually reveals a mild to moderate amount of arm edema. On occasion, mild cyanosis of the hand and fingers as well as dilated collateral veins over the arm and chest is observed.

More commonly, deep venous thrombosis of the upper extremity occurs in patients who have or have had indwelling central venous catheters or pacemakers.[10] The majority of cases are asymptomatic and are diagnosed when patients present with catheter malfunction. Alternatively, the catheter may function normally and the patient develops arm pain and swelling. Shoulder pain is not uncommon, and this may be due to local inflammatory reaction. With long-standing thrombosis, collateral veins will develop and are visualized as dilated veins on the involved side of the chest wall.

As with deep venous thrombosis of the lower extremities, clinical presentation of upper extremity thrombosis is nonspecific. Identical signs and symptoms may occur in patients with thoracic outlet venous obstruction from tumor mass or adenopathy, without associated deep venous thrombosis. Clinically significant pulmonary emboli have been reported with upper limb deep venous thrombosis in patients who do not have local symptoms.

Superficial Thrombophlebitis

Superficial thrombophlebitis is uncommon in the upper extremities. It usually occurs in association with local inflammation or infection secondary to venipuncture, catheter insertion, or chemical phlebitis. It is manifested as a tender, red, warm cord beneath the skin that follows the course of the superficial vein. Swelling of the involved arm is not a typical feature of isolated superficial thrombophlebitis; its presence suggests that there may be underlying deep venous thrombosis.

Chronic Venous Insufficiency

Chronic venous insufficiency that follows an episode of thrombosis is less frequent in the upper extremities than in the legs, and it is a more common complication in patients who have had primary thrombosis than in those with catheter-related thrombosis.[11] The typical features are heaviness and swelling of the involved arm that are exacerbated with exercise. Dilated superficial veins are often observed in the arms or chest wall. The clinical findings are indistinguishable from those of patients with chronic lymphedema, which can occur after nodal dissection of the axilla in breast cancer surgery.

Central Veins

Inferior Vena Cava Thrombosis

Patients with thrombosis affecting the inferior vena cava may present with bilateral leg swelling, vague abdominal pain, and increasing girth from ascites. Men may also complain of scrotal edema. Over time, dilated superficial veins will develop on the abdominal wall, representing venous flow in collaterals. All of these symptoms result from the increased venous pressure and venous congestion of the leg veins and mesenteric vessels. Depending on the degree of obstruction of the inferior vena cava, symptoms may be mild or severe. Depending on the location of the thrombus, organ damage of the kidneys or liver may result secondary to ischemia from venous congestion. Like thrombi in the leg and pelvic veins, thrombi in the inferior vena cava are sources of clinically significant pulmonary emboli. These emboli can be life-threatening because of their large size.

Superior Vena Cava Syndrome

As with the inferior vena cava, thrombosis of the superior vena cava may be manifested with fulminant symptoms. Patients may develop a sudden or gradual onset of periorbital edema, facial swelling, and plethora, with or without swelling of the neck and arms. Dilated superficial veins on the chest wall are usually prominent. Many cases are associated with thoracic malignant disease and occasionally develop as a complication of an indwelling central venous catheter.[12] Thrombus in the superior vena cava may extend directly into the right atrium and can serve as a source of potentially fatal pulmonary emboli.

DIAGNOSTIC TECHNIQUES

Veins of the Lower Extremities

Deep Venous Thrombosis

Patients with deep venous thrombosis may have minimal or atypical symptoms, and clinical features that are generally considered diagnostic can be found in nonthrombotic disorders.[13] Only about 25% of patients who present with compatible symptoms have deep venous thrombosis confirmed on objective testing. On the other hand, imaging techniques can produce false-positive or false-negative results. Therefore, both clinical assessment and diagnostic imaging are essential to make an accurate diagnosis and to avoid the risks of either untreated thrombosis or unnecessary anticoagulation.

A proper clinical assessment includes a careful evaluation of the patient's signs, symptoms, and risk factors for venous thromboembolism. Alternative diagnoses should be considered, especially if the patient has atypical symptoms or no risk factors. To improve the consistency and accuracy of the clinical examination, a clinical prediction rule for determining the pretest likelihood of deep venous thrombosis has been developed and validated (Table 14.4).[14] On the basis of the total score given for the presenting clinical features, patients are stratified into low-, intermediate-, or high-probability categories for having deep venous thrombosis. The most subjective and problematic item in this 9-point clinical model is the identification of an alternative diagnosis. Nonetheless, the model has been proved to be robust and helpful in multiple medical settings, including outpatient clinics, emergency departments, and in-hospital services.

The currently available imaging technologies available for diagnosis of acute deep venous thrombosis include venous ultrasonography, contrast venography, computed tomographic scanning, and magnetic resonance imaging. Impedance plethysmography and scanning with fibrinogen labeled with iodine 125 are outdated methods and are considerably less accurate. Magnetic resonance imaging is not widely used, and evidence of its accuracy remains limited. In addition to

WELLS' CLINICAL ASSESSMENT MODEL FOR THE PRETEST PROBABILITY OF LOWER EXTREMITY DEEP VENOUS THROMBOSIS

	Score*
Active cancer (treatment ongoing or within previous 6 months or palliative)	1
Paralysis, paresis, or recent plaster immobilization of the lower extremities	1
Recently bedridden >3 days or major surgery within 4 weeks	1
Localized tenderness along the distribution of the deep venous system	1
Entire leg swollen	1
Calf swelling >3 cm asymptomatic side (measured 10 cm below tibial tuberosity)	1
Pitting edema confined to the symptomatic leg	1
Collateral superficial veins (nonvaricose)	1
Previously documented deep venous thrombosis	1
Alternative diagnosis as likely as or greater than that of deep venous thrombosis	−2

*In patients with symptoms in both legs, the more symptomatic leg is used. Pretest probability is calculated as the total score: high ≥ 3; moderate, 1 or 2; low ≤ 0.

Table 14.4 Wells' clinical assessment model for the pretest probability of lower extremity deep venous thrombosis.

these imaging techniques, testing of D-dimer levels in the blood has been established as a reliable test for exclusion of acute deep venous thrombosis in symptomatic patients.

Although contrast venography remains the reference standard technique for diagnosis of deep venous thrombosis, the most popular test is venous ultrasonography. The compression technique in combination with real-time B-mode imaging has proved to be sensitive (95%) and highly specific (96%) for diagnosis of symptomatic, proximal deep venous thrombosis.[15] This involves the application of direct pressure on the transverse diameter of the vein with the ultrasound transducer. Inability to fully compress the vessel is considered diagnostic for deep venous thrombosis. In many centers, three-point compression at the inguinal region, mid thigh, and popliteal fossa is the standard approach to detect deep venous thrombosis in the leg. Other strategies involve compression along the length of the femoral vein and the popliteal vein, below the calf trifurcation, and into the calf veins. The addition of Doppler or color imaging does not substantially add to the accuracy of compression ultrasonography but is sometimes helpful for identifying the vessel and assessing the amount of residual blood flow (Fig. 14.6). In addition to imaging of the veins, the ultrasound examination is useful for detecting conditions that can mimic deep venous thrombosis, such as ruptured Baker's cyst or an abscess. The entire examination usually takes no longer than 10 to 15 minutes.

The major advantages of ultrasonography are that it does not use ionizing radiation and is noninvasive, readily available, and relatively inexpensive. Portable ultrasound machines are also available for examination in the hospital of patients who are too ill to be transported to the radiology department. The clinical limitations of ultrasonography are its poor ability to diagnose isolated calf vein thrombosis and its reduced sensitivity in patients with asymptomatic disease. The variability in the diagnostic accuracy of ultrasonography in detecting calf vein thrombosis may be related to the small size of the thrombus, the experience of the sonographers, and the differences in populations of patients. The usefulness of ultrasonography is also somewhat reduced in patients with significant leg edema or morbid obesity because of the inability of the ultrasound beam to adequately penetrate the tissues and to visualize the veins. Any equivocal findings on ultrasonography should be confirmed with contrast venography. When venography is not available or is contraindicated because of medical reasons (e.g., allergy to the contrast material, renal failure), serial ultrasonography is recommended. This requires the patient to return to the ultrasound department for one or two repeated ultrasound examinations during the next 5 to 10 days. Serial ultrasonography will help detect potential proximal extension of a calf thrombus if one is missed on initial presentation. Proximal extension into the larger veins of the leg may occur in 20% to 30% of patients who present with isolated calf vein thrombosis. Untreated calf vein thrombosis may spontaneously resolve in 20% of cases and is considered to be less significant in terms of the risk of clinically important sequelae.[16]

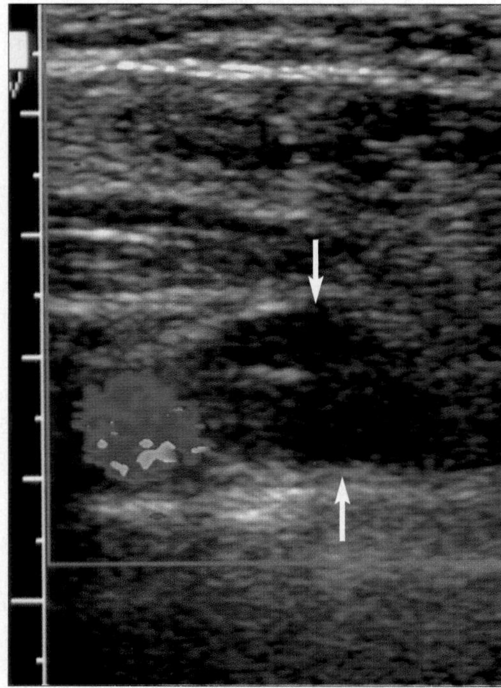

Figure 14.6 Doppler ultrasound appearance of deep venous thrombosis. The superficial femoral vein is filled with echogenic material representing thrombus, and no flow can be identified in the vein on Doppler evaluation. Flow can be identified in the adjacent artery on color Doppler evaluation *(arrows)*.

Venography is more reliable than ultrasonography in detecting smaller thrombi in the calf veins, but it is an invasive study that requires the injection of iodinated contrast material into a small vein in the foot and visualization of the venous flow by fluoroscopy. An intraluminal filling defect on two or more views is considered diagnostic of acute deep venous thrombosis. Other findings, such as nonfilling of veins and abrupt cutoff of contrast dye, are less reliable as diagnostic criteria. Phlebitis or allergic reactions to the contrast material occur in up to 2% of patients. The examination is uncomfortable for patients and is technically demanding. Many centers do not have the expertise to perform adequate venography. The contrast load is also contraindicated in patients with renal insufficiency or severe congestive heart failure.

Magnetic resonance imaging has a limited role for diagnosis of acute deep venous thrombosis but is a valuable tool in detecting cerebral venous thrombosis.[17,18] Its ability to differentiate old versus new thrombus on the basis of signal characteristics of the thrombus is also an advantage over ultrasonography. This feature is particularly important for diagnosis of recurrent deep venous thrombosis, which remains difficult to diagnose by ultrasonography and venography. Acute thrombi are usually hypoechoic and expand the caliber of the vessel on ultrasonography. As the thrombus matures, it usually contracts and becomes more echogenic. However, these criteria are difficult to apply in individual patients and are unreliable in diagnosis of recurrent thrombosis, especially in patients without previous studies for comparison. Contrast-enhanced computed tomographic scanning of the lower extremities has been used to detect deep venous thrombosis in combination with scanning of the chest for pulmonary emboli. There are reports exhibiting the high accuracy of this double imaging technique used in patients thought to have acute pulmonary embolism.[19,20] However, critics have pointed to the large dose of radiation from this approach and the limited accuracy of the venous imaging portion. Venography is considered the current standard for diagnosis of recurrent deep venous thrombosis, but it is limited by availability and the expertise required to perform the test and to interpret the findings.

D-dimer testing is a useful tool to exclude acute deep venous thrombosis.[21] D-dimer assays were developed about 2 decades ago to measure this degradation product of cross-linked fibrin. D-dimers are generated when a thrombus undergoes physiologic breakdown through the process of fibrinolysis. To date, many different assays have been evaluated for their accuracy in diagnosis of deep venous thrombosis, but not all are clinically useful.[21,22] Currently, all D-dimer assays are based on enzyme-linked immunosorbent assay, latex agglutination, or whole blood red cell agglutination techniques. The enzyme-linked immunosorbent assays provide quantitative results and have a sensitivity of more than 95% but a specificity of 30% or less. New-generation quantitative latex agglutination assays have comparable sensitivities and marginally higher specificities. The whole blood red cell agglutination assay has a sensitivity of about 85% and specificity ranging from 30% to 60%.[22] Older latex agglutination tests are not useful for diagnosis of deep venous thrombosis because of poor sensitivity and low specificity, but they are reasonable for crude measurements of D-dimer, as in cases of disseminated intravascular coagulopathy. The lack of specificity of D-dimer testing is due to the elevation of D-dimer levels in nonthrombotic situations, such as infection, inflammation, pregnancy, and malignant disease. In general, a positive D-dimer test result is not useful because the test lacks specificity, whereas a negative result helps exclude acute deep venous thrombosis in selected clinical situations. However, the results of D-dimer assays should not be used alone in the assessment of suspected deep venous thrombosis.

Because of the lack of specificity of the D-dimer testing, it should be used only in conjunction with another diagnostic test or a validated clinical prediction rule. Management studies have shown that it is safe to withhold anticoagulant therapy in patients with a negative D-dimer assay result in combination with either a normal finding on ultrasound examination or a low probability of deep venous thrombosis.[23] The likelihood for development of deep venous thrombosis in such patients during the next 3 months is less than 2%. Therefore, the appropriate use of D-dimer testing can reduce the need for ultrasound examinations to investigate patients with a suspected first episode of deep venous thrombosis.

By the combination of clinical assessment with the available technologies, deep venous thrombosis can be reliably diagnosed in almost all patients on initial presentation.[24,25] A reasonable diagnostic strategy for suspected lower extremity deep venous thrombosis is shown in Figure 14.7. Although this strategy simplifies the diagnostic process and reduces the cost associated with investigations, it does not replace the physician's clinical judgment, which should be appropriately exercised in all cases.

Superficial Thrombophlebitis

Superficial thrombophlebitis is mainly diagnosed on the basis of the clinical examination. A palpable red and tender cord representing the thrombosed vessel is characteristic.

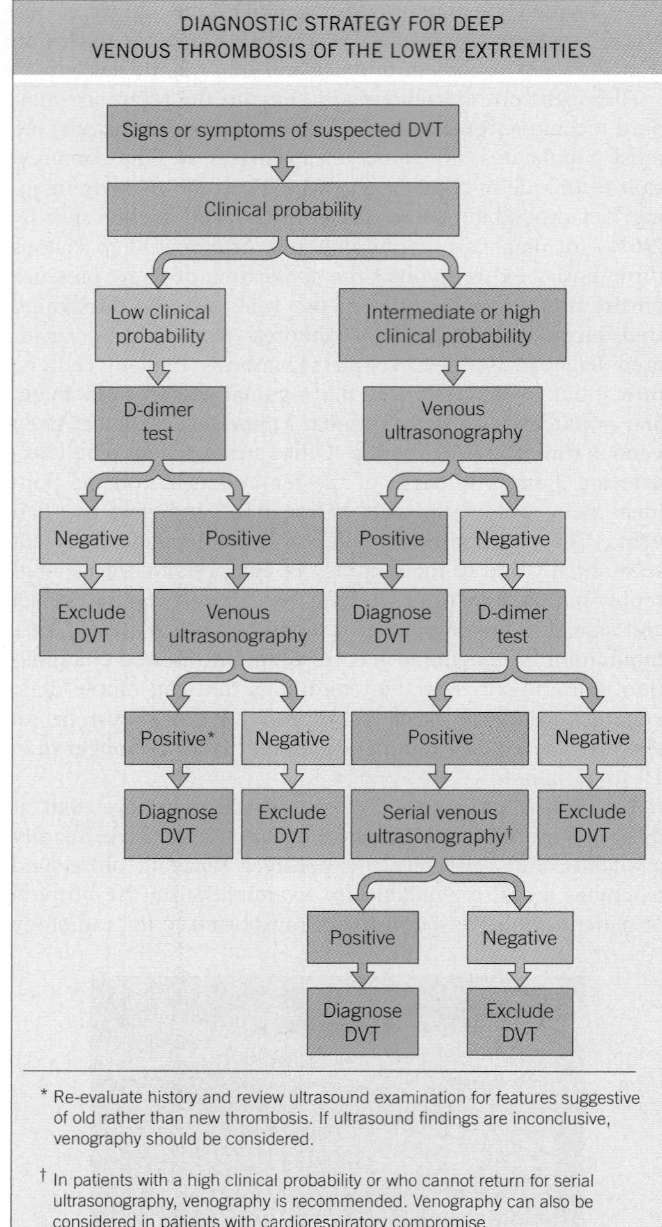

Figure 14.7 Diagnostic strategy for deep venous thrombosis (DVT) of the lower extremities.

Confirmation can be obtained with venous ultrasonography. Thrombosis is detected with the same ultrasound criteria as are used for deep venous thrombosis.

Venous Insufficiency

The sine qua non of venous insufficiency is incompetent venous valves. In patients with varicose veins, the incompetent valves are in the superficial veins, resulting in reflux and venous stasis of these small vessels. In patients with deep venous thrombosis, damage to the valves may result in the development of postphlebitic syndrome.

Doppler ultrasonography is the test of choice to identify the presence and location of refluxing venous segments. Retrograde flow of blood in superficial, communicating, and deep veins can readily be identified, particularly with color Doppler study. Venous reflux of more than 0.5 second is considered abnormal.[26]

Other studies that aid in the diagnosis of venous insufficiency include photoplethysmography and direct measurements of venous pressure, which is typically elevated in this condition. Photoplethysmography relies on color changes to assess refilling rates of small skin veins after exercise. These rates are substantially reduced in patients who have significant venous insufficiency. Direct venous pressure measurements require the placement of a small needle with a pressure transducer in a vein in the foot.

Veins of the Upper Extremities

As it is for lower extremity deep venous thrombosis, venous ultrasonography is the favored initial screening test; contrast venography remains the reference standard for diagnosis of deep venous thrombosis of the upper limbs. However, because the proximal sections of the subclavian and innominate veins are poorly visualized and cannot be compressed under the clavicle, ultrasonography is not as accurate in this setting compared with detection of deep venous thrombosis of the legs.[27] In patients with central venous catheters or pacemaker wires, visualization of the entire vein may also be obscured. Large thrombi are usually identified, but small thrombi can be missed (Fig. 14.8). Use of dampening or absence of Doppler signals alone as the criterion for diagnosis of deep venous thrombosis is unreliable because extrinsic venous compression from central masses or strictures can produce the same results. Therefore, contrast venography should be used if the ultrasound findings are equivocal and the clinical features are compatible with upper extremity thrombosis.

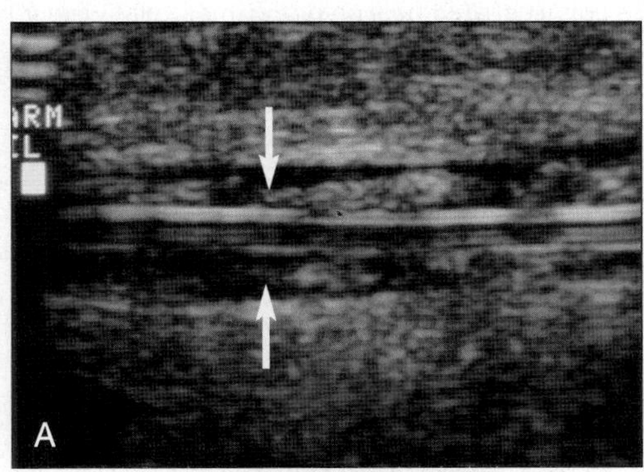

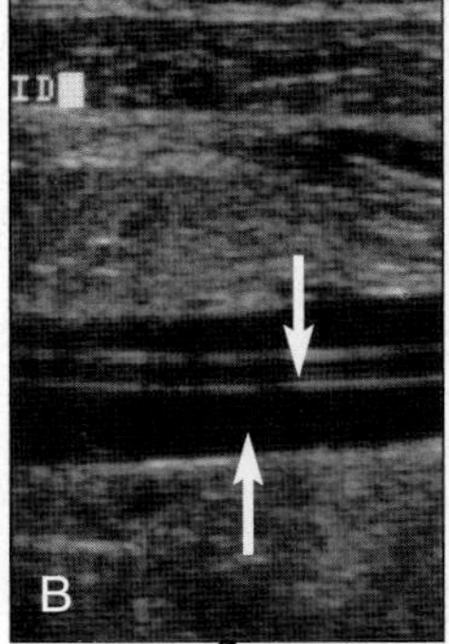

Figure 14.8 Thrombus surrounding a central venous catheter. This 29-year-old man with Crohn's disease presented with arm swelling. **A,** Echogenic thrombus *(arrows)* surrounding the catheter in the basilic vein. **B,** The catheter can be seen to extend more proximally through the subclavian vein into the superior vena cava. No thrombus surrounds the more proximal portion of the catheter *(arrows)* in the subclavian vein.

Central Veins

Inferior Vena Cava Thrombosis

Doppler ultrasonography can diagnose venous thrombosis in the inferior vena cava or the iliac veins in the pelvis either directly by visualizing the thrombus or indirectly by detecting dampening of the Doppler spectrum in the common femoral veins in the legs. Visualization of the inferior vena cava and iliac veins is sometimes difficult because of their greater depth and overlying bowel gas, which frequently blocks the ultrasound beam. Obstruction of the hepatic veins or the adjacent inferior vena cava (Budd-Chiari syndrome) can be easily identified by ultrasound examination because the liver frequently serves as a good acoustic window in transmitting the ultrasound beam.

Computed tomography and magnetic resonance imaging are other alternative studies that can demonstrate masses and thrombosis that obstruct either the pelvic veins or the inferior vena cava. Contrast agents are required in these tests to help delineate thrombus from surrounding soft tissue structures.

Superior Vena Cava Thrombosis

Doppler ultrasonography can be used initially to diagnose superior vena cava obstruction. Central thrombus extending into the subclavian or more distal vessels can be readily detected. However, isolated central thrombi in the superior vena cava and other conditions obstructing central venous return (e.g., masses or fibrosis) are not well visualized by ultrasonography because the bony thorax blocks the ultrasound beam.

The normal variations that occur from transmitted pressure changes related to respiration and atrial contractions may be reduced or completely eliminated. In most instances, contrast-enhanced computed tomography is the test of choice in investigating a patient with symptoms of superior vena cava syndrome (Fig. 14.9). This study can detect thrombosis in the central vasculature and may also provide an

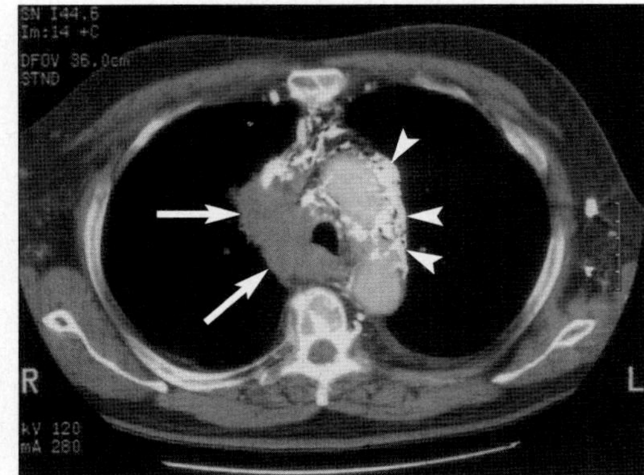

Figure 14.9 Obstruction of the superior vena cava caused by mediastinal adenopathy. In this 55-year-old man with lung carcinoma, a lymph node mass *(arrows)* is obstructing the superior vena cava. Multiple collateral vessels are demonstrated *(arrowheads)*.

alternative diagnosis for the symptoms of venous congestion (e.g., bronchogenic carcinoma).

Magnetic resonance imaging is also being used to evaluate conditions that obstruct the central veins within the thorax. It can demonstrate venous patency as well as identify thrombi, masses, strictures, or fibrosis, which can obstruct the veins. Intravascular contrast agents are useful in differentiating thrombus from other pathologic processes. Magnetic resonance imaging can also be useful in patients who are not able to receive iodinated contrast media because of severe allergic-type reactions or renal insufficiency. However, patients who receive gadolinium-based contrast agents can also have allergic-type reactions, particularly if they have been demonstrated to have a previous allergic reaction to iodinated contrast material. Pacemakers and many types of cerebral aneurysm clips preclude patients from undergoing this test.

A reasonable diagnostic imaging strategy for suspected deep venous thrombosis in the upper extremity, neck, or superior vena cava is shown in Figure 14.10.

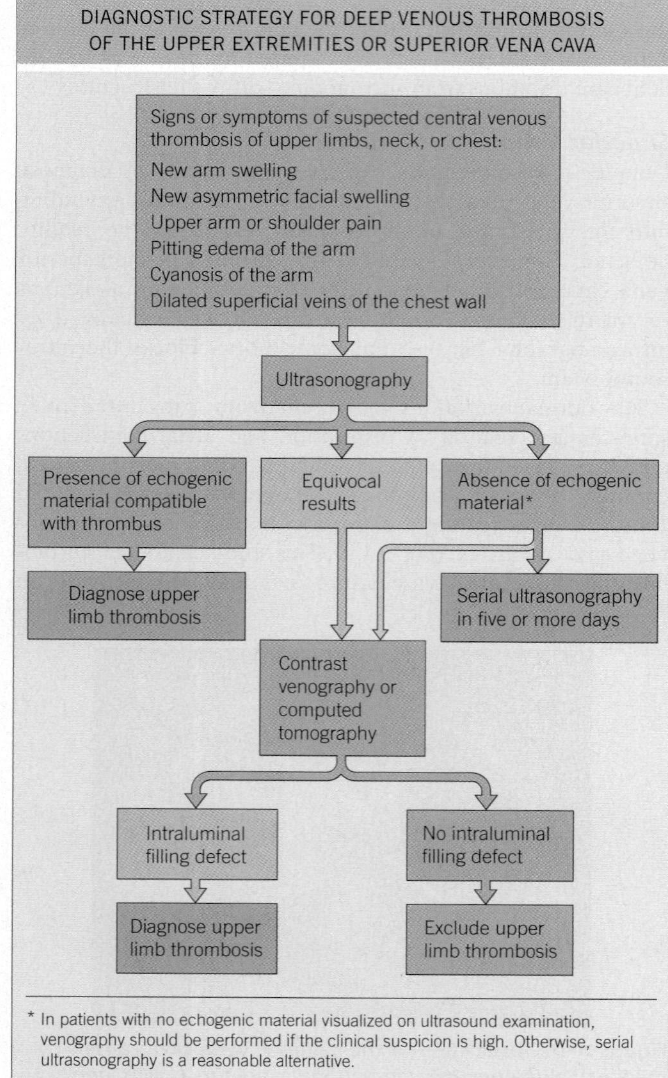

Figure 14.10 Diagnostic strategy for deep venous thrombosis of the upper extremities or superior vena cava.

MANAGEMENT

Veins of the Lower Extremities

Deep Venous Thrombosis

The most effective way of reducing the frequency of venous thrombosis is to use prophylaxis in appropriate clinical situations. Low-, moderate-, and high-risk situations can be identified on the basis of the patient's inherent risk of venous thromboembolism and the external factors that can heighten the risk of thrombosis (see Tables 14.1 and 14.2). In high-risk situations, up to 50% to 60% of the patients may develop venous thromboembolism, and approximately 2% to 4% of them will experience fatal pulmonary embolism.[28] Although prophylaxis is effective in reducing the risk by 50% to 80%, a substantial number of patients with high risk will still develop deep venous thrombosis. The options for prophylaxis are mechanical (e.g., compression stockings, pneumatic compression devices) and pharmacologic (e.g., subcutaneous unfractionated or low-molecular-weight heparin). The decision to use either or both mechanical and chemical prophylaxis should take into consideration the patient's risk factors for bleeding and the ability of the patient to tolerate lower extremity compression. Table 14.5 outlines the general recommendations for prophylaxis in various medical and surgical settings.[28] Prophylaxis should be continued as

GENERAL RECOMMENDATIONS FOR PROPHYLAXIS OF DEEP VENOUS THROMBOSIS
General medical disorders
Low-dose unfractionated heparin or low-molecular-weight heparin
Elastic compression stockings may be added to pharmacologic agents
Acute spinal cord injury
Low-molecular-weight heparin
If anticoagulation is contraindicated, intermittent pneumatic compression with elastic compression stockings
General surgery
Early ambulation
For low- or moderate-risk surgery, low-dose unfractionated heparin or low-molecular-weight heparin
For high-risk surgery (e.g., cancer), low-molecular-weight heparin
For patients with active or a high risk of bleeding, intermittent pneumatic compression
Orthopedic surgery
For total hip replacement: warfarin, low-molecular-weight heparin, fondaparinux, or adjusted-dose unfractionated heparin
For total knee replacement: warfarin, low-molecular-weight heparin, fondaparinux, or intermittent pneumatic compression
For hip fracture: warfarin, low-molecular-weight heparin, or fondaparinux
Neurosurgery
Intermittent pneumatic compression or low-molecular-weight heparin with elastic stockings

Table 14.5 General recommendations for prophylaxis of deep venous thrombosis.

long as the patient remains at risk for thrombosis, and studies suggest that prophylaxis should be extended beyond hospital discharge in certain populations of patients, such as those having hip replacement or cancer surgery.

The standard treatment of symptomatic deep venous thrombosis is systemic anticoagulant therapy with a heparin followed by a coumarin derivative.[29,30] Many new anticoagulants are being developed, and some have the potential to replace traditional agents.[31] In the past decade, the use of low-molecular-weight heparins has largely replaced the traditional standard of unfractionated heparin for the initial treatment of venous thromboembolism, and more recently, a synthetic, indirect activated factor X inhibitor, fondaparinux, was shown to be comparable to heparins for initial treatment.[32,33] In comparison with unfractionated heparin, low-molecular-weight heparins and fondaparinux have more predictable anticoagulant effects, require no laboratory monitoring, can be given subcutaneously, and are associated with a lower risk of heparin-induced thrombocytopenia. Large meta-analyses have also shown that unmonitored, weight-adjusted subcutaneous low-molecular-weight heparin is safer and more effective than unfractionated heparin administered by continuous infusion guided by laboratory monitoring of the activated partial thromboplastin time.[34] Low-molecular-weight heparins and fondaparinux also have the advantage of being available on an outpatient basis, thereby improving the patient's general quality of life and leading to substantial cost savings by reducing hospitalization.

Once a diagnosis of deep venous thrombosis has been confirmed, a low-molecular-weight heparin can be started with weight-based dosing. Laboratory monitoring is not required routinely, but it is recommended in patients with renal insufficiency, with morbid obesity, or who are pregnant. The peak anti-Xa levels at 3 to 4 hours after an injection should be measured in these patients because the pharmacokinetics and pharmacodynamics of these drugs have not been well studied in these special populations of patients. Similarly, the distribution and clearance of these drugs may be different in patients who have extensive iliofemoral deep venous thrombosis or who are hemodynamically unstable because of accompanying pulmonary emboli. These patients require hospitalization and are usually treated with unfractionated heparin. Unfractionated heparin should be given as an initial bolus followed by a continuous intravenous infusion. A weight-based or standard nomogram should be used to adjust the dose of unfractionated heparin according to the activated partial thromboplastin time to ensure that therapeutic levels are reached as soon as possible and are maintained.[35] Like low-molecular-weight heparins, fondaparinux is given subcutaneously once daily in doses adjusted for the patient's weight, and it is cleared by the renal route. Unlike the heparins, fondaparinux can cross the placental barrier; it has been used in pregnant women with heparin hypersensitivity, but the safety data are very limited. These parenteral agents should be given for a minimum of 5 days in patients with uncomplicated thrombosis and for 7 days or longer in those who have extensive disease. These agents must also be continued until the anticoagulant level achieved by the coumarin derivative is therapeutic for at least 2 days.

Oral anticoagulant therapy with use of a coumarin derivative or vitamin K antagonist is usually given within 24 to 48 hours of starting a heparin or fondaparinux. In North America, the most common agent used is warfarin. Because of the narrow therapeutic window, the anticoagulant response must be measured and monitored on a regular basis to adjust the warfarin dose to maintain therapeutic levels.[36] An international normalized ratio of 2.0 to 3.0 is considered the acceptable therapeutic range for oral anticoagulation in deep venous thrombosis. The ratio is calculated on the basis of the measured prothrombin time and the sensitivity of the specific reagent used to measure the prolonged clotting time. This standardization of the prothrombin time measurement allows direct comparisons of results from different laboratories.

Low-molecular-weight heparin is now the preferred therapy for initial and long-term treatment of deep venous thrombosis and pulmonary embolism in patients with cancer.[37,38] It is more efficacious than the traditional regimen with heparin followed by a coumarin derivative and does not require laboratory monitoring.

The optimal duration of anticoagulation after an episode of deep venous thrombosis is dependent on a number of factors. Clinical trials have shown that a minimum of 3 months is required, but longer periods of anticoagulation are recommended for patients with ongoing risk factors, such as active cancer, or who have had previous episodes of thrombosis.[39,40] Continuing vitamin K antagonist therapy is highly effective and will reduce the risk of recurrent thrombosis by more than 80%, but this is accompanied by a risk of major bleeding of 1% to 12% per year. Therefore, the decision to continue or to stop anticoagulant therapy should be based on the risk of recurrent thrombosis versus the risk of major, serious bleeding in each individual patient. Preliminary data have suggested that D-dimer levels may be useful in stratifying patients into different risk groups for recurrent thrombosis.[41] Some general recommendations for the duration of therapy are outlined in Table 14.6.

Second-line therapies for acute treatment of deep venous thrombosis include thrombolytic therapy and inferior vena cava filter placement. Unfortunately, the efficacy and safety of these modalities have not been sufficiently investigated in clinical trials. Catheter-directed or systemic thrombolysis to treat extensive proximal lower extremity deep venous thrombosis has been advocated by some, particularly if the thrombus extends into the iliac veins in the pelvis. Although there is evidence that radiographic thrombus resolution is accelerated by thrombolytic therapy, significant improvement in clinical recovery or a reduction in the risk of postphlebitic syndrome has not been demonstrated.[42] Furthermore, the risk of major bleeding, especially intracranial bleeding, is approximately 2% in patients who receive thrombolysis.[43] A recent randomized trial comparing unfractionated heparin alone with different thrombolysis regimens showed venographic improvement with thrombolysis but a substantially higher rate of major bleeding and pulmonary embolism.[44] Clearly, risk assessment tools are necessary to identify those patients who may benefit from thrombolysis. Limited evidence is available for the use of inferior vena cava filters. A multicenter, randomized clinical trial demonstrated that inferior vena cava filters can reduce the risk of early pulmonary embolism in patients with proximal deep venous thrombosis who were also treated with anticoagulant therapy; but after 2 years, this benefit was lost, and the patients who received a filter were more likely to develop recurrent deep venous thrombosis.[45] Furthermore, there was no difference in the long-term mortality between patients with a filter and those without. On the basis of current evidence, the insertion of an inferior vena cava filter should be reserved for settings in which anticoagulation is contraindicated.[46,47] One possible approach to provide early protection against pulmonary embolism without increasing the risk of recurrent deep venous thrombosis is to use a temporary or retrievable filter. Further studies are required to evaluate this potential option.

Venous Insufficiency

Graduated compression stockings remain the first line of treatment for venous insufficiency. Although frequently useful for reducing swelling and providing pain relief, stockings do not address the underlying problem of valvular insufficiency. Compliance also tends to be poor because of cost, unattractiveness, and difficulty with putting the stockings on. In patients who are not responsive to conservative measures, more invasive treatment methods are available. In patients who have venous insufficiency that is isolated to the superficial system, the injection of sclerosing agents into the involved veins may be beneficial in mild cases. More extensive reflux can be dealt with by stripping, if possible, all of the incompetent veins. Laparoscopic techniques have now been developed as an alternative to open surgical methods in suitable patients.[48] These measures to deal with reflux of the superficial veins are not successful if there is also reflux of the deep veins. Simply stripping or sclerosing the refluxing superficial venous segments can exacerbate limb swelling by eliminating collateral pathways. Several surgical techniques are available for reflux of the deep veins, including direct repair of the valves and transposition of venous segments with competent valves. Success rates are disappointing. Patients with skin ulcerations are treated with local wound care. Skin grafting and plastic surgery may be required in severe cases.

Superficial Thrombophlebitis

Superficial thrombophlebitis, without accompanying deep venous thrombosis, usually does not require treatment with systemic anticoagulation. Warm compresses, nonsteroidal anti-inflammatory agents, and leg elevation are usually effective methods of providing symptomatic relief. Patients who do not respond to these conservative measures will usually respond rapidly to a short course of subcutaneous unfractionated or low-molecular-weight heparin therapy.[49] Recurrent or refractory cases should prompt the physician to look for an underlying cause, such as malignant disease or inherited thrombophilia.

Veins of the Upper Extremities

Deep Venous Thrombosis

Very little research has been done to study the optimal treatment for deep venous thrombosis of the upper extremities. For patients with either primary (or effort-related) thrombosis or catheter-related thrombosis of the subclavian or axillary vein, conventional treatment consists of initial therapy with either low-molecular-weight or unfractionated heparin, followed by long-term oral anticoagulant therapy.[50] Anticoagulation should be continued for a minimum of 3 months, longer if a catheter remains in place. As it is for lower extremity deep venous thrombosis, the use of thrombolysis or other more aggressive interventions is controversial.

Many vascular surgeons consider catheter-directed thrombolysis to be the preferred initial treatment of selected patients with primary upper extremity deep venous thrombosis. The risk of recurrent thrombosis and postphlebitic syndrome may be reduced, but long-term evidence to support this is lacking. Post-lysis venography may allow better visualization of the involved anatomy to test for positional, extrinsic venous compression at the thoracic outlet, thereby facilitating plans for more aggressive intervention, if indicated. Venous angioplasty and subsequent stenting can correct underlying strictures, although surgical decompression has been found to be necessary to maintain long-term venous patency in patients with significant thoracic outlet obstruction.

Catheter-related thrombosis should be treated conservatively with anticoagulant therapy. Removal of the catheter is not necessary and has not been shown to improve outcomes. If the catheter is functioning, routine use should continue. If the catheter is blocked, patency sometimes returns after a few days of anticoagulation, and the catheter can

GENERAL RECOMMENDATIONS FOR THE DURATION OF ANTICOAGULATION FOR DEEP VENOUS THROMBOSIS

Patient Characteristics Associated with Thrombotic Event	Risk of Recurrence	Duration of Anticoagulant Therapy
Reversible major risk factor (major surgery, pelvic or leg trauma, major medical illness)	<5% per year	3 months
Weak risk factor (estrogen use, long-distance travel, minor trauma) and no inherited or acquired thrombophilia identified	5%-10% per year	3-6 months
Unprovoked thrombotic event with no inherited or acquired thrombophilia identified Unprovoked thrombotic event with heterozygous factor V Leiden or prothrombin G20210A mutation	~10% per year	3-6 months*
Recurrent unprovoked events with or without thrombophilic state identified Unprovoked thrombotic event with antithrombin, protein C, or protein S deficiency; homozygous factor V Leiden; double heterozygosity; antiphospholipid antibody syndrome; advanced malignant disease	>10% per year	Extended or indefinite therapy*

*May consider longer duration of therapy on the basis of the patient's preference and risk of bleeding.

Table 14.6 General recommendations for the duration of anticoagulation for deep venous thrombosis.

be salvaged for use. Previously, prophylaxis with low-dose warfarin was recommended, but more studies have shown that low-dose anticoagulant prophylaxis with either warfarin or low-molecular-weight heparin is not effective.

Central Veins

Thrombosis of the inferior or superior vena cava requires systemic anticoagulation to prevent clinically significant pulmonary emboli and to relieve venous obstruction. Interventional radiologic techniques can be used to instill thrombolytic agents directly into the thrombi in certain patient subsets. This may result in faster lysis of thrombi and control of local symptoms. In patients who cannot tolerate anticoagulant therapy, placement of a vena caval filter is indicated because of the high incidence of pulmonary embolism.

PROGNOSIS

Prognosis depends on the etiology of the venous disease. Overall, anticoagulant therapy is effective in treating uncomplicated deep venous thrombosis of the upper or lower extremities. The most common complications are pulmonary embolism, recurrent deep venous thrombosis, and postphlebitic syndrome. Pulmonary embolism occurs in 40% of patients who present with deep venous thrombosis, but most of these cases are asymptomatic, and treatment does not differ. The risk of recurrent thrombosis after a 3-month course of anticoagulant therapy is approximately 2% to 5% per year in patients with provoked or secondary deep venous thrombosis and 10% to 15% per year in those with idiopathic thrombosis. About 5% of the recurrent thrombotic events are fatal. Postphlebitic syndrome occurs in up to 50% of patients, but the majority of the cases are mild and manageable with conservative treatment. Anticoagulant-related bleeding must also be considered in patients receiving long-term anticoagulation. The risk of major bleeding is approximately 1% to 3% per year, but it varies considerably, depending on a number of patient-related factors. Approximately 20% of all major bleeding events are fatal.

Patients with poor prognosis after an episode of deep venous thrombosis are those with underlying malignant disease or aggressive thrombophilia (e.g., antiphospholipid antibody syndrome). Cancer patients have a substantial risk of recurrent thrombosis despite conventional anticoagulation with heparin and vitamin K antagonist therapy. These patients also have a higher risk of bleeding due to thrombocytopenia, invasive procedures, and other comorbid conditions. Low-molecular-weight heparins are more effective and probably safer than vitamin K antagonist therapy in patients with cancer. Although extended or indefinite anticoagulant therapy is generally recommended in patients with metastatic disease, quality of life and life expectancy are important issues to consider in deciding on how long to treat these patients with anticoagulant therapy. Indefinite anticoagulant therapy may also be indicated in some patients with symptomatic antiphospholipid antibody syndrome. Some of these patients are also resistant to conventional anticoagulant therapy, and a combination of antithrombotic and antiplatelet agents may be necessary to prevent recurrent thrombotic events.

SUMMARY

Venous thromboembolism is the most common disease affecting the veins. It affects approximately 0.1% of persons per year, and the incidence rises dramatically with increasing age. The basic pathophysiologic process involves perturbation of the hemostatic balance to favor thrombosis. This can result from venous stasis, vessel wall damage or endothelial dysfunction, or hypercoagulability from excessive activation of the coagulation pathway. Although many patients develop deep venous thrombosis in the presence of risk factors, deep venous thrombosis can also occur without obvious provocation. Some of the patients with idiopathic thrombosis have an inherited or acquired thrombophilic condition, whereas the remainder have no identifiable biochemical or genetic abnormality. Many noninvasive methods are now available to diagnose deep venous thrombosis, but contrast venography remains the reference standard. Compression ultrasonography is the initial test of choice in evaluating a patient with suspected deep venous thrombosis of the extremities, but equivocal or conflicting results require further confirmatory testing. The cornerstone of deep venous thrombosis prevention and treatment is systemic anticoagulant therapy, which is highly effective but somewhat burdensome. To reduce the incidence of thrombosis, prophylaxis should be used in appropriate medical and surgical settings. In patients with confirmed deep venous thrombosis, outpatient low-molecular-weight heparin therapy is the initial treatment of choice, but these agents must be given as subcutaneous injections. Long-term therapy with a vitamin K antagonist is needed to prevent recurrent thrombosis, but laboratory monitoring is necessary to ensure adequate anticoagulant levels and to minimize the risk of bleeding. Monotherapy with low-molecular-weight heparin is preferred to vitamin K antagonists in patients with cancer. The long-term prognosis of most patients with venous thrombosis is favorable, provided the diagnosis is accurate and adequate treatment is instituted without significant delay. Serious morbidity and mortality can result from misdiagnosis, delayed treatment, or treatment-related complications.

chapter 15

Surgery for Vascular Disease

Henrik Sillesen

Surgery is indicated or necessary only for a minority of patients with manifestations of vascular disease. The majority of patients, even those who are symptomatic, may be managed by lifestyle changes and medical therapy. Therefore, the vascular physician sees many more patients than are eventually treated by either endovascular or open surgery. In the author's institution, there are almost 6000 outpatient visits for 1100 procedures annually.

Surgery for vascular disease is performed to treat symptoms (intermittent claudication, rest pain, ischemic ulcers, abdominal angina), to prevent strokes (carotid disease), to prevent amputation (critical limb ischemia), or to save the life of the patient (to prevent death from ruptured abdominal aortic aneurysm). In asymptomatic patients with atherosclerotic disease, surgery may be performed to prevent stroke (asymptomatic carotid disease) or death from a ruptured abdominal aortic aneurysm or to treat severe hypertension (renal artery disease).

In common for all vascular operations are the following facts:

- The operation does *not* cure the underlying disease.
- There is considerable comorbidity in the majority of cases.
- For many procedures, the rate of complications is considerable.
- Many patients are not managed properly with respect to medical therapy and changes in lifestyle.

Surgery for vascular disease has evolved dramatically during the last 25 years. In Denmark, the number of procedures has increased sixfold in this period. Interestingly, endovascular therapy was developed for peripheral arterial disease more than 40 years ago, and today approximately 25% to 50% of procedures employ this technique. In contrast, it was much later that endovascular techniques were undertaken for treatment of coronary artery disease, for which the majority of patients are managed today by percutaneous coronary intervention.

There are a number of reasons for this considerable difference. First, the length of the lesions responsible for chronic lower limb ischemia is often 20 to 30 cm in addition to tandem lesions. Second, flow is low in the resting state, which for most patients is the majority of the time. These conditions predispose to treatment failure; even primary failure to pass the lesion with a guide wire is not uncommon.

Vascular surgery was among the first surgical specialties to have level I and level II evidence to guide management decisions. Endarterectomy for carotid stenosis became evidence based in 1991, and resection of abdominal aortic aneurysm was later shown to be beneficial. A number of trials have demonstrated the value of other procedures; however, newer trials have shown that not all procedures benefit patients because of the major comorbidity in some of these patients. More recently, some (including this author) have questioned the validity of older trials comparing best medical treatment with medical treatment plus surgery. The trials showing the benefit of carotid endarterectomy randomized patients 20 years ago (before the use of statins, today's antihypertensive drugs, and newer antiplatelet agents); thus, "best medical" treatment has developed tremendously since then and most certainly provides much greater prevention compared with medical treatment at that time (see later discussion).

Owing to the limitations of a chapter on surgery for vascular disease in a cardiology textbook, this chapter focuses on the main three areas covering more than 90% of surgery for arterial vascular disease: peripheral arterial disease, aortic aneurysms, and carotid disease (Fig. 15.1). Surgical management of mesenteric artery and renovascular disease is also covered. A short section on management of acute deep venous thrombosis is also included.

PERIPHERAL ARTERIAL DISEASE

Peripheral arterial disease, like atherosclerosis in other vascular beds, is a chronic condition that develops during decades. On average, symptoms from the lower limbs develop 5 to 10 years later than from the coronary circulation. Acute ischemia may develop because of thrombosis in a vessel with preexisting atherosclerotic plaques or stenosis, be due to embolism (i.e., from mural thrombus in the heart or an arterial lesion upstream), or be a result of trauma.

Peripheral arterial disease is traditionally divided into four stages (Fontaine):

- asymptomatic: ankle-brachial index (ABI) <0.9;
- functional pain (claudication);
- rest pain; and
- nonhealing ulcers or gangrene.

INCIDENCE

In the most recent population-based studies in western Europe, the incidence of symptomatic peripheral arterial disease is 3% to 4% among 60- to 65-year-olds, increasing to

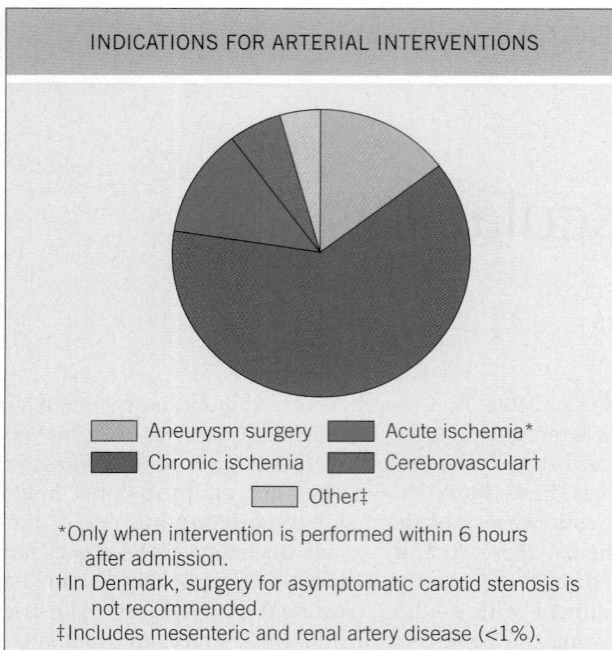

Figure 15.1 Indications for arterial interventions.

15% to 20% in persons 85 to 90 years of age.[1-3] Similar findings have been reported in the United States. Looking at asymptomatic cases (ABI <0.9), the incidence is much higher, approximately 20% of all persons older than 65 years, ranging from 10% in persons 60 to 65 years old to almost 50% of those 85 to 90 years old.[1-3]

Critical limb ischemia, defined as ABI of less than 0.4, rest pain, or nonhealing ulcers, occurs in 1% of persons aged 65 years or older.

PATHOPHYSIOLOGY

The asymptomatic stage is especially interesting because it is associated with an approximately threefold increased mortality compared with matched controls,[4,5] yet the condition can be identified by a simple test: measurement of ankle blood pressure. This test takes only a few minutes and is expressed as the ABI, whereby the ankle pressure is divided by the highest of the two arm blood pressures. In this manner, variations in blood pressure between measurements do not influence the test result. Not only is an ABI below 0.9 associated with increased mortality from cardiovascular causes, but also the level of ABI reduction is predictive: the lower the ABI, the worse the prognosis.[4]

Identification of an asymptomatic person with an ABI of less than 0.9 is not a case for evaluation with respect to revascularization of the lower limbs but a case for preventive cardiovascular medicine.

Claudication is experienced by the patient as pain in lower limb muscles appearing after walking, most often in the calf, the thigh, and more rarely the buttocks. The walking distance eliciting the pain is variable (e.g., beginning after 10 to 15 meters in severe cases, whereas other patients will report pain only when walking fast uphill for 500 meters). It is important for both the patient and the treating physician to understand that claudication, although it may be incapacitating for a few and troublesome for many, signals severe vascular disease systemically and that cardiovascular morbidity and mortality are high (elevated three to five times compared with matched controls).

Rest pain typically begins at night when the patient is in the horizontal position. The positive effect of gravity on lower limb perfusion is then abolished. The patient typically complains about pain in the toes or feet during the night, and most have experienced that standing or sitting up relieves the pain. Many patients will sleep sitting in a chair.

Nonhealing ulcers often begin after minor trauma (e.g., hitting a toe against a chair or by wearing shoes that are too small). In some cases, the ulcers develop without any trauma, and those will often progress to gangrene if they are not treated. Ischemic ulcers develop on toes or on the foot, typically at points where shoes are in firm contact. Thus, they are usually easy to discriminate from venous ulcers, which are located at the level of the ankles or lower calf.

Rest pain, nonhealing ulcers, and gangrene are often referred to as critical ischemia.

PROGNOSIS

The risk of amputation is only 1% to 2% at 5 years. Twenty-five percent of claudicants will experience a worsening of their symptoms from the lower legs; however, 75% will be unchanged or improve without revascularization.[6] In contrast, the "systemic" risk is huge. Mortality in 5 years will be 15% to 25%, and many more will suffer nonfatal myocardial infarction and stroke.

TREATMENT

Treatment of patients with intermittent claudication therefore involves two aspects:

- treatment of symptoms from the lower limb, and
- prevention of cardiovascular complications.

The treatment of symptoms includes lifestyle modification, medical therapy, and interventional therapy by either percutaneous transluminal angioplasty (PTA) or open surgery. The prevention of cardiovascular complications includes lifestyle modification and preventive medical therapy.

It is outside the scope of this chapter to go into detail on all aspects of lifestyle modification and preventive medical therapy. It is, however, extremely important for the reader to understand that patients with peripheral arterial disease derive as much benefit, or more, from lifestyle modification and aggressive preventive medical therapy as any other group of patients does. In this chapter, only details of lifestyle modification and medical therapy important to how and when PTA and surgery are indicated are mentioned.

Treatment of Symptoms from the Lower Limb

Most patients should be managed without PTA or surgery. Because the risk of cardiovascular complications is much higher than the risk of amputation, the main focus should be on preventive measures to halt the atherosclerotic process.

Exercise therapy has proved effective for improvement of walking distance, and regular exercise for 3 months can be expected to improve walking distance by 200% to 250%.[7] Exercise also reduces cardiovascular morbidity and mortality, and it cannot be stressed enough (for both the patient and the physician) that this is extremely important. Because the effect on walking distance is so good, and because it is important for survival, exercise therapy should be tried before interventional treatment is considered. There are only a few exceptions in which interventional treatment may be considered early: patients with very short walking distance not able to carry out important daily responsibilities such as their work and, of course, patients at risk of amputation.

The dilemma of explaining to the patient that the symptoms being experienced from the lower limb are signaling high cardiovascular risk rather than lower limb risk is very challenging. First, there is (or has been) a general perception that atherosclerosis in the limb is less dangerous than in other locations. The author hopes that the introductory remarks in this chapter change this potential misperception for the reader.

Medical therapy for claudication includes cilostazol and statins. Treatment with both may be expected to improve walking distance by 30% to 50%, and the statins furthermore reduce the cardiovascular risk. Other drugs have not proved useful with respect to significant improvement in walking distance.

Interventional Therapy

Interventional treatment (endovascular or open surgery) for peripheral arterial disease is indicated when

1. exercise and other lifestyle modifications have failed to improve symptoms to an acceptable state;
2. claudication is incapacitating; and
3. critical limb ischemia is present (rest pain, nonhealing ulcers, or gangrene).

The choice between PTA and open surgical management depends on the location and extent of disease. In general, endovascular treatment can be expected to perform well in cases of shorter lesions, whereas surgery is preferred in case of extensive occlusive disease. Obviously, whenever comparable results can be obtained, PTA is preferred for the simple reason that it is less invasive and associated with fewer complications compared with open arterial reconstructions. In patients with severe comorbidity that might complicate the outcome of open surgery, PTA is preferred, even though surgery theoretically would be the treatment of choice if only patency of the revascularization procedure were considered.

The arterial lesions causing obstruction of blood supply to the lower limb are most often located in the distal abdominal aorta just proximal to the aorta-iliac bifurcation, in the common iliac arteries, and in the common and superficial femoral arteries. The arteries in the calf, the anterior and posterior tibial and the peroneal arteries, are often involved in cases with critical ischemia and in diabetics. In general, when patients suffering diabetes present with symptoms, they have a more distal involvement (i.e., open vessels to the level of the popliteal artery and then occlusive disease of the calf vessels and sometimes also of the arteries in the foot). Because all reconstructions yield better results with respect to patency the more centrally located the lesions, this explains the worse results of revascularization for diabetics with toe or foot ulcers.

Percutaneous Transluminal Angioplasty

PTA can in principle be performed anywhere between the heart and the feet. The more centrally located the lesions being treated, the better the results, especially with PTA. Also, the shorter the stenosis or occlusion, the better the results, and stenting improves patency in most cases. Endovascular-treated common iliac arteries, as an example, remain patent in 60% to 80% of cases after 5 years, and thereafter they may often be redilated. Primary stenting has become the preferred treatment in most cases. Obviously, because complications are rare and this procedure is associated with the best results, the tendency to offer PTA for iliac artery obstruction is greater than for occlusive disease more peripherally located.

PTA of the common femoral artery may be performed when the superficial femoral artery is occluded from the origin and runoff is only in the profound femoral artery. Otherwise, the risk of causing damage to the femoral bifurcation mandates that these lesions be treated by endarterectomy, as described later. PTA of the superficial femoral artery (Fig. 15.2) may relieve symptoms, but the results depend on the extent of disease. The longer the lesion, the worse is the prognosis. Stenting appears to improve patency, at least for longer lesions (Table 15.1).[8] When the indication for PTA is claudication, patency is superior compared with the indication of critical ischemia. This difference, of course, relates to the more extensive nature of the disease in the case of critical limb ischemia and maybe also to the poor runoff vessels. The 3-year patency is 48%, which may be improved to 64% if stenting is added. In the case of critical limb ischemia, the results at 3 years show a patency of 30% without stenting and 63% with stenting (see Table 15.1).[8]

PTA of crural vessels is also feasible; however, the long-term results are not good. Data on limb salvage with PTA of crural vessels alone are scarce.

Another endovascular technique for treatment of long superficial femoral artery occlusions is that of subintimal angioplasty. Here, the guide wire intentionally is manipulated into the subintimal space, where a new lumen is created. Re-entry is attempted distal to the occlusion. Results for limb salvage have been reported to be excellent from a few centers,[9] whereas others have had less impressive experience.[10]

Adjunctive medical therapy to improve patency after PTA and stenting with anticoagulation or antiplatelet therapy has been tested in only a few trials. Antiplatelet drugs improve patency, and the combination of aspirin and clopidogrel may be beneficial.[11]

Open Surgical Revascularization

Open surgical revascularization still dominates as the choice of treatment in cases of critical limb ischemia because of the extensive nature of the atherosclerotic lesions in these patients. For claudication, open surgical treatment is rarely performed; however, for extensive disease of the distal aorta and iliac arteries, the aortobifemoral bypass remains the

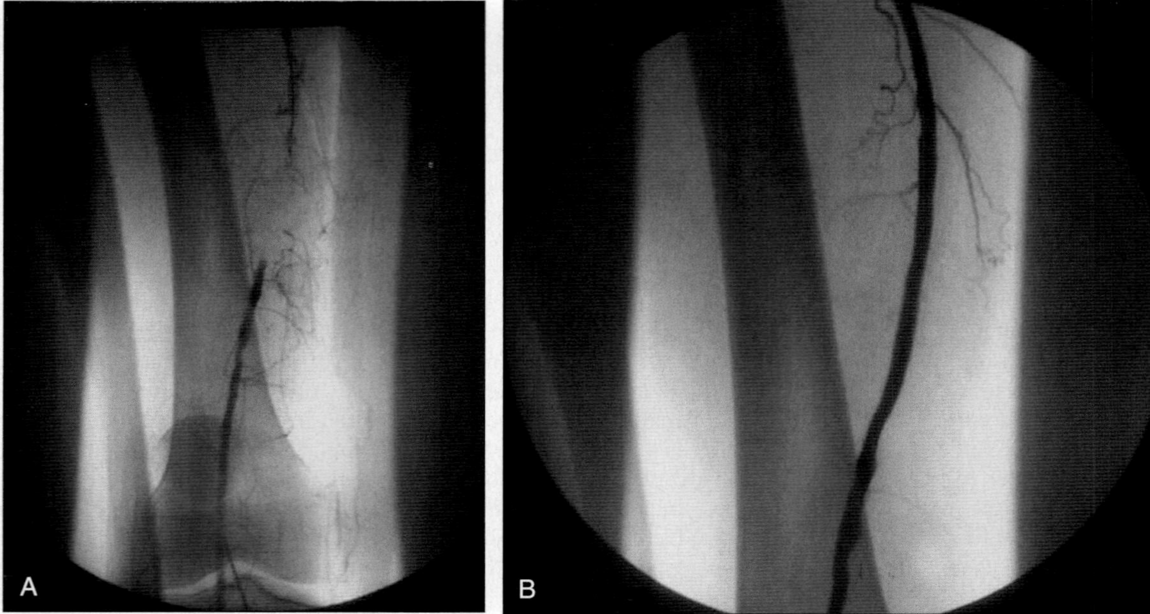

Figure 15.2 **Short occlusion of the superficial femoral artery (A) treated with PTA and stenting (B).**

POOLED PATENCY OF ENDOVASCULAR PROCEDURES (TASC II)

	1 year (%)	3 years (%)	5 years (%)
Iliac artery	86	82	71
Femoropopliteal stenosis: PTA	77	61	55
Femoropopliteal occlusion: PTA	65	48	42
Femoropopliteal stenosis: PTA + stent	75	66	
Femoropopliteal occlusion: PTA + stent	73	64	

Inter-Society Consensus for the Management of Peripheral Arterial Disease (TASC).
PTA, percutaneous transluminal angioplasty.

Table 15.1 Pooled patency of endovascular procedures (TASC II).

procedure with the best long-term outcome. Endarterectomy, as described later, may also be an option for treatment of claudication. Only one trial has compared open surgery with endovascular treatment of critical limb ischemia, the Bypass versus Angioplasty in Severe Ischemia of the Leg (BASIL) trial. The primary efficacy parameter was amputation-free survival, but because approximately two thirds of the endpoints were deaths, only one third of the endpoints really determined which procedure was best. Within 6 months postoperatively, there was no difference in the primary endpoint, but thereafter bypass patients seemed to do better.[12]

In general, two surgical techniques are used: endarterectomy and bypass. Endarterectomy is performed by separating the intima from the media, and in this manner the atherosclerotic lesion can be removed. Endarterectomy can be used in cases with severely occlusive lesions of limited anatomic extension (Fig. 15.3), such as severe atherosclerosis around the aortic bifurcation, in the external iliac, or in the common femoral artery. The advantage of this technique is that it often can be performed without the use of artificial graft material, and patency is excellent. However, in the case of smaller arteries (i.e., the femoral or carotid), a patch may be inserted when the arteriotomy is sewn (Fig. 15.4).

Bypass is preferred when the obstructive or occlusive lesions are extensive, for example, total superficial femoral artery occlusion or multiple serial lesions warranting a femoral-crural bypass (Fig. 15.5). Bypass surgery can be performed with artificial materials or with autologous veins. For bypass of aortic or iliac artery origin, artificial grafts are almost always used. This is because there is no easily removable vein with similar dimensions that can be used in these locations. Dacron or polytetrafluoroethylene (PTFE) grafts also perform very well in the aortoiliac-femoral

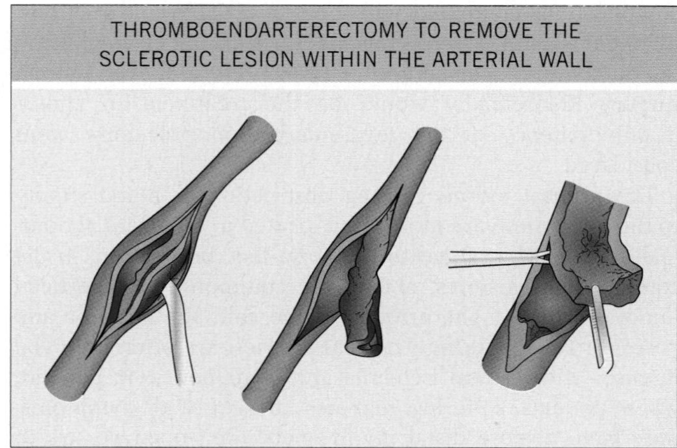

Figure 15.3 **Thromboendarterectomy to remove an atherosclerotic lesion from within the arterial wall.**

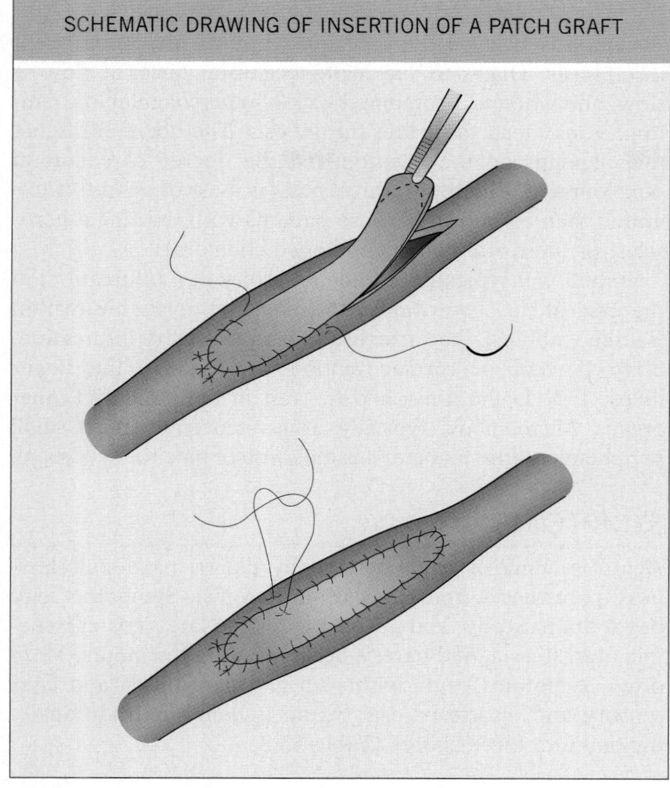

Figure 15.4 Insertion of a patch graft.

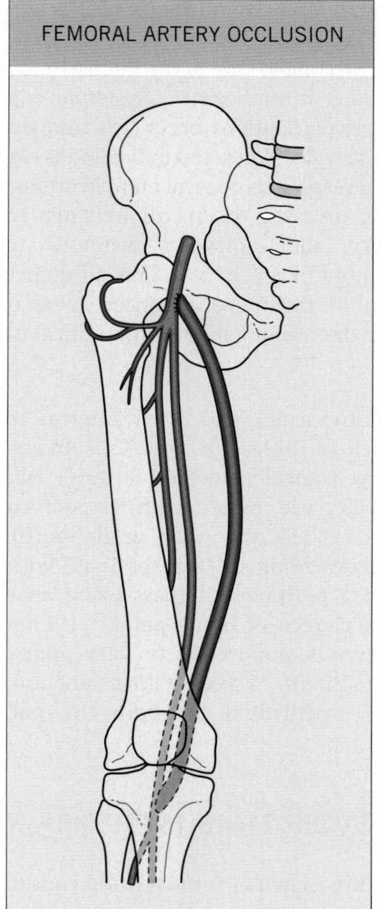

Figure 15.5 Long superficial femoral artery occlusion treated with femoropopliteal bypass.

region. For peripheral bypasses, typically originating from the common femoral artery, autologous vein grafts are preferred for two reasons: they last longer (much better patency), and they carry less risk of infection (Table 15.2). For longer bypasses, such as from the common femoral to the popliteal artery below the knee, a saphenous bypass is performed, leaving the vein in situ. This means that the vein is left in its original anatomic location, but proximally and distally anastomosed to the arterial system. The venous valves are cut with a knife mounted on a catheter, and side branches are occluded. In this manner, the vein retains its nervous innervations and native vascularization.

Complications

Complications of endovascular treatment relate mainly to the site of puncture and the risk of peripheral embolization. "Systemic" cardiovascular complications are rare. Hematoma in the access groin is common; however, it only rarely requires that any action be taken. Development of an iatrogenic pseudoaneurysm is seen in 0.5% to 1% of cases and can easily be treated with ultrasound-guided compression or ultrasound-guided thrombin injection.

Complications of open surgical treatment can be divided into local and systemic categories. The local complications relate to the actual incisions and dissections, including wound healing and infections. Whereas complications due to accidental damage to other organs or structures are very rare, wound healing problems and infections are unfortunately common. Especially, surgery on the lower limb involving the groin and peripheral incisions may have wound complications in 10% to 20% of cases (hematoma, lymph oozing, or necrosis of the wound).[13] Infections are seen in 3% to 5% of cases, approximately one third involving the vascular reconstruction. Infection of the vascular reconstruction is more frequent when artificial graft material is used.[13]

POOLED PATENCY OF BYPASS PROCEDURES (TASC II)

	5 years (%)	10 years (%)
Aortobifemoral		
Limb based	91	86
Patient based	85	79
Femorofemoral crossover		75
Femoropopliteal vein		80*
Femoropopliteal PTFE		30-75*

Inter-Society Consensus for the Management of Peripheral Arterial Disease (TASC).
*Secondary patency.

Table 15.2 Pooled patency of bypass procedures (TASC II).

Systemic complications to open surgical revascularization relate to the surgical trauma and to the stress response. In vascular reconstructions involving the aorta and other central arteries, the cardiopulmonary complication rate is considerable. Implantation of an aortobifemoral bypass graft is associated with a 30-day mortality of 2% to 5% and a rate of "general" complications of 10% to 15% (pulmonary, cardiac, renal; prolonged stay in the intensive care unit; stroke; and deep venous thrombosis).[13] Systemic complications to peripheral revascularizations occur less frequently; however, they are considerable. When the indication is claudication, the morbidity with respect to general complications is low, 2% to 4%; however, in cases of critical ischemia and peripheral bypass surgery, the morbidity increases to 10% with a 30-day mortality of 3% to 5%. This difference in morbidity is a reflection of the more advanced level of generalized atherosclerotic disease in patients with critical ischemia.

Results

Results of endovascular and open surgical reconstructions are summarized in Tables 15.1 and 15.2. In general, in treatment of more centrally located arterial obstruction, the long-term results are better with respect to patency. In peripheral reconstructions, vein grafts perform better. It may seem unrewarding to treat patients with critical limb ischemia with a peripheral bypass using an artificial graft having a 50% chance of being patent at 1 year. However, if the alternative is amputation or very poor quality of life (i.e., severe rest pain), 1 year with a functioning graft may very well be worthwhile for both the patient and the surgeon.

ACUTE LOWER LIMB ISCHEMIA

Acute lower limb ischemia is most often caused by thrombosis in existing atherosclerosis, that is, a patient with previous symptoms of chronic peripheral arterial disease. Another common cause is thrombosis of a popliteal aneurysm.

Embolism remains a common cause, although not as often as in the past as a result of better anticoagulant therapy for patients with atrial fibrillation. Eighty percent of emboli are of cardiac origin; however, aneurysms of the aorta or peripheral aneurysms may give rise to peripheral emboli.

Other causes include trauma and iatrogenic lesions (e.g., from arteriography with puncture of the femoral artery). Aortic dissection may cause lower limb ischemia as well as acute deep venous thrombosis (phlegmasia cerulea dolens).

The incidence in western Europe is 300 to 400 per million per year.

PATHOPHYSIOLOGY

Thrombosis is caused by plaque rupture and subsequent thrombosis. Distal to the acute occlusion, arterial flow is slow, and when it is combined with a hypercoagulable condition, it may lead to further thrombosis. The degree of ischemia depends on the location and the degree of collateral development. Therefore, thrombosis is most often better tolerated than embolism because patients with existing atherosclerosis most often have developed collaterals.

Emboli will typically occlude an artery at a bifurcation; in the case of the lower limbs, this is at the aortic bifurcation (saddle embolus), iliac artery, and femoral artery bifurcation. Sixty percent of cardiac emboli will end in the lower limbs, 15% in the arms, and the rest in the brain and other organs. Microemboli, typically from aneurysms, affect small peripheral arteries and are thus the cause of blue toe syndrome.

SYMPTOMS

Acute ischemia is characterized by pallor, pain, pulselessness, paresthesia, and paresis (the five *p*'s). Symptoms may begin dramatically, and in some cases the late signs of ischemia, paresthesia, and paresis occur within a few hours. More often, symptoms begin with pain and paresthesia and later sensory and muscle paresis. Acute ischemia is traditionally divided into three classes (Table 15.3).

DIAGNOSIS

Diagnosis is often easy with typical clinical signs. ABI will be low, if it is measurable at all. Duplex ultrasonography, magnetic resonance imaging, or digital subtraction angiography is possible but may delay treatment. In the case of thrombosis, it is most often desirable to perform arteriography with subsequent thrombolysis to visualize the underlying pathologic process causing the thrombosis.

PROGNOSIS

If revascularization is possible before irreversible ischemia has occurred, the limb can be salvaged and normal function regained. Comorbidity is high in the case of acute ischemia. When acute revascularization is needed, the procedure-related mortality is 10% to 20% due to release of toxic substances from ischemic tissue combined with existing cardiac disease.

SEPARATION OF THREATENED FROM VIABLE EXTREMITIES

		Findings		Doppler Signals	
Category	**Description and Prognosis**	**Sensory Loss**	**Muscle Weakness**	**Arterial**	**Venous**
I. Viable	Not immediately threatened	None	None	Audible	Audible
II. Threatened					
a. Marginal	Salvageable if promptly treated	Minimal (toes) or none	None	(Often) inaudible	Audible
b. Immediate	Salvageable with immediate revascularization	More than toes, associated with rest pain	Mild, moderate	(Usually) inaudible	Audible
III. Irreversible	Major tissue loss or permanent nerve damage inevitable	Profound, anesthetic	Profound, paralysis (rigor)	Inaudible	Inaudible

Table 15.3 Separation of threatened from viable extremities.

TREATMENT

Thrombosis in existing atherosclerotic lesions may be treated by endovascular or open surgery. Endovascular repair is preferred if revascularization is not imminent. By catheter-directed, intra-arterial thrombolysis, the underlying atherosclerotic lesions will be exposed and may in some cases be treated by PTA or stenting. In other cases, bypass surgery may be needed. Inoperable cases may be converted into operable cases by thrombolysis because distal thrombosis most often makes surgery (and PTA) useless when there are no runoff vessels. However, another advantage of thrombolysis is that emergency surgery is converted into a less urgent intervention.

Emboli can be treated by embolectomy by insertion of a balloon catheter in the femoral or popliteal artery and retraction of the emboli after the balloon is inflated. Some cases of embolism may also be treated by thrombolysis.

PREVENTION

Arterial emboli have a high recurrence rate, so if possible, the underlying case should be treated—corrective treatment for atrial fibrillation and resection or exclusion of aneurysms. If the source of the embolism cannot be eliminated, anticoagulation must be considered.

ATHEROSCLEROSIS OF RENAL AND MESENTERIC ARTERIES

Renal artery obstruction may cause severe hypertension and renal failure, and interventional treatment may improve both conditions. Today, open surgical management is only rarely performed because endovascular management is much less invasive and is feasible in the majority of cases. Open surgery, thromboendarterectomy or bypass, is performed when renal artery disease is combined with other disease, such as aortic occlusion or abdominal aortic aneurysm.

Mesenteric artery occlusive disease may cause abdominal angina. Just like atherosclerotic lesions in other locations, many cases are asymptomatic and probably do not need intervention with regard to the obstructive disease. However, lifestyle changes and medical preventive treatment are indicated.

Patients with classic symptoms, postprandial pain occurring 10 to 20 minutes after a meal and weight loss, often benefit from revascularization. However, many patients have less obvious symptoms, and the mere co-occurrence of a lesion on one of the three main vessels supplying blood to the gastrointestinal tract (celiac trunk, superior and inferior mesenteric artery) does not warrant interventional treatment. In general, a single lesion in one of the three arteries is seldom thought to be able to cause ischemia.

Diagnosis is possible by ultrasound examination of the suprarenal vessels in most cases. Otherwise, computed tomographic or magnetic resonance angiography or digital subtraction angiography may be needed.

Interventional treatment today is mainly balloon angioplasty and stenting. Long occlusions of the superior mesenteric artery or occlusive mesenteric disease combined with other disease of the aorta may be treated by open surgery (i.e., aortomesenteric bypass).

ISCHEMIA OF THE ARMS

Atherosclerosis and ischemia of the arm are much less common than in the lower limb.

The most common location for development of atherosclerosis in the arteries supplying the upper extremity is in the brachiocephalic trunk and subclavian arteries central for the origin of the vertebral arteries. Rarely, occlusive lesions are located more peripherally in the subclavian or axillary arteries. Takayasu's vasculitis may also cause upper extremity ischemia.

Typical symptoms of chronic arm ischemia include "claudication," that is, pain when the arm is used. In typical cases, pain is encountered on performing tasks with the arms elevated, such as hanging laundry, or other physical use of the arm. Critical ischemia with rest pain or gangrene is rare but may occur.

Diagnosis is easy with lack of pulses at palpation. Measurement of bilateral blood pressure and ultrasound examination may locate and quantitate the stenotic lesion. If blood pressure cannot be measured by auscultation, a Doppler device may be used as for measurement of ankle blood pressure. In addition, or in the case of severe ischemia, finger pressure may be measured by strain-gauge technique. Upper arm evaluation by computed tomographic or magnetic resonance angiography or digital subtraction angiography may be supplemental.

The prognosis is often good because development of critical ischemia with the necessity for amputation is rare. Vasculitis should be suspected in patients with finger gangrene.

Treatment of upper extremity atherosclerosis is similar to that of atherosclerosis in other vascular distributions: risk factor reduction by lifestyle changes and preventive medications for all, and revascularization for some. In fact, only rarely is interventional treatment indicated; however, in case of incapacitating functional pain or critical ischemia, revascularization should be considered. Endovascular treatment dominates because of its less invasive nature for lesions near the origin of the brachiocephalic trunk and subclavian arteries. For lesions that cannot be treated by endovascular techniques, such as long lesions or lesions that cannot be crossed by a guide wire, bypass surgery is indicated (carotid-subclavian bypass). Peripheral bypass of the upper extremity (e.g., at the level of the brachial artery) is rare, and patency is poor.

Acute arm ischemia is most often due to embolization but alternatively can be due to thrombosis in an existing stenosis, such as of the subclavian artery. Whereas the embolism may be treated easily by embolectomy through a small incision in the cubital fossa, the thrombosis may be more complex to treat, perhaps requiring intra-arterial thrombolysis before vascular reconstruction. Embolism is most often of cardiac origin, due to atrial fibrillation, mural thrombus in the heart, or valve disease. Vascular causes include a subclavian aneurysm or stenosis. Microemboli may occur peripherally and present as gangrene of one or more fingers. Obviously, eradication of the embolic source is crucial, if possible. Treatment of the peripheral ischemia may include thrombolysis; however, in most cases, collaterals develop, and amputation does not become necessary.

ABDOMINAL AORTIC ANEURYSMS

This section focuses on abdominal aortic aneurysms (AAAs). Thoracic aortic aneurysms are discussed in Chapter 11.

Aneurysm of the aorta is a common condition in the elderly, especially in the infrarenal aorta. An artery per definition becomes aneurysmal when the diameter increases more than 50% locally compared with the "normal" diameter proximal or distal to this site. In the infrarenal aorta, an aneurysm is present when the diameter exceeds 30 mm.

The prevalence of AAA is approximately 5% in men older than 70 years; however, only a minority of them will have a size that mandates surgery (diameter of more than 5 to 6 cm). In patients with other atherosclerotic manifestations, such as peripheral arterial disease or carotid disease, the incidence of AAA is two to three times greater than in persons without atherosclerotic disease. Also, there is a 2:1 ratio of AAA occurring in men compared with women. Finally, the tendency to develop AAA is partly inherited; the risk for a man with a father or brother with AAA is approximately 20%.

PATHOPHYSIOLOGY

Arteries enlarge with age, and the diameter of the infrarenal aorta is normally less than 20 mm in a 70-year-old man. If the wall weakens locally, an aneurysm develops. A true aneurysm develops when all three layers in the arterial wall are involved and dilate, as in the case of the typical infrarenal AAA. False aneurysms or pseudoaneurysms develop after iatrogenic trauma, such as by PTA or other transfemoral procedures and at arterial anastomotic sites. Dissection occurs when a rupture of the intima allows blood to enter between the layers of the artery wall.

Aortic aneurysms may rupture, leading to almost certain death. It is estimated that 80% to 90% of patients with an AAA rupture die before they get to a hospital. Ruptured AAA causes an estimated 2% to 3% of all deaths among men; the number for women is 1%.

In most AAAs, there is an atherosclerotic degeneration of the vessel wall, which dilates; however, it is unclear why atherosclerosis results in occlusive disease in some patients and in aneurysm development in others. Accelerated breakdown of elastin plays a role in AAA development. Simultaneous presence of both occlusive and aneurysmatic disease is common in many patients. Inflammatory aneurysms are present in 5% to 10% of AAAs in which the aortic wall is thickened as part of perianeurysmal or retroperitoneal fibrosis.

SYMPTOMS

Symptoms from AAA are rare, so most cases are asymptomatic. Diagnosis is often made coincidentally, as when a patient complains of slight upper gastric pain and has an ultrasound examination of the gallbladder, which discloses the AAA. Also typically, a patient may complain of back pain, and the AAA is discovered on a lumbar radiograph. Whether the patient's pain was really related to the AAA or to gallstones or to the back is often difficult to ascertain.

Some patients will sense a pulsation in the abdomen; however, large aneurysms may cause discomfort or compress surrounding organs, mainly the gastrointestinal tract. The main risk, off course, is rupture, which most often leads to immediate death when it is intraperitoneal. If rupture is into the retroperitoneal space, a hematoma may be contained, and the patient may survive for hours. Rupture and development of a hematoma lead to pain in the abdomen or back. Chronic rupture is rare because almost all cases will be fatal within hours.

Aneurysms may cause peripheral embolization. A cyanotic or gangrenous toe is the first symptom.

DIAGNOSIS

Diagnosis of AAA is easy. Ultrasonography is accurate in making the diagnosis and estimating the diameter of the aneurysm. In the few cases in which ultrasound examination is inconclusive, a primary computed tomographic scan may be necessary. Otherwise, computed tomographic or magnetic resonance scanning is performed only when the size of the AAA dictates that intervention should be considered. Arteriography is rarely performed for AAA; however, in the case of both AAA and symptoms of peripheral arterial disease, arteriography may be warranted for planning of the revascularization procedure.

Ruptured AAA should always be suspected in a patient with acute abdominal pain in preshock.

PROGNOSIS

The risk of rupture relates to the size of the aneurysm. When the diameter exceeds 6 cm, the annual risk of rupture is 10% to 20%; the risk of rupture of an AAA with a diameter of 3 to 4 cm is less than 1%. Aneurysms tend to expand; small aneurysms dilate 1 to 2 mm per year, whereas larger aneurysms may expand two to three times faster. Smoking and hypertension seem to increase the rate of growth.

Rupture is associated with 90% mortality. The survival for those who reach the hospital and have immediate surgery is approximately 50%.

TREATMENT

Treatment of AAA involves, in addition to surgery for some, the same preventive treatment that is given to other patients with atherosclerotic manifestations: lifestyle changes and medical therapy with platelet inhibitors, statins, and blood pressure control.

Treatment of ruptured AAA is always interventional (surgical or endovascular) unless the patient's overall condition is considered too poor to attempt rescue. In some cases, a fatal AAA may be a dignified death, for example, in an elderly patient suffering both end-stage renal failure and heart failure. Symptomatic, nonruptured aneurysms should be treated acutely or subacutely because of the risk of imminent rupture.

Treatment of large, asymptomatic AAAs reduces mortality.[14] Elective interventional treatment should be offered in the case of asymptomatic AAAs if the risk of rupture exceeds the risk of the procedure, if the patient is fit for the procedure and expected to have some good-quality years remaining. Because any procedure for treatment of AAA either carries a considerable perioperative risk or involves a very long postoperative period with potential reinterventions, the decision to offer interventional treatment is not always easy, and it is almost always a decision made with the patient and the patient's family.

The choice between treatment modalities is made keeping these facts in mind: open surgery is a well-proven procedure with known risks and long-term results, including an overall 3% to 5% perioperative mortality but almost no further AAA-related morbidity after the procedure. In contrast, endovascular aneurysm repair (EVAR) has been shown to have lower perioperative morbidity: 1.5% for EVAR compared with 4.5% for open surgery.[15,16] On the other hand, EVAR is still a procedure under development. The number of reinterventions due to either migration or failure of the implanted device, both leading to endoleak (blood reentering the excluded aneurysm sac, which is thereby again at risk of rupture), is 20% to 40% after 3 years. This means that most EVAR cases need to have lifelong surveillance with repeated ultrasound and computed tomographic scans. For instance, a 65-year-old man with a 6-cm AAA and no other known comorbidity should be offered treatment, preferentially open surgery, because his perioperative risk will be low (i.e., 2% to 3%), whereas the annual risk of rupture is approximately 10%. At the other end of the spectrum is the 80-year-old man with previous coronary artery bypass surgery and chronic obstructive pulmonary disease with a similar-sized AAA of 6 cm. His risk with open surgery includes more than 10% 30-day mortality in addition to a considerable risk of other complications. Endovascular treatment could be a good alternative for this patient if the patient is expected to live at least 3 to 5 years.

EVAR has been thought to be a treatment alternative for patients unfit for open surgery. The EVAR 2 trial tested the hypothesis that patients found unfit for open repair could be randomized to either conservative management or EVAR. Survival was not improved by EVAR, and it was poor in both groups; approximately 50% of patients in both groups were dead at 3 years, and only one quarter of deaths were aneurysm related.[17] Thus, being found unfit for surgery in this study indicated a poor prognosis in general that EVAR did not affect.

Open surgical treatment with resection of the aneurysm and replacement of the diseased part of aorta with an artificial graft has been performed for more than 40 years. With the aorta clamped either above or below the renal arteries and the iliac arteries similarly clamped, a Dacron or PTFE graft can be implanted either end-to-end to the aorta or as a bifurcated aorto–bi-iliac or aortobifemoral graft, depending on the condition of the iliac arteries, which are often aneurysmatic as well (Fig. 15.6). Complications of open surgical repair relate to the considerable surgical trauma of this major procedure. Cardiac, pulmonary, and renal complications dominate, and in the Danish National Vascular registry, which includes more than 99% of all procedures performed in the last 10 years, approximately 20% develop general complications, which include prolonged stay in the intensive care unit and stroke.

Endovascular treatment of AAA involves inserting a collapsed prosthesis through the femoral artery, placing it below the renal arteries, and deploying and fixing it (stenting) under radiographic guidance. The technique mostly used today involves insertion of a bifurcated graft from one femoral artery and then placement of the other limb through the contralateral femoral artery (Fig. 15.7). In some cases, the latter part of the procedure is impossible (i.e., chronic iliac artery occlusion); thus, an aorto–uni-iliac graft is supplemented by an open surgical femorofemoral crossover bypass graft (see Fig. 15.7). Complications of EVAR are few in the perioperative period, but a considerable number of patients will need repeated interventions, which in most cases can be performed by endovascular techniques. These include placement of another proximal stent as a result of endoleak, embolization of inferior mesenteric or internal iliac arteries, and more.

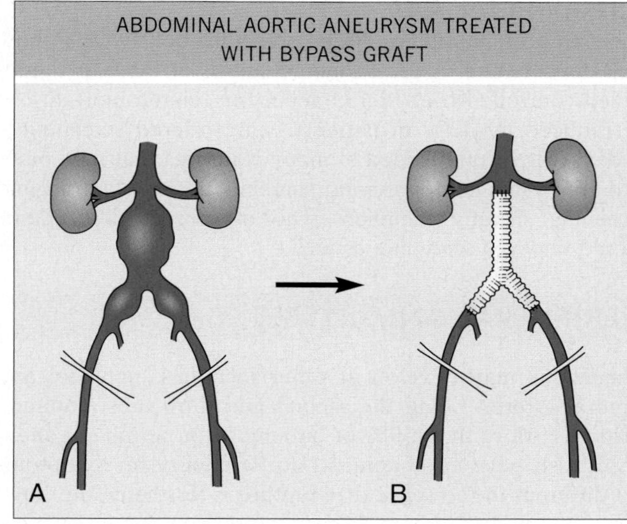

Figure 15.6 Abdominal aortic aneurysm treated by resection and implantation of aorto–bi-iliac bypass graft.

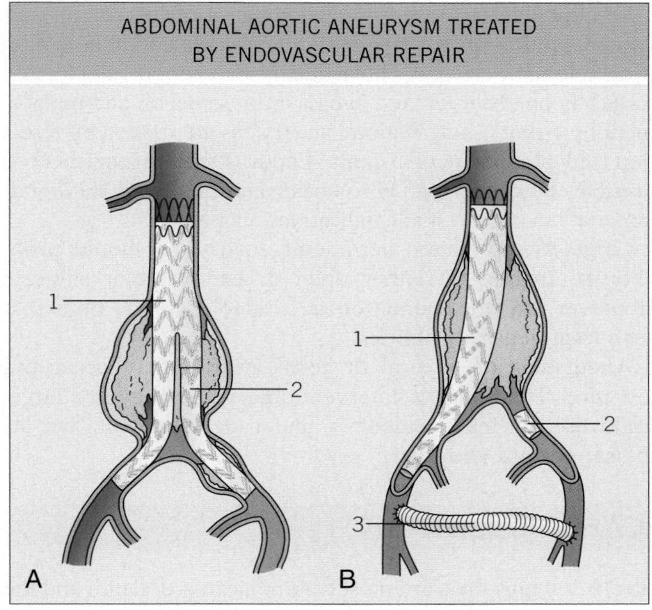

Figure 15.7 Abdominal aortic aneurysm treated by endovascular repair. A, First the bifurcated graft is inserted through the right femoral artery and fixed by stenting at the proximal and distal ends of the graft. The left limb is inserted through the left femoral artery and connected to the main graft. **B,** Insertion of an aorto–uni-iliac endograft combined with a femorofemoral bypass graft is used when one of the iliac arteries cannot be passed.

Screening for AAA

The value of population-based screening for AAA is now well documented. A recent meta-analysis of the four randomized controlled trials found aneurysm-related mortality to be reduced by 43% in patients being offered screening.[18] Today, it is recommended in many countries that men older than 65 years and previous smokers undergo ultrasound screening. Family members who are direct descendants should undergo screening as well.

PERIPHERAL ANEURYSMS

Aneurysms may develop at other locations, popliteal and femoral arteries being the second and third most common locations. More than 50% of patients with peripheral aneurysms also have an abdominal aortic aneurysm. Symptoms are different in the sense that rupture is less common; however, symptoms derived from compression (popliteal vein thrombosis, pain, and other symptoms of nerve compression), peripheral embolization, or thrombosis of the vein most often bring the patient to medical attention.

Treatment is the same as for abdominal aortic aneurysm: general prevention against atherosclerotic disease and intervention in symptomatic cases. Popliteal aneurysms are generally treated surgically by exclusion and bypass or by resection and replacement by a short graft. Femoral aneurysms are treated by resection and placement of a graft. Endovascular management is possible; however, graft thrombosis and failure of stent-graft material have so far made indications unclear.

Large asymptomatic peripheral aneurysms should probably be treated by either open or endovascular surgery. However, no documentation is available at this time that such treatment is beneficial.

Aneurysms of visceral or renal arteries may occur but are rare. Treatment is interventional when they are large. Endovascular management is under development, but its indications are unsettled.

CAROTID DISEASE

Stroke remains the third most common cause of death and the most common cause of disability, at least in the Western world. The relationship to atherosclerosis for many stroke patients is well documented, although stroke, unlike other ischemic conditions, has other common pathogenetic mechanisms. This section focuses on stroke in relation to carotid artery disease and especially prevention of stroke in these patients.

It is very important to discriminate between symptomatic disease and asymptomatic cases. Patients with recent cerebrovascular symptoms and an ipsilateral stenosis are comparable to patients with a recent acute coronary event: the risk of a new thromboembolic event is very high, and diagnostic work-up and treatment should be started immediately. The pathogenetic mechanism is very similar to that of an acute coronary event with plaque rupture and subsequent thrombosis. However, in the case of the carotid, embolization into a cerebral artery is much more common than thrombotic occlusion of the carotid artery itself. Perhaps the larger diameter of the carotid artery explains this difference.

The prevalence of carotid stenosis is high. Among patients with acute cerebrovascular symptoms, an ipsilateral stenosis of more than 50% diameter reduction is found in 15% to 20% of cases. In patients with other clinical atherosclerotic manifestations, a carotid stenosis is found in 20% to 30%.

PATHOPHYSIOLOGY AND SYMPTOMS

Refer to Chapter 10.

PROGNOSIS

The risk of stroke is increased in the presence of carotid stenosis. For asymptomatic patients with a carotid stenosis exceeding 60% diameter reduction, the annual risk of ipsilateral stroke is approximately 2%. When carotid stenosis is related to recent ipsilateral cerebral ischemic symptoms (symptomatic stenosis), the risk is much higher, especially just after the first event. The 30-day risk of stroke in patients with previous cerebrovascular symptoms is as high as 10% when an ipsilateral carotid stenosis is present. Thereafter, the risk gradually declines, and after a year, it is approximately 2% to 3% annually, similar to asymptomatic carotid stenosis. The 3-year risk of ipsilateral stroke is 25% to 30% in symptomatic patients with a stenosis greater than 70% diameter reduction.

TREATMENT

Treatment of patients with carotid stenosis is like that of any other condition related to atherosclerosis: treatment of the atherosclerotic disease itself and treatment of local manifestations. Risk factor reduction, including changes in lifestyle, is exactly the same as for patients with other clinical manifestations of atherosclerosis, although there may be regional variation in the choice of antiplatelet agents. Aggressive lipid lowering reduces both the risk of recurrent stroke and the risk of coronary events.[19]

Any intervention for carotid stenosis is performed to prevent future "local" events (stroke). Thus, the risk of the intervention itself should be weighed against the absolute risk of an event. Furthermore, the most common complication of surgery and stenting is ipsilateral stroke, the event that the procedure is supposed to prevent. Most important, the overall risk of the patient should be weighed against the absolute risk reduction derived from the procedure.

Diagnosis of carotid disease should be done with duplex ultrasound scanning (Fig. 15.8). The accuracy of the method is well documented for both identification and quantification of degree of stenosis. Many surgeons will perform endarterectomy based only on ultrasound examination.

Symptomatic patients with carotid stenosis benefit from endarterectomy when the stenosis is greater than 50% to 70% diameter reduction and neurologic symptoms are within 6 months of surgery.[20,21] The North American Symptomatic Carotid Endarterectomy Trial (NASCET) and the European Carotid Surgery Trial (ECST) randomized simultaneously, but independently, symptomatic patients with carotid stenosis to best medical treatment (at that time—see discussion later) or best medical treatment plus endarterectomy. Both trials showed significant benefit (50% relative risk reduction) in patients with greater than 70% stenosis (diameter reduction), whereas the group with 50% to 69% stenosis had only a marginal effect. Patients with stenoses of less than 50% had no benefit.[20,21]

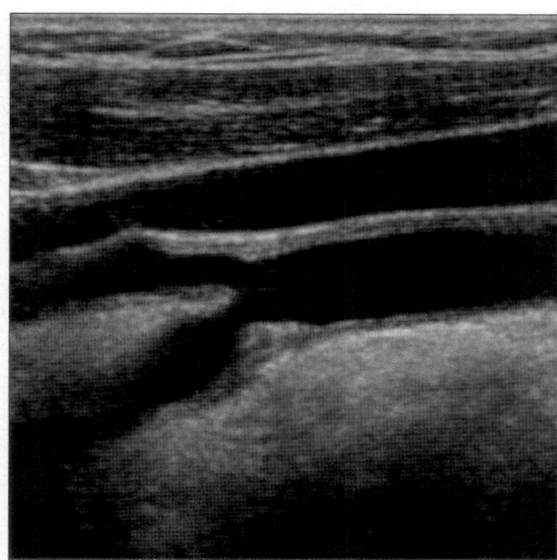

Figure 15.8 B-mode ultrasound image of carotid stenosis.

However, recent reanalysis of the pooled data from these two trials showed that the time interval between onset of neurologic symptoms and surgery was the most important predictive factor of benefit for the patient.[22] The earlier the operation, the greater the benefit. The overall absolute risk reduction of approximately 15% conveyed by endarterectomy could be doubled when patients were operated on within 2 weeks of symptoms. With the knowledge gained during the last 10 to 15 years concerning the vulnerable plaque and plaque rupture, this finding does not come as a great surprise. However, when these trials were designed, this pathogenetic mechanism of acute ischemia was unknown.

Also, sex, age, and degree of stenosis are factors that influence the benefit of surgery.[22] Male sex, older age, and severity of stenosis all increase the risk of future stroke in patients with stenosis without any increased risk of the surgical procedure; thus, the overall benefit is greater.

Asymptomatic carotid stenosis is more controversial, although two major trials have shown a small but statistically significant benefit of surgery. First, the Asymptomatic Carotid Atherosclerosis Study (ACAS) trial showed a 50% relative risk reduction of ipsilateral stroke. However, the absolute risk reduction was marginal, only 1% per year.[23] Later, the Asymptomatic Carotid Surgery Trial (ACST) reproduced these findings.[24] Taking into consideration that the average annual mortality during the trial was 3% to 4%, in addition to other ischemic events that were unaffected by the procedure, it may be questioned whether the cost-benefit is reasonable both for the patient and for society. As discussed later, the medical treatment offered during these trials was much poorer than what is recommended today; thus, the outcomes of these trials may not be reflective of the risk in these patients today.

If better criteria for selection of patients at higher risk become available, selective surgery for high-risk cases of asymptomatic carotid stenosis may yield greater or even much greater benefit.

Technical Considerations

Carotid endarterectomy may be performed in two ways: classic endarterectomy (see Fig. 15.3) or eversion endarterectomy. In eversion endarterectomy, the internal carotid artery is divided from the bifurcation, and endarterectomy is performed by everting the vessel wall, thereby removing the carotid lesion. After the stenosis has been removed, the bifurcation is reconstructed by reanastomosis of the internal carotid to the bifurcation.

Carotid endarterectomy may be performed under general or local anesthesia. Classically, general anesthesia has been preferred; however, this has carried the challenge of monitoring cerebral circulation during clamping of the carotid artery. A variety of methods have been used, including electroencephalographic monitoring, stump pressure, distal internal carotid artery pressure, evoked potentials, near-infrared spectroscopy, transcranial Doppler imaging, and more. None of these methods has proved ideal, so some surgeons use a shunt on a selective basis whenever their method for monitoring indicates risk of cerebral ischemia during clamping, whereas others use a shunt routinely. However, performing endarterectomy under local anesthesia gives the surgeon the opportunity to communicate with the patient during clamping. Having the patient awake and responsive during surgery may be the best monitoring of cerebral function during clamping. Also, local anesthesia may carry less cardiac and pulmonary risk. Smaller trials and a recent meta-analysis indicate superiority of local anesthesia; however, large trials are necessary to show a difference in a procedure with 3% to 6% risk of complications.[25] The general anesthetic versus local anesthetic for carotid surgery (GALA) trial, designed to answer this question, randomized 3526 patients to one type of anesthesia or the other between 1999 and 2007. The primary endpoint, a composite of stroke (including retinal infarction), myocardial infarction or death between randomization and 30 days after surgery, occurred in 4.8% of the general and 4.5% of the local anesthesia patients, a trend that was not statistically significant.[26]

Carotid stenting has not yet been proved in randomized clinical trials to prevent ipsilateral ischemic events. Seven randomized controlled trials have been published to compare stenting with endarterectomy; however, they have focused so far only on comparison of perioperative complications. The two most recent trials, the Endarterectomy versus Angioplasty in Patients with Symptomatic Severe Carotid Stenosis (EVA-3S) and the Stent-Protected Angioplasty versus Carotid Endarterectomy (SPACE) trials, failed to show an advantage of the less invasive carotid stenting method with respect to perioperative events. In fact, the EVA-3S trial was stopped early because of excess complications in the stenting group. A recent Cochrane meta-analysis, including all seven randomized controlled trials, favors surgery with respect to the primary outcome parameter: perioperative death and ipsilateral stroke.[27] It is, however, important to acknowledge that technology does develop rapidly, and some of the trials may have used devices or technologies that are already outdated. Similarly, there may be differences in trial design, and criticism has been raised specifically as to the training of investigators in some studies. Interestingly, stenting appears to be associated with higher complication rates when it is performed early after neurologic symptoms and in the elderly—the two strongest indications.

Finally, stenting should be evaluated in long-term studies and compared not only with endarterectomy but also with medical therapy, which has improved dramatically in the last 10 to 20 years (see discussion later).

Carotid revascularization before coronary artery bypass surgery has been practiced in some places, whereas others have not found it useful. The potential advantage is avoidance of cerebral ischemia during the relative hypotension on-pump; however, the complications of carotid revascularization have outweighed the gains, as evaluated by recent reviews.

Is the Evidence for Endarterectomy Outdated?

Three of the four major trials proving endarterectomy to be of value for symptomatic and asymptomatic surgery were performed when the only fairly constant preventive medication given was aspirin. The last trial randomized 8 to 10 years ago, and only 30% of patients were taking statins. It is stated in the design of these trials that hypertension and hypercholesterolemia were treated when present; however, in that era, the treatment goals for both hypertension and hypercholesterolemia were much more lax than they are now. Also, new drugs have been introduced and their benefit documented since these trials randomized patients: statins, newer antiplatelet agents, dual antiplatelet therapy, and newer antihypertensive drugs. It may be speculated that if these drugs were used systematically, the risk in patients with carotid stenosis would be much less, not least in those with vulnerable plaques. Therefore, new trials are needed to test if today's medical therapy compared with intervention plus best medical therapy remains inferior to surgery or stenting. New trials are *not* unethical—it is unethical not to undertake new trials.

DEEP VENOUS THROMBOSIS OF THE LOWER LIMB

Deep venous thrombosis (DVT) occurs most frequently in the lower limb and the clinical picture is variable, from no symptoms to severe swelling with intense pain and, in the worst case, amputation. The annual incidence is estimated to be 1 per 500 inhabitants in Western countries. This section is included because catheter-directed thrombolysis is a treatment modality that shows great promise in removing the thrombus and preventing post-thrombotic syndrome.

ETIOLOGY AND PATHOPHYSIOLOGY

DVT occurs during a combination of stagnant blood flow, injury to the venous vessel wall, and activation of the patient's coagulation system (Virchow's triad). The risk is especially high in the perioperative period in patients undergoing lower abdominal surgery and orthopedic surgery, in patients with low cardiac output (either after myocardial infarction or in patients with heart failure), in postpartum women, and in women taking estrogens. The risk of DVT is increased in patients with previous DVT. A number of conditions leading to hypercoagulability also increase the risk of DVT: protein C or protein S deficiency, factor V Leiden, and others.

The clinical course depends on the balance between progressive thrombosis and recanalization of the vein. The final outcome, including patency of the vein and function of venous valves, is a balance between organization of the thrombus, thrombolysis, progression of thrombosis, and rethrombosis. Venous reflux due to injured venous valves is the main mechanism that results in chronic venous hypertension leading to the post-thrombotic syndrome.

SYMPTOMS

Symptoms of DVT depend on the extent of the thrombus. The patient may be asymptomatic, but pain or swelling is common. Many patients will describe localized pain days before swelling occurred (e.g., in the groin in the case of thrombosis of the femoral vein). If the iliac vein is thrombosed, the whole leg is swollen; DVT of the distal femoral–popliteal vein causes swelling of the calf. The leg is most often red and warm, and sensory and motor functions are normal. Therefore, the condition is easy to distinguish from acute arterial obstruction.

In the worst case, the tissue perfusion can become so poor that amputation is necessary (cerulea dolens), which is rare and mainly seen in patients with malignant disease.

DIAGNOSIS

Diagnosis is made by ultrasonography or venography. D-dimer assay may exclude DVT; however, imaging is needed to locate and to evaluate the extent of the thrombosis. Thus, a D-dimer test can be used as a screening tool in patients with unilateral swelling of a leg or with unexplained pain. Finding of an elevated D-dimer level mandates imaging.

Ultrasound duplex scanning should be the method of choice. Contrast venography should be the second choice or used when ultrasound examination is inconclusive.

COMPLICATIONS AND CLINICAL COURSE

Untreated DVT may progress and spread to other venous segments. Pulmonary embolism is common (up to 50%); however, the majority of pulmonary emboli are asymptomatic. Pulmonary symptoms with dyspnea or hemoptysis are seen in some cases, and fatal embolism occurs only in 1% today. Venous gangrene may develop in the case of extensive thrombosis with so severe edema that arterial inflow is compromised.

Prospective studies have shown that already 40% of the thrombosed venous segments are recanalized after 7 days, increasing to 90% after 9 months. Rethrombosis or new DVT within 3 months is seen in 5%, even when it is treated adequately with warfarin; the rate is much higher if treatment is insufficient with too low an international normalized ratio.

Chronic venous insufficiency only rarely develops in the case of crural thrombosis, but the incidence increases the more central the DVT is. In the case of iliac vein thrombosis, approximately 50% will develop post-thrombotic syndrome after 5 to 10 years.

One third of patients with DVT remain asymptomatic, whereas two thirds will develop venous reflux within 1 year.

Secondary varicose veins are common in patients with previous DVT and may be a sign of collateral development.

TREATMENT OF ACUTE DEEP VENOUS THROMBOSIS

When DVT is suspected, low-molecular-weight heparin should be administered immediately; and when the diagnosis is confirmed, anticoagulant therapy with a vitamin K antagonist should be started. If interventional treatment is considered, anticoagulant therapy is postponed until this has been either undertaken or eliminated as an option. For details of anticoagulant therapy, refer to Chapter 145.

Anticoagulant therapy is given for 3 to 6 months to prevent further thrombosis or rethrombosis. If the patient has a coagulation disorder, such as factor V Leiden, lifelong therapy should be considered.

Thrombolytic therapy is given by catheter directed into the thrombosed vein, in most cases supplemented by balloon angioplasty and stenting after lysis is complete. Almost all fresh thrombi (<2 weeks) can be lysed. Fast recanalization preserves venous valve function by preventing destruction, and the primary success rate is high; 80% to 90% of thrombi can be lysed, and patients can be discharged with normal functioning veins.[28] Intermediate results are good; however, the long-term results are unknown. The main purpose of thrombolysis is to prevent development of post-thrombotic syndrome; thus, treatment is indicated only for central DVT (femoroiliac) and in patients with an expected survival of 10 to 15 years.

Systemic thrombolysis is obsolete today.

Venous thrombectomy has largely been replaced by catheter-directed thrombolysis because results are better and the procedure is less invasive and therefore has fewer local complications (Fig. 15.9). One of the reasons for the disappointing results of thrombectomy was probably

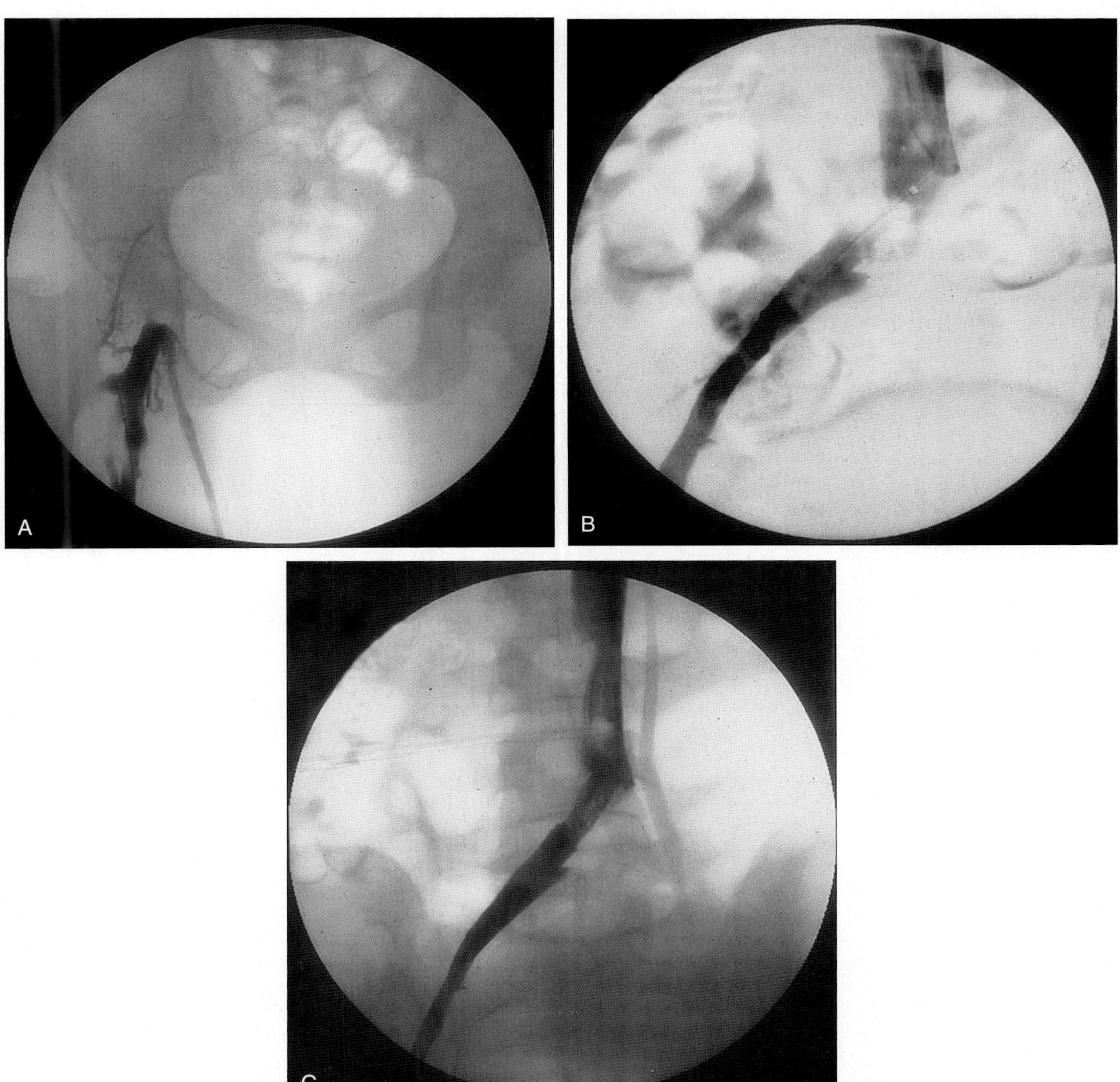

Figure 15.9 **A,** Venogram showing iliac deep venous thrombosis. **B,** After thrombolysis, the iliac vein is open, but a severe stenosis remains. **C,** After stenting of the proximal iliac vein.

that although the thrombosis could be removed, the underlying iliac vein stenosis, which is present in 50% to 70% of iliac DVT, was not corrected. Thus, the recurrence rate was suboptimal.

Pulmonary embolism may theoretically be prevented in patients with DVT by insertion of a filter in the vena cava. However, the method is used only in certain parts of the world because of the very good medical prophylaxis and lack of convincing data proving benefit.

PREVENTION

Any patient with DVT should be screened for abnormalities in the coagulation system. Prophylaxis is important in patients at risk undergoing major surgery by the use of mechanical or pharmaceutical methods, compression stockings, or low-molecular-weight heparin.

chapter 16

Special Problems in Vascular Disease

a. Compromise of an Internal Thoracic Artery to Coronary Artery Graft by Subclavian Artery Disease

Michael H. Crawford and Mark Langsfeld

DEFINITION OF PROBLEM

The internal thoracic artery is the preferred coronary artery bypass graft and conduit because of its relative resistance to atherosclerosis and its long-term maintenance of patency. However, flow in this vessel can be compromised by disease of the subclavian artery proximal to the origin of the internal thoracic artery. Because evaluation of the subclavian arteries by angiography is often not done, potential problems can develop after coronary artery bypass graft surgery because of preexisting disease, progression of preexisting minor disease, or subsequent development of subclavian atherosclerosis.

TYPICAL CASE

A 66-year-old man presented with angina pectoris associated with left arm exertion but not with right arm exertion. He had undergone coronary artery bypass graft surgery 3 years previously, with a left internal thoracic artery graft to the left anterior descending coronary artery and a vein graft to the distal right coronary artery. He had been pain free until recently. His hypertension was under treatment with beta blockers and a diuretic, but with intermittent difficulty in blood pressure control, possibly related to differences in blood pressure between his two arms. Physical examination showed blood pressure of 160/90 mm Hg in the right arm and 130/80 mm Hg in the left arm. Angiography demonstrated a 90% stenosis of the left subclavian artery proximal to the internal thoracic artery takeoff (Fig. 16A.1). The internal thoracic artery and saphenous vein grafts to the heart were patent, and there were no new native coronary artery lesions. Mild left arm exertion in the catheterization laboratory produced retrograde blood flow from the internal thoracic artery to the distal subclavian artery. At that time, the patient developed chest pain and electrocardiographic ST depression in the anterior precordial leads. The patient underwent left subclavian artery stenting with complete relief of his symptoms.

DIFFERENTIAL DIAGNOSIS

The major differential diagnostic entities in this case include progression of native coronary artery disease, vein graft disease, and technical problems with the internal thoracic artery graft. Vein graft disease is very common, especially in patients who do not control their risk factors for atherosclerosis, but it usually becomes evident later after bypass surgery. Anastomotic problems with the internal thoracic artery usually cause difficulties earlier after surgery and would be an unlikely cause in this patient. Atherosclerosis of the internal thoracic artery is quite unusual and would not be a common cause of recurrent angina after bypass surgery. The general incidence of significant subclavian stenoses found in patients undergoing cardiac catheterization is less than 5%. However, a study of patients with peripheral vascular disease who underwent a cardiac catheterization reported 18.7% of these patients with more than 50% stenosis of the left subclavian artery. Because of the excellent collateral network, lesions of the subclavian artery requiring arterial reconstruction are relatively uncommon. However, the cardiovascular physician must be aware of the potential for subclavian disease before using the internal thoracic artery for coronary revascularization. Signs and symptoms of subclavian-innominate occlusive disease include ischemic digits secondary to emboli, arm claudication, and vertebrobasilar symptoms associated with arm exercise. Measurement of bilateral upper extremity blood pressures must be performed. Patients who are thought to have subclavian disease should undergo arch aortography at the time of the cardiac catheterization. In the patient who has already undergone internal thoracic artery coronary revascularization, development of chest pain with left arm exertion and a blood pressure discrepancy of greater than 20 mm Hg are suggestive of the development of proximal subclavian artery occlusion.

TREATMENT OPTIONS

The traditional approach to subclavian artery obstruction is surgery. The intrathoracic approach involves thoracotomy and then either subclavian endarterectomy or aortosubclavian

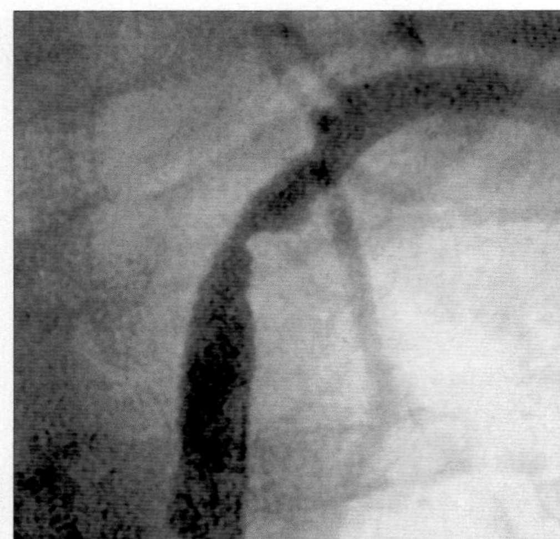

Figure 16A.1 Subclavian artery disease. Angiogram of the left subclavian artery showing the critical stenosis proximal to the origin of the internal thoracic artery.

grafting. This is a technically demanding operation, with mortality reported to be as high as 18% and morbidity up to 23%. Because of these high rates of associated mortality and morbidity, the extrathoracic approach is usually recommended. The most common extrathoracic operation is the carotid-subclavian bypass graft using a synthetic conduit (Fig. 16A.2). It is also possible in some patients to transpose the ipsilateral subclavian artery to the carotid artery, which avoids use of a synthetic conduit (Fig. 16A.3). More recently, angioplasty and stenting have been used to treat subclavian stenosis or short occlusions. Good results can be obtained with percutaneous therapy, with very low morbidity and mortality rates. Initial treatment failures and higher restenosis rates usually occur in patients with total occlusions. Percutaneous

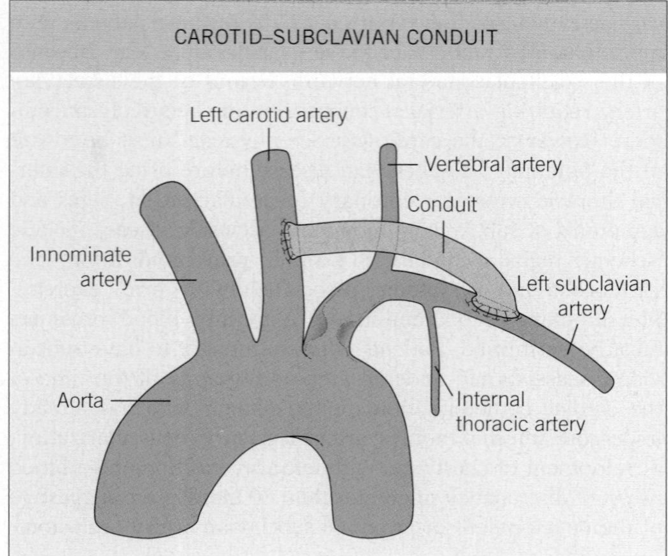

Figure 16A.2 Surgery for subclavian artery disease. Course of the carotid-subclavian conduit to bypass a critical obstruction in the left subclavian artery.

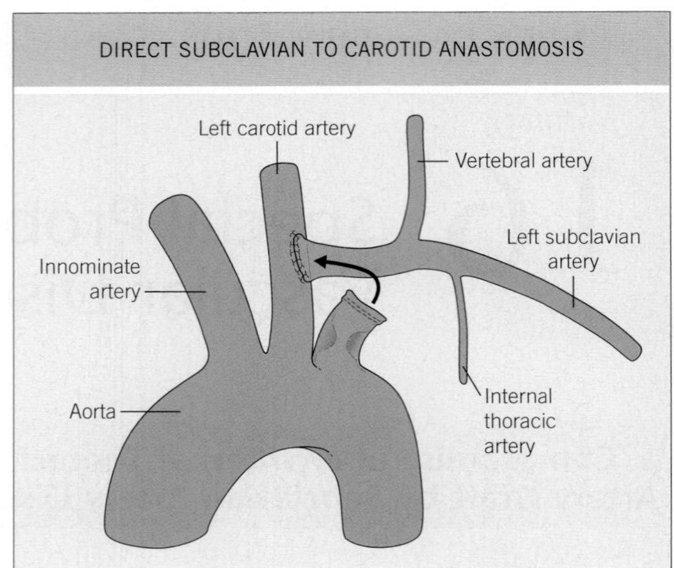

Figure 16A.3 Direct subclavian to carotid anastomosis.

treatment series report primary patency rates up to 95% at 5 years. Overall, percutaneous therapy for arch branch occlusive disease can be considered a viable initial treatment option as it has good results and does not preclude later surgical reconstruction if it is needed. The role of stent placement at the time of angioplasty has not been defined. However, most centers routinely employ stents, particularly in treating patients with total occlusions.

SUMMARY

Recurrent angina after internal thoracic artery coronary bypass surgery caused by significant proximal subclavian artery stenosis is an unusual complication of bypass surgery. Significant preoperative problems with the subclavian artery can be suspected if patients have symptoms of digital ischemia, arm numbness, weakness, paresthesias, or vertebral-basilar symptoms. All patients undergoing coronary artery bypass graft procedures should have bilateral preoperative blood pressure measurement. If the systolic blood pressure between the two arms differs by more than 20 mm Hg, such patients should undergo angiography of the subclavian artery preoperatively. Routine assessment of subclavian artery and internal thoracic artery patency by angiography is not recommended if the blood pressures are symmetric. If subclavian artery stenosis or occlusion is detected, the standard extrathoracic surgical approach of carotid to subclavian artery revascularization is the "gold standard," but angioplasty and stenting can be considered an acceptable initial form of treatment.

b. Localized Lymphedema

Michael H. Crawford and Mark Langsfeld

DEFINITION OF PROBLEM

Localized lymphedema results in a swollen extremity. Lymphedema is caused by lymphatic obstruction, which can be a result of developmental abnormalities (primary) or secondary to damage to lymph vessels or lymph nodes. In addition to the cosmetic issues of a swollen limb, local discomfort, limb mobility impairment, and susceptibility to infection are potential problems.

TYPICAL CASE

A 28-year-old woman was admitted to the hospital with pain and swelling of the left leg. She had noted progressive painless swelling of the left leg during the past 2 years after her first pregnancy. Elevation and support hose reduced the swelling, but it was never completely relieved. During the past 2 days, she had noted red streaks arising from the ankle ascending to the lower leg, pain, and increased foot swelling. On the morning of the day of admission, she had a chill. Otherwise, she was in good health. Physical examination showed a temperature of 100°F (37.8°C), a heart rate of 98 beats per minute, and a normal blood pressure. Her left leg was markedly swollen but did not indent easily because of thickened skin with a "peau d'orange" appearance at the ankle. Erythematous streaks at the ankle were confirmed, and there was considerable swelling of the foot and toes. Also, her right leg showed mild edema. There were no enlarged lymph nodes palpated, and abdominal-pelvic examination findings were normal. Duplex Doppler examination of the extremities showed normal arterial and venous vessels. Lymphoscintigraphy showed reduced deep lymph vessels in the left lower extremity and prominent superficial lymph vessels (Fig. 16B.1). The patient was treated with oral antibiotics, and the lymphangitis recovered quickly. She was fitted with a graduated elastic support stocking with 50 mm Hg compression at the ankle, which reduced the swelling in her left leg.

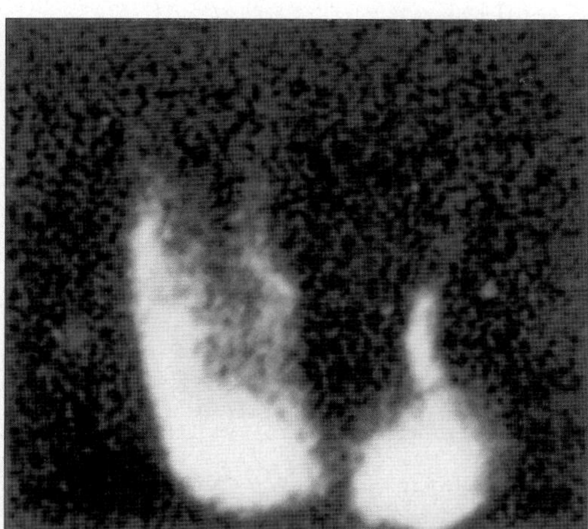

Figure 16B.1 Localized lymphedema. Bilateral lymphoscintigram of the lower legs, posterior view, showing main central lymph flow from the pool of isotope injected into the distal right foot and diffuse superficial channel flow in the swollen left leg.

DIFFERENTIAL DIAGNOSIS

The differential diagnosis of localized edema is inflammation, venous obstruction, or lymphatic obstruction (Table 16B.1). Inflammation can be due to angioneurotic edema or to infection. In both cases, the extremity is warm, red, and often painful. Angioneurotic edema is characterized by the typical history of repeated episodes of erythematous skin lesions, pruritus, and edema. Infection often is manifested with evidence of lymphangitis and signs of systemic infection such as fever. Venous disease is the most common cause of lower extremity edema and can be due to a variety of causes. Localized swelling along the course of the greater or lesser saphenous vein is caused by superficial thrombophlebitis. More diffuse edema, especially in the calf, is usually secondary to deep venous thrombosis. Thrombosis of the inferior vena cava or iliac veins will cause the entire lower extremity to be markedly swollen. Patients who are at risk for deep venous thrombosis include hospitalized or bedridden patients, those with recent major surgery, hypercoagulable patients, cancer patients, obese patients, and those suffering trauma to the lower extremity. Swelling secondary to venous disease is greatly improved in a short time (<24 hours) with bed rest and leg elevation. Confirmation of venous disease is accomplished with venous duplex scanning (compression ultrasonography combined with analysis of Doppler flow).

Lymphatic obstruction is most frequently caused by damage to the lymphatic vessels and enlarged lymph nodes from a variety of causes, the most important of which is neoplasm in the pelvis or lymphoma. In a man with lower extremity lymphedema, prostate cancer should be suspected. Because of the types of disease that cause lymphatic obstruction and damage, this condition usually has its age at onset after 35 to 40 years. By contrast, primary lymphedema, which is due to congenital lymphatic malformation, occurs at younger ages. About 15% of such patients present shortly after birth (Milroy's disease, MIM 153100). Another form, called lymphedema praecox or Meige's lymphedema (MIM 153200), presents in young women, with a frequency of nine times that in men, often starting at menarche or after the first pregnancy. Lymphedema praecox represents 75% of cases of localized lymphedema. It usually involves the lower extremities, with predominance of the left leg, but it can be bilateral. In this condition, lymphoscintigraphy shows absent or a diminished number of superficial leg lymphatics.

DIFFERENTIAL DIAGNOSIS OF LOCALIZED EDEMA		
Diagnosis **Inflammatory**	**Clinical Features**	**Lymphoscintigraphy**
Infection	Hot, red, lymphangitis	Hypoplasia
Angioneurotic	Localized edema, red	Normal
Venous obstruction		
Thrombophlebitis	Increased skin pigmentation Dilated superficial veins	Normal
Increased pressure	Pitting edema at ankles	Normal
Compression	Pitting edema at ankles	Normal
Lymphatic obstruction		
Enlarged nodes	Palpable lymphadenopathy	Obstructed, dilated with collaterals
Postsurgical	Evidence of surgery	Obstructed, dilated with collaterals
Filariasis	History of exposure	Obstructed, varicose
Lymphatic absence or obliteration		
Radiation	History of exposure	Hypoplasia
Dysplasia	Nonpitting edema to toes	↓Deep channels ↑Superficial channels

Table 16B.1 Differential diagnosis of localized edema.

The remainder of patients with primary lymphedema have either proximal occlusion in the aortoiliac or inguinal lymph nodes (lymphedema is usually unilateral and involves the entire lower extremity) or hyperplasia and incompetence of the lymph vessels (men with bilateral lymphedema).

Lymphoscintigraphy, involving the injection of radiocolloids into the foot of the affected extremity, is the most commonly used modality for evaluation of lymphedema. After injection, visible tracer activity is noted to ascend the anteromedial leg, with normal lymph flow seen in the inguinal nodes by 1 hour. Abnormal findings, such as tracer accumulation, presence of a cutaneous pattern, and reduced uptake by proximal nodes, are similar in both primary and secondary forms of lymphedema. In secondary forms, presence of malignant disease must be ruled out. Computed tomographic scans of the abdomen and pelvis are useful for diagnosis of proximal tumors. Magnetic resonance imaging scans are also used in the diagnosis of extremity soft tissue tumors or congenital vascular malformations, both of which can cause leg swelling.

TREATMENT OPTIONS

Treatment of primary lymphedema involves a comprehensive local management strategy for the extremity. Elevation can help reduce the amount of swelling, but it is not feasible to maintain this except for short periods during the day. Graduated compression is highly effective, but the elastic hose must have approximately 40 to 50 mm Hg of compression at the ankle and then be graduated cephalad, and it must be fitted properly so that it is comfortable for the patient. Sequential compression devices also have a role in long-term management. However, physical therapy or massage therapy currently is used most frequently in lymphedema treatment centers to help reduce swelling and to maintain normal tissues in lymphedema patients.

It is important to pay meticulous attention to the status of the skin in the affected extremity. Overlooked dermatophytosis is often the source of skin breakdown and a portal for bacteria to enter the extremity. All fungal infections should be aggressively treated. Any evidence of bacterial infection should be treated with oral antibiotics, and in patients with recurrent episodes, prophylactic antibiotics should be used.

SUMMARY

Localized lymphedema in older individuals is usually caused by obstruction or obliteration of lymphatics because of neoplasm or surgery or radiation therapy for neoplasm. In younger women, it is often a developmental abnormality that does not manifest itself until menarche or first pregnancy. The major differential diagnoses are thrombophlebitis and the postphlebitic limb. Treatment focuses on local measures such as massage therapy to reduce the swelling and to prevent secondary infections. In extreme cases, surgery to reduce the amount of subcutaneous tissue can be considered.

SECTION 2

ISCHEMIC HEART DISEASE

chapter 17

Physiology of Coronary Circulation

Eric O. Feigl and Wolfgang Schaper

Key Factors

- Because the left ventricle compresses its own vascular bed in systole, coronary blood flow is phasic, with maximal flow during diastole.
- The left ventricle extracts about 75% of the oxygen delivered by the coronary arteries. Thus, there is limited oxygen extraction reserve in the coronary circulation.
- Active coronary artery autoregulation maintains a constant coronary flow until coronary blood pressure drops below about 60 mm Hg.
- Vasodilator reserve is the difference between prevailing coronary flow and flow after maximal coronary artery dilatation.

Clinical implications

- At coronary artery lumen diameter reductions of 85% at rest and 45% at maximum exercise, vasodilator reserve is exhausted, resulting in inadequate perfusion pressure distal to the stenosis, which may result in rest or exertional myocardial ischemia, respectively.
- Repeated ischemic episodes can lead to chronic, but sometimes reversible, depression of cardiac contraction and collateral vessel growth.

The coronary circulation is unique in that it perfuses the heart, which is the organ responsible for generating the pressure and flow that enables all of the organs in the body, including the heart, to be perfused. This simple convergence has profound consequences because compromise of the coronary circulation attenuates cardiac pumping, which will further compromise coronary blood flow and lead to a downward spiral. Two reviews provide more information than is presented in this brief chapter.[1,2]

The left ventricular myocardium normally extracts about 75% of the oxygen (O_2) delivered by arterial coronary blood flow, resulting in a coronary venous O_2 tension at rest of approximately 18 mm Hg. Thus, there is a very limited O_2 extraction reserve. Because mammalian myocardium has little anaerobic capacity, any increase in myocardial O_2 consumption must be promptly matched by an increase in O_2 delivery through coronary blood flow. As discussed later, coronary blood flow is subject to both feedback and feed-forward control mechanisms that result in excellent matching of coronary flow to myocardial O_2 consumption.

PHYSIOLOGY

Pressure-Flow Relationships

The coronary circulation manifests active autoregulation. This means that within the autoregulatory range of perfusion pressure (usually about 60 to 140 mm Hg), coronary blood flow is fairly constant despite changes in arterial perfusion pressure (Fig. 17.1). The level of autoregulated coronary blood flow depends on the ongoing rate of myocardial O_2 consumption, being greater for high levels of O_2 consumption than for low levels. Autoregulation is not observed clearly when aortic blood pressure is changed because the aortic pressure represents the afterload on the left ventricle, and increases in afterload increase myocardial O_2 consumption and thus coronary flow (see later). It is necessary to hydraulically separate the aorta and the coronary circulation (usually with a pump) to observe autoregulation.

The mechanisms responsible for the active change in vascular resistance that keeps coronary flow constant with a change in perfusion pressure are poorly understood. There are two postulated mechanisms: myogenic control and local metabolic control. The myogenic hypothesis is based on the observation that stretching vascular smooth muscle is a stimulus for it to contract. An increase in intracoronary arterial pressure not only increases the perfusion pressure (arterial pressure minus venous pressure), but also increases the distending pressure in the coronary vascular tree. Thus, the pressure distention of the vessels results in an active constriction that increases vascular resistance and maintains a relatively constant flow. As discussed later, the coronary circulation exhibits strong local metabolic control, and another hypothesis states that coronary autoregulation is simply a manifestation of the feedback between myocardial metabolism and coronary blood flow (i.e., the constancy of coronary flow during autoregulation is secondary to the constancy of myocardial metabolism). Because both myogenic responses and local metabolic control can be demonstrated in the coronary circulation, many investigators conclude that both mechanisms are involved in coronary autoregulation.

Autoregulation is lost at pressures below approximately 60 mm Hg, and coronary blood flow becomes pressure dependent (i.e., decreasing coronary perfusion pressure decreases coronary flow). Below the autoregulatory range, coronary vasodilator reserve is said to be exhausted. The loss of

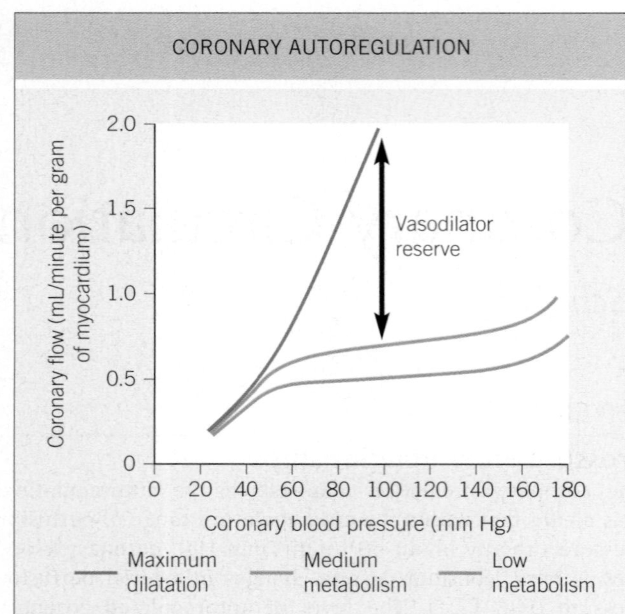

Figure 17.1 Coronary autoregulation. Note that coronary blood flow is reasonably constant despite changes in coronary artery pressure. Below the autoregulatory range (approximately 60 mm Hg), flow is strongly pressure dependent. Vasodilator reserve is the increase in flow between the prevailing flow and a specified "maximum" vasodilator stimulus. Below the autoregulatory range, vasodilator reserve is exhausted.

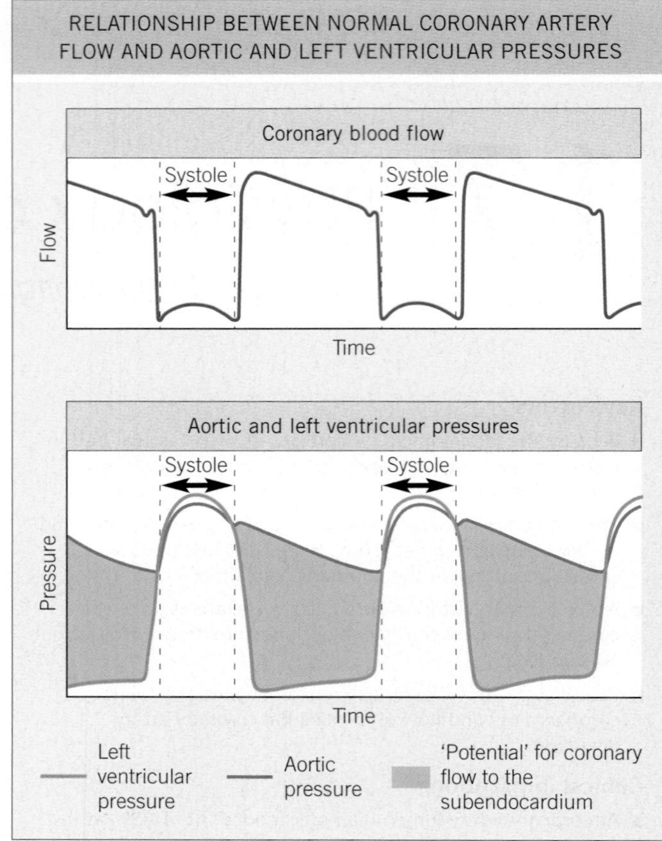

Figure 17.2 Relationship between normal coronary artery flow and aortic and left ventricular pressures. Coronary blood flow is low during systole because of systolic compression of intramyocardial coronary vessels. The "potential" for coronary flow to the subendocardium is the difference between diastolic aortic and left ventricular pressures multiplied by the diastolic period. A low aortic pressure or a brief diastolic period (tachycardia) may compromise subendocardial blood flow.

autoregulation at low coronary pressure is a critical element in producing angina pectoris (see later).

Vasodilator reserve is a useful concept frequently used to characterize the status of the coronary circulation. A stimulus or stress is administered, and the increase in coronary blood flow is determined. If the coronary pressure distal to a stenosis is close to or below the lower limit of autoregulation, vasodilator reserve will be compromised (see later).

Formally stated, vasodilator reserve is the increase in flow between the prevailing flow and maximal coronary vasodilatation. The "maximal" vasodilatation may be produced by drugs (e.g., adenosine, dipyridamole) or by exercise that increases myocardial O_2 consumption. Although vasodilator reserve is a useful concept, maximal vasodilatation is an inexact quantity. For example, the maximal coronary blood flow observed during exercise can be augmented by an infusion of adenosine. For this reason, vasodilator reserve is usually evaluated with a standardized protocol, and the true maximal level is not reached because to do so would overstress the patient. Note that when the coronary circulation is pharmacologically dilated, flow is strongly pressure dependent (i.e., there is no autoregulation), and coronary vasodilator reserve varies as a function of arterial pressure (see Fig. 17.1).

Phasic Flow

During each systole, the left ventricle compresses its own vascular bed, which results in phasic coronary artery inflow that is small during systole and large during diastole (Fig. 17.2). The flow in epicardial coronary veins has the opposite phase, with outflow being large during systole and small during diastole. Thus, the intramyocardial coronary vascular volume is low during systole and high during diastole. The myocardial compressive force is much greater in the subendocardium than in the subepicardium. Direct observation of microvessels in the inner layer of the left ventricle reveals that subendocardial vessels are narrowed but not completely closed during systole.[3] During systole, there is retrograde outward flow in arterial vessels that penetrate from the epicardium to the endocardium of the left ventricle. With the onset of ventricular relaxation, there is a rush of antegrade flow in the penetrating arteries as they refill. The result of the large compressive forces in the subendocardium and the oscillating flow that it produces is that the innermost layers of the left ventricle are perfused only during diastole.

Myocardial systolic compression of left ventricular subendocardial vessels is an example of a vascular "waterfall" (an unfortunate, misleading term), in which arterial pressure minus tissue pressure determines flow rather than the usual arterial pressure minus venous pressure. The compressive tissue pressure in the inner layer of the left ventricle is approximately equal to the blood pressure in the left ventricular cavity. Thus, it is possible to describe the driving pressure for subendocardial flow as the coronary artery pressure minus the left ventricular cavity pressure. During systolic ejection, when the aortic valve is open, the left ventricular pressure and the coronary artery pressure are essentially equal, and there is no flow to the subendocardium. During diastole, when the aortic valve is closed, the left ventricular pressure is low and the driving pressure for subendocardial flow is the coronary (aortic) pressure minus the left ventricular pressure. The time integral of aortic pressure minus left ventricular pressure during the diastolic period represents the "potential" for subendocardial flow (see Fig. 17.2). Any intervention that shortens the diastolic period (tachycardia) or decreases the pressure difference between the coronary arteries and the left ventricle (e.g., coronary stenosis or aortic valve stenosis) will jeopardize flow to the inner layer of the left ventricle (see later).

A second factor that places the subendocardium at risk is that the inner layer is at the distal end of the coronary arterial tree. The coronary arteries branch from the aorta just distal to the aortic valve and course over the surface of the heart like a crown (hence the name "coronary") before branching and penetrating the myocardium from outside to inside. If coronary flow is restricted, the most distal area will be most compromised. This is analogous to the patient who has ischemic symptoms in the foot as a result of an arterial stenosis in the femoral artery of the thigh.

Despite the fact that the left ventricular subendocardium is at the greatest risk of underperfusion, the inner layers of the heart normally receive greater blood flow than the outer layers. The normal ratio of subendocardial to subepicardial flow (the "endo-epi" ratio) is approximately 1.1. This is because the myocardial O_2 consumption is slightly greater in the inner layers than in the outer layers of the left ventricle. An endo-epi flow ratio of less than 0.8 is clear evidence of disease.

Myocardial Oxygen Consumption

Anaerobic metabolic capacity is small in the myocardium, and the heart is dependent on O_2 supply on a beat-to-beat basis. Cardiac hypoxia stimulates anaerobic glycolysis, but during ischemia, this effect is blunted by the buildup of hydrogen ions that are not washed away. The fuel for energetic reactions in the heart is adenosine triphosphate (ATP), which is required for muscle contraction, ion pumping, and other cellular functions. The myocardium is omnivorous and will metabolize glucose, lactate, pyruvate, and fatty acids, depending on what is available in arterial blood. The number of ATP molecules that can be generated from the oxidation of substrates varies. Complete oxidation of glucose will yield 3.17 ATP molecules per molecule of O_2 (the P/O_2 ratio), whereas complete oxidation of the fatty acid palmitate will yield 2.83 ATP molecules, about a 12% difference. Normally, the heart oxidizes a mixture of substrates, and even shifting to glucose alone will result in only a modest increase in the P/O_2 ratio. Thus, the total metabolism of the myocardium may be determined by measuring the rate of myocardial O_2 consumption, often expressed as microliters O_2/minute per gram of myocardium. Myocardial O_2 consumption is the major determinant of coronary blood flow; therefore, it is useful to consider the factors that influence O_2 consumption (see later).

Resting myocardial O_2 consumption is about 70 μL O_2/minute per gram of left ventricle, depending on how slow the heart rate is in the resting state. If the heart is arrested with a high potassium ion (K^+) concentration solution, the myocardial O_2 consumption falls to about 25% of the resting value. The arrested "basal" myocardial O_2 consumption represents the basic "housekeeping" O_2 requirements for cellular integrity, independent of the energy needs associated with cardiac contraction. Thus, about 75% of resting myocardial O_2 consumption is related to cardiac contraction and the associated ion pumping that is needed for the action potential and excitation-contraction coupling. During strenuous exercise, myocardial O_2 consumption may increase fourfold to fivefold over the resting value.

A simple way of relating cardiac contraction and myocardial O_2 consumption is to correlate O_2 consumption with external cardiac work. However, it has been repeatedly observed that left ventricular stroke work and O_2 consumption are poorly correlated. What has been found is that the development of tension by the left ventricle is also an important determinant of myocardial O_2 consumption. This can be nicely demonstrated in an experimental preparation in which the left ventricle beats isovolumically. During this condition, there is no ejection and thus no external cardiac work, yet the myocardial O_2 consumption is high. Thermodynamically, work costs energy, but work alone is a poor correlate of myocardial O_2 consumption.[4]

The tension in cardiac fibers in the wall of the left ventricle depends on the size (radius) of the ventricle and the thickness of the wall. The average tangential tension (hoop stress) in a thick-walled cylinder is approximately given by the law of Laplace

$$T = \Delta Pr/h$$

where T is the tension (dynes/cm^2), r is the inside radius (cm), ΔP is the transmural pressure difference (dynes/cm^2), and h is the wall thickness (cm). Therefore, the wall tension needed to generate an afterload systolic blood pressure of 120 mm Hg is greater for an acutely dilated left ventricle than it is for a normal ventricle. Thus, acute cardiac dilatation may increase myocardial O_2 consumption and the need for coronary blood flow without a change in blood pressure. In chronic cardiac hypertrophy with thickening of the ventricular wall, the thickening tends to normalize the wall tension and the coronary flow per gram. However, total O_2 consumpton and coronary flow will increase with hypertrophy.

It is apparent that tachycardia will augment myocardial O_2 consumption because of the increased frequency of the heartbeat. An additional factor that influences myocardial O_2 consumption is cardiac contractility. Augmenting contractility with catecholamines increases myocardial O_2 consumption, primarily by increasing the development of cardiac tension and the cardiac work, but there is probably an additional component related to the contractility change.[4]

Numerous indices have been developed for estimating myocardial O_2 consumption from hemodynamic variables. The observation that several indices that contain very different hemodynamic variables can provide reasonable estimates of myocardial O_2 consumption emphasizes that the indices are correlative descriptions and do not reveal fundamental physiologic mechanisms.[4] The simplest and most clinically useful index of myocardial O_2 consumption is the product of left ventricular systolic blood pressure and heart rate.

This index is useful within a single subject during physiologic or pharmacologic changes, but it is less accurate for comparison of different subjects because of varying ventricular size.

In summary, the major determinants of left ventricular myocardial O_2 consumption are heart rate and the development of tension in the ventricular wall. The tension depends on left ventricular systolic pressure and size, as can be estimated with the law of Laplace. Augmented cardiac contractility also adds to myocardial O_2 consumption.

Control of Coronary Blood Flow

Local Metabolic Feedback Control

An intrinsic local mechanism controls coronary blood flow to match changes in myocardial O_2 consumption. The hypothesis is that cardiac myocyte O_2 tension (or a closely related variable) is the regulated variable kept at the operating point by a local metabolic negative feedback control mechanism. Therefore, when myocardial O_2 consumption increases, there is an incipient decrease in cardiac O_2 tension, which results in a local vasodilator signal that increases coronary blood flow and O_2 delivery to the myocardium. The augmented O_2 delivery restores myocardial O_2 tension toward the normal operating point in a negative feedback manner. There have been several hypotheses about local metabolic control of coronary blood flow; three are discussed:

- the adenosine hypothesis;
- the role of K^+_{ATP} channels; and
- the role of O_2 and carbon dioxide (CO_2).

Adenosine Hypothesis

The adenosine hypothesis proposes that adenosine is released by cardiac myocytes as an inverse function of myocardial O_2 tension. Therefore, if myocardial O_2 tension falls, additional adenosine is released from cardiac myocytes. Adenosine then crosses the interstitial space to act on adenosine receptors on coronary vascular smooth muscle cells to initiate coronary vasodilatation. According to this hypothesis, adenosine acts as a classic transmitter by which information from one cell (cardiac myocyte) is transmitted to another cell (coronary smooth muscle). It is well established that adenosine is a coronary vasodilator, and the initial studies of the adenosine hypothesis demonstrated that cardiac hypoxia or ischemia resulted in the release of adenosine from the myocardium and in coronary vasodilatation. However, it has been difficult to establish that adenosine is involved in physiologic control of coronary blood flow. Recent investigations using adenosine receptor blockade and adenosine measurements indicate that adenosine is not involved in coronary hyperemia when myocardial O_2 consumption is increased by cardiac pacing or exercise.[5] However, it is well established that ischemic or hypoxic myocardium releases adenosine, which acts as a pathophysiologic vasodilator.

Role of K^+_{ATP} Channels

K^+_{ATP} channels are found in the membranes of cardiac and coronary vascular smooth muscle cells and have been postulated to be involved in local metabolic control of coronary blood flow. Blocking of K^+_{ATP} channels with glibenclamide results in a decrease in coronary blood flow and coronary venous O_2 tension. The initial experiments demonstrated that coronary vasodilatation during hypoxia or ischemia was blunted by glibenclamide. However, glibenclamide also blocks adenosine coronary vasodilatation, which indicates that K^+_{ATP} channels are involved in coronary dilatation caused by adenosine. Therefore, the experiments with hypoxia and ischemia are most parsimoniously interpreted as glibenclamide blunting the vasodilatory effects of adenosine because adenosine is known to be released during cardiac hypoxia and ischemia. Even though glibenclamide decreases resting coronary blood flow, it does not blunt the increase in coronary blood flow when myocardial O_2 consumption is augmented during pacing tachycardia or exercise.[6,7]

In summary, blockade of K^+_{ATP} channels with glibenclamide lowers resting coronary blood flow but does not blunt the increase in flow when myocardial O_2 consumption is increased. Thus, K^+_{ATP} channels are not an important element in local metabolic feedback control of coronary blood flow.

Role of Oxygen and Carbon Dioxide

A seemingly simple hypothesis for local metabolic control of coronary blood flow is that coronary vascular smooth muscle dilates with hypoxia and hypercapnia without an intermediate mediator such as adenosine. The difficulty with this hypothesis is that blood flow is primarily controlled by precapillary arterioles upstream from where the bulk of O_2 and CO_2 exchange occurs. Thus, the blood inside the arteriole has O_2 and CO_2 tensions that are close to the arterial level, and it is difficult to understand how arteriolar smooth muscle could be very sensitive to the rates of myocardial O_2 consumption and CO_2 production. Coronary blood flow certainly responds to changes in arterial blood O_2 content. For example, anemia (low arterial O_2 content, normal O_2 tension) increases coronary blood flow, but coronary venous O_2 tension is little changed, demonstrating a good match between O_2 delivery and myocardial O_2 consumption by local metabolic control.

There is an interesting synergism between O_2 and CO_2 when low O_2 and high CO_2 levels combine to produce a substantial coronary vasodilatation that is more than a simple summation of the independent O_2 and CO_2 effects.[8] A correlation between coronary blood flow and the synergistic effects of O_2 and CO_2 can be made when myocardial O_2 consumption is increased by cardiac pacing, but this accounts for only about 40% of the increase in coronary flow.[8] Of course, the correlation does not establish that O_2 and CO_2 are acting directly on coronary vascular smooth muscle without some unidentified intermediate mediator.

Nitric Oxide

There has been much interest in the role of nitric oxide (NO) produced by vascular endothelial cells in the control of blood flow. Several agents, such as acetylcholine and bradykinin, cause coronary vasodilatation in an endothelium-dependent manner, whereby receptors on endothelial cells are activated; this leads to an intracellular signal (calcium ion) to activate the enzyme NO synthase, which converts L-arginine and O_2 to the NO radical and L-citrulline. Nitric oxide is a gas that readily diffuses to the adjacent smooth muscle in the vascular wall. The NO activates guanylyl cyclase, which in turn forms cyclic guanosine monophosphate from guanosine triphosphate. Increased levels of cyclic guanosine monophosphate lead to vascular smooth muscle relaxation, probably by reducing intracellular calcium ion concentration.

An important aspect of the role of NO is that flow-induced shear stress on endothelial cells activates NO synthase, and this is the mechanism by which downstream arteriolar vasodilatation produces an upstream arterial dilatation.[9] This is a very nice adaptation by which the total coronary resistance is adjusted according to the prevailing local metabolic control occurring at the arteriolar level, and upstream diameter is adjusted to the endothelial shear rate. In effect, the shear rate at the endothelial lining of proximal coronary arteries is adjusted so as not to be too low (causing stasis thrombosis) or too high (causing endothelial damage).

Nitric oxide is not stored in cells, and it is rapidly inactivated by other free radicals; therefore, the prevailing NO level is dependent on the rate of synthesis by NO synthase. L^{ω}-Nitro-L-arginine and other analogues of arginine have been used as false substrates for NO synthase to inhibit NO production and to test the physiologic role of NO. Infusion of L^{ω}-nitro-L-arginine during rest and exercise has a minor effect on coronary blood flow, but it does slightly lower coronary venous O_2 tension, indicating that the balance between coronary O_2 delivery and myocardial O_2 consumption has been decreased.[10] Thus, NO is not important in local metabolic control of total coronary blood flow, but it does adjust the shear stress in the coronary arterial tree.

Intracoronary injection of acetylcholine in normal subjects produces an endothelium-dependent (NO) coronary vasodilatation and an increase in coronary blood flow. Patients who have coronary atherosclerosis have a diminished acetylcholine response or even coronary vasoconstriction as a result of acetylcholine acting directly on vascular smooth muscle. Patients who have risk factors for atherosclerosis have a diminished coronary vasodilatation response to acetylcholine before any coronary atherosclerosis is detectable. These observations raise the interesting question of the roles of the endothelium and NO in atherosclerosis. At this time, it is not clear whether the loss of endothelial NO function is part of the pathogenesis of atherosclerosis or whether the diminished acetylcholine response is an incidental indicator of endothelial dysfunction.

In summary, although local metabolic control of coronary blood flow is the dominant controller, the mechanism for this effect is unknown. Blockade of adenosine receptors, K^{+}_{ATP} channels, or NO synthesis modestly reduces coronary venous O_2 tension but does not impede the increase in flow during cardiac pacing or exercise.

Autonomic Control of Coronary Blood Flow

α-Adrenoceptor Vasoconstriction

Activation of the sympathetic innervation of the heart results in tachycardia and augmented cardiac contractility, both of which increase myocardial O_2 consumption, which in turn results in local metabolic vasodilatation and an increase in coronary blood flow. The local metabolic vasodilatation occurs primarily in small arterioles; at the same time, there is direct activation of α-adrenoceptors on proximal medium and large coronary arterial vessels. The activation of α-adrenoceptors causes vasoconstriction, which modestly restricts the overall increase in coronary flow. Such a sympathetic relative vasoconstriction seems paradoxical because flow must increase to allow the increase in myocardial O_2 consumption secondary to sympathetic fiber activation. The relative α-adrenoceptor vasoconstriction has been observed whenever there is sympathetic activation of the heart (e.g., during baroreceptor reflexes, emotion, and exercise).[11]

However, the paradoxical relative α-adrenoceptor–mediated coronary vasoconstriction does have a beneficial effect. There is phasic backflow in the penetrating coronary arteries during systole and a rush of forward flow at the beginning of diastole to refill the arterial tree before nutritive flow in microcirculation of the subendocardium can begin. This to-and-fro flow oscillation is wasted flow, but this is not a problem at rest because the duration of diastole is long and the demand for coronary flow is low. However, when the diastolic period is brief during tachycardia and coronary blood flow is high, as occurs during exercise with strong sympathetic activation of the heart, the subendocardium may become inadequately perfused. Activation of α-adrenoceptor vasoconstriction in proximal portions of the coronary arterial tree stiffens these vessels and reduces the magnitude of the wasted to-and-fro flow during the cardiac cycle.[12] The effect is to adjust the frequency-dependent complex input impedance of the coronary circulation to the heartbeat frequency so that flow to the left ventricular subendocardium is maintained during exercise.[13] The effect of α-adrenoceptor vasoconstriction on transmural flow is important only during tachycardia and high coronary flow demand, as occurs during exercise, because there is an adequate diastolic perfusion time at normal heart rates.

β-Adrenoceptor Vasodilatation

At the same time as activation of cardiac sympathetic fibers is causing α-adrenoceptor–mediated vasoconstriction of medium and large coronary arteries, there is an active β-adrenoceptor–mediated vasodilatation of the coronary arterioles. The arterioles are the dominant site of coronary vascular resistance, and the β-adrenoceptor vasodilatation increases coronary blood flow. During exercise, about 25% of the increase in coronary blood flow is due to norepinephrine (noradrenaline) from cardiac sympathetic nerves acting directly on arteriolar α-adrenoceptors.[14] The remaining vasodilatation during exercise is due to the undefined local metabolic vasodilator mechanism discussed before.

Characteristics of Feedforward Control

Both the α- and β-adrenoceptor–mediated control of coronary blood flow are examples of feedforward control, which does not require an error signal to activate the control mechanisms. Feedforward control may also be called parallel (or yoked) control because activation of adrenergic receptors in the coronary circulation occurs in parallel with activation of adrenergic receptors in the myocardium. The distinguishing characteristic of feedforward control is that it does not operate on an error signal, unlike feedback control. Two variables, such as flow and metabolism, can be closely matched because the same control signal is directed at both variables. Therefore, during exercise, sympathetic discharge to the heart increases the heart rate and the cardiac contractility, and thus the myocardial O_2 consumption, while simultaneously causing β-adrenoceptor–mediated coronary vasodilatation to help match O_2 delivery to O_2 metabolism.

The advantage of a feedforward system is that two variables can be modulated together without lag or error. The disadvantage of a feedforward system is that it is not self-checking, and if an error develops, there is no way of correcting it. A system with combined feedback and feedforward control has many of the advantages of both systems, and this is how coronary blood flow is controlled.

In summary, feedforward α-adrenoceptor–mediated vasoconstriction of medium and large coronary arteries reduces wasteful to-and-fro flow oscillations and helps maintain flow to the subendocardium during exercise, when both heart rate and myocardial O_2 consumption are high. Feedforward β-adrenoceptor–mediated vasodilatation of coronary arterioles helps match flow to metabolism during exercise.

PATHOPHYSIOLOGY

Coronary Stenosis

An atherosclerotic lesion in an epicardial coronary artery is a hydraulic resistor in series with the arteriolar resistance in the coronary microcirculation. Flow through a stenosis is very different from laminar flow in a uniformly smooth vessel. Blood must accelerate through the narrow stenosis, where there is a large loss of viscous energy caused by the high shear rate. There is also a large loss of energy at the exit of the stenosis, where there is highly disturbed flow with whirls and eddies. These losses of energy result in a large pressure drop across the stenosis so that the pressure downstream from a stenosis may be too low for adequate perfusion of the distal microvascular bed.

In contrast to a smooth, uniform vessel, in which the drops in flow and pressure along the vessel are linearly related to each other, the pressure-flow relation in a stenosis is markedly nonlinear. The pressure difference required to force blood through a stenosis rises exponentially as a function of flow (Fig. 17.3). This approximately quadratic function has serious consequences for the coronary circulation.

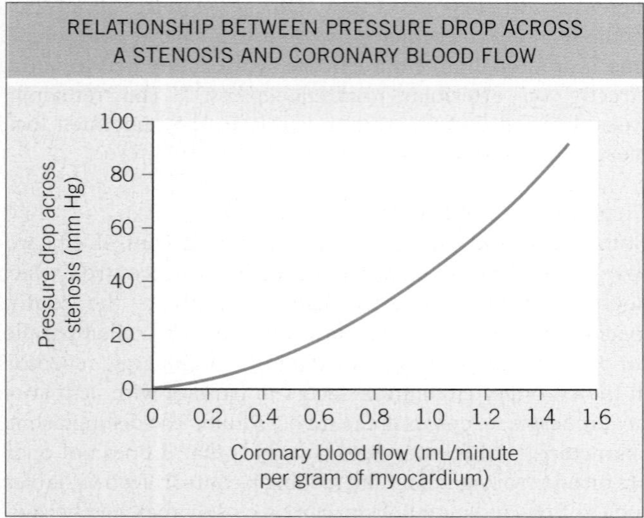

Figure 17.3 Relationship between pressure drop across a stenosis and coronary blood flow. The pressure drop is that which might be seen across an 80% diameter stenosis of a coronary artery. If the aortic pressure is 100 mm Hg and the flow 1.0 mL/min per gram of myocardium, the pressure distal to the stenosis will be below the lower limit of autoregulation (approximately 60 mm Hg) and the patient will probably experience angina, even though flow is greater than an initial resting value of approximately 0.5 mL/min per gram of myocardium.

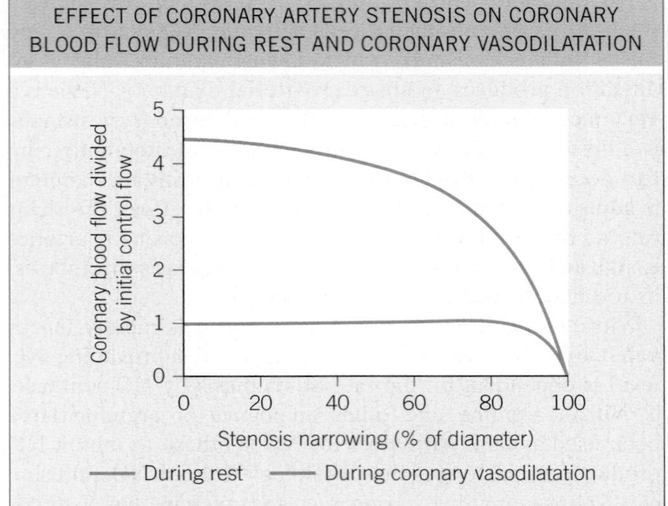

Figure 17.4 Effect of coronary artery stenosis on coronary blood flow during rest and coronary vasodilatation. Because of the nonlinear resistance characteristics of stenoses, the critical narrowing is about 85% at resting flows but about 45% during hyperemia. (From Gould et al. ©1994, with permission of Excerpta Medica Inc.)

The effects of different stenoses on coronary blood flow are shown in Figure 17.4. When coronary blood flow is at a normal resting value (i.e., low), a diameter narrowing of the coronary artery of approximately 85% is necessary to reduce flow. This critical narrowing changes from about 85% to about 45% when unrestricted flow is increased fourfold by exercise or drugs.

Angina Pectoris and Subendocardial Ischemia

All of the aspects of coronary physiology discussed in the preceding sections may be put together in an understanding of why a patient who has coronary atherosclerosis may develop angina pectoris on exertion.

The atherosclerotic stenosis in an epicardial coronary artery is a nonlinear resistor in series with the downstream arterioles in the coronary circulation. When myocardial O_2 consumption is low during resting conditions, the corresponding coronary blood flow is also low but not restricted by the stenosis. This is because the pressure drop across the stenosis is modest at low flow (nonlinear stenosis resistance). During rest, the pressure distal to the stenosis (but proximal to the coronary arterioles) is above the critical lower level for autoregulation (approximately 60 mm Hg). If coronary pressure available to the coronary arterioles is in the autoregulatory range, arteriolar autoregulation (vasodilatation) keeps coronary blood flow in balance with the prevailing myocardial O_2 consumption by a poorly understood local metabolic control mechanism. Despite the pathologic upstream stenosis resistance, the in-series downstream arteriolar vasodilatation keeps total coronary vascular resistance and coronary blood flow normal at rest.

When a patient who has angina begins to exercise, myocardial O_2 consumption increases and local metabolic arteriolar vasodilatation ensues. However, this also draws a higher blood flow rate through the coronary stenosis, but this can be accomplished only by a more and more drastic exponential pressure drop across the stenosis. Although aortic pressure increases during exercise, the increase is not enough to offset the loss of pressure across the stenosis, and the pressure distal to the stenosis falls below the autoregulatory range (i.e., coronary arteriolar vasodilator reserve becomes exhausted). When coronary pressure distal to the stenosis is below the autoregulatory range, flow is strongly pressure dependent, and a small decrease in pressure results in a steep fall in flow.

Recall that the systolic myocardial compressive force is large in the subendocardium and small in the subepicardium and that the innermost layers of the left ventricle are perfused only during diastole. With exertion, heart rate increases with only a slight decrease in the duration of systole, and thus the diastolic interval between beats for subendocardial perfusion becomes very brief. The combination of the augmented myocardial O_2 consumption caused by the tachycardia plus the diminished diastolic time places the subendocardium at risk of underperfusion, and the pressure-robbing stenosis completes the pathophysiologic process.

An additional factor that compromises subendocardial flow is that the subendocardium is at the distal end of the coronary vascular tree because the coronary arteries penetrate the myocardium from epicardium to endocardium. The ischemic manifestations of an upstream stenosis are found in the distal vasculature; for example, a patient who has a femoral artery stenosis in the thigh will have ischemic symptoms in the foot.

In summary, several factors combine to produce subendocardial ischemia in the presence of an epicardial coronary artery stenosis during exertion. The stenosis acts as a nonlinear resistor that drastically lowers coronary pressure to a level below the autoregulatory range. Blood flow to the subendocardium occurs only during diastole, and the tachycardia during exertion abbreviates diastole. Finally, the subendocardium is at the distal end of the coronary arterial tree.

Beyond Physiologic Regulation

When the vasodilatory reserve of the coronary system is exhausted, as with exercise in the presence of a stenosis, myocardial ischemia develops. This can be measured by the breakdown of glucose and glycogen to lactate, by the fall of phosphocreatine and ATP, and by the increase in adenosine and hydrogen ion concentrations. If such situations recur, adaptive mechanisms become operative; the myocardium develops increased tolerance toward ischemia (ischemic preconditioning), and collateral blood vessels grow to compensate for the increase in total resistance (arteriogenesis).

Hibernating and Stunned Myocardium

Another type of adaptation is believed to exist in so-called hibernating myocardium, a most baffling clinical syndrome in which noncontracting myocardium, subtended by a heavily stenosed coronary artery, resumes normal function after coronary artery bypass surgery.[15] It is believed that the classic dogma of coronary flow regulation is reversed—not "flow follows function" but rather "function follows flow." The new concept of hibernating myocardium states that in contrast to the acutely ischemic myocardium, the chronically underperfused myocardium can reduce its energy requirements to the existing flow and reduce function accordingly without signs of ischemia or infarction. This situation has been reported to exist for months in patients who do not have ultrastructural signs of damage and degeneration. If true, this observation would shatter the classic dogma, and a new model of coronary blood flow regulation would be needed. The difficulty with the new concept is that it cannot be studied in laboratory animals because dogs and pigs do not tolerate a stable underperfusion for a prolonged time; either they develop a collateral circulation and revert to normal regulation or the tissue undergoes necrosis. The structural alterations found in the myocardium of patients have not been elicited in experimental animals. However, a close look at the published human data shows that only a small fraction of patients thought to have hibernation had a structurally normal noncontracting myocardium.[16] Most other patients showed various degrees of advanced degeneration, fibrosis, and apoptotic death among myocytes. Blood flow studies with positron emission tomography scanning demonstrated that patients with hibernating myocardium did not have reduced resting blood flow but only limited dilatory capacity.[17] It is, therefore, highly probable that patients who have noncontracting left ventricular areas and normal blood flow were studied while they were experiencing the syndrome of "stunned myocardium" (i.e., a long-lasting contractile dysfunction following a brief period of acute ischemia caused by exertion, as after an anginal attack). It is likely that when such episodes occur frequently, the myocardium can never recover from stunning and so remains in a permanent state of contractile failure. Because stunned myocardium consumes less O_2 than normal myocardium does, it is understandable that this is tolerated for some time without much damage. However, constant stretching alternated with brief periods of ischemia causes ultrastructural and molecular changes, such as loss of sarcomeres, accumulation of glycogen, increased expression of transforming growth factor β, fibrosis, and decreased capillary density, all of which are typical for hibernating myocardium.[16] Finally, DNA damage is no longer repaired, and the cells die of apoptosis. The original hypothesis that hibernating myocardium is able to down-regulate O_2 consumption to the available O_2 supply is untenable. Although the classic signs of acute ischemia are not present, the myocardium shows all of the symptoms of chronic degeneration and does not even react transcriptionally to the repeated ischemic stimulus (see later).

A molecular switch that could act in chronic ischemia by forcing the myocyte into reduced contractility would be the up-regulation of the phospholamban gene. Phospholamban reduces the release of calcium by the sarcoplasmic reticulum and would therefore reduce the force of contraction and, with it, the O_2 requirements. Targeted disruption and inactivation of the phospholamban gene in mice cause the heart to beat continuously at maximal contractility.[18] Overexpression would result in the loss of contraction. However, hibernating myocardium in patients exhibits extremely low levels of phospholamban mRNA, close to the levels in knockout mice.[19] This means that not only does the heart not try to down-regulate O_2 consumption, but also it tries in vain to increase contractility by allowing an excess of calcium, released by the sarcoplasmic reticulum, to enter the cytoplasm.

The conclusion is that the classic dogma of coronary physiology still stands, flow follows function; but when flow cannot rise to match O_2 demand, the myocytes die. Depending on the degree of the flow deficit, myocytes die slowly when the deficit exists occasionally and rapidly when the deficit is large and permanent. The original hypothesis predicted that hibernating myocardium, which represents a stable down-regulation of the O_2 requirements, is not in need of immediate revascularization procedures. New research refutes this hypothesis and emphasizes the need for speedy revascularization to salvage the myocardium at risk of degeneration.

Arteriogenesis and Collateral Development

The coronary arteries of most mammals including humans (with the exception of rats and pigs) are not anatomic end-arteries; rather, they are interconnected on the arteriolar level. This means that acute occlusion of one artery does not lead to complete cessation of flow; the interconnecting collateral network is able (in the canine heart) to deliver up to 30% of the normal resting flow. If coronary occlusion proceeds more gradually for days or weeks, a fraction of these interconnecting collateral vessels develop into small arteries that are able to deliver about 30% of maximum flow. The molecular mechanism of this adaptation is called arteriogenesis, in contrast to angiogenesis, which describes the formation of capillaries. Whereas angiogenesis is initiated by tissue hypoxia or ischemia, arteriogenesis is probably not.

In 1965, Fulton[20] demonstrated that the stem parts of epicardial collateral vessels in the human heart are surrounded by nonischemic muscle. In the dog, enlarged epicardial collateral vessels are never in contact with ischemic myocardium for most of their course. Experiments by Gregg[21] in chronically instrumented dogs showed no change in contractility of the epicardial myocardium during the course of slowly progressing coronary artery occlusion and subsequent collateral vessel development, meaning that this region was not ischemic. The epicardial myocardium of collateralized canine hearts exhibits good autoregulation (relatively lesser flow increase for any pressure increase), and this is not changed by a bypass graft. Moreover, the ischemic canine subendocardium does not produce collateral arteries. After the ischemia has long abated, the formation of collateral vessels continues for weeks and may be complete about 6 months after occlusion. It is therefore very unlikely that arteriogenesis is caused by tissue hypoxia.

Fluid shear stress may be the initiating event in arteriogenesis. If a coronary artery becomes stenosed to a degree that the pressure distal to the stenosis is lower than the pressure proximal to the stenosis, this differential is then also transmitted within the interconnecting arteriolar network that connects adjacent vascular territories. This causes flow in the most conductive routes of this network toward the distal distribution system of the occluded artery. The increased flow increases the fluid shear stress markedly, which leads to the expression of monocyte chemoattractant protein 1. At the same time, intercellular adhesion molecule 1 is also expressed on the endothelial surface, which leads to monocyte adherence. These cytokines become activated and produce growth factors as well as proteases. The growth factors initiate mitosis of the endothelial and smooth muscle cells. The proteases lead to the digestion of the extracellular matrix proteins that keep the cells glued together. Protease action leads to thinning of the arteriolar wall, and the smooth muscle cells can now slide past each other, which gives the collateral artery the appearance of a thin-walled vein. These vessels become leaky, and thrombin and fibrin accumulate in the adventitia, a process that initiates a perivascular inflammation with invasion of T lymphocytes. Because these collateral arteries markedly increase in size (up to 20 times the initial diameter in the canine heart), space must be generated to accommodate them. To achieve this, the surrounding myocardium is attacked by T lymphocytes and dies. Digestion of the matrix leads to greater smooth muscle cell mobility, and a significant proportion of smooth muscle cells migrate from the media to the intima, where they continue to proliferate and create intimal cushions similar to those found in certain stages of atherosclerosis.

Excessive intima formation may be the cause of disappearance of the majority of collateral arteries some time after growth stimulation. Initially, about 24 vessels in the canine heart and about 30 in the rabbit hind leg will participate in the growth process, but only four of these vessels will mature into much larger collateral arteries. The others disappear again, and closure by excessive intima formation is probably the mechanism. The process of collateralization consumes collateral arterioles; because most of them occlude after recruitment, fewer are available for a new round of adaptation.

The collateral circulation restores autoregulation; when flow conductance of collateral vessels increases as a result of growth, the arterioles of the recipient vascular bed resume autoregulation. This can be demonstrated by measuring the time course of the peripheral coronary pressure distal to the stenosis, which falls for a short time during progressive coronary occlusion but quickly resumes values near aortic pressure. If autoregulation is then abolished by infusion of vasodilators, the peripheral pressure falls again because the increase in blood flow through the incompletely adapted collateral vessels leads to a fall in pressure. The peripheral coronary pressure is a good index of the degree of adaptation by collateral vessels. It rises in an S-shaped function over time, and the steepest phase is completed in less than 3 days. In the best cases (dog epicardial collateral vessels), peripheral coronary pressure reaches a final value around 50% of aortic perfusion pressure under maximum vasodilatation. It is not known why collaterals do not reach the full potential of the artery they have replaced. It may have something to do with the tortuosity of collateral vessels. Collateral arteries have a tortuous appearance perhaps because of the twists and turns of the arcade-like network from which they originate but also because the arterial growth occurs not only in a radial direction but also in a longitudinal direction. Collateral arteries are up to two times longer than needed, even when the fact that they have to be long enough not to be stretched during diastole is taken into account. The tortuous course has serious consequences—the increase in length increases resistance, and the curvature causes additional pressure losses. On the other hand, helical flows can be advantageous up to a point; they prevent turbulence and reduce shear stress, which may be the reason that the growth process stops before a complete restitution is reached.[22] Markedly tortuous vessels may exhibit extremely low shear rates at the inner curvature, which will up-regulate the expression of growth factors (such as platelet-derived growth factor) and increase intima formation.

Early restoration of autoregulatory blood flow and normalizaton of fluid shear stress by radial expansion of collateral vessels leading to a premature termination of the growth process are factors that limit the function of collateral circulation. A new experiment in the vascular periphery of rats was reported[23] in which the collateral blood flow, after femoral artery occlusion, was rerouted directly into the venous system, thereby dramatically increasing flow and shear stress. When the arteriovenous fistula was closed 1 to 4 weeks later, the collateral vessels had expanded in number and size to such an extent that their maximal conductance had reached that of the normal femoral artery bed by 1 week and exhibited twice the maximal physiologic conductance after 4 weeks. This experiment supports the controlling influence of fluid shear stress. Collateral vessels obtained from this experiment were used for genome-wide screening for genes that are regulated by shear stress.[24]

An experiment of nature in which collateral vessels enlarge to enormous dimensions, showing that they are not inherently growth restricted, is the White-Garland syndrome. In this syndrome, the left coronary artery originates from the pulmonary artery (a condition known as ALCAPA, anomalous left coronary artery–pulmonary artery connection). After birth, when the pressure in the normal right coronary artery exceeds that in the pulmonary artery, collateral vessels begin to grow between the right and left coronary arteries to such an extent that a left-right shunt develops. This causes an audible pansystolic-diastolic murmur because of the turbulent flow. Despite the enormous dimensions of the collateral vessels, the subtended myocardium becomes ischemic because the actual perfusion pressure is only slightly higher than the pulmonary artery pressure. A maintained large pressure difference along collateral vessels with high shear stress is apparently necessary for optimal morphogenesis of collateral vessels. What we can learn from this situation is that the reestablishment of coronary autoregulation by the arterioles of the recipient bed restricts the further potential for growth of collateral vessels in the usual case of collaterals between coronary arteries in which both arteries are fed from the aorta.

Hypoxia and Blood Vessel Growth

Hypoxia is a potent vasodilator; its role in the regulation of coronary blood flow is discussed earlier. Hypoxia is also known to play a role in angiogenesis, the formation of capillaries. The molecular pathway that originates with tissue hypoxia and leads to the growth of new capillaries is relatively well known. Hypoxia-inducible factor is a nuclear protein that is activated or transcribed when tissue O_2 tension falls; hypoxia-inducible factor binds to a DNA sequence in the promoter of the vascular endothelial growth factor (VEGF) gene, which encodes an endothelial-specific mitogen that leads to the sprouting of new capillaries.[25] The mRNA of VEGF is present in normal myocardium. Targeted disruption of the hypoxia-inducible factor 1α gene is lethal not because VEGF cannot be transcribed but rather because of the apoptotic cell death of mesoderm-derived cells. Targeted disruption of the VEGF gene is also lethal because the embryonic formation of blood vessels is disturbed.[26]

In the adult heart, brief coronary occlusions up-regulate the VEGF mRNA within a very short time (30 minutes to 2 hours), but this is largely due to the stabilizing influence of another protein that also becomes active under hypoxic conditions. The stabilizing protein binds to the 3′ untranslated region of the mRNA and retards its degradation. The 3′ untranslated region of many mRNAs contains regions rich in adenine-uracil that target the mRNA for rapid degradation and thereby shortens the half-life of the message, making sure that the translation remains temporally controlled. Cytoplasmic proteins that bind to the region that is rich in adenine-uracil retard degradation, thereby making a more efficient use of the mRNA strand, which can enter the ribosome again for another round of translation. The low-level constitutive transcriptional activity of the VEGF gene leads to a rise in the intracellular mRNA concentration when degradation is reduced by the hypoxic activation of the stability-conferring protein. The nature of this protein is currently under intense investigation. It appears certain that more than one protein is involved, possibly with several different proteins being specific for specific RNAs. The von Hippel–Lindau protein, which is overexpressed in hypervascularized kidney tumors, is a known VEGF-binding protein, which leads to VEGF overexpression. The stability-conferring proteins of some cytokines and growth factors are localized in the cytoplasm and become activated by phorbolesters, which suggests an involvement of protein kinase C for intracellular signaling. The transcriptional and post-transcriptional hypoxic regulation of gene activity is shared with other genes whose products are known to exert functions during hypoxic conditions, such as lactate dehydrogenase and glutamic acid phosphodehydrogenase.[27] Furthermore, VEGF enjoys the privilege that its mRNA can enter a protected site of the ribosome that is repressed for most other RNAs during hypoxia, a condition that is known to inhibit translation. Despite these many advantages (high physiologic cardiac concentrations and sensitive transcriptional, post-transcriptional, and translational up-regulation), hypoxic angiogenesis in the heart is not particularly active and appears to be repressed in chronically hypoxic hibernating myocardium. In the adult mammal, VEGF-induced angiogenesis is probably only a sideline of the main VEGF action, which is in the stress response. Acute stresses such as brief coronary occlusions, mild right ventricular pressure overload or stretch, tissue-specific activation of the renin-angiotensin system, and glucose deprivation rapidly increase myocardial VEGF mRNA without subsequent angiogenesis. However, the increased expression of VEGF results in a rapid up-regulation of endothelial tissue factor, which induces a hypercoagulative state.

SUMMARY

Coronary blood flow is closely matched to myocardial O_2 consumption by a combination of feedback and feedforward control mechanisms. The dominant factors are local metabolic feedback control by a poorly understood mechanism and feedforward coronary vasodilatation mediated by sympathetic β-adrenoceptors. The normal coronary circulation exhibits strong autoregulation. The myocardial ischemia that develops during exertion in patients who have coronary atherosclerosis is caused by coronary artery pressure distal to a stenosis falling below the autoregulatory range when vasodilator reserve is exhausted.

Repeated ischemic episodes with myocardial stunning lead to the syndrome of myocardial hibernation, in which cardiac contraction is chronically impaired, usually with myocardial degeneration. Coronary artery stenosis also leads to arteriogenesis and the development of collateral vessels, a process that involves several cytokines and that stimulates hypertrophy of previously existing arteriolar collateral vessels.

chapter

18 Coronary Artery Anomalies

Allen J. Taylor and Renu Virmani

Definition

- Coronary artery anomalies encompass abnormalities in the origin, course, or distribution of the coronary arterial circulation.

Key Features

- Coronary artery anomalies are a rare form of congenital heart disease affecting approximately 1% of the population.
- Coronary anomalies are the second most common cause of sports-related sudden cardiac death in the young.
- Many coronary artery anomalies are benign, but some, particularly origin of the left or right coronary artery from the contralateral coronary cusp, are potentially serious.
- Clinical presentations of coronary anomalies range from asymptomatic to angina, myocardial infarction, congestive heart failure, and sudden cardiac death.
- Tomographic imaging techniques (cardiac computed tomography or cardiac magnetic resonance imaging) are the preferred methods to define the anatomic course of anomalous coronary arteries.

Therapy

- Surgical correction is generally indicated for serious anomalies when they cause symptoms or when they are identified in youth.
- Surgical reimplantation or "unroofing" is generally preferred to coronary bypass surgery when possible, although outcomes data for all methods are sparse.

Coronary artery anomalies are rare. Because estimates of the prevalence of coronary artery anomalies are derived from autopsy or angiographic series, their true incidence is unknown. Coronary artery anomalies are found in approximately 1% of patients undergoing coronary angiography[1-3] and in approximately 0.3% of autopsy specimens.[4] The majority of coronary artery anomalies (81%) identified in angiographic series do not pose major threats to myocardial perfusion and therefore are benign.[3] These primarily consist of minor variations in the location of coronary artery origin, including origin of the left anterior descending artery from a separate ostium in the left sinus of Valsalva and origin of the left circumflex coronary artery from the right coronary artery or right sinus of Valsalva. Thus, potentially serious coronary anomalies are very uncommon.

Although uncommon, some coronary anomalies are well described as a cause of cardiovascular morbidity and mortality. The described spectrum of symptoms arising from coronary anomalies includes angina, syncope, congestive heart failure, myocardial infarction, and sudden death.[5] Sudden cardiac death is the most dramatic presentation for a coronary anomaly. Particularly prevalent among young patients with sports-related sudden cardiac death, these anomalies account for 12%[6] to 19%[7] of such cases compared with 1.2% (i.e., similar to the background prevalence in the population) in cases of non–sports-related sudden death.[6] As a cardiovascular cause of sudden death in the young, coronary anomalies rank second, behind hypertrophic cardiomyopathy.

ANATOMY AND PATHOLOGY

The normal positions of the origin and distribution of the coronary arteries are highly variable. Normally (85% of cases), the right coronary artery arises from the right sinus of Valsalva as the "dominant" artery of the heart, defined as the artery of origin for the posterior descending artery. The left main coronary artery normally arises in the left sinus of Valsalva and divides into the left anterior descending coronary artery and the left circumflex coronary artery. The left circumflex coronary artery is the dominant vessel of the heart in approximately 10% of cases, whereas the remaining 5% of hearts show a codominant circulation (i.e., the posterior descending artery supplied by both the right and left circumflex coronary arteries). Variations of the origin and course of the coronary arteries beyond this general description are considered abnormal.

Various classification schemes for congenital coronary artery anomalies have been proposed.[8-11] These include variants of the origin, course, and distribution of the major epicardial vessels that occur in the absence of other congenital heart defects. A detailed classification of known isolated coronary anomalies is shown in Table 18.1.

Congenital coronary artery anomalies occur sporadically. Thus, there is no known genetic predisposition of coronary artery anomalies, beyond that arising from their occasional association with other forms of congenital heart disease. In a series of 1000 cases of coronary artery anomalies identified during cardiac catheterization at the Cleveland Clinic, only 10.1% had another congenital heart defect.[12] The coronary anomalies were most commonly of ectopic coronary arterial origin. Associated congenital heart defects (in decreasing order of prevalence) included mitral valve prolapse, bicuspid aortic valve, tetralogy of Fallot, corrected and uncorrected transposition of the great vessels, univentricular heart, and aortic

The opinions and assertions contained herein are the private views of the authors and are not to be construed as official or as reflecting the views of the Department of the Army or Department of Defense.

ANOMALIES OF CORONARY ARTERIAL ORIGIN, ASSOCIATED CONGENITAL CORONARY ANOMALIES, AND HEART DISEASES
Origin of one or more coronary arteries from the pulmonary trunk and one or more coronary arteries from the aorta
Left main from pulmonary trunk
Right from pulmonary trunk
Left anterior descending from pulmonary trunk
Left circumflex from pulmonary trunk
Accessory coronary artery from pulmonary trunk
Origin of one or two coronary arteries from the pulmonary trunk without origin of a coronary artery from the aorta
Right and left main from pulmonary trunk
"Single coronary artery" from pulmonary trunk
Anomalous origin of one or more coronary arteries from the aorta
Left main and right from right aortic sinus
Left main and right from left aortic sinus
Left main and right from posterior aortic sinus
Right and left circumflex from right aortic sinus (or left circumflex from right) and left anterior descending from left sinus
Right and left anterior descending from right aortic sinus (or left anterior descending from right) and left circumflex from left sinus
Right from posterior aortic sinus and left main from left sinus
Left main from posterior aortic sinus and right from right sinus
Left anterior descending and left circumflex from separate ostium in left aortic sinus and right from right aortic sinus
Origin of only one coronary artery from the aorta without origin of a coronary artery from the pulmonary trunk (single coronary ostium)
From the right aortic sinus
From the left aortic sinus
From the posterior aortic sinus
Modified from Roberts WC. Major anomalies of coronary arterial origin seen in adulthood. Am Heart J 1986;111:941-963.

Table 18-1 Anomalies of coronary arterial origin, associated congenital coronary anomalies, and heart diseases.

coarctation (Table 18.2). In particular, tetralogy of Fallot is associated with anomalous origin of the right coronary artery, and transposition of the great vessels is associated with single coronary artery.

The developmental origin of coronary artery anomalies involves variations in the persistence and involution of coronary artery anlagen.[13] Originally, six coronary artery anlagen appear, three from the aorta and three from the pulmonary artery. Under normal conditions, the coronary arteries arise from two persistent anlagen, and the others, including all three pulmonary anlagen, undergo rapid involution. Anomalous origin of one or both coronary arteries could result from the combination of abnormal persistence of one or more of the normally involuted pulmonary artery or coronary artery anlagen or abnormal involution of one or more of the normally persistent coronary anlagen.

PATHOPHYSIOLOGY

Anomalous coronary arteries are believed to cause reduced regional myocardial blood flow through mechanisms other than atherothrombosis. The mechanism of abnormal blood flow differs, depending on the particular anomaly. In origin of one or more coronary arteries from the pulmonary trunk, marked intercoronary shunting has been identified, and regional ischemia arises from a steal phenomenon.[14] Ischemic changes on a resting electrocardiogram (most often seen in children) and on exercise stress tests have been described. Chronic ischemia in these cases is also present, and patients with congestive heart failure may show improved left ventricular systolic function after myocardial revascularization.

Ectopic origin of the coronary artery causes regional myocardial ischemia due to impaired coronary flow reserve. In these anomalies, the initial coronary artery course is abnormal; findings include acute angulation of the aortocoronary junction, presence of a slit-like coronary ostium, ostial tissue flaps (valve-like ridge), and initial coronary arterial course within the aortic wall. Although the anomalous vessel can course between cardiac structures (e.g., between the aorta and pulmonary trunk), a common misconception is that the coronary artery is "compressed" between these structures. This is physiologically implausible, given that mean pulmonary artery pressure is lower than coronary perfusion pressure (diastolic aortic pressure). More likely, and consistent with the predilection for exercise-related deaths, is that additional distortion of the proximal coronary artery through

ASSOCIATED CONGENITAL CORONARY ANOMALIES AND HEART DISEASE[9,12]

Congenital Heart Defect	Congenital Coronary Anomaly
Mitral valve prolapse	Left circumflex from right coronary artery or aortic sinus Separate orifice for left anterior descending and left circumflex Ectopic origin of right coronary artery Coronary artery fistula
Bicuspid aortic valve	Separate orifice for left anterior descending and left circumflex Ectopic origin of left circumflex in right aortic sinus Ectopic origin of right coronary artery Single coronary artery
Tetralogy of Fallot	Ectopic origin of right coronary artery Ectopic origin of left main from right aortic sinus
Transposition of the great vessels	Single coronary artery
Univentricular heart	Extended anterolateral distribution of the right coronary artery
Coarctation of the aorta	Separate orifice for left anterior descending and left circumflex Ectopic origin of left circumflex in right aortic sinus

Table 18-2 Associated congenital coronary anomalies and heart disease.

hemodynamic aortic expansion accentuates the anomaly-related anatomic limitations to coronary flow reserve.[15,16] The importance of slit-like orifice and acute-angle takeoff is suggested by several observations: (1) their frequent pathologic description in patients dying suddenly in the setting of anomalous coronary arteries[5,17]; (2) the prevalence of abnormalities of the proximal coronary artery is increased threefold to fourfold in cases of sudden cardiac death of unknown cause, even in the absence of a coronary artery anomaly[18]; and (3) surgical revision of the coronary artery ostium can result in relief of symptoms, as reported in a surgical series of eight cases of anomalous right coronary artery with slit-like orifice.[19] Another important variable is the amount of myocardium at risk. Sudden death is more common when the anomalous vessel is dominant.[20]

Whether coronary artery anomalies create a predisposition for early atherosclerosis because of altered coronary flow has been controversial. Large angiographic series suggest against such an association.[2,21] In an analysis of 76 anomalous coronary arteries contained in the Coronary Artery Surgery Study registry, the degree of atherosclerosis was compared with control arteries.[21] A trend for increased stenosis in anomalous left circumflex vessels was seen, although the difference in mean percentage of stenosis between cases and controls was of no clinical significance. Registries of patients in a symptomatic coronary disease age group, like the Coronary Artery Surgery Study, have not found a higher incidence of coronary anomalies. In young patients dying with coronary anomalies, only 1% are found to have significant atherosclerotic arterial narrowing.[5] In total, it seems unlikely that coronary anomalies create a major predisposition for accelerated atherosclerosis.

CLINICAL PRESENTATIONS

In general, coronary artery anomalies may be manifested with symptoms that include angina, shortness of breath, and syncope. More severe presentations include the clinical syndromes of myocardial infarction, congestive heart failure, and sudden cardiac death, generally occurring during or shortly after strenuous physical exertion. Overall, symptoms are present in approximately one third of patients. In the Armed Forces Institute of Pathology (AFIP) series,[5] the majority of cases with sudden death (62%) were asymptomatic. Symptoms were most commonly reported in cases of ectopic origin of the left main coronary artery from the right aortic sinus (50%). In comparison, no patients with ectopic origin of the right coronary artery were symptomatic. This suggests that a greater extent of myocardium at risk, such as in cases of anomalous left main origin or when the anomalous vessel is dominant in the coronary circulation,[20] can determine symptoms and outcomes.

Tomographic imaging procedures, such as cardiac computed tomography and cardiac magnetic resonance imaging, are the tests of choice for diagnosis. Cardiac computed tomography has been shown to be more accurate than invasive angiography and fully defines anatomic details with high temporal and spatial resolution.[22-26] Cardiac magnetic resonance imaging is a second choice based on lower spatial and temporal resolution. The growing use of high-resolution, tomographic imaging techniques such as cardiac computed tomography is leading to increased incidental identification of coronary artery anomalies. Thus, in the future, it is anticipated that a greater number of asymptomatic or atypically symptomatic patients will be identified with coronary anomalies, leading to better understanding of their natural history and more informed decision making. In the interim, clinical decision making for these patients will be challenging; there are no optimal means of risk stratification for uncommon outcomes such as sudden cardiac death.

CORONARY ANOMALY SUBTYPES

Anomalous Origin of One or More Coronary Arteries from the Aorta

Left Main and Right Coronary Artery from the Right Aortic Sinus (Figs. 18.1 and 18.2)

Anatomy and Sudden Cardiac Death

Anomalous origin of the left main coronary artery from the right aortic sinus is classified further on the basis of the course of the anomalous artery: between the aorta and pulmonary trunk; anterior to the pulmonary trunk; posterior to the aorta; and posterior to the right ventricular outflow tract within the interventricular septum. In 60% of cases, the anomalous left main most commonly courses between the aorta and pulmonary trunk.[5] This anomaly accounts for 2.8% of serious coronary anomalies and occurs with an incidence of 1 in 12,500.[3] Although this anomaly is relatively uncommon in angiographic

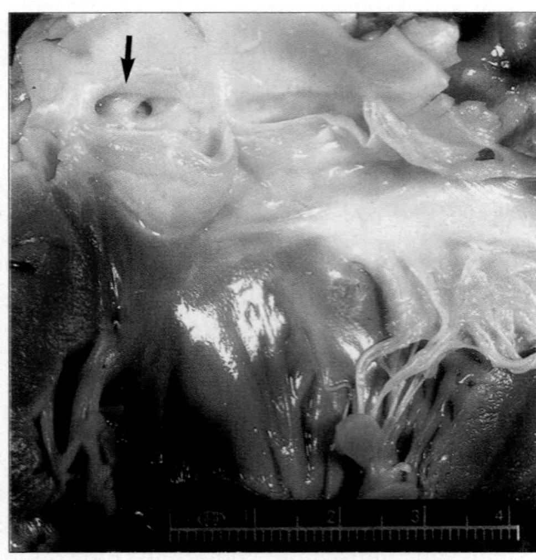

Figure 18.1 View of the left ventricular outflow tract and aorta showing left and right coronary ostia arising from the right coronary sinus of a 14-year-old boy who died suddenly while playing soccer.

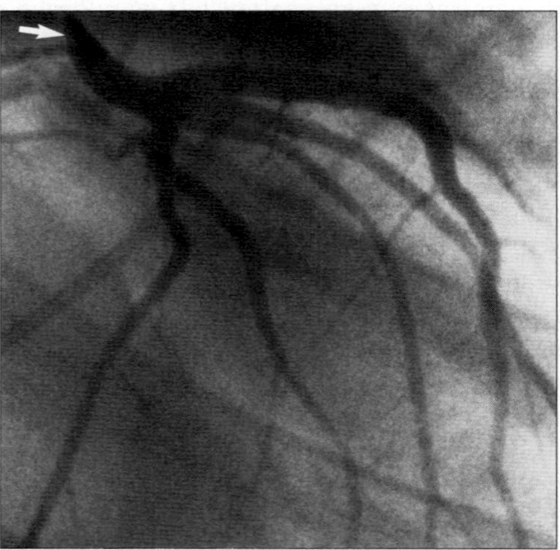

Figure 18.2 Left coronary angiogram (right anterior oblique projection) of an anomalous left main coronary artery from the right coronary sinus. The crescent-shaped orifice *(arrow)* suggests the presence of an ostial ridge. (From Taylor AJ, Farb A, Ferguson M, Virmani R. Myocardial infarction associated with physical exertion in a young man [clinical conference]. Circulation 1997;96:3201-3204. Reproduced with permission of the American Heart Association.)

series, it is significantly overrepresented in pathology series because of its clear association with sudden cardiac death (Table 18.3). In the AFIP series, 28 of 49 cases (57%) died suddenly, usually in association with exercise. Sudden death is most common (82%) when the anomalous artery courses between the aorta and pulmonary trunk.[5]

Left Main and Right Coronary Artery from the Left Aortic Sinus (Figs. 18.3 and 18.4)

Anomalous origin of the right coronary artery from the left aortic sinus is classified further on the basis of the course of the anomalous artery. In the majority of cases, the anomalous vessel courses between the aorta and pulmonary trunk (67%); the remainder usually course posterior to the aorta.[5] This anomaly is the most common, potentially serious, coronary artery anomaly, accounting for 8.1% of serious coronary anomalies,[3] more than twice as common as anomalous origin of the left main or left anterior descending artery. Initially, this anomaly was believed to be benign; however, accumulating reports have now clearly associated this anomaly with sudden cardiac death. Sudden death is observed in approximately 25% of cases, with roughly half of these in association with exercise.[5]

Left Circumflex and Right Coronary Artery from the Right Aortic Sinus (Fig. 18.5)

The left circumflex can arise either as an initial branch of the right coronary artery or from a separate ostium in the right aortic sinus. This is the most common anomaly of coronary arterial origin, accounting for 28% of anomalies identified by cardiac catheterization[3] and with an incidence of 1 in 300. This anomaly is generally considered benign, although sudden deaths have been uncommonly reported.[9,27] The high prevalence of this anomaly and low incidence of sudden death (see Table 18.3) support the suggestion that this anomaly is probably benign. Awareness of this anomaly is important during cardiac surgery to avoid problems with myocardial protection or during prosthetic valve placement.

Diagnosis of Coronary Arteries Arising from the Contralateral Coronary Sinus

The diagnosis of these coronary artery anomalies has been traditionally performed by coronary arteriography. Certain arteriographic clues can be useful in fully defining their course.[3,28] Of particular importance is identification of cases in which the course of anomalous right or left main coronary artery from the contralateral coronary sinus is between the aorta and pulmonary trunk. This particular course is angiographically distinct in the right anterior oblique projection when the left main forms a cranial-posterior loop (Fig. 18.6).[28] An alternative method is to perform simultaneous pulmonary and coronary arteriography[29] or, more practically, to insert a pulmonary artery catheter as an angiographic marker for the location of the pulmonary vessels.

More recently, noninvasive imaging modalities have been reported for the identification of coronary arterial anomalies. Standard two-dimensional echocardiography has been reported as a screening procedure for coronary anomalies in athletes. An echocardiographic screening study[30] of 3650 athletes found three cases of anomalous right (n = 2) and left (n = 1) coronary artery from the contralateral aortic sinus. However, the specificity of transthoracic echocardiography is insufficient for this test to serve as an accurate screening tool.[31] Alternative noninvasive procedures in the case of inadequate screening echocardiography include transesophageal echocardiography[32-43] and magnetic resonance imaging.[33,44-46] Each can be used to identify the origin and course of an anomalous coronary artery. Optimal diagnostic details are provided by cardiac computed tomography, with accuracy exceeding invasive techniques; however, requirements for administration of intravenous iodinated contrast material and exposure to ionizing radiation limit the application of this technique as a screening procedure.[22-26,47,48] These noninvasive imaging modalities will ultimately be valuable tools to overcome the selection bias within angiography or pathology studies of coronary anomalies.

RELATIVE FREQUENCY OF CORONARY ARTERY ANOMALIES IN ANGIOGRAPHY AND PATHOLOGY SERIES		
Anomaly	**Angiography* (%) N = 799**	**Pathology (%) N = 242**
Anomalous origin of one or more coronary arteries from pulmonary trunk		
Left main coronary artery or left anterior descending from pulmonary trunk	1.4	15.3
Both coronary arteries from pulmonary trunk		1.2
Right coronary artery from pulmonary trunk	0.2	0.4
Anomalous origin of one or more coronary arteries from aorta		
Left main coronary artery and right coronary artery from right aortic sinus	2.8	20.2
Right coronary artery and left main coronary artery from left aortic sinus	17.0	21.5
Left circumflex and right coronary artery from right aortic sinus	58.4	8.7
Right coronary artery and/or left main coronary artery from posterior aortic sinus	0.6	7.0
Right coronary artery and left anterior descending from right aortic sinus	4.8	0.4
Single coronary artery ostium from aorta		
Single right coronary artery ostium	3.1	9.1
Single left coronary artery ostium	3.9	9.1
Other coronary artery anomalies		
Hypoplastic coronary artery		5.4
Coronary artery fistula	7.8	1.7

*Relative frequency of coronary artery anomalies in adults as an isolated finding, without other congenital heart disease.
Data from Yamanaka and Hobbs[3] and Taylor et al.[5]

Table 18-3 Relative frequency of coronary artery anomalies in angiography and pathology series.

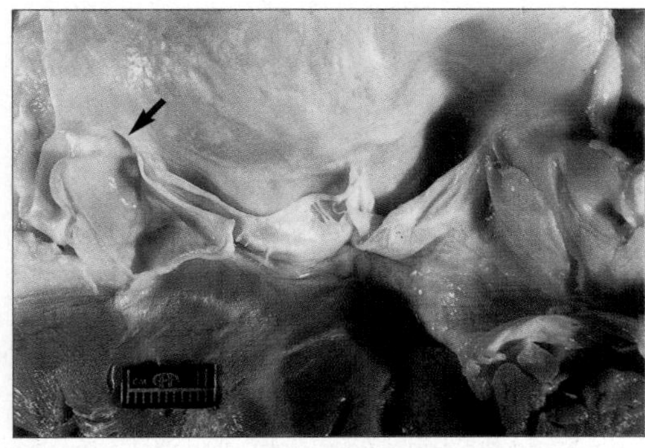

Figure 18.3 View of the left ventricular outflow tract and aorta showing left and right coronary arteries arising from the left coronary sinus. A slit-like coronary orifice and ostial ridge are present at the right coronary ostium *(arrow)*.

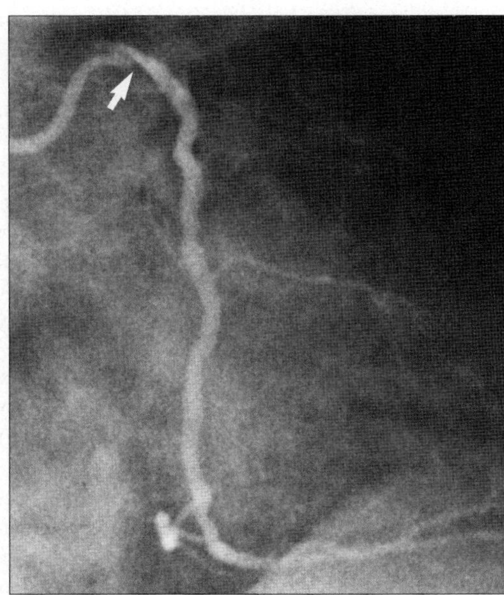

Figure 18.4 Left coronary angiogram (right anterior oblique projection) showing an anomalous right coronary artery from the left coronary sinus. The proximal right coronary artery is visibly narrowed *(arrow)* from the slit-like coronary orifice and aortic intramural course.

Pathophysiology

Limited data are available on the physiologic consequences of abnormalities in the initial coronary artery course in cases of ectopic coronary origin. One case report details an intraoperative evaluation at the time of coronary bypass for treatment of ectopic origin of the right coronary artery from the left aortic sinus.[49] Impaired coronary flow reserve in response to transient coronary occlusion was successfully resolved by coronary bypass grafting. We reported[45] the case of a 20-year-old man who presented with syncope, chest pain, and an extensive anterolateral myocardial infarction and ultimately died. Before death, diagnostic coronary angiography revealed an anomalous left main coronary artery arising from the right coronary cusp. Important angiographic features included a superior and anterior course of the anomalous left main coronary artery in the right anterior oblique projection, suggesting that the left main passed between the aorta and pulmonary trunk (Fig. 18.7). The crescent-like shape of the coronary ostium indicated the presence of

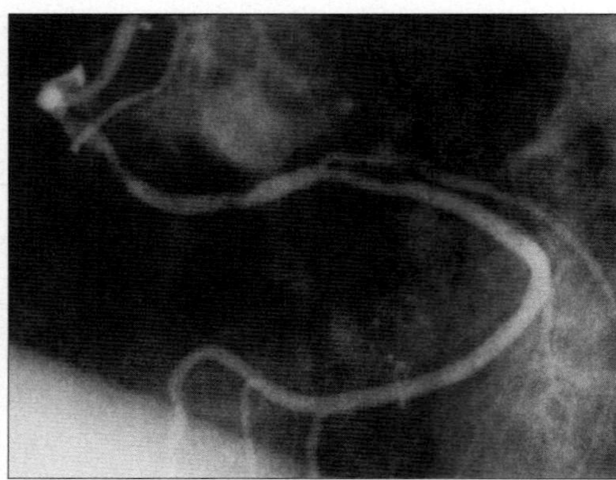

Figure 18.5 Right coronary angiogram (right anterior oblique projection) showing an anomalous left circumflex from the right coronary artery, coursing posterior to the aorta (demonstrated by the U-shaped appearance of the coronary artery).

an ostial valve–like ridge (see Figs. 18.2 and 18.7). Angiographic gray banding of the left main coronary artery suggested arterial narrowing along the aortic intramural course. The coronary arteries were otherwise normal. Examination of the coronary arteries at autopsy revealed an anomalous origin of the left main coronary artery from the anterior portion of the right sinus of Valsalva (Fig. 18.8a, b). No thrombi or intimal disruptions were found. Features of the initial coronary artery course included an acute-angle takeoff and an ostial ridge of aortic wall tissue overlying and partially obstructing the left main orifice. The left main artery coursed anteriorly between the aorta and main pulmonary artery. The heart was perfusion fixed through the aortic stump. Gross examination after perfusion fixation disclosed a large region of poor fixation, corresponding to the perfusion bed supplied by the left main coronary artery (Fig. 18.8c). The myocardial sections were then fixed by immersion in formalin for 24 hours (Fig. 18.8d). Further gross examination showed an acute, near-circumferential, focally transmural myocardial infarction extending from base to apex involving both papillary muscles with relative sparing of the posterior left ventricular wall. The regions of poor perfusion fixation and myocardial infarction were identical.

The regional myocardial pattern of the initial perfusion fixation suggests the relative significance of the acute-angle takeoff and ostial ridge. Distention of the aortic root by perfusion fixation at physiologic pressure resulted in fixation only of the epicardial surface (outer third) of the interventricular septum, anterior wall, and lateral wall; the subendocardial and mid-myocardial walls in these areas were nonperfused and non-fixed. These myocardial regions of no flow during perfusion fixation were consistent with the vascular bed of the left main coronary artery and corresponded precisely with the areas of infarction seen after further immersion fixation. This finding indicates that compression of the left main by the pulmonary trunk (not pressurized during perfusion fixation), which is a proposed mechanism for reduced coronary blood flow in this anomaly, is not necessary to reduce myocardial blood flow. Rather, abnormalities in the initial coronary artery course that are subject to aortic pressure are of greater relative importance. However, sudden cardiac death can occur without any obvious abnormalities in the proximal coronary artery course,

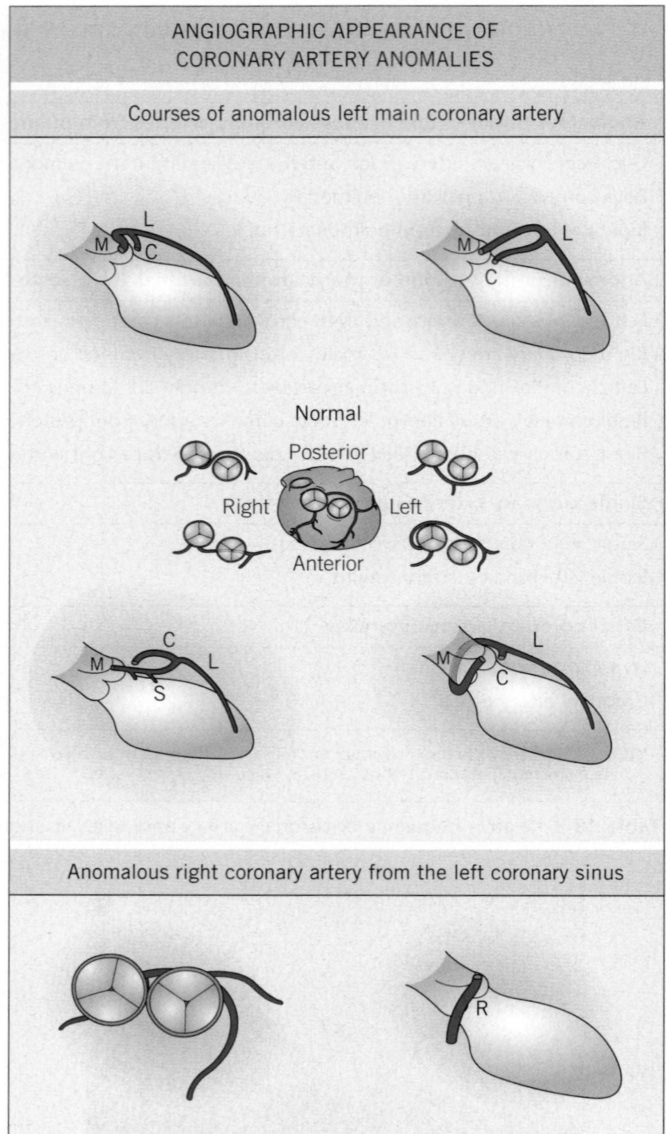

Figure 18.6 Angiographic appearance of coronary artery anomalies. Schematic representations of the four different angiographic courses of the anomalous left main from the right coronary sinus and the anomalous right coronary artery from the left coronary sinus. (From Kern MJ. The Cardiac Catheterization Handbook. St. Louis, Mosby–Year Book, 1991.)

suggesting that in a minority of patients, mechanisms beyond those arising from abnormalities of the initial coronary artery course, such as accentuation of proximal coronary abnormalities from hemodynamic expansion of the compliant aortic root or abnormal coronary vasomotor tone associated with endothelial dysfunction, may play a role in sudden cardiac death.

There are a number of candidate pathologic variables of significance in cases of an anomalous coronary artery arising from the contralateral coronary sinus and coursing between the great vessels.[50] These include the size of the slit-like coronary orifice (transverse ostial dimension), the angle at which the anomalous coronary artery arises from the aorta, the distance that the coronary artery is contained within the aortic wall, the fibrous ridges at the coronary ostium, and the degree

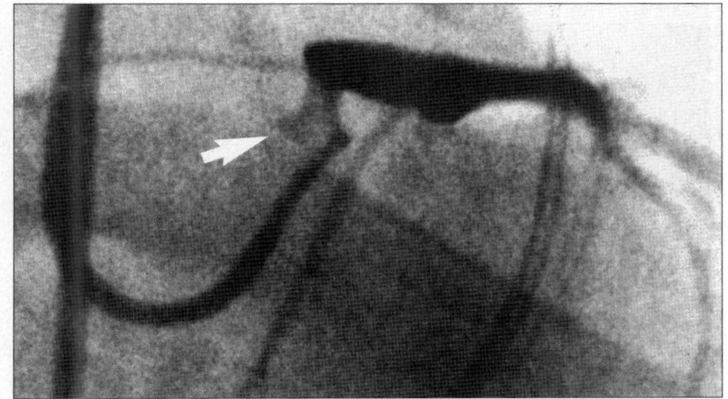

Figure 18.7 Left coronary angiogram (right anterior oblique projection) showing the angiographic appearance of an anomalous left main coronary artery arising from the right coronary sinus. The coronary ostium has a crescent-like appearance created by the ostial valve–like ridge *(arrow)*. The proximal coronary artery courses in a superior and anterior direction, indicating that the left coronary traverses between the aorta and pulmonary trunk. Attenuation of the angiographic density of contrast material within the left main coronary artery (so-called gray banding) is suggestive of arterial narrowing along the aortic intramural course. (From Taylor AJ, Farb A, Ferguson M, Virmani R. Myocardial infarction associated with physical exertion in a young man [clinical conference]. Circulation 1997;96:3201-3204. Reproduced with permission of the American Heart Association.)

of displacement of the anomalous artery from the appropriate coronary sinus. Theoretically, some of the variables, if more severe, could predispose patients to sudden cardiac death and therefore provide insight into prognosis. However, a study found no differences in the severity of these variables in patients with and without anomaly-related sudden cardiac death.[46] Furthermore, these pathologic features showed a high degree of variability between patients (Fig. 18.9). Thus, it is likely that plasticity of these features under changing hemodynamic conditions (such as increased cardiac output and blood pressure leading to aortic wall expansion and accentuation of coronary ostial abnormalities) also plays a role. The role of aortic compliance provides a unifying theme between the predilection for exercise-related death and adverse outcomes in the young (putatively with more compliant great vessels). In sum, the accurate identification of patients at increased risk of sudden cardiac death will be difficult at best.

Origin of One or More Coronary Arteries from the Pulmonary Trunk

These anomalies are particularly uncommon, accounting for less than 1% of congenital coronary anomalies.[3]

Total Anomalous Origin of the Coronary Arteries from the Pulmonary Trunk

This rare anomaly (approximately 30 reported cases) is associated with other major congenital cardiac anomalies 68% of the time. Symptoms, primarily congestive heart failure or myocardial ischemia, begin within the first few days of life as coronary flow diminishes with declining pulmonary vascular resistance. Survival beyond 2 weeks of age is uncommon[51] because of myocardial infarction due to myocardial perfusion with deoxygenated blood at low pressure. Attempts at surgical repair have been unsuccessful, probably because of preexisting severe myocardial damage.

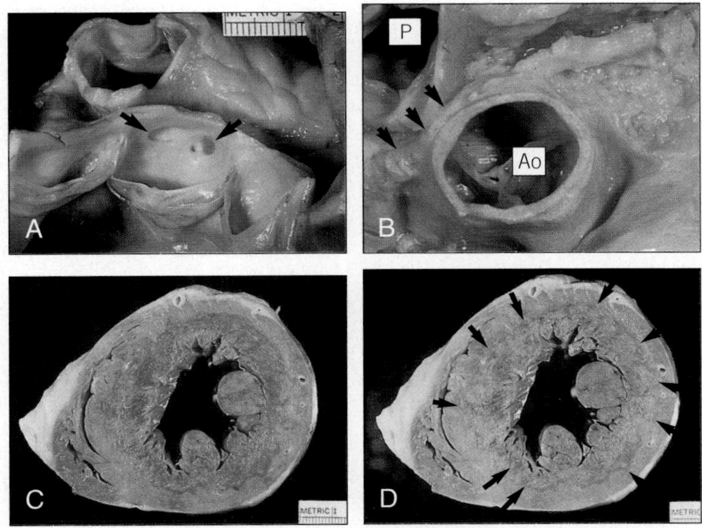

Figure 18.8 Fatal case of anomalous left main coronary artery from the right aortic sinus. A, Opened aortic root showing left main ostium *(left arrow)* arising from the anterior portion of the right coronary sinus. An ostial ridge is present, and the left main artery has an acute-angle takeoff. The normal right coronary ostium and the conus branch *(right arrow)* are seen. **B,** Aortic root viewed from above demonstrating the initial course of the anomalous left main artery *(arrowheads)* traversing between the aorta (Ao) and pulmonary (P) arteries. **C,** Mid-myocardial section after 15 minutes of perfusion fixation through the aortic stump at 100 mm Hg. Circumferential nonfixation (red myocardium) in the septum and the anterior and lateral walls corresponds to the poor perfusion in the distribution of the anomalous left main coronary artery. **D,** Mid-myocardial section (same section as in Fig. 18.8C) after 24 hours of immersion fixation shows transmural acute myocardial infarction (pale myocardium) in the anterior and lateral walls *(arrowheads)*. Both papillary muscles are infarcted. The areas of infarction correspond precisely with the areas of poor perfusion and fixation in Figure 18.8C.

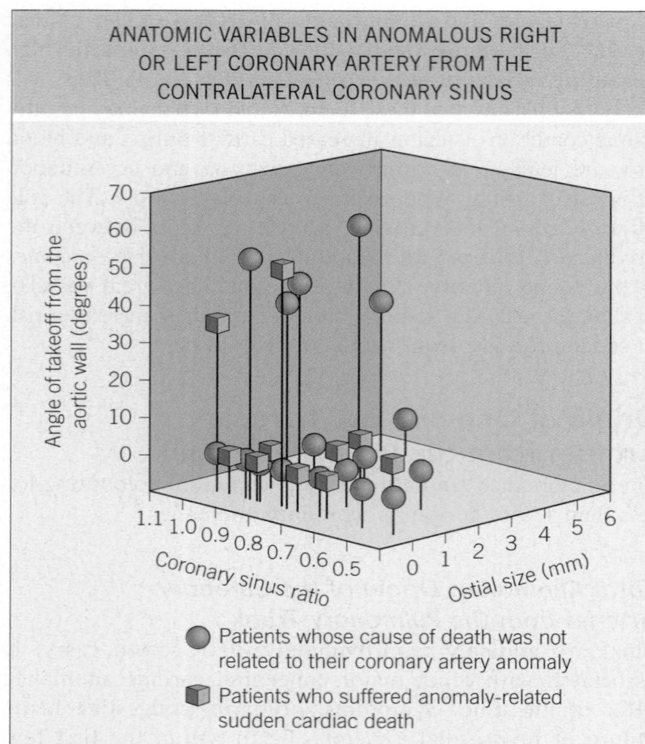

Figure 18.9 Three-dimensional plot of the anatomic variables ostial size (mm), length of aortic intramural segment (mm), and angle takeoff from the aortic wall (degrees) for all cases of anomalous right or left coronary artery from the contralateral coronary sinus. Spheres represent patients with non–anomaly-related cause of death; cubes represent patients with anomaly-related sudden cardiac death. (From Taylor AJ, Byers JP, Cheitlin MD, Virmani R. Anomalous right or left coronary artery from the contralateral coronary sinus: "high-risk" abnormalities in the initial coronary artery course and heterogeneous clinical outcomes. Am Heart J 1997;133:428-435.)

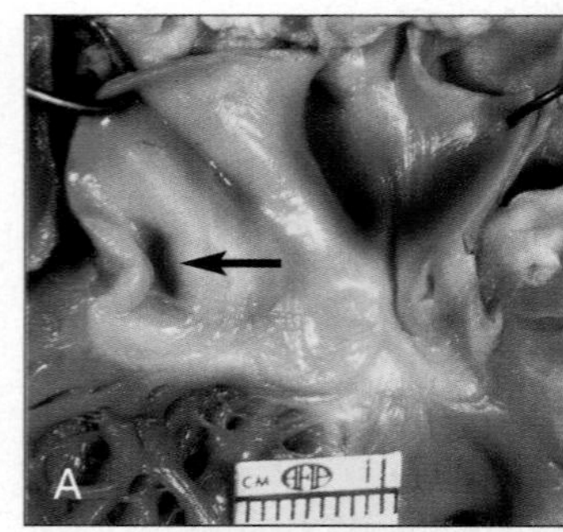

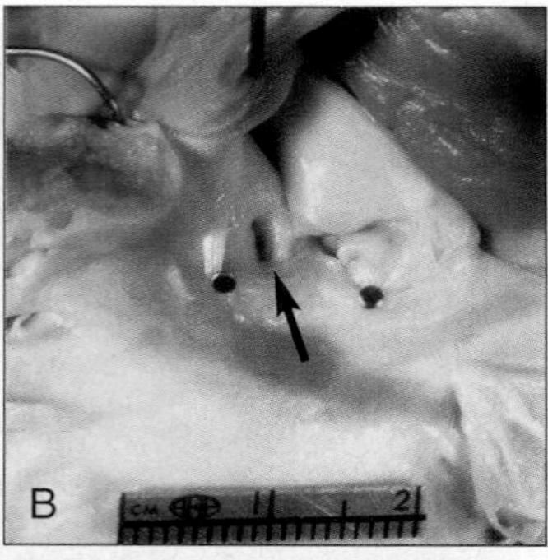

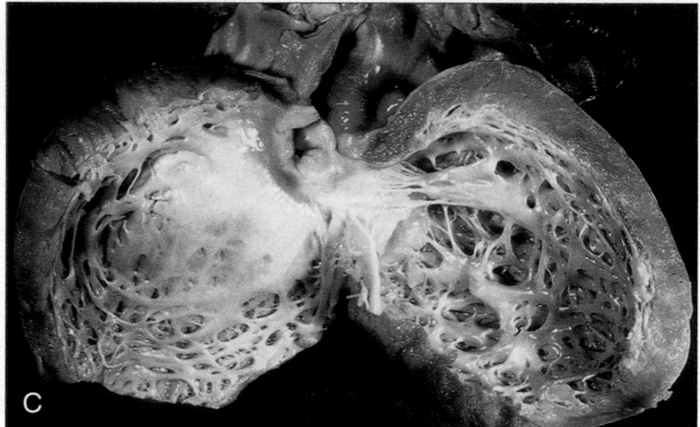

Figure 18.10 Heart at autopsy from a 6-month-old boy who died of severe congestive heart failure. A, Left main coronary artery arises from the pulmonary trunk. **B,** Aortic valve orifice illustrates the presence of a single, dilated right coronary orifice. **C,** Endocardial fibroelastosis of the left ventricle with dilatation. Note scarring of the anterolateral papillary muscle.

Origin of the Left Main Coronary Artery from the Pulmonary Trunk (Fig. 18.10)

This anomaly has been frequently reported (more than 500 cases, incidence approximately 1/300,000)[8] and is the most common anomaly involving a coronary artery arising from the pulmonary trunk. It is many times more common than anomalous origin of either the left anterior descending or right coronary artery from the pulmonary trunk in both angiographic[3] and autopsy[5] series. This anomaly is very commonly fatal,[9] including a predominance of death during early childhood from myocardial ischemia and systolic dysfunction resulting in congestive heart failure and sudden death. Electrocardiographic findings, including broad, deep Q waves, can aid in the differentiation of this anomaly from myocarditis or dilated cardiomyopathy.[52] In a minority of cases (approximately 20%), sufficient myocardial collaterals develop from the normally arising right coronary artery, and survival into adulthood may occur. In these cases, a continuous murmur may be present, and symptoms (angina pectoris, myocardial infarction, dyspnea, syncope, and sudden death) generally are present.[53-56] Angiography accurately diagnoses this anomaly, with the demonstration of collateral channels from the right coronary artery to the left coronary system with drainage to the pulmonary trunk. Ischemia arises from either shunting of blood into the pulmonary trunk or insufficient myocardial blood flow from some other mechanism.[56] Echocardiography can also diagnose this anomaly through demonstration of an enlarged right coronary artery relative to the aortic size[57] and by abnormal flows on Doppler echocardiography.[58,59] Treatments for this anomaly involve surgical closure of the left main artery with or without a concomitant bypass graft to the left anterior descending artery. An alternative procedure is primary reanastomosis of the anomalous artery from the pulmonary trunk to the aorta or subclavian artery.[53] Because of a persistent risk for late cardiac death after left main artery ligation alone, the definitive approach for long-term survival involves establishment of a two–coronary artery system with reimplantation techniques. Long-term results from these procedures appear favorable.[60]

Origin of the Right Coronary Artery from the Pulmonary Trunk

This anomaly is much less common (approximately 30 reported cases) than anomalous origin of the left main artery from the pulmonary trunk. The intercoronary shunt[14] from the left main to the vein-like[61] right coronary artery in this anomaly leads to dilatation of the left coronary artery,[62] but it is usually asymptomatic and not associated with myocardial ischemia. Most patients with this anomaly are asymptomatic, although angina and cardiac enlargement have been reported.[63-65] Because of this, surgical correction of this anomaly has been recommended.[9] Surgical correction of this anomaly is accomplished by either end-to-side anastomosis of the right coronary artery to the aorta or reimplantation techniques. Creation of a two–coronary artery system is preferred to simple ligation of the anomalous vessel.

Origin of the Left Anterior Descending Coronary Artery from the Pulmonary Trunk

This anomaly is much less common than anomalous origin of the left main artery from the pulmonary trunk and has been reported in fewer than 20 patients ranging in age from childhood to middle age. In general, this anomaly generally is manifested early in life with intercoronary shunting leading to a murmur and myocardial ischemia[66,67] with congestive heart failure[68] or cardiac enlargement.[69] Surgical correction of this anomaly is advised. The optimal operation for this anomaly is not well defined, but options include reimplantation techniques[69] and coronary bypass surgery.[67,70] With successful surgical revascularization, relief of ischemic symptoms and improvement of ejection fraction can occur.[67]

Other Anomalous Coronary Arteries from the Pulmonary Trunk

A single adult case of origin of the left circumflex from the pulmonary trunk as an isolated anomaly has been described.[71] The patient was symptomatic (angina), had normal ventricular function, but did not have a dilatation of the coronary arteries or a detectable left-to-right shunt. Another uncommon anomaly is origin of a small, accessory coronary artery from the pulmonary trunk, with otherwise normal origin and distribution of the left and right coronary arteries. Although one case report found this anomaly in association with symptoms in an elderly patient,[72] this anomaly is of no functional consequence. It is usually unrecognized at autopsy and has not been reported in large angiographic series.

OTHER CORONARY ARTERY ANOMALIES

Single Coronary Artery

The coronary circulation may be entirely supplied by a single coronary artery arising from the right, left, or posterior aortic sinus. The course of the coronary arteries can be highly variable, with 23 different courses described by Roberts.[9] Several classification schemes have been proposed, with subgroups based on either the site of origin and course of the anomalous vessel from an angiographic perspective[10,73] or descriptive anatomic terminology.[9] In general, single coronary artery is described according to the sinus in which it arises and the course of the coronary artery (anterior to the right ventricle or pulmonary trunk, between the aorta and pulmonary trunk, or posterior to the aorta).

Single coronary artery is uncommon as an isolated congenital coronary anomaly, occurring in 1 in 2250 patients undergoing angiography.[3] In a compilation of 142 cases, there was an approximately equal distribution of origin from the right and left coronary sinus.[73] (Of note, a single coronary artery may also arise from the posterior aortic sinus.) Associated anomalies of the heart and great vessels were seen in 68% of patients younger than 20 years and included transposition of the great vessels and bicuspid aortic valve. In comparison, few of the adult cases (6%) had other associated congenital heart defects. Since the publication of this large series, there have been numerous additional smaller series of this anomaly. Single coronary artery can be associated with sudden death (6 of 44 cases [14%] in the AFIP series),[5] with a greater incidence of sudden death when the single coronary artery arises from the right aortic sinus. Because there is no currently available option for surgical correction of this anomaly, the use of medications to treat ischemic heart disease should be considered.

Hypoplastic Coronary Arteries

Hypoplastic coronary arteries are diagnosed when neither the right nor the left circumflex coronary artery extends beyond the lateral border of the heart to the midportion of the posterior atrioventricular groove. The coronary arteries serving the posterior portion of the heart are small in caliber. This anomaly has been primarily described in autopsy specimens and not in angiographic series. Roberts identified hypoplastic coronary arteries in 8 of 3400 autopsy hearts, but a definitive association with sudden death could not be shown.[74] However, seven cases with sudden death described by Zugibe and colleagues[75] showed myocardial abnormalities (patchy fibrosis or myocardial infarction). Thirteen cases were described in the AFIP series, including five (38%) with sudden death. Thus, although uncommon, hypoplastic coronary arteries are underrecognized during life and are associated with ischemic myocardial injury. Because there are no current options for surgical correction of this anomaly, therapy with anti-ischemic medications should be considered.

Coronary Artery Fistula (Fig. 18.11)

Coronary artery fistulas have been commonly described and can be congenital (persistence of embryonic arterioluminal sinusoids) or acquired (usually traumatic or postoperative) anomalies. There is a slight predominance for coronary artery fistulas involving the right coronary artery,[76] and multiple fistulas have been reported.[77] The usual site of termination is one or more low-pressure structures in the heart or great vessels (right or left atrium, right ventricle, coronary sinus, pulmonary artery, superior vena cava).[76,78] Angiographic series have found a predominance of fistulas terminating in the pulmonary artery,[78] whereas these may be overlooked in autopsy series, in which the right-sided cardiac structures are most common. Typically, they appear as dilated, tortuous communications between the coronary artery and a cardiac chamber or pulmonary trunk (Fig. 18.12). Echocardiography can accurately diagnose coronary artery fistulas but may be limited for the detection of fistulas associated with small shunts.[79-81] In selected cases, myocardial contrast echocardiography may better define the drainage of fistulas or be useful in confirming the success of operative repair.[82]

Most patients are asymptomatic, and many fistulas are incidentally discovered during cardiac catheterization. Myocardial ischemia[77] and angina pectoris can occur, but myocardial infarction is rare. Other complications (e.g., compression of other cardiac structures, infective endocarditis, rupture) are very rare. Large fistulas may cause symptoms of volume overload and present as a continuous murmur heard best at the base of the heart (coronary–pulmonary artery fistulas) or lower

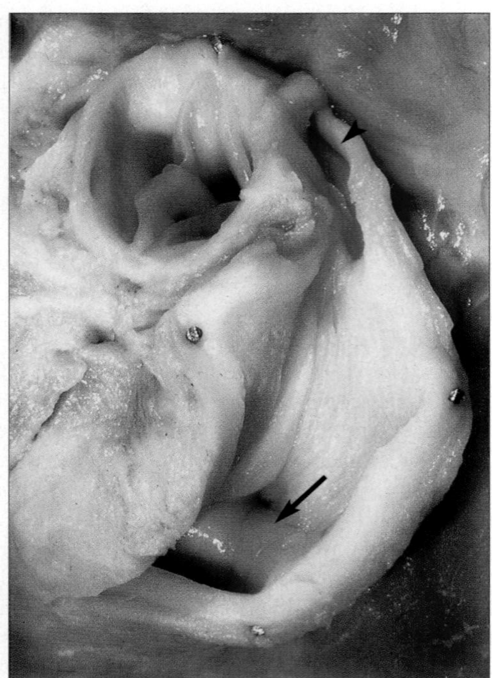

Figure 18.11 Autopsy specimen showing a coronary artery fistula. The left coronary artery *(arrowhead)* is dilated with thickening of arterial wall *(arrow),* with drainage into the right ventricle.

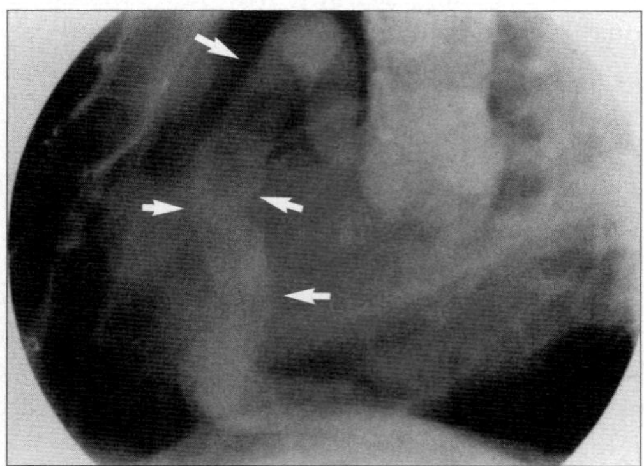

Figure 18.12 Coronary angiogram (right anterior oblique projection) showing a right coronary artery to right ventricle fistula. The right coronary artery is markedly enlarged.

sternal borders (coronary–right atrium fistulas). Coronary arteriovenous and coronary-cameral fistulas may also be manifested with a widened pulse pressure from the presence of a runoff lesion from the aorta. Fistulas with large shunts are generally surgically repaired with good success.[83,84] Successful treatment of coronary artery fistulas with transcatheter closure devices has been reported.[85]

MANAGEMENT

In the past, the diagnosis of a coronary artery anomaly was most frequently made in symptomatic patients or as an autopsy finding in cases of sudden death. In the future, it is reasonable to anticipate that an increasing number of patients will be prospectively and coincidentally identified with these anomalies by cardiovascular tomographic imaging procedures such as cardiac computed tomography (Fig. 18.13). The management of these cases will be difficult in the absence of controlled data to guide treatment decisions. For example, when should patients undergo surgical correction of coronary anomalies? Surgically correctable anomalies include anomalous origin of one or more coronary arteries from the pulmonary trunk and ectopic origin of a coronary artery from the aorta. All patients with origin of a coronary artery from the pulmonary trunk should be strongly considered for surgical correction. In contrast, management decisions in cases of ectopic coronary arterial origin can be difficult. Case series clearly document heterogeneity in the clinical course of patients with anomalous right or left coronary artery. Thus, whereas some patients die suddenly, others can live a normal life span with an unrepaired anomalous coronary artery.[86,87] The precise risk for sudden cardiac death in an individual patient is difficult to determine, and thus management decisions should be highly individualized. In the asymptomatic patient, considerations in the decision on "prophylactic" correction include the known risk for sudden cardiac death, the inability to risk stratify the patient by morphologic criteria, and the patient's age. Whereas the need for prophylactic surgical correction is most compelling in a young patient, there is little question that anomaly-related sudden cardiac death can occur regardless of the patient's age. However, this risk does appear to decrease with advancing age and is clearly lower (and perhaps quite low overall) for anomalous origin of the right coronary artery from the left coronary cusp. Overall, it is likely that the risk for sudden cardiac death attributable to the coronary anomaly in an older patient is low, although the precise magnitude of risk is unknown because of the influence of selection bias and unknown denominator size in an autopsy series. How to relate this risk to the risk of surgical correction with coronary bypass surgery is unknown and should be a highly individualized decision in an older, asymptomatic patient,[19,88] in part because age is a reflection of the individual's benign natural history and the possible influence of age-related changes in aortic compliance. The impact of symptoms on risk for sudden cardiac death is unknown. When symptoms are present, the argument supporting surgical correction is aided by the goal of symptom relief.

Recommendations for the patient with an uncorrected coronary artery anomaly arising from the contralateral coronary sinus and coursing between the aorta and pulmonary trunk include the avoidance of strenuous activity, given the known propensity for sudden cardiac death to occur in relation to exercise. Otherwise, anatomic correction can be attempted through a variety of means including percutaneous stenting, coronary bypass procedures, and anatomic revisions such as coronary reimplantation or "unroofing." Surgical correction is preferred; however, coronary bypass procedures are limited by technical graft failures and problems with graft maturation due to competitive coronary blood flow in the native circulation. Thus, reimplantation or unroofing (particularly feasible with a long aortic intramural segment of the anomalous artery) is the present preferred technique with favorable early results.[15,89-92] Cardiac computed tomography is important in presurgical planning to determine the feasibility of reimplantation (e.g., limited when the coronary artery takes an early intramyocardial course) or unroofing.

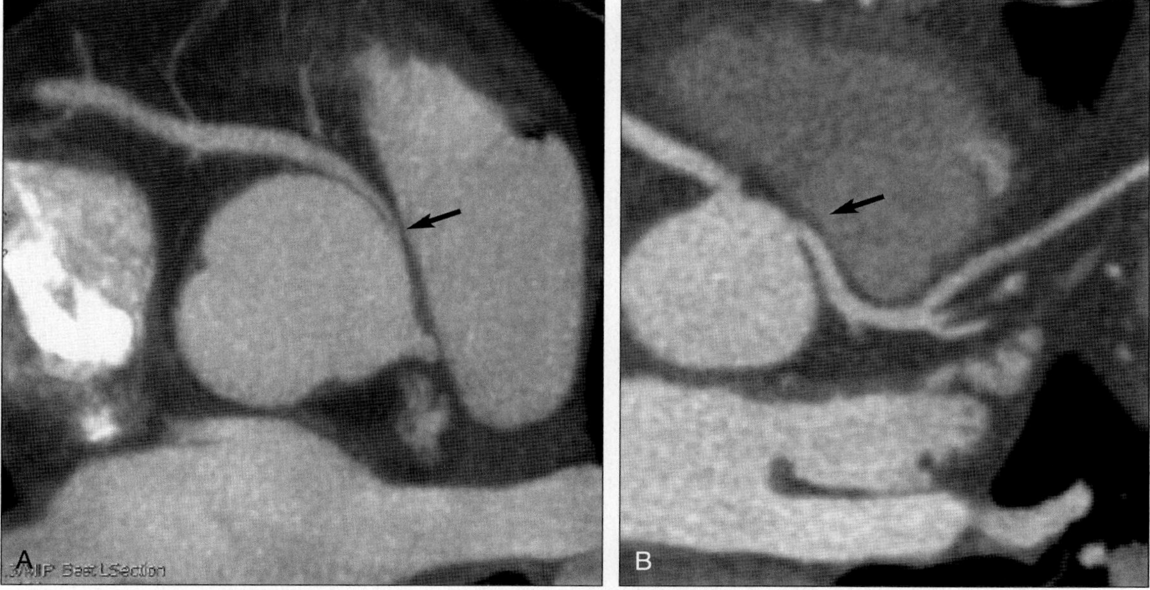

Figure 18.13 Contrast-enhanced coronary computed tomographic angiogram showing *(arrows)* anomalous right coronary artery from the left coronary artery cusp **(A)** and anomalous left coronary artery from the right coronary artery cusp **(B)**.

Screening for Coronary Anomalies in Athletes

Coronary artery anomalies are among the least common identified cardiac abnormalities that cause sudden cardiac death. However, they are found with an increased prevalence in cases of sports-related death, leading to heightened awareness and interest disproportionate to their impact as a public health issue. Should athletes undergo preparticipation cardiovascular screening, and what should that screening consist of? Medicolegally, most states in the United States require at least some medical screening before athletic participation, but the nature of this process is highly variable. Italy has used routine echocardiography in screening for more than 30 years.[93] Screening history and physical examinations alone are insufficient to detect many abnormalities, such as coronary anomalies. Nonetheless, this is the recommended procedure.[94] To improve effectiveness, screening programs are likely to require resource-intensive, noninvasive screening tests such as electrocardiography and echocardiography. Impediments to the acceptance of such tests as cost-effective strategies include the low incidence of abnormalities and problems with false-positive and false-negative test results.

SUMMARY

Coronary artery anomalies are a rare form of congenital heart disease affecting approximately 1% of the population. They encompass a wide range of abnormalities in the origin, course, or distribution of the coronary arterial circulation. Most coronary anomalies are benign, but some, including origin of a coronary artery from the pulmonary trunk, ectopic origin of a coronary artery, and single coronary artery, can result in cardiovascular symptoms and even sudden cardiac death. The pathophysiologic mechanism of symptoms lies in abnormalities in coronary flow including shunting (origin of a coronary artery from the pulmonary trunk) and dynamic limitations to coronary flow reserve (ectopic coronary arterial origin). Surgical correction is generally indicated for patients with symptoms or when these anomalies are identified in youth.

chapter 19

Pathophysiology of Myocardial Ischemia

Prediman K. Shah and Erling Falk

Definition

- Myocardial ischemia is a condition characterized by inadequate myocardial perfusion.

Key Features

- Coronary atherosclerosis, with or without thrombosis superimposed, is by far the most frequent cause of ischemic heart disease.
- Myocardial ischemia may result from an increase in myocardial oxygen demand in the setting of a flow-limiting coronary stenosis (reduced flow reserve, the predominant mechanism in stable angina) or a primary reduction in coronary blood flow due to thrombosis or vasoconstriction (dynamic flow obstruction, the predominant mechanism in the life-threatening acute coronary syndromes).
- In ischemic heart disease, many ischemic episodes remain clinically silent.
- Transient noninfarctional myocardial ischemia may give rise to postischemic contractile dysfunction (stunning).
- Chronic or repetitive myocardial ischemia may lead to chronic but potentially reversible contractile dysfunction (hibernation).

Clinical Implications

- Myocardial ischemia may be prevented or mitigated by reducing the myocardial oxygen consumption (targeting heart rate, wall tension, and contractility) or increasing the blood supply (targeting atherosclerosis, endothelial dysfunction, thrombosis, vasoconstriction, and collaterals).
- Myocardial ischemia is one of the determinants of morbidity and impaired quality of life in patients with coronary artery disease.

Myocardial ischemia is a condition that is characterized by inadequate myocardial perfusion relative to the metabolic needs of the myocardium (Fig. 19.1). Ischemia is therefore associated with a reduced delivery of oxygen and metabolic substrates along with a reduced ability to wash out products of metabolism. Myocardial hypoxia and consequent anaerobic metabolism are two of the cardinal features of ischemia. Myocardial ischemia is one of the major consequences of atherosclerotic coronary artery disease and contributes to the various clinical syndromes associated with coronary artery disease (stable angina, acute coronary syndromes, and silent ischemia). Although, traditionally, medical terminology has equated myocardial ischemia with angina pectoris, it may occur without symptoms (silent ischemia).[1]

Patients often differ in the severity of clinical manifestations and the frequency with which symptoms accompany episodes of myocardial ischemia. Even in the same patient, some episodes of ischemia may remain clinically silent, whereas others are accompanied by symptoms. In addition to limiting effort tolerance and quality of life, myocardial ischemia may presage a more serious clinical outcome, such as acute myocardial infarction and sudden death, especially in patients with unstable angina.[2] It has also been suggested that repeated episodes of symptomatic or silent ischemia or a state of chronic myocardial ischemia may lead to chronic left ventricular dysfunction.[3] A proper understanding of the mechanisms that contribute to the production of myocardial ischemia provides a rational basis for the selection of appropriate therapeutic intervention. Relief of myocardial ischemia remains one of the important goals of intervention in ischemic heart disease.

ANATOMY

Angiographic studies have demonstrated that in patients with symptomatic or asymptomatic myocardial ischemia, a flow-limiting stenosis (>50% to 75% reduction in cross-sectional area) of one or more epicardial coronary arteries can be demonstrated in 80% to 90% of cases.[4] In large angiographic series, approximately equal incidence of one-, two-, and three-vessel disease is found, with 6% to 12% incidence of left main stem stenosis. Ischemia in the absence of demonstrable coronary stenosis may also occur and result from vasospasm, as in many cases of Prinzmetal's variant angina, and from microcirculatory disease or dysfunction, as in syndrome X and in hypertrophic heart disease accompanying hypertension, aortic stenosis, and hypertrophic cardiomyopathy.

Several investigators have shown that there are qualitative differences in the culprit coronary lesions on angiography and angioscopy between patients who present with unstable angina and those with stable angina, even though traditional angiographic markers of severity of coronary artery disease (number of vessels with flow-limiting stenoses, percentage diameter of stenosis, minimal diameter of stenosis, length of stenosis, presence and absence of collaterals) do not differ between the two groups (Figs. 19.2 to 19.4).[5] The coronary stenosis tends to be more eccentric or irregular, with overhanging and irregular margins and with intraluminal haziness and filling defects, in patients who have unstable angina. These angiographic features are consistent with a ruptured plaque with or without a superimposed thrombus as demonstrated by angioscopic and anatomic findings. These complex lesions are observed in about 70% of patients with unstable angina in a culprit lesion, whereas similar features are much less prevalent (<25%) in patients with stable angina. These

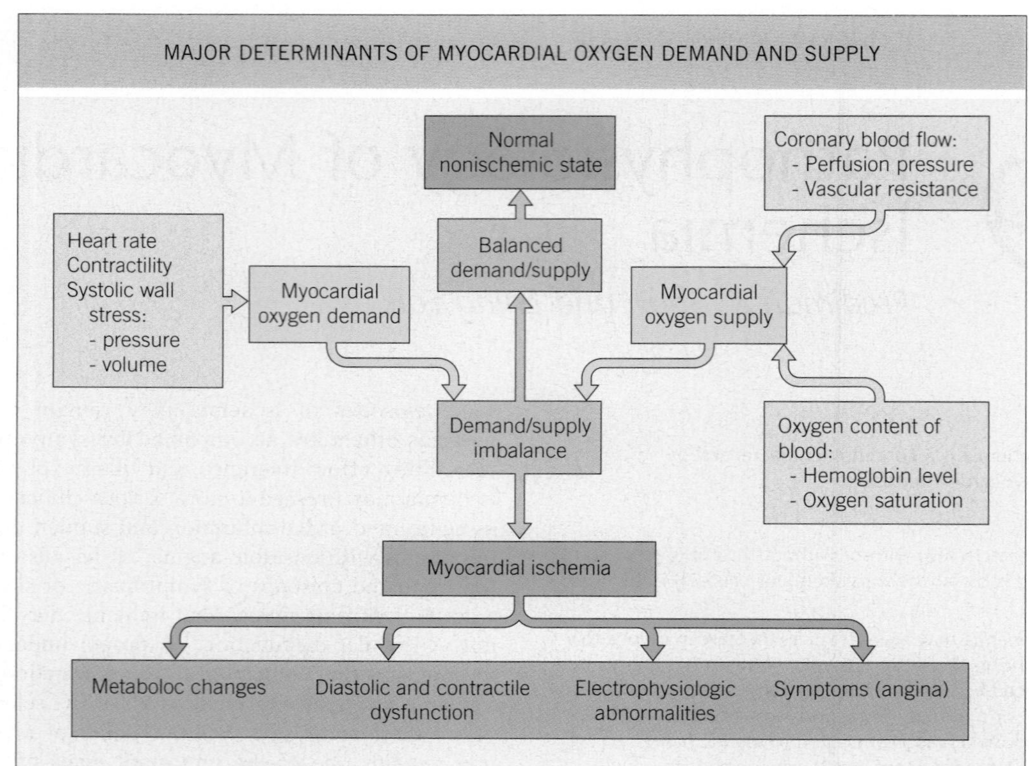

Figure 19.1 Major determinants of myocardial oxygen demand and supply. The consequences of an imbalance between demand and supply (ischemia) are shown.

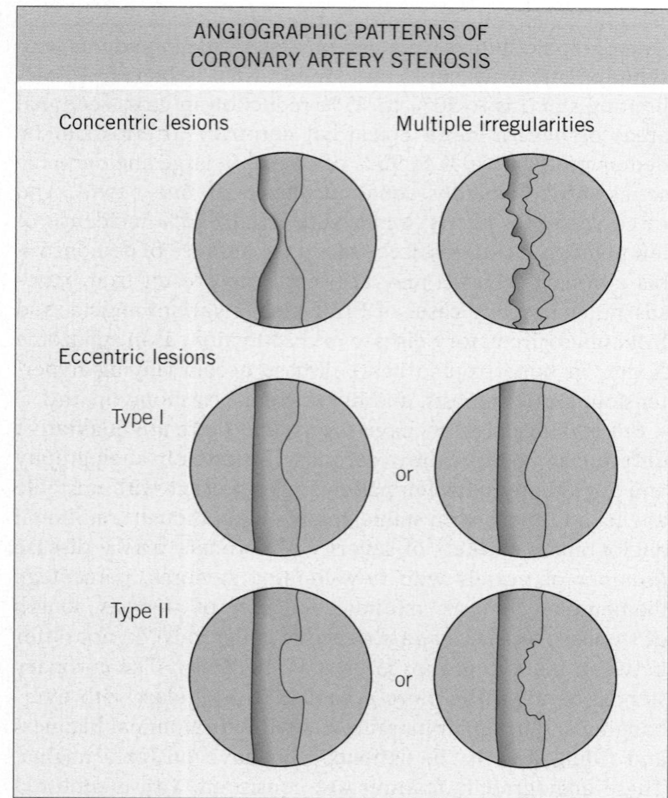

Figure 19.2 Angiographic patterns of coronary artery stenosis. (Modified from Ambrose JA, Winters SL, Stern A, et al. Angiographic evolution of coronary artery morphology and pathogenesis of unstable angina pectoris. J Am Coll Cardiol 1985;5:609-616. © American College of Cardiology.)

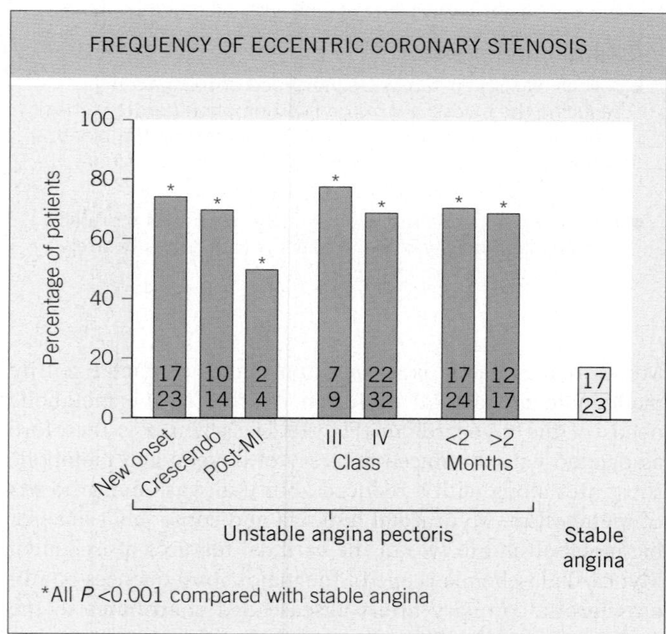

Figure 19.3 Differences between culprit coronary lesions in patients with stable and unstable angina. Frequency of eccentric coronary stenosis with scalloped or overhanging margins (Ambrose type II eccentric lesion). MI, myocardial infarction. (Modified from Ambrose JA, Winters SL, Stern A, et al. Angiographic evolution of coronary artery morphology and pathogenesis of unstable angina pectoris. J Am Coll Cardiol 1985;5:609-616. © American College of Cardiology.)

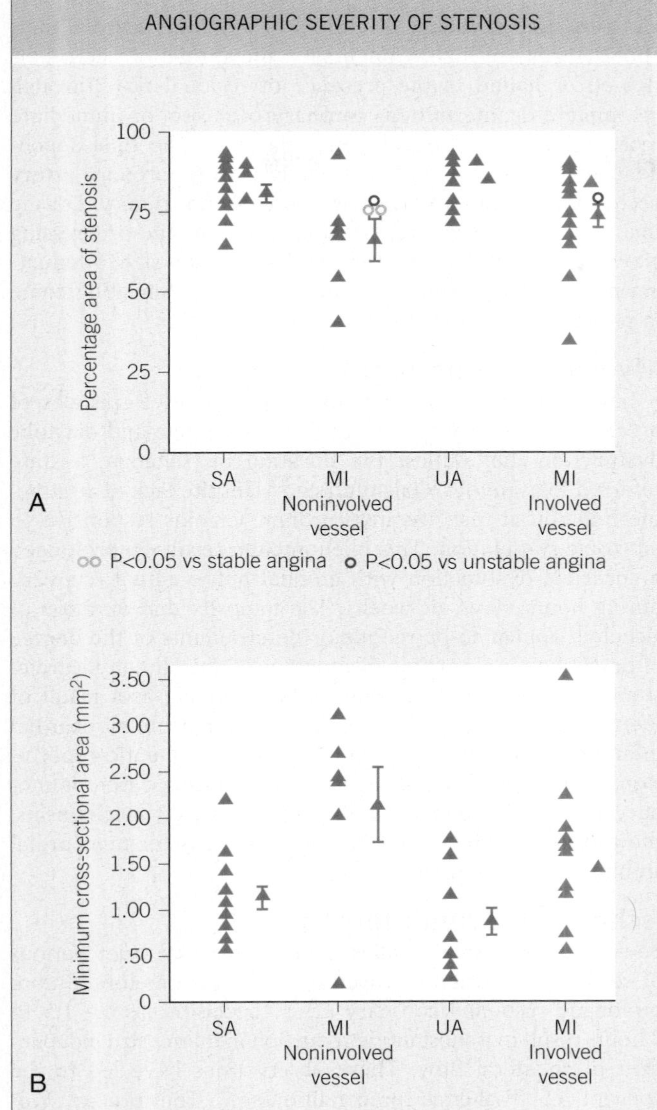

Figure 19.4 Angiographic severity of stenosis. Percentage diameter of stenosis **(A)** and minimum cross-sectional area **(B)** in the culprit coronary artery are contrasted among patients with stable angina (SA), unstable angina (UA), and acute myocardial infarction (MI). Note the significant overlap between clinical categories. (Modified from Wilson RF, Holida MD, White CW. Quantitative angiographic morphology of coronary stenoses leading to myocardial infarction or unstable angina. Circulation 1986;7:286-293.)

angiographic, angioscopic, and anatomic findings are consistent with the current view that plaque rupture with superimposed thrombosis has a key role in the pathophysiologic process and complications (acute myocardial infarction, sudden death, unstable angina.)[2]

PHYSIOLOGY

Determinants of Myocardial Oxygen Consumption

Myocardium derives its energy predominantly from oxidative metabolism. Myocardial oxygen demand is regulated mainly by ventricular pressure developed during contraction, extent of myocardial shortening (stroke volume), heart rate, and contractile state. The oxygen consumption of a noncontracting canine heart averages 1.5 mL/min per 100 g of tissue, whereas a beating canine heart consumes 8 to 15 mL/min per 100 g of tissue. Myocardial oxygen consumption is also influenced by the fraction of energy derived from the metabolism of fatty acids, which in turn varies directly with circulating levels of fatty acids and inversely with glucose concentration.

Determinants of Coronary Blood Flow

Coronary blood flow is related directly to the driving pressure within the coronary arteries and inversely to the coronary vascular resistance and cardiac compressive forces. Coronary vascular resistance is regulated by metabolic, neurohormonal, and endothelial factors. Because myocardium is predominantly an aerobic organ with high oxygen extraction at rest, any increase in myocardial oxygen consumption in a normal heart is met predominantly by an immediate increase in coronary blood flow, thus closely coupling oxygen consumption with flow. Increased blood flow in response to increased metabolic demand has been attributed to increased production of adenosine, a potent vasodilator, although vasoactive substances such as nitric oxide and others may also contribute to increased blood flow.[6,7]

Coronary Blood Flow Autoregulation

Under carefully controlled experimental conditions in which all other variables are kept constant, coronary blood flow in the dog remains relatively constant over a mean arterial pressure ranging from 60 to 130 mm Hg. This phenomenon, called autoregulation, also has an important role in humans, maintaining normal resting perfusion to the myocardium distal to a severe stenosis despite a reduced poststenotic coronary pressure. Autoregulation of blood flow is achieved by varying the caliber of the arterioles. Thus, arteriolar vasodilatation tends to maintain normal flow in the face of epicardial coronary stenosis until the severity of stenosis reaches the point at which all of the vasodilator reserve is exhausted; at that point, any further increase in stenosis or a decrease in upstream arterial pressure actually decreases blood flow. Because coronary collaterals do not exhibit autoregulation, flow through collaterals varies directly with the driving pressure.

Autoregulation has been attributed both to nitric oxide, a potent vasodilator released by vascular endothelium in response to a variety of signals including changes in stretch and shear rate, and to direct myogenic control.

Cardiac Compressive Forces

With each ventricular systole, an increase in intracavitary pressure and the throttling effect of myocardial contraction essentially shut off systolic blood flow, especially through the subendocardium, where flow remains predominantly diastolic in nature. This compressive phenomenon is exaggerated when the compressive force exceeds the aortic pressure (in valvular or subvalvular left ventricular outflow tract obstruction). In such conditions, tachycardia with shortening of diastole and relative prolongation of systole or arteriolar vasodilatation induced by exercise or drugs may precipitate subendocardial ischemia even in the absence of coronary artery stenosis. In contrast to that in the left ventricle, right ventricular perfusion tends to occur both in diastole and in systole because of a considerably lower systolic compressive force in the right side of the heart; however, in the presence of right ventricular systolic hypertension, the perfusion pattern resembles that of the left ventricle, making the right ventricle more susceptible to ischemic insult.

Metabolic Consequences of Myocardial Ischemia

When coronary blood flow decreases below metabolic needs, there is a rapid decrease in cellular adenosine 5′-triphosphate (ATP) and creatine phosphate, as use continues in the face of reduced synthesis. Furthermore, because of insufficient oxidative phosphorylation, breakdown of adenosine 5′-diphosphate eventually leads to the formation of adenosine, inosine, hypoxanthine, and xanthine. Ischemia is accompanied by a reduced extraction of free fatty acids, reduced lactate extraction, and increased lactate production. It results in a decline in the pH of myocardium and an increase in extracellular potassium concentration. With severe and prolonged ischemia, cellular ability to maintain volume and ionic integrity and the ability to generate high-energy phosphates are lost when the ATP stores are depleted by 80% or more.[8] As a consequence, cell swelling and damage to the sarcolemma occur, with increased accumulation of intracellular calcium, and irreversible myocyte damage ensues.

Hemodynamic and Functional Consequences of Myocardial Ischemia

Because the heart is an aerobic organ, a decrease in coronary blood flow results in a rapid decline in delivery of oxygen to the myocardium, with immediate loss of regional contractile function. Depending on the magnitude of myocardial involvement and the adequacy of compensatory hyperfunction of the nonischemic myocardium, regional dysfunction results in a global decline in myocardial function, with ventricular dilatation and a decline in ejection fraction and stroke volume. In addition to contractile dysfunction, ischemia also produces regional and global myocardial diastolic dysfunction as indicated by decreased relaxation and increased diastolic stiffness, both of which contribute to an increased left ventricular filling pressure and heart failure. Changes in systolic and diastolic function are followed by electrocardiographic changes and eventually by symptoms of angina; however, angina may not follow all episodes of myocardial ischemia. During regional myocardial ischemia, nonischemic segments may demonstrate compensatory hyperfunction, preserving global ventricular function.[9]

Wavefront of Ischemia and Necrosis

When coronary blood flow declines, the subendocardium bears the brunt of ischemic injury because of poor collateral flow and increased metabolic needs. The innermost few cell layers of the myocardium remain resistant to flow deprivation, however, because of direct diffusion of oxygen from cavitary blood. Subendocardial ischemic necrosis (myocardial infarction) begins to develop within about 20 minutes after cessation of blood flow, and the necrosis spreads from subendocardium toward subepicardium in a time-dependent wavefront manner.[10,11] This endocardium-to-epicardium spread of necrosis is accelerated when residual blood flow is limited, because of lack of collateral flow or complete and persistent coronary occlusion, or when myocardial metabolic needs are high. Conversely, the spread of necrosis is slowed or halted in the presence of residual flow through incomplete or intermittent coronary occlusion or immediate recruitment of well-developed collaterals. The time-dependent evolution of myocardial necrosis after coronary artery occlusion provides a narrow window of opportunity. During this period, successful reperfusion can abort the progressing wavefront of necrosis, thereby limiting infarct size, attenuating myocardial dysfunction, and improving clinical outcome in patients with evolving myocardial infarction.

Myocardial Stunning

It has been repeatedly demonstrated that brief episodes of severe ischemia can lead to prolonged systolic and diastolic dysfunction that outlast the duration of ischemia, a state referred to as myocardial stunning.[12] Despite lack of contractile function at rest, the myocardium remains responsive to inotropic stimulation. This phenomenon results in prolonged myocardial dysfunction with gradual but eventual recovery during hours, days, or weeks. The intensity and duration of ischemia appear to be the major determinants of the degree of postischemic reversible dysfunction. Clinically, myocardial stunning is often seen during unstable angina as a result of intermittent episodes of ischemia at rest, in acute myocardial infarction followed by spontaneous or therapeutic reperfusion, and after ischemic cardiac arrest during cardiopulmonary bypass. Despite a number of postulated mechanisms, the precise metabolic and biochemical basis for myocardial stunning is poorly understood.[13]

Ischemic Preconditioning

Several experimental studies have shown that brief periods of coronary occlusion followed by reperfusion before a more prolonged sustained coronary artery occlusion lasting 1.5 to 3 hours result in a substantive reduction in infarct size independent of collateral flow. These observations have led to the concept of "ischemic preconditioning." The precise biochemical mediators of this interesting phenomenon are not fully understood; potential mediators include activation of an energy-sparing ATP-activated potassium channel, slowing of glycolysis with attenuation of intracellular acidosis, and molecular adaptation with induction of heat shock protein.[13-15]

Evidence for the existence of the phenomenon of ischemic preconditioning in humans is mostly indirect. For example, infarct size is reduced, ventricular function is better preserved, and mortality is lower in patients with Q-wave acute myocardial infarction in whom the infarction was preceded by preinfarction angina (clinical surrogate for brief periods of ischemia) than in those without antecedent preinfarction angina. This may be an example of ischemic preconditioning.[16]

Similarly, angina early during exercise necessitating a brief rest followed by resumption of activity without further angina (so-called warm-up phenomenon) may represent yet another clinical manifestation of ischemic preconditioning.

PATHOPHYSIOLOGY

Myocardial ischemia in coronary artery disease results from an imbalance between myocardial energy requirements (myocardial oxygen demand) and myocardial oxygen and substrate delivery (myocardial oxygen supply) (see Fig. 19.1). Normally, epicardial coronary arteries serve predominantly as conduits, offering little resistance to blood flow. With a progressive increase in the severity of coronary artery stenosis, the resting myocardial blood flow is maintained until the stenosis is about 90% of the diameter (Fig. 19.5).[17] However, the peak hyperemic response (flow reserve) to brief total occlusion or in response to an arteriolar dilator stimulus such as papaverine or dipyridamole is reduced at a stenosis diameter of about 50% to 60%.

Maintenance of resting blood flow in the face of an increasing severity of epicardial stenosis has been attributed by some to progressive resting arteriolar dilatation downstream from the stenosis, thereby using up the flow reserve to maintain resting flow (autoregulation). Gould[18] has provided an alternative explanation for this phenomenon (Fig. 19.6). According to Gould, resting coronary flow is determined primarily by the ratio of aortic pressure and the sum of resistance of the epicardial stenosis (R_s) and the downstream arteriolar resistance (R_b) in series (see Fig. 19.6). When the downstream arteriolar resistance is large compared with the epicardial resistance, large changes in epicardial stenosis have little effect on total coronary flow. However, when the epicardial stenosis becomes sufficiently severe that its resistance matches that of downstream arteriolar resistance, vasodilatation occurs and resting blood flow decreases. When the stenosis resistance exceeds that of the downstream arteriolar resistance, autoregulation of coronary flow is lost, and total coronary blood flow is primarily determined by stenosis resistance alone.

During the stable phase of coronary artery disease, in which ischemia occurs mostly during physical or emotional stress, increases in determinants of myocardial oxygen demand (heart rate, contractile state, and wall tension) frequently trigger ischemia by increasing myocardial oxygen requirements. An increase in myocardial oxygen requirement leads to an absolute reduction in blood flow to the subendocardial region with an endocardium-to-epicardium flow redistribution (endo-epi steal) because of a much more limited vasodilator flow reserve in the subendocardium than in the subepicardium. Normally, the subendocardial layers of the left ventricle have a 25% greater blood flow than the subepicardium because of greater systolic compressive forces and wall stress and a greater level of vasodilatation in the region. Because of the greater degree of vasodilatation at rest, the flow reserve in the subendocardium is reduced, accounting for the greater susceptibility of the subendocardium to ischemia when there is a reduction in the subendocardial driving pressure (difference between the coronary perfusion pressure and the ventricular diastolic pressure) or an increase in heart rate.

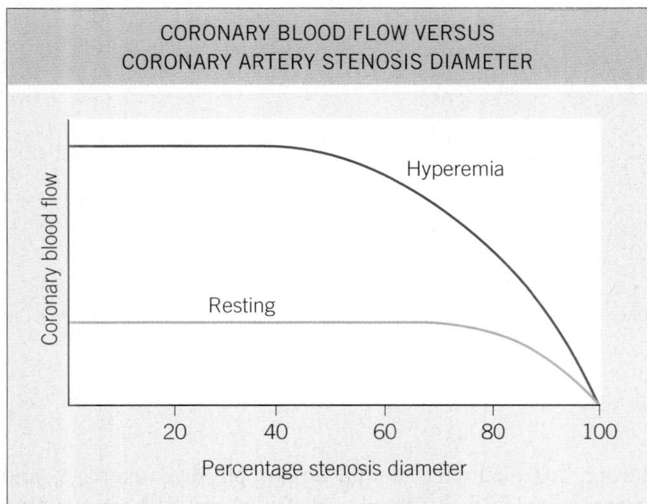

Figure 19.5 Relationship between percentage diameter of coronary artery stenosis and blood flow at rest and under hyperemic conditions. Note that at rest, blood flow remains essentially unchanged (because of arteriolar vasodilatation–mediated autoregulation) until the stenosis is greater than about 80%. However, under hyperemic stress, the autoregulatory reserve is exhausted much earlier, and flow begins to decline when the diameter stenosis exceeds 50%.

Dynamic Nature of Coronary Artery Stenosis

Passive Changes in Stenosis Severity

Autopsy studies have demonstrated that many coronary stenoses are caused by eccentric atherosclerotic plaques that involve only a portion of the arterial wall, sparing a variable arc of the vessel wall.[19] In such compliant coronary stenoses, changes in distending pressure have been shown to produce changes in stenosis severity. Increased blood flow velocity in the stenosis or a decrease in upstream aortic pressure can result in a decrease in distending pressure, which in turn results in the passive collapse of the pliable segment of the vessel wall, contributing to an increased severity of stenosis.[20]

Role of Endothelial Dysfunction

Since the landmark study of Furchgott and Zawadski[21] in 1980, it has become well known that endothelium plays a critical part in modulating vascular tone in large conduit arteries as well as in the microcirculation.[21-23] Several studies have shown that the vasoactive effects of acetylcholine, serotonin, norepinephrine (noradrenaline), thrombin, substance P, adenine nucleotides, bradykinin, and endothelin result from a balance between their direct vasoconstrictor effects on the vascular smooth muscle and their indirect endothelium-dependent vasodilator effects.[22,23] When endothelium is intact and healthy, a net vasodilator effect predominates; however, when endothelium is structurally damaged or functionally abnormal, vasodilator responses to these endothelium-dependent vasodilators are attenuated, and paradoxical vasoconstriction can occur (Fig. 19.7). Reduced vasodilator or paradoxical vasoconstrictor responses to these endothelium-dependent vasodilators have now been demonstrated in atherosclerotic coronary arteries (with stenosis or luminal irregularities) as well as in nonatherosclerotic large vessels (brachial artery) and the coronary and forearm microcirculation in patients with atherosclerotic coronary artery disease (Fig. 19.8).

In contrast, vasodilator response to nitroglycerin and nitroprusside is usually normal because these agents are endothelium-independent vasodilators that produce direct vasodilator effects on the vascular smooth muscles without the requirement of endothelium. Abnormal vasoconstrictor

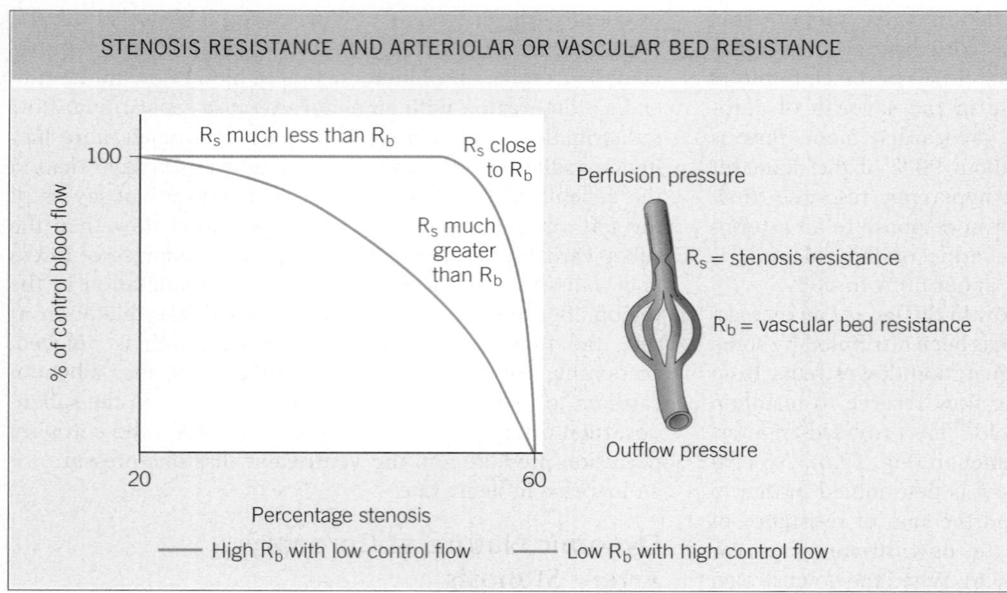

Figure 19.6 Influence of stenosis resistance and arteriolar or vascular bed resistance on the relationship between percentage diameter stenosis and coronary blood flow. Coronary blood flow is determined mainly by R_b if R_b is large compared with R_s. When R_s approaches or exceeds R_b, then R_s has a greater effect. (Modified from Gould KL. Quantification of coronary artery stenosis in vivo. Circ Res 1985;57:341-353.)

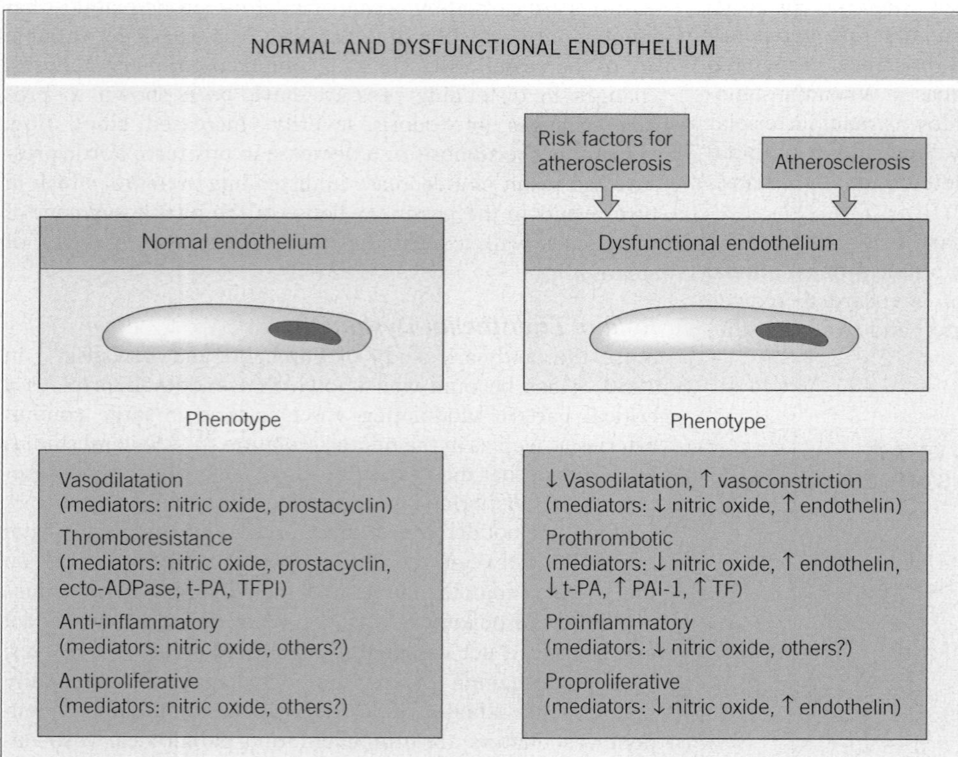

Figure 19.7 Normal and dysfunctional endothelium. Note that healthy endothelium promotes vasodilatation, resists platelet attachment and thrombosis, repels leukocyte adhesion, and inhibits proliferation of vascular smooth muscle cells. This phenotype is altered when endothelial health is disturbed by risk factors for atherosclerosis and atherosclerotic process. PAI-1, plasminogen activator inhibitor 1; TFPI, tissue factor pathway inhibitor; TF, tissue factor; t-PA, tissue plasminogen activator.

responses to acetylcholine and other humoral mediators are also generally associated with abnormal vasoconstrictor responses to physiologic stimuli, such as physical exercise, mental stress, cold exposure, and increased shear stress.[22-26]

Thus, abnormal vasoconstriction in response to physical or mental stress superimposed on a coronary stenosis may contribute to transient worsening of the severity of coronary stenosis. This effect, coupled with a reduced microvascular vasodilator function, may thus trigger myocardial ischemia during, for example, mental stress, physical exercise, and exposure to cold. Reduced endothelial vasodilator function has been demonstrated in the presence of risk factors for atherosclerotic vascular disease (advancing age, dyslipidemia, cigarette smoking, hypertension, diabetes, hyperhomocysteinemia, estrogen deficiency), even in the absence of structural abnormalities in the vessel wall. This suggests that endothelial dysfunction may antedate the development of atherosclerotic lesions.

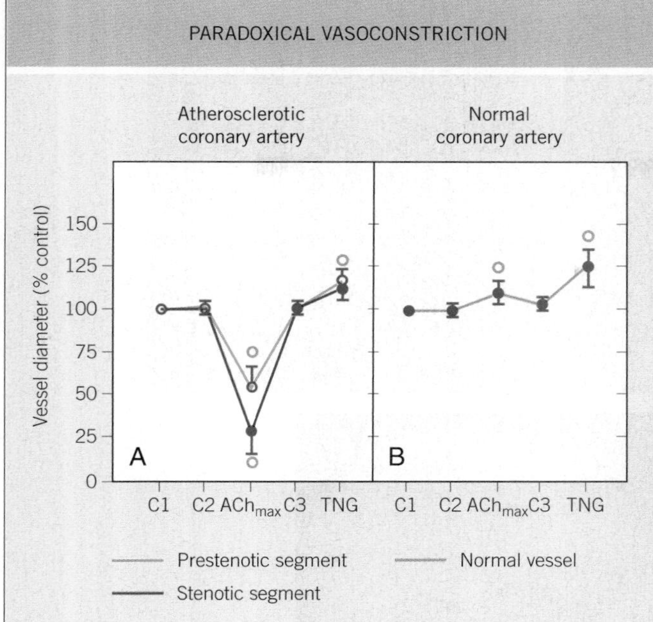

Figure 19.8 Paradoxical vasoconstriction. Quantitative coronary angiography demonstrates paradoxical vasoconstriction, reflecting endothelial dysfunction, in response to intracoronary injection of acetylcholine (ACh), an endothelium-dependent vasodilator, in atherosclerotic human coronary artery. In contrast, the normal coronary artery shows a vasodilator response to ACh. C, control; TNG, nitroglycerin. (Modified from Ludmer P, Selwyn AP, Shook TL, et al. Paradoxical vasoconstriction induced by acetylcholine in atherosclerotic coronary arteries. N Engl J Med 1986;315: 1046-1051. © Massachusetts Medical Society.)

Normal endothelium synthesizes several vasoactive molecules, including vasodilators, such as nitric oxide, prostacyclin, and a hyperpolarizing factor, and vasoconstrictors, such as endothelin, angiotensin II, and vasoconstricting prostanoids.[27-30] Reduced vasodilator responses in atherosclerosis and in the presence of risk factors for atherosclerosis have largely been attributed to reduced production or increased inactivation of nitric oxide, which is one of the key vasodilator signaling molecules produced by healthy endothelium.[22,23] Several studies have demonstrated that endothelium constitutively produces small amounts of nitric oxide from arginine through the action of an enzyme called nitric oxide synthase.[22,23] Nitric oxide rapidly diffuses into the vascular media, where it increases the concentrations of cyclic guanylic acid (cGMP) in smooth muscle cells. cGMP serves as a substrate for cGMP–dependent protein kinase, which is essential for the intracellular calcium-lowering effects of cGMP, which cause relaxation of the vascular smooth muscle cells.[23] Nitric oxide also produces other biologic effects, including a reduction in endothelial adhesivity for inflammatory cells, an antiplatelet effect, and an antiproliferative effect on vascular smooth muscle cells.[22,23]

In addition, the enhanced smooth muscle cell responsiveness and an increased production of the vasoconstrictor peptide endothelin may have a contributory role. Several studies have demonstrated an improvement in endothelium-mediated vasodilator function with aggressive modification of risk factors, accompanied by a reduction in the frequency of both symptomatic and silent myocardial ischemia (Fig. 19.9).[31,32]

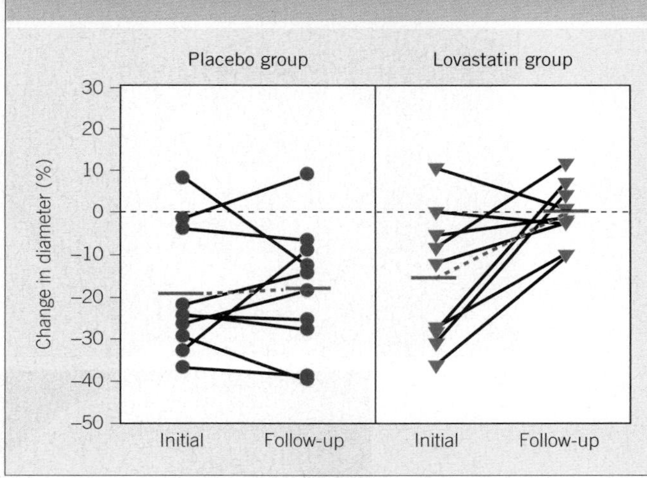

Figure 19.9 Improvement in the endothelium-dependent vasodilator response of coronary arteries to acetylcholine 6 months after lipid-lowering therapy with lovastatin. (Modified from Treasure CB, Klein JL, Weintraub WS, et al. Beneficial effects of cholesterol-lowering therapy on the coronary endothelium in patients with coronary artery disease. N Engl J Med 1995;332: 491-497. © Massachusetts Medical Society.)

Plaque Disruption and Thrombosis

It is now generally accepted that myocardial ischemia in unstable angina is predominantly triggered by dynamic coronary thrombosis, resulting in an abrupt and episodic increase in coronary stenosis with a resultant decrease in coronary blood flow (Fig. 19.10).[2,33,34] Coronary thrombi tend to be dynamic, with episodic growth, lysis, incorporation into the plaque, and downstream embolization contributing to the episodic effects on coronary blood flow. Coronary thrombus generally evolves from disruption of an atherosclerotic plaque (Fig. 19.11).

Disruption of an atherosclerotic plaque occurs in two main forms: classic plaque rupture (or fissuring), accounting for 70% to 80% of coronary thrombi, and so-called plaque erosion, accounting for the remaining 20% to 30%.[33,35] Rupture is a deep plaque injury in which the highly thrombogenic lipid-rich atheromatous core is exposed to the flowing blood. In contrast to plaque rupture, plaque erosion is a poorly defined superficial injury; the term is, in fact, used for all but rupture-related plaque changes found beneath coronary thrombi, whether or not actual plaque “erosion” or inflammation can be identified microscopically. Plaque rupture is a more frequent cause of coronary thrombosis in men compared with women (80% versus 60%), but otherwise, risk factors for atherosclerosis do not appear to be related to a particular type of thrombosis.[33,35]

Plaques that rupture and produce coronary thrombi are generally large but may not be severely obstructive on angiography before their rupture.[2,33,34] Such plaques tend to be lipid rich, with increased inflammatory cell infiltration (macrophages, T cells, mast cells), increased neovascularity, fewer smooth muscle cells, and thinned-out fibrous caps.[2,33-36] Plaques with these compositional attributes have, by inference, been considered to be vulnerable plaques before their rupture, although there are no prospective studies that have demonstrated such a transition.

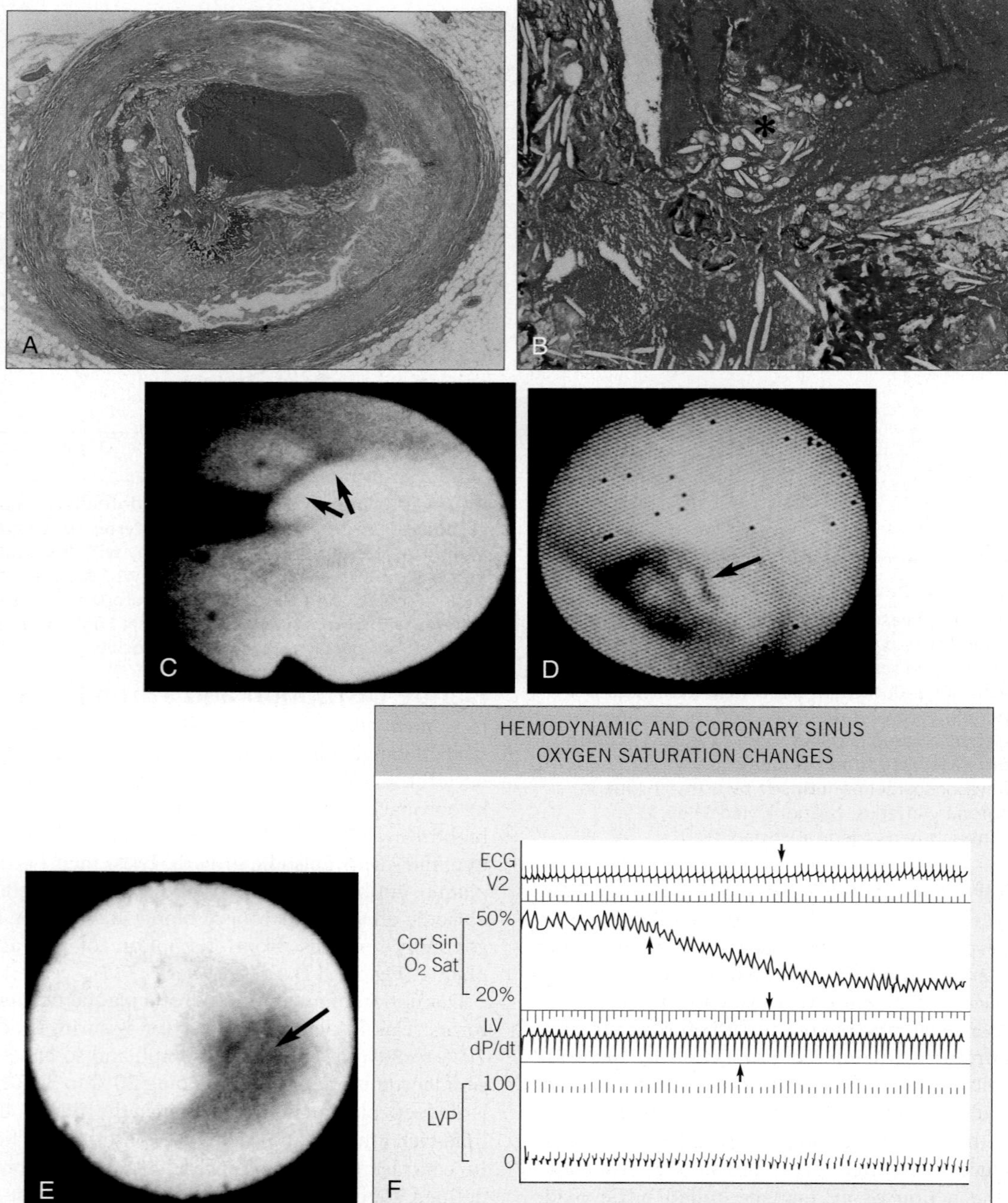

Figure 19.10 Plaque disruption and thrombosis. A, Coronary artery plaque demonstrating rupture of the fibrous cap (blue) with superimposed thrombus (dark red). **B,** A higher magnification shows lipid components of the plaque *(asterisk)* extruding into the lumen at the site of plaque rupture with superimposed thrombus. **C-E,** In vivo angioscopic views of culprit coronary stenosis. Arrows show a smooth intact plaque in stable angina **(C)**, a disrupted plaque in unstable angina **(D)**, and partially occlusive intraluminal thrombus in unstable angina **(E)**. (Modified from Sherman CT, Litvack F, Grundfest W, et al. Coronary angioscopy in patients with unstable angina pectoris. N Engl J Med 1986;315:913-915.) **F,** Hemodynamic and coronary sinus oxygen saturation (Cor Sin O_2 Sat, a surrogate for coronary blood flow) changes recorded continuously during an episode of rest angina in a patient with unstable angina. The episode of ischemia is initiated by a primary reduction in coronary blood flow *(first arrow),* which is later followed by alterations in left ventricular function, hemodynamic state, and the electrocardiogram (ECG). LV, left ventricular; LVP, left ventricular pressure. (Modified from Chierchia S, Brunelli C, Simonetti L, Lazzari M, Maseri A. Sequence of events in angina at rest: primary reduction in coronary blood flow. Circulation 1980;61:759-768.)

The precise mechanisms that lead to plaque rupture are not well understood. It has been hypothesized that excessive degradation of extracellular matrix through the release of a family of matrix-degrading enzymes (matrix-degrading metalloproteinases and cysteine proteases such as cathepsins) expressed by inflammatory cells (mostly macrophages), in addition to increased death of matrix-synthesizing vascular smooth muscle cells through apoptosis, may deplete the collagen framework in the fibrous cap.[2,33,34] The collagen content of the fibrous cap is largely responsible for the plaque's tensile strength; its depletion would result in cap thinning and, eventually, its mechanical failure (rupture), either spontaneously or in response to hemodynamic stresses.

Activation of inflammatory cells by various cytokines, immune mechanisms and immunomodulatory molecules such as CD40, mast cell–derived proteases, oxidant stress,

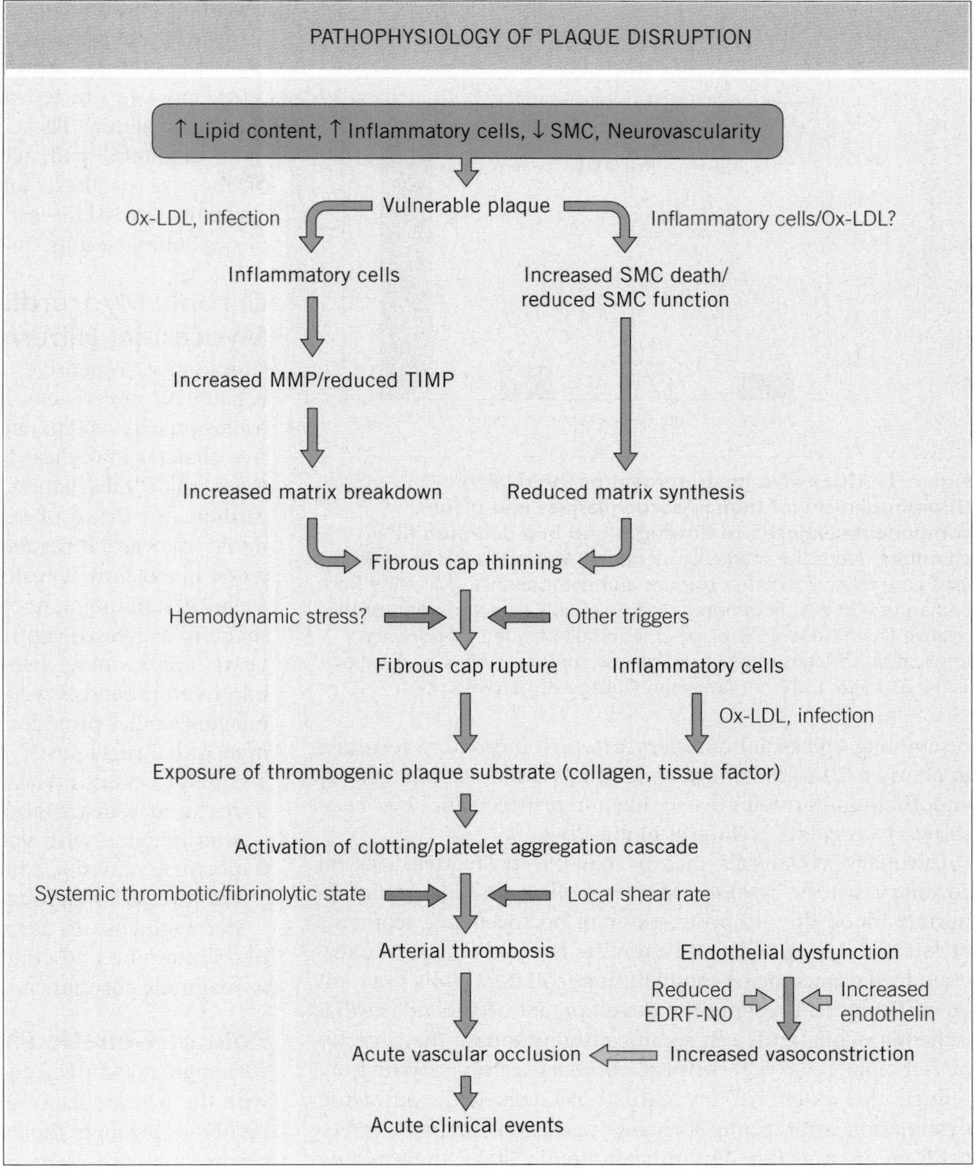

Figure 19.11 Pathophysiology of plaque disruption and consequent thrombosis responsible for acute ischemic syndromes. EDRF-NO, endothelium-derived relaxing factor–nitric oxide; MMP, matrix metalloproteinase; Ox-LDL, oxidized low-density lipoprotein; SMC, smooth muscle cells; TIMP, tissue inhibitor of metalloproteinase.

oxidized lipids, and matrix molecules such as tenascin C produced by macrophages in the plaque may contribute to a net increase in matrix-degrading activity by up-regulation of matrix metalloproteinases in atherosclerotic lesions.[2,33,34] In addition, activated inflammatory cells and toxic components of oxidized lipids in the plaque may further contribute to plaque disruption by reducing the matrix content through stimulation of smooth muscle cell death by apoptosis. In the past few years, several putative murine models of atherosclerotic plaque rupture or coronary vaso-occlusive disease have been reported, but in general, several limitations exist in these models as faithful indicators of human disease.[37-39]

The magnitude and the duration of the thrombotic response after plaque disruption are probably determined by the thrombogenicity of the plaque constituents, the local rheology related to severity of stenosis and consequent shear rate, and the systemic thrombotic-antithrombotic and fibrinolytic-antifibrinolytic balances.[2,33,34] Among the plaque components, the lipid-rich core appears to be highly thrombogenic because of its high tissue factor content; tissue factor, in turn, is predominantly produced by the inflammatory cells (mostly the macrophages) in the plaque (Fig. 19.12).[40]

Role of Collaterals

Collaterals are vascular channels that connect epicardial coronary arteries, providing alternative sources of blood flow distal to a coronary artery obstruction. These interconnecting vascular channels, which are present in normal hearts, range in diameter from 20 to 200 μm, and their density varies greatly among different individuals and species.[41,42] These collateral channels, although anatomically present, remain functionally closed under normal circumstances because of lack of a pressure gradient between the donor and recipient arteries. However, when a coronary artery obstruction is imposed, the poststenotic decline in pressure creates an immediate gradient for flow from the high-pressure donor vessel to the low-pressure recipient vessel, opening up the collateral channels. After opening, the thin-walled collateral channels undergo several anatomic changes that transform them into three-layer structures

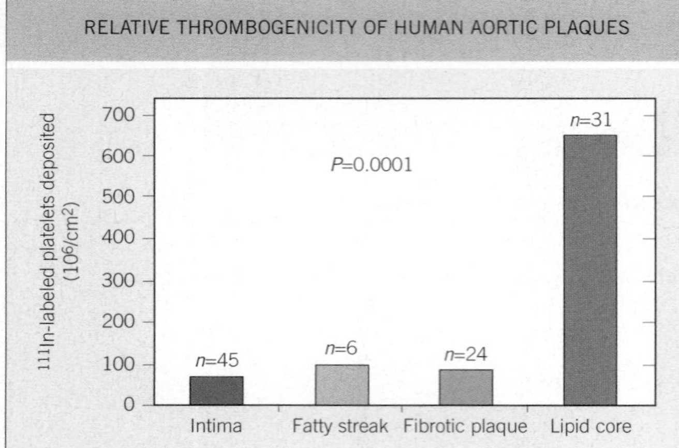

Figure 19.12 Ex vivo measurement of the relative thrombogenicity of human aortic plaques and plaque components exposed to flowing blood in a Badimon flow chamber. Note the markedly increased thrombogenicity of the lipid core relative to other plaques and components. (Modified from Fernandez-Ortiz A, Badimon JJ, Falk E, et al. Characterization of the relative thrombogenicity of atherosclerotic plaque components: implication for consequences of plaque rupture. J Am Coll Cardiol 1994;23:1526-1529. © American College of Cardiology.)

resembling epicardial coronary arteries, ultimately resulting in nearly a 10-fold increase in luminal diameter. Endogenous endothelium-derived nitric oxide and prostacyclin have been shown to regulate collateral blood flow.

Coronary collaterals clearly have a protective role in coronary artery disease. Mature collaterals can maintain normal blood flow to poststenotic or postocclusive segments at rest and during moderate exercise; but with maximal exercise or pharmacologic vasodilatation, collateral flow may not be sufficient to preclude the development of subendocardial ischemia. Collaterals can significantly attenuate the severity of ischemia related to critical coronary artery obstruction, reduce the extent of myocardial necrosis and contractile dysfunction after acute coronary occlusion, maintain myocardium in a viable but noncontractile state (hibernating myocardium) after coronary occlusion, and, in some cases, completely prevent the development of myocardial infarction and ventricular dysfunction in the face of total coronary artery occlusion. The density and extent of coronary collateral circulation vary according to

- species: pigs, rats, and black Russian rabbits have little preexisting collateral circulation, whereas guinea pigs have extensive preexisting collaterals; dogs, New Zealand white rabbits, and humans have an intermediate level of collaterals; and
- severity of obstruction: in humans, angiographic evidence of functional collaterals is rarely observed until coronary stenosis is more than 70% diameter; this highlights the importance of a pressure gradient for opening up of preexisting collateral channels.

A number of studies have examined the effects of chronic exercise on coronary collateral development in animals and humans, but the overall results have not been encouraging. In recent years, local or systemic administration of angiogenic growth factors such as fibroblast growth factor and vascular endothelial growth factor, using recombinant forms of these proteins, naked DNA encoding these proteins, or viral vectors carrying the DNA encoding these proteins, has been tested in experimental models of limb and cardiac ischemia. These strategies have been shown to promote collateral and neovascular growth.[43] Human studies of the use of these angiogenic factors in peripheral and coronary arterial disease have yielded inconsistent, marginal, or conflicting results.[44]

Chronic Myocardial Ischemia and Myocardial Hibernation

Chronic or repetitive reduction of myocardial perfusion because of severe coronary stenoses or collateralized total occlusion may lead to depressed contractile function and adaptive changes in myocardial metabolism, resulting in a state of myocardial "hibernation," with noncontractile but viable myocardium.[3,12] Proof of viability is provided if these nonfunctional myocardial segments recover their contractile function when blood flow is restored through revascularization. From a clinical standpoint, patients with coronary artery disease with severely depressed ventricular function and chronic congestive heart failure may benefit symptomatically and have an improved prognosis with revascularization when noninvasive imaging studies provide evidence of viability in noncontractile myocardial segments.[45] A number of noninvasive techniques are used to assess myocardial viability. They include[46]

- rest and redistribution or reinjection myocardial perfusion imaging with various radioactive perfusion tracers;
- positron emission tomography using radiolabeled ammonia to assess myocardial blood flow and radiolabeled deoxyglucose to assess myocardial metabolism;
- dobutamine and contrast echocardiography; and
- magnetic resonance imaging.

Role of Genetic Factors

Although no known genetic factors are directly associated with the occurrence of myocardial ischemia, they are clearly involved through their influence on the predisposition to coronary atherosclerosis and thrombosis, which are the anatomic determinants of myocardial ischemia.[47] These genetic factors involve both mutations and polymorphisms of various genes that are associated with lipoprotein metabolism, the hemostatic system, inflammation and matrix regulation, homocysteine metabolism, iron metabolism, insulin resistance, hypertension, the renin-angiotensin system, endothelial nitric oxide synthesis, and the cellular redox state.[47,48] In addition to these factors, genetic influences may also be among the determinants of the extent and adequacy of coronary collateral circulation, which has an important part to play in mitigating the consequences of coronary artery disease. Observations in murine models have identified a role for key membrane channel genes in the regulation of vascular tone; mutations in these genes have produced ischemic syndromes simulating Prinzmetal's angina in humans.[49,50]

CLINICAL IMPLICATIONS

An improved understanding not only of the role of the fixed coronary stenosis caused by atherosclerosis but also of endothelial dysfunction, vasoconstriction, and plaque disruption with thrombosis has led to improved therapeutic options for alleviation of myocardial ischemia. Thus, myocardial ischemia may be alleviated by interventions that

- prevent plaque progression, disruption, and thrombosis through plaque stabilization (lipid-lowering and risk factor–modifying therapies) and antithrombotic activity (antiplatelet and anticoagulant drugs in acute coronary syndromes);
- reduce the severity of coronary stenosis (percutaneous coronary intervention);
- circumvent the stenosis (bypass surgery);
- reduce myocardial oxygen demand (beta blockers, heart rate–slowing calcium channel blockers, nitrates);
- reduce coronary vasomotor tone directly (nitrates, calcium channel blockers); and
- improve endothelial function (lipid lowering, risk factor–modifying therapies, oral L-arginine).

In addition:

- Partial inhibition of fatty acid oxidation and prevention of myocyte calcium overload through inhibition of the late phase of the inward sodium current (late I_{Na}) during cardiac repolarization have been demonstrated by novel compounds (ranolazine).[51]
- Enhanced external counterpulsation has been shown to reduce refractory angina. Both reduced myocardial oxygen demand and improved perfusion have been implicated, but precise reasons for clinical benefit remain uncertain.[52]
- Spinal cord stimulation has been shown to be particularly useful, safe, and effective treatment in the management of patients with refractory angina pectoris and those unsuitable for percutaneous or surgical revascularization. Clinical and experimental research has shown that it decreases myocardial ischemia without masking the clinical symptoms of its imminent development. Potential mechanisms that have been implicated include placebo effects, primary antinociceptive effects, involvement of endogenous opiates, anti–sympathetic nervous system effects, increases in coronary blood flow, and redistribution of myocardial blood flow.[53]
- Therapeutic angiogenesis by use of growth factors, gene therapy, and cell therapy to improve collateral flow and to improve perfusion remains an attractive concept that is continuing to be evaluated.

Persistent or repetitive ischemia leading to myocardial hibernation may be an important contributor to the syndrome of chronic severe left ventricular dysfunction and congestive heart failure in subsets of patients with coronary artery disease; restoration of perfusion by invasive treatment may improve quality of life and survival. An improved understanding of the protective role of collaterals and factors that regulate collateral growth has led to the concept of therapeutic angiogenesis, which may provide a novel approach to improving myocardial perfusion and quality of life in patients with end-stage symptomatic ischemic heart disease that is not amenable to invasive revascularization. Finally, the phenomenon of ischemic preconditioning opens up the possibility of yet another potential target for therapeutic exploitation.

SUMMARY

Myocardial ischemia results from a dynamic interplay between several pathophysiologic processes that determine coronary blood flow and myocardial oxygen and energy needs. A fixed coronary stenosis caused by buildup of an atherosclerotic plaque reduces coronary flow reserve, whereas vasoconstriction in the coronary lesion and impaired vasodilator capacity of the microcirculation, as a result of endothelial dysfunction, contribute a dynamic component. Together, these factors lead to episodic reduction in coronary flow and endocardium-to-epicardium flow redistribution, which leads to myocardial ischemia. In acute coronary syndromes, coronary thrombus superimposed on a disrupted plaque creates yet another mechanism for additional dynamic coronary obstruction, which has a critical role in mediating episodic flow reductions and myocardial ischemia. In addition to episodic chronic or acute myocardial ischemia, a chronic state of myocardial ischemia (hibernation) also exists that can contribute to ventricular dysfunction and congestive heart failure. Finally, brief episodes of ischemia may attenuate the extent of necrosis after a subsequent prolonged but not permanent coronary occlusion through the phenomenon of ischemic preconditioning.

chapter 20

Noninvasive Diagnosis of Ischemic Heart Disease

Jamieson M. Bourque and George A. Beller

Problem

- Detection of significant coronary artery stenoses can be accomplished by a variety of noninvasive techniques. The strengths and weaknesses of these methodologies must be appreciated by clinicians evaluating patients with suspected or known coronary artery disease to maximize cost-effectiveness and to minimize future adverse cardiac outcomes.

Key Features

- Computed tomographic coronary calcium scoring and angiography can detect atherosclerosis and identify patients at high risk for future cardiac events who are in need of more intensive medical therapy or further diagnostic testing.
- Physiologic stress testing with perfusion imaging and functional wall motion assessment provides greater diagnostic and prognostic information than exercise electrocardiographic testing alone.

Clinical Implications

- Noninvasive approaches to the diagnosis of coronary artery disease and prognostic assessment assist in the management of patients who have undiagnosed chest pain or stable angina or who have had an uncomplicated myocardial infarction.

The sequelae of coronary artery disease (CAD) continue to impose significant clinical and economic burdens, and identification of those at highest risk of major adverse cardiac events is imperative to maximize the benefits of revascularization and intensive medical therapy. A large variety of noninvasive techniques are available for the detection of CAD. Atherosclerosis follows a steady progression from subtle changes in the vessel wall to lesions causing luminal obstruction, which progress until myocardial ischemia ensues or a plaque ruptures, causing an acute coronary syndrome. Ischemia is associated with a cascade of events starting with perfusion abnormalities and then progresses to electrocardiographic (ECG) changes with exercise and symptoms. Myocardial injury is also a consequence of this ischemic cascade (Fig. 20.1). Noninvasive techniques can be separated into two main types: those that provide anatomic assessment of the coronary vasculature, assessing the presence of calcium, atherosclerotic plaque, and luminal obstruction; and those that provide functional information, assessing the impact of obstructive lesions on the perfusion and regional and global function of the myocardium. The different modalities available are listed in Table 20.1.

ANATOMIC ASSESSMENT

X-ray coronary angiography remains the principal means for assessment of anatomic obstruction of the coronary vessels by atherosclerotic plaque. However, this technique is invasive, has infrequent but significant possible complications, and is expensive. Moreover, x-ray coronary angiography provides only an outline of the coronary lumen. Calcification and nonobstructive coronary plaque are underappreciated because of the Glagov phenomenon, in which the vessel dilates in response to increasing obstruction to maintain lumen size.[1] There have been advances in noninvasive angiographic techniques that can diagnose and provide prognostic information for CAD through assessment of coronary calcium content, identification of plaque through visualization of the entire vessel wall, and potentially even characterization of plaque composition with a lower cost and decreased risk of complications than with invasive x-ray angiography.

Coronary Calcification Imaging

Individualized risk assessment for the likelihood of CAD is a key first step in the prevention of adverse cardiac outcomes. Early diagnosis of coronary atherosclerosis can guide necessary increases in the intensity of medical therapy provided and can guide further testing. Clinical risk scores, such as the Framingham risk score, provide useful discrimination of the need for further evaluation and treatment. However, there is significant room for improved characterization, and coronary artery calcium scoring (CACS) provides a low-cost, low-radiation, highly reproducible method to further identify who is at higher risk for cardiac events.

Atherosclerosis formation ultimately results in vessel wall calcification, and CACS by use of computed tomography can directly measure this. Because it measures the last stage of atherosclerosis, CACS misses soft plaque. However, the extent of calcified plaque directly correlates with the amount of noncalcified plaque and cardiac events.[2]

The incidence of coronary calcium varies by age, gender, and ethnicity. Fifty percent of those older than 65 years have a score above 400, whereas those middle-aged have only a 5% incidence.[3] In women, the peak incidence occurs 10 to 15 years later than in men.[2,3] Studies such as the MESA study have shown the average score to be 22% less in African American and intermediate in Hispanic patients.[2] These differences underscore the need for age-, gender-, and potentially even ethnicity-specific cutpoints for risk assessment.

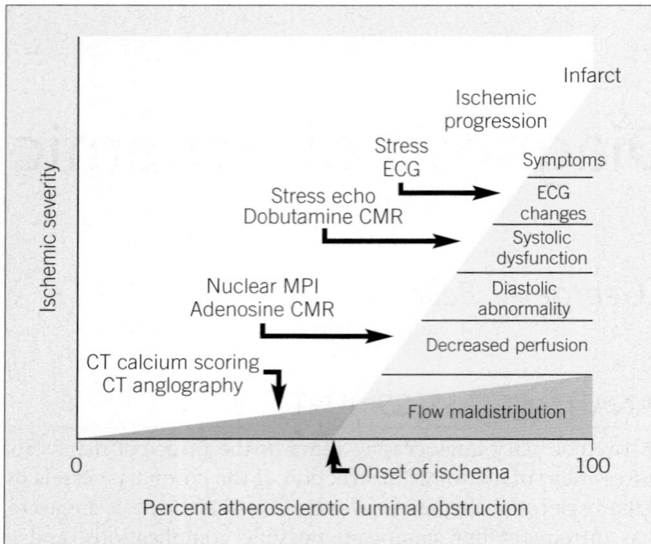

Figure 20.1 Relationship of noninvasive imaging modalities to the progression of atherosclerosis and ischemia. Atherosclerosis causes worsening coronary luminal obstruction (blue shaded area). When sufficient obstruction occurs, ischemia ensues (yellow shaded area), which progresses from flow maldistribution to decreased perfusion and eventually infarct. The arrows point to the stage of this atherosclerotic-ischemic process assessed by each noninvasive imaging study. CMR, cardiovascular magnetic resonance perfusion imaging; CT, computed tomography; ECG, electrocardiography; MPI, myocardial perfusion imaging;

NONINVASIVE METHODS FOR THE ASSESSMENT OF CORONARY ARTERY DISEASE
Anatomic
Computed tomographic coronary artery calcium scoring (CACS) Computed tomographic coronary angiography (CTCA) Magnetic resonance coronary angiography (MRCA)
Functional
Exercise Stress electrocardiography Nuclear myocardial perfusion imaging (MPI) Stress echocardiography Pharmacologic Nuclear myocardial perfusion imaging (MPI) Single-photon emission computed tomography (SPECT) Positron emission tomography (PET) Stress echocardiography Cardiovascular magnetic resonance perfusion imaging (CMR) CMR stress functional imaging (for wall motion assessment) Computed tomographic perfusion imaging (currently experimental)
Hybrid
Combination SPECT and CTCA (SPECT-CT) Combination PET and CTCA (PET-CT)

Table 20.1 Noninvasive methods for the assessment of coronary artery disease.

Description of Procedure

CACS was originally performed by electron beam computed tomography, but multidetector computed tomography used for coronary angiography is now the primary method and shows highly comparable results.[3] Scoring is performed with the Agatston method, a semiquantitative, semiautomatic, highly reproducible technique that sums the products of calcified plaque area and a density coefficient based on Hounsfield units.

Although there is a lack of standardization, a score of 100 is considered clinically significant by many; 400 typically represents a high-risk scan. Quantitative scoring can be performed though measurement of the true volume and absolute calcium mass, but this is time-consuming and not currently clinically feasible.

Diagnostic and Prognostic Accuracy of Test

CACS is ideal for asymptomatic patients with intermediate clinical risk scores. Those with low Framingham risk scores have lower event rates and thus a low positive predictive value even with a higher calcium score. Patients with high Framingham risk scores should already be treated aggressively with medical therapy and probably warrant further imaging irrespective of their calcium score. Although significant information can be gleaned for symptomatic patients, they too require additional testing for obstructive disease beyond calcium scoring.

There is growing evidence of the strong diagnostic and prognostic power of CACS. Symptomatic patients have an odds ratio of 20 for any calcium and 50 for stenosis of 70% or more. With a CACS cutpoint of 100, two studies showed the sensitivity for an x-ray angiographic obstruction of more than 50% at 87% to 95%, with a specificity of 79% in both.[2] A score below 100 was associated with a 3% risk of significant stenosis, and the negative predictive value was 96% to 100%. Myocardial perfusion imaging provides complementary information, but a CACS below 10 decreases the risk of an abnormal finding on myocardial perfusion imaging to 2%. CACS alone is still deemed insufficient if symptoms are present but can provide useful information, especially if physiologic testing is indeterminate or not possible. The data on use of CACS to examine regression of atherosclerosis are insufficient and contradicting, and thus it is not recommended because of the questionable efficacy, cost, and radiation exposure.

Extensive data exist for prognosis with CACS in asymptomatic cohorts. It is a strong predictor of cardiovascular death and nonfatal myocardial infarction, with a relative risk of 4.3 (95% CI, 3.5, 5.2) for any detectable calcium. Likewise, the 3- to 5-year event rate without calcium is 0.4%.[2] CACS provides additional prognostic information when it is broken down into ranges. The relative risk for cardiovascular death or nonfatal myocardial infarction ranges from 1.9 for mild calcification (CACS < 100) to 7.2 for moderate calcification (CACS 400 to 1000) and 10.8 for severe calcification (CACS > 1000) (Fig. 20.2). CACS provides incremental prognostic information over the Framingham risk scores, especially when the Framingham risk score is intermediate. A CACS above 400 confers the same risk of events as a cardiac disease equivalent (like diabetes mellitus).[2] Survival is also proportional to the presence of coronary calcium in the three major coronary arteries adjusted for age and CAD risk factors. Patients with coronary artery calcification in all three major arteries have a worse event-free survival

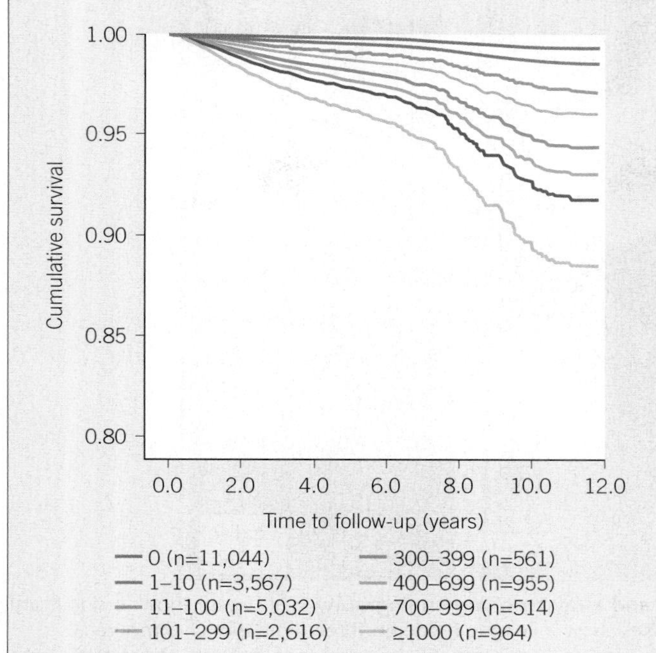

Figure 20.2 Cox proportional hazards adjusted 12-year survival curves for all-cause mortality stratified by coronary artery calcium score. Increasing calcium scores were associated with worsening survival ($P < .0001$). (Reprinted with permission from Budoff MJ, Shaw LJ, Liu ST, et al. Long-term prognosis associated with coronary calcification. J Am Coll Cardiol 2006;49:1860-1870.)

compared with those with coronary artery calcification in one or two of the major vessels.[4]

CACS has additional prognostic value in diabetes mellitus, with a greater increase in mortality for every corresponding calcium score. The 3-year relative risk of death is 58 with a CACS above 1000. Moreover, a CACS of 0 confers a long-term survival for patients with diabetes mellitus similar to those without the disease.[5] Thus, a CACS of 0 can provide good patient reassurance, but no data suggest that we should subsequently decrease the aggressiveness of treatment. Given the high rates of asymptomatic cardiac events in patients with diabetes mellitus, CACS could potentially be used for screening in this population to identify those at higher risk, with additional testing only for those reaching a threshold CACS of 100 or 400.

Summary

As stated in an American College of Cardiology/American Heart Association expert consensus document, establishment of baseline risk is very important, and CACS is a highly reproducible, excellent marker of atherosclerosis, with the presence of calcium confirming plaque. Unfortunately, reimbursement issues currently limit its clinical use. CACS is useful for risk stratification in asymptomatic individuals with an intermediate Framingham risk score, not for general screening for the overall population. It can provide useful information in symptomatic patients, but even those with atypical symptoms should have further anatomic or physiologic testing. The extent and localization of calcified plaques with CACS do not correlate with the degree and location of coronary artery stenoses.[6] Moreover, CACS cannot identify culprit lesions, differentiate stable from unstable plaques, or assess soft plaque. The true plaque burden is underestimated. For these reasons, information on the degree and localization of obstruction and the burden of soft plaque requires luminal evaluation as with multidetector computed tomographic coronary angiography.

Cardiac Computed Tomography

Noninvasive evaluation of the coronary arteries has been limited by their small size, tortuous nature, and rapid and significant movement during the cardiac cycle. However, computed tomography of the coronary arteries (CTCA) increasingly offers the temporal resolution (speed) and high spatial resolution required to image these vessels successfully. Moreover, CTCA allows viewing of the entire vessel and surrounding tissue so that nonobstructive plaque is appreciated early, before the luminal encroachment assessed by x-ray coronary angiography (Fig. 20.3).

Description of Procedure

CTCA was previously limited by slower scan times that necessitated heart rates below 60 through beta-blocker use. The scanners also had low spatial resolution because of their 4- or 16-slice capabilities, and up to 27% of coronary segments were unevaluable, greatly reducing the diagnostic accuracy of CTCA. Multidetector-row computed tomography (MDCT) devices are currently available that obtain 64 slices with a high spatial resolution (collimation) of 0.6 mm. Gantry rotation times have markedly improved, increasing the temporal resolution and thus minimizing motion artifact. Moreover, dual source/dual energy scanners are now available with two sources placed orthogonally that scan simultaneously, further reducing the gantry rotation time by 50%, increasing temporal resolution and allowing higher heart rates, frequently precluding the use of beta blockers. Dual-source MDCT showed positive (81%) and negative (99%) predictive values for the detection of stenoses of 50% or more for patients with heart rates above 65/minute comparable to those for patients with heart rates below 65/minute.[7] Sublingual nitroglycerin is given to induce vasodilatation for improved vessel visualization.

Up to 150 mL of iodinated contrast material is injected to provide contrast of the coronary vessels, at the expense of contrast allergy and nephropathy risk, especially in high-risk patients, such as those with diabetes or a serum creatinine concentration above 2.0 mg/dL. The heart is imaged during multiple phases of the cardiac cycle as identified by ECG gating, with the clearest pictures typically obtained during late diastole, the time of least cardiac motion. Breath-holds of up to 15 to 20 seconds are used to minimize respiratory motion. However, irregular heart rhythms and inadvertent changes in body position can create misregistration artifacts that reduce image quality and create visible gaps in the coronary segments. Assessing the phases consecutively can provide an estimate of cardiac function.

Despite these improvements, other limitations still restrict CTCA use. Highly radiodense materials such as calcium and metal cause blooming artifacts that can falsely obscure the coronary lumen and artificially inflate lesion sizes. Thus, coronary stents and severe calcification, as often seen in older patients and those with diffuse disease or chronic renal

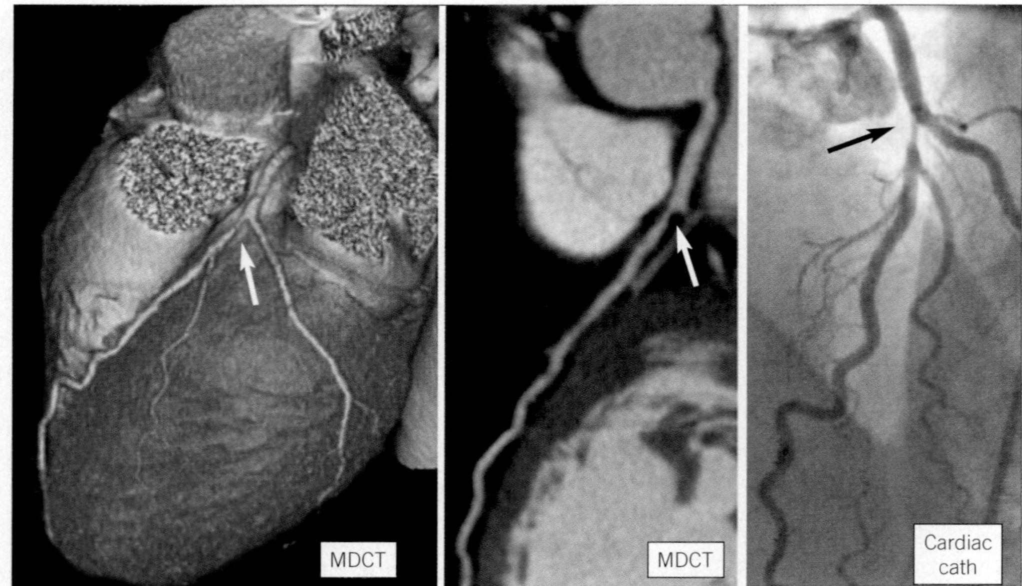

Figure 20.3 Significant coronary stenosis on computed tomography and x-ray coronary angiography. This figure shows a significant left anterior descending coronary artery stenosis. The left and middle boxes show a volume-rendered three-dimensional computed tomography angiogram and a single planar computed tomography angiographic view, respectively; the arrows illustrate the stenosis from soft plaque. Note that the entire extent of the lesion can be assessed, not just the portion obstructing the coronary lumen. These images correlate well visually with the reference angiogram from cardiac catheterization, with the arrow showing the same significant stenosis. (Reprinted with permission from Miller JC, Abbara S, Achenbach S, et al. Utilization Rounds of the MGH: Coronary CT Angiography. Journal of the American College Radiology, 2006;3:560–564.)

insufficiency, can preclude the use of CTCA. Stents of less than 3 mm in diameter are not routinely evaluable. Even without other confounding problems, the spatial resolution is currently insufficient to image coronary segments with diameters of less than 1.5 mm, and many distal coronary segments and side branches remain indeterminate. As the technology improves from increased scanner rotational speed, more slices acquired simultaneously, and better image reconstruction algorithms, these limitations will be further reduced, and CTCA will become an increasingly viable alternative to invasive assessment of CAD in select populations of patients.

Radiation Effects

A significant concern with CTCA is the radiation dose provided. Unlike nuclear myocardial perfusion imaging, in which the radiation dose is spread out over the entire body, CTCA focuses the radiation burden on the chest, where the breasts and lungs are highly sensitive to radiation. The average radiation exposure from CTCA is currently 10 to 18 mSv (which describes the effective dose, an estimate of the biologic effects of absorbed radiation) versus 3 to 5 mSv for selective x-ray coronary angiography. In comparison, the annual exposure in the United States from background sources is 3.6 mSv. This focused radiation dose provides a small but quantifiable absolute increased risk of cancer that is as high as 1/143 (0.7%) for 20-year-old women but only 1/2017 (0.02%) in 80-year old men because of their shortened life expectancy.[8] The risk is significantly higher with combination coronary-aortic scans, as with the emergency department "triple rule-out" through assessment for coronary disease, pulmonary embolism, and aortic dissection. Higher detector numbers only increase the dose. Techniques such as ECG-dependent tube current modulation and tube voltage reduction can reduce the radiation dose by as much as 50% to 65% but adversely affect imaging quality.

Indications and Selection of Patients

Indications for CTCA have not yet been fully optimized, and its many current limitations and radiation exposure require careful selection of patients for suitable clinical questions. Current indications include the following.

Assessment of Possible Coronary Artery Disease

CTCA should be limited to those with a lower likelihood of disease and intervention, in whom identification of CAD would affect medical management. This includes patients with atypical symptoms and intermediate risk factors or an inconclusive presentation, such as with prior equivocal test results. In this group, CTCA can lead to a definitive diagnosis and identify need for further testing. Patients with definitively positive stress test results or typical anginal symptoms with moderate to high risk of disease should proceed directly to cardiac catheterization. CTCA is optimal in younger patients without stents or extensive calcification, although it should be avoided in young women if possible because of their higher risks of breast cancer with radiation exposure.

Assessment with Known Prior Coronary Artery Disease

The role of CTCA in this population is less well defined. Given the frequent need for subsequent coronary angiography and physiologic assessment, CTCA can bring unnecessary added cost, time, and radiation exposure. Moreover, patients with prior CAD have a higher likelihood of vessel calcification and prior stent placement, limiting interpretation and systematically underestimating corresponding lumen size.

Bypass Graft Assessment

CTCA is particularly good for evaluating the lumens of coronary artery bypass grafts because of their larger diameters and decreased susceptibility to cardiac motion. However, CTCA is not good at assessing the graft distal anastomosis site or distal native coronary vessels because of the high rate of vessel calcification and stenting. Moreover, the large field of view required to image the mammary artery grafts leads to high radiation exposure. These factors currently limit CTCA usefulness in this population.

Presurgical Coronary Assessment

A developing indication for CTCA is coronary artery assessment before cardiothoracic surgery to assess for coronary obstruction and to identify the precise course and topography of the left anterior descending coronary artery, branching of the intrathoracic arteries, and relationship of target vessels to intercostal spaces to minimize surgical trauma, especially for repeated procedures.[6] The role of CTCA in these instances is still uncertain.

Diagnostic and Prognostic Accuracy of Test

The number of uninterpretable segments has decreased with corresponding improved diagnostic accuracy with 64-slice scanners. For CAD assessment, the largest series to date reveals 86% of segments interpretable with a sensitivity of 95% and a specificity of 93%.[6,9] The overall diagnostic accuracy falls between 91% and 100%, depending on the study group. In symptomatic patients in one study, CTCA had the ability to identify the cause of chest pain in the majority of cases (75%), but 25% required additional testing.[10] In comparison to nuclear perfusion imaging, CTCA has high sensitivity, with normal studies correlating well with the absence of inducible ischemia. However, the specificity for ischemia detection remains poor; only 50% of those with positive CTCA findings have defects on myocardial perfusion imaging. This suggests that some patients may have needless additional invasive testing and inappropriate treatment that could be potentially harmful, given the potential for stent thrombosis and complications of anticoagulation. However, the corollary to this is that myocardial perfusion imaging identifies only functional defects and may falsely reassure patients with subclinical CAD who might benefit from aggressive medical therapy. Fifty-two percent had coronary plaques despite normal myocardial perfusion imaging.[9] The two tests are complementary, but concurrent use leads to cost and radiation dose issues.

There are no good data evaluating diagnostic accuracy of 64-slice MDCT in patients with known prior CAD. One of the biggest remaining obstacles to the use of CTCA in patients with known CAD is the evaluation of coronary stents. A meta-analysis of 807 patients with coronary stents by 16- or 64-slice CTCA revealed a sensitivity of 84%, specificity of 91%, positive likelihood ratio of 12.2, and negative likelihood ratio of 0.23. Thirteen percent of segments were uninterpretable. Small stent diameter was probably the biggest culprit; only stents with a diameter of more than 3 mm were able to be interpreted reliably. CTCA had an excellent sensitivity and specificity for bypass graft stenosis (99% and 96%, respectively), but issues with graft anastomosis site obstruction and downstream vessels remain.[11]

Limited information exists for the prognosis of patients undergoing CTCA as it remains a relatively new technique. One study observed 100 patients for 1 year (stenoses of more than 50% were considered significant). Those with a normal study had no events, and patients with at least one lesion of 50% or greater had a 9% risk of cardiac death, nonfatal myocardial infarction, or unstable angina, with a 63% total event rate including revascularization.[6] These data are promising, but longer follow-up is needed. Multiple studies are currently under way.

Vessel Wall Imaging (Plaque Characterization)

CTCA has the potential for vessel wall imaging, plaque characterization, and possibly even perfusion. A key aspect of our goal to reduce cardiovascular events is the identification of unstable plaques with a higher likelihood of imminent or ongoing rupture. Vulnerable plaques have been shown to contain lipid-laden cores, thin fibrous caps, and limited calcium. The increasing spatial resolution of MDCT is now allowing visualization of the different regions within the vessel wall. Plaque characterization is essential, as there is a direct correlation between the number of mixed plaques and the number of cardiac events. Moreover, survival was shown to be directly related to amount of plaque in the left anterior descending coronary artery by CTCA.[12] However, this application is still limited, with lipid cores and fibrosis often being confused, and further technologic advances are necessary before clinical use.

Summary

Advances in technology have allowed noninvasive assessment of the coronary arteries through CTCA with excellent sensitivity and negative predictive value but relatively poor specificity and positive predictive value. Specific indications are still being determined, and its role in symptomatic evaluation is currently unknown because of the overestimation of coronary stenosis severity, as confirmed by recently published appropriateness criteria.[13] CTCA may be best suited for younger patients with atypical symptoms who come to the emergency department or for presurgical cardiothoracic assessment. However, the radiation risks are not trivial, and alternative testing should be considered for women younger than 40 years, with additional disease protocols avoided if possible. Prognostic information is currently limited but should be available in the next several years. Vessel wall imaging for plaque identification, computed tomographic perfusion, and combined myocardial perfusion–CTCA imaging to assess for hemodynamically significant lesions represent exciting areas of ongoing research.

Magnetic Resonance Coronary Angiography

An alternative noninvasive angiographic approach is magnetic resonance coronary angiography (MRCA). This technology is not ready for clinical use, but significant progress has been made. Compared with CTCA, MRCA has a lower spatial resolution and has imaging times longer than one cardiac cycle, requiring multiple breath-holds.[14]

MRCA uses specific electrical frequencies to cause protons to resonate, emitting energy that is captured by receiver coils and converted into an image. ECG and respiratory gating are used to minimize motion artifact. Unlike all other angiographic methods at this time, MRCA uses special sequences to enhance the intrinsic contrast of the coronary tissue to enhance their viewing. The left anterior descending and right coronary arteries can be seen more easily and for longer lengths than the left circumflex because of their closer proximity to the surface imaging coils.

Although MRCA has the potential for good soft tissue characterization and high spatial resolution, many limitations remain, including those found with CTCA, such as arrhythmias, respiratory motion, and metallic artifact from stents. Advantages of MRCA include the lack of radiation exposure and lack of nephrotoxic contrast agents.

Analysis is currently limited to the proximal vessels (for anomalous coronary artery origins and proximal vessel disease), with variable sensitivity and specificity as high as 100% and 85%, respectively, but with wide variation.[14] Minimal prognostic information is available. Thus, MRCA is insufficient as an independent diagnostic modality in symptomatic patients at this time.[13] New sequences and 3 Tesla scanners will likely enhance signal-noise ratio and decrease scan times. The higher magnet strength does increase steady-state free precession artifacts and gating difficulty. Coronary vessel wall imaging is improving, but current results are variable. High tissue contrast through novel MRCA sequences should ultimately lead to superior results compared with CTCA.

PHYSIOLOGIC ASSESSMENT

Anatomic identification of atherosclerosis is important for the diagnosis of coronary disease and guidance of revascularization decisions. However, to fully evaluate symptoms and to optimize treatment, the physiology of obstructive coronary lesions must be determined. Current methods compare the perfusion and function of the myocardium at rest to a stress state, induced by exercise or pharmacologic agents, in which the heart's compensatory mechanisms are overwhelmed and defects are unmasked.

Coronary segments with obstructive plaques vasodilate to maintain appropriate flow and thus decrease their coronary flow reserve. Perfusion imaging takes advantage of this phenomenon and uses a stress agent to produce heterogeneity of blood flow between myocardial regions supplied by normal coronary arteries and those with decreased cardiac flow reserve from physiologically significant coronary artery stenoses. Studies that examine myocardial function, on the other hand, use rest studies to identify noncontractile, likely infarcted myocardium and stress studies to induce wall motion abnormalities that suggest ischemia.

Functional testing can be used to diagnose CAD but will miss nonobstructive disease and thus some patients who could benefit from aggressive medical therapy and lifestyle modification. The strength of functional testing, however, is the excellent prognostic information it provides, especially with more established techniques, although emerging modalities are quickly establishing their own prognostic information. The current functional modalities are presented in Table 20.1.

Exercise Stress Electrocardiography

Exercise ECG stress testing is a well-established procedure that has been used for the detection of CAD and assessment of prognosis for many years. Exercise testing is an exceptionally safe procedure in appropriate patients (Table 20.2), with the incidence of myocardial infarction or death occurring at a rate of 1 in 2500 tests. All protocols for diagnostic exercise testing involve a warm-up, low-load phase followed by progressive uninterrupted exercise at increasing levels of cardiac workload with a subsequent recovery period. The most popular incremental exercise protocol is the Bruce protocol, which increases treadmill speed and incline every 3 minutes.

Although angina-type chest pain produced by progressive exercise during testing is strongly predictive of CAD, the definition of a positive test endpoint for ischemia is 1.0 mm or more of horizontal or downsloping ST-segment depression for at least 80 ms in the presence of a normal resting ECG recording (Fig. 20.4). Rapid upsloping ST-segment depression (known as J-point depression) is a normal ECG response to exercise. Several ECG stress test findings have been associated with a high risk of future cardiac events (Table 20.3). Some abnormal ST-segment responses occur only during the recovery period, which means that monitoring must be

CONTRAINDICATIONS TO EXERCISE TESTING
Absolute contraindications
Acute myocardial infarction (within 2 days)
High-risk unstable angina*
Uncontrolled cardiac arrhythmias causing symptoms or hemodynamic compromise
Symptomatic severe aortic stenosis
Uncontrolled symptomatic heart failure
Acute pulmonary embolus or pulmonary infarction
Acute myocarditis or pericarditis
Acute aortic dissection
Relative contraindications†
Left main coronary stenosis
Moderate stenotic valvular heart disease
Electrolyte abnormalities
Severe arterial hypertension‡
Tachyarrhythmias or bradyarrhythmias
Hypertrophic cardiomyopathy and other forms of outflow tract obstruction
Mental or physical impairment leading to inability to exercise adequately
High-degree atrioventricular block

*Braunwald E, Antman EM, Beasley JW, et al. ACC/AHA 2002 guideline update for the management of patients with unstable angina and non–ST-segment elevation myocardial infarction: a report of the American College of Cardiology/American Heart Association Task Force on Practice Guidelines (Committee on the Management of Patients with Unstable Angina). 2002. Available at: http://www.acc.org/clinical/guidelines/unstable/unstable.pdf.

†Relative contraindications can be superseded if the benefits of exercise outweigh the risks.

‡Defined as systolic blood pressure above 200 mm Hg or diastolic blood pressure above 110 mm Hg.

(From Gibbons RJ, Balady GJ, Beasley JW, et al. ACC/AHA guidelines for exercise testing. A report of the American College of Cardiology/American Heart Association Task Force on Practice Guidelines (Committee on Exercise Testing). J Am Coll Cardiol 1997;30:260-311; after Fletcher GF, Balady G, Froelicher VF, et al. Exercise standards: a statement for healthcare professions from the American Heart Association Writing Group. Circulation 1995;91:580-615. Copyright © 2002 by the American College of Cardiology Foundation and the American Heart Association, Inc.

Table 20.2 Contraindications to exercise testing.

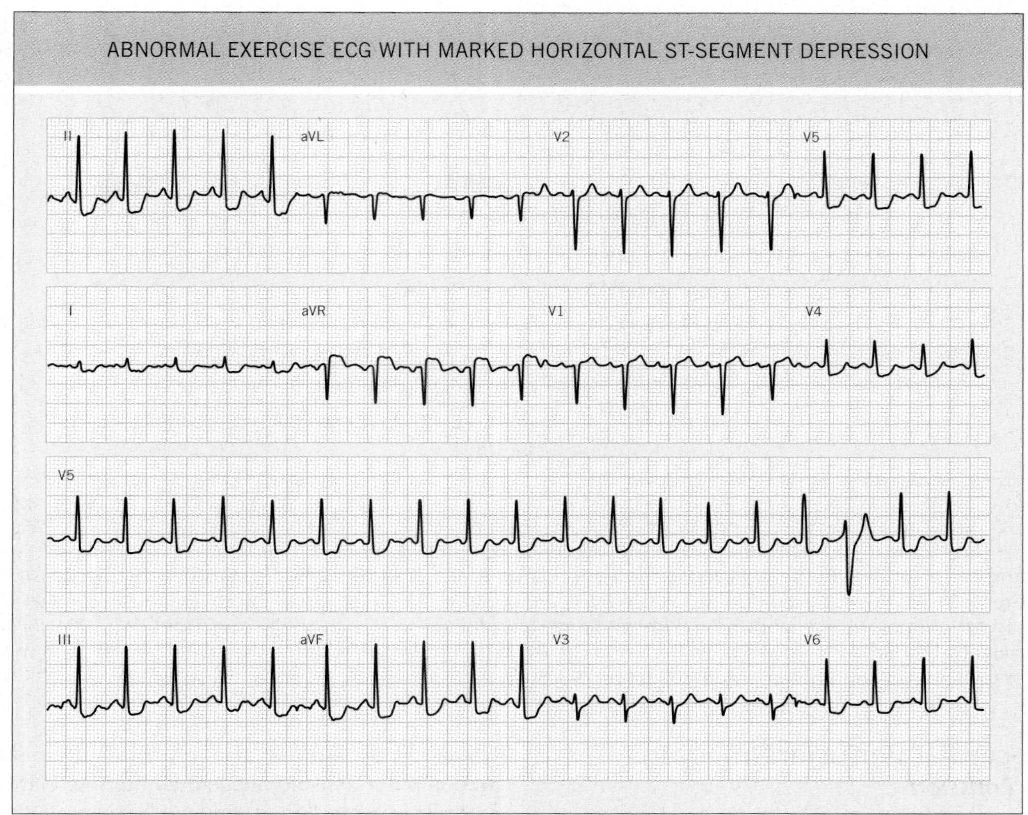

Figure 20.4 Abnormal exercise ECG recording with marked horizontal ST-segment depression.

HIGH-RISK EXERCISE ECG STRESS TEST VARIABLES
Failure to achieve >6 metabolic equivalents of workload
Failure to exceed systolic blood pressure of >120 mm Hg, or ≥10 mm Hg decrease in blood pressure with exercise
ST-segment depression ≥2.0 mm at low workload (stage 1)
ST-segment depression ≥1.0 mm in 5 leads or more
ST-segment depression ≥1.0 mm lasting ≥5 minutes into the recovery period
Exercise-induced ST-segment elevation in leads without Q waves
Limiting angina
Nonsustained or sustained ventricular tachycardia

Table 20.3 High-risk exercise ECG stress test variables.

continued for a minimum of 5 minutes after exercise or until ST-segment abnormalities have resolved. Slow upsloping ST-segment depression is not diagnostic of CAD.

The overall sensitivity and specificity were 68% and 77% in the largest meta-analysis of exercise testing (147 studies), with a predictive accuracy of 73%. Other studies show a positive predictive value of 44% and a negative predictive value of 98%.[15] False-positive ST-segment depression responses can be observed in patients receiving digoxin or who have concomitant left ventricular hypertrophy, Wolff-Parkinson-White syndrome, electrolyte abnormalities, bundle branch blocks, hyperventilation syndromes, or microvascular angina.

In general, the lower prevalence of CAD in women (particularly premenopausal women) results in a lower specificity of the ST-segment depression response to exercise, yielding a higher rate of false-positives.[15] Exercise tolerance is lower in women than in men, which may also contribute to a lower diagnostic accuracy of the exercise ECG stress test.

A normal exercise stress ECG test confers a low risk of adverse cardiac events (0.7% to 0.9% at 6 months). A positive result imparts a significantly increased risk of adverse cardiac outcomes (1.7% to 2.3% at 6 months).[15]

Exercise Workload and Heart Rate Response

Exercise testing imparts significant prognostic information through several parameters, including ST changes as discussed before. However, two additional parameters that correlate well with clinical risk are exercise workload attained and abnormal heart rate recovery after exercise completion. The maximum attained exercise stage was found to predict 4-year survival and the likelihood of three-vessel proximal stenoses in the Coronary Artery Surgery Study.[16] However, the most predictive variable in prior studies has been the number of metabolic equivalents completed; each 1-MET increase improves survival by 12% to 18% (Fig. 20.5).[17]

Another important prognostic factor with exercise testing is an abnormal heart rate recovery. It is a predictor of mortality independent of clinical risk factors, ventricular function, and severity of CAD, with a hazard ratio of 1.6 (95% CI, 1.2-2.0).[18]

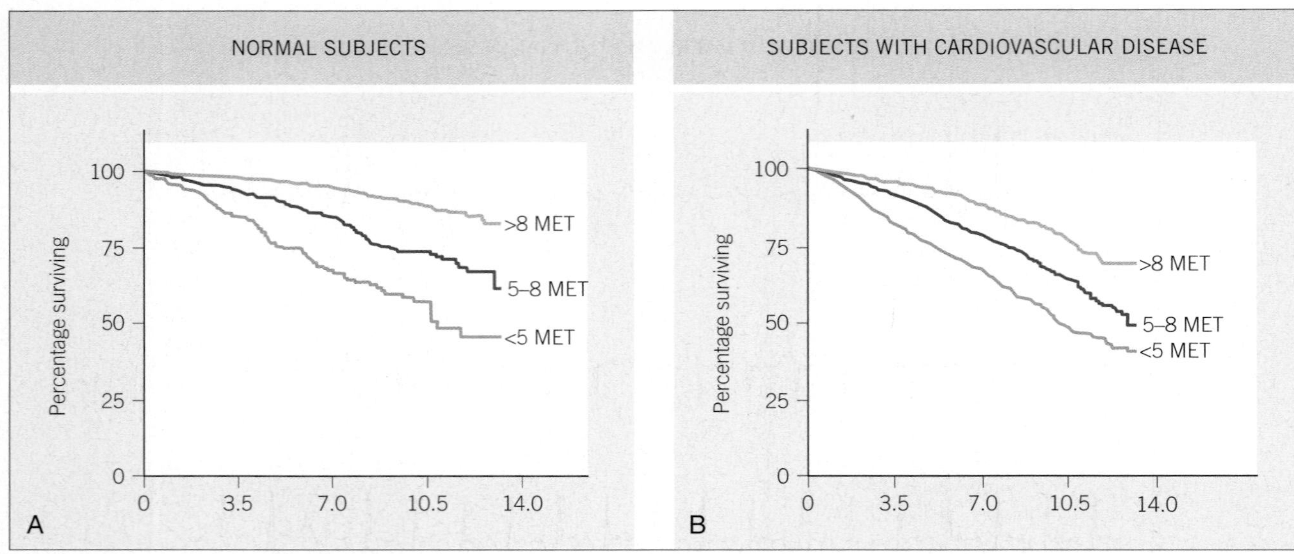

Figure 20.5 Long-term survival by peak exercise capacity. Panels **A** and **B** show survival curves out to 14 years stratified on the basis of initial exercise capacity achieved during stress electrocardiography. The large visual improvements in survival with increasing exercise workload for normal subjects and those with cardiovascular disease were statistically significant ($P < .001$ for both). MET, metabolic equivalent. (Modified with permission from Myers J, Prakash M, Froelicher V, et al. Exercise capacity and mortality among men referred for exercise testing. N Engl J Med 2002;346:793-801.)

Nuclear Myocardial Perfusion Imaging

Single-Photon Emission Computed Tomography

Nuclear myocardial perfusion imaging by single-photon emission computed tomography (SPECT) has been available longer than any other of the major modalities used today. It has been invaluable in the detection of CAD and myocardial ischemia and in the assessment of prognosis.

Description of Procedure

Nuclear myocardial perfusion imaging can be accomplished with exercise or pharmacologic stress and gated imaging employing technetium Tc 99m–labeled sestamibi or tetrofosmin or thallium Tl 201. Most laboratories use one of the ^{99m}Tc-labeled perfusion agents for stress imaging because of their improved specificity for CAD detection compared with ^{201}Tl. Resting perfusion is assessed with a lower dose of the tracer for the same-day imaging protocol, whereas for obese subjects, a 2-day imaging protocol is used whereby high doses of the tracers are administered for both stress and rest imaging. For the dual imaging approach, rest imaging is performed with ^{201}Tl followed immediately by stress testing with one of the ^{99m}Tc-labeled agents.

Exercise is the preferred method of stress because of its direct physiologic effects and the significant additional data it provides (see the earlier section on exercise workload). Pharmacologic stress imaging is performed with a vasodilator such as adenosine or dipyridamole or with dobutamine for patients with active wheezing due to pulmonary disease. Whenever possible, low-level exercise is performed simultaneously with vasodilator stress except for patients with complete left bundle branch block, in whom only vasodilator stress is used. This improves image quality and may provoke true ischemia, thereby increasing the CAD detection rate. The principle behind stress SPECT imaging is that these agents are taken up by myocardial tissue in proportion to blood flow, yielding defects in uptake that can be identified visually and with use of computer-assisted image quantitation. Gating of the images permits quantitation of regional function, determination of left ventricular ejection fraction, and assessment of left ventricular volumes.[19] Typically, short-axis, vertical long-axis, and horizontal long-axis images are obtained. Stress-induced defects that improve or disappear on resting imaging are referred to as reversible defects, which represent ischemia, whereas defects that persist on stress and rest images are referred to as fixed defects, which are most often representative of scar due to myocardial infarction.

Indications and Selection of Patients

Exercise and pharmacologic stress SPECT imaging are invaluable in assessing prognosis and selecting patients who will benefit most from further invasive evaluation with an eye toward revascularization. Patients with symptoms and an intermediate pretest likelihood of CAD have the largest benefit. Those with highly atypical symptoms and minimal cardiac risk factors have a low pretest probability of disease and a decreased positive predictive value. This leads to higher rates of false-positive studies, exposing the patients to the unnecessary added cost and complications of additional work-up and treatment. Similarly, those with high pretest likelihood of CAD from typical symptoms and high Framingham risk scores should be referred directly to invasive coronary angiography unless complicating factors exist. Use of SPECT myocardial perfusion imaging in those with an intermediate pretest probability maximizes the study benefit.

Use of nuclear myocardial perfusion imaging for screening in asymptomatic patients is not cost-effective. Exceptions to this include some high-risk patients with poor functional status for whom intermediate or high-risk surgery is planned. Other patients who may benefit from stress SPECT imaging for ischemia detection are those with chronic renal disease who are going to undergo dialysis or be considered for transplantation and patients who have had coronary artery bypass grafting 5 years or more earlier. Further research may show subsets of diabetics who may benefit from screening, as this population has worse outcomes and higher rates of asymptomatic ischemia because of their neuropathic abnormalities.

Diagnostic and Prognostic Accuracy of Test

In a pooled analysis of studies published in the literature comprising 8964 patients, the sensitivity for stress SPECT perfusion imaging for CAD detection was 86% with a 74% specificity and an 89% normalcy rate.[20] The normalcy rate is a surrogate for specificity and represents the percentage of normal stress perfusion images in patients with a less than 5% pretest likelihood of CAD. Specificity determination requires referral for coronary angiography and thus has an inherent referral bias because patients with true negative study results are not referred to catheterization. For SPECT imaging, false-positive study results are most often due to artifacts such as breast attenuation in women and posterobasal wall attenuation in both men and women. These sources of artifact can be diminished with ECG gating of the images and use of attenuation correction algorithms. Fixed defects due to artifact will show preserved wall thickening from end-diastole to end-systole on gated images, whereas such defects due to scar will most often show hypokinesis or akinesis.

One of the limitations of SPECT perfusion imaging is that the perfusion tracers show a plateau in myocardial uptake with hyperemic flows above 2.0 mL/min per gram, which reduces the detection rate of mild coronary stenoses (50% to 70%). In addition, only relative flow from one area of the myocardium to another area rather than absolute flow in milliliters per minute per gram can be determined. Some patients with three-vessel disease have balanced ischemia with a uniform decrease in coronary flow reserve in the distribution of all three coronary arteries. In patients with this phenomenon, the tracer uptake on the stress perfusion scan can appear normal or nearly normal, resulting in underestimation of the extent of disease. If wall motion abnormalities are observed in the absence of perfusion defects, this enhances the identification of high-risk coronary anatomy, as does the presence of transient left ventricular cavity dilatation from stress to rest images.[21] Similarly, left main coronary stenoses may be missed because of this phenomenon. In one study, high-risk disease with moderate or severe defects was seen in only 59% of patients with left main coronary disease by quantitative SPECT imaging.[22]

From multiple studies published in the literature, it is clear that patients with a normal stress perfusion scan have an excellent outcome. In a pooled analysis comprising 58,424 patients undergoing exercise SPECT, the annual death or myocardial infarction rate was 0.7% in patients with a low-risk scan versus 5.6% for patients with a moderately or severely abnormal scan.[23] For 11,231 patients who underwent pharmacologic stress imaging, the annual event rate was 1.2% for patients with a low-risk scan and 8.3% for patients with an abnormal scan. The more severe the perfusion abnormalities, the higher the subsequent event rate, which increases from 3.0% annually for patients with a mildly abnormal pharmacologic stress SPECT study to 10.9% annually for patients with a severely abnormal study.[24] In another large study comprising 14,273 patients without documented CAD, the annual overall mortality for patients with normal images was 1.9% during a 10-year period. In this study, a normal SPECT study was an effective gatekeeper for coronary angiography in that only 1.3% of these patients with normal images were referred for early angiography.[25]

Figure 20.6 from the pooled analysis by Shaw and Iskandrian[23] shows that diabetics with normal or abnormal scans had a significantly higher death or nonfatal myocardial infarction rate compared with that of nondiabetics. Female diabetics had an annual hard event rate of almost 3% with a normal scan and more that 10% with an abnormal scan, compared with male diabetics, whose event rates were significantly lower. Diabetics who present with dyspnea may benefit from stress SPECT perfusion imaging. Such patients have more than a 50% prevalence of abnormal stress SPECT images. The diabetics who presented with dyspnea rather than angina had a 3.3% annual death or infarction rate during follow-up with a normal scan and a 13.2% event rate

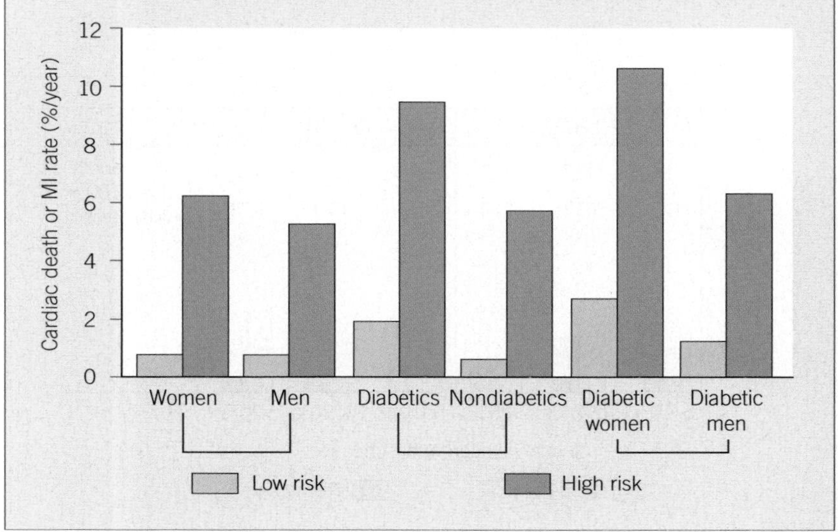

Figure 20.6 Annual risk of cardiac death or nonfatal myocardial infarction (MI) in subsets of patients referred for nuclear myocardial perfusion imaging, including both women and men and diabetics and nondiabetics. (Reprinted with permission from Shaw LJ, Iskandrian AE. Prognostic value of gated myocardial perfusion SPECT. J Nucl Cardiol 2004;11:171-185.)

with an abnormal imaging study, both higher event rates than those of diabetic patients with normal or abnormal scans who presented with angina. Totally asymptomatic diabetics with a high-risk stress SPECT scan have a 61% prevalence of left main CAD, three-vessel CAD, or two-vessel CAD with a proximal left anterior descending coronary artery stenosis.[26]

The addition of abnormal wall thickening or wall motion on stress gated SPECT images improves the detection of proximal left anterior descending coronary artery and multivessel disease compared with evaluation of perfusion defects alone.[27] It also enhances risk stratification. The survival free of death or nonfatal infarction in patients with abnormal perfusion or function in three coronary supply regions is substantially lower at 30 months (70%) compared with that of patients with such abnormalities in one or two coronary supply regions.[28] The worse the wall motion score and the lower the left ventricular ejection fraction (LVEF) on gated SPECT, the higher the event rate. Travin and colleagues[29] showed that in patients with an ejection fraction of 30% to 39%, the annual event rate was 7.6% compared with 1.8% for patients with LVEF of 50% or greater. At 2 years of follow-up, patients with extensive ischemia by perfusion defect criteria and a SPECT LVEF of less than 40% had a 20% cardiac event rate, compared with patients with a LVEF of 40% or greater with the same degree of ischemia, who had an approximate 8% 2-year event rate. Thus, the combination of the presence of inducible ischemia and post-stress functional abnormalities identifies a higher risk subgroup of patients.

The percentage of the myocardium rendered ischemic on stress SPECT imaging can assist in identifying which patients might benefit the most from an invasive strategy.[19] Figure 20.7 shows that for patients with LVEF of less than 60%, only those with ischemia of more than 20% of the left ventricle had a better outcome with revascularization compared with medical therapy. Those with 5% to 10% ischemia and those with 10% to 20% ischemia had similar cardiac death rates with medical therapy or revascularization. In patients with LVEF greater than 60%, the mortality rate during follow-up was superior for revascularization in patients with 10% to 20% and more than 20% of the total left ventricular myocardium rendered ischemic, respectively. Patients with mild ischemia (5% to 10% of the left ventricle) had similar low mortality rates for medical therapy versus revascularization.

Summary

Patients with an intermediate- or high-risk pretest probability of CAD and chest pain are candidates for exercise or pharmacologic stress SPECT perfusion imaging as summarized in the American College of Cardiology Foundation/ American Society of Nuclear Cardiology appropriateness criteria.[30] Patients with a normal or nearly normal scan have an excellent prognosis. Some patients with a normal perfusion scan, particularly on vasodilator stress imaging, may have balanced ischemia and underlying left main or three-vessel disease. Some of these patients may have transient ischemic left ventricular cavity dilatation, in which the stress image shows a larger cavity size than the corresponding rest image. This is attributed to diffuse subendocardial ischemia. Such patients may also have multiple wall motion abnormalities with uniform tracer uptake, which suggests disease of higher risk than is obvious from the SPECT perfusion pattern alone. If patients with diffuse CAD and normal perfusion studies undergo exercise stress, they may manifest poor exercise tolerance and exhibit ischemic ST-segment changes. Diabetics with normal perfusion studies have a higher event rate than that of nondiabetics with a normal scan, and any diabetic patient with even mild reversibility should probably undergo coronary angiography because the extent of anatomic disease may still be substantial. Patients with moderately or severely abnormal scans should probably be referred for invasive evaluation if 10% or greater ischemia is identified. The COURAGE trial nuclear substudy showed that such patients did better with optimal medical therapy and percutaneous intervention compared with optimal medical therapy alone (unpublished, presented at the American Heart Association Scientific Sessions, 2007).

Positron Emission Tomography

Positron emission tomography (PET) is an additional nuclear perfusion modality with some advantages over SPECT imaging, but availability, cost, and other issues limit it to a secondary stress modality.

PET imaging uses positron-emitting isotopes of fluorine, rubidium, oxygen, nitrogen, and other elements to assess

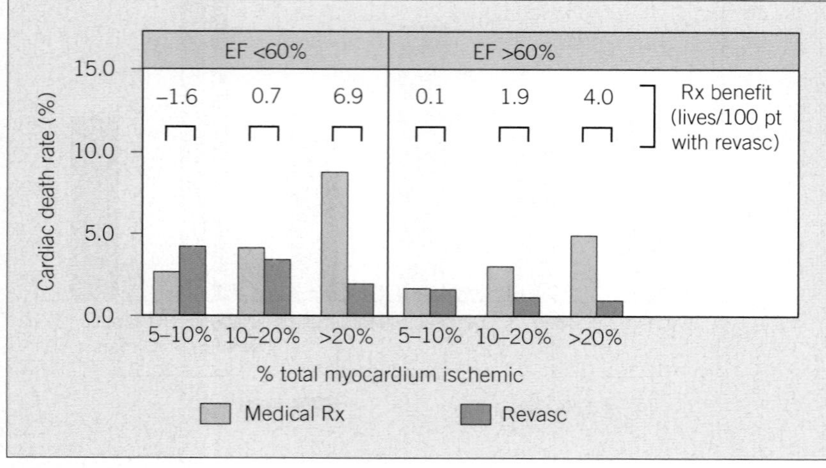

Figure 20.7 Predicted cardiac death rates by Cox proportional hazards modeling stratified by both ejection fraction (<60% and ≥60%) and percentage of the left ventricle ischemic (<10%, 10% to 20%, >20%). Rates of cardiac death are shown separately for medical therapy versus surgical revascularization. The percentage of lives saved per 100 patients treated with early revascularization is shown above the bars. (Reprinted with permission from Germano G, Berman D. Clinical Gated Cardiac SPECT. Armonk, NY, Futura, 1999.)

regional blood flow, metabolism, and function. Positron annihilation causes emission of photons at 180 degrees that are registered together. This coincidence detection improves the spatial resolution of PET (5 to 7 mm versus 10 to 14 mm for SPECT) and decreases attenuation with more accurate correction.[31] This allows the absolute quantification of flow and thus coronary flow reserve. Absolute flow determination gives PET an advantage over SPECT in identifying balanced ischemia, diffuse nonocclusive narrowing, or occlusive lesions in the zone of highest radiotracer uptake. It also allows assessment of preclinical atherosclerosis and microvascular endothelial dysfunction.[31] PET has increased sensitivity that shortens scan time and further increases spatial resolution. ECG gating allows measurement of ventricular function.

PET isotopes have shorter half-lives than SPECT agents, and most must be produced with a cyclotron close to the scanner, which limits their use to major academic institutions. However, the primary agent used in PET stress imaging is rubidium Rb 82, a ^{201}Tl analogue that can be generated offsite, but it does not have improved resolution over ^{99m}Tc SPECT and has an uptake plateau at stress levels.[32] Its short half-life allows complete studies in 1 hour but limits stress to only pharmacologic agents.

In a cohort of 663 patients pooled from the literature, PET myocardial perfusion imaging had an 89% sensitivity and an 86% specificity for CAD detection.[20] The largest prospective comparison of ^{82}Rb PET versus ^{99m}Tc SPECT in different patient groups showed improved diagnostic accuracy (89% versus 79%) and improved interpretive confidence (96% versus 81%) primarily from the improved recognition of normal scans. There was a trend toward increased sensitivity with PET (87% versus 82%), and specificity is improved (93% versus 73%).[33] The largest improvement over SPECT occurs in the diagnosis of multivessel disease, with 71% diagnosed correctly with PET versus 48% with SPECT. There are scant prognostic data available for PET stress imaging.

A lack of widespread availability, the exclusion of exercise testing with its significant ancillary information, and increased cost limit the use of PET stress imaging. Consequently, it is typically used only in patients with conflicting or inconclusive results. Of note, PET also has the potential to directly image hypoxia and inflamed atherosclerotic plaques, and active research is under way to further develop these applications.

Metabolic Ischemia Imaging

Metabolic imaging of the myocardium has previously been limited to glucose and fatty acid assessment by PET. However, iodine 123–labeled 15-(*p*-iodophenyl)-3R,*S*-methylpentadecanoic acid (BMIPP) is a fatty acid analogue that can be imaged by SPECT and has been used in Japan for more than 10 years. Abnormal BMIPP uptake occurs when ischemic tissue switches from fatty acid to glucose use, leaving a defect on SPECT imaging. This metabolic switch lasts at least 30 hours after the ischemia has resolved (and possibly up to 14 days), and thus BMIPP serves as an "ischemic memory" agent. It can identify coronary lesions in patients with unstable angina with a sensitivity of 86% and specificity of 95%.[34] Major adverse cardiac events directly correlate with the extent and severity of BMIPP lesions. BMIPP does not work well for identifying chronic ischemia (48% sensitivity) or differentiating ischemia from infarct, however, and more traditional tracers should be used in these settings.[34] Trials in the United States are ongoing.

Stress Echocardiography

An alternative to perfusion assessment to assess the physiology of CAD is functional imaging with exercise or dobutamine stress echocardiography.

Description of Procedure

Baseline cardiac function is assessed with rest echocardiography before stress. Exercise or pharmacologic stress is then performed. Exercise stress imaging is performed immediately after treadmill exercise or during supine bicycle exercise. Pharmacologic stress can be obtained with dobutamine or vasodilators (dobutamine is the preferred method). Dobutamine is given intravenously starting at 5 to 10 μg/kg per minute up to a maximum of 40 μg/kg per minute to increase inotropy and chronotropy and thus myocardial oxygen demand to induce ischemia. A common limitation with dobutamine stress is the failure to reach 85% or more of the maximum predicted heart rate, and atropine to a maximum dose of 2 mg can be given to augment the heart rate if necessary. Dobutamine can induce anxiety, palpitations, flushing, arrhythmias (rarely life-threatening), and paradoxical hypotension.

A positive response is defined as the appearance of a new regional wall abnormality as a consequence of stress.[35] Diagnostic accuracy depends on high study quality, experienced sonographers, and high-resolution scanners. Images should be stored in digital format, and pre- and post-stress views should be compared side by side.

Indications and Selection of Patients

The indications for stress echocardiography are similar to those for nuclear myocardial perfusion imaging. Patients with symptoms and an intermediate pretest likelihood of CAD derive the most benefit. Stress echocardiography adds incremental clinical value and may be more cost-effective compared with exercise testing alone in this population.[36]

Echocardiography is significantly limited in certain groups, such as obese patients and those with chronic lung disease, in whom the ultrasonographic windows may be poor. When endocardial visualization is poor, intravenous administration of contrast material has been used to improve border definition. However, because of increased cases of anaphylactoid cardiopulmonary collapse, the Food and Drug Administration has placed a black-box warning on these agents in which use with unstable angina, worsening heart failure, or acute myocardial infarction is contraindicated.

Diagnostic and Prognostic Accuracy

Stress echocardiography has a sensitivity 5% to 10% lower than that with nuclear stress perfusion imaging, ranging from 80% to 86%.[36,37] However, as with perfusion imaging, the sensitivity increases in patients with multivessel disease, prior infarction, and greater stenosis severity. Important adverse effects on sensitivity are elapsed time from end exercise until images are completely acquired and incomplete visualization of all myocardial segments. The specificity is high with stress echocardiography, ranging from 80% to 95%.[36,37] Nonischemic cardiomyopathy can cause asymmetric myocardial dysfunction that can be misinterpreted.

Exercise stress echocardiography has a higher overall sensitivity and comparable specificity versus pharmacologic stress for obstructive CAD (dobutamine performs better than vasodilator stress). Sensitivity can be increased if absence of hyperdynamic segmental response is considered a positive result. Beta blockade may attenuate dobutamine-induced ischemia, and this effect can be only partially negated by atropine use. Numerous studies show that exercise echocardiography and dobutamine echocardiography have high positive predictive values (ranges, 86% to 100% and 85% to 100%) and lower negative predictive values (ranges, 57% to 93% and 38% to 94%), reflecting the lower sensitivity. The overall diagnostic accuracy is 85% with exercise echocardiography and 83% with dobutamine echocardiography.[36]

Stress echocardiography (especially exercise) is a significant predictor of prognosis incrementally over exercise ECG and clinical risk stratification including rest echocardiography (Fig. 20.8). This is especially the case when adjunctive variables such as change in left ventricular end-systolic volume and exercise ejection fraction are considered.

A meta-analysis of exercise echocardiography showed a high negative predictive value for cardiac death or nonfatal myocardial infarction (98.4%; 95% CI, 98.5, 99.0). The annual event rate was 0.54% after a normal exercise stress echocardiogram.[38] Prognosis with an abnormal exercise echocardiogram is comparable between men and women. A 0.5-unit increase in an indexed score of wall motion increased the risk of events by approximately 50% in both genders.[39] This score and the presence of ischemia were the strongest predictors of events in a study by Olmos and coworkers.[40] This study showed comparable prognostic ability between exercise echocardiography and exercise ^{201}Tl scintigraphy in 248 patients receiving both studies. Marwick and associates[41] showed a relative risk of 5.06 with positive ischemia on exercise echocardiography for subsequent cardiac events through Cox multivariable proportional hazards analysis.

Dobutamine stress echocardiography also has good prognostic ability. In 1734 consecutive patients, stress-induced ischemia had a hazard ratio of 3.3 for cardiac death or nonfatal myocardial infarction.[42] The number of ischemic segments predicted late cardiac events. These two variables were also independent predictors of cardiac death along with age and heart failure in another cohort of patients (Fig. 20.9).[43] Prognostic ability extends to risk stratification in symptomatic women with no known CAD. In a group of 456 women, the 3-year survival free of hard cardiac events was 99.5% versus 69.5% for the cohorts with negative and positive results, respectively.[44]

In similar fashion to SPECT perfusion imaging, preoperative dobutamine stress echocardiography can stratify patients into low-, medium-, and high-risk subgroups, with one study showing 0%, 9%, and 43% postoperative event rates, respectively.[45] The benefit of this testing appears highest with an intermediate clinical risk profile. The recommended algorithm for noninvasive preoperative testing has recently been updated in an American College of Cardiology/American Heart Association guideline.[46]

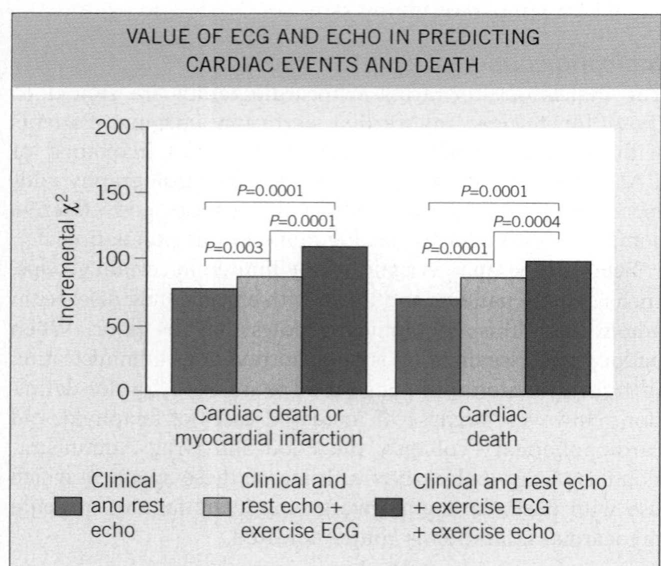

Figure 20.8 Incremental value of exercise electrocardiography (ECG) and exercise echocardiography (echo) in predicting cardiac events *(left)* and cardiac death *(right)*. The addition of exercise ECG variables to the clinical and rest echocardiographic models significantly improved the models. The addition of exercise echocardiographic variables further improved both models. (From Arruda AM, Das MK, Roger VL, et al. Prognostic value of exercise echocardiography in 2,632 patients ≥65 years of age. J Am Coll Cardiol 2001;37:1036-1041, with permission of the American College of Cardiology.)

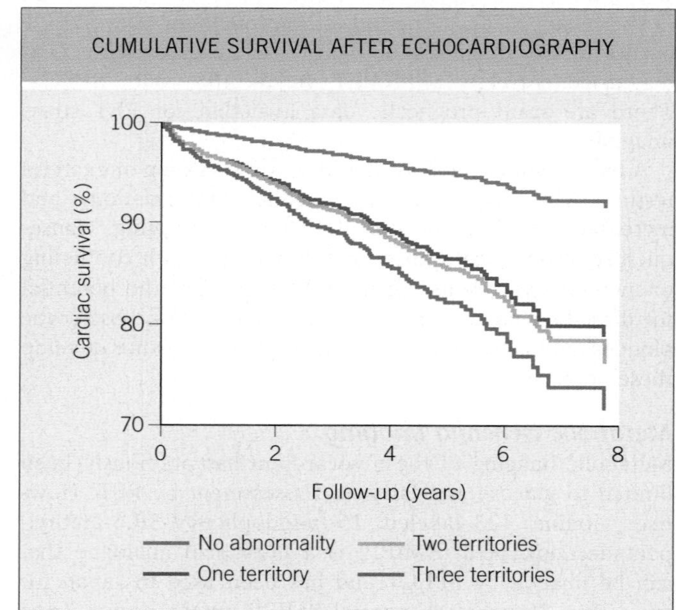

Figure 20.9 Cumulative survival after dobutamine echocardiography. Survival curves derived from the Cox model showing the relation of extent of abnormal function at peak stress to outcome. The outcome of patients with a normal scan was significantly different from the outcome of those with functional abnormalities of increasing severity ($P < .0001$). (From Marwick TH, Case C, Sawada S, et al. Prediction of mortality using dobutamine echocardiography. J Am Coll Cardiol 2001;37:754-760.)

Cardiac Magnetic Resonance Stress Imaging

Cardiovascular magnetic resonance (CMR) stress imaging is a relatively new technique made possible by significant technologic advances that can examine myocardial perfusion and inducible myocardial dysfunction. Although only available in a select few centers, it is becoming an alternative to traditional perfusion and functional testing with some definite advantages and limitations.

Description of Procedure

All CMR perfusion studies require pharmacologic stress at this time, although exercise methods are in development. Dobutamine CMR uses inotropy and chronotropy to increase myocardial oxygen demand and to induce myocardial dysfunction. Wall motion is analyzed in the same fashion as in stress echocardiography, comparing resting and stress images to identify areas of hypokinesis or dyskinesis that are likely to represent ischemia. The biggest advantage of this technique over echocardiography is that poor ultrasound windows do not occur as in certain echocardiography patients.

CMR perfusion imaging, like similar modalities, measures coronary blood flow reserve by the ratio of stress to rest perfusion. Fast data acquisition is crucial as images are taken during the static diastolic phase (through ECG gating), which is markedly reduced at increased heart rates. Parallel imaging and breath-holding are used to increase the temporal and spatial resolution. Blood flow is made visible through the administration of gadolinium, a contrast agent that shortens a property of magnetic resonance imaging, the T1 relaxation time, causing a brighter signal. Areas with poor perfusion have less gadolinium enhancement and are seen as dark.[47,48] This initial approach was limited by artifactual decreased signal during both rest and stress that was often confused with infarct. Therefore, additional late gadolinium enhancement (LGE) imaging was added, which shows infarcted myocardium as bright because of increased gadolinium uptake across disrupted cell membranes and delayed washout.[47] This has reduced but not eliminated artifactual problems.

Importantly, CMR stress images are obtained without the use of ionizing radiation, and patients benefit from shorter examination times than with other perfusion modalities (although D-SPECT will likely erase this disparity). However, the patient is relatively inaccessible during a small portion of the examination.

Image interpretation can be done both quantitatively and qualitatively through a 16-segment model that lacks the 17th apical segment used in nuclear imaging. The quantitative approach provides absolute blood flow in milliliters per minute per gram of myocardium but requires extensive, time-consuming postimage processing. PET is the only other modality that can currently give this information. Qualitative interpretation of these images is made significantly easier by the increased spatial resolution (43 mm^3 versus 1000 mm^3 for nuclear SPECT). This also provides the potential to discern endocardial from epicardial flow and thus provide information on the microcirculation.[47,48]

CMR also provides improved identification and measurement of perfusion defects through an absolute comparison of the abnormal area with the remaining normal tissue in that segment rather than a relative comparison to the reference myocardial segment (with the highest uptake on the scan). Moreover, flow differences can be measured across the entire spectrum of coronary dilatation and flow, as the signal intensity increases linearly with tissue perfusion rather than reaching a plateau, allowing more accurate assessment.[47,48]

Indications and Selection of Patients

As with the other stress imaging modalities, stress CMR imaging was recommended by an American College of Cardiology Foundation 2006 consensus panel for patients with an intermediate probability of CAD or for determination of the physiologic significance of indeterminate lesions found on angiography. It can also be considered a more definitive test in patients with poor ultrasound windows for echocardiography. However, its limited prognostic information should be kept in mind, and the appropriateness criteria list the role of CMR as uncertain for symptomatic patients or for equivocal other imaging results.[13] The high resolution of this technique makes it superior for the assessment of microvascular obstruction as seen in syndrome X and hypertrophic obstructive cardiomyopathy. This is especially important given the increasing prevalence of microvascular dysfunction with the metabolic syndrome. Stress CMR is an especially good option for young women as there is no radiation exposure.

CMR is contraindicated in patients with implantable cardioverter-defibrillators, although future ones may be MRI compatible. Intracoronary stents are generally considered safe, especially more than 2 weeks after implantation. CMR is contraindicated in patients with significant renal dysfunction because of the possibility of nephrogenic systemic fibrosis, a potentially fatal condition, after gadolinium administration. There are several other populations of patients in which other modalities should be considered. Patients with arrhythmias, especially when they are irregular, can disrupt ECG gating and lead to a considerable reduction in resolution. Likewise, patients with shortness of breath or difficulty following commands may have significant respiratory motion artifact. Stress agent use can enhance claustrophobia from the close confines of the scanner. Finally, patients with any risk of instability would be inaccessible for a short but defined time.

Diagnostic and Prognostic Accuracy of Test

Early studies of CMR stress imaging were limited by small, heterogeneous samples with varying protocols examined retrospectively. In a meta-analysis of 2191 patients, the sensitivity and specificity of stress perfusion CMR imaging for the detection of CAD were 91% and 81%, respectively, compared with 83% and 86% with CMR dobutamine stress wall motion analysis.[49] Despite improved sensitivity with CMR perfusion imaging, poor specificity remained. However, Kim and associates[47] from Duke described a multicomponent analysis that has markedly improved specificity and has become the standard CMR stress imaging protocol (Fig. 20.10). CMR perfusion imaging is performed to examine for defects at stress and rest, and then LGE is used to identify areas of infarct. Perfusion deficits on stress but not on rest signify areas of ischemia. Matched defects on rest and stress may represent artifacts or infarct. These perfusion images are compared with the LGE images, which either confirm or refute infarction. If the perfusion defects are larger than the areas of LGE, there

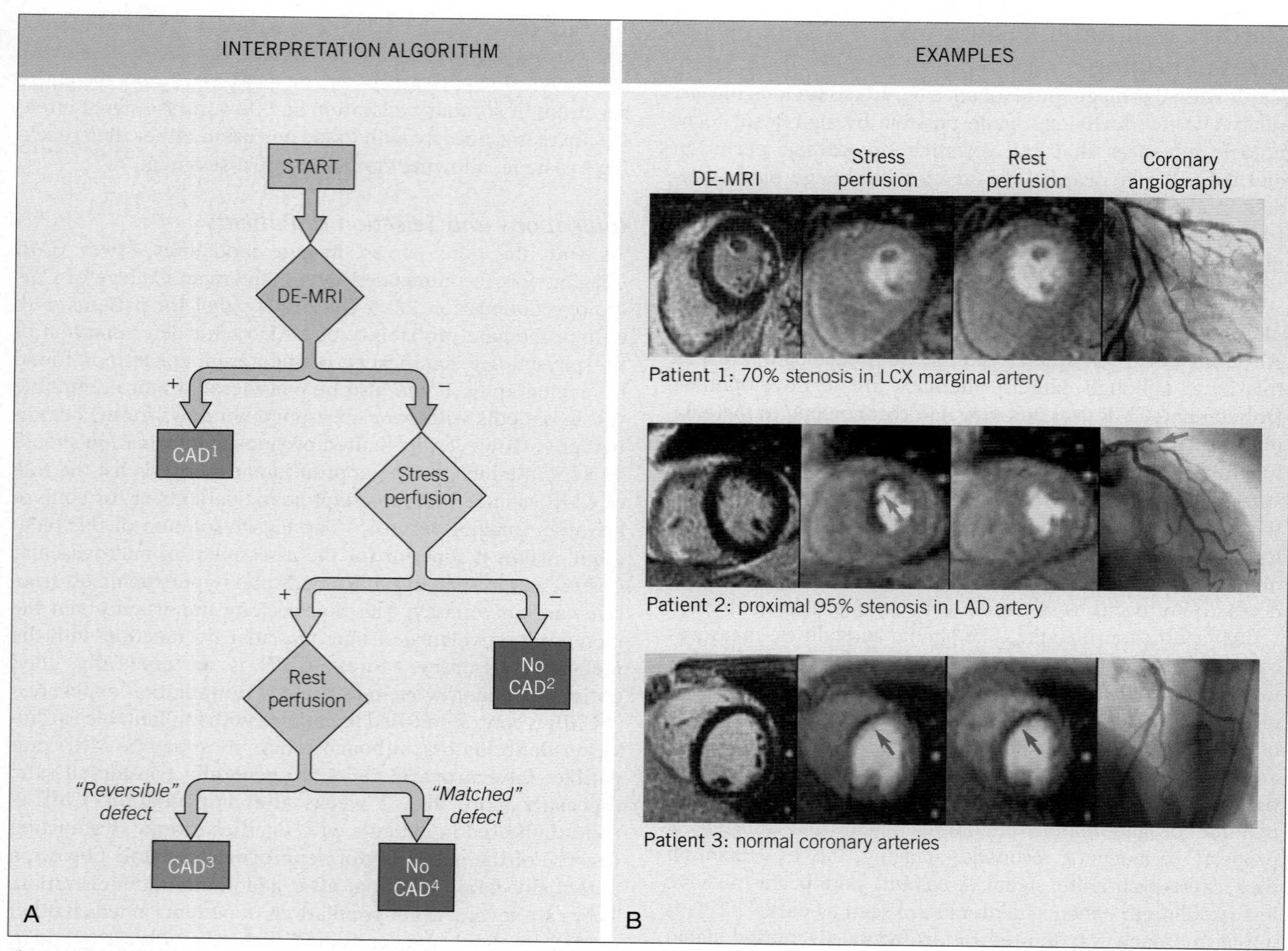

Figure 20.10 Perfusion cardiac magnetic resonance algorithm for the diagnosis of coronary artery disease. Panel **A** shows the interpretation algorithm. Panel **B** shows three examples. Patient 1 shows inferolateral increased signal on late gadolinium enhancement imaging (delayed enhancement, DE-MRI) with no perfusion abnormalities consistent with a prior infarct, with obtuse marginal disease on x-ray angiography. Patient 2 shows a normal DE-MRI with an anteroseptal reversible defect consistent with ischemia caused by the 95% proximal left anterior descending artery stenosis. Patient 3 has a matched stress-rest perfusion defect but no late gadolinium enhancement on DE-MRI, which is appropriately judged to be artifact as confirmed by the normal coronary angiogram. (Reprinted with permission from Kim HW, Klem I, Kim RJ. Detection of myocardial ischemia by stress perfusion cardiovascular magnetic resonance. Cardiol Clin 2007;25:57-70.)

is likely peri-infarct ischemia. In their analysis, this approach yielded an excellent sensitivity of 89%. The specificity markedly improved from 58% with perfusion alone to 87% with the addition of LGE imaging. The overall diagnostic accuracy was 88% for stenoses greater than 70% (50% for the left main coronary artery).[47]

Limited data are available on the prognosis of stress CMR, given its recent development. One study of 513 patients compared adenosine perfusion CMR with dobutamine stress wall motion imaging. Both techniques added significant incremental value over risk factors and resting wall motion.[50] In a multivariable model, ischemia identified by dobutamine CMR was highly predictive of cardiac events with a hazard ratio of 5.42 (95% CI, 2.18-13.50), and ischemia on adenosine CMR had an even stronger association (hazard ratio, 12.51; 95% CI, 3.64-43.03). With abnormal CMR perfusion, the 3-year rate of cardiovascular death and nonfatal myocardial infarction was 16.3%.[50]

Summary

Stress CMR imaging can be performed to examine both inducible wall motion abnormalities with dobutamine stress and perfusion defects through adenosine or dipyridamole stress. Both have good sensitivity, specificity, and diagnostic accuracy, but adenosine perfusion with the addition of delayed hyperenhancement imaging provides the best diagnostic accuracy. Increasing prognostic data reveal a high correlation between abnormal stress CMR images and major adverse cardiac events.

Future directions include improved magnetic resonance pulse sequences to reduce artifacts, standardization of definitions and procedures for analysis, and combination stress CMR and magnetic resonance angiography with plaque characterization once these techniques have improved. Use of a stronger 3 Tesla magnet will provide improved image resolution, but the resultant increased magnetic field and gadolinium distribution homogeneities may limit its use in stress CMR imaging.

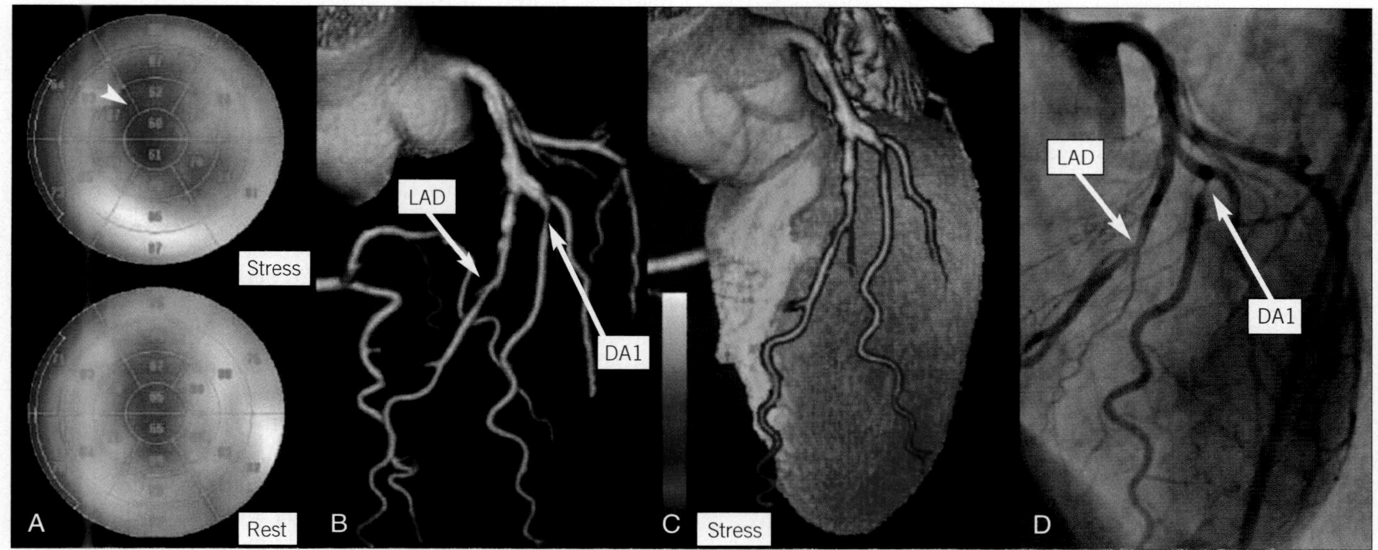

Figure 20.11 Fused SPECT-CT image of the heart. **A,** Standard stress and rest perfusion maps reveal a predominantly reversible anteroapical defect *(arrowhead)*. **B,** A three-dimensional volume-rendered CTCA image reveals a proximal first diagonal (DA1) stenosis and myocardial bridging of the mid left anterior descending (LAD) coronary artery. **C,** Fused SPECT-CT image clearly shows the perfusion defect associated with the DA1 stenosis. **D,** The CTCA findings are confirmed with invasive x-ray coronary angiography. (Reprinted with permission from Gaemperli O, Schepis T, Valenta I, et al. Cardiac image fusion from stand-alone SPECT and CT: clinical experience. J Nucl Med 2007;48:696-703.)

Hybrid Imaging

Hybrid imaging, currently combining CTCA with PET or SPECT perfusion imaging, allows the identification of CAD, perfusion, viability, and ventricular function, all with one imaging study (Fig. 20.11). Computed tomography provides information on the presence and extent of luminal obstruction. However, less than 50% of the obstructive lesions on CTCA have associated perfusion defects on PET.[51] PET and SPECT perfusion imaging identify ischemia with high sensitivity, but they underestimate the true extent of CAD (even PET with absolute quantitation) and thus may miss important opportunities for more aggressive medical therapy. Its multiple approaches make hybrid imaging especially good at informing revascularization decisions. Use of combination scanners allows spatial alignment and full assessment in a single imaging session. Moreover, computed tomography allows improved attenuation correction. An important limitation is the radiation dose, typically 10 to 18 mSv for CTCA and approximately 5 to 6 mSv for ^{82}Rb PET.[31]

Combining SPECT perfusion imaging with CTCA relies on relative flow rather than absolute quantification but is more readily available and significantly improves the positive predictive value of lesions on CTCA (31% to more than 77% in one study) with continued high negative predictive value.[9] SPECT myocardial perfusion imaging adds incremental information to CTCA on lesion severity that could affect treatment decisions in up to 29% of patients. This is especially true in multivessel disease and branch vessel involvement. Further research and development are needed in this burgeoning area.

DIAGNOSTIC STRATEGY

In this era of increasing medical costs, rational use of expensive noninvasive technology is critically important, and corresponding appropriateness criteria address this important issue.[13,30,52] Some suggest that imaging studies are overused, particularly when they are ordered in conjunction with treadmill exercise testing in patients with low (<10%) pretest likelihood of CAD. Symptom-limited treadmill ECG testing alone may suffice to exclude significant underlying CAD as the cause of atypical chest pain. This would certainly be the case in patients whose resting ECGs are normal and who are judged to have a low pretest likelihood of disease (Fig. 20.12). Patients who have an intermediate pretest likelihood of disease (≥10%, <85%) can undergo exercise ECG testing as the first step if the resting ECG is normal.

However, many observers would combine the exercise ECG with an imaging procedure at the outset to enhance both the diagnostic and prognostic value of the assessment

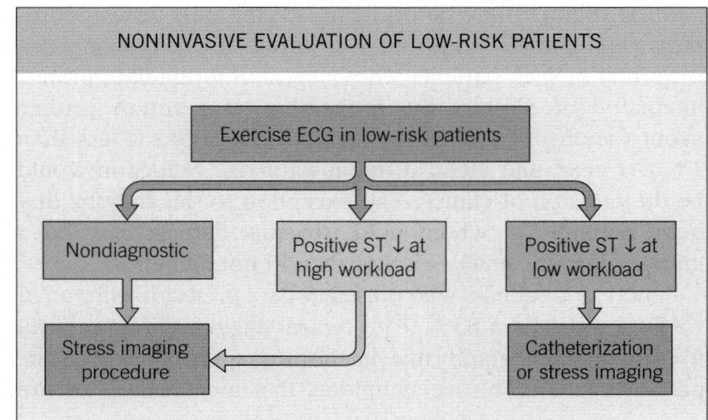

Figure 20.12 The noninvasive evaluation in patients at low pretest risk for coronary artery disease and who have a normal resting electrocardiogram. This would include patients with nonanginal chest pain but for whom a stress test of some sort is required to rule out coronary artery disease as the cause of atypical symptoms.

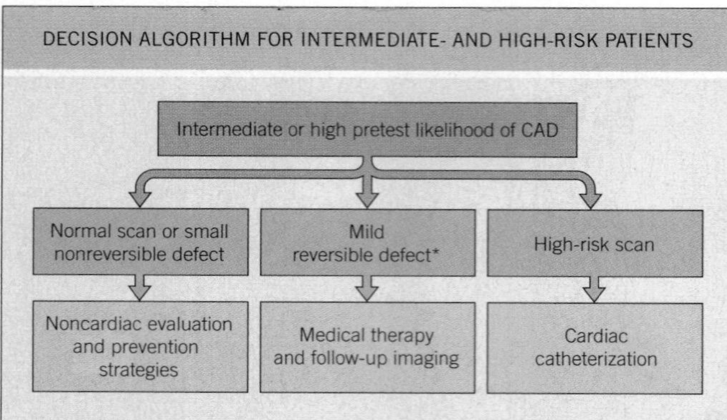

Figure 20.13 Algorithm for decision making regarding stress testing in patients with an intermediate or high pretest likelihood of coronary artery disease. Such patients would benefit from combined stress exercise ECG with an imaging procedure. In this example, single-photon emission computed tomographic (SPECT) imaging is employed. For this algorithm, it is assumed that patients with only a mild reversible defect, particularly when it is confined to one coronary supply region, can be managed medically with aggressive lipid-lowering therapy and anti-ischemic drugs. However, such patients would be candidates for an invasive strategy if symptoms that interfered with quality of life persisted or progression of disease was reflected by more extensive or severe defects on follow-up imaging (see text for explanation). CAD, coronary artery disease. *Non–high-risk SPECT scan with no multivessel disease pattern or extensive defect in the left anterior descending coronary artery region. (Modified from Beller GA, Zaret BL. Contributions of nuclear cardiology to diagnosis and prognosis of patients with coronary artery disease. Circulation 2000;101:1465-1478.)

(Fig. 20.13). This is because of the added sensitivity for CAD detection and the incremental prognostic value when perfusion imaging or functional testing is added to the clinical and ECG stress test information. When a patient with an intermediate pretest likelihood of disease has an abnormal scan, particularly if multiple reversible perfusion or functional defects are noted or a multivessel scan pattern is identified, coronary angiography should be considered. If, however, the scan shows a mild to moderate defect, particularly if this is confined to a single vascular region, aggressive medical therapy may be prudent. If symptoms persist, coronary angiography would be warranted. If the imaging test is normal in such patients who have an intermediate pretest likelihood of disease, the probability of a future cardiac event (death or nonfatal myocardial infarction) is less than 1% per year, and medical therapy for risk reduction would be the decision of choice. The exception to this may be diabetic patients, in whom mild ischemic defects may be a marker of more severe disease than in nondiabetics.

Finally, for patients who present with a pretest likelihood of CAD of more than 85% (e.g., typical angina), direct referral to coronary angiography may be the most appropriate decision, particularly if there are symptoms that are unstable or are limiting quality of life. If such patients have mild angina, ECG stress testing combined with a stress imaging procedure may be the best approach for further risk stratification. Patients who have mild defects, particularly when these are confined to a single vascular region, might safely be managed medically rather than with revascularization. In contrast, patients who have high-risk imaging variables would be candidates for coronary angiography with a view to revascularization.

Physiologic testing with stress perfusion or functional imaging may be valuable even when it is performed after coronary angiography. One indication for noninvasive testing after catheterization is in the instance of intermediate-grade stenosis (50% to 70%) with uncertain physiologic significance.

The strengths and weaknesses of the different imaging modalities, the prognostic information currently available, and the specific clinical situation should be used to guide which test is optimal (Table 20.4). The direct identification of ischemia with physiologic testing and the wealth of diagnostic and prognostic data available make these the primary noninvasive tests performed. However, anatomic imaging can identify disease and guide need for aggressive medical therapy at a much earlier stage. The roles of CACS and CTCA are not fully defined, with limited prognostic data. More research is needed and is under way. Current testing decisions should be guided by recently written and updated American College of Cardiology/American Heart Association guidelines and appropriateness criteria.[2,13,15,30,36,46,52]

SUMMARY

Noninvasive imaging for ischemic heart disease in a cost-effective manner is essential to avoid unnecessary invasive testing and to decrease adverse cardiac outcomes. We currently have excellent modalities that can provide important information about the anatomic presence and physiologic significance of CAD. Both nuclear perfusion imaging and stress echocardiography have excellent negative predictive values for identifying patients with a low risk (<1% annually) for cardiac events. Conversely, patients with abnormal scans have a sevenfold increase in annual risk of death or infarction. Combination multimodality testing will likely play an increased role with anatomic localization of ischemia and functional significance assessment of indeterminate obstructive coronary lesions. Additional imaging modalities are under active investigation, including magnetic resonance coronary angiography, computed tomographic perfusion, and ischemic memory agents such as BMIPP. There is a strong future in molecular imaging that will allow direct plaque visualization with evaluation of stability and other important characteristics. We must also look more closely at specific subgroups, especially those with diabetes and other high-risk conditions. A screening approach, possibly using calcium scoring, may prove beneficial for decreasing future cardiac events. We need further research to see if this sort of method will ultimately prove effective.

ADVANTAGES AND LIMITATIONS OF THE VARIOUS DIAGNOSTIC IMAGING MODALITIES		
Modality	**Advantages**	**Limitations**
CT calcium scoring	Early diagnosis of CAD High sensitivity Linear correlation with cardiac events	Insufficient testing for symptomatic patients Low specificity Not currently reimbursed
CT coronary angiography	Noninvasive visualization of coronary atherosclerosis Good for presurgical cardiac risk assessment and surgical planning in low-risk patients High negative predictive value and hence useful in patients with a low to intermediate likelihood of CAD Can help avoid invasive testing	Diagnostic and prognostic role not fully defined Lesion functional information not provided Poor specificity and positive predictive value for CAD Calcification and stents can cause lesion overestimation Potential for additional unnecessary testing Limited assessment of smaller vessels <2 mm Breath-holding and ECG gating required Radiation and contrast risks
Exercise electrocardiography	Inexpensive With good cardiac workload, provides a high negative predictive value Useful for high-risk occupations or before vigorous exercise in older patients	Insufficient sensitivity and specificity in most patients Baseline ECG abnormalities limit usefulness Requires achieving $\geq$85% of the maximum predicted heart rate for age
SPECT myocardial perfusion imaging	Very high sensitivity and good specificity for myocardial ischemia Wealth of prognostic data available Readily accessible Few absolute or relative contraindications	Assesses only functionally significant CAD Balanced ischemia can be missed Tissue attenuation and high visceral radioactivity can confound diagnosis
Positron emission tomography	Absolute quantification of blood flow and flow reserve rather than relative flow Improved specificity and interpretive confidence over SPECT perfusion imaging Improved sensitivity for balanced ischemia Good for patients with inconclusive noninvasive results	Limited availability Higher cost Exercise stress is not currently possible Extensive prognostic data are not available
Stress echocardiography	Less expensive than perfusion imaging High specificity Equivalent negative predictive value versus SPECT	Less sensitivity than perfusion imaging Poor acquisition in many patients Nonischemic dysfunction can be misinterpreted
Stress cardiovascular magnetic resonance	Excellent sensitivity and specificity when delayed hyperenhancement imaging is in use Excellent spatial resolution Good for microvascular dysfunction and hypertrophic obstructive cardiomyopathy No radiation provided Absolute quantification available, but qualitative assessment is still primarily used	Prognostic value not fully determined Contraindicated with implantable cardioverter-defibrillators Limited availability Exercise stress not currently possible Gadolinium can be toxic in renal disease Breath-holding and ECG gating required Can exacerbate claustrophobia

CAD, coronary artery disease; CT, computed tomography; ECG, electrocardiography; SPECT, single-photon emission computed tomography.

Table 20.4 Advantages and limitations of the various diagnostic imaging modalities.

chapter 21

Invasive Diagnosis of Ischemic Heart Disease

William F. Fearon

Coronary angiography has been the traditional reference standard for invasive diagnosis of coronary artery disease. It continues to play an integral role in detecting critical coronary narrowings, but adjunctive methods using a coronary pressure wire to assess the physiologic impact or an intravascular ultrasound catheter to identify the anatomic characteristics of a specific lesion have now replaced angiography as the most sensitive tool for invasive evaluation of coronary disease.

This chapter briefly reviews the indications, technique, and complications of coronary angiography. The role of the coronary pressure wire and intravascular ultrasonography in the catheterization laboratory is detailed. Finally, other less commonly used and in some cases experimental methods for invasive investigation of the coronary arteries are introduced.

CORONARY ANGIOGRAPHY

Historical Perspective

Coronary angiography is defined as the visualization of the coronary arteries after injection of contrast media. In 1958, the first selective coronary angiography was performed by F. Mason Sones, Jr.[1] At the time, there was great concern that injection of contrast media into one coronary artery would result in asymmetric hypoxia and development of ventricular tachycardia; but after the accidental selective injection of a right coronary artery at the time of aortic root angiography demonstrated no adverse sequelae, Sones began intentional selective coronary angiography.[2] Soon thereafter, Melvin P. Judkins and Kurt Amplatz introduced preformed catheters to facilitate coronary ostia engagement.[3,4] In addition, a truly percutaneous approach through the modified Seldinger approach to the femoral artery became commonplace. Both advancements made the procedure simpler and safer and likely increased its widespread adaptation.

Current Indications

As the safety of coronary angiography has improved and the complication rates have fallen, the indications for angiography have broadened. In any given patient, multiple considerations must be made in determining whether to perform a procedure. The same tenet holds true with coronary angiography, and the following represents a review of the commonly accepted reasons for performing coronary angiography. In all cases, it is important to balance the benefit of the information obtained from the angiographic evaluation against the risks, although relatively low, and the expense, which is relatively high.

The primary clinical reasons for performing coronary angiography are to diagnose the presence and severity of coronary atherosclerosis when noninvasive imaging fails to do so, to determine whether revascularization with percutaneous coronary intervention or coronary artery bypass surgery is warranted and feasible, and to measure the effects of a particular treatment for research purposes.[5]

In patients who have known or suspected coronary artery disease, whether asymptomatic or with stable angina, class I indications for angiography based on the American College of Cardiology/American Heart Association guidelines include severe angina (Canadian Cardiovascular Society class III or IV), high-risk noninvasive stress test (e.g., significant resting or exercise-induced left ventricular dysfunction, high-risk treadmill score, or large amount of ischemia based on echocardiographic or nuclear imaging), and regardless of the presence of angina, successful resuscitation from cardiac death, sustained monomorphic ventricular tachycardia, or unsustained polymorphic ventricular tachycardia.[5]

In patients with non–ST-segment elevation acute coronary syndromes, some controversy exists about the role of coronary angiography; but most investigators agree that in patients with high-risk features, as defined by a clinical score such as the TIMI risk score, or in patients with low-risk features but a high-risk noninvasive stress imaging study, diagnostic angiography should be performed.[6] In the setting of ST-segment elevation myocardial infarction, emergent coronary angiography should be performed if it is available in a timely fashion and at a center experienced in performing primary percutaneous coronary intervention.[7]

Preoperative coronary angiography is generally performed in patients with cardiac risk factors who are scheduled for cardiac surgery, such as valve replacement. In those undergoing noncardiac surgery, angiography is generally recommended in those with high-risk noninvasive stress imaging studies or in those with angina refractory to medical therapy or unstable angina.

A number of centers perform routine coronary angiography after cardiac transplantation or before kidney, liver, or lung transplantation in patients with multiple cardiac risk factors or abnormal noninvasive stress imaging studies. In this group of pretransplantation patients, traditional angiography may be replaced by noninvasive coronary imaging with multislice computed tomographic coronary angiography as this technique continues to be refined and experience with it grows.

There are no absolute contraindications to coronary angiography, particularly in the setting of an acute ST-segment elevation myocardial infarction. However, a number of relative contraindications must be considered (Table 21.1).

Technique

Coronary angiography is currently performed by the modified Seldinger technique to obtain arterial access in the femoral, radial, or brachial artery with use of a 4 to 6 French vascular sheath. Preprocedure aspirin is given, but periprocedural heparin is generally not necessary. Local anesthesia and conscious sedation are administered before vascular access is obtained. In most centers, a Judkins left 4 catheter (4 to 6 French in size) is used to engage the left coronary ostium. It is advanced over an angle-tipped 0.35-inch guide wire under fluoroscopic guidance. In most cases, the catheter requires little manipulation to engage the left coronary ostium. Hand or automated injections of 5 to 10 mL of radiographic contrast media are made, and cineangiograms are recorded in multiple projections. The left coronary catheter is removed, and a Judkins right 4 catheter is advanced in a similar fashion to the root of the aorta. To engage the right coronary ostium, the catheter requires clockwise torquing. Once it is engaged, cineangiograms are repeated after injection of contrast material. At the end of the procedure, the vascular sheath is removed, and manual pressure is applied or a vascular closure device is inserted to facilitate hemostasis.

Complications

The overall complication rate for diagnostic coronary angiography is believed to be less than 2%; the most common complication is related to vascular injury (Table 21.2). Other complications, such as death, myocardial infarction, and stroke, are extremely rare, although the patient's clinical risk for a complication is an important determinant of the frequency. For example, left main coronary stenosis may increase the risk of a complication twofold. Cardiogenic shock, acute myocardial infarction, significant valvular disease, renal insufficiency, and advanced age all contribute to an increased complication rate.[5]

RELATIVE CONTRAINDICATIONS TO CORONARY ANGIOGRAPHY
Active infection
Active bleeding
Coagulopathy
Acute renal failure
Acute stroke
Severe anemia
Decompensated congestive heart failure
Severe uncontrolled hypertension
Severe electrolyte imbalance
Severe concomitant illness drastically shortening life expectancy
Severe lack of cooperation by the patient

Modified from Scanlon PJ, Faxon DP, Audet AM, et al. ACC/AHA guidelines for coronary angiography: executive summary and recommendations. A report of the American College of Cardiology/American Heart Association Task Force on Practice Guidelines (Committee on Coronary Angiography) developed in collaboration with the Society for Cardiac Angiography and Interventions. J Am Coll Cardiol 1999;33:1756-1824.

Table 21.1 Relative contraindications to coronary angiography.

COMPLICATIONS OF CORONARY ANGIOGRAPHY

Complication	Rate (%)
Death	0.11
Myocardial infarction	0.05
Stroke	0.07
Vascular complication	0.43
Contrast reaction	0.37
Arrhythmia	0.38
Hemodynamic complication	0.26
Perforation of heart chamber	0.03
Other complications	0.28
Total	1.70

Modified from Scanlon PJ, Faxon DP, Audet AM, et al. ACC/AHA guidelines for coronary angiography: executive summary and recommendations. A report of the American College of Cardiology/American Heart Association Task Force on Practice Guidelines (Committee on Coronary Angiography) developed in collaboration with the Society for Cardiac Angiography and Interventions. J Am Coll Cardiol 1999;33:1756-1824.

Table 21.2 Complications of coronary angiography.

Angiographic Diagnosis of Coronary Artery Disease

Typically, the angiographic diagnosis of coronary artery disease is made subjectively by the cardiologist who performed the procedure. In general, a visual estimation of the severity of a coronary narrowing is reported. Classification systems aimed at standardizing the interpretation of an angiogram have been created that incorporate lesion characteristics such as degree of calcification, length, eccentricity, tortuosity, and location at a bifurcation. These techniques, however, are inherently limited by interobserver variability.[8]

Quantitative coronary angiography is a computer-assisted method of measuring lesion length and stenosis severity. By use of an object of known size, such as the catheter, to calibrate the system, quantitative coronary angiography ideally is less subjective and more accurate. Unfortunately, it too is prone to error and subjectivity due to operator technique.

A number of limitations to angiography hamper its ability to accurately diagnose coronary disease, particularly in the setting of moderate narrowing or diffuse disease. First, because the angiogram is a two-dimensional representation of a three-dimensional object, an eccentric narrowing can be missed if the correct angle is not used to image the vessel.[9] Second, because a diseased area of a coronary artery is generally compared with an adjacent "normal" area, patients with diffuse disease, without any focal component, can be incorrectly classified as having normal coronary arteries. Finally, the angiogram highlights the lumen of the coronary artery but provides no information about the wall of the vessel. Positive remodeling of the artery at the site of atherosclerotic plaque development can result in preservation of the lumen and a nearly normal angiogram, which hides the atherosclerosis from the angiographer. Because of these limitations, a number of adjunctive techniques have been developed to improve the invasive diagnosis of ischemic heart disease. The remainder of this chapter focuses particularly on the use of the coronary pressure wire and the intravascular ultrasound catheter in diagnosis of coronary artery disease.

CORONARY PRESSURE WIRE

Historical Perspective

Gould and colleagues[10] first introduced the concept of coronary flow reserve (CFR) more than 30 years ago. CFR is defined as the ratio between the maximum achievable coronary flow during hyperemia and the resting coronary flow. Because coronary velocity is proportional to coronary flow, CFR can be estimated by measuring the coronary velocity at rest and during maximal vasodilatation. In the early 1990s, it became possible to measure CFR in the catheterization laboratory by use of a standard angioplasty guide wire, with a Doppler transducer mounted at its tip, and by administration of a vasodilatory agent, such as adenosine or papaverine. A number of studies demonstrated the utility of measuring CFR in patients with intermediate coronary lesions.[11-13]

However, CFR by definition interrogates the status of the entire coronary circulation, both the epicardial vessel and the microcirculation. In patients with microvascular dysfunction, for example, from diabetes or a past myocardial infarction, CFR will be abnormal, limiting its application for identifying ischemia-producing epicardial disease.[14] In addition, because CFR incorporates resting flow in its definition, it is affected by changes in resting hemodynamics, limiting its reproducibility.[15,16] Finally, CFR does not have a clear normal value; in general, a CFR above 2 is "normal," but this may vary from patient to patient. In an attempt to overcome these limitations and to provide a more accurate invasive physiologic assessment of epicardial coronary disease, Pijls and De Bruyne introduced the concept of myocardial fractional flow reserve.[17]

Fractional Flow Reserve

Fractional flow reserve (FFR) is defined as the maximum flow down a vessel in the presence of a stenosis compared with the maximum flow in the theoretical absence of the stenosis (i.e., in the normal artery).[17] During maximum flow in a coronary artery, resistance is minimized and flow becomes proportional to pressure. Thus, the equation for FFR can be changed to the ratio of coronary pressure in the presence of a stenosis compared with its theoretical absence. In a normal vessel, proximal coronary pressure is equal to distal coronary pressure. Therefore, in a diseased vessel, the proximal coronary pressure is a reflection of what the distal pressure would be in the theoretical absence of the disease. FFR can then be calculated by measuring distal pressure in a diseased artery and dividing it by proximal pressure, during maximal flow or vasodilatation (Fig. 21.1).[17]

Unlike CFR, FFR is independent of the systemic blood pressure and heart rate and is very reproducible.[15,16] It has a clear normal value, 1.0, and a well-established abnormal value of less than 0.75 as discussed later. FFR can be measured accurately in patients with microvascular disease. Because achieving maximal hyperemia in measuring the pressure gradient across a stenosis is critical to accurate assessment of FFR, a dysfunctional microcirculation secondary to, for example, myocardial infarction can impair its vasodilatory capacity. This can result in a decrease in the transstenotic pressure gradient and in what one initially might consider an overestimation of the FFR. However, unlike CFR, as long as the microvascular dysfunction is assumed to be a chronic issue, the FFR measurement continues to provide useful information about the epicardial lesion in this setting; an FFR above 0.75 implies the absence of myocardial ischemia and the lack of need for

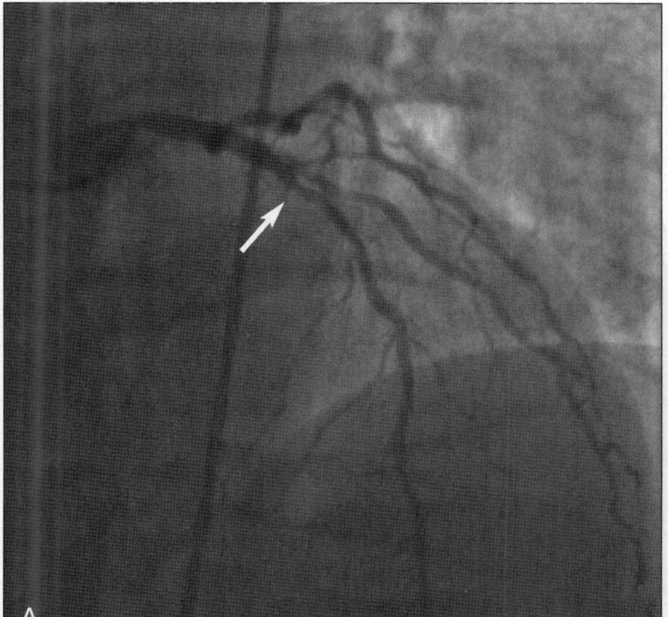

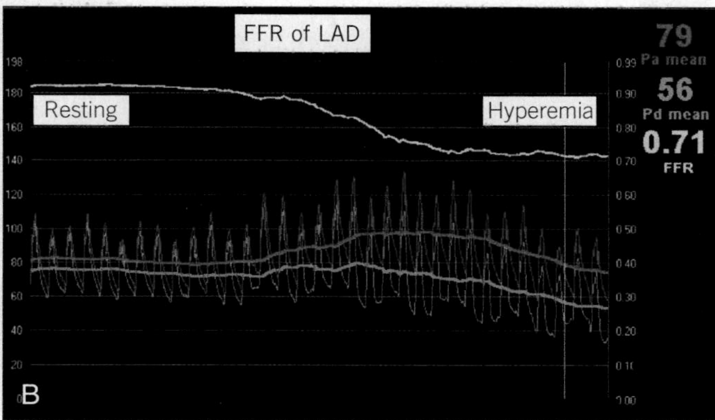

Figure 21-1 A, Angiogram in the cranial angulation displaying an intermediate left anterior descending lesion (*arrow*). **B,** Tracing of the fractional flow reserve (FFR) of the intermediate left anterior descending (LAD) lesion in **A**.

revascularization.[18] In patients with acute ST-segment elevation myocardial infarction, in which there may be some degree of reversible microvascular dysfunction as a result of myocardial stunning, FFR may not be accurate.

Fractional Flow Reserve Technique

The coronary pressure wire is a 0.014-inch coronary guide wire with a miniaturized, high-fidelity pressure sensor mounted 3 cm from the tip of the wire at the junction of the radiopaque and radiolucent segments. Currently, there are two manufacturers of the pressure wire (Radi Medical Systems and Volcano Therapeutics), each of which has its own consoles that analyze and display the pressure recordings.

After administration of 50 to 70 units/kg of heparin and 100 to 200 μg of intracoronary nitroglycerin to maximally dilate the epicardial coronary vessel, a coronary pressure wire is connected to a commercially available analyzer and calibrated outside of the body. The pressure wire is then advanced typically through a guiding catheter, and the pressure sensor is positioned near the ostium of the guiding catheter where the pressure signal from the wire is equalized to the pressure signal from the catheter. The wire is then advanced to the distal third of the vessel of interest, beyond the stenosis of interest. Maximal coronary hyperemia is induced generally with a bolus of intracoronary adenosine (50 to 100 μg) or with intravenous adenosine (140 μg/kg per minute) infusion. FFR is measured as the mean distal pressure measured with the wire divided by the mean proximal coronary or aortic pressure measured with the guide catheter. In the presence of diffuse disease or sequential stenoses, the wire can be pulled slowly back to the ostium of the coronary during maximal hyperemia to identify whether there is a focal area responsible for the bulk of the pressure gradient in the case of diffuse disease or to identify which lesion is most responsible for the gradient in the case of sequential stenoses (Fig. 21.2). In this way, FFR is not only a vessel-specific method for identifying ischemia but also lesion specific.[19] This concept explains why many think that FFR is a more accurate determinant of ischemic heart disease than noninvasive stress imaging.[20]

Complications from measuring FFR are rare and include those typical with placement of a Doppler guide wire down a vessel.[21] Rarely, dissection, clot formation, or spasm can occur. Complications with the hyperemic agents are more common. Intracoronary adenosine can cause transient bradycardia in 10% or more of cases, depending on the dose and the vessel (dominant right coronary artery being more common), but clinically relevant bradycardia is extremely rare with intracoronary administration. Intravenous adenosine infusion commonly causes benign chest discomfort or dyspnea, and as long as the patient is forewarned, it is well tolerated. In patients with significant obstructive lung disease, intravenous adenosine infusion should be used with caution because it can exacerbate this condition. Bradyarrhythmias can occur with intravenous adenosine infusion but typically resolve once the infusion is discontinued.[19] Intracoronary papaverine can cause ventricular arrhythmias in approximately 1% of cases, and therefore it is not commonly used anymore.[22]

There are some potential pitfalls to measurement of FFR. The most important is achieving inadequate hyperemia. With intravenous adenosine administered through the femoral vein, this is very unlikely; however, with intracoronary adenosine, if the guide catheter is not well seated in the ostium of the coronary, some adenosine may be injected into the aorta. For this same reason, guide catheters with side holes should not be used. On occasion, the pressure wire pressure reading can "drift," resulting in inaccurate pressure recordings. This is usually only a small amount, but after FFR is measured, it is useful to do a pullback of the pressure wire to confirm that the pressure reading from the wire with the sensor near the ostium of the guide catheter is still equal to the guide catheter pressure reading. Finally, if there is ostial coronary disease, the guide catheter can contribute to further ostial narrowing and impair maximal flow down the vessel, resulting in an FFR that is falsely elevated. Ventricularization of the proximal pressure tracing can be a clue that this is occurring. If intravenous adenosine is being administered, this pitfall can be avoided by unseating the guide catheter. When intracoronary adenosine is administered, once the medication has been injected, quickly unseating the guide catheter will allow more accurate FFR measurement.[23]

Fractional Flow Reserve in Intermediate Lesions

A number of studies have compared FFR with noninvasive stress tests to identify ischemia-producing intermediate lesions in a variety of populations.[24-29] The landmark study, performed by Pijls and colleagues,[30] measured FFR in 45 patients with chest pain and moderate coronary narrowings. All patients underwent exercise stress testing, nuclear

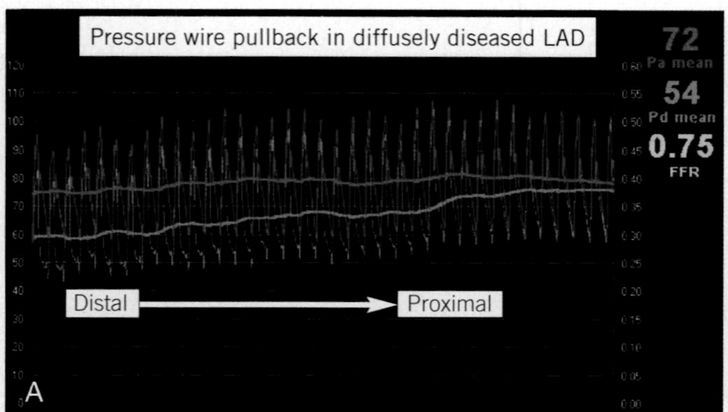

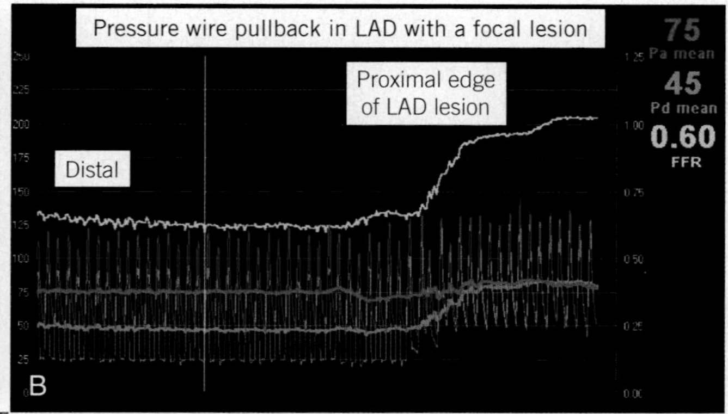

Figure 21.2 A, Tracing of the gradual change in pressure gradient as the pressure wire is slowly pulled proximal in a vessel with diffuse atherosclerosis. **B,** Tracing demonstrating the sudden change in pressure gradient as the pressure wire is slowly pulled proximal in a vessel with focal high-grade narrowing.

perfusion scanning, and stress echocardiography, and if any one of these was abnormal, the lesion was classified as ischemia producing. The sensitivity of FFR with use of a cutoff of less than 0.75 for identifying reversible ischemia was 88%, the specificity was 100%, and the accuracy was 93%. Since this publication, a number of other studies have been reported in patients with intermediate lesions and multivessel coronary disease, after recent acute myocardial infarction, or in the setting of non–ST-segment elevation acute coronary syndromes.[18,31,32] In all cases, an FFR cutoff between 0.75 and 0.80 correlated best with noninvasive evaluation for ischemia. On the basis of these data, it is unlikely that significant ischemia is present if the FFR is above 0.80, and it is extremely likely if the FFR is below 0.75. In patients who have an FFR in the so-called gray zone, it is recommended that the operator determine the need for revascularization on the basis of the clinical situation as well as the FFR result.

The safety of deferring intervention if the FFR is 0.75 or less has been investigated in a multicenter, randomized study.[33] At 2-year follow-up, patients with intermediate coronary lesions and chest pain in whom FFR was 0.75 or higher had lower event rates (although not statistically significant) when randomized to deferral of percutaneous coronary intervention (PCI) compared with the group randomized to performance of PCI. At 5-year follow-up, the cardiac death and myocardial infarction rate in the group randomized to deferral of PCI was 3.3% compared with 7.9% in those randomized to performance of PCI (Fig. 21.3).[34] A large, multicenter, international study comparing FFR guidance with angiographic guidance for PCI in patients with multivessel coronary disease is currently under way.[35]

The cost-effectiveness of measuring FFR in patients with intermediate lesions has also been studied.[32,36] Leesar and colleagues[32] randomized 70 patients who were admitted with non–ST-segment elevation acute coronary syndromes and were found to have intermediate coronary lesions to either measurement of FFR at the time of diagnostic coronary angiography or to nuclear perfusion imaging. If the FFR suggested ischemia, PCI was performed; otherwise, patients in this arm were managed medically. In the nuclear perfusion imaging arm, if the stress test was abnormal, patients returned to the catheterization laboratory for PCI; otherwise, they were managed medically. The duration and cost of hospitalization were significantly less in the FFR arm. At roughly 1 year of follow-up, there was no difference in clinical events between the two groups.

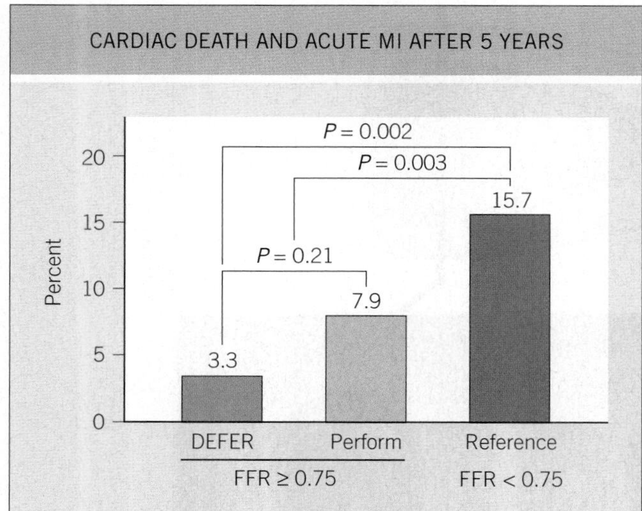

Figure 21.3 Graph from the DEFER study demonstrating the favorable outcome after 5 years in patients in whom the FFR was 0.75 or higher and PCI was deferred compared with those in whom PCI was performed anyway. MI, myocardial infarction. (From Pijls NH, van Schaardenburgh P, Manoharan G, et al. Percutaneous coronary intervention of functionally nonsignificant stenosis: 5-year follow-up of the DEFER Study. J Am Coll Cardiol 2007; 49:2105-2111.)

Fractional Flow Reserve in Left Main Disease

Because of the potential significance of a left main coronary narrowing and because the left main coronary supplies blood to a large amount of myocardium, some have thought that FFR would not be valid in this setting or that a different cutoff value should be used. However, a number of studies have now been completed in which FFR was measured; below 0.75, patients were referred for coronary artery bypass surgery, and at 0.75 and above, the left main lesion was managed medically.[37-39] During follow-up of more than 2 years, outcomes in those patients with an intermediate left main stenosis and a nonischemic FFR were excellent and as good as if not better than the outcomes in patients with ischemic FFRs who underwent surgery. These data suggest that FFR can be used safely to guide decision making in patients with intermediate left main lesions and that a cutoff value of 0.75 still applies.

Fractional Flow Reserve in Diffuse Disease

A significant number of patients with chest pain and abnormal stress tests undergo coronary angiography and are diagnosed with "normal" coronary arteries. A proportion of these patients are likely to have diffuse epicardial coronary artery disease that is contributing to the symptoms and stress test abnormality. Measurement of FFR can be a useful method for identifying diffuse epicardial disease responsible for ischemia. In one study, De Bruyne and colleagues[40] performed FFR in 106 adjacent angiographically normal-appearing vessels of 62 patients undergoing PCI in another stenotic vessel. The average FFR was 0.89 in these angiographically normal-appearing vessels, with 8% having an FFR below 0.75. In contrast, the FFR was 0.97 on average in 37 truly normal vessels in 10 patients without atherosclerosis.

In another study evaluating FFR in 53 cardiac transplant recipients with angiographically normal or mild disease, the average FFR was 0.88 ± 0.07, and 15% of cases had an FFR of 0.80 or less.[41] Intravascular ultrasonography confirmed mild to moderate diffuse atherosclerosis in these patients. Moreover, the FFR correlated significantly with the degree of plaque burden detected by intravascular ultrasonography ($r = 0.55$; $P < .0001$). These studies highlight the prevalence of angiographically silent diffuse coronary disease and the importance of adjunctive methods beyond angiography for diagnosis of ischemic coronary disease. The role of FFR after PCI is not discussed, nor is the use of FFR to guide multivessel intervention, although both are areas of great clinical interest.[35,42,43]

INTRAVASCULAR ULTRASONOGRAPHY

Historical Perspective

Intravascular ultrasonography (IVUS) is another adjunctive technique beyond angiography for assessing the epicardial coronary artery. It is complementary to FFR in that it provides anatomic information instead of physiologic information. In the late 1980s and early 1990s, Yock, Fitzgerald, and others introduced and validated IVUS as a method for obtaining detailed information of vessel size, plaque burden and morphologic character, and lesion length.[44] Since that time, advances in technology have resulted in improved image resolution and smaller catheters. IVUS has played a critical role in our understanding about coronary artery disease. Not only has it made us aware of angiographically silent coronary disease, but it has allowed us to better understand the pathophysiologic process of coronary disease.[45] In particular, IVUS has been instrumental in our understanding about vascular remodeling, the normal and abnormal response to atherosclerosis and percutaneous coronary intervention, and the pathophysiologic process of acute coronary syndromes (Fig. 21.4).[46]

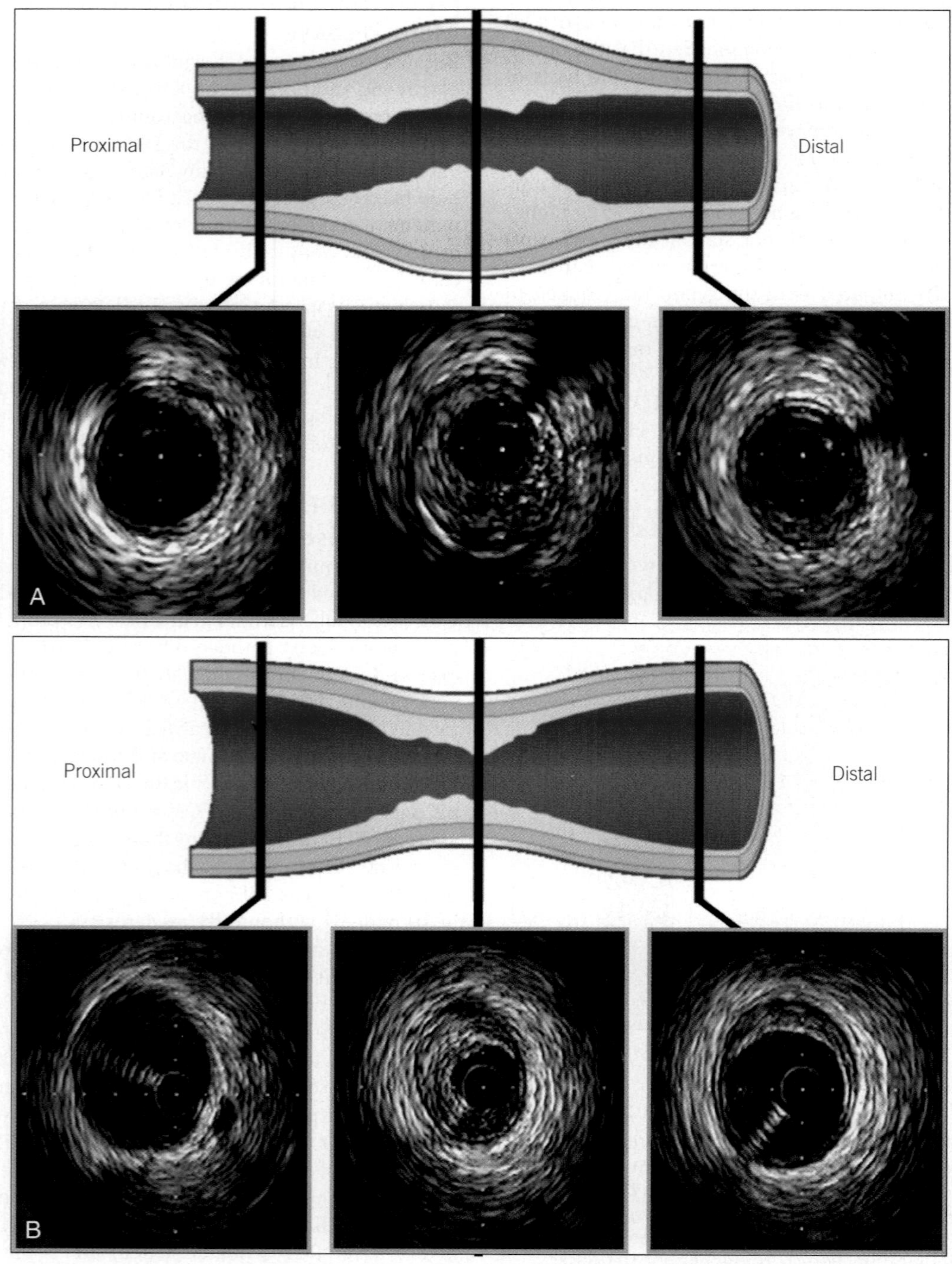

Figure 21.4 A, A coronary artery with positive remodeling and the corresponding cross-sectional IVUS images. **B,** A coronary artery with negative remodeling and the corresponding cross-sectional IVUS images.

Intravascular Ultrasonography Technique

IVUS systems consist of two major components, a catheter that is equipped with a miniaturized transducer and a console that processes electronic signals into cross-sectional images. Current IVUS catheters use the monorail design and are available in 2.5 to 3.5 French sizes, allowing the use of a 6 French guiding catheter. IVUS images are generated by either mechanical or solid-state technology.[47]

After administration of intravenous heparin and intracoronary nitroglycerin, the IVUS catheter is passed over a standard angioplasty guide wire. The transducer is positioned in the vessel beyond the area of interest and then slowly pulled back either manually or with a mechanical pullback device. The advantage of the latter technique is that it allows precise calculation of length and reconstruction of the two-dimensional images into a three-dimensional structure, providing volumetric data.

Major complications of IVUS are rare, occurring in less than 0.5%.[48] The most common complication is transient spasm, which occurs in approximately 3% of cases.

Intravascular Ultrasonography in Intermediate Lesion Assessment

Although the primary role of IVUS is to help guide PCI by providing detailed preintervention information about lesion characteristics and by assessing optimal stent deployment, it has also been applied as a method for assessing the need for PCI in patients with intermediate coronary lesions. For example, Nishioka and colleagues[49] compared IVUS parameters measured in 70 de novo coronary lesions (the majority classified as intermediate) with the results of nuclear perfusion imaging. The authors found that a minimum lumen cross-sectional area defined as 4 mm^2 or less had a sensitivity of 88% and a specificity of 90% for predicting a reversible perfusion defect on the nuclear perfusion imaging study. Others have found that the follow-up event rate is low in patients with intermediate lesions and an IVUS-derived minimum lumen area of 4 mm^2 or more (Table 21.3).[50]

More recently, IVUS parameters have been compared with FFR for determining the functional significance of moderate stenoses.[51] Takagi and colleagues[51] performed IVUS in 51 coronary lesions (approximately half were considered intermediate) and compared the IVUS-derived minimum lumen cross-sectional area and percentage area stenosis with the FFR result. They found a strong positive correlation between the minimum lumen area and FFR (r = 0.79; $P < .0001$) and negative correlation between percentage area stenosis and FFR (r = −0.77; $P < .0001$). Using a cutoff of less than 3.0 mm^2 to define an abnormal minimum lumen cross-sectional area and less than 0.75 to define an abnormal FFR, the investigators found that IVUS had a sensitivity of 83% and a specificity of 92% for detecting ischemia-producing lesions based on FFR. Defining an abnormal percentage area stenosis based on IVUS as more than 60% resulted in a sensitivity of 92% and a specificity of 89% for predicting an abnormal FFR. In every lesion in which either the minimum lumen area or the percentage area stenosis was abnormal, the FFR was below 0.75.

ROLE OF INTRAVASCULAR ULTRASONOGRAPHY AND FRACTIONAL FLOW RESERVE IN VARIOUS SETTINGS

	Intravascular Ultrasonography	Fractional Flow Reserve
Significant intermediate lesion	MLD <1.8 mm MLA <4.0 mm^2	<0.75-0.80
Significant left main lesion	MLD <2.8 mm MLA <5.9 mm^2	<0.75-0.80
Serial lesions	Assesses anatomic severity along the length of the artery	Relative contribution of each stenosis on pullback method
Saphenous vein graft	Identifies lesion severity, plaque characteristics, and need for distal protection	No data available
Ostial lesions	Helps locate ostial-aorta juncture and correct stent position	<0.75-0.80
Acute STEMI	Can identify ruptured plaque, lesion, and vessel characteristics	May not be accurate because of microvascular stunning
Bifurcation lesions	Assesses size of main and side branch, adequacy of result	<0.75-0.80

MLA, minimum lumen area; MLD, minimum lumen diameter; STEMI, ST-segment elevation myocardial infarction.
Modified from Tobis J, Azarbal B, Slavin L. Assessment of intermediate severity coronary lesions in the catheterization laboratory. J Am Coll Cardiol 2007;49:839-848.

Table 21.3 Role of intravascular ultrasonography and fractional flow reserve in various settings.

Intravascular Ultrasonography in Left Main Disease

IVUS has also been applied to further assess the significance of left main coronary disease when the angiogram is equivocal. Various cutoff values have been proposed for determining whether a left main lesion requires revascularization.[52-54] A study compared IVUS findings with FFR in 55 patients with angiographically ambiguous left main lesions.[38] Using FFR as the reference standard, the investigators found that an IVUS-derived minimum lumen area of 5.9 mm^2 had a sensitivity and specificity of 93% and 95%, respectively, and an IVUS-derived minimum lumen diameter of 2.8 mm had a sensitivity and specificity of 93% and 98%, respectively, for predicting a significant stenosis.

IVUS, however, is inherently limited in assessing the functional significance of coronary narrowings because it provides anatomic information only. Thus, a specific IVUS minimum lumen diameter or area might be quite significant in one patient but not in another, or in one location in a vessel but not in another.[52] For this reason, it is recommended that IVUS be used to assess lesion characteristics and to guide technical considerations with respect to PCI and that FFR be employed to determine the physiologic significance of coronary narrowings and the need for PCI.[55]

OTHER TECHNIQUES

Invasive Assessment of the Coronary Microvasculature

Traditional coronary angiography provides limited information about the status of the coronary microcirculation (vessels smaller than 500 μm). Yet, appreciation of the importance of the microvasculature in determining patient outcomes both in the setting of acute coronary syndromes and in stable patients continues to grow.[56] For this reason, a number of invasive techniques for evaluation of the microcirculation have been proposed.

The TIMI myocardial perfusion grade is an angiographic method for assessing microvascular function, particularly in the setting of ST-segment elevation myocardial infarction. Gibson and colleagues[57] demonstrated a significant 30-day mortality gradient in 762 patients with ST-segment elevation myocardial infarction treated with fibrinolysis, based on the microvascular function assessed at angiography 90 minutes after reperfusion therapy. Those with preserved microvascular function (TIMI myocardial perfusion grade 3) had the lowest mortality (2%), whereas those with the worst microvascular function (grade 0/1) had the highest mortality (6.0%). The TIMI myocardial perfusion grade has been well validated and is readily available in the catheterization laboratory, but it is qualitative and subjective, and some question its utility in individual patients.[58]

CFR is another method that has been applied in the catheterization laboratory to invasively assess microvascular function.[59] CFR, as mentioned previously, is limited by the fact that epicardial disease affects its value. In addition, it is not as reproducible as other measures and has a wide range of normal values. Other Doppler wire parameters, such as deceleration time and flow reversal, have been shown to be useful indicators of microvascular function and powerful predictors of outcome in patients with ST-segment elevation myocardial infarction.[60,61] The simultaneous measure of distal coronary pressure and Doppler wire–derived flow to calculate microvascular resistance may also be a useful Doppler wire–derived method for assessing the microvasculature.[62]

The index of microcirculatory resistance (IMR) is a relatively new method for interrogating the microcirculation by use of the coronary pressure wire.[63] With commercially available software, the shaft of the pressure wire can act as a proximal thermistor, and the pressure sensor can act as a distal thermistor; the transit time of an injectate can be determined by a validated thermodilution technique.[64,65] IMR is calculated by dividing the mean distal pressure by the inverse of the hyperemic mean transit time or, more simply, by multiplying the mean distal pressure by the hyperemic mean transit time. IMR is unique compared with CFR because it is independent of the epicardial vessel and specific for the microvasculature.[66,67] It is more reproducible compared with CFR because it is not affected by resting hemodynamics.[16] In a study in patients treated with primary PCI for ST-segment elevation myocardial infarction, IMR measured immediately after PCI predicted peak creatine kinase, whereas other measures including CFR and TIMI myocardial perfusion grade did not.[68] IMR was the only significant predictor of recovery of left ventricular function at 3 months after PCI.

Angioscopy

Angioscopy is a method that allows direct visualization of the epicardial vessel. It has been shown to be useful for determination of the morphologic character of plaque and

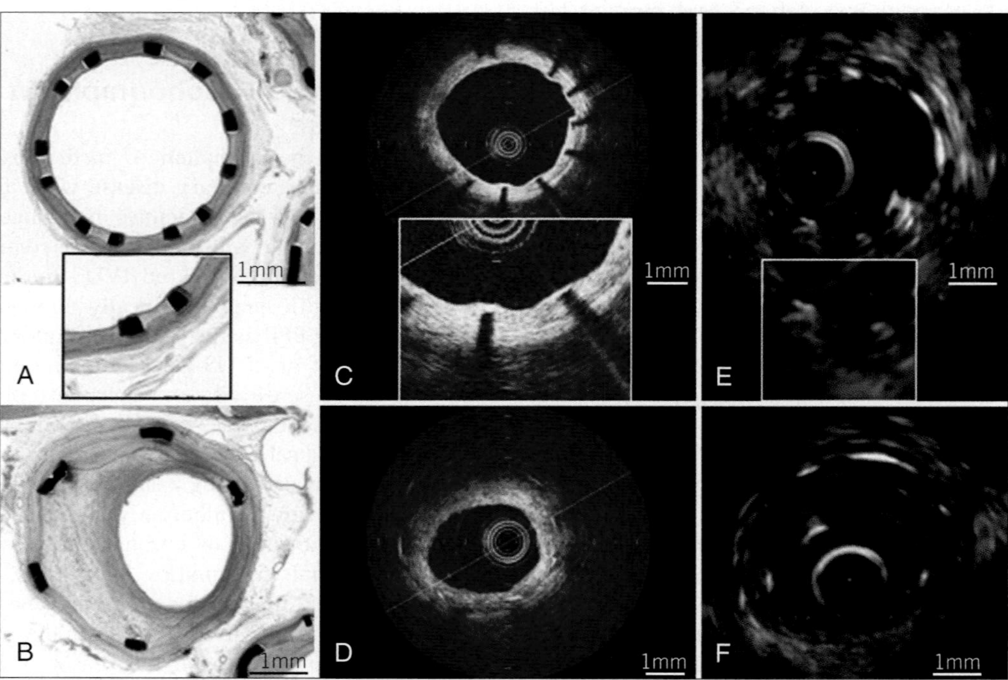

Figure 21.5 A and **B,** Histologic sections of a porcine coronary artery 1 month after stenting show very little neointima **(A)** and more substantial neointima **(B)**. **C** and **D,** The corresponding optical coherence tomography images at the same cross section. Note the resolution of optical coherence tomography (*inset* in **C**) in comparison to the corresponding IVUS images displayed in **E** and **F**.

may have a role in identifying vulnerable plaques.[69] It requires occlusion of the vessel and a saline infusion to replace blood, which have limited its clinical applicability and relegated it to being primarily a research tool.

Optical Coherence Tomography

Optical coherence tomography is a new wire-based method for interrogation of the epicardial vessel. It is analogous to IVUS, but instead of using reflected sound waves, it uses reflected light waves (Fig. 21.5). This provides superior resolution, on the order of 10 to 20 μm (compared with roughly 150 μm with IVUS). Preliminary work suggests that it might be useful for identifying vulnerable plaques.[70,71]

chapter

22 Chronic Stable Angina Pectoris

Udho Thadani

Definition

- Chronic stable angina pectoris is experienced as transsternal or retrosternal pressure or a choking sensation or pain that may radiate to the left arm, jaw, neck, or back. It is brought on in a predictable manner by exertion or by emotional upset. Sublingual nitroglycerin or cessation of exertion relieves the discomfort.

Key Features

- The underlying lesion responsible for angina pectoris and myocardial ischemia is often a severe narrowing of one or more coronary arteries.
- Underlying left ventricular systolic function at rest, extent of coronary artery disease, and comorbid conditions determine the long-term prognosis.
- Most patients can be managed with medical treatment.

Therapy

- Treatment is targeted at relief of symptoms with antianginal medications or revascularization procedures and at reduction of adverse clinical outcomes (myocardial infarction and coronary death) with lifestyle modifications and pharmacotherapy.

Chronic stable angina pectoris refers to the predictable occurrence of pressure or a choking sensation in the chest or adjacent areas caused by myocardial ischemia in association with physical or emotional stress and prompt relief of these symptoms with rest or sublingual nitroglycerin (glyceryl trinitrate).[1-3] An imbalance between myocardial oxygen (O_2) demand and supply is responsible for myocardial ischemia and anginal pain.[4] In most patients who have chronic stable angina, the underlying lesion responsible for reduced myocardial blood flow (O_2 supply) during periods of increased demand is severe atherosclerotic narrowing of one or more coronary arteries,[2,3,5] which paradoxically constrict during exercise owing to endothelial dysfunction.[6] Noninvasive stress testing[7-10] and coronary angiography permit identification of severe coronary stenotic lesions responsible for myocardial ischemia and anginal pain. In addition to severe obstructive atherosclerotic lesions, coronary arteries of patients with stable angina contain many more nonobstructive lesions. These lesions grow at a variable rate and rupture unpredictably and thus may remain clinically silent or be manifested as an acute coronary syndrome.[3,5,11,12] Therefore, treatment strategy should include

- relief of symptoms and increase in angina-free walking time by increasing myocardial O_2 supply or decreasing myocardial O_2 consumption, or both; and
- reduction in cardiac mortality and incidents of myocardial infarction by lifestyle modification, aspirin, and stabilization of atherosclerotic plaques with pharmacotherapy.[3,5,11]

ANATOMY AND PATHOLOGY

In patients who have chronic stable angina, severe atherosclerotic narrowing of one or more epicardial arteries is often found at autopsy. These severe lesions are composed of complex atherosclerotic material, which is usually not prone to plaque rupture.[5,11] In the remaining coronary tree, however, atheromas are often present at various stages, and these nonobstructive lesions are rich in lipid content, are prone to fissuring or disruption,[3,5,11,12] and account for the unpredictable occurrence of acute coronary syndromes in these patients.[3,5,11]

PATHOPHYSIOLOGY

In most patients who have stable angina, myocardial ischemia results from an increased myocardial O_2 demand that cannot be met by an increase in coronary blood flow because of a flow-limiting atherosclerotic obstructive lesion (>70% of the vessel diameter) of one or more coronary arteries.[2,5,11] The exact mechanism that triggers anginal pain is unknown.[4,13] The coronary arteries of a patient who has stable angina have dysfunctional endothelium,[14] which accounts for paradoxical constriction of epicardial stenotic atherosclerotic arteries during exercise[6] and emotional stress and thus further reduction in blood flow to the ischemic myocardium. The endothelial dysfunction and paradoxical vasoconstriction of the atherosclerotic plaque is probably responsible for the variable anginal threshold and resting chest pain that are often mentioned by patients who have stable angina.[15] During ambulatory monitoring, it has been shown that myocardial ischemia without angina (silent ischemia) is a far more frequent manifestation of coronary artery disease in these patients.[16] The incidence of ambulatory ischemia is the greatest in the early morning between 6:00 and 10:00 AM, and it is multifactorial in origin.

Myocardial ischemia may occasionally occur in the presence of normal coronary arteries because of

- a marked increase in myocardial O_2 demand;
- increased vasoconstriction of epicardial coronary arteries;
- thrombosis;
- increased blood viscosity;
- a hypercoagulable state;
- small-vessel disease; or
- coronary artery embolization.

Most patients who have stable angina have reproducible symptoms, which, by arbitrary definition, are usually stable during a period of 3 to 6 months.[2,11] However, patients may experience worsening of their angina with a diminished exercise threshold either through progression of the disease or because of a pathophysiologic state such as thyrotoxicosis, supraventricular tachycardia, aortic stenosis, uncontrolled hypertension, or severe anemia.

The factors that determine myocardial O_2 consumption and that influence coronary blood flow must be appreciated to understand the rationale of treatment in stable angina.

The heart is an aerobic organ that needs O_2 to oxidize substances that produce energy for contraction and other functions. Heart work consists of pressure work and kinetic work. In normal circumstances, pressure work, which approximates peak systolic pressure and cardiac output, is the major component of the work performed by the heart; kinetic work, which depends on the cardiac output, blood viscosity, cross-sectional area of the major resistance site (the aortic valve), and ejection time, contributes little to total work.[4,13] The most important determinants of myocardial O_2 demand are heart rate, wall stress (tension), and contractility. Each cardiac cycle requires a certain amount of O_2. More O_2 is required as the heart beats faster. A rapid heart rate also increases the force of myocardial contraction (treppe phenomenon or Bowditch staircase phenomenon), which increases myocardial O_2 consumption.[4,13] Thus, tachycardia of any cause increases myocardial O_2 needs. Wall stress is a more appropriate term than tension, although the terms are used interchangeably. According to the law of Laplace, wall stress can be expressed as

$$\text{Wall stress} = \frac{P \infty R}{h}$$

where P is intraventricular pressure, R is the radius, and h is the wall thickness. In a spherical or ellipsoidal model (e.g., the human heart), wall stress is more accurately expressed as

$$\text{Wall stress} = \frac{P \infty R_i}{2h(1 + h/2R_i)}$$

where R_i is the internal radius.

Sarnoff and colleagues included time in the equation and used the "tension time index" (i.e., the area under the ventricular pressure curve) as the major determinant of O_2 consumption of the contracting heart.[4,13] Without knowledge of the radius or chamber size and wall thickness, however, the pressure time index is more accurate than the tension time index.[4,13] In clinical situations, it is often difficult to measure the radius and wall thickness of the ventricle, and therefore pressure time index is often used as the determinant factor for myocardial O_2 uptake. Furthermore, wall stress does not take into account the effects of myocardial contractility, which under increased inotropic stimulation such as physical or mental stress may be the major determinant of myocardial O_2 demand.[4,13]

Myocardial O_2 requirements vary widely, depending on the physical state of the individual. The variation in mechanical work of the heart is most obvious during physical activity, which enhances sympathetic tone and leads to an increase in heart rate, contractility, and blood pressure. These changes augment myocardial performance at the cost of increased myocardial O_2 uptake, which in normal subjects is balanced by a parallel increase in coronary blood flow and hence in myocardial O_2 supply (Fig. 22.1).[13] However, in pathophysiologic states such as coronary artery stenosis, the increased demand may outstrip the supply, with detrimental consequences (see Fig. 22.1).[13]

The most important determinant of coronary blood flow is myocardial O_2 demand. This autoregulation of flow helps maintain variable blood supply and therefore O_2 supply to the myocardium.[4,13] Under basal conditions, myocardial O_2 extraction is near maximum, as indicated by very low coronary sinus blood O_2 saturation. Therefore, an increase in myocardial O_2 supply can be achieved primarily by an increase in coronary blood flow. It has been proposed that the myocardium communicates its O_2 requirements to the coronary arteries by the rate of production of adenosine. The breakdown of high-energy phosphate compounds during increased myocardial O_2 demand produces adenosine, which in turn produces coronary vasodilatation and therefore an increase in coronary blood flow.[4,13] The other proposed mediators for coronary dilatation are prostaglandins, protons, and other vasoactive compounds such as potassium and lactate.[4,13] However, none is as important as adenosine.[4,13]

In the normal heart, there are more than 2000 capillaries/mm^3; in normal circumstances, only 60% to 80% of these are functioning. When myocardial O_2 tension falls, more capillaries are recruited. This capillary recruitment is important in meeting the increased myocardial O_2 requirements.

In the left ventricle, the throttling effect of the myocardium on the penetrating coronary vessels during systole severely impairs coronary blood flow.[4,13] The epicardial blood flow is less impaired than the subendocardial blood flow because the intramyocardial pressure is maximal in the subendocardial region. Therefore, blood flow occurs in the left coronary artery predominantly in diastole and to a small extent in systole. In contrast, in the right coronary artery, because the right ventricular intramyocardial pressure is low, blood flow occurs both in systole and in diastole except in pathophysiologic conditions associated with pulmonary hypertension, when diastolic blood flow in the right coronary artery becomes predominant. Subendocardial blood flow in the left ventricle is also influenced by the end-diastolic pressure in the left ventricle, which, if high, can impede blood flow to the subendocardial regions. The net coronary blood flow during diastole is determined by the perfusion pressure, which in the case of the left coronary artery is the difference between the diastolic coronary artery pressure (or aortic diastolic pressure in the absence of coronary stenosis) and the coronary sinus pressure, which in turn is influenced by the right atrial pressure. In the case of the right coronary artery, the perfusion pressure is the difference between the right coronary artery systolic or diastolic pressure and the right ventricular systolic or diastolic pressure. In the left ventricle, coronary blood flow is determined by the diastolic pressure time index, which is the area under the aortic pressure curve during diastole.[4,13]

Because the coronary blood flow occurs predominantly in diastole, the duration of diastole assumes greater importance; the longer the diastole, the greater the flow. Thus, tachycardia not only increases myocardial O_2 requirement but can also decrease coronary blood flow during each cardiac cycle.

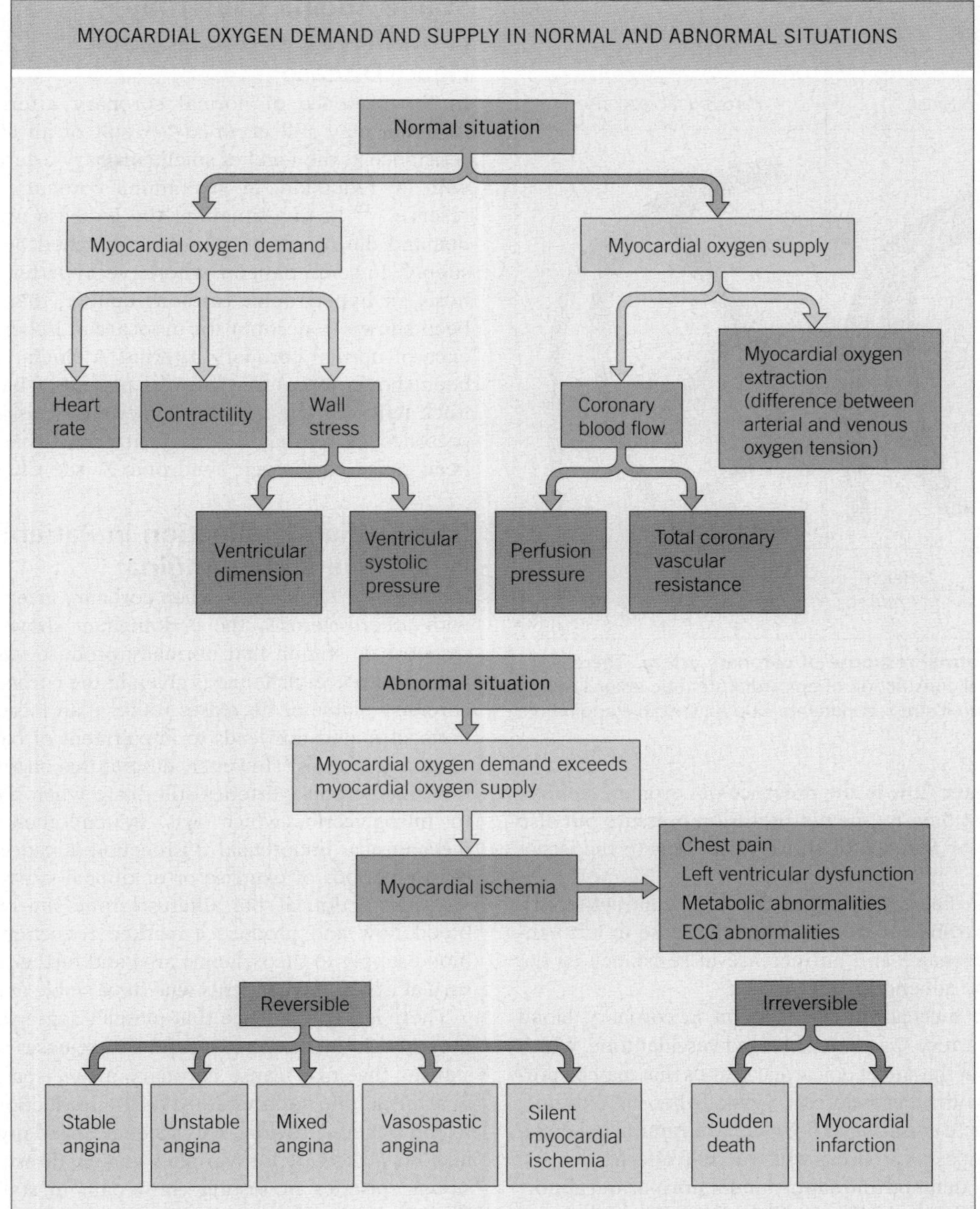

Figure 22.1 Myocardial oxygen demand and supply in normal and abnormal situations. Relative increase in myocardial oxygen demand or actual reduction in coronary blood flow produces myocardial ischemia. (From Thadani U, Olson EG, Hamilton SF. Pathophysiology of myocardial ischemia. In Abrams J, Pepine CE, Thadani U, eds. Medical Therapy of Ischemic Heart Disease. Nitrates, Beta-Blockers and Calcium Antagonists. Boston, Little, Brown, 1992:1-36.)

In patients who have stable angina, severe atherosclerotic narrowing of the coronary arteries increases the resistance to blood flow across the stenosis. The resistance increases by a power of 4 as the radius decreases (Poiseuille's law), so that reducing the internal diameter by 70%, 80%, or 90% dramatically elevates the resistance. Basal coronary blood flow falls when the luminal area is reduced by 90% or more. With the reduction in coronary blood flow, there is a compensatory vasodilatation in the ischemic bed. However, the maximum vasodilatory reserve is impaired in the presence of coronary stenosis, producing a 50% or greater reduction in the lumen area.[4,13]

The length of the stenosis also plays an important role in determining coronary blood flow. A stenosis of more than 5 mm and multiple stenoses in the same artery have more profoundly deleterious effects on coronary blood flow than does a single stenosis of less than 5 mm. When atherosclerosis is eccentric, a normal portion of coronary artery can undergo dynamic changes in tone, which, if augmented, can produce critical stenosis (Fig. 22.2).[13]

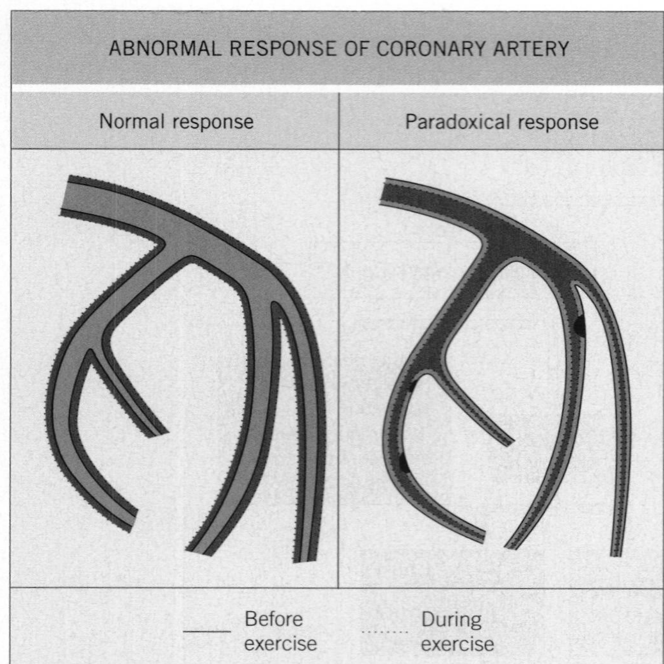

Figure 22.2 Abnormal response of coronary artery. There is often a paradoxical constriction of epicardial stenotic lesions during exercise or emotional stress in patients who have stable angina pectoris.

The net coronary flow in the presence of coronary stenosis is determined not only by the net perfusion pressure but also by the presence or absence of collateral vessels to the ischemic region.[4,13]

Severe myocardial ischemia also leads to contractile failure of the myocardium, with a resulting increase in left ventricle diastolic pressure and an increase in resistance to the blood flow in the subendocardial tissue.[4,13]

An alternative mechanism of reduction in coronary blood flow is coronary artery spasm or increased vascular tone, which occurs primarily at the site of epicardial vessels that may be normal or involved with atherosclerosis. Spasm, when it is extreme, may cause complete cessation of flow with transmural ischemia, but gradation of spasm can occur with variable effects.

Myocardial O_2 demand and supply under normal and abnormal situations is shown in Figure 22.1. A relative imbalance between myocardial O_2 demand and supply caused by either an increase in myocardial O_2 demand or a reduction in coronary blood flow produces myocardial ischemia (see Fig. 22.1).

The results of myocardial ischemia are determined by the territories supplied by the stenotic coronary arteries and the extent of collateral vessels. Because collateral vessels are not always visible and because there is an overlap of flow by the two adjacent branches of coronary arteries, the ischemic area produced by coronary obstruction is always less than the area supplied by the obstructed vessel.[4,13] Because subendocardial regions are more vulnerable, ischemia initially starts in the subendocardial region and eventually advances to the subepicardial region. With branch artery narrowing, subendocardial blood flow falls at about a 25% occlusion, with metabolic changes developing at about a 60% occlusion and contractility and electrocardiographic changes at a 75% occlusion. With major artery occlusion, such changes occur at about 20% to 45% flow reduction.[4,13]

Stable Angina Caused by Nonatherosclerotic Ischemic Heart Disease

In the presence of normal coronary arteries, myocardial ischemia may still occur as a result of an abnormally high resistance at the level of small coronary arteries or arterioles with a reduction in maximum coronary vascular flow reserve.[4,13] In this situation, the increase in myocardial O_2 demand during stress cannot be matched by an increase in supply. In some patients who have hypertension, aortic stenosis, or hypertrophic cardiomyopathy, this mechanism has been shown to account for myocardial ischemia in the presence of normal coronary arteries. A similar mechanism has been shown to operate in some patients who do not have a thick left ventricle but who experience classic angina in the presence of normal coronary arteries. This syndrome has been called cardiologic syndrome X (see Chapter 24).

Endothelial Dysfunction in Patients Who Have Stable Angina

Studies have shown that when coronary arteries are involved with atherosclerosis, the endothelium shows a paradoxical response to stimuli that normally produce vasodilatation.[6,14] Thus, when acetylcholine is given in the coronary arteries, the coronary diameter decreases rather than increases at the stenotic sites, and this leads to impairment of blood flow in the coronary arteries. However, despite this endothelial dysfunction, the coronary arteries still dilate when they are exposed to nitroglycerin, which acts by endothelium-independent mechanisms. Endothelial dysfunction is especially important during periods of exercise or emotional stress as paradoxical vasoconstriction at the atherosclerotic site can compromise blood flow and produce a marked reduction in myocardial blood supply to the ischemic area and further aggravate myocardial ischemia in patients who have stable angina.

There is also evidence that platelet aggregation at the atherosclerotic or damaged vessel site releases vasoactive substances that may cause coronary artery spasm or a change in arterial tone and therefore further reduction of blood flow to the ischemic region. This mechanism of myocardial ischemia may account for variable angina thresholds and occasional episodes of resting chest pain in stable angina.[13,15] The mechanism by which chest pain (angina) is produced is not known, but it may be related to stretching of the ischemic myocardium or stimulation of the nerve endings caused by accumulation of metabolites or changes in the pH.[4,13]

During an episode of angina, there is often evidence of subendocardial ischemia manifested by ST-segment depression; when the territory of ischemia is large, changes in systolic and diastolic left ventricular function may be seen. Depending on the extent of ischemia, left ventricular global ejection fraction may or may not decrease, but regional left ventricular function often shows some abnormality.

CLINICAL PRESENTATIONS

Patients with stable exertional angina often give a history of a strangling feeling or a pressure-like sensation localized in the retrosternal and substernal region (Table 22.1).[1-3,5,11] If the pressure sensation is severe, it is experienced by the

CLINICAL PRESENTATIONS OF CHRONIC STABLE ANGINA		
Symptoms	**Precipitating Factors**	**Relief of Symptoms**
Transsternal or retrosternal tightness, heaviness, pressure, or pain	Effort (walking or other exercise) Emotional stress (occasionally at rest)	Rapid relief with discontinuation of effort or after sublingual nitroglycerin
Radiation to or only localization to left arm, neck, jaw, back, or epigastric region		
Angina equivalents: dyspnea, fatigue, belching, eructations	Effort (walking or other exercise)	

Table 22.1 Clinical presentations of chronic stable angina.

patient as chest pain, which is usually intermittent and often precipitated by activity. The discomfort may radiate to the neck or the left arm and sometimes to the right arm or the back. Some patients experience pain or discomfort only in these areas and not in the chest. The pain is usually precipitated by activity or emotional upset and is relieved on discontinuation of activity or ingestion of sublingual nitroglycerin. By definition, the frequency of anginal episodes will have been stable without deterioration for at least a period of 3 to 6 months. The symptoms are often reproducible by identical physical activity. Some patients who have classic exertional angina have a variable angina threshold,[2,3,15] and nearly 30% to 40% of patients give a history of intermittent chest pain at rest that is rapidly relieved with sublingual nitroglycerin.[3,11,15] Some patients who have stable angina may give a history of breathlessness, fatigue, nausea, or recurrent belching on exertion rather than chest discomfort, and this is especially encountered in the elderly and in patients who have diabetes mellitus.[3,5,11] This is known as angina equivalent. The angina equivalent symptoms are rapidly relieved by discontinuation of the physical activity or by sublingual nitroglycerin.

Patients who have stable angina may experience deterioration in their walking distance with early onset of chest pain as a result of progression of coronary artery disease or because of environmental or emotional factors that produce changes in the coronary vasomotor tone and reduce the coronary blood flow (see Fig. 22.2).[13] Many patients who have stable angina give a history of worsening symptoms during activity, especially after a heavy meal. This postprandial decrease in angina threshold must be appreciated because many of these patients are often labeled as having indigestion rather than angina.

Ventricular arrhythmias are uncommon during episodes of angina in patients who have stable angina. Rarely, patients may present with exercise-induced dizziness or syncope during exercise as a result of severe underlying coronary artery disease.

DIAGNOSTIC TECHNIQUES

Diagnostic techniques are outlined in Table 22.2.

History

Despite the vast array of sophisticated diagnostic techniques that are available, a detailed history is most important and usually provides important diagnostic clues. The history must include detailed evaluation of symptoms and precipitating factors. Location, quality, severity, and chronology must be elicited. In addition to chest discomfort during exertional or emotional stress, dyspnea, nausea, fatigue, faintness, and recurrent belching associated with exertion (angina equivalents) should also be noted.[3,11,17]

DIAGNOSTIC TECHNIQUES IN CHRONIC STABLE ANGINA	
Method	**Comments**
History	Most important Risk factor assessment
Examination	For functional assessment Comorbid conditions
12-lead ECG	Q waves for previous myocardial infarction but limited value otherwise
Exercise ECG	Very useful in men High false-positive rates in women Provides prognostic information
Echocardiogram at rest	Global and regional LVEF provides prognostic information
Exercise echocardiogram	Localizes site and severity of ischemia
Radionuclide ventriculography	Global and regional LVEF provides prognostic information at rest
Stress radionuclide perfusion imaging	Localizes site and severity of ischemia Better correlation with coronary angiography than standard ECG Increased lung uptake and left ventricular cavity dilatation have prognostic implications
Coronary angiography	Accurately defines anatomic disease but not its physiologic significance
Left ventriculography	LVEF provides prognostic information
Right atrial pacing	Limited usefulness
ECG, electrocardiography; LVEF, left ventricular ejection fraction.	

Table 22.2 Diagnostic techniques in chronic stable angina.

The past medical history with regard to myocardial infarction or valvular heart disease also helps in reaching a diagnosis. A detailed family history and risk assessment (smoking, family history of premature coronary artery disease, lipid abnormalities, diabetes, and hypertension) may point to the correct diagnosis. However, the location of the chest pain, the precipitating factors, and the duration of the pain do not correlate well with prognosis or angiographic extent of coronary artery disease.

Physical Examination

The physical examination can provide some clues to the presence of underlying coronary disease; but in patients who have stable angina, it often does not provide any diagnostic information. The findings of hypertension, peripheral vascular disease, carotid artery disease, or signs of hypercholesterolemia (such as xanthoma or xanthelasma) often raise the possibility of underlying coronary artery disease as the etiology for stable angina. One must also examine for the presence or absence of valvular heart disease; this is especially important in aortic stenosis, which could account for chest pain on exertion. During an episode of angina, a finding of mitral regurgitation indicates papillary muscle ischemia, whereas presence of basal rales suggests left ventricular dysfunction.

MANAGEMENT

The goals of treatment in stable angina are shown in Table 22.3:

- to decrease the frequency and severity of angina symptoms and to increase the duration of angina-free exercise (functional capacity); and
- to prolong life and to reduce incidence of acute coronary syndrome (unstable angina, myocardial infarction, and coronary death).

Recently, the emphasis of treatment has been on reducing the frequency and severity of ambulatory myocardial ischemic episodes,[16] but the usefulness of this approach needs to be confirmed in larger clinical trials.[11]

The relief of symptoms and the increase in angina-free walking time are achieved by increasing myocardial O_2 supply or decreasing myocardial O_2 consumption, or both. The reduction of cardiac mortality and incidents of myocardial infarction is achieved by pharmacotherapy and stabilization of atherosclerotic plaques (see Table 22.3). Comorbid, treatable conditions that could aggravate angina (e.g., anemia, thyrotoxicosis) must be sought and treated in all patients who have chronic stable angina.[3,5,11,17] Lifestyle changes, especially smoking cessation and risk factor modification, must be stressed to all patients.[3,11,17]

MANAGEMENT OF CHRONIC STABLE ANGINA	
Goal	**How to Achieve the Goal**
Abolish or reduce anginal episodes	Trial of antianginal drugs Coronary revascularization
Increase angina-free walking or exercise	Antianginal drugs Coronary revascularization
Prolong life and reduce acute coronary events (unstable angina, myocardial infarction, coronary death)	Lifestyle modification Modify or correct risk factors Daily aspirin Pharmacotherapy of dyslipidemia Control of hypertension Beta blockers, ACE inhibitors, and CABG surgery in special situations

ACE, angiotensin-converting enzyme; CABG, coronary artery bypass graft.

Table 22.3 Management of chronic stable angina.

The three options for treatment of stable angina are

- drug therapy;
- coronary balloon angioplasty; and
- coronary artery bypass graft (CABG) surgery.

Therapy should be individualized, and consideration should be given to the risks as well as to the benefits of each therapeutic option with regard to symptom relief and longevity.

Coronary angiography is not always indicated in stable angina.[3,11,17] It is indicated in patients who remain symptomatic despite optimal medical therapy. It should also be considered in patients who have an early positive exercise test result and in those with poor left ventricular function to exclude left main coronary artery or triple-vessel disease and to assess the suitability of coronary artery anatomy for revascularization procedures.

Prolonging Life and Preventing Myocardial Infarction and Other Acute Ischemic Syndromes

Smoking Cessation

Smoking cessation is essential in all patients who have stable angina because it reduces the risk of coronary artery disease mortality by 50% in 1 year; after 5 to 10 years, the coronary mortality risk reaches that of nonsmokers.[18] The use of transdermal nicotine patches or bupropion is safe and superior to placebo in helping people to stop smoking.[11] Stopping smoking not only prolongs survival and reduces morbidity but also has a positive effect on exercise performance in patients who have stable angina.

Aspirin

Daily use of aspirin has been shown to reduce the incidence of sudden death and acute myocardial infarction in stable angina. In the Swedish Angina Pectoris Aspirin Trial (SAPAT), daily use of aspirin was associated with a 34% reduction in the incidence of sudden death and acute myocardial infarction, with an absolute reduction of 12 sudden deaths for every 1000 patients treated during the 15-month period.[19] The relative reduction in secondary endpoints (vascular events, vascular death, all-cause mortality, and stroke) ranged from 22% to 32%. There was no difference in major bleeding episodes, including hemorrhagic strokes, between the aspirin and placebo groups. On the basis of these data and available data of the usefulness of aspirin in acute myocardial infarction and unstable angina, it is mandatory that aspirin be used in all patients with stable angina unless they are unable to tolerate the medication because of either an allergic reaction or intolerable gastrointestinal side effects.[5,20]

Ticlopidine and Clopidogrel

There are no data to suggest that these agents improve survival in stable angina.[3,5,11] Given the risk of rare leukopenia and the thrombotic thrombocytopenic purpura that is observed with ticlopidine, this agent cannot be recommended for routine use in stable angina. Patients who are intolerant to aspirin therapy may be treated with clopidogrel. Although there are no data specifically relating to patients who have stable angina, clopidogrel has been shown to be safe and possibly effective in survivors of myocardial infarction.[5] Clopidogrel was shown to be as effective as aspirin.

Long-term treatment with a combination of aspirin plus clopidogrel is not superior to aspirin treatment alone and increases the risk of bleeding,[21] and it is not recommended for treatment of patients with stable angina. However, combination of aspirin plus clopidogrel for up to 3 to 12 months after coronary artery stenting reduces adverse clinical outcomes and is indicated in this group of patients.

Lipid-Modifying Therapy

In coronary artery disease, effective lipid lowering results in plaque stabilization, regression of coronary lesions, and, in some studies, reduced total and cardiovascular mortality, reduced need for revascularization, and reduced episodes of ambulatory ischemia.[3,11]

Patients who have elevated low-density lipoprotein (LDL) cholesterol should be considered for lipid-lowering therapy. Dietary therapy for 2 to 3 months to lower fasting total cholesterol and LDL-cholesterol levels should be tried initially. However, most patients need drug therapy with 3-hydroxy-3-methylglutaryl coenzyme A (HMG-CoA) reductase inhibitors, which have been shown in studies to be safe and effective.[3,5,11]

Although trials with the lipid-lowering agents have not specifically evaluated patients who have stable angina,[3] the results of these trials are nevertheless applicable to stable angina because most of these patients have underlying coronary artery disease. A reduction in mortality, stroke risk, and cardiovascular morbidity with statins in post–myocardial infarction patients and in asymptomatic patients who have elevated LDL-cholesterol levels has been well documented in numerous large trials.[3,5,11] In the Scandinavian Simvastatin Survival Study (4S) trial,[22] 4444 patients with either a previous myocardial infarction or stable angina and an elevated total and LDL-cholesterol level were randomized to either simvastatin or placebo. After a mean follow-up of 5.4 years, simvastatin therapy was shown to provide

- a 38% reduction in LDL-cholesterol levels;
- a 30% reduction in all-cause mortality;
- a 42% reduction in coronary events; and
- a 37% reduction in the need for revascularization procedures.

The mortality reduction in the simvastatin group became apparent at 1 year of follow-up. The 6-year follow-up probability of survival for the placebo group was 87.6%; for the simvastatin group, it was 91.3%. In this study, reduction of mortality in the simvastatin group was observed in both men and women and in those younger and older than 65 years. More aggressive reduction of LDL-cholesterol with high-dose atorvastatin (80 mg) compared with less aggressive reduction of LDL-cholesterol with atorvastatin (10 mg daily) reduces cardiovascular morbidity and mortality but not total mortality.[23-25]

In a study of patients with mildly symptomatic coronary artery disease and exertional angina, an aggressive lipid-lowering regimen using atorvastatin was shown to reduce adverse outcomes compared with balloon angioplasty.[26] Taking these trials together with available trials of other lipid-lowering agents (lovastatin and pravastatin), one can recommend lipid-lowering therapy with HMG-CoA reductase inhibitors in patients who have stable angina and LDL-cholesterol levels above 120 to 135 mg/dL.[3,5,11] The aim of therapy in stable angina should be to reduce the fasting LDL-cholesterol level to below 100 mg/dL, especially in patients who have had CABG surgery.

In men who have normal LDL-cholesterol levels but low high-density lipoprotein cholesterol level, treatment with gemfibrozil has been shown to reduce cardiovascular morbidity and mortality.[27] Nicotinic acid is an alternative in this group of patients.[3,5,24,25]

Combinations of lipid-modifying agents are widely used. However, at present, there are inadequate data to recommend combination of statins plus fibrates or nicotinic acid to treat dyslipidemia in patients with stable angina.[3,24,25]

There are no published trials of omega-3 fatty acid in stable angina,[3] but secondary prevention trials in post–myocardial infarction patients have shown a significant reduction in cardiovascular morbidity and mortality with omega-3 fatty acids. In clinical practice, omega-3 fatty acid is often combined with a statin when triglyceride levels are high. What is not known is whether omega-3 fatty acids exert further additional benefits when they are added to aspirin and statins or are equally effective as or more effective than these agents.[3]

Treatment of Hypertension

Hypertensive patients who have stable angina need to have their blood pressure controlled to below 140 mm Hg systolic and 90 mm Hg diastolic. Control of high blood pressure reduces the stroke incidence, all-cause mortality, and coronary artery disease mortality.[28] In the published trials, a regimen of diuretics and beta blockers plus add-on therapy to lower blood pressure has been used.[3,5,17] In a recent trial, long-acting dihydropyridine calcium channel blockers were also shown to reduce coronary morbidity and stroke rate by 42%. The totality of available data suggests that blood pressure must be adequately controlled in patients who have stable angina and hypertension to influence the outcome favorably.[5,11,28]

Hormone Replacement Therapy

No outcome trials have been performed of estrogen replacement therapy in stable angina.[3,5,24,25] Observational studies suggested that estrogen replacement therapy given to women with postmenopausal symptoms had a favorable influence on the risk of mortality. However, a large randomized trial in postmenopausal women was terminated because hormone replacement therapy (0.625 mg conjugated equine estrogen plus 2.5 mg medroxyprogesterone) increased the incidence of coronary heart disease, stroke, pulmonary embolism, and risk of breast cancer compared with treatment with placebo.[29] Thus, hormone replacement therapy to prevent cardiovascular mortality cannot be routinely recommended in postmenopausal women.

Testosterone Replacement Therapy

No outcome trials are available to recommend testosterone replacement therapy in patients with stable angina. Initial results suggest that testosterone may exert anti-ischemic effects in men with angina who have low testosterone levels.

Revascularization Procedures

In patients who have reduced left ventricular function and three-vessel disease and in those who have left main coronary artery disease, there is evidence that CABG improves prognosis for the first 10 years.[30-33] This mode of therapy is therefore recommended in this group of patients. However, CABG surgery by itself does not reduce the incidence of myocardial infarction in patients who have stable angina.[3,24,25,30-32] There are no data to suggest that CABG surgery improves survival in patients who have good left ventricular function, nor does it reduce the overall risk of myocardial infarction in patients who have good or poor left ventricular function.[3,25,30-32] Therefore, it should be offered as initial therapy only to patients who remain symptomatic despite medical therapy or to those who are unwilling to take medications.[3,5,11,17,24,25]

There are no data to suggest that percutaneous intervention with either balloon angioplasty or stent placement improves survival or reduces the incidence of myocardial infarction in stable angina.[3,5,11,24,25,32,34-37] On the contrary, the use of balloon angioplasty and stent placement is associated with immediate leak of cardiac markers (non–Q wave myocardial infarction).[3] Published results show that angioplasty is not superior to medical therapy,[3,24,25,34-37] and a study showed that aggressive medical treatment that included lipid-lowering therapy in mildly symptomatic patients with stable angina and one- or two-vessel coronary artery disease was superior to balloon angioplasty with or without stent placement.[26]

Angiotensin-Converting Enzyme Inhibitors

Angiotensin-converting enzyme (ACE) inhibitors improve outcome in patients with ischemic heart disease who have reduced left ventricular function.[38,39] They are therefore indicated in patients with reduced left ventricular function who have stable angina.

Outcome data in patients with chronic coronary artery disease and preserved left ventricular function are controversial. Beneficial effects were reported in the EUROPA trial[40] but not in the PEACE trial.[41] In the PEACE trial, all patients had documented coronary artery disease and left ventricular ejection fraction above 40%. Thus, at present, routine use of ACE inhibitors in patients with stable angina and left ventricular ejection fraction above 40% cannot be recommended.

Antianginal Drugs

Outcome studies of antianginal drugs (beta blockers, nitrates, and calcium channel blockers) have not been performed in patients who have stable angina.[3,5,11,25] Recent trials have shown that beta blockers reduce mortality in patients with ischemic cardiomyopathy who are receiving concomitant therapy with digoxin, diuretics, and ACE inhibitors.[3,42] Therefore, beta-blocker therapy is indicated in patients with stable angina who have reduced left ventricular function.[3,5] Furthermore, beta blockers reduced mortality and morbidity in post–myocardial infarction patients and in mildly symptomatic patients with stable angina who had evidence of exercise and ambulatory ischemia.[43] Therefore, beta-blocker therapy should be used in stable angina unless it is contraindicated.

Antioxidants

The role of antioxidants in improving survival or reducing adverse outcome in patients with stable angina is unclear,[3,11] and routine use is not recommended.[3,5] In the Cambridge Heart Antioxidants Study (CHAOS), vitamin E (800 mg administered once daily) was shown to reduce adverse outcomes.[44] However, in another study, α_1-tocopherol and beta-carotene had no effect on survival in patients with stable angina.[45]

Moderate Alcohol Intake

Studies have shown that a low to moderate consumption of alcohol (up to one or two glasses of wine per day) reduces mortality in patients who have coronary artery disease. Therefore, such patients may use alcohol in moderation, although there are no data that relate specifically to stable angina.[3]

Exercise Training

Exercise training and continued medical treatment have been shown to be superior to percutaneous coronary angioplasty in patients with stable angina.[46] However, the results of this study need to be confirmed in large randomized trials of exercise training compared with no exercise training with or without coronary intervention.

At present, it is recommended that patients should exercise or walk on a regular basis for at least 30 minutes five times a week or more.

Decreasing the Frequency and Severity of Symptoms and Improving Exercise Performance

Drug Therapy

Three classes of drugs are available for initial treatment of patients with stable angina (Fig. 22.3):

- nitrates;
- beta blockers; and
- calcium channel blockers.

Nitrates

Organic nitrates have a well-established role in drug therapy for angina.[47] Nitrates are coronary vasodilators and they are anti-ischemic, although the antianginal effects are more far-reaching. Nitrates produce venodilatation, thereby reducing preload, and high doses of nitrates also reduce afterload through arterial vasodilatation. The reduction of preload is secondary to reduced venous return, which in turn reduces ventricular volume and intracavitary pressure and ventricular wall stress. Nitrates can produce dilatation of the site of stenotic coronary lesions and thus increase perfusion to the ischemic myocardium. Nitrates also increase collateral blood flow to ischemic areas (Fig. 22.4).

Several large well-designed trials of intermittent dosing regimens or special formulations have shown that nitrates can improve angina-free walking times and total exercise duration and that they can reduce exercise-induced ST-segment

INITIAL ANTIANGINAL THERAPY FOR STABLE ANGINA		
Nitrate	Beta blocker	Calcium antagonist
First choice if left ventricular function is depressed or if angina is infrequent	First choice in previous myocardial infarction and in hypertension, left ventricular systolic or diastolic dysfunction, or supraventricular tachyarrhythmias	First choice if beta blocker is contraindicated or not tolerated Avoid short-acting dihydropyridine calcium antagonists Avoid in post–myocardial infarction patients who have evidence of heart failure (although amlodipine may be used with caution)

Figure 22.3 Initial antianginal therapy for stable angina.

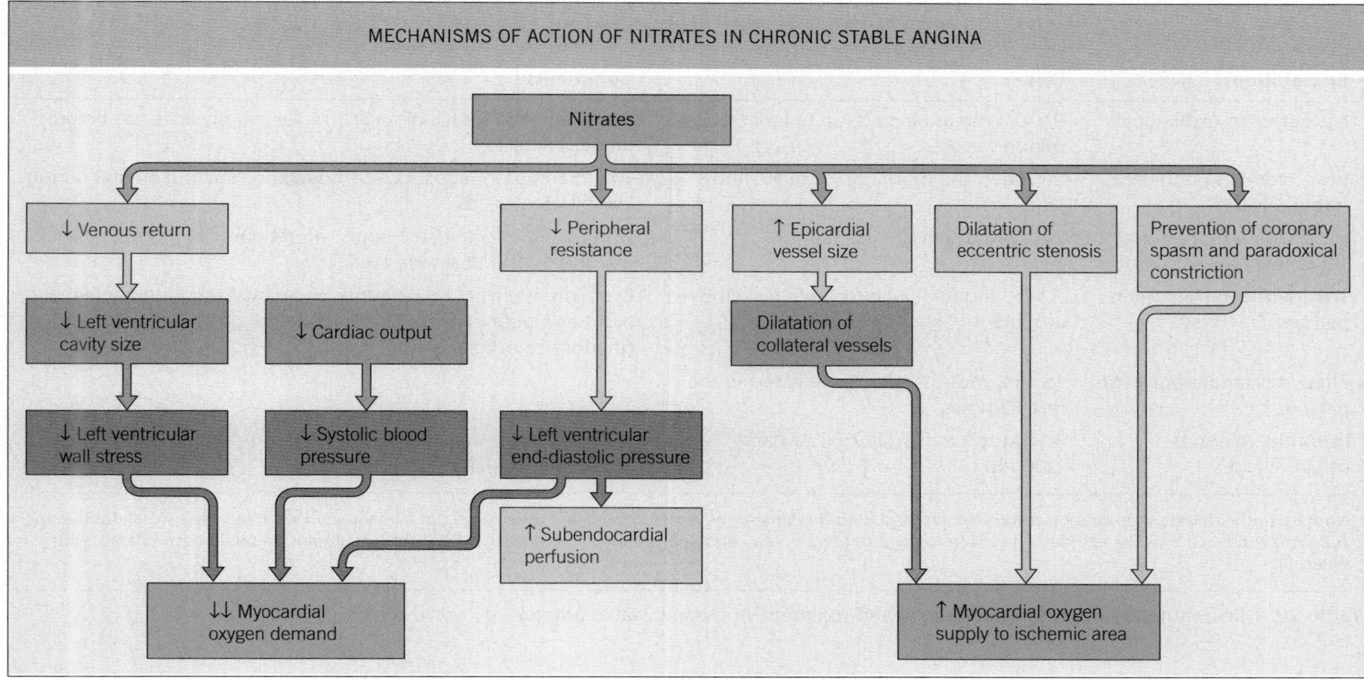

Figure 22.4 Mechanisms of action of nitrates in chronic stable angina.

depression.[48-50] An established attack of angina can be relieved with sublingual nitroglycerin. Use of prophylactic sublingual nitroglycerin also prolongs angina-free walking performance.

Nitrates are inexpensive, well tolerated, and effective, and they are thus often the first-line therapy for angina. The main problems with their use are the following[5,47]:

- Some patients will not take nitrates, irrespective of their effectiveness for angina relief, because of adverse effects such as headaches, flushing, and, rarely, syncope or aggravation of angina.
- Education of the patient is important because sublingual nitroglycerin tablets lose their potency over time and need to be replaced every 2 months.
- The effective long-term use of nitrates is hampered by the development of tolerance to these agents.

Continuous or intermittent around-the-clock use of nitrates for a 24-hour period leads to development of tolerance and to ineffectiveness with time.[50] The mechanism by which nitrate tolerance develops is unclear, and therefore concomitant therapy with agents that may avoid nitrate tolerance cannot be recommended at present.[50]

Intermittent administration with eccentric regimens or formulations that allow a gradual decrease in plasma nitrate concentrations at night (Table 22.4) is a proven way of preventing tolerance and is recommended at present. Tolerance can be successfully prevented by the administration of rapid-release isosorbide mononitrate at 7-hour intervals or of extended-release isosorbide mononitrate once daily. The choices are to use

- intermittent therapy with a transdermal nitroglycerin patch that releases at least 7.5 to 10 mg of nitroglycerin in a 12-hour period and to remove the patch after 12 hours; or
- standard or long-acting formulation of isosorbide mononitrate.

However, these regimens leave patients unprotected in the night and early hours of the morning, and nocturnal or early morning angina is a problem in 7% to 10% of patients during intermittent nitroglycerin patch therapy.[49] This phenomenon has not been reported with oral isosorbide mononitrate treatment.[48,50] Furthermore, exercise tolerance may be reduced before patch renewal in the mornings, a phenomenon known as the zero-hour effect.[49,50] Isosorbide dinitrate is widely used, but there are few data to suggest efficacy of the second dose, even when it is administered in an eccentric dosage regimen.[48]

The most common adverse effect associated with nitrates is headaches. In about 10% of patients, headaches preclude the use of long-acting nitrates because they cause poor compliance.[5,47] Concomitant use of aspirin may prevent headaches and coronary events. Another serious adverse effect of nitrates in sensitive patients is severe hypotension and syncope.[5] Patients who experience syncope after a sublingual dose of nitroglycerin should not be prescribed long-acting nitrates. Hypotension and reflex tachycardia may aggravate angina in some patients.

Beta Blockers

Beta blockers are very effective in the management of stable angina.[51] These agents decrease myocardial work and improve exercise tolerance. The primary mechanism of this benefit is through a competitive blockade of β-adrenergic receptors that reduces heart rate and contractility and therefore myocardial O_2 demand (Fig. 22.5). In addition, beta blockers decrease exercise-induced vasoconstriction and blunt the rise in systolic blood pressure during exercise. Beta blockers also increase coronary perfusion by prolonging diastolic perfusion time.

Numerous beta blockers are available for clinical use (Table 22.5). They have the common property of blocking

RECOMMENDED NITRATE PREPARATIONS AND REGIMENS IN CHRONIC STABLE ANGINA		
Preparation	**Dose**	**Comments**
Nitroglycerin (sublingual)	0.3-0.4 mg as needed (up to four tablets 5 minutes apart)	For established attack of angina or for prophylactic use before physical activity
Isosorbide-5-mononitrate (rapid release)	20 mg in the morning; 20 mg 7 hours later	Total duration of effect, 12-14 hours; no rebound angina during low-nitrate periods
Isosorbide-5-mononitrate (sustained release)	120-240 mg in the morning	Duration of effect, 10-12 hours; no rebound angina; 30- and 60-mg doses are ineffective
Transdermal nitroglycerin patches	7.5-10 mg for 12 hours; patches removed at night	Duration of effect, 10-12 hours; occasional rebound angina at night and poor exercise tolerance before patch renewal (predose zero-hour effect)
Phasic-release nitroglycerin patches	15 mg, most of which is released in the first 12 hours	
Isosorbide dinitrate (rapid release)	30 mg twice daily at 7:00 AM and 1:00 PM	Effective for up to 6 hours after morning dose; no data about after the afternoon dose

Note that other nitrate preparations or formulations and dosing regimens are either ineffective or the subject of inadequate data. Headaches may limit therapy, and nitrate-induced syncope caused by hypotension, although rare, is a contraindication to nitrate therapy. Nitrates should not be used concomitantly with sildenafil.

Table 22.4 Recommended nitrate preparations and regimens in chronic stable angina.

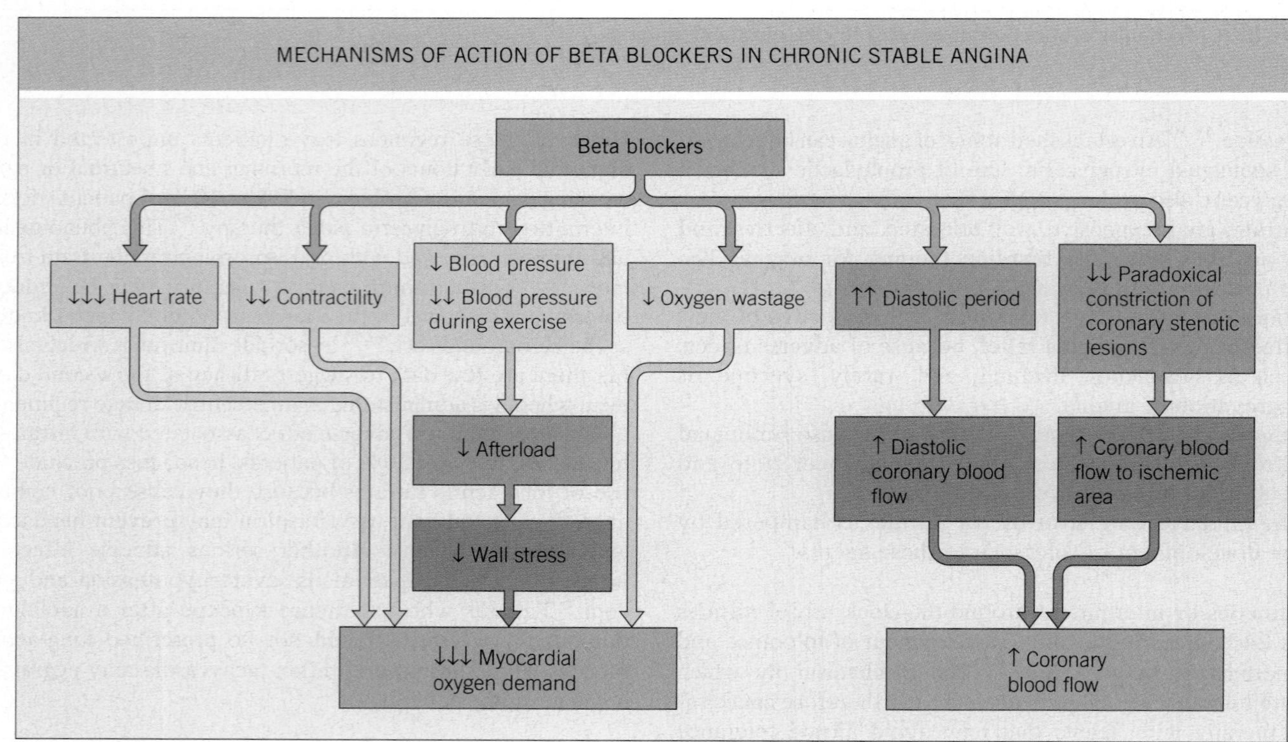

Figure 22.5 Mechanisms of action of beta blockers in chronic stable angina.

β_1-adrenergic receptors. Nonselective beta blockers block both β_1 and β_2 receptors. Some agents additionally block α_1 receptors or directly dilate blood vessels. Irrespective of the individual differences of beta blockers, they are all equally effective in patients who have stable angina.[51] Selection of an individual agent is based on the duration of effects, the presence of concomitant disease state, and other considerations.

Beta blockade is the most effective means of reducing myocardial ischemia, both during exercise and at rest. Beta blockers may be advantageously combined with other antianginal drugs such as nitrates or dihydropyridine calcium channel blockers.[3,5,11,17,24,25]

The common use of beta blockers, the dosage and frequency of administration, and the possible adverse effects are shown in Table 22.5. The adequacy of dosing is best judged by evaluating the effects of beta-blocker therapy on exercise performance and heart rate during exercise.[52]

When beta blockers are used, one must consider safety considerations.[5] The common adverse effects are directly related to beta blockade. These include

BETA BLOCKERS USED IN CHRONIC STABLE ANGINA		
Preparation	**Dose**	**Comments**
Atenolol	50-100 mg q24h	Cardioselective
Metoprolol (rapid release)	50-100 mg q8h or q12h	Cardioselective
Metoprolol (long acting)	50-200 mg q24h	Cardioselective
Betaxolol	10-20 mg q24h	Cardioselective
Bisoprolol	5-10 mg q24h	Cardioselective
Acebutolol	200-400 mg q8h	Cardioselective, with ISA
Propranolol (rapid release)	40-80 mg q8h or q12h	Not cardioselective
Propranolol (long acting)	80-320 mg q24h	
Oxprenolol	40-80 mg q8h	Not cardioselective, with ISA
Timolol	5-15 mg q8h	Not cardioselective
Nadolol	80-240 mg q24h	Not cardioselective
Carvedilol	25-50 mg q12h	Not cardioselective, with α-blocking activity
Labetalol	100-200 mg q8h	Not cardioselective, with vasodilation activity
Pindolol	2.5-7.5 mg q8h	Not cardioselective, with ISA
Celiprolol	400 mg q24h	Cardioselective, with ISA and β_2-stimulating activity

Note that beta blockers are contraindicated in asthma, severe chronic obstructive pulmonary disease, high-grade atrioventricular block, and peripheral vascular disease with leg pain at rest. They may cause fatigue, bronchospasm, central nervous system side effects, coldness of the extremities, impotence, bradycardia, and hypotension.

ISA, intrinsic sympathomimetic activity.

Table 22.5 Beta blockers used in chronic stable angina.

- bradycardia;
- hypoperfusion;
- reduction in left ventricular contractility;
- bronchospasm; and
- an inhibitive response to hypoglycemia.

Adverse effects unrelated to beta blockade include

- lethargy;
- depression;
- vivid dreams;
- constipation; and
- impotence.

In general, beta blockers are contraindicated in patients who have bronchospastic disorders. However, cardioselective blockers of β_1 receptors may be used in low doses. Agents that have intrinsic sympathomimetic activity or added effects on α receptors may also be used with caution.

In patients who have diabetes mellitus and are taking insulin, the symptoms of hypoglycemia may be masked by nonselective beta-blocker therapy. There is less risk of this effect with cardioselective agents. Mild glucose intolerance may occur with any beta blocker, especially if it is used in conjunction with a diuretic. However, beta blockers have been used safely and effectively in patients who have type 2 (non–insulin-dependent) diabetes mellitus and stable angina.

Beta blockade is dangerous in patients with conduction system abnormalities, especially sick sinus syndrome. Beta blockers are also contraindicated in patients with peripheral vascular disease who have resting leg pain. However, beta blockers can be used effectively and safely in patients who have intermittent claudication as a result of peripheral vascular disease.

Dose alterations in renal failure may be required, especially for water-soluble agents excreted by the kidney (e.g., atenolol, acebutolol, timolol, and sotalol).

Calcium Channel Blockers

Calcium channel blockers are commonly used for treatment of stable angina and hypertension.[53,54] They act mainly by vasodilatation and reduction of peripheral vascular resistance (Figs. 22.6 and 22.7). The nondihydropyridine agents (verapamil and diltiazem), a T-channel blocker (mibefradil), and bepridil inhibit the sinoatrial and atrioventricular nodes and thus also reduce myocardial O_2 demand. The dihydropyridine agents (e.g., nifedipine, amlodipine, felodipine, and nisoldipine) do not affect the sinoatrial or atrioventricular nodes in humans; their mechanism of action is primarily by dilating the coronary arteries and reducing peripheral vascular resistance (and thus reducing myocardial O_2 demand) and by increasing coronary blood flow. Calcium channel blockers block the entry of calcium into the calcium channels in both smooth muscle and myocardium so that less calcium is available to the contractile apparatus. The net result is vasodilatation and a decrease in myocardial contractility. The decrease in contractility is usually modest because of the unloading effect of peripheral vasodilatation. Diltiazem and verapamil affect the sinoatrial and atrioventricular nodes, and these agents are especially useful in patients who have a history of supraventricular tachycardia and stable angina.

All calcium channel blockers inhibit L-type calcium current in arterial smooth muscle at low concentration and therefore dilate coronary arteries. A major antianginal effect is coronary vessel dilatation and prevention of exercise-induced vessel constriction. Afterload reduction and,

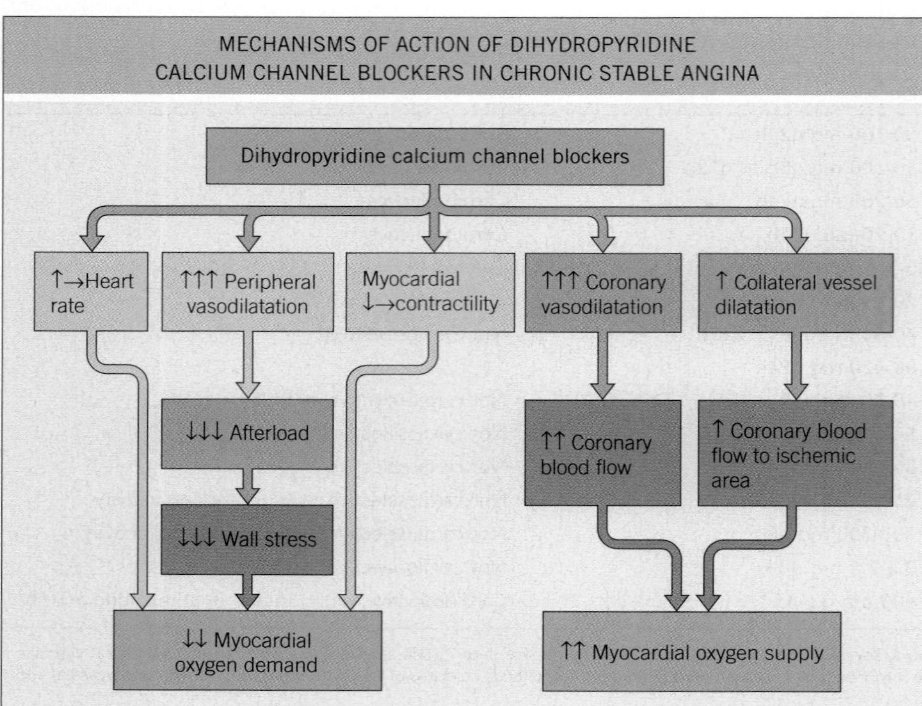

Figure 22.6 Mechanisms of action of dihydropyridine calcium channel blockers in chronic stable angina. Note that in some patients, increased coronary blood flow to nonischemic areas may cause coronary steal.

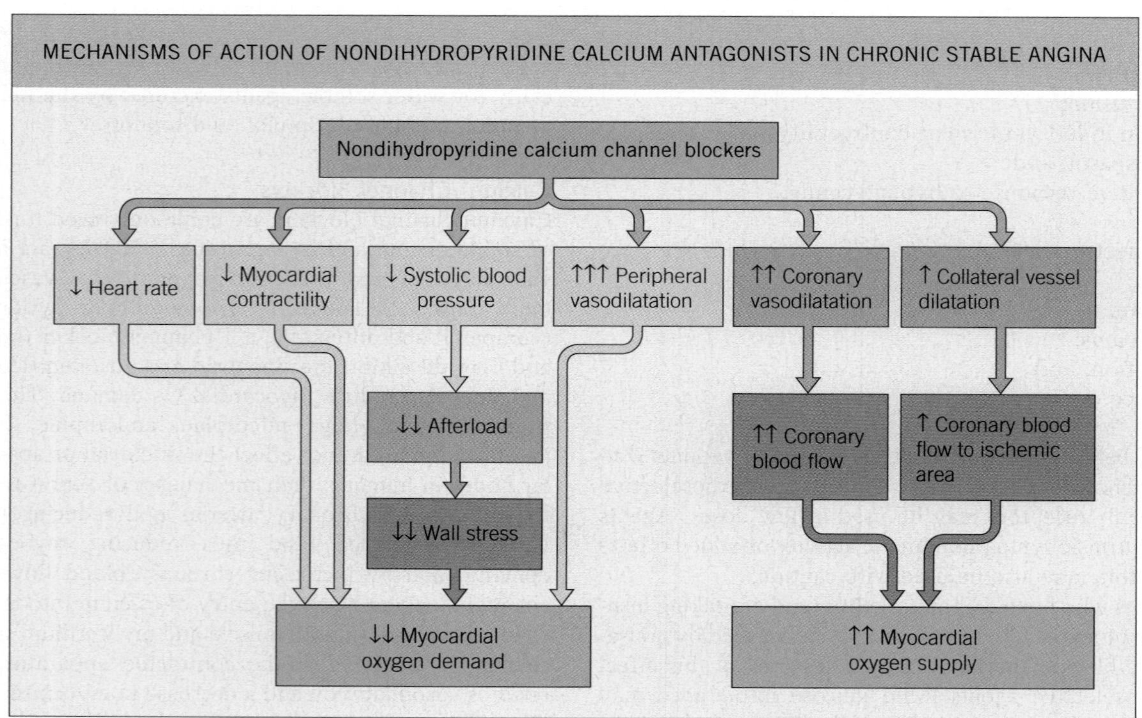

Figure 22.7 Mechanisms of action of nondihydropyridine calcium channel blockers in chronic stable angina. Note that in patients who have systolic left ventricular dysfunction, the left ventricle may dilate further because of negative inotropic effects with worsening of heart failure.

in the case of nondihydropyridine channel blockers, the suppressant effects on the sinoatrial node and myocardium also contribute to antianginal efficacy.

Despite the recent controversy surrounding calcium channel blockers, studies of the long-acting dihydropyridine and nondihydropyridine agents have shown that they are safe and effective in ischemic heart disease.[3,54,55] Monotherapy with amlodipine, diltiazem, or verapamil increases exercise tolerance and time to reach 1 mm of ST-segment depression.[56-60] The current doses and regimens of different calcium channel blockers that are recommended for treatment of stable angina are shown in Table 22.6.

CALCIUM CHANNEL BLOCKERS USED IN CHRONIC STABLE ANGINA		
Preparation	Dose	Comments
Diltiazem (rapid release)	60-120 mg q6h	Contraindicated in second- and third-degree AV block and left ventricular systolic dysfunction
Diltiazem (slow release)	80-240 mg q12h	Contraindicated in second- and third-degree AV block and left ventricular systolic dysfunction
Diltiazem (long acting)	120-420 mg q24h	240-360 mg is the most effective dose
Verapamil (rapid release)	80-120 mg q8h	Contraindicated in second- and third-degree AV block and left ventricular systolic dysfunction; constipation a problem in elderly
Nifedipine (slow release)	30-120 mg q24h	Avoid in aortic stenosis
Amlodipine	5-10 mg q24h	Avoid in aortic stenosis
Nisoldipine (long acting)	20-40 mg q24h	Avoid in aortic stenosis
Felodipine	10-20 mg q24h	Avoid in aortic stenosis

Note that there is a higher incidence of ankle edema with the nondihydropyridine agents.
AV, atrioventricular.

Table 22.6 Calcium channel blockers used in chronic stable angina.

Combination Therapy

Optimal antianginal therapy with a single antianginal agent is often as effective as combination therapy with two or three agents.[2,3,5,11,17,25] Published data show that maximal triple therapy is not superior to combination therapy with two agents.[3,11,60]

In patients who are receiving beta blockers but are still symptomatic, the addition of a dihydropyridine calcium channel blocker or a long-acting nitrate is often useful and reduces evidence of myocardial ischemia.[54,55,59-63] Efficacy and safety of the combination therapy of a beta blocker plus amlodipine[60,62,63] or atenolol plus diltiazem[60,63] have been established. However, the latter combination is associated with more severe adverse outcomes.[5] Therefore, a combination of a beta blocker and a dihydropyridine calcium channel blocker is recommended to avoid the adverse effect of the combination therapy on the sinoatrial and atrioventricular nodes.[3,5,11,25,60] Although no data exist on the combined use of a calcium channel blocker and a long-acting nitrate, such therapy is often used in clinical practice and is well tolerated.[3,5,11,24,60]

The most common adverse effects of the calcium channel blockers are facial flushing and headaches. The dihydropyridine group of drugs causes a higher incidence of ankle edema than the nondihydropyridine agents do. Constipation is more of a problem with verapamil, and this is especially important in treating elderly patients (see Table 22.6).

Nicorandil

Nicorandil is a nitrate-moiety nicotinamide ester and adenosine triphosphate–sensitive potassium channel opener. In several European countries and in Japan, this agent is widely used to treat patients with stable angina.[64] Earlier studies reported antianginal and anti-ischemic effects.[3] Studies in the United States and Australia, however, failed to confirm the superiority of nicorandil over placebo.[3,65] Nicorandil is not available for clinical use in North America.

Lipid-Lowering Agents

Improvement of myocardial ischemia during ambulatory monitoring has been described in several studies; both the number of ischemic episodes and the duration of episodes decreased with pravastatin and lovastatin, which are HMG-CoA reductase inhibitors.[66] However, it is not known whether these agents improve exercise performance. Lipid-lowering agents are recommended for patients with stable angina who have dyslipidemia because these agents have an important influence on prognosis in these patients.

Angiotensin-Converting Enzyme Inhibitors

Conflicting results have been published about the use of ACE inhibitors in stable angina. Despite their beneficial effects on endothelial function, no definite recommendation for their routine use can be made for patients with angina unless they have poor left ventricular function.[3,5,11,25]

A large trial in patients with stable angina failed to show superiority of quinalapril compared with placebo on either the treadmill walking time or ambulatory myocardial ischemia.[67]

Ranolazine

Ranolazine (500 to 1000 mg twice daily) has been approved in the United States for treatment of patients with angina either as MDNP therapy or as additional therapy in patients who remain symptomatic despite treatment with either a beta blocker or amlodipine.

Ranolazine is an effective antianginal and anti-ischemic agent, and the slow-release formulation increases exercise duration in a dose-related fashion.[68] Combination of ranolazine plus atenolol (50 mg daily) or diltiazem (180 mg daily) or amlodipine (5 mg daily) also increases angina-free exercise duration.[69] Reduction in angina frequency has been reported when ranolazine (500 to 1000 mg twice daily) was added to amlodipine (10 mg daily) to treat patients with stable angina.[70]

Despite the documented antianginal efficacy of ranolazine, the drug at first was not approved for initial treatment of patients with stable angina as the drug increases QT interval by 4 to 6 ms.[68,69] New labeling has lifted this restriction, the clinical significance of this degree of QT prolongation remains unclear, and there have been no reports of torsades de pointes during ranolazine therapy. In a study in patients with acute coronary syndrome, ranolazine reduced the incidence of ventricular arrhythmia but did not decrease cardiovascular morbidity or mortality.[71]

The cytochrome P450 3A4–mediated pathway accounts for the majority of ranolazine biotransformation. Potent inhibitors of CYP3A4, such as ketoconazole, and intermediate inhibitors, such as diltiazem, significantly increase ranolazine concentration and should be used concomitantly with caution.

Ranolazine is a substrate and an inhibitor of P-glycoprotein; verapamil, a drug that inhibits P-glycoprotein and increases ranolazine absorption and plasma concentration, therefore should not be concomitantly used with ranolazine. Ranolazine increases digoxin concentration and should be used with caution in patients who are taking digoxin.

The exact mechanism by which ranolazine exerts anti-ischemic and antianginal effects remains unknown.[3,25] The drug does not exert any hemodynamic effects and thus does not significantly change either the heart rate or blood pressure.

Earlier studies suggested that ranolazine inhibits free fatty acid oxidation.[3] However, there is only minimal inhibition of free fatty acids at therapeutic concentrations of ranolazine. It is therefore unlikely that ranolazine exerts antianginal or anti-ischemic effects primarily by metabolic modulation.

Studies in isolated myocytes and in animals show that ranolazine inhibits late sodium inward current during periods of ischemia and thus reduces intracellular calcium overload.[72] This leads to improvement in ischemia-induced mechanical dysfunction, reduction in abnormal contraction and relaxation, and reduction in diastolic tension.[72] These effects of ranolazine may thus reduce myocardial O_2 demand and improve coronary blood flow during diastole.

Common side effects include dizziness, nausea, asthenia, and constipation. Syncope is a very rare complication and appears to be related to the central effects of ranolazine.

Metabolic Modulators

Trimetazidine is available for clinical use in many European countries but not in the United States as an adjunct therapy for angina.[3,25] The exact mechanism by which trimetazidine exerts antianginal effects is unknown. It is considered to be a metabolic modulator by partially inhibiting free fatty acid oxidation and thus increasing glucose use.

In patients who remain symptomatic despite treatment with beta blockers, calcium channel blockers, and long-acting nitrates, trimetazidine decreased angina frequency without exerting any effect on heart rate or blood pressure.[73-76] Side effects reported are nausea, vomiting, fatigue, and myalgia.

Rho Kinase Inhibitor

This class of drugs is promising. The Rho kinase inhibitor fasudil is a potent anti-ischemic agent. When it is given in addition to a beta blocker, it reduces exercise-induced ischemia, but its anti-anginal effects are yet to be established.[77]

Sinus Node–Blocking Agents

Ivabradine

There is a lot of interest in drugs that specifically lower heart rate without affecting the blood pressure or pulmonary function. At present, ivabradine, which blocks funny inward current (I_f) in the sinus node, is under active investigation. Ivabradine has been shown to increase exercise duration and to reduce exercise-induced myocardial ischemia,[78] but its approval is awaiting the results of a large ongoing outcome trial. Ivabradine can rarely cause marked slowing of sinus rate and visual disturbances.[3,25,76]

Revascularization Procedures

Percutaneous Coronary Interventions

Balloon coronary angioplasty with or without stent placement is effective in reducing angina frequency and exercise-induced ischemia (see Chapter 35).[3,24,25,34,37] Both balloon angioplasty and stents are, however, associated with the problem of restenosis. The restenosis rate is greatest in the first 6 months after therapy and is lower with drug-eluting stents than with angioplasty or with bare metal stents. A main concern after the placement of drug-eluting stents in coronary arteries is the risk of in-stent thrombosis, with a reported incidence of 0.6% to 1.8%. This may be manifested as a heart attack or even sudden cardiac death.[79,80] Although early in-stent thrombosis can be markedly reduced with dual antiplatelet treatment with aspirin plus clopidogrel, late and very late thrombosis remains a concern, and how to prevent it from occurring remains elusive at present.[80] There is also a concern of in-stent thrombosis when dual antiplatelet treatment needs to be discontinued for elective surgery.

Although this mode of therapy is widely used in North America for initial treatment of stable angina, it should be reserved for patients who do not respond adequately to antianginal therapy, patients in whom lifestyle is still impaired despite adequate medical therapy, and patients who refuse to take medical therapy. Neither angioplasty nor stents prolong survival or reduce the incidence of myocardial infarction compared with medical therapy.[11,24,25,36,37] Furthermore, a study showed the superiority of medical therapy to angioplasty or stent placement with regard to serious adverse outcomes, although relief of angina was experienced by more patients with angioplasty.[26]

The long-term success rate of percutaneous coronary interventions is lower in diabetic patients owing to higher restenosis rates.

Coronary Artery Bypass Surgery

Coronary artery bypass surgery relieves angina and reduces myocardial ischemia in nearly 80% of patients (see Chapter 36). However, in the United States, a 20-year follow-up in the Veterans Affairs cooperative study of CABG surgery for stable angina showed that the initial antianginal therapy was correlated with a significantly higher probability of remaining free of myocardial infarction (57% versus 41%; $P = .02$) and of being alive without myocardial infarction (18% versus 11%; $P = .00031$).[30] This small trial of 686 patients indicated that the initial CABG surgery did not improve survival of low-risk patients (those who had good left ventricular function) and did not reduce overall risk of myocardial infarction.[11] Furthermore, despite an early survival benefit of up to a decade with surgery in high-risk patients (those with impaired left ventricular function), long-term survival rates were similar in both treatment groups. In total, twice as many CABG procedures were performed in the group assigned to surgery without any long-term survival or symptomatic benefits.

A review of published data showed that revascularization with CABG surgery is not superior to medical therapy,[3,11] the only exception being patients with left main coronary artery disease, who were excluded from the randomized trials; these patients are candidates for CABG surgery. Moreover, the benefit of up to 10 years on survival but not on the incidence of myocardial infarction has been shown with CABG surgery in patients with diminished left ventricular function and three-vessel coronary artery disease. Therefore, CABG surgery should be reserved for this group of patients and for those who do not respond to medical therapy.[11] Long-term outcome is improved by CABG surgery compared with balloon angioplasty in patients who have diabetes mellitus.

One study showed that revascularization strategy was superior to pharmacologic treatment that targeted angina relief or myocardial ischemia, but the revascularization mortality from different institutes in this study was only 1.2%.[16] The reported average mortality in the United States is 3.2% (range, 1% to 12%). Thus, large trials are needed to address the issue of whether revascularization strategy is superior to strategies that target relief or reduction of ambulatory ischemia.[3,11] On the basis of the available data, initial medical therapy should be considered in all patients who have stable angina.

Choice of Drug Therapy for Chronic Stable Angina

The choice of initial drug therapy for chronic stable angina should depend on the presence or absence of concomitant disease (Table 22.7).[2,3,5,11,24,25,76] The proposed treatment of patients with stable angina (Table 22.8), which has been modified from recent publications,[5,11] outlines preference of therapeutic strategy in different patient groups with stable angina.

Treatment of Refractory Chronic Stable Angina

Many patients who have stable angina remain symptomatic despite adequate medical therapy as they are not candidates for revascularization because of unsuitable anatomy, previous revascularization procedures, or concomitant disease. These patients pose a medical dilemma, and special measures may be needed to relieve the angina.[3,5,11,25,76]

Bepridil

Bepridil is a calcium channel blocker, but it prolongs the QT interval and produces torsades de pointes.[5,11] It is a very effective antianginal agent, but it should be used only in patients who remain symptomatic despite maximal medical therapy and who are not candidates for revascularization procedures.[3,5,11,25,76]

Laser Revascularization

Transmyocardial laser revascularization can improve the functional class of angina, but this procedure is associated with higher initial mortality[3,81,82] and is not therefore routinely recommended.[3,82] The newer technique of transcutaneous myocardial laser revascularization is being investigated; initial data looked promising, but recent placebo (sham treated) controlled trials have been disappointing.[3,25,76,82,83] Percutaneous myocardial laser revascularization is therefore not recommended to treat patients with stable angina.

Enhanced External Counterpulsation

Several trials have shown the usefulness of noninvasive enhanced external counterpulsation in improving exercise performance and time to ischemia and in reducing myocardial ischemia in chronic stable angina.[3,82,84,85] Although the trials have been small, this therapy may be worth a trial in patients who do not respond to conventional medical therapy.[3,82]

Spinal Cord Stimulation

Patients who are refractory to antianginal therapy and are not candidates for revascularization have been shown to

ANTIANGINAL TREATMENT OPTIONS IN PATIENTS WITH AND WITHOUT CONCOMITANT DISEASE

			Calcium Channel Blockers	
Concomitant Disease	Long-acting Nitrates	Beta Blockers	Long-acting Dihydropyridines	Nondihydropyridines (verapamil and diltiazem)
None	+++	+++	++	+++
Hypertension	+	+++	++	+++
Recent myocardial infarction	+++	+++	–	+
Reduced left ventricular function	+++	+++	–	–
Supraventricular tachycardia	+	+++	–	+++
Mild chronic obstructive pulmonary disease	+++	+	+++	+++
Severe chronic obstructive pulmonary disease or asthma	+++	–	+++	+++
Peripheral vascular disease	++	++	+++	++
Type 1 (insulin-dependent) diabetes mellitus	+++	+	+++	+++
Type 2 (non–insulin-dependent) diabetes mellitus	+++	++	+++	+++
Chronic renal disease	+++	++	+++	+++
Sinus bradycardia (heart rate below 50 bpm or second- or third-degree AV block)	+++	–	+++	–

Note that diltiazem is the nondihydropyridine agent used in non–Q wave myocardial infarction in the absence of congestive heart failure.
AV, atrioventricular; +++ very effective and desirable; ++ moderately effective and desirable; + effective but less desirable; – should be avoided.

Table 22.7 Antianginal treatment options in patients with and without concomitant disease.

PROPOSED TREATMENT FOR STABLE ANGINA PECTORIS	
Patient Characteristics	**Treatment**
All patients	Daily aspirin Smoking cessation Treat dyslipidemia Control of high blood pressure to levels ≤140/90 mm Hg (to 130/80 mm Hg in diabetes mellitus)
Left main or three-vessel coronary artery disease with decreased left ventricular function	CABG surgery (if feasible) ACE inhibitor and beta blockers when ejection fraction <40%
One-, two-, or three-vessel disease with normal left ventricular function	Antianginal drug treatment Percutaneous transluminal coronary angioplasty or CABG surgery if symptoms are not controlled with drug treatment
Refractory angina, very poor left ventricular function, or not a candidate for revascularization	Consider bepridil, external enhanced counterpulsation, transmyocardial laser revascularization, spinal cord stimulation, transthoracic sympathetic denervation, or heart transplantation

ACE, angiotensin converting enzyme; CABG, coronary artery bypass graft.

Table 22.8 Proposed treatment for stable angina pectoris.

PARAMETERS ASSOCIATED WITH POOR PROGNOSIS IN CHRONIC STABLE ANGINA	
Parameter	**Comments**
Diminished global left ventricular function at rest	Most important, best correlation with long-term survival
Comorbid conditions	Very important
Marked symptom-limited exercise capacity	Failure to complete stage 2 of the Bruce protocol or equivalent (workload ≤6.5 METs)
Time at onset, magnitude, morphologic features, and persistence of ST-segment depression in the postexercise period	Useful when changes occur at low workload (≤6.5 METs)
Fall in systolic blood pressure during exercise	Often indicates poor left ventricular function or severe coronary artery disease
Left ventricular cavity dilatation, increased lung uptake	Requires exercise echocardiography or radionuclide perfusion imaging; suggests left ventricular failure caused by severe ischemia

MET, metabolic equivalent of task.

Table 22.9 Parameters associated with poor prognosis in chronic stable angina.

improve their functional class of angina with spinal cord stimulation.[3,25,82,86] The technique is performed in only a few centers, and larger trials are needed before this procedure can be recommended as routine therapy.[3,82]

Transcutaneous Electrical Nerve Stimulation

Transcutaneous electrical nerve stimulation has been shown to be effective in patients who are refractory to standard medical therapy and are not candidates for revascularization procedures.[3,11,82]

Angiogenic Gene Therapy

This mode of treatment is under active investigation, but published results to date have been discouraging.[3,82,87] In a recent trial, intracoronary angiogenic gene therapy was not superior to placebo and failed to improve exercise duration or to improve outcome in symptomatic patients with angina pectoris.[88]

PROGNOSIS

The annual death rate of patients with stable angina is 1.6% to 3.2%.[89] The principal determinants of prognosis are (Table 22.9)

- left ventricular systolic function;
- extent of coronary artery disease;
- exercise duration or effort tolerance; and
- comorbid conditions.

The ability to complete stage 3 of the standard Bruce protocol and normal left ventricular function denote a relatively good prognosis. The published data on natural history and prognosis have not taken into consideration medical therapy, which has incorporated aspirin and lipid-lowering agents (drugs that reduce mortality and morbidity in coronary artery disease). Therefore, it is conceivable that the natural prognosis of stable angina might be very different from the published data.[5,11]

SUMMARY

Stable chronic angina pectoris refers to a strangling feeling, pain, or discomfort that is due to underlying myocardial ischemia. The location of discomfort is usually substernal, retrosternal, or transsternal, and it may radiate to the neck or the left arm and sometimes to the right arm and the back. The pain is usually precipitated by activity or emotional upset and relieved by discontinuation of activity or ingestion of sublingual nitroglycerin. By definition, the frequency of angina episodes has been stable without deterioration for at least a period of 3 to 6 months. A well-taken history will document this fact. Some patients may present with angina equivalent (dyspnea or fatigue on exertion). Severe atherosclerotic narrowing of one or more coronary arteries is responsible for myocardial ischemia and angina in most patients who have stable angina. Noninvasive stress tests permit identification of severe stenotic lesions but do not predict acute coronary events. The coronary arteries of a patient who has stable angina also contain many nonatherosclerotic plaques, which are prone to fissuring or rupture in an unpredictable manner, resulting in presentation of acute coronary syndromes (unstable angina, myocardial infarction, and sudden ischemic death). The important determining factors of prognosis in stable angina are underlying resting systolic left ventricular function, severity and extent of coronary artery disease, duration of exercise on the treadmill, left ventricular cavity dilatation during exercise, and increased radionuclide lung uptake during exercise as well as the presence of serious comorbid conditions. The annual death rate of patients who have stable angina is 1.6% to 3.2%. Long-term prognosis for patients with stable angina who have good left ventricular function despite severe coronary artery disease is similar with medical treatment and surgical revascularization procedures. There are no data to show that percutaneous intervention, such as balloon angioplasty or stent placement, improves prognosis of patients with stable angina. There are also no data to suggest that CABG surgery reduces the incidence of myocardial infarction, which is invariably due to fissuring or rupture of nonobstructive lesions (which are often not bypassed).

In addition to symptomatic relief of symptoms and an increase in angina-free walking time with antianginal drugs or revascularization procedures, emphasis of treatment must be on reducing adverse clinical outcomes (unstable angina, coronary death, and myocardial infarction). The role of smoking cessation, daily use of aspirin, and treatment of dyslipidemias and of high blood pressure in all patients together with the use of beta blockers and ACE inhibitors in patients who have diminished systolic left ventricular function in reducing adverse outcome has been well established. It is not known whether antianginal drugs have an effect on adverse outcomes in patients who have stable angina. All three groups of drugs (nitrates, beta blockers, and calcium channel blockers) and Ranolazine are effective antianginal and anti-ischemic agents. All patients with stable angina should be advised to carry sublingual nitroglycerin and to use it for relief of an established attack. Initial therapy with antianginal agents should take into consideration comorbid conditions and incorporate adequate monotherapy before a trial of combination with different classes of antianginal drugs. Triple therapy may be more deleterious than treatment with two agents. Patients who remain symptomatic despite adequate medical therapy and those who cannot tolerate or are not willing to take medical treatment should be considered for revascularization procedures. Coronary balloon angioplasty, coronary stents, and CABG surgery all provide symptomatic relief. CABG surgery is indicated in patients who have diminished left ventricular function plus three-vessel disease, those who have left main coronary artery disease, and those who have multivessel disease and diabetes mellitus. Patients who have refractory angina despite medical therapy and who are not candidates for revascularization procedures may be candidates for newer techniques of enhanced external counterpulsation, spinal cord stimulation, bepridil therapy, or transmyocardial revascularization.[40]

chapter 23

Variant Angina Pectoris

Juan Carlos Kaski and Ramón Arroyo-Espliguero

Definition

- Variant angina pectoris is typically defined as angina at rest associated with transient ST-segment elevation, both of which resolve spontaneously or with the administration of nitrate.

Key Features

- Chest pain at rest is typical of transient myocardial ischemia.
- Pain episodes are more common at night or in the early morning.
- Exercise capacity is preserved.
- Coronary artery spasm is the most common underlying mechanism.

Therapy

- Response to calcium channel blockers, nitrates, or both is excellent.

The first clear description of variant angina pectoris was given by Prinzmetal and colleagues[1] in 1959. They reported findings in a group of patients who presented with chest pain at rest and transient ST-segment elevation in the electrocardiographic (ECG) recording. Paradoxically, despite angina at rest, most of these patients had a preserved exercise capacity. Prinzmetal and colleagues speculated that variant angina was caused by a reduction in coronary blood supply that was due to transient increases in "coronary tonus" at the site of atheromatous lesions. Later, it became apparent that coronary artery spasm responsible for variant angina can occur in both angiographically normal and diseased vessels. The true prevalence of variant angina pectoris is unknown, but it is clearly less common than typical chronic stable angina pectoris or unstable angina. Coronary artery spasm is the most common pathogenic mechanism in variant angina pectoris.

ANATOMY AND PATHOLOGY

Little information is available about morphologic changes in the coronary arteries of patients with variant angina that may lead to spasm. In one of the original patients described by Prinzmetal and colleagues,[1] all "major coronary arteries were markedly sclerotic." Subsequently, during the past few decades, the majority of autopsy studies in patients with transient ST-segment elevation associated with angina at rest showed the presence of some degree of coronary artery disease at the spastic sites. However, coronary spasm resulting in cardiac death has been reported by El-Maraghi and Sealey[2] to occur in the absence of atherosclerotic plaques or other coronary lesions. Other authors have observed endothelial erosion, fibromuscular dysplasia, and increased concentration of mast cells in the arterial adventitia in the coronary arteries of patients with vasospastic angina.

Controversial data exist about whether coronary vasospasm may injure the vessel wall and result in the development or progression of organic stenoses.[3,4] The histologic features of plaque have been shown to be similar in patients with variant angina and in patients showing restenosis after coronary angioplasty.[5]

PATHOPHYSIOLOGY

Prinzmetal and colleagues[1] intuitively suggested that the newly described "variant" form of angina was caused by an increased coronary arterial tone. Their hypothesis was actually confirmed when coronary spasm was observed by selective coronary arteriography during chest pain attacks in patients with Prinzmetal's variant angina.[6,7]

"Physiologic" Coronary Artery Constriction, Coronary Atheroma, and Spasm

The coronary arteries have a basal tone and are able to contract further or to relax in response to different stimuli. The coronary arteries of experimental animals constrict in response to appropriate stimuli and show a 20% to 30% uniform reduction in diameter compared with baseline.[8] Similarly, in patients with chronic stable angina, the reduction in epicardial coronary artery diameter in response to coronary constrictors is usually diffuse and mild (<30%) even at the site of atheromatous plaques. This rather uniform and only mild or moderate vasoconstriction represents a vasomotor response that can be considered to be within the "physiologic" range.[8] In variant angina, however, vasoconstriction becomes a dominant force and causes chest pain and myocardial ischemia.

Coronary artery spasm very often occurs at the site of atheromatous plaques, particularly in white patients but not necessarily so in Japanese patients. It has been suggested that atheromatous plaques could magnify the lumen diameter reduction caused by physiologic vasoconstriction (geometric theory).[9] However, studies have shown that the degree of vasoconstriction measured at the spastic site is greater than that predicted by geometric considerations,[10,11] thus confirming that patients with variant angina truly have hyperreactive coronary artery segments.[11,12] In patients with variant angina, constrictor stimuli cause a lumen reduction that is several orders of magnitude greater in spastic segments

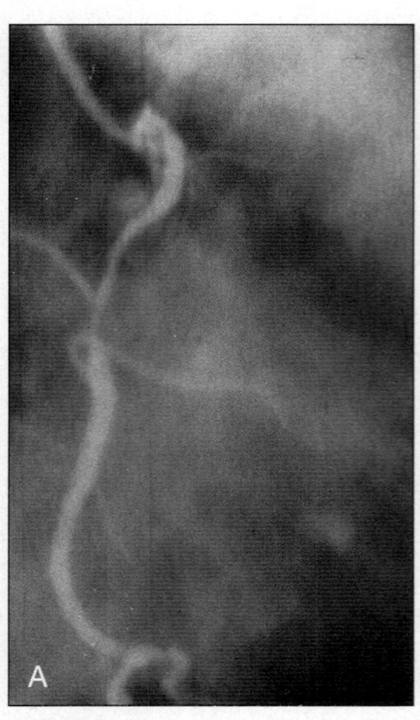

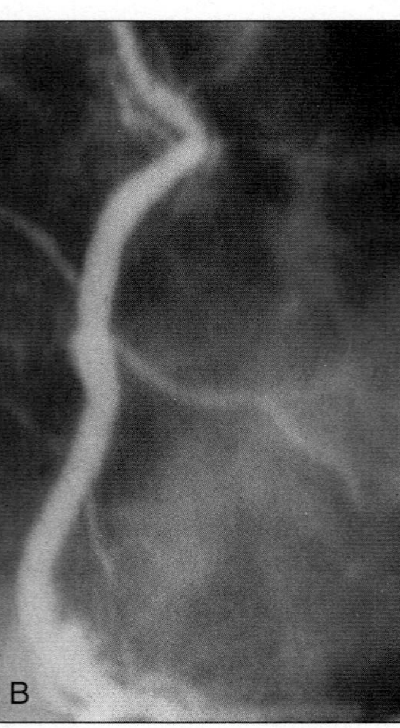

Figure 23.1 Segmental coronary artery spasm. A, The spasm involves the proximal segment of the right coronary artery. **B**, Administration of intracoronary nitrate resulted in significant vasodilatation of the coronary artery and abolished the spasm.

compared with nonspastic segments. This local coronary hyperreactivity has also been documented during spontaneous coronary spasm in patients with typical variant angina.[12] Severe segmental spasm often results in coronary occlusion and reduced blood flow (Fig. 23.1).

The definition of coronary spasm is arbitrary, but cardiologists agree that coronary artery spasm is a severe, abnormal vasoconstriction of the large epicardial arteries that often leads to transmural myocardial ischemia. It is usually transient and resolves spontaneously or is promptly relieved by nitrates. However, spasm may be long lasting and refractory to treatment. There is no agreed limit as to the magnitude of lumen diameter reduction that is required for the diagnosis of spasm. However, in patients with variant angina and angiographically normal coronary arteries who develop ischemia during spasm, the lumen diameter reduction exceeds 70%. By use of angiographic criteria, it would seem reasonable to define epicardial coronary spasm as coronary artery constriction leading to total or subtotal vessel occlusion. This definition applies to spasm that occurs in normal arterial segments or in segments with organic stenosis. However, it is difficult to distinguish lesser degrees of constriction from true spasm when the constriction occurs in segments with severe atherosclerotic lesions (i.e., >80% stenosis).

Epicardial Coronary Artery Hyperreactivity

Current evidence suggests that coronary spasm is likely to result from a local nonspecific coronary hyperreactivity to constrictor stimuli. Kaski and associates[11] have shown that patients with variant angina have an enhanced coronary artery reactivity to a variety of vasoconstrictor agents and that coronary spasm often results from a focal coronary hyperreactivity to generalized stimuli.[12] The cause of the local hyperreactivity cannot be attributed simply to the presence of atherosclerotic plaques in the arterial intima at sites of coronary spasm. Coronary atheroma is extremely common both in patients with angina and in asymptomatic subjects, whereas coronary spasm is far less common. Moreover, ergonovine testing very rarely elicits coronary spasm in patients with chronic stable angina despite the presence of coronary disease.

Coronary spasm has a multitude of possible triggers (Table 23.1), which indicates that coronary hyperreactivity in patients with variant angina is likely to be nonspecific. Indeed, coronary spasm can be caused by a variety of agents that act on different arterial receptors,[11] that is, ergonovine, histamine, dopamine, acetylcholine, norepinephrine (noradrenaline), and serotonin; it can also be caused by increasing the arterial blood pH to 7.65 to 7.70 with the hyperventilation test. A primary neural origin for spasm is unlikely as spasm has been observed in human transplanted hearts and in explanted, perfused hearts in the miniature pig model. However, changes in autonomic tone, especially vagal withdrawal,[13] may act as a trigger of epicardial artery spasm. The local coronary hyperreactivity seen in patients with spasm persists for months and even years in some patients, suggesting that the pathogenesis of coronary spasm, as seen in variant angina, is compatible with a postreceptor

FACTORS THAT CONTRIBUTE TO THE DEVELOPMENT OF CORONARY ARTERY SPASM
Cigarette smoking
Cocaine use
Hypomagnesemia
Insulin resistance
Vitamin E deficiency
Administration of sumatriptan and ergotamine (migraine treatment)
Hyperventilation
Cold stimulation

Table 23.1 Factors that contribute to the development of coronary artery spasm.

alteration of signal transduction in vascular smooth muscle cells rather than an alteration in the local endothelial lining or an unusual response of resident cells in the wall of the spastic coronary artery. Experimental molecular studies seem to confirm this notion. Phosphorylation of regulatory subunits of myosin light chain (rMLC) promotes cross-bridge cycling by increasing affinity of myosin for actin. The level of rMLC phosphorylation is determined by the balance between the myosin light chain kinase and the myosin light chain phosphatase. Vascular smooth muscle contraction is initiated by calcium/calmodulin-activated myosin light chain kinase with subsequent phosphorylation of rMLC. Contractions of smooth muscle are dependent not on the concentration of intracellular calcium alone but also on the sensitivity of the contractile apparatus to calcium. Rho kinase, activated by the upstream guanosine triphosphatase RhoA, reduces myosin light chain phosphatase activity by phosphorylating the myosin-binding subunit of the enzyme and thus augments vascular smooth muscle contraction at a given calcium concentration (calcium sensitization).[14]

Several studies using animal models have provided strong evidence that alterations in the RhoA/Rho kinase pathway mediate hypercontractility to vasoactive substances. It has been shown that Rho kinase is up-regulated at the spastic site (at all levels, including mRNA, protein, and activity), causing the increase in myosin light chain phosphorylations.[15] In the Sur2 and Kir6.1 knockout mice, a Prinzmetal variant angina–like phenotype has been reported.[16,17] The adenosine triphosphate (ATP)–dependent potassium (K_{ATP}) channels are an octameric functional complex consisting of the sulfonylurea receptor (Sur1 or Sur2) subunit and an inward rectifier potassium channel subunit (Kir6.1 or Kir6.2). The occurrence of this phenotype may explain the beneficial antianginal effects of the vasodilator nicorandil, which preferentially activates Sur2 and Kir6.1 channels. Potentially, an increased susceptibility to vasospasm could result from the administration of sulfonylurea agents, which are known to close Sur2 K_{ATP} channels.[18]

Endothelial Dysfunction and Vasospasm

The potential pathogenic role of endothelial dysfunction in coronary spasm deserves consideration. A close correlation between spastic sites and histologically documented atheromatosis was observed in experimental animals, even when the coronary lesions could not be detected with angiography. Endothelial dysfunction is associated with abnormalities in vasomotor tone that in the presence of coronary artery stenosis may lead to myocardial ischemia (mixed angina or dynamic coronary artery stenosis).[19] Several abnormalities in endothelial function may be implicated in the pathogenesis of coronary vasospasm, including increased release and activity of the vasoconstrictor peptide endothelin,[20] oxidative stress, and impairment of flow-dependent coronary dilatation due to decreased production of nitric oxide (NO).[21] Decreased production and reduced activity of NO in some patients may be the result of a mutation in the endothelial NO synthase gene (eNOS). However, it is unlikely that endothelial dysfunction alone is responsible for coronary spasm in patients with variant angina.

Kugiyama and coworkers[22] have suggested that coronary spasm is linked to a deficiency in endothelial NO availability, but other authors[23] have shown preserved endothelium-dependent vasodilatation at the vasospastic site in patients with Prinzmetal's variant angina. It has also been shown that inhibition of NO alone was not enough to produce coronary vasospasm.[24] These studies support the notion that vascular hyperreactivity plays a major pathogenic role in variant angina and that hyperreactivity is not necessarily mediated by endothelial dysfunction.

Although decreases in NO-mediated function may not directly determine the hypercontractile status of a blood vessel, it is possible that alterations in NO may indirectly alter the contractile apparatus. NO increases cyclic guanosine monophosphate (cGMP) and activates cGMP-dependent protein kinase, which inhibits RhoA-induced calcium sensitivity of the contractile apparatus. Thus, decreased NO production or bioavailability could potentially shift the balance in favor of RhoA and Rho kinase activation and enhanced vascular contractility.[14]

Inflammation and Vasospasm

Several proinflammatory molecules have been reported to be elevated in patients with variant angina and associated with the severity of vasospastic attacks. Plasma levels of intercellular adhesion molecule 1, type II phospholipase A_2, fibrinogen, and high-sensitivity C-reactive protein have been associated with coronary artery spasm, suggesting the presence of an inflammatory process in spastic coronary arteries.[25] Moreover, circulating activated T lymphocytes were significantly higher in patients with variant angina than in patients with chronic stable angina. Anatomic-pathologic studies of coronary arteries of patients with variant angina showed infiltration of T lymphocytes, macrophages, and mast cells and diffuse intimal thickening. It is particularly interesting to note the association reported between vasospastic angina and allergic hypersensitivity, probably mediated by mast cells, histamine, and leukotrienes.[26]

Drugs and Coronary Vasospasm

Illicit Drugs

Coronary spasm is responsible for a large proportion of cases of acute myocardial infarction with normal coronary arteries (approximately 20% of all myocardial infarctions in individuals younger than 35 years). Coronary spasm–related infarctions in the younger are associated with drug abuse, cocaine being the most frequent cause.[27] However, most of the commonly used illicit substances have been reported to cause intense coronary vasospasm when they are used alone or in combination.[28] Vasodilator therapy may be lifesaving in the treatment of patients with cocaine-induced coronary spasm, whereas thrombolytic drugs and propranolol have been reported to have deleterious effects in these cases.[29]

Pharmacologic Agents

Coronary spasm leading to acute myocardial infarction has also been reported with the use of antimigraine agents, chemotherapy, anesthetics, and antibiotics.[27] Ephedrine, ergonovine, ergotamine, sumatriptan, bromocriptine, 5-fluorouracil, propofol, and amoxicillin have been linked to cases of severe vasospasm. Selective serotonin type 1 (5-$HT_{1B/D}$) agonists (both oral and subcutaneous 5-$HT_{1B/D}$ agonists, such as sumatriptan) have also been implicated in spasm-induced myocardial infarction, and use in patients with variant angina may be problematic.[30-33]

Genetic Abnormalities

The syndrome of variant angina does not have a familial component. However, coronary spasm is more prevalent in the Japanese than in the white population, suggesting that genetic factors may be implicated in its pathogenesis. In Japanese patients, it was demonstrated that the missense Glu298Asp variant in exon 7 and the T−786C mutation in the 5′ flanking region of the eNOS gene are significantly associated with coronary spasm. The missense Glu298Asp mutation affects the function of eNOS protein, and the T−786C mutation in the 5′ flanking region reduces promoter activity of the eNOS gene. These findings suggest that the eNOS gene variants impair endothelial NO synthesis and predispose those patients that carry the mutant allele to coronary spasm.[34] It is therefore conceivable that variant angina may arise from the interaction of genetic and environmental factors.

Other genetic abnormalities have recently been associated with the development of variant angina in a Korean population. Functional polymorphisms of the α- and β-adrenergic receptors (α_{2C}Del322-325 allele carrier state and β_2Gln27 allele homozygote state) were reported to be significant predictors of variant angina. The functional impairment of the α_{2C}-adrenergic receptor due to Del322-325 polymorphism is known to result in increased α-adrenergic activation leading to vasoconstriction and increased susceptibility to vasospasm. Decreased β_2-adrenergic activity associated with β_2Gln27 homozygote may result in impaired vessel dilatation.[35]

CLINICAL PRESENTATION

Prevalence

The true prevalence of coronary spasm is not known, but men and women are equally affected. Patients with variant angina tend to be younger than patients with chronic stable angina, and although many do not exhibit classic cardiovascular risk factors, cigarette smoking has been reported to be associated with spasm.[36] Variant angina has also been shown to be associated with an increased prevalence of migraine and Raynaud's syndrome, aspirin-induced asthma,[37] and cocaine abuse.[38]

Chest Pain and Electrocardiographic Changes

Characteristically, patients with variant angina pectoris experience angina at rest that is typical in character and radiation, but they have a preserved exercise capacity. Chest pain is typically associated with transient ST-segment elevation in the ECG recording (Fig. 23.2) and tends to occur mainly at night or in the early morning hours (Fig. 23.3). Both chest pain and ECG changes usually subside spontaneously or can be relieved rapidly by sublingual or intravenous nitrate. Hyperventilation, emotional stress, exposure to cold, and occasionally exercise can precipitate attacks of vasospastic angina. In approximately 30% of patients, spasm develops during exercise or, more typically, 1 to 5 minutes after effort. Although coronary spasm tends to last only a few minutes before it resolves spontaneously, prolonged episodes of vasospastic angina are not uncommon and may lead to subendocardial or transmural myocardial infarction, arrhythmias, and sudden cardiac death.[39,40] Patients with variant angina may present with syncope caused by complete atrioventricular block and asystole or ventricular tachyarrhythmias.

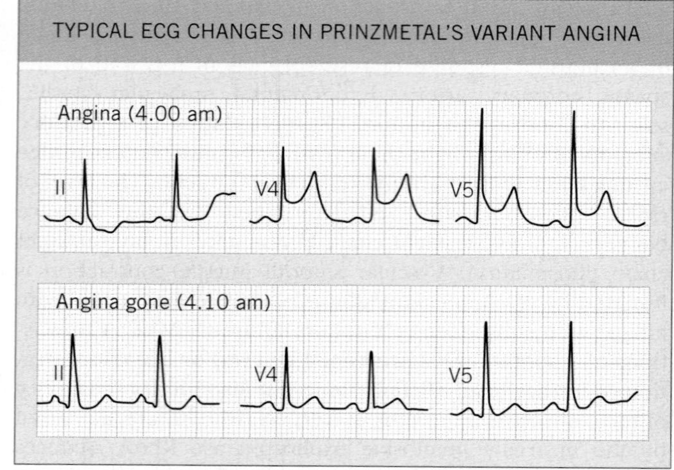

Figure 23.2 Typical ECG changes in Prinzmetal's variant angina. This man had completely normal coronary arteriograms. The vasospastic episode recorded here occurred while the patient was asleep. He was awakened by angina, which subsided after the administration of sublingual nitrate, and the ST segment returned to baseline within minutes after the nitrate treatment.

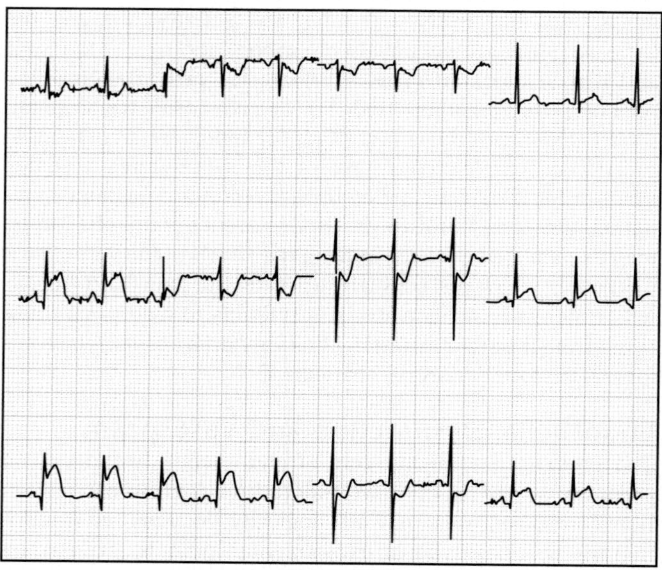

Figure 23.3 Severe transient ST-segment elevation in Prinzmetal's variant angina in the absence of chest pain (silent myocardial ischemia). This episode was recorded at 9:28 AM. In a sizable proportion of patients, occlusive coronary spasm and ST-segment elevation develop in the absence of chest pain (silent ischemia).

Arrhythmias are a frequent finding during occlusive coronary vasospasm and may be life-threatening, that is, atrioventricular block (often associated with right coronary artery spasm) and ventricular tachycardia. Patients with variant angina who develop life-threatening arrhythmias have a greater degree of baseline QT dispersion,[41] indicating heterogeneity of repolarization that is present even in the absence of ischemia.

Although ST-segment elevation is the hallmark of variant angina, coronary spasm may also be associated with ST-segment depression, T-wave inversion, and pseudonormalization of the T wave. ST-segment depression is often seen during subocclusive spasm or with occlusive spasm in the presence of collateral circulation. During spastic episodes, QT-interval prolongation and T-wave pseudonormalization have been described.

Angiographic Features

Coronary spasm is a dynamic process in which the severity, location, and appearance of the spastic vessel (or vessels) may vary from patient to patient and also within patients. It is often a focal process that affects only one segment of an artery, with other segments of the spastic artery as well as the other coronary arteries remaining relatively unaffected (Fig. 23.4; see also Fig. 23.1). In some patients, however, coronary spasm is a generalized process that results in diffuse coronary artery narrowing, a finding that is more common in Japanese patients. The number of spastic obstructions in one artery or the number of arteries involved in the spastic process may vary dramatically from patient to patient. Coronary spasm usually involves a major artery or its large branches (lumen diameter $\geq$ 1.5 mm) and rarely affects the distal portions of the vessel. However, coronary microvascular spasm[42] has also been described, mainly in Japanese patients, and this may be responsible for at least some cases of variant angina, preferentially in women who present with both typical and prolonged anginal pain.[43]

In patients who have normal or mildly abnormal coronary arteriograms, a segment that is subtotally obstructed by spasm usually has a tapered appearance (see Fig. 23.4). The length of the spastic segment may vary from 2 mm to more than 2 cm. Severe coronary spasm may affect more than one coronary segment simultaneously. Multivessel spasm has been reported to occur in approximately 9% of cases and is more common in patients with angiographically normal coronaries or atheromatous stenoses of less than 50%.[44] Approximately 60% of patients with vasospastic angina have severe coronary artery disease, and the other 40% have normal or mildly abnormal coronary arteriograms. A higher proportion (60%) of normal coronary arteriograms has been reported in Japanese studies. Even when a coronary arteriogram can be considered normal, microscopic examination of the artery or intravascular ultrasonography may reveal underlying atherosclerotic disease. Intravascular ultrasonography has disclosed the presence of

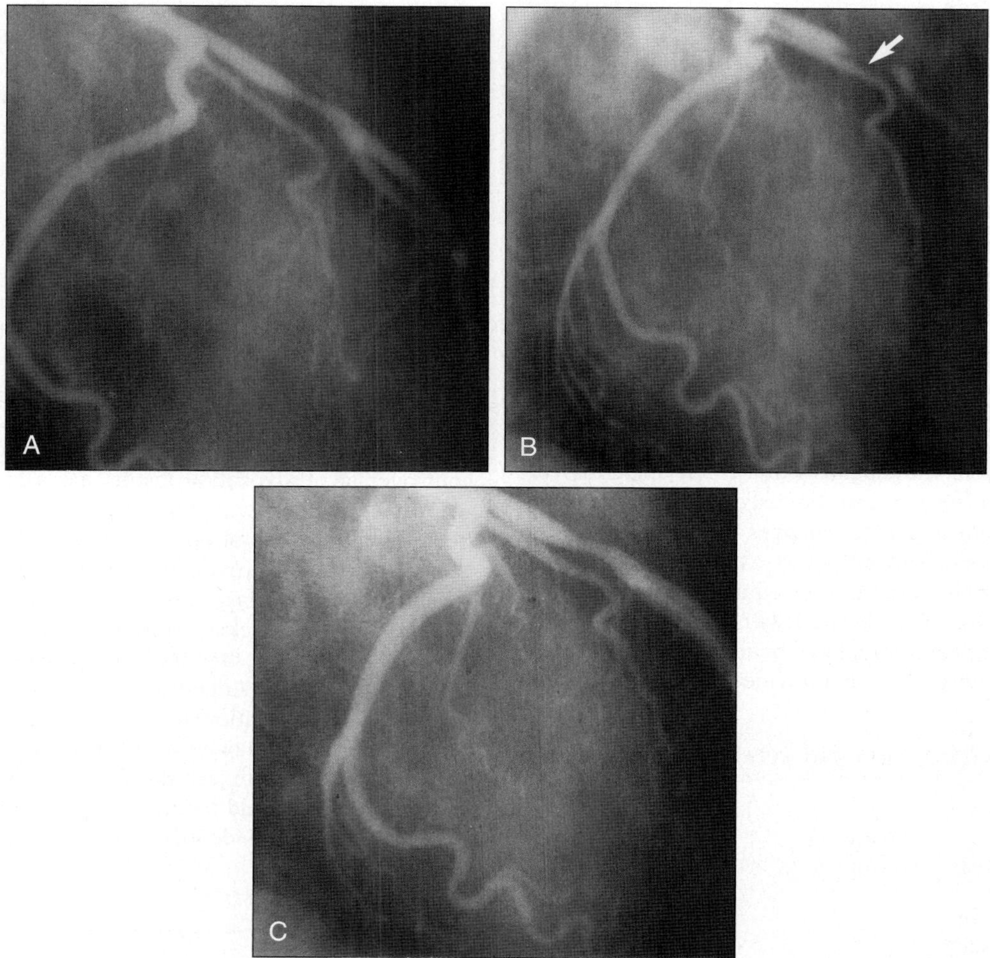

Figure 23.4 Characteristic appearance of focal coronary artery spasm occurring spontaneously during cardiac catheterization. These angiograms are from a patient who had symptoms typical of variant angina. **A**, Cardiac catheterization; baseline left coronary artery injection. **B**, Coronary artery spasm developed spontaneously at a site of a "smooth" fixed stenosis located in the midportion of the left anterior descending coronary artery *(arrow)*. **C**, The administration of intracoronary nitrates relieved coronary spasm but had no effect on the atheromatous narrowing.

diffuse intimal thickening in spastic coronary arteries, and this finding was independent of the presence or absence of traditional risk factors of coronary disease.[45]

Catheter-Induced Spasm

Catheter-induced spasm usually refers to coronary spasm caused by stimulation of the vessel wall by the catheter tip at angiography. It occurs more commonly in the proximal segment of the right coronary artery and is very rarely associated with chest pain or myocardial ischemia. On occasions in patients with variant angina, catheter stimulation of a coronary artery may precipitate spasm with angina and ST-segment elevation. However, catheter-induced coronary spasm is not a marker of disease activity in patients with variant angina. The clinical significance of catheter-induced coronary spasm is still largely unknown.

DIAGNOSTIC TECHNIQUES

In a sizeable proportion of patients, symptoms and ECG changes are typical and the diagnosis is straightforward. On most occasions, however, the diagnosis of coronary spasm is elusive and requires a high degree of suspicion (Table 23.2).

Exercise Testing and Ambulatory Electrocardiographic Monitoring

Although a proportion of patients have exercise-induced spasm, exercise treadmill testing is of limited diagnostic value in variant angina. Thallium Tl 201 scintigraphy combined with exercise stress seems to have a higher sensitivity than treadmill testing alone for detection of myocardial ischemia.[46] True silent or "clandestine" ischemia, defined as a normal result of exercise stress testing but with perfusion defects in the ^{201}Tl tomographic study, has been described in these patients but is uncommon.[47]

Prolonged (24 to 48 hours) ambulatory monitoring of the ST segment is an extremely valuable tool, particularly in patients with nocturnal angina episodes.

Provocation Testing

In patients in whom the diagnosis of variant angina is elusive, provocation testing can be used to reproduce the patient's chest pain and ECG changes (Fig. 23.5).[48] These tests should always be carried out by experienced personnel with the appropriate resuscitative equipment to minimize the obvious risk that is associated with the provocation of coronary spasm. Several tests have been used with different degrees of sensitivity. The ergonovine test is perhaps the most sensitive and specific.[49] A positive result is defined as the induction of spasm that replicates the patient's symptoms or associated ST-segment shifts. Although the ergonovine test is safe in experienced hands,[50] refractory spasm and life-threatening conduction disturbances may occur. Ergonovine has been administered safely under ECG and echocardiographic monitoring. The development of regional wall motion abnormalities due to transmural ischemia resulting from induced vasospasm can be detected by echocardiography before any ECG changes occur. However, the safety of ergonovine testing performed outside the catheterization laboratory has been questioned on the basis that it may be difficult to promptly reverse spasm by sublingual or intravenous nitrates as opposed to intracoronary nitrates. In a study of 1372 patients who had no evidence of significant obstructive coronary artery disease,[51] ischemia-independent side effects were seen in 0.9%. Sensitivity and specificity for the diagnosis of vasospasm, as assessed angiographically, were 93% and 91%, respectively. None of the patients died or developed myocardial infarction, but arrhythmias occurred in 1.9% of patients. Whether carried out in the catheterization laboratory or in the noninvasive setting, these tests should be carried out by trained personnel. Ergonovine should be administered gradually and the test promptly terminated when chest pain or ECG or echocardiographic abnormalities are detected. Intracoronary acetylcholine is also used as a provocative test of spasm, and this test has been reported to be sensitive and relatively safe (incidence of serious complications, 0.6%).[52] The hyperventilation test, 5 minutes of vigorous respirations, has a sensitivity and specificity of 62% and 100%, respectively. Compared with patients with a negative hyperventilation test result, those with a positive test result had a higher frequency of anginal attacks ($\geq$5 per week), multivessel spasm, and high-degree atrioventricular block or ventricular tachycardia during an attack.[53] The sensitivity of the hyperventilation test is higher when the test is performed in the early morning (from 6:00 AM to 8:00 AM), and it can also be performed in association with the cold pressor stress to increase its sensitivity further.[54]

The clinical role of provocation testing for coronary spasm is controversial. Provocation testing has a high sensitivity for identifying patients with clinically active vasospastic angina, but such patients can often be diagnosed clinically. However, the clinical role of provocation tests for diagnosis of a vasospasm etiology in a large population with undiagnosed chest pain syndromes is unclear. Moreover, it is not known whether altering therapy on the basis of provocation test results modifies prognosis. Adlam and coworkers[55] suggested that noninvasive provocation testing, such as ergonovine stress echocardiography, may be useful to rule out spasm in patients with intermediate clinical suspicion of variant angina, and invasive testing should be limited to patients with refractory vasospastic angina to identify a target for coronary stenting.[55]

DIAGNOSTIC TOOLS IN CORONARY ARTERY SPASM
Careful clinical history
24-hour ambulatory ECG monitoring
Provocation tests (e.g., with ergonovine, hyperventilation, or acetylcholine)
Exercise stress testing
Coronary angiography
The combination of typical chest pain at rest, transient ECG changes (usually ST-segment elevation), myocardial perfusion or wall motion abnormalities, and a preserved exercise capacity virtually confirm the diagnosis of coronary artery spasm.

Table 23.2 Diagnostic tools in coronary artery spasm.

MANAGEMENT

Acute Attacks

Coronary spasm can be a life-threatening condition, and physicians should bear in mind that attacks of variant angina are potentially lethal. Thus, treatment of acute episodes should be prompt and effective. Sublingual nitrate preparations are the agents of choice in ambulatory patients and usually relieve

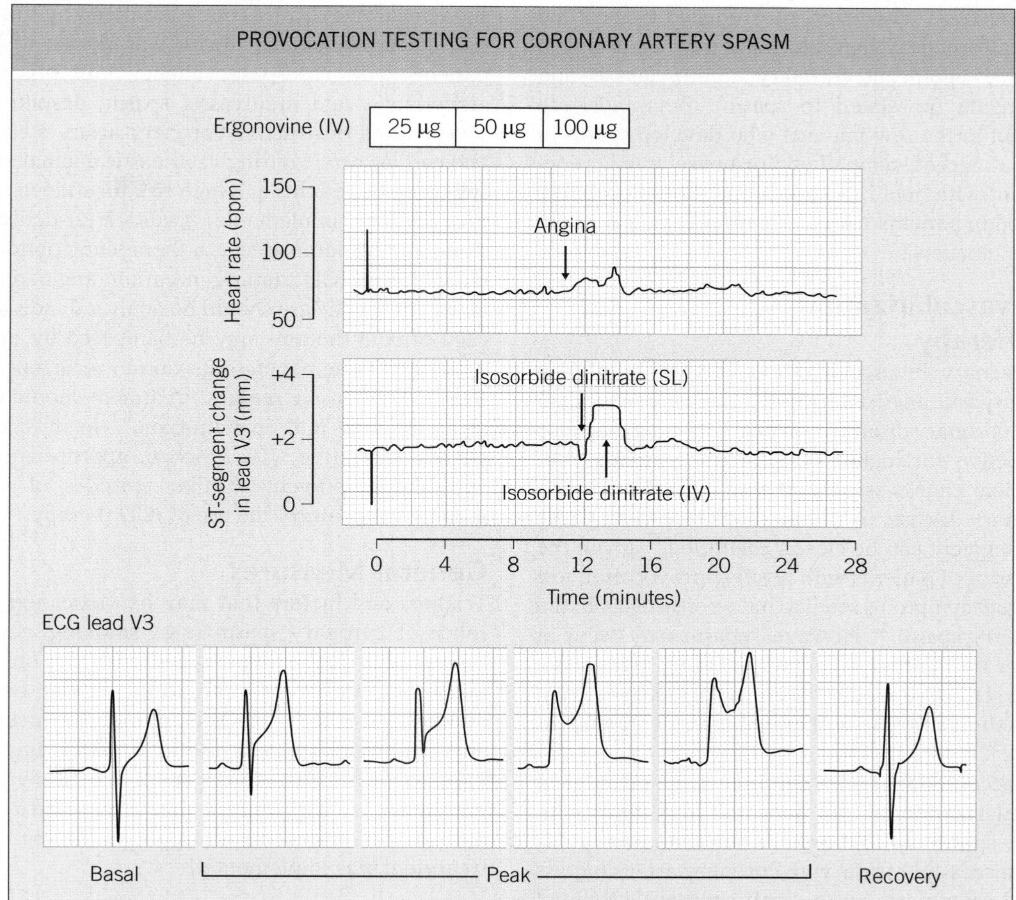

Figure 23.5 Provocation testing for coronary artery spasm. ST-segment elevation and chest pain developed in this patient during the administration of intravenous (IV) ergonovine. Both the typical ECG changes and the angina subsided after the administration of intravenous isosorbide dinitrate. SL, sublingual.

the chest pain and the ECG changes within minutes. Patients should be carefully instructed to use these agents promptly after the onset of chest pain. In patients who have frequent or prolonged episodes or spasm refractory to sublingual nitrates, admission to the hospital is required for ECG monitoring and the administration of intravenous nitroglycerin or isosorbide dinitrate. In the catheterization laboratory, intracoronary nitrate preparations can be used to relieve spasm that is refractory to conventional forms of nitrate administration.

Long-term Therapy to Prevent Attacks

Long-term therapy is aimed at reducing chest pain and preventing coronary spasm and associated myocardial ischemia, whether painful or silent, and also at reducing cardiac events (i.e., unstable angina, myocardial infarction, and death).

Calcium channel blockers and oral or buccal nitrates (and combinations of these) are effective long-term therapy. Calcium channel blockers are now considered to be the agents of choice in therapy for vasospastic angina. During the past 15 years, the efficacy of these agents has been well documented by numerous studies, including several randomized controlled trials. Newer sustained-release or long-acting formulations of calcium channel blockers are also effective.[56]

Calcium channel blockers and nitrates should be administered at doses that are clinically effective. High doses are usually required during the first 3 to 4 months of treatment. The dose can be individually titrated to minimize side effects and to avoid hypotension.

Treatment with α-receptor blockers may be of some benefit, especially in patients with an incomplete response to calcium channel blockers and nitrates.

Duration of Treatment

Serious cardiac events in patients with variant angina occur within the initial 3 to 6 months, and therefore therapy should be kept at a high dose at least during this period. Withdrawal from antianginal agents should be tailored to the individual. In patients who do not have serious arrhythmias or syncopal episodes during attacks, therapy may be discontinued gradually after a prolonged asymptomatic period of approximately 12 to 18 months. In patients who have refractory spasm or a troublesome symptom, therapy should be continued longer term. In every case, careful assessment of disease activity (i.e., by symptoms, Holter monitoring, nitrate consumption, provocation testing) is necessary before therapy is discontinued.

Beta Blockers and Coronary Spasm

Available data seem to indicate that beta blockade as sole therapy may be deleterious in patients with vasospastic angina, particularly in those who have normal coronary arteries or mild coronary atherosclerosis. However, the reduced myocardial oxygen demand afforded by beta blockade may be useful in patients who have significant coronary atherosclerosis and effort-induced angina (unrelated to spasm). Beta blockade may also be useful in the few patients who develop spasm in association with a marked sympathetic response or migraine. Even so, treatment with beta blockade alone should probably be contraindicated in patients with coronary spasm, especially nonselective beta blockers.

Coronary Revascularization and Brachytherapy

Percutaneous coronary revascularization may be helpful in patients with vasospastic angina if hemodynamically significant fixed obstructive coronary disease is present. Stenting may also be clinically effective for highly symptomatic patients with uncontrolled anginal attacks associated with mild to moderate obstructive coronary disease, in whom a localized vasospastic coronary artery segment can be clearly identified,[57] given the fact that the majority of patients with positive provocation test results and recurrent symptoms seem to have consistency in the location of coronary spasm.[58] However, spasm may recur at sites distinct from the treated segment, including multivessel spasm. Therefore, effective medical therapy including calcium channel blockers should not be withdrawn after percutaneous revascularization.[59]

It is generally accepted that both percutaneous and surgical coronary revascularization are not indicated in patients with isolated coronary spasm without organic coronary artery disease. However, successful results with coronary artery bypass grafting (internal mammary artery graft, without proximal ligation of the native coronary artery) have been reported in two patients with life-threatening refractory vasospastic angina with normal coronary arteries. Concerns have been raised, however, about the long-term internal mammary artery graft patency because of competitive flow.[60] Spasm occurring distal to the anastomosis or at the site of the internal mammary artery graft is also a potential problem.

High-dose intravascular beta irradiation, as used in intracoronary brachytherapy, can cause severe and prolonged coronary artery spasm.[61] In this setting, spasm may be due to acute radiation-induced endothelial dysfunction or the release of vasoconstrictive mediators from activated platelets or the endothelium. However, despite this immediate increase of vasoconstriction and spasm induced by brachytherapy, a loss of vasomotion several weeks after the application of the intracoronary irradiation may occur, suggesting the potential benefit of this technique in patients with refractory and highly symptomatic variant angina.[62] Despite the initial success of these preliminary studies, further trials are required to confirm the usefulness of this intervention in patients with variant angina pectoris.

Implantable Cardioverter-Defibrillator Therapy

Arrhythmias are a frequent finding during occlusive coronary vasospasm and may be life-threatening, that is, atrioventricular block (often associated with right coronary artery spasm) and life-threatening ventricular arrhythmias. However, despite improvements in clinical symptoms and prognosis with vasodilator therapy, the prevention of ventricular arrhythmias or sudden cardiac death is not guaranteed by this treatment. The risk of cardiac sudden death was shown to be increased in patients with vasospastic angina with syncope and serious arrhythmias and multivessel spasm, despite the absence of severe fixed obstructive coronary artery stenoses.[63] Syncope and cardiac arrest during vasospastic anginal attacks identify a subgroup of patients at a high risk for sudden cardiac death. In this setting, implantable cardioverter-defibrillators (ICDs) should be contemplated as a therapeutic option. However, the indication of ICD therapy in variant angina is not straightforward, and each case should be analyzed individually. The efficacy of ICD therapy may be hampered by the occurrence of prolonged ischemic episodes due to recurrent vasospasm, and therefore intensive medical treatment should be administered in addition to ICD implantation.[64] In most cases of variant angina presenting with syncope, appropriate treatment with vasodilators prevents further episodes of vasospasm, thus making unnecessary the use of ICD therapy.

General Measures

Triggers and factors that may be associated with the recurrence of coronary spasm (e.g., smoking, cocaine addiction, high alcohol intake, hypomagnesemia, use of serotonin uptake inhibitors, and hyperventilation) should be identified and avoided. In certain patients, avoidance of exposure to cold and emotional stress is useful in reducing the incidence of vasospastic attacks. A very small pilot study of 15 postmenopausal women with variant angina reported a decrease in anginal attacks induced by hyperventilation when estradiol treatment was implemented.[65]

Refractory Spasm

The term *refractory coronary spasm* implies that symptoms recur despite "optimal" therapy. However, as suggested by Conti,[66] both *refractoriness* and *optimal* are relative terms. Refractory coronary spasm may evolve toward myocardial infarction, sudden death, or recurrent postinfarction angina. The key to successful therapy for "refractory" patients lies in the identification of factors responsible for spasm. Associated "trigger" mechanisms (e.g., hyperventilation, use of drugs able to cause spasm, and exposure to cold) should be investigated. In some instances, rest angina and ST-segment elevation refractory to conventional variant angina treatment are noted in patients who have severe coronary artery stenosis. In these cases, it may be appropriate to act aggressively to reduce platelet aggregation and myocardial oxygen demand and to improve endothelial dysfunction.

Although various calcium channel blockers appear to have similar efficacy for treatment of variant angina, a combination of calcium channel blockers from different "families" is sometimes required for treatment of refractory forms of coronary spasm. In some patients, significant single-vessel coronary stenosis and recurrent coronary spasm at the stenotic segment may be successfully treated with percutaneous transluminal coronary angioplasty and stenting. However, the incidence of restenosis and acute reocclusion after angioplasty is higher in patients with vasospastic angina than in patients with typical exertional angina pectoris. Bypass surgery is very rarely effective in the treatment of variant angina, but the association of this procedure with sympathetic denervation (plexectomy) has been reported to be effective in refractory variant angina patients with significant coronary disease.[67] Brachytherapy is also an emerging possibility for prevention of recurrence of vasospasm in patients with highly symptomatic refractory variant angina.[62]

Recent Developments and Future Advances

Studies in vitro demonstrated that Rho and Rho kinase are involved not only in smooth muscle contraction but also in cell proliferation, differentiation, migration, and invasion. Moreover, regression of atherosclerosis has been reported in a porcine model with long-term inhibition of Rho kinase by fasudil.[68] It was recently found that fasudil, a Rho kinase inhibitor, dose dependently inhibited serotonin-induced coronary hypercontraction and enhanced myosin light chain phosphorylations in the spastic coronary segment in the interleukin-1β porcine model.[69] Fasudil was also effective in selectively preventing acetylcholine-induced coronary artery spasm and resultant myocardial ischemia in patients with vasospastic angina.[70] Compared with calcium channel blockers, this Rho kinase inhibitor may be a more suitable choice for patients with vasospastic angina because of its selective spasmolytic effect. Selective effects reducing calcium sensitivity in hyperreactive coronary segments may prevent vasospasm. Effective management of the condition requires a better understanding of the molecular mechanisms responsible for spasm.

PROGNOSIS

Prognosis is good in patients with variant angina and normal coronary arteriograms who respond to treatment with calcium channel blockers or nitrates. The incidence of acute myocardial infarction, malignant arrhythmias, and sudden death is extremely low in this patient cohort. In a large series of 277 patients with a median follow-up of 7.5 years, recurrent angina was common (39%), but cardiac death and myocardial infarction were relatively infrequent and occurred in 3.5% and 6.5% of patients, respectively.[71] Very often, infarction occurs in the first few months after diagnosis, and iatrogenic factors should be carefully investigated. Cardiac death in patients who have variant angina is often sudden, suggesting an arrhythmic origin that is most likely linked to acute myocardial ischemia. Patients with variant angina in whom serious arrhythmias develop during spontaneous episodes of pain have a higher risk of sudden death, and QT dispersion appears to be a marker of increased mortality risk.

Predictive factors of poorer outcome should be investigated in patients with variant angina and include coronary artery stenosis, risk factors of coronary disease (particularly smoking), and persistent or recurrent refractory spasm.[71] Variant angina patients with severe coronary artery disease are more likely to develop myocardial infarction. Interestingly, in these patients, the presence of severe stenoses increases the risk of myocardial infarction but not that of ventricular arrhythmias.[72]

Long-term follow-up studies have shown that episodes of variant angina may persist despite treatment with calcium channel blockers and nitrates. Persistent symptoms are associated with continuing to smoke, insufficient dosage of antianginal agents, and continuing exposure to triggers of spasm. Long-term remissions are also common and have been reported in as many as 60% to 80% of patients.

SUMMARY

Prinzmetal's variant angina is typically caused by focal coronary spasm, which characteristically triggers chest pain at rest and ST-segment elevation. Studies have shone light into the molecular mechanism of coronary vasospasm, which involves the RhoA and Rho kinase systems. Coronary spasm may develop in atheromatous segments but also in angiographically normal coronary segments. Triggers have been identified, and these should be specifically avoided. Calcium channel blockers and nitrates are useful for successful management of the patient. Although variant angina has a relatively good prognosis, prolonged coronary spasm may lead to myocardial infarction and sudden cardiac death.

chapter 24

Microvascular Angina Pectoris and Cardiac Syndrome X

Hans Erik Bøtker

Definition

- Cardiac syndrome X is characterized by angina pectoris caused by coronary microvascular dysfunction in patients who have nonstenotic epicardial arteries on coronary angiography.

Key Features

- Microvascular angina pectoris is most frequently secondary to cardiac or generalized diseases that impair the coronary microcirculation and provoke myocardial ischemia.
- Patients with cardiac syndrome X have angina pectoris and ischemia-like ST-segment depression during exercise stress testing in the absence of specific cardiac or generalized disease. Approximately 40% of patients have evidence of microvascular dysfunction, but the disorder is not restricted to a microvascular abnormality. Syndrome X is a heterogeneous disorder with various underlying mechanisms that involve both cardiac and noncardiac elements.

Therapy

- In patients who have microvascular angina pectoris secondary to a specific cardiac or generalized disorder, therapy is directed toward the underlying disease.
- An attempt must be made to classify patients who have cardiac syndrome X according to the underlying pathophysiologic process so that therapy can be instituted on rational grounds.

Between 10% and 30% of patients who undergo coronary angiography because of angina pectoris have normal-appearing epicardial coronary arteries on angiography. Patients who have persistent angina pectoris and normal findings on coronary angiography may benefit from additional diagnostic procedures that are able to demonstrate disturbances of the microcirculation because these abnormalities are accessible for treatment in some cases. Disturbances of the microcirculation are frequently secondary to specific heart diseases or to generalized disorders that affect the coronary circulation. The disturbances may also be manifested without concomitant diseases, as occurs in patients who have cardiac syndrome X.

Cardiac syndrome X is characterized by angina pectoris, ST-segment depression suggestive of myocardial ischemia during stress testing, and normal coronary angiograms. The entity has been considered equivalent to microvascular angina because of the microcirculatory disturbances demonstrated in some of the patients. However, the cardiac syndrome X is not restricted to a microvascular disease. Rather, it is a heterogeneous disorder with various underlying mechanisms.

ANATOMY AND PHYSIOLOGY

The microvascular bed consists of a proximal and a distal compartment. The proximal compartment is composed of the prearterioles interposed between the large conduit arteries; the distal compartment is composed of the arterioles and the capillaries. The main function of the prearterioles is to maintain optimal perfusion pressure at the origin of the arterioles. This is achieved by constriction of the prearterioles when aortic pressure increases and relaxation when aortic pressure decreases. The responsible mechanisms are neural, humoral, and local vasoactive factors. Prearterioles are extensively innervated by sympathetic nervous fibers.

In contrast, arterioles, which have a diameter of 100 μm or less, are sparsely innervated. Their muscle fibers are controlled almost entirely by the local humoral environment, in particular the concentration of oxygen. The function of the arterioles is to regulate blood flow at the capillary level and to ensure optimum equilibrium between the supply of nutrients and the washout of waste products.

Through these microvascular mechanisms, coronary blood flow is regulated almost exactly in proportion to the need of the myocardium for oxygen, which is closely related to cardiac work. The mechanisms ensure coronary autoregulation, which maintains coronary flow over a wide range of perfusion pressures (Fig. 24.1).

In the absence of coronary stenosis, the contribution of the large epicardial arteries to coronary resistance is negligible compared with that of the microvascular component. In healthy subjects, the microvasculature allows an increment of myocardial blood flow between three and six times its basal level. The amount by which coronary blood flow increases in response to maximal arteriolar dilatation is defined as the coronary flow reserve and reflects the vasodilator capacity of the heart (see Fig. 24.1). Age, sex, heart rate, and blood pressure affect the magnitude of the coronary flow reserve.[1] However, as illustrated in Figure 24.1, the coronary flow reserve does not result from a simple one-dimensional comparison of two flow values; rather, it results from the area limited by the pressure-flow relationships that occur in the presence and in the absence of arteriolar tone.

PATHOPHYSIOLOGY

A reduction in the cardiac vasodilator capacity may cause inadequate coronary blood flow in relation to the metabolic demand of the heart. Several factors can reduce blood flow

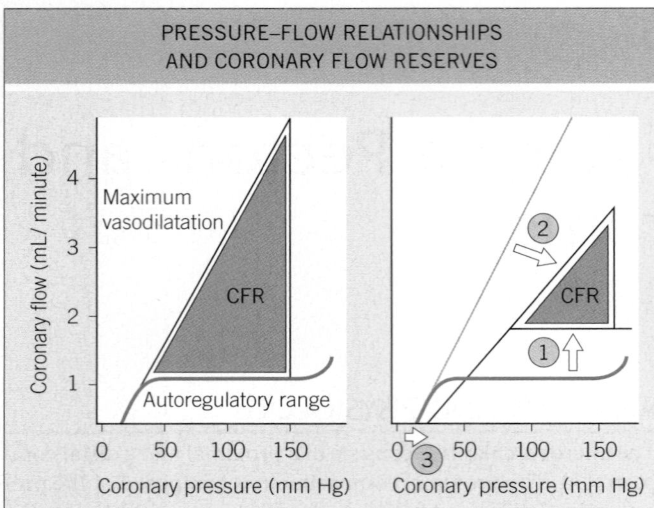

Figure 24.1 Pressure-flow relationships. The coronary flow reserve (CFR) is the amount by which coronary flow increases in response to maximal arteriolar dilatation; it is dependent on blood pressure. Mechanisms for reduction of the coronary flow reserve: 1, upward shift of autoregulation curve, as in conditions with an increase in metabolic demand; 2, decreased slope in the absence of arteriolar tone; and 3, increase in the pressure value at zero flow (i.e., the critical closing pressure) with vascular abnormalities.

at the microvascular level (Table 24.1). These abnormalities are frequently secondary to specific cardiac or generalized vascular or nonvascular diseases, among which the most common are arterial hypertension, valvular diseases, cardiomyopathies, and diabetes mellitus. Frequently, the impairment of the coronary flow reserve is not caused by a single mechanism in these disorders but involves both vascular and myocardial components. In arterial hypertension, medial wall thickening is considered to be the most important mechanism for microvascular dysfunction because angina pectoris and the impairment of the coronary flow reserve can be present in the absence of myocardial hypertrophy.[2] On the other hand, aortic stenosis with ventricular enlargement and dilatation results in increased wall tension such that the myocardial component reduces coronary flow reserve.[2]

The underlying pathophysiologic mechanism of cardiac syndrome X has not been established. The syndrome is heterogeneous by nature and contains both cardiac and noncardiac components. One unifying mechanism cannot be identified in all patients. Even though the coronary arteries appear smooth and nonstenotic on the coronary angiogram, intracoronary ultrasound studies have revealed that the coronary arteries may exhibit atheromatous disease and intimal thickening in up to 60% of the patients.[3] These morphologic abnormalities may affect coronary vasomotion.[3] It has been hypothesized that epicardial disease may underlie insufficient release of endothelium-derived relaxing factor and attenuated dilatation at the prearteriolar level in some patients who have syndrome X.[4]

Approximately 40% of patients with syndrome X have an abnormally reduced capacity to increase coronary flow in response to stimuli such as exercise, atrial pacing, and pharmacologic vasodilatation.[5] The abnormality is evident as slow coronary flow on coronary angiography in a subset of patients.[6] Skin capillary rarefaction has been demonstrated in patients with syndrome X,[7] but no morphologic abnormalities are found in the coronary microcirculatory vessels, so the disturbance is considered to be functional.[8] Several mechanisms have been suggested to account for this abnormality (Table 24.2). The link between coronary microvascular dysfunction and myocardial ischemia is attractive. Even though evidence for myocardial ischemia in terms of metabolic and functional consequences of the reduced coronary flow reserve may not be demonstrable in the majority of patients with syndrome X by many methods, positron emission tomography,[9] nuclear magnetic resonance spectroscopy, and magnetic resonance imaging indicate that heterogeneity of perfusion may lead to patchily distributed ischemia[10] rather than subendocardial ischemia.[11]

SOURCES OF DISTURBED CORONARY MICROCIRCULATION
Vascular abnormalities
Hypertrophy of the tunica media, remodeling and dysplasia of arterioles
Arterial hypertension
Hypertrophic cardiomyopathy
Diabetic microangiopathy
Inadequate growth of microvessels in relation to hypertrophied myocytes
Hypertrophic and dilated cardiomyopathy
Insudation and accumulation of proteins in the vascular wall
Amyloidosis
Immunocomplex diseases
Endothelial dysfunction of the coronary microcirculation
Myocardial abnormalities
Hypertrophy of myocytes
Arterial hypertension
Aortic stenosis
Hypertrophic cardiomyopathy
Abnormal composition of the myocardium
Deposit disorders
Infiltrating interstitial processes
Collagen
Amyloidosis
Parasitosis
Inflammatory processes
Vasculitis
Myocarditis
Metabolic abnormalities
Increased oxygen consumption
Increased ventricular wall stress
Hyperthyroidism
Rheologic abnormalities
Increased blood viscosity
Paraproteinemia
Polyglobulia and polycythemia
Hyperlipidemia

Table 24.1 Sources of disturbed coronary microcirculation.

MECHANISMS THAT CONTRIBUTE TO A REDUCED CORONARY FLOW RESERVE IN CARDIAC SYNDROME X
Mechanisms with demonstrated myocardial ischemia
Microvascular spasm Endothelial dysfunction
Mechanisms not necessarily associated with myocardial ischemia
Endothelial dysfunction Coronary artery hyperreactivity Increased circulating endogenous vasoconstrictor peptides Estrogen deficiency Increased adrenergic tone Prearteriolar constriction and patchy release of adenosine Abnormal interstitial release of potassium Increased pain perception

Table 24.2 Mechanisms that contribute to a reduced coronary flow reserve in cardiac syndrome X.

However, mechanisms other than ischemia may be responsible for the symptoms in a considerable number of cases, and two mechanisms validate cardiac causes of nonischemic angina pectoris in patients who have cardiac syndrome X. A patchy prearteriolar constriction may lead to compensatory release of adenosine, which mediates coronary arteriolar dilatation by stimulating adenosine A_2 receptors to ensure adequate perfusion in these areas (Fig. 24.2).[4] Because adenosine also acts as a pain messenger, the resulting increase in adenosine concentrations in the myocardial interstitium causes pain by stimulation of adenosine A_1 receptors. Interstitial adenosine accumulation may also induce ST-segment changes by shortening the action potential of the myocytes and by negative chronotropic effects.

The other mechanism that may cause angina pectoris and ST-segment changes in the absence of ischemia involves interstitial accumulation of potassium caused by abnormalities in potassium metabolism. Patients who have cardiac syndrome X have excessive potassium efflux from skeletal muscle during exercise.[12] These findings may account for the high prevalence of generalized fatigue in the skeletal muscles of these patients. Also, potassium acts as a pain messenger when it is retained in the myocardial interstitium. Because potassium also modifies systemic and coronary vasoreactivity, the myocardial accumulation of potassium may account for all of the features of cardiac syndrome X, including angina pectoris, ST-segment changes, reduced coronary flow reserve (in some cases), and a good prognosis. This abnormality may be linked to the adenosine abnormality because adenosine alters potassium flux.

Angina-like chest pain involves noncardiac mechanisms, including behavioral or psychiatric disorders, esophageal pain, and musculoskeletal diseases.[13] Abnormal handling of afferent messages from the heart by the central nervous system has been recognized in patients who have syndrome X. Frontal lobe activation is necessary for the sensation of pain in patients who have classic coronary artery disease and in patients who have syndrome X, but patients with syndrome X also have activation of the right insula.[14] This cortical cerebral region may be the substrate of abnormal visceral pain perception.

CLINICAL PRESENTATION

Angina pectoris caused by microvascular dysfunction is manifested as chronic stable angina pectoris, which is comparable to angina pectoris caused by epicardial coronary stenosis.

In contrast to angina pectoris secondary to classic coronary artery disease, syndrome X is characterized by 70% to 80% of the patients being women.[15] The age at onset is similar in patients with syndrome X and patients with coronary atherosclerosis. The anginal attacks may be of prolonged duration and with a poor response to sublingual nitrates. Traditional prophylactic antianginal medication is often insufficient in syndrome X. In addition to angina pectoris, many patients suffer from generalized fatigue in skeletal muscles.[16] The symptoms are similar to those seen in patients who have fibromyalgia.

Risk factors such as hyperlipidemia and insulin resistance are more frequent in patients with syndrome X than in healthy control subjects.[17] Confusion about syndrome X has been created on terminologic grounds because a metabolic entity characterized by obesity, dyslipidemia, insulin resistance, and arterial hypertension has also been termed syndrome X. The two X syndromes must be clearly separated, and metabolic syndrome X is now preferentially called the insulin resistance syndrome.

Panic disorders, anxiety neuroses, and neuroticism are encountered with a more than average frequency in patients who have syndrome X and are considered to be important components of the syndrome. An abnormal psychiatric background may help explain the enhanced sensitivity to pain and the unjustified anxiety about prognosis. Organic and psychological mechanisms of pain production overlap and interact. It is not always possible to clarify whether a primary psychological disturbance initiated the chest pain syndrome, but abnormal beliefs and illness worries can act as maintaining factors. For this reason, it is important to look for evidence of psychiatric disorder or abnormal psychological processes and to address them early.

DIAGNOSTIC TECHNIQUES

Additional diagnostic procedures are essential in patients who have persistent angina pectoris and normal coronary angiograms

- to establish the diagnosis;
- to clarify whether the symptoms are part of a cardiac disorder or a generalized disorder, which has therapeutic consequences; and
- to clarify whether the patient has microvascular dysfunction.

Before these procedures are undertaken, make sure that the coronary angiograms are of excellent quality and that they contain multiple and angulated views so that the question of "missed" significant coronary artery disease can be eliminated.

A thorough medical history and clinical examination are of importance because they will frequently point toward the diagnosis of generalized disorders that affect the coronary microcirculation. In addition, an exercise stress test is required to clarify whether ST-segment depression is present. Epicardial spasms must be excluded by provocative spasm tests, such as the hyperventilatory test or intracoronary injection of acetylcholine or ergonovine during angiography.

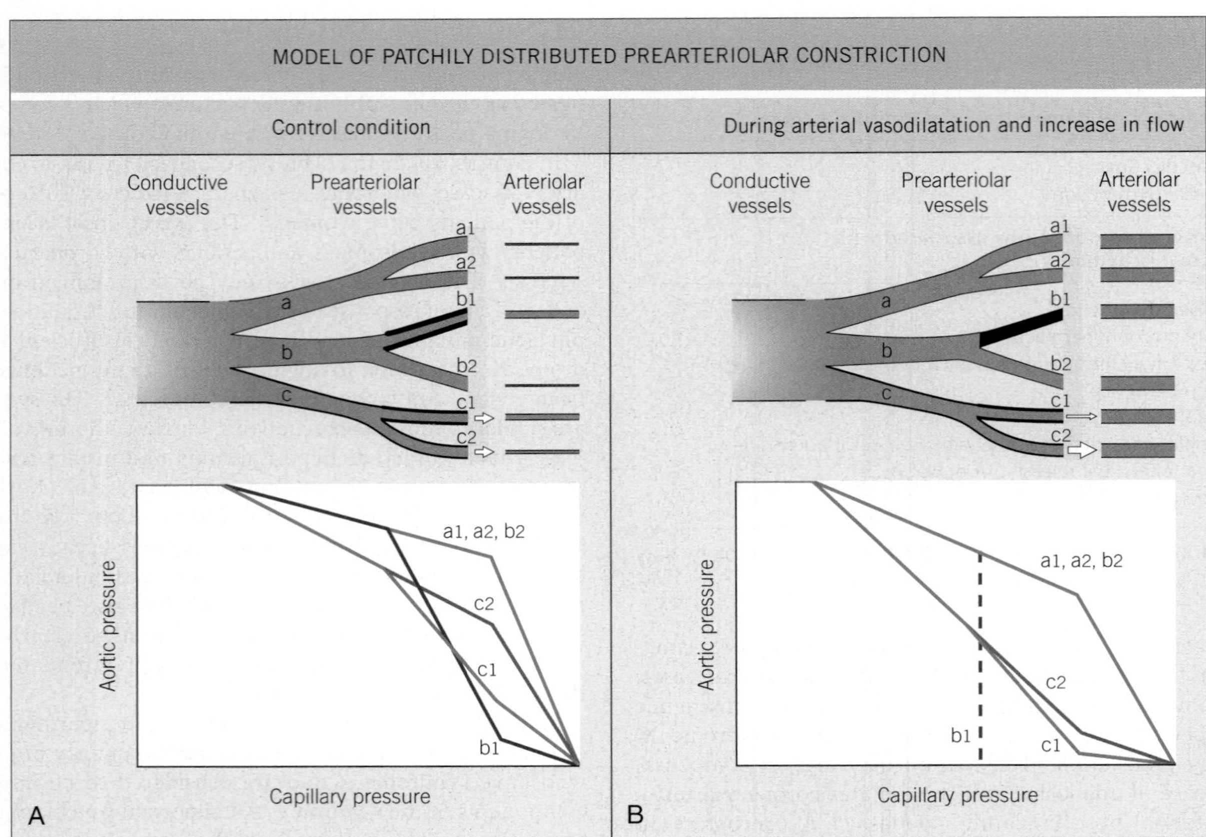

Figure 24.2 Model of patchily distributed prearteriolar constriction. A, Control condition, during which conduit coronary arteries have no significant flow resistance and the pressure in the conduit artery remains identical to the aortic pressure. Across the prearterioles, the pressure decreases progressively in proportion to their degree of constriction. The major pressure drop across the resistance vessels usually takes place in the arterioles (a1, a2, b2). In cases with prearteriolar constriction, significant pressure drop is moved from the arterioles to the prearterioles (b1, c1, c2). **B,** During arteriolar vasodilatation and increase in flow, such as with metabolic (exercise) or pharmacologic (dipyridamole) stimuli. The vasodilatory reserve of the arterioles distal to the constricted prearterioles is reduced because the arterioles are already dilated to preserve resting flow. The coronary arteriolar dilatation is mediated by compensatory release of adenosine. During metabolic or pharmacologic arteriolar vasodilatation, the pressure drop across the prearterioles increases only slightly because vasodilatation of the prearterioles compensates almost completely for the increased flow (a1, a2, b2). In cases with constricted prearterioles, the pressure drop across the prearterioles will increase because no vasodilatation is generated (b1, c1, c2). The pressure drop increases in proportion to basal prearteriolar constriction. Steal can develop when an increase in flow through c2 causes a pressure decrease at the branching point distal to the constricted segment c, so that the driving pressure becomes insufficient to perfuse the most constricted branch, c1, adequately. Consequently, blood flow (indicated by arrows) can decrease compared with the basal condition. At the end of the prearteriole with the most marked constriction (b1), intravascular pressure may become insufficient to maintain lumen patency, resulting in vessel collapse. (Modified from Maseri A, Crea F, Kaski JC, Crake T. Mechanisms of angina pectoris in syndrome X. J Am Coll Cardiol 1991;17:499-506, with permission from the American College of Cardiology.)

Echocardiography can clarify whether specific cardiac diseases, such as valvular disease, cardiomyopathies, deposit diseases, and pericardial diseases, are present.

The demonstration of a microvascular dysfunction relies on measurement of the coronary flow reserve. Evidence of myocardial ischemia is not necessarily required because microvascular abnormalities may be responsible for angina pectoris in the absence of ischemia. Three coronary vasodilator compounds are currently used in humans to achieve maximal coronary vasodilatation: dipyridamole, papaverine, and adenosine. Dipyridamole is administered intravenously, adenosine can be administered either intravenously or into the coronary arteries, and papaverine has to be injected into the coronary arteries. Dipyridamole administration reveals a higher frequency of abnormal coronary flow reserve than adenosine and papaverine do.

The coronary flow reserve can be measured by invasive and noninvasive techniques. Intracoronary Doppler measurements, intracoronary thermodilution, and positron emission tomography can be used for measurement of coronary flow reserve in patients who have syndrome X. A coronary flow reserve of less than 2.5 is most frequently considered abnormal.

Doppler catheters or thermodilution wires placed in the coronary arteries well beyond their origin from the aorta can measure mean coronary flow velocities in individual vessels. The catheter and wire sizes are small and do not limit the flow in the major coronary arteries. Pharmacologic agents used for the determination of coronary flow reserve may influence epicardial diameter directly. In addition, the diameter of epicardial vessels may increase through an endothelium-mediated mechanism when flow velocity increases. This phenomenon can be prevented by nitroglycerin-induced dilatation of coronary vessels before measurements are made.

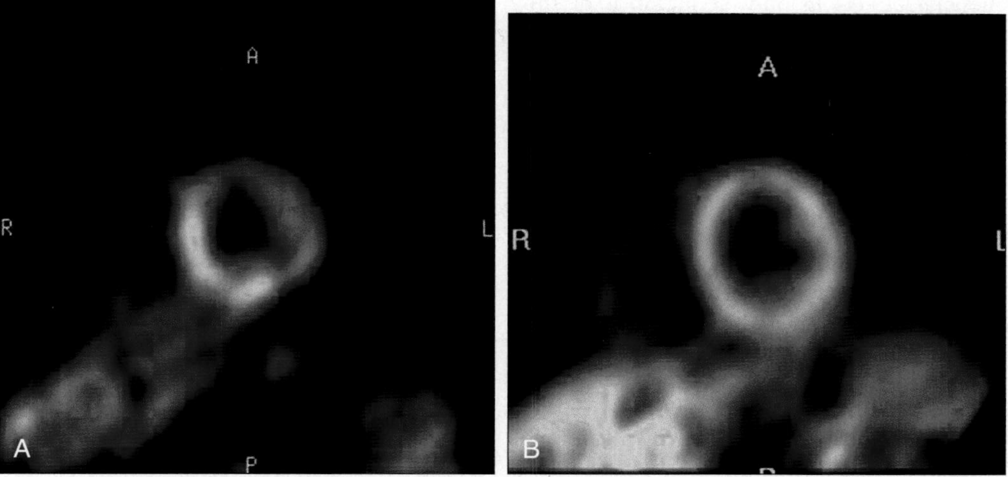

Figure 24.3 A, Heterogeneity of myocardial perfusion in a patient with syndrome X studied with positron emission tomography and [^{13}N]ammonia as perfusion tracer. **B,** Healthy control subject with homogeneous myocardial perfusion shown for comparison. A, anterior; R, right; L, left; P, posterior.

Myocardial blood flow can be quantified noninvasively with positron emission tomography using perfusion markers such as [^{13}N]ammonia, rubidium Rb 82, and [^{15}O]water. Tracer kinetic models describing the myocardial kinetics of [^{13}N]-ammonia have been established. In the case of syndrome X, positron emission tomography can be used for semiquantitative purposes to clarify whether a patient has a heterogeneous distribution of blood flow in the heart (Fig 24.3) and for quantitative purposes to measure the magnitude of coronary flow reserve. Most recently, noninvasive evaluation of coronary flow reserve by echocardiography and pulse-wave Doppler study of peak diastolic left anterior descending flow has been shown to provide reliable information on the severity of microvascular impairment in patients with syndrome X.[18]

Myocardial perfusion scintigraphy may show regional perfusion defects during exercise stress testing in patients who have syndrome X. The highest percentage is observed with thallium Tl 201 scintigraphy, by which up to 98% of the patients have detectable perfusion defects.[19] This is in contrast to positron emission tomography, by which these findings are inconsistently described. The discrepancy may be explained by the fact that ^{201}Tl is a potassium analogue. The abnormalities observed with thallium may reflect abnormalities in myocardial potassium handling rather than flow disturbances.

TREATMENT STRATEGIES FOR CARDIAC SYNDROME X
Traditional antianginal medication
Nitrates
Beta blockers
Calcium channel blockers
Unconventional medical treatment
Aminophylline
α_1-Adrenoceptor blockers
Angiotensin-converting enzyme inhibitors
17β-estradiol
Imipramine
Analgesics
Nonmedical treatment
Spinal cord stimulation
Thoracic sympathectomy

Table 24.3 Treatment strategies for cardiac syndrome X.

MANAGEMENT

In patients who have microvascular dysfunction secondary to specific cardiac or generalized disease, the goal is treatment of the underlying disease because the cardiac symptoms and the microvascular dysfunction are often reversible.[2] If treatment of the primary disease is not possible or is insufficient, treatment with traditional antianginal drugs should be undertaken.

In patients who have cardiac syndrome X, rational therapy relies on the demonstration of the pathogenetic mechanism. Until progress is made in subclassification of the patients according to the underlying mechanisms, the clinical approach must be empiric and individualized (Table 24.3). Because the prognosis is good, the goal of therapy is a reduction in the frequency and the severity of pain. Common to all patients who have normal ventricular function and absence of left bundle branch block is that the cornerstone of therapy remains reassurance. The need for hospitalization is reduced when a diagnostic angiogram reveals normal coronary arteries.[20] For many patients, reassurance helps them to bear the pain, but a substantial number need additional medical therapy, which may be difficult to accomplish because the efficacy is less than in angina pectoris caused by classic coronary artery disease. Thus, treatment of patients who have cardiac syndrome X must be based on a good physician-patient relationship. It requires not only great patience but also time.

Nitrates

Nitrates dilate large epicardial coronary arteries but influence the microvasculature to a limited extent. In contrast to patients with flow-limiting epicardial coronary stenoses, nitrates have beneficial effects in only about 50% of the patients and may even have adverse effects in some patients during exercise stress testing.[21] Clinical experience indicates that patients who have pain relief by sublingual nitroglycerin usually benefit from nitrate preparations with prolonged duration, but no trials have been conducted on the chronic administration of nitrates in patients who have syndrome X.

Beta Blockers

Beta blockers produce improvement in exercise-induced angina pectoris in patients who have evidence of enhanced sympathetic tone[21] that can be detected by a rapid increase in rate-pressure product during exercise stress testing.

Calcium Channel Blockers

A reduction in attacks of angina has been detected with verapamil as well as with nifedipine. These agents are recommended for patients who have no evidence of enhanced sympathetic activity.

Aminophylline

Treatment with aminophylline is a rational treatment for patients who have abnormal adenosine metabolism. Unfortunately, no specific test allows identification of this subgroup. Some indication of abnormal adenosine metabolism or disturbed effects of adenosine on coronary vasodilatation may be obtained from information about impairment of coronary flow reserve with use of dipyridamole or adenosine as a vasodilator. Several studies have demonstrated that aminophylline may have beneficial effects on angina pectoris in patients who have syndrome X. Because discrepancy between the anginal symptoms and the ST-segment depression exists in some studies,[22] the mode of action may be an analgesic effect mediated through blockade of the adenosine A_1 receptors.

α_1-Adrenoceptor Blockers

Doxazosin increases the coronary flow reserve in patients who have cardiac syndrome X, but neither doxazosin nor prazosin has demonstrated an effect on angina pectoris in patients.

Angiotensin-Converting Enzyme Inhibitors

Enalapril may improve effort tolerance in patients who have syndrome X.

Estrogen

Like aminophylline, 17β-estradiol has beneficial influence on exercise-induced angina pectoris but no effect on ST-segment depression in women who have syndrome X. The mechanism of action may be an analgesic effect. Estrogen is recommended for postmenopausal women who have syndrome X.[23]

Imipramine

Imipramine is a tricyclic antidepressant that reduces the sensitivity to pain through mechanisms in the central nervous system. Imipramine reduces anginal episodes in patients who have normal coronary angiograms irrespective of the presence of ST-segment depression, psychological state, gastrointestinal disorders, and musculoskeletal disorders.[24] Side effects are not quite negligible. The most frequent is sedation, but tachycardia, arrhythmia, and prolongation of atrioventricular conduction time are also seen. The drug is recommended for patients for whom other agents are without effect.

Analgesics

Non-narcotic analgesics may be used in patients who have cardiac syndrome X, but their efficacy is usually insufficient. Owing to addiction and because the disorder has a good prognosis, narcotic analgesic agents should be used infrequently for pronounced anginal attacks that are not relieved by other treatment.

Other Treatments

Spinal cord stimulation reduces exercise-induced angina in patients who have syndrome X. The long-term effect is unknown. Because the efficacy appears to decrease with time after implantation, the device should be offered only to selected patients. Thoracic sympathectomy has been used in a few patients. The experiences are too few to allow general recommendations. Patients with syndrome X benefit from physical training in terms of exercise capacity and quality of life[25] and should be highly advised to avoid a sedentary lifestyle.

PROGNOSIS

The prognosis of microvascular angina in cardiac and generalized diseases is entirely dependent on the primary disease.

The prognosis of patients who have cardiac syndrome X is good with regard to mortality and incidence of myocardial infarction. Patients who have evidence of ischemia by ST-segment depression have the same benign prognosis as the larger group of patients who have angina and normal coronary arteries in the absence of ST-segment depression (Fig. 24.4). In contrast to this benign somatic prognosis, the social prognosis is poor in many patients, who suffer from persistent anginal symptoms and a poor response to available medical therapy. The associated anxiety is only temporarily relieved by reassurance. Studies suggest, however, that some patients[26,27] and in particular those with a previous myocardial infarction[28] despite normal coronary angiograms may have coronary atherosclerosis to an extent that may compromise prognosis. These patients should be treated with conventional risk-modifying medication including antithrombotic and lipid-lowering drugs.

A small subgroup of patients initially classified as having syndrome X may experience deterioration in left ventricular function over time. These patients often present with left bundle branch block at rest or during exercise stress testing. In contrast to most patients without left bundle branch block, patients who have left bundle branch block demonstrate myocardial ischemia by myocardial lactate production

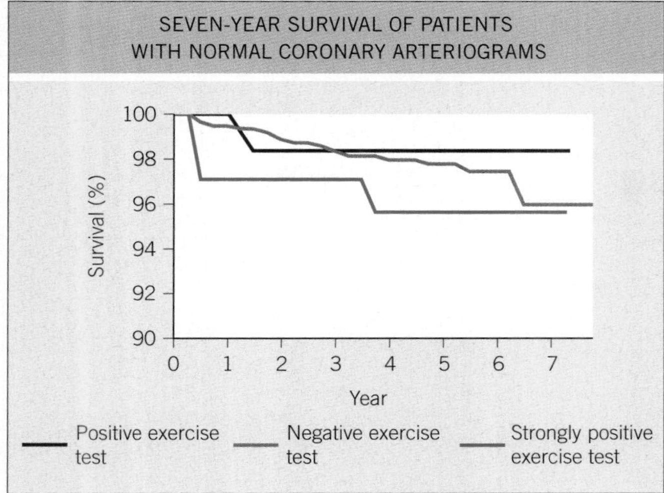

Figure 24.4 Seven-year survival of patients with normal coronary arteriograms. Negative, positive, and strongly positive exercise test results are compared. (Modified from Kemp HG, Kronmal RA, Vlietstra RE, Frye RL; the Coronary Artery Surgery Study [CASS] participants. Seven year survival of patients with normal or near normal coronary angiograms. A CASS registry study. J Am Coll Cardiol 1986;7:479-483, with permission from the American College of Cardiology.)

during rapid atrial pacing. These patients are considered to be suffering from an early form of cardiomyopathy.

SUMMARY

Microvascular dysfunction may cause angina pectoris in a number of cardiac and generalized disease states because a reduced coronary flow reserve leads to myocardial ischemia. Treatment of the underlying disease is the first step in therapy. Cardiac syndrome X has been considered to be a "primary form" of microvascular angina. The entity may include microvascular abnormalities, but it also involves abnormalities in central processing of afferent pain messages from the heart. It is important to recognize cardiac syndrome X because it leads to human discomfort and consumes medical resources, rather than because it carries a poor prognosis. Treatment is difficult because the importance of each of several underlying mechanisms varies between patients and may even be unknown in some cases. Careful classification according to these mechanisms is a major goal for establishing rational therapy. We must avoid disregarding these patients because of our own ignorance about the condition and inability to provide rational therapy.

chapter 25

Asymptomatic Myocardial Ischemia

Prakash C. Deedwania

Definition

- Asymptomatic myocardial ischemia is the objective evidence of myocardial ischemia (as inferred from transient ECG changes) in the absence of chest pain or other anginal equivalents.

Key Features

- Asymptomatic ischemia can be encountered in asymptomatic patients with no known coronary artery disease and in patients with coronary artery disease.
- Asymptomatic ischemia is the most prevalent form of myocardial ischemia that occurs during routine daily activities in patients with known coronary artery disease.
- Asymptomatic ischemia frequently occurs despite control of anginal symptoms with medical treatment.
- Most episodes result from an increase in myocardial oxygen demand.
- The presence of ischemia, regardless of associated symptoms, is associated with adverse prognosis and poor clinical outcome.

Therapy

- Although all antianginal drugs are useful, treatment with beta blockers is most effective in suppressing asymptomatic ischemia.

Myocardial ischemia is generally accepted as a common expression of coronary artery disease (CAD), and angina has been considered the hallmark symptom of CAD and myocardial ischemia. Studies suggest, however, that angina is a relatively insensitive and nonspecific predictor of significant CAD.[1] Furthermore, it has been shown that a lack of anginal symptoms does not imply the absence of severe and potentially lethal coronary stenosis. Even in patients who have significant CAD, the absence of angina does not predict benign prognosis.[2] Moreover, the severity of anginal symptoms does not correlate well with the extent of CAD or long-term prognosis (Fig. 25.1).[3] Ambulatory electrocardiographic monitoring (AEM) in patients with angina pectoris and stable CAD has demonstrated frequent episodes of asymptomatic ischemia during daily life.[4] Asymptomatic myocardial ischemia is defined as the presence of ST-segment depression without associated chest pain. The presence of myocardial perfusion abnormalities during episodes of ST-segment depression recorded on AEM provides strong evidence of the ischemic nature of the ST-segment changes.[4]

It is estimated that as many as 9 million Americans have chronic CAD, and of these, 4 to 5 million might have asymptomatic ischemia. Several studies have shown that asymptomatic ischemia occurs frequently (Fig. 25.2), despite control of symptoms,[5,6] and the presence of such residual asymptomatic ischemia is associated with an adverse clinical outcome and increased risk of death.[7] Advanced obstructive CAD may exist with minimal or no symptoms and can progress rapidly, leading to myocardial infarction or death with little warning. In some cases, sudden death may be the initial manifestation of CAD,[8] and it has been estimated that 18% of coronary events occur with sudden death as the first event[8]; more than 50% of sudden cardiac deaths occur without a previous history of CAD. Detection of myocardial ischemia during exercise testing in asymptomatic people has been shown to predict a greater risk of subsequent coronary events and death.[9]

Traditionally, management of patients who have CAD has consisted of treatment prescribed for the control of symptoms; however, recent data suggest that this strategy does not abolish all ischemic events. As many as 40% of patients with stable angina who are treated with one or more antianginal drugs have episodes of asymptomatic ischemia during daily life (Fig. 25.3).[5,6] In various subsets of patients with CAD, the presence of residual asymptomatic ischemia regardless of the presence or absence of associated symptoms has been shown to predict a greater risk of coronary events and cardiac death.[7]

PATHOPHYSIOLOGY

Myocardial ischemia generally develops as a result of an imbalance between coronary blood flow and myocardial oxygen demand. In the presence of fixed obstructive lesions of the coronary arteries, there may be an insufficient increase in the coronary blood flow or maldistribution of flow during periods of increased demand due to limited coronary reserve. The coronary flow may also be reduced as a result of heightened vasomotor tone at the site of an occlusive plaque. The area of a coronary artery that is affected by an atherosclerotic plaque is particularly susceptible to vasospasm because of the associated endothelial dysfunction and reduced bioavailability of nitric oxide in response to vasodilatory stimuli. Additional factors that may play a part in reducing the coronary blood flow include platelet aggregation and transient clot formation with partial occlusion at the site of an atherosclerotic plaque, which tend to develop fissures or fractures during periods of increased stress.

Although the pathophysiologic process responsible for the genesis of asymptomatic ischemic episodes used to be not well understood, studies have provided considerable insight. Earlier studies suggested that a reduction in coronary blood

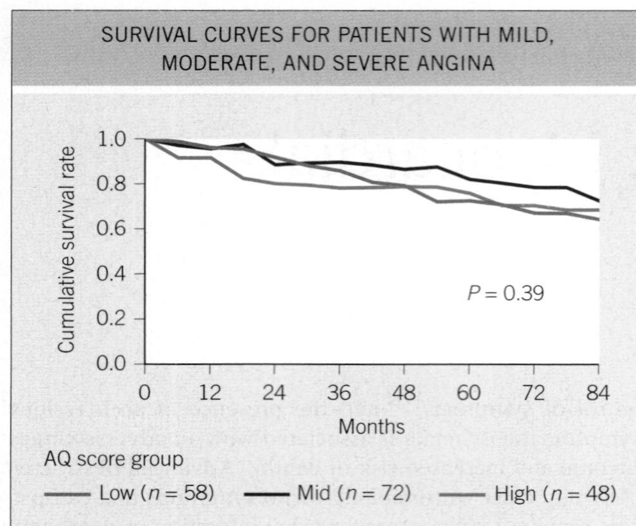

Figure 25.1 Survival curves for patients with mild, moderate, and severe angina. Cumulative survival rates during the 7-year follow-up in relation to the severity of symptoms in the medical arm of the Veterans Administration cooperative study of surgery for coronary artery occlusive disease. AQ, angina questionnaire. (Modified with permission from Hultgren H, Peduzzi P; participants of the Veterans Administration cooperative study of surgery for coronary arterial occlusive disease. Relation of severity of symptoms to prognosis in stable angina pectoris. Am J Cardiol 1984;54:988-993.)

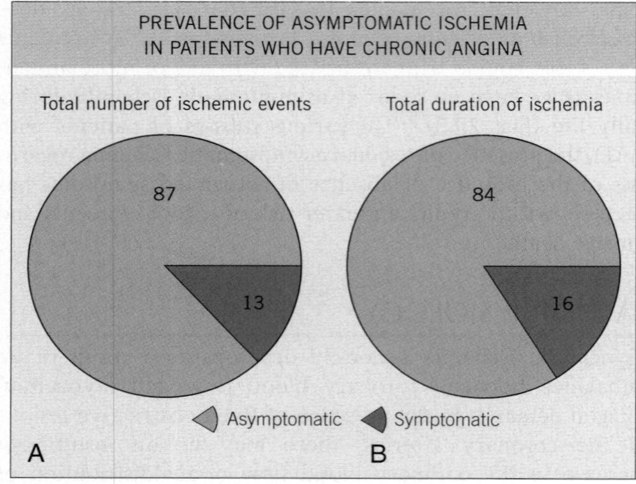

Figure 25.2 Prevalence of asymptomatic ischemia in patients who have chronic angina. A, The total number of ischemic events shows that most transient ischemic events were without symptoms. **B,** Similarly, the duration of asymptomatic events accounted for most (84%) of the total ischemic time during 24-hour ambulatory electrocardiographic monitoring. (Modified with permission from Deedwania P, Carbajal E. Prevalence and patterns of silent myocardial ischemia during daily life in stable angina patients receiving conventional antianginal drug therapy. Am J Cardiol 1990;65:1090-1096.)

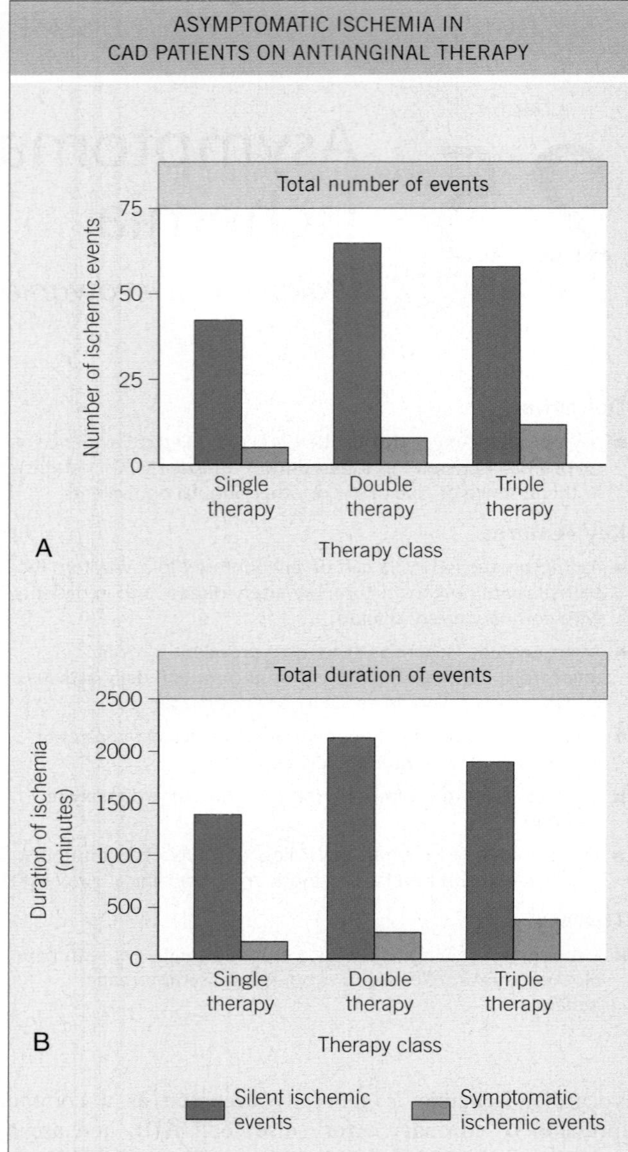

Figure 25.3 Asymptomatic ischemia in patients with coronary artery disease (CAD) receiving antianginal therapy. Total number **(A)** and total duration **(B)** of silent and symptomatic ischemic events during ambulatory electrocardiographic monitoring in patients receiving single, double, and triple antianginal drug regimens. There was no statistical difference between the three groups. (Modified with permission from Deedwania P, Carbajal E. Prevalence and patterns of silent myocardial ischemia during daily life in stable angina patients receiving conventional antianginal drug therapy. Am J Cardiol 1990;65:1090-1096.)

flow had a dominant role. This concept was based primarily on relatively small increases in the heart rate immediately preceding asymptomatic ischemic episodes during daily life.[10] This idea was further supported by data that showed that the magnitude of the increase in the heart rate preceding asymptomatic ischemic episodes during daily life was significantly smaller than the increase observed during exercise-induced ischemia in the same patient.[11] Moreover, because most asymptomatic episodes occur either during minimally strenuous activity or at times of no strenuous activity, it had been postulated that an increase in myocardial oxygen demand was unlikely to play a significant part. None of these explanations, however, provided any direct evidence for a reduction in coronary blood flow as a primary mechanism responsible for asymptomatic myocardial ischemia.

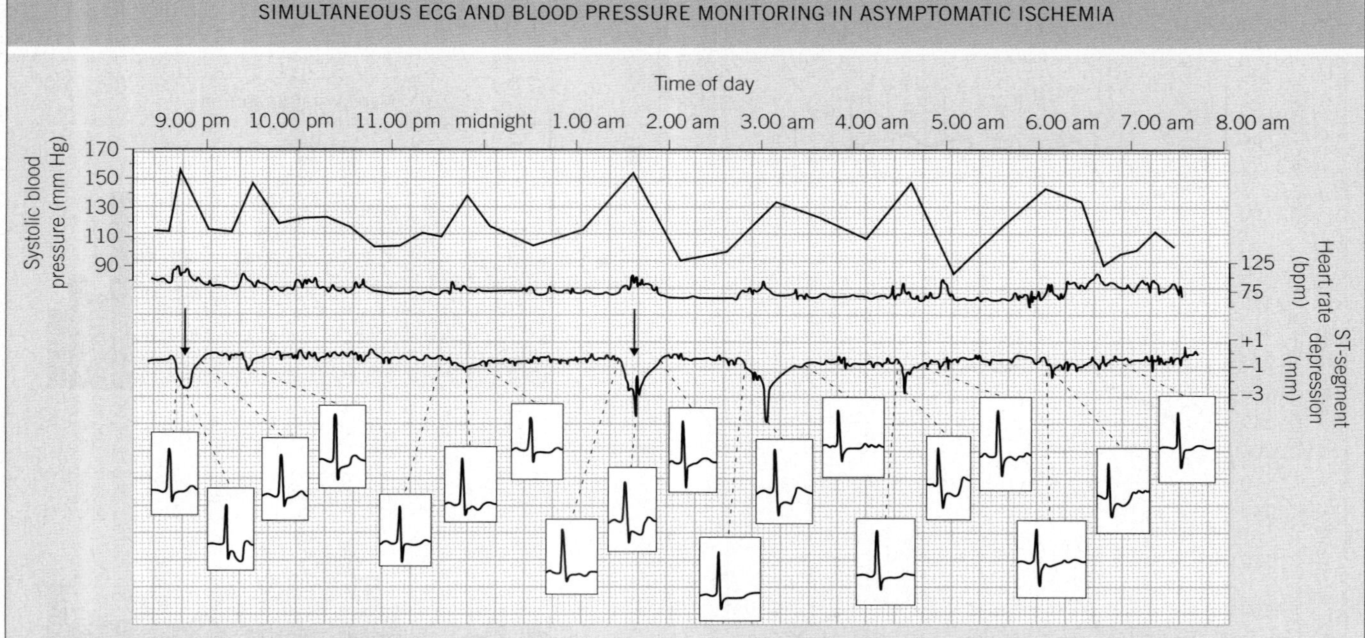

Figure 25.4 Simultaneous electrocardiographic (ECG) and blood pressure monitoring in asymptomatic ischemia. Simultaneous ambulatory ECG and blood pressure monitoring data reveal an increase in heart rate and systolic blood pressure both before and during most events. (Modified with permission from Deedwania P, Nelson J. Pathophysiology of silent myocardial ischemia during daily life: hemodynamic evaluation by simultaneous electrocardiographic and blood pressure monitoring. Circulation 1990;82:1296-1304.)

An increase in myocardial oxygen demand plays a significant part in the pathophysiologic process of asymptomatic myocardial ischemia.[12] In a study of 25 patients with CAD, stable angina, and a positive exercise treadmill test (ETT) result, simultaneous AEM and blood pressure monitoring were performed for 24 to 48 hours (Fig. 25.4).[12] The results of this study demonstrated that significant increases in heart rate and systolic blood pressure frequently preceded the onset of asymptomatic ischemic episodes during routine daily activities. This study also demonstrated a morning surge in the frequency of asymptomatic ischemic episodes, which was similar to that reported previously; this paralleled the morning increases in heart rate and systolic blood pressure (Fig. 25.5). These circulatory changes observed before the onset of asymptomatic ST-segment depression during Holter monitoring closely resemble those involved in the pathophysiologic process of angina pectoris.[12] On the basis of these data and the results of several other studies, it seems reasonable to consider that both an increase in myocardial demand and a decrease in coronary blood supply are involved in the genesis of asymptomatic myocardial ischemia.

Although the precise mechanism that is responsible for the lack of chest pain during asymptomatic ischemic episodes has not been established, several hypotheses have been proposed. In patients undergoing percutaneous transluminal coronary angioplasty (PTCA), data obtained during coronary artery balloon occlusion show that chest discomfort is the last event in the sequence of ischemic changes and that, in general, it is preceded by abnormalities of left ventricular function and by ischemic electrocardiographic (ECG) changes. Therefore, it seems reasonable to assume that during an asymptomatic episode, myocardial ischemia evolves to the point of ECG changes but fails to reach the pain threshold. It has also been suggested that during asymptomatic episodes, myocardial ischemia may be less severe and last for a shorter time than symptomatic episodes in the same patient.

Results of some studies suggest that patients with asymptomatic ischemia may have a higher threshold for pain or a generalized defective perception of painful stimuli.[13] Pain perception can also be altered by psychological factors and cultural background. A role of endorphins in exercise-induced asymptomatic ischemia has been proposed.[11] In the light of these findings, it can be concluded that different mechanisms might be operative in different patients. It is not easy, however, to quantify the contribution of different mechanisms in an individual patient. Whatever the underlying mechanism may be, it is generally accepted that cardiac ischemia may be asymptomatic because of a defective anginal warning system.

It is well known that cardiovascular events tend to cluster in the early hours of the morning.[14,15] A number of studies have shown that myocardial infarction, sudden cardiac death, and cerebrovascular accidents demonstrate a circadian pattern (Fig. 25.6), with a preponderance in the morning hours. Studies in patients who have stable CAD have shown that asymptomatic ischemia detected during Holter monitoring also has a circadian pattern, with increased ischemic activity in the morning hours.[14,15] This circadian pattern of both symptomatic and asymptomatic ischemia is very similar to that observed for acute myocardial infarction and sudden death, and it may be an important substrate for these events. In patients with variant angina, a circadian variation in the coronary artery tone has been demonstrated by reduced ischemic threshold during exercise in the morning

PATHOPHYSIOLOGIC BASIS OF THE CIRCADIAN PATTERN OF ASYMPTOMATIC ISCHEMIA
Heart rate (bpm)
Systolic blood pressure (mm Hg)
Double product (heart rate × systolic blood pressure × 10⁻²)
Number of events
01 am
02 am
03 am
04 am
05 am
06 am
07 am
08 am
09 am
10 am
11 am
noon
01 pm
02 pm
03 pm
04 pm
05 pm
06 pm
07 pm
08 pm
09 pm
10 pm
11 pm
midnight
P < .05
P < .01
P < .005
Asymptomatic myocardial ischemia
Symptomatic myocardial ischemia

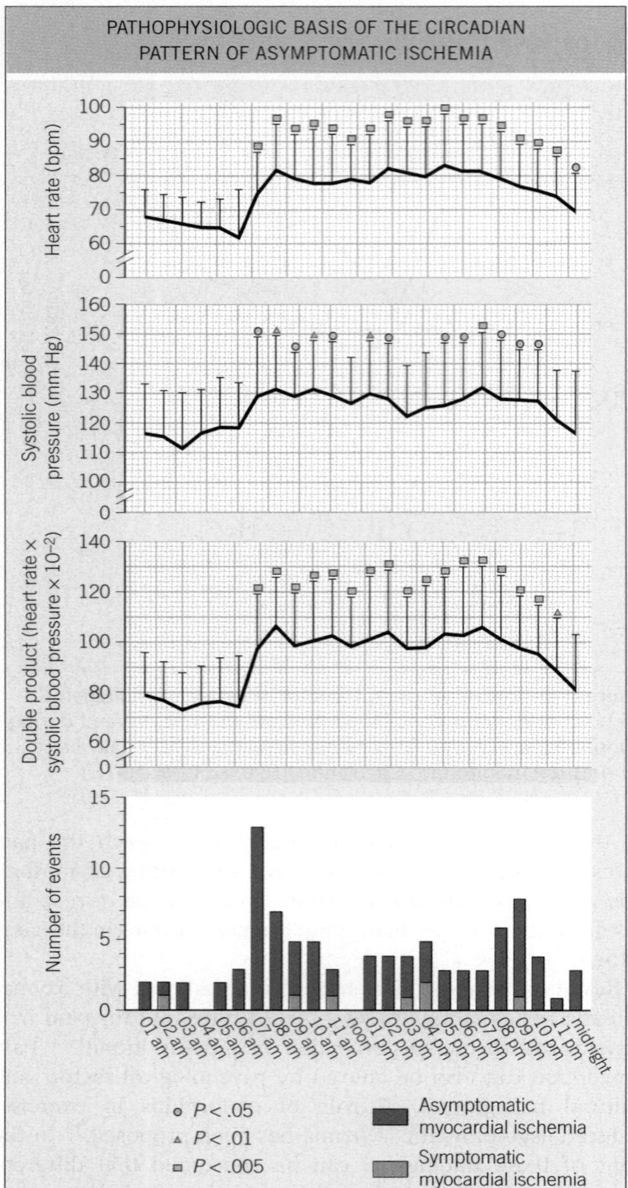

Figure 25.5 Pathophysiologic basis of the circadian pattern of asymptomatic ischemia. The 24-hour distribution of silent ischemic events during continuous electrocardiographic monitoring parallels the circadian pattern of heart rate and systolic blood pressure. Note the simultaneous and significant increases in both the circulatory changes and silent ischemic events between 6:00 AM and 7:00 AM. (Modified with permission from Deedwania P, Nelson J. Pathophysiology of silent myocardial ischemia during daily life: hemodynamic evaluation by simultaneous electrocardiographic and blood pressure monitoring. Circulation 1990;82:1296-1304.)

compared with the threshold in the afternoon.[14,15] The circadian rhythms of physiologic changes, such as a surge in systemic arterial pressure, enhanced coronary vasomotor tone, increased platelet aggregability, and reduced fibrinolytic activity, may play a significant part in the genesis of ischemic episodes during the morning hours.[14,15] The simultaneous increases in ischemic episodes, heart rate, and blood pressure at this time of day suggest that increased levels of sympathetic activity must contribute to the morning surge of these events

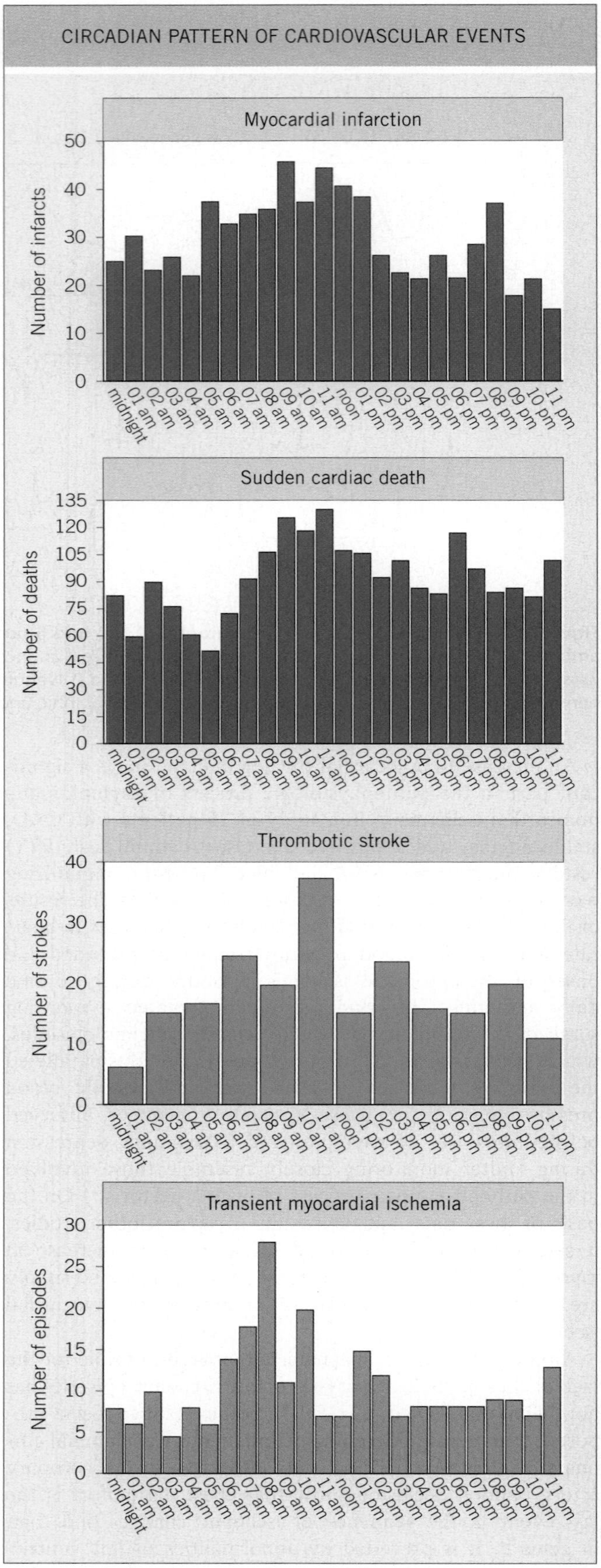

CIRCADIAN PATTERN OF CARDIOVASCULAR EVENTS
Myocardial infarction
Number of infarcts
Sudden cardiac death
Number of deaths
Thrombotic stroke
Number of strokes
Transient myocardial ischemia
Number of episodes
midnight
01 am
02 am
03 am
04 am
05 am
06 am
07 am
08 am
09 am
10 am
11 am
noon
01 pm
02 pm
03 pm
04 pm
05 pm
06 pm
07 pm
08 pm
09 pm
10 pm
11 pm

Figure 25.6 *See legend on opposite page.*

Figure 25.6 Circadian pattern of cardiovascular events. Time of day at onset of myocardial infarction, sudden cardiac death, stroke, and transient myocardial ischemia in four different groups of patients. Each of the disorders exhibits a prominent increase in frequency of onset in the period from 6:00 AM to noon. (Modified with permission from Muller JE, Tofler GI, Stone PH. Circadian variation and triggers of onset of acute cardiovascular disease. Circulation 1989;79:733-743.)

(see Fig. 25.5). It is also possible that a combination of factors, such as increased coronary vasomotor tone and enhanced sympathetic activity, might render the atherosclerotic plaque unstable, and plaque fissuring could result from a surge in blood pressure. Increased platelet aggregability and decreased intrinsic fibrinolytic activity could facilitate thrombus formation at the site of plaque rupture, or they could predispose a nonocclusive mural thrombus to extend and so worsen obstruction of the lumen of a vessel. This sequence of physiologic changes could trigger an acute ischemic episode, which could potentially lead to an acute coronary event such as myocardial infarction or sudden cardiac death.

DEFINITION

Asymptomatic myocardial ischemia is defined as the objective evidence of myocardial ischemia in the absence of chest pain or other anginal equivalents. Myocardial ischemia is inferred from

- transient ST-segment changes;
- myocardial perfusion defects; or
- reversible abnormalities in regional wall motion.

Although asymptomatic ischemia was defined a number of years ago, the concept has received considerable attention in recent years because of technologic advances in ECG monitoring that allow continuous monitoring to detect myocardial ischemia.[1,2,16] Whereas previous work was limited to ECG monitoring in cardiac care units and the exercise laboratory, electrocardiograms can now be recorded for 24 to 72 hours by Holter monitoring, and this provides an opportunity for continuous monitoring during routine daily activities. In addition, asymptomatic ischemia is also detected during cardiac imaging studies, such as stress perfusion scintigraphy, stress echocardiography, and dobutamine or dipyridamole stress imaging studies.

DIAGNOSTIC TECHNIQUES

Several diagnostic tools are available for the evaluation of asymptomatic ischemia. ETT and AEM are commonly used in clinical practice and are suitable as the initial tests for most patients. Exercise testing is an established and widely available technique for diagnosis of myocardial ischemia in the laboratory. In people with a normal ECG recording, the development of horizontal or downsloping ST-segment depression of 1 mm or more during a standard ETT is well-accepted evidence of exercise-induced ischemia. On the basis of the available data, ETT appears to be the most suitable and readily available initial diagnostic test with which to document myocardial ischemia in patients with CAD in addition to those without clinically manifested CAD. Exercise testing has been used to screen high-risk, asymptomatic people to identify those with asymptomatic CAD. Although conventional ST-segment analysis during ETT is moderately sensitive in detecting CAD, it yields an unacceptably high rate (10% to 35%) of false-positive responses, particularly in asymptomatic people. Because of this, diagnosis of myocardial ischemia during ETT in asymptomatic people should be confirmed by one of the radionuclide imaging techniques (e.g., perfusion scintigraphy or exercise ventriculography) or by stress echocardiography before the person is labeled as having CAD.

In recent years, Holter monitoring has frequently been used for the detection of asymptomatic ischemia.[1] Holter monitoring has the advantage of providing long-term ECG recording of the out-of-hospital ischemic and arrhythmic events. Episodes of asymptomatic ischemia on Holter monitoring are diagnosed by a sequence of ECG changes, including a flat or downsloping ST-segment depression of at least 1 mm with a gradual onset and offset that lasts for at least 1 minute.[1] A new episode is defined whenever it is separated from another episode by at least 1 minute. Although ST-segment depression during AEM has not always been accepted as unequivocal evidence of myocardial ischemia, studies have shown an excellent correlation between ambulatory ST-segment depression and other simultaneous objective evidence of ischemia during perfusion scintigraphy, radionuclide ventriculography, and hemodynamic monitoring.[15] These findings have confirmed the association between myocardial ischemia and ST-segment depression on the ECG recording during Holter monitoring in patients who have CAD.

Currently, three types of AEM recorders are available for evaluation of transient ischemic ST-segment changes:

- amplitude-modulated recorders;
- frequency-modulated recorders; and
- solid-state digital recorders.

Although frequency-modulated recorders have been considered the "gold standard" for assessment of myocardial ischemia, studies comparing the current available amplitude-modulated and frequency-modulated monitoring systems have demonstrated that newer amplitude-modulated devices with improved recording of low-frequency signals and playback features can reliably reproduce ST-segment changes recorded with frequency-modulated systems. The availability of digital recording devices provides yet further sophistication of ECG recording and should allow greater opportunity for accurate differentiation of artifacts and false-positive ST-segment changes from the true episodes of asymptomatic ischemia.

Although previous studies primarily used ECG changes on stress electrocardiography or AEM for the evaluation of asymptomatic myocardial ischemia, a number of cardiac imaging modalities have been used more recently. These include myocardial scintigraphy during physical exercise on a treadmill or during pharmacologic stress with adenosine or dipyridamole, exercise radionuclide ventriculography, and stress echocardiography. Because of the greater sensitivity of the imaging techniques, the reported prevalence of asymptomatic ischemia in these studies is generally greater than that reported with ECG monitoring. There is, however, little available information from well-controlled, large, prospective clinical trials about the prognostic importance of asymptomatic ischemia detected by the imaging methods. Until such information becomes available (and also because of their high cost), these techniques cannot be recommended for routine evaluation of asymptomatic myocardial ischemia.

MANAGEMENT

Traditionally, the management of patients with CAD has been focused on the relief of anginal symptoms. As the presence of myocardial ischemia rather than associated symptoms appears to determine the prognosis, it has been suggested that all episodes of myocardial ischemia should be abolished, regardless of associated symptoms. Although the benefit of such treatment is not fully established, the results of several large-scale clinical trials provide considerable support for abolishing all episodes of ischemia.

Because of the recent concern about asymptomatic ischemia, most conventional antianginal drugs have been evaluated in a more objective manner for their anti-ischemic effects outside the exercise laboratory. These agents have been used either as monotherapy or in combinations of two or more drugs. Although most antianginal drugs seem to be effective in reducing the frequency and severity of anginal attacks, their efficacy in suppressing asymptomatic ischemia is variable. Several studies, both in patients with acute ischemic syndromes and in patients with CAD and stable angina, have revealed that drug treatment aimed at control of symptoms does not eliminate or adequately suppress episodes of asymptomatic ischemia that are recorded during AEM. As mentioned before, it is the presence of residual ischemia regardless of associated symptoms that determines the prognosis and clinical outcome. On the basis of these findings, it has been suggested that anti-ischemic therapy should be targeted at abolishing symptomatic and asymptomatic ischemia.

The following sections discuss the effects of the most commonly used anti-ischemic therapies in the treatment of patients with CAD and their ability to suppress asymptomatic ischemia. The elimination or reduction in the episodes and duration of ST-segment depression on AEM has been frequently used as evidence of anti-ischemic efficacy.

Nitrates

Nitrates have been used for their antianginal effects for more than a century. Although nitrates have been used extensively in the management of patients who have angina and CAD, limited data are available to help evaluate the effect of treatment with nitrates on episodes of asymptomatic ischemia that are detected during AEM. Review of the available data suggests that treatment with nitrates is effective in reducing the frequency and duration of ischemic episodes (Fig. 25.7) and that treatment with nitrates results in total suppression of ischemic activity in approximately 35% of patients (Fig. 25.8).[17,18] Findings from some studies that have evaluated the effect of nitrates on asymptomatic ischemia suggest that compared with placebo, nitrate therapy may be relatively ineffective in reducing the magnitude of asymptomatic ischemia during daily life, particularly when longer acting nitrates are used.[18] This may be partially due to nitrate tolerance, which has frequently been reported as occurring with long-acting nitrates unless eccentric dosing schedules are used.

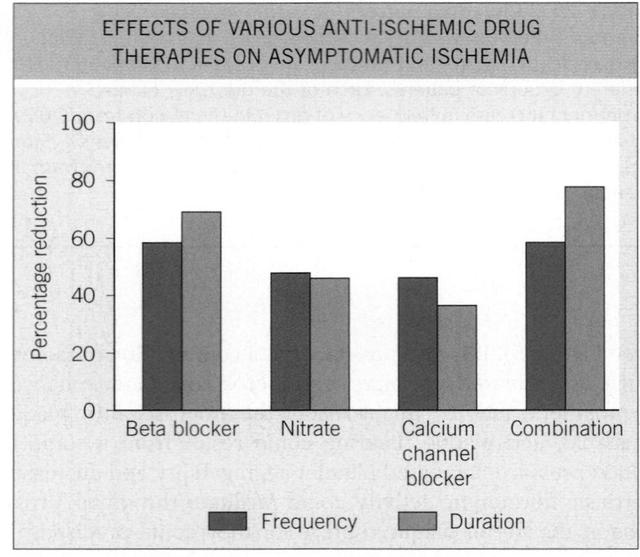

Figure 25.7 Effects of various anti-ischemic drug therapies on asymptomatic ischemia. The percentage reduction in frequency and duration of silent ischemic events achieved by treatment with different classes of antianginal drugs.

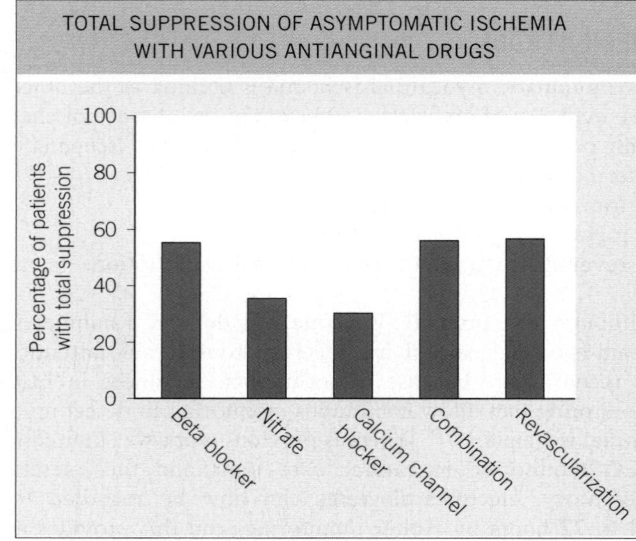

Figure 25.8 Total suppression of asymptomatic ischemia with various antianginal drugs. Comparison of the percentage of patients who achieve complete suppression of ischemia during Holter monitoring in response to different classes of antianginal agents or coronary revascularization.

β-Adrenergic Blockers

It is well known that beta blockers have an important role in the management of patients with stable CAD as well as of patients with acute ischemic syndromes. Beta blockers primarily decrease myocardial oxygen demand by several actions, including reduction of the heart rate at rest, attenuation of the heart rate response to exercise, decrease of the blood pressure, and diminishment of the force of ventricular contraction. These drugs exert their actions through binding to specific receptors in cardiac muscle (particularly β_1 receptors), and by doing so, they competitively inhibit the binding of catecholamines, with a resultant attenuated cardiac response to sympathetic stimulation.

A number of studies have evaluated the effect of beta blockers on asymptomatic ischemia.[19-21] They appear to be more effective than other antianginal agents.[20,21] Pooled analysis of the available data indicates that treatment with beta blockers in patients who have CAD is associated with a 59% reduction in the frequency of asymptomatic ischemia during daily life and a 69% reduction in its duration (see Figs. 25.7 and 25.8). Several beta blockers have been evaluated for their efficacy in modifying the frequency and duration of ischemic episodes (Fig. 25.9). The available data indicate that treatment with beta blockers results in total suppression of ischemia in approximately 55% of patients (see Figs. 25.8 and Fig. 25.9).[19-21] In addition to these beneficial effects, treatment with beta blockers also attenuates the morning increase (circadian variation) in asymptomatic ischemia in patients who have CAD, which might contribute to reduction of the risk of acute myocardial infarction and sudden cardiac death in the morning hours.[21]

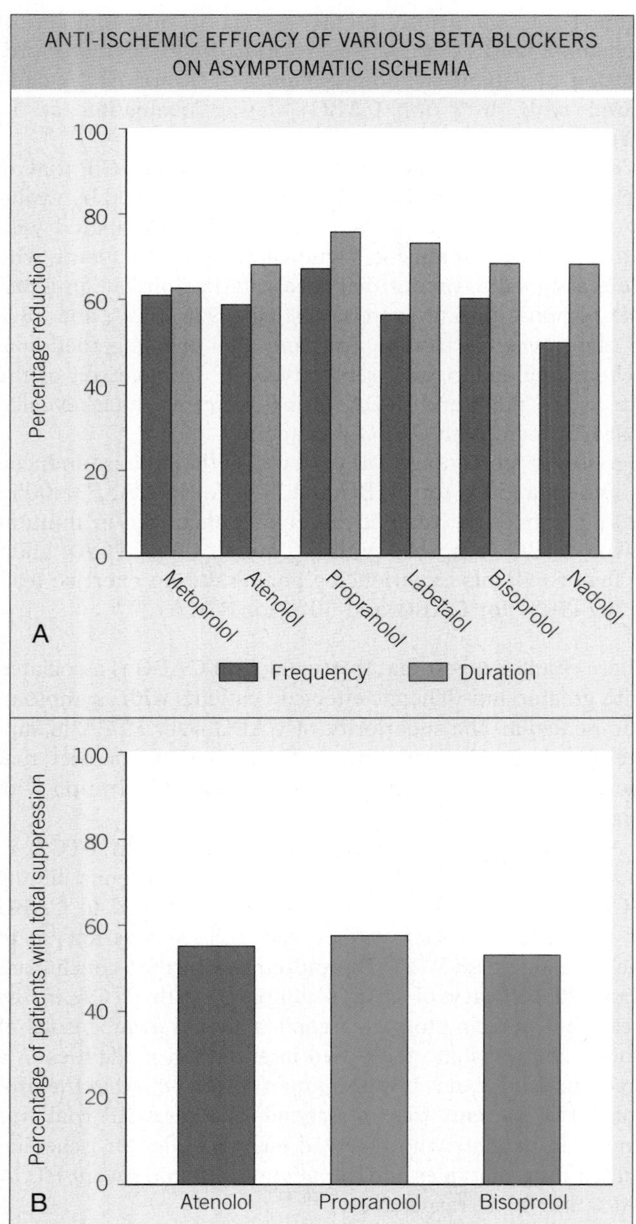

Figure 25.9 Anti-ischemic efficacy of various beta blockers on asymptomatic ischemia. A, Comparison of the effect of treatment with various beta blockers on reduction in frequency and duration of silent ischemic events. **B,** Comparison of the effect of treatment with beta blockers on complete suppression of ischemic activity during Holter monitoring.

Calcium Channel Blockers

Several studies have evaluated the effects of treatment with calcium channel blockers on asymptomatic ischemia during AEM in patients with CAD.[21-24] Pooled analyses of these studies have shown a reduction in the frequency and duration of asymptomatic ischemia by approximately 46% and 36%, respectively (see Fig. 25.7). Although relatively few studies have evaluated the efficacy of calcium channel blockers in completely suppressing ischemic episodes, the available data indicate that, in general, these agents are not very effective in totally suppressing myocardial ischemia (see Fig. 25.8).[21,22] It has also been suggested that treatment with certain calcium channel blockers, particularly short-acting dihydropyridines, might lead to reflex tachycardia and an increase in catecholamines secondary to profound episodic peripheral vasodilatation, which can result in proischemic effects. However, the newer, more vasoselective and long-acting agents, such as amlodipine and felodipine, do not seem to produce such adverse effects.[22]

Combination Drug Therapy

Combination therapy of anti-ischemic drugs might allow treatment with lower doses of each drug, which can help reduce side effects and improve compliance.[21-24] In general, an appropriate combination should cancel or dampen undesirable actions from specific drugs and prevent any increase in myocardial oxygen demand. A useful combination might be a nitrate preparation (with a nitrate-free period of 10 to 12 hours) plus a long-acting beta blocker. Another possibility is a calcium channel blocker (e.g., diltiazem or verapamil) plus a nitrate, or a beta blocker plus a calcium channel blocker (e.g., amlodipine). When combination therapy is being evaluated in an individual patient, treatment of other associated medical conditions should be taken into consideration as part of the therapeutic strategy.

Limited data are available from studies that have evaluated the effects of combination anti-ischemic treatment on asymptomatic ischemia.[21-26] The combination of a beta blocker, atenolol, and a calcium channel blocker, nifedipine or amlodipine, has been found to have greater anti-ischemic effect than treatment with either agent alone. The anti-ischemic effects of combination therapy have been characterized by a reduced frequency and a shorter duration of asymptomatic ischemic episodes (see Fig. 25.7) and a greater rate of total suppression of ischemia during ECG monitoring (see Fig. 25.8). In some studies, the use of combination therapy resulted in total suppression of ischemia in more than 75% of the patients. In the U.S. National Institutes of Health Asymptomatic Cardiac Ischemia Pilot (ACIP) study, two drug combination schedules were used for patients who were allocated randomly to groups to receive angina-guided or ischemia-guided treatments.[20,26,27] The combination of atenolol and nifedipine or the combination of diltiazem and isosorbide dinitrate resulted in a modest degree of total suppression rates of 48% and 33%, respectively.[20] However, the relatively modest effects of combination therapy on total suppression of ischemia in the ACIP study could be partly explained by the fact that the drugs used were not given in optimal doses.[26] It is wholly conceivable that higher dosages would have resulted in better rates of suppression. Regardless of the findings from these studies, it is generally believed that combination therapy is usually needed in patients who have advanced CAD and asymptomatic ischemia.

Myocardial Revascularization

Compared with the numerous clinical trials with anti-ischemic drugs, there are few studies that have evaluated the effects of myocardial revascularization by coronary artery bypass grafting (CABG) or PTCA on asymptomatic ischemia. Most studies have been uncontrolled and conducted in an unsystematic manner in a variety of clinical settings. In some cases, ischemia was detected in the exercise laboratory; in others, it was detected during AEM; in yet others, the only evidence of ischemia was noted on nuclear imaging studies.

In the retrospective evaluation from the Coronary Artery Surgery Study (CASS) of patients who underwent evaluation by an ETT before CABG and again a few months after CABG, there was, overall, a similar percentage of patients who showed evidence of asymptomatic ischemia during the ETT before CABG (29.8%) and after CABG (29.3%).[28] In another study of patients who underwent evaluation by AEM before and after CABG, myocardial revascularization resulted in a reduction in the frequency and duration of asymptomatic ischemic episodes, and approximately 33% of patients had no evidence of ischemia during AEM that was performed 3 months after bypass surgery.[29] Another study after CABG showed that a fairly large proportion (70% to 80%) of patients were free of asymptomatic ischemia during the early follow-up (1 to 3 months) and late follow-up (12 months) evaluations.[30] The results of these studies suggest that CABG is highly effective in reducing the risk of asymptomatic ischemia. However, because of the lack of a proper randomization scheme and comparison with other forms of treatment, it has not been possible to assess the relative superiority, if any, of CABG in the treatment of asymptomatic ischemia.

The studies evaluating the effect of PTCA in patients with asymptomatic ischemia have largely concentrated on evaluation of findings during exercise testing. It has been reported that PTCA results in 60% to 70% suppression of asymptomatic ischemia during exercise testing performed soon after the procedure.[31,32] However, in some of these studies, patients were preselected on the basis of the presence of single-vessel CAD, and many studies were retrospective and nonrandomized. In general, it is now believed that surgical myocardial revascularization with CABG is more effective than PTCA in suppressing ischemia during daily life.

Drug Treatment Versus Revascularization

Only one large, randomized, prospective study has compared the effects of treatment with combination drug therapy and those of myocardial revascularization on asymptomatic ischemia detected during exercise testing and during AEM. In the ACIP trial, patients were allocated randomly to groups to receive stepped medical treatment with one of two different drug combination schedules (titrated to control symptoms or to suppress myocardial ischemia) or to undergo myocardial revascularization by CABG or PTCA.[20,27] The results of the ACIP study revealed that treatment with myocardial revascularization was more effective than either angina-guided or ischemia-guided drug treatments in reducing the frequency and duration of ischemic events and that it was associated with a greater percentage of patients who were free of ischemia during AEM at 1-year follow-up.[33]

Further evaluation of the effects of CABG or PTCA on ischemia during AEM revealed that treatment with CABG achieved a significantly greater reduction in magnitude of ischemia than PTCA and was associated with a greater proportion of patients without ischemia (70% for PTCA compared with 46% for CABG) during evaluation at 12 weeks.[26,33]

The efficacy of randomized treatments in the ACIP trial on ischemia detected during AEM was also confirmed by evaluation of the results obtained during ETTs. Compared with either medical treatment, significantly fewer patients who were assigned to myocardial revascularization had an ischemic response during exercise testing (69%, 85%, and 88% in the revascularization arm and the angina-guided and ischemia-guided groups, respectively).[33] Comparison of the effects of CABG and PTCA during exercise testing revealed that treatment with CABG resulted in

- a lower percentage of patients with exercise-induced ischemia (54% for CABG and 77% for PTCA; $P = .005$);
- longer exercise time to onset of ischemia (7.6 minutes for CABG compared with 6.5 minutes for PTCA); and
- fewer patients experiencing angina during exercise testing (10% for CABG and 30% for PTCA).[26,33]

These results suggest that treatment with CABG is associated with greater anti-ischemic effects in patients with asymptomatic ischemia. The superiority of CABG over PTCA in suppressing ischemia might be partly related to the fact that there was more complete myocardial revascularization with bypass surgery.[26,34]

Although CABG appeared to be superior to PTCA in reducing the magnitude of asymptomatic ischemia in the ACIP trial, patients were not randomly assigned to CABG or PTCA in this study; rather, the decision was left up to the investigators.[19,26,33] Therefore, any further conclusions about the efficacy of CABG compared with PTCA in the treatment of asymptomatic ischemia should await results of studies that evaluate these two intervention modalities in a randomized manner. It is also important to note that the proportion of patients free of ischemia in the ACIP trial was similar in patients who received angina-guided or ischemia-guided drug therapies and in patients who underwent PTCA (40% and 46%, respectively).[26,33]

Although few data are available with which to evaluate the efficacy of medical treatment and myocardial revascularization on asymptomatic ischemia, the available information suggests that treatment with an effective dose of beta blocker alone or a drug combination that includes a beta blocker can result in a degree of suppression of ischemia similar to that achieved with myocardial revascularization. Estimates suggest that revascularization strategies will cost more than medical treatment initially, but within 10 years, the costs will be equal because of subsequent ischemic events.[35]

Effect of Anti-Ischemic Therapy on Clinical Outcome in Stable Coronary Artery Disease

Because it is the presence of myocardial ischemia, regardless of the associated symptoms, that predicts the adverse clinical outcome, it would seem logical to think that total suppression of ischemia might be associated with a better clinical outcome. On the basis of this concept, it has been suggested that the goal of antianginal therapy should be the suppression of all ischemic episodes, whether they are painful or painless. Although this concept appears attractive, there is little evidence to support the hypothesis that complete suppression of ischemia with aggressive anti-ischemic therapy results in better clinical outcome.

A few well-controlled, randomized, and large-scale studies have evaluated the impact of ischemia-guided therapy on clinical outcome in patients with stable CAD. In the Atenolol Silent Ischemia Study (ASIST), evaluation of clinical outcome during the 1-year follow-up revealed that compared with those given placebo, patients treated with atenolol experienced fewer unfavorable events (11% compared with 25%, respectively; $P < .001$) and a longer event-free survival (120 days compared with 79 days, respectively), with a relative risk reduction of 56% ($P = .001$) (Fig. 25.10).[19] The Swiss Interventional Study on Silent Ischaemia type I (SWISSI I) compared antianginal drug therapy and risk factor control with risk factor control only and demonstrated a reduction in cardiac events with antianginal therapy. All the patients in SWISSI I had myocardial ischemia confirmed by stress imaging, and there was less ischemia during an average follow-up of 11 years. Also, left ventricular ejection fraction remained unchanged on antianginal therapy, whereas it decreased significantly on risk factor control only.[53]

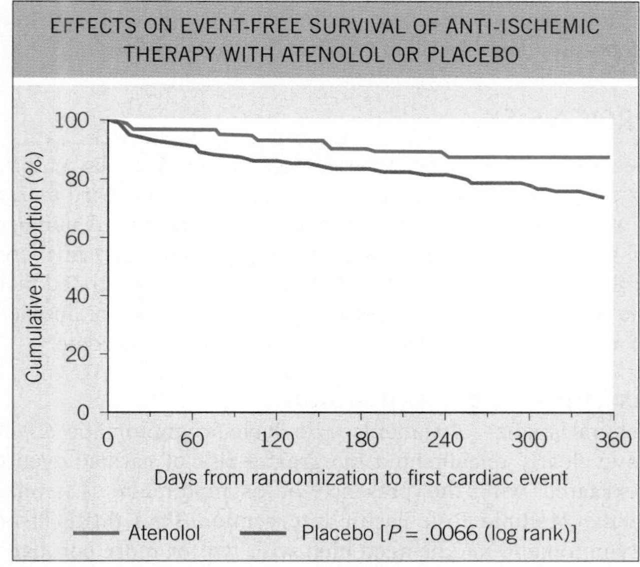

Figure 25.10 Effects on event-free survival of anti-ischemic therapy with atenolol or placebo. Kaplan-Meier curves comparing the cumulative probabilities of patients who have silent ischemia on ambulatory ECG monitoring not experiencing an adverse event during follow-up after random allocation to groups to receive atenolol or placebo. The risk reduction was 56% (95% CI, 25% to 74%; $P = .001$). (Modified with permission from Pepine C, Cohn P, Deedwania P, et al. Effects of treatment on outcome in mildly symptomatic patients with ischemia during daily life: the Atenolol Silent Ischemia Study. Circulation 1994;90:762-768.)

In the ACIP study, myocardial revascularization (especially CABG) appeared to be a more effective anti-ischemic treatment than either combination drug therapy (atenolol plus nifedipine or diltiazem plus isosorbide dinitrate).[20,26,33] The evaluation of clinical events (secondary endpoints) in the ACIP study revealed that compared with titrated combination drug therapies (angina guided or ischemia guided), patients who were randomly assigned to myocardial revascularization (predominantly CABG) experienced a lower rate of coronary events (Fig. 25.11). Most of the benefit secondary to revascularization was noted in the patients who underwent CABG, and patients treated with PTCA did not have an outcome significantly different from the outcome of those who received antianginal drug treatment.[33] In SWISSI II, a more recent study that included coronary artery stenting, patients with a recent myocardial infarction, stress imaging–confirmed silent ischemia, and one- or two-vessel coronary artery disease were randomized to percutaneous coronary intervention or anti-ischemic medical therapy. During a mean follow-up of 10 years, major adverse coronary events were reduced by percutaneous coronary intervention (hazard ratio, 0.33; 95% CI, 0.20-0.55; $P < .001$). Also, there was less evidence of ischemia in the percutaneous coronary intervention patients, and left ventricular ejection fraction was maintained, whereas it decreased significantly in the drug therapy group.[54]

Although the results from this pilot study indicate that surgical myocardial revascularization is most effective in suppressing myocardial ischemia and that it improves clinical outcome compared with medical treatment, there were some limitations to this study that preclude definite conclusions. The drug treatments were not optimized, and thus the effects of drugs on clinical outcome might have been minimized. Also, there was a potential physician-referral bias toward increased frequency of revascularization procedures in patients who were assigned to medical treatments.

Although not specifically designed for evaluation of the effect of therapy on asymptomatic ischemia, a study compared the effects of conservative medical therapy with those of myocardial revascularization in 1000 survivors of acute myocardial infarction who had evidence of myocardial ischemia on exercise testing (56% had asymptomatic ischemia). Although overall mortality after a medical follow-up at 2.4 years was the same in the two groups, those treated aggressively with revascularization had fewer reinfarctions and admissions for unstable angina.[36] However, as with the ACIP study, the medical treatment was not optimized in this trial either, raising the question of potential bias against medical treatment. To determine whether complete suppression of ischemia will translate into improved clinical outcome, long-term, large-scale studies need to be conducted with various therapeutic strategies to achieve the desired anti-ischemic effects.[20,26,33,36]

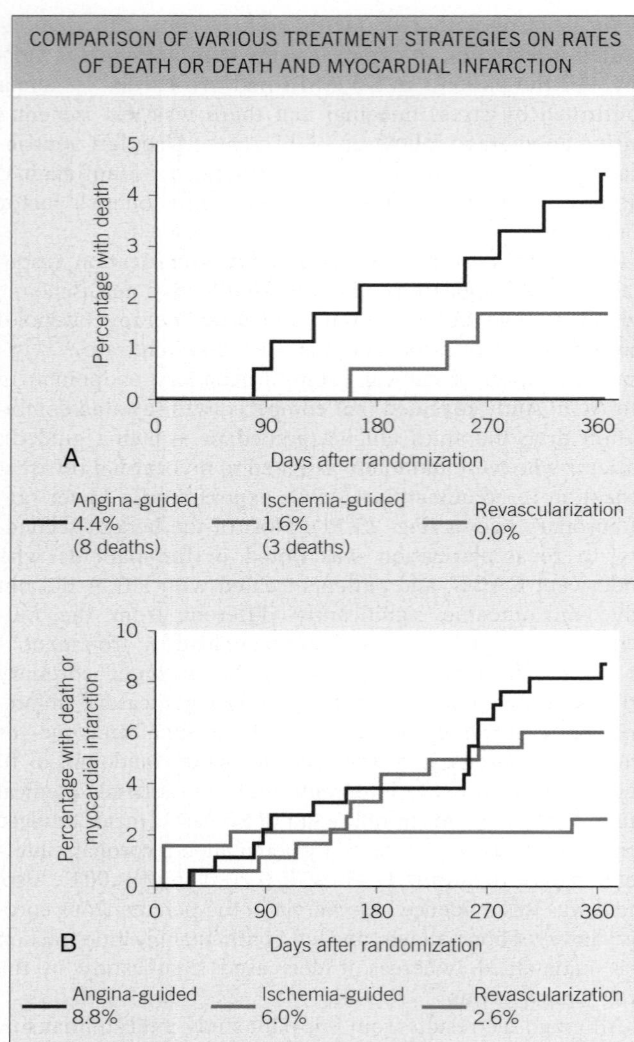

Figure 25.11 Comparison of various treatment strategies on rates of death or death and myocardial infarction. A, Although the number of fatal events was small, the percentage of patients who died during the 1-year follow-up was significantly lower for patients assigned to the revascularization strategy than for those assigned to the angina-guided strategy. The mortality rate was similar between the angina-guided and ischemia-guided strategies. **B,** The combination of death and myocardial infarction was significantly less common among patients assigned to the revascularization strategy than among those assigned to the angina-guided strategy but not less common than among those assigned to the ischemia-guided strategy. (Modified with permission from Rogers W, Bourassa M, Andrews T, et al. Asymptomatic Cardiac Ischemia Pilot study: outcome at 1 year for patients with ischemia randomized to medical therapy or revascularization. J Am Coll Cardiol 1995;26:594-605.)

Another important point to consider in the overall context of previous studies is that in none of these studies was risk factor modification considered part of the therapeutic strategy. The available data from studies evaluating the effects of risk factor modification indicate that such treatment can improve endothelial function, reduce the risk of ischemia, and stabilize the plaques.[37,38] Recent data indicate that lipid-decreasing treatment can be effective in reducing the episodes of ischemia and improving myocardial perfusion (Fig. 25.12).[37] Future studies designed to evaluate the best therapeutic approach for

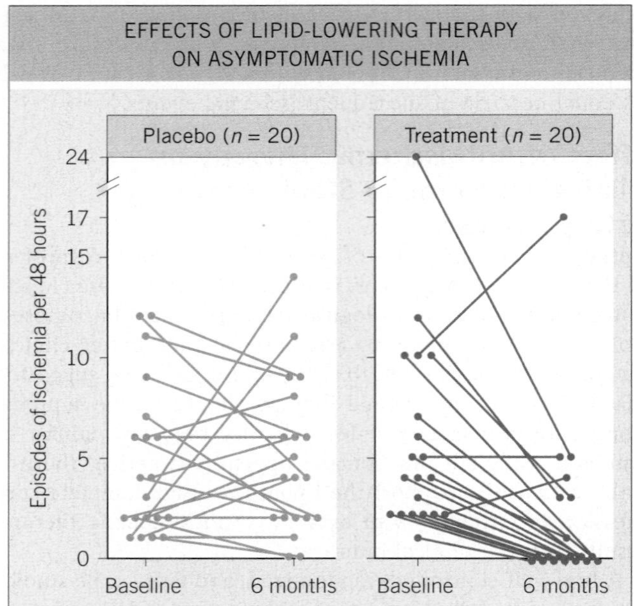

Figure 25.12 Effects of lipid-lowering therapy on asymptomatic ischemia. Effects of decreasing cholesterol during 6 months on the number of episodes of ischemic ST-segment depression in individual patients who have coronary artery disease. These patient-by-patient data show that 2 patients of 20 in the placebo group compared with 13 patients of 20 in the treatment group exhibited resolution of ischemia. (Modified with permission from Andrews TC, Raby K, Barry J, et al. Effect of cholesterol reduction on myocardial ischemia in patients with coronary disease. Circulation 1997;95:324-328.)

patients with asymptomatic ischemia should include aggressive risk factor modification and lipid-decreasing treatment to achieve maximum success in reducing the risk of ischemia and decreasing the risk of related adverse outcome.[38]

PROGNOSIS

Because asymptomatic ischemia does not produce discomfort, its presence would not be of much clinical consequence unless it were associated with an adverse clinical outcome. A number of studies in previously asymptomatic patients and in those with clinically manifested CAD have clearly demonstrated that the presence of ischemia, regardless of the presence or absence of symptoms, is associated with adverse clinical outcome.

Asymptomatic Individuals

Several studies of patients who have asymptomatic CAD have clearly documented the greater risk of cardiac events associated with the presence of asymptomatic ischemia. In the Multiple Risk Factor Intervention Trial (MRFIT) of asymptomatic middle-aged men with two or more coronary risk factors, the presence of ischemia during exercise testing was highly predictive of cardiac death (risk ratio, 3.4) compared with those without ischemia.[9] The Lipid Research Clinic Primary Prevention Trial (LRCPPT) study of 3600 men without previous evidence of CAD who underwent a submaximal ETT showed a significantly greater age-adjusted cardiovascular mortality among men with exercise-induced ischemia compared with those without ischemia (mean follow-up, 8.4 years).[39]

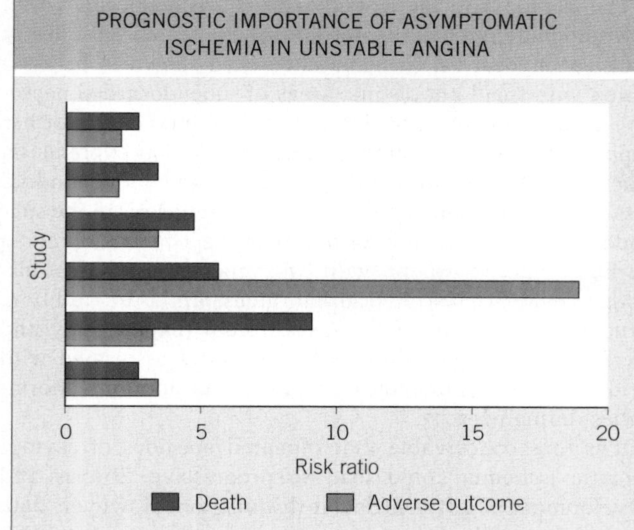

Figure 25.13 Prognostic importance of asymptomatic ischemia in unstable angina. Bar graph showing influence of silent ischemia, as detected by ambulatory monitoring, on risk of death or adverse outcome (death or nonfatal myocardial infarction, or both) in patients with unstable angina. Data are from six studies involving approximately 500 patients, with follow-up ranging from "in-hospital" to 24 months. The increased risk for adverse outcome that is associated with detectable ischemia ranges from about 2-fold to 19-fold; that for death ranges from about 3-fold to 9-fold. (Modified with permission from Pepine C. Is silent ischemia a treatable risk factor in patients with angina pectoris? Circulation 1990;82[Suppl II]:II135.)

Patients Who Have Acute Myocardial Infarction and Unstable Angina

The prognostic significance of asymptomatic ischemia is well established in survivors of acute myocardial infarction. The results of predischarge exercise testing in these patients have revealed that the presence of ischemia with or without pain during exercise testing is associated with an increased risk of future cardiac events and death. Asymptomatic ischemia during AEM also portrays a poor prognosis in survivors of myocardial infarction. Several studies have shown that 10% to 30% of patients with a recent myocardial infarction have asymptomatic episodes during AEM. The presence of asymptomatic ischemia has been shown to predict increased risk of future coronary events and cardiac death.

Asymptomatic myocardial ischemia in patients with unstable angina is also associated with adverse prognosis (Fig. 25.13). Patients with unstable angina who have asymptomatic ischemia during continuous ECG monitoring have an increased risk of experiencing an acute myocardial infarction or cardiac death or of needing CABG during the subsequent follow-up period.[1,16,40]

Patients Who Have Stable Coronary Artery Disease

The increased risk of coronary events and cardiac mortality has been well documented in patients who have stable CAD and evidence of asymptomatic ischemia during exercise testing or AEM. As an example, in a report from CASS in 880 patients with CAD who underwent exercise testing,[41] a significantly greater probability of experiencing myocardial infarction or

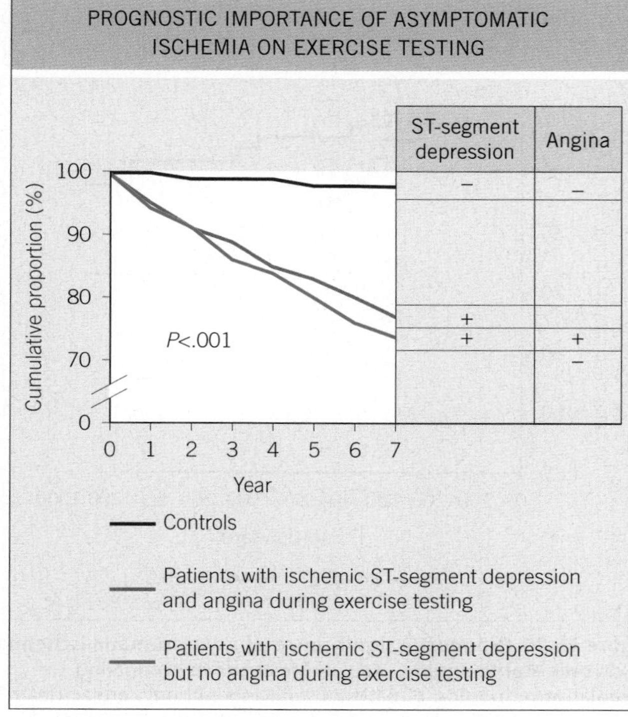

Figure 25.14 Prognostic importance of asymptomatic ischemia on exercise testing. Cumulative 7-year probability of remaining free of myocardial infarction and sudden death among patients with ischemic ST-segment depression but no angina during exercise testing, patients with both ischemic ST-segment depression and angina during exercise testing, and 1019 controls without coronary artery disease and without either ischemic ST-segment depression or angina during exercise testing. There was no statistically significant difference between the rates for the two groups of patients, but the control group had substantially fewer events. (Modified with permission from Weiner D, Ryan T, McCabe C, et al. Risk of developing an acute myocardial infarction or sudden coronary death in patients with exercise-induced silent myocardial ischemia. A report from the Coronary Artery Surgery Study [CASS] registry. Am J Cardiol 1988;62:1155-1161.)

sudden death during the 7-year follow-up was found in patients with exercise-induced asymptomatic ischemia (26%) or symptomatic ischemia (23%) than in patients without exercise-induced ischemia (2%) (Fig. 25.14). Asymptomatic ischemia during ambulatory monitoring in studies of patients with stable angina, most of whom were free of symptoms, was associated with a greater risk of future coronary events and cardiac death (Figs. 25.15 and 25.16).[5] Multiple regression analyses comparing several established clinical, ECG, and exercise test parameters revealed that symptomatic ischemia during AEM was the most powerful predictor, and an independent predictor, of adverse clinical outcome and cardiac mortality.[7]

In the ACIP trial of 558 patients, death, myocardial infarction, or admission to the hospital occurred in 13% of patients with asymptomatic ischemia within 12 months. Multivariate analysis indicated that only the number of ischemia episodes on the entry AEM predicted outcome, although the effect was small (odds ratio, 1.06).[27] An angiographic study from the ACIP trial found no correlation between the severity of coronary disease or the presence of a complex plaque and adverse outcome at 12 months.[42]

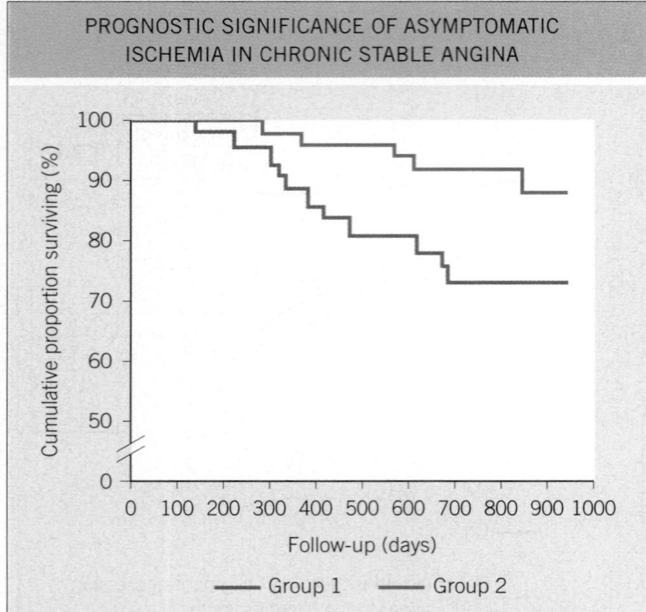

Figure 25.15 Prognostic significance of asymptomatic ischemia in chronic stable angina. Kaplan-Meier curves comparing cumulative proportion of patients surviving without cardiac death during mean follow-up of 2 years for 46 patients with silent ischemia (group 1) and 61 patients without ischemia (group 2) during ambulatory ECG monitoring (*P* = .02). (Modified with permission from Deedwania P, Carbajal E. Silent ischemia during daily life is an independent predictor of mortality in stable angina. Circulation 1990;81:748-756.)

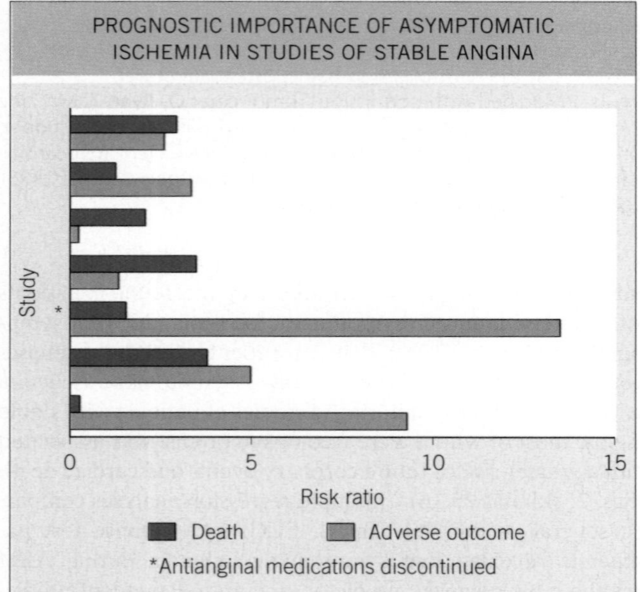

Figure 25.16 Prognostic importance of asymptomatic ischemia in studies of stable angina. Influence of silent ischemia, as detected by ambulatory ECG monitoring, on risk of death or adverse outcome (death or nonfatal myocardial infarction, or both) in patients with stable angina or stable coronary artery disease. Data are from seven studies involving more than 500 patients, with follow-up ranging from 6 months to 36 months. The increased risk for adverse outcome associated with detectable ischemia ranges from about 2-fold to 14-fold, and that for death ranges from about 2-fold to 4-fold. (Modified with permission from Pepine C. Is silent ischemia a treatable risk factor in patients with angina pectoris? Circulation 1990;82[Suppl II]:II135.)

The reason for the adverse prognosis associated with asymptomatic ischemia is not known. Repeated episodes of transient myocardial ischemia have been shown to be associated with small but distinct areas of subendocardial necrosis in an animal model.[43] These findings are further supported by studies demonstrating myocardial hypokinesia associated with abnormalities of nuclei and mitochondria, loss of myocytes, and increased interstitial fibrosis in the subendocardial areas on myocardial biopsy specimens obtained during surgery in patients with CAD; there was no gross histologic evidence of myocardial infarction.[43] In addition, structural alterations of the myocardium (hypertrophy and increased interstitial non-muscle tissue) are associated with evidence of ischemia-induced regional wall motion abnormalities during exercise.[44]

It is thus conceivable that repeated episodes of asymptomatic ischemia could lead to progressive fibrosis and development of left ventricular dysfunction. However, data are lacking on the long-term consequences of repeated episodes of asymptomatic ischemia on left ventricular function in patients with CAD. Serial evaluations by radionuclide angiography or echocardiography are needed to determine the effects of asymptomatic ischemia on left ventricular ejection fraction. It is also conceivable that prolonged episodes of asymptomatic ischemia lead to changes in electrophysiologic properties of myocardium, which in turn produce a milieu that is prone to life-threatening ventricular arrhythmias. Finally, silent ischemia may simply be a marker of increased risk for CAD progression, plaque disruption, and thrombosis.

PREVALENCE

Asymptomatic Individuals

Asymptomatic myocardial ischemia by definition implies absence of symptoms. Thus, it is difficult to define the true prevalence of asymptomatic ischemia in the population at large. However, results from several screening studies have been used to estimate the prevalence of asymptomatic CAD.[1,9,39,45,46]

Data from two large studies, one in the United States (N = 1390) and another in Norway (N = 2014) in asymptomatic middle-aged men undergoing screening with exercise testing, revealed that asymptomatic ischemia during exercise with significant angiographic CAD was detected in approximately 2.5%.[45,46] In a smaller study of 129 asymptomatic men (mean age, 46 years) undergoing ETT and fluoroscopy to seek coronary artery calcification, 13 had both exercise-induced myocardial ischemia and calcification of at least one coronary artery; coronary angiography revealed that 12 of the 13 men had significant CAD.

However, whereas evaluation of coronary artery calcification may be suitable for screening purposes in selected individuals, it is not an established diagnostic criterion for CAD, despite a great deal of enthusiasm by some to perform electronic beam computed tomography for identification of patients with CAD. More recently, an Italian study evaluated 4842 asymptomatic men aged between 40 and 59 years with a three-stage diagnostic procedure; patients were advanced to subsequent stages if they were suspected of having asymptomatic ischemia or infarction in each stage.[47] The first stage included ECG monitoring at rest, hyperventilation test, exercise ECG test, and 24-hour Holter ECG monitoring; the second stage included echocardiography, thallium 201 scintigraphy in conjunction with exercise testing or dipyridamole test, exercise radionuclide ventriculography, and ergonovine test; the third stage consisted of coronary angiography. The final diagnosis of asymptomatic myocardial ischemia or infarction was reached in 25 patients (adjusted prevalence, 0.89%).[47]

An additional group comprises people who suffer from clinically asymptomatic or unrecognized myocardial infarction and those who have survived an episode of sudden cardiac death. In the Framingham study of 5127 asymptomatic individuals who underwent routine ECG evaluation, 28% of the men and 35% of the women developed ECG evidence of myocardial infarction during the 30-year follow-up. In another study of previously asymptomatic survivors of sudden cardiac death, asymptomatic ischemia was found in 80% of the patients.[48] These results are further supported by findings from a study evaluating autopsy data in 23,996 persons (aged between 30 and 69 years) who were not known to have CAD. This study showed evidence of significant CAD in 6.4% of the men examined.[49]

On the basis of these data, it has been estimated that 2% to 4% of apparently healthy asymptomatic middle-aged men have significant coronary disease. Furthermore, asymptomatic men with two or more major coronary risk factors (e.g., smoking, obesity, family history of heart disease, age older than 45 years, diabetes mellitus, hypertension, and hypercholesterolemia) have an incidence of significant disease that may approach 10%. The data in women are inconclusive because of a greater incidence of false-positive ECG recordings.

Patients Who Have Known Coronary Artery Disease

A larger segment of the population affected by asymptomatic ischemia consists of people who are known to have CAD. This includes patients who have had a previous myocardial infarction and those who have angina pectoris. Reviews of available data indicate that 15% to 30% of survivors of acute myocardial infarction have asymptomatic ischemia.[40,50] Studies in patients who have unstable angina have revealed that asymptomatic ischemia occurs in 30% to 40% of these patients, despite aggressive medical treatment.

The prevalence of asymptomatic ischemia in the nearly 6 million people in the United States who have chronic CAD is estimated to be between 40% and 50%.[1] This makes asymptomatic ischemia the most common manifestation of CAD. Several studies, including data in patients who have CAD and stable angina undergoing ETT and AEM evaluation, have shown that asymptomatic ischemia is far more common than symptomatic ischemia.[1,41] Pooled data from several reports have revealed an incidence of asymptomatic ischemic ST-segment changes during exercise of up to 50%.[1,16] In patients who have CAD and stable angina who undergo AEM, asymptomatic ST-segment depression has been observed during 80% of ischemic episodes in 25% to 40% of those who are asymptomatic but who have evidence of ischemia in daily life.[1,4-6] On the basis of these data, it can be estimated that between 2 and 3 million people in the United States with stable CAD have evidence of asymptomatic myocardial ischemia.[1]

Studies in patients with CAD clearly show that conventional or intensive antianginal drug treatment aimed at symptom control does not eliminate asymptomatic ischemic episodes. In a study of 105 patients with stable angina and CAD who were considered adequately treated with one or more antianginal drugs, more than 40% had asymptomatic ischemia (see Figs. 25.1 and 25.2) during AEM.[5] Most ischemic episodes occurred during minimal or no physical activity, and the majority of patients were free of symptoms during the monitoring period.[5]

SUMMARY

Asymptomatic ischemia occurs frequently both in patients who have acute CAD and in those who have stable CAD. The data that are available from a number of studies indicate that the presence of asymptomatic ischemia identifies patients who are at greater risk of coronary events and cardiac death. Although all anti-ischemic treatments are useful, beta blockers appear to be the most effective drugs for the treatment of asymptomatic ischemia, particularly in suppressing the morning surge of ischemic activity. Whether treatment of asymptomatic ischemia can alter the associated adverse prognosis is not yet fully established. Although there are some interesting data indicating that additional suppression of asymptomatic ischemia beyond manifest angina will be helpful, it is clear that additional large-scale trials are required. Revascularization, particularly if it is complete, may be more effective than medical treatment in reducing asymptomatic ischemia. In addition, it is now clear that reduction of risk factors leads to improved perfusion, including reduction of asymptomatic ischemia. Because risk factor reduction can improve endothelial dysfunction, it is presumed that this mechanism is responsible for reducing ischemia. This further emphasizes the importance of aggressive risk factor reduction in patients who have known coronary artery disease.[51-54]

chapter 26 Special Problems in Myocardial Ischemia

a. Diagnostic Procedures in Stable Patients with Symptoms Suggestive of Myocardial Ischemia

Harvey S. Hecht

DEFINITION OF PROBLEM

Physicians are confronted with a multiplicity of diagnostic procedures for the evaluation of stable patients with symptoms of myocardial ischemia. Unlike acute coronary syndrome, in which catheterization is the procedure of choice, a stable clinical situation permits a number of options ranging the entire gamut of technology, from exercise to pharmacologic, function to anatomy, and noninvasive to invasive (Table 26A.1).

TYPICAL CASE

A 64-year-old man, with hypertension treated with an angiotensin-converting enzyme inhibitor and hypercholesterolemia treated with a statin, presented with a 2-month history of substernal pressure always related to moderate exertion, relieved within 2 to 3 minutes by rest. He underwent treadmill nuclear stress testing with a same-day rest and stress technetium protocol, with an exercise duration of 10 minutes on a standard Bruce protocol, achieving a maximum heart rate of 148 beats per minute (95% predicted maximal heart rate) and blood pressure of 198/84 mm Hg, accompanied by mild typical chest discomfort. There was 1.5 mm of horizontal ST-segment depression in leads II, III, AVF, and V_4 through V_6, which was interpreted as an ischemic response. However, the myocardial perfusion images (Fig. 26A.1) demonstrated normal perfusion. The mismatch of electrocardiographic and perfusion findings prompted the cardiologist to order multidetector computed tomographic coronary angiography (CTA). Significant disease in the left anterior descending coronary artery as well as a 50% distal left main stenosis was noted (Fig. 26A.2). Cross-sectional analysis revealed a critical left main minimum luminal area of 3.5 mm^2, well below the 6.0 mm^2 lower limits of normal (Fig. 26A.3). The patient was referred for coronary angiography, which confirmed the significant left anterior descending disease but revealed only mild narrowing in the left main coronary artery (see Fig. 26A.2). Intravascular ultrasonography (IVUS) was performed and confirmed the CTA findings (see Fig. 26A.3); bypass surgery was performed.

DIAGNOSTIC TEST DATA REQUIREMENTS

In this clinical scenario, the presenting symptoms were typical for stable angina, and the diagnosis of ischemic heart disease was apparently confirmed by the abnormal exercise electrocardiogram. However, the normal myocardial perfusion imaging raised significant doubt, suggesting that the electrocardiographic response was falsely positive and that the symptoms may have been an atypical presentation of a noncardiac etiology. A second diagnostic test was therefore required, and CTA was chosen to provide the anatomic information that until the advent of CTA could be provided only by invasive coronary angiography. The CTA presented unequivocal angiographic evidence of severe left anterior descending disease and critical left main disease. Selective coronary angiography was then performed and also revealed severe left anterior descending disease. IVUS was required because of the borderline angiographic appearance (<50% stenosis) of the left main; it confirmed the diagnosis, and the patient was referred for bypass surgery.

This sequence of events is particularly instructive because it demonstrates the qualitatively different data provided by the different diagnostic modalities and the apparent problems that can arise, even in this classic clinical scenario. A variety of data are often required to make appropriate clinical decisions because the characteristics of stable angina do not allow differentiation between the extremes of critical left main or triple-vessel coronary disease, which may require percutaneous or surgical intervention, and small branch vessel disease, which may be treated medically, as well as all stages in between.

The diagnostic test data that are required for appropriate decision making encompass the following.

1. Sensitivity, specificity, and predictive value for obstructive coronary disease. The accuracy of any diagnostic test is dependent on the prevalence of disease in the test population (Bayes' theorem). In the setting of classic angina, the pretest likelihood (prevalence) is greater than 80%, and a positive diagnostic test result does

not add significantly to the already high pretest likelihood. However, confirmation is essential; a negative test result would pose a significant problem because despite the classic symptoms, the diagnosis cannot be validated and treatment cannot be initiated without objective evidence of disease. In the current case, the initial diagnostic test yielded conflicting results and gave no clue to the severity of the disease, if any. The second test, CTA, has a higher sensitivity, specificity, and predictive value than nuclear stress testing.

DIAGNOSTIC PROCEDURES IN STABLE PATIENTS WITH SYMPTOMS OF MYOCARDIAL ISCHEMIA			
Perfusion	**Anatomy**	**Ischemia**	**Plaque**
Nuclear stress testing: exercise, pharmacologic		x	
Positron emission tomography perfusion imaging		x	
Magnetic resonance perfusion imaging		x	
Fractional flow reserve*		x	
Function			
Stress electrocardiography		x	
Stress echocardiography: exercise, pharmacologic		x	
Anatomy			
Selective coronary angiography*	x		
Multidetector computed tomographic coronary angiography	x		x
Intravascular ultrasound* (IVUS)	x		x
*Invasive.			

Table 26A.1 Diagnostic Procedures in Stable Patients with Symptoms of Myocardial Ischemia.

2. Extent of ischemic myocardium. Determination of the amount of ischemic myocardium, irrespective of the anatomic data, has the advantage of a large prognostic database but is very much dependent on variables that may limit its utility. The accuracy of all stress tests depends on achieving adequate disparities between supply and demand with exercise or dobutamine or creating differential blood flow with adenosine or dipyridamole to identify all segments that are supplied by potentially flow-limiting stenoses. All too often, only the most severe stenosis is identified, and the extent of potential ischemic myocardium may be underestimated. The first test in the current case, nuclear stress testing, is designed to evaluate ischemic myocardium but yielded normal results.
3. Extent of anatomic disease. Tests that provide anatomic data without associated functional information cannot assess the ischemic burden; but by defining the course of the vessels distal to a stenosis, they can delineate the amount of myocardium at potential risk and confirm the diagnosis of coronary artery disease. They are not dependent on the vagaries of achieving adequate flow differentials, and they display all lesions in all arterial segments. The choice of CTA as the second test was designed to provide anatomic data without measurement of ischemic burden.

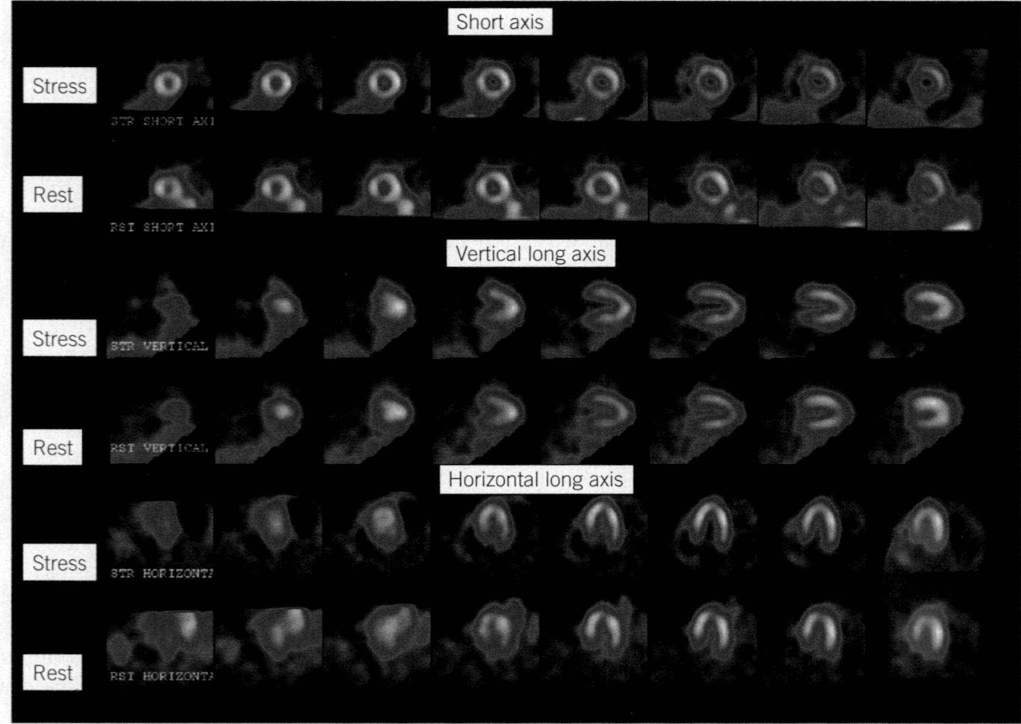

Figure 26A.1 Nuclear stress test reveals uniform perfusion both with stress and at rest in the short-axis, vertical axis, and horizontal long-axis views.

4. Plaque burden and characterization. Modalities that can both quantitate the amount of plaque and characterize plaque vulnerability by identification of low-density lipid–laden areas adjacent to the lumen (thin-cap fibroatheroma), plaque ulceration, and rupture may offer a unique approach to risk stratification and treatment. CTA and IVUS can provide this information, which in this case was needed for the appropriate clinical decision. Measurement of minimum luminal area, which was critical in assessing the left main stenosis, is unique to these modalities.

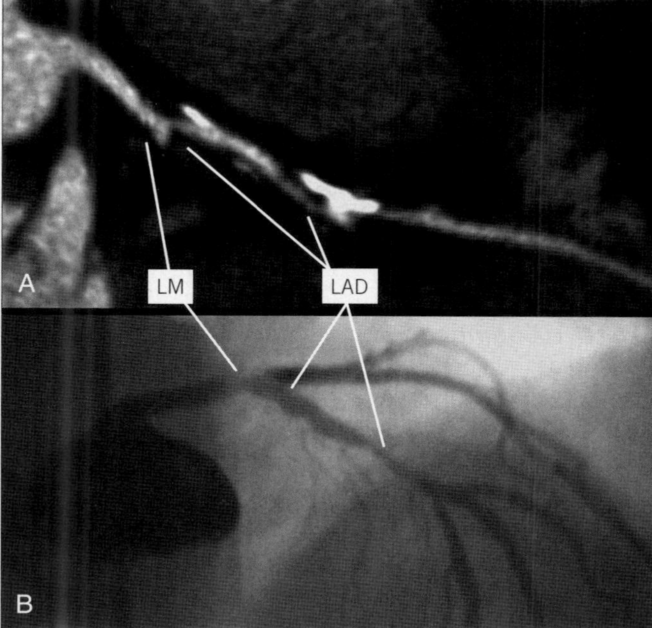

Figure 26A.2 **A,** Multidetector computed tomographic coronary angiography of the left coronary artery demonstrating 50% distal left main (LM) stenosis as well as significant ostial and proximal left anterior descending (LAD) disease. **B,** On the corresponding selective coronary angiogram, only the proximal left anterior descending stenosis appears significant.

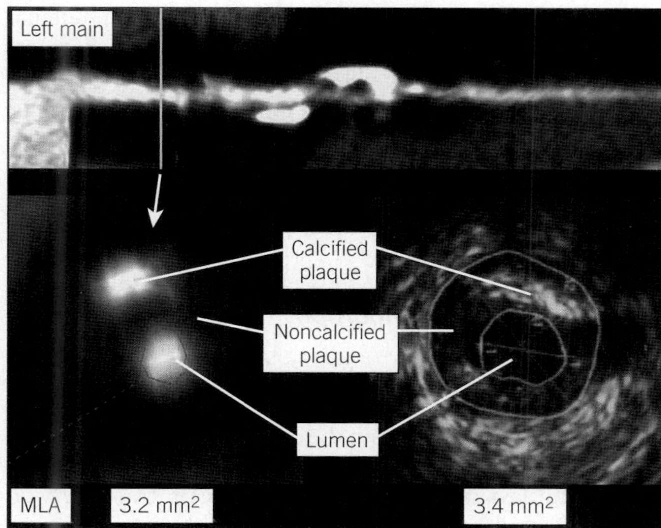

Figure 26A.3 *Top,* Straightened reconstruction of the left anterior descending coronary artery, with a cursor drawn through the left main stenosis. *Left,* Cross section of the distal left main stenosis revealing the calcified and noncalcified plaques and the contrast-filled lumen with a minimum luminal area (MLA) of 3.2 mm^2. *Right,* Corresponding intravascular ultrasound image revealing the same components and a minimum luminal area of 3.4 mm^2.

DIAGNOSTIC OPTIONS

With a plethora of diagnostic tests offering different data sets, the appropriate choice requires an understanding of their advantages and disadvantages in the specific clinical setting.

Perfusion Tests

Nuclear Stress Testing

Advantages

Myocardial perfusion imaging (MPI) with technetium or thallium is performed with either exercise or pharmacologic stress. It has become the most frequently used diagnostic test and has accumulated an extraordinary database relating prognosis to the amount of ischemia in thousands of patients. In the patient with stable angina, in addition to confirming the presence of disease, it can lead to invasive angiography with a view to catheter-based or surgical intervention if the ischemic burden is sufficiently large (>30% of the left ventricular myocardium). With lesser degrees of ischemia, aggressive medical therapy would be indicated, with intervention reserved for uncontrolled symptoms.

Disadvantages

Because MPI is abnormal only in the setting of a stenosis greater than 50% and never presents direct evidence of atherosclerosis, a normal test result in the setting of classic stable symptoms presents the alternatives of assuming the patient does not have what the clinical presentation overwhelmingly indicates or performing a second diagnostic test to confirm the diagnosis of coronary artery disease. In addition, MPI may underestimate the ischemic burden in advanced disease: 40% of patients with triple-vessel disease and 15% of those with left main disease will have images that are normal or consistent with only single-vessel disease, as illustrated by the present clinical scenario. This is representative of a problem common to all the perfusion imaging modalities: the unavoidable designation of the best perfused area as normal will consistently lead to underdiagnosis of ischemia in the vascular bed with the least obstructive disease. In addition, the radiation dose ranges from 14 to 32 mSv, higher than with typical selective coronary angiography.

Positron Emission Tomography Stress Testing

Advantages

Positron emission tomography (PET) imaging with pharmacologic stress and rubidium as a flow tracer has the highest sensitivity and specificity of all the perfusion modalities, provides ischemic burden data, and is considered by many to be the diagnostic test of choice.

Disadvantages

The relative paucity of PET scanners performing MPI and their absence from the private cardiology office, as well as the greater expense, have significantly limited its application. As with all perfusion imaging, it designates the best perfused segments as normal, even if they are subserved by diseased vessels. The superior sensitivity renders a normal test result less likely but may still be problematic. Radiation exposure is in the range of 16 mSv.

Fractional Flow Reserve

Advantages

Fractional flow reserve (FFR) is used to evaluate the significance of intermediate stenoses at the time of invasive angiography by measuring flow proximal and distal to the stenosis in response to adenosine infusion. Values below 0.75 connote sufficient flow limitation to warrant intervention. It offers the unique opportunity to evaluate the significance of a single stenosis, as opposed to all other modalities that allow, at best, evaluation of a single arterial system.

Disadvantages

FFR is invasive and presupposes that the patient has already been sent for invasive angiography. Moreover, the validation of this technology by comparison with MPI subjects it to the limitations of MPI.

Functional Tests

Electrocardiographic Treadmill Testing

Advantages

The oldest of the diagnostic options, electrocardiographic treadmill testing provides electrocardiographic evidence of inducible ischemia as well as a measure of exercise capacity, both of which have significant prognostic implications.

Disadvantages

Electrocardiographic treadmill testing has the lowest sensitivity of all the options, is not reliable in the setting of underlying electrocardiographic abnormalities, and will require an additional confirmatory test if the results are normal in the setting of stable angina. Moreover, it does not provide information other than inferential evidence for the presence or absence of obstructive disease; ischemic burden cannot be evaluated.

Stress Echocardiography

Advantages

Exercise or dobutamine induction of wall motion abnormalities provides sensitivity, specificity, and prognostic data similar to MPI, as well as a sense of the amount of jeopardized myocardium, and is free of radiation. Unlike MPI, each myocardial segment serves as its own reference, and provided sufficient stress has been achieved, stress echocardiography should be more accurate in detecting left main and triple-vessel disease.

Problems

Although it is purportedly equivalent to MPI, it is perceived outside of university centers as being far less sensitive and more subject to variations in study quality and interpretation. As with all the options, a normal test result belies the diagnosis of angina, and a second test may be required.

Magnetic Resonance Dobutamine Stress Imaging

Advantages

Magnetic resonance imaging of adenosine and dobutamine-induced wall motion abnormalities has diagnostic power similar to that of stress echocardiography. It represents a viable alternative.

Disadvantages

As with PET imaging, it is not readily available in the private sector and is much more expensive than stress echocardiography.

Anatomic Tests

Selective Coronary Angiography

Advantages

Selective coronary angiography (SCA) has long been regarded as the "gold standard" for coronary evaluation, with an extensive prognostic database. Arguments have been made for proceeding directly to SCA in the patient with classic angina because the diagnosis is not in doubt and all that remains is to define the extent of disease. Decisions to intervene are based on the number of diseased vessels and the extent of the disease, which is not apparent from MPI. Intermediate stenoses can be further evaluated with FFR or IVUS.

Disadvantages

SCA is invasive, and the prognostic data are not superior to those based on noninvasively obtained ischemic burden derived from MPI. Moreover, the parameter on which SCA interpretation is based (i.e., percentage diameter stenosis) is devoid of physiologic significance; the minimum luminal area, rather than a single minimum luminal diameter, determines flow and cannot be obtained from SCA. In addition, if similar anatomic information can be obtained from a noninvasive alternative (i.e., CTA), the patient is spared the possible morbidity, mortality, and greater expense inherent in SCA. In the present case, the left main disease was not apparent on SCA, and IVUS was required to confirm the CTA left main findings.

Intravascular Ultrasonography

Advantages

IVUS may be used as an adjunct to SCA to determine the significance of intermediate stenoses that may not appear sufficiently severe to explain the symptoms of stable angina. Minimum luminal areas of less than 4 mm^2 in the proximal vessels and less than 6 mm^2 in the left main correlate well with MPI evidence for ischemia and with untoward outcomes and are used as criteria for intervention. The ability to measure the minimum luminal area as well as to provide plaque burden and characterization may give the truest picture of the atherosclerotic process. Through the use of radiofrequency backscatter analysis, the thin-cap fibroatheroma may be identified and, pending the results of ongoing studies, may be a target for interventional treatment.

Disadvantages

IVUS is invasive. Despite its correlation with MPI, it does not provide direct evidence for ischemia. As with FFR, it presupposes invasive angiography.

Multidetector Computed Tomographic Coronary Angiography

Advantages

CTA has the highest sensitivity and specificity of all the noninvasive diagnostic tests and possesses all of the advantages of SCA, without being invasive. Of equal importance, it can display the arterial wall as well as the lumen and allows minimum luminal area measurement and plaque characterization on cross-sectional images, unlike perfusion imaging and SCA.

Disadvantages

CTA, similar to SCA, does not provide evidence of ischemia. However, minimum luminal area measurements provide IVUS-like guidance. Radiation is, in general, similar to or less than that of MPI but greater than with the typical SCA.

SUMMARY

The diagnostic tests are interrelated in an often contradictory manner. SCA serves as the gold standard for CTA, MPI, PET, electrocardiographic treadmill testing, and stress echocardiography, but it does not correlate well with IVUS and is intrinsically flawed by reliance on the nonphysiologic percentage diameter stenosis. IVUS and FFR were validated by comparison with MPI, which in turn was validated by SCA, which does not correlate well with IVUS. It is clear that there is no gold standard, and decision making based on a single test result will invariably overlook some physiologic or anatomic data. Nonetheless, it is increasingly unrealistic and cost prohibitive to perform multiple diagnostic tests in the patient with stable angina. Because there is no single test that can consistently supply *all* the data necessary for appropriate decision making, and because the quality of each modality may vary greatly from one facility to another, the physician must choose the best available resource and not rely on accuracies published at academic centers. In the patient with stable angina, the diagnosis would have been obvious if the first test had been CTA, a test not affected by the potential of MPI for underestimation of multivessel or left main disease.

Although CTA is the latest addition to the diagnostic armamentarium, it appears to provide the requisite combination of sensitivity and specificity, coronary anatomy, and plaque burden and characterization to serve as the initial diagnostic test. If CTA does not yield sufficient diagnostic information, MPI may follow to provide ischemic burden data.

b. Sexual Activity and the Cardiac Patient

Jonathan Abrams

DESCRIPTION OF PROBLEM

Sexual activity has achieved a new prominence with the advent of sildenafil citrate and two other remarkably effective drugs for impotence or erectile dysfunction (ED). The availability of these agents has stimulated a dialogue relating to the potential risks of sex in cardiac patients and whether it is safe to use one of these drugs (sildenafil, vardenafil, and tadalafil). This commentary reviews the physiologic energy requirements of sexual activity as well as the actions and potential hazards of ED therapy and provides guidelines for a safe and practical approach to sex in the cardiac patient.

It is estimated that 20 to 30 million American men have experienced some degree of ED. The most important association with ED is increased age; the incidence of ED rises dramatically in men as they get older. Many factors that are common to cardiac patients correlate with disturbed sexual function. Smoking, diabetes, hypertension, and hyperlipidemia are frequently found in cardiac subjects, and each is associated with endothelial dysfunction. Depression in the post–myocardial infarction or post–coronary bypass patient is often associated with decreased libido and sexual performance. Recent surveys suggest that up to 40% to 50% of men between the ages of 40 and 70 years experience some degree of ED at one time or another. Smokers have a twofold increased likelihood of having impaired sexual performance. The development and marketing of the phosphodiesterase type 5 (PDE-5) inhibitors created intense interest in use of these drugs to improve or to reverse sexual dysfunction. Thus, hundreds of thousands of men have used or will use these agents; some may be engaging in sexual relations to a greater degree than ever or enjoying sex for the first time in years. The latter is important, as there is a real risk, although uncommon, for individuals engaged in new or increased sexual activity. Such behavior can impart a hazard in the presence of severe underlying coronary disease, particularly if it is occult. It remains unclear if the PDE-5 inhibitors, in the absence of nitrate consumption, impart any specific hazard. However, recent data are reassuring.

TYPICAL CASE

A 53-year-old man developed severe chest pain during sexual intercourse. In the emergency department, he was diagnosed with an acute anterior myocardial infarction and given thrombolytic therapy. Left ventricular function was severely impaired, with an ejection fraction of 25% to 30%. He developed mild congestive heart failure, which improved with an angiotensin-converting enzyme inhibitor and diuretics. After hospital discharge, he participated in a cardiac rehabilitation program. Medications included aspirin, lisinopril, metoprolol, and furosemide. He was overtly depressed, and this persisted in spite of counseling and sertraline therapy. He complained of mild anginal chest discomfort that was effort related but refused to undergo coronary angiography. He was reluctant to resume regular sexual activity because of fear of another heart attack. He was given sildenafil to aid his sexual function as he reported classic symptoms of ED. Four months later, he developed severe chest pain 90 minutes after sex. Emergency rescue personnel gave him a dose of nitroglycerin spray. He promptly became extremely dizzy and was found to have a blood pressure of 80/60 mm Hg., with a heart rate of 62 beats per minute.

DIFFERENTIAL DIAGNOSIS

In a patient with documented coronary artery disease (CAD) and abnormal left ventricular function, a variety of factors could have precipitated chest pain and the resulting hypotension that followed sexual activity. These include a severe anginal episode and even an acute myocardial infarction. The hypotension could reflect low stroke volume related to acute infarction, perhaps with a mechanical complication such as severe mitral regurgitation. Another possibility is extensive ischemia-induced myocardial dysfunction alone or superimposed on preexisting left ventricular systolic dysfunction. Marked vagotonia with or without bradycardia or heart block could produce this picture. Another possibility is a sildenafil-nitroglycerin interaction, resulting in marked hypotension (see later).

Cardiovascular Physiologic Response to Sexual Activity

A number of studies have provided information about the physiologic "costs" of sexual intercourse. These data, using heart rate and blood pressure responses and usually employing ambulatory recording technology, suggest that sexual activity is equivalent to mild to moderate exercise (Table 26B.1). The actual energy costs of sex appear to range between 2 and 6 metabolic equivalents. Cardiovascular responses to sexual stimulation and activity are also affected by the atmosphere or excitement level surrounding the sexual activity; use of medications, recreational drugs, cigarettes, or alcohol; the presence or absence of known or occult CAD; and other factors, such as a recent large meal. Thus, it is difficult to predict the precise level of energy cost of sexual activity for a given individual. The physiologic and hemodynamic effects of sexual activity are also related to the fitness level of the individual; physically fit subjects have lower energy requirements than do those who are sedentary (Table 26B.2). Thus, intelligent use of exercise testing to evaluate a subject's functional capacity, the presence or absence of ischemia, and the level of work at which ischemia or arrhythmia (if any) occurs can assist the physician and patient in making appropriate decisions about the safety of sexual activity. In particular, a stress test (see later) can help define recommendations and precautions that might be prudent (including *no* sexual intercourse in highly symptomatic or vulnerable individuals). Some drugs should be used with caution.

ENERGY COSTS OF SOME COMMON ACTIVITIES	
Activity	**METs**
Walking (2–3 mph)	2–3
Light housework	3–4
Heavy housework	5–6
Stair climbing, walk up hill	4–5
Painting, masonry	4–5
Sexual activity	2–6
Cycling (10 mph)	6–7
Moderate recreation (golf, bowling, doubles tennis, dancing)	5–7
Shoveling	10
Strenuous sports (swimming, singles tennis, skiing, basketball)	>10

METs, metabolic equivalents.

Table 26B.1 Energy costs of some common activities.

PHYSIOLOGIC RESPONSE TO SEXUAL ACTIVITY		
	Estimated Hemodynamic Responses to Sexual Activity	
	Younger	**Older**
Maximal heart rate	115-180 beats/minute	80-185 beats/minute
Systolic blood pressure	≤190 mm Hg	≤150 mm Hg

Note: Individual responses are highly variable. Physically fit individuals have lower energy costs and heart rate and blood pressure responses.

Table 26B.2 Physiologic response to sexual activity.

In general, the dictum for the safety of PDE-5 drugs is to use common sense. Individuals with cardiovascular disease who would not be proscribed from sexual activity need no admonition about sexual intercourse or medication use. Figure 26B.1 outlines a risk assessment algorithm to guide the physician's advice about sexual activity and sildenafil, tadalafil, or vardenafil. Individuals at intermediate or questionable CAD risk should be carefully evaluated by the physician; when in doubt, or if symptoms suggest a potential hazard, an exercise test may be useful. In high-risk patients, a cardiovascular stress test and a careful history are mandatory. For instance, general health and well-being, frequency of cardiovascular symptoms and the lowest level of physical activity to precipitate such symptoms, frequency of sexual activity, intensity of sexual intercourse, and prescription drug history should all be evaluated.

Figure 26B.2 outlines the molecular structure of the PDE-5 drugs. Table 26B.3 demonstrates clinical pharmacology of PDE-5 agents.

Drugs and Erectile Dysfunction

Many pharmacologic therapies used in middle-aged men can contribute to or even cause sexual dysfunction. Table 26B.4 lists some common drugs that may contribute to ED. In combination with underlying impaired endothelial function or overt vascular disease, these pharmacologic agents may contribute an important component to ED. It is not always easy to withdraw or to switch drugs prescribed for specific conditions. Nevertheless, it is critical for the individual with ED and his physician to review and to assess the patient's medication list with a specific focus on the issue of sexual dysfunction (see Table 26B.4).

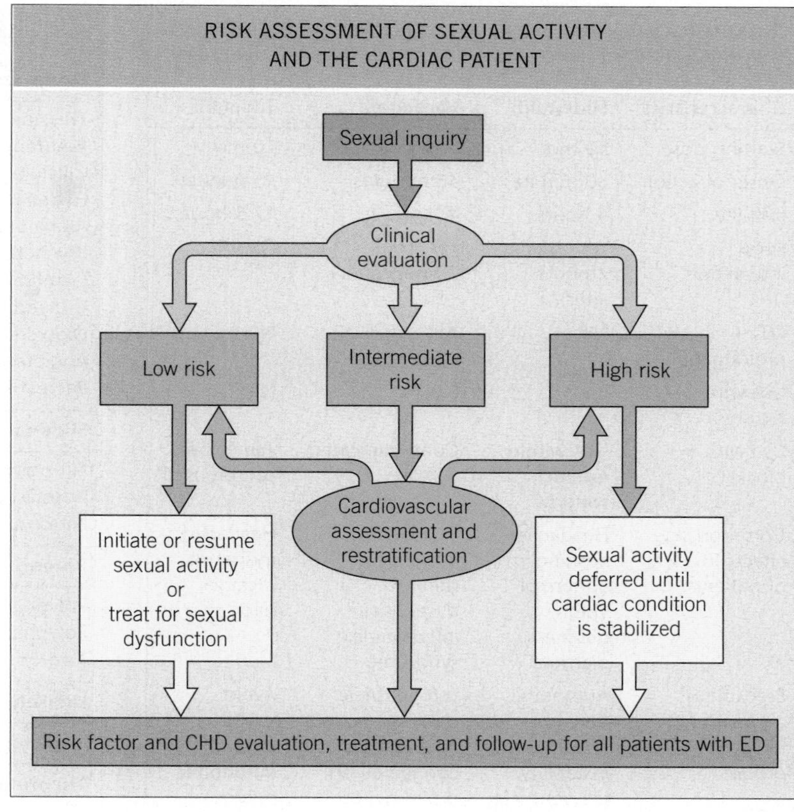

Figure 26B.1 Risk assessment of sexual activity and the cardiac patient. Risk assessment algorithm to guide the physician's advice about sexual activity and sildenafil, tadalafil, or vardenafil. CHD, coronary heart disease; ED, erectile dysfunction. (From Kostis JB, Jackson G, Rosen R, et al. Sexual dysfunction and cardiac risk [the Second Princeton Consensus Conference]. Am J Cardiol 2005;96:313-321.)

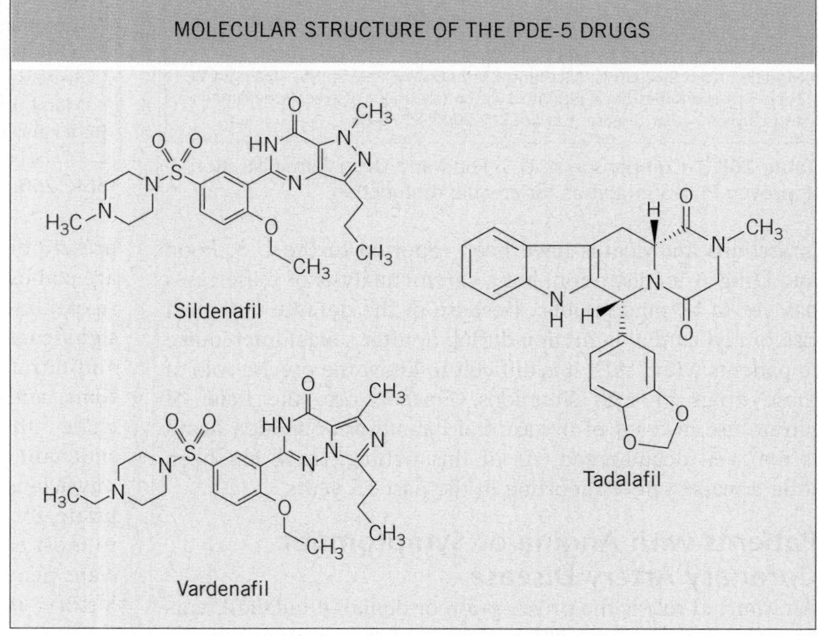

Figure 26B.2 Molecular structure of the PDE-5 drugs. (From Ravipati G, McClung J, Aronow W, Peterson S, Frishman W. Type 5 phosphodiesterase inhibitors in the treatment of erectile dysfunction and cardiovascular disease. Cardiol Rev 2007;15:76-86.)

TREATMENT OPTIONS

Guidelines for Sildenafil, Tadalafil, or Vardenafil Administration

In 1999, the American College of Cardiology and the American Heart Association published a consensus document relating to the use of the PDE-5 drugs in patients with cardiovascular disease. Guidelines and recommendations are provided to guide physicians as to how to deal with potential adverse events. It is likely that the same guidelines apply to all three ED agents and are still appropriate. In 2005, the report "Sexual Dysfunction and Cardiac Risk" from the Second Princeton Consensus Conference was published, outlining much of this discussion in detail. Although relatively conservative in outlook, these reports are a valuable overview of the subject (see Fig. 26B.1). A number of myocardial

COMPARISON OF U.S. FOOD AND DRUG ADMINISTRATION–APPROVED PDE-5 INHIBITORS FOR ERECTILE DYSFUNCTION			
Characteristics	Sildenafil	Vardenafil	Tadalafil
Starting dose	50 mg	5 mg	10 mg
Onset of action	60 minutes	45 minutes	45 minutes
Half-life	4 hours	4 hours	17.5 hours
Food interaction	Yes (take 2 hours after)	Yes (take 2 hours after)	No
QT prolongation	No	Yes	No
Use with nitrates	No	No	No
Use with α_1 blockers	Not within 4-hour window	Contraindicated	Tamsulosin can be used
Common side effects in >2% of patients	Headache, flushing, abnormal vision, dizziness, diarrhea	Headache, flushing, rhinitis, dyspepsia, influenza-like syndrome	Headache, dyspepsia, myalgia, back pain
Precautions and warnings in special groups	Autonomic nervous system instability, left ventricle outflow obstruction	Left ventricle outflow obstruction, congenital QT prolongation taking class IA and III antiarrhythmic agents	Avoid excess alcohol, autonomic nervous system instability, left ventricle obstruction

Modified from Ravipati G, McClung J, Aronow W, Peterson S, Frishman W. Type 5 phosphodiesterase inhibitors in the treatment of erectile dysfunction and cardiovascular disease. Cardiol Rev 2007;15:76-86.

Table 26B.3 Comparison of U.S. Food and Drug Administration–approved PDE-5 inhibitors for erectile dysfunction.

DRUGS AND SILDENAFIL
Drugs associated with erectile dysfunction
Thiazides β-Adrenergic blockers Calcium channel antagonists Hydralazine Alpha blockers Psychotropic agents Gemfibrozil Cimetidine Digoxin Angiotensin-converting enzyme inhibitors Recreational drugs: alcohol, cocaine, heroin, marijuana
Sildenafil-drug interactions: Dangerous
Nitroglycerin Isosorbide dinitrate, 5-mononitrate Nitroprusside
Potential problem
Polypharmacy for hypertension Polypharmacy for congestive heart failure Two or more vasoactive drugs
Unlikely problem
Single-drug therapy for hypertension
Theoretical problem (use lower doses)
Concomitant cytochrome P450 3A4 inhibitors (prolong sildenafil half-life) Macrolide antibiotics (e.g., erythromycin) Cimetidine Antifungals Protease inhibitors Many other drugs Renal and hepatic dysfunction

Table 26B.4 Drugs and sildenafil.

infarctions and deaths have been reported to the U.S. Food and Drug Administration, but a careful analysis of these cases has yet to be made public. Because of the definite but small risk of myocardial infarction during or after sexual intercourse in patients with CAD, it is difficult to know the precise role of these drugs in such situations. Furthermore, the issue of nitrate use in cases of myocardial infarction or sudden death is not well documented. As of this writing, there has been little adverse safety reporting in the past 15 years.

Patients with Angina or Symptomatic Coronary Artery Disease

An ironclad rule is the proscription or denial of tadalafil, vardenafil, or sildenafil to any patient likely to experience anginal chest pain with modest physical activity. Thus, individuals with chronic stable angina should probably not be given a PDE-5 inhibitor as there is always a chance that the patient will be exposed to or be given nitroglycerin, often by emergency or hospital personnel. Such individuals may be counseled to engage in sexual activity but emphatically warned against the concomitant use of nitroglycerin or long-acting nitrates if a PDE-5 inhibitor is used. It is naive to assume that men with coronary disease will not be able to obtain these drugs, even if the physician refuses to provide a prescription. Patients with heart failure or hypertension who are stable with pharmacologic therapy may safely engage in sexual intercourse and use PDE-5 inhibitors in the absence of significant cardiovascular symptoms, recent hospitalization, and nitrate use. Polypharmacy, class III heart failure symptoms, and low blood pressure are factors that should preclude the administration of tadalafil, vardenafil, or sildenafil (Fig. 26B.3). Dialogue with male patients and their physicians demands a careful sexual history as being appropriate for any individual interested in sildenafil use. Many to most cardiac patients will experience ED at times; physicians need to alter their mindset to initiate a sexual activity history, not only when a PDE-5 inhibitor is the issue but for more general counseling and guidance. The Second Princeton Consensus Conference report goes into more detail about risk factor modification to treat ED as well as to increase safety of the PDE-5 agents and is recommended to physicians interested in the subject.

Physiology of Erectile Dysfunction

Normal erectile function involves a complex interplay of neurogenic, vascular, and humoral-hormonal phenomena. In brief, the corpus cavernosum becomes engorged as the extensive venous sinusoids serve as reservoirs for storage

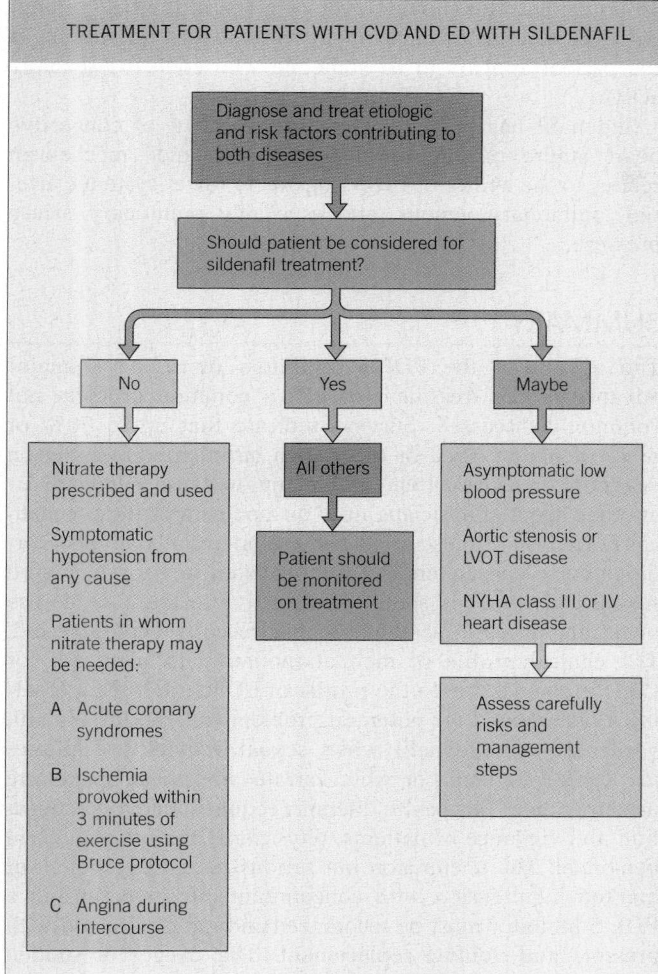

Figure 26B.3 Algorithm for treatment of patients with cardiovascular disease (CVD) and erectile dysfunction (ED) with sildenafil. LVOT, left ventricular outflow tract; NYHA, New York Heart Association (class of functional capacity on a grading scale of I to IV).

of blood during the erectile process. Compression of the venous drainage is critical to maintenance of erection and engorgement. The erectile process is modulated in part by noncholinergic, nonadrenergic neurons in the corpus cavernosum that release nitric oxide. Smooth muscle vasodilatation of the cavernosal arteries induced by nitric oxide results in venous sinusoid engorgement and tumescence. ED may be a result of hormonal, vascular, neurogenic, psychogenic, or pharmacologic factors, often in combination. In general, impaired nitric oxide availability from a variety of causes results in ED. Sildenafil or either of the other two agents enhances the physiologic activity of nitric oxide by decreasing the breakdown or metabolism of cyclic guanosine monophosphate (cGMP) through PDE-5 inhibition (Fig. 26B.4). Studies suggest that tadalafil, vardenafil, and sildenafil are effective for most causes of ED, with remarkable consistency no matter what the underlying etiology.

Coronary Risk Factors and Erectile Dysfunction

It is well known that classic coronary risk factors may signal underlying or occult CAD in subjects without a history of

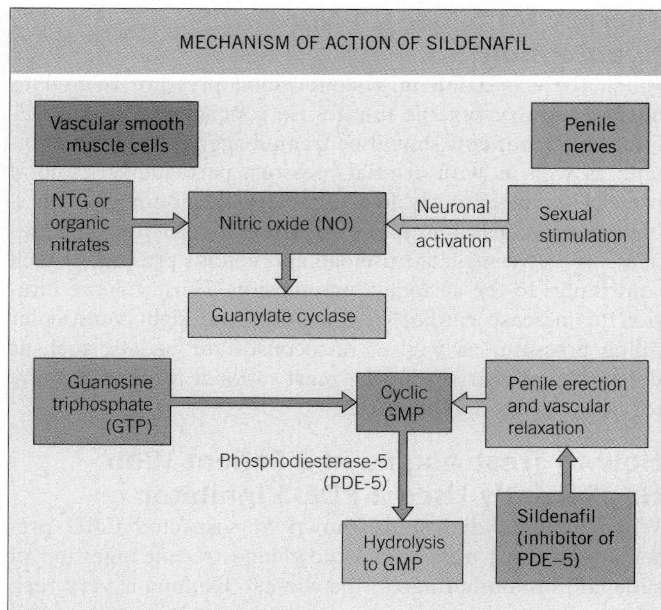

Figure 26B.4 Mechanism of action of sildenafil. GMP, guanosine monophosphate; NTG, nitroglycerin.

chest pain. Thus, endothelial dysfunction and latent coronary atherosclerosis may become clinically manifested in subjects with clinical ED but no evidence of CAD. It is recommended that the development of ED in middle-aged men should heighten awareness and suspicion that the individual may also have "the other" ED, that is, endothelial dysfunction caused by coronary disease. The Second Princeton Consensus Conference's detailed appropriate approach to men with ED is important reading for physicians who prescribe PDE-5 inhibitors.

The Nitrate Interaction

Nitroglycerin and the long-acting nitrates are nitric oxide donors that act at the vascular smooth muscle cell and platelet by increasing cGMP through activation of guanylate cyclase (see Fig. 26B.4). The combination of an exogenous nitrate and a PDE-5 inhibitor results in a significant increase in cGMP availability. The nitrate delivers more nitric oxide into the vasculature, whereas sildenafil and the other agents prevent breakdown of cGMP, the second messenger that directly initiates vascular smooth muscle relaxation and vasodilatation. Thus, enhanced hemodynamic action of organic nitrates occurs when sildenafil and the other agents are administered in the presence of a nitrate; blood pressure may fall dramatically.

Because of the potential of this adverse drug interaction, it is imperative to warn all patients with CAD never to take sublingual nitroglycerin or to use long-acting nitrates while taking sildenafil, tadalafil, or vardenafil. At least 24 hours should elapse between prior nitrate use and administration of sildenafil and vardenafil and 2 days with tadalafil. No data are available that adequately elucidate the duration of the "danger period" after PDE-5 administration when a nitrate is given other than the average duration of action as provided by the pharmaceutical companies.

Therapy for Sildenafil-Nitrate Hypotension

When there is a fall in systolic blood pressure related to nitroglycerin or organic nitrate use concomitant with PDE-5 ingestion, patients should be treated aggressively with volume as well as with arterial pressors, particularly if blood pressure is dangerously low. The Trendelenburg position is obligatory. Physicians often do not recognize that nitrates decrease left ventricular preload and venous pressure, which contributes to the systemic hypotension. Thus, volume infusion to increase cardiac preload (left and right ventricular filling pressure) as well as vasoconstrictor agents, such as dopamine, appears to be the most rational form of therapy for acute severe hypotension.

How to Treat Angina in a Patient Who Has Recently Used a PDE-5 Inhibitor

When an individual with known or suspected CAD presents with chest pain and acknowledges recent ingestion of sildenafil or another agent, the clinical dilemma is very real; *nitrates must not be used in such circumstances*. A rapid-acting beta blocker is a reasonable choice for ischemia control in these patients, if blood pressure is not excessively low. Careful administration of intravenous metoprolol or esmolol is appropriate if sustained chest pain is present. Intravenous diltiazem is another option. Small doses of narcotics should be used, if necessary. Once the angina abates, continued therapy with any of these agents remains appropriate, depending on the clinical situation and the physician's judgment.

Emergency Personnel and PDE-5 Agents

It is imperative that ambulance and emergency department personnel as well as coronary care unit nurses and physicians *always* ask a new male patient with recent-onset chest pain if he has used sildenafil or another agent within the past 24 to 36 hours. Nitrates should never be given in the field, ambulance, or emergency department without such questioning if the patient appears to be someone who could be sexually active.

Sildenafil has been effective in treatment of congestive heart failure in some studies. The presumed mechanism relates to the ability of PDE-5 agents to lower systemic arterial, pulmonary venous, and especially pulmonary artery pressure.

SUMMARY

The advent of the PDE-5 inhibitors represents a major advance in the treatment of ED, a common problem not commonly discussed. Surveys indicate that up to 50% or more of middle-aged or older men may experience ED on occasion or more often, and many will use sildenafil or another agent. Physicians need to understand the mechanisms of action of these drugs and the potentially adverse cardiovascular consequences resulting from new or increased sexual activity; they should be sensitive to the possible use of nitrates if a PDE-5 inhibitor has recently been ingested. The clinical profile of men at moderate to high risk for CAD is comparable to the profile of ED in adult men, creating a background for potential problems related to tadalafil, vardenafil, or sildenafil when sexual activity precipitates myocardial ischemia or when nitrates and these agents are used together. This health dilemma requires increased education and vigilance of patients, physicians, and other medical personnel. The uncommon but serious potential problem of marked hypotension with concomitant nitroglycerin and a PDE-5 inhibitor must be recognized and rapidly treated with pressors and volume replacement. The danger of sudden death and acute myocardial infarction related to tadalafil, vardenafil, or sildenafil, if any, remains unclear; further data are required to resolve this question.

c. The Diagnosis of Coronary Artery Disease in Patients Being Considered for Renal Transplantation

Anuradha Tunuguntula and Rajni Rao

CASE

A 49-year-old African American man was referred to the cardiology service for left-sided heart catheterization before renal transplantation. The patient has end-stage renal disease due to poorly controlled hypertension as well as hyperlipidemia (total cholesterol level, 210 mg/dL; high-density lipoprotein concentration, 38 mg/dL; low-density lipoprotein concentration, 120 mg/dL) and a history of tobacco use. The patient reported having intermittent, nonradiating chest tightness for 3 months as well as dyspnea on exertion. His functional capacity was judged to be less than 4 metabolic equivalents. The physical examination was significant for hypertension (160/100 mm Hg) and a fourth heart sound. The electrocardiogram revealed sinus rhythm and left ventricular hypertrophy. The echocardiogram showed mild left atrium enlargement, mitral annular calcification, moderate mitral regurgitation, moderate concentric left ventricular hypertrophy, and a left ventricular ejection fraction of 50%. An adenosine nuclear perfusion scan showed mild ischemia of the proximal half of the anterolateral wall and mild scarring of the inferior wall. Therefore, coronary angiography was performed. The patient had normal left main, left anterior descending, left circumflex, and right coronary arteries, and there was a mild 30% stenosis of the ramus intermedius. Aggressive medical management of coronary artery disease risk factors was recommended while awaiting renal transplantation.

DISCUSSION

Renal transplant recipients die of cardiovascular disease at an accelerated rate compared with the general population. There is general agreement among transplant programs that

PATIENTS AT HIGH RISK FOR POST-TRANSPLANTATION CARDIOVASCULAR EVENTS
Diabetics
Men >45 years
Women >55 years
Previous ischemic heart disease
Peripheral vascular disease
Abnormal electrocardiogram
Echocardiographic evidence of left ventricular dysfunction
Left ventricular ejection fraction <40%
Left ventricular hypertrophy
Smokers
Duration of dialysis >2 years
Fasting total cholesterol level >200 mg/dL
High-density lipoprotein cholesterol level <35 mg/dL

Table 26C.1 Patients at high risk for post-transplantation cardiovascular events.

cardiovascular assessment is required for many patients awaiting transplantation, with more intense evaluation for "high-risk" patients (Table 26C.1).[1] There is no consensus, however, on who should be screened or the optimal method and frequency of screening for occult cardiovascular disease.

Diabetics have a markedly elevated risk of cardiovascular disease compared with nondiabetics, and they have greater mortality after acute coronary syndromes than do patients with other causes of end-stage renal disease. One third of the cardiac deaths are attributed to acute myocardial infarction, and the poorest survival after acute myocardial infarction occurred in patients with diabetic end-stage renal disease.[2] Similarly, patients with a prior history of ischemic heart disease have been shown to be at high risk for the development of coronary events after transplantation.

In dialysis patients, traditional factors account for some of the increased risk of coronary artery disease, however the use of Framingham-based equations underestimates the real risk because risk factors such as hyperhomocysteinemia, increased C-reactive protein levels, calcium phosphate deposition, and anemia, all common in patients with end-stage renal disease, are not included. Pretransplantation echocardiographic measures of left ventricular mass and function have been shown to be independent predictors of cardiovascular death, with increased mortality in those with systolic dysfunction or concentric left ventricular hypertrophy.[3] Dialysis patients are susceptible to progressive cardiomyopathy, coronary artery disease, and accelerated aortic stenosis.

Cardiovascular disease often progresses rapidly in patients on maintenance hemodialysis, and at least 5% of patients on the waiting list die each year.[4] The duration of dialysis is an important risk factor for cardiovascular death after transplantation.[4] Patients transplanted preemptively before the development of end-stage renal disease have a better cardiac prognosis than do those who had been receiving hemodialysis. While a patient awaits availability of a suitable kidney, all potentially reversible risk factors for coronary artery disease should be addressed: hyperlipidemia, hypertension, diabetes mellitus, smoking, obesity, and sedentary lifestyle.[5] To reduce unnecessary cardiac evaluations, patients can be stratified according to their likelihood of cardiovascular events, with screening recommended for those at highest risk (see Table 26C.1). Initial evaluation with resting echocardiography and myocardial perfusion studies or stress echocardiography is recommended for high-risk patients. Coronary angiography is reserved for those in whom screening test results are positive for ischemia.[1] However, patients with symptomatic coronary artery disease may proceed directly to coronary angiography. Any change in clinical status (e.g., new cardiac event, worsening congestive heart failure) should be reported to the transplant center and mandates reevaluation.

There is no optimal strategy for ongoing cardiac surveillance of patients on the renal transplant waiting list. Guidelines for regular cardiac reevaluation of patients on the waiting list have been proposed (Fig. 26C.1).[6]

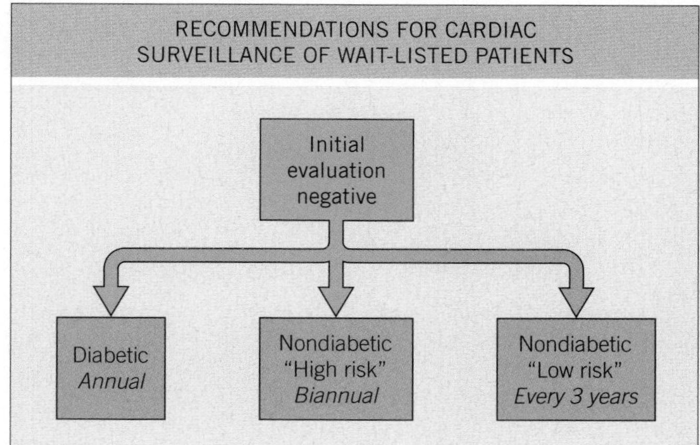

Figure 26C.1 Recommendations for cardiac surveillance of wait-listed patients. (From Herzog CA, Ma JZ, Collins AJ. Comparative survival of dialysis patients in the United States after coronary angioplasty, coronary artery stenting, and coronary artery bypass surgery and impact of diabetes. Circulation 2002;106:2207–2221.)

chapter 27

Diagnosis of Acute Myocardial Ischemia and Infarction

Sharif A. Halim, L. Kristin Newby, and E. Magnus Ohman

Definition

- The diagnosis of acute myocardial ischemia and infarction has important therapeutic and prognostic implications.

Key Features

Myocardial infarction or ischemia is diagnosed by these findings:

- History of chest discomfort or clinical equivalents.
- Electrocardiographic evidence of ischemia or infarction.
- Elevation of biomarkers in the serum consistent with myocardial necrosis.
- Imaging evidence of new loss of viable myocardium or regional wall motion abnormalities.

Clinical Implications

- Early and rapid diagnosis of myocardial ischemia or infarction identifies a group that may achieve maximum benefit from evidence-based therapies.

During the last several years, there has been considerable debate as to what should constitute the definition of myocardial infarction (MI). Not only does the diagnosis of MI have clinical implications, it also carries with it epidemiologic, economic, and psychosocial ramifications. However, distinguishing between acute coronary syndromes without myocardial injury and those with a small component of cardiac injury was often difficult, with challenges created by evolution of increasingly sensitive diagnostic assays for serum markers of necrosis and the variable precision of these assays. In an attempt to standardize the definition of MI, including incorporation of the use of troponins, in 2000 the European Society of Cardiology/American College of Cardiology Committee for the Redefinition of Myocardial Infarction proposed a redefinition of MI that incorporated small amounts of cardiac injury in which troponin effectively replaced creatine kinase (CK) MB as the "gold standard" for MI diagnosis in the appropriate clinical circumstances.[1] Despite this document, questions and concerns remained about application of the "new" definition of MI in various clinical situations (including percutaneous coronary intervention [PCI], coronary artery bypass graft [CABG] surgery, sudden death), the interrelationship of troponin results with other diagnostic tools (electrocardiography, imaging), and the application of the new parameters for MI not only in clinical practice but also in clinical research.[2] To address these lingering issues, a Global Task Force was assembled to establish consensus for a universal definition of MI.[3] This most recent definition has expanded on the prior document to include more specific recommendations, with the integration of multiple modalities for diagnosis and parameters for other less recognized forms of MI (Table 27.1).

Based on the new universal definition, there are three categories of diagnostic tools:

- electrocardiography;
- biomarkers; and
- imaging.

DESCRIPTION OF DEVICE, TECHNIQUE, AND PROCEDURE

Electrocardiography

Electrocardiography (ECG) is a cost-effective and integral test for the diagnosis of myocardial ischemia and infarction.[1,3-6] It is widely available and can easily be recorded at the time a patient presents with symptoms, including by paramedics and other medical personnel in the field. Clinicians are trained in rapid interpretation of this diagnostic modality; thus, it is usually the first objective test performed when myocardial ischemia or infarction is suspected. The presence of acute changes in the ST segments or T waves and evolution of Q waves potentially allow clinicians to estimate timing of the ischemic event or infarction and the amount of myocardium at risk as well as suggest the infarct-related artery in the case of ST-segment elevation.[7] Whereas there are certain stereotypical patterns of acute MI, other changes are less specific and require interpretation by cardiologists and additional testing to distinguish a diagnosis of MI from ischemia. There are also a number of ECG abnormalities that are observed in conditions other than acute MI that mimic changes seen in acute MI. These include conditions such as acute pericarditis, left ventricular hypertrophy, left bundle branch block, Brugada syndrome, and early repolarization patterns (Table 27.2).[8] Typical appearances of these abnormalities on ECG are demonstrated in Figures 27.1 and 27.2.

In general, there are four categories of ECG findings during suspected acute coronary syndrome: ST-segment elevation, ST-segment depression, confounding ECG patterns, and T-wave inversion or nonspecific patterns. ST-segment elevation is underpinned by a pathophysiologic process different from that of non–ST-segment elevation patterns and typically indicates a greater degree of thrombus burden with total occlusion of an epicardial coronary vessel. The ST-segment elevation, or current of injury, on the ECG is

ESC/ACCF/AHA/WHF UNIVERSAL DEFINITION OF MYOCARDIAL INFARCTION
Criteria for acute MI
1. Detection of rise and/or fall of cardiac biomarkers (preferably troponin) with at least one value above the 99th percentile of the upper reference limit (URL) together with evidence of myocardial ischemia with at least one of the following: Symptoms of ischemia ECG changes indicative of new ischemia (new ST-T changes or new left bundle branch block [LBBB]) Development of pathological Q waves in the ECG Imaging evidence of new loss of viable myocardium or new regional wall motion abnormality
2. Sudden unexpected cardiac death, involving cardiac arrest, often with symptoms suggestive of myocardial ischemia, and accompanied by presumably new ST elevation, or new LBBB, and/or evidence of fresh thrombus by coronary angiography and/or at autopsy, but death occurring before blood samples could be obtained, or at a time before the appearance of cardiac biomarkers in the blood.
3. For percutaneous coronary interventions (PCI) in patients with normal baseline troponin values, elevations of cardiac biomarkers above the 99th percentile URL are indicative of periprocedural myocardial necrosis. By convention, increases of biomarkers greater than 3 × 99th percentile URL have been designated as defining PCI-related myocardial infarction. A subtype related to a documented stent thrombosis is recognized.
4. For coronary artery bypass grafting (CABG) in patients with normal baseline troponin values, elevations of cardiac biomarkers above the 99th percentile URL indicative of periprocedural myocardial necrosis. By convention, increases of biomarkers greater than 5 × 99th percentile URL plus either new pathological Q waves or new LBBB, or angiographically documented new graft or native coronary artery occlusion, or imaging evidence of new loss of viable myocardium have been designated as defining CABG-related myocardial infarction.
5. Pathological findings of an acute myocardial infarction
Criteria for prior MI
Any one of the following criteria satisfies the diagnosis for prior MI: 1. Development of new pathological Q waves with or without symptoms 2. Imaging evidence of a region of loss of viable myocardium that is thinned and fails to contract, in the absence of a nonischemic cause 3. Pathological findings of a healed or healing myocardial infarction
ESC/ACCF/AHA/WHF, European Society of Cardiology, American College of Cardiology Foundation, American Heart Association, World Heart Federation. From Thygesen K, Alpert JS, White HD; Joint ESC/ACCF/AHA/WHF Task Force for the Redefinition of Myocardial Infarction. Universal definition of myocardial infarction. Circulation 2007;116:2634-2653.

Table 27.1 ESC/ACCF/AHA/WHF universal definition of myocardial infarction.

COMMON ELECTROCARDIOGRAPHIC PITFALLS IN DIAGNOSIS OF MYOCARDIAL INFARCTION
False positives
Benign early repolarization Left bundle branch block Preexcitation Brugada syndrome Pericarditis, myocarditis Pulmonary embolism Subarachnoid hemorrhage Metabolic disturbances (i.e., hyperkalemia)
False negatives
Prior MI with Q waves and/or persistent ST elevation Paced rhythm Left bundle branch block
From Thygesen K, Alpert JS, White HD; Joint ESC/ACCF/AHA/WHF Task Force for the Redefinition of Myocardial Infarction. Universal definition of myocardial infarction. Circulation 2007;116:2634-2653.

Table 27.2 Common electrocardiographic pitfalls in diagnosis of myocardial infarction.

associated with total occlusion of an epicardial coronary artery and is directed toward the region of infarct, resulting in the ability to localize ECG findings to regions of myocardium affected and origin of blood supply.

Non–ST-segment elevation refers to a broader range of ECG findings that may be nonspecific and difficult to interpret. These findings include ST-segment depression and T-wave changes that in contrast to ST-segment elevation are not reliable for localizing the area of myocardial ischemia.[9,10] These changes may be transient, present only during chest pain episodes in unstable angina, or may be more persistent in many patients with non–ST-segment elevation MI. These changes are usually indicative of an acute or evolving process; Table 27.3 summarizes ECG findings indicative of prior or old MI. In addition to the diagnostic utility of assessing for Q waves, there is evidence that suggests the prognostic importance of identifying new small Q waves in non–ST-segment elevation acute coronary syndrome. In a retrospective evaluation of 10,500 patients presenting with non–ST-segment elevation acute coronary syndrome who had repeated ECG 30 days after the initial event, new Q waves of 40 ms or more in duration were associated with mortality rates almost double those without new Q waves.[11]

Beyond these categories of ECG changes during myocardial ischemia or infarction, confounding ECG abnormalities deserve particular attention as their presence may obscure ST-segment changes and make interpretation of the ECG difficult. These include right and left bundle branch blocks, left ventricular hypertrophy, and ventricular paced rhythms (see Table 27.2). Interpretation of ECGs in these settings requires the use of several strategies: knowledge of the ST-segment and T-wave

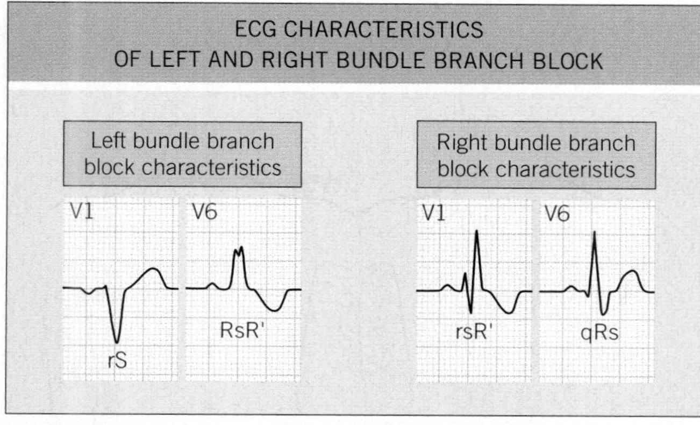

Figure 27.1 ECG characteristics of left and right bundle branch block.

changes associated with these patterns, performance of serial ECGs, and comparison with previous ECGs if they are available.[12,13] In conjunction with certain criteria developed for interpretation of ECGs in these settings, these strategies make it possible to make the diagnosis of myocardial ischemia or infarction in the setting of such confounding patterns. Regarding right bundle branch block, ST-segment changes occurring in leads other than V_1 through V_3 are reliable for the detection of MI. In addition, if the ECG demonstrates upright T waves in a scenario concerning for MI, T-wave pseudonormalization may be present, in which case it becomes imperative to obtain prior ECGs if they are available.

There has been a recent movement aimed at optimizing the ECG identification of MI. Consequently, there are various techniques in development to improve the diagnostic accuracy of the ECG. Currently, body surface mapping, a technique that uses numerous leads on a patient's anterior

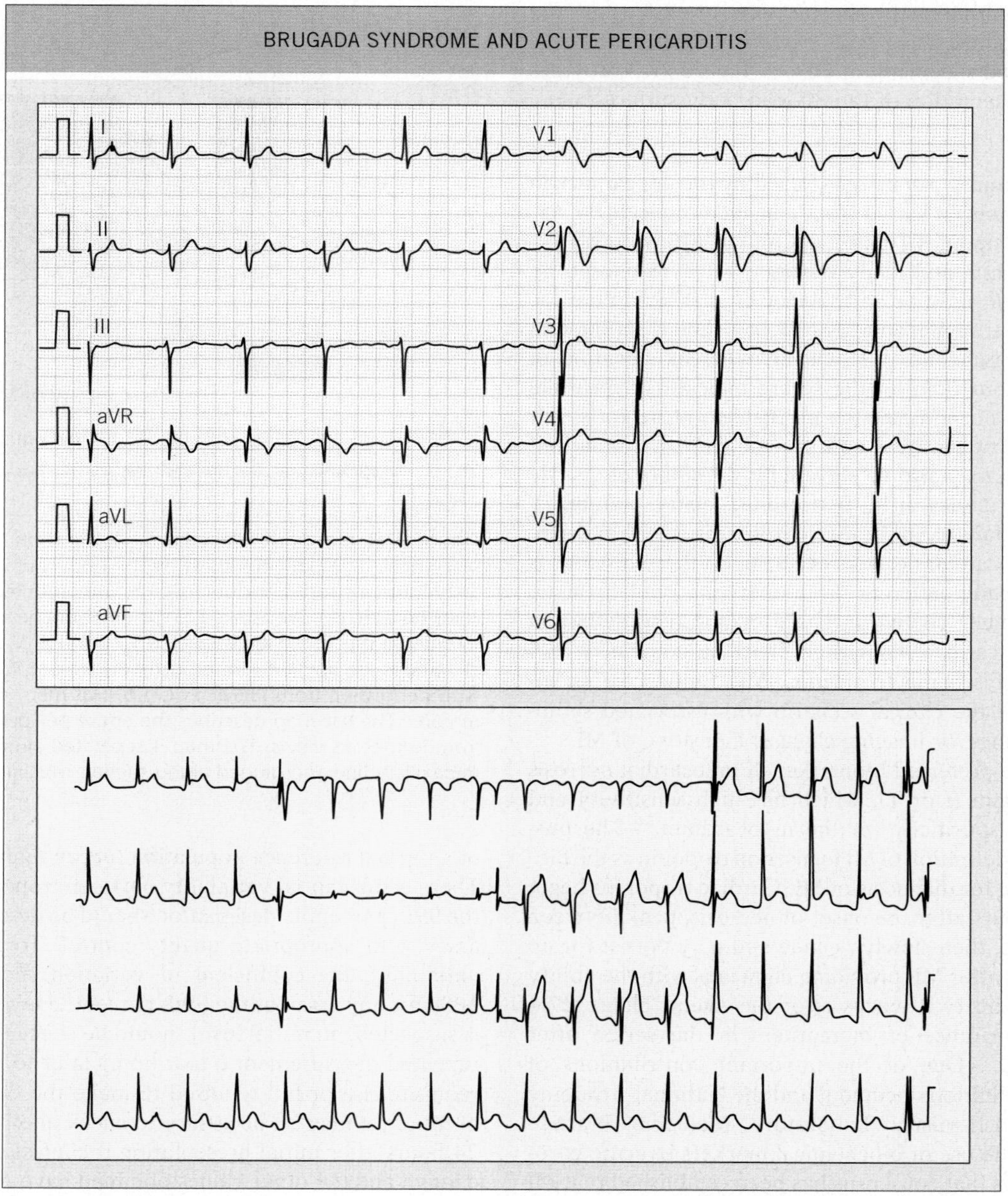

Figure 27.2 ECG findings in Brugada syndrome *(top)* and acute pericarditis *(bottom)*.

ELECTROCARDIOGRAPHIC CHANGES ASSOCIATED WITH PRIOR MYOCARDIAL INFARCTION
Any Q wave in leads V_2-V_3 ≥0.02 s or QS complex in leads V_2 and V_3
Q wave ≥0.03 s and ≥0.1 mV deep or QS complex in leads I, II, aVL, aVF, or V_4-V_6 in any two leads of a contiguous lead grouping (I, aVL, V_6; V_4-V_6; II, III, aVF)
R wave ≥0.04 s in V_1-V_2 and R/S ≥1 with a concordant positive T wave in the absence of a conduction defect
From Thygesen K, Alpert JS, White HD; Joint ESC/ACCF/AHA/WHF Task Force for the Redefinition of Myocardial Infarction. Universal definition of myocardial infarction. Circulation 2007;116:2634-2653.

Table 27.3 Electrocardiographic changes associated with prior myocardial infarction.

and posterior chest, is receiving more attention. This system provides a more detailed visualization of cardiac electrical activity than the standard 12-lead ECG.[14] Recent evidence suggests that combining physicians' interpretations of the ECG with algorithms using body surface mapping improves the sensitivity and specificity of ECG.[15] Figure 27.3 provides a pictorial representation of the 80-lead body surface map.

Biomarkers

Myocardial cell injury can be recognized by the appearance in the blood of proteins released from damaged myocytes: myoglobin, cardiac troponins T and I, CK and its MB isoform, lactate dehydrogenase, and many others.[16] MI is diagnosed by the appearance of sensitive and specific biomarkers in the circulation, such as troponin and CK-MB, in a clinical setting that is suggestive of ischemia.[1,3] However, whereas elevation of these cardiac biomarkers in the serum indicates myocardial necrosis, it does not indicate the mechanism of necrosis. For example, the most sensitive and specific cardiac biomarker, troponin (I or T), may also be elevated in a number of disease states, such as myocarditis, pericarditis, acute pulmonary embolism, renal failure, infiltrative cardiac disorders, and sepsis.[16,17] The myocardial necrosis occurring in these diseases is pathophysiologically different from that observed in acute coronary syndrome. Therefore, based on the new definition of MI, elevated cardiac biomarkers must be combined with some evidence of ischemia to diagnose MI.[3] Evidence of ischemia may include the clinical scenario with associated symptoms, ECG findings, or imaging changes indicative of MI.

Currently, the preferred biomarker of myocardial necrosis is cardiac troponin (I or T), which has high sensitivity and nearly absolute specificity for the myocardium.[16] The proposed universal definition of MI focuses on troponin as the biomarker of choice for diagnosis of MI. Cardiac troponins begin to rise 3 to 4 hours after the onset of necrosis, peak between 18 and 36 hours, then slowly decline and may persist for up to 10 to 14 days after MI, providing clinicians with the ability to diagnose MI up to 2 weeks after the event. Figure 27.4 details the appearance of biomarkers in the serum after symptom onset.[18] One of the important contributions of the universal definition document and the National Academy of Clinical Biochemistry Laboratory Medicine Practice Guidelines for the use of biochemical markers in acute coronary syndrome is that consensus has been established that MI is indicated when troponin values exceed the 99th percentile

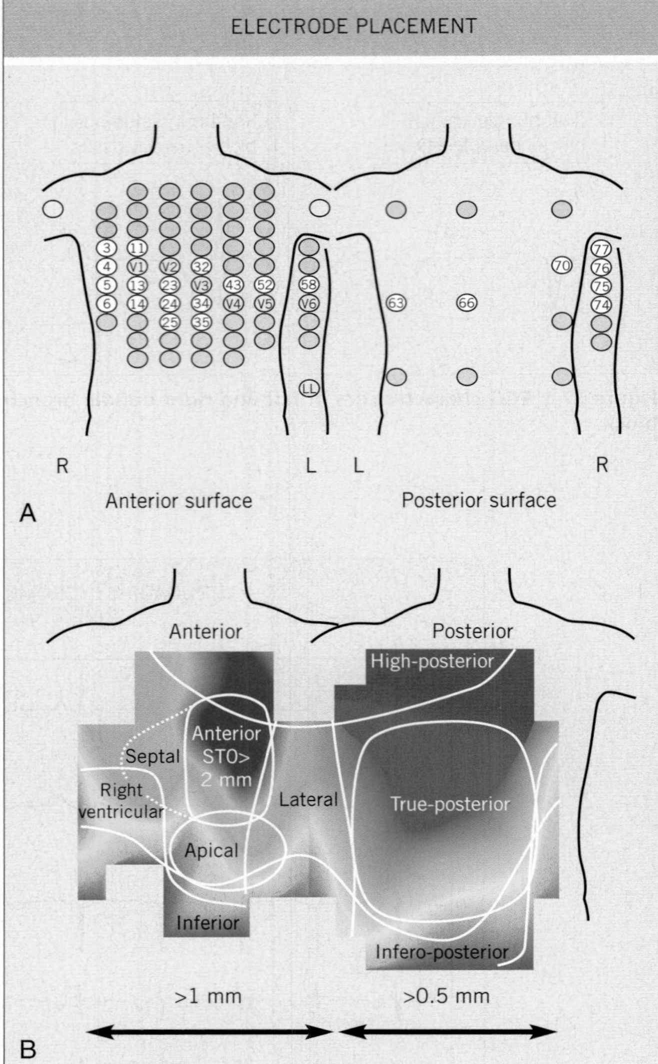

Figure 27.3 Electrode placement. A, Location of electrode placement on a patient's chest by the body surface mapping vest. Sixty-four electrodes, including three unnumbered proximal limb leads (RA, LA, LL), are applied to the anterior chest surface. Note the traditional precordial leads labeled V_1 through V_6. Sixteen electrodes are applied to the posterior chest surface. (Reproduced with permission from PRIME ECG.) **B,** Flat map with anatomic regions. The flat map describes the entire perspective of the heart from numerous views. The map is separated along the right midaxillary line and hinged along the left midaxillary line.[14]

of a normal reference population (upper reference limit).[19,20] There is substantial variability between troponin assays; thus, the 99th percentile designation should be determined for each assay with appropriate quality control. To account for this variability, the coefficient of variation should not exceed 10% for any assay at the 99th percentile level.[19,21] When MI is suspected, an initial level should be checked, followed by a repeated measurement 6 to 9 hours later to demonstrate the requisite rise or fall required to make the diagnosis.[22,23] On occasion, it may be necessary to check another sample 12 to 24 hours after initial presentation if clinical suspicion is high enough and the other values obtained have not exceeded the 99th percentile of the upper reference limit.[23]

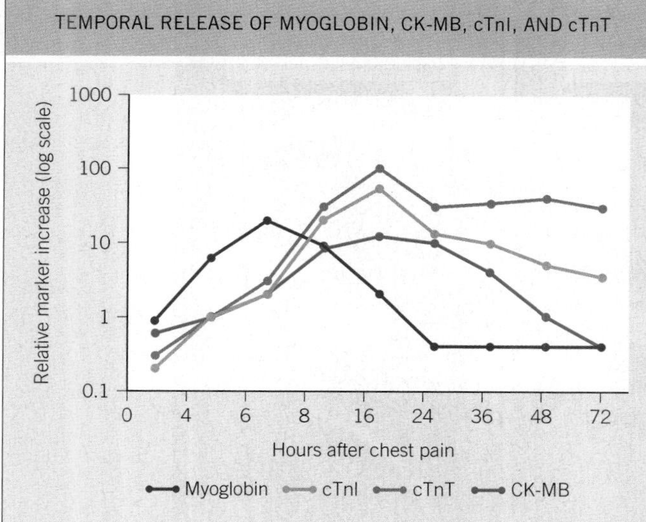

Figure 27.4 Temporal release of myoglobin, CK-MB, and cardiac troponins I (cTnI) and T (cTnT). (With permission from Christenson RH, Azzazy HME. Biomarkers of necrosis: past, present and future. In Morrow DA, ed. Cardiovascular Biomarkers: Pathophysiology and Clinical Management. New York, Humana Press, 2006:3-24).

Imaging

Noninvasive imaging techniques play many roles in establishing the diagnosis of MI. In addition, they are frequently used to provide prognostic information and to guide medical therapy, such as in the setting of impaired left ventricular function. The appropriate use of these techniques during the workup of MI has yet to be fully described, and debate exists between experts. Based on the universal definition of MI, demonstrating the loss of viable myocardium or wall motion abnormalities by various imaging modalities is one of the criteria for diagnosis of MI.[3] In the inpatient or outpatient setting, these modalities can also be used for stress identification of ischemia in combination with exercise treadmill or pharmacologic stress (i.e., dobutamine, adenosine, or dipyridamole). Common imaging techniques in acute and chronic MI include echocardiography, radionuclide imaging, and magnetic resonance imaging.[24] Other less commonly used imaging modalities include positron emission tomography and x-ray computed tomography. The American College of Cardiology recommends use of echocardiography or radionuclide imaging when the diagnosis of MI is unclear at presentation.[4] In addition, these imaging modalities, along with cardiac magnetic resonance imaging, can be used to estimate infarct size and residual left ventricular function during the index hospitalization. Furthermore, at time of discharge, these modalities may be useful in guiding future medical and interventional therapies by assessing other areas of inducible ischemia and viability.[4,6] Our discussion focuses on the commonly used modalities.

Echocardiography

Echocardiography is a simple, readily available noninvasive imaging technique. It has moderate spatial and temporal resolution. In considering the diagnosis of MI or ischemia, echocardiography is primarily used to assess left ventricular function and wall motion. When it is combined with Doppler study, information also can be obtained about valvular abnormalities and for estimation of pressure gradients. In the setting of acute MI, echocardiography may be helpful in evaluating the extent of myocardium at risk based on the degree of left ventricular dysfunction and wall motion abnormalities.[25,26] However, its utility is limited in the setting of known left ventricular dysfunction and prior MI with residual wall motion abnormalities. Another limitation is the inability of echocardiography to distinguish between MI and ischemic myocardium with hibernation.

Cardiac Magnetic Resonance Imaging

Cardiovascular magnetic resonance imaging (MRI) has excellent spatial resolution and moderate temporal resolution. It has been validated as a standard for assessing myocardial function and even provides detailed information about myocardial fibrosis that occurs in specific patterns according to etiology.[27,28] Resting perfusion imaging with late gadolinium enhancement clearly delineates subendocardial and transmural infarction. Myocardial ischemia is detected by use of stress first-pass contrast-enhanced myocardial perfusion MRI, and studies have demonstrated the high diagnostic accuracy of stress myocardial perfusion MRI for detecting significant coronary artery disease.[29] Examples of cardiovascular MRI images obtained after ST-segment elevation MI (STEMI) and non–ST-segment elevation MI (NSTEMI) are depicted in Figure 27.5. Images demonstrating myocardial ischemia with stress testing are shown in Figure 27.6. Unfortunately, this modality is not readily available at many medical centers and is impractical in the acute setting.

Radionuclide Imaging

Several radionuclide tracers are available and allow direct imaging of viable myocytes or ischemia. These include thallium Tl 201, technetium Tc 99m sestamibi or tetrofosmin, and [^{18}F]2-fluorodeoxyglucose.[30-32] Perfusion imaging, particularly with sestamibi, is widely available and can diagnose acute MI early. These agents can also be used to image severely hypoperfused myocardium, providing an estimate of myocardial area at risk or infarct size. Furthermore, radionuclide imaging may be used to assess the extent of salvageable myocardium and to evaluate left ventricular function and wall motion when it is combined with gated three-dimensional tomographic slice reconstruction of the available images.[33,34]

INDICATIONS AND OBJECTIVES

Acute coronary syndrome (ACS) defines a spectrum of diagnoses from unstable angina to NSTEMI to STEMI. Patients are grouped into these categories on the basis of clinical presentation (i.e., symptoms suggestive of ischemia or infarction), ECG findings, and cardiac biomarker evaluation. For the purposes of this discussion, we combine unstable angina and NSTEMI into a grouping of non–ST-segment elevation ACS.

The classic description of myocardial ischemia as a crushing or pressure-like substernal discomfort combined with adrenergic symptoms (i.e., diaphoresis, nausea, vomiting, lightheadedness, anxiety) is often cited[35,36]; however, this constellation of symptoms is often absent, particularly in certain groups, such as women, the elderly, and patients with

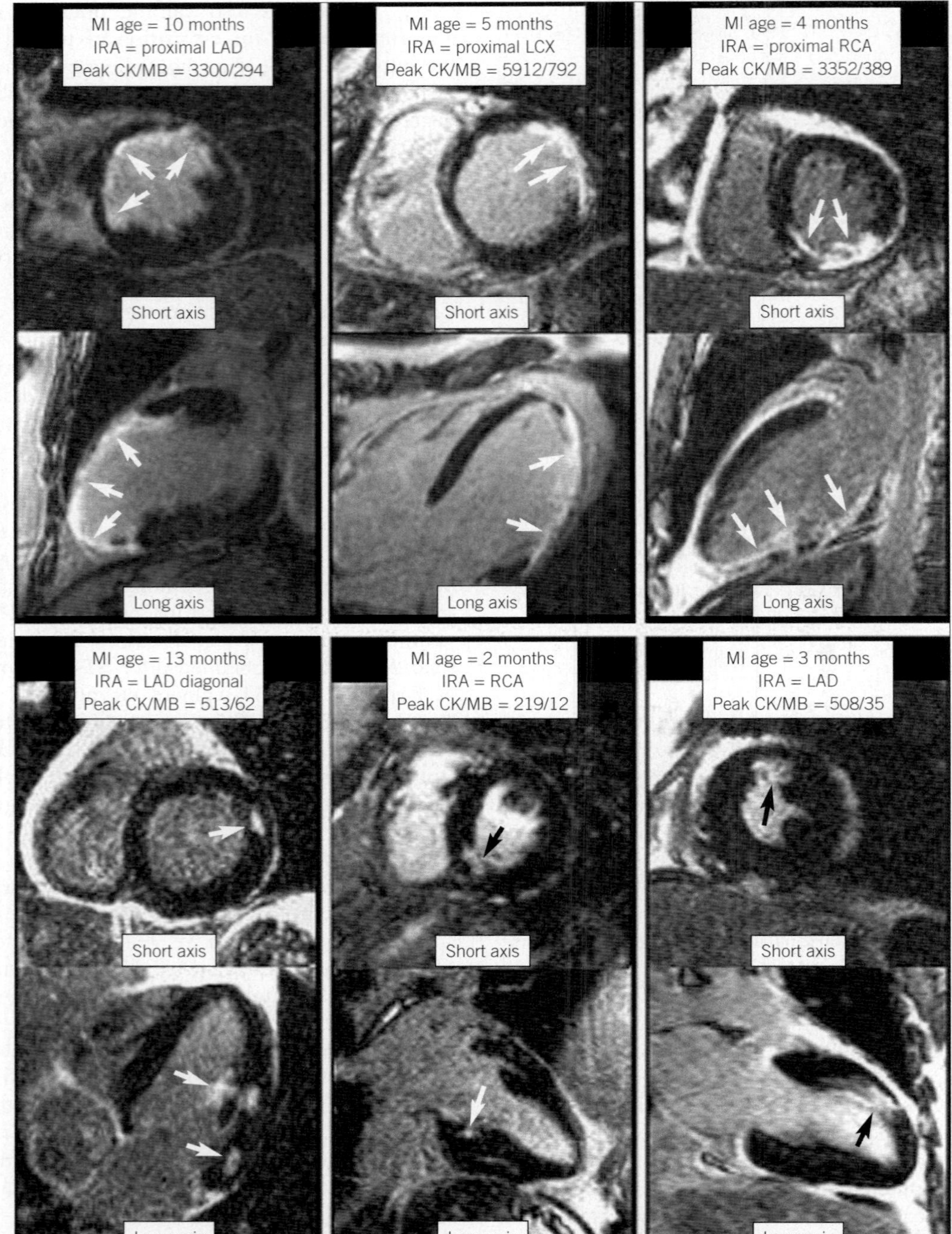

Figure 27.5 Cardiac MRI demonstrating transmural infarction *(top)* based on infarct-related artery (IRA) in the case of STEMI and subendocardial infarction *(bottom)* in the case of NSTEMI. LAD, left anterior descending; LCX, left circumflex; RCA, right coronary artery. (With permission from Wu E, Judd RM, Vargas JD, Klocke FJ, Bonow RO, Kim RJ. Visualisation of presence, location, and transmural extent of healed Q-wave and non–Q-wave myocardial infarction. Lancet 2001;357:21-28.)

diabetes.[37,38] In fact, up to 25% of patients who sustain an MI are asymptomatic during the acute event, and the diagnosis is often made retrospectively. Nonetheless, clinicians rely on certain clinical presentations that suggest myocardial ischemia or infarction to accurately assess for the presence of disease. The National Heart Attack Alert Group Program suggests that patients with the following symptoms receive an evaluation for possible MI: (1) chest pain, pressure, tightness or heaviness, or radiating pain in the neck, jaw, shoulder, back, or arms; (2) indigestion, heartburn, nausea, and vomiting—these symptoms commonly occur in patients with acute MI; (3) shortness of breath; (4) and weakness, dizziness, lightheadedness, or syncope or loss of consciousness.[39] As one can imagine, this creates a diagnostic burden for

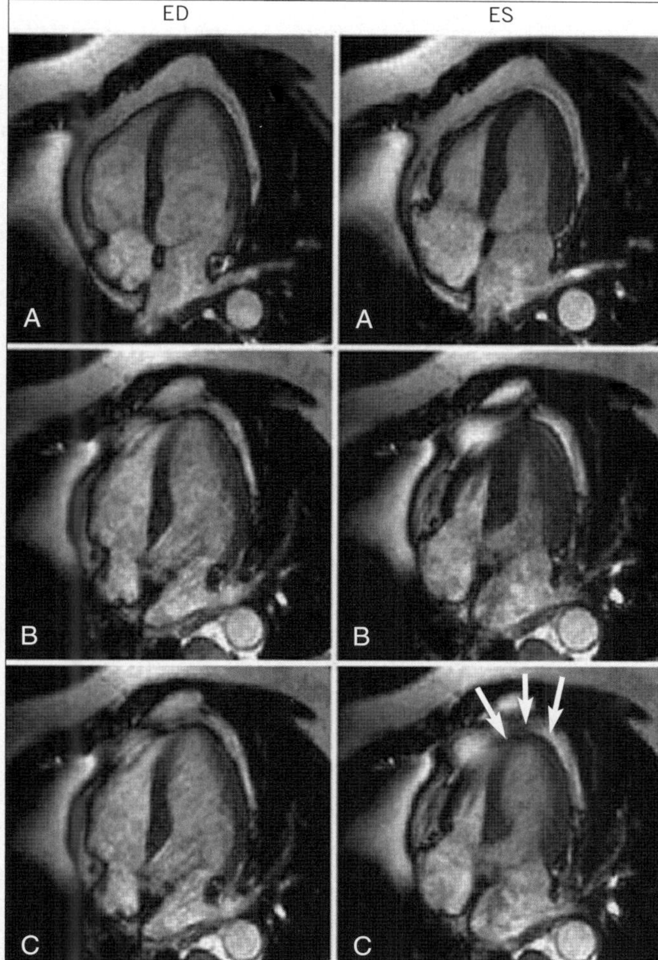

Figure 27.6 Four-chamber magnetic resonance images (SENSE b-SSFP) at rest **(A),** at intermediate-dose dobutamine (20 μg/kg per minute) **(B),** and at peak-dose dobutamine (40 μg/kg per minute) **(C)** showing both end-diastolic (ED, *left column*) and end-systolic (ES, *right column*) phases: 45-year-old man with atypical chest pain. Intermediate-dose dobutamine MRI displayed adequate increase of endocardial inward movement and wall thickening compared with rest. At peak-dose dobutamine, the patient developed a pronounced akinesis *(arrows)* in the apex indicative of stress-induced ischemia. Coronary angiography revealed a high-grade stenosis of the distal left anterior descending artery. (With permission from Strach K, Meyer C, Schild H, Sommer T. Cardiac stress MR imaging with dobutamine. Eur Radiol 2006;16:2728-2738.)

clinicians, and this is where the supporting diagnostic modalities are applied. The remainder of this section focuses on the application of each of these diagnostic tools to specific clinical scenarios.

ST-Segment Elevation Myocardial Infarction

The development of ST-segment elevation signifies impending or current infarction and requires immediate attention and intervention. The distinction of STEMI from other forms of ACS is important as this is a branch point in therapy; STEMI requires quick and accurate assessment, as time to revascularization is an important predictor of outcome.[40]

The clinical presentation is often dramatic and has classic features of MI. However, the key step in establishing the diagnosis of STEMI is the ECG. Therefore, to ensure timely detection and reperfusion of STEMI, the ECG should be obtained within 10 minutes of presentation in all patients with symptoms of suspected ACS.[4,6]

Figure 27.7 illustrates progression of the ECG during STEMI. ST-segment elevations also localize the infarct-related artery with relatively high certainty.[9,10] In general, ST-segment elevations in the inferior leads (II, III, aVF) represent inferior MI and correspond to right coronary artery occlusion; elevations in the anterior precordial leads (V_1 through V_4) represent anterior wall MI and correspond to left anterior descending coronary occlusion; and elevations in the lateral leads (I, aVL, V_5 and V_6) reflect lateral wall MI and correspond to left circumflex coronary occlusion (see Figures 27.8 to 27.11 for examples). If the left circumflex

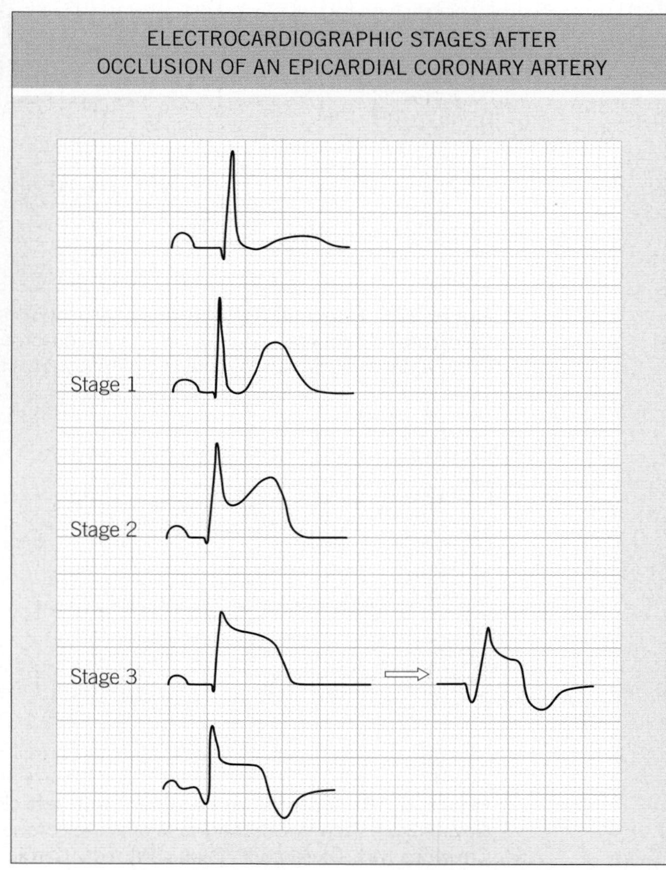

Figure 27.7 Electrocardiographic stages after occlusion of an epicardial coronary artery. The earliest changes (stage 1) are observed in the amplitude and shape of the T wave with no changes in the level of the ST segment. Thus, the T wave becomes taller and more symmetric (i.e., the ascending and descending limbs). In stage 2, the degree of ST-segment elevation is less than 50% of the R-wave amplitude if there is a QR configuration of the QRS or if the ST-segment elevation is accompanied by disappearance of the S wave in cases of an RS configuration of the QRS. In stage 3, the ST-segment elevation is already more than 50% of the R wave. Shortly, the T wave becomes negative and the Q waves appear. (With permission from Veldkamp RF, Simoons ML, Pope JE, Krucoff MW. Continuous multilead monitoring in acute myocardial infarction. In Clements IP, ed. The Electrocardiogram in Myocardial Infarction. Armonk, NY, Futura, 1998:1-30.)

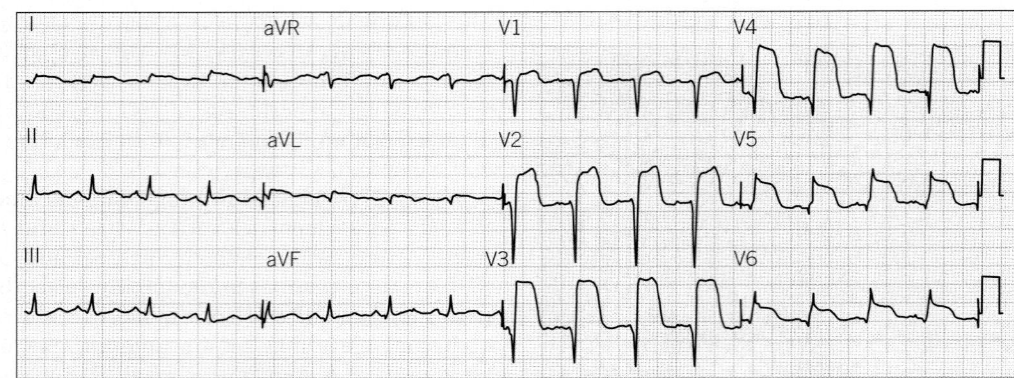

Figure 27.8 Proximal left anterior descending coronary occlusion.

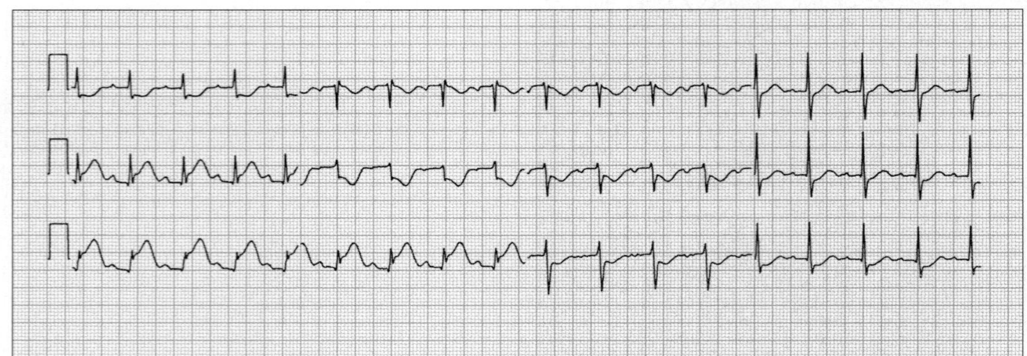

Figure 27.9 Proximal right coronary artery occlusion. (With permission from Jaffe AS, Davidenko J, Clements I. Diagnosis of acute coronary syndromes including acute myocardial infarction. In Crawford MH, DiMarco JP, Paulus WJ, eds. Cardiology. St. Louis, Mosby, 2004:311-328.)

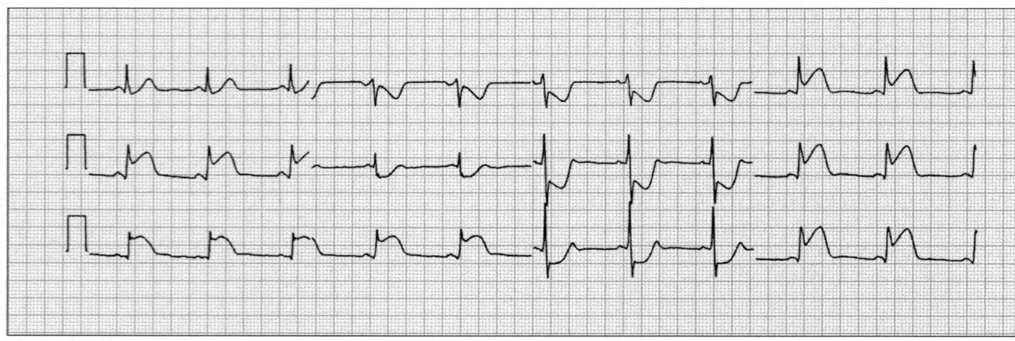

Figure 27.10 Occlusion of dominant mid left circumflex artery. (With permission from Jaffe AS, Davidenko J, Clements I. Diagnosis of acute coronary syndromes including acute myocardial infarction. In Crawford MH, DiMarco JP, Paulus WJ, eds. Cardiology. St. Louis, Mosby, 2004:311-328.)

coronary artery is dominant, supplying blood flow to the inferior wall, ST-segment elevations may occur in leads II, III, and aVF as well. Unfortunately, the diagnosis of left circumflex occlusion is challenging as it often has an electrocardiographically silent presentation. It is in the case of clinical suspicion of left circumflex occlusion that posterior ECG leads (V_7 to V_9) or, potentially, body surface mapping may have the greatest utility.

On occasion, depending on the timing of the presentation, ST-segment elevation may be preceded by hyperacute T waves characterized by increased T-wave amplitude with prominent symmetry. Another unique scenario is that of posterior wall MI, which may be manifested as ST-segment depression in leads V_1 and V_2 that would appear as ST-segment elevations if the ECG were to be "flipped over" or if posterior leads (V_7 to V_9) were applied.[41,42] In addition, in the case of inferior MI, it is advisable to record right precordial leads (V_3R and V_4R), seeking concomitant presence of right ventricular infarction.[43] Clinicians must be able to recognize the presence of right ventricular infarction as there are certain treatment and prognostic implications. For example, nitrates are contraindicated as reduction of preload may result

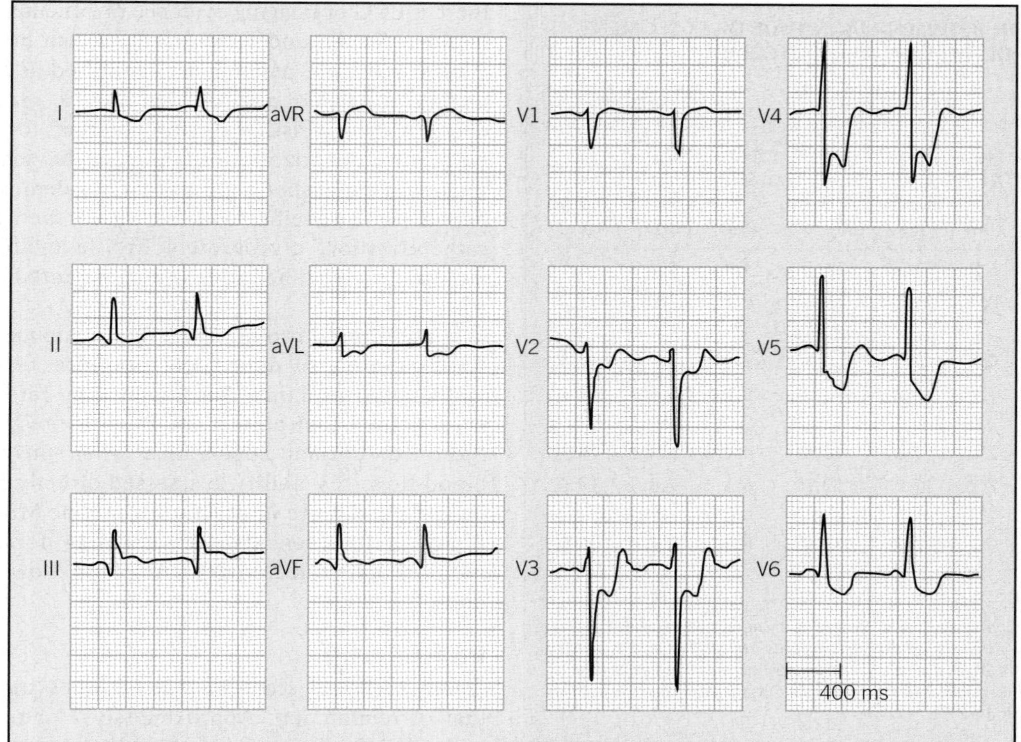

Figure 27.11 Left main coronary disease. (With permission from Jaffe AS, Davidenko J, Clements I. Diagnosis of acute coronary syndromes including acute myocardial infarction. In Crawford MH, DiMarco JP, Paulus WJ, eds. Cardiology. St. Louis, Mosby, 2004:311-328.)

ELECTROCARDIOGRAPHIC MANIFESTATIONS OF ACUTE MYOCARDIAL ISCHEMIA (IN ABSENCE OF LEFT VENTRICULAR HYPERTROPHY AND LEFT BUNDLE BRANCH BLOCK)
ST elevation
New ST elevation at the J-point in two contiguous leads with the cutoff points: $\geq$0.2 mV in men or $\geq$0.15 mV in women in leads V_2-V_3 and/or $\geq$0.1 mV in other leads
ST depression and T-wave changes
New horizontal or downsloping ST depression $\geq$0.05 mV in contiguous leads; and/or T inversion $\geq$0.1 mV in two contiguous leads with prominent R wave or R/S ratio $>$1
From Thygesen K, Alpert JS, White HD; Joint ESC/ACCF/AHA/WHF Task Force for the Redefinition of Myocardial Infarction. Universal definition of myocardial infarction. Circulation 2007;116:2634-2653.

Table 27.4 Electrocardiographic manifestations of acute myocardial ischemia (in absence of left ventricular hypertrophy and left bundle branch block).

in profound hypotension. In addition, large-volume fluid resuscitation is the treatment of choice for hypotensive patients suspected of having right ventricular infarction.

Table 27.4 lists ECG criteria for the diagnosis of MI. The other diagnostic tools previously mentioned do not have a major role in the diagnosis of STEMI; ECG findings are usually enough to warrant either immediate fibrinolysis or coronary angiography with or without intervention. However, biomarkers and imaging are often used in a complementary role to estimate infarct size and left ventricular function and thus play a role in guiding adjunctive treatment and assessing prognosis.[26,44]

Non–ST-Segment Elevation Acute Coronary Syndrome

The non–ST-segment elevation ACS has many clinical presentations. The symptomatic presentation of the patient may be as convincing as that of someone with STEMI or may even be completely "silent." In non–ST-segment elevation ACS, clinicians rely heavily on multiple diagnostic tools. The ECG may demonstrate myriad abnormalities, none of which is specific for MI. The ST-segment and T-wave changes indicative of myocardial ischemia are described in Table 27.4.[45] As mentioned previously, these changes are less reliable in localizing specific arterial territories that are involved as they represent subendocardial rather than transmural ischemia. However, the number of leads involved does correlate with the extent of myocardial ischemia and mortality,[46] as does the magnitude of ST-segment depression if it is present.[47,48] Table 27.5 details the correlation between magnitude of ST-segment depression and outcomes, particularly death and recurrent MI. Figure 27.12 illustrates ECG changes that may occur during NSTEMI.

The primary tool used to make the diagnosis of NSTEMI is cardiac biomarker evaluation. Any patient with symptoms of ischemia and elevation of cardiac-specific biomarkers, particularly troponin, above the 99th percentile with a characteristic rise or fall pattern has had an MI. As described in the universal definition of MI, the identification of MI in the absence of clearly ischemic symptoms may also be made if

CORRELATION BETWEEN MAGNITUDE OF ST-SEGMENT DEPRESSION AND OUTCOMES

	PARAGON-A			GUSTO-IIb		
Outcome	No ST ↓ (%)	ST ↓ 1 mm (%)	ST ↓ ≥2 mm (%)	No ST ↓ (%)	ST ↓ 1 mm (%)	ST ↓ ≥2 mm (%)
(Re) MI 30 days	6.8	11.2	14.1	4.9	6.0	8.5
(Re) MI 6 months	8.4	14.1	16.3	6.1	7.8	11.3
Death 30 days	0.7	2.8	6.3	2.0	2.7	8.3
Death 6 months	1.1	6.2	12.0	3.6	5.6	12.1
Death 1 year	2.0	7.8	13.4	4.4	6.9	14.1
Death/MI 30 days	7.2	12.1	17.1	6.5	7.8	14.6
Death/MI 6 months	9.2	16.7	23.9	8.9	11.7	19.9

From Kaul P, Fu Y, Chang WC, et al. Prognostic value of ST segment depression in acute coronary syndromes: insights from PARAGON-A applied to GUSTO-IIb. PARAGON-A and GUSTO IIb Investigators. Platelet IIb/IIIa Antagonism for the Reduction of Acute Global Organization Network. J Am Coll Cardiol 2001;38:64-71.

Table 27.5 Correlation between magnitude of ST-segment depression and outcomes.

there is ECG or imaging evidence of ischemia.[3] If cardiac biomarkers remain undetected in the serum in the appropriate clinical scenario, patients are identified as having unstable angina. Unstable angina identifies a group of patients deemed at high risk or having potential for infarction. The NSTEMI categorization qualifies as having an infarction; thus, it distinguishes a group that has demonstrated proven benefit with specific evidence-based therapies (i.e., early catheterization, glycoprotein IIb/IIIa inhibitors, and low-molecular-weight heparins as demonstrated in Figures 27.13 and 27.14).[49-52]

In addition to providing further evidence of MI, imaging is often used to detect the presence of hibernating or viable myocardium. This distinction refers to zones of myocardium that appear infarcted by resting imaging but return to normal appearance when provided increased blood flow.[53] Viability is assessed directly by radionuclide imaging and more indirectly by cardiac MRI. Echocardiography is less sensitive at assessing for viability as it requires larger differences in blood flow to detect wall motion changes.

Reinfarction

Another clinical scenario that deserves some discussion is that of reinfarction. Approximately 2% to 8% of patients with STEMI suffer a reinfarction.[54,55] Accordingly, clinicians should have a high index of suspicion and suspect reinfarction on the basis of indicative symptoms. Also, there are particular instances when reinfarction should be considered

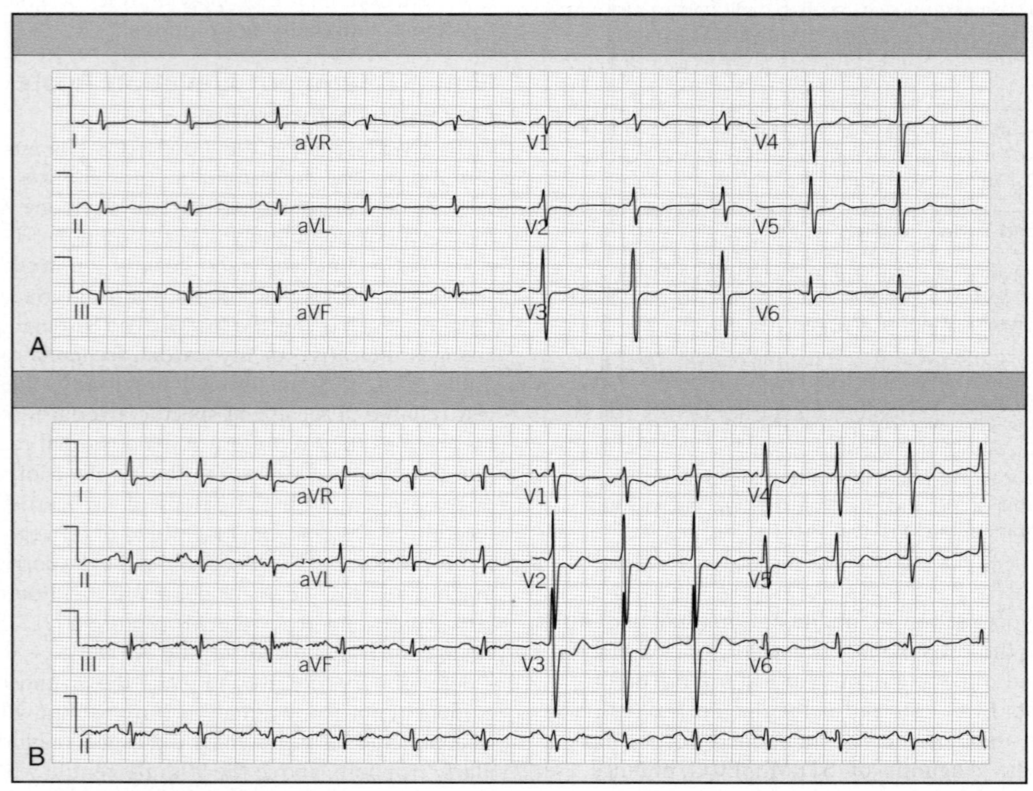

Figure 27.12 ECG findings in NSTEMI. A, Baseline. **B,** During acute event. (With permission from Jaffe AS, Davidenko J, Clements I. Diagnosis of acute coronary syndromes including acute myocardial infarction. In Crawford MH, DiMarco JP, Paulus WJ, eds. Cardiology. St. Louis, Mosby, 2004:311-328.)

in the absence of classic symptoms of ischemia. These include cardiac arrest, hemodynamic instability, and profound hyperglycemia. The first two should prompt an immediate evaluation, and after appropriate resuscitative measures, evaluation should include an ECG and continuous cardiac rhythm monitoring. The ECG diagnosis of reinfarction may be confounded by initial ECG changes or those of ST-segment and T-wave evolution. However, reinfarction should be suspected when ST-segment elevation of 0.1 mV or more recurs in a patient with a lesser degree of ST-segment elevation on a previous ECG obtained in the absence of symptoms or new pathognomonic Q waves develop in at least two contiguous leads, especially in association with clinical symptoms of ischemia present for at least 20 minutes.[3] Of note, ST-segment elevation may also be seen in the post-MI period occurring in the presence of left ventricular aneurysm formation or threatening myocardial rupture. These scenarios require further attention, particularly imaging, to assess the extent of the pathologic process.[26]

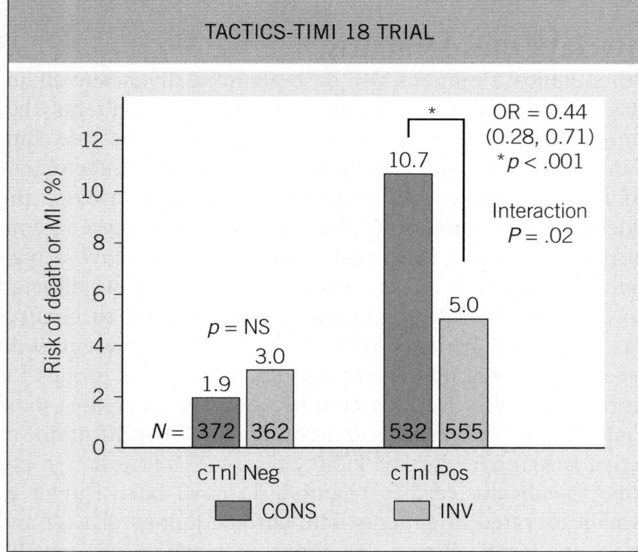

Figure 27.13 Benefit of an early invasive (INV) versus conservative (CONS) management strategy on the risk of death and new or recurrent MI at 6 months in patients with non–ST-segment elevation acute coronary syndrome enrolled in the TACTICS–TIMI 18 trial. The early invasive strategy consisted of routine cardiac catheterization within 48 hours of presentation and revascularization when appropriate regardless of clinical course. The conservative strategy included coronary angiography and revascularization only when prompted by recurrent spontaneous or provoked ischemia. Neg, negative; Pos, positive. (Data from Morrow DA, Cannon CP, Rifai N, et al. Ability of minor elevations of troponins I and T to predict benefit from an early invasive strategy in patients with unstable angina and non–ST elevation myocardial infarction: results from a randomized trial. JAMA 2001;286:2405-2412.)

Biomarkers also have a role in evaluating for reinfarction. Traditionally, CK-MB has been used to detect reinfarction. CK-MB is detected in the serum 3 to 12 hours after an ischemic event that leads to infarction, peaks at approximately 24 hours, and returns to normal at 48 to 72 hours. Troponin differs in that it may remain elevated up to 10 to 14 days (cardiac troponin T remains elevated longer than cardiac troponin I) after the initial event, making the diagnosis of reinfarction difficult.[16,17] There are some recent data to suggest that troponin values may be used in this scenario as well; however, these data come from a small sample size and only compare cardiac troponin I with CK-MB in a setting in which all patients had reinfarction by CK-MB.[56] Appropriate biomarker evaluation of reinfarction requires immediate measurement of the employed biomarker at the time reinfarction is suspected, as assessed by ECG changes, clinical signs and symptoms, or both. A second sample should be obtained 3 to 6 hours later. Recurrent infarction is diagnosed if there is a 20% or more increase of the value obtained in the second sample above the first and if the value exceeds the 99th percentile, which defines MI.[3]

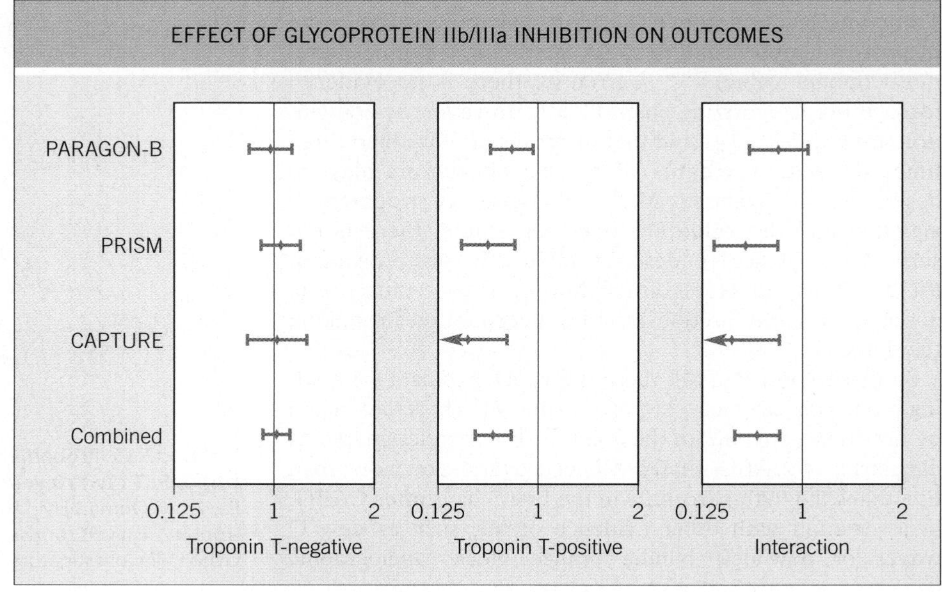

Figure 27.14 Effect of glycoprotein IIb/IIIa inhibition on outcomes based on troponin status. (With permission from Newby LK, Ohman EM, Christenson RH, et al. Benefit of glycoprotein IIb/IIIa inhibition in patients with acute coronary syndromes and troponin T–positive status: the PARAGON-B Troponin T Substudy. Circulation 2001;103:2891-2896.)

Myocardial Infarction Associated with Revascularization Procedures

Periprocedural MI is an entity that has received greater attention the last several years and has been described in the consensus statement released by the European Society of Cardiology, the American College of Cardiology, and the World Heart Federation.[3] This entity is different from spontaneous MI because periprocedural MI is associated with direct instrumentation of the heart during procedures such as PCI and CABG. During PCI, myocardial necrosis may result from various mechanisms including side branch occlusion, disruption of collateral flow, distal embolization, coronary dissection, slow flow or no-reflow phenomenon, and microvascular plugging. Despite current antithrombotic and antiplatelet therapies as well as protective devices, the embolization of atherosclerotic plaque or debris cannot be completely prevented. Myocardial injury during CABG may result from direct myocardial trauma, coronary dissection, ischemia related to inadequate cardiac protection, microvascular events related to reperfusion, graft failure, or failure to reperfuse myocardium not subtended by graftable vessels. Cardiac MRI has demonstrated new areas of myocardial necrosis after PCI as well as evidence of diffuse subendocardial injury after CABG.[57,58] The other imaging modalities are less sensitive at identifying smaller areas of injury or infarct; thus, they do not have a major role in postprocedure MI diagnosis unless a relatively large area of myocardium is suspected to be involved.

There have been standard diagnostic criteria created to identify PCI-related MI and CABG-related MI. In the setting of PCI, ECG changes are similar to those seen with spontaneous MI, which have been discussed previously. After CABG, new ST-segment and T-wave abnormalities are common but not necessarily diagnostic of MI.[59] However, if new Q waves are identified in territories other than those suspected before surgery, MI should be considered, especially in conjunction with cardiac biomarker elevation or new wall motion abnormalities.

Myocardial necrosis after PCI may be detected by measuring biomarkers immediately after the procedure, at 6 to 12 hours, and again at 18 to 24 hours after intervention. Troponin elevation above the 99th percentile is indicative of post-PCI myocardial necrosis (assuming a normal baseline troponin value).[60-62] Currently, there is no evidence for a cutoff categorizing post-PCI MI. However, by convention, it has been suggested that increases of more than three times the 99th percentile of cardiac biomarkers may be designated PCI-related MI.[3] Otherwise, if troponin is elevated and the value has not been stable, there is not sufficient evidence to describe its use in postprocedural MI. If biomarker levels are falling or stable, the criteria described for reinfarction may be incorporated in making the diagnosis.

Similar to post-PCI MI, there is a paucity of data for guiding biomarker diagnosis of post-CABG MI. Therefore, again by arbitrary convention, the Joint Task Force designated as diagnostic of CABG-related MI an elevation of more than five times the 99th percentile in the first 3 days after CABG, in association with other evidence of MI, such as new Q waves or new left bundle branch block, angiographic evidence of native or graft vessel occlusion, or imaging evidence of loss of previously viable myocardium.[3] Whereas diagnosis of PCI- or CABG-related MI is challenging, data support that elevations of biomarkers, both CK-MB and troponin, are associated with overall worse prognosis and clinical outcomes.[63-66]

Special Considerations

Other clinical situations also pose potential diagnostic dilemmas. In particular, there are populations of patients that more commonly present atypically, requiring the astute clinician to consider the diagnosis of myocardial ischemia or infarction: diabetes mellitus, chronic kidney disease, the elderly, and women.[37,38] These groups often present with atypical symptoms and require the clinician to have a high index of suspicion for MI. Then, attention may be directed toward use of ECG, biomarkers, and imaging to confirm the diagnosis. Patients with diabetes often present with "silent" ischemia and are among the highest risk groups for coronary disease. Another clinical scenario that creates some confusion in emergency departments is identification of active ischemia in chronic kidney disease. The cardiac troponins, specifically cardiac troponin T, have been shown to remain elevated in patients with chronic kidney disease and end-stage renal disease, as these biomarkers are renally cleared. Therefore, clinicians may be tempted to downplay elevated troponins in this setting. Unfortunately, this generates the potential for failure to identify active ischemia in an already high-risk group. Furthermore, data suggest that regardless of the presence of classic ACS, elevated troponin in this setting is a marker for worse prognosis.[67-69] Figures 27.15 and 27.16 relate troponin positivity as well as magnitude of troponin elevation with mortality. In addition, this group, given their higher risk for adverse cardiac outcomes, may achieve greater benefit from application of evidence-based therapies in non–ST-segment elevation ACS.

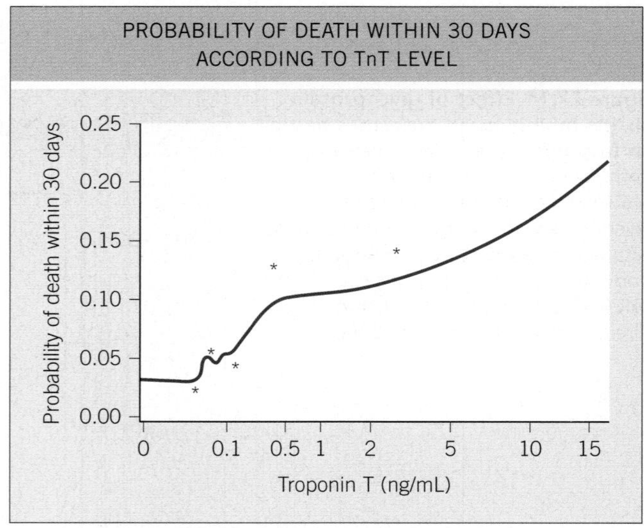

Figure 27.15 Probability of death within 30 days according to troponin T (TnT) level at hospital admission. (Data from GUSTO-IIa. From Ohman EM, Armstrong PW, Christenson RH, et al. Cardiac troponin T levels for risk stratification in acute myocardial ischemia. GUSTO IIa Investigators. N Engl J Med 1996;335:1333-1341.)

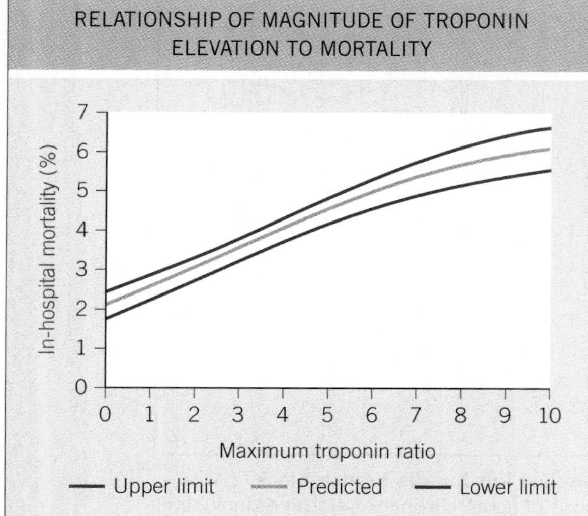

Figure 27.16 Relationship of magnitude of troponin elevation to mortality. (Data from CRUSADE, Roe MT, Peterson ED, Li Y, et al. Relationship between risk stratification by cardiac troponin level and adherence to guidelines for non–ST-segment elevation acute coronary syndromes. Arch Intern Med 2005;165:1870-1876.)

Another scenario that deserves mention is distinguishing chest pain secondary to ACS from non-ACS chest pain. Emergency departments worldwide are faced with this decision numerous times a day, and it may often be quite difficult to make this distinction. Whereas the cardiac biomarkers, particularly troponin, have become the gold standard for detecting myocardial necrosis, the identification of myocardial ischemia by use of serum or plasma markers has not yet been fully validated. Currently, there are two assays approved by the Food and Drug Administration for the detection of myocardial ischemia: ischemia-modified albumin and myeloperoxidase. Both of these markers have been shown to be elevated early when myocardial ischemia occurs[70,71]; however, they are neither sensitive nor specific for diagnosis of ACS when they are used alone. If these tests are combined with ECG and cardiac biomarkers mentioned previously, they do have the ability to rule out ACS with a high degree of certainty, provided they are used in an appropriate clinical scenario.[70,72]

ACCURACY

Electrocardiography

Depending on the presence or absence of ST-segment elevation and other changes, ECG has varying levels of sensitivity and predictive accuracy for detecting MI. For example, 76% of patients meeting criteria for ST-segment elevation of at least 1 mm in two contiguous limb leads or 2 mm in the precordial leads had MI.[45] In contrast, only 21% of patients with ST-segment depression, nonspecific ST-segment changes, or T-wave changes indicative of ischemia ultimately were found to have MI. Table 27.6 summarizes sensitivities and positive predictive values for various ECG findings.[45]

As mentioned earlier, there are certain scenarios that limit the diagnostic potential of ECG in identifying myocardial ischemia or infarction. Table 27.2 lists common situations that result in both false-positive and false-negative ECGs. In the case of left bundle branch block, criteria have been established that may aid in the ECG identification of MI. These criteria are listed in Table 27.7, and Figure 27.17 depicts an ECG demonstrating these diagnostic changes. A score of 3 or higher has 90% specificity for the diagnosis of MI.[73]

SUMMARY OF SENSITIVITIES AND POSITIVE PREDICTIVE VALUES FOR VARIOUS ELECTROCARDIOGRAPHIC FINDINGS

ECG Finding	Positive Predictive Value (%)	Sensitivity (%)
≥1-mm ST elevation or Q waves in ≥2 leads	461/605 (76)	461/1024 (45)
New ischemia or strain ≥1 mm, ST depression in ≥2 leads	203/531 (38)	203/1024 (20)
Other new ST- or T-wave changes of new ischemia or strain	147/693 (21)	147/1024 (14)
Old infarction, ischemia, or strain	50/644 (8)	50/1024 (5)
Other new or old abnormality	56/1147 (5)	56/1024 (5)
Nonspecific ST-T changes only	72/1433 (5)	72/1024 (7)
Normal	35/2062 (2)	35/1024 (3.4)

From Rouan GW, Lee TH, Cook EF, Brand DA, Weisberg MC, Goldman L. Clinical characteristics and outcome of acute myocardial infarction in patients with initially normal or nonspecific electrocardiograms (a report from the Multicenter Chest Pain Study). Am J Cardiol 1989;64:1087-1092.

Table 27.6 Summary of sensitivities and positive predictive values for various electrocardiographic findings.

ELECTROCARDIOGRAPHIC FEATURES IN LEFT BUNDLE BRANCH BLOCK

Criterion	Odds Ratio (95% CI)	Score
ST-segment elevation ≥1 mm and concordant with QRS complex	25.2 (11.6 to 54.7)	5
ST-segment depression ≥1 mm in lead V_1, V_2, or V_3	6.0 (1.9 to 19.3)	3
ST-segment elevation ≥5 mm and discordant with QRS complex	4.3 (1.8 to 10.6)	2

From Sgarbossa EB, Pinski SL, Barbagelata A, et al. Electrocardiographic diagnosis of evolving acute myocardial infarction in the presence of left bundle-branch block. GUSTO-1 (Global Utilization of Streptokinase and Tissue Plasminogen Activator for Occluded Coronary Arteries) Investigators. N Engl J Med 1996;334:481-487.

Table 27.7 Electrocardiographic features in left bundle branch block.

Biomarkers

The preferred biomarker for the diagnosis of MI is troponin I or troponin T, although CK-MB by mass assay is acceptable and may be preferred in some situations. Table 27.8

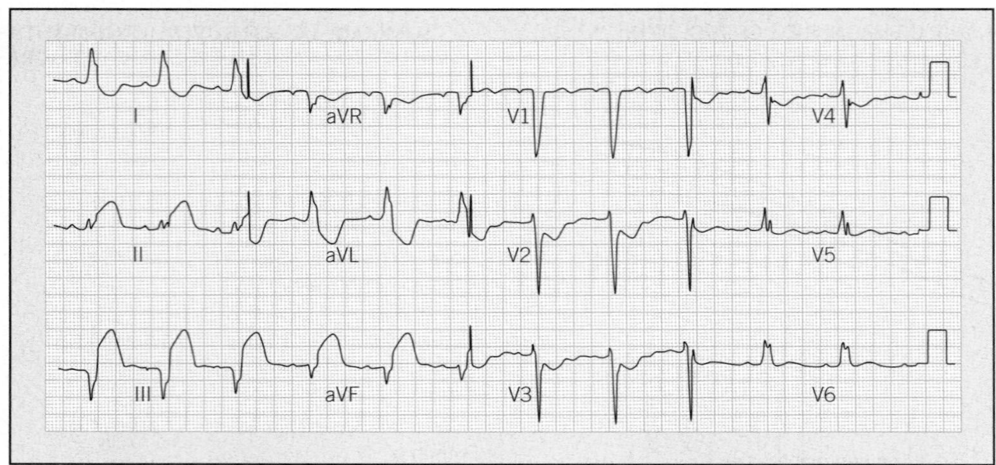

Figure 27.17 ECG findings indicative of STEMI with baseline left bundle branch block. (With permission from Jaffe AS, Davidenko J, Clements I. Diagnosis of acute coronary syndromes including acute myocardial infarction. In Crawford MH, DiMarco JP, Paulus WJ, eds. Cardiology. St. Louis, Mosby, 2004:311-328.)

PROPERTIES OF BIOMARKERS OF MYOCARDIAL NECROSIS

Biochemical Marker	Molecular Weight (g/mole)	Cardiac Specific?	Advantage	Disadvantage	Duration of Elevation
Myoglobin	18,000	No	High sensitivity and negative predictive value Useful for early detection of MI and reperfusion	Low specificity in presence of skeletal muscle injury and renal insufficiency Rapid clearance after necrosis	12-24 hours
h-FABP	15,000	+	Early detection of MI	Low specificity in presence of skeletal muscle injury and renal insufficiency	18-30 hours
CK-MB, mass assays	85,000	+++	Ability to detect reinfarction Large clinical experience Previous gold standard for myocardial necrosis	Lowered specificity in skeletal muscle injury	24-36 hours
CK-MB isoforms	85,000	+++	Early detection of MI	Lack of availability and experience	18-30 hours
cTnT	37,000	++++	Tool for risk stratification Detection of MI up to 2 weeks High specificity for cardiac tissue	Not an early marker of myocardial necrosis Serial testing needed to discriminate early reinfarction	10-14 days
cTnI	23,500	++++	Tool for risk stratification Detection of MI up to 7 days High specificity for cardiac tissue	Not an early marker of myocardial necrosis Serial testing needed to discriminate early reinfarction No analytical reference standards	4-7 days

Times of first increase for the markers are 1 to 3 hours for myoglobin, 3 to 4 hours for CK-MB mass, 3 to 4 hours for cardiac troponin T (cTnT), and 4 to 6 hours for cardiac troponin I (cTnI). h-FABP, heart fatty acid–binding protein; MI, myocardial infarction.

Modified from Christenson RH, Azzazy HME. Biomarkers of necrosis: past, present and future. In Morrow DA, ed. Cardiovascular Biomarkers: Pathophysiology and Clinical Management. New York, Humana Press, 2006:3-24.

Table 27.8 Properties of biomarkers of myocardial necrosis.

describes characteristics of various biomarkers that have been used to evaluate for MI. The troponins and CK-MB have demonstrated high specificity and sensitivity in detecting myocardial necrosis, particularly cardiac troponin.[16,20] A prospective study comparing cardiac troponin I, cardiac troponin T, and CK-MB in 54 patients presenting with symptoms concerning for MI demonstrated that the cardiac troponins had nearly 100% specificity and positive predictive value. All three biomarkers had comparable sensitivity (90%), and the negative predictive values were 97.8%, 97.6%, and 97.6% for cardiac troponin I, cardiac troponin T, and CK-MB, respectively.[74]

Imaging

A normal echocardiogram or resting ECG-gated nuclear scintigram has a 95% to 98% negative predictive value for excluding MI.[25,26,75-77] A prospective study evaluating echocardiography for the diagnosis of MI in the emergency department demonstrated a sensitivity of 93% but a specificity of only 59% because echocardiography is unable to distinguish old versus new wall motion abnormalities.[78] In addition, the interpretation of echocardiography requires highly trained technicians or physicians and is largely dependent on the quality of the images obtained. Radionuclide imaging, on the other hand, is almost always technically adequate for interpretation. However, this modality suffers from the same limitation in distinguishing old from new infarction. Compared with biomarkers, both techniques are less specific and sensitive for the diagnosis of MI. In the case of echocardiography, injury involving more than 20% of myocardial wall thickness is required before a segmental wall motion abnormality can be detected[79]; with regard to radionuclide imaging, more than 10 g of myocardial tissue must be injured before a perfusion defect can be identified.[80] In contrast, cardiac troponin can be detected in the bloodstream above the 99th percentile when less than 1 g of myocardial tissue has undergone necrosis.[1]

Cardiac MRI is a new imaging technique that is receiving more and more attention. Its use in the acute setting has not yet been validated, but it has proven efficacy for evaluation of myocardial viability as well as structure and function.[27] Cardiac MRI is also beneficial in differentiating cardiac infiltrative disorders, which may also result in elevated cardiac biomarkers, from myocardial necrosis associated with ACS.[81,82]

COMPLICATIONS

There are few complications associated with the diagnostic tools used for detection of myocardial ischemia and infarction. ECG is a noninvasive test that may be performed quickly. Beyond the complications associated with venipuncture, checking for biomarker elevation in the blood is also a safe and easily performed test. Inherent to all tests is the possibility of a false-positive result and unnecessary further testing. In the case of suspected MI, the potential of undergoing diagnostic coronary angiography is the most invasive next step, and there are inherent risks to this procedure. The imaging modalities used in the work-up of MI are generally safe and do not have any major complications. Although radiation exposure occurs with the use of radionuclide imaging, the actual risk is quite minimal.[83] However, there has been recent evidence to suggest that patients with end-stage renal disease or advanced chronic kidney disease are sensitive to gadolinium received during MRI. In these patients, this contrast agent may result in the rare disease entity nephrogenic fibrosing dermopathy, resulting in diffuse thickening of the skin, more commonly on the extremities, that may be devastating.[84] Otherwise, clinicians may rest assured that the tools described are safe and effective methods to diagnose MI.

DIAGNOSTIC STRATEGY

The appropriate evaluation of myocardial ischemia and infarction requires the use of a combination of diagnostic tools. The initial assessment is made by clinical signs or symptoms of MI, and as it is readily available, ECG is usually the first objective test. If there are findings suggestive of STEMI, further diagnostic work-up is unnecessary, and intervention with angiography or primary PCI (preferred) or fibrinolytic therapy is undertaken. On the other hand, if the ECG demonstrates ST-segment depression, T-wave changes, other nonspecific ST-segment abnormalities, or even no abnormalities, the focus shifts to the use of cardiac biomarkers and in some cases imaging to establish the diagnosis of MI. Figure 27.18 illustrates a diagnostic strategy for assessment of patients with suspected myocardial ischemia or infarction.

SUMMARY

Clinicians have a variety of tools at their fingertips when evaluating a patient for myocardial ischemia and infarction. During the past decade, there has been a transition to a focus on evidence of myocardial necrosis in the serum detected through the use of sensitive and specific troponin assays in conjunction with symptoms, the ECG, and, in some cases, imaging modalities. Importantly, broad consensus for how to define MI has now been established among clinicians, clinical trialists, epidemiologists, imagers, electrocardiographers, and laboratorians. It is on this foundation that continuing advances in technology will be evaluated and considered.

There is a definite trend toward improving the accuracy of tools used in the diagnosis of MI. The 80-lead ECG vest, or body surface mapping, is drawing increasing attention and has been incorporated into clinical use at some medical centers for use in the emergency department. However, additional research will be needed to understand the incremental contribution of this technology in clinical practice. Furthermore, the ischemia markers are available to aid in the distinction between cardiac and noncardiac chest pain as well as in the early identification of ACS not yet identified by standard biomarkers. The application of "omic" technology (metabolomics, proteomics, and genomics) to the diagnosis of ischemia and infarction is a developing area of research. Recent early work has indicated that these technologies may offer promise in distinguishing patients with ischemia from those without evidence of ischemia.[76,77]

Finally, ultrasensitive troponin assays are currently being developed that may detect extremely small amounts of myocardial necrosis, perhaps on the picomolar (10^{-12}) or even femtomolar (10^{-15}) levels.[85,86] As these assays become readily available in clinical practice, it will be the responsibility of clinicians and researchers to determine how they should best be used and interpreted. For example, troponin elevation has been demonstrated in patients with chronic heart failure in the outpatient setting, indicating ongoing myocardial necrosis.[87] The mechanism of this necrosis seems to be related to apoptosis as opposed to the ischemia-driven necrosis seen in ACS. The ultrasensitive assays will undoubtedly detect this degree of myocardial necrosis; thus, clinicians must be able to interpret the results appropriately within the context of the testing scenario. Furthermore, these assays will almost certainly once again redefine "normal" with respect to circulating biomarkers of myocardial necrosis, and understanding the prognostic implications of such low-level detection of troponin will be critical.

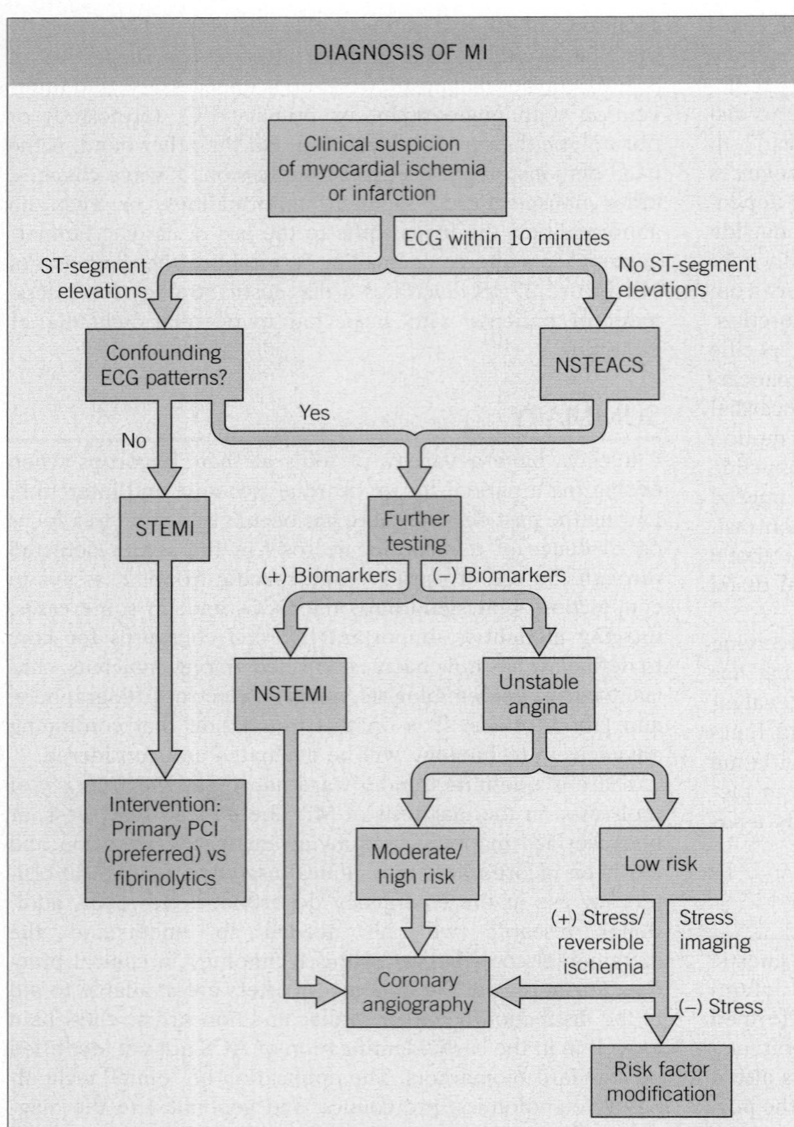

Figure 27.18 Diagnosis of myocardial infarction (MI): flow chart. This diagram details the approach to the diagnosis of MI. In the case of STEMI, biomarkers and imaging are not necessary to make the diagnosis as ST-segment elevations warrant angiographic evaluation if it is available. However, biomarkers are used in this setting to confirm the diagnosis as well as to provide prognostic and therapeutic information. Imaging is used to identify ventricular dysfunction, valvular abnormalities, and other mechanical complications of acute MI. ECG, electrocardiography; NSTEACS, non–ST-segment elevation acute coronary syndrome; NSTEMI, non–ST-segment elevation myocardial infarction; PCI, percutaneous coronary intervention; STEMI, ST-segment elevation myocardial infarction.

chapter 28

Pre-Hospital Phase of Acute Coronary Syndrome

Christian Juhl Terkelsen

Definition

- The pre-hospital phase of acute coronary syndrome comprises the time from onset of symptoms until admission to hospital.

Key Features

- One third of patients with acute myocardial infarction die in the pre-hospital phase without receiving medical help.
- Advanced life support or basic life support (layman) is essential.
- Easy access to traditional defibrillators or automated external defibrillators (layman) is of paramount importance.
- Patients with ST-segment elevation myocardial infarction (STEMI) or bundle branch block myocardial infarction (BBBMI) should receive reperfusion therapy by primary percutaneous coronary intervention (PPCI) or fibrinolysis.
- A 1-hour reduction in delay before initiation of reperfusion therapy translates into approximately 20 extra lives saved per 1000 treated.
- Pre-hospital diagnosis is recommended and should be combined with rerouting of STEMI patients directly to catheterizations laboratories for PPCI if the anticipated delay used to perform PPCI instead of on-site fibrinolysis (PCI-related delay) is below 120 minutes.
- In case of a PCI-related delay above 120 minutes, pre-hospital fibrinolysis may be a valuable alternative to PPCI.
- Pharmacologic therapy in the acute phase constitutes aspirin, clopidogrel, heparin, nitroglycerin, morphine, and beta blocker.

Acute coronary syndrome comprises unstable angina pectoris and acute myocardial infarction (AMI). Patients with unstable angina pectoris have symptoms of myocardial ischemia (angina) at rest but no rise in markers of myocardial necrosis. The electrocardiogram may be normal or with negative T waves, ST-segment depression (Fig. 28.1a), or even intermittent ST-segment elevation. The diagnosis of AMI mandates a typical rise in biochemical markers of myocardial necrosis combined with symptoms of ischemia, electrocardiographic changes indicative of new ischemia (ST changes or new bundle branch block), development of pathologic Q waves, or imaging evidence of new loss of viable myocardium or new regional wall motion abnormality. The diagnosis of AMI can also be established in case of sudden, unexpected cardiac death at a time before blood sampling or before the appearance of cardiac biomarkers in the blood if it is accompanied by presumably new ST elevation or bundle branch block or evidence of fresh thrombus by coronary angiography or autopsy.[1]

EPIDEMIOLOGY

The prognosis has steadily improved in patients with AMI during the last decades. One third of patients with AMI, however, still die suddenly in the pre-hospital phase without receiving medical help (Fig. 28.2).[2,3] Among patients admitted to the hospital, 1-year mortality is still above 20% in unselected cohorts and around 10% in patients selected for reperfusion therapy.[4,5]

ACUTE MYOCARDIAL INFARCTION CATEGORIES

AMIs are categorized according to the presenting electrocardiogram (see Fig. 28.1) into ST-elevation myocardial infarction (STEMI), non–ST-elevation myocardial infarction (NSTEMI), and bundle branch block myocardial infarction (BBBMI). STEMI can be further divided into inferior (ST elevation in II, III, aVF), lateral (ST elevation in I, aVL, V_5-V_6), posterior (reciprocal ST depression in V_1-V_4), and anterior (ST elevation in I, V_1-V_6). The diagnosis of STEMI is fairly accurate on the basis of symptoms and electrocardiographic findings. Posterior STEMI, however, is often missed or misinterpreted as NSTEMI. The diagnosis of BBBMI is also difficult because it may be difficult to establish whether the bundle branch block is newly developed. It has previously been considered that STEMI patients suffered total occlusion of epicardial coronary arteries by thrombus and seldomly spasm, whereas NSTEMI patients suffered a subocclusion of epicardial coronary arteries. Later studies have documented that also in NSTEMI, the majority of patients have total occlusion in the early hours.[6]

INITIAL ASSESSMENT AND THERAPY

Depending on the qualifications of attending personnel, the initial assessment and treatment of patients with symptoms of acute coronary syndrome involve advanced life support or basic life support. Securing airway, breathing, and circulation is of paramount importance. In case of out-of-hospital cardiac arrest, bystanders should call the emergency medical services immediately and then initiate cardiopulmonary resuscitation. Bystander cardiopulmonary resuscitation doubles the chance of survival. Immediate access to emergency medical services is essential. In the pre-hospital phase, ventricular fibrillation or pulseless ventricular tachycardia is the dominant arrhythmia in patients with cardiac arrest (Fig. 28.3). Prompt defibrillation is essential, and for each

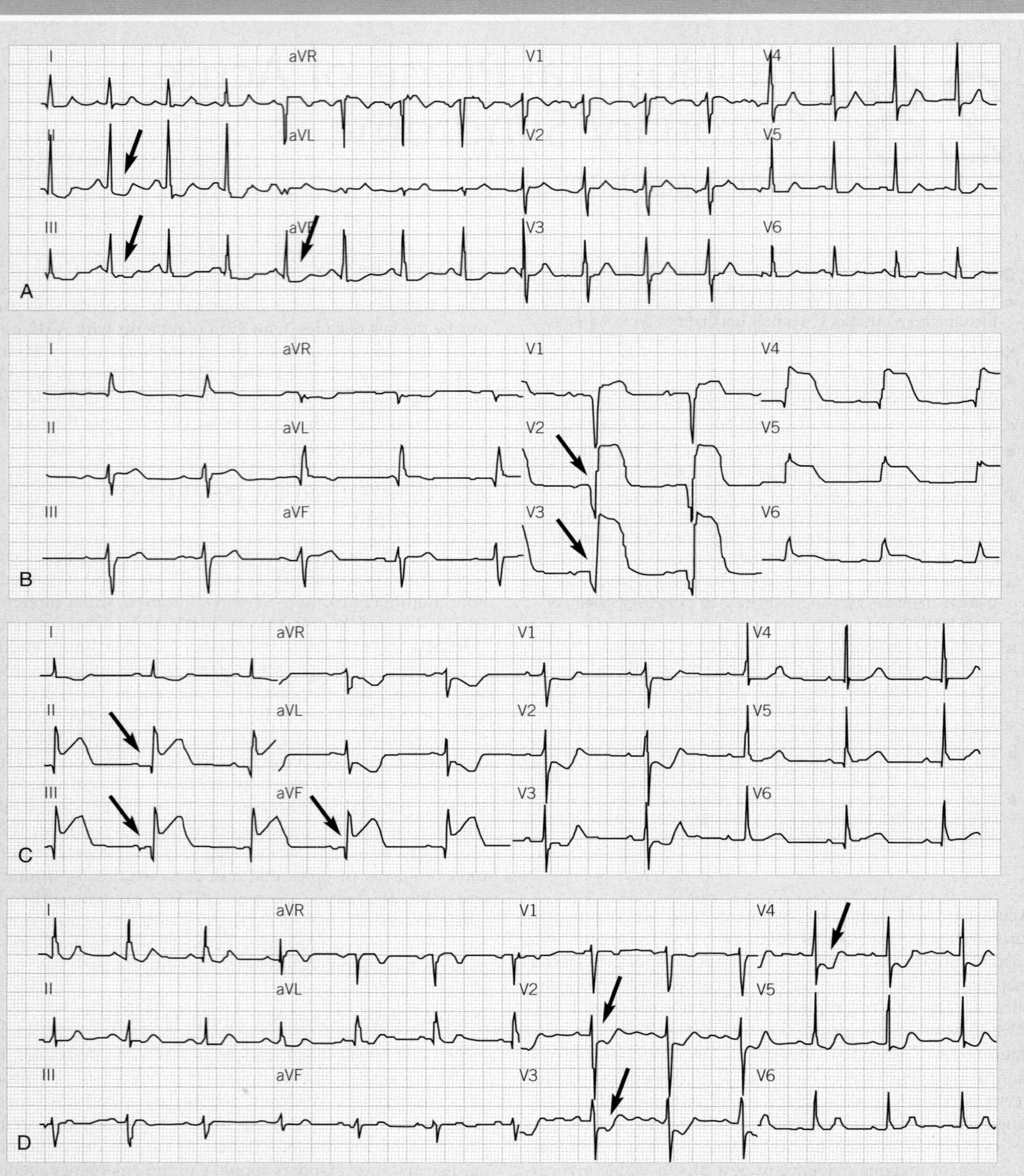

Figure 28.1 Electrocardiographic findings for unstable angina pectoris (UAP) and ST-segment elevation myocardial infarction (STEMI). A, Unstable angina pectoris or non–ST-elevation myocardial infarction (NSTEMI). **B,** Anterior STEMI. **C,** Inferior STEMI. **D,** Posterior STEMI.

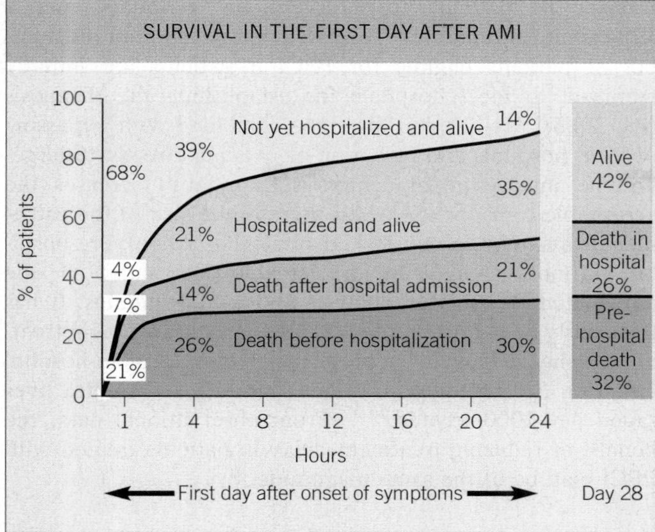

Figure 28.2 Survival in the first day after acute myocardial infarction. (From Löwel H, Lewis M, Hörmann A. Prognostic significance of the pre-hospital phase in acute myocardial infarction: results of the Augsburg Myocardial Infarct Registry, 1985-1988 [in German]. Dtsch Med Wochenschr 1991;116:729-733.)

minute delay in defibrillation, the chance of a successful outcome falls about 7% to 10%. The goal is to deliver a shock within 5 minutes of the emergency medical services call.

The pre-hospital acquisition and interpretation of the electrocardiogram by ambulance physicians, paramedics, or general practitioners is recommended. If the attending health personnel are unable to establish the diagnosis of STEMI, the use of telemedicine should be considered (e.g., transmission of the electrocardiogram to a hospital) to allow a hospital-based physician to evaluate the diagnosis. This would allow the majority of citizens transported by ambulance to have the diagnosis of STEMI established in the pre-hospital phase.[7]

During the initial assessment, patients should have an intravenous line established and receive oxygen; if AMI is suspected, aspirin should be given. Administration of aspirin results in approximately 12 extra lives saved per 1000 treated.[8] Additional pharmacologic therapy constitutes nitrates for angina and congestive heart failure, furosemide for congestive heart failure, beta blockers for angina, opioids for pain and pulmonary congestion, atropine in case of bradycardia or even asystole, epinephrine during cardiac arrest, and antiemetics for nausea and vomiting. In case of AMI, heparin

Figure 28.3 Advanced life support algorithm. CPR, cardiopulmonary resuscitation; PEA, pulseless electrical activity; VF, ventricular fibrillation; VT, ventricular tachycardia. (Modified from The pre-hospital management of acute heart attacks. Recommendations of a Task Force of the European Society of Cardiology and the European Resuscitation Council. Eur Heart J 1998;19:1140-1164.)

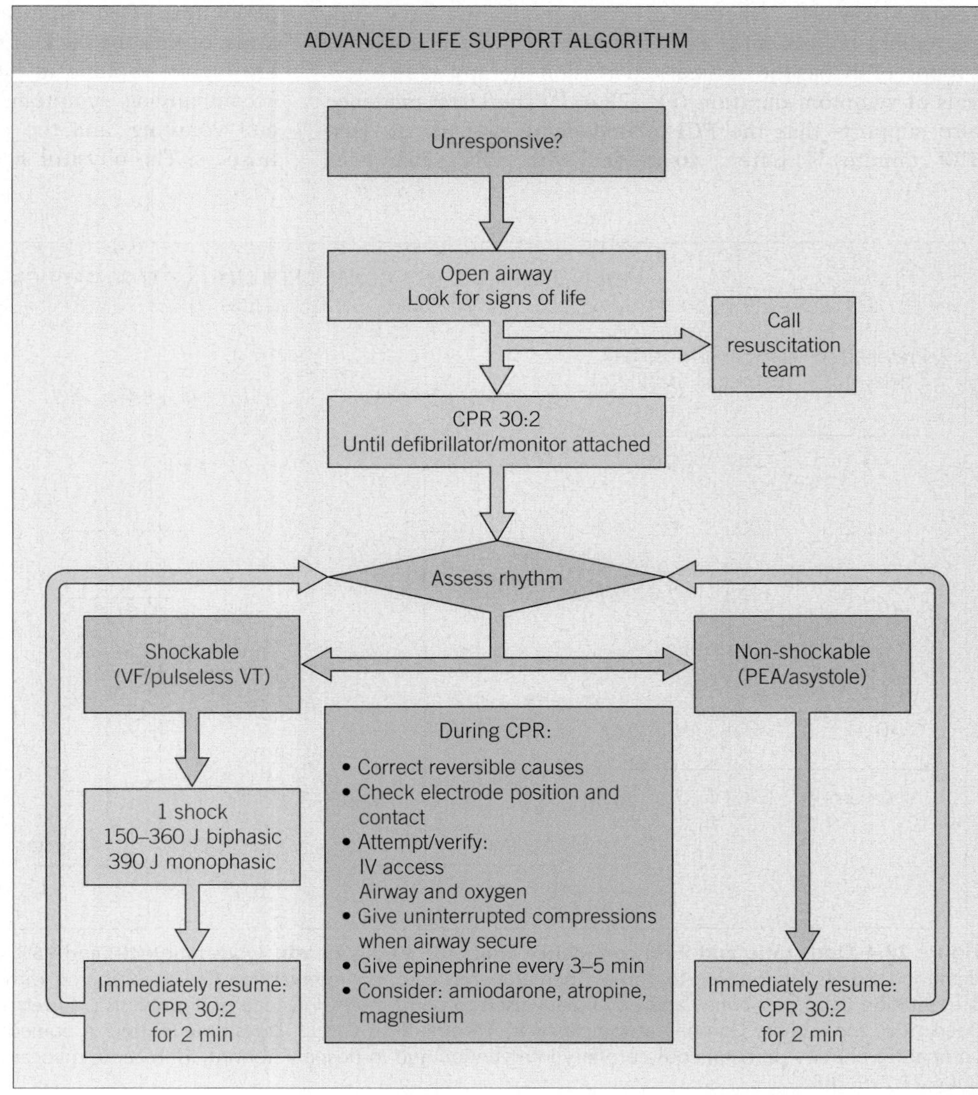

should be considered (unfractionated or fractionated according to local recommendation). In case of hypotension, volume substitution may be relevant in right ventricular infarction, whereas inotropics may be preferable in anterior infarctions. Pharmacologic treatment of tachyarrhythmias may comprise beta blocker, digoxin, amiodarone, and lidocaine.

CHOICE AND TIMING OF REPERFUSION THERAPY

In patients with STEMI or BBBMI, reperfusion therapy is essential to restore epicardial blood flow and to improve outcome. Previous studies have documented that fibrinolysis instead of placebo saves 23 to 40 extra lives per 1000 treated.[8,9] In previous randomized controlled trials comparing primary percutaneous coronary intervention (PPCI) with fibrinolysis, PPCI treatment saved an additional 26 lives per 1000 treated with PPCI instead of fibrinolysis.[10] PPCI, however, is not a universally available treatment modality, and there must be an extra delay used to perform PPCI instead of administering on-site fibrinolysis (PCI-related delay) beyond which the beneficial effect of PPCI is outweighed by the harmful effect of postponing reperfusion therapy. The choice of reperfusion strategy may vary from region to region. However, whereas previous guidelines have supported fibrinolysis in the early incomers,[11,12] recent evidence supports PPCI as the optimal reperfusion therapy at all intervals of symptom duration (Fig. 28.4).[10] The latest evidence also supports that the PCI-related delay may be at least 120 minutes.[10] Often, treatment with PPCI mandates transfer of patients to interventional hospitals, and a 120-minute acceptable PCI-related delay may limit the number of patients eligible for PPCI if patients are initially admitted to local hospitals for establishing the diagnosis (Fig. 28.5). Pre-hospital diagnosis combined with bypassing of local hospitals and rerouting of patients directly to large-volume interventional centers substantially increases the acceptable transport time and thereby the size of the catchment areas to interventional hospitals (Fig. 28.5e). Pre-hospital fibrinolysis may be a valuable alternative if the anticipated PCI-related delay is above 120 minutes. It has previously been documented that a 1-hour reduction in treatment delay achieved by pre-hospital instead of in-hospital initiation of fibrinolysis translates into 15 to 21 extra lives saved per 1000 treated.[13-15] From observational data, the benefit of reducing treatment delay in patients treated with PPCI may be of the same magnitude.[16]

CLINICAL PRESENTATION

Chest pain or discomfort is observed in most of the patients who present with acute coronary syndrome. The nature of the discomfort may be pressing, crushing, constricting, or just itching. The usual location is mid retrosternal. The pain or discomfort often radiates into the throat, into one or both arms, or into the back or the upper abdomen. The symptoms are highly variable in intensity and nature. There may be accompanying symptoms in the form of anxiety, nausea, and vomiting, and the patients often complain of breathlessness. The physical signs in patients with AMI may vary

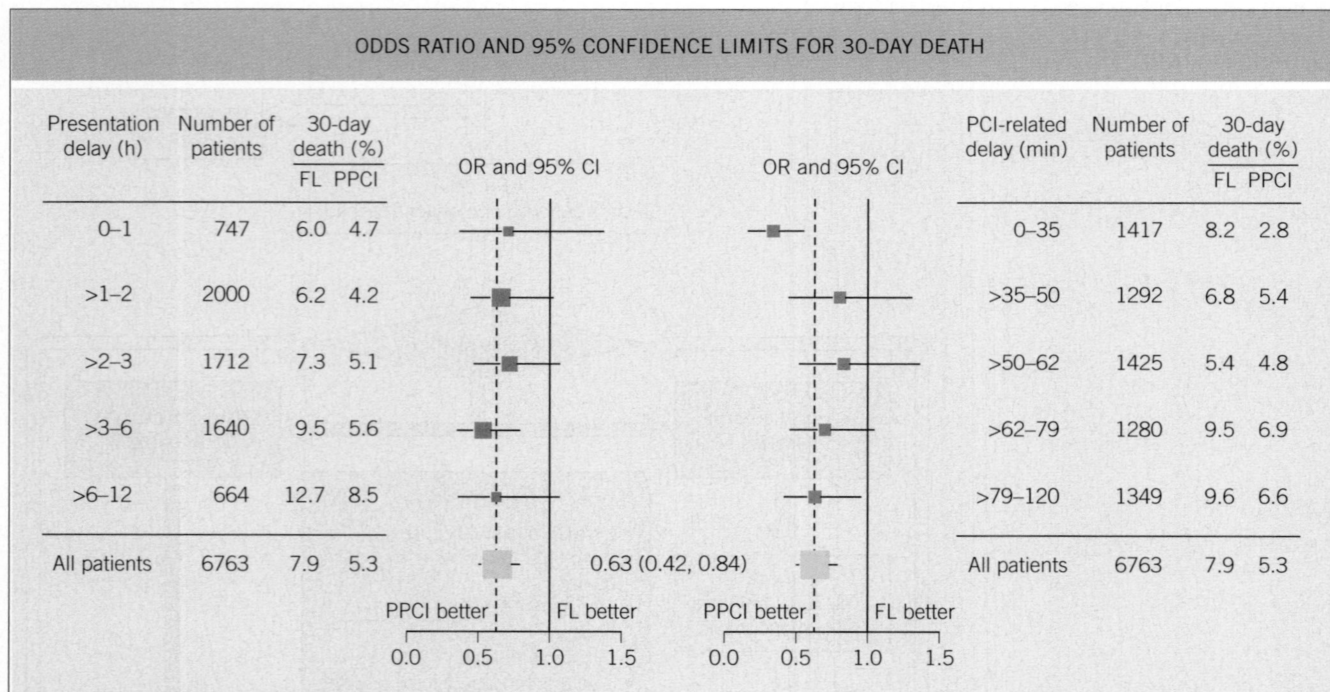

Figure 28.4 Odds ratio and 95% confidence limits for 30-day death. Odds ratio (OR) and 95% confidence intervals (CI) for 30-day death in patients randomized to primary percutaneous coronary intervention (PPCI) compared with fibrinolysis (FL) according to presentation delay *(left panel)* and extra delay used to perform PPCI instead of fibrinolysis (PCI-related delay) *(right panel)*. (From Boersma E; the Primary Coronary Angioplasty vs. Thrombolysis Group. Does time matter? A pooled analysis of randomized clinical trials comparing primary percutaneous coronary intervention and in-hospital fibrinolysis in acute myocardial infarction patients. Eur Heart J 2006;27:779-788.)

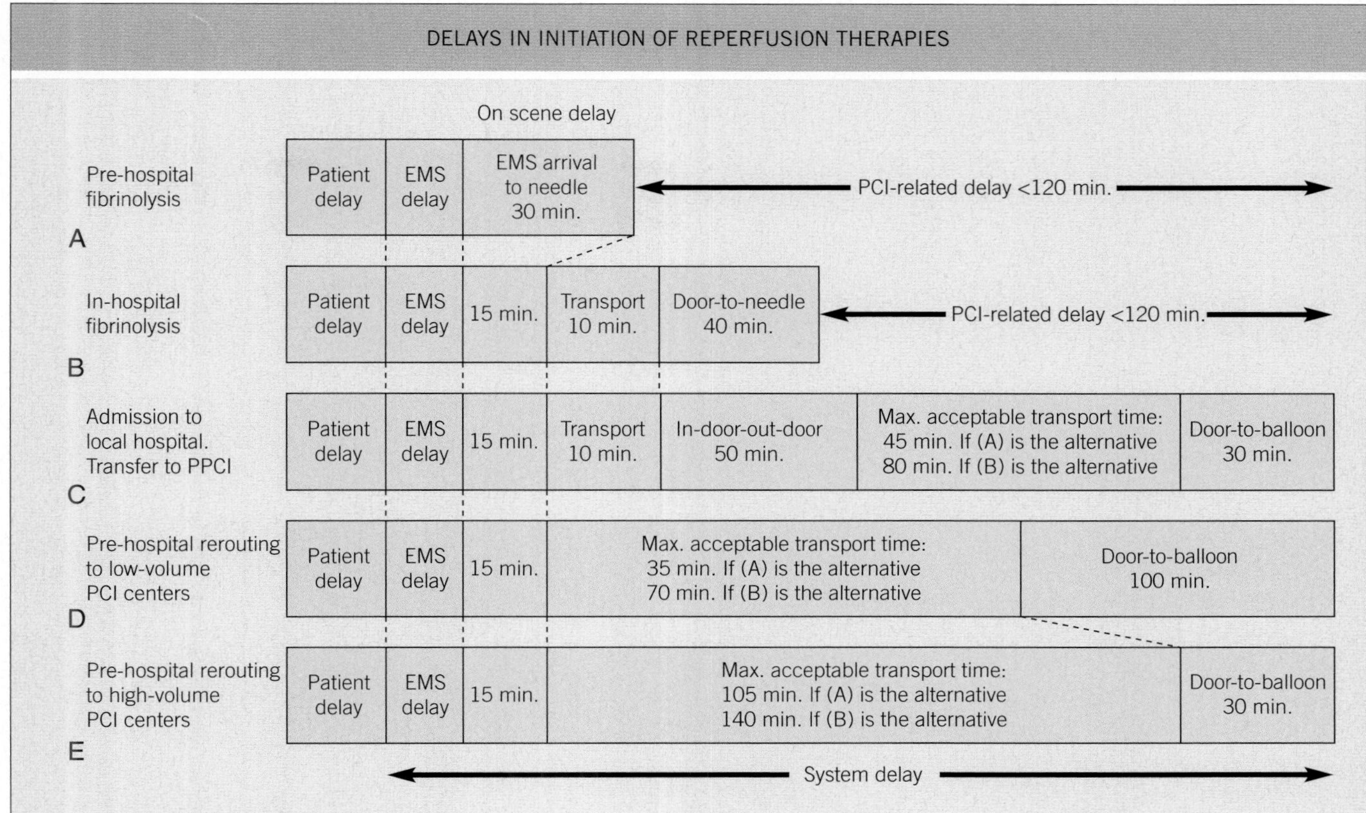

Figure 28.5 Delays in initiation of in-hospital fibrinolysis or pre-hospital fibrinolysis *(top)* and acceptable transportation delay to interventional hospital in considering pre-hospital diagnosis combined with rerouting for primary percutaneous coronary intervention (PPCI). EMS, emergency medical system; PCI-related delay: extra delay used to perform PPCI instead of administering on-site fibrinolysis. (Modified from Terkelsen CJ; Treatment delays in ST elevation myocardial infarction. BMJ 2008;336(7641):401-402.)

according to the presence or absence of early left ventricular failure. In patients with acute left-sided heart failure, rales can be heard over the lungs. In patients who have inferior myocardial infarction with right ventricular involvement, there may be low blood pressure and elevated central venous pressure.

SUMMARY

AMI is still the major cause of death in the Western world. However, its incidence is declining. Still, one third of patients with AMI die in the pre-hospital phase without being treated by health personnel. In the pre-hospital phase, advanced life support and basic life support are essential, and easy access to traditional or automated external defibrillators is of paramount importance. Pre-hospital diagnosis is essential in patients with STEMI or BBBMI, who will benefit from pre-hospital rerouting to large-volume PCI centers for PPCI in case of a PCI-related delay below 120 minutes. Pre-hospital fibrinolysis may be a valuable alternative in remaining patients, whereas in-hospital fibrinolysis should be considered only in self-presenters at hospitals without easy access to catheterization laboratories.

chapter 29 In-Hospital Phase of Unstable Angina and Non–ST-Segment Elevation Myocardial Infarction

Lars Wallentin, Bertil Lindahl, and Agneta Siegbahn

Definition

- Unstable coronary artery disease describes unstable angina and non–ST-segment elevation myocardial infarction.

Key Features

- Unstable coronary artery disease is the most common cause (30% to 50%) of admission to coronary care units.
- The lesion is elicited by coronary artery plaque rupture or erosion, or both, with a superimposed thrombus.
- Initial evaluation is by history, ST-T changes on electrocardiography at rest, and measurement of troponin.

Therapy

- Initial treatment is with aspirin, $P2Y_{12}$ inhibition, intravenous or subcutaneous anticoagulation, beta blockade, nitrates, and, with high risk and if an early invasive procedure is planned, platelet glycoprotein IIb/IIIa blockade.
- Early risk stratification is performed by monitoring ischemia, markers of myocardial damage, myocardial dysfunction, renal dysfunction, anemia, and inflammation.
- Moderate- to high-risk patients should be managed with early coronary angiography and, if suitable, revascularization; low-risk patients are further evaluated by stress test and echocardiography.
- Long-term prevention is with aspirin, $P2Y_{12}$ inhibition, beta blockade, angiotensin-converting enzyme inhibitor, and cholesterol lowering by statins.

Acute coronary syndrome comprises all conditions caused by sudden impairment of blood flow in a coronary artery that leads to ischemia in the corresponding area of the myocardium. The acute coronary syndrome therefore includes acute myocardial infarction, unstable angina pectoris, and even sudden death resulting from an arrhythmia caused by sudden myocardial ischemia. The borderline between acute myocardial infarction and unstable angina pectoris is arbitrary and depends on the methods and definitions used to prove myocardial necrosis. Clinically and pathologically, there is a spectrum of acute coronary syndromes ranging from ST-segment elevation myocardial infarction through non–ST-segment elevation myocardial infarction to unstable angina pectoris with or without minor myocardial damage.[1-5] ST-segment elevation myocardial infarction, which often develops into a Q-wave myocardial infarction, is often explained by a persisting total occlusion in a coronary artery that is not compensated for by collateral flow and that leads to a transmural myocardial infarction in the area supplied by the occluded artery. If the blood flow is not reestablished within the first few hours, a remaining regional left ventricular dysfunction with an associated risk of congestive heart failure and ventricular arrhythmia will develop. Non–ST-segment elevation myocardial infarction, which often develops into a non–Q wave myocardial infarction, and unstable angina are most often caused by a thrombotic stenosis of a coronary artery that leads to either severe impairment or transient interruption of coronary blood flow. These conditions are merged into the concept of unstable coronary syndrome or unstable coronary artery disease. The term *unstable coronary artery disease* is preferred by us because it emphasizes that the risk and instability in all these conditions reside in the underlying thrombotic coronary lesions rather than in the transient symptoms.[2] Table 29.1 summarizes the characteristics of the acute coronary syndromes.

EPIDEMIOLOGY AND RISK FACTORS

Unstable coronary artery disease (CAD) is currently the major cause of admission to coronary care units and explains 30% to 50% of all such admissions. For every patient who has ST-segment elevation myocardial infarction, there are three patients who have unstable coronary syndrome. Thus, in a population with an annual admission rate for myocardial infarction of 2500 per million, there will be around 3500 to 4000 admissions for unstable coronary syndrome.[3] The risk factors for the development of unstable CAD are the same as those for any manifestation of atherosclerotic CAD. In addition to age and male sex, the dominating risk factors are diabetes mellitus, hypertension, dyslipidemia, and smoking. There are also influences from geography, psychosocial factors, and low physical activity. Other conditions that might contribute to clinical manifestations are life crises, acute or chronic stress, sudden unusual strenuous physical activity, and other diseases and surgical procedures.[3]

ANATOMY AND PATHOLOGY

The rapid development of a reduction in blood flow is related to fissuring of atherosclerotic plaques and the formation of thrombi. The thrombi may cause a flow-limiting stenosis or an occlusion, but they may also embolize to the peripheral coronary circulation. The flow limitation may fluctuate owing to both the continuous formation and dissolution of the thrombus and the phenomenon of distal platelet emboli.[6-11] Flow

ACUTE CORONARY SYNDROMES						
Concept	**ECG**	**Myocardial Damage**	**Coronary Lesion**	**Treatment**	**Myocardial Lesion**	**Prognosis**
ST-segment elevation myocardial infarction	ST-segment elevation New Q wave	Large	Persistent thrombotic total occlusion	Reperfusion Aspirin Beta blockade	Transmural myocardial infarction	Congestive heart failure Arrhythmia
Unstable coronary disease or unstable coronary syndrome	ST-segment depression or T-wave inversion No ST-segment elevation No new Q wave	Minor or none	Transient thrombotic occlusion Coronary thrombus with distal emboli Thrombotic severe stenosis	Aspirin $P2Y_{12}$ inhibitor GpIIb/IIIa inhibitor Fondaparinux LMW heparin Heparin Bivalirudin Beta blockade PCI, CABG	Non–Q wave infarction or unstable angina	Reinfarction or recurrent ischemia
CABG, coronary artery bypass grafting; ECG, electrocardiography; LMW, low molecular weight; PCI, percutaneous coronary intervention.						

Table 29.1 Acute coronary syndromes.

fluctuations may also be related to the development of collateral flow, to changes in vasomotor tone, and to vasospasm.[9,12] Many patients who have unstable CAD are elderly and often have preformed collateral vessels as a result of older stenotic lesions and occlusions.

The diseased coronary arteries are also prone to a vasospastic response because of the loss of the protective function of the normal endothelium.[12] Thus, the pathologic anatomy of the coronary arteries in unstable CAD often shows widespread atherosclerosis and several stenotic lesions and occlusions.[6,13] In the acute phase of the disease, it is often possible to demonstrate one culprit lesion with the most severe stenosis, a recent plaque fissure, and a fresh coronary thrombus (Fig. 29.1).[7-10,13,14] At other locations in the coronary arteries, there may simultaneously exist more plaque erosions and fissures, even with superimposed thrombotic material, but without an influence on the dynamics of coronary blood flow. However, such lesions may give rise to distal embolization of fragile platelet aggregates. Therefore, the myocardium of patients who have unstable CAD, even in the absence of a diagnosis of myocardial infarction, may show minor patchy areas of cellular necrosis because of recent embolization (see Fig. 29.1).[8]

Although the typical myocardial infarction in unstable CAD is nontransmural and subendocardial at autopsy, the myocardial damage may be quite variable. Thus, from unstable CAD to ST-segment elevation–Q-wave myocardial infarction, there is a continuum of fairly similar lesions in the coronary arteries and the myocardium. Even so, the dominating finding in unstable CAD is a severe stenosis in about 75% of patients; in the remainder, there is a total occlusion with nontransmural, less extensive diffuse myocardial damage because of blood supply from collaterals. This contrasts with the findings in 80% to 90% of cases of typical ST-segment elevation–Q-wave myocardial infarction of a total coronary occlusion, usually with no collateral supply, and the development of a transmural myocardial necrosis corresponding to the area of blood supply.[6,13]

PATHOPHYSIOLOGY

Atherosclerosis

Accumulating evidence indicates that the process of atherosclerosis is a chronic inflammatory disease (Fig. 29.2).The lesions represent a series of highly specific cellular and molecular responses.[15,16] The disease is basically a degenerative process in which the vessel wall is damaged by long-lasting exposure to mechanical injury and to different toxic substances. The damage depends on a combination of factors that are associated with well-known risk factors for atherosclerosis, such as

- elevated and modified low-density lipoprotein (LDL) cholesterol;
- hypertension;
- diabetes mellitus; and
- cigarette smoking.

In the response-to-injury hypothesis, which was first presented more than 20 years ago, endothelial denuding was proposed as the first step in the process. Today, endothelial dysfunction rather than denuding is emphasized.[15] In addition to the risk factors listed, the endothelial dysfunction may possibly be caused by gene mutations or polymorphisms, homocysteinemia, or infections with microorganisms and a combination of these factors.[15,17] Initiation of lesions occurs when endothelial cells, which are activated by different risk factors, express adhesion molecules. Vascular cell adhesion molecule 1 binds to monocytes and T lymphocytes that are found in early human atheroma.[2,18,19] On binding to the endothelium, leukocytes penetrate into the intima. Monocyte chemoattractant protein 1 (MCP-1), a chemotactic molecule secreted by the activated endothelial cells, appears responsible for the directed migration of monocytes into the intima at sites of plaque formation.[20] The activation of endothelial cells leads to increased permeability and to increased influx of LDL-cholesterol and inflammatory cells, monocytes-macrophages, and T lymphocytes.[2,18,19] Proliferation, migration, and synthesis of new matrix by intimal smooth muscle cells and activation of macrophages and T lymphocytes resulting in secretion of cytokines and growth

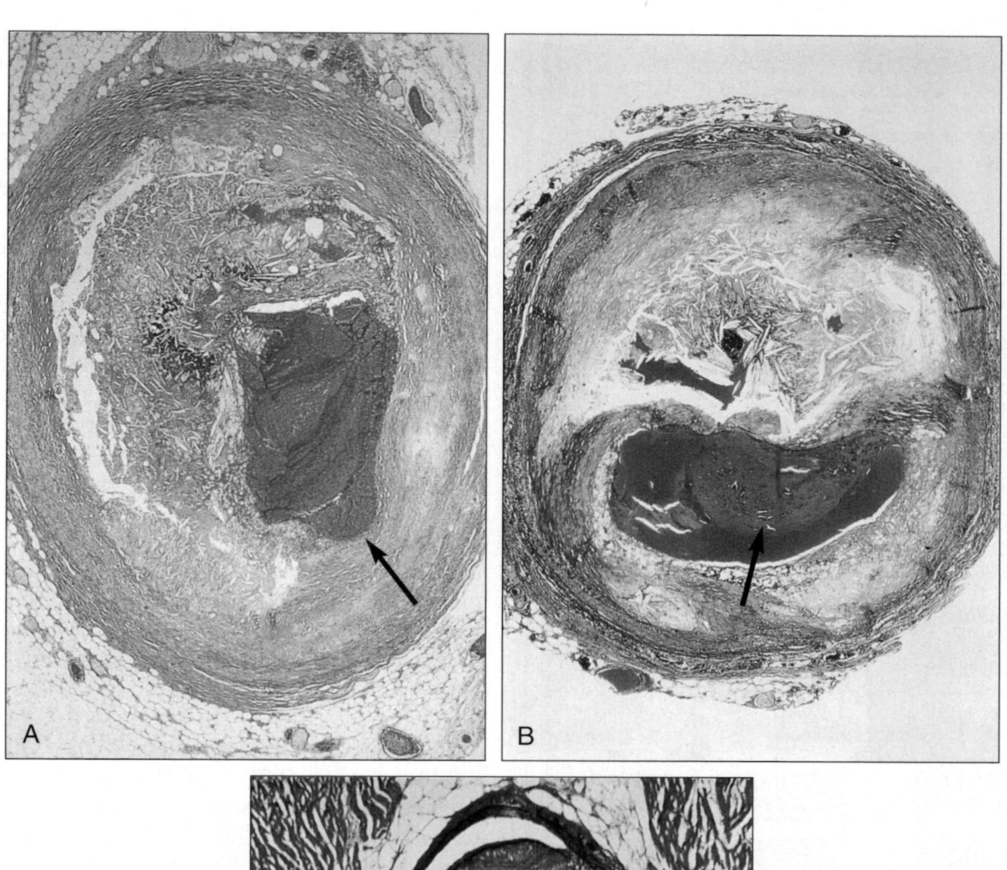

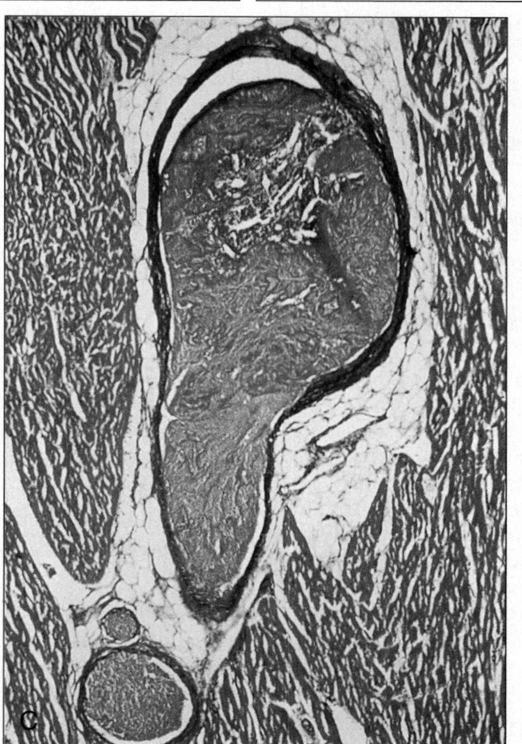

Figure 29.1 Coronary thrombosis. Coronary thrombosis is a dynamic process that is usually superimposed on a disrupted plaque. **A,** Lipid-rich plaque with ruptured surface and occlusive luminal thrombosis *(arrow)* superimposed. **B,** Disrupted plaque with platelet-rich nonocclusive thrombosis *(arrow)* superimposed. **C,** Small artery occluded by aggregated platelets (microembolus) found in the myocardium downstream of an evolving coronary thrombus. Such downstream embolization is often associated with microinfarcts in the myocardium. (Courtesy of Professor Erling Falk.)

factors give rise to the mature atherosclerotic plaque.[2,15,16,18,19] As a consequence of the chronic inflammation, the intima layer becomes fibrotic. In the plaque, a combination of proliferation of smooth muscle cells and matrix formation and degeneration with LDL-cholesterol accumulation and cell death (probably caused by apoptosis) takes place.[2,18-21] Small plaque ruptures are common; these are usually clinically silent but contribute to the progression of atherosclerosis.

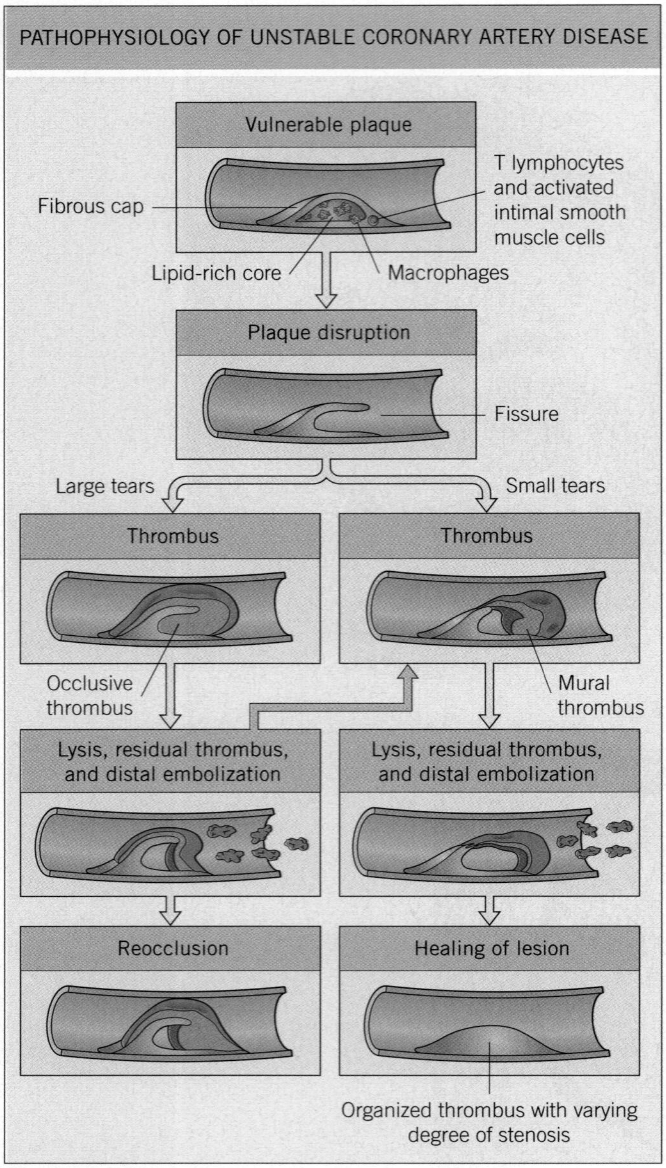

Figure 29.2 Pathophysiology of unstable coronary artery disease. Disruption of an atherosclerotic plaque results in a thrombus, which partially or totally occludes the lumen of the vessel. The outcome of the injury and the healing process may range from a total occlusion to minor plaque stenosis. (Modified from Fuster V, Lewis A. Conner Memorial Lecture. Mechanisms leading to myocardial infarction: insights from studies of vascular biology. Circulation 1994;90:2126-2146.)

Plaque Disruption and Thrombosis

Two main components can be identified in the mature atherosclerotic plaque[10,11]:

- soft lipid-rich atheromatous gruel; and
- hard collagen-rich sclerotic tissue—the so-called fibrous cap.

Two forms of damage to the plaque can induce thrombosis in the coronary vessel:

- a rupture of the fibrous cap; and
- a superficial erosion of the endothelium that covers the plaque.

About 75% of coronary thrombi are precipitated by plaque rupture and 25% by plaque erosion.[18] Plaques that are regarded as vulnerable and at high risk for rupture or fissuring are lipid rich and have a necrotic core, which occupies a high proportion of the plaque volume, and a thin fibrous cap.[10] These plaques have a high content of macrophages, which are often localized in the so-called shoulder region between the normal vessel wall and the atherosclerotic wall; increased expression of procoagulant activity, that is, tissue factor; and low densities of smooth muscle cells in the fibrous cap.

The vulnerability of the plaque, that is, its predisposition to rupture, is determined by the mechanical strength of the fibrous cap to resist circumferential tensile stress and intrinsic forces.[18] The process of plaque rupture is, however, not only mechanical. Activated T lymphocytes stimulate macrophages in the plaques to secrete a number of extracellular matrix–degrading enzymes (e.g., plasminogen activators and matrix metalloproteinases).[22] By weakening the fibrous cap, these substances can predispose to rupture of the plaque. Recent work provides evidence for a central role of the CD40-CD40L pathway and interleukin (IL)–18 in these inflammatory processes of atherosclerosis.[22,23]

CD40-CD40L Interaction and IL-18 in Vascular Cell Crosstalk

CD40 ligand (CD40L, CD154), a member of the tumor necrosis factor gene superfamily, is expressed in a number of cells (activated $CD4^+$ T lymphocytes, monocytes and macrophages, endothelial cells, vascular smooth muscle cells, activated basophils) and recently also was demonstrated in activated platelets.[24,25] Its receptor, CD40, is expressed predominantly by B lymphocytes but also by a variety of other cells including smooth muscle cells, endothelial cells, and monocytes and macrophages.[26] Colocalization of both receptors and ligand on atheroma-associated endothelial cells, smooth muscle cells, and macrophages has been shown in vitro as well as in situ.[24] Coupling of CD40L to CD40 mediates various proatherogenic processes, including expression of adhesion molecules and secretion of matrix metalloproteinases, chemokines, cytokines, and growth factors. The CD40-CD40L–mediated signals also induce tissue factor expression and procoagulant activity in monocytes-macrophages and in vascular smooth muscle cells.[24,27] In a model of atherosclerosis using hyperlipidemic mice, CD40L interference by a specific antibody reduced the size and the lipid content of the initial atherosclerotic lesions as well as the number of infiltrating leukocytes.[28] Furthermore, in established atherosclerosis, delayed anti-CD40L antibody treatment inhibited further progression and induced a more stable plaque phenotype.[29]

IL-18 is a proinflammatory cytokine and member of the IL-1 cytokine family.[30] It is produced by a variety of cells, in particular by activated macrophages and dendritic cells. IL-18 induces the production of a number of proinflammatory factors, such as IL-1β, IL-8, adhesion molecules, and metalloproteinases. IL-18 also stimulates interferon γ production in T_H1 cells, macrophages, and NK cells.[31] IL-18 also plays an important role in the atherosclerotic process, by interferon γ production and up-regulation of the scavenger receptor–chemokine CXCL16. IL-18 is abundant in atherosclerotic plaques and associated with plaque destabilization and vulnerability.[32,33] Animal models support this role and further demonstrate the beneficial effects of inhibiting IL-18 on plaque progression.[34]

Rupture of these vulnerable coronary plaques is probably the most important mechanism underlying the sudden onset of acute coronary syndromes.[11] The vessel wall injury at the site of plaque rupture exposes collagen and induces rapid activation of platelets. Moreover, rupture of lipid-rich coronary plaques exposes the highly thrombogenic core to the circulating blood, thus setting off the coagulation cascade and the formation of a fibrin-rich thrombus (see Fig. 29.2). In plaque erosion, the overlying endothelium undergoes denudation with exposure of collagen and tissue factor, and thrombus formation occurs on the surface of the plaque.[11] These plaques lack a superficial lipid core but are rich in smooth muscle cells that have the capacity to express tissue factor.[35] When smooth muscle cells are exposed to thrombin and other products released during thrombosis, such as growth factors (platelet-derived growth factor), they also produce the inflammatory mediator IL-6, which can induce an acute-phase response.[36] In addition to these erosions, accumulation of macrophages and lymphocytes is observed.[37] Plaque erosions seem to be relatively more common in younger patients and in women, and they are also frequently seen in patients who suffer sudden death as a result of coronary thrombosis.[35]

Platelets

Platelets play a pivotal role in thrombosis after plaque rupture or plaque erosion (Fig. 29.3). At the time of vascular injury, the subendothelial matrix, including collagens, laminin, fibronectin, and von Willebrand factor, is exposed to the flowing blood. The platelets adhere to subendothelial structures, and they undergo changes in shape, aggregate, and release intracellular substances, which enhance the thrombotic process.[38] The property of the platelets to adhere and to aggregate is mediated through a specific glycoprotein (Gp) expressed on the platelet surface.[39] Adhesion to subendothelial structures is mediated mainly through the binding of collagen to GpIa and GpVI receptors and by the binding of von Willebrand factor to GpIb receptors.[40] In atherosclerotic, stenosed blood vessels with increased "shear rate," the binding of von Willebrand factor is enhanced. Adherence of platelets does not involve previous activation of the cells.

Platelets express on their surface specific glycoprotein receptors, namely, GpIIb/IIIa receptors, which belong to the integrin receptor family. The GpIIb/IIIa receptor is the most abundant platelet glycoprotein—there are about 80,000 receptors on each cell. In the resting state, the affinity of GpIIb/IIIa for fibrinogen is low. On agonist stimulation, so-called inside-out signaling induces conformational changes of the receptor, leading to a marked increase in affinity for fibrinogen and substantial receptor occupancy. Platelet aggregation is mainly mediated by fibrinogen that is bonded to GpIIb/IIIa. To a lesser extent, other substances may bind to the receptor (e.g., vitronectin, fibronectin, and von Willebrand factor). It has been shown that prothrombin can bind to these receptors, and when bound, it can be activated to thrombin.[41] Some of the most important agonists for platelet stimulation are adenosine diphosphate, epinephrine (adrenaline), thrombin, collagen, and serotonin. In addition to aggregation of the platelets, fibrinogen binding induces outside-in signaling, leading to secretion of a number of substances that

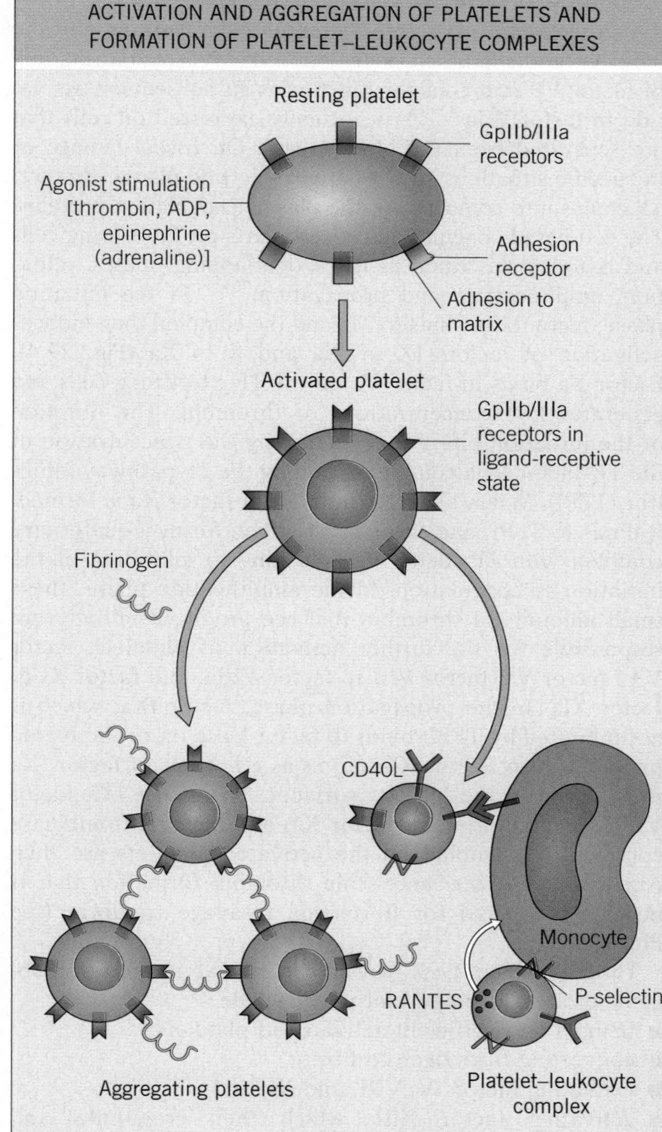

Figure 29.3 Activation and aggregation of platelets and formation of platelet-leukocyte complexes. Stimulation of platelets by adhesion or agonist receptors induces transition of glycoprotein IIb/IIIa receptors to active ligand-binding receptors. Glycoprotein IIb/IIIa receptors occupied by fibrinogen support aggregation through formation of bridges between adjacent platelets. Activated platelets express P-selectin and CD40 ligand (CD40L) on their surface. These receptors mediate the binding of leukocytes, thus forming complexes between the cells. ADP, adenosine diphosphate.

are stored in the platelets. Examples of these factors are platelet-activating factors (e.g., adenosine diphosphate, thromboxane A_2, and serotonin), growth factors (e.g., platelet-derived growth factor), cytokines (RANTES), coagulation factors (factor V and von Willebrand factor), and plasminogen activator inhibitor 1. On secretion, P-selectin and CD40L are exposed on the platelet surface.[25,42,43] These structures mediate binding of platelets to leukocytes, which may induce cytokine release from the leukocytes and tissue factor expression in monocytes.[42-44] Secretion from the platelets, however, need not be preceded by aggregation (see Fig. 29.3).

Cell-Based Coagulation Process

Tissue factor (TF) is a transmembrane glycoprotein and the main initiator of blood coagulation in vivo by the binding of factor VII and cofactor function in its subsequent activation to factor VIIa.[45] TF is normally expressed on cells that are separated from the bloodstream. On tissue damage or in specific situations such as atherosclerotic plaque rupture, TF comes into contact with the plasma coagulation proteins. The cell-based coagulation process starts on TF-bearing cells and is today described in three overlapping phases: initiation, amplification, and propagation.[45,46] In the initiation phase, factor VIIa binds to TF, and the complex then induces activation of factors IX to IXa and X to Xa (Fig. 29.4). Factor Xa binds to factor Va on the TF-expressing cells and generates low concentrations of thrombin. The duration of the initiation phase is regulated by the concentration of the TF–factor VIIa complexes and by the TF pathway inhibitor (TFPI). When a certain amount of factor Xa is formed, it binds to TFPI, and this complex than forms a quaternary complex with TF–factor VIIa, leading to inhibition of the initiation of coagulation. In the amplification phase, these small amounts of thrombin that are produced initially are responsible for the further activation of platelets, factor V to factor Va, factor VIII to factor VIIIa, and factor XI to factor XIa. In the propagation phase, factor IXa, which is not inhibited by TFPI, binds to factor VIIIa on the activated platelets. Also, factor XIa serves as a booster of factor IXa production on the platelet surfaces. The factor IXa–factor VIIIa complex provides factor Xa, and the prothrombinase complexes assembled on the activated platelets are then responsible for the large-scale thrombin formation that is necessary in vivo for fibrinogen cleavage to fibrin (see Fig. 29.4).[47]

Thrombin (Fig. 29.5) plays a central role in the thrombogenic process. Its important roles include

- being a most efficient activator of platelets;
- converting fibrinogen to fibrin;
- activating factors V, VIII, and XI; and
- activating factor XIII, which then cross-links and stabilizes fibrin.

On binding to thrombomodulin, the thrombin-thrombomodulin complex activates the protein C anticoagulation system and activates carboxypeptidase thrombin-activable fibrinolysis inhibitor.

Thrombin also has a number of other cell-activating properties. It induces proliferation and migration of smooth muscle cells and fibroblasts.[48] Thrombin is also able to induce secretion of a number of cytokines and growth factors from endothelial cells and circulating monocytes.[49] Moreover, thrombin can induce procoagulant activity in endothelial cells by up-regulation of TF expression (see Figs. 29.4 and 29.5).

Tissue Factor and Coronary Artery Disease

TF antigen has been identified in the necrotic core of coronary atherosclerotic plaques and in the extracellular matrix of the arterial wall in atherosclerosis.[50-52] Macrophages, smooth muscle cells, and endothelial cells are the principal cells that express TF. It has recently been demonstrated that TF in plaque is functionally active and correlates with platelet deposition.[53] Platelet deposition and thrombus formation on the lipid-rich atheromatous core that is exposed to flowing blood can be up to six times as much as that on the adventitia and collagen-rich matrix.[54] TF antigen and TF activity seem to be significantly higher in plaques from patients who have unstable angina and myocardial infarction than in plaques from patients who have stable angina.[55] TF in the lipid-rich core is largely derived from macrophages that are present in the plaque.

However, the TF content within the plaques varies according to the clinical syndrome. In patients who have stable angina, TF is located predominantly in the acellular component of the plaque. In contrast, in patients who have unstable angina, TF correlates with macrophage and smooth muscle cell areas.[55] Furthermore, a high correlation has been found between TF and macrophages in thrombus areas in tissue from patients who have unstable angina. Oxidized LDL and different cytokines, such as IL-1, tumor necrosis factor, MCP-1, and platelet-derived growth factor

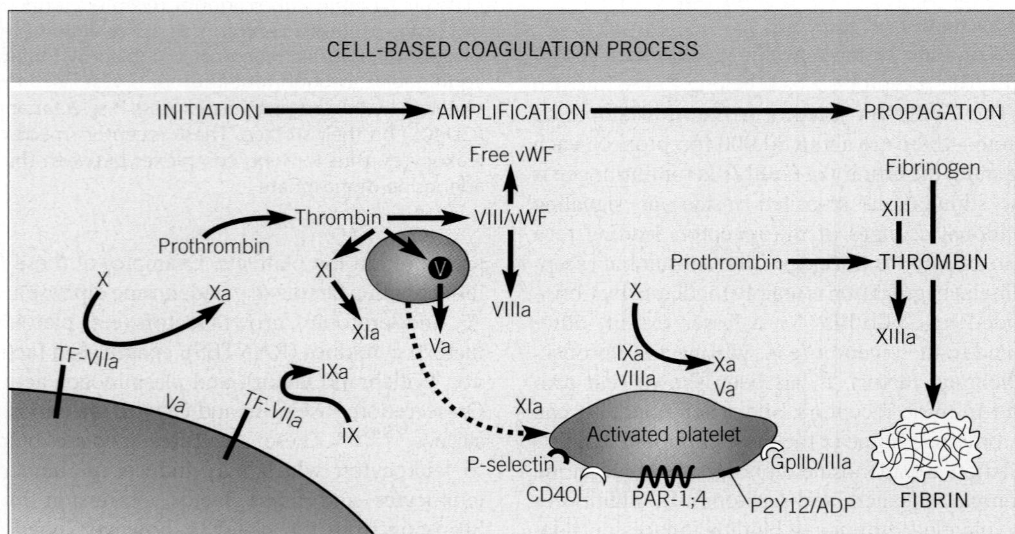

Figure 29.4 Cell-based coagulation process.

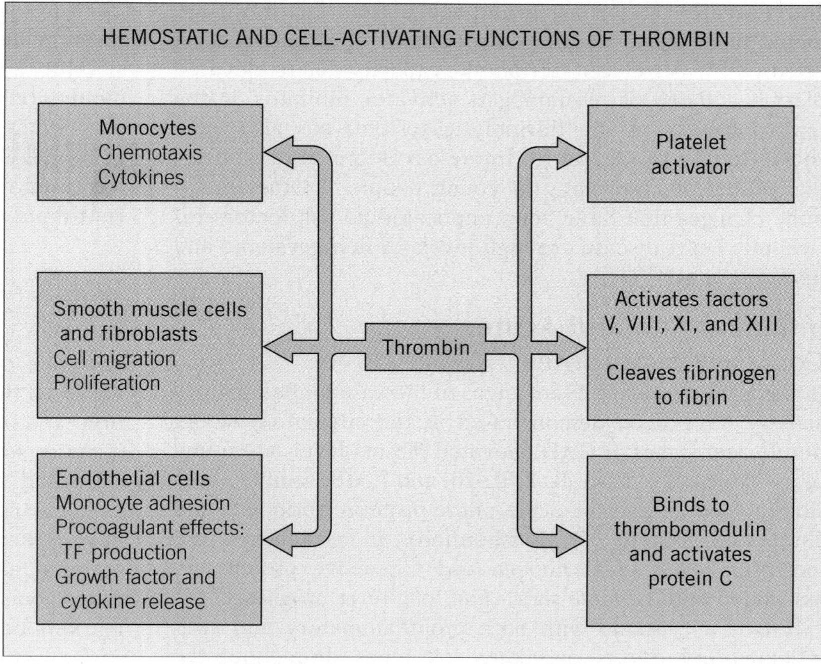

Figure 29.5 Hemostatic and cell-activating functions of thrombin.

BB, that are present in the plaques can stimulate the cells to express functional TF.[56,57] Moreover, CD40-CD40L interaction contributes to TF induction in macrophages and in smooth muscle cells.[22,24] Studies have demonstrated that variations in the TF gene may regulate the expression and activity of TF in monocytes-macrophages and predict uneventful outcome in acute coronary syndromes.[58,59] Thus, all of these observations indicate that TF is an important determinant of the thrombogenicity in unstable CAD. Finally, TF–factor VIIa induces intracellular signaling that promotes cell migration and plays a role in the development of vasa vasorum neovascularization in coronary arteries.[60,61]

Local Factors That Contribute to Thrombogenesis

A number of local and systemic factors decide whether the plaque rupture will lead to a small mural thrombus or an obstructive thrombus that significantly interferes with the blood flow (Table 29.2; see also Fig. 29.1). Most plaque ruptures are asymptomatic but induce growth of the plaque and varying degrees of stenosis of the vessel due to superimposed thrombus formation.[10] The degree of plaque rupture, fissure, or ulcer and the tissue substrate exposed to the blood are the most important local factors that determine thrombus formation. The degree of arterial stenosis also influences the development of the thrombus. Deposition of platelets is directly correlated to the degree of stenosis and to the severity of vasoconstriction. Thrombus-promoting factors can be summarized as[10]

- large tears;
- lipid extrusion;
- high TF expression;
- high grade of stenosis; and
- low blood flow.

LOCAL AND SYSTEMIC FACTORS THAT CONTRIBUTE TO THROMBOGENESIS
Local factors
Severity of vessel wall injury (area and depth correlated to size and stability of thrombus)
Degree of stenosis (correlated to platelet deposition)
Vasoconstriction (correlated to platelet deposition)
Tissue substrate (lipid rich, collagen rich)
Residual thrombus formation (surface thrombin)
Systemic factors
Elevated levels of fibrinogen and factor VII
Fibrinolysis (plasminogen activator inhibitor 1)
Activated platelets and coagulation (soluble tissue factor, prothrombin fragment F1+2, fibrinopeptide A)
Inflammatory activity (C-reactive protein, cytokines, activated leukocytes)
Homocystinemia
Lipoprotein(a)

Table 29.2 Local and systemic factors that contribute to thrombogenesis.

Another local cause of major importance for the thrombotic process is residual mural thrombus, which is a highly thrombogenic substrate. The main reason for this is that a residual thrombus has high local thrombin activity on its surface.

Systemic Factors That Promote Thrombogenesis

The balance between the coagulation and fibrinolytic systems at the time of plaque rupture influences the outcome. A number of epidemiologic studies of large-scale populations have clearly established that increased levels and activities of fibrinogen and coagulation factor VII are major risk factors for the development of ischemic heart disease.[62,63] A reduced fibrinolytic capacity due to elevated plasma activity of plasminogen activator inhibitor 1 (the main inhibitor of the fibrinolytic system) has also been shown to be a risk factor for future development of myocardial infarction, especially in young people.[64] Other metabolic changes that have been implicated as risk factors for ischemic heart disease are high levels of homocysteine and lipoprotein(a).[65,66]

Inflammation and Acute Coronary Syndromes

In the acute coronary event, signs of increased inflammatory activity have been demonstrated in the circulating blood. In different stages of CAD, elevated plasma levels are found of cytokines IL-1, IL-6, IL-8, IL-10, and IL-18; soluble adhesion molecules; and the acute-phase proteins fibrinogen and C-reactive protein.[67,68] Furthermore, in unstable CAD, increased levels of fibrinogen and C-reactive protein are associated with a worse short- and long-term prognosis.[69-72]

IL-6 is a cytokine with both proinflammatory and anti-inflammatory effects on many cell types throughout the body. Large, prospective studies of healthy populations have demonstrated that elevated plasma levels of IL-6 are associated with an increased risk of premature death or future myocardial infarction, independent of other cardiovascular risk factors.[73] In the FRISC II trial, comprising patients with acute coronary syndrome, IL-6 was shown to be a powerful marker for identifying unstable CAD patients with increased risk of death in a 6- and 12-month perspective. IL-6 was independent of other risk indicators, including C-reactive protein. This risk was significantly reduced by an early invasive treatment strategy.[74]

Accumulating data have demonstrated systemic activation of coagulation and of platelets and leukocytes in unstable CAD. Increased concentrations of soluble TF and increased thrombin generation and activity indicate a procoagulable state.[75-77] Circulating lymphocytes and monocytes are activated in unstable CAD.[78] Circulating monocytes have increased expression of TF on their surface and may therefore contribute to the systemic activation of coagulation.[78] With use of whole blood flow cytometry, increased levels of platelet activation, platelet microparticles, and expression of P-selectin were found in unstable CAD.[79,80] Patients with unstable CAD also have a significant increase in amounts of platelet-granulocyte and platelet-monocyte complexes in the circulation.[81,82] Women with unstable CAD have remarkably raised levels of circulating platelet-monocyte complexes compared with men with the same syndrome and also with women with stable angina.[82] These complexes are formed by activated cells and have been shown to induce further activation of these cells, that is, production and secretion of TF and a number of proinflammatory cytokines (IL-1, IL-8, and MCP-1), thereby promoting inflammation and coagulation. CD40L, in addition to the cell-associated form, also occurs in a soluble, biologically active form (sCD40L) that is rapidly released from activated T lymphocytes.[83] Patients with unstable CAD have higher concentrations of sCD40L than do patients with stable angina or healthy volunteers.[84-86] The association of a novel gene variation in the *CD40LG* gene and plasma concentrations of sCD40L was recently demonstrated. Increased plasma concentration of sCD40L was associated with a higher risk of future myocardial infarction, but not to death, in patients with acute coronary syndrome.[86] Finally, circulating inflammatory factors, acute-phase reactants, and cytokines not only may mark increased risk for future cardiovascular events but also can contribute to their pathogenesis.

CLINICAL PRESENTATIONS

Unstable CAD is a heterogeneous clinical syndrome. An adequate operational definition of unstable CAD must be based on the information at the time of the initial presentation and evaluation. Hence, this operational definition includes some patients who will subsequently be found to have had an acute Q-wave myocardial infarction as well as some patients who will be found subsequently not to have ischemic heart disease. Unstable angina and non–ST-segment elevation myocardial infarction can be differentiated only with certainty when the results of cardiac markers become available.

The history is the most important tool for establishing the diagnosis of unstable CAD. There are three principal presentations (Table 29.3):

- new-onset angina;
- increasing angina; and
- angina at rest.

These presentations are not always distinct in clinical practice. Prolonged chest pain at rest or during slight exertion is the condition that most often causes the patient to seek medical attention. Because many conditions can cause chest pain, it is important to elucidate the character of the symptoms to distinguish myocardial ischemia from nonischemic or noncardiac chest pain. The chest pain in unstable CAD usually has the same qualities as the chest pain in typical stable angina (see Chapter 22), except that the episodes often are more severe and prolonged, occur at rest, and have no obvious relation to exertion or stress. The complaint is most often characterized as a deep, poorly localized chest or arm discomfort, often described as pressure, squeezing, or fullness.

PRINCIPAL PRESENTATIONS OF UNSTABLE CORONARY ARTERY DISEASE	
New-onset angina	Angina that gives marked limitations of ordinary physical activity (CCSC class ≥III) with onset within 2 months
Increasing angina	Angina on effort with a change in a previous stable pattern: distinctly more frequent, longer in duration, or lower in threshold (i.e., increased by at least one CCSC class to at least class III within 2 months)
Angina at rest	Angina occurring at rest and usually prolonged for more than 15 minutes; occurring within 1 week of presentation

CCSC, Canadian Cardiovascular Society Classification.

Table 29.3 Principal presentations of unstable coronary artery disease.

The discomfort often radiates to the shoulders, neck, jaw, and arms. Some patients have no chest pain but present solely with discomfort in the jaw, neck, or arms. Administration of sublingual nitrate often provides only temporary or incomplete relief. Associated symptoms during attacks, such as dyspnea, diaphoresis, nausea, and anxiety, are common. On occasion, patients present with unexplained, new-onset, or worsened effort dyspnea as the sole manifestation of unstable CAD. In particular, elderly patients and patients who have diabetes mellitus may present with little or no chest pain.

Other important aspects of the patient's history are

- the previous manifestations of heart disease (e.g., effort angina, previous myocardial infarction, congestive heart failure, or previous revascularization);
- peripheral or cerebrovascular atherosclerotic disease;
- a family history of premature CAD; and
- the presence of coronary risk factors (i.e., diabetes mellitus, hypertension, smoking, and hyperlipidemia).

A history that includes any of these factors, especially previous manifestations of coronary heart disease, supports the diagnosis and adversely affects the prognosis. The likelihood of coronary heart disease also increases with age and with male sex. It is also important to be aware of conditions outside the coronary vascular bed that may precipitate unstable CAD by increasing the myocardial oxygen demand or decreasing the oxygen supply (e.g., fever, infection, arrhythmias, thyrotoxicosis, anemia, or hypoxemia).

The findings on physical examination are commonly normal, and physical examination plays no major role in diagnosis of unstable CAD. However, the examination may reveal findings that increase the likelihood of significant CAD, such as signs of left ventricular dysfunction, hypertension, and peripheral or cerebrovascular atherosclerotic disease. Furthermore, the examination may reveal signs of noncoronary heart disease or extracardiac disease, which may mimic unstable CAD.

Differential diagnosis includes esophageal pain (e.g., reflux, abnormal motility, or rupture), musculoskeletal pain, pericarditis, hypertrophic cardiomyopathy, gastritis, peptic ulceration or perforation, biliary colic or cholecystitis, pleurisy, aortic dissection, pulmonary embolism, and pneumothorax. However, these conditions may coexist with coronary heart disease (e.g., esophageal pain and musculoskeletal pain).

DIAGNOSIS AND RISK STRATIFICATION

Early diagnosis and risk assessment are essential for the application of appropriate treatment and further management in the patient with suspicion of unstable CAD. For establishing the diagnosis, symptoms and markers indicative of myocardial ischemia together with markers of myocardial damage are critical. For risk assessment, a number of additional factors reflecting different aspects of the pathophysiologic process provide additional information. However, the predictive abilities of the different factors differ considerably between different endpoints. In general, more factors are predictive of mortality than of subsequent myocardial infarction (Table 29.4).

EARLY AVAILABLE FACTORS ASSOCIATED WITH A WORSE PROGNOSIS IN UNSTABLE CORONARY DISEASE

	Death	Myocardial (Re-)infarction
Factors from patient's history		
High age	x	x
Diabetes mellitus	x	x
Previous myocardial infarction	x	x
Previous angina	x	x
Previous or ongoing heart failure	x	—
Markers of ischemia		
ST-segment depression on electrocardiogram	x	x
ST-segment episodes at ST monitoring	x	x
Markers of acute myocardial damage		
Troponin T or I elevation	x	x
Markers of inflammation		
C-reactive protein	x	—
Markers of cardiac performance		
Depressed left ventricular ejection fraction	x	—
Brain (or B-type) natriuretic peptide (BNP) or NT-proBNP elevation	x	—
Markers of renal dysfunction		
Decreased creatinine clearance	x	—
Increased cystatin C elevation	x	—

Table 29.4 Early available factors associated with a worse prognosis in unstable coronary disease.

Factors Derived from the Patient's History and Examination

In the era of advanced technology, the importance of data derived from the patient's history and the examination of the patient must not be forgotten.[1] The age of the patient is a strong and independent prognostic indicator. Other important prognostic factors are a history of previous myocardial infarction, congestive heart failure, angina pectoris, and diabetes mellitus (Fig. 29.6a).[87] Furthermore, data from the patient's examination, such as pulse rate, blood pressure level, and presence of rales on lung auscultation, provide prognostic information. Thus, the risk assessment of a patient with suspicion of unstable CAD should always start by taking a good clinical history and performing a careful physical examination.

Markers of Ischemia

Electrocardiography

The 12-lead electrocardiogram (ECG) provides important diagnostic and prognostic information. Thus, a 12-lead ECG at rest should be obtained on admission and, whenever possible, during an episode of chest pain in patients who are suspected of having an acute coronary syndrome. Comparison with a previous ECG, if available, facilitates the interpretation. Because as much as two thirds of all ischemic episodes in unstable CAD are silent (i.e., not associated with chest pain), continuous multiple-lead ECG monitoring might increase the possibility of detecting transient ischemic episodes. The diagnosis of acute ischemia is based primarily on changes in the ST segment and the T wave. ST-segment elevation strongly suggests the diagnosis of an acute myocardial infarction, although transient ST-segment elevation may be seen during attacks of chest pain in severe unstable angina and in the rare condition of variant angina (see Chapter 23). The most characteristic finding in unstable CAD is ST-segment depression with or without associated T-wave changes. However, marked ST depression in leads V_1-V_3 may indicate a true posterior transmural infarction that should be handled and treated as ST-segment elevation myocardial infarction (see Chapter 30). Very widespread ST-segment depression (in seven or more leads) has a high specificity for acute myocardial infarction.[88] Isolated T-wave inversion is less specific, but it too may indicate ischemia; in particular, deep symmetric anterior (leads V_2-V_4) T-wave inversion suggests ischemia caused by a stenosis in the proximal left anterior descending artery. The prevalence of minor T-wave inversion (<1 mm) or T-wave flattening, especially in lateral leads (leads V_5-V_6), is not higher among unstable CAD patients than in the emergency department population overall, and thus it is of limited diagnostic value.[89] Transient episodes of bundle branch block may occasionally be seen during ischemic attacks. Presence of older pathologic Q waves, which are indicative of a previous myocardial infarction, gives circumstantial support to a diagnosis of unstable CAD. Importantly, a normal ECG on admission does not exclude unstable CAD. However, a completely normal ECG recorded during an episode of significant chest pain should turn the attention to other possible causes of the patient's complaints.

The ECG findings on admission contain prognostic information. Patients whose ECGs show ST-segment depression have a higher risk of subsequent cardiac events than do those whose ECGs show no ST-segment depression (Fig. 29.6b).[90-92] The risk of adverse events also increases with increasing degree of ST-segment depression.[88] Furthermore, patients who have episodes of ST-segment changes during continuous monitoring, whether silent or not, have an increased risk of subsequent cardiac events.[93] The treatment benefit from an early invasive approach is larger in patients who have ST-segment depression than in patients without ST-segment depression.[91,92]

Stress Testing

In recent years, focus has changed from late risk assessment, performed at or after discharge, to early risk stratification performed within the first 6 to 12 hours after admission. Therefore, the role for additional stress testing has become limited to patients at low risk according to the early risk assessment and especially if the diagnosis of unstable CAD is uncertain. An exercise test with continuous ECG recording, which is inexpensive and widely available, can in general be recommended as the standard mode of stress testing. However, in patients who have persisting widespread anterior ST deviations or bundle branch block in the ECG at rest, an imaging technique, such as stress echocardiography or perfusion scintigraphy, is required. Furthermore, in patients who are unable to exercise because of physical limitations, a pharmacologic stress together with an imaging technique is necessary. For a thorough discussion of stress testing, see Chapter 20.

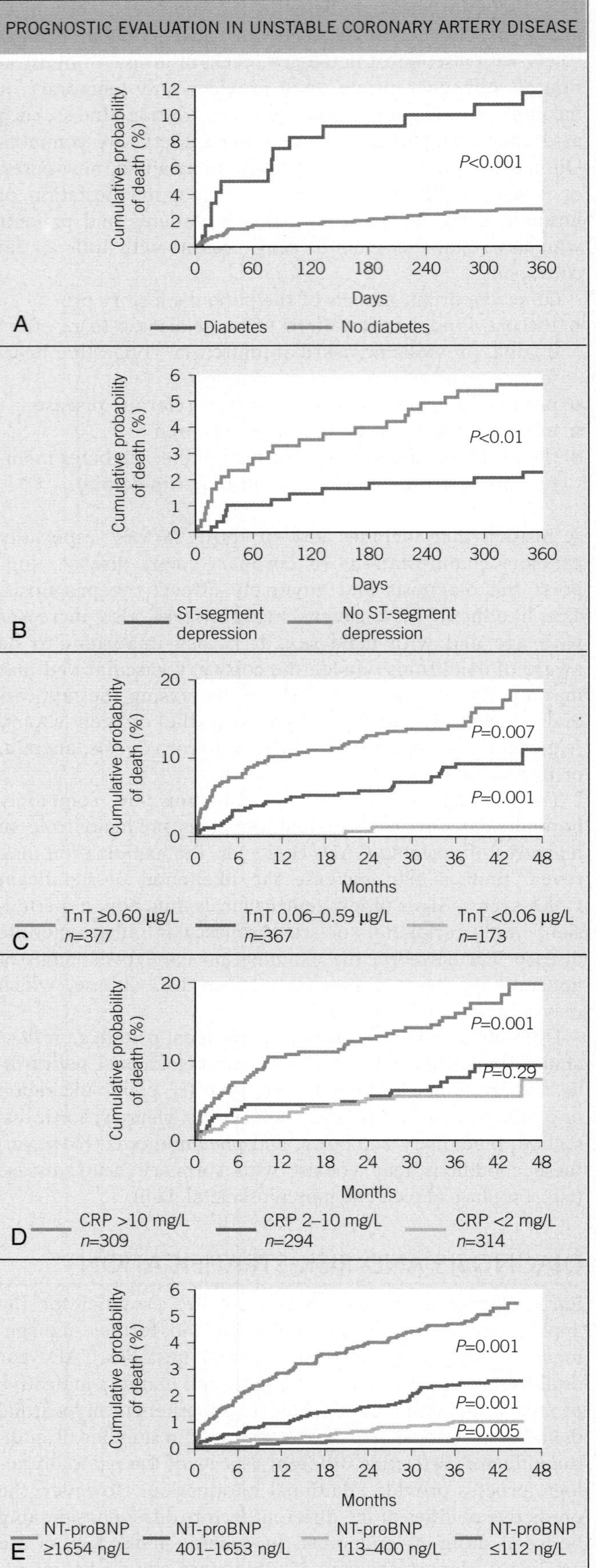

Figure 29.6 *See legend on opposite page.*

Figure 29.6 A to F, Prognostic evaluation in unstable coronary artery disease. CRP, C-reactive protein; GFR, glomerular filtration rate; TnT, troponin T. (Modified from Jernberg T, Lindahl B, James S, Larsson A, Hansson LO, Wallentin L. Cystatin C: a novel predictor of outcome in suspected or confirmed non–ST-elevation acute coronary syndrome. Circulation 2004;110:2342-2348.)

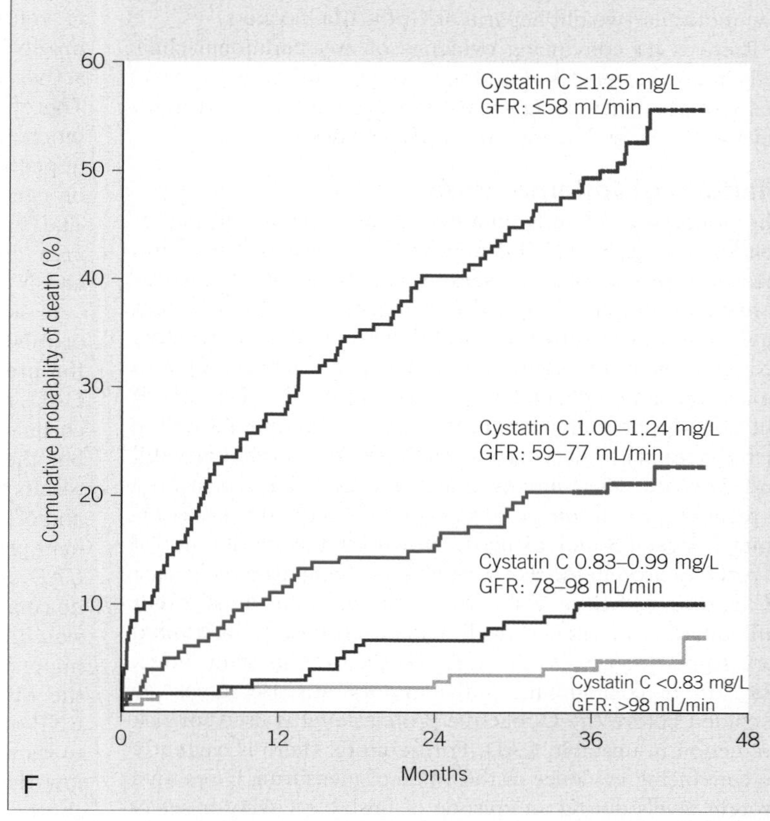

Markers of Acute Myocardial Damage ("Cardiac Markers")

The separation of a non–ST-segment elevation myocardial infarction from unstable angina is dependent on the ability to show myocardial necrosis by measurements of markers of myocardial damage. Cardiac troponin T and cardiac troponin I are the preferred biochemical markers for detection of myocardial necrosis because of their high sensitivity and specificity and their wide time window (i.e., there is a long duration of elevated plasma levels after myocardial damage) (see Chapter 27).[5] These properties make the troponins especially suitable for detection of small myocardial damage in unstable patients who have repeated episodes of ischemia of different intensity and of several days' duration. Furthermore, the recently introduced "high sensitivity" troponin assays allow reliable detection of even smaller amounts of myocardial damage, leading to a diagnosis of myocardial infarction in a large proportion of patients who previously were diagnosed with unstable angina. For the diagnosis of acute myocardial infarction, there is now universal consensus that the 99th percentile troponin level of healthy subjects, provided the total coefficient of variation is below 10% for the particular assay at that level, should be used as the decision level.[5] However, the development of very sensitive troponin assays also makes it even more important to be familiar with and, in the individual case, to consider other possible causes of myocardial damage and minor troponin elevation (see Chapter 27) before making the diagnosis of non–ST-segment elevation myocardial infarction.

Because of the delay between the time of myocardial damage and the rise of troponin level in the circulation, it is not possible to exclude myocardial infarction or damage with certainty on admission. Therefore, repeated blood sampling and measurements are required during the first 6 hours after admission and after any new prolonged episode of chest pain during hospitalization. Several manufacturers now provide rapid and accurate tests for point-of-care measurements. These tests are capable of a substantial reduction in the time between blood sampling and the availability of the analytical result, thereby facilitating the early diagnostic and prognostic evaluation.

Patients with elevation of troponin, compared with those without, have an increased risk of new cardiac events, both short and long term. Meta-analyses of published studies have demonstrated a two to nine times higher mortality and two to four times higher risk of death and myocardial infarction in patients with elevated troponin.[94,95] The risk of a new myocardial infarction is substantially increased as soon as a troponin elevation is detectable, whereas the risk of death seems to increase gradually with increasing troponin levels (Fig. 29.6c).[71,96] The prognostic value of troponins in unstable CAD can be attributed to underlying severe coronary stenosis, culprit lesion thrombosis, downstream embolization with microinfarction, and, in some patients, total coronary occlusion and a large myocardial infarction and reduced left ventricular function.[96]

The identification of patients who have elevated troponin levels is useful for selecting treatment in patients who have unstable CAD. Patients who have elevated troponin levels, in contrast to those who do not, derive the largest benefit from an early invasive approach[92,97] and from treatment with low-molecular-weight heparin or GpIIb/IIIa blockers.[98,99]

There is no convincing evidence of any additional clinically relevant benefit of adding another marker of myocardial damage when a high-sensitivity troponin assay is used, neither for early diagnosis nor for risk assessment.

Markers of Inflammation

The importance of inflammatory mechanisms in the pathogenesis of unstable CAD is now well established. Therefore, measurements of plasma markers of inflammation, such as C-reactive protein, IL-6, and fibrinogen, for risk assessment have gained increasing interest. Of these markers, C-reactive protein is the most extensively studied and has been found to be a strong and independent predictor of death[71](Fig. 29.6d) but not of a new myocardial infarction. The optimal timing of measurement and cutpoint of C-reactive protein are still under debate. Most studies in unstable CAD have measured C-reactive protein on or close to admission and used a cutpoint between 3 and 15 mg/L. However, the routine use of C-reactive protein for risk assessment is hampered by its lack of cardiospecificity. C-reactive protein, and most other inflammatory markers as well, rise in response to inflammatory stimuli regardless of origin. Therefore, an acute infection or a concomitant inflammatory disease must be excluded before the C-reactive protein level is used for risk prediction in unstable CAD. Furthermore, there is currently no convincing evidence of the value of measuring C-reactive protein levels during an episode of unstable CAD for selection of treatment.[100]

Markers of Cardiac Performance

Echocardiography at Rest

For diagnostic purposes, two-dimensional echocardiography at rest has limited value, although it may show transiently hypokinetic or akinetic segments of the left ventricle wall as evidence of ongoing myocardial ischemia or stunning in patients who have unstable angina. However, neither the existence nor the absence of abnormalities of wall motion is diagnostic. Some patients (at least 30%) will have had a previous myocardial infarction to explain a hypokinetic or akinetic area. Other patients may have perfectly normal wall motion between the episodes of ischemia. For assessment of the global and regional left ventricular systolic function, two-dimensional echocardiography at rest is very useful. Because left ventricular systolic function is one of the most important and powerful prognostic variables, it should be determined in most cases of unstable CAD. Around 10% of an unstable CAD population will have at least moderately depressed left ventricular systolic function (ejection fraction < 0.40), and the long-term mortality is approximately three times higher among these compared with those with normal left ventricular systolic function.[101] However, for the very early risk assessment, echocardiography has some disadvantages. It is rather time-consuming and requires a certain amount of personal skill and is therefore difficult to perform on admission of every patient with a suspicion of an unstable CAD.

Natriuretic Peptides

Brain (or B-type) natriuretic peptide (BNP) belongs to the family of natriuretic peptides and is released in response to ventricular stretch to the circulation as a prohormone, proBNP, which is immediately split into the physiologically active form, BNP, and the inactive form, NT-proBNP. Therefore, both BNP and NT-proBNP are useful as biochemical measurements of cardiac performance. The upper reference level in healthy individuals is dependent on gender and age for both BNP and NT-proBNP. The upper reference level is higher in women than in men and increases by age. The absolute levels of BNP and NT-proBNP are assay specific.

In acute and chronic heart failure, both BNP and NT-proBNP have been shown to be valuable for diagnosis and for prediction of death.[102] During an episode of unstable CAD, not only does the BNP or NT-proBNP level reflect the chronic and acute ischemic systolic and diastolic dysfunction, but there is also evidence that myocardial ischemia per se results in increased levels. Thus, it is not surprising that BNP and NT-proBNP have been shown to be strong and independent predictors of death (Fig. 29.6e) in patients with unstable CAD or suspicion of unstable CAD.[103,104] There is currently no consensus on the optimal timing of measurement and decision limits of BNP and NT-proBNP. It will be difficult if not impossible to define a single decision limit, applicable to all the different clinical situations in which measurement of BNP or NT-proBNP is warranted. However, it is reasonable to state that a level below the upper reference level implies a low risk; above that level, there is a continuous increase in short- and long-term mortality with increasing levels. The few studies that have evaluated the use of BNP or NT-proBNP levels for therapeutic decision making have yielded conflicting results, and therefore it is currently not possible to make any recommendations for selection of treatment based on BNP or NT-proBNP levels.[100]

Markers of Renal Dysfunction

Renal dysfunction has important implications for the choice of drug treatment and how to dose many drugs. Therefore, assessment of renal function is part of the routine evaluation of all hospitalized patients. In patients with unstable CAD, renal dysfunction is common; at least 25% will have renal dysfunction, defined as a calculated creatinine clearance below 60 mL/min. Furthermore, renal dysfunction has convincingly been shown to be independently associated with an increased mortality in a number of studies (Fig. 29.6f).[105,106] Despite this, measurement of renal function has been underused for risk assessment in clinical practice. There are several alternative methods for estimation of the renal function. The plasma creatinine level is influenced by the muscle mass and age of the patient and is thus a relatively poor estimate of the renal function. Therefore, the calculated creatinine clearance (Table 29.5) reflects the renal function much more accurately.[107] An alternative method of estimation of the renal function is determination of cystatin C, which is an inhibitor of cytokine-activated elastolytic cysteine proteases. After filtration by the glomeruli, cystatin C undergoes catabolization by the tubular cells without reabsorption to the blood flow. The level is not dependent on muscle mass or protein intake. Several studies have demonstrated that cystatin C mirrors

ESTIMATED GLOMERULAR FILTRATION RATE: THE FOUR-VARIABLE MODIFICATION OF DIET IN RENAL DISEASE (MDRD) STUDY EQUATION
GFR = 175 × SCr$^{-1.154}$ × age$^{-0.203}$ × 0.742 (if female) × 1.212 (if black)
GFR expressed as mL/min/1.73m^2
Standardized serum creatinine expressed as mg/dL

Table 29.5 Estimated Glomerular Filtration rate: the Four-Variable Modification of Diet in Renal Disease (MDRD) Study Equation.[108]

the glomerular filtration rate more adequately than creatinine does and at least as well as calculated creatinine clearance. Furthermore, there is evidence that cystatin C provides prognostic information in unstable CAD at least as strong as calculated creatinine clearance.[106]

An Integrated Approach to Early Risk Stratification

The process of risk stratification should start on admission by taking a careful history, performing a regular clinical examination, and obtaining a 12-lead ECG and a few blood tests (troponin I or T, creatinine for calculation of creatinine clearance [or cystatin C], and possibly NT-proBNP/BNP), followed by repeated measurements of troponin for another 6 hours. Patients with a history suggestive of an acute coronary syndrome and in whom two or more of these factors are positive have a high risk of new cardiac events and should therefore be treated and handled aggressively.[108] On the other hand, patients without any of these factors being positive are at low risk and can preferably be treated conservatively. In these patients, the diagnosis of non–ST-segment elevation acute coronary syndrome should be questioned; the diagnosis needs to be substantiated by a positive stress test result.

Several alternative models for such an integrated risk assessment have been presented, of which the Thrombolysis in Myocardial Infarction (TIMI) risk score is the most well known (Fig. 29.7).[109] Although the individual factors in the different scoring systems may vary somewhat, some clinical factors, findings on the ECG, and cardiac markers are included. The TIMI risk score seems also useful for selection of treatment, including invasive versus noninvasive therapy and antiplatelet therapy.[110]

Coronary Angiography

Coronary angiography can be performed for diagnostic and prognostic purposes or as a prelude to revascularization procedures. Findings at coronary angiography are dependent on the population studied. In two separate studies,[111,112] the proportion of patients who had no significant stenosis and those with one-, two-, or three-vessel disease varied, being 9% to 19%, 26% to 38%, 29% to 29%, and 15% to 37%, respectively. Patients who presented with ST depression, compared with those who had either T-wave inversions alone or no ST-T changes, had a higher proportion (70% versus 42%) of high-risk coronary lesions (defined here as three-vessel disease or two-vessel disease with proximal left anterior descending artery stenosis or left main coronary artery stenosis). The proportion of patients who had no significant stenosis was less

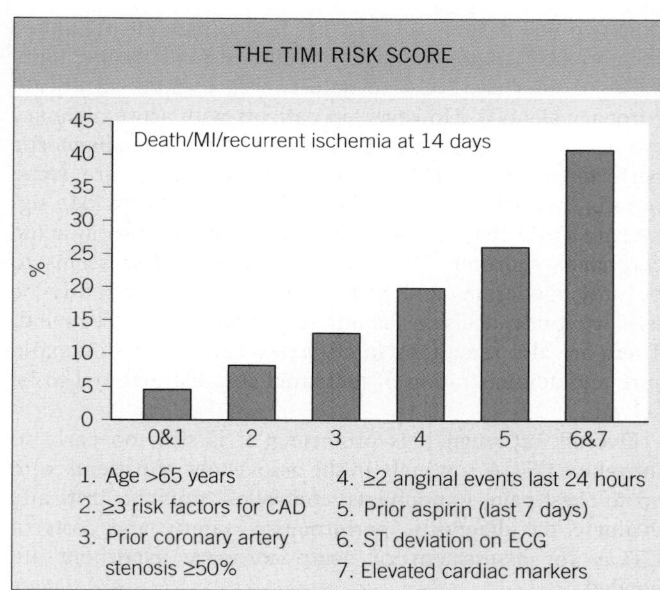

Figure 29.7 The TIMI risk score. One point is scored for each applicable item. CAD, coronary artery disease; ECG, electrocardiography; MI, myocardial infarction.

than half of the proportion in those who did not have ST-T changes (7% versus 17%).[112] Complex plaque morphology and coronary artery thrombi are more commonly seen in patients who have unstable angina than in patients who have stable angina (Fig. 29.8). In prognostic evaluations of patients with ischemic heart disease, an increasing number of coronary vessels with significant stenoses has been shown to be associated with an adverse outcome. In the study by Luchi and colleagues,[113] the 2-year mortality in medically treated patients with unstable angina was 5% in those who had one-vessel disease, 8% in those who had two-vessel disease, and 11% in those who had three-vessel disease.

Multislice Computed Tomographic Coronary Angiography

Multislice computed tomographic coronary angiography (CTCA) is a new noninvasive method that determines the

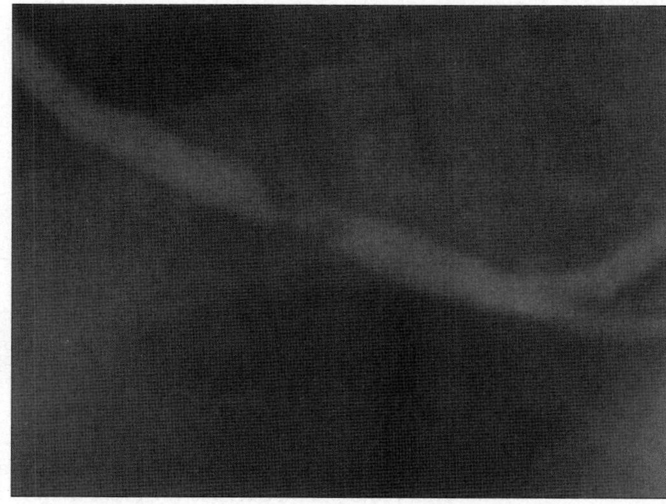

Figure 29.8 Coronary artery disease. Severely stenotic and ulcerated anterior descending artery in a patient with unstable coronary artery disease.

presence and extent of CAD. Studies in patients scheduled for coronary angiography have demonstrated the potential value of 64-slice CTCA to detect or to exclude significant coronary stenosis. However, in patients with acute coronary syndrome, the available information about the diagnostic performance of CTCA is very limited. There are some reports suggesting the ability of CTCA to safely exclude significant CAD (high negative predictive value) also in acute coronary syndrome.[114] However, the specificity seems to be only moderate, and hence CTCA cannot currently be used to guide decisions about revascularization treatment. There are also remaining safety issues about radiation exposure and administration of iodinated contrast material to be solved.

Overall, although it is promising, it is still too early to introduce CTCA routinely in the assessment of patients with acute chest pain. Randomized controlled trials that critically evaluate the diagnostic performance, safety, and costs of CTCA for assessment of acute coronary syndrome are needed.

MANAGEMENT

An overview of management is given in Figure 29.9. The main aims of treatment are to reduce symptoms, to prolong life, to reduce myocardial damage, and to prevent recurrence. This is usually accomplished by a combination of anti-ischemic medications, platelet inhibitory medications, and anticoagulant medications and, in most cases, early revascularization by percutaneous coronary intervention (PCI) or coronary artery bypass grafting (CABG).[3,4] Thus, for patients admitted with suspected or definite unstable coronary syndrome, the treatment alternatives in the PATCH regimen (the name of which is taken from the initial letters of its components) should be considered:

- **P**ain relief (opioids, oxygen, nitrates).
- **A**nti-ischemic treatment (beta blockers, nitrates, calcium channel blockers).
- **T**hrombosis treatment (platelet inhibition with aspirin, $P2Y_{12}$ receptor inhibition, GpIIb/IIIa receptor antagonism, and coagulation inhibition with factor Xa and factor IIa inhibition).
- **C**oronary revascularization (PCI or CABG).
- **H**eart failure treatment (diuretics, nitrates, angiotensin-converting enzyme [ACE] inhibitors).

All patients are primarily treated with a combination of platelet inhibition and anticoagulant treatment under close monitoring of the symptoms and laboratory signs of ischemia (by ECG monitoring), myocardial damage (by troponin levels), left ventricular dysfunction (by NT-proBNP levels or echocardiography), renal dysfunction (by creatinine clearance), anemia (by hemoglobin concentration), and inflammation (by C-reactive protein level). The continued management is based on risk stratification by the clinical history and the occurrence of indicators of a raised risk for future events. The moderate- to high-risk patients, as indicated by refractory symptoms or recurrent or persisting episodes of ischemia or by several indicators of raised risk for future events, are taken to early coronary angiography

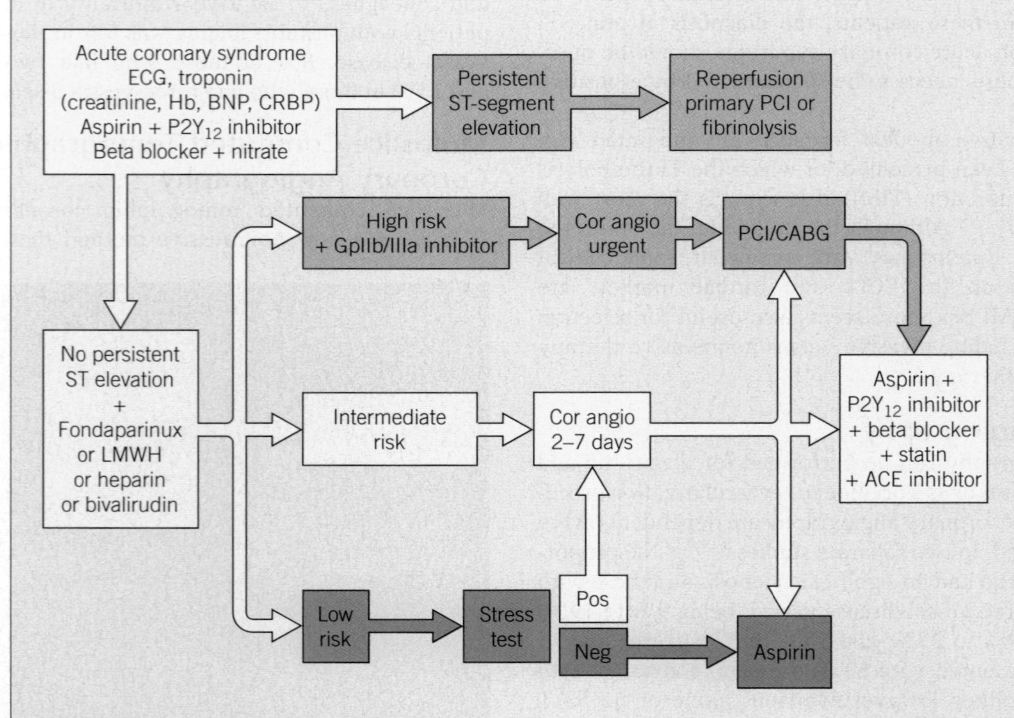

Figure 29.9 An early invasive strategy is associated with a reduction in myocardial infarction and hospital readmission because of severe angina and an improved long-term survival. BNP, brain (or B-type) natriuretic peptide; CABG, coronary artery bypass grafting; cor angio, coronary angiography; CRBP, cellular retinol-binding protein; ECG, electrocardiography; Hb, hemoglobin; LMWH, low-molecular-weight heparin; PCI, percutaneous coronary intervention.

and, if appropriate, revascularization.[3,4] The lower risk patients should be evaluated by a stress test before discharge and, in case of signs of severe ischemia, also be considered for early coronary angiography and revascularization. The lower risk patients without signs of stress-induced ischemia have a very low risk for subsequent coronary events and could rapidly be discharged.[3,4]

By use of this approach, the patient's condition will rapidly be stabilized and allow discharge within 2 to 7 days. The long-term treatment aims to prevent recurrence of new episodes of angina and infarction and to avoid progression of the CAD. Therefore, the long-term strategy conforms with the conventional ABCD regimen:

- antiplatelet treatment with aspirin and $P2Y_{12}$ inhibition;
- beta blockade;
- cholesterol lowering with statins; and
- dilatation with ACE inhibitors.

Of course, other general measures, such as control of hypertension, abstaining from smoking, and lifestyle changes, are as important after an episode of instability as in other manifestations of CAD.[3,4]

Initial Treatment

Of the large group of patients who arrive at the emergency department because of chest pain, about two thirds need to be admitted to the hospital because of a suspicion of myocardial infarction or an unstable coronary syndrome. About 5% to 10% of those who are sent home will later develop a myocardial infarction. With use of the modern methods of monitoring and early diagnosis (i.e., multiple-lead ischemia monitoring, frequent blood sampling for biochemical markers of myocardial damage, and echocardiography), most patients who have an unstable coronary syndrome will be identified within the first 2 to 6 hours. Hence, the availability of this technology considerably increases the safety of patients.

The combination of the clinical history, physical examination, 12-lead ECG at rest, and tests of troponin is used for the primary evaluation for admission and the intensity of primary treatment. This initial evaluation is, thereafter, supplemented with the continuous observation of symptoms, ECG monitoring for ischemia, and further laboratory tests (i.e., creatinine, hemoglobin, and NT-proBNP during the first 6 to 12 hours). Patients who have a jeopardized circulation as well as other patients at very high risk are provided with an indwelling venous catheter and ECG monitoring and immediately taken to the coronary care unit or directly to the catheterization laboratory for definite diagnosis by urgent coronary angiography and an opportunity for simultaneous PCI.[3,4] Transient or persisting ST depression with or without T-wave inversion in association with chest pain is a reliable indicator of unstable CAD and is almost always associated with severe coronary lesions. In patients with isolated T-wave inversion, the likelihood of a thrombotic process is considerably increased by elevated troponin. Therefore, all patients with ST-segment dynamics or troponin elevations should be directly transferred to the coronary care unit.[3,4] In remaining patient categories, supplementary investigations with chest radiography, echocardiography, computed tomography, or magnetic resonance imaging of the chest may be necessary to establish the diagnosis and optimal treatment strategy.

Treatment Strategy in the Hospital

All patients who are suspected of having ischemia should urgently be started on a combination of anti-ischemic and antithrombotic treatment. If the patient has persistent severe pain, opioids can be used as needed together with nasal oxygen and nitrates. Platelet inhibition with aspirin and $P2Y_{12}$ inhibition should be started immediately. In addition, parenteral anticoagulant treatment is given either as infusion of unfractionated heparin or bivalirudin or as subcutaneous administration of fondaparinux once daily or low-molecular-weight heparin twice daily. If there are repeated episodes of ischemia or the patient demonstrates criteria of moderate to high risk with troponin elevation, the addition of intravenous GpIIb/IIIa blockade should be considered. In such patients, early coronary angiography and, if appropriate, PCI should also be performed under the continuous protection of aspirin, $P2Y_{12}$ inhibition, anticoagulation, and GpIIb/IIIa blockade. This strategy of treatment of unstable coronary syndromes is based on evidence from several large-scale clinical trials and recent treatment guidelines.[3,4] Anti-ischemic treatment with intravenous beta blockers followed by oral beta blockers should be used in all patients who have a systolic blood pressure above 100 mm Hg and a pulse rate above 60 beats per minute and in whom beta blockers are not contraindicated. As an alternative, anti-ischemic therapy with calcium channel blockers such as diltiazem or verapamil can be used. Beta blockers can also be combined with calcium channel blockers, in which case the dihydropyridines (nifedipine, felodipine, or amlodipine) are preferred to avoid the combination of several drugs with a negative chronotropic effect. Finally, ACE inhibition should be initiated in all patients with symptoms or signs of left ventricular dysfunction. The early initiation of effective cholesterol-lowering treatment by statins is also indicated in the majority of patients.[3,4]

Antithrombotic Treatment

Platelet Inhibition

To provide adequate platelet inhibition, several platelet inhibitory agents are combined, especially in the acute phase of unstable CAD. Currently, the following principles are used in this setting:

- inhibition of platelet cyclooxygenase by aspirin;
- inhibition of the platelet $P2Y_{12}$ receptor by clopidogrel or prasugrel; and
- inhibition of the platelet GpIIb/IIIa receptor.

Aspirin

Aspirin attenuates platelet aggregation by a nonreversible acetylation of the cyclooxygenase in the platelet, which inhibits the production of thromboxane A_2, thereby reducing the likelihood of formation of arterial thrombi at sites of plaque erosions and fissures.[115] In the 1980s, four large-scale clinical trials showed that aspirin, in daily doses of 75 to 1200 mg, reduces the relative risk of death and myocardial infarction in patients with unstable CAD by at least 50%.[116] During long-term treatment, the lowest aspirin dose is as effective as higher doses but has fewer side effects. However, to obtain platelet inhibition within the initial hours of treatment, the first dose needs to be higher (300 to 500 mg); the recommended maintenance dose currently is 75 to 100 mg/day.[117]

$P2Y_{12}$ Inhibition

The thienopyridines clopidogrel and prasugrel are irreversible $P2Y_{12}$ receptor inhibitors that inhibit adenosine diphosphate–induced platelet aggregation during the lifespan of the platelet. Both compounds are orally absorbed prodrugs. The metabolic activation of clopidogrel is slow, and maximal inhibition of platelet activity is not reached until 2 to 6 hours after ingestion of loading doses of 300 to 600 mg. In addition, the metabolic activation of clopidogrel is variable between patients and associated with 20% to 40% of poor responders who have an inadequate protection against new events on the maintenance dose of 75 mg daily. Prasugrel is a later developed thienopyridine with a more rapid and complete metabolic activation associated with onset of a maximal inhibition of platelet activity 30 to 60 minutes after an oral loading dose of 60 mg and no low responders at a maintenance dose of 10 mg daily.[115,118,119] As aspirin mainly inhibits collagen-induced aggregation, the simultaneous inhibition of the adenosine diphosphate–induced platelet aggregation by clopidogrel will have a synergistic inhibitory effect on platelet aggregation. However, the combination of $P2Y_{12}$ inhibition with aspirin increases the risk of bleeding,[120] and this risk is further increased by use of the more effective inhibitor prasugrel in comparison to clopidogrel.[121]

In the first large-scale clinical trial of patients with unstable CAD (CURE), treatment with the combination of clopidogrel and aspirin for 3 to 12 months versus aspirin alone reduced the rate of cardiovascular death, reinfarction, and stroke by 20% (absolute reduction, 2%) compared with aspirin alone (Table 29.6).[120,122] The combination of clopidogrel and aspirin is associated with a raised risk of bleeding (absolute increase, 1% of major bleeding), especially at CABG procedures. It is therefore recommended that clopidogrel treatment be terminated 5 days before planned CABG procedures.[123] To obtain a rapid onset of the effect, clopidogrel should be started with a loading dose of 600 mg followed by 75 mg daily.[124] In the recent large-scale trial comparing prasugrel and clopidogrel on top of aspirin in patients with unstable CAD accepted for PCI procedures after coronary angiography, there was a further 20% relative (2% absolute) reduction in myocardial infarction, half of which occurred within 3 days of the procedure and half during the 6 to 15 months of long-term treatment. Simultaneously, however, there was a significant further increase in bleeding (absolute 1% increase in major bleeding or requirement for transfusion). There was also a pronounced increase in bleeding risk in patients requiring CABG, emphasizing the need for termination of prasugrel at least 7 days before surgical procedures.[121]

Glycoprotein IIb/IIIa Inhibition

Glycoprotein IIb/IIIa inhibition (Table 29.7) influences the common pathway of platelet activation, which is the expression of the platelet surface receptor for fibrinogen—the GpIIb/IIIa receptor. The first clinically available compound was the GpIIb/IIIa monoclonal chimeric humanized antibody (abciximab), which irreversibly binds to the receptor.[115,118] Several large-scale trials have shown that an intravenous

RANDOMIZED CONTROLLED TRIALS OF HEPARIN AND LMW HEPARIN IN ADDITION TO ASPIRIN IN UNSTABLE CORONARY ARTERY DISEASE.?

Study	Test Treatment	Comparator Treatment	Basic Treatment	Death + AMI, Test/Comparator, 30 days (*P*)	More than Moderate Bleeding, Test/ Comparator (*P*)
Heparin and LMW heparin versus placebo					
Theroux[134] (1988) N = 243	Heparin infusion	Placebo	Aspirin	3.3%/6.6%	
RISC[134] (1990) N = 399	Heparin	Placebo	Aspirin	3.8%/4.8%	
ATACS[134] (1994) N = 214	Heparin infusion + warfarin	Placebo	Aspirin	8.5%/10% at 3 months	
FRISC[139] (1996) N = 1498	Dalteparin	Placebo	Aspirin	8.0%/10.7% (.07)	1.1%/0.8% (NS)
LMW heparin versus heparin					
FRIC[134] (1997) N = 1482	Dalteparin	Heparin infusion	Aspirin	4.3%/4.7% (NS)	1.6%/1.4% (NS)
ESSENCE[140] (1997) N = 3171	Enoxaparin	Heparin infusion	Aspirin probably	6.1%/7.7% (NS)	3.3%/6.5% (NS)
TIMI 11B[141] (1999) N = 3910	Enoxaparin	Heparin infusion	Aspirin	7.4%/8.3% (NS)	1.0%/0.6% (NS)
FRAX.I.S.[134] (1999) N = 2317	Fraxiparin	Heparin infusion	Aspirin	8.6%/7.9% (NS) (3 months)	1%/1% (NS)
INTERACT[144] (2003) N = 746	Enoxaparin	Heparin infusion	Aspirin Eptifibatide	5.0%/9.0% (.03)	2.0%/3.1% (NS)
A to Z[143] (2004) N = 3629	Enoxaparin	Heparin infusion	Aspirin	7.4%/7.9% (NS)	1.0%/0.8% (NS)
SYNERGY[142] (2004) N = 9978	Enoxaparin	Heparin infusion	Aspirin Clopidogrel	14.0%/14.5% (NS)	13.0%/13.6% (NS)

*Including more than 100 patients in each group.
AMI, acute myocardial infarction; LMW, low molecular weight.

Table 29.6 Randomized controlled trials of heparin and LMW heparin in addition to aspirin in unstable coronary artery disease.

RANDOMIZED CONTROLLED TRIALS OF PLATELET INHIBITION WITH GLYCOPROTEIN IIB/IIIA BLOCKADE IN UNSTABLE CORONARY DISEASE.?						
Study	**Test Treatment**	**Comparator Treatment**	**Basic Treatment**	**Death + AMI, Test/Comparator, 1-5 days (*P*)**	**Death + AMI, Test/Comparator, 30 days (*P*)**	**More than Moderate Bleeding, Test/Comparator (*P*)**
PARAGON A[128] (1998) N = 1513	Lamifiban infusion, low dose	Heparin infusion	Aspirin		10.6%/11.7% (.48)	6.0%/5.5% (NS)
PARAGON A[128] (1998) N = 1527	Lamifiban infusion, high dose	Heparin infusion	Aspirin		12.0%/11.7% (.89)	10.7%/0.5% (.002)
PRISM[130] (1998) N = 3232	Tirofiban infusion	Heparin infusion	Aspirin	1.2%/1.6% (NS)	5.8%/7.1% (.11)	2.5%/2.4% (NS)
PRISM-PLUS[129] (1998) N = 695	Tirofiban infusion	Heparin infusion	Aspirin	10.4%/7.7% (NS)	13.6%/11.7% (NS)	
PRISM-PLUS[129] (1998) N = 1570	Tirofiban infusion	Placebo	Aspirin + heparin infusion	4.3%/8.9% (.006)	8.7%/11.9% (.03)	4.0%/3.0% (NS)
PURSUIT[131] (1998) N = 9461	Eptifibatide infusion	Placebo	Aspirin + heparin infusion	7.6%/9.1% (.01)	14.2%/15.7% (.04)	5.2%/2.0% (< .001)
CAPTURE[126] (1997) N = 1265	Abciximab infusion	Placebo	Aspirin + heparin infusion	0.6%/2.1% (.03)	4.8%/9.0% (.003)	7.1%/3.4% (.005)
GUSTO IV[132] (2001) N = 2498 + 5202	Abciximab infusion	Placebo	Aspirin + heparin infusion	2.1%/1.5% (NS)	8.0%/8.7% (NS)	0.8%/0.3% (.005)

*Containing more than 100 patients in each group.
AMI, acute myocardial infarction.

Table 29.7 Randomized controlled trials of platelet inhibition with glycoprotein IIb/IIIa blockade in unstable coronary disease.

bolus followed by 24 hours' infusion of abciximab in addition to aspirin and heparin will provide a 50% relative reduction in procedure-related myocardial infarction.[125,126] Even in unstable CAD patients pretreated with a combination of aspirin and clopidogrel at a PCI procedure, the addition of abciximab was associated with a further reduction in event rate in the patients at higher risk as identified by elevated troponin levels.[127]

At present, two synthetic reversible inhibitors of the GpIIb/IIIa receptor are available for intravenous use. In clinical trials of unstable coronary syndromes, infusion for 72 hours of these compounds has been shown to reduce the rates of both spontaneous and procedure-related myocardial infarction when added to aspirin and heparin.[128-131] Also, these substances have their main effect in patients with elevated troponin levels and a PCI performed during GpIIb/IIIa antagonist infusion. However, in meta-analyses of all trials on unstable CAD without scheduled PCI, routine GpIIb/IIIa inhibition provides no clinically important benefits.[132,133]

Treatment with GpIIb/IIIa antagonists in combination with aspirin and heparin gives a pronounced inhibition of the platelet activity and the coagulation activity, and this necessarily increases the risk of bleeding. As major bleedings in unstable CAD are associated with a worse long-term outcome, it is important to reduce the bleeding rate. This can be accomplished by the use of fondaparinux instead of heparins as the routine anticoagulant in unstable CAD and by use of low heparin doses at the PCI procedures. The decision to start GpIIb/IIIa blockade should be associated with planned coronary angiography and PCI while the treatment is still ongoing, as mainly patients who have early PCI will obtain any long-term gains of this treatment.[3]

Coagulation Inhibition

In unstable CAD, the formation of intracoronary thrombi is associated with both an activation of coagulation and platelets. Therefore, both platelet inhibition with oral aspirin and oral $P2Y_{12}$ inhibition and coagulation inhibition by parenteral treatment is today the routine treatment in unstable coronary syndromes. The oral platelet inhibition is maintained for a long-term period; the anticoagulant treatment usually is given until an eventual early revascularization procedure or hospital discharge.[3,4]

Currently, there are several options to provide coagulation inhibition in unstable CAD[134]:

- indirect inhibition of factors IIa and Xa by intravenous unfractionated heparin;
- direct inhibition of factor IIa by bivalirudin;
- indirect inhibition of factors Xa and IIa by low-molecular-weight heparin (enoxaparin); and
- indirect inhibition of factor Xa by fondaparinux.

Indirect Inhibition of Factor IIa and Factor Xa with Unfractionated Heparin

Unfractionated heparin (Table 29.8) attenuates the coagulation cascade as a cofactor to antithrombin, inhibiting both factor Xa and thrombin.[134] In a series of small studies performed around 20 years ago, the addition of intravenous

RANDOMIZED CONTROLLED TRIALS OF $P2Y_{12}$ INHIBITION IN ADDITION TO ASPIRIN IN UNSTABLE CORONARY ARTERY DISEASE.?					
Study	**Test Treatment**	**Comparator Treatment**	**Basic Treatment**	**Death + AMI + Stroke, Test/Comparator (*P*)**	**More than Moderate Bleeding, Test/Comparator (*P*)**
CURE[120] (2001) N = 12,563	Clopidogrel 75 mg daily	Placebo	Aspirin	9.3%/11.5% (.00005) 3-12 months of follow-up	3.6%/2.7% (.003)
TRITON[121] (2007) N = 13,608	Prasugrel 10 mg daily	Clopidogrel 75 mg daily	Aspirin Heparin GpIIb/IIIa inhibitor	9.9%/12.1% 6-15 months of follow-up	5.0%/3.8% (.002)

*Including more than 100 patients in each group.

Table 29.8 Randomized controlled trials of $P2Y_{12}$ inhibition in addition to aspirin in unstable coronary artery disease.

unfractionated heparin to aspirin provided an around 50% further relative reduction in the risk of death and myocardial infarction in the acute phase of unstable CAD. In addition, the treatment ameliorated both the symptoms (episodes of chest pain and ischemia). It is currently recommended that the unfractionated heparin dose in unstable CAD be a weight-adjusted intravenous bolus (60 IU/kg; maximal dose, 4000 IU) followed by an infusion (12 IU/kg; maximal dose, 1000 IU/h). Further dosing is adjusted to achieve an activated partial thromboplastin time of 50 to 70 seconds. The therapeutic range is relatively narrow, with a risk of inadequate therapeutic effect at levels below and above this range and also of bleeding at high levels. Therefore, the activated partial thromboplastin time needs to be measured 6 hours after the start of the infusion and at least twice daily thereafter. Furthermore, because of a risk of thrombocytopenia, platelet counts need to be obtained at least once before, during, and after treatment.[134]

Direct Factor IIa Inhibition with Bivalirudin

Direct thrombin inhibition provides a more predictable anticoagulant response than unfractionated heparin does. Bivalirudin has a short half-life and is given as an intravenous infusion (0.75 mg/kg bolus followed by 1.75 mg/kg per hour).[134] When given during elective or urgent PCI, it provides protection from acute ischemic events similar to that of a regimen of unfractionated heparin plus planned GpIIb/IIIa inhibition, with significantly fewer bleeding complications.[135] In a recent large-scale trial of patients with unstable CAD managed with an invasive strategy, bivalirudin alone was compared with combination treatment with either unfractionated heparin or enoxaparin together with GpIIb/IIIa inhibitor or bivalirudin together with GpIIb/IIIa inhibitor on top of aspirin and clopidogrel. The results showed no difference in ischemic events (death, myocardial infarction, or unplanned revascularization) but a lower bleeding rate with bivalirudin alone compared with the other regimens. Therefore, bivalirudin is as least as effective and as safe as unfractionated heparin with and without GpIIb/IIIa inhibition in moderate- to high-risk patients with non–ST-segment elevation acute coronary syndrome.[136-138]

Indirect Inhibition of Factor Xa and Factor IIa with Low-Molecular-Weight Heparin

Low-molecular-weight heparin, which consists mainly of smaller molecules of around 5000 kDa, mainly is active through its inhibition of factor Xa activity. In contrast to unfractionated heparin, low-molecular-weight heparin is almost completely absorbed after subcutaneous administration and has a more predictable dose-effect relationship by subcutaneous injections every 12 to 24 hours without laboratory monitoring.[134] In a trial performed around 15 years ago, it was shown that the addition of 5 days of subcutaneous low-molecular-weight heparin to aspirin will provide around 50% further relative reduction in the risk of death and myocardial infarction in unstable CAD.[139] In direct comparison to 48 hours of unfractionated heparin infusion, 3 to 8 days of low-molecular-weight heparin was associated with a slight (9% relative) reduction in ischemic events without any significant increase in major bleeding.[140-144] Therefore, low-molecular-weight heparin is usually preferred to unfractionated heparin because of higher efficacy and more convenient twice-daily subcutaneous administration without the need for laboratory monitoring.[3,4] At present, two low-molecular-weight heparins are approved for use in the acute phase of unstable CAD—dalteparin (120 IU/kg body weight every 12 hours) and enoxaparin (1 mg/kg body weight every 12 hours).[140,141,145,146] However, the superiority to unfractionated heparin and the safety and efficacy at PCI procedures and in combination with clopidogrel and GpIIb/IIIa inhibitors are shown only with enoxaparin. Therefore, enoxaparin currently is the preferred low-molecular-weight heparin in unstable CAD.[3,4]

Indirect Factor Xa Inhibition with Fondaparinux

Fondaparinux inactivates factor Xa by binding to antithrombin but without any effect on thrombin activity. The compound produces a predictable anticoagulant response at once-daily subcutaneous injection without any need for coagulation monitoring.[134,147] In a very large trial of patients with unstable CAD, a regimen of subcutaneous injection of fondaparinux, 2.5 mg once daily, was compared with subcutaneous injection of enoxaparin, 1 mg/kg body weight twice daily, for a mean of 6 days.[148,149] The results showed no difference in ischemic events (death, myocardial infarction, or refractory ischemia) at 9 days. However, the rates of major bleeds were halved with fondaparinux (2.2%) compared with enoxaparin (4.1%). Major bleeding was also shown to be an independent predictor of long-term mortality, which was lower with fondaparinux. At PCI procedures, fondaparinux was associated with a slightly increased risk of catheter-related thrombi, a complication that seemed avoidable by pretreatment with unfractionated heparin at the procedure. Thus, compared with the enoxaparin regimen, fondaparinux reduces the risk of bleeding, lowers long-term morbidity, and improves survival.

Anti-Ischemic and Heart Failure Treatment

Patients who have unstable coronary syndromes benefit from the same supportive treatment for ischemia and heart failure as for other CAD patients. Although beta blockers have not specifically been shown to reduce the rates of myocardial infarction and mortality in unstable CAD, their routine use is recommended on the basis of their preventive effects on recurrence of symptoms and on mortality in patients with myocardial infarction left ventricular failure. In patients in whom beta blockers are contraindicated, the calcium channel blockers verapamil and diltiazem may be used for their preventive effects against reinfarction and episodes of angina in unstable patients who do not have signs of heart failure. If the symptom relief produced by beta blockade is inadequate, vasodilating calcium channel blockers (e.g., nifedipine, felodipine, or amlodipine) and long-acting nitrates can be added.[3,4,150] In patients who have heart failure or left ventricular dysfunction, ACE inhibitors have been found to reduce mortality and new episodes of myocardial infarction and unstable angina. In several trials, ACE inhibition has been associated with reduction in mortality, myocardial infarction, and stroke in patients with CAD. Therefore, also in patients with unstable CAD, the use of ACE inhibitors is generally recommended.[151,152]

Treatment of Hyperlipidemia and Diabetes Mellitus

As in other manifestations of CAD, dyslipidemia is a common finding and occurs in the majority of patients. There is now overwhelming evidence that statin treatment will reduce mortality and the rate of coronary events in patients with established CAD or risk factors for CAD regardless of their lipid levels. Recently, three randomized clinical trials have shown reduction in ischemic events and mortality by starting high doses of statin treatment immediately in association with the index event in patients with unstable CAD. Thus, the early use of statins in patients with LDL-cholesterol above 2.0 mmol/L (80 mg/dL) is currently recommended.[153-155]

Diabetes mellitus occurs in about 20% of patients and is an independent risk factor for new events in unstable coronary syndromes as well as in myocardial infarction.[87,156-158] Therefore, close attention to optimal metabolic control and wide indications for insulin treatment are recommended.[3,4]

Revascularization by Percutaneous Coronary Intervention or Coronary Artery Bypass Grafting

Severe coronary lesions can be demonstrated at coronary angiography in about 80% to 90% of patients who have unstable coronary disease. Because of the presence of a recent plaque fissure and a fresh thrombus and sometimes a recent myocardial infarction, the risk of complications at revascularization procedures is higher than in stable patients. However, this risk has been reduced in the past few years by the use of stenting and GpIIb/IIIa blockade.[4,159] Previously, there was discussion of whether early invasive procedures should focus only on the culprit lesion or aim for "complete" revascularization. Currently, immediate complete revascularization in a one-stage procedure is the recommended approach, which also has been documented in the randomized clinical trials. In these trials, procedures on one or two lesions were generally performed by PCI, whereas procedures on three or more lesions and on left main CAD were managed by CABG.[97,160-165]

For many years, there was debate about the benefits of routine early invasive intervention compared with a noninvasive intervention in unstable CAD based on three large-scale randomized trials of an early invasive versus a noninvasive treatment strategy in unstable CAD (FRISC II, TACTICS–TIMI 18, and RITA 3).[97,160-164] An early invasive strategy is associated with a reduction in myocardial infarction and hospital readmission because of severe angina and an improved long-term survival (Fig. 29.10 and Table 29.9). Between the trials, there was a gradient of larger benefit in the trial with the largest contrast in proportion of patients revascularized between the two arms. Within the trials, the largest benefits were consistently seen in patients at higher

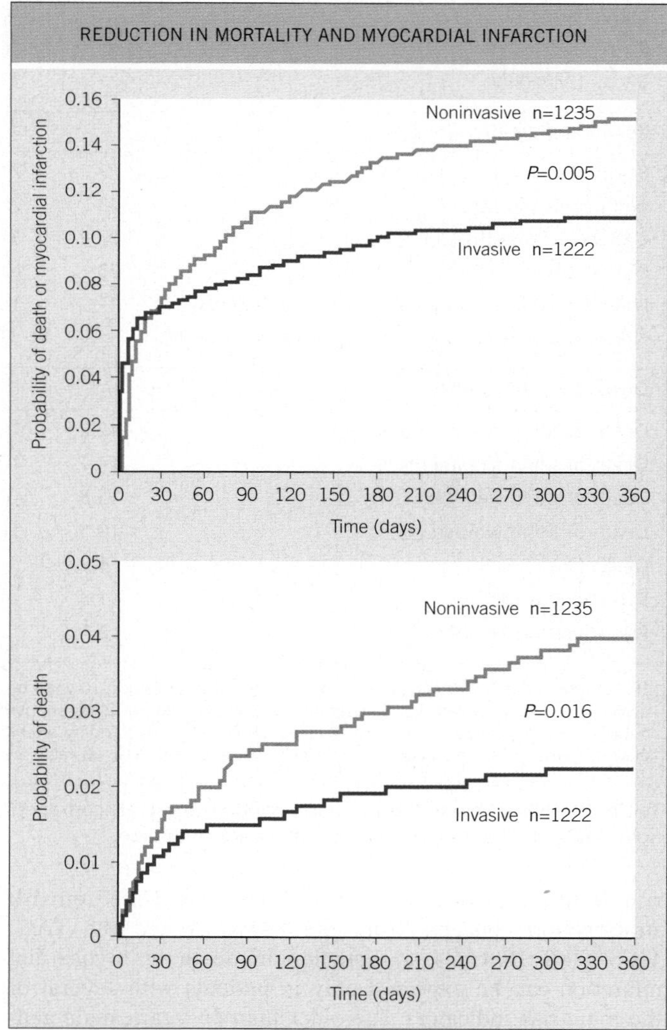

Figure 29.10 Effects of a noninvasive versus an invasive strategy in unstable CAD in the FRISC II trial.

OVERVIEW OF THE FOUR LARGE RANDOMIZED TRIALS COMPARING AN EARLY INVASIVE WITH AN EARLY NONINVASIVE STRATEGY IN UNSTABLE CORONARY ARTERY DISEASE.?								
	FRISC II[160]		TACTICS[97]		RITA 3[164]		ICTUS[165]	
N	2457		2220		1810		1200	
Time period	1996-1998		1997-1999		1997-2001		2001-2003	
Baseline findings on admission								
Inclusion diagnosis	NSTEMI/UA		NSTEMI/UA		UA		NSTEMI	
Median age (years)	65		62		62		62	
Female (%)	31		34		38		27	
Diabetes mellitus	12		28		13		13	
Previous MI	22		39		28		23	
ST depression	46		39		37		48	
Biochemical marker elevation	57		37		18		82	
Angiography	Ninv	Inv	Ninv	Inv	Ninv	Inv	Ninv	Inv
Before discharge–7 days (%)	10	96	51	97	16	96	53	98
6-12 months (%)	47	98	61	98	48	97	67	99
Extent of CAD (invasive group)								
0 v.d. (%)		14		13		22		
1 v.d. (%)		30				33		
2 v.d. (%)		26				24		
3 v.d., LMD (%)		31		43		22		
Revascularization								
Before discharge–10 days (%)	9	71	36	60	10	44	40	76
Within 6-12 months (%)	43	78	44	61	28	57	54	79
CABG 6-12 months (%)	23	37	16	22	12	21	14	18
PCI 6-12 months (%)	20	41	28	40	16	36	40	61
Non-revascularization with 1-3 v.d., 10 days (%)		15		27		34		
Non-revascularization with 1-3 v.d., 12 months (%)		8		26		21		
Outcome 6-12 months								
Death or MI or severe angina (%)	42.2	13.2	19.4	15.9	14.5	9.6	21.2	22.7
Death or MI in all patients (%)	14.1	10.4	9.5	7.3	8.3	7.6		
Death or MI in men (%)	15.8	9.6			10.1	7.0		
Death or MI in women (%)	10.5	12.4			5.1	8.6		
Death (%)	3.9	2.2	3.5	3.3	3.9	4.6	2.5	2.5
Spontaneous MI (%)	11.3	4.2			5.7	3.3	4.6	3.7
Procedure-related MI (%)	2.1	5.4			0.4	1.7	5.4	11.3

*Including more than 1000 patients and performed during the last 10 years by baseline treatment with aspirin, heparin, or low-molecular-weight heparin and with availability of glycoprotein IIb/IIIa inhibitors and stents followed by thienopyridine.

CAD, coronary artery disease; Inv, invasive; LMD, left main coronary artery disease; MI, myocardial infarction; Ninv, noninvasive; NSTEMI, non–ST-segment elevation myocardial infarction; v.d., coronary vessel disease; UA, unstable angina.

Table 29.9 Overview of the four large randomized trials comparing an early invasive with an early noninvasive strategy in unstable coronary artery disease.

risk, with no gains in patients at lower risk. Based on risk stratification concepts from the FRISC II and the TACTICS–TIMI 18 trials, a reduction in death or myocardial infarction can be expected only in patients with several of the main risk indicators: age older than 65 years, male gender, occurrence of coronary risk factors (e.g., diabetes mellitus), previous myocardial infarction, previous severe angina or coronary lesions, ST-segment depression, reduced creatinine clearance, or elevation of troponin and NT-proBNP or C-reactive protein on admission.[161,166,167] In the more recent ICTUS trial,[165] strategy with revascularization based on clinical symptoms and a predischarge exercise test for selection of patients for an early invasive strategy provided results similar to that of bringing all patients with troponin elevation to an early catheterization. Early revascularization is associated with early hazard because of procedure-related events. This early in-hospital risk is, however, compensated by a lower risk of events after revascularization and eventually also by a reduced event rate while waiting for the invasive procedure.[162] Early procedure-related deaths are more common in patients treated with CABG. Thus, only patients with a risk profile that indicates gains from early revascularization should be referred for early CABG.[168] Therefore, early coronary angiography and revascularization should not be used routinely in all patients with unstable CAD. Instead, the decision for early invasive procedures should be based on risk stratification with use of information from clinical history and presentation, signs of ischemia, and biochemical markers—and eventually in clinically stabilized patients, a predischarge stress test. Thus, early coronary angiography and, if appropriate, complete revascularization should be used selectively and be reserved for patients at moderate to high risk of future complications of the acute coronary syndrome.[3,4]

PROGNOSIS

Until the beginning of the 1980s, unstable angina or non–Q wave myocardial infarction carried a 5% to 10% absolute risk of death or myocardial infarction during the first week and another 20% risk of the same events during the following 6 to 12 months. In the second half of the 1980s, long-term treatment with aspirin was shown to halve this complication rate. In the first half of the 1990s, it was demonstrated that intravenous unfractionated heparin or subcutaneous low-molecular-weight heparin further reduced the risk of recurrent symptoms and reinfarction in the acute phase, with some remaining long-term benefit. Recently, it was shown that the inherent raised risk of bleeding by combining different antithrombotic agents can be halved by the use of subcutaneous fondaparinux instead of any of the heparins. The combination of aspirin with clopidogrel for 3 to 12 months in the beginning 2000s was shown to provide a further 20% relative risk reduction. Its replacement with the more effective $P2Y_{12}$ inhibitor prasugrel carries the promise of another 20% relative reduction in ischemic events. During the last decade, early revascularization with PCI or CABG has been documented as an effective additional treatment that improves survival, reduces reinfarction, and improves symptoms and quality of life in moderate- to high-risk patients. The risks associated with early revascularization have during the last decade been further reduced by the use of GpIIb/IIIa inhibitors or bivalirudin in association with PCI procedures. With use of the currently recommended short- and long-term pharmacologic treatments and an early invasive strategy in moderate- to high-risk patients, unstable CAD carries a low mortality and complication rate. Still, the condition is demanding on the health care resources because of the need for acute care in a coronary care unit environment, immediate risk stratification with ECG and biochemical markers, intense antithrombotic medication, and performance of early revascularization procedures. However, in comparison to a noninvasive approach, the invasive strategy is cost-effective as it provides important benefits to the patient without incremental costs.[169,170]

SUMMARY

Unstable CAD comprises the clinical conditions of unstable angina and non–ST-segment elevation myocardial infarction, which are related to a sudden impairment of blood flow because of a thrombotic stenosis or occlusion in a coronary artery, leading to ischemia in the corresponding area of the myocardium. The amount of myocardial damage is related to the duration of the coronary occlusion, the availability of collateral arteries, and the occurrence of distal emboli. The underlying cause of the coronary thrombus is a process of lipid infiltration, inflammation, and collagen degradation that leads to plaque erosion or rupture, which causes platelet and coagulation activation. The treatment strategy in unstable CAD in relation to risk evaluation is summarized in Figure 29.9.

The classic symptoms of the disease are episodes of angina of increasing intensity at effort or at rest, or both, during the previous 4 weeks, usually with an episode of chest pain during the previous 24 to 48 hours. The early diagnosis is established by signs of ischemia or minor myocardial damage as recorded by the ECG at rest (ST depression or T-wave inversion) and by elevation of cardiac markers (troponin). Patients with unstable CAD are heterogeneous and have differing contributions from the different pathophysiologic mechanisms and differing prognoses. Therefore, an early evaluation of possible underlying mechanisms and an assessment of the prognosis are important in attempts to tailor the treatment to the individual patient. This evaluation should start at admission and thereafter be reassessed repeatedly throughout the hospitalization period. The early risk stratification is usually accomplished by the clinical history and ECG and by monitoring for myocardial damage with blood samples for biochemical markers (troponin), myocardial dysfunction (NT-proBNP, echocardiography), renal dysfunction (creatinine clearance), anemia (hemoglobin), and inflammation (C-reactive protein).

To reduce oxygen demand to the myocardium, all patients should be treated with a combination of anti-ischemic drugs, such as beta blockers and nitrates and, as needed, calcium channel blockers. As a thrombotic process causes the condition in the majority of patients, a combination of dual platelet inhibition by aspirin and $P2Y_{12}$ inhibition and short-term (2 to 8 days) anticoagulant treatment by subcutaneous fondaparinux or low-molecular-weight heparin is currently standard treatment of all unstable CAD patients. Patients with continuing symptoms, as well as those with a modest to high risk as indicated by the occurrence of several of the risk indicators, should have early coronary angiography within the first 24 to 48 hours. In the high-risk patients, intravenous treatment with GpIIb/IIIa inhibition should be used in association to reduce the risk of periprocedural events. After coronary angiography, all patients with significant coronary lesions are revascularized either immediately by PCI or, as appropriate, within the next few days by CABG.

After stabilization of the condition by invasive procedures or by medication, there still remains a raised risk of new events during the next 3 to 6 months. This risk can be mitigated by long-term treatment by dual platelet inhibition with aspirin and $P2Y_{12}$ inhibition, beta blockade, cholesterol lowering with statins, and ACE inhibition.

chapter 30

Subacute In-Hospital Phase of ST-Segment Elevation Myocardial Infarction

Jayanta Das and Sanjay Kaul

HYPOTENSION

Definition

- Reduced blood pressure

Key Features

- Blurry vision, confusion, dizziness, syncope, lightheadedness, lethargy

Therapy

- Clinical evaluation, fluids, sodium chloride, inotropes, vasopressor therapy, fludrocortisone

PULMONARY EDEMA

Definition

- Fluid accumulation in the lungs

Key Features

- Dyspnea, tachypnea, hemoptysis, diaphoresis, anxiety, orthopnea, pallor

Therapy

- Mechanical or noninvasive ventilation, inotropes, vasopressor therapy, nitrates, loop diuretics

CARDIOGENIC SHOCK

Definition

- Inadequate organ perfusion secondary to ventricular failure

Key Features

- Hypotension, anxiety, alterations in mental status, jugular venous distention, oliguria, tachypnea, pulmonary edema, mottled skin

Therapy

- Revascularization, inotropic agents, vasopressor therapy, intra-aortic balloon pump, ventricular assist device

RIGHT VENTRICULAR INFARCTION

Definition

- Right ventricular failure and elevated right-sided filling pressure despite normal left ventricular function
- Associated with inferior wall myocardial infarction

Key Features

- Jugular venous distention, clear lung fields, and hypotension
- High-grade atrioventricular block, tricuspid regurgitation, right ventricular free wall rupture, and tamponade can also be seen.

Therapy

- Maintenance of right ventricular preload (volume infusion), inotropic therapy, afterload reduction, revascularization

MITRAL VALVE REGURGITATION

Definition

- Pathologic escape of blood from the left ventricle to the left atrium secondary to an incompetent mitral valve

Key Features

- Acute pulmonary edema, hypotension
- Associated with inferior myocardial infarction and chordae tendineae or papillary muscle rupture

Therapy

- Urgent surgical intervention, intra-aortic balloon pump, afterload reduction (nitrates)

VENTRICULAR SEPTAL RUPTURE

Definition

- Necrosis and fissure of the ventricular septum

Key Features

- Loud systolic murmur over region between left sternal border and apex, acute heart failure, hypotension, pulmonary edema

Therapy

- Emergent surgical intervention
- Intra-aortic balloon pump, inotropic therapy, and afterload reduction

LEFT VENTRICULAR FREE WALL RUPTURE

Definition

- Rupture of the myocardial wall at a junction of necrotic and normal myocardium

Key Features

- Cardiac tamponade

Therapy

- Emergent surgical intervention
- Intra-aortic balloon pump, inotropic therapy, fluid infusion

PERICARDITIS

Definition

- Inflammation of the fibrous sac surrounding the heart
- Exudate may be serous, purulent, fibrinous, or hemorrhagic.

Key Features

- Chest pain worsened when supine, improved with sitting forward
- Cough, fever, lethargy, and anxiety
- Friction rub on auscultation

Therapy

- Nonsteroidal anti-inflammatory drugs
- Pericardiocentesis, antibiotics, colchicine, steroids, or surgery may be necessary, depending on underlying etiology.

VENTRICULAR FIBRILLATION

Definition

- Chaotic uncoordinated contraction of the ventricles secondary to disorganized electrical activity.

Key Features

- Cardiac arrest, sudden cardiac death

Therapy

- Emergent defibrillation, implantation of cardioverter-defibrillator, precordial thump

VENTRICULAR TACHYCARDIA

Definition

- Three or more beats of ventricular origin in succession at a rate greater than 100 beats per minute

Key Features

- May lead to ventricular fibrillation and sudden death

Therapy

- Electrical cardioversion-defibrillation, amiodarone, procainamide

ACCELERATED IDIOVENTRICULAR RHYTHM

Definition

- Ventricular tachycardia occurring secondary to an ectopic focus
- Slightly faster than underlying sinus rhythm

Key Features

- Associated with recanalization of a coronary artery

Therapy

- Observation

ATRIAL FIBRILLATION

Definition

- Chaotic and irregular contraction of bilateral atria
- Sinoatrial conduction is overwhelmed by disorganized electrical activity originating in the pulmonary veins and atria.

Key Features

- Palpitations, dyspnea, lethargy

Therapy

- Rate control: beta blockers, calcium channel blockers, cardiac glycosides (digoxin)
- Anticoagulation: coumadin, aspirin
- Cardioversion, ablation

BRADYARRHYTHMIAS

Definition

- Reduced heart rate
- May occur secondary to conduction block or disordered automaticity

Key Features

- Syncope, fatigue, lethargy, dizziness

Therapy

- Atropine; transcutaneous, transvenous, or permanent pacemaker

The purpose of this chapter is to focus on key issues relating to the management of patients with ST-segment elevation myocardial infarction (STEMI) during the subacute in-hospital phase. Recommended indications for diagnostic and therapeutic intervention based on clinical trial evidence and expert opinion are summarized. An overview of the management of the patient with STEMI is presented with special emphasis on triage, risk stratification, pharmacologic therapy, complications, and education of the patient.

TRIAGE

After initial management and stabilization, patients with STEMI should be triaged to either the coronary care unit (CCU) or the step-down unit. Continuous electrocardiographic (ECG) monitoring and pulse oximetry should be established in addition to ready access to hemodynamic monitoring and defibrillation.[1] On initial presentation to the unit, patients should be assessed for cardiac ischemia and heart failure and should be administered aspirin and beta blockers if they were not received previously. Intravenous nitroglycerin may be administered for control of recurrent chest pain, blood pressure control, or heart failure symptoms. Hypoxia should be corrected, especially if oxygen saturation is less than 90%. Once the patient is stable for 6 hours and oxygen saturation is greater than 90%, supplemental oxygen can be discontinued. Serum cardiac biomarkers, complete blood count, international normalized ratio, activated partial thromboplastin time, electrolyte levels, blood urea nitrogen concentration, creatinine concentration, glucose concentration, and serum lipid levels should be determined to help risk stratify the patient. A complete lipid profile should be obtained in all STEMI patients at time of admission or within 24 hours of presenting symptoms. Low-density lipoprotein (LDL) cholesterol is known to rapidly decrease within the first 48 hours after an acute event.[2] The CCU should be equipped and staffed for monitoring of intra-arterial blood pressure and pulmonary artery catheter pressure. STEMI patients should have ECG monitoring for a minimum of 24 hours or until they are event free for 12 to 24 hours. Continuous monitoring allows assessment of the culprit artery after fibrinolysis and detection of reocclusion after percutaneous coronary intervention (PCI), recurrent ischemia, infarct extension, and arrhythmia.[3]

Low-risk STEMI patients who have demonstrated clinical stability in the CCU or have undergone successful PCI may be triaged to the step-down unit. Provided patients are on continuous monitoring and the ward is equipped for defibrillation, it is reasonable to triage patients with symptomatic but stable heart failure or well-tolerated arrhythmias to step-down. Progression from CCU to step-down to hospital ward is dictated by the patient's risk and clinical course.

EARLY MEASURES

Activity

Physical activity should be limited in STEMI patients. By reducing exertional activity and sympathetic stimulation, myocardial oxygen demand can be decreased.[4] It is important to accomplish this goal without deconditioning the patient. Deconditioning occurs when patients have undergone long periods of bed rest without upright posture. The absence of work against gravity impairs the ability of the cardiovascular system to regulate blood pressure, thus increasing risk of orthostatic hypotension and syncope. To combat these risks, it is reasonable to allow patients to have bedside commode privileges after 12 to 24 hours of hemodynamic stability and freedom from ischemia.[1,5]

Diet

Patients should be given "nothing by mouth" (NPO status) until stable. If at that time they are considered for early cardiac catheterization or surgical revascularization, they can be prescribed a clear liquid diet extended to NPO status before the intervention. STEMI patients should receive the National Cholesterol Education Program Adult Treatment Panel III–recommended therapeutic lifestyle change (TLC) diet (<7% of total calories as saturated fats, <200 mg of cholesterol per day, increased omega-3 fatty acids, and appropriate calorie intake for energy needs).[6] Sodium intake should be restricted to a maximum of 2 g per day in STEMI patients with concurrent hypertension or heart failure.[1] Docusate sodium may be used as a stool softener to reduce performance of the Valsalva maneuver.

Altered Mentation and Anxiolysis

STEMI patients should be monitored for increased anxiety or alterations in behavior once they are in the CCU. Mental status change in patients after thrombolysis should be taken seriously, and computed axial tomography or magnetic resonance imaging should be considered to rule out intracerebral hemorrhage.[1] Untreated anxiety has been associated with an increase in adverse cardiac events.[7] It is reasonable to manage anxiety with behavioral interventions, liberalized visiting rules, or anxiolytic medications (diazepam, oxazepam) if necessary.[1]

Education of the Patient

Once hospitalized, the patient should continue to be educated about his or her diagnosis, plan for inpatient treatment, and projected length of stay. Effort should be made to explain coronary artery disease and its risk factors in addition to therapies that can decrease risk (smoking cessation, diet, exercise, rehabilitation, and medication compliance). The patient should be oriented to his or her surroundings and to what tests, procedures, and daily nursing care to expect.[1] Finally, patients should be made aware of how to recognize symptoms and how to contact the medical staff.

EARLY RISK STRATIFICATION

Risk stratification is used to estimate the patient's prognosis and to plan management. There are several tools used commonly for risk stratification (Table 30.1). Validated in GUSTO-I, the Killip system classifies patients according to clinical signs of heart failure, with higher scores correlating with increased risk of mortality.[8] Hemodynamic assessment through invasive monitoring may also be used for prognostication.[9] The Forrester-Diamond classification scale uses data from Swan-Ganz catheter readings (cardiac index, pulmonary capillary wedge pressure) to estimate in-hospital risk of mortality. Several risk prediction scores (e.g., TIMI, Selker) have been developed to aid in risk stratification.[10,11] These tools incorporate past history of coronary artery disease, risk factors for coronary artery disease, ECG changes, biomarker elevations, signs of congestive heart failure, and hemodynamic or electrical instability to approximate likelihood of early (30-day) mortality as well as major adverse cardiac events after STEMI.

PHARMACOTHERAPY

Trial evidence in support of therapeutic interventions is summarized in Table 30.2. The dosing recommendations are summarized in Table 30.3.

Initial Phase

Antithrombotic Agents

Activation of platelets and the coagulation cascade plays a vital role in the pathogenesis of coronary thrombosis, the proximate cause of STEMI. A number of antiplatelet and anticoagulant agents have been developed to inhibit platelet function and coagulation. The major objective of antithrombotic therapy is establishment and maintenance of patency of the infarct-related artery, thereby promoting myocardial salvage and consequently improved morbidity and survival.

Antiplatelet Agents

Aspirin is one of the most effective and widely used therapies in the management of acute and nonacute coronary artery disease. Aspirin inhibits platelet cyclooxygenase, the rate-limiting enzyme in the synthesis of thromboxane A_2, a potent platelet agonist. A collaborative meta-analysis of 15 randomized trials in nearly 20,000 patients showed a 27% risk reduction in mortality in patients with acute myocardial infarction (MI) treated with aspirin.[12] In the ISIS-2 trial, treatment with aspirin alone was as effective as streptokinase in reducing early mortality.[13] On the basis of these data, aspirin is now considered essential during initial management for all STEMI patients. Nonenteric aspirin should be given early at a dose between 162 and 325 mg (for rapid bioavailability) and continued indefinitely at a daily dose of 75 to 162 mg (preferably enteric formulation) regardless of administration of additional antiplatelet medications.[12] Aspirin suppositories may be used in patients with nausea, vomiting, or other upper gastrointestinal tract disorders in response to oral treatment.

The thienopyridine derivatives ticlopidine and clopidogrel are suitable alternatives in patients intolerant to aspirin; ticlopidine exhibits reduced tolerability (excess rash, diarrhea, and adverse hematologic outcomes) compared with

RISK STRATIFICATION SYSTEMS USED IN CLASSIFICATION OF ST-SEGMENT ELEVATION MYOCARDIAL INFARCTION SEVERITY			
Killip classification (clinical parameters)[8]			
Level	**Definition**		**Clinical findings**
Class I	No heart failure		No clinical signs of cardiac decompensation
Class II	Heart failure		S_3 gallop, rales up to half of lung fields
Class III	Severe heart failure		Pulmonary edema with rales throughout lung fields
Class IV	Cardiogenic shock		Hypotension (BP <90 mm Hg), oliguria, cyanosis, and diaphoresis
Forrester-Diamond classification (hemodynamic parameters)[9]			
Level	**Definition**		**Hemodynamic Findings**
Class I	Normal hemodynamics		PCWP <18, CI >2.2
Class II	Pulmonary congestion		PCWP >18, CI >2.2
Class III	Peripheral hypoperfusion		PCWP <18, CI <2.2
Class IV	Pulmonary congestion and peripheral hypoperfusion		PCWP >18, CI <2.2
TIMI risk score[10]			
Factor	**Points per Factor (total, 0-14)**	**Total Additive Score**	**30-Day Mortality Rate (per InTIME II)**
History		0	0.8%
Age 75 years and older	3	1	1.6%
Age 65-74 years	2	2	2.2%
Diabetes, HTN, or angina	1	3	4.4%
Physical examination		4	7.3%
Systolic BP <100 mm Hg	3	5	12%
Heart rate >100 bpm	2	6	16%
Killip class II-IV	2	7	23%
Weight <67 kg (150 pounds)	1	8	27%
Presentation		>8	36%
Anterior ST-segment elevation or LBBB	1		
Time to reperfusion therapy >4 hours	1		

In both the Killip and Forrester classification systems, prognosis worsens with increasing class. The TIMI risk score categorizes clinical findings with regard to history, physical examination, and presenting signs. Each finding is attributed a point value, and the accumulated score estimates likelihood of mortality. BP, blood pressure; CI, cardiac index; HTN, hypertension; LBBB, left bundle branch block; PCWP, pulmonary capillary wedge pressure.

Table 30.1 Risk stratification systems used in classification of ST-segment elevation myocardial infarction severity.

clopidogrel. Both these agents inhibit platelets through a mechanism independent of aspirin by blocking the adenosine diphosphate P2Y receptor. Treatment with clopidogrel in patients with STEMI is recommended in the American College of Cardiology/American Heart Association guidelines for patients intolerant to aspirin,[1] and the adjunctive use of clopidogrel plus aspirin during fibrinolytic therapy for STEMI was recently approved on the basis of the results of the COMMIT/CCS-2 trial.[14] Although the role of combined therapy in catheter-based reperfusion, the preferred strategy in most centers in the United States, has not been explored directly, a nonrandomized subgroup analysis of Clopidogrel as Adjunctive Reperfusion Therapy (CLARITY) suggested that more than half of the benefit observed with clopidogrel at 30 days occurred in patients undergoing PCI (1.5% of 2.5% absolute risk difference).[15] Ticlopidine is not currently approved for adjunctive use with aspirin in STEMI.

On the basis of these findings, a daily maintenance dose of 75 mg of clopidogrel is recommended without a loading dose for a minimum of 1 month in patients treated with thrombolysis. In patients who have undergone primary PCI, clopidogrel should be continued for at least 1 month after bare-metal stent implantation or for a minimum of 12 months after drug-eluting stent implantation, especially in patients at low risk for bleeding.[16] Clopidogrel treatment has been shown to significantly increase bleeding in patients who undergo urgent or emergent coronary artery bypass graft (CABG) surgery.[17] Thus, the American College of

Cardiology/American Heart Association guidelines recommend stopping clopidogrel at least 5 days (and preferably 7 days) before CABG surgery.[18]

The glycoprotein IIb/IIIa receptor inhibitors have been the subject of extensive investigation, during both forms of reperfusion therapy—fibrinolysis and primary PCI. Glycoprotein inhibitors appear useful for preventing thrombotic complications in patients with STEMI undergoing PCI but do not provide any benefit and may potentially cause harm (bleeding, including intracranial bleeding, in patients older than 70 years) in patients treated with fibrinolytic therapy. A meta-analysis of eight trials reported improved survival with these agents with use during primary PCI.[19] On the basis of these findings, the guidelines give a class IIa (level B)

CLINICAL TRIALS OF THERAPEUTIC INTERVENTIONS FOR ST-SEGMENT ELEVATION MYOCARDIAL INFARCTION				
Intervention	**Trial**	**Sample Size**	**Treatment Groups**	**Outcomes**
Fibrinolytics				
Fibrinolytics	Fibrinolytic Therapy Trialists' (FTT)[67] Collaborative Group (follow-up: 5 weeks)	43,976 acute MI patients	Fibrinolytics vs placebo	All-cause death OR, 0.78 95% CI, 0.70-0.87
Primary percutaneous coronary intervention				
Primary PCI	Keeley meta-analysis of 23 trials[68] (follow-up: 4-6 weeks)	7793 acute MI patients	Primary PCI vs fibrinolytics	Death, MI, or stroke OR, 0.53 95% CI, 0.45-0.63 All-cause death OR, 0.73 95% CI, 0.62-0.86 Hemorrhagic stroke OR, 0.05 95% CI, 0.01-0.35
Antiplatelets				
Aspirin, initial phase	The Second International Study of Infarct Survival (ISIS-2)[13] (follow-up: 5 weeks)	17,187 acute MI patients	Aspirin vs control	CV death OR, 0.23 95% CI, ***
Aspirin, long term	Antithrombotic Trialists' Collaboration[12] (follow-up: 2 years)	59,395 high-risk patients	Aspirin vs control	CV death, MI, or stroke RR, 0.81 95% CI, 0.79-0.84
Clopidogrel	Clopidogrel and Metoprolol in Myocardial Infarction Trial (COMMIT/CCS-2)[14] (follow-up: 28 days)	45,852 patients presenting with suspected acute MI (majority received fibrinolytics)	Clopidogrel + ASA vs placebo + ASA	Death, MI, or stroke OR, 0.91 95% CI, 0.86-0.97 All-cause death OR, 0.93 95% CI, 0.87-0.99 Major bleeding OR, 1.07 95% CI, 0.84-1.37
	Clopidogrel as Adjunctive Reperfusion Therapy (CLARITY)–Thrombolysis in Myocardial Infarction (TIMI) 28 study[15] (follow-up: 3.5 days)	3941 patients with STEMI (54% received fibrinolytics)	Clopidogrel + ASA vs placebo + ASA	Death, recurrent MI, or occluded infarct-related artery OR, 0.64 95% CI, 0.53-0.76 Major bleeding OR, 1.2 95% CI, 0.65-2.22
Glycoprotein IIb/IIIa inhibitors	Meta-analysis (De Luca et al[19]) (follow-up: 30 days)	3949 patients with acute MI	Primary PCI + glycoprotein inhibitor vs primary PCI + control	Death OR, 0.68 95% CI, 0.47-0.99 MI OR, 0.56 95% CI, 0.33-0.94 Major bleeding OR, 1.16 95% CI, 0.85-1.59

(Continued)

Anticoagulants				
Unfractionated heparin	Meta-analysis (Collins et al,[20] 26 trials) (follow-up: 30 days)	68,090 patients with acute MI	UFH + ASA vs ASA	Death RR, 0.95 95% CI, 0.9-0.996 MI RR, 0.92 95% CI, 0.84-0.996 Major bleeding RR, 1.46 95% CI, 1.24-1.73
LMWH (enoxaparin)	Enoxaparin and Thrombolysis Reperfusion for Acute Myocardial Infarction Treatment (ExTRACT–TIMI 25)[22] (follow-up: 30 days)	20,506 STEMI patients undergoing fibrinolysis	Enoxaparin vs UFH	Death or MI RR, 0.83 95% CI, 0.77-0.9 Death RR, 0.92 95% CI, 0.84-1.02 Severe bleeding RR, 1.53 95% CI, 1.23-1.89
LMWH (reviparin)	Clinical Trial of Reviparin and Metabolic Modulation in Acute Myocardial Infarction Treatment Evaluation (CREATE)[23] (follow-up: 7 days)	15,570 patients with STEMI or new LBBB	Reviparin vs placebo	Death, MI, or stroke RR, 0.87 95% CI, 0.79-0.95 Death RR, 0.87 95% CI, 0.79-0.96 Recurrent MI RR, 0.77 95% CI, 0.62-0.95 Severe bleeding RR, 2.49 95% CI, 1.61-3.87
Anti-Xa agent (fondaparinux)	Organization for the Assessment of Strategies for Ischemic Syndromes (OASIS-6)[24] (follow-up: 30 days)	12,092 patients with STEMI	Fondaparinux vs UFH or placebo	Death or MI RR, 0.86 95% CI, 0.77-0.96 Death RR, 0.87 95% CI, 0.77-0.98 Severe bleeding RR, 0.79 95% CI, 0.58-1.09
Antithrombin agent (bivalirudin)	Harmonizing Outcomes with Revascularization and Stents in AMI (HORIZONS AMI)[25] (follow-up: 30 days)	3602 patients with STEMI	Bivalirudin vs UFH + glycoprotein IIb/IIIa inhibitor during primary PCI	Death, MI, TVR, stroke, or major bleeding HR, 0.75 95% CI, 0.62-0.92 Death, MI, TVR, or stroke HR, 1.00 95% CI, 0.75-1.32 Death RR, 0.66 95% CI, 0.44-1.00 Major bleeding RR, 0.59 95% CI, 0.45-0.76
Beta blockers				
Beta blockers, initial phase	First International Study of Infarct Survival Collaborative Group (ISIS-1)[26] (follow-up: 7 days)	16,027 patients with acute MI	IV, then oral atenolol for 7 days vs placebo	Death RR, 0.79 95% CI, 0.58-1.09
	Metoprolol in Acute Myocardial Infarction (MIAMI)[27] (follow-up: 15 days)	5778 patients with acute MI	IV, then oral metoprolol for 15 days vs placebo	Death RR, 0.85 95% CI, 0.64-1.15

	Clopidogrel and Metoprolol in Myocardial Infarction Trial (COMMIT/CCS-2)[30] (follow-up: 15 days)	45,852 patients with acute MI	IV, then oral metoprolol for 15 days vs placebo	Death, MI, or cardiac arrest OR, 0.96 95% CI, 0.9-1.01 All-cause death OR, 0.99 95% CI, 0.92-1.05 Ventricular fibrillation OR, 0.83 95% CI, 0.75-0.93 Cardiogenic shock OR, 1.30 95% CI, 1.19-1.41
Beta blockers, long term	Beta Blocker Heart Attack Trial (BHAT)[31] (follow-up: 30 months)	3837 patients 5 to 21 days post MI	Oral propranolol vs placebo	Mortality RR, 0.74
	Carvedilol Post-Infarct Survival Control in LV Dysfunction (CAPRICORN)[32] (follow-up: 1.3 years)	1959 patients with left ventricular dysfunction post MI (EF <40%)	Oral carvedilol vs placebo	All-cause death HR, 0.77 95% CI, 0.6-0.98 Death or MI HR, 0.71 95% CI, 0.57-0.89
Renin-angiotensin-aldosterone system inhibitors				
ACE inhibitors, short term	Meta-analysis (ACE Inhibitor Myocardial Infarction Collaborative Group[34]) (follow-up: 30 days–6 months)	92,433 patients with acute MI	ACE inhibitor vs placebo	Death OR, 0.92 95% CI, 0.88-0.97
ACE inhibitors, long term	Meta-analysis (ACE Inhibitor Myocardial Infarction Collaborative Group[34]) (follow-up: >6 months)	13,612 patients with acute MI	ACE inhibitor vs placebo	Death RR, 0.79 95% CI, 0.65-0.96
Angiotensin receptor blocker	Valsartan in Acute Myocardial Infarction Trial (VALIANT)[36] (follow-up: 2.1 years)	577 patients with acute MI and heart failure	Valsartan vs captopril	All-cause death RR, 1.00 95% CI, 0.90-1.11
Aldosterone receptor blocker	Eplerenone Post–Acute Myocardial Infarction Heart Failure Efficacy and Survival Study (EPHESUS)[37] (follow-up: 16 months)	6632 patients with acute MI and heart failure	Eplerenone vs placebo	All-cause death RR, 0.85 95% CI, 0.75-0.96 Cardiac death or cardiac rehospitalization RR, 0.87 95% CI, 0.79-0.95

ACE, angiotensin-converting enzyme; ASA, aspirin; CI, confidence interval; CV, cardiovascular; EF, ejection fraction; HR, hazard rate; IV, intravenous; LBBB, left bundle branch block; MI, myocardial infarction; LMWH, low-molecular-weight heparin; OR, odds ratio; PCI, percutaneous coronary intervention; RR, risk ratio; STEMI, ST-segment elevation myocardial infarction; TVR, target vessel revascularization; UFH, unfractionated heparin.

Table 30.2 Clinical trials of therapeutic interventions for ST-segment elevation myocardial infarction.

recommendation for abciximab and class IIb (level C) for eptifibatide and tirofiban during treatment with primary PCI.[1]

Anticoagulants

The standard anticoagulant agent used in clinical practice is unfractionated heparin (UFH).[1,20] However, there is some controversy about its efficacy in improving coronary artery patency and mortality when it is used with some fibrinolytic agents.[21] It appears that UFH may have more convincing evidence of benefit with fibrin-specific (alteplase, reteplase, and tenecteplase) compared with non–fibrin-specific (streptokinase, anistreplase, urokinase) lytic therapy.[1] The recommended dose of UFH is an initial bolus of 60 IU/kg (maximum, 4000 IU) followed by an initial infusion of 12 IU/kg per hour (maximum, 1000 IU/h). The activated partial thromboplastin time during maintenance therapy should be 1.5 to 2 times the control value. In the absence of any ongoing indication (atrial fibrillation, thromboembolism), there is no evidence of benefit in prolonging UFH infusion beyond 48 hours.

Recent trials have evaluated the role of four alternative anticoagulant agents for STEMI: one involving enoxaparin (a low-molecular-weight heparin) versus UFH as adjunctive therapy

PHARMACOLOGIC MANAGEMENT OF ST-SEGMENT ELEVATION MYOCARDIAL INFARCTION ACCORDING TO THERAPEUTIC AGENT AND CLINICAL COURSE			
Medication	**First 24 hours**	**During Hospitalization**	**Hospital Discharge and Long Term**
Antiplatelet	ASA 162-325 mg + Clopidogrel 300-mg load	ASA 75-162 mg/day Clopidogrel 75 mg/day	ASA 75-162 mg/day indefinitely Clopidogrel 75 mg, 4 weeks (at least 1 year with DES)
Anticoagulant	IV UFH 60 IU/kg bolus 12 IU/kg/h infusion to aPTT 1.5-2 × control *or* Enoxaparin 1 mg/kg SC *or* Fondaparinux 2.5 mg SC	Continue UFH infusion × 2 days *or* Enoxaparin × 8 days *or* Fondaparinux × 8 days	Warfarin in atrial fibrillation, large MI with mural thrombus, or VTE
Beta blocker	IV followed by oral beta blockade in patients without contraindication	Oral daily (titrate metoprolol to 100 mg twice daily if tolerated)	Oral daily (continue full dose)
ACE inhibitor	Patients presenting with anterior MI, pulmonary edema, or EF <0.40 but stable hemodynamics (SBP >100 mm Hg)	Oral daily	Oral daily indefinitely
Angiotensin receptor blocker	ACE intolerant, heart failure, or EF <0.40	Oral daily	Oral daily indefinitely
Aldosterone antagonist	NA	Patients with history of heart failure, diabetes mellitus, or LVEF <0.40 Treat on background of ACE inhibitors Contraindicated in patients with history of renal dysfunction, K^+ <5.0 mEq/L	Same as during hospitalization
Statin	Measure lipid profile within 24 hours	Initiate statin therapy regardless of LDL level; target TG elevation with niacin or fibrates	Indefinitely LDL at least <100 mg/dL and ideally <70 mg/dL

ACE, angiotensin-converting enzyme; aPTT, activated partial thromboplastin time; ASA, aspirin; DES, drug-eluting stent; EF, ejection fraction; IV, intravenous; LDL, low-density lipoprotein; LVEF, left ventricular ejection fraction; MI, myocardial infarction; NA, not applicable; SBP, systolic blood pressure; SC, subcutaneous; TG, triglyceride; UFH, unfractionated heparin; VTE, venous thromboembolism.

Table 30.3 Pharmacologic management of ST-segment elevation myocardial infarction according to therapeutic agent and clinical course.

with primarily fibrin-specific fibrinolysis (ExTRACT–TIMI 25)[22]; a second involving reviparin (a low-molecular-weight heparin) versus UFH as adjunctive therapy with primarily non–fibrin-specific fibrinolysis (CREATE)[23]; a third involving fondaparinux (an anti-Xa agent) versus enoxaparin as adjunctive therapy with primarily non–fibrin-specific fibrinolysis (OASIS-6)[24]; and the fourth involving bivalirudin (direct antithrombin) versus UFH plus platelet glycoprotein IIb/IIIa inhibitor as adjunctive therapy during primary PCI.[25] The results indicate that therapy with both enoxaparin and reviparin was associated with significantly superior efficacy outcomes, but risk of serious bleeding was significantly increased compared with UFH. In contrast, treatment with fondaparinux was associated with significantly reduced risk of ischemic outcomes, including mortality, especially in patients undergoing fibrinolytic therapy, without increasing major bleeding.[24] However, a significant number of catheter-related thromboses were seen in patients undergoing primary PCI. The unpublished results of the HORIZONS AMI appear to be favorable for bivalirudin, with significant advantage in major bleeding without increase in ischemic outcomes.[25]

Enoxaparin is given as an initial 30-mg intravenous bolus, followed 15 minutes later by subcutaneous injections of 1.0 mg/kg every 12 hours; if the patient is older than 75 years, the initial intravenous bolus is eliminated and the subcutaneous dose is reduced to 0.75 mg/kg every 12 hours. Maintenance dosing with enoxaparin should be continued for the duration of the index hospitalization, up to 8 days. Unfractionated and low-molecular-weight heparins can both be used in STEMI patients undergoing PCI. The dose recommendations for fondaparinux and bivalirudin await an update of the guidelines.

β-Adrenoreceptor Blockers

The 2004 American College of Cardiology/American Heart Association guidelines recognize a beneficial clinical impact of both early and late beta-blocker therapy in the management of STEMI.[1] Beta blockade reduces the frequency of ventricular tachyarrhythmias, the incidence of reinfarction in subjects receiving fibrinolytics, and the size and complications of infarction including mortality in those not treated with fibrinolytic therapy. Beta blockade appears to decrease myocardial oxygen demand by reducing heart rate, systemic arterial pressure, and contractility and improves myocardial perfusion by prolonging diastole and redistributing blood flow from epicardium to the subendocardium.[1]

A large part of the evidence supporting beta-blocker use in STEMI therapy comes from pre–reperfusion era studies. Both ISIS-1[26] and MIAMI[27] trials provided evidence of a mortality benefit at 7 and 15 days with intravenous atenolol and metoprolol, respectively. A number of trials have subsequently questioned the mortality benefit of early beta blockade[28,29]; the most recent trial, the COMMIT/CCS-2,[30] failed to demonstrate benefit in all-cause death or composite of death, reinfarction, or cardiac arrest. Although allocation to the metoprolol arm resulted in reductions in reinfarction and ventricular fibrillation from day 2 onward, a 30% relative increase in cardiogenic shock was seen in the treatment arm, especially on day 1 of therapy. In view of the recent evidence, it is reasonable to initiate oral beta-blocker therapy in the first 24 hours for patients who do not have any of the following contraindications: signs of heart failure; evidence of a low-output state; increased risk for cardiogenic shock; or other relative contraindications to beta blockade (PR interval greater than 0.24 second, second- or third-degree heart block, active asthma, or reactive airway disease). It may be appropriate to use a short-acting intravenous beta blocker in patients with refractory tachycardia or hypertension who are not at high risk for cardiogenic shock (age $>$ 70 years, systolic blood pressure $<$ 120 mm Hg, or Killip class $>$ I). Long-term oral beta blockers are strongly recommended (class I, level of evidence A) for secondary prevention in the highest risk patients, such as those with low ejection fraction, heart failure, or post shock, once they have stabilized, with gradual dose titration.[31-33]

Inhibition of the Renin-Angiotensin-Aldosterone System

Inhibition of the renin-angiotensin-aldosterone system prevents ventricular remodeling and collagen formation in patients with left ventricular dysfunction after acute MI and affects a number of pathophysiologic mechanisms that are thought to be important in the prognosis of patients with acute MI.

Angiotensin-converting enzyme (ACE) inhibition affects numerous cell processes by reducing the interaction of angiotensin II with AT_1 receptors and by inhibiting the metabolism of bradykinin, a potent vasodilator. Cardioprotective effects of ACE inhibitors are related to reduction in salt and water retention, peripheral vasoconstriction, myocardial and vascular hypertrophy, and central sympathetic outflow. A number of randomized controlled trials have established the benefit of early ACE inhibitor therapy in the setting of STEMI. A meta-analysis of 13 trials in nearly 100,000 patients reported a significant reduction in mortality.[34] Benefit was largest in subgroups with prior infarction, heart failure, depressed ejection fraction, or tachycardia. It is recommended that ACE inhibitors be administered within the first 24 hours of STEMI to patients with anterior infarction, pulmonary congestion, or left ventricular ejection fraction less than 0.40, in the absence of contraindications (e.g., hypotension, allergy).[1] Treatment should begin with a low dose of a short-acting ACE inhibitor (such as captopril) and be titrated up slowly to full dose within the first 2 days. Treatment should be continued long term, preferably with a long-acting once-daily oral ACE inhibitor.

Studies have shown angiotensin receptor blockers to be safe alternatives to ACE inhibitors in patients with ischemic heart disease and heart failure. OPTIMAAL (Optimal Trial in Myocardial Infarction with Angiotensin II Antagonist Losartan), a randomized trial, compared treatment of post-STEMI patients with captopril or losartan.[35] Follow-up revealed no difference in mortality. VALIANT (Valsartan in Acute Myocardial Infarction Trial) randomized post-MI patients with poor left ventricular function to captopril, valsartan, or a combination of both.[36] No statistically significant difference in mortality was seen between treatment arms, although side effects were most common in the combination therapy group. Current guidelines recommend the use of angiotensin receptor blockers in patients who are intolerant of ACE inhibitors and have post-MI left ventricular dysfunction (frank congestive heart failure or left ventricular ejection fraction $\leq$40%).[1]

Clinical investigation has established a role for aldosterone-blocking agents in patients after STEMI. The EPHESUS study showed that addition of eplerenone to optimal medical therapy reduces morbidity and mortality among patients with acute MI complicated by left ventricular dysfunction and heart failure.[37] Aldosterone-blocking agents are indicated as long-term therapy in STEMI patients with reduced left ventricular function but without renal dysfunction (creatinine clearance $<$50 mL/min) or hyperkalemia (potassium concentration $>$5.9 mEq/L).[1]

Miscellaneous Agents

Oxygen

Oxygen is universally used as initial treatment in patients with ischemic events to ameliorate associated hypoxemia.[1,38] Although there are few side effects with oxygen therapy, excess treatment can lead to systemic vasoconstriction, thereby unfavorably altering the demand-supply balance; and in patients with chronic obstructive pulmonary disease, it can result in reduced respiratory drive. Patients with oxygen saturation above 90% should be weaned from supplemental oxygen after the first 6 hours, if possible.

Nitroglycerin

Nitrates improve preload and afterload through peripheral arterial and venous dilatation.[1] Improved myocardial perfusion may also be due to dilatation of epicardial and collateral arteries. Evidence for mortality benefit was observed in the pre–reperfusion therapy era.[39] However, the benefits of routine use of intravenous nitroglycerin are less obvious in the contemporary reperfusion therapy era, in which β-adrenoceptor blockers and ACE inhibitors are routinely prescribed for patients with STEMI.[40] STEMI patients with ongoing ischemia should receive sublingual nitroglycerin (0.4 mg) every 5 minutes for a total of three doses. Intravenous nitroglycerin may be used for relief of ischemia, control of hypertension, or management of pulmonary congestion.[1] Nitroglycerin should not be used in ischemic patients with bradycardia, tachycardia, recent phosphodiesterase inhibitor use, right ventricular infarction or failure, and systolic blood pressure below 90 mm Hg or more than 30 mm Hg below baseline.[41]

Calcium Channel Blockers

The routine use of calcium antagonists cannot be recommended. Multiple trials of calcium antagonists have failed to establish a role for these agents in the treatment of most patients with STEMI.[1]

Lidocaine

Lidocaine is no longer recommended for use as a prophylactic agent in the prevention of ventricular arrhythmia in the setting of STEMI because of the risk of bradyarrhythmias and asystole.[1]

Morphine Sulfate

Currently, morphine sulfate (2 to 4 mg intravenously with increments of 2 to 8 mg intravenously repeated at 5- to 15-minute intervals) is the analgesic of choice for management of pain associated with STEMI. However, recent retrospective data have shown an increase in mortality in non-STEMI patients treated with morphine for pain relief.[42] Given this evidence, the role of morphine sulfate in acute coronary syndrome appears to be uncertain.

Magnesium Supplementation

The routine use of magnesium supplementation cannot be recommended as the largest controlled trial, MAGIC, failed to establish its role during fibrinolytic treatment of patients with STEMI. However, serum magnesium concentration should be measured in all patients on admission, and any demonstrated deficits should be corrected to minimize the risk of arrhythmias.[43]

Glycemic Control

Tight glucose control in diabetics during and after STEMI has been shown to lower acute and long-term (mean, 3.4 years) mortality.[44] Hypoglycemic therapy should be initiated to achieve hemoglobin A_{1c} concentration of less than 7%. Thiazolidinediones should not be used in patients recovering from STEMI who have New York Heart Association class III or class IV heart failure because of fluid retention.

Chronic Phase (Secondary Prevention)

Aspirin

The Antithrombotic Trialists' Collaboration evaluated 18,788 MI patients and reported a 25% reduction in the risk of recurrent infarction, stroke, or vascular death in patients receiving prolonged antiplatelet therapy. A daily dose of aspirin (75 to 162 mg orally) should be given indefinitely to patients recovering from STEMI.[1,12]

Beta Blocker

All patients after STEMI except those at low risk (normal or nearly normal ventricular function, successful reperfusion, absence of significant ventricular arrhythmias) and those without contraindications should receive beta-blocker therapy. Treatment should begin within a few days of the event, if it has not been initiated acutely, and continue indefinitely. Patients with moderate or severe left ventricular failure should receive beta-blocker therapy with a gradual titration scheme.[1]

Inhibition of the Renin-Angiotensin-Aldosterone System

An ACE inhibitor should be prescribed at discharge for all patients without contraindications after STEMI. If an ACE inhibitor cannot be tolerated, an angiotensin receptor blocker should be prescribed.[34]

Cholesterol Management

Although there has been no direct evaluation of lipid-modifying therapy initiated acutely in the setting of STEMI, the treatment guidelines recommend that lipid-lowering therapy be initiated before discharge in these patients.[1] This recommendation is based on the pronounced impact on major cardiovascular outcomes (including cardiovascular and all-cause mortality) in secondary prevention and acute coronary syndrome studies.[45,46] Currently, the guidelines recommend starting drug therapy if the LDL-cholesterol level is above 100 mg/dL, with the target LDL-cholesterol level being less than 100 mg/dL and ideally less than 70 mg/dL.[1] Combination therapy is recommended if a single-drug regimen does not allow one to reach target. If triglyceride levels are 200 to 499 mg/dL in the setting of normal LDL concentration, the non–high-density lipoprotein cholesterol target is less than 130 mg/dL, with further reduction to less than 100 mg/dL thought to be reasonable. Therapeutic options include increased statin therapy, addition of niacin, or fibrate therapy. If triglyceride levels are 500 mg/dL or higher, therapeutic options indicated to prevent pancreatitis are fibrate and niacin before LDL-lowering therapy.

Implantable Cardioverter-Defibrillator Implantation

Poor outcomes are associated with ventricular fibrillation (VF) or hemodynamically unstable ventricular tachycardia (VT) if it is present more than 2 days after STEMI.[1] A meta-analysis comparing implantable cardioverter-defibrillator (ICD) placement with antiarrhythmics in such a population demonstrated a significant reduction in both arrhythmic and all-cause death in favor of ICD implantation.[47] On the basis of these findings, an ICD is recommended for patients with VF or hemodynamically significant sustained VT more than 2 days after STEMI, provided the arrhythmia is not judged to be due to transient or reversible ischemia or reinfarction.[1]

Patients with inducible sustained VT and poor left ventricular function are also at higher risk for adverse cardiac events. Two trials, MADIT and MUSTT, demonstrated advantage for ICD compared with medical antiarrhythmic therapy in patients with low ejection fraction, nonsustained VT, and electrophysiology study–inducible ventricular tachyarrhythmias.[48,49] The MADIT II trial randomized 1232 post-MI subjects with ejection fraction of less than 30% to receive ICD implantation or not. At 20 months, ICD placement significantly reduced mortality.[50] On the basis of these studies, the guidelines support ICD therapy in coronary artery disease patients with poor left ventricular function (ejection fraction <30%) at high risk of life-threatening ventricular arrhythmias.[1]

Education

Education of the patient should focus on lifestyle modification with particular attention to the recommendations summarized in Table 30.4.[51]

COMPLICATIONS AND THEIR MANAGEMENT

Hypotension

Hypotension may be due to hypovolemia, ventricular failure, arrhythmia, mechanical complications, or other causes such as sepsis or pulmonary embolism.[1] Hypovolemia may also occur from poor oral intake, vomiting, diaphoresis, diuresis, medications, peripheral vasodilatation, or bleeding. All patients without evidence of volume overload should be given a fluid bolus. Hemoglobin concentration should be determined and

EDUCATION RECOMMENDATIONS FOR POST-STEMI PATIENTS IN THE CONVALESCENT STAGE	
Long-term management	
Smoking	Assess tobacco use; encourage discontinuation of smoking and avoidance of secondhand smoke exposure. Provide counseling and pharmacologic therapy. Refer for formal cessation programs, if indicated.
Hypertension	Encourage lifestyle modification: weight control, physical activity, alcohol moderation, moderate sodium restriction, and emphasis on fruits, nuts, vegetables, and low-fat dairy products. Provide pharmacologic therapy. Blood pressure control goal is <140/90 mm Hg or <130/80 mm Hg if chronic kidney disease or diabetes.
Physical activity	Assess risk, preferably with exercise test, to guide prescription. Encourage minimum of 30 to 60 minutes of activity, preferably daily but at least 3 or 4 times weekly (walking, jogging, cycling, or other aerobic activity), supplemented by an increase in daily lifestyle activities (e.g., walking breaks at work, gardening, household work). Cardiac rehabilitation programs are recommended for patients with STEMI.
Weight management	Goal: BMI 18.5 to 24.9 kg/m^2 Waist circumference: women: <35 inches; men: <40 inches
Diabetes management	Goal: $HgbA_{1c}$ <7%
Hormone therapy	Hormone therapy with estrogen plus progestin should not be given de novo to postmenopausal women after STEMI for secondary prevention of coronary events.
Antioxidant therapy	Antioxidant vitamins, such as vitamin E and vitamin C supplements, should not be prescribed to patients recovering from STEMI to prevent cardiovascular disease.
Air travel	Post MI: NYHA I, 6 to 8 weeks; NYHA II-IV, only if medically necessary and accompanied by physician
Sexual intercourse	May resume a few weeks post MI if there are no severe complications Patients capable of briskly walking a few blocks or climbing two flights of stairs without chest discomfort or severe shortness of breath should be able to resume sexual activity with very minimal risk. Regular physical activity, defined as expenditure of at least 6 METs 3 times per week, decreases the likelihood of adverse cardiovascular events during or shortly after sexual intercourse.

BMI, body mass index; $HgbA_{1c}$, hemoglobin A_{1c} level; METs, metabolic equivalents; NYHA, New York Heart Association; MI, myocardial infarction; STEMI, ST-segment elevation myocardial infarction.
From Smith S, Allen J, Blair SN, et al. AHA/ACC guidelines for secondary prevention for patients with coronary and other atherosclerotic vascular disease: 2006 update. Circulation 2006;113:2363-2372.

Table 30.4 Education recommendations for post-STEMI patients in the convalescent stage.

electrocardiography and echocardiography performed to screen for conduction abnormality or mechanical etiology. If the patient needs pressure support, dopamine is the first agent of choice, given its inotropic and vasoconstrictive properties. Norepinephrine may be given for more potent vasoconstriction in cases of severe hypotension. Once systolic arterial pressure reaches 80 mm Hg, conversion to dopamine at a rate of 2.5 to 5 μg/kg per minute and titration as needed to 5 to 15 μg/kg per minute should be considered. If arterial pressure stabilizes around 90 mm Hg with pressors, intravenous administration of dobutamine may be started with concomitant weaning of dopamine.

Pulmonary Edema

Acute coronary occlusion can result in myocardial ischemia, leading to systolic as well as diastolic dysfunction and eventually culminating in pulmonary edema. Pulmonary edema is associated with significantly increased mortality rate.[1] Early management should consist of oxygenation if oxygenation saturation is below 90% and identification of fluid status and pressure. Echocardiography can be useful in rapidly diagnosing the cause of pulmonary edema (systolic or diastolic dysfunction, mechanical complication). Patients with hypotension and ventricular failure may need inotropic and vasopressor support. Intra-aortic balloon counterpulsation (IABP) may also be used to improve cardiac output. If reperfusion is attempted in this scenario, PCI is preferred to fibrinolytics. Patients presenting with left ventricular dysfunction and hypervolemia will benefit from preload reduction through administration of nitrates, morphine, or diuretics.[52] Sublingual or spray nitroglycerin has a faster onset of action compared with intravenous treatment. Patients presenting with elevated systemic pressures should be administered intravenous nitroglycerin with a 10- to 20-μg bolus, followed by a 10-μg/min infusion. Dosing is then titrated up by 5 to 10 μg/min every 5 minutes until dyspnea relief, 10% decrease in arterial pressure, or increase in heart rate by 10 beats per minute.[1] Intravenous diuretics may also be used to reduce preload (e.g., furosemide, 20 to 80 mg intravenously). If blood pressure permits, use of ACE inhibitors may be preferred because of their proven mortality benefit. Captopril, a short-acting agent, may be used initially. Begin with 3.125 to 6.25 mg and double the dose up to 25 to 50 mg every 8 hours. Once tolerated, a long-acting agent may be substituted.

Cardiogenic Shock

Echocardiography with color-flow Doppler study is useful in both diagnosing the cause of cardiogenic shock (ventricular failure, mechanical complication) and differentiating it from hypovolemic, obstructive, distributive, or endocrine forms of shock. Cardiogenic shock occurs in 5% to 20% of patients after MI. Intra-arterial monitoring is indicated, and IABP is recommended for STEMI-related shock not quickly reversed with medical therapy.[1] Emergency revascularization has emerged as a beneficial treatment strategy in patients suffering cardiogenic shock secondary to STEMI. The SHOCK trial tested 302 such patients with either acute mechanical reperfusion or initial medical stabilization and delayed revascularization as needed.[53] At 12-month follow-up, a statistically significant reduction in mortality was seen in patients undergoing acute recanalization. On the basis of this finding, emergency revascularization is the strategy of choice in ischemic cardiogenic shock patients younger than 75 years. It is recommended that patients with severe three-vessel or left main coronary artery disease be sent for CABG within the first 18 hours of presentation.[1] For moderate three-vessel disease, it is recommended to proceed with PCI of the infarct-related artery and delayed CABG in stabilized patients.

Right Ventricular Infarction

Right ventricular MI occurs in 30% to 40% of inferoposterior MIs and 5% to 10% of anterior MIs; isolated right ventricular infarction is rare. Clinically significant right ventricular infarction presents with signs of severe right ventricle failure (jugular venous distention, Kussmaul's sign, hepatomegaly) and clear breath sounds with or without hypotension. The infarction may be manifested on ECG as lack of reciprocal ST-segment depression in leads V_1 to V_3, a 1-mm ST-segment elevation in lead V_1 and the right-sided precordial leads, especially V_4R; it should be screened for in all patients with inferior STEMI presenting with hypotension.[54] Two-dimensional echocardiography is helpful in determining the degree of right ventricular dysfunction. Catheterization of the right side of the heart often reveals a distinctive hemodynamic pattern resembling a "square root" sign (steep right atrial *y* descent and an early diastolic dip and plateau in right ventricular waveforms). Therapy consists of volume expansion to maintain adequate right ventricular preload and inotropic therapy with dobutamine to improve cardiac performance with attendant reduction in pulmonary capillary wedge and pulmonary arterial pressures.[55] If possible, fibrinolysis or PCI should be performed to achieve coronary reperfusion. Afterload-reducing agents or IABP may be useful in unloading the left ventricle and increasing right ventricular output.[56] If atrioventricular dyssynchrony or heart block is seen, atrioventricular sequential pacing should be started to improve output and to reverse shock.[57]

Mitral Valve Regurgitation

Papillary muscle rupture presenting as acute mitral regurgitation should be high in the differential diagnosis of a patient presenting with inferior STEMI, pulmonary edema, and shock.[1] It occurs in 1% of patients with acute MI. Transthoracic or transesophageal echocardiography is used to confirm the diagnosis. Interventions to reduce regurgitant volume include IABP, inotropic support, and afterload reduction to improve left ventricular output while the patient is sent for angiography and urgent surgery.

Ventricular Septal Rupture

Ventricular septal rupture occurs in 1% to 2% of patients with acute MI. The GUSTO-I and SHOCK trials demonstrated that ventricular septal rupture is most often due to thrombolysis within the first 24 hours of STEMI.[53,58] Patients often present with pulmonary edema and shock, with a harsh systolic murmur and a palpable thrill in the third to fourth left intercostal space along the left sternal border being the prominent finding on physical examination. Diagnosis is confirmed by Doppler examination on echocardiography. Management includes placement of IABP, with inotropes and nitrates carefully titrated to maintain mean arterial pressure. Regardless of stability, patients with ventricular septal rupture should be sent for emergency surgical repair as mortality with medical therapy alone approaches 95%.[1,59]

Left Ventricular Free Wall Rupture

Left ventricular free wall rupture is a rare event (0.8% to 6.2% of cases), often occurring in either the first 24 hours of MI or 3 to 5 days later.[60] Risk factors include first MI, anterior infarct, Q-wave infarct, increased age (especially elderly women), lack of collaterals, and recent use of thrombolytics, corticosteroids, or nonsteroidal anti-inflammatory drugs. Immediate fluid replacement and surgical correction are vital. CABG should be performed at the same time as repair. Prognosis is poor.[1]

Pericarditis

Pericarditis is an acute inflammation of the pericardium associated with transmural MI extending to the epicardium.[1] Early pericarditis (1 to 4 days) occurs in 10% of acute MI patients; late pericarditis (1 to 8 weeks) occurs in 1% to 3% of acute MI patients. Clinical findings include pleuritic chest discomfort and positional pain exacerbated when supine and relieved when upright. Pain may radiate to the left shoulder, scapula, or trapezius muscle, and auscultation may reveal a friction rub. The classic ECG finding is of diffuse concave upward ST-segment elevation in all leads except aVR and V_1 (usually depressed) and diffuse PR depression. Symptoms may begin weeks after STEMI. Treatment begins with a 162- to 325-mg oral daily dose of aspirin; however, doses as high as 650 mg orally every 4 to 6 hours may be needed.[61] Colchicine (0.6 mg every 12 hours) and acetaminophen are safe alternative treatments. Scar thinning and myocardial rupture are associated with ibuprofen and corticosteroid treatment, so they should not be used. Detection of an effusion or clinical deterioration in the setting of pericarditis is a contraindication to anticoagulant therapy.

Arrhythmias

Arrhythmias frequently complicate STEMI early on. The mechanisms responsible for infarction-related arrhythmias include autonomic nervous system imbalance, electrolyte disturbances, ischemia, and slowed conduction in zones of ischemic myocardium.

Ventricular Fibrillation

Risk factors for VF include age older than 75 years, elevated sympathetic tone, hypercalcemia, hypokalemia, hypomagnesemia, acidosis, and possibly free radical formation after ischemic reperfusion.[62,63] After immediate treatment, acid-base and electrolyte status should be normalized (keep potassium concentration above 4.0 mEq/L and magnesium concentration above 2.0 mEq/L). Post-STEMI VF occurs most often within the first 4 hours of an event. Intravenous beta blockade followed by oral therapy has been associated with a reduced incidence of early VF.[1] Acute treatment of VF or pulseless VT begins with an immediate unsynchronized electrical shock with a monophasic shock energy of 200 J. If it is unsuccessful, a second shock of 200 to 300 J and, if necessary, a third shock of 360 J is indicated.[1] Amiodarone (300 mg or bolus of 5 mg/kg) between shocks is the antiarrhythmic of choice in patients with shock-resistant VF.

Ventricular Tachycardia

Sustained VT is defined as that either lasting more than 30 seconds or immediately resulting in circulatory failure. No prophylactic therapy is indicated for nonsustained VT.[1] The preponderance of events occur within the first 48 hours of STEMI; if VT or VF occurs outside of this period, an electrophysiology study may be warranted. VT is characterized as monomorphic or polymorphic on the basis of QRS appearance. Sustained symptomatic VT of either kind requires urgent treatment. Rapid, polymorphic VT or pulseless VT is treated like VF, with an initial unsynchronized shock of 200 J, with further shocks at higher energies as needed. Symptomatic monomorphic VT, however, should be treated with an initial 100-J synchronized discharge, again followed by increasing energies as needed.[64] A small dose of midazolam or other sedative may be given before shock if blood pressure tolerates. If the patient is hemodynamically stable and heart rate is below 150 beats per minute, amiodarone or procainamide may be used instead of cardioversion[65]; 150 mg of amiodarone should be infused during 10 minutes and repeated every 10 to 15 minutes as needed. The cumulative dose should be less than 2.2 g during 24 hours. As in VF, attempts should be made to improve ischemia and to normalize electrolyte concentrations.

Accelerated Idioventricular Rhythm

Accelerated idioventricular rhythm (AIVR, "slow ventricular tachycardia"), a ventricular rhythm with a rate of 60 to 100 beats per minute, occurs in 25% of patients with STEMI. It is often a marker of successful reperfusion, with the rate of AIVR usually similar to that of the sinus rhythm that precedes and follows it. For the most part, AIVR is benign and does not develop into classic VT. Most episodes of AIVR do not require treatment if the patient is monitored carefully; degeneration into a more serious arrhythmia is rare.

Atrial Fibrillation

Atrial fibrillation is commonly seen after STEMI. Sympathetic stimulation, atrial stretch secondary to ventricular dysfunction, ischemia of the circumflex or right coronaries, hypokalemia, and hypoxia can all lead to atrial fibrillation.[1] Treatment requires addressing the underlying causes, such as electrolytes, ischemia, hypoxia, or other causes (e.g., hyperthyroid state). If the patient is clinically unstable, immediate synchronized cardioversion should be performed. Conscious sedation with a short-acting anesthetic should be given before discharge if tolerable. Shock should be synchronized with the QRS complex, so the R wave should be monitored with an appropriate lead to allow triggering. Begin with a monophasic shock at 50 J for atrial flutter. Atrial fibrillation will require an initial monophasic shock energy of 200 J. Increase by 100 J until a maximum of 400 J is reached.[66] Intravenous amiodarone or digoxin (especially in patients with heart failure) may be used if an unstable patient does not respond to cardioversion. If the patient is hemodynamically stable, rapid ventricular rate can be slowed with intravenous beta blockade (metoprolol, 2.5 to 5.0 mg every 2 to 5 minutes to a maximum of 15 mg within 10 to 15 minutes). Alternative rate-slowing agents can be used if beta blockers are contraindicated. Clinical risk for post-STEMI stroke will dictate anticoagulation. Unfractionated or low-molecular-weight heparin should be started if anticoagulation is indicated. Warfarin may also be started concurrently and heparin discontinued once the international normalized ratio reaches therapeutic threshold.

Bradyarrhythmia

Bradycardia is commonly associated with inferior STEMI as a result of increased vagal tone or release of adenosine.[1] Other causes of bradyarrhythmias include hyperkalemia, medication side effects, and metabolic abnormalities. Advanced atrioventricular block due to ischemic dysfunction of the conduction system is more common with large anterior infarction. Permanent ventricular pacing is indicated if such heart block is associated with bundle branch block or third-degree atrioventricular block is noted. Pharmacologic treatment includes use of atropine, epinephrine, and aminophylline. Glucagon is useful if beta blockers or calcium channel blockers are responsible for bradycardia.

POSTINFARCTION RISK STRATIFICATION AND MANAGEMENT

STEMI patients treated with fibrinolysis and deemed to be at high risk for further cardiac events should be referred for coronary angiography. New-onset congestive heart failure, ejection fraction below 40%, and recurrent ischemia at rest or with minimal exertion are indications for catheterization and revascularization if suitable.[1] All STEMI survivors should undergo an evaluation of left ventricular function before discharge. If the patient has an interpretable ECG, he or she may undergo a submaximal exercise test before discharge. If the ECG is uninterpretable (left bundle branch block, digitalis toxicity, resting ST and T-wave changes), the patient may undergo stress echocardiography or stress radionuclide myocardial perfusion scintigraphy. Those who cannot undergo exercise testing should undergo a pharmacologic stress test. Adenosine or dipyridamole myocardial perfusion scintigraphy or dobutamine stress echocardiography is indicated in this instance. If the patient is found to have clinically significant ischemia on testing (>2 mm ST-segment depression, ST-segment elevation >1 mm, moderate to severe angina, or poor exercise capacity) or resting ejection fraction below 40%, the patient should be referred to coronary angiography. In the absence of these findings, it is reasonable to treat patients with aggressive medical therapy.[1]

SUMMARY

The current best practice for the diagnosis and management of STEMI requires the clinician to focus on prevention, diagnosis, acute intervention, and long-term treatment of the disease. Prompt recognition and care directed at emergent reperfusion with fibrinolytic agents or PCI followed by appropriate risk stratification, the use of disease-modifying therapies (such as aspirin, beta blockers, cholesterol-lowering agents, and ACE inhibitors), defibrillators, lifestyle modification, and education of the patient have led to a marked decline in in-hospital and long-term fatality rates during the last 2 decades.

chapter 31

Complications of Acute Myocardial Infarction

Bojan Cercek and Prediman K. Shah

Definition

- Acute myocardial infarction results from ischemic necrosis of myocardium. It is associated with a number of hemodynamic complications that result from alterations in contractile and diastolic performance of the left and right ventricles, changes in mitral valve function, and mechanical complications with rupture of various cardiac structures.

Key Features

- The clinical manifestations of pump failure in acute myocardial infarction result from decreases in cardiac output and arterial blood pressure, which leads to signs and symptoms of organ hypoperfusion.
- At the same time, elevations in pulmonary capillary wedge pressure, resulting from altered left ventricular systolic and diastolic function and the superimposition of mitral regurgitation, lead to signs and symptoms of pulmonary congestion and edema.

Therapy

- Treatment of pump dysfunction in acute myocardial infarction involves general supportive care to sustain vital organ perfusion and function, limitation of ongoing ischemia and infarction with aggressive reperfusion-based interventions, and surgical revascularization and correction of mechanical complications in selected patients.

Myocardial infarction is associated with a number of complications that involve the cardiac conduction system (various degrees of atrioventricular and intraventricular block): the propensity for ventricular and supraventricular arrhythmias; a variety of hemodynamic disturbances that result from contractile and diastolic ventricular dysfunction; and the mechanical disruption of intracardiac structures that leads to papillary muscle rupture with mitral regurgitation, septal rupture with left-to-right shunt, and cardiac free wall rupture with cardiac tamponade or pseudoaneurysm formation. In addition, thromboembolic events, pericarditis, and recurrent ischemia or reinfarction also constitute important complications of acute myocardial infarction (AMI). Before the introduction of coronary care units, ventricular arrhythmias (ventricular tachycardia and fibrillation) used to be the leading causes of death in hospitalized patients with AMI. However, with the introduction of coronary care units and the availability of cardioversion-defibrillation, arrhythmic deaths have become less frequent, and hemodynamic disturbances resulting in pump failure and cardiac rupture have emerged as the leading causes of death in AMI. One or more complications occur in 20% to 25% of patients with AMI. The overall in-hospital mortality of patients with AMI still ranges from 5% to 15%.

ANATOMY AND PATHOLOGY

AMI is most commonly the consequence of acute coronary artery occlusion resulting from superimposition of a thrombus on a disrupted atherosclerotic plaque (Fig. 31.1).[1] Uncommon causes of AMI include aortic or coronary artery dissection, coronary artery vasculitis, and coronary embolism. After coronary artery occlusion, the myocardial area at risk begins to undergo necrosis within 20 to 25 minutes, beginning in the subendocardial layers and progressing in a subepicardial direction in time-dependent wavefronts (Fig. 31.2).[2,3] Transmural necrosis within the risk area is often complete within 4 to 6 hours after the onset of coronary artery occlusion, although this time frame may be slower or faster, depending on the availability of residual blood flow through collaterals or spontaneous changes in the severity of coronary artery occlusion. The overall extent of necrosis ultimately depends on the size of the risk area, the duration of coronary artery occlusion, and the residual collateral flow. In nearly two thirds of patients with cardiogenic shock, there is evidence of extensive acute transmural myocardial necrosis; in the remaining third, shock results from smaller areas of necrosis superimposed on previous infarcts or large areas of ischemic nonfunctioning but viable myocardium (hibernating and stunned myocardium), resulting in ischemic paralysis with only modest areas of myocardial infarction. Regional thinning and expansion of the transmurally infarcted zone, a process known as infarct expansion, is frequently observed in patients with large anterior infarction, and this leads to ventricular dilatation and further hemodynamic compromise, contributing to the syndrome of pump failure. Nearly 70% of patients with shock demonstrate extensive and severe multivessel coronary obstructive disease. Contrary to previous reports that suggested predominance of anterior infarction in shock, GUSTO-I and the international SHOCK registry reported anterior infarction in only half of the patients with cardiogenic shock. Whereas cardiogenic shock is more common in patients presenting with ST elevation (4.5%), it does occur in patients with non–ST elevation acute coronary syndrome (2.5%).[4,5]

In patients with infarction resulting from an occlusion of the right coronary artery, necrosis of a variable portion of the right ventricular myocardium is common (30% to 40% of cases) in association with infarction of the posterior third of the interventricular septum and the inferior-posterior wall of the left ventricle. All of these areas share a common blood supply from the right coronary artery, which is often occluded proximal to the right ventricular branches. In only 6% of patients with evidence of right ventricular

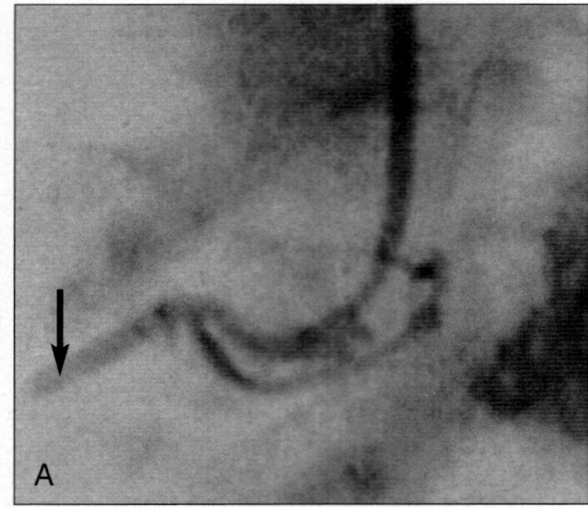

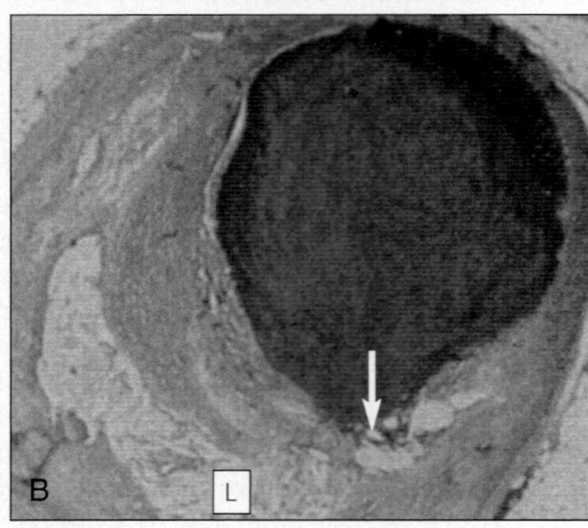

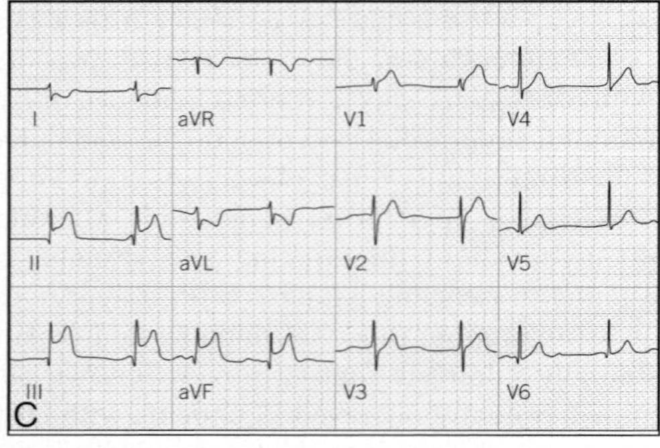

Figure 31.1 Coronary occlusion. A, Coronary angiogram showing an occluded coronary artery in a patient with acute myocardial infarction *(arrow)*. **B,** Pathologic basis of acute coronary occlusion shown in a coronary artery with plaque and plaque rupture *(arrow)* with a superimposed occlusive thrombus. **C,** An electrocardiogram showing ST-segment elevation in a patient with acute evolving myocardial infarction.

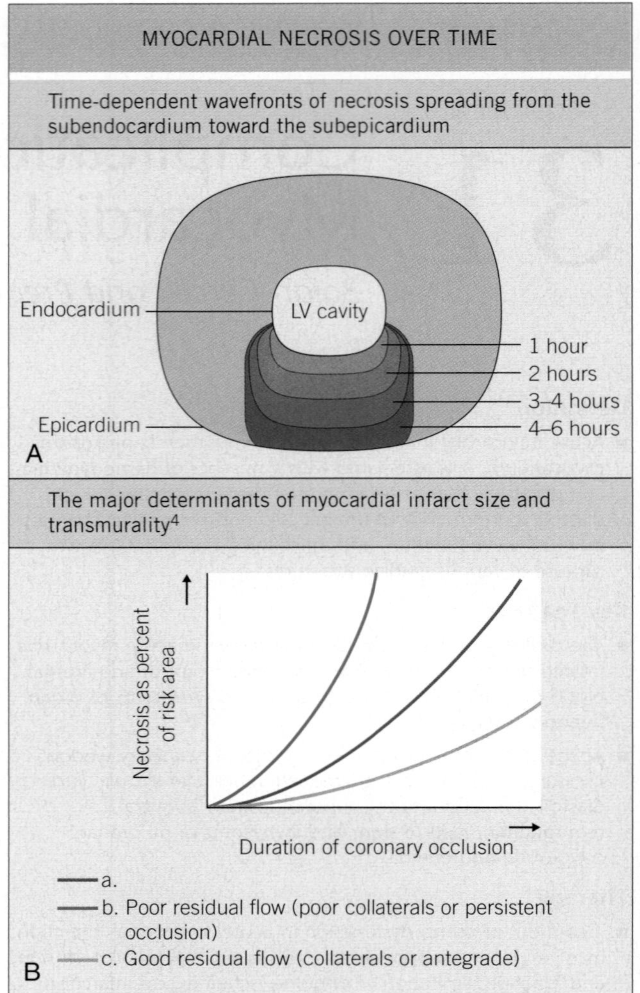

Figure 31.2 Myocardial necrosis over time. A, Time-dependent wavefronts of necrosis spreading from the subendocardium toward the subepicardium after coronary occlusion. LV, left ventricular. **B,** Time-dependent nature of the evolution of myocardial necrosis after acute coronary artery occlusion and the modulating influence of residual flow.

infarction is the culprit artery the left circumflex coronary artery.[6,7] Right ventricular infarction related to occlusion of the left anterior descending coronary artery is rare.

Myocardial infarction can result in acute mitral regurgitation due to

- papillary muscle and left ventricular dysfunction, with annular dilatation and incomplete coaptation of mitral leaflets;
- rupture of the tip or, less commonly, the trunk of the papillary muscle; and
- rarely, rupture of chordae tendineae.

In one report of 47 patients with acute mitral regurgitation, 31 cases were due to papillary muscle rupture and 16 were from other causes.[8] The high propensity of papillary muscles for ischemia and infarction is related partly to their disadvantaged blood supply at the terminus of cardiac arterial circulation. In addition, papillary muscles are subjected to a high degree of tension development during systole, with high oxygen need similar to that of subendocardial myocardium. In many cases, mitral regurgitation results from papillary muscle dysfunction when papillary muscle contraction occurs along an abnormal axis. The axis is shifted inappropriately by coexistent ventricular dilatation and dyssynergy, and the mitral leaflets are unable to coapt appropriately in systole. The anterolateral papillary muscle receives blood supply from the left anterior descending coronary artery and from the left circumflex coronary artery. For the posteromedial papillary muscle, the perfusion is predominantly from the posterior descending branch of the dominant coronary artery (commonly the right but occasionally the left circumflex coronary artery). Both papillary muscles receive chordal attachment from both mitral leaflets. Ischemia, infarction, and rupture are 5 to 10 times more common in the posteromedial papillary muscle than in the anterolateral papillary muscle because of more inconsistent blood supply to the posteromedial papillary muscle. In patients with papillary muscle rupture, the right coronary artery tends to be the culprit artery in about 70% and the circumflex in about 30% of patients. In patients with non–rupture-related mitral regurgitation, the culprit artery tends to be the right in 27%, circumflex in 33%, right and circumflex in 33%, and left anterior descending in 6% of patients. Likewise, the extent of coronary artery disease is also variable, with single-vessel disease occurring in 44% of patients with rupture compared with 13% of patients without papillary rupture. Papillary muscle rupture may even occur with small infarcts with minor electrocardiographic and enzyme abnormalities. The left ventricular ejection fraction may be higher in patients with acute mitral regurgitation from papillary muscle rupture compared with that in patients without rupture.[8] Rupture of papillary muscle tends to occur between 2 and 9 days after infarction; but in up to 35% of cases, it may occur within 24 hours of onset of infarction, particularly in patients who received thrombolytic therapy.[9] The most frequent form of papillary muscle rupture involves one of the smaller heads of the papillary muscle, whereas rupture of the main trunk of the papillary muscle is less common (Fig. 31.3a). In a series of 22 patients, 15 (68%) had partial rupture of the body or one or more tips of the papillary muscle, and complete rupture was found in 7 (32%) patients.[9]

Interventricular septal rupture is another rare complication and occurs in 0.5% to 2% of cases of AMI. It is responsible for 1% to 5% of all infarct-related deaths (Fig. 31.4a).[10] Septal rupture occurs equally frequently in anterior and inferior or posterior infarction. In a series of patients from our institution, 45% of septal ruptures occurred with anterior infarction, 45% occurred with inferior-posterior infarction, and 10% occurred with combined anterior and posterior-inferior infarction.[11] Septal rupture is associated with infarction of the interventricular septum as well as a variable extent of the left or right ventricular myocardium. The rupture is located basally in patients with inferior infarcts and apically in patients with anterior infarcts. Simple septal rupture is a discrete defect with direct through-and-through communication. The entrance and exit of the defect are at the same level of the septum. In contrast, complex septal rupture consists of irregular, serpiginous, often multiple tears in the necrotic myocardium. The inferiorly located defects are more often of the complex type; apical defects are more often discrete.[12] Single-vessel disease is found in 40% to 55% of patients, with 62% having right coronary artery and 38% having left anterior descending involvement. Rupture of the septum may occur within the first 24 hours of onset of infarction or as late as 2 weeks. In non-reperfused infarcts, septal rupture mostly (89%) tends to occur between 3 and 7 days after infarction, on an average

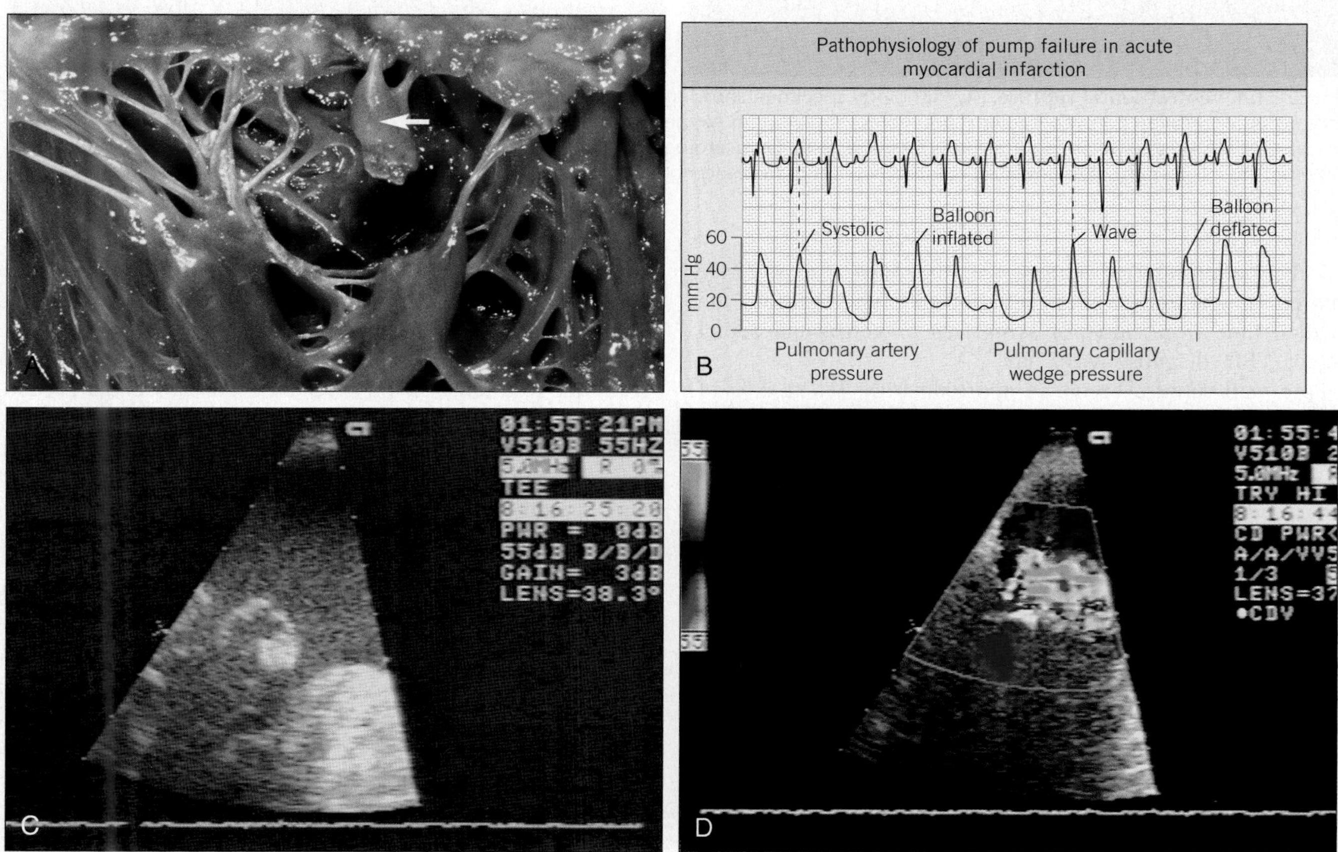

Figure 31.3 Papillary muscle rupture. A, Pathology specimen showing a ruptured papillary muscle. **B,** Hemodynamic findings in acute severe mitral regurgitation showing a large *v* wave in the wedge pressure tracing reflected onto the pulmonary artery pressure tracing. **C** and **D,** Transesophageal echocardiographic Doppler findings in papillary muscle rupture showing the triangular head of the papillary muscle attached to the flail mitral leaflet **(C)** and anteriorly directed color-flow jet of severe mitral regurgitation **(D)**.

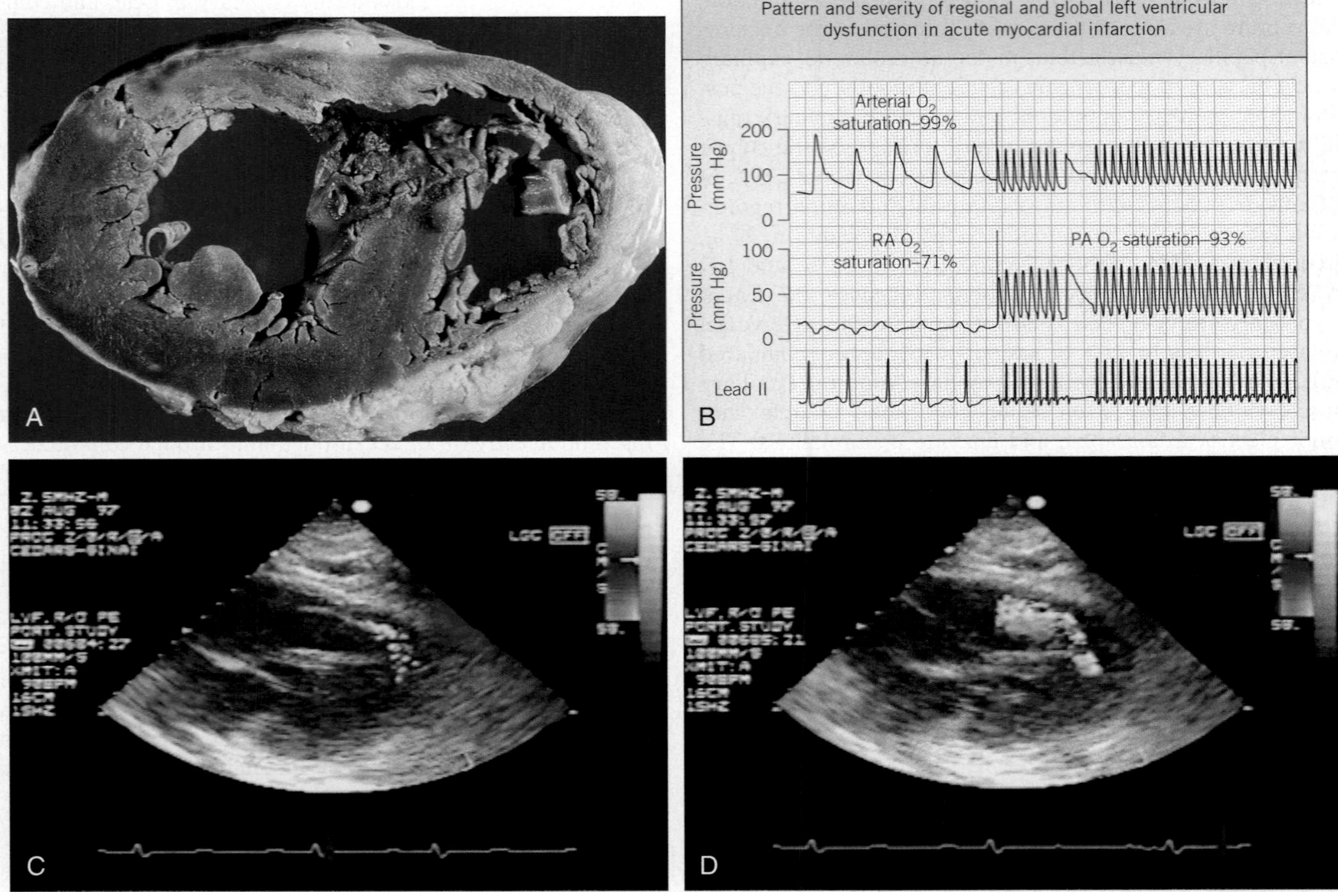

Figure 31.4 Ventral septal rupture. A, Pathology specimen showing an acute posterior interventricular septal rupture. **B,** Hemodynamic findings in a postinfarction ventricular septal defect showing an oxygen saturation step-up in the blood from the pulmonary artery (PA) compared with that from the right atrium (RA). **C** and **D,** Echocardiographic Doppler findings in a postinfarction ventricular septal defect showing the left-to-right shunt–related color-flow jet and a dilated right ventricle.

2.2 days after inferior infarcts and 6.2 days after anterior infarcts. In patients treated with thrombolytic therapy, the median time from onset of symptoms to ventricular septal defect (VSD) diagnosis was 1 day.[13]

Free wall rupture occurs in approximately 1% to 8% of patients and accounts for 7% to 24% of infarction-related deaths (Fig. 31.5). It accounts for a larger percentage of death in patients who have received thrombolytic therapy (12.1%) compared with those who have not (6.1%).[14] Up to 40% of ruptures occur within 24 hours of onset of symptoms, and most occur within 1 week.[10] The infarction is transmural, with persistently occluded infarct-related artery and sparse collaterals. The extent of the infarct can be variable, and even very small transmural infarcts can lead to rupture. The anterior and inferior walls of the left ventricle are equally frequently involved, whereas rupture of the right ventricle is very rare. Left ventricular hypertrophy may be protective. Three types of rupture have been described: slit-like tear within the infarcted area, erosion of the infarcted myocardium at the border of infarcted and viable myocardium, and early pseudoaneurysm formation.[15,16]

In a minority of patients, free wall rupture is followed by the formation of a pseudoaneurysm when rupture is followed by containment of the hemopericardium by circumferential adhesions between the pericardium and the epicardium or scar tissue (Fig. 31.6a). Left ventricular pseudoaneurysm occurs in 0.5% of patients referred for cardiac catheterization. In a recent review, 55% of pseudoaneurysms were due to myocardial infarction, 15% were the result of surgery, 7% were due to trauma, and 5% resulted from infection. Pseudoaneurysms were posterior in 43% and anteroapical in 42%.[17] Rare examples of a variant of pseudoaneurysm in which a thin layer of epicardium remains intact over an area of intramyocardial rupture of an infarct have been reported (pseudo-pseudoaneurysm); this can simulate a pseudoaneurysm on various noninvasive imaging techniques.

Infarct expansion is a fixed, permanent, regional thinning and expansion of the infarct zone that predisposes to true aneurysm formation and rupture.[18] Free wall rupture occurs in only 1% to 2% of patients without significant infarct expansion. Infarct expansion is caused by defective infarct healing or increased left ventricular wall stress with slippage of necrotic myofibrils, causing regional thinning and expansion. It occurs in 35% to 42% of transmural anterior or anteroapical infarcts and less often with other sites of infarction.

A true left ventricular aneurysm occurs in 3.5% to 38% of patients surviving acute transmural myocardial infarction. In one prospective series, dyskinesis and aneurysm were observed with anterior infarction in 77% and with

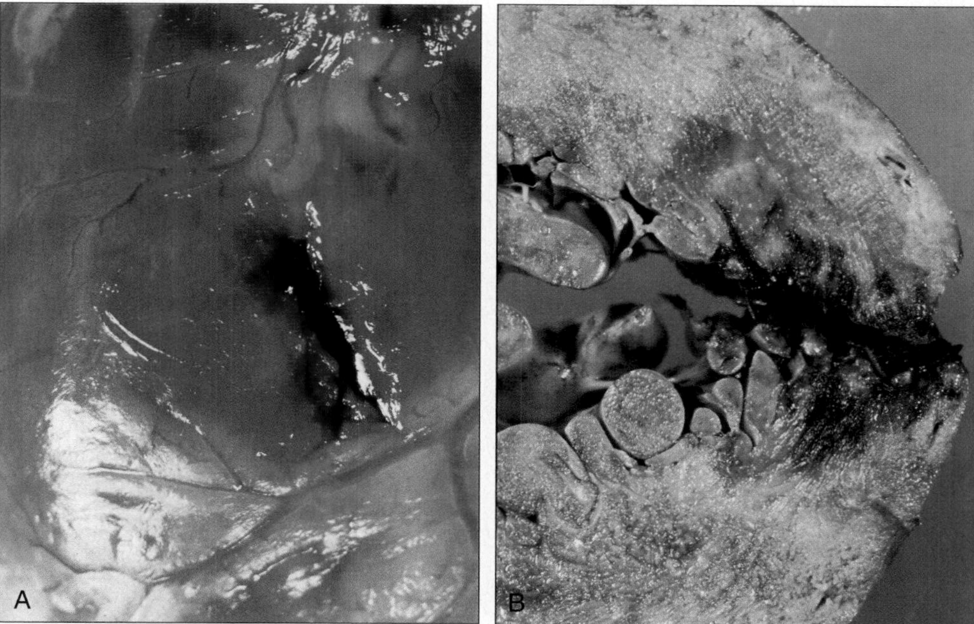

Figure 31.5 Free wall rupture. A and **B,** Pathology specimen of an acute postinfarction free wall rupture.

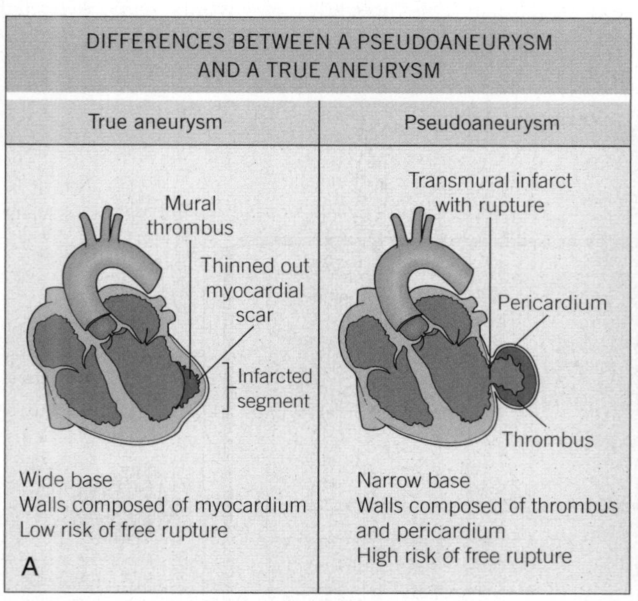

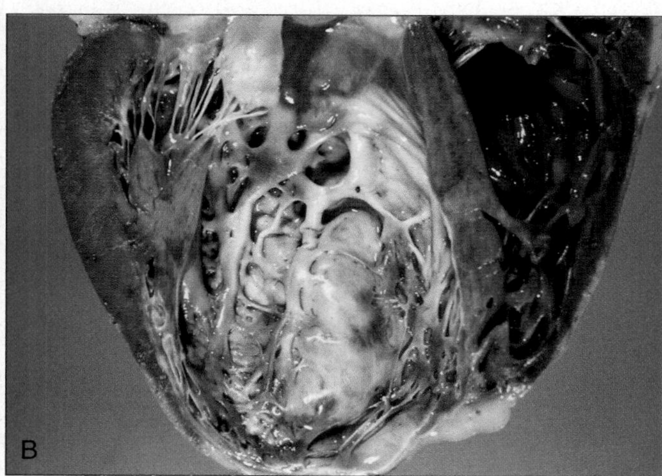

Figure 31.6 Pseudoaneurysm and true aneurysm. A, The features of a true ventricular aneurysm compared with those of a false ventricular aneurysm. **B,** A pathologic specimen of a true ventricular aneurysm.

inferoposterobasal infarction in 17% of patients.[19] The aneurysm is a circumscribed, noncontractile outpouching of the left ventricle. It forms when the necrotic tissue stretches, thins, and expands. Initially, the aneurysm contains necrotic tissue, but the walls become densely fibrotic and may even calcify (Fig. 31.6b). The aneurysms vary in size, have a wide base, and are frequently lined by thrombus. Anterior aneurysms were first observed within days in 12 of 27 patients who eventually developed aneurysms. These early observations were made by use of echocardiography and probably represented examples of regional myocardial dyskinesia, which generally precedes the development of aneurysms in anterior infarction. Regional dyskinesia is rarely observed in patients with posterior infarcts, who develop aneurysms generally within 3 months after the acute infarction. A ventricular aneurysm puts the entire ventricle at a mechanical disadvantage by splinting adjacent normal myocardium as well as by predisposing to malalignment of papillary muscles with consequent mitral regurgitation. Contractile energy expended by normal myocardium is wasted by the aneurysm during its passive systolic outward bulging. Progressive congestive heart failure and cardiomegaly can thus develop after aneurysm formation. In spite of the high frequency of associated mural thrombosis in ventricular aneurysms (15% to 77% at necropsy or surgery), the frequency of clinically recognized systemic embolism is low (2% to 5%). Ventricular aneurysms also tend to predispose to late ventricular arrhythmias and sudden death. The arrhythmias are thought to originate from re-entry circuits at the junction of aneurysm to normal myocardium. In contrast to a pseudoaneurysm, free rupture of a true aneurysm is extremely rare.

PATHOPHYSIOLOGY OF PUMP FAILURE IN ACUTE MYOCARDIAL INFARCTION

The classic pathophysiologic paradigm of pump failure in AMI is shown in Figure 31.7a. The clinical syndrome of pump failure in AMI results chiefly from contractile (systolic) and diastolic dysfunction of the left ventricle.[10,20,21] In some patients, however, the syndrome of pump failure may result from other complications of AMI, such as predominant right ventricular dysfunction, acute mitral regurgitation, left-to-right interventricular shunt from septal rupture, or cardiac tamponade from free wall rupture.[10,21] Pump failure may be precipitated, worsened, or perpetuated by additional factors, such as sustained or recurrent supraventricular or ventricular arrhythmias, severe bradyarrhythmias including complete heart block, relative or absolute hypovolemia, inappropriate use of negative inotropic drugs, infection, or blood loss.

Contractile dysfunction in AMI ranges from regional hypokinesis (reduced contraction) and akinesis (lack of contraction) to dyskinesis (paradoxical systolic expansion).[10,21] Progressive abnormalities of regional myocardial function and increasing extent of involved myocardium result in increased left ventricular end-systolic volume with a consequent decrease in stroke volume and ejection fraction (Fig. 31.7b). In general, with involvement of 10% of the left ventricle, the left ventricular ejection fraction declines with minimal decrease in stroke volume; on the other hand, fatal cardiogenic shock is usually associated with involvement of 40% or more of the left ventricular myocardium.[22] Infarct expansion also contributes to an overall deterioration of ventricular function. Infarct expansion is caused by defective infarct healing or increased left ventricular wall stress, with slippage of necrotic myofibrils causing regional thinning and expansion.[23] It occurs in 35% to 42% of transmural anterior or anteroapical infarcts, with a lower incidence for other sites of infarction.[23] The expansion begins within hours of an infarction and progresses during the first week. The expansion distorts left ventricular shape, imposing additional stress on undamaged myocardium. Eventually, regional expansion contributes to global left ventricular remodeling associated with an increase in left ventricular size and volume, with compensatory hypertrophy and decrease in ejection fraction. This cascade of events can eventually

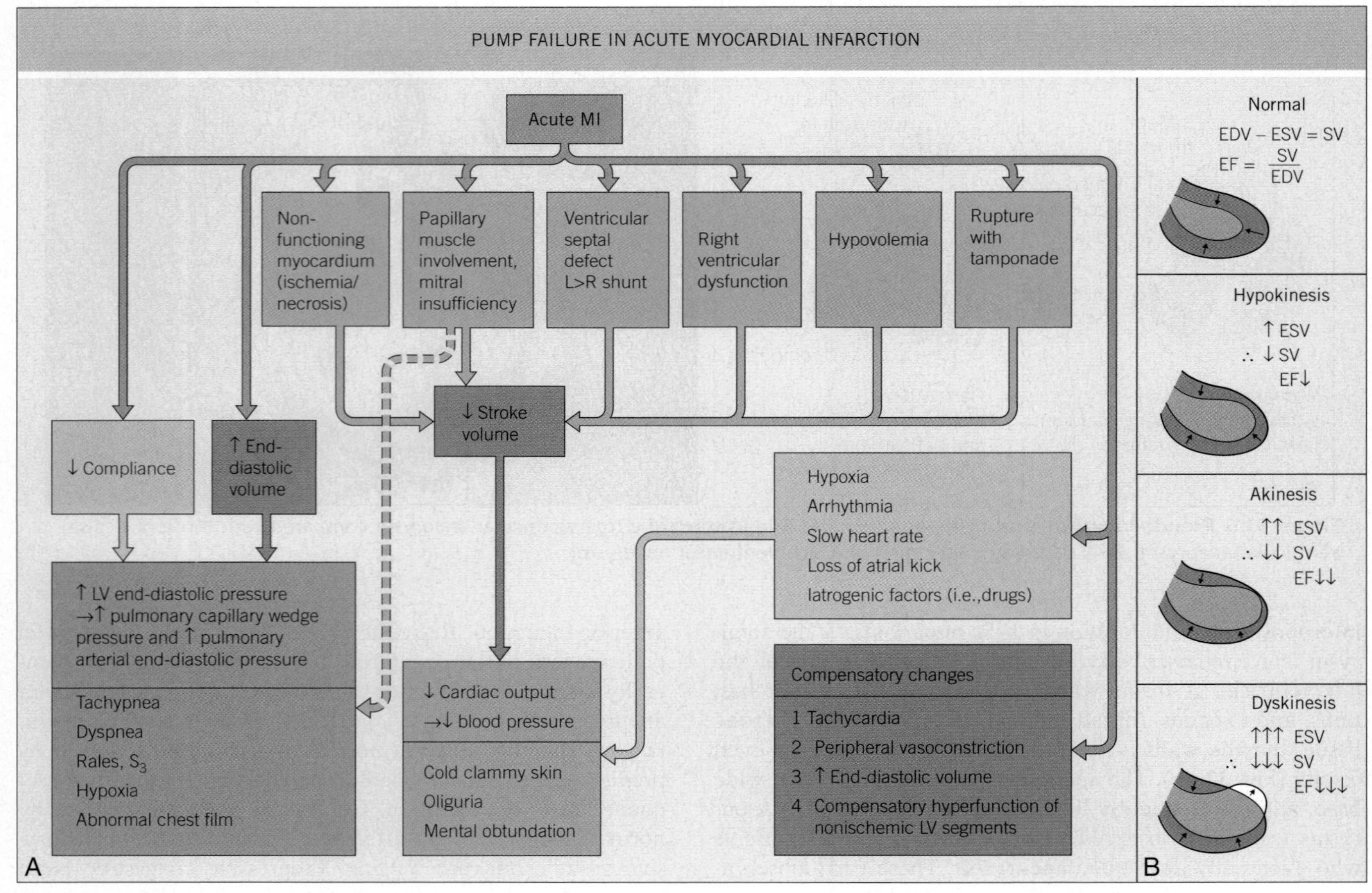

Figure 31.7 Pump failure in acute myocardial infarction. A, Pathophysiology of pump failure in acute myocardial infarction (MI). **B,** Pattern and severity of regional and global left ventricular dysfunction in acute myocardial infarction. EDV, end-diastolic volume; EF, ejection fraction; ESV, end-systolic volume; LV, left ventricular; SV, stroke volume.

precipitate or worsen congestive heart failure.[23] The noninfarcted regions may exhibit compensatory hyperkinesis, thereby attenuating decline in overall ejection fraction; however, in patients with multivessel coronary artery disease, noninfarcted regions could become ischemic with associated contractile dysfunction, contributing to a decline in overall left ventricular ejection fraction. Clinical evidence of left ventricular failure is frequently observed when contractile dysfunction involves more than 25% of the left ventricle. Other compensatory mechanisms that are activated to attenuate adverse hemodynamic consequences of left ventricular dysfunction include ventricular dilatation, sympathoadrenal activation with increase in heart rate, and peripheral vascular resistance; however, these adaptive mechanisms eventually contribute to further compromise of ventricular and mitral valve function, arrhythmias, and peripheral perfusion.

Left ventricular diastolic compliance is generally reduced in AMI and may be detectable even with the limited extent of infarction. It reflects alterations in viscoelastic properties of the ischemic and necrotic tissue from cellular and interstitial edema in the acute phase and healing with fibrosis in the subacute and chronic phases.[10,20,21] Acute right ventricular dilatation and dysfunction may also contribute to the decreased left ventricular compliance through leftward bulging of interventricular septum and an increase in intrapericardial pressure.[24]

A new paradigm that includes the role of a systemic inflammatory response syndrome has been proposed.[25] Patients with large infarcts have elevation of body temperature, elevated white blood cell count, increased levels of C-reactive protein, and interleukins as markers of inflammation. Inflammatory mediators (like tumor necrosis factor α, interleukins 1 and 6) induce inducible nitric oxide synthase in many cell types, which leads, at least in experimental models, to increased toxic levels of nitric oxide and cytotoxic nitric oxide–derived species. The presence of these high levels of nitric oxide and related species leads to inhibition of myocardial contractility, reduced catecholamine responsivity, and induction of systemic vasodilatation. The exact role and significance of this paradigm have not yet been established. Initial clinical attempts at inhibition of the inflammatory response were promising. The recent larger trial with a nonselective nitric oxide synthase inhibitor has not been successful.[26] The role of inflammatory response or systemic inflammatory response syndrome in genesis of cardiogenic shock remains nevertheless intriguing. The average ejection fraction in the SHOCK trial was 31%. Similar systolic impairment is often seen in uncomplicated myocardial infarction, and survivors of cardiogenic shock have good functional status at follow-up. These observations do suggest a reversible temporary vascular component of cardiogenic shock, in addition to the classic paradigm of progressive myocardial ischemia and necrosis.[27]

The clinical syndrome of pump failure and shock in AMI may also result from mechanical complications, such as acute mitral regurgitation (resulting from papillary muscle rupture, severe left ventricular dysfunction with annular dilatation, and papillary muscle dysfunction), interventricular septal rupture with a resultant acute VSD and a left-to-right shunt, and subacute or acute free wall rupture leading to hemopericardium and cardiac tamponade.

Acute mitral regurgitation after myocardial infarction can further contribute to hemodynamic abnormalities, leading to clinical manifestations of pump failure. Depending on the severity of regurgitation as well as the overall compliance of the left atrium, acute mitral regurgitation results in increases in left atrial and pulmonary capillary wedge and pulmonary arterial pressures, leading to pulmonary congestion or pulmonary edema. Reduced forward flow contributes to a reduction in cardiac output and blood pressure. Acute unloading effects of mitral regurgitation may paradoxically increase left ventricular ejection fraction, especially in patients with papillary muscle rupture. Thus, patients with papillary muscle rupture rapidly develop pulmonary congestion and pulmonary edema and progress to hypotension and shock. In a series of 22 patients, 19 of 22 (86%) presented with pulmonary edema or shock.[9]

Rupture of the septum results in an acute left-to-right shunt with right ventricular volume overload, increased pulmonary blood flow, and reduced systemic blood flow. Reduction in systemic blood flow results in a low-output hypotensive syndrome that frequently progresses to shock. In one series of patients, cardiogenic shock was present in 50% and pulmonary congestion in 23% of patients.[11] The left ventricular ejection fraction is variably depressed or normal, depending on the magnitude of associated infarction. The right ventricular ejection fraction may also be depressed secondary to right ventricular volume overload and increased pulmonary arterial pressure or because of concomitant ischemic damage of the right ventricle in patients with inferior-posterior myocardial infarction.

Free wall rupture occurs when myocardial necrosis is transmural with persistently occluded infarct-related artery and sparse or no collaterals. Loss of structural integrity of the infarcted area, leading to rupture, may result not only from myocyte necrosis but also from the additive effects of acute proteolytic degradation of interstitial collagen matrix of the heart due to activation of matrix-degrading metalloproteinases.[10,28] Free wall rupture in some series occurred more often after first infarction, in the elderly, in women, and in those with a history of systemic hypertension or hypertension complicating myocardial infarction. Early ambulation and short-term use of anti-inflammatory drugs (steroids, indomethacin) and anticoagulants have also been associated with increased risk of rupture in some studies. In the National Registry of Myocardial Infarction, there was a clustering of ruptures during the first 24 hours in patients treated with thrombolytic therapy. In these patients, death occurred nearly 4 days earlier than in patients not receiving thrombolytic therapy and dying of other causes (2.7 versus 6.3 days).[29,30] It is conceivable that thrombolytic therapy, if it is administered late, more than 11 hours after onset of symptoms, after transmural necrosis is complete, may increase the risk of cardiac rupture or hemopericardium. Thrombolytic therapy may contribute to cardiac rupture in transmural infarcts through plasmin generation and plasmin-induced activation of matrix-degrading metalloproteinases in the myocardium. In contrast, timely reperfusion therapy, within 6 to 7 hours of symptom onset, before transmural spread of the necrotic wavefront, may actually halt transmural spread of necrosis and reduce the risk of free wall rupture by preserving a viable shell of epicardial tissue.

Free wall rupture results in acute or subacute hemopericardium with cardiac tamponade, which compromises cardiac filling and leads to subacute or acute reduction in cardiac output and arterial blood pressure.[31] In contrast, primary percutaneous coronary intervention was shown to consistently reduce the risk of cardiac rupture. There were no cases of rupture among 103 patients with primary percutaneous coronary intervention compared with 2.8% in 1162 patients treated with thrombolytic therapy and 2.4% in 1112 patients who did not receive reperfusion therapy.[32]

Ischemia and infarction of the right ventricle occur in as many as 30% to 40% of patients with acute inferior or posterior myocardial infarction.[10,21,33,34] The ischemia and necrosis also involve the posterior septum and variable degrees of inferoposterior wall of the left ventricle. Although some patients with right ventricular infarction may have little or only subclinical hemodynamic compromise, many develop hypotension and a low-output syndrome often accompanied by bradycardia and atrioventricular block.[10,21,33] The predominant mechanism by which acute right ventricular infarction leads to a low-output hypotensive state is by reduction of left ventricular end-diastolic volume and filling. This results from reduced right ventricular stroke output as well as an increase in intrapericardial pressure due to acute right ventricular dilatation.[33] Accompanying bradycardia and atrioventricular block and loss of synchronized atrial kick, a result of increased vagal tone or ischemia of the sinus or atrioventricular node, contribute to the hemodynamic compromise in this condition.

CLINICAL PRESENTATION OF PUMP FAILURE

Isolated Pulmonary Congestion

Pulmonary congestion without overt manifestations of hypotension or vital organ hypoperfusion is present in 15% to 20% of patients with AMI and results from an elevated pulmonary capillary wedge pressure (usually 18 to 25 mm Hg) due to decreased left ventricular diastolic compliance or increased end-diastolic volume, or both. Mitral regurgitation may also contribute to elevation of pulmonary capillary wedge pressure. Clinical manifestations include dyspnea, orthopnea, tachypnea, bibasilar post-tussive pulmonary rales or a palpable or audible S_3 gallop, mild to moderate hypoxemia, and radiologic evidence of mild to moderate pulmonary congestion.

Acute Pulmonary Edema without Hypotension

Acute pulmonary edema is a more severe form of pulmonary congestion that results from a rapid increase in lung water content. It is characterized by acute respiratory distress, bilateral pulmonary rales with or without wheezing, impaired pulmonary gas exchange, and signs of sympathetic overactivity such as cool, clammy, and diaphoretic skin, often with increased heart rate and blood pressure; however, in some patients, there may be bradycardia due to associated atrioventricular or intraventricular conduction block and hypotension due to severe reduction in cardiac output. Acute pulmonary edema complicating myocardial infarction is associated with a high mortality of 10% to 25%.

Pulmonary edema results from a rapid increase in the pulmonary capillary wedge pressure, usually greater than 25 mm Hg. Patients with pulmonary edema are frequently severely hypoxemic and may also exhibit acidosis resulting from carbon dioxide retention and lactic acidosis. Acute pulmonary edema generally occurs with extensive left ventricular systolic dysfunction resulting from extensive AMI or from cumulative effects of previous and new myocardial infarction, although reduced diastolic compliance may occasionally be the chief culprit. In some patients, profound global myocardial ischemia in association with relatively small or modest myocardial necrosis may also result in pulmonary edema (ischemic paralysis). Acute pulmonary edema may also complicate severe acute mitral regurgitation regardless of the severity of left ventricular infarction or systolic dysfunction.

Shock Syndrome (Cardiogenic Shock)

Cardiogenic shock is a syndrome of acute, severe, and prolonged tissue hypoperfusion with markedly reduced cardiac output and blood pressure. The syndrome is usually diagnosed as the presence of sustained hypotension (usually systolic blood pressure of less than 90 mm Hg) and signs and symptoms of vital organ hypoperfusion, such as oliguria, clouded sensorium, and cool and clammy skin. The shock syndrome in AMI may result from one or more of the following:

- severe contractile dysfunction of the left ventricle with a markedly reduced ejection fraction (ventriculopenic shock);
- severe contractile dysfunction of the right ventricle; and
- mechanical complications, such as acute mitral regurgitation, VSD, or cardiac free wall rupture with cardiac tamponade.[10,20,22,35]

In the SHOCK prestudy registry, postinfarction shock was due to left ventricular pump failure in 85%, acute VSD or acute mitral insufficiency in 8%, right ventricular failure in 2%, and concurrent illness in 5% of patients.[5] Cardiogenic shock occurs in 5% to 7% of patients who present with ST elevation and often develops several hours after admission.[4,5,35,36] In the National Registry of Myocardial Infarction, shock was present in 1% of the patients at the time of hospital admission and in up to 2.9% in randomized trials of patients with non–ST elevation acute coronary syndrome.[37]

Types of Shock in Acute Myocardial Infarction

Ventriculopenic Shock

The clinical manifestations of cardiogenic shock due to extensive left ventricular damage include cool and clammy skin, with evidence of organ hypoperfusion (i.e., oliguria), and impaired mental status. Pulse is generally thready and rapid with a narrow pulse pressure. Supraventricular and ventricular arrhythmias are commonly observed in patients with shock. Heart sounds are often feeble, and evidence of left ventricular dysfunction, such as atrial or ventricular gallops and pulmonary rales of varying distribution, is frequently present. Hemodynamic evaluation generally demonstrates a markedly reduced cardiac index (generally below 2.2 L/min per m^2), an elevated pulmonary capillary wedge pressure (often exceeding 18 mm Hg), and an elevated systemic vascular resistance with systolic blood pressure of 90 mm Hg or less. Noninvasive assessment of left ventricular function by two-dimensional echocardiography or radionuclide ventriculography generally reveals a dilated left ventricle with extensive wall motion abnormalities and a reduced ejection fraction (often below 30%).

Shock from Mechanical Complications

Acute Papillary Muscle Rupture

The incidence of mitral regurgitation is high after AMI and varies considerably (3.4% to 74%) according to the method of detection and the reported severity.[38,39] The causes of mitral regurgitation after myocardial infarction include papillary muscle rupture, chordal rupture, ischemia or scar of the papillary muscle, mitral annulus dilatation, tethering of the mitral leaflets due to change in left ventricular geometry, and preexisting mitral regurgitation. It is the severe acute mitral regurgitation that occurs with papillary muscle rupture that is of most clinical significance. Acute mitral regurgitation is associated with the development of a new apical systolic murmur of variable intensity, duration, and radiation; in some patients, however, the murmur may even be completely absent (silent mitral regurgitation).[10,21] A palpable thrill is rare and occurs in less than 2% of cases. The chest radiograph shows pulmonary congestion or edema, occasionally preferentially distributed to right upper lung lobes, simulating pulmonary infiltrate. This preferential location is due to a regurgitant jet directed toward the orifice of the right upper lobe pulmonary vein. Diagnosis can be established at the bedside with echocardiography and Doppler studies, which show a flail mitral leaflet, inferoposterior wall motion abnormalities, and the presence of severe mitral regurgitation. The characteristic echo of the ruptured tip of the papillary muscle can sometimes be demonstrated by transesophageal echocardiography only (see Fig. 31.3c, d). Nevertheless, normal or hyperdynamic left ventricular wall motion with mitral regurgitation in a postinfarction patient with pulmonary edema and shock should suggest the diagnosis. The majority of patients, though, have reduced left ventricular function (average ejection fraction, 37%).[40] Pulmonary capillary wedge pressure is elevated, with tall v waves sometimes reflected onto the pulmonary arterial tracing as well (see Fig. 31.3b).

Acute Ventricular Septal Rupture

Acute ventricular septal rupture is characterized by a new loud holosystolic precordial murmur with widespread radiation with a palpable systolic thrill in about 50% of cases. Right ventricular volume overload secondary to the shunt, concomitant right ventricular ischemic damage, and tricuspid regurgitation may produce signs of systemic venous congestion out of proportion to those of pulmonary venous congestion. Symptoms often include chest pain and shortness of breath, followed by progressive hypotension and shock.[41,42] The diagnosis can be confirmed rapidly at the bedside by echocardiography and Doppler studies (see Fig. 31.4c, d).[10,21] Bedside right-sided heart catheterization can also be used to establish the diagnosis by right-sided heart blood oximetry, which permits an approximate calculation of the degree of left-to-right shunt (see Fig. 31.4b). The incidence of acute septal rupture has decreased from 1% to 3% in the pre-reperfusion era to only 0.2% to 0.4% in patients treated with thrombolytic therapy.[13] In the Should We Emergently Revascularize Occluded Coronaries for Cardiogenic Shock registry, only 3.9% of patients had ventricular septal rupture. The GUSTO-I study suggested that ventricular septal rupture is more common in patients with anterior myocardial infarction, whereas previous experience was that the incidence is equal in patients with anterior and inferior infarcts. Septal rupture occurs more often in patients with unsuccessful reperfusion[13] and inadequate collateral circulation. It occurs earlier in the course in patients treated with thrombolytic therapy, with a median time of approximately 1 day, compared with almost a week in patients who do not receive thrombolytic therapy.[43]

Cardiac Free Wall Rupture

Free wall rupture can present as a catastrophic syndrome with sudden onset of tearing chest pain, rapidly followed by hypotension, distention of neck veins, and pulseless electrical activity. Vagal stimulation is prominent, with junctional or sinus bradycardia. Patients may exhibit agitation and confusion. Death ensues rapidly because of hemopericardium and tamponade (see Fig. 31.5).

In some patients, free wall rupture develops with intermittent chest pain and progressive tamponade that evolves during several hours to days before death results from the syndrome of subacute cardiac rupture.[10,21,44,45] Patients usually have episodes of chest pain, with minimal or no additional electrocardiographic changes. Prompt clinical suspicion allows the diagnosis to be confirmed by echocardiography and subsequent diagnostic pericardiocentesis. Although long-term survival without repair has been reported, prompt surgical repair has been shown to be feasible with excellent long-term survival.[36]

In a minority of patients, free wall rupture is followed by the formation of a pseudoaneurysm when rupture is followed by containment of the hemopericardium by circumferential adhesions between the pericardium and the epicardium or scar tissue. Almost 90% of patients with pseudoaneurysms are symptomatic, with symptoms of congestive heart failure being common. Rarely, systolic and diastolic murmurs, presumably related to oscillation of blood across the narrow neck of the aneurysm, may be present, thus simulating valvular heart disease.[10,21] The chest radiograph is usually abnormal, with an enlarged or distorted cardiac silhouette, and persistent ST-segment elevation may be noted in about 20% of cases. Echocardiography shows some abnormality in 90% of patients but is diagnostic in only one third of patients. The diagnostic echocardiographic features are pericardial effusion and the demonstration of an aneurysm with a narrow neck and discontinuation of the endocardial lining at the site of the aneurysmal communication with the left ventricle. Pericardial effusion was present in 75% of the patients with free wall rupture or tamponade in the SHOCK trial registry[31] and was generalized in only two thirds of the patients. López-Sendón reported that presence of an effusion of more than 5 mm was 100% sensitive for the diagnosis of subacute ventricular wall rupture.[46] It does appear that in some patients, the acquisition of adequate images is impossible or the effusion is so small that it is not easily detectable by echocardiography but may still produce substantial hemodynamic effects. Other diagnostic techniques, such as transesophageal echocardiography, magnetic resonance imaging, radionuclide ventriculography, and contrast left ventriculography, may also be helpful in establishing the diagnosis. Unlike true aneurysm, the pseudoaneurysm is prone to rupture with an invariably fatal outcome.[17] The incidence of free wall rupture in the reperfusion era is between 2% and 3%, accounting for 10% to 15% of mortality.[31,46] The rupture is more likely in patients older than 70 years, with anterior infarct, and when patients are treated more than 2 hours after onset of the symptoms. Thrombolytic therapy also increases the risk of rupture compared with primary angioplasty.[47] This is likely due to the lower incidence of successful reperfusion with thrombolytic therapy compared with primary angioplasty.[48] Late thrombolytic therapy, more than 12 hours after onset of symptoms, was suggested to increase the incidence of myocardial rupture, which was not substantiated in the LATE trial.[49]

Right Ventricular Infarction

Right ventricular infarction is shown in Figure 31.8. Significant right ventricular dysfunction should be considered in any patient with acute inferior or posterior myocardial infarction with elevated jugular venous pressure or increased jugular venous pressure during inspiration (Kussmaul's sign) or during abdominal compression (abdominojugular reflux) with little evidence of pulmonary congestion. These findings are present in nearly 50% to 70% of cases. In about 30% of patients, however, jugular venous pressure may not show any detectable abnormalities, or the patient may have pulmonary congestion due to concomitant significant involvement of the left ventricle or mitral regurgitation. A murmur of tricuspid regurgitation secondary to right ventricular papillary muscle dysfunction or pulsus paradoxus simulating cardiac tamponade may occur but is uncommon. The electrocardiogram, in addition to the changes of acute inferior infarction, frequently shows ST-segment elevation in V_1 and right-sided precordial leads (rV_3 or rV_4). Less commonly, ST-segment elevation involves left-sided precordial leads up to V_5, in decreasing magnitude. Such precordial ST elevations may create confusing electrocardiographic patterns that simulate concomitant left anterior descending coronary occlusion but are most likely due to dilatation of the infarcted right ventricle.[33]

Hemodynamic abnormalities in acute right ventricular infarction may vary. Elevated right atrial and right ventricular end-diastolic pressure can be equal to or above the pulmonary capillary wedge pressure. Steep right atrial *y* descent with paradoxical increase in right atrial pressure during inspiration (Kussmaul's sign) and dip and plateau during diastole in the right ventricular pressure tracing are similar to those of cardiac tamponade, constrictive pericarditis, or restrictive myocardial disease.[10,21,31] Right-to-left shunt through a stretched patent foramen ovale may occur when the right atrial pressure is markedly elevated, resulting in arterial desaturation that does not improve with increased fractional inspired oxygen (FIO_2) or mechanical ventilation. Echocardiography demonstrates right ventricular dilatation, right ventricular free wall motion abnormalities, and depressed ejection fraction (<0.39). The left ventricles generally have only mildly depressed ejection fraction (>0.45). Patients with severe biventricular dysfunction should be assessed separately and managed like those with predominantly severe left ventricular dysfunction.

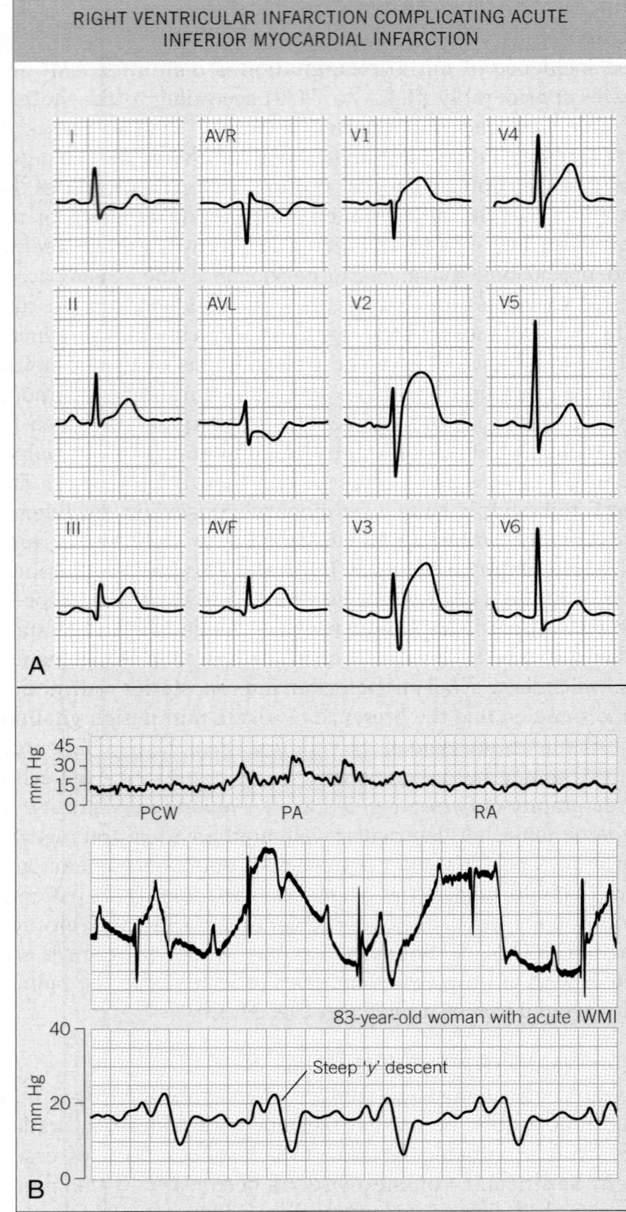

Figure 31.8 Findings in right ventricular infarction complicating an acute inferior myocardial infarction. A, Electrocardiogram showing concomitant ST-segment elevation in V_1 through V_3 due to right ventricular involvement. (From Geft IL, Shah PK, Rodriguez L, et al. ST elevations in leads V_1 to V_5 may be caused by right coronary occlusion and acute right ventricular infarction. Am J Cardiol 1984;53:991–996.) **B,** Hemodynamics showing an elevated right atrial pressure (with a steep *y* descent) and its equalization with the pulmonary wedge pressure, simulating the hemodynamic findings of cardiac tamponade. IWMI, inferior wall myocardial infarction; PA, pulmonary artery pressure; PCW, pulmonary capillary wedge diastolic pressure; RA, right atrial pressure. (Modified from Shah PK, Swan HJC. Predominant right ventricular dysfunction in acute myocardial infarction. Med Rounds 1984;3:6.)

DIAGNOSTIC TECHNIQUES

In addition to clinical assessment, a variety of other techniques are used to diagnose and to assess the severity of hemodynamic compromise, the extent of left and right ventricular regional and global dysfunction, and the presence and location of mechanical complications in patients with AMI. These techniques include bedside hemodynamic assessment with the Swan-Ganz pulmonary artery balloon flotation catheter, echocardiography and Doppler techniques, radioisotope ventriculography, and left-sided heart catheterization.

DIAGNOSTIC TECHNIQUES FOR ASSESSMENT OF PATIENTS WITH HEMODYNAMIC COMPLICATIONS AFTER ACUTE MYOCARDIAL INFARCTION	
Diagnostic Technique	**Useful For**
Bedside hemodynamic monitoring	Clarifying role of hypovolemia versus LV failure Diagnosis of acute mitral regurgitation, acute VSD, RV infarction, and tamponade Assessment of prognosis Selection of appropriate therapy for pump failure Rapid assessment of response to therapy
Left-sided heart catheterization and coronary angiography	Assessment of extent and location of LV regional and global dysfunction, size, shape, and remodeling Assessment of severity of mitral regurgitation Diagnosis and assessment of left-right shunt with a VSD Diagnosis of true aneurysm versus pseudoaneurysm Diagnosis of cardiac rupture Diagnosis of a mural thrombus
Echocardiography and Doppler flow studies	Assessment of regional and global LV/RV dysfunction and size Diagnosis of papillary muscle rupture and mitral regurgitation Diagnosis of acute VSD Diagnosis of true aneurysm, pseudoaneurysm, and mural thrombus Assessment of infarct expansion and LV remodeling Diagnosis of RV infarction and atrial level right-left shunt Diagnosis of pericardial fluid or blood and cardiac tamponade Diagnosis of free wall rupture
Radionuclide imaging Radionuclide ventriculography	Assessment of regional and global LV/RV dysfunction and size Assessment of infarct expansion and remodeling Diagnosis of RV infarction Diagnosis of left-to-right shunt in a VSD (first-pass technique) Diagnosis of true aneurysm and pseudoaneurysm Detection of intrapericardial bleeding in subacute cardiac rupture
Perfusion imaging	Diagnosis of ischemic nonfunctional but viable myocardium Assessment of extent of infarction and prognosis
Infarct-avid imaging	Diagnosis of LV/RV infarction Assessment of infarct size and prognosis

LV, left ventricular; RV, right ventricular; VSD, ventricular septal defect.

Table 31.1 Diagnostic techniques for assessment of patients with hemodynamic complications after acute myocardial infarction.

Table 31.1 summarizes the value of various diagnostic techniques in the assessment of patients with hemodynamic complications after AMI. In the diagnosis of mechanical complications of AMI, echocardiography has largely replaced catheterization as the preferred diagnostic tool. In the GUSTO-I study, echocardiography alone was the most commonly used diagnostic tool to confirm VSD in 25% of the patients.[13]

MANAGEMENT OF HEMODYNAMIC COMPLICATIONS OF ACUTE MYOCARDIAL INFARCTION

General Principles

The overall goals in the management of patients with AMI are as follows:

- Terminate ongoing ischemia, limit myocardial infarct size, and preserve ventricular function. This overall goal is predominantly achieved by restoring and maintaining full infarct-related artery patency (TIMI grade 3 flow) and myocardial perfusion (TIMI myocardial blush grade 3) by use of one or more reperfusion strategies (thrombolytic therapy or direct coronary angioplasty, stenting with adjunctive antithrombotic therapy; rarely, urgent coronary artery bypass surgery).
- Prevent and treat complications with appropriate supportive and definitive therapy.

Thus, in patients with AMI who present with or develop pump failure, reperfusion strategies and supportive therapy must be considered concurrently. Reperfusion therapy is not discussed any further in this chapter because it is discussed in Chapter.[34]

Treatment of Isolated Pulmonary Congestion and Acute Pulmonary Edema

The object of therapy is to ensure adequate arterial oxygenation with the help of supplemental oxygen, to relieve pulmonary venous congestion and edema by rapidly reducing pulmonary capillary wedge pressure, and to maintain an adequate arterial pressure and a stable cardiac rate and rhythm (Table 31.2). Rapid reduction of pulmonary capillary wedge pressure is generally achieved by use of rapidly acting intravenous diuretics such as furosemide (frusemide) or ethacrynic acid along with intravenous vasodilators such as nitroglycerin.[10,21,50] In

MANAGEMENT GUIDELINES FOR ACUTE PULMONARY EDEMA
Immediate objectives
Maintain adequate gas exchange (supplemental oxygen, intubation, CPAP) Restore and maintain normal cardiac rate and rhythm Retard lung fluid filtration and facilitate lung fluid removal by rapidly reducing PCW by ■ redistributive measures (nitrates, other vasodilators, morphine) ■ depletive measures (diuretics, ultrafiltration, improving renal function) ■ improving LV function and reducing MR (vasodilators, inotropes, IABP, reperfusion) ■ maintaining adequate arterial pressure for organ perfusion in hypotensive patients (inotropes, IABP)
Identify and treat precipitating or aggravating factors
Reperfusion and adjunctive IABP to limit ongoing ischemia and necrosis Coronary intervention or surgery for recurrent ischemia and mechanical complications
CPAP, continuous positive airway pressure; IABP, intra-aortic balloon pump; LV, left ventricular; MR, mitral regurgitation, PCW, pulmonary capillary wedge pressure.

Table 31.2 Management guidelines for acute pulmonary edema.

addition, small intravenous doses of morphine sulfate are useful to calm the usually anxious and agitated patient and to reduce dyspnea in patients with severe pulmonary edema by reducing pulmonary capillary wedge pressure. Use of morphine can be associated with hypotension, bradycardia, and respiratory depression. In the retrospective analysis of the CRUSADE database, morphine use was associated with increased risk of in-hospital death.[51] In severely hypertensive patients, infusion of sodium nitroprusside or repeated doses of intravenous enalaprilat may also be extremely useful.[10,21,52] Nitrates reduce pulmonary congestion by preload reduction from venodilatation, by afterload reduction from arteriolar dilatation, and by directly improving left ventricular compliance. When nitrates or other potent vasodilators are used, special care should be taken to prevent hypotension. Excessive diuresis should also be avoided because that may result in electrolyte depletion (notably hypokalemia) as well as hypotension and a low-output state from underfilling of the left ventricle.

In addition to reducing elevated pulmonary capillary wedge pressure, maintaining adequate pulmonary gas exchange requires supplemental oxygen by nasal cannulas or facemask. Endotracheal intubation and mechanical ventilation should be considered in patients who appear moribund, are unable to maintain an arterial partial oxygen tension (Po_2) of at least 60 mm Hg or oxygen saturation above 92%, or develop progressively rising Pco_2 or declining arterial pH. Use of positive end-expiratory pressure with mechanical ventilation may be necessary to maintain adequate systemic oxygenation and allow the use of relatively safe concentrations of oxygen (i.e., $Fio_2 < 60$); such therapy may, however, compromise cardiac output. Meta-analysis of studies evaluating efficacy and safety of noninvasive ventilation—continuous positive airway pressure ventilation and noninvasive positive-pressure ventilation—have suggested that both techniques decrease the need for intubation and that continuous positive airway pressure ventilation is also associated with a reduced mortality in patients with acute pulmonary edema.[53,54] Inotropic vasopressor therapy, intra-aortic balloon pumping, and acute reperfusion in acute pulmonary edema in selected patients are discussed later.

Treatment of Ventriculopenic Shock

Reperfusion-based therapies that limit ongoing myocardial necrosis and prevent reinfarction were shown to reduce mortality. When successful myocardial reperfusion is achieved, the in-hospital mortality is reduced from 80% to 20%. The management that improves ventricular performance and cardiac output to maintain adequate perfusion to vital organs while reducing pulmonary congestion and maintaining adequate pulmonary gas exchange in itself does not affect mortality. Overall, the mortality of ventriculopenic shock remains high, about 50% in-hospital mortality.[22,35,36]

General supportive measures include relief of pain, maintenance of adequate oxygenation and ventilation, correction of electrolyte and acid-base abnormalities, treatment of nausea and vomiting, control of cardiac dysrhythmias, and maintenance of an adequate heart rate, when necessary with atrioventricular synchrony. Specific therapy for "cardiogenic shock" was initially facilitated by bedside hemodynamic monitoring with the Swan-Ganz pulmonary artery balloon flotation catheter.[47] In recent years, Doppler echocardiography has evolved into an excellent bedside tool for guiding the therapy.[55] In the Euro-Heart Survey of acute coronary syndromes, 68% of patients with cardiogenic shock had an echocardiographic evaluation, most within 24 hours, compared with 20.2% who had right-sided heart catheterization.[56]

Specific therapeutic interventions are summarized in Table 31.3. Maintenance of a minimum arterial pressure of 90 to 100 mm Hg and cardiac output sufficient to preserve vital organ function requires the use of pharmacologic agents as well as, in many cases, mechanical circulatory assist. Dopamine, dobutamine, amrinone or milrinone, and less frequently vasoconstrictor agents such as norepinephrine (noradrenaline) are used to maintain arterial blood pressure and cardiac output. Intravenous dopamine exerts its cardiovascular effects by direct stimulation of β-adrenergic and dopaminergic-specific receptors and by release of endogenous norepinephrine from sympathetic nerve endings. At relatively low doses of 2 to 5 μg/kg per minute, a majority of patients demonstrate significant increases in stroke volume and cardiac output mediated by β-adrenergic stimulant effects on myocardial contractility. Also, renal blood flow increases with redistribution toward the inner third of the renal cortex, an effect that is mediated by interaction with dopaminergic-specific receptors. At this dosage, chronotropic and peripheral vasoconstrictor effects tend to be relatively minimal. With increasing doses, there are dose-dependent increases in chronotropic, arrhythmogenic, and α-adrenergic vasoconstrictor and vasopressor effects. These may result in a decrease in tissue perfusion and an increase in pulmonary arterial and left ventricular filling pressures secondary to elevated afterload. Myocardial ischemia may also be provoked by inotropic, chronotropic, and vasopressor effects at higher doses.[10,21] Dobutamine, a synthetic catecholamine, has predominantly β-adrenergically mediated positive inotropic and

LOW-OUTPUT STATE AND SHOCK AFTER ACUTE MYOCARDIAL INFARCTION				
	Recognition			
Underlying Abnormality	Clinical	Hemodynamic	Others	Guide to Management
Ventriculopenic shock	Shock syndrome Rales, S_3 Abnormal chest radiography	Elevated PCW Depressed CI High SVR Low BP	Markedly depressed LVEF (i.e., $\leq$0.30)	Inotropes-pressors to maintain systolic BP approximately 90 mm Hg and CI of > 2 L/m^2 Vasodilators added to keep PCW 12–15 mm Hg IABP if no response to above + general supportive care Consider acute reperfusion with PTCA and/or thrombolysis
Acute severe mitral regurgitation	Shock syndrome Rales, S_3, abnormal radiography Holosystolic murmur; occasionally murmur not heard or soft and brief	Elevated PCW with tall *v* waves Depressed CI High SVR Low BP	LVEF may be normal, elevated, or variably depressed, depending on extent of necrosis of LV Echo shows flail leaflet Doppler shows regurgitation	Vasodilators + inotropes to maintain systolic BP approx. 90, PCW 12–15 mm Hg, and CI > 2 L/m^2 IABP followed by early catheterization and surgery + general supportive care
Acute VSD	Shock syndrome Rales, S_3 Holosystolic murmur with precordial thrill in 50%	O_2 step-up from RA to RV or PA Thermodilution curve shows evidence of shunt	First-pass radionuclide study shows left–right shunt LVEF and RVEF are variable as in mitral regurgitation and depend on extent of necrosis 2D echo visualizes defect Shunt seen on Doppler	Same as above + general supportive care
Hypovolemia	Shock syndrome Lungs and radiographs do not show signs of LV failure (but in some patients may show persistent signs of LV failure if hypovolemia is superimposed on a patient with prior LV failure, generally from overdiuresis) Orthostatic ↑ in HR and/or ↓ in BP	PCW generally <12–15 mm Hg CI depressed SVR may be high BP may be low Some patients with this profile have RV infarction		If patient has clinical evidence of hypoperfusion, then rapid but careful volume expansion until PCW is approximately 15 mm Hg, but no higher than 18 mm Hg
Predominant acute right ventricular infarction	Shock syndrome in a patient with inferior infarction JVD or HJR in 70% of cases Lungs and radiographs generally clear with minimal or no signs of LV failure Occasionally pulsus paradoxus and Kussmaul's sign Rarely severe hypoxia from right–left shunt across a PFO	RA pressure $\geq$ PCW Reduced PA and RV pulse pressure Depressed CI 30% may have normal RA pressure (Volume challenge may bring out occult findings)	Dilated RV with ↓ RVEF (<0.39) LVEF generally >0.45 Some patients have severely depressed LVEF, and such patients should be categorized differently	Increase volume if PCW < 15 mm Hg until PCW is approx 15 mm Hg If no improvement, add inotropic agent and/or vasodilator, depending on BP

BP, blood pressure; CI, cardiac index; 2D, two-dimensional; HJR, hepatojugular reflex; HR, heart rate; IABP, intra-aortic balloon pumping; JVD, jugular venous distention; LV, left ventricular; LVEF, left ventricular ejection fraction; PA, pulmonary artery; PCW, pulmonary capillary wedge pressure; PFO, patent foramen ovale; PTCA, percutaneous transluminal coronary angioplasty; RA, right atrium; RV, right ventricular; RVEF, right ventricular ejection fraction; SVR, systemic vascular resistance; VSD, ventricular septal defect.

Table 31.3 Low-output state and shock after acute myocardial infarction.

chronotropic effects. Dose-related increases in stroke volume, cardiac output, and reduction in left ventricular filling pressures are notable effects of intravenous infusion of dobutamine in both acute and chronic heart failure. Inappropriate increases in heart rate are uncommonly observed at infusion rates below 15 to 20 μg/kg per minute. Dobutamine is generally preferred to dopamine because it tends to produce equivalent increases in cardiac output but with lesser increments in heart rate, a lower risk of arrhythmias, no vasoconstrictor effects, and a more consistent reduction in left ventricular filling pressures. However, relatively modest pressor effect compared with dopamine makes dobutamine, as the sole agent, inappropriate when systemic blood pressure is very low (i.e., <80 mm Hg).[10,21] Norepinephrine is a naturally occurring catecholamine with potent α-adrenergic receptor–stimulating effects and relatively modest β-adrenergically mediated myocardial inotropic and chronotropic effects. The peripheral vasoconstrictor effects of norepinephrine make it a potent pressor agent to maintain adequate arterial pressure in severely hypotensive patients who are unresponsive to dopamine. Little increase or an actual decrease in cardiac output and compromise of peripheral organ blood flow result in later deterioration. Thus, as soon as it is feasible, norepinephrine should be replaced by dopamine or dobutamine. In some patients, noncatecholamine inotropic agents such as milrinone and amrinone may be useful in producing a short-term improvement in cardiac performance. Levosimendan is among a new class of inotropic agents.[57] It sensitizes the contractile apparatus to calcium ions. In addition to positive inotropic effects, levosimendan also has vasodilating effects through the opening of adenosine triphosphate–sensitive potassium channels in vascular smooth muscle cells. Because of this effect, levosimendan is not recommended as a stand-alone agent. It may be used in combination with other vasoactive drugs; however, the experience is quite limited.[58]

The judicious use of vasodilators such as nitrates, nitroprusside, and α-adrenergic receptor–blocking agents, often in combination with positive inotropic agents, may further improve left ventricular performance by reducing ventricular afterload and preload. However, worsening hypotension must be avoided.[10,21]

The use of *N*-monomethyl-l-arginine, a nitric oxide inhibitor, is predicated on the hypothesis that systemic inflammatory response plays a significant role in cardiogenic shock.[59] In a limited study of 11 patients with refractory cardiogenic shock, it significantly increased urine output and blood pressure and was associated with a 72% 30-day survival. In the TRIUMPH study, tilarginine was planned to be evaluated in a randomized fashion in 658 patients with refractory cardiogenic shock after successful reperfusion.[26] The study was prematurely terminated because of lack of effect in an interim analysis. In the 398 enrolled patients, the primary endpoint of 30-day mortality occurred in 48% of the patients treated with tilarginine and in 42% who received placebo. Similarly, a complement-blocking monoclonal antibody, pexelizumab, directed against complement protein C5 appeared to reduce mortality but had no effect on the primary endpoint of infarct size in a trial of 960 patients with ST elevation myocardial infarction undergoing primary percutaneous intervention.[60] In the larger APEX trial of 5745 patients with ST elevation myocardial infarction, pexelizumab had no effect on 30-day mortality (4.06% in the active treatment group and 3.93% in the placebo group; P =.78).[61]

Mechanical Circulatory Assist Devices in Cardiogenic Shock

Intra-aortic Balloon Pump

The intra-aortic balloon pump (IABP) is the most commonly used assist device in the management of patients with cardiogenic shock (Fig. 31.9).[10,21,62-66] Electrocardiographically triggered inflation of the balloon at the onset of diastole in the aorta just distal to the left subclavian artery increases the diastolic pressure and thus the coronary perfusion pressure, augmenting subendocardial blood flow (diastolic augmentation). Presystolic deflation reduces the afterload to the left ventricle as it allows ejection of the stroke volume into the virtually empty space in the descending aorta instead of through the resistance peripheral vessels (presystolic unloading). The combined effects tend to reduce myocardial ischemia and reduce left ventricular diastolic pressures and mitral regurgitation; the forward stroke volume is modestly improved. Most patients with cardiogenic shock demonstrate initial stabilization with IABP, and the SHOCK registry data suggested a 20% risk reduction in mortality with the use of IABP. In the only randomized trial examining the use of IABP with thrombolysis, only 57 patients were randomized, but the 6-month mortality was 39% compared with 80% in patients who received thrombolysis alone (P <.05).[10,21,63] The use of IABP may increase the rate of final infarct-related artery patency after failed thrombolysis or angioplasty and reduce the rate of the composite endpoint of death, reinfarction, revascularization, and ischemia (13% versus 24%).[64,65]

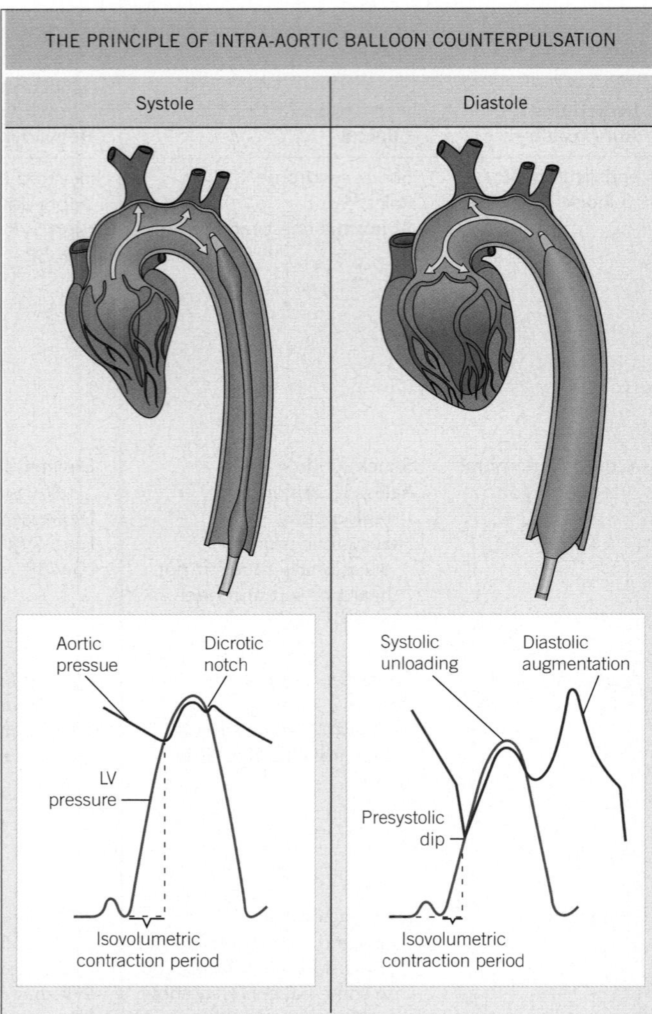

Figure 31.9 The principle of intra-aortic balloon pump. Initiation of balloon inflation is timed to the arterial dicrotic notch, producing an augmentation in proximal aortic diastolic pressure. Deflation of the balloon is timed to begin just before the onset of the next ventricular systole, which produces the systolic unloading effect (presystolic dip). LV, left ventricular.

In the PAMI-2 study, routine IABP use with angioplasty in high-risk patients with AMI reduced the incidence of recurrent ischemia or need for repeated invasive procedure.[66]

In the SHOCK trial, IABP was used in 87% of patients and did not affect mortality at 12 months of follow-up. Complications of IABP include lower extremity ischemia, which is especially likely in the elderly, in women, and in patients with diabetes or peripheral vascular disease.[67] Other complications include aortic dissection, thrombocytopenia, and infection.[68] Although the use of IABP is recommended in current guidelines, IABP is largely underused.[69]

Ventricular Assist Devices

Several assist devices that can take over the function of the left or the right ventricle have been developed for patients unable to maintain hemodynamic function with pharmacologic measures and IABP.[70-74] External devices such as the pneumatically driven Thoratec system can be used as intermediate-term support for either the left or right ventricle or both ventricles. As a bridge to transplantation, their use is associated with survival rates as high as 76%. Implantable devices (HeartMate, Novacor) are more suitable for longer term support. Currently, the assist devices are primarily used in patients with end-stage heart disease awaiting cardiac transplantation. For short-term support in the cardiac catheterization laboratory during complex procedures in unstable patients, percutaneous cardiopulmonary bypass technique can provide hemodynamic support pending definitive therapy. The Hemopump consists of a turbine in a catheter that is introduced into the femoral artery and passed into the left ventricle. It decompresses the left ventricle and augments cardiac output, providing short-term hemodynamic support.[70] The percutaneously inserted left ventricular assist devices TandemHeart and Impella 2.5 LP have been tested in small clinical trials with evidence of significant hemodynamic improvement in patients with cardiogenic shock; however, no effect on clinical outcomes has been proved.[71]

Role of Reperfusion and Revascularization in Cardiogenic Shock

Observational studies have suggested that an aggressive interventional approach aimed at mechanical or surgical revascularization can improve survival in patients with cardiogenic shock. Some studies have reported 1-year mortality rates as low as 4% to 20% after successful angioplasty.[75] In an observational study of patients with cardiogenic shock in the international SHOCK registry, the patients selected for cardiac catheterization and subsequent revascularization after development of shock had in-hospital mortality of 51% compared with 85% in patients who did not undergo angiography and subsequent revascularization.[4] In the SHOCK registry, the patients selected for the revascularization 1 to 3 days after the onset of shock did not experience worse outcome than that of patients revascularized within 8 hours after the onset.[4] The numbers of patients in each group were small, but data nevertheless suggest that even late revascularization may be beneficial compared with no revascularization. In the GUSTO-I trial of thrombolysis in AMI, cardiogenic shock occurred in 7.2%. The 30-day mortality of 38% was lower in 406 patients undergoing early angiography leading to revascularization if indicated, compared with a mortality of 62% in patients who did not.[5] In the Duke database, the mortality was 33% in shock patients with patent infarct-related arteries and 75% in patients with an occluded artery, irrespective of the mode of recanalization.

Most of the studies evaluating the role of acute coronary intervention in patients with cardiogenic shock were done before the widespread availability of coronary stenting. Webb[76] reported that in patients with cardiogenic shock, bail-out stenting for failed balloon angioplasty was associated with low (27%) mortality. These results compare favorably with the previous reports of 70% mortality in patients with failed balloon angioplasty.[77] Coronary stents are currently used in a substantial number of patients with AMI. In a series of 66 patients, stenting was associated with lower incidence of death, myocardial infarction, or infarct-related artery revascularization at 6 months compared with percutaneous transluminal coronary angioplasty alone (20% versus 67%).[78] Similarly, the new glycoprotein IIb/IIIa antagonists are now routinely used during procedures in patients with AMI. Preliminary data and extrapolation from other settings suggest that these potent platelet inhibitors will be a desirable addition to the therapeutic interventions, such as thrombolysis, coronary angioplasty, and stenting, by facilitating coronary clot lysis and reducing reocclusion and microvascular plugging.

In the GUSTO trial, a more aggressive use of resources in U.S. patients enrolled in the GUSTO-I study compared with Europe (angiography, 58% versus 23%; IABP, 35% versus 7%; pulmonary catheter placement, 57% versus 22%; ventilatory support, 54% versus 38%; and revascularization by percutaneous transluminal coronary angioplasty, 26% versus 8%, or coronary artery bypass grafting, 16% versus 9%) was associated with lower 30-day mortality in the U.S.-treated patients (50% versus 66%) compared with patients randomized in Europe.[79] These data suggest that an aggressive approach to treatment of patients with cardiogenic shock or at high risk for development of cardiogenic shock may be justified. In a prospective randomized trial (SHOCK trial) comparing aggressive interventional revascularization with aggressive medical therapy supported by IABP in patients with cardiogenic shock after AMI,[80] the primary endpoint of 30-day mortality did not appear to be improved by acute coronary intervention (possibly, in part, because of the small number of patients enrolled). Longer term survival, especially in the younger cohort, was significantly better with coronary intervention, confirming the benefit of an aggressive revascularization-based strategy in the management of patients with cardiogenic shock; however, the absolute and relative magnitude of benefit was less than that observed in nonrandomized trials.[80] On the basis of these data, current guidelines recommend immediate invasive coronary intervention as the preferred modality of treatment of younger (<75 years) patients with cardiogenic shock. The analysis of the subgroup of elderly patients, nevertheless, suggested that early revascularization was associated with lower mortality (48% versus 81%; P =.003).[81] Recent analysis of percutaneous revascularization from the SHOCK trial suggested that early restoration of flow is a major determinant of outcome and that revascularization benefits patients even beyond the 12-hour postinfarction time window.[82] In the Global Registry of Acute Coronary Events (GRACE) study, percutaneous revascularization with stenting was the best predictor of hospital survival in patients with cardiogenic shock (odds ratio, 3.99; 95% CI,

2.41–6.62).[83] In patients with non–ST elevation myocardial infarction in the SHOCK registry, revascularization was not associated with significant survival benefit.[84]

In contrast to percutaneous transluminal coronary angioplasty and stenting, the role of thrombolysis in patients with established cardiogenic shock is far less clear. A number of uncontrolled studies reported marked clinical improvement and lower mortality than expected with thrombolytic therapy.[85,86] In the early studies of intracoronary streptokinase, the patients who were successfully reperfused had lower mortality than those with persistent coronary occlusion (42% versus 84%). These early studies suggested that the patency of the infarct-related artery is the mechanism of the beneficial effect. On the other hand, in a placebo-controlled trial in patients with established cardiogenic shock, intravenous thrombolysis was not associated with improved outcome.[87] The number of patients with shock in these studies was low, and the beneficial effect might have been missed.[88] A meta-analysis by the Fibrinolytic Therapy Trialists of the placebo-controlled trials of thrombolytic therapy in AMI in patients with systolic blood pressure of less than 100 mm Hg showed an apparent 29% to 35% reduction in the 1-month mortality compared with placebo. In the same analysis, thrombolytic therapy given to patients with hypotension and tachycardia above 100 beats per minute reduced the mortality from 61% to 54%. The differences were not statistically significant, probably because of the small number of patients.[89] In two larger studies of thrombolytic agents, GUSTO-I and the International Study Group, the mortality in patients with shock was lower with streptokinase than with tissue plasminogen activator (t-PA): 65% versus 78% and 51% versus 57%, respectively.[5,90] The mechanism of the potential advantage of streptokinase over t-PA in this setting is unknown. The rate of successful reperfusion with thrombolytic therapy is less in patients with shock compared with nonshock patients,[76] possibly because of decreased diffusion of the thrombolytic agent into the thrombus with decreased pressure gradient across the coronary bed. There is evidence to suggest that the adjunctive use of an IABP with thrombolytic therapy may increase the rate of successful recanalization of the infarct-related artery and improve outcome.[49]

In contrast to the inconsistent or modest effects of thrombolytic therapy in patients with established cardiogenic shock, thrombolytic therapy with either streptokinase or t-PA, compared with placebo, appears to reduce the likelihood of subsequent development of cardiogenic shock by 25% to 43%.[89,90]

Emergency coronary artery bypass grafting during the acute phase of myocardial infarction is associated with increased mortality compared with elective procedures (7% to 8% versus 2% to 3%).[91] In a small series of patients with cardiogenic shock operated on within 24 hours, hospital mortality ranging from 20% to 26% has been reported. Improvements in technology and the aggressive use of coronary interventions (angioplasty, stenting, adjunctive potent antithrombotic drugs) have reduced the need for urgent surgical revascularization in patients with cardiogenic shock. Acute surgical intervention is mostly reserved for patients who are not amenable to coronary intervention or when intervention fails, in patients with severe concomitant multivessel disease with ongoing ischemia, and in patients with mechanical complications.

Treatment of Papillary Muscle Rupture

Management of patients with papillary muscle rupture involves supportive therapy for pulmonary congestion and edema as outlined earlier, supportive therapy for hemodynamic stabilization with use of vasoactive medications and IABP support, and urgent surgical intervention. In a case series from the Mayo Clinic, all but 3 of 22 patients were treated surgically within 3 weeks after AMI, with an overall surgical mortality of 27%; however, the mortality was 42% in patients with left ventricular ejection fraction below 45%.[9] Long-term survival was 64% in patients who survived the operation. In 5 patients with valve repair or replacement only, without coronary revascularization, the early and late mortality was high: 80% and 100%, respectively.[9] This contrasts with an earlier report of 100% mortality from the same institution in medically treated patients with postinfarction papillary muscle rupture. In the SHOCK trial registry, only 46% of patients with cardiogenic shock and severe acute mitral regurgitation underwent surgical treatment.[40] In-hospital mortality was 40% in the group that was operated on, compared with 71% mortality of patients who did not have valve surgery. Some patients in the registry received percutaneous coronary intervention rather than valve surgery. In spite of reports of sporadic favorable response of acute mitral regurgitation to percutaneous coronary intervention,[92] others were unable to observe reversal of acute mitral regurgitation with thrombolysis or percutaneous coronary intervention.[93] These data underscore that clinicians caring for these patients are often unduly conservative when selecting these patients for mitral valve surgery. Early recognition of severe mitral regurgitation may lead to surgical treatment before cardiogenic shock develops and improve prognosis.

Treatment of Ventricular Septal Rupture

The prognosis is ominous in the absence of urgent surgical intervention. In older series, medical management carried a virtually 100% long-term mortality.[10,13,21] With early surgical repair, the survival was 64% at 1 month, 59% at 1 year, and 47% at 5 years.[11,13,80] Early mortality was increased in patients with diabetes and elevated preoperative right atrial pressure. Patients who died had a mean right atrial pressure of 16 mm Hg compared with 10 mm Hg in survivors.[11] This supports the notion that right ventricular dysfunction negatively influences outcome, which may in part account for the observed worse outcome of patients with inferior infarction and VSD compared with anterior infarcts with VSD.[11,80]

Inotropic and vasopressor drug therapy as well as IABP support is often necessary to sustain arterial blood pressure and vital organ perfusion pending cardiac catheterization and surgical intervention. Surgery involves repair of the defect and, whenever necessary, may also involve infarctectomy, mitral valve repair or replacement for associated mitral regurgitation, and coronary artery bypass grafting. Residual shunting after VSD repair has been observed in as many as 28% of patients with repair. The results of surgery appear to be less favorable for inferior-posterior VSDs compared with anterior VSDs, possibly because of technical problems with repair as well as coexistent mitral regurgitation and ischemic right ventricular dysfunction in inferior-posterior infarcts.[11,13,94] In the SHOCK trial registry, only 56% of patients with acute VSD underwent surgical repair, with

19% in-hospital survival in patients who underwent surgical repair and only 5% in medically treated patients.[95] Interestingly, 13% had associated free wall rupture. These outcomes are worse than in recently reported series with 52% mortality in 22 subjects[96] and suggest that early surgical intervention should be attempted in all patients, before the onset of shock. The development of shock in these patients is unpredictable and makes delay of surgery for infarct healing and improved surgical outcomes unwarranted. Urgent early surgery remains the best therapeutic option.

Successful percutaneous closure of acute peri-infarct VSD has recently been reported, and several devices are undergoing clinical testing.[97] In the initial experience at our institution in eight patients with postinfarction VSD who were deemed to be poor surgical candidates, percutaneous closure was successful in five patients. However, despite successful closure of VSD, only one of five patients was still alive 1 month after the procedure. Percutaneous closure of a postinfarction VSD is technically demanding, and serpiginous channels of VSD, adjacent infarcted myocardium with the possibility of additional tears, and perforations of the infarcted free wall pose major hurdles against a successful outcome.[98]

Treatment of Free Wall Rupture

Free wall rupture after AMI usually presents with abrupt and catastrophic hemodynamic collapse from acute hemopericardium, resulting in rapid electromechanical dissociation and death. Most such patients cannot be salvaged, although rare examples of salvage with heroic measures (bedside thoracotomy followed by surgery) have been reported. However, with subacute free wall rupture, prompt diagnosis and surgical treatment can lead to gratifying results with good long-term survival (Table 31.4).[36] Of the 28 patients in the SHOCK trial registry, 40% survived. Of the 6 patients who were treated with pericardiocentesis alone, 50% survived, compared with 38% survival in 21 patients who had surgical repair.[31] These data are similar to survival of 48%, reported previously.[46] Surgical treatment consists of closure with either prosthetic patch with pledged sutures or patch adhered with biologic glue.

Attenuation of Infarct Expansion and Adverse Remodeling

Experimental as well as clinical studies have suggested that reperfusion therapy, angiotensin-converting enzyme inhibitors, and nitroglycerin may attenuate adverse remodeling, especially in patients with large anterior infarction, contributing to an improved prognosis.[99] Interestingly, recanalization of the infarct-related artery late after onset of chest pain, when significant salvage of myocardium is unlikely, may also attenuate adverse left ventricular remodeling. The proposed mechanisms include increased healing of the myocardium and increased stiffness of the reperfused necrotic myocardium, resulting in a smaller left ventricular cavity and lesser wall stress.[99] In contrast, routine angiography and recanalization more than 3 days after myocardial infarction in patients with persistently occluded infarct-related artery did not reduce either death or reinfarction compared with conservative management.[100]

Treatment of Left Ventricular Aneurysm

The outcome of patients who develop a true left ventricular aneurysm after AMI tends to be poor. Surgical resection of the aneurysm, often combined with coronary artery bypass grafting (because more than 50% have multivessel disease) and mitral valve repair or replacement if the papillary muscles are involved, is indicated when aneurysm development is associated with severe heart failure.[101] This procedure can lead to gratifying results, particularly when the noninvolved myocardium has good contractile function. Surgical resection guided by electrophysiologic mapping is also performed when an aneurysm produces refractory and recurrent life-threatening arrhythmias. In patients with mural thrombus and systemic embolism, anticoagulant therapy or surgical removal is often advised. However, no controlled studies have been reported to document the efficacy of any treatment in the prevention of embolic events in this setting.

SEVERITY OF PUMP FAILURE AND HOSPITAL MORTALITY IN ACUTE MYOCARDIAL INFARCTION

		Equivalent Clinical Subsets		
Clinical Category	Pathophysiologic Basis	Killip*	Cedars-Sinal	Equivalent Hemodynamic Subsets
Subclinical	Minimal or compensated LV dysfunction	I (1%–3%)	I (1%)	I (CI >2.2, PCW <18) (3%)
Pulmonary congestion	Systolic and/or diastolic LV dysfunction and/or mitral regurgitation or VSD	II (3%–5%)	II (3%–5%)	II (CI > 2.2, PCW > 18) (9%)
Pulmonary edema	As above but more severe	III (5%–25%)	II (5%–25%)	II (CI > 2.2, PCW > 18) (9%)
Low-output state or shock	As above	IV (30%–60%)	IV (50%–60%)	IV (CI <2.2, PCW > 18) (51%)
With pulmonary congestion or edema	Hypovolemia	None	III (18%)	III (CI <2.2, PCW <18) (23%)
Without pulmonary congestion	Predominant RV infarction Brady-tachyarrhythmias Cardiac rupture or tamponade			

*Updated data. Percentage in-hospital mortality in different subsets is shown in parentheses. CI, cardiac index (L/min per m^2); LV, left ventricular; PCW, pulmonary capillary wedge pressure (mm Hg); RV, right ventricular; VSD, ventricular septal defect.

Table 31.4 Severity of pump failure and hospital mortality in acute myocardial infarction.

In contrast to the true left ventricular aneurysm, postinfarction pseudoaneurysm carries a relatively high risk of free rupture with invariably fatal outcome.[10,21] Therefore, surgical resection is often advised, even in an asymptomatic subject.[102,103]

Shock Syndrome without Pulmonary Congestion

Hypovolemia

A minority of patients with AMI may develop hypotension and shock state without evidence of pulmonary congestion. Left ventricular filling pressures are low or only minimally elevated, and rapid volume expansion may improve the clinical and hemodynamic state.[10,17,74] The hypovolemic state may result from overdiuresis, excessive use of vasodilators, possible reflex-mediated inappropriate peripheral vascular pooling, and in some cases fluid and blood loss. These patients can be recognized when low-output state or shock is associated with collapsed neck veins, lack of signs of pulmonary congestion on physical examination and chest radiography, and absence of S_3 gallop. In some patients, the diagnosis can be made with certainty only by invasive hemodynamic monitoring. The hemodynamic profile of these patients is typified by a reduced cardiac index (often less than 2.2 L/m^2 per minute) and pulmonary capillary wedge pressure (<18 mm Hg but usually considerably lower). Some patients with predominant right ventricular dysfunction complicating an acute inferior infarction may have a similar hemodynamic profile.[33]

The treatment of these patients requires rapid volume infusion with aliquots of 50 to 100 mL of fluid (colloid or crystalloid) under close clinical observation to avoid pulmonary congestion due to excessive increase in pulmonary capillary wedge pressure. In some patients, particularly those receiving crystalloid infusions, pulmonary congestion and edema may occur at lower pulmonary capillary wedge pressure, possibly because of dilutional hypoalbuminemia that results in a reduction of intracapillary oncotic pressure. In patients with severely reduced left ventricular systolic function, pump function often fails to improve despite restoration of pulmonary capillary wedge pressure to seemingly adequate levels. Also in patients with markedly abnormal ventricular compliance, volume loading may elevate pulmonary capillary wedge pressure without a real increase in left ventricular preload or end-diastolic volume. Thus, volume loading should be performed with careful clinical or hemodynamic monitoring to avoid pulmonary congestion.

Right Ventricular Infarction

The low-output hypotensive syndrome in patients with predominant right ventricular infarct results from reduced left ventricular diastolic filling. The reduction in left ventricular filling results from reduced right ventricular systolic function and an increase in intrapericardial pressure secondary to right ventricular dilatation. This situation is somewhat analogous to that of cardiac tamponade. Bradyarrhythmias, including advanced atrioventricular block, are frequent and may contribute significantly to the low-output syndrome, particularly in association with loss of appropriately timed atrial contraction.

Volume infusion alone is rarely successful in improving the hemodynamics in hypotensive patients with right ventricular infarction. Concomitant use of inotropic drug therapy with dobutamine or dopamine is required.[10,21,33] Restoration of atrioventricular synchrony with pacing may also improve the hemodynamic state in patients with advanced atrioventricular block.[10,21] However, reperfusion therapy in evolving right ventricular infarction can rapidly reverse hemodynamic abnormalities and improve clinical outcome and therefore must be considered the primary therapeutic option.[105-107]

The overall hospital outcome is generally favorable in this subset of patients, especially in younger patients when left ventricular function is preserved and no mechanical complications supervene. In the elderly, right ventricular involvement with acute inferior myocardial infarction is associated with worse prognosis compared with no right ventricular involvement.[108] The favorable outcome is probably because of frequent spontaneous improvement in the right ventricular function over time. This is probably due to more favorable oxygen supply-demand characteristics and rapid development of collaterals in the right ventricle.[10,21,33]

Higher risk is primarily determined by the extent of the left ventricular involvement or extent of the infarction.[33,105,109] Mortality tends to be high in elderly patients or in patients with unsuccessful reperfusion of the infarct-related artery.[7,108] In a large randomized trial, the 30-day mortality in patients with successful reperfusion was 5.9%. The reperfusion was successful in only 54% of patients. In a study of primary angioplasty, successful recanalization of the right coronary artery was achieved in 91%, but successful reperfusion of the right ventricular branches was achieved in only 77%.[6] Reperfusion of the right ventricular branches resulted in immediate improvement of right ventricular function. Although the in-hospital mortality was unusually high (58% in patients with unsuccessful reperfusion), right ventricular function in survivors was almost normal at 1-month follow-up.[6] Inhaled nitric oxide has been tried in severe right ventricular dysfunction after infarction. In our limited experience, the effect has not been very significant or persistent. With a significant increase in right atrial pressure and a patent foramen ovale, a right-to-left shunt may occur and cause hypoxemia. A successful treatment by percutaneous closure with a septal occluder has been reported.[110]

PROGNOSIS

The outcome of patients with hemodynamic complications after AMI is predominantly determined by the severity of clinical and hemodynamic compromise, the extent and severity of left and right ventricular dysfunction, the presence or absence of mechanical complications, and the aggressiveness of therapeutic interventions. The overall outcome of different subsets of patients is summarized in Table 31.4.

chapter 32

Surgery for Complications of Myocardial Infarction

Aziz Ghaly and Gregory P. Fontana

Mechanical complications of acute myocardial infarction are rare but rapidly fatal if they are not treated expeditiously. They include postinfarction ventricular septal defect (VSD), myocardial free wall rupture, and ischemic acute mitral regurgitation. These complications arise from transmural infarction with resultant ventricular muscle rupture. Acute rupture of the free ventricular wall usually results in immediate death, and few patients survive this condition.[1] Postinfarction rupture of the interventricular wall results in VSD and acute deterioration.[2] A similar clinical situation occurs when the papillary muscle ruptures, resulting in acute mitral regurgitation.

The cornerstone in the management of such complications is the prompt diagnosis of the condition and early surgical consultation as some of these cases present true surgical emergencies. Most of these patients will die within 6 weeks if they are left with medical treatment only. Advances in surgical techniques and technology in cardiac surgery have improved the results of such procedures. Yet, these procedures still carry high mortality rates and pose significant technical challenges.

These patients are usually critically ill, and early diagnosis and early surgical intervention can only positively affect the outcome. The introduction of thrombolytic therapy has markedly decreased the incidence of such complications. However, these complications appear to occur earlier in the course of the acute myocardial infarction than before the era of thrombolytic therapy as shown in the GUSTO-I study. The incidence of postinfarction VSD reported in the literature was about 1% to 2%, whereas in the GUSTO-I study, it was reduced to just 0.2%.[3,33]

POSTINFARCTION VENTRICULAR SEPTAL DEFECT

Rupture of the left ventricular wall is responsible for one third of the deaths from acute myocardial infarction. Free wall rupture results in immediate death and accounts for about 85% of fatality from postinfarction VSD; rupture of the interventricular wall with the resultant postinfarction VSD accounts for the rest of the cases.[4] Typically, postinfarction VSD occurs in patients with complete occlusion of a single coronary vessel with poor collateral circulation. Deja and colleagues[5] confirmed in a relatively recent study the observations previously made by Hill and coworkers,[6] in which single-vessel coronary disease was found in 64% of cases of postinfarction VSD. It appears that there is a slight male predominance, and the mean age of patients is 65 years. Anterior VSD results from occlusion of the left anterior descending coronary artery; posterior VSD results from occlusion of the posterior descending artery, which arises from either the right coronary artery in right-dominant hearts or from the circumflex in left-dominant hearts. Postinfarction VSD can be a simple defect connecting the right and left ventricles or more commonly a complex defect with serpiginous course. It is not uncommon to see multiple defects at the time of operation with friable septal tissue.

DIAGNOSIS

The most common presentation is that of a patient 2 to 4 days after myocardial infarction, with sudden hemodynamic deterioration, shortness of breath, and sometimes associated chest pain. The presentation can be as early as a few hours or as late as a few weeks after acute myocardial infarction. The clinical picture and presentation of postinfarction VSD are similar to those of acute mitral regurgitation, and the two conditions must be properly identified and differentiated. In postinfarction VSD, the murmur is best heard to the left of the sternum and is associated with a thrill. New conduction defects are a common feature in postinfarction VSD. The right-sided heart catheterization shows oxygen saturation step-up indicating a left-to-right intracardiac shunt. Echocardiography, particularly transesophageal, provides definitive diagnosis as well as valuable information about wall motion, size and location of the defect, and any other associated valvular abnormalities. On the other hand, mitral valve regurgitation has a soft systolic murmur, usually is not associated with a thrill, and is not associated with intracardiac shunt. As in the case of postinfarction VSD, the echocardiogram is diagnostic of this condition. In rare cases, the patient may have VSD and rupture of the papillary muscle as well. In this scenario, the patient should have the mitral valve replaced at the time of VSD repair.

MANAGEMENT

In medically treated patients, the mortality rate is 60% to 70% in the first 2 weeks; only 9% survive 3 months.[7] Thus, the goal of the initial medical management is to achieve reasonable hemodynamic stability for the patient to tolerate the surgical repair. Surgery should be performed expeditiously, usually within the first 24 hours of presentation. Medical therapy includes intravenous fluids and intravenous vasopressor support. The use of vasodilators, such as sodium nitroprusside, decreases the afterload and hence decreases the cardiac work and increases the forward flow. However, this class of medication is often poorly tolerated because of severe hypotension. Milrinone seems to be better tolerated as it has an inotropic effect as well as a vasodilator effect. Tachycardia is common in such patients; it acts as a compensatory mechanism to increase the cardiac output. An attempt to treat this tachycardia can have a detrimental effect on hemodynamics. Almost invariably, these patients require an intra-aortic balloon pump (IABP), which has been found to be an important tool to hemodynamically stabilize the patient before surgical repair. IABP increases cardiac output, increases coronary perfusion, and decreases cardiac work by decreasing the afterload. Left-sided heart catheterization is usually needed for evaluation of these patients before surgical repair and delineates the coronary anatomy, as coronary bypass grafting of the occluded or stenotic vessels may be necessary at the time of repair. This, however, should not delay the operative repair, and the surgery can proceed without performance of coronary angiography when the patient is hemodynamically unstable.

Experience with surgical repair of postinfarction VSD during the last few decades has shown that early surgical repair of these critically ill patients before the development of end-organ dysfunction provides the best chance for survival.[8,9] Again, the initial medical management is aimed at stabilization of the patient enough to tolerate surgery and to prevent end-organ failure. Patients who continue to be hemodynamically unstable with evidence of end-organ failure are poor surgical candidates and rarely survive the operation. A multidisciplinary approach including the participation of the cardiologist, the cardiac surgeon, the patient's advocate, and the patient's family should be implemented to have a realistic expectation of the outcome and to make the appropriate decisions.

Operative management of these patients is very important and should include the active participation of the surgeon with the anesthesiologist and the perfusionist. Severe hypotension and cardiac arrest can occur during induction; therefore, the surgical team should be in the operating room and ready when anesthesia is administered. Transesophageal echocardiography is an invaluable adjunct to the procedure and should be used whenever possible.

Operative Procedures

There has been an evolution of the operative techniques during the last few decades since Cooley described the first procedure in 1956.[4] The surgical approach depends on the location of the postinfarction VSD and on the concurrent planned procedures. Postinfarction VSD is classified into three types on the basis of the location of the septal rupture: apical, anterior, and posterior VSDs. The anterior septal rupture is the most common and the easiest to repair. The posterior septal rupture is more difficult to repair because of its location and its proximity to the mitral valve, which makes the exposure unfavorable. The apical rupture is a rare type of VSD and can be repaired by amputation of the distal portions of the left ventricle, septum, and right ventricle and then direct closure of the right and left ventricles against the septum.

Detailed description of the different surgical approaches is beyond the scope of this chapter; however, we describe the current concept of surgical repair that has the most favorable result. These procedures are always performed through median sternotomy with establishment of cardiopulmonary bypass through bicaval cannulation, moderate hypothermia, and cold blood cardioplegia. The incision is made in the center of the infarcted area and then extended proximally and distally to an area of viable myocardium. In the case of anterior VSD, this incision is usually 1 to 2 cm to the left and parallel to the left anterior descending artery. In the case of posterior VSD, the incision is made 1 to 2 cm to the left and parallel to the posterior descending artery.

The relatively new concept of endocardial patch repair with infarct exclusion (Fig. 32.1) allows the exclusion of the infarcted myocardium from the high ventricular pressure rather than excision of the infarcted muscle. This technique was described by David and coworkers[10,35] and entails placement of a glutaraldehyde-fixed bovine pericardium patch to the endocardium of the ventricle wall over the infarcted septum. The incision in the ventricle is then closed over the pericardial patch. This helps in preservation of myocardial geometry, remodeling of the acutely infarcted ventricle, and preservation of ventricular function. This type of repair has significantly improved the mortality rate for such procedures.

After weaning from cardiopulmonary bypass, the patients frequently require continuation of the IABP support for the immediate postoperative period. Intraoperative transesophageal echocardiography is used to detect any residual VSD and to assess the competency of the mitral valve. A small amount of residual shunt is not uncommon; however, any significant VSD needs to be repaired. If concomitant mitral regurgitation due to papillary muscle rupture is present, the valve should be replaced.

Outcome of Surgical Repair

Table 32.1 shows some of the results of surgical repair of postinfarction VSD at different institutions.[7] The in-hospital mortality rate for patients undergoing repair of postinfarction VSD is reported in most series between 27% and 50%.[11-18] David and Armstrong[19] reported operative mortality of 19% in a series of 44 patients. In the GUSTO-I study, the 30-day mortality for those patients who did not undergo surgery was 94%. The long-term results for the survivors of surgical repair have been encouraging. The 5-year actuarial survival in most series ranges from 40% to 72%, with most of the patients in New York Heart Association (NYHA) functional class I and class II. In the series of Daggett and colleagues,[20] long-term follow-up showed that 75% of patients are in NYHA functional class I and another 12.5% in class II. Dalrymple-Hay and associates[13] reported 10-year survival of 39%.

Perioperative cardiogenic shock and right ventricular failure have been identified as independent risk factors for mortality for postinfarction VSD repair. Posterior VSD repair is associated with a less favorable outcome in many series; however, this has not been a consistent finding. One explanation why posterior repair might have a less favorable outcome is the difficult surgical exposure and the associated right ventricular failure resulting from infarcted right-sided myocardium. Many other risk factors have been identified as poor predictors of survival, including age and renal dysfunction.[21-23] Early postinfarction rupture and time from

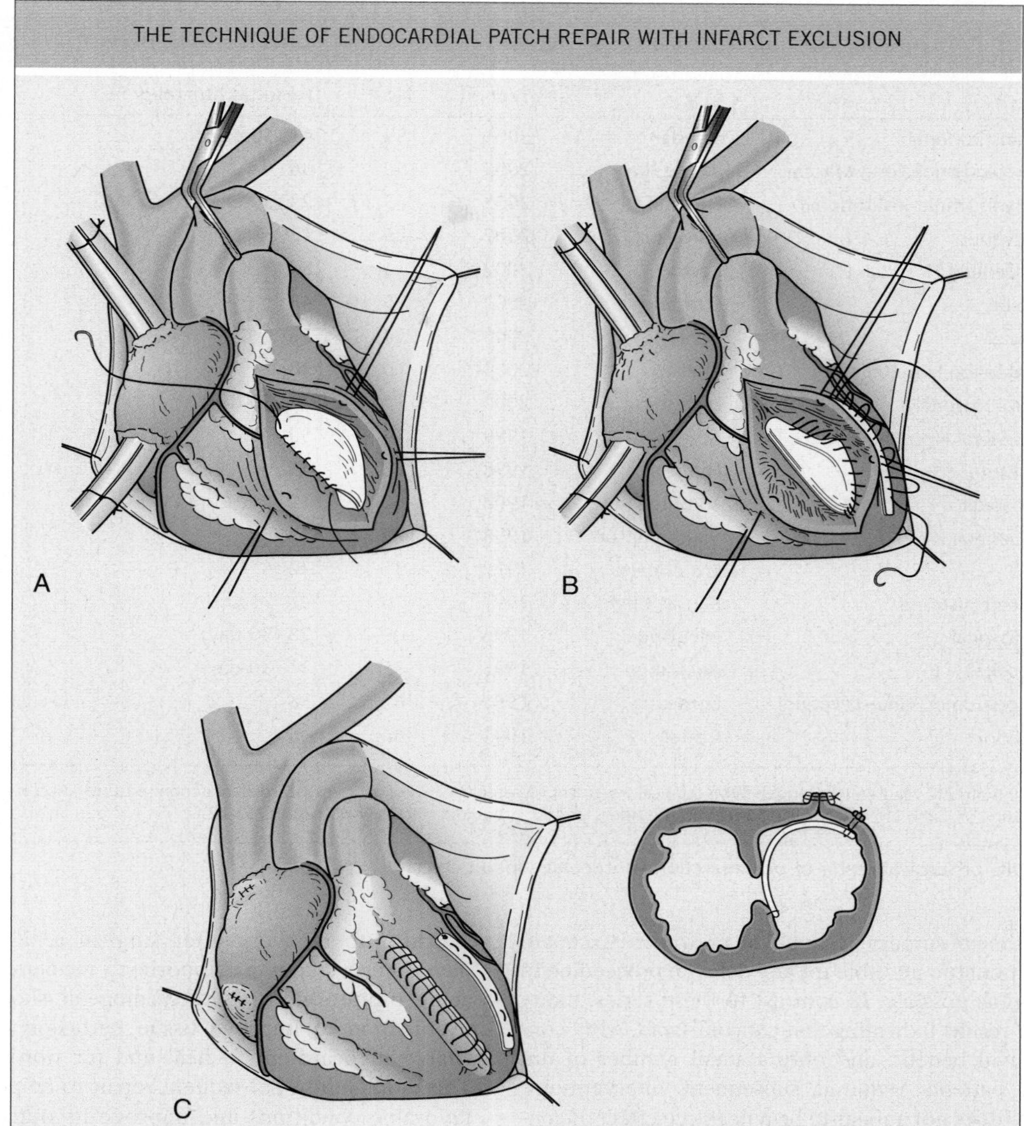

Figure 32.1 Technique of endocardial patch repair with infarct exclusion. A vertical ventriculostomy is made (**A**), and glutaraldehyde-fixed pericardium is sutured to the endocardium (**B**). The completed repair will exclude the infarcted area from the circulation (**C**).

infarction to rupture have also been shown to be predictors of poor survival after repair. The poor outcome in this group of patients can be explained by the fact that patients who develop myocardial rupture early tend to have more extensive myocardial infarction. Concomitant coronary artery bypass grafting (CABG), the patch material used, and residual VSD have not been found to have an impact on survival.

Residual VSD is not an uncommon finding, and it was as high as 42% in one series. Only 12% of such patients required reoperation. The high incidence of postrepair VSD may be due to development of a new VSD as a result of progression of the infarction missed, multiple VSDs, or failure of repair. Small, asymptomatic VSDs should not be repaired; they are well tolerated by those patients, and the risk of reoperation is very high. However, symptomatic large VSD with Qp/Qs of more than 1.5 should be repaired or undergo transcatheter closure.

The use of IABP has failed to show survival benefit. Some reports have shown peak improvement in 24 hours of use, with no further benefit for longer use. In addition, there are some data to suggest increased mortality with IABP use. Despite that, the widespread belief is that IABP is an important adjunct to achievement of hemodynamic stability in the perioperative period of those critically ill patients.

Most centers advocate performing CABG during repair of postinfarction VSD in patients with significant coronary artery disease.[24-26] Multiple reports have shown short- and long-term survival benefit for concomitant coronary revascularization with no added risk to the procedure. In a multicenter observational study of 65 consecutive patients who underwent repair of acute postinfarction VSD, the adjusted freedom from death in concomitant CABG patients at 30 days and 1, 2, and 4 years was 96.2%, 91.6%, 88.8%, and 82.8%, respectively. The non–concomitant CABG patients showed freedom of death of 79.15%, 58.8%, 49.1%, and 32.2%, respectively. Many argue against the idea of performing coronary revascularization at the time of VSD repair; however, there is no evidence that this is true. Although preoperative left-sided heart angiography

RESULTS OF SURGICAL REPAIR OF POSTINFARCTION VENTRICULAR SEPTAL DEFECT					
Institution	**City**	**Year**	**No.**	**Hospital Mortality %**	**5-Year Survival %**
Sweden (multi-institutional)	Sweden	2005	189	41 (30-day)	38
Ospedale di Circolo-Fondazione Macchi	Varese, Italy	2005	50	36	47
Northwest England (multi-institutional)	England	2003	65	23 (30-day)	
Hôpital Haut-Lévêque	Bordeaux	2002	85	42	33
Massachusetts General Hospital	Boston	2002	114	37	45
Papworth Hospital	Cambridge	2002	25	48	
University Hospital	Zurich	2000	54	26	52
Sakurabashi Watanabe Hospital	Osaka	2000	16	38	
Glenfield General Hospital	Leicester	2000	117	37 (30-day)	46
Evangelismos General Hospital	Athens	1999	14	50	
Texas Heart Institute	Houston	1998	126	46	
The Toronto Hospital	Toronto	1998	52	19	65
Southampton General	Southampton	1998	179	27	49
Cedars-Sinai	Los Angeles	1998	31	32	
Mid America Heart Institute	Kansas City	1997	76	41	41
St. Anthonius Hospital	Nieuwegein	1996	109	28 (30-day)	
Green Lane Hospital	Auckland	1995	35	31 (30-day)	60
Hôpital Cardiologique du Haut-Lévêque	Bordeaux	1991	62	38	44
CHU Henri Mendor	Cretell	1991	66	45	44

Modified from Agnihotri AK, Madsen JC, Daggett WM. Surgical treatment of complications of acute myocardial infarction: postinfarction ventricular septal defect and free wall rupture. In Cohn LH, ed. Cardiac Surgery in the Adult, 3rd ed. New York, McGraw-Hill, 2008:753-784.

Table 32.1 Results of surgical repair of postinfarction ventricular septal defect.

may delay the time of surgery, it should be performed except in the case of a patient too unstable for any delay in proceeding to surgery as soon as possible. In contrast to these series, many have published results indicating that concomitant CABG conferred no survival benefit, and only a small number of unrevascularized patients required subsequent interventions. However, there does not appear to be a negative effect of concomitant CABG in this setting.

Role of Percutaneous Device Closure

The role of catheter closure devices in postinfarction VSD is expanding.[27-29] Initial reports showed very high rates of device failure and mortality due to expansion of the area of friable and infarcted septum. However, the closure devices have been successful in treating patients with residual and recurrent postinfarction VSD. Another role for the transcatheter closure devices is to provide temporary hemodynamic relief until the time of surgical repair. Holzer and coworkers[30] reported successful deployment of the Amplatz occluder device in 16 of 18 patients, with five deaths after 332 days of follow-up. In their series, there were only two cases with residual VSD. The transcatheter closure of postinfarction VSD is expected to increase in the future with the constant improvement and development of devices.

Role of Ventricular Assist Devices

Ventricular assist devices can reduce left ventricular systolic pressure, reduce interventricular shunt, and improve right ventricular function. Ventricular assist devices have been used in severely hemodynamically compromised patients as a bridge to recovery after surgical repair.[31,32] Also, they have been used as a temporizing measure in patients after acute rupture with severe cardiogenic shock and end-organ dysfunction to improve tissue perfusion and to allow the friable myocardium to heal and for fibrosis to take place. This would allow subsequent repair to be performed in more favorable conditions and improve its outcome. There have been some reports of successful placement of percutaneous assist devices in patients with postinfarction VSD as a bridge for transplantation. However, there have been some cases of device failure as a result of device occlusion with friable infarcted myocardium. The use of ventricular assist devices in the treatment of patients with cardiogenic shock is increasing as the experience with the wide variety of new and less invasive devices expands.[33]

FREE VENTRICULAR WALL RUPTURE

Free ventricular wall rupture is classified into three types: acute, subacute, and chronic. It results from transmural myocardial infarction. As discussed before, acute rupture is much more common and usually results in immediate death. The subacute type can present with a picture similar to that of cardiac tamponade, with chest pain and acute deterioration of the hemodynamics in a patient with acute myocardial infarction. The chronic type, which is rare, usually results in ventricular false aneurysm. The acute deterioration in a patient's condition with new onset of chest pain and the finding of hemopericardium on echocardiography is diagnostic. Urgent surgical repair is the treatment of such conditions and is performed through median sternotomy and with the use of cardiopulmonary bypass. It entails closure of the defect either primarily or with the use of patch material after removal of the necrotic myocardium. There are some reports of successful closure with fibrin glue.[34]

ACUTE ISCHEMIC MITRAL REGURGITATION

Mitral regurgitation complicates about 18% of cases after acute myocardial infarction; more than 3% of patients develop severe mitral regurgitation and congestive heart failure. By definition, ischemic mitral regurgitation is a functional regurgitation with normal valve leaflets. The mitral valve is a complex structure consisting of leaflets, chordae tendineae, the valve annulus, papillary muscles, the left ventricle, and the left atrium. Normal function of the valve is the result of interaction of all of these structures, and any change of these structures can result in valve dysfunction.[38]

Papillary muscle rupture is a rare complication and is responsible for 1% to 5% of deaths from acute myocardial infarction. Those patients are usually acutely ill and hemodynamically unstable, requiring intravenous inotropic support and IABP support. The posteromedial papillary muscle is supplied by the right coronary artery and is the most common one to rupture. The anterolateral papillary muscle is supplied by the left anterior descending artery and the posterior descending artery and is responsible for about one third of cases of papillary muscle rupture.

However, acute ischemic mitral regurgitation can result from multiple acute and subtle changes, other than papillary muscle rupture, that render the valve incompetent. Mitral valve annulus dilatation is an important cause of valve incompetence.[36] Many animal studies have identified a variety of subvalvular geometric changes that participate in the pathophysiologic process of ischemic mitral regurgitation.

Clinical Presentation

Patients with acute ischemic mitral regurgitation due to papillary muscle rupture present with symptoms similar to the ones described for postinfarction VSD. They develop cardiogenic shock and symptoms of congestive heart failure that is usually unresponsive to inotropic and IABP support. The murmur of mitral regurgitation is a pansystolic murmur localized to the apex of the heart. Unlike in postinfarction VSD, heart block is uncommon, and there is no evidence of left-to-right shunt. Transesophageal echocardiography is diagnostic and helps determine the pathology of the mitral valve. Such information is important to decide on the type of repair and whether to repair or to replace the mitral valve.

Management

The preoperative management should focus on optimizing cardiac and end-organ function. This can be achieved by proper use of afterload reduction agents, beta blockers, and diuretics and optimization of the preload. Many patients will require preoperative IABP. Most of the patients are brought to the operating room after left-sided heart catheterization to determine the type of revascularization required with the mitral valve repair or replacement. However, obtaining left-sided heart catheterization should not delay the surgery or jeopardize the patient's condition.

Surgical therapy provides the best chance for survival for those patients with cardiogenic shock and severe congestive heart failure secondary to papillary muscle rupture. Early revascularization with percutaneous transluminal coronary angioplasty and thrombolytic therapy in a few highly selected, stable patients with acute ischemic mitral regurgitation, not due to papillary muscle rupture, has provided excellent results.

Surgical Treatment

Surgical treatment consists of mitral valve repair or replacement with complete coronary artery revascularization when indicated. Most surgeons agree on performing CABG for a lesion identified by preoperative cardiac catheterization, as revascularization of completed myocardial infarction will positively affect ventricular remodeling. The decision either to replace or to repair the mitral valve is based on the intraoperative transesophageal echocardiographic findings. A simple central jet, no papillary muscle rupture, and minimal tethering of the leaflets suggest successful repair. Most surgeons will replace the mitral valve with ruptured papillary muscle. Complex prolonged repair of the mitral valve is poorly tolerated by those very ill patients and should be substituted by expeditious valve replacement. The goal of the operation is to provide myocardial revascularization and mitral valve competence with minimal time of myocardial ischemia.[38,39] The procedure is performed with a standard median sternotomy, bicaval cannulation, and cardiopulmonary bypass. In the rare case of isolated mitral valve repair in a patient with previous sternotomy, the right thoracotomy approach can be used. Mitral valve replacement should be performed with preservation of the infravalvular structures. Preservation of the subvalvular integrity is essential for the ventricular function after valve replacement. Amputation of the chordae and papillary muscle will lead to serious ventricular changes affecting the ventricular geometry, wall thickness, loss of normal systolic torsional deformity, and ventricular wall stress. Chordal preservation with mitral valve replacement will provide improved ventricular geometry and augments ventricular function.

Placement of a low-profile mitral valve is important in the ischemic myocardium. Mechanical valves have the lowest profile, but they require lifelong anticoagulation. The bioprosthetic valves are more appealing as they require no anticoagulation and have a relatively long durability profile. Mitral valve repair should be performed whenever feasible.[37] Many techniques have been developed for mitral valve repair, with excellent results. The principle of valve repair is augmentation of the zone of coaptation with placement of a circumferential annuloplasty ring to undersize and to overcorrect the mitral valve annulus (Fig. 32.2). In the event of papillary muscle rupture, papillary muscle relocation or reimplantation have proven effective. This will prevent progressive mitral annulus dilatation during the process of remodeling and restores the normal geometry and the ellipsoid shape of the left ventricle.

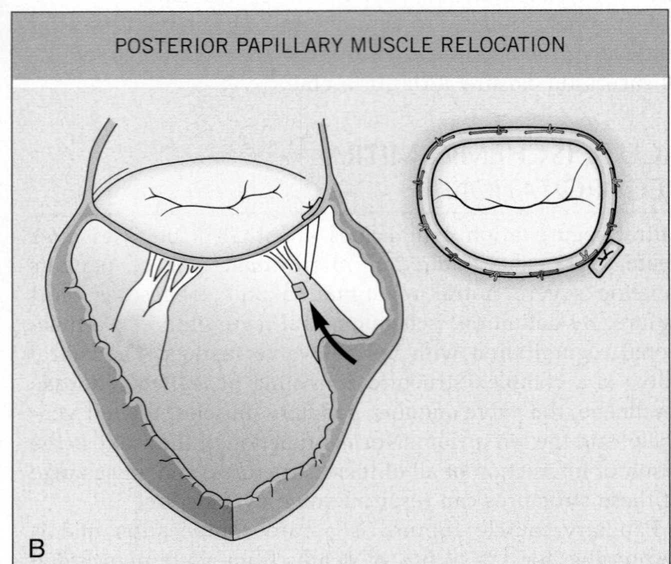

Figure 32.2 Some of the surgical techniques used in mitral valve repair. A, Placement of ring annuloplasty to achieve proper coaptation of the valve leaflets by annular reduction. **B**, Posterior papillary muscle relocation.

Results of Surgical Treatment

The results of repair of acute mitral valve replacement are unfavorable. Hospital mortality in this group of patients has been reported between 30% and 70%. Recent results have shown improvements with the adoption of chordal preserving techniques after valve replacement, geometric mitral reconstruction, and complete coronary revascularization. The 5-year survival for such patients, even in the recent results, is still in the 50% range.

SUMMARY

Patients requiring urgent surgical therapy for complications of myocardial infarction continue to challenge cardiologists and surgeons alike. The development of new surgical and transcatheter options has had a positive impact on acute and late survival.

chapter 33

Post-Hospital Phase of an Acute Coronary Syndrome

Emily E. Hass and Sidney C. Smith, Jr.

Definition and Description

- Several treatments have been shown to reduce the risk of recurrent coronary events and mortality in clinical trials among patients who have survived acute coronary syndromes (ACS).

Key Features

- Early and long-term use of daily antiplatelet therapy with aspirin, clopidogrel, or both as indicated.
- Early use of beta-blocking agents after ACS, continued long term.
- Treatment with angiotensin-converting enzyme inhibitors.
- Comprehensive management of lipid-lowering therapies, with initiation of treatment in the hospital and a goal of decreasing low-density lipoprotein cholesterol to 100 mg/dL (2.6 mmol/L) and the optional goal of 70 mg/dL or less after ACS.
- Smoking cessation.
- Initiation of a cardiac rehabilitation program.

Clinical Implications

- Secondary prevention therapies after ACS have contributed to an impressive decline in subsequent cardiovascular events and mortality.

Coronary heart disease (CHD) is the leading cause of death in the United States, with approximately 1.2 million acute myocardial infarctions each year. Of these patients, roughly 38% will die of the event.[1] Rates of mortality from CHD peaked around 1968 but have markedly declined since then, with age-adjusted rates decreasing by 50% by the turn of the century (Fig. 33.1).[1,2] The in-hospital mortality for myocardial infarction patients younger than 70 years decreased from more than 20% in 1965 to approximately 5% to 6% in 1990 and 4.6% in 2004.[1,3,4] The development of specialized coronary care units, direct current defibrillators, improved hemodynamic monitoring, and acute reperfusion therapies have all contributed to this impressive decline in mortality. A recent statistical analysis of U.S. deaths from coronary disease from 1980 to 2000 looked at the effectiveness of specific cardiac treatments and changes in risk factors contributing to the reduction in CHD mortality. Treatments such as secondary prevention therapy, initial treatments for acute coronary syndrome (ACS) and heart failure, and revascularization accounted for approximately 47% of the decline. Forty-four percent of the decline was attributed to risk factor reduction, such as reduction in lipid levels, hypertension, and smoking.[2] During this period, there has also been a dramatic improvement in late survival after myocardial infarction; between 1990 and 1996, the average annual rate of decline in mortality from CHD was 2.6% in the United States.[3] The development of post–myocardial infarction risk stratification to identify patients who are at high risk for recurrent myocardial infarction and death and the reduction of risk factors with secondary prevention techniques have been important components of this improvement.[5]

The clinical designation "acute coronary syndromes" includes ST-segment elevation myocardial infarction, non–ST-segment elevation myocardial infarction, and unstable angina. Although there may be certain differences in the initial treatment of patients with ACS (e.g., thrombolytic therapy for ST-segment elevation myocardial infarction but not for non–ST-segment elevation myocardial infarction or unstable angina), the underlying atherothrombotic process is similar. Thus, the long-term secondary prevention therapies outlined here for the three entities composing ACS differ little.

Several factors influence prognosis after ACS, and risk stratification after myocardial infarction is crucial in helping to determine long-term survival. Tools such as the Global Registry of Acute Coronary Events (GRACE) Prediction and Score card and nomogram can be useful in estimating the risk of 6-month postdischarge mortality after hospitalization for ACS.[6] Factors related to the extent of myocardial damage during ACS include left ventricular function, recurrent ischemia, and persistent cardiac arrhythmias.[7] Patients who have depressed left ventricular function, as measured by left ventricular ejection fraction (LVEF), or clinical signs of congestive heart failure (CHF) are at increased risk of increased morbidity and mortality after ACS. An LVEF of less than 30% on predischarge assessment is associated with a mortality as high as 45% at 1 year[8,9]; therefore, evaluation of left ventricular function is crucial before a post–myocardial infarction patient is discharged from the hospital. Echocardiography is an ideal method for determining left ventricular function because it can provide additional information about valve function, regional contractility, and the presence of thrombi. Radionuclide ventriculography may also be used to determine ventricular function and to provide an objective assessment of LVEF. The goals of post-hospital management for ACS patients include reducing mortality and improving quality of life by preserving left ventricular function. More recently, cardiac magnetic resonance imaging has become a valuable tool for assessment of function, perfusion, and viability of the myocardium.

Residual ischemia, as demonstrated by objective electrocardiographic findings during symptoms, is also a prognostic

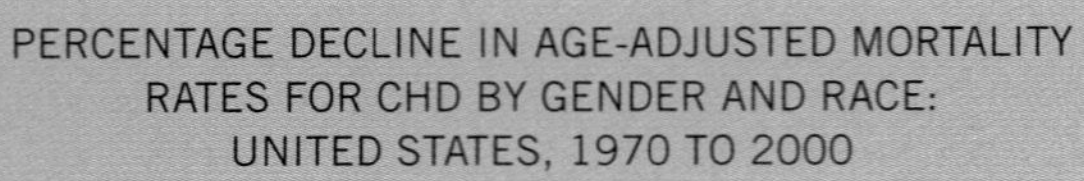

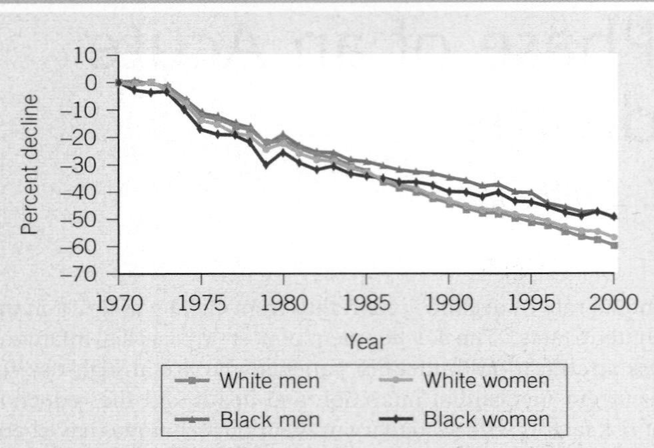

Figure 33.1 Percentage decline in age-adjusted mortality rates for CHD by gender and race: United States, 1970 to 2000. (From Chobanian AV, Bakris GL, Black HR, et al. Seventh report of the Joint National Committee on Prevention, Detection, Evaluation, and Treatment of High Blood Pressure. Hypertension 2003;42:1206-1252.)

marker for recurrent myocardial infarction and increased mortality after ACS. Recurrent myocardial infarction is strongly associated with increased early mortality, although the presence of post–myocardial infarct angina alone is not as clearly associated with decreased survival. There is evidence that patients who have a normal early exercise electrocardiogram have a low 1-year mortality rate,[10] and thus it is reasonable to recommend predischarge symptom-limited electrocardiographic exercise testing or early postdischarge (2 to 4 weeks) exercise electrocardiographic testing to evaluate for recurrent ischemia. Secondary prevention therapies, including the use of aspirin, beta blockers, angiotensin-converting enzyme (ACE) inhibitors, and lipid-lowering therapy, can significantly minimize and reduce the occurrence of ischemia after ACS.

Cardiac arrhythmias, such as nonsustained ventricular tachycardia, ventricular ectopy, or new atrial fibrillation, are also poor prognostic markers after myocardial infarction. These are often manifestations of poor left ventricular function or recurrent ischemia, or both. The goals of post-hospital care and secondary prevention are to maintain and to improve left ventricular function, to eliminate ischemia, and, in the process, to minimize the risk of sudden cardiac death secondary to arrhythmias.

This chapter outlines techniques of risk reduction for future myocardial infarction in patients after ACS. The secondary prevention measures presented herein represent pharmacologic and behavioral methods that have been shown to reduce the risk of recurrent myocardial infarction and death in patients who have CHD. These therapies largely involve improvement or control of impaired left ventricular function and the broad treatment of risk factors associated with atherosclerosis to reduce future ischemic events and to stabilize underlying disease. In 1996, the American Heart Association (AHA) and the American College of Cardiology (ACC) issued a comprehensive statement outlining current understanding of the best treatments with which to reduce risk in patients who have CHD; in 2001 and 2006, the statement was updated to reflect the results of subsequent clinical trials and patient studies (Table 33.1).[11]

AHA/ACC SECONDARY PREVENTION FOR PATIENTS WITH CORONARY AND OTHER VASCULAR DISEASE*: 2006 UPDATE

	Intervention Recommendations with Class of Recommendation and Level of Evidence
SMOKING Goal Complete cessation. No exposure to environmental tobacco smoke.	■ Ask about tobacco use status at every visit. **I (B)** ■ Advise every tobacco user to quit. **I (B)** ■ Assess the tobacco user's willingness to quit. **I (B)** ■ Assist by counseling and developing a plan for quitting. **I (B)** ■ Arrange follow-up, referral to special programs, or pharmacotherapy (including nicotine replacement and bupropion). **I (B)** ■ Urge avoidance of exposure to environmental tobacco smoke at work and home. **I (B)**
BLOOD PRESSURE CONTROL Goal <140/90 mm Hg or <130/80 mm Hg if patient has diabetes or chronic kidney disease	**For all patients:** ■ Initiate or maintain lifestyle modification—weight control; increased physical activity; alcohol moderation; sodium reduction; and emphasis on increased consumption of fresh fruits, vegetables, and low-fat dairy products. **I (B)** **For patients with blood pressure ≥140/90 mm Hg (or ≥130/80 mm Hg for individuals with chronic kidney disease or diabetes):** ■ As tolerated, add blood pressure medication, treating initially with beta blockers and/or ACE inhibitors, with addition of other drugs such as thiazides as needed to achieve goal blood pressure. **I (A)** [For compelling indications for individual drug classes in specific vascular diseases, see Seventh Report of the Joint National Committee on Prevention, Detection, Evaluation, and Treatment of High Blood Pressure (JNC 7).][92]

LIPID MANAGEMENT Goal LDL-C <100 mg/dL If triglycerides are ≥200 mg/dL, non–HDL-C should be <130 mg/dL[†]	**For all patients:** ■ Start dietary therapy. Reduce intake of saturated fats (to <7% of total calories), *trans* fatty acids, and cholesterol (to <200 mg/d). **I (B)** ■ Adding plant stanol/sterols (2 g/d) and viscous fiber (>10 g/d) will further lower LDL-C. ■ Promote daily physical activity and weight management. **I (B)** ■ Encourage increased consumption of omega-3 fatty acids in the form of fish[‡] or in capsule form (1 g/d) for risk reduction. For treatment of elevated triglycerides, higher doses are usually necessary for risk reduction. **IIb (B)** **For lipid management:** Assess fasting lipid profile in all patients, and within 24 hours of hospitalization for those with an acute cardiovascular or coronary event. For hospitalized patients, initiate lipid-lowering medication as recommended below before discharge according to the following schedule: ■ LDL-C should be <100 mg/dL **I (A), and** ■ Further reduction of LDL-C to <70 mg/dL is reasonable. **IIa (A)** ■ If baseline LDL-C is ≥100 mg/dL, initiate LDL-lowering drug therapy.[§] **I (A)** ■ If on-treatment LDL-C is ≥100 mg/dL, intensify LDL-lowering drug therapy (may require LDL-lowering drug combination[‖]). **I (A)** ■ If baseline LDL-C is 70 to 100 mg/dL, it is reasonable to treat to LDL-C <70 mg/dL. **IIa (B)** ■ If triglycerides are 200 to 499 mg/dL, non–HDL-C should be <130 mg/dL **I (B), and** ■ Further reduction of non–HDL-C to <100 mg/dL is reasonable. **IIa (B)** ■ Therapeutic options to reduce non–HDL-C are: ⇒ More intense LDL-C–lowering therapy **I (B),** or ⇒ Niacin[¶] (after LDL-C–lowering therapy) **IIa (B),** or ⇒ Fibrate therapy[#] (after LDL-C–lowering therapy) **IIa (B)** ■ If triglycerides are ≥500 mg/dL,[#] therapeutic options to prevent pancreatitis are fibrate[¶] or niacin[¶] before LDL-lowering therapy; and treat LDL-C to goal after triglyceride-lowering therapy. Achieve non–HDL-C <130 mg/dL if possible. **I (C)**
PHYSICAL ACTIVITY Goal 30 minutes, 7 days per week (minimum 5 days per week)	■ For all patients, assess risk with a physical activity history and/or an exercise test, to guide prescription. **I (B)** ■ For all patients, encourage 30 to 60 minutes of moderate-intensity aerobic activity, such as brisk walking, on most, preferably all, days of the week, supplemented by an increase in daily lifestyle activities (e.g., walking breaks at work, gardening, household work). **I (B)** ■ Encourage resistance training 2 days per week. **IIb (C)** ■ Advise medically supervised programs for high-risk patients (e.g., recent acute coronary syndrome or revascularization, heart failure). **I (B)**
WEIGHT MANAGEMENT Goal Body mass index: 18.5 to 24.9 kg/m^2 Waist circumference: men <40 inches, women <35 inches	■ Assess body mass index and/or waist circumference on each visit and consistently encourage weight maintenance/reduction through an appropriate balance of physical activity, caloric intake, and formal behavioral programs when indicated to maintain/achieve a body mass index between 18.5 and 24.9 kg/m^2. **I (B)** ■ If waist circumference (measured horizontally at the iliac crest) is ≥35 inches in women and ≥40 inches in men, initiate lifestyle changes and consider treatment strategies for metabolic syndrome as indicated. **I (B)** ■ The initial goal of weight loss therapy should be to reduce body weight by approximately 10% from baseline. With success, further weight loss can be attempted if indicated through further assessment. **I (B)**
DIABETES MANAGEMENT Goal HbA_{1c} <7%	■ Initiate lifestyle and pharmacotherapy to achieve near-normal HbA_{1c}. **I (B)** ■ Begin vigorous modification of other risk factors (e.g., physical activity, weight management, blood pressure control, and cholesterol management as recommended above). **I (B)** ■ Coordinate diabetic care with patient's primary care physician or endocrinologist. **I (C)**
ANTIPLATELET AGENTS/ ANTICOAGULANTS	■ Start aspirin 75 to 162 mg/d and continue indefinitely in all patients unless contraindicated. **I (A)** ⇒ For patients undergoing coronary artery bypass grafting, aspirin should be started within 48 hours after surgery to reduce saphenous vein graft closure. Dosing regimens ranging from 100 to 325 mg/d appear to be efficacious. Doses higher than 162 mg/d can be continued for up to 1 year. **I (B)** ■ Start and continue clopidogrel 75 mg/d in combination with aspirin for up to 12 months in patients after acute coronary syndrome or percutaneous coronary intervention with stent placement (≥1 month for bare metal stent, ≥3 months for sirolimus-eluting stent, and ≥6 months for paclitaxel-eluting stent). **I (B)**

(Continued)

AHA/ACC SECONDARY PREVENTION FOR PATIENTS WITH CORONARY AND OTHER VASCULAR DISEASE*: 2006 UPDATE—Cont'd	
	Intervention Recommendations with Class of Recommendation and Level of Evidence
ANTIPLATELET AGENTS/ ANTICOAGULANTS—Cont'd	⇒ Patients who have undergone percutaneous coronary intervention with stent placement should initially receive higher-dose aspirin at 325 mg/d for 1 month for bare-metal stent, 3 months for sirolimus-eluting stent, and 6 months for paclitaxel-eluting stent. **I (B)** ■ Manage warfarin to international normalized ratio = 2.0 to 3.0 for paroxysmal or chronic atrial fibrillation or flutter, and in post–myocardial infarction patients when clinically indicated (e.g., atrial fibrillation, left ventricular thrombus). **I (A)** ■ Use of warfarin in conjunction with aspirin and/or clopidogrel is associated with increased risk of bleeding and should be monitored closely. **I (B)**
RENIN-ANGIOTENSIN-ALDOSTERONE SYSTEM BLOCKERS	**ACE inhibitors:** ■ Start and continue indefinitely in all patients with left ventricular ejection fraction ≤40% and in those with hypertension, diabetes, or chronic kidney disease, unless contraindicated. **I (A)** ■ Consider for all other patients. **I (B)** ■ Among lower-risk patients with normal left ventricular ejection fraction in whom cardiovascular risk factors are well controlled and revascularization has been performed, use of ACE inhibitors may be considered optional. **IIa (B)** **Angiotensin receptor blockers:** ■ Use in patients who are intolerant of ACE inhibitors and have heart failure or have had a myocardial infarction with left ventricular ejection fraction ≤40%. **I (A)** ■ Consider in other patients who are ACE inhibitor intolerant. **I (B)** ■ Consider use in combination with ACE inhibitors in systolic-dysfunction heart failure. **IIb (B)** **Aldosterone blockade:** ■ Use in post–myocardial infarction patients, without significant renal dysfunction** or hyperkalemia,†† who are already receiving therapeutic doses of an ACE inhibitor and beta blocker, have a left ventricular ejection fraction ≤40%, and have either diabetes or heart failure. **I (A)**
BETA BLOCKERS	■ Start and continue indefinitely in all patients who have had myocardial infarction, acute coronary syndrome, or left ventricular dysfunction with or without heart failure symptoms, unless contraindicated. **I (A)** ■ Consider chronic therapy for all other patients with coronary or other vascular disease or diabetes unless contraindicated. **IIa (C)**
INFLUENZA VACCINATION	■ Patients with cardiovascular disease should have an influenza vaccination. **I (B)**

*Patients covered by these guidelines include those with established coronary and other atherosclerotic vascular disease, including peripheral arterial disease, atherosclerotic aortic disease, and carotid artery disease. Treatment of patients whose only manifestation of cardiovascular risk is diabetes will be the topic of a separate AHA scientific statement. ACE indicates angiotensin-converting enzyme.

†Non–HDL-C = total cholesterol minus HDL-C.

‡Pregnant and lactating women should limit their intake of fish to minimize exposure to methylmercury.

§When LDL-lowering medications are used, obtain at least a 30% to 40% reduction in LDL-C levels. If LDL-C <70 mg/dL is the chosen target, consider drug titration to achieve this level to minimize side effects and cost. When LDL-C <70 mg/dL is not achievable because of high baseline LDL-C levels, it generally is possible to achieve reductions of >50% in LDL-C levels by either statins or LDL-C-lowering drug combinations.

‖Standard dose of statin with ezetimibe, bile acid sequestrant, or niacin.

¶The combination of high-dose statin + fibrate can increase risk for severe myopathy. Statin doses should be kept relatively low with this combination. Dietary supplement niacin must not be used as a substitute for prescription niacin.

#Patients with very high triglycerides should not consume alcohol. The use of bile acid sequestrant is relatively contraindicated when triglycerides are >200 mg/dL.

**Creatinine should be <2.5 mg/dL in men and <2.0 mg/dL in women.

††Potassium should be <5.0 mEq/L.

From Smith SC Jr, Blair SN, Criqui MH, et al. Preventing heart attack and death in patients with coronary disease. Consensus panel statement. Circulation 1995;92:2-4.

Table 33.1 AHA/ACC Secondary Prevention for Patients with Coronary and Other Vascular Disease: 2006 Update.

ANTIPLATELET AND ANTICOAGULANT THERAPY

Mechanisms of Action

Aspirin (acetylsalicylic acid) inhibits platelet aggregation by blocking the synthesis of thromboxane A_2, which causes vasoconstriction and promotes platelet aggregation. The benefit of aspirin as an inhibitor of platelet aggregation and thrombosis in the setting of ACS has been well documented.

The Second International Study of Infarct Survival (ISIS-2) examined more than 17,000 patients with suspected acute myocardial infarction in 16 countries; these patients were allocated randomly to groups to receive intravenous streptokinase, aspirin, both treatments, or neither treatment within 24 hours of the onset of symptoms.[12] Among the 8587 patients who received 162.5 mg of aspirin, there were 804 (9.4%) vascular deaths, compared with 1016 (11.8%) vascular deaths among the 8600 patients who received placebo ($2P < .00001$). This

23% reduction in vascular mortality was highly significant compared with placebo, and the benefit was maintained during a mean of 15 months of follow-up. There were also significant reductions in nonfatal reinfarction and nonfatal stroke with aspirin. On the basis of the results of this trial, it was estimated that 1 month of low-dose aspirin, when started immediately in 1000 patients suspected of having suffered acute myocardial infarction, would lead to 25 fewer deaths and 10 to 15 fewer nonfatal reinfarctions or strokes. Continuation of such treatment for longer would prevent even more deaths and nonfatal events.

The Antiplatelet Trialists' Collaboration meta-analysis of 25 trials estimated reductions of 30% for nonfatal myocardial infarction and 15% for vascular death in patients receiving antiplatelet therapy who had a previous history of unstable angina or myocardial infarction. The studies examined had treatment periods ranging from 1 to 6 years.[13] Findings of this study are summarized in Table 33.2. In a follow-up study by the same group that examined the effect of prolonged aspirin use, more than 70,000 high-risk patients (those with a history of some type of vascular disease) and 30,000 low-risk patients were included in the analysis. Among 20,000 patients who started to take aspirin after myocardial infarction, 10% suffered a repeated vascular event while receiving antiplatelet therapy compared with 14% of control patients; in about 20,000 patients with a history of myocardial infarction, there was a 13% incidence of repeated vascular events with antiplatelet treatment compared with a 17% incidence in those with no such history. There was a combined reduction of about 33% in the incidence of nonfatal myocardial infarction and in vascular death when all high-risk patients were taken together. The antiplatelet regimen most often used was "medium-dose" aspirin (75 to 325 mg/day), and dosage within this range seemed to provide similar benefit.[14]

Another meta-analysis that calculated the approximate "number needed to treat" with aspirin to prevent one cardiovascular morbidity during the course of the study found this to range from 45 to 455 patients, although most studies tended toward the lower figure.[15] The number needed to treat in the Antiplatelet Trialists' Collaboration, the most important analysis to date, was approximately 83 patients. All reviewed studies showed some benefit in reducing future morbidity associated with CHD, and two studies had significant reductions in the endpoints of cardiovascular death and nonfatal myocardial infarction.

Other antiplatelet agents have also been evaluated for secondary prevention. Ticlopidine and clopidogrel are thienopyridine derivatives that inhibit platelet aggregation by blocking the binding of adenosine diphosphate, leading to inhibition of the binding process between fibrinogen and glycoprotein IIb/IIIa.[16] Because of their efficacy in medical therapy for patients with ACS as well as in the prevention of stent thrombosis in combination with aspirin, these agents have come under greater scrutiny within the past 2 decades. Ticlopidine was studied in the Studio della Ticlopidina nell'Angina Instabile (STAI) trial,[17] in which the incidence of atherothrombotic events among patients with unstable angina was compared between those receiving 250 mg of ticlopidine twice daily and controls. There was a significant decrease of 46% in the incidence of nonfatal myocardial infarction and vascular death in the treated group at 6-month follow-up; however, ticlopidine was not compared with aspirin, and thus it is not clear whether the benefit represents an improvement over aspirin.

Clopidogrel, which is also a thienopyridine derivative, was compared with aspirin in the Clopidogrel versus Aspirin in Patients at Risk of Ischemic Events (CAPRIE) trial.[18] In this study of more than 19,000 high-risk patients, three groups were defined: those who had recent myocardial infarction, those who had had a recent stroke, and those with significant peripheral arterial disease. Patients were randomly assigned to receive aspirin (325 mg/day) or clopidogrel (75 mg/day) for a mean follow-up of 1.9 years. Clopidogrel-treated patients had an 8.7% relative reduction in myocardial infarction, stroke, or vascular death (5.32%, compared with 5.83% with aspirin). Most of the benefit observed with clopidogrel was in those with peripheral arterial disease. In a subset analysis of the CAPRIE trial, there was no benefit for clopidogrel over aspirin among patients enrolled because of previous myocardial infarction. On the basis of the results of the CAPRIE trial, it was concluded that although clopidogrel could not be recommended as being superior to aspirin, it would be an acceptable alternative to aspirin in those who are unable to take aspirin.

Subsequent to CAPRIE, two trials investigated the benefit of clopidogrel for patients with ACS. The Clopidogrel in Unstable angina to prevent Recurrent ischemic Events (CURE) trial[19] randomly assigned 12,562 patients with ACS who presented within 24 hours to clopidogrel and aspirin or to clopidogrel and placebo, with follow-up for 3 to 12 months. The combined endpoint of cardiovascular death, myocardial infarction, or stroke was reduced by 20% (from 11.5% to 9.3%; $P < .001$) when clopidogrel was given in combination with aspirin (Fig. 33.2). Clopidogrel treatment was also associated with a reduction in the rate of in-hospital severe ischemia and revascularization. The benefits of clopidogrel were seen broadly among low-, intermediate-, and high-risk groups. Major bleeding was increased in the clopidogrel group compared with the placebo group (3.7% compared with 2.7%; $P = .003$) and also occurred in those undergoing coronary bypass graft surgery performed within the first 5 days after clopidogrel was stopped. Importantly, the benefits of clopidogrel persisted for up to 9 months when it was given for treatment of ACS. In the Percutaneous

SECONDARY PREVENTION OF VASCULAR DISEASE WITH PROLONGED ANTIPLATELET THERAPY

Endpoint	Percentage Reduction in Vascular Disease
Nonfatal myocardial infarction	32 ± 5
Nonfatal stroke	27 ± 6
Important vascular event	25 ± 3
Cardiovascular mortality	15 ± 4

A meta-analysis of 25 trials involving patients with a history of cardiovascular disease.

Modified from Antiplatelet Trialists' Collaboration. Secondary prevention of vascular disease by prolonged antiplatelet treatment. BMJ 1988;296:320-331. With permission from the BMJ Publishing Group.

Table 33.2 Secondary prevention of vascular disease with prolonged antiplatelet therapy.

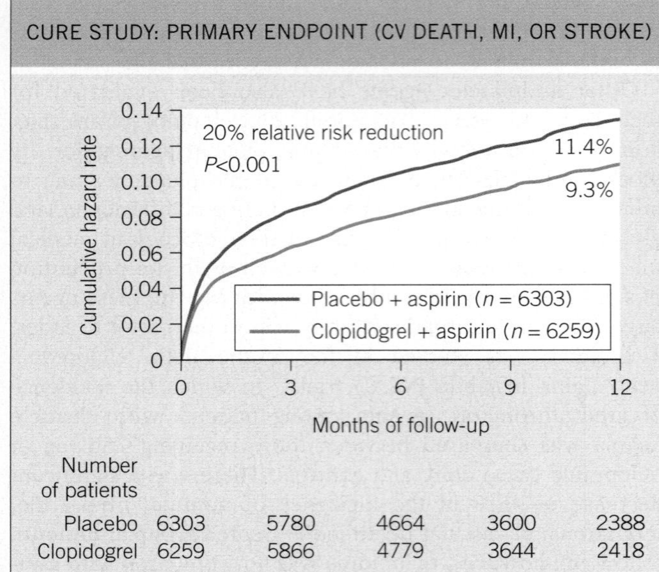

Figure 33.2 CURE study: primary endpoint of cardiovascular (CV) death, myocardial infarction (MI), or stroke. In combination with standard therapy. (From the CURE Trial Investigators; Yusuf S, Zhao F, Mehta SR, Chrolavicius S, Tognoni G, Fox KK. Effects of clopidogrel in addition to aspirin in patients with acute coronary syndromes without ST-segment elevation. N Engl J Med 2001;345:494-502.)

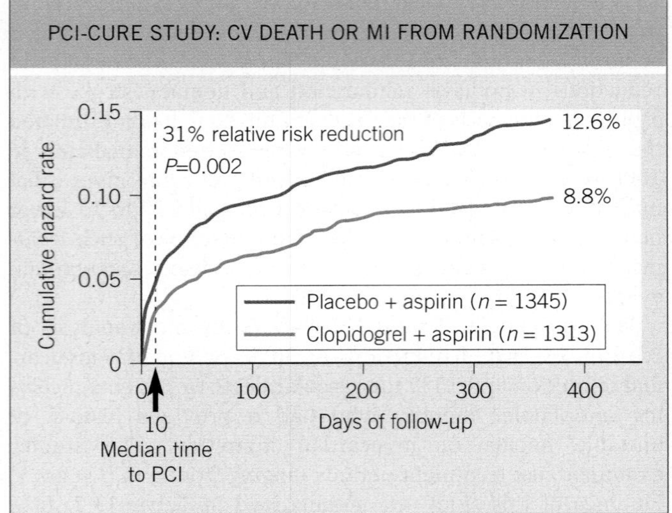

Figure 33.3 PCI-CURE study: cardiovascular (CV) death or myocardial infarction (MI) from randomization. In combination with standard therapy. PCI, percutaneous coronary intervention. (From Mehta SR, Yusuf S, Peters RJ, et al. Effects of pretreatment with clopidogrel and aspirin followed by long-term therapy in patients undergoing percutaneous coronary intervention: the PCI-CURE study. Lancet 2001;358:527-533.)

Coronary Intervention (PCI)–CURE study, a subset of the CURE trial,[20] 2658 patients undergoing percutaneous coronary intervention were randomly assigned to clopidogrel or placebo treatment. A reduction in the primary endpoint (cardiovascular death, myocardial infarction, or urgent target vessel revascularization within 30 days of percutaneous coronary intervention) of 30% was noted (4.5% compared with 6.4%; $P = .03$) and an overall 31% (8.8% compared with 12.6%; $P = .002$) reduction in cardiovascular death or myocardial infarction when clopidogrel was given (Fig. 33.3). The benefits persisted for 9 months.

Further studies regarding optimal duration of clopidogrel use have become important because of concern about risk for early and late stent thrombosis, myocardial infarction, and death associated with its premature discontinuation. The Clopidogrel for the Reduction of Events During Observation (CREDO) study addressed the effectiveness of clopidogrel at 28 days and at 1 year in patients who underwent percutaneous coronary intervention. In a randomized, blinded, placebo-controlled trial, 2116 patients with symptomatic coronary disease who were likely candidates for stent placement were allocated to a clopidogrel loading dose followed by 75 mg/day for 28 days. After 28 days, the placebo group reverted to placebo; the clopidogrel group continued the 75-mg dose. All subjects received 81 to 325 mg of aspirin for 1 year. The first main outcome measure (composite death, myocardial infarction, and stroke at 1 year) showed a 26.9% relative reduction in the clopidogrel group (95% confidence interval, 3.9%-44.4%; $P = .02$). The second main outcome (composite death, myocardial infarction, or urgent revascularization at 28 days) was not reduced by clopidogrel pretreatment.[21]

Other more recent trials that have influenced the duration of clopidogrel therapy are those focused on outcomes associated with bare-metal and drug-eluting stents. In particular, drug-eluting stents have been implicated in a higher rate of late stent thrombosis (approximately 1.2% by 30 days of follow-up).[22] Premature discontinuation of antiplatelet agents was associated with both subacute and late stent thrombosis in 29% of patients treated with drug-eluting stents in a large observational cohort study.[23] Such results prompted specific recommendations for minimum durations of combined clopidogrel and aspirin therapy. Two publications of pooled data published in 2007 looked at outcomes for bare-metal and drug-eluting stents, with similar conclusions.[22,24] The first, a cumulative analysis of studies comparing drug-eluting versus bare-metal stents involving almost 20,000 patients in 4-year follow-up, concluded the following: a nonsignificant increased frequency of stent thrombosis at 1 year with drug-eluting stents, no difference in endpoints of death or death and infarction, but a significant reduction in target lesion revascularization.[22] The second, a meta-analysis of 38 trials (18,023 patients), looked at outcomes comparing bare-metal stents with sirolimus-coated and paclitaxel-coated stents; all three groups were associated with similar overall mortality and cardiac mortality, sirolimus stents with the least risk of myocardial infarction, and paclitaxel stents with the highest risk of late stent (>30 day) thrombosis.[24]

On the basis of these and other studies, in 2007, the AHA/ACC issued a science advisory regarding the recommended duration of dual platelet therapy.[25] These recommendations are reflected in the 2007 AHA/ACC guidelines for unstable angina and non–ST-segment elevation myocardial infarction (UA/NSTEMI), which recommend continuation of clopidogrel (75 mg/day) for at least 1 year in patients receiving drug-eluting stents. The 2007 ACC/AHA/NSTEMI also recommend that at a minimum, patients should be treated with dual antiplatelet therapy (aspirin, 162-325 mg, plus clopidogrel, 75 mg) for 1 month for bare-metal stents, 3 months for sirolimus stents, and 6 months for paclitaxel stents. However, the guidelines emphasize the importance of at least 12 months of dual antiplatelet therapy with drug-eluting stents if hazards to its use (such as bleeding) do not exist.

Indications, Contraindications, and Objectives

The effective dosage of aspirin has been debated, and although most of the early trials used doses of aspirin of more than 325 mg/day, more recent studies have shown similar benefit and fewer adverse side effects with smaller doses (75 to 160 mg/day). In a subset of the CURE trial, ACS patients were randomized to clopidogrel or placebo for up to 1 year. All patients received aspirin but were randomized to one of three doses (≤100 mg, 101 to 199 mg, or ≥200 mg). Results showed each dose to be similarly effective in reducing the combined endpoint of cardiovascular death, myocardial infarction, or stroke when given in combination with clopidogrel. However, the larger the aspirin dose, the larger the incidence in major bleeding (3.0%, 3.4%, and 4.9%; $P = .0009$). These data suggest that the optimal aspirin dose that produces benefit with reduced bleeding risk is 75 to 100 mg/day.[26]

In a 2007 systematic review of eight prospective, randomized, controlled trials and three prospective observational studies with clinical endpoints evaluating varying doses of aspirin in cardiovascular disease, results showed that aspirin doses greater than 75 to 81 mg do not enhance efficacy but do increase risk of gastrointestinal bleeding.[27] On the basis of the data that have been presented, which show a 20% to 30% reduction in cardiovascular deaths and recurrent myocardial infarction, even with lower doses of aspirin, current recommendations are for aspirin use to start immediately during admission to the hospital with ACS and to continue indefinitely. Clopidogrel and ticlopidine may be good alternatives for those who have aspirin intolerance. In addition to their association with an increase in bleeding, the thienopyridine-derivative antiplatelet agents have several potentially serious side effects, such as neutropenia and thrombotic thrombocytopenic purpura.[28] On the basis of the results of CURE and PCI-CURE demonstrating improved outcomes for both lower and higher risk patients with non–ST-segment elevation ACS, it is recommended that these patients, regardless of risk or the need for interventional procedures, be treated with clopidogrel and continued on this therapy for up to 9 months. In accordance with the 2007 AHA/ACC science advisory, in patients who have received bare-metal stents or drug-eluting stents, in the absence of risks for bleeding or other contraindications, dual antiplatelet therapy is recommended for at least 12 months. Accordingly, elective surgeries should be delayed until the patient has finished a recommended duration of antiplatelet therapy. If emergent surgery requiring discontinuation of clopidogrel is needed, aspirin should be continued, if possible, to decrease the risk of stent thrombosis.[25]

ANTICOAGULATION

The use of anticoagulation either alone or combined with antiplatelet treatment to reduce risk after ACS has also been evaluated and has been found to have benefit in reducing cardiac mortality and nonfatal myocardial infarction when the dosage of warfarin was carefully controlled. In many studies, the benefit of warfarin anticoagulation has been demonstrated or offset by the incidence of significant major bleeding complications or embolic events as a result of inadequate dosing or poor control of the international normalized ratio (INR).[29-32] The WArfarin Re-Infarction Study (WARIS) II trial provides evidence supporting the use of warfarin in combination with aspirin or given alone after myocardial infarction in 3630 patients younger than 75 years who were randomly assigned to aspirin (160 mg daily), aspirin (75 mg daily) combined with warfarin (INR, 2.0 to 2.5), or warfarin alone (INR, 2.8 to 4.2).[33] The primary outcome of death, nonfatal reinfarction, or thromboembolic cerebral stroke occurred more frequently in those receiving aspirin (20.0%) than in those receiving warfarin and aspirin (15.0%) or warfarin alone (16.7%). The difference between the two groups receiving warfarin was not statistically significant, but both were significantly better than aspirin alone. The major benefit from the warfarin treatments was to reduce the occurrence of nonfatal reinfarction and nonfatal thromboembolic stroke, whereas no reduction in mortality was observed among the three groups. Unfortunately, the use of warfarin was associated with a higher risk of bleeding, with approximately four times as many major bleeding episodes in the two groups receiving warfarin than in the group receiving aspirin alone.

Indications and Contraindications

Long-term anticoagulation with warfarin after myocardial infarction is recommended for patients with left ventricular thrombus, large akinetic left ventricular segments, or persistent atrial fibrillation and for those unable to take daily aspirin. In patients with large anterior myocardial infarction or left ventricular thrombus, warfarin should be started immediately and continued for a minimum of 6 months, maintaining an INR of 2 to 3. There are no randomized, controlled trials that have demonstrated a clear benefit of warfarin over aspirin for reducing stroke, reinfarction, and mortality, and in most, there have been increased bleeding complications observed among those receiving warfarin treatment. The key to successful treatment with warfarin after ACS appears to reside in the selection of high-risk patients and careful control of INR, with lower target INR values if aspirin (preferably low-dose) or clopidogrel is given along with warfarin therapy. Particular caution is warranted in patients requiring dual antiplatelet therapy along with warfarin, such as those with stent placement in whom chronic anticoagulation is required for atrial fibrillation or a prosthetic valve. An algorithm of recommendations for antiplatelet therapy and anticoagulation in unstable angina and non–ST-segment elevation myocardial infarction is presented in the 2007 AHA/ACC guidelines (Fig. 33.4).[34]

β-ADRENERGIC BLOCKERS

Mechanisms of Action

β-Adrenergic blocking agents benefit post–myocardial infarction patients by decreasing myocardial oxygen demand, heart rate, systemic blood pressure, and contractility. In addition, they reduce both ventricular and supraventricular arrhythmias after myocardial infarction. There is also evidence that beta blockers may slow the progression of coronary atherosclerosis.[35]

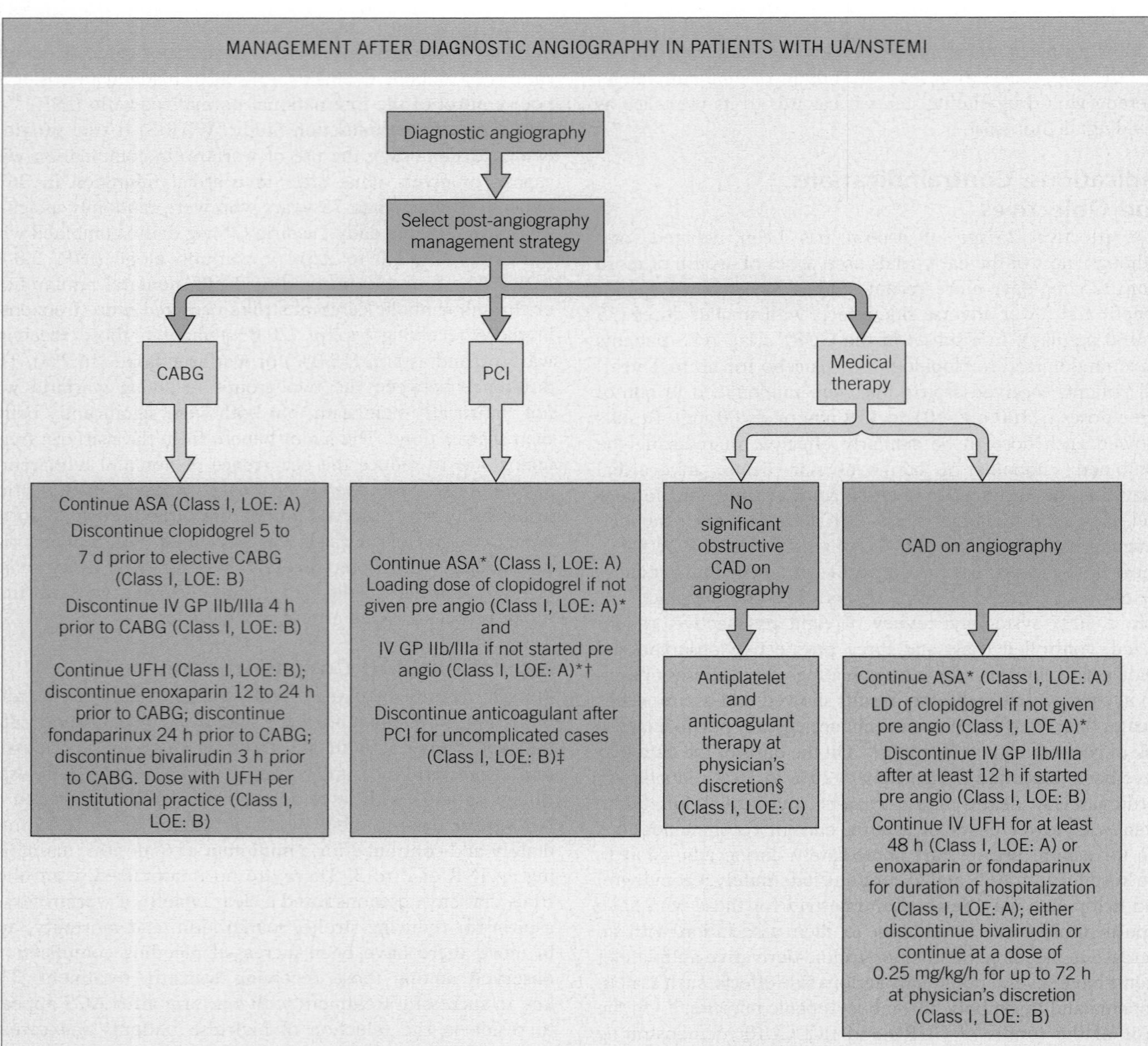

Figure 33.4 Long-term anticoagulant therapy at hospital discharge in patients with unstable angina and non–ST elevation myocardial infarction (UA/NSTEMI). *See dosing Table 13. †Evidence exists that glycoprotein IIb/IIIa inhibitors may not be necessary if the patient received a preloading dose of at least 300 mg of clopidogrel at least 6 hours earlier (Class I, Level of Evidence B for clopidogrel administration) and bivalirudin is selected as the anticoagulant (Class IIa, Level of Evidence B). ‡Additional bolus of unfractionated heparin is recommended if fondaparinux is selected as the anticoagulant (see dosing Table 13). §For patients in whom the clinician believes coronary atherosclerosis is present, albeit without any significant, flow-limiting stenoses, long-term treatment with antiplatelet agents and other secondary prevention measures should be considered. ASA, aspirin; CABG, coronary artery bypass graft; CAD, coronary artery disease; GP, glycoprotein; IV, intravenous; LD, loading dose; PCI, percutaneous coronary intervention; pre angio, before angiography; UA/NSTEMI, unstable angina/non–ST elevation myocardial infarction; UFH, unfractionated heparin. (From Anderson JL, Adams CD, Antman EM, et al. ACC/AHA 2007 guidelines for the management of patients with unstable angina/non–ST elevation myocardial infarction: a report of the American College of Cardiology/American Heart Association Task Force on Practice Guidelines [Writing Committee to Revise the 2002 Guidelines for the Management of Patients with Unstable Angina/Non–ST-Elevation Myocardial Infarction] developed in collaboration with the American College of Emergency Physicians, the Society for Cardiovascular Angiography and Interventions, and the Society of Thoracic Surgeons endorsed by the American Association of Cardiovascular and Pulmonary Rehabilitation and the Society for Academic Emergency Medicine. J Am Coll Cardiol 2007;50:e1-e157.)

Several trials have confirmed the benefit of beta-blocker therapy after ACS. The first major trial to document this benefit was the Norwegian timolol trial, published in 1981, in which 1884 patients were started on timolol or placebo at 7 to 28 days after myocardial infarction and then observed for up to 33 months. There was a 39% relative reduction in the mortality rate in the treated group (21.9% for placebo compared with 13.3% for timolol) at 33 months and a 28% reduction in reinfarction rate.[36]

TRIALS OF BETA BLOCKERS IN POST–MYOCARDIAL INFARCTION PATIENTS								
Trial	No. of Patients	Entry into Study	Therapy	Dose	Follow-up	Mortality (%) Treated	Untreated	Risk Reduction
Hjalmarson et al.[39]	1395	<48 hours	Metoprolol	15 mg IV, then 200 mg/day	24 months	13.2	17.2	23.3
First International Study of Infarct Survival Collaborative Group[38]	16,027	<12 hours	Atenolol	5-10 mg IV, then 100 mg/day	12 months	10.7	12.0	10.8
The Norwegian Multicenter Study Group[36]	1884	7-28 days	Timolol	20 mg/day	17 months	10.6	17.5	39.9
Beta-Blocker Heart Attack Trial Research Group[37]	3837	5-21 days	Propranolol	180-240 mg/day	25 months	7.2	9.8	26.5

Table 33.3 Trials of beta blockers in post–myocardial infarction patients.

The Beta Blocker Heart Attack Trial (BHAT) revealed a 28% reduction in sudden death among post–myocardial infarction patients treated with propranolol compared with those treated with placebo (3.3% compared with 4.6%) and an overall mortality reduction of 27% (7.2% compared with 9.8%); the average follow-up period was 25 months.[37]

The ISIS-1 and Gothenburg metoprolol trials similarly showed a significant benefit with use of beta blockers early after myocardial infarction.[38,39] The ISIS-1 trial revealed that early use of atenolol reduced 7-day mortality, decreasing it from 4.3% to 3.7% in the treated group. This benefit was believed to be primarily related to a reduction in the incidence of cardiac rupture.[38]

The majority of studies involving beta-blocker therapy were conducted in the era before the use of thrombolytic therapy for acute myocardial infarction, and until recently, data have been lacking to substantiate the benefits of beta-blocker therapy given after myocardial infarction among patients treated acutely with thrombolytic therapy. The Thrombolysis in Myocardial Infarction (TIMI) II trial evaluated metoprolol treatment in a subset of 1390 patients who were receiving thrombolysis plus either early intravenous metoprolol started within 2 hours of hospital admission followed by oral metoprolol or oral metoprolol started only 6 days after admission. Although the overall mortality was similar in both groups, there was a significant decrease in the incidence of nonfatal myocardial infarction and recurrent ischemia in the group that received early intravenous and oral metoprolol.[40]

In contrast to these observations, a study involving the use of intravenous atenolol after thrombolytic therapy in myocardial infarction seemed to show conflicting data about the early use of intravenous beta blockers.[41] A group of more than 18,000 patients who received immediate intravenous atenolol followed by oral atenolol was compared with a group of 12,500 who received only early oral atenolol after thrombolysis. Both groups enjoyed a survival benefit compared with patients who did not receive beta-blocker treatment, but the use of early intravenous atenolol was associated with a greater incidence of heart failure, shock, recurrent ischemia, and pacemaker use, leading to a significantly greater mortality rate than in those who received only early oral treatment. The researchers concluded that the use of oral atenolol as soon as the patient's condition was stable was the safest and most effective beta-blocker regimen.

A summary of important trials of beta blockers is presented in Table 33.3.

Additional evidence is now available regarding the beneficial effect of beta blockers on coronary atherosclerotic lesions. In a 2007 pooled analysis from four intravascular ultrasound studies including 1515 patients with established coronary disease, the average atheroma volume was significantly less in those receiving beta blockers ($P <.001$) versus those who did not ($P =.86$).[35] This finding was independent of statin use, ACE inhibitor use, and low achieved levels of low-density lipoprotein (LDL), seeming to implicate beta blockers in regression or decreasing progression of coronary artery disease. Postulated mechanisms of this regression include reduced heart rate, reduced endothelial permeability to lipoproteins, and reduced proclivity of LDL-cholesterol to the vessel wall. Beta blockers also decrease the incidence of sudden cardiac death during the acute and postinfarction phase. In a meta-analysis of 16 studies, involving more than 19,000 patients, that assessed the benefit of beta-blocker therapy on total mortality and sudden death after myocardial infarction, 333 patients suffered sudden death after receiving beta blockers, compared with 480 patients who did not receive therapy.[42] This 34% decrease in sudden death was highly significant. The possible actions by which beta blockers may effect this improvement include a reduction in early cardiac rupture (within 24 hours) and a reduction in the incidence of ventricular fibrillation.

Notable exception to the use of beta blockers in acute myocardial infarction is in the event of cocaine-induced myocardial infarction, in which the unopposed beta blockade may precipitate coronary vasospasm by α-adrenergic stimulation. If used, labetalol, which has both alpha- and beta-blocking properties, is recommended.[34]

Indications and Contraindications

In spite of the evidence of their benefit, beta blockers remain underused after myocardial infarction. The low overall use of these drugs can be partially explained by physicians' fear of their adverse effects or the presence of contraindications. In the Cooperative Cardiovascular Project, beta-blocker therapy after myocardial infarction was reviewed in more than 200,000 records of Medicare patients.[43] Administration of beta blockers increased from 48% in 1992 to 68% in 1995 among patients who had no contraindications to their use. Medicare and Medicaid data pooled from 3558 hospitals during the first half of 2004 indicated that 84% of patients received a beta blocker at discharge.[44] For those who had relative contraindications, as defined by the 1996 ACC recommendations,[45] there was a 45% rate of use in 1995.

The commonly listed relative contraindications to the use of beta blockers include the following[45]:

- bradycardia;
- severe unstable left ventricular failure or hypotension;
- signs of peripheral hypoperfusion;
- PR prolongation on electrocardiography of more than 0.24 second;
- second- or third-degree atrioventricular block;
- severe chronic obstructive pulmonary disease;
- a history of asthma;
- a history of severe peripheral vascular disease; and
- type 1 (insulin-dependent) diabetes mellitus.

In the study of beta-blocker use in Medicare patients, records revealed a beneficial effect from the drugs, even in those with one or more relative contraindications.[43] In fact, there was an overall reduction in mortality of 40% in higher risk patients who were discharged receiving beta blockers compared with those who were not. Every subgroup analyzed, including those with diabetes mellitus, chronic obstructive pulmonary disease, or CHF, experienced benefit. This reduction was greater than that shown in a meta-analysis of beta-blocker use, in which overall mortality was reduced by 22%.[46] An additional subgroup analysis of 115,000 patients aged 65 years or older also showed a 14% lower mortality risk at 1 year.

The ACC/AHA guidelines recommend that beta-blocker therapy should begin within 12 hours of myocardial infarction, regardless of the use of thrombolytic agents, and they also recommend that it should be continued in the long term, although there are no significant data about the efficacy of beta blockers beyond 2 to 3 years. For patients who require early intravenous beta-blocker therapy because of continuing or recurrent ischemia or tachyarrhythmias, such as atrial fibrillation or rapid ventricular response, oral therapy should be initiated as soon as the stability of the patient allows.[45]

ANGIOTENSIN-CONVERTING ENZYME INHIBITORS

Mechanisms of Action

ACE inhibitors have also taken their place as effective treatment after myocardial infarction, alongside other pharmacologic methods designed to reduce cardiovascular morbidity and mortality. Although the use of thrombolytics, antiplatelet agents, and beta blockers has improved post–myocardial infarction mortality and reinfarction rates, a significant number (up to 14%) of patients who survive myocardial infarction still develop signs or symptoms of left ventricular dysfunction.[47] The development of left ventricular dysfunction is a poor prognostic marker, and it is strongly correlated with an increased risk of subsequent nonfatal or fatal cardiovascular events. The use of ACE inhibitors in the immediate post–myocardial infarction setting to prevent left ventricular dysfunction has been closely examined because they have been shown to be of great benefit in those patients with chronic heart failure.

Acute myocardial infarction results in the activation of neurohormonal systems that may lead to increasing myocardial oxygen demand and infarct extension or left ventricular dilatation. The release of epinephrine (adrenaline) and norepinephrine (noradrenaline) increases with the pain and anxiety associated with an acute infarct, and this leads to an increased heart rate and workload for the heart. A decrease in blood pressure or cardiac output can lead to increased peripheral sympathetic activation, thereby activating the renin-angiotensin system. Increased production and release of angiotensin II lead to increasing vasoconstriction, myocardial workload, and myocardial oxygen demand. Coronary vascular tone is also increased, leading to reduced coronary blood flow.[48] Compensatory left ventricular hypertrophy and subsequent dilatation may also develop as a result of this early neurohormonal activation. Left ventricular failure, arrhythmias, and death have been associated with neurohormonal activation. Renin and angiotensin concentrations are increased, even in patients who have uncomplicated myocardial infarction, and they are much greater in patients who develop heart failure in the acute setting. ACE inhibitors block this neurohormonal activation, particularly the higher concentrations associated with left ventricular dysfunction, thereby reducing concentrations of circulating catecholamines and angiotensin II.[48]

Ventricular remodeling is a name given to the pathologic dilatation that occurs after myocardial infarction. The degree of remodeling, or dilatation, is directly related to the size and duration of the infarct. In the immediate setting of myocardial infarction, inflammation and edema are followed by fibroblast proliferation and collagen deposition, leading to thinning, scar formation, and dilatation. This left ventricular dilatation causes left ventricular performance to suffer. Early studies in the rat model revealed that the early and chronic use of captopril could attenuate left ventricular remodeling and the resulting left ventricular dysfunction.[49]

ACE inhibitors have been shown to decrease morbidity and mortality in patients after myocardial infarction. Several large trials have demonstrated improved survival, although the populations studied and the timing of ACE inhibitor therapy have remained controversial.

In the Survival And Ventricular Enlargement (SAVE) trial, 2231 patients with ACS and reduced LVEF (<40%) received captopril at a mean of 11 days (range, 3 to 16 days) after myocardial infarction, with an approximately 20% reduction in mortality.[50] The overall reduction in mortality was seen after 12 months and was significant after an average follow-up of 42 months. The target dose of captopril was 25 mg three times daily during the stay in hospital, increasing to 50 mg three times daily after discharge. Similarly, the Acute Infarction Ramipril Efficacy (AIRE) trial studied 2006 patients with clinical heart failure who were allocated randomly to groups to receive ramipril or placebo from 2 to 9 days (mean, 5 days) after myocardial infarction. They were observed for an average of 15 months. There was a 27% risk reduction in all-cause mortality in patients with heart failure who received ramipril.[51] In the Studies Of Left Ventricular Dysfunction (SOLVD) trial,[52] 4200 asymptomatic patients with LVEF of less than 35%, of whom 80% had had a previous myocardial infarction, had a 20% risk reduction in combined endpoints of death and CHF requiring admission to the hospital with enalapril at a mean dose of 16.7 mg/day. Similarly, in the Trandolapril Cardiac Evaluation (TRACE) study,[53] 1749 patients with LVEF of approximately 35% or less were allocated randomly to groups to receive trandolapril or placebo 3 to 7 days after myocardial infarction and continued for 24 to 50 months. There was a significant reduction (22%) in total mortality and cardiovascular mortality. A progression to more severe heart failure was reduced, as was the incidence of sudden death. Another more contemporary study looking at ACE inhibition in stable coronary disease contradicted the TRACE study results. In the Prevention of Events with Angiotensin-Converting Enzyme Inhibition (PEACE) trial, almost 8300 patients with stable coronary disease and normal left ventricular function were blindly randomized to a 4-mg dose of trandolapril versus placebo with the hypothesis that these patients would also experience a decrease in the composite endpoint of cardiovascular death, myocardial infarction, and revascularization. Interestingly, no benefit was observed. The investigators theorized that the population of their study patients, who at baseline were healthier, with no left ventricular dysfunction, with more intense risk factor modification, were at lower cardiovascular risk for events and therefore did not derive the benefits seen in the less healthy populations in the previous studies.[54]

In all these long-term studies except for PEACE, ACE inhibitors initiated within several days showed benefit in cardiovascular mortality and morbidity, especially in patients who developed heart failure as the result of myocardial infarction. More recently, an effort to examine the effect of earlier initiation of ACE inhibitor treatment on long-term cardiovascular events has been undertaken. The Survival of Myocardial Infarction Long-Term Evaluation (SMILE) trial sought to determine the efficacy of the early use of zofenopril on total mortality, CHF, and nonfatal recurrent myocardial infarction in 1556 patients who suffered acute anterior myocardial infarction but who were not eligible for thrombolysis.[55] ACE inhibitor treatment or placebo was started within 24 hours and continued for 6 weeks, and patients were observed for 1 year. There was a trend toward reduced mortality at 6 weeks, which persisted and was significant at 1 year, with a 25% reduction in mortality. The Cooperative New Scandinavian Enalapril Survival Study (CONSENSUS II) offered conflicting data, however, in a trial that enrolled patients to placebo or intravenous enalapril within 15 hours of the onset of symptoms of myocardial infarction. Treatment with oral medication was started 6 hours later and continued for 6 months. The mortality rate was actually higher in the enalapril group, particularly among the elderly, and this was thought to be at least partially attributable to early hypotension after the intravenous administration of enalapril was begun.[56] One interesting finding from a subgroup analysis of the CONSENSUS II trial was that there seemed to be an aspirin–ACE inhibitor interaction, which led to attenuation of the effect of enalapril in patients who were receiving aspirin before their myocardial infarction.[57] The mortality benefit for patients receiving the combination was not as great as for patients who received enalapril alone. ACE inhibitors stimulate increased prostaglandin release, leading to prostaglandin-mediated vasodilatation. Researchers hypothesized that aspirin may antagonize the effects of ACE inhibitors by its antiprostaglandin effects, thereby inhibiting vasodilatation. Since then, several studies have determined that the benefit of ACE inhibitors is independent of the concomitant use of aspirin. A systematic review of six randomized, placebo-controlled trials of more than 22,000 patients sought to identify whether the benefit of ACE inhibitors on primary outcome (composite death, myocardial infarction, stroke, hospitalization for CHF, or revascularization) was affected by aspirin's presence. Although with a marginally significant *P* value (.07), the data confirmed that ACE effects against major vascular events remained substantial in both the presence and absence of aspirin. The marginal *P* value does raise the possibility of some interaction between the two medications but should not alter recommendations to continue the concomitant use of both medications in the study population.

ACE inhibitor therapy may also exert beneficial effects in patients who have CHD by a direct effect on the coronary vasculature. ACE inhibition has been shown to improve endothelium-dependent vasodilatation in coronary epicardial and resistance arteries in patients who have CHD. It is believed that ACE inhibition exerts its favorable effect on the coronary vasculature by increasing nitric oxide bioreactivity.[58] Presumably, these actions are secondary to ACE inhibitor–associated improvement in endothelial function.

In an attempt to identify definitively those subgroups of patients who would benefit most from ACE inhibition after ACS and to determine conclusively whether early treatment was beneficial, the ACE Inhibitor Myocardial Infarction Collaborative Group reviewed individual data from four recent large trials. Data were available from more than 98,000 patients enrolled in the CONSENSUS II, Gruppo Italiano per lo Studio della Sopravvivenza nell'Infarto Miocardico (GISSI-3), ISIS-4, and Chinese Cardiac Study (CCS-I) trials.[59] These trials used captopril, enalapril, or lisinopril given within 36 hours of the onset of symptoms of myocardial infarction. Overall, there was a significant 7% reduction in mortality at 30 days for patients receiving ACE inhibitors (7.11%) compared with those taking placebo (7.59%). Most of this mortality benefit was seen in the first week after myocardial infarction. Younger patients tended to have a greater mortality benefit, as did patients with myocardial infarction (14% risk reduction). ACE inhibitor therapy significantly reduced the incidence of nonfatal CHF and was very beneficial in patients with previous myocardial infarction, diabetes, and hypertension. Treatment with ACE inhibitors was associated with a significantly greater incidence of hypotension after ACS, an effect that increased with increasing age of the patient. The overall mortality benefit from the early use of ACE inhibitors that was continued for 1 month was approximately five lives saved per 1000 patients treated.

Data from the Heart Outcomes Prevention Evaluation (HOPE) trial suggest that ACE inhibitors given to post–myocardial infarction patients with normal LVEF may also improve survival and decrease major adverse cardiovascular events, including stroke and the need for revascularization procedures.[60]

Similar data were derived from the EUROPA study. Patients who were slightly healthier at baseline but still with cardiovascular risk saw a 20% reduction in the primary outcome of cardiovascular death, nonfatal myocardial infarction, or cardiac arrest when administered perindopril versus placebo.[61]

The 2006 updates to the ACC/AHA guidelines for secondary prevention in patients with cardiovascular disease recommend ACE inhibition as first-line therapy in post–myocardial infarction patients with left ventricular dysfunction but endorse the second-line use of an angiotensin receptor blocker if the patient is ACE intolerant on the basis of data showing noninferiority of angiotensin receptor blockers in a similar population. The VALIANT trial included more than 14,000 patients with recent myocardial infarction complicated by heart failure or left ventricular dysfunction. Valsartan or combination valsartan and captopril was administered in an effort to determine if valsartan alone or the combination of the ACE inhibitor and angiotensin receptor blocker reduced mortality compared with captopril alone. Results showed that valsartan alone was similar to captopril alone for all-cause mortality but increased adverse events without benefit in the combination.[62] Similarly, the CHARM-Alternative study looked at 2028 patients with symptomatic heart failure and left ventricular dysfunction who were ACE inhibitor intolerant. Candesartan administration reduced cardiovascular mortality and morbidity in these patients.[63] The data suggest that angiotensin receptor blockers are a good alternative to those intolerant of ACE inhibitors. In addition, studies have also reconfirmed the recommendation for aldosterone use in post–myocardial infarction patients with LVEF below 40% and heart failure.[11]

Despite the benefits of ACE inhibitors, their implementation in patients after ACS remains low as documented by several reports, although statistics for use have been slowly improving. A 1998 review of 190,000 patients in the National Registry of Myocardial Infarction 2 (NRMI-2) revealed that only 42.6% of those deemed to benefit most from ACE inhibitors (i.e., those with CHF or an LVEF of less than 40%) were discharged receiving ACE inhibitors, and overall only 27.6% received ACE inhibitors.[64] In 1998, data from the Cooperative Cardiovascular Project, which reviewed indicators of secondary prevention in Medicare patients who were discharged after ACS, found that less than 60% of ideal candidates were discharged with ACE inhibitors.[65] More recent National Medicare and Medicaid data collected as part of the Hospital Quality Alliance Program between July 2004 and June 2005 indicated that 82.4% of post–myocardial infarction patients with left ventricular dysfunction were discharged on an ACE inhibitor or an angiotensin blocker. Similar rates were found in the National Veterans Health Administration data and the AHA Get With the Guidelines data.[1]

Indications, Contraindications, and Objectives

On the basis of published data, the following recommendations can be made for the use of ACE inhibitors in the ACS setting. Patients with poor left ventricular function or CHF, those who have large anterior myocardial infarctions, and those with hypertension or diabetes mellitus receive particular benefit from the ACE inhibitors. These patients should be prescribed therapy early, starting with low doses and increasing expeditiously to maximum tolerated doses. These patients should be continued on therapy in the long term (at least 2 to 3 years) and in most cases indefinitely. There is also benefit from the use of ACE inhibitors in patients with uncomplicated myocardial infarction in the absence of left ventricular dysfunction, diabetes, or hypertension, and it is reasonable to start ACE inhibitor therapy in this group of patients during hospitalization.

Cardiogenic shock and hypotension in the setting of ACS are contraindications to the immediate commencement of ACE inhibitor therapy; so too are known hypersensitivity to ACE inhibitors and azotemia. Care should be taken in initiating ACE inhibitors in the elderly because elderly people may be more prone to hypotension. Angiotensin receptor blockers are an acceptable alternative with similar beneficial effects if ACE intolerance is an issue. In general, the long-term benefit of ACE inhibitor therapy is proportionate to the disease-related risk, with those patients at lowest risk (i.e., normal left ventricular function, normal blood pressure, no diabetes mellitus, and a history of recent revascularization) benefiting least.

LIPID-DECREASING TREATMENT

Mechanisms of Action

All patients should be evaluated and treated for dyslipidemia after ACS. An ever-growing body of evidence proves that lipid-decreasing treatment reduces total mortality, cardiac mortality, the need for revascularization, subsequent cardiac events, and stroke. 3-Hydroxy-3-methylglutaryl coenzyme A (HMG-CoA) reductase inhibitors (the "statins") have become the mainstays for lipid lowering, particularly in those with CHD with increased LDL concentrations as defined by the National Cholesterol Education Program (NCEP) guidelines. At the advent of the statins' clinical use, when their power to lower cardiovascular risk was just beginning to be discovered, studies primarily focused on the effects of a statin compared with a placebo to assess beneficial outcomes in patients with CHD. In particular, three large randomized clinical trials using statins confirmed the benefits of decreasing the concentrations of LDL-cholesterol in patients who have known CHD.

In 1994, the first large trial to demonstrate the beneficial effect of statin drugs on cardiovascular morbidity and mortality was the Scandinavian Simvastatin Survival Study (4S).[66] In this trial, 4444 men and women with a diagnosis of CHD and hypercholesterolemia (range, 213 to 310 mg/dL [5.5 to 8.0 mmol/L]; mean, 260 mg/dL [6.7 mmol/L]) were observed for 5.4 years. Simvastatin treatment resulted in a 25% reduction in total cholesterol and a 35% reduction in LDL-cholesterol levels. During this study, 256 patients (12%) in the placebo group died, compared with 182 patients (8%) in the simvastatin group, corresponding to a 30% reduction in total mortality. Of these deaths, there were 189 deaths from CHD in the placebo group and 111 deaths from CHD in the treatment group, yielding a highly significant 42% reduction in CHD mortality. There was also a reduction of 37% in revascularization procedures and a reduction of 28% in stroke. The benefits were seen among elderly patients in addition to the young.

Whereas the 4S evaluated the benefits of lipid decreasing in patients who had increased lipid concentrations, in 1996, the Cholesterol And Recurrent Events (CARE) trial extended the findings of the 4S to patients with normal total cholesterol concentrations, concentrations that are consistent with the levels of total cholesterol and LDL-cholesterol found in the majority of patients with CHD and ACS. Patients were randomized to treatment with pravastatin or placebo. The study broadly confirmed the benefit of statin drugs in reducing LDL-cholesterol concentrations and subsequent cardiac events.[67] In this study of more than 4000 subjects, patients treated with pravastatin had a 32% reduction in mean LDL-cholesterol concentration to 98 mg/dL (2.5 mmol/L), which was maintained during the follow-up period of 5 years. A significant risk reduction of 24% in the incidence of fatal and nonfatal coronary events was observed in patients treated with statin therapy (274 patients with placebo compared with 212 patients with pravastatin). The benefits of lipid reduction became apparent within 1.5 years after treatment started, a finding that was also seen in the 4S. The CARE study was not powered to detect a decrease in total mortality.

Published in 1998, the Long-term Intervention with Pravastatin in Ischemic Disease (LIPID) trial also investigated the benefit of lipid decreasing on mortality in patients who had a history of myocardial infarction or unstable angina with a wide range of cholesterol concentrations (155 to 271 mg/dL [4 to 7 mmol/L]).[68] Mortality from CHD in patients receiving pravastatin compared with that in patients receiving placebo was studied in 9014 patients who were observed for a mean of 6.1 years. Patients in the treatment arm achieved an 18% reduction in total cholesterol. There was a 24% relative risk reduction in the primary endpoint of death from CHD in treated patients compared with placebo patients. Overall, there was a 22% decrease in mortality in patients receiving pravastatin. Secondary endpoints included relative reductions of 29% in the incidence of myocardial infarction, 19% in the incidence of stroke, 22% in the rate of coronary artery bypass graft surgery, 19% in the rate of percutaneous transluminal coronary angioplasty, and 22% in the rate of admission to the hospital for unstable angina.

These three large randomized, controlled trials of statins formed the cornerstone of recommendations for statin use and lipid lowering. Mortality and morbidity data with statin use having been established, more specific questions about timing and dosing of statins, statins in percutaneous coronary intervention, combination therapies, and head-to-head statin comparisons were posed in the late 1990s and into the turn of the millennium. In 2001, the Adult Treatment Panel III (ATP III) of the NCEP issued a set of guidelines for lipid management based on the studies available to date.

Several studies have addressed the question of whether patients with ACS would benefit from early initiation of lipid-decreasing treatment. In the Myocardial Ischemia Reduction with Aggressive Cholesterol Lowering (MIRACL) trial,[69] aggressive lipid reduction with atorvastatin was compared with placebo therapy for 3086 patients with ACS. Treatment was started early, within 24 to 96 hours after admission to the hospital. Within 16 weeks after the treatment was started, the primary endpoint (death, nonfatal myocardial infarction, resuscitated cardiac arrest, or recurrent severe myocardial ischemia) was reduced from 17.4% to 14.8% (placebo compared with atorvastatin; $P = .048$). Significant reductions in recurrent ischemia and stroke were observed for those treated with atorvastatin; however, no significant differences occurred in the risk of death, nonfatal myocardial infarction, cardiac arrest, or worsening heart failure between the two groups. The results of initiating lipid-decreasing treatment at the time of admission to the hospital for acute myocardial infarction were reported by the Swedish Registry of Cardiac Intensive Care involving 19,599 men and women younger than 80 years admitted to the hospital in 58 Swedish hospitals during the period 1995-1998. A 25% reduction in the adjusted relative risk of mortality was observed in patients in whom statin therapy was initiated before discharge from the hospital (Fig. 33.5). In the largest study of the effects of early statin treatment in acute myocardial infarction, the NRMI-4 investigators included more than 170,000 patients with acute myocardial infarction, of whom 22% received statin treatment within the first 24 hours of hospitalization, and looked at the rate of complications as well as in-hospital mortality. New or continued administration of statin compared with no statin significantly reduced mortality (4.0% and 5.3% compared with 15.4%) and lowered the incidence of cardiogenic shock, arrhythmias, cardiac arrest, and rupture but not recurrent myocardial infarction.[70] The data accumulated from these evolving studies support the recommendation that statin therapy be initiated during the stay in the hospital in patients admitted for ACS.

The Heart Protection Study (HPS) trial, which included more than 20,536 men and women with coronary disease, other vascular disease, diabetes, or hypertension,[71] addressed the issue of whether patients would benefit from statin therapy irrespective of their initial cholesterol concentrations. The

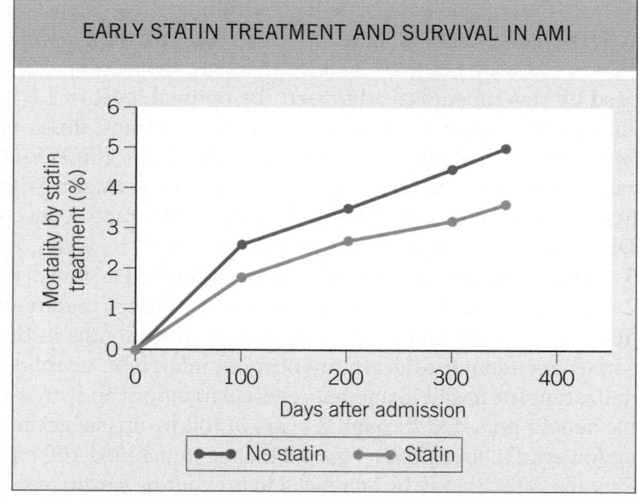

Figure 33.5 Early statin treatment and survival in acute myocardial infarction (AMI). From a study of 19,599 men and women younger than 80 years discharged after acute myocardial infarction from 58 Swedish hospitals between 1995 and 1998. A total of 5528 (28%) received statin, and 14,071 (72%) received no statin. Highest hospital rates of use, 48%; lowest, 12%. (Modified from Stenestrand U, Wallentin L. Early statin treatment following acute myocardial infarction and 1-year survival. JAMA 2001;285:430-436.)

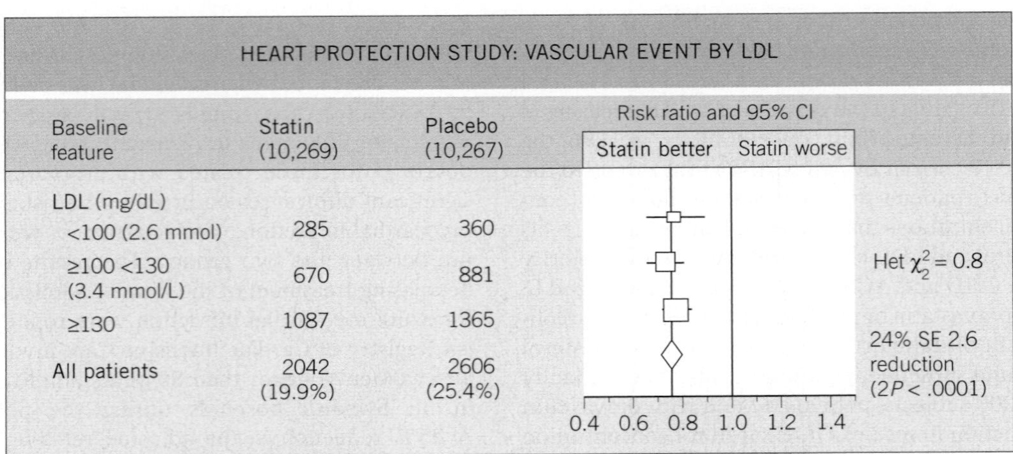

Figure 33.6 Heart Protection Study: vascular event by low-density lipoprotein (LDL) concentration. CI, confidence interval; Het, heterogeneity coefficient; SE, standard error.

study reported results among patients aged 40 to 80 years who were allocated randomly to receive daily simvastatin (40 mg) or placebo. Previous myocardial infarction was reported for 41% of the patients in the study. A highly significant 18% reduction occurred in coronary mortality among those treated with statin therapy (5.7% compared with 6.9%; P =.0001), and total mortality, after a mean follow-up of 5 years, was also significantly reduced among those receiving statin treatment. Importantly, significant reductions in major cardiovascular events and mortality were seen at all starting concentrations of LDL, even for patients whose LDL concentration was less than 100 mg/dL when therapy was initiated (Fig. 33.6). The findings were observed among major cardiovascular events for all important prespecified subgroups, including women and among patient age groups. These findings lend support to the thesis that lipid-decreasing treatment should be initiated among all patients with atherosclerotic cardiovascular disease and suggest that all those admitted with ACS should be started on statin therapy unless a specific contraindication exists.

Given that lipid lowering with statins reduces cardiovascular risk across a wide range of cholesterol levels, the next question posed by several studies addressed the optimal level of LDL-cholesterol by treating with intense versus standard doses of statin. In 4162 patients hospitalized for ACS, the PROVE-IT trial compared a standard dose of 40 mg of pravastatin with intensive treatment with 80 mg of atorvastatin. Each reduced LDL levels; the pravastatin group achieved a mean of 95 mg/dL, and the atorvastatin group achieved a mean of 62 mg/dL. The benefits of the intensive therapy emerged after only 30 days and became significant at 4 months in the composite endpoint of death, myocardial infarction, or rehospitalization for unstable angina, revascularization, and stroke. This benefit persisted through 2 years of follow-up, suggesting that lower LDL levels even beyond the recommended 100 mg/dL by the ATP III may be beneficial in preventing cardiovascular death and events after ACS.[72] Another large trial of intensive lipid lowering corroborated the benefits of low LDL concentrations shown in PROVE-IT using a population of patients with stable coronary disease. The Treating to New Targets (TNT) investigators enrolled 10,001 patients with clinically stable CHD with LDL levels below 130 mg/dL to receive either 10 mg or 80 mg of atorvastatin. These doses reduced mean LDL levels to 101 mg/dL and 77 mg/dL, respectively. Primary outcomes were a major cardiovascular event (death from CHD, nonfatal myocardial infarction, resuscitation after cardiac arrest, stroke). The intensively treated group had 22% relative reduction in the primary outcome (P <.001).

The REVERSAL study also looked at intensive versus moderate lipid lowering but was designed to measure its effect on atheroma burden by intravascular ultrasonography. Approximately 650 patients were randomized to receive either moderate lipid-lowering therapy (pravastatin, 40 mg) or intensive lipid-lowering therapy (atorvastatin, 80 mg) and had intravascular ultrasound examinations performed at baseline and after 18 months of treatment. Efficacy was measured as change in atheroma volume between the two intravascular ultrasound studies. Results demonstrated progression of coronary atherosclerosis in the pravastatin arm but no progression in the atorvastatin group, providing further evidence to reduce LDL levels below the recommended level of 100 mg/dL.[73]

The growing body of evidence proving that LDL reduction is paramount to decreasing cardiovascular risk prompted an update to the ATP III recommendations issued in 2001.[74,75] The 2004 changes added a new optional LDL goal of less than 70 mg/dL for those at very high risk for CHD and modified the intensity of LDL lowering in patients with multiple (2+) CHD risk factors to more aggressive lipid standards based on their calculated 10-year risk for a CHD event. In those with elevated triglyceride levels (>200 mg/dL), a new secondary target of therapy, non–high-density lipoprotein (HDL) cholesterol (goal 30 points higher than LDL measurement), was added to diminish the influence of intermediate lipoproteins on atheroma progression (see Table 33.1, lipid management).[11]

In 2005, the Cholesterol Treatment Trialists' (CTT) Collaborators presented the results of a large meta-analysis of more than 90,000 patients in 14 randomized trials of statins, which further bolstered the decision to intensify recommended LDL reduction. The large number of subjects boosted the power to examine mortality data, and the unique analysis used weighted estimates to determine the effect of a decrease of 39 mg/dL (1.0 mmol/L) of LDL on individual clinical outcomes.[76] The results showed a 19% reduction in cardiac mortality per 39 mg/dL-reduction in LDL as well as a 21% reduction in major vascular events (P <.0001) (Fig. 33.7). Importantly, the absolute reduction in LDL corresponded to a proportional reduction in events (P <.0001) (Fig. 33.8). Notably, these effects were seen early in

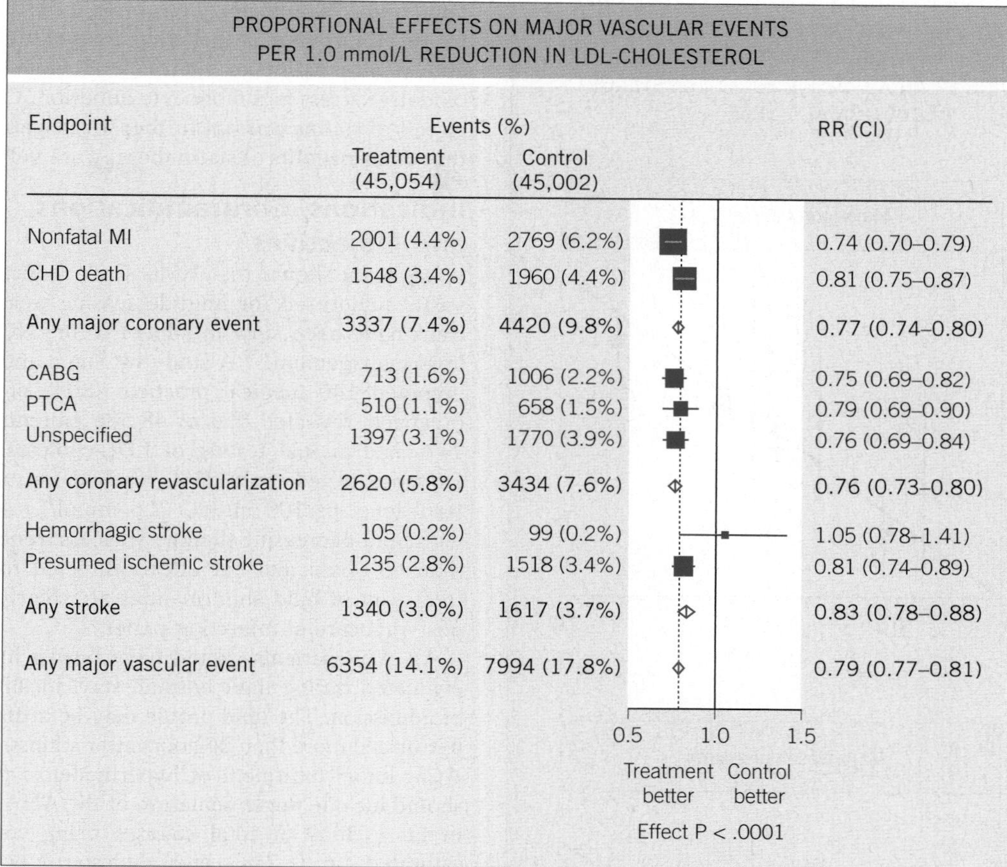

Figure 33.7 Proportional effects on major vascular events per 1.0 mmol/L reduction in LDL-cholesterol concentration. CABG, coronary artery bypass grafting; CHD, coronary heart disease; CI, confidence interval; MI, myocardial infarction; PTCA, percutaneous transluminal coronary angioplasty; RR, relative risk. (From Baigent C, Keech A, Kearney PM, et al. Efficacy and safety of cholesterol-lowering treatment: prospective meta-analysis of data from 90,056 participants in 14 randomised trials of statins. Lancet 2005;366:1267-1278.)

treatment but persisted or enhanced throughout the 5-year duration. Other important results in this study showed no increased risk of nonvascular causes of death and no increased incidence of cancer as a result of LDL lowering.

The mechanisms by which lipid decreasing benefits patients who have CHD have yet to be fully elucidated, but they include reduced progression of lesions and, to a lesser degree, increased regression of lesions. Meta-analyses of studies of patients treated with lipid-decreasing treatments show that although dramatic regression of lesions is uncommon, treated patients had a 1% to 2% regression in the degree of stenosis compared with a 3% increase in the control group. There was also a reduction in the incidence of lesion progression in the treated patients (about 25% in these patients compared with a 50% progression in untreated patients).[77] These changes are much less impressive than the overall reduction in cardiac risk offered by lipid reduction, and they do not account for all of the benefit seen with aggressive lipid management. It is also believed that an increased atherogenic state leads to vasorelaxant dysfunction as a result of an impairment in the release of endothelium-derived relaxing factor, a product of the normally functioning endothelium. Patients who have CHD may in fact have coronary vasoconstriction in response to endothelium-derived relaxing factor, a paradoxical response that contributes to luminal narrowing.

Most important, lipid-decreasing treatment may lead to stabilization of plaques and prevention of plaque disruption. It has been found that plaques that tend to rupture and lead to coronary artery occlusion generally have a greater core lipid content and that plaque disruption more commonly occurs at areas of the plaque that are rich in lipids. More recently, the ARMYDA (Atorvastatin for Reduction of Myocardial Damage During Angioplasty) investigators published three studies providing evidence of beneficial effects of statins beyond their lipid-lowering potential. The first trial enrolled 152 patients with chronic stable angina who were to have elective percutaneous coronary intervention. Subjects were pretreated with a 40-mg dose of atorvastatin 7 days before the procedure. Results showed an impressive 81% risk reduction of periprocedural myocardial infarction.[78] The second trial, ARMYDA-ACS, enrolled 171 patients with non–ST-segment elevation myocardial infarction who were to undergo nonemergent angioplasty. Treatment subjects were loaded with 80 mg of atorvastatin 12 hours before percutaneous coronary intervention, with another 40-mg dose 2 hours before the procedure. At 30 days, the primary endpoint (death, myocardial infarction, and repeated coronary vascularization) was significantly reduced in the treatment compared with the placebo group (5% versus 17%; $P = .01$).[79] Both of these studies support the use of statins

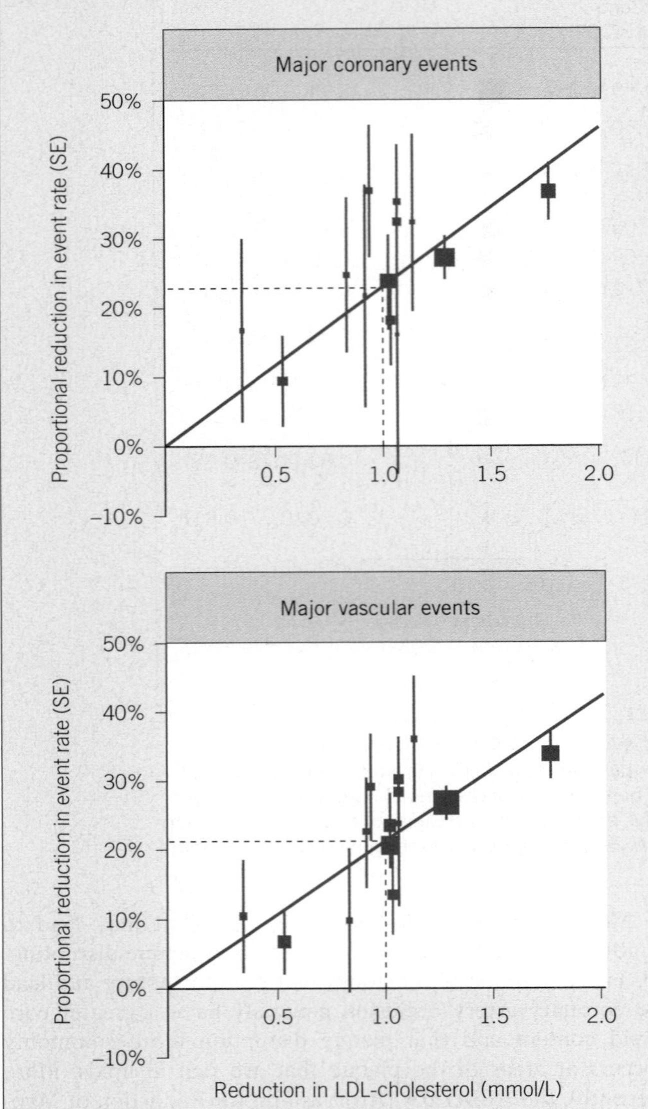

Figure 33.8 Relation between proportional reduction in incidence of major coronary events and major vascular events and mean absolute LDL-cholesterol reduction at 1 year. SE, standard error. (From Baigent C, Keech A, Kearney PM, et al. Efficacy and safety of cholesterol-lowering treatment: prospective meta-analysis of data from 90,056 participants in 14 randomised trials of statins. Lancet 2005;366:1267-1278.)

before coronary intervention but, more important, indicate that the statins' immediate benefits are not due to a lipid-lowering effect, raising the possibility of a pleiotropic effect of the therapy. The third trial, ARMYDA-CAMs, has indeed demonstrated evidence for the endothelial effect of statins. In this subset of the first ARMYDA trial, markers of inflammatory endothelial activation were measured in those subjects who had received atorvastatin or placebo before undergoing percutaneous coronary intervention as previously described. Results showed an attenuation of the rise in intercellular adhesion molecule 1 and E-selectin levels, indicating a decreased endothelial inflammatory response.[80] Postulated mechanisms for this improvement include increased nitric oxide bioavailability, attenuation of ventricular remodeling, or decreased oxidative stress and monocyte adhesion. Clearly, pleiotropic effects of statins warrant further investigation, and it is likely that other benefits of statin therapy are yet to be elucidated.

Indications, Contraindications, and Objectives

It has been shown that HMG-CoA reductase inhibitors are vastly underused for lipid-decreasing treatment, and physicians have been slow to adhere to the NCEP guidelines for lipid management.[77] A study by Sueta and colleagues[81] that involved 140 medical practices (80% of them cardiologic practices) revealed that of 48,586 patients with CHD, only 44% had annual testing of LDL-cholesterol concentration. Of those tested, only 25% reached the target LDL-cholesterol level of 100 mg/dL (2.6 mmol/L) or less. Treatment with lipid-decreasing therapy was less frequent in those older than 65 years. Further efforts directed toward widespread treatment of lipid abnormalities are clearly indicated among post–myocardial infarction patients.

All ACS patients should have fasting lipid concentrations evaluated during their hospital stay, ideally within 24 hours of admission. The lipid profile may be artifactually low if it is performed more than 24 hours after admission in patients with ACS. Initial treatment of hyperlipidemic patients after ACS should include implementation of the AHA diet, which is low in fat (<30% of total calories being contributed by fat), saturated fat (<7%), and cholesterol (<200 mg/day [5.2 mmol/L]).[45] Dietary emphasis should also be placed on intake of fruits and vegetables, and patients should be encouraged to pursue a Mediterranean-style diet.[82] Pharmacotherapy with HMG-CoA reductase inhibitors should be initiated with the goal of reducing LDL-cholesterol concentrations to less than 100 mg/dL (2.6 mmol/L), with an optional goal of less than 70 mg/dL in very high risk individuals. Ongoing lipid studies may eventually prompt recommendations for further LDL goal reduction as suggested by the PROVE-IT, CTT, and TNT trials; but until the optimal level is definitely established, current NCEP guidelines recommend these stated levels. On the basis of the results of the HPS trial, many would advocate starting lipid-decreasing treatment in all patients after ACS, even among those whose LDL concentration is less than 100 mg/dL without treatment. On the basis of the NRMI-4 and MIRACL studies, statins should be started early in the hospitalization. In addition to improvement of outcomes when they are administered early, the initiation of a lipid-lowering agent during hospitalization was shown to be a strong predictor of continued use at 6 months in a retrospective analysis.[83] HDL-cholesterol concentrations should be more than 40 mg/dL, and nonpharmacologic methods (such as weight reduction and exercise) should be implemented if the HDL-cholesterol concentration is less than this. Hypertriglyceridemia is also frequently associated with increased plasma cholesterol concentrations. The NCEP goal for triglycerides in patients who have CHD is less than 150 mg/dL.[84]

With increasing emphasis on improvement of the quality of health care in the United States, health care provider performance goals have been developed to aid in the adoption and standardization of proven, cost-effective preventive techniques. In the United States since July 1999, the National Committee for Quality Assurance Health Plan Employer Data and Information Set performance measures require documentation of LDL-cholesterol concentration in all patients after ACS, percutaneous coronary intervention, or coronary artery bypass surgery.[85] Starting in 2000, the performance measures state that patients should have documented LDL-cholesterol concentrations of less than 130 mg/dL (3.3 mmol/L). As more rigorous performance measures are instituted, it is expected that the National Committee for Quality Assurance will identify the NCEP goal of LDL-cholesterol concentration of less 100 mg/dL (2.6 mmol/L) as a performance measure.

SMOKING CESSATION

Mechanisms of Action

Among the secondary prevention strategies available to patients with cardiovascular disease, smoking cessation has been associated with the greatest reduction in total mortality. Patients who stop smoking can reduce their rates of death and myocardial infarction during the first year after smoking cessation; after 3 years, their risk matches that of CHD patients who have never smoked.[86] The mechanisms by which cigarette smoking increase the risk of primary and recurrent cardiovascular events are related to the damage to the endothelium and resultant dysfunction. Available smoking cessation therapies include nicotine replacement, which by itself is rarely efficacious in long-term cessation. Bupropion, an antidepressant, acts as a weak inhibitor of neuronal uptake of neurotransmitters, which may enhance smoking cessation by acting on the "reward center" of the brain. A newer agent, varenicline, is a partial agonist at the $\alpha_4\beta_2$ subtype of the nicotinic acetylcholine receptor in the brain, the receptor thought to be responsible for the dependence-forming properties of nicotine. Its largest side effect produced in approximately 24% of users is nausea, and nicotine replacement is contraindicated with its use.[87]

Indications and Contraindications

Smoking cessation should be considered mandatory, especially for patients admitted with ACS, in addition to those who have a diagnosis of CHD or previous myocardial infarction. Organized smoking cessation programs that include predischarge education and follow-up after discharge from the hospital, by a person trained in cessation techniques, can be very effective in helping patients with ACS abstain from smoking.[88] Medical treatment with bupropion for 7 weeks was associated with cessation rates of 28.8% for those taking 100 mg daily and 44.2% for dosages of 300 mg daily, compared with 12.4% for those taking placebo.[89] In a randomized, controlled trial of 1027 patients, varenicline yielded a 23% 1-year continuous abstinence from smoking compared with 14.6% for bupropion and 10.3% for placebo. All subjects underwent smoking cessation counseling.[87] Unfortunately, smoking cessation programs are not widely available or are underused. Pharmacologic methods, such as nicotine patches or gum and medications such as bupropion and varenicline, can increase the chances of success and should be used as part of an overall strategy.

HYPERTENSION CONTROL

Mechanisms of Action

Systemic hypertension can contribute to the development of CHF and ischemia in the post–myocardial infarction setting. In addition, left ventricular hypertrophy is associated with increased first-year mortality after nontransmural (non–Q wave) myocardial infarction.[90,91] Although no controlled trials have shown an unequivocal improvement in mortality after myocardial infarction as a result of control of hypertension alone, there are data indicating that patients who have preexisting hypertension have a worse prognosis, and there is evidence that control of hypertension may improve survival after ACS.[7]

Indications and Contraindications

In hypertensive patients with left ventricular dysfunction after myocardial infarction, ACE inhibitors are the agents of choice because they may control blood pressure and minimize left ventricular remodeling or dilatation, thereby preventing the development of CHF and its associated morbidity and mortality. In post–myocardial infarction patients who do not have significant left ventricular hypertrophy or CHF, beta blockers should be the first agents used to control hypertension because they also independently improve post–myocardial infarction survival. Cardioselective beta blockers may also be used in patients who have reduced left ventricular function, particularly if they are started at low doses and very gradually increased. In patients in whom beta blockers are contraindicated or in those who need additional medical treatment to control hypertension, ACE inhibitors or calcium channel blockers may be useful. However, studies that have examined the use of calcium channel blockers after myocardial infarction have not shown clear evidence of an improvement in mortality. Information to help guide specific hypertensive therapy can be found in the seventh report of the Joint National Committee on hypertension.[92]

CARDIAC REHABILITATION

Mechanisms of Action

Concepts about the care of patients who have CHD and post–myocardial infarction patients have changed dramatically through the years. In the early years of the 20th century, post–myocardial infarction rehabilitation consisted of several weeks of bed rest; current standards include early in-hospital ambulation and discharge from the hospital within a few days. The progress that has allowed the early effective treatment of ACS and subsequent early hospital discharge presents a challenge to physicians to implement secondary prevention measures to reduce subsequent morbidity and mortality associated with ACS.

It is estimated that only 11% to 20% of patients who have known CHD participate in some form of cardiac rehabilitation. A recent analysis of the use of cardiac rehabilitation by Medicare beneficiaries after myocardial infarction or coronary bypass surgery found that cardiac rehabilitation was used by only 13.9% of post–myocardial infarction patients and by 31% of patients after coronary artery bypass grafting.[93] This is in spite of studies indicating that cardiovascular death and all-cause mortality after myocardial infarction may be reduced by 20% to 25% in patients who undergo cardiac rehabilitation.[94,95] Although most rehabilitation programs have tended to focus on exercise and conditioning, the goals have more recently broadened to include assistance in stopping smoking, more aggressive lipid management, and psychosocial counseling.

An article on guidelines for cardiac rehabilitation in the United Kingdom outlined three elements of a thorough rehabilitation program, and it is useful to consider these[96]:

- The first element is for post–myocardial infarction patients to have an explanation and understanding of what has happened to them, of the possible causes, and of the implications for their future health.
- The second element is specific rehabilitation intervention that emphasizes secondary prevention techniques, exercise training, and psychological support.
- The third element is the provision of assistance in the long-term process of readaptation to a normal life, which may include education and counseling about employment.

The role of exercise training and conditioning has been a prominent aspect of most rehabilitation programs. Possible mechanisms by which exercise may improve heart function and reduce symptoms and cardiac mortality after myocardial infarction include the decreases in myocardial work and oxygen demand that occur with conditioning, increased myocardial oxygen supply, and improved myocardial and endothelial function.[97] Supervised exercise may also restore the patient's confidence and improve levels of activity more quickly. It may also help reverse adverse risk factors and contribute to secondary prevention. Patients who begin an exercise program after ACS have fewer visits to physicians and hospitals and are more likely to return to work; patients who have angina also gain greater symptomatic benefit from an exercise program. An aggressive exercise program is contraindicated in those patients who are susceptible to exercise-induced arrhythmias and in those who have unstable angina.[96]

Indications and Contraindications

An important goal for patients after ACS is the return to previous levels of activity and employment. In low-risk patients who have preserved LVEF, a return to work or previous levels of activity within 2 weeks can be safely encouraged.[45,98] In this group, air travel, sexual intercourse, and driving can all be safely undertaken within 2 weeks, although care should be taken to avoid excessively stressful situations soon after ACS. For patients who recover from a complicated myocardial infarction, air travel, driving, and other potentially physically or emotionally stressful situations should not be undertaken until at least 2 to 3 weeks after all symptoms have resolved.[45]

ANTIOXIDANT THERAPY AND DIETARY MODIFICATION

Mechanisms of Action

An area of preventive cardiology that attracted considerable attention in the 1990s is the question of the benefit of the so-called antioxidants. Vitamins A, C, and E and beta-carotene have been the most studied of the antioxidants, and of these, vitamin E (alpha-tocopherol) currently is the most widely used. The theory behind the use of antioxidants, although it is not yet fully elucidated, holds that the oxidation of the LDL particle is associated with the presence and growth of atherosclerotic lesions. Oxidized LDL particles that are incorporated into atherosclerotic plaques interact with macrophages, promoting inflammation at the site of the plaques and thereby potentially increasing instability of the plaque. Oxidized LDL particles are also involved with endothelial damage and interference with normal vascular tone.[99] It has been reasoned that substances that inhibit the oxidation of LDL-cholesterol particles should lead to less atherogenic burden and should yield more stable plaques that are less likely to rupture and lead to ACS.

Several studies have indicated that there is no significant benefit for cardiovascular mortality conferred by beta-carotene.[100,101] Vitamin E has been associated with some favorable studies with regard to reducing the risk of complications of CHD. Several epidemiologic studies have indicated a reduction in deaths from CHD in patients who have greater intakes of vitamin E.[102] Vitamin E has been studied in three large clinical trials, with apparently conflicting results. The first of these trials was the Cambridge Heart Antioxidant Study (CHAOS), in which the benefit of either 400 IU/day or 800 IU/day of vitamin E (2002 patients) compared with placebo (967 patients) was examined in patients who had angiographic evidence of coronary atherosclerosis.[103] The rate of nonfatal myocardial infarction was significantly reduced with vitamin E (14 of 1035 patients) compared with placebo (41 of 967 patients). This benefit became apparent after only 200 days of treatment. There were slight but not statistically significant increases in cardiovascular deaths in the vitamin E group (27 patients) compared with the placebo group (23 patients).

A study from the National Public Health Institute in Finland that examined the effects of beta-carotene and vitamin E on male smokers found no significant difference in the number of major coronary events between treatment and placebo groups. There were significantly more deaths from fatal CHD in the beta-carotene and combination (beta-carotene and vitamin E) groups compared with the placebo group. No increase in mortality was noted in the vitamin E–alone group compared with the placebo group.[104] A follow-up study by the same group of researchers concluded that there was no significant difference in the recurrence of angina or other CHD in groups taking vitamin E alone or vitamin E plus beta-carotene compared with placebo.[105]

Although the CHAOS study concluded that there was a benefit for the incidence of recurrent myocardial infarction in patients with CHD, this was not seen in the Finnish study, and neither study demonstrated a decrease in cardiovascular mortality.[103,104] The differences noted in the rate of cardiovascular events may be explained by the dosages of vitamin E used in the two studies. The dose in the Finnish study (vitamin E supplements of 50 IU/day) was much lower than the doses in the earlier CHAOS trial (400 IU/day and 800 IU/day). Trials examining vitamins A and C have been disappointing and have shown no clear benefit to date.

In the HPS trial of antioxidant vitamin supplementation, 20,536 adults aged 40 to 80 years with cardiovascular disease or diabetes were randomly allocated to groups to receive combined vitamin E (600 mg), vitamin C (250 mg), and beta-carotene (20 mg) daily or placebo.[106] Compliance with treatment was 83% among both groups for the 5-year period of therapy. There were no significant differences in all-cause mortality (14.1% compared with 13.5%) or other cardiovascular endpoints. Thus, the largest available experience from a randomized controlled study demonstrates no benefit for several antioxidant vitamins at the specified doses. An antioxidant study particularly focused on women corroborated the lack of cardioprotection for vitamin C, vitamin E, or beta-carotene. In the study, 8171 women with a history of cardiovascular events or with 3+ risk factors for cardiovascular disease were assigned to receive each of three vitamins or placebo. After a follow-up of 9.4 years, no benefit was seen with treatment in cardiovascular mortality, myocardial infarction, revascularization, or stroke.[107]

Dietary supplementation with n-3 polyunsaturated fatty acids, which are found in fish oil, has also received much attention for their possible role in secondary prevention of CHD. The large GISSI-Prevenzione trial examined the benefit of fish oil alone or in combination with vitamin E in more than 11,000 survivors of myocardial infarction.[108] Patients were randomly assigned to groups to receive fish oil, vitamin E, a combination of fish oil and vitamin E, or placebo, and they were observed for 42 months. Patients who received 1 g of n-3 polyunsaturated fatty acid supplements per day had a 15% decrease in the combined endpoints of death, nonfatal myocardial infarction, and stroke and a 17% reduction in the risk of cardiovascular death compared with those assigned to placebo on two-way analysis. The decrease in cardiovascular deaths, particularly sudden deaths, accounted for the overall benefit seen in the combined endpoint with n-3 polyunsaturated fatty acids. No additional beneficial effect in the combined endpoint was seen for those patients who received vitamin E in combination with n-3 polyunsaturated fatty acids or in those who received vitamin E alone.[108] Further study of omega-3 supplementation is warranted.

Another study examined the role of the Mediterranean-type diet in reduction of CHD deaths during a mean follow-up time of 46 months.[109] Patients who ate the Mediterranean diet (which consisted of greater amounts of breads, legumes, vegetables, and margarine made from rapeseed oil and less butter, cream, cheese, and meat) were compared with those who followed a "prudent Western diet." Cardiovascular deaths, in addition to the combined endpoints of recurrent myocardial infarction and cardiac deaths, were significantly reduced in people following the Mediterranean diet. The rate of cardiac deaths and nonfatal myocardial infarction in the experimental group was 1.24 per 100 patients/year, compared with 4.07 per 100 patients/year in the control group. The benefits seen with the Mediterranean diet were not associated with any change in lipid concentrations. Antioxidant effect and reduction of tendency toward unstable arrhythmias have been proposed as the reason for these benefits. Further studies are needed to confirm these results, but this study suggests that physicians need to counsel post–myocardial infarction patients on dietary modification much more aggressively.[109]

Indications, Contraindications, and Objectives

Because of the lack of strong clinical data indicating an improvement in mortality, in addition to the potential for toxicity of the lipid-soluble vitamins, routine administration of vitamins with antioxidant properties after ACS cannot be recommended. However, early evidence suggests that the use of n-3 polyunsaturated fatty acids (in the form of fish oil) and adherence to a Mediterranean diet may reduce the risk of recurrent myocardial infarction in patients with CHD.

HORMONE REPLACEMENT THERAPY

Mechanisms of Action

Early observational studies suggested a mortality and morbidity benefit of hormone replacement therapy in postmenopausal patients with or without CHD. However, the Heart and Estrogen/Progestin Replacement Study (HERS) trial evaluated 2763 postmenopausal women younger than 80 years who had a history of CHD treated with estrogen and medroxyprogesterone.[110] The primary outcome was nonfatal myocardial infarction or CHD death. Secondary outcomes included CHF, unstable angina, coronary revascularization, stroke, and peripheral vascular disease. The groups treated with estrogen replacement and those receiving placebo did not differ significantly in primary or secondary cardiovascular outcomes, despite an 11% decrease in the LDL-cholesterol concentrations and a 10% increase in HDL concentrations in those receiving estrogen treatment. Cardiovascular events occurred more frequently within 1 year in the hormone-treated women but less frequently at 4 and 5 years. More venous thromboembolic events and gallbladder disease occurred in the hormone-treated group. There was no difference in total mortality.

Indications and Contraindications

Because of the lack of a positive effect on mortality and overall cardiovascular events in women treated with hormone replacement therapy, and because of an increase in venous thromboembolic events, hormone replacement therapy cannot now be routinely recommended for secondary prevention in women and should not be given as therapy after ACS.

INFLUENZA VACCINATION

In 2006, the AHA/ACC guidelines for secondary prevention[4] included a recommendation for annual influenza vaccination in individuals with cardiovascular disease. Through an unknown mechanism, cardiovascular disease more than any other chronic condition predisposes individuals to the risk of influenza-related death.[111] Only one randomized trial of influenza vaccination in cardiovascular disease exists. In 2002, the FLUVACS study enrolled 301 patients who were hospitalized either for myocardial infarction or to undergo elective percutaneous coronary intervention. Patients were randomly assigned to vaccine or no vaccine. Results showed a 1-year relative risk for cardiovascular mortality of 2% in the vaccinated group versus 8% in the unvaccinated group. Composite endpoint (cardiovascular death, myocardial infarction, or severe ischemia) was also significantly lower in the vaccinated group at 11% versus 23%.[111] On the basis of these findings, annual influenza vaccination for all individuals with cardiovascular disease is recommended.

SUMMARY

As guidelines for the use and implementation of secondary prevention strategies have been issued after large clinical trials, there has been increased recognition of the value of these techniques. Benefits have clearly been shown for post–myocardial infarction risk reduction conferred by early aspirin use; the use of beta blockers, ACE inhibitors, and lipid-decreasing strategies; and smoking cessation. The use of secondary prevention techniques has not kept pace with the documentation of their benefit, although improvements are being made. The Cooperative Cardiovascular Project examined the use of secondary prevention strategies in the charts of more than 13,000 Medicare patients during the period 1992-1993 and compared it with a follow-up chart review in 1995-1996. During the study period, there were significant increases in aspirin use during hospital stay, aspirin prescription at discharge, beta blocker use during ACE inhibitor use, and smoking cessation counseling. Most important, these changes were associated with decreased early and late mortality during the study period. These improvements were noted even though the duration of hospital stay decreased by almost 2 days during the course of the study.[65]

The Cardiac Hospitalization Atherosclerosis Management Program (CHAMP) trial initiated at the University of California, Los Angeles, provides a striking example of how use of critical pathways during hospital stay and initiation of therapies at the time of admission to the hospital can improve use of secondary prevention therapeutic strategies.[112] The use of lipid-decreasing medications, ACE inhibitors, beta blockers, and aspirin was significantly increased with implementation of the CHAMP program. For example, the prescription of statins at the time of discharge increased from 6% before CHAMP to 86% after CHAMP, and the percentage of patients with LDL concentration of less than 100 mg/dL at 12 months increased from 6% to 58%. Associated with the implementation of CHAMP was an improvement of all outcome parameters in comparison with results of the pre-CHAMP era (Fig. 33.9).

On the basis of the success of CHAMP, the AHA has initiated a nationwide program named Get With The Guidelines to improve use of secondary prevention therapies and thereby contribute to the goal of reducing the national burden of heart disease and stroke by 25% by the year 2010. The five key performance measures targeted in the Get With The Guidelines program are discharge with aspirin, beta blocker, and ACE inhibitor therapy; lipid lowering therapy if LDL concentration is above 100 mg/dL; and smoking cessation counseling. Data collected regarding 74,143 patients admitted to one of 376 hospitals participating in the Get With The Guidelines program indicated improvement in quality of care for secondary preventive measures. Although not at goal, these statistics indicate increased awareness by physicians in treating risks for CHD (Table 33.4).[1]

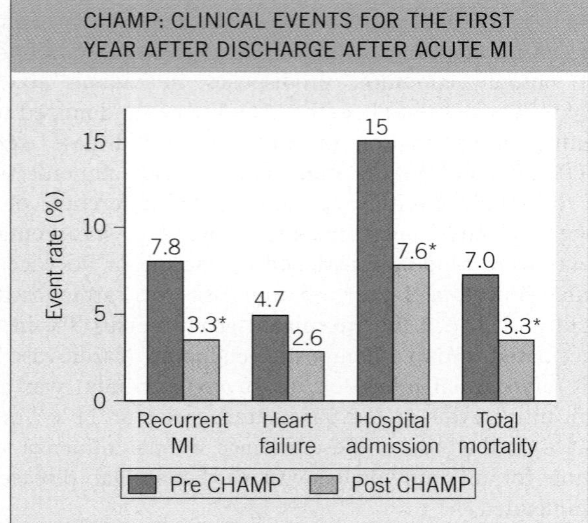

Figure 33.9 CHAMP: clinical events for the first year after discharge after acute myocardial infarction (MI). (Modified from Fonarow GC, Gawlinski A, Moughrabi S, Tillisch JH. Improved treatment of coronary heart disease by implementation of a Cardiac Hospitalization Atherosclerosis Management Program [CHAMP]. Am J Cardiol 2001;87:819-822.)

AHA GET WITH THE GUIDELINES—CORONARY ARTERY DISEASE PROGRAM

Performance Indicator	Percentage of Inpatients
Aspirin within 24 h of admission	94.6%
Aspirin at discharge*	94.2%
Beta blocker at discharge*	90.5%
ACE inhibitor at discharge	66.0%
ACE inhibitor at discharge for acute MI patients*	68.2%
ACE inhibitor in left ventricular systolic dysfunction patients	79.2%
Lipid therapy at discharge	72.1%
Lipid therapy at discharge if LDL >100 mg/dL*	78.1%
BP control (to <140/90 mm Hg) at discharge	78.8%
Smoking cessation counseling*	90.0%
Referral to cardiac rehabilitation	70.3%
Composite quality-of-care measure†	86.3%

Get With The Guidelines (GWTG)—Coronary Artery Disease is an AHA program for the improvement of quality of care. Participating hospitals are involved in initiatives specifically designed to increase adherence to key quality indicators in patients admitted with a cardiovascular event. The table summarizes performance on the selected quality-of-care indicators. These were collected from 74,143 patients who were admitted to 376 hospitals participating in the GWTG–Coronary Artery Disease program from January 1, 2005 through December 31, 2005.

ACE, angiotensin-converting enzyme; BP, blood pressure; LDL, low-density lipoprotein; MI, myocardial infarction.

In-hospital mortality was 4.7%, and mean length of hospital stay 5.3 days (median, 4.0 days). (Note: This excludes transfer-out patients. If discharge status is missing, "no" is assumed.)

*Indicates the 5 key performance measures targeted in GWTG–Coronary Artery Disease.

†The composite quality-of-care measure indicates performance on the provision of several elements of care. It is computed by summing the numerators for each key performance measure across the population of interest to create a composite numerator (all the care that was given), summing the denominators for each measure to form a composite denominator (all the care that should have been given), and reporting the ratio (the percentage of all the needed care that was given).

ACE, angiotensin-converting enzyme; BP, blood pressure; LDL, low-density lipoprotein; MI, myocardial infarction.

From Rosamond W, Flegal K, Friday G, et al. Heart disease and stroke statistics—2007 update: a report from the American Heart Association Statistics Committee and Stroke Statistics Subcommittee. Circulation 2007;115:e69-e171.

Table 33.4 AHA Get With The Guidelines—Coronary Artery Disease Program.

Another initiative sponsored by the ACC designed to measure improved adherence to secondary preventive measures for patients with acute myocardial infarction is the Guidelines Applied in Practice initiative. In 2002, ten participating hospitals documented adherence to measures in 735 patients at baseline, followed by implementation of the Guidelines Applied in Practice project. After 4 months, adherence to evidence-based therapies was measured in 914 patients. On comparison of baseline and postintervention samples, significant increases in adherence were noted in the use of aspirin and beta blockers on admission to the hospital and with the administration of aspirin and smoking cessation counseling on discharge. A trend toward adherence was seen in other treatment goals but was nonsignificant.[113] In 2005, the impact of the Guidelines Applied in Practice project was assessed by looking at mortality rates in Medicare patients in 33 participating hospitals. Mortality rates were assessed in the hospital, at 30 days, and at 1 year. Results showed a significant 21% to 26% decrease in mortality rates for each interval assessed.[114] These data provide further evidence that implementation of programs that enhance adherence to national guidelines improves outcomes after acute myocardial infarction.

Recognizing their important contribution to patient outcomes, the Joint Commission on Accreditation of Healthcare Organizations has made secondary prevention therapies after myocardial infarction an important component of its hospital measures program.

MORTALITY BENEFIT FROM RISK REDUCTION STRATEGIES IN PATIENTS WITH ESTABLISHED CARDIOVASCULAR DISEASE

Intervention	Reduction Total Mortality (%)
Smoking cessation	43
Lipid lowering	30
Angiotensin-converting enzyme inhibitors	20
Beta blockers	27
Aspirin	15
Anticoagulants	10
Hypertension control	12

Table 33.5 Mortality benefit from risk reduction strategies in patients with established cardiovascular disease.

Although there is much room for improvement in the rate of use of effective secondary prevention therapies, the recent trends toward their increased use for survivors of ACS are encouraging.[115] Their combined benefits of reducing total mortality (Table 33.5), recurrent admission to the hospital, and need for revascularization and of improving overall quality of life hold tremendous promise for patients who have cardiovascular disease.

chapter

34 Special Problems in Acute Myocardial Infarction

a. Right Ventricular Infarction

Peter Clemmensen and Michael Dilou Jacobsen

DEFINITION OF PROBLEM

Acute myocardial infarction (AMI) usually refers to infarction of the left ventricle. Involvement of the right ventricle is, however, quite common. Autopsy studies demonstrate biventricular involvement of the AMI in approximately 50% of patients who have had an AMI. Isolated right ventricular AMI is rare, being found in less than 3% of AMI autopsies. Right ventricular involvement is associated with an adverse outcome and has been shown to be an independent predictor of prognosis. Right ventricular AMI can result in hemodynamic compromise, and because the clinical findings and therapeutic options differ from those of routine treatment of AMI (see Chapter 30), it is important to recognize and to be familiar with the invasive and noninvasive tests that can help establish the diagnosis.

TYPICAL CASE

A 76-year-old caucasian woman was awoken by substernal chest pain radiating to the back and left arm. She experienced vomiting and an episode of near-fainting. There was no previous history of cardiac disease; risk factors for coronary artery disease included her age and smoking. She demanded ambulance assistance and arrived at the local emergency department 1.5 hours after the onset of her symptoms, still in pain but without dyspnea. The physical examination revealed a pale patient, and despite elevated jugular venous pressure, there were no rales or pathologic heart murmurs. Her blood pressure was low, at 100/55 mm Hg initially and declining to 75/50 mm Hg on arrival in the coronary care unit. The chest radiograph showed clear lung fields, the presenting electrocardiogram (ECG) showed only slight changes in the inferior leads, and thrombolytic therapy was deferred.

Because of sustained hypotension in this patient, who had typical symptoms of AMI but insignificant inferior ST-segment changes, right ventricular AMI was anticipated, and a second ECG that included the right-sided precordial leads was recorded (Fig. 34A.1). Right ventricular AMI was diagnosed, and the patient received intravenous tenecteplase (7000 units during 10 seconds) in combination with subcutaneous enoxaparin (70 mg). Saline infusion was administered slowly during a 2-hour period, starting with 250 mL during 30 minutes and repeated after 1 hour, resulting in a blood pressure rise to 100/70 mm Hg.

The next day, the patient remained without chest pain and was normotensive, but she suddenly developed repeated ventricular fibrillation and finally asystole and could not be resuscitated. Autopsy showed massive right ventricular AMI with some involvement of the left ventricle (Fig. 34A.2).

DIFFERENTIAL DIAGNOSIS

Findings of hypotension and elevated jugular venous pressure, possibly Kussmaul's sign, in a patient without rales and with clear lung fields are characteristic of right ventricular AMI. The ECG often shows ST-segment elevation in leads II, III, and aVF (diagnostic of inferior wall AMI), but ST-segment elevation is additionally found in the right-sided precordial leads. When the ST-segment elevation is 1 mm or greater, these changes are both highly specific and sensitive for right ventricular AMI. The right-sided ECG leads V_3R through V_7R should therefore be used in all patients who have complicated inferior AMI. On occasion, ST-segment elevation can be seen in leads V_1 through V_3. Examples of ECG findings in relation to anatomic location and the extent of right ventricular AMI are shown in Figure 34A.2.

Echocardiography in the acute phase is of utmost importance because it can be performed at the bedside to assess right ventricular size and regional wall motion. Also, it can exclude major differential diagnoses, namely, pericardial effusion with or without cardiac rupture and tamponade. The echocardiographic examination also provides information about the extent of left ventricular AMI and concomitant valve disease. Other noninvasive methods, such as myocardial scintigraphy, are impractical and are rarely used.

Invasive hemodynamic monitoring is helpful in establishing the diagnosis of right ventricular AMI, and furthermore it can be used to guide therapy. Hemodynamic findings suggestive of right ventricular infarction include

- elevated right atrial pressure (to more than 10 mm Hg);
- equalization of right atrial and pulmonary artery wedge pressures; and
- a right ventricular pressure curve that displays a dip-plateau.

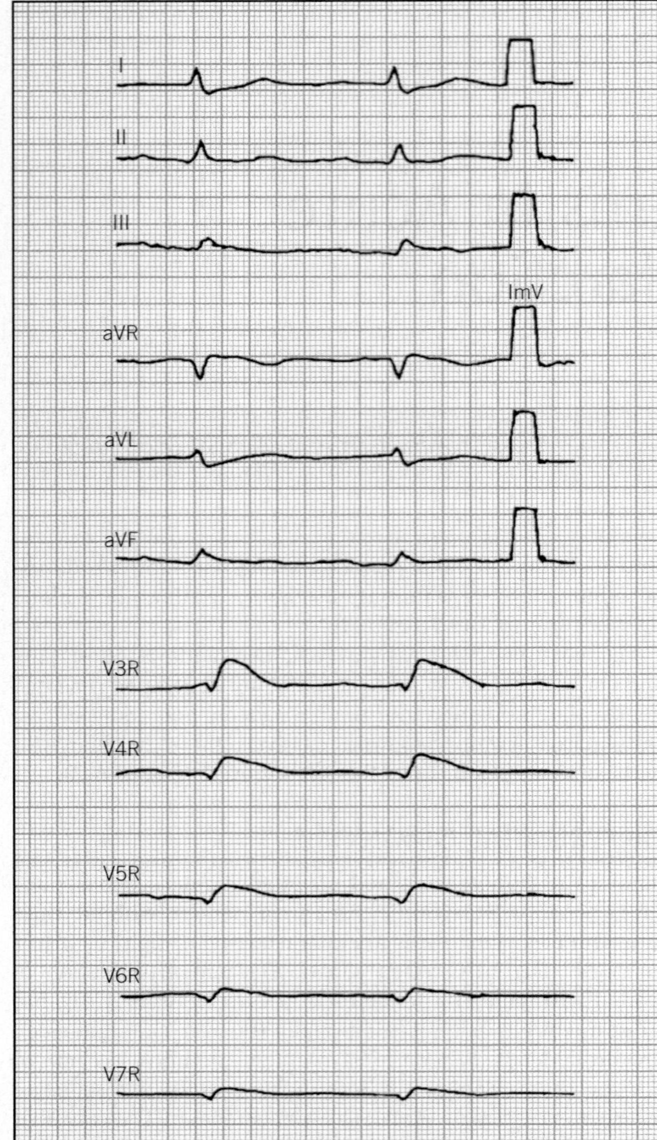

Figure 34A.1 Right ventricular acute myocardial infarction. The ECG shows the three standard leads, the three unipolar extremity leads, and five right-sided precordial leads. Note the almost normal ST-T pattern in leads II, III, and aVF. ST-segment elevation and developing Q waves are observed in leads V_3R through V_7R. The paper speed was 50 mm/s. (Courtesy of Dr. Henning Rud Andersen.)

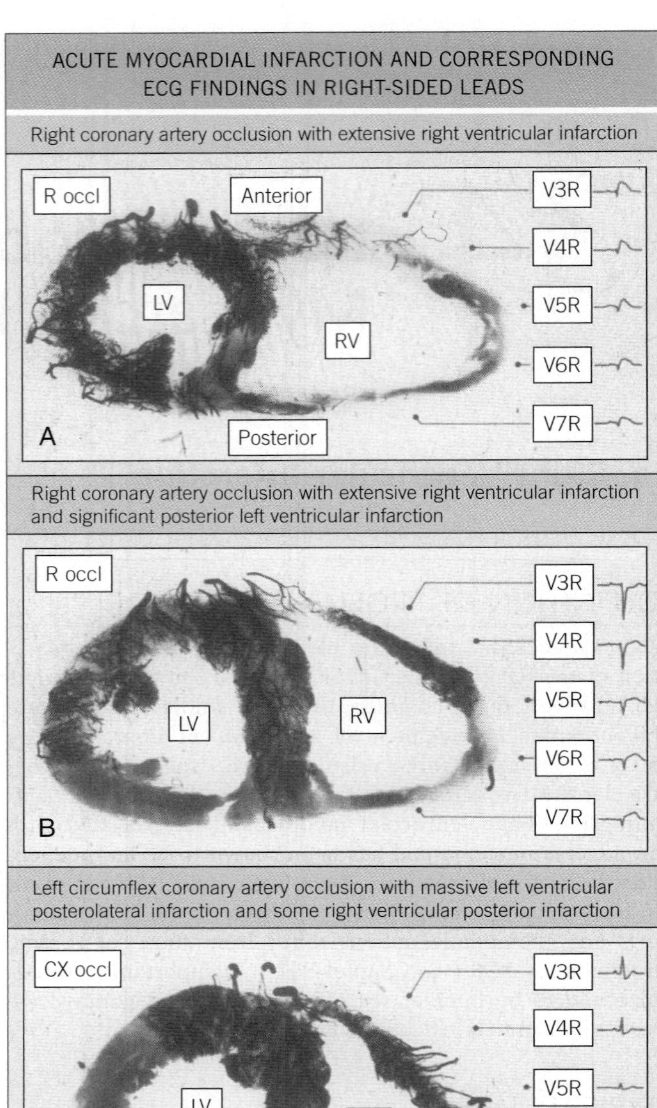

Figure 34A.2 Acute myocardial infarction and corresponding ECG findings in right-sided leads. Transventricular angiographic slices illustrating lack of contrast in the areas of acute myocardial infarction associated with coronary artery occlusion and the corresponding ECG findings in the right-sided precordial leads. **A**, The fatal case presented in the text, with right coronary artery occlusion resulting in extensive right ventricular infarction. **B**, Right coronary artery occlusion with extensive right ventricular infarction but also with significant posterior left ventricular infarction. **C**, Left circumflex coronary artery occlusion with massive left ventricular posterolateral infarction and some right ventricular posterior infarction. LV, left ventricle; RV, right ventricle. (Courtesy of Dr. Henning Rud Andersen.)

Because the dip-plateau shape of a right ventricular pressure curve can be interpreted as a sign of compromised diastolic ventricular function, as seen with constriction and tamponade, echocardiography is mandatory to avoid attempts at pericardiocentesis.

TREATMENT OPTIONS

The acute treatment should follow AMI treatment guidelines. In the rare instances in which isolated ST-segment elevation is seen in the right-sided chest leads, the role of reperfusion therapy is not fully elucidated but should be considered, especially in hypotensive patients and in those who are in shock. Avoid preload-reducing drugs such as diuretics, nitrates, and even morphine. Optimize hemodynamics in the hypotensive patient by volume infusion with 250 mL of saline repeated up to 1000 mL. Dobutamine is the drug of choice to maintain adequate blood pressure and to increase cardiac output. Fluid infusion warrants frequent monitoring for pulmonary edema because the left ventricle is most often involved in the infarction. Special attention should be paid to saline overload in volume-sensitive patients, such as those who have

- a left ventricular ejection fraction that is known to be low;
- aortic stenosis; and
- significant mitral regurgitation.

Pulmonary capillary wedge pressure should not exceed 15 mm Hg, and right atrial pressure should be maintained at 15 mm Hg or greater. Mechanical hemodynamic support with an intra-aortic balloon pump can be used to sustain reperfusion after primary or rescue angioplasty and in patients who are in shock.

Complete heart block is not uncommon, even after reperfusion therapy, and temporary pacing should be instituted as needed. The right ventricle is thin, and when infarcted, it is even more vulnerable, with the risk of electrical instability and perforation during placement of pulmonary or pacing catheters.

SUMMARY

The incidence of right ventricular infarction in patients with inferior AMI ranges from 15% to 50% in various studies. Clinically important right ventricular infarctions are those that are associated with hypotension and cardiogenic shock, but they are readily diagnosed by obtaining right-sided precordial ECG leads and by echocardiography. Prompt diagnosis of right ventricular AMI in complicated inferior AMI is important because the treatment options differ from those of routine AMI management. In mild cases, cautious infusion of saline may reverse hypotensive episodes, but patients who have refractory hypotension or shock should be considered for invasive monitoring and treatment.

b. Acute Myocardial Infarction and Normal Coronary Arteries

Peter Clemmensen, Michael Dilou Jacobsen, and Peer Grande

DEFINITION OF PROBLEM

Angiographic studies have shown that even in patients who have acute myocardial infarction (AMI) with ST-segment elevation, total coronary occlusion is not always present. Some patients have “minimal lesions” obstructing 30% to 50% of the lumen of the coronary artery; there may even be angiographically normal coronary arteries. Table 34B.1 summarizes the extent of coronary artery disease in patients who have AMI.

TYPICAL CASE

A 44-year-old caucasian man who had no previous cardiovascular history suddenly felt nauseated with sweating on his way to an early morning meeting. Soon afterward, he developed chest pain. Risk factors for coronary artery disease included gender and a 24-year history of cigarette smoking. The man continued to drive but left the highway to present himself at the emergency department of a nearby hospital. The electrocardiogram showed ST-segment elevation in the inferior leads, and he was treated with 300 mg of aspirin, intravenous beta blockade, and nitroglycerin. After 15 minutes without improvement in the ST-segment changes, repeated intravenous doses of reteplase (10 units) were administered, first in the emergency department and, after 30 minutes, on arrival in the coronary care unit. The in-hospital course was uneventful. Total cholesterol concentration was 4.6 mmol/L. A predischarge cardiac catheterization was performed on day 6; it showed no significant coronary artery disease (Fig. 34B.1). Global left ventricular ejection fraction was preserved at 51% despite some inferior wall hypokinesia. The patient was discharged on aspirin (75 mg every 24 hours) and metoprolol (100 mg every 24 hours). He was scheduled for outpatient follow-up, including exercise testing and rehabilitation, especially smoking cessation class.

NUMBER OF DISEASED CORONARY VESSELS IN ACUTE MYOCARDIAL INFARCTION

Number of Vessels or Type of Lesion	Percentage of Patients
Minimal lesion	10
One vessel	55
Two vessels	20
Three vessels	10
Left main coronary artery	5

*Number of coronary arteries in acute myocardial infarction with significant atherosclerosis, as determined by coronary angiography. The numbers are adapted from the studies in the Further Reading list at the end of the chapter. Minimal lesion usually refers to atherosclerosis with a residual stenosis of less than 50% after acute myocardial infarction.

Table 34B.1 Number of diseased coronary vessels in acute myocardial infarction.

DIFFERENTIAL DIAGNOSIS

Probably the most common cause of AMI associated with normal coronary arteries is acute thrombosis in the presence of minimal-lesion atherosclerosis. If the patient is a smoker and is older than about 40 years, one might choose to accept this pathophysiologic mechanism. Angiographically normal coronary arteries can show extensive atherosclerosis when they are examined by intravascular ultrasonography or on autopsy; both methods have shown that atherosclerosis in the coronary arteries is often diffuse and involves long segments of the diseased vessel. The symptoms and clinical findings associated with AMI can be mimicked by several other

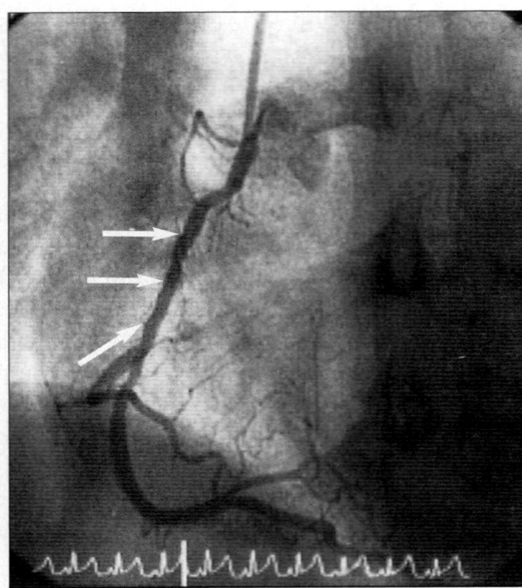

Figure 34B.1 Coronary arteriogram obtained on day 6 after acute myocardial infarction with ST-segment elevation that was treated with fibrinolytic therapy. The left anterior descending and left circumflex coronary artery (not shown) were completely normal. The right coronary artery has some irregularities *(arrows)* but no significant coronary artery disease. Acute thrombosis at the site of minor coronary atherosclerosis is likely to have occurred.

disease states; furthermore, many of these result in abnormal electrocardiographic findings and elevated biochemical markers of myocardial injury (troponin T, troponin I, creatine kinase MB, creatine kinase, and myoglobin). The electrocardiogram can be falsely positive with regard to signs of ischemia, whether or not there are concomitant complaints of chest pain (Table 34B.2).

Of greater clinical importance are those conditions that cannot be easily discerned from AMI with underlying significant coronary artery disease (Table 34B.3). These conditions are often treated like conventional AMI initially and become correctly diagnosed only if coronary angiography is performed. Although most of these conditions are rare, it is important to recognize them because subsequent treatment

CONDITIONS ASSOCIATED WITH ELECTROCARDIOGRAPHIC CHANGES THAT CAN BE INTERPRETED AS ISCHEMIA
Pericarditis
Pneumothorax
Hyperkalemia
Hypocalcemia
Digitalis use
Quinidine use
Hypothermia
Benign repolarization
Intracranial catastrophe
*There is no chest discomfort except in the first two conditions, and the biochemical markers of myocardial injury are normal.

Table 34B.2 Conditions associated with electrocardiographic changes that can be interpreted as ischemia.

DIFFERENTIAL DIAGNOSIS OF ACUTE MYOCARDIAL INFARCTION WITH NORMAL CORONARY ARTERIES.*
Minimal-lesion coronary artery disease
Pericarditis or myocarditis
Cocaine intake
Hematologic disorders (e.g., protein C or protein S deficiency)
Coronary embolism
Arteritis
Hyperparathyroidism
Trauma
Coronary artery spasm
*These conditions are associated with chest discomfort, electrocardiographic changes, and myocardial injury but angiographically normal coronary arteries.

Table 34B.3 Differential diagnosis of acute myocardial infarction with normal coronary arteries.*

requires multidisciplinary collaboration. The patient should be asked about cocaine abuse or recent viral infections that might suggest pericarditis or myocarditis. Embolism is diagnosed primarily by echocardiography, but more extensive ultrasound or magnetic resonance imaging examinations are warranted in patients who may have right-to-left shunting resulting in paradox embolism to a coronary artery. Hematologic and autoimmune diseases are diagnosed from appropriate blood samples.

TREATMENT OPTIONS

As mentioned in the case presentation, the acute treatment is often conventional, including fibrinolytic therapy or percutaneous coronary intervention in patients who have ST-segment elevation AMI. The rare conditions listed in Table 34B.3 should be treated by specific interventions and the precipitating factor eliminated.

The majority of patients who have AMI and normal coronary arteries do not have any of these conditions. No clinical, randomized studies have evaluated the different treatment options in this category of patients. The prognosis in these patients is excellent, which renders the evaluation of post-AMI medical therapy difficult. Revascularization is not necessary, but some experts believe that coronary artery spasm is the underlying pathophysiologic stimulus for thrombus formation and start treatment with calcium channel blockers or nitrates. In the absence of randomized data, it is suggested that standard post-AMI medical regimens not be diverged from and that treatment with aspirin and beta blockers be continued. It is essential that patients stop smoking, and hyperlipidemia should be treated (see Chapter 8).

SUMMARY

AMI is usually the result of acute thrombosis at the site of significant coronary atherosclerosis. Pathologic and angiographic studies have documented the occurrence of AMI in patients who do not have significant coronary obstruction and even in patients who have angiographically normal coronary arteries. The pathogenesis is likely to be in situ thrombosis with or without embolization and possibly superimposed coronary spasm. Although the prognosis in these patients is good, with the death rate below 2% per year and the rate of recurrent AMI below 3% per year during long-term follow-up, post-AMI medical management should follow normal routines (see Chapter 33). Sometimes it is appropriate to question the diagnosis of AMI, especially in very young (i.e., those younger than 40 years) nonsmokers and in those who have completely normal coronary arteries. The important differential diagnoses that should be considered are presented in Table 34B.3.

c. Non-Reperfused Acute Myocardial Infarction after Thrombolytic Therapy

Peter Clemmensen and Michael Dilou Jacobsen

DEFINITION OF PROBLEM

Thrombolytic therapy for acute myocardial infarction (AMI) was introduced as routine treatment after large, placebo-controlled clinical trials demonstrated a significant decrease in mortality with thrombolysis. Thrombolytic therapy is effective because most patients with AMI have a thrombotic occlusion of a major coronary artery that is lysed by the fibrinolytic drug. Because reestablishment of coronary patency and myocardial reperfusion were believed to be essential for therapeutic success, immediate coronary arteriography was often carried out after intravenous thrombolytic therapy. This allowed patients who had persistent coronary thrombi or severe residual stenosis to have additional intracoronary thrombolytic therapy or percutaneous coronary intervention (PCI). Furthermore, patients with three-vessel disease or left main stem stenosis would be identified and could be transferred for acute or subacute coronary artery bypass surgery. This clinical approach, when tested in randomized trials, was not associated with improved mortality and morbidity and could even have serious adverse effects—especially bleeding. Additional drawbacks associated with acute coronary angiography include its cost, its unavailability to the majority of patients, and the fact that it provides only a “snapshot” of coronary patency. Immediate routine coronary angiography after full-dose fibrinolytic therapy is referred to as facilitated PCI but is presently considered contraindicated on the basis of both older and recent clinical trials. Trials are still being conducted in this field to identify drugs or combinations thereof as well as the timing of procedures to broaden the indication for facilitated PCI in subsets of patients. However, rescue PCI after thrombolysis is recommended by the American College of Cardiology and the American Heart Association in unstable patients with cardiogenic shock, pulmonary edema, hemodynamically compromising ventricular arrhythmias, persistent ischemic symptoms, or failure of ST-segment resolution. Finally, subacute post-thrombolysis coronary angiography—and PCI, if applicable—performed within 24 hours is recommended by the European Society of Cardiology. Current American College of Cardiology/American Heart Association guidelines suggest an invasive strategy with PCI of hemodynamically significant stenoses in patent infarct arteries more than 24 hours after ST-segment elevation myocardial infarction.

A patent infarct-related coronary artery after intravenous thrombolytic therapy remains one of the major determinants of both short- and long-term outcomes for patients, thus creating a need for noninvasive methods for evaluation of therapeutic success after intravenous thrombolytic therapy for AMI. Several methods have been proposed during the past 2 decades, including monitoring of chest pain severity and arrhythmias; but with the exception of accelerated idioventricular rhythm, these are neither specific nor sensitive enough for clinical use. The most widely studied noninvasive methods for monitoring reperfusion after intravenous thrombolytic therapy are based on determination of the blood concentration of macromolecules that are released from infarcted myocardium and monitoring of electrocardiographic ST-segment resolution.

TYPICAL CASE

A 50-year-old man was admitted 4 hours after the onset of chest pain. The electrocardiogram showed ST-segment elevation (Fig. 34C.1), and there were no contraindications to fibrinolytic therapy. The blood pressure was 150/85 mm Hg, and the creatine kinase MB level on admission was 35 μg/L. Intravenous alteplase and heparin were administered. Despite intravenous beta blockade and morphine, the patient continued to be in pain, and the degree of ST-segment elevation was unchanged. After 2 hours, the patient was in Killip class II and the blood pressure had dropped to 95/50 mm Hg. Intravenous furosemide was administered. Acute cardiac catheterization showed a normal left but occluded right coronary artery (Fig. 34C.2a). Rescue PCI was performed, and the infarct-related coronary artery was reopened (Fig. 34C.2b). The blood pressure quickly normalized, and the intra-aortic balloon pump was not necessary. The rest of the patient’s stay in the hospital was uneventful.

DIFFERENTIAL DIAGNOSIS

It is important to appreciate the limited specificity of myocardial reperfusion as assessed clinically. If acute coronary angiography is undertaken, the infarct-related coronary artery will be found to be open at the epicardial level in some cases. The electrocardiogram probably reflects the true reperfusion status of the myocardium and distal embolization; no reflow or misinterpreted timing of symptom onset can explain the apparent discrepancy when there are pronounced electrocardiographic abnormalities but an open infarct-related coronary artery.

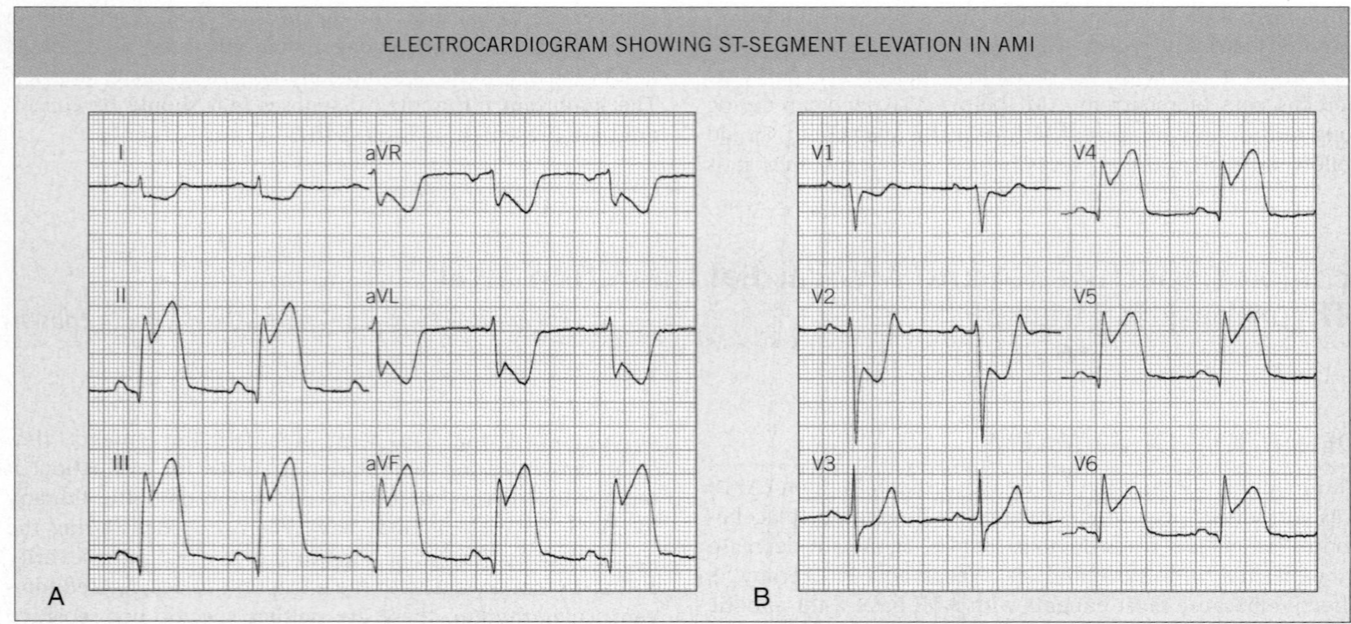

Figure 34C.1 Electrocardiogram showing ST-segment elevation in acute myocardial infarction (AMI). There is 9- to 10-mm ST-segment elevation in leads II, III, and aVF **(A)** but also ST-segment elevation in the apical leads V_4-V_6 **(B)** and ST-segment depression in leads I, aVL, and V_1-V_3. Note the positive terminal T wave in V_1-V_3 indicating extensive inferolateral infarction.

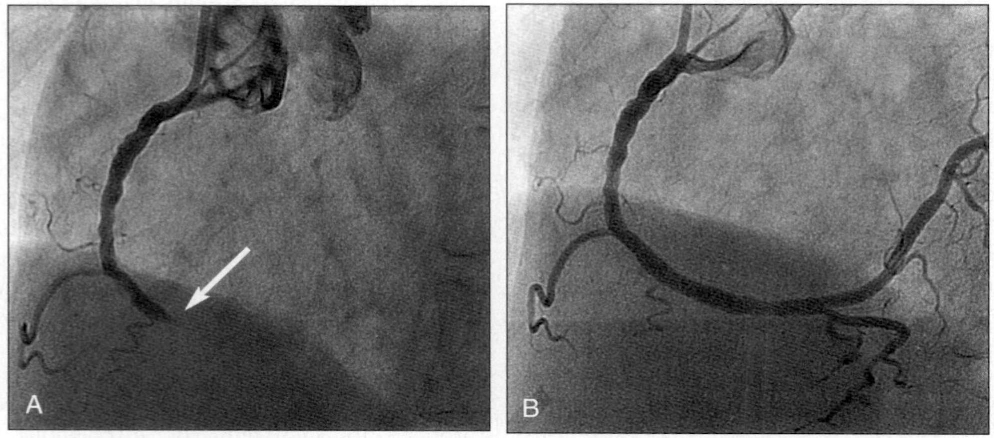

Figure 34C.2 Cardiac catheterization in a patient with acute myocardial infarction and inferior ST-segment elevation on the electrocardiogram. **A**, Owing to continued pain without signs of improvement in ST-segment elevation and early signs of heart failure, acute coronary arteriography was undertaken. It shows occlusion *(arrow)* of the mid right coronary artery. **B**, After rescue angioplasty, the vessel is open with TIMI grade 3 flow.

If left ventricular wall motion and the coronary arteries are normal, the differential diagnoses listed in Tables 34B.2 and 34B.3 should be considered.

TREATMENT OPTIONS

Primary PCI is associated with a higher acute patency of the infarct-related coronary artery. When failure of fibrinolysis in AMI is suspected, there are limited treatment options. Even with conservative treatment, some patients may experience later opening of the infarct-related artery and derive benefit, even though myocardial salvage has not occurred. The symptoms should be monitored closely for heart failure, angina, and ischemia on a predischarge exercise test. If any of these variables are positive, the patient should be referred for invasive evaluation. Repeated thrombolytic therapy is probably used to some extent, particularly in hospitals without cardiac catheterization facilities, but there are no convincing data to suggest a wider use of this approach. Mechanical revascularization with either rescue PCI or coronary artery bypass grafts must be considered in the hemodynamically unstable patient. Although this strategy has not been formally proved in randomized clinical trials, this patient subset is at high risk, and further treatment should be decided promptly after characterization of the coronary anatomy. Patients who are in Killip class III or class IV should be considered candidates for receiving intra-aortic balloon counterpulsation or a percutaneous heart assist device (Impella) (see Chapter 31).

SUMMARY

Intravenous fibrinolytic therapy fails to lyse the occluding coronary thrombus effectively in approximately 20% of patients. Reperfusion failure is recognized clinically by lack of ST-segment resolution, persistence of pain, and hemodynamic instability of the patient. Stable patients and those who have small inferior AMI have a low fatality risk and should be treated conservatively. Patients with large anterior AMI and those who have signs of heart failure, regardless of the location of the AMI, should be considered for transfer to a tertiary medical center for invasive evaluation and treatment.

d. Suspected Myocardial Ischemia in the Emergency Department

James A. Goldstein

DEFINITION OF PROBLEM

Acute chest pain prompts 6 million patients annually to undergo emergency department evaluation to exclude acute coronary syndrome (ACS). The diagnosis is straightforward in those whose initial electrocardiogram (ECG) or cardiac enzyme levels clearly indicate ACS. Although more than 50% of acute chest pain cases represent noncardiac conditions, symptomatic clinical presentations frequently overlap, contributing to the challenge of rapidly and efficiently establishing the correct diagnosis. An initially normal ECG and cardiac enzymes do not exclude ACS or other potentially life-threatening causes of chest pain, including aortic dissection, pulmonary embolism, and pericardial disease. Alarmingly, up to 8% of patients with ACS are misdiagnosed and inappropriately discharged home. However, only a minority of patients whose initial ECGs and cardiac studies are normal are actually suffering from ACS. Nevertheless, because the consequences of diagnostic failure are so serious with respect to both medical and malpractice considerations, it is routine practice to evaluate nearly all such patients through "rule out myocardial infarction" protocols employing serial ECGs, cardiac enzyme determinations, and stress imaging modalities. This approach has reduced diagnostic error but is resource-intensive and time-consuming, incurs an estimated cost of $10 to $12 billion annually in this country alone, and often is not definitive.

Multislice computed tomographic coronary angiography (CTA) provides high-resolution coronary angiograms noninvasively. Previous studies have now established that CTA is highly accurate for delineation of the presence and severity of coronary atherosclerosis. Its high negative predictive value for exclusion of significant coronary artery stenoses makes it potentially attractive for evaluation of a low-risk chest pain population (i.e., those with initially normal ECG and enzyme levels and a low likelihood of atherosclerosis). Recent observations from a randomized study comparing CTA with traditional nuclear stress testing for such "low-risk" acute chest pain patients demonstrate that CTA, based on its ability to rapidly and accurately delineate the absence of coronary artery disease, immediately established a diagnosis in 75% of cases; importantly, the strategy of "first-line" CTA facilitated more rapid discharge and was associated with lower costs. CTA also has the capability to delineate other potentially life-threatening causes of chest pain, including aortic dissection, pulmonary embolism, and pericardial disease, and thus may be used, in appropriate cases, for a rapid "triple rule-out" chest pain evaluation. However, CTA has limitations, particularly with regard to cases with inadequate image quality and its inability to determine the physiologic significance of coronary lesions judged to be of intermediate severity.

A TALE OF TWO CASES

The following two cases illustrate the potential power and applicability of CTA in the evaluation of low-risk acute chest pain patients.

A 55-year-old man without prior cardiovascular disease presented to the emergency department in the late morning with intermittent vague upper chest and shoulder discomfort for 24 hours. His major risk factor was smoking. The physical examination findings and the initial ECG and cardiac enzyme levels were normal. The patient underwent CTA (Fig. 34D.1), which documented a tight mid right coronary artery stenosis, mild disease in the proximal circumflex, and normal left anterior descending artery. He was treated with aspirin, heparin, beta blockers, and intravenous nitroglycerin; he then underwent successful percutaneous revascularization the following day.

A 48-year-old man without prior cardiovascular disease presented to the emergency department in the early evening with 4 hours of squeezing substernal chest pain. Major risk factors included obesity and hyperlipidemia. The physical examination findings and the initial ECG and cardiac enzyme levels were normal. Overnight, the patient underwent a traditional rule-out protocol including serial ECGs and enzyme determinations, which were normal. The next day, a stress nuclear study showed good exercise tolerance without symptoms or ECG changes, but imaging suggested a subtle reversible defect in the inferior-apical region. The patient underwent CTA (Fig. 34D.2), which documented completely normal coronary arteries. He was immediately discharged home.

EVALUATION STRATEGIES

Accurate and efficient diagnosis of acute chest pain is a challenging clinical problem. The traditional rule-out protocol for myocardial infarction employing serial ECGs and enzyme determinations followed by rest-stress imaging is reasonably accurate, safe, and widely available; one major advantage is that it provides myocardial perfusion data, thereby offering

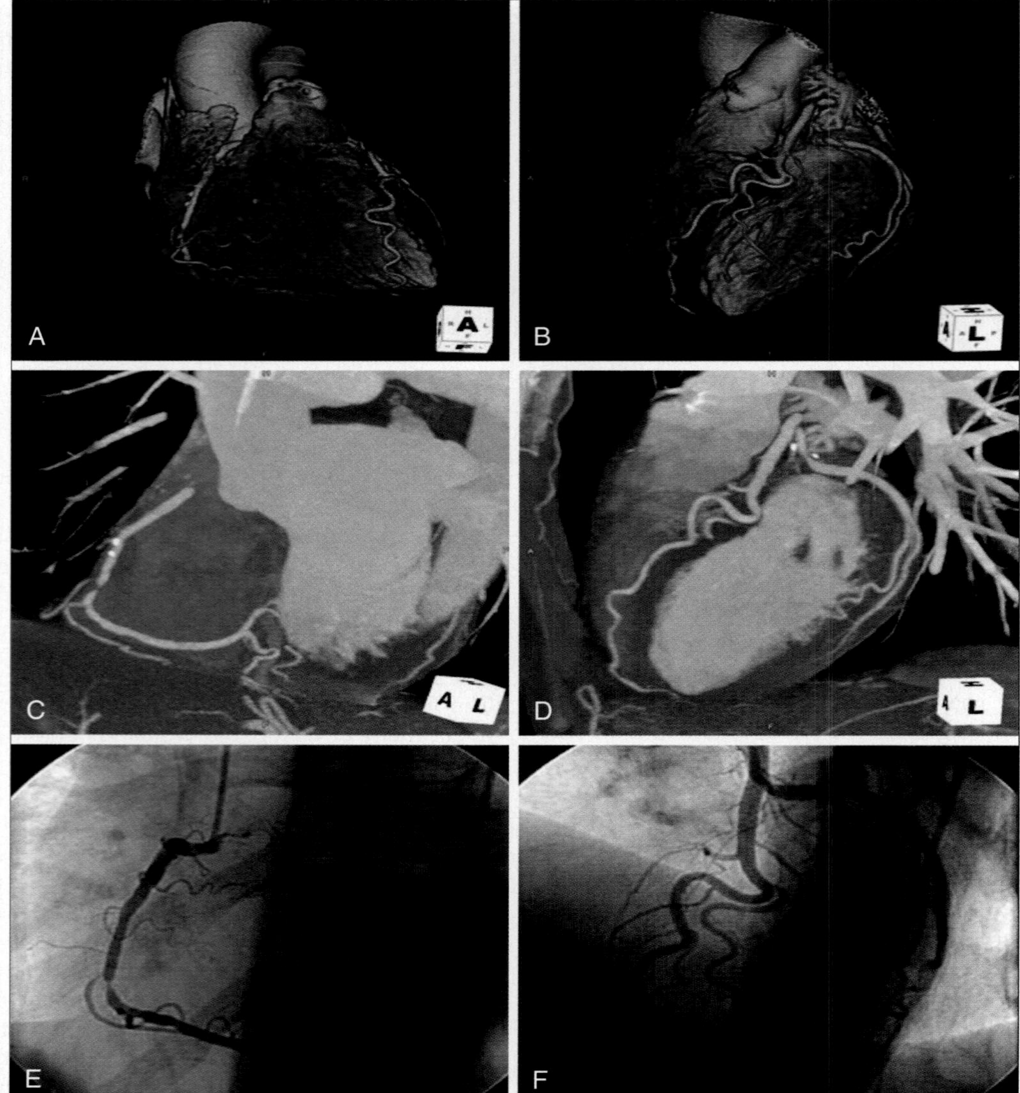

Figure 34D.1 Visualization of soft and hard coronary arteriosclerotic plaques by 64-slice multislice computed tomography. **A** and **B**, Volume rendering technique demonstrates stenosis of right coronary artery below the acute marginal branch as well as nodular coronary calcifications largely extrinsic to the right coronary lumen **(A)** and normal left coronary artery **(B)**. **C** and **D**, Maximum-intensity projection of the same arteries demonstrates severe soft plaque stenosis of the right coronary artery and superficial calcific plaque. **E** and **F**, Invasive coronary angiography of the same arteries.

insights into the physiologic significance of coronary stenoses. However, this strategy is time-consuming, expensive, and not always definitive. CTA is an attractive approach to adjudicate acute chest pain, based on its capability to rapidly and noninvasively image the coronary vasculature with excellent accuracy for the presence and severity of luminal stenoses; CTA can also delineate other serious sources of acute chest pain, including aortic dissection, pulmonary embolism, and pericardial disease. However, CTA has significant limitations, including the fact that it delineates anatomy only and cannot yet provide physiologic coronary blood flow data; thus, coronary lesions judged moderate in severity and of unclear hemodynamic significance require further interrogation to determine their relationship to the index chest pain episode. This limitation has led to legitimate concerns not only in regard to the need for further noninvasive testing to establish the physiologic significance of the lesion but also about the possibility of unnecessary invasive procedures. Other disadvantages of CTA include inadequate diagnostic quality scans in approximately 10% of cases because of motion, coronary calcification, or obesity and exposure to radiation and iodinated contrast material.

Although recent observations demonstrate the potential attractiveness of CTA as the first-line diagnostic strategy to accurately, rapidly, and efficiently establish the cause of chest pain, this approach is not applicable to all patients with acute chest pain. CTA is perhaps most powerful in defining the presence or absence of disease; accordingly, this test is particularly well suited for low-risk chest pain patients, that is, those with a low pretest likelihood of harboring coronary atherosclerosis. However, when the pretest probability of atherosclerosis is high (American College of Cardiology criteria including known vascular disease, age older than 70 years, and diabetes), physiologic stress testing may be

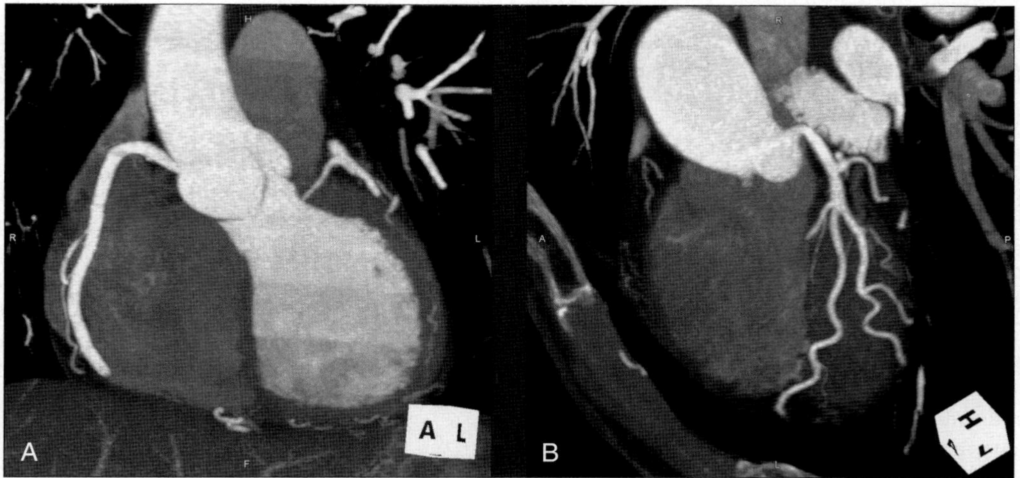

Figure 34D.2 CTA demonstrating completely normal right (A) and left (B) coronary arteries.

more effective in solving clinical questions. On the basis of these considerations, the patient-based algorithm in Figure 34D.3 may be applicable to various acute chest pain scenarios:

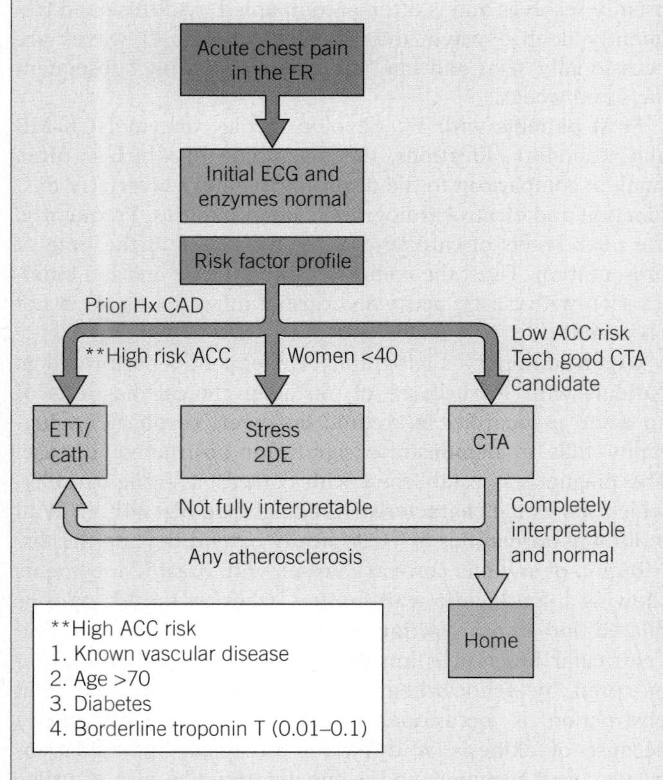

Figure 34D.3 Diagnostic algorithm for acute chest pain in the emergency department. ACC, American College of Cardiology; Cath, catheterization; CTA, computed tomographic coronary angiography; ECG, electrocardiogram; ETT, exercise tolerance test; Hx CAD, history of coronary artery disease; Stress 2DE, two-dimensional stress echocardiography.

- In patients with acute chest pain and high clinical suspicion for ACS based on initially abnormal ECG and enzyme levels, therapy for ACS should be instituted and patients hospitalized for consideration of further invasive evaluation and therapy.
- In those with acute symptoms and initially normal ECG and enzyme levels but prior documented coronary disease or with a moderate to high pretest likelihood of manifest coronary atherosclerosis (not low risk by American College of Cardiology criteria), a physiologic stress test is most appropriate as the initial testing strategy, with invasive catheterization after an abnormal result.
- In those low-risk patients with initially normal ECG and enzyme levels, CTA is an attractive initial strategy (excluding those with contraindications to the administration of contrast material or younger women, in whom breast irradiation is undesirable). Patients in whom CTA demonstrates normal or nearly normal vessels can be safely discharged; those with severe disease require hospitalization. The remaining small number of cases with coronary lesions of intermediate severity (25% to 70%) will require subsequent stress imaging study to ascertain physiologic ischemia.

SUMMARY

These results illustrate the strengths and weaknesses of traditional noninvasive stress imaging approaches and CTA as strategies to evaluate patients with acute chest pain. In the majority of cases, CTA definitively and noninvasively establishes or excludes coronary artery disease as the cause of chest pain. However, this approach has significant limitations, particularly with regard to its inability to determine the physiologic significance of coronary lesions judged to be of intermediate severity as well as in cases with inadequate image quality.

e. Tako-Tsubo Cardiomyopathy

David Singh and Prediman K. Shah

DEFINITION OF PROBLEM

Tako-tsubo cardiomyopathy (TC) has recently been recognized as a distinct clinical entity characterized by transient left ventricular (LV) apical ballooning and systolic dysfunction. The disorder is usually brought about by psychological or physiologic stress. TC was first recognized in Japan in 1990 in patients who presented with signs and symptoms of acute myocardial infarction but were found to have nonobstructed epicardial coronary arteries on coronary angiography. The term *tako-tsubo* was used because left ventriculograms consistently revealed a morphologic appearance that resembled a Japanese octopus trap (Fig. 34E.1). Since that time, other terms have been used to describe TC, including stress cardiomyopathy, apical ballooning syndrome, broken heart syndrome, and ampulla cardiomyopathy.

The incidence of TC has not been well established, but it may account for 1% to 2% of patients who present with the signs and symptoms of an acute myocardial infarction. The disorder is predominantly seen in postmenopausal women but has also been described in younger patients as well as in men. Although the classic description of TC involved patients with preceding emotional stress (such as death of a spouse, friend, or close relative and on occasion even good news), it is likely that physiologic stress (such as surgery, general anesthesia, sepsis, metabolic disturbances, sudden cardiac death, acute pulmonary disease, and cardiac exercise stress testing) can trigger the disorder with similar frequency. In one prospective study of 92 noncardiac patients admitted to a medical intensive care unit, 20 patients (22%) were found to have LV apical ballooning on admission. LV function recovered after an average of 7 days in these patients.

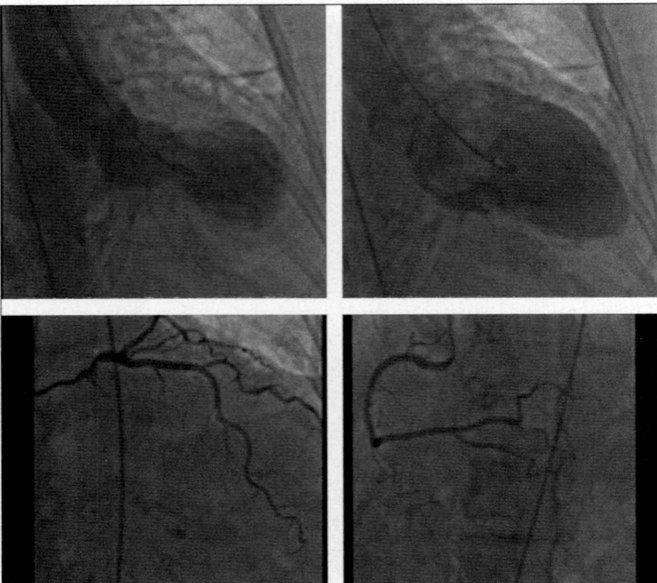

Figure 34E.1 The term *tako-tsubo* describes a morphologic appearance that resembles a Japanese octopus trap on left ventriculograms.

The clinical presentation of patients with TC is frequently indistinguishable from that of patients with an acute myocardial infarction. Whereas the majority of patients present with ischemic-like chest pain, other presenting symptoms can include acute dyspnea, syncope, cardiogenic shock, palpitations, and nonspecific symptoms such as fatigue and malaise.

Electrocardiographic changes in the acute phase frequently resemble those of an acute myocardial infarction (Fig. 34E.2). ST-segment elevation is frequently present in precordial leads but can be seen in limb leads as well. In the absence of ST elevation, a wide variety of electrocardiographic changes may be seen, including ST depression, nonspecific T-wave abnormalities, prolongation of the QT interval, and right or left bundle branch block. The electrocardiogram typically evolves during a period of 2 to 3 days. ST-segment elevation usually resolves and is often accompanied by diffuse and frequently deep T-wave inversions. Pathologic Q waves are occasionally seen and may even resolve during subsequent days and weeks.

Most patients with TC develop cardiac enzyme (CK-MB and troponin) elevations, the magnitude of which is often small in comparison to the disproportionately severe LV dysfunction and electrocardiographic abnormalities. Frequently, the peak levels of cardiac enzyme are noted at the time of presentation. Thus, the common temporal rise and fall kinetics seen with classic acute myocardial infarction is often not observed.

Urgent coronary angiography is frequently performed in patients with TC because of mistaken clinical diagnosis of an acute myocardial infarction; however, coronary angiography fails to demonstrate significant obstructive disease. The diagnosis is established with contrast LV angiography, which shows the characteristic findings (see Fig. 34E.1). Wall motion abnormalities in TC typically extend beyond the distribution of any one coronary vessel, with basal LV segments showing hyperkinetic wall motion, whereas the LV apex is dilated and shows dyskinesis or akinesis. On occasion, mid ventricular function is impaired as well. These findings are mirrored by echocardiography. A dynamic outflow tract obstruction is occasionally seen with echocardiography because of akinesis or dyskinesis of apical and mid ventricular wall segments and a hypercontractile base. Cardiac magnetic resonance imaging may be helpful in excluding myocardial infarction as delayed contrast enhancement is not usually seen in patients with TC.

The LV dysfunction associated with TC is transient, and most patients show dramatic improvement, including normalization of wall motion and ejection fraction, within 2 weeks. The overall prognosis for TC is excellent in the absence of comorbid conditions, and most patients survive

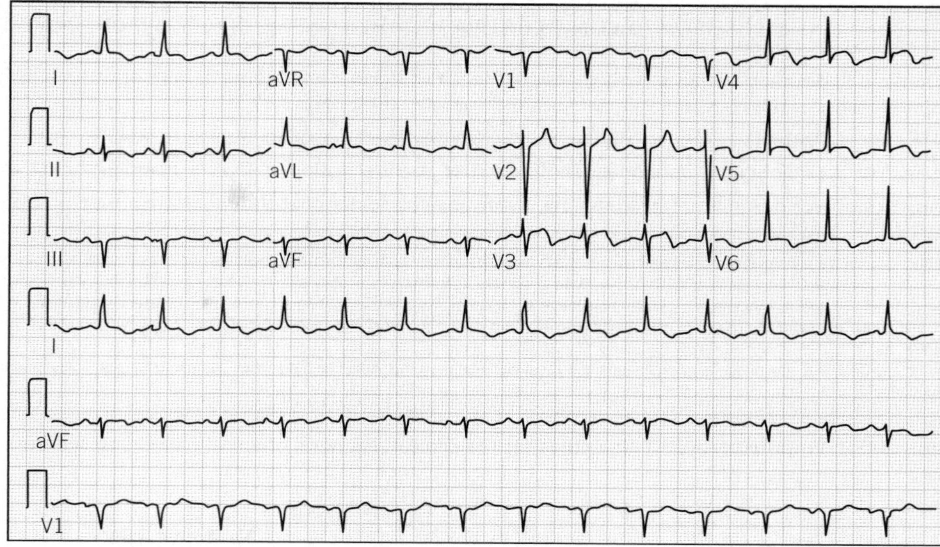

Figure 34E.2 Electrocardiographic changes in the acute phase frequently resemble those of an acute myocardial infarction.

their index hospitalization. Four-year survival for patients presenting with TC is similar to that of an age-, gender-, and race-matched population. In a longitudinal case series of 100 TC patients, recurrence was found to be relatively infrequent, with a 4-year mean recurrence rate of 11%. In this series, almost one third of patients continued to have chest pain. None of the patients who underwent coronary angiography for continued chest pain were found to have progression of coronary atherosclerosis.

The pathophysiologic mechanism of TC remains elusive. Although the precise mechanism has not been elucidated, it is likely that alterations in sympathetic tone contribute to the pathogenesis of the disorder. ^{123}I-labeled metaiodobenzylguanidine (^{123}I-MIBG) myocardial scintigraphy performed in TC patients suggests the presence of sympathetic hyperactivity in regions of the heart with impaired function. In addition, there is strong evidence that elevated catecholamines play a role in the development of TC. In one study, patients presenting with TC were found to have plasma catecholamine levels several times higher than those of patients who were comparably ill from classic acute myocardial infarction.

Microvascular dysfunction has also been proposed as a potential culprit in the development of TC. Patients with TC have been shown to have abnormally high TIMI frame counts (in all three epicardial coronary arteries) and apical perfusion defects on myocardial contrast echocardiography, both of which suggest the presence of microvascular dysfunction. Another marker of microvascular function, coronary flow reserve, has been shown to be impaired during the acute phase of TC. In one study, TC patients with reduced coronary flow reserve had normalization of their microvascular function at 3-week follow-up. These findings further support the possibility that microvascular dysfunction may contribute to the LV dysfunction in TC. However microvascular dysfunction as a consequence rather than as a cause cannot be ruled out. Other theories that have been proposed include coronary vasospasm and spontaneous recanalization of an acute atherothrombotic coronary occlusion.

TYPICAL CASE

A 73-year-old woman with end-stage renal disease underwent semielective thrombectomy for a clotted arteriovenous fistula. Several hours after her operation, the patient developed retrosternal chest pain associated with shortness of breath. The electrocardiogram was notable for QT prolongation and ST elevation in the anterior precordial and lateral leads (see Fig. 34E.2). Out of concern for a possible atherothrombotic acute coronary syndrome, emergent coronary angiography was performed, which revealed no epicardial coronary occlusion and minimal atherosclerotic change. Left ventriculography revealed a tako-tsubo pattern with apical ballooning and preserved basal function (see Fig. 34E.1). Echocardiography revealed akinesis of the mid-distal LV walls and LV apex and an estimated LV ejection fraction of 30% to 35%. Troponin I level peaked at 10.8 ng/mL. The patient was monitored in the intensive care unit for several days and did not require inotropic or vasopressor support. Follow-up echocardiography performed several months later demonstrated normalization of the LV ejection fraction and wall motion.

DIFFERENTIAL DIAGNOSIS

The differential diagnosis of TC includes acute coronary syndrome as well as several other conditions that may produce ST-segment changes and apical ballooning (Table 34E.1). Because TC can be indistinguishable from classic acute myocardial infarction, coronary angiography is needed to rule out epicardial coronary occlusion. Additional conditions that might resemble TC include myocarditis, intracerebral hemorrhage, coronary artery spasm, and spontaneously recanalized left anterior descending artery occlusion.

TREATMENT OPTIONS

Treatment of TC is largely supportive. At least one fifth of patients with TC present with pulmonary edema and may require diuretic and other supportive therapy. Patients with

PROPOSED MAYO CLINIC CRITERIA FOR THE CLINICAL DIAGNOSIS OF APICAL BALLOONING SYNDROME
Transient hypokinesis, akinesis, or dyskinesis of the left ventricular mid segments with or without apical involvement. The regional wall motion abnormalities extend beyond a single epicardial vascular distribution.*
Absence of obstructive coronary disease or angiographic evidence of acute plaque rupture†
New electrocardiographic abnormalities (either ST-segment elevation or T-wave inversion) or elevated cardiac troponin
Absence of recent significant head trauma, intracranial bleeding, pheochromocytoma, myocarditis, hypertrophic cardiomyopathy

*There are rare exceptions to these criteria, such as those patients in whom the regional wall motion abnormality is limited to a single coronary territory.

†It is possible that a patient with obstructive coronary atherosclerosis may also develop apical ballooning syndrome. However, this is very rare in our experience and in the published literature, perhaps because such cases are misdiagnosed as an acute coronary syndrome.

In both of these circumstances, the diagnosis of apical ballooning syndrome should be made with caution, and a clear stressful precipitating trigger must be sought.

Reprinted with permission from Prasad A. Apical ballooning syndrome: an important differential diagnosis of acute myocardial infarction. Circulation 2007;115: e56-e59.

Table 34E.1 Proposed Mayo Clinic criteria for the clinical diagnosis of apical ballooning syndrome.

severe LV dysfunction or cardiogenic shock may require inotropic support or mechanical circulatory support with an intra-aortic balloon pump. The role of beta blockade during the acute and postrecovery phases has not been rigorously studied. Some have advocated for the use of beta blockade after LV function has recovered to protect against recurrence, but this practice needs to be substantiated by further studies.

A variety of arrhythmias have been associated with TC, including atrioventricular block, atrial fibrillation, and ventricular tachycardia or fibrillation, which may require additional supportive therapy. Because most patients demonstrate dramatic improvement in LV ejection fraction within 1 to 2 weeks, decisions about prophylactic implantable cardioverter-defibrillator placement should not be hastily made during the acute phase.

SUMMARY

Tako-tsubo cardiomyopathy is characterized by transient LV dysfunction that is usually brought about by psychological or physiologic stress. The LV dysfunction seen in TC typically involves akinesis or dyskinesis of the LV apex with preserved or hypercontractile basal function. LV function usually normalizes within 2 weeks of presentation. TC may be indistinguishable from acute coronary syndrome on presentation. However, coronary angiography performed in TC patients demonstrates no significant epicardial coronary stenoses or atherosclerotic burden. Postulated mechanisms include catecholamine-mediated cardiotoxicity, microvascular dysfunction, coronary spasm, and spontaneous recanalization of an acutely occluded coronary artery. Treatment is mainly supportive, and the prognosis for TC patients is generally excellent.

chapter 35

Catheter-Based Techniques to Treat Ischemic Heart Disease

Pim J. de Feyter

Definition

- Catheter-based treatment is aimed at restoration of coronary blood flow by mechanical dilatation of a coronary stenosis by balloon inflation or stent implantation.

Key Features

- Catheter-based treatment is currently preferred to coronary artery bypass grafting in a ratio of 3:1.
- Balloon angioplasty and stent implantation are the key techniques.
- Bare-stent implantation has significantly reduced major procedural complications but is associated with a 15% to 30% in-stent restenosis rate.
- Drug-eluting stents have a low (<10%) in-stent restenosis rate but require long-term dual antiplatelet treatment (aspirin and clopidogrel) to prevent late stent thrombosis.
- Adjunctive treatment with platelet glycoprotein IIb/IIIa antagonists, in addition to aspirin and heparin, is recommended to reduce procedural complications in high-risk patients.
- Early invasive strategy is superior to conservative strategy in patients with high-risk unstable coronary artery disease.
- Drug-eluting stents are recommended to treat in-stent restenosis after bare-metal stent implantation.

Therapy

- Patients who have stable or unstable angina, or non–ST-segment elevation myocardial infarction, and focal stenosis in one or two coronary vessels are candidates for catheter-based treatment.
- Primary catheter-based treatment is superior to thrombolytic treatment in patients with acute ST-segment elevation myocardial infarction.
- Catheter-based treatment is preferred in elderly patients with severe comorbidity.
- Unprotected left main disease or three-vessel disease is referred to catheter-based therapy only if it is not suitable for coronary artery bypass grafting.
- Catheter-based treatment must be followed by lifestyle changes, aspirin, and lipid-modifying drugs.

Catheter-based techniques to treat coronary artery narrowing or occlusion have revolutionized the management of patients who have chronic or acute ischemic heart disease.

The percutaneous catheter technique has found widespread acceptance and now constitutes a viable strong option among the available medical and surgical treatments of ischemic heart disease. The first procedure was performed in 1977 by Gruentzig; it was a success, and 10 years later, repeated coronary angiography showed that the artery was still widely patent. Initially, the balloon catheter was large, stiff, and not very steerable or trackable. During the years, significant improvements in interventional equipment and technique have been accomplished so that today we have very low profile, highly steerable and trackable balloon catheters and a wide variety of guide wires that are able to negotiate complex calcific lesions or chronic total occlusions.

In addition to balloon catheters, intracoronary stent implantation has emerged as a second major breakthrough technique, and rotational atherectomy has been developed to treat severe calcific stenoses.

A prerequisite for correct performance of percutaneous coronary intervention is the availability of sophisticated radiographic equipment. Currently, image acquisition with a matrix size of 512 × 512 pixels is considered a minimum, and 1024 × 1024 pixels is preferred. Digital image enhancement, zooming, cine loops, and quantitative coronary angiography are invaluable.

Radiation exposure to operating personnel can be reduced by the use of

- pulsed fluoroscopy;
- gap filling to allow reduced frame rate acquisition (7.5 to 12 frames per second);
- optimal filtering; and
- projections other than the left superior oblique projection.

Adjunctive therapy, in addition to standard treatment with aspirin and heparin, with platelet glycoprotein IIb/IIIa antagonists has significantly reduced the frequency of major adverse coronary events related to the procedure in high-risk patients.

All these technical advances and increased operator experience have made catheter-based coronary therapy relatively safe and effective. Major remaining problems are

- occurrence of death or myocardial infarction during the procedure of approximately 4%;
- treatment of left main disease;
- treatment of bifurcation lesions;
- catheter-based treatment in diabetic patients;
- treatment of chronic total occlusion of arteries;
- occurrence of in-stent restenosis (bare-metal stents or drug-eluting stents); and
- occurrence of very late stent thrombosis.

These limitations have prompted the many current studies that aim to make the technique safer and more acceptable as a first-choice option to treat coronary obstructions.

BALLOON ANGIOPLASTY

Description of Technique

Balloon angioplasty is a percutaneous coronary intervention technique. Access to the vascular system is achieved by puncture of the right femoral artery. Alternative sites of puncture are the left femoral artery, the brachial artery, and the subclavian artery. Recently, the radial artery approach has been used; this allows quick mobilization of the patient after the procedure so that outpatient catheter-based treatment is possible.

Basic tools for the performance of percutaneous coronary intervention are the guiding catheter, the guide wire, and the balloon catheter.

The guiding catheter has a specific preshaped curve that makes engagement of the ostium of the right coronary artery or left main stem relatively easy. Its tip is soft and atraumatic to prevent damage to the ostia. Guiding catheters have different diameters, ranging from 4 French (1.2 mm) to 8 French (2.7 mm). The guiding catheter is inserted through an introducer sheath into the artery.

The guide wire is a long wire with a soft, floppy tip that is shapeable (J curve). The guide wire is steerable ("torqueable") so that the wire can be maneuvered into the tortuous coronary vessels and across the lesion into the distal vessel segment. The diameter of a standard wire is 0.014 inch (0.36 mm). The wire is used as a rail over which the balloon catheter slides into the coronary vessel and is placed precisely across the coronary lesion.

The balloon catheter consists of a long catheter with an inflatable balloon at its distal end. Modern balloon catheters have a very low crossing profile and good trackability and pushability, and they can be rapidly inflated or deflated. The balloons vary in length; they are usually 2 cm, but they may be as short as 1 cm or as long as 6 cm.

The balloon inflation pressures vary from 1 up to 20 atmospheres or, rarely, 25 atmospheres, depending on the characteristics of the coronary lesion. The inflated balloon diameter ranges from 1.5 to 5 mm; in the majority of the cases, a 3- to 3.5-mm balloon is used. In a conventional over-the-wire balloon catheter, the guide wire lumen runs through the entire shaft of the balloon. The monorail balloon catheter has a short, distally located guide wire lumen that allows easy and quick introduction or changing of balloon catheters.

The balloon angioplasty technique consists of five basic steps (Fig. 35.1):

- placement of guiding catheter;
- introduction and steering of the guide wire into the coronary artery and crossing of the coronary lesion;
- introduction of the balloon catheter over the guide wire into the coronary vessel and precise placement across the lesion;
- inflation of the balloon during a short period (30 seconds to 3 minutes or longer, depending on the ischemic electrocardiographic changes, blood pressure, and pain tolerance); and
- deflation of the balloon and removal of the balloon catheter.

Mechanism

The two key mechanisms of enlargement of the lumen by balloon angioplasty are dissection of intima and media and increase in total vessel circumference. Unfortunately, the extent of barotrauma to the vessel wall that is induced by balloon inflation is largely uncontrolled, and such barotrauma may sometimes cause excessive damage and abrupt coronary occlusion as a result of an occlusive dissection. In addition, disruption to the vessel wall may trigger intensive platelet adhesion and aggregation; subsequent occlusive coronary thrombosis, which is not always prevented by adjunctive pharmacotherapy, may develop. Abrupt coronary occlusions are the cause of major morbidity and mortality of catheter-based treatment during the procedure[1]; they occur in 4% to 8% of procedures when only balloon angioplasty is used. Abrupt occlusion can safely be treated by immediate stent implantation.

Restenosis after Balloon Angioplasty

Restenosis typically occurs within 6 months of a successful coronary intervention; the majority occur within 3 to 4 months. The incidence of restenosis is reported to be between 30% and 50%. The restenosis rate is higher in the presence of

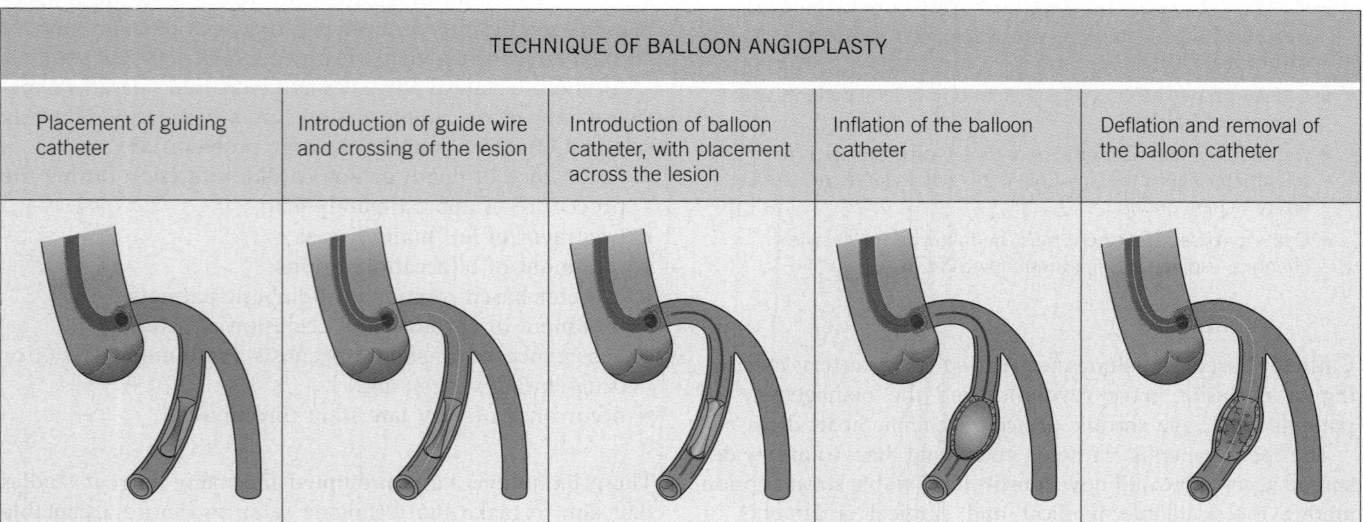

Figure 35.1 Technique of balloon angioplasty.

- a long lesion (>20 mm), an ostial lesion, a chronic total occlusion, or a bifurcation lesion; and
- lesions in small vessels (<2.5 mm) and in patients with diabetes mellitus.

Two processes may play a role in restenosis:
- neointimal hyperplasia, which is considered to be a response to vessel injury and which consists of proliferation of smooth muscle cells and synthesis of extracellular collagen and proteoglycan matrix; and
- early elastic recoil and, more important, late restrictive remodeling, which result in a decrease in the total vessel circumference and, consequently, in a reduction of the vessel lumen.

Neointimal hyperplasia accounts for roughly one third of the lumen loss and restrictive remodeling for about two thirds. Stents were devised to reduce the process of restenosis.

INTRACORONARY STENT IMPLANTATION

Intracoronary stent implantation is the second major breakthrough (after balloon angioplasty) in percutaneous interventional cardiology. Stents have various diameters (between 2.5 mm and 5 mm) and various lengths (between 8 mm and 32 mm). Stents are premounted on a balloon catheter (balloon-expandable stents) and are delivered by inflation of the balloon at the site of the lesion (Fig. 35.2).

Mechanism

The intracoronary stent is an extremely useful device for scaffolding disrupted or friable atherosclerotic material and for eliminating acute and chronic recoil of the vessel wall, thus optimizing the coronary lumen and coronary flow hemodynamics (Figs. 35.3 and 35.4).

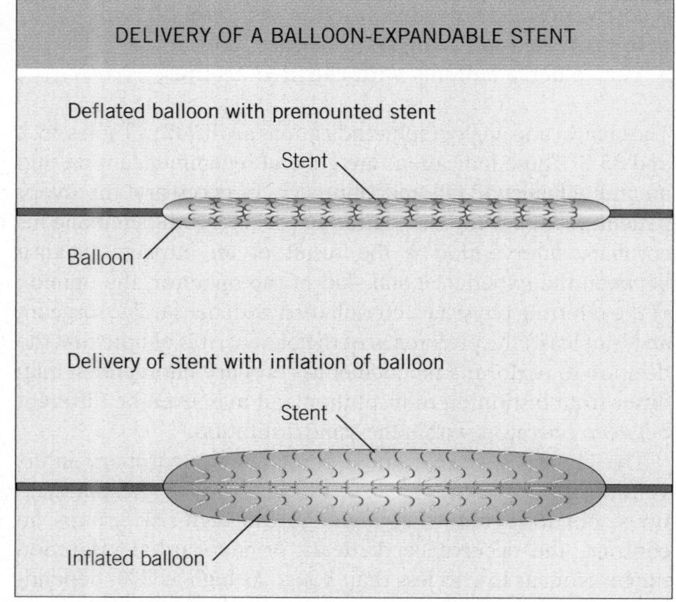

Figure 35.2 Delivery of a balloon-expandable stent. When the stent is delivered, the balloon is inflated so that the stent is "pushed" against the wall of the artery. The stent does not recoil after the balloon is deflated and removed.

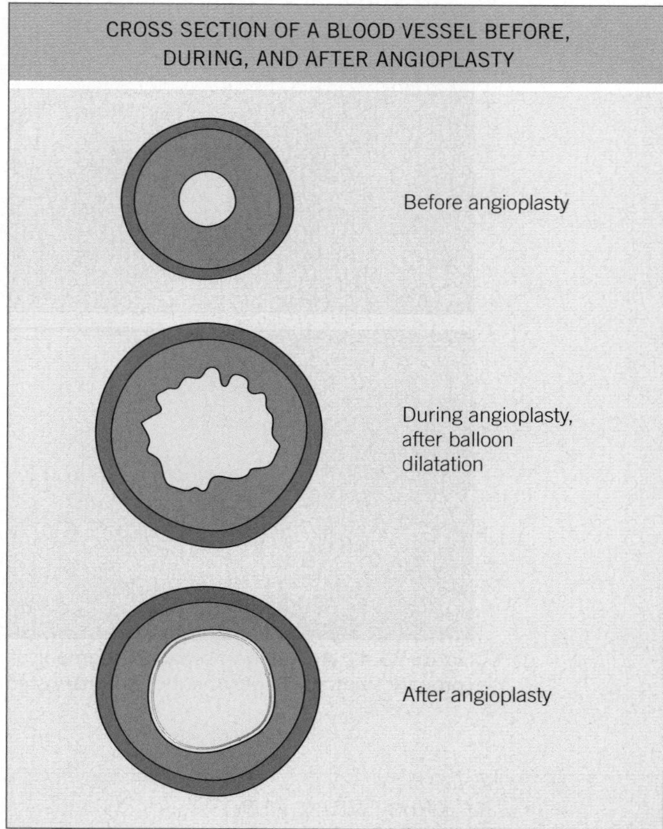

Figure 35.3 Cross section of a blood vessel before, during, and after angioplasty. After balloon dilatation, the lumen is irregular because of fracture and rupture of plaque; however, the total vessel area has increased. After stent implantation, the lumen is regular and round, and dissections are tacked against the vessel wall.

Intracoronary stenting has improved the safety of percutaneous coronary intervention and has significantly reduced the need for bailout bypass surgery. Intracoronary stenting is associated with two major problems:
- acute or subacute stent thrombosis; and
- late in-stent restenosis.

The frequency of acute and subacute stent thrombosis is greatly reduced after aggressive antiplatelet treatment with the combination of aspirin and clopidogrel to less than 1.5%.[2] In high-risk patients, adjunctive treatment with glycoprotein IIb/IIIa inhibitors has significantly reduced major complications during stenting (5.3% for the abciximab group compared with 10.8% for the placebo group).[3]

Restenosis after Bare-Metal Stent Implantation

Stent implantation has eliminated vessel recoil (as was seen after balloon angioplasty) and thereby is associated with a significant reduction in restenosis rate. However, stent implantation exacerbates the neointimal proliferation response; this results in an in-stent restenosis rate of 15% to 25%, which may even be higher in lesions in small vessels, long lesions, ostial lesions, bifurcational lesions, and obstructions in venous bypass grafts or in patients with diabetes mellitus.

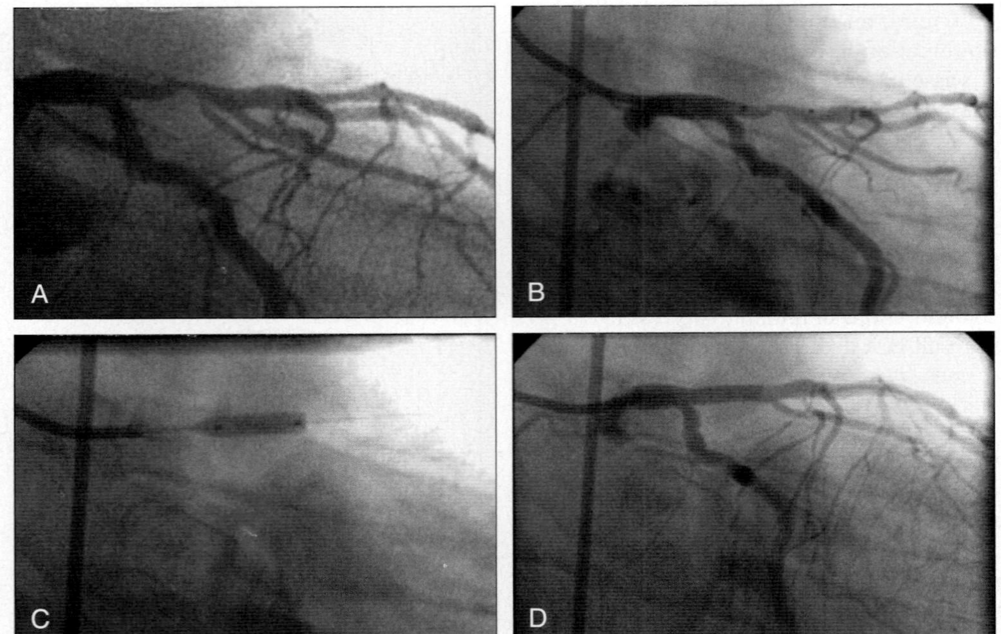

Figure 35.4 **A,** Lesion in proximal segment of left anterior descending artery. **B,** Exact position of coronary stent. **C,** Deployment of coronary stent (balloon inflation). **D,** After stent implantation.

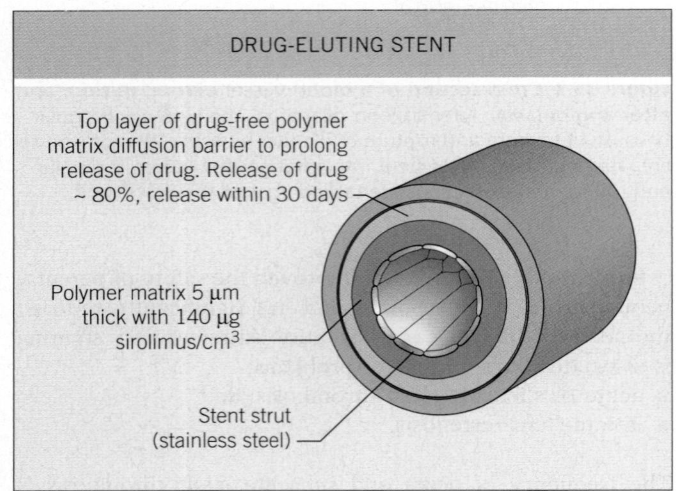

Figure 35.5 Drug-eluting stent.

Drug-Eluting Stents

The neointimal hyperplasia causing in-stent restenosis may be limited or prevented by local delivery of antiproliferative drugs. Drug-eluting stents are metallic scaffolds that are covered with polymers from which less than 0.1 mg of a cytotoxic or anti-inflammatory compound is progressively released during the first weeks after stent implantation (Fig. 35.5). The most frequently used compounds are paclitaxel and sirolimus.

INDICATIONS FOR PERCUTANEOUS CORONARY INTERVENTION

An evaluation scheme of patients referred for percutaneous coronary intervention is provided in Figure 35.6. In general, the patients should be symptomatic and have signs of objective ischemia. The relative risks and benefits of catheter-based treatment should be carefully balanced against the risks and benefits of medical and surgical treatment. A risk stratification for percutaneous interventions can be developed on the basis of clinical, angiographic, and lesion characteristics, which allow stratification into low or high risk for death or myocardial infarction or cerebral bleeding (Table 35.1). Patients at high risk for death have the following characteristics:

- last remaining vessel;
- large area of myocardium at risk;
- left ventricular ejection fraction less than 30%;
- unprotected left main stem disease; and
- very elderly patients with calcified arteries.

The clinical and angiographic indications are listed in Tables 35.2 and 35.3. These indications are general recommendations, and an individualized, tailored approach is necessary for every patient. A final recommendation to proceed with percutaneous coronary intervention is the result of an intricate balance between the experience and skill of the operator, the opinion of the referring physician, consultation with the cardiac surgeon, and (not least) the preference of the patient. It is of note that the decision to perform a percutaneous coronary intervention may differ from institution to institution and may even be different between operators within the same institution.

The clinical success rate of percutaneous coronary intervention is well above 95% in the majority of these indications, but it is somewhat lower in the high-risk groups; in contrast, the occurrence of death or myocardial infarction ranges from as low as less than 3% to as high as 8%, depending on the risk profile of the patient (see Table 35.1). Lesions that have a decreased success rate are

- chronic total coronary occlusions; and
- lesions situated in a heavily calcific, tortuous vessel.

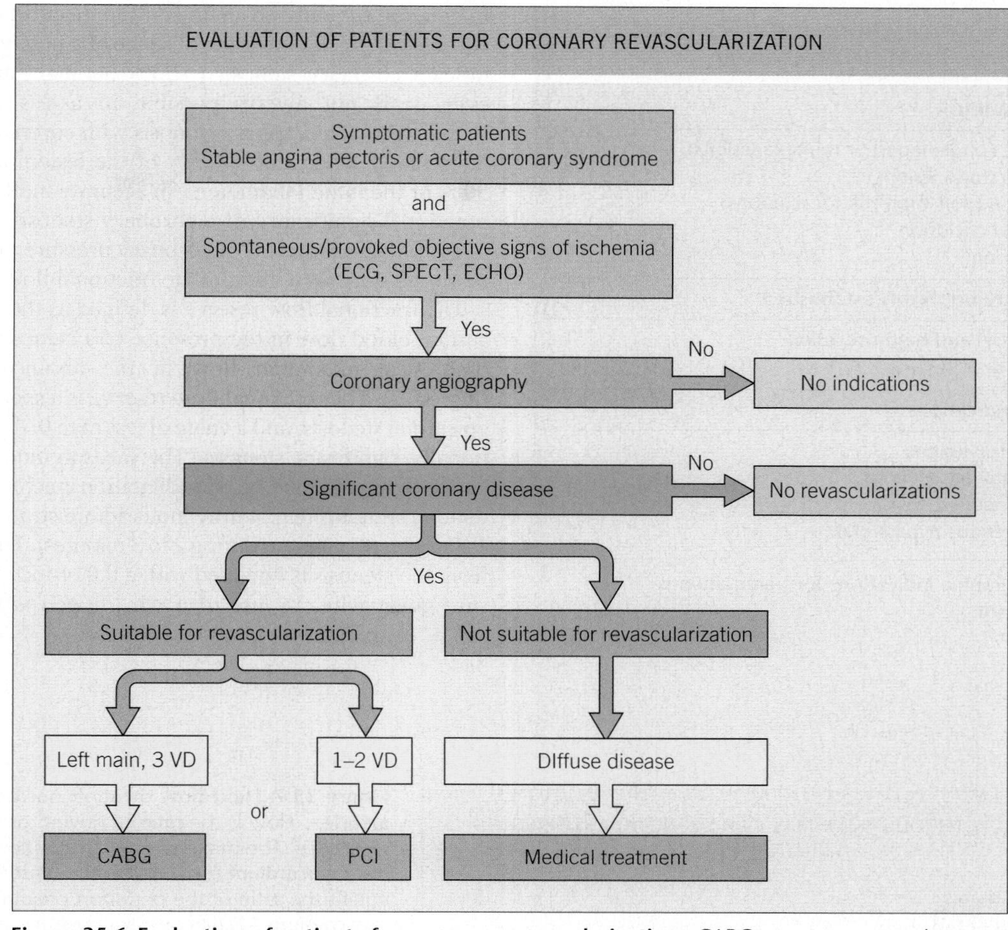

Figure 35.6 Evaluation of patients for coronary revascularization. CABG, coronary artery bypass grafting; ECHO, echocardiography; ECG, electrocardiography; PCI, percutaneous coronary intervention; SPECT, single-photon emission computed tomography; VD, vessel disease.

RISK STRATIFICATION FOR PERCUTANEOUS INTERVENTIONS

	Low Risk (death or MI < 3%)	High Risk (death or MI > 3%)
Clinical	Stable angina and acute coronary syndromes LVEF >30%	After MI or unstable angina pectoris LVEF <30% Very elderly (>80 years) Severe comorbidity
Angiography	One, two, or three vessels with focal disease Ostial/mid left main disease	Distal left main disease Diffuse disease Severe calcification Tortuous vessels Old vein grafts Bifurcation lesion

LVEF, left ventricular ejection fraction; MI, myocardial infarction.

Table 35.1 Risk stratification for percutaneous interventions.

CLINICAL INDICATIONS FOR PERCUTANEOUS CORONARY INTERVENTION

Established indications
Moderate to severe stable angina (if evidence of reversible ischemia)
High-risk unstable angina or non–ST-segment elevation myocardial infarction
Acute ST-segment elevation myocardial infarction
Indications that are not firmly established
Rescue percutaneous coronary intervention after failed thrombolysis
Cardiogenic shock after myocardial infarction
Revascularization after successful resuscitation (sudden death)
Patients who have diabetes mellitus

Table 35.2 Clinical indications for percutaneous coronary intervention.

ANGIOGRAPHIC INDICATIONS FOR PERCUTANEOUS CORONARY INTERVENTION
Established indications
One-vessel disease (single lesion or multiple lesions) Two-vessel disease (focal lesions) Three-vessel disease (non–high-risk focal lesions) Single chronic total occlusion Focal vein graft lesion
Indications that are not firmly established
Last remaining vessel and high-risk lesion Diffuse, long vein graft disease
Not first-choice indications
Three-vessel high-risk lesions Left main stem distal bifurcation Two chronically occluded vessels Totally occluded venous bypass graft

Table 35.3 Angiographic indications for percutaneous coronary intervention.

In general, the only absolute contraindication to percutaneous coronary intervention is the absence of a hemodynamically significant coronary stenosis (>50% luminal narrowing). However, it is not always possible to assess the physiologic significance of a coronary stenosis with coronary angiography, particularly when the severity of the lesion is approximately 50% of the lumen diameter. An accurate method to assess the functional significance of a coronary stenosis has been developed, the measurement of coronary pressure proximal and distal to the stenosis, to derive the fractional flow reserve.[4]

The fractional flow reserve is defined as the maximum myocardial blood flow in the presence of a stenosis divided by the theoretical maximum flow in the absence of a stenosis (Fig. 35.7). The fractional flow reserve is a specific index for an epicardial stenosis, and a value of less than 0.75 indicates a functionally significant stenosis. The measurements are relatively easily obtained. Maximal vasodilatation is achieved with a vasodilating stimulus (e.g., intravenous administration of adenosine, 140 μg/kg per minute, during 2 to 3 minutes). The pressure distal from the stenosis is obtained with a 0.014-inch (0.36-mm) pressure guide wire, by use of a wire tipped with an electronic

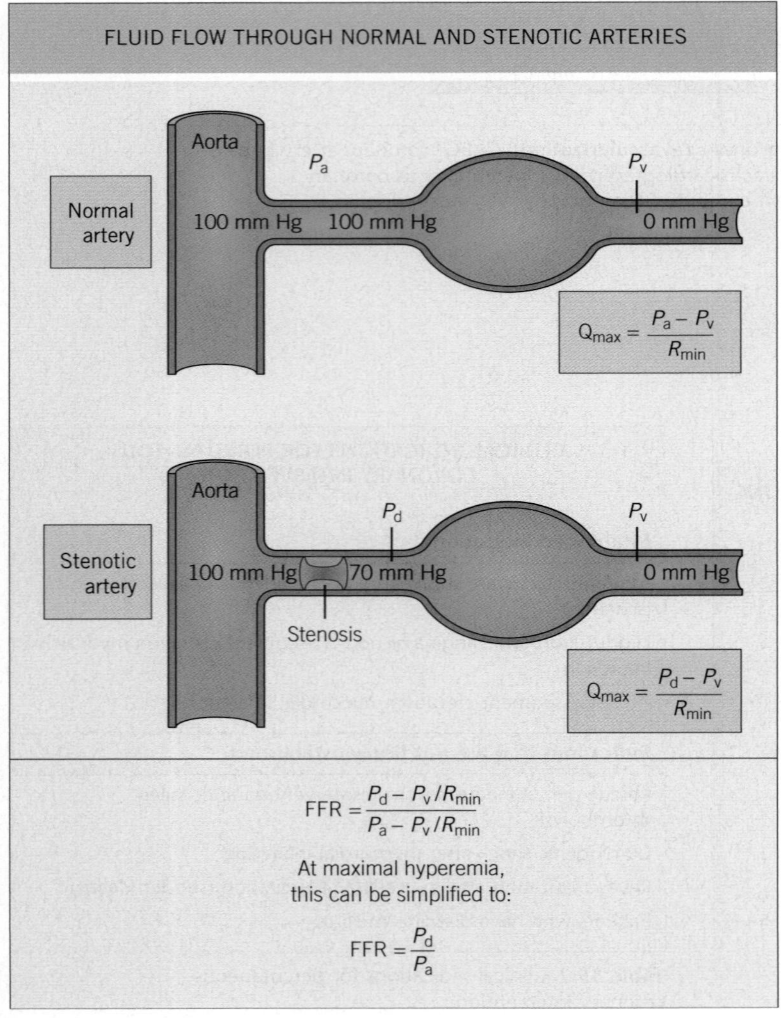

Figure 35.7 Fluid flow through normal and stenotic arteries. Flow is the ratio of driving pressure to resistance. The maximum attainable flow (Q_{max}) through the myocardium (obtained with a vasodilating stimulus) equals the ratio of the perfusion pressure across the myocardium (distal coronary pressure, P_d, minus central venous pressure, P_v) and the resistance (R_{min}). If there is no stenosis, the perfusion pressure is the mean aortic pressure, P_a, minus P_v; in the case of a stenosis, this becomes P_d minus P_v. The fractional flow reserve (FFR) can be calculated. At maximum hyperemia, R_{min} is minimal and constant, and the venous pressure is usually normal; therefore, the equation can be simplified to give FFR as the ratio of P_d to P_a. In this example, FFR is 0.7.

sensor. It has been shown that if an angiographically suspected significant lesion appears to be functionally insignificant, it is justifiable not to dilate the lesion. The DEFER study investigated the appropriateness of intracoronary stenting of functionally nonsignificant stenoses that were on visual assessment judged to have a stenosis severity of more than 50%.[5] The patients were randomized to deferral (N = 91) or performance (N = 90), that is, stent implantation. Five-year follow-up data showed no difference in the event-free survival between the deferral and performance groups: 80% and 73%, respectively ($P = .52$). The composite rate of cardiac death and acute myocardial infarction was 3.3% and 7.9%, respectively ($P = .21$), and the frequency of patients free from chest pain at 5-year follow-up was not different between the two groups.

PERCUTANEOUS CORONARY INTERVENTION

Stent implantation has emerged as the predominant percutaneous strategy in symptomatic patients with coronary artery disease. Stent implantation has replaced balloon angioplasty because the treated lesion shows greater stability after stenting, which has made the procedure safer and predictable; it has significantly reduced the restenosis rate and the necessity for repeated percutaneous coronary intervention, but it has not reduced the mortality and procedural myocardial infarction rate (Table 35.4).[6] Yet, the rate of angiographic restenosis in patients who received bare-metal stents was on average 27% at 6 months. Implantation of drug-eluting stents has further reduced the restenosis rate. In a meta-analysis, the safety and efficacy of drug-eluting stents (sirolimus and paclitaxel drug-eluting stents) reduced the target vessel revascularization and restenosis rates, but the mortality and myocardial infarction rates remained similar (Table 35.5).[7] A question has been raised whether there were differences in safety or efficacy between sirolimus and paclitaxel drug-eluting stents. A meta-analysis of randomized head-to-head clinical trials compared the safety and efficacy of sirolimus and paclitaxel drug-eluting stents (Table 35.6).[8] There were no differences in the frequency of mortality, myocardial infarction, or stent thrombosis, but sirolimus-eluting stent implantation was associated with a lower need for target vessel revascularization.

BALLOON ANGIOPLASTY VERSUS BARE-METAL STENT IMPLANTATION (N = 9918 PATIENTS)

	Balloon Angioplasty (5190)	Bare-Metal Stent (4728)	Odds Ratio	95% CI
Death or MI (%)	5.4	4.9	0.9	0.72-1.11
Repeated PCI (%)	17	11	0.59	0.50-0.68
Restenosis* (%)	40	27	0.52	0.37-0.69

*Angiographic restenosis.
PCI, percutaneous coronary intervention.
From Brophy JM, Belisle P, Joseph L. Evidence for use of coronary stents. A hierarchical bayesian meta-analysis. Ann Intern Med 2003;138:777-786.

Table 35.4 Balloon angioplasty versus bare-metal stent implantation (N = 9918 patients).

SAFETY AND EFFICACY OF BARE-METAL STENTS VERSUS DRUG-ELUTING STENTS

	DES (2641)	BMS (2449)	Odds Ratio	95% CI
Death (%)	0.9	0.9	1.1	0.61-2.06
MI (%)	2.7	2.9	0.92	0.65-1.25
TVR (%)	4.2	13.2	0.26	0.14-0.45
MACE (%)	7.8	16.4	0.42	0.32-0.53
Restenosis (%)	8.9	29.3	0.18	0.06-0.40

BMS, bare metal stent; DES, drug-eluting stent; MACE, major adverse cardiovascular events; MI, myocardial infarction; TVR, target vessel revascularization.
From Babapulle MN, Joseph L, Bélisle P, Brophy JM, Eisenberg MJ. A hierarchical Bayesian meta-analysis of randomised clinical trials of drug-eluting stents. Lancet 2004;364:583-591.

Table 35.5 Safety and efficacy of bare-metal stents versus drug-eluting stents.

SIROLIMUS-ELUTING STENTS VERSUS PACLITAXEL-ELUTING STENTS

	SES (1845)	PES (1824)	Odds Ratio	95% CI
TVR (%)	5.1	7.8	0.64	0.49-0.84; $P = .001$
Stent thrombosis (%)	0.9	1.1	0.85	0.46-1.59
Death (%)	1.4	1.6	0.85	0.50-1.46
Death or MI (%)	4.9	5.8	0.84	0.63-1.12

MI, myocardial infarction; PES, paclitaxel-eluting stents; SES, sirolimus-eluting stents; TVR, target vessel revascularization.
From Kastrati A, Dibra A, Eberle S, et al. Sirolimus-eluting stents vs paclitaxel-eluting stents in patients with coronary artery disease. JAMA 2005;294:819-825.

Table 35.6 Sirolimus-eluting stents versus paclitaxel-eluting stents.

Drug-eluting stents have been shown to be safe and effective not only in selected patients with uncomplicated, simple coronary lesions but also in "real-world" patients who underwent drug-eluting stent treatment for a wide variety of lesions and clinical situations (Fig. 35.8).[9] Importantly, the data from the registry showed that the efficacy of drug-eluting stents was better in various subgroups: in the elderly; in patients with stable angina, acute coronary syndrome, acute myocardial infarction, and multivessel disease; in short, long, and complex lesions; and in patients with diabetes mellitus. There has been concern about the higher occurrence of late stent thrombosis after implantation of drug-eluting stents compared with bare-metal stents, particularly in patients with complex lesions. However, current evidence suggests that there are no convincing data demonstrating a difference in the frequency of stent thrombosis between bare-metal stents and drug-eluting stents, nor is there a difference in the mortality rate (Table 35.7).[10]

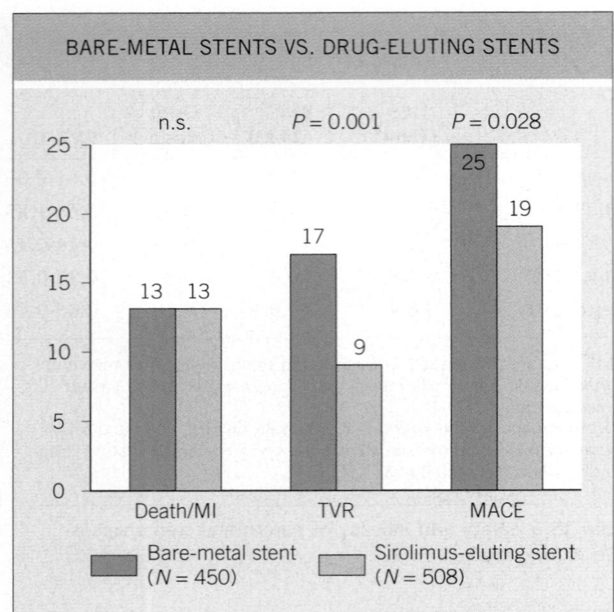

Figure 35.8 Bare-metal stents versus drug-eluting stents in "real world" patients research registry, 3 years of follow-up. MACE, major adverse cardiovascular events; MI, myocardial infarction; TVR, target vessel revascularization.

STENT THROMBOSIS, MORTALITY, AND NONFATAL MYOCARDIAL INFARCTION IN DRUG-ELUTING STENTS VERSUS BARE-METAL STENTS			
	DES (2486)	BMS (2472)	HR (95% CI)
Death or MI (%)	5.9	6.0	1.03 (0.80-1.30)
TVR (%)	9.7	10.2	0.97 (0.81-1.16)
MACE (%)	5.4	5.6	1.0 (0.80-1.26)

BMS, bare-metal stents; DES, drug-eluting stents; HR, hazard ratio; MACE, major adverse cardiac events; MI, myocardial infarction; TVR, target vessel revascularization.

From Kastrati A, Dibra A, Eberle S, et al. Sirolimus-eluting stents vs paclitaxel-eluting stents in patients with coronary artery disease. JAMA 2005;294:819-825.

Table 35.7 Stent thrombosis, mortality, and nonfatal myocardial infarction in drug-eluting stents versus bare-metal stents.

PERCUTANEOUS CORONARY INTERVENTION IN SPECIAL SITUATIONS

Elderly Patients

Percutaneous intervention in elderly patients is more challenging because of the presence of peripheral atherosclerosis and the resulting difficulties of catheterization. The immediate success rate of approximately 90% is acceptable, but the mortality rate and the rate of procedure-induced myocardial infarction are higher than in the younger population. Stent implantation in elderly patients appears to increase the safety of coronary intervention, but it is still associated with greater rates of procedural complications and worse 6-month outcomes than in younger patients. A randomized, prospective, multicenter trial enrolled patients 75 years of age or older who had chronic angina despite taking at least two antianginal drugs. The trial compared an invasive approach with optimal medical treatment, assigning 155 patients to invasive treatment and 150 to medical therapy. Symptom relief and quality of life were significantly better with revascularization treatment.[11] Percutaneous transluminal coronary angioplasty (PTCA) may be preferred to coronary artery bypass grafting (CABG) in high-risk elderly patients, who are more susceptible to the side effects of general anesthesia, major surgery, and use of mechanical heart-lung circulation.

Elderly patients with an acute myocardial infarction often present the physician with a treatment dilemma. A series of patients older than 75 years were randomly allocated to groups to receive intravenous streptokinase or primary angioplasty.[12] The primary endpoint, a composite of death, reinfarction, or stroke at 30 days, occurred in 9% of the patients in the angioplasty group compared with 29% in the thrombolysis group. Thus, primary angioplasty is preferred strategy in elderly patients with an acute myocardial infarction.

Primary Percutaneous Coronary Intervention for Acute ST-Segment Elevation Myocardial Infarction

Primary percutaneous coronary balloon angioplasty for acute ST-segment elevation myocardial infarction (STEMI) is superior to treatment with thrombolytic agents (Fig. 35.9).[13] However, primary balloon angioplasty was limited by recurrent ischemia in 10% to 15% of patients, reinfarction in 5% to 10%, late restenosis in 25% to 40%, and reintervention in 10% to 20%. These limitations were reduced by primary coronary stent implantation. A meta-analysis including 4433 patients demonstrated that stenting is superior to primary balloon angioplasty (Table 35.8).[14] The mortality was similar for both techniques, but reinfarction, target vessel revascularization because of reocclusion, and restenosis were lower in stented patients.

Recently, drug-eluting stents have been used for the treatment of STEMI. A meta-analysis comparing drug-eluting stents with bare-metal stents showed that drug-eluting stents were superior to bare-metal stents, with a reduction in target vessel revascularization and major adverse coronary events (Table 35.9).[15] Adjunctive treatment with abciximab, a glycoprotein IIb/IIIa inhibitor, further reduced the mortality and 30-day reinfarction rate in patients undergoing primary percutaneous coronary intervention compared with a control group. The 30-day mortality was 2.4% versus 3.4% ($P = .047$), the 6-month mortality was 4.4% versus 6.2% ($P = .01$), and the 30-day reinfarction rate was 1.0% versus 1.9% ($P = .03$). Abciximab did not result in an increased risk of intracranial bleeding or other major bleeding complications.[16]

Although primary percutaneous coronary intervention is the first-choice option for the treatment of STEMI, fibrinolytic treatment remains a very useful and common treatment. In case of failure of fibrinolytic treatment, it has been shown that rescue percutaneous coronary intervention did not reduce all-cause mortality but was associated with significant reductions in heart failure and reinfarction compared with conservative treatment (Table 35.10).[17] Repeated fibrinolytic therapy was not associated with significant clinical improvement.

Emergency revascularization was associated with clinical improvement in patients with STEMI and cardiogenic shock in the SHOCK trial,[18] in which 152 patients were assigned

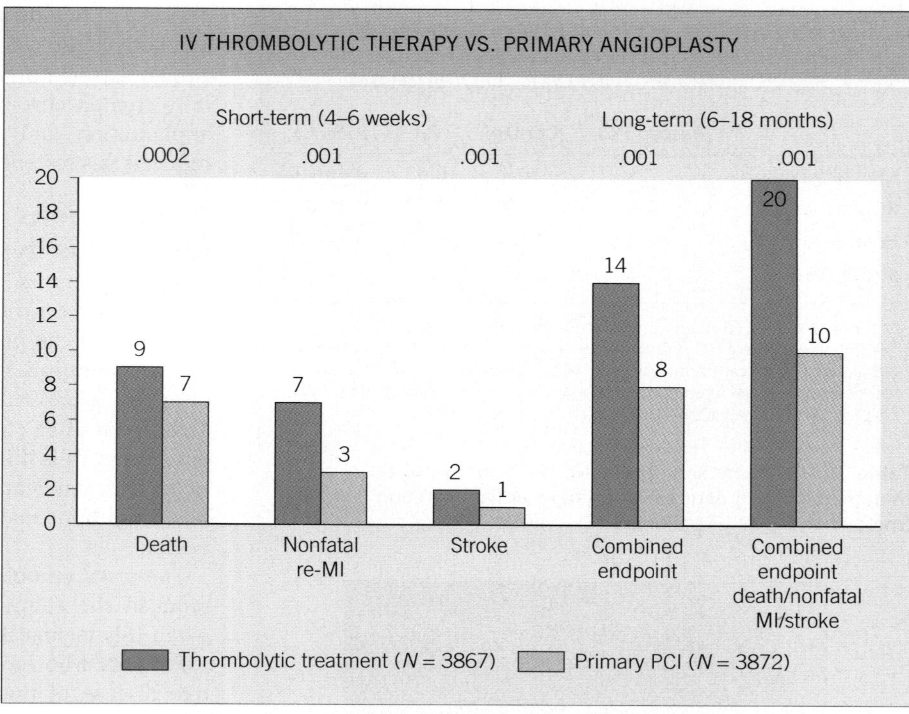

Figure 35.9 Intravenous thrombolytic therapy versus primary angioplasty for treatment of acute ST-segment elevation myocardial infarction. MI, myocardial infarction; PCI, percutaneous coronary intervention.

PRIMARY STENTING VERSUS BALLOON ANGIOPLASTY FOR TREATMENT OF ACUTE ST-SEGMENT ELEVATION MYOCARDIAL INFARCTION (N = 4433)

1-Year follow-up	Odds Ratio	95% CI
Mortality	1.09	(0.80-1.50)
Reinfarction	0.67	(0.45-0.99)
Target vessel revascularization	0.76	(0.39-0.59)

From Nordmann AJ, Hengstler P, Harr T, Young J, Bucher HC. Clinical outcomes of primary stenting versus balloon angioplasty in patients with myocardial infarction: a meta-analysis of randomized controlled trials. Am J Med 2004;116:253-262.

Table 35.8 Primary stenting versus balloon angioplasty for treatment of acute ST-segment elevation myocardial infarction (N = 4433).

DRUG-ELUTING STENTS VERSUS BARE-METAL STENTS FOR TREATMENT OF ACUTE ST-SEGMENT ELEVATION MYOCARDIAL INFARCTION (N = 2357)

Follow-up 8-12 months	DES (1177)	BMS (1180)	RR	95% CI
Death or MI (%)	5.8	6.9	0.84	0.62-1.15
Stent thrombosis (%)	2.3	2.6	0.87	0.53-1.45
TVR (%)	4.8	12.6	0.40	0.30-0.54
MACE (%)	9.3	17.6	0.53	0.43-0.66

BMS, bare-metal stents; DES, drug-eluting stents; MACE, major adverse cardiac events; MI, myocardial infarction; RR, relative risk; TVR, target vessel revascularization.

From Pasceri V, Patti G, Speciale G, Pristipino C, Richichi G, Di Sciascio G. Meta-analysis of clinical trials on use of drug-eluting stents for treatment of acute myocardial infarction. Am Heart J 2007;153:749-754.

Table 35.9 Drug-eluting stents versus bare-metal stents for treatment of acute ST-segment elevation myocardial infarction (N = 2357).

to emergency revascularization and 150 patients to initial medical treatment. The 30-day all-cause mortality was not different between the revascularization group and the medical group (46.7% versus 56.0%), but the 6- and 12-month mortality was lower in the revascularization group than in the medical group (50.3% versus 63.1% and 55% versus 70%, respectively).

In conclusion, primary percutaneous coronary intervention for STEMI is first-choice treatment and should be performed in patients for whom there is direct and easy access to coronary intervention facilities or who have a contraindication to thrombolytic treatment; optimal thrombolytic treatment should be offered to all other patients. Rescue percutaneous coronary intervention after failed thrombolysis is useful, and patients in cardiogenic shock benefit from primary percutaneous coronary intervention.

Percutaneous Coronary Intervention for Chronic Total Occlusion

Chronic total coronary vessel occlusions are notoriously difficult to treat with percutaneous coronary intervention techniques. Chronic total coronary vessel occlusions are found in as many as one third of patients with significant vessel disease, and they account for 10% of all percutaneous coronary interventions. The rate of success in opening these vessels ranges from about 50% to 70% (Fig. 35.10). The success rate depends on certain characteristics of a chronic occlusion: it is lower with long duration of occlusion, long length of occlusion, missing stump, presence of bridging collaterals, and underdeveloped or absent collateral circulation.[19]

RESCUE ANGIOPLASTY FOR FAILED THROMBOLYTIC THERAPY FOR ST-SEGMENT ELEVATION MYOCARDIAL INFARCTION (META-ANALYSIS, 1117 PATIENTS)				
	Rescue PCI	Control	RR	95% CI
Mortality (%)	7.3	10.4	0.69	0.46-1.05
Reinfarction (%)	6.1	10.7	0.58	0.35-0.97
Heart failure (%)	12.7	17.8	0.73	0.54-1.0
Stroke (%)	3.4	0.7	4.98	1.10-22.5

PCI, percutaneous coronary intervention; RR, relative risk.
From Wijeysundera HC, Vijayaraghavan R, Nallamothu BK, et al. Rescue angioplasty or repeat fibrinolysis after failed fibrinolytic therapy for ST-segment myocardial infarction: a meta-analysis of randomized trials. J Am Coll Cardiol 2007;49:422-430.

Table 35.10 Rescue angioplasty for failed thrombolytic therapy for ST-segment elevation myocardial infarction (meta-analysis, 1117 patients).

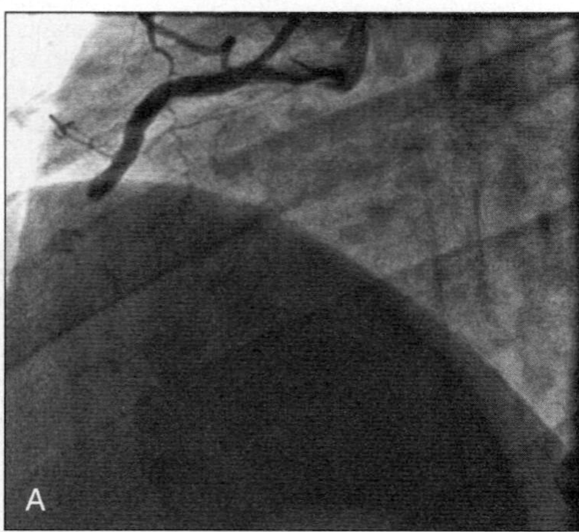

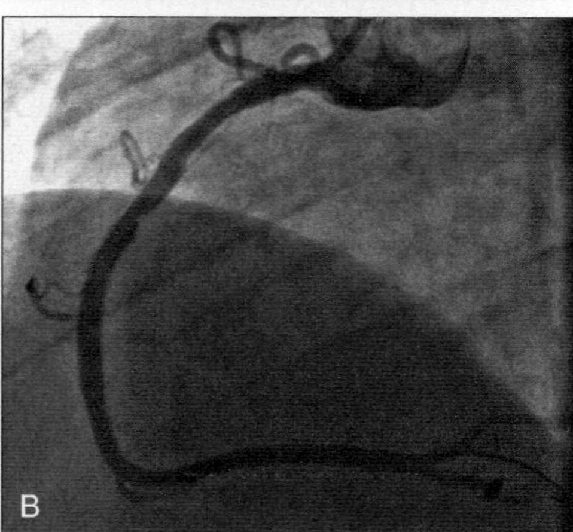

Figure 35.10 Chronic total coronary vessel occlusion. A, Chronic total occlusion, right coronary artery. **B,** Opening of chronic total occlusion.

The recent introduction of sophisticated guide wires that have a hydrophilic coating and special wires with a stiff tip has increased the success rate. However, these wires have the disadvantage that they easily cause wire perforation of the coronary artery. This is usually without adverse clinical sequelae, but it may be associated with ischemia if the healthy distal vessel segment is damaged or with the development of pericardial hemorrhage or tamponade, particularly with the adjunctive use of glycoprotein IIb/IIIa platelet receptor antagonists. Unfortunately, the rate of restenosis of a successfully treated chronic total occlusion is high, although stent implantation and very recently drug-eluting stents have reduced this restenosis rate significantly to less than 20%.[20]

Percutaneous Coronary Intervention for Venous Bypass Graft Obstruction

Deterioration of saphenous vein grafts occurs over time and may lead to recurrent ischemia. Percutaneous catheter-based intervention can be performed as an alternative to repeated bypass operation. Focal obstructions in the bypass graft can often be successfully treated, but the rate of restenosis is high, even after stent implantation.[21] Diffuse disease of an old vein graft is difficult to treat and is often associated with ischemic complications resulting from embolization of friable, thrombotic material from the graft to the distal coronary vessel.

The distal embolization protection device has significantly reduced the sequelae of embolization. It should be used when it is technically possible.[22,23]

Patients who have recurrent ischemia caused by obstructive disease of their saphenous vein grafts pose a difficult dilemma for the treating physician. In general, focal disease may be treated with a catheter-based technique; but in the presence of extensive diffuse disease, repeated surgery may be the preferred strategy, particularly if the degenerated venous bypass graft will be replaced by an arterial graft.

The prognosis of symptomatic patients after bypass grafting is rather poor because of the high rate of in-stent restenosis and progression of disease in native coronary arteries and other sites in the bypass grafts.

PERCUTANEOUS CORONARY INTERVENTION AND OTHER INTERVENTIONS: ASSESSED AND COMPARED

Medical Treatment versus Percutaneous Transluminal Coronary Angioplasty

Two recent large-scale trials have investigated the efficacy of drug treatment in comparison with percutaneous coronary intervention in patients who have stable coronary artery disease (Table 35.11).[24,25] The second Randomised Intervention Treatment of Angina (RITA 2) trial demonstrated that death and myocardial infarction occurred in 6.3% of the patients treated with percutaneous coronary intervention compared with 3.3% of those treated medically.[24] The number of revascularizations was slightly greater in the medical group than in the percutaneous coronary intervention group. However, percutaneous coronary intervention was again associated with greater symptomatic improvement, especially in patients who had more severe angina. The COURAGE trial compared optimal medical therapy with or without percutaneous coronary intervention in patients with stable coronary artery disease.[25] The COURAGE trial randomized 2287 patients who had objective evidence of myocardial ischemia and significant coronary artery disease (two thirds had significant multivessel disease). The primary outcome, death from any cause and

MEDICAL TREATMENT COMPARED WITH PTCA AND PCI IN PATIENTS WITH STABLE CORONARY ARTERY DISEASE				
	RITA 2		COURAGE	
Follow-up (median)	2.7 years		4.6 years	
	Medical (N = 514)	PTCA (N = 504)	Medical (N = 1138)	PCI (N = 1149)
Death (%)	1.4	2.2	6.5	5.9
MI (%)	1.9	4.2	11.3	12.5
Repeated PCI or CABG (%)	25.5	19	30.6	19.9

CABG, coronary artery bypass grafting; PCI, percutaneous coronary intervention; PTCA, percutaneous transluminal coronary angioplasty.

Table 35.11 Medical treatment compared with PTCA and PCI in patients with stable coronary artery disease.

nonfatal myocardial infarction during follow-up (2.5 to 7.0 years), was 19% in the percutaneous coronary intervention group and 18.5% in the medical therapy group ($P = .62$). The percutaneous coronary intervention group had lower rates of angina and repeated revascularization.

These trials confirm the general opinion that patients with stable angina should be managed initially with medical treatment (including lipid-decreasing treatment, which in the majority of cases offers adequate relief of symptoms) and that percutaneous coronary intervention is required only if these patients fail to respond adequately to medical treatment.

Percutaneous Coronary Intervention for Unprotected Left Main Disease

Percutaneous coronary intervention for unprotected left main disease is not recommended as first-choice treatment and should be considered only if severe comorbidity (for instance, in elderly patients) contraindicates revascularization by CABG.

Percutaneous Coronary Intervention in Patients at High Surgical Risk

The AWESOME trial demonstrated that percutaneous coronary intervention is a relatively safe and effective alternative to CABG for patients unresponsive to intensive medical treatment who are at high risk for CABG. In particular, percutaneous coronary intervention is a better alternative than repeated CABG in these high-risk patients.[26]

Percutaneous Coronary Intervention in Patients with Small Vessels

The role of percutaneous stent implantation in small vessels remains controversial. Some studies showed reductions in restenosis (compared with balloon angioplasty), and some studies did not show any difference. Restenosis remains high, around 40%, and suggests that careful judgment is required before such patients are treated percutaneously.

Percutaneous Coronary Intervention in Patients with Diabetes Mellitus

Diabetic patients represent almost one quarter of all those undergoing revascularization. Percutaneous coronary intervention in diabetic patients was associated with a higher incidence of myocardial infarction and repeated revascularization compared with CABG. Bare-metal stent implantation has reduced the incidence of revascularization, but this rate is still higher than after CABG. In the Arterial Revascularization Therapy Study (ARTS) trial, the event-free survival at 1 year in diabetic patients treated with stenting was 63.4% compared with 84.4% treated with CABG ($P < .001$). This was mainly driven by the higher need for repeated revascularization in stented diabetic patients.[27] The 5-year outcomes of the ARTS trial showed that stented diabetic patients did significantly less well than surgically treated diabetic patients and overall that diabetics did less well than nondiabetics irrespective of treatment by stenting or CABG (Table 35.12).[28] The role of drug-eluting stents, with the promise of a further reduction in the incidence of repeated percutaneous coronary intervention, may further improve percutaneous coronary intervention outcomes for diabetics and reduce the gap of repeated revascularization between percutaneous coronary intervention and CABG.

Adjunctive Treatment of Abciximab in Diabetics

The adjunctive treatment with abciximab, a glycoprotein IIb/IIIa inhibitor, demonstrated a survival advantage conferred by abciximab in diabetics from 4.5% to 2.5% ($P = .03$).[29] Diabetic patients undergoing percutaneous coronary intervention for non-STEMI acute coronary syndrome had a lower 30-day mortality with the use of a glycoprotein IIb/IIIa inhibitor.[30]

Percutaneous Coronary Intervention for In-Stent Restenosis

In-stent restenosis is difficult to treat because it is associated with a high recurrence rate. Implantation of a drug-eluting stent for in-stent restenosis within the previous implanted bare-metal stent is now the best option but, according to a meta-analysis concerning 1230 patients, still is associated with a recurrence rate of 17%.[31]

Percutaneous Transluminal Coronary Angioplasty versus Coronary Artery Bypass Grafting

The outcome of PTCA compared with CABG was recently reported in a meta-analysis of 13 randomized trials of 7964 patients.[32] CABG was associated with lower 5-year mortality, less angina, and fewer revascularization procedures. There was no difference in the myocardial infarction rate. CABG provided a better survival at 5 to 8 years in patients with multivessel disease. Coronary stenting has significantly reduced the need for repeated revascularization, and the 5-year outcomes after coronary stenting versus CABG for the treatment of multivessel disease have recently been reported (Table 35.13).[28] The ARTS trial demonstrated that at 5 years, there was no difference in mortality between stenting and CABG, whereas the incidence of stroke or myocardial infarction also was not

ARTS TRIAL: 5-YEAR OUTCOMES IN DIABETICS AND NONDIABETICS TREATED WITH STENTING OR CORONARY ARTERY BYPASS GRAFTING					
	Stented Diabetics	Nondiabetics		CABG Diabetics	Nondiabetics
Mortality (%)	13.4	6.8	($P = .03$)	8.3	7.5
Repeated revascularization (%)	42.9	27.5*	($P = .002$)	10.4	8.4
MACE (%)	54.5	38.7*	($P = .003$)	25	21.2

*Stented nondiabetics versus CABG nondiabetics: $P < .001$.
CABG, coronary artery bypass grafting; MACE, major adverse cardiovascular events.

Table 35.12 ARTS trial: 5-year outcomes in diabetics and nondiabetics treated with stenting or coronary artery bypass grafting.

ARTS TRIAL: 5-YEAR OUTCOMES OF CORONARY STENTING VERSUS CABG FOR MULTIVESSEL DISEASE				
	Stent	CABG	Relative Risk (95% CI)	*P* Value
Death (%)	8.0	7.6	1.05 (0.71-1.6)	.83
CVA (%)	3.8	3.5	1.10 (0.62-1.97)	.76
Q-wave MI (%)	6.7	5.6	1.19 (0.76-1.85)	.47
Non–Q wave MI (%)	1.8	0.8	2.22 (0.78-6.35)	.14
Repeated revascularization (%)	30.3	8.8	3.46 (2.61-4.6)	< .001
MACE (%)	41.7	21.8	1.91 (1.60-2.28)	< .001

CABG, coronary artery bypass grafting; CVA, cerebrovascular accident; MACE, major adverse cardiovascular event; MI, myocardial infarction.

Table 35.13 ARTS trial: 5-year outcomes of coronary stenting versus CABG for multivessel disease.

different. The overall major adverse event rate was higher in the stent group, which was mainly caused by the need for repeated revascularization.

In conclusion, it appears that CABG is associated with a slightly more favorable long-term outcome in terms of lower mortality at 5 years and fewer repeated revascularization procedures compared with coronary stenting. The use of drug-eluting stents may further reduce the disadvantage. However, it remains to be seen whether the same outcomes can be accomplished in real-world patients with multivessel disease including complex left main disease.

GRACE RISK SCORE		
Risk Category	GRACE Risk Score	In-Hospital Deaths (%)
Low	≤108	<1
Intermediate	109-140	1-3
High	>140	>3
		Post-Discharge Deaths (%)
Low	≤88	<3
Intermediate	89-118	1-3
High	>118	>8

Table 35.14 GRACE risk score.

Early Invasive versus Conservative Strategy in Patients with Unstable Coronary Artery Disease

Patients who are admitted with unstable coronary artery disease (either unstable angina or non–ST-elevation myocardial infarction) and having refractory angina, profound or dynamic electrocardiographic changes, and major arrhythmic or hemodynamic instability should undergo coronary angiography and revascularization as soon as possible. Patients without these characteristics should undergo risk assessment to identify those at high or low risk. The GRACE risk score is recommended; it is based on assessable variables, such as age, heart rate, systolic blood pressure, serum creatinine level, Killip class at admission, presence of ST depression, and elevated cardiac biomarkers.[33] According to the GRACE risk score, three risk categories have been developed (Table 35.14). The score should be determined at admission, during admission if the clinical situation changes, and at discharge. The score can be easily determined with use of a computer or PDA software of a simplified nomogram (freely available at *http://www.outcomes.org/grace*). On the basis of the evidence shown in a recent meta-analysis of seven contemporary trials with 8375 patients available for analysis, an early (within 72 hours) invasive strategy is recommended in patients at high risk (Table 35.15).[34] It is notable that only patients with elevated troponins at admission benefited from an invasive strategy, whereas troponin-negative patients did not. Early revascularization was associated with a sustained long-term beneficial effect. Of the patients who were revascularized, about 10% underwent CABG and about 90% percutaneous coronary intervention. An early invasive strategy was associated with a lower 5-year cardiovascular event rate. In the RITA 3 trial,

EARLY INVASIVE STRATEGY VERSUS CONSERVATIVE STRATEGY IN PATIENTS WITH NON-STEMI ACUTE CORONARY SYNDROME (N = 8375)			
Mean follow-up 2 years	**Early Invasive Strategy (N = 4178)**	**Conservative Strategy (N = 4197)**	**Relative Risk (95% CI)**
All-cause mortality (%)	4.9	6.5	0.75 (0.63-0.90)
Nonfatal myocardial infarction (%)	7.6	9.1	0.83 (0.72-0.96)
From Bavry A, Kumbhani D, Rassi A, Bhatt D, Askari A. Benefit of early invasive therapy in acute coronary syndromes. J Am Coll Cardiol 2006;48:1319-1325.			

Table 35.15 Early invasive strategy versus conservative strategy in patients with non-STEMI acute coronary syndrome (N = 8375).

16.6% of patients with an intervention died or had nonfatal myocardial infarction compared with 20% with conservative treatment.[35] In the FRISC II trial, this was 19.9% versus 24.5%, respectively.[36]

A conservative strategy is recommended in patients at low risk. However, in these low-risk patients, a stress test to provoke ischemia is recommended before discharge. In case of ischemia, revascularization is recommended. The Danish trial in Acute Myocardial Infarction (DANAMI) unequivocally demonstrated that patients who had inducible ischemia within 1 week of a first myocardial infarction that had been treated with thrombolytic agents and who were revascularized (PTCA, 53%; CABG, 30%; no revascularization, 17%) fared significantly better during a medium-term follow-up period of 2.4 years than did patients who were treated conservatively.[37] The combined endpoint of death, reinfarction, and hospital admission for unstable angina was 26.9% in the invasive arm compared with 40.4% in the conservative arm ($P < .001$).

Thus, it may be concluded that an early invasive strategy is both safe and effective for high-risk patients who have unstable angina coronary artery disease and that a conservative, ischemia-guided strategy is preferable in patients who do not have a high-risk profile and no provocable myocardial ischemia.

SUMMARY

Catheter-based treatment of chronic and acute ischemic heart disease has evolved into a worldwide accepted method of revascularization. This procedure is now performed more often than coronary artery bypass grafting. Percutaneous coronary intervention is based on balloon angioplasty and intracoronary stent implantation. Platelet glycoprotein IIb/IIIa antagonists, as adjunctive treatment to aspirin and heparin, should be administered to minimize the major complication rate and to increase the safety of the procedure in high-risk patients. Patients with focal one-vessel or two-vessel disease and a few patients with three-vessel disease and lesions suitable for percutaneous techniques are candidates for catheter-based treatment. Patients with three-vessel disease (and lesions not suitable for percutaneous coronary intervention) and left main stem disease should undergo surgical revascularization.

Problems related to percutaneous intervention are

- the persisting albeit low major procedural complication rate, which should initiate further improvements in the technique to increase the safety;
- the obstinate 6-month restenosis rate, which is reduced, although not eradicated, by stent implantation (including drug-eluting stents);
- the occurrence of early, late, and very late stent thrombosis in bare-metal stents or drug-eluting stents;
- the low success rate of opening chronic occluded arteries (currently approximately 80% of cases) and methods to keep these vessels open;
- the treatment of long, diffuse disease and disease in small arteries, which are associated with high rates of restenosis; and
- relatively high major adverse event rate in patients with diabetes mellitus.

Catheter-based treatment of ischemic heart disease is just one step in the management of these patients. All these patients should have a risk profile assessment, with subsequent appropriate counseling, and the great majority of patients should receive long-term aspirin and cholesterol-decreasing medication.[38]

chapter

36 Surgery for Ischemic Heart Disease

Amgad E. Elsherif and Kenton J. Zehr

Definition

- Direct coronary artery revascularization is the principal surgical therapy for ischemic heart disease. Randomized studies have demonstrated improved survival among several cohorts of surgical patients compared with those treated medically or with percutaneous transluminal coronary angioplasty.

Key Features

- During the past 3 decades, advances in surgical methodology have improved event-free survival, decreased the morbidity and mortality of coronary artery bypass surgery, and facilitated postoperative care.

Therapy

- Less invasive techniques for coronary artery bypass allow surgeons to provide direct revascularization to patients whose medical conditions might prohibit standard operation with cardiopulmonary bypass and to patients with less severe coronary disease who have previously been treated with catheter intervention.

There are nearly 1,000,000 coronary artery bypass graft (CABG) operations performed per year. Roughly one half are performed in North America, one quarter in western Europe, and the remainder in the rest of the world. This chapter presents relevant history, procedures, indications, results, and recent innovations of surgical coronary revascularization.

Before CABG, many innovative ideas were designed to augment blood flow to ischemic myocardium. Some were partially successful, but most were not, and all have been abandoned in their original form.[1-4] The forerunner of direct revascularization was the Vineberg procedure, in which the left internal thoracic artery (LITA) was tunneled into the myocardium.[5] Although most such operations were not successful, the procedure was instrumental in stimulating subsequent methods of direct coronary revascularization.

The development of cine coronary arteriography by Sones and Shirey[6] of the Cleveland Clinic in the late 1950s provided the foundation for CABG. Detailed angiographic studies permitted accurate placement of bypass grafts, and Favaloro and colleagues[7,8] reported a series of 951 patients having direct coronary revascularization between May 1967 and June 1970. In these early operations, only the right coronary artery was bypassed; but with evidence of good short-term patency, surgeons applied the technique to the left coronary artery circulation. In 1969, Johnson and coworkers[9] reported successful bypass to left-sided coronary arteries in 301 patients. The mortality rate of 12% was a vast improvement over previously published mortality rates of nearly 50% involving operative procedures on the left coronary artery circulation.

The next significant advancement was the introduction of direct anastomosis of the LITA to the left anterior descending (LAD) coronary artery. A Russian surgeon, Kolessov,[10] performed the operations in dogs and later in patients. Green and asssociates[11] performed the LITA-to-LAD bypass in patients at New York University using optical magnification and extracorporeal circulation. These early series established the feasibility of the procedure, and the development of safe extracorporeal circulatory support systems and the introduction of cardioplegia heralded the modern era of coronary revascularization.

Long-term efficacy of coronary revascularization was established by three randomized studies.[12-14] The European study[12] randomized 768 men to medical or surgical treatment. In follow-up extending to 8 years, survival was significantly improved by surgery in patients with significant three-vessel disease and in patients with significant stenoses in the proximal LAD coronary artery who had two- or three-vessel disease. Compared with medically treated patients, late mortality was reduced by 53% at 5 years in surgically treated patients, and among those with three-vessel disease, the 5-year mortality rate was lowered by 66%. In the subgroup of patients with significant narrowing of the proximal LAD coronary artery, the 5-year mortality rate was lowered 60% by surgery (Fig. 36.1).

The Veterans Administration study[13] evaluated long-term survival after CABG in 686 patients with stable angina, and patients were observed for an average of 11.2 years. The 7-year survival curves for the total population of patients showed a statistically significant survival benefit of 77% with surgical therapy compared with 70% survival with medical treatment. This benefit diminished by 11 years of observation, but a survival advantage persisted 11 years in surgical patients with three-vessel disease and impaired left ventricular function and in those at high clinical risk defined by preoperative ST-segment depression, history of myocardial infarction, or hypertension (Fig. 36.2).

The Coronary Artery Surgery Study (CASS)[14] reported survival data of 780 patients with stable angina and ejection fractions greater than 35% who were assigned to receive medical or surgical therapy. At 8 years of follow-up, 87% of surgically treated patients were alive compared with 84% of those receiving medical therapy. Although not statistically significant, the trend favored surgical therapy.

Of note, the subgroup with three-vessel disease and a reduced ejection fraction of less than 50% but greater than 35% had a significant survival benefit in the surgical group at 7 years of 88% compared with 65% in the medical therapy group (Fig. 36.3).

These randomized studies comparing coronary artery bypass surgery with medical therapy included different patient populations with regard to symptomatic status, left ventricular function, degree of coronary artery stenosis, and distribution of disease. During the years of study enrollment, there were rapidly evolving technical changes, improvements in medical therapy, and improvements in postoperative care, with resultant marked changes in perioperative mortality. Despite the differences in study design, the trials resulted in a common theme that direct revascularization afforded a survival benefit in those patients with advanced occlusive coronary artery

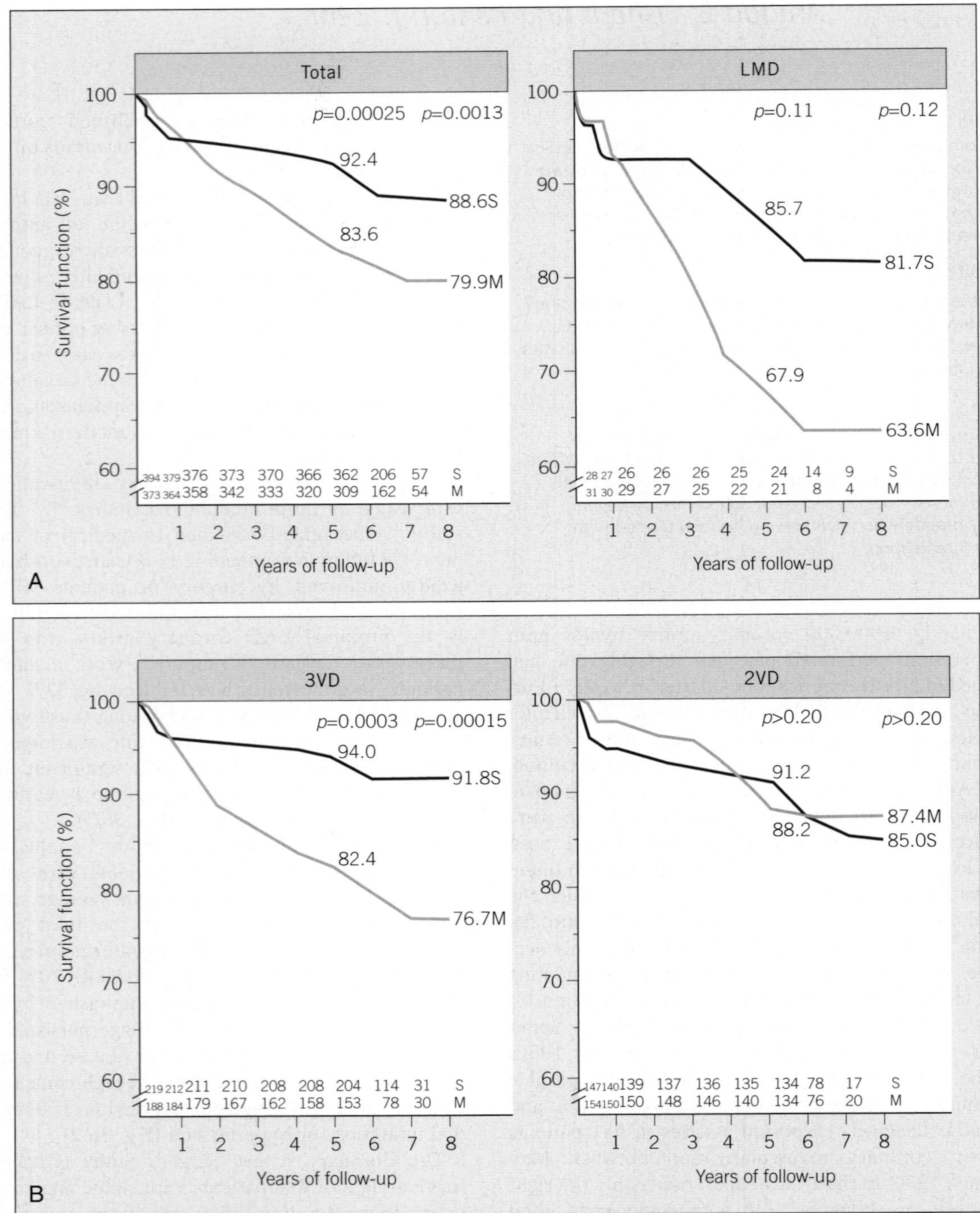

Figure 36.1 Survival curves from the prospective, randomized study of coronary artery bypass surgery and stable angina pectoris by the European Coronary Surgery Study Group. A, Survival curve for the patients randomized to the medical (M) or surgical (S) group in the total population, and those with left main coronary artery disease (LMD). **B,** Survival curves for those with three vessel disease (3VD) and two vessel disease (2VD). *(Continued)*

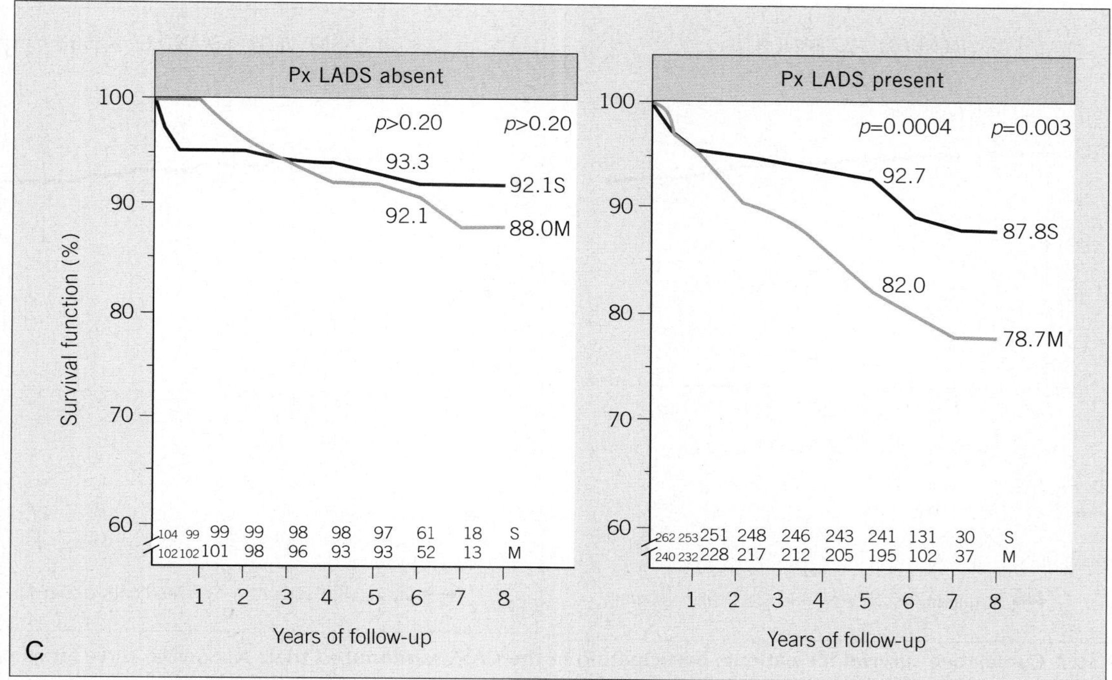

Figure 36.1—cont'd **C,** Survival curves for those without proximal left anterior descending disease (Px LADS absent) and those with Px LADS present. (From European Coronary Surgery Study Group. Long-term results of prospective randomized study of coronary artery bypass surgery in stable angina pectoris. Lancet 1982;2:1173–1180.)

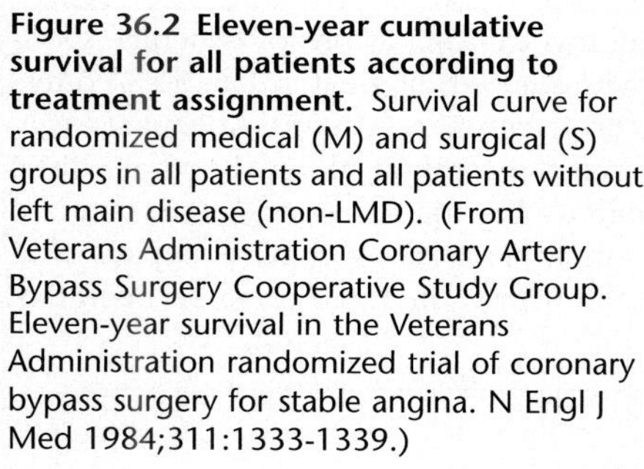

Figure 36.2 Eleven-year cumulative survival for all patients according to treatment assignment. Survival curve for randomized medical (M) and surgical (S) groups in all patients and all patients without left main disease (non-LMD). (From Veterans Administration Coronary Artery Bypass Surgery Cooperative Study Group. Eleven-year survival in the Veterans Administration randomized trial of coronary bypass surgery for stable angina. N Engl J Med 1984;311:1333-1339.)

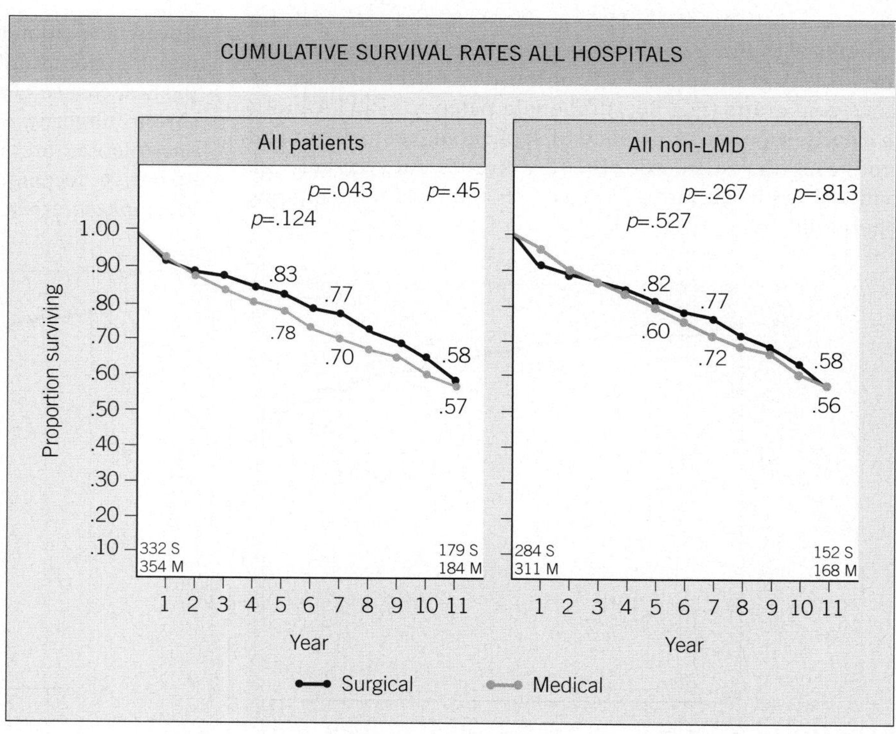

disease that placed large areas of myocardium at risk, particularly in patients with reduced ventricular function.

The survival benefit of surgery versus medical therapy diminishes over time, largely because of development of occlusive disease in saphenous vein grafts. LITA grafts appear resistant to atherosclerosis, and the improved late patency of these bypasses improves survival of patients. Loop and colleagues[15] compared outcome of 2306 patients who received a LITA-to-LAD graft alone or combined with one or more saphenous grafts with outcome of 3625 patients who received only saphenous vein bypass grafts. The 10-year actuarial survival rate significantly favored those

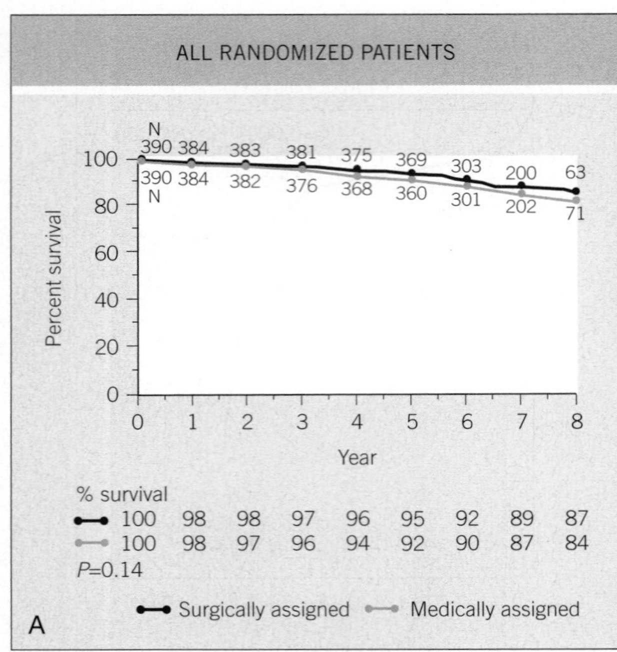

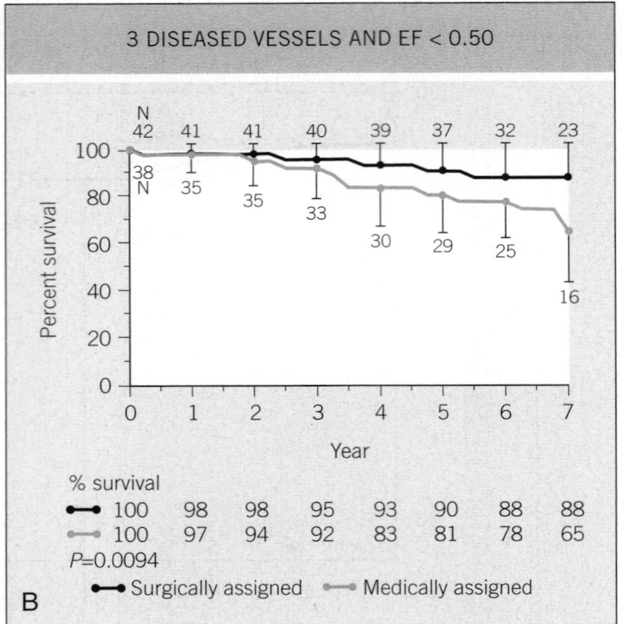

Figure 36.3 Cumulative survival for patients participating in the CASS randomized trial. A, Survival curve for all patients assigned to medical or surgical therapy. **B,** Survival curve for patients with three diseased vessels and ejection fractions (EF) less than 0.50 assigned to medical or surgical therapy. (From Killip T, Passamani E, Davis K; the CASS Principal Investigators and their associates. Coronary Artery Surgery Study [CASS]: a randomized trial of coronary bypass surgery. Circulation 1985;72[Suppl V]:V102-V109.)

with one-vessel disease, two-vessel disease, or three-vessel disease receiving the LITA graft. Actuarial survival for patients with three-vessel disease was 82.6% in those receiving a LITA graft versus 71% in those receiving only saphenous vein grafts (Fig. 36.4). The late patency of LITA grafts is clearly superior to patency of saphenous vein grafts. This study set the standard of LITA bypass for virtually all patients with occlusive disease of the LAD undergoing operation.

DESCRIPTION OF TECHNIQUE

Revascularization of all myocardium at risk of ischemia (grafting all major arteries with stenoses of greater than 50%) offers the best chance of success in coronary surgery. Adequate exposure to target vessels and the creation of widely patent distal anastomoses are required. For these reasons, the standard operative technique employs cardiopulmonary bypass with cardioplegic arrest of the heart. The most common operation

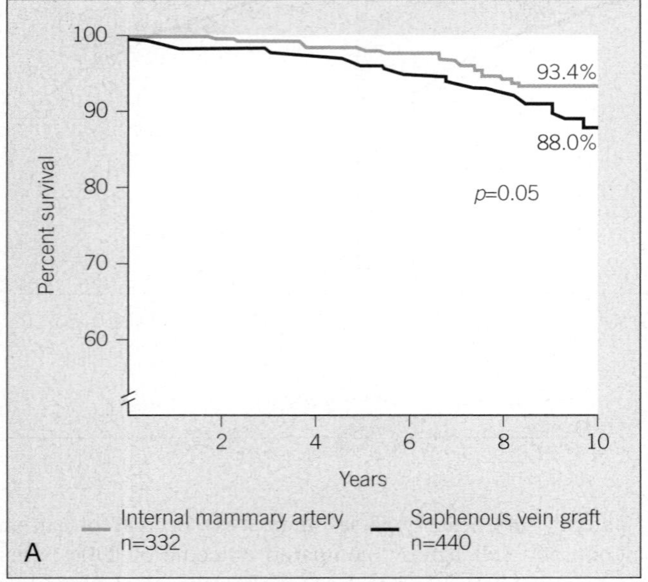

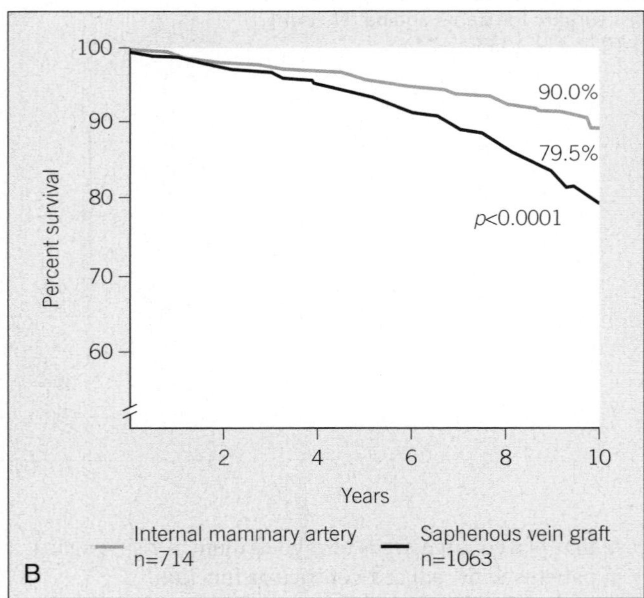

Figure 36.4 Survival curves of patients who received internal mammary artery grafts compared with those who received only saphenous vein grafts. A, Ten-year survival of patients with one-vessel (anterior descending artery) disease who had either an isolated internal mammary artery graft or a vein graft. **B,** Ten-year survival of patients with two-vessel disease, including those with lesions of the proximal anterior descending artery.

(Continued)

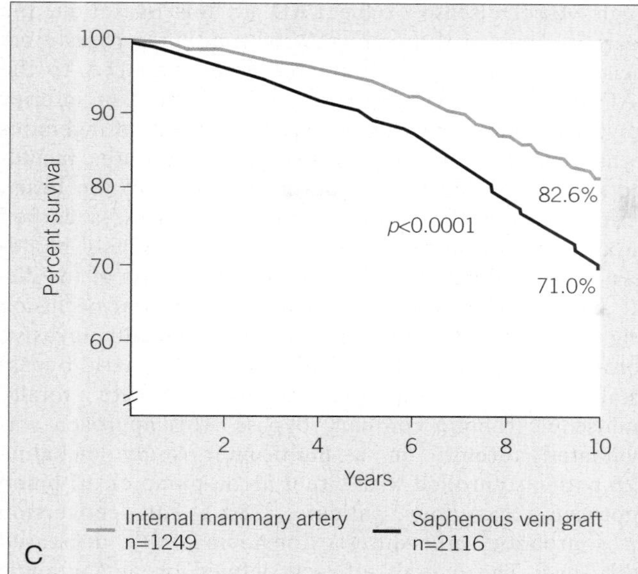

Figure 36.4—cont'd C, Ten-year survival of patients with three-vessel disease. The internal thoracic artery group received one arterial graft and one or more saphenous vein grafts. The saphenous vein graft group received all vein grafts. (From Loop FD, Lytle BW, Cosgrove DM, et al. Influence of the internal-mammary artery graft on 10-year survival and other cardiac events. N Engl J Med 1986;314:1-6.)

has been LITA bypass of the LAD and saphenous vein bypass grafting to all other distal targets. Recently, there has been interest in the use of other arterial conduits, primarily the right internal thoracic artery and the radial artery, to improve long-term patency of all of the bypass grafts.

Setup and Establishment of Cardiopulmonary Bypass

The operation is performed through median sternotomy with cannulation of the ascending aorta and right atrium (Fig. 36.5). Careful inspection and palpation of the aorta at the anticipated site of cannulation are necessary to avoid embolization of calcified, atherosclerotic debris; epiaortic ultrasonography may be helpful in visualizing the aortic wall if plaque is suspected.

Most centers use high-flow cardiopulmonary bypass (blood flow index of 2.0 to 2.4 L/min) at normothermia or mild hypothermia with a mean perfusion pressure of 55 to 65 mm Hg. Pressures should be maintained at 75 mm Hg in patients with renal insufficiency or carotid artery occlusive disease. Distal graft-to-coronary anastomoses are performed after the aorta is clamped and the heart arrested with cold blood cardioplegia (Fig. 36.6). After completion of all distal anastomoses, the aortic clamp is removed, and the proximal saphenous vein bypass graft anastomoses are created with a partial occlusion clamp placed on the ascending aorta to allow the heart to be reperfused through the native coronaries and the LITA-to-LAD graft (Fig. 36.7). Some surgeons prefer to complete the proximal graft anastomoses with the aorta clamped.

Radial Artery Grafts

There has been renewed interest in the radial artery as a conduit for the coronary artery. In early series, stenotic lesions and occlusion were observed in as many as 35% of patients,

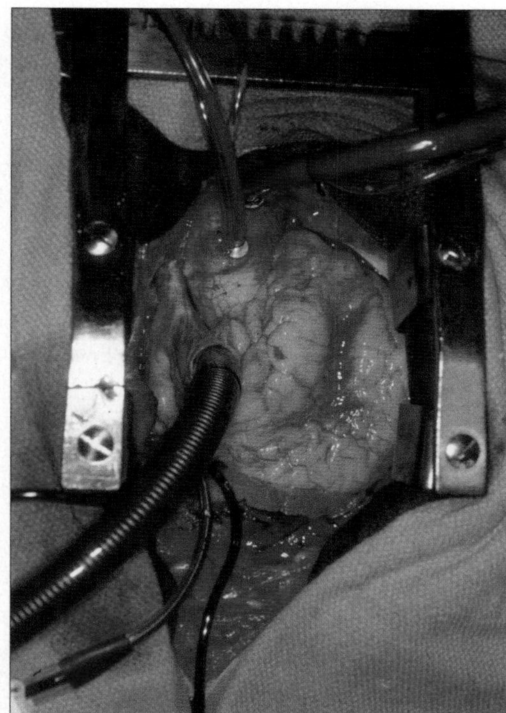

Figure 36.5 Typical surgical setup and cannulas for cardiopulmonary bypass and coronary artery bypass grafting. The patient's head is toward the top.

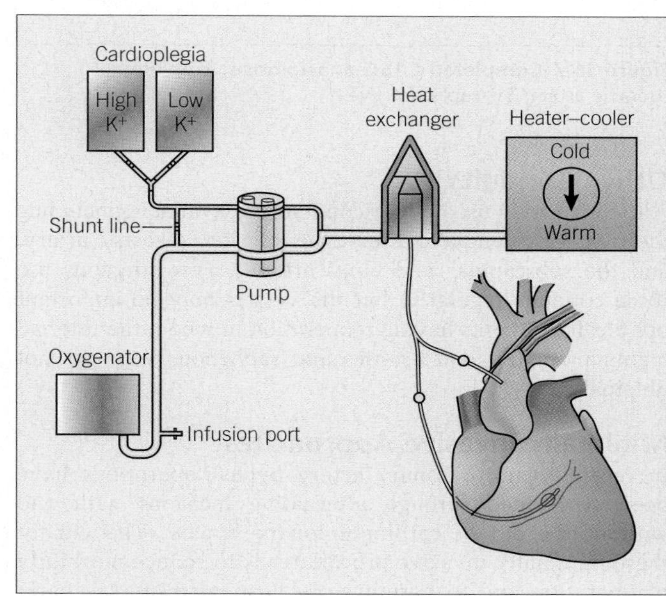

Figure 36.6 Cardioplegia.

but it appears that many of these unsatisfactory angiographic findings were caused by spasm of this muscular vessel. Indeed, 20-year patency of radial artery bypass grafts has been documented.[16] Nitrovasodilators or calcium channel blockers may prevent spasm; use of these drugs perioperatively and during the first 6 months postoperatively, coupled with atraumatic harvest techniques, results in patency rates of radial artery bypass grafts that are similar to those of free internal thoracic artery (ITA) grafts.

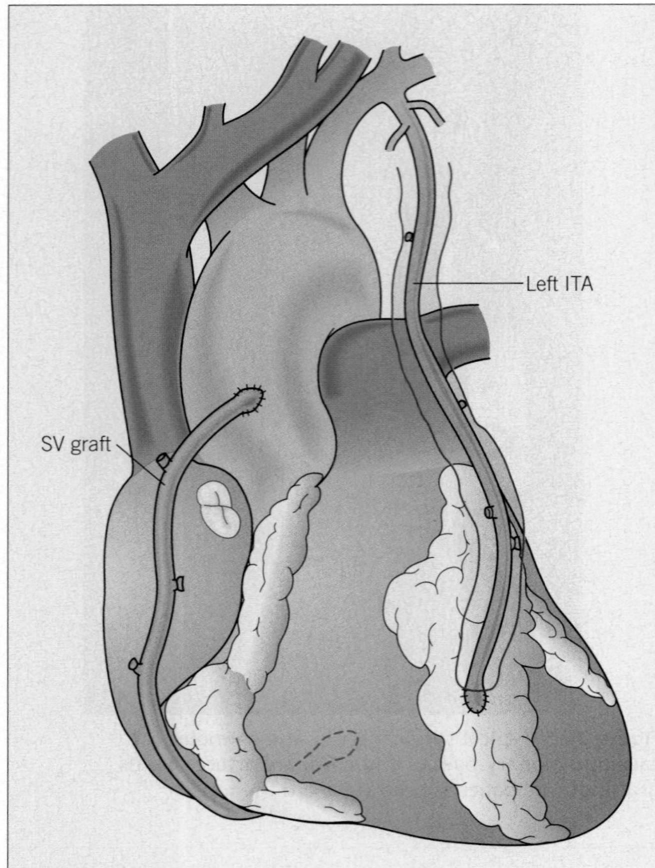

Figure 36.7 Completed CABG anastomosis. ITA, internal thoracic artery; SV, saphenous vein.

Other Conduits

Although rarely used, other conduits are available, including the right gastroepiploic artery, the inferior epigastric artery, and the subscapular and ulnar arteries. Few surgeons use these conduits regularly, but the vessels may be important options for patients having reoperation in whom the internal mammary and radial arteries and saphenous vein are not obtainable.

Minimally Invasive Approaches

In recent years, coronary artery bypass operations have been performed through alternative incisions with and without the aid of cardiopulmonary bypass. The aim of these minimally invasive procedures is to reduce morbidity of operation and to permit early hospital dismissal, early return to work, and normal activities. Such methods are not entirely new; Kolessov constructed LITA-to-LAD anastomoses without the aid of cardiopulmonary bypass, but the method was abandoned because of the improved operative conditions provided by extracorporeal circulation. Ironically, avoidance of the deleterious effects of cardiopulmonary bypass is now being promoted as the reason to embrace the minimally invasive direct coronary artery bypass procedure.[17-19]

The minimally invasive direct coronary artery bypass procedure has been proposed as an alternative to percutaneous transluminal coronary angioplasty (PTCA) for single-vessel disease of the LAD. In this operation, the heart is exposed through a 10-cm transverse parasternal incision, and a bypass is created from the LITA to the LAD directly or with an interposed segment of inferior epigastric artery or radial artery.[20] A variety of ingenious techniques aid in beating heart surgery procedures, including stabilizing devices to minimize motion of the heart, ventricular apical suction positioning devices, a carbon dioxide blower-mister to keep the field relatively bloodless, and intraluminal shunts to allow perfusion of the distal artery during periods of temporary arterial occlusion (Fig. 36.8). Some surgeons advocate minimally invasive coronary surgery with use of cardiopulmonary bypass established by peripheral cannulation with totally endoscopic robotic coronary bypass. This approach was evaluated recently in a multicenter study including 228 patients enrolled with either an on-pump or off-pump approach. Sixty-four patients (28%) had conversion to nonrobotic procedures. Conversion rate decreased with time. The overall efficacy defined by angiographic patency or lack of ischemic signs on stress electrocardiography was 97%. The incidence of major adverse cardiac events within 6 months was 5%. This method, port access (Fig. 36.9) or port coronary artery bypass, has the advantage of operation on an arrested heart and allows small incisions.[21,22]

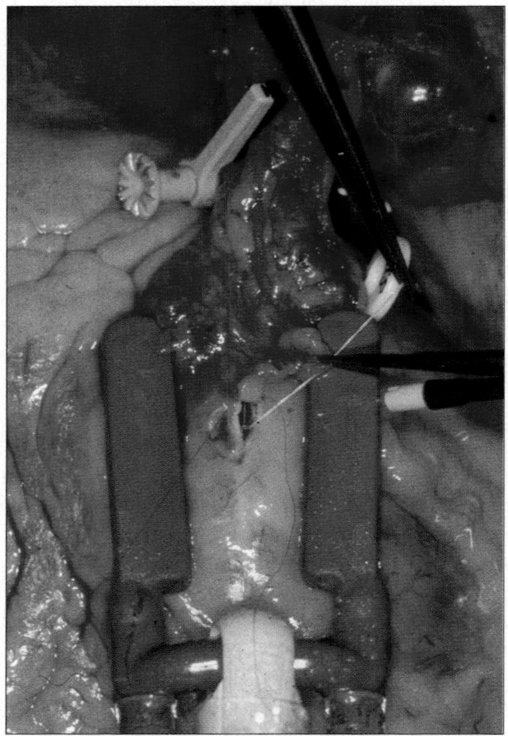

Figure 36.8 Off-pump coronary artery bypass setup for a left internal thoracic artery to left anterior descending coronary artery anastomosis. The anastomosis is half completed. The patient was very dependent on the anterior wall and required intraluminal shunting for the anastomosis to be performed safely. The indication for off-pump coronary artery bypass was severe chronic obstructive pulmonary disease. Bullous emphysematous changes are readily observed.

Figure 36.9 Port access.

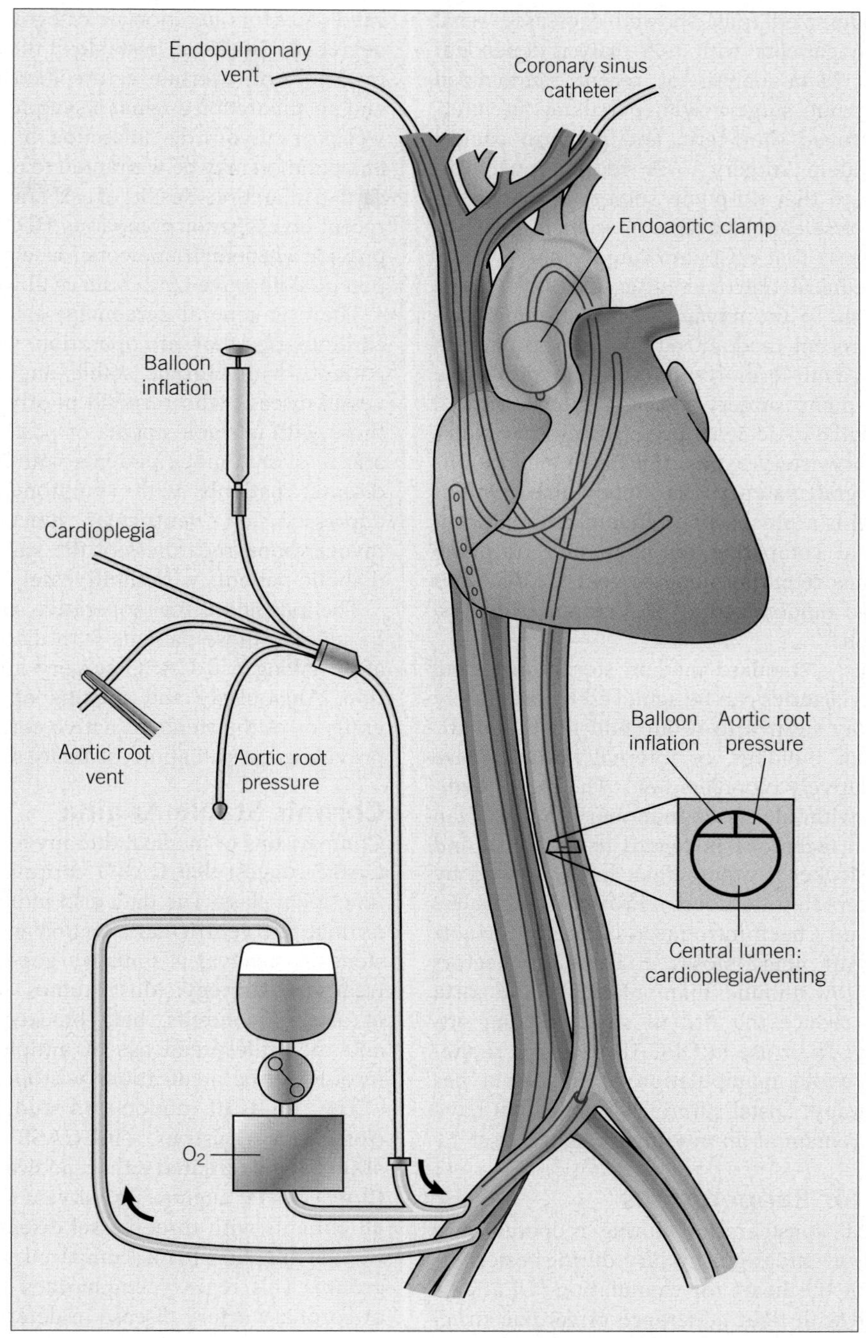

Off-Pump Coronary Artery Bypass

Historically, coronary revascularization without extracorporeal circulation has been used in situations in which cardiopulmonary bypass technology is not readily available or is prohibitively expensive. The interaction between the blood components and synthetic services of the cardiopulmonary bypass system results in activation of complement and neutrophils, causing a systemic inflammatory response syndrome. Although this response may cause significant morbidity, the long-term sequelae of the inflammatory response result in little mortality in most patients undergoing routine coronary artery bypass. Proponents of this technique cite the experience of 1761 cases of Buffolo and Gerola,[23] 1420 cases of Benetti and colleagues,[24] and 2052 cases of Tasdemir and associates[25] performed in a situation with limited resources in which clinical outcome has been good. Of note, three-vessel revascularization was rarely performed in these series. Certainly, CABG without cardiopulmonary bypass has allowed more patients to benefit from an operation in medical environments where conventional methods are not feasible on a large scale. There is a growing body of literature suggesting a reduction in perioperative morbidity in patients at higher risk for complications related to cardiopulmonary bypass. This includes elderly patients and patients with calcified ascending aortas, carotid disease, previous stroke, or CABG. Another relative indication for off-pump bypass grafting is severe pulmonary disease or renal disease, in which cardiopulmonary bypass may impair postoperative pulmonary or renal function. Recent randomized trials showed decreased renal morbidity in diabetic patients with non–dialysis-dependent renal insufficiency.[26] Meta-analysis of recent randomized trials comparing off-pump surgery with percutaneous intervention showed improved short-term and midterm clinical outcomes with off-pump surgery.[27] A recent review of 11,413 patients showed that off-pump surgery is associated with fewer major adverse cardiac events in women. This retrospective study suggests that off-pump surgery narrows the gender disparity in clinical outcomes after CABG.[28] Some controversy remains as to the advantages of off-pump surgery. Results from a recent randomized trial of 150 patients showed excellent medium-term results with no difference between on- and off-pump surgery.[29] Conventional wisdom suggests that the potential to decrease perioperative morbidity with off-pump coronary artery bypass (OPCAB) may be offset by less favorable graft patency. The Randomized On/Off Bypass (ROOBY) trial is a prospective randomized multicenter single-blinded trial comparing on-pump and off-pump techniques for veterans requiring nonemergent CABG. This includes 2200 patients randomized at 17 Veterans Administration medical centers.[30]

The procedure uses a standard median sternotomy, and access to the coronary arteries can be achieved by accurately placing pericardial stay sutures to rotate and lift the heart. Silastic tapes, vascular bulldogs, or internal occluders are used to provide a relatively bloodless field. The use of pedicled arterial grafts without cardiopulmonary bypass can allow a true no-touch technique in regard to the aorta and may reduce risk of stroke or other organ injury caused by embolization of atherosclerotic debris. Proximal sutureless connectors have recently been introduced clinically for aortosaphenous vein graft anastomoses.[31] These connectors were introduced to allow minimal manipulation of the aorta and theoretically to reduce the risk of stroke during off-pump bypass grafting. Their use in OPCAB to attach saphenous vein grafts to avoid manipulation of the aorta has become standard therapy. Distal sutureless connectors have been introduced but remain at an investigational stage.[32]

Considerations for Reoperations

The primary technical consideration during reoperation is avoidance of cardiac or patent graft injury during resternotomy and dissection of the heart for cannulation.[33] Patients at high risk are those with tight adherence of cardiac structures to the posterior sternum as seen on lateral chest radiography and angiography, patients with patent ITA grafts crossing the midline, and artery or vein grafts closely adherent to the sternotomy as seen on lateral angiography. Patients who have previously received mediastinal irradiation are at risk. Patients with aortic aneurysms or patients with high right-sided pressures and enlarged right atria or ventricles are at risk for cardiac injury during sternal reentry. In these patients, it is wise to expose and, on occasion, to cannulate the femoral vessels before opening the sternum.

INDICATIONS FOR SURGERY

Most patients come to medical attention because of angina pectoris or equivalent symptoms, and symptom relief is an important issue in considering operation. Traditionally, candidates for operation are categorized as stable with variable degrees of disability; unstable, if the symptoms occur at rest or randomly on exertion or are increasingly severe over time; and postinfarction angina, if symptoms develop within several weeks of a myocardial infarction. In addition to symptom relief, an operation may be warranted to reduce risk of death or myocardial infarction. Results of early randomized studies and more recent investigation comparing PTCA procedures with CABG provide a general framework for selection of patients who have potential improvement in survival with CABG.

There is general agreement among cardiac surgeons and cardiologists that an operation should be considered for patients with chronic stable angina and significant three-vessel disease who respond poorly to medical management; those with unstable angina or postinfarct angina; asymptomatic or symptomatic patients with left main coronary artery disease; patients with symptomatic three-vessel disease, depressed left ventricular function, and known viable myocardium, regardless of the stability of their angina; and diabetic patients with multivessel disease.

The indications for reoperative surgery are much less clear. In general, those patients with disabling recurrent symptoms after having had CABG surgery are considered for reoperation. Angioplasty and stenting of stenosed saphenous vein grafts or of the stenosed native coronary artery culprit lesion provide good palliation for many such patients.

Chronic Stable Angina

Comparisons of medical therapy and CABG or of PTCA and CABG suggest that CABG improves event-free survival and functional class. The data also indicate that for patients with normal left ventricular function without left main coronary stenosis, survival is similarly good, regardless of the initial treatment strategy. Most studies antedated the routine use of arterial conduits, beta blockers, the advent of PTCA, and the widespread use of antiplatelet agents and cholesterol-lowering medications postoperatively.

The results of randomized studies are supported by data from large registries. The CASS registry observed nearly 4000 patients treated either medically or surgically with class III or class IV angina.[34] Five-year survival was improved for all patients with three-vessel disease, regardless of left ventricular function (87% compared with 65% for the medical group). This registry emphasized the importance of extent of coronary artery disease in determining outcome. Patients with proximal lesions and three-vessel disease had increased survival benefit with surgical therapy. The CASS registry also showed a decrease in late infarction in patients with three-vessel disease undergoing early surgery.

The Duke University registry[35] collected approximately 4000 patients from 1969 to 1984. Their results confirmed the CASS registry results and identified left ventricular dysfunction to be the most important negative determinant of long-term survival.

Proudfit and colleagues[36] reported a registry of 408 medical and 390 coronary artery bypass patients operated on at the Cleveland Clinic from 1975 to 1979; these patients had mild angina or myocardial infarction without angina. The significance of this study was the ability to compare the 10-year survival of patients who underwent coronary bypass surgery with an ITA bypass with that of patients having only saphenous vein grafts. Although the survival was higher for the saphenous vein subset compared with the medical group through 7 years (90% and 82.5%, respectively), this difference was eliminated by 10 years (76% in each group). Survival at 10 years was 92% in those who received ITA grafts (179 patients). This study proved that the ITA-to-LAD graft improved long-term survival. By comparing this study with the previous randomized multicenter trials, which used only vein, the 10-year results of the medically versus surgically treated patients with vein were nearly identical.

More recent studies have entered patients with stable angina into randomized trials of interventional therapies, PTCA, and CABG. The Medicine, Angioplasty or Surgery Study (MASS)[37] randomized 214 patients with stable angina and single severe proximal stenosis of the LAD; 70 patients underwent ITA bypass grafting, and there were 72 in the angioplasty or medical therapy groups each. At 5-year follow-up, the cumulative event-free survival was 98.6% for CABG patients, 63.9% for PTCA patients, and 88.9% for patients treated medically.[38] There were no differences in mortality or infarction rates at the 3- or 5-year reporting. Both interventional techniques provided greater relief of anginal symptoms than did medical treatment alone.

The Asymptomatic Cardiac Ischemia Pilot (ACIP) study[39] was designed to assess three treatment strategies for 558 patients with cardiac ischemia on electrocardiography or treadmill testing. Patients were assigned to an angina-guided medical strategy (n = 184), ischemia-guided medical strategy (n = 182), or revascularization intervention (n = 192). At 3 months postoperatively, ischemia as seen on the electrocardiogram was suppressed in 70% of bypass patients versus 46% of the PTCA patients. Of patients with a positive exercise treadmill test result preoperatively, 46% had normal test results after bypass grafting versus 23% of patients after PTCA. In addition, angina was alleviated in 91% of surgical patients versus 68% of angioplasty patients. These results persisted during the first year of follow-up, confirming that inducible myocardial ischemia is significantly reduced in patients undergoing a more aggressive revascularization approach.

The trial of invasive versus medical therapy in elderly patients (TIME) randomized 148 patients aged 75 years or older to medical therapy and 147 to invasive therapy.[40] The patients all suffered from chronic stable angina. Of the 147 patients undergoing catheterization, 79 underwent PTCA, 30 underwent CABG, and 43 were treated medically. Major adverse cardiac events occurred in 49% of the patients in the noninvasive limb and 19% in the invasively diagnosed or treated group. This study showed that patients with higher risk profiles should be offered invasive assessment and revascularization if appropriate.

Unstable Angina

The question of medical versus revascularization management in the treatment of unstable angina is no longer an issue because of the ability of revascularization procedures to reduce anginal symptoms. These patients are clinically difficult to manage. Their pharmaceutical regimen often calls for intravenous nitrates and heparin to stabilize their angina. There is controversy as to the appropriate intervention required.

Two large randomized studies[41,42] initiated in the 1970s compared medical versus surgical management in patients with unstable angina; survival of surgical and medical patients was similar, but relief of angina was improved in patients having coronary artery bypass. Importantly, a large percentage of medically treated patients crossed over into surgical therapy during early follow-up. The National Cooperative Study Group[41] enrolled 288 patients into medicine or surgical limbs from 1972 to 1976. The crossover rate to surgical therapy was 36% at median follow-up of 30 months. There was an increased incidence of nonfatal myocardial infarction in the surgery group because of a 17% perioperative infarction rate. The prevalence of late infarction was no different. In the largest prospective randomized trial, the Veterans Administration Cooperative Study,[42] 468 patients were enrolled between 1976 and 1982. Although the 10-year survival rate for medically treated patients was 62% compared with 61% for the surgical patients, survival in patients with impaired left ventricular function was 51% for medically treated patients and 59% for surgically treated patients. Although the differences were significant at 5 years of follow-up, these differences at 10 years were no longer significant. This was similar for the subgroup of patients with three-vessel disease. Initially, the crossover rate to surgery from the medically treated group was 34% at 2 years. This percentage increased to 50% at 10 years of follow-up.

Diminishing benefits were again interpreted to be the result of progressive vein graft disease and the absence of arterial conduit grafting. Kaiser and associates[43] reviewed 14 studies that evaluated CABG for unstable angina. Ten-year survival was noted to be 80%, and 80% of those patients remained free of angina.

Percutaneous Transluminal Coronary Angioplasty versus Coronary Artery Bypass Graft for Stable or Unstable Angina

There have been a large number of randomized trials designed to assess the efficacy of PTCA versus CABG in patients with anginal syndromes. These studies have enrolled nearly 5000 patients since 1993 with multivessel disease with variable proportions of stable and unstable angina.

The largest of these trials was the Bypass Angioplasty Revascularization Investigation (BARI),[44] which compared 1829 patients from 18 clinical centers with a follow-up of 5.4 years. Of those assigned to the PTCA group, 54% required additional revascularization procedures, compared with 8% of those in the CABG group. At 5-year follow-up, 86% of the patients who had bypass were angina free compared with 78% of those who underwent PTCA. A significant survival advantage was noted in the subgroup of patients with diabetes mellitus. In those patients undergoing CABG, the survival rate was 80.6% compared with 65.5% in those patients who underwent PTCA. This survival advantage in the diabetic group was even more pronounced at 7-year follow-up; survival was 76.4% for the CABG group and 55.7% for the PTCA group.[45]

At 7 years, the nondiabetics had virtually identical survival (CABG, 86.4%; PTCA, 86.8%). However, the PTCA group continued to have a higher subsequent revascularization rate than the CABG group (59.7% versus 13.1%). The BARI investigators have also reported a significant protective effect of CABG compared with PTCA in preventing death after subsequent spontaneous Q-wave myocardial infarction in diabetic patients eligible for the BARI study. This protective effect was not true for nondiabetic patients.[46] The BARI results were corroborated by Niles and coworkers.[47] The authors analyzed a cohort of 2766 diabetic patients in a large regional database who were similar to patients randomized in the BARI trial. Initial revascularization strategies were PTCA in 736 and CABG in 2030. After adjustment for risk factors, diabetic patients with two- or three-vessel disease undergoing a PTCA initial revascularization strategy were 49% (hazard ratio, 1.49) more likely to die during the 5-year follow-up period than those undergoing initial bypass surgery. In the group with three-vessel disease, the hazard ratio was 2.02 favoring CABG.

The Coronary Angioplasty versus Bypass Revascularization Investigation (CABRI)[48] reported 1-year results of 1054 patients presenting with an average angina class III or greater. Only 15% of each limb was designated unstable angina. Mortality was similar; 33.6% of those assigned to the PTCA group required additional intervention within 1 year compared with 6.5% of those randomized to CABG. The patients receiving PTCA required significantly more antianginal medication and had a significant increase in the prevalence of clinically significant angina. The CABRI study patients were analyzed at 4 years to determine if diabetics benefited from a particular revascularization mode.[49] Although diabetics had a 2.19 relative risk for mortality compared with nondiabetics (17.8% versus 8.1%), the absolute risk of death comparing CABG and PTCA in diabetics did not reach significance (12.5% versus 22.6%).

The Randomised Intervention Treatment of Angina trials were companion trials, RITA-1[50] and RITA-2.[51] The first compared CABG with PTCA, and the second compared PTCA with medical therapy. Patients with stable and unstable angina were eligible for the RITA-1 trial. In the RITA-2 trial, only 10% had unstable angina. The trial was geared toward mild anginal grades. In RITA-1, 1011 patients were randomized to PTCA or CABG. There was no difference in the primary endpoints of death or nonfatal myocardial infarction (17% and 16%, respectively). There was a crossover rate of 26% in the PTCA group, and 19% required an additional PTCA. After 3 years of follow-up, the reintervention rate was 4% per year in the PTCA group compared with 2% per year in the CABG group. In addition, there was 10% excess of clinically significant angina in the PTCA group compared with the CABG group. The RITA-2 trial randomized 1018 patients to medical or PTCA therapy with a median follow-up of 2.7 years. Death or myocardial infarction occurred in 6.3% of those treated with PTCA compared with 3.3% in the medical group. This difference was significant and related to procedural complications. Of the patients who underwent PTCA, 19% required an additional bypass procedure or repeated PTCA compared with 23% in the medically treated group. There was a 16.5% excess of clinically significant angina in short-term follow-up. This decreased to 7.6% after 2 years. There was clear symptomatic benefit noted in either mild or severe chronic stable angina or unstable angina in the CABG groups compared with those receiving PTCA or medical management.

The Emory Angioplasty versus Surgery Trial (EAST)[52] randomized 392 patients, of whom 80% had class III or class IV angina. Mortality and myocardial infarction rates at 3-year follow-up were similar. However, 20% of the PTCA patients suffered from recurrent angina compared with 12% of the bypass patients, and 54% of the PTCA patients required repeated procedures compared with 13% of the bypass patients. The EAST study was analyzed again at 8 years. Survival was 79.3% in the PTCA group and 82.7% in the CABG group. At 8 years, 2.4% of the CABG patients had undergone repeated CABG, whereas 29.3% of the PTCA-treated patients had undergone CABG. The data regarding diabetics was analyzed. At 8 years, surgery was favored with 75.5% survival compared with 60.1% in PTCA-treated diabetics. This curve did not reach significance, but there were only 30 patients in the surgery group and 29 in the PTCA group. These results further corroborate the BARI results.

The German Angioplasty Bypass Surgery Investigation (GABI)[53] randomized 359 patients. The patients were weighted toward a milder degree of angina, with 14% of those having unstable angina. There was no difference in in-hospital or postoperative mortality. Patients who underwent CABG were more likely to have a perioperative myocardial infarction compared with those who underwent PTCA (8.1% versus 2.3%, respectively). In the PTCA group, 44% required further intervention versus only 6% in the CABG group at 1-year follow-up. There was no difference in anginal recurrences, but the PTCA group required more antianginal medication.

The Argentine Randomized Trial of Percutaneous Transluminal Coronary Angioplasty Versus Coronary Artery Bypass Surgery in Multivessel Disease (ERACI)[54] randomized 127 patients to PTCA or CABG. Freedom from all cardiac events (death, infarction, angina, or repeated procedures) was significantly greater for those undergoing bypass surgery compared with the PTCA group (77% versus 47%, respectively). Mortality or the frequency of myocardial infarction was similar, and again, patients who had coronary artery bypass surgery were free of angina 79% of the time compared with 57% of those having PTCA. The reintervention rate for those initially undergoing bypass was 6.3% versus 37% for those having coronary angioplasty.

The ERACI II trial is one of the first trials to compare present-day percutaneous techniques of PTCA and stenting with CABG[55]; 450 patients were randomized to percutaneous intervention (225) or CABG (225). This study has been widely quoted, emphasizing the freedom from death and myocardial infarction at 1-year follow-up in the PTCA and stenting group (96.9% and 97.7%, respectively) compared with the CABG group (92.5% and 93.4%). However, the perioperative mortality and myocardial infarction rates in the surgery group (5.7% and 5.7%) were higher than the rates observed in all the other comparison studies. The perioperative events account for most of the events occurring in the surgical group. The reintervention rate was 16.8% in the PTCA and stenting group compared with 4.8% in the CABG group.

Another trial comparing PTCA and stenting with CABG was the Arterial Revascularization Therapies Study (ARTS).[56,57] A total of 1205 patients were randomized (605 stenting, 600 CABG). At 1-year follow-up, mortality was 2.8% in the CABG group and 2.5% in the stenting group. Repeated revascularization was required in 3.5% of CABG patients compared with 16.8% of stented patients. Overall event-free survival was 87.8% for those undergoing CABG compared with 73.8% in the stenting group. This study also confirmed the presence of diabetes mellitus as a negative predictor of outcome in the stenting group. Complete revascularization was accomplished in 84.1% of the CABG patients compared with 70.5% of the stenting patients. At 1-year follow-up, 10% of the incompletely revascularized patients in the stenting group required subsequent bypass surgery compared with 2% of the completely revascularized patients.[57]

A third prospective randomized trial compared stenting with internal mammary artery grafting for proximal, isolated de novo left anterior coronary artery stenosis (SIMA)[58]; 59 patients underwent CABG, and 62 underwent stenting. Event-free survival, including death, myocardial infarction, and the need for repeated revascularization, was 93% in the CABG group and 79% in the stenting group at 2.4 ± 0.9 years. The difference was all due to the need for repeated revascularization.

These nine trials consistently failed to show a difference in mortality or follow-up myocardial infarction rates. However, all nine studies showed a high incidence of need for repeated revascularization procedures in the PTCA groups compared with the CABG groups. Overall, the trials demonstrated that CABG results in a marked reduction in recurrence of angina or the need for repeated revascularization procedures in the follow-up period. Recently, closer analysis of the diabetic subgroup in several of these comparison studies has shown a survival benefit favoring CABG. The BARI II trial was designed to further analyze the diabetic subgroup with multivessel coronary artery disease and is now under way.

CLINICAL AND ANGIOGRAPHIC CHARACTERISTICS OF STUDY PATIENTS WHO UNDERWENT CORONARY ARTERY BYPASS GRAFTING

	Study Period*			
Variable	**Time I**	**Time II**	**Time III**	***P***
No. of patients	2250	2705	2144	—
No. of procedures	2264	2275	2209	—
Age (yr) (mean ± SD)	61.6 ± 9.3	64.4 ± 9.4	65.8 ± 9.5	<.001
Male (%)	30.6	77.6	75.7	<.001
Age ≥65 yr (%)	40.4	54.4	60.8	<.001
Age ≥75 yr (%)	7.1	12.8	17.4	<.001
EF (%) (mean ± SD)	55 ± 13	56 ± 14	60 ± 15	<.001
NYHA (%)	55 ± 13	56 ± 14	60 ± 15	<.001
I	1	2	2	
II	6	7	6	
III	62	49	42	
IV	29	35	23	
Unknown	2	8	27	
Acute MI (%)	5.0	6.9	13.1	<.001
Prior MI (%)	57.0	55.6	50.7	<.001
Prior PTCA (%)	0.9	9.4	15.8	<.001
No. of prior CABG (%)				
One	9	10	9	NS
Two	1	1	0	NS
No. of vessels diseased (%)				
One	12.0	10.4	12.1	
Two	33.1	32.5	34.2	
Three	54.9	57.1	53.7	
Left main disease (%)	18.6	24.0	28.3	<0.001

*The 10-year study period was divided into three equal intervals: I, January 1, 1982, to April 30, 1985; II, May 1, 1985, to August 31, 1988; and III, September 1, 1988, to December 31, 1991.

CABG, coronary artery bypass grafting; EF, ejection fraction; MI, myocardial infarction; NS, nonsignificant; NYHA, New York Heart Association; PTCA, percutaneous transluminal coronary angioplasty; SD, standard deviation.

From Harris WO, Mock MB, Orszulak TA, Schaff HV, Holmes DR Jr. Use of coronary artery bypass surgical procedure and coronary angioplasty in treatment of coronary artery disease: changes during a 10-year period at Mayo Clinic Rochester. Mayo Clin Proc 1996;71:927-935.

Table 36.1 Clinical and angiographic characteristics of study patients who underwent coronary artery bypass grafting.

During the past decade, the number of patients being treated with revascularization by percutaneous catheter techniques has increased markedly. This is largely due to the lower cost of a PTCA procedure and the decreased level of invasion associated with catheterization and angioplasty. This is apparent in a series of patients treated with CABG and PTCA during a 10-year period at the Mayo Clinic from 1982 to 1991 (Tables 36.1 and 36.2).[59] The 7099 patients were divided into three equal periods. Use of PTCA increased from 784 procedures in period I to 3516 procedures in period III. The number of CABG procedures remained constant, in the region of 2200. The use of the ITA increased from 23% in period I to 84% of patients in period III. During the same period, the perioperative myocardial infarction rate declined from 5.7% to 2%. Multivessel coronary angioplasty was observed to increase from 10% of the cases in period I to 15% in period III. Mortality for both procedures remained stable throughout the study. More recently, patients in both groups were more likely to be older, to have increased comorbidities, to have undergone previous revascularization procedures, and to be referred for emergency revascularization. The surgical patients were older, had a higher percentage of left main disease, and had more previous myocardial infarctions than did the PTCA cohort. These observations demonstrate the increased use of PTCA during a 10-year period before the availability of any randomized data. This probably represents a continued national trend. More clear-cut guidelines for various subgroups are needed.

Drug-Eluting Stents

The introduction of drug-eluting stents (DES) was recently studied. A retrospective study[60] evaluated the use of DES (sirolimus or paclitaxel) in patients with severe left ventricular dysfunction; 220 patients with an ejection fraction below

CLINICAL CHARACTERISTICS OF STUDY PATIENTS WHO UNDERWENT CORONARY ARTERY ANGIOPLASTY				
	Study Period*			
Variable	Time I	Time II	Time III	*P*
No. of patients	636	1804	2497	—
No. of segments	784	2528	3516	—
Male (%)	75	74	71	NS
Age (yr) (mean ± SD)	58 ± 11	62 ± 11	65 ± 14	<.001
Age ≥65 yr (%)	28	43	54	<.001
Age ≥75 yr (%)	4	12	20	<001
Diabetes (%)	8	14	18	<.001
Hypertension (%)	38	48	47	<.001
Smoker (%)	34	22	19	<.001
CHAC (%)				NS
1	1	1	1	
2	17	13	15	
3	29	31	21	
4	26	23	27	
5	17	18	17	
Unknown	10	15	18	
Prior MI (%)	44	45	51	NS
Recent MI (%)	19	16	18	NS
Prior PTCA (%)	8	16	23	<.001
Prior CABG (%)	6	12	14	<.001

*The 10-year study period was divided into three equal intervals: I, January 1, 1982, to April 30, 1985; II, May 1, 1985, to August 31, 1988; and III, September 1, 1988, to December 31, 1991.

CABG, coronary artery bypass grafting; CHAC, Canadian Heart Association classification; MI, myocardial infarction; NS, nonsignificant; PTCA, percutaneous transluminal coronary angioplasty; SD, standard deviation.

From Harris WO, Mock MB, Orszulak TA, Schaff HV, Holmes DR Jr. Use of coronary artery bypass surgical procedure and coronary angioplasty in treatment of coronary artery disease: changes during a 10-year period at Mayo Clinic Rochester. Mayo Clin Proc 1996;71:927-935.

Table 36.2 Clinical characteristics of study patients who underwent coronary artery angioplasty.

30% underwent revascularization with either DES or CABG. The primary outcome of the study was all-cause mortality. Secondary endpoints included major adverse cardiac and cerebrovascular events (MACCE): a combination of all-cause death, ST-segment elevation myocardial infarction, stroke, or target vessel revascularization with either bypass surgery or repeated percutaneous coronary intervention of the target vessel. The New York Heart Association (NYHA) functional class was determined before percutaneous coronary intervention or CABG and at follow-up. The combined endpoint (MACCE) of all-cause mortality, myocardial infarction, stroke, or target vessel revascularization occurred in 14 patients (11%) in the DES group and in 15 patients (16%) in the CABG group (P = NS). The MACCE-free survival at 2 years was 76% for the DES group and 79% for the CABG patients (P = NS). Three patients (2%) in the DES group and two patients (2%) in the CABG cohort had repeated percutaneous coronary intervention during the follow-up for target vessel or graft failure (P = NS). However, eight more patients (6%) in the DES cohort required further revascularization with percutaneous coronary intervention in a vessel different from the index artery. After adding those patients in the DES group requiring any revascularization during the 2 years of follow-up, no difference in MACCE-free survival was noted between the two groups (16% in DES and 16% in CABG; P = NS). No patient required CABG. Three patients in the CABG group suffered from a myocardial infarction (all ST-segment elevation myocardial infarctions) postoperatively. No CABG patient had an acute myocardial infarction during follow-up. One patient in the DES cohort had an ST-segment elevation myocardial infarction for late stent thrombosis during follow-up, but there were no in-hospital acute myocardial infarctions or deaths as result of the DES procedures. This study showed that DES implantation in patients with severe left ventricular dysfunction yields similar long-term survival benefit compared with coronary bypass surgery, although a definitive statement for revascularization of patients with severe ischemic cardiomyopathy cannot be made because of the observational and retrospective nature of the study.

Another retrospective study[61] compared the outcome of CABG versus DES in diabetic patients with multivessel disease; 205 patients were included. The primary clinical endpoints were freedom from major adverse cardiac events at 30 days and 1 year. At 1 year, the mortality rate was similar in the CABG and DES groups (8% versus 10%; $P = .6$). The major adverse cardiac events rate was lower in the CABG group (12% versus 27%; $P = .006$) because of less repeated revascularization with CABG (3% versus 20%; $P < .001$). Stroke occurred only in the CABG group (4% versus 0%; $P = .04$). Angiographically documented stent thrombosis after DES occurred in 3%. CABG was associated with fewer major adverse cardiac events primarily because of the higher repeated revascularization rate with DES and is therefore superior to DES.

DES appear to be safe and feasible for selected patients with multivessel disease; the reintervention gap was narrowed in the era of DES. However, restenosis and progression of disease need to receive substantial emphasis in randomized trials.[62]

Hybrid vascularization combines minimally invasive coronary surgery with catheter-based coronary intervention. This concept is gaining renewed interest because totally endoscopic left internal mammary artery to LAD placement has become feasible and because DES in non-LAD targets may be competitive even for arterial grafts.[63] Multiple recent case reports[63,64] and retrospective series evaluated this integrated intervention. Selected elderly patients with multivessel coronary disease and severe concomitant diseases have excellent early and good midterm results. They may benefit from this procedure by avoiding cardiopulmonary bypass.[65] This technique may minimize surgical trauma; however, so far, long-term results are limited by the results of percutaneous coronary intervention.[66] The choice of suitable vessel, the type of stent, and the timing of intervention must be carefully considered.[67]

Coronary Artery Bypass Graft after Acute Myocardial Infarction

Surgical revascularization soon after acute myocardial infarction carries a small but definite increase in operative risk compared with CABG in stable patients, and this risk is determined by the extent of myocardial damage and acuteness of the myocardial infarction. Perioperative mortality rates in early series ranged as high as 30% to 40% for patients having bypass within the first week after myocardial infarction and nearly 20% for patients operated on 2 to 4 weeks after infarction.

Improved revascularization techniques and improved methods of myocardial protection have ameliorated this risk; Applebaum and colleagues[68] reported a mortality rate of 6.7% in 406 patients operated on within 30 days of acute myocardial infarction. In this study, three factors influenced perioperative mortality: ejection fraction of less than 30%, preoperative shock, and age older than 70 years. Late results were good, with an 88% survival at 3 years and 84% survival 5 years after operation. Indeed, the data suggest that patients younger than 70 years with an ejection fraction greater than 30% in the absence of cardiogenic shock can be operated on relatively early after acute myocardial infarction with little increase in early mortality. This was corroborated in a study by Kaul and associates,[69] in which 642 patients underwent CABG within 30 days of an acute myocardial infarction. Early mortality was 5.9% for the entire series but 26% for the subset of patients with a left ventricular ejection fraction less than 30%. In the report of Lee and coworkers[70] of 316 patients having CABG within 21 days of a myocardial infarction, in-hospital mortality was 5.1% compared with a 2.5% mortality among patients without recent myocardial infarction at the same institution. Again, increased mortality was associated with preoperative status and ranged from 1.2% in patients with stable angina after myocardial infarction to 26% in patients with cardiogenic shock. Multivariant logistic regression analysis identified requirement of preoperative intra-aortic balloon pumping, decreased left ventricular function, and renal insufficiency as independent correlates of mortality. They concluded that bypass surgery can safely be performed in stable patients at any time after an acute myocardial infarction with an operative mortality similar to that of elective surgery.

The Danish Trial in Acute Myocardial Infarction (DANAMI) study[71] compared revascularization with conservative strategy in patients with myocardial ischemia after thrombolytic treatment for first acute myocardial infarction. Patients were randomized to either PTCA (n = 266) or CABG (n = 147) within 2 to 10 weeks of a myocardial infarction; 505 patients were randomized to the conservative treatment group. At median follow-up of 2.4 years, mortality was 3.6% in the invasive treatment group and 4.4% in the conservative treatment group. PTCA and CABG resulted in a lower incidence of acute myocardial infarction (5.6% versus 10.5%) and a lower incidence of readmission for an unstable anginal syndrome (17.9% versus 29.5%). This randomized trial suggested that patients with inducible ischemia after myocardial infarction treated by PTCA or CABG had a reduction in reinfarction, fewer hospital admissions for unstable angina, and a lower prevalence of stable angina.

Frequently, PTCA is employed as initial therapy for reperfusion. In other patients, selection of PTCA versus CABG depends on the patient's age and general medical condition, the presence of angina or inducible ischemia, and the extent of coronary artery disease and left ventricular function. For patients with preserved left ventricular function, multivessel involvement, and no serious complicating conditions, CABG performed early (within the first 3 weeks) after myocardial infarction offers the best chance for avoidance of ischemic events and return to normal activities.

Patients with Left Ventricular Dysfunction

Patients with moderate to severe left ventricular dysfunction and severe coronary artery disease have long-term survival benefit with CABG according to the CASS study.[72] Patients with a left ventricular ejection fraction greater than 35% and less than 50% had a survival benefit from an initial surgical strategy. At 10-year follow-up,[72] survival was 75% compared with 58% for the medically treated group. This also held for event-free survival (63% and 49%, respectively). These results were disputed in the meta-analysis by Yusuf and colleagues[73] in the Coronary Artery Bypass Graft Surgery Trialists Collaboration. This study failed to show a reduction in mortality in patients with normal or abnormal left ventricular function at 5 or 10 years.

Because of these discrepancies, numerous articles have appeared in the literature attempting to sort out which patients with left ventricular dysfunction have long-term benefit from CABG. In a unique series from Moshkovitz and colleagues,[74] 75 patients with an ejection fraction less than 35% underwent OPCAB; perioperative mortality was 2.7%, and 4-year actuarial survival was 73%. This series contained an inordinate number of high-risk patients; 18 patients were emergencies, and of these, six patients were in cardiogenic shock. Chan and associates[75] performed stress thallium studies in 37 of 57 patients with ejection fractions of 28% ± 4%. Operative mortality was 1.7%. The adjusted odds ratio was 15 in predicting improvement of left ventricular function in patients who had large reversible thallium defects. Di Carli and associates[76] used positron emission tomography to look at the extended perfusion metabolic mismatch; 50 patients were treated medically, and 43 patients underwent CABG. Patients with a mismatch at 4-year follow-up had a survival of 75% versus 30% with medical management. If there was no mismatch, CABG improved symptoms and survival in patients with severe angina (100% versus 60%). The presence of angiographic coronary collaterals may be important. Kozman and coworkers[77] showed an improved recovery of regional and global myocardial function after coronary artery bypass in those patients with ejection fractions of 25% with a higher number of collaterals to ischemic regions. Allman and colleagues[78] reported a meta-analysis of 24 studies comparing survival of patients with severe coronary artery disease and left ventricular dysfunction undergoing revascularization versus medical management. All 3088 patients underwent viability testing by thallium perfusion imaging, [^{18}F]fluorodeoxyglucose metabolic imaging, or dobutamine echocardiography. Follow-up was 25 ± 10 months. In patients who demonstrated viability, there was a 79.6% reduction in annual mortality compared with medically treated patients (16% versus 3.2%). The magnitude of benefit in patients with viability was related to the degree of left ventricular dysfunction. These studies suggest that patients with significantly dysfunctional left ventricles and large areas of hibernating myocardium shown by viability studies, those with unstable angina, or patients extensively collateralized in bypassable regions are greatly benefited by CABG.

Left Main Disease

All three randomized studies, the Veterans Affairs cooperative study,[13] the European study,[12] and the CASS study,[72] showed a survival benefit in patients with a greater than 50% narrowing of the left main coronary artery. This was particularly evident in patients with higher grade stenoses and left ventricular dysfunction. Rittenhouse and colleagues[79] also showed that patients with severe left main coronary artery disease and concomitant right coronary artery occlusion benefited from bypass graft surgery. Chaitman and associates[80] showed a 5-year survival benefit in CASS study patients with left main disease receiving surgery compared with those receiving medical therapy (85% and 55%, respectively). Surgically treated patients had significantly less angina and need for antianginal drugs. Because angioplasty and stenting, procedures of the left main coronary artery, would place an inordinate amount of myocardium at risk should a complication occur, left main coronary artery lesions are treated nearly exclusively by CABG.

Extracorporeal Membrane Oxygenation and Ventricular Assist Devices

The mortality rate for patients presenting with cardiogenic shock remains high. A number of techniques have been proposed for circulatory support in these patients. Patients presenting with cardiogenic shock may benefit from extracorporeal membrane oxygenation (ECMO) or a ventricular assist device (VAD) as a temporary bridge to recovery or a bridge to transplantation. Randomized comparison favored VAD over intra-aortic balloon support in patients with revascularized acute myocardial infarction complicated by cardiogenic shock.[81] Cardiac power index as well as other hemodynamic and metabolic variables could be improved more effectively with VAD support. However, complications of severe bleeding and limb ischemia were encountered more frequently after VAD, whereas 30-day mortality was the same.[81]

Another recent retrospective report evaluated the bridge-to-bridge concept in 131 patients presenting with heart failure. All patients were initially supported with ECMO. In 28 patients, subsequent VAD implantation was necessary (bridge-to-bridge concept); 14 bridge-to-bridge patients (50%) became long-term survivors with a mean follow-up of 39 months. Complications after ECMO and VAD were bleeding and thromboembolic events.[82]

Other case reports evaluated early percutaneous VAD implantation in humans for acute right ventricular failure.[83,84] Future trials are needed to assess the effectiveness of the percutaneous VAD in patients with right ventricular failure. The TandemHeart is a recently introduced percutaneous VAD. It has been used for assisting the left ventricle in a variety of high-risk percutaneous interventions, in helping the left ventricle recover from myocarditis, in cardiomyopathies, and in cardiogenic shock after acute coronary syndromes.[85] Limited data exist on its applications in patients with right ventricular failure.[85]

Transmyocardial Laser Revascularization and Stem Cell Therapy

Transmyocardial laser revascularization (TMR) is a technique for the treatment of patients with chronic angina that is refractory to medical therapy and who are not eligible for surgical intervention.[86] Six prospective randomized clinical trials have been performed with TMR. All trials showed a significant improvement in angina class; however, results for improved survival, increased exercise tolerance, improved ejection fraction, and improved myocardial perfusion were less definitive.[86] TMR has also been used as an adjunct to CABG. A recent randomized multicenter study evaluated TMR with CABG versus CABG alone. There were no significant intergroup differences in the number of intraoperative or in-hospital adverse events. Both groups had improved angina and functional status at 1 and 4 years, with no significant differences in cumulative 4-year mortality. The incidence of repeated revascularization was 24% after CABG alone versus none after CABG plus TMR.[87] More recently, TMR was used with cell therapy for patients with severe ischemic disease. Eight patients with refractory angina were enrolled. This resulted in a reduction in ischemic score by magnetic resonance imaging as well as a reduction in functional class of angina.[88] The guidelines for clinical use of TMR were recently reported according to the format of the American Heart Association and the American College of Cardiology.[89] There are class I indications for sole TMR therapy and class IIa indications for TMR as an adjunct to CABG.[89]

CONTRAINDICATIONS

There are no absolute contraindications to CABG, but multiple factors may predispose a patient to a poor outcome. These factors must be weighed to determine the appropriateness of surgical revascularization versus less invasive procedures. Whereas advanced age is not a contraindication to surgery, it is well known that mortality is higher in elderly patients. Older patients have increased organ system disease. At the Mayo Clinic,[90] 159 patients older than 80 years undergoing CABG had an overall mortality rate of 10%. In patients without other organ system disease, the mortality rate was 4%, and 5-year survival was 80%. In a study of nearly 12,000 patients older than 60 years, Craver and associates[91] found that operative mortality for CABG was significantly higher among patients 80 years and older (9.1%) compared with patients in the age group 60 to 69 years (3.4%). The frequency of stroke rose from 2.6% at age 60 to 69 years, to 4.7% at 70 to 79 years, to 5.7% in octogenarians.[91]

LATE RESULTS AND GRAFT PATENCY

Many long-term data are presented in previous portions of this chapter. Several studies take a retrospective look at large consecutive series. Rahimtoola and colleagues[92] reviewed a cohort of patients who had their initial procedures during the years 1974 to 1988 (n = 7026). These patients had a 2.1% operative mortality and a 10- and 15-year survival probability of 74% ± 1% and 55% ± 2%, respectively. Sergeant and coworkers[93] reviewed a consecutive series of 9600 patients for up to 20 years. The freedom from reintervention at 1, 10, and 15 years was 99%, 89%, and 72%, respectively. Sergeant and coworkers concluded that patients were relatively free of the need for reintervention within the first decade after coronary artery bypass, but approximately 50% of patients surviving more than 10 years required reintervention.

Stahle and colleagues[94] examined survival of 4661 patients having CABG and related the observed survival to that expected in the general Swedish population. The relative hazard compared with the general population was 0.72 at 3 years postoperatively, and this increased to 3.36 during the 10th year. This study showed that for the first 7 or 8 years after CABG, the survival rate was similar to that in the population at large. After that, the surgical effect diminished, and mortality from the coronary disease process increased substantially.

The largest CABG database is the Society of Thoracic Surgeons (STS) database.[95] In data collected for more than 646,000 patients from 1990 to 1996, the annual observed operative mortality has decreased from 3.5% in 1990 to 3.1% in 1996. Of data collected in 1996 for more than 170,000 patients, there was a 1.8% mortality for initial operations performed electively. For first operations performed under emergency conditions, the mortality was 5.7%. In reoperations, the respective mortalities were 5.4% and 13%. The highest risk category was those undergoing salvage procedures. In these patients, the observed mortality was 25.9%. If mortality was categorized by gender in these same patients, the mortality was 4% for women compared with 2.5% for men. If age was taken into account, the mortality was 1.1% in those patients aged 20 to 50 years, with a nearly linear progression from 50 to 90 years of age ranging from 1.6% to 7.2%.

The patency rate for saphenous vein bypass grafts ranges from 40% to 50% at 10 years. The patency rate of various free or pedicled arterial conduits is less well known. Lytle and associates[96] retrospectively studied a consecutive series of 100 patients receiving a LITA graft and a consecutive series of 100 patients receiving saphenous vein grafts. Forty-six patients in the ITA group were catheterized at a mean catheterization interval of 22 months; 91% of these grafts were patent. Fifty-six patients in the saphenous vein graft group were catheterized at a mean interval of 20 months; 79% of these grafts were patent. In a follow-up publication looking at these same patients at 18 to 20 years of follow-up, 29 patients were catheterized at more than 10 years of follow-up for a 10% graft occlusion rate compared with 32 grafts studied in the saphenous vein group for a 50% occlusion rate.

In current practice, arterial grafts to arteries other than the LAD are used with increasing frequency. In a study from the Mayo Clinic,[97] the right internal thoracic artery (RITA) was compared with the LITA with regard to patency. In 413 patients undergoing bilateral ITA grafts, 67 patients had graft angiography performed up to 97 months after the operation. The patency of the RITA graft was 86% versus 89% for the LITA graft. When the ITA graft was used to bypass vessels other than the LAD, the patency rate was 76%. Tatoulis and colleagues[98] analyzed 1454 patients who had a free RITA graft. In 71 patients who were angiographically studied at a mean follow-up of 4.5 years, 94.5% of the grafts were widely patent. Ura and colleagues[99] evaluated long-term patency of pedicle RITA bypasses through the transverse sinus. Early angiography was performed shortly after surgery in 114 consecutive surviving patients. The patency was 97.1% for the RITA and 95.4% for the LITA grafts to the LAD in the same patients. Seventy-three patients consented to have a late angiographic study at a mean follow-up of 59 months; 89.9% of the RITA grafts and 92.3% of the LITA grafts were patent.

Tatoulis and colleagues[100] reported on a 5-year experience of use of radial artery grafts in 6646 patients (4872 single radial artery and 1774 bilateral radial artery). Angiography was performed on a small proportion, mostly for patients returning with symptoms. Patency was 90.2% (333 of 369 grafts).

Thus, there is continuing evidence that arterial conduits can achieve good early and late patency rates, irrespective of the region of myocardium being revascularized. Arterial conduits should be preferentially used when the targets are good and the myocardium is viable.

PERIOPERATIVE AND EARLY RESULTS OF OFF-PUMP CORONARY ARTERY BYPASS GRAFTING

The conduct of OPCAB surgery has been greatly facilitated by new techniques of stabilization, cardiac positioning, and sutureless anastomotic techniques. Recently, the OPCAB has become the preferential technique for revascularization by a subset of surgeons. It is estimated that 10% to 15% of all CABG procedures are currently being performed as OPCABs in the United States. Several large nonrandomized studies have compared perioperative results of OPCAB versus conventional CABG. Hernandez and colleagues[101] compared 1741 OPCAB patients with 6126 conventional CABG patients. Mortality rates, incidence of stroke, mediastinitis, and return to the operating room for bleeding were similar between the groups. Magee and associates[102] showed an increased mortality of 3.5% among 6466 patients undergoing conventional CABG compared with 1.8% in 1983 patients undergoing OPCAB. Cleveland and associates[103] analyzed the STS database from 1998 to 1999. A total of 126 centers performed 118,140 CABG procedures. The number of OPCABs was 11,717 (9.9%). The risk-adjusted mortality was 2.3% compared with 2.9% in the conventional CABG group. The risk-adjusted major complication rate was 14.2% in the conventional CABG group compared with 10.6% in the OPCAB group. These studies show that perioperative results are comparable if not better in the OPCAB groups, but none of the studies addresses graft patency or long-term results.

Several studies have shown that the elderly subgroup may benefit from off-pump surgery. OPCAB has been associated with decreases in mortality, stroke rate, transfusion requirements, time spent in the intensive care unit, and length of hospital stay in this higher risk group.[104-107] One caveat of these retrospective studies is that few demonstrate equal numbers of grafts placed in the OPCAB patients. In general, 0.5 to 1.0 fewer grafts have been placed in the OPCAB patients compared with conventional CABG patients. In a small randomized trial, Czerny and colleagues[108] described 40 patients undergoing OPCAB compared with 40 undergoing conventional CABG. The specific emphasis was on the ability to completely revascularize patients with each technique. Only 65% of OPCAB patients were completely revascularized; 12.5% had vessels that were not grafted for technical reasons, and 22.5% were converted to conventional CABG because of intramyocardial vessels or hemodynamic instability. In the CABG group, 85% were completely revascularized. This study emphasized the importance of selection of patients based on coronary artery anatomy.

There have been few large randomized trials. In the Beating Heart Against Cardioplegic Arrest Studies (BHACAS 1 and 2), analyses showed risk decreases with OPCAB (n = 200) compared with conventional CABG (n = 201). Atrial fibrillation was reduced by 25%, mediastinitis by 12%, inotropic requirement by 18%, transfusion of red blood cells by 31%, and hospital stay longer than 7 days by 13%. Four patients (2%) in the OPCAB group died, compared with seven patients (3%) in the conventional CABG group (hazard ratio, 0.57). In this study, OPCAB significantly reduced in-hospital morbidity without compromising outcome in the first 1 to 3 years after surgery compared with conventional CABG. van Dijk and colleagues[109,110] enrolled 142 OPCAB patients and 139 conventional CABG patients into a randomized controlled trial. There was no perioperative mortality. There were two mortalities in each group at 1 year of follow-up. Perioperative results were similar, except that OPCAB patients required less transfusion compared with the conventional CABG patients (3% versus 13%). CK-MB release was 41% less in the OPCAB patients. Cognitive decline occurred in 21% of the OPCAB group compared with 29% in the conventional CABG group at 3 months. However, these differences were not discernible at 12 months. These few randomized studies emphasize the potential benefit that can be gained by avoiding cardiopulmonary bypass.

Several studies have looked at graft patency in an organized consecutive fashion. Puskas and coworkers[111] catheterized 167 of 200 consecutive OPCAB patients at discharge. Of 421 grafts, 416 (98.8%) were patent, with only 23 (5.5%) having FitzGibbon B appearance. Lund and colleagues[112] catheterized 103 consecutive patients at discharge. Patency was 95.3%, 91.8%, and 85.3% in the left anterior descending, circumflex, and right coronary artery distributions, respectively. Zehr and coworkers[113] did immediate postoperative angiography in 50 consecutive OPCAB patients. Patency was 90.2% for ITA grafts, 88.2% for radial artery grafts, and 96.1% for saphenous vein grafts. Although perioperative graft patency appears comparable to conventional CABG, long-term patency studies have yet to be reported in the literature.

It appears that OPCAB surgery in experienced hands results in a modest perioperative benefit compared with conventional CABG. These benefits may include quicker recovery, reduced need for transfusions, decreased short-term neurocognitive decline, and overall decreased costs. Higher risk subgroups appear to benefit the most, particularly the elderly. Proof of good long-term graft patency is required to justify widespread use in low-risk patients.

COMPLICATIONS

The most important perioperative complications are stroke, wound infection, and myocardial infarction. Neurologic complications can be divided into the categories of permanent stroke, transient ischemic events, and delirium. Incidence of permanent neurologic deficit ranges from 0.8% to 5.2%, and the associated mortality rate may be as high as 38%. The two main causes of stroke are low-flow phenomenon, resulting from associated carotid stenosis and poor crossover within the circle of Willis, and embolic events because of the application of a cross-clamp in an atherosclerotic aorta or embolic particles released from arterial cannulation and perfusion.

Patients at high risk for stroke after CABG include those with previous stroke, carotid bruit, history of hypertension, advanced age, and diabetes mellitus.[114] The association between perioperative stroke, cervical bruits, and asymptomatic carotid artery stenosis is complex. Studies of routine carotid artery ultrasound screening show that approximately 20% of patients undergoing coronary artery bypass will have more than 50% stenosis of one or both carotid arteries.[115] In the report of Schwartz and associates,[115] overall risk of stroke or death in patients with positive findings on preoperative carotid ultrasound screening was 2.1%, but risk of stroke increased to 5.3% in patients with unilateral or bilateral carotid stenosis of 80% or greater. These data and accumulated clinical experience suggest that such patients may benefit from CABG with simultaneous carotid endarterectomy.

Intraoperative ultrasonographic scanning of the ascending aorta is advocated by some as a method to reduce stroke caused by embolism of atherosclerotic debris during cannulation and aortic clamping. Patients in whom severe atherosclerosis of the ascending aorta is identified can be managed by altering the location of arterial cannulation, avoiding aortic cross-clamping, or, in extreme cases, excision and replacement of the ascending aorta. We use epiaortic echocardiography selectively in patients suspected of having aortic atheroma. An alternative revascularization strategy for patients with severe atherosclerotic involvement of the ascending aorta is OPCAB grafting with the use of bilateral ITAs and T-graft radial artery grafts to eliminate aortic manipulation.

Deep sternal wound infections and mediastinitis are infrequent but devastating complications that prolong hospital stay and increase risk to the patient of further complications of septicemia and multisystem organ failure. Wound infections of all types occur in approximately 2% of patients having coronary artery bypass surgery, and half of these involve the sternum and mediastinum. Jones and colleagues[116] reviewed the cases of 409 patients with deep sternal infections and found that hospital mortality was 8.1%.

Problems with sternal wound healing and infection appear to be increased in diabetic patients undergoing bilateral ITA grafting. Borger and colleagues[117] reported mediastinal infection in 14.3% of diabetic patients having bilateral ITA grafts. Data from Grossi and colleagues[118] suggest that the use of double ITA grafts in patients with diabetes mellitus increases the risk of deep sternal infection 13.9-fold, and the use of bilateral ITAs doubled the risk compared with a single ITA graft. Sternal wound infections occurring early after operation can be managed by thorough débridement, reclosure, and irrigation with antimicrobial solutions in conjunction with systemic antibiotics. More extensive infections may require sternectomy to cure the sepsis, and various methods of chest wall reconstruction have been described.

The reported occurrence of perioperative myocardial infarction varies widely according to definition and thoroughness with which it is sought. In the STS database (Table 36.3), 1.1% of patients having CABG in 1996 were identified as having perioperative myocardial infarction.

Rao and associates[119] attempted to isolate independent predictors of low cardiac output syndrome in 4558 patients undergoing isolated coronary artery bypass. The presence of postoperative low cardiac output syndrome was 9.1%. In addition to poor preoperative cardiac function and severe coronary artery disease, risk factors included reoperation,

POSTOPERATIVE COMPLICATIONS OF CORONARY ARTERY BYPASS: STS CARDIAC SURGERY DATABASE 1997

Patient Population	174,806
Operative Survivors	169,976 (97.24%)
Operative Mortalities	4,830 (2.76%)

Risk Variable	Count	% of Population	Mortality with Variable Present		Mortality with Variable Absent		Relative Risk	x^2 value
Operative								
Reoperation for bleeding	4170	2.39%	468/4170	11.22%	4362/170,636	2.56%	4.39	.0000
Perioperative myocardial infarction	2177	1.25%	427/2177	19.61%	4403/172,629	2.55%	7.69	.0000
Infection								
Sternum, superficial	1279	0.73%	37/1279	2.89%	4793/173,527	2.76%	1.05	.7762
Sternum, deep	1099	0.63%	107/1099	9.74%	4723/173,707	2.72%	3.58	.0000
Leg	2228	1.27%	84/2228	3.77%	4746/172,578	2.75%	1.37	.0035
Neurologic								
Stroke, permanent	2947	1.69%	757/2947	25.69%	4073/171,859	2.37%	10.84	.0000
Stroke, transient	1319	0.75%	53/1319	4.02%	4777/173,487	2.75%	1.46	.0052
Delirium	4697	2.69%	328/4697	6.98%	4502/170,109	2.65%	2.64	.0000
Continuous coma, 24 hours	800	0.46%	564/800	70.50%	4266/174,006	2.45%	28.76	.0000
Pulmonary								
Ventilation 1 day	10,261	5.87%	2131/ 10,261	20.77%	2699/164,545	1.64%	12.66	.0000
Pulmonary embolism	566	0.32%	99/566	17.49%	4731/174,240	2.72%	6.44	.0000
Pulmonary edema	3933	2.25%	544/3933	13.83%	4286/170,873	2.51%	5.51	.0000
ARDS	1655	0.95%	453/1655	27.37%	4377/173,151	2.53%	10.83	.0000
Pneumonia	4530	2.59%	715/4530	15.78%	4115/170,276	2.42%	6.53	.0000
Renal								
Renal failure	5765	3.30%	1510/ 5765	26.19%	3320/169,041	1.96%	13.34	.0000
Dialysis required	1610	0.92%	711/1610	44.16%	4119/173,196	2.38%	18.57	.0000
Other								
Heart block (requiring permanent pacemaker)	1430	0.82%	93/1430	6.50%	4737/173,376	2.73%	2.38	.0000
Cardiac arrest	2838	1.62%	1728/ 2838	60.89%	3102/171,968	1.80%	33.75	.0000
Tamponade	699	0.40%	151/699	21.60%	4679/174,107	2.69%	8.04	.0000
Gastrointestinal complication	4382	2.51%	651/4382	14.86%	4179/170,424	2.45%	6.06	.0000
Multisystem failure	1148	0.66%	823/1148	71.69%	4007/173,658	2.31%	31.07	.0000
Atrial fibrillation	33,764	19.32%	1246/ 33,764	3.69%	3584/141,042	2.54%	1.45	.0000

Table 36.3 Postoperative complications of coronary artery bypass: STS Cardiac Surgery Database 1997.

emergency operation, female gender, diabetes, and age older than 70 years.

Reoperation for bleeding remains a significant operative complication and occurred in 2.2% of the 1996 STS database patients. The Karolinska Hospital[120] reviewed more than 8500 procedures to study reoperation for bleeding during a 25-year period. In patients having an ITA harvested, the most common cause of bleeding was the ITA bed in 43%. Reoperation for bleeding occurred in 8.6% of patients older than 80 years. The risk factors for reoperation were advanced age, need for combined procedure, earlier era of surgery, and use of an ITA. Moulton and coworkers,[121] in an analysis of 6015 patients undergoing cardiopulmonary bypass procedures, found four risk factors associated with re-exploration: increased age, preoperative renal insufficiency, operation other than CABG, and prolonged bypass time. Re-exploration was a risk factor for postoperative mortality, renal failure, prolonged mechanical ventilation, adult respiratory distress syndrome, sepsis, and atrial arrhythmias. These data were corroborated by the Northern New England Cardiovascular Disease Study Group,[122] which analyzed 8586 patients undergoing isolated CABG between 1992 and 1995; 3.6% underwent re-exploration for bleeding. Their in-hospital mortality was 9.5% versus 3.3% in patients not requiring reoperation. In addition, the average duration of stay was increased by 6 days. These studies emphasized the importance of reducing postoperative bleeding by antifibrinolytic agents and close attention to hemostasis.

Atrial fibrillation after CABG occurs with marked regularity. It has been shown by Leitch and coworkers[123] to be related to age, and the incidence ranged from 3.7% in patients younger than 40 years to 27.7% in patients 70 years of age or older in a consecutive series of 5807 patients. Although there is a risk of embolism occurring because of atrial fibrillation, hemodynamic compromise is a more common associated problem. Because of the increase in heart rate, there is decreased diastolic filling time and thus decreased cardiac output. Thus, control of the ventricular response is the foremost concern. Digitalis and calcium channel blockers remain acute rate control medications. For longer term rate control and atrial fibrillation prophylaxis, amiodarone has been reported to be an effective therapy and is replacing the use of procainamide and quinidine.

SUMMARY

Surgery for coronary artery disease has matured during the past 25 years. Direct coronary artery bypass yields predictable relief of angina in 80% to 90% of patients and improves survival of patients. The current trend to revascularization with multiple arterial grafts should further improve patient outcome, both length and quality of survival. New surgical methods, including less invasive approaches and operation without the use of cardiopulmonary bypass, may decrease early morbidity and mortality of operation, but the ultimate role of these techniques is yet unknown. Although percutaneous methods are favored for patients with less advanced coronary atherosclerosis, coronary artery bypass is still preferred for the majority of patients with multivessel disease, especially for those with left main coronary artery stenosis, poor left ventricular function, and diabetes mellitus.

chapter 37

Special Problems in Nonpharmacologic Therapy

a. Unprotected Left Main Coronary Angioplasty

Michael Ragosta

DEFINITION OF PROBLEM

Atherosclerotic narrowing of the left main coronary artery occurs in approximately 5% of patients who have angina pectoris, congestive heart failure, or myocardial infarction. The presence of significant narrowing (>50%) of the left main coronary artery is a high-risk finding with a poor prognosis if it is treated medically. The randomized, controlled trials of coronary artery bypass grafting (CABG) compared with medical treatment have shown 3-year survival rates exceeding 90% in patients treated with surgery and less than 70% survival in patients treated medically. For this reason, CABG has evolved as the dominant treatment mode for significant left main coronary artery lesions in appropriate patients.

Percutaneous coronary intervention (PCI) of left main coronary disease is an alternative to CABG; this option has been contemplated since the balloon angioplasty era. Compared with disease in other arteries, left main coronary lesions offer unique challenges to the interventional cardiologist. One of the important differences between PCI involving the left main stem compared with other sites lies in the size of the vascular territory supplied by the left main coronary artery. From an interventional cardiologist's perspective, left main coronary artery disease is classified as either protected or unprotected. Left main coronary PCI may be performed without great fanfare when a significant left main stenosis exists in the setting of previous CABG with patent grafts to either the left anterior descending artery or the left circumflex system (Fig. 37A.1). This constitutes a protected left main intervention because only a portion of the vascular territory defined by the left main coronary artery is at risk from the intervention; the remaining arterial supply is protected by the patent bypass graft.

The relatively large diameter of the left main stem and its proximal location on a straight segment are favorable features for PCI. However, there are several features that can make PCI more challenging in an unprotected left main stem than in other vessels:

- Disease may be located at the ostium, potentially leading to technical difficulties in positioning of the guide catheter and in precise positioning of the balloon catheter or stent.
- Left main stenoses often involve the distal segment and are therefore bifurcation lesions with an associated greater degree of procedural difficulty and risk and poorer long-term outcome. Lesions of the distal left main treated with PCI require great care to protect the two major branches, the left circumflex artery and the left anterior descending artery.
- The risk of unprotected left main angioplasty is substantially greater than that of angioplasty in other vessels, predominantly because of the size of the myocardium subtended by the left main coronary artery.

Even transient occlusion can cause dramatic hemodynamic collapse or life-threatening arrhythmia, leading to a fatal outcome during the procedure. Similarly, if abrupt vessel closure or subacute stent thrombosis occurs, the consequence will probably prove fatal before the patient can return to the catheterization laboratory and undergo a repeated procedure to restore patency of the vessel. Thus, percutaneous intervention of an unprotected left main coronary artery represents a substantial challenge to the modern-day interventional cardiologist.

TYPICAL CASE

A 36-year-old man with no previous cardiac history presented with an acute anterolateral myocardial infarction. Thrombolytic therapy 2 hours after the onset of symptoms resolved his pain and electrocardiographic changes. Twenty-four hours later, he developed recurrent chest pain and ST-segment elevation with tachycardia and hypotension consistent with cardiogenic shock. Emergency cardiac catheterization demonstrated significant stenosis in the distal right coronary artery and an acutely occluded left main coronary artery (Fig. 37A.2). The patient's condition rapidly deteriorated, with progressive hypotension despite intravenous pressor agents and intra-aortic balloon counterpulsation. The cardiothoracic surgeons were emergently consulted, and while the operating room was being prepared, balloon angioplasty of the left main coronary artery occlusion was performed in the hope that restoration of blood flow would allow him to survive until CABG. Balloon dilatation of the distal left main coronary artery was easily and quickly performed, restoring blood flow to the left circumflex artery

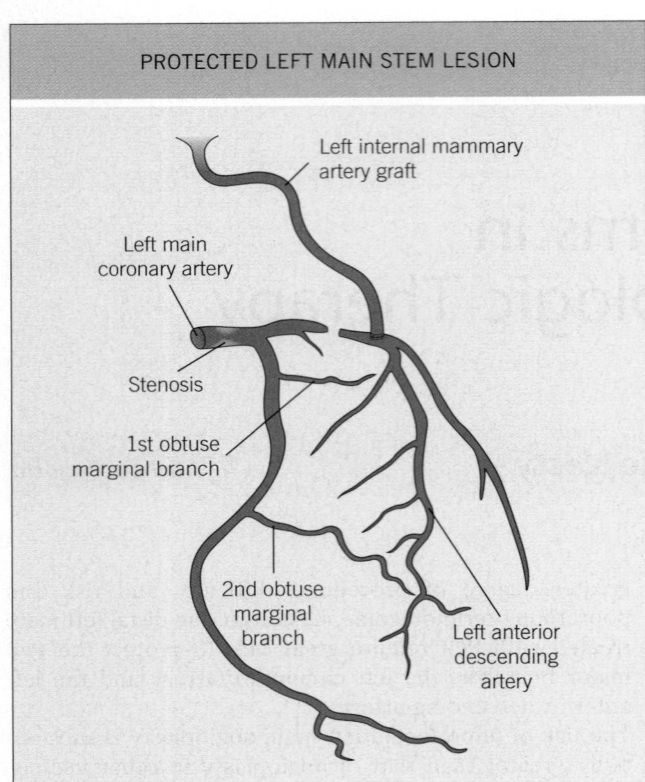

Figure 37A.1 Protected left main stem lesion. The patent left internal mammary artery graft supplies the left anterior descending artery, thus "protecting" a portion of the left main stem vascular territory.

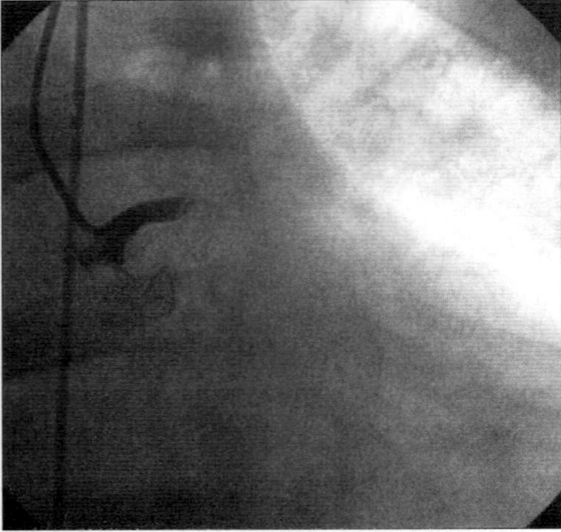

Figure 37A.2 Complete occlusion in the distal portion of the left coronary artery.

and left anterior descending artery and rapidly improving his hemodynamic status (Fig. 37A.3). Because the lesion involved the bifurcation of the distal left main stem, it was thought that CABG would provide a better result than stenting. The patient underwent emergency CABG and had an uneventful postoperative course, with predischarge echocardiography showing only moderate left ventricular dysfunction.

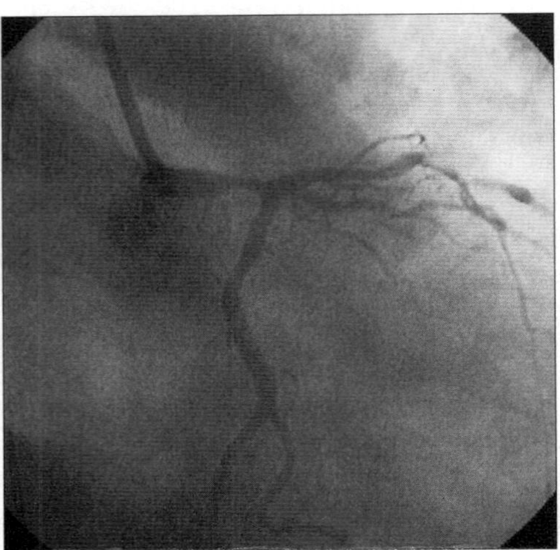

Figure 37A.3 Restoration of blood flow in the circumflex and left anterior descending artery branches after balloon angioplasty. A significant narrowing of the distal left main stem remains.

DIFFERENTIAL DIAGNOSIS

Cardiologists faced with the decision between CABG and an unprotected left main PCI must first categorize the patient along the spectrum of possible clinical presentations. At one end of the spectrum are patients in cardiogenic shock or acute myocardial infarction, similar to the case presented here, in whom there is no time to contemplate bypass surgery. In such cases, PCI is often applied as a lifesaving measure. Similarly, PCI is often performed in patients with severe left main disease who are not candidates for CABG because of the presence of significant comorbid illness, such as end-stage lung or kidney disease, malignant disease, or advanced age. Left main PCI is sometimes performed in patients suitable for CABG but who refuse this surgery because of personal preferences. The final group of patients in whom there is great controversy at present includes those with left main disease who are agreeable and appropriate candidates for CABG.

Important factors determining the risk and likelihood of success of a percutaneous intervention in an unprotected left main include the acuity of the patient's presenting syndrome, the location of the lesion (i.e., ostial versus midportion versus distal), the status of the right coronary artery, and the left ventricular function. Elective intervention in an unprotected left main coronary lesion in a stable patient is associated with the greatest success and the best outcome. Many published series report procedural success rates close to 100% and an in-hospital mortality between 0% and 10%, depending on the patient's comorbidity. Not surprisingly, patients undergoing unprotected left main coronary PCI presenting with acute myocardial infarction or shock have the worst outcome, with in-hospital mortality ranging from 25% to greater than 50%. Furthermore, patients undergoing nonemergent coronary intervention who are considered "good" candidates for CABG have substantially better outcomes with left main interventions than do patients considered to be "poor" candidates for bypass surgery, reflecting the higher rate of comorbidities affecting prognosis in the poor surgical candidate group.

TREATMENT OPTIONS

CABG remains the treatment of choice for unprotected left main coronary artery disease in patients suitable for surgery. In certain circumstances, as described here, a PCI may be contemplated. It is often prudent to involve cardiothoracic surgeons in such decisions.

Percutaneous intervention in an unprotected left main coronary artery requires careful planning. The hemodynamic sequelae of transient occlusion of the left main coronary artery should be anticipated. The size and status of the right coronary artery as well as left ventricular function are important variables, and the procedural complication rate is substantial if there is severe left ventricular dysfunction. The in-hospital mortality for elective patients with preserved ejection fractions is typically around 2% compared with an in-hospital mortality of 20% to 30% for patients with reduced ejection fraction. Patients who have reduced ventricular function or an occluded right coronary artery, or both, may require placement of an intra-aortic balloon pump or a percutaneous support device as a prophylactic measure during the procedure.

A variety of techniques have been used to treat unprotected left main coronary disease. Stents are currently the favored method. Debulking procedures, such as directional atherectomy with adjunctive stenting, may sometimes prove useful in the presence of eccentric lesions. Similarly, rotational atherectomy has a niche role as an adjunctive treatment in some calcified left main lesions and for the treatment of some ostial lesions. Balloon angioplasty alone is generally not an acceptable treatment. Early experience with balloon angioplasty alone revealed high procedural mortality, high restenosis rates, and poor long-term survival. The results for stenting are substantially better, with low procedural mortality and acceptable long-term survival (Table 37A.1).

Restenosis after bare-metal stenting of an unprotected left main coronary artery occurs in at least 25% of patients within 6 to 12 months of the intervention. Patients typically present with recurrent angina, but a disturbing number may present as sudden death, with no antecedent symptoms. This observation has led to the common clinical practice of performing routine angiography at 2 to 4 months in these high-risk patients as a method of surveillance and identification of asymptomatic restenosis.

Drug-eluting stents reduce rates of restenosis compared with bare-metal stents, but the safety and efficacy of drug-eluting stents have not been thoroughly evaluated in left main coronary disease. Initial reports observed restenosis rates as low as 2%; however, studies involving patients with distal left main stem disease and disease involving the bifurcation of the left main found much higher restenosis rates, usually because of recurrent stenosis of the ostium of the left circumflex (see Table 37A.1). Currently, there are few randomized studies comparing drug-eluting stents with bare-metal stents in left main coronary disease; in one study, only 2% of patients treated with paclitaxel-eluting stents had clinical restenosis at 6 months compared with 16% of patients treated with bare-metal stents. Additional work is necessary to establish the role of drug-eluting stents in the treatment of left main coronary disease.

RESULTS OF UNPROTECTED LEFT MAIN INTERVENTION

Study	No. of Patients	In-Hospital Deaths	Long-Term Deaths	Restenosis
Bare-metal stent studies				
Tan et al. (2001)				
Low risk*	89	0%	3.4% at 1 year	1 year: 11.4% CABG 20.4% PCI
Overall	279	13.7%	24.2% at 1 year	1 year: 9.4% CABG 24.2% PCI
Black et al. (2001)	92	4.3%	10.9% at 6 months	6.5% at 6 months
Silvestri et al. (2000)				
"Good" candidates	93	0%	0% at 6 months	21% at 6 months
"Poor" candidates	47	0%	10.6% at 6 months	10.5% at 6 months
Drug-eluting stent studies				
Park et al. (2005)	102	0%	0% at 1 year	2% at 1 year
Price et al. (2006)	50*	0%	10% at 9 months	38% TLR at 9 months
Chieffo et al. (2006)	107*	0%	2.8% at 1 year	19.6% TLR
Erglis et al. (2007)	103	0%	2.0% at 6 months	
50 BMS			16% at 6 months	
53 DES			2% at 6 months	

*Most lesions involved the distal left main.

BMS, bare-metal stent; CABG, coronary artery bypass grafting; DES, drug-eluting stent; PCI, percutaneous coronary intervention; TLR, target lesion revascularization.

Table 37A.1 Results of unprotected left main intervention.

SUMMARY

PCI of unprotected left main coronary disease provides unique challenges to the interventional cardiologist. Patients with significant left main stem disease who are suffering cardiogenic shock or acute myocardial infarction or those who either refuse or are not candidates for CABG can be treated by percutaneous techniques. Stenting is the preferred treatment modality. The procedural risks are high, particularly in clinically unstable patients. Restenosis rates with bare-metal stents are similar to those seen in other coronary arteries; however, restenosis may present as sudden death, thereby requiring increased vigilance for its presence after successful procedures. Drug-eluting stents may lower restenosis rates in this subgroup of patients, but their ultimate role in treatment of this condition remains unclear at present.

b. Chronic Total Occlusion

Michael Ragosta

DEFINITION OF PROBLEM

All the current percutaneous techniques used to treat coronary stenoses depend on the successful placement of a guide wire into the distal portion of the coronary artery. Inability to cross a lesion with a guide wire remains the most common cause of a failed intervention. With modern equipment and techniques, the overwhelming majority of subtotally narrowed coronary stenoses are successfully crossed with a guide wire, but the same high success rate cannot be applied to arteries with total (100%) occlusion.

Total coronary occlusions observed in the setting of an acute myocardial infarction are usually easy to cross with a guide wire because the infarct-related artery is occluded with a soft thrombus. Angioplasty guide wires easily cross more than 90% of these occlusions. Similarly, there is also a high likelihood of successful guide wire placement when an artery is occluded from a well-defined acute coronary event occurring within 4 to 6 weeks. However, when the total occlusion is chronic (>3 months or of an unknown duration), successful angioplasty is possible in less than 70% of patients. Chronic total occlusions are fairly common, observed in one third of patients undergoing catheterization, and remain an important reason for referral of patients with multivessel coronary disease to coronary bypass surgery instead of a less invasive, percutaneous approach as the revascularization strategy. Patients undergoing successful percutaneous intervention of chronic total occlusion have greater freedom from angina and less need for bypass surgery. A large, nonrandomized study found that successful treatment of a chronic total occlusion leads to a 10-year survival advantage compared with failed treatment of a chronic total occlusion. Thus, methods to improve the success of percutaneous intervention for chronic total occlusion are desirable.

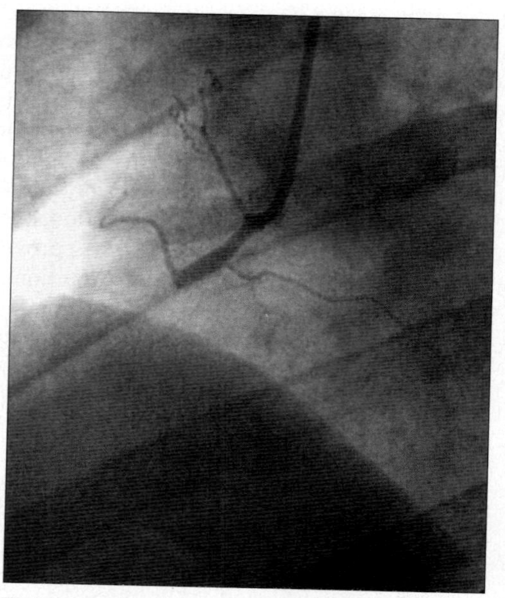

Figure 37B.1 Complete occlusion of the proximal right coronary artery.

TYPICAL CASE

A 60-year-old man with dyslipidemia presented with a 6-month history of classic anginal pain with minimal exertion. A stress test reproduced angina at a low workload; perfusion imaging demonstrated a large, reversible defect in the inferior and posterolateral walls. Coronary angiography revealed a normal left coronary artery and complete occlusion of a dominant right coronary artery with collateral filling from the left (Fig. 37B.1). Several angiographic characteristics suggested that the occlusion might be amenable to percutaneous approaches, including the absence of bridging collateral vessels and a short length of occlusion as determined by analysis of collateral vessels from the left coronary artery. A floppy-tip guide wire failed to cross the occluded segment. A tapered-tip stiff guide wire successfully entered the true lumen beyond the stenosis, confirmed by visualization of the collateral vessel from contralateral injection of the left coronary artery. Balloon angioplasty restored anterograde flow, and two sirolimus-eluting stents were deployed at the site of the occlusion, with an excellent angiographic result and resolution of the patient's angina (Fig. 37B.2).

DIFFERENTIAL DIAGNOSIS

Once total coronary occlusion is demonstrated by angiography, several features help predict success. Occlusions less than 3 months old are more likely to be treated successfully than are those of longer duration. Careful analysis of the angiogram provides further assistance in estimating the likelihood of success. Angiographically evident thrombus is a feature of a recent occlusion, and its presence may be helpful when the precise duration of occlusion is unknown.

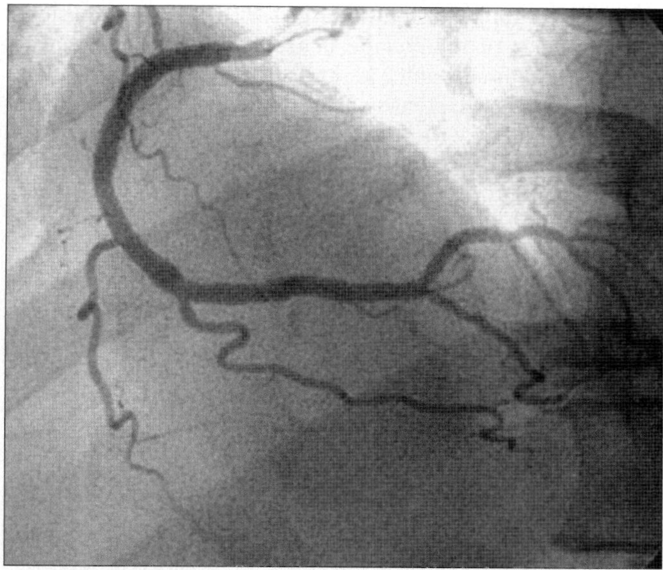

Figure 37B.2 Excellent angiographic appearance after successful angioplasty and stenting. This study is from the same patient as in Figure 37B.1.

CHRONIC TOTAL OCCLUSION: CLINICAL AND ANGIOGRAPHIC FEATURES THAT PREDICT SUCCESS OF PERCUTANEOUS INTERVENTION
Favorable features
Tapered occlusion
Absence of branch at occlusion site
Recent occlusion (less than 6 weeks ago)
Presence of thrombus
Short occlusion as assessed by collateral vessels
Absence of bridging collateral vessels
Lack of proximal vessel tortuosity
Unfavorable features
Abrupt occlusion
Presence of side branch at site of occlusion
Occlusion for longer than 6 weeks
Long occlusion as assessed by collateral vessels
Bridging collateral vessels

Table 37B.1 Chronic total occlusion: clinical and angiographic features that predict success of percutaneous intervention.

A tapering entry point into the occluded segment directs the guide wire to the site of occlusion and may improve the chances of successful crossing. The collateral vessels from the contralateral artery should be carefully analyzed. The precise length of the occlusion can often be ascertained by review of angiographic collateral vessels. Histologic studies performed on arteries shown to be completely occluded by angiography have found that tapered and short occluded segments are composed primarily of loose fibrous areas. These segments provide a potential route for successful transit of the guide wire, whereas arteries with abrupt occlusions over long segments have a greater proportion of dense fibrous tissue that is unlikely to provide easy passage of a guide wire. Bridging collateral vessels represent dilated vasa vasorum, which form around the occluded site and reconstitute the vessel distally (Fig. 37B.3). Although bridging collaterals do not by themselves necessarily predict failure, their presence implies greater chronicity of the occlusion and thus a lower likelihood of success. In addition, the operator may be unable to steer the guide wire away from these vessels and fail to find the path to the true lumen. Table 37B.1 summarizes the clinical and angiographic variables that are useful for predicting successful angioplasty in chronic total occlusion.

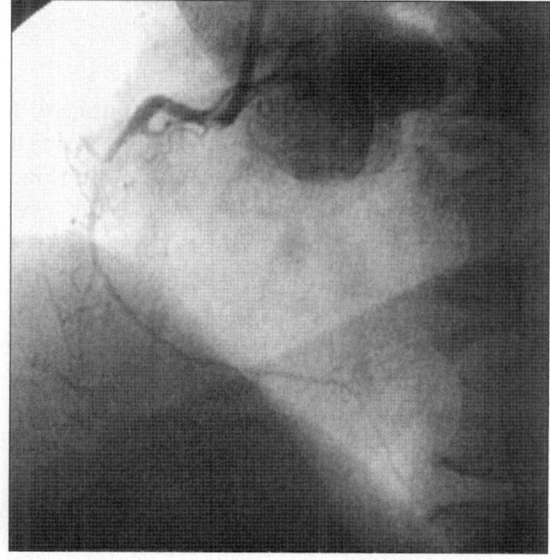

Figure 37B.3 Chronic occlusion of the right coronary artery, with a fine network of vessels spanning the occlusion and reconstituting the distal vessel (bridging collaterals).

TREATMENT OPTIONS

The major obstacle lies in the inability to pass a guide wire through the occlusion. Although several clever devices to penetrate the occluded site have been approved, such as a blunt microdissection catheter and an infrared laser, they have met with limited clinical success. Improvements in guide wire technology and the development of novel techniques, such as visualization of the collateral vessel by contralateral injection of contrast material and the parallel wire technique, are the source of the most recent wave of success. Although procedural success for the treatment of chronic occlusion has improved, it has stagnated at around 70% for the past decade.

When conventional floppy-tipped guide wires fail, specialized guide wires providing greater torque control with stiffer and more tapered tips designed to optimize successful crossing may be tried. Great care must be taken to be sure the wire remains within the lumen. Perforations and subintimal wire positioning can easily occur with aggressive attempts at crossing the lesion, but they usually do not result in injury to the patient unless the incorrect wire position goes unrecognized. It is of paramount importance that balloon catheter advancement and balloon inflation should not proceed unless the operator is sure that the wire has gained access to the true lumen of the distal artery. Once anterograde flow is established, coronary stents are usually employed to obtain an optimal angiographic result. Drug-eluting stents appear safe and effective in this subgroup, significantly lowering the previously observed high restenosis rate in patients treated with bare-metal stents.

It is sometimes believed that attempted angioplasty of a chronically occluded artery is without risk because the vessel is already completely occluded and therefore it is not possible to further jeopardize the coronary circulation. This is clearly incorrect. In addition to the possible hazards of left main coronary artery dissection during attempts at intervention of a chronically occluded left anterior descending or circumflex artery or the risk of coronary perforation and tamponade, angioplasty of chronically occluded arteries may result in acute ischemia from embolization to collateralized myocardium or from loss of side branches. Importantly, collateral vessels present before the intervention may quickly regress when anterograde flow is restored and may not be available to protect the myocardium in the event of abrupt occlusion. In large series of total occlusions, the incidence of tamponade is around 1%, acute myocardial infarction is about 2%, and the in-hospital death rate is around 1%. Restenosis rates of chronically occluded arteries treated with balloon angioplasty or bare-metal stents are high; restenosis may be manifested as reocclusion. Drug-eluting stents appear effective in this group, with restenosis rates of 5% to 10%.

SUMMARY

Chronically occluded coronary arteries are commonly seen and difficult to treat with percutaneous techniques, predominantly because of limited success at crossing the occlusion with a guide wire. Several clinical and angiographic features assist in determining the likelihood of successful angioplasty.

c. Saphenous Vein Graft Interventions

Michael Ragosta

DEFINITION OF PROBLEM

The recurrence of angina after successful coronary artery bypass grafting (CABG) may be caused by either progression of coronary disease in the native vessels or atherosclerotic narrowing or occlusion of the saphenous vein grafts. In the first year after CABG, up to 20% of saphenous vein grafts occlude. By 10 years, nearly half of all vein grafts are occluded and nearly half of those that are patent have atherosclerotic narrowing. Treatment of saphenous vein graft disease may prove difficult. Repeated CABG carries a substantially greater mortality and a lower likelihood of symptom relief than for a first bypass operation. Percutaneous coronary interventional techniques have been applied to vein grafts but are associated with a high complication rate, primarily from distal embolization, and high restenosis rates.

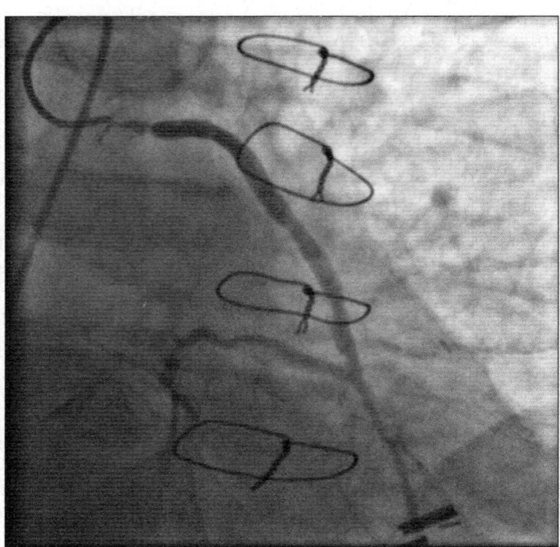

Figure 37C.1 Stenosis involving the ostium and proximal segment of a 16-year-old saphenous vein graft to the ramus intermedius.

TYPICAL CASE

A 72-year-old man developed recurrent, stable angina during several weeks, culminating in a prolonged episode of rest chest pain that prompted hospital admission. He became pain free with nitroglycerin. The electrocardiogram on presentation showed no diagnostic changes, and an initial troponin determination was mildly elevated at 0.11 ng/dL. Past history is notable for diabetes mellitus and CABG, 16 years earlier, consisting of a saphenous vein graft to a large ramus intermedius branch and a left internal mammary graft to the left anterior descending artery. Cardiac catheterization revealed proximal occlusion of the mid right coronary and left main coronary arteries. The left internal mammary graft to the left anterior descending artery was widely patent. Selective angiography of the saphenous vein graft to the ramus intermedius revealed severe narrowing of the graft involving the ostium and proximal segment (Fig. 37C.1). After administration of a bolus plus infusion of bivalirudin, distal protection was accomplished by positioning a FilterWire EX (Boston Scientific Corporation) in the distal portion of the vein graft (Fig. 37C.2). Balloon angioplasty followed by insertion of a 4.0-mm bare-metal stent resulted in an excellent result with normal angiographic flow (Fig. 37C.3). The patient suffered no adverse in-hospital events and remained symptom free at follow-up.

DIFFERENTIAL DIAGNOSIS

Stenotic lesions in bypass grafts reflect a variety of pathophysiologic processes, depending on the location of the stenosis and the temporal relationship to CABG. Narrowings seen during the first year after CABG often represent fibrocellular plaque from neointimal formation. Stenoses occurring later than 12 months after CABG are usually atheromatous and resemble native coronary artery atherosclerotic lesions. When the saphenous vein graft is noted to have severe disease throughout the graft, it is known as a

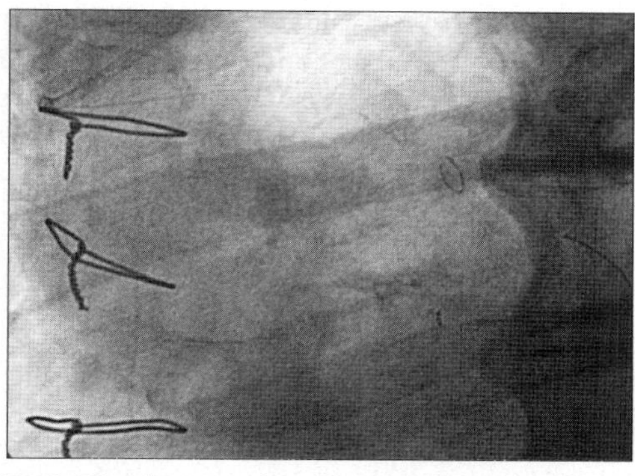

Figure 37C.2 Distal protection by use of a FilterWire placed in the distal portion of the vein graft.

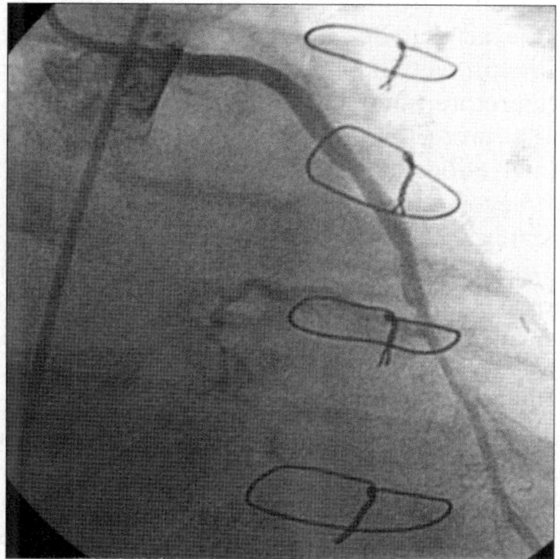

Figure 37C.3 Saphenous vein graft after balloon angioplasty and placement of a bare-metal stent. This is the same graft as in Figure 37C.1.

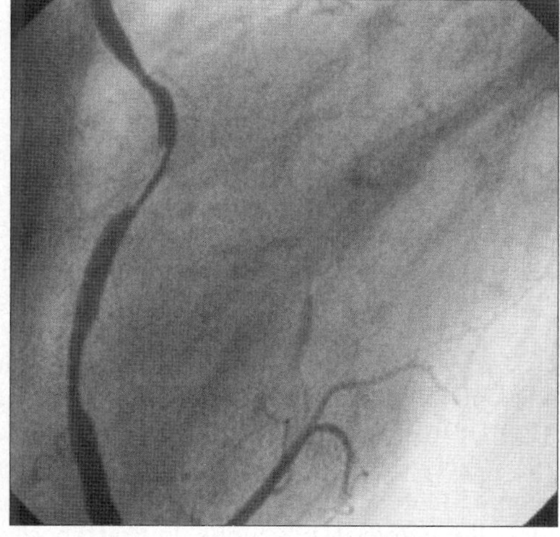

Figure 37C.4 Severely diseased, degenerated saphenous vein graft with bulky atheroma. Such lesions carry a high risk of embolic events during percutaneous intervention.

degenerated graft (Fig. 37C.4). Saphenous vein graft lesions may occur at the aortic ostium, within the midportion of the graft, or distally at the anastomosis of the vein graft to the native coronary artery.

TREATMENT OPTIONS

Repeated coronary bypass surgery is not an attractive option because of a twofold to threefold greater risk of death compared with either a first bypass procedure or a percutaneous intervention. In addition, reoperation may injure the coexisting, healthy internal thoracic artery conduit already grafted to the left anterior descending artery.

Saphenous vein graft lesions are readily amenable to a variety of percutaneous techniques. Early experiences with balloon angioplasty alone found acceptable procedural success rates but restenosis rates in excess of 50%. Directional atherectomy failed to reduce rates of restenosis and was quickly abandoned for this condition because of high rates of distal embolization and periprocedural myocardial infarction. Bare-metal stents have improved angiographic success rates and lowered restenosis rates compared with balloon angioplasty, but the acute complication rate, restenosis rate, and long-term event rate after bare-metal stenting of vein graft disease remain unacceptably high.

The most important risk of a saphenous vein graft intervention is the occurrence of distal embolization of atheromatous debris or development of the "no-reflow" phenomenon, both of which may lead to a periprocedural myocardial infarction. These complications are rarely seen after balloon angioplasty or stenting of native coronary arteries but complicate at least 10% to 15% of saphenous vein graft interventions. Distal embolization is particularly common in vein grafts more than 3 years old, with lesions that appear bulky and eccentric, and in degenerated or diffusely diseased vein grafts; it is rare with stenoses at the anastomotic sites in the first year after bypass or when there is in-stent restenosis. Importantly, this complication is associated with increased morbidity and mortality. One study found that patients with a major rise in creatine kinase MB (CK-MB) level (more than five times normal) after saphenous vein graft interventions have a 1-year mortality of 11.7% compared with 4.8% for those who had a normal CK-MB level after intervention.

Pharmacologic measures to improve the outcome of saphenous vein graft interventions have been largely unsuccessful. Although platelet glycoprotein IIb/IIIa receptor antagonists reduce ischemic complications in high-risk patient and lesion subsets undergoing intervention of native coronary arteries, these drugs are not effective in improving acute outcomes for interventions involving saphenous vein grafts. Similarly, although intracoronary adenosine or intracoronary verapamil often improves no-reflow or slow flow complicating an intervention on a native coronary lesion, these agents appear less effective when they are applied to slow-flow states occurring after vein graft intervention, reflecting the greater role of macroembolization of debris as the underlying pathophysiologic mechanism of this problem.

Several novel devices intended to improve the acute outcome of saphenous vein graft interventions by reducing distal embolization have been proposed. Exclusion of the atheroma by covering the plaque with a polytetrafluoroethylene-covered stent led to a higher rate of distal embolization compared with conventional stents in several

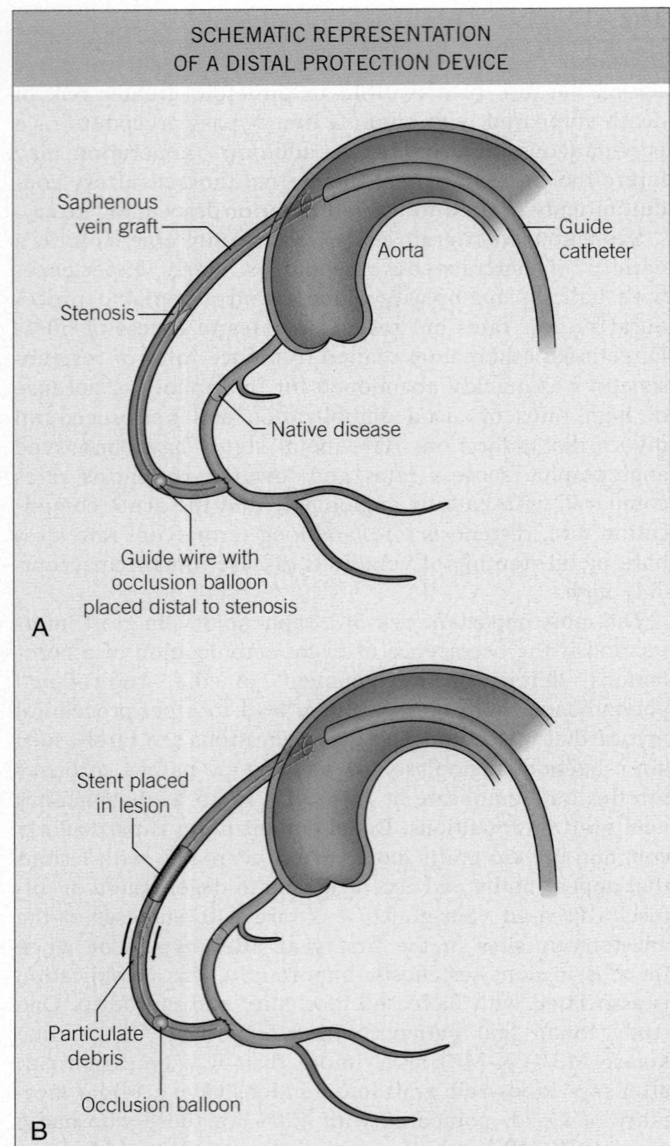

Figure 37C.5 Example of a distal protection device.

disappointing, randomized controlled trials. To date, the distal protection devices have emerged as the most successful means of reducing the risk of embolization and subsequent myocardial infarction. The Saphenous vein graft Angioplasty Free of Emboli Randomized (SAFER) trial randomly allocated 801 patients with saphenous vein graft lesions to stenting with a distal balloon occlusive protection device or to stenting without this device and showed a 42% reduction in major adverse cardiac events with distal protection (Fig. 37C.5). Another device, consisting of a distal, retrievable filter on an angioplasty guide wire (FilterWire), has shown outcomes similar to those achieved with distal balloon occlusive protection. The FilterWire is currently the more widely embraced protection device among practicing interventional cardiologists primarily because it provides several advantages to the distal balloon occlusive protection device. These include (1) the ability to continually inject contrast material during protection, allowing adequate visualization of the vessel to guide the intervention; (2) the allowance of continued blood flow, thereby avoiding ischemia during protection; and (3) the relative ease of device delivery. Distal protection devices have become important adjuncts and should be routinely used whenever possible during the percutaneous treatment of saphenous vein graft lesions.

Even if distal protection devices are employed, percutaneous intervention of saphenous vein grafts should still be considered high risk. Angiographically evident macroembolization of debris is seen in about 2% of cases despite distal protection, and about 10% of protected vein graft interventions are associated with a periprocedural rise in CK-MB. This may be explained by either failure of the device to collect all debris or the fact that the very act of vein graft instrumentation to place the protection device may result in some embolization. Furthermore, some vein graft lesions may not allow the use of distal protection. The currently used devices are best for proximal lesions and require several centimeters of healthy vein graft beyond the stenosis for optimal use. Thus, stenoses in the distal part of the vein graft are usually not protectable. With the exception of acute occlusions, totally occluded vein grafts should not be approached with percutaneous techniques because of a very low success and unacceptably high complication rate.

The use of bare-metal stents in saphenous vein grafts is associated with a high rate of repeated revascularization procedures. These events consist of both in-stent restenosis and progression of saphenous vein graft disease at other sites within the graft. Limited data involving small numbers of patients suggest that drug-eluting stents are effective at reducing the 6-month rate of in-stent restenosis in saphenous vein graft disease compared with bare-metal stents; however, there remains some concern about the risk of late stent thrombosis and the long-term safety of these devices in this patient subset.

SUMMARY

Stenoses in saphenous veins are a common cause of recurrent angina after CABG. Many of these lesions can be successfully treated by percutaneous techniques. The major risk of intervention on a vein graft arises from distal embolization resulting in acute myocardial infarction. Degenerated grafts and vein grafts more than 3 years old with bulky, large-volume atheromatous plaques carry the greatest risk of adverse events. Lesions developing early after CABG at the distal anastomosis of the graft and native artery carry the lowest risk and have the best long-term outcome. Coronary stents improve outcome compared with balloon angioplasty alone, but restenosis is common, and the efficacy and safety of drug-eluting stents in this subset remain unclear. Distal protection devices have become the standard of care and should be used whenever possible to reduce the occurrence of distal embolization and subsequent infarction.

d. Percutaneous Intervention of Cardiac Allograft Vasculopathy

Michael Ragosta

DEFINITION OF PROBLEM

Cardiac allograft vasculopathy is an important problem limiting long-term survival after cardiac transplantation. The reported prevalence of cardiac allograft vasculopathy varies, depending on the technique used to define its presence. With use of routine coronary angiography, the prevalence of any atherosclerosis has been found to be between 10% and 15% at 1 year and up to 50% by 5 years. Angiography is specific for identification of coronary disease but is not very sensitive for this process, particularly in the early stages when cardiac allograft vasculopathy affects only the arterial wall and does not yet compromise the lumen, a requirement for detection by angiography. In addition, cardiac allograft vasculopathy may affect the coronary arteries in a diffuse manner. Angiography assesses only the arterial lumen and requires an uninvolved "normal" segment to serve as a reference for luminal narrowing to be appreciated. For this reason, diffuse disease may escape detection by angiography. Intravascular ultrasonography is a more sensitive method to detect cardiac allograft vasculopathy. It can detect the disease very early when it involves only the arterial wall and before it narrows the lumen. When intravascular ultrasonography is used, the frequency of finding atherosclerotic disease is greater. In one study involving 132 patients 1 to 9 years after transplantation, the prevalence of atherosclerosis by intravascular ultrasonography (defined as an intimal thickness greater than 0.5 mm) was 80% for the first 3 years after transplantation and 92% in years 4 to 9.

The lesions of cardiac allograft vasculopathy have been historically described as diffuse, obliterative, and primarily affecting the mid-sized and distal coronary arteries. Studies using intravascular ultrasonography have found a greater proportion of atherosclerotic lesions in the proximal segments of the artery and a greater frequency of focal lesions than previously believed, with 64% of proximal segments, 43% of mid segments, and 26% of distal segments demonstrating atherosclerosis; more than half of these lesions were focal. The risk of a cardiac event in patients who have focal stenoses in a proximal segment or a mid-vessel segment is very high. The mortality 2 years after the angiographic identification of a moderate or severe stenosis exceeds 50%. Thus, there is a great deal of interest in methods of treating these lesions in the hope of improving allograft and patient survival.

TYPICAL CASE

A 52-year-old man underwent routine coronary angiography 6 years after orthotopic heart transplantation. Angiography performed 2 years earlier showed only mild luminal irregularities of the right coronary artery. At the time of the present angiographic evaluation, he remained asymptomatic with no functional limitation. Left ventricular function and right-sided heart hemodynamics were normal. Coronary angiography, however, demonstrated severe narrowing in the proximal segment and midportion of a dominant right coronary artery (Fig. 37D.1). This was successfully treated with balloon angioplasty followed by the placement of two rapamycin-eluting coronary stents. An excellent angiographic result was obtained (Fig. 37D.2).

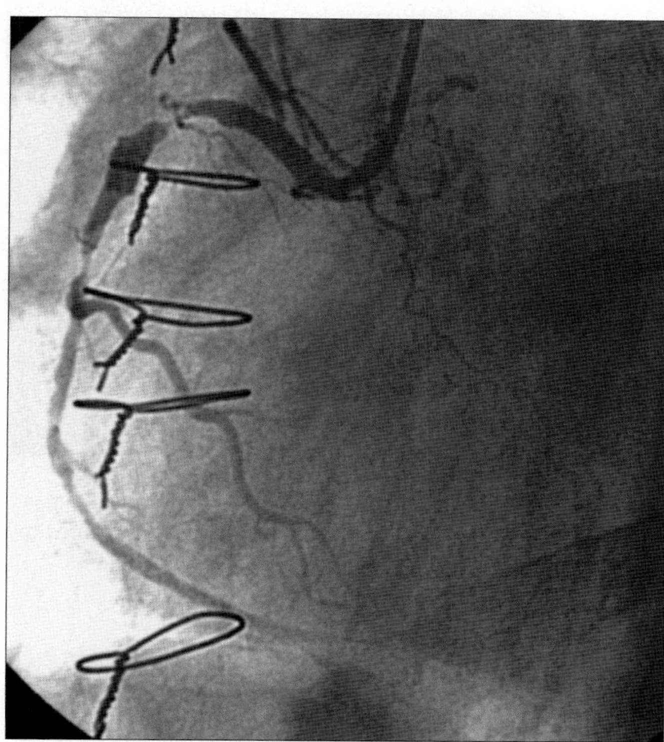

Figure 37D.1 Severe, multiple atherosclerotic lesions in a dominant right coronary artery 6 years after orthotopic heart transplantation.

DIFFERENTIAL DIAGNOSIS

Patients who have cardiac allograft vasculopathy are usually asymptomatic. The atherosclerotic lesions are typically found by routine coronary angiography. Most transplant centers perform this procedure every 12 months after cardiac transplantation for the specific purpose of identifying atherosclerotic lesions. If symptoms are present, they usually are due to progressive left ventricular dysfunction and congestive heart failure caused by the obstructive coronary lesions. Symptoms may mimic an episode of acute rejection. Arrhythmias and sudden death are other possible manifestations. Chest pain syndromes are unusual because of cardiac denervation but have been described.

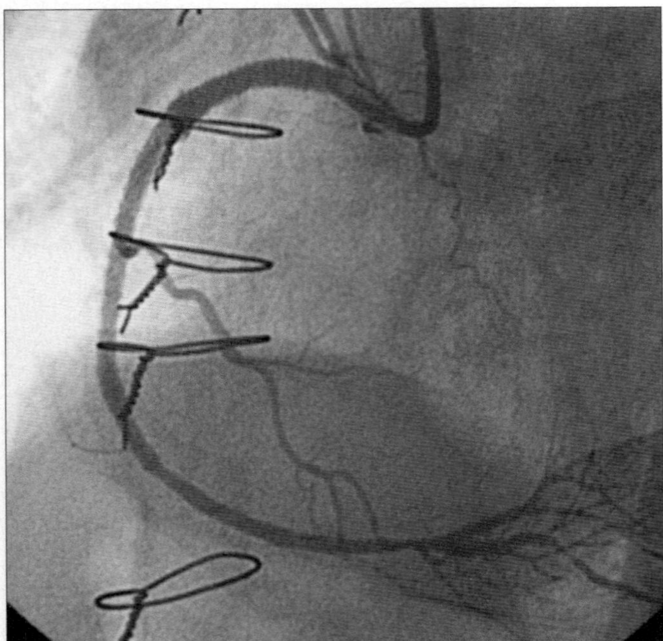

Figure 37D.2 Improvement in angiographic appearance after successful stenting of the vessel. Two rapamycin-eluting stents totaling 61 mm in length were inserted and post-dilated to 3.5 mm in diameter. This study is from the same patient as in Figure 37D.1.

Cardiac allograft vasculopathy characteristically appears by angiography as diffuse, distal obliterative lesions. There is often a "pruned" appearance to the angiogram with a paucity of small branches noted. These angiographic observations, however, are not specific for cardiac allograft vasculopathy. Other conditions, such as diabetes mellitus, may cause similar angiographic findings. Furthermore, focal lesions in proximal segments are commonly observed and are indistinguishable from "garden-variety" atherosclerosis. In some cases, these lesions may represent donor-transmitted atherosclerosis.

TREATMENT OPTIONS

Strategies to prevent or to treat transplant-associated vasculopathy are limited. Simvastatin initiated early after transplantation can improve survival and lower the rate of development of transplant-associated vasculopathy but does not eliminate the problem. Once the disease has developed, the only definitive treatment is retransplantation. Retransplantation, however, is greatly limited by the availability of donors and the observation that the outcome after retransplantation for severe cases of cardiac allograft vasculopathy is substantially worse than for initial transplants, with 4-year survival of only 50%.

Coronary revascularization procedures may be performed in appropriate patients with the unproven intention of reducing the high event rate. In the presence of extensive disease not amenable to percutaneous approaches, coronary artery bypass grafting has been performed, but it carries significant risk and worse outcomes than coronary artery bypass grafting in native atherosclerotic coronary disease. Percutaneous interventional techniques, including balloon angioplasty and stenting, have been used (Table 37D.1). There are no randomized controlled studies, and most reported series are small. On the basis of these reports, it can be concluded that percutaneous coronary intervention is safe, with success rates above 90%. Restenosis rates for balloon angioplasty are quite high and may exceed 50%. Whereas stents clearly lower restenosis rates when they are used to treat traditional atherosclerotic lesions, the restenosis rates with bare-metal stents in patients with cardiac allograft vasculopathy are very high. Small studies suggest lower restenosis rates with drug-eluting stents compared with balloon angioplasty or bare-metal stents; however, there are few data on the safety and efficacy of drug-eluting stents in this condition.

Revascularization procedures should be considered palliative procedures. It is not clear that these techniques have a favorable impact on the natural history of the disease or that they salvage the allograft. Although it is well recognized that the outcome without revascularization for patients who have focal lesions is poor, patients who undergo percutaneous coronary intervention are likely to require

SELECTED REPORTS DESCRIBING THE OUTCOME OF PERCUTANEOUS INTERVENTIONS IN PATIENTS WITH TRANSPLANT-ASSOCIATED VASCULOPATHY

Reference	No. of Patients	Success	Long-Term Outcome	Technique and Restenosis
Halle et al. (1995)	66	94%	61% 19-month survival	POBA = 55%
Simpson et al. (2005)	33	99%	61% 2-year survival	POBA = 53% BMS = 46%
Jonas et al. (2006)	25	100%	Not available	BMS = 38%
Tanaka et al. (2006)	65	93%	56% 5-year survival	POBA = 56% BMS = 31% DES = 19%

BMS, bare-metal stent; DES, drug-eluting stent; POBA, percutaneous transluminal coronary balloon angioplasty.

Table 37D.1 Selected reports describing the outcome of percutaneous interventions in patients with transplant-associated vasculopathy.

numerous repeated interventions, and a large proportion develop heart failure, require retransplantation, or die.

An important variable that predicts outcome is the presence of distal disease. In a multicenter report of the outcome of revascularization in transplant vasculopathy, 56% of patients who had distal arteriopathy died or underwent retransplantation, compared with only 18% who did not have distal arteriopathy. Thus, although treatment of proximal and mid-vessel stenoses may improve the short-term outcome of patients who have transplant-associated vasculopathy, long-term outcome will probably best be improved by methods directed at preventing the development and progression of the disease.

SUMMARY

Atherosclerotic disease affecting the coronary arteries of the transplanted heart is common and limits the long-term survival of the allograft. There is no effective medical treatment, and retransplantation is the only definitive treatment. Percutaneous techniques such as balloon angioplasty and coronary stenting can be safely applied to these lesions but are associated with a high rate of restenosis. It is unclear whether aggressive revascularization by percutaneous techniques improves allograft survival and provides any long-term benefit other than palliation.

e. In-Stent Restenosis

Michael Ragosta

DEFINITION OF THE PROBLEM

Coronary stents have dramatically improved clinical outcomes after percutaneous coronary interventions. Stents have markedly reduced the frequency of life-threatening complications of coronary interventions, such as abrupt vessel closure, and have nearly eliminated the need for emergency coronary artery bypass grafting due to dissection or threatened vessel closure. Importantly, coronary stents have also reduced the incidence of restenosis compared with balloon angioplasty. Although stents have improved long-term outcomes compared with balloon angioplasty, initial clinical implementation of the first generation of coronary stents relied on bare-metal stents; rates of target vessel revascularization after bare-metal stenting range from 10% to 40%, with the higher rates of restenosis particularly evident among patients with diabetes, in small-diameter arteries (<3.0 mm), and in long stent lengths (>25 mm). Treatment of bare-metal stent restenosis has traditionally been associated with a high rate of additional recurrence (30% to 70%).

Two basic angiographic patterns of in-stent restenosis are typically observed:

1. focal restenosis, accounting for roughly 50% of cases and consisting of discrete narrowing either within the stent or at the edges of the stent; and
2. diffuse restenosis, accounting for the remaining cases of in-stent restenosis and manifested as severe narrowing along the entire length of the stented segment. This subset of in-stent restenosis is particularly difficult to treat and is associated with a very high rate of recurrence when it is treated with conventional interventional techniques.

The mechanism of in-stent restenosis has been explored by use of intravascular ultrasonography. Although stent recoil, poor initial stent deployment, and plaque prolapse contribute to some cases of in-stent restenosis, the great majority of cases are due to intimal proliferation. Drug-eluting stents represented a major breakthrough in prevention of in-stent restenosis. The currently approved drug-eluting stents release an antiproliferative agent (sirolimus or paclitaxel), inhibiting intimal proliferation and reducing the rate of in-stent restenosis to only 5% to 10%.

TYPICAL CASE

Recurrent stable angina developed 4 months after a 3.0-mm × 28-mm-long bare-metal stent was used to treat a high-grade proximal left anterior descending coronary artery stenosis in a 56-year-old diabetic man. Repeated coronary angiography showed severe, diffuse narrowing within the entire stented segment. The lesion was successfully treated with balloon angioplasty followed by placement of a 3.0-mm × 32-mm-long sirolimus-eluting stent. The patient's angina resolved, with no recurrence during follow-up.

DIFFERENTIAL DIAGNOSIS

In-stent restenosis typically presents as recurrent stable or rest angina 2 to 6 months after the initial procedure, but it may present as late as 12 months. Chest pain syndromes after successful coronary intervention are fairly common and may be due to causes other than ischemia. Chest pain syndromes within the first month of an intervention are rarely due to in-stent restenosis; this is explainable by the fact that several months are typically required for intimal proliferation to progress to the extent that there is enough luminal narrowing to cause symptoms. Patients who have abrupt onset of symptoms in the first few weeks after a successful intervention should be evaluated for subacute stent thrombosis, which is usually a dramatic clinical event presenting as an ST-segment elevation, acute myocardial infarction, or acute coronary syndrome in the first 2 to 4 weeks after stenting. When subacute thrombosis is excluded, noncardiac causes of chest pain become more likely in this early time frame because in-stent restenosis is rare during the first month after intervention. Chest pain syndromes occurring later than 12 months after a successful stenting procedure are due to in-stent restenosis in only a minority of patients. Many of these cases are attributable to new stenoses at other coronary artery sites. Rarely, cases of "late" stent thrombosis may present months to years after stenting, particularly when antiplatelet therapy is prematurely discontinued after placement of a drug-eluting stent, but late stent thrombosis may also rarely complicate bare-metal stents.

TREATMENT OPTIONS

It is very easy to achieve an excellent angiographic result with little risk of complication by any of the conventional percutaneous techniques to eliminate the stenosis of in-stent restenosis. However, the treatment of in-stent restenosis is challenging because of the very high recurrence rates. This is particularly true with diffuse in-stent restenosis. For example, the rate of target vessel revascularization after balloon angioplasty of focal in-stent restenosis is approximately 20%, whereas rates as high as 60% have been reported when balloon angioplasty is applied to diffuse in-stent restenosis.

The first effective method of treating in-stent restenosis involved the use of vascular brachytherapy. Both beta and gamma irradiation delivered by a catheter-based technique at the time of repeated intervention for in-stent restenosis have been shown effective at reducing the rate of target vessel revascularization by about 50%. The benefits of vascular brachytherapy were consistent among several important subgroups, including patients with diabetes, long lesion length, and saphenous vein grafts. Vascular brachytherapy introduced several unique problems, however. The phenomenon of late stent thrombosis (>2 months and up to at least 12 months), probably due to impaired re-endothelialization of the stent, became apparent. This often devastating problem was associated with the placement of a new stent at the time of vascular brachytherapy and with the short-term use of dual antiplatelet agents. The second problem unique to brachytherapy was the occurrence of the "edge" or "candy wrapper" effect. This problem was attributed to inadequate dosing of radiation throughout the extent of the injured area, known as geographic miss, with underdosing of radioactivity at the edges leading to promotion of intimal proliferation rather than inhibition. These stenoses occurring at the edge of the stent were the major cause of brachytherapy "failure," often leading to target vessel revascularization events after brachytherapy.

The widespread introduction of drug-eluting stents rapidly led to the decline of vascular brachytherapy for two reasons. First, drug-eluting stents markedly decreased in-stent restenosis, thereby nearly eliminating the problem vascular brachytherapy was designed to treat. Second, drug-eluting stents have also been found effective at reducing recurrent restenosis when they are used to treat in-stent restenosis of bare-metal stents, obviating the need for performance of the often cumbersome, personnel-intensive, and time-consuming radiation-based procedure. Thus, much to the delight of interventional cardiologists, vascular brachytherapy has been relegated to the history books as an obsolete albeit one-time useful therapy.

At present, the rare occurrences of in-stent restenosis are treated by one of several methods. If the original stent was a bare-metal stent, the interventionalist may choose to insert a drug-eluting stent. If restenosis occurs within a drug-eluting stent, optimal treatment depends on the location and type of restenosis. Most commonly, in-stent restenosis of drug-eluting stents consists of a focal, discrete lesion within the stent. These may be treated simply with balloon dilatation. Focal and discrete lesions may also occur at the edges of the stent, involving a segment of unstented coronary artery. These lesions are often treated by placing an additional stent (either drug eluting or bare metal). Diffuse in-stent restenosis within a drug-eluting stent is unusual but is a particularly disappointing event with a high long-term adverse event rate. Optimal percutaneous therapy is unclear and includes simple balloon dilatation versus repeated stenting with another drug-eluting stent. Coronary bypass surgery may be the best revascularization treatment for severe and diffuse in-stent restenosis of a drug-eluting stent involving a major coronary artery such as the left anterior descending.

In addition to drug-eluting stents, methods of preventing in-stent restenosis include the use of the stents with the shortest length and greatest lumen diameter possible. Intravascular ultrasonography may be useful in guiding stent deployment and assist in achieving the greatest possible luminal diameter. The safety and efficacy of drug-eluting stents have been well established primarily in the selected patients enrolled in the initial randomized trials of drug-eluting stents versus bare-metal stents. The safety and efficacy for "off-label" indications involving complex patient and lesion subsets are not clear and a focus of intense study. In addition, there is concern that the risk of late stent thrombosis, although very low, may be greater for drug-eluting stents compared with bare-metal stents, particularly when there is premature cessation of dual antiplatelet therapy. In the future, it is hoped that newer generation drug-eluting stents using different compounds or platforms for drug delivery will eliminate in-stent restenosis without increasing the risk of thrombosis or other adverse event, thereby forever removing one of the few remaining limitations of percutaneous coronary interventions.

f. Acute and Late Stent Thrombosis

Gautam Kedia and Sanjay Kaul

DEFINITION OF PROBLEM

Stent thrombosis is a rare but potentially life-threatening adverse event after percutaneous coronary intervention with either bare-metal stents (BMS) or drug-eluting stents (DES). In the United States, the two most commonly used types of DES are paclitaxel-eluting stents and sirolimus-eluting stents. In clinical trials, the cumulative incidence of stent thrombosis with DES at 9 to 12 months has ranged from 0.5% to 0.7%, roughly comparable to the incidence with BMS.[1] By contrast, the rate in registries more representative of clinical practice has been reported to be twofold to threefold higher.[2-5] In addition, a key difference is the temporal pattern of stent thrombosis. Whereas early (<30 days) and late (30 days to 1 year) stent thrombosis occur with similar frequency with BMS and DES, very late (beyond 1 year) stent thrombosis is somewhat more common with DES. Very late stent thrombosis has been reported to occur at a rate of 0.2% per year in clinical trials[6] and 0.5% to 0.6% per year with broader use of DES in clinical practice.[7] Although it is rare, stent thrombosis can result in death in almost one third to one half of cases and death or myocardial infarction in 70% to 100% of cases (Table 37F.1).[3-5,8-11]

Although much about the pathophysiologic process of stent thrombosis associated with DES remains unresolved, many contributing factors have been identified (Fig. 37F.1). Recent observations based on necropsy studies,[12] clinical investigations using angioscopy,[13] and assessment of endothelial function studies[14] implicate delayed healing and impaired re-endothelialization to be a key mechanism. Intravascular ultrasound studies show a higher incidence of incomplete stent apposition with evidence of vessel remodeling after DES implantation.[15] In addition, drugs released from the drug-polymer combination may exert a thrombogenic effect as both paclitaxel and sirolimus enhance endothelial tissue factor expression, the principal activator of the extrinsic pathway of the coagulation cascade.[16]

Several procedural factors may also translate into increased risk for thrombus formation, including small vessel size, increased stent length,[17] incomplete deployment of the stent,[18] stenting of bifurcation lesions,[3,4] and late stent malapposition.[15]

Certain subgroups of patients may also be more susceptible to stent thrombosis. This includes patients presenting with acute myocardial infarction and those with diabetes mellitus, depressed ejection fraction, and chronic renal failure.[3] In addition, patients with complex coronary disease, including longer lesions and multivessel, bifurcation,[19] left main, and vein graft disease, may also be at greater risk for stent thrombosis.

Impact of Antiplatelet Therapy

Dual antiplatelet therapy with aspirin and a thienopyridine, most commonly clopidogrel, is generally recommended after stent implantation to mitigate the risk of stent thrombosis. Because the window of thrombotic risk with BMS is thought to be short (it takes 2 to 4 weeks for re-endothelialization or healing to be completed), aspirin and clopidogrel therapy is recommended for only 30 days after implantation of BMS.[20] For DES, for which healing is delayed, dual antiplatelet therapy was initially recommended for a minimum of 3 months with the sirolimus-eluting stents and 6 months with the paclitaxel-eluting stents, with extension to 12 months in both types of DES, particularly in patients at low risk of

CLINICAL IMPORTANCE OF STENT THROMBOSIS

Study	Stent Type	Confirmation of Stent Thrombosis	Duration	Death (%)	Death or MI (%)
Iakovou et al.[3] (2005) N = 2229	DES	Angiogram or clinical	9 months	45	93
Ong et al.[4] (2005) N = 2016	DES	Angiogram plus clinical	1 months	25	100
Kuchulakanti et al.[5] (2006) N = 2974	DES	Angiogram	6 months	31	72*
Cutlip et al.[8] (2001) N = 6186	BMS	Angiogram or clinical	6 months	21	70
Heller et al.[9] (2001) N = 1855	BMS	Angiogram plus acute MI	9 months	17	100
BASKET-LATE[10] (2006) N = 746	DES	Angiogram plus clinical	18 months	19†	88†
Mauri et al.[11] (2007) N = 4545	DES	Angiogram plus clinical	4 years	31	84*

*Only MI rates reported.
†Cardiac death.
BMS, bare-metal stent; DES, drug-eluting stent; MI, myocardial infarction.

Table 37F.1 Clinical importance of stent thrombosis.

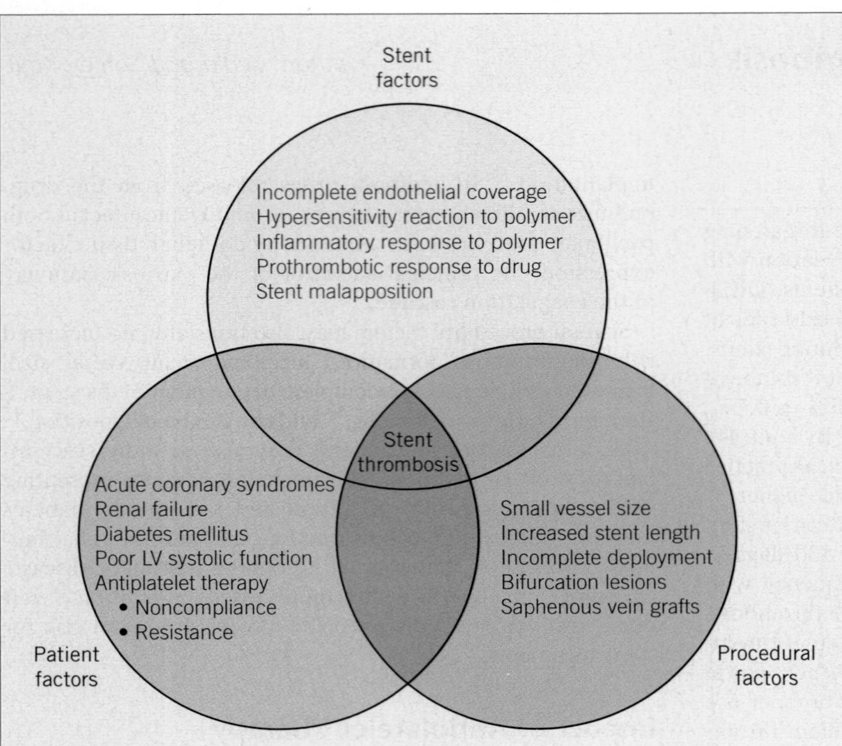

Figure 37F.1 Factors contributing to drug-eluting stent thrombosis. LV, left ventricle.

bleeding.[20] A large observational study from Duke University reported that clopidogrel use at both 6 and 12 months was associated with a significantly lower rate of death and myocardial infarction at 24 months.[21] Several additional observational studies have demonstrated a correlation between discontinuation of clopidogrel and occurrence of stent thrombosis.[3-5] These cases of stent thrombosis occur at variable time points, often months after the deployment of the stent or after discontinuation of dual antiplatelet therapy.[4,10] Thus, the true window of risk for stent thrombosis with DES, and therefore the need for dual antiplatelet therapy, is currently unknown.

Based on these findings, the Food and Drug Administration Advisory Panel[22] and a science advisory by five major professional societies (American College of Cardiology, American Heart Association, Society for Cardiovascular Angiography and Interventions, American College of Surgeons, and American Dental Association) endorsed the recommendation that treatment with aspirin and clopidogrel for up to 1 year after DES implantation (in patients not at high bleeding risk) may be warranted to mitigate the increased risk for late stent thrombosis.[23] However, patients often are not able to continue with dual antiplatelet therapy. Some patients may experience adverse bleeding with dual antiplatelet therapy, whereas others may be noncompliant because of either intrinsic factors or the excess cost of clopidogrel.

Still other patients may require surgical procedures that necessitate discontinuation of dual antiplatelet therapy to prevent major bleeding. For such patients, some institutions have developed "bridging" protocols for prevention of stent thrombosis. These protocols typically involve treatment with short-acting antithrombotic agents as a temporary bridge between discontinuation and reinitiation of dual antiplatelet therapy. Such bridging treatment protocols should be routinely incorporated into the preoperative assessment, with the benefit-risk profile of this strategy clearly communicated between the surgeons, anesthesiologists, referring physicians, and cardiologists.

Although important, discontinuation of dual antiplatelet therapy is not the sole determinant of stent thrombosis. Registry data of 3021 patients from Italy and Germany suggest that discontinuation of clopidogrel therapy was not an independent predictor of thrombosis (9 of 16 cases of thrombosis after 6 months occurred while the patients were receiving clopidogrel therapy).[24] This was further highlighted in an autopsy study of patients with stent thrombosis, the majority of whom actually were receiving dual antiplatelet therapy at the time of the event.[12] These patients may be "resistant" or "hyporesponsive" to antiplatelet therapy,[25] which may be associated with stent thrombosis.[26,27] Genetic patient variability in the hepatic CYP3A4 pathway may be contributing to insufficient levels of the active metabolite of clopidogrel.[28] Having standardized laboratory assays to assess adequate platelet reactivity would be helpful, but none has yet been validated to be reliable and reproducible. These findings call into question the assertion that extending dual antiplatelet therapy to 12 months will mitigate or ameliorate the risk of stent thrombosis.[29] Thus, the risk-benefit-cost of dual antiplatelet therapy is not clear enough to warrant definitive recommendations.

TYPICAL CASE

A 65-year-old diabetic man presents with unstable angina and on catheterization is found to have a 75% stenosis of the left anterior descending artery. He subsequently receives a DES to the lesion and is discharged home on aspirin and clopidogrel (Plavix) for 6 months, with which he remains compliant.

However, 9 months after the procedure, the patient is readmitted with chest pain and an electrocardiogram demonstrating ST-segment elevation in the anterior precordial leads. The patient is emergently taken to the cardiac catheterization laboratory and is found to have acute thrombus within the previously placed DES in the left anterior descending artery.

DIFFERENTIAL DIAGNOSIS

Patients with known coronary artery disease and prior stent implantation may present with acute myocardial infarction or death. In an acute myocardial infarction, stent thrombosis should be suspected, particularly in cases with recent stent implantation or antiplatelet therapy discontinuation. Stent thrombosis should also be suspected if a patient with prior stent implantation presents with sudden death. However, diagnosis of these cases can be problematic because sudden death can occur for a variety of reasons, and autopsy studies are frequently unavailable. For example, sudden-onset cardiac events in patients with cancer or intercurrent infection (both prothrombotic states) may truly be related to stent thrombosis and yet adjudicated as noncardiac.

Recognizing these issues and in an attempt to establish the precise incidence of stent thrombosis, the Academic Research Consortium—a roundtable of investigators, industry representatives, and regulators—has proposed a new standardized hierarchical definition to categorize stent thrombosis.[30] Studies have compared stent thrombosis by this definition with protocol definitions (Table 37F.2).[11] By the Academic Research Consortium criteria, stent thrombosis is classified as definite (angiographic or pathologic confirmation of acute thrombosis in acute coronary syndromes), probable (any unexplained death within 30 days or a target vessel myocardial infarction without angiographic confirmation of thrombosis or other identified culprit lesion), or possible (any unexplained death after 30 days).

In addition to difficulties in diagnosis of a stent thrombosis, it remains unclear whether the increase in stent thrombosis in DES compared with BMS truly translates into increased incidence of adverse clinical events. For example, using adverse cardiovascular events such as myocardial infarction and death as surrogates for stent thrombosis, studies have reached conflicting conclusions as to whether DES is responsible for worse outcomes.[6,31]

One possible explanation may be related to insufficient pooled sample size because stent thrombosis is a rare event, thus resulting in a beta (false-negative) error of about 60% to 70%.[29] Thus, an adequately powered study would require a sample size of more than 10,000 patients to permit detection of differences in risk. An alternative explanation may lie in the fact that the increased risk of adverse consequences due to late stent thrombosis may be offset by a corresponding reduction in risk due to a reduced rate of restenosis and a reduced need for reintervention (the so-called offsetting hypothesis).[32] Restenosis is a far less serious although more frequent complication than stent thrombosis but may be associated with some risk, especially when interventions known to induce thrombotic complications, such as vascular brachytherapy, are used for its treatment.[29,32]

CUMULATIVE INCIDENCE OF STENT THROMBOSIS ACCORDING TO VARIOUS DEFINITIONS AND TIME INTERVALS

Definition	SES	BMS	*P*	PES	BMS	*P*
Early (<1 month)						
Protocol	4 (0.5%)	1 (0.1%)		7 (0.5%)	7 (0.5%)	
ARC definite	3 (0.3%)	0 (0%)		5 (0.4%)	6 (0.4%)	
ARC definite or probable	4 (0.5%)	3 (0.3%)		7 (0.5%)	7 (0.5%)	
Late (1 month to 1 year)						
Protocol	1 (0.1%)	4 (0.5%)		3 (0.2%)	2 (0.1%)	
ARC definite	1 (0.2%)	4 (0.5%)		5 (0.3%)	3 (0.2%)	
ARC definite or probable	1 (0.1%)	8 (1.0%)		5 (0.4%)	4 (0.3%)	
Very late (>1 year)						
Protocol	5 (0.6%)	0 (0%)		6 (0.6%)	1 (0.2%)	
ARC definite	6 (0.7%)	3 (0.3%)		6 (0.6%)	5 (0.5%)	
ARC definite or probable	8 (0.9%)	4 (0.4%)		10 (0.9%)	7 (0.6%)	
Overall						
Protocol	10 (1.2%)	5 (0.6%)	.20	16 (1.3%)	10 (0.8%)	.24
ARC definite	10 (1.2%)	7 (0.8%)	.47	16 (1.3%)	14 (1.1%)	.71
ARC definite or probable	13 (1.5%)	15 (1.7%)	.70	22 (1.8%)	18 (1.4%)	.52

ARC, Academic Research Consortium; ARC definite, angiographic or pathologic confirmation of acute thrombosis in acute coronary syndromes; ARC probable, any unexplained death within 30 days or a target vessel myocardial infarction without angiographic confirmation of thrombosis or other identified culprit lesion; BMS, bare-metal stent; PES, paclitaxel-eluting stent; SES, sirolimus-eluting stent.

Modified from Mauri L, Hsieh WH, Massaro JM, et al. Stent thrombosis in randomized clinical trials of drug-eluting stents. N Engl J Med 2007;356:1020-1029.

Table 37F.2 Cumulative incidence of stent thrombosis according to various definitions and time intervals.

TREATMENT OPTIONS

The occurrence of stent thrombosis is catastrophic; it often leads to acute myocardial infarction or sudden death due to the abrupt occlusion of a coronary artery. Furthermore, optimal treatments are lacking. The use of balloon angioplasty and repeated stenting has been associated with a high rate of major adverse events, probably due to residual thrombus and distal embolization.[33] Thrombolytic therapy has also been associated with poor success and high complication rates.[33] Whereas the use of platelet glycoprotein IIb/IIIa inhibitors has been shown to reduce ischemic events after stenting, their use in the treatment of acute stent thrombosis is limited.[34] A treatment strategy involving optimal thrombus removal by thrombectomy devices, preferably under intravascular ultrasound guidance and combined with a platelet glycoprotein IIb/IIIa inhibitor, may be a potential therapeutic option, especially in those presenting without cardiogenic shock.[35] Because of the lack of an ideal treatment strategy, however, prevention of stent thrombosis is essential. This includes careful selection of patients who receive DES, such as those without diabetes, chronic kidney disease, or multivessel disease. In addition, complex lesions including bifurcation disease should be avoided. It is also extremely important to ensure that patients are compliant with dual antiplatelet therapy. Even then, stent thrombosis may occur, and definitive therapy is limited.

SUMMARY

Stent thrombosis is a complex vascular event mediated by several patient and procedural factors. Although rare, it is often catastrophic, leading to events such as acute myocardial infarction and death in a high percentage of cases. Furthermore, late stent thrombosis appears to be more prevalent yet less predictable with DES compared with BMS. Thus, it is important to carefully select the patients who receive DES. These patients must have few comorbidities and single isolated coronary lesions easily amenable to stenting. In addition, the interventionalist must confirm full stent deployment with little malapposition. Finally, compliance with dual antiplatelet therapy must be ensured.

SECTION

3

HYPERTENSIVE HEART DISEASE

chapter 38

Etiology and Pathogenesis of Systemic Hypertension

Eduardo Pimenta, David A. Calhoun, and Suzanne Oparil

Definition

- Essential hypertension refers to elevated systemic blood pressure without a clear etiology.

Key Features

- Essential hypertension accounts for approximately 90% of all hypertension cases.
- Essential hypertension clusters in families and results from a complex interaction of genetic and environmental factors.
- Other common factors related to essential hypertension include increased sympathetic activity, fluid and electrolyte imbalance, disorders of the renin-angiotensin-aldosterone system, obstructive sleep apnea, diabetes, obesity, and alterations in ion transport.
- Endothelial dysfunction, increased vascular reactivity and vascular remodeling may also contribute to blood pressure elevation.
- Increased vascular stiffness contributes to systolic hypertension in the elderly.

Clinical Implications

- Essential hypertension is a multifactorial disorder in which several factors in the same patient interact to produce to the clinical finding of elevated blood pressure.

Blood pressure (BP) is a quantitative trait that is highly variable. In population studies, BP has a normal distribution that is slightly skewed to the right. There is a strong positive and continuous correlation between BP and the risk of cardiovascular (CV) disease (stroke, myocardial infarction, heart failure), renal disease and mortality, even in the normotensive range.[1] Treatment with any commonly used regimen reduces CV risk, and larger reductions in BP are associated with larger reductions in risk.[2]

Essential, primary, or idiopathic hypertension is high BP in which secondary causes, such as aldosteronism, renovascular disease, renal failure, or pheochromocytoma, are not present. Essential hypertension accounts for 90% of all cases of hypertension, and it is a heterogeneous disorder, with different patients having different predisposing factors that lead to high BP. The BP phenotype in any individual depends on the expression of a set of genes that tend to raise or lower BP, interacting with a variety of environmental and demographic factors, such as high alcohol intake, diets high in salt and low in potassium and calcium, aging, sedentary lifestyle, socioeconomic status, and stress.[3]

A large number of pathophysiologic factors have been implicated in the genesis of essential hypertension (Box 38.1). Further, the novel concept that structural and functional abnormalities in the vasculature, including endothelial dysfunction, increased oxidative stress, vascular remodeling, and decreased compliance, may antedate hypertension and contribute to its pathogenesis has gained strength in recent years. This concept has important implications for the targeting of antihypertensive therapy to achieve benefits beyond BP lowering.

ANATOMY AND PHYSIOLOGY

Systemic BP is the product of cardiac output and peripheral resistance (Fig. 38.1). Peripheral resistance is almost entirely determined by the properties of the small distal arteries, those with diameters of 1 mm or less. The large central arteries are primarily conduits for blood flow, but their compliance properties may affect BP during the early phase of systole. Increased stiffness of these vessels in older individuals is responsible for selective increases in systolic BP in this age group. The phenotype of smooth muscle in the walls of the resistance vessels is controlled by perivascular nerves and by humoral mediators circulating systemically or produced locally by endothelial cells. Contraction of vascular smooth muscle is regulated by the extent of phosphorylation of the myosin light chain. Calcium is released into the cytosol and combines with calmodulin to activate myosin light chain kinase and effect phosphorylation. Local regulation of arteriolar resistance permits appropriate distribution of blood flow to local tissue beds.

Genetics

Genes clearly contribute to variation in BP. Studies suggest that genetic factors account for 40% to 50% of BP variance and environment accounts for 10% to 30%.[3] Evidence for genetic influence on BP comes from a variety of sources: twin studies document greater concordance of BP in monozygotic than dizygotic twins, and population studies show greater similarity in BP within than between families. The latter observation is not attributable to a shared environment only, because adoption studies demonstrate greater concordance of BP among biological siblings than adoptive siblings living in the same household. Further, single genes can have large effects on BP, accounting for the rare mendelian forms of high and low BP.[4]

Mutations in several genes have been shown to raise BP through a common pathway, by increasing or decreasing salt and water reabsorption in the nephron (Fig. 38.2). Mendelian forms of BP deviation (hypertension and hypotension) are summarized in Table 38.1. These mutations affect

PATHOPHYSIOLOGIC FACTORS IMPLICATED IN THE GENESIS OF ESSENTIAL HYPERTENSION

- Increased sympathetic nervous system activity
- Heightened exposure and/or response to psychosocial stress
- Overproduction of sodium-retaining hormones and vasoconstrictors
- Chronically elevated sodium intake
- Inadequate dietary intakes of potassium and calcium
- Increased or inappropriate renin secretion
- Deficiencies of vasodilators, such as prostaglandins and nitric oxide
- Congenital abnormalities of the resistance vessels
- Diabetes mellitus and insulin resistance
- Obesity
- Increased activity of vascular growth factors
- Altered cellular ion transport

Box 38.1 Pathophysiologic factors implicated in the genesis of essential hypertension.

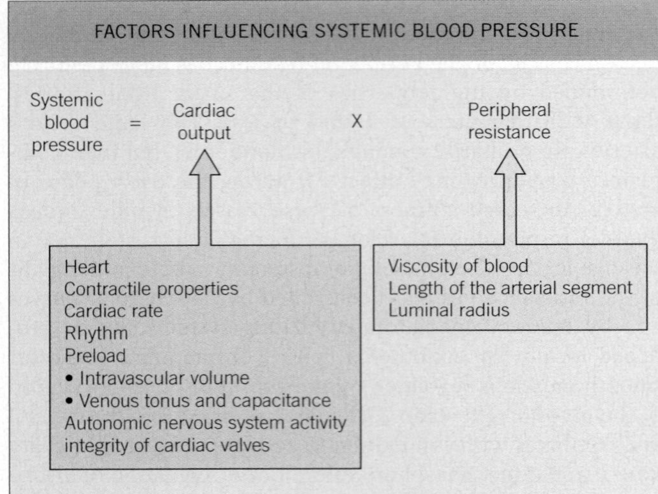

Figure 38.1 Factors influencing systemic blood pressure.

BP by altering renal salt handling, reinforcing the hypothesis of Guyton that the development of hypertension is dependent on genetically determined renal dysfunction with resultant salt and water retention (see Fig. 38.2).[5] Although identifiable single-gene mutations account for only a very small percentage of cases of hypertension, study of these rare disorders may elucidate pathophysiologic mechanisms that predispose to more common forms of hypertension and may suggest novel therapeutic approaches.[3]

For example, mutations in genes encoding Wnk1 (lysine deficient protein kinase 1) and Wnk4 (lysine deficient protein kinase 4) that are found in pseudohypoaldosteronism type II, a rare hypertensive disorder in which renal NaCl absorption is increased and K^+ secretion is impaired, may be related to essential hypertension. Wnk1 and Wnk4 are expressed in the distal nephron (distal convoluted tubule and collecting duct) and play a role in regulating renal tubular Na^+ excretion. Studies using transgenic mice have

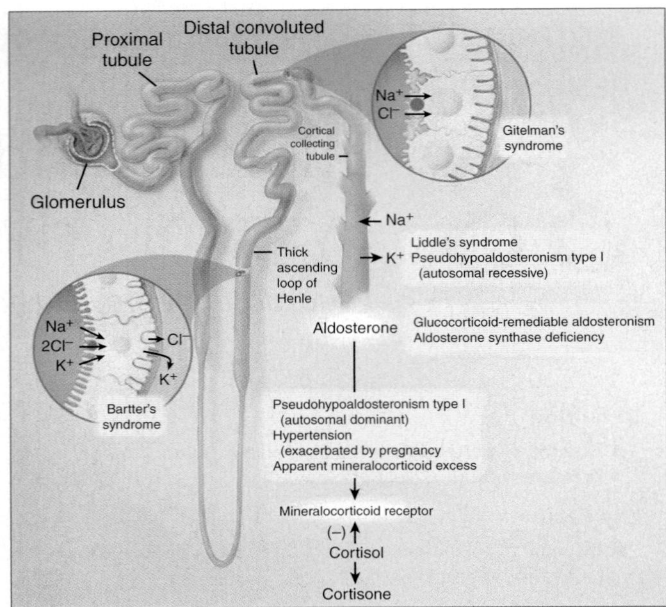

Figure 38.2 Molecular mechanisms mediating salt reabsorption in the kidney and associated monogenic hypertensive diseases. (From Lifton RP, Ghavari AG, Geller DS. Molecular mechanisms of human hypertension. Cell 2001;104:545-556.)

demonstrated that Wnk4 is a molecular switch that regulates the balance between NaCl reabsorption and K^+ secretion by altering the mass and function of the distal convoluted tubule through its stimulatory effect on the Na-Cl cotransporter (NCC) and the Na^+ channel ENaC and its inhibitory effect on the renal outer medullary K^+ channel (ROMK).[6,7]

The candidate gene approach typically compares the prevalence of hypertension or the level of BP among individuals of contrasting genotypes at candidate loci in pathways known to be involved in BP regulation. Given the complex physiologic determination of BP, the list of candidate genes is potentially enormous, and the effect of one gene is likely to be small and inconsistent across different genetic and environmental studies.[4] Many polymorphisms in and around a large range of candidates (Box 38.2) have been associated with BP but almost every published positive result has been followed by a negative result.[8]

Polymorphisms in the renin-angiotensin-aldosterone system (RAAS) genes for renin (-5312T), angiotensinogen (AGT M235T), angiotensin-converting enzyme (ACE I/D), angiotensin II type 1 receptor (AT1 A1166C), and aldosterone synthase (CYP11B2-344T/C) have been major targets for genetic investigation in essential hypertension. However, the influence of these genetic factors on BP in diverse population groups is still uncertain and controversial.[9]

Hypertension is a polygenetic condition with multiple interactions of networked genes, strongly influenced by environmental factors. Improved techniques of genetic analysis, in particular, genome-wide linkage analysis, have enabled a search for genes that contribute to the development of primary hypertension in the population.[8,10,11] The approach relies on studies of single nucleotide polymorphic (SNP) markers, in most cases derived from experimental rodent models. Recent advances in molecular genetics, genomics, and bioinformatics have facilitated the design and analysis of genome-wide

KNOWN MAJOR GENETIC CAUSES OF HIGH AND LOW BLOOD PRESSURE		
Disease	**Phenotype**	**Genetic Cause**
Glucocorticoid remediable hyperaldosteronism	Autosomal dominant, hypertension-variable hyperaldosteronism	Chimeric 11β-hydroxylase/aldosterone synthase gene
Syndrome of apparent mineralocorticoid excess	Autosomal recessive, volume expansion, hypokalemia, low renin and aldosterone	Mutations in the 11β-hydroxysteroid dehydrogenase gene
Liddle's syndrome	Autosomal dominant, hypertension, volume expansion, hypokalemia, low renin and aldosterone	Mutation subunits of the epithelial Na^+ channel *SCNN1B* and *SCNN1G* genes
Pseudohypoaldosteronism type 2 (Gordon's syndrome)	Autosomal dominant, hypertension, hyperkalemia, volume expansion, normal glomerular filtration rate	Linkage to chromosomes 1q31-q42 and 17p11-q21
Gitelman's syndrome	Autosomal recessive, low blood pressure, hypokalemic alkalosis, hypocalciuria	Mutations in the Na^+/Cl^- cotransporter *NCCT* gene
Bartter's syndrome	Autosomal recessive, low blood pressure, hypokalemic alkalosis, hypercalciuria	Mutations in the $Na^+/K^+/2Cl^-$ cotransporter *NKCC2* gene or mutations in the K^+ channel *ROMK* gene
Bartter's syndrome type III	Autosomal-recessive, low blood pressure, hypokalemic alkalosis, hypercalciuria without nephrocalcinosis	Mutations in the Cl^- channel *CLCNKB* gene
Pseudohypoaldosteronism type 1 (severe)	Autosomal recessive, low blood pressure, renal salt wasting, hyperkalemia and metabolic acidosis, elevated aldosterone levels	Mutation subunits of the epithelial Na^+ channel *SCNN1B* and *SCNN1G* genes
Pseudohypoaldosteronism type 1 (mild)	Autosomal dominant, low blood pressure, renal salt wasting, hyperkalemia and metabolic acidosis, elevated aldosterone levels that remit with age	Mutations in mineralocorticoid receptor gene
Polycystic kidney disease	Autosomal dominant, renal cysts, hypertension and renal failure, liver cysts, cerebral aneurysms and valvular heart disease	Mutations in the *PKD1* and *PKD2* genes
Pheochromocytoma	Multiple endocrine neoplasia type 2A: autosomal dominant, medullary thyroid carcinoma, pheochromocytoma and hyperaldosteronism	Mutations in the *RET* proto-oncogene
	von Hippel-Lindau disease: autosomal dominant, retinal angiomas, hemangioblastoma of the cerebellum and spinal cord, renal cell carcinomas, adrenal pheochromocytomas	Mutations in the *VHL* tumor supressor gene
	Neurofibromatosis type I: autosomal dominant, multiple neurofibromas, café au lait spots, Lisch's nodules of the iris and pheochromocytomas	Mutations in the *NF1* tumor supressor gene
	Nonsyndromic pheochromocytomas	Mutations in *RET, VHL, SDHB, SDHD* genes
Hypertension exacerbated in pregnancy	Autosomal dominant, early onset, severe hypertension with low aldosterone levels, exacerbated in pregnancy	Missense mutation resulting in substitution of leucine for serine at codon 810 (MR_{L810})

From Harrap SB. Blood pressure genetics. In Oparil S, Weber MA, eds. Hypertension: A Companion to Brenner & Rector's The Kidney, 2nd ed. Philadelphia, Elsevier, 2005:39-59.

Table 38.1 Known major genetic causes of high and low blood pressure.

GENETIC POLYMORPHISMS ASSOCIATED WITH BLOOD PRESSURE

- Angiotensin-converting enzyme
- Angiotensinogen
- Glucocorticoid receptor
- Insulin receptor
- Complement C3F
- β_2-Adrenergic receptor
- Lipoprotein lipase
- Type 1A dopamine receptor
- Alpha-adducin
- α_{1B}-Adrenergic receptor
- Endothelial nitric oxide synthase
- Pancreatic phospholipase A_2
- α_2-Adrenergic receptor
- SA gene
- Angiotensin II type 1 receptor
- G protein β3 subunit
- 6-Phosphogluconate dehydrogenase
- Prostacyclin synthase
- Growth hormone
- $Na^+/K^+/2Cl^-$ cotransporter
- Alpha(1) Na^+/K^+ ATPase
- GPR10

Box 38.2 Genetic polymorphisms associated with blood pressure.

association studies directed toward identifying the genetic basis of many common human diseases, including hypertension.[12-14] These include the availability of the International HapMap resource, which documents patterns of genome-wide variation and linkage disequilibrium in four population samples; the availability of dense genotyping chips, containing sets of hundreds of thousands of SNPs that provide good coverage of much of the human genome; and the availability of appropriately large and well-characterized clinical samples for many common diseases.

Utilizing these techniques, the Wellcome Trust Case Control Consortium carried out a genome-wide association study of 2000 individuals and 3000 controls in the United Kingdom, attempting to identify genes involved in seven common human diseases, including hypertension.[12] None of the variants previously associated with hypertension showed evidence for association in this study. There are several possible explanations for this finding. (1) Hypertension may have fewer common risk alleles of larger effect sizes than some of the other complex phenotypes. If so, identification of susceptibility variants for hypertension will likely depend on the synthesis of findings from multiple large-scale studies. (2) This study could have failed to detect genuine common susceptibility variants of large effect size because they were poorly tagged by the set of SNPs genotyped. For example, at least one of the variants that has been associated with hypertension, the promoter of the *Wnk1* gene, was not well tagged by the Affymetrix chip used in this study. Further rounds of genotyping using resources that offer increased density (or complementary SNP sets), and/or improved analytical methods (for example, imputation-based) should improve genotyping. (3) A further limitation of this study is the susceptiblity of the hypertension phenotype to the diluting effects of misclassification bias due to the presence of hypertensive individuals in the control samples. This could be dealt with in future studies by use of controls specifically screened to exclude individuals with elevated BP.

Pharmacogenomics explores the genome-based variations among individuals in response to therapeutic agents. Specifically in relation to hypertension, pharmacogenomics tries to identify genetic polymorphisms involved in the BP lowering response and clinical outcomes relating to the pharmacokinetics and pharmacodynamics of antihypertensive therapy. Although polymorphisms in a variety of genes, such as α-adducin, ACE, and angiotensinogen, have been implicated as determinants of BP responses to various antihypertensive agents,[15-21] these results have generally not been reproducible in multiple studies involving different population groups.[8] None of the associations described was strong enough to justify genetic analysis in clinical practice. The inconsistent findings are related, in part, to biases from patient selection and analyses that combined different alleles, different therapeutics, and different endpoints.[22]

Hypertension and Other Inherited Cardiovascular Risk Factors

Genetic and epidemiologic studies have shown that CV risk factors, including hypertension, tend to cosegregate more commonly than would be expected by chance. The clustering of metabolic risk factors in relation to hypertension has been referred to as the metabolic syndrome.[23] The involved risk factors are most commonly hypertension, dyslipidemia, insulin resistance, and obesity. Other associated abnormalities include microalbuminuria, high uric acid levels, hypercoagulability, and accelerated atherosclerosis. The American Heart Association definition for metabolic syndrome requires any three of five criteria: elevated waist circumference, elevated triglycerides, reduced high-density lipoprotein (HDL) cholesterol, elevated BP, and elevated fasting glucose.[24]

Whether obesity, particularly abdominal obesity, or insulin resistance is the root cause of the metabolic syndrome is a matter of debate. Multiple metabolic pathways have been proposed to link insulin resistance and compensatory hyperinsulinemia to the other CV or cardiometabolic risk factors.[25] However, only about half to two thirds of persons with the metabolic syndrome are insulin resistant, and a smaller proportion of those with insulin resistance meet the criteria for metabolic syndrome.[26] Obesity is largely associated with metabolic syndrome, and 50% to 80% of patients with body mass index (BMI) of 30 kg/m^2 or greater have the metabolic syndrome.

Both insulin resistance and/or compensatory hyperinsulinemia and obesity contribute to BP elevation by promoting renal sodium reabsorption and sympathetic nervous system activation.[23] In addition, abdominal obesity contributes to hypertension by activating the RAAS, increasing intrarenal compression and promoting sleep disturbances.[27] Although the Seventh Report of the Joint National Committee on Prevention, Detection, Evaluation, and Treatment of High Blood Pressure (JNC 7) does not provide specific treatment guidelines for patients with the metabolic syndrome, 2007 European guidelines emphasize the benefits of RAAS inhibitors in these patients.[28] Until a common etiology is identified, physicians must assess and treat each individual component of the metabolic syndrome, recognizing that many patients with essential hypertension also have or will develop insulin resistance and/or dyslipidemia.

Uric Acid and Hypertension

Uric acid is a risk factor for hypertension and CV disease. Whether uric acid plays a pathogenic role in CV disease or is only a marker for associated risk factors, such as insulin resistance, obesity, diuretic use, hypertension, and renal disease, is unclear.[29] Hyperuricemia in humans is associated with renal vasoconstriction and is positively correlated with plasma renin activity in hypertensive subjects, suggesting that uric acid could have adverse effects that are mediated by an activated RAAS. The Losartan Intervention for Endpoint Reduction in Hypertension (LIFE) trial showed that baseline serum uric acid level was associated with increased risk for CV disease events in women, even after adjustment for concomitant risk factors, including use of thiazide diuretics.[30] Treatment with the uricosuric angiotensin receptor blocker (ARB) losartan attenuated the time-related increase in serum uric acid in the LIFE trial, and 20% of the treatment effect on the composite CV endpoint among women was attributed to this effect. These provocative findings point to a need for further studies of the role of uric acid in the pathogenesis of hypertension and CV disease in humans.

Sympathetic Activation

Increased sympathetic nervous system activity is a major determinant of BP elevation. The mechanisms of increased sympathetic nervous system activity in hypertension are complex and involve alterations in baroreflex and chemoreflex pathways at both peripheral and central levels (Fig. 38.3). Sympathetic nervous system activation raises BP in both normotensive and hypertensive subjects through stimulation of the heart, kidney, and peripheral vasculature, causing, respectively, increases in cardiac output, fluid retention, and vascular resistance. Autonomic imbalance (increased sympathetic tone accompanied by reduced parasympathetic tone) has been associated with many metabolic, hemodynamic, trophic, and rheologic abnormalities that result in morbidity and mortality.[31] Increased sympathetic activation probably contributes to the development of hypertension. Over time, however, sympathetic activation seems to subside, suggesting that it plays a lesser role in maintaining established hypertension.

Population-based studies demonstrate a positive correlation between heart rate and future development of hypertension. The multicenter longitudinal Coronary Artery Risk Development in Young Adults (CARDIA) study followed 4762 black and white men and women, initially aged 18 to 30 years, over a 10-year period.[32] Heart rate was an independent predictor of diastolic hypertension in white men and women and black men. Since heart rate is, in large part, under sympathetic control, these results support the concept that chronic sympathetic overactivity induces hypertension. Diastolic BP relates more closely to vascular resistance than to cardiac function per se, and these results also suggest that increased sympathetic tone may increase diastolic BP by causing vascular smooth muscle cell (VSMC) proliferation and vascular remodeling.

Reflex and behavioral control of BP is integrated in the rostral ventrolateral nucleus of the medulla oblongata (RVLM), sometimes referred to as the vasomotor control center.[33] The most critical RVLM input comes from the adjacent nucleus tractus solitarius (NTS), which receives afferent fibers from stretch-sensitive mechanoreceptors in the carotid sinus and aortic arch (aortocarotid baroreflexes) and the cardiac atria and ventricles (cardiopulmonary baroreflexes). Activation of the central and peripheral sympathetic nervous system mediates salt sensitivity of BP: the mechanism of neurally mediated salt-sensitive hypertension has been elucidated in studies carried out in spontaneous hypertensive rats (SHR).[34] In this model, dietary salt increases BP by reducing norepinephrine release from nerve terminals in the anterior hypothalamic area, reducing activation of local sympathoinhibitory neurons. This results in increased sympathetic outflow and higher BP. In hypertensive humans, neurovascular compression of the RVLM is associated with increased sympathetic nerve activity.[35]

Levels of sympathetic nervous activity in hypertensive patients differ according to BMI and gender. Using single fiber recording methodology, a technique that records the firing patterns in individual vasoconstrictor sympathetic fibers, patterns of sympathetic activation have been shown to differ in normal-weight and obesity-related hypertension in both the firing characteristics of individual sympathetic fibers and global sympathetic outflow.[36] Microneurography studies have also shown gender difference in the regulation of sympathetic nervous activity.[37] Muscle sympathetic nerve activity was significantly higher in hypertensive than in normotensive women, but it was not higher in hypertensive than in normotensive men. Further, increased muscle sympathetic nerve activity was related to BMI in men but not in women.[37]

Norepinephrine spillover is a technique of estimating norepinephrine release, which is thought to be a more sensitive index of sympathetic activity than measurement of circulating plasma norepinephrine levels. Whole body norepinephrine spillover is elevated in young hypertensive subjects compared with normotensive controls.[38] Regional studies suggest that this increased sympathetic activity is primarily attributable to greater sympathetic outflow to the musculature, kidneys, and heart. Measurements of norepinephrine spillover in normotensive offspring of hypertensive parents suggest that increases in sympathetic activity that predispose to the development of hypertension are, in large part, genetic in origin.

Microneurography, a technique of using microelectrodes to directly measure peripheral or muscle sympathetic nerve activity (usually in the peroneal nerve), is also a more sensitive and specific index of sympathetic activity than measurement of plasma norepinephrine levels. Using this technique, investigators have generally found muscle sympathetic nerve activity to be increased in hypertensive versus normotensive subjects.[39] Muscle sympathetic nerve activity has also been associated with left ventricular mass in hypertensive patients. Using cardiac magnetic resonance imaging, a positive correlation has been found between sympathetic nerve activity, analyzed by microneurography, and left ventricular mass in hypertensive patients.[40]

Stress

Exposure to stress increases sympathetic outflow, and it has been hypothesized that repeated stress-induced vasoconstriction results in vascular hypertrophy, leading to progressive increases in peripheral resistance and BP. Laboratory stress

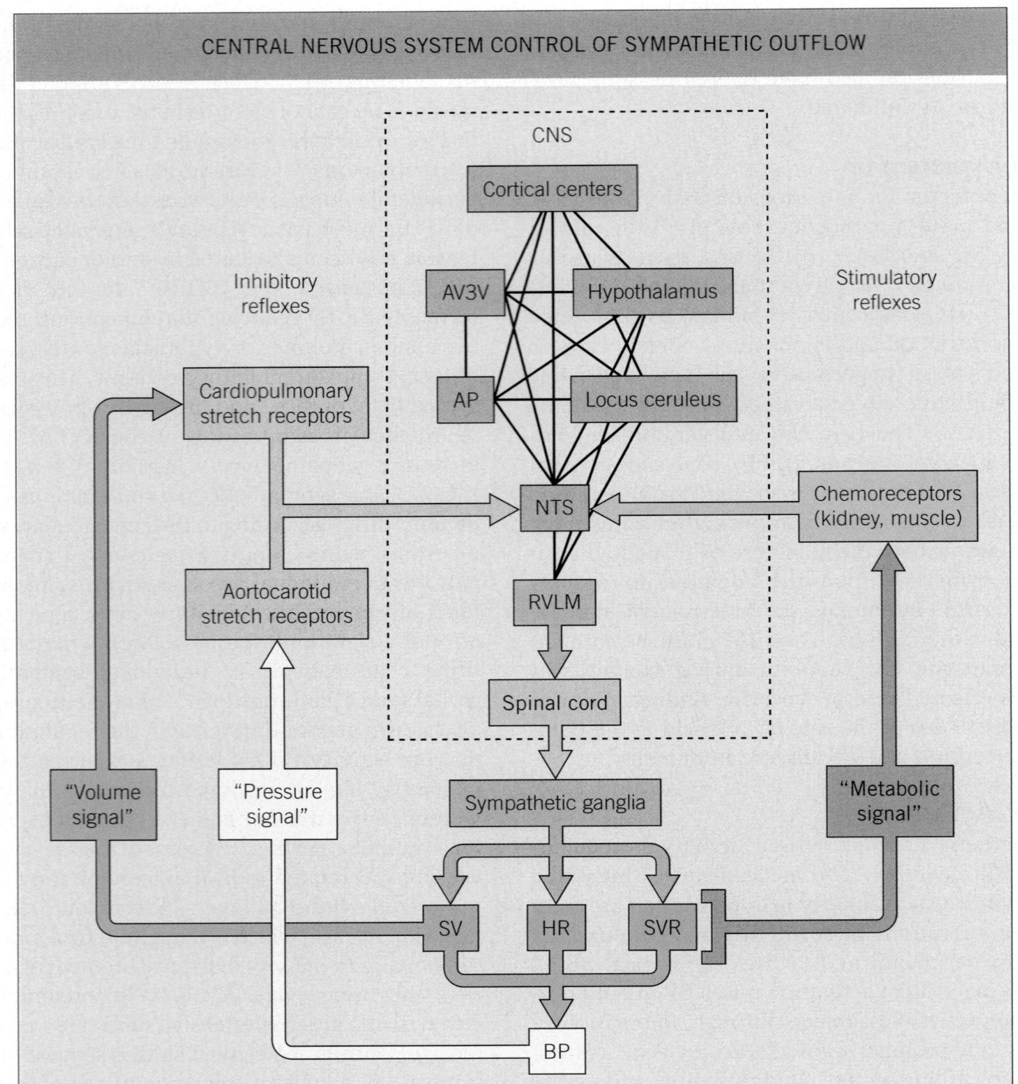

Figure 38.3 Central nervous system control of sympathetic outflow. Efferent sympathetic nervous system (SNS) output is the result of integrated actions of several central nervous system (CNS) centers, including many areas of the cortex as well as lower centers in the hypothalamus, basal ganglia (especially the locus ceruleus), and circumventricular regions, including the area postrema (AP) and anterolateral third ventricular (AV3V) area of the brain. The critical integrator region is the nucleus tractus solitarius (NTS) in the medulla oblongata. The NTS receives inhibitory afferent signals from the baroreflexes (volume and pressure signals) and stimulatory afferent signals from renal and muscular chemoreceptors (metabolic signals). SNS outflow is ultimately dependent on stimulation of the rostral ventrolateral medulla (the RVLM or vasomotor center), which is tonically inhibited by the adjacent NTS. Circumventricular regions such as the AP have no blood-brain barrier, and stimulation of the AP by circulating angiotensin II blunts the inhibitory effects of the NTS. RVLM stimulation sends signals via the spinal cord and sympathetic ganglia to regulate blood pressure (BP) levels. (From Izzo JL Jr. The sympathetic nervous system in acute and chronic blood pressure elevation. In Oparil S, Weber MA, eds. Hypertension: A Companion to Brenner & Rector's The Kidney, 2nd ed. Philadelphia, Elsevier, 2005:60-76.)

testing suggests that persons with a family history of hypertension manifest augmented vasoconstrictive responses to laboratory stressors, such as cold pressor testing and mental stress, that may predispose them to the development of hypertension.[41] This is particularly true for young African American subjects. Using microneurography, muscle sympathetic nerve activity responses to cold pressor testing have been found to be greater in young African American subjects with a positive family history of hypertension compared with white subjects with or without a family history of hypertension.[41] This suggests that greater stress-induced increases in sympathetic activity, in combination with the greater socioeconomic stress that black people must endure, may contribute to the significantly greater incidence of hypertension in African Americans compared with American white subjects.

Stress reduction through nonpharmacologic means, such as yoga, meditation, or slow breathing exercises, can successfully reduce BP. Device-guided slow breathing exercises have been shown to reduce BP in hypertensive patients.[42] A randomized study in 149 hypertensive patients reported reductions of

15.0 mm Hg in systolic BP with use of a device to assist with slow breathing more than 22 minutes/week over 8 weeks.[43] However, larger multicenter, double-blind studies with longer follow-up are needed to provide answers about the suitability and efficacy of slow breathing exercises in the clinical management of hypertensive patients.[44]

Acupuncture, an ancient technique anchored in traditional Chinese medicine, has been reported to be useful for treating CV diseases, including arterial hypertension. A randomized study in 160 hypertensive patients reported significant BP reduction in patients treated with active compared to sham acupuncture, but the effect disappeared after cessation of acupuncture treatment.[45] Clearly, more evidence is needed before acupuncture can be accepted as a chronic treatment for BP elevation.

Peripheral vascular resistance is characteristically elevated in hypertension because of alterations in structure, mechanical properties, and function of small arteries. Remodeling of these vessels contributes to the development of high BP, and it is associated with target organ damage. Peripheral resistance is determined at the level of the precapillary vessels, including the arterioles (arteries containing a single layer of VSMC) and the small arteries (lumen diameters <300 μm). The elevated resistance seen in hypertensive subjects is related to a combination of rarefaction (decrease in number of parallel-connected vessels) and an increased wall-to-lumen ratio, resulting in narrowing of the lumen of resistance vessels. Examination of specimens obtained from gluteal fat biopsies of patients with untreated essential hypertension has uniformly revealed reduced lumen areas and increased media-to-lumen ratios without an increase in medial area in resistance vessels (inward, eutrophic remodeling) (Fig. 38.4).

ACE inhibitors, ARBs, and calcium channel blockers (CCBs) induce vasodilation, which may contribute to the correction of small artery remodeling.[46] Studies have consistently shown that beta-blocker therapy does not reverse small artery structural remodeling as effectively as RAAS blockers and CCBs, even with similar BP reduction.[47-49] Short-term benefit of RAAS blocker and CCB treatment is principally derived from BP lowering, but in the longer run, vascular protection may be the major mechanism by which these agents prevent target organ damage and CV events. However, further study is needed to establish the relation between normalization of resistance vessel structure and reduced CV morbidity and mortality with antihypertensive treatment.

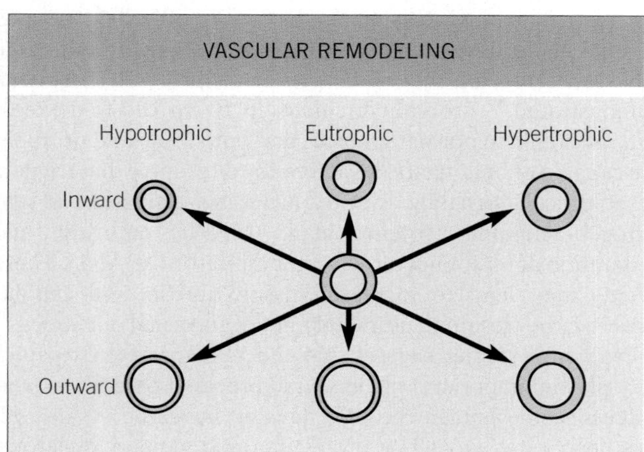

Figure 38.4 Vascular remodeling. The starting point is the vessel at the center. Remodeling can be hypertrophic (e.g., increase of cross-sectional area, vessels in right column), eutrophic (no change in cross-sectional area, vessels in center column), or hypotrophic (e.g., decrease of cross-sectional area, vessels in left column). These forms of remodeling can be inward (e.g., reduction in lumen diameter, vessels in top row) or outward (e.g., increase in lumen diameter, vessels in bottom row). (From Mulvany MJ. Vascular remodelling of resistance vessels: can we define this? Cardiovasc Res 1999;41:9-13.)

Arterial Stiffness

Arterial stiffness (reduction of elasticity) and altered wave reflection are important determinants of increased systolic and pulse pressure (PP). Alterations in the load-bearing media of elastic arteries, including progressive loss of the orderly arrangement of elastic fibers and laminae and thinning, splitting, fraying, and fragmenting of elastin fibers, are involved in the stiffening process.[50] Aging and increased BP are the two major determinants of arterial stiffness. The two-phase (elastin and collagen) content of load-bearing elements in the media is responsible for the behavior of these vessels under stress. At low pressures, stress is borne almost entirely by the distensible elastin lamellae, whereas at higher pressures, less distensible collagenous fibers are recruited, and the vessel appears stiffer.

Increased arterial stiffness contributes to the wide PP commonly seen in elderly hypertensive patients, in part by increasing the pulse wave velocity (PWV). With each ejection of blood from the left ventricle, a pressure (pulse) wave is generated and travels from the heart to the periphery at a finite speed that depends on the elastic properties of the conduit arteries. The pulse wave is reflected at any point of discontinuity in the arterial tree and returns to the aorta and left ventricle. The timing of the wave reflection depends on both the elastic properties and the length of the conduit arteries. Pulse wave analysis (PWA) provides the augmentation index (AIx) that is a surrogate of wave reflection and is defined as augmented pressure (magnitude of wave reflection) divided by PP.[51]

In younger persons (Fig. 38.5, top panel), PWV is sufficiently slow (approximately 5 m/s) that the reflected wave reaches the aortic valve after closure, leading to a higher diastolic BP and enhancing coronary perfusion by providing a "boosting" effect. In older persons, particularly if they are hypertensive, PWV is greatly increased (approximately 20 m/s) because of central arterial stiffening. At this speed, the reflective wave reaches the aortic valve before closure, leading to a higher systolic BP, PP, and afterload and a decreased diastolic BP, in some cases compromising coronary perfusion pressure (see Fig. 38-5, bottom panel). This phenomenon accounts for the increase in systolic BP and PP and the fall in diastolic BP that is seen in the elderly population, and is exaggerated in the presence of antecedent hypertension. The increase in systolic BP increases cardiac metabolic requirements and predisposes to the development of left ventricular hypertrophy and heart failure. PP is closely related to systolic BP and is linked to advanced atherosclerotic and CV events, such as fatal and nonfatal myocardial infarction and stroke. PP is a better predictor of CV

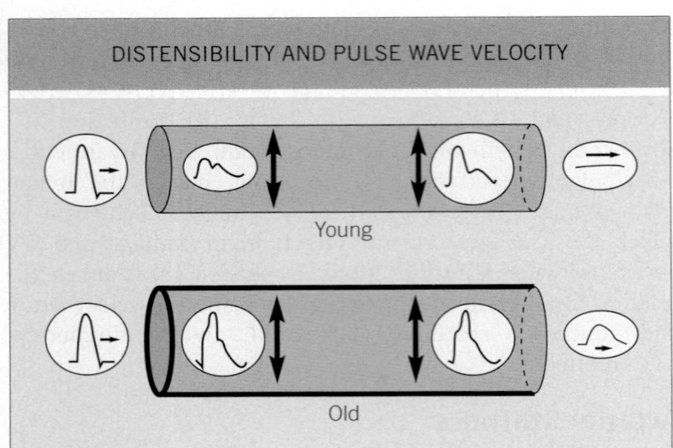

Figure 38.5 Distensibility and pulse wave velocity. Simple tubular models of the arterial system, connecting the heart *(left)* to the peripheral circulation *(right)*. Normal distensibility and normal pulse wave velocity in a young subject *(top)* and decreased distensibility with increased pulse wave velocity in an old subject *(bottom)*. (From O'Rourke MF, Hashimoto J. Mechanical factors in arterial aging: a clinical perspective. J Am Coll Cardiol 2007;50:1-13.)

disease risk than systolic or diastolic BP alone in patients who are over 50 years old. Aortic stiffness has also been shown to be an independent predictor of all-cause and CV mortality, fatal and nonfatal coronary events, and fatal strokes in patients with essential hypertension, type 2 diabetes, and end-stage renal disease.[52]

Changes in arterial stiffness and wave reflection have been evaluated after therapeutic interventions. Nonpharmacologic treatments, including exercise training, weight loss, dietary changes (e.g., low-salt diet, moderate alcohol consumption, garlic powder, α-linoleic acid, dark chocolate, and fish oil), and menopausal hormone therapy, have been shown to reduce arterial stiffness in hypertensive subjects.[50] Pharmacologic antihypertensive treatment with diuretics, beta blockers, ACE inhibitors, ARBs, and CCBs also reduce arterial stiffness, but beta blockers and diuretics are less effective than the newer drug classes.[50] In CAFE (Conduit Artery Functional Endpoint Study), a substudy of ASCOT (Anglo-Scandinavian Cardiac Outcomes Trial), the reductions in central systolic BP and PP were greater in the treatment group that received amlodipine with or without perindopril than in the treatment group that received atenolol with or without bendroflumethiazide, despite similar reductions in brachial systolic BP and PP.[53] However, because central PP and AIx were not assessed at baseline, but only after 1 year of treatment in the CAFE study, it is not possible to determine the absolute magnitude of the central PP and AIx reductions, and thus their influence on CV events.

In a study of 101 patients with stage 1 hypertension randomized to treatment with enalapril or indapamide, brachial BP was reduced similarly in both groups, but aortic systolic BP and PP were significantly lower in patients treated with enalapril compared to indapamide.[54] Whether this effect on arterial stiffness, which has been reported in other studies,[55] is responsible for the "benefit beyond BP lowering" that has been attributed to ACE inhibitor therapy remains to be determined.

Renin-Angiotensin-Aldosterone System

The RAAS is an important modulator of BP and volume regulation in both normotensive and hypertensive persons. The development of pharmacologic antagonists to its various components has proved useful in the treatment of hypertension and related target organ damage. Renin, which is synthesized and released predominantly from the juxtaglomerular cells in the kidney, catalyzes the formation of angiotensin I (Ang I) from angiotensinogen. Ang I, in turn, is processed by ACE and other proteases to form Ang II (Fig. 38.6).

The major physiologic and pathophysiologic effects of the pathway are mediated by Ang II. These include constriction of resistance vessels, stimulation of aldosterone synthesis and release, stimulation of renal tubular sodium reabsorption (directly and indirectly via aldosterone), inhibition of renin release, and neural effects, including stimulation of thirst, release of antidiuretic hormone and increases in sympathetic output. In addition, Ang II is a potent growth hormone and mitogen, inducing both cell hyperplasia and hypertrophy.

Two major receptor subtypes for Ang II have been cloned and characterized. Stimulation of the Ang II type 1 receptors (AT1R) mediates the above responses (Fig. 38.7). Stimulation of Ang II type 2 receptors (AT2R) appears to play a counterregulatory role to that of the AT1R, mediating vasodilator, antiproliferative, and perhaps anti-ischemic effects. In addition to the circulating RAAS, local production of Ang II occurs in a variety of tissues, including blood vessels, heart, adrenal glands, and brain. Local production of Ang II, particularly under pathologic conditions, may not be ACE dependent but may rely instead on alternative pathways. The serine protease chymase, in particular, contributes significantly to the formation of Ang II in heart and blood vessels.[56]

The RAAS is classically described as a circulating system in which renin generated in the kidney initiates a cascade of events with a single endpoint, the generation of Ang II. However, local generation of angiotensins independent of circulating renin and angiotensinogen has been described in eye, adrenal gland, testis, ovaries, and brain, organs in which de novo synthesis of the renin precursor prorenin has been demonstrated.[57] Prorenin circulates in 10- to 100-fold excess of active renin in normal subjects, and both renin and prorenin are capable of binding to and activating a receptor that triggers a set of cell signaling events, including activation of the mitogen-activated protein kinase (MAPK) pathway, and generation of plasminogen activator inhibitor 1 (PAI-1). These events may lead to increased tissue fibrosis and cellular hypertrophy, resulting ultimately in CV and renal outcomes.[58]

Preclinical studies suggest that the renin/prorenin receptor may play an important role in CV and renal disease. Rats overexpressing the human receptor develop increased systolic BP and heart rate, as well as proteinuria and glomerulosclerosis, and these alterations worsen progressively with aging.[59,60] Infusion of a renin/prorenin receptor blocking peptide significantly inhibited the renal changes.[60] Activation of renin/prorenin receptors has also been shown to increase transforming growth factor β (TFG-β) synthesis by human and rat mesangial cells, thus potentially leading to glomerular and interstitial transforming renal disease.[61] Although these mechanisms have not yet been identified in humans,

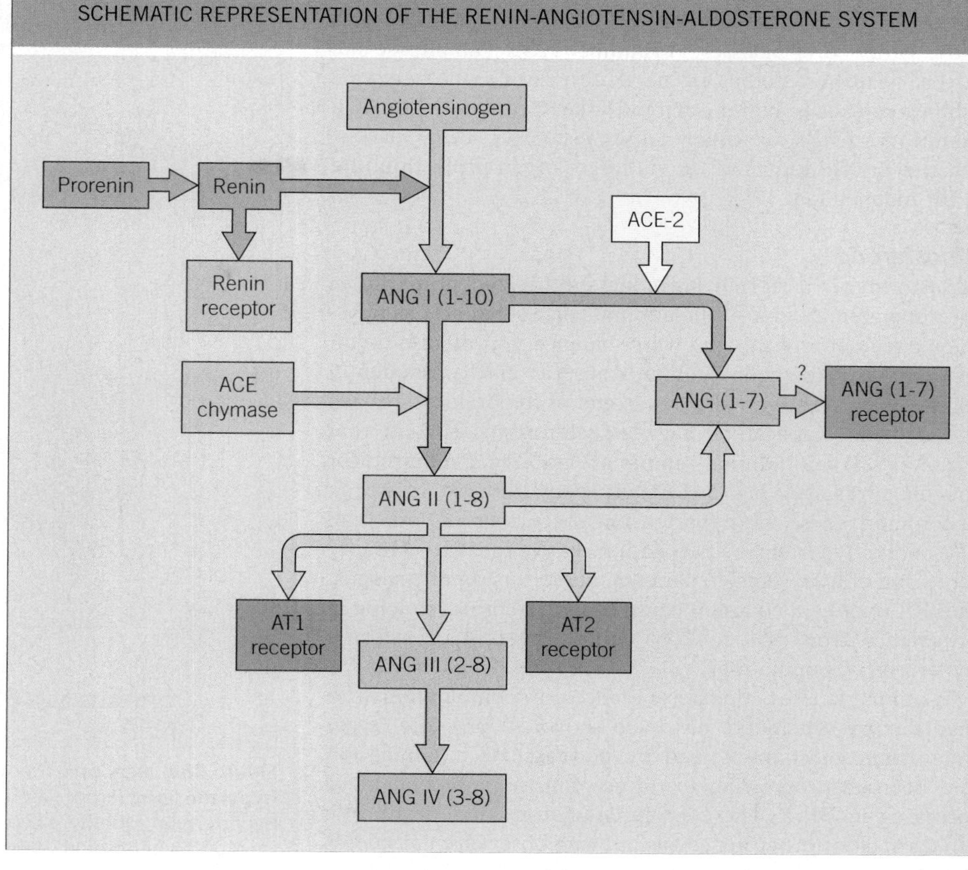

Figure 38.6 Schematic representation of the renin-angiotensin-aldosterone system. ACE, angiotensin-converting enzyme; ANG, angiotensin (roman numerals refer to the nomenclature for the peptide; numbers in parentheses refer to the amino acid positions in the peptide relative to ANG I, which has 10 amino acids); AT1, angiotensin II type 1 receptor; AT2, angiotensin II type 2 receptor. (Modified from Reudelhuber TL. Renin. In Oparil S, Weber MA, eds. Hypertension: A Companion to Brenner & Rector's The Kidney, 2nd ed. Philadelphia, Elsevier, 2005:89-94.)

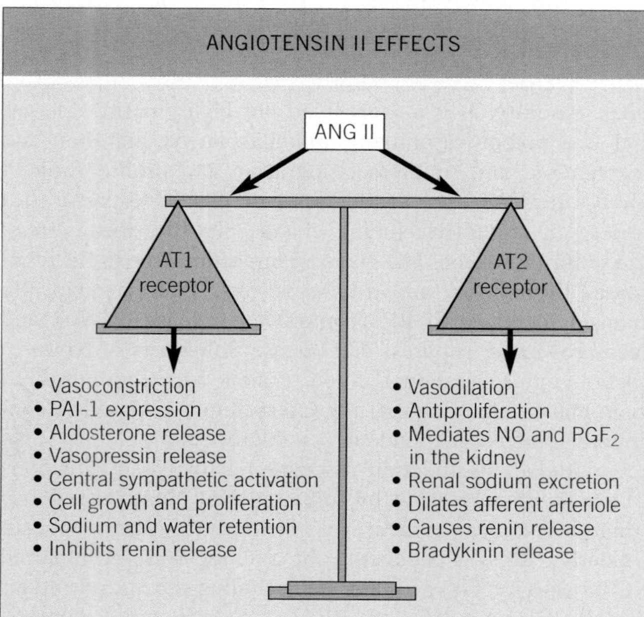

Figure 38.7 Angiotensin II effects at receptors subtype 1 (AT1) and subtype 2 (AT2). NO, nitric oxide; PGF_2, prostaglandin F_2; PAI-1, plasminogen activator inhibitor 1.

discovery of a functional renin prorenin receptor has demonstrated for the first time that renin has a function beyond catalytic activity and angiotensin generation that may have as yet unidentified clinical significance.

Activation of the RAAS may contribute to the development and/or progression of CV disease, including hypertension, left ventricular hypertrophy, heart failure, and atherosclerosis. Hypoperfusion of the kidney is a strong stimulus for renin release, and evidence from animal models indicates that enhancement of renin secretion from a kidney perfused by a stenosed renal artery and the concomitant increase in circulating Ang II levels are the major causes of hypertension after functional stenosis of a renal artery. These increases, however, are transient, and most patients with renal artery stenosis have normal or only slightly elevated plasma renin and Ang II levels.

Independent of pretreatment renin levels, beta blockers (which inhibit renin release), direct renin inhibitors, ACE inhibitors, and ARBs are effective in treating hypertension. The development of direct renin inhibitors has been intensively pursued for decades since blocking the cascade at its first step could theoretically lead to more complete RAAS inhibition. The direct renin inhibitor that has been approved for use in the United States has been shown to reduce BP as effectively as most other antihypertensive agents and to have BP lowering effects that are additive with most other drug classes, including ACE inhibitors and ARBs.[62] Further studies are needed to clarify whether renin inhibition leads to better outcomes than treatment with ACE inhibitors, ARBs or other antihypertensive drug classes, whether by BP reduction or via target organ protection that is BP independent.

Aldosterone

Aldosterone is a steroid hormone synthesized primarily in the zona glomerulosa of the adrenal cortex that acts as physiologic regulator of salt and water balance. It promotes unidirectional transepithelial sodium transport and consequently retains water. The modern syndrome of hyperaldosteronism differs from classical primary aldosteronism (PA) in that hypokalemia and adrenal tumors are no longer required for the diagnosis. PA has historically been thought to be an uncommon cause of hypertension, occurring in less than 1% of the hypertensive population. However, with broader screening of hypertensive patients, numerous reports suggest that PA may be a common cause of hypertension, ranging in prevalence from 8% to 20% among general or selected hypertensive populations.[63]

In animal studies, aldosterone excess in combination with high dietary salt intake has been shown to promote target organ damage characterized by perivascular inflammation and necrosis progressing to diffuse fibrosis independent of increases in BP.[64] These proinflammatory and profibrotic effects of aldosterone are consistent with observational studies of patients with PA, who have an increased likelihood of left ventricular hypertrophy,[65] proteinuria,[66] and endothelial dysfunction,[67] each of which independently predicts increased CV risk. Clinical studies suggest that the sodium and fluid retaining effects of aldosterone excess may also contribute to target organ damage in patients with PA. Patients with hyperaldosteronism have more albuminuria, higher glomerular filtration rate (GFR), greater left ventricular hypertophy, and larger left atrial volumes than patients with essential hypertension who have similar office BPs.[68,69] In addition, patients with PA show greater reduction in left ventricular hypertrophy and left atrial volume with spironolactone treatment compared to patients with essential hypertension.[69] The pathologic processes by which aldosterone promotes target organ damage is complex, but these findings suggest that intravascular volume retention can contribute to aldosterone-induced proteinuria and cardiac hypertrophy in humans. Patients with PA showed greater decreases in albuminuria and GFR after adrenalectomy or aldosterone blocker treatment than patients with essential hypertension, despite similar BP reductions.[66] These findings suggest that aldosterone-induced proteinuria in humans is related, at least in part, to intravascular volume retention and subsequent increases in GFR.

There is an association between aldosterone excess, obesity, and obstructive sleep apnea (OSA).[70,71] Stimulation of aldosterone release by visceral fat, excessive sodium retention stimulated by sympathetic activation, and hypoxemia are possible mechanisms that may account for this association.[70] Sympathetic activity is increased in patients with hypertension and OSA, suggesting that intermittent hypoxemia could contribute to adrenergic activation.[72] Obesity and/or sleep-disordered breathing also may stimulate the adrenal glands to produce excessive amounts of aldosterone. However, the pathogenic mechanisms of hypertension in persons with OSA are not well understood (Fig. 38.8).

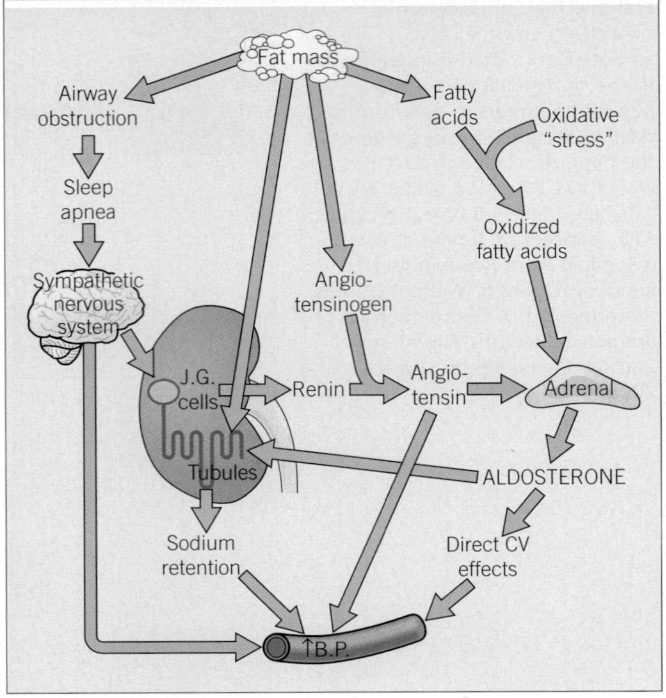

REAL AND THEORETICAL LINKS CONNECTING OBESITY TO HYPERTENSION

Figure 38.8 Real and theoretical links connecting obesity to hypertension. (From Goodfriend TL, Calhoun DA. Resistant hypertension, obesity, sleep apnea, and aldosterone: theory and therapy. Hypertension 2004;43:518-524.)

Endothelial Dysfunction

Nitric Oxide

Nitric oxide (NO) is a short lived but highly permeable gas that is a potent vasodilator, inhibits platelet adhesion and aggregation, and suppresses migration and proliferation of VSMC. It is released by endothelial cells in response to a variety of stimuli, including changes in BP, shear stress, and pulsatile stretch. NO plays an important role in BP regulation, thrombosis, and atherosclerosis. Pharmacologically induced increases in BP promote the release of NO, and decreases in BP suppress NO release. Inhibitors of NO production induce sustained hypertension when administered to animals, suggesting that the CV system is exposed to continuous tonic NO-dependent vasodilator tone.[73]

Endothelial dysfunction associated with essential hypertension is characterized by impaired NO bioactivity determined by measurement of reactive oxygen species. Oxidative stress is believed to be a major cause of impaired NO bioactivity. Oxygen radicals, including superoxide anions (O_2^-), scavenge NO effectively, reducing its bioavailability. Reactive oxygen species can be generated by nonenzymatic and enzymatic sources: NAD(P)H oxidase and cyclooxygenases are the major sources of O_2^-.[74] Consequently, the vasoconstrictive effect of Ang II is mediated by reactive oxygen species, mainly O_2^-, and their interaction with endothelium-derived NO.

Some antihypertensive agents, such as nebivolol (beta blocker), ACE inhibitors, ARBs, and CCBs can improve endothelial function, thus increasing NO bioavailability or decreasing oxidative stress.[74] A potential antihypertensive effect has also been attributed to statins. Pharmacologic inhibition of 3-hydroxy-3-methylglutaryl coenzyme A (HMG-CoA) reductase leads to potent stimulation of endothelial NO synthase, attenuating the expression of caveolin-1 and reducing the abundance of caveolae in endothelial cells.[75] Caveolin plays a role in endothelial function, binding directly to and inhibiting endothelial NO synthase, thus decreasing NO availability.[76] This mechanism may explain the potential BP reducing effect of statins.

Endothelin

Endothelin (ET) is a potent vasoactive peptide produced by endothelial cells that has both vasoconstrictor and vasodilator properties. The family of endothelins includes three isoforms. ET-1 plays the prominent role in the CV system, producing vasoconstriction via ET-A and ET-B receptors on VSMC, whereas activation of ET-B receptors on endothelial cells leads to vasodilation.[77]

ET receptor antagonists reduce BP and peripheral vascular resistance in both normotensive persons and hypertensive patients,[78,79] supporting the interpretation that ET plays a role in the pathogenesis of systemic hypertension. Most studies support a predominant role for ET-A receptors in mediating the vasoconstrictor effects of ET-1 in hypertension, but others report vasoconstriction mediated through the ET-B receptor as well.[80] Circulating ET levels are increased in some hypertensive patients, particularly African Americans and persons with transplant hypertension, endothelial tumors, and vasculitis.[81]

Both nonselective and selective ET receptor antagonists have been evaluated in clinical trials in patients with systemic hypertension. The nonselective ET-A/-B receptor antagonist bosentan has been shown to reduce BP significantly, but is associated with considerable risk of liver toxicity.[78,82] Darusentan, a selective ET-A antagonist, has been tested in 115 patients with resistant hypertension. Darusentan decreased systolic BP by 11.5 and diastolic BP by 6.3 mm Hg compared to placebo after 10 weeks of follow-up.[83] The most common adverse events were mild to moderate edema and headache. Long-term studies are needed to compare the efficacy and safety/tolerability of ET receptor antagonists alone or added to established antihypertensive drug treatment in patients with systemic hypertension. More data on BP effects, hypertension-related target organ damage, CV events, and safety are needed if these agents are to enjoy widespread use in this large patient group.

Vasodilators

Natriuretic Peptides

Since the seminal observation of de Bold and colleagues[84] that atrial extracts have potent natriuretic and BP-lowering effects, natriuretic peptides have been the most thoroughly studied endogenous antihypertensive mediators. Natriuretic peptides play an important role in the integrative control of CV and renal function and in the pathogenesis of hypertension and related target organ damage, promoting natriuresis, vasodilation, vascular remodeling, inhibition of cell proliferation, and modulation of sympathetic nervous system and RAAS function.[85]

Five distinct natriuretic peptides have been identified and characterized: atrial natriuretic peptide (ANP), brain natriuretic peptide (BNP), C-type natriuretic peptide (CNP), dendroaspis natriuretic peptide (DNP), and urodilatin. ANP is expressed in and released from atrial myocytes in response to stretch and a variety of neurohumoral stimuli. ANP has renal, hemodynamic, and neurohumoral effects that reduce extracellular volume and systemic vascular resistance and thus lower BP. In addition, ANP inhibits growth and proliferation of critical cell types in the heart and vasculature. Relative ANP deficiency, reflected in a blunted increase or a paradoxical decrease in plasma ANP in response to high dietary salt intake, has been demonstrated in humans with salt-sensitive hypertension and in children of hypertensive parents.[85] We have also demonstrated that patients with resistant hypertension have lower ANP levels than normotensive and mild hypertensive patients.[86]

Genetic studies have associated polymorphisms in the ANP gene with hypertension in some populations. Using the candidate gene approach, Rutledge and coworkers[87] have demonstrated that an Hpa II variant within a polymorphic region in intron 2 of the ANP gene is more common among hypertensive African Americans than among normotensive controls. This study supports the hypothesis that a deficit of ANP secretion or augmented metabolism may be genetically determined and contribute to salt sensitivity and hypertension in African Americans. Thus, experimental and clinical studies suggest a role for ANP in the regulation of BP and the pathogenesis of some forms of hypertension and their associated target organ damage.

Kallikrein-Kinin System

The kallikrein-kinin system operates in parallel with the RAAS but has many functions that oppose the actions of Ang II and aldosterone. The kinins, peptides that contain the sequence of bradykinin, stimulate release of a variety of vasodilator/natriuretic/antitrophic mediators through the B_2 receptors. B_2 receptors also form heterodimers with the AT1R, activating AT1R signaling, and form a complex with endothelial NO synthase that inhibits NO generation, thus accounting for a large variety of sometimes opposing CV effects.[88]

Decreased activity of the kallikrein-kinin system has been linked to human hypertension in that low urinary kallikrein excretion has been described in normotensive children of hypertensive parents, whereas high urinary kallikrein has been associated with a decreased risk of essential hypertension.[89] However, animal models with genetic deletion of components of the kallikrein-kinin system do not develop hypertension, suggesting that the kinins are not fundamental in the pathogenesis of that disorder, at least in mice.[90]

Kinins mediate some of the CV and renal effects of the ACE inhibitors and ARBs, as well as some of the adverse effects of the former drug class. Kininase inhibition may contribute to the antihypertensive effect of ACE inhibitors. Experimental studies have reported that the acute antihypertensive effect of ACE inhibitors may be due to an increase in tissue kinins, which regulate vascular resistance via the release of NO and/or prostaglandins.[89] Kinins may also mediate the vasoprotective, infarct reducing, and heart failure preventing effects of ACE inhibitors. Because blockade of the AT1R increases Ang II levels, which in turn may activate the AT2R, the CV benefits of ARBs may be mediated in part by kinins via activation of AT2R. Bradykinin also appears to play an important role in mediating the counterregulatory/protective effects of AT2R, which oppose the effects of AT1R.[90]

Adipocytokines

Adipocytokines are bioactive substances secreted by the adipose tissue. Leptin and adiponectin are proteins synthesized and secreted by adipocytes, up-regulated in obesity, whose primary function is energy balance control. Leptin plays an important role in the pathophysiology of obesity-related atherogenesis through multiple mechanisms, including proliferative, proinflammatory, prothrombotic, and pro-oxidant actions. In contrast, adiponectin, which is down-regulated in obese subjects, protects against atherosclerotic CV disorders.[91]

Several reports have suggested either a vasodilator or vasconstrictor action of leptin. Chronic hyperleptinemia increases BP via impaired vasodilation and/or enhanced vasoconstriction.[91,92] Clinical studies have shown elevated plasma leptin in patients with essential hypertension and a significant positive correlation between leptin and BP independent of adiposity in both normotensive and hypertensive individuals. However, a cause-effect relationship between leptin levels and hypertension in humans has not been demonstrated directly. Leptin also appears to be involved in the CV complications of obesity, including arterial hypertension, left ventricular hypertrophy, retinopathy and nephropathy, independent of BP regulation.[93] Leptin levels are positively related to CV outcomes, including myocardial infarction and stroke, in humans independent of traditional CV risk factors and BMI.[94]

In contrast to leptin, plasma levels of adiponectin correlate negatively with BMI, and hypertensive persons have been reported to have significantly lower plasma adiponectin levels than normotensives.[91] There is evidence from both preclinical and clinical studies that Ang II plays a role in suppressing adiponectin levels. Infusion of Ang II into Wistar rats increased BP and decreased plasma adiponectin levels, and olmesartan partially restored these changes, suggesting that adiponectin acts via signaling through the AT1R.[95] Further, in patients with essential hypertension, ACE inhibitor or ARB treatment has been shown to increase circulating adiponectin concentrations without affecting BMI.[96] The precise molecular mechanisms whereby Ang II signaling reduces adiponectin expression and the role of adiponectin per se in regulating BP remain to be determined.[91]

Adiponectin may have vasoprotective effects beyond BP lowering. Evidence obtained from animal models has demonstrated that adiponectin protects against the development of obesity-related vascular pathology, including atherosclerosis and vascular remodeling,[97] endothelial dysfunction,[98] and thrombosis formation.[99] Adiponectin treatment also inhibits apoptosis of cardiac myocytes and fibroblasts exposed to hypoxia-reoxygenation stress,[100] suggesting the possibility that adiponectin administration might have a practical clinical application in the treatment of acute myocardial infarction.

SUMMARY

Many factors contribute to the development of essential hypertension. Because these factors are rarely known in any given patient, treatments are now empirical. It is highly likely that, in the third millennium, advances in understanding of the etiology of hypertension will lead to more effective, highly selective, individualized pharmacogenomic approaches to hypertension prevention and treatment. Although syndromes exist in which hypertension is determined by a single abnormal gene, in most patients, interactions among various genetic and environmental factors contribute to the development of hypertension. Appropriate treatment strategies for such patients require broadly based approaches that address more than one factor.

chapter 39

Epidemiology of Hypertension

Hirotsugu Ueshima

Issues/Problems

- The definition of hypertension is arbitrary, because blood pressure has a unimodal distribution in the population as well as a continuous relationship with cardiovascular risk.
- The rise in blood pressure with age, which varies substantially across populations and within populations over time, is determined largely by environmental factors and is therefore preventable.

Key Findings

- Obesity, physical inactivity, heavy alcohol consumption, high dietary salt and low potassium consumption are among the most important factors in the emergence of hypertension as a mass phenomenon.
- Obesity is becoming a global epidemic, and obesity-related hypertension has increased in both children and adults.
- Reducing salt intake, increasing potassium intake, and following the guidelines of the DASH diet have emerged as effective strategies for lowering blood pressure.
- Extensive research on the relationship between genetic abnormality and blood pressure in populations has been done, but none of various genetic abnormalities have been shown to be responsible for any applicable portion of hypertension nor blood pressure level in the general population.

Clinical Implications

- The usual levels of blood pressure are directly and continuously related to the risks of both stroke and coronary heart disease across the entire distribution of blood pressure.
- Thus, a small downward shift in mean population blood pressure, achievable by public policy and lifestyle changes, should lead to sizeable reduction in the incidence of stroke and coronary heart disease.

Blood pressure is a continuous, normally distributed variable in the population. Hypertension is therefore a quantitative phenomenon in which the definition of abnormality is arbitrary and pragmatic. It is reported that among persons 35 to 64 years old, 30% in North America and 50% in six European countries have hypertension.[1] The prevalence of hypertension increases with advancing age to the point where more than half of people aged 60 to 69 years old and 70% of people 70 years or older are hypertensive.[2] Data from prospective observational studies and from randomized controlled trials of antihypertensive agents have shown a consistent, continuous linear relation between usual blood pressure levels and the risk of coronary heart disease (CHD) and stroke.[3,4] Stroke is more strongly related to blood pressure level than CHD. Elevated blood pressure is also a major predictor of heart failure and of end-stage renal failure.[5] Furthermore, the fundamental problem in hypertension is the tendency for blood pressure to rise with age, but this varies considerably both within[6] and between populations worldwide[7] and over time.[8] Thus hypertension is as much a disorder of populations as of individuals.

It is accepted that the development of hypertension reflects a complex and dynamic interaction between genetic and environmental causal factors. However, we have made limited progress in identifying important markers of genetic susceptibility to hypertension. Differences in environmental factors largely determine the substantial variation in blood pressure levels between and within populations.[9]

DIAGNOSTIC CRITERIA

The classification of adult blood pressure from the Seventh Report of the Joint National Committee on Detection, Evaluation and Treatment of High Blood Pressure (JNC 7) (Table 39.1)[10] and from the 2007 Guidelines of the European Society of Hypertension (ESH) and of the European Society of Cardiology (ESC)[11] is well known and referred to in many countries. As a definition and classification of blood pressure, hypertension is defined as systolic blood pressure (SBP) of greater than 140 mm Hg and diastolic blood pressure (DBP) of greater than 90 mm Hg. Normal blood pressure was defined for SBP less than 120 mm Hg and DBP less than 80 mm Hg, and the new category of "prehypertension" for SBP 120 to 139 mm Hg/DBP 80 to 89 mm Hg was created in the JNC 7 report. On the other hand, the categories of "high normal" (SBP 130-139 mm Hg/DBP 85-89 mm Hg), "normal" (SBP 120-129 mm Hg/DBP 80-84 mm Hg), and "optimal" (SBP <120 mm Hg and DBP <80 mm Hg) in the ESH/ESC guidelines were defined. For the category of hypertension, "stage 1" and "stage 2" were defined in the JNC-7 report, whereas "grade 1," "grade 2," and "grade 3" were given together with "isolated systolic hypertension" in ESH/ESC guidelines (see Table 39.1). In the 1999 World Health Organization–International Society of Hypertension (WHO/ISH) guidelines, the same definition and classification of blood pressure levels are proposed, although the terms "mild" and "moderate" hypertension are retained.[5]

The risk of cardiovascular disease increases with SBP at every level of DBP,[12] and current classification systems are based on both systolic and diastolic levels. The concept of isolated systolic hypertension (defined as SBP ≥140 mm Hg and DBP <90 mm Hg) is promoted in current international guidelines, reflecting the data from trials reported over the past decade.[11]

CLASSIFICATION OF BLOOD PRESSURE FOR ADULTS AGED 18 YEARS AND OLDER							
						Management Initial Drug Therapy	
BP Classification	Systolic BP (mm Hg*)		Diastolic BP (mm Hg*)	Lifestyle Modification	Without Compelling Indication	With Compelling Indication
Normal	<120	and	<80	Encourage		
Prehypertension	120-139	or	80-89	Yes	No antihypertensive drug indicated	Drug(s)for the compelling indications†
Stage 1 hypertension	140-159	or	90-99	Yes	Thiazide-type diuretics for most; may consider ACE inhibitor, ARB, beta blocker, CCB, or combination	Drug(s) for the compelling indications Other antihypertensive drugs (diuretics, ACE inhibitor, ARB, beta blocker, CCB) as needed
Stage 2 hypertension	≥160	or	≥100	Yes	2-Drug combination for most (usually thiazide-type diuretic and ACE inhibitor or ARB or beta blocker or CCB)‡	Drug(s) for the compelling indications Other antihypertensive drugs (diuretics, ACE inhibitor, ARB, beta blocker, CCB) as needed

Optimal blood pressure with respect to cardiovascular risk is less than 120/80 mm Hg. However, unusually low readings should be evaluated for clinical significance. The diagnosis of hypertension was based on the average of two or more readings taken at each of two visits after an initial screening. Note that stage 3 and stage 4 hypertension have been combined, owing to the relative infrequency of stage 4 hypertension.

*Treatment determined by highest BP category.

†Treat patients with chronic kidney disease or diabetes to BP goal of less than 130/80 mm Hg.

‡Initial combined therapy should be used cautiously in those at risk for orthostatic hypotension.

ACE, angiotensin-converting enzyme; ARB, angiotensin-receptor blocker; BP, blood pressure; CCB, calcium channel blocker.

From The Seventh Report of the Joint National Committee on Prevention, Detection, Evaluation, and Treatment of High Blood Pressure. JAMA 2003;289:2560–2572.

Table 39.1 Classification of blood pressure for adults aged 18 years and older.

In the presence of other cardiovascular risk factors, clinical cardiovascular disease or target organ disease (Table 39.2),[10] the risk of cardiovascular disease is substantially increased regardless of the blood pressure level. Thus the presence or absence of hypertensive target organ disease and the additional risk factors should be recorded in specific detail. There is therefore increasing emphasis on the use of formal risk scoring systems that incorporate, in addition to blood pressure measurements, information on end-organ damage and the presence of additional risk factors such as diabetes. The Framingham CHD score was first introduced, and then country-specific cardiovascular prediction charts and WHO/ISH prediction charts have prevailed.[13] The use of such risk scoring systems, which is likely to increase with the widespread availability of appropriate computer software,[14] allows the clinician to base therapy decisions on the absolute annual risk of a major cardiovascular disease event, estimated at the individual patient level.

PREVALENCE AND INCIDENCE

The magnitude of the rise in blood pressure with age varies markedly in different geographic regions and over time. A number of isolated rural communities have been identified in which blood pressure does not rise with age.[15] When individuals from these communities enter the army or migrate to the city their blood pressure rises.[16] Even within an industrialized country such as the United Kingdom, there is a pronounced north-south gradient in blood pressure, with higher levels in the north of the country. In the British Regional Heart Study (BRHS), age-adjusted blood pressure varied by

MAJOR RISK FACTORS AND TARGET ORGAN DAMAGE
Hypertension†
Cigarette smoking
Obesity (BMI ≥30)†
Physical activity
Dyslipidemia†
Diabetes mellitus†
Microalbuminuria or estimated GFR <60 mL/min
Age (>55 years for men, >65 years for women)
Family history of premature cardiovascular disease (men <55 years or women ≤65 years)
Heart
Left ventricular hypertrophy
Angina or prior myocardial infarction
Prior coronary revascularization
Heart failure
Brain
Stroke or transient ischemic attack
Chronic kidney disease
Peripheral arterial disease
Retinopathy

*BMI indicates body mass index calculated as weight in kilograms divided by the square of height in meters.

†Component of the metabolic syndrome.

GFR, glomerular filtration rate.

From JNC 7, JAMA 2003;289:2560–2572.

Table 39.2 Major risk factors and target organ damage.

9 mm Hg across 24 towns in England, Wales, and Scotland,[6] which is only partially explained by differences in the proportion of the population that has lower socioeconomic status (associated with higher blood pressure), or by differences in the prevalence of obesity or other factors linked with the development of hypertension. Similarly, blood pressure differences between northern and southern Chinese populations were explained by multiple dietary factors, including sodium, in an International Study on Macronutrients and Blood Pressure (INTERMAP).[17] In the United States, favorable secular trends were observed in the mean blood pressure of the population and in the age-adjusted prevalence of hypertension in a series of nationally representative cross-sectional surveys conducted over several decades.[8] The annual national trends in blood pressure levels by age and sex are reported from Japan (Fig. 39.1).[18] After the peak of the SBP in 1965, steep lowering trends in general were observed for both men and women with a concomitant great decline in stroke mortality and morbidity.[18] Geographic and temporal variation in blood pressure of this magnitude attests to the importance of environmental factors in the development of this hypertension.

Prevalence

The prevalence of hypertension in the general population clearly depends on the arbitrary criteria used for definition, on the sampling strategy, and on the techniques and conditions for blood pressure measurement. It must also be emphasized that the relationship between blood pressure and disease risk is continuous and that much of the burden of blood pressure–related cardiovascular and renal disease in the population can be attributed to blood pressures within the so-called normotensive range.

Data on the prevalence of hypertension in the U.S. adult civilian, noninstitutionalized population, based on the National Health and Nutrition Examination Survey 1988-2000 (NHANES) are presented in Table 39.3.[19] Hypertension was defined on the basis of the USA Joint National Committee Guidelines (JNC-VI) criteria (mean SBP $\geq$140 mm Hg, mean DBP $\geq$90 mm Hg, or current treatment for hypertension) for 5448 participants, aged 18 years and older. On the basis of these data, it was estimated that 29% of the U.S. adult population have hypertension.[19] In most age groups the prevalence of hypertension is greater in non-Hispanic blacks than in non-Hispanic white and Mexican American populations. Men have a higher prevalence of hypertension than women in the younger age groups, whereas in the older age groups this trend is reversed. Most of the hypertension in young adults results from elevations in DBP, whereas in later life isolated elevations in SBP account for more than 60% of the hypertension seen in men and 70% of the hypertension seen in women.

It is difficult to compare precisely the prevalence of hypertension among populations and/or countries without any high standardization procedure. The INTERMAP study makes it possible to compare the prevalence of blood pressure categories among 17 populations for men and women aged 40 to 59 years old, randomly selected in a given population of Japan, China, United Kingdom, and United States in 1996-1999 (Table 39.4).[20] In this international study, the prevalence of hypertension for the Japanese population was not different from those of Americans. The prevalence of "optimal" was rather higher in Japan, the United Kingdom, and the United States.

The comparison of North America (U.S. and Canada) with six European countries for persons aged 35 to 64 years old with a standard procedure showed that the prevalence of hypertension for six European countries was higher than those of North America (39% vs. 25%).[1]

Trends in the Prevalence of Hypertension

Data from four separate nationally representative cross-sectional surveys on the prevalence of hypertension in the adult U.S. population are available from the years 1960 to 1991.[8] A dramatic fall in age-adjusted prevalence rates was seen between the 1976 to 1980 survey and the 1988 to 1991 survey in men and women and in blacks and whites. Hypertension awareness, treatment, and control rates also appear to have improved dramatically between the periods of 1976 to 1980 and 1988 to 1991. These changes contributed to equally dramatic reductions in morbidity and mortality attributable to hypertension between the early 1960s and the late 1980s, with declines in age-adjusted stroke and CHD mortality of approximately 60% and 53%, respectively. However, in the early part of the 1990s, this decline in hypertension prevalence leveled off, and the prevalence of hypertension in 1999 to 2000 was rather increased (see Table 39.3). Improvements in hypertension awareness, treatment, and control rates have slowed markedly, as evidenced in the comparison between NHANES II phase 1 (1988-1991) and phase 2 (1991-1994).[10] In this context it is noteworthy that, since 1993, U.S. age-adjusted stroke mortality rates have risen slightly, and the slope of the age-adjusted rate of decline in mortality from CHD has leveled. Similarly, the prevalence of hypertension in Japan has decreased greatly during 1965 to 1990 with a similar trend of blood pressure level. An approximately 80% decline of stroke mortality was recorded during this period.[18]

Incidence

There is a paucity of data on the incidence of hypertension in the general population. Changing definitions and differences in measurement techniques have impeded comparative examination of the incidence of hypertension in different populations. The incidence of hypertension increases sharply with age, with higher rates in men than in women in the early decades of life and the reverse in later decades. Data from the Framingham Heart Study have allowed analysis of incidence and trends in definite hypertension during 30 years of follow-up in a group of 5209 subjects.[21] Hypertension incidence increased from 3.3% in men and 1.5% in women at ages 30 to 39 years to 6.2% in men and 8.6% in women at ages 70 to 79 years, with no consistent secular trend in 2-year incidence rates evident for either sex during the 30-year study period between the 1950s and the 1970s. The Framingham study revealed that the residual lifetime risks for developing hypertension and stage 1 high blood pressure or higher ($\geq$140/90 mm Hg, regardless of treatment) were 90% in both 55- and 65-year-old participants.[22]

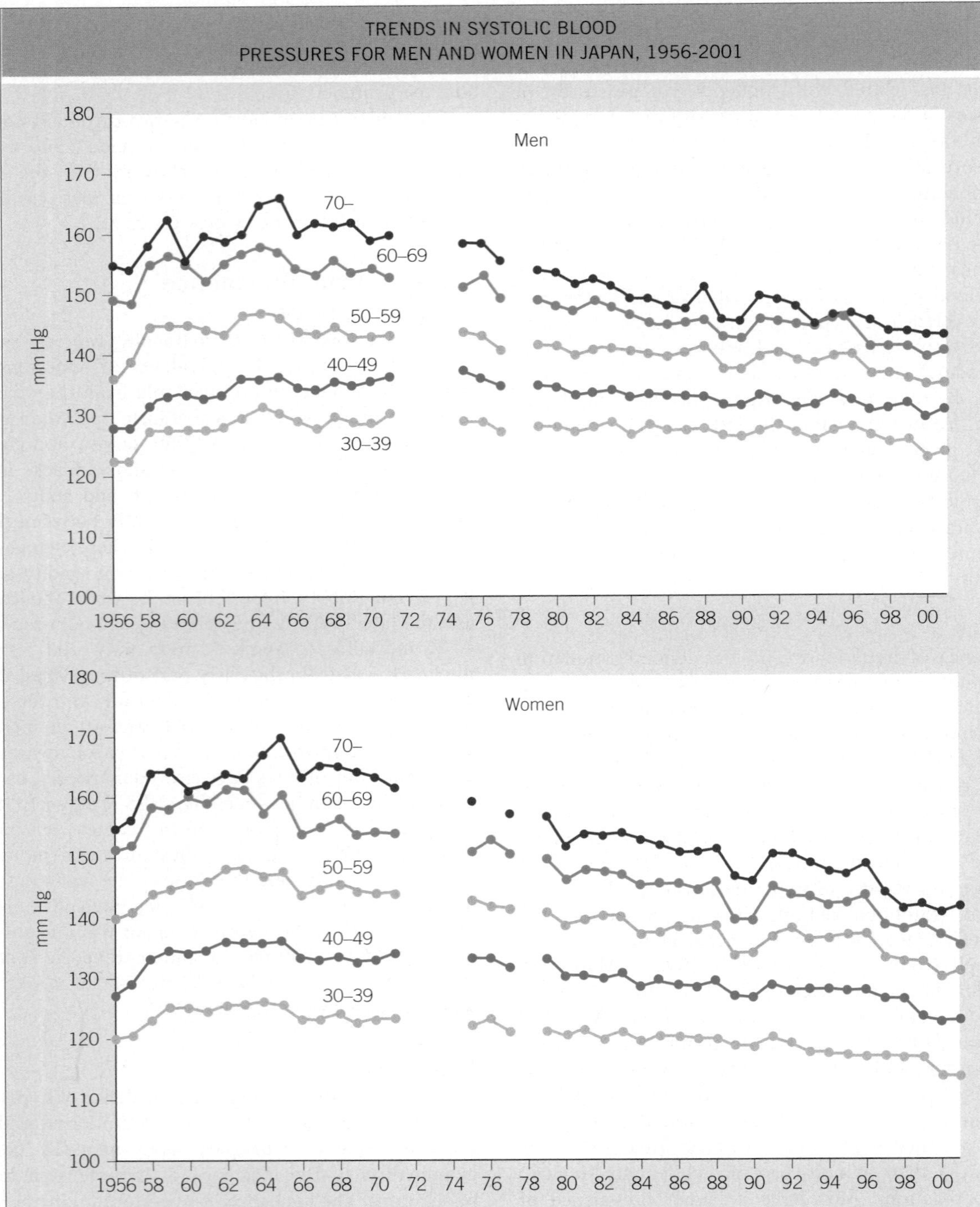

Figure 39.1 Trends in systolic blood pressures for men and women in Japan, 1956-2001. Systolic blood pressure levels for men and women have declined substantially since around 1965, whereas the rate of stroke mortality was highest in Japan. Especially, blood pressure in men and women older than 60 years was much larger and evident than that for men and women in their 30s to 50s. The lowering trend in systolic blood pressure slowed down since around 1990 and is compatible with that of the similar slowdown phenomenon of stroke mortality. (From Ueshima H. Explanation for the Japanese paradox: prevention of increase in coronary heart disease and reduction in stroke. J Athero Thrombo 2007;14:278-286.)

RISK FACTORS

Increasing age is the dominant risk factor for hypertension. Predictably, baseline blood pressure is also a major risk factor for later hypertension in longitudinal studies. High normal blood pressure has also consistently been found to be one of the strongest predictors for the later development of hypertension.[23]

The issue of blood pressure tracking in childhood (the stability over time of an individual's blood pressure level relative to that of his or her peers) has been extensively investigated.

AWARENESS, TREATMENT, AND CONTROL AMONG PARTICIPANTS WITH HYPERTENSION IN THE U.S. POPULATION, 1988-2000					
	Prevalence of, % (SE)			Change, 1988 to 2000	
	1988-1991 (n = 3045)	1991-1994 (n = 3017)	1999-2000 (n = 1565)	% (95% CI)	*P* Value
	69.2 (1.3)	67.8 (1.8)	68.9 (1.5)	−0.3 (−4.2 to 3.6)	0.58
	52.4 (1.4)	52.0 (1.0)	58.4 (2.0)	6.0 (1.2 to 10.8)	0.007
Among those treated	46.9 (2.2)	43.6 (1.7)	53.1 (2.4)	6.2 (0 to 12.6)	0.03
Among all with hypertension	24.6 (1.4)	22.7 (1.1)	31.0 (2.0)	6.4 (1.6 to 11.2)	0.004
<140/90 mm Hg (among treated hypertensive diabetic individuals)	53.1 (4.5)	41.6 (5.8)†	46.9 (4.7)	−6.2 (−19.0 to 6.6)	0.83
<130/85 mm Hg (among treated hypertensive diabetic individuals)	28.5 (4.2)	17.2 (4.2)	17.2 (4.2)†	−3.1(−14.5 to 8.3)	0.70

*Data are weighted to the U.S. population.
†Estimates are unreliable because of National Health and Nutrition Examination Survey minimum sample size criteria or coefficient of variation of at least 0.30.
CI, confidence interval.

Table 39.3 Awareness, treatment, and control among participants with hypertension in the U.S. population, 1988-2000*.

PERCENTAGE OF PARTICIPANTS BY BLOOD PRESSURE CATEGORY BY MEN AND WOMEN, INTERMAP STUDY, 1996-1999						
Sample	Number	Optimal (%)	Normal (%)	High Normal (%)	Hypertension Stage 1 (%)	Hypertension Stages 2 and 3 (%)
Men						
Japan	574	49	24	15	11	2
People's Republic of China	416	54	21	11	10	4
United Kingdom	266	36	27	14	18	5
United States	1103	48	27	15	9	2
Women						
Japan	571	70	17	8	6	0
People's Republic of China	423	54	19	13	10	4
United Kingdom	235	63	18	10	8	1
United States	1092	62	18	12	7	1

*Blood pressure categories:
Optimal: SBP <120 mm Hg and DBP <80 mm Hg; normal (not optimal): SBP <130 mm Hg, DBP <85 mm Hg (exclusive of optimal)
High normal: SBP 130-139 mm Hg or DBP 85-89 mm Hg; hypertension stage 1: SBP 140-159 mm Hg or DBP 90-99 mm Hg
Hypertension stages 2 and 3: SBP 160 mm Hg or DBP 99-100 mm Hg, SBP ≥180 mm Hg or DBP ≥110 mm Hg
From Stamler J, Elliott P, Chan Q, for the INTERMAP Research Group. INTERMAP Appendix Tables. J Hum Hypertens 2003;17:665-775.

Table 39.4 Percentage of participants by blood pressure category by men and women, INTERMAP study, 1996-1999*.

In general, correlation coefficients for replicate measures of blood pressure over time in childhood are moderately impressive, with replicate tracking correlations in excess of 0.4 after 8 years of follow-up.[24] High blood pressure in children and adolescents is often associated with positive history of hypertension or cardiovascular diseases. It is also frequently associated with overweight.[25]

Smoking caused an acute rise in blood pressure and heart rate for more than 15 minutes; however, most epidemiologic studies considering the effects of alcohol drinking found that blood pressure levels among cigarette smokers were the same as, or lower than, those in nonsmokers. Smoking cessation is necessary for reducing cardiovascular disease risk and other smoking-related diseases; however, it does not lower blood pressure.[26]

Major Lifestyle and Environmental Risk Factors: Overview

Elucidation of lifestyle-related and environmental risk factors for hypertension holds the promise of prevention. Work in recent decades has identified an important role in the development of hypertension for a small number of interrelated lifestyle and environmental risk factors, of which the most important are[9,10,11,27-29]

- calorie excess (as manifested by obesity);
- high dietary salt;
- low potassium consumption;
- excess alcohol consumption; and
- physical inactivity.

Therefore, lifestyle modifications shown in Table 39.5 from the USA Joint National Committee Guidelines (JNC 7) are important and effective measures for all persons to prevent hypertension and/or to lower blood pressure.[9,10] Among them, weight control is an important issue, considering rapid increase in obese persons in the world. Dietary sodium reduction is also a core measure for lowering blood pressure not only in individuals but also in populations. No more than 4 to 6 g/day of sodium chloride intake is recommended for hypertensive persons.[9-11,27-29] Salt reduction is specifically sensitive for reducing blood pressure in black and older people.

A large number of additional factors have been investigated in studies of the etiology of hypertension, including psychosocial stress, dietary calcium, magnesium, omega-3 fatty acids, fish oil and other dietary fats, coffee, protein, fiber, and specific dietary patterns such as vegetarianism.[29]

Current observational and clinical trial data suggest that dietary calcium, magnesium, fish oil, and coffee make relatively small contributions to the population burden of hypertension.[28-30] We now have clear evidence to support a major role in the prevention and control of hypertension for specific dietary patterns such as the Dietary Approaches to Stop Hypertension (DASH) diet (essentially a "prudent" diet that emphasizes fruits, vegetables, and low-fat dairy products).[31,32] Miscellaneous environmental factors associated with adverse effects on blood pressure include environmental temperature (cold), noise exposure, and trace elements, including lead, cadmium, copper, and zinc.

Work on the role of psychosocial stress in hypertension is beset with problems of definition and measurement. However, this is a potentially important area, particularly in the broader societal context of social and economic inequalities, which are fundamental determinants of health.

Obesity

Obesity control is now a major global population health challenge. An association between obesity and hypertension, independent of other potential confounding factors (including measurement artifact), is well documented in children,[33] adolescents, and adults. An increase in body weight from childhood to young adulthood is a major predictor of adult hypertension.[34] In prospective studies, obesity, whether expressed as body mass index (BMI), relative weight, skinfold thickness, or waist-to-hip ratio, has consistently emerged as a significant predictor of incident hypertension. However, it is unclear how the obesity epidemic increased the prevalence of hypertension and/or blood pressure level in children over the last few decades.[35] In addition, there is no definite evidence for a connection, primarily because of the limitation of blood pressure measurement without standardized methods determining the trends in blood pressure over time.

Obesity, especially abdominal obesity, is correlated with hypertension, dyslipidemia, and hyperglycemia. A phenomenon of risk factor clustering together with obesity is termed metabolic syndrome.[36] There are two pathophysiologic pathways for metabolic syndrome; one is that insulin resistance[37] is a primary cause of the risk factor cluster including abdominal obesity; and the other pathway is that abdominal obesity is a primary cause for the metabolic syndrome including insulin resistance. Obesity control is critically important even though neither one is a true cause, because such risk factor clustering as metabolic syndrome increases risk for cardiovascular diseases.

There is substantial clinical trial evidence that weight loss lowers blood pressure in both normotensives and hypertensives.[38] In a systematic review of the effects of sustained weight reduction on blood pressure, based on randomized

LIFESTYLE MODIFICATIONS TO MANAGE HYPERTENSION.*

Modification	Recommendation	Approximate Systolic BP Reduction, Range
Weight reduction	Maintain normal body weight (BMI, 18.5-24.9)	5-20 mm Hg/10 kg weight loss
Adopt DASH eating plan	Consume a diet rich in fruits, vegetables, and low-fat dairy products with a reduced content of saturated and total fat	8-14 mm Hg
Dietary sodium reduction	Reduce dietary sodium intake to no more than 100 mEq/L (2.5 g sodium or 6 g sodium chloride)	2-8 mm Hg
Physical activity	Engage in regular aerobic physical activity such as brisk walking (at least 30 minutes per day, most day of the week)	4-9 mm Hg
Moderation of alcohol consumption	Limit consumption to no more than 2 drinks per day (1 oz or 30 mL ethanol [e.g., 24 oz beer, 10 oz wine, or 3 oz 80-proof whiskey]) in most men and no more than 1 drink per day in women and lighter weight persons	2-4 mm Hg

*For overall cardiovascular risk reduction, stop smoking. The effects of implementing these modifications are dose and time dependent and could be higher for some individuals.

BMI, body mass index calculated as weight in kilograms divided by the square of height in meters; *BP,* blood pressure; *DASH,* Dietary Approaches to Stop Hypertension.

Source: from JNC 7. Hypertension 2003;42:1206-1252.

Table 39.5 Lifestyle modifications to manage hypertension.*

controlled trials with at least 6 months of follow-up, significant pooled net changes in SBP and DBP of −5.2/−5.2 mm Hg and −2.8/−2.3 mm Hg were found in hypertensive and normotensive participants, respectively.[39] It should be noted that the contributions of concurrent changes in salt and alcohol consumption and levels of physical activity were not addressed in these trials. In practice it is extremely difficult to isolate the independent effects of weight loss on blood pressure. In practice, however, this is an issue of limited clinical or population health relevance.

Physical Activity

There is consistent evidence from observational studies of a strong inverse association between habitual exercise levels and blood pressure.[40] There is clear and consistent evidence from observational epidemiologic studies that physical activity reduces the risk of heart attack and stroke.[41] The beneficial effects of exercise on vascular endpoints are probably mediated, at least in part, via effects of exercise on blood pressure. A meta-analysis involving 72 trials, 105 study groups (normal blood pressure, prehypertension, and hypertension), and 3936 participants.[48] The meta-analysis shows that endurance training induced significant net reduction of resting and daytime ambulatory blood pressure of, respectively 3.0/2.4 mm Hg and 3.3/3.5 mm Hg.[42] The reduction of resting blood pressure was more pronounced in the 30 hypertensive study groups (−6.9/−4.9 mm Hg) than others.[42] Systemic vascular resistance decreased by 7.1%, plasma norepinephrine by 29%, and plasma renin activity by 20%. Concomitantly, body weight decreased by 1.2 kg and waist circumference by 2.8 cm, and the homeostasis model assessment index of insulin resistance by 3.1 U. On the other hand, high-density lipoprotein (HDL)-cholesterol increased by 0.032 mmol/L. This meta-analysis shows that aerobic endurance training decreases blood pressure through a reduction of vascular resistance, in which the systemic nervous system and the renin-angiotensin system appear to be involved, and favorably affects concomitant cardiovascular risk factors.[42]

Thus sedentary patients should be advised to take up exercise of moderate intensity on a regular basis, such as 30 to 45 minutes daily.[43] The type of exercise should be primarily endurance physical activity (walking, jogging, swimming) supplemented by resistance exercise.[43] However, intensive isometric exercise such as heavy weight lifting can have a marked pressor effect and should be avoided.[11]

Alcohol

In cross-sectional studies, a consistent positive association between alcohol consumption and blood pressure has been observed, which is independent of age, obesity, cigarette smoking, social class, and sodium excretion.[44] Since the positive relationship between alcohol consumption and blood pressure, regardless of the type of alcoholic beverage, is observed worldwide in different cultures and populations, it shows that alcohol itself raises blood pressure. In the BRHS, it was estimated that approximately 10% of hypertension, defined as blood pressure at or above 160/95 mm Hg, could be attributed to moderate or heavy drinking.[45] A Japanese nationwide study in 1980 showed that 32% of hypertension (≥160/95 mm Hg) for men aged 30 to 69 years old was attributable to alcohol consumption. Another Japanese study in 1990 also showed that 34% of hypertension defined as SBP/DBP ≥140/90 mm Hg in men aged 30 years and over was attributable to drinking alcohol.[46] In the U.S. nurses cohort, a prospective study involving 58,218 female registered nurses, of whom 3275 reported a diagnosis of hypertension over 4 years' follow-up, alcohol was an independent predictor of hypertension, with an approximately twofold increased risk among women who consumed more than 35 g of alcohol (about three standard drinks) daily.[47] In this study (as in most cross-sectional studies) there was evidence of a threshold effect, whereby a daily alcohol intake up to about 20 g did not increase the risk of hypertension, but beyond this level the risk increased progressively.

The data from interventional studies are consistent with an important causal role for heavy alcohol consumption in the etiology of hypertension. In a meta-analysis of 15 randomized controlled trials of alcohol and blood pressure in which alcohol reduction was the only intervention, alcohol reduction was associated with a significant reduction in mean (95% confidence interval [CI]) systolic and diastolic blood pressures of −3.31 mm Hg (−2.52 to −4.10 mm Hg) and −2.04 mm Hg (−1.49 to −2.58 mm Hg), respectively. A dose-response relationship was observed between mean percentage of alcohol reduction and mean blood pressure reduction.[48] The mechanism for the putative effects of alcohol on blood pressure are unclear; possibilities include

- a direct pressor effect of alcohol;
- sensitization of resistance vessels to pressor substances;
- stimulation of the sympathetic nervous system (possibly due to fluctuating blood alcohol levels); and
- increased production of adrenocorticoid hormones.

The effect of alcohol on blood pressure is rapidly reversible.[48,49] In a study of 577 factory workers, high recent alcohol intake (within the previous 3 days) but not previous intake was associated with significantly elevated blood pressure, which suggests that the association between alcohol intake and blood pressure may largely reflect a subacute chronic withdrawal phenomenon. Also, 15 previous intervention studies show that the effect of alcohol on blood pressure is refractory.[49] This hypothesis may be relevant to the well-documented phenomenon of variation in blood pressure levels according to the day of week, with higher levels on Mondays.[50]

Dietary Salt

The contribution of dietary factors such as salt to the rise in blood pressure with age and the development of essential hypertension have been difficult to elucidate because of the poor precision (or reliability) with which dietary exposures are measured in free-living subjects and the limited range of dietary exposures in most populations.[7,30] There is also the problem of multicollinearity (i.e., the tendency for dietary elements, such as sodium, potassium, and fat, to be intercorrelated at both the individual and population level). Despite these difficulties, the evidence that salt intake plays a critical role in blood pressure regulation is now overwhelming.[27,28,51,52] The evidence from diverse sources, including observational epidemiologic studies, animal models, and randomized controlled trials in hypertensive and normotensive subjects, all points in the same direction.[51,52] In the International Study of Salt and Blood Pressure (INTERSALT), which included over 10,000 subjects (men and women aged 20 to 59 years) in 52 different population groups in 32 countries, positive associations between urinary sodium excretion (a marker of salt intake) and blood pressure were observed within and between populations.[7,51] Within populations, those with higher sodium excretion tended to have higher blood pressure; in the across-population, ecologic analyses, populations with higher mean sodium excretion had higher mean blood pressures. In men and women at all ages, it was estimated that a 100 mmol/day increase in sodium intake was associated with an average increase in systolic blood pressure of up to 6 mm Hg.[7,51,52] Estimates of association were larger for older people (aged 40 to 59 years) than for younger people (aged 20 to 39 years). One of the key findings from this study was a consistent and highly significant association of sodium excretion across populations with the slope or rise of blood pressure with age.

It is argued that in INTERSALT the magnitude of the effect on blood pressure over a substantial range of sodium excretion (100 mmol/day—approximately 6 g) was small and was further attenuated on adjustment for BMI. However, measurement imprecision affecting both exposure and outcome is undoubtedly a critical issue in observational studies of diet and blood pressure, and the findings from INTERSALT, which is essentially a cross-sectional snapshot of the relation between salt and blood pressure, are supported by evidence from animal and experimental studies.[53] In addition, if a cross-sectional study of the INTERSALT negates confounding factors and a cause-effect relationship is also assured, it is rather reflecting the effect of long-term dietary habit on blood pressure.

In one randomized controlled trial that involved 500 newborn infants in the Netherlands, it was found that infants who were given formula milk and solids with reduced salt content had significantly lower blood pressure at 6 months of age relative to a control group on a standard infant diet.[54] Intriguingly, on re-examination of a subgroup of these children at age 15 years, there was evidence that the beneficial effects of early salt restriction on blood pressure persisted into adolescence.[55] Law and colleagues,[53] in a meta-analysis of 78 trials of the effect of sodium intake on blood pressure, reported that the effects of sodium restriction of at least 5 weeks' duration were consistent with the observational epidemiologic data.

A well-designed clinical trial for testing the effects on blood pressure of reduced dietary sodium and the Dietary Approaches to Stop Hypertension (DASH) diet revealed that the reduction of sodium intake to levels below the current recommendation of 100 mmol (about 6 g salt) per day and the DASH diet both lower blood pressure substantially.[32,56] The magnitude of sodium reduction on systolic blood pressure of the DASH study was compatible with the INTERSALT findings (Fig. 39.2). A meta-analysis based on 17 trials with 734 hypertensive subjects estimated that in people with median age of 50 years old, a reduction in daily salt intake of about 3 g, attainable by moderate dietary salt reduction, will lower SBP by an average of 5 mm Hg. If the group examined contained all individuals, including normotensives, the estimated reduction in SBP/DBP was −2.9/−1.7 mm Hg.[57]

It is estimated from major U.S. and U.K. population studies that a 2 mm Hg reduction in SBP will lower CHD and stroke death by 4% and 6%, respectively.[28] Thus the potential clinical and public health impact of relatively modest salt restriction is substantial. As an example, Japanese people had the highest stroke mortality in the world in 1965, and it is recorded that salt consumption in the 1950s, estimated by 24-hour urine collection, was around 14 to 27 g/day with the highest prevalence of hypertension.[18,58,59] This highest stroke mortality of Japan in the world was reduced dramatically by 80% during 1965 to 1990, with a marked decline in the prevalence of hypertension and in the population blood pressure level following a substantial reduction of salt consumption.[18,59]

Nowadays, the average salt consumption of Japanese people is around 12 g/day.[60] Reductions in salt intake may be of particular benefit in the elderly. In a randomized controlled trial involving men and women aged 60 to 78 years, a reduction in daily salt intake from 10 to 5 g for a period of 1 month was associated with an average fall in SBP of 7 mm Hg.[61] These effects, which were seen in normotensive and hypertensive subjects, translate into an estimated 36% reduction in stroke risk over a 5-year period in this age group. Given the high underlying incidence of stroke in the elderly, a reduction in stroke incidence of this magnitude (more than one third) would represent a public health triumph. In this study, as in similar studies, there was no evidence of a distinct subgroup of so-called salt-sensitive subjects. This concept (much favored by the salt industry) that a minority of the population may be salt sensitive, with the rest of the population being relatively unaffected, has now been discredited.[27]

In addition to the data on salt and blood pressure there is substantial evidence that high salt intake predicts left ventricular hypertrophy.[62] There is also accumulating evidence that in overweight persons, higher dietary salt intake is associated with increased risk of CHD, stroke, and overall mortality.[63,64] Thus, patients who have diagnosed hypertension or who have high normal blood pressure can be advised, on the basis of good evidence, to reduce their salt intake. Most salt in our diet is hidden in processed foods, such as bread, biscuits, and breakfast cereals. Indeed, the salt concentration of many processed foods approaches or exceeds that of seawater.

Potassium

The relation between sodium intake, potassium intake, and blood pressure is complex and has not been completely resolved. The possibility that sodium and potassium are interdependent has been emphasized by the demonstration of consistent associations between the sodium-to-potassium ratio and blood pressure in studies such as INTERSALT.[7] The interventional studies on the relationship between potassium and blood pressure in adults are encouraging and supportive of a causal relation.[65] In a meta-analysis of 33 trials of potassium supplementation (from which one extremely positive study was excluded), Whelton and colleagues[65] observed a significant reduction in mean (95% CI) systolic and diastolic blood pressure of −3.11 mm Hg (−1.91 to −4.31 mm Hg) and −1.97 mm Hg (−0.52 to −3.42 mm Hg), respectively. The effect of potassium supplementation appeared to be enhanced in studies in which participants were concurrently exposed to a high intake of sodium.[65] Preferred strategy to increase potassium intake is to consume foods such as fruits and

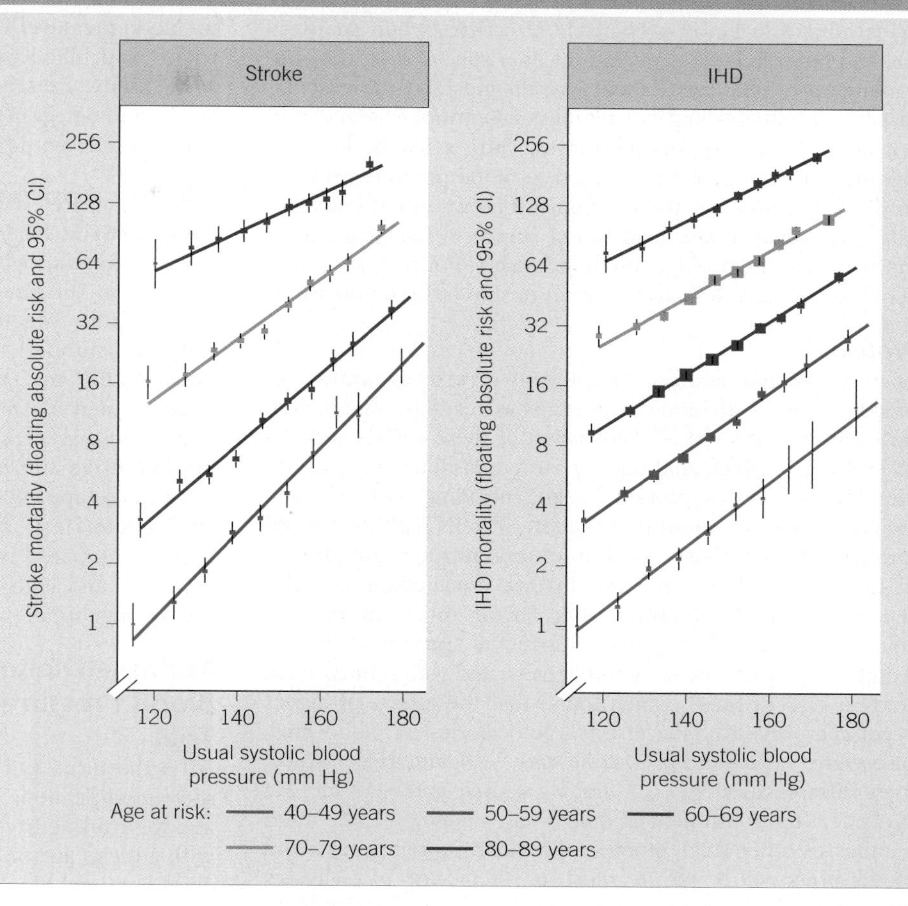

Figure 39.2 Stroke and ischemic heart disease (IHD) mortality rates in each decade of age versus usual systolic blood pressure at the start of that decade. Rates are plotted on a floating absolute scale, and each square has area inversely proportional to the effective variance of the log mortality rate. (From Prospective Studies Collaboration. Lancet 2002;360:1903-1913.)

vegetable that are rich in potassium, rather than supplementation.[29] The DASH diet provides around 4.7 g/day (120 mmol/day) of potassium. The average intake of potassium in the United States from NHANES III is 2.9 to 3.2 g/day (74 to 82 mmol/day) in adult men and 2.1 to 2.3 g/day (54 to 59 mmol/day) in adult women. In the generally healthy population with normal kidney function, an increase in potassium intake is not risky, although high potassium intake may cause adverse cardiac effects due to hyperkalemia in patients with impaired kidney function. Thus, most people with normal renal function will be advised to increase potassium intake through fresh fruits and vegetables.[9,10,29]

Calcium and Magnesium

An inverse association between calcium intake and blood pressure has been reported among women and blacks, and less commonly among white men.[66] The data from clinical trials of the effect of calcium supplementation on blood pressure are inconsistent, and the overall effect, as estimated in meta-analyses of controlled trials, is small (albeit significant) with an average fall in blood pressure of 1.4/0.8 mm Hg.[67]

There is also a weak relationship between magnesium intake and blood pressure in observational studies.[68] As with calcium, trials of the effect of magnesium supplements on blood pressure have been disappointing, with small average falls in blood pressure of limited clinical and population health significance. Overall, data are insufficient to recommend either supplemental calcium or magnesium as a means to lower blood pressure.[10,11,29]

Other Dietary Factors

Fat

Diets varying in total fat and ratios of saturated to unsaturated fat have shown little if any effect on blood pressure with the exception of omega-3 fatty acids from fish oils. Meta-analyses of clinical trials indicate that supplementation with relatively large doses of omega-3 fatty acids lowers blood pressure, although the effect is largely confined to hypertensive people.[69] In the Trials of Hypertension Prevention, however, omega-3 fatty acids did not prevent hypertension in those with high normal blood pressure.[70] The INTERMAP study on macronutrient and blood pressure surveyed 17 diverse population samples from 4 countries (Japan, China, United Kingdom, and United States) for 4680 men and women aged 40 to 59 years old.[30,71] The study was cross-sectional but has a large sample size with high quality of standardized methods. Recently, the INTERMAP study revealed that omega-3 fatty acid intake (total of marine and vegetable source) was weakly and inversely related to SBP and DBP after adjustment for 17 variables.[71] This was observed in both hypertensive and in nonhypertensive individuals. This finding may suggest that 70 g of fatty fish may contribute to lowering SBP by 1 mm Hg.[71]

Dietary intake of omega-6 fatty acids has little effect on blood pressure. The INTERMAP study also found a nonsignificant weak and inverse relationship of linoleic acid (main source of polyunsaturated fatty acids and omega-6 fatty acids) intake to blood pressure.[72] However, when analyzed for "nonintervened" subjects (not on a special diet, not consuming nutritional supplements, no diagnosed cardiovascular disease or diabetes and not taking medication), dietary linoleic acid intake and polyunsaturated fatty acids intake were significantly and inversely related to blood pressure. Several studies have assessed the relationship between monounsaturated fatty acid intake and blood pressure. However, most of the studies did not find any relationship. For saturated fatty acid intake, there was also no relationship to blood pressure.

Protein

In observational studies, a significant inverse association of blood pressure with intake of protein has been reported in multiple adjusted analyses.[73] The largest of these studies was the INTERSALT, which analysed the stored 24-hour urinary samples for markers of protein intake, including total nitrogen excretion, urea-N, and urinary sulfate. The INTERSALT study found significant inverse relation of total nitrogen and urea-N in urine with blood pressure. Inverse associations are also reported from the Multiple Risk Factor Intervention Trial cohort and the Dietary and Nutritional Survey of British Adults. The most recent comprehensive and well standardized study is INTERMAP, which found that the effects of higher vegetable protein intake of 2.8% kilocalories on blood pressure were −2.1 mm Hg systolic and −1.4 mm Hg diastolic; these differences were −1.1 mm Hg systolic and −0.7 mm Hg diastolic after adjustment of height and weight.[74] There are a number of other small studies addressing protein intake and blood pressure; however, most of them are inconclusive because of their methodologies. There are six reports from cohort studies and the results are also inconclusive.

In contrast, recent clinical trials with supplementation of soybean protein found blood pressure lowering effect with some inconsistency. Therefore recent data from both observational studies and clinical trials support the concept that eating vegetable protein lowers blood pressure to some extent. If it is confirmed, this concept will have important public health consequences for lowering population blood pressure and preventing cardiovascular diseases.[72]

Fiber

Some observational studies suggest that dietary fiber intake is inversely related to blood pressure. Recent meta-analysis of 20 randomized controlled clinical trials showed that dietary fiber intake was associated with a significant −1.65 mm Hg reduction in DBP and nonsignificant −1.15 mm Hg reduction in SBP.[75] Effects of dietary fiber intake were stronger in hypertensive subjects than in nonhypertensive subjects. Overall, data are still insufficient for concluding that an increase in dietary fiber intake can lower blood pressure.[29,75,76]

Complex Dietary Patterns

Blood pressure in vegetarians is generally lower than in nonvegetarians. In trials of vegetarian diets it has been shown that substitution of animal with vegetable products reduces blood pressure.[77] In the DASH study,[31,32] the positive effect of vegetarian diets on blood pressure probably reflects the cumulative and synergistic effect of a number of individual nutrients (such as vegetable proteins, potassium, magnesium, and calcium), which in isolation exert relatively small effects on blood pressure. The relationship between dietary micronutrients and blood pressure is being explored in the INTERMAP Study. Presently, it is reported that vegetable protein intake and omega-3 fatty acid intake were related significantly and inversely with blood pressure in the INTERMAP study.[71]

Dietary Approaches to Stop Hypertension (DASH) Trial

The DASH trial (which involved adults with an average SBP of less than 160 mm Hg and a DBP of 80 to 95 mm Hg, a diet rich in fruit, vegetables, and low-fat dairy products with reduced saturated and total fat) lowered SBP by 5.5 mm Hg and DBP by 3.0 mm Hg more than a control diet.[31] In a subsequent DASH-Sodium trial, addressing the separate and combined effects of the DASH diet and salt restriction, normotensive subjects assigned to the DASH diet and low salt intake (approximately 3 g per day) reduced systolic BP by 7.1 mm Hg (7.2 mm Hg for blacks and 6.9 mm Hg for others) compared to those assigned to the control, standard U.S. diet and high salt intake (approximately 9 g per day, the average intake in developed countries).[32]

Multiple Dietary Changes to Lower Blood Pressure—The PREMIER Clinical Trial

After the success of the DASH study, effects of multiple lifestyle modifications to lower blood pressure were examined and their feasibility was also tested for 810 men and women with a mean age of 50 years. The participants' eligibility was above-optimal blood pressure, including stage 1 hypertension (120-159 mm Hg systolic and 80-95 mm Hg diastolic) and who were not taking antihypertensive medications.[78] The PREMIER clinical trial had three arms: a group with long-established recommendation ("established"), established plus DASH diet group, and advise only (control) group. The multibehavioral intervention included weight reduction, increase in moderate intensity physical activity, salt restriction, and alcohol moderation. The trial continued for 18 months. The two intervention groups at the end of 18 months had lower prevalence of hypertension than the control group. Blood pressure was reduced largely in the two intervention groups than in the control group; however, the blood pressure difference was not significant. This well-designed controlled study shows a possibility that multiple and long-term lifestyle modifications may be feasible and effective in lowering blood pressure and preventing hypertension.[78]

Caffeine

Caffeine raises blood pressure acutely, and there is now considerable evidence that chronic coffee consumption raises blood pressure. In a meta-analysis, based on 11 controlled trials in which coffee consumption was the only difference between intervention and control groups, systolic and diastolic blood pressure increased by 2.4 (range, 1.0-3.7) mm Hg and 1.2 (range, 0.4-2.1) mm Hg, respectively, with coffee treatment compared with control. There was an independent, positive relationship between cups of coffee consumed and subsequent change in systolic blood pressure, and the effect of coffee drinking on blood pressure was greater in trials with younger participants.[79] Another recent meta-analysis of 16 randomized controlled trials comprising 1010 subjects also found similar effects of caffeine or coffee on blood pressure rise.[80] When coffee trials and caffeine trials were analyzed separately, blood pressure elevation appeared to be larger for caffeine than for coffee.[80]

Psychosocial Factors

Although there is increasing evidence that psychosocial factors contribute to the development of hypertension, the importance of these factors relative to other dietary and behavioral factors remains uncertain. Although research has focused on possible direct effects of psychosocial "stress" on blood pressure, one must also consider the effect of "stressors," such as poverty, unemployment, and poor education, on aspects of lifestyle that are linked to hypertension, including overeating, a high salt diet, and physical inactivity.[81] In considering psychosocial issues, it is also helpful to distinguish between general features of the environment, such as "social solidarity," and social support and aspects of behavior at the individual level, such as the predominant individual response (or coping) patterns and expression of anger.[82] The former are more likely to be related to blood pressure differences between populations, and the latter may contribute to blood pressure differences within populations.

Acculturation and migrant studies broadly support a role for psychosocial factors in hypertension, although the potential for confounding needs to be considered carefully, especially in relation to changes in body weight, salt intake, and physical activity.[82] In particular, it has been suggested that there may be an important interaction between salt intake and psychosocial stress in the development of hypertension. It may be that high salt sensitizes the vasculature to neurohumoral stimuli.

The role of anxiety and depression as risk factors for incident hypertension was examined in the NHANES I Epidemiologic Follow-up Study. A cohort of 2992 men and women who did not have evidence of hypertension at baseline, were followed for between 7 and 16 years.[83] Anxiety and depression were found to be independent predictors of incident hypertension in both blacks and whites in analyses adjusted for a wide range of potential confounding factors. A population-based, prospective, observational study using participant data from the Coronary Artery Risk Development in Young Adults (CARDIA) study showed that higher two type A behavior patterns, that is, hostile attitudes (hostility) and time urgency/impatience, were significantly associated with risk of developing hypertension at 15-year follow-up for a total of 3308 black and white adults aged 18 to 30 years.[84]

Predictably, the intervention data on psychosocial stress and hypertension are sparse and unhelpful. In a recent meta-analysis of trials that involved stress management techniques, such as meditation and biofeedback with at least 6 months of follow-up, only eight trials that met the inclusion criteria were identified and the findings were inconsistent.[39]

Intrauterine Growth and Hypertension

Barker and Clark[85] have developed the hypothesis that hypertension and related cardiovascular risk factors, including central obesity, hyperlipidemia, glucose intolerance, and type 2 diabetes, originate through impaired growth and development during fetal life and infancy. Based on data from a series of historic cohort studies, it is suggested that low birth weight and other indices of abnormal growth in utero and during early life, including an elevated ratio of placental to birth weight and low Ponderal index (height divided by the cube of the weight, a marker of thinness), are associated with higher blood pressure, glucose intolerance, other cardiovascular risk factors, and increased risk of cardiovascular disease events and mortality in adult life.[85] A recent meta-analysis from 20 Nordic cohorts (birth years 1910-1987) revealed an inverse association between birth weight and SBP, irrespective of adjustment for concurrent body mass index. The estimated effect of birth weight on SBP at age 50 years was −1.52 mm Hg/kg (95% CI, −2.27 to −0.77) in men and −2.80 mm Hg/kg (95% CI, −3.85 to −1.76) in women.[86]

Hypertension and related cardiovascular disease risk factors may be consequences of "programming," whereby a stimulus or insult at a specific, critical, sensitive period of early life results in long-term changes in specific aspects of physiology and metabolism.[85] This is an important and exciting hypothesis, which has shifted the focus of work on the environmental origins of hypertension and related cardiovascular risk factors from middle age to early life.[86]

Genetic Study for Hypertension

A large number of investigations for searching genetic factors of hypertension have been done, and some rare genetic disorders that raise blood pressure and are also related to hypertension were found. In addition, genetic association studies have identified polymorphisms in several candidate genes for raising blood pressure. However, none of these genetic abnormalities has been shown to be responsible for any influence on blood pressure level and also the prevalence of hypertension in the general population.[11]

PROGNOSIS

Data from prospective observational studies for participants with no past history of stroke or CHD suggest that usual systolic blood pressure levels are directly and continuously related to the risk of both stroke and CHD (CHD is expressed as IHD in the figure) (Fig. 39.2).[87] Throughout middle age, a SBP 20 mm Hg lower than usual in associated with a greater than twofold difference in the risk of stroke death and a twofold difference in the risk of CHD death, although the strength of the association between the risk of stroke and CHD death and usual SBP declines to some extent with increasing age at death. This association is as strong in the normotensive as in the hypertensive range of blood pressure in subjects who have no previous history of CHD or stroke. Even as the lowest levels of blood pressure are approached, the incidence of both stroke and CHD continues to decline. Thus, for populations with a high prevalence of cardiovascular disease, small shifts in mean population blood pressure should lead to sizeable reductions in the incidence of stroke and CHD. It is also estimated from epidemiologic studies in the United States and United Kingdom that 2 mm Hg SBP reduction in the population would result in a 5% reduction of stroke mortality and 4% reduction of CHD mortality.[28] A similar estimation has been obtained in Japanese cohort studies.[18]

In meta-analyses, the pooled effects from a large number of trials indicate that a reduction in DBP of 5 to 6 mm Hg that is maintained for a few years reduces the risk of stroke by approximately 38% and the risk of CHD by approximately 16%.[4]

SUMMARY

Hypertension represents a major global public health challenge. There is no threshold for the graded relationship between blood pressure level and cardiovascular disease (CVD) morbidity and mortality. Therefore it is very important for reducing population blood pressure level by means of lifestyle modification: salt restriction, prevention of obesity epidemic, moderation of alcohol consumption, and prevention of physical inactivity. Other dietary approaches, such as increased intake of vegetables, fruits, and vegetable protein; reduction of fat intake in the most developed countries; and increased intake of omega-3 fatty acids may also contribute to the reduction in blood pressure level and prevalence of hypertension in a population. In general, the effect of each dietary modification on reducing blood pressure is small; however, their additive effects may result in a substantial fall in population blood pressure and in CVD mortality and morbidity. If the population systolic blood pressure were lowered by 2 mm Hg, it is estimated that around 6% reduction of stroke and 4% reduction of CHD may result. This is called a "population strategy" by Rose.[88] On the other hand, "high risk strategy" detection, and treatment and control of hypertension is also important for the prevention of CVD in hypertensive people, although this approach does not contribute as much as a population approach, as a whole, for reducing CVD morbidity and mortality in a population. Therefore, as a public health measure, it is very important to suggest appropriate lifestyle guidelines that people can easily follow. In this context, food labeling of salt content may be an effective and useful measure for salt reduction within a population. The action for reducing population salt intake, such as "World Action of Salt and Health" by MacGregor and Sever,[89] may be an important and effective public health leadership for reducing high salt intake in a population through raising awareness of the importance of salt reduction in the world. For future studies, not only the epidemiologic observational studies on lifestyles, especially dietary habits and nutrients and food intake, but also interventional studies are important for making and implementing useful public health policy and treatment measures for patient education.

chapter 40

Clinical Recognition of Hypertension

Shawna D. Nesbitt, Wanpen Vongpatanasin, and Ronald G. Victor

Issue/Problems

- Early clinical recognition of hypertension is the first step in improving control.

Key Findings

- The proper technique of blood pressure measurement is the cornerstone of early hypertension detection.
- The initial evaluation of the hypertensive patient should focus on not only the level of blood pressure, but also the presence and severity of target organ damage and the presence of other cardiovascular risk factors and comorbidities.
- Appropriate treatment thresholds and goals should be established.

Clinical Implications

- Individualized treatment strategy for the hypertensive patient should be predicated on assessment of overall cardiovascular risk.

Nearly 30% of adults in the United States suffer from hypertension.[1] It is the most common reason for a physician office visit.[1] A meta-analysis of 1 million persons worldwide demonstrated the risk of fatal heart attack and stroke doubled with every increase of 20 mm Hg in systolic and/or 10 mm Hg in diastolic blood pressure (BP) from an initial blood pressure of 115/75 mm Hg (Fig. 40.1).[2] Similarly hypertension bears a strong relationship to peripheral vascular disease, aortic dissection, chronic renal failure, and dementia. Despite these known facts, hypertension remains poorly treated in the majority of affected individuals in all countries.[3] Although hypertension awareness is increasing in all U.S. ethnic groups, treatment and control rates lag far behind.[1] Inadequate treatment of hypertension is a major factor contributing to some of the adverse secular trends in the last decade, including an increased incidence of stroke, heart failure, and renal failure, as well as a reduction in the decline in coronary heart disease mortality.

Early recognition is critical since the estimated lifetime risk of developing hypertension is 90%.[4] Additionally, hypertension is frequently accompanied by other comorbidities, such as dyslipidemia, overweight and obesity, and diabetes.[5-7] Because hypertension is largely asymptomatic for years, clinical recognition of hypertension rests on the accurate measurement of blood pressure accompanied by an accurate history and physical examination.

It is essential to determine

- the duration and staging of blood pressure elevation;
- the presence of target organ damage;
- the presence of other comorbidities; and
- the likelihood of secondary hypertension.

DIAGNOSTIC CRITERIA

Although the relationship of blood pressure to cardiovascular risk is continuous, expert panels have designated treatment guidelines based on epidemiologic and clinical trial data assessing the risk-benefit ratio of treatment to assist clinicians in management. For example, the Framingham study demonstrated that high normal blood pressure carries higher risk of cardiovascular disease than optimal blood pressure.[8] For the general population, hypertension is defined as blood pressures of 140 mm Hg or higher systolic or 90 mm Hg diastolic. There are five major sets of guidelines: the Seventh Report of the Joint National Committee on Prevention, Detection, Evaluation and Treatment of High Blood Pressure (JNC 7), the Hypertension African American Working Group Consensus Statement (HAAWG), the American Heart Association (AHA) Cardiovascular guidelines 2007, the British Hypertension guidelines, and the European Society of Hypertension guidelines. Table 40.1[9-13] shows the JNC 7 classification for adults. The most prominent change to this classification is the newly defined "prehypertension" stage and that normal blood pressure is considered less than 120/80 mm Hg. This is in recognition of the continuous relationship of blood pressure to cardiovascular death. This classification applies to individuals aged 18 years and over who are not taking antihypertensive medications and who are not acutely ill. Although not all of the guidelines have adopted the same terminology of classification, all clearly acknowledge the progression of cardiovascular risk with increasing blood pressure even below the threshold of 140/90 mm Hg.

The emergence of the class of prehypertension highlights the importance of the progression of blood pressure. The recent Trial of Preventing Hypertension (TROPHY) showed that 63% of the upper 50th percentile of prehypertension (BP 130-139/85-89 mm Hg) will develop clinical hypertension in 4 years (Fig. 40.2),[14] whereas the Framingham study shows that the lower 50th percentile of prehypertension (BP 120-129/80-85 mm Hg) will develop clinical hypertension at a rate of 5% to 25% over 4 years, depending on age.[15] When a person's systolic and diastolic pressures fall into different stages, the higher stage should apply.

The initial evaluation for hypertension should focus on (1) staging the blood pressure; (2) assessing the patient's overall cardiovascular risk; and (3) detecting clues indicating potential identifiable causes of hypertension that require further evaluation. A thorough history and physical examination; routine laboratory studies for urinalysis, complete blood cell count,

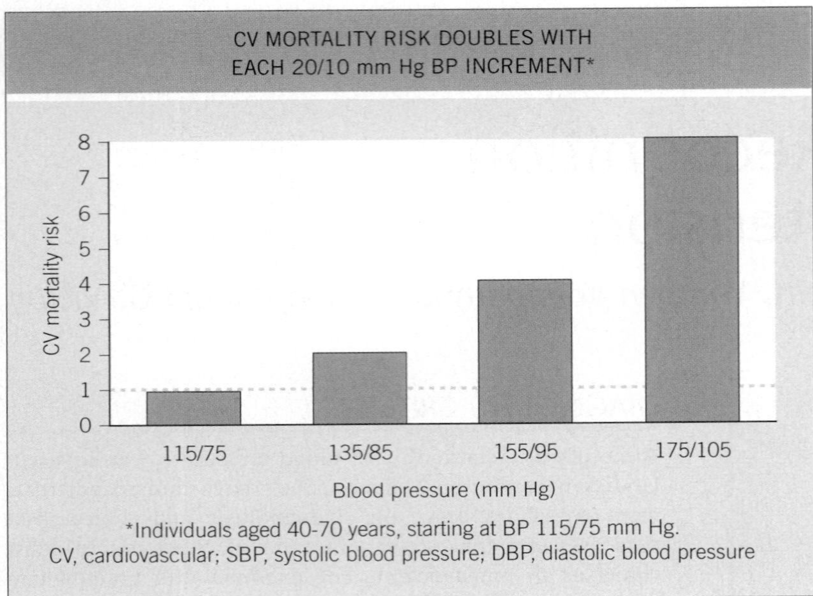

Figure 40.1 A meta-analysis of 1 million persons worldwide demonstrated that the risk of fatal heart attack and stroke doubled with every increase of 20 mm Hg in systolic and/or 10 mm Hg in diastolic blood pressure from an initial blood pressure of 115/75 mm Hg. (From Chobanian AV, Bakris GL, Black HR, et al, for the Joint National Committee. The Seventh Report of the Joint National Committee on Prevention, Detection, Evaluation, and Treatment of High Blood Pressure. The JNC-7 Report. JAMA 2003;289:2560-2572.)

STAGING OF OFFICE BLOOD PRESSURE

Blood Pressure Stage	Systolic (mm Hg)	Diastolic (mm Hg)
Normal	<120	<80
Prehypertension	120-139	80-89
Hypertension		
Stage 1	140-159	90-99
Stage 2	≥160	≥100

Modified from Chobanian AV, Bakris GL, Black HR, et al, for the Joint National Committee. The Seventh Report of the Joint National Committee on Prevention, Detection, Evaluation, and Treatment of High Blood Pressure: the JNC 7 report. JAMA 2003;289:2560-2572.

Table 40.1 Staging of office blood pressure.

potassium, sodium, creatinine, fasting glucose, total cholesterol, and high-density lipoprotein cholesterol; and a resting 12-lead electrocardiogram are necessary to obtain the initial clinical data needed to accomplish these goals. Other useful tests include microalbuminuria (albumin:creatinine ratio) and blood levels of calcium, uric acid, fasting triglycerides, low-density lipoprotein cholesterol, glycosylated hemoglobin, and thyroid stimulating hormone. In some patients an echocardiogram may provide helpful additional data about the burden of blood pressure on the cardiovascular system.

Twenty-four hour variability is inherent to blood pressure. Therefore a proper assessment of blood pressure must include multiple measurements on at least two visits. Blood pressure should be taken at least twice after a 5-minute quiet rest period while the patient is comfortably seated, with the feet on the floor and back supported (Fig. 40.3). The arm should be supported at heart level and the cuff should be appropriately sized for the arm of the individual. Patients should be instructed not to use tobacco or caffeine within 30 minutes of measurement. To minimize the possibility of missing the true systolic blood pressure in patients who may have an auscultatory gap, the radial artery pulse should be palpated while inflating the cuff on the upper arm until the pulse disappears. This approximates the systolic blood pressure. Then the cuff should be inflated to 20 mm Hg above this pressure and deflated at a rate of 2 to 3 mm Hg per second while auscultating over the brachial artery. The systolic blood pressure and diastolic blood pressures correspond to the Korotkoff sounds I and V, respectively. To assess postural changes and anatomic abnormalities, blood pressure should be measured in both arms while seated as well standing after 5 minutes.[9] During the initial assessment, blood pressures should be measured in both upper extremities and in the lower extremities for comparison, because unequal blood pressures are suggestive of coarctation of the aorta.

Blood pressures are often higher in the physician's office than when measured at home; this has been described as the "white coat" or "office only" elevation. This condition is defined as daytime (out of office) blood pressures less than 130/80 mm Hg, with office readings greater than 140/90 mm Hg and no evidence of target organ damage. The prognostic importance of white coat hypertension remains unresolved, but increasing evidence suggests that this condition may not be benign.[16] The opposite condition, so-called masked hypertension, reverse hypertension, or home hypertension, is defined as daytime out-of-office blood pressures greater than 130/80 mm Hg with office readings less than 140/90 mm Hg.[17]

Home self-monitoring of blood pressure not only assists in the evaluation of this effect for therapeutic choices but importantly also actively engages a patient in his or her own health care. However, the devices need to be checked for accuracy in the office. Patients should be instructed to

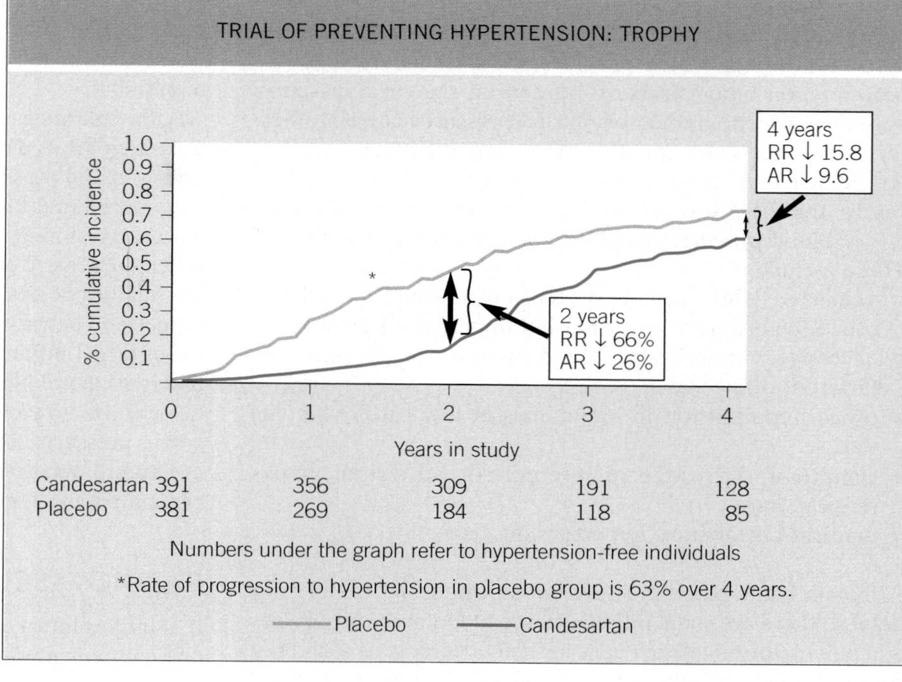

Figure 40.2 The recent Trial of Preventing Hypertension (TROPHY) showed that 63% of the upper 50th percentile of prehypertension (BP 130-139/ 85-89 mm Hg) will develop clinical hypertension in 4 years. (From Julius S, Nesbitt SD, Egan BM, et al. Feasibility of treating prehypertension with an angiotensin-receptor blocker. N Engl J Med 2006;354:1685-1697.)

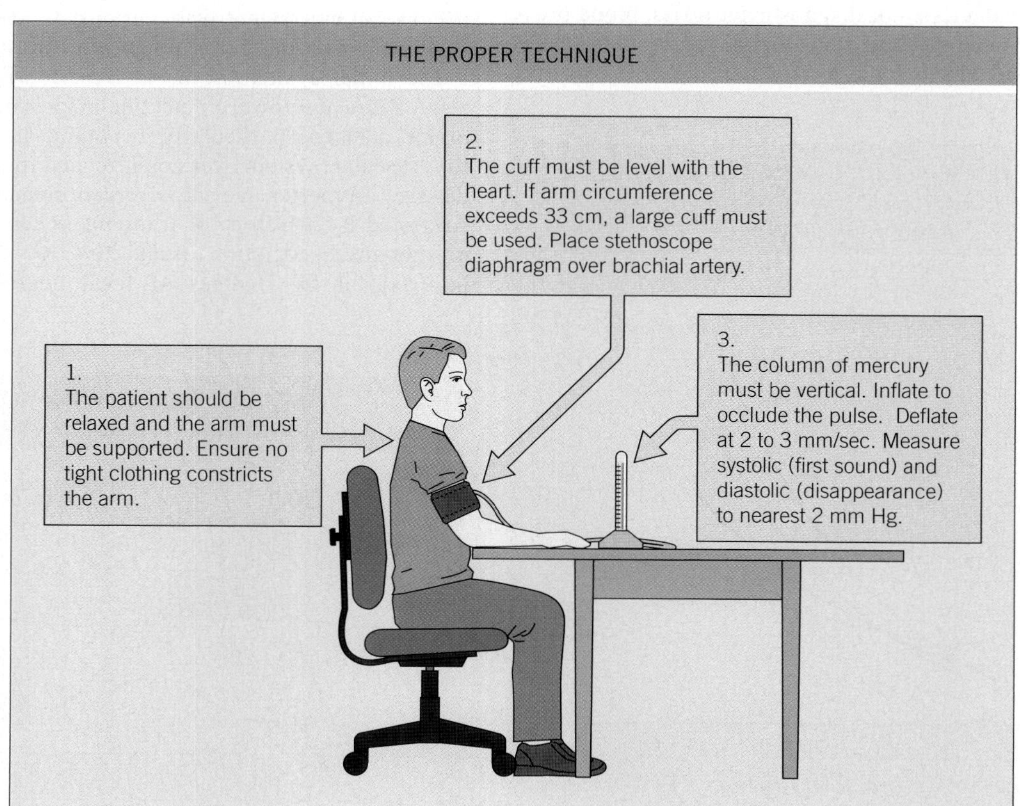
THE PROPER TECHNIQUE
1.
The patient should be relaxed and the arm must be supported. Ensure no tight clothing constricts the arm.
2.
The cuff must be level with the heart. If arm circumference exceeds 33 cm, a large cuff must be used. Place stethoscope diaphragm over brachial artery.
3.
The column of mercury must be vertical. Inflate to occlude the pulse. Deflate at 2 to 3 mm/sec. Measure systolic (first sound) and diastolic (disappearance) to nearest 2 mm Hg.

Figure 40.3 The proper technique of blood pressure measurement. (Modified from Kaplan NM. Measurement of Blood Pressure. In Kaplan NM, ed. Kaplan's Clinical Hypertension, 8th ed. Philadelphia, Lippincott Williams & Wilkins, 2002:pp38.)

record their blood pressures at various times. An even more reliable diagnostic tool is 24-hour ambulatory blood pressure monitoring, which provides the best measure of the time-integral blood pressure burden on the cardiovascular system. As such, ambulatory blood pressures correlate better than office readings with target organ damage, such as left ventricular hypertrophy (LVH) (Fig. 40.4).[16,18] Currently, there are several situations in which home or ambulatory blood pressure monitoring is particularly useful.[19,20] These include

- suspected white coat hypertension, defined as isolated office hypertension with normal home blood pressure;
- excessive variability of blood pressure at the same or different office visits;
- office hypertension in individuals at low cardiovascular risk;
- symptoms suggestive of intermittent orthostatic hypotension; and
- medication-resistant hypertension.

Although home blood pressure monitoring is in general very helpful, there are some pitfalls. Home blood pressure devices and ambulatory monitors vary in their accuracy; as such they should be periodically validated, ideally against a mercury column to ensure accuracy. However such mercury devices are increasingly more difficult to acquire, given tighter occupational health standards. Therefore in most cases home devices are calibrated in the doctor's office against aneroid or oscillometric devices. For diagnostic purposes, blood pressure readings need not be taken more often than twice weekly. Occasionally a patient may become obsessed and anxious about the normal variability of blood pressure readings; to minimize these responses all patients need to be instructed on the appropriate use of home blood pressure monitors.

Although measurements of clinic or ambulatory blood pressures are typically obtained from the brachial or radial artery, blood pressure in the central aorta may differ greatly from peripheral blood pressure in the same subject, depending on the timing of forward pressure waveform relative to reflected wave from the peripheral vasculature. An increasing number of observational studies in hypertensive patients suggested central aortic blood pressure as a stronger predictor of target organ damage and cardiovascular complications than peripheral blood pressure.[21,22] A variety of noninvasive devices are now clinically available for estimation of central aortic pressure. Reliability of these devices and usefulness of routine measurement of central aortic blood pressure in clinical practice remain to be determined.

CARDIOVASCULAR RISK ASSESSMENT

It is important to emphasize that blood pressure level is only one component of the overall cardiovascular risk. The risk of cardiovascular disease is directly related to the number of risk factors in an individual.[23] Furthermore, most hypertensive individuals have concomitant risk factors even in the prehypertensive range of blood pressure (Fig. 40.5).[24,25] Thus comorbidity and target organ damage contribute to the overall assessment of hypertensive disease and likewise have an impact on the treatment decisions that follow.[9]

The initial evaluation of the hypertensive patient should also be directed toward detecting evidence of existing target organ damage, particularly in brain, heart, kidney, and the vascular system (retinopathy and peripheral vascular disease). Hypertensive target organ damage in the brain is suggested by a history of transient ischemic attack, stroke, or impaired cognition (suggestive of repeated lacunar infarcts), or by findings of focal neurologic deficits on

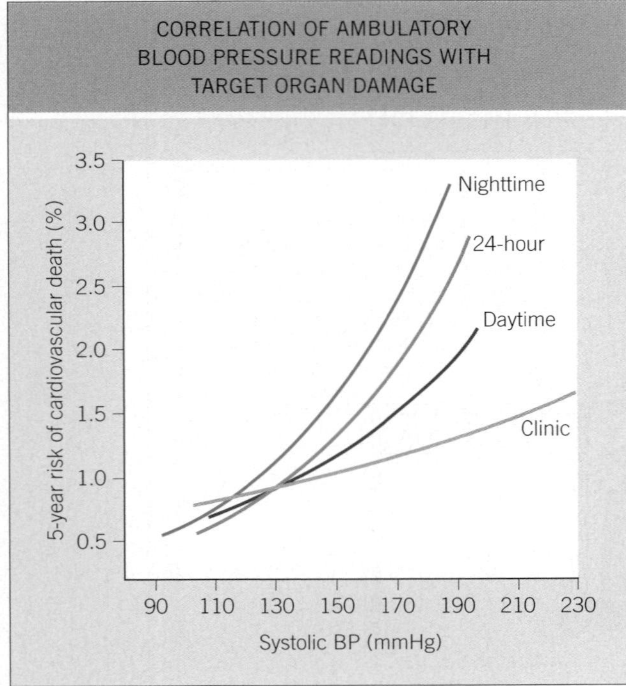

Figure 40.4 Ambulatory blood pressures correlate better than office readings with target organ damage, such as left ventricular hypertrophy (LVH).

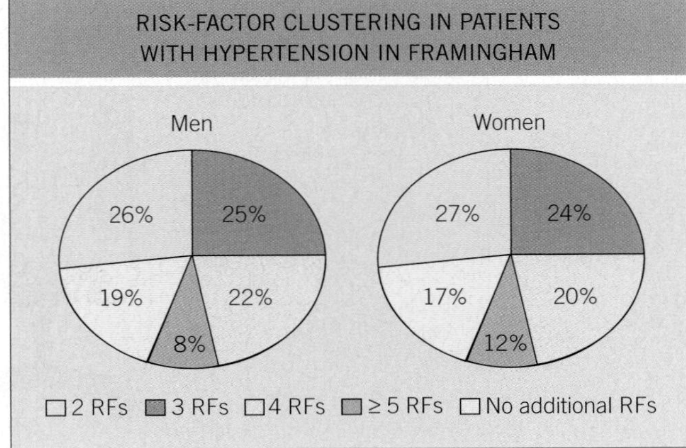

Figure 40.5 The risk of cardiovascular disease is directly related to the number of risk factors (RFs) in an individual. Furthermore, most hypertensive individuals have concomitant risk factors even in the prehypertensive range of blood pressure.

physical examination. A history of heart failure, angina, prior myocardial infarction or revascularization procedures, or electrocardiographic findings of left ventricular hypertrophy suggest hypertensive target organ damage in the heart. Routine echocardiography would be optimal, if available, because it has greater sensitivity in detecting left ventricular hypertrophy and it provides additional information about left ventricular geometry and diastolic and systolic ventricular function. As many as half of patients who present for their initial evaluation of hypertension will already have echocardiographic evidence of left ventricular hypertrophy.[26] Recent studies suggest not only that left ventricular mass is a powerful predictor of subsequent cardiovascular events, but also that reduction in LVH through treatment will reduce cardiovascular events.[27]

An elevated serum creatinine level or the presence of proteinuria suggests hypertensive target organ damage in the kidney. Hypertensive target organ damage in the peripheral arterial circulation is suggested by a history of intermittent or rest claudication, by findings of abdominal or carotid bruits, reduced peripheral pulses on physical examination or ultrasound, or radiologic confirmation of peripheral atherosclerotic plaque. Finally, during every initial evaluation of the hypertensive patient, the pupils should be dilated for careful assessment of the retinal manifestations of hypertension.

High-Risk Hypertension

The recommendations for high-risk populations have broadened to include more special groups. In 2003 with the publication of the JNC 7 and HAAWG guidelines, only diabetics and patients with renal disease were identified as high risk. However, in 2007 the AHA Council for High Blood Pressure issued recommendations that expanded the high-risk populations to include patients with stable angina, unstable angina, non–ST elevation myocardial infarction (NSTEMI), ST elevation myocardial infarction (STEMI), left ventricular dysfunction (LVD), peripheral arterial disease, carotid artery disease, patients with a 10-year Framingham risk score of coronary artery disease of 10% or greater, and heart failure. Pharmacologic therapy should be initiated at blood pressure of 130/80 mm Hg for these high-risk populations (Table 40.2).[11]

HIGH-RISK POPULATIONS WITH TREATMENT THRESHOLD AND GOAL BP ≤130/80 mm Hg
Diabetes
Renal disease
10-year Framingham risk ≥10%
Unstable or stable angina
NSTEMI or STEMI
Peripheral arterial disease
Aortic vascular disease
Carotid artery disease
CHF
LV dysfunction (goal <120/80)

BP, blood pressure; CHF, congestive heart failure; LV, left ventricular; NSTEMI, non–ST elevation myocardial infarction; STEMI, ST elevation myocardial infarction.

From Chobanian AV, Bakris GL, Black HR, et al, for the Joint National Committee. The seventh report of the Joint National Committee on prevention, detection, evaluation, and treatment of high blood pressure. JAMA 2003;289:2560-2572; Douglas JG, Bakris GL, Epstein M, et al, for the Hypertension in African Americans Working Group. Management of high blood pressure in African Americans. Consensus Statement of the Hypertension in African Americans Working Group of the International Society on Hypertension in Blacks. Arch Intern Med 2003;163:525-541; Rosendorff C, Black HR, Cannon CP et al. Treatment of Hypertension in the Prevention and Management of Ischemic Heart Disease: A Scientific Statement From the American Heart Association Council for High Blood Pressure Research and the Councils on Clinical Cardiology and Epidemiology and Prevention. Circulation 2007;115:2761-2788.

Table 40.2 High-risk populations with treatment threshold and goal BP ≤130/80 mm Hg.

Secondary Hypertension: Identifiable Causes

It is not clinically indicated to perform screening tests on every hypertensive individual for secondary causes of hypertension, because these entities account for only 5% of all cases of hypertension. Although rare, secondary causes are important to identify because they are potentially curable forms of hypertension. However, evaluation is clearly indicated when historical clues and physical examination findings are suggestive of secondary hypertension (Table 40.3). The major causes of secondary hypertension are summarized in Table 40.4.[28]

Other behavioral factors and concomitant conditions may affect the diagnosis of hypertension. The recent increase in the prevalence of overweight has an important effect on blood pressure and cardiovascular risk. Treatment for blood pressure clearly includes weight management strategies; thus recognition is essential. In addition, other conditions such as sleep apnea have an effect on blood pressure, and importantly, diagnosis and treatment of sleep apnea may improve blood pressure considerably.[29,30] Ingestion of excess alcohol, over-the-counter drugs, recreational drugs, herbal products, licorice (glycyrrhetinic acid), and other prescription drugs may affect the presentation of blood pressure (Table 40.5).[31,32]

WHO SHOULD BE SCREENED FOR SECONDARY HYPERTENSION? HISTORICAL CLUES*
■ Resistance to ≥3 drug therapy
■ Young age of onset of HTN (<30 years)
■ Worsening of hypertension
■ Episodes of extreme BP elevation
■ Low potassium and muscle cramps
■ Daytime sleepiness, snoring, poor sleep habits

*For physical examination clues, see Table 40.4.
BP, blood pressure; HTN, hypertension.

Table 40.3 Who should be screened for secondary hypertension? Historical clues.

GUIDE TO EVALUATION OF SECONDARY HYPERTENSION		
Suspected Dx	**Clinical Features**	**Diagnostic Testing**
Renal parenchymal hypertension	Elevated serum creatinine or abnormal urinalysis	24-hr urine creatinine and protein, renal ultrasound
Renovascular disease	New elevation in serum creatinine, marked elevation in serum creatinine with initiation of ACEI or ARB, refractory hypertension, flash pulmonary edema, abdominal bruit	MR or CT angiogram, invasive angiogram
Coarctation of the aorta	Arm pulses > leg pulses, arm BP > leg BP, chest bruits, rib notching on CXR	MRA, aortogram
Primary aldosteronism	Hypokalemia, refractory hypertension	Plasma renin and aldosterone, 24-h urine potassium, 24-h urine aldosterone and potassium after salt loading, saline suppression testing
Cushing's syndrome	Truncal obesity, purple striae, muscle weakness	Plasma cortisol, urine cortisol after dexamethasone, adrenal CT scan
Pheochromocytoma	Spells of tachycardia, headache, diaphoresis, pallor, and anxiety	Plasma-free metanephrines, 24-h urine fractionated metanephrines, adrenal CT scan, MIBG scan
Obstructive sleep apnea	Loud snoring, daytime somnolence, obesity	Sleep study

BP, blood pressure; CXR, chest X-ray; CT, computerized tomography; MR, magnetic resonance; MIBG, metaiodobenzylguanidine scan.
Modified from Kaplan NM. Kaplan's Clinical Hypertension, 8th ed. Philadelphia, Lippincott Williams & Wilkins, 2002.

Table 40.4 Guide to evaluation of secondary hypertension.

BEHAVIORAL FACTORS ASSOCIATED WITH THE RECOGNITION OF HYPERTENSION
Obesity
Sleep apnea
Alcohol intake
Herbal supplements
OTC drugs: NSAIDs, nasal decongestants, appetite suppressants, immunosuppressants, British licorice (glycyrrhetinic acid)
Concomitant drugs: immunosuppressants, erythropoietin, hormonal replacement therapy, beta-agonist inhalers
Recreational drugs: (e.g., cocaine, crystal methamphetamine)

OTC, over-the-counter; NSAIDs, nonsteroidal anti-inflammatory drugs.

Table 40.5 Behavioral factors associated with the recognition of hypertension.

SUMMARY

Early clinical recognition of hypertension is the first step in improving hypertension control rates. Accurate assessment of blood pressure is a critical feature in the assessment of hypertensive risk. Yet, the prognosis depends not only on the level of blood pressure, but also on the presence and severity of other risk factors, target organ damage, and comorbidity. Currently, risk factor assessments use the presence of clinically manifest end-organ disease. Implementing prevention maneuvers at an earlier point in the development of hypertensive disease may have a resounding effect on the rates of subsequent cardiovascular disease.

chapter 41

Complications of Hypertension: The Heart

Chim C. Lang, Henry Krum, and Gregory Y. H. Lip

Definition

- The clinical cardiac complications of persistently and abnormally increased systemic blood pressure include increased left ventricular (LV) mass, with or without chamber dilatation, left atrial abnormalities, myocardial ischemia, systolic and diastolic LV dysfunction, atrial and ventricular arrhythmias, and sudden death.

Key Findings

- The cardiac complications of hypertension result from the interaction of hemodynamic, vascular, cardiac, and neurohumoral pathogenetic processes, including increased LV wall stress, alterations in myocardial gene expression, endothelial dysfunction, and activation of the adrenergic and renin-angiotensin systems.
- Left ventricular hypertrophy (LVH), whether diagnosed by electrocardiography or by echocardiography, is a major contributor to the major cardiac complications.
- Heart failure related to hypertension is characterized by ventricular remodeling and may progress from asymptomatic diastolic LV dysfunction to symptomatic systolic dysfunction, according to the degree of blood pressure control and the extent of any myocardial ischemia.
- Concurrent atherosclerotic coronary heart disease and hypertension increase the risk of all cardiovascular events and the likelihood of complications of the acute coronary syndromes.
- Arrhythmias and sudden cardiac death are increased in hypertensive patients, especially those with LVH and myocardial ischemia.

Clinical Implications

- Decreasing blood pressure to optimal levels is paramount.
- Reducing total absolute cardiovascular disease risk by treating risk factors, such as diabetes, dyslipidemia, cigarette smoking, and physical inactivity, is a critical component of treatment.
- Regression of LVH is associated with most antihypertensive agents (except direct-acting vasodilators). The regression of LVH reduces overall cardiovascular risk and atrial fibrillation and improves outcomes.
- Selection of antihypertensive therapy that is also appropriate for the treatment of concomitant cardiac complications (i.e., angiotensin-converting enzyme inhibitors and/or angiotensin receptor antagonists for LV systolic dysfunction; angiotensin receptor antagonists for LV diastolic dysfunction; beta blockers for angina pectoris, post–myocardial infarction, and atrial or ventricular arrhythmias) is essential.

The heart is responsible for the pathogenesis of hypertension, yet it also suffers its consequences. The earliest changes in cardiac hemodynamics are largely compensatory in nature, but if a patient's hypertension is untreated or uncontrolled, these invariably lead to compromise of cardiac structure and function. In particular, it has been well recognized that the presence of left ventricular hypertrophy (LVH) is an adverse feature in hypertension, with affected patients having a substantially greater risk of cardiovascular events, including mortality and morbidity from heart failure, atrial fibrillation, sudden death, and stroke. Indeed, LVH is probably the most visible manifestation of hypertensive target organ damage. However, hypertension is a complex disease in which several genetic and demographic factors, comorbid diseases (e.g., diabetes and obesity), pathophysiologic processes, and environmental influences interact to produce a wide array of target organ damage. The major clinical consequences of hypertension stem not only from the effects of increased blood pressure but also from pathophysiologic, functional, and structural responses to hypertension (Table 41.1).

PATHOPHYSIOLOGY OF HYPERTENSIVE HEART DISEASE

The presence of hypertension more than doubles the risk for coronary artery disease, including myocardial infarction and sudden death, and more than triples the risk of congestive heart failure.[1-3] Although hypertension, coronary artery disease, and heart failure are separate disease processes with their distinct natural histories, they are clinically linked and their courses critically affect one another.[4,5] For example, coronary hemodynamics may be altered, with reduced coronary flow reserve, in hypertension. This may reflect a reduction in the density of resistance coronary arterioles, an increase in wall thickness-to-lumen ratio, a reduction in coronary vasodilator capacity, and an increase in the systolic impediment to coronary flow in hypertrophy.[6] These coronary alterations may directly contribute to impaired ventricular function. However, in the late stages of hypertension, there may be marked interstitial fibrosis and structural remodeling of the LV chamber, which will also result in reduced contractile efficiency.

These findings underpin the concept of "hypertensive heart disease" as a distinct entity, which is independent of other common associated diseases such as atheromatous coronary artery disease.[4,5] Hypertensive heart disease has been defined as the response of the heart to the afterload imposed on the left ventricle by the progressively increasing arterial pressure and total peripheral resistance produced by the hypertensive vascular disease.[7] Specifically, hypertensive heart disease is characterized by altered coronary hemodynamics and reserve, cardiac dysrhythmias, LVH and

CARDIAC COMPLICATIONS OF SYSTEMIC HYPERTENSION

Left ventricular Hypertrophy +/− Chamber Dilation	Left Atrial Abnormalities
Heart failure	Diastolic dysfunction Asymptomatic left ventricular dysfunction Asymptomatic left ventricular dilatation Symptomatic heart failure
Coronary heart disease	Angina pectoris Acute coronary syndromes
Arrhythmias and sudden death	Atrial arrhythmias Ventricular arrhythmias Sudden cardiac death

Table 41.1 Cardiac complications of systemic hypertension.

enlargement, ventricular fibrosis, diastolic dysfunction, and cardiac failure.

Hypertensive heart disease develops in response to mutually shared genetic determinants, environmental risk factors, and hemodynamic and nonhemodynamic mechanisms (Fig. 41.1). Because the heart and conduit vessels are integral components of a pulsatile pumping system, the hemodynamic mechanisms that lead to hypertensive heart disease include both cardiac elements (myocardial contractility and wall stress,[8] stroke volume[9]) and vascular factors (peripheral resistance and vascular compliance[10]), which undergo complex, interrelated adaptive and degenerative changes in response to the chronic increase in mean and pulsatile hemodynamic load (Table 41.2).

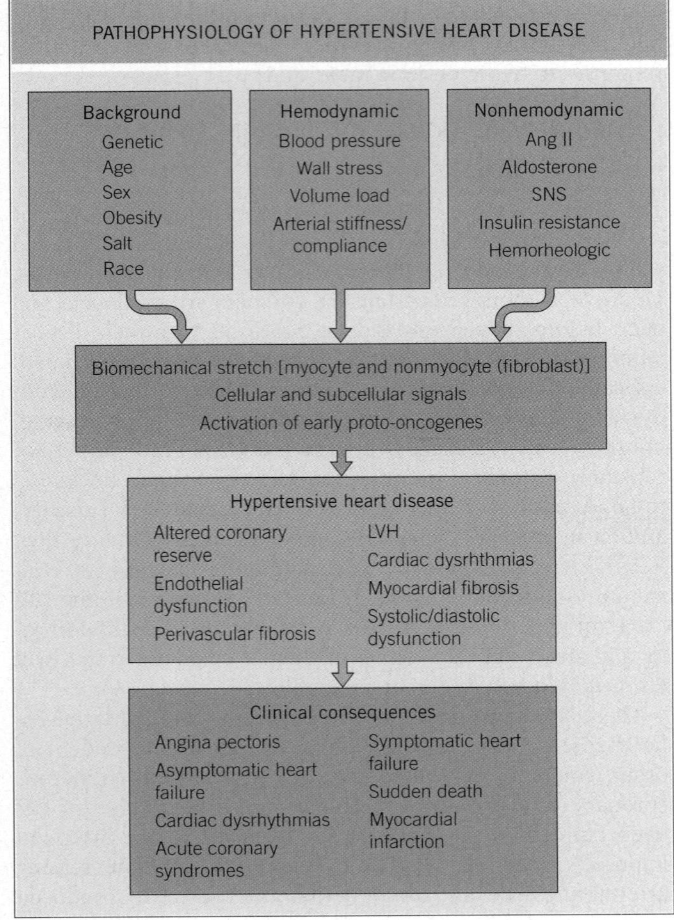

Figure 41.1 Pathophysiology of hypertensive heart disease. Ang II, angiotensin II; LVH, left ventricular hypertrophy; SNS, sympathetic nervous system.

Although hemodynamic load is the basic initial stimulus to begin the sequence of biological events leading to the development of hypertensive heart disease, nonhemodynamic factors may also influence and contribute to the cascade of molecular changes that eventually yield the adverse structural remodeling that begets hypertensive heart disease. These nonhemodynamic factors include age, race, genetic contributions, obesity, salt intake, insulin resistance,[11-13] and a number of neuroendocrine factors (such as angiotensin II, aldosterone, sympathetic tone, endothelin) and hemorheologic factors (blood viscosity, plasma volume).[14,15] Abnormalities in one or more of these factors may antedate the development of sustained clinical hypertension, but may be pathogenetically operative in the preclinical stages of systemic hypertension.

Indeed, despite blood vessels being exposed to high pressures, the complications of hypertension (e.g., myocardial infarction and stroke) are paradoxically thrombotic rather than hemorrhagic; this is now referred to as the thrombotic paradox of hypertension or the Birmingham paradox. Certainly, abnormalities of hemostasis, platelets, and endothelial damage/dysfunction are present in hypertension, contributing to a prothrombotic or hypercoagulable state.[15] These abnormalities have also been associated with hypertensive target organ damage, including LVH; furthermore, they can be beneficially improved with antihypertensive treatment.

The sequence of events that leads from these multiple hemodynamic and nonhemodynamic factors to hypertensive heart disease is only beginning to be elucidated.[16] Both

PATHOGENETIC PROCESSES UNDERLYING CARDIAC DAMAGE FROM SYSTEMIC HYPERTENSION

Neurohormonal	Activation of the renin-angiotensin-aldosterone system Enhanced adrenergic activity Increased production or reduced degradation of biologically active molecules (e.g., angiotensin II, cytokines)
Hemodynamic	Increased peripheral resistance Increased circumferential and meridional wall stress Decreased coronary reserve
Vascular	Endothelial dysfunction Vascular remodeling Decreased vascular compliance Exaggerated vascular reactivity Coronary and peripheral vascular atherosclerosis
Myocardial	Left ventricular remodeling Fetal gene expression Myocyte hypertrophy Alterations in extracellular matrix

Table 41.2 Pathogenetic processes underlying cardiac damage from systemic hypertension.

myocytes (cardiac and vascular) and nonmyocytes (fibroblast) are direct biomechanical sensors of hemodynamic load. Their activation leads to a series of cellular and subcellular signals that regulate the expression of proto-oncogenes and other genes that regulate cell growth, apoptosis, phenotype, and matrix turnover. In hypertensive heart disease, tissue homogeneity gives way to heterogeneity and a disproportionate involvement of noncardiomyocyte cells, which accounts for the adverse structural remodeling of both myocardial and vascular tissue structure.[17,18] These alterations in tissue structure are responsible for the pathologic LVH and medial thickening of intramural coronary arteries and arterioles of hypertensive heart disease and contribute to its enhanced risk of adverse cardiovascular events, including myocardial infarction, diastolic and/or systolic dysfunction, and arrhythmias.

CARDIAC COMPLICATIONS OF HYPERTENSION: LEFT VENTRICULAR HYPERTROPHY

Epidemiologic data convincingly show that cardiovascular and cerebrovascular risk increase with increasing blood pressure, with a "dose-response" relationship (see Chapter 39). Even though LVH, heart failure, coronary disease, and cardiac arrhythmias occur in the nonhypertensive patient, when these conditions are accompanied by high blood pressure they are associated with greater target organ damage, increased risk of nonfatal cardiac events, premature cardiovascular death, and a worse overall prognosis. Simply decreasing the blood pressure may be inadequate, and a focus on multiple risk factor modification and reduction in total cardiovascular disease risk "burden" may be necessary.

Although LVH may be defined by an increase in LV mass, quantified by measurements of postmortem LV weight, by electrocardiographic (ECG) criteria, or by echocardiography, it is complicated by the marked variability in LV size in the normal adult population. LV mass is strongly related to body size, with components attributable to lean body mass and obesity. Criteria for LVH are therefore based on values that have been indexed to height, weight, or body surface area.

Upper limits of normal LV mass indexed to body surface area, established using M-mode echocardiography in a healthy subset of the Framingham Heart Study population are 131 g/m^2 in men and 100 g/m^2 in women (Table 41.3).[19] Using these criteria, LVH was present in 12% of men and 14% of women in the Framingham study. In normotensive adults, LVH is directly related to the risk of developing later hypertension,[20] raising the possibility that LVH may also be involved in the development of hypertension.

Increased blood pressure greatly increases the risk of having LVH: there is a 43% increase in the relative risk of having LVH in men and a 25% increase in women for each 20 mm Hg increase in systolic pressure.[21] The prevalence of LVH in secondary forms of hypertension owing to renovascular or endocrinologic disease is similar to that in essential hypertension.[22]

Prognostic Implications of LVH

Left ventricular hypertrophy established by ECG or by echocardiography is a strong and independent risk factor for cardiovascular morbidity and mortality in the general population, in hypertensive patients, and in patients with coronary artery disease.[23,24] Echocardiographic LVH predicts an increased risk of cardiovascular morbidity and death, even after adjustment for other major risk factors (age, blood pressure, pulse pressure, treatment of hypertension, cigarette use, diabetes, obesity, cholesterol profile, and electrocardiographic evidence of LVH). LVH significantly increases the risk of coronary artery disease, congestive heart failure, cerebrovascular accidents, ventricular arrhythmias, and sudden death. It increases the relative risk of mortality by twofold in individuals with coronary artery disease and by fourfold in those with normal epicardial coronary arteries. In otherwise healthy individuals followed for 4 years in whom LVH was defined as an LV mass adjusted for height of 143 g/m in men and greater than 102 g/m in women, the relative risk of developing cardiovascular disease was 1.49 in men and 1.57 in women for each increment of 50 g/m in LV mass. Although the ECG is a much less sensitive measure for LVH, presence of LVH on the ECG increases the risk of cardiovascular diseases from threefold to sevenfold, depending on the age and sex of the patient.

It had been suggested that the pattern of LV geometry may be related to the risk for cardiovascular morbidity and mortality. Four different LV geometric patterns have been identified: normal LV geometry, concentric remodeling, eccentric LVH, and concentric LVH. Longitudinal studies have shown that the risk of cardiovascular disease was highest in patients with concentric geometry.[25,26] However, it should be noted that the LV mass tends to be greater in concentric LVH. Consequently, the prognostic impact of LV geometry may be reduced or abolished because of the overwhelming prognostic value of LV mass itself.

ECHOCARDIOGRAPHIC CRITERIA FOR UPPER LIMITS OF LV MASS*

	Men	Women
Number	347	517
Age (yr)	42 ± 12	43 ± 12
LV mass, absolute (g)	259	166
LV mass, corrected for BSA (g/m^2)	131	100
LV mass, corrected for height (g/m)	143	102

LV mass was calculated using the formula: $LVM = 0.8 \times (1.04 \times [LVID + LVPWT + IVST]^3 - LVID^3)$ where LVID = LV internal diameter, LVPWT = LV posterior wall thickness, and IVST = intraventricular septal thickness.

*Criteria for upper limits of LV mass in adult men and women are set at two standard deviations above the mean values for healthy populations derived from the cohort and offspring subjects of the Framingham Heart Study.

BSA, body surface area.

Modified with permission from Levy D, Savage DD, Garrison RJ, et al. Echocardiographic criteria for left ventricular hypertrophy: the Framingham Heart Study. Am J Cardiol 1987;59:956-960.

Table 41-3 Echocardiographic criteria for upper limits of LV mass.

Pathophysiology

Genetic and nongenetic influences on hemodynamic and nonhemodynamic factors that eventually cause intracellular stimulation of protein synthesis may influence the development of LVH (see Fig. 41.1). There are several lines of evidence that support the genetic influences on the development of LVH. Ravogli and colleagues[27] found an increased LV mass in normotensive offspring of hypertensive parents. Other studies documenting a possible genetic factor include twin studies[28] and racial studies comparing white and black patients with hypertension. The African American ancestry has been identified as an independent risk factor for LVH.[29] Finally, a number of candidate genes have been studied, including angiotensin-converting enzyme (ACE) gene insertion/deletion polymorphism and the aldosterone synthase gene.[30,31]

Both pressure and volume are implicated in the development of LVH. For instance, diastolic blood pressure is more closely related to LV wall thickness, and will correspond to a pure pressure load, whereas systolic blood pressure is more closely related to LV mass, suggesting an influence of both pressure and load. Reduced arterial compliance in hypertension will also increase pulsatile load, and provides a further stimulus to LVH.[32] Some cross-sectional studies have suggested that an increase in blood pressure variability may be better correlated with the presence of LVH.[33] Nonhemodynamic risk factors for the development of LVH include trophic factors mediated by the renin-angiotensin-aldosterone system, sympathetic tone, and insulin. Angiotensin II promotes myocyte growth, and aldosterone may increase collagen content and stimulate the development of myocardial fibrosis.[17,18] Insulin has trophic effects, and hypertensive LVH is often associated with high insulin levels and insulin resistance.[34] Obesity, which is associated with increased plasma volume and cardiac output, is also a determinant of LV mass.[35]

In response to hemodynamic overload and associated increases in systolic wall stress, specific hypertension-related growth factors are activated and produced.[36] Both myocytes and nonmyocytes (vascular and fibroblast) may respond as direct biomechanical sensors of the hemodynamic load. The biomechanical signal transduction that has been observed in animal models shows that it is often accompanied by recruitment of the G protein–coupled neurohormones, activation of which likely serves to amplify the growth signaling triggered by the mechanical event itself. Table 41.4 shows some of the stimuli of ventricular hypertrophy that have been identified that are either of a neuroendocrine origin (e.g., catecholamines) or are synthesized and released locally by the myocytes and nonmyocytes (e.g., angiotensin II). The signaling pathways responsible for the hypertrophic growth have been actively studied, and it is likely that reversible protein phosphorylation and dephosphorylation are involved. Three signaling pathways show potential as regulators of the response: protein kinase C, mitogen-activated protein kinase cascades, and calcineurin.[37] Oxidative stress may also contribute to LVH.[38]

Besides myocyte hypertrophy, there is also nonmyocyte growth in LVH that leads to an adverse structural remodeling of the myocardium and vasculature. An exaggerated interstitial and perivascular accumulation of collagens type I and type III has been found in the hypertensive heart.[17,18] Thus it has been suggested that it is not the quantity but the quality of the myocardium that distinguishes the LVH in hypertension from adaptive hypertrophy in the athlete. Structural homogeneity of cardiac tissue is governed by a balanced equilibrium existing between stimulator and inhibitor signals that regulate cell growth, apoptosis, phenotype, and matrix turnover (Fig. 41.2). Stimulators are normally counterbalanced by inhibitors (see Fig. 41.2). Loss of this reciprocal regulation accounts for connective tissue remodeling in LVH.

STIMULI AND SIGNALS OF VENTRICULAR MYOCYTE HYPERTROPHY

Agonist Type	Examples	Point of Action
Vasoactive peptides	ET-1, Ang II	$G\alpha_q/G\alpha_{11} \rightarrow$ PIP2 hydrolysis $\rightarrow$ nPKCs
α_1-Adrenergic agonists	Norepinephrine Epinephrine	$G\alpha_q/G\alpha_{11} \rightarrow$ PIP2 hydrolysis $\rightarrow$ nPKCs?
Direct activators of PKC	Tumor-promoting phorbol esters	nPKCs/cPKCs
Peptide growth factors	Fibroblast growth factors Insulin-like growth factor 1	Receptor protein tyrosine kinases
Cytokines	Cardiotrophin-1	Gp130/interleukin-6 receptor
Arachidonate metabolites	Prostaglandin $F_{2\alpha}$	JNKs
Mechanical stretch	Autocrine/ paracrine factors (ET-1, Ang II)	PIP2 hydrolysis/ PKC? JNKs?
Cell contact	Not known	Not known

Stimuli and signals of ventricular myocyte hypertrophy. Ang II, angiotensin II; ET-1, endothelin-1; $G\alpha_q$, $G\alpha_{11}$, G proteins; Gp130, glycoprotein 130; JNK, c-Jun N-terminal kinase; PIP2, phosphatidylinositol bisphosphate; cPKC, nPKC, cytoplasmic and nuclear protein kinase C.

With permission from Sugden PH. Signaling in myocardial hypertrophy. Life after calcineurin? Circ Res 1999;84:633-646.

Table 41.4 Stimuli and signals of ventricular myocyte hypertrophy.

The mechanisms by which LVH is associated with the increased risk of cardiovascular sequelae are not fully understood. The development of LVH is associated with myocardial fibrosis and subsequent diastolic dysfunction, an important factor in the evolution of congestive heart failure. The reduced coronary reserve in LVH increases the risk of myocardial ischemia—which may in turn promote potentially lethal arrhythmias—and the possibility of suffering from myocardial infarction. The increase in myocardial fibrosis may lead to disturbed repolarization of the myocardium, potentially leading to malignant arrhythmias and subsequent sudden death. Finally, more prothrombotic abnormalities have been found in association with LVH, contributing to the increased risk of thrombotic complications.[15]

Clinical Presentation and Diagnosis

Pathologic hypertrophy may be associated with an absence of symptoms for many years before the development of congestive heart failure or unexpected sudden death. Thus, in contemporary clinical practice, the diagnosis depends predominantly on ECG or echocardiographic measurements. Nevertheless, physical examination may reveal some clues. Pulsations lateral to the medioclavicular line are a sensitive but nonspecific sign. A thrusting apex greater than 2 cm in

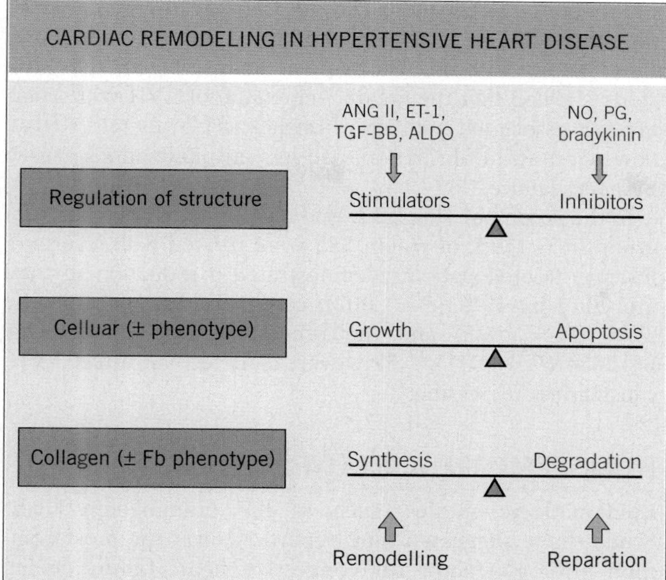

Figure 41.2 Cardiac remodeling in hypertensive heart disease. Homogeneity in myocardial structure is preserved by a balanced equilibrium between stimulators and inhibitors that respectively regulate cell growth and death (or apoptosis) and fibroblast (Fb) collagen turnover (and/or cell phenotype). In hypertensive heart disease, an adverse structural remodeling is related to an imbalance in this equilibrium in favor of an absolute increase in stimulators or a relative increase secondary to a paucity of inhibitors. ALDO, aldosterone; ANG II, angiotensin II; ET-1, endothelin-1; NO, nitric oxide; PG, prostaglandin; TGF, transforming growth factor. (With permission from Weber KT. Cardioreparation in hypertensive heart disease. Hypertension 2001;38:588-591.)

diameter suggests LV enlargement; if it is more than 3 cm in diameter in the left cubitus position, it is considered an accurate sign. A chest x-ray is of limited value for the determination of LVH, as the picture will show the outer contour of the heart but will not specifically delineate the heart.

The ECG is a readily available and specific diagnostic procedure. A negative P wave in the precordial leads reflects an increased load on the left atrium. Large QRS amplitude with deep S in the anterior leads and high R in the lateral leads reflects an enlarged LV diameter; prolonged ventricular activation time, such as wide QRS complex, and ST-T changes reflect altered myocardial depolarization and repolarization as a result of an increased wall thickness. Furthermore, it appears that an anterolateral hemiblock in hypertensive patients is a finding suggestive of LVH. Various combinations of these criteria have been suggested to identify LVH by ECG. However, a recent systematic review involving 21 studies (n = 5608 patients) by Pewsner and colleagues[39] assessed the accuracy of ECG in screening in hypertensive patients and highlighted the low sensitivity of the ECG in detecting LVH when compared with the echocardiogram.

Echocardiography can provide accurate measurements of the intraventricular septum, the posterior LV wall thickness, and the LV diameter in diastole. Echocardiographic determination of LVH is characterized by high specificity (80% or greater) and sensitivity (80% or greater). In addition, echocardiography can reveal other reasons for LVH (e.g., valvular diseases, hypertrophic cardiomyopathy) and can provide information on the existence of different patterns of LV geometry and of systolic and diastolic function and the possible detection of collagen deposition in LVH. Tissue Doppler imaging is also increasingly used for assessing global ventricular function in systole and diastole.[40]

New three-dimensional techniques for imaging the heart include magnetic resonance imaging, advanced computed tomography techniques, and three-dimensional echocardiography.[41] All these techniques can measure myocardial mass more accurately than conventional echocardiographic techniques and may thus offer an advantage. However, their role in the routine clinical assessment of the hypertensive patient remains to be established.

Management

Because LVH is such an important independent risk factor in hypertension, there is general agreement that it is beneficial to prevent and to regress LVH. Regression is associated with such potential benefits as improved cardiac performance and diastolic filling, enhanced coronary flow reserve, and decreased ventricular arrhythmias. Many studies have reported reduced LV mass and wall thickness as a result of antihypertensive treatment. Blood pressure reduction by means of all classes of antihypertensive agents, with the possible exception of pure vasodilators such as minoxidil and hydralazine, reduces LVH. In long-term follow-up, the cumulative incidence of nonfatal cardiovascular events is significantly greater among treated hypertensive patients without LVH regression when compared with those with significant LVH regression.[42]

Several meta-analyses have suggested that certain classes of antihypertensive agents may be more effective than others in promoting regression of LVH.[43,44] These analyses are complicated by inherent demographic, biological, or pharmacologic variables, because the studies in these analyses included patients of dissimilar sex, race, age, and number who were treated for varying periods, using unlike doses and with different compounds of the same therapeutic class (perhaps having dissimilar physiologic, pharmacodynamic, and pharmacokinetic actions), and who had varying treatment histories (in which past therapeutic effects may be of extreme importance). It should, however, be noted that although there have been a number of intervention trials that have compared the effects of single antihypertensive agents on LVH, most of these trials have turned out to be comparisons of combination therapies, because most patients needed to take more than one drug. Therefore, we do not know at present whether changes induced directly by prior pharmacologic treatments or indirectly by the biological effects of treatment have a prolonged effect mediated by biologically altered cellular memory.

There is increasing evidence of improved prognosis associated with LVH regression. Much of this evidence comes from the LIFE study.[43] The Losartan Intervention for Endpoint Reduction in Hypertension (LIFE) study was the first double-blind, randomized, parallel-group trial in patients with essential hypertension and ECG evidence of LVH, who were randomly allocated to losartan-based (n = 4605) or atenolol-based (n = 4588) treatment (Fig. 41.3).[43] The primary composite endpoint (cardiovascular mortality, stroke, and myocardial infarction) was in favor of losartan [11% event rate, compared with 13% for atenolol; adjusted

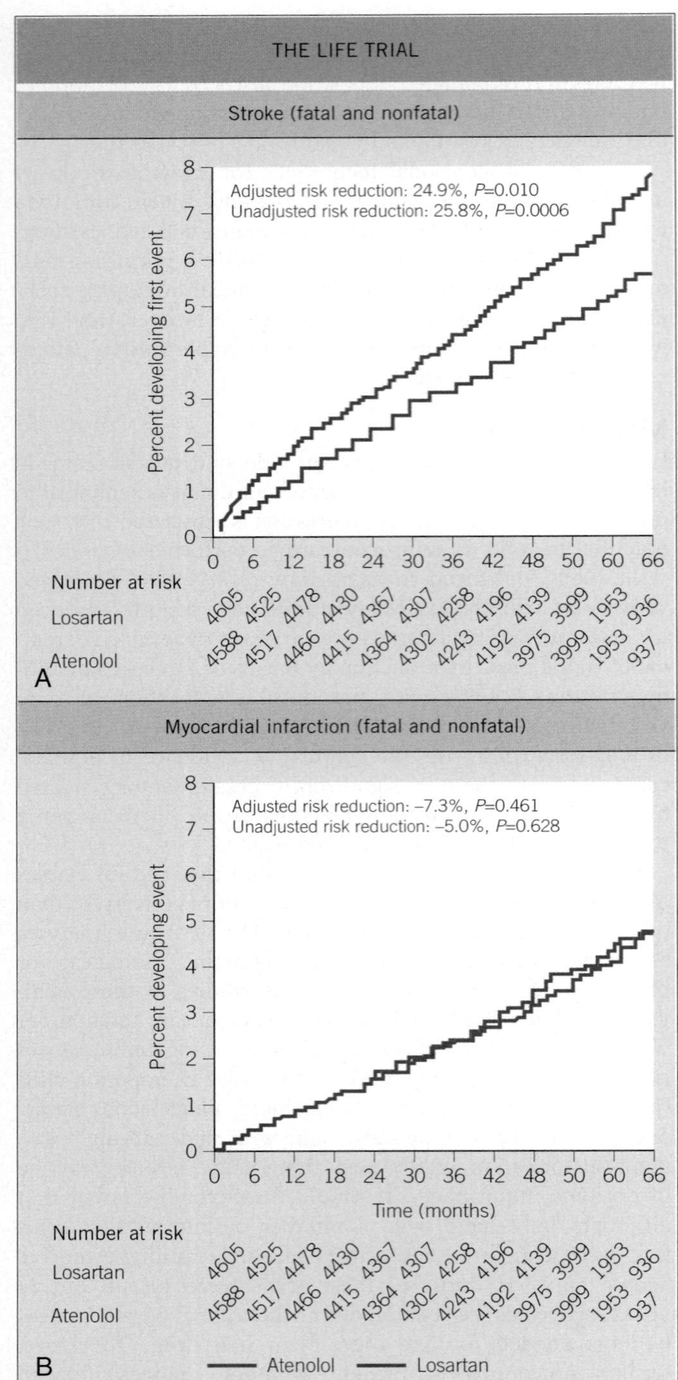

Figure 41.3 The LIFE trial. Comparison of effects of losartan and atenolol on stroke (**A**) and myocardial infarction (**B**).

hazard ratio, 0.87 (95% confidence interval [CI], 0.77-0.98; *P* =.021)] and was attributable to a 25% reduction in stroke by losartan [5%, compared with atenolol, 7%; adjusted hazard ratio, 0.75 (95% CI, 0.63-0.89; *P* < .001)]. The rates of myocardial infarction, cardiovascular mortality, admission to hospital because of heart failure, and revascularization were not significantly different between the two treatment groups. In addition, there was a 25% reduction in cases of new diabetes in patients treated with losartan compared with those given atenolol. Even among "low-risk" patients in the LIFE study—that is, those without vascular disease or diabetes—there was an 18% reduction in the primary endpoint in those taking losartan. Subsequent analysis from the LIFE study showed that the greater regression of LVH with losartan was associated with fewer cardiovascular events, stroke, new-onset atrial fibrillation, and less hospitalizations caused by heart failure.[44-48]

In the accompanying LIFE study paper on the diabetic subgroup (n = 1195, of whom 585 were treated with losartan), losartan-treated patients demonstrated a reduction in total mortality by 39% (*P* = .002), cardiovascular mortality by 37% (*P* = .028) and the primary composite endpoint by 24% (*P* = .031).[49] However, diabetes can affect LVH, causing less regression.[50]

HEART FAILURE AND HYPERTENSION

Epidemiologic studies, such as the Framingham Heart Study, have suggested that hypertension is the most common etiologic factor for congestive heart failure, being present in 50% of cases. Nevertheless, contemporary studies suggest that ischemic heart disease is now the most common cause, especially as the treatment of myocardial infarction is improving, resulting in more survivors. Furthermore, hypertension may itself result in heart failure because of underlying coronary artery disease and arrhythmias, such as atrial fibrillation, in addition to diastolic dysfunction.

The apparent underestimation of the role of hypertension in heart failure may indeed be the result of changes in blood pressure at clinical presentation, from heart failure itself or coronary artery disease. Indeed, blood pressure may no longer be increased at clinical presentation with heart failure, because of impaired LV pump function or because of reduced blood pressure after superimposed but unrecognized coronary events.[40]

Unlike heart failure caused by coronary artery disease, in which heart failure progresses after a discrete event (myocardial ischemia or infarction) that damages the heart muscle, LV dysfunction in the hypertensive patient may progress gradually through several functional and morphologic stages (Fig. 41.4)[51]:

- LV diastolic dysfunction with concentric remodeling;
- asymptomatic LV systolic dysfunction with concentric LVH;
- asymptomatic LV dilatation with eccentric LVH; and
- symptomatic LV systolic dysfunction with eccentric LVH and greater dilatation.

This progression may be changed by loading conditions (e.g., extremely high blood pressures) or superimposition of myocardial ischemia or infarction, which may transform the course from an insidious but incremental process to a precipitous conversion to symptomatic congestive heart failure, arrhythmias, or sudden death.

Pathophysiology

Diastolic Dysfunction

In hypertensive LVH, the ventricle cannot relax normally in diastole. Thus, to produce the necessary increase in ventricular input, especially during exercise, there is an increase in left atrial pressure rather than the normal reduction in

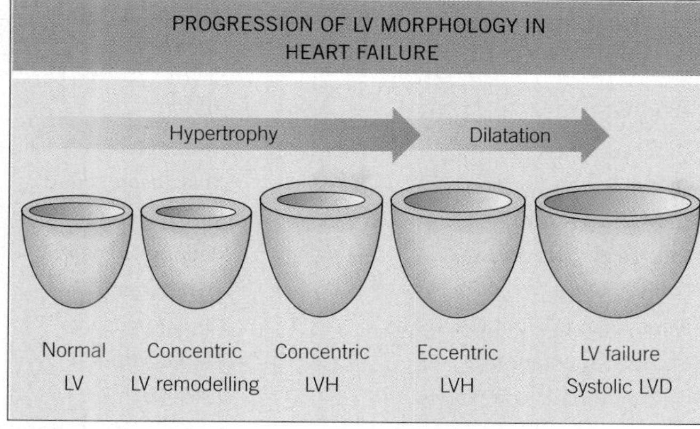

Figure 41.4 Progression of LV morphology in heart failure. LVD, left ventricular dysfunction; LVH, left ventricular hypertrophy. (Modified from Lopez-Sendon J. Regional myocardial ischemia and diastolic dysfunction in hypertensive heart disease. Eur Heart J 1993;14(Suppl J):110-113.)

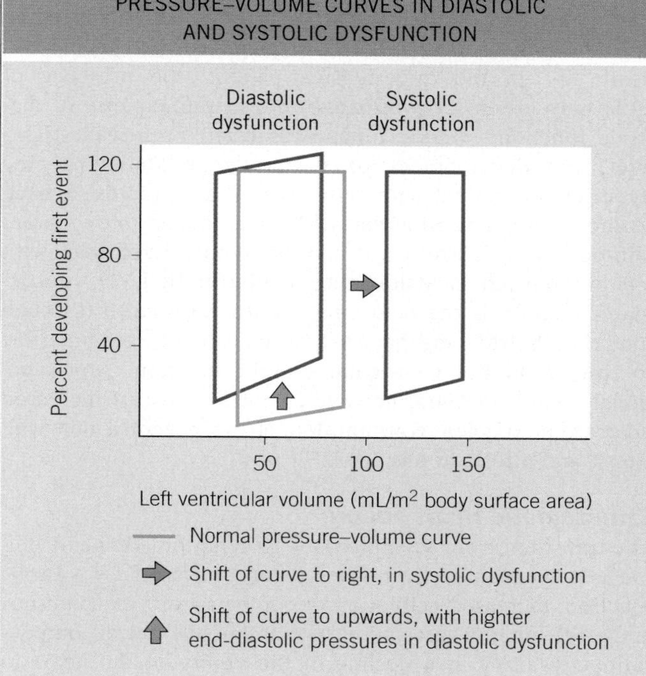

Figure 41.5 Pressure-volume curves in diastolic and systolic dysfunction.

ventricular pressure, which produces a "suction effect." This can lead to an increase in pulmonary capillary pressure that is sufficient to induce pulmonary congestion. Diastolic dysfunction and the increase in atrial pressure can also lead to atrial fibrillation,[51a] and in hypertrophied ventricles dependent on atrial systole, the loss of atrial transport can result in a significant reduction in stroke volume and pulmonary edema. Exercise-induced subendocardial ischemia can also produce an "exaggerated" impairment of diastolic relaxation of the hypertrophied myocardium.

In hypertensive patients, diastolic abnormalities may be the most common and earliest manifestations of ventricular dysfunction. Abnormalities of LV diastolic relaxation and compliance usually occur even before evidence of systolic dysfunction, most often in conjunction with LVH, although the syndrome can occur even in the absence of LVH. Diastolic dysfunction is commonly clinically silent and may only be recognized during the course of echocardiographic detection of LVH (Fig. 41.5) or as part of the evaluation of ventricular function. Indeed, diastolic dysfunction may be the sole abnormality of ventricular hemodynamics detected in approximately 40% of patients with clinical signs and symptoms of heart failure. The overall prevalence of normal systolic function in patients with symptoms of congestive heart failure ranges from 11% to 83% in hypertensive patients and from 5% to 67% in patients with coronary artery disease (see Chapter 73).

Hypertension may cause alterations in the major determinants of diastolic function, ventricular relaxation and compliance. Rather than being a passive phenomenon, ventricular relaxation is an active, energy-requiring process that occurs at the onset of ventricular diastole when atrial pressure exceeds ventricular pressure. Ventricular relaxation is also particularly sensitive to loading conditions, ischemia, ATP availability, cytosolic calcium availability, and other alterations in calcium handling by the sarcoplasmic reticulum. Left ventricular compliance, in contrast, is a more passive process that occurs later in diastole, and its determinants include increased LV wall thickness, increased chamber stiffness, and increased total myocardial collagen content. Abnormal arterial compliance may potentially contribute to the development of LV diastolic dysfunction in hypertensive heart disease.[52]

Clinically, diastolic dysfunction can present with all the typical signs and symptoms of congestive heart failure. Although the symptoms of heart failure may be exacerbated by concomitant ischemia and arrhythmias, there is evidence that hypertension per se can exacerbate diastolic dysfunction and pulmonary edema. Studying patients hospitalized with hypertensive pulmonary edema, Gandhi and colleagues[53] demonstrated the dramatic acute effects of acute elevations in systolic blood pressure in reducing diastolic performance. These patients did not have transient LV systolic dysfunction. This study emphasizes the role of hypertension in producing and exacerbating diastolic dysfunction.

Asymptomatic LV Systolic Dysfunction

Depressed LV systolic function is the most potent risk factor for the development of overt congestive heart failure, and in hypertensive patients this can develop secondary to coronary artery disease. It is also a risk factor for a late stage of hypertensive heart disease. A reduction in LV systolic performance predicts the progressive dilatation of the heart and confers a markedly adverse prognosis. If left untreated, even minimally depressed systolic function eventually progresses to symptomatic heart failure. In the hypertensive patient, accurate assessment of ventricular function is therefore essential, and if reduced systolic function is confirmed, even in the absence of symptoms, aggressive therapy is imperative.

In asymptomatic patients with abnormal LV systolic function, progression to ventricular dilatation appears to be slower and clinical events, including death, less common. Nonetheless, in asymptomatic patients with LV systolic dysfunction, survival at 2 years is significantly reduced (15% to 18%), compared with patients who have normal systolic function.[54,55]

Asymptomatic Left Ventricular Dilatation

Left ventricular dilatation is a precursor of heart failure and an indication of increased risk of major cardiac events and death.[56,57] In the hypertensive patient, the presence of LVH may lessen LV wall stress, but at the expense of diastolic function, systolic function is often preserved. However, the development of ventricular dilatation in the hypertensive patient with LVH, even if asymptomatic, is an ominous sign, indicating that LVH is no longer able to maintain normal wall stresses. It may be hypothesized that, with loss of the mechanical advantage conferred by LVH, ventricular dilatation is the next compensatory response (through the Frank-Starling mechanism), which is invoked in an effort to restore normal ventricular systolic function. Any functional benefit derived, however, is at the cost of increased myocardial oxygen consumption, greater ventricular wall stress, and afterload mismatch.

Symptomatic Heart Failure

The transition from asymptomatic to symptomatic heart failure is accompanied by further deterioration of LV systolic function, increased activation of compensatory mechanisms, and more rapid progress along the path to cardiac decompensation, resulting in a decline in the ability of the heart to deliver enough oxygen to enable tissues to function optimally. In the hypertensive patient, it is unclear whether neurohormone-induced increases in peripheral vascular resistance initially exceed a threshold of afterload mismatch and cause a decline in cardiac pumping capacity, or whether the factors that lead to increases in peripheral resistance also exert an independent parallel effect on the heart, leading to remodeling of the LV, microvascular dysfunction, and a decline in pumping capacity.

The compensatory mechanisms (i.e., activation of the renin-angiotensin-aldosterone system, catecholamines, cytokines, and molecular vasodilatory systems) become more maladaptive, with fluid retention, vasoconstriction, progressive cardiac dilatation, and further impairment. Myocyte hypertrophy, cellular contractile dysfunction, apoptosis, and associated changes in collagen composition, extracellular matrix, and chamber geometry have long-term deleterious effects on cardiac energy balance and contractile function.

Clinical Presentations

Although useful in understanding pathophysiology, categorization of the clinical features of heart failure according to diastolic or systolic dysfunction is inappropriate, because both these mechanisms may be active in an individual patient.

The signs and symptoms of heart failure in the hypertensive patient are similar to those of patients with heart failure of other etiology (Table 41.5). Dyspnea is the most consistent symptom, whether heart failure is due primarily to systolic or to diastolic dysfunction. The hypertensive patient may present with a combination of symptoms, some classically attributable to systolic dysfunction, such as fatigue, exercise intolerance, and muscle weakness; and others typical of diastolic dysfunction and pulmonary congestion, including breathlessness, persistent cough, and pulmonary edema. Exacerbation of pulmonary symptoms by tachycardia or loss of sinus rhythm (with the development of atrial fibrillation) may suggest diastolic dysfunction.

COMMON PRESENTING SYMPTOMS AND SIGNS OF CONGESTIVE HEART FAILURE IN HYPERTENSION

Symptoms	Signs
Dyspnea at rest	Resting tachycardia
Dyspnea with exertion	Third heart sound
Effort intolerance	Vascular congestion
Fatigue and weakness	Peripheral edema
Orthopnea	Hypotension
Paroxysmal nocturnal dyspnea	Organomegaly
Impaired mentation	Pleural effusion
Gastrointestinal complaints	Cachexia

Table 41.5 Common presenting symptoms and signs of congestive heart failure in hypertension.

Diagnostic Techniques

The diagnostic approach to hypertensive heart failure is no different from that of congestive heart failure, in general (see Chapter 42). The history and physical examination may provide important clues in clinical differential diagnosis, but are of limited value in establishing a definitive pathophysiologic diagnosis. Because coronary disease often coexists with hypertension, a careful clinical history, physical examination, or laboratory evidence of myocardial ischemia or infarction may be important in establishing the underlying cause(s) of heart failure. Physical findings, including jugular venous distention, third or fourth heart sound, pulmonary rales or pedal edema, would not reliably differentiate heart failure caused by diastolic dysfunction from that caused by systolic dysfunction. Indeed, diastolic dysfunction may lead to decreased cardiac output (a cardinal finding in systolic dysfunction), and systolic dysfunction may lead to increased LV filling pressures (a cardinal finding in diastolic dysfunction) (Fig. 41.6).

The ECG and chest radiograph may provide important information, but do not differentiate diastolic from systolic dysfunction. Echocardiography[58] and radionuclide ventriculography are useful for documentation of the presence, type, and severity of LV dysfunction and may play a crucial role in the differential diagnosis, staging, and management of heart failure. In addition to assessing LV function, the echocardiogram with Doppler is

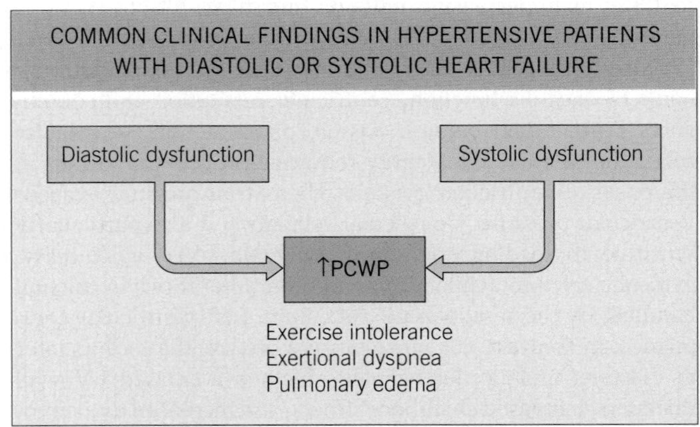

Figure 41.6 Common clinical findings in hypertensive patients with diastolic or systolic heart failure. PCWP, pulmonary capillary wedge pressure.

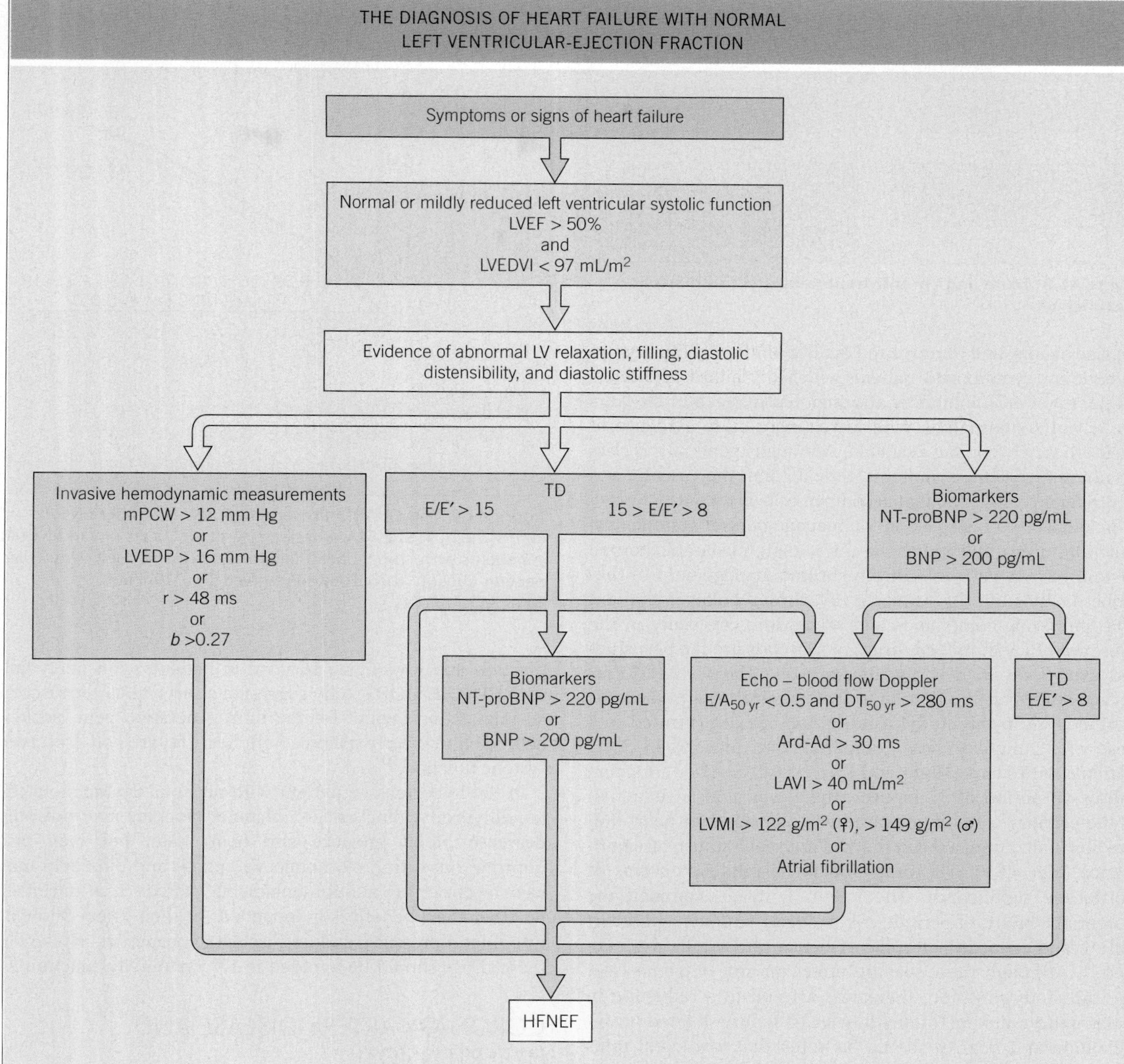

Figure 41.7 The diagnosis of heart failure with normal left ventricular ejection fraction (LVEF). As recommended by the Heart Failure and Echocardiography Associations of the European Society of Cardiology. (From Paulus WJ, Tschope C, Sanderson JE, et al. How to diagnose diastolic heart failure: a consensus statement on the diagnosis of heart failure with normal left ventricular ejection fraction by the Heart Failure and Echocardiography Associations of the European Society of Cardiology. Eur Heart J 2007;28:2539-2550.)

helpful in excluding the presence of valvular, pericardial, infiltrative, or congenital heart disease. A recent consensus statement supports the use of B-type natriuretic peptide (BNP) determination, and tissue Doppler imaging should be used in the diagnosis of diastolic heart failure (Fig. 41.7).[59]

Magnetic resonance imaging (MRI) has recently emerged as a useful imaging modality that can provide an extremely accurate assessment of LV chamber dimensions and function.[60]

Management

The approach to management of heart failure in the hypertensive patient should, in general, follow principles similar to those for congestive heart failure. High blood pressure should be treated and controlled. Concomitant cardiac ischemia and arrhythmias should be managed accordingly. As regards treatment of acute heart failure, little is to be gained by differentiating diastolic from systolic dysfunction; in chronic heart failure, aggressive blood pressure control, rate/rhythm control, and LVH regression are important aims in diastolic heart failure. In addition to relief of symptoms, therapeutic approaches should aim to slow the course of ventricular remodeling and prevent progression of cardiac and vascular damage (Fig. 41.8).

Angiotensin-converting enzyme inhibitors are the first-line treatment of chronic heart failure[61,62]; they prevent or slow the progression of heart failure, decrease the risk of major

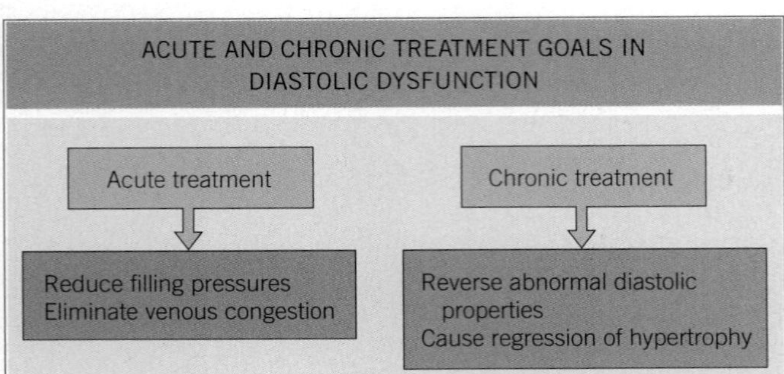

Figure 41.8 Acute and chronic treatment goals in diastolic dysfunction.

cardiac events, and improve the quality of life, in both asymptomatic and symptomatic patients with heart failure. In patients intolerant of ACE inhibitors, the angiotensin receptor blockers are a viable alternative, with increasingly more evidence of their efficacy becoming available. Although agents of this class do not relieve acute symptoms, they do limit the vascular and ventricular remodeling that accompanies heart failure.

In addition to their role in the management of systolic dysfunction, drugs that target the renin-angiotensin-aldosterone system may have a role in the chronic management of diastolic dysfunction, by reducing myocardial collagen content and improving compliance and relaxation, especially in the presence of LVH. Indeed, drugs of this class are the best studied drug class in diastolic dysfunction. The CHARM-Preserved study[63] is the first large scale clinical trial in diastolic dysfunction. In this study, candesartan cilexitil (titrated to a dose of 32 mg/day) was compared with placebo in 3031 patients with heart failure and LVEF >40%. After a median follow-up period of 37 months, there was a 11% reduction in the primary endpoint of cardiovascular death or heart failure hospitalization, a result that did not reach statistical significance (Fig. 41.9). The reduction in hospitalization was of borderline significance. The PEP-CHF trial examined the potential benefits of perindopril in elderly patients with heart failure and echocardiographic evidence of diastolic dysfunction.[64] Although there was no effect on any outcome over the full study duration, there was a trend to a reduction in the primary outcome of death or heart failure–related hospitalization at 1 year. It should be noted that low event rates and low recruitment rate resulted in a considerable loss of statistical power to show an effect of perindopril. There are two ongoing large trials in diastolic dysfunction, one involving another angiotensin receptor blocker[65] and the other will investigate the potential beneficial effects of spironolactone.[66] In patients in whom ACE inhibitors (or angiotensin receptor blockers) are not well tolerated or are contraindicated, the combination of hydralazine and isosorbide dinitrate may be a suitable alternative, although the survival benefit is greater with ACE inhibitors.[67] This combination may have particular benefits for hypertensive Afro-Caribbean patients with heart failure.[68] The addition of incremental doses of loop diuretics to ACE inhibitors is required for the management of fluid retention, edema, or pulmonary congestion, but is symptomatic rather than diagnostic.

Beta blockers have proved to be effective antihypertensive agents; they also slow heart rate and are effective in treating myocardial ischemia, in addition to improving LV

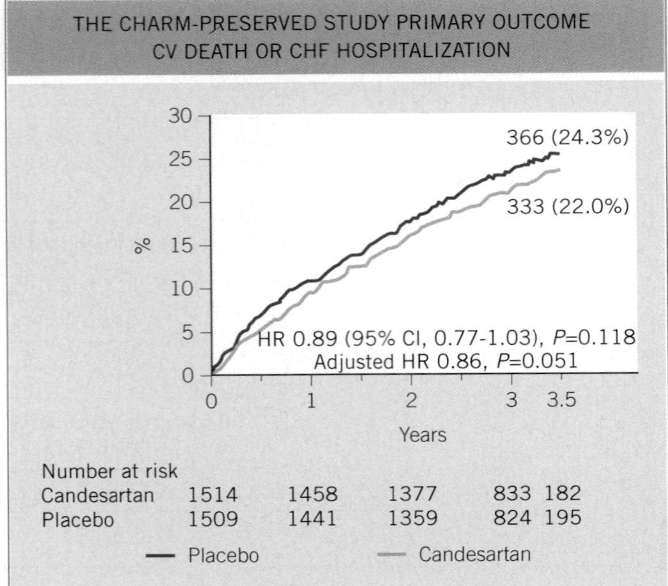

Figure 41.9 The CHARM-Preserved study. (With permission from Yusuf S, Pfeffer MA, Swedberg K, et al. Effects of candesartan in patients with chronic heart failure and preserved left ventricular ejection fraction: the CHARM-Preserved Trial. Lancet 2003;362:777-781.)

function and prolonging survival in patients with heart failure.[69] The SENIORS study suggested a survival/cardiovascular hospitalization benefit for the third-generation beta blocker, nebivolol, in elderly patients with heart failure and preserved systolic function.[70]

In the hypertensive patient with diastolic dysfunction, the nondihydropyridine calcium channel blockers may not only decrease blood pressure and heart rate, but may also improve relaxation. Although verapamil and diltiazem may have a direct "relaxation-enhancing" effect, it is uncertain whether their benefit is independent of their effect on heart rate, blood pressure, and anti-ischemic properties. However, these drugs should be avoided in LV systolic dysfunction.

CORONARY ARTERY DISEASE AND HYPERTENSION

There is a close relationship between hypertension and risk of coronary artery disease. The risk for development of a cardiovascular event is approximately doubled in the hypertensive patient, and this is irrespective of sex or age, or whether systolic or diastolic blood pressure is increased.[71] Indeed, there is almost a "dose-response" relationship between coronary heart disease risk and increasing blood pressure, greater blood pressures being associated with greater risk (see Chapter 39). In a study of 5000 patients with chronic angina pectoris, more than 50% had history of hypertension.[72] In one study evaluating the effects of normal blood pressure (BP), prehypertension, and hypertension on progression of coronary atherosclerosis by intravascular ultrasound, uncontrolled blood pressures contributed to greater disease progression and atheroma volume, whereas the most favorable rate of progression of coronary atherosclerosis was observed in patients whose BP fell within the

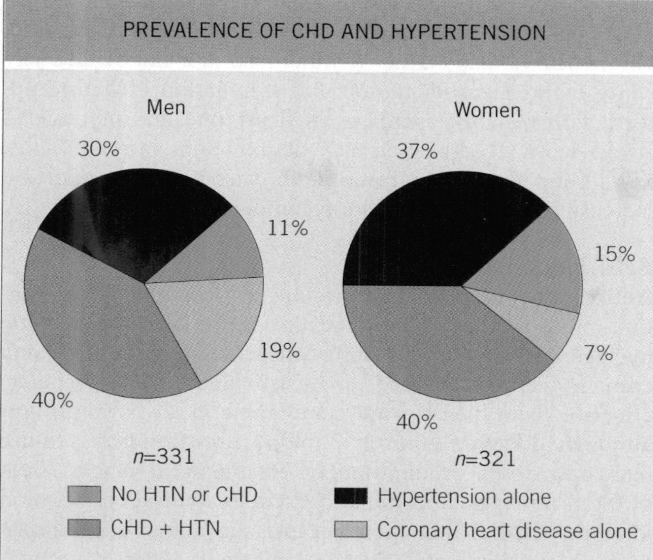

Figure 41.10 Prevalence of coronary heart disease (CHD) and hypertension (HTN), alone and in combination, among Framingham Heart Study patients with congestive heart failure.

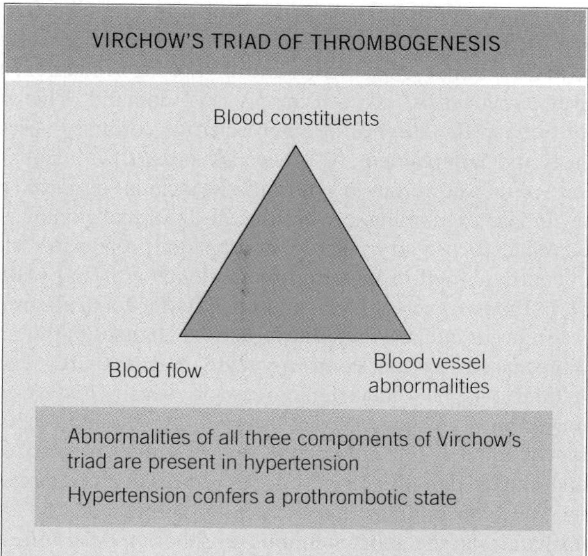

Figure 41.11 Virchow's triad of thrombogenesis: the Birmingham paradox.

"normal" range (i.e., systolic BP <120 mm Hg and diastolic BP <80 mm Hg).[73]

Furthermore, patients with hypertension have an increased incidence of unrecognized myocardial infarction, a greater likelihood of complications from acute coronary syndromes, and, compared with normotensive patients, worse acute and 5-year survival after myocardial infarction (Fig. 41.10).

Pathophysiology

Hypertension not only contributes to the development of atherosclerosis in the epicardial arteries, but is also important in the genesis of structural and functional abnormalities of the microvascular endothelium (atheromatous plaques do not occur in the microvasculature).

There is growing evidence that the atherosclerotic process is a response to injury of the vascular endothelium and to consequential changes in the production and release of vasodilator and vasoconstrictor substances. Nitric oxide, the most important of the endothelium-derived relaxing factors, is integral to the modulation of the atherogenic process. Other processes, such as platelet aggregation and adhesion, proliferation of smooth muscle cells, and leukocyte adhesion, are also important.[74] Whether abnormalities in endothelial structure and function (and associated atherogenesis?) that occur in hypertension are the cause or the consequence of increased blood pressure remains an area of active investigation.[75]

Increasing evidence suggests that patients with hypertension also demonstrate (Fig. 41.11) abnormalities of

- vessel walls (endothelial dysfunction or damage);
- blood constituents (abnormal concentrations of hemostatic factors, platelet activation and fibrinolysis); and
- blood flow (rheology, viscosity, and flow reserve).

The fulfillment of the three components of Virchow's triad for thrombogenesis suggests that hypertension confers a prothrombotic or hypercoagulable state, which appears to be related to the degree or severity of target organ damage. These abnormalities can be related to long-term prognosis and, in addition, may be altered by antihypertensive treatments. As the process of thrombogenesis is intimately related to atherogenesis, the prothrombotic state in hypertension may contribute to the increased risk of (atherosclerotic) coronary artery disease and thrombus-related complications, such as unstable angina and myocardial infarction.[76,77] Additional myocardial ischemia can be caused by reduction in coronary blood flow in the large conduit arteries or reduced coronary reserve resulting from an inadequate coronary blood flow response to increased myocardial oxygen demand (often related to microvascular dysfunction).[15]

Finally, hypertension may also result in changes in mechanical and hemodynamic forces that can influence plaque composition, the potential for plaque erosion, and the likelihood of plaque disruption. Hypertension-related increases in transmural pressure, wall tension, and shear stresses induce excess proliferation, hypertrophy, and hyperplasia of vascular smooth muscle cells; increased vascular wall thickness; reduced vascular dilatory capacity; and accelerated plaque formation. Perivascular fibrosis may also contribute to impaired coronary flow reserve. Schwartzkopff and colleagues[78] demonstrated that perivascular collagen volume formation correlated inversely with coronary flow reserve in hypertensive individuals. Indeed, myocardial ischemia caused by abnormalities in endothelial function and coronary vascular reactivity has also been reported in hypertensive patients, independent of coronary atherosclerosis or LVH and hypercholesterolemia.

Clinical Presentations

The spectrum of clinical presentations of coronary artery disease and hypertension, with angina, acute coronary syndromes and myocardial infarction, are discussed in detail in Chapter 40.

Chronic angina pectoris is related to myocardial ischemia secondary to luminal encroachment by one or more atherosclerotic plaques in an epicardial artery. However, in the hypertensive patient there also appear to be functional and structural alterations in the coronary microvasculature, resulting in an imbalance between myocardial oxygen supply and demand. This may occur even in the absence of atherosclerotic coronary vascular disease and independent of other risk factors.[79,80] This syndrome, often referred to as syndrome X, includes atypical chest pain, female predominance, occasional abnormal noninvasive tests, reduced coronary reserve, and benign prognosis—which has been described in hypertensive patients with and without LVH. In the presence of LVH, endothelial functional abnormalities also occur and are linked to structural changes in the myocardium, such as increased myocyte hypertrophy, excess interstitial collagen, reduced microvascular density and external compression of intramyocardial arterioles. In the hypertensive patient without LVH, myocardial ischemia may be attributed to endothelial damage produced by increased blood pressure alone, by concomitant hypercholesterolemia, or by basic abnormalities in the neurohumoral control of vascular tone.

Hypertension, especially in the presence of LVH, increases the risk of complications after myocardial infarction, including infarct expansion, reinfarction, and cardiac rupture. In hypertensive patients with LVH, the clinical manifestations of atherosclerotic epicardial coronary disease may overlap with the clinical features of nonatherosclerotic vascular dysfunction and ventricular remodeling, such as arterial vasospasm, impaired ventricular performance, reduced coronary reserve, and electrical instability.

Diagnostic Techniques

In the hypertensive patient, it may be difficult to distinguish the secondary ST-T wave changes (ST segment depression and T wave inversion) that is associated with LVH or microvascular disease from the primary ST-T wave depression that is associated with unstable angina and non–Q wave infarction. These differences may be difficult to distinguish, even during exercise stress testing, as the baseline ST-T changes associated with LVH and hypertension may limit the specificity of these findings. Detailed diagnosis and investigations for coronary artery disease are summarized in Chapters 19 and 20.

Management

Management of the patient with hypertension and either documented or suspected coronary disease requires

- control of hypertension;
- avoidance of symptoms of myocardial ischemia;
- prevention of coronary complications (unstable angina, infarction, heart failure, or death); and
- prevention of other cardiovascular disease through management of risk factors.

Blood pressure reduction is the critical element of management. The purported superiority of specific drug classes is still debated.[81] Irrespective of the differences, combination of drugs is frequently required to achieve blood pressure targets.[82]

In choosing an antihypertensive medication for a patient with possible or confirmed coronary disease, it is important to consider not only the blood pressure–decreasing efficacy of the drug, but also its value or limitations in reducing myocardial ischemia and limiting total cardiovascular disease risk.[83] Some antihypertensive agents may aggravate myocardial ischemia even though blood pressure is decreased. Direct-acting vasodilators (hydralazine and minoxidil) may cause marked vasodilatation and stimulation of baroreceptors, with resulting increases in heart rate and myocardial stroke work. Hydralazine may directly stimulate the heart, in addition to its potent peripheral vasodilatory properties, increasing contractility and oxygen demand.

Beta Blockers

Although beta blockers are no longer recommended as routine initial therapy,[84] they are the agents of choice for the management of patients with concurrent hypertension and coronary artery disease or heart failure. Anti-ischemic effects of beta blockers are comparable in all racial groups, although effective control of blood pressure may require increased doses or duration of treatment in blacks. Beta blockers are also recommended for secondary prevention after myocardial infarction because they have been shown to reduce infarct size, decrease mortality after infarction, decrease the incidence of nonfatal ischemic complications, and reduce arrhythmias and sudden death.[85]

Nitrates

Glyceryl trinitrate and other organic nitrates, administered sublingually, transdermally or orally, have long been a mainstay of treatment for angina pectoris. However, although nitrates may variably decrease blood pressure through venodilatation and reductions in arteriolar tone, they have no use in the management of chronic systemic hypertension and are used primarily for the management of acute anginal episodes (administered sublingually) and for chronic angina pectoris (long-acting preparations).

Angiotensin-Converting Enzyme Inhibitors

Evidence from clinical trials has established this class of agent as effective for the treatment of hypertension and heart failure and for the prevention of renal insufficiency in diabetic patients. Recent studies of ACE inhibitors in humans with chronic ischemic coronary disease have not shown that these drugs have substantial anti-ischemic action, and they are of limited value in the treatment of angina or the acute coronary syndromes. They have also been shown to prevent myocardial remodeling and heart failure and to decrease death rates in patients with myocardial infarction and LV dysfunction.

Calcium Channel Blockers

The impact of dihydropyridine calcium channel blockers on myocardial infarction had been the subject of controversy.[86] However, these drugs have been shown to be effective in the treatment of acute severe coronary spasm and Prinzmetal's variant angina. There is data that long-acting dihydropyridine calcium channel blockers, such as nifedipine GITS in the ACTION trial, are safe in patients with stable angina.[87] Although it had no effect on major cardiovascular mortality, it reduced the need for coronary angiography and coronary interventions. After myocardial infarction, the dihydropyridine calcium channel blockers have been shown to have a negative impact on reinfarction and mortality rates, and are not recommended in the management of acute myocardial infarction, especially with LV dysfunction. In contrast, nondihydropyridine calcium channel blockers may be of considerable utility in patients with hypertension and active ischemic heart disease. The INVEST study demonstrated equal efficacy of a verapamil-based regimen in comparison to a beta blocker–based regimen in such patients.[88]

In patients who cannot tolerate beta blockers, ivabradine may provide an alternative antianginal agent that lowers heart rate exclusively by selectively inhibiting the I(f) channel.[89] This agent has no negative inotropy, unlike calcium channel blockers, and is currently being investigated in patients with active ischemia and systolic LV dysfunction.[90]

Drug Combinations for Hypertension and Coronary Artery Disease

Although available data are limited, combination therapy may prove advantageous in selected circumstances. For example, low-dose combinations of beta blockers and dihydropyridine calcium channel blockers may effectively control both angina and hypertension with reduced adverse side effects. Because of their negative inotropic and chronotropic effects, beta blockers should not be combined with nondihydropyridine calcium channel blockers in patients at risk for bradycardia (e.g., long PR interval, atrioventricular nodal disease) or with ventricular dysfunction with dilatation. Calcium channel blockers (e.g., amlodipine or felodipine) may be added to ACE inhibitors and diuretics for more effective control of angina and blood pressure.

ARRHYTHMIAS AND SUDDEN DEATH

Hypertension is an important risk factor for the development of atrial and ventricular arrhythmias and sudden cardiac death.[4,91] Hypertension may play a direct part in the development of these rhythm disturbances by contributing to the development of LVH, atherosclerotic disease, and microvascular dysfunction. The risk of arrhythmias is greatest with evidence of LVH and/or left atrial abnormality on echocardiography and ECG, even in patients with no clinical history of coronary disease.[92] Hypertensive individuals are predisposed to arrhythmias even with normal cardiac chamber size.[93]

Atrial Arrhythmias

Atrial fibrillation is the most common and most serious of the atrial tachyarrhythmias because of its association with fatal and nonfatal stroke and heart failure.[94] Indeed, hypertension accounts for more atrial fibrillation in the population than does any other risk factor,[95] especially if associated hypertensive LVH is present.[96] Other than diabetes, hypertension is the only cardiovascular risk factor that independently predicts the development of atrial fibrillation, even after adjustment for age and associated comorbidity. A high pulse pressure is a particularly strong predictor of subsequent atrial fibrillation.[97]

The presence of hypertension adds to the risk of stroke and thromboembolism in atrial fibrillation, which is reduced by anticoagulation; among anticoagulated atrial fibrillation patients, good blood pressure control reduces the risk of stroke and thromboembolism.[98]

The evaluation and management of the hypertensive patient with atrial fibrillation should include

- appropriate selection of antihypertensive drug;
- identification of prognostic markers;
- exclusion of intrinsic cardiac disease;
- maintenance of sinus rhythm; and
- anticoagulation if there is persistent atrial fibrillation.

The use of renin-angiotensin blocking antihypertensive agents in ameliorating atrial fibrillation is attracting much interest. For example, Madrid and colleagues[99] have shown that agents such as angiotensin receptor blockers prolong the atrial effective refractory period and this translates into beneficial clinical effects. A large-scale clinical trial is currently evaluating whether these beneficial effects may result in fewer major cardiac events.[100]

Ventricular Arrhythmias

Premature ventricular ectopy and complex ventricular tachyarrhythmias are common in hypertensive individuals, but are more prevalent in patients with hypertension and LVH than in those without hypertrophy or in normotensive individuals.[101] The arrhythmic risk of hypertensive patients has been shown to markedly increase if microvolt level T wave alternans is present.[102] Arrhythmias in hypertensive patients have been shown to be related to LVH, but are independent of coexisting coronary artery disease or LV dysfunction. Increased risk of sudden death appears to be due primarily to coincident myocardial ischemia and concomitant subendocardial fibrosis and collagen deposition, with impaired coronary vasodilator reserve, subendocardial ischemia, and cellular electrophysiologic abnormalities related to cardiac hypertrophy.

In the treatment of ventricular arrhythmias, the use of beta blockers as antihypertensive agents is desirable because of their role as anti-ischemic and antiarrhythmic agents. Low-dose diuretic treatment also reduces cardiovascular events in hypertensive patients. Conversely, use of high-dose diuretics and hypokalemia or hypomagnesemia during drug treatment of hypertension must be avoided because of the increased risk of arrhythmias in the presence of electrolyte imbalance.

Sudden Cardiac Death

Hypertension-induced LVH is a risk factor for spontaneous ventricular arrhythmias and is associated with a greater risk of sudden cardiac death.[103] Some 80% of individuals who experience sudden cardiac death have coronary heart disease.[104] It should be remembered that not all sudden death is arrhythmia-related, as autopsy studies confirm the presence of thrombus in the left main coronary artery, in keeping with the prothrombotic state seen in hypertension.[15]

Although hypertension, LVH, hypercholesterolemia, glucose intolerance, smoking, and excess weight are risk factors for coronary artery disease, these factors also identify individuals at risk for sudden cardiac death. Advanced LV dysfunction is also an independent predictor of sudden cardiac death in patients with ischemic and nonischemic cardiomyopathy.

For patients who have suffered myocardial infarction and for those with heart failure, beta blockers are the drugs of choice. However, the implantable cardioverter-defibrillator appears to be the best current therapeutic modality for prophylaxis against sudden cardiac death, and should be used in high-risk populations.[105]

chapter 42

Complications of Hypertension: The Kidney

Domenic A. Sica

Definition

- Hypertensive nephrosclerosis is a blood pressure–related pathologic process marked by a progressive decline in renal function.

Key Features

- Hypertensive nephrosclerosis is in most instances a slowly progressive disease with few, if any, clinical symptoms.
- Biochemical markers of renal function, such as serum creatinine level, are insensitive indicators of the onset or rate of progression of hypertensive nephrosclerosis unless it is at an advanced stage.

Therapy

- Careful control of blood pressure is needed to slow the progression of hypertensive nephrosclerosis.
- Most antihypertensive medications can effectively reduce blood pressure in this disease, although diuretics are predictably needed to maximize the effect of other medications. Angiotensin-converting enzyme inhibitors and angiotensin receptor blockers are considered important elements in nearly all treatment regimens for this disease.

The impact of hypertension on highly vascular organs such as the kidney can be particularly devastating. Irrespective of the form of hypertension (essential or secondary), once a hypertensive state is present the kidney becomes a target organ for hypertension-related damage. Although the specific means by which hypertension produces renal structural damage is still open to conjecture, it is now well recognized that if hypertension is left untreated, there is a certain inexorability to the renal failure process, with the frequent development of end-stage renal disease (ESRD). Even with treatment there is no guarantee that the kidney is necessarily shielded. The optimum blood pressure (BP) for the preservation of renal function and which antihypertensive medication (or medications) optimizes renal protection are still being debated.

Furthermore, hypertension and progressive renal disease may be influenced by (and in their own right) influence a number of other cardiovascular (CV) illnesses, including heart failure (HF) and coronary artery disease (CAD). In the presence of HF, senescence-related change in renal function accelerates. In the presence of atherosclerotic CAD, a similar vascular change occurs in the renal vascular bed. This latter phenomenon can be present as either renal artery stenosis or microvascular disease (or both), and if vascular involvement is extreme enough the kidney is overly sensitized to certain forms of antihypertensive therapy, such as angiotensin-converting enzyme (ACE) inhibitors and angiotensin receptor blockers (ARBs).

A final consideration relative to hypertension and progression of renal disease is the observation that left ventricular hypertrophy (LVH) and CAD are often present and progressive in patients with chronic kidney disease (CKD). Patients who have renal insufficiency do not usually die of their renal failure; rather, their demise is most commonly linked to a CV event.

The costs of managing hypertension, renal failure, and associated CV conditions are significant and typically represents a major component of health care expenditures for many industrialized countries. Fortunately, effective preventive and treatment modalities for CKD are increasingly available. Most strategies now involve administration of an ACE inhibitor or an ARB. However, treatment of hypertension alone may be of only modest value unless the entire spectrum of disease-accelerating factors is suitably modified. Such additional treatment measures now are recognized to include cessation of smoking, lowering of low-density lipoprotein (LDL) cholesterol, tight blood glucose control, control of calcium/phosphate homeostasis, and elimination of platelet effect(s).

ANATOMY AND PATHOLOGY

The number of patients who develop ESRD secondary to hypertension-associated nephrosclerosis is increasing and it is considered as one of the most common causes of ESRD as reported in all national registries in Europe and the United States. Hypertension-associated nephrosclerosis now accounts for 24.6% of new dialysis patients in the United States.[1] Hypertensive nephrosclerosis began to stand out as a recognized cause of ESRD only in the early 1980s, coinciding with what was a steady increase in the mean age of new dialysis patients. Although these numbers suggest an important role for hypertensive nephrosclerosis in progression to ESRD, the mere fact that hypertension is present in an ESRD patient (who does not have diabetes and/or significant proteinuria) does not automatically mean they have hypertensive nephrosclerosis. It is likely that there exists an assignment bias to this category when this constellation of symptoms is present. Such an assignment bias typically ignores the pre-ESRD course that may not be at all compatible with a diagnosis of hypertensive nephrosclerosis.

The mechanisms that initiate the process of glomerulosclerosis are not static. Once these processes are set in

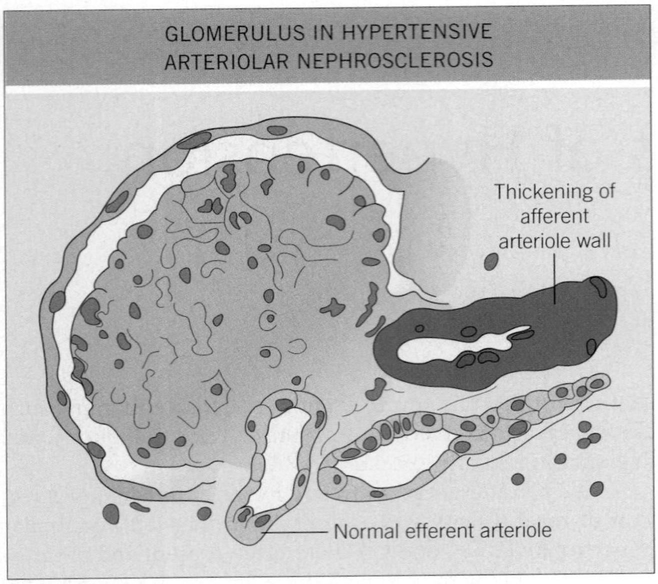

GLOMERULUS IN HYPERTENSIVE ARTERIOLAR NEPHROSCLEROSIS

Thickening of afferent arteriole wall

Normal efferent arteriole

Figure 42.1 Glomerulus in hypertensive arteriolar nephrosclerosis. There is thickening of the afferent arteriolar wall caused by the deposition of hyaline material, resulting in a narrowing of the lumen. The efferent arteriole appears normal.

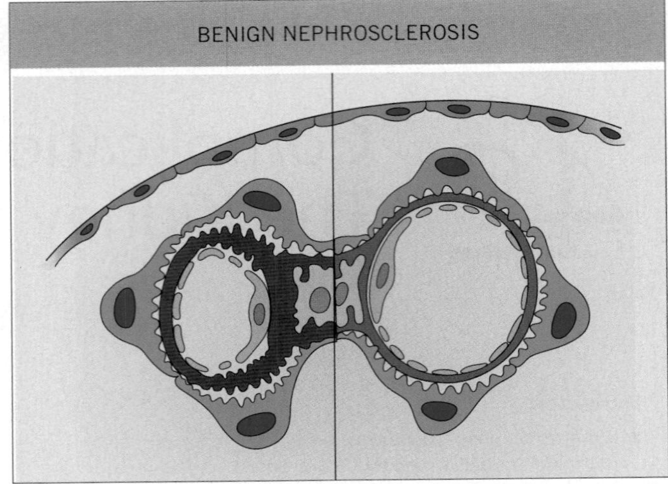

Figure 42.2 Ischemic glomerulus in benign nephrosclerosis. The major change is wrinkling and thickening of the glomerular basement membrane, particularly adjacent to the mesangium.

motion, glomerulosclerosis is typically progressive in nature, often paralleling the severity of hypertension. In humans, it has been repeatedly observed that the renal vessels that are most susceptible to pathologic change in hypertension are the small renal arteries (the arcuate and interlobular arteries) and arterioles. The preglomerular blood vessels (afferent arterioles) are more prominently affected than are the post-glomerular circulation (efferent arterioles) (Fig. 42.1). The vascular pathology of the small arteries and arterioles can be assigned to three general categories:

- hyaline arteriolar sclerosis;
- myointimal hypertrophy and hyperplasia; and
- fibrinoid necrosis.

Hyperplastic vasculopathy and/or necrotizing arteriolitis/fibrinoid necrosis are key pathologic features of malignant hypertension, as compared to the more nonspecific hyaline arteriolar sclerosis, which is seen in all forms of hypertension.

The sequelae of arterial narrowing are related to the degree and the rate at which such narrowing takes place. Statistically significant relationships exist between the prevailing diastolic pressure and the degree to which afferent renal arteriolar thickening and narrowing occurs.[2] The term nephrosclerosis is literally defined as hardening of the kidneys and has been used to describe the renal pathologic lesions that arise in conjunction with essential hypertension. Because the vascular lesions of hypertension primarily affect the small preglomerular arteries, downstream elements such as the glomeruli and postglomerular structures are subject to the changes of ischemic deprivation (Fig. 42.2). In mild hypertension, most glomeruli remain structurally normal; moreover, there is little evidence of tubular atrophy or interstitial fibrosis. As hypertension progresses in severity or duration, the same structures begin to demonstrate direct hypertensive injury in addition to ischemic changes. Global sclerosis, tubular atrophy, interstitial fibrosis, and, on occasion, an interstitial inflammatory cell infiltrate all surface at this stage of renal involvement with hypertension.

Although small vessel disease in the kidney is probably the most important vascular complication, from a functional viewpoint the larger renal arteries are also subject to considerable pathologic change. Atheromatous disease of the major renal arteries develops at an earlier stage in patients who have already been hypertensive. When such atheromatous disease is present, it is often associated with a more rapidly progressive form of renal insufficiency. Physiologically significant occlusive renal artery disease can accelerate any adverse renal consequences of the hypertensive process. In essential hypertension, the more severe the elevation in BP, the more prominent the small vessel lesions. In renal artery stenosis, despite the sometimes rather aggressive nature of the hypertension, small vessels—typically downstream from the stenotic lesion—are protected from the full brunt of hypertensive change. The deterioration in renal function observed under these circumstances more commonly relates to a form of diffuse ischemic atrophy.

PATHOPHYSIOLOGY

An important risk factor that contributes to acceleration of renal disease is systemic hypertension, which may be both cause and consequence of chronic renal disease (Fig. 42.3). The relationship between BP and serum creatinine level is progressive and gradual even across "normal" values of each, and there is no evidence of a threshold.[3] This pattern resembles the continuous pattern of risk for stroke and CV disease that is observed across BP values; it suggests that even modest BP elevations may bring about a rise in serum creatinine if they are sustained over a sufficiently long period of time. In patients with senescence-related renal disease, hypertension also accelerates the more moderate loss of renal function that occurs with normal aging.

Patients who have CKD demonstrate both higher daytime BP values and often a loss of the characteristic nocturnal BP

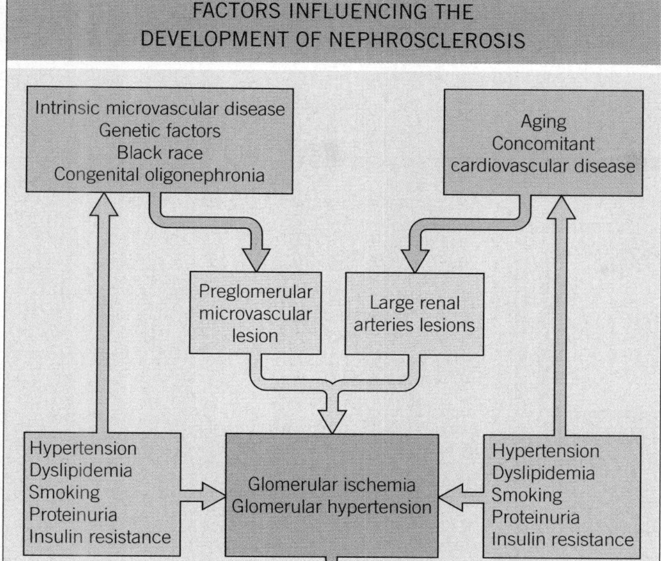

Figure 42.3 Factors influencing the development of nephrosclerosis. (Modified from Marin R, Gorostidi M, Fernandez-Vega F, Alvarez-Navascues R. Systemic and glomerular hypertension and progression of chronic renal disease: the dilemma of nephrosclerosis. Kidney Int 2005;68(Suppl 99):S52-S56.)

decline (i.e., they show a "nondipping" pattern of BP), so that the mechanisms of hypertensive injury are more continuously operable in these patients. The significance of a lack of decline in nocturnal BP as a renal and a CV risk factor has only recently emerged; a nocturnal nondipping BP pattern is now known to be associated with more severe LVH and a higher prevalence rate of microalbuminuria as well as an accelerated decline in the rate of loss of renal function.[4] This nocturnal nondipping pattern is more common in black people. Furthermore, an elevation in serum creatinine (to 1.7 mg/dL or more) has been shown to be a potent and independent risk factor for increased mortality (primarily due to CV and cerebrovascular events),[5] which suggests that the presence of hypertensive nephrosclerosis is an indication of a more generalized systemic atherosclerotic process.[6,7]

In essential hypertension, glomerular damage occurs either because of ischemia secondary to narrowing of the preglomerular vessels by arteriosclerosis or because of direct damage by increased transmural pressures in glomerular capillaries. The latter occurs as the result of an inability of the preglomerular vessels to autoregulate normally and typically leads to glomerular capillary hyperperfusion. It is probable that the extent of such injury partially dictates the degree of proteinuria seen in the various stages of nephrosclerosis, although direct glomerular capillary damage is more likely to account for the higher protein excretion rates (more than 1 g/24 h) that are occasionally observed in hypertensive patients.[8] More recently, the notion has arisen that proteinuria in hypertensive nephrosclerosis may reflect generalized systemic transvascular leakiness, possibly mediated by endothelial dysfunction. In most hypertensive patients, renal insufficiency is typically mild, although progression to ESRD has been observed to occur with some regularity. Whether hypertension can, of itself, cause ESRD, or whether a preexisting glomerular lesion is a needed component of the disease process is still vigorously debated.

The true incidence of hypertensive nephropathy has proven difficult to determine because, in the absence of a renal biopsy, the diagnosis of hypertensive nephropathy is often a presumptive rather than a definitive diagnosis. Certain groups, including African Americans, appear to have a particular susceptibility to hypertension (albeit occurring at a lower relative rate) as a cause of ESRD, even after accounting for differences in severity of BP and a lower socioeconomic status.[1,9]

Several explanations have been proposed for this phenomenon. This tendency for hypertensive patients of African American origin to develop ESRD has been associated with a familial clustering,[10,11] birth weights of less than 2500 g,[12] higher systolic BP values, and a lower socioeconomic status.[9] To date, two chromosomal regions have demonstrated linkage or association with ESRD in the American black population. These are the plasma prekallikrein gene and the human homologue of the rodent renal failure 1 gene.[11] Further considerations have included inadequate treatment, renal damage that is present before the inception of therapy, the existence of intrinsic renal processes refractory to conventional therapies, and the observation that daytime BP measurements fail to capture the fact that African Americans more frequently demonstrate a nondipping nocturnal BP pattern.[13] It is likely that many of these processes are linked to dietary sodium (Na^+) intake, salt sensitivity, and variable degrees of insulin resistance, and the way in which these processes independently and collectively exaggerate the risk of hypertensive renal injury.

It has long been believed that the kidneys of African American and white hypertensive patients behave in a physiologically and pathologically different fashion. For example, African American hypertensive patients typically exhibit much higher renal vascular resistance than whites, and they excrete smaller amounts of renal kallikrein. Furthermore, there has been speculation about racially specific forms of hypertensive nephropathy. In support of a significant incidence of hypertensive nephrosclerosis in African Americans are the findings from the pilot phase of the African-American Study of Kidney Diseases (AASK), wherein nondiabetic hypertensive African Americans with mild to moderate renal insufficiency (glomerular filtration rate [GFR], 51.7 ± 13.6 mL/min/1.73 m^2) in the absence of marked proteinuria underwent percutaneous renal biopsy. In this study 35 of the 39 biopsy specimens contained pathologic vascular lesions supporting a clinical diagnosis of hypertensive nephrosclerosis.[14]

Angiotensin II is critically involved in hypertension-related renal failure, a finding underscored by the effectiveness of therapies, such as ACE inhibitors and/or ARBs, that aim to inhibit its varied actions.[15] Angiotensin II has direct parenchymal and/or arterial effects (Fig. 42.4). For example, either circulating or locally produced angiotensin II (or both) increase systemic and, in many instances, intraglomerular pressures. Angiotensin II factors in the trapping of macromolecules in the mesangium lead to selective defects in glomerular barrier function and promote glomerular hypertrophy.

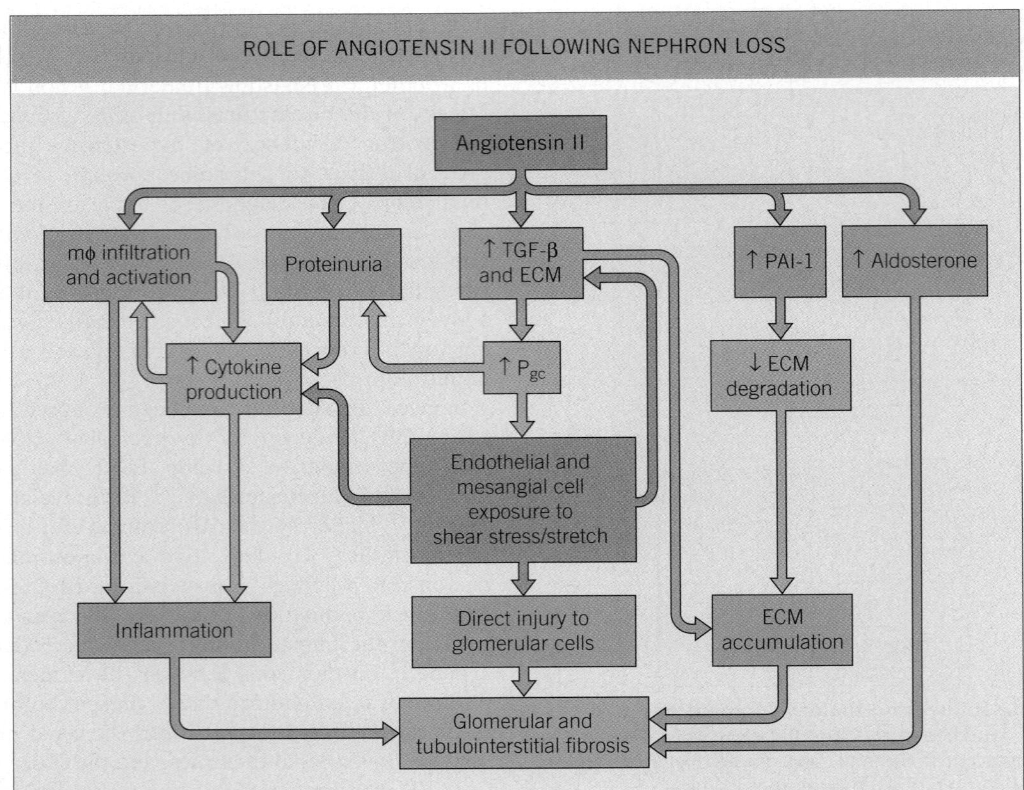

Figure 42.4 Role of angiotensin II following nephron loss. ECM, extracellular matrix; mϕ, macrophage; PAI-1, plasminogen activator inhibitor 1; P_{gc}, glomerular capillary hydraulic pressure; TGF-β, transforming growth factor-β.

Angiotensin II is indirectly profibrotic, acting through overexpression of the fibrogenic cytokine transforming growth factor-β (TGF-β) and/or the expression/secretion of endothelin. Angiotensin II also induces tubulointerstitial fibrosis by stimulating the angiotensin type 1 (AT_1) receptor. Another mechanism that can be offered for the observed racial difference in hypertensive nephrosclerosis is that endothelin 1 concentrations are higher in blacks, which can amplify glomerular damage, perhaps through induction of TGF-β. Renal fibrosis can be induced by TGF-β, which is overexpressed in blacks.[16] In turn, TGF-β induces endothelin 1 expression and stimulates renin release, which through generation of angiotensin II can sustain TGF-β synthesis.

CLINICAL PRESENTATION

Benign nephrosclerosis (also known as hypertensive nephropathy or hypertensive nephrosclerosis) is an insidious disease with no apparent symptoms. It usually begins by the age of 50 years and is more common in males and in African Americans and more often than not occurs coincident to essential hypertension (Table 42.1). In many cases of hypertensive nephrosclerosis, the onset of the disease proves difficult to date, because office-based assessment of renal function is not routinely performed, and when it is, it proves diagnostically insensitive for this disease. Thus, although this disease is present and progressive, the perception of "normal renal function" hangs on well beyond its time. It is noteworthy that the aging process is marked by deterioration in several facets of renal function. This senescence-related deterioration in renal function is accelerated by elevated BP and progresses at a faster rate than does the renal functional loss occurring in normotensive age-matched controls.[17]

In the early stages of benign nephrosclerosis, there is no apparent reduction in renal function. The early stages of this disease may be characterized by increased cardiac output, LVH, and glomerular hyperfiltration, not unlike the

FACTORS THAT SUPPORT A DIAGNOSIS OF HYPERTENSIVE NEPHROSCLEROSIS
■ Absence of any cause of primary renal disease
■ Family history with onset of hypertension between 25 and 45 years of age
■ African American race
■ Long-standing or stage 2 hypertension
■ Onset of hypertension before the development of proteinuria
■ Presence of left ventricular hypertrophy
■ Evidence of hypertensive retinal damage
■ Low-level hyperuricemia
■ Existence of a blunted renal hemodynamic response to protein loading or amino acid infusion
■ Biopsy evidence, degree of glomerular ischemia and fibrosis compatible with degree of arteriolar and small artery vascular disease

Table 42.1 Factors that support a diagnosis of hypertensive nephrosclerosis.

beginning stages of diabetic nephropathy.[18] When confounding variables such as age, sex, weight, and BP are controlled for, no racial disparities are detected between matched black and white patients with early-stage hypertension findings.[19] In hypertensive nephrosclerosis, the urinary sediment is typically bland, though on occasion it may reveal hyaline and granular casts and, rarely, red blood cells. Small amounts of protein, in the microalbuminuria range (20 to 200 μg/min), may be found in the urine, particularly when BP is poorly controlled. The earliest detectable abnormality is a decrease in renal blood flow (RBF), with a reduction in GFR occurring sometime later. The maintenance of a normal GFR despite a decrease in RBF has been attributed to increased efferent arteriolar resistance. In turn, this appears to be linked to an excessive effect of angiotensin II, which is seemingly poorly suppressible with an increase in salt intake.[20] The fall in RBF that is observed in hypertensive patients correlates with the extent of renal vascular damage and with the severity and duration of the disease. The fall in RBF in hypertensive nephrosclerosis is typically greater in African American hypertensive patients.

As the renal injury of hypertensive nephrosclerosis progresses, serum creatinine values slowly rise, although often in an imperceptible fashion. This picture is similar to that seen with the senescent kidney, where the greatest age-related functional change is observed in those with BP in the hypertensive range. The presence of significant proteinuria (more than 1 g per 24 hours) should cause one to entertain a diagnosis other than hypertensive nephrosclerosis. It should be stressed that a noteworthy elevation in the serum creatinine value may not occur until the GFR has fallen to less than 30% of normal and thereby is a late finding in benign nephrosclerosis (and in other renal diseases).

DIAGNOSTIC TECHNIQUES

Diagnosing hypertensive nephrosclerosis before the onset of clinical signs and symptoms is a challenging task since this diagnosis can be considered only after having systematically eliminated other forms of progressive renal insufficiency. The presentation of hypertensive nephrosclerosis is often difficult to differentiate from that of parenchymal renal disease, atheroembolic renal disease, and renovascular hypertension with renal insufficiency. A noninvasive technique does not exist for the accurate diagnosis of hypertensive nephrosclerosis. As such, a definitive diagnosis relies on the findings of a renal biopsy. Even in the case of renal biopsy, the severity of clinical hypertension does not correlate well with the histopathologic changes of hypertensive nephrosclerosis. Because of the absence of a "defining" test and the limited sensitivity of existing testing methods, many patients who are thought to have hypertensive nephropathy may, in fact, have other causes of renal dysfunction.

Renal imaging studies, such as intravenous pyelography and renal ultrasound (more commonly used), may show cortical thinning or smaller kidneys, particularly as measured in their longitudinal axis. The urine sediment does not have any defining characteristics. Low-grade proteinuria, often in the microalbuminuria range, is often present but seldom reaches the nephrotic range. Other components of the "hypertensive work-up," such as an automated chemistry profile or an ECG, do not provide any meaningful indication of the level of renal involvement attributable to hypertension. An exception to this may be the uric acid level, in that the hyperuricemia accompanying nephrosclerosis is commonly greater than that observed in patients with primary renal diseases. The difficulty in determining the presence or extent of hypertensive nephrosclerosis primarily resides in an inability to accurately establish either its onset or its rate of progression. Hypertensive nephrosclerosis is often insidious in its progression, with a major loss of renal function often having been sustained despite the serum creatinine (significantly influenced by muscle mass) being only nominally above the "normal" value for a patient. An understanding of the limitations of the serum creatinine value (as well as other renal function measurements) is essential for the early diagnosis of hypertension-related renal dysfunction. These renal function measurements are also encumbered with similar interpretive difficulties when they are used to gauge success (or failure) of various therapies used to slow progressive renal failure.

The GFR in adults with CKD can be approximated from a plasma creatinine value (provided it is greater than 2 mg/dL) with the aid of additional demographic and biochemical variables. Gender, height, weight, age, and race should be taken into account. Serum creatinine values may best describe renal function when values are obtained at the time of a carefully performed 24-hour creatinine clearance; therein they can be indexed to a measured value for creatinine clearance. This will establish the prevailing relationship between serum creatinine and the creatinine clearance and in that way validate any subsequent interpretation of changes in serum creatinine values.

The renal clearance of creatinine derives from a combination of filtration and tubular secretion. The contribution of tubular creatinine secretion to total urinary creatinine is not constant, varying based on circadian factors and degree of renal insufficiency. Under normal circumstances, tubular creatinine secretion is responsible for 10% of daily urine creatinine excretion; thus a creatinine clearance can be expected to overestimate "true" GFR by the same amount (10%). With progressive renal failure, as much as 40% of excreted urine creatinine can derive from tubular secretion and therefore seriously undermine the use of creatinine clearance as a measure of renal function. Moreover, this tendency for tubular creatinine secretion to increase in the face of declining renal function keeps serum creatinine values from increasing as much as might be expected in the face of progressive renal disease.

The difficulty in interpreting a serum creatinine may be overcome by the measurement of GFR, which can provide a more quantitative assessment of filtration capacity. GFR begins to decline relatively early in the course of renal disease. Although GFR cannot be directly measured in humans, it can be indirectly estimated by determining endogenous creatinine clearance. This method has considerable limitations, not the least of which is the need for accurate timing of urine collections; 24-hour creatinine clearance measurements are routinely subject to patient error in the collection process. Because of this, carefully timed (2 to 4 hours in duration), water-loaded creatinine clearance measurements are seen as a preferred alternative. Overnight creatinine clearance measurements can simplify the issue of urine collections. Unfortunately, nighttime creatinine clearance values systematically exceed daytime values in that nocturnal creatinine secretion routinely exceeds that observed in the daytime. In addition to the timing inaccuracies for creatinine clearance measurements, body weight and surface area (which are indicative of the amount of muscle mass) and intrinsic day-to-day variation in renal function will influence results. These factors contribute to a variability of up to 30% in creatinine clearance values on repeat measurements. In light of this, a number of authorities in the field now view the measurement of creatinine clearance as an anachronism. As such, the sensitivity of creatinine clearance measurements is sufficiently weak that early renal involvement from benign nephrosclerosis may go unrecognized. The same appears to apply to the predictive performance of renal function equations.[21]

An alternative approach to measurement of renal function relates to the manner in which creatinine is tubularly secreted. Creatinine is eliminated via the organic cation secretory pathway, a process that can be inhibited by other organic cations, such as the H_2 receptor antagonist cimetidine and the antibiotic trimethoprim. Upon receipt of either of these compounds, serum creatinine values can rise by as much as 1 to 2 mg/dL (thereby invalidating serum creatinine as a measure of renal function) without a corresponding change in blood urine nitrogen (BUN) values. A true change in renal function would typically be characterized by a simultaneous rise in both serum creatinine and BUN values. This competition for tubular secretion of creatinine can be used to good effect in the measurement of renal function. If creatinine secretion is intentionally blocked with cimetidine, a subsequently obtained creatinine clearance more closely approximates a patient's true GFR obtained by a gold standard measure such as an inulin clearance.[22] Although the optimal dose and timing of cimetidine for this purpose is still undecided, a single 1200-mg dose 2 hours before beginning urine collection is probably suitable.

Microalbuminuria, which can be found in approximately 15% of patients who have uncomplicated essential hypertension, is held to be a marker of generalized endothelial dysfunction and not nephrosclerosis. Moreover, it does not automatically predict the development of nephrosclerosis. As of yet, the effect of various antihypertensive drugs in reducing microalbuminuria cannot be taken as evidence of renal protection in benign nephrosclerosis. Proteinuria exceeding 1 g per 24 hours is occasionally observed in benign nephrosclerosis. Dasgupta and colleagues[23] observed protein excretion of 2.3 ± 2.4 g/day in a cohort of 60 patients with biopsy proven benign nephrosclerosis; thus, although proteinuria of this magnitude should generally prompt a search for alternative causes, it can be consistent with benign nephrosclerosis alone.

MANAGEMENT

Hypertensive nephrosclerosis is usually slowly progressive provided that BP is adequately controlled, although some patients progress to ESRD. Those factors associated with progression to ESRD include age, African American ethnicity, level of proteinuria, systolic BP values, and coexistent CV disease. Nephrosclerosis is being increasingly diagnosed in older individuals with CV disease; thus a multifactorial approach involving smoking cessation and taking lipid-lowering and antiplatelet agents would seem to offer the best chance at improving CV and renal outcomes in patients with benign nephrosclerosis.[24]

ACE inhibitors (at least in black people) seem to cause a differential slowing in the progression of classic hypertensive nephrosclerosis (see the following section on ACE inhibitors) when compared with either a beta blocker or a dihydropyridine calcium channel blocker (CCB).[25] The selection of a particular antihypertensive agent or combination of agents should address the possibility of renal and/or cardiac counterregulatory responses to antihypertensive therapy early in the course of therapy. The major pathways by which the kidney influences BP include renin release and Na^+ retention, acting together or separately, but additional nonrenal mechanisms such as tachycardia may also be a contributing counterregulatory process. When Na^+ intake is overly restrictive or diuresis excessive, the accompanying change in renin-angiotensin-aldosterone system (RAAS) activity can limit the BP fall. Nonspecific vasodilators (such as minoxidil) or agents that block the sympathetic nervous system (such as clonidine or beta blockers) when given in high doses are particularly prone to causing Na^+ retention.

In the treatment of hypertensive nephrosclerosis, an important feature of an antihypertensive compound is its ability to consistently reduce BP (particularly systolic BP) throughout a 24-hour dosing interval. Blood pressure control becomes especially critical in the presence of proteinuria in excess of 1 g per 24 hours. Blood pressure should be controlled to a value of 130/85 mm Hg or lower (125/75 mm Hg) in patients who have proteinuria in excess of 1 g per 24 hours, with whatever antihypertensive therapy is necessary. Typically, when BP is effectively controlled, the decline in GFR that accompanies this type of renal failure can be expected to slow noticeably (see the following section on ACE inhibitors). On occasion, renal function continues to deteriorate despite effective BP control.[26] Such reports are possibly explained by variable renal effects of different classes of antihypertensive medications (such as diuretics or beta blockers) and/or unrecognized large or small vessel renal arterial disease, inadequate reduction in systolic and diastolic BP (an adequate reduction being considered to be below 140/90 mm Hg), or failure to identify an out-of-office BP pattern that differs from that obtained in the course of routine office visits. On a practical basis, most office visits occur at the time of peak medication effect and can miss the fact that the medication effect has faded at the later stages of the dosing interval.

Although ACE inhibitor therapy appears to be the preferred treatment for hypertensive nephrosclerosis, monotherapy with ACE inhibitors is often inadequate to control BP. The selection of additional antihypertensive agents depends largely on the volume status of the patient and the additional underlying determinants of hypertension. Sodium restriction and diuretic therapy remain a crucial element in the treatment of hypertensive nephrosclerosis, particularly as creatinine clearance drops below 60 mL/min. Thiazide diuretics are effective as long as the creatinine clearance is above 30 mL/min or the serum creatinine is less than 2 to 2.5 mg/dL. As renal function further declines, loop diuretics (furosemide [frusemide], bumetanide, or torsemide) frequently become necessary. Pronounced Na^+ retention is uncommon in hypertensive nephrosclerosis irrespective of the severity of the renal insufficiency. If edema is a dominant finding in a patient who has hypertensive nephrosclerosis, it generally derives from a renal stimulus to Na^+ retention (as occurs with drugs such as minoxidil, clonidine, or beta blockers) or the coexistence of HF. Combination diuretic therapy with a loop diuretic and a thiazide diuretic (such as metolazone) is occasionally required in the treatment of these patients.

Patients who have hypertensive nephrosclerosis are generally not prone to developing hyperkalemia except possibly in the case of the elderly. Thus there is a wider margin of safety with potassium-sparing diuretics, such as spironolactone, amiloride, and triamterene, in patients who have pure hypertensive renal disease than is the case, for example, in patients with diabetic nephropathy, where hyperkalemia becomes a relevant consideration much earlier in the renal failure process. CCBs are used with some regularity in these patients. Heterogeneity for renal effects exists among the CCBs. Compounds such as verapamil and diltiazem exhibit different renal effects (such as their being antiproteinuric) than dihydropyridine CCBs. Moreover, on the basis of the AASK results, amlodipine should not be used in African American patients with hypertensive nephrosclerosis unless accompanied by either an ACE inhibitor or an ARB. At this time it is unclear what level of protection is afforded the kidney when an ACE inhibitor or an ARB is given together with a dihydropyridine CCB.[25]

Renin-Angiotensin System Inhibitors

Multiple drugs are typically needed to control BP in hypertensive nephrosclerosis. There is increasing recognition that the RAAS is integrally involved in hypertensive change in the kidney (Fig. 42.5). Recent evidence (particularly in hypertensive patients who have diabetic nephropathy) has established that agents that act on this system (i.e., ACE inhibitors and ARBs [and possibly direct renin inhibitors]) provide renal benefits that extend beyond those achieved with BP reduction alone.[27] The experimental basis for RAAS blockade in the treatment of progressive renal failure is strong.[28]

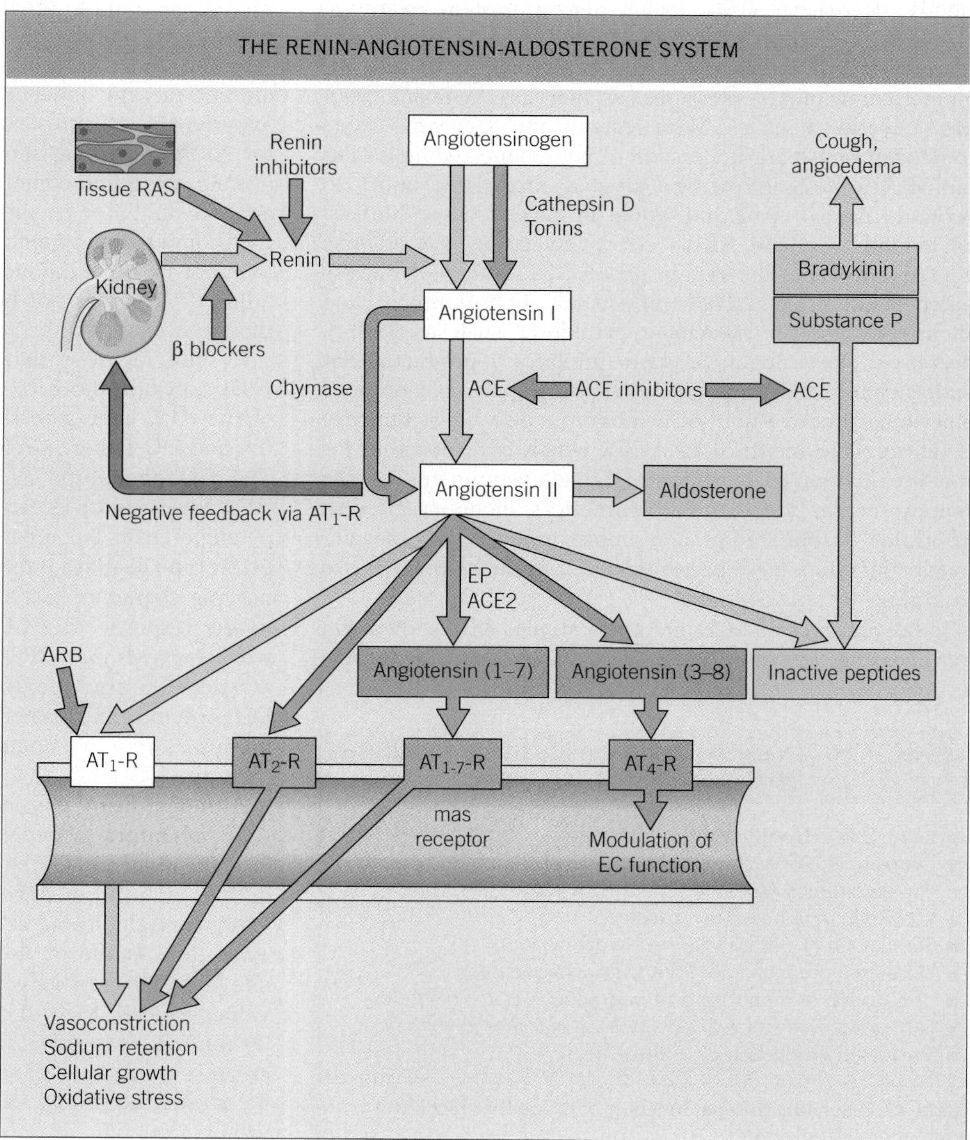

Figure 42.5 The renin-angiotensin-aldosterone system. Darker arrows show stimulation and lighter arrows show inhibition. β blockers, renin inhibitors, inhibitors of angiotensin-converting enzyme (ACE), and angiotensin II type-1 receptor blockers (ARB) reduce the activity of the renin-angiotensin system (RAS). AT-R, angiotensin receptor; EP, endopeptidases; EC, endothelial cells. (From Staessen JA, Li Y, Richart T. Oral renin inhibitors. Lancet 2006;368:1449-1456.)

Of the different classes of antihypertensive agents postulated to slow the progression rate of renal failure, ACE inhibitors (and more recently ARBs) have been most extensively studied.[29,30] Several ACE inhibitors have been shown to slow the progression of renal failure, including

- captopril, 12.5 to 50 mg/day;
- enalapril, 5 to 40 mg/day;
- benazepril, 10 mg/day;
- ramipril, 1.25 to 5 mg/day; and
- cilazapril, 2.5 to 5 mg/day.

ACE inhibitors are predominantly renally cleared; therefore in these studies it is likely that renal failure increased the systemic exposure (and thereby effect) to these medications.[31] The renoprotective effect of ACE inhibitors is most evident in patients who have heavy proteinuria (more than 3 g per 24 hours), who, if left untreated, generally see their renal failure progress more rapidly.[29] Blood pressure control becomes even more important under these circumstances.[30]

ACE inhibitors (and ARBs) have several renal effects that can be viewed as being renoprotective, including (but not limited to) decreasing efferent arteriolar resistance, transiently decreasing GFR, and reducing protein excretion (Table 42.2). Early opinion highlighted these hemodynamic features of ACE inhibitors, in light of their ability to decrease glomerular capillary pressures, as their predominant renoprotective mechanisms. More recently the RAAS has come to be viewed as part of a system of interconnected molecules biologically designed to be activated after tissue injury to promote tissue repair and, when in excess, tissue fibrosis. ACE inhibitors (and ARBs) effectively curtail the adverse consequences of this repair process by hemodynamically independent effects. These effects are importantly linked to a reduction in fibrogenic cytokines, such as TGF-β, decreased plasminogen activator inhibitor 1 production by endothelial and vascular smooth muscle cells, and reduced macrophage activation. ACE inhibitors also block kininase II (an enzyme identical to ACE), which is responsible for the breakdown of bradykinin. Some components of the renoprotective effects of ACE inhibitors, including efferent arteriolar vasodilatation and improvement in glomerular barrier function, have been attributed to the associated rise in kinins.[32,33]

In the presence of ACE inhibition, studies have shown that various other enzymes, including chymase and other serine proteases, are capable of generating angiotensin II. These non-ACE enzymes have been held accountable for the return of angiotensin II values to baseline levels (so-called angiotensin II escape) during chronic ACE inhibition. Although angiotensin II escape is of poorly defined clinical significance, it has led to speculation that the more complete blockade of angiotensin II effect with ARBs may separate these two drug classes in favor of ARBs. To date, this is an unproven hypothesis, because no head-to-head studies have been undertaken that compare ACE inhibitors to ARBs in nephropathic states.[33] Since chronic ACE inhibition is accompanied by angiotensin II escape, alternative explanations have been sought for the persistence of BP effect and the manifest organ protection properties with this drug class. In this regard, kinin-mediated effects of ACE inhibition have been proposed. The kinin hypothesis for the nephroprotection of ACE inhibitors, although interesting, awaits confirming studies in humans (Fig. 42.6).

BENEFITS TO RENAL FUNCTION OF DRUGS THAT BLOCK THE RENIN-ANGIOTENSIN SYSTEM
■ Reduction in blood pressure
■ Decrease in glomerular capillary pressures from a decrease in efferent arteriolar tone
■ Reduction in urine protein excretion
■ Stimulation of extracellular matrix degradation
■ Decreased production of fibrogenic cytokines such as TGF-β
■ Attenuation of monocyte and macrophage tissue infiltration
■ Decreased production of plasminogen activator inhibitor 1
■ Decreased production of aldosterone

Table 42.2 Benefits to renal function of drugs that block the renin-angiotensin system.

The renoprotective effects of ACE inhibitors can vary greatly. In some patients ACE inhibition shows little or no initial effect on the rate of renal functional decline. In other instances, for unclear reasons, an antiproteinuric effect may be confined only to the initial treatment period.[34] Three factors can be considered as potential modifiers of the renal response to ACE inhibitors. First, a low Na^+ intake or diuretic therapy enhances both the antiproteinuric and antihypertensive effects of ACE inhibitors, which is also the case for ARBs.[35] Second, short-term studies suggest that dietary protein restriction complements the antiproteinuric effect of an ACE inhibitor in patients with nephrosis, implying that this combination might prove more effective than ACE inhibitor treatment alone in slowing the progression of renal failure.[36] This has not been comparably studied with ARB therapy.

A third factor is that of an inherited insertion/deletion (I/D) polymorphism for ACE activity. Two common forms of the ACE gene give rise to three potential genotypes: II, ID, and DD (where I refers to insertion and D to deletion). The DD phenotype is associated with higher circulating ACE levels and a greater pressor response to the infusion of angiotensin I compared with the II phenotype; the ID phenotype displays intermediate characteristics. These phenotypic characteristics have been suggested to be relevant to the response to ACE inhibition. In this regard, recent work suggests that GFR declines more rapidly and there is a reduced antiproteinuric effect in patients exhibiting the DD polymorphic pattern who are treated with an ACE inhibitor; this phenomenon is not observed with ARB therapy.[37]

Although many physicians view it as unsafe to administer ACE inhibitors to patients with reduced renal function, in fact, the renal and CV benefits of ACE inhibition are greatest in this patient type. Accordingly, ACE inhibitors are not formally contraindicated at any level of renal function.[38] However, they should be used cautiously, starting at low doses and then progressively titrated up when serum creatinine values exceed 3 mg/dL (or creatinine clearance values are 30 mL/min or below), because the risk of hyperkalemia is greatest at this level of renal function. ACE inhibitors should be titrated according to tolerability and action on BP and proteinuria.

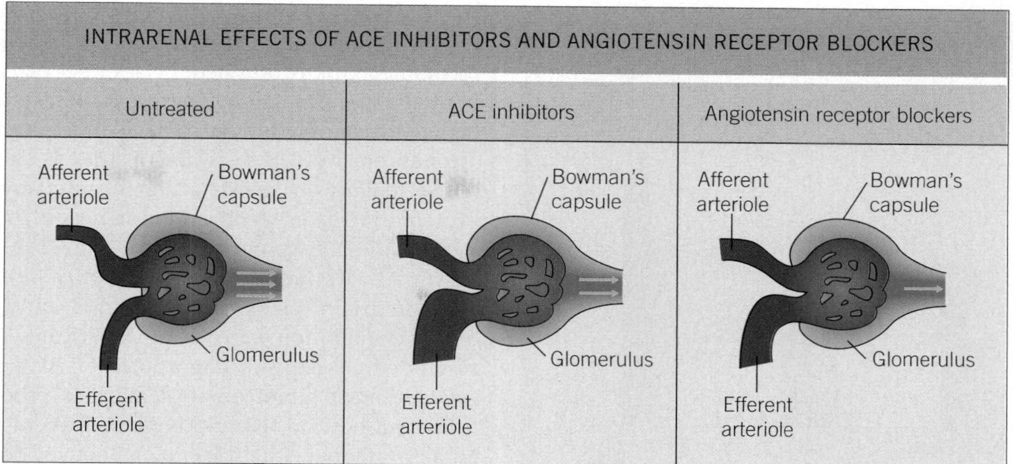

Figure 42.6 Intrarenal effects of angiotensin-converting (ACE) inhibitors and angiotensin receptor blockers (ARBs). In the untreated state efferent arteriolar tone is presumably increased and glomerular hyperfiltration exists *(left panel)*. The change in the diameter of the efferent arteriole is greater with ACE inhibition, reflecting the combined effect of increased bradykinin and decreased angiotensin II concentrations on efferent arteriolar tone *(middle)*. A proposed consequence of this change is a somewhat greater drop in the glomerular filtration rate with an ACE inhibitor. In the case of ARBs the absence of a direct effect on bradykinin limits any decrease in efferent arteriolar tone to what might occur with a reduction in angiotensin II effect *(right)*. Although this scenario has been demonstrated experimentally, confirming evidence of this process is still not available in humans.

The manner in which renal function changes when an ACE inhibitor is started depends on the treatment circumstances. In most instances there is little to no change in serum creatinine value (or the level of renal function) when an ACE inhibitor is started. This is typically the case when hypertension alone is being treated. Occasionally, renal function declines (by 10% to 20%) shortly after an ACE inhibitor is started, a process that arises from a resetting of renal hemodynamics and is fully reversible when the drug is discontinued. This pattern is observed in patients with underlying renal disease. The magnitude of this early drop in renal function may, in fact, identify those patients likely to benefit most from ACE inhibitor therapy.[39] Concern engendered by this change in renal function is unfounded. A more substantial drop in renal function is occasionally seen in patients who are being treated with an ACE inhibitor. This occurs most commonly in patients who are either volume contracted and/or have bilateral large or small artery disease in the renal vascular bed. Correction of any volume deficit typically returns renal function to baseline values. In the instance of renal arterial disease, reducing the dosage of an ACE inhibitor (or, if necessary, discontinuing it) will restore renal function to its baseline level.[40] The change in renal function with ARBs given to patients with or without renal disease appears to differ little from that seen with ACE inhibitors (see Fig. 42.6).

AFRICAN-AMERICAN STUDY OF KIDNEY DISEASES

The support for the use of ACE inhibitors in the patient with hypertensive nephrosclerosis has until recently been somewhat speculative. The African-American Study of Kidney Disease and Hypertension (AASK) has retired the issue of appropriateness of ACE inhibitor use in hypertensive nephrosclerosis (at least in black people).[25] The AASK trial evaluated 1094 self-identified African Americans with hypertension, aged 18 to 70 years, with a GFR between 20 and 65 mL/min/1.73 m^2. The trial was carried out in nondiabetic African Americans who had a urinary protein-to-creatinine ratio of <2.5 and did not have significant ongoing systemic illness.

This trial employed a 3 × 2 factorial design with patients randomized to a usual mean arterial pressure (MAP) goal of 102 to 107 mm Hg or to a low MAP goal of 92 mm Hg. Patients were randomly assigned to one of three antihypertensive agents: a beta blocker, metoprolol (50 to 200 mg/day [Toprol XL]); an ACE inhibitor, ramipril (2.5 to 10 mg/day [Altace]); or the dihydropyridine calcium channel blocker (DHP-CCB), amlodipine (5 to 10 mg/day [Norvasc]). If BP did not reach the assigned goal with maximum tolerated doses of the blinded drug, additional open-label drug could be added in the following suggested order: furosemide, doxazosin, clonidine, hydralazine, or minoxidil. The scheme for this study was an uneven block design with a 2:2:1 randomization ratio for metoprolol, ramipril, and amlodipine, respectively. Thus 441 patients were assigned to metoprolol, 436 patients to ramipril, and 217 to amlodipine. GFR was measured by iothalamate clearance twice at baseline; thereafter, it was measured at 3 and 6 months and every 6 months for the remainder of the study.[25]

The analysis in this study rather convincingly demonstrated a renoprotective effect in African Americans with ramipril as compared to amlodipine. The results of this trial were particularly prominent in those subjects with proteinuria beyond the threshold of clinically significant "dipstick positive" proteinuria (UP/Cr >0.22 or >300 mg/day). This conclusion is supported by several of the findings from the AASK trial, including a significant reduction in risk of the clinical composite outcome, a slower decline in GFR, and a reduction in

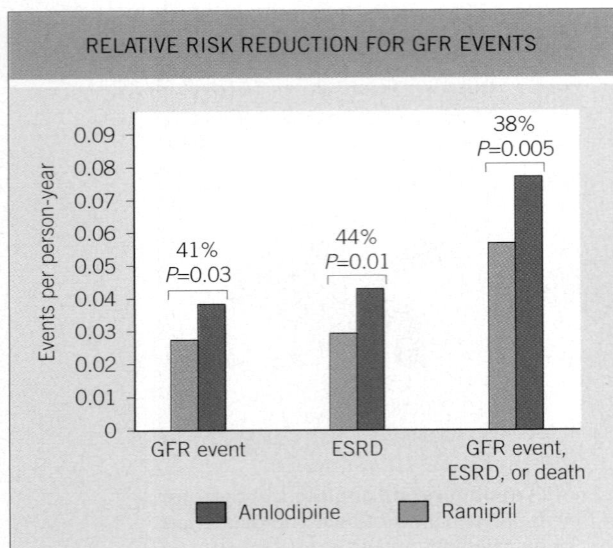

Figure 42.7 Relative risk reduction for GFR events.

urinary protein excretion with ramipril as compared to amlodipine (Fig. 42.7). In addition, a 37% risk reduction (favoring metoprolol) was observed when metoprolol-treated patients were compared with those receiving amlodipine. These findings resulted in an early termination of the amlodipine treatment limb of this study. The findings in the nonproteinuric study participants, although more subtle, in no way offer dissenting information to the superiority of ACE inhibitor–based regimens in African American patients with hypertensive nephrosclerosis.[25]

In nonproteinuric African American patients with hypertensive nephrosclerosis, several observations supported the claim of superiority for ramipril. First, there was a reduction in the time to event in the entire group as well as a reduction in urinary protein excretion. Second, this group also experienced a 56% reduction in the progression to clinically significant proteinuria (UP/Cr > 0.22 or > 300 mg/day) on ramipril compared with amlodipine. It is of interest that prior recommendations of a beneficial effect of ACE inhibition in both diabetic and nondiabetic renal insufficiency targeted higher levels of proteinuria per day as the threshold where a renoprotective effect is demonstrated. This analysis of the AASK data set suggests a significantly lower threshold of proteinuria for an ACE inhibitor benefit but cannot define the specific breakpoint per se.[25,41]

The AASK study is also noteworthy in that it is the first outcome trial to demonstrate a significantly beneficial effect of ACE inhibition in African Americans. Moreover, these results emphasize the importance of ACE inhibitors in the prevention of target organ damage, a process that appears to extend beyond the positive benefit(s) of mere BP control alone, although there remains active debate as to the BP-independent effects of RAAS blockade.[42] The AASK trial was not mechanistically driven, so one can only speculate on the reasons behind the benefits of ramipril in these studies. Changes in angiotensin II effect have been proffered as at least a partial explanation for these findings. It should be stressed that the capacity of an ACE inhibitor to reduce urinary protein excretion is an important additional mechanism capable of retarding progression of renal disease. Because microalbuminuria and frank proteinuria are risk factors for cardiovascular as well as renal disease, reduction in urinary protein excretion is generally viewed as a desirable attribute of a compound. The AASK trial was not designed to specifically address the mechanistic bridge between the observed improved renal and cardiovascular outcomes and a reduction in protein excretion. Its findings, though, should be viewed as providing additional support to the therapeutic maxim that if urinary protein excretion is increased it should be reduced, however possible (Table 42.3).[43]

Finally, the literature is replete with statements that suggest ACE inhibitor monotherapy is not as effective in hypertensive African Americans. This has influenced clinical prescription practice such that hesitancy exists to use these

BENEFITS TO RENAL FUNCTION OF DRUGS THAT BLOCK THE RENIN-ANGIOTENSIN SYSTEM
Key points of the African American study of kidney disease and hypertension
■ Treatment with ramipril was significantly better than amlodipine in slowing the progression of renal disease in patients with a baseline urine protein-to-creatinine ratio >0.22 (300 mg protein/day). ■ In the entire cohort, after adjusting for prespecified baseline covariates, ramipril was associated with risk reduction in time of progression to the following clinically relevant endpoints as compared to amlodipine: 41% risk reduction for ESRD or death, and 38% risk reduction for GFR events, ESRD, or death. ■ The reduction in risk of the combined endpoints of ESRD, death, or GFR was influenced heavily by the subgroup of patients with baseline proteinuria; this subgroup contributed 63% of the events, although it represented only 33% of the cohort. ■ Treatment with amlodipine increased proteinuria by 58% in the first 6 months, whereas ramipril decreased proteinuria by 20%. The rate at which UP/Cr <0.22 progressed to >0.22 was 56% lower in the ramipril-treated group than in the amlodipine group. ■ At the end of the follow-up, there was no difference in the decline of GFR among patients with no baseline proteinuria or a GFR of at least 40 mL/min/1.73 m^2, which was related to the fact that those in the amlodipine treatment group experienced an acute rise in GFR shortly after beginning therapy. ■ Achieved BP averaged (SD) 128/78 (12/8) mm Hg in the lower BP group and 141/85 (12/7) mm Hg in the usual BP group did not improve the rate at which GFR changed, and the lower BP did not significantly reduce the rate of the clinical composite outcome.
ESRD, end-stage renal disease; GFR, glomerular filtration rate.

Table 42.3 Benefits to renal function of drugs that block the renin-angiotensin system.

drugs as monotherapy in hypertensive African Americans. This hesitancy also appears to carry over to the use of ACE inhibitors in this population as part of a multidrug regimen. The findings from the AASK trial should dispel this myth. As the AASK trial demonstrated, when an ACE inhibitor is used in combination with a diuretic and other agents, BP control is achieved and maintained and renoprotection is readily evident. Moreover, AASK demonstrated that the number of drugs, the percentage of participants on diuretics, and the achieved BP (133/82 mm Hg) were similar for participants randomized to amlodipine and ramipril, strengthening the argument that the renoprotective effect of ramipril as compared to amlodipine is independent of the achieved BP readings.[37]

PROGNOSIS

Hypertensive nephrosclerosis is considered to be one of the most common causes of ESRD in the United States and Europe, with a greater prevalence in African Americans and the elderly. The increasing incidence of ESRD as a result of this disease is somewhat paradoxical, considering the recent emphasis on the treatment of hypertension. Its rising incidence may relate in part to the inability to differentiate hypertensive nephrosclerosis from other renal diseases, such as ischemic nephropathy in association with renal arterial disease or parenchymal disease, which can itself raise BP. There is no reason to believe that there will be a dramatic decline in the foreseeable future in either the "perceived" or the actual incidence of hypertensive nephrosclerosis. This is particularly so in light of the increasing diagnosis of nephrosclerosis in the aging population with CV diseases.

The prognosis for patients who have established hypertensive nephrosclerosis does not strictly parallel the level of renal function. For example, a serum creatinine level in the 115 μmol/L (1.3 mg/dL) range in many patients aged more than 60 years reflects at least a 50% loss of GFR, as does a level greater than 133 μmol/L (1.5 mg/dL) in a younger patient. The adverse renal consequences of these modest functional changes are not immediately apparent, since they lie in an early onset of anemia, secondary hyperparathyroidism, and most importantly in a much higher rate of CV disease. For example, the Hypertension Detection and Follow-up Program showed that baseline serum creatinine had a significant prognostic value for the 8-year mortality rate. In those with serum creatinine values over 151 μmol/L (1.7 mg/dL), mortality was more than three times higher than in those with more normal levels of renal function.[5] These data indicate that an elevated serum creatinine is a potent independent risk factor for mortality, as are both microalbuminuria and macroproteinuria.

True hypertensive nephrosclerosis is slowly progressive, and its rate of progression is probably related to the degree to which systolic and diastolic BP are effectively controlled. Unfortunately, the optimum BP for maximum slowing of the rate of renal functional decline has to date not been established. Further confusing the issue is the fact that hypertensive nephrosclerosis may have different mechanisms (or rates of progression) that are the result of race. In blacks, renal biopsy findings are more severe with a solidified form of global glomerulosclerosis, segmental sclerotic lesions, tubular atrophy, and interstitial fibrosis being more common. Blood pressure levels and proteinuria appear not to account for these morphologic lesions, suggesting that other factors may play a role.[44] This is not to say that tight BP control may not favorably influence the course of this disease in blacks.

Alternatively, the most effective class of antihypertensive agents for treatment of hypertensive nephrosclerosis appears to be ACE inhibitors (at least in blacks). Many of the studies conducted to answer these questions (other than the AASK trial) have been underpowered or have not had adequate controls, making their interpretation difficult and limiting the generalizability of the findings. Furthermore, the therapeutic response to an antihypertensive class in a patient who has essential hypertension, without discernable renal dysfunction, has been taken to automatically represent the response of patients who have hypertensive nephrosclerosis. This is a presumption that requires careful consideration and more definitive proof.[45]

SUMMARY

Our understanding of hypertensive nephrosclerosis is in a state of flux, partly because hypertension can be both a cause and a consequence of progressive renal insufficiency. So-called essential hypertension can also turn into renovascular hypertension, which can be a subtle occurrence. When renovascular disease exists, with or without hypertension, a form of "ischemic nephropathy" arises, and the rate of decline in renal function accelerates even with what appears to be good BP control.

Irrespective of the form of hypertension, meticulous control of BP is likely to afford patients with hypertensive nephrosclerosis the most benefit. In the past, diastolic BP control was perceived as being the most important treatment goal, whereas systolic BP control is now considered to be as important, if not more so. The goal systolic and diastolic BP values in hypertensive nephrosclerosis are not yet firmly established. As a point of reference, JNC-7 suggests that BP in CKD (whatever the type) should be controlled to 130/80 mm Hg, particularly in the presence of proteinuria, with whatever antihypertensive therapy is necessary.[46] Goal BP readings in this disease may ultimately be determined by demographic subsetting of patients; for example, African American hypertensive patients "may" require a lower BP than whites to best slow the decay in renal function attributable to hypertension. With this in mind, in the recently concluded AASK trial, "kidney protection" did not differ between the two goal BP groups (mean arterial pressure of either 92 or 102 to 107 mm Hg).[41] This study did not include whites, so no conclusion can be drawn concerning racial differences in goal BP for hypertensive nephrosclerosis.

The treatment plan for the hypertension of progressive nephrosclerosis should take into account the stage of the disease (i.e., the lower the GFR, the more important it is that salt balance is maintained with dietary Na^+ restriction, diuretic use, or both). To a backdrop of Na^+ balance can then be added any number of different antihypertensive drug classes, with an emphasis on the use of ACE inhibitors or ARBs (as of yet not formally studied in this disease), particularly if proteinuria is present (Table 42.4).

CLINICAL USE OF ACE INHIBITORS IN HYPERTENSIVE NEPHROSCLEROSIS
■ ACE inhibitors can effectively lower BP in hypertensive nephrosclerosis, but often a diuretic must be co-administered to obtain optimal BP reduction. ■ A low-sodium diet, diuretic therapy, and/or protein restriction enhances the antiproteinuric effect of ACE inhibitors. ■ Glomerular filtration rate tends to decline more rapidly in ACE inhibitor–treated patients who have the DD genotype for ACE, although there is substantial environmental-genotypic interference for this phenomenon. ■ ACE inhibitors are not contraindicated at any particular level of renal function unless their use results in clinically significant hyperkalemia. ■ ACE inhibitor initiation can be accompanied by a 10%-25% decline in GFR, a phenomenon exaggerated by the presence of volume contraction. This decline in renal function is typically reversible and does not necessitate discontinuation of the ACE inhibitor. ■ ACE inhibitor use can occasionally be accompanied by a dramatic (50% or greater) decline in GFR, in which case large vessel renal artery or extensive renal microvascular disease is often present. ■ ACE inhibitors can worsen the anemia of chronic kidney disease, requiring that their use include periodic monitoring of hemoglobin levels. This anemia will respond to exogenous erythropoietin administration.

Table 42.4 Clinical use of ACE inhibitors in hypertensive nephrosclerosis.

An evolving understanding of the actions of each of the components of the RAAS provides the basis for specific targeting of this system to optimize effects on end-organ injuries. ACE inhibitors and ARBs are important drugs for treatment of this disease, although they will ultimately need to be compared with each other. Of late, aldosterone receptor antagonist therapy is assuming an important role in the treatment of this disease (at least in experimental models). To date, little difference has been detected in animal studies comparing various ACE inhibitors to ARBs. It should be noted that equivalent final sums of injury do not necessarily reflect the identity of intervening mechanisms, because these drug classes are fundamentally different in their mechanisms of action.

chapter 43

Complications of Hypertension: Stroke

Tom Robinson, Fiona Brodie, and Efstathios Manios

Definition

- Stroke is defined clinically as a rapidly developing focal neurologic deficit lasting longer than 24 hours or causing death, which is attributable to a vascular cause.

Key Features

- Hypertension is a significant risk factor for first stroke.
- Hypertension acutely post-stroke is associated with poor short-term and long-term outcomes.

Therapy

- The benefit of hypertension treatment for primary prevention of stroke is clear. However, the choice of a specific regimen must be individualized and will be guided by the patient's clinical situation.
- Despite its high prevalence, the optimal management of arterial hypertension during the acute stroke stage has not been established and remains an issue of long-standing debate and little consensus.
- Antihypertensive treatment is recommended for the prevention of recurrent stroke. The benefit has been associated with an average reduction of 10/5 mm Hg, whereas normal blood pressure levels have been defined as less than 120/80 mm Hg by JNC-7.

Stroke is defined clinically as a rapidly developing focal neurologic deficit lasting greater than 24 hours or causing death, which is attributable to a vascular cause.[1] Stroke is common, remaining the third commonest cause of death worldwide with approximately 20% of patients being dead within 1 month of first stroke[2] and a significant cause of disability and health resource use in the developed world.

The incidence of stroke varies between populations and increases with age, but community-based studies suggest an age-standardized annual incidence for first-ever stroke of between 238 and 627 per 100,000.[3]

Hypertension is a significant risk factor for stroke, along with increasing age, cigarette smoking, atrial fibrillation, diabetes mellitus, and obesity. While these risk factors are common to other vascular diseases including ischemic heart disease and peripheral vascular disease, the relation between blood pressure and stroke mortality is stronger than that for mortality due to ischemic heart disease, as shown in a meta-analysis including one million adults.[4] Hypertension is established to be a significant risk factor for ischemic stroke due to both small and large vessel disease and for stroke due to cerebral hemorrhage.[5,6] This association has been shown for both systolic and diastolic blood pressure (BP), and appears to be a continuous risk across BP values (Fig. 43.1).[7] A reduction in systolic BP of 10 mm Hg is associated with a one third reduction in risk of stroke, with an increased risk reduction for larger reductions in systolic BP.[8] Relative risk of stroke (all-cause) with a usual diastolic BP >110 m Hg is of the order of 10 to 12 times that of someone with a usual diastolic BP of <79 mm Hg.

ANATOMY AND PATHOLOGY

Stroke encompasses a range of clinical syndromes, and it is important to establish the underlying etiology, because this has implications for prognosis, future stroke risk, and optimization of subsequent management. Neuroimaging allows reliable distinction between cerebral infarction and cerebral hemorrhage, and may be helpful in determining etiology in some cases.

Ischemic Stroke

Cerebral infarction accounts for 80% to 85% of all strokes. Previously ischemic stroke has been considered a single disease; however, it has become increasingly clear that there is a spectrum of clinical and pathologic subtypes, for which different risk factors may play an important role. The Trial of Organon 10172 in acute stroke treatment (TOAST) classification was developed to improve classification of ischemic stroke into clinically relevant subtypes, and shows good inter-rater reliability.[9] Unlike the Oxfordshire Community Stroke Project classification,[10] which uses clinical features to predict the likely site/size of the corresponding brain lesion as well as outcome, the TOAST classification takes into account not only clinical information but also the results of relevant investigations, including brain CT/MRI, ECG/echocardiography, carotid artery imaging, and hematologic investigation for prothrombotic states (such as anticardiolipin antibodies) (see Table 43.1). Broadly speaking, ischemic stroke may be classified as being due to large artery atherosclerosis, cardioembolism, small vessel occlusive disease, or other rarer causes. Hypertension is an important factor in the development of atherosclerosis, which leads to the development of plaques within large and medium-sized artery walls. Necrosis or rupture of these plaques leads to thrombus formation, which can cause either direct vessel occlusion or embolization. Small vessel disease is characterized by occlusion of a single cortical perforating artery, giving rise to a "lacunar" syndrome. This may occur in isolation or may be associated with more widespread small vessel arteriopathy or leukoariosis. Hypertension is associated with small vessel

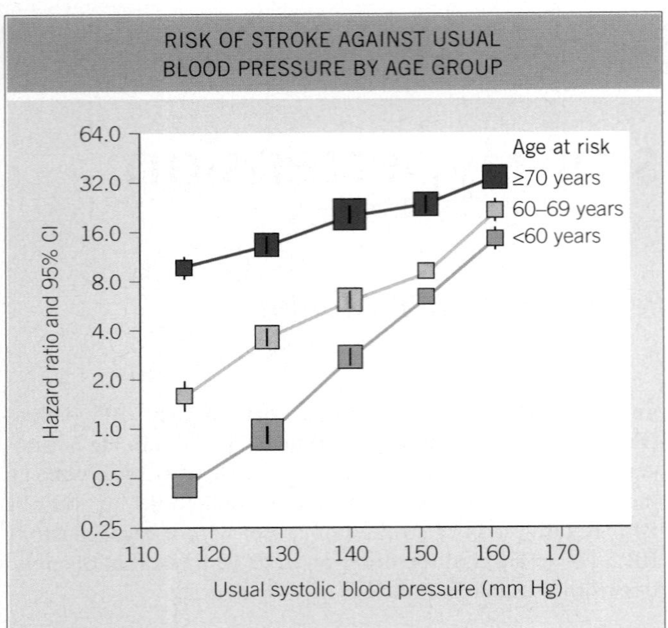

Figure 43.1 Risk of stroke against usual BP by age group. (From Lawes CM, Rodgers A, Bennett DA, et al. Blood pressure and cardiovascular disease in the Asia Pacific region. J Hypertens 2003;21:707-716.)

disease, and this association appears to be stronger than for large artery atherosclerosis A recently published study of small vessel disease, large vessel disease, and controls found an odds ratio of 3.43 (95% confidence interval [CI], 2.32-5.07; $P < .001$) for the presence of hypertension in small vessel compared to large vessel stroke.[11] In addition, hypertension is a risk factor for the development of atrial fibrillation[12] and ischemic heart disease, both of which are commonly implicated in cardioembolic stroke. The TOAST classification of ischemic stroke is presented in Table 43.1.[9]

Stroke due to Hemorrhage

Intracerebral hemorrhage accounts for around 10% to 15% of first strokes, and confers a worse prognosis than ischemic stroke, with 30-day mortality reaching up to 50% and half of these deaths occurring within the first 48 hours (subarachnoid hemorrhage tends to occur in a younger age group and in those with saccular aneurysms in the circle of Willis; it is not considered in further detail in this chapter).

Intracerebral hemorrhage is usually defined as being lobar (arising in the temporal, parietal, occipital, or frontal lobes), or deep (arising around the basal ganglia or brainstem). It has traditionally been thought that hypertension is more associated with deep hemorrhage, and a recent meta-analysis found hypertension to be almost twice as common in patients

TOAST CLASSIFICATION OF ISCHAEMIC STROKE

TOAST Stroke Subtype Classification*	Clinical Features	Neuroimaging	Supporting Features	Other
Large artery atherosclerosis	Cortical impairment (e.g., dysphasia, neglect) or cerebellar or brainstem signs	Significant stenosis or occlusion of major brain artery, cortical/cerebellar infarct or subcortical infarct >1.5 cm	Carotid artery stenosis >50% History of same-territory TIA Peripheral vascular disease	No evidence of cardioembolic cause
Cardioembolism	May be similar to above	May be similar to above	History of TIA in a different territory or history of a systemic occlusive vascular event Identifiable high or medium risk source of cardioembolus	No evidence of large artery atherosclerosis as cause
Small vessel occlusion (lacunae)	Lacunar syndrome (motor/sensory/sensorimotor involvement affecting ≥2 out of arm/face/leg, ataxic hemiparesis)	Subcortical or brainstem infarction <1.5 cm	History of hypertension, diabetes	No evidence of large artery atherosclerosis or cardioembolic cause
Other determined etiology	Clinical features of acute ischemic stroke	CT/MRI consistent with acute ischemic stroke	Diagnostic evidence of a rare cause, e.g., vasculopathy, hematologic disorder, procoaguable state	No evidence of large artery atherosclerosis or cardioembolic cause
Undetermined etiology	Clinical features of acute ischemic stroke	CT/MRI consistent with acute ischemic stroke	Lack of diagnostic evidence, or diagnostic evidence for >1 subtype	No likely cause identified, or more than one possible cause (e.g., atrial fibrillation and ipsilateral carotid stenosis >50%)

*The first four categories are further classified as possible or probable, depending on results of further investigations.

Table modified from Adams HP Jr, Bendixen BH, Kappelle LJ, et al. Classification of subtype of acute ischemic stroke. Definitions for use in a multicenter clinical trial. TOAST. Trial of Org 10172 in Acute Stroke Treatment. Stroke 1993;24:35-41.

Table 43.1 TOAST classification of ischaemic stroke.

with deep compared to lobar hemorrhage in studies including around 4000 patients[13] with intracerebral hemorrhage.

Along with hypertension, other important risk factors for intracerebral hemorrhage include excess alcohol consumption, male gender, increasing age, and anticoagulant use. Cerebral amyloid angiopathy is also a risk factor for intracerebral hemorrhage, and the association appears to be stronger for lobar than deep intracerebral hemorrhage.[14] Cerebral amyloid angiopathy is characterized pathologically by amorphous fibrillar protein (amyloid) deposition in the walls of small and medium cerebral arteries, which predisposes to vessel rupture. It is strongly associated with increasing age, but not specifically with hypertension. Intracerebral hemorrhage secondary to cerebral amyloid angiopathy tends to be recurrent, lobar, and multifocal, and although the diagnosis is pathologic, gradient echo MRI may now allow a "probable" diagnosis to be made ante mortem.[15]

PATHOPHYSIOLOGY

Cerebral Autoregulation in Hypertension

Cerebral autoregulation is the mechanism by which cerebral blood flow may be maintained despite changes in cerebral perfusion pressure, and can be defined as being static (responding gradually to long-term changes) or dynamic (responding to acute changes). Under normal physiologic conditions, cerebral blood flow is around 50 mL/100 g/minute, and this can usually be maintained across a wide range of blood pressures (mean arterial pressure [MAP] of 60 to 160 mm Hg).

There appears to be adaptation of cerebral autoregulation in patients with hypertension, and the lowest MAP before symptoms of cerebral hypoperfusion appear is also higher in patients with hypertension than in normotensive patients[16]; this is illustrated in Figure. 43.2.[17] This resetting of autoregulation appears to be reversible to some extent when hypertension is treated, but it is likely that hypertension over a long time leads to permanent changes in vascular structure, some of which may be irreversible. It is important that an awareness of altered cerebral autoregulation in hypertension does not lead to a reticence to treat, but initial treatment of severe hypertension should be aimed at a gradual reduction rather than a sudden fall to levels considered normotensive, as this may precipitate symptoms of cerebral ischemia (or infarction).

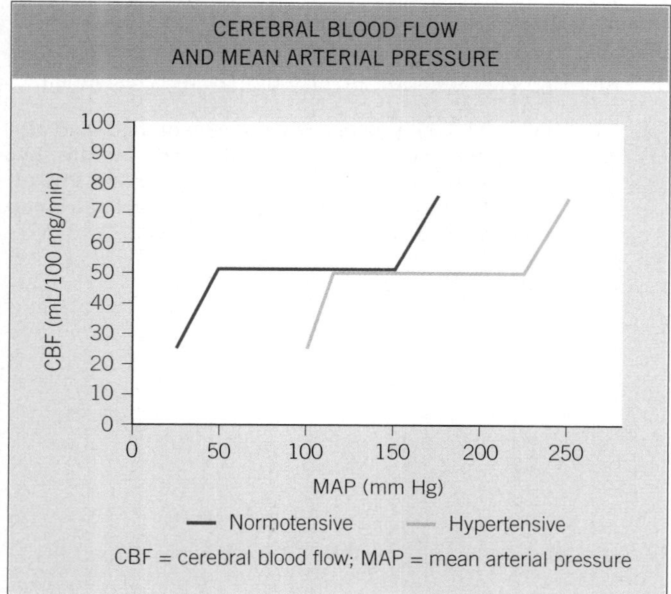

Figure 43.2 Cerebral blood flow and mean arterial pressure. (From Ruland S, Aiyagari V. Cerebral autoregulation and blood pressure lowering. Hypertension 2007;49:977-978.)

Cerebral Autoregulation in Acute Stroke

Dynamic cerebral autoregulation has been shown to be impaired following acute stroke, with a reduced ability to maintain constant cerebral blood flow in response to sudden fluctuations in BP,[18] whereas static autoregulation does not appear to be affected in the same way. Autoregulation is impaired not only in the affected hemisphere, but globally. It remains unclear to what extent dynamic cerebral autoregulation recovers following acute stroke, and this issue may be confounded in part by the number of patients who in addition to stroke disease are also hypertensive. It therefore seems likely that as a direct result of the neurologic insult there is some derangement of factors that usually maintain constant cerebral blood flow, and thus cerebral blood flow may become critically dependent on systemic blood pressure. This clearly has implications for how and when hypertension should be managed in the acute post-stroke period, and this is considered in further detail in the following section on blood pressure management in acute stroke.

CLINICAL PRESENTATIONS

Hypertension as a Risk Factor for Stroke

Arterial hypertension affects from 20% to 30% of the world population and is the most prevalent modifiable risk factor for stroke.[19] There is a continuous and consistent association between both systolic and diastolic BP and the risk of cerebrovascular disease,[20] which is independent of other risk factors. The higher the BP, the greater the risk of stroke. The JNC-7 Report considered that vascular risk begins with BP values of 115/75 mm Hg, and the risk doubles with each increase of 20/10 mm Hg.[21] The Framingham Heart Study showed that BP values of greater than 120/80 mm Hg were associated with a higher risk of cardiovascular disease.[22] A recent meta-analysis of more than 40 randomized, controlled trials of BP lowering, which included more than 188,000 participants, indicated that a 10 mm Hg reduction in systolic BP would be associated with a 31% reduction in risk of stroke.[8] Initial evidence of the positive and continuous association between BP and the risk of stroke came from North American and European populations.[23] More recently, a similar association has been demonstrated in Asian populations, although the slope of the relationship appears to be somewhat steeper for Asian than white populations,[7,24] possibly because of, at least in part, the relatively higher incidence of hemorrhagic stroke in Asian populations. The relationship between BP and stroke risk has been demonstrated for all age groups studied. Although the strength of the association becomes attenuated with increasing age, it is still strong and continuous among those aged 70 years or more.[24]

Historically, BP treatment has focused on diastolic BP control, but more recently at least equal attention is being paid to the control of systolic BP. This is especially relevant in the prevention of stroke, where the continuum of systolic BP rise is the most relevant risk factor.[25] As age increases, systolic BP continues to rise at least into the 70s, whereas diastolic BP reaches a plateau in the early 50s then declines. Systolic BP level is directly related to the risk of stroke, particularly after age 65 years. In the Framingham study, elderly men with isolated systolic hypertension had twice the risk of stroke, and women, 1.5 times the risk.

There has been considerable debate over the shape of the association curve between BP and stroke. Some cohort data appear to demonstrate a J-shaped curve,[26,27] and it has been suggested that this relationship indicates that BP has been lowered too far and that cerebral blood flow is compromised, leading to ischemia. It is more likely to reflect deteriorating health, accounting perhaps for both falling BP and a greater likelihood of a cardiovascular event. Trials such as PROGRESS[28] and HOPE[29] have found no evidence of a J-curve association across a wide range of BP levels. The majority of BP-lowering studies support a log-linear association and indicate that a potential J-curve relationship should not detract attention from the major benefits of BP lowering.

Blood pressure control is also related to the risk of stroke and systemic embolic events in patients with atrial fibrillation (AF) who are taking anticoagulants. In an analysis from the Stroke Prevention by Oral Thrombin Inhibitor in Atrial Fibrillation (SPORTIF) trial,[30] there was an increasing rate of stroke and Systemic Embolic Events (SEE) with increasing quartiles of systolic BP in patients with AF. For the top quartile of systolic BP compared with the lowest quartile, the hazard ratio (HR) for stroke and SEE was 1.83 (95% CI, 1.22-2.74), whereas mortality was lower in the top quartile (HR, 0.64; 95% CI, 0.49-0.83). Event rates for stroke/SEE increased markedly at mean systolic BP of less than 140 mm Hg, emphasizing the importance of good BP control in such patients.

Acute Stroke Blood Pressure

Several observational studies have illustrated the change in blood pressure following admission with acute stroke. Around 46% of patients with acute stroke have a history of hypertension, but around 69% will have a systolic BP of 170 mm Hg or greater at the time of admission,[31] and around 80% will have a BP considered hypertensive by World Health Organisation (WHO) criteria (>140/90 mm Hg). The mechanism for this is not entirely clear, nor is it clear whether this is a physiologic response to improve perfusion to adjacent ischemic tissue, or whether it is a detrimental side effect with the potential to worsen cerebral edema. BP levels tend to fall spontaneously over 4 to 7 days even without treatment, returning to pre-stroke levels in around two thirds of patients.[32]

It has been postulated that very high BP immediately post-stroke may be detrimental; equally, very low BP may be thought to worsen outcome. In fact both are true. In a review of 17,398 ischemic stroke patients enrolled in the International Stroke Trial, a U-shaped curve of systolic BP versus both early mortality (at 14 days) and late death and dependency (at 6 months) is demonstrated.[32] For each 10 mm Hg systolic BP below 150 mm Hg there was a 17.9% increase in early death, and for every 10 mm Hg systolic BP above 150 mm Hg there was a 3.8% increase in early mortality, as shown in Figure 43.3. A systematic review of BP post-stroke (ischemic and hemorrhagic) and outcome is in keeping with this observation, adding that high systolic BP, mean arterial BP (MAP), and diastolic BP are all associated with increased death and dependency.[33]

In addition to the effect of BP on mortality, several authors have investigated potential relationships between BP and other outcomes, including stroke recurrence and functional outcome. It has been shown that higher diastolic BP and higher pulse pressure on 24-hour monitoring post-stroke are associated with an increased risk of stroke recurrence, and also that higher systolic BP following acute ischemic stroke is associated with poorer early (10 day) and late (6 month) functional outcome in terms of modified Rankin scores (though this latter finding was not independent of initial stroke severity).[34] Another study demonstrated that patients with higher systolic and diastolic BP following acute ischemic stroke actually had a *better* functional outcome at 90 days, but patients with a baseline systolic BP greater than 185 mm Hg or diastolic BP of 110 mm Hg were excluded.[35]

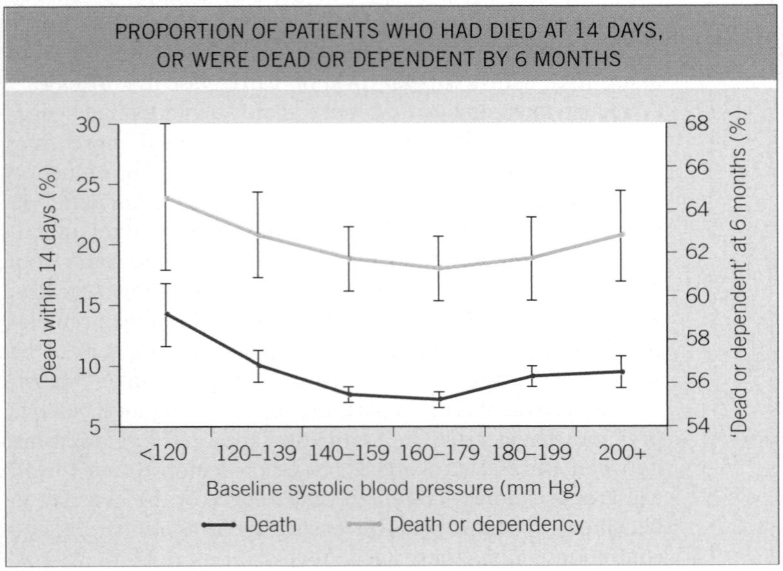

Figure 43.3 Proportion of patients who had died at 14 days or were dead or dependent at 6 months, by blood pressure. (From Leonardi-Bee J, Bath PM, Phillips SJ, Sandercock PA. Blood pressure and clinical outcomes in the International Stroke Trial. Stroke 2002;33:1315-1320.)

The relationship between BP and outcome following intracerebral hemorrhage appears to be less clear. Most studies have been relatively small, often retrospective, and without standardized BP treatment. One retrospective review of 87 patients with intracerebral hemorrhage found that patients with lower MAP of 145 mm Hg or less and 125 mm Hg or less between 0 and 6 hours had more favorable outcomes in terms of death or severe morbidity at 30 days[36]; the majority received some antihypertensive therapy (usually nifedipine or sodium nitroprusside). A larger series (1701 patients) found MAP to be higher for those who had fatal versus nonfatal intracerebral putaminal or thalamic hemorrhage, but no such association in cerebellar, subcortical, or pontine hemorrhage.[37]

The volume of intracerebral hemorrhage is an important determinant of outcome,[38] and there is increasing evidence that hyperacute hematoma expansion is also associated with increased mortality,[39] but these factors do not appear to be directly related to BP.

Post-Stroke Blood Pressure

It is established that hypertension is a major risk factor for first stroke, and that lowering BP reduces this risk. The association, however, for effect of BP on recurrent stroke has been a matter of some debate, and concerns regarding effects on cerebral autoregulation or carotid stenosis have led to uncertainty regarding subsequent management of hypertension following a stroke.

In an analysis of 675 patients in the Oxfordshire Community Stroke Project, 180 experienced recurrent stroke (of whom 135 were first recurrence), and it was found that the only significant factor relating to recurrence risk was smoking status at the time of stroke, and that BP at baseline and at 1 month post-stroke were not associated with risk of recurrence.[40] The authors postulated, however, that the lack of a statistically significant association may have been due to low absolute numbers of recurrent stroke. In an observational study in Pennsylvania, which enrolled 662 patients within 1 month of stroke and followed them up at 4- to 6-month intervals (mean 24 months), there were 81 recurrent strokes; those with a diastolic BP of 95 mm Hg or more had a recurrence rate of 43%, whereas those with diastolic BP less than 95 mm Hg had a recurrence rate of 19% ($P = .005$). There was not a clear association between systolic BP and recurrence risk, but BP values were dichotomized, and the upper limit of "normal" chosen was 150 mm Hg, perhaps too high a threshold to observe a significant effect.[41]

The effects of BP following stroke on other outcomes such as mortality are less clear, with little observational data on the subject. Several interventional trials of antihypertensive therapy following stroke have been carried out in the last few years, with the introduction of therapy between 1 week and 3 months after stroke, and these have studied a number of endpoints, including vascular and all-cause mortality, stroke recurrence, and occurrence of vascular events; the individual trials are considered in more detail later in the section on management and prognosis.

DIAGNOSTIC TECHNIQUES

Neuroimaging

Neuroimaging in acute stroke should be able to reliably exclude hemorrhage and nonstroke diagnoses, to identify potentially viable ischemic tissue (i.e., tissue that may benefit from thrombolytic therapy), and to identify major extracranial or intracranial arterial occlusion.[42]

CT shows early signs of ischemia, but it may take 2 to 3 hours before these are apparent. MR T2 imaging shows infarction but does not distinguish reliably between acute and old changes. MR diffusion imaging, however, can detect ischemia within a few minutes from onset, with ischemic areas showing reduced apparent diffusion constant (ADC). MR diffusion imaging can also detect ischemia up to 3 days after transient ischemic attack, with CT appearing normal.

Given the speed and availability of unenhanced CT, along with its ability to reliably detect or exclude hemorrhage, this has tended to be the imaging of choice in acute stroke, particularly when a timely decision regarding thrombolysis is required.[43] There has been controversy regarding means of interpreting hyperacute CT scans, and the "one third if the MCA" rule (if more than one third of the area supplied by the MCA is involved) and hyperdense MCA sign have been used to guide decisions on thrombolysis, but their validity and reproducibility are imperfect. The Alberta Stroke Program Early CT Score (ASPECTS)[44] is a scoring system used to grade extent of ischemic MCA territory infarcts, but has not been validated for clinical use.

CT and MR angiography can be used to identify arterial occlusion, and MR angiography has better sensitivity than ultrasound at detecting internal carotid artery stenosis and occlusion. CT perfusion and MRI perfusion-diffusion mismatch can also identify ischemic penumbra.[45]

MANAGEMENT AND PROGNOSIS

Primary Prevention

There is now strong and widely accepted evidence that BP-lowering treatment reduces the risk of stroke not only in hypertensive individuals but also in high-risk individuals with BP below 140/90 mm Hg. Several trials have compared the effects of antihypertensive agents from five major classes (diuretics, beta blockers, angiotensin-converting enzyme inhibitors [ACEIs], calcium antagonists, angiotensin II type 1 receptor blockers [ARBs]) on lowering BP and the risk of stroke (Fig. 43.4).[46]

The ALLHAT study[47] enrolled a population of 33,357 hypertensive patients, older than 55 years with one or more coronary risk factors, and compared chlorthalidone (12.5 to 25 mg/day) with amlodipine (2.5 to 10 mg/day) or lisinopril (10 to 40 mg/day), over 4 to 8 years' follow-up. No significant differences were observed between the treatment arms with respect to the combined primary outcome (MI or death from cardiovascular disease). There was also no difference between the diuretic and amlodipine groups for stroke risk. However, the lisinopril group had a 15% higher risk of stroke than the diuretic group. Further analysis showed that this effect was largely attributable to a 40% higher stroke risk in black participants assigned lisinopril. The HOPE study[20] enrolled 9297 patients older than 55 years with a history of cardiovascular disease or diabetes and at least one other cardiovascular risk factor. Patients were randomized to either ramipril (10 mg/day) or matching placebo for a mean of 5 years. Only 46% of the study population were hypertensives. A significant relative risk reduction of 32% for stroke was observed among patients allocated to ramipril

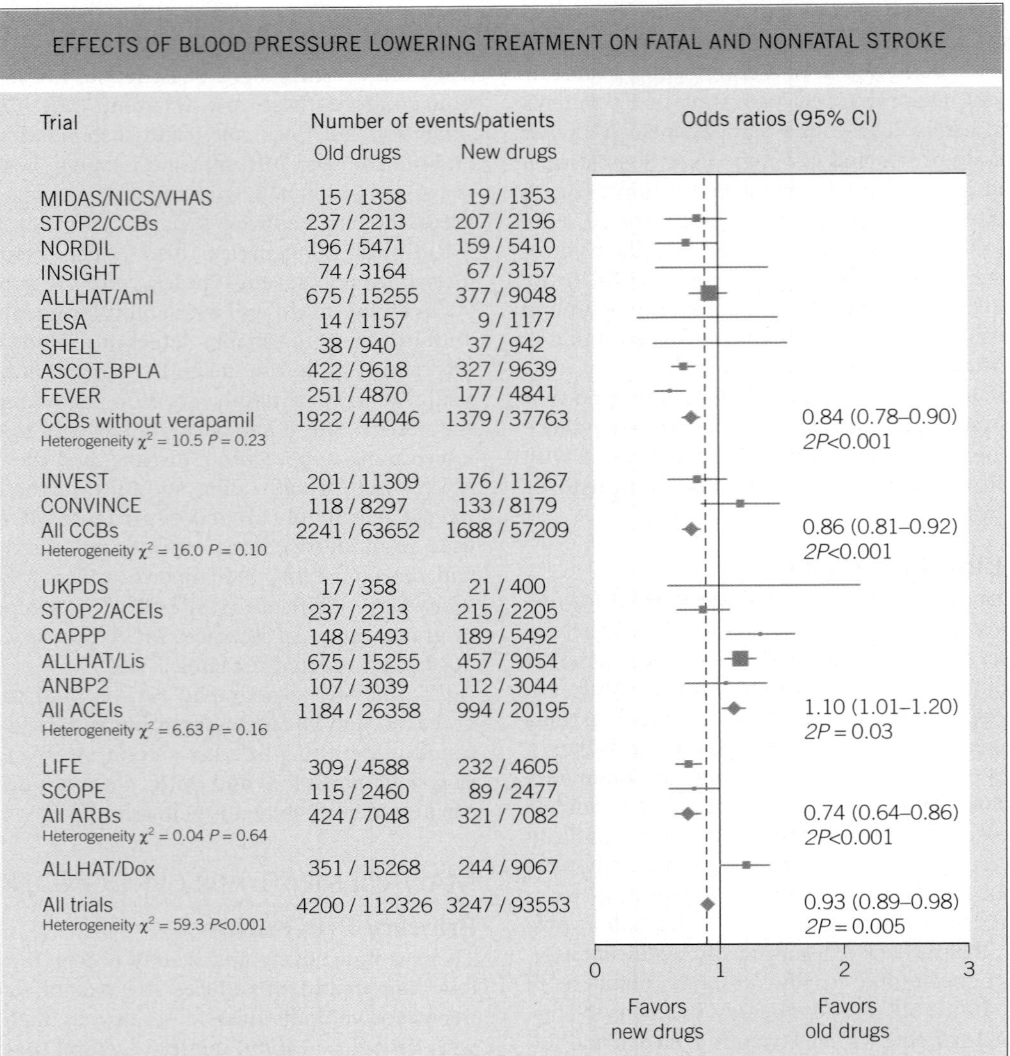

Figure 43.4 Effects of blood pressure lowering treatment on fatal and nonfatal stroke in actively controlled trials comparing new with old (diuretics and/or beta blockers) antihypertensive drugs. Dox indicates the alpha blocker doxazosin. ■, Odds ratios in individual trials with a size proportional to the inverse of the variance of the odds ratios; – and ◆, 95% CIs for individual trials and summary statistics, respectively. (From Zhang H, Thijs L, Staessen JA. Blood pressure lowering for primary and secondary prevention of stroke. Hypertension 2006;48:187-195.)

compared with placebo, as well as a 20% relative risk reduction for myocardial infarction.

The ASCOT-BPLA study[48] randomly allocated 19,257 individuals aged 40 to 79 years with hypertension and at least three other cardiovascular risk factors to an amlodipine-based (amlodipine, 5 to 10 mg; adding perindopril, 4 to 8 mg, as required) as compared to an atenolol-based drug regimen (atenolol, 50 to 100 mg; adding bendroflumethiazide, 1.25 to 2.5 mg, and potassium as required). After 5.5 years' median follow-up, the amlodipine-based regimen was associated with a 23% stroke risk reduction and 14% decrease in coronary events. The INSIGHT study,[49] which compared nifedipine with a diuretic in hypertensive patients with at least one vascular risk factor, did not show any significant differences in benefit. The NORDIL study[50] compared diltiazem with diuretic plus a beta blocker. A significant benefit was observed, in the prevention of the first stroke in the diuretic plus beta-blocker group. Finally, two studies with verapamil compared to atenolol (INVEST)[51] and compared to a diuretic plus BB (CONVINCE)[52] did not show conclusive data in favor of verapamil in preventing first stroke.

The LIFE study[53] enrolled 9193 hypertensive patients, aged 55 to 80 years with left ventricular hypertrophy, who were randomly assigned to losartan (50 to 100 mg/day) or atenolol (50 to 100 mg/day). Over 4 years of follow-up, those assigned to losartan had a 25% lower risk of fatal or nonfatal stroke than those assigned to atenolol, despite similar reductions in BP in both groups. Additionally, in the SCOPE study,[54] 4937 elderly patients with mild to moderate hypertension were randomized to treatment with candesartan 8 to 16 mg daily or placebo (double-blind). Open-label antihypertensive therapy was added as needed to control BP. Allocation to candesartan was associated with a 28% significant reduction in the risk of nonfatal stroke. The VALUE study[55] compared valsartan (80 to 160 mg/day) with amlodipine in 15,245 hypertensive patients with a high risk for myocardial infarction, peripheral arterial disease, or stroke/TIA. The results did not show statistically significant differences in the prevention of primary cardiac episodes or overall stroke.

In primary prevention of stroke, ACEIs (except in the ethnic black population) and ARBs have shown greatest efficacy. Treatment benefit is greater compared with best conventional treatment in patients with high vascular disease risk (ramipril), in elderly hypertensive patients (candersartan), in hypertensive patients with left ventricular hypertrophy (losartan), and in hypertensive patients with at least three vascular risk factors (amlodipine better than atenolol). However, in most hypertensive patients, the choice of drug will be guided by the patient's clinical situation, including the presence of target organ damage, diabetes, established vascular or kidney disease, or other comorbidities. Finally, the absolute target BP level is uncertain and should be individualized, but benefit has been associated with an average reduction of 10/5 mm Hg, and normal BP levels have been defined as less than 120/80 mm Hg by JNC-7.[21]

Blood Pressure Management in Acute Stroke

As discussed, elevated BP values (>140/90 mm Hg) are present in up to 80% of patients with acute stroke,[56,57] whereas nearly one in four patients presents with markedly raised systolic BP of more than 180 mm Hg. The elevation in BP may be secondary to the stress of the cerebrovascular event, a full bladder, nausea, pain, preexisting hypertension, a physiologic response to hypoxia, or a response to increased intracranial pressure. In a majority of patients, a decline in BP occurs within the first hours after stroke even without any specific medical treatment.[58] The BP often falls spontaneously when the patient is moved to a quiet room, is allowed to rest, the bladder is empty, or the pain is controlled.

However, the optimal management of arterial hypertension during the acute stroke stage has not been established and remains an issue of ongoing debate. Theoretical reasons for lowering BP include reducing the formation of brain edema, lessening the risk of hemorrhagic transformation of the infarction, preventing further vascular damage, and forestalling early recurrent stroke. Conversely, aggressive treatment of BP may lead to neurologic worsening by reducing perfusion pressure to ischemic areas of the brain.[59]

Unfortunately, data from randomized controlled trials are limited and inconclusive when considering whether lowering BP during the first hours of ictus is beneficial in stroke patients (Fig. 43.5).[60] The Acute Candesartan Cilexetil Therapy in Stroke Survivors (ACCESS), a prospective, double-blind, placebo controlled, randomized phase II trial, evaluated the use of an angiotensin II receptor blocker in acute ischemic stroke patients with severely elevated BP levels (systolic BP >180 mm Hg and/or diastolic BP >105 mm Hg). Preliminary data from 432 patients demonstrated that oral candesartan reduced a composite secondary outcome (all-cause mortality and vascular events) by 52.5%.[61] It should be noted, though, that the trial was stopped prematurely with a neutral finding for its primary outcome (total mortality and disability at 3 months). In a small randomized study, Eames and colleagues[62] found no major reduction in BP among patients treated with bendrofluazide, and they concluded that this agent was not effective in treating hypertension after stroke. In contrast, beta blockers, such as propranolol and atenolol, achieve a greater BP fall compared to placebo. However, both beta blockers have resulted in a nonsignificant increase in mortality and decrease in neurologic and functional outcome at 6 months compared to placebo.[63,64] The safety and feasibility of labetalol, a combined β- and α-adrenergic antagonist, in rapidly and effectively reducing BP has been demonstrated in the NINDS thrombolysis trial.[65] The administration of calcium channel antagonists during the acute stage of ischemic stroke has neutral effect on functional outcome or survival, according to the conclusions of a review from the Blood Pressure in Acute Stroke Collaboration (BASC).[63] In addition, the INWEST trial demonstrated that the functional outcome was worsened in parallel with the degree by which BP was reduced.[66] Finally, large, well-designed trials are needed to clarify the management of arterial hypertension after acute stroke. The results of currently ongoing trials (CHHIPS,[67] COSSACS,[68] ENOS,[69] and SCAST) may provide some answers to some of the former unresolved issues.

The European Stroke Initiative (EUSI)[70] and the Stroke Council of the American Stroke Association[71] have released updated scientific statements and guidelines regarding the management of hypertension in the setting of acute ischemic stroke. Both authorities recommend that BP should not be lowered in ischemic stroke patients who are not otherwise candidates for thrombolysis (grade C recommendation). Threshold BP values demanding immediate medical interventions are recommended by consensus. More specifically, pharmacologic intervention is indicated if repeated BP readings reveal systolic BP values greater than 220 mm Hg and diastolic BP greater than 120 mm Hg. In patients eligible for thrombolytic therapy, systolic BP values higher than 185 mm Hg or diastolic BP values higher than 110 mm Hg should be actively treated and maintained at desired levels (<185/110 mmHg) during and after thrombolysis infusion. Situations that might require urgent antihypertensive therapy independent of BP levels include acute myocardial infarction, severe left ventricular heart failure, aortic dissection, acute renal failure, acute pulmonary edema, and hypertensive encephalopathy.

In cases where acute therapeutic manipulation of BP is indicated, BP lowering should be done cautiously at a clinically significant and relevant degree (target BP reduction ranging from 10% to 15%), to avoid profound (>20%) BP reductions that have been associated with neurologic and functional worsening.[66] Parenteral agents, such as labetalol, nicardipine, and urapidil, that are easily titrated and have minimal vasodilatory effects on cerebral blood flow are preferred. In certain cases with excessive diastolic BP levels (>140 mm Hg), intravenous administration of sodium nitroprusside is recommended for adequate BP control despite possible adverse effects, such as reflex tachycardia and coronary artery ischemia (Table 43.2). Finally, the use of sublingual nifedipine should be avoided because of the risk of abrupt BP reduction and possible ischemic steal.[70,71]

Current recommendations for treatment of elevated BP levels in patients with intracerebral hemorrhage are more aggressive than those for cases with ischemic stroke (Table 43.3).[72] Accordingly, systolic and diastolic BP levels should be maintained below 180 and 105 mm Hg, respectively. Blood pressure levels should be lowered carefully with close and continuous observation of BP values, using an easily titrated, short-acting agent, such as labetalol,

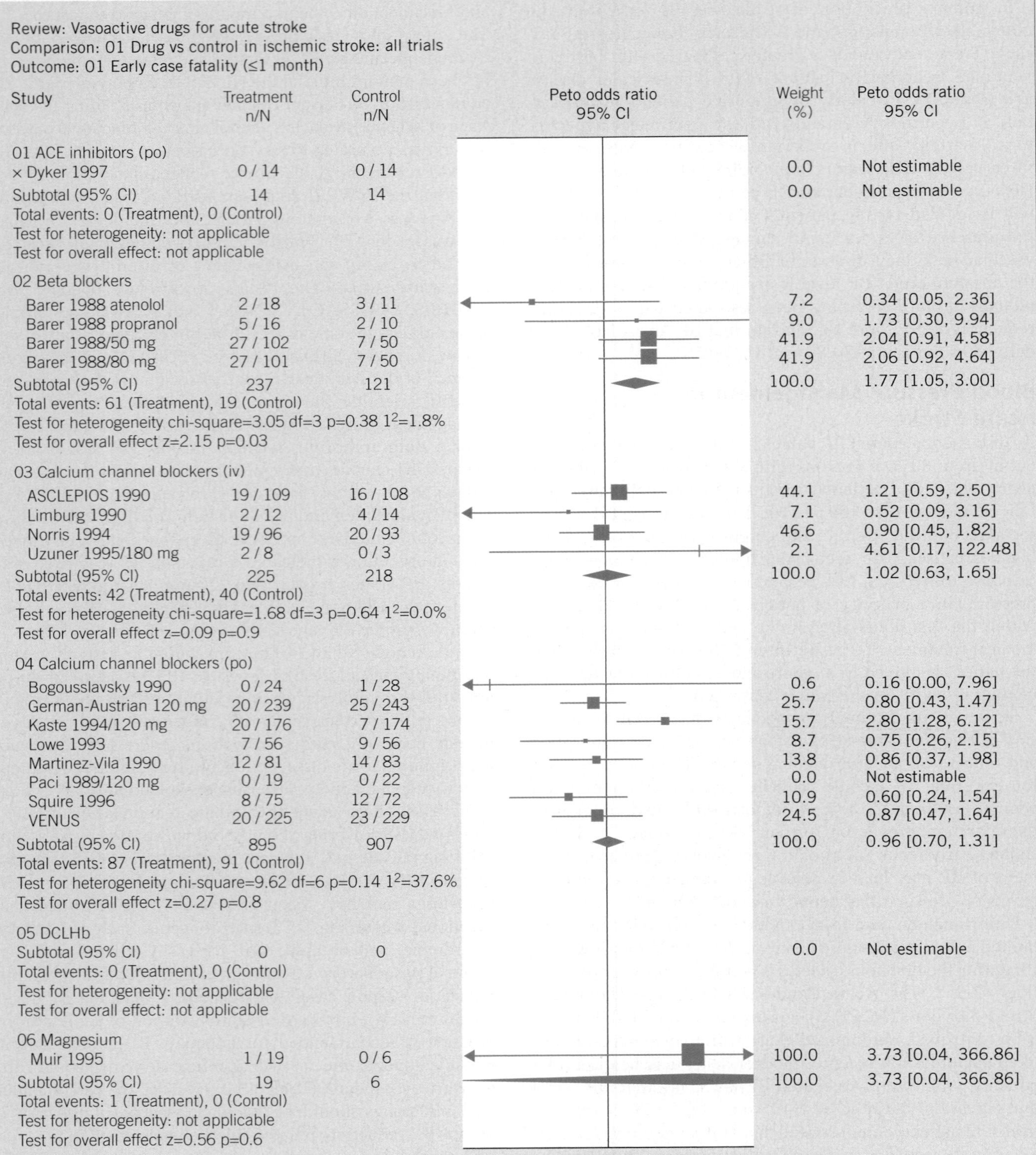

Figure 43.5 Analysis 01.01. Comparison 01 drug versus control in ischemic stroke: all trials, outcome 01 early case fatality (≤1 month). (From Blood Pressure in Acute Stroke Collaboration (BASC). Vasoactive drugs for acute stroke. Cochrane Database Syst Rev 2000;(4):CD002839.)

(Continued)

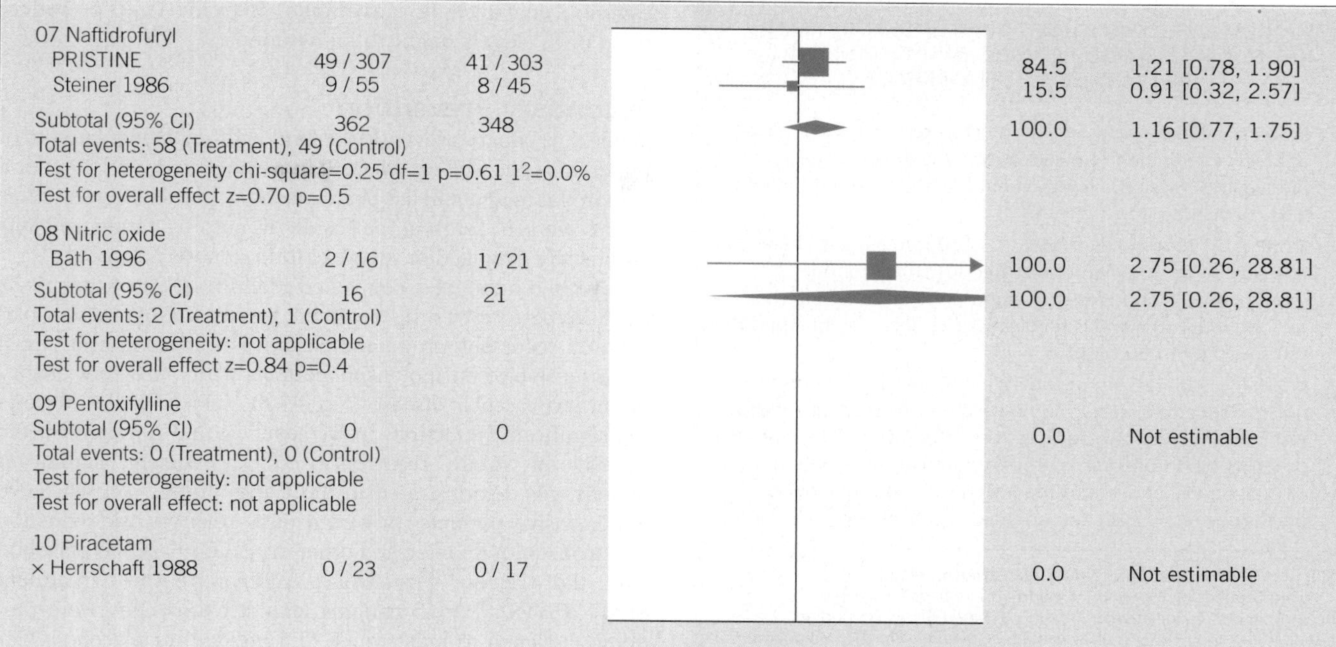

Figure 43.5—cont'd.

APPROACH TO ARTERIAL HYPERTENSION IN ACUTE ISCHEMIC STROKE

Indication that patient is eligible for treatment with intravenous rtPA or other acute reperfusion intervention
- Blood pressure level
  - Systolic >185 mm Hg or Diastolic >110 mm Hg
    - Labetalol 10 to 20 mg IV over 1 to 2 minutes, may repeat x 1;
    - or
    - Nitropaste 1 to 2 inches;
    - or
    - Nicardipine infusion, 5 mg/h, titrate up by 2.5 mg/h at 5- to 15-minute intervals, maximum dose 15 mg/h; when desired blood pressure attained, reduce to 3 mg/h
  - If blood pressure does not decline and remains >185/110 mm Hg, do not administer rtPA

Management of blood pressure during and after treatment with rtPA or other not acute reperfusion intervention
- Monitor blood every 15 minutes during treatment and then for another 2 hours, then every 30 minutes for 6 hours, and then every hour for 16 hours
- Blood pressure level
  - Systolic 180 to 230 mm Hg or diastolic 105 to 120 mm Hg
    - Labetalol 10 mg IV over 1 to 2 minutes, may repeat every 10 to 20 minutes, maximum dose of 300 mg;
    - or
    - Labetalol 10 mg IV followed by an infusion at 2 to 8 mg/min
  - Systolic >230 mm Hg or diastolic 121 to 140 mm Hg
    - Labetalol 10 mg IV over 1 to 2 minutes, may repeat every 10 to 20 minutes, maximum dose of 300 mg;
    - or
    - Labetalol 10 mg IV followed by an infusion at 2 to 8 mg/min;
    - or
    - Nicardipine infusion, 5 mg/h, titrate up to desired effect by increasing 2.5 mg/h every 5 minutes to maximum of 15 mg/h
  - If blood pressure not controlled, consider sodium nitroprusside

From Adams HP Jr, Del Zoppo G, Alberts MJ, et al. Approach to Arterial Hypertension in Acute Ischaemic Stroke. Guidelines for the early management of adults with ischemic stroke: a guideline from the American Heart Association/American Stroke Association Stroke Council, Clinical Cardiology Council, Cardiovascular Radiology and Invervention Council, and the Atherosclerotic Peripheral Vascular Disease and Quality of Care Outcomes in Research Interdisciplinary Working Groups: the American Academy of Neurology affirms the value of this guideline as an educational tool for neurologists. Stroke 2007;38:1655-1711.

Table 43.2 Approach to arterial hypertension in acute ischemic stroke.

SUGGESTED RECOMMENDED GUIDELINES FOR TREATING ELEVATED BLOOD PRESSURE IN SPONTANEOUS INTRACEREBRAL HEMORRHAGE

1. If SBP is >200 mm Hg or MAP is >150 mm Hg, then consider aggressive reduction of blood pressure with continuous intravenous infusion, with frequent blood pressure monitoring every 5 minutes.
2. If SBP is >180 mm Hg or MAP is >130 mm Hg and there is evidence of or suspicion of elevated ICP, then consider monitoring ICP and reducing blood pressure using intermittent or continous intravenous medications to keep cerebral perfusion pressure >60 to 80 mm Hg.
3. If SBP is >180 mm Hg or MAP is >130 mm Hg and there is not evidence of or suspicion of elevated ICP, then consider a modest reduction of blood pressure (e.g., MAP of 110 mm Hg or target blood pressure of 160/90 mm Hg) using intermittent or continuous intravenous medications to control blood pressure, and clinically reexamine the patient every 15 minutes.

SBP, systolic blood pressure; MAP, mean arterial pressure.
From Broderick J, Connolly S, Feldmann E, et al. Suggested Recommended Guidelines for Treating Elevated Blood Pressure in Spontaneous Intracerebral Haemorrhage. Guidelines for the management of spontaneous intracerebral hemorrhage in adults: 2007 update: a guideline from the American Heart Association/American Stroke Association Stroke Council, High Blood Pressure Research Council, and the Quality of Care and Outcomes in Research Interdisciplinary Working Group. Stroke 2007;38: 2001-2023.

Table 43.3 Suggested recommended guidelines for treating elevated blood pressure in spontaneous intracerebral hemorrhage.

esmolol, enalapril, or nicardipine. Extreme (>20%) reductions in BP levels ought to be avoided.

Secondary Prevention

While the primary prevention of stroke through the treatment of hypertension is well established, the issue of lowering BP after a cerebrovascular event has been uncertain, particularly since this might worsen cerebral perfusion if autoregulation remains chronically damaged or severe carotid stenosis is present.

Several randomized, controlled trials investigated the effects of antihypertensive drug treatment versus no treatment or placebo on recurrent stroke and cardiovascular complications in hypertensive or normotensive patients with a previous history of cerebrovascular disease (Fig. 43.6).[46] Two studies, despite the significant reductions in BP levels, could not confirm the benefit on stroke recurrence.[73,74] Conversely, significant benefit was demonstrated in the Carter study,[75] in which 96 hypertensive patients showed a 66% relative risk reduction for stroke with thiazide and other drugs compared to placebo.

In the Chinese Post-stroke Antihypertensive Treatment Study (PATS),[76] 5665 patients with stroke or TIA were randomly assigned to indapamide (2.5 mg/day) or placebo. Over a 2-year follow-up, indapamide decreased BP by 5 mm Hg systolic and 2 mm Hg diastolic and reduced stroke recurrence by 29%. In the HOPE trial,[29] 1013 patients with a previous history of stroke were randomized to ramipril (up to 10 mg/day) or matching placebo given on top of unspecified background therapy. Compared with placebo, the ACE inhibitor reduced BP by

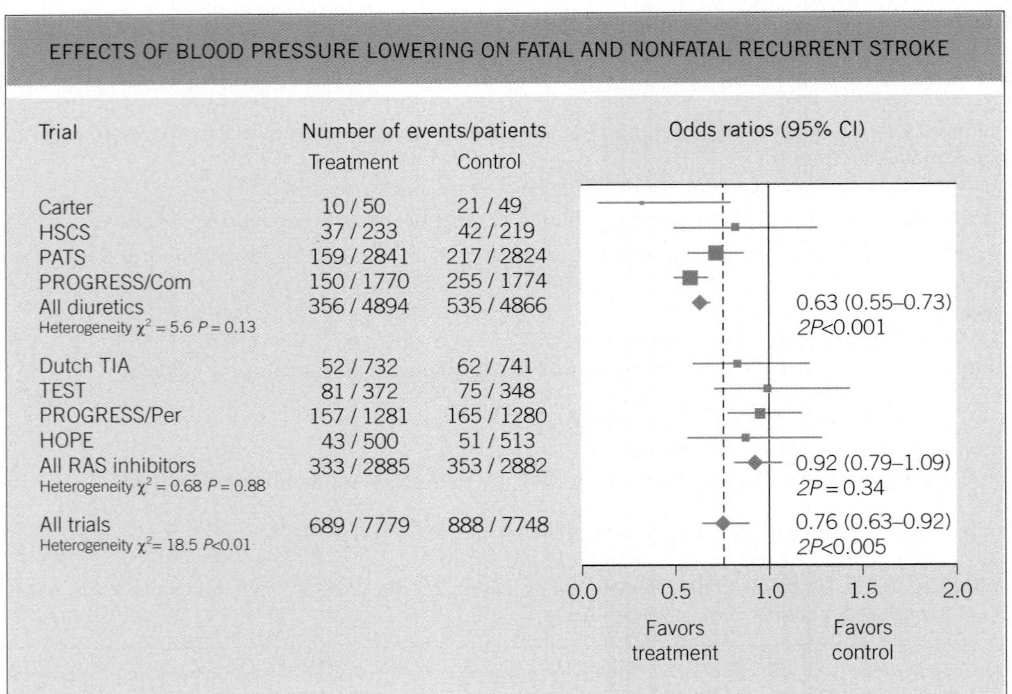

Figure 43.6 Effects of blood pressure lowering on fatal and nonfatal recurrent stroke. ■, Odds ratios in individual trials with a size proportional to the inverse of the variance of the odds ratios; – and ◆, 95% CIs for individual trials and summary statistics, respectively. (From Zhang H, Thijs L, Staessen JA. Blood pressure lowering for primary and secondary prevention of stroke. Hypertension 2006;48:187-195.)

3.1 mm Hg systolic and 1.7 mm Hg diastolic, but the relative risk reduction of 15% was not significant.

The PROGRESS study[77] included 6105 patients with a history of cerebrovascular disease. Patients in the active treatment group received perindopril (4 mg/day) either alone or together with indapamide (2.5 mg/day). Combination therapy lowered systolic and diastolic BP by 12.3 mm Hg and 5.0 mm Hg, respectively, and reduced stroke recurrence by 43%. Monotherapy with perindopril lowered systolic BP by 5.0 mm Hg and diastolic BP by 2.0 mm Hg, but the relative risk reduction was only 4%.

In addition to these trials, the MOSES study[78] included 1405 high-risk hypertensive patients with cerebral event during the last 2 years who were randomized to eprosartan (600 mg/day) or nitrendipine (10 mg/day) and followed for a period of 2.5 years. The eprosartan arm achieved a significant relative risk reduction benefit of 21% for the composite endpoint and 25% for stroke recurrence, although the final mean BP levels were unchanged.

The meta-analysis of Rashid and associates,[79] which does not include the MOSES study, showed that the combination of ACE inhibitors and diuretics was the only scheme that achieves a benefit after stroke or TIA, with a reduction in all adverse vascular events, including stroke and myocardial infarction.

On the basis of PATS and PROGRESS trials and the quoted meta-analysis, the treatment which achieves the greatest benefit following stroke or TIA is ACE inhibitors combined with a thiazide diuretic. Additionally, according to the MOSES study, treatment with eprosartan is effective and better than nitrendipine. These drugs are indicated when attempting to achieve a gradual reduction in BP levels following the acute phase of stroke, administered according to tolerance and the patient's concomitant diseases (myocardial infarction, heart failure, renal artery stenosis, diabetes mellitus, etc.).

In the Early Use of Existing Preventive Strategies for Stroke (EXPRESS) study,[80] early initiation of existing optimized medical therapy after TIA or minor stroke—including optimization of BP—was associated with an 80% reduction in the risk of early recurrent stroke. In EXPRESS the treatment protocol recommended was tailored to the individual patient but generally included aspirin or clopidogrel; simvastatin (40 mg daily); BP lowering unless systolic BP was below 130 mm Hg on repeated measurement (either by increases in existing medication, or by commencement of perindopril 4 mg daily, with or without indapamide 1.25 mg daily); and anticoagulation as required.

SUMMARY

Stroke is a common and important consequence of hypertension, and there is robust evidence that treatment of hypertension reduces risk of first stroke and recurrent stroke, as well as the occurrence of other major vascular events. BP following acute stroke follows a U-shaped curve in relation to mortality, but at present there is no consensus regarding early management of hypertension after acute stroke, except in a few circumstances (e.g., thrombolysis).

chapter 44

Nonpharmacologic Prevention and Management of Hypertension

Francesco P. Cappuccio, Alfonso Siani, and Saverio Stranges

- The first step in the management of patients of any age who have hypertension should be a reduction in salt intake (from 9 to 6 g/day), either alone or in combination with anti-hypertensive drugs, should be the first step for the management of patients with hypertension.
- A high potassium diet with an increase in the consumption of fruit, vegetables, and legumes is also recommended.
- Weight reduction, regular dynamic exercise, and restriction of alcohol consumption should be included in management plans for the prevention and nonpharmacologic treatment of hypertension.
- Limited evidence supports the roles of calcium and magnesium, or stress management for the prevention and management of hypertension.

Cardiovascular diseases (CVDs) represent the leading cause of mortality, morbidity, and disability worldwide.[1] In the past several decades, there has been an increasing burden of CVDs in many developing countries. Indeed, 70% of the total number of cardiovascular deaths occurs in developing countries, albeit CVDs are still proportionally more relevant in developed countries. The strategy for the primary prevention of CVDs resides in the detection and management of major risk factors. Seventy-five percent of the global burden of CVD results from smoking, high blood cholesterol levels, high blood pressure, or their combination. In particular, high blood pressure is the most powerful predictor of stroke and other cardiovascular events. Specifically, hypertension affects approximately 1 billion individuals worldwide, thus representing the most common cardiovascular condition in the world as well as the number one attributable risk for death.[2] In addition, about 62% of cerebrovascular disease and 49% of ischemic heart disease are attributable to suboptimal blood pressure levels (systolic blood pressure >115 mm Hg).[1]

The burden of hypertension-related diseases is likely to increase as the population ages, as suggested by recent data from the Framingham Heart Study, whereby normotensive individuals at 55 years of age have a 90% lifetime risk of developing hypertension.[3] Therefore prevention and treatment of hypertension are increasingly regarded as a public health priority. In developed countries, it is a priority because of the magnitude of the incidence of CVD and the potential benefits of hypertension prevention; in developing countries, because of the rising magnitude of CVD incidence.[4]

Nonpharmacologic interventions, also termed lifestyle modifications, represent an essential approach to the primary prevention of high blood pressure and an important component of the treatment of hypertension. They represent as well cost-effective measures in the context of a multifaceted public health strategy to reduce blood pressure at a population level. The current lifestyle modifications that effectively lower blood pressure include weight reduction if overweight or obese; reduction of dietary salt (sodium) intake; increased potassium intake; moderation of alcohol consumption; adoption of a dietary plan based on the DASH (Dietary Approaches to Stop Hypertension) diet, which is a diet rich in fruit, vegetables, and low-fat dairy products with a reduced content of saturated and total fat; and regular aerobic exercise.[5] These lifestyle modifications are effective in reducing blood pressure, increasing the efficacy of pharmacologic therapies, and reducing the global risk of CVD.

We will review the available literature and discuss the importance of these nonpharmacologic measures in light of the current evidence regarding their efficacy in lowering blood pressure. We will also evaluate the appropriateness of recommendations at a population level regarding some of these measures (e.g., reduction of dietary salt intake) and the different approaches to intervention needed to successfully prevent hypertension in developing and developed countries.

WEIGHT REDUCTION

The prevalence of obesity has increased worldwide.[6] Data from the U.S. National Health and Nutrition Examination Survey (NHANES) indicate that 32.2% of American adults (20 years or older) are obese (body mass index [BMI] $\geq$30 kg/m^2), whereas only one third (33.7%) are in the range of normal weight (BMI <25 kg/m^2).[7] Obesity and overweight are becoming increasing public health issues in many developing regions as well (e.g., Latin America, Middle East) and represent major contributors to the global burden of disease.[8]

Obesity is an independent risk factor for coronary heart disease, stroke, and total cardiovascular morbidity and mortality, and is strongly associated with other cardiovascular risk factors. Specifically, the relationship between obesity and hypertension is very well documented. Blood pressure is strongly correlated with BMI. The prevalence of obesity-related hypertension varies with age, ethnicity, and sex of the population studied.[9] Approximately one third of cases of hypertension are attributable to obesity, although in young adults and children the figures may be substantially higher.[10] Likewise, weight gain, even of a modest magnitude, is itself an important risk factor for the development of hypertension in adulthood. This effect is present in both genders, stronger in young adults and weaker in people of black African ancestry; conversely, weight loss reduces the risk of hypertension.[11,12]

Recent investigations have also emphasized the importance of body fat distribution in the association between obesity and blood pressure. Specifically, abdominal adiposity with central fat accumulation has been reported as a stronger determinant of hypertension risk than relative weight.[13,14]

Based on the large body of evidence on the relationship between body weight and blood pressure, weight reduction has been proposed as a measure to reduce blood pressure in both clinical and public health guidelines.[5] Over the past 3 decades, several randomized controlled clinical trials have reported on the beneficial effects of weight loss interventions on the prevention and treatment of hypertension. In the latest published meta-analysis of 25 randomized, controlled trials, which included only trials based on weight reduction through energy restriction, increased physical activity or both, average reductions of 4.4/3.6 mm Hg for systolic and diastolic blood pressure, respectively, were reported for a 5-kg weight loss (Fig. 44.1).[15] A dose-response was observed, meaning that the greater the weight loss, the greater the blood pressure reduction. Furthermore, the lowering effect of weight reduction on blood pressure was independent of age, gender, and initial BMI, although the effect appeared greater in patients on antihypertensive medication. This meta-analysis also highlights the problem of lack of compliance during long-term interventions, because the maximal effect was reached before the end of the trials. Additionally, the long-term effects of weight reduction on blood pressure are not fully understood; however, they seem to be in magnitude less than those reported in short-term trials. In fact, a recent systematic review, based on studies with follow-up of 2 years or longer, demonstrated decreases of 6.0/4.6 mm Hg for systolic and diastolic blood pressure, respectively, for 10-kg weight loss, about half of that predicted from the short-term trials.[16] Several factors such as initial blood pressure, length of follow-up, medication changes, and physiologic restrictions may contribute to this reduced effect in the long-term studies. Nevertheless, weight loss programs represent an essential component of a multifaceted nonpharmacologic intervention to manage hypertension; in addition, they are adjuvant measures to pharmacologic therapies, because they decrease the dosage of antihypertensive medication needed to reach blood pressure control.[17]

Many biological mechanisms have been proposed to explain the link among obesity, weight change, and blood pressure. For example, an overactive renin-angiotensin-aldosterone system is likely to be a key mechanism of the hypertensive response in obese individuals, whose circulating levels of renin activity and aldosterone are higher than in nonobese subjects.[18] Further mechanisms may reside in inhibition of the natriuretic peptides system, which is critical to prevent excess salt and water retention, promote vascular relaxation, and inhibit sympathetic outflow; increased activity of the sympathetic nervous system; and reduced insulin sensitivity and hyperinsulinemia.[19]

In summary, the current evidence from clinical trials strongly supports the notion that prevention of weight gain in normal-weight individuals and weight loss in overweight and obese individuals, in combination with other lifestyle modifications, are highly effective strategies for the prevention and management of hypertension both in individuals and the community at large.[5]

DIETARY SALT (SODIUM) REDUCTION

Epidemiologic Evidence

The importance of salt (sodium chloride) intake in determining blood pressure and the incidence of hypertension is well established. Furthermore, randomized, controlled clinical trials of moderate reductions in salt intake show a dose-dependent cause-effect relation and lack of a threshold effect within usual levels of salt intake in populations worldwide.[20] The effect is independent of age, sex, ethnic origin, baseline blood pressure, and body mass. Thus, the reduction of dietary sodium intake is one of the most important and effective lifestyle modifications to reduce blood pressure and control hypertension.[5,21]

The INTERSALT study, a large epidemiologic investigation on 10,079 men and women, aged 20 to 59 years, in 52 centers from 32 countries around the world, was one of the first epidemiologic studies to examine this question.[22] This study tested both the within- and cross-population association between 24-hour urinary sodium excretion, reflecting the amount of sodium intake, and blood pressure levels. The within-center results showed a significant, positive, independent, and linear association between 24-hour urinary sodium excretion and blood pressure levels. Specifically, a 100 mmol per day higher sodium intake (about 2.3 g/day) would predict a 3 to 6 mm Hg higher systolic and up to 3 mm Hg higher diastolic blood pressure. Similar results were obtained in different subgroup analyses: men, women, young, elderly, and participants without hypertension. In the cross-population analysis, significant, independent relations were found between 24-hour urinary sodium excretion and median systolic and diastolic blood pressure, prevalence rate of hypertension, and rise of systolic and diastolic blood pressure with age.

Besides the epidemiologic observational evidence, over 50 randomized clinical trials have supported a role of salt intake reduction in the prevention and management of high blood pressure (Fig. 44.2). In the largest of these trials, the Dietary Approaches to Stop Hypertension (DASH) trial, 412 participants were randomly allocated to two dietary regimens: one following a control diet, which was representative of the average diet in the United States; one following the DASH diet—a diet rich in fruits, vegetables, and low-fat or fat-free diary products and reduced in saturated and total fat content. Inside each arm of the trial, participants were randomly assigned to three groups with increasing amounts of sodium intake. As estimated from 24-hour urinary collections, the three sodium levels (lower, intermediate, and higher) provided 65, 107, and 142 mmol per day, respectively, which correspond approximately to intakes of 1.5, 2.5, and 3.3 g of sodium per day, respectively.[23] In this trial, a sodium reduction alone from a high to a low level was associated with a blood pressure reduction of 8.3/4.4 mm Hg among hypertensive individuals and 5.6/2.8 mm Hg among normotensive individuals. Moreover, the combination of this amount of sodium reduction and the DASH diet further

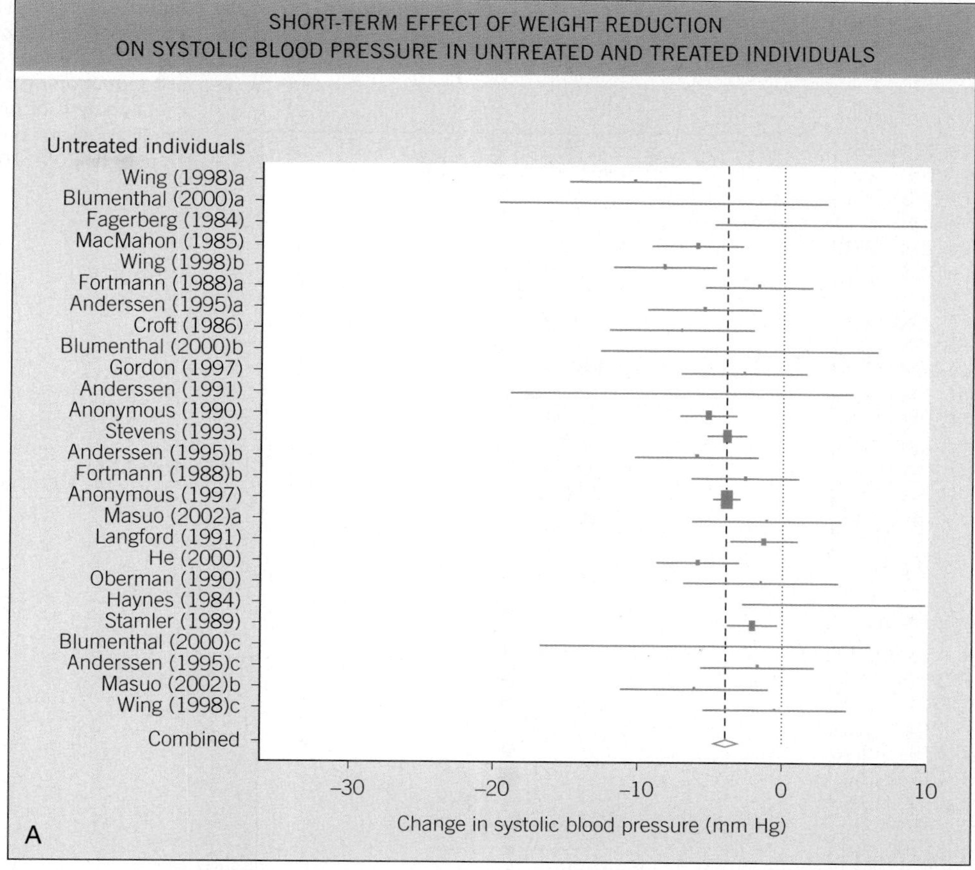

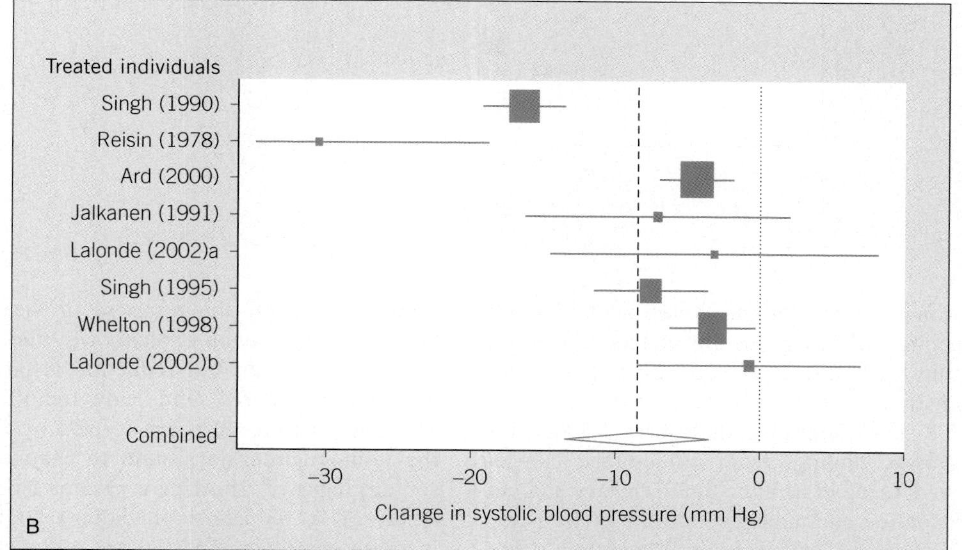

Figure 44.1 Short-term effect of weight reduction on systolic blood pressure in untreated and treated individuals. (From Neter JE, Stam BE, Kok FJ, Grobbee DE, Geleijnse JM. Influence of weight reduction on blood pressure: a meta-analysis of randomized controlled trials. Hypertension 2003;42:878-884.)

reduced blood pressure by 11.5/5.7 mm Hg and 7.1/3.7 mm Hg, respectively, among those with and without hypertension. Significant effects of sodium reductions on blood pressure levels were present in both genders, all racial and age groups, though they were more marked among African Americans, women (for systolic blood pressure), and persons older than 45 years.[24]

Pooled estimates from meta-analyses of clinical trials on the effects of salt reduction on blood pressure levels indicate a fall in systolic and diastolic blood pressure of 7.1/3.9 mm Hg, respectively, in hypertensive individuals and 3.6/1.7 mm Hg in normotensive individuals per 100 mmol reduction of 24-hour urinary sodium excretion (about 6 g salt/day). In the latest published meta-analysis of 40 randomized trials,

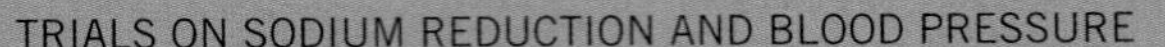

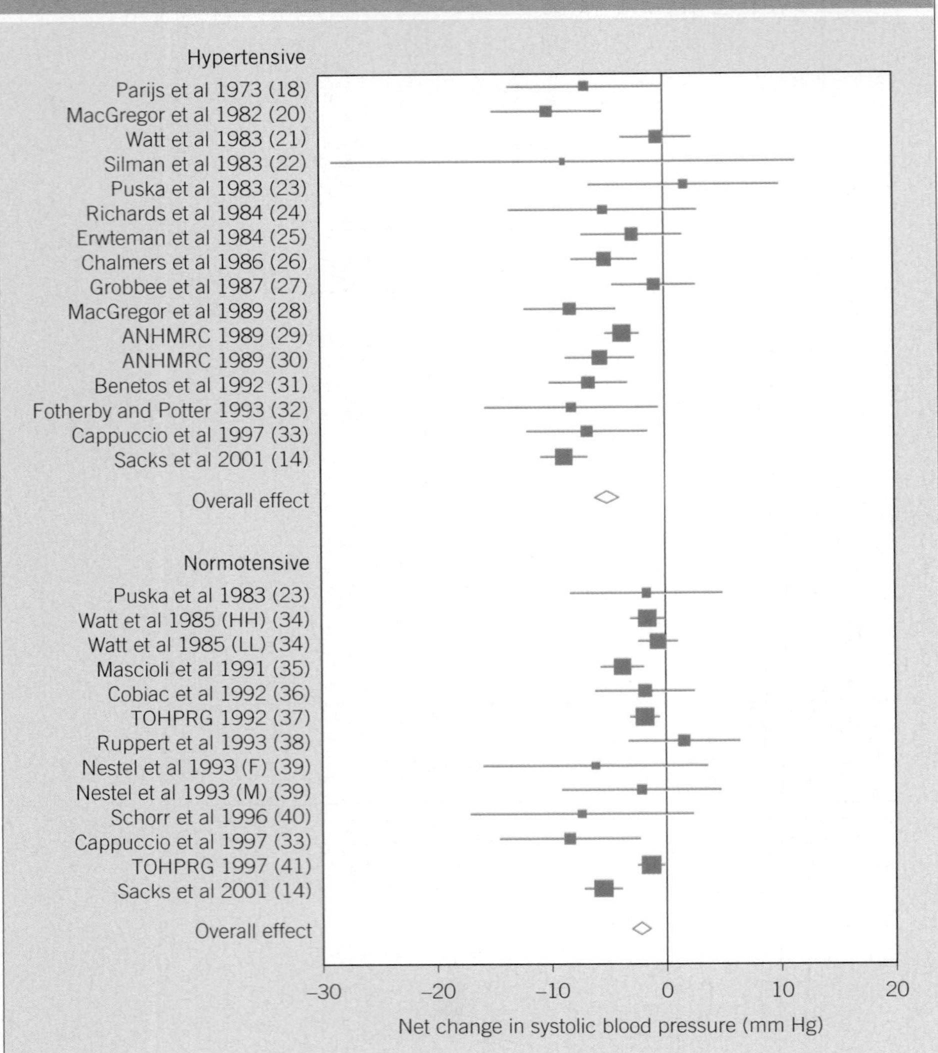

Figure 44.2 Trials on sodium reduction and blood pressure. (From He FJ, MacGregor GA. Effect of modest salt reduction on blood pressure: a meta-analysis of randomized trials. Implications for public health. J Hum Hypertens 2002:16:761-770.)

an average reduction in urinary sodium excretion of 77 mmol per day was associated with a reduction in blood pressure levels of 2.5/2.0 mm Hg.[25] Blood pressure response was significantly larger in hypertensive than normotensive individuals (systolic: −5.2 vs −1.3 mm Hg; diastolic: −3.7 vs −1.1 mm Hg). Furthermore, findings from randomized clinical trials have supported a role of a reduction in dietary sodium in the primary prevention and management of hypertension. For example, in the Trials of Hypertension Prevention, phase II, a sodium reduction of 100 mmol per day, alone or combined with weight loss, prevented hypertension by 20% throughout 48 months of intervention in overweight adults.[26]

Recently, compelling evidence has become available to support a reduction in salt intake in children and adolescents as well, to prevent the rise in blood pressure with age and the ensuing risk of hypertension.[27,28]

The interindividual variability in terms of blood pressure response to dietary changes in sodium intake has been termed salt sensitivity,[29] and it is likely to be due to the degree of response of the renin-angiotensin system.[30] The weaker the response of this system to a change in sodium intake, the larger the response of the blood pressure will be. This phenomenon explains why the blood pressure lowering effect of sodium reduction is larger in hypertensive individuals, elderly, and "low-renin" black populations. These groups are all characterized by weaker responses of the renin-angiotensin system to changes in the amount of sodium ingested, showing a greater blood pressure fall as a result of a reduction of dietary sodium. This response increases with age and is largest in the elderly. For example, in a double-blind, randomized trial, a modest reduction in sodium intake in people over the age of 60 induced a significant reduction in blood pressure without untoward effect, irrespective of the initial blood pressure.[31] These observations are relevant to the prevention of hypertension-related diseases in developed countries, where the majority of strokes occur in the elderly and individuals with blood pressure levels below the treatment threshold for hypertension.[32]

People of black African origin show a greater blood pressure response when dietary salt is reduced. For example, the efficacy of a moderate reduction in salt intake has recently been tested in two short-term trials in both urban and rural areas of West Africa, namely Nigeria and Ghana, where the prevalence of hypertension is increasing.[33,34] In both studies a moderate reduction in salt intake was associated with a significant reduction in blood pressure comparable to that seen in white populations. In areas such as sub-Saharan Africa, the prevalence of hypertension is increasing, the health care resources are scarce, and thus the identification of people with hypertension is still haphazard. The effectiveness of a reduction in salt intake at a population level might prove extremely important for policymakers.

Despite the large body of evidence supporting the efficacy of dietary sodium reduction in the prevention and management of hypertension, the long-term outcome benefits as well as the appropriateness of a population-wide strategy to reduce dietary salt intake are still controversial issues. The major benefit of sodium reduction is the lowering of blood pressure. It has been argued that the blood pressure reduction realistically achievable at a population level (i.e., 1 to 3 mm Hg in systolic blood pressure) is small, not clinically significant, and lacking clear long-term benefits.[35] However, in a meta-analysis of 61 prospective studies, it has been estimated that even a reduction of 2 mm Hg in systolic blood pressure would determine a 10% reduction in stroke mortality and a 7% reduction in mortality from coronary heart disease or other cardiovascular causes, meaning a large number of premature deaths and disabilities would be avoided.[36] In addition, in a recent published paper, Cook and colleagues[37] reported the long-term effects of reduced dietary sodium on cardiovascular disease in people participating in the controlled randomized trials of hypertension prevention follow-up studies (TOHP I and II) (Fig. 44.3). More than 3000 participants without hypertension were randomized to a reduced sodium intake for 18 months (TOHP I) or 36 to 48 months (TOHP II), or to a control arm. The reductions in sodium intake were 44 mmol/day and 33 mmol/day (equivalent to about 2.6 g and 2.0 g of salt, respectively). The results show that people originally allocated to either sodium reduction group had a 30% lower incidence of cardiovascular events in the next 10 to 15 years, irrespective of sex, ethnic origin, age, body mass, and blood pressure. The benefits exceed those estimated by the published meta-analysis.[36] The study by Cook and colleagues[37] is the first to report a beneficial effect of dietary salt reduction on cardiovascular outcomes based on randomized trial data. The study strengthens the support for dietary recommendations for lower salt intake to prevent cardiovascular disease in the general population.

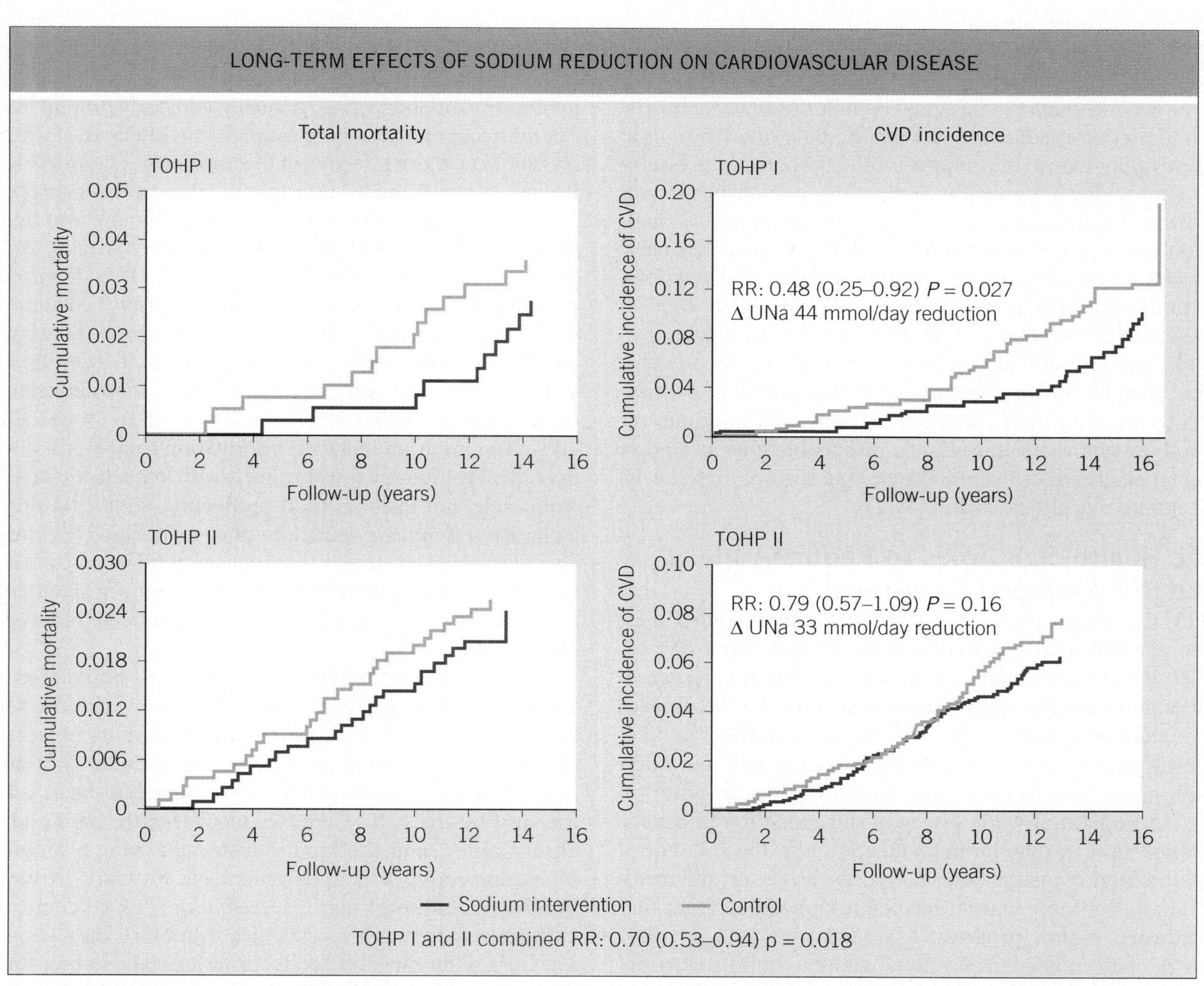

Figure 44.3 Long-term effects of sodium reduction on cardiovascular disease. (From Cook NR, Cutler JA, Obarzanek E, et al. Long-term effects of dietary sodium reduction on cardiovascular disease outcomes: observational follow-up of trials of hypertension prevention. Br Med J 2007;334:885-888.)

PRACTICAL ADVICE ON HOW TO REDUCE SALT INTAKE AND ACHIEVE A MODERATE BUT SUSTAINED REDUCTION IN SALT INTAKE	
1. Never add salt to a meal	
Do not use rock salt and sea salt. They are just the same as table salt! Most sauces contain salt (e.g., tomato ketchup, soy sauce, HP sauce).	Use pepper, garlic, lemon, and herbs instead!
2. Do not add salt to the cooking	
Do not use stock cubes, gravy browning, soy sauce, or salted dry fish. Take care with curry powders and prepared mustards.	Try other flavorings! Any fresh, frozen, or dried herbs; all spices; lemon or lime; vinegar; wine, beer, or cider; onions, garlic, shallots, ginger, and chili peppers
3. Avoid manufactured or processed foods with added salt	
Read food labels. Salt is sodium chloride. At the moment most food labels only report sodium as grams per 100 grams of food. To convert to salt, multiply by 2.5. 1 g sodium per 100 g food is equivalent to the saltiness of sea water! Most breads are high in salt. Many cereals contain too much salt. All ready soups, all processed meats, take-away pizzas, ready-made foods, etc., are often very high in salt. Avoid Chinese take-out and some mineral waters. Target daily salt intake should not exceed 5 grams per day.	Ideally you should only choose food items with no more than 0.3 g sodium per 100 g food (equivalent to ~0.75 g salt per 100 g food).

Table 44.1 Practical advice on how to reduce salt intake and achieve a moderate but sustained reduction in salt intake.

Moreover, although the principal benefit of salt reduction is the blood pressure reduction, it is not the only one. There is a large body of evidence that supports other benefits: regression of left ventricular hypertrophy, reduction in proteinuria and glomerular hyperfiltration, reduction in osteoporosis and bone mineral loss with age, protection against stomach cancer and stroke, protection against asthma attacks, and possibly protection against cataracts.[38]

In summary, reduction of dietary salt intake appears a plausible population-wide recommendation for the prevention and treatment of hypertension.[5,21] A decrease of dietary sodium to no more than 100 mmol per day (2.3 g sodium or 5.8 g sodium chloride) represents a reasonable goal at a population level, given the current dietary patterns of high levels of salt intake worldwide (Table 44.1).

Public Health Strategies to Reduce Salt Intake in Developed Countries

In 1985, the World Health Organization recommended that the average salt intake should be reduced to 5 g per day or less. However, few countries have policies for targeted reduction in salt intake. Differences exist between developed and developing countries. In westernized countries, people derive salt mostly from bread and processed food, and only a small proportion comes from discretionary use (up to 20%).[39] A population-wide policy of salt reduction in developed countries can only be implemented with the collaboration of the food industry. Over the years, however, the need to sustain a profitable market has led to opposition from the food industry or slow progress.[40]

In developed countries a sustained and long-term reduction in salt intake based on educational and behavioral interventions only is likely to be unsuccessful in reducing blood pressure at a population level, because the majority of an individual's salt intake is not added by the person but is already present in foods. Therefore a population-wide strategy involving the food industry would be more effective in the long term. The North Karelia Project is a meaningful example to support this concept. This program was launched in 1972 in Finland to prevent noncommunicable diseases and, primarily, to reduce mortality and morbidity from cardiovascular diseases.[41] The interventions implemented during this trial were extensive: collaborations with the community, health services, and food industry were added to a mass media campaign. The results have been outstanding. Over 25 years, the age-adjusted mortality rate from cardiovascular disease among men aged 25 to 64 years fell by 73%. The program included information campaigns, development of new industry food products with less salt, welfare losses from taxes/subsidies on food production with little salt, and, assuming a 2 mm Hg reduction of systolic blood pressure, the cost of avoided treatment for myocardial infarction and stroke, cost of avoided antihypertensive treatment, hospital costs in additional life-years, and productivity gains from reduced morbidity and mortality.

A recent global and regional analysis of population interventions including government cooperation with food industry and change of legislation on salt content of processed food consistently showed their cost-effectiveness in limiting cardiovascular diseases.[42] This strategy has been adopted recently by the U.K. Department of Health, the Food Standard Agency, and the food industry, showing a simple way of implementing a nonpharmacologic measure to limit the burden of cardiovascular diseases in developed countries.

Future options are to establish voluntary target levels of salt for a wide range of foods, or to legislate so that the food industry has to comply. The "voluntary" option would support existing work, but it is unlikely to achieve the set targets. The recent position of the industry in rejecting the "traffic light" proposal for labeling, whereby highly salted foods would carry a red alert warning, is one measure of the gap still remaining. The legislation option would require the food industry to reduce the salt content of processed food to within set levels. The experience in Finland suggests that legislation has added value to the previous option and at this stage is necessary and justified.

In conclusion, doctors and health professionals have long used dietary counseling to deliver nonpharmacologic management of hypertension. However, advising patients to reduce salt intake with a lifestyle package quickly delivered in a busy primary care setting is ineffective.[43] Therefore, without considerably modifying the environment by allowing greater availability of low salt foods, people in developed countries will find it difficult to exercise their "choice" when trying to reduce dietary salt.[44]

Public Health Strategies to Reduce Salt Intake in Developing Countries

Worldwide, stroke is second only to ischemic heart disease as a cause of death, and most of these deaths occur in developing countries.[8] For example, in areas like sub-Saharan Africa the prevalence of hypertension is elevated and comparable to figures from developed regions.[2,45] Moreover, the burden of diseases attributable to hypertension (e.g., stroke, heart, and renal failure) is much greater in sub-Saharan Africa than in the Western societies because competing risk factors like tobacco smoking and high serum cholesterol are not highly prevalent yet.[8]

Salt consumption in developing countries is becoming more common as urbanization increases. However, interventions to reduce salt intake at a population level have not been extensively studied in these countries. The population approach to reduce salt consumption is particularly relevant in developing countries because of the cost-effectiveness of these measures.[42] Furthermore, in countries of sub-Saharan Africa where effective health care provision for chronic diseases is haphazard, a population strategy to limit salt consumption might prove extremely effective. It can be predicted that the same reduction in salt intake obtained with a behavioral intervention will be more effective in black African origin populations than in white populations because of the higher salt sensitivity of black African origin populations and because most of the salt ingested is added to food by the consumer, whereas processed food is used relatively scarcely compared to developed countries.[32]

Two short-term trials in sub-Saharan Africa have confirmed that simple, cost-effective, and culturally adapted behavioral and educational interventions to reduce blood pressure can be successfully implemented (Fig 44.4).[33,34] Concerns about population-wide strategies to limit salt consumption in developing countries pertain to the perceived risk of counteracting worldwide policies directed to the prevention of iodine deficiency disorders (IDD) through universal salt iodization. There is an urgent need to consider alternative vehicles for the deliveries of iodine to populations. In the meantime, an increase in the proportion of iodine fixed to salt could be considered.

A reduction in salt intake that prevented 10% of hypertension would have a greater impact in a sub-Saharan population than in a Western population. In fact, in sub-Saharan Africa 11 times more strokes are estimated to be prevented

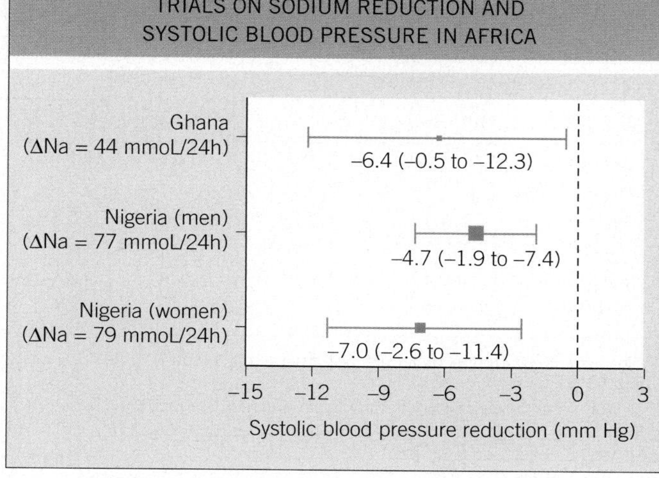

Figure 44.4 Trials on sodium reduction and systolic blood pressure in Africa. (From Adeyemo AA, Prewitt TE, Luke A, et al. The feasibility of implementing a dietary sodium reduction intervention among free-living normotensive individuals in south west Nigeria. Ethn Dis 2002;12:207-212; Cappuccio FP, Kerry SM, Micah FB, Plange-Rhule J, Eastwood JB. A community programme to reduce salt intake and blood pressure in Ghana (ISRCTN 88789643). BMC Public Health 2006;6:13.)

in people under 65 of age when compared with developed countries. The benefit of a public health intervention aimed at reducing salt intake, thereby reducing the prevalence of hypertension, would be substantial in developing countries (almost a 20% reduction in the incidence of stroke in people under 65 years old). Given the size of the populations in sub-Saharan Africa, and considering that the incidence of stroke in people under 65 is estimated to be approximately seven times greater in this region compared with developed countries, one might expect the benefits of such an intervention to be significantly greater in this region than in developed countries.

In conclusion, in many developing countries, like those of sub-Saharan Africa, where the main source of salt is still discretionary, community-based and context-specific initiatives can be effective and should be pursued,[34] given the increasing burden of cardiovascular disease related to hypertension.

DIETARY POTASSIUM INCREASE

Increased potassium intake is inversely related to blood pressure levels. The evidence is supported by findings of animal studies, observational epidemiologic investigations, and clinical trials. Moreover, meta-analyses of randomized controlled trials on the efficacy of potassium supplementation in reducing blood pressure levels in both normotensive and hypertensive individuals consistently demonstrate this inverse relationship.

The INTERSALT cooperative study was one of the earlier epidemiologic investigations to estimate the effect of potassium intake on blood pressure levels. This study tested both the within- and cross-population association between 24-hour urinary sodium, potassium, and sodium-to-potassium ratio, reflecting the amount of dietary intake of these micronutrients, and blood pressure levels. Within the

META-ANALYSES OF POTASSIUM SUPPLEMENTATION*				
	Systolic Blood Pressure		Diastolic Blood Pressure	
All Trials	Net Change	95% CI	Net Change	95% CI
Cappuccio et al (1991)	−5.9	−5.2 to −6.6	−3.4	−2.8 to 4.0
Whelton et al (1997)	−3.1	−1.9 to −4.3	−2.0	−0.5 to −3.4
Geleijnse et al (2003)	−2.4	−3.1 to −3.7	−1.6	−0.5 to −2.6

*Results are reported as mean net systolic/diastolic blood pressure changes and 95% CI.

Data from Geleijnse et al,[25] Cappuccio and MacGregor,[46] and Whelton et al.[47]

Table 44.2 Meta-analyses of potassium supplementation.

centers, a reduction in systolic and diastolic blood pressure of 3.4/1.9 mm Hg was related to a higher potassium intake of 50 mmol per day. Furthermore, the sodium-to-potassium ratio was positively and significantly related to the blood pressure levels of individuals in both men and women. These relationships were more marked with increasing age.[22]

Numerous clinical trials have reported on the effect of potassium supplementation on blood pressure levels in both normotensive and hypertensive individuals. Although results have not always been consistent, pooled estimates from meta-analyses support a significant inverse association between potassium intake and blood pressure levels[25,46,47] in both normotensive and hypertensive individuals (Table 44.2).

In an early meta-analysis including 19 clinical trials with both normotensive and hypertensive individuals, an overall effect of potassium supplementation of −5.9 mm Hg (95% CI, −6.6 to −5.2) and −3.4 mm Hg (95% confidence interval [CI], −4.0 to −2.8) was reported for systolic and diastolic blood pressure, respectively. The magnitude of the blood pressure lowering effect of potassium supplementation was greater in individuals with high blood pressure (−8.2 mm Hg [−9.1 to −7.3 mm Hg] for systolic, and −4.5 mm Hg [−5.2 to −3.8 mm Hg] for diastolic blood pressure) and appeared to be more pronounced the longer the duration of the supplementation.[46] Likewise, in a later meta-analysis including 33 randomized controlled trials, potassium supplementation was associated with a significant reduction in mean systolic and diastolic blood pressure of −3.1 mm Hg (−1.9 to −4.3 mm Hg) and −2.0 mm Hg (−0.5 to −3.4 mm Hg), respectively.[47] The average effect size was larger in trials conducted in hypertensive individuals (−4.4/−2.5 mm Hg for systolic and diastolic blood pressure, respectively). Finally, a recent meta-analysis by Geleijnse and colleagues[25] including 27 potassium trials showed a significant inverse association between increased potassium intake (median: 44 mmol/24 h) and blood pressure levels, although the effect size reported was slightly smaller than that previously published, that is, a decrease in systolic and diastolic blood pressure of 2.4 mm Hg (95% CI, 1.1 to 3.7) and 1.6 mm Hg (95% CI, 0.5 to 2.6), respectively. Consistent with the two previously published meta-analyses, blood pressure response was larger in hypertensive than normotensive individuals.

The lowering effect of potassium supplementation on blood pressure levels is independent of the baseline potassium status; it appears similar in women and men, whereas it is stronger among hypertensive individuals and individuals of black African origin, as also confirmed by pooled estimates of a published meta-analysis.[47] Furthermore, the lowering effect of potassium supplementation on blood pressure is dependent on the concurrent intake of dietary sodium and vice versa. This means that this effect is larger in individuals on a high-sodium diet and smaller in individuals on a low-sodium diet; conversely, the lowering effect of a reduction in dietary sodium intake on blood pressure is larger in individuals on a low-potassium diet and smaller in individuals on a high-potassium diet.[21] Accordingly, the ratio of sodium to potassium excreted in urine is more closely related to changes in blood pressure levels than either urinary sodium or potassium excretion individually.[22,47]

Fruit, vegetables, legumes, and nuts are the main sources of dietary potassium in the form of inorganic or organic salts. These foods, especially fruit and vegetables, are rich in potassium as well as in other essential micronutrients; therefore diet is a suitable strategy to increase the levels of potassium intake and prevents the need for supplements. Several randomized controlled trials have reported on the lowering effects on blood pressure of dietary interventions providing large intakes of potassium. For example, in the Dietary Approaches to Stop Hypertension (DASH) trial, the two groups that increased fruit and vegetable consumption, with consequently larger amounts of potassium, experienced significant reductions in blood pressure levels.[23]

The increase in potassium intake from natural dietary sources may represent a feasible and effective measure to reduce the need for antihypertensive medication. For example, Siani and colleagues[48] found that after dietary advice, which was specifically aimed at increasing potassium intake, the intervention group increased their potassium intake compared to the control group. More importantly, as a result of the dietary intervention, blood pressure could be controlled using less than 50% of the initial pharmacologic therapy in 81% of the patients in the intervention group, compared with 29% of the patients in the control group.[48]

The mechanisms responsible for the lowering effect of increased potassium intake on blood pressure are not fully understood. Several hypotheses have been put forward.[49] High potassium intake might exert a vascular protective effect and reduce the development of atherosclerosis. It may also reduce arteriolar thickening in the kidney. Moreover, potassium infusion increases acetylcholine-induced vasodilatation, and this effect is inhibited by the consequent infusion of the nitric oxide synthase inhibitor L-NMMA (L-nitromonomethylarginine). This suggests that potassium could lower blood pressure by a nitric oxide–dependent vasodilatation. Conversely, potassium depletion in humans is accompanied by sodium retention and calcium depletion and also by an altered response to vasoactive hormones. These metabolic effects together with the direct vasoconstrictive effects of hypokalemia might be the cause of the augmentation in blood pressure during a decrease of potassium intake.

In summary, the adoption of a high-potassium diet is a reasonable, effective nonpharmacologic measure to improve blood pressure control in hypertensive individuals and to prevent the risk of hypertension in the general population. The level of intake that should be recommended is dependent on the levels of potassium status in a specific population, as well as on the presence of conditions or drug therapies that can impair potassium excretion. A recent statement from the American Heart Association sets the recommended level of potassium intake, among healthy individuals, as 4.7 g/day (120 mmol/day).[21] This level of intake has been based primarily on findings from clinical trials and the potassium content of the DASH diet.[23] In the Western populations the current levels of potassium intake are generally lower than this recommended level. In individuals affected by disease conditions impairing potassium excretion (e.g., diabetes, chronic renal insufficiency, end-stage renal disease, severe heart failure, and adrenal insufficiency) or on drug therapies that may interfere with potassium excretion (e.g., angiotensin-converting enzyme inhibitors, angiotensin receptor blockers, nonsteroidal anti-inflammatory agents, and potassium-sparing diuretics), a lower level of intake (i.e., <4.7 g/day [120 mmol/day]) is recommended to prevent the risk of hyperkalemia.[50]

MODERATION OF ALCOHOL CONSUMPTION

Heavy alcohol consumption has been consistently associated with elevated blood pressure and increased risk of hypertension in epidemiologic studies.[51-54] The increased risk of hypertension occurs at levels of consumption above approximately two drinks per day in men and one drink per day in women and lighter-weight individuals.[5,21] The observational data have been corroborated by findings of randomized controlled trials showing a blood pressure–raising effect of alcohol, which is reversible in both normotensive and hypertensive individuals. Specifically, in a meta-analysis of 15 randomized controlled trials, the authors estimated a reduction in systolic and diastolic blood pressure of 3.3/2.0 mm Hg, respectively, for a median 76% reduction in alcohol consumption from a baseline of 3 to 6 drinks per day (Fig. 44.5).[55] Blood pressure reductions were similar in hypertensive and normotensive individuals. Importantly, the relationship between reduction in mean percentage of alcohol and decline in blood pressure was dose dependent. Findings from this meta-analysis also suggest that the reduction in blood pressure following a

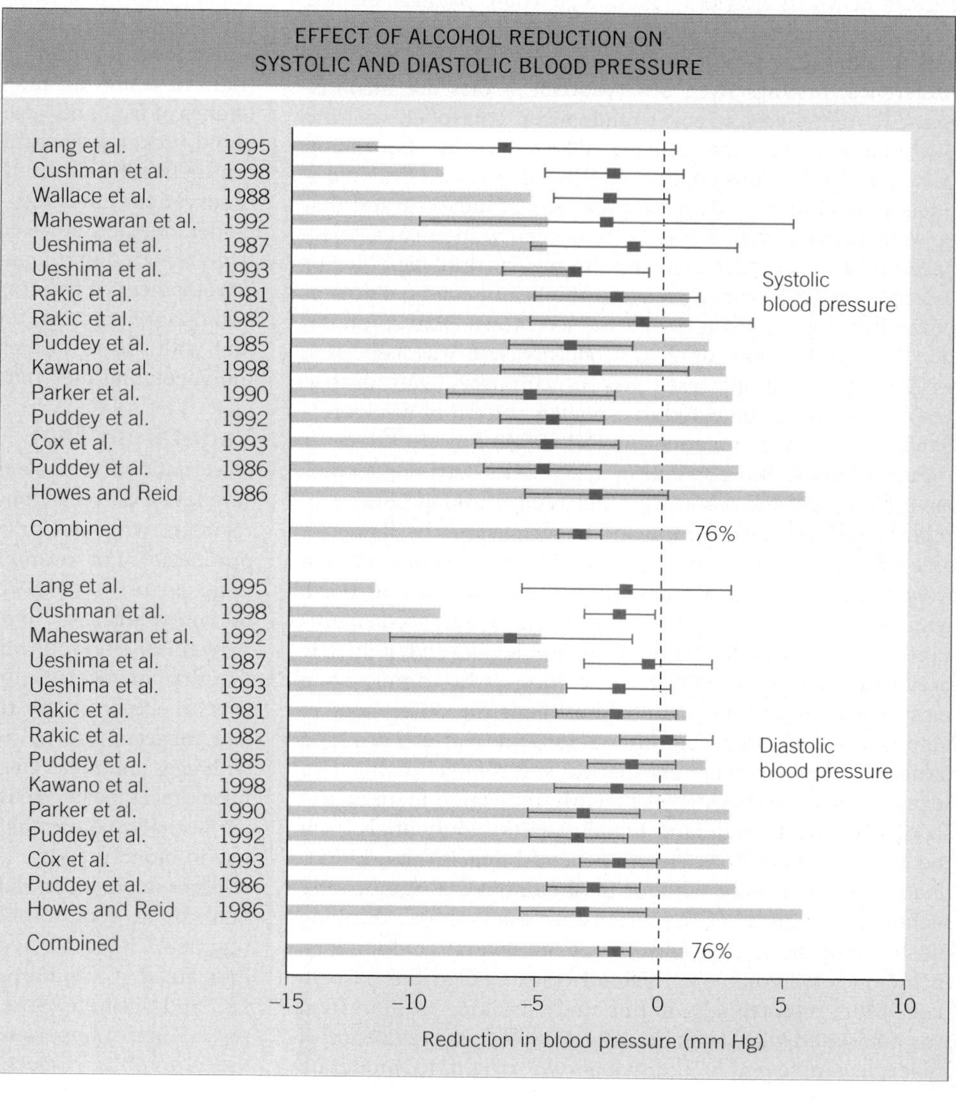

Figure 44.5 Effect of alcohol reduction on systolic and diastolic blood pressure. (From Xin X, He J, Frontini MG, Ogden LG, Motsamai OI, Whelton PK. Effects of alcohol reduction on blood pressure: a meta-analysis of randomized controlled trials. Hypertension 2001;38:1112-1117.)

reduction in alcohol intake can be sustained over time. Altogether, these results reinforce recommendations for moderation of alcohol consumption to prevent and treat hypertension.

Several issues on the association between alcohol consumption and blood pressure are still controversial. For example, it remains unclear whether, in the range of low-to-moderate alcohol consumption, the association is linear or J-shaped and whether there is a threshold effect. In the Kaiser-Permanente Study,[51] there was no difference in the hypertension-related hospitalization between nondrinkers and light drinkers (i.e., <2 drinks/day), which suggests a threshold effect. On the other hand, findings from the INTERSALT study suggest a continuous relationship between alcohol consumption and blood pressure in men and, if anything, a weaker relation at levels below 300 mL per week.[52] However, findings from the Nurses' Health Study II showed a J-shaped association between alcohol consumption and risk of developing hypertension, with light drinkers demonstrating a modest decrease in risk and more regular heavy drinkers demonstrating an increase in risk.[53]

Increasing evidence suggests that the association between alcohol consumption and blood pressure levels is a function not only of the average quantity consumed but also of the pattern in which alcohol is consumed. These patterns include beverage preference, frequency and intensity of consumption, and drinking in relation to food consumption. For beverage preference, findings from observational studies are inconsistent[53,54]; moreover, a recent randomized controlled trial did not detect a beverage-specific effect on the association between alcohol consumption and blood pressure.[56] For frequency and intensity of consumption, some studies suggest that episodic heavy drinking may be associated with greater differences in blood pressure compared to regular drinking.[52,57] For example, findings from a study on the health consequences of binge drinking in 1154 men and women showed that consumption of eight or more drinks on one occasion was associated with a significant increased risk of coronary heart disease and hypertension compared to a regular pattern of drinking.[57] Similar results were found in the INTERSALT study.[52]

Furthermore, two population-based cross-sectional studies have examined the association between drinking pattern in relation to food consumption and hypertension.[54,58] Trevisan and colleagues,[58] in a large sample of adult men and women from the Italian Nine Communities Study, found that those who drank wine with and without meals experienced significantly higher systolic blood pressure levels and a higher prevalence of hypertension than those who drank wine mostly with food, even after adjustment for differences in volume of alcohol consumption among the various drinking pattern categories. This association was similar in the two sexes.[58] These findings were recently replicated in an analysis of 2609 white male and female healthy individuals from the Western New York Health Study.[54] Specifically, individuals drinking mostly without food exhibited a significantly higher prevalence of hypertension than those drinking mostly with food, after adjustment for several confounders, including total volume of alcohol consumed in the past 30 days. More interestingly, in this study drinking without food was associated with a significantly 45% higher prevalence of hypertension, even in individuals with light to moderate alcohol intake (i.e., <2 drinks/day). This finding suggests that drinking without food may counteract the benefits associated with moderate alcohol use on the cardiovascular system. However, prospective studies are needed to support these findings and clarify the role of drinking pattern in the relationship between alcohol consumption and blood pressure.

In summary, moderation of alcohol consumption is a well-documented and effective recommendation to lower blood pressure among habitual drinkers. Currently, the recommended threshold is two or fewer alcoholic drinks per day in men and one or less per day in women and lighter-weight persons.[5,21] Extended recommendations should pertain to the way in which alcohol is consumed among habitual drinkers. Specifically, a regular consumption versus a heavy episodic drinking pattern, preferably in relation to mealtime, appears a reasonable, additional lifestyle behavior that should be adopted by habitual drinkers.

IMPORTANCE OF DIETARY PATTERNS

Diet is one of the most important determinants of blood pressure levels in both individuals and populations. There are large variations in dietary patterns across populations that are likely to contribute to the observed differences in mean blood pressure levels, with populations consuming mostly plant-based diets having lower blood pressure than populations in industrialized countries. Moreover, even within industrialized countries, individuals consuming diets with elevated intakes of fruit and vegetables tend to have, on average, lower blood pressure than individuals following more typical Western diets with elevated intake of saturated fats.[59] Ecological observations have been corroborated by findings of numerous epidemiologic studies and randomized controlled trials, which have reported on the important role of dietary patterns in the development of hypertension. In this section, we will focus on two dietary patterns, for which the current evidence is consistent with regard to their efficacy in lowering blood pressure: the vegetarian diet and the DASH diet.

Vegetarian Diet

Observational data clearly support the benefits on blood pressure levels derived from the adherence to a vegetarian dietary regimen with no or very little amount of animal-based products.[59] For example, in a cross-sectional analysis on a large cohort of 34,192 California Seventh-day Adventists, the prevalence of hypertension was nearly double among Adventists who followed a diet similar to a typical American diet than in vegetarian Adventists.[60] The Seventh-day Adventists are expected, by religious belief, to abstain from alcohol and tobacco, and to follow a vegetarian diet supplemented with eggs and milk. Overall, they tend to have lower mortality from cancer, heart disease, and diabetes than non-Adventists living in the same communities. Furthermore, the age-dependent rise in blood pressure levels, typically experienced by individuals living in industrialized countries, may be largely attenuated by a long-term adherence to a vegetarian dietary regimen.[61] Overall, available data from observational studies indicate that vegetarians have lower systolic (3 to 14 mm Hg) and diastolic (5 to 6 mm Hg) blood pressure, and lower prevalence of hypertension than nonvegetarians (2% to 40% vs 8% to 60%, respectively).[59]

Randomized controlled trials have corroborated the blood pressure lowering effects of vegetarian diets in both normotensive and hypertensive individuals. Specifically, a recent meta-analysis of 24 randomized placebo-controlled trials to estimate the effect of fiber supplementation on blood pressure levels showed a moderate but significant reduction in blood pressure levels.[62] In particular, fiber supplementation (average dose, 11.5 g/day) changed systolic blood pressure by −1.1 mm Hg (95% CI, −2.5 to 0.2) and diastolic blood pressure by −1.3 mm Hg (95% CI, −2.0 to −0.5), with larger reductions in older individuals (>40 years) and in hypertensive subgroups.

Vegetarian diets include higher intakes of fiber, potassium, and polyunsaturated and monounsaturated fatty acids, and lower intakes of alcohol, animal proteins, and saturated fats, which are all plausible contributors to the lower mean blood pressure levels in vegetarians, as compared to the general population. However, the lowering effects on blood pressure derived from a vegetarian diet may be additionally caused by other nondietary factors (e.g., increased physical activity) that tend to cluster with dietary components as part of a comprehensive "vegetarian" lifestyle.

Dietary Approach to Stop Hypertension Diet

Recent reports emphasize the importance of adopting a dietary regimen similar to the DASH diet as one major lifestyle modification to prevent and treat hypertension.[5,21] The DASH dietary plan provides large intakes of fruit, vegetables, and low-fat dairy products; comprises whole grains, poultry, fish, and nuts; and includes limited amounts of red meat, sweets, and sugar-containing beverages. Thus, in comparison with habitual diets of Western societies, the DASH dietary pattern provides higher intakes in potassium, magnesium, calcium, fiber, and proteins and lower intakes in total fat, saturated fat, and cholesterol.

The blood pressure lowering effect of this diet is the result of the combined effects of these nutrients when consumed together in food, rather than of the specific effect of a single nutrient. Indeed, the DASH trial was designed to test the effects on blood pressure of a change in dietary patterns, rather than the effects of a change in a single nutrient, as generally tested in previous trials.[63] This trial was an 11-week feeding program including 459 adults with (n = 133) and without hypertension (n = 326). For 3 weeks, participants followed a control diet that was low in fruit, vegetable, and dairy products. The fat content was representative of the average consumption in the United States. Then, for the next 8 weeks, participants were randomly allocated in three groups and each group was fed three different diets. One group was fed the same control diet, the second group a diet richer in fruit and vegetables but similar to the control diet for other nutrients, and the third group was fed the DASH diet, that is, a diet rich in fruits, vegetables, and low-fat or fat-free dairy products and low in saturated and total fat content, in other words a high potassium, magnesium, calcium, fiber, and protein diet. The sodium intake was held constant in the three groups. Alcohol intake and body weight did not change during the trial or among the groups. Overall, findings indicated a gradient in the reduction in blood pressure among the diets. The DASH diet significantly reduced systolic and diastolic blood pressure by 5.5/3.0 mm Hg, respectively, compared to the control diet, whereas the "fruit and vegetables" diet significantly reduced systolic and diastolic blood pressure by 2.8/1.1 mm Hg, respectively, compared to the control diet. Among subjects with hypertension, the blood pressure reductions in the DASH group were more marked, that is 11.4/5.5 mm Hg for systolic and diastolic blood pressure, respectively, compared to the control diet. Interestingly, the blood pressure lowering effects of the DASH diet occurred within the first 2 weeks of the trial. Further subgroup analyses showed significant effects of the DASH diet in all major subgroups (e.g., sex, race, age, body mass index, etc.), although the effects were more marked among African Americans (reduced 6.9/3.7 mm Hg) than in whites (reduced 3.3/2.4 mm Hg).[64]

In a further analysis from the same trial, the authors examined the blood pressure effects of the DASH trial in combination with a reduction in sodium intake.[23] A total of 412 participants were randomly allocated to two dietary regimens, one following a control diet representative of the average diet in the United States and one following the DASH diet. Within these two dietary regimens, participants were randomly assigned to 3 decreasing levels of salt consumption, defined as high (150 mmol per day, 3.5 g of sodium per day, reflecting typical consumption in the United States), intermediate (100 mmol per day, 2.3 g of sodium per day, reflecting the upper limit of the current recommendations), and low (50 mmol per day, 1.6 g of sodium per day). Each feeding period lasted 30 consecutive days. Findings showed that (a) the DASH diet may lower blood pressure independent from the level of sodium intake; (b) the blood pressure lowering effect of a reduction in sodium intake may occur by reducing the sodium intake even to levels below the currently recommended limit (i.e., 100 mmol per day); (c) the effects of sodium reductions are observed in all major subgroups; and (d) greater lowering effects on blood pressure may derive from the combination of the two interventions than from adopting either the DASH diet or low sodium diet individually. In fact, the difference of systolic blood pressure between the DASH–low sodium group and the control–high sodium group was a substantial reduction of 7.1 mm Hg in participants without hypertension and 11.5 mm Hg in participants with hypertension. The last finding resembles the effect of a single drug therapy in hypertensive individuals. Thus the combination of the DASH diet and reduced sodium intake represents an alternative to drug therapy for individuals who have mild hypertension and are willing to comply with long-term dietary changes.

The Optimal Macronutrient Intake Trial to Prevent Heart Disease (OmniHeart) has extended the observations derived from the DASH trials by examining the effects of three dietary patterns with documented lowering effects on blood pressure and serum lipids, among 164 adults with prehypertension or stage 1 hypertension.[65] One diet, resembling the DASH diet, was rich in carbohydrates (58% of total calories); the other two dietary regimens partially replaced carbohydrates with either a higher content of proteins (about half from plant sources) or a higher content of unsaturated fats (predominantly monounsaturated fats). The feeding periods lasted 6 weeks, and body weight was held constant.

Systolic blood pressures were lowered in each of the three intervention groups compared with baseline. However, blood pressures were further lowered in the two dietary regimens providing a partial substitution of carbohydrates (10% of total kcal) with either proteins or unsaturated fats (1.4 and 1.3 mm Hg, respectively). Thus these findings indicate that, along with known determinants of blood pressure (i.e., micronutrients [sodium and potassium], body weight, alcohol consumption, and the DASH diet), macronutrients and the qualitative composition of diet are also important factors to consider for the prevention and management of hypertension.

REGULAR AEROBIC EXERCISE

Regular aerobic exercise is an important part of current recommendations for the prevention and treatment of high blood pressure. Specifically, at least 30 minutes per day of aerobic activity of moderate intensity (e.g., quick walking) on five or more occasions per week is the recommended level set by current guidelines.[5] In a meta-analysis of 54 randomized controlled trials including 2419 participants, aerobic exercise was associated with a significant reduction in systolic and diastolic blood pressure of 3.8/2.6 mm Hg, respectively (Fig. 44.6).[66] Blood pressure reductions induced by aerobic exercise were observed in both normotensive and hypertensive individuals and in normal-weight and overweight subgroups. Although the blood pressure lowering effect of aerobic exercise can be considered clinically moderate, it constitutes, however, a valuable public health strategy for the prevention and treatment of high blood pressure. In fact, a modest reduction in the population's blood pressure levels would translate into a significant decrease in the incidence of hypertension-related diseases.

Aerobic exercise comprises activities like walking, running, cycling, and swimming. Although all forms of dynamic exercise seem to be effective in reducing blood pressure, adherence to the intervention program is crucial to be successful in achieving and maintaining the benefit.

On the other hand, resistance training, also known as isometric or static exercise (e.g., weight training or body building), is not included in current recommendations for the prevention and management of high blood pressure because of the lack of conclusive evidence on its effectiveness in lowering blood pressure and the potential for long-term hypertensive effects. However, two meta-analyses of randomized controlled trials indicate that resistance training is not associated with chronic elevations of blood pressure and, instead, may induce a moderate reduction of blood pressure levels in healthy adults; but its efficacy in lowering blood pressure in hypertensive and elderly individuals is still controversial.[67,68] Currently, the evidence suggests that moderate-intensity resistance training could be performed in combination with aerobic exercise in the context of a comprehensive exercise program to prevent CVD in healthy adults.[69]

Recent evidence emphasizes the efficacy of the simultaneous implementation of current lifestyle recommendations, such as regular exercise, to prevent and treat high blood pressure. Specifically, the PREMIER clinical trial examined the combined effects of the DASH diet with "established" recommendations, comprising weight loss, exercise, and restriction of sodium and alcohol.[70] Participants were 810 adults with above-optimal blood pressure, including stage 1 hypertension (120-159 mm Hg systolic and 80-95 mm Hg diastolic), and who were not on antihypertensive medications. They were randomly allocated to one of three intervention groups: (a) "established," a behavioral intervention that implemented established recommendations; (b) "established plus DASH," which also implemented the DASH diet; and (c) an "advice only" control group. At the end of the trial (after 6 months), in the group assigned to lifestyle modification only, the established group, the mean net reduction in blood pressure was 3.7/1.7 mm Hg, compared to the control group, whereas for the group that followed the established recommendations together with the DASH diet, the mean net reduction in blood pressure was 4.3/2.6 mm Hg, compared to the control group. Thus these findings point to the feasibility of comprehensive lifestyle modifications and their lowering effects on blood pressure for both nonhypertensive individuals with above-optimal blood pressure and hypertensive individuals who are not receiving medication therapy.

Many plausible biological mechanisms may explain the blood pressure lowering effects induced by regular exercise.[71] For example, a "hemodynamic" mechanism would involve the reduction of both resting cardiac output and peripheral vascular resistance. Furthermore, a "humoral" mechanism would determine the reduction of the activity of the renin-angiotensin-aldosterone system and of the sympathetic nervous system activity and an increase in prostaglandins with vasodilator effect. Finally, recent findings suggest that an enhancement in insulin sensitivity may represent a further mechanism for the beneficial effects of physical activity on blood pressure and hypertension risk.[72]

CONCLUSIONS

The current lifestyle modifications that effectively lower blood pressure include weight reduction if overweight or obese, reduction of dietary sodium intake, increased potassium intake, moderation of alcohol consumption among regular drinkers, adoption of a dietary plan based on the DASH diet, and regular aerobic exercise.

In the clinical setting, a comprehensive lifestyle intervention represents a cost-effective therapeutic option among nonhypertensive individuals with above-optimal blood pressure levels as well as among hypertensive individuals who are not receiving medication therapy and are compliant with sustained lifestyle changes. In addition, comprehensive lifestyle modifications represent an essential adjuvant therapy in hypertensive individuals who are already on drug treatment.

In the public health arena, there is an urgent need to develop and implement population-wide strategies aimed at substantial "societal" changes to tackle the current epidemic of hypertension in both developed and developing countries. However, these changes will be realistic if collaborative initiatives are implemented at multiple levels: governments, manufacturers, health care providers, researchers, and the general public. In particular, the increasing burden of hypertension is a serious public health challenge in developing countries because of the lack of resources. Nevertheless, community-based strategies of health promotion (e.g., salt reduction) are warranted in these settings.

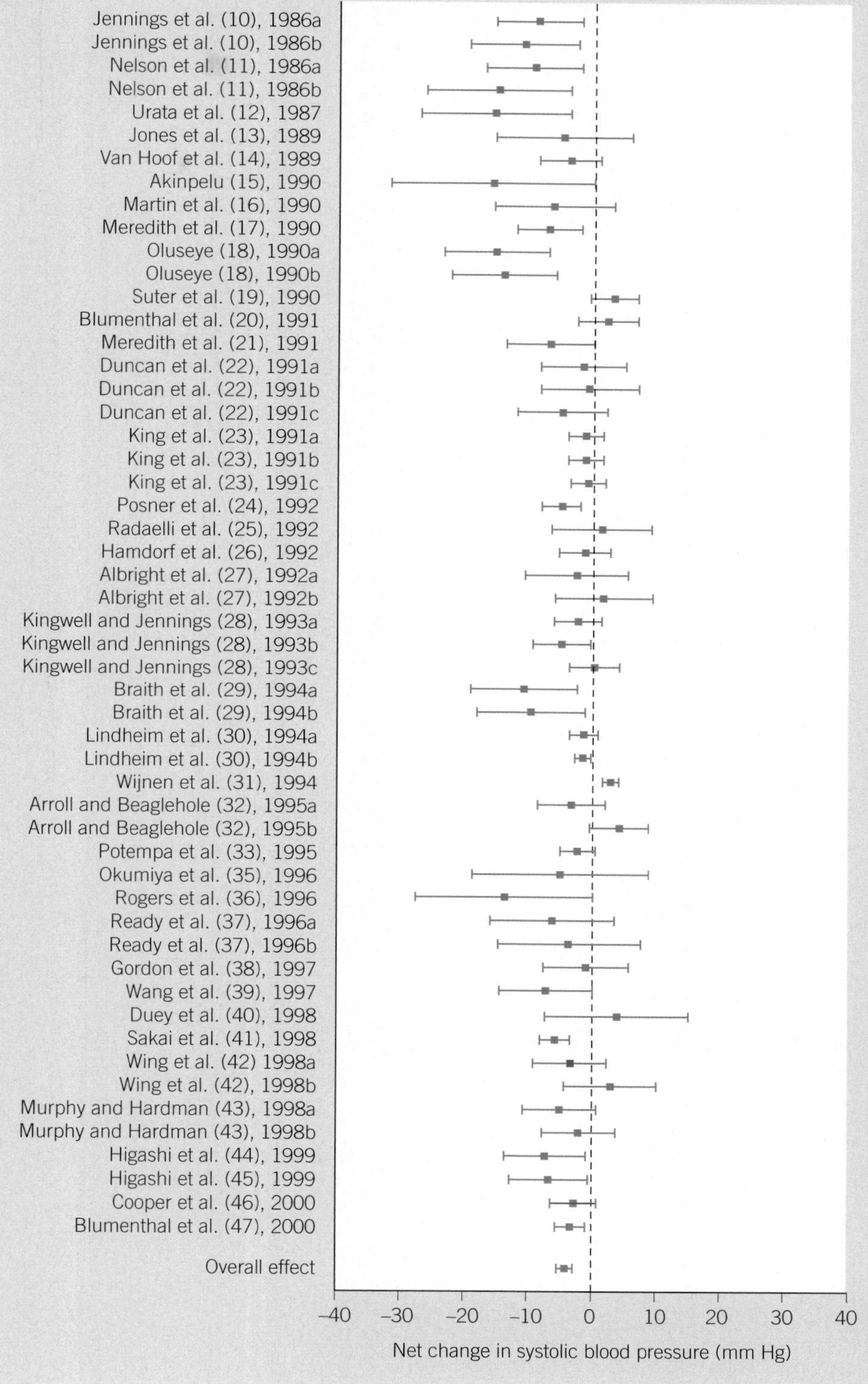

Figure 44.6 Effect of aerobic physical activity on systolic blood pressure. (From Whelton SP, Chin A, Xin X, He J. Effect of aerobic exercise on blood pressure: a meta-analysis of randomized, controlled trials. Ann Intern Med 2002;136:493-503.)

chapter

45 Pharmacologic Treatment

George S. Stergiou and George L. Bakris

Definition

- Pharmacologic therapy provides the most effective way to lower blood pressure (BP) that in turn markedly reduces cardiovascular and renal morbidity and mortality.

Key Features

- All contemporary antihypertensive drugs exert similar effect on blood pressure; some drug classes may have benefits beyond their blood pressure lowering effect in certain subpopulations of patients.
- Both systolic and diastolic BP levels should be effectively controlled. However, after the age of 50 years systolic blood pressure is a much stronger cardiovascular risk factor, and systolic hypertension is far more difficult to control than diastolic.
- Individualization of therapy—evaluation for the presence of cardiovascular risk factors other than hypertension and the extent of preexisting target organ damage is a key factor in a patient's global risk assessment and facilitates the selection of appropriate therapy and treatment targets.

Therapy

- Most of the patients with hypertension are untreated or undertreated.
- Multidrug regimens are needed in more than 75% of patients to achieve target BP goals recommended by guidelines; early use of fixed-dose combination therapy may improve medication adherence.
- Physicians should inform patients early on about BP goals, benefits of achieving such goals, and complications if such goals are not met as well as requirements of intensive hypertension regimens. Educated patients with realistic expectations are more likely to achieve the goals of BP therapy with fewer side effects.

Hypertension is one of the most prevalent health problems worldwide. In the United States, it is one of the most common reasons to see a physician in the outpatient settings. Numerous observational studies as well as meta-analyses of pooled data have demonstrated conclusively that untreated hypertension is associated with increased risk of cardiovascular (CV) morbidity and premature death in both Western[1-5] and Eastern[6] populations. A meta-analysis of 61 prospective studies including 1 million adults showed that for each 20/10 mm Hg increase in blood pressure (BP) starting from the level of 115/75 mm Hg, the CV risk is doubled.[7] The incidence of renal insufficiency and subsequent end-stage renal disease is also increased in patients with poorly controlled blood pressure.[8,9] Similar associations have been established for other steadily increasing cardiovascular conditions, such as left ventricular hypertrophy, congestive heart failure, peripheral vascular disease, and carotid atherosclerosis. Improved understanding of the impact of hypertension on CV health and increasing availability of effective, safe, and better tolerated drugs can significantly improve hypertension control rates and thereby reduce the CV morbidity and mortality.

Antihypertensive therapy contributes in a major way to a significant reduction in the rates of stroke and heart disease seen over the last 4 decades in the United States. Despite all this progress, the number of patients achieving satisfactory BP control in the United States remains low. Only 37% of adult hypertensive Americans in 2003-2004 had their BP controlled to less than 140/90 mm Hg, the level recommended as the target for uncomplicated hypertension.[10] The BP control rates are still worse for the elderly, in whom isolated systolic hypertension predominates, and for some high-risk populations, such as those with diabetes and/or renal disease with proteinuria. Similar reports from other countries reveal an even worse record of BP control, regardless of populations studied, accessibility to or cost of medical care, or the treatment settings.[11-15]

Over the past several years, it has become increasingly clear that the risk we attribute to hypertension is better correlated with the level of systolic rather than diastolic BP, especially in those over the age of 50 years. Pulse pressure, the difference between systolic and diastolic BP, may be a better predictor of risk than systolic BP, although the available data on this subject are still incomplete. Franklin and coworkers,[16] using data from the Framingham Heart Study cohort, has shown that at all levels of systolic BP (even as low as 110 to 130 mm Hg), risk is smaller with higher diastolic BP.[16,17] Meta-analyses of studies suggested that pulse pressure has strong predictive value for CV events, specifically in subjects older than 55 years.[7,18] However, other investigators note that this predictive effect of pulse pressure is eliminated when adjustment for systolic BP is performed.[19]

As the Western societies age, the prevalence of isolated systolic hypertension is expected to increase. This type of hypertension is more difficult to control and is associated with the higher risk of target organ damage. Thus more patients will require prolonged, intensive, multidrug regimens to reach the recommended BP goals. This projection is already confirmed by the report from Vasan and colleagues[20] who, using data from the Framingham Heart Study cohort, predicted the lifetime risk of developing hypertension to be 90%. In addition, over 60% of U.S. adults are expected to use BP-lowering medications in their lifetime.[20] Various interventions, both pharmacologic and nonpharmacologic, can effectively lower BP; of these, pharmacologic therapy seems to be more effective than lifestyle modifications and has a better rate of long-term adherence to prescribed regimen. In the studies where quality of life was measured, patients in the active drug treatment groups who achieved lower BP felt better and reported fewer symptoms.[21]

OBJECTIVES OF PHARMACOLOGIC THERAPY FOR HYPERTENSION

Hypertension is rarely an isolated condition. Coexisting abnormalities like diabetes, dyslipidemia, obesity, and proteinuria are present in many hypertensive patients.[22] The number of concomitant risk factors is directly proportional to the global risk of the future cardiovascular and renal events. The recognition of this association forms the basis of the recommendation for initiation of drug therapy in the Joint National Committee on Prevention, Detection, Evaluation, and Treatment of High Blood Pressure (JNC-7),[23] the American Heart Association (AHA),[24] the European Society of Hypertension and European Society of Cardiology (ESH-ESC),[25] the International Society of Hypertension and World Health Organization (ISH-WHO),[26] and the British NICE guidelines.[27] The JNC-7 strategy for the classification and the management of hypertension in adults is shown in Table 45.1.[23]

Pharmacologic therapy of hypertension is initiated only after the initial evaluation of a patient is completed, the diagnosis of hypertension confirmed, and the patient has failed lifestyle modification in the presence of stage 1 hypertension (Table 45.2). Note that lifestyle changes *must* accompany all pharmacologic treatments. Several BP measurements performed according to accepted procedural guidelines are necessary for the diagnosis of hypertension. The initial assessment should include focused medical history, especially personal and family history of hypertension and antihypertensive drug use. In addition, the presence of risk factors for CV disease or overt CV disease/target organ damage is evaluated both by clinical history and physical examination as well as limited laboratory evaluation. Secondary forms of hypertension need to be excluded and are discussed elsewhere in this book. Special attention to rule out commonly acquired causes of BP elevation, such as sleep apnea and drug-induced hypertension, is important; common causes are summarized in Table 45.3.[28]

Blood pressure, both in an individual and in populations, is a continuously distributed variable and the decision to classify a patient as hypertensive is necessarily arbitrary. Various schemes of global CV risk assessment have been developed and incorporated in the hypertension treatment guidelines endorsed by national and international panels of experts (see Table 45.1).[23-27] Moreover, different BP values are now recommended as thresholds for pharmacologic therapy in different risk groups and special subpopulations (Table 45.4).[23-27] The major concern with pursuing some of the aggressive goals is the possibility of a harmful effect of excessively low BP, especially diastolic BP—the so-called J-curve hypothesis. However, the results of the Hypertension Optimal Treatment (HOT)[29] and United Kingdom Prospective Diabetes Study (UKPDS)[30] suggest no excessive mortality in groups assigned to lower BP targets. Moreover, in both studies, diabetics with the lowest achieved BP had the lowest event rates. Similarly, in the Systolic Hypertension in the Elderly Program (SHEP) study, individuals in the active treatment group who achieved the average diastolic BP of 68 mm Hg had better overall outcomes and fewer coronary events compared to controls with an average diastolic BP of 72 mm Hg.[31] However, recent data suggest that in the elderly and those with coronary heart disease the reduction of diastolic BP to less than 60 mm Hg is associated with increased CV risk.[32,33]

CLASSIFICATION AND MANAGEMENT OF BLOOD PRESSURE FOR ADULTS

BP Classification	SBP* mm Hg	DBP* mm Hg	Lifestyle Modification	Initial Drug Therapy: Without Compelling Indication	Initial Drug Therapy: With Compelling Indications (See Table 45.8)
Normal	<120	and <80	Encourage	No antihypertensive drug indicated	Drug(s) for compelling indications‡
Prehypertension	120-139	or 80-89	Yes		
Stage 1 hypertension	140-159	or 90-99	Yes	Thiazide-type diuretics for most May consider ACEI, ARB, BB, CCB, or combination	Drug(s) for the compelling indications‡ Other antihypertensive drugs (diuretics, ACEI, ARB, BB, CCB) as needed
Stage 2 hypertension	≥160	or ≥100	Yes	Two-drug combination for most† (usually thiazide diuretic and ACEI or ARB or BB or CCB)	

*Treatment determined by highest BP category.
†Initial combined therapy should be used cautiously in those at risk for orthostatic hypotension.
‡Treat patients with chronic kidney disease or diabetes to BP goal of <130/80 mm/Hg.
DBP, diastolic blood pressure SBP, systolic blood pressure. ACEI, angiotensin-converting enzyme inhibitor; ARB, angiotensin receptor blocker; BB, beta blocker; CCB, calcium channel blocker.
From Chobanian AV, Bakris GL, Black HR, et al; Joint National Committee on Prevention, Detection, Evaluation, and Treatment of High Blood Pressure; National Heart, Lung, and Blood Institute; National High Blood Pressure Education Program Coordinating Committee. Seventh report of the Joint National Committee on Prevention, Detection, Evaluation, and Treatment of High Blood Pressure. Hypertension 2003;42:1206-1252.

Table 45.1 Classification and management of blood pressure for adults.

LIFESTYLE MODIFICATIONS THAT LOWER BLOOD PRESSURE
1. **Reduction of body weight** (5 kg threshold; 10 kg reduces BP ~10/8 mm Hg) 2. **Increased consumption of fruits and vegetables** (at least 4 servings/day, with low-fat dairy products and decreased saturated and total fat can lower BP ~6/3 mm Hg, and often helps reduce salt consumption) 3. **Reduction in dietary salt consumption** (target 100 mmol/day; can lower BP ~12/10 mm Hg, but individual responses vary) 4. **Increase physical activity** to at least 30 minutes per day, most days of the week (can lower BP 8/4 mm Hg, and often helps control weight) 5. **Moderation of alcohol consumption** (target 10 g ethanol—1 drink/day for women; 20 g—2 drinks/day for men; can lower BP by up to 8/4 mm Hg in those who drink more than 5 drinks/day) 6. **Stress management** (randomized clinical trials outside the workplace have been unconvincing, but many psychologists still recommend the approach, despite a lack of detailed protocols that uniformly lower BP) Other lifestyle modifications that are routinely recommended: 1. **Tobacco avoidance** (lowers cardiovascular risk independently of any effect on BP) 2. **Fish consumption** (improves lipid profiles and cardiovascular risk, more than expected if just BP effect alone was operative) 3. **Increasing dietary fiber** (improves lipid profiles and cancer risk, independently of effect on BP)
Adapted from Chobanian AV, Bakris GL, Black HR, et al; Joint National Committee on Prevention, Detection, Evaluation, and Treatment of High Blood Pressure; National Heart, Lung, and Blood Institute; National High Blood Pressure Education Program Coordinating Committee. Seventh Report of the Joint National Committee on Prevention, Detection, Evaluation, and Treatment of High Blood Pressure. Hypertension 2003;42:1206-1252.

Table 45.2 Lifestyle modifications that lower blood pressure.

The 2007 AHA[24] and ESH-ESC guidelines[25] recommend a lower BP goal, which is below 130/80 mmHg for all hypertensive patients at high CV risk. The key initial element to succeed in achieving BP goals is acceptance by the patient that they have a disease that will require lifelong attention to diet and lifestyle as well as need for medication to keep BP within a certain range.

DRUGS KNOWN TO ELEVATE BLOOD PRESSURE
■ Nonsteroidal anti-inflammatory drugs ■ Sympathomimetic amines (e.g., phenylpropanolamines) ■ Estrogen and estrogen analogues (e.g., oral contraceptive pills and hormone replacement therapy) ■ Methylxanthines (e.g., theophylline, caffeine, theobromine) ■ Cyclosporine and tacrolimus ■ Erythropoietin ■ Sibutramine ■ Ergotamine ■ Cortisone and other steroids (corticosteroids, mineralocorticoids, anabolic steroids, and ACTH) ■ Cocaine ■ Nicotine ■ Licorice ■ Phencyclidine ("angel dust") ■ "Herbal ecstasy" (and other ephedrine-containing substances) ■ Withdrawal from certain drugs (e.g., beta blockers, alpha agonists, cocaine, nicotine, opioids, ethanol, calcium antagonists)

Table 45.3 Drugs known to elevate blood pressure.

Other factors that contribute to improving adherence with medication regimens are summarized in Table 45.5. In addition to these factors, several considerations regarding medication selection, in addition to compelling indications, need to be considered. The JNC-7[23] and ESH-ESC[25] have proposed individualization of BP therapy based on coexisting conditions (Table 45.6).

Multiple recent trials have compared the traditional diuretic or beta-blocker–based treatment strategies to those based on angiotensin-converting enzyme inhibitors (ACEIs), calcium channel blockers (CCBs), or angiotensin receptor blockers (ARBs). In general, all major groups of antihypertensive agents have similar capacity to lower BP. A meta-analysis of 29 clinical trials that encompass 162,341 participants by the Blood Pressure Lowering Treatment Trialist's Collaboration group supports the concept that all agents that lower BP will reduce CV risk.[34] However, some differences in the specific outcomes, such as strokes (favoring diuretics and CCBs) and coronary events (favoring ACEIs and beta blockers), exist between certain groups.

The potential benefit of ACEIs independent of BP control, was initially suggested in the HOPE trial, where ramipril significantly reduced CV events compared to placebo in

GOAL BLOOD PRESSURE BY GUIDELINE COMMITTEES (mm Hg)

Guidelines	Year of Publication	Hypertension without Diabetes or Renal Disease	Diabetes or Kidney disease	Proteinuria >1g	All High-Risk Hypertensives
JNC-7[23]	2003	<140/90	<130/80	<125/75	—
ESH-ESC[25]	2007	<140/90 at least and lower values if tolerated	<130/80	even lower than <130/80	<130/80
AHA[24]	2007	<130/80	<130/80	—	<130/80
ADA[51]	2007	<140/90	<130/80	—	—
NKF[52]	2007	—	<130/80	<125/75	—

ADA, American Diabetes Association; AHA, American Heart Association; ESH-ESC, European Society of Hypertension—European Society of Cardiology; JNC, Joint National Committee; NKF, National Kidney Foundation.
Data from Chobanian et al,[23] Rosendorff et al,[24] Mancia et al,[25] Buse et al,[51] and KDOQI.[52]

Table 45.4 Goal blood pressure by guideline committees (mm Hg).

STRATEGIES TO IMPROVE MEDICATION ADHERENCE
■ Educate the patient regarding the proper use of medications
■ Improve patient's social support network (e.g., spouse or caretaker)
■ Increase patient's autonomy and involvement in making decisions (when appropriate)
■ Remove barriers to compliance with taking pills
■ Integrate into activities of daily living (e.g., brushing teeth)
■ Avoid large ("horse") pills
■ Avoid bad-tasting formulations (e.g., lactulose, quinine)
■ Simplify the therapeutic regimen
■ Minimize the number of pills—prefer fixed-dose combinations
■ Minimize the frequency of taking pills—prefer once-daily dosing with drugs with full 24-hour action
■ Minimize the inconvenience of taking pills
■ Provide a positive attitude and positive reinforcement about achieving therapeutic goals
■ Use self-monitoring of blood pressure by patients at home
■ Maintain continuity of care with the same practitioner
■ Use well-tolerated antihypertensive drug therapy, individualized for each patient

Table 45.5 Strategies to improve medication adherence.

CONSIDERATIONS FOR INITIAL ANTIHYPERTENSIVE DRUG THERAPY	
Compelling Indications Unless Contraindicated Indication	**Drug Therapy**
Diabetes mellitus, types 1 and 2	ACEIs, ARBs
Diabetes and nondiabetic proteinuria	ACEIs, ARBs
Diabetes and microalbuminuria	ACEIs, ARBs
Renal insufficiency, diabetic and nondiabetic (up to creatinine 3 mg/dL)	ACEIs, ARBs
Heart failure (systolic)	ACEIs, ARBs, beta blockers, aldosterone antagonists, diuretics
Myocardial infarction	Beta blockers (non-ISA), ACEIs, ARBs, aldosterone antagonists
Coronary heart disease	ACEIs
Isolated systolic hypertension (older patients)	Diuretics, CCBs
May have favorable effects on comorbid conditions	
Recurrent atrial fibrillation	ACEIs, ARBs
Angina	Beta blockers, nondihydropyridine CCBs
Atrial tachycardia and fibrillation	Beta blockers, nondihydropyridine CCBs
Cyclosporine-induced hypertension	CCBs (caution with the dose of cyclosporine)
DM (types 1 and 2) with proteinuria	CCBs (nondihydropyridine), low-dose diuretics
Peripheral vascular disease	Alpha blockers, CCBs
Pregnancy	Labetalol hydrochloride, methyldopa, dihydropyridine CCBs
Dyslipidemia	Alpha blockers
Migraine	Beta blockers (noncardioselective), CCBs (nondihydropyridine)
Osteoporosis	Thiazide diuretics
Preoperative hypertension	Beta blockers
Prostatism (benign prostatic hyperplasia)	Alpha blockers
May have unfavorable effects on comorbid conditions	
Bronchospastic disease	Beta blockers
Depression	Beta blockers, central α-agonists, reserpine
DM, types 1 and 2	Beta blockers, moderate- to high-dose diuretics
Dyslipidemia	Beta blockers (non-ISA), diuretics (high-dose)
Gout	Diuretics
Second- or third-degree heart block	Beta blockers, CCBs (nondihydropyridine)
Renal insufficiency—bilateral renovascular disease	ACEIs, ARBs, renin inhibitors

ACEIs, angiotensin-converting enzyme inhibitors; ARBs, angiotensin receptor blockers; CCBs, calcium channel blockers; DM, diabetes mellitus; ISA, intrinsic sympathomimetic activity.
Modified from Chobanian AV, Bakris GL, Black HR, et al; Joint National Committee on Prevention, Detection, Evaluation, and Treatment of High Blood Pressure; National Heart, Lung, and Blood Institute: National High Blood Pressure Education Program Coordinating Committee. Seventh Report of the Joint National Committee on Prevention, Detection, Evaluation, and Treatment of High Blood Pressure. Hypertension 2003;42:1206-1252.

Table 45.6 Considerations for initial antihypertensive drug therapy.

participants with multiple CV risk factors who had an average BP of 138/78 mm Hg.[35] However, the group receiving ramipril did have a slightly lower BP (3/2 mm Hg) and somewhat skewed distribution in risk factors potentially favoring the active treatment group.[35] Additionally, ramipril was dosed at night, which may have also contributed to the benefit, if a large proportion of patients were nondippers. A meta-analysis, however, supports the contention that ACEIs might have a BP-independent effect on the risk of major coronary disease events when compared to ARBs.[36]

The ALLHAT study was prematurely stopped because of excessive rates of stroke and heart failure with the alpha blocker doxazosin as compared to the diuretic chlorthalidone.[37] However, in the ALLHAT, chlorthalidone appeared as effective as the CCB amlodipine and the ACEI lisinopril on the primary endpoint of the study, which was preventing fatal coronary heart disease events or nonfatal myocardial infarction.[38] Regarding the secondary endpoints, chlorthalidone was superior to amlodipine in preventing heart failure and superior to the ACEI lisinopril in preventing combined CV events, stroke, and heart failure.[38] It should be mentioned, however, that BP was higher in the lisinopril group, which explains, at least in part, the higher CV events rate in this group.[38] On the contrary, in the second Australian BP study, elderly patients with hypertension randomized to the thiazide diuretic hydrochlorothiazide had fewer cardiovascular events compared to those randomized to lisinopril.[39]

In the VALUE study the ARB valsartan was as effective as amlodipine in reducing cardiac disease events (primary endpoint) despite a higher BP in the valsartan group.[40] However, in the LIFE study the ARB losartan was more effective than the beta blocker atenolol in CV protection (particularly stroke) in hypertensive patients with electrocardiographic left ventricular hypertrophy.[41] Furthermore, in the ASCOT study, hypertensive subjects randomized to amlodipine (and if needed, perindopril) had fewer CV events than those randomized to atenolol and if needed, bendrofluazide.[42] The difference in CV protection in this ASCOT study is largely attributed to the greater BP reduction in the amlodipine group.

A meta-analysis of outcome studies of beta-blocker–based therapy in hypertension showed limited stroke protection compared to that achieved by other drugs.[43] Because of these data and the consistent evidence showing increased risk of new-onset diabetes with beta blockers, particularly combined with diuretics,[38,40-42,44,45] in the recent NICE, AHA, and ISH-WHO hypertension guidelines, beta blockers are not regarded as first-line drugs.[24,26,27] However, the ESH-ESC guidelines recommend beta blockers as first-line drugs, apart from hypertensive patients with metabolic syndrome or glucose intolerance.[25]

Meta-analyses of the large prospective outcome trials suggested that the achieved cardiovascular protection is mainly attributed to the treatment-induced BP decline and there might be little difference among the commonly used drugs, such as CCBs, alpha blockers, ACEIs, and ARBs.[36,46] These data emphasize the need for strict control of BP, which is not achieved in the majority of patients in clinical practice.[47]

Any discussion on the pharmacologic therapy of hypertension needs to recognize that multidrug treatment strategies are needed in sicker people (those with diabetes, renal insufficiency, obesity, sleep apnea, and related conditions) with higher BPs to achieve the lower BP targets (see Table 45.4).[34] A paradigm initially developed by the U.S. National Kidney Foundation and recently updated by members of both U.S. and European Blood Pressure Guideline committees, provides an approach to both help achieve BP goals with medications proven to reduce CV risk and renal disease progression and have additive BP-lowering effects when used in combination (Fig. 45.1).[9,48] Drug classes with compelling indications for certain conditions are outlined in Table 45.1 and used in the figure. This paradigm takes advantage of existing fixed-dose combinations to improve medication adherence (see Fig. 45.1).

To reduce the number of pills a given patient takes and help improve medication adherence, a number of fixed-dose combination medications are available throughout the world (Table 45.7). Furthermore, less than half of hypertensive patients achieve BP targets with monotherapy with no or minimal side effects.

It is clear that multiple medications in a reasonable combination are needed to reduce not only CV risk but also kidney disease progression risk, as shown in a variety of clinical trials that have randomized to various levels of BP (Fig. 45.2). A reduction in BP of 10 mm Hg can have a major impact on CV outcomes[7] and in renal disease progression (Fig. 45.3). Systolic BP goals are generally more difficult to achieve, even when forced titration is used, as observed in many recent randomized controlled trials[49] where the average of three to four agents in moderate doses were needed to achieve BP goals.[48] The JNC-7 and more recently the AHA and the ESH-ESC recommended that treatment initiation with a combination of two drugs should be considered if BP is more than 20 mm Hg systolic or 10 mm Hg diastolic above the recommended goal.[23-25] A multicenter study including hypertensive individuals with type 2 diabetes showed that treatment initiation with a fixed-dose combination increased the percentage of patients reaching the recommended BP goal compared to initiation with monotherapy and addition of a second drug at 2 months (Fig. 45.4).[50] When BP goals are achieved, it is more likely that CV events will be reduced and renal function will be preserved (see Fig. 45.3).

ANTIHYPERTENSIVE AGENTS

Table 45.8 summarizes all the classes of BP-lowering agents.

Diuretics

Indications and Contraindications

Diuretics primarily in the form of thiazides are indicated as a first-line therapy for uncomplicated hypertension. They are proven to reduce cardiovascular complications of stroke and coronary heart disease particularly in older patients with isolated systolic hypertension.[31,34,38,46] They are safe and effective in low doses in patients with type 2 diabetes[34] and are recommended as add-on drugs to ACEIs or ARBs in these patients.[25,51,52] They are widely available, inexpensive, and cause minimal undesirable metabolic effects when low-dose schemes are employed. If an alternative first-line agent is used, they should be considered as a second-choice agent, particularly in patients who are considered salt sensitive, such as elderly, obese, and diabetic patients and possibly African American and Hispanic patients. It is now accepted that in most patients the addition of a diuretic is necessary to achieve the target BP goal.

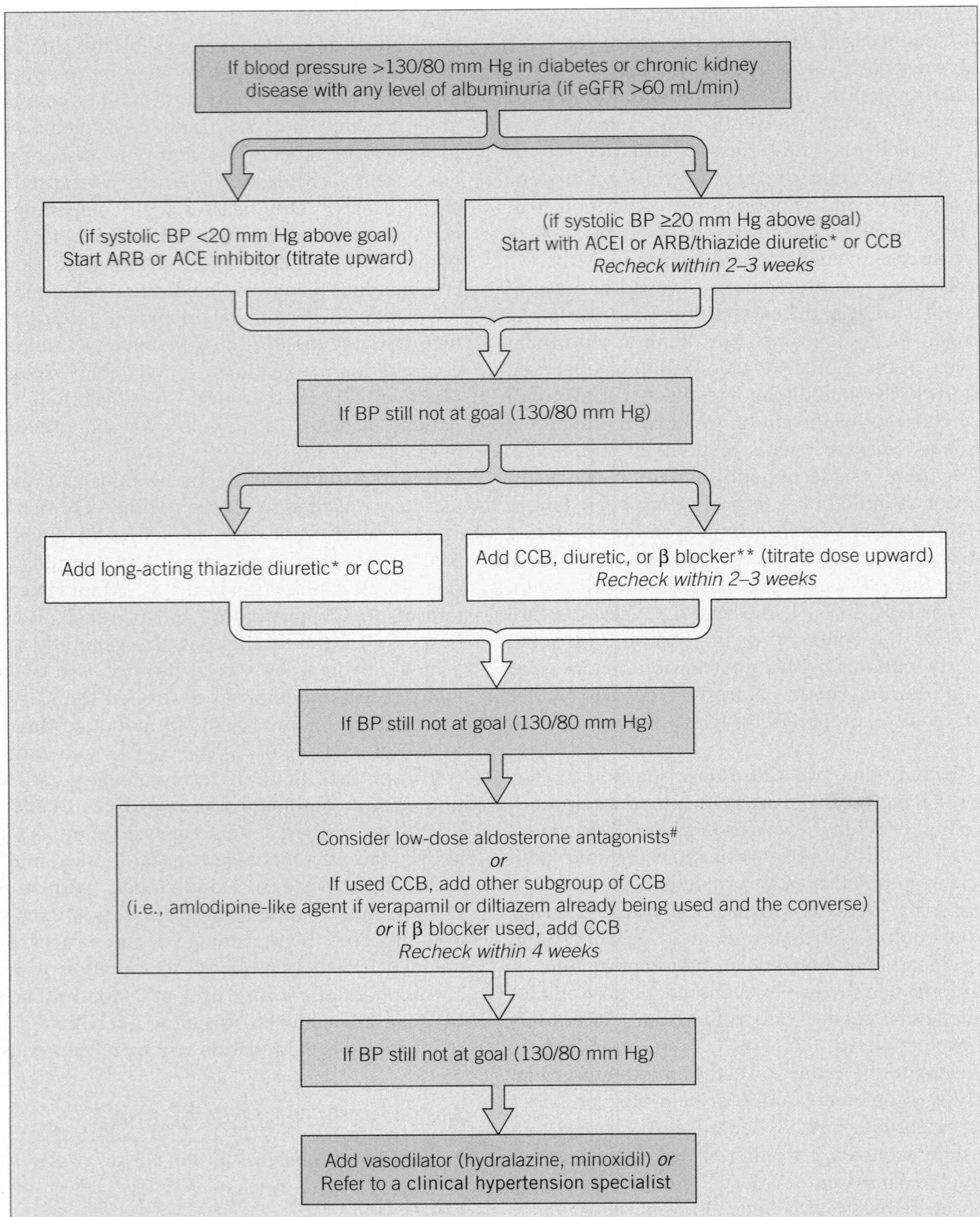

Figure 45.1 *Chlorthalidone (dose of 25-50 mg) is the thiazide used in almost all outcome trials that show reduction in CV events. **If a beta blocker is used for hypertension, the vasodilating beta blockers are preferred because they have fewer adverse effects and generally do *not* exacerbate preexisting diabetes or promote new-onset diabetes. #Aldosterone blockade is useful in sleep apnea and obese African American women. Caution should be used if baseline potassium on a well-dosed diuretic is >4.8 mEq/L, because the risk of hyperkalemia will be increased. (Modified from Ruilope L, Kjeldsen S, De La Sierra A, et al. The kidney and cardiovascular risk—implications for management: a consensus statement from the European Society of Hypertension. Blood Pressure 2007;16:72-79; Bakris GL, Williams M, Dworkin L, et al, for the National Kidney Foundation Hypertension and Diabetes Executive Committees Working Group. Preserving renal function in adults with hypertension and diabetes: a consensus approach. Am J Kidney Dis 2000;36:646-661.)

Side Effects

Because of the mechanism of action, aggressive therapy with diuretics can lead to significant volume depletion and prerenal azotemia. Dose-dependent electrolyte abnormalities and metabolic effects are not uncommon. Hypokalemia and hypomagnesemia are the most significant and may predispose patients to malignant arrhythmias and sudden cardiac death. Small and usually transient increase in total cholesterol and triglycerides may be seen. Thiazides have also been implicated in worsening glycemic control in diabetes, which might be ameliorated but not eliminated if co-administered with ACEIs or ARBs.[53] Hyperuricemia leading to precipitation of

COMBINATION DRUGS FOR HYPERTENSION	
Drug	**Trade Name**
Beta-adrenergic blockers and diuretics	
Atenolol, 50 or 100 mg/chlorthalidone, 25 mg	Tenoretic
Bisoprolol fumarate, 2.5, 5, or 10 mg/hydrochlorothiazide, 6.25 mg	Ziac*
Metoprolol tartrate, 50 or 100 mg/hydrochlorothiazide, 25 or 50 mg	Lopressor HCT
Nadolol, 40 or 80 mg/bendroflumethiazide, 5 mg	Corzide
Propranolol hydrochloride, 40 or 80 mg/hydrochlorothiazide, 25 mg	Inderide LA
Propranolol hydrochloride (extended release), 80, 120, or 160 mg/hydrochlorothiazide, 50 mg	Inderide
Timolol maleate, 10 mg/hydrochlorothiazide, 25 mg	Timolide
ACE inhibitors and diuretics	
Benazepril hydrochloride, 5, 10, or 20 mg/hydrochlorothiazide, 6.25, 12.5, or 25 mg	Lotensin HCT
Captopril, 25 or 50 mg/hydrochlorothiazide, 15 or 25 mg	Capozide*
Enalapril maleate, 5 or 10 mg/hydrochlorothiazide, 12.5 or 25 mg	Vaseretic
Lisinopril, 10 or 20 mg/hydrochlorothiazide, 12.5 or 25 mg	Prinzide, Zestoretic
Fosinopril 10, 20 mg/hydrochlorothiazide 12.5 mg	Monopril/HCT
Moexipril 7.5 or 15 mg/hydrochlorothiazide 12.5 or 25 mg	Uniretic
Quinapril 10, 20 mg/hydrochlorothiazide 12.5 or 25 mg	Accuretic
Angiotensin II receptor blockers and diuretics	
Losartan potassium, 50 or 100 mg/hydrochlorothiazide, 12.5 or 25 mg	Hyzaar
Valsartan, 80, 160, or 320 mg/hydrochlorothiazide, 12.5 or 25 mg	Diovan/HCT
Irbesartan, 150 or 300 mg/hydrochlorothiazide, 12.5 or 25 mg	Avalide
Candesartan, 16 or 32 mg/hydrochlorothiazide, 12.5 mg	Atacand HCT
Telmisartan, 40 or 80 mg/hydrochlorothiazide, 12.5 mg	Micardis HCT
Eprosartan, 600 mg/hydrochlorothiazide, 12.5 or 25 mg	Teveten HCT
Olmesartan, 20 or 40 mg/hydrochlorothiazide, 12.5 or 25 mg	Benicar HCT
Angiotensin II receptor blockers and calcium channel blockers	
Valsartan, 160 or 320 mg/amlodipine, 5 or 10 mg	Exforge
Olmesartan, 20 or 40 mg/amlodipine, 5 or 10 mg	Azor
Calcium channel blockers and ACE inhibitors	
Amlodipine besylate, 2.5 or 5 mg/benazepril hydrochloride, 10 or 20 mg	Lotrel
Verapamil hydrochloride (extended release), 180 or 240 mg/trandolapril, 1, 2, or 4 mg	Tarka
Felodipine, 5 mg/enalapril maleate, 5 mg	Lexxel
Other combinations	
Triamterene, 37.5, 50, or 75 mg/hydrochlorothiazide, 25 or 50 mg	Dyazide, Maxide
Spironolactone, 25 or 50 mg/hydrochlorothiazide, 25 or 50 mg	Aldactazide
Amiloride hydrochloride, 5 mg/hydrochlorothiazide, 50 mg	Moduretic
Guanethidine monosulfate, 10 mg/hydrochlorothiazide, 25 mg	Esimil
Hydralazine hydrochloride, 25, 50, or 100 mg/hydrochlorothiazide, 25 or 50 mg	Apresazide
Methyldopa, 250 or 500 mg/hydrochlorothiazide, 15, 25, 30, or 50 mg	Aldoril
Reserpine, 0.125 mg/hydrochlorothiazide, 25 or 50 mg	Hydropres
Reserpine, 0.10 mg/hydralazine hydrochloride, 25 mg/hydrochlorothiazide, 15 mg	Ser-Ap-Es
Clonidine hydrochloride, 0.1, 0.2, or 0.3 mg/chlorthalidone, 15 mg	Combipres
Methyldopa, 250 mg/chlorothiazide, 150 or 250 mg	Aldochlor
Reserpine, 0.125 or 0.25 mg/chlorthalidone, 25 or 50 mg	Demi-Regroton, Regroton
Reserpine, 0.125 or 0.25 mg/chlorothiazide, 250 or 500 mg	Diupres
Prazosin hydrochloride, 1, 2, or 5 mg/polythiazide, 0.5 mg	Minizide

*Approved as first-line agents for lowering blood pressure by Food and Drug Administration, United States.

Table 45.7 Combination drugs for hypertension.

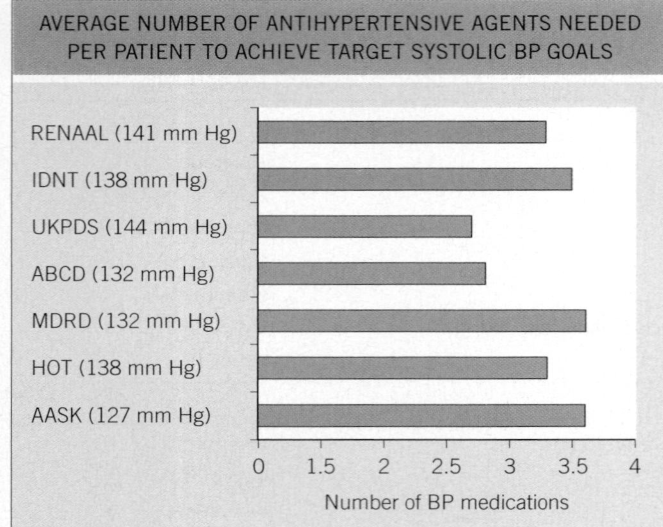

Figure 45.2 Average number of antihypertensive agents needed per patient to achieve target BP goals in various outcome trials. (Modified from Bakris GL. Maximizing cardiorenal benefit in the management of hypertension: achieve blood pressure goals. J Clin Hypertens (Greenwich) 1999;1(2):141-147.)

acute gout attack has been reported. Compared to other antihypertensives, higher rates of erectile dysfunction are seen in male patients treated with long-term diuretics.[21,54] Potassium-sparing agents may cause hyperkalemia and hypermagnesemia, particularly in patients with decreased renal function and heart failure. Impotence and gynecomastia are frequent side effects specific to spironolactone therapy and less so with the newer aldosterone antagonist eplerenone.

β-Adrenergic Receptor Blockers

Mechanism of Action

This class of drugs exerts its effect by selective inhibition of β-adrenergic receptors in a variety of tissues. Their specific mechanism of antihypertensive effect is unknown. Most likely their BP-lowering effect is a combination of reduced cardiac output and heart rate, inhibition of central nervous system sympathetic outflow, inhibition of renin release at the kidney level, and resetting of baroreceptor sensitivity. The agents in this class differ in their β_1-receptor selectivity, membrane stabilizing activity, and intrinsic sympathetic activity. Some of the beta blockers, notably labetalol and carvedilol, possess varying degrees of α-adrenergic receptor blocking properties and hence, unlike most agents of the class, are vasodilators. Nebivolol, the newest approved beta blocker, vasodilates through a mechanism that potentiates nitric oxide. All beta-blocking agents appear to be equally effective BP-lowering medications in equipotent doses.

Indications and Contraindications

As mentioned previously, the recent NICE, AHA, and ISH-WHO hypertension guidelines do not recommend beta blockers as a first-line therapy for uncomplicated hypertension, because they provide less CV protection and cause metabolic disturbances,[24,26,27] whereas the JNC-7 and the ESH-ESC still regard beta blockers as first-line drugs.[23,25] However, their effectiveness post–myocardial infarction, in angina pectoris, and in heart failure is well established. In this population, they prevent recurrent ischemia, myocardial infarction, progression of heart failure, and sudden cardiac death. Beta blockers are indicated in the hypertensive patient with symptomatic ischemic heart disease, survivors of myocardial infarction, patients with ventricular arrhythmias and certain atrioventricular node–dependent supraventricular arrhythmias, and patients with compensated congestive heart failure. In diabetic patients the American Diabetes Association (ADA) and the AHA guidelines recommend the use of beta blockers as third-line drugs after ACEIs or ARBs and diuretics.[24,51] In hypertensives with left ventricular hypertrophy, the elderly, and those with metabolic syndrome or glucose intolerance, beta blockers are not the preferred therapy.[25,41,43] Beta blockers are relatively contraindicated in patients with reactive airway disease, as well as in patients with significant bradyarrhythmia or second- or third-degree atrioventricular block. Concerns as to worsening glycemic control and precipitation of diabetes during beta-blocker therapy are documented.[55] There is evidence that carvedilol, which has α_1-antagonistic and antioxidant properties, does not worsen insulin resistance as the beta-one blocker metoprolol does.[56]

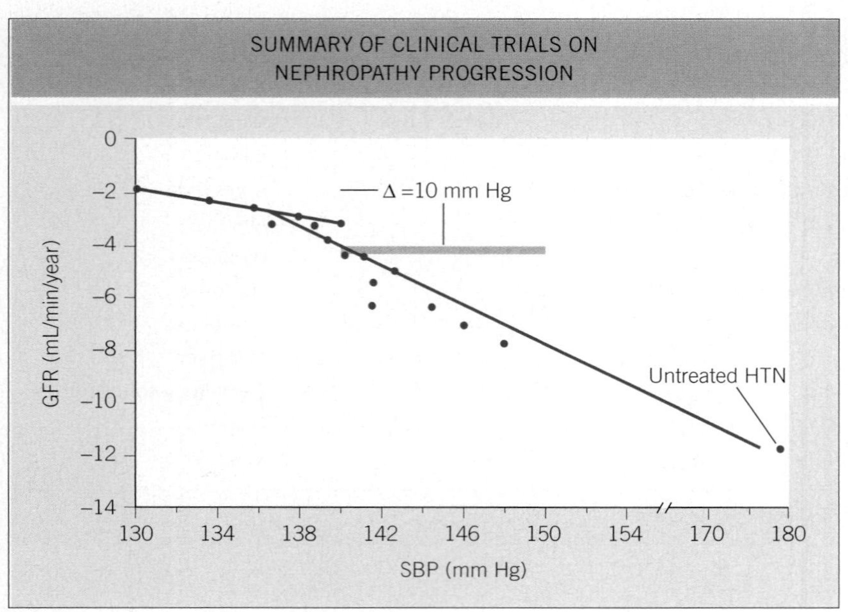

Figure 45.3 Summary of clinical trials on nephropathy progression.

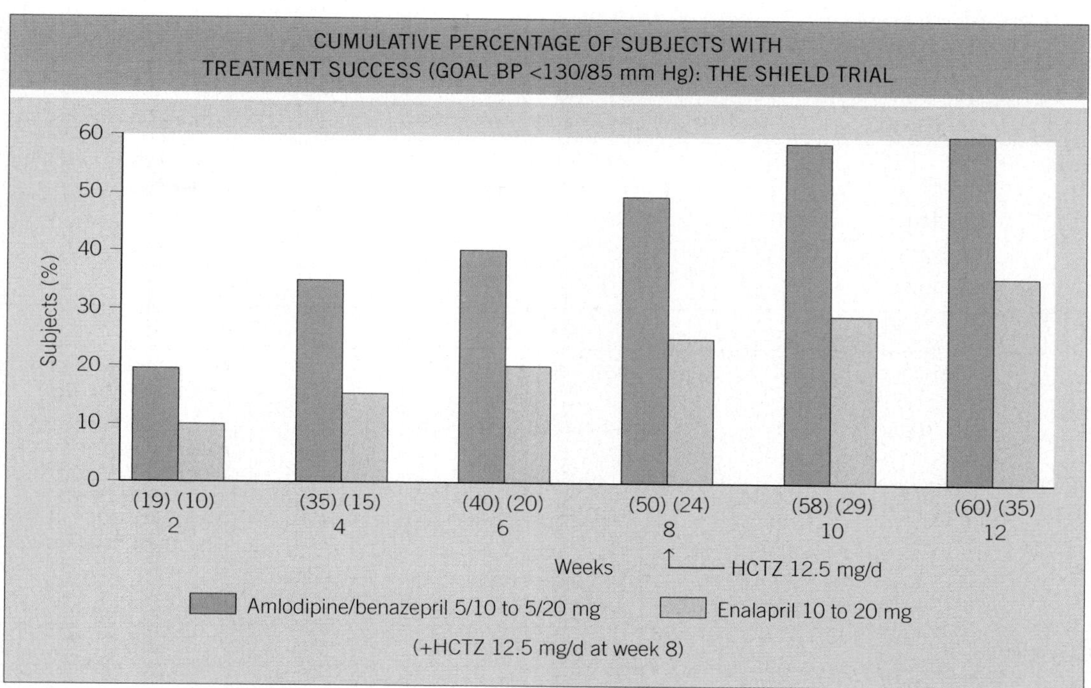

Figure 45.4 Cumulative percentage of subjects with treatment success (goal BP <130/85 mm Hg): the SHIELD trial. (Data from Buse JB, Ginsberg HN, Bakris GL, et al; American Heart Association; American Diabetes Association. Primary prevention of cardiovascular diseases in people with diabetes mellitus: a scientific statement from the American Heart Association and the American Diabetes Association. Diabetes Care 2007;30:162-172.)

PHARMACOLOGIC PROPERTIES OF COMMONLY USED ANTIHYPERTENSIVE AGENTS

Drug	Dosage (mg/day)	Doses/Day	Mechanisms of Action	Special Considerations
Diuretics				
Thiazides and related drugs				
Hydrochlorothiazide	12.5-25	1	Decrease body sodium and extracellular fluid volume, also vasodilation	More effective antihypertensive agents than loop diuretics, unless serum creatinine is >2.0 mL/min or creatinine clearance <50 mL/min
Loop diuretics				
Furosemide	20-320	2	Inhibit 2Cl-Na pump ascending loop of Henle	Effective even in patients with advanced renal or congestive heart failure
Bumetanide	0.5-5	2		
Ethacrynic acid	25-100	2		
Torasemide	5-20	1		
Fixed-dose diuretics				
Potassium sparing			Increase K^- reabsorption	Weak diuretics
HCTZ/amiloride				
HCTZ/triamterene				
Spironolactone	25-50	2-3	Aldosterone antagonist	May cause hyperkalemia in with serum creatinine >2.5 mg/dL particularly when combined with ACE inhibitors, K^+ supplements, or NSAIDs
Triamterene	50-100	2		
Eplerenone	50-100	1		
Adrenergic inhibitors				
Beta Blockers				
Cardioselective			Inhibit β_1-receptors, decrease CO	In higher doses, will also inhibit β_2-receptors
Atenolol	25-100	1	Increase SVR, decrease plasma renin activity (PRA)	
Metoprolol	50-200	1-2		

Table 45.8

(Continued)

PHARMACOLOGIC PROPERTIES OF COMMONLY USED ANTIHYPERTENSIVE AGENTS—CONT'D				
Drug	**Dosage (mg/day)**	**Doses/Day**	**Mechanisms of Action**	**Special Considerations**
Noncardioselective			Inhibit β_1- and β_2-receptors	More likely to cause metabolic side effects
Nadolol	20-240	1		
Propranolol	40-240	1-2		
Timolol	20-40	2		
Vasodilating				
Carvedilol	6.25-25	2	α-β_1 and β_2 (ratio 1:3)	No exacerbation of diabetes, reduces new-onset diabetes
Carvedilol CR	20, 40, 80	1	α-β_1 and β_2 (ratio 1:3)	Same as regular carvedilol but once daily
Labetalol	200-800	2-3	α-β_1 and β_2 (ratio 1:7)	
Nebivolol	5-10	1	Highest selectivity for β_1 in the class Vasodilates through increases in nitric oxide effect	No exacerbation of diabetes, reduces new-onset diabetes
Antiadrenergic agents				
Centrally acting				
α-Methyldopa	250-1500	2	Stimulate α_2-adrenergic receptors in the brainstem, resulting in inhibition of efferent sympathetic activity; decrease SVR	Sudden withdrawal may result in hypertensive crisis
Clonidine	0.1-0.6	2		
Clonidine TTS	0.1-0.3	Once/week		
Guanfacine	1-3	1		
Peripherally acting				
Guanethidine	10-100	1	Inhibit norepinephrine release from sympathetic nerve terminals; decrease SVR	Frequently cause orthostatic hypotension and sexual dysfunction
Reserpine	0.05-0.25	1	Depletion of norepinephrine	Causes frequent neurologic symptoms
α_1-Receptor blockers				
Doxazosin	2-16	1	Inhibit α_1-adrenergic receptors	First-dose effect; postural hypotension Useful for prostatic hypertrophy
Prazosin	2-20	1-2	Decrease SVR; CO same or increases	
Terazosin	1-20	1		
ACE inhibitors*				
Benazepril	10-40	1-2	Block conversion of angiotensin I to angiotensin II; decrease aldosterone; may increase bradykinin and vasodilatory prostaglandins; decrease SVR; no change in CO	When added to diuretics may cause hypotension; may cause hyperkalemia in patients with renal failure, those with hypoaldosteronism, those receiving K-sparing diuretics or NSAIDs
Captopril	12.5-100	2-3		
Cilazapril	2.5-5	1-2		
Enalapril	2.5-40	1-2		
Fosinopril	10-40	1		
Lisinopril	5-40	1		
Benazepril	10-40	1		
Captopril	25-100	2		
Enalapril	5-40	1-2		
Fosinopril	10-40	1		
Lisinopril	10-40	1		
Moexipril	7.5-30	1		
Perindopril	4-8	1		
Quinapril	10-80	1		
Ramipril	2.5-20	1		
Trandolapril	1-4	1		

Table 45.8

PHARMACOLOGIC PROPERTIES OF COMMONLY USED ANTIHYPERTENSIVE AGENTS—CONT'D				
Drug	**Dosage (mg/day)**	**Doses/Day**	**Mechanisms of Action**	**Special Considerations**
Angiotensin receptor blockers*				
Losartan	50-40	1-2	Selectively block AT_1 receptors of angiotensin II	As for ACEIs
Valsartan	80-320	1		Do not cause cough
Irbesartan	150-300	1	Decrease aldosterone	
Candesartan	8-32	1	Decrease SVR	
Telmisartan	40-80	1	No change in CO	
Olmesartan	20-40	1		
Eprosartan	400-800		1-2	
Calcium channel blockers				
Non-dihydropyridines				
Diltiazem	90-360	3-4	Blocks entry of calcium into smooth muscle cells resulting in vasodilation Decrease SVR	
Diltiazem CD	180-360	1	Blunt increases in exercise heart rate.	
Verapamil	80-480	2-3		May cause heart block, particularly when combined with beta blocker
Verapamil SR	120-480	1-2		
Verapamil-Covera HS	180-240	1 (at bedtime)		
Dihydropyridines				
Amlodipine	2.5-10	1	Same as diltiazem and verapamil	More potent vasodilators than diltiazem and verapamil; may cause dizziness, headache, tachycardia, flushing, edema
Felodipine	5-20	1	Do not blunt increase in exercise heart rate	
Isradipine	2.5-10	2		
Nicardipine	60-120	3		
Nifedipine	30-120	3		
Nifedipine (GITS)	30-120	1		
Nisoldipine	10-10	1-2		
Direct vasodilators				
Hydralazine	50-200	2-4	Direct relaxation of smooth muscle cells, causing arteriolar vasodilation secondary to opening [K+] channels	Limited efficacy if given alone due to fluid retention and reflex vasodilation. Should be combined with a diuretic and a beta blocker to prevent edema and tachycardia
Minoxidil	2.5-80	1		

*NOTE: With both ACEIs and ARBs, a rise in serum creatinine of 30% that remains stable over the span of a couple of months and is not associated with hyperkalemia (i.e. >6 mEq/L) should result in sustained maintenance of this agent, because renal and CV outcome will be better.[52,62]
CO, cardiac output; HCTZ, hydrochlorothiazide; NSAIDs, nonsteroidal anti-inflammatory drugs; SVR, systemic vascular resistance.

Table 45.8 Pharmacologic properties of commonly used antihypertensive agents.

Side Effects

Beta blockers are usually well tolerated even in higher doses. In the younger patients, treatment with a beta blocker may lead to decreased exercise capacity. Most of the beta blockers are known to exacerbate dyslipidemia. Carvedilol has been shown to have no negative metabolic effects and may be a preferred beta blocker in patients with type 2 diabetes or severe lipid abnormalities. Erectile dysfunction, especially in middle-aged and older patients, is another unwanted effect.

Angiotensin-Converting Enzyme Inhibitors

Mechanism of Action

ACEIs inhibit the generation of angiotensin II from angiotensin I. They also inhibit the degradation of bradykinin and other vasoactive peptides. Acute administration of ACEIs rapidly reduces angiotensin II levels. This effect, however, is transient, with angiotensin II levels returning to baseline in several weeks. Given that ACEIs display sustained effect on BP despite the "angiotensin escape phenomenon," other mechanisms of long-term antihypertensive effect have been proposed. Increased levels of bradykinin and resulting increase in production of nitric oxide and vasodilator prostaglandins are some of the mechanisms implicated in the long-term antihypertensive effect of ACEIs. From a hemodynamic standpoint, administration of ACEIs results in a fall in systemic vascular resistance, balanced decrease in preload and afterload, as well as mild increase in stroke volume and cardiac output, which are not accompanied by reflex tachycardia. Renal blood flow is usually increased, which together with decreased efferent arteriolar resistance results in no significant change in glomerular filtration rate.

All commercially available ACEIs have similar capacity to reduce BP. No significant changes between the members of the class are observed, except for absorption, half-life, and elimination, which dictate dosing. Additionally, all ACEIs have tissue penetrating properties, when used in doses documented from clinical trials to show a risk reduction. Thus the favorable effects of ACE inhibition are considered a class effect. ACEIs are effective in patients in all subgroups and all ethnic groups if given in sufficiently high doses.

Indications and Contraindications

In published guidelines, ACEIs are considered as first-line therapy for hypertension and are particularly indicated in all subjects with type 2 diabetes and in patients with diabetic and nondiabetic nephropathy.[24,25,51,52] In addition, ACEIs are recommended post–myocardial infarction, in heart failure, and in left ventricular dysfunction and appear to be especially useful in treating hypertensives with diabetic and nondiabetic renal disease.[23-25,57] Lewis and colleagues[58] showed that captopril reduces the risk of combined endpoint of dialysis and transplantation in type 1 diabetics by 50% compared to other agents when similar levels of BP control are attained. The AASK study indicated that ramipril retarded renal disease progression in patients with hypertensive renal disease and proteinuria when compared to amlodipine.[59] A meta-analysis of 43 randomized controlled trials in patients with diabetic nephropathy showed that ACEIs significantly reduced renal outcomes and all-cause mortality.[60] Jafar and associates[61] published a meta-analysis of 11 randomized controlled trials where they examined the efficacy of ACEIs in treatment of nondiabetic renal disease and concluded that ACEI-based treatment was more effective than other drugs in slowing the progression of renal damage. The beneficial effect of ACEIs was over and beyond the BP-lowering effect and was greater in patients with proteinuria. Based on these data, ACEIs are regarded as preferred therapy for hypertensive patients with coexisting renal disease.[23-25,51,52]

Side Effects

ACEIs are usually well tolerated. However, up to 20% of patients develop side effects necessitating termination of therapy. Cough is the most often reported side effect, and hyperkalemia may occur particularly in subjects with decreased renal function. Cough is a complication seen in administration of all agents of this class. It might appear in the first days or even months after treatment initiation and usually resolves up to 2 weeks after discontinuation of therapy. Angioedema is uncommon but prevalent in African Americans and smokers, with rates up to 5% reported in African American participants in any given clinical trial. It is not a dose-dependent effect and can occur at any time during the therapy. It is more common in multiracial populations. Acute renal dysfunction that is induced or mediated by ACEIs is a problem commonly seen in clinical practice and often results in inappropriate discontinuation of ACEI therapy, despite its proven benefits in improving cardiovascular and renal outcomes. Although ACEIs acutely reduce the glomerular filtration rate by 5% to 15% with corresponding increase in serum creatinine levels, no long-term renal function loss occurs. An overview of 12 randomized renal disease progression trials where ACEIs were initiated in patients with preexisting renal insufficiency found that a strong trend exists toward acute increase in serum creatinine up to 30%.[62] This acute increase usually stabilizes within the first 3 to 4 months of ACEI administration and is accompanied by long-term preservation of renal function.[63] On a practical level, creatinine and potassium levels should be checked within the first week or two following the initiation of ACEI therapy in patients with renal insufficiency. Withdrawal of ACEI should occur only when the creatinine rise exceeds 30% above baseline within the first 3 to 4 months of therapy or if persistent hyperkalemia develops in a patient who is euvolemic. Transient withdrawal of diuretics may be needed in patients with suspected hypovolemia. In patients with continuous rise of creatinine level and persistent hyperkalemia, ACEIs should be stopped and the assessment for bilateral renal artery disease should be considered. It is recognized that continued treatment with ACEIs despite rising creatinine levels may lead to chronic and irreversible renal failure. Since ACEIs can cause birth defects, they are absolutely contraindicated in pregnancy.

Angiotensin II Receptor Blockers

Mechanism of Action

Angiotensin II receptor blockers selectively inhibit AT_1 receptors and, thus, the vasoconstriction and growth promoting actions of angiotensin II. Several types of angiotensin II receptors have been described; of these, the AT_1 receptor mediates the common physiologic effects of angiotensin II. All currently available drugs in this group selectively block the AT_1 receptor. Activation of the AT_2 receptors during AT_1 blockade appears to play a role in vascular regulation, although their role is not completely understood at this time. All agents in this class have similar efficacy and BP-lowering effect. Also, all agents in this class have fairly flat dose-response curve, and higher doses typically provide little additional BP-lowering effect. It has been suggested that higher doses of ARBs may have better antiproteinuric effect, which is associated with long-term renal function preservation.[63]

Indications and Contraindications

ARBs and ACEIs affect similar physiologic mechanisms and seem to offer comparable clinical benefits. In the VALUE study in high-risk hypertensive patients, the ARB valsartan was as effective as the CCB amlodipine in reducing the primary combined CV endpoint, despite the higher BP in the valsartan group.[40] In the LIFE study in hypertensive patients with left ventricular hypertrophy, losartan was more effective than atenolol in preventing CV events and stroke.[41] Two studies in patients post–myocardial infarction with heart failure showed similar CV protection with ARBs and ACEIs.[64,65] Furthermore, studies in heart failure showed that ARBs improve CV morbidity and mortality when administered alone or with ACEIs.[66-68]

Both the Reduction of End Point in Non–insulin dependent type 2 diabetes with the Angiotensin II Antagonist Losartan study (RENAAL)[69] and the Irbesartan in Diabetic Nephropathy Trial (IDNT)[70] showed that ARBs reduced the risk of primary endpoint of doubling serum creatinine, need for dialysis or transplantation, and death compared to placebo when similar BP control is achieved. Therefore, as with ACEIs, current guidelines recommend the use of ARBs as first-line treatment of uncomplicated hypertension with specific indication in diabetics, in patients with diabetic and nondiabetic nephropathy, and in patients with coronary heart disease and heart failure.[23-25,51,52] Interestingly, a combination of ARBs and ACEIs provides additional renoprotective effects.[71] A large ongoing outcome study (ONTARGET) is investigating the value of the ACEI-ARB combination in CV protection.[72]

Side Effects

ARBs are remarkably well tolerated. In clinic trials their side effects profile is equal or better than placebo. Unlike ACEIs, they do not cause cough. They have rarely been associated with angioedema. Like ACEIs, they may induce progressive renal insufficiency in patients with renovascular disease. They are also contraindicated in pregnancy.

Calcium Channel Blockers

Mechanism of Action

CCBs are a family of drugs sharing the same site of action—inhibition of L-type voltage-gated channel. They are most commonly classified as dihydropyridines, such as nifedipine and amlodipine, and nondihydropyridines, such as diltiazem and verapamil. Despite differences in the chemical structure, the efficacy of all members of this family in lowering BP is very similar. Both dihydropyridines and nondihydropyridines are primarily arterial vasodilators. These agents have differential effects on the kidney and sympathetic system (Table 45.9).[73] Both classes are known to produce vasodilatation of coronary arteries, with nondihydropyridines slowing heart rate as well.

FACTORS THAT HELP EXPLAIN THE DIFFERENTIAL EFFECTS OF CALCIUM CHANNEL BLOCKERS ON KIDNEY AND CV OUTCOMES

	CCB Effect	
	DHPCCBs	Non-DHPCCBs
Parameter	(Amlodipine-like)	(Verapamil, diltiazem)
Albuminuria/proteinuria	→	→ ↓*
Mesangial volume expansion (diabetes)	→	↓
Glomerular scanning†	→	↓
Renal autoregulation ‡	Abolished	Partially abolished
Sympathetic tone	→↓	↓

→No effect, ↓decrease.
*Decreased only if blood pressure reduced and on low-salt diet.
†Data from animal models. Note, however, that renal autoregulatory mechanisms are not affected by ACE inhibitors.
‡Data from both animal and human experiments.
CCB, calcium channel blocker; DHPCCBs, dihydropyridines.
Modified from Bakris GL, Weir MR, Secic M, Campbell B, Weis-McNulty A. Differential effects of calcium antagonist subclasses on markers of nephropathy progression. Kidney Int 2004;65(6):1991-2002.

Table 45.9 Factors that help explain the differential effects of calcium channel blockers on kidney and CV outcomes.

Indications and Contraindications

Dihydropyridine CCBs were studied against placebo in elderly hypertensive patients, where they were found to confer significant CV benefits, especially protection from cerebrovascular events.[74,75] This effect was seen in patients of both white and Asian descent. Several reports based on case control studies suggested excessive rates of myocardial infarction and coronary disease mortality in hypertensives treated with short-acting dihydropyridines. These concerns were not confirmed in trials where long-acting dihydropyridine CCBs were a primary treatment strategy[29] or in trials where they were tested against therapy based on diuretics,[38,76] beta blockers,[42] ACEIs,[38] or ARBs.[40] However, dihydropyridine CCBs were inferior to ACEIs or ARBs in trials assessing the renoprotective effects.[59,63] Therefore dihydropyridine CCBs are a reasonable first-line strategy for patients with uncomplicated hypertension, whereas in patients with coronary artery disease or renal impairment they are administered on top of renin-angiotensin system blockers.[25,51,52] In diabetic patients the ADA and the AHA guidelines recommend the use of CCBs as third-line drugs after ACEIs or ARBs and diuretics.[24,51]

Regarding the nondihydropyridine CCBs, the NORDIL study[77] suggested that diltiazem-based therapy confers similar protection from stroke, myocardial infarction, and CV death in patients with uncomplicated hypertension as compared to conventional diuretic and beta-blocker–based therapy. Nondihydropyridine CCBs may have a role in treatment of hypertensive patients with renal insufficiency where they seem to confer an additive antiproteinuric effect when used with ACEIs or ARBs (see Table 45.9).[73,78] The INVEST study with 22,576 hypertensive patients with coronary artery disease showed that the mortality and morbidity of the verapamil-trandolapril–based therapy were similar to those of the atenolol-hydrochlorothiazide–based therapy.[79]

Side Effects

The most common side effects of dihydropyridine CCBs are headache, flushing, and peripheral edema, which is typically exacerbated by high-salt diet and improved with coadministration of ACEIs or ARBs. Constipation, bradycardia, and peripheral edema are the most frequent side effects of nondihydropyridine CCBs.

Renin Inhibitors

Renin inhibitors block the renin-angiotensin system at the point of its activation. They act through the reduction of plasma renin activity (PRA), which is increased with ACEIs and ARBs.[80,81] The first orally active inhibitor, aliskiren, is available for clinical use in several countries. Aliskiren has a dose-dependent BP-lowering effect in daily dose range from 150 to 300 mg. Clinical trials have shown additive antihypertensive effects with thiazide diuretics and also ACEIs and ARBs. Interestingly, aliskiren has been shown to neutralize the diuretic-induced renin increase. Studies using ambulatory BP monitoring demonstrate 24-hour efficacy.[80,81] There are promising data from short-term trials in diabetic proteinuria, left ventricular hypertrophy, and heart failure. As is the case with ARBs, aliskiren has minimal adverse effects.[80,81] Aliskiren appears to have the same contraindications as ACEIs and ARBs, in pregnancy and bilateral renal artery stenosis. The long-term effects of this drug on CV and renal endpoints are currently being investigated in outcome trials. Until these data become available, aliskiren should be used as a second-line drug when first-line drugs are ineffective or poorly tolerated.

α-Adrenergic Receptor Antagonists

See Table 45.8.

Other Agents

Other currently approved agents including clonidine, reserpine, methyldopa, moxonidine, hydralazine, and minoxidil are associated with higher incidence of side effects and should not be used as first-line therapy. Their role as add-on agents is also questionable given the plethora of other safe and effective choices available. Occasionally, they may be needed in situations where the more contemporary drugs are ineffective, poorly tolerated, or considered unsafe, such as in the treatment of hypertension in pregnancy where methyldopa and hydralazine are still preferred by many obstetricians. Agents used to treat hypertensive urgencies are summarized in Table 45.9.

HYPERTENSIVE EMERGENCIES

Agents used to treat hypertensive emergencies are summarized in Table 45.10.[82] Hypertensive emergencies are those when end-organ damage is present and clinical symptomatology is present, such as a seizure, loss of feeling or movement in the arm, rupturing abdominal aneurysm, or renal failure.

SUMMARY

Hypertension should and can be effectively treated with the combination of physician and patient perseverance, lifestyle modifications, and currently available medications. One of the main challenges in pharmacologic therapy is widespread therapeutic inertia or apathy. We certainly need new, more effective, and well tolerated drugs, which would reignite excitement about hypertension control. Several new classes of drugs are currently in different phases of clinical trials. Their role in therapy of hypertension and ability to reduce cardiovascular and renal endpoints is not defined as yet. Given its proven benefits, pharmacologic therapy will remain the mainstay of treatment for the 1.2 billion hypertensive individuals estimated to be living in the world by 2010.

TYPES OF HYPERTENSION CRISES, WITH SUGGESTED DRUG THERAPY AND BLOOD PRESSURE TARGETS

Type of Crisis	Drug of Choice	BP Target
Neurologic		
Hypertensive encephalopathy	Nitroprusside*	25% reduction in mean arterial pressure over 2-3 h
Intracranial hemorrhage or acute stroke in evolution	Nitroprusside* (controversial)	0%-25% reduction in mean arterial pressure over 6-12 h (controversial)
Acute head injury/trauma	Nitroprusside*	0%-25% reduction in mean arterial pressure over 2-3 h (controversial)
Subarachnoid hemorrhage	Nimodipine	Up to 25% reduction in mean arterial pressure in previously hypertensive patients, 130-160 systolic in normotensive patients
Cardiac		
Ischemia/infaction	Nitroglycerin or nicardipine	Reduction in ischemia
Heart failure	Nitroprusside* or nitroglycerin	Improvement in failure (typically 10%-15% decrease in BP)
Aortic dissection	Beta blocker + nitroprusside*	120 mm Hg systolic in 30 minutes (if possible)
Renal		
Hematuria or acute renal impairment	Fenoldopam	0%-25% reduction in mean arterial pressure over 1-12 h
Catecholamine excess states		
Pheochromocytoma	Phentolamine	To control paroxysms
Drug withdrawal	Drug withdrawn	Typically only one dose necessary
Pregnancy-related		
Eclampsia	$MgSO_4$, methyldopa, hydralazine	Typically <90 mm Hg diastolic, but often lower

*Some physicians prefer an intravenous infusion or either fenoldopam or nicardipine, neither of which has potentially toxic metabolites, over nitroprusside. Recent studies have also shown improvements in renal function during therapy with the former as compared to nitroprusside.

Modified from Elliott WJ, Black HR. Hypertension crises. In Parillo JE, Bone RC, eds. Clinical Care Medicine: Principles of Diagnosis and Management. Philadelphia, Mosby Year Book Publishers 1990:565-576.

Table 45.10 Types of hypertension crises, with suggested drug therapy and blood pressure targets.

chapter 46 Hypertensive Crisis

Ehud Grossman and Gregory Y. H. Lip

Definition

- Hypertensive crises are acute, life-threatening medical conditions that are usually associated with very high blood pressure.

Key Features

- Hypertensive crises occur most commonly in patients with known previous hypertension, although some can present with hypertensive crises de novo, with no previous history of hypertension.
- Severe hypertension in an otherwise relatively symptomless patient does not constitute a hypertensive emergency, and is best classified as an "urgency."
- The true hypertensive emergencies are acute aortic dissection, gross left ventricular failure with very high blood pressures, eclampsia or preeclampsia, and hypertensive encephalopathy.

Therapy

- In the vast majority of severely hypertensive patients, blood pressure should be reduced gradually with orally active drugs, and long-term control of blood pressure is probably the most important factor influencing prognosis.
- In true hypertensive emergencies, parenteral therapy is often required in the early phase.

Hypertensive crisis is defined as a severe elevation in blood pressure (BP), such as a diastolic BP above 120 to 130 mm Hg, and can be subclassified into either a "hypertensive emergency" or "hypertensive urgency."[1]

Hypertensive emergencies are relatively rare and defined as such only when there is an immediate threat to the integrity of the cardiovascular system (Table 46.1). Patients with a hypertensive emergency require an immediate reduction in BP to avoid serious end-organ damage, generally by intravenous therapy in an intensive care setting.[2]

Unlike a hypertensive emergency, patients with severe elevation in BP who have no evidence of progressive end-organ injury are classified as having a hypertensive urgency and require only a gradual reduction in BP over 12 to 24 hours.[3]

It has been estimated that approximately 1% of patients with hypertension will develop a hypertensive crisis at some point during their lives.[3] The incidence of hypertensive crisis has increased over the past four decades. Hospital admissions for hypertensive emergency in the United States more than tripled between 1983 and 1990 from 23,000 per year to 73,000 per year.[3] The prevalence of hypertensive crises is unknown. A wide variety of results have been reported. For example, Zampaglione and colleagues[4] found that hypertensive crises accounted for more than 25% of all patient visits to a medical section of an emergency department, with hypertensive emergencies accounting for one third of these cases. In a recent study done in an emergency department, hypertensive crisis was the reason for referral in 1.7% of all clinical emergencies. Out of 452 patents with hypertensive crises, 179 (39.6%) had the criteria of hypertensive emergency. Most cases of hypertensive emergency corresponded to cerebrovascular events.[5]

Before the effective treatment of accelerated-malignant hypertension, survival was 20% and 1%, at 1 and 5 years, respectively. During the last two decades, survival has improved, with a 10-year survival rate of 67% and mean survival of 18 years being reported.[6] Therapy has dramatically reduced immediate deaths from hypertensive encephalopathy, acute renal failure, hemorrhagic strokes, and congestive heart failure.

Hypertensive crises still occur most commonly in patients with known previous hypertension. Nevertheless, some patients can present with a hypertensive crisis de novo, with no previous history of hypertension.[7] Secondary causes of hypertension are more common in patients presenting with hypertension emergency than in those who have hypertension urgency, with the underlying secondary causes including renovascular disease, primary renal diseases, pheochromocytoma, connective tissue disorders, and primary hyperaldosteronism.[8] Approximate entropy (ApEn) of BP based on software analysis of 24-hour ambulatory BP monitoring (ABPM) may predict the development of hypertensive crisis.[9]

In about 50% of patients with hypertensive emergency there may be an underlying cause, but underlying primary renal diseases will be missed unless all patients are subjected to renal biopsy.

With the diversity of clinical presentations of hypertensive crises, it is important to both understand the underlying mechanisms and have coherent management strategies for these conditions. The mortality in untreated patients can be very high, but the over-rapid treatment of the condition itself may also be hazardous. For example, the mortality in untreated malignant phase hypertension is around 88% in 2 years.[10] There is also a high rate of progression to renal dysfunction necessitating long-term dialysis if the disease is managed inappropriately.

ANATOMY AND PATHOPHYSIOLOGY

In severe hypertension, there may be intense constriction and thickening of the arteriolar walls, causing a high peripheral resistance. In most cases, this is mediated by high circulating concentrations of renin and angiotensin II. With mild-to-moderate increases in BP, the initial physiologic

DEFINITION OF A HYPERTENSIVE EMERGENCY
Moderate to severe elevation of arterial pressure associated with: 1. Malignant hypertension* 2. Intracranial hemorrhage 3. Atherothrombotic cerebral infarction 4. Acute congestive heart failure 5. Acute coronary insufficiency 6. Acute renal insufficiency 7. Acute aortic dissection 8. Eclampsia
*Malignant hypertension: a syndrome characterized by elevated BP accompanied by encephalopathy or nephropathy or by papilledema and/or microangiopathic hemolytic anemia.

Table 46.1 Definition of a hypertensive emergency.

response is arteriolar vasoconstriction to maintain relatively constant tissue perfusion and prevent the high BP from being transmitted to small distal vessels. The brain, kidneys, and heart have these protective autoregulatory mechanisms that maintain a stable blood flow.

In the malignant phase (usually with severe retinal involvement), severe BP elevation above the autoregulatory threshold leads to transmission of the pressure to small distal vessels, causing endothelial injury. The endothelial dysfunction leads to increased vascular wall permeability, cell proliferation, and activation of the coagulation cascade and platelets, resulting ultimately in fibrinoid necrosis of small blood vessels, release of vasoconstrictor substances, and tissue ischemia. This process leads to a vicious cycle of further vascular injury, tissue ischemia, and release of more vasoconstrictor substances.[11]

Autoregulation is particularly important in the brain. With normal cerebral autoregulation, vasodilatation occurs in response to a decrease in the perfusion pressure, whereas vasoconstriction occurs when the BP increases, thus allowing cerebral blood flow to be relatively constant during fluctuations in the systemic mean arterial pressure, from approximately 70 to 150 mm Hg. This regulatory process is believed to be due to a myogenic response controlled by stretch receptors in the cerebral arterioles, although hypoxia and the local (cerebrovascular) or circulating renin-angiotensin systems may also play a part. Within the brain, the breakthrough vasodilatation from failure of autoregulation—for example, in chronic hypertension or severe BP elevation—leads to disruption of the blood-brain barrier, the development of cerebral edema, and the clinical picture of hypertensive encephalopathy.

CLINICAL PRESENTATIONS

Hypertensive Emergency (Includes Malignant Phase Hypertension)

Hypertensive emergency has replaced the old term malignant hypertension, by including all cases of acute rise in BP associated with acute target organ damage, in addition to malignant hypertension per se.[1]

Malignant phase hypertension is usually defined clinically as an increased BP in association with bilateral retinal linear or flame-shaped hemorrhages, cotton-wool exudates, hard exudates, or a combination of these three, with or without papilledema. This definition includes both Keith, Wagener, and Barker grades 3 and 4 retinopathy (Fig. 46.1). The differentiation between grades 3 and 4 retinopathy is unhelpful, because the presence of papilledema is an unreliable sign, and both retinopathy categories carry an equally bad prognosis; thus both should be considered to be malignant hypertension.[12,13] A recent review on hypertensive retinopathy suggests that hemorrhage, microaneurysm, cotton-wool spot, hard exudate, or a combination of these signs plus swelling of the optic disk indicate malignant hypertension.[14]

Clinical Epidemiology

The incidence of malignant hypertension is 1 to 2 per 100,000 population per year.[15] There were no specific trends seen over the period from 1970 to 1993 with respect to the number of new cases, the mean duration of known hypertension before presentation, presenting BPs, or the number of antihypertensive drugs that were being used. Despite reports that this disease is generally becoming less frequent in the Western world,[16] there has been no reduction in its incidence in the west of Birmingham, England (Fig. 46.2).[15] In some developing countries, malignant hypertension remains a common problem and is an important cause of end-stage renal failure.[17,18]

Although malignant hypertension often occurs in patients with long-standing uncontrolled hypertension, many of whom have discontinued antihypertensive therapy, the condition can present de novo in patients without a previously known history of hypertension. Essential hypertension is usually the most common underlying cause of hypertensive emergency,[15,19,20] but secondary causes are generally more prevalent than in nonmalignant hypertension, especially among younger patients.[21] Underlying renal artery stenosis is also commonly present, particularly in white patients.[22]

Malignant hypertension can present in both young and old patients.[23] Risk factors for hypertensive emergency include a history of hypertension during pregnancy,[24] oral contraceptive use,[25] smoking,[23,26] stress,[27] diabetes mellitus,[5] the ACE DD genotype,[28] and less effective control of systolic BP on an outpatient basis.[29]

In patients of African origin, the prognosis of malignant hypertension is significantly worse than in whites, but this difference has been shown to be entirely attributable to later clinical presentation, with higher BPs and a greater prevalence of renal dysfunction, rather than a true racial difference.[30,31] Thus Afro-Caribbean patients fared badly, not because of their ethnic origin, but because of their higher BPs and greater renal impairment.

Clinical Features

A proportion of patients with malignant hypertension are asymptomatic or present at a late stage in their disease. This proportion can range from 10%[15] to 75%.[19] Complications associated with hypertensive emergency can include neurologic syndromes, myocardial ischemia and infarction, acute left ventricular dysfunction, aortic dissection, acute renal failure, microangiopathic hemolytic anemia, and eclampsia. The predominant presenting symptoms are central nervous system abnormalities. In one study, types of end-organ damage associated with hypertensive emergencies included cerebral infarction (24%), acute pulmonary edema (23%),

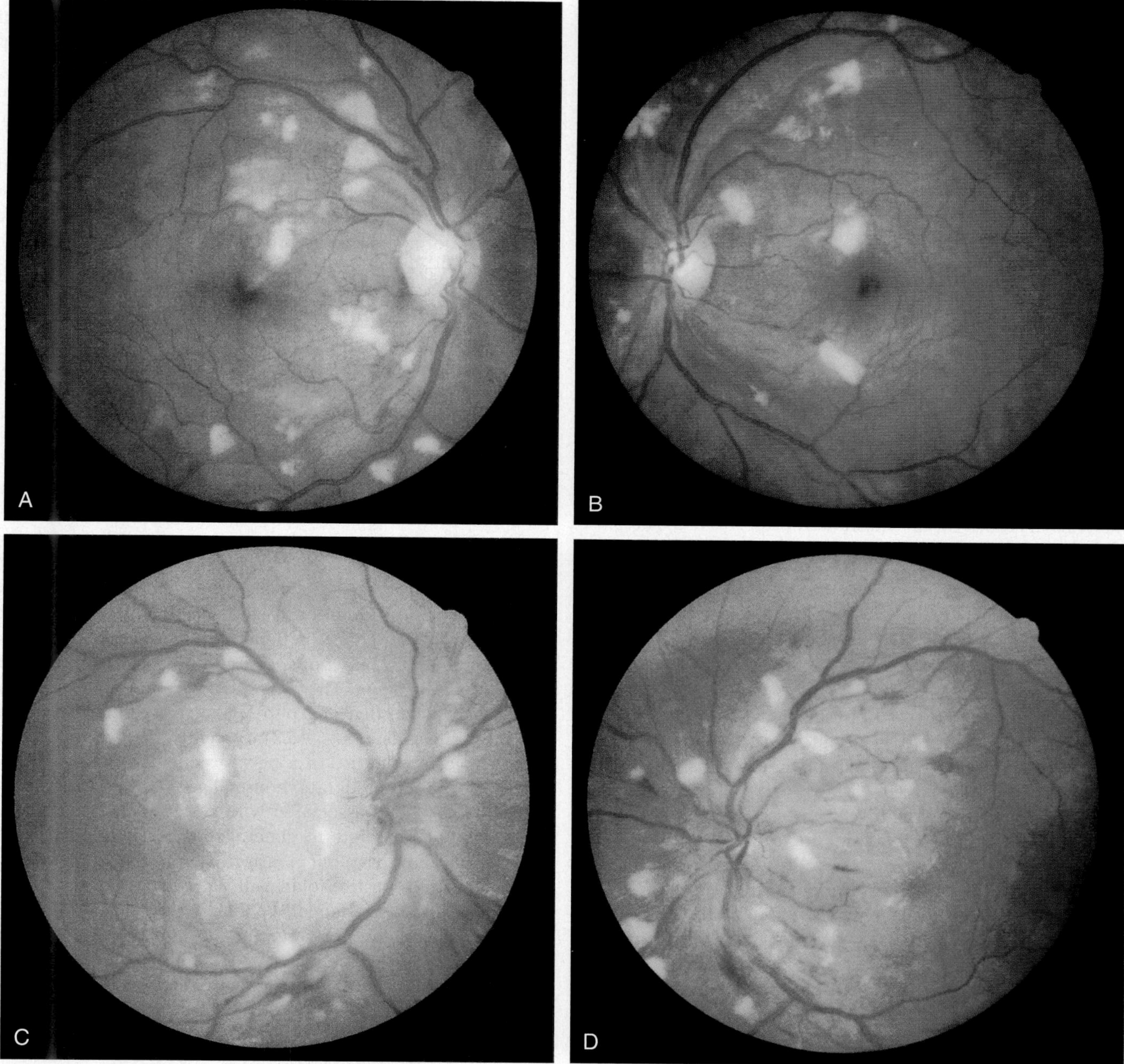

Figure 46.1 Keith, Wagener, and Barker grades 3 and 4 hypertensive retinopathy. A, B, Grade 3 retinopathy, showing attenuated arterioles and venous dilatation. Multiple widespread, large, cotton-wool spots, suggesting ischemic fundi. **C, D,** Grade 4 retinopathy, showing bilateral optic disk swelling (papilledema) and widespread cotton-wool spots, macula stars, and flame-shaped hemorrhages, with attenuated arterioles. (From Lip PL, Lip GY, Beevers, DG et al. Fundal changes in malignant hypertension. J Hum Hypertens 1997;11:395-396.)

hypertensive encephalopathy (16%), and cerebral hemorrhage, which accounted for only 4.5%. In another study, visual disturbance with or without headaches were the presenting symptoms in 48% of cases, and angina or myocardial infarction were complicating features in approximately 20%.[15] A high proportion of patients have cardiomegaly (47%) on their chest radiograph and left ventricular hypertrophy (77%) on their electrocardiogram (ECG),[15] although some appear to have normal ECGs or echocardiograms, despite their very high BPs at presentation,[7,32,33] suggesting that the malignant hypertension may have been of acute onset in a proportion of patients.

Renal Involvement in Malignant Hypertension

Renal involvement in malignant hypertension has been referred to as malignant nephrosclerosis, leading to acute renal failure, hematuria, and proteinuria. Renal biopsy usually reveals the pathologic hallmark of hypertensive emergency—fibrinoid necrosis in the arterioles and capillaries—but histologic changes can be similar to those seen in the hemolytic-uremic syndrome and progressive systemic sclerosis. Renovascular disease in the setting of malignant hypertension can lead to glomerular ischemia and activation of the renin-angiotensin system, and further exacerbation of hypertension.

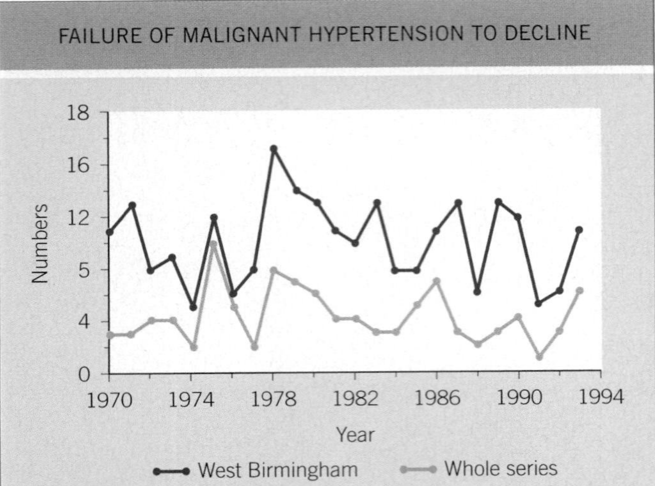

Figure 46.2 Failure of malignant hypertension to decline. Numbers of patients with malignant hypertension presenting each year in the west Birmingham malignant hypertension series, with data presented for the whole series and those residing within the immediate catchment area of the hospital. (With permission from Lip GY, Beevers M, Beevers DG. Do patients with de novo hypertension differ from patients with previously known hypertension when malignant phase hypertension occurs? Am J Hypertens 2000;13(8):934-939.)

Isles[34] suggested that patients with malignant hypertension can be considered in three groups, each with a different renal prognosis with respect to renal outcome: (1) patients whose serum creatinine is less than 300 μmol/L (3.4 mg/dL) at presentation, who do well with effective antihypertensive therapy; (2) patients with chronic renal failure (serum creatine >300 μmol/L) who do not require renal dialysis immediately, but often progress to end-stage renal failure; and (3) a small group with acute renal failure.

This suggests that in malignant hypertension, irreversible renal damage will usually have occurred if the serum creatinine is 300 μmol/L or higher, unless acute renal failure is superimposed. Nevertheless, other series have not seen such a division,[35] with patients with hypertensive emergency and a serum creatinine less than 300 μmol/L at presentation still showing a deterioration in overall renal function after long-term follow-up (mean 70 months), despite good BP management.

Renal failure was the most common cause of death in the west Birmingham series, and presenting urea and creatinine concentrations were independent predictors of survival.[23] The Aberdeen Hypertension Clinic report also found that serum creatinine at referral was an independent predictor of survival.[21] Unlike the urea and creatinine serum, urate levels do not appear to be predictive of the deterioration in renal function or overall survival.[36]

Retinopathy Changes in Hypertensive Emergency

The first and most widely used classification of hypertensive fundus changes is that of Keith, Wagener, and Barker (Table 46.2).[10] The strength of this classification was the correlation between clinical findings and prognosis, in which groups 3 and 4 had a poor prognosis compared with groups 1 and 2 (Fig. 46.3).

Dodson and coworkers[13] suggested a simpler system, dividing patients into two groups (Table 46.3). Group 1 patients were those with arteriolar tortuosity, silver and copper wire changes, and arteriolar-venous nipping (or "nicking"). These features are closely related to age and general arterial disease in addition to the BP, and the prognosis is good. Group 2 includes patients with retinal flame-shaped hemorrhages, cotton-wool spots, and hard exudates with or without papilledema. The prognosis of this group is substantially worse than that of group 1, and changes correlate well with prognosis (see Fig. 46.3). Recently, Wong and Mitchell[14] suggested the use of a new system that includes three categories: mild, moderate, and malignant retinopathy. Mild retinopathy that is associated with a modest risk for cardiovascular disease refers to generalized arteriolar narrowing, focal arteriolar narrowing, arteriovenous nicking, opacity (copper wiring) of arteriolar wall, or a combination of these signs. Moderate retinopathy that is strongly associated with cardiovascular morbidity and mortality refers to hemorrhage (blot, dot, or flame-shaped), microaneurysm, cotton-wool spot, hard exudate, or a combination of these signs.

KEITH, WAGENER, AND BARKER CLASSIFICATION

	Group 1 (benign hypertension)	Group 2 (more marked hypertension retinopathy)	Group 3 (mild angiospastic retinopathy)	Group 4 (malignant hypertension)
Retinal findings	Mild narrowing or sclerosis of the retinal arterioles	Moderate to marked sclerosis of the retinal arterioles Exaggerated arterial light reflex Venous compression at arteriovenous crossings	Retinal edema, cotton-wool spots and hemorrhages Sclerosis and spastic lesions of retinal arterioles Hard exudates including a macular star	All of the findings for groups 1-3, plus optic disk edema
Clinical features	No symptoms General good health	Blood pressure higher and more sustained than group 1 (asymptomatic) Good general health	Blood pressure high and sustained (symptomatic)	Cardiac and renal functions may be impaired Reduced survival

From Keith NM, Wagener HP, Barker NW. Some different types of essential hypertension: their course and prognosis. Am J Med Sci 1974;268(6):336-345.

Table 46.2 Keith, Wagener, and Barker classification.

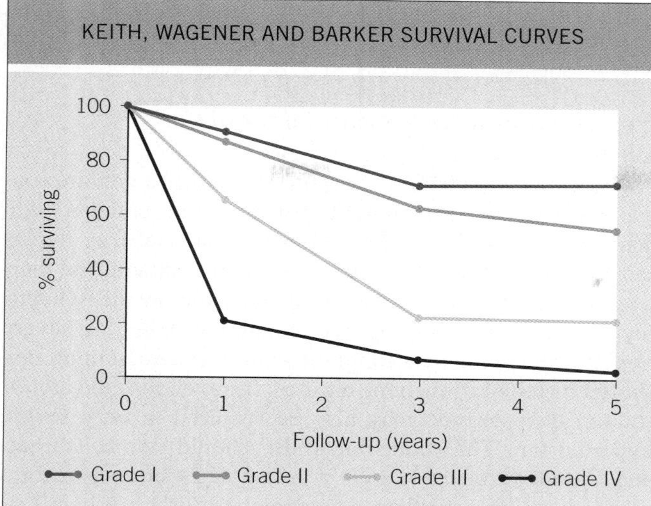

Figure 46.3 Keith, Wagener, and Barker survival curves according to grade of hypertensive retinopathy. (With permission from Keith NM, Wagener HP, Barker NW. Some different types of essential hypertension: their course and prognosis. Am J Med Sci 1974;268(6):336-345.)

REVISED GRADING SYSTEM FOR HYPERTENSIVE RETINOPATHY

Grade	Retinal Changes	Prognosis
I (nonmalignant)	Generalized arteriolar narrowing or tortuosity Focal constriction	May depend on blood pressure, but age and other concomitant cardiovascular risk factors equally important
II (malignant or accelerated)	Hemorrhages, hard exudates, cotton-wool spots, +/− optic disk swelling	Most cases die within 2 years if untreated In treated patients, median survival is now over 12 years

From Dodson PM, Lip GY, Eames SM, Gibson JM, Beevers DG. Hypertensive retinopathy: a review of existing classification systems and a suggestion for a simplified grading system. J Hum Hypertens 1996;10(2):93-98.

Table 46.3 Revised grading system for hypertensive retinopathy.

Malignant retinopathy that is strongly associated with death refers to signs of moderate retinopathy plus swelling of the optic disk. It should be noted that similar retinal appearances with hemorrhages and even papilledema can be seen in patients with severe anemia, connective tissue disease, and infective endocarditis. Furthermore, benign intracranial hypertension may cause bilateral papilledema, but is usually self-limiting and minimally symptomatic. Nevertheless, severe hypertension and lone bilateral papilledema may represent a variant of malignant hypertension, with similar clinical features and prognosis.[22]

Hypertensive Encephalopathy

Hypertensive encephalopathy refers to the presence of symptoms or signs of cerebral edema caused by breakthrough hyperperfusion from very severe hypertension or sudden increases in BP. This hypertensive emergency has to be distinguished from neurologic symptoms associated with high BP, including intracerebral or subarachnoid bleeding or lacunar infarcts.

Hypertensive encephalopathy is usually characterized by high BP and the onset of headache, nausea, and vomiting, followed by visual disturbances and fluctuating nonlocalizing neurologic symptoms, such as restlessness, confusion, and, if the hypertension is not treated, seizures and coma.[37] Severe retinopathy is frequently, although not universally, present. Hypertensive encephalopathy is usually associated with a history of hypertension that has been inadequately treated or in which previous treatment has been discontinued. Hypertensive encephalopathy is often indistinguishable from other acute neurologic complications of hypertension, including cerebral infarction, subarachnoidal bleeding, or intracerebral hemorrhage. The only definite criterion to confirm diagnosis of hypertensive encephalopathy is a prompt improvement in the patient's condition in response to antihypertensive therapy.[38] This syndrome is now considered to be very rare, partly because of the more efficient detection and management of hypertension. The increasing use of computed tomography (CT) and magnetic resonance imaging (MRI) has demonstrated that many patients believed initially to have encephalopathy had instead cerebral infarcts, hemorrhages, or space-occupying intracranial lesions.

Severe Hypertension with Acute Stroke

The approach to the management of severe hypertension during the acute phase of stroke has been less well researched. This is not an uncommon problem, because up to 80% of patients admitted with acute stroke will have increased BP. However, by day 10 after an ischemic stroke, two thirds of these patients will be normotensive, even without treatment. This therefore presents a problem on how best to identify patients who are truly in need of antihypertensive treatment, and to provide benefit rather than harm.[39] It is possible that the increase in BP may actually have a protective role in the acute phase of stroke. In healthy people, cerebral blood flow is usually kept constant by autoregulatory mechanisms. After a stroke, these "usual" autoregulatory mechanisms are lost, or at least impaired, which means that the perfusion in the ischemic areas at risk of stroke progression become pressure-dependent, and the areas surrounding the area of infarct are most at risk. It is therefore imperative that rapid reduction in BP and hypotension be avoided in the acute period after stroke.

The hazards of aggressive treatment of hypertension after a stroke are well documented. In a randomized, placebo-controlled trial comparing nimodipine with placebo in stroke patients, no benefits were found from active treatment, and there was a trend for this drug to be harmful.[40] The consensus therefore is that, in acute stroke, patients with hypertension should be watched and not treated. Current national guidelines recommend lowering blood pressure during stroke only if end-organ damage is present or if systolic/diastolic blood pressures exceed 220/120 or 185/110 mm Hg in patients ineligible and in those eligible to receive thrombolytic drug therapy, respectively.[41,42]

The Acute Candesartan Cilexetil Therapy in Stroke Survivors (ACCESS) study assessed the safety of modest BP reduction by candesartan cilexetil in the early treatment of stroke. The trial was stopped prematurely when 342 patients (339 valid) had been randomized, because the cumulative 12-month mortality and the number of vascular events differed significantly in favor of the candesartan cilexetil group (odds ratio, 0.475; 95% confidence interval [CI], 0.252-0.895). The study showed that early antihypertensive therapy with candesartan cilexetil is a safe therapeutic option when there is need for lowering BP.[43] Only two randomized trials addressing the value of antihypertensive treatment after a stroke are available. Carter[44] studied 97 stroke patients with severe hypertension (BP >160/110 mm Hg) within 2 weeks of admission to hospital who were subsequently randomly assigned to active or no treatment. Mortality in the treated group was significantly decreased, 20.4% at the end of the 2- to 5-year follow-up, compared with 43.8% in the control limb, although no benefit was seen for those aged 65 years or more. In the multicenter Hypertension-Stroke Cooperative Study,[45] 452 hypertensive stroke survivors were randomly assigned to receive an antihypertensive agent or placebo, but total mortality and stroke rates were unchanged in the two arms; in a subgroup analysis, African Americans did, however, appear to have some benefit from treatment. Meta-analysis of these intervention studies in hypertensive stroke survivors, together with two other studies with atenolol in patients with transient ischemic attacks, showed a borderline significant reduction in stroke recurrence in the active treatment group.[46]

The Perindopril Protection Against Recurrent Stroke Study (PROGRESS) study[47] investigated the value of indapamide with or without perindopril in stroke survivors, some of whom had a very recent stroke (see Chapter 43). Over-rapid decreases in BP were avoided, but these drugs were associated with fewer second strokes in both normotensive and hypertensive individuals.

Severe Hypertension with Intracerebral Hemorrhage

As a result of intracerebral hemorrhage, intracerebral pressure rises and higher intra-arterial pressure is required to perfuse the brain adequately. In this condition, hypertension may be a result of increased intracerebral pressure and may resolve spontaneously within 48 hours.[38]

Rapid reduction in BP may indeed prevent further bleeding, but at the risk of cerebral hypoperfusion.[48]

Thus there is no consensus on the advisability of reducing BP in these patients.[49] Two prospective studies, the Antihypertensive Treatment in Acute Cerebral Hemorrhage (ATACH) pilot study and the Intensive Blood Pressure Reduction in Acute Cerebral hemorrhage (INTERACT) study will answer the question of whether aggressive control of BP during the first hours after onset of intracerebral hemorrhage can improve outcome. In the meantime, BP reduction should not exceed 20% of pretreatment BP level.[50] If BP is extremely elevated (diastolic pressure greater than 140 mm Hg) for more than 20 minutes, intesintravenous treatment is recommended.

Hypertensive Left Ventricular Failure

Hypertension can lead to heart failure by a number of mechanisms (see Chapter 41). Severe hypertension results in a significant increase in afterload and causes decompensation of the failing heart. These factors are accompanied by myocardial fibrosis, probably related to activation of angiotensin II and aldosterone.

Hypertension with Myocardial Infarction or Unstable Angina

An excessively high BP (>180/110 mm Hg) is a definite contraindication to thrombolytic treatment in patients with acute myocardial infarction. After exclusion of true hypertensive emergencies by examination of the patient, the therapeutic strategy should be focused on protecting the ischemic myocardium. The appropriate initial treatment of severe hypertension with a concomitant acute myocardial infarction should include intravenous nitrates. Intravenous labetalol or sodium nitroprusside may also be required in very severe hypertension. The reduction of BP should not be abrupt, and a gradual reduction over a period of 24 hours is recommended, so that further myocardial or brain ischemia is avoided. Once the systolic BP is reduced to less than 180 mm Hg, thrombolytic therapy may be administered. Alternatives such as primary percutaneous transluminal coronary angioplasty should be considered in suitable patients.

Hypertension with Aortic Dissection

Aortic dissection occurs from an intimal tear that allows the passage of blood into the media, creating a false subintimal channel contained externally by the outer medial and adventitial layers of the aorta (Fig. 46.4). With each systolic pulse, the shear stresses extend the dissection either proximally or distally, potentially leading to cardiac tamponade, aortic regurgitation, aortic rupture, or occlusion of side branches, with end-organ ischemia.

Predisposing factors include hypertension, atherosclerosis, cystic medial necrosis, and Marfan's syndrome. The majority of patients are men who are older than 50 years, but pregnant women can also be affected in labor, particularly if they have Marfan's syndrome. Typically, dissection presents with a sudden, severe, retrosternal chest pain that radiates posteriorly to the interscapular region or the base of the neck. Signs may include new aortic regurgitation, a difference in BP between the two arms, absent pulses, or evidence of hemorrhage. The condition may also present with an acute

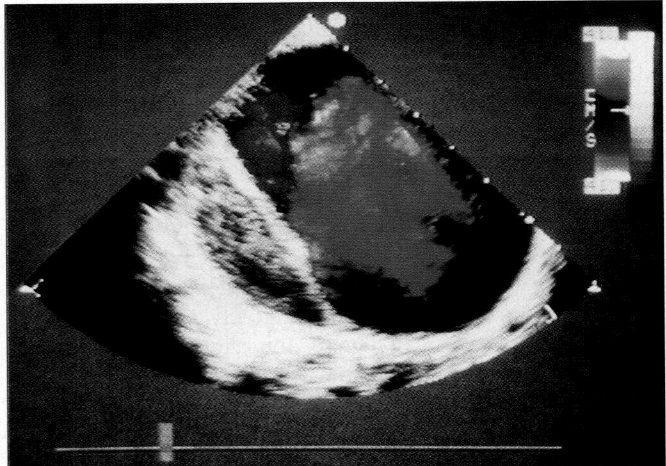

Figure 46.4 Transesophageal echocardiogram showing dissecting aortic aneurysm.

abdomen, stroke, or myocardial infarction. Most untreated patients with acute aortic dissection die within 1 year, and most of the deaths occur within 2 weeks. Once diagnosis is suspected, attempts should be made to decrease the shear stress to the aortic wall with suitable agents. BP should be reduced within 15 to 30 minutes to the lowest tolerated level that preserves adequate organ perfusion.

Severe Preeclampsia or Eclampsia

Preeclampsia

Pregnancy-induced hypertension (BP >140/90 mm Hg) after the 20th week of pregnancy that is associated with proteinuria (>300 mg/L) is often referred to as preeclampsia. This commonly occurs in primigravidas and marks a severe, acute change in the mother's condition. Although preeclampsia is defined as presenting after 20 weeks, it may occur earlier or become evident only after delivery. The incidence of proteinuric preeclampsia in the United Kingdom is of the order of 1 in 20 to 30 pregnancies, with higher rates in women with prepregnancy hypertension.

Clinical symptoms are common, with generalized puffiness, frontal headaches, visual symptoms (jagged, angular flashes at the periphery of the visual fields; loss of vision in areas) caused by cerebral edema. There may be epigastric pain because of hepatic edema. On examination, the BP may be high with a sharp increase in proteinuria. Usually, hypertension precedes proteinuria, but the converse is occasionally encountered. Blood pressures are usually unstable at rest, and circadian rhythm is altered, first with a loss of physiologic nocturnal dipping and, in severe cases, "reverse dipping" with the BPs seen at night. Papilledema may be seen on funduscopy. There may be brisk reflexes and ankle clonus. Edema is less reliable because mild pretibial and facial edema are commonly found in normal pregnancy. Urgent antihypertensive and anticonvulsant treatment is needed.

Eclampsia

Eclampsia is a hypertensive emergency that is associated with a high incidence of both maternal and fetal death. Eclampsia occurs in approximately 1 pregnancy in 500. The condition resembles other forms of hypertensive encephalopathy, with the similar symptoms of headaches, nausea, vomiting, and convulsions. Blood pressures are invariably high and proteinuria (>300 mg/L) is almost always present. There may be gross edema and convulsions, and when they occur they usually develop in labor or in the puerperium. Convulsions may be preceded by auras, epigastric pain, apprehension, and hyperreflexia, although there is little or no warning in many cases. After intense tonic-clonic seizures, the patient may become stuporous or comatose. Another complication common to eclampsia and hypertensive encephalopathy is cortical blindness, which results in visual loss caused by petechial hemorrhages and focal edema in the occipital cortex. Other complications include pulmonary edema, renal failure, hepatic failure, papilledema, retinal hemorrhages or even detachment, and cerebrovascular accidents.

DIAGNOSTIC TECHNIQUES

Diagnostic tests in hypertensive crises are dependent upon the condition and the clinical state of the patient. In severe hypertensive emergencies, such as aortic dissection, hypertensive left ventricular failure, and hypertensive encephalopathy, the patient may be far too ill to undertake all the "routine" investigations for hypertension, and the strategy is to stabilize the patient, make the diagnosis, and correct the problem. In contrast, many patients with hypertensive emergency present with only mild symptoms of visual disturbance, headaches, or dizziness, allowing full investigation and exclusion of secondary causes of hypertension. All patients will need urine analysis, ECG, and tests of renal function. Otherwise, the general "work-up" of all patients with hypertensive crises (after stabilization) should include investigation of their hypertension, which has been discussed in Chapter 40. In particular, secondary causes of hypertension may be more common in hypertensive emergency and should thus be excluded in such patients.

Evaluation of Patients with Hypertensive Crisis

Early triage is critical in an effort to assure the most appropriate therapy for each patient.[51] A brief but thorough history should address the duration as well as the severity of hypertension, all current medications, including prescription and nonprescription drugs, and the use of recreational drugs. Direct questioning regarding the level of compliance with current antihypertensive medications may establish inadequacy of therapy. Information regarding neurologic, cardiovascular, and renal symptoms and specific manifestations, such as headache, seizures, chest pain, dyspnea, and edema, is important for the correct diagnosis. A history of other comorbid conditions and prior cardiovascular or renal disease is critical for the initial evaluation.

Physical assessment should start with BP measurement in both arms, with an appropriate size cuff. A careful cardiovascular examination as well as a thorough neurologic examination, including mental status, should be conducted. A careful funduscopic examination should be performed to detect hemorrhages, exudates, and papilledema.

Initial laboratory evaluation should include urinalysis with sediment examination, an immediate chemistry profile, blood count, and an ECG. Laboratory results together with a complete history and thorough physical examination should enable a clinical assessment of the degree of target organ involvement and should facilitate the selection of an appropriate antihypertensive agent for initial treatment.

Proteinuria, red blood cells, and/or cellular casts in the urine are suggestive of renal parenchymal disease. Anemia with fragmented red blood cells suggests microangiopathic hemolytic anemia. Electrolyte abnormalities and evidence of renal dysfunction may suggest secondary hypertension. The ECG should identify evidence of coronary ischemia and left ventricular hypertrophy, and pulse deficits should raise the question of aortic dissection. A CT scan of the head should be considered when the clinical examination suggests cerebrovascular ischemia or hemorrhage or when the patient is comatose. The initial evaluation should help to decide whether to treat the patient with hypertensive crisis as an emergency or urgency. The decision to treat as an emergency should prompt immediate admission to an intensive care unit for intravenous treatment and continuous BP monitoring.

MANAGEMENT

The urgency of interventions in hypertensive crises depends on the clinical syndrome. For example, uncomplicated malignant phase hypertension is associated with target organ damage, which occurs over days or weeks rather than minutes, and can be referred to as a hypertensive urgency rather than an emergency. By contrast, hypertensive encephalopathy, hypertensive left ventricular failure, and aortic dissection can be immediately life-threatening and are more typical hypertensive emergencies. Similarly, eclampsia (or severe preeclampsia) can result in a high maternal and fetal morbidity and mortality if immediate and effective antihypertensive therapy is not initiated.

In hypertensive urgencies, in which acute target-organ damage is absent, immediate and rapid reduction of BP with parenteral drugs is rarely indicated, and oral antihypertensive therapy can be given. Indeed, aggressive treatment with parenteral drugs may place the patient at unnecessary risk, as serious and sometimes fatal complications of treatment have been reported. Parenteral therapy requires intensive care monitoring and should be restricted to severe hypertensive emergencies, in which complications such as hypertensive encephalopathy, left ventricular failure, and aortic dissection are present. Some of the commonly used parenteral drugs are discussed further in the following sections. Sublingual nifedipine, which was once considered as a first-line drug, should not be used in view of the negligible oral absorption, the unpredictable hypotensive effects, and an increased risk of arrhythmias, stroke, or worsening cardiac ischemia or infarction.[52] With other more effective agents available, clonidine is now a less popular choice for the treatment of hypertensive crises.

Sodium Nitroprusside

Sodium nitroprusside is a potent direct-acting vasodilator that acts on both arteriolar and venous vessels, reducing cardiac afterload and preload. It is a potentially dangerous drug and should be administered only in the intensive care unit where cardiac monitoring and constant, preferably invasive, BP monitoring are available. The major limitation to the use of nitroprusside is its metabolism to a toxic metabolite, thiocyanate, potentially leading to the development of cyanide or, rarely, thiocyanate toxicity, which may be fatal. This problem, which is manifested by clinical deterioration, altered mental status, and lactic acidosis, can be minimized by treatment for as short a time as possible using the lowest dose possible and by careful monitoring of the patient. Treatment for a prolonged period (>24 to 48 hours), underlying renal insufficiency, and the use of doses that exceed the capacity of the body to detoxify cyanide (more than 2 μg/kg/min) increase the risk of cyanide accumulation. Thiocyanate accumulates during prolonged infusion, and concentrations should be measured after 48 hours to ensure that they do not exceed 1.7 mmol/L. Thiocyanate psychosis occurs above this concentration, and the infusion should therefore be stopped. An infusion of sodium thiosulfate can be used in affected patients to provide a sulfur donor to detoxify cyanide into thiocyanate. Nitroprusside should not be given to pregnant women.

The drug is administered as a continuous titrated infusion, with a rapid onset of action (1 to 2 minutes) and short duration of action (1 to 5 minutes). It is inactivated by light and should therefore be protected during the infusion. The recommended starting dose of nitroprusside is 0.25 to 0.5 μg/kg/min. This can be increased as necessary to a maximum dose of 8 to 10 μg/kg/min, although use of these higher doses should generally be avoided or limited to a maximum duration of 10 minutes. The aim is to achieve a diastolic BP of 90 to 110 mm Hg over 2 to 3 hours.

Labetalol

Labetalol is a combined alpha and beta blocker that can be administered either by bolus injection or by intravenous infusion. It may produce severe and unpredictable hypotension and is contraindicated in patients with asthma, chronic obstructive lung disease, congestive heart failure, bradycardia, and atrioventricular block. Nevertheless, labetalol is safe in patients with active coronary disease, because it does not increase the heart rate. Its rapid onset of action (5 minutes or less) makes it the only beta blocker that is useful in the treatment of hypertensive emergencies. Labetalol can be given as an intravenous bolus or infusion. The bolus dose is 20 mg initially, followed by 20 to 80 mg every 10 minutes to a total dose of 300 mg. The infusion rate is 0.5 to 2 mg/min.

Nitrates

Intravenous nitrates (e.g., glyceryl trinitrate) cause venous dilatation at low doses and both arteriolar and venous dilatation at higher doses. They are of limited value in hypertensive encephalopathy, because of headache, which frequently occurs with the high doses required to reduce BP. Nitrates are most useful in patients with symptomatic coronary disease and in other situations, such as postoperative hypertension or hypertensive heart failure. The initial dose of glyceryl trinitrate is 5 μg/min, which can be increased as necessary to a maximum of 100 μg/min. The onset of action is 2 to 5 minutes, and the duration of action is 5 to 10 minutes. Headache (as a result of direct vasodilatation) and tachycardia (resulting from reflex sympathetic activation) are the primary side effects.

Fenoldopam

Fenoldopam is a selective postsynaptic dopaminergic (DA_1) receptor agonist with weak α_2-antagonistic properties. Fenoldopam is a natriuretic agent that has a potent vasodilator activity affecting primarily the renal vasculature.[53]

The onset of action is within 5 minutes, with the maximal response being achieved by 15 minutes. The duration of action is 30 to 60 minutes with the pressure gradually returning to pretreatment values without rebound upon termination of the drug. Several clinical trials showed the effectiveness of intravenous fenoldopam in the treatment of severe hypertension and hypertensive crisis. At a dose of 0.2 to 0.5 μg/kg/min, fenoldopam decreases BP to desired levels within 5 to 40 minutes. Side effects include headache, flushing, and dizziness. Tachycardia has occasionally been noted, and a dose-related increase in intraocular pressure has been observed in normotensive and hypertensive patients. It seems that fenoldopam is comparable to sodium nitroprusside and can be the drug of choice in severely hypertensive patients with impaired renal function.

Nicardipine

Nicardipine is a dihydropyridine calcium antagonist with high vascular selectivity that can be administered intravenously.[54] The onset of action of intravenous nicardipine is between 5 and 10 minutes with duration of action of 15 to 90 minutes. It is an effective antihypertensive agent that decreases afterload by reducing total peripheral resistance without reducing cardiac output. Nicardipine improves left ventricular ejection fraction and pumping activity, both in normal and failing hearts. The drug dilates more selectively the cerebral and coronary arteries than the remainder of the arterial tree, without changing heart rate. It may preserve tissue perfusion and therefore may be advantageous in patients with ischemic disorders, such as coronary, cerebrovascular, and peripheral vascular disease. The drug is given as a continuous infusion at a starting dose of 5 mg/h followed by increments of 2.5 mg/h every 5 minutes until either reaching a maximal dose of 30 mg/h or achieving the desired reduction in BP. Side effects include headache, hypotension, and nausea. Nicardipine is as effective as sodium nitroprusside in patients with severe postoperative hypertension. Patients receiving intravenous nicardipine can then be easily switched to oral medication.

Esmolol

Esmolol is an ultra-short-acting β_1-selective adrenergic blocker. The onset of action of this agent is within 60 to 120 seconds, and the duration of action is extremely short, about 10 to 30 minutes. This characteristic provides a significant advantage because it is possible to titrate esmolol easily to the desired effect. The drug can be administered either as a bolus injection or as a continuous intravenous infusion. The recommended loading dose is a bolus of 250 to 500 μg/kg/min followed by an infusion of 50 to 100 μg/kg/min. Esmolol is frequently combined with direct vasodilators to provide a more desirable hemodynamic profile. The negative chronotropic effect produced by esmolol may be beneficial in patients with ischemic heart disease.

Urapidil

Urapidil is a selective postsynaptic α_1-adrenoreceptor antagonist with strong vasodilating properties. The fact that it also antagonizes the presynaptic $5HT_1A$ (hydroxytryptamine) receptors explains the lack of reflex tachycardia in response to peripheral vasodilatation. Urapidil has a rapid onset of action, with a response rate of 81% to 100% in hypertensive emergencies.[55] Urapidil is given as an intravenous bolus at a dose of 12.5 to 25 mg followed by a continuous infusion at a rate of 5 to 40 mg/h. It has no effect on coronary sinus blood flow, myocardial oxygen consumption, and myocardial lactate extraction, and it does not increase intracranial pressure. Adverse effects occur in 2% of all patients and include hypotension, headache, and dizziness. Urapidil is safe and efficient in intraoperative hypertensive crisis. Urapidil is equally effective compared to sodium nitroprusside with fewer adverse effects. Therefore urapidil is a reasonable alternative to sodium nitroprusside in the treatment of hypertensive emergency, especially in intraoperative hypertensive crisis.

Enalaprilat

Enalaprilat is the only available angiotensin-converting enzyme (ACE) inhibitor that can be administered intravenously. Enalaprilat lowers BP within 15 to 30 minutes, but the BP response in hypertensive emergencies is unpredictable, in part because of variable degrees of plasma volume expansion. The initial recommended dose for enalaprilat is 0.625 to 1.25 mg administered over 5 minutes. The maximal single dose should not exceed 5 mg for patients receiving diuretics and 1.25 mg for patients with renal impairment.[2] The initial dose can be repeated after 1 hour if clinical response is inadequate. The total daily dose should not exceed 20 mg. In patients with severe renal insufficiency the dose should be decreased, because the compound is excreted primarily by the kidney.

Enalaprilat may induce a dramatic fall in BP in patients who are volume depleted by prior dietary sodium restriction or diuretic use. Because enalaprilat may induce severe hypotension in volume-depleted patients, it should be used with caution in patients who are at risk for cerebral hypotensive episode. A low dose of 0.625 mg may be adequate for initial treatment of hypertensive crisis.

The most common adverse effect is hypotension. The risk for hypotension increases in patients with evidence of renal hypertension, volume-depleted patients, and patients with prior use of diuretics. Enalaprilat is contraindicated in patients with evidence of bilateral renal artery stenosis or in patients with unilateral stenosis of a single kidney.[56] Thus enalaprilat is particularly useful in hypertensive emergencies associated with congestive heart failure or high renin levels, and can be easily replaced by oral enalapril for long-term maintenance therapy.

Arterial Vasodilators

Diazoxide and hydralazine, both arterial vasodilators, were previously popular in the management of hypertensive crises. Diazoxide used to be administered by rapid bolus injection, but this led to a number of cases of cerebral infarction and death. It can be given by smaller and more regular bolus doses or by intravenous infusion, but this is rarely indicated. A beta blocker such as propranolol or labetalol is usually given concurrently to block reflex tachycardia. It is recommended that diazoxide should not be used in patients with angina pectoris, myocardial infarction, pulmonary edema, or a dissecting aortic aneurysm. Diazoxide can also cause marked fluid retention, and a loop diuretic may need to be added if edema or otherwise unexplained weight gain is noted. Diazoxide is also longer acting and, in the currently recommended doses, requires less monitoring than nitroprusside, because the peak effect is seen within 15 minutes and lasts for 4 to 24 hours.

Hydralazine, like diazoxide, is a direct arteriolar vasodilator with little or no effect on the venous circulation. Reflex tachycardia is associated with both diazoxide and hydralazine, so the same precautions apply in patients with underlying coronary disease or a dissecting aortic aneurysm, and a beta blocker should be given concurrently. Hydralazine remains the agent of choice in the management of severe preeclampsia, but should be avoided in patients with known or suspected coronary disease. The hypotensive response to hydralazine is less predictable than that seen with other parenteral agents, and its current use is mainly limited to pregnant women. The initial dose is 5 to 10 mg intravenously, with a maximum dose of 20 mg. The decrease in BP begins within 10 to 30 minutes and lasts 2 to 4 hours.

Phentolamine

Phentolamine is a parenteral nonspecific α-adrenergic blocking agent with rapid onset and short-lasting hypotensive effect. It is given intravenously in boluses of 5 to 10 mg as necessary. Adverse effects include tachycardia, vomiting, and headache. In patients with coronary artery disease phentolamine may induce angina pectoris or myocardial infarction. It is specifically useful in treatment of catecholamine-mediated hypertensive crises.[56] However, it is not consistently effective in other types of hypertensive emergencies.

Hypertensive Urgencies

The initial aim of treatment in hypertensive urgency is to decrease the BP by 20% to 25% during the first 24 hours and to a target diastolic BP of around 100 mm Hg over the next few days, using combination therapy if necessary. The maximum initial decrease in BP should not exceed 25% of the presenting value, to avoid underperfusion of the brain, heart, and kidneys.[6,57] Blood pressure should be lowered gradually over the first few days with oral therapy alone. Parenteral therapy is rarely required. A gradual reduction in BP will allow adaptation of disordered cerebral autoregulation and avoid target organ ischemia.

The first-line oral antihypertensive agent is either a calcium channel blocker (such as nifedipine retard) or a beta blocker (e.g., bisoprolol) (Fig. 46.5). An appropriate dose is nifedipine retard 10 to 20 mg in the tablet formulation, and the dose can be repeated or increased at intervals of 4 to 6 hours to bring about a gradual reduction in BP. Sublingual nifedipine capsules should not be used, because they are associated with unpredictable decreases in BP, visual loss, cerebral infarction, and myocardial infarction, although these can be minimized if the tablet formulation is used.[52,58,59] The dihydropyridine calcium channel blocker nicardipine has also been used safely in hypertensive urgencies, possibly with less risk of over-rapid BP reduction.

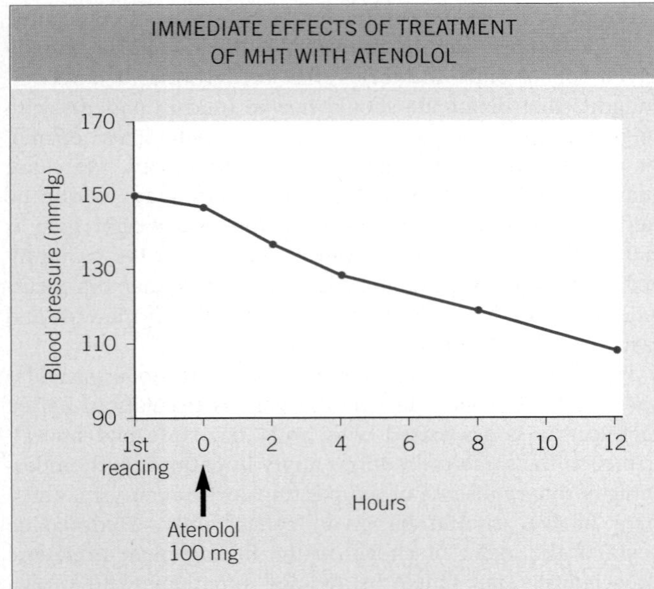

Figure 46.5 Immediate effects of treatment of malignant hypertension with 100 mg atenolol.

Beta blockers are useful alternatives, but should be avoided in patients with asthma, bradycardia, and left ventricular failure. It is sensible to start with small doses, such as 25 mg daily of atenolol, increasing the dose as necessary.[58] The combination of oral atenolol and nifedipine is often a well-tolerated and effective regimen.

Diuretics should be restricted to patients with evidence of fluid overload. Many patients are mildly volume depleted, presumably secondary to pressure-related diuresis and activation of the renin-angiotensin system. The ACE inhibitors may produce rapid and dangerous decreases in BP, particularly in patients with renovascular disease,[60] which may be undiagnosed in the acute situation, and these drugs are therefore not recommended as first-line therapy in hypertensive urgency.

Hypertensive Encephalopathy

Sodium nitroprusside is the drug of choice when neurologic damage is believed to be imminent. Parenteral labetalol, fenoldopam, nicardipine, urapidil, and nitrates have also been successfully used in the treatment of hypertensive encephalopathy. Rarely, diazoxide and hydralazine have been used, albeit with some caution. It must be stressed, however, that this syndrome is very rare, and when the diagnosis is suspected, CT or MRI scanning frequently reveals evidence of cerebral infarction or hemorrhage.

Hypertension with Stroke

Cerebral autoregulation is commonly disturbed after an acute stroke, and excessive antihypertensive treatment may only serve to worsen the cerebral damage. Antihypertensive treatment may lead to rapid and dangerous decreases in BP and should be administered only in the case of very severe increases in BP (diastolic BP greater than 130 mm Hg). In these cases, oral treatment with small doses of nifedipine or atenolol may be required. Parenteral treatment is almost always contraindicated. The calcium channel blocker, nimodipine, has beneficial effects on cerebral vasospasm after subarachnoid hemorrhage, but these effects do not appear to be related to the small decrease in BP with this drug (see Chapter 43).

Hypertensive Left Ventricular Failure

In addition to the conventional management of hypertensive left ventricular failure with opioids and loop diuretics, intravenous sodium nitroprusside or fenoldopam can be used to reduce preload and afterload when the BP is very high. Nitrates may also be used but are less potent.

Hypertension with Acute Coronary Syndromes

An increase in the systemic vascular resistance leads to an increase in left ventricular wall tension and myocardial oxygen demand. In patients with severe hypertension and angina, intravenous nitrates are valuable because they reduce systemic vascular resistance and improve coronary perfusion. Beta blockers are of proven prognostic value in acute myocardial infarction. In severe hypertension, an intravenous infusion may be necessary, and labetalol has been successfully used. Sodium nitroprusside should be reserved for resistant cases, as it may exacerbate coronary ischemia. Nifedipine (especially in the short-acting capsule form) must not be used in unstable angina or recent acute myocardial infarction.

Hypertension with Aortic Dissection

The treatment of choice in type B aortic dissection (distal to the subclavian artery) is prompt and effective control of BP. All patients should be treated pharmacologically to reduce the BP to a systolic pressure of around 100 mm Hg, to reduce the heart rate to 60 to 70 beats per minute, to reduce the force of systolic ejection and aortic shear stress, and to limit the size of the dissection. Initial treatment should consist of labetalol or a combination of intravenous nicardipine or fenoldopam or sodium nitroprusside with intravenous beta-blocking agent, most commonly metoprolol or esmolol. Used alone, sodium nitroprusside increases the velocity of ventricular contraction so that simultaneous beta blockade is obligatory (see Chapter 11).

Preeclampsia and Eclampsia

The main aim of antihypertensive treatment is to reduce the risk of maternal cerebral hemorrhage. In the majority of cases, delivery of the baby leads to an improvement in the clinical state, although this can take up to 1 week. Eclampsia has been reported to occur postnatally and intensive monitoring should continue for up to 1 week after delivery.

The aim of antihypertensive treatment should be to reduce the diastolic BP to between 90 and 105 mm Hg. Prolonged periods of hypotension and precipitous decreases in BP may lead to a reduction in uteroplacental blood flow. In milder cases, BP can be reduced with oral agents. Nifedipine tablets (10 to 20 mg), hydralazine (25 to 50 mg), and atenolol (50 to 100 mg) have all been used, if necessary in combination. Hydralazine remains the most commonly used parenteral agent in the urgent management of severe preeclampsia and eclampsia. However, reflex tachycardia often leads to sustained high levels of systolic pressure in the presence of acceptable levels of diastolic pressure. This is a more dangerous situation, because a high systolic BP may lead to cerebral hemorrhage. Beta blockade will help to prevent this effect, and is to be recommended when intravenous hydralazine is used. Intravenous labetalol is effective in reducing and maintaining acceptable BP, although fetal and neonatal bradycardia may result from fetal β-adrenergic blockade. In addition to management of the hypertensive emergency, it may be necessary to control seizures. Magnesium sulfate is the drug of choice in this instance and is of proven benefit in preventing recurrent seizures.

PROGNOSIS

There has been a significant improvement in median survival time in patients with hypertensive emergency presenting after 1980, compared with earlier cases. The median 5-year survival was 28.2% for those presenting before 1970, 49.3% for those presenting between 1970 and 1979, and 74.0% for those presenting after 1980 (Fig. 46.6).[31]

This finding parallels the advent of effective antihypertensive therapy, resulting in an improvement in the prognosis,

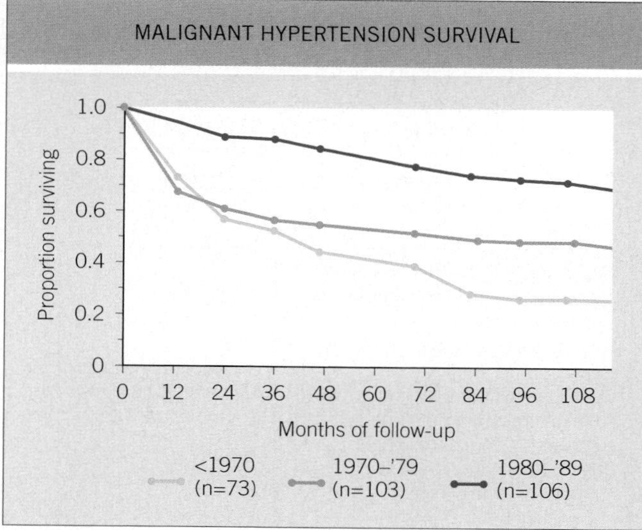

Figure 46.6 Survival of patients with malignant hypertension presenting before 1970 and during 1970-79 and 1980-89 in the west Birmingham malignant hypertension series. (With permission from Lip GY, Beevers M, Beevers DG. Does renal function improve after diagnosis of malignant phase hypertension? J Hypertens 1997; 15(11):1309-1315.)

especially with the prevention of strokes, renal failure, and heart disease. Nevertheless, the mortality remains high in black patients (especially males), who tended to have higher BPs and more renal impairment at presentation. In most series, renal failure was the most common cause of death, followed by cardiovascular complications such as strokes and heart attacks. The duration of previously known hypertension, age at first referral, and renal function (presenting urea and creatinine concentrations) are independent predictors of survival.[20,31] Better BP control, defined as mean diastolic BP less than 100 mm Hg at follow-up, improves prognosis on univariate analysis (Fig. 46.7).

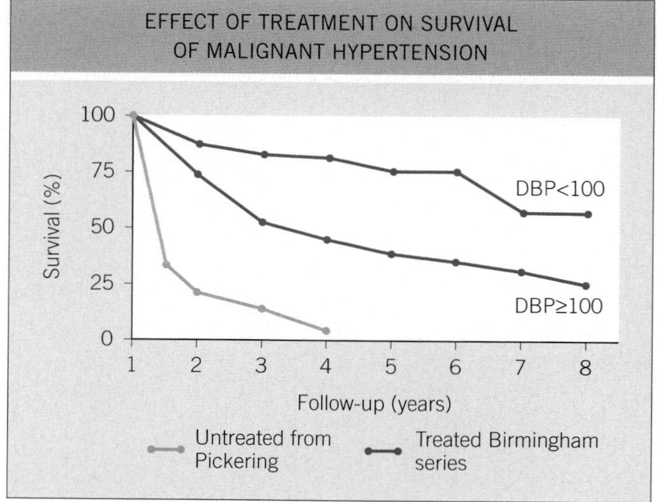

Figure 46.7 Survival of patients with malignant hypertension. Untreated patients (Pickering) are compared with treated Birmingham patients according to diastolic BP (DBP) control (i.e., last recorded diastolic BP <100 mm Hg compared with ≥100 mm Hg).

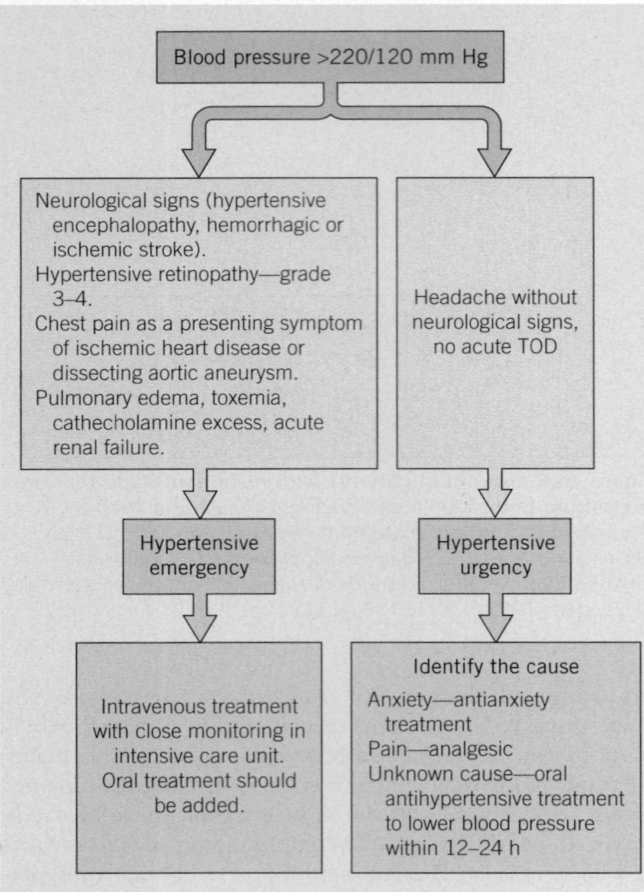

Figure 46.8 Algorithm that details the difference between a hypertensive urgency and a hypertensive emergency. Severe hypertension does not constitute a hypertensive emergency, and is best classified as an urgency. The true emergencies are acute aortic dissection, gross left ventricular failure with very high BPs, eclampsia or preeclampsia, and hypertensive encephalopathy.

SUMMARY

Severe hypertension in a relatively symptomless patient does not constitute a hypertensive emergency, and is best classified as an urgency. In such patients, parenteral drugs should not be used, as they may cause cerebral or myocardial ischemia, especially with overenthusiastic reduction of BP. The true emergencies are acute aortic dissection, gross left ventricular failure with very high BPs, eclampsia or preeclampsia, and hypertensive encephalopathy. In the vast majority of severely hypertensive patients, the BP should be reduced gradually with orally active drugs, and long-term control of BP is probably the most important factor influencing prognosis (Fig 46.8).

chapter 47

Diagnosis and Treatment of Secondary Hypertension

David Martins and Keith C. Norris

Definition

- Secondary hypertension refers to those cases of hypertension in which a cause is known for the elevated blood pressure.

Key Features

- Although the precise mechanism for the elevation in blood pressure is unknown in many of the cases, abnormalities of renal and neuroendocrine systems have been observed in most cases of secondary hypertension.
- Many atypical clinical and laboratory features characterize cases of secondary hypertension. Many of these features are relatively specific for some of the cases and should guide the diagnostic evaluation for secondary hypertension.

Treatment

- Cases of secondary hypertension are often refractory to empirical antihypertensive drug therapy. Treatment targeted to underlying abnormalities usually alleviates and may even cure the hypertension depending on the cause and duration of elevated blood pressure.

The estimated proportion of the cases of secondary hypertension among patients with systemic hypertension ranges from about 5% to 10% depending on the study setting. The results of 3783 patients reported by Sinclair and colleagues[1] and 665 patients by Rudnick and coworkers[2] who were studied in primary care settings are shown in Table 47.1. The 4429 patients studied by Anderson and associates,[3] also shown in Table 47.1, were consecutively referred to a blood pressure clinic for possible secondary hypertension. These studies indicate few patients with systemic hypertension will have a specific identifiable cause for the elevated systemic blood pressure. Many of that subset will exhibit suggestive signs and/or symptoms on initial evaluation and should undergo further evaluation for a definitive etiology of their hypertension. The diseases more commonly known to be associated with systemic hypertension are listed in Table 47.2. The identification of an underlying cause is important because directed therapy can cure or better control the "secondary hypertension" in many of these patients.

ETIOLOGY

Renal Disorders

Renal Parenchymal Disease

Renal parenchymal disease is the most common cause of secondary hypertension in adults. It accounts for 2% to 5% of cases. Renal parenchymal disease can be acute or chronic, unilateral or bilateral, and is often but not always associated with reduced glomerular filtration, commonly termed renal insufficiency. Several mechanisms have been proposed for the elevated blood pressure in renal parenchymal disease. However, in patients with coexisting renal insufficiency the inability of the reduced functional renal mass to excrete salt and water in adequate amounts to maintain normal intravascular volume has been advanced as the most probable reason for the elevation in blood pressure, although additional neurohormonal factors including renin-angiotensin-aldosterone system, erythropoietin, adrenergic system, and baroreceptor activity may play a role. Thus with progressive renal disease, blood pressure becomes dependent on the abnormal fluid homeostasis leading to a volume-dependent hypertension. In patients on maintenance hemodialysis, elevated predialysis blood pressure levels tend to fall synchronously with ultrafiltration during a dialysis treatment, remaining depressed during the ensuing 24 hours before rising again during the second day.[4]

It has also been suggested that the accumulation of endogenous inhibitors of nitric oxide synthesis may play a pathogenetic role in this progressive rise in blood pressure on days in between dialysis in these patients.[5] Thus the pathophysiologic processes responsible for the elevation of blood pressure in patients with renal parenchymal disease without significant reduction in renal function are complex and remain poorly defined. The activation of the renin-angiotensin-aldosterone system is the best studied of the presently proposed neurohormonal contributors, and there may well be many other yet unknown mechanisms.

Renovascular Disease

Renovascular disease accounts for 1% to 2% of adult cases of secondary hypertension. It is, however, the most common cause of curable hypertension. Most cases of renovascular hypertension develop from a partial obstruction of one main renal artery, but only a branch need be involved and even segmental arterial obstruction has been reported to cause hypertension in over 10% of cases of renovascular disease.[6] Bilateral renovascular disease is less common, occurring only in 25% of the subjects in the Cooperative Study on Renovascular Hypertension.[7]

The elevated blood pressure in renovascular disease arises from a reduction in renal blood flow and the activation of the renin-angiotensin-aldosterone system, as shown in Figure. 47.1. When the degree of stenosis markedly impairs renal perfusion and glomerular filtration, particularly in bilateral cases, excessive intravascular volume may contribute to the resulting

THE PROPORTION OF THE VARIOUS DIAGNOSES IN PATIENTS WITH SECONDARY HYPERTENSION			
Diagnoses	**Rudnick et al (%)**	**Sinclair et al (%)**	**Anderson et al (%)**
Essential hypertension	94.0	92.1	89.5
Chronic renal disease	5.0	5.6	1.8
Renovascular disease	0.2	0.7	3.3
Cushing's syndrome	0.2	0.1	0.6
Oral contraceptive–induced	0.2	1.0	
Primary hyperaldosteronism		0.3	1.5
Pheochromocytoma		0.1	0.3
Coarctation of aorta	0.2		
Data from Sinclair et al,[1] Rudnick et al,[2] and Anderson et al.[3]			

Table 47.1 The proportion of the various diagnoses in patients with secondary hypertension.

hypertension. The partial obstruction of a main renal artery in adult patients with renovascular hypertension is most commonly caused by atherosclerosis or fibromuscular dysplasia. The other causes of renovascular obstruction are less common. Atherosclerotic disease is more preponderant in older men, in whom it accounts for about two thirds of the cases and tends to affect the proximal third of the main renal artery. Fibromuscular dysplasia is more common in young females. It accounts for about one third of the cases and tends to affect the distal two thirds and/or branches of the renal artery.

Renovascular hypertension was once reported to be less common in black than in white hypertensive individuals. It is now believed that the high prevalence of essential hypertension in the hypertensive blacks may mitigate the clinical decision to search for secondary causes, thereby masking the true prevalence of renovascular hypertension in this population. When cases are carefully selected and properly assessed, with arteriography performed in all subjects, the prevalence of renovascular hypertension in blacks approaches that in white hypertensives.[8]

Liddle's Syndrome

Liddle's syndrome is an autosomal dominant disorder that results from a mutation in the gene for the amiloride-sensitive sodium channel in the collecting duct of the kidney. Liddle's syndrome represents the prototype for a direct genetic linkage in hypertension. The resulting defective sodium channel is unresponsive to the mineralocorticoids and remains constitutively open, leading to unregulated sodium reabsorption and potassium secretion. The hypertension in these patients is a direct consequence of sodium retention and volume overload.

CAUSES OF SECONDARY HYPERTENSION			
Systolic and diastolic hypertension			
Renal Disorders	**Endocrine Disorders**	**Neuropsychologic Disorders**	**Other**
Renal parenchymal disease	Acromegaly	Intracranial hypertension	Coarctation of the Aorta
Acute and chronic	Hyperthyroidism	Brain tumor	Pregnancy-induced hypertension
glomerulonephritis	Hyperparathyroidism	Encephalitis	Polycythemia vera
Polycystic kidney disease	Adrenal	Respiratory acidosis	**Drugs**
Diabetic nephropathy	Cortical hyperfunction	Sleep apnea	Cyclosporin
Obstructive uropathy	Cushing's syndrome	Spinal cord transection	Erythropoietin
Neoplasms	Congenital adrenal hyperplasia	Quadriplegia	Phenylpropanolamine
Renal trauma	Primary hyperaldosteronism	Acute porphyria	
Radiation nephritis	Glucocorticoid-remediable	Polyneuritis	**Alcohol**
Pyelonephritis	aldosteronism	Diencephalic syndrome	**Substance abuse (e.g., cocaine,**
Renovascular disease	Mineralocorticoid hypertension	Familial dysautonomia	**amphetamines)**
Renal artery stenosis	Medullary hyperfunction	(Riley-Day)	
Renal artery thrombosis	Pheochromocytoma	Acute stress	
Renal artery embolism	Exogenous hormones	Postoperative	**Systolic hypertension**
Intrarenal vasculitis	Glucocorticoids	Postresuscitation	
Renal artery aneurysms	Mineralocorticoids	Sickle-cell crisis	**Increased cardiac output**
Renal artery	Sympathomimetics	Alcohol withdrawal	Aortic insufficiency
compression	Tyramine-containing foods	Pancreatitis	Arteriovenous fistula
Primary sodium retention	on MAOIs	Burns	Paget's disease
Liddle's syndrome	Oral contraceptives	Pain	Beriberi
Gordon's syndrome		Hypoglycemia	Rigidity of the aorta
Renin-producing tumors		Psychogenic hyperventilation	
MAOI, monoamine oxidase inhibitor.			

Table 47.2 Causes of secondary hypertension.

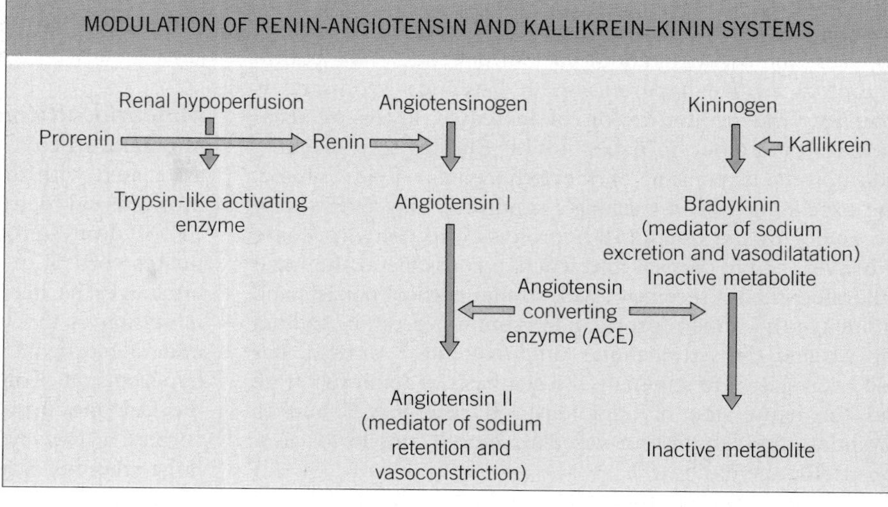

Figure 47.1 The pivotal role of angiotensin-converting enzyme (ACE) in the modulation of the renin-angiotensin system and the kallikrein-kinin system. Note the simultaneous activation of a vasoconstricting sodium-retaining system and deactivation of a vasodilatating sodium-excreting system by ACE.

Endocrine Disorders

Acromegaly

Acromegaly is a disorder of excessive growth hormone with significant cardiovascular manifestations. Although acromegaly is a relatively rare cause of secondary hypertension, 25% to 50% of patients with acromegaly will exhibit elevated blood pressure if they retain normal function of the rest of the pituitary gland.

The precise mechanism for the elevated blood pressure in patients with acromegaly is poorly defined. The administration of growth hormone has been shown to produce sodium retention, expansion of the extracellular fluid volume, and abnormalities in white blood cell sodium transport.[9] The presence of an increase in glomerular filtration rate, renal plasma flow, and sodium space, and a decrease in plasma renin activity (PRA) in patients with acromegaly suggest an apparent increase in the extracellular fluid. The increase in left ventricular mass and cardiac stroke volume frequently encountered in acromegaly as well as the associated obesity and insulin-resistant state may also play a role in the development of hypertension.

Hypothyroidism

Hypothyroidism is a thyroid hormone deficiency disorder that is often associated with clinically apparent cardiovascular signs and symptoms. The cardiovascular manifestations of hypothyroidism depend on the stage of the disease. In mild to moderate hypothyroidism there is an increased frequency of hypertension, particularly diastolic hypertension. Blood pressure drops as the disease progresses and hypotension supervenes in severe hypothyroidism.[10]

The pathophysiologic basis for the hypertension in hypothyroidism is unknown. Reduced cardiac output and increased total peripheral resistance have been documented in hypothyroidism. There is also a reduction in the total blood volume and a redistribution of blood flow, with mild reductions in cerebral and renal flow and significant reductions in cutaneous flow, which may lead to counterregulatory responses to increased systemic blood pressure.

Hyperthyroidism

Hyperthyroidism is a disorder of thyroid hormone excess and is also commonly associated with cardiovascular manifestations. An increase in systolic blood pressure is a common finding in hyperthyroidism.

Although the precise mechanism for hypertension in hyperthyroidism is unclear, a reduction in the systemic vascular resistance[11] and an increase in cardiac output, stroke volume index, mean systolic ejection rate, and velocity and extent of wall shortening have been reported.[12] Many of these changes in cardiac functions were once attributed to the high metabolic demand placed on the heart by peripheral tissues in hyperthyroidism. However, the increase in cardiac output is greater than would be expected on the basis of increased metabolic demand alone, suggesting thyroid hormones exert a direct cardiac stimulant effect that is independent of their effects on peripheral tissue metabolism.[13]

Hyperparathyroidism

Hyperparathyroidism is a disorder of parathyroid hormone excess. Hypertension is more common among patients with hyperparathyroidism than in the general population.[14] The pathophysiologic basis for this hypertension is multifactorial. The results of several studies evaluating the possible roles of hypercalcemia and renal function are conflicting. An increase in plasma renin activity and aldosterone levels has been reported in hyperparathyroidism. A close correlation has been demonstrated between parathyroid hormone and intracellular calcium, indicating that parathyroid hormone may act as an ionophore for calcium entry into the cells. However, correlation between blood pressure and intracellular calcium in patients with primary hyperparathyroidism has not been proved. The expression of a parathyroid hypertensive factor in hypertensive primary hyperparathyroid patients may be responsible for the elevated blood pressure in these patients.[15]

Adrenocortical Causes

Adrenocortical causes of secondary hypertension account for less than 1% of adult cases of secondary hypertension. Neoplastic and hyperplastic lesions of the adrenal cortex are associated with abnormal synthesis and secretion of adrenocortical androgens, glucocorticoids, and mineralocorticoids.

Cushing's Syndrome

Cushing's syndrome is a disorder of glucocorticoid excess. Hypertension occurs in about 80% of patients.[16] The pathophysiology of the hypertension in Cushing's syndrome is complex. The demonstration of increased levels of atrial natriuretic hormone in patients with Cushing's syndrome[17] indicates the expansion of the extracellular fluid volume. The excess cortisol in Cushing's syndrome may overwhelm the ability of the renal 11β-hydroxysteroid dehydrogenase to convert active cortisol into inactive cortisone at the renal mineralocorticoid receptor level, so that cortisol persists and stimulates the mineralocorticoid receptors to retain sodium and expand the extracellular fluid volume.[18] Cortisol has also been shown to stimulate the synthesis of renin substrate and the expression of angiotensin II receptors,[19] and to potentiate the response of vascular smooth muscle to vasoconstrictor agents.[20]

Congenital Adrenal Hyperplasia

Congenital adrenal hyperplasia is a collection of enzyme deficiencies that interfere with the synthesis of cortisol. Deficiencies in 11β-hydroxylase and 17α-hydroxylase are associated with hypertension. The pathophysiology of hypertension in these enzyme deficiency states involves the accumulation of the substrates for the deficient enzymes proximal to their sites of action.

The low level of cortisol stimulates the release of the pituitary adrenocorticotropic hormone (ACTH) and increases the accumulation of these cortisol precursors. One of these precursors, deoxycorticosterone, is active at the mineralocorticoid receptor site and is responsible for the hypertension that occurs in patients with 11β-hydroxylase deficiency[21] and 17α-hydroxylase deficiency.[22]

Primary Hyperaldosteronism

Primary hyperaldosteronism is a disorder of mineralocorticoid excess. Aldosterone is the major mineralocorticoid produced by the human adrenal cortex. Hyperaldosteronism is the syndrome associated with aldosterone excess. Hypertension is a common manifestation of primary hyperaldosteronism and is a direct consequence of increased renal sodium reabsorption with the expansion of the extracellular fluid volume.[23] Although the volume excess abates somewhat under the influence of the natriuretic peptides and pressure natriuresis, the hypertension persists, perhaps by an increase in systemic vascular resistance partially due to augmented sympathoadrenal activity.[24]

Glucocorticoid-Remediable Aldosteronism

Glucocorticoid-remediable aldosteronism is an autosomal dominant disorder that is characterized by hypertension and variable degrees of aldosterone excess.

This disorder results from a mutation in the chimeric 11β-hydroxylase/aldosterone synthase gene. This mutation fuses the promoter region of the 11β-hydroxylase gene to the coding region of the aldosterone synthase gene, and leads to the expression of aldosterone synthase in the zona fasciculata under the control of pituitary ACTH. The disease is characterized by an ectopic synthesis and secretion of aldosterone and a shift in the control of aldosterone production from the renin-angiotensin system to pituitary ACTH. It is the ability of glucocorticoids to suppress the pituitary production of ACTH that makes the aldosterone excess of this disease and its associated hypertension glucocorticoid-remediable.[25,26]

Mineralocorticoid Hypertension

Mineralocorticoid hypertension refers to a group of disorders associated with the deficiency or inhibition of the 11β-hydroxysteroid dehydrogenase enzyme in the renal tubule. 11β-Hydroxysteroid dehydrogenase is the enzyme that inactivates cortisol at the renal mineralocorticoid receptor and minimizes its mineralocorticoid activity. The deficiency or inhibition of this enzyme leaves cortisol active at the renal mineralocorticoid receptor, leading to salt retention and hypertension. Congenital deficiency[27] and the inhibition of this enzyme, usually by glycyrrhetinic acid (3β-D-monoglucuronyl-18β-glycyrrhetinic acid) following the ingestion of large amounts of licorice,[28] have been described in the literature. Similar enzyme inhibition has been described with ingestion of tobacco, some red wines, and carbenoxolone.

Pheochromocytoma

The adrenal medulla provides the adrenal link of the sympathoadrenal system. This system is responsible for the synthesis, secretion, and circulating of catecholamines.

Pheochromocytoma is a catecholamine-producing tumor of the sympathoadrenal system with several cardiovascular manifestations. Hypertension is the major manifestation of pheochromocytoma. Although paroxysmal attacks are the hallmark of pheochromocytomas, more than half of the patients have sustained hypertension and about 10% are normotensive. The hypertension of pheochromocytoma is largely attributed to the release of active catecholamines that induce peripheral vasoconstriction and increase total peripheral resistance.

Exogenous Hormones

Exogenous hormones are important causes of secondary hypertension. Glucocorticoid therapy is associated with Cushing's syndrome. Mineralocorticoid and sympathomimetic therapy may be associated with elevated blood pressure. The ingestion of tyramine-containing foods (e.g., cheese, yogurt, sour cream, broad beans, beer, and wines, particularly Chianti and sherry) while on treatment with monoamine oxidase inhibitors impairs the oxidative deamination of tyramine, an exogenous catecholamine, and may precipitate a hypertensive crisis.

Many women who take estrogen-containing oral contraceptive pills exhibit a slight rise in blood pressure, and about 5% develop hypertension within 5 years of oral contraceptive use.[29] The exact mechanism for the hypertension on the oral contraceptive pill is unclear. Estrogens and the synthetic progestogens used in oral contraceptives have all been reported to cause sodium retention.[30] Plasma insulin levels are increased after the start of oral contraceptive pill use,[31] suggesting insulin resistance may contribute to the associated rise in blood pressure.

Neuropsychologic Disorders

Neuropsychologic disorders are commonly recognized as causes of secondary hypertension. The mechanisms of elevated blood pressures in many of these disorders are poorly defined.

The central nervous system plays a pivotal role in the regulation of blood pressure. Many cortical and subcortical regions that have marked cardiovascular effects have been described. The cardiovascular impulses of the central nervous system are carried by the preganglionic autonomic neurons and are relayed to the postganglionic autonomic neurons in the autonomic ganglia. The distribution of these autonomic postganglionic neurons to the heart, blood vessels, kidneys, and adrenals allows the central nervous system to alter major determinants of blood pressure, such as contractile force, heart rate, venous capacitance, peripheral resistance, and extracellular fluid volume.[32] Abnormalities in the cardiovascular reflexes modulated by the central nervous system may contribute to the elevated blood pressures observed in neuropsychologic disorders.

Coarctation of the Aorta

Coarctation of the aorta is a congenital narrowing of the aorta. It may occur at any level of the aorta but is usually found just beyond the origin of the left subclavian artery or distal to the insertion of the ligamentum arteriosum. A spectrum of anatomic lesions exists, ranging from a localized constriction of the lumen to a diffuse narrowing of the aorta. Hypertension in the arms and diminished femoral pulses are the classic features of coarctation. The mechanical obstruction created by the coarctation contributes to the hypertension. Augmented norepinephrine and renin output in response to maximal exercise has also been reported in these patients and may play a role in the reported elevation in blood pressure immediately following surgical correction.[33]

Pregnancy-Induced Hypertension

Pregnancy-induced hypertension occurs in about 10% of first pregnancies. The diagnosis is usually based on a rise in blood pressure of 30/15 mm Hg or more above baseline or to a level above 140/90 mm Hg during the second half of pregnancy or immediately after delivery.

Although the precise mechanism for pregnancy-induced hypertension is unknown, there is an increased frequency of the disease in primigravid women and in subsequent pregnancies with a different father, whereas the frequency of the disease decreases with repeated exposure to semen of the father before conception. These findings suggest an immunologic mechanism for the disease.[34] Trophoblastic antigens have been shown to provoke an immune response that prevents the normal invasion of the uterus by the trophoblast.[35] The failure of extravillous cytotrophoblast cells to invade the maternal uterine spiral arteries to a sufficient depth in early pregnancy compromises the uteroplacental perfusion and predisposes the placenta to ischemia in late pregnancy. The compensatory mechanisms that are activated by the ischemia of the placenta may contribute to the elevated blood pressure in patients with pregnancy-induced hypertension.[36]

Hematologic Disorders

Hematologic disorders that are associated with increased number of red blood cells are frequently associated with secondary hypertension.[37] The abnormal blood rheology associated with the increased blood viscosity in patients with increased number of red blood cells may contribute to the elevated blood pressures observed in these patients.[38]

Minerals and Vitamins

There is accumulating evidence of association of elevated blood pressure with low levels of certain minerals and vitamins. Low levels of potassium and calcium have been associated with elevated blood pressure and optimizing the levels of these minerals has been shown to lower blood pressure. Hypertension and cardiovascular disease are prominent features of thiamine deficiency (vitamin B_6). Otherwise known as beriberi, thiamine deficiency is relatively rare in the United States because most foods are now fortified with minerals and vitamins. However, recent immigrants, alcoholics, and patients with genetic beriberi remain at significant risk for this secondary cause of hypertension. Vitamin D deficiency is becoming increasingly associated with hypertension and cardiovascular disease in spite of the fortification of milk and dairy products with vitamin D. The current recommended daily allowances of vitamin D may not support optimal serum levels of vitamin D. However, the optimization of serum levels of vitamin D has not been shown to lower blood pressure and alleviate the risk of hypertension associated with vitamin D deficiency.[39]

Drugs

Drugs that are known to cause sustained hypertension are few and include cyclosporin A and erythropoietin. Many more stimulant drugs, including cocaine, amphetamines, methylphenidate, and phenmetrazine, cause transient elevations in blood pressure and may interfere with the efficacy of blood pressure medications, but rarely cause sustained hypertension unless prolonged ischemia and/or secondary anatomic changes are induced.

Cyclosporin A is a primary immunosuppressive agent given to patients after solid organ transplantations. The use of cyclosporin A has been associated with widespread vasoconstriction and decreased renal blood flow thought to evolve from vascular injury. The resulting increase in peripheral resistance and decrease in the glomerular filtration rate underlie the pathophysiology of cyclosporin-induced hypertension.[40]

Erythropoietin is a recombinant hematopoietic growth factor given primarily to patients with anemia of chronic kidney disease, malignancy, or other causes of chronic anemia. Reports of hypertension are common in patients on erythropoietin, and the mechanism is thought to include an increase in blood volume and a decrease in the hypoxic vasodilatation by the perpetual correction of anemia with erythropoietin administration.[41]

Alcohol

The intake of large amounts of alcohol has been associated with secondary hypertension.[42] Although the precise mechanism by which alcohol raises the blood pressure is unknown, oral alcohol has been associated with increased sympathetic activity and elevation in blood pressure in normotensive humans.[43]

PATHOPHYSIOLOGY

Although the etiology of secondary hypertension includes a long and lengthening list of abnormalities of renal function, neuroendocrine function, and many other factors that are

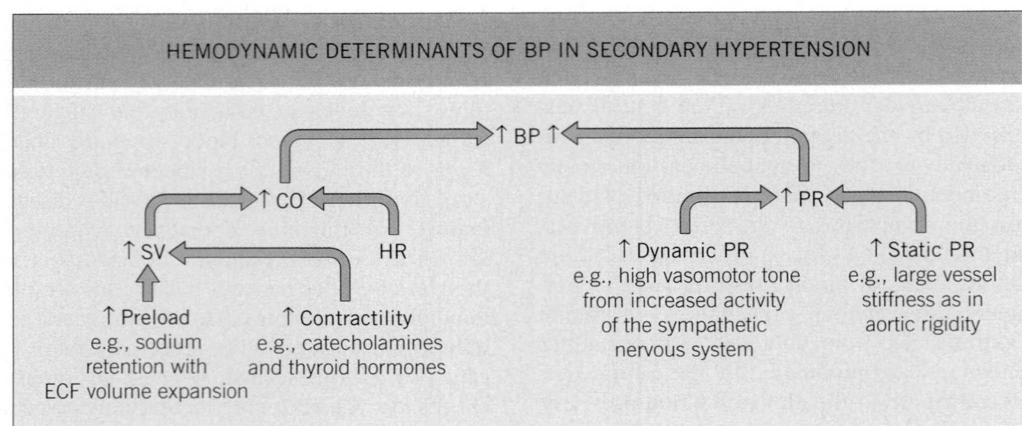

Figure 47.2 Hemodynamic determinants of blood pressure (BP) in secondary hypertension. CO, cardiac output; ECF, extracellular fluid; HR, heart rate; PR, peripheral resistance; SV, stroke volume.

not completely understood, the basic pathophysiology of the elevation of blood pressure in secondary hypertension revolves around the relationship between blood pressure and its hemodynamic determinants (Fig. 47.2). An increase in cardiac output is consistently associated with an initial rise in blood pressure and a fall in peripheral resistance. With the exception of patients with hyperdynamic circulation, the cardiac output eventually returns to normal with a secondary rise in peripheral resistance, indicating that it is the rise in peripheral resistance that maintains the elevated blood pressure.[44]

The peripheral resistance is modulated by a complex interaction of local humoral factors with systemic neurohormonal changes that modify the characteristics of the vessel wall and alter luminal diameter. Some of the secretory factors involved in this modulation are listed along with their effects in Table 47.3. Many of these factors can cause both functional contraction and structural remodeling of the blood vessel, including hypertrophy.[45] It has been suggested that repeated dynamic functional vasoconstriction under the influence of these pressor-growth promoters may lead to static structural changes that sustain the elevated peripheral resistance and blood pressure.[46]

The findings from the study of certain pure forms of hormonally induced hypertension has led to the hypothesis that most forms of secondary hypertension have two pressor processes: an initial rapid and reversible primary process that initiates the hypertension, and a final slow and stable secondary process that maintains the hypertension even after the removal of the primary cause.[47]

It is noteworthy that the predominant process responsible for initiation and maintenance of hypertension in any specific patient with secondary hypertension will not be easily discernible because of the complex interactions among the processes that control blood pressure. The understanding of the determinants of blood pressure and the basic pathophysiology of hypertension provides a good theoretic framework for the accurate interpretation of the clinical signs and symptoms of the patient that may provide an insight into the probable predominant mechanism for the elevation in blood pressure.

SOME OF THE AGENTS INVOLVED IN THE HUMORAL AND NEUROHORMONAL MODULATION OF PERIPHERAL RESISTANCE

Agents that Induce Vasoconstriction and Initiate Vascular Smooth Muscle Growth and ECM Production	Agents that Induce Vasodilation and Inhibit Vascular Smooth Muscle Growth and ECM Production
Vasopressin	Atrial natriuretic factor
Endothelin	Nitric oxide
Angiotensin II	Prostacyclin
Catecholamines	Heparinoids

ECM, extracellular matrix.

Table 47.3 Some of the agents involved in the humoral and neurohormonal modulation of peripheral resistance. Under normal conditions there is a balance between the vasoconstricting growth-promoting factors and the vasodilatory growth-inhibiting factors.

CLINICAL PRESENTATION

Several clinical and laboratory features will suggest the diagnosis of secondary hypertension on initial evaluation (Table 47.4). In view of the low frequency of secondary diagnoses in patients with hypertension and the high cost and relative risk of diagnostic evaluation, the selection of patients for further evaluation should be based on reasonable and reliable clinical indices.

History

The onset of hypertension before age 25 years or after age 55 years is suggestive of, but not specific for, secondary hypertension. Primary hypertension is still more common than secondary hypertension in adolescents, particularly in the presence of a family history of hypertension, obesity, and poor physical fitness. Most patients diagnosed with hypertension after age 55 years exhibit no identifiable cause and probably represent late diagnoses of primary hypertension. However, if the onset of hypertension can be shown to be after age 55 years, then the diagnosis of secondary hypertension will be more likely. The presence of multiple system complaints, particularly on initial evaluation, is suggestive of a secondary cause for the hypertension. Many of the endocrine disorders and vasculitides that affect the kidneys are systemic diseases and often produce multiple system complaints. A history of weakness, fatigue, polyuria,

FEATURES SUGGESTIVE OF SECONDARY HYPERTENSION
■ Onset of hypertension before age 25 or after age 55 years
■ Severe hypertension; blood pressure level >180/100 mm Hg at baseline
■ Sudden onset; change from normal blood pressure to severe hypertension in less than a year
■ Refractory hypertension; blood pressure refractory to standard therapy
■ Poor response to prior effective drug therapy
■ Paroxysmal attacks of hypertension with palpitations, pallor, perspiration, and tremor
■ Multiple system complaints on initial evaluation
■ Asymmetry of the peripheral pulses with lower blood pressures in the lower extremities
■ Abdominal bruit, particularly over the renal artery with a diastolic component
■ Bilateral flank masses
■ Presence of end-organ damage
– Grade 2 or more retinopathy
– Left ventricular hypertrophy
– Serum creatinine >1.5 mg/dL
■ Laboratory abnormalities
– Hyperglycemia
– Hypokalemia
– Hypercalcemia

Table 47.4 Features suggestive of secondary hypertension.

and cramps suggesting hypokalemia may signal mineralocorticoid hypertension. A history of panic attack and palpitation may suggest the diagnosis of pheochromocytoma. The presence of multiple system complaints should raise the index of suspicion for a probable systemic cause for the hypertension.

The medication history of all patients with a recent diagnosis of hypertension should be thoroughly reviewed to exclude the ingestion of exogenous hormones and the use of both prescribed and nonprescribed drugs that are known to cause hypertension. The list should include medications that are obtainable over-the-counter and nonprescription natural products. Many over-the-counter medications are known to interfere with the efficacy of antihypertensive medications and may mimic a refractory hypertensive state. Some natural products are now known to contain hormonal products, and a few have been associated with hypertension.

A history of chronic kidney disease in a patient with hypertension is difficult to interpret because hypertension is a common cause of kidney disease and kidney disease is the most common cause of secondary hypertension. If it can be reliably ascertained that the kidney disease antedates the hypertension, then the diagnosis of secondary hypertension can be established.

A family history of subarachnoid hemorrhage and kidney disease in a patient with hypertension may suggest polycystic kidney disease as a possible cause for the hypertension. Patients with a history of early-onset hypertension in first-degree relatives should be screened for glucocorticoid-remediable aldosteronism. A history of illicit drug use, especially cocaine, amphetamines, excessive consumption of alcohol, or a combination, in a patient with hypertension may suggest the diagnosis of secondary hypertension.

Physical Examination

Morbid obesity, especially in a patient with a history of snoring and excessive daytime sleepiness, may suggest sleep apnea as a possible cause for the hypertension. Obesity with truncal emphasis, cutaneous striae, buffalo hump, and moon facies are some of the clinical signs of cortisol excess that should suggest adrenal hyperfunction as a probable cause for the hypertension, particularly in a patient with hypokalemia and hyperglycemia.

Abnormal secondary sexual characteristics are common manifestations of patients with the 11β-hydroxylase deficiency type of congenital adrenal hyperplasia. Male patients demonstrate advanced masculinization, whereas female patients exhibit cystic acne, increased facial hair, and male pattern baldness with prominent recession of the anterior hairline. Patients with 17α-hydroxylase deficiency usually exhibit no secondary sexual characteristics, with eunuchoid body proportions.

Markedly variable blood pressure readings may suggest the diagnosis of pheochromocytoma, especially in a patient with paroxysms of pallor, palpitation, and perspiration. Palpable purpura is suggestive of vasculitis and should prompt the exclusion of an intrarenal vasculitis as a probable cause for the hypertension. Severe hypertension with florid signs of end-organ damage, especially hypertensive retinopathy, at baseline may suggest the diagnosis of secondary hypertension. Systolic hypertension particularly in a relatively young patient with a resting tachycardia may signal the diagnosis of hyperthyroidism. Diastolic hypertension and a relative bradycardia should prompt evaluation for hypothyroidism. Orthostatic blood pressure changes, especially in patients receiving no blood pressure medications, may signal autonomic dysfunction and suggest a neurologic basis for the hypertension. Asymmetry of the peripheral pulses with lower blood pressures in the lower extremities and a systolic murmur in the middle of the back should suggest coarctation of the aorta as the probable cause for the hypertension. The persistence of the Korotkoff sounds to zero during manual blood pressure measurement may suggest aortic regurgitation, particularly in a patient with collapsing peripheral pulses, systolic hypertension, diastolic murmurs, and a soft single second heart sound.

Bilateral flank masses that move with respiration in a patient with hypertension should suggest the diagnosis of polycystic kidney disease. Auscultatory abdominal bruit heard over the renal areas with a diastolic component may suggest the diagnosis of renovascular hypertension. Enlarged prostate on rectal examination of an elderly male patient with hypertension may suggest the diagnosis of an obstructive uropathy. Large extremities with coarse facial features, protruding jaw, and wide spacing of the teeth should suggest the diagnosis of acromegaly.

DIAGNOSTIC TECHNIQUES

The laboratory tests for the initial evaluation for hypertension should include a urinalysis, a complete blood count, and a serum chemistry that includes potassium, blood urea nitrogen, creatinine, calcium, and fasting glucose levels. In patients with multiple system complaints, the initial evaluation should also include an erythrocyte sedimentation rate, thyroid function tests, and serologic tests for immune complex–mediated intrarenal vasculitis. Suggestive clinical and laboratory features on initial examination should prompt further diagnostic evaluation for secondary hypertension.

Hypokalemia

An unprovoked and persistent hypokalemia in a patient with a recent diagnosis of hypertension is a common laboratory manifestation of mineralocorticoid excess and should prompt the measurement of urine chloride and potassium concentrations. A urine chloride level less than 15 mmol/L and a urine potassium level greater than 25 mmol/L in a patient with hypokalemia and hypertension support a mineralocorticoid excess state and should prompt the measurement of plasma renin activity (PRA) and plasma aldosterone (PA) level, preferably in the morning with the patient upright. It is recommended that all blood pressure medications be withheld for at least 2 weeks before the measurement of PRA and PA.

A high PRA with a high PA level is indicative of a renin-angiotensin system–dependent aldosterone-mediated mineralocorticoid excess that implicates renal artery stenosis, renin-secreting tumor, or both as the probable causes for the hypertension. There are several diagnostic tests that can be employed for the initial evaluation of patients with features that are suggestive of renovascular hypertension. The sensitivity and specificity of some of these radiologic tests are depicted in Table 47.5. The gold standard for the diagnosis of renal artery stenosis is renal arteriography. Renin-secreting tumors may be identified on renal arteriograms performed for suspected renal artery stenosis, but they require a guided renal biopsy and a histopathologic examination for definitive diagnosis. Extrarenal renin-secreting tumors should be suspected in the setting of a normal renal arteriogram and features suggestive of renovascular hypertension.[48]

A low PRA with a high PA level is indicative of a renin-angiotensin system–independent aldosterone-mediated mineralocorticoid excess that may implicate primary hyperaldosteronism as the likely cause for the hypertension. The low PRA actually lends little support to the diagnosis of primary hyperaldosteronism, because some patients with essential hypertension exhibit low PRA, but the high plasma aldosterone level is strongly suggestive of primary hyperaldosteronism. In fact, a PA level greater than 20 ng/mL with PA/PRA ratio greater than 30 may yield a sensitivity of 90%, a specificity of 91%, a positive predictive value of 69%, and a negative predictive value of 98%. The definitive biochemical diagnosis of hyperaldosteronism can be made by determining aldosterone excretion rate during salt loading. An aldosterone excretion rate above 14 mg/day in a 24-hour urine sample that contains more than 250 mmol/L of sodium after 3 days of salt loading identifies patients with primary hyperaldosteronism with a sensitivity of 96% and a specificity of 93%.[49] The salt loading can be achieved by infusion of 25 mL/kg of 0.9% saline over 4 hours for 3 days or addition of 10 to 12 g of sodium chloride tablets to the diet daily for 3 days. The serum potassium level must be monitored closely, because salt loading promotes kaliuresis and may further lower the serum potassium. The 24-hour urinary sodium excretion should be measured daily to ensure adequate salt loading. Saline infusion is contraindicated in patients with severe hypertension, hypertensive emergencies, and congestive heart failure. Blood pressure medications should be discontinued at least 2 weeks before the determination of aldosterone excretion rate.

RADIOLOGIC TESTS FOR THE EVALUATION OF RENOVASCULAR HYPERTENSION		
Diagnostic Test	**Sensitivity (%)**	**Specificity (%)**
Renal artery arteriography	99	99
Magnetic resonance angiography	97	95
Captopril renal scan	93	95
Renal artery duplex sonography	86	93
Intravenous digital subtraction angiography	88	89
Rapid-sequence intravenous pyelography	74	86

Table 47-5 Radiologic tests for the evaluation of renovascular hypertension.

A low PRA and a low plasma aldosterone is indicative of a renin-angiotensin system–independent, non–aldosterone-mediated mineralocorticoid excess that may suggest the diagnosis of congenital adrenal hyperplasia or 11β-hydroxysteroid dehydrogenase deficiency. Bilateral adrenal enlargement on CT or MRI of the abdomen and elevated levels of blood and 24-hour urinary deoxycorticosterone are supportive, but the specific diagnosis of congenital adrenal hyperplasia is usually established by genetic analysis and the pattern of elevations in blood and urine levels of adrenal steroids and the cortisol precursors of the impeded pathways.[50] Patients with 11β-hydroxysteroid dehydrogenase deficiency exhibit a high urinary cortisol-to-cortisone ratio, but the specific diagnosis requires genetic confirmation.

A normal PRA in a patient with hypokalemia and hypertension does not exclude the possibility of a secondary cause for the hypertension. In fact, many patients with renovascular hypertension do not exhibit a high PRA. The predictive value of PRA can be increased by a captopril test. The test involves the measurement of PRA 60 minutes after an oral administration of captopril (50 mg diluted in 10 mL of water) in a patient on normal salt intake and preferably on no antihypertensive medications for at least 2 weeks before the test. The diagnosis of renovascular hypertension requires a stimulated PRA of at least 12 ng/mL per hour, an absolute increase of 10 ng/mL per hour or more in PRA, and a 150% or more increase in PRA. The inhibition of the angiotensin-converting enzyme (ACE) by captopril in a patient with renovascular disease precipitates an acute ischemia in the kidney with the stenotic artery and provides a stimulus for the release of renin into the plasma. The captopril test identifies patients with renovascular hypertension with a sensitivity of 74% and a specificity of 89%. The captopril test may be less useful in African American patients because of the higher prevalence of low PRA.

Hyperglycemia

An elevated fasting serum glucose level in a patient with a recent diagnosis of hypertension is not uncommon. Diabetes mellitus and essential hypertension commonly coexist in the same patient and may represent the association between hypertension and insulin resistance, particularly with accompanying obesity.[51] Moreover, diabetic nephropathy is a recognized cause of hypertension. In addition, many endocrine causes of hypertension, notably acromegaly, pheochromocytoma, and Cushing's syndrome, are also associated with an elevation in the fasting serum glucose.

Acromegaly can be evaluated by obtaining a serum level of insulin-like growth factor I (IGF-I). IGF-I is a peptide produced by the peripheral tissues and is dependent on growth hormone (GH) production. IGF-I level in serum has been shown to correlate very well with the integrated GH secretion over a 24-hour period. The interpretation of serum levels of IGF-I should be based on a range defined for specific age groups, because IGF-I concentrations show a significant decline with advancing age. The level of serum IGF-I may be elevated at puberty and in pregnancy and depressed in hypoproteinemic conditions like cirrhosis, malnutrition, and nephrotic syndrome, because IGF-I is largely bound by specific binding proteins.

The most reliable test for the diagnosis of acromegaly is the oral glucose tolerance test. In normal subjects an oral glucose load will suppress the serum GH to a nadir of less than 2 μg/mL, but in acromegaly the serum GH level remains unchanged in response to a glucose load and may even rise. Random serum GH levels have very little role in the evaluation of acromegaly because of the short plasma half-life of GH and the pulsatile nature of its secretion.

Pheochromocytoma is best initially evaluated by the measurement of plasma epinephrine and norepinephrine levels and 24-hour urinary levels of metanephrine and normetanephrine. It is most desirable to measure the level of both catecholamines in plasma and the level of one of the two metabolites, preferably metanephrine, in urine. The blood sample for these plasma catecholamine levels must be obtained from a patient who has been resting for at least 30 minutes in a supine position after an overnight fast and at least 3 hours after smoking or chewing tobacco. A combined level of plasma epinephrine and norepinephrine in excess of 2000 pg/mL establishes the diagnosis of pheochromocytoma. Levels below 2000 pg/mL but above 1000 pg/mL should be followed by the clonidine suppression test, during which plasma catecholamine levels are obtained at baseline and hourly for 3 hours after 0.3 mg of clonidine by mouth. The blood pressure and pulse rate should be monitored every 30 minutes during the clonidine suppression test, because profound and prolonged hypotension has been reported in some patients during this test. The normal response to clonidine is suppression of plasma catecholamine level by at least 50% from baseline or to a level below 500 pg/mL. Nonsuppression of elevated plasma catecholamines by clonidine is strongly suggestive of pheochromocytoma.

Plasma catecholamine levels of 1000 pg/mL or less in a patient with clinical features suggestive of pheochromocytoma is about the only indication left for the glucagon stimulation test, during which plasma catecholamine levels are obtained at baseline and 3 minutes after an intravenous bolus injection of 2 mg of glucagon. The intravenous access should be maintained and blood pressure monitored and recorded every minute for 5 minutes after glucagon injection because life-threatening pressor crises have been reported following this injection in some patients with pheochromocytoma. Intravenous phentolamine 5 mg bolus after a 0.5-mg test dose should be readily available to terminate a life-threatening pressor response. Glucagon has little or no effect on blood pressure or plasma catecholamine levels in normal subjects, but may cause an increase in the blood pressure and circulating catecholamine levels in patients with pheochromocytoma. A threefold increase in plasma catecholamine levels or an absolute level higher than 2000 pg/mL in response to glucagon injection is required for the diagnosis of pheochromocytoma with this test. A blood pressure rise of at least 20/15 mm Hg is desirable but not essential to confirm the diagnosis. The glucagon stimulation test in a normotensive patient is potentially dangerous and rarely indicated.

Computed tomography and MRI of the abdomen are used to localize pheochromocytoma after the diagnosis of the tumor is established by biochemical tests. Radiolabeled ^{131}I-metaiodobenzylguanidine (MIBG) scan provides both anatomic localization and functional characterization. It is less sensitive but more specific than both CT and MRI, and should be reserved for patients with biochemical diagnosis of pheochromocytoma and negative localization studies. The agent of MIBG scan (^{131}I-MIBG) requires active concentration in the sympathoadrenal tissues by the catecholamine reuptake mechanisms for efficient localization of the tumor, so the use of drugs that block catecholamine reuptake (e.g., tricyclic antidepressants, cocaine, etc.) may result in false-negative results.

The initial screening for Cushing's syndrome can be by the measurement of 24-hour urinary free cortisol (UFC) or the overnight dexamethasone suppression test. UFC has no validity in patients with renal insufficiency, and the overnight dexamethasone suppression test may give false-positive results in patients with psychiatric illness, obesity, alcoholism, or high stress level; patients who are pregnant; and patients who are taking phenobarbital, phenytoin, or estrogen. A 24-hour UFC higher than 100 mg or morning serum cortisol level greater than 5 mg/dL after a 1.0 mg dose of dexamethasone given at 11:00 PM the night before the test should suggest cortisol excess and prompt the measurement of plasma ACTH, preferably at 8:00 AM.

A low level of plasma ACTH is suggestive of an adrenal tumor or hyperplasia and should be evaluated further by an abdominal CT. A high level of plasma ACTH, greater than 200 pg/mL, is suggestive of an ectopic ACTH production and should prompt a search for ACTH-producing tumors, such as carcinoid tumors, small cell carcinoma of the lungs, and so on. Elevated plasma ACTH levels that are less than 200 pg/mL will require the standard dexamethasone suppression test, during which dexamethasone is administered to the patient first at 0.5 mg orally every 6 hours for 48 hours, and then at 2.0 mg orally every 6 hours for 48 hours. The 24-hour UFC and morning serum cortisol are measured at baseline and on the second day on each dose.

Nonsuppression on low-dose dexamethasone and suppression on high-dose dexamethasone with at least 50% reduction in plasma cortisol and 90% reduction in UFC from baseline support the diagnosis of a pituitary tumor or hypothalamopituitary dysfunction. Nonsuppression on both low- and high-dose dexamethasone is suggestive of ectopic production of ACTH.

A normal level of plasma ACTH in a patient with cortisol excess will require a corticotropin-releasing hormone (CRH)

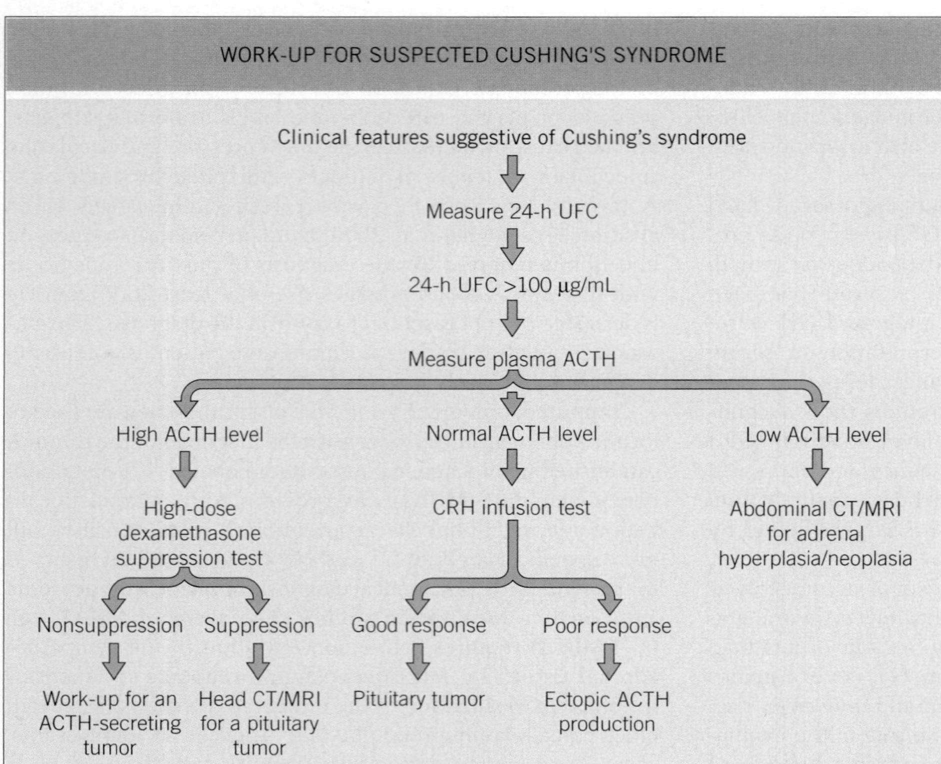

Figure 47.3 Suggested work-up for a patient suspected of having Cushing's syndrome. A good response to CRH is defined as a 20% increase in serum cortisol and a 50% increase in plasma ACTH. ACTH, adrenocorticotropic hormone; CRH, corticotropin-releasing hormone; UFC, urinary free cortisol.

infusion test. The CRH test involves the measurement of serum cortisol and plasma ACTH in response to bovine CRH infusion. An increase in plasma ACTH in response to CRH is suggestive of the diagnosis of a pituitary tumor or hypothalamopituitary dysfunction, whereas a lack of response will suggest an ectopic production of ACTH (Fig. 47.3).

Hypercalcemia

Elevated serum calcium in a patient with a recent diagnosis of hypertension may suggest parathyroid hormone (PTH) excess, but the many non–PTH-mediated causes of hypercalcemia, including malignancy, vitamin D toxicity, increased bone turnover, and milk alkali syndrome, must be considered in the evaluation of the patient before the diagnosis of primary hyperparathyroidism is considered.

Serum calcium levels can also be affected by diuretic therapy in patients with hypertension. Thiazide diuretics can raise serum calcium and mimic primary hyperparathyroidism, whereas loop diuretics can lower serum calcium and mask the diagnosis of primary hyperparathyroidism. Elevated serum calcium that cannot be explained by clinical data should prompt the measurement of the intact PTH molecule in serum, and an elevated PTH level in a patient with an unexplained hypercalcemia establishes the diagnosis of primary hyperparathyroidism.

MANAGEMENT

In many patients with secondary hypertension, the elevated blood pressure will fall with the identification and control of the underlying disease, hence the need for prompt and proper evaluation of patients with clinical and laboratory features suggestive of secondary hypertension. The blood pressure may not fall within normal range, and blood pressure control measures may be required in addition to the treatment of the underlying disease.

Lifestyle modifications and antihypertensive medications should be given equal emphasis in the management of the hypertension. Lifestyle modifications that have been shown to be effective in blood pressure control, overall improvement in cardiovascular health, or both include weight reduction, aerobic exercise, limitation of alcohol intake, smoking cessation, stress reduction, and reduction in sodium, cholesterol, and dietary fat intake.

Although antihypertensive medications are generally effective in lowering blood pressure in most patients with hypertension, the selection of a drug for initial therapy should be made with due consideration for the underlying disease in patients with secondary hypertension. Some classes of antihypertensives have been shown to improve the clinical outcome for some forms of secondary hypertension better than others, and some causes of secondary hypertension call for caution with the use of some classes of antihypertensives. Some of the etiologies of secondary hypertension and the preferred classes of antihypertensives for initial therapy are listed in Table 47-6. Drugs from other classes may be added to drugs from the preferred class as required for blood pressure control, provided that they have no adverse effect on the underlying disease.

Treatment should begin with the minimum effective dosage to minimize side effects and prevent a sudden reduction in blood pressure. Drug and dosage should not be adjusted more often than every 4 weeks, except in patients with stage III hypertension, because most long-acting antihypertensives take 4 to 6 weeks to exert their maximum effect in lowering blood pressure.

SELECTION OF ANTIHYPERTENSIVE MEDICATION FOR SECONDARY HYPERTENSION	
Causes of Hypertension	**Preferred Class of Antihypertensive Drug**
Diabetic nephropathy	ACE inhibitors Nondihydropyridine calcium channel blockers
Obstructive uropathy from an enlarged prostate	Alpha blockers
Renal parenchymal disease	ACE inhibitors
Renovascular hypertension	ACE inhibitors*
Liddle's syndrome	Sodium channel blockers (e.g., amiloride)
Hyperthyroidism	Beta blockers
Primary hyperaldosteronism	Potassium-sparing diuretic therapy
Pheochromocytoma	Alpha blockers
Acute stress	Beta blockers
Cyclosporin-induced hypertension	Calcium channel blockers
Isolated systolic hypertension	Diuretics

Drugs may be added as required for blood pressure control but due consideration must be given to the interaction of the drug class with the cause of the hypertension.

*ACE inhibitors may aggravate renal ischemia with a compromise in renal function in patients with high-grade unilateral renal artery stenosis.

Table 47.6 Selection of antihypertensive medication for secondary hypertension.

The use of antihypertensive medications should be carefully monitored for efficacy and side effects, especially in cases where the class of antihypertensive drug is more likely to have adverse effects due to the cause of secondary hypertension. Whenever possible, office blood pressure measurements should be supplemented with home readings. Blood pressure readings in the morning before the dose for the day tend to reflect the duration of blood pressure control, whereas readings in the evenings or late afternoon are more indicative of the degree of blood pressure control.

The target blood pressure level depends on the cause of the hypertension and the existing comorbidity. For most patients with hypertension the target level will be below 140/90 mm Hg. In patients with diabetes mellitus and renal insufficiency, lower target levels, usually below 130/85 mm Hg, have been shown to better preserve renal function and protect against stroke and cardiac events. However, in patients with a history of ischemic heart disease, there may be a critical level of diastolic blood pressure beyond which further reduction may compromise coronary circulation and increase the patient's risk of an adverse cardiovascular event.

A good control of blood pressure after the treatment of the underlying disease should prompt a gradual decrease in the number and dosage of antihypertensive drugs. Patients who maintain normal blood pressures on low-dose single-drug antihypertensive therapy can be taken off medication and observed periodically to ensure that blood pressure remains normal. The probability that the patient will be successfully taken off medication depends on the cause of hypertension and the degree of compliance with lifestyle modification. Most patients with drug-induced hypertension do not require long-term antihypertensive drug therapy, and can be taken off medication soon after the discontinuation of the offending drug. Patients who make and keep to the recommended lifestyle changes are more likely to maintain normal blood pressure after the discontinuation of antihypertensive medication. The failure to successfully discontinue therapy for hypertension after the treatment of the cause may reflect the onset of an insidious and likely irreversible secondary process that maintains the hypertension even after the removal of the primary cause.

PROGNOSIS

The prognosis of secondary hypertension depends on the outcome of the complex interaction among the underlying disease and its response to therapy, the duration of the hypertension and its response to blood pressure control measures, and the patient's risk for cardiovascular mortality. Many of the causes of secondary hypertension will respond to prompt and appropriate treatment with favorable outcomes, but the response of blood pressure to the treatment of the underlying disease frequently depends on the duration of hypertension. Timely diagnosis and treatment of the underlying disease will shorten the duration of hypertension and may abort the slow pressor mechanism(s) that perpetuates the hypertension. A high number of cardiovascular risk factors and comorbid conditions will have an adverse effect on the prognosis of secondary hypertension. The goal of therapy is to minimize the contribution of hypertension and its cardiovascular complications to the overall morbidity and mortality of the patient with secondary hypertension. The extent to which that can be achieved will depend on the prompt identification of the patient at risk and institution of appropriate treatment for the underlying disease, blood pressure control, and cardiovascular risk reduction through lifestyle modifications and evidence-based pharmacologic therapies.

SUMMARY

Secondary hypertension is uncommon in the adult hypertensive population. Selection of cases for further diagnostic evaluation should be limited to those with clinical and laboratory features that are suggestive of a specific secondary cause. Specific therapy for some secondary causes of hypertension may obviate the need for long-term empirical treatment. Strategies for blood pressure control should be initiated promptly with equal emphasis on drug therapy and lifestyle modifications.

chapter

48 Difficult Hypertension Management Issues

a. Hypertension and Ethnicity

Gregory Y. H. Lip and Bernard Cheung

DEFINITION OF PROBLEM

There are well-described ethnic variations in the pathophysiology and management of hypertension that are important in black or African-origin populations. Black patients with essential hypertension are at greater risk of developing cardiovascular complications, particularly strokes and renal failure. This is manifested by a threefold increase in overall cardiovascular mortality in comparison with whites, a sixfold to sevenfold increase in mortality under the age of 50 years, the earlier development of hypertensive nephrosclerosis, and a 5- to 18-fold rise in the incidence of end-stage renal disease, especially in the 25- to 45-year age group. There is less information on hypertension in Indo-Asian populations, but emerging data on Asian populations have informed our management strategies.

TYPICAL CASES

Case 1: A 48-year-old Afro-Caribbean man presented with a long history of resistant hypertension. He was a nonsmoker and drank 30 to 40 units of alcohol per week. He was taking lisinopril 2.5 mg and atenolol 25 mg, and his blood pressure was 186/104 mm Hg. There was a left ventricular heave but examination was otherwise normal. His fundi showed bilateral arteriovenous nicking, arteriolar narrowing, and silver wiring. The electrocardiogram (ECG) showed sinus rhythm with evidence of left ventricular hypertrophy (LVH). Urinalysis showed trace protein only and his serum biochemistry revealed a potassium level of 4.0 mmol/L, urea level of 6.0 mmol/L, and creatinine level of 100 μmol/L. Echocardiography confirmed the presence of LVH.

The patient's atenolol was stopped in view of the lack of beta-blocker synergism with angiotensin-converting enzyme (ACE) inhibitors. The dose of the latter was increased to lisinopril 40 mg, and bendrofluazide 2.5 mg and (later) amlodipine 10 mg daily were added to his therapy, resulting in blood pressure of 142/84 mm Hg at follow-up.

Case 2: A 53-year-old businessman of Chinese ethnicity was referred for further management of hypertension. He was intolerant of a thiazide diuretic and a beta blocker, and was recently switched to perindopril 4 mg daily but noticed a dry cough. He disliked the idea of taking Western medications for life, and occasionally tried herbal remedies. He had a high salt and low alcohol intake. His blood pressure was 159/87 mm Hg, body mass index (BMI) 40 kg/m^2, and urinalyis results were normal. ECG findings were normal. Fasting glucose level was 8.5 mmol/L (153 mg/dL), and total cholesterol was 7.7 mmol/L (300.3 mg/dL). The patient was given lifestyle advice, including smoking cessation, low-salt weight-reducing diet, and regular physical activity. Valsartan 80 mg daily was prescribed to replace perindopril. However, his blood pressure remained high (159/98 mm Hg); because a blood pressure target of 130/80 mm Hg was adopted in view of his diabetes, amlodipine 5 mg daily was added.

DIFFERENTIAL DIAGNOSIS

Patients should have renal function, serum biochemistry, and dipstick urinalysis initially. Renal impairment carries a bad prognosis, whereas a normal serum potassium makes a diagnosis of Conn's syndrome less likely. Dipstick proteinuria of + or more indicates protein excretion of 0.3 g/L. This is a useful screening test in the clinic and may point to further investigation of renal disease as an underlying cause of hypertension. Rarely, the chest radiograph may indicate unusual causes of hypertension, such as rib notching in coarctation of the aorta.

The ECG is useful as a screening test for LVH. The presence of LVH has important prognostic implications, because hypertensive patients with LVH have an increased risk of cardiovascular events, cardiac dysfunction, atherosclerotic vascular disease, arrhythmias (e.g., ventricular arrhythmias and atrial fibrillation), and sudden death. A hypertensive patient with LVH also has a fourfold increased risk of stroke compared with a patient who has similar blood pressure levels but no LVH.

The presence of hypercholesterolemia adds to the cardiovascular risk of hypertension. If urinalysis indicates proteinuria, it would be important to quantify the degree of proteinuria with a 24-hour urinary protein excretion test. In severe hypertension with paroxysmal symptoms such as pallor or palpitations, urinary catecholamine levels would be useful as a screening test for rare causes such as pheochromocytoma. Echocardiography would be a second-line investigation and would be the best noninvasive method for studying cardiac structure and function. It is also superior to the ECG in confirming LVH. An abdominal ultrasound may help in excluding renal artery stenosis (unilateral small kidney), adrenal tumors, and chronic renal disease (bilateral small, shrunken kidneys).

Secondary causes of hypertension should be considered in hypertensive patients younger than 35 years, patients with abnormal baseline investigations, those presenting with malignant hypertension, and those with drug-resistant hypertension.

TREATMENT OPTIONS

Nonpharmacologic Management

Lifestyle and nonpharmacologic interventions in hypertensive blacks may result in a significant blood pressure reduction, thereby avoiding or reducing the need for antihypertensive therapy. For example, there is evidence that sodium restriction is particularly beneficial in the management of mild to moderate hypertension in black patients, and the effects are equivalent to those of low-dose thiazide diuretics. In view of the greater tendency for "sodium sensitivity" in hypertensive blacks, moderate sodium restriction, reducing sodium intake to less than 100 mmol/day, should always be initiated.

Dietary modifications, including weight loss, have been shown to reduce blood pressure. There is evidence that a high potassium diet with more fruits and vegetables also lowers blood pressure. Although the blood pressure reduction in hypertensive blacks that is due to weight loss may be less pronounced than in white hypertensives, weight control should be positively encouraged. Chronic high alcohol ingestion (three to five drinks daily) is associated with higher blood pressure levels in black and white patients, and advice regarding alcohol moderation is appropriate.

In case 2, the family history (hypertension in parents and siblings) is often useful because older Asians often come from large families. The most important environmental cause of hypertension in Chinese patients is obesity. The obese person often has the metabolic syndrome (abdominal obesity, raised blood pressure, raised blood glucose level, raised triglyceride levels, and low high-density cholesterol (HDL) level). Therefore the management of the hypertensive patient should include a comprehensive assessment of cardiovascular risk and the management of modifiable cardiovascular risk factors. In particular, Asians have a propensity to develop type 2 diabetes. The patient in case 2 was obese, had hypertension, elevated fasting glucose level, high triglyceride levels, and low HDL levels—all the components of the metabolic syndrome. It is worth noting that Asians have lower cutpoints for obesity; BMI higher than 25 is considered obese, and abdominal obesity is present if the waist circumference is 90 cm or greater in men and 80 cm or greater in women.

A calorie-controlled diet and regular physical activity are very important lifestyle measures that will help to not just lower blood pressure, but also improve blood glucose level and the lipid profile. The sodium intake varies tremendously in Asia. High sodium intake in Chinese patients is related to the use of soy sauce, marinated and salt-preserved foods, and fast foods. It is possible to cut the sodium intake drastically by eating at home, choosing fresh ingredients, and refraining from dipping foods in soy sauce. Smoking is not uncommon among Chinese men. Stopping smoking is important, not because it is the cause of the hypertension, but because it adds to the cardiovascular risk in the hypertensive patient. Alcohol is an uncommon cause of hypertension in many parts of Asia where few people are regular drinkers. Physical inactivity is a problem in Asia because it is a sign of seniority and affluence. Tai chi or yoga, although healthy for many reasons, is not strenuous enough to have any impact on obesity or cardiovascular fitness.

Pharmacologic Management

In an Afro-Caribbean patient (case 1), antihypertensive agents such as beta blockers and ACE inhibitors generally tend to be less effective than calcium channel blockers or diuretics. This is because of the tendency toward a low-renin, salt-sensitive state and a lower cardiac output, with increased peripheral resistance. Younger black patients may be more responsive than the elderly, because they tend to have renin levels closer to normal. These differences in therapeutic effects are likely to be related to the increased salt sensitivity, low renin activity, reduced Na^+/K^+-ATPase activity, and relative, expansion of plasma volume.

A comparison of the antihypertensive response between black and white patients suggests that black patients require between two and four times the dose of ACE inhibitor or beta blocker to achieve a response similar to that observed in white patients. This difference is generally eliminated by the addition of a diuretic, but low doses of either ACE inhibitors or beta blockers as monotherapy should be avoided in blacks. In one study, for example, enalapril alone produced only a minimal antihypertensive effect, whereas combination therapy with 12.5 mg/day hydrochlorothiazide lowered the mean blood pressure from 157/101 to 132/86 mm Hg. This reduced efficacy is a particular problem in the elderly black hypertensive patient. However, numerous studies have demonstrated the beneficial effects of ACE inhibitors in nephropathy, particularly in the presence of proteinuria, and these agents remain first-line antihypertensive therapy in this group of patients, irrespective of ethnic origin.

Importantly, the potentially life-threatening complication of ACE inhibitor–induced angioedema is more common in black patients, with an adjusted relative risk of 4.5 in African Americans. A plausible mechanism for this adverse effect involves the vasoactive peptide bradykinin, and the increased risk in black patients may occur as a result of racial differences in the kallikrein-kinin system, with increased sensitivity to bradykinin. Angioedema normally occurs within the first few weeks of therapy, and patients should be advised to report urticarial symptoms and to stop the ACE inhibitor immediately in the event of swelling of the lips, face, or tongue. The incidence of dry cough is very high in Chinese patients (up to 44%), although angioedema is surprisingly uncommon. For those who need a blocker of the renin-angiotensin system, an ARB should be considered in those who are intolerant of ACE inhibitors. More information is required regarding the efficacy and tolerability of the angiotensin II receptor antagonists in black hypertensive patients, but a few cases of angioedema have been reported.

In Chinese, the beta blockers are very well tolerated. As monotherapy, they do not control blood pressure well, and they seem to be inferior in terms of stroke protection; however, they are useful in people with ischemic heart disease and heart failure. In Chinese, the dose for a beta blocker is usually lower because of either lower body weight or slower hepatic metabolism.

Calcium channel blockers are highly effective antihypertensive agents in black and Asian patients. Edema and flushing are common side effects, especially in hot weather. Headaches and palpitations are also commonly encountered. Nevertheless, none of these side effects are dangerous nor do they require regular monitoring of blood chemistry. Calcium channel blockers are effective in the prevention of stroke, which is the major complication of hypertension in Asians. One comparison of the antihypertensive effects of verapamil, atenolol, and captopril in hypertensive blacks demonstrated that verapamil was the superior agent for blood pressure reduction. The response to these drugs is enhanced by a low renin state and a high dietary salt intake, which are common features in the black hypertensive population.

Alpha-receptor blocking agents reduce peripheral vascular resistance and therefore reduce blood pressure in black hypertensive patients. In ALLHAT, there was an increase in heart failure admissions, so these drugs are no longer first-line.

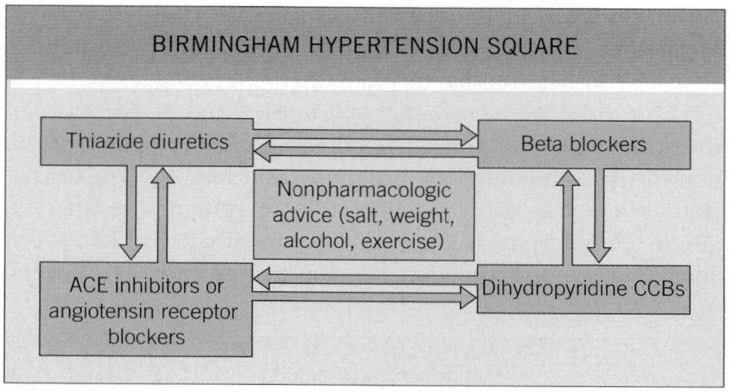

What To Do If the Therapy Doesn't Work

There are logical add-on therapies and less logical combinations. For example, beta blockers work well with the dihydropyridine calcium channel blockers and, by offsetting tachycardia and sympathetic stimulation, they may actually reduce side effects. There is good evidence of synergy between the thiazide diuretics and beta blockers, ACE inhibitors, and angiotensin II receptor antagonists. Similarly, calcium channel blockers work well in combination with the classes of drug that block the generation or effects of angiotensin II.

On the other hand, there are some drug combinations that are not particularly effective and some are unsafe. There is little synergy between thiazide diuretics and the dihydropyridine calcium channel blockers. The addition of an ACE inhibitor to a beta blocker also tends to be less effective because the beta blockers will already have blocked renin release. To aid sensible prescribing we have developed the Birmingham Hypertension Square for add-in drugs in the management of hypertension (Fig. 48A.1). The clinician should opt to approach the square from any corner, with first-line drugs chosen logically. The optimal second-line agents are immediately adjacent and indicated by the arrows. Multidrug therapy is often required in patients with moderate to severe hypertension, which occurs with increased frequency in blacks.

Figure 48A.1 Combination effects of hypertensive drugs. The Birmingham Hypertension Square for the optimum choice of add-in or synergistic drugs in the management of hypertension.

The optimal blood pressure in black patients is still uncertain. Most studies suggest that a diastolic blood pressure of 85 mm Hg may maximally decrease the incidence of stroke and congestive heart failure in blacks and whites. However, hypertensive blacks can occasionally continue to develop progressive renal insufficiency despite seemingly adequate control, suggesting that even lower pressures may be required for optimal renal protection.

Finally the physician needs to ensure that there is good drug compliance. Deterioration in blood pressure control is often related to the kidney, such as renal impairment or renal artery stenosis. The patient should be asked about other concurrent medicines, such as licorice, herbal medicines, and over-the-counter medicines.

SUMMARY

In view of the high prevalence of salt sensitivity in hypertensive blacks, advice regarding dietary sodium restriction is important and should be combined with other nonpharmacologic measures, including weight control, alcohol moderation, and regular exercise. Low-dose thiazide diuretics remain effective, inexpensive first-line agents in blacks, as are the calcium channel blockers. Beta blockers, ACE inhibitors, and angiotensin II receptor antagonists are less effective when used as monotherapy, especially when used in low doses, although the combination of one of these with a diuretic eliminates some of the ethnic differences between blacks and nonblacks.

b. Hypertension in Pregnancy: Preeclampsia

David Churchill

DEFINITION OF PROBLEM

In pregnancy the definition of hypertension is a systolic blood pressure of 140 mm Hg or higher, or a diastolic pressure of 90 mm Hg or higher on two occasions, 4 or more hours apart. In the classical diagnosis of preeclampsia, hypertension has to occur in combination with proteinuria, the latter at a level of 300 mg or higher in 24 hours. It also occurs only after 20 weeks' gestation, with one exception, in the presence of a hydatidiform mole. Although preeclampsia has an incidence of 2% to 4%, it accounts for a large proportion of all low- and very-low-birthweight babies and is a significant cause of maternal morbidity and mortality.

Preeclampsia is a multisystem disorder with a diverse pathophysiology and has a variety of clinical presentations (Fig. 48B.1). This has led to some researchers widening the criteria for diagnosis to include hypertension and one or more of the following: proteinuria, renal insufficiency, liver disease, neurologic or hematologic problems, and fetal growth restriction. When the liver and hematologic systems are affected alone, the syndrome is known by the mnemonic HELLP, which stands for hemolysis, elevated liver enzymes, and low platelets.

ETIOLOGY

The true cause of preeclampsia remains unknown. However it is believed that the abnormality lies in the decidual segments of the vascular tree and is characterized by endothelial damage. This ultimately results in vascular thrombotic episodes and placental ischemia. This inadequate maternal vascular response to placentation becomes clinically evident in the second and third trimesters but probably has its root much earlier in the first trimester.

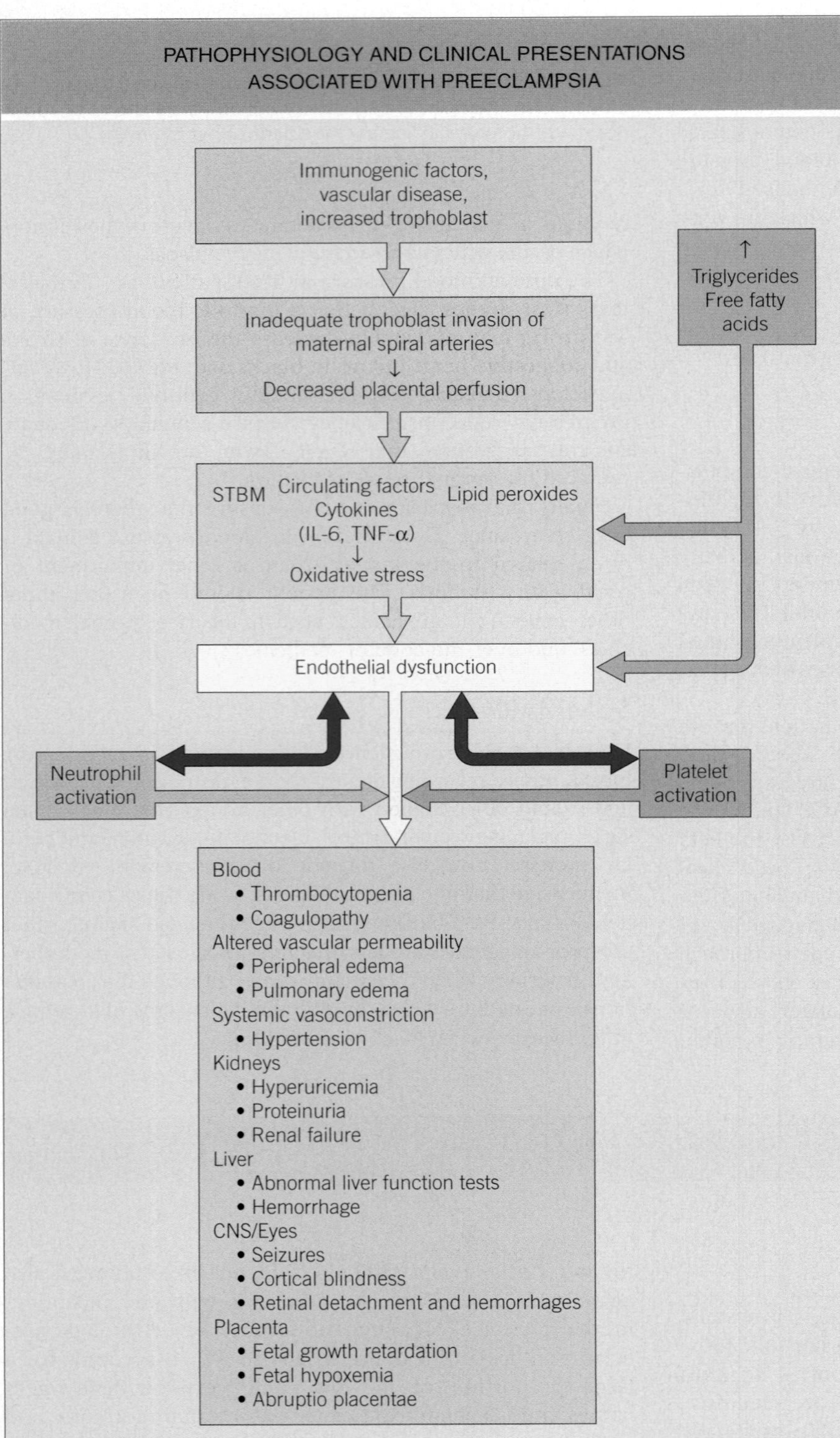

Figure 48B.1 Pathophysiology and clinical presentations associated with preeclampsia. (From Karthikeyan VJ, Lip GYH. Hypertension in pregnancy: pathophysiology and management strategies. Curr Pharm Des 2007; 13:2567-2579.)

TYPICAL CASE

A 34-year-old primigravid woman with essential hypertension was referred to the obstetric day assessment unit at 26 weeks of gestation by her midwife. She was complaining of a 24-hour history of visual disturbances, nausea, and frontal headaches unrelieved by simple analgesics. Her blood pressure was 150/100 mm Hg and dipstick analysis of her urine sample revealed 2+ of protein in a clean midstream specimen. Investigations showed a moderately low platelet count and a raised serum uric acid level. The serum albumin level was also low, and a 24-hour urine collection for total protein quantified the loss at 1.5 g/day. The diagnosis of preeclampsia was made. Fetal biometry was performed with an ultrasound scan and a severely growth-restricted fetus was discovered; the abdominal circumference was below the third percentile for gestational age. In addition it was noted that the amniotic fluid volume was reduced and Doppler ultrasound of the umbilical artery showed absent end-diastolic flow (Fig. 48B.2). However, a cardiotocograph showed a normal fetal heart rate pattern, and so no immediate action was required. The patient was kept in the hospital with both the fetal and maternal conditions being closely monitored over the following 4 days. She was given methyldopa 250 mg three times a day orally to control her blood pressure and intramuscular betamethasone to accelerate surfactant production in the fetal lung. Repeated measures of the platelet count and serum albumin showed a continuing fall in these values. The uric acid level continued to rise, and on day 5 the liver enzymes became mildly elevated. On day 6 she complained of severe frontal headaches, visual disturbances, nausea, and uncontrollable vomiting. Examination demonstrated generalized edema, right hypochondrial tenderness, hyperreflexia, and clonus. The blood pressure was measured at 180/120 mm Hg. The decision was taken to end the pregnancy. She was given a loading dose (4 g over 30 minutes) of magnesium sulfate and maintained on an infusion of 1 g per hour. Her blood pressure was stabilized with 20 mg oral nifedipine, given in two doses 15 minutes apart. A cesarean section was performed to deliver the fetus and placenta. Over the next 72 hours the patient slowly recovered but was left with mild hypertension of 140/90 mm Hg. At follow-up 6 weeks after delivery, her blood pressure, hematologic, and biochemical indices had all returned to normal.

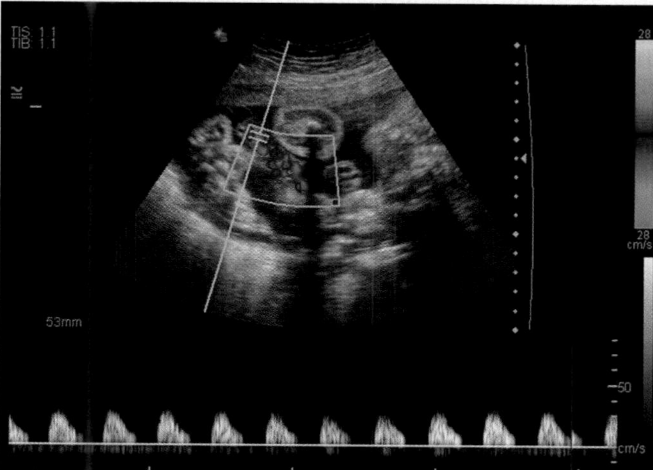

Figure 48B.2 An umbilical artery Doppler waveform showing absence of forward flow in the umbilical cord in late diastole.

TREATMENT OPTIONS

Conservative management of preeclampsia is acceptable in moderate to severe cases at a very early gestation, but when the acute phase is reached the only cure is to end the pregnancy, delivering the baby and placenta. Antihypertensive treatment allows prolongation of pregnancies, with the beneficial effect of enabling greater fetal maturity and allowing time for the maternal administration of corticosteroids to reduce the effects of respiratory distress syndrome in the infant. However, close maternal and fetal monitoring is mandatory, and if any signs of an impending maternal or fetal crisis develop, the pregnancy should be ended.

Methyldopa has been the mainstay antihypertensive for use in pregnancy for many years. Its safety profile is well recognized. Unfortunately, methyldopa has a poor side effect profile, with up to 20% of patients needing to discontinue the drug. Many obstetricians have turned to beta blockers, such as oxprenolol or labetalol as first-line treatment agents. Oxprenolol has been compared with methyldopa in a small randomized controlled trial and was found to be an acceptable drug to use. The oxprenolol group did have a better outcome in terms of perinatal mortality, but the trial was too small to be conclusive.

However, a meta-analysis of drug trials for the treatment of hypertension in pregnancy found that a fall in blood pressure, as measured by the mean arterial pressure, was associated with a reduction in the infant birth weight, and that the fall in weight appeared to be proportional to the reduction in pressure.

Overall, the aim of oral antihypertensive therapy should be to maintain a level of blood pressure that avoids undue stress on the maternal circulation and has no detrimental effect on the uteroplacental unit. The levels of blood pressure that require treatment remain unclear. The majority of obstetricians will treat patients when the diastolic pressure exceeds 100 mm Hg and tolerate levels between 90 mm Hg and 100 mm Hg. Others would treat at much lower levels of diastolic pressure (e.g., 90 to 95 mm Hg). Whichever level the clinician chooses to treat, it is important to be consistent and to lower the blood pressure smoothly and slowly. It should also not be lowered too far, because a raised blood pressure may in fact be a compensatory mechanism to achieve an adequate blood flow through an already compromised placental circulation.

Given the current evidence, it is probably prudent to reserve treatment for those patients who will derive a real benefit. They are likely to be those at very early gestations and/or with the most severe form of the disease.

In situations where either methyldopa or one of the beta blockers fails to have the desired effect in lowering blood pressure, a second-line agent may be used. Although the published evidence is not as great as for the other two drugs, the calcium channel blocker nifedipine is widely used and is believed to be safe in these circumstances.

Nifedipine can also be used when patients reach crisis point. The symptoms and signs of a crisis may include clonus, nausea, vomiting, and right hypochondrial pain. Eclampsia or some other serious complication is a very real risk and there is an urgent need to control severe hypertension. Oral nifedipine can be used in the first instance. This will often be sufficient to control the patient's blood pressure in preparation for delivery. Care must be taken when using nifedipine in patients who are also receiving magnesium sulfate. The effects can be additive and precipitous falls in blood pressure can occur. If oral treatment is ineffective or is not suitable, intravenous hydralazine can be used. Bolus doses of 5 to 10 mg are given in the first instance, but if no appreciable effect is noted after three doses at intervals of 15 minutes, an infusion should be administered.

One drawback with hydralazine is the reflex tachycardia, which can result in the systolic pressure remaining at dangerously high levels. The addition of small intravenous doses of a beta blocker such as labetalol (25 mg) will prevent this.

Cerebral autoregulation breaks down at blood pressures in excess of 170/110 mm Hg and the cerebral circulation becomes prone to disruption, leading to strokes. Therefore it is important to maintain the maternal systolic blood pressure below 160 mm Hg, giving a margin of safety. A fall in blood pressure that is too great can compromise the uteroplacental circulation, resulting in fetal hypoxia. During treatment a cardiotocograph should be performed to look for any abnormal fetal heart rate patterns. Maintaining the diastolic pressure between 90 and 100 mm Hg and a systolic pressure less than 160 mm Hg is good control and should be aimed for in all acute crises.

Fluid management needs rigorous attention in the acute situation. The endothelial damage caused by the disease process results in capillary leakage of fluid into the extracellular space, causing generalized edema. Administration of large volumes of fluid can precipitate pulmonary edema, which, if not recognized early enough and treated promptly with diuretics and fluid restriction, will result in adult respiratory distress syndrome.

Magnesium sulfate is the drug of choice to prevent and treat eclampsia. Magnesium levels can be monitored biochemically, clinically, or both by observing the respiratory rate and tendon reflexes. Absence of patellar tendon reflexes is an early warning sign of toxicity, which if left unrecognized could lead to respiratory depression. The antidote to toxicity is 1 g of intravenous calcium gluconate solution.

For many years the only practically useful predictive test for preeclampsia was to identify women by their clinical risk factors (e.g., those with preexisting essential hypertension, renovascular hypertension, antiphospholipid syndrome, and early-onset preeclampsia in a previous pregnancy). However, a technique visualizing Doppler waveforms in the uterine artery at around 20 weeks of gestation has shown that the presence of a raised resistance or a "notch" in the waveform in early diastole (Fig. 48B.3) is specific and sensitive for predicting the development of preeclampsia later in the pregnancy. Those with abnormal waveforms need more intensive antenatal surveillance and may possibly be prescribed low-dose aspirin. A recent systematic review has concluded that low-dose aspirin (60 to 150 mg) reduces the incidence of preeclampsia by 17% in high-risk pregnancies. However, questions remain over when is the best time to start treatment, but on balance the evidence tends to favor treatment starting in early gestation.

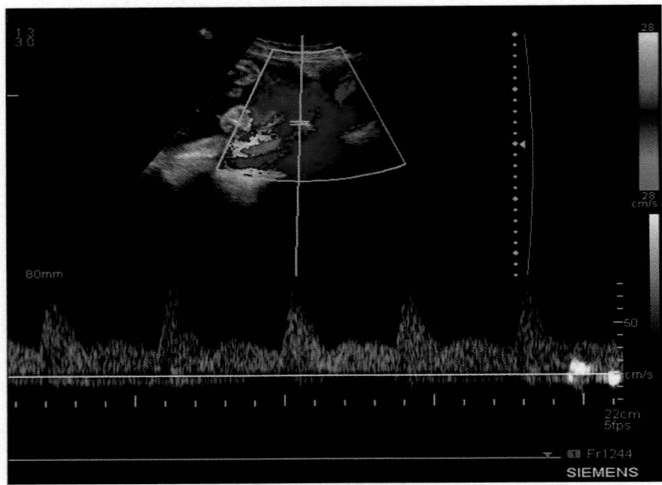

Figure 48B.3 A Doppler waveform of a maternal uterine artery showing a notch in early diastole.

SUMMARY

Hypertension in pregnancy is a common problem. But it is in the form of preeclampsia that it is at its most dangerous. Maternal complications of preeclampsia include eclamptic seizures, renal failure, retinal detachment, disseminated intravascular coagulopathy, and myocardial infarction as well as significant fetal morbidity and mortality from intrauterine growth retardation and iatrogenic prematurity. Treatment requires attention to detail, good blood pressure control, and constant vigilance to detect the early signs of significant complications.

c. Perioperative Hypertension

William J. Elliott

DEFINITION OF PROBLEM

Perioperative hypertension is sustained elevated blood pressure (BP) (BP typically ≥140/90 mm Hg in the United States, or ≥160/95 mm Hg in many other countries) immediately before, during, or after a surgical procedure. The specific BP level that increases perioperative risk and should be treated is unclear; the American Society of Anesthesiologists (ASA) uses 180/100 mm Hg as the cutoff. Although randomized clinical trials with morbidity or mortality endpoints have not been done, lowering BP in these settings is recommended by recent guidelines. Preexisting hypertension is found in about 80% to 90% of patients who develop perioperative hypertension. Because the prevalence of hypertension, the need for surgery, and poorer outcomes are all directly correlated with increasing age, control of perioperative hypertension is most important in older individuals. Perioperative hypertension is more common with coronary artery bypass, carotid endarterectomy, aortic aneurysm repair, intracranial exploration, and pheochromocytoma surgery.

TYPICAL CASE

A 74-year-old man with a 30-year history of hypertension and dyslipidemia was scheduled for an elective total knee replacement. A dobutamine echocardiogram was normal 6 days before the scheduled procedure. Despite having taken all of his usual medications (amlodipine, aspirin, atorvastatin, lisinopril, and chlorthalidone) 4 hours beforehand, the procedure was cancelled because his BP was 220/128 mm Hg. Seven days after beginning atenolol, the procedure was successfully performed with an estimated blood loss of 750 mL. Intraoperatively, he had a nadir BP of 108/42 mm Hg; 3 L of saline were given. On the second postoperative day, after two units of autotransfused blood, his BP reached 190/106 mm Hg, his serum creatinine level increased by 50%, and intravenous fenoldopam was administered. Narcotics were given for incisional pain, resulting in lowered (but not quite normal) BPs for about 4 hours after each injection. Over the next 3 days, relative oliguria was treated with serial doses of furosemide, and his BP decreased to an average of 138/86 mm Hg during the next 3 days. During 7 days of rehabilitation, normal BPs were recorded. He was discharged from the hospital 10 days after the operation, and the atenolol was discontinued 18 days later. BPs remained well controlled thereafter, with the same antihypertensive drug regimen as before the procedure.

DIFFERENTIAL DIAGNOSIS

The most easily remedied causes of acute hypertension related to surgery are pain, stress, anxiety, and/or bladder distention. Hypertension on the second or third postoperative day may occur because the patient's usual oral antihypertensive medications were withheld; this is most common with alpha agonists or beta blockers, but has been reported for diuretics and calcium antagonists. Other agents (monoamine oxidase inhibitors, cocaine, large intravenous salt loads during/after surgery) may also elevate BP. Rarely, perioperative hypertension may be the presenting sign of a pheochromocytoma; norepinephrine production by these tumors typically surges with the induction of general anesthesia.

TREATMENT OPTIONS

Although there are more than 100 oral medications for hypertension, the roster of options for other routes of administration is limited, but may soon grow. The onset of action for transdermal clonidine is usually too long for it to be useful in this setting. Intravenous options in the United States include several diuretics (chlorothiazide, furosemide), several beta blockers (atenolol, esmolol, metoprolol, labetalol, propranolol), an alpha agonist (methyldopa), an angiotensin-converting enzyme (ACE) inhibitor (enalaprilat), several calcium antagonists (verapamil, diltiazem, nicardipine), and several other drugs (hydralazine, diazoxide, or clevidipine). Nitroprusside, fenoldopam, and nitroglycerin are currently the three most commonly used drugs for hypertensive emergencies. Each drug has situations for which it can be recommended (Fig. 48C.1).

PREOPERATIVE ASSESSMENT

The preoperative assessment of patients at risk for cardiovascular complications has been addressed by recent guidelines. Apart from preoperative testing for asymptomatic coronary disease, preoperative evaluation includes three important issues (Fig. 48C.2). Successful oral antihypertensive drug therapy should be continued up to and including the day of surgery. Some authorities recommend withholding both angiotensin converting-enzyme inhibitors and angiotensin II receptor blockers on the morning of surgery, because of an excess risk of hypotension after induction of anesthesia. Although no clinical trial evidence exists, several decades of experience have shown that intraoperative hypertension and postoperative complications are less frequent and less severe when most long-term antihypertensive drug therapy is uninterrupted. Most anesthesiologists have a low threshold for postponing elective procedures if the immediate preoperative BP is "high;" many use 180/100 mm Hg or higher as the criterion. Ethical constraints prohibit "proof" of the wisdom of this policy, as it has become standard practice. Whether a beta blocker should be part of the antihypertensive regimen for those undergoing major (and other noncardiac) surgery is still controversial. Several meta-analyses of various subsets of the 17 randomized trials reported through 2007, a cohort study comparing outcomes in 119,362 people receiving beta blockers versus 663,635 controls, and several case-control studies all suggested significant reduction in myocardial infarction and death in those receiving a preoperative beta blocker. The PeriOperative Ischemic Evaluation (POISE) trial randomized 8351 high-risk patients undergoing noncardiac surgery to placebo or metoprolol succinate, started 2-4 hours preoperatively, and continued for 30 days. Although metoprolol was associated with a significantly lower risk of cardiac events and of myocardial infarction, there was an unexpected significant **increase** in stroke and a non-significant **increase** in death. A subsequent meta-analysis of 33 trials involving 12,306 subjects (with POISE accounting for about 80% of the endpoints) concluded that "evidence does not support . . . beta blocker therapy . . . in patients having non-cardiac surgery." This will likely cause the current American College of Cardiology/American Heart Association guidelines to be revisited.

INDUCTION AND MAINTENANCE OF ANESTHESIA

The risk of hypertension is greatest during laryngoscopy, intubation, and the induction of anesthesia. Systolic BP elevations of 30 mm Hg in normotensive patients and up to 90 mm Hg in uncontrolled hypertensive patients are common. Preoperative stress and anxiety often exacerbate this

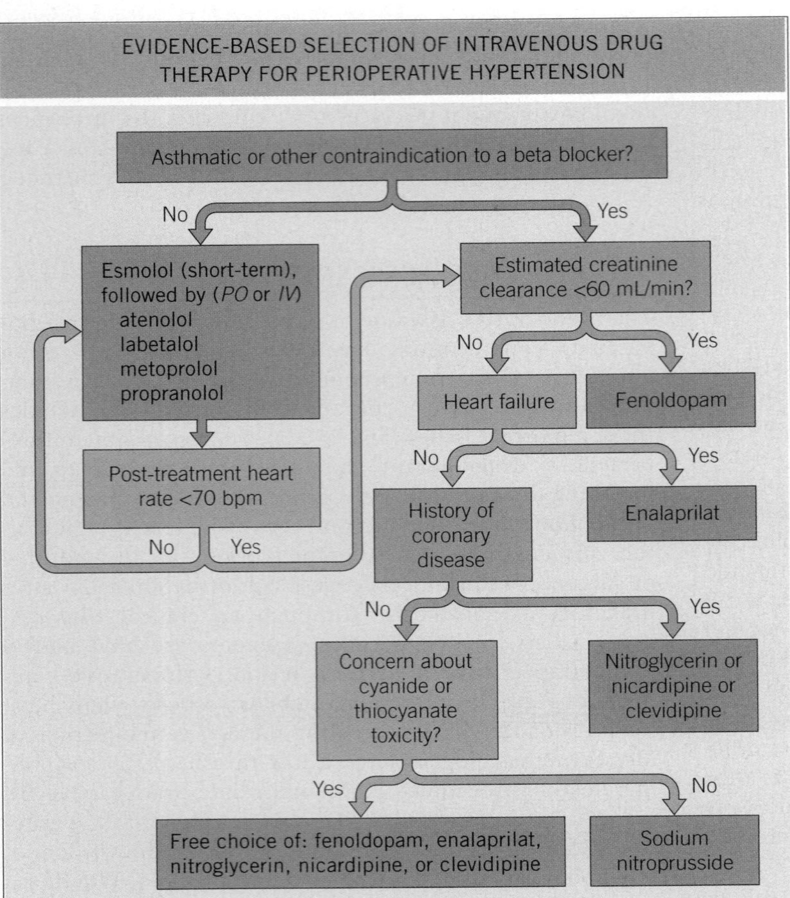

Figure 48C.1 Evidence-based selection of intravenous drug therapy for perioperative hypertension. Although there is a long tradition and many pharmacokinetic reasons for using nitroprusside as the drug of choice, other drugs chosen earlier in the hierarchy of these questions have proven benefits in reducing morbidity and mortality. Esmolol is suggested as an initial beta blocker because of its short duration of effect (and therefore reversibility); a longer-acting agent is often used after initial beta blockade with esmolol.

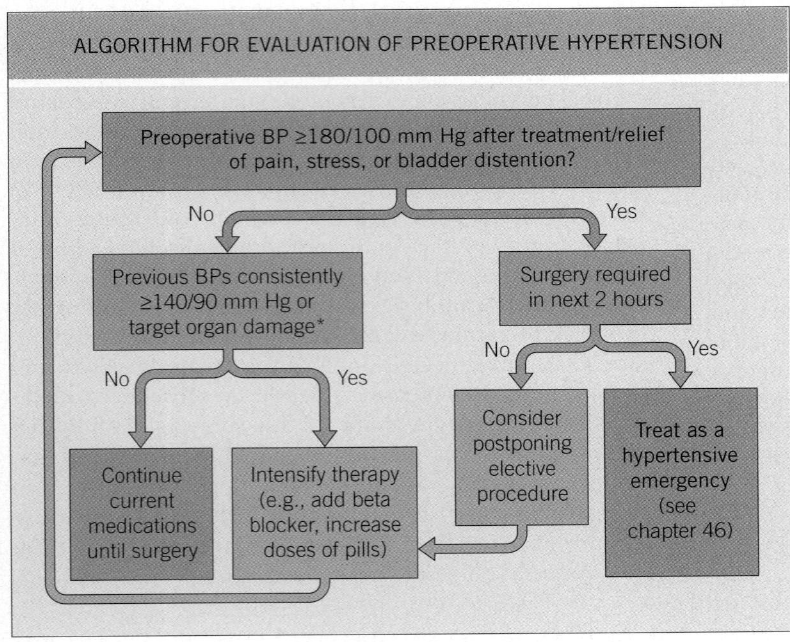

Figure 48C.2 Road map for evaluation of preoperative hypertension. *Target organ damage includes (but is not limited to) known atherosclerotic disease (e.g., coronary heart disease, previous stroke, or transient ischemic attack), electrocardiographic changes consistent with ischemia or left ventricular hypertrophy, and/or renal impairment (elevated serum creatinine, albumin/creatinine ratio, or proteinuria). BP, blood pressure.

response, and prophylactic anxiolytic agents are often given to prevent it. These brief periods of hypertension are important to avoid or minimize, especially for patients who are at higher risk (ASA class III or IV). Perioperative soothing music (administered by headphones to the patient) may reduce preoperative stress and BP.

Loss of venous tone during induction of anesthesia and during the operative procedure is more common in hypertensive than normotensive patients, and increases the risk of acute hypotension. This is often best managed by physical measures (e.g., Trendelenburg position) and judicious intravenous infusion of fluids.

INTRAOPERATIVE HYPERTENSION

Prospective studies have shown an increased incidence of both myocardial ischemia and renal dysfunction among patients with abnormal intraoperative BPs. When BP changes by more than 20% (or even less in vascular or neurosurgery), there is concern, often followed by treatment. Short-acting, easily titrated drugs (e.g., nitroprusside) are preferred for acute treatment of hypertension. An initial fluid bolus is generally given for hypotension, although vasoconstrictors are occasionally needed.

POSTOPERATIVE HYPERTENSION

An increase in BP due to pain (35% of hypertensive cases), sympathetic stimulation of emerging from anesthesia (16%), and/or hypercarbia (15%) is common in the recovery room, especially after myocardial revascularization. It is standard procedure (despite no clinical trial evidence) to survey for and treat these causes of hypertension before giving antihypertensive drug therapy. Exceptions exist in vascular and neurosurgery, where even brief elevations in BP in the postoperative period have been associated with poorer outcomes.

TREATMENT AND MONITORING

Many episodes of perioperative hypertension qualify as hypertensive emergencies or urgencies (see Chapter 46). Oral medications are usually not an option, and intravenously administered drugs are preferred (see Fig. 48C.1). In many centers, nitroprusside is the drug of choice for short-term control of BP, especially intraoperatively and on the first postoperative day. Toxicity of its metabolites, thiocyanate and cyanide, is the chief concern; these accumulate at high dose or during prolonged infusion (typically >8 hours). Nitroglycerin infusions are commonly used during and after cardiac and cardiovascular surgery, but can be technically challenging. Intravenous nicardipine is sometimes given when an antianginal arteriolar dilator is preferred. An ultra–short acting dihydropyridine calcium antagonist, clevidipine, has been recently approved, and is especially useful for perioperative use. The peripheral dopamine-1 agonist, fenoldopam, has some clinical trial evidence to support its preferential use in major vascular procedures (e.g., coronary artery bypass, aortic aneurysm repair), presumably because it increases renal blood flow and improves several measures of renal function. These attributes may be more important for patients with preexisting renal impairment or diabetes. Esmolol is the beta blocker with the shortest elimination half-life and is often used initially to control tachycardia; other beta blockers can be used, but their effects linger for many hours. Enalaprilat is the only ACE inhibitor available for intravenous use, and it also has prolonged effects after acute administration. Phentolamine is generally useful only for pheochromocytoma. Diuretics are usually given only if there is fluid overload, iatrogenic or not. Other intravenous antihypertensive drugs, including hydralazine, methyldopa, diazoxide, propranolol, metoprolol, atenolol, diltiazem, or verapamil, are less commonly used.

For many patients, the risk of hypotension and organ hypoperfusion after a long-acting antihypertensive agent is probably higher than the acute risk of a few minutes of hypertension. As a result, short-acting, easily titrated drugs are generally preferred for the shortest possible duration. Prospective monitoring of a patient's BP, urinary output, serum creatinine, and cardiac enzymes allow the physician to minimize BP deviations and watch for and avoid target organ damage.

SUMMARY

Although clinical trials have not been done to demonstrate morbidity or mortality reduction with preventing or treating hypertension in the perioperative setting, this is generally accepted as standard medical practice. The addition of a beta blocker to the antihypertensive regimen decreases the risk of cardiac events in patients undergoing noncardiac surgery, but its routine use is controversial. Continuation of long-term antihypertensive medications, postponement of surgery for those with preoperative hypertension, and careful control of BP both intraoperatively and postoperatively are thought to increase the likelihood of uneventful recovery after an otherwise successful surgical procedure.

d. Ambulatory Blood Pressure Monitoring

Apurv Khanna and William B. White

DEFINITION OF THE PROBLEM

The key parameter defining hypertension in clinical medicine is the office blood pressure (BP) value, typically measured by a nurse or physician using a mercury column sphygmomanometer or an aneroid manometer. However, the doctor's office BP has many pitfalls, including observer bias, miscuffing, and measurements that may not be representative of the average daily pressure for a given patient. Monitoring the BP outside the medical care environment has become a useful part of clinical hypertension assessment and management. There are two forms of out-of-office BP monitoring: (1) self or home monitoring, usually performed by the patient (or a relative) with a portable semiautomatic device or aneroid manometer plus stethoscope; and (2) ambulatory BP monitoring, which uses automatic devices for repeated determinations during an extended time period, typically 24 hours so that both awake and sleep periods are captured. Both techniques have been shown to substantially improve our understanding of BP behavior in patients and aid in diagnosis and therapeutic decision making.

CIRCADIAN VARIABILITY OF BLOOD PRESSURE

The circadian rhythm of BP has been recognized since the mid-1960s, but its clinical importance in the management of hypertension has only been fully realized in the 21st century. Arterial BP has a daily variation characterized by a rapid rise upon awakening, increased variability during the awake period in ambulant normal subjects and hypertensive patients, and a substantial reduction in BP during sleep. Increases in the incidence of sudden death, nonfatal myocardial infarction (MI), unstable angina, and stroke in the morning indicate that a patient's physiologic status may play an important role in the onset of cardiovascular events. Additionally, the loss of the nocturnal decline in BP has been associated with increased risk of cardiac, renal, and vascular target organ injury compared with patients whose decline in BP at night is normal. Additionally, patients with hypertension who exhibit a nocturnal BP increase compared with daytime BP (so-called risers) have the worst prognosis for stroke and cardiac events. There is also some evidence that patients with marked nocturnal BP declines (extreme dippers) are at risk of lacunar strokes and silent myocardial ischemia. A recent cohort analysis by Boggia and coworkers demonstrated the importance of nocturnal BP in predicting prognosis. In fact, the BP at night was more robust than the BP during the daytime for predicting fatal endpoints, and the night-to-day ratio predicted total, cardiovascular, and noncardiovascular mortality. The confirmation that correcting 24-hour BP profiles results in clinical outcomes benefit will require clinical trials that specifically test this hypothesis. In the future, however, if the use of ambulatory blood pressure monitoring is validated from such trials, we will likely see an exponential growth in its application in clinical medicine.

DEVICES AND VALIDATION

Over the past 25 years, noninvasive automatic devices have been developed for hypertension management and clinical research. In recent years, the ambulatory BP monitors have become much more practical to use in patient care. The devices are much smaller than in the past (less than 1 pound in most instances), simple to apply by a nurse or technician, and precise. These fully automatic, programmable recorders are capable of 100 to 200 BP and pulse measurements from an energy source of two to four small batteries. The devices measure BP either by oscillometry or auscultation of Korotkoff sounds. Oscillometric measurement is derived from oscillations emanating from the brachial artery into the BP cuff—the amplitude of the oscillations are related to a standard form of BP (usually mercury column measurements by auscultation) and an algorithm is then developed. The oscillometric methodology is accurate in patients who have midrange BPs and hold their arms still during cuff inflation and deflation. In some studies, oscillometric BP determination is less accurate in older patients or those with extremely low or high pressures compared to midrange BP values. Auscultatory measurements mimic those of clinicians and use a microphone for detection of the Korotkoff sounds. Auscultatory devices are also subject to noise artifact when the patient has excessive arm motion during the actual BP measurement. Ambulatory BP recorders used in clinical research or practice should be independently validated using established criteria.

HOW DO AMBULATORY BPs COMPARE WITH MEASUREMENTS IN THE DOCTOR'S OFFICE?

It is helpful to develop a frame of reference for the values derived from the ambulatory BP recordings, because most practicing physicians would naturally compare these BPs with those obtained in their office. The recorders are usually programmed to measure 50 to 100 BPs in 24 hours. In about 80% of patients with hypertension, there is a reproducible diurnal and nocturnal pattern in BP during a 24-hour period of measurement characterized by high and more variable pressures while awake (with the highest during work) and lower and less variable values during sleep. Once a recording has been completed in an individual patient, the data are expressed as the mean 24-hour, awake, and sleep systolic and diastolic pressures. Blood pressure during sleep is usually lower than the office pressure, whereas BP during wakefulness is similar to the values obtained in the office. One must keep these differences in mind when trying to interpret ambulatory BP recordings. Most consensus groups have used a 24-hour BP higher than 130/80 mm Hg and an awake BP higher than 135/85 mm Hg as abnormal based on several new outcome studies comparing ambulatory versus clinic BP in patients with hypertension.

AMBULATORY BLOOD PRESSURE AND TARGET ORGAN DISEASE

Nearly all cross-sectional studies published to date have shown the ambulatory BP to be superior to office BP in predicting target organ involvement. The most striking evidence has come from assessment of the relations among office pressure, ambulatory BP, and indexes of left ventricular hypertrophy. Using intra-arterial pressure measurements (thus beat-to-beat BP values are obtained), it has been shown that variability of BP may be a predictor of morbidity in hypertension. However, this has not been confirmed by numerous studies using noninvasive BP measurements. Numerous studies have now also shown that ambulatory BP is an independent predictor of cardiovascular risk. Most of these studies have also demonstrated that a loss of nocturnal decline in BP (so-called nondippers) conveys excessive risk for stroke and myocardial infarction.

CLINICAL DIAGNOSES OR PROBLEMS IN WHICH NONINVASIVE AMBULATORY BLOOD PRESSURE MONITORING MAY BE USEFUL
■ Office or white coat hypertension ■ Borderline hypertension with or without target organ involvement ■ Evaluation of patients refractory to antihypertensive therapy ■ Episodic hypertension ■ Hypotensive symptoms associated with antihypertensive medications ■ Autonomic dysfunction/nocturnal hypertension ■ Exclusion of placebo reactors when determining efficacy of antihypertensive drug therapy in controlled clinical trials
Modified from National High Blood Pressure Education Program Working Group report on ambulatory blood pressure monitoring. Arch Intern Med 1990;150:2270-2280.

Table 48D.1 Clinical diagnoses or problems in which noninvasive ambulatory blood pressure monitoring may be useful.

USEFULNESS OF AMBULATORY BLOOD PRESSURE IN CLINICAL PRACTICE

Several subsets of hypertensive diagnoses have been elucidated as a result of ambulatory BP monitoring (Table 48D.1). Clinical problems seen most often by practicing physicians that are appropriate for ambulatory BP monitoring include the assessment of possible "white coat" hypertension, borderline hypertension (with and without evidence for target organ damage), and evaluation of refractory hypertension in patients on complex antihypertensive regimens. A number of well-performed studies show that these patients might benefit when the ambulatory BP is known in addition to the measurements made in the medical care environment. It is not uncommon that refractory patients (regardless of age) on antihypertensive drugs have a pressor response in the medical care environment that brings them into hypertensive ranges, yet their out-of-office values are normal. Conversely, it is not unusual to perform ambulatory BP monitoring in a hypertensive patient with reasonably good office pressures and find that BP levels are not well-controlled late in the dosing period of the medication (Fig. 48D.1). In an assessment of a physician's practice habits associated with ambulatory BP recordings, about 30% to 40% of the patients were prescribed more medications to

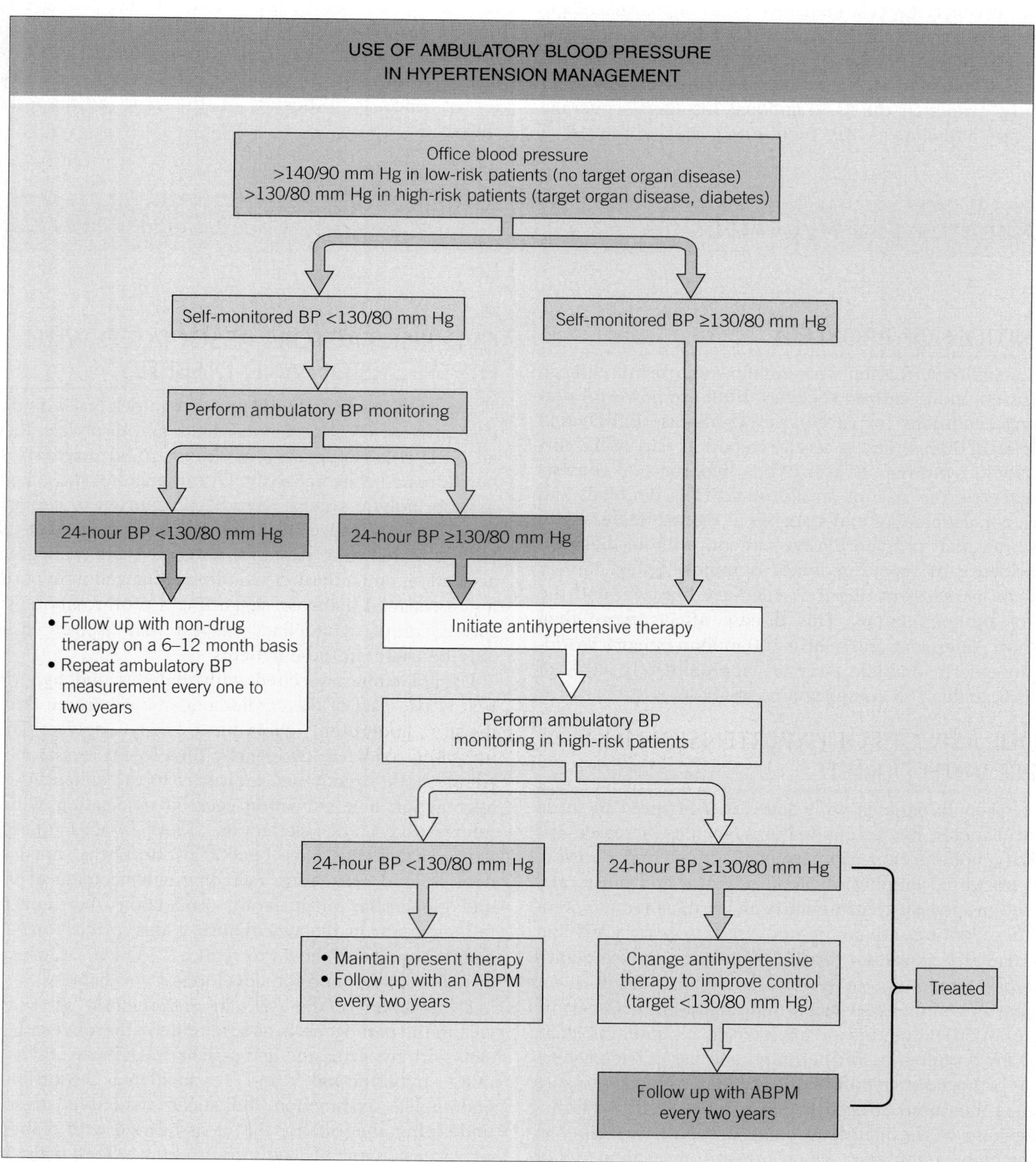

Figure 48D.1 Algorithm for using ambulatory blood pressure monitoring (ABPM) in clinical practice.

improve BP control. These types of findings have resulted in an algorithm for the utility of ambulatory blood pressure monitoring in clinical practice (see Fig. 48D.1).

COST AND COVERAGE CONSIDERATIONS

Ambulatory BP monitoring may cost the physician, hospital, or heart station several thousand dollars to provide one or two adequate recorders and software for data analysis and report generation. While more costly than self-monitoring, ambulatory BP monitoring is still useful because it may identify those who truly require antihypertensive therapy as well as those who may be best managed with nonpharmacologic therapy. Furthermore, ambulatory BP is the only means that we have to obtain BP measurements during sleep. During 2001, the Center for Medicare and Medicaid Services independently evaluated the U.S. national insurance coverage policy for ambulatory BP monitoring and approved a national policy that would pay for the study when it is used in the diagnosis of white coat hypertension. Other diagnoses considered, such as episodic hypertension, refractory hypertension, and evaluation of antihypertensive therapy were not covered in the policy.

SUMMARY

Ambulatory BP measurement has become a helpful tool in hypertension management, especially for the assessment of white coat hypertension in untreated patients and the white coat effect in the older, treated patient. Virtually all observational cohort studies have shown that ambulatory BP is superior to the doctor's office pressure in predicting cardiovascular events. Finally, drug development for hypertension mandates that ambulatory BP studies are performed to properly evaluate the pharmacodynamics of once-daily dosing of the new antihypertensive therapies.

e. Diabetes and Hypertension

Samy I. McFarlane, Guido Lastra, and James R. Sowers

DEFINITION OF PROBLEM

Diabetes and hypertension are common comorbid diseases in westernized, industrialized societies. Both are powerful predisposing conditions for cardiovascular disease (CVD) and chronic renal disease and generally coexist as part of the cardiometabolic syndrome (CMS). When hypertension coexists with diabetes, the risk of stroke or CVD is doubled, and the risk for developing end-stage renal disease increases to 5 to 6 times that of hypertensive patients without diabetes. The incidence of type 2 diabetes is rapidly rising, largely related to increases in obesity, sedentary lifestyle, and the aging of the population. This disease affects more than 22 million Americans and nearly 300 million persons worldwide. In elderly diabetic patients, approximately 80% of death is secondary to complications of CVD.

UNIQUE ASPECTS OF HYPERTENSION IN PEOPLE WITH DIABETES

Hypertension in patients with diabetes, compared to those without diabetes, has unique features, such as increased salt sensitivity, volume expansion, isolated systolic hypertension, loss of nocturnal dipping of blood pressure and pulse, and increased propensity to proteinuria and orthostatic hypotension. These features are considered risk factors for CVD and are particularly important for selecting the appropriate antihypertensive therapy, for example, low-dose diuretics for treatment of volume expansion and angiotensin-converting enzyme (ACE) inhibitors or angiotensin receptor blockers (ARBs) for proteinuria. Furthermore, because of the propensity to orthostatic hypotension, standing blood pressure should be measured at each patient's office visit. Additionally, because of the increased blood pressure variability in these patients, ambulatory blood pressure measurements or home blood pressure monitoring may be particularly useful.

CVD RISK FACTORS ASSOCIATED WITH HYPERTENSION AND DIABETES

The goal of lowering blood pressure in persons with diabetes is to prevent CVD-associated death and disability; therefore all CVD risk factors such as smoking and inactivity should be addressed concomitantly. Disturbances of the coagulation and fibrinolytic system have been reported in persons with hypertension, especially those with concomitant glucose abnormalities and vascular disease. Platelet aggregation, activation, and adhesion are often enhanced in hypertension and associated diabetes, suggesting a prothrombotic state in this condition. Guidelines suggest that aspirin 75 mg/day may be useful in these patients.

Dyslipidemia associated with diabetes and hypertension that is also part of the cardiometabolic syndrome (low high-density lipoprotein cholesterol, high triglycerides, and increased oxidized low-density lipoprotein levels) may contribute both directly and indirectly to the enhanced platelet aggregation and activation seen in association with these interrelated CVD risk factors. There is accumulating evidence that statins have beneficial effects that are independent of lipid reductions, including enhancement of vascular and glomerular nitric oxide production and reduction in inflammation in the vasculature, kidney, and bones. These agents have been shown to reduce CVD events, progression of nephropathy, and the development of diabetes.

Dysfunction of the vascular endothelium plays a major role in the pathogenesis of accelerated atherosclerosis in persons with hypertension and associated diabetes. Hyperglycemia, hypertension, and dyslipidemia contribute to endothelial dysfunction. Enhanced oxidative stress is an underlying abnormality that is associated with diabetes and hypertension and probably contributes to both diabetic renal disease and CVD. Altered redox state and associated

DIETARY AND LIFESTYLE MODIFICATIONS RECOMMENDED FOR MANAGEMENT OF HYPERTENSION
1. Weight loss 2. Exercise (aerobic physical activity) 30-45 min at least 3 times a week 3. Reduced sodium intake to 100 mmol (2.4 g) per day 4. Smoking cessation 5. Adequate intake of dietary potassium, calcium, and magnesium 6. Reduced alcohol intake to <1 oz (30 mL) of ethanol (24 oz [720 mL]) per day 7. Diet rich in fruits and vegetables but low in fat

Table 48E.1 Dietary and lifestyle modifications recommended for management of hypertension.

endothelial dysfunction may also help explain the observation that albuminuria is a good predictor for the development of CVD (stroke and myocardial infarction) and renal disease.

TREATMENT OPTIONS

The consensus blood pressure goal in diabetic persons with hypertension is less than 130/80 mm Hg. Pharmacologic therapy should be initiated simultaneously with dietary and lifestyle modifications as outlined in Table 48E.1. Based on the results of the Dietary Approaches to Stop Hypertension (DASH) study, reducing sodium intake to levels below 100 mmol per day and following the DASH diet both lower blood pressure substantially, with greater effects in combination than singly. Diabetic patients will generally require three medications on average for adequate blood pressure control. Data from the U.K. Prospective Diabetes Study and other studies indicate that three or more antihypertensive medications are usually required to achieve blood pressure goal in people with diabetes.

According to the current recommendations, ACE inhibitors, ARBs, low-dose diuretics, beta blockers, and calcium channel antagonists can be used for pharmacologic therapy of hypertension in diabetic patients (Fig. 48E.1). However, based on relatively recent data, ARBs and ACE inhibitors are preferred first-line therapy in patients with proteinuria, because they have been shown to provide renal and CVD protection. However, since combination therapy is usually necessary for adequate blood pressure control, combination of an ACE inhibitor or ARB and low-dose diuretic or a dihydropyridine calcium channel blocker is useful in this patient population as an initial therapy.

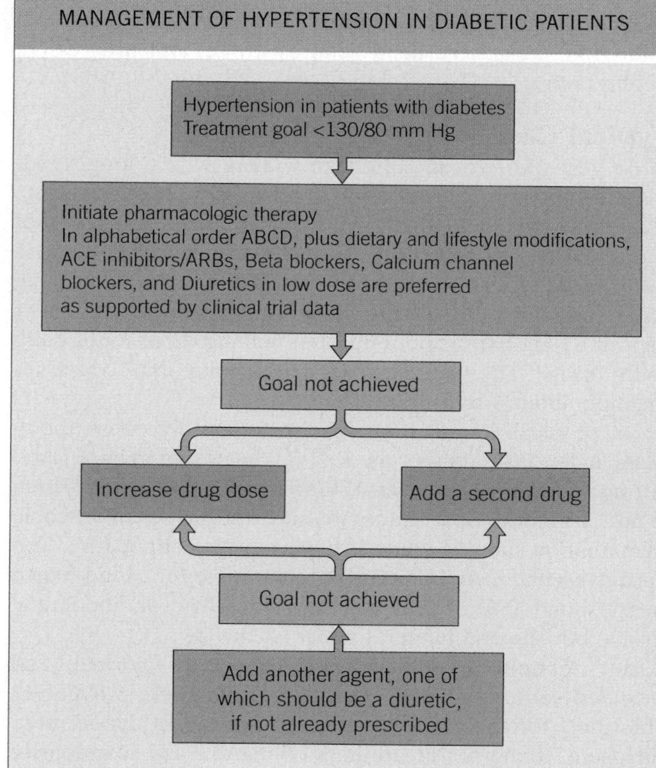

Figure 48E.1 Management of hypertension in patients with diabetes. In patients with >1g proteinuria and renal insufficiency the treatment goal is BP <125/75 mm Hg. ARBs, angiotensin receptor blockers.

SUMMARY

Hypertension is twice as common in people with diabetes and it accounts for up to 80% of CVD complications. Control of blood pressure to levels below 130/80 mm Hg in persons with diabetes has been shown to reduce CVD morbidity and mortality and is currently the recommended goal of therapy. This may require combination of antihypertensive agents. Medications that have been shown to reduce both the renal and CVD risk, such as ACE inhibitors and ARBs, are the preferred first line of treatment in these patients.

f. Resistant Hypertension

Peter D. Hart and George L. Bakris

DEFINITION OF THE PROBLEM

Resistant hypertension is defined as blood pressure (BP) of 140/90 mm Hg or higher or 130/80 mm Hg or higher in patients with diabetes or chronic kidney disease (i.e., serum creatinine of >1.5 mg/dL or urine albumin creatinine ratio >300 mg/g of creatinine), despite adherence to therapy with maximum doses of at least ***three*** antihypertensive agents including a diuretic.

The exact incidence of resistant hypertension is not well defined in the literature, but it may be more common than previously thought, based on estimates derived from recent large outcome trials, such as ALLHAT, VALUE, and CONVINCE. Resistant hypertension is more common in patients 60 years and above and is associated with increased long-term risk of cardiovascular events, such as myocardial infarction, congestive heart failure, stroke, and progressive nephropathy.

Typical Case

A 65-year-old African American woman with a long-standing history of hypertension, coronary artery disease, hyperlipidemia, and osteoarthritis is referred for resistant hypertension. Her medications include hydrochlorothiazide 12.5 mg daily, enalapril 20 mg twice daily, atenolol 100 mg daily, nifedipine XL 60 mg daily, simvastatin 40 mg daily, aspirin 81 mg daily, and ibuprofen 600 mg three times daily with meals. The patient does not smoke, but consumes alcohol, about 4 to 5 drinks daily.

On physical examination she is moderately obese (body mass index 32), pulse rate was 84 beats per minute, and sitting blood pressure was 170/95 mm Hg, measured three times, 5 minutes apart and without orthostasis. Fundoscopic examination showed grade II hypertensive retinopathy. The cardiovascular examination was remarkable for a loud fourth heart sound (S4). There were no epigastric or abdominal bruits, but she had bilateral pedal edema 2+.

Her laboratory studies were generally normal and included serum sodium, 138 meq/L; potassium, 3.8 meq/L; chloride, 105 meq/L; bicarbonate, 26 meq/L; blood urea nitrogen, 30 mg/dL; creatinine, 1.5 mg/dL; and low-density lipoprotein (LDL) cholesterol, 125 mg/dL; and spot urine albumin creatinine ratio, 500 mg/g.

Diagnosis

This patient meets the JNC 7 criteria for diagnosis of resistant hypertension. The suggested approach for the management of this condition is largely based on clinical experience and observational data from hypertension specialty clinics and is summarized in Figure 48F.1.

Factors to consider before truly giving a diagnosis of resistant hypertension include:

(1) Pseudoresistance: A white coat phenomenon defined as persistently elevated blood pressure in the physician's clinic or office but normal blood pressure at home must be excluded with repeated home blood pressure measurements or 24-hour ambulatory blood pressure monitoring. These patients typically have no evidence of target organ damage. Also in older patients, pseudo-hypertension due to severely calcified and sclerotic arteries could present as resistant hypertension and should be suspected by the presence of palpable radial pulse while the brachial artery is occluded by the cuff (the Osler maneuver). An intra-arterial blood pressure measurement confirms this condition.

(2) Patient adherence: Adherence to lifestyle modifications and drug therapy must be carefully evaluated and confirmed. Although difficult to recognize, suggestive symptoms include missed clinic appointments, lack of use of medication refills, and presence of normal heart rate in patients taking beta blockers.

(3) Physician inaction (inertia): Some patients receive inadequate or insufficient antihypertensive drug dose titration despite multiple clinic visits. In other patients, noninitiation or use of inappropriate diuretics, such as thiazide, in a patient with an estimated glomerular filtration rate (GFR) that is less than 30 mL/min, may be an important reason for the poorly controlled blood pressure.

(4) Drug-drug interaction or exogenous substances: A detailed drug history, including over-the-counter pain medicines, herbal preparations, and nutritional supplements must be obtained routinely in these patients. Nonsteroidal anti-inflammatory drugs (NSAIDs) will antagonize the effects of some antihypertensive agents secondary to local prostaglandin inhibition and impairment of sodium excretion, which induces volume expansion. This is relevant in the patient described previously.

(5) Secondary hypertension: True secondary hypertension is uncommon but must be evaluated if the conditions discussed above have been excluded. Of note, chronic kidney disease, renovascular disease, hyperaldosteronism, pheochromocytoma, and sleep apnea are conditions that must be screened for and if detected should be managed appropriately (Table 48F.1).

TREATMENT OPTIONS

The JNC 7 recommends lifestyle modifications in all patients with hypertension and they should be strongly encouraged to reduce sodium intake (<2 g per day), consume no more than 3 drinks per day, and engage in regular physical exercise such as walking for 30 to 45 minutes daily. Each of these approaches produces a modest but clinically important reduction in BP of about 2 to 8 mm Hg on the average. Patient adherence is important and can be enhanced by involvement of nurses or physician assistants, use of telephone contacts, and clinic follow-up reminders.

Appropriate diuretic therapy is the cornerstone for the management of resistant hypertension because volume retention is common. Thiazide diuretics are effective for lowering blood pressure at doses of 12.5 to 25 mg daily in patients with normal renal function. However, if renal function is impaired, loop diuretics must be used; and for short-acting loop diuretics, such as furosemide and bumetinide, the frequency should be increased to two or three times daily. Torasemide is longer acting and can be given once daily, although in some cases it should be given twice daily. It has been observed that adequate diuretic therapy may lead to blood pressure control in many of these patients.

Logical combination of BP agents from different classes is another useful strategy. In general adding a medication with a different mechanism of action compared to the drugs the patient is already receiving may overcome the adverse compensatory effects caused by the initial drug(s). For example, addition of an angiotensin-converting enzyme (ACE) inhibitor or angiotensin receptor blocker (ARB) may ameliorate the diuretic-induced stimulation of the renin-angiotensin system because of volume contraction. Addition of beta blockers and loop diuretics to patients on direct vasodilators, such as hydralazine, minoxidil, or both, counteracts the reflex tachycardia and edema associated with these agents.

A new and very effective treatment paradigm is the use of low-dose aldosterone antagonists for the control of resistant hypertension. Recent studies demonstrate that addition of low doses of spironolactone (12.5 to 50 mg daily) to a

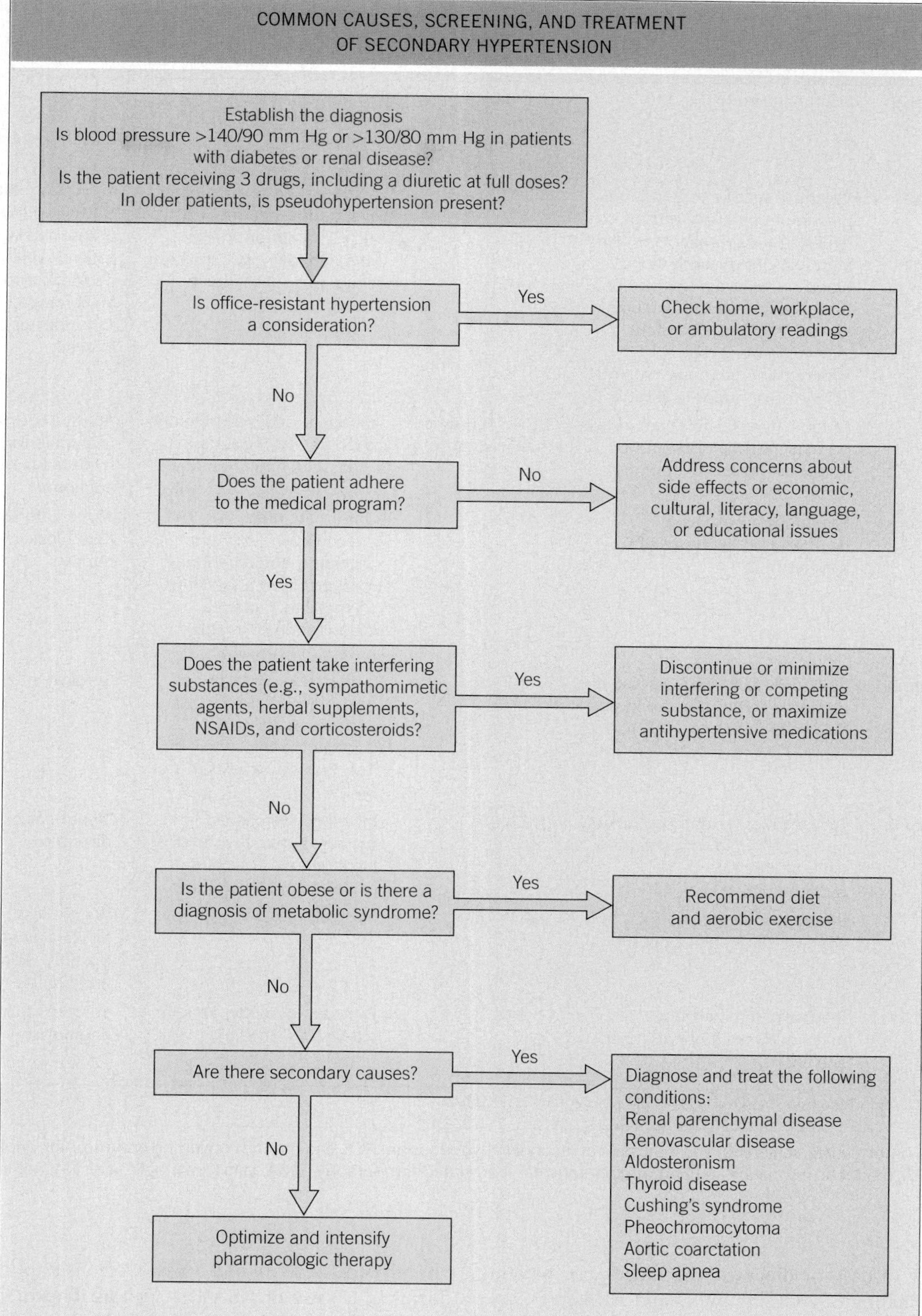

Figure 48F.1 Approach to the management of resistant hypertension. (Modified with permission from Moser M, Setaro JF. Resistant or difficult to control hypertension. N Engl J Med 2006;355:385-392.)

multidrug regimen that includes ACE inhibitors or ARBs and diuretics produces a marked blood pressure reduction seemingly in excess of what would be expected of other BP agents. Spironolactone is especially useful in obese females with sleep apnea. This observation occurred in patients with or without aldosterone excess. Indeed dual diuretic therapy with spironolactone and a loop diuretic was associated with a reduction in systolic blood pressure of 20 to 25 mm Hg and diastolic blood pressure of 10 to 12 mm Hg. At low doses, aldosterone antagonists are relatively safe and well tolerated, but hyperkalemia is an important complication that must be closely monitored, especially in patients with

COMMON CAUSES, SCREENING, AND TREATMENT OF SECONDARY HYPERTENSION				
Secondary Cause	**Symptoms and Signs**	**Estimated Prevalence (%)**	**Screening Tests or Findings**	**Treatment**
Renal parenchymal disease	Nocturia, edema	(1.0-8.0) (depending on the creatinine level)	Proteinuria, cells, and casts; elevated levels of serum creatinine	ACE inhibitor or ARB plus loop diuretic; beta blocker; calcium channel blocker
Renal artery disease	Recent onset of elevated blood pressure in older patients or hypertension in patients under 5 yr; loss of previously good blood pressure control; use of tobacco; widespread vascular disease; multidrug-resistant hypertension; severe hypertension in young patients epigastric or abdominal bruit	3.0-4.0	Increased serum creatinine level during treatment with an ACE inhibitor or ARB; MRA; Doppler; ACE inhibitor renography; disparity in kidney size	Angioplasty with stenting in patients with unilateral disease and in selected patients with bilateral disease; balloon angioplasty for fibromuscular dysplasia; ACE inhibitor or ARB with diuretic
Aldosteronism	Fatigue: hypokalemia (not always present); lack of response to potassium supplementation	1.5-15.0 (higher in recent series)	Abnormal ratio of aldosterone to renin (> 25:1); abnormal response to sodium loading; imaging studies (CT or MRI)	Aldosterone antagonists; ACE inhibitor or ARB with hyperplasia; surgery for adenoma
Pheochromocytoma	Palpitations; headache; diaphoresis; paroxysms of hypertension	< 0.5	Abnormal urinary catecholamine excretion (including norepinephrine > 80 pg/24hr, and VMA >5 mg/24hr): plasma metanephrines; imaging studies (CT or MRI)	Alpha-adrenergic inhibitor; beta blocker; surgical removal
Cushing's syndrome	Obesity: striae; muscle weakness; increased serum glucose level; fluid retention	< 0.5	Increased levels of urinary cortisol (> 55 pg/24 hr); positive results on a dexamethasone suppression test; imaging studies (CT or MRI)†	Surgical intervention
Hyperthyroidism or hypothyroidism	Tachycardia; weight loss; anxiety (in hyperthyroidism); weight gain; fatigue (in hypothyroidism)	1.0-3.0	Increased systolic blood pressure (hyperthyroidism); increased diastolic blood pressure (hypothyroidism)	Treatment of underlying disorders
Sleep apnea	Interrupted sleep; snoring; daytime somnolence obesity	NA	Sleep studies	Weight loss; continuous positive airway pressure; possibly, aldosterone antagonists
Coarctation of the aorta	Brachial or femoral pulse differential; systolic bruits (back and chest)	< 1.0	Echocardiography; imaging studies (CT or MRI)	Surgery; balloon angioplasty

Data adapted with permission from Moser et al. N Engl J Med 2006;355:385-392.

Table 48F.1 Common causes, screening, and treatment of secondary hypertension. ACE, angiotensin converting enzyme; ARB, angiotensin receptor blocker; MRI/MRA, magnetic resonance imaging/angiography; CT, computed tomography; VMA, vanillylmandelic acid; NA, not available.

chronic kidney disease or diabetes, the elderly, or patients taking a combination of ACE inhibitors and ARBs.

Lastly, new drugs on the horizon for treatment of resistant hypertension are selective endothelin-A receptor antagonists. Studies are ongoing to evaluate the role of these agents being added as fourth or fifth line in the context of achieving blood pressure goals. These studies will be completed in late 2008 and thus are not available at this time.

In the current patient, pseudoresistance was excluded with home blood pressure readings that were similar to the clinic blood pressure and secondary causes of resistant hypertension were considered less likely. The major problems identified were (1) poor adherence to lifestyle modifications (i.e., no physical activity and excessive consumption of alcoholic drinks); (2) use of NSAIDs, such as ibuprofen, which most likely antagonized the ACE inhibitor and also contributed to volume retention; (3) inappropriate and inadequate use of thiazide diuretics. In this patient with impaired renal function and an estimated GFR of <60 mL/min, use of loop diuretics is preferred; and (4) poor medication adherence, especially to the beta blocker, atenolol, is suggested by the patient's heart rate of 88 beats per minute. Use of fixed-dose combinations reduces pill number, drug-related adverse reactions, and has been shown to improve adherence.

The patient was counseled and encouraged to implement lifestyle changes, and her medicines were modified as follows. The ibuprofen was discontinued, and acetaminophen 1 g three to four times daily initiated. Enalapril and nifedipine was stopped, and a fixed-dose combination of amlodipine and benazepril (Lotrel) 10/40 mg daily was started. The thiazide diuretic was switched to furosemide (short-acting loop diuretic) 40 mg twice daily, and statin, atenolol, and aspirin were continued. Her clinic follow-up blood pressure at 4 and 8 weeks were 155/90 mm Hg and 145/85 mm Hg, respectively. At 8 weeks, spironolactone 12.5 mg twice daily was added, and within 4 weeks her BP was controlled at 130/70 mm Hg. After 2 years the patient's blood pressure has remained at the goal of less than 130/80 mm Hg without drug-related adverse effects. The new, more selective aldosterone antagonist eplerenone has a better side effect profile than spironolactone and could be substituted in similar patients but increased cost may not justify its use.

SUMMARY

Patients with suspected resistant hypertension must be carefully evaluated for pseudoresistance, adherence to lifestyle modifications, and adequate medication therapy. Use of logical multidrug combinations in appropriate doses is effective for blood pressure control. Diuretics remain the cornerstone for the treatment of resistant hypertension, and low-dose aldosterone antagonists are very effective therapeutic agents for optimal blood pressure management.

g. Hypertension in the Context of Acute Coronary Syndromes and Acute Coronary Interventions

Hung-Fat Tse and Gregory Y. H. Lip

DEFINITION OF PROBLEM

Patients presenting with acute coronary syndrome (ACS) and severe hypertension are commonly encountered (Table 48G.1). Very often, the cardiologist is called to decide whether antithrombotic or coronary reperfusion therapy should be instituted. In patients with ST-segment elevation myocardial infarction (STEMI), a decision has to be made on the type of coronary reperfusion used. Unless the primary percutaneous coronary intervention (PCI) facilities are readily available, thrombolytic therapy is still the most commonly prescribed treatment in many hospitals for patients with STEMI. Unfortunately, in patients presenting with severe uncontrolled hypertension, thrombolytic therapy is either delayed or avoided because of the potential risk of disabling stroke. According to current guidelines, refractory hypertension (systolic blood pressure >180 mm Hg) is a relative contraindication to thrombolytic therapy. Nevertheless, such a decision may result in an increased risk of cardiac complications related to STEMI, including severe cardiac dysfunction and arrhythmias. Furthermore, recurrent chest pain in these patients will pose more management problems, because the symptoms may represent ongoing ischemia or even reinfarction. An abnormal baseline electrocardiogram (ECG), with lateral ST-T segment depression ("strain" pattern) typically seen in some patients with left ventricular hypertrophy (LVH) may cause diagnostic uncertainty for ongoing cardiac ischemia.

ACUTE MYOCARDIAL INFARCTION AND SEVERE HYPERTENSION—IMPLICATIONS
1. Thrombolytic therapy and glycoprotein IIb/IIIa inhibitor use may be delayed or contraindicated because of higher risk of cerebral hemorrhage.
2. True malignant hypertension may coexist.
3. Abnormal baseline ECGs may cause diagnostic uncertainty and mask ongoing ischemia.
4. LVH results in more cardiac complications or sudden cardiac death.
5. Secondary causes should be considered (e.g., aortic dissection, renal artery stenosis, pheochromocytoma).
6. Higher risk of catheter-induced dissection of the aorta or coronary artery.

Table 48G.1 Acute myocardial infarction and severe hypertension—implications.

TYPICAL CASE

A 65-year-old, overweight, recently retired businessman presented at midnight to the casualty department with a 6-hour history of severe central chest pain associated with vomiting. He was a nonsmoker but was told by his family doctor that he had asthma and mild hypertension, for which he had been taking bendrofluazide 2.5 mg daily for a number of years. On examination, the patient was anxious, sweaty, and dyspneic; pulse was 102 beats/minute regular; and blood pressure was 250/145 mm Hg, similar in both arms. A fourth heart sound and a grade 3/6 systolic murmur were heard over the precordium, and scattered, fine crepitations were heard over the lung bases. Fundi were difficult to visualize for papilledema, but there were no obvious exudates or hemorrhages. Chest x-ray revealed mild pulmonary edema and cardiomegaly. His ECG showed an anterior myocardial infarction with LVH and strain pattern also present.

In view of his high blood pressure, thrombolytic therapy was withheld and this was discussed and agreed with the patient. He was given aspirin (300 mg), clopidogrel (300 mg immediately then 75 mg daily), and intravenous 80 mg furosemide (frusemide) and 5 mg diamorphine with antiemetic. An intravenous nitrate infusion was also started and titrated every 5 minutes to slowly reduce blood pressure to lower than 180/110 mm Hg. In view of his asthma and pulmonary edema, intravenous beta blockers were not used. His chest pain resolved while in the coronary care unit (CCU), but he developed frequent runs of ventricular tachycardia (VT) and an amiodarone infusion was therefore added. An echocardiogram revealed concentric LVH and a hypokinetic aneurysmal anteroapical segment of the left ventricle.

Because the patient developed recurrent chest pain the following day, cardiac catheterization was performed, which revealed a severe 95% stenosis in the proximal left anterior descending (LAD) artery. Successful PCI of the LAD lesion was performed, with the bare metal stent deployed at the dilated lesion. His blood pressure was better controlled over the next few days, and he was discharged 7 days later. The following regimen was prescribed: aspirin 75 mg once daily, clopidogrel 75 mg once daily, ramipril 5 mg twice daily, atenolol 50 mg once daily, and simvastatin 40 mg once daily. When discharged, his blood pressure was 140/85 mm Hg.

DIFFERENTIAL DIAGNOSIS

The psychological stress of the symptoms and the likelihood of a heart attack, plus the need to be treated in hospital, with a busy emergency department or an intimidating CCU environment, would certainly raise one's blood pressure. This transient elevation of blood pressure may gradually lower with time when the patient settles and pain is resolving.

For someone who usually has preexisting hypertension on medication or when there is evidence of hypertensive target organ damage, for example, with ECG criteria of LVH criteria, the very high blood pressure reading could be indicative of a true "hypertensive crisis" accompanying the ACS. Occasionally, some patients may have no known history of hypertension (or it is possibly undiagnosed). Clinically, accelerated/malignant hypertension is diagnosed by the presence of severe hypertension with bilateral retinal hemorrhages and exudates, with or without papilledema. The types of hypertensive emergencies in patients admitted with ACS are listed in Table 48G.2.

An acute dissecting thoracic aortic aneurysm secondary to severe hypertension may mimic or even present as an ACS event, especially when the dissection involves the coronary ostia. In this case, thrombolytic therapy is contraindicated and CT or MRI scan would be required to confirm the underlying pathology. Similarly, patients with acute myocardial infarction (AMI) may also have atherosclerotic renal artery stenosis, which may induce a hypertensive crisis later. More unusual secondary causes of severe hypertension, such as pheochromocytoma, are not unknown in the context of an ACS. Indeed, recent reports demonstrated that transient left ventricular apical ballooning syndrome, which can mimic STEMI, can complicate patients with pheochromocytoma or emotional stress. Conversely, it is not uncommon for hypertensive patients with LVH to present with an ACS, but only minimal or mild coronary artery disease is present on coronary angiography.

TYPES OF HYPERTENSIVE EMERGENCIES IN PATIENTS WITH ACUTE MYOCARDIAL INFARCTION

- Hypertensive encephalopathy
- Cerebral infarction
- Intracranial hemorrhage, subarachnoid hemorrhage
- Myocardial ischemia
- Left ventricular failure and acute pulmonary edema
- Aortic dissection
- Acute renal insufficiency
- Microangiographic hemolytic anemia

Table 48G.2 Types of hypertensive emergencies in patients with acute myocardial infarction.

TREATMENT OPTIONS

A patient presenting with ACS and very high blood pressure represents a clinical conundrum for the reasons discussed earlier. Because thrombolysis is relatively contraindicated in the presence of very high blood pressure (>180/110 mm Hg), the treatment would initially be directed to control the blood pressure. On the other hand, it should be emphasized that malignant hypertension can cause arteriolar damage and thus impairment of organ perfusion and loss of local autoregulation of blood flow.

Thus, while treatments are instituted to lower blood pressure, one should avoid inducing an abrupt reduction of pressure because this may precipitate renal failure or stroke or exacerbate ongoing myocardial ischemia. The aim, therefore, should be to lower the blood pressure gradually to less than 180/110 mm Hg. However, the treatment plan should be individualized according to the patient's age and comorbidity.

There are a range of intravenous drugs that can be used to lower blood pressure in patients with severe hypertension presenting with an ACS or needing coronary intervention. In these patients, nitroglycerine (NTG) infusion probably has the safest profile and advantages and is recommended as first-line treatment, with beta blockers and other nitrates (isosorbide dinitrate, etc.) as alternatives. Nitrates lower the cardiac preload and afterload as well as induce coronary vasodilation at the ischemic area, thus improving both heart failure and myocardial perfusion. An alternative would be to give a beta blocker, either orally or intravenously, in the absence of contraindications such as bronchospasm or acute pulmonary edema. Esmolol is an intravenous beta blocker with a short half-life (9 minutes), and its infusion rate (50 to 200 μg/min) can be titrated according to clinical response. Its fast onset and offset of action has advantages if there is concern over the patient's ability to tolerate beta blockers. Other alternatives are intravenous labetalol (50 mg over 1 min, repeated after 5 min) or metoprolol (5 mg every 2 min, to a maximum of 15 mg, followed by 50 mg orally every 6 h). Beta blockers are also useful in treating concurrent cardiac ischemia and tachyarrhythmias, but some caution is needed if the patient is hypotensive. In the COMMIT (ClOpidogrel and Metoprolol in Myocardial Infarction Trial), however, the use of intravenous followed by oral administration of metoprolol had a neutral effect on mortality, because the reduction of reinfarction and ventricular fibrillation were counterbalanced by a higher incidence of cardiogenic shock.

As mentioned earlier, alternative reperfusion strategies for STEMI, such as primary PCI, should be a more preferable option in this case if access to such therapy is available. Primary PCI is generally preferred if skilled catheterization laboratory facilities are readily available (door-to-needle time less than 1 hour); the patient has a high risk of STEMI (cardiogenic shock; Killip class III or above; large anterior infarction); contraindications to thrombolysis are present; presentation is late (e.g., longer than 3 hours); and STEMI is unconfirmed. Nevertheless, a thrombolytic agent may still be considered when the blood pressure is reduced, preferably to less than 160/100 mm Hg (to minimize bleeding risks) and still well within the beneficial window (12 hours from the onset of chest pain).

All hypertensive patients who sustain a STEMI should be considered for an antihypertensive therapy regimen that should include a beta blocker and an angiotensin-converting enzyme (ACE) inhibitor, in addition to low-dose aspirin unless otherwise contraindicated. In patients who are intolerant to ACE inhibitors, angiotensin receptor blockers (valsartan, candesartan) can be used. Furthermore, the use of clopidogrel can be considered in patients with STEMI and is mandatory for some months after PCI with stent placement. Short-acting dihydropyridine calcium antagonist agents can induce reflex tachycardia, which may be detrimental. In particular, sublingual nifedipine can cause an unpredictable sudden drop of blood pressure (which is dangerous during ACS), in addition to the fact that there is no absorption of the drug from the buccal mucosa. Rate-limiting calcium antagonists (verapamil, diltiazem) may be useful in the absence of heart failure or left ventricular dysfunction, especially if beta blockers are contraindicated and atrial tachyarrhythmias are present. Many hypertensive patients may be taking diuretics at presentation and the volume depletion and hypokalemia may increase the risk of cardiac arrhythmias and sudden death. In addition, aldosterone blockade (spironolactone, eplerenone) can be used in patients without significant renal dysfunction or hyperkalemia and whose blood pressure cannot be adequately controlled with therapeutic doses of ACE inhibitors and beta blockers. The target blood pressure in hypertensive patients after STEMI should be lower than 130/80 mm Hg.

Furthermore, the use of anticoagulants will require frequent monitoring, and if blood pressure remains uncontrolled, agents such as low-molecular-weight heparin, bivalirudin (a direct thrombin inhibitor), and glycoprotein IIb/IIIa antagonists (e.g., abciximab, tirofiban) should be used with some caution.

The occurrence of ventricular arrhythmias, such as VT, are common in STEMI. Effective treatment of myocardial ischemia with reperfusion therapy and beta blockers, and correction of electrolyte disturbances (potassium, magnesium) help to prevent VT. Patients with hemodynamically unstable VT should be treated with electrical cardioversion, whereas amiodarone infusion is the recommended first-line treatment for hemodynamically stable VT.

SUMMARY

A patient presenting with ACS and very high blood pressure constitutes a clinical conundrum, because thrombolytic therapy is delayed and sometimes contraindicated, and thus valuable viable myocardium is lost, which determines both short- and long-term prognosis. Such a presentation may also be part of a true hypertensive urgency or emergency, leading to rapid macrovascular and microvascular damage. Fortunately, this is rare but still remains a major problem for both patient and physician.

In most cases, treatment should be aimed at relieving symptoms, achieving a smooth reduction of blood pressure over a period of 24 to 48 hours, and protecting the ischemic but potentially viable myocardium and reducing mortality. Thrombolytic therapy can still be given when blood pressure is reduced, preferably to lower than 160/100 mm Hg, and still within the treatment window. Primary angioplasty is an option if thrombolytic therapy is unacceptable and such service is available. An intravenous nitrate infusion, perhaps with a beta blocker (either orally or intravenously), should be used to achieve smooth reduction of blood pressure (Fig. 48G.1).

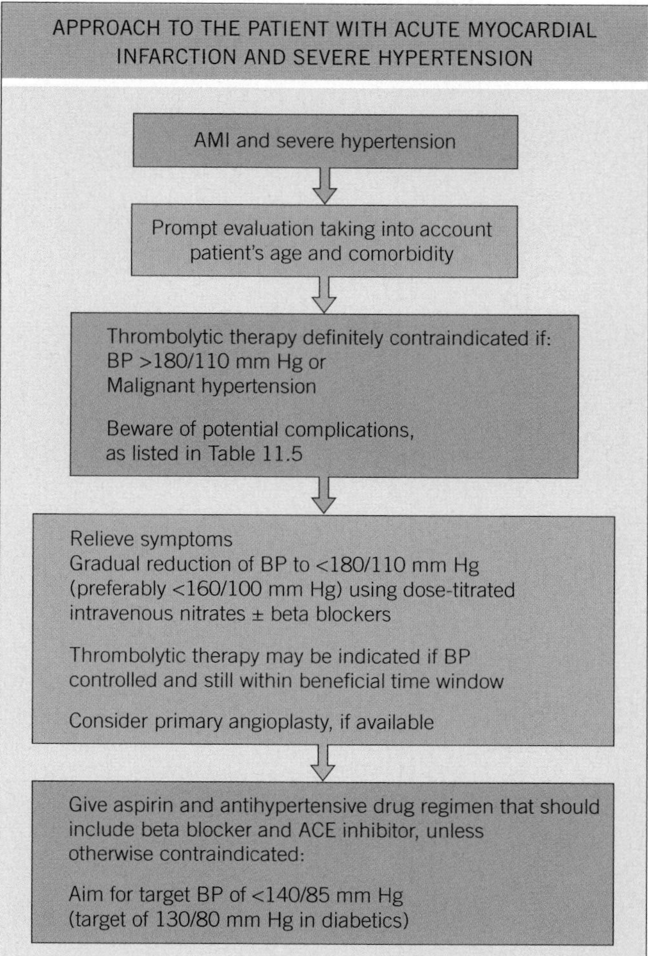

Figure 48G.1 Approach to the patient with acute myocardial infarction and severe hypertension.

SECTION 4

CARDIAC ARRHYTHMIAS

chapter 49

Basic Cardiac Electrophysiology and Anatomy

Mark E. Anderson and Dan M. Roden

Definition

- The fundamental electrical events in the heart are generation and propagation of an action potential, the process whereby the cell membrane potential becomes positive (depolarizes) from a negative resting potential and then repolarizes back to the resting level.

Key Features

- Specialized ion channel proteins in the cell membrane open and close to generate the action potential.
- Differential expression or function of ion channels is responsible for electrophysiologic heterogeneity in cardiac tissues.
- Specialized proteins called connexins make up gap junctions for cell-cell conduction.

Clinical Implications

- Genetic differences in ion channel function result in characteristic arrhythmia syndromes.
- Normal and abnormal cardiac rhythms are subject to the effects of drugs and disease on ion channels and structural proteins.

Recent advances in molecular biology and ion channel physiology have provided a new understanding of the mechanisms that underlie normal and abnormal cardiac electrophysiology. These advances have led to a growing realization that heterogeneity of ion channel expression or function is responsible for a wide range of electrophysiologic and pathophysiologic effects, such as

- action potential prolongation in midmyocardial cells;
- variable responses to drugs that prolong the action potential;
- dispersion of refractoriness in cardiomyopathies and other settings; and
- congenital arrhythmias.

This chapter summarizes basic cardiac electrophysiology to enable a better understanding of these processes.

ANATOMY AND BIOCHEMISTRY

Conduction System

The specialized cardiac conduction system contains the site of initiation of the normal heartbeat and serves to guide the sequence of electrical activation temporally and spatially over the entire heart. Initiation of the normal heartbeat occurs in the sinoatrial node (Fig. 49.1; see Chapter 53). From this position in the high right atrium, activation proceeds along preferential routes to the left atrium (Bachman's bundle) and to the atrioventricular (AV) node located in the basal interatrial septum through the crista terminalis (see Fig. 49.1).

The precise borders of the compact AV node are controversial, but the general area of interest for the AV node and its atrial insertions is the triangle of Koch (see Fig. 49.1). The triangle of Koch is bounded by the tendon of Todaro (cephalad), the tricuspid valve annulus (caudad), and the coronary sinus ostium (posteriad). The distal AV node is continuous with the bundle of His, which bifurcates into the right and left bundle branches. The right bundle branch continues as a single structure before it arborizes into histologically distinct Purkinje fibers that contact individual ventricular myocytes. After crossing the membranous interventricular septum, the left bundle branch trifurcates into anterior, posterior, and middle fascicles, all of which give rise to Purkinje fibers. Action potentials recorded from each of these areas have distinct morphologic appearances that are attributable to the presence of different ion channel populations, as discussed later (see Fig. 49.1).

Myocardium

Recent work has elucidated the ionic basis for variation in the duration and shape of action potentials recorded in different parts of the ventricular myocardium, as discussed later (see Fig. 49.1). The left ventricular free wall is composed of three functionally distinct but histologically similar cell types:

- the epicardial layer, which is the outermost layer;
- the endocardial layer, which lines the ventricular cavities and contains the terminal components of the specialized conduction system; and
- the midmyocardial cell layer.

The midmyocardial cell layer makes up approximately 30% of the total left ventricular mass and is characterized by longer resting action potentials compared with action potentials in the epicardial and endocardial cells. The action potentials of the midmyocardial cells are also disproportionately prolonged in heart failure, during slow heart rates, and by a variety of drugs that prolong the action potential (see Chapter 63).[1] The resultant increased heterogeneity in action potential duration under these conditions is believed to contribute to reentrant excitation that causes torsades de pointes and other arrhythmias. Although they are histologically similar to the other cell layers, the midmyocardial cells contract more rapidly and vigorously than the other layers.

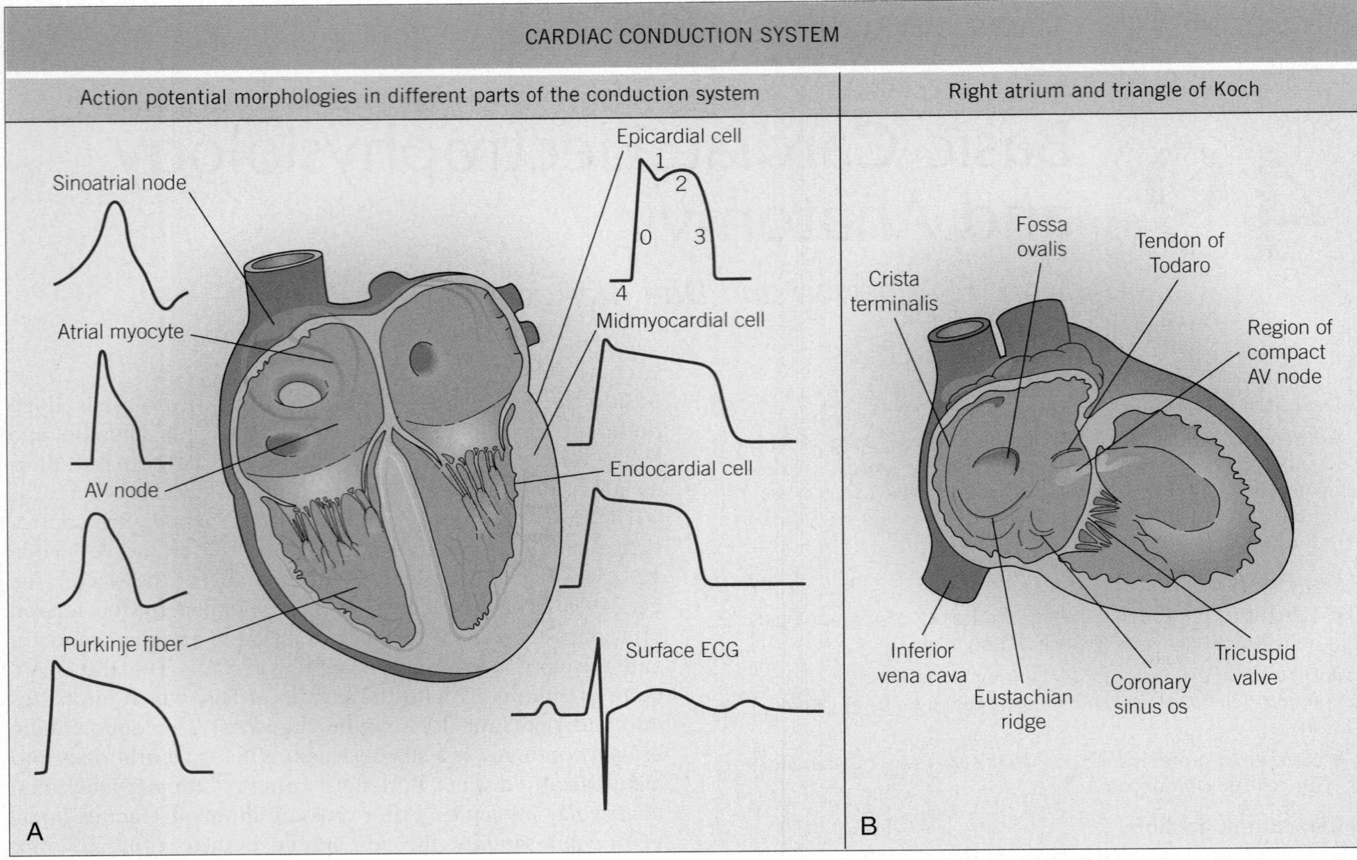

Figure 49.1 Cardiac conduction system. A, Action potentials in different parts of the conduction system have different morphologic appearances. The sinoatrial node has an action potential with a prominent phase 4 and a slow phase 0. Action potential phases are numbered for the example of the epicardial cell. Action potentials from atrial myocytes are shorter than those from ventricular myocytes owing to a prominent transient outward current. Action potentials from ventricular epicardial, midmyocardial, and endocardial ventricular myocytes also differ in shape. A surface electrocardiogram (ECG) is shown to illustrate the hypothesized relationship of these ventricular action potentials to the T and U waves.[1] **B,** The right atrium and the triangle of Koch in greater detail. AV, atrioventricular.

PHYSIOLOGY

Electrical activation of the myocardium occurs to release calcium ions (Ca^{2+}) from intracellular stores (the sarcoplasmic reticulum) to generate mechanical systole. Long-lasting (L-type) Ca^{2+} current ($I_{Ca\text{-}L}$) is the primary signal that evokes release of sarcoplasmic reticulum Ca^{2+} in heart muscle (so-called Ca^{2+}-induced Ca^{2+} release), and the action potential plateau functions to increase $I_{Ca\text{-}L}$, at least in part for this reason.

The sequential activation and inactivation of the various ion channel proteins allows repetitive action potential generation and is due to gating, a process of transition through open, closed, and inactive conformational states that permits ion currents to flow. For many of the cardiac ion channels, the gating process is driven by the cell membrane potential (voltage-dependent gating), but it is also influenced by the state of ion channel phosphorylation and ligand binding and by direct, cell membrane–delimited, G protein–coupled receptor interactions with ion channels. The state of ion channel phosphorylation is tightly controlled by anchoring protein complexes, which act to couple kinases and phosphatases together in the immediate vicinity of their ion channel targets.

Cell Membrane Potential

The cell membrane potential derives from an unequal distribution of ions across this semipermeable membrane. The unequal distribution of sodium ions (Na^+; greater concentration outside the cell) and potassium ions (K^+; greater concentration inside the cell) is generated by the Na^+-K^+ exchanger, an energy-requiring pump. Ions distribute across the cell membrane and reach their electrochemical equilibrium only to the extent allowed by the semipermeable nature of the cell membrane. Individual ionic currents are generated when ion channels open, selectively increasing the cell membrane permeability, and allow passage of ions across the cell membrane.

The physiologist Nernst[2] described the relationship between electrical and chemical equilibria for individual ions according to the following equation:

$$E_X = \frac{RT}{nF} \ln \frac{[X]_o}{[X]_i}$$

where E_X is the cell membrane potential at which ion X is in electrical and chemical equilibrium, R is the gas constant, T is the absolute temperature, n is the valence of the ion in question, F is Faraday's constant, and ln $[X]_o/[X]_i$ is the natural

PHYSIOLOGIC REVERSAL POTENTIALS				
Ion	Intracellular Concentration (mmol/L)	Extracellular Concentration (mmol/L)	Ratio of Extracellular to Intracellular Concentration	Reversal Potential (mV)
Calcium	1×10^{-7}	1.5	15,000	+129
Sodium	12	145	12	+67
Chloride	4.2	123	29	−90
Potassium	155	4	0.026	−98

Table 49.1 Physiologic reversal potentials

log of the ratio of the concentration of ion X on the outside to that on the inside of the cell membrane.

Table 49.1 shows equilibrium potentials for individual ions under physiologic conditions of temperature and ionic activities. The Nernst equation indicates that there will be no net movement of ion X across a completely permeable membrane at the stated ratio of concentrations if the membrane is at potential *E* (physiologically or by command in a voltage clamp experiment). At rest, the cell membrane is most permeable to K^+, and so the resting cell membrane potential approaches the E_K (i.e., about −90 mV). At this potential, the resting membrane is not permeable to Na^+, and so there is no Na^+ movement despite electrical and chemical gradients that would drive Na^+ into the cell. During phase 0 depolarization, the cell membrane rapidly increases permeability to Na^+ because Na^+ channels open, and the cell membrane potential approaches E_{Na} (about +55 mV) as Na^+ moves along its electrochemical gradient (Fig. 49.2). These changes in the permeability of the cell membrane to specific ions are due to the gating processes of the individual ion channel proteins.

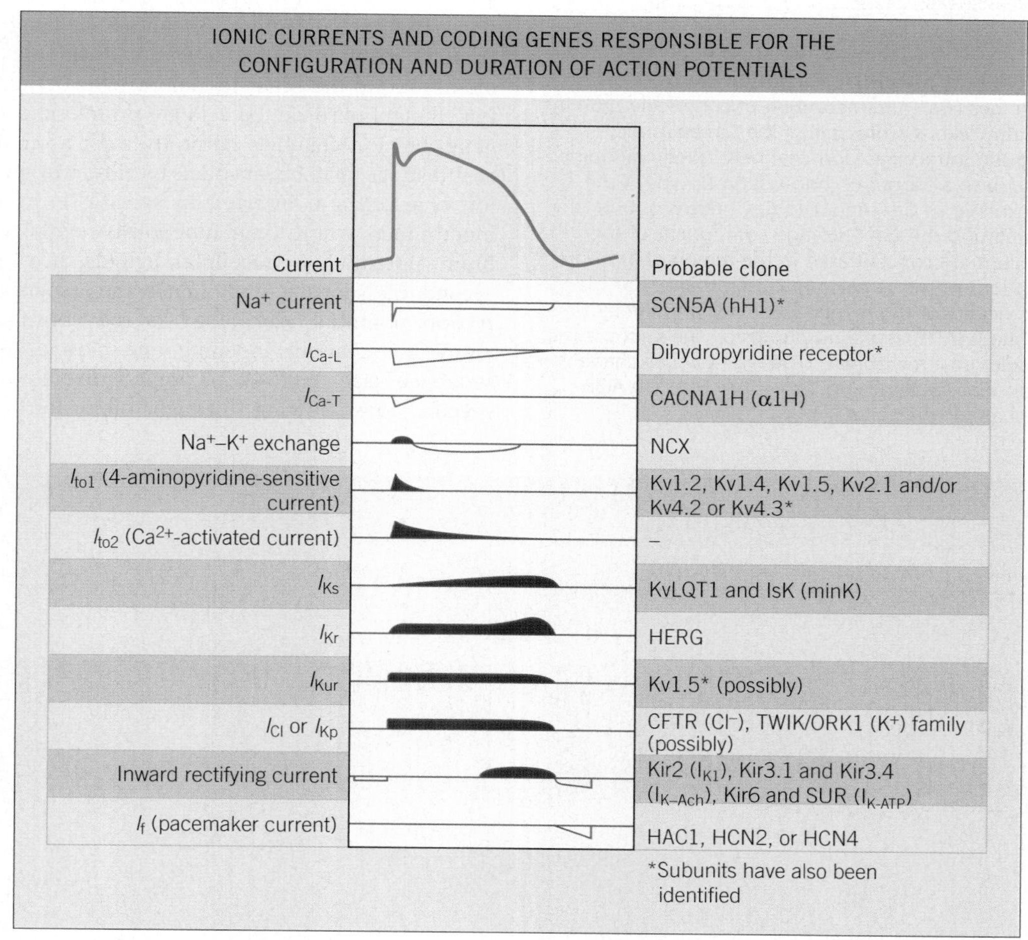

Figure 49.2 Ionic currents and coding genes responsible for the configuration and duration of action potentials. The relative magnitude of the currents is approximately proportional to the excursion from baseline. Outward currents are shown above the baseline; inward currents are shown below the baseline. Na^+, sodium ion; $I_{Ca\text{-}L}$, long-lasting (L-type) calcium (Ca^{2+}) current; $I_{Ca\text{-}T}$, transient (T-type) Ca^{2+} current; NCX, Na^+-Ca^{2+} exchanger; I_{to1}, first component of the transient outward current; I_{to2}, second component of the transient outward current; I_{Ks}, slow component of the delayed rectifier current; I_{Kr}, rapid component of the delayed rectifier current; I_{Kur}, ultrarapid component of the delayed rectifier current; I_{Cl}, chloride current; I_{Kp}, plateau potassium current; I_f, hyperpolarization activated (funny) current.

Excitation-Contraction Coupling

The purpose of electrical excitation of the cardiac cell membrane is to trigger muscle shortening by the myofilament proteins in response to increased intracellular Ca^{2+} concentration ($[Ca^{2+}]_i$). The process by which mechanical shortening is transduced from an electrical signal is called excitation-contraction coupling (Fig. 49.3). Cardiac muscle is unique in that it principally uses a calcium-induced calcium release (CICR) mechanism for excitation-contraction coupling, as first described by Fabiato and Fabiato.[3] CICR occurs when a transsarcolemmal Ca^{2+} "trigger" stimulates the ryanodine receptor release channels on the sarcoplasmic reticulum so that they open and release a larger amount of myofilament activator Ca^{2+} to initiate contraction. The primary trigger for CICR is $I_{Ca\text{-}L}$,[4] but transsarcolemmal Ca^{2+} influx from T-type Ca^{2+} current ($I_{Ca\text{-}T}$)[5] and the Na^+-Ca^{2+} exchanger (NCX)[6,7] can also support CICR. (T-type indicates transient, to distinguish it from L-type, long-lasting.). The $[Ca^{2+}]_i$ results in feedback on repolarizing currents, presumably to control the duration of the action potential plateau for purposes of grading cellular Ca^{2+} entry. The multifunctional Ca^{2+}/calmodulin-dependent protein kinase II (CaMKII) is an important second messenger for coupling changes in $[Ca^{2+}]_i$ to repolarizing currents because mice with genetic CaMKII inhibition show truncated ventricular action potentials due to reductions in the fast component of the transient outward current and the inward rectifier K^+ currents.[8]

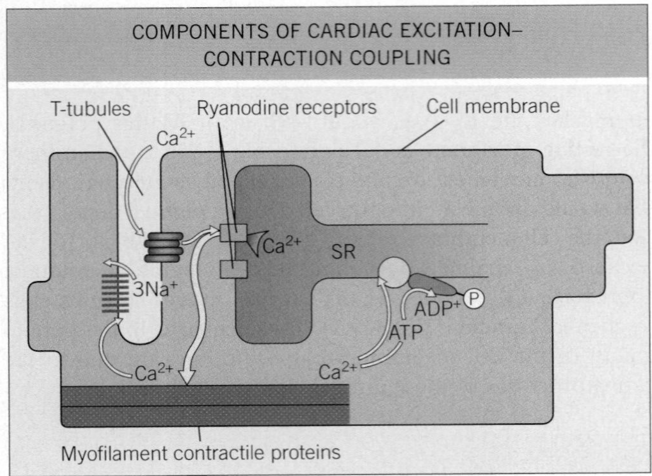

Figure 49.3 Components of cardiac excitation-contraction coupling. Calcium ions (Ca^{2+}) for activation of contractile proteins are released from intracellular stores called the sarcoplasmic reticulum (SR) through intracellular ion channels called ryanodine receptors, in response to a trigger of long-lasting (L-type) Ca^{2+} current (a process known as Ca^{2+}-induced Ca^{2+} release). Both the L-type Ca^{2+} channels and the Ca^{2+} storage component of the sarcoplasmic reticulum are concentrated in the region of T-tubules, which are invaginations of the sarcolemmal membrane. Ca^{2+} is removed from the vicinity of the myofilaments for diastole by adenosine triphosphate (ATP)–requiring pumps on the sarcoplasmic reticulum and sarcolemmal membrane. The Na^+-Ca^{2+} exchanger protein is also important for removing Ca^{2+} from the cell. ADP, adenosine diphosphate; P, phosphate.

Ion Channel Currents

Ion channels are the fundamental units of cardiac excitation (Fig. 49.4; see Chapters 50 and 63). They are the pores through which individual ions move from one side of the cell membrane to the other to generate the action potential. The ion channel pore can be a single protein encoded by a single gene, but ion channels naturally exist as complexes of several distinct proteins encoded by different genes. Translated ion channels are inserted in specific locations in the cell membranes, where their function is regulated by cell membrane potential, extracellular ligands, $[Ca^{2+}]_i$, intracellular second messengers, and membrane-associated G proteins. Action potential physiology is the coordinated result of many ion channels opening and closing together and in sequence (see Fig. 49.2). Ionic currents are created by specific ions flowing through open ion channels along

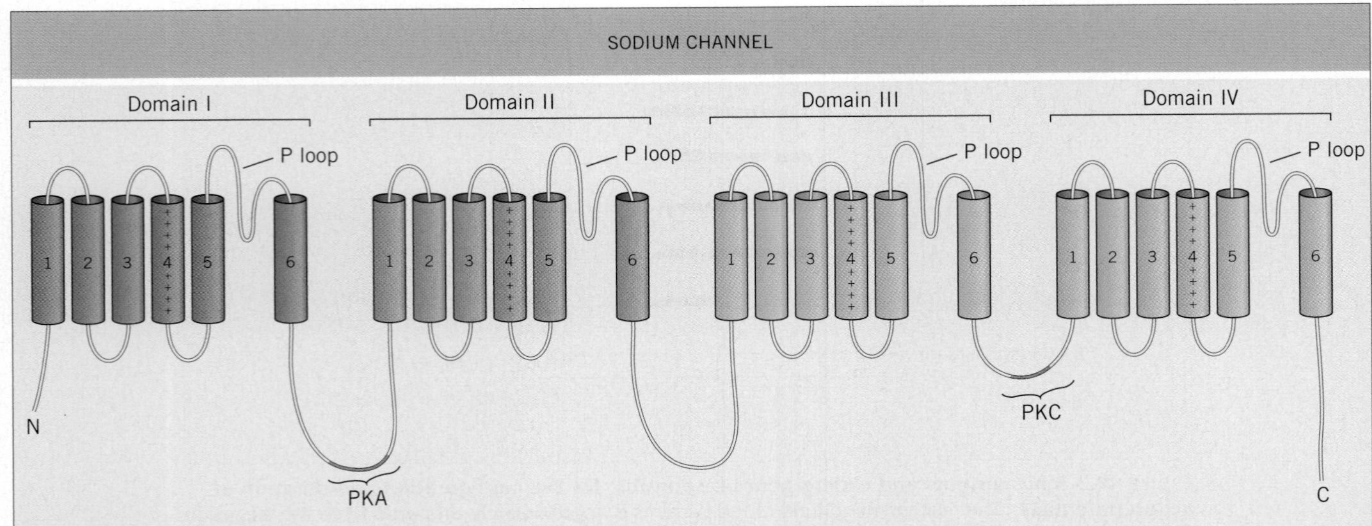

Figure 49.4 Sodium channel, a member of the six membrane–spanning voltage-gated superfamily of ion channels. The transmembrane-spanning segments (1-6) are shown for each domain (I-IV). A large intracellular linker between domains I and II and a smaller linker between domains III and IV contain consensus sites for phosphorylation by protein kinase A (PKA) and protein kinase C (PKC), respectively. Segment 4 is enriched in positively charged amino acids, moves in and out of the membrane in response to changes in cell membrane potential, and acts as the voltage sensor. The P loop connects segments 5 and 6, which interact between all four domains to form the ion channel pore.

energetically favorable electrical and chemical gradients. Major cardiac ionic currents and the probable ion channels that underlie these currents are described here.

Sodium Current

The Na^+ channel, responsible for the sodium current (I_{Na}), was the first cloned member of the six membrane–spanning segment, voltage-gated superfamily of ion channels.[9] The relationship between structure and function in this and other members of the superfamily has been studied in detail. Functional components of ion channel gating, hypothesized from mathematical models developed by Hodgkin and Huxley[10] in the 1940s and 1950s, have now been assigned to specific regions of protein structure. In each tissue in which I_{Na} can be recorded (e.g., brain, heart, skeletal muscle), a different Na^+ channel gene (encoding a slightly different protein) is expressed; the predominant cardiac Na^+ channel is encoded by the *SCN5A* gene. Other genes encode structurally similar proteins; they include the L-type Ca^{2+} channel and the T-type Ca^{2+} channel. Shaker and related voltage-gated K^+ channels are one-quarter the size of the Na^+ and Ca^{2+} channels and are believed to assemble as tetramers to form a channel.

The basic structure of the Na^+ and Ca^+ channels is shown in Figure 49.4 and includes four domains, each containing six transmembrane segments. The fourth transmembrane-spanning segment of each domain includes positively charged lysine or arginine residues at every third amino acid position and is believed to serve as the "voltage sensor," which accounts for the opening and closing of the channel that are dependent on the cell membrane potential. The ion channel pore is formed by the interaction between the linking region, which lies between the fifth and sixth transmembrane-spanning segments of each of the four domains of the channel, and the four individual proteins that assemble as a tetramer to form a K^+ channel.

Activity of the Na^+ channel is further modulated by association with auxiliary β subunits, although the role of these proteins in modulating cardiac I_{Na} is uncertain; both changes in gating (e.g., opening and inactivation rates) and changes in cell surface channel expression have been proposed. Phosphorylation by serine-threonine kinases, such as protein kinase A (PKA) and protein kinase C (PKC),[11] also affects I_{Na} in vitro, although, again, the role of these modifications in situ is uncertain. Recent work has shown that the cardiac Na^+ channel is regulated by $[Ca^{2+}]_i$ and the $[Ca^{2+}]_i$-sensing protein calmodulin. Na^+ channels are enriched in the vicinity of intracellular Ca^{2+} release sites, and so it is logical that $[Ca^{2+}]_i$ may play a part in the regulation of I_{Na} and cardiac excitability. In this first report, Ca^{2+}/calmodulin was found to bind to an "IQ" domain on the Na^+ channel C terminus (see Fig. 49.4), where it enhances a gating process termed slow inactivation.[12]

The Na^+ channel is present in all cardiac myocytes and specialized conduction cells except the clear cells of the sinus node and cells in the compact AV node, where phase 0 of the action potential is dependent on Ca^{2+} current. Single Na^+ channel recordings reveal brief openings[13] and a single channel conductance of approximately 27 pS. Whole-cell currents activate and inactivate quickly. In general, the kinetics of activation are so fast that I_{Na} has to be recorded at reduced temperature or in decreased Na^+ concentrations to achieve accurate measurements. Sodium current activates at cell membrane potentials up to about −50 mV. It is thought that inactivated channels must move to a different conformation (the rested state) before they again become available for excitation. Recovery from inactivation occurs at negative cell membrane potentials, and if inactivation is reduced by experimental shifting of the cell membrane potential negatively to −90 mV, I_{Na} is increased. This indicates that a population of Na^+ channels remains inactive even at the resting cell membrane potential.

The Na^+ channel is the site of action of all three subclasses of the Na^+ channel–blocking antiarrhythmic agents. The magnitude of I_{Na} directly determines the rate of rise of phase 0 (see Figs. 49.1 and 49.2) and is the major factor that determines the rate of conduction in all cardiac myocytes and in most cells of the specialized conduction system. Mutations in *SCN5A* cause two diseases associated with sudden death: one form of the congenital long QT syndrome and the Brugada syndrome (see Chapter 63).

4-Aminopyridine–Sensitive Current and Calcium-Activated Chloride Ion Current Components of the Transient Outward Current

In humans, the 4-aminopyridine–sensitive (first) component of the transient outward current (I_{to1}) is believed to be encoded by the Kv4.3 gene, now termed *KCND3*.[14] Like other Shaker-type K^+ channel genes, *KCND3* makes a protein product that forms tetramers to produce a functional ion channel. The I_{to1} is present in the atria and the ventricles and is a voltage-activated K^+ current with rapid activation and inactivation kinetics (Fig. 49.5). Inactivation accumulates as a function of heart rate, which means that I_{to1} is reduced at faster heart rates. The I_{to1} is identified in experimental preparations using the blockers 4-aminopyridine and tetraethylammonium, but it is also inhibited by quinidine. It is important for shaping phase 1 of the action potential (see Figs. 49.1 and 49.2); thus, if I_{to1} is reduced, the end of phase 1 of the action potential is more positive, and therefore the flow of Ca^{2+} and other currents may be altered. The transient outward current (I_{to}) is prominent throughout the atrial and ventricular epicardium, and I_{to1} is reduced both in patients who have terminal heart failure and in myopathic ventricular myocytes,[15] which partly explains the prolonged action potentials found in these cells. Reduction of I_{to1} under certain conditions thus may contribute to arrhythmias in patients who have heart failure. I_{to} displays variability in its density and its gating among species and specific cell layers.[16] This may reflect expression of different K^+ channel subunits, 18 different function-modifying subunits,[17] or other poorly understood factors.

L-Type Calcium Current

L-type Ca^{2+} current is a voltage-gated current. It is activated at cell membrane potentials that are positive to −40 mV, and it is present throughout the specialized conduction system, atria, and ventricles. The α_{1C} subunit is the major protein subunit comprising the cardiac L-type Ca^{2+} channel. It was cloned and expressed in 1989 by Mikami and coworkers,[18] shortly after this group cloned the Na^+ channel. The α_{1C} subunit was found to have a motif similar to that of other members of the six membrane–spanning voltage-gated superfamily of ion channel proteins. Single-channel recordings are usually made in the absence of Ca^{2+}, with barium ions (Ba^{2+}) substituted

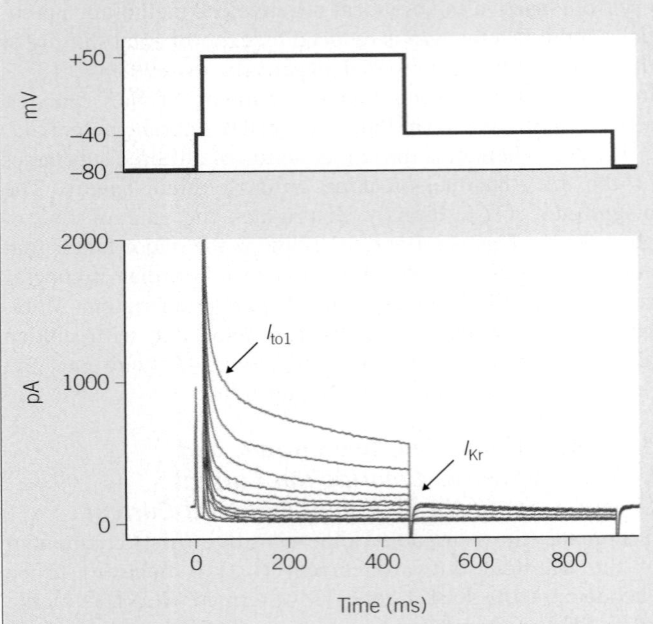

Figure 49.5 Whole-cell potassium currents from ventricular myocytes in response to voltage clamp command steps from −80 mV to +50 mV. Voltage command steps were performed in 10-mV increments, and each step was followed by a return to −40 mV to measure the rapid component of the delayed rectifier current (I_{Kr}). A brief (30-ms) step to −40 mV was used to inactivate sodium and calcium currents. The first components of the transient outward current (I_{to1}) and I_{Kr} are indicated by arrows. I_{to1} activates and inactivates quickly (as seen by the decay in outward current). I_{Kr} is seen after the cell membrane potential is stepped back down to −40 mV. (Data courtesy of Drs. Yuejin Wu and Mark Anderson.)

as the charge carrier to reduce Ca^{2+}-dependent inactivation. Single-channel conductance in Ba^{2+} is typically 20 pS, but it is smaller and of shorter duration when Ca^{2+} is present.

Whole-cell currents activate at cell membrane potentials that are positive to −40 mV and inactivate slowly compared with I_{Na}, which was the basis for an early nomenclature denoting $I_{Ca\text{-}L}$ as the "slow inward" current (Fig. 49.6). The designation L-type stands for long-lasting, in contrast to the faster activation and inactivation kinetics of I_{Na}. L-type Ca^{2+} current inactivation is complicated because it is dependent on

- cell membrane potential;
- $[Ca^{2+}]$, calmodulin, and calmodulin kinase; and
- time.

L-type Ca^{2+} channels are the main portals for Ca^{2+} entry into cardiac myocytes. Ca^{2+} is a critical regulator of diverse cellular functions, so it is not surprising that $[Ca^{2+}]_i$ also regulates I_{Ca}. At least two calmodulin-binding domains on the L-type Ca^{2+} channel C terminus are involved in transducing the Ca^{2+}-bound calmodulin[19,20] signal into changes in I_{Ca}. Mutation in one of these calmodulin-binding domains (an IQ domain that is homologous to a similar region on the Na^+ channel C terminus) increases I_{Ca} and eliminates $[Ca^{2+}]_i$-dependent I_{Ca} inactivation,[19] whereas a short peptide modeled after the IQ domain induces L-type Ca^{2+} channels to

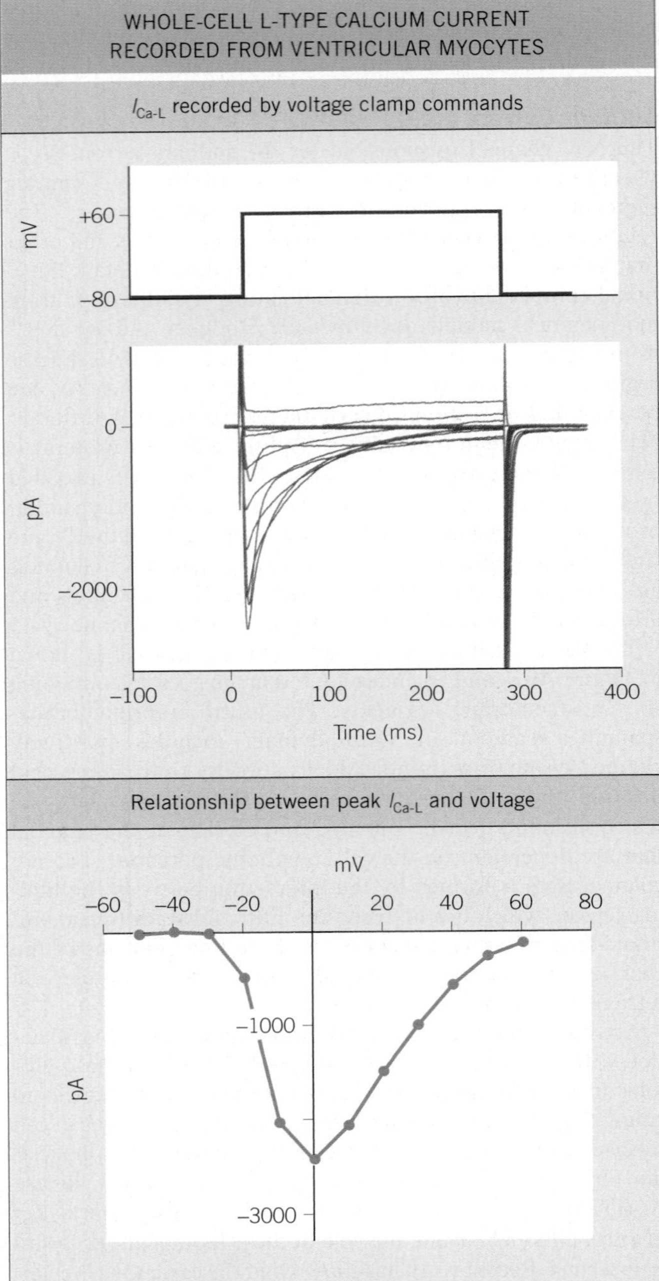

Figure 49.6 Whole-cell L-type calcium current ($I_{Ca\text{-}L}$) recorded from ventricular myocytes. $I_{Ca\text{-}L}$ was recorded by voltage clamp commands from −80 mV to +60 mV for 250 ms in steps of 10 mV. $I_{Ca\text{-}L}$ quickly activates (although this process is slower than for sodium current) and then slowly inactivates (as seen by the current decay from peak negative values toward 0 pA during most voltage clamp steps). Ionic conditions of solutions inside and outside the cell were chosen to eliminate sodium and potassium currents. For the relationship between peak $I_{Ca\text{-}L}$ and voltage, data are plotted as the peak value of the inward current (i.e., the maximum negative value) against the voltage command potential. Peak $I_{Ca\text{-}L}$ current occurs at a cell membrane potential of 0 mV. (Data courtesy of Drs. Yuejin Wu and Mark Anderson.)

open with increased probability.[21] Ca^{2+}-bound calmodulin also activates CaMKII, and CaMKII induces L-type Ca^{2+} channels to enter a gating mode with prolonged openings.[22] An auxiliary β subunit protein has a highly conserved CaMKII phosphorylation site, and two of the four major cardiac β subunit isoforms have a CaMKII binding motif.[23] CaMKII phosphorylation of the β subunits, rather than the pore-forming α subunit, appears to be necessary and sufficient for CaMKII effects on I_{Ca}.[24] The physiologic and pathophysiologic significance of Ca^{2+}/calmodulin and calmodulin kinase regulation is yet to be fully understood, but these signals and Ca^{2+} channel gating behaviors are already linked to end-stage cardiomyopathy,[25] cell survival,[26] excitation-contraction coupling,[27] and cardiac arrhythmias.[28]

Three classes of ligands each contain clinically important members:

- dihydropyridines (nifedipine and nitrendipine);
- phenylalkylamines (verapamil); and
- benzodiazepines (diltiazem).

All the clinically used agents are antagonists,[22] but agonist ligands exist and are used experimentally.

L-type Ca^{2+} channels are concentrated in T-tubule membranes,[29] close to the sarcoplasmic reticulum Ca^{2+} release channels.[25] This Ca^{2+} is most important for triggering the secondary release of Ca^{2+} (i.e., the CICR) from the sarcoplasmic reticulum. Sarcoplasmic reticulum Ca^{2+} activates the myofilaments to produce contraction and also influences Ca^{2+}-dependent ionic currents on the sarcolemma, such as the second component of the transient outward current (I_{to2}) and NCX, in addition to $I_{Ca\text{-}L}$ itself.

The effects of $I_{Ca\text{-}L}$ on the action potential waveform are complex; it may directly lengthen the action potential (because it is an inward current) but indirectly shorten the action potential by activating I_{to2}, or it may lengthen the action potential by activating NCX, and $[Ca^{2+}]_i$ can increase or decrease $I_{Ca\text{-}L}$. In addition to the α_1 subunit, other auxiliary components of the L-type Ca^{2+} channel are the β, γ, and $\alpha_2\delta$ subunits, which act to modify the response of $I_{Ca\text{-}L}$ to the cell membrane potential and other signaling molecules. Because $[Ca^{2+}]_i$ is of central importance to the function and survival of cardiac myocytes, it is not surprising that regulation of $I_{Ca\text{-}L}$ is both complex and sometimes, apparently, redundant.

T- and D-Type Calcium Currents

The gene *CACNA1* encodes the ion channel protein α_{1G}, which is responsible for $I_{Ca\text{-}T}$ and was first cloned in the brain. More recently, the cardiac T-type Ca^{2+} channel α_{1H} was identified.[30] The protein α_{1H} is encoded by the gene *CACNA1H*, and it also exists in noncardiac tissues. Both α_{1G} and α_{1H} are homologous to other six membrane–spanning voltage-gated ion channels.

T-type Ca^{2+} current is prominent in atrial myocardium and in the portions of the specialized conduction system in the AV node, the bundle of His and the Purkinje fibers. In these sites, it may increase the duration of the action potential and contribute to the release of intracellular activator Ca^{2+} from the sarcoplasmic reticulum. T-type Ca^{2+} current is not apparently present in ventricular myocardium, and it is insensitive to $I_{Ca\text{-}L}$ antagonists at clinically relevant concentrations.[31] T-type Ca^{2+} current is voltage gated and activated over a more negative cell membrane potential range than $I_{Ca\text{-}L}$ (between −80 mV and −50 mV). Single-channel conductances are smaller and of shorter duration than $I_{Ca\text{-}L}$, and these properties are the basis for the designation T-type, which indicates tiny or transient. The macroscopic current activates more rapidly than $I_{Ca\text{-}L}$.

In contrast to $I_{Ca\text{-}L}$, $I_{Ca\text{-}T}$ is not facilitated or inactivated by intracellular Ca^{2+} or β-adrenergic stimulation. Mibefradil, a $I_{Ca\text{-}T}$ antagonist, was marketed for a short time for clinical uses (its inhibitory concentration for 50% of peak current [IC_{50}] is 1.4 μmol/L in a heterologous expression system), but it was withdrawn because of multiple drug interactions. Blockade of $I_{Ca\text{-}T}$ remains a viable therapeutic goal because it may allow control of rapid ventricular response in atrial fibrillation (or other supraventricular tachycardias; see Chapters 57 to 59) without producing a significant negative inotropic effect owing to the absence of this channel in ventricular myocardium.

Until recently, only Ca^{2+} channels encoded by α_{1C}, α_{1G}, and α_{1H} (each the product of a different gene) were believed to populate the myocardium, although a much wider variety of related Ca^{2+} channel types are present in other tissues. However, a knockout mouse lacking a neuronal L-type calcium channel, encoded by the α_{1D} subunit, has been engineered. Surprisingly, these mice exhibited reduced heart rates and slowed AV nodal conduction.[32,33] Although no clinically useful D-type Ca^{2+} channel antagonists are available, D-type Ca^{2+} channels now represent a potential pharmacologic target for modulation of cardiac impulse formation and AV nodal conduction.

Ultrarapid, Rapid, and Slow Components of the Delayed Rectifier Current

Rectification is the property by which ionic current deviates from ohmic conductance (i.e., equal conductance for inward and outward currents) and instead flows preferentially in one direction. Delayed rectifier K^+ currents are activated by cellular depolarization, with a delay after phase 0. The delayed rectifier current increases as a function of time during the plateau, but the inward current (primarily through L-type Ca^{2+} channels) is inactivating. The net result is that outward current through delayed rectifier channels eventually exceeds inward current, and repolarization is accomplished.

Three major subtypes of delayed rectifier current (generically termed I_K) have been identified in cardiac tissue. They have different rates of activation, different cellular localizations, and different pharmacologies, and they are the result of different ion channel proteins encoded by different genes.

Ultrarapid Component of the Delayed Rectifier Current

The ultrarapid component of the delayed rectifier current (I_{Kur}) activates, as its name suggests, within milliseconds of a depolarizing pulse. Outward current increases as the extent of depolarization increases, and with very long depolarizations, the current displays slow inactivation.[34] In rats, I_{Kur} is present in the atria and ventricles; in humans, it is readily detected in atrial cells but not in ventricular cells. It is blocked by many K^+ channel–blocking agents, such as quinidine and tetraethylammonium, but it appears to be more sensitive than most K^+ channels to 4-aminopyridine, with IC_{50} values often less than 100 μmol/L. A channel with characteristics that are very similar to native I_{Kur} can be reconstituted by expression of the Kv1.5 gene.[35] In addition, Kv1.5 mRNA is far more abundant in human atrium than in human ventricle,[36] and antisense inhibition of Kv1.5 inhibits I_{Kur} in human atrial cells but not in human ventricular cells.[37] These findings, taken together, provide strong evidence that Kv1.5 underlies I_{Kur}. Ancillary β subunits that appear to associate with Kv1.5 and that modify its function in vitro have been described, but the extent to which these protein-protein interactions play a role in cardiac tissue remains uncertain. PKA activation increases I_{Kur}, whereas activation of PKC reduces it. It is also reduced in atrial fibrillation, through unknown mechanisms.[38] Kv1.5/I_{Kur} blockers are currently in development as potentially useful agents in atrial fibrillation (that would be predicted to lack ventricular proarrhythmic effects); the first of these, vernakalant (which also blocks I_{Kr} [see later] and sodium current), received a recommendation for approval from a Food and Drug Administration advisory panel in late 2007.

Rapid Component of the Delayed Rectifier Current

The rapid component of the delayed rectifier current (I_{Kr}) and the slow component (I_{Ks}) were first dissected in guinea pig ventricular cells, in which I_{Kr} was defined as the component blocked by D-sotalol and by the methanesulfonanilide (QY1) E-4031.[39] The rapid component activates rapidly (within tens of milliseconds) and displays the unusual property that with increasing depolarization, outward current actually decreases. This is a manifestation of very rapid inactivation that the channel undergoes with depolarizing pulses. One result is that although I_{Kr} flows during the plateau of the action potential, it actually increases as the cell begins to repolarize, thus further hastening final repolarization. Contrary to the prediction of the Nernst equation, it also displays the unusual property that its magnitude decreases when extracellular K^+ concentration ($[K^+]_e$) is decreased.[40] This finding may well underlie the prolongation of action potentials that occurs in hypokalemia.

The I_{Kr} is encoded by the human ether-a-go-go–related gene (*HERG*, now termed *KCNH2*).[41] As discussed further in Chapter 63, *KCNH2* mutations are one cause of the congenital long QT syndrome, and most drugs that have been associated with the acquired long QT syndrome are I_{Kr} blockers. Low $[K^+]_o$ not only reduces I_{Kr} but also potentiates drug block of the current,[42] providing another explanation for the mechanism by which hypokalemia constitutes a risk factor for drug-induced long QT–related arrhythmias. Although KCNH2 protein includes a cyclic nucleotide–binding domain in its C terminus, its function in heart is at present not known to be modulated by activation of second messengers.

Slowly Activating Component of Delayed Rectifier Current

The slowly activating component of delayed rectifier current is known as I_{Ks}. Even with very long voltage clamp pulses, the current does not reach steady state. The amplitude of I_{Ks} is markedly increased by a variety of intracellular signaling systems, including PKA and (in some species) PKC. Specific adapter proteins that bring the kinase and the channel in proximity to allow this regulation have now been identified.[43] Both I_{Ks} and I_{Kr} are recorded in human atrium and ventricle. The K^+ channel, expression of which underlies I_{Ks}, is *KvLQT1* (now termed *KCNQ1*). However, when *KvLQT1* is expressed alone, a small current with very rapid activation kinetics is observed. When *KCNQ1* is coexpressed with the ancillary subunit encoded by *KCNE1* (originally termed *minK*), a current with the physiologic characteristic of I_{Ks} is observed.[44] Mutations in *KCNQ1* or *KCNE1* also cause the congenital long QT syndrome. Specific blockers of I_{Ks} that have been developed are not undergoing clinical trials because of the justified concern for proarrhythmia. β-Adrenergic receptor activation increases Ca^{2+} current, and other things being equal, it should prolong cardiac action potentials. Activation of β-mediated I_{Ks} is an important mechanism limiting this action potential prolongation under conditions of adrenergic stress. Deactivation of I_{Ks} is believed to be sufficiently slow that unless the heart rate is very slow, current will "accumulate" at fast rates. The clinical importance of this finding is that I_{Ks} has a greater role in repolarization of cardiac tissue at fast rates than at slow rates, when I_{Kr} is relatively more predominant. Thus, I_{Kr} blockade leads to exaggerated action potential prolongation at slow rates, a risk factor for long QT arrhythmias. Conversely, a reduction in I_{Ks} (through genetic mutations or drug block) would be predicted to result in marked QT prolongation at rapid rates, and indeed arrhythmias in the congenital long QT syndrome due to loss of I_{Ks} function occur when the underlying rate is rapid. In this situation, arrhythmias may result from intracellular calcium overload.[45]

Adenosine Triphosphate–Sensitive Potassium Current

An adenosine triphosphate (ATP)–sensitive K^+ current ($I_{K\text{-}ATP}$) was originally identified in heart cells.[46] $I_{K\text{-}ATP}$ is detected in a wide variety of tissues (brain, pancreas, muscle), and its diverse pharmacology and gating properties probably reflect variable subunit compositions among tissues. In heart, $I_{K\text{-}ATP}$ is reconstituted by coexpression of a K^+ channel (Kir6.2) and an auxiliary protein (SUR) that acts as the sulfonylurea receptor. Specific cardiac forms of SUR-Kir6.2 exist, which suggests that cardiac-specific therapeutic agents might be developed. Similarly, other members of the Kir6.x family (a group of inward rectifiers) may associate with specific SURs to generate tissue-specific $I_{K\text{-}ATP}$s. Knockout of the Kir6.1 subunit results in premature death from Prinzmetal's angina, indicating that this channel is also expressed in coronary vasculature.[47]

The $I_{K\text{-}ATP}$ is tonically suppressed by the presence of ATP, with an IC_{50} of 10 μmol/L, and it opens when the intracellular ATP concentration is reduced.[46] Thus, $I_{K\text{-}ATP}$ activity is coupled to the cellular metabolic state. It is controversial whether this current operates under basal conditions to influence the cardiac action potential, although metabolic oscillations within the cardiomyocyte may result in concomitant $I_{K\text{-}ATP}$ activity,[48] and this current appears to be critical for ischemic preconditioning.[49] It is thought that $I_{K\text{-}ATP}$ shortens the duration of action potential under conditions in which ATP concentration is reduced, such as ischemia. Agents that activate (or open) $I_{K\text{-}ATP}$ include glibenclamide and pinacidil, and these agents result in decreased blood pressure through their action at arterial smooth muscle. One potential application of these agents is to shorten the action potential duration in congenital long QT syndromes to prevent torsades de pointes (see Chapter 63). Quinidine inhibits $I_{K\text{-}ATP}$.

Sodium-Calcium Exchanger

The cardiac Na^+-Ca^{2+} exchanger protein (NCX1) was cloned in 1990 and is part of an exchanger superfamily of genes.[50] It is believed to exist as a single protein with 11 transmembrane-spanning segments including a large intracellular loop linking S5 and S6.[50] The intracellular loop contains peptides important for the regulation of NCX activity. A so-called XIP region is present near the N terminus of the loop, and this region is important for activation of the exchanger by intracellular Ca^{2+}.[51] The NCX is present throughout the heart.

Current occurs because the NCX is electrogenic: it exchanges one Ca^{2+} for three Na^+ and thus transports a net positive charge with each exchange cycle. Typically, the NCX current is inward (i.e., the net result of transporting three Na^+ in and one Ca^{2+} out), and this acts as an important extrusion mechanism to prevent $[Ca^{2+}]_i$ overload; this inward current is termed forward-mode Na^+-Ca^{2+} exchange. Forward-mode Na^+-Ca^{2+} exchanger activity results in a transient inward current that is likely to underlie arrhythmia-triggering delayed after-depolarizations in $[Ca^{2+}]_i$ overload conditions.[52,53] The NCX may also act in reverse mode and produce an outward current that brings Ca^{2+} into the cell for CICR.[7] The ability of the NCX to reverse itself may be important for the configuration and physiology of the cardiac action potential. A reduction in NCX inward current may contribute to the positive inotropy that follows cardiac glycoside therapy. This reduction may follow partial dissipation of the Na^+ gradient (i.e., increased intracellular Na^+) after inhibition of the Na^+,K^+-ATPase. Surprisingly, NCX knockout mice are viable but appear to survive by a coordinated compensation of excitation-contraction coupling, in which reduction of I_{Ca} is predominant.[54]

Na^+,K^+-ATPase

The Na^+,K^+-ATPase generates the physiologic gradient of Na^+ and K^+ across the cell membrane. It is a heteromeric protein complex that consists of the catalytic and cardiac glycoside-binding α subunit and an auxiliary β subunit. Three separate isoforms of the Na^+,K^+-ATPase catalytic subunit are present in human heart (α_1, α_2, and α_3 isoforms). These isoforms are differentially distributed in the sarcolemma: the α_1 isoform is preferentially expressed in the T-tubules,[55] near the site of Ca^{2+} release. The Na^+,K^+-ATPase requires ATP and magnesium ions to pump Na^+ out of the cell and K^+ into it against their electrical and chemical gradients. For each ATP, three Na^+ are transported out of the cell and two K^+ are transported into the cell, and the pump is thus electrogenic (with the net current being outward).

The Na^+,K^+-ATPase is the only known receptor for clinically used digitalis glycosides. The Na^+-K^+ current is regulated by PKA, PKC, $[Ca^{2+}]_i$, and calmodulin kinase, and it may affect both the action potential configuration and the resting cell membrane potential as a persistent inward current.

Hyperpolarization-Activated (Pacemaker or "Funny") Current

Unlike other currents, this displays a "funny" behavior: activation by hyperpolarization. The channel protein responsible for the hyperpolarization-activated current, or the funny current (I_f), was recently cloned from brain[56] and heart[57] and was found to be phylogenetically related both to Shaker-type K^+ voltage–gated ion channels and to cyclic nucleotide (ligand)–gated ion channels. Two isoforms, HCN2 and HCN4, have been identified in heart. The I_f is an inward current that is activated at cell membrane potentials that are negative to −60 mV.

As one of several currents that contribute to phase 4 depolarization and thereby help determine the sinus rate, I_f has been called the pacemaker current. A recently described defect in I_f in zebrafish results in sinus bradycardia and impaired heart rate response to sinus node stimulation, highlighting the role of I_f in determining sinus rate.[58] The current is also expressed in ventricular myocytes (although it is ordinarily activated at very negative potentials), and it may play a part in the generation of arrhythmias in heart failure[59] and hypertrophy.[60] Cyclic nucleotide–gated channels respond to cyclic nucleotides such as cyclic adenosine monophosphate (cAMP), after binding to a cyclic nucleotide–binding domain, with increased channel opening. Presumably, the response of I_f to cAMP binding or a phosphorylation event explains the well-known modulation of sinus rate caused by adrenergic and cholinergic stimulation, and it may be responsible for adrenergic-dependent arrhythmias.

Inward Rectifier Current

The equilibrium potential for K^+ under physiologic conditions, predicted by the Nernst potential, is approximately equal to the resting potential of cardiac cells. This, in turn, implies that channels exist in the resting cell membrane that allow K^+ to move along its electrochemical gradients to achieve this equilibrium. These are inward rectifier channels. At potentials that are negative to the equilibrium potential, inward rectifier channels pass a large inward current (I_{K1}) to bring the potential back to the equilibrium potential. In contrast, at potentials that are positive to the equilibrium potential, inward rectifier channels pass a much smaller outward I_{K1} to repolarize the cell. This characteristic of passing current more effectively in one direction than in another is termed rectification. In the case of inward rectifier channels, it is thought that intracellular magnesium and polyamines act as a plug in the inner mouth of the channel pore to prevent K^+ from leaving the cell, whereas no such mechanism is present to prevent K^+ from entering the cell at potentials that are negative to the resting potential. Inward rectifier channels are expressed in many excitable and nonexcitable cells. The channel with biophysical characteristics and expression pattern that appears best to match that of the cardiac inward rectifier K^+ current is Kir2.1, occasionally termed hIRK.[61] The genes whose expression leads to I_{K1} include *KCNJ2* and *KCNJ4*. As with other channels, varying I_{K1} behaviors may reflect variable subunit compositions in a species- and chamber-specific fashion.

No specific blockers of the inward rectifier current have been developed, although the current is inhibited by quinidine and Ba^{2+}.

Calcium-Activated Nonselective Current

A Ca^{2+}-activated nonselective cation channel clone (mNSC1) has been isolated from a mouse pancreatic beta-cell line and found to be present in heart.[62] The channel had three or four predicted transmembrane-spanning regions and may be responsible for previously studied cardiac currents. Evidence for this current exists in a variety of mammalian species,[63] and it has been implicated in the initiation of triggered arrhythmias.[64] This current has not been documented in humans. Single-channel conductances recorded from heart are 15 pS, and the probability of channel opening increases with increasing $[Ca^{2+}]_i$, but the channel is not voltage gated. Neither single-channel nor whole-cell records show inward or outward rectification, but whole-cell Ca^{2+}-

activated nonselective cation currents showing inward rectification have been described. The channel is impermeable to anions and is termed nonselective because once it is activated by increased $[Ca^{2+}]_i$, it is permeable to a variety of monovalent cations. Although no specific antagonists are available to measure the effect of blockade on action potential configuration, the outward current, which is present at positive cell membrane potentials, would shorten the action potential, and the inward current, which is present at negative cell membrane potentials, would lengthen the action potential and could contribute to triggered arrhythmias.

Cell-Cell Communication through Gap Junctions

Gap junctions are structures that are located primarily at the ends of cardiac myocytes. They allow intracellular contents to be transported from one cell to another and also facilitate propagation of electrical impulses. Gap junctions are formed by expression of connexin genes.[65] As with the inward rectifier current, connexins are ubiquitously expressed throughout most cell types in the body that require cell-cell communication.

The control of the specific conductances is afforded by expression of specific connexin subtypes in specific tissues. The connexin genes expressed in the heart are Cx40, Cx43, and Cx45. Connexin proteins form hexamers that are hemichannels in each cell. Each hemichannel "finds" a corresponding hemichannel in a neighboring cell to form a gap junction. It is unknown whether heteromeric gap junctions can be formed. The gene Cx43 is expressed throughout the heart, whereas Cx45 is thought to encode an atrial gap junction channel; Cx40 is expressed in the conduction system.

Altered function of connexin gene products or altered distribution (e.g., a uniform distribution across the myocyte rather than a concentration at the ends) may underlie abnormal impulse propagation in diverse diseases, such as healing myocardial infarction or atrial fibrillation.[66] Interestingly, a number of other cardiac ion channels are also localized at the ends of cardiac myocytes. These include Kv1.5 and SCN5A. The significance of this striking channel localization has not been determined.

Ion Channel Gating

Gating refers to the process whereby an ion channel protein undergoes transitions among conformations that correspond to open, closed, and inactivated states (Fig. 49.7). Inactivated and closed states do not allow conduction of ionic current. Transitions between different gating states are driven by cell membrane potential and by permeant ion concentrations on either side of the membrane in voltage-gated ion channels and by ligand binding in ligand-gated ion channels. Other factors, such as ion channel phosphorylation, $[Ca^{2+}]_i$, and time, also influence the gating state of many ion channel proteins.

Second Messengers

Second messengers are produced intracellularly after agonist binding to a receptor on the cell membrane. The function of many ion channels is influenced by second-messenger signaling cascades, chiefly through actions on ion channel protein phosphorylation and $[Ca^{2+}]_i$, both of which may affect gating transitions. A common example is the β-adrenergic signaling

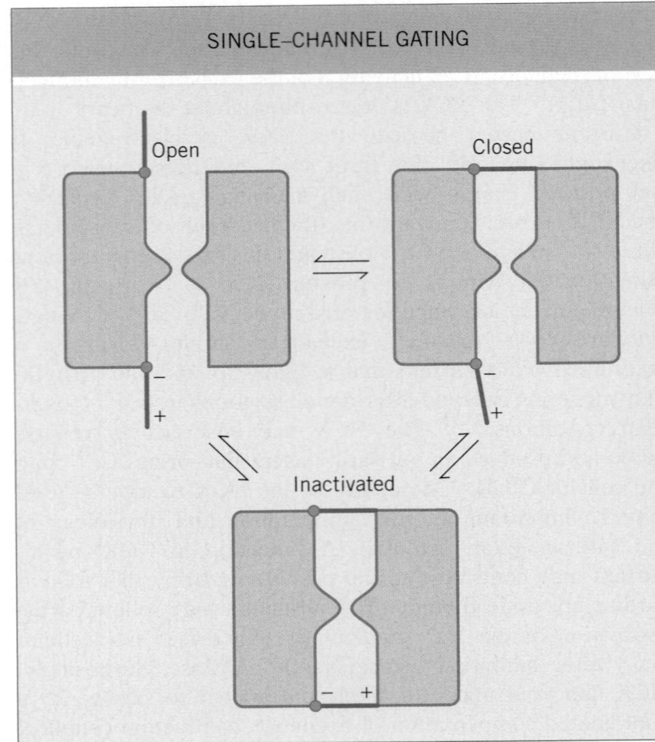

Figure 49.7 Single-channel gating. Voltage-gated ion channel proteins move between open, closed, and inactivated states by a process termed gating. The channel pore is depicted with a critical narrowing that serves as the ion selectivity filter and makes the ion channel permeable only to certain ions. The inactivation gate is an electric dipole, and it opens and shuts in response to sensed cell membrane potentials. Movement of this dipole can be measured when the larger ionic current is blocked.

cascade that influences many different ion channels, but its effect on $I_{Ca\text{-}L}$ is perhaps the best studied (Fig. 49.8).

Agonist binding to the β_1 receptor activates the membrane-associated enzyme adenylate cyclase. This enzyme catalyzes the production of the second messenger cAMP, which binds to the regulatory domain of PKA to release the active catalytic subunit. PKA phosphorylates L-type Ca^{2+}, Na^+, Cl^-, and K^+ channels. Phosphorylation of L-type Ca^{2+} channels by PKA increases the probability of a gating transition to the open state and also favors long channel openings (termed mode 2 gating), which increase $I_{Ca\text{-}L}$.[67]

Agonist binding to β-adrenergic receptors activates the membrane-associated enzyme phospholipase C, which catalyzes key steps in the generation of two second messengers: inositol 1,4,5-triphosphate and diacylglycerol.[68] Although inositol 1,4,5-triphosphate is an important signal for the mobilization of intracellular Ca^{2+} in most cell types, including vascular smooth muscle, its role in cardiac myocytes is unclear. Diacylglycerol activates many PKC isoforms by binding to the regulatory domain and exposing the catalytic site.[69] As with PKA phosphorylation, PKC phosphorylation is known to modulate the gating properties of a number of ion channels, including the Na^+ channel and the L-type Ca^{2+} channel, and some K^+ currents, such as I_{to1}.

An important body of recent findings has highlighted the fact that the actions of a variety of kinases, including PKA and PKC, are spatially regulated by specific anchoring proteins.[43,70]

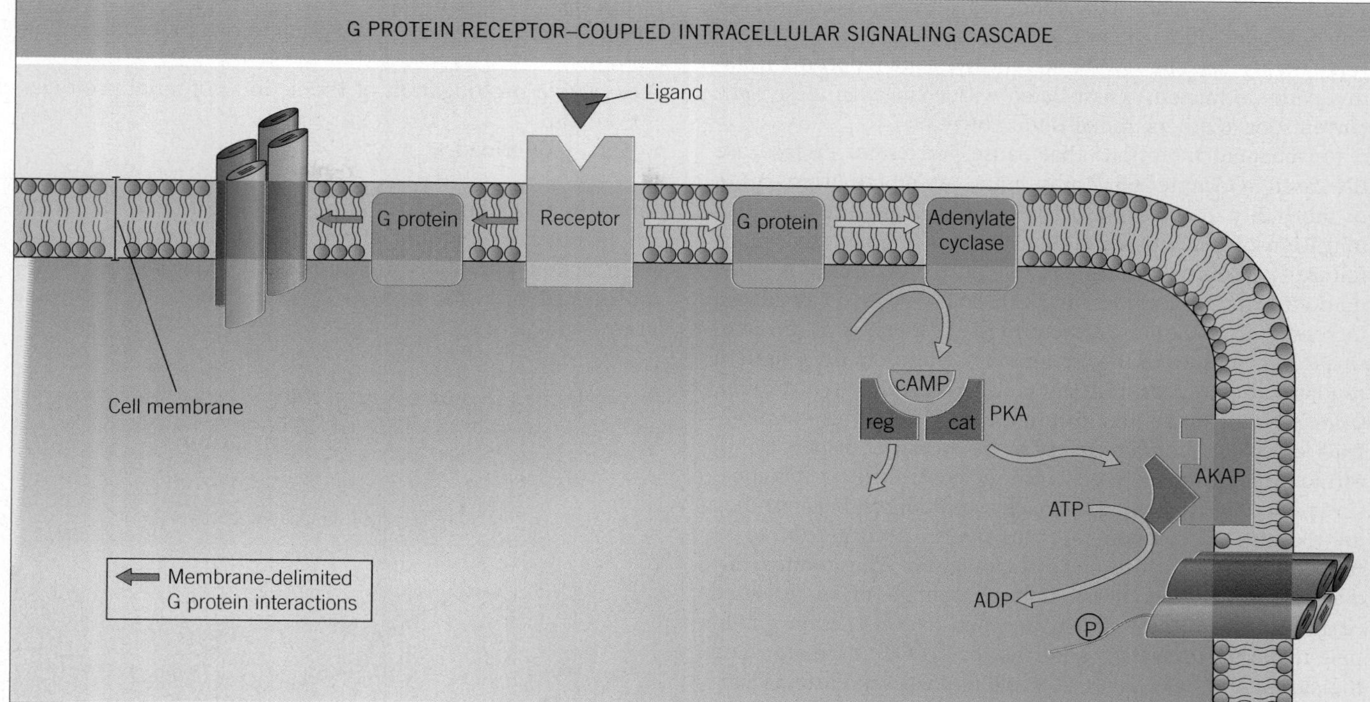

Figure 49.8 G protein receptor–coupled intracellular signaling cascade. The G protein–coupled receptor is activated by the binding of an agonist ligand. Such receptors may affect ion channel behavior directly through membrane-delimited G protein interactions *(leftward arrows)* or by activation of intracellular signaling cascades. In this example, G proteins activate the membrane-bound enzyme adenylate cyclase. This enzyme catalyzes production of the second-messenger molecule, cyclic adenosine monophosphate (cAMP), which in turn binds to protein kinase A (PKA) and releases the active catalytic subunit (cat) from the constraining regulatory subunit (reg). Actions of the PKA catalytic subunit are localized to specific intracellular targets by anchoring proteins (A kinase–anchoring proteins, AKAPs). After localization to an ion channel protein target, PKA catalyzes phosphorylation of the ion channel, which affects channel behavior. ADP, adenosine diphosphate; ATP, adenosine triphosphate; P, phosphate.

The anchoring proteins for PKA are called A kinase–anchoring proteins, and those for PKC are called receptors for activated C kinase. This distinction is not absolute, as some PKC isoforms may also bind to A kinase–anchoring proteins. Anchoring proteins act to position kinases in the vicinity of their protein substrates, including ion channels, and also to partner kinases with phosphatases, enzymes that reverse kinase actions by catalyzing the dephosphorylation reaction. Thus, anchoring proteins are the scaffold for coregulating kinase and phosphatase actions on ion channel proteins.

G Protein–Coupled Receptors

G proteins are heteromeric, membrane-associated proteins that bind guanine nucleotides. They couple activation of receptors at the cell membrane to effector molecules, including ion channel proteins. G proteins can affect ion channel function by[71]

- activating second-messenger systems (e.g., by activating adenylate cyclase to stimulate cAMP or by activating the PKA signaling cascade);
- increasing $[Ca^{2+}]_i$ (e.g., by activating phospholipase C to generate inositol 1,4,5-triphosphate); or
- directly interacting with ion channel proteins through cell membrane–delimited pathways.

One of myriad examples is the L-type Ca^{2+} channel: after agonist binding to β-adrenergic receptors, this channel is activated through the action of G proteins, both directly (through a membrane-delimited pathway) and more indirectly (through activation of the PKA signaling cascade).[72] G protein signaling is also essential for muscarinic receptor–mediated inhibition of $I_{Ca\text{-}L}$.[73]

PATHOPHYSIOLOGY

Electrophysiologic Remodeling

Electrophysiologic remodeling refers to changes in electrophysiology that arise as a result of the disease process itself. It often reflects disease-related changes in expression or function of ion channel genes (or other genes) that then determine arrhythmias in disease. The expression and function of ion channels and resultant ionic currents can be affected by heart rate. One example is the prolongation of repolarization seen with bradycardia and complete AV node block that is manifested on the surface electrocardiogram as prolongation of the QT interval.[74] This prolongation of the QT interval reflects prolongation of the action potential and is an important predisposing factor for torsades de pointes.

Recently, there has been increasing recognition of the fact that sustained rapid heart rates may contribute to arrhythmogenic changes in ionic currents and electrophysiologic properties in the atrium[75] and ventricle.[76] Atrial fibrillation results in an acute change in the effective refractory period (a function of the rapidity of action potential repolarization), which is mediated by $I_{Ca\text{-}L}$ and, presumably, by $[Ca^{2+}]_i$. Experimental tachycardia-induced cardiomyopathy results in decreased ventricular $I_{Ca\text{-}L}$ and NCX, abnormal sarcoplasmic reticulum function and intracellular Ca^{2+} homeostasis,[77] and reduced repolarizing current.[76] Whether tachycardia-induced cardiomyopathy in humans is associated with changes in these ionic currents, or in others, remains unknown.

Ion channel mutations that cause congenital disease are discussed in Chapter 63. Arrhythmias are an important cause of morbidity and mortality in acquired heart diseases. Prolongation of the action potential is seen in congestive heart failure, cardiomyopathies, and hypertrophy. This is most marked in the midmyocardial cell layer, where it results in increased dispersion of refractoriness. Dispersion of refractoriness is a measure of the maximum variation in the length of repolarization across different cell types in the myocardium. Clinically, the maximum difference in QT intervals in the 12-lead electrocardiogram is used to measure dispersion of refractoriness. Purkinje cells do not contribute to this measurement, despite having long action potentials, because they are too minor a component of the overall myocardium to be reflected in the surface electrocardiogram. The midmyocardial cell layer, in contrast, is large enough to be reflected on the surface electrocardiogram, and its long action potentials make an important contribution to QT dispersion and the terminal T wave and U wave.[78] Two repolarizing currents, I_{to1} and I_{K1}, are reduced in cardiomyopathy, and this reduction probably accounts for the observed increase in action potential duration and dispersion of refractoriness.[79] Reduced I_{to}[80] and disordered intracellular Ca^{2+} homeostasis[81] are features of cells isolated from the border zone of myocardial infarcts, and this suggests that disordered ion channel function may contribute to the electrophysiologic changes and propensity for arrhythmias that are present in patients who have coronary artery disease. Disordered cell-cell communication caused by altered distribution, expression, or function of connexin channels, in addition to interstitial fibrosis, is also likely to contribute to these arrhythmias.

CLINICAL IMPLICATIONS

Arrhythmia Mechanisms

Three basic mechanisms are responsible for cardiac arrhythmias:

- abnormal automaticity;
- triggering of arrhythmias; and
- re-entry.

In some clinical situations, several mechanisms may coexist; for example, enhanced automaticity may generate re-entrant excitation.

Abnormal Automaticity

Abnormal automaticity occurs when phase 4 repolarization becomes accelerated or manifested in either

- tissue that is normally associated with automatic behavior (e.g., the sinoatrial node); or
- myocardial tissue that is not normally associated with spontaneous phase 4 depolarization.

In either case, enhanced automaticity is often associated with increased adrenergic tone, which affects currents such as I_f that are responsible for the slope of phase 4 depolarization.

Triggered Arrhythmias

Triggered arrhythmias typically occur in two (often coexisting) settings:

- excessive prolongation of the action potential prolongation; and
- $[Ca^{2+}]_i$ overload.

Early after-depolarizations (Fig. 49.9) are oscillations in the cell membrane potential during repolarization. They arise when action potentials are prolonged (e.g., by I_{Kr} block) and inward currents, such as $I_{Ca\text{-}L}$ and NCX, then become larger.

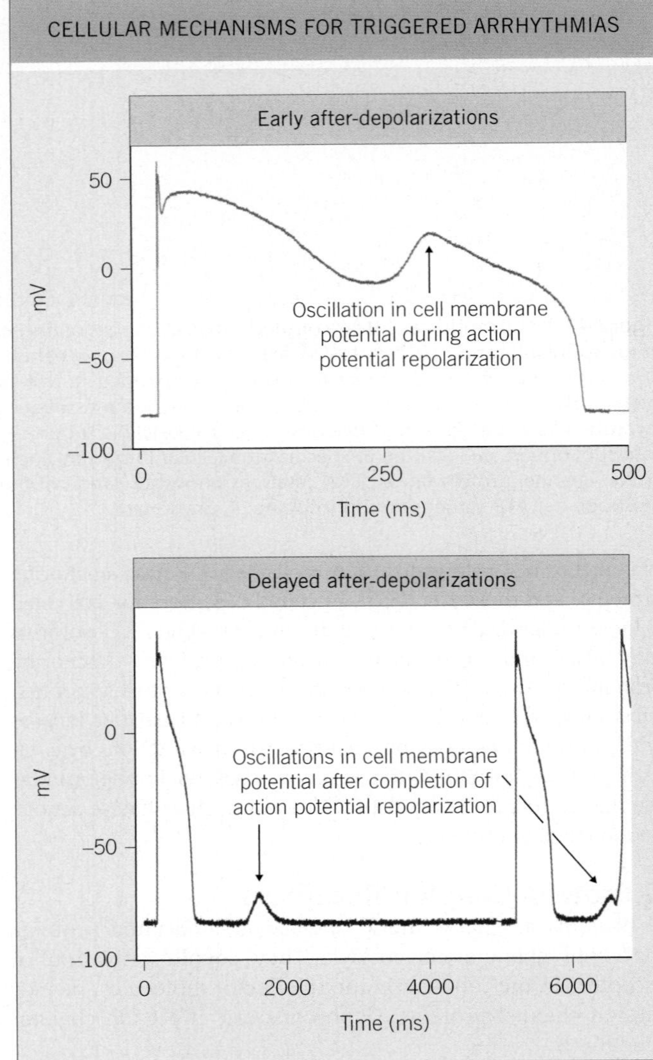

Figure 49.9 Cellular mechanisms for triggered arrhythmias. Early after-depolarizations, induced by hypokalemia and slow stimulation, are seen as oscillations in the cell membrane potential during action potential repolarization. Delayed after-depolarizations, induced by digoxin toxicity, are oscillations in the cell membrane potential that occur after completion of action potential repolarization. The second delayed after-depolarization leads to a triggered action potential. Early and delayed after-depolarizations both lead to triggered arrhythmias when the cell membrane potential repolarizes to threshold for activation of sodium channels and generation of repetitive action potentials. (Data courtesy of Drs. Yuejin Wu and Mark Anderson.)

Delayed after-depolarizations are oscillations in the cell membrane potential that occur after completion of action potential repolarization (see Fig. 49.9). Increased $[Ca^{2+}]_i$ probably facilitates both early[82,83] and delayed after-depolarizations[45]; but in delayed after-depolarizations, increased $[Ca^{2+}]_i$ directly activates a transient inward current, which causes the after-depolarization.

Both early and delayed after-depolarizations trigger arrhythmias when they are of sufficient magnitude to depolarize the cell membrane to the threshold needed for the generation of action potentials. Early after-depolarizations are facilitated in vitro by slow heart rates and K^+ channel block and are thus most often implicated in arrhythmias related to a prolonged QT interval (torsades de pointes). Delayed after-depolarizations, in contrast, are generated in vitro at rapid rates and by agents that enhance intracellular Ca^{2+} loading (e.g., digitalis, catecholamines). Delayed after-depolarizations have classically been implicated in digitalis toxicity and probably play a role in other settings of intracellular calcium overload (like the congenital arrhythmia syndromes discussed in Chapter 63). As described before, recent thinking about mechanisms of arrhythmias with I_{Kr} or I_{Ks} block suggests overlap between the two mechanisms. Both mechanisms may also operate in acute ischemia.

Re-entrant Arrhythmias

Re-entrant arrhythmias occur when an activation wavefront repetitively follows an anatomic or functional circuit within the myocardium or specialized conduction system. Requirements for tachycardia caused by anatomic re-entry are

- a circuit with an entrance and exit to the greater mass of myocardium; and
- a zone of slow conduction that facilitates the excitable gap (i.e., a region of nonrefractory tissue within the re-entrant circuit).

From the standpoint of ion channel pathology, functional re-entry may occur in the setting of increased dispersion of refractoriness, whereas anatomic re-entry is often dependent on slow conduction (e.g., through infarct border zone tissue or the AV node).

SUMMARY

Ion channel structure and function, structural proteins, and anatomic factors determine the electrical activity of the heart. This new information not only has revolutionized our understanding of the fundamental basis of cardiac electrical activity but forms the basis for current efforts to improve selectivity, specificity, and safety of therapies used to treat cardiac arrhythmias.

chapter 50

Antiarrhythmic Drug Therapy

Arnold Pinter, Wendy Lau, David Newman, and Paul Dorian

Definition

- Antiarrhythmic drugs, for the purposes of this section, are drugs that exert their antiarrhythmic effect by acting on one or more ion channels in the cell. They have been classified according to their predominant electrophysiologic effects on the action potential (Vaughan Williams classification) or their action on the "vulnerable parameter" of a particular arrhythmia (Sicilian Gambit). Some other drugs may exert direct or indirect antiarrhythmic activity by other means (e.g., drugs that alter fibrosis, gap junctions, inflammation) and may prevent or reduce arrhythmias, but they are considered only briefly in this section.

Key Features

- Agents with predominantly class I mechanism of action (sodium channel blockers) are effective at converting and suppressing supraventricular tachyarrhythmias and ventricular ectopy; however, they are associated with increased mortality in patients with structural heart disease.
- Agents with class II mechanism of action (beta blockers) reduce the incidence of sudden death in a variety of patient populations and should be considered in patients in the setting of left ventricular dysfunction or coronary artery disease. They are useful in the prevention of recurrent atrial fibrillation and slowing of the ventricular response in this arrhythmia and in the treatment of exercise-related atrial and ventricular arrhythmias. They may also increase the efficacy of class I and class III agents in suppressing inducibility or recurrence of ventricular tachycardia.
- Agents with predominantly class III mechanism of action (potassium channel blockers) are probably the most effective antiarrhythmic therapy for a wide range of supraventricular and ventricular tachyarrhythmias. The success of complex agents such as amiodarone and sotalol has prompted the development of newer class III agents, some of which block more than one ion channel.
- Agents with class IV mechanism of action (calcium channel blockers) are useful for re-entrant rhythms involving the atrioventricular node and for slowing the ventricular response to atrial fibrillation and flutter.

Clinical Implications

- Antiarrhythmic drug efficacy may be predicted by use of surrogate measures, such as programmed electrical stimulation, to assess variables such as prolongation of refractory period, prolongation of ventricular tachycardia cycle length, and suppression of tachycardia inducibility. Electrophysiologic studies to assess antiarrhythmic drug efficacy are no longer conducted routinely because of their limited predictive value. An antiarrhythmic drug may not alter or may even increase mortality despite effective suppression of an arrhythmia by electrophysiologic testing.
- The proarrhythmic potential of antiarrhythmic drugs must always be considered in selecting antiarrhythmic therapy, especially for suppression of a non–life-threatening arrhythmia.

Despite advances in nonpharmacologic therapies (e.g., implantable cardioverter-defibrillators and radiofrequency ablation), many patients will continue to require pharmacologic therapy to alleviate symptoms or to prolong life. Antiarrhythmic agents are increasingly used as adjunctive therapy to decrease device discharges in patients with implantable cardioverter-defibrillators.

Arrhythmias occur unpredictably (although they may not be randomly distributed over time) and may be dangerous. The usual therapeutic paradigm of administering a treatment, assessing the results, and modifying the treatment on the basis of the clinical response may not be easily applied to patients with arrhythmias. Because episodes may be asymptomatic, there may be no event to indicate the efficacy of a drug. The variables that govern the relationship between drug dosing and outcomes are complex. They can be broken down into

- pharmacokinetic variables, which govern the relationship between drug dose and the concentration achieved by that dose at the effector site; and
- pharmacodynamics, which govern the relationship between effector site concentration and cellular effects (Fig. 50.1).

These parameters influence the physiologic effects, which represent the responses of the affected tissues as modulated, for example, by interacting drugs or neurohumoral variables. This in turn results in a particular clinical outcome modulated by the severity of the underlying illness, by time-dependent alterations in the substrate, and by factors external to the patient (e.g., the probability of being resuscitated from a serious arrhythmia). Predicting a particular clinical outcome from a particular drug dose is subject to extraordinary variability and complexity.

MECHANISMS OF ACTION

General Principles of Pharmacokinetics

Antiarrhythmic agents normally have a narrow toxic-therapeutic relationship. Alterations in the rate of any of the four processes of absorption, distribution, metabolism, and elimination can result in important variations (between and within patients) in plasma concentrations.

Drugs exist in plasma both in the free form and bound to plasma proteins. Virtually all assays for drug concentration in the blood measure both free and protein-bound drugs. Only a free drug is capable of distributing into tissues and

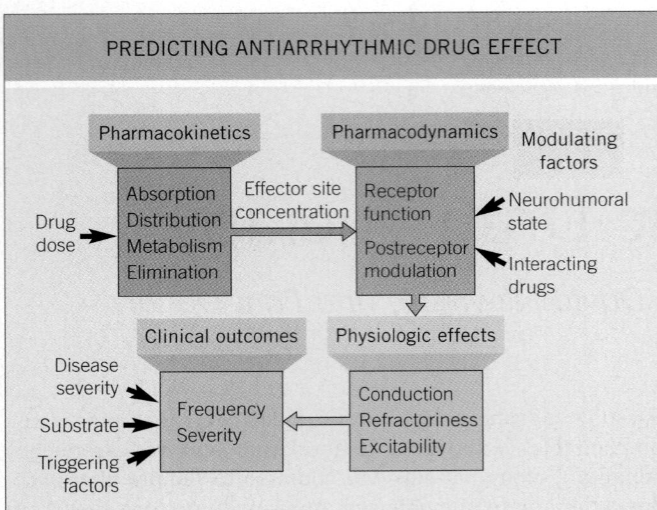

Figure 50.1 Predicting antiarrhythmic drug effect.

exerting a pharmacologic action. The fraction of drug that is bound varies greatly among different antiarrhythmic agents but is fairly constant for individual drugs over the clinically relevant range of plasma concentrations. Exceptions are phenytoin, lidocaine (lignocaine), propafenone, and disopyramide, for which binding sites become saturated at high concentrations. Therefore, a doubling of total drug concentration at this level represents more than doubling of unbound drug. Total plasma concentrations of a given drug generally correlate reasonably with electrophysiologic effects, and it has not been necessary to develop assays to measure free drug concentrations for antiarrhythmic agents.

The rate and extent of metabolism of a drug can vary greatly from patient to patient owing to genetics, environment, age and disease states, and the influence of drugs given concomitantly. The genetically determined activity of hepatic *N*-acetyltransferase regulates the development of antinuclear antibodies and the development of the lupus syndrome in response to procainamide. Slow acetylator phenotypes appear more prone than rapid acetylators to development of lupus. Similarly, genetically determined differences in metabolism of propafenone result in a small proportion of patients (approximately 7%) who are slow metabolizers, resulting in very high blood levels. Cimetidine and ranitidine may affect drug metabolism by inhibition of hepatic P450 enzymes.

Some drugs have metabolites that add to or alter the effects of the parent compound by exerting similar actions, by competing with the parent compound, or by mediating drug toxicity. Quinidine has at least four active metabolites, but none with potency that exceeds that of the parent drug and none primarily implicated in causing torsades de pointes. About 50% of procainamide is metabolized to *N*-acetylprocainamide. Only the parent drug blocks cardiac sodium channels and slows impulse propagation in the His-Purkinje system. *N*-acetylprocainamide prolongs repolarization. However, it competes with procainamide for renal tubular secretory sites and can increase the parent drug's elimination half-life and accumulate in high concentrations with renal impairment. Drug interactions with a channel, receptor, or enzyme may depend on the three-dimensional geometry (stereoselectivity) of the drug. Many drugs have stereoisomers (molecules with the same atomic composition but different spatial arrangement) that can influence drug effects, metabolism, binding, clearance, and excretion. Most drugs are prescribed as 50/50 mixtures of their two forms (racemates), which may make 50% of the dose ineffective for some drugs. Except for timolol, virtually all beta blockers are racemates. D-Propranolol exerts antiarrhythmic actions that are unrelated to β-adrenoceptor blockade, whereas L-propranolol blocks the β receptor. Both enantiomers (mirror images) of sotalol block the potassium channel to prolong action potential duration, but the L-isomer is responsible for virtually all the beta-blocking activity.

Other drugs with notable stereoselective differences include disopyramide, one form of which [*S* (+)] prolongs repolarization and has greater antiarrhythmic effects than the other form [*R* (−)], which shortens repolarization. The latter form has less anticholinergic effects. The *S* enantiomer of verapamil is at least eight times more active than the *R* enantiomer in slowing atrioventricular conduction. The systemic concentrations of *R* and *S* enantiomers are dependent on route of administration; with oral administration, there is rapid stereoselective biotransformation during the first pass of verapamil through the portal circulation, resulting in a twofold greater bioavailability of the *R* enantiomer compared with the more active *S* enantiomer. This accounts for the difference in efficacy between oral and intravenous routes of administration of the drug. Stereoselectivity affects sodium channel–blocking drugs less than β-adrenoceptor blockers, potassium channel blockers, and calcium channel blockers.

The pharmacokinetics of antiarrhythmic drugs in current clinical use are summarized in Table 50.1; the dose regimens are summarized in Table 50.2.

Some patients have unusually high sensitivity to a given blood concentration of certain antiarrhythmic drugs; for example, they may have QT intervals that fall within the normal limits but may have some degree of genetic defect in their repolarization currents that predisposes them to unexpectedly large effects on repolarization after any drug with class III effects, leading to an increased risk of the torsades de pointes type of proarrhythmia.

Electrophysiologic Effects of Antiarrhythmic Drugs

There are two putative causes of arrhythmias:

- alterations in impulse formation leading to enhanced or abnormal automaticity, or triggered activity; and
- alterations in impulse conduction resulting in re-entry phenomena.

These mechanisms are described in detail in Chapter 49.

Effect of Antiarrhythmic Agents on Automaticity

Most antiarrhythmic agents suppress automaticity by

- decreasing the slope of phase 4 spontaneous depolarization (see Chapter 49 and Fig. 50.1);
- shifting the threshold voltage to a less negative level; or
- hyperpolarizing the resting membrane potential.

Although these effects also decrease the frequency of discharge of normal pacemaker cells, they have a more pronounced action on ectopic activity. The relatively selective

PHARMACOKINETICS OF ANTIARRHYTHMIC DRUGS							
Drug	Bioavailability (%)	Vd (L/kg)	Protein Binding (%)	Elimination Half-Life (h)	Therapeutic Range (μg/mL)	Biotransformation and Excretion	Metabolites
Quinidine	75	2-3	75-90	4-8	2-6 (7.3-21.9 μmol/L)	Liver: 80% Kidney: 10%-20% unchanged	Hydroxyquinidine: slight activity
Procainamide	75-95	1.5-2.5	15-25	2-4	4-10 (17-42.5 μmol/L)	Liver: acetylation Kidney: 60% unchanged	*N*-Acetylprocainamide: class III activity
Disopyramide	90	0.5-1.5	35-95	6-9	2-5	Liver: 25%-35% inactive Kidney: 50% unchanged	*N*-Dealkyldisopyramide: less active than parent compound
Lidocaine		1-2	65-75	0.3-2	1.5-5 (5.7-21.3 μmol/L)	Liver: 90% dealkylated	Monoethylglycylxylidine, glycine xylidine: relatively inactive
Mexiletine	90	5-9	75	9-12	0.5-2	Liver: 90% Kidney: 10% unchanged (↑with acid urine)	Inactive
Phenytoin	Variable	0.5-1	90	18-36	10-20 (39.6-79.2 μmol/L)	Liver: 95% hydroxylated to inactive compound	Inactive
Flecainide	95	9	50	16-20	0.2-1 (0.42-2.11 μmol/L)	Liver: >70%	Inactive
Propafenone	5-12, dose dependent	3	>95	3-5	0.5-1	Liver: >99% genetic variation in biotransformation	Hydroxypropafenone: active
Propranolol	25-50	3-4	85-95	3-6	0.05-0.1 (0.19-0.39 μmol/L)	Liver: High first-pass extraction	4-Hydroxypropranolol: slight activity
Amiodarone	20-50	Very large	>96	≥60 days	0.5-3	Liver: de-ethylation	Desethylamiodarone: active
Sotalol	>95	1.5	Negligible	13	1-2 (3.7-7.4 μmol/L)	Kidney: 100% unchanged	None
Dofeltide	90%	3	60-70%	8-12	4-8	Kidney: 80% Liver: 20%	Inactive
Verapamil	15-30	4-5	90	3-7	0.1-0.15	Liver: high first-pass extraction	Norverapamil: moderately active

Table 50.1 Pharmacokinetics of antiarrhythmic drugs.

USUAL DOSE RANGES FOR ANTIARRHYTHMIC DRUGS					
	Intravenous		Oral (mg)		Time (h) to Peak Plasma Concentration (Oral)
Drug	Loading	Maintenance	Loading	Maintenance	
Quinidine	5-10 mg/kg at 0.3-0.5 mg/kg/min	0.25 mg/kg/min	300-600 q6h	200-300 q6-8h	1.5-3
Procainamide	6-13 mg/kg at 0.2-0.5 mg/kg/min	2-6 mg/min	500-1000	350-1000 q3-6h (50 mg/kg/day)	1
Disopyramide	1-2 mg/kg during 15-45 minutes*	1 mg/kg/h	300	100-400 q6-8h	1-2
Lidocaine	1-3 mg/kg at 20-50 mg/min	1-4 mg/min			
Mexiletine	500 mg*	500-1000 mg q24h	400-600	150-300 q6-8h	2-4
Tocainide	750 mg*		400-600	400-600 q8-12h	0.5-2
Phenytoin	100 mg q5min for ≤1000 mg		1000	100-400 q12-24h	8-12
Flecainide	2 mg/kg*	100-200 mg q12h		50 q12h; maximum recommended dose, 300/day	3-4
Propafenone	1-2 mg/kg*		600-900	150-300 q8-12h	1-3
Propranolol	0.25-0.5 mg q5min for ≤0.15-0.2 mg/kg			10-200 q6-8h	4
Ibutilide	1-2 mg				
Amiodarone	5 mg/kg during 10-30 minutes	720-1000 mg q24h	For VT: 1200-1600 qd for 1-2 weeks, then 600-800 qd for 2-4 weeks For SVT: 600-800 qd for 2 weeks	For VT: 200-400 qd For SVT: 200 qd	
Sotalol	0.5-1.5 mg/kg during 10 minutes*			80 mg q12h to start, incrementing gradually to 320 mg/day as needed	2.5-4
Verapamil	10 mg during 1-2 minutes	0.005 mg/kg/min		80-120 q6-8h	1-2
Adenosine	6-12 mg (rapidly)				
Dofetilide				125 qd to 500 q12h	2

*Not available (approved) in North America for intravenous use.
SVT, supraventricular tachycardia; VT, ventricular tachycardia.

Table 50.2 Usual dose ranges for antiarrhythmic drugs.

suppression of ectopic foci may abolish an arrhythmia caused by abnormal automaticity at doses that have little effect on normal sinus node function. Suppression of phase 4 depolarization may result in a reduction of the heart rate or, possibly, asystole in the presence of sinus node dysfunction.

Triggered activity, another form of abnormal automaticity (see Chapter 49), may occur with digitalis toxicity or may be induced by drugs that prolong repolarization. These oscillations in membrane potential can be suppressed by calcium channel blockers or magnesium, by restoring electrolyte balance to the cell milieu, or by increasing heart rate.

Effect of Antiarrhythmic Agents on Re-entry

Re-entry is a common cause of ventricular tachycardia (VT), atrial flutter, atrioventricular (AV) node re-entry, and AV re-entry (see Chapters 57 to 60). Antiarrhythmic agents abolish re-entry by slowing conduction (impairing or halting propagation in the circuit), increasing refractoriness so that the re-entrant wavefront impinges on refractory tissue, or both.

Use Dependence and Reverse Rate Dependence

Use dependence describes a greater effect at more rapid rates of stimulation and after longer periods of stimulation. It usually is manifested as a greater drug-induced slowing of conduction at rapid heart rates.

Use-dependent phenomena are best explained by the modulated receptor hypothesis for sodium channel blockers. In this model, sodium channel–blocking agents attach to their receptor on the sodium channel during the open or inactivated state of the sodium channel. Drug attachment blocks channel function (i.e., slows conduction and the rate of rise of phase 0 [V_{max}] of the action potential) in a fashion that is both time and voltage dependent. The effect increases with

CLASSIFICATION OF ANTIARRHYTHMIC MECHANISMS		
Class	**General Mechanism**	**Examples**
I	Sodium channel blockade	
Ia	↓↓Phase 0 upstroke rate Delay conduction Prolong repolarization	Quinidine, procainamide, disopyramide
Ib	Little effect on phase 0 in normal tissue ↓Phase 0 upstroke rate in abnormal tissue Shorten repolarization or little effect	Lidocaine, mexiletine, tocainide, phenytoin
Ic	↓↓↓Phase 0 upstroke rate Markedly slow conduction Slight effect on repolarization	Flecainide, propafenone, encainide, moricizine
II	Beta blockade	Propranolol, metoprolol, esmolol, and many others
III	Marked prolongation of repolarization	Amiodarone, sotalol, bretylium, ibutilide, dofetilide, azimilide, tedisamil
IV	Calcium channel blockers	Verapamil, diltiazem

Table 50.3 Classification of antiarrhythmic mechanisms.

each action potential and dissipates during diastole. Drugs also dissociate from the channel in a time- and voltage-dependent manner so that the net effect is residual slowed conduction; this results in an enhanced drug effect at faster rates because there is less time for drug unblocking. Some sodium channel blockers with slow kinetics of channel block and unblock (especially class Ic drugs) can possess marked use dependence with widening of the QRS during exercise resembling VT.

Some drugs exert greater effects at slow rates, with progressive loss of effect at rapid rates, a phenomenon termed reverse rate dependence. This occurs with drugs that lengthen repolarization (potassium channel–blocking drugs), especially those that block the rapidly activating component of the delayed rectifier potassium channel (I_{Kr}). Amiodarone is an important exception as it prolongs action potentials relatively uniformly at different heart rates.[1] Reverse rate dependence may be due to a relatively greater contribution of I_{Ks}, a slowly activating outward potassium current, as rate increases, causing more rapid repolarization at rapid rates than at slower rates.

During short diastolic intervals, I_{Ks} may be incompletely deactivated, resulting in a greater net repolarizing current. However, in some species, including humans, I_{Ks} deactivates rapidly and may not be the cause of reverse rate dependence. In an experimental model, I_{Ks} blockade increased the reverse rate dependence of I_{Kr} blockade by dofetilide.[2] Reverse rate dependence has two disadvantages:

- at rapid rates, wavelength is hardly prolonged, diminishing the likelihood of preventing re-entrant tachycardias; and
- at slow heart rates, the occurrence of early after-depolarizations and torsades de pointes is promoted.

CLASSIFICATION

The most widely accepted classification of antiarrhythmic drug action was proposed by Vaughan Williams[3] and later modified. In this classification, the actions of various agents are separated according to their predominant electrophysiologic effects on the action potential recorded largely from Purkinje fibers in vitro (Table 50.3). This classification is descriptive and describes antiarrhythmic drug actions rather than antiarrhythmic drugs. Many antiarrhythmic drugs have actions that relate to more than one class or subclass in the classification, and many have metabolites with a different class of action from that of the parent drug. Not all drugs with uniform mechanism of action have identical effects, whereas some with different mechanisms have overlapping actions. Nevertheless, the Vaughan Williams classification continues to be widely used.

Class I Mechanism of Action

Class I action relates to slowing the rate of rise of phase 0 (V_{max}) of the action potential by blocking membrane fast sodium channels. This action may be divided into three subgroups based on the time constants (τ) for recovery of the sodium channel from block. This parameter is a measure of use dependence and predicts the extent to which a drug will decrease conduction velocity in sodium-dependent cardiac tissue. Different effects on repolarization are also seen between the class I subgroups.

Class Ia Mechanism of Action

Class Ia action results in reduced V_{max} and delayed conduction. Drugs with class Ia action also prolong repolarization. Kinetics of onset and offset in blocking the sodium channel are of intermediate rapidity ($\tau = 300$ to 1500 ms).

Class Ib Mechanism of Action

Class Ib action results in shortened action potential duration and reduced V_{max} in abnormal tissue (especially if it is partially depolarized) but not in normal tissue. Onset and offset kinetics are fast ($\tau < 300$ ms).

Class Ic Mechanism of Action

Class Ic action results in markedly reduced V_{max}, markedly slowed conduction, and minimal prolongation of refractoriness. Onset and offset kinetics are slow ($\tau = 3$ to 12 s).

Class II Mechanism of Action

Drugs with class II mechanism of action competitively block β-adrenergic receptors and depress phase 4 depolarization (normal automaticity).

Class III Mechanism of Action

Class III drugs block one or more of a variety of repolarizing potassium channels and thus prolong action potential duration and refractory periods. Drugs with predominantly class Ia mechanism of action (e.g., quinidine) also block potassium channels.

Class IV Mechanism of Action

Drugs with class IV mechanism of action block the slow calcium channel, decreasing the inward current carried by calcium across the cell membrane. In the sinus node, this results in less net inward (depolarizing) current during the latter part of spontaneous diastolic depolarization. The net result is a decrease in the rate of rise (slope) of phase 4 spontaneous depolarization and a slowing of the heart rate. In addition, these drugs slow conduction in tissues dependent on calcium currents (e.g., the AV node), prolonging the PR interval.

The Sicilian Gambit

Given the limitations of the commonly used, modified Vaughan Williams classification of antiarrhythmic drug action, a new approach to classification of drugs with potential antiarrhythmic activity, termed the Sicilian Gambit, has been proposed.[4,5] In this approach, a number of potential targets for drug action are identified; these targets include

- various ion-conducting channels (sodium, potassium, calcium, chloride);
- receptors (α-adrenergic, β-adrenergic, muscarinic, purinergic); and
- pumps (Na^+,K^+-ATPase).

All antiarrhythmic drugs or substances that affect cardiac electrophysiology would then be characterized by their actions on each of these channels, receptors, or pumps.[5] The actions of the drugs may be activation or inhibition with varying kinetics and intensity. The Sicilian Gambit (Fig. 50.2) attempts to

- identify the mechanisms of a particular arrhythmia;
- determine the "vulnerable parameter" of the arrhythmia most susceptible to modification;
- define the target most likely to affect the vulnerable parameter; and then
- select a drug that will modify the target.

Unfortunately, the precise mechanisms of arrhythmias and the specific consequences of actions on particular channels or receptors are poorly understood. In particular, the subtle and delicate interaction between the trigger for an arrhythmia and its maintenance is usually not well understood. Nevertheless, the Sicilian Gambit is a useful conceptual framework for describing the currently known effects of antiarrhythmic drugs, and it aids in the understanding of the multiplicity of drug actions.

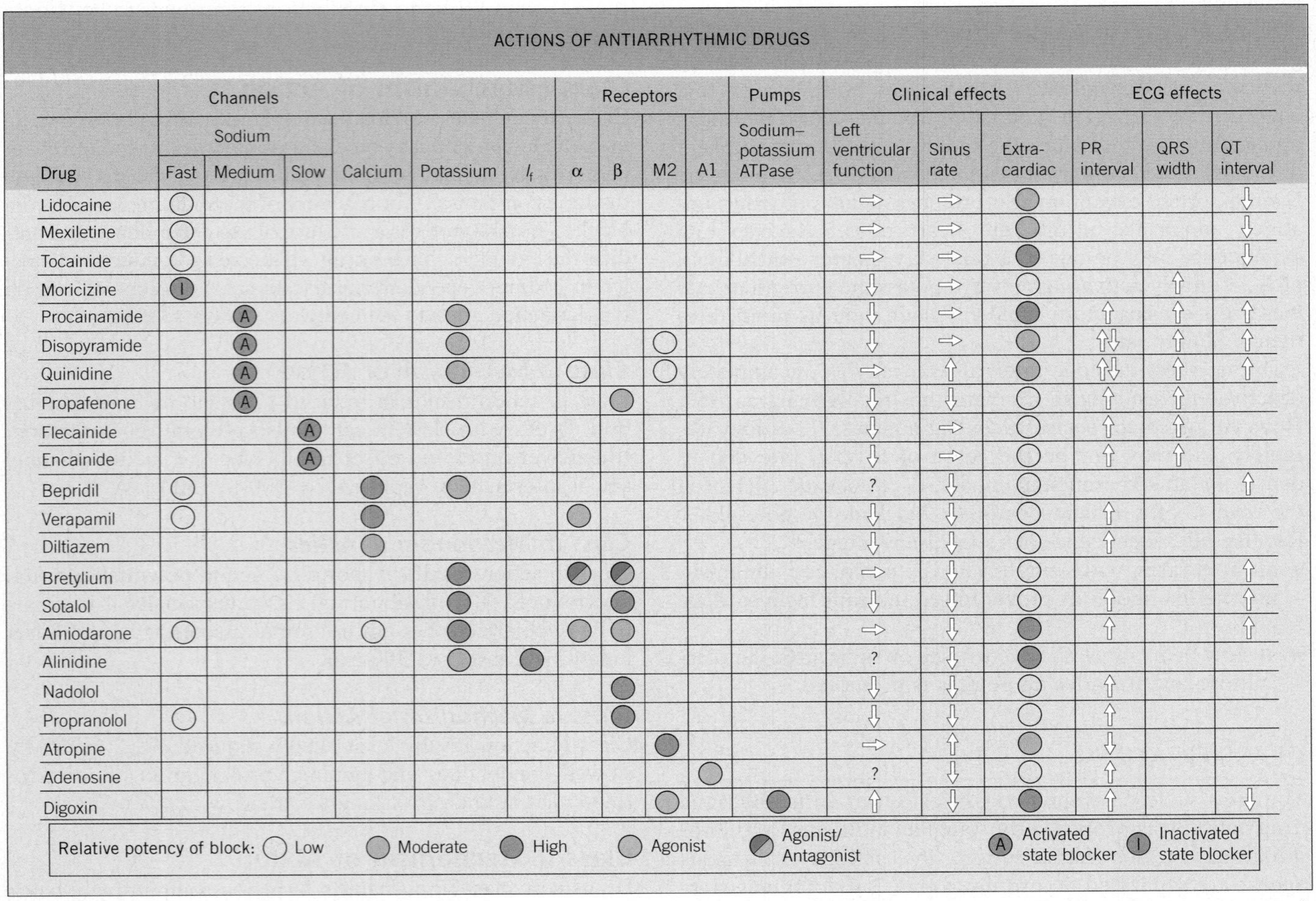

ACTIONS OF ANTIARRHYTHMIC DRUGS

	Channels						Receptors				Pumps	Clinical effects			ECG effects		
	Sodium										Sodium–potassium ATPase	Left ventricular function	Sinus rate	Extra-cardiac	PR interval	QRS width	QT interval
Drug	Fast	Medium	Slow	Calcium	Potassium	I_f	α	β	M2	A1							
Lidocaine	Low											→	→	Moderate			↓
Mexiletine	Low											→	→	Moderate			↓
Tocainide	Low											→	→	High			↓
Moricizine	I (inactivated state blocker)											↓	→	Low		↑	
Procainamide		A (activated state blocker)			Moderate							↓	→	High	↑	↑	↑
Disopyramide		A (activated state blocker)			Moderate				Low			↓	→	Moderate	↑↓	↑	↑
Quinidine		A (activated state blocker)			Moderate		Low		Low			→	↑	High	↑↓	↑	↑
Propafenone		A (activated state blocker)						Moderate				↓	↓	Low	↑	↑	
Flecainide			A (activated state blocker)		Low							↓	→	Low	↑	↑	
Encainide			A (activated state blocker)									↓	→	Low	↑	↑	
Bepridil	Low			High	Moderate							?	↓	Low			↑
Verapamil	Low			High			Moderate					↓	↓	Low	↑		
Diltiazem				Moderate								↓	↓	Low	↑		
Bretylium					High		Agonist/Antagonist	Agonist/Antagonist				→	↓	Low			↑
Sotalol					High			High				↓	↓	Low	↑		↑
Amiodarone	Low			Low	High		Moderate	Moderate				→	↓	High	↑		↑
Alinidine					Moderate	High						?	↓	High			
Nadolol								High				↓	↓	Low	↑		
Propranolol	Low							High				↓	↓	Low	↑		
Atropine									High			→	↑	Moderate	↓		
Adenosine										Agonist		?	↓	Low	↑		
Digoxin									Agonist		High	↑	↓	High	↑		↓

Relative potency of block: ○ Low; Moderate; High; Agonist; Agonist/Antagonist; (A) Activated state blocker; (I) Inactivated state blocker

Figure 50.2 Actions of antiarrhythmic drugs. (From Rosen MR. Consequences of the Sicilian Gambit. Eur Heart J 1995;16[Suppl G]:32-36).[5]

DRUGS WITH CLASS Ia MECHANISM OF ACTION

Quinidine

Pharmacokinetics

Quinidine sulfate is rapidly and nearly completely absorbed after oral administration; the gluconate salt is absorbed more slowly and less completely. An intravenous preparation is available, but it can cause severe hypotension and must be administered with caution; nevertheless, it may be very useful clinically in the setting of amiodarone-refractory storms of VT and ventricular fibrillation (VF). Approximately 80% of a dose is hydroxylated in the liver through the P450 cytochrome system (isoenzyme CYP3A4); the metabolites are cardioactive. The remainder of the drug is excreted unchanged by the kidney. Quinidine is approximately 80% bound to plasma proteins, including albumin and α_1-acid glycoprotein.

During heart failure, the total clearance of quinidine decreases and its half-life increases. Left ventricular dysfunction (left ventricular ejection fraction below 35%) results in altered drug concentration–effect relationships, with less efficacy for VT.[6]

Electrophysiologic Effects

Quinidine slows the rapid sodium current, decreasing the rate of rise of phase 0 of the action potential (V_{max}). It also decreases the slope of phase 4 spontaneous depolarization, tending to inhibit ectopic rhythms due to automaticity. Quinidine suppresses ventricular arrhythmias caused by increased normal but not abnormal automaticity. Quinidine may also abolish re-entrant arrhythmias; it produces bidirectional block by depressing membrane responsiveness and by prolonging the effective refractory period. Prolongation of refractoriness is more prominent at slow heart rates (reverse rate dependence) owing to block of I_K, whereas faster rates result in more block of sodium channels ([positive] use dependence). Quinidine produces early after-depolarizations, which may be responsible for torsades de pointes.

Quinidine may cause an increase in heart rate either by a reflex increase in sympathetic activity or by a decrease in vagal tone. The drug may produce severe sinus bradycardia in patients who have sick sinus syndrome.

In therapeutic concentrations, quinidine has little effect on the PR interval but prolongs the QRS complex and QTc. These effects become more pronounced with increasing plasma concentrations.

Cardiovascular and Hemodynamic Effects

Quinidine has minimal negative inotropism. Administered intravenously, quinidine may produce vasodilatation and marked hypotension as a result of its α-adrenergic receptor–blocking effects.

Indications, Contraindications, and Objectives

Quinidine is useful in atrial, AV junctional, and ventricular tachyarrhythmias.

Quinidine is associated with long-term maintenance of sinus rhythm in about 50% of patients converted from atrial flutter or fibrillation. It may cause an increase in the ventricular rate by slowing atrial flutter rate, allowing 1:1 conduction over the AV node, and shortening AV nodal refractoriness through its anticholinergic effect. Patients should receive AV node–blocking drugs (e.g., digitalis, beta blockers, or calcium channel blockers) before quinidine is administered. A meta-analysis of six studies of quinidine versus placebo showed that quinidine-treated patients remained in sinus rhythm longer but had increased total mortality.[7]

In Wolff-Parkinson-White syndrome, quinidine prolongs the effective refractory period of the accessory pathway, preventing reciprocating tachycardias and slowing the ventricular response from accessory pathway conduction during atrial flutter or fibrillation. One report suggests that quinidine effectively prevents induction of VF in patients with Brugada syndrome and may also suppress spontaneous arrhythmias.[8]

Quinidine may be combined with other antiarrhythmic agents for increased efficacy (see later). Empiric therapy with quinidine or procainamide is associated with increased frequency of sudden death in patients with coronary artery disease resuscitated after cardiac arrest.[9] Quinidine crosses the placenta and can be used to treat arrhythmias in the fetus. Quinidine sulfate is currently no longer routinely available because the manufacturer decided to stop its production in 2006.[10]

Complications

Gastrointestinal symptoms (nausea, vomiting, diarrhea, abdominal pain, and anorexia) are common but possibly milder with the gluconate form. Large doses of the drug may produce cinchonism, characterized by a spectrum of central nervous system symptoms including blurred vision, tinnitus, hearing loss, visual disturbances, headache, confusion, delirium, and psychosis. Drug fever and rare idiosyncratic reactions, such as thrombocytopenia secondary to antiplatelet antibodies, have been reported. Side effects preclude long-term administration in 30% to 40% of patients.

With increasing plasma levels of quinidine, the risk of AV block or asystole increases. Quinidine-induced cardiac toxicity can be treated with isomolar sodium lactate. Toxic concentrations may also induce abnormal automaticity and VT. Torsades de pointes may occur at therapeutic plasma concentrations of quinidine in patients who exhibit excessive QT prolongation. This occurs in 1% to 3% of patients receiving quinidine; it can be treated acutely with intravenous magnesium.

Quinidine can interact with other drugs. It will cause a twofold increase in serum digoxin concentration in patients at steady state as a result of decreased renal and nonrenal clearance of digoxin and the displacement of digoxin from tissue-binding sites by the quinidine molecule. Verapamil inhibits quinidine metabolism. Drugs that induce hepatic enzyme production, such as phenobarbital and phenytoin, can shorten the duration of action of quinidine by increasing its rate of elimination, whereas inhibitors of cytochrome P450 CYP3A4 (such as erythromycin) decrease quinidine total clearance and may lead to toxicity. Quinidine is a potent inhibitor of CYP2D6 and can alter the pharmacokinetics of other drugs that undergo extensive CYP2D6-mediated metabolism (e.g., propafenone, metoprolol, and mexiletine). Approximately 90% of the population express the 2D6 isozyme and are extensive metabolizers. Coadministration of quinidine with other drugs that undergo extensive CYP2D6-mediated metabolism can convert extensive metabolizers into poor metabolizers.

Procainamide

Pharmacokinetics

Procainamide is more than 75% bioavailable after oral administration. It can be given by the intravenous or intramuscular route. The intravenous preparation can cause hypotension if it is rapidly administered. Procainamide has a relatively short half-life of 2 to 3 hours. A prolonged-release form of the drug given every 6 hours provides adequate steady-state plasma levels.

A variable proportion of the drug is acetylated in the liver to *N*-acetylprocainamide (NAPA). Unlike the parent drug, NAPA has little effect on V_{max} of Purkinje fibers but prolongs the duration of the action potential, that is, class III drug action. The concentration-response relationship for NAPA is different from that for procainamide.

The NAPA metabolite is eliminated primarily through the kidneys. Hence, the patient's acetylation status and renal function are important in determining the plasma concentration at steady state, and dosages need to be adjusted in patients with renal impairment. Age also appears to affect both procainamide clearance and the NAPA:procainamide concentration ratio independently of the decline in renal function that occurs in elderly patients.

Electrophysiologic Effects

The antiarrhythmic effects of procainamide are similar to those of quinidine. Like quinidine, procainamide prolongs the effective refractory period more than it prolongs the duration of the action potential. Early responses arising from less negative resting potentials, which might conduct slowly or block and cause an arrhythmia, are prevented from occurring. When procainamide is combined with sotalol, greater antiarrhythmic efficacy is achieved than with either agent alone.[11] Procainamide at high concentrations can elevate defibrillation thresholds.

Cardiovascular and Hemodynamic Effects

Procainamide is comparable to quinidine in its minimal negative inotropic effects at usual oral clinical doses. It lacks quinidine's vagolytic and α-adrenergic–blocking activity and is better tolerated when it is given intravenously. Intravenous administration may still produce peripheral vasodilatation and hypotension, possibly through ganglionic blockade or central nervous system sympathetic inhibition, or both.

Indications, Contraindications, and Objectives

Procainamide is used to treat both supraventricular and ventricular arrhythmias. It is particularly useful in the treatment of atrial fibrillation associated with rapid conduction over an accessory pathway. Intravenous procainamide can be used for chemical cardioversion of recent-onset atrial fibrillation or flutter, especially in North America, where the available intravenous drugs for this purpose are limited. Intravenous procainamide can be used to substitute ajmaline in the diagnostic testing (unmasking) of Brugada electrocardiographic pattern.

Procainamide is more effective than lidocaine in preventing the induction of VT by programmed stimulation and in terminating sustained monomorphic VT.[12]

The electrophysiologic response to intravenous procainamide predicts the response to the drug given orally. Patients who have a left ventricular ejection fraction of 40% or greater and whose VT is rendered noninducible by intravenous procainamide have a high likelihood of responding to the drug given orally. Procainamide slows the rate of induced VT, a change correlated with the increase in QRS duration. Adding amiodarone to procainamide slows the VT cycle length further but only slightly increases noninducibility rate.[13]

Complications

Excessive concentrations of procainamide markedly impair conduction, resulting in asystole or ventricular arrhythmias similar to those seen with quinidine. NAPA can also induce QT prolongation and torsades de pointes. Hypersensitivity reactions include occasional drug fever and, rarely, agranulocytosis. Gastrointestinal intolerance is less frequent than with quinidine, and central nervous system side effects, including depression, hallucinations, and psychosis, occur less frequently than with lidocaine.

A more common and troublesome reaction is the development of a syndrome resembling systemic lupus erythematosus (SLE), which presents with arthralgia, fever, hepatomegaly, and pleuropericardial inflammation. The SLE phenomenon is dose and time related and is more likely to occur in patients who exhibit slow hepatic acetylation and higher plasma drug concentrations. The drug-induced SLE may be accompanied by lupus erythematosus cells in the blood smear. Between 60% and 70% of patients receiving procainamide on a chronic basis develop antinuclear antibodies, with clinical symptoms occurring in 20% to 30%. Positive serologic test results are not sufficient to discontinue the drug unless they are accompanied by symptoms or the presence of anti-DNA antibody. SLE usually disappears on withdrawal of the drug. Corticosteroid administration may alleviate the symptoms. In contrast to naturally occurring SLE, the brain and kidney are spared, and there is no predilection for women.

Disopyramide

Pharmacokinetics

Disopyramide is 80% to 90% absorbed after oral administration, and bioavailability exceeds 80%. At least 50% of the orally ingested drug is excreted unchanged by the kidneys. Approximately 30% of the drug is converted to the less active mono-*N*-dealkylated metabolite by the liver.

Electrophysiologic Effects

The electrophysiologic properties of disopyramide are similar to those of quinidine: it slows the rate of rise of phase 0 (V_{max}) of the action potential and causes a concentration-dependent decrease in the slope of phase 4 depolarization. Disopyramide also slows sinus rate and may cause bradyarrhythmias in patients with sinus node dysfunction. The drug exerts greater anticholinergic effects than quinidine and does not appear to affect α- or β-adrenoceptors.

Cardiovascular and Hemodynamic Effects

Disopyramide exerts a marked negative inotropic effect, especially in patients with left ventricular dysfunction. It is generally contraindicated in patients with a history of congestive heart failure. The negative inotropic and anticholinergic effects of disopyramide have suggested utility for idiopathic hypertrophic cardiomyopathy and vasodepressor syncope.

Indications, Contraindications, and Objectives

Disopyramide appears comparable to quinidine and procainamide in preventing recurrence of VT or atrial fibrillation in selected patients. It is especially attractive in patients with atrial fibrillation that occurs predominantly at nighttime or at rest (vagally mediated atrial fibrillation).[14]

Complications

Most side effects with disopyramide relate to anticholinergic activity (e.g., dry mouth, urinary hesitancy or retention, blurred vision, and constipation). Patients who demonstrate an excessively prolonged QT interval with disopyramide are at risk for development of torsades de pointes.

DRUGS WITH CLASS Ib MECHANISM OF ACTION

Lidocaine

Pharmacokinetics

Lidocaine is administered intravenously because extensive first-pass transformation by the liver prevents clinically effective plasma concentrations orally. The drug is dealkylated and eliminated almost entirely by the liver; therefore, dosage adjustments are necessary in the presence of hepatic disease or dysfunction. Lidocaine clearance exhibits the time dependency common to high-clearance agents. With a continuous infusion lasting more than 24 hours, there is a decrease in total lidocaine clearance and an increase in elimination half-life compared with a single dose. Lidocaine free plasma levels can vary in certain patients owing to binding with albumin and the acute-phase reactant α_1-acid glycoprotein. Levels of α_1-acid glycoprotein are increased in patients after surgery or acute myocardial infarction, whereas levels of both α_1-acid glycoprotein and serum albumin are decreased in chronic hepatic disease or heart failure and in those who are malnourished. This is an essential consideration because it is the unbound fraction that is pharmacologically active.

Electrophysiologic Effects

Lidocaine causes a modest reduction in V_{max} (phase 0) of the action potential at normal hyperpolarized (−60 to −90 mV) potentials. It also shortens the duration of the action potential and the effective refractory period of normal Purkinje fibers and ventricular myocardial cells. The shortening effect on the action potential is greater than that on the effective refractory period, a phenomenon termed postrepolarization refractoriness. Lidocaine has little effect in atrial tissue.

Lidocaine may occasionally cause sinus node depression in patients with preexisting sinus node dysfunction. The drug slows conduction most in hypoxic or ischemic tissues, which are partially depolarized, and at high rates of stimulation (use-dependent effect). Lidocaine can elevate defibrillation thresholds.

Cardiovascular and Hemodynamic Effects

Lidocaine has little or no negative inotropic effect. Unlike drugs with class Ia action, lidocaine does not alter autonomic function.

Indications, Contraindications, and Objectives

Experimentally, lidocaine has been found to prevent VF arising during myocardial ischemia or infarction by preventing the fragmentation of organized large wavefronts into heterogeneous wavelets. Although lidocaine is of proven benefit in preventing VF early after clinical myocardial infarction, there is no evidence that it reduces mortality. To the contrary, lidocaine may increase mortality after myocardial infarction by approximately 40% to 60%.[15] There are no controlled studies of lidocaine in secondary prevention of recurrence of VT or VF.

Lidocaine terminates organized monomorphic spontaneous VT or induced sustained VT in only approximately 20% of cases and is less effective than many other antiarrhythmic drugs.[16] In a blinded, randomized study of intravenous lidocaine versus intravenous amiodarone in out-of-hospital VF resistant to defibrillation, lidocaine was associated with half the likelihood of survival to hospital admission compared with amiodarone.[17]

Complications

Central nervous system side effects such as drowsiness, slurred speech, paresthesias, agitation, and confusion predominate. These symptoms may progress to convulsions and respiratory arrest with higher plasma concentrations. A rare adverse effect is malignant hyperthermia.

Cimetidine significantly reduces the systemic clearance of lidocaine as well as the volume of distribution at steady state and the degree of plasma protein binding. Beta blockers also reduce lidocaine clearance owing to a decrease in hepatic blood flow. For the same reason, clearance is reduced in congestive heart failure or low-output states.

Amiodarone may also influence the pharmacokinetics of lidocaine. In patients receiving amiodarone, single doses of intravenous lidocaine do not influence the pharmacokinetics of either agent. When amiodarone treatment is started in patients who are already receiving lidocaine infusion, there is a decrease in lidocaine clearance, which can result in toxic lidocaine levels.

Mexiletine

Pharmacokinetics

Mexiletine is an orally effective structural analogue of lidocaine. It is well absorbed and biotransformed by the liver to inactive metabolites; the half-life is relatively long (about 12 hours).

Electrophysiologic Effects

Mexiletine has electrophysiologic effects similar to those of lidocaine; it shortens the duration of the action potential in normal tissues but slows conduction, especially in diseased tissues. Mexiletine also suppresses abnormal automaticity in Purkinje fibers. There is no prolongation of the QT interval.

Cardiovascular and Hemodynamic Effects

Very little negative inotropic effect is seen.

Indications, Contraindications, and Objectives

Like lidocaine, mexiletine is effective in the treatment of ventricular arrhythmias. Success rates vary from 6% to 60% and may be increased in some patients if mexiletine is combined with another antiarrhythmic agent such as procainamide, a beta blocker, quinidine, disopyramide, propafenone, or amiodarone. Like other drugs with predominantly class I mechanism of action, mexiletine may increase mortality in post–myocardial infarction patients.[18]

Mexiletine, when added to amiodarone, was effective in the treatment of very frequent ventricular tachyarrhythmia in a patient with an implantable defibrillator.[19]

Complications

Gastrointestinal (nausea, vomiting, dyspepsia, anorexia) and central nervous system side effects (tremor, ataxia, dizziness, dysarthria, diplopia, insomnia, confusion) are common and respond to a decrease in dose. Proarrhythmia is uncommon.

Phenytoin

Pharmacokinetics

Orally administered phenytoin (diphenylhydantoin) is incompletely absorbed, and the degree of absorption varies with the brand. Therapeutic serum concentrations (10 to 20 μg/mL) are similar for treatment of both cardiac arrhythmias and epilepsy. More than 90% of a dose is hydroxylated in the liver to presumably inactive compounds. Capability for hydroxylation is genetically determined; hence, there is wide variation in phenytoin metabolism between patients.

Electrophysiologic Effects

The antiarrhythmic properties of phenytoin generally resemble those of lidocaine.

Cardiovascular and Hemodynamic Effects

Clinically useful doses of phenytoin produce little or no alteration in left ventricular function.

Indications, Contraindications, and Objectives

Phenytoin is rarely used as an antiarrhythmic agent in adults, with the possible exception of the treatment of arrhythmias secondary to digitalis toxicity. It is more often used in children with ventricular arrhythmias.

Complications

Central nervous system effects (nystagmus, ataxia, drowsiness) are the most common manifestations of phenytoin toxicity and are directly related to increases in plasma drug concentration. Gastrointestinal symptoms (nausea, dyspepsia, anorexia) are also relatively common.

A large number of drugs may affect the plasma concentration of phenytoin. For example, drugs such as isoniazid, chloramphenicol, and phenothiazines, which compete with phenytoin for hepatic enzymes, may increase phenytoin levels. The enzyme system that metabolizes phenytoin becomes saturated at plasma concentrations within the therapeutic range, resulting in an increasing half-life with increasing phenytoin load.

DRUGS WITH CLASS Ic MECHANISM OF ACTION

Flecainide

Pharmacokinetics

Flecainide has a long half-life of 16 to 20 hours after oral administration. It undergoes partial biotransformation to less active metabolites. Both parent and metabolites are renally eliminated.

Electrophysiologic Effects

The drug is a potent suppressant of V_{max} in Purkinje and myocardial fibers, causing marked slowing of conduction in all cardiac tissues in a use-dependent fashion. It shortens the duration of the action potential in Purkinje fibers but prolongs it in ventricular muscle. Prolongation of refractoriness is more marked in atrial tissues. Anterograde and retrograde refractoriness in accessory pathways can increase significantly. Automaticity is reduced by an elevation in threshold potential rather than by a decrease in the slope of phase 4 depolarization.

Flecainide causes a dose-dependent increase in PR and QRS intervals and QRS duration with minimal effect on QTc.

Cardiovascular and Hemodynamic Effects

Flecainide is negatively inotropic and can cause worsening of left ventricular function.

Indications, Contraindications, and Objectives

Like other class Ic agents, flecainide is effective in a wide variety of supraventricular and ventricular arrhythmias. It is a potent suppressant of ventricular ectopy. Flecainide increases mortality in patients with frequent premature ventricular contractions after myocardial infarction and is contraindicated in patients with coronary artery disease. Flecainide is highly effective in slowing conduction over accessory AV pathways. It is also effective in restoring and maintaining sinus rhythm in atrial fibrillation and flutter. Flecainide may be more effective than procainamide in acute termination of atrial fibrillation.[20]

Complications

The most common side effects include dizziness, blurred vision, headache, and nausea. Proarrhythmia occurs infrequently but is more common in patients with preexisting sustained VT or cardiac decompensation and with higher doses of the drug. The Cardiac Arrhythmia Suppression Trial (CAST) showed that in patients with frequent premature ventricular contractions after myocardial infarction, flecainide increased mortality by more than twofold compared with placebo.[21] Serious adverse effects occur in less than 2% of patients without structural heart disease treated for atrial arrhythmias. Flecainide may aggravate preexisting sinus or AV conduction disturbance. Pacing and defibrillation thresholds are increased by flecainide.

Flecainide increases serum concentrations of digoxin (by 15% to 25%) and propranolol (by 30%). Conversely, propranolol, quinidine, and amiodarone may increase flecainide serum concentrations.

Propafenone

Pharmacokinetics

Propafenone undergoes extensive first-pass transformation to a hydroxylated metabolite with reduced electrophysiologic effects. Bioavailability increases as the dose increases, and plasma concentration increases nonlinearly with dose. A 3-fold increase in dosage results in a 10-fold increase in plasma concentration, presumably as a result of saturation of hepatic metabolic mechanisms. There is marked variability of pharmacokinetics and pharmacodynamics between patients because of genetically determined differences in metabolism. About 93% of the population are extensive metabolizers and exhibit short elimination half-lives, low plasma concentrations of the parent compound, and high concentrations of metabolites. In poor metabolizers, propafenone causes a relatively greater β-adrenergic receptor–blocking effect.

Electrophysiologic Effects

Like flecainide, propafenone slows conduction in all cardiac tissues in a use-dependent manner. It also modestly prolongs the duration of the action potential in atrial and ventricular tissues, prolonging refractoriness. It decreases the slope of phase 4 depolarization in Purkinje fibers but has little effect on sinus node automaticity. The drug causes an increase in all electrocardiographic intervals, including PR, QRS, QT, and QTc intervals.

Cardiovascular and Hemodynamic Effects

Negative inotropism may worsen preexisting left ventricular dysfunction and congestive heart failure.

Indications, Contraindications, and Objectives

Like flecainide, propafenone is a "broad-spectrum" antiarrhythmic agent that is effective in a wide variety of arrhythmias. It has been used effectively in children. Propafenone increases the pacing threshold but not the defibrillation threshold. It is less effective than implantable defibrillators after cardiac arrest.[22] The drug has been combined effectively with mexiletine in the treatment of sustained VT.[23] Because of similarity with flecainide, it should be used cautiously in patients who have had a myocardial infarction or who have heart failure. Propafenone is safe and effective in restoring sinus rhythm and preventing recurrences of atrial fibrillation in patients without significant heart disease. Single-dose oral propafenone has a high cardioversion rate when it is used within 48 hours of onset of atrial fibrillation, making the drug, along with flecainide, suitable for the so-called pill-in-the-pocket approach.[24]

Complications

Propafenone is usually well tolerated, but it can cause nausea, weakness, dizziness, blurred vision, and a metallic taste in about 15% of patients. Exacerbation of bronchospasm may occur as a result of its beta-blocking actions. The incidence of proarrhythmia with propafenone is probably comparable to that with flecainide. Both flecainide and propafenone can convert atrial fibrillation into slow atrial flutter with 1:1 conduction to the ventricle, leading to an increase in the ventricular rate; therefore, both drugs should be used in combination with an AV node–blocking agent in this setting.

Moricizine

Moricizine hydrochloride is a phenothiazine derivative used for ventricular tachyarrhythmias. It has class Ia, Ib, and Ic electrophysiologic properties.

Pharmacokinetics

Moricizine undergoes extensive first-pass metabolism after oral ingestion, resulting in a bioavailability of 35% to 40%. The drug is 95% bound to α_1-acid glycoprotein and albumin. The concentrations of pharmacologically active metabolites, of which there are at least two, are small. Excretion is by the fecal route (slightly more than 50%) and the renal route (slightly less than 50%).

Electrophysiologic Effects

Moricizine blocks the fast inward sodium channel predominantly in the inactivated state, with a resultant decrease in V_{max}, the amplitude and duration of the action potential. The drug also blocks the slow calcium channel and I_K and prolongs AV nodal and His-Purkinje conduction time and QRS duration. Sinus node automaticity is not affected. Moricizine raises the defibrillation threshold minimally.

Cardiovascular and Hemodynamic Effects

Moricizine has minimal negative inotropic effects.

Indications, Contraindications, and Objectives

Moricizine suppresses ventricular ectopy and nonsustained VT in 60% to 80% of patients in both short- and long-term studies. It was as effective for the suppression of ventricular arrhythmias as quinidine and more effective than propranolol or disopyramide.[25] Results from CAST II suggest that moricizine should not be given to post–myocardial infarction patients with left ventricular dysfunction and asymptomatic ventricular ectopy. Moricizine was found to increase mortality in this context during initial but not long-term therapy.[26]

Complications

Moricizine is usually well tolerated. Central nervous system effects (tremor, headache, vertigo, nystagmus, and dizziness) or gastrointestinal side effects (nausea, vomiting, and diarrhea) may occur. Proarrhythmia occurs in 3% to 15% of patients, especially in older patients and those with severe ventricular arrhythmias.

Summary of Drugs with Class I Mechanism of Action

Agents with class Ia or Ic action are effective in treating a wide variety of supraventricular tachyarrhythmias. Despite their efficacy against ventricular arrhythmias, drugs with class I action are ineffective at reducing mortality and are likely to increase mortality with sustained VT or cardiac arrest. Although treatment in individual patients may prevent VT or VF, class I action drugs should be used with reservation or not at all for this purpose. Individual and meta-analytic studies strongly indicate that suppression of premature ventricular contractions and nonsustained VT by class I action agents can be associated with unacceptably high mortality (Fig. 50.3). However, class I antiarrhythmic drugs may be used as adjunctive therapy to prevent frequent recurrences of ventricular tachyarrhythmia in patients with an implantable defibrillator, especially if amiodarone is ineffective or was not tolerated.[27]

DRUGS WITH CLASS II MECHANISM OF ACTION

Propranolol and Other Beta Blockers

Examples of other beta blockers are acebutolol, atenolol, bisoprolol, carvedilol, metoprolol, nadolol, oxprenolol, timolol, and xamoterol.

The antiarrhythmic actions of beta blockers are considered to be a "class effect." Most of the discussion here concentrates on propranolol as a prototypical beta blocker.

Pharmacokinetics

Many different beta-blocking agents are available for clinical use. A description of the individual pharmacokinetic profiles is beyond the scope of this chapter.

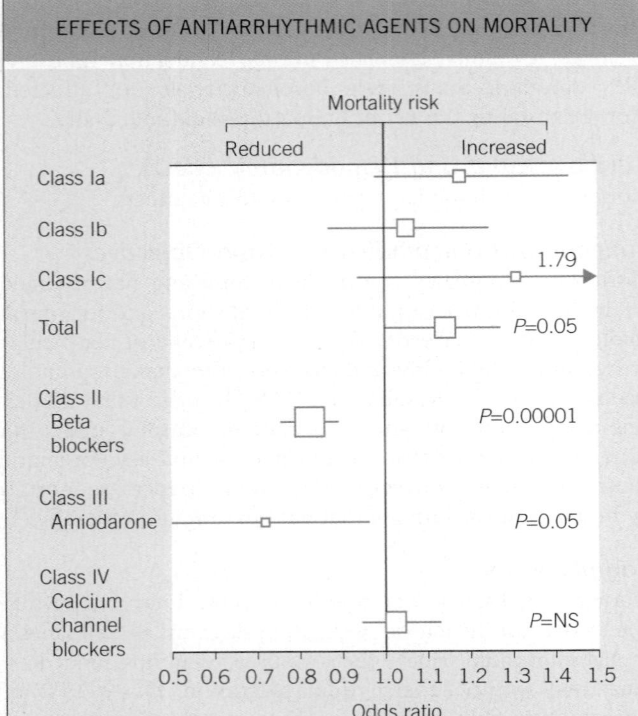

Figure 50.3 Effects of antiarrhythmic agents on mortality. Typical odds ratio by classes and subclasses. The areas of the squares are proportional to the variance for each trial or group of trials; the bars indicate 95% confidence interval. Portions to the left of the vertical line indicate reduced risk with treatment; portions to the right of the vertical line indicate increased risk with treatment. Note that in the trials of class I agents, there was an overall increased risk (with excesses observed in classes Ia, Ib, and Ic). The use of classes II and III significantly reduced risk; with class IV, there was a nonsignificant trend toward excess risk. In the total for the class I drugs, data from a small trial of three class I agents (quinidine, disopyramide, and mexiletine), which were excluded from data for the individual subclasses, have been included. (From Teo KK, Yusuf S, Furberg CD. Effects of prophylactic antiarrhythmic drug therapy in acute myocardial infarction. An overview of results from randomized controlled trials. JAMA 1993;270:1589-1595. ©1993, American Medical Association.)

Electrophysiologic Effects

Propranolol exerts its major antiarrhythmic effect through competitive inhibition of β-adrenoceptors, which also results in a relative prominence of vagal effects on the heart. Although the drug also possesses local anesthetic (membrane-stabilizing) action, this does not contribute to its role as an antiarrhythmic agent in therapeutic doses. The drug also reduces the amplitude of digitalis-induced delayed after-depolarizations and suppresses triggered activity in Purkinje fibers. Propranolol decreases the slope of phase 4 depolarization of the sinus node, resulting in sinus bradycardia. The PR interval lengthens, but not refractoriness and conduction in the normal His-Purkinje system. There is no effect on the QRS complex. With sympathetic stimulation, propranolol limits or prevents β-adrenergic–mediated shortening of action potential duration and refractoriness and increased automaticity.

Indications, Contraindications, and Objectives

All antiarrhythmic effects (class I, class III) are antagonized by catecholamine or sympathetic neural stimulation.[28] As a result, the addition of a beta blocker to most antiarrhythmic regimens is generally desirable. When catecholamine excess is responsible for generating autonomous ectopic rhythm disturbances (e.g., pheochromocytoma, exercise-induced VT), propranolol is useful in abolishing the arrhythmia. Beta blockers may be more effective than placebo in preventing recurrences of paroxysmal atrial fibrillation. Beta blockers are more effective than digoxin in controlling ventricular rate in atrial fibrillation or flutter. They are especially useful in preventing and controlling the rate of atrial fibrillation or atrial flutter after cardiac surgery.[29]

Propranolol may slow or terminate AV node or AV re-entry and may be used prophylactically to prevent a recurrence. It is also useful for treating inappropriate sinus tachycardia.

Combining a beta blocker with digoxin, quinidine, or a variety of other agents with class I or class III action may be effective when the first drug has failed (Fig. 50.4).[30] Metoprolol and esmolol may be useful in patients with multifocal atrial tachycardia.

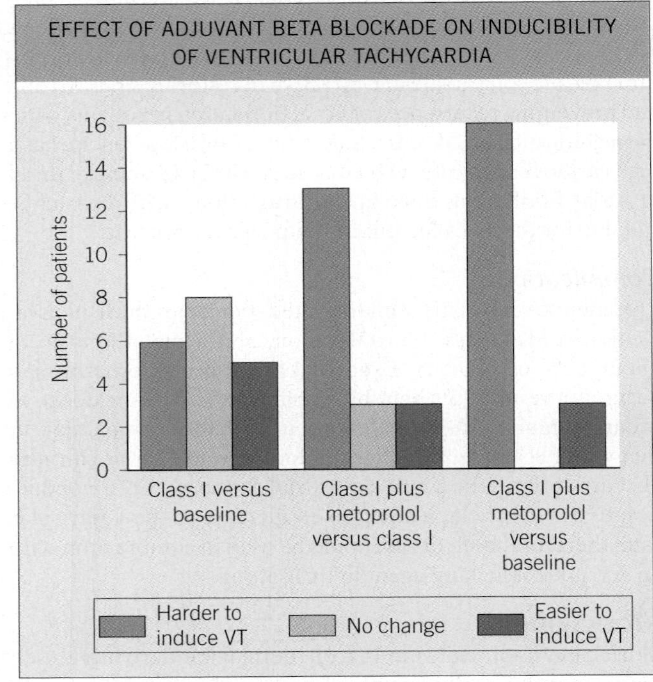

Figure 50.4 Effect of adjuvant beta blockade on inducibility of ventricular tachycardia. Nineteen patients with clinical ventricular tachycardia (VT) and baseline inducible sustained monomorphic VT were evaluated. Compared with baseline, therapy with class I drugs (quinidine, procainamide, mexiletine, tocainide, flecainide, propafenone, or a combination of these agents) made six patients more difficult to induce, caused no change in eight patients, and made five patients easier to induce. Addition of metoprolol to class I drug therapy resulted in 68% of the patients being more difficult to induce compared with class I drug therapy alone and 84% of the patients being more difficult to induce compared with the baseline state ($P < .05$). Eight patients (42%) became noninducible with the addition of metoprolol to class I drug therapy. (Modified from Brodsky MA, Chough SP, Allen BJ, et al. Adjuvant metoprolol improves efficacy of class I antiarrhythmic drugs in patients with inducible sustained monomorphic ventricular tachycardia. Am Heart J 1992;124:629-635.)

Propranolol may be effective for digitalis-induced arrhythmias, such as atrial tachycardia, nonparoxysmal AV junctional tachycardia, and VT. It is also useful in preventing ventricular arrhythmias associated with the most common form of familial prolonged QT syndrome.

Although beta blockers are not potent suppressants of premature ventricular contractions, they have been shown to reduce sudden death after myocardial infarction.[18] This may be due to a direct antiarrhythmic effect or an indirect anti-ischemic effect of chronic β-adrenoceptor blockade, or both. In patients with symptomatic heart failure, beta blockade decreases mortality, at least in part through a reduction in the risk of sudden death.

Complications and Hemodynamic Effects

The adverse cardiac effects of β-adrenergic blockers are generally predictable, the most important being left ventricular failure, hypotension, sinus bradycardia, and, rarely, AV block.

Summary of Drugs with Class II Mechanism of Action

Most antiarrhythmic agents may be combined with a beta blocker because antiarrhythmic effects are antagonized by catecholamine or sympathetic neural stimulation. Beta blockers are the only drugs that have been unequivocally shown to reduce cardiac and sudden death mortality in a variety of patient populations (see Fig. 50.3). Unless beta blockers are contraindicated, all patients at risk of serious ventricular arrhythmias, especially if they have left ventricular dysfunction, should receive beta-blocker therapy.

DRUGS WITH CLASS III MECHANISM OF ACTION

Amiodarone

Amiodarone is a complex and incompletely understood drug originally introduced as an antianginal agent.

Pharmacokinetics

Amiodarone is slowly, variably, and incompletely absorbed after oral administration. It has a very large steady-state volume of distribution due to its extensive uptake by tissues, especially fatty tissues. The drug is extensively (>96%) bound to albumin and α_1-acid glycoprotein, and it has a half-life of 60 days or longer after long-term administration. The drug is extensively de-ethylated in the liver to *N*-desethylamiodarone, which has significant electrophysiologic effects.

Full clinical effects may not be achieved for up to 6 weeks after initiation of treatment, with a slower onset for some effects (e.g., increases in refractoriness) than for others (e.g., slowing of AV nodal conduction). Loading doses are almost always recommended when oral amiodarone is prescribed because of the large volume of distribution (see Table 50.2).

Electrophysiologic Effects

Amiodarone has complex effects and possesses class I, II, III, and IV actions. The electrophysiologic and electrocardiographic effects associated with short-term intravenous administration of amiodarone differ from those with long-term oral therapy, yet both methods of administration produce defined and potent antiarrhythmic actions in patients. In general, the predominant electrophysiologic effects of intravenous amiodarone occur in sinus and AV nodal tissue. Intravenous amiodarone slows heart rate and increases sinus node recovery times; the PR interval, the AH interval, and the AV nodal effective refractory period are prolonged with little effect on the HV interval. It also has a profound antiadrenergic action that differs from that seen during long-term oral therapy.

Intravenous amiodarone also demonstrates heart rate–dependent effects that suggest class I (sodium channel–blocking) activity at rapid stimulation frequencies, although the sodium channel–blocking effects are modest compared with the antiadrenergic effects. Some studies show modest action potential and refractory period prolongation after intravenous use. Experiments showing a decrease in the slope of diastolic depolarization and a decrease in the sinus action potential amplitude are consistent with an effect on slow (calcium) channel conductance.

The dominant effect of oral amiodarone is probably through prolongation of the duration of the action potential and of refractoriness of all cardiac fibers, which increases progressively over time; this effect is mediated by block of multiple potassium currents. Amiodarone slows conduction at fast rates more than at slow rates (use dependence), not only by depressing V_{max} but also by increasing resistance to passive current flow. It does not prolong repolarization more at slow rates than at fast rates (i.e., it does not exhibit reverse rate dependence), but it does exert time-dependent effects on refractoriness.

The high iodine content of amiodarone exerts an antithyroid action, which may in itself have antiarrhythmic effects.

Oral amiodarone also has weak, noncompetitive β-adrenergic–blocking properties and blocks inward calcium current.

N-Desethylamiodarone has class I and class III activity and probably contributes significantly to antiarrhythmic efficacy. The delay before adequate concentrations of this metabolite are built up may explain in part the delay in the antiarrhythmic action of amiodarone.

Amiodarone causes an increase in the QT interval and smaller increases in the PR and QRS intervals. It slows the sinus rate by 20% to 30% and can slow the rate of monomorphic tachycardia to a similar extent. Defibrillation thresholds may be increased by oral amiodarone.

Cardiovascular and Hemodynamic Effects

The drug is a peripheral and coronary vasodilator and an effective antianginal agent. Although it has modest negative inotropic properties, it rarely causes clinically evident hemodynamic impairment, even in patients with severe left ventricular dysfunction.

Indications, Contraindications, and Objectives

In patients with frequent episodes of sustained VT or VF (electrical storm), intravenous amiodarone is effective and has relatively few adverse effects. In patients who had out-of-hospital cardiac arrest due to refractory ventricular arrhythmias, treatment with intravenous amiodarone as an adjunct to advanced cardiac life support measures led to significantly improved survival to hospitalization compared with placebo (ARREST study).[31] Compared with lidocaine, intravenous amiodarone resulted in substantially higher rates of survival to hospital admission in patients with shock-resistant out-of-hospital VF (ALIVE study).[17] On the basis of this and other investigations, intravenous amiodarone is now among the first-line drugs in the Guidelines 2006 for Cardiopulmonary Resuscitation and Emergency Cardiovascular Care as an agent to be considered for hemodynamically stable monomorphic VT, prolonged polymorphic VT without QT prolongation, and VF or pulseless VT.

Oral amiodarone can be used in the treatment of virtually any clinical tachyarrhythmia. It has been used

- to control a wide spectrum of supraventricular tachyarrhythmias, including recurrent paroxysmal supraventricular tachycardias;
- to slow the ventricular response in atrial fibrillation and flutter;
- to maintain sinus rhythm after chemical or electrical conversion; and
- to prevent recurrence of VT.

Amiodarone is effective in the conversion of chronic and recent-onset atrial fibrillation and orally or intravenously for atrial fibrillation after cardiac surgery. For acute conversion of atrial fibrillation (within 24 hours), amiodarone is similarly effective to flecainide, quinidine, racemic sotalol, and propafenone. It was more effective than sotalol or propafenone for the prevention of recurrences of atrial fibrillation during long-term use (CTAF and SAFE-T trials).[32,33] Most studies suggest a moderate reduction of atrial fibrillation episodes after coronary artery bypass surgery or valve surgery by perioperative oral amiodarone.[34,35]

The drug exerts a powerful suppressant effect on premature ventricular contractions and nonsustained VT and provides control in 60% to 80% of recurrent sustained VT and VF when continuous oral therapy with conventional drugs has failed.[36] Amiodarone is also safe and effective in controlling refractory tachyarrhythmias in infants. In the OPTIC trial, amiodarone, when used in combination with a beta blocker, was more effective than sotalol or other beta blockers alone in the reduction of recurrent ventricular tachyarrhythmia episodes in patients with an implantable defibrillator.[37]

The role of oral amiodarone in improving survival has been the subject of intense investigation. The CASCADE trial found that compared with standard antiarrhythmic agents, the use of amiodarone was associated with less cardiac mortality, cardiac arrest, or syncope in those resuscitated from out-of-hospital VF.[38] Several large primary prevention trials have examined its effect on life-threatening arrhythmias and mortality. Two key post–myocardial infarction trials, EMIAT[39] and CAMIAT,[40] demonstrated that amiodarone reduced arrhythmic but not overall mortality. The GESICA[41] and EPAMSA[42] trials showed survival benefit of amiodarone in heart failure, whereas CHF-STAT[43] did not. A subsequent meta-analysis of published randomized controlled trials in patients with recent myocardial infarction or congestive heart failure showed that amiodarone reduced the risk of arrhythmic or sudden death by 29%, resulting in an overall reduction of 13% in total mortality (Fig. 50.5).[44] Amiodarone appeared

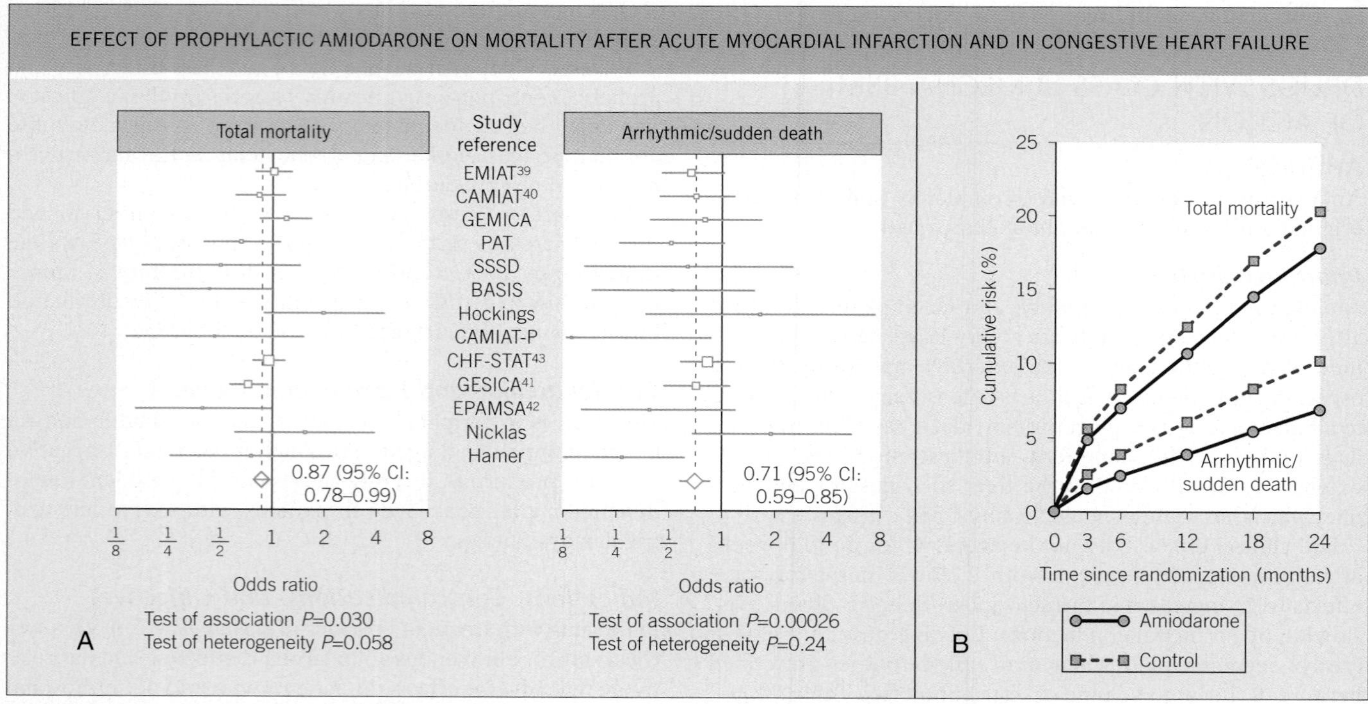

Figure 50.5 Effect of prophylactic amiodarone on mortality after acute myocardial infarction and in congestive heart failure. Results from 13 randomized controlled trials. **A,** Total mortality and arrhythmic or sudden death mortality. The areas of the squares are proportional to the amount of information; the lines represent 95% confidence interval. The combined results of the 13 trials show a statistically significant odds ratio for total mortality in favor of amiodarone (0.87; 95% CI, 0.78-0.99; $P = .03$), indicating a 13% relative reduction in risk. The odds ratios for individual studies show some variation, and the formal test of heterogeneity was of borderline statistical significance ($P = .058$). **B,** The effect of amiodarone treatment over time. The curves reflect the cumulative risk of death computed from pooled control and amiodarone-treated patients. Amiodarone continues to exert a beneficial effect over time. (From Amiodarone Trials Meta-Analysis Investigators. Effect of prophylactic amiodarone on mortality after acute myocardial infarction and in congestive heart failure: meta-analysis of individual data from 6500 patients in randomised trials. Lancet 1997;350:1417-1424. © The Lancet Ltd 1997).[44]

to be more effective when it was used in combination with a beta blocker. In the SCD-HeFT trial, however, amiodarone did not reduce mortality compared with placebo in patients with left ventricular dysfunction (ejection fraction <35%) and NYHA class II-III heart failure.[45]

To date, the evidence for survival benefit with amiodarone is insufficient to advise routine empiric use of the drug in patients who have mildly reduced left ventricular ejection fraction, asymptomatic ventricular arrhythmias after myocardial infarction, or hypertrophic cardiomyopathy. In a trial of post–myocardial infarction patients with nonsustained VT and a depressed ejection fraction (MADIT[46]), implantable cardioverter-defibrillators statistically improved survival compared with the antiarrhythmic drug arm, in which most patients were taking amiodarone. Three secondary prevention trials, AVID, CIDS, and CASH,[47] directly compared implantable cardioverter-defibrillator therapy with amiodarone in patients with sustained VT or VF and showed superior benefit of implantable cardioverter-defibrillators compared with empiric amiodarone in improving overall survival. The results of all these studies were somewhat confounded by the fact that many of the defibrillator patients received concomitant beta blockers throughout and sotalol or amiodarone during follow-up.

On the basis of these findings, amiodarone is safe to use in post–myocardial infarction and congestive heart failure patients who need antiarrhythmic therapy. Although amiodarone is probably the most effective of all the antiarrhythmic drugs in preventing sudden arrhythmic death, rarely causing serious proarrhythmia, high-risk patients should be considered for an implantable cardioverter-defibrillator as frontline therapy.

Complications

Amiodarone has a very wide spectrum of toxic effects. In case series, adverse effects are reported by about 75% of patients treated with amiodarone for 5 years; these adverse effects necessitate stopping of the drug in 18% to 37%. However, serious adverse effects leading to discontinuation occur less frequently in placebo-controlled trials, being about 15% at 2 years in excess of placebo discontinuation rates. Adverse effects become more frequent when therapy is continued long term, but most are reversible with dose reduction or cessation of treatment.

Some of the more common effects include gastrointestinal intolerance, weight loss, corneal microdeposits (invariable) with disturbance of night vision (occasional), photosensitivity, and blue-gray facial discoloration. During acute loading, central nervous system symptoms such as tremor, ataxia, fatigue, insomnia, and vivid dreams may occur; these may also develop slowly and appear late after initiation of therapy. During long-term treatment, an insidious peripheral neuropathy may develop in approximately 1% of patients.

Although asymptomatic elevations of hepatic enzymes are commonly observed, liver toxicity necessitating cessation of amiodarone is rare. The drug does not have to be stopped unless liver enzymes exceed two or three times normal in a patient who had normal values before starting treatment with amiodarone.

Alterations in levels of thyroid-stimulating hormone or thyroid hormone are found in up to 30% of patients taking amiodarone, but symptomatic hypothyroidism is not common (2% to 4%) and hyperthyroidism is even less so (1% to 2%). These complications are not dose related. Amiodarone blocks the peripheral conversion of thyroxine (T_4) to triiodothyronine (T_3), resulting in a slight increase in T_4, reverse-T_3, and thyroid-stimulating hormone and in a slight decrease in T_3. No therapy is required for mild elevations of thyroid-stimulating hormone (<20 mIU/mL). If overt hypothyroidism develops, amiodarone therapy may be continued if it is clinically indicated, with concomitant thyroid hormone replacement. Amiodarone-induced hyperthyroidism is more difficult to treat and usually requires drug discontinuation as well as antithyroid medications.

The most dangerous side effect is pulmonary toxicity, reported in up to 5% to 10% of patients; it may occur at any time after therapy is begun. In blinded controlled studies, excess pulmonary toxicity over placebo is less frequent, approximately 1% per year,[44] supporting the fact that the diagnosis of amiodarone-induced pulmonary dysfunction is often obscured by congestive heart failure. Pulmonary toxicity may be fatal in 5% to 10% of patients.

Reported pulmonary complications have included phospholipidosis, alveolitis, and fibrosis. The mechanism is unclear but may involve direct cellular toxicity, phospholipidosis with disordered surfactant turnover and handling, immune (hypersensitivity) reaction, and oxidation or destabilization of the cell membrane. Dyspnea, nonproductive cough, and fever are common symptoms, whereas other patients may present with acute respiratory failure.

Clinical and laboratory findings include pulmonary crepitations, hypoxia, abnormality on gallium scan, and reduced diffusion capacity. The typical radiographic appearance involves diffuse bilateral pulmonary infiltrates, although alveolar patterns, interstitial patterns, and pleural effusions have also been noted. The drug must be discontinued if such pulmonary inflammatory changes occur. Corticosteroids can be tried, but no controlled studies have been performed to support their use.

The incidence of pulmonary toxicity increases with higher doses and increasing age; it is uncommon at maintenance doses of less than 300 mg daily. Recommended practices for screening and detection of pulmonary, hepatic, and thyroid adverse effects with amiodarone include careful clinical follow-up, annual chest radiography, and twice-yearly monitoring of aspartate aminotransferase and thyroid-stimulating hormone concentrations.

Another rare but potentially serious adverse event reported after amiodarone use is optic neuropathy (although a definite causal link has not been established), which can cause blindness.

Cardiac side effects include symptomatic bradycardia in approximately 2% of patients, which may be aggravated by the concurrent administration of beta blockers or calcium channel blockers. Drug-induced tachyarrhythmia is rare.

Important interactions with other drugs occur. Amiodarone interferes with cytochrome P450-mediated drug biotransformation. The dose of warfarin, phenytoin, digoxin, and many class I action antiarrhythmic drugs should be reduced by one third to one half when these drugs are given concomitantly with amiodarone, and plasma drug levels or other therapeutic indices (e.g., international normalized ratio for warfarin) should be monitored closely until a new steady state has been attained.

Sotalol

Sotalol is a competitive, nonspecific β-adrenoceptor blocker that also prolongs action potential duration and refractoriness in all cardiac tissues.

Pharmacokinetics

Sotalol is completely absorbed and has a half-life of about 12 hours after oral administration. It is largely eliminated by the kidneys, and doses need to be reduced substantially in patients with renal insufficiency.

Electrophysiologic Effects

The drug suppresses phase 4 spontaneous depolarization and may produce severe sinus bradycardia. It also slows AV nodal conduction. The duration and refractoriness of action potentials in atrial and ventricular myocardium are prolonged because of blockade of I_{Kr}. In most studies but not all, this class III effect is greater at slow rates and is reduced or absent at very rapid rates (reverse rate dependence). Both D- and L-isomers have similar effects on prolonging repolarization, whereas the L-isomer is responsible for virtually all the beta-blocking activity. Sotalol prolongs the QT interval.

Cardiovascular and Hemodynamic Effects

Worsening of left ventricular function can occur in patients with preexisting left ventricular enlargement and congestive heart failure. Asymptomatic left ventricular dysfunction is not an absolute contraindication to its use.

Indications, Contraindications, and Objectives

The combination of β-adrenoceptor blockade and prolongation of the duration of the action potential may be especially effective in preventing sustained VT. Sotalol appears to be more effective than most class I antiarrhythmic drugs in treating ventricular tachyarrhythmias. It is superior to lidocaine for acute termination of sustained VT[16] and is useful in patients with arrhythmogenic right ventricular dysplasia.[48] It reduces defibrillation energy requirements[49]; in patients with implanted cardioverter-defibrillators, the combined endpoint of time to therapy for VT or VF or death is significantly prolonged over placebo, although it is less effective than amiodarone and only slightly better than other beta blockers.[37,50] After acute myocardial infarction, sotalol reduces mortality, although not significantly and not to a greater degree than beta blockers that do not have direct antiarrhythmic effect.

In the Electrophysiologic Study versus Electrocardiographic Monitoring (ESVEM) trial, which involved patients who had sustained VT or VF, sotalol was superior to six agents with class I action, individually and collectively, with respect to total mortality, sudden death, cardiac death, and especially VT recurrence.[51]

Sotalol is also useful in a wide variety of supraventricular tachycardias, including atrial fibrillation and flutter, atrial tachycardia, AV nodal re-entry, and AV re-entry. It slows the ventricular rate in the event of arrhythmia recurrence as a result of its beta-blocking effect. It is effective in preventing atrial fibrillation after coronary surgery.[52]

Complications

Adverse effects commonly seen with other beta blockers (e.g., fatigue and dizziness, insomnia) occur with sotalol. Drug-induced polymorphic VT (torsades de pointes) develops with excessive QT prolongation, especially if hypokalemia is present. This proarrhythmia is dose dependent and is more common in women, in patients with renal dysfunction, and in patients who have structural heart disease.

Bretylium

Bretylium is a drug with class III activity formerly available for intravenous use. It is no longer available.

Ibutilide

Ibutilide is available only as an intravenous agent, specifically for the acute termination of atrial fibrillation and flutter.

Pharmacokinetics

Ibutilide is rapidly distributed to a very large volume, so that its electrophysiologic effects dissipate rapidly after initial intravenous administration. The drug undergoes extensive metabolism in the liver, first using an oxidation reaction and then a hydroxylation reaction. Its metabolites are not thought to add significantly to its electrophysiologic effects.

Electrophysiologic Effects

Ibutilide increases the slow inward movement of sodium during the plateau phase, thus prolonging the duration of the action potential and the QT interval. Although this is the predominant theory, evidence indicates that the drug also blocks I_{Kr}. Because ibutilide is rapidly distributed, the effect on the QT interval is transient. The risk of ventricular proarrhythmia is greatest within the first hour of the initial drug infusion. Ibutilide significantly reduces atrial and ventricular defibrillation energy requirements.

Cardiovascular and Hemodynamic Effects

Ibutilide does not have a negative hemodynamic effect and does not precipitate congestive heart failure. It also does not affect other parameters of cardiovascular performance, such as peripheral vascular resistance, arterial pressure, or left ventricular end-diastolic pressure.

Indications, Contraindications, and Objectives

Ibutilide is useful for the rapid conversion of recent-onset atrial fibrillation and flutter to sinus rhythm. Pretreatment with ibutilide enhances the efficacy of transthoracic electrical cardioversion of atrial fibrillation.[53]

Complications

Ibutilide does not undergo any pharmacokinetic interactions with other frequently used cardiac drugs, such as beta blockers, calcium channel blockers, warfarin, and diuretics. Slowing of the heart rate is likely to increase the incidence of torsades de pointes. Ibutilide has an additive effect on the QT interval when it is used in patients with hypokalemia or when it is combined with other drugs that cause QT prolongation. The incidence of torsades de pointes in patients treated with ibutilide in clinical trials is 4% to 5% and may be lower in patients who have good left ventricular function and higher heart rates.[54]

Dofetilide

Dofetilide was approved for general use in late 1999. It represents the first orally administered drug with relatively pure class III antiarrhythmic properties to be widely released.

Pharmacokinetics

Orally administered dofetilide is well absorbed and has a bioavailability of more than 90%. Maximal plasma concentrations occur about 2 hours after oral dosing, and the drug's elimination half-life from plasma is 8 to 10 hours. Approximately 70% to 80% of the drug is excreted unchanged through the kidneys; the remainder is metabolized in the liver to inactive metabolites. Total dofetilide clearance in patients without severe renal insufficiency is proportional to creatinine clearance. The dose of dofetilide should be adjusted for renal function and QT response to therapy. Despite its hepatic metabolism, dofetilide does not appear to interact with digoxin, propranolol, or warfarin. Cimetidine prolongs the half-life of dofetilide by inhibiting renal tubular dofetilide secretion, whereas ranitidine does not. Verapamil increases peak plasma concentrations after oral ingestion, primarily by increasing intestinal blood flow. Ketoconazole decreases the nonrenal clearance of dofetilide, an interaction that may become significant in patients with renal dysfunction.

Electrophysiologic Effects

Dofetilide blocks the I_{Kr} repolarizing current in all myocardial tissues with high potency. The drug prolongs the duration of the action potential in both the atria and the ventricles, thus leading to a dose-dependent increase in refractory periods and QT interval. No changes have been observed in the RR, PR, AH, or HV intervals or in sinus node function. Dofetilide block of I_{Kr} increases as extracellular potassium concentration is reduced. Thus, correction of hypokalemia is of crucial importance in treating QT prolongation and torsades de pointes caused by I_{Kr} blockade. The drug exhibits reverse rate dependence, with rate-related reductions in its capacity to prolong action potential duration and effective refractory period. Dofetilide lowers defibrillation energy requirements.

Cardiovascular and Hemodynamic Effects

The drug is well tolerated. Cardiovascular side effects appear to be virtually absent, even in patients with impaired left ventricular function.

Indications, Contraindications, and Objectives

Dofetilide is effective in the conversion and maintenance of sinus rhythm in patients who have atrial fibrillation or flutter. Intravenous dofetilide was more effective than amiodarone in restoring sinus rhythm in patients with atrial fibrillation or flutter, although a significant incidence (8%) of torsades de pointes was noted.[55]

The effect of dofetilide on mortality and morbidity was studied in the Danish Investigators of Arrhythmia and Mortality on Dofetilide (DIAMOND) trials. This involved high-risk patients with either congestive heart failure (DIAMOND-CHF)[56] or recent myocardial infarction (DIAMOND-MI).[57] These trials showed a neutral effect on mortality, a relatively low incidence of torsades de pointes, and a beneficial effect in maintaining sinus rhythm in patients with atrial fibrillation and those developing arrhythmia during follow-up. This contrasts with the results of the SWORD study,[58] in which there was increased total mortality in patients who had had a myocardial infarction and who were treated with D-sotalol. In one study, dofetilide was better tolerated than sotalol and was equally effective in the prevention of VT inducibility.[59] The initial dosage of dofetilide should be based on the patient's creatinine clearance (Table 50.4) and should be conducted during in-hospital electrocardiographic monitoring. The QTc should be checked 2 to 3 hours after each dose. If the change in QTc is 15% or more or if the QTc is more than 500 ms, reduction in dose is recommended. All patients should be monitored in the hospital for 3 days during drug initiation.

DOSAGE OF DOFETILIDE ADJUSTED FOR CREATININE CLEARANCE

Creatinine Clearance (mL/min)	Dofetilide Dose: Initial	Dofetilide Dose: Adjustment for QTc ≥15% or QTc >500 ms
>60	500 μg bid	250 μg bid
40-60	250 μg bid	125 μg bid
20-39	125 μg bid	125 μg daily
<20	Not recommended	—

Table 50.4 Dosage of dofetilide adjusted for creatinine clearance.

Complications

In placebo-controlled trials, the incidence of noncardiac adverse events in patients receiving dofetilide (e.g., headache, muscle cramps) has been similar to that in the placebo groups. The major cardiovascular adverse events have been directly related to the electrophysiologic properties of the drug: QT prolongation and torsades de pointes. The overall incidence of torsades de pointes in both oral and intravenous studies of dofetilide has generally been less than 3%, with a substantially lower incidence reported after adjustment of dosage for creatinine clearance and QTc.

Investigational Drugs

Azimilide

Azimilide is a novel antiarrhythmic agent that blocks both the rapidly activating (I_{Kr}) and slowly activating (I_{Ks}) components of the delayed rectifier cardiac potassium current. Many existing and experimental potassium channel blockers (e.g., sotalol, dofetilide, E-4031) are derivatives of methanesulfonamide and block only I_{Kr}. In contrast, azimilide, a chlorophenylfuranyl compound, has the unique ability to block both I_{Kr} and I_{Ks}. The clinical importance of this multiple potassium channel blockade is not known. However, I_{Ks} has been implicated in the repolarization process at higher (tachycardic) heart rates, under sympathetic stimulation, and with increased stretch. Thus, under conditions of tachycardia and β-adrenergic stimulation, when conventional I_{Kr} blockers lose their efficacy, azimilide has the potential to be effective.

Pharmacokinetics
Azimilide pharmacokinetics are very predictable. The oral drug is completely absorbed, with peak plasma levels occurring 5 to 7 hours after ingestion. Steady-state azimilide levels have been rapidly attained with use of a well-tolerated 3-day loading-dose regimen. The drug has a long terminal half-life of 4 days, which permits once-daily dosing and significantly limits major fluctuations in blood levels. The bulk of drug clearance is through hepatic metabolism, with about 10% renal metabolism. Only one of the metabolites has any class III activity. Clinical data suggest that dose adjustments are not required for differences in age, sex, hepatic or renal function, or concomitant use of digoxin or warfarin.

Electrophysiologic Effects
Azimilide produces a concentration-dependent inhibition, with similar potency, of both I_{Kr} and I_{Ks} in isolated human atrial and ventricular myocytes. It increases the duration of the action potential and of the effective refractory period in isolated cardiac tissues and myocytes. In intact animal models, the drug suppresses both atrial and ventricular arrhythmias. Azimilide causes QT prolongation in a dose-dependent manner but has no significant effect on the PR or QRS intervals. Its in vivo effects appear to be rate independent and are maintained under ischemic or hypoxic conditions. Reduced reverse rate dependence may make azimilide less likely to be associated with polymorphic VT (torsades de pointes) than other specific I_{Kr} blockers are.

Cardiovascular and Hemodynamic Effects
Azimilide appears to be well tolerated, producing no clinically significant changes in heart rate or blood pressure.

Current Clinical Status
The safety and efficacy of azimilide in prolonging the time to recurrence of atrial fibrillation or atrial flutter and paroxysmal supraventricular tachycardia were evaluated in the three trials of the Azimilide Supraventricular Arrhythmia Program (SVA-3). Results showed a dose-dependent prolongation of time to first recurrence.[60] In the SVA-4 trial, however, 125 mg daily of azimilide did not significantly increase the time to recurrent supraventricular tachycardia.[61] The Azimilide Postinfarction Survival Evaluation (ALIVE) study showed identical mortality in the placebo and azimilide-treated groups in high-risk patients (those with depressed ejection fraction) after a recent myocardial infarction.[62] The randomized controlled SHIELD trial showed that azimilide significantly reduced VT and VF events requiring shock or antitachycardia pacing in patients with an implantable defibrillator.[63] Azimilide is not currently approved for use by regulatory authorities.

Complications
Both oral and intravenous azimilide appear to be well tolerated, even in patients who have structural heart disease. The incidence of serious adverse events, including torsades de pointes, is low (<1%). An early (within 6 months) reversible neutropenia may rarely occur.

Dronedarone
Dronedarone is an investigational agent, structurally related to amiodarone, with multiple electrophysiologic actions. Like amiodarone, it possesses all four Vaughan Williams class effects, with a predominantly class III effect. Its main advantage over amiodarone is that it lacks the iodine moiety of amiodarone, and it is expected that it will have a better side effect profile.

Dronedarone has antiadrenergic effects and has been shown to prolong atrial and ventricular refractory periods, AV node conduction, and the paced QRS complex. It has also been shown to decrease ischemia-induced ventricular arrhythmias in animal models. Most of the clinical studies with dronedarone assessed its efficacy in the treatment of atrial fibrillation. The identical ADONIS and EURIDIS trials were reported together.[64] In those trials, dronedarone increased the time to first recurrence of symptomatic atrial fibrillation and reduced the ventricular rate during atrial fibrillation compared with placebo. Dronedarone was well tolerated, and there was no difference in any of the potential side effects compared with placebo with the exception of a higher incidence of elevated serum creatinine levels in the dronedarone group.

However, a study of high-risk patients with congestive heart failure and ventricular dysfunction (ANDROMEDA) was prematurely terminated because of increased mortality in the dronedarone treatment group compared with placebo.

Dronedarone has not been approved by regulatory authorities.

Vernakalant
Vernakalant (RSD1235) is a mixed frequency-dependent Na^+ and atria-preferential K^+ channel blocker (I_{to} and I_{Kur}). It was specifically designed for the treatment of atrial fibrillation. In several studies, RSD1235 has been shown to selectively prolong atrial refractory periods without significant effects on ventricular refractoriness or QT intervals, thus potentially reducing the risk of torsades.[65] In clinical studies, intravenous vernakalant was more effective than placebo in the cardioversion of recent-onset atrial fibrillation or atrial flutter.[66] Among the adverse events, neurologic side effect, especially dysgeusia, was common. Vernakalant has not been approved yet by the Food and Drug Administration.

Summary of Drugs with Class III Mechanism of Action
Complex class III action agents such as amiodarone and sotalol are extremely effective in the treatment of recurrent sustained VT and VF. The side effect profile of these agents has led to the search for agents with simpler ion channel–blocking properties. However, the isolated block of I_{Kr} has been found to have either a neutral effect (e.g., dofetilide) or a deleterious effect (e.g., D-sotalol) on mortality in patients after myocardial infarction. On the other hand, such agents have been shown to exert beneficial antifibrillatory effects in patients with atrial fibrillation and may have a role after cardiac surgery. Drugs that block more than one ion channel, such as azimilide and dronedarone, are under active study.

DRUGS WITH CLASS IV MECHANISM OF ACTION

Verapamil and Diltiazem

Pharmacokinetics

Verapamil and diltiazem are described in greater detail in Chapter 45.

Electrophysiologic Effects

Verapamil and diltiazem block the inward current carried by calcium and exert their main antiarrhythmic action by slowing AV nodal conduction and by prolonging its effective refractory period. They slow the ventricular response to atrial fibrillation. Phase 0 of the action potential is not altered, and neither is the duration of the action potential. The slope of phase 4 depolarization is decreased, and the heart rate is slightly reduced. The PR interval may increase, but QRS duration and the QT interval are unaltered.

Cardiovascular and Hemodynamic Effects

Verapamil and, to a lesser extent, diltiazem have negative inotropic properties and may worsen left ventricular dysfunction. The drugs also cause peripheral vasodilatation with a resultant fall in blood pressure.

Indications, Contraindications, and Objectives

Verapamil and diltiazem can prevent AV node or AV re-entry. They slow the ventricular response over the AV node during atrial fibrillation or flutter but are not effective in establishing and maintaining sinus rhythm. Verapamil is not effective for VT, although it may suppress some forms of idiopathic VT without associated structural heart disease, such as left fascicular VT and right ventricular outflow tract VT. Verapamil and diltiazem could also be useful in patients with ventricular arrhythmias caused by coronary artery spasm.

Complications

Both verapamil and diltiazem cause bradycardia, and asystole has been reported, particularly if the drugs are used in combination with a beta blocker. Side effects include gastrointestinal intolerance and constipation. Diltiazem may cause headache, flushing, and ankle swelling. Verapamil increases serum digoxin levels by decreasing its excretion by approximately 30%.

Intravenous verapamil may accelerate the ventricular response over the accessory pathway in patients with atrial fibrillation associated with the Wolff-Parkinson-White syndrome. This effect is due to reflex sympathetic stimulation as a result of peripheral vasodilatation and transient hypotension.

Summary of Drugs with Class IV Mechanism of Action

Verapamil and diltiazem are useful in the treatment of AV node and AV re-entry and for slowing the ventricular response to atrial fibrillation and flutter. They are also indicated for treatment of ventricular arrhythmias associated with coronary artery spasm.

OTHER DRUGS WITH ANTIARRHYTHMIC ACTION

Digoxin

Although it is described in detail in Chapter 72, some aspects of digoxin are worthy of consideration in the management of arrhythmias. Digoxin prolongs the effective refractory period and diminishes conduction velocity in Purkinje fibers while shortening the refractory period in atrial and ventricular myocardial cells. Prolongation of the effective refractory period of the AV node causes prolongation of the PR interval in the presence of sinus rhythm and permits digoxin to control the ventricular response rate in atrial fibrillation and flutter, its most important antiarrhythmic action.

There is no evidence that digoxin increases the likelihood of conversion to sinus rhythm in paroxysmal or persistent atrial fibrillation or that it prevents the recurrence of atrial fibrillation after cardioversion. It is relatively ineffective at reducing the ventricular rate in atrial fibrillation during exercise; but at rest, digoxin improves hemodynamics to a similar extent as intravenous diltiazem does.[67] Digoxin also increases vagal activity and thus slows the sinus rate.

If it is present in toxic serum concentrations, digoxin causes increased abnormal automaticity with resultant VT. This may be potentiated by hypokalemia. Arrhythmias caused by digoxin toxicity have traditionally been treated with lidocaine or phenytoin.

Adenosine

Adenosine is a naturally occurring substance that attaches to receptors in the AV and sinus nodes. Intravenously administered adenosine is inactivated in the blood within seconds and has a very short duration of action. At therapeutic doses, AV nodal conduction is markedly slowed or interrupted in a use-dependent fashion, producing transient AV block. This makes adenosine almost universally effective for re-entrant arrhythmias that use the AV node as a portion of the circuit. It is considered to be first-choice therapy for AV nodal and AV re-entrant arrhythmias. It can also be used to produce transient AV block during atrial flutter or fibrillation, thereby facilitating the diagnosis by exposing the atrial rhythm.

Adenosine may be useful in the differential diagnosis of wide QRS tachycardias because it terminates many supraventricular tachycardias or reveals the underlying atrial rhythm with generally no effect in VT. However, it can accelerate the ventricular response or precipitate VF in pre-excited atrial fibrillation.[68] In addition, adenosine can terminate some VTs, such as idiopathic right ventricular outflow VT.

Transient bradycardia, flushing, dyspnea, chest pressure, and slight hypotension may occur, although serious side effects are very rare. Acute asthmatic attacks can be precipitated in patients with asthma.

Magnesium

Although it is not directly antiarrhythmic in most models of arrhythmia, intravenous magnesium effectively abolishes polymorphic ventricular arrhythmias that occur in the context of QT prolongation (i.e., torsades de pointes VT caused by drugs). It interferes with calcium transfer across the cell membrane and within the cell, and at high doses, it reduces heart rate and slows AV nodal conduction and may slow intraventricular conduction. Despite promising evidence from in vitro studies and small trials, intravenous magnesium therapy did not reduce mortality in a large randomized study of patients with suspected acute myocardial infarction.[69]

ANTIARRHYTHMIC EFFECTS OF NON-ANTIARRHYTHMIC DRUGS

Although this subject is beyond the scope of this chapter, it is worth mentioning that several agents not considered to be antiarrhythmic drugs (i.e., they do not directly affect ion channels) appear to have direct antiarrhythmic effects. These include angiotensin-converting enzyme inhibitors and angiotensin receptor blockers, fish oil (omega-3 fatty acid), statins, and steroids, all of which demonstrated atrial antifibrillatory effect.[70]

The angiotensin-converting enzyme inhibitors and angiotensin receptor blockers reduce blood pressure, which itself has antifibrillatory effect in the atria, but their benefit in preventing atrial fibrillation goes beyond that. In the LIFE study,[71] for example, losartan and atenolol reduced blood pressure equally, yet losartan was better than atenolol in the prevention of atrial fibrillation. Irbesartan, in combination with amiodarone, was superior to amiodarone alone in preventing atrial fibrillation recurrence after cardioversion.[72]

There is observational evidence that statins reduce the risk for development of atrial fibrillation, possibly because of their anti-inflammatory effects. That hypothesis is supported by the evidence that low-dose glucocorticoid therapy, used in adjunction to propafenone in patients with persistent atrial fibrillation and normal left ventricular function, produced dramatic reduction in atrial fibrillation recurrence.[73]

Fish oil (which is rich in n-3 polyunsaturated fatty acids) is believed to have anti-inflammatory properties and antiarrhythmic effects. It has been shown to reduce the development of atrial fibrillation.[74]

ANTIARRHYTHMIC DRUG COMBINATIONS

Multiple antiarrhythmic effects, particularly prolongation of repolarization, β-adrenergic blockade, and modest prolongation of conduction, may be useful for an antiarrhythmic regimen. This is supported by the success of amiodarone, a compound that exhibits antiarrhythmic properties from all Vaughan Williams classes, in the prevention of sudden death.[44] Randomized clinical trials of device therapy versus pharmacotherapy have consistently used amiodarone as the drug of choice in prospective comparisons. In addition to increased drug efficacy, there would theoretically be decreased proarrhythmia if repolarization were not excessively prolonged at slow heart rates.

Interest in combining antiarrhythmic drugs has been prompted by the lack of efficacy of monotherapies and the toxicity resulting from high doses of individual agents. For most drugs, persistently inducible VT, even if it is slowed, is associated with a high rate of VT recurrence and sudden death.[75] Antiarrhythmic effectiveness may be obtained by combining antiarrhythmic drugs with complementary mechanisms of action to alter the ventricular tachyarrhythmia substrate. Combinations that have been investigated include class Ia with class Ib action,[76] class I with class II action,[77] and class I with class III action.[11,13,78] The best-studied combination of drugs with primarily class I mechanism of action is quinidine plus mexiletine, whose benefit is best correlated with enhanced prolongation of refractoriness over each drug alone (a class III effect).[76,79]

Sotalol, like amiodarone, also prolongs ventricular refractoriness, and the racemate (D,L-sotalol) has significant beta-blocking effects. However, reverse rate dependence can be a problem, with the promotion of proarrhythmia at slow heart rates (see earlier). A regimen consisting of sotalol, which prolongs ventricular repolarization and has beta-blocking properties, and quinidine or procainamide, which prolongs refractoriness and slows cardiac conduction modestly, has been shown to be useful in suppressing VT inducibility and recurrence of arrhythmia.[11] There were no incidences of proarrhythmia, particularly torsades de pointes, with this combination.[11] The absence of torsades de pointes may have been due to the low doses of sotalol and quinidine or procainamide used in the study, thereby minimizing the potential for toxicity of each individual drug. Moreover, it appeared that reverse rate dependence, as judged by an attenuation of refractory period prolongation with successive extrastimuli, a characteristic of sotalol alone, was attenuated by its combination with quinidine or procainamide (Fig. 50.6).[80]

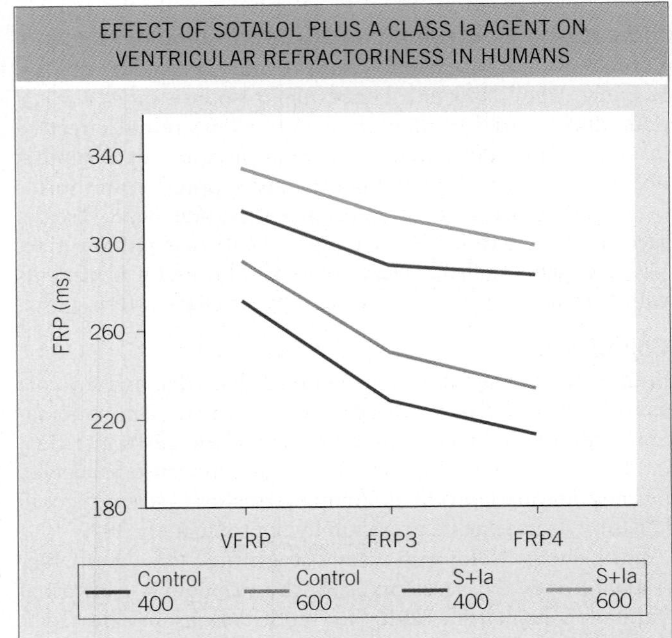

Figure 50.6 Effect of sotalol plus a class Ia agent on ventricular refractoriness in humans. Thirty-two patients with spontaneous sustained ventricular tachycardia were studied with programmed extrastimulation in the drug-free state and after treatment with sotalol and a class Ia agent (quinidine or procainamide). The curves show the ventricular functional refractory period (VFRP, which is the V_1 upstroke to the V_2 upstroke), the shortest interval for the V_2 to V_3 upstroke (FRP3), and the shortest interval for the V_3 to V_4 upstroke (FRP4) with no antiarrhythmic drug regimen and cycle lengths of 400 ms (control 400) and 600 ms (control 600) and during therapy with sotalol and a class Ia agent at cycle lengths of 400 ms (S + Ia 400) and 600 ms (S + Ia 600). Progressive shortening of FRP with repetitive extrastimuli, seen in the control groups, is attenuated with therapy. (From Lee SD, Newman D, Ham M, et al. Electrophysiologic mechanisms of antiarrhythmic efficacy of a sotalol and class Ia drug combination: elimination of reverse use dependence. J Am Coll Cardiol 1997;29:100-105. Reprinted with permission from the American College of Cardiology.)

Interactions between drug effect and autonomic state may alter potassium currents and promote reverse rate dependence. Adrenergic stimulation can shorten the duration of the action potential by

- increasing the heart rate;
- enhancing repolarizing currents, such as the transient outward potassium current, the I_{Ks} component of the delayed rectifier; and
- altering the chloride current and the sodium-potassium pump current.

In patients receiving class I or class III antiarrhythmic therapy, drug-mediated prolongation of the action potential and refractoriness is attenuated by isoproterenol in the electrophysiology laboratory.[28] As a result, beta blockade may have additive benefit combined with any antiarrhythmic drug, particularly in states with high adrenergic tone, such as sustained VT. In the substudy analysis of both CAMIAT and EMIAT, there were substantial additive benefits of amiodarone and beta blockers, as opposed to amiodarone alone.[81] It is also not surprising that β-adrenergic antagonists used in combination with class I drugs decrease the incidence of VT and couplets on ambulatory electrocardiographic monitoring and on exercise testing. When metoprolol is added to class I drugs, noninducibility is increased significantly compared with class I monotherapy regimens, with success rates ranging from 30% to more than 60% when sustained VT induction is used as a study endpoint (see Fig. 50.4).[30,80]

PROARRHYTHMIA

All currently available antiarrhythmic drugs that act by altering cardiac electrical properties have the potential to cause proarrhythmia, defined as either the worsening of preexisting arrhythmias or the induction of new forms of arrhythmia in a given patient. Other drugs not considered antiarrhythmic may have channel-blocking properties that may also cause fatal proarrhythmia in susceptible individuals. Proarrhythmic reactions can take a variety of forms:

- an increased number of premature atrial or ventricular complexes;
- an increase in the ventricular response rate to atrial fibrillation or flutter;
- the induction or facilitation of sustained ventricular tachyarrhythmias;
- the alteration of ventricular tachyarrhythmia properties such that they become resistant to direct current electrical cardioversion; and
- sinus bradycardia or AV block.

Perhaps the most disturbing manifestation of proarrhythmia is one in which overt tachyarrhythmias may not even be evident—specifically, an increase in the mortality rate in treated patients. In studies involving patients after myocardial infarction or patients who have atrial fibrillation, an excess in sudden or presumed arrhythmic death rates was responsible for increases in mortality, pointing directly to proarrhythmic mechanisms.[82] Drugs involved include those with class Ia, Ib, Ic, and III mechanisms of action. This is important especially for an arrhythmia such as atrial fibrillation, which is rarely lethal on its own.

Mechanisms of Proarrhythmia

Postulated mechanisms include excessive slowing of conduction and excessive action potential prolongation.[82,83]

Proarrhythmia Related to Sodium Channel Blockade

A major effect of sodium channel blockade is conduction slowing, which is usually more prominent in diseased or abnormal tissue than in normal tissue. This conduction slowing appears to be responsible for proarrhythmia during sodium channel blocker therapy. In patients with ventricular scarring caused by remote myocardial infarction (a substrate with depressed conduction), the addition of a sodium channel blocker may facilitate re-entrant VT by further depressing conduction, especially in the presence of superimposed ischemia. Such VT can be manifested as incessant, very wide complex VT that is resistant to electrical cardioversion.

Similarly, in patients with atrial flutter, conduction slowing by sodium channel–blocking drugs can slow the flutter rate. With slowed atrial flutter, 1:1 AV nodal conduction may result from previous 2:1 or higher AV block. Increased frequency of VT and atrial flutter with 1:1 conduction has been most commonly recognized with drugs such as flecainide and propafenone but can also occur with quinidine and similar compounds.

Organic heart disease, particularly in association with coronary artery disease, has been found to be an important risk factor for class Ic proarrhythmia.[84] Acute myocardial ischemia produces a variety of important electrophysiologic derangements (including profound alterations in excitability and impulse propagation) that greatly predispose to malignant ventricular tachyarrhythmias. Sodium channel blockers may promote ischemic VF by their effects on cellular excitability and impulse propagation.[82] It has also been suggested that spatially heterogeneous effects on action potential repolarization may result from the combination of acute ischemia and sodium channel blockade and contribute significantly to the genesis of ventricular tachyarrhythmias.[85]

Acute ischemia may be the central factor promoting class I drug–associated mortality in studies such as CAST.[21] This speculation is supported by an analysis of nonfatal ischemic events and sudden death in CAST,[86] which found that patients treated with encainide or flecainide had the same number of endpoint events as placebo-treated patients when nonfatal ischemic events and sudden death were combined as endpoints. The excess of sudden death in drug-treated patients was balanced by a reduced incidence of nonfatal ischemic events, suggesting that encainide and flecainide transformed what would otherwise have been nonfatal acute myocardial ischemia into lethal ischemic arrhythmias.

Drugs with class I action may also cause proarrhythmia in the absence of cardiac disease, but the incidence is lower and the mechanisms are less clear than in the setting of acute ischemia or previous myocardial infarction.

Proarrhythmia Related to Action Potential Prolongation

Torsades de pointes, polymorphic VT associated with prolonged QT interval, is most common for drugs whose major effect is the prolongation of cardiac action potentials, specifically class Ia and class III agents. The incidence of torsades de pointes complicating therapy with these drugs is about

1% to 3%. Proarrhythmia with class Ic drugs typically is manifested as incessant VT but not torsades de pointes.

Many other types of drugs have been associated with the development of torsades de pointes. Erythromycin, certain nonsedating antihistamines (e.g., terfenadine and astemizole), cisapride, and tricyclic antidepressants have been reported as inducing this proarrhythmia.

QT prolongation with incipient torsades de pointes has a number of highly characteristic features. The QTU interval is markedly prolonged, often ending with very large U waves. The syndrome is facilitated by hypokalemia, hypomagnesemia, bradycardia, and drugs that prolong the action potential. When exposed to these conditions, both Purkinje fibers and midmyocardial cells (so-called M cells) frequently develop early after-depolarizations (EADs) and triggered upstrokes arising from EADs. These abnormalities are generally thought to contribute to the initiation of torsades de pointes and perhaps to its maintenance.

Prolongation of the action potential is a direct result of decreased outward potassium (or increased inward) current during the plateau. EADs may be a manifestation of the same changes, although the discontinuity in the ordinarily smooth course of repolarization that they represent suggests that other mechanisms may be operative. For example, prolongation of the action potential might cause increases in intracellular calcium, and the resultant increase in sodium-calcium exchange might then provide an additional inward current that causes the EAD.[87] The triggered upstroke is clearly a manifestation of an inward current (e.g., through slow calcium channels). Even so-called pure potassium channel–blocking drugs with no other pharmacologic actions can produce EADs and triggered activity in vitro (and torsades de pointes in vivo). Thus, it seems likely that action potential prolongation itself results in a series of secondary changes (including EADs and triggered activity) that then cause torsades de pointes.

The rate-dependent effects of drugs that prolong the action potential may exacerbate the risk of EADs, triggered activity, and torsades de pointes. Specifically, many drugs that prolong the action potential appear to exert their greatest effects at very slow rates (when torsades de pointes is a risk) and to exert much less effect at rapid rates (when the effects of prolonging the action potential and the refractory period are desirable), a phenomenon termed reverse rate dependence.

Antiarrhythmic drugs with class III mechanism of action are particularly likely to produce EADs in Purkinje fibers that survive in a region of myocardial infarction.[88] Such regional EADs might result in VT without prolongation of the QT interval or the typical features of torsades de pointes, and they could underlie the increased mortality risk of patients who had had a myocardial infarction and who were treated with D-sotalol in the SWORD trial.[58]

Prevention and Management of Proarrhythmia

Although the development of adverse effects from antiarrhythmic drugs is for the most part unpredictable, general guidelines for the prevention and management of drug-induced arrhythmias may be offered:

- Identify patients at risk for proarrhythmia.
- Use the smallest effective dose of a drug, especially in patients likely to have decreased drug clearance.
- Use combinations of antiarrhythmic drugs with caution.
- Avoid exacerbating factors for proarrhythmia (e.g., bradycardia, hypokalemia, and hypomagnesemia); this is especially important in patients taking concomitant diuretic therapy.
- Monitor patients carefully for evidence of excess drug effect or excessive drug concentrations (if facilities are available).
- Discontinue a possibly toxic drug immediately and rechallenge under careful observation only if necessary.
- Treat arrhythmias associated with delayed repolarization by correcting electrolyte abnormalities.

Most of the early experience with risk factors for torsades de pointes came from experience with quinidine for atrial fibrillation.[89] With this drug, torsades de pointes were most commonly observed after cardioversion from atrial fibrillation to normal sinus rhythm with a slow rate. Information (before administration of the drug) obtained from the surface electrocardiogram that may possibly predict an increased likelihood of marked drug-induced QTc interval prolongation includes a marked increase in the QT interval after a pause, post-extrasystolic T-wave abnormality, and failure of the QT interval to shorten appropriately during autonomic stimulation maneuvers such as the Valsalva maneuver or during exercise.

Identification of patients receiving antiarrhythmic drug therapy at risk for torsades de pointes is aided not only by measurement of the QT interval (QTc and QT dispersion) but also by observing the appearance of prominent U waves, the amplitude of which can be equal to or greater than that of the T wave, or abnormal QTU prolongation and distortion after pauses.[90]

A paradoxical increase in the QTc interval was observed during exercise in 11 patients taking class Ia antiarrhythmic drugs who developed polymorphic VT compared with patients taking these drugs who did not develop this arrhythmia.[91] Although no particular QT interval separates "therapeutic" from "proarrhythmic" prolongation, a QT or QTc interval of more than 550 ms probably indicates a risk for subsequent proarrhythmia.

In addition, a number of risk factors for torsades de pointes from sotalol have been identified. These risk factors include[92]

- a serum potassium level of less than 4.0 mmol/L at baseline;
- female sex;
- a history of sustained ventricular arrhythmia or congestive heart failure; and
- a sotalol regimen of more than 320 mg daily.

ANTIARRHYTHMIC DRUGS IN PREGNANCY

An increased incidence of maternal cardiac arrhythmias is observed during pregnancy, explained in part by the metabolic, hormonal, and hemodynamic changes of pregnancy. In addition, advances in cardiac surgery have allowed an increased number of women with congenital cardiac malformations to reach reproductive age. Arrhythmias may also be the initial presentation of a serious cardiovascular condition that develops or is discovered during pregnancy, such as peripartum cardiomyopathy. Alternatively, maternal administration of drugs may be required to treat fetal arrhythmias.

Physiologic changes that occur during pregnancy include an increment in cardiac output by 30% to 50% and in blood volume by 40% to 50%, a fall in serum protein concentration, an alteration in gastric secretion and motility, and the hormonal stimulation of liver enzymes. These changes can affect the absorption, bioavailability, and elimination of most drugs. Because the magnitude of the changes varies with different stages of pregnancy, closer drug monitoring and more frequent dose adjustment are necessary in comparison to the nonpregnant condition, with particular attention paid to the clinical and electrophysiologic response to the particular agent.

Therapy should be avoided, if possible, during the first weeks of gestation, when the risk for development of congenital malformations is greatest. Because all antiarrhythmic medications have potential side effects to both the mother and the fetus, the smallest recommended dose should be used initially. The patient should be monitored regularly with evaluation of clinical response and with measurement of serum drug levels (when available), along with reassessment for continued need for medication. Adverse effects, especially proarrhythmia, must be considered in the mother and fetus, and antiarrhythmic drugs with class I or class III mechanism of action should be initiated during inpatient cardiac monitoring. The majority of antiarrhythmic drugs are U.S. Food and Drug Administration category C, which means that there are either animal studies suggesting risks but no confirmatory human studies or no controlled studies in either humans or animals (Table 50.5).

DEFINITION OF FOOD AND DRUG ADMINISTRATION PREGNANCY CATEGORIES

Pregnancy Category	Definition
A	Controlled studies show no risk. Adequate, well-controlled studies in pregnant women have failed to demonstrate risk to the fetus in any trimester of pregnancy.
B	No evidence of risk in humans. Adequate, well-controlled studies in pregnant women have not shown increased risk of fetal abnormalities despite adverse findings in animals, or, in the absence of adequate human studies, animal studies show no fetal risk. The chance of fetal harm is remote but remains a possibility.
C	Risk cannot be ruled out. Adequate, well-controlled human studies are lacking, and animal studies have shown a risk to the fetus or are lacking as well. There is chance of fetal harm if the drug is administered during pregnancy, but the potential benefits outweigh the risk.
D	Positive evidence of risk. Studies in humans have shown evidence of fetal risk. Nevertheless, the potential benefits from the use of the drug in pregnant women outweigh the risk.
X	Contraindicated in pregnancy. Studies in animals or humans have shown fetal risk, which clearly outweighs any possible future benefit to the patient.

From Physician's Desk Reference. Montvale, NJ, Medical Economics, Inc, 1999.

Table 50.5 Definition of Food and Drug Administration pregnancy categories.

Table 50.6 lists the specific antiarrhythmic drugs in order of their Vaughan Williams class and summarizes their experience during pregnancy.

ANTIARRHYTHMIC DRUGS IN RENAL FAILURE

In comparison to patients with normal renal function, any dose or dosage schedule of an antiarrhythmic agent in a patient with renal failure may produce higher plasma concentrations of the drug and for a longer duration. Patients with renal failure can also react unpredictably and atypically to pharmacologic agents; thus, the adverse effects of a drug in this clinical setting are often related to factors other than plasma drug concentration. For example, the effects of many antiarrhythmic agents are exacerbated by abnormalities in serum concentrations of potassium, magnesium, and calcium; hypoxemia; and the hyperadrenergic state of renal disease and dialysis.

Renal failure often modifies the pharmacokinetics and pharmacodynamics of a drug (Table 50.7). In addition to a simple reduction in renal function and glomerular filtration rate, there is a greater variability in drug absorption, protein binding, metabolism, receptor affinity, sensitivity, and responsiveness. Lower protein binding may be related to hypoproteinemia or hypoalbuminemia, an alteration of the protein molecule, or competition for protein-binding sites by endogenous substances and other types of chronic renal failure therapy. Patients with renal failure are commonly treated with several agents; drug-drug interactions can affect gastrointestinal absorption, protein binding, tissue distribution, drug metabolism and clearance, and pharmacodynamic properties.

For drugs cleared by the kidney, dosing is adjusted for renal function. Three dosing modifications can be employed: the dosing interval can be lengthened without altering the dose amount, the dose amount can be lowered without changing the dosing schedule, or a combination of both. The second approach is preferable in most patients because it avoids wide swings in plasma drug concentrations. Dose adjustment information for the use of dofetilide in renal disease is presented in Table 50.4.

SUMMARY

Despite recent advances in our knowledge of arrhythmogenesis and the mechanisms of antiarrhythmic drug action, truly "rational" antiarrhythmic therapy is still elusive. When choosing antiarrhythmic therapy, the physician must consider not only pharmacokinetic and pharmacodynamic variables that may affect drug efficacy but also various modulating factors, such as the patient's neurohumoral state and potential drug interactions.

There is no ideal method of predicting antiarrhythmic drug efficacy, although electrophysiologic studies may be useful.

All antiarrhythmic drugs with primarily sodium channel–blocking (class I) action, when carefully studied in large randomized trials of high-risk patients, have caused increased mortality. In contrast, beta blockers are the only drugs that have been unequivocally shown to reduce cardiac and sudden death mortality in a variety of patient populations. Beta blockers have additive benefit in that they suppress

EXPERIENCE WITH ANTIARRHYTHMIC DRUGS DURING PREGNANCY					
Drug	**FDA Category***	**Potential Adverse Effects**	**Best Indication**	**Use During Lactation**	**Comments**
Quinidine	C	Maternal and fetal thrombocytopenia, eighth nerve toxicity, torsades de pointes	Variety of maternal and fetal arrhythmias	Generally compatible, but caution advised	Long record of safety
Procainamide	C	Lupus-like syndrome with long-term use, torsades de pointes	Drug of choice for acute treatment of undiagnosed, wide complex tachycardia	Compatible, but long-term therapy should be avoided	Has the advantage of intravenous dosing, long record of safety
Disopyramide	C	Induction of uterine contractions, torsades de pointes	Limited experience; other alternatives available	Compatible	Limited experience
Lidocaine	B	Central nervous system adverse effects, bradycardia	Maternal VT, arrhythmias due to digoxin toxicity	Compatible	Long record of safety; avoid with fetal distress
Mexiletine	C	Central nervous system adverse effects, fetal bradycardia, low APGAR score	VT	Compatible	Limited experience
Phenytoin	D	Mental and growth retardation, fetal hydantoin syndrome	Arrhythmias due to digoxin toxicity	Generally compatible, but caution advised	Better alternatives available; avoid if possible
Flecainide	C	Increased mortality in patients with previous myocardial infarction; generally safe in structurally normal hearts	Variety of maternal and fetal VT and SVT	Compatible	First-line option for treating fetal SVT with hydrops
Propafenone	C	Same concerns as with flecainide; mild beta-blocker effects	Variety of maternal and fetal VT and SVT	Unknown	Limited experience
Beta blockers	C/D	Intrauterine growth retardation, fetal bradycardia, hypoglycemia, fetal apnea	Maternal SVT, idiopathic VT, AF rate control	Avoid atenolol; metoprolol and propranolol are compatible	Generally safe; avoid during first trimester; cardiac-selective agents are preferred
Amiodarone	D	Fetal hypothyroidism, prematurity, low birth weight, congenital malformations	Life-threatening ventricular arrhythmias	Avoid; a large amount of drug is absorbed by the infant	Avoid if possible, especially during first trimester
Sotalol	B	Torsades de pointes, beta-blocker effects	Maternal VT and SVT, hypertension in the past	Generally compatible, but caution advised	Limited experience
Ibutilide	C	Torsades de pointes	Acute termination of atrial fibrillation or flutter	Unknown	No experience in pregnancy
Verapamil	C	Maternal hypotension, fetal bradycardia, and heart block	Maternal and fetal SVT, idiopathic VT, AF rate control	Compatible	Relatively safe, but safer options are available
Diltiazem	C	Limited experience; same concerns as with verapamil	Maternal SVT, AF rate control	Compatible	Verapamil preferred because of longer record in pregnancy
Adenosine	C	Dyspnea, bradycardia	Acute termination of maternal SVT	Unknown, but probably safe	First option for acute treatment of SVT
Digoxin	C	Low birth weight	Fetal and maternal SVT, AF rate control	Compatible	Long record of safety

*Food and Drug Administration risk category. See Table 50.5.
AF, atrial fibrillation; SVT, supraventricular tachycardia; VT, ventricular tachycardia.
From Joglar JA, Page RL. Antiarrhythmic drugs in pregnancy. Curr Opin Cardiol 2001;16:40-45.

Table 50.6 Experience with antiarrhythmic drugs during pregnancy.

ANTIARRHYTHMIC DRUGS IN RENAL FAILURE							
	Half-life (h)		Protein Binding (%)				
Drug	Normal	Renal Failure	Normal	Renal Failure	Adjustment for Renal Failure	Removal by Dialysis	Comments
Quinidine	6	5-14	80-85	↑	No	Yes, hemodialysis	May increase serum digoxin levels
Procainamide	3-4	11-20	15-20	Unchanged	Yes	Yes, hemodialysis	Some patients require higher plasma concentrations (10-25 μg/mL)
Disopyramide	5-7	10-18	40-90	—	Yes	Yes, hemodialysis	Protein binding concentration dependent
Lidocaine	1.2-2.2	1.3-3	60-66	Unchanged	No	No	Protein binding may be concentration dependent
Mexiletine	7-11	↑	57-69	—	Yes	—	—
Tocainide	15	—	10	—	Yes	—	—
Phenytoin	24	May be shorter	90-95	70-85	No	No	Protein binding decreased in renal failure
Flecainide	8-14	↑	50-70	—	Yes	—	—
Propafenone	2-10	—	85-87	—	—	—	—
Propranolol	2-4	2-4	90-95	—	No	Yes, hemodialysis	Active metabolites may accumulate
Atenolol	6-9	15-35	<5	—	Yes	Yes, hemodialysis	Significant accumulation in renal failure
Metoprolol	2.5	4.5	12	—	No	Yes, hemodialysis	—
Bretylium	6.0	13.6	—	—	Yes	—	Avoid when creatinine clearance <10 mL/min
Amiodarone	≥60 days	—	>95	—	—	—	—
Sotalol	8	15-50	50	—	Yes	Yes, hemodialysis	—
Verapamil	3	?7	90	~90	No	Yes	—
Diltiazem	2	?8	83	—	No	—	—
Digoxin	45	72-96	25	18	Yes	No	Radioimmunoassay may overestimate serum levels in renal failure

Modified from Leier CV, Boudoulas H. Cardiovascular Disorders and Diseases. Armonk, NY, Futura, 1992.

Table 50.7 Antiarrhythmic drugs in renal failure.

inducibility and recurrence of VT when they are combined with antiarrhythmic agents from other classes, particularly class I and class III, as a result of attenuation of antiarrhythmic effect with sympathetic stimulation. This provides a rationale for combinations of antiarrhythmic drugs that also avoid side effects and increase antiarrhythmic efficacy.

Agents with class III mechanism of action are the most effective drugs for the treatment of recurrent supraventricular and ventricular tachyarrhythmias. Recent attention has focused on compounds that have the propensity to block more than one ion channel, and the results of randomized controlled trials as to the safety and efficacy of these agents are awaited.

chapter

51 Principles of Catheter Ablation

David E. Haines

Definition

- Catheter ablation therapy is controlled delivery of destructive energy through an intravascular catheter, resulting in irreversible damage to a critical anatomic substrate that is responsible for arrhythmia initiation or propagation.

Key Features

- Many anatomic substrates for many arrhythmias may be approached with intravascular catheters guided by electrophysiologic mapping techniques or, in some cases, by anatomic guidance.
- Radiofrequency energy delivery through an electrode catheter effectively creates thermal injury and ablates the myocardial tissue with which it is in contact.

Clinical Implications

- Catheter ablation is an effective curative treatment for a wide variety of symptomatic arrhythmias.

The concept of ablation therapy for the treatment of arrhythmias was based on the hypothesis that all arrhythmias, no matter what their mechanism, are dependent on some critical anatomic substrate in the heart for their initiation or propagation. After initial success with surgical techniques for ablation in patients with arrhythmias, Scheinman and coworkers[1] and Gallagher and colleagues[2] reported in 1982 that delivery of high-energy direct current shocks through transvenous electrode catheters could produce complete heart block in patients with atrial fibrillation and poorly controlled ventricular response rates. Although this transcatheter technique was effective, energy delivery was difficult to titrate and to control. In 1985, a new technique was described whereby high-frequency alternating current was passed through an electrode catheter and the contiguous tissue was cauterized.[3] Soon thereafter, radiofrequency catheter ablation was attempted in patients with arrhythmias. A feature of catheter ablation with radiofrequency energy was that the lesions created were very controllable but relatively small. Therefore, high success rates with ablation were not achieved until techniques for mapping were improved and the anatomic-electrophysiologic relationships of arrhythmic substrates were better understood.

Today, radiofrequency catheter ablation has evolved into one of the most successful interventions in medicine. In most cases, symptomatic arrhythmias are the result of an abnormal anatomic structure (such as a bypass tract in Wolff-Parkinson-White syndrome) or a normal structure with unfavorable electrophysiologic properties (such as a slow atrioventricular [AV] nodal pathway in AV nodal re-entrant tachycardia). By selectively destroying the arrhythmogenic tissue, the interventional cardiac electrophysiologist can truly cure the patients of their diseases. With procedure success rates exceeding 95% and significant complication rates less than 1%, radiofrequency catheter ablation has evolved into a dominant therapeutic modality for a wide variety of arrhythmias. Pulmonary vein isolation and atrial substrate modification procedures are now an excellent option for selected patients with atrial fibrillation. New ablation technologies, such as cryothermic, laser, and high-intensity focused ultrasound ablation, may improve procedure efficacy and safety.

DESCRIPTION OF THE DEVICES AND TECHNIQUES

Biophysics of Radiofrequency Catheter Ablation

Lesions are created with radiofrequency catheter ablation by the conduction of alternating electrical current through tissue, which in turn heats the tissue and causes thermal injury (Fig. 51.1). Whenever electricity is passed through a resistive medium, the energy is dissipated as heat (similar to what is observed with passage of household electrical current through an incandescent light bulb filament). In the case of catheter ablation, the electrode catheter is a low-impedance conduction line, and the myocardial tissue is the high-impedance "load" of the electrical circuit. The current passes from the electrode catheter tip, through the myocardium, through the chest, and into a dispersive electrode placed on the patient's skin. Direct tissue heating occurs in the shallow tissue layers close (1 to 4 mm) to the electrode, then heat is passively conducted to deeper tissue layers.[4] The greatest heating occurs in regions where the radiofrequency electrical current is most concentrated. In the case of catheter ablation, that region is within 1 to 4 mm of the electrode-tissue interface. Because the dispersive electrode has a large surface area, relatively little heat is generated in its area of contact with the skin. High-frequency alternating current is used to avoid nerve and muscle stimulation that could result in pain and arrhythmias. Temperature is usually measured at the catheter tip during the energy delivery to avoid excessive heating that can result in boiling at the electrode tip when temperatures exceed 100°C, with associated thrombus and char formation.[5] Most operators select a target temperature of 70°C or lower during routine catheter ablation because of inhomogeneity of heating along electrodes[6] and potential

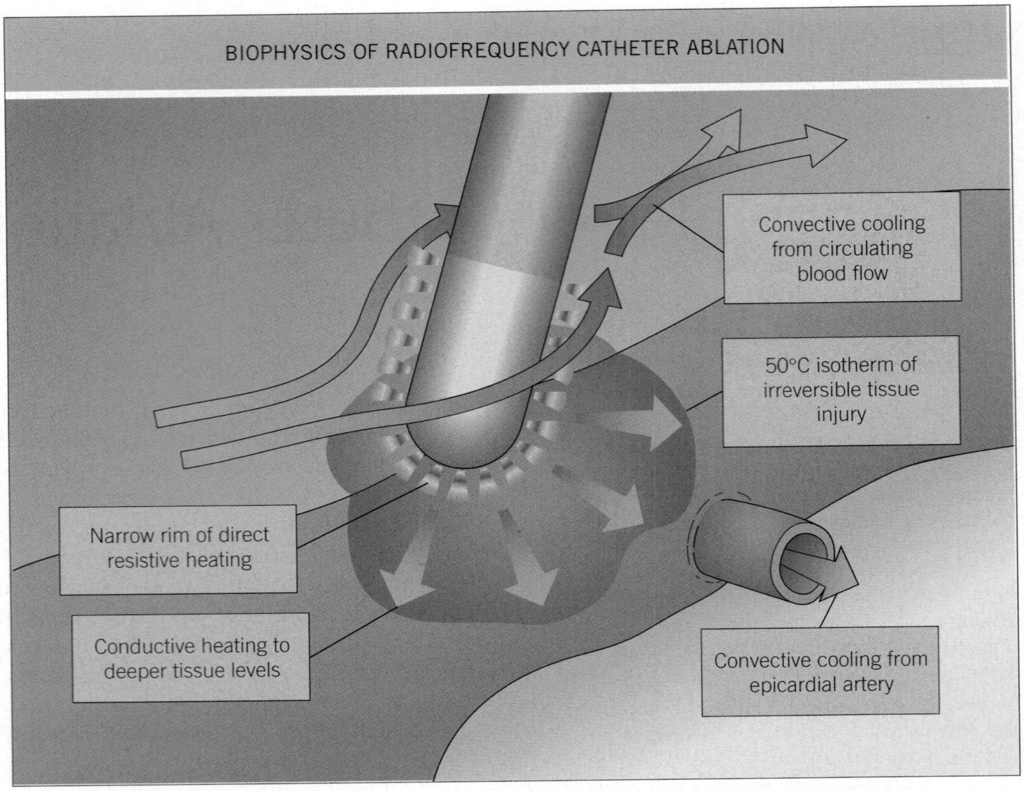

BIOPHYSICS OF RADIOFREQUENCY CATHETER ABLATION

Convective cooling from circulating blood flow

50°C isotherm of irreversible tissue injury

Narrow rim of direct resistive heating

Conductive heating to deeper tissue levels

Convective cooling from epicardial artery

Figure 51.1 Radiofrequency catheter ablation from the tip of an electrode catheter to the endocardial surface. The cutaway view shows the narrow rim of direct resistive heating and heat conduction to deeper tissue layers to create the pathologic lesion. Convective cooling on the endocardial surface by circulating blood flow cools the electrode and decreases the lesion diameter on the endocardium. The convective cooling from epicardial arterial blood flow protects those vessels from excessive heating.

underestimation of the peak temperature from a single sensor. In opposition to tissue heating is the tissue cooling that occurs from convective heat loss into the circulating blood pool. If there is too much convective cooling, as is sometimes the case with ablation in regions of high blood flow, tissue heating may be inadequate. Paradoxically, surface convective cooling by circulating blood or perfusion of the catheter tip with saline may allow the use of higher ablation power without excessive surface heating and yield a larger and deeper ablative lesion (Fig. 51.2).[7]

At present, ablation catheters have

- characteristics of high torsional stiffness for excellent torque delivery;
- deflectable distal sections of the catheter that give the operator the ability to steer the catheter tip to the desired location; and
- large (4- to 10-mm) electrode tips with embedded thermistors or thermocouples for temperature monitoring.

The handle of the catheter has the control actuator, usually a thumb wheel or a thumb slide that controls the degree of tip deflection. The operator is able to maneuver the catheter tip along the endocardial surface by a combination of translational motion, torque, and tip deflection. Achievement of stable electrode-tissue contact is important for successful delivery of energy to the tissue. Therefore, catheters that reliably allow the operator to attain a stable tip position at a wide variety of sites are the most useful. To facilitate site access, different curve shapes and curve radii are available for most catheters. Also, long guiding sheaths having distal segments with various curves and shapes help in the placement and stability of ablation electrodes in selected cases.

New Tools for Catheter Ablation

Radiofrequency Catheter Ablation with Large Electrodes

For complex arrhythmia substrates, larger lesions with greater depth are desirable. It has been demonstrated that lesion size and geometry are related to the size and geometry of the ablation electrode.[8] Therefore, large and deep lesions are best created by large electrodes and long lesions by long electrodes. Early attempts at catheter ablation that used catheters with 2-mm electrode tips had low success rates and long procedure times. With the introduction of a 4-mm electrode tip ablation catheter, results improved significantly.[9] The larger electrode size produced larger ablative lesions that in turn allowed ablation of deeper anatomic targets and increased likelihood of procedure success. At present, large electrodes measuring 8 mm and 10 mm in length are used for ablation of difficult anatomic substrates and have higher efficacy in atrial flutter ablation compared with 4-mm tip catheters.[10] Unfortunately, the constraint provided by the requirement of vascular access limits the diameter of electrode that can be reasonably used. Novel catheter designs are being tested with use of an inflatable balloon that have ultrasound or radiofrequency energy sources to achieve larger volumes of tissue heating.

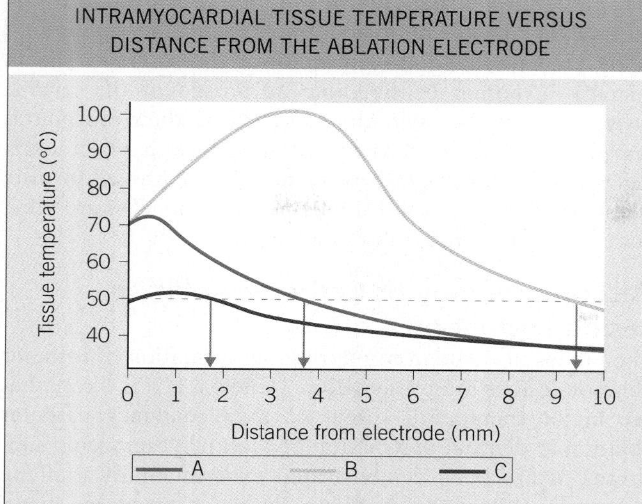

Figure 51.2 Intramyocardial tissue temperature versus distance from the ablation electrode during delivery of radiofrequency energy in steady-state conditions. Line A shows the radial temperature profile from a typical ablation with good electrode-tissue contact and good tissue heating. The peak tissue temperature is close to the surface and crosses the 50°C isotherm (the threshold of irreversible tissue injury) at a depth of approximately 3.7 mm. Line B represents a case in which there is significant convective cooling of the endocardial surface (because of saline perfusion of the catheter tip or sliding catheter contact with the endocardium). In this case, the delivered power is much greater, but there is no sudden increase in electrical impedance because the temperature at the endocardial surface is 70°C. The high power results in deeper resistive heating, and the peak temperature may be achieved 3 to 4 mm from the endocardial surface. The radial temperature gradient is shifted rightward, and the critical temperature of 50°C is achieved at a depth of 9.3 mm. Note that the peak intramyocardial temperature approaches 100°C in this example. If 100°C is significantly exceeded, a vapor bubble may form and explode out of the tissue ("pop lesion"). Line C represents a case of significant convective cooling on the endocardial surface, but in this case, the magnitude of the delivered radiofrequency power is limited. Thus, deep tissue heating is modest, and the anticipated lesion depth is small (<2 mm).

Cooled-tip or Irrigated-tip Catheter Ablation

Convective cooling of a catheter tip during radiofrequency catheter ablation allows the operator to deliver high power without the surface temperature exceeding 100°C (the temperature at which boiling and charring occur). Tip cooling has been accomplished with two methods:

- saline irrigation through small holes drilled in the tip of the electrode[7]; and
- closed saline perfusion through the catheter tip by an infusion and return line.[11]

A randomized trial was performed to compare irrigated-tip with conventional radiofrequency ablation in 50 patients with atrial flutter. The procedures were ultimately successful with both techniques, but the total duration of the procedure, duration of exposure to fluoroscopy, and number of deliveries of radiofrequency energy were significantly lower in patients treated with the irrigated catheter system.[12] The potential disadvantage of cooled-tip or irrigated-tip ablation is that temperature monitoring at the electrode tip cannot be used as a guide for power titration, and it is possible to superheat the tissue, with resultant formation of intramyocardial, expanding steam bubbles that can, in the worst case, vent through the myocardial wall, resulting in perforation. In addition, the greater depth of lesion formation can potentially lead to injury to deep structures, such as coronary arteries, phrenic nerve, and esophagus. Therefore, this technology is reserved for ablation of refractory arrhythmias with large and deep arrhythmogenic substrates or atrial fibrillation ablation in which transmural lesion formation is paramount for procedural success.

Microwave Catheter Ablation

An alternative approach to increasing the depth or diameter of catheter ablative lesions is to use an energy source different from standard radiofrequency energy. Higher frequency electromagnetic radiation does not conduct electrically in tissue but can radiate through tissue if it is transmitted from a properly designed radiative source built in the form of a catheter. Microwave energy oscillating at 915 or 2450 MHz causes dielectric heating of the water in tissue and can achieve deeper heating than conventional radiofrequency ablation. A helical antenna catheter has been tested in vivo and reliably produces lesions 9 mm in depth.[13] These are slightly deeper than standard radiofrequency ablative lesions but not as deep as those created with irrigated-tip catheters. Clinically, microwave probes have been used to create linear atrial ablative lesions during open heart surgery in patients with atrial fibrillation, with modest success.[14] However, there are many technical limitations of microwave antenna catheter design that to date have limited the broad application of this technique.

Laser Catheter Ablation

In a higher electromagnetic radiation frequency range, tissue is ablated by optical heating. Depending on the frequency, laser energy can achieve tissue heating very superficially (higher frequencies) or very deep (lower frequencies). The geometry of laser ablation from an end-fire ablation catheter is unfavorable because the lesion is narrow at the endocardial contact point and then spreads to greater width in the midmyocardium. It has been used with some success with intraoperative epicardial ablation of sources of ventricular tachycardia,[15] but this has not translated into a commercially successful end-fire laser catheter. Laser ablation has been coupled with a unique balloon-tipped catheter for pulmonary vein isolation. With this system, the balloon contact with the atrial wall can be visualized with a cardioscope, and an arc of laser energy can be delivered to the targeted tissue. Preliminary clinical studies have shown the benefit of this technology, but durable value of this approach remains to be demonstrated.[16]

Ultrasound Catheter Ablation

In contrast to heating with electromagnetic energy, ultrasound energy heats through mechanical heating with sound waves. The possible advantages of heating with ultrasound energy are that

- there is a 10:1 ratio of tissue to blood absorption;
- the depth of heating can be controlled by the frequency of ultrasound energy selected; and

- the ultrasound beam can potentially be focused to a specific depth on a specific target.

Clinical ablation systems have been developed that use a cylindrical ultrasound transducer mounted within a saline-filled balloon at the tip of a catheter. Ablation in a circumferential pattern was tested for pulmonary vein isolation in patients with paroxysmal atrial fibrillation. This approach failed to target the critical extraostial atrial tissue that is important in successful elimination of atrial fibrillation, and results were disappointing.[17] A newer design uses a second gas-filled balloon contiguous to the saline-filled balloon. The fluid-gas interface is reflective and allows generation of a forward-firing circular energy beam that can be focused 2 mm from the balloon surface, thus maximizing tissue heating.[18] This technology has been effective in eliminating atrial fibrillation in pilot trials, but with deeper tissue heating comes concerns about risks of collateral damage to contiguous anatomic structures. The ultimate utility of ultrasound as an energy source for catheter ablation of atrial fibrillation or other arrhythmias remains to be determined.

Cryothermic Catheter Ablation

For some decades, cryothermy has been used in the surgical suite to ablate arrhythmogenic substrates. Myocardium is typically frozen with a probe cooled to −70°C by liquid nitrogen or other coolants. The deep freezing of the tissue results in the formation of an intracellular ice matrix, with cytoskeletal disruption, and in the formation of an extracellular ice matrix, with damage to the sarcolemmal membrane. The resultant lesions are homogeneous and well demarcated. More recently, investigators have succeeded in cooling the tips of intracardiac catheters and producing a cooling effect sufficient to achieve effective ablative lesions. Cryothermic ablation has the advantage of being able to confirm the optimal ablation site by reversibly cooling the tissue to confirm the desired physiologic effect before an irreversible ablative lesion has been produced. Although cryothermic ablation is effective, tissue temperatures below −30°C must be achieved for success, and a long duration of tissue freezing (>5 minutes) is required to maximize the depth of the lesion.[19] Studies have demonstrated the utility of cryothermic ablation in patients with a variety of arrhythmias. It is particularly useful, in light of its safety profile, in catheter ablation in the pediatric population.[20] Recently, cryoablation through a cryoballoon catheter has been employed in the treatment of paroxysmal atrial fibrillation.[21]

Robotic Navigation

Manipulation of catheters to various targets for successful ablation requires considerable technical skill and experience. That requirement has limited catheter ablation of challenging arrhythmias, such as atrial fibrillation and ventricular tachycardia, to specialized referral centers and may represent a barrier against patient access to optimal therapy. Robotic navigation may allow less experienced operators to achieve similar results by transferring the actual movement of the catheter to a computer-driven system guided by the operator's manipulation of a joystick or computer mouse. This is technically accomplished by a pair of large external magnets that move the magnetic tip of the catheter in the direction selected by the operator and actuated by the computer[22] or by a computer-controlled motor-driven steerable sheath system.[23] Another considerable advantage of the robotic systems is that the operators can perform their procedures seated at a computer console and away from harmful ionizing radiation. Although these systems are approved for use, it remains to be determined whether their benefits are great enough to offset their substantial costs.

Pathophysiology of Catheter Ablation Lesion Formation

The modes of tissue injury during the formation of catheter ablation lesions are presented in Table 51.1. It is likely that the major therapeutic effect of radiofrequency catheter ablation is thermal destruction of the arrhythmogenic substrates. It has been demonstrated experimentally that the isotherm of irreversible tissue injury assessed by histochemical staining techniques is 52°C to 55°C. Studies of isolated tissue preparations indicate a loss of electrophysiologic function at temperatures above 50°C.[24,25] In the clinical setting, a variety of patterns of measured temperatures and physiologic effects are observed. In general, greater tissue temperatures correlate with larger anatomic lesions and increased likelihood of ablation success. However, because of the profound effect of convective cooling by the circulating blood pool at the electrode-tissue contact point, the temperature measured by a catheter-mounted temperature sensor often underestimates the peak tissue temperature.[7]

The tissue effects of radiofrequency catheter ablation are consistent with thermal coagulation of tissue with, acutely, central coagulative necrosis and a hemorrhagic border zone. This viable border to the acute lesion has significant electrophysiologic and ultrastructural derangements[24-26] and may either recover or progressively necrose in the hours after ablation. Chronically, lesions are contracted and fibrotic, with a clearly demarcated border between the ablated and unaffected myocardium. The absence of patchy border zone fibrosis accounts for the relative absence of proarrhythmia attributed to catheter ablation procedures. Because of the effect of convective cooling from the high-velocity blood flow within the large epicardial coronary arteries, there is usually sparing of the vessel wall from the effects of nearby catheter ablation.

MODES OF TISSUE INJURY DURING CATHETER ABLATION
Tissue effects
Desiccation Coagulative necrosis Microvascular injury
Cellular effects
Membrane poration with depolarization and calcium overload Protein inactivation Cytoskeleton disruption Nuclear degeneration

Table 51.1 Modes of tissue injury during catheter ablation.

INDICATIONS, CONTRAINDICATIONS, AND OBJECTIVES

The technique of catheter ablation is constantly evolving, with broadening indications and increasing procedure success rates. To understand the specific applications of this technology, it is important to consider it in the context of the specific arrhythmia mechanisms being treated (Table 51.2). For a detailed discussion of the epidemiology, pathophysiology, natural history, and options for treatment of these arrhythmias, refer to Chapters 57 to 62.

Paroxysmal Supraventricular Tachycardia

Paroxysmal supraventricular tachycardias are most commonly due to AV nodal re-entrant tachycardia or AV reciprocating tachycardia. The anatomic substrate for AV nodal re-entrant tachycardia is an array of atrial conduction pathways inserting into the AV node. Typically, the atrial insertion into the AV node that is located anteriorly and superiorly on the interatrial septum has properties of relatively fast conduction and hence is termed the fast pathway. The atrial insertion that is located inferiorly and posteriorly along the tricuspid valve annulus near the coronary sinus os typically has slower anterograde conduction properties and is called the slow pathway (see Chapter 57). Either pathway may be ablated, but the much preferred target is the slow pathway. Both radiofrequency energy and cryothermy have been used with high success in the elimination of the slow pathway. A desire for curative treatment and a drug-free lifestyle has become the most common indication for the procedure. Success rates of 95% are routinely achieved with AV nodal modification, and success rates approaching 100% are reported from experienced centers.[27,28] After a successful initial procedure, the reported risk of recurrence of arrhythmia is 2% to 8%. In such patients, a repeated ablation procedure has a very high likelihood of curing the arrhythmia.

The anatomic substrate for AV reciprocating tachycardia is an accessory pathway (bypass tract, bundle of Kent) that is an additional electrical connection between the atrium and the ventricle. It creates a re-entrant circuit down the AV node, through the ventricle, up the pathway, through the atrium, then down the node again (orthodromic); less commonly, the arrhythmia follows the circuit in the opposite direction (antidromic). Elimination of the accessory pathway eliminates the arrhythmia (see Chapter 60). Mapping around the AV valve annulus identifies the location of early activation from the pathway. In many cases, a small high-frequency potential can be observed between the local atrial and ventricular electrograms; it represents accessory pathway activation and is a highly specific marker for successful sites of ablation (Fig. 51.3). Technical factors that increase the difficulty of the procedure include the presence of several accessory pathways, anatomic abnormalities such as Ebstein's anomaly, and epicardial or posteroseptal location of the pathway. The primary indication for catheter ablation is the elimination of symptoms from recurrent supraventricular tachycardia. An additional indication for accessory pathway ablation is to reduce the risk of sudden death in patients who have rapidly conducting pathways and thereby may suffer a cardiac arrest in the setting of atrial fibrillation with very rapid ventricular rates. At present, successful ablation of accessory pathways can be achieved in more than 90% of patients, with success rates exceeding 98% in experienced laboratories.[29] After initial procedural success, the risk of recurrence of an accessory pathway is 3% to 5%. In these cases, it is typically recommended that the patient undergo a repeated procedure because permanent cure can be achieved more than 90% of the time.

CLINICAL ARRHYTHMIAS TREATED WITH CATHETER ABLATION

Arrhythmias	Ablation Target	Success Rate (%)	Recurrence Rate (%)
AV reciprocating tachycardia	Accessory pathway	>95	3-5
AV nodal re-entrant tachycardia	Slow AV nodal pathway	>98	2-8
Atrial flutter	Tricuspid–inferior vena cava isthmus	>90	10
Atrial fibrillation (palliative)	Compact AV node	>99	5
Atrial fibrillation (curative)	Focal—pulmonary veins	>70	30-40
	Re-entrant—linear lesions	>60 (approximately)	>40
Automatic (ectopic) atrial tachycardia	Focus of abnormal automaticity	>80	5
Sinoatrial re-entrant tachycardia	Sinus node region	>95	5
Inappropriate sinus tachycardia terminals	Broad region of superior crista	>75	>50
Idiopathic ventricular tachycardia	Focus of abnormal automaticity or insertion of abnormal fascicle	>90	5
Re-entrant ventricular tachycardia	Slow conduction zone at border of healed infarction	60-70	30-40

AV, atrioventricular.

Table 51.2 Clinical arrhythmias treated with catheter ablation.

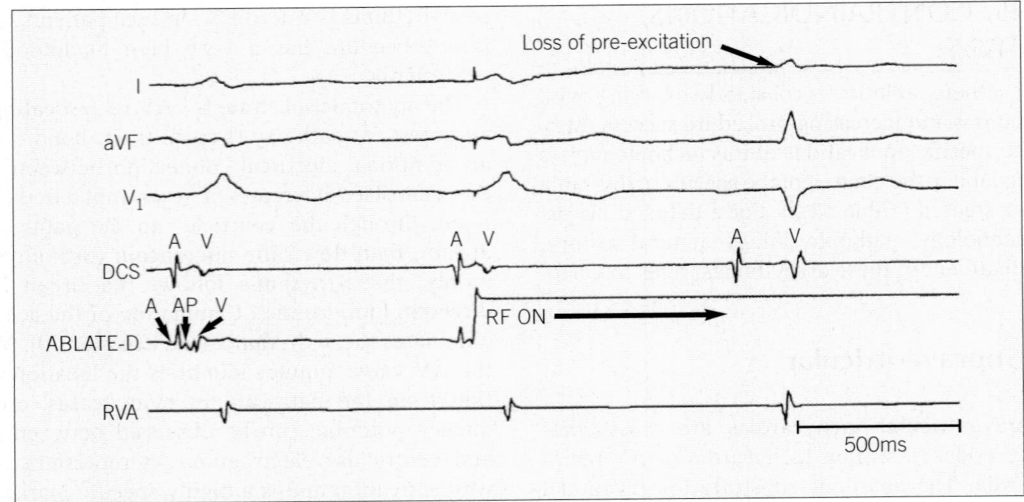

Figure 51.3 Accessory pathway ablation. Surface electrocardiogram leads I, aVF, and V_1 and intracardiac electrograms from the distal coronary sinus (DCS), the distal bipole of an ablation electrode positioned contiguous to the site of the accessory pathway (ABLATE-D), and the right ventricular apex (RVA). Before the onset of radiofrequency energy delivery (RF ON), the atrial (A) to ventricular (V) conduction time on the left free wall was very short as a result of conduction down an accessory pathway. A high-frequency potential between the atrial and ventricular deflections can be seen on the ablation catheter electrogram representing accessory pathway (AP) activation. Within 1 second of onset of radiofrequency energy, the pattern of pre-excitation is lost on the surface electrocardiogram and the atrial-to-ventricular interval suddenly increases, indicating successful ablation of anterograde accessory pathway conduction.

Atrial Arrhythmias

The mechanisms of atrial arrhythmias include atrial flutter, atrial fibrillation, and focal atrial tachycardia. Typical atrial flutter is a macroreentrant rhythm that has a circuit around the tricuspid annulus. Because this arrhythmia depends on intact conduction through the isthmus of tissue between the tricuspid annulus and the inferior vena cava–eustachian valve, linear ablation across this isthmus terminates the arrhythmia and prevents recurrence. One can confirm successful bidirectional isthmus conduction block with pacing maneuvers (Fig. 51.4). At present, typical atrial flutter can be successfully ablated acutely in more than 90% of patients.[30] Procedure time and number of lesions required to achieve success may be reduced by the use of an irrigated-tip radiofrequency ablation catheter.[12] With confirmation of bidirectional conduction block in the tricuspid–inferior vena cava isthmus, the likelihood of recurrence of late atrial flutter is approximately 10%.[31] A randomized trial comparing catheter ablation versus amiodarone drug therapy as first therapy for new-onset atrial flutter showed a higher success rate (96% versus 71%; $P < .0001$) and a lower complication rate (0% versus 10%; $P = .03$) with catheter ablation.[32] Thus, ablation therapy should be strongly considered for anyone with this arrhythmia. Patients who have undergone open heart surgery requiring an atriotomy are at risk of having atrial tachycardia that is related to the atriotomy scar. In these cases, the surgical scar acts as an anatomic barrier around which a re-entrant wavefront travels. In many cases, the scar-related tachycardia coexists with typical type I atrial flutter. Ablation between the atriotomy scar and a contiguous anatomic structure (e.g., the inferior vena cava) will result in interruption of the circuit. Ablation success can be achieved in more than 90% of these patients by means of these techniques.[33]

Atrial fibrillation is a complex rhythm that has varying mechanisms among the spectrum of patients with this disorder. At one end of the scale are patients who may be younger, have normal hearts and normal atrial size, and have frequent brief paroxysms of atrial fibrillation. These individuals have atrial fibrillation that is caused by a rapidly firing focus or foci, typically arising from the muscular sleeve of the pulmonary veins.[34,35] Conduction of the rapid impulses to the remainder of the heart cannot maintain a 1:1 relationship at those high rates, and therefore the propagating waves break up into fibrillatory activity of typical appearance. When the focal activity stops, the fibrillation usually stops soon thereafter. If the patient has frequent atrial ectopy or short bursts of atrial tachycardia, it may be possible to map the earliest sites of atrial activation, then directly ablate these foci with standard radiofrequency ablative techniques (Fig. 51.5). However, the arrhythmia may originate from multiple veins or the transition tissue outside of the vein orifice. Therefore, the present-day accepted ablation approach is an anatomically guided four-vein extraostial pulmonary vein isolation procedure. The location and morphologic features of the pulmonary veins are typically delineated by one or more imaging technologies including cardiac magnetic resonance imaging,[36] computed tomographic angiography,[37] and intracardiac echocardiography.[38] During the procedure, movement of the ablation catheter within the left atrium is guided by fluoroscopy, intracardiac echocardiography, and electroanatomic mapping systems that employ a "global positioning system" to track the movement of the catheter in a three-dimensional computer-rendered geometry.[39,40] The result of ablation is electrical isolation of the pulmonary vein myocardial sleeve from the remainder of the heart. The acute success rate of pulmonary vein isolation approaches 100%, but if any tissue along the ablation line is damaged but not destroyed, there may be recovery of electrical conduction along this

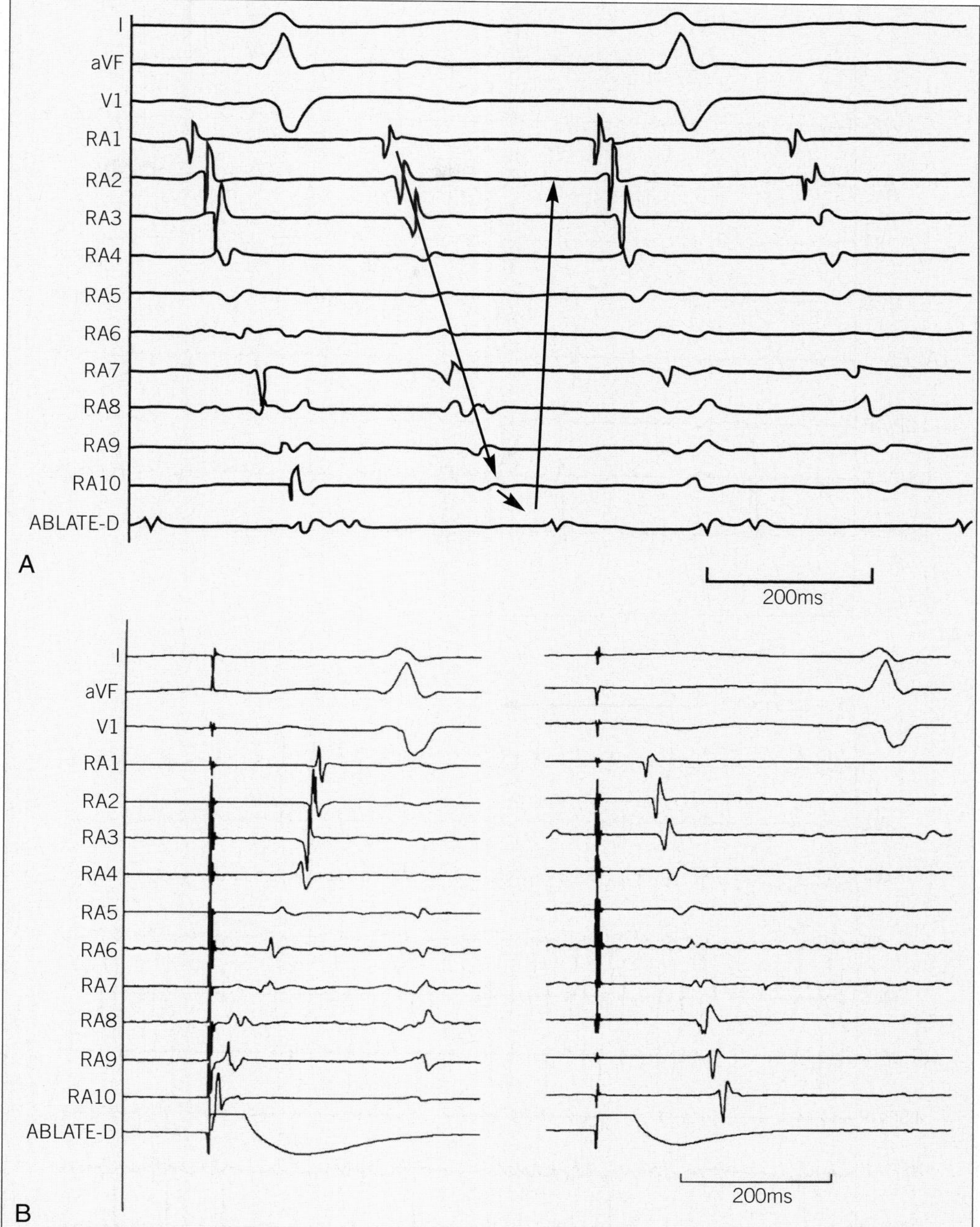

Figure 51.4 Ablation of atrial flutter. Surface leads I, aVF, and V_1 and intracardiac electrograms from a 10-bipole electrode positioned in the right atrium around the tricuspid annulus. The distal electrodes (RA1) are positioned at the low lateral right atrium, electrode pairs RA2 to RA9 are along the free wall and roof of the right atrium, and the proximal electrodes (RA10) are positioned near the interatrial septum. A roving mapping-ablation catheter (ABLATE-D) is located in the tricuspid–inferior vena cava isthmus. **A,** The activation pattern of ongoing type I (counterclockwise) atrial flutter is indicated by the arrows. **B,** After successful linear ablation in the tricuspid–inferior vena cava isthmus, bidirectional isthmus block is confirmed. *Left,* Intra-atrial conduction from low septal pacing. Note that the interatrial septum and high atrial free wall are activated early, and activation of the low lateral atrium (RA1) is late despite anatomic proximity (on opposite sides of the ablation line) of the RA1 and the pacing electrode. *Right,* Atrial activation during low lateral pacing. In this case, the atrial free wall activation is low to high, and the septal activation is latest.

line as the tissue heals, resulting in electrical reconnection of the pulmonary vein to the atrium.[41] This accounts for the recurrence rates after a single procedure of 30% to 60%. With two or more ablation procedures, however, long-term success can be achieved in 70% to 86% of patients, depending on selection criteria.[42-44]

The opposite end of the spectrum of atrial fibrillation is characterized by patients who have a pattern of chronic or persistent atrial fibrillation, tend to be older, and have structural heart disease with left atrial enlargement. It is hypothesized that the dominant mechanism of atrial fibrillation in these patients is re-entry. During this arrhythmia, one or

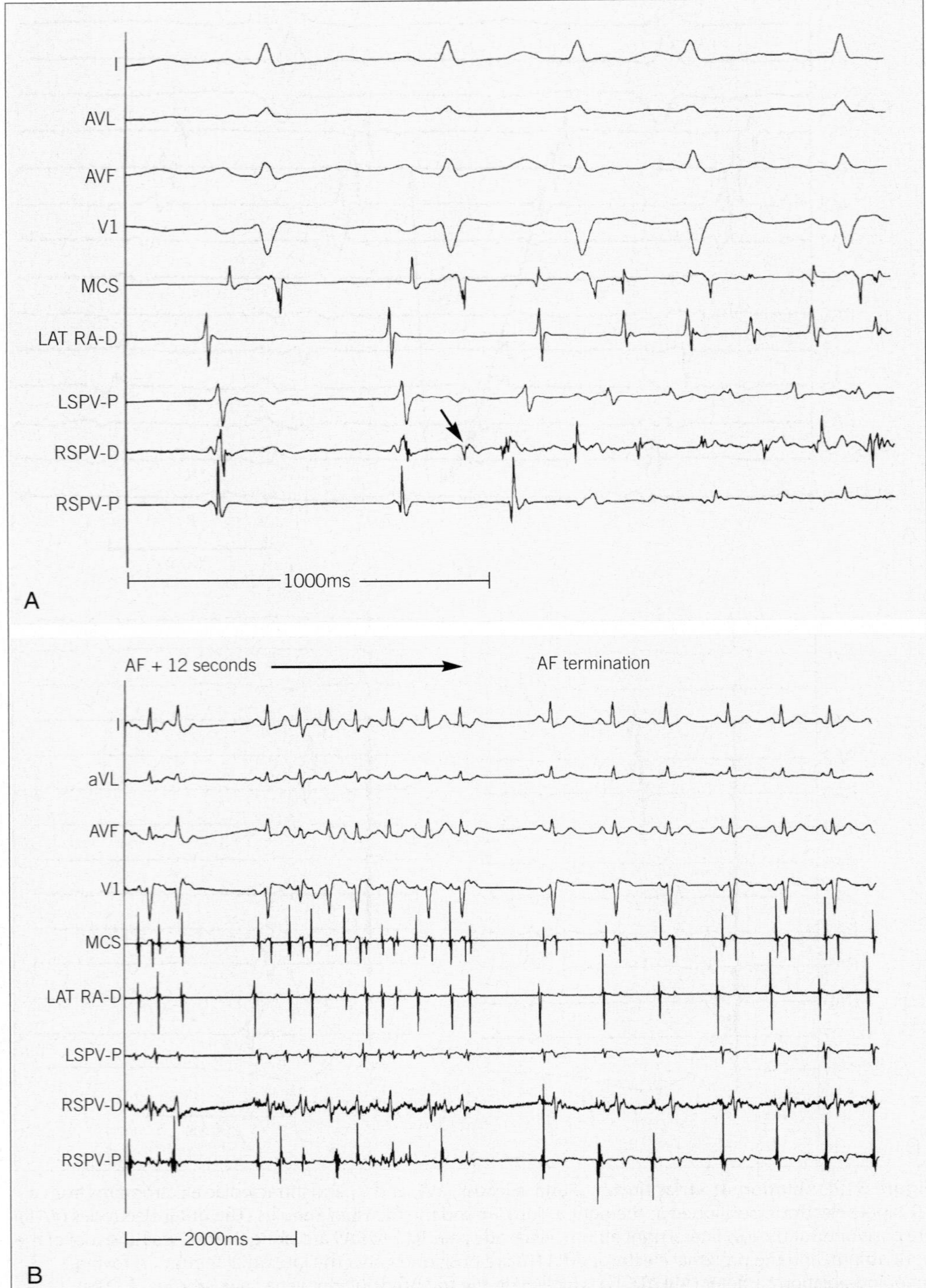

Figure 51.5 Ablation of atrial fibrillation of focal origin. Surface leads I, aVL, aVF, and V_1 and intracardiac electrograms from the middle coronary sinus (MCS), the lateral right atrium (LAT RA-D), the proximal bipole of a quadripolar catheter positioned in the left superior pulmonary vein (LSPV-P), and the distal and proximal bipoles of a catheter in the right superior pulmonary vein (RSPV-D and RSPV-P, respectively). **A,** Initiation of atrial fibrillation from a focal source in the RSPV as indicated by earliest atrial activation near to the distal bipole of the catheter in this position *(arrow)* and a spread of activation to the remaining atrial recording sites. **B,** Application of radiofrequency energy to this site results in termination of this arrhythmia and clinical cure. AF, atrial fibrillation.

more vortex-like waves of electrical activity called rotors activate the atria at high rates. Similar to the response to focal firing, the propagating waves break into fibrillatory conduction. The heterogeneity of conduction and block, in turn, creates reactivation wavefronts and stimulates formation of new rotors.[45] Treatment of this type of arrhythmia with ablation requires extraostial pulmonary vein isolation in addition to aggressive modification of broad regions of atrial myocardium that participate in the propagation of the re-entrant wavefronts. Areas with patterns of complex fractionated atrial electrograms are hypothesized to correlate with the location of the rotor drivers and are specifically targeted for ablation.[46] Autonomic modulation may play an important role in suppressing atrial fibrillation with ablation. Several ganglionic plexuses are anatomically situated at the base of the pulmonary veins. Ablation of these regions may reduce vagal stimulation of the atria and reduce vagally mediated atrial fibrillation.[47] With use of an aggressive stepwise ablation approach, persistent and chronic atrial fibrillation can be cured in 50% to 74% of patients.[44,48,49]

When patients are not candidates for curative catheter ablation and standard treatments such as suppressive antiarrhythmic drugs and rate-controlling drugs are unsuccessful, effective rate control can be achieved with catheter ablation of the AV junction and creation of complete heart block. Although the resultant junctional escape rhythm is usually adequate to prevent hemodynamic embarrassment, it is not adequate to maintain normal hemodynamics and exercise tolerance. For that reason, AV junctional ablation is always accompanied by placement of a rate-responsive permanent pacemaker. Of note, despite restoration of a regular resting and exercise heart rate with this approach, the atria continue to fibrillate, and therefore chronic anticoagulation is still required.

Automatic atrial tachycardia (also ectopic or focal atrial tachycardia) is a tachycardia of focal origin from the left or right atrial chamber. The most common sites of origin of these arrhythmias are the crista terminalis in the right atrium and the pulmonary veins in the left atrium. Limited clinical series of catheter ablation of these arrhythmias report success rates of 80% to 96%.[50] Atrial arrhythmias that have a P-wave morphology identical to that seen during normal sinus rhythm most likely have their origin from the sinoatrial node or its surrounding tissue. The arrhythmia mechanism can be re-entrant or automatic. Sinoatrial re-entrant tachycardia may be eliminated with focal ablation in more than 95% of cases.[51] In contrast, the automatic tachycardia termed inappropriate sinus tachycardia does not have a discrete focal origin and instead appears to be a disorder of enhanced responsiveness to normal sympathetic stimulation (see Chapters 53 and 57).[52] Ablation may be considered in patients who are refractory to drug treatment, but extensive ablation of the sinus node region and the superior portions of the crista terminalis is required to achieve any modification of the sinus node activity.[53] Unfortunately, the high rate of recurrence of arrhythmia and the significant risk of excessive sinus node ablation requiring permanent pacemaker implantation limit the utility of this procedure.

Ventricular Arrhythmias

Ventricular tachycardia may sometimes be found in patients with no underlying structural heart disease. The most common sites of origin are the ventricular outflow tract (right more common than left) and the left ventricle in the area of the left posterior fascicle. Outflow tract tachycardias usually have a left bundle branch block morphology and inferior electrocardiographic axis and are focal in origin. They have a relatively high cure rate (>90%) with focal endocardial ablation techniques.[54] When these arrhythmias arise from the left ventricular outflow tract, catheter access is more challenging because they are usually subepicardial in location. Success can be achieved with ablation by way of a transthoracic pericardial puncture, from the coronary venous system, or from the aortic root with ablation through the aortic valve leaflet to the summit of the ventricle.[55] In addition to these patients, some presenting with very symptomatic high-density or complex premature ventricular contractions (>20,000 in a 24-hour period) are good candidates for focal catheter ablation of outflow tract premature ventricular complex sites. Left ventricular fascicular tachycardias are unusual in that they are re-entrant in mechanism and are usually verapamil sensitive. They typically have a right bundle branch block morphology and a leftward axis. During mapping, the site of arrhythmia origin shows a high-frequency potential preceding the local ventricular activation that represents local fascicular activation. Catheter ablation at that location results in successful elimination of the tachycardia in more than 90% of cases.[56]

In the setting of structural heart disease and ventricular scar, slowed electrical conduction through regions of patchy fibrosis is the substrate for re-entry and leads to the common form of ventricular tachycardia.[57] Catheter ablation is one of several therapeutic options in patients with re-entrant ventricular tachycardia. In patients with severely depressed ventricular function, it is most commonly used in conjunction with an implantable cardioverter-defibrillator. During ablation procedures, sites critical for arrhythmia propagation can be identified by mapping the circuit of electrical activation during induced tachycardia and identifying the critical slow conduction zone (Fig. 51.6). If the tachycardia is not hemodynamically tolerated, the substrate can be mapped with a three-dimensional computerized mapping system that identifies regions of low-voltage scar. Ablation at the border zone of scar or across a narrow isthmus of tissue between contiguous scars will usually favorably modify the clinical tachycardia.[58] Ventricular tachycardia ablation has been shown to be very successful as palliative therapy in the setting of frequent implantable cardioverter-defibrillator discharges[59] and has also been proved to reduce clinical occurrence of ventricular tachycardia when it is used prophylactically in patients with implantable cardioverter-defibrillators.[60]

COMPLICATIONS

Catheter ablation is generally safe and effective for treatment of patients with symptomatic arrhythmias. However, as with any procedure that requires catheter placement and manipulation in the heart, complications may occur. When decisions are being made about referral of a patient for curative catheter ablation, particularly when the indication for the procedure is the desire for a drug-free lifestyle, the risks of the procedure must be carefully weighed relative to the anticipated benefit, and patients should be fully informed.

The overall risk of complications is approximately 3%, with a risk of serious, irreversible complications of 0.5% to 1%. These risks include heart block, stroke, and valve injury. The reported risk of death due to catheter ablation ranges from 0% to 0.06%. In addition, significant reversible complications have been reported, including vascular injury (0.6%), pericardial tamponade (0.21% to 0.6%), and pulmonary embolism (0% to 0.13%).[61,62] A rare but devastating complication of atrial fibrillation ablation is esophageal injury with atrioesophageal fistula.[48,63]

The final risk to patient and operator alike is that of exposure to radiation. Whereas fluoroscopy time with diagnostic

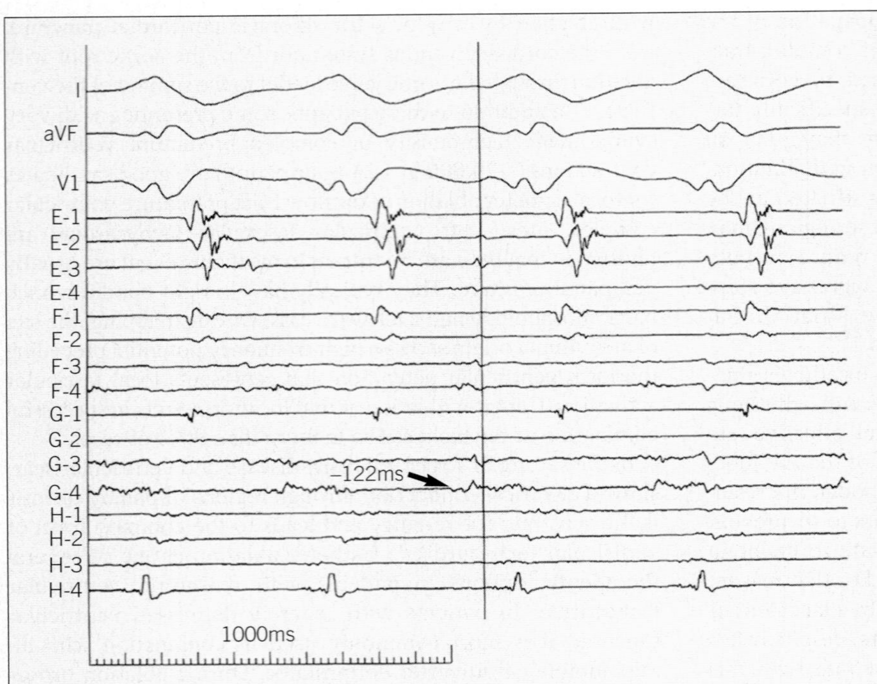

Figure 51.6 Cardiac recordings in ventricular tachycardia. Surface leads I, aVF, and V_1 and intracardiac electrograms from one half of a 64-pole basket electrode catheter positioned in the left ventricle during ongoing ventricular tachycardia. Bipolar recordings from each electrode pair (1-4, distal to proximal) on each of splines E to H are displayed. The mapping site from the proximal bipole of the G spline (G-4) shows local fractionated diastolic activity that precedes the onset of the surface QRS complex by 122 ms and corresponds with the slow conduction zone of the re-entrant circuit.

electrophysiologic procedures is usually less than 10 minutes, manipulation of catheters to ablation targets can result in prolonged exposure, occasionally exceeding 1 hour. Studies have translated this exposure into a lifetime risk of radiation-induced fatal malignant disease of 0.03% for every hour of fluoroscopic exposure and a risk of genetic defects of 20 per 1 million births.[64] As many patients undergoing catheter ablation are young, this risk must be considered.

SUMMARY

Catheter ablation has established itself as one of the most effective treatment modalities in cardiology today. Unlike most therapies for most diseases, catheter ablation is truly curative in many cases. This, coupled with a low rate of procedure-related complications, has led to a dramatic growth in its use during the past decade. Experienced operators can achieve successful ablation of the common forms of paroxysmal supraventricular tachycardia in more than 95% of cases. This success has led to expansion of the list of indications for this procedure, including focal atrial tachycardia, atrial flutter, idiopathic ventricular tachycardia, and re-entrant ventricular tachycardia in the setting of structural heart disease. Catheter ablation has most recently been pursued as a curative strategy in patients with atrial fibrillation, with improving outcomes as experience increases and ablation tools improve. It may become first-line therapy in selected patients, but its long-term durability remains to be proved. New techniques, new technologies, and new insights into the mechanisms of arrhythmia will continue to expand the horizons of catheter ablation in the years to come.

chapter 52

Syncope

Andrew D. Krahn, Raymond Yee, Allan C. Skanes, Lorne J. Gula, and George J. Klein

Definition

- Syncope is the transient loss of consciousness associated with loss of postural tone, with spontaneous recovery that does not require intervention.

Key Features

- Syncope is difficult to diagnose because the underlying cause is often transient, infrequent, and unpredictable. A diagnosis is obtained in only 75%, even after extensive testing.
- Testing is divided into baseline clinical assessment, passive monitoring tests, and active provocative testing to reproduce an episode.
- The majority of causes are cardiac, with neurocardiogenic and arrhythmias the leading diagnoses.
- Detection of significant underlying heart disease is important for assessing risk and directing investigations because of risk of ventricular arrhythmias.

Therapy

- Once a diagnosis is obtained, therapy directed at the cause is usually effective, including lifestyle modification, pharmacologic therapy, pacing, or an implantable defibrillator.

To a historical purist, the word *syncope* was originally meant for transient loss of consciousness due to reduced cardiac output. The term has evolved and has become synonymous with transient loss of consciousness regardless of ultimate etiology. Syncope is a common disorder, affecting 30% of adults at some point during their life.[1] Syncope is responsible for 1% to 6% of emergency department visits and 0.6% to 1.0% of hospital admissions.[2-4] This has a large impact on health care costs, influenced by the extent of investigation and the nature of treatment. There is a bimodal pattern of age at presentation: a peak during adolescence and early adulthood that is predominantly neurocardiogenic syncope; and a second peak in the sixth and seventh decades reflecting arrhythmias from organic or degenerative heart disease.[1] Patients who suffer from syncope may experience significant morbidity from the trauma related to the episode, or they may experience indirect adverse effects from loss of employment or personal freedom related to inability to drive a vehicle or to perform their jobs. Syncope is a marker of risk for sudden death in patients with structural heart disease.

Syncope is a complex clinical entity with multiple causes that can be difficult to diagnose. The major obstacles to diagnosis are the periodic and unpredictable nature of events and the high spontaneous remission rate. The cause of recurrent syncope is often difficult to determine if the diagnosis is not evident from initial clinical and laboratory investigations.[5,6] Physiologic monitoring during spontaneous syncope constitutes the "gold standard" for diagnosis of cardiovascular causes of syncope. This is frequently unattainable. Clinicians often rely on clinical assessment and abnormal laboratory results to make an inferential diagnosis and subsequent therapeutic decision. Advances in long-term cardiac monitoring techniques have added a powerful tool to the diagnostic armamentarium.

ANATOMY AND PHYSIOLOGY

Syncope is a symptom that can arise from a number of pathophysiologic substrates. In the majority of cases, syncope is caused by transient loss of neurologic function due to loss of cerebral blood flow. Sudden reduction or cessation of cerebral blood flow results in reduced activity in the reticular activation center. If this process is of sufficient severity and duration, the patient will experience presyncope followed by syncope. During sustained episodes of hypotension, patients may experience other manifestations of altered neurologic function, including urinary or fecal incontinence and seizure activity. Primary neurologic dysfunction without an alteration in cerebral blood flow can also cause loss of consciousness that is usually accompanied by other evidence of neurologic dysfunction.

PATHOPHYSIOLOGY

The underlying pathophysiologic mechanism that leads to loss of consciousness covers a wide range of disease processes (Table 52.1). The unifying feature in the majority of syncopal episodes is a sudden reduction in cerebral blood flow. Sudden cessation of cerebral blood flow results in loss of consciousness within 4 to 10 seconds, based on a study testing rapid inflation of a neck cuff to 600 mm Hg.[7] Varying degrees and duration of reduction of blood flow may result in presyncope or syncope.

Pathophysiologic Approach

One conceptual approach to the underlying cause of syncope is presented in Figure 52.1. Rather than listing all potential causes of syncope, it is easier to consider broad categories based on the underlying pathophysiologic process, including vasomotor causes, arrhythmias, other cardiovascular causes, and noncardiovascular causes. One large series examined 433 patients presenting with syncope to the emergency department, to a primary care setting, or during hospitalization.[8] The cause of syncope was assigned after initial investigation and 40 months

PATHOPHYSIOLOGIC CLASSIFICATION OF SUDDEN LOSS OF CONSCIOUSNESS		
Cardiovascular		
Arrhythmias	Bradycardia	Sinus bradycardia or pause
		Atrioventricular block
	Tachycardia	Supraventricular tachycardia
		Ventricular tachycardia
	Mixed	Bradycardia-tachycardia syndrome
		Torsades de pointes
		Long QT syndrome
Obstruction	Left ventricular	Aortic stenosis
		Hypertrophic cardiomyopathy
		Rare forms, such as subvalvular web
	Other	Intracardiac tumors
		Mitral stenosis
Vasomotor		Neurocardiogenic (vasovagal)
		Postural tachycardia syndrome
		Postural hypotension
		Carotid sinus hypersensitivity
		Situational syncope (e.g., micturition, cough, defecation)
Noncardiovascular		
Neurologic		Seizure disorder
		Cerebrovascular accident
		Autonomic neuropathy
Endocrine (hypoglycemia)		
Pulmonary embolism		
Psychogenic		

Table 52.1 Pathophysiologic classification of sudden loss of consciousness.

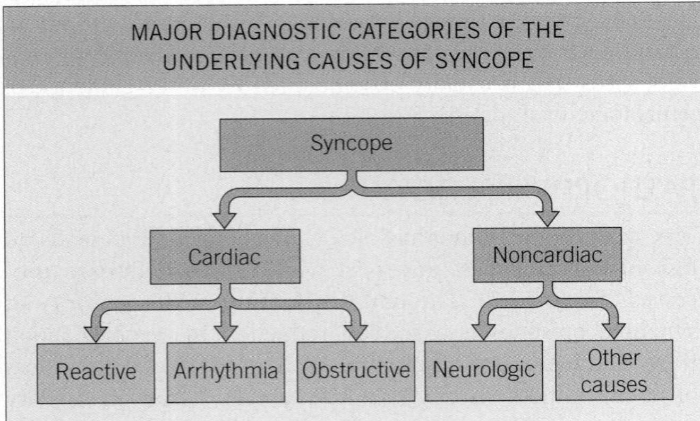

Figure 52.1 Major diagnostic categories of the underlying causes of syncope. The most common diagnoses are vasomotor or reactive syncope and arrhythmias.

THE CAUSE OF SYNCOPE IN 254 PATIENTS DIAGNOSED DURING INITIAL ASSESSMENT AND FOLLOW-UP*		
Cause	N	%
Cardiovascular	**229**	**90.2**
Arrhythmias	87	34.3
Bradycardia	30	11.8
Sinus bradycardia or pause	4	1.6
Bradycardia-tachycardia syndrome	15	5.9
Atrioventricular block	8	3.2
Pacemaker malfunction	3	1.2
Tachycardia	57	22.4
Supraventricular	8	3.2
Ventricular	47	18.5
Torsades de pointes	2	0.8
Other	14	5.5
Aortic stenosis	8	3.2
Myocardial infarction	5	2.0
Dissecting aortic aneurysm	1	0.4
Vasomotor	128	50.4
Neurocardiogenic (vasovagal)	35	3.8
Drug induced	9	3.5
Postural hypotension	43	16.9
Carotid sinus hypersensitivity	5	2.0
Situational syncope	36	14.2
Noncardiovascular	**25**	**9.8**
Neurologic	18	7.1
Seizure disorder	7	2.8
Cerebrovascular	8	3.2
Other	3	1.2
Pulmonary embolism or hypertension	4	1.6
Psychogenic	3	1.2

*A cause for syncope was not established in 179 patients (41%).
Modified from Kapoor WN. Evaluation and outcome of patients with syncope. Medicine (Baltimore) 1990;69:160-175. See text for discussion.

Table 52.2 The cause of syncope in 254 patients diagnosed during initial assessment and follow-up.

of follow-up in 254 patients (58.7%; Table 52.2). Cardiovascular causes accounted for 90.2% of diagnosed cases, with vasomotor or reactive causes by far the most common, accounting for 50.4% of patients. This included neurocardiogenic syncope with or without a clinical precipitant in 28.0% and orthostatic hypotension in 16.9%. Arrhythmias accounted for 34.3% of causes, with a high incidence of nonsustained ventricular tachycardia (19.3%). This series was reported before the use of prolonged monitoring strategies with external or implantable loop recorders. Because bradycardia is often intermittent, it may have been detected less frequently than with current diagnostic techniques. This series was biased toward diagnosis of ventricular tachycardia, accepting nonsustained ventricular tachycardia as diagnostic in 39 patients (15.4%). Nonetheless, these data highlight the fact that syncope is usually a cardiovascular disorder and that vasomotor and arrhythmic causes predominate in those patients who are ultimately diagnosed.

Arrhythmias

Either bradyarrhythmias or tachyarrhythmias may cause syncope. In situations in which a symptom-rhythm correlation can be obtained, bradyarrhythmias are more common, particularly in the elderly. Excessively rapid or slow rates are often associated with hemodynamic compromise, but the majority of nonsustained and even sustained arrhythmias are surprisingly well tolerated. The rate of heart rate change is often more important than the absolute heart rate, with symptoms often most pronounced immediately after the onset of an arrhythmia. The adaptation of the peripheral vasculature to a sudden change in heart rate with attendant fall in cardiac output strongly influences the severity of symptoms.

Neurocardiogenic Syncope

The underlying pathophysiologic mechanism of neurocardiogenic syncope is incompletely understood. This is reflected in the many synonyms used to describe it, including vasovagal syncope, neurally mediated syncope, and vasodepressor syncope. When an individual stands, there is gravity-mediated displacement of blood resulting in a fall in venous return to the heart. The resultant fall in cardiac output and blood pressure is sensed by arterial baroreceptors, primarily located in the carotid sinus and aortic arch. These baroreceptors send afferent signals to the medulla, resulting in a centrally mediated increase in sympathetic tone. Myocardial C fibers respond to stretch or pressure by sending afferent projections centrally to the medulla, also influencing vagal output. As a result of these adaptive responses, there is often little postural change in blood pressure in normal individuals.

Although the exact nature of the "misfire" in neurocardiogenic syncope is unknown, several postulates have been suggested.[9] One hypothesis involves excessive venous pooling with a marked reduction in venous return. The resultant ventricular volume reduction combined with a reflex increase in sympathetically mediated contractility exerts a marked pressure effect on myocardial C fibers. This triggers a paradoxical overshoot of sympathetic withdrawal and increase in vagal activity. Another explanation suggests a disorder of central sympathetic regulation because a reduction in sympathetic nerve traffic has been observed just before syncope in patients undergoing tilt testing.[10] This decrease may be abrupt or gradual and is associated with a baseline alteration in the response of sympathetic baroreflex mechanisms to orthostatic stress. Central factors that may play a role in this include serotonin, opiates, and cerebrovascular autoregulation.

There are several variants of neurocardiogenic syncope in which a specific precipitant can be identified. This is termed situational syncope, which includes a number of triggers for a "vasovagal" type of reaction. These are likely to represent a family of forms of reflex syncope, in which the afferent stimulus is variable with a similar efferent. Specific triggers include micturition, cough, defecation, deglutition, and the sight of blood. The mechanism in these settings is presumed to relate to abrupt changes in venous return and autonomic tone.

There is substantial overlap between the clinical features of neurocardiogenic syncope and chronic fatigue syndrome. Bou-Holaigah and associates[11] compared tilt test results of 23 patients with chronic fatigue syndrome with those of 14 healthy controls. A positive response was observed in 22 of 23 chronic fatigue patients and 4 controls (96% versus 29%; p = .0001). Typical symptoms in chronic fatigue patients were aggravated or reproduced by tilting, including chronic lightheadedness, nausea, and diaphoresis. This study suggests a link between chronic fatigue syndrome and neurocardiogenic syncope, although the underlying pathophysiologic process of chronic fatigue syndrome remains ill defined.

Several variants of autonomically mediated syncope and presyncope exist. This includes postural tachycardia syndrome, which is characterized by exaggerated sinus tachycardia during standing associated with a minimal fall in blood pressure.[12] These patients are more likely to experience presyncope than syncope and often complain of chronic fatigue, dizziness, and exercise intolerance. This syndrome may represent an early form of autonomic dysfunction that shares many characteristics with chronic fatigue syndrome and inappropriate sinus tachycardia. Altered norepinephrine reuptake is a genetically mediated disease caused by a point mutation on chromosome 18 that leads to failure to reuptake norepinephrine in the postsynaptic cleft, leading to initial hypertension and subsequent failure to maintain blood pressure as norepinephrine levels drop, with attendant presyncope or syncope.[13-15] This uncommon condition is diagnosed by measurement of supine and upright catecholamine levels.

Orthostatic Hypotension

Standing invokes a series of adaptations that compensate for gravitational pooling of blood in the abdomen and lower limbs. When venous return and blood pressure fall, carotid and aortic arch baroreceptor stimulation results in peripheral vasoconstriction and venoconstriction, and cardiac mechanoreceptors are inhibited. The ability to maintain blood pressure in the face of prolonged standing is largely dependent on the carotid baroreceptor and to some degree on neurohormonal mechanisms. Primary chronic autonomic failure associated with other idiopathic neurologic defects was initially described by Shy and Drager.[16] It has more recently been termed multiple system atrophy. This condition is marked by postural hypotension associated with multiple manifestations of autonomic dysfunction. Secondary autonomic dysfunction leading to orthostatic hypotension can be caused by a number of disorders including diabetes, Parkinson's disease, and multiple sclerosis. It is also seen in elderly patients in the absence of a primary process. The most common cause of postural hypotension is drug induced. This is often seen in patients receiving antihypertensive therapy who have labile blood pressure. Agents well known to cause or to exacerbate hypotension include diuretics, vasodilators, angiotensin-converting enzyme inhibitors, calcium channel blockers, and alcohol.

Neurologic Causes of Loss of Consciousness

Seizures may present as unexplained loss of consciousness, particularly with a first event. In general, it is not difficult to distinguish seizures from syncope on the basis of a clinical assessment including an interview of an observer. The exception to this is the atonic seizure (drop attack) or akinetic seizure, most commonly seen in children with transient loss of consciousness without a postictal state. The electroencephalogram is frequently abnormal in this setting. The frequency of seizures as an explanation for syncope in published series is highly variable but probably represents a small proportion of cases.[1]

Cerebrovascular disease is a rare cause of syncope. Isolated syncope due to cerebral ischemia without other neurologic manifestations on history and physical examination is unlikely. Nonetheless, transient or sustained vertebrobasilar ischemia may lead to vertigo, dizziness, syncope, speech changes, and memory loss. Vascular disease other than atherosclerosis, including various forms of arteritis and subclavian steal syndrome, may also cause these changes. Autonomic disorders leading to hypotension are discussed under orthostatic hypotension (see earlier).

CLINICAL PRESENTATION

History

Syncope represents a collection of symptoms and signs that may be caused by a number of different underlying disease processes. Patients with syncope may use a number of different terms to describe their episodes, including dizziness, fainting, lightheadedness, and blackouts. A prodrome is seen in many patients, which may last from less than a second to several minutes. Sheldon and colleagues[17] have developed a structured set of syncope questionnaires to discriminate mechanisms of syncope on the basis of historical features. A simple 9-point questionnaire generates a score that can be very useful in discriminating mechanism of loss of consciousness, particularly for primary care physicians (Table 52.3). The typical characteristics of the three most common mechanisms of syncope are summarized in Table 52.4.

Patients with neurocardiogenic syncope typically report feeling warm with diaphoresis and a sense of "graying out" before loss of consciousness. Although this is classically described in neurocardiogenic syncope, any patient who is experiencing a fall in blood pressure may report it. The majority of episodes occur in the upright posture, occasionally while sitting and very rarely in the supine position. Patients often report additional presyncopal episodes, with the ability to avert syncope by sitting or lying down quickly. Patients are usually unresponsive for less than a minute, are often fatigued after an episode, but are oriented and responsive within minutes.[17] Patients may complain of fatigue for hours or even days after an episode.

The classic Stokes-Adams attack is seen in patients who develop sudden bradycardia, originally described in patients with atrioventricular (AV) block.[18,19] Similar features would be expected with a transient tachycardia. Patients describe sudden collapse with minimal or no warning, with consciousness resuming within seconds to minutes. Patients will often suffer injury if attacks occur while standing. Patients presenting with this historical "profile" should undergo investigations tailored to detection of an arrhythmic cause. The key historical clue to detection of a cardiac cause for syncope is the presence of previous heart disease by history, often confirmed by physical examination and laboratory testing.

Additional important historical clues may point the clinician in the direction of other diagnoses (see Table 52.4). A history of palpitations may suggest an underlying tachycardia. Patients with irregular palpitations may be describing atrial fibrillation, which is often associated with sinus node disease in the bradycardia-tachycardia syndrome. The typical episode of syncope or presyncope occurs when atrial fibrillation terminates, followed by a prolonged pause (see Chapter 53). Seizure activity including incontinence, tonic-clonic movements, tongue biting, and a prolonged postictal state characterized by confusion and somnolence strongly suggests a primary seizure disorder. Patients who suffer prolonged hypotension may develop secondary seizure activity, which can be mistaken for epilepsy. In the Framingham study, the risk factors for syncope were hypertension, cardiac medication, and previous stroke or transient ischemic attack,[20] probably reflecting an aging population with transient hypotension causing symptoms.

Finally, syncope may present as a secondary diagnosis in patients whose primary complaint is related to the trauma suffered from the syncopal episode. This includes patients with unexplained motor vehicle accidents, orthopedic injury such as hip fracture in the elderly secondary to a fall, and soft tissue injuries including burns and lacerations.

DIAGNOSTIC QUESTIONS DIFFERENTIATING SEIZURE DISORDER FROM SYNCOPE

Historical Question	Diagnostic Score for Positive Response
At times do you wake with a cut tongue after your spells?	2
At times do you have a sense of déjà vu or jamais vu before your spells?	1
At times is emotional stress associated with losing consciousness?	1
Has anyone ever noted your head turning during a spell?	1
Has anyone ever noted that you are unresponsive, have unusual posturing or have jerking limbs during your spells, or have no memory of your spells afterward?	1 for any positive response
Has anyone ever noted that you are confused after a spell?	1
Have you ever had lightheaded spells?	−2
At times do you sweat before spells?	−2
Is prolonged sitting or standing associated with your spells?	−2

Diagnostic score ≥ 1: diagnosis of seizure disorder.
Diagnostic score < 1: diagnosis of syncope.
Modified from Sheldon R, Rose S, Ritchie D, et al. Historical criteria that distinguish syncope from seizures. J Am Coll Cardiol 2002;40:142-148.

Table 52.3 Diagnostic questions differentiating seizure disorder from syncope.

KEY FINDINGS DURING CLINICAL ASSESSMENT OF LOSS OF CONSCIOUSNESS			
History	**Arrhythmic**	**Neurocardiogenic**	**Seizure**
Character of prodrome	Short palpitations	Warm, diaphoresis, nausea, darkening vision	Aura; may be none
Duration of loss of consciousness	Seconds to minutes	Usually <60 seconds	Variable
Seizure activity	Unlikely	Rare	Always
Time to complete recovery	Seconds to minutes	Minutes	Minutes to hours
Presyncopal spells without syncope	Sometimes	Often	Rare
Relationship of episodes to posture	None; may be worse upright	Usually upright	None
Associated palpitations	Sometimes	Sometimes	None
Physical examination			
Postural blood pressure changes	No	Often	No
Physical signs of obstructive cardiac etiology	No	No	No
Evidence of other structural heart disease	Often	No	No
Neurologic deficit	No	No	Often
Maneuvers			
Valsalva	No effect	No effect	No effect
Carotid sinus massage	May see bradycardia	May see bradycardia	No effect

Table 52.4 Key findings during clinical assessment of loss of consciousness.

Physical Examination

The key purpose of the physical examination is to identify comorbidities that remain evident after the episode and that may explain or contribute to syncope. This process is frequently not productive. Blood pressure and heart rate should be checked lying, immediately after standing, and after 3 minutes of standing. The cardiovascular examination should focus on detection of structural heart disease, in particular conditions that could lead to obstruction of blood flow. These include aortic stenosis, hypertrophic cardiomyopathy, and intracardiac tumors. More common forms of structural heart disease, such as coronary artery disease, left ventricular dysfunction, and hypertrophy, may not contribute directly to a diagnosis but are important for assessing risk and directing investigations based on clinical index of suspicion. A neurologic assessment is useful to detect deficits that suggest seizures or to document the postictal state if assessment is performed soon after a seizure.

Adjuncts to the Physical Examination

Several tests or maneuvers have been suggested to enhance the diagnostic yield of the physical examination. Postural change in blood pressure has already been mentioned. The Valsalva maneuver is useful to bring out latent left ventricular outflow tract obstruction. Carotid sinus massage is useful when carotid sinus syncope (or hypersensitivity) is suspected. This is a form of neurally mediated syncope characterized by syncope or presyncope associated with sinus bradycardia, arrest, or AV block that can be reproduced by applying pressure to the carotid sinus. Before carotid sinus massage is performed, the artery should be auscultated. If a bruit is heard, carotid sinus massage is contraindicated. After the carotid is palpated, firm pressure should be applied at the level of the carotid bifurcation in the direction of the vertebra for 5 seconds. Some clinicians advocate constant pressure, whereas others use a massaging motion. This can be performed on the opposite side after a 30-second rest period. The test is normally performed with electrocardiographic and blood pressure monitoring in the supine position. Performance of carotid sinus massage in the upright position enhances the sensitivity of the test.[21,22] The risk of neurologic complications from carotid sinus massage is 0.28%.[23]

The normal response to carotid sinus massage is slowing of the sinus rate (and at times AV conduction); a 3-second pause represents the upper limit of normal. A positive test response is defined as cardioinhibitory when there is a pause longer than 3 seconds or vasodepressor when there is a fall in blood pressure of 50 mm Hg that is not associated with bradycardia. There is often a component of both vasodepression and inappropriate low heart rate or pause. Because asymptomatic pauses can be seen in patients with a history of syncope from other causes and in asymptomatic healthy elderly persons, carotid sinus syncope should be diagnosed only when a positive test response reproduces symptoms or there is strong clinical suspicion that the observed changes reflect the underlying cause of syncope.

DIAGNOSTIC TECHNIQUES

The history and physical examination remain the cornerstone of the diagnostic process. In many patients, the underlying cause of syncope is intermittent and infrequent, or it may be constant but its manifestation may be infrequent. The sporadic nature of syncope makes a simple profile of the patient at the time of presentation unlikely to provide a certain diagnosis. The clinician must integrate the patient's profile, the description of the syncopal event, the findings on physical examination, and the results of subsequent diagnostic testing to arrive at a clinical diagnosis.

Testing in syncope patients may be considered under three broad categories. The first involves acquiring a profile of the patient at the time of presentation, including clinical assessment, resting electrocardiogram, and investigations that characterize the patient's cardiac and neurologic status. This includes tests such as short-term electrocardiographic monitoring, echocardiography, electroencephalography, and blood work. This phase of investigation will provide a presumptive diagnosis when the presentation is typical for a clinically recognized disorder such as neurocardiogenic syncope or a persistent abnormality is detected that is inferred to have caused the syncopal episode, such as persistent AV block that was presumed to be associated with a prolonged pause causing the index syncopal event. The profile is also useful to estimate prognosis.

The second category involves provocative testing in an attempt to reproduce a syncopal episode or to detect an abnormal physiologic response that can be inferred to explain the preceding syncopal episode. This includes tests such as tilt table testing, electrophysiologic study, and sleep-deprived electroencephalography. These tests are often useful when initial testing is not productive but require considerable clinical judgment to be interpreted because they represent an "artificial" physiologic response. The induced abnormality may not be observed (sensitivity) or may be incidental to the real cause of syncope (specificity).

The final form of testing involves physiologic monitoring in the hope that the patient will experience a spontaneous episode of syncope that can be correlated with the physiologic parameter being monitored. At present, this is possible for electrocardiographic monitoring with Holter monitoring and external and implantable loop recorders. The ideal test for syncope (which does not exist) would involve comprehensive physiologic monitoring during a spontaneous episode, including cardiac, vascular, and neurologic function. This strategy is limited by the reliance on a recurrence of syncope, which may be associated with risk of injury and even death, particularly when the patient is at risk for ventricular arrhythmias.

Electrocardiographic Monitoring

Assessment of the resting electrocardiogram with short-term electrocardiographic monitoring is the most common initial investigation and should be performed in all patients. This is typically performed in the emergency department immediately after presentation or in a primary care setting. This yielded a diagnosis in 6.9% of patients in one series,[8] with ongoing episodes of bradycardia or AV block in 40% of those 6.9% of patients, tachycardia in 43%, and acute myocardial infarction in 17%. The observed abnormalities on electrocardiography must be carefully correlated with the clinical presentation because the findings may be asymptomatic or unrelated to the actual cause of syncope.

Ambulatory monitoring by Holter monitoring or in-patient telemetry is performed in the majority of patients who present with syncope. A critical review of published data on the utility of this approach suggests that it should play a more limited role. Syncope recurred in 4% of patients during monitoring from various series (range, 1% to 26%),[24,25] suggesting a low likelihood of establishing a symptom-rhythm correlation. This is not surprising, given the infrequent sporadic nature of syncope. In contrast, some form of asymptomatic arrhythmia, such as sinus pauses, AV block, or nonsustained ventricular tachycardia, occurred in 13% of cases. These findings may provide clinically useful information that contributes to a diagnosis but must be interpreted with caution. Presyncope is more likely to recur than syncope during any form of monitoring but is much less likely to be associated with an arrhythmia.[26,27] In addition, the "presyncope" may not necessarily be of the same cause as the clinical syncope. Nonetheless, short-term monitoring is useful in some patients in whom a rhythm profile is sought, even though symptoms are unlikely to recur during monitoring. In a primary care setting, ambulatory monitoring plays a role as a "rule-out" test in patients with frequent symptoms in whom sinus rhythm is documented.

Myocardial Imaging

Myocardial imaging with echocardiography or radionuclide ventriculography rarely suggests a cause of syncope. Routine imaging is associated with low diagnostic yields (1% to 3%).[28] Rarely, clinically unsuspected obstructive causes, such as hypertrophic cardiomyopathy and intracardiac tumors, are detected. The major use of cardiac imaging is as a prognostic tool to detect the presence of significant structural heart disease. Patients with previous myocardial infarction or reduced left ventricular function are at increased risk for life-threatening ventricular arrhythmias. The presence of significant structural heart disease should prompt the clinician to pursue a cause for syncope that addresses the risk of life-threatening ventricular arrhythmias (see later).

Tilt Table Testing

There is currently no gold standard for the diagnosis of neurocardiogenic syncope. In the past, the diagnosis was purely a clinical one based on clinical presentation and laboratory evidence excluding other causes. Head-up tilt table testing was devised to provide a form of provocative orthostatic stress resulting in venous pooling in the hope of prompting the hemodynamic changes and symptoms that occur in neurocardiogenic syncope in susceptible individuals.[29,30] It has subsequently been applied to patients with suspected neurocardiogenic syncope.

Tilt table testing is typically performed in a setting in which hemodynamic monitoring is available, such as an electrophysiology laboratory or dedicated testing room. The patient initially lies supine on a motorized table with a footplate that allows rapid elevation and (more important) lowering from 0 to 90 degrees (Fig. 52.2). The electrocardiogram and blood pressure are monitored throughout the test. Digital plethysmography that displays continuous blood pressure is ideal for rapid detection of blood pressure changes. A less convenient alternative is an automated arm pressure cuff. After the patient is monitored, an intravenous line is inserted. Monitoring before intravenous line insertion is important because some patients will develop symptoms at that time. A restraining strap is attached around the patient's waist and chest to

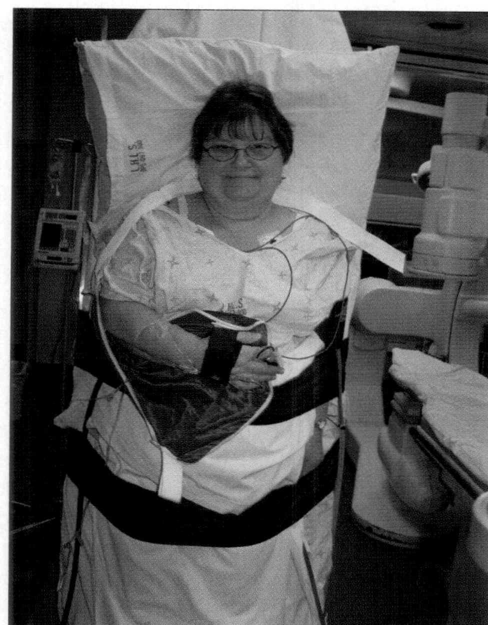

Figure 52.2 Patient undergoing a tilt table test. Note that the patient appears upright but is strapped to the motorized table at 80 degrees. There is continuous electrocardiographic and blood pressure monitoring, with intravenous administration of isoproterenol if the passive phase of the test is normal. See text for discussion.

prevent falling off the table in the event of syncope during the upright phase. The patient is then observed for 5 to 15 minutes to establish a supine steady state.

Several protocols for tilt testing have been devised, varying the duration of observation, the angle of upright tilt, and the use of pharmacologic adjuncts.[31-33] Not surprisingly, more aggressive protocols that use a longer observation period, a steeper tilt angle, and pharmacologic adjuncts are associated with improved sensitivity while sacrificing specificity. In a typical tilt test, the patient is raised to 60 to 80 degrees and monitored for 15 to 45 minutes. During this passive phase of the test, the room is often relatively quiet; some testing facilities even dim the overhead lights. If symptoms do not recur during this period, the patient is returned to the supine position and a pharmacologic adjunct is added to enhance the sensitivity of the test (active phase). The patient is then re-tilted, and monitoring continues for another 15 to 45 minutes.

Isoproterenol (1 to 4 mg/min) is given by infusion to enhance the hypercontractile state that contributes to sudden sympathetic withdrawal. Nitroglycerin is also used to potentiate venous pooling and vasodilatation. Less common adjuncts include edrophonium and adenosine. An alternative orthostatic stressor to tilt testing is lower body negative pressure resulting in venous pooling, which is not widely used. If symptomatic hypotension and bradycardia occur, the patient is promptly returned to the supine position to prevent injury, and the test is concluded.

The response to tilt testing has been divided into three forms[33]:

1. Cardioinhibitory—the primary response is a fall in heart rate, which usually precedes or coincides with the fall in blood pressure. This slowing may be profound, with rare episodes of 30 seconds or more of asystole. Rarely, this slowing may be associated with life-threatening bradycardia-dependent arrhythmias, including torsades de pointes and ventricular fibrillation. For this reason, cardiac resuscitation equipment should be kept in the room.
2. Vasodepressor—the primary response is a fall in blood pressure before any change in heart rate. Patients with a vasodepressor response will often have oscillations in blood pressure before a more marked fall.
3. Mixed response—there is simultaneous fall in blood pressure and heart rate, although the relative contribution of each is variable, even in the same patient from episode to episode.

Most patients fall into the mixed category. A pure cardioinhibitory response is infrequent, so that vasodilatation plays a part in most episodes. Conversely, even in the absence of marked bradycardia, the heart rate is usually inappropriately "normal" during a fall in blood pressure, so that an inappropriate chronotropic response is present to some degree in most patients.

Neurocardiogenic syncope remains a clinical diagnosis that is supported by the results of tilt testing. In a review of 33 studies of tilt testing, a positive response was seen in 49% of passive tests and 66% of active tests in patients with prior syncope.[34] Test results are reproducible in 71% to 87% of patients. It is important to note the patient's symptoms during the test, paying particular attention to whether the test reproduces the patient's spontaneous symptoms. This is particularly relevant in considering the false-positive rate of tilt testing, 9% for passive testing and 27% for active testing, based on the rate of inducing a vagal response with syncope in a well person without a history of syncope. When it is applied to a patient with an undiagnosed syncopal episode, a false-positive tilt test response indicates that although the patient may have inducible vasovagal physiology, it may be unrelated to the real cause of syncope.

Tilt testing is indicated in patients who have recurrent syncope in whom there is a suggestion that neurocardiogenic syncope may be the cause. It may also be indicated after a single episode when the patient is in a high-risk setting (pilot, heavy machinery operator) or has organic heart disease with symptoms suggestive of neurocardiogenic syncope. In the latter patient, it is important also to investigate other causes of syncope, including life-threatening arrhythmias. This is particularly relevant given the false-positive rate of tilt testing. Similar to the use of Bayes theorem as it applies to the use of exercise testing, tilt testing is most useful in patients with an intermediate pretest probability of disease, for whom a positive test response that reproduces the symptoms provides a solid clinical diagnosis and a negative test response focuses investigations elsewhere (Fig. 52.3). For example, tilt testing adds little to establish a diagnosis in a classic presentation of fainting at the sight of blood in an adolescent with a typical prodrome. In this situation, the pretest and post-test probabilities of disease are comparable, regardless of test result.

Loop Recorders

Conventional ambulatory monitoring techniques including Holter monitoring and telemetry are limited by the unpredictability and infrequency of recurrent symptoms, leading

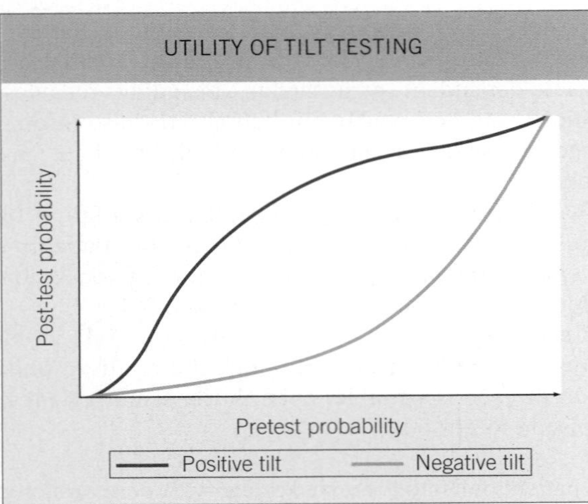

Figure 52.3 Schematic illustrating the utility of tilt testing, similar to the application of Bayes theorem to exercise testing and coronary artery disease. Tilt testing is best applied to those patients with an intermediate pretest probability of disease (curves are most divergent), for whom a positive test response confirms the diagnosis and a negative test response focuses the clinician on other testing strategies. The false-positive and false-negative rates of tilt testing suggest that it has little role when the diagnosis of neurocardiogenic syncope is unlikely (bottom left corner) or very likely (top right corner).

to a low diagnostic yield. Extended monitoring permits a longer sampling period to correlate spontaneous symptoms with rhythm, improving diagnostic yield dramatically. The external loop recorder continuously records and stores an external single modified limb lead electrocardiogram with a 4- to 18-minute memory buffer (Fig. 52.4). After spontaneous symptoms occur, the patient activates an event button that stores the previous recorded information, which can subsequently be downloaded and analyzed. This system can be used for weeks or even months at a time. The recording device is worn like a pager, with two leads attached to chest electrodes, which must be removed for bathing or showering. The captured rhythm strip can be downloaded by a dial-in method to a base station or when the device is returned. The resultant rhythm strip is usually adequate to determine heart rate, but p waves may be difficult to see (Fig. 52.5).

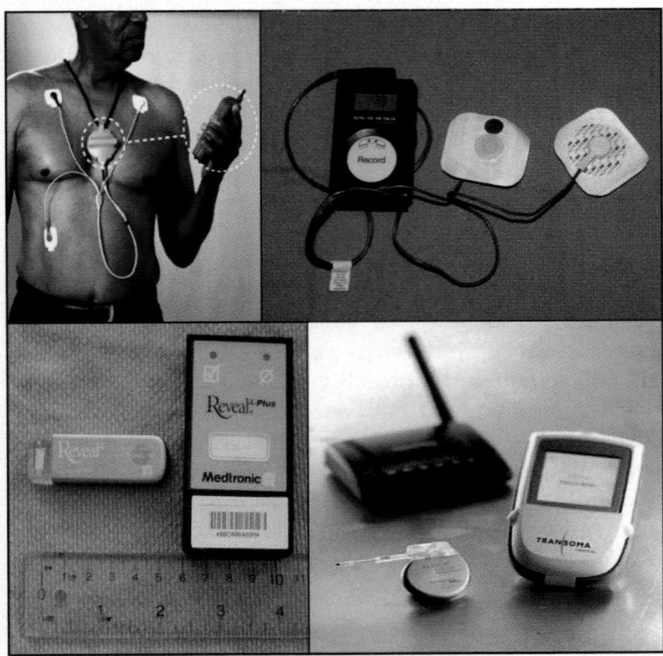

Figure 52.4 Mobile outpatient telemetry *(upper left),* external loop recorder *(upper right),* and implantable loop recorders (Medtronic, *lower left;* Transoma, *lower right*). See text for discussion.

Long-term compliance with this device can be problematic because of electrode- and skin-related problems and waning motivation of the patient in the absence of a recurrence. Compliance can be enhanced by education of the patient and careful follow-up. Compliance is also more likely when patients require a definitive diagnosis and treatment before being permitted to drive or to return to work. Linzer and coworkers[27] reported the use of a patient-activated loop recorder in 57 patients with syncope and nondiagnostic findings on history, physical examination, and 24-hour ambulatory monitoring. A diagnosis was obtained in 14 of 32 patients who had a recurrence of symptoms. Device malfunction, noncompliance of the patient, or inability to activate the recorder was responsible for the lack of diagnosis in the remaining 18. Brown and coworkers[35] have reported similar results. A randomized study in 100 patients with unexplained syncope or presyncope compared diagnostic utility of Holter monitors with external loop recorders and found a 55% diagnostic yield with loop recorders compared with 19% with Holter monitoring,[36] confirming the superior yield of loop recorders in a prospective fashion. Recent addition of automatic activation during high and low heart rate events has further enhanced the utility of the external loop recorder.[37] This device appears to have its greatest role in highly motivated patients with frequent syncope in whom spontaneous symptoms are likely to recur within 2 to 4 weeks. Continuous Holter-type monitoring systems that collect and transmit electrocardiographic data via the Internet or satellite are emerging as intermediate forms of monitoring that provide a wealth of continuous electrocardiographic data.[38,39] Once again, they are limited by compliance of the patient and frequency of symptoms, but they do not require the patient's activation to capture an event.

The implantable loop recorder permits prolonged monitoring without external electrodes that is ideally suited to patients with infrequent recurrent syncope.[40] At present, implanted loop recorders are manufactured by Medtronic and Transoma Medical. Both are smaller than a conventional pacemaker generator, record a single-lead electrocardiogram with no transvenous lead, and have the potential to deliver 30 months or more of battery life. The device is inserted in

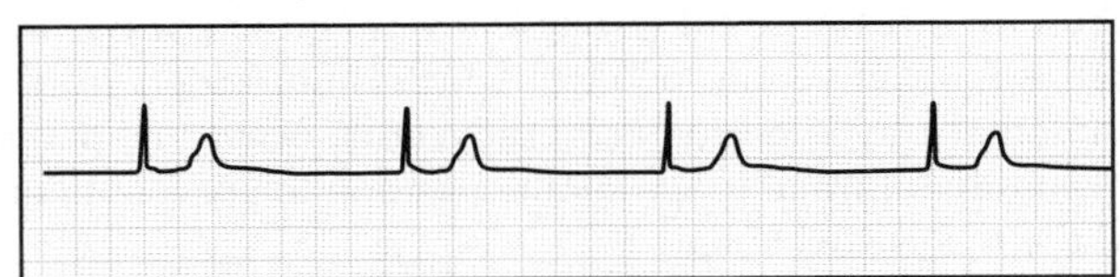

Figure 52.5 Rhythm strip obtained with an external loop recorder during presyncope in a 58-year-old woman with recurrent syncope and presyncope. Junctional rhythm at 44 beats per minute is noted. Syncope and presyncope resolved after permanent pacemaker implantation.

the left side of the chest with use of local anesthetic. The recorded bipolar electrocardiographic signal is stored in a loop buffer that stores the recorded electrocardiogram in several programmable memory bin configurations. Devices have the ability to automatically detect high and low heart rate and pause events, and features that promise to recognize atrial fibrillation, ventricular ectopy, and various autonomic and risk-stratifying factors such as heart rate variability have recently been developed. Manual activation is also possible after the patient experiences syncope or presyncope. Data retrieval is influenced by the manufacturer platform; Medtronic uses retrieval after interrogation with a standard pacemaker programmer, and Transoma uses a patient activator that downloads daily events by a Web-based service with an analog phone line (Fig. 52-6).

The implant procedure is similar to a small pacemaker pocket creation. An adequate signal can be obtained anywhere in the left thorax, without the need for cutaneous mapping. Mapping is often helpful to maximize signal size and the R to T wave ratio for optimal automatic detection. The patient along with a spouse, family member, or friend is instructed in the use of the activator at the time of implantation. Use of prophylactic antibiotics is recommended because local wound infection has occurred in some patients who did not receive antibiotics.

Several studies have demonstrated the feasibility of the implantable loop recorder in establishing a symptom-rhythm correlation during long-term monitoring.[41-45] The largest of these studies combined data from 206 patients from three centers.[46] The majority of patients studied had previous noninvasive testing and selective invasive testing including tilt testing and electrophysiologic studies. An arrhythmia was detected in 22% of patients and was excluded in 42% of patients; symptoms resolved without recurrence in 31%. Bradycardia was detected more frequently than tachycardia (17% versus 6%), usually leading to pacemaker implantation. Of importance, 4% of patients failed to properly activate the device after spontaneous symptoms, thus failing to obtain a symptom-rhythm correlation. Multivariate modeling did not identify any significant preimplantation predictors of subsequent arrhythmia detection other than a weak association with advancing age and bradycardia. Unfortunately, no age group had an incidence of bradycardia greater than 30%, suggesting a limited role for empiric pacing in the population with unexplained syncope.

Additional studies of the implantable loop recorder have focused on the utility of prolonged cardiac monitoring in select populations. Zaidi and colleagues[47] performed cardiac assessment in 74 patients with ongoing seizures despite anticonvulsant therapy or unexplained recurrent seizures, including tilt testing and carotid sinus massage in all patients and monitoring with an implantable loop recorder in 10 patients. Tilt testing response was positive in 27% of patients, and carotid sinus massage was positive in 10%. Two of the 10 patients with implantable loop recorder demonstrated marked bradycardia preceding seizure activity. This study suggested that seizures that are atypical in presentation or response to therapy may have a cardiovascular cause and that long-term cardiac monitoring plays a role in select patients.

The ISSUE (International Study on Syncope of Uncertain Etiology) investigators implanted loop recorders in 111 patients with syncope who underwent tilt testing, regardless of tilt result.[48] Syncope recurred in 34% of patients in both the tilt-positive and tilt-negative group, with marked bradycardia or asystole the most common recorded arrhythmia during follow-up (46% and 62%, respectively). In a second study, 52 patients with syncope and bundle branch block with normal electrophysiologic test results underwent implantation of loop recorders.[38] Syncope recurred in 22 of

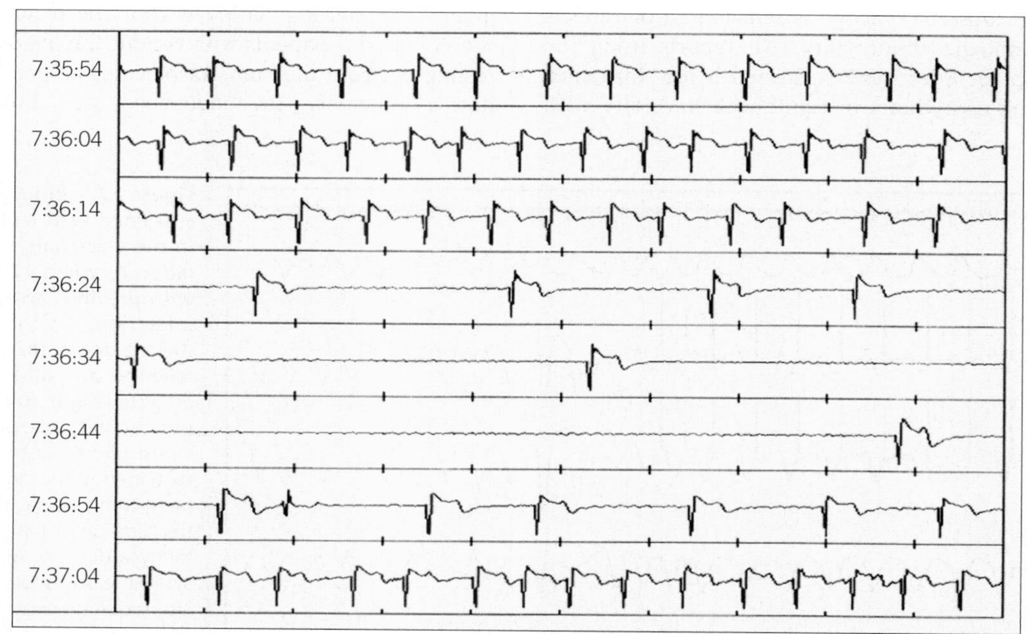

Figure 52.6 Rhythm strip obtained with an implantable loop recorder in a 69-year-old man with two syncopal episodes in the previous 18 months. Each line represents 10 seconds of a single-lead rhythm strip. Note marked bradycardia with a 14-second pause. Syncope resolved after permanent pacemaker implantation.

the 52 patients. Long-term monitoring demonstrated marked bradycardia mainly attributed to complete AV block in 17, whereas it excluded AV block in 2. This study confirmed the previous view that normal electrophysiologic test results do not exclude progression to complete AV block and that prolonged monitoring or consideration of permanent pacing is reasonable in this population. ISSUE 2 performed loop recorder implantation in 443 patients with recurrent syncope in the absence of structural heart disease who were presumed to have vasovagal syncope.[49] Syncope recurred in 143 patients, with a symptom-rhythm correlation in 102 patients. In those 102 patients, loop recorder–directed therapy (predominantly pacing for bradycardia) was associated with a lower risk of syncope recurrence (10% versus 41%; $P = .0005$). This was not a randomized assessment of the benefit of pacing, but it raises the possibility that spontaneous cardioinhibitory syncope recorded with prolonged monitoring may identify a subgroup of patients with vasovagal syncope who benefit from pacing. This hypothesis is being tested in the ISSUE 3 trial, which follows the same algorithm but randomizes patients with loop recorder–documented pauses.

Finally, two prospective randomized trials have compared early use of the loop recorder for prolonged monitoring with conventional testing in patients undergoing a cardiac work-up for unexplained syncope who did not have significant structural heart disease.[42,50] Both studies showed a higher diagnostic yield with use of loop recorders and also showed that the apparent up-front cost of a somewhat invasive strategy was actually cost-effective compared with conventional testing because of the dramatic improvement in diagnostic yield.[50,51] These data highlight the limitations of conventional diagnostic techniques. In patients who have infrequent syncope, the implantable loop recorder is the diagnostic tool of choice when noninvasive testing is negative and an arrhythmia is suspected.

Syncope resolves in almost one third of patients despite frequent episodes before implantation of the device. This suggests that the cause of syncope is self-limited or reflects a transient physiologic abnormality. All reports using the implantable loop recorder have suggested a low incidence of life-threatening arrhythmia or significant morbidity with a prolonged monitoring strategy. Selection bias of clinicians appears to identify patients at low risk of sudden death in whom it is appropriate to implant the device. In patients with significant structural heart disease, an implantable cardioverter-defibrillator (ICD) or electrophysiologic testing should be considered before a long-term monitoring strategy.

Electrophysiologic Testing

Electrophysiologic testing for syncope has previously been considered the final arbiter when the result of noninvasive testing is negative or inconclusive.[52] This arises from the assumption that electrophysiologic testing has a high sensitivity and specificity for determination of the cause of syncope. Electrophysiologic testing involves insertion of temporary transvenous pacing and recording catheters through the right femoral vein. Measurement of the AH and HV intervals assesses the potential for AV block. The sinus node recovery time and sinoatrial conduction time assess sinus node function and conduction into and out of the sinus node; these two tests have a low sensitivity and specificity and have limited clinical utility. Finally, extrastimulus testing is performed in the atrium and ventricle to induce tachycardias.

The role of electrophysiologic testing in patients with syncope has been extensively studied. The overall likelihood of a positive test result is 53%, with a wide range of reported values.[53-63] The definition of a positive test result is highly variable. A review of these studies suggests that electrophysiologic testing is best applied to patients with structural heart disease, in particular patients with previous myocardial infarction or left ventricular dysfunction.[52] Testing in this context is primarily directed at induction of ventricular tachycardia, which is possible in up to 70% of patients with this history (Fig. 52.7). The variability in diagnostic yield in different series is largely explained by the prevalence of structural heart disease. In patients with syncope, coronary artery disease, and inducible ventricular tachycardia, appropriate ICD discharge is common.[64] A second population in whom electrophysiologic testing is considered is patients with conduction abnormalities on the resting electrocardiogram. As indicated before, long-term monitoring in patients with conduction system disease and normal

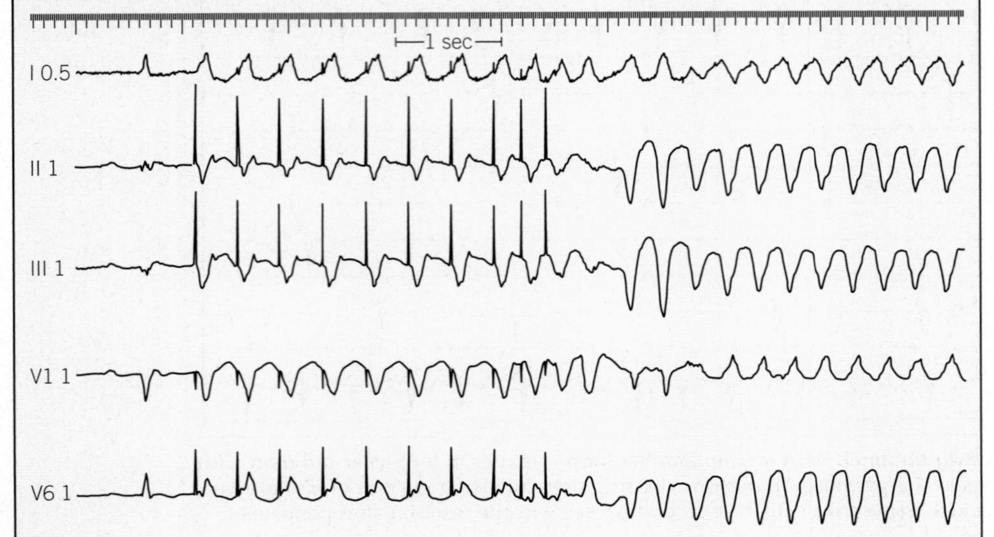

Figure 52.7 Induction of rapid, sustained ventricular tachycardia in the electrophysiology laboratory in a 72-year-old man with previous anterior infarction. A single sinus beat on the left side of the tracing is followed by a drive train of 8 beats at cycle length 400 ms (150 beats per minute), followed by two ventricular extrastimuli that induce sustained monomorphic ventricular tachycardia at a cycle length of 300 ms (200 beats per minute). This tachycardia was associated with a systolic blood pressure of 50 mm Hg, requiring urgent cardioversion, and was presumed to be the cause of syncope.

electrophysiologic test results suggests that the negative predictive value of the test is not good,[65] calling into question the routine use of electrophysiologic testing in this population of patients.

Electrophysiologic testing is limited by the need to extrapolate from abnormal test results to a cause of spontaneous syncope. Such results as the induction of nonsustained ventricular arrhythmias, ventricular fibrillation induced by multiple closely coupled extrastimuli, and sustained bradyarrhythmias and tachyarrhythmias that do not reproduce the patient's spontaneous symptoms may be difficult to relate to the clinical syncope. The negative predictive value of electrophysiologic testing in dilated cardiomyopathy is well known to be unacceptably low. The difficulty correlating induced abnormalities with previous syncope is borne out by the 5% to 32% recurrent syncope risk after a positive electrophysiologic test result when therapy is directed at the abnormality detected at electrophysiologic testing. In addition, electrophysiologic testing has a low sensitivity in patients with documented intermittent bradyarrhythmias associated with syncope.[66,67]

Finally, syncope in a patient with left ventricular dysfunction often leads to consideration of a primary prevention ICD, regardless of the mechanism of syncope. This precludes the need for electrophysiologic testing, which in many ways has been relegated to the population of patients with intermediate left ventricular function and a worrisome symptom presentation. It is not certain to what degree an abnormal study reflects the true cause of syncope or is merely a marker of higher mortality.

Other Tests

Additional testing is often performed when the initial clinical assessment suggests a cause other than an arrhythmia or vasomotor syncope. Myocardial infarction causing syncope as an isolated presentation is very rare, and the routine evaluation for infarction has been questioned.[68] Neurologic investigation is best performed when there is a suspicion from the initial clinical evaluation that seizure or cerebral ischemia may have caused loss of consciousness. The routine use of brain imaging with computed tomography or magnetic resonance imaging, electroencephalography, or carotid Doppler blood flow assessment has a very low yield in the absence of clinical suspicion and should be reserved for patients whose history suggests seizure activity, whose physical examination demonstrates neurologic abnormalities, or when recurrent syncope is unexplained after cardiac evaluation, particularly once an arrhythmia has been ruled out.[69] Metabolic causes such as hypoglycemia should be investigated in those patients who complain of altered levels of consciousness (versus sudden loss of consciousness).

Development of a simple routine approach to the patient with syncope will inevitably fail to take into account the nuances of each individual case. The key direction in investigation is set by the initial clinical assessment. In those patients with recurrent unexplained syncope or a single episode that is worrisome in its description, investigations should be performed on the basis of clinical index of suspicion. One simplistic approach to this population is illustrated in Figure 52.8. Note the emphasis on less invasive and inexpensive testing early, shifting to higher yield but invasive testing if a diagnosis is not obtained. Ambulatory monitoring is not performed because of the low yield unless symptoms are frequent or an abnormality is detected on the resting electrocardiogram.

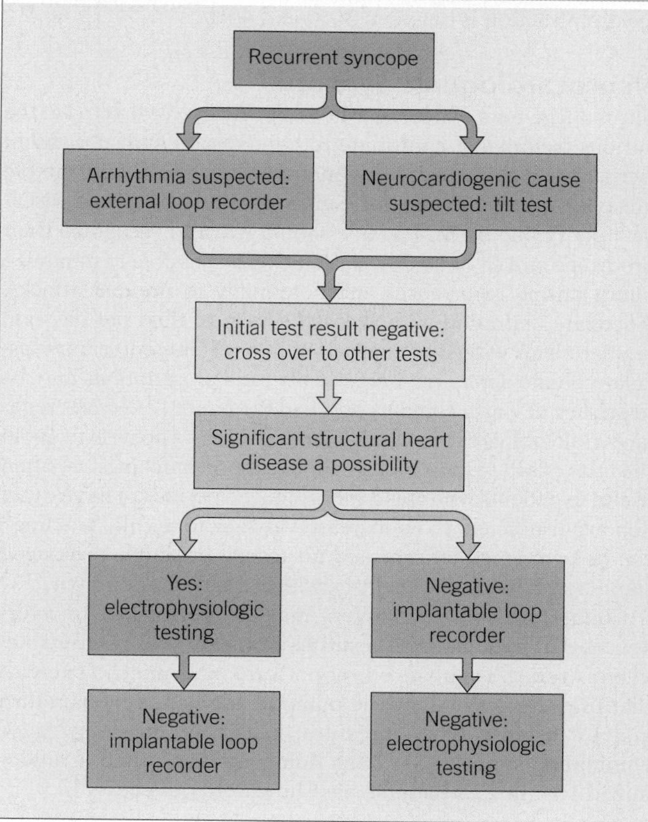

Figure 52.8 Flow diagram illustrating the diagnostic approach to the patient with recurrent syncope or a single worrisome episode. In the patient with significant structural heart disease, an implantable cardioverter-defibrillator or electrophysiologic testing should be considered early in the diagnostic process if ventricular tachycardia is suspected.

MANAGEMENT

Arrhythmias

Once a diagnosis is established, therapy directed at the underlying cause is usually successful. Pacemaker implantation is effective at resolving symptoms related to bradycardia[70] unless bradycardia is a component of neurocardiogenic syncope with a predominant vasodepressor component (see later). Antiarrhythmic drug therapy, catheter ablation, and ICD use are usually effective in eliminating syncope in patients whose symptoms have been correlated with a tachyarrhythmia. Link and associates[64] have reported frequent appropriate ICD discharges in patients with syncope who have structural heart disease and inducible ventricular arrhythmias, supporting the use of ICDs in this population. Mittal and coworkers[71] examined electrophysiologically guided therapy in 67 patients with syncope and coronary artery disease and found frequent appropriate ICD discharges. Despite the apparent prevention of sudden death, mortality from coronary artery disease and noncardiac causes resulted in a 45%

2-year survival. Given its role in primary prevention, an ICD is likely to be indicated in any patient with syncope and an ejection fraction less than 30% and should be considered if the ejection fraction is between 30% and 40%.[72]

Neurocardiogenic Syncope

The management of neurocardiogenic syncope is directed at the various factors that contribute to hypotension and subsequent symptoms. The majority of patients will improve with simple lifestyle measures to maximize intravascular volume and vascular tone (Table 52.5). Patients should learn to recognize their prodrome and sit or lie down as quickly as possible to minimize injury during recurrences and potentially to prevent attacks. Adequate hydration with at least 2 liters of fluid per day and regular meals with sufficient salt intake will minimize intravascular volume depletion. Larger daily fluid prescriptions may be necessary in warm climates or when the patient exercises regularly. Salt tablets can be used in those patients who wish to avoid the taste of salt in their food. Venous support stockings are often useful in patients who stand for prolonged periods or have overt venous insufficiency. To increase vascular tone, tilt "training" can be performed by repeated tilt testing or simple prolonged standing while leaning against a wall in a safe environment.[73-75]

Counterpressure maneuvers may be performed to avert syncope in patients with a sufficient prodrome. In principle, venous return is enhanced by performing isometric exercise that uses the skeletal muscle pump to augment venous return and to increase blood pressure. Feasibility in reducing or eliminating syncope has been demonstrated,[76] and a randomized trial in 223 patients has shown effectiveness.[77]

THERAPY FOR NEUROCARDIOGENIC SYNCOPE	
Therapy	**Mechanism of Benefit**
Lifestyle	
Increase fluid intake (2-3 liters/day)	Increases intravascular volume
Increase salt intake	Increases intravascular volume
Regular meals	Avoids dehydration
Exercise	Increases vascular tone
Avoid triggers (i.e., prolonged standing)	
Pharmacologic	
Beta blockers	Blunts cardiac mechanoreceptor activation
Fludrocortisone	Increases intravascular volume
Midodrine, etilefrine	Prevents venous pooling
Theophylline	
Fluoxetine, sertraline	Central serotonin reuptake inhibition
Nonpharmacologic	
Venous support stockings	Prevents venous pooling
Tilt training	Prevents venous pooling
Dual-chamber pacemaker	Prevents cardioinhibitory component of abnormal reflex

Table 52.5 Therapy For Neurocardiogenic Syncope.

Pharmacologic therapy for neurocardiogenic syncope suffers from a lack of rigorous randomized clinical trial data to direct treatment. Most series that employed a pharmacologic intervention after a diagnosis is established (usually with tilt testing) have shown a reduction in frequency of episodes compared with the period before diagnosis. However, syncopal events are often clustered before diagnosis and may well diminish in frequency or resolve once a diagnosis is established. Agents used most commonly include beta blockers, adrenocorticosteroids, and vasoconstrictors.[78-83] Disopyramide has been used in the past but was ineffective in a placebo-controlled randomized trial.[84] Small studies using beta blockers have been inconclusive.[81,83] The Prevention of Syncope Trial (POST) was a prospective randomized trial comparing metoprolol with placebo.[78] This showed no benefit in the overall population of 208 patients. Interestingly, the prespecified age subgroup analysis suggested a benefit in patients older than 42 years and an increased recurrence risk in those younger than 42 years. This trial suggests that beta blockers may play a role in management of neurocardiogenic syncope with advancing age, particularly in patients with hypertension. Vasoconstrictors such as midodrine and etilefrine have also been used to prevent venous pooling and to counteract arterial dilatation. A multicenter randomized placebo-controlled trial by the VASIS investigators has shown no benefit with etilefrine,[82] although a second small study showed a benefit with midodrine.[85] Finally, a single placebo-controlled trial of paroxetine has shown a reduction in syncopal events.[86] During a 2-year follow-up period, 53% of placebo patients experienced recurrence compared with 18% of paroxetine patients ($P < .0001$). These studies have improved a once empiric climate of pharmacotherapy for neurocardiogenic syncope. A summary of largely empiric decision making for neurocardiogenic syncope is presented in Figure 52.9.

Pacing has been considered in neurocardiogenic syncope because absolute or relative bradycardia typically accompanies both spontaneous neurocardiogenic syncope and tilt-induced syncope in the majority of patients. It is reasonable to presume that pacing will have a benefit in those patients with a profound cardioinhibitory response. However, in most cases, the bradycardia is accompanied by varying degrees of peripheral vasodilatation and hypotension that may be independent of any change in heart rate. An exaggerated pacing rate response to sudden deceleration is used to offset the sudden bradycardia or inappropriate "normal" heart rate seen in patients with a vasodilatory response.

Several studies have examined the long-term impact of pacing in series of patients with recurrent neurocardiogenic syncope.[87-90] The benefit of pacing was evident compared against medical or no therapy or when the trials were not rigorously blinded. There was no evidence of benefit when both patients and physicians were unaware of whether pacemaker programming was to an active or inactive mode.[91,92] A recent meta-analysis strongly suggested that the primary mechanism of benefit of pacemaker insertion is an expectation response, suggesting that the physiologic benefit is small.[93] Although these trials have dramatically reduced enthusiasm for pacing, the ISSUE 2 trial has raised concern that tilt testing is not suited to select patients who may benefit from pacing and that a rigorous trial in the spontaneous cardioinhibitory subgroup is warranted.

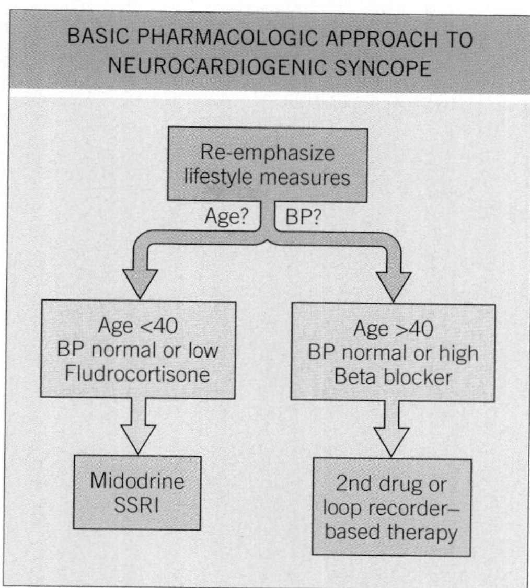

Figure 52.9 Simplified algorithm summarizing a basic pharmacologic approach to neurocardiogenic syncope. Note that lifestyle measures with hydration, increased salt intake, and counterpressure maneuvers cannot be overemphasized before pharmacologic adjuncts are considered. Treatment is influenced by age and blood pressure (BP). SSRI, selective serotonin reuptake inhibitor.

PROGNOSIS

Mortality

The outcome of patients with syncope is strongly influenced by the presence of underlying heart disease.[1,8,52] Several studies have examined the outcome of patients with syncope, noting that annual mortality was 19% to 30% in patients with a cardiac cause, 0% to 12% with a noncardiac cause, and 6% with unexplained syncope. Patients with neurocardiogenic syncope had a prognosis similar to that of those free of syncope, consistent with the presumed benign nature in all but rare circumstances. Sudden death is extremely uncommon in the absence of heart disease, suggesting a good prognosis in this subgroup. Conversely, the presence of a cardiac cause of syncope or known underlying heart disease suggests a relatively high risk of sudden death. It is the adverse prognosis of those patients with heart disease that drives their aggressive investigation to prevent sudden death.

SUMMARY

Syncope remains a challenging puzzle despite significant advances in our diagnostic armamentarium. The differential diagnosis of syncope is extensive because of the large number of conditions that can lead to loss of consciousness. Careful clinical assessment and directed testing often lead to a presumptive diagnosis. Advances in prolonged monitoring technology have significantly enhanced our ability to diagnose arrhythmias. Treatment of an arrhythmia usually eliminates syncope when a symptom-rhythm correlation is obtained.

Future development in the field of syncope is likely to see improved implantable monitoring technology with a wider range of monitoring parameters. Clinical predictors of the underlying cause of syncope may permit focusing of invasive and costly diagnostic and therapeutic resources on those patients most likely to benefit. Finally, enhanced understanding of the interaction of the neurologic and cardiovascular systems is likely to provide insight into the mechanism of reactive syncope, leading to rigorously tested treatment strategies.

chapter 53

Sinus Node Dysfunction

John P. DiMarco

Definition

- Heart rates during sinus rhythm are inappropriate for current physiologic demands and result in symptoms or arrhythmias.

Key Features

- Both intrinsic disease of the sinus node and extrinsic factors may result in sinus node dysfunction.
- Intrinsic sinus node disease may occur in all types of heart disease and in the elderly even without heart disease.

Therapy

- Permanent pacing is indicated if transient and easily reversible causes are not identified. Pacing should be tailored to preserve normal ventricular activation when possible.

The sinus node serves as the primary cardiac pacemaker, and as such, its activity controls heart rate in normal individuals. Both intrinsic disease and a variety of extrinsic factors can have an effect on sinus node function. Sinus node dysfunction (SND) may result in symptoms ranging from minor palpitations that are of little clinical significance to life-threatening bradyarrhythmias.

ANATOMY AND PATHOLOGY

The sinus node is composed of a collection of specialized pacemaker cells embedded in a fibrous matrix that lies in the sulcus terminalis between the superior vena cava and the right atrial appendage.[1] In adults, the center of the sinus node measures approximately 1 to 2 cm by 0.5 cm. When examined by light microscopy, the cells in the center of the node appear as small fusiform cells, which are smaller than normal atrial myocytes (Fig. 53.1). In the periphery of the node and along the crista terminalis, transitional cells can be found that may also have a pacemaker function. The sinoatrial nodal artery provides the primary blood supply to the region, but other atrial or bronchial arterial branches may also contribute. The sinoatrial nodal artery is a proximal branch of the right coronary artery in 55% to 60% of the population. In the remaining patients, it arises from the left coronary system as a branch of the circumflex artery. The sinus node communicates with the parasympathetic nervous system by afferent and efferent fibers that pass through the pulmonary vein fat pad from both the right and left vagus nerves. The entire sinus node region is richly innervated with muscarinic nerve endings. Sympathetic stimulation occurs either directly through the right stellate cardiac nerve or indirectly from circulating catecholamines. In normal individuals at rest, parasympathetic tone predominates. Thus, the intrinsic heart rate—the heart rate seen during full pharmacologic autonomic blockade or in denervated sinus nodes in transplant recipients—is usually 90 to 100 beats per minute, which is significantly higher than the normal resting heart rate in adults. Secretion of endogenous substances, including adenosine and sphingosine, can also influence sinus node activity.

Several ionic currents contribute to the action potential of the sinus node, and several patterns are present in different portions of the node.[2-4] At rest, the membrane potential is less negative than that seen in atrial or ventricular myocytes (see Chapter 49). The action potential upstroke is mediated by L-type calcium channels. The background inward rectifying K^+ current, I_{K1}, which is responsible for the stable resting potential in working myocardium, is not present in the sinus node. During the action potential, the rapid and slow delayed rectifier K^+ currents are activated, and their decay during diastole unmasks the inward pacemaker currents. As the membrane potential becomes more negative, a pacemaker current carried by sodium and potassium ions (I_f) is activated and depolarizes the cell until threshold is reached; this current is mediated by a hyperpolarization-activated, cyclic nucleotide–gated (HCN) channel thought to be composed of six transmembrane segments, a pore loop between the fifth and sixth segments, and a cyclic nucleotide–binding domain in the C-terminal region. The T-type calcium current is also involved in pacemaking and may contribute to the second half of the action potential. The Na^+-Ca^+ exchanger and the inward sodium current also can influence pacemaker activity. Conduction velocities within the sinus node are much slower than those in atrial or ventricular muscle or in the His-Purkinje system, probably because of low expression of the connexins Cx43 and Cx40. Conduction failure within the node, leading to sinoatrial exit block, is possible. Pacemaker shifts to subsidiary cells within the node may occur, and this may be detected by minor changes in P-wave morphology on the surface electrocardiogram.

PATHOPHYSIOLOGY

Both intrinsic and extrinsic factors may result in clinically important abnormalities of sinus node function (Table 53.1). Intrinsic factors are defined as those that change the anatomy or functional integrity of the pacemaker cells in the node. Extrinsic factors are usually transient phenomena that may intermittently depress sinus node automaticity or conduction but are not associated with structural changes in the node itself. Some patients may have both intrinsic and extrinsic causes for clinically significant arrhythmias.

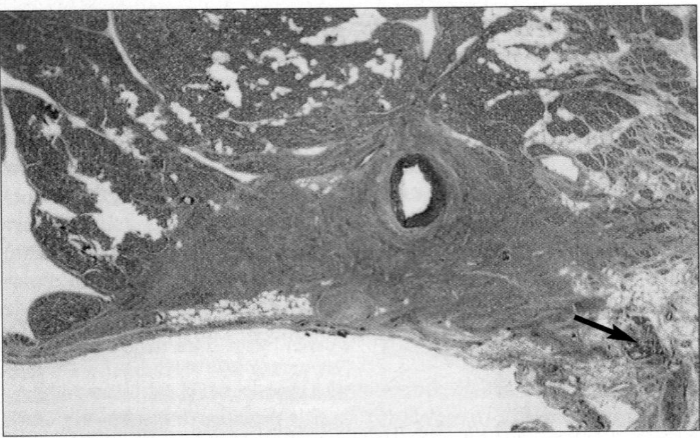

Figure 53.1 Histology of the sinus node. The small cells of the sinus node surround the sinus node artery on the endocardial surface of the right atrium. The darker cells of the crista terminalis are seen toward the bottom right *(arrow)*. Masson trichrome stain. (Courtesy of Dr. C. Guiraudon, University of Western Ontario, London, Ontario, Canada.)

SINUS NODE DYSFUNCTION	
Intrinsic causes	**Extrinsic causes**
Idiopathic degeneration	Autonomically mediated syndromes
Chronic ischemia	■ Neurocardiac syncope
Infiltrative disease	■ Carotid sinus hypersensitivity
Inflammatory disease	■ Situational, e.g., sneezing, coughing, micturition, vomiting
Musculoskeletal disease	Drugs
Connective tissue disorders	Endocrinopathy, e.g., hypothyroidism
Surgical trauma	Intracranial hypertension
Familial diseases	Electrolyte disturbance

Table 53.1 Sinus node dysfunction.

Intrinsic Factors

The pathologic finding most commonly noted in patients with SND is replacement of normal pacemaker cells in the region of the sinus node with fibrous tissue.[1] Diseases associated with this replacement are listed in Table 53.1. SND is also commonly seen after cardiac surgical procedures that involve incisions in the right atrium. Ion channel mutations in the genes encoding the sodium channel, *HCN4* and ankyrin-B, have been described in rare families with inherited SND.[3,5,6] Heart failure and electrical remodeling during rapid atrial rates (e.g., in atrial fibrillation) are other potential causes of SND.

Extrinsic Factors

The autonomic nervous system exerts profound effects on sinus node function, and symptomatic sinus bradyarrhythmias occur frequently in patients with sinus nodes that are completely normal in structure and intrinsic function.[7] Neurocardiac syncope occurs when peripheral venous pooling and decreased left ventricular filling results in hypotension with inappropriate sinus slowing or atrioventricular block. Autonomically mediated sinus arrest may occur for many seconds.[8] Other neurally mediated syndromes that can result in abnormal sinus node function include carotid sinus hypersensitivity, glossopharyngeal neuralgia, and physiologically inappropriate sinus tachycardia, either as a continuous finding or as a response to orthostatic stress. Common physical maneuvers or everyday life situations, such as sneezing, coughing, swallowing, or vomiting, may serve as triggers for reflex-mediated sinus bradycardia or sinus arrest in susceptible individuals (see Chapter 52).

DRUGS ASSOCIATED WITH SINUS NODE DYSFUNCTION
Antiarrhythmic drugs
β-Adrenergic blocking agents: systemic and ophthalmologic
Calcium channel–blocking agents: verapamil and diltiazem
Antihypertensive agents
Cardiac glycosides
Other drugs: lithium, cimetidine, among others

Table 53.2 Drugs associated with sinus node dysfunction.

Drug therapy is another important cause of symptomatic SND (Table 53.2). Antiarrhythmic drugs, sympatholytic agents used as antihypertensives, calcium channel blockers, β-adrenergic blockers including systemically absorbed ophthalmic preparations, lithium, and several other agents may suppress sinus node activity in susceptible individuals. Drug-induced bradycardia may be mild or extreme, depending on individual sensitivities to the drug involved. A thorough drug history should be obtained in all patients who present with SND because discontinuation of the offending agent may be the only intervention required.

Sinus bradycardia may also be a benign and completely physiologic finding, particularly in physically trained individuals, during sleep, or in asymptomatic elderly patients. For this reason, caution must be exercised before SND is treated in any asymptomatic individual.

Patients with extrinsically mediated SND or with physiologic sinus bradycardia may be distinguished from those with intrinsic sinus node disease because the former group will usually have normal responses to invasive tests of sinus node function.[9,10]

Electrocardiographic Features

Physiologic or pathologic disturbances in sinus node function may present with a variety of electrocardiographic patterns.

Sinus arrhythmia is a normal and very common physiologic phenomenon characterized by a wide variation in sinus cycle length. The variation most often occurs in phase with respiration. Although some patients may become aware of their irregular pulse, sinus arrhythmia is benign and of little clinical import.

Sinus tachycardia is usually a normal physiologic response to a perceived need for an increase in cardiac output due to stimuli such as exercise, fever, and mental stress. The maximum achievable sinus heart rate varies inversely with age. A frequently used estimate of an individual's "predicted maximal heart rate" is 220 minus the age in years. Inappropriate sinus tachycardia is said to be present when the sinus rate is elevated out of proportion to metabolic demand, either intermittently or continuously. Sinus tachycardia, whether appropriate or inappropriate, is an automatic rhythm and therefore typically exhibits "warm-up" and "cool-down" phases rather than the abrupt onset and termination that are characteristics of re-entrant arrhythmias.

Sinus node re-entry is caused by re-entry within atrial tissue in or near the sinus node region. Except for abrupt onset and termination, sinus node re-entrant tachycardia resembles sinus tachycardia on electrocardiography.

Sinus bradycardia is defined as any stable sinus rate below 50 beats per minute. Sinus bradycardia may be either a normal or a pathologic finding, depending on whether the sinus rate is appropriate for current demand. When automaticity in the junctional region becomes greater than that of the sinus node, a junctional rhythm will be observed (Fig. 53.2).

Sinus arrest occurs when there is a sudden, unexpected pause in sinus node activity (Fig. 53.3). This may be due to either decreased automaticity or blocked conduction of impulses out of the node.

Sinoatrial conduction block is often described in a manner similar to that used to describe atrioventricular block. In type I sinoatrial exit block, the P-P intervals before the pause progressively lengthen with a Wenckebach-type periodicity. In type II sinoatrial exit block, the P-P intervals remain constant before the dropped P waves (see Fig. 53.3). In high-grade sinoatrial exit block, several P waves will be dropped, but the total pause should be a multiple of the sinus cycle length.

Wandering atrial pacemakers are commonly observed in asymptomatic individuals. The electrocardiogram in these patients shows variations in P-wave morphology, with an irregular atrial cycle length. The changes in P-wave morphology are due to shifts in pacemaker activity to subsidiary atrial sites.

SND may contribute to or coexist with atrial tachyarrhythmias, usually atrial fibrillation or atrial flutter, in what is commonly referred to as the bradycardia-tachycardia syndrome.[10] Sinus pauses may be particularly prolonged when the tachyarrhythmia terminates (Fig. 53.4). SND is commonly associated with atrioventricular nodal conduction problems.[11,12] The presence either of marked first-degree atrioventricular block

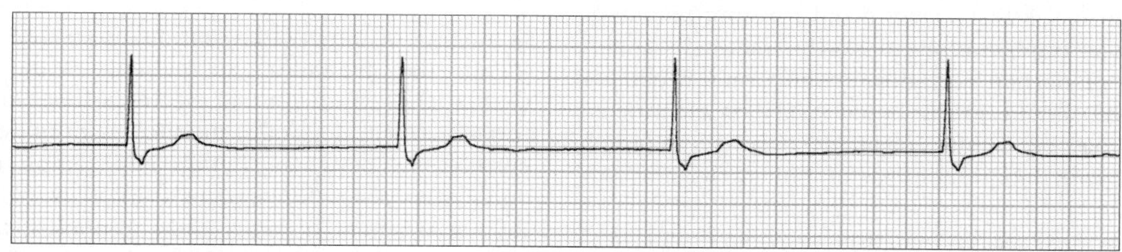

Figure 53.2 Junctional escape rhythm in a patient with sinus node disease. This tracing was obtained in a 68-year-old hypertensive woman during a dizzy spell. A junctional escape rhythm at 40 beats per minute without obvious atrial activity is shown.

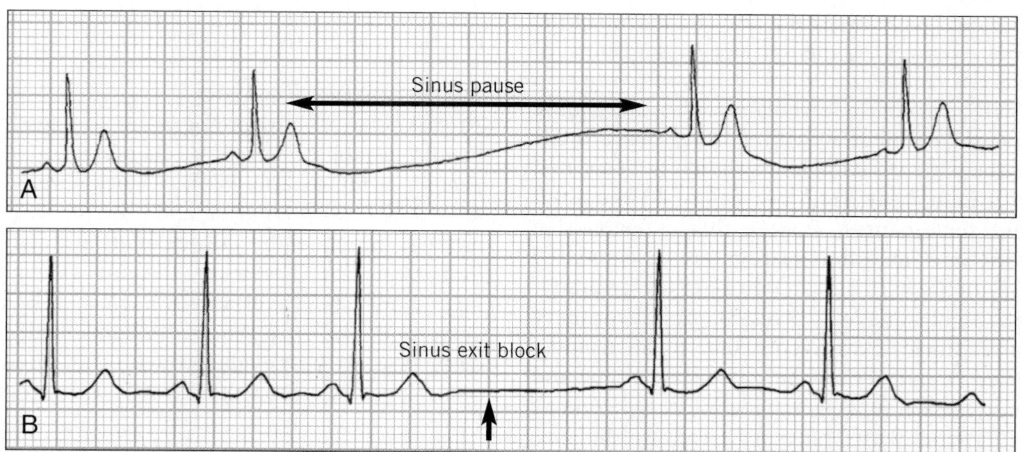

Figure 53.3 Sinus arrest and sinoatrial exit block. A, The sudden pause in sinus rate is characteristic of sinus arrest. **B**, The pause is twice the P-P interval, indicating sinoatrial exit block.

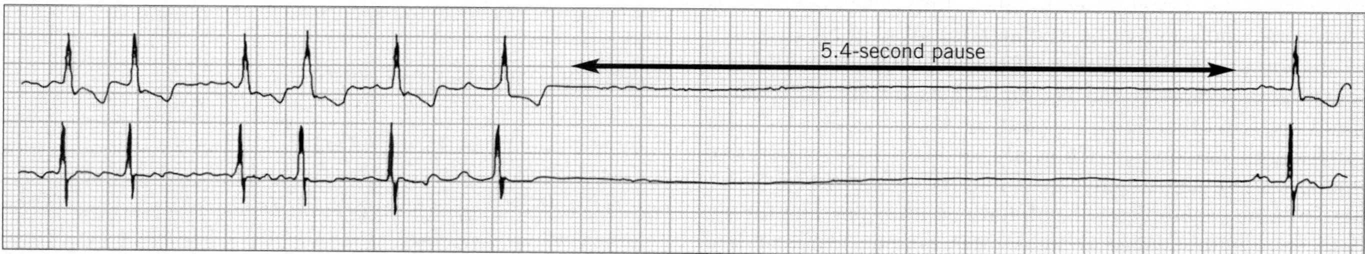

Figure 53.4 Bradycardia-tachycardia syndrome. This ambulatory electrocardiographic recording was obtained in a 79-year-old man with near-syncope. The beginning of the tracing shows atrial fibrillation. When the atrial fibrillation terminates, a 5.4-second pause occurs until the sinus node recovers.

at long sinus cycle lengths or of slow ventricular rates in the absence of drugs during intermittent atrial flutter or fibrillation should alert one to the presence of diffuse conduction system disease.

Chronotropic incompetence is a term used to describe the situation in which the resting sinus rate is not clearly abnormal but there is only a limited ability to increase the heart rate in response to an increase in metabolic demand. Chronotropic incompetence may exist even if the resting sinus rate is not greatly depressed.[13]

CLINICAL PRESENTATIONS

Ferrer[14] popularized the term *sick sinus syndrome* to describe patients with a variety of symptoms associated with abnormalities in sinus node function. SND may occur at any age, but symptomatic SND that will require therapy is much more common in the elderly. The prevalence of SND has been estimated to be as high as 1 in 600 elderly individuals. Sick sinus syndrome is the reason listed for approximately 50% of pacemaker implantations in North America.[15] Given the wide range of normal variation in sinus rate, a clinical diagnosis of SND should not be based solely on electrocardiographic findings but should be made only if symptoms that correlate with abnormalities in sinus rhythm are documented.[16]

Syncope is the most serious symptom associated with bradycardic SND and may be seen when the SND is due to either extrinsic or intrinsic factors. Sudden slowing or cessation of sinus node activity will produce hypotension and loss of consciousness unless an adequate lower pacemaker takes over. Other symptoms of bradycardia may be more subtle. Fatigue, dizziness, changes in mental status, shortness of breath, and exercise intolerance are commonly seen in patients with SND, but these complaints also commonly occur in the general population with normal heart rates. Other causes for the patient's complaints should be suspected unless sustained waking heart rates are below 40 beats per minute, there are sinus pauses of more than 3 seconds in duration, or symptoms and bradycardia are documented simultaneously. Patients with sinus node re-entry or bradycardia-tachycardia syndrome may present with a primary complaint of palpitations. If atrioventricular nodal conduction is not affected, rapid ventricular rates may occur and cause chest pain, dyspnea, and lightheadedness. Syncope or near-syncope in patients with bradycardia-tachycardia syndrome may occur either as a result of rapid heart rates during tachycardia or because of pauses after the tachycardia stops. Stroke and systemic embolism occur at an increased frequency in patients with the bradycardia-tachycardia syndrome and may be the first manifestation of the disorder.

Inappropriate sinus tachycardia is a poorly defined disorder that is characterized by sinus rates during exercise or mild exercise that are in excess of those needed to meet physiologic demands.[17] Clinically, at least three patterns of inappropriate sinus tachycardia may be encountered. Some patients may complain of palpitations and, on monitoring, will have wide swings in sinus rates ranging from marked sinus bradycardia during sleep or rest to exaggerated tachycardia during minor exercise and stress. These patients have intrinsically normal sinus node function. Psychiatric disorders such as anxiety, neuroses, and panic attacks must be considered in the differential diagnosis. The palpitations themselves are best managed with reassurance. Some patients will have tachycardia reproducibly in response to moderate orthostatic stress. This syndrome has been called the postural orthostatic tachycardia syndrome, and affected patients may be severely disabled.

Continuous inappropriate sinus tachycardia is much less common. These patients have persistently elevated heart rates during both rest and exercise. Average resting heart rates of 110 to 130 beats per minute are not uncommon. Atrial tachycardias from a site adjacent to the sinus node must be considered in the differential diagnosis. Autonomic nervous system testing in these patients shows depressed cardiovagal reflexes, β-adrenergic hypersensitivity, and a high intrinsic heart rate after pharmacologic blockade with atropine and propranolol.

DIAGNOSTIC TECHNIQUES

A number of noninvasive and invasive tests may prove useful in the evaluation of patients with suspected SND (Table 53.3). Both routine electrocardiography and ambulatory electrocardiographic monitoring provide the most direct correlations between rhythm and symptoms and are the "gold standards" for diagnosis. Exercise testing, pharmacologic assessment of sinus node responses, and head-up tilt testing may also be useful in selected individuals. Several invasive tests of sinus node function have been described and may be of value in difficult cases. All of these tests must be interpreted in the context of the patient's underlying cardiac condition, so other investigations to evaluate cardiac function and anatomy are frequently important.

Noninvasive Testing

Ambulatory electrocardiography is the usual first step toward establishment of a diagnosis in patients with suspected symptomatic SND. Sinus bradycardia between 40 and 60 beats per minute and sinus pauses of up to 3 seconds are not infrequently documented in totally asymptomatic individuals.[16,18] Therefore, the goal of ambulatory recordings should be to establish a clear relationship between symptoms and arrhythmia. Patients with symptoms on a daily basis are best evaluated with continuous 24- to 48-hour recordings, whereas those with less frequent symptoms

TESTS OF SINUS NODE FUNCTION
Noninvasive tests
Ambulatory electrocardiographic monitoring, continuous or intermittent
Response to physiologic maneuvers
Exercise testing
Autonomic pharmacologic blockade
Invasive tests
Sinus node recovery time
Sinoatrial conduction time, direct and indirect

Table 53.3 Tests of sinus node function.

would be best evaluated with external or implantable loop recorders, which can store multiple short rhythm "snapshots."[19] Documentation of simultaneous symptoms and arrhythmia is necessary to confirm a diagnosis of SND that justifies therapy. Asymptomatic disturbances of sinus rate are of little diagnostic value unless extreme findings, such as sustained rates below 30 beats per minute or pauses of longer than 3 seconds, are recorded. Even these findings may not be sufficient to justify intervention, especially if they only occur during sleep.[16]

If ambulatory monitoring is normal or inconclusive and SND is still suspected to be the cause of the patient's symptoms, other noninvasive tests may be appropriate. Exercise testing is useful in patients with exercise-induced palpitations or in those with suspected chronotropic incompetence. A normal heart rate response to exercise may also help differentiate well-trained individuals with severe resting bradycardia from those with true SND.

Sinus node function during pharmacologic stress or neural activity may be studied in a number of ways. Heart rate responses to carotid sinus massage or the Valsalva maneuver may be assessed at the bedside. Upright tilt or vasodilator-induced hypotension can be used to test for the normal response of tachycardia. Autonomic nervous system influences on the sinus node may be studied by use of β-adrenergic blockade or stimulation or parasympathetic blockade with atropine. The intrinsic heart rate, defined as the heart rate after full β-adrenergic and muscarinic receptor blockade, is one measure of sinus node function that is also commonly used.

Invasive Testing

Although several invasive measures of sinus node function have been described, they are not commonly used in isolation for clinical decision making. The most commonly used invasive test of sinus node function is the sinus node recovery time (SNRT), an assessment of the response of the sinus node to overdrive atrial stimulation.[20] The SNRT is based on the principle that when a cardiac tissue with spontaneous depolarization is repetitively stimulated by impulses from another source, its intrinsic automaticity will be suppressed transiently after stimulation is discontinued. This phenomenon is termed overdrive suppression, and a quantitative assessment of overdrive suppression is often used as a measure of intrinsic sinus node function.

The SNRT is measured by placement of a pacing catheter in the high right atrium with delivery of 30- to 60-second trains of fixed-rate pacing over a range of cycle lengths. The interval from the last paced stimulus to the first spontaneous sinus beat is defined as the SNRT (Fig. 53.5). Because the duration of the SNRT depends on the spontaneous sinus cycle length (SCL), the most common measurement used is the corrected sinus node recovery time (CSNRT), which is calculated by subtracting the SCL that preceded pacing from the SNRT (CSNRT = SNRT − SCL). Values for a corrected CSNRT greater than 550 ms are considered to be abnormal, and values greater than 1000 ms are almost always associated with symptomatic SND.

Measurement of the SNRT in this fashion assumes that each paced impulse conducts into the sinus node and depolarizes it. However, conduction block into the node may

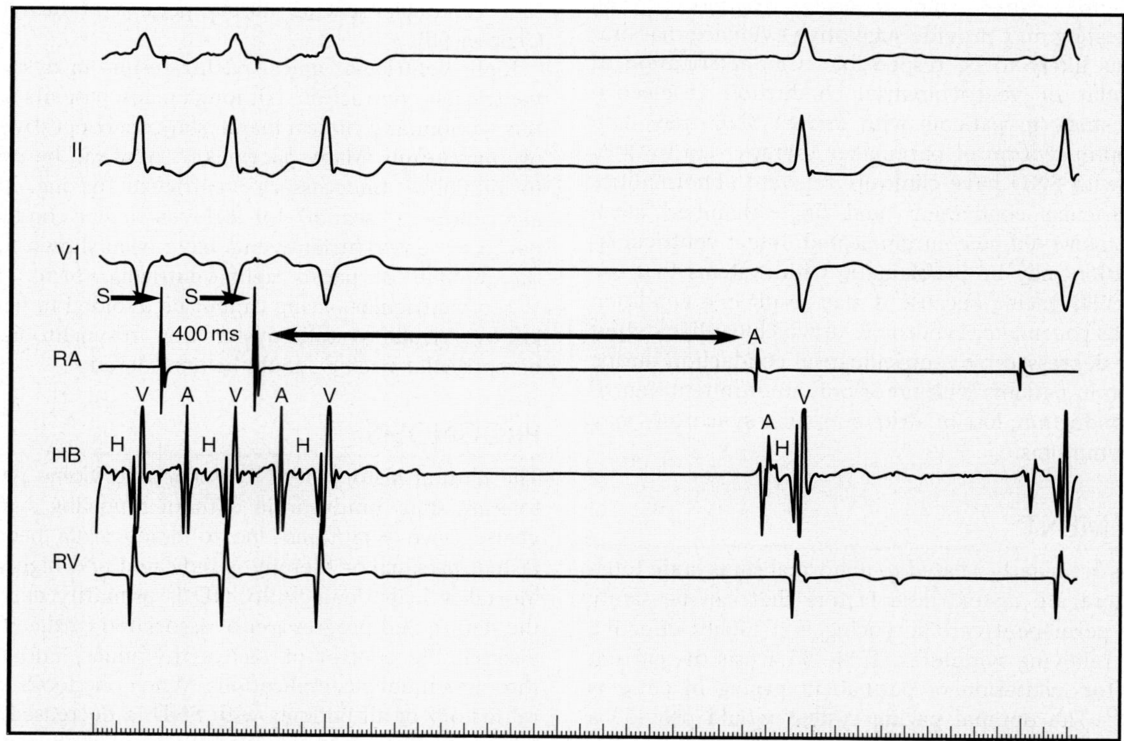

Figure 53.5 Abnormal sinus node recovery time. The tracings shown are surface electrocardiogram leads II and V_1 and intracardiac recordings from the right atrium (RA), His bundle (HB), and right ventricle (RV). After pacing for 30 seconds at a cycle length of 400 ms, stimulation is stopped and a sinus node recovery time (SNRT) of 2148 ms is measured. The preceding sinus cycle length was 990 ms, giving an abnormal corrected recovery time of 1158 ms. A, atrium; H, His; S, stimulus; V, ventricle.

occur, resulting in an artificially short SNRT. In such cases, the secondary pause after the first recovery beat may be greatly prolonged and serve as a qualitative marker of abnormal sinus node recovery.

Conduction delay or block into and out of the sinus node may lead to arrhythmias. Both indirect and direct techniques for measurement of sinoatrial conduction are available. Indirect methods use premature atrial stimulation (Strauss method) or short runs (≤8 beats) of atrial pacing (Narula method) to measure increments in the reset interval over the basic sinus cycle length.[20] The interval between the last paced atrial stimulus and the next sinus beat should be a measure of three variables: conduction into the node, the sinus cycle length, and conduction out of the node. Conduction is usually assumed to be equal in both directions, so the interval measure after pacing minus the sinus cycle length divided by 2 is used to estimate the one-directional sinoatrial conduction time. Indirect measures of sinoatrial conduction agree reasonably well with estimates made by direct sinus node electrogram recordings.

It is only rarely necessary to perform invasive testing of sinus node function. The correlation of symptoms with spontaneous arrhythmias remains the cornerstone of diagnosis of SND. Results of invasive testing should be positive only in patients with intrinsic SND.[17,20] These individuals will typically have frequent episodes of SND during routine monitoring, and the clinical diagnosis will be obvious. However, invasive tests may be of value during the comprehensive invasive evaluation of patients with unexplained syncope or other known cardiac arrhythmias. In patients with intermittent symptoms, it may be difficult to distinguish between several potential causes, and abnormal responses during sinus node testing may provide suggestive evidence that bradycardia was likely to be responsible. Characterization of atrioventricular or ventriculoatrial conduction at electrophysiologic study in patients with known SND may help select the optimal form of pacemaker therapy. Up to 20% of patients with SND have clinically relevant abnormalities in atrioventricular conduction, and single-chamber, atrial pacing systems would be contraindicated. Intact ventriculoatrial conduction may be problematic with systems that use only ventricular pacing because it may result in a condition referred to as pacemaker syndrome, in which cardiac output is markedly depressed by ventriculoatrial conduction during pacing. Even in patients with no or only intermittent ventriculoatrial conduction, loss of atrioventricular synchrony may still cause symptoms.

MANAGEMENT

If symptoms are clearly related to abnormal sinus node function and there are no extrinsic factors that can be safely eliminated, permanent cardiac pacing is a highly effective method for relieving symptoms. Table 53.4 lists the current indications for institution of permanent pacing in patients with SND.[21] The optimal pacing system would provide a normal chronotropic response to exercise or stress and maintain atrioventricular synchrony. Atrial pacing or a system that preferentially allows normal conduction should be used if possible.[22,23] A sensor-based, rate-adaptive atrial or dual-chamber pacing system should be employed in patients with SND. In patients with bradycardia-tachycardia syndrome, atrial pacing may delay or prevent episodes of atrial fibrillation or atrial flutter. The ability to switch to a ventricular-based pacing mode during atrial tachyarrhythmias will prevent high-rate ventricular pacing during periods of tachycardia (see Chapter 55).

Right ventricular apical pacing results in dyssynchronous ventricular contraction. Although many patients will tolerate this without any clinical manifestations, congestive heart failure may result. Many pacemakers now can be programmed to minimize unnecessary ventricular pacing. Proprietary algorithms to "search" for atrioventricular conduction after paced or sensed atrial events have been shown to minimize the number of paced right ventricular beats (Fig. 53.6). When ventricular pacing cannot be avoided in patients with left ventricular systolic dysfunction, resynchronization with biventricular pacing should be considered.

INDICATIONS FOR PERMANENT PACING IN SINUS NODE DYSFUNCTION

Class	Indications
I (indicated)	Documented symptomatic bradycardia and/or chronotropic incompetence even if these result from required drug therapy
IIa (reasonable)	Heart rate of less than 40 bpm when a clear association between symptoms consistent with bradycardia and documented bradycardia has not been established; and Syncope of unexplained origin and clinically significant abnormalities of sinus node function during electrophysiologic testing
IIb (may be considered)	Minimally symptomatic patients with chronic heart rates less than 40 bpm while awake
III (not indicated)	Symptomatic patients; and Symptomatic patients where symptoms have been clearly documented to occur in the absence of bradycardia

Modified from Epstein AE, DiMarco JP, Ellenbogen KA, et al. ACC/AHA/HRS 2008 guidelines for device-based therapy of cardiac rhythm abnormalities: executive summary. Heart Rhythm 2008;5:934-955.

Table 53.4 Indications for permanent pacing in sinus node dysfunction.

PROGNOSIS

The natural history of SND is variable. Some patients may tolerate sinus bradycardia without reporting symptoms for years. Once symptoms due to bradycardia become manifested, pacemaker therapy is indicated and highly effective. Mortality in patients with SND is primarily determined by the nature and progression of associated cardiac or systemic disease, the control of tachyarrhythmias, and the risk of thromboembolic complications. When one looks at the natural history of all patients with SND, a decreased life expectancy is observed. In one study of 148 patients who received pacemakers for SND, the observed survival at 1, 5, and 10 years was 84%, 57%, and 27%, respectively, compared with age- and sex-adjusted actuarial survival rates for the general population of 94%, 70%, and 45%.[24] However,

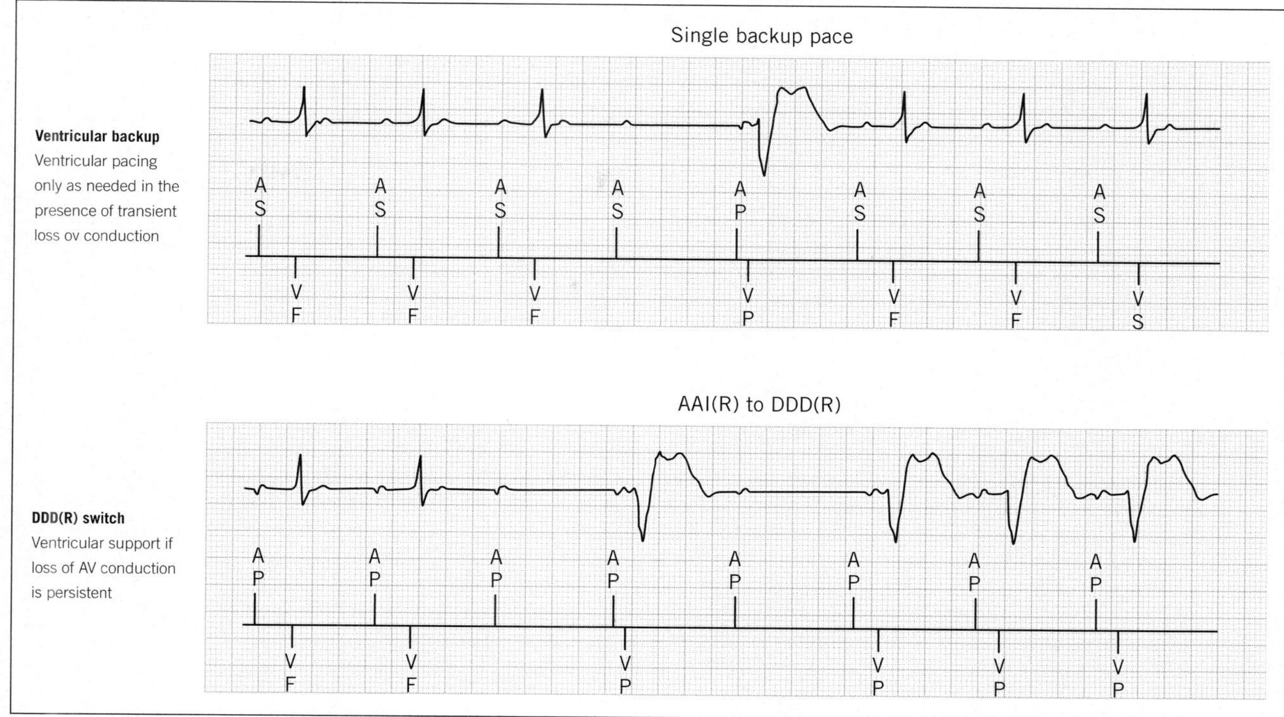

Figure 53.6 Algorithm to decrease ventricular pacing. In the top panel, the first three beats are atrially sensed (AS) with sensed conducted ventricular beats (VF). If a P wave blocks, backup ventricular pacing after the next atrial beat occurs. In the bottom panel, when the next beat is again blocked, the mode changes to DDD(R). The pacemaker will then periodically check at programmed intervals for the return of intrinsic conduction.

among those patients without identifiable structural heart disease, the survival rate was as expected. In the Mode Selection in Sinus-Node Dysfunction Trial[25] that included 2010 elderly patients observed for a median of 33.1 months, 20.5% of those randomized to ventricular pacing and 19.7% of those randomized to dual-chamber pacing died (P = NS), with most deaths due to noncardiac causes. Two meta-analyses have examined the benefits of atrial-based, usually dual-chamber versus single-chamber pacing in patients with SND and atrioventricular block.[26,27] Both identified trends in favor of atrial-based pacing for the prevention of stroke, congestive heart failure, and death and significant benefits in atrial fibrillation and pacemaker syndrome. As more pacemakers become capable of minimizing unnecessary right ventricular pacing, these patterns should become more pronounced. Even with older devices, atrial-based pacing systems are relatively cost-effective.[28]

SUMMARY

Disorders of sinus node function are common causes of symptoms that may be due to the inappropriate rate itself, concomitant changes in blood pressure, or associated tachycardias. When SND is due to extrinsic causes, attempts to prevent or to treat the primary cause should be the first step in therapy. When SND is due to intrinsic disease affecting the sinus node itself, or when an extrinsic cause cannot be controlled, permanent pacing is indicated.

chapter 54

Atrioventricular and Intraventricular Conduction Disorders

Decebal-Gabriel Laţcu and Nadir Saoudi

Definition

- Atrioventricular and intraventricular conduction disorders are characterized by delays during impulse propagation in the specialized conduction system of the heart.

Key Features

- PR interval prolongation to more than 200 ms.
- Failure to conduct all atrial impulses to the ventricles.
- Widening of the QRS complex due to delays in the His-Purkinje system.
- Associated with many types of structural heart disease.

Therapy

- Conduction disorders that result in symptoms of hemodynamic compromise and are irreversible require therapy, usually cardiac pacing.

The efficacy of cardiac performance depends critically on precise timing of depolarization in interdependent structures. Under physiologic conditions, this involves the spontaneous (automatic) formation of an impulse in the sinus node, which is then conducted in a serial and synchronized way to the atria, the atrioventricular (AV) node, and then on to the different parts of both ventricles. Excitation and contraction of the atria are almost synchronous and are completed before contraction of the ventricles. This is ensured by an AV conduction delay.[1]

Furthermore, ventricular contraction proceeds in a way to ensure that closure of the AV valves is followed by waves of excitation and contraction spreading from the ventricular apices toward the outflow tracts and orifices. The nodes, tracts, and networks of tissue that ensure this function constitute the cardiac conduction system.

ANATOMY AND PHYSIOLOGY

The human AV node is an oval or elliptical structure made of specialized muscular tissues (Fig. 54.1). It is subendocardial and contained exclusively within the atrial component of the triangle of Koch (Fig. 54.2).[2]

The triangle of Koch is delineated by

- the sinus septum (which harbors the tendon of Todaro);
- the membranous septum (as part of the central fibrous body); and
- the line of attachment of the septal leaflet of the tricuspid valve.

Two main preferential routes of entrance into the AV node have been described on the basis of electrophysiologic[3] and anatomic[4,5] observations:

- the fast pathway, which is anterosuperior to the main body of the AV node; and
- the slow pathway, which is inferior to the main body of the AV node.

However, as early as 1906, Tawara[6] described posterior extensions of the node. Mines[7] had in 1913 the intuition of a division of the atrioventricular connection. The first evidence of functional longitudinal dissociation within the AV node was provided by Moe's animal experimentations.[8] The fast pathway has fast conduction and a longer refractory period, whereas the slow pathway has slow conduction and a shorter refractory period. It has been suggested that these areas are composed histologically of ordinary atrial myocardial cells and that the difference in the speed of conduction may be related solely to a different orientation of the myocardial fibers (Fig. 54.3).[9] It has also recently been shown in humans that a right atrial posterior extension of the AV node is present in almost all hearts, and the AV node has never been found to have a "blunt" posterior ending. The cellular makeup of this extension is similar to that of the compact node, and this may provide the substrate for the slow pathway.[10]

The cellular component of the AV junctional area is made up mainly of transitional myocytes and to a lesser extent, of nodal myocytes. The large population of slow-conducting transitional myocytes is thought to be responsible for the AV conduction delay as a result of decremental impulse propagation. However, studies are inconsistent with theories of decremental conduction and prove the existence of a conduction barrier between the atrium and the AV node that is an important determinant of AV node delay.[11,12]

The AV node receives most of its blood supply from a dedicated ascending branch of the right coronary artery in about 90% of people. In the remaining 10%, the supply is provided by the left anterior coronary artery.

The AV bundle (or the bundle of His) is formed by tracts of myocytes converging at the anteroinferior pole of the AV node, at the apex of the triangle of Koch, from where they penetrate into the AV membranous septum. The bundle of His is surrounded by fibrous tissue as it passes through the central fibrous body (Fig. 54.4). After a short course of 1 to 2 cm, it divides into right and left bundle branches. The bundle of His receives most of its blood supply from both the AV nodal artery and branches of the left anterior descending artery.

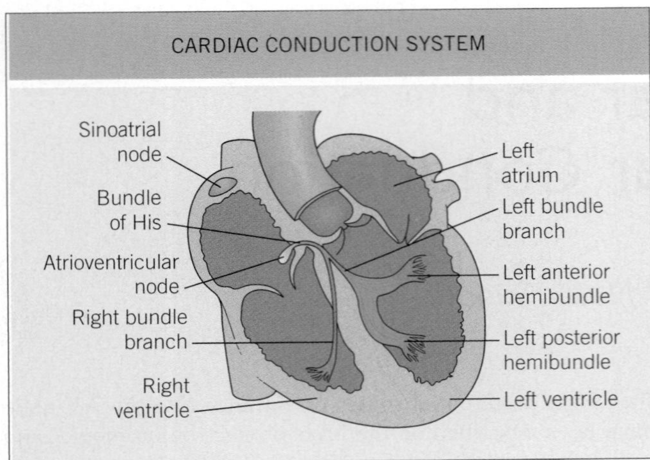

Figure 54.1 The cardiac conduction system.

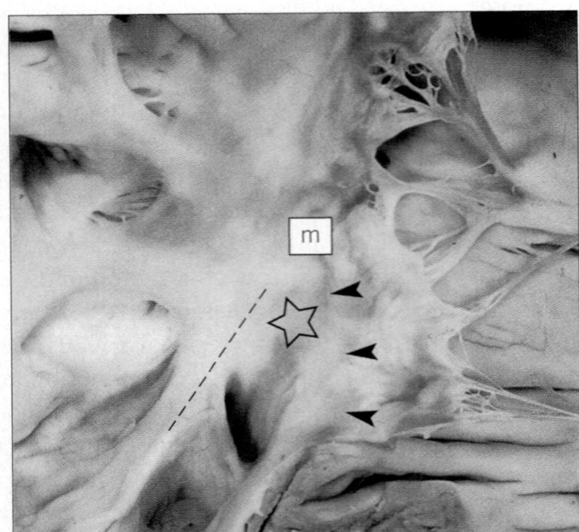

Figure 54.2 Right atrial view of the AV node within the triangle of Koch. The right side of the heart is opened to show the triangle of Koch delimited by the tendon of Todaro *(broken line)*, the membranous septum (m), and the attachment of the tricuspid valve *(arrowheads)*. The location of the AV node is indicated by the star. (From Anderson RH, Ho SY, Becker AE, Lang M. Living Anatomy. Ghent, Biosense, 1997.)

The right branch of the bundle of His continues as a narrow, discrete round group of cord-like fascicles running first inside the myocardium and then subendocardially to emerge beneath the medial papillary muscle of the right ventricle (Fig. 54.5). The left bundle branch is composed of a sheet of fascicles that diverge apically and subendocardially across the left aspect of the interventricular septum and then soon separate into anterior and posterior sheets to the corresponding papillary muscles (Fig. 54.6). Both bundle branches are insulated as they descend toward the apex. Fine branches leave the sheets, forming subendocardial networks, which first encompass the papillary muscles and then spread subendocardially to form an interweaving network that supplies all parts of the ventricle.

It has been clinically useful to consider the division of the left branch into two subdivisions (or hemibranches or fascicles), one anterior and a larger one posterior. Pathologic studies, however, show that in some people, a third intermediate fascicle (also called a medial or septal fascicle) emerges from the left bundle itself or its posteroinferior division; in other people, the subdivision of the left branch resembles a syncytium more than a discrete fascicle fanning out over the left septal surface. The left branch has blood supply from the AV nodal artery, the posterior descending artery, and the circumflex artery.

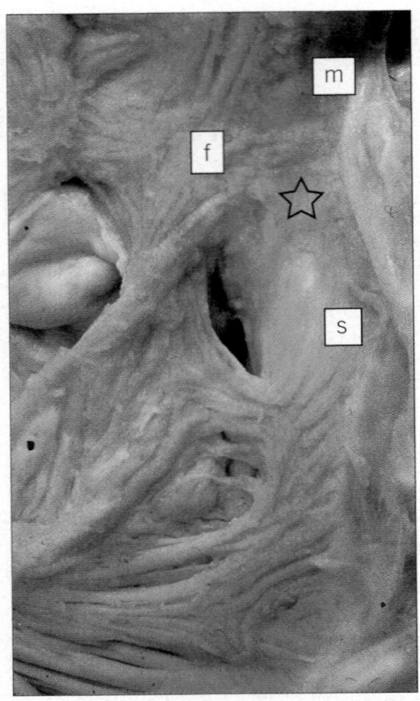

Figure 54.3 Right atrial view of the location of the slow (s) and fast (f) pathways of entrance into the AV node. A close-up view of the arrangement of the subendocardial fibers in and around the triangle of Koch. The location of the AV node is indicated by the star. The slow pathway encompasses a relatively large area between the coronary sinus ostium and the attachment of the tricuspid valve. Note that in the slow pathway, these superficial subendocardial fibers tend to run obliquely with respect to the tricuspid annulus; in the fast pathway, they tend to run perpendicularly with respect to the tricuspid annulus. Anisotropic conduction due to fiber orientation may also be related to deeper fibers. m, membranous septum. (From Anderson RH, Ho SY, Becker AE, Lang M. Living Anatomy. Ghent, Biosense, 1997.)

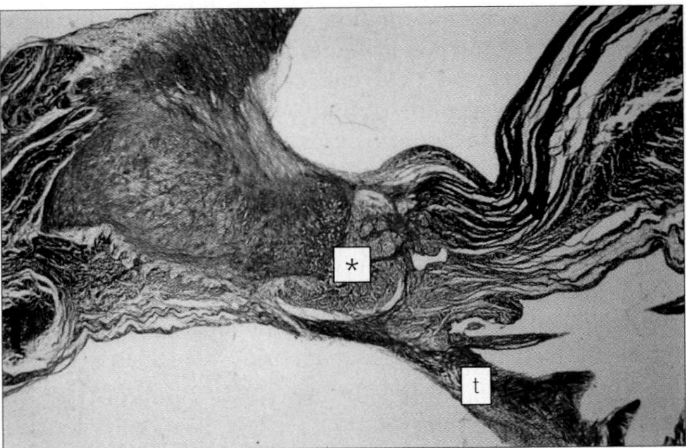

Figure 54.4 Penetrating AV bundle surrounded by fibrous tissue as it passes through the central fibrous body. The position of the bundle of His is indicated by the asterisk. t, tricuspid valve. Photomicrograph stained with Masson trichrome; original magnification ×40. (From Anderson RH, Ho SY, Becker AE, Lang M. Living Anatomy. Ghent, Biosense, 1997.)

Figure 54.5 Right bundle branch surrounded by fibrous tissue passing under the medial papillary muscle. The position of the right bundle branch is indicated by the asterisk. V, ventricular myocardium. Photomicrograph stained with Masson trichrome; original magnification ×100. (From Anderson RH, Ho SY, Becker AE, Lang M. Living Anatomy. Ghent, Biosense, 1997.)

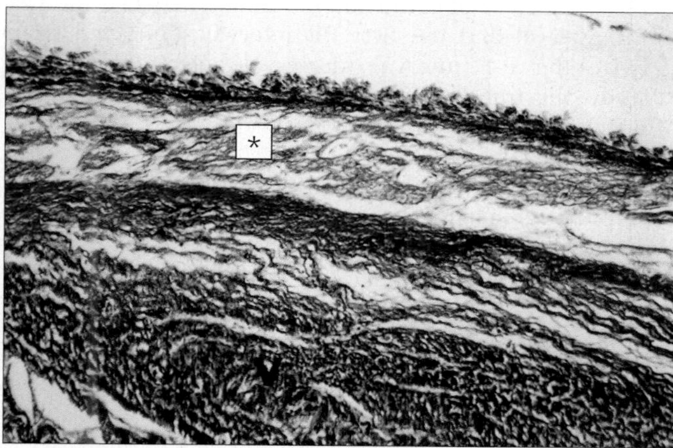

Figure 54.6 Left bundle branch as it passes like a sheet between fibrous tissue in the subendocardium of the ventricular septum. The position of the left bundle branch is indicated by the asterisk. Photomicrograph stained with Masson trichrome; original magnification ×100. (From Anderson RH, Ho SY, Becker AE, Lang M. Living Anatomy. Ghent, Biosense, 1997.)

The conduction system of the heart is influenced by both the parasympathetic and the sympathetic nervous systems, the effect being by far more pronounced at the level of the AV node than at the level of the His-Purkinje network. In canines, parasympathetic nerves are in the vicinity of the coronary sinus ostium. They act by releasing acetylcholine in the central region of the AV node and by modulating the amount of norepinephrine (noradrenaline) release at the prejunctional and postjunctional sites. Sympathetic stimulation (e.g., from the left stellate ganglion) shortens AV nodal conduction time, whereas left vagal stimulation lengthens it.

PATHOLOGY

Apart from the numerous intrinsic diseases that affect the conduction system, conduction disorders can be seen in any condition that affects the blood supply or neural inputs to the conducting tissues. In addition, a number of drugs and chemical agents also result in conduction abnormalities. Some of the common causes that can lead to AV and interventricular conduction disturbances are listed in Table 54.1.

COMMON CAUSES OF ATRIOVENTRICULAR AND INTRAVENTRICULAR CONDUCTION DISTURBANCE
Intrinsic causes
Congenital
Sclerodegenerative
Ischemia
Trauma (surgical)
Connective tissue disorders
Tumors
Sarcoidosis
Extrinsic causes
Drugs
Autonomic disorders
Hypothyroidism

Table 54.1 Common causes of atrioventricular and intraventricular conduction disturbance.

PATHOPHYSIOLOGY

Atrioventricular Conduction Disturbances

On the basis of the surface electrocardiogram (ECG), AV conduction disturbances can be divided into three types:

- first-degree AV block;
- second-degree AV block; and
- third-degree (complete) AV block.

First-degree Atrioventricular Block

First-degree AV block refers to prolongation of conduction time between the atria and the ventricles, in other words, a prolongation of the PR interval on the ECG. The normal PR interval measures between 0.12 and 0.2 second in an adult who has a heart rate within physiologic range (60 to 100 beats per minute) and 0.18 second in children younger than 14 years. In first-degree AV block, each P wave is followed by a QRS complex with a PR interval that exceeds 0.20 second (usually between 0.21 and 0.4 second). Longer PR intervals may be observed, but they are usually associated with second-degree AV block.

First-degree AV block is due to a true anatomic or functional impairment of conduction. It can be permanent or transient and may be located at the level of the AV node, the bundle of His, or the bundle branches. An example of an ECG from a patient in first-degree AV block is shown in Figure 54.7.

First-degree AV block is rarely accompanied by clinical sequelae except for prolongation of the time between the *a* and the *c* waves of the jugular venous pulse. Prolongation of the PR interval can itself give rise to a deterioration in cardiac function,[13] especially in cardiac insufficiency patients, because of loss of atrioventricular synchrony and shortening of the ventricular filling time.[14]

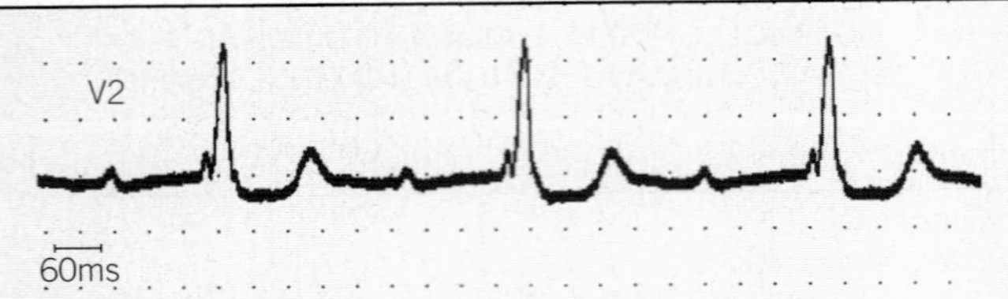

Figure 54.7 First-degree AV block. The PR interval is particularly prolonged, to 320 ms. Major prolongation of the PR interval is almost always due to a delay within the AV node. In this case, associated right bundle branch block is observed.

Second-degree Atrioventricular Block

In second-degree AV block, conducted atrial beats are interspersed with nonconducted beats. However, one of the additional prerequisites for this definition is the regularity of the atrial rhythm. Atrial premature contractions that fail to conduct to the ventricles because of normal AV node refractoriness are not considered to be the result of AV block. Similarly, the atrial rate is of prime importance.

Second-degree AV block is considered abnormal when it occurs in the physiologic heart rate range. At faster rates, it is considered a normal response to atrial tachycardia. Again, the lesion that is responsible for impairment of conduction may be located at the level of the AV node, the bundle of His, or the bundle branches. Second-degree block is further classified into

- Möbitz (type I, Wenckebach) AV block;
- type II second-degree AV block;
- 2:1 AV block;
- multilevel AV block;
- reverse alternate Wenckebach AV block; and
- high-grade AV block.

Möbitz Atrioventricular Block

Möbitz (type I or Wenckebach) AV block was first described by Wenckebach long before the invention of the ECG. He described it as a form of conduction disturbance characterized by a progressive lengthening of the interval between the *a* and the *c* waves of the jugular pulse, terminating in a dropped *c* wave.[15] Later, the ECG features were characterized by Möbitz as a progressive prolongation of the PR interval until there was a dropped ventricular beat (Fig. 54.8).[16] The phenomenon is usually repetitive.

Wenckebach and Winterberg[17] further characterized this phenomenon by describing other characteristics (Fig. 54.9), including

- progressive lengthening of the PR interval;
- the increment between the first and the second conducted beats being the largest;
- progressive decrease in the R-R intervals because of decrease in the PR increment; and
- a short ventricular pause produced by the nonconducted P wave that is equal to the difference between the last PR interval and the first PR interval subtracted from twice the P-P interval (during an electrophysiologic study, this translates into an increase in the AH interval, which parallels the PR prolongation).

The term *typical Wenckebach periodicity* has been applied to second-degree block that shows all of these characteristics. When P wave activity is not clearly discernible on the

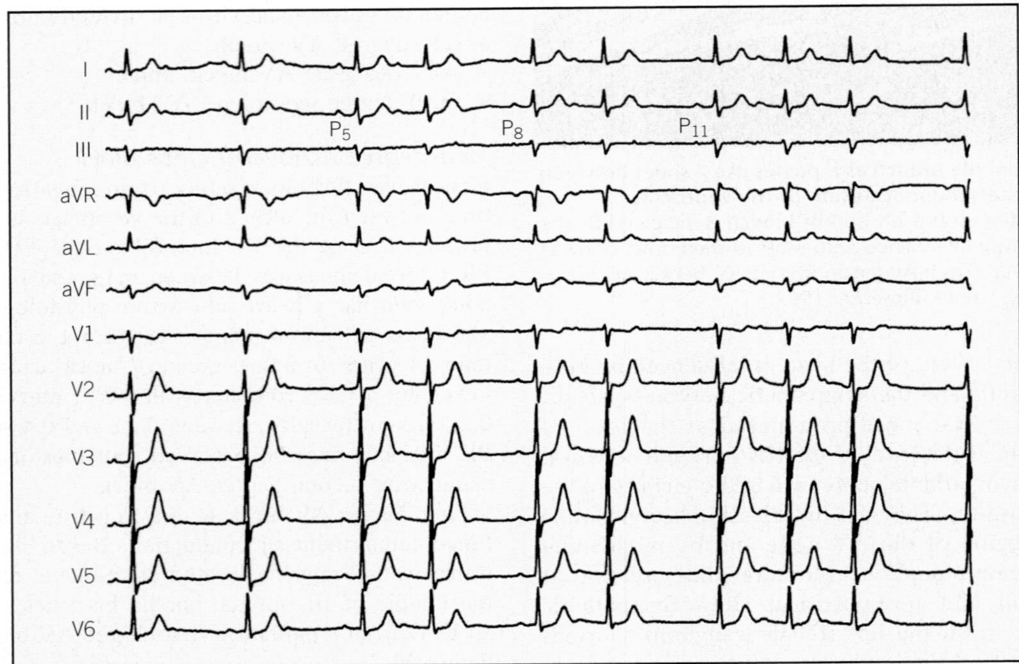

Figure 54.8 Second-degree type I AV block and 2:1 AV block. Three periods of Wenckebach-type AV block are shown starting with the fifth, eighth, and eleventh P waves. In the first two periods of block, only one PR is prolonged before the dropped beat, and they are described as 3:2 Wenckebach periods. In the third period of block, after a major PR prolongation after the second P wave of the period, the subsequent PR prolongation is less marked. This is described as a 4:3 Wenckebach block. Note that the P-P interval is constant. In the right part of the tracing, there is intermittent 2:1 PR relation. Alternating 2:1 AV block with 3:2 and 4:3 Wenckebach sequences suggests that the lesion responsible for this pattern of AV block is located within the AV node.

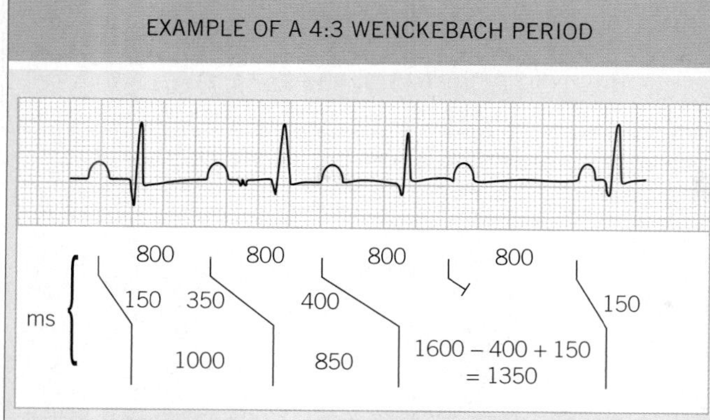

Figure 54.9 Typical theoretical example of a 4:3 Wenckebach period. The baseline sinus rhythm is 75 beats per minute, which corresponds to a cycle length of 800 ms. The first PR interval of the sequence is 150 ms. The second P wave is conducted with a PR interval of 350 ms, which is due to an increment of 200 ms in the AV nodal conduction time. The third PR is longer, but because the increment is decreasing, the PR interval is prolonged by only an additional 50 ms and is now 400 ms. The fourth P wave is blocked. Analysis of the QRS sequences shows group beating of the three conducted beats that tend to cluster toward the end of the period, which always ends with a long diastole.

surface ECG, Wenckebach periodicity can be recognized because of one of its aftereffects, resultant "group beating." The regular appearance of grouped QRS complexes has been called the footprints of Wenckebach. However, in clinical situations, it is now generally recognized that all of the features are found in perhaps less than 50% of cases.

Type II Second-degree Atrioventricular Block

In type II second-degree AV block, the PR interval remains constant before sudden block of the P wave. The PR interval may be normal or slightly prolonged, although not as much as in first-degree AV block. The first PR interval after the pause is always the same as the other PR intervals. According to the accepted current terminology, only one P wave is blocked (Fig. 54.10). However, in the early description by Möbitz, several consecutive P waves could be blocked. This is now generally described as high-degree AV block (see later).

Clinical Applications of the Type I and Type II Second-degree Atrioventricular Block

The subclassification of second-degree AV block into types I and II has important clinical applications. Type I AV block with a normal QRS configuration usually denotes conduction disturbance in the AV node, and such a disturbance does not generally progress rapidly to higher grades and clinically severe forms of AV block. If this form of block is seen with bundle branch block, the site of block could be in the AV node or in the His-Purkinje system.

Type II block in the absence of any abnormality of the QRS complex can be due to intra-His AV block, but the block is more likely to be due to AV nodal block. On the other hand, when type II block is accompanied by a bundle branch block, the disturbance is usually localized to the His-Purkinje system and is very likely to progress to symptomatic third-degree AV block.

2:1 Atrioventricular Block

2:1 AV block cannot be readily classified into any of the types of second-degree block discussed before. It is therefore preferable to refer to this conduction disturbance separately as 2:1 AV block. This pattern often alternates with other types of second-degree block, thus suggesting the level of the lesion (see Fig. 54.8). When this is associated with normal sinus rhythm, the P-P interval that encompasses the QRS complex may be shorter than one that does not. This phenomenon is referred to as ventriculophasic sinus arrhythmia. A similar phenomenon modulates AV nodal conduction time in patients with 2:1 AV block at the intra-His level; this is referred to as ventriculophasic AV nodal conduction. Both observations are thought to depend on phasic baroreflex activation.[18]

Multilevel Atrioventricular Blocks

Multilevel AV blocks are commonly observed during regular atrial tachycardias or flutter. They are not conventionally referred to as blocks but rather as alternate Wenckebach periodicity. In the typical form of alternate Wenckebach conduction, two levels of blocks are in series within the AV node. The upper level allows 2:1 AV conduction, whereas the conducted beat (i.e., every other beat) is conducted with the progressive typical prolongation of the Wenckebach phenomenon (Fig. 54.11).[19]

Reverse Alternate Wenckebach Block

Reverse alternate Wenckebach block has been described as a particular form of incomplete 2:1 AV block that is characterized by a gradual decrease in the PR interval interrupted by 1:1 conduction with a typical Wenckebach phenomenon. We and Castellanos and coworkers have found that this is a frequent pattern observed within a range of atrial rates and sandwiched between 3:2 and 2:1 AV conduction (Fig. 54.12).[20,21]

High-grade Atrioventricular Block

High-grade AV block may be defined as the intermittent blockade of two or more supraventricular impulses (Fig. 54.13). In case of slow atrial rate, it is often associated with a dissociated junctional escape rhythm, with which it interferes. The blocked impulses are followed by a pause, allowing the emergence of an escape rhythm. This may continue because of the concealed retrograde AV nodal conduction that prohibits further anterograde propagation of the supraventricular impulse for a short period, until anterograde capture shortens the VV (ventricular) cycle and reinitiates the phenomenon. Periodic anterograde capture by the sinus P wave may lead to emergence of regular patterns. For example, if the first QRS complex of the escape rhythm is followed by anterograde capture through the normal conduction pathway, the phenomenon is called escape capture bigeminy.

Third-degree Atrioventricular Block

Third-degree (complete) AV block is the most advanced state of AV block, in which there is complete absence of conduction of impulses from the atria to the ventricles. The atria and the ventricles are asynchronously controlled by independent pacemakers, resulting in AV dissociation. Note that high-grade or complete AV block is not synonymous with AV dissociation, as patients who have complete AV block

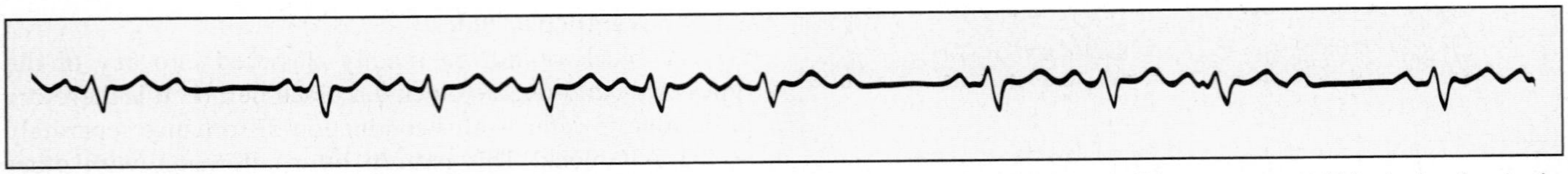

Figure 54.10 Möbitz type II second-degree AV block. ECG lead II in a patient with intermittent sudden unexpected blockade of a single P wave, without discernible increase in the preceding PR interval.

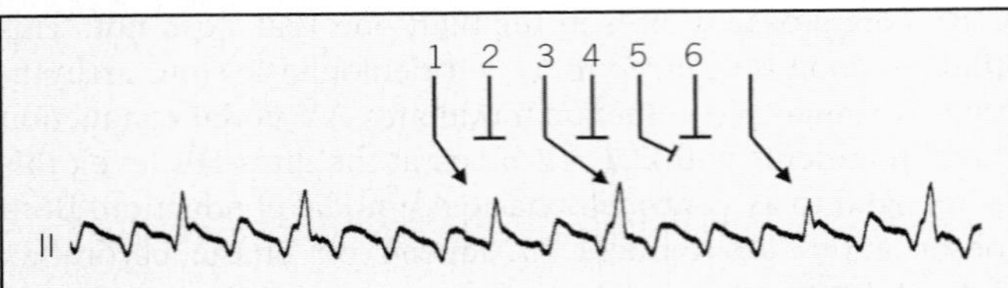

Figure 54.11 Alternate Wenckebach periods. In this example, which was observed during typical atrial flutter, there is a 6:2 relationship between the paced *a* waves and the resulting QRS complex. The ladder diagram shows what occurs in a model of dual level of block within the AV node when the upper block is of the 2:1 type and the lower block is of the Wenckebach type. The first impulse crosses both levels with the usual AV nodal delay. The second impulse blocks in the zone of 2:1. The third impulse is conducted across both areas with a longer distal delay. The fourth impulse blocks in the zone of 2:1, but the fifth impulse blocks because it is the third beat of the distal 3:2 Wenckebach sequence. The sixth impulse blocks in the zone of 2:1, and the period resumes. This can be described by the formula $2n + (2/n)$, where n is the number of observed QRS complexes within a given period. This can be indirectly diagnosed by the observation of "group beating" that is typical of Wenckebach periods.

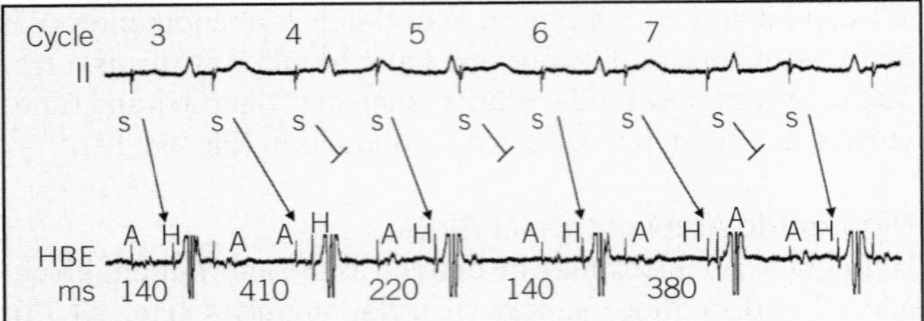

Figure 54.12 Reverse alternating Wenckebach periodicity during fixed-rate atrial pacing at a cycle length of 400 ms. The three first atrial pacing spikes capture the atrium, resulting in a 3:2 Wenckebach AV nodal sequence. This is followed by a sequence of 2:1 AV block during which AH of the conducted beat measures 220 ms. The sixth AH is then shorter than the 2:1 period, and this is now 140 ms. It is the first beat of a new 3:2 period, and the subsequent (seventh) AH is 380 ms; this precedes the dropped beat. If this period is again followed by a single 2:1 period of AV conduction, it bears the name of reverse alternating Wenckebach period. It is best described by the sum of the atrial beats of both periods (3 + 2) divided by the number of resulting ventricular beats (2 + 1) (i.e., 5:3). S, electrical pacing spike; HBE, His bundle electrogram; numerical values are those of AHs.

have complete AV dissociation, but patients who have complete AV dissociation (e.g., in ventricular tachycardia) may or may not have AV block (Fig. 54.14).

In complete AV block, the atrial rate is faster than that of the escape pacemaker, which can be idionodal or ventricular. Long recordings fail to reveal any captured beat, except for rare captures due to supernormality.[22] Sometimes retrograde ventriculoatrial conduction may be observed. The QRS width

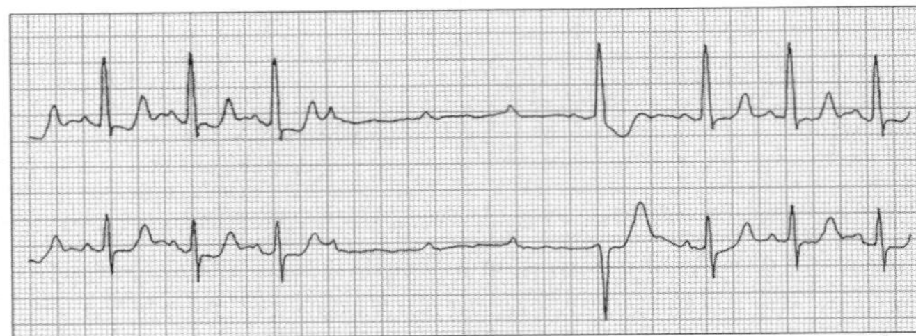

Figure 54.13 High-grade AV block. During a Holter recording, the first three P waves are conducted with a normal PR interval. The fourth, fifth, sixth, and seventh P waves are blocked, and normal AV conduction resumes with the sixth P wave. The fourth QRS complex is an escape beat of ventricular origin.

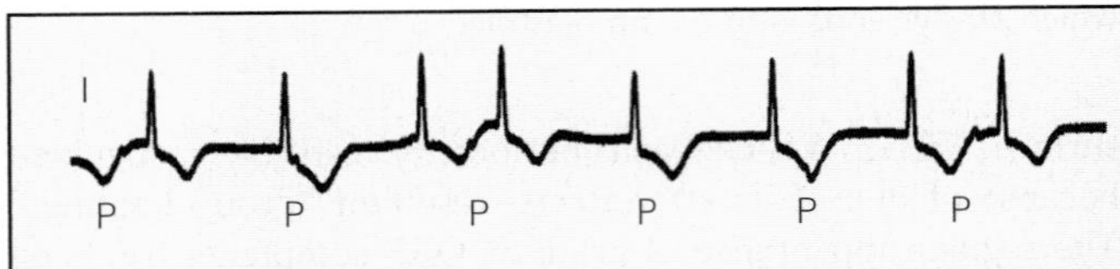

Figure 54.14 AV dissociation without AV block. During an episode of sinus bradycardia, a junctional escape rhythm emerges at a rate faster than that of sinus rhythm. An episode of AV dissociation ensues, which is periodically interrupted by anterograde sinus capture if the P wave falls late enough after the preceding junctional beat to allow anterograde propagation of impulses. In this case, the two first QRS complexes are junctional escape beats. The first P wave falls immediately after the second QRS complex and cannot cross the AV node, which is refractory as a result of the preceding QRS complex. The second P wave falls later and is able to propagate through the normal pathway to capture the ventricle and thereby reset the escape rhythm. After another three junctional escape QRS complexes, the phenomenon repeats. The primary mechanism responsible for AV dissociation here is the sinus bradycardia with a faster junctional escape. There is no sign of accompanying AV block.

and morphology can give reliable clues as to whether the block is occurring at the level of the AV node or the bundle of His or distal to the bundle of His (Figs. 54.15 and 54.16). Prolonged periods of asystole at initiation of conduction interruption or because of exit block of the subsidiary pacemakers may result in cardiac arrest and sudden arrhythmic death (Fig. 54.17). A particular form of complete AV block is the one observed during a severe vagal state. It is not due to structural lesion of the AV conduction system; rather, it is merely functional. It is associated with bradycardia and is usually not life-threatening, although the quality of life of the patients suffering from this condition may be severely impaired.

Intraventricular Conduction Defects

Conduction disturbances that are recognized as bundle branch block on the surface ECG are usually related to structural and less commonly, physiologic reasons. The bundle

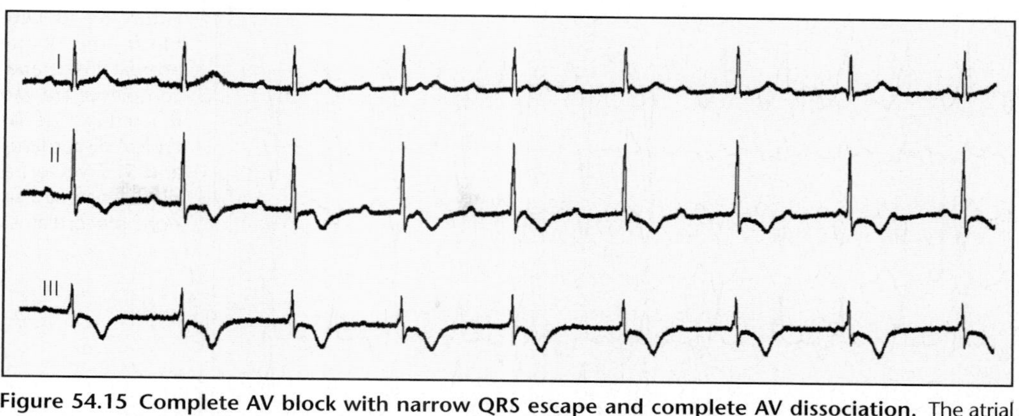

Figure 54.15 Complete AV block with narrow QRS escape and complete AV dissociation. The atrial rate is slightly more than twice as fast as the ventricular escape rate. None of the sinus P waves is able to penetrate the escape focus and depolarize it. The normal shape of the QRS complex suggests that the escape focus originates in the AV node. In contrast to Figure 54.14, the AV dissociation here is the direct result of AV block.

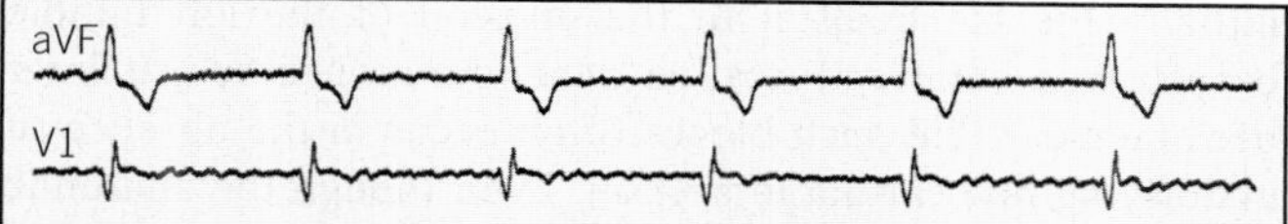

Figure 54.16 Complete AV block with wide QRS escape rate. During ongoing atrial fibrillation, there is AV dissociation and a slow, regular, and wide QRS ventricular escape rate. The simple observation of a regular ventricular rate during ongoing atrial fibrillation strongly suggests associated complete AV block.

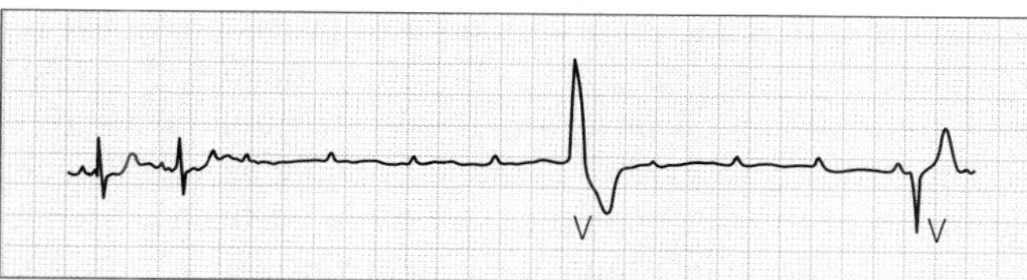

Figure 54.17 Paroxysmal complete AV block during a Holter recording. The first two beats are normally conducted, narrow QRS complexes. All subsequent P waves are blocked. The two subsequent ventricular QRS complexes are of ventricular origin and may represent ventricular escape. This explains why syncope and cardiac arrest may occur at initiation of complete block, although they are reversible as a result of the emergence of a ventricular escape rhythm. On arrival at the hospital, a rhythm analogous to that shown in Figures 54.15 and 54.16 may then be recorded. This occurs here without discernible change in the rate of the P waves, but it is sometimes associated with acceleration or deceleration of the sinus rate.

branch block patterns have conventionally been thought to represent conduction disturbance in the corresponding bundle branch or fascicle.[23] Theoretically, similar ECG patterns can also be produced by conduction delay more distally in the Purkinje network, at the junction of the Purkinje network and the myocytes, and in the working myocardium.[24] Experimental and clinical evidence for production of similar patterns as a result of more proximal longitudinal dissociation (in the AV node or the bundle of His) has also been reported.[25]

Left Bundle Branch Block

Left bundle branch block (LBBB) corresponds to situations in which severe slowing or complete interruption of conduction occurs in the left branch or its fascicles. In this condition, the left ventricle is activated after the right ventricle. The impulse descends within the right branch to activate the right ventricle while simultaneously crossing the interventricular septum to activate the left ventricle. During this phase, impulse propagation is no longer mediated by the specialized conduction system and is therefore slow, which explains the widening of the QRS complex (up to 0.12 to 0.18 second). An upright, notched, or slurred R wave in leads I, aVL, and V_6 reflects the change in the main direction of ventricular activation, which is now right to left.[26]

Because of reversal of septal activation, which also occurs from right to left, an important ECG feature of LBBB is the frequent absence of normal septal waves (R wave in lead V_1 and Q wave in lead V_6). As a result, the QRS complex tends to be a monophasic R wave in leads I and aVL and the left precordial leads and a QS complex in the right precordial leads. There are, however, many variations in the LBBB pattern, one of the most common being the persistence of a small r wave in the right precordial leads (Fig. 54.18).

The frontal QRS axis in LBBB may be either normal (11%) or more frequently direct to the left (between −30 and −90 degrees), but a marked left axis deviation is almost always due to left anterior hemiblock. Among patients with LBBB, those with a left axis deviation have a greater incidence of myocardial dysfunction, more advanced conduction disease, and greater cardiovascular mortality than those with a normal axis.[27]

Another important feature is the QRS and ST-T vectors opposition. In leads in which the QRS complex is positive (leads I and aVL and the left precordial leads), the ST segment is depressed and the T wave is negative. Sometimes there is no discordance between the vectors of the QRS complex and the ST segment–T wave, and this has been proposed as suggesting associated myocardial ischemia. On occasion, the appearance of bundle branch block may be rate dependent; this is then termed aberration (see later).

In the incomplete form of LBBB, the initial vectors of septal activation remain abnormal; but because the left branch still conducts, there is little delay in the left ventricular activation. Thus, the QRS complex is slightly prolonged (it does not exceed 0.12 second), but the septal R and Q waves are absent. Associated axis shift and discordance of QRS and ST-T vectors are observed in the majority of cases.

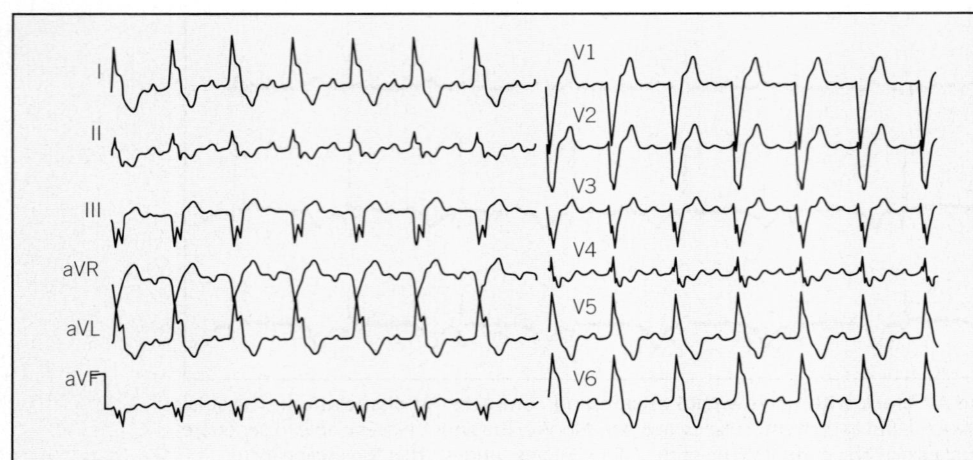

Figure 54.18 Left bundle branch block. The PR interval is within normal limits, and the QRS complexes are wide and without marked axis deviation. Note the typical discordance between QRS and ST-T vectors and the atypical persistence of a small r wave in the right precordial leads.

Right Bundle Branch Block

In normal intraventricular conduction, most of the electrical forces are due to left ventricular activation, and the right ventricle contributes little to the QRS morphology. However, when the right branch conduction is interrupted or severely delayed, right ventricular activation follows left ventricular activation, again coming after transseptal impulse propagation.

As a result, in complete right bundle branch block (RBBB), the QRS complex is wide (>0.12 second), with terminal forces representing right ventricular activation. Because the early forces that represent septal activation are unaltered, the initial small r wave in the right precordial leads and the q wave in leads V_5 and V_6 remain. The typical distortion of the QRS complex in RBBB is recorded in lead V_1 with a monophasic, double-peaked R wave separated by an S wave of variable amplitude (rR′ or rsR′ or rSR′). The R′ wave is larger than the r wave in both amplitude and duration.[28] The delayed right ventricular activation also accounts for the S wave in leads I, aVL, V_5, and V_6, which is usually marked and wide (Fig. 54.19). As in LBBB, the QRS complex and ST-T wave vectors are discordant in RBBB, yielding a T wave that is negative in leads V_1 and V_2.

Criteria defining the existence of incomplete RBBB are controversial. It is often diagnosed when a late R′ wave is recorded in lead V_1 but with a QRS complex width that does not exceed 0.12 ms.

Fascicular Blocks

In addition to block involving the main trunk of the left bundle, conduction abnormalities can occur separately in either of the two divisions or fascicles of the left bundle. Although initially the block distal to the division of the left bundle branch was incorrectly called peri-infarction block, it later became clear that such blocks often occur in the absence of underlying myocardial infarction. Even though the anatomic division of the left branch is inconstant, the concept has received support from experimental data and clinical experience. The common features of fascicular blocks (or hemiblocks) are the alteration in the morphology of the QRS complex and the axis shift without major QRS widening.

Left Anterior Hemiblock

Left anterior hemiblock (or left anterior fascicular block) is a conduction disturbance that can be either functional or structural and that can occur at any level (proximal or distal) of the anterosuperior division of the left bundle branch. The initial forces of the QRS complex are oriented from the endocardium to the epicardium (i.e., rightward, inferiorly, and anteriorly), which is responsible for the small q waves in leads I and aVL as well as the r wave in the inferior leads. However, immediately afterward, the posteroinferior division region of the left endocardium starts being activated abnormally before the anterosuperior region. This results in a marked left axis shift. As a result, the ECG picture of left anterior hemiblock is characterized by a qR wave in leads I and aVL, with leads II, III, and aVF showing a small r wave followed by a deep S wave. The frontal plane QRS axis is between −45 and −90 degrees (Fig. 54.20).

The degree of abnormal left axis deviation required for the diagnosis of left anterior hemiblock has been the subject of

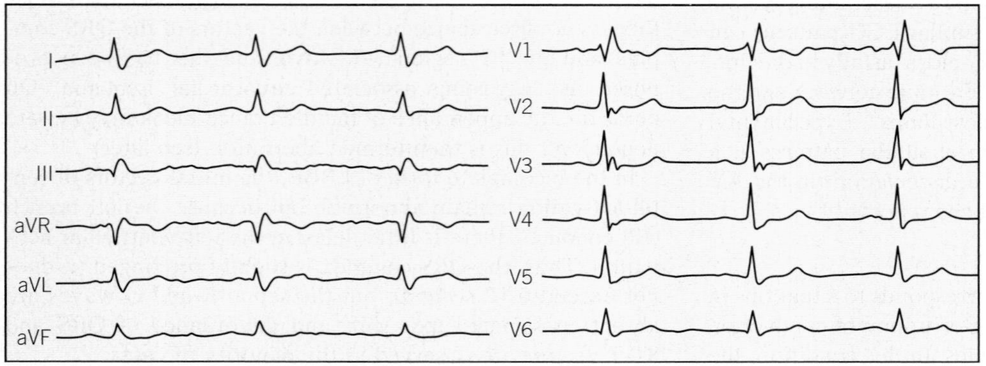

Figure 54.19 Complete right bundle branch block. The typical pattern of rSR′ is best seen in lead V_1. The QRS axis is slightly deviated on the right (at 90 degrees).

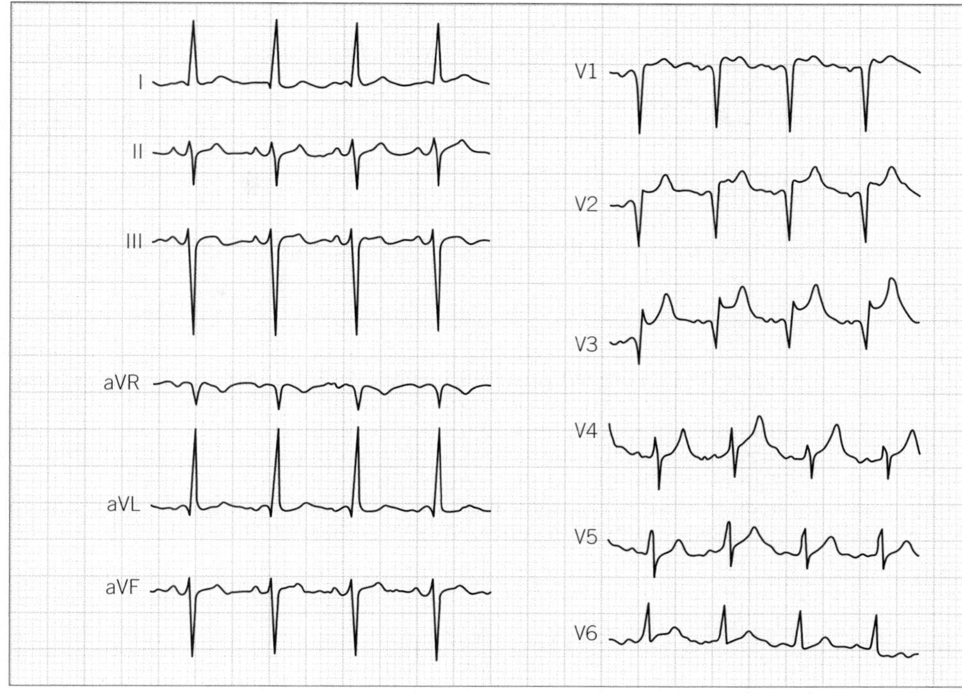

Figure 54.20 Left anterior hemiblock during acute anteroseptal myocardial infarction. The QRS axis is about −50 degrees, with tall R waves in leads I and aVL and tall S waves in the inferior leads. This pattern is frequently observed after occlusion of the left anterior descending coronary artery.

debate and speculation.[29] We consider that if the electrical axis lies between −30 and −60 degrees, left anterior hemiblock is probably present; but if it lies between −60 and −90 degrees, it is almost certainly present. If the axis is close to −30 degrees, it is useful to record the ECG during a deep breath (which produces an inferior shift of the diaphragm) to test axis stability.

A frequent additional observation is the displacement of the precordial transitional zone to the left, and the appearance of marked S waves in the left precordial leads, reflecting the superior orientation of the left ventricular forces.

Left Posterior Hemiblock

Left posterior hemiblock (or left posterior fascicular block) is a conduction disturbance that can be functional or structural. It can occur at any level (proximal or distal) of the posteroinferior division of the left bundle branch, resulting in a delay of activation of this region, which now occurs significantly after the anterosuperior region.

In pure left posterior hemiblock, the initial forces of the QRS will be oriented from the endocardium to the epicardium (i.e., leftward, superiorly, and somewhat anteriorly), which is responsible for the small r waves in leads I and aVL as well as the q wave in the inferior leads. The activation then proceeds over the electrically preponderant left ventricle through the other hemibranch (i.e., inferiorly, posteriorly, and slightly rightward), resulting in a marked clockwise rotation of the electrical QRS axis. As a result, there is a small r wave followed by a deep S wave in leads I and aVL. The inferior leads (II, III, and aVF) show a narrow initial q wave followed by a large R wave. The frontal plane QRS axis varies from +90 to +120 degrees. The magnitude of the right axis deviation in pure left posterior hemiblock is less than the magnitude of the left axis deviation in left anterior hemiblock. Indeed, the hallmark of left posterior hemiblock is an inferior axis shift more than a right axis deviation.

Although the classic criteria for left posterior hemiblocks require an electrical axis of +120 degrees or more, incomplete left posterior hemiblock has also been observed and is associated with stepwise right shifts (Fig. 54.21). Therefore, some degree of left posterior hemiblock might be present even if the axis does not exceed +120 degrees. Other authors have suggested that an axis shift beyond +90 or even +80 degrees may be sufficient in the absence of right ventricular hypertrophy.[30] This pattern is particularly rare and often accompanies RBBB. In Rosenbaum's classic definition, other causes of right axis deviation should be excluded, and this further renders the diagnosis difficult.

Bifascicular Block

The term *bifascicular block* is sometimes used to describe complete LBBB or, more commonly, RBBB that is associated with block of either of the two fascicles of the left bundle branch.

The most common combination is RBBB and left anterior hemiblock. The superimposition of complete RBBB on left anterior hemiblock does not further affect the initial QRS forces. It is diagnosed when marked left axis deviation with an rS pattern in the inferior leads is associated with a late wide R′ wave in lead V_1 and a QRS widening to more than 0.12 second (Fig. 54.22).

The combination of RBBB and left posterior hemiblock is rare; but in the initial series in which left posterior hemiblock was reported, RBBB was present in the majority of the cases. This combination is recognized when a typical RBBB pattern in the right precordial leads is associated with a large rS complex in leads I and aVL.

RBBB associated with alternating anterior and posterior left hemiblock is the mark of severe intraventricular conduction disturbances that are usually associated with Möbitz type II AV conduction block. The term *trifascicular block*

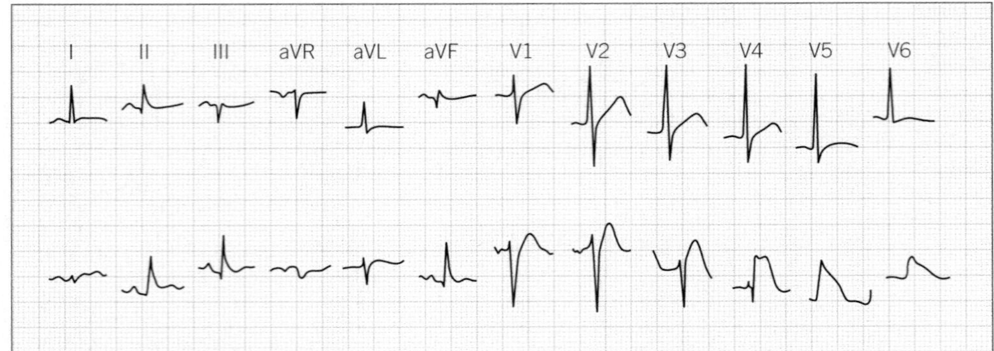

Figure 54.21 Pure left posterior hemiblock. The control tracing (upper strip) shows an old posteroinferior myocardial infarction with an electrical QRS axis of 0 degrees. Three weeks later, an acute apicolateral injury is accompanied by a right axis shift to 90 degrees with slight QRS enlargement and the appearance of qR waves in the inferior leads, which obscure the previous ECG signs of myocardial infarction. (From Castellanos A, Agha AS, Beteler B, Castillo CA, Berkovitz BV. A study of arrival of excitation at selected ventricular sites during human bundle branch block using close bipolar catheter electrodes. Anaesthesiology 1973;63:208-213.)

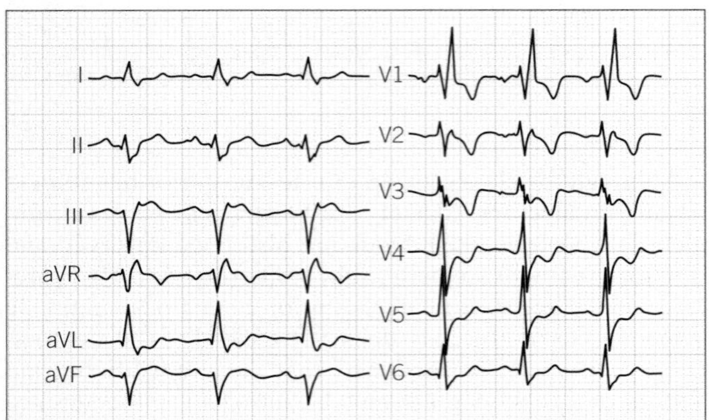

Figure 54.22 Right bundle branch block associated with left anterior hemiblock. The typical pattern of RBBB is easily recognizable in lead V_1. However, the QRS axis is shifted leftward to 45 degrees, and there is associated block of the left anterior hemibranch. This pattern is also referred to as bifascicular block. In this example, the PR interval is normal. Association with first-degree AV block has sometimes been mislabeled as trifascicular block; but in such a situation, the PR prolongation is most often due to an AV nodal delay associated with the intraventricular conduction block.

has been used when RBBB and left anterior hemiblock are associated with a prolonged PR interval. In fact, the increase in the PR interval is due to a delay of conduction in the AV node more often than to slowing of conduction in the left posterior fascicle.

Nonspecific Intraventricular Conduction Disturbances

Block that occurs distal to the main division of the bundle branches has been referred to by a large variety of names, such as focal block, arborization block, reticular block, parietal block, intrainfarction block, peri-infarction block, postinfarction block, and diffuse intraventricular block. Several factors, including hyperkalemia, acidosis, intoxication with antiarrhythmic drugs, injection of contrast medium into the coronary artery, diffuse myocardial fibrosis, and large scars or infarcted areas, may be responsible for this widening of the QRS complex, which does not fulfill the criteria for RBBB or LBBB. The presence of a normal Q wave supports delay in the peripheral Purkinje fibers, in the junction of the Purkinje fibers and the muscle, or in the ordinary myocardial fibers themselves as the cause of the prolongation of the QRS complex. Marked left axis deviation indicates the presence of associated left anterior hemiblock.

Aberration

Aberration refers to intraventricular conduction abnormalities (frequently bundle branch block) that are related to changes in heart rate or other functional factors, in the absence of "fixed" structural conduction defects. The most common example is block occurring after premature atrial excitation has encroached on the relative or effective refractory period of one of the bundle branches (most often the right). The resulting QRS complex is wide and exhibits a bundle branch block pattern.[31]

The so-called Ashman phenomenon (aberrancy after a "long-short" cycle sequence) differs from that just described in that the abnormal conduction is a function of an altered duration of the refractory period rather than of changing prematurity of stimulation. As it was initially described, it is frequently observed during atrial arrhythmias when the constant changes in the atrial cycle length result in variations in the RR cycle, which produces parallel changes in the refractory period of the bundle branches.[32]

Another common observation is the fast rate–dependent aberration that may be observed at the initiation of a supraventricular tachycardia. This has also been termed phase 3 block or aberrancy, and it is also due to refractory period encroachment. Once the phenomenon has been initiated, it is perpetuated by retrograde invasion of the blocked branch by the impulse that has propagated transseptally. This occurs late in the QRS complex and results in a delayed activation of the blocked branch with respect to the QRS. Therefore, the subsequent impulse arrives relatively early, and the phenomenon is maintained (Fig. 54.23).

The opposite phenomenon, in which the appearance of the block is linked to a decrease in heart rate, has been termed bradycardia-dependent block or phase 4 block.[33]

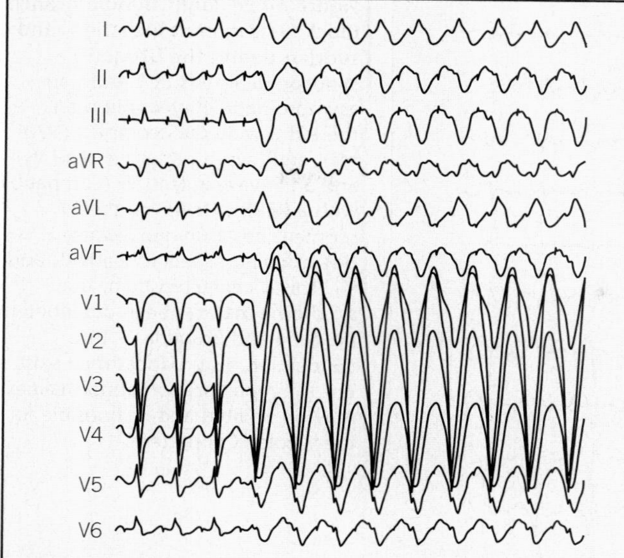

Figure 54.23 Rate-dependent LBBB during an electrophysiologic study. In this patient, who was treated with oral cibenzoline for paroxysmal atrial fibrillation, a subtle shortening of the atrial pacing cycle length is accompanied by emergence of complete LBBB with marked left axis deviation. Whereas in the right half of the ECG, the QRS complex exhibits only incomplete LBBB with normal QRS axis, the sixth QRS complex suddenly widens with abrupt left axis rotation and discordance of QRS-T vectors.

CLINICAL PRESENTATIONS

The symptoms produced by disturbances in AV or intraventricular conduction are generally attributable to the resultant bradycardia as well as to consequences of the loss of AV or intraventricular and interventricular synchrony.[34] The severity of symptoms is dependent on the age of the patient, the presence or absence of organic heart disease, and the degree of physical activity. The symptoms range from decrease in effort tolerance to giddiness, presyncope, and frank syncope. About half of the patients who present with syncope have an abnormal ECG, with the most common abnormalities being bundle branch block and bifascicular block.[35] Arrhythmias as a cause of syncope are diagnosed by ECG in 2% to 11% of patients who present with syncope. In patients who have underlying heart disease, the onset of conduction block may result in worsening of symptoms of heart failure and ischemia. Children who have congenital AV block are often asymptomatic.

The only physical signs detectable in first-degree AV block are a prolongation of the time between the *a* and the *c* waves of the jugular venous pulse and a softening of the first heart sound. In patients with dilated cardiomyopathy, shortening of the AV delay by dual-chamber pacing may increase left ventricular filling time and may have therapeutic potential, even in the absence of conventional indications for pacemaker implantation.[36]

In second-degree AV block, there is a mismatch in the number of *a* and *c* waves in the venous pulse, and the arterial pulse may be irregular. Type I second-degree AV block is frequently encountered during acute inferior infarction, is often transient, does not necessarily require temporary pacing, and has a good prognosis.[37] It also occurs during intoxication by drugs that act on AV node conduction, such as digitalis, calcium channel blockers, and beta blockers. It may also be chronic in a large variety of situations (see Table 54.1). In such cases, type I AV block is generally due to impairment of conduction in the AV node, is associated with narrow QRS, may be clinically silent or mildly symptomatic, and usually does not rapidly progress to more advanced forms of AV block. The only exception is the rare patient who has type I second-degree intra-His AV block.

In contrast, type II AV block is often located within the His-Purkinje system, is associated with a wide QRS, and precedes the development of Adams-Stokes syncope and complete AV block. It is almost never seen during inferior infarction, and when it does occur in this context, it is associated with impaired prognosis.[37]

Third-degree AV block is accompanied by a host of physical signs, including cannon *a* waves in the venous pulse, wide arterial pulse pressure, and varying intensity of the first heart sound. Complete AV block has variable clinical presentations, depending on the site of block. Block at the level of the AV node is generally accompanied by a relatively fast escape rate (40 to 60 beats per minute) with narrow QRS because its origin is in or near the bundle of His. It usually speeds up with atropine or exercise. The most typical example is the congenital form of AV block.[38] AV blocks occurring below the level of the bundle of His are accompanied by slower escape rates with wide QRS and carry a much poorer prognosis.

Both forms of complete AV block are often initially paroxysmal. Paroxysmal AV block can be due to hypersensitivity of the AV node to vagal reflexes, surgery, electrolyte disturbances, degenerative processes, coronary artery disease, myocarditis, tumors, Chagas' disease, rheumatoid nodules, calcified aortic stenosis, myxedema, polymyositis, infiltrative processes, and many other pathologic conditions.

Bundle branch blocks affect the second heart sound, with LBBB producing reverse splitting. In the absence of clinically overt cardiac disease, the presence of LBBB or RBBB is not associated with increased overall mortality. However, isolated LBBB is associated with an increased risk for development of overt cardiovascular disease and with increased cardiac mortality.[39] During acute myocardial infarction, the overall incidence of bundle branch block has been reported to be 23.6%, RBBB being twice as frequent as LBBB. Patients with bundle branch block have lower ejection fractions, more left anterior descending artery–related infarctions, higher peak creatine kinase levels, more diseased vessels, and higher mortality rates.[40] Poor R-wave progression and LBBB are commonly observed in dilated cardiomyopathy.

In 1992, Brugada and Brugada[41] described the association of RBBB pattern, ST-segment elevation in right precordial leads, and sudden death in otherwise apparently healthy subjects. The QRS complex in the Brugada syndrome in V_1 and V_2 leads ends by a positive deflection followed by an elevated downsloping ST segment with a negative T wave (Fig. 54.24). These abnormalities may be transient and are unmasked by the injection of Vaughan Williams class I antiarrhythmic drugs, thereby identifying patients at risk. Available data suggest that in 30% of cases, mutations in the cardiac sodium channel gene *SCN5A* are responsible for the loss of the dome of the action potential in the right ventricular epicardium.[42,43]

This is to be differentiated from the early repolarization syndrome, which is also characterized by ST-segment elevation but is not associated with arrhythmias.[44] In this

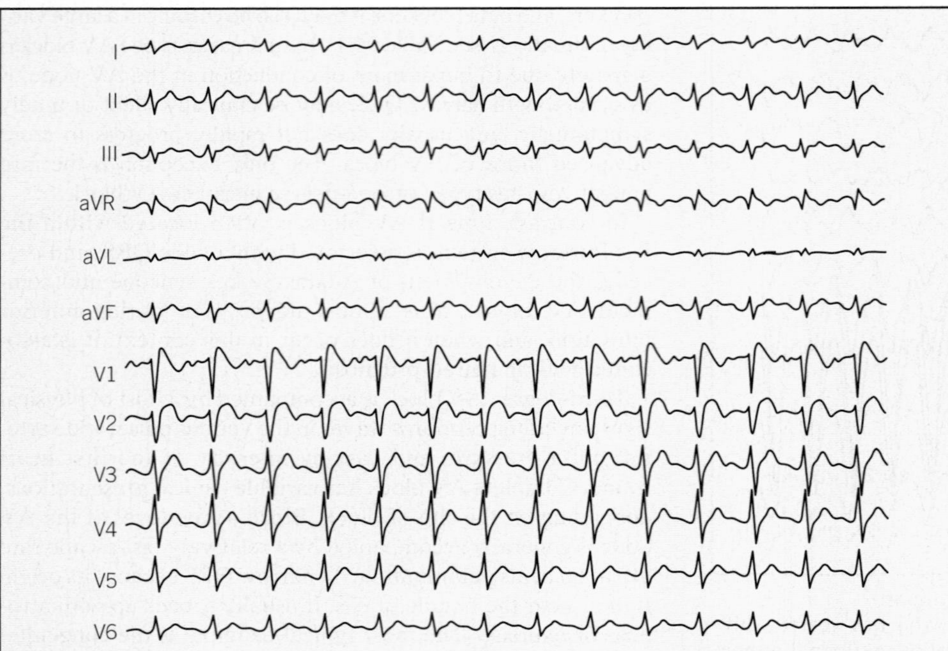

Figure 54.24 Right bundle branch block, ST-segment elevation, and sudden death: the Brugada syndrome. In this ECG from an asymptomatic 40-year-old man, there is a wide QRS complex (120 ms), an R′ wave pattern in lead V_1, and an S wave in lead V_6 (compatible with a RBBB). However, the ST segment has a unique, bizarre downsloping aspect in leads V_1 and V_2. This is characteristic of the syndrome that has been described by Brugada and Brugada.[41] True conduction disturbances may exist, but the repolarization abnormalities may be isolated and responsible for the whole ECG pattern.

syndrome, the ST segment is elevated in leads V_2 to V_4, with an upward concavity with a positive T wave. Studies in patients with spinal cord injury in whom the ECG is altered in a similar fashion suggest that in these cases, cardiac sympathetic control may be altered in the presence of normal parasympathetic function.[45]

Another form of right ventricular conduction delay has been described in patients who have arrhythmogenic right ventricular dysplasia. The delayed activation is inscribed in the form of a sharp deflection (the epsilon wave) after termination of the QRS, during either the ST segment or the upstroke of the T wave.[46]

There is vast evidence that intraventricular conduction disturbances may alter interventricular and intraventricular contraction synchrony, left ventricular systolic function, and filling, resulting in impairment of cardiac output (left ventricular dyssynchrony–induced cardiomyopathy[47]). Signs of heart failure may appear or worsen, especially in patients with preexisting cardiac insufficiency.

DIAGNOSTIC TECHNIQUES

The cornerstone test for the diagnosis of conduction disturbance is ECG documentation of the block. However, very often, these blocks are transient or intermittent. This is the reason that prolonged and repeated heart rate monitoring may be performed and other tests may be needed to identify the presence and severity of a conduction disturbance.

Noninvasive Tests

Ambulatory ECG monitoring is an important tool, not only for documenting the occurrence of conduction blocks but also for establishing the relationship between the heart block and symptoms. Such monitoring often has to be done for more than 24 hours. In some instances, a patient-activated event recorder may be more helpful. First-degree AV block and type I second-degree AV block can occur in otherwise normal young adults, especially athletes.[48] A recently reported diagnostic test is the use of intravenous adenosine for identification of patients with syncope caused by paroxysmal AV block (see Chapter 52).[49]

Invasive Electrophysiologic Testing

Invasive electrophysiologic tests are used to test the integrity of AV node and His-Purkinje system conduction. This is routinely done by measuring baseline conduction intervals after having inserted two or three catheters under local anesthesia, most often through the venous femoral route (Fig. 54.25). The AH interval is measured from the beginning of the atrial deflection as recorded in the bundle of His electrogram, and the HV interval is measured from the beginning of the H deflection to the earliest ventricular activity, whether intracardiac or on the surface ECG. The AH interval recorded in the bundle of His electrogram measures 54 to 130 ms, and the HV interval measures 31 to 55 ms (see Fig. 54.25). If the baseline intervals are normal or nondiagnostic, provocative maneuvers such as overdrive pacing or drugs can be used to unmask underlying conduction system disease.[50]

In patients who have conduction disease, it is important to localize the site of block; blocks that are proximal to the bundle of His have a better prognosis than those in which the disease is more distal.[51] The value of electrophysiologic studies in patients with bifascicular block has been a matter of much investigation and debate. Some studies have found a prolonged HV interval to be a predictor of future complete heart block, whereas others have found no such correlation (Fig. 54.26).[52-54] From the available literature, it appears that an HV interval of more than 70 ms predicts a high chance for development of high-grade AV block in patients with bifascicular block, especially in the presence of symptoms of syncope or presyncope and underlying coronary or

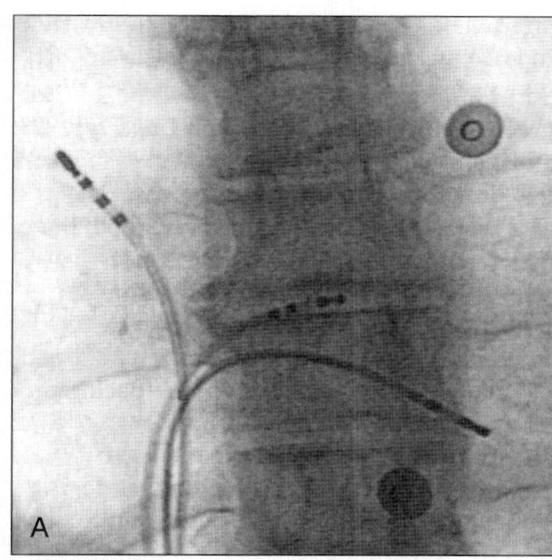

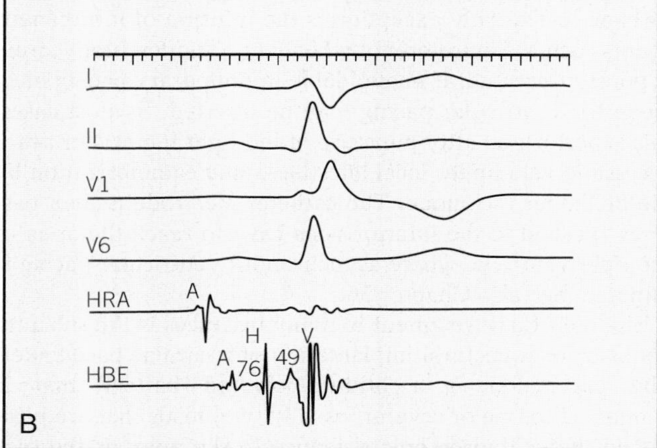

Figure 54.25 Electrophysiologic studies for the evaluation of AV conduction disturbances. A, Example of electrode positioning. In this anteroposterior fluoroscopic view, three sensing and pacing quadripolar leads can be seen. They have been introduced through the venous femoral approach and are positioned in the high right atrium, against the septal leaflet of the tricuspid valve in the area of the bundle of His and in the right ventricle close to the apex. Each lead is able to record local intracavitary ECGs, and pacing is usually performed from the high right atrium and the apex of the right ventricle. **B,** Normal intracavitary electrical recording. Despite a typical RBBB pattern on the surface ECG, the intracardiac time intervals are normal, proving the integrity of the AV node and the remaining branches of the bundle of His. HRA, high right atrium; HBE, His bundle electrogram.

cardiac muscle disease. HV block, induced by incremental atrial pacing in the basal state or under pharmacologic provocation, is also a rare but useful predictor of impending AV block in these patients (Fig. 54.27).[51,55] This does not apply when block below the H deflection is recorded after a premature atrial depolarization because the latter may be due to normal His-Purkinje system refractoriness.

Invasive electrophysiologic testing may also be used to differentiate proximal block from distal block in cases of bundle branch block.[56] This may have some clinical implication, especially in postoperative bundle branch block. An RR index has been proposed[57] as being useful to predict the site of block during incremental pacing. This was done by calculating the numeric difference between the R-R interval

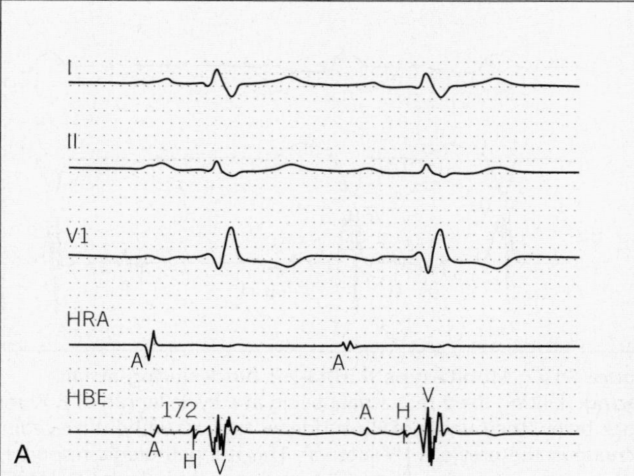

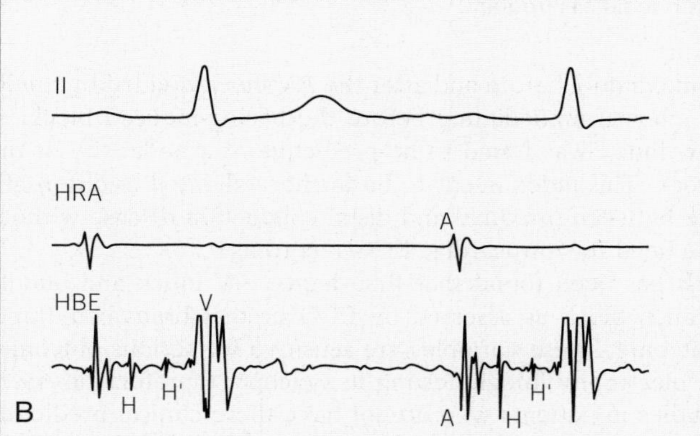

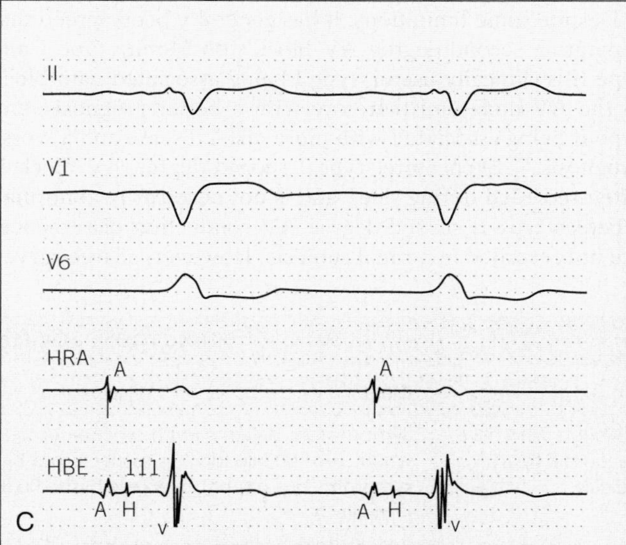

Figure 54.26 Electrophysiologic studies. A, Delay within the AV node (supra-His). The slight prolongation of the PR interval on the surface ECG is due to an increase in the AV nodal conduction time to 172 ms. **B,** Intra-His first-degree AV block. The normal potential of the bundle of His is narrow, and its duration does not exceed 25 ms. Here, there is a split potential with a frank interspike interval, indicating delay within the AV node itself. This does not usually translate into a discernible delay in the PR interval on the surface ECG. **C,** Infra-His first-degree block. In this example, the HV conduction time is prolonged to 111 ms. Even in asymptomatic patients, this condition is an accepted indication for pacemaker implantation. HRA, high right atrium; HBE, His bundle electrogram.

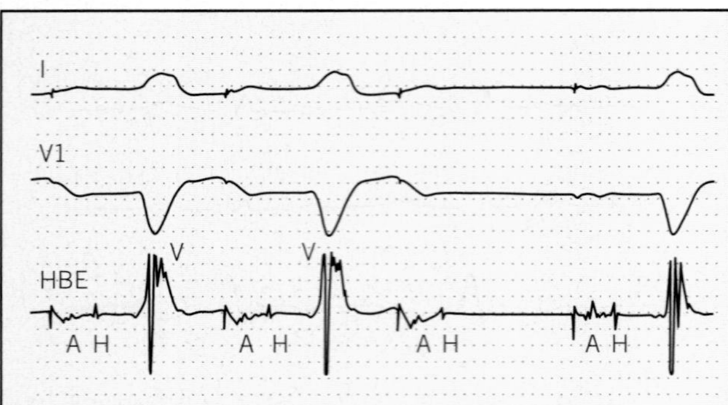

Figure 54.27 Möbitz type II infra-His block during atrial pacing. During fixed-rate atrial pacing at a cycle length of 800 ms, block below the bundle of His suddenly appears without preceding increase in the previous HV interval. This is a pathologic response, and it is an accepted indication for pacemaker implantation. HBE, His bundle electrogram.

immediately before and after the AV block divided by the R-R interval immediately before the pacing-induced block. A low index was found to be predictive of a nodal site of the block. This index needs to be further validated to differentiate between proximal and distal conduction disease without the need for intracardiac ECG recording.

It has been found that first-degree AV block and bundle branch block as assessed by ECG predict bradyarrhythmic outcome. These variables are sensitive for serious outcomes of electrophysiologic testing in syncope; therefore, invasive studies in patients who do not have these clinical predictors are likely to be of very low diagnostic yield.[58]

Despite some limitations, it has generally been agreed that separating second-degree AV block into Möbitz type I and type II is clinically useful, type I being associated with block in the AV node and therefore with a better prognosis, and type II being associated with more distal disease and a worse prognosis.[59] Even more, type I second-degree AV block is often recorded during sleep and is not necessarily abnormal, whereas type II second-degree AV conduction disturbances are not recorded in normal subjects. However, a large survey has reported that prognosis is similar in patients with Möbitz type I and Möbitz type II AV block.[60] This report has also shown that pacing produces a similar degree of prognostic improvement in both groups. Therefore, second-degree AV block in an asymptomatic patient constitutes an additional indication for electrophysiologic testing so that decision on pacemaker implantation may be made on the basis of the site of conduction disturbance.

The current guidelines from the American Heart Association and the American College of Cardiology for the performance of invasive electrophysiologic testing in patients with conduction disturbances are given in Table 54.2.[61]

MANAGEMENT

Except for transient, reversible causes of AV block, drugs do not have any significant role to play in the long-term management of patients with AV or intraventricular conduction disturbances. The only exception is the infusion of intravenous agents such as isoproterenol whenever a sudden bradycardia is poorly tolerated. If unavoidable, a temporary pacing electrode for ventricular pacing may be inserted. In most cases, this is performed after puncture of the right femoral or other accessible vein under local anesthesia and catheterization by the Seldinger technique. The catheter electrode is then passively pushed in the inferior vena cava to reach the apex of the right ventricle, where asynchronous ventricular pacing is initiated. See also Chapter 56.

The only final treatment in many instances is the subcutaneous or retropectoral implantation of a cardiac pacemaker. The pacemaker is a lithium-powered battery that is connected to one or several (usually two) leads that are positioned under fluoroscopic guidance to the apex or the septum of the right ventricle or the right atrial wall or appendage. Permanent pacemaker implantation is clearly indicated in all symptomatic patients who have advanced degrees of heart block. It is also indicated in patients with forms of heart block or intraventricular conduction defects that are considered to cause a high risk for development of higher grades of AV block. The current guidelines from the

INDICATIONS FOR ELECTROPHYSIOLOGIC STUDIES

	Class I	Class II
Patients who have acquired heart block	Symptomatic patients (with syncope or near-syncope) in whom His-Purkinje block is suspected to be a cause of symptoms but has not been established with ECG recordings	Patients with second- or third-degree AV block in whom knowledge of the site or mechanism of block, or both, may help direct therapy or assess prognosis
	Patients with second- or third-degree AV block treated with a pacemaker who remain symptomatic (with syncope or near-syncope) in whom another arrhythmia is suspected as a cause of symptoms	Patients with concealed junctional extrasystoles suspected as a cause of second- or third-degree AV block pattern (i.e., pseudo-AV block)
Patients who have chronic intraventricular block	Symptomatic patients in whom the cause of symptoms is unknown	Asymptomatic patients with bundle branch block in whom pharmacologic therapy that could increase conduction delay or produce heart block is contemplated

American Heart Association–American College of Cardiology guidelines.
Modified from Zipes DP, DiMarco JP, Gillette P, et al. Guidelines for clinical intracardiac electrophysiologic studies and catheter ablation procedures. AHA/ACC Task Force report. Circulation 1995;92:673-691.

Table 54.2 Indications for electrophysiologic studies.

American Heart Association, the American College of Cardiology, and the former North American Society for Pacing and Electrophysiology (now Heart Rhythm Society) for pacemaker implantation in patients with conduction disorders are given in Chapter 55.[62] Essentially, these include

- all symptomatic cases of AV block;
- asymptomatic cases of third-degree AV block; and
- asymptomatic cases of second-degree AV block, when these blocks have an intra-His or infra-His bundle origin or are associated with bundle branch block or bifascicular block.

Single-chamber ventricular-demand pacing (VVI pacing) prevents the ventricular rate from decreasing below a preset rate. If the spontaneous rate decreases below this preset rate, the pacemaker paces at a cycle length that is appropriate to maintain the preset rate. This type of pacemaker is ideal for paroxysmal AV block. It is simple to implant and to program and is easy to follow, and its cost is relatively low because of its long life expectancy. Its major disadvantage is AV desynchronization, which may be a clinically relevant problem in permanent AV block. At times, the ventricular pacing rate can be increased as a function of a nonphysiologic sensor. These so-called VVIR pacemakers are particularly useful in young, otherwise active patients who have permanent complete AV block and coexisting permanent atrial arrhythmias.

In general, preservation of normal AV synchrony will be favored by implantation of an AV sequential pacemaker whenever required. The most frequently implanted pacemakers operate in the DDD mode (i.e., they pace and sense in both the atrium and the ventricle) (Fig. 54.28). They are more complex to implant as they require two separate leads in the majority of cases; they are also more expensive and more difficult to fine-tune, but their diagnostic and therapeutic capabilities are far superior.[63] Various algorithms have been developed for paroxysmal AV block to minimize right ventricular pacing, such as a pacemaker that functions as an atrial pacemaker and switches to classic DDD mode only when block occurs.

In the last decade, attention has been drawn to the alteration of impulse propagation yielding loss of ventricular synchronization in patients with heart failure and wide QRS (mostly left bundle branch block). Cardiac resynchronization therapy has developed as a complement to medical treatment of heart failure. A third lead to stimulate the left ventricle provides a "triple-chamber pacemaker." This lead is generally positioned in an epicardial vein through the coronary sinus. Many studies have shown improvement in clinical signs of heart failure[64-66] and in overall mortality[67] with ventricular resynchronization in selected patients.

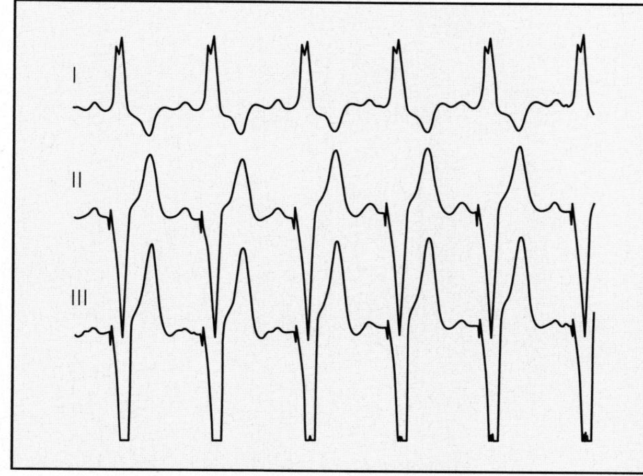

Figure 54.28 Paced beats with a dual-chamber pacemaker. Because the pacing electrode is located at the apex of the right ventricle, the paced beats always have a left bundle branch block aspect and a left axis deviation. Synchronization with the sinus P waves implies atrial detection, which (in the majority of cases) occurs by an additional lead positioned in the right atrial appendage or the right lateral free wall.

SUMMARY

Atrioventricular and intraventricular conduction disturbances are frequently observed in a variety of clinical situations during the routine practice of cardiology. Their ECG expression is variable, and clinical severity ranges from the most benign to the rapidly life-threatening condition. They are usually but not invariably related to underlying heart disease, the prognosis of which they often alter. Modern pacemaker therapy is usually the only effective treatment and has allowed tremendous progress in the relief of symptoms of the affected patients.

chapter 55

Cardiac Pacing

Jens Cosedis Nielsen and Henning Rud Andersen

Definition

- Cardiac pacemakers are instruments that are used for treatment of bradyarrhythmias and related conditions.

Key Features

- Pacemaker therapy abolishes bradycardia-related symptoms effectively, improves quality of life, reduces morbidity and may reduce mortality, and is cost-effective.
- Physiologic pacing that maintains atrioventricular synchrony, enables rate-adaptive pacing, and preserves intrinsic atrioventricular conduction, if appropriate, should be the standard.
- Optimal pacemaker therapy requires careful selection of pacemaker type and pacing mode for each patient, individual programming of available pacemaker features, and careful pacemaker follow-up with individual optimization of the pacemaker system.

Clinical Implications

- Correct pacemaker therapy is the treatment of choice for cardiac bradyarrhythmias.

Within the past decades, the rates of pacemaker implantation have increased steadily,[1] and every year more than 400,000 new pacemakers are implanted at more than 7000 centers worldwide, the majority in the United States and Europe.[2-4] In 2002, the rate of primary pacemaker implantation was estimated at 612 per million population in the United States[1]; in 1997, the implantation rate was 275 per million population in Europe, varying from 57 to 585 per million between countries.[3] It is estimated in the United States that approximately 450,000 patients or 2.6 per 1000 persons live with cardiac pacemakers.[5] Most pacemaker patients are elderly; 85% are 65 years or older, and mean age at implantation is approximately 75 years.[3]

The early pacemakers were single-chamber devices connected to a lead implanted in the right ventricle and able to deliver asynchronous paced impulses. In the 1960s, demand pacing was introduced, and in the 1980s, systems acting more physiologically with dual-chamber pacing and rate-adaptive function as the most important advances were more widely accepted. The use of dual-chamber systems has increased during the last decade, and today, dual-chamber pacemakers with rate-adaptive abilities are the most commonly used pacemakers for new implants.[1,3,4] Evolution in pacemaker technology is continuing; the latest innovations are pacemakers with advanced algorithms promoting intrinsic ventricular conduction, semiautomatic devices, and devices with features for remote monitoring.

Since 1997, the first randomized trials of pacing mode have been published. In two studies, both with relatively small sample size, single-chamber atrial pacing was found to be associated with a significantly better long-term outcome than single-chamber right ventricular (VVI) pacing in patients with sick sinus syndrome,[6] whereas no convincing differences were observed between dual-chamber pacing and VVI pacing in elderly patients who had atrioventricular (AV) block or sick sinus syndrome.[7] Since then, three large randomized trials of pacing mode selection have been reported, indicating that although dual-chamber pacing reduces the incidence of atrial fibrillation compared with VVI pacing, selection of dual-chamber pacing has no beneficial effect on mortality, heart failure, or quality of life.[8-10] A high proportion of ventricular pacing has been associated with atrial fibrillation and heart failure. Recently, the use of new algorithms minimizing ventricular pacing has been found to reduce the occurrence of atrial fibrillation compared with traditional dual-chamber pacing maintaining AV synchrony at the cost of a larger proportion of ventricular pacing.[11]

DESCRIPTION OF DEVICES, TECHNIQUES, AND PROCEDURES

Permanent Pacemakers

Pacemakers and Leads

A pacemaker system for permanent pacing consists of a pacemaker and one lead (single-chamber pacemaker) or two leads (dual-chamber pacemaker) implanted in the right atrium or right ventricle, or both (Fig. 55.1). The pacemaker contains a battery, the power source, and a pulse generator, the electronic unit controlling the behavior of the pacemaker.

Battery

The power source is usually a constant-voltage lithium-iodine battery that has a predictable voltage behavior over time; the battery voltage remains relatively constant throughout most of its discharge. The potentials delivered by antibradycardia pacemakers are monophasic. Battery current drain is highly dependent on pacemaker programming. A pacemaker with 6 years of battery longevity under nominal pacing parameters may reach its replacement time at 2 years at one extreme or at more than 10 years at the other extreme. Expected battery longevity is 5 to 10 years for dual-chamber pacemakers and 7 to 12 years for single-chamber pacemakers. In modern pacemakers, an elective replacement indicator is activated when battery depletion is near. The clinical indicators of battery depletion vary between

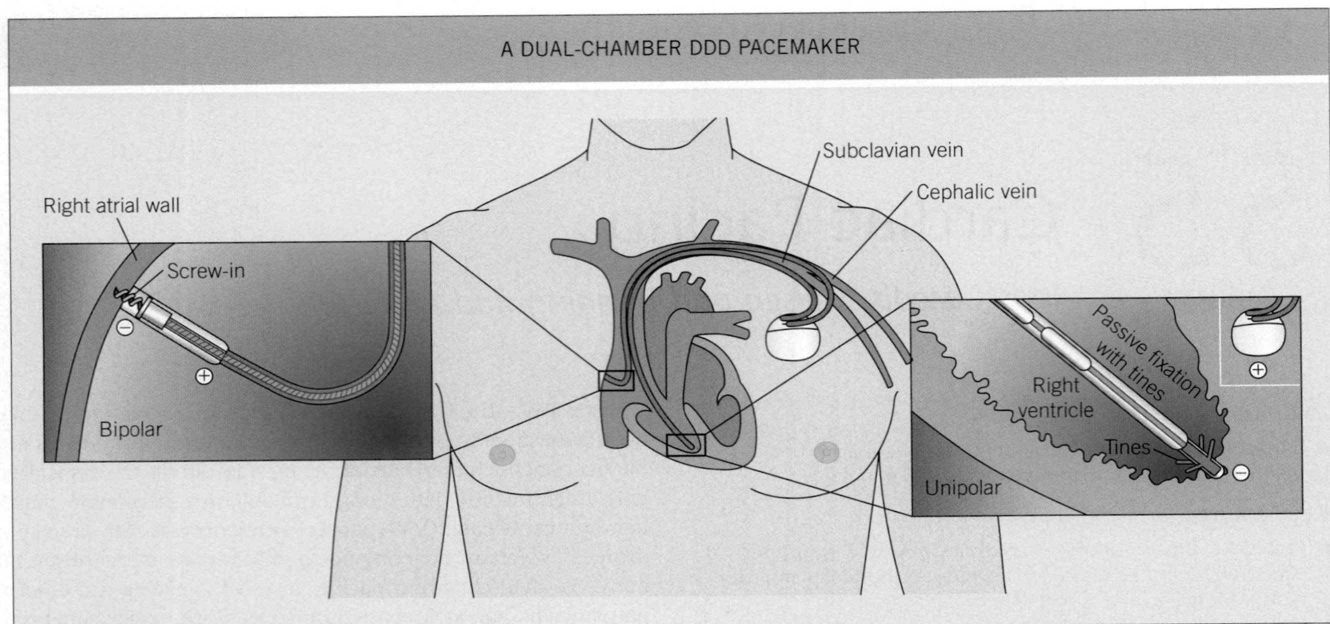

Figure 55.1 A dual-chamber pacemaker (DDD). It is implanted in the left pectoral region. The atrial bipolar lead is implanted through the left cephalic vein and actively fixated in the right atrium. The ventricular unipolar lead is implanted through the left subclavian vein and passively fixated with tines captured in the right ventricular myocardial trabeculae.

manufacturers and models, the most common being stepwise changes in telemetered battery voltage and battery impedance, pacing rate or magnet rate, and change in pacing mode (e.g., DDDR→VOO). The elective replacement indicator indicates that the pacemaker should be replaced. In determining time of replacement, it also should be considered what consequences loss of capture will have in each particular patient; replacement should be done sooner in pacemaker-dependent patients.

Pacemaker Leads

Pacemaker leads are unipolar or bipolar. In a unipolar system, a single electrode (the cathode) is located at the lead tip, and the pacemaker can act as the other electrode (the anode). Bipolar systems have both electrodes near the distal end of the lead, the tip electrode acting as the cathode and the more proximal ring electrode as the anode (see Fig. 55.1). Bipolar leads reduce the risk of myopotential oversensing, far-field sensing, crosstalk, and local skeletal muscle stimulation, and they allow programmable switching between bipolar and unipolar configurations. Because of these advantages, bipolar leads should be used as the standard in both the atrium and the ventricle. Earlier generations of bipolar leads had a higher rate of lead failures during long-term follow-up than did unipolar leads owing to the more complex design, but high long-term reliabilities have been documented for newer bipolar leads. The stimulus artifact size on the electrocardiogram is large in unipolar pacing, whereas it is small and sometimes difficult to see in bipolar pacing. However, the polarity of bipolar leads can be changed temporarily during pacemaker testing.

Endocardial fixation of leads can be either passive or active (see Fig. 55.1). Passive fixation is obtained by use of leads with tines or wings, which are trapped in the trabeculae of the right atrium or ventricle. Active fixation is done by screwing a fixed- or retractable-tip screw into the atrial or ventricular myocardium. Active fixation reduces the frequency of atrial lead dislodgements and is therefore recommended as standard in the right atrium. In the right ventricle, leads with active fixation can be implanted more easily in localities other than the apex, such as the outflow tract or the septum. Epicardial leads are used most commonly in pediatric pacing, but they can be used also in adults if there is no venous access.

Most modern leads have a small tip surface area with a porous surface, promoting low thresholds, low current drain, and good sensing. Steroid-eluting leads have a little reservoir of glucocorticoids, which diminishes the inflammatory reaction at the electrode-endocardial interface and thus improves acute and chronic pacing thresholds and sensing.

Pacemaker Features

Definitions of common terms used in cardiac pacing are listed in Table 55.1 and discussed in detail here.

Threshold and Strength-Duration Relationship

The pacing threshold is defined as the minimum stimulus amplitude at any given pulse width required to consistently achieve myocardial depolarization (myocardial capture) outside the heart's refractory period. Threshold should be measured in volts (V). Threshold can be measured by increasing stimulus amplitude until capture occurs or by decreasing amplitude until loss of capture occurs. At pacing rates below 150 beats per minute, there is no significant difference between thresholds measured by these two methods. At implantation, an atrial threshold of 1.5 V or lower and a ventricular threshold of 1.0 V or lower at pulse width 0.5 ms should be obtained. In most patients, the threshold rises during the first 2 to 4 weeks after implantation, reaches a peak, and then decreases to reach a chronic level after 6 to 8 weeks slightly higher than the acute threshold. At the initial programming after implantation, an output of between

DEFINITIONS OF SELECTED PACEMAKER FEATURES	
Threshold	The minimum stimulus amplitude at any given pulse width required to consistently achieve myocardial depolarization (capture) outside the heart's refractory period[15]
Impedance	The sum of all forces opposing the flow of current in an electric circuit In pacemaker systems, the impedance is determined by the resistance of the leads, the tissue between the electrodes, and the electrode-tissue interfaces.
Sensing	The peak-to-peak amplitude in millivolts (mV) of the intracardiac signal (P wave or R wave)
Slew rate	The change in intracardiac electrogram voltage over time (dV/dt)
Sensitivity	The level in millivolts (mV) that an intracardiac electrogram has to exceed to be sensed by the pacemaker; acts as a filter for noise
Rate-adaptive function	The pacemaker is able to change paced heart rate in response to a sensor indicating alteration in activity; indicated for patients with chronotropic incompetence
Mode switch	Automatic change of the pacing mode from DDD or VDD to a nonatrial tracking mode: VVI, VDI, or DDI in case of atrial fibrillation, atrial flutter, or other supraventricular tachyarrhythmia
Rate hysteresis	Delaying onset of ventricular pacing to preserve normal physiologic activation and contraction, e. g., starting ventricular pacing with a rate of 110 beats per minute in case of decrease in heart rate below 50 beats per minute in patients with recurrent vasovagal syncope
Rate-adaptive AV delay	Automatic shortening of the AV delay in case of increasing heart rate
AV hysteresis	Automatic search scan for spontaneous ventricular events during a prolonged AV interval; in case of spontaneous ventricular events, the AV interval remains extended to preserve intrinsic AV conduction

Table 55.1 Definitions of selected pacemaker features.

three and five times the acute threshold and a pulse duration of 0.4 to 0.5 ms should be programmed. At subsequent follow-up after 2 to 3 months, output should be reduced to minimize current drain. This is done by reducing voltage output, not by reducing pulse duration. Reducing voltage output is more energy efficient because the battery current drain varies as the square of voltage. During follow-up, the output of the pacemaker should be programmed to no less than twice the chronic voltage threshold at the pulse duration used to achieve an adequate safety margin (2:1). Some new devices have the capability of automatically measuring pacing thresholds and adjusting output thereafter according to a programmable safety margin, so-called auto-capture.

Sensing, Sensitivity, and Impedance

Sensing is defined as the peak-to-peak amplitude in millivolts (mV) of the intracardiac electrogram. The amplitude of the ventricular R-wave electrogram is larger than the size of the atrial P-wave electrogram. At implantation, an atrial electrogram above 1.5 mV and a ventricular electrogram above 6 mV should be obtained. After implantation, the amplitude of the electrogram usually declines during the first weeks, then increases and reaches a chronic value slightly lower than that noted at implantation. At implantation, the slew rate, defined as the change in intracardiac electrogram voltage over time (dV/dt), should be above 0.5 V/s in both atrium and ventricle. Both the amplitude of the electrogram and the slew rate are important determinants of whether an electrical signal will be sensed by the pacemaker.

Immediately after lead implantation, the sensed electrogram is distorted by an "injury current," an ST elevation after the initial R-wave spike in the ventricular electrogram or an elevation after the P-wave spike in the atrial electrogram. This injury current is thought to result from damage of the endocardial surface produced by contact with or pressure from the lead and thus reflects good endocardial contact. The injury current disappears after a few days.

Sensitivity is the level in millivolts (mV) that an intracardiac electrogram has to exceed to be sensed by the pacemaker. Sensitivity is programmable and acts as a filter for noise, ensuring that small electrical signals caused, for example, by skeletal muscle movements are not sensed by the pacemaker and interpreted as cardiac electrograms. Sensitivity should be programmed after measurement of the intracardiac electrogram. Sensitivity should not exceed half that of the sensed electrogram. Sensitivity must be larger with unipolar leads than with bipolar leads because noise signals are larger in unipolar leads.

Impedance can be defined as the sum of all forces opposing the flow of current in an electric circuit. Impedance is measured in ohms (Ω). In pacemaker systems, the lead impedance is determined by the resistance of the conducting lead (or leads), the tissue between the electrodes, and the electrode-tissue interface (which is largely influenced by the electrode surface area and the electrode surface composition). Normal lead impedance is 250 to 1200 Ω at output 5.0 V, most often 500 to 800 Ω. Usually, lead impedance remains stable or decreases slightly after implantation. A very low impedance (<250 Ω) may indicate failure of lead insulation, whereas a high impedance (>2000 Ω) accompanied by a high pacing threshold indicates lead fracture.

The Pacemaker Code

In 2002, the North American Society of Pacing and Electrophysiology and the British Pacing and Electrophysiology Group revised the five-letter code for antibradycardia pacing that explains the basic pacemaker mode and function (Table 55.2).[12] The first letter indicates the chambers paced, and the second letter indicates the chambers sensed: V, ventricle; A, atrium; and D, dual (both A and V). The third letter indicates the response to sensing: I if a sensed signal inhibits pacemaker discharge; T if a sensed signal triggers pacemaker discharge (e.g., sensed atrial electrogram triggers ventricular pacing in a patient with AV block and a dual-chamber pacemaker); and D if both functions are available. The fourth letter indicates the presence (R) or absence (O) of rate-adaptive function. The fifth letter indicates multisite pacing: in none of the chambers (O); in one or both of the atria (A), that is, with stimulation sites in each atrium, more than one stimulation site in either atrium, or any combination of the two; in one or both of the ventricles (V), that is, with stimulation sites in each ventricle, more than one stimulation site in either ventricle, or any combination of the two; or in any combination of A and V (D). Some manufacturers use the letter S in positions one and two

THE REVISED NASPE/BPEG GENERIC CODE FOR ANTIBRADYCARDIA PACING					
Position	I	II	III	IV	V
Category	Chambers Paced	Chambers Sensed	Response to Sensing	Rate Modulation	Multisite Pacing
Letters	O = None A = Atrium V = Ventricle D = Dual (A + V)	O = None A = Atrium V = Ventricle D = Dual (A + V)	O = None T = Triggered I = Inhibited D = Dual (T + I)	O = None R = Rate modulation	O = None A = Atrium V = Ventricle D = Dual (A + V)
Manufacturer's designation only	S = Single (A or V)	S = Single (A or V)			

Modified from Bernstein AD, Daubert JC, Fletcher RD, et al. The revised NASPE/BPEG generic code for antibradycardia, adaptive-rate, and multisite pacing. North American Society of Pacing and Electrophysiology/British Pacing and Electrophysiology Group. Pacing Clin Electrophysiol 2002;25:260-264. Reproduced with permission.

NASPE, North American Society of Pacing and Electrophysiology; BPEG, British Pacing and Electrophysiology Group.

Table 55.2 The revised NASPE/BPEG generic code for antibradycardia pacing.

to indicate a single-chamber device, which can be connected to a lead implanted in the atrium or in the ventricle.

Different Pacing Modes

Dual-Chamber Pacing

DDD Pacing

A DDD pacemaker paces and senses in both the atrium and the ventricle, and DDD pacing includes both inhibited and triggered function. The fundamental function of a simple DDD pacemaker (with ventricular-based lower rate timing, which is the most common) can be explained by four timing intervals (Fig. 55.2)[13]:

- lower rate interval (LRI);
- atrial escape interval (AEI);
- atrioventricular interval (AVI); and
- ventricular refractory period (VRP).

The LRI is the interval starting with a sensed or paced ventricular event and ending with a paced stimulus delivered to the ventricle. This interval is determined by the lower rate; a lower rate programmed to 60 beats per minute equals LRI of 1 second. The LRI can be divided into two sections: the AEI, which is the first part of the LRI and ends with an atrial paced event; and the AVI, which starts with a sensed or paced atrial event and ends with a paced ventricular event. A sensed atrial event that occurs before completion of the AEI terminates this interval and initiates the AVI. A sensed ventricular event terminates the LRI and AVI. A sensed or paced ventricular event initiates the VRP, which prevents ventricular channel sensing of the evoked potential and the T wave and also initiates the postventricular atrial refractory period (PVARP), which prevents atrial sensing of retrograde P waves and far-field ventricular events. The total atrial refractory period (TARP) is the PVARP plus the AVI. Both the AVI and the PVARP are programmable. The TARP determines the maximum rate of atrial sensing followed by ventricular pacing (maximum tracking rate) that the DDD pacemaker can achieve. For example, an AVI of 200 ms and a PVARP of 300 ms equals a TARP of 500 ms and a maximum tracking rate of 120 beats per minute (i.e., 60,000 ms per minute or 500 ms).

Crosstalk is inappropriate sensing of the atrial stimulus by the ventricular channel (which thereby is inhibited). In patients who do not have intrinsic ventricular rhythm, crosstalk may cause potentially catastrophic asystole. To prevent crosstalk, a ventricular blanking (refractory) period of 10 to 60 ms starts with each paced atrial stimulus. In addition, a ventricular safety pacing feature incorporated in the pacemaker's electronic unit helps prevent crosstalk.

Other Dual-Chamber Pacing Modes

These modes are most easily understood as DDD systems that lack one or more of its functions. They are used most often in cases when a DDD pacemaker must be downgraded because of complications. A modern DDD pacemaker can be programmed to several different modes.

VDD Pacing

VDD pacing can be programmed if atrial pacing is not necessary. Special single leads that sense only in the atrium and pace and sense in the ventricle are available for this purpose. This option can be useful for patients with AV block and normal sinus node function. If there is no sensed atrial activity, a VDD system will function as a VVI pacemaker.

DDI Pacing

The DDI pacing mode is not able to increase ventricular paced activity in response to increased atrial rate (lacks atrial tracking) and therefore always paces the ventricle at the programmed lower rate. It is not recommended as the primary chosen mode.

DVI Pacing

Like DDI, DVI pacing lacks atrial tracking. Moreover, during DVI pacing, there is no sensing of the atrial electrograms, which results in asynchronous atrial pacing. This might precipitate atrial fibrillation, and it should not be recommended as the primary chosen pacing mode.

Single-Chamber Pacing

VVI Pacing

The function of a single-chamber ventricular pacemaker can be explained by only two timing intervals, the LRI given by the programmed lower rate and the VRP (Fig. 55.3). VVI pacing disturbs normal AV synchrony, and therefore it

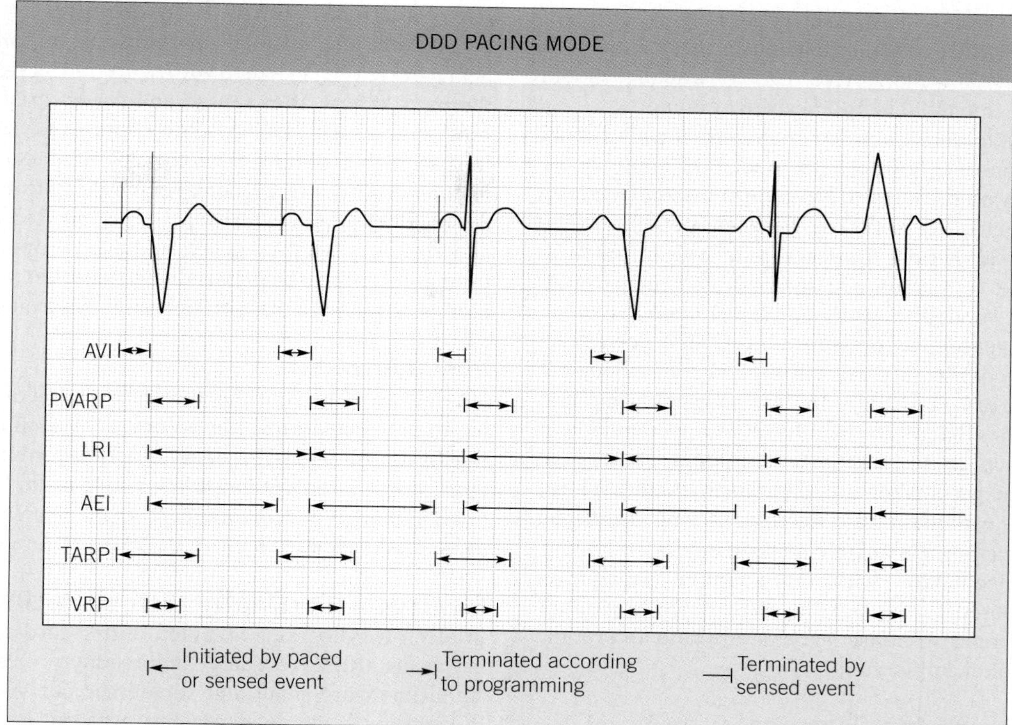

Figure 55.2 DDD pacing mode. The two first beats with dual-chamber pacing, the third beat with atrial pacing and ventricular sensing, the fourth beat with atrial sensing and ventricular pacing, the fifth beat with a spontaneous and normal P wave and QRS complex, and the sixth beat with a ventricular premature complex followed by a retrograde P wave.Timing intervals are as follows: The lower rate interval (LRI) starts with a sensed or paced ventricular event and ends with a paced stimulus delivered to the ventricle and is determined by the lower rate. The LRI can be divided into two sections: the atrial escape interval (AEI), which is the first part of the LRI and ends with an atrial paced event; and the atrioventricular interval (AVI), which starts with a sensed or paced atrial event and ends with a paced ventricular event. An atrial sensed event that occurs before completion of the AEI terminates this interval and initiates the AVI. A sensed ventricular event terminates the LRI and AVI. A sensed or paced ventricular event initiates the postventricular atrial refractory period (PVARP), which prevents atrial sensing of retrograde P waves and far-field ventricular events. The PVARP + AVI is the total atrial refractory period (TARP). The TARP determines the maximum tracking rate. A paced or sensed ventricular event initiates a ventricular refractory period (VRP), which prevents ventricular channel sensing of the evoked potential and the T wave. To prevent crosstalk, a ventricular blanking (refractory) period of 10 to 60 ms starts with each paced atrial stimulus.

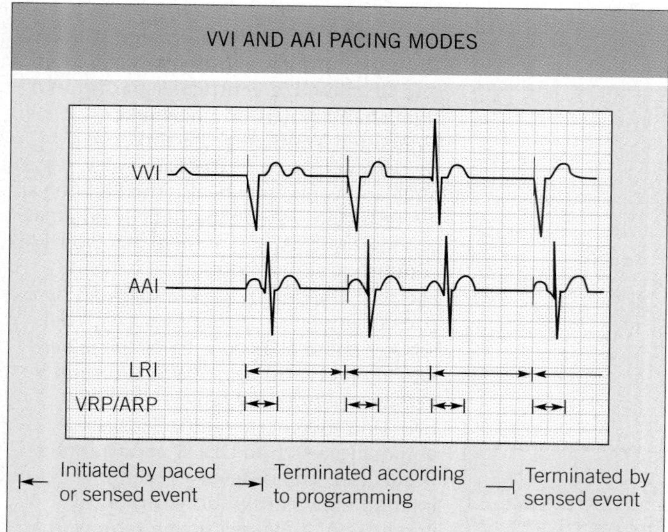

Figure 55.3 Single-chamber ventricular (VVI) and atrial (AAI) pacing modes. The first two and the fourth beats are paced beats; the third beat is a sensed beat. The function of a single-chamber VVI or AAI pacemaker can be explained by only two timing intervals: a lower rate interval (LRI), starting with a sensed or paced event and ending with a paced stimulus; and a refractory period, ventricular refractory period (VRP) in a VVI pacemaker and atrial refractory period (ARP) in an AAI pacemaker. The LRI is determined by the programmed lower rate.

should be recommended only for patients who have chronic atrial fibrillation or flutter.

AAI Pacing

The function of the AAI pacemaker can be understood from the LRI and the atrial refractory period, analogous to the VVI pacemaker (see Fig. 55.3). AAI pacing can be used for patients with sick sinus syndrome and no signs of AV conduction disturbances. Optimal function of the AAI pacemaker is best achieved with use of a bipolar lead and a low sensitivity because of the low amplitude of the atrial electrograms.

Rate-Adaptive Function and Sensors

Normally, the increase in heart rate provides the majority (75%) of increment in cardiac output during exercise, whereas maintenance of AV synchrony and increase in contractility account for the remaining 25%.[14] Probably around 40% of pacemaker patients exhibit some degree of chronotropic incompetence,[15] defined as an insufficient increase in heart rate in response to exercise. Patients with chronotropic incompetence should receive pacemakers with rate-adaptive function, enabling the pacemaker to increase the paced heart rate in response to the activity or exercise that is accompanied by an insufficient intrinsic rise in heart rate. Rate-adaptive single-chamber or dual-chamber pacing is superior to fixed-rate pacing in these patients.[16,17] Many pacemaker patients are elderly and often unable to perform bicycle ergometry or treadmill exercise tests. Chronotropic function in these patients is best evaluated by a walking test. Casual walking should increase the heart rate to 90 to 100 beats per minute.

The sensor used to detect activity or exercise ideally should mimic the function of a normal sinus node. Different sensor types are currently used. The most common of these are activity sensors—piezoelectric crystals or accelerometers, which although not physiologically ideal act quite well in practice. Sensors of minute ventilation, QT interval, and temperature are used in other models. Sensors of central venous oxygen saturation, right ventricular pressure and its first derivative, pH, and cardiac contractility are currently being evaluated. Sensor activity is programmable. In new pacemaker models, sensor combinations that automatically adjust upper and lower rate and sensor activity (e.g., activity and minute ventilation sensors in the same pacemaker and self-adjusting sensors) have been introduced. Automatic rate decrease during nighttime, so-called sleep function, is available in some models.

In general, pacemakers with rate-adaptive capabilities should be considered for all but the most inactive patients because chronotropic response may deteriorate over time also after pacemaker implantation.

Other Programmable Features

Mode Switching

Mode switching is the ability of a dual-chamber pacemaker to change the pacing mode automatically and reversibly to a non-atrial tracking mode, in practice to VVI, VDI, or DDI mode, during atrial fibrillation or flutter or other supraventricular tachyarrhythmia. Mode switching prevents ventricular pacing at the upper rate limit in case of such arrhythmias. The algorithms used for mode switching differ between pacemaker models.[18]

Atrioventricular Delay Programming

In modern dual-chamber pacemakers, a rate-adaptive AV delay, decreasing in length with heart rate increase and that furthermore differs after sensed and paced atrial events, can be programmed. This facility allows a more physiologic action of the pacemaker with respect to the AV conduction. The opposite feature, AV hysteresis, increases AV delay to promote intrinsic AV conduction and ventricular activation. Recently, algorithms allowing very long AV delays and even dropout of single ventricular beats have been introduced to further minimize ventricular pacing in patients with sick sinus syndrome (Fig. 55.4).

Rate Hysteresis

Making use of an algorithm that delays onset of ventricular pacing to preserve normal physiologic activation and contraction, rate hysteresis is used for patients with recurrent vasovagal syncope, starting ventricular pacing with a faster than normal rate (e.g., 110 beats per minute) in case of a decrease in rate below some predetermined level (e.g., 50 beats per minute).

Electrocardiography during Pacing

In electrocardiograms obtained during cardiac pacing, unipolar pacing artifacts are large and readily visible, whereas bipolar artifacts are small and sometimes not visible (Fig. 55.5). If capture is obtained, pacing artifacts in the atrium are followed by paced P waves, which are different from intrinsic P waves. Ventricular pacing with capture alters the ventricular activation dramatically, and when the lead is implanted in the right ventricular apex, paced ventricular beats resemble the left bundle branch pattern (see Fig. 55.5). Ventricular fusion beats occur when the ventricles are activated simultaneously by the paced impulse and an intrinsic depolarization. Fusion beats are different from the spontaneous QRS complexes and often narrower than paced complexes with full capture.

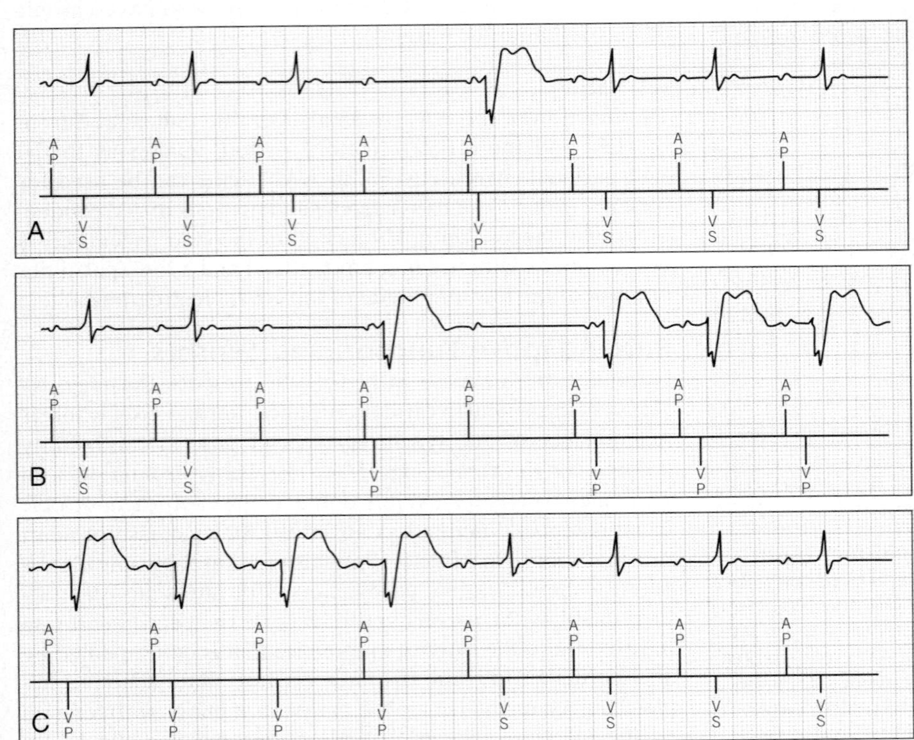

Figure 55.4 Example of an algorithm to promote intrinsic ventricular activation and to minimize ventricular pacing in a dual-chamber (DDD) pacemaker (Managed Ventricular Pacing, Medtronic). Initially, the pacemaker senses atrial and ventricular beats. The PR intervals are restricted only by the underlying atrial or sensor rate (**A,** *left*). If the patient loses AV conduction, dropout of one R wave is allowed. The next P wave is followed by a paced ventricular backup beat **(A)**. The longest pause allowed is twice the lower rate interval + 80 ms. If AV conduction is not present after the sensed atrial beat following the paced ventricular backup, automatic switch to DDDR pacing mode occurs **(B)**. The pacemaker then intermittently checks for return of AV conduction. If AV conduction returns, the device returns to act as an AAIR pacemaker, sensing also the ventricular beats **(C)**.

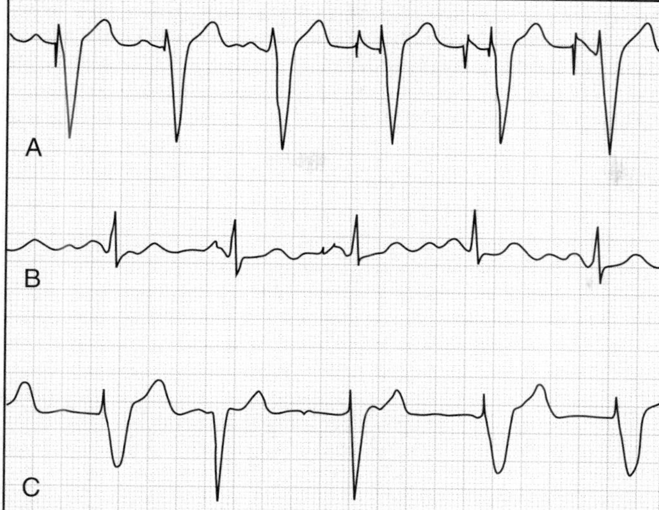

Figure 55.5 Electrocardiography during pacing. A, DDD pacing: to the left, spontaneous P waves followed by ventricular pacing; to the right, pacing in both atrium and ventricle. **B,** Bipolar AAI pacing. **C,** Unipolar VVI pacing. Note the small pacing artifacts caused by bipolar pacing **(B)** in contrast to the large pacing artifacts caused by unipolar pacing **(A, C)**.

Programmers

The function of pacemakers can be altered by noninvasive programming. Each pacemaker manufacturer provides a programmer for its pacemakers. Electromagnetic waves are used for the communication between programmer and pacemaker.

Hemodynamics during Pacemaker Treatment

Maintenance of AV synchrony, a normal activation and contraction pattern of the ventricles, and rate adaptation during exercise are the three most important considerations in pacemaker hemodynamics.[14,19-21]

During VVI pacing, AV synchrony is lost, and the activation and contraction sequence of the ventricles is disadvantageously altered.[21] VVI pacing therefore is associated with a lower cardiac output, a lower exercise tolerance, and a higher incidence of pacemaker syndrome (see later) than with either DDD or AAI pacing. DDD pacing preserves AV synchrony but also changes the activation and contraction sequence of the ventricles, as VVI pacing does, and is consequently associated with a lower cardiac output than sinus rhythm or AAI pacing with intrinsic ventricular activation.[21] Acutely, right ventricular pacing in VVI or DDD pacing mode reduces left ventricular ejection fraction and changes the distribution of the myocardial blood flow.[22] Long-term ventricular pacing furthermore causes left atrial dilatation[23,24] and may, at least in a subset of patients, induce or precipitate congestive heart failure.[24-26] The disadvantageous effect of ventricular pacing has been called ventricular desynchronization. DDD pacing is associated with a lower incidence of congestive heart failure than is VVI pacing.[9] Traditionally, the ventricular lead has been implanted in the right ventricular apex. Theoretically, pacing from the right ventricular septum or outflow tract may cause less desynchronization and has been found to improve acute hemodynamics compared with apical pacing. No studies, however, have indicated a better clinical outcome of the patients using pacing sites other than the right ventricular apex, and no recommendation could be proposed concerning the location of the right ventricular pacing site in the 2007 European Society of Cardiology guidelines for pacing.[27] From a hemodynamic point of view, VVI pacing is quite suboptimal, may even be harmful to long-term ventricular performance, and should probably be avoided except in patients with chronic atrial fibrillation or flutter.

Pacemaker Implant and Follow-up

The recommendations for permanent pacemaker implantation are shown in Table 55.3.[28] It is important that the implanter verify the indication for permanent pacemaker implantation, both the symptoms of the patient and the documentation of bradyarrhythmia, to select the correct pacemaker system. As a rule, cephalic vein cutdown should be the first choice for lead introduction because it has a lower complication rate than subclavian vein puncture. During the implantation procedure, thresholds, amplitude of sensed values, and impedances are obtained by use of a pacing system analyzer. Implanters of pacemakers should not perform fewer than 12 operations per year.[29]

The recommendations for complete ambulatory follow-up of pacemaker patients are listed in Table 55.4.[30] During the first week after implantation, motion of the ipsilateral arm and shoulder should be limited, but complete range of motion should be resumed 2 or 3 weeks postoperatively. For legal reasons, it is frequently recommended to wait

GENERAL RECOMMENDATIONS FOR PERMANENT PACEMAKER IMPLANTATION
Pacemaker implantation
The indication for permanent pacemaker implantation should be verified
Left-sided implantation (if the patient is right-handed)
Sterility
Prophylactic systemic antibiotics[68]
Sedation and analgesics and local anesthesia
Electrode placement (guided by fluoroscopy) after cephalic vein cutdown (first choice) or subclavian venipuncture (second choice); should be tested for mechanical stability and diaphragmatic stimulation
Ventricular electrodes: threshold, $\leq$1.0 V; sensed R, >6 mV; slew rate, >0.5 V/s
Atrial electrodes: threshold, $\leq$1.5 V; sensed P, >1.5 mV; slew rate, >0.5 V/s
Pocket formation and placement of pacemaker in pocket
Pacemaker programming and testing
Full pacemaker testing including thresholds, sensed values, and impedances
Output settings in atrium and ventricle: voltage, 3 to 5 times the threshold; pulse duration, 0.4-0.5 ms
Sensitivity according to sensed P and R waves
Individual programming of the pacemaker
Chest radiograph if pneumothorax suspected

Table 55.3 General recommendations for permanent pacemaker implantation.

PACEMAKER FOLLOW-UP	
Patient assessment	
History	Dizziness, syncope, palpitations, dyspnea, fatigue, chest pain, medication review
Physical examination	Blood pressure
	Heart rate and rhythm (electrocardiographic rhythm with and without magnet)
	Respiratory rate and effort
	Heart sounds, breath sounds
	Edema
	Skin color
	Wound and site assessment
	Neck veins for cannon waves
Device assessment	
Device history	Age of the lead and the pulse generator
	Specific operating characteristics of pulse generator and leads
	Previous clinical complications
	Previous hardware complications (e.g., advisory hardware, lead fracture, abandoned leads)
	Known reliability of implanted hardware
Available telemetry	Programmed settings including last programmed date
	Date stamping of changes in battery status
	Model number
	Patient information and implantation date
	Battery status (cell impedance, voltage, energy, charge, current drain)
	Lead information (type of lead, lead impedance, polarity)
Available diagnostic data	Heart rate counters including user-defined high rate counters
	Counter of ventricular arrhythmias and atrial tachycardia
	Sensor rate histograms
	Intracardiac electrogram and telemetered marker channel
	Diagnostics specific to therapies, such as heart rate drop and mode switching
	Lead impedance trends over time
	Capture and sensing thresholds over time
	Indicators of the percentage of pacing and sensing in each chamber
	Automatic features including automatic rate sensor changes, pacing thresholds, and changes in device output
Direct programming	Capture and sensing threshold assessment
	Atrioventricular conduction and ventriculoatrial conduction measurements when appropriate

Complete ambulatory follow-up of pacemaker patients should be performed routinely after 2 to 3 months and subsequently at least every year after implantation.
Modified from Fraser JD, Gillis AM, Irwin ME, et al. Guidelines for pacemaker follow-up in Canada: a consensus statement of the Canadian Working Group on Cardiac Pacing. Can J Cardiol 2000;16:355-363.

Table 55.4 Pacemaker follow-up.

1 week postoperatively before car driving is resumed. We do routine follow-up at 3 months and 12 months and subsequently every year after implantation. At the first follow-up visit, the voltage output of the pacemaker is reduced if threshold is low. The patient's safety has higher priority than saving battery current drain, and the safety margin (the voltage output to threshold ratio) should not be less than 2:1.

Several new devices have abilities for remote monitoring that automatically sends information from the device to the pacemaker clinic by the telephone network, potentially reducing the need for routine ambulatory follow-up in the future.

INDICATIONS AND CONTRAINDICATIONS

Permanent Pacing

The indications reported for permanent pacemaker implantation vary widely between countries (Table 55.5). The two most common indications for implantation are sinus node dysfunction and AV block.

In 2002, the 1998 guidelines of the American College of Cardiology (ACC) and the American Heart Association (AHA) for the implantation of cardiac pacemakers were updated.[31,32] In 2007, new guidelines for cardiac pacing and cardiac resynchronization therapy were published by the European Society

INDICATIONS FOR PRIMARY PACEMAKER IMPLANTATION IN THE UNITED STATES AND EUROPE		
Indication for Primary Pacemaker Implantation	**United States**	**Europe**
Sinus node dysfunction	59%	27% (16%-41%)*
AV block	39%	44% (21%-57%)*
Atrial fibrillation and bradycardia	NR	17% (8%-24%)
Ablation-induced AV block	2%	1.4% (0.5%-3.2%)
Hypersensitive carotid sinus or neurally mediated syncope	1%	2.4% (0.4%-7.5%)

*Estimated means and range are reported.
NR, not reported.
Data from the 1990-2002 survey in the United States[1] and from the 1997 European cardiac pacing survey based on national registers in 20 European countries.[3]

Table 55.5 Indications for primary pacemaker implantation in the United States and Europe.

of Cardiology (ESC)[27]; these vary slightly from the ACC/AHA guidelines as discussed in the text. The indications for pacing in AV block, sinus node dysfunction, and other special conditions are listed in Tables 55.6 and 55.7. In considering the indication for cardiac pacing in a patient, both the ACC/AHA guidelines and the ESC guidelines are useful. Guidelines for temporary pacing are given in Chapter 56.

Recommended pacemaker modes are presented in Table 55.8.

Acquired Atrioventricular Block

All adult patients, whether symptomatic or asymptomatic, who have permanent third-degree AV block or Möbitz type II second-degree AV block should be treated with permanent pacing (see Table 55.6). In these patients, survival is compromised without a pacemaker, and pacemaker treatment probably improves survival.[33,34] For patients who have Möbitz type I second-degree AV block, the ACC/AHA guidelines recommend no pacing if the patient is asymptomatic. An observational study from 1985 indicates that elderly patients who have chronic Möbitz type I AV block have a prognosis similar to that of those who have Möbitz type II block. Both types of block were associated with excess mortality if patients were left unpaced, whereas paced patients had a survival similar to that expected for the normal population.[34] No studies have contradicted these findings. In the new ESC guidelines, permanent pacing is recommended also for asymptomatic patients who have Möbitz type I second-degree AV block that is not known to be a supra-Hisian conduction block (which can be diagnosed only by an invasive electrophysiologic study).[27]

Nocturnal Möbitz type I AV block in a young, asymptomatic subject is associated with high vagal tone and is not an indication for pacemaker implantation.

Isolated first-degree AV block should be considered an indication for permanent pacing only if temporary pacing alleviates symptoms or improves hemodynamics in patients who have left ventricular dysfunction.[35] In all cases of severe left ventricular dysfunction with an indication for permanent pacing, cardiac resynchronization therapy should be considered to avoid deterioration of left ventricular function due to pacing-induced desynchronization (see Chapter 74).

Bundle Branch Block (Bifascicular and Trifascicular Block)

Isolated bifascicular or trifascicular block without symptoms is associated with heart disease, most often coronary artery disease, but the risk of progression to higher grade AV block is low and does not indicate prophylactic pacing. Patients who have bifascicular or trifascicular block and syncope without apparent second- or third-degree AV block should undergo evaluation including an invasive electrophysiologic study because ventricular tachycardia is the cause of syncope in a considerable proportion of the patients. In those in whom no cause of syncope is detected during this evaluation, permanent pacemaker treatment is recommended. In the 2007 ESC guidelines, the finding on electrophysiologic study of markedly prolonged HV interval (≥100 ms) or pacing-induced infra-His block in patients with symptoms is a class I indication for pacing; neuromuscular disease with any degree of fascicular block is a class IIa indication for pacing.[27]

Congenital Atrioventricular Block

Permanent pacing is indicated (class I) in pediatric patients who have congenital complete AV block with any of the following conditions[27]:

- symptoms (syncope or presyncope, congestive heart failure, exercise intolerance);
- heart rate below 50 to 55 beats per minute in infants (<70 beats per minute in congenital heart disease);
- ventricular dysfunction;
- wide QRS escape rhythm;
- complex ventricular ectopy;
- abrupt ventricular pauses more than two or three times the basic cycle length;
- prolonged QTc time; or
- presence of maternal antibody–mediated block.

Children who have congenital heart block should be referred for expert evaluation and treatment. Acquired symptomatic AV block or sinus node dysfunction also may indicate permanent pacing in children. However, the decision to initiate permanent pacing in children always should be an expert decision. Congenital heart block in adults should probably be considered an indication for permanent pacing, even in asymptomatic patients.[36]

INDICATIONS FOR PACING IN AV CONDUCTION DISEASE

Acquired AV block in adults

Class I

- Third-degree and advanced second-degree AV block associated with any one of the following conditions:
  a. Bradycardia with symptoms (including heart failure) presumed to be due to AV block. (C)
  b. Arrhythmias and other medical conditions that require drugs that result in symptomatic bradycardia. (C)
  c. Documented periods of asystole ≥3.0 seconds or any escape rate <40 bpm in awake, symptom-free patients. (B, C)
  d. After catheter ablation of the AV junction. (B, C)
  e. Postoperative AV block that is not expected to resolve after cardiac surgery. (C)
  f. Neuromuscular diseases with AV block, with or without symptoms. (B)
- Second-degree AV block with associated symptomatic bradycardia. (B)

Class IIa

- Asymptomatic third-degree AV block with average awake ventricular rates of ≥40 bpm, especially if cardiomegaly or left ventricular dysfunction is present. (B, C)
- Asymptomatic type II second-degree AV block with a narrow QRS. When type II second-degree AV block occurs with a wide QRS, pacing becomes a Class I recommendation. (B)
- Asymptomatic type I second-degree AV block at intra- or infra-His levels found at electrophysiological study performed for other indications. (B)
- First- or second-degree AV block with symptoms similar to those of pacemaker syndrome. (B)

Class IIb

- Marked first-degree AV block (>0.30 second) in patients with LV dysfunction and symptoms of congestive heart failure in whom a shorter AV interval results in hemodynamic improvement, presumably by decreasing left atrial filling pressure. (C)
- Neuromuscular diseases with any degree of AV block (including first-degree AV block) with or without symptoms. (B)

Class III

- Asymptomatic first-degree AV block. (B)
- Asymptomatic type I second-degree AV block at the supra-His level or not known to be intra- or infra-Hisian. (B, C)*
- AV block expected to resolve and unlikely to recur (e.g., drug toxicity, Lyme disease, or during hypoxia in sleep apnea syndrome in absence of symptoms). (B)

Chronic bifascicular and trifascicular block

Class I

- With intermittent third-degree AV block. (B)
- With type II second-degree AV block. (B)
- With alternating bundle-branch block. (C)

Class IIa

- Syncope not demonstrated to be due to AV block when other likely causes have been excluded, specifically ventricular tachycardia (electrophysiological study). (B)
- Incidental finding at electrophysiological study of markedly prolonged HV interval (≥100 milliseconds) in asymptomatic patients. (B)*
- Incidental findings at electrophysiological study of pacing-induced infra-His block that is not physiological. (B)*

Chronic bifascicular and trifascicular block—cont'd

Class IIb

- Neuromuscular diseases with any degree of fascicular block with or without symptoms. (B)*

Class III

- Fascicular block without AV block or symptoms. (B)
- Fascicular block with first-degree AV block without symptoms. (B)

AV block associated with acute myocardial infarction

Class I

- Persistent second-degree AV block in the His-Purkinje system with bilateral bundle-branch block or third-degree AV block within or below the His-Purkinje system after AMI. (B)
- Transient advanced (second- or third-degree) infranodal AV block and associated bundle-branch block. If the site of block is uncertain, an electrophysiological study may be necessary. (B)
- Persistent and symptomatic second- or third-degree AV block. (C)

Class IIb

- Persistent second- or third-degree AV block at the AV node level. (B)

Class III

- Transient AV block in the absence of intraventricular conduction defects. (B)
- Transient AV block in the presence of isolated left anterior fascicular block. (B)
- Acquired left anterior fascicular block in the absence of AV block. (B)
- Persistent first-degree AV block in the presence of bundle-branch block that is old or indeterminate in age. (B)

Class I: Conditions for which there is evidence and/or general agreement that a given procedure or treatment is beneficial, useful, and effective.
Class II: Conditions for which there is conflicting evidence and/or a divergence of opinion about the usefulness/efficacy of a procedure or treatment.
Class IIa: Weight of evidence/opinion is in favor of usefulness/efficacy.
Class IIb: Usefulness/efficacy is less well established by evidence/opinion.
Class III: Conditions for which there is evidence and/or general agreement that a procedure/treatment is not useful/effective and in some cases may be harmful.
Level of evidence is indicated in parentheses (see text).
*Indications given in the 2007 ESC guidelines[27] differ as discussed in the text.
ACC/AHA guidelines and indications for permanent pacing.[31,32] Reproduced with permission.

Table 55.6 Indications for pacing in AV conduction disease.

Atrioventricular Block Associated with Acute Myocardial Infarction

Transient AV block is a common complication of acute myocardial infarction, especially inferior wall myocardial infarction. Such a situation may necessitate temporary pacing in the acute phase to alleviate symptomatic bradycardia (see later). Permanent pacing is very rarely needed in patients who have inferior wall myocardial infarction and narrow QRS complex.[37] Permanent pacing should be instituted only if a second- or third-degree AV block persists for more than 8 to 10 days after the acute myocardial infarction.[37]

INDICATIONS FOR PACING IN SINUS NODE DYSFUNCTION
Class I
■ Sinus node dysfunction with documented symptomatic bradycardia, including frequent symptomatic sinus pauses. Bradycardia may be iatrogenic and occur as a consequence of essential long-term drug therapy for which there are no acceptable alternatives. (C)
■ Symptomatic chronotropic incompetence. (C)
Class IIa
■ Sinus node dysfunction occurring spontaneously or as a result of necessary drug therapy, with heart rates <40 bpm when a clear association between significant symptoms consistent with bradycardia and the actual presence of bradycardia has not been documented. (C)
■ Syncope of unexplained origin when major abnormalities of sinus node function are discovered or provoked in electrophysiological studies. (C)*
Class IIb
■ In minimally symptomatic patients, chronic heart rate <40 bpm while awake. (C)
Class III
■ Sinus node dysfunction in asymptomatic patients, including those in whom substantial sinus bradycardia (heart rate <40 bpm) is due to long-term drug treatment.
■ Sinus node dysfunction in patients with symptoms suggestive of bradycardia that are clearly documented not to be associated with a slow heart rate.
■ Sinus node dysfunction with symptomatic bradycardia due to nonessential drug therapy.
Hypersensitive carotid sinus and neurally mediated syndromes
Class I
■ Recurrent syncope caused by carotid sinus stimulation; minimal carotid sinus pressure induces ventricular asystole of more than 3-second duration in the absence of any medication that depresses the sinus node or AV conduction. (C)
Class IIa
■ Recurrent syncope without clear, provocative events and with a hypersensitive cardioinhibitory response. (C)
■ Significantly symptomatic and recurrent neurocardiogenic syncope associated with bradycardia documented spontaneously or at the time of tilt-table testing. (B)
Class IIb
■ Neurally mediated syncope with significant bradycardia reproduced by a head-up tilt with or without isoproterenol or other provocative maneuvers. (B)*
Class III
■ A hyperactive cardioinhibitory response to carotid sinus stimulation in the absence of symptoms or in the presence of vague symptoms such as dizziness, lightheadedness, or both. (C)
■ Recurrent syncope, lightheadedness, or dizziness in the absence of a hyperactive cardioinhibitory response.
■ Situational vasovagal syncope in which avoidance behavior is effective.

Class I: Conditions for which there is evidence and/or general agreement that a given procedure or treatment is beneficial, useful, and effective.
Class II: Conditions for which there is conflicting evidence and/or a divergence of opinion about the usefulness/efficacy of a procedure or treatment.
Class IIa: Weight of evidence/opinion is in favor of usefulness/efficacy.
Class IIb: Usefulness/efficacy is less well established by evidence/opinion.
Class III: Conditions for which there is evidence and/or general agreement that a procedure/treatment is not useful/effective and in some cases may be harmful.
Level of evidence is indicated in parentheses (see text).
*Indications given in the 2007 ESC guidelines[27] differ as discussed in the text.
ACC/AHA guidelines and indications for permanent pacing.[31,32]
Reproduced with permission.

Table 55.7 Indications for pacing in sinus node dysfunction.

RECOMMENDED PACEMAKER MODES

Diagnosis	Optimal	Alternative	Inappropriate
Sinus node dysfunction	AAIR	AAI	VVI, VDD, VDI, DDI
	DDDR + MVP*	DDDR	
AV block	DDD	VDD VVIR†	AAI, DDI
Sinus node dysfunction and AV block	DDDR	DDD	AAI, VVI†
Chronic AF with AV block	VVIR†	VVI	AAI, DDD, VDD
Hypersensitive carotid sinus and neurally mediated syndromes	DDI	DDD VVI‡	AAI, VVI,‡ VDD

The optimal pacing mode should be considered for each patient. The alternative mode should be regarded as less satisfactory but acceptable in some groups of patients. The inappropriate modes should not be used. AF, atrial fibrillation or flutter, AV; atrioventricular.
*MVP: algorithm to minimize ventricular pacing.
†VVIR pacing may be an alternative for patients who have a low level of physical activity and in those with a short expected life span.
‡VVI pacing should be used only in case of chronic atrial fibrillation or other chronic atrial tachyarrhythmia.

Table 55.8 Recommended pacemaker modes.

Patients who have acute myocardial infarction and intraventricular conduction defects, with the exception of isolated left anterior fascicular block, have an unfavorable prognosis and an increased incidence of sudden death.[38,39] This poor prognosis is associated with extensive myocardial necrosis and mainly caused by malignant arrhythmia, pump failure, and electromechanical dissociation, not by progressive AV block. However, transient high-degree AV block in the acute phase of myocardial infarction in these patients seems to be associated with a high risk of recurrent AV block and sudden death, which may be reduced by pacemaker treatment. This risk is particularly high in patients who have right bundle branch block and left anterior hemiblock.[38] Permanent pacing can be recommended for patients who already have or develop permanent bundle branch block and had transient AV block in the acute phase of myocardial infarction. In such patients, echocardiography should be done to evaluate the indication for treatment with an implantable defibrillator, maybe in combination with cardiac resynchronization therapy (see Chapter 74).

Selection of Pacing Modes in AV Block

Bradycardia caused by AV block requires ventricular pacing, which may be VVI pacing or dual-chamber pacing. AV synchrony is lost in VVI pacing and preserved in dual-chamber pacing. Dual-chamber pacing has been found to be superior to VVI pacing in several small studies, being associated with better "general well-being," exercise capacity, functional status,[40] and quality of life.[16,41] VVI pacing is associated with an increased risk of pacemaker syndrome,[42,43] and it has been suggested that many apparently asymptomatic patients with VVI pacemakers suffer from a subclinical form of pacemaker syndrome and may benefit from upgrading to dual-chamber pacing.[44] Observational analyses have indicated that in patients who have coexisting congestive heart failure, VVI pacing increases mortality compared with dual-chamber pacing.[45,46] In the first large-scale randomized trial, the Canadian Trial of Physiological Pacing (CTOPP), comparing VVIR (n = 1474) and physiologic (DDD) pacing (n = 1095), there was no difference in the primary endpoint, cardiovascular death or stroke, between treatment groups after 3.5 years of follow-up.[10] Atrial fibrillation was significantly reduced (relative risk reduction, 18%) in the physiologically paced group. After an extended follow-up to a mean of 6 years after pacemaker implantation, this difference in occurrence of atrial fibrillation persisted, but no significant differences in other clinical endpoints had emerged.[47] In CTOPP, 52% of the patients had AV block. In a later subgroup analysis of data from the CTOPP trial, patients with an unpaced heart rate below 60 beats per minute had a significantly worse outcome with VVI pacing.[48] In the randomized UK-PACE trial comparing VVI and DDD pacing in 2000 elderly patients with AV block, no differences in overall or cardiovascular mortality, atrial fibrillation, or heart failure were observed between treatment groups.[8] Although DDD pacing does not improve survival compared with VVI pacing, the higher incidence of atrial fibrillation and pacemaker syndrome with VVI pacing and the improved well-being associated with DDD pacing indicate that DDD pacing should be recommended as the optimal pacing mode in AV block, with single-lead VDD pacing a reasonable alternative for those with normal sinus node function. VVIR pacing should be used in patients with chronic atrial fibrillation and bradycardia (Fig. 55.6). As indicated by the UK-PACE trial, VVIR pacing may be an alternative for patients who have a low level of physical activity and in those with a short expected life span.[27] The use of algorithms promoting intrinsic ventricular conduction may rarely cause bradycardia-related ventricular tachyarrhythmia in patients with AV block, and there is no documentation that the use of such algorithms is beneficial for this group of patients.

Sinus Node Dysfunction (Sick Sinus Syndrome)

Sinus node dysfunction includes sinus arrest, sinoatrial block, and sinus bradycardia and is associated with paroxysmal atrial fibrillation or flutter (bradycardia-tachycardia syndrome) in at least 50% of patients at the time of pacemaker implantation (see Chapter 53). Sinus node dysfunction is a relatively benign condition and is not associated with any significant excess mortality compared with the normal population. Pacemaker treatment in sinus node dysfunction is

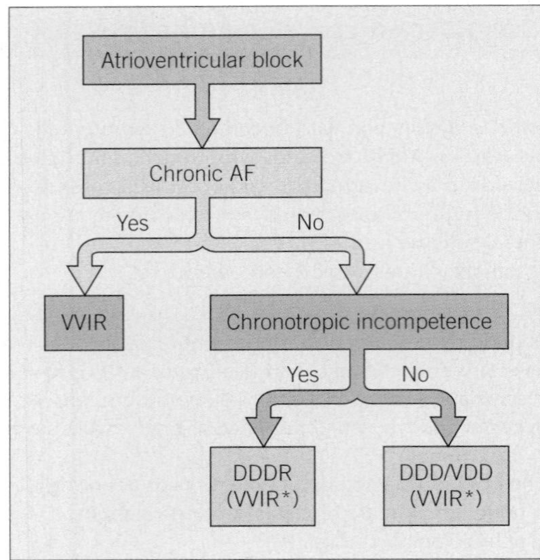

Figure 55.6 Flow chart for selection of pacing mode in patients with AV block. *VVIR pacing may be an alternative for patients who have a low level of physical activity and in those with a short expected life span. In case of chronotropic incompetence, rate-adaptive pacing should be chosen. AF, atrial fibrillation.

effective in relieving bradycardia-related symptoms but does not necessarily improve survival. However, pacing is the treatment of choice for patients who have symptomatic sinus node dysfunction because there are currently no acceptable pharmacologic alternatives.[49] In the recent ESC guidelines, sinus node disease induced at electrophysiologic study is a class I indication for pacing, and the finding of a corrected sinus node recovery time of more than 800 ms is a class IIa indication for pacing in patients with otherwise unexplained syncope.[27] Only very rarely is it indicated to perform an invasive electrophysiologic study to decide whether a patient should receive a permanent pacemaker for sinus node disease.

Selection of Pacing Modes in Sinus Node Dysfunction

Bradycardia caused by sinus node dysfunction in patients who have normal AV conduction can be treated with AAI, VVI, or DDD pacing. Several observational studies have indicated that VVI pacing is associated with an increased mortality and morbidity compared with AAI pacing.[50] This was confirmed in a long-term follow-up in the first randomized comparison of AAI and VVI pacing in patients who have sinus node dysfunction. After a mean follow-up of 5.5 years, VVI pacing was associated with significantly higher overall mortality, cardiovascular mortality, atrial fibrillation, arterial thromboembolism, and heart failure compared with AAI pacing.[6,24] In the CTOPP trial, 34% of the patients had isolated sinus node dysfunction. As in the whole CTOPP population, atrial fibrillation was significantly reduced with physiologic pacing in the subgroup with sinus node dysfunction; however, no significant differences were observed in other clinical endpoints at end of follow-up.[10] This finding was supported by the results of the MOST (Mode Selection Trial in Sinus Node Dysfunction) trial, comparing DDDR and VVIR pacing in 2010 patients who had sinus node dysfunction. In the MOST trial, atrial fibrillation was significantly reduced in the DDDR group, whereas no differences were observed in the primary endpoint (death or nonfatal stroke) or in the secondary endpoints (all-cause mortality and stroke).[9] The incidence of congestive heart failure was lower in the DDDR group than in the VVIR group.[9] In a subgroup analysis of data from the MOST trial, an increasing percentage of ventricular pacing was found to be correlated with increasing occurrences of both atrial fibrillation and hospitalization for heart failure.[25] Recently, the SAVE PACe (Search AV Extension and Managed Ventricular Pacing for Promoting Atrioventricular Conduction) trial documented that reducing ventricular pacing by means of special algorithms promoting intrinsic ventricular conduction reduces the occurrence of atrial fibrillation in patients with sinus node dysfunction and DDD pacemaker (see Fig. 55.4).[11]

AAI pacing is the only pacing mode without any ventricular pacing and desynchronization; it is the pacing mode so far found to be associated with the lowest risk of atrial fibrillation[6,51] and furthermore with less thromboembolism and a better survival than by VVI pacing.[6] The incidence of AV block requiring upgrading of the pacemaker in patients primarily treated with an AAI or AAIR pacemaker is approximately 1.7% per year.[52,53] Because DDD pacing protects patients from AV block, it has been used routinely for all patients with sinus node dysfunction in many implanting centers. At present, the recommended pacing mode for patients who have sinus node dysfunction is either AAIR or DDDR with programming of an algorithm promoting intrinsic ventricular conduction (Fig. 55.7; see also Fig. 55.4).[11] AAIR pacing is appropriate only in patients without compromised AV conduction (PQ ≤220 ms, no second- or third-degree AV block, no bradycardia <40 beats per minute or R-R intervals >3 seconds during atrial fibrillation), without bundle branch block (QRS width <120 ms), without concomitant hypersensitive carotid sinus (see later), and with one-to-one AV conduction at a paced rate of 100 beats per minute measured at time of implantation. As some degree of chronotropic incompetence is common among patients who have sinus node dysfunction, they should receive rate-adaptive pacemakers. VVI pacing is not appropriate in sinus node dysfunction. If DDDR pacing is used, mode switch should be active. There is no documentation that patients with sinus node dysfunction and paroxysmal atrial fibrillation profit from the presently available antitachycardia pacemaker algorithms.[54]

During AAIR pacing, a paradoxical prolongation of the spike-R interval during exercise occurs in a minority of patients and may be associated with such symptoms as chest pain, dyspnea, and lightheadedness, the so-called AAIR pacemaker syndrome.[55] This phenomenon is probably the result of an inadequate balance between the pacemaker sensor activity and the level of sympathetic tone during initial exercise, and it tends to correct itself as sympathetic tone progressively increases during exercise.[55,56] The paradoxical prolongation of the spike-R interval during exercise most often occurs in patients receiving drugs that depress AV conduction. The risk of AAIR pacemaker syndrome is low, especially if the maximum sensor rate is programmed to approximately 90 to 100 beats per minute, which is appropriate in most elderly patients during normal daily activities. In the clinical setting, the AAIR pacemaker syndrome is rarely significant.[53]

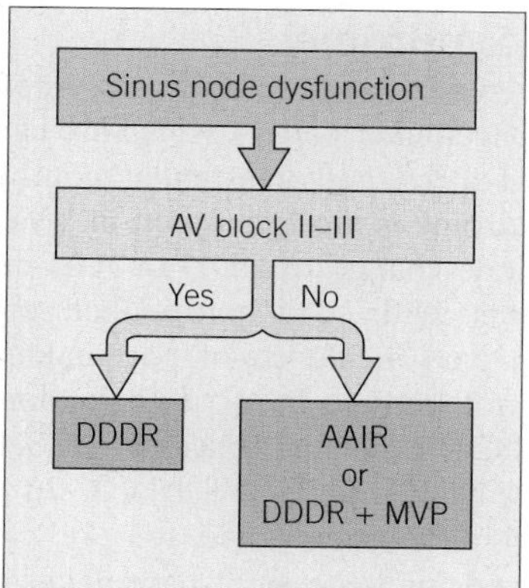

Figure 55.7 Flow chart for selection of pacing mode in patients with sick sinus syndrome. AAIR pacing is appropriate in patients without compromised AV conduction (PQ ≤220 ms, no bradycardia <40 beats per minute or R-R intervals >3 seconds during atrial fibrillation or flutter), without bundle branch block (QRS width <120 ms), without concomitant hypersensitive carotid sinus, and with one-to-one AV conduction at a paced rate of 100 beats per minute measured at time of implantation. MVP, algorithm to minimize ventricular pacing.

Pacing in Hypersensitive Carotid Sinus and Neurally Mediated Syncope

Hypersensitive carotid sinus and neurally mediated syncope account for an unknown but probably not minor proportion of syncopal attacks leading to hospital referral. Pacemaker implantation rates for these diagnoses have increased recently. In northeastern England, they were the indication in 23% of the total implantations after the opening of a dedicated syncope and falls clinic, which focused attention on these diagnoses.[57]

The diagnosis of hypersensitive carotid sinus (carotid sinus syndrome) is made by reproducing symptoms by means of carotid sinus massage in a syncopal patient in whom there is considered to be no other cause of syncope after extensive investigation.[58] Symptomatic asystole lasting at least 3 seconds caused by sinus arrest or AV block must be documented during carotid sinus massage. Patients who have hypersensitive carotid sinus are predominantly male (the male-to-female ratio is 2:1) and older than 70 years. Dual-chamber pacing has been found to effectively reduce recurrent syncope in such patients, although it does not completely abolish it.[59] Only patients with recurrent syncope should be considered candidates for permanent pacing.[27] DDD and DDI pacing with rate hysteresis (in which a decrease in the rate below 50 beats per minute, for example, triggers pacing at a rate of 100 beats per minute) are the preferred pacing modes. AAI or VVI pacing should not be used.[58]

Neurally mediated or vasovagal syncope is common, and only a minor subset of patients with recurrent, severe "malignant" vasovagal syncopal attacks should be considered candidates for pacing. Compared with patients with hypersensitive carotid sinus, patients with vasovagal syncope often are younger, and their syncopal attacks more often are preceded by an identifiable set of warning symptoms that the patient can recognize. In patients in whom syncope and a predominantly cardioinhibitory component (defined as a heart rate below 40 beats per minute for more than 10 seconds or asystole for more than 3 seconds) can be documented by electrocardiographic recording or reproduced by tilt table testing, and in whom other therapeutic options have failed, cardiac pacing can be recommended. According to the 2007 ESC guidelines, pacing should be considered only for carefully selected patients older than 40 years.[27] DDD and DDI pacing with rate hysteresis are the recommended pacing modes.

Pacing in Other Patients

Permanent pacing is recommended for patients with long QT syndrome who have coincidence of AV block or evidence of symptomatic bradycardia. In high-risk patients with long QT syndrome, especially those with aborted sudden death or a strong family history of sudden cardiac death, an implantable cardioverter-defibrillator should be recommended.[27]

In patients who have hypertrophic obstructive cardiomyopathy, DDD pacing with a short AV delay that ensures complete myocardial capture from the right ventricular apex reduces the left ventricular outflow tract gradient. Small studies have indicated a symptomatic effect of DDD pacing in patients with hypertrophic obstructive cardiomyopathy.[60] However, no large randomized trials have confirmed these results, and there is no evidence to suggest that pacing alters disease progression or reduces mortality. Therefore, the indication for pacing is controversial. In the 2007 ESC guidelines, pacing is recommended for patients with hypertrophic obstructive cardiomyopathy with symptomatic bradycardia due to beta blockade when alternative therapies are unacceptable; it can be considered for patients with drug-refractory hypertrophic obstructive cardiomyopathy and contraindications to septal ablation or myectomy.[27]

In patients with congestive heart failure, bundle branch block, and depressed left ventricular function, cardiac resynchronization therapy has been found to reduce mortality and morbidity (see Chapter 74).

Pacing for Atrial Fibrillation

Several studies on the efficacy of pacing on suppression of paroxysmal atrial fibrillation have been done. In patients with sinus node dysfunction, AAI pacing and DDD pacing with algorithms promoting intrinsic ventricular conduction both are better than traditional DDD pacing, which again is superior to VVI pacing[6,9-11] in this context. Any clinically significant superiority of atrial overdrive pacing, rate-adaptive atrial pacing, or special atrial fibrillation–depressing algorithms as well as of selective site atrial pacing in suppression of atrial fibrillation remains to be proved.[54]

Contraindications to Permanent Pacing

To prevent pacemaker pocket infection, a permanent pacemaker should not be implanted in patients who have ongoing systemic or local infection. If pacing is necessary during the course of the infection, temporary pacing should be maintained, and a permanent pacemaker can be implanted when the infection has resolved. Bleeding diathesis is a relative contraindication to pacemaker implantation, and in anticoagulated patients, the international normalized ratio (INR) level should not exceed 2 to 2.5 at the time of implantation.

Obviously, temporary and reversible causes of conduction disorders must be considered to be contraindications to permanent pacing. Such temporary conditions include myocarditis, drug intoxication, electrolyte disturbances, and inferior myocardial infarction. Other indications listed under class III indications in the ACC/AHA and ESC guidelines[27,32] should also be considered contraindications to permanent pacing.

Cost-effectiveness of Permanent Pacing

Permanent pacing is clinically effective, and there are no acceptable alternatives to pacemaker implantation in most patients. The cost-effectiveness of permanent pacing cannot therefore be compared with alternative treatments or with no treatment. The costs of different pacing modes in permanent pacing have been evaluated. Taking into account both the costs of pacemaker products and implantation and the costs of adverse outcomes after pacemaker implantation, VVI pacing is associated with higher costs than are both AAI pacing (in sinus node dysfunction) and DDD pacing (in sinus node dysfunction or AV block). The magnitude of this cost difference ranges from 24% to 27% in comparing VVI with DDD pacing mode and from 34% to 35% in comparing VVI with AAI pacing mode.[61] Another analysis has found that in both sinus node dysfunction and AV block, DDD pacing is cost-effective compared with VVI pacing, and in the third year after implantation, the cumulative costs of DDD pacing are lower than the cumulative costs of VVI pacing.[62] The initially lower price of a VVI pacemaker and one lead compared with a DDD pacemaker and two leads is outweighed by the costs associated with the higher incidences of adverse events—pacemaker syndrome, atrial fibrillation, thromboembolism, and heart failure—that are seen during VVI pacing.

COMPLICATIONS

By far the most common pacemaker complication is erroneous or inappropriate programming of the pacemaker, which results in a less than optimal device function.

Pacemaker Syndrome

The pacemaker syndrome is defined as "symptoms and signs present in the pacemaker patient which are caused by inadequate timing of atrial and ventricular contraction."[43] The pacemaker syndrome is most common in VVI pacing. Reoperation with mode change to DDD or AAI must be considered in patients with VVI pacemaker and pacemaker syndrome. The true incidence of pacemaker syndrome in VVI pacing is not known. In the two randomized trials of VVIR versus DDDR pacing (Pacemaker Selection in the Elderly [PASE] trial[7] and MOST trial[9]), 26% and 16.5%, respectively, of patients assigned to VVIR pacing crossed over to DDDR pacing because of pacemaker syndrome during follow-up.[7] Crossover, however, was easily done, as all patients included in these two trials had DDDR pacemakers implanted, and the crossover rate does not reflect the incidence of necessary upgradings due to pacemaker syndrome in patients with VVIR pacemakers. In the CTOPP study, in which mode change from VVI to DDD required a reoperation, only 4.3% of patients in the VVI group had crossed over to physiologic pacing at 5 years.[10] One study indicates that 75% of patients with VVI pacemakers who have no complaints of pacemaker syndrome benefit from upgrading to DDD pacing, which suggests the existence of a "subclinical" pacemaker syndrome.[44]

Pacemaker and Lead Complications

Complications may occur in relation to or shortly after the implantation procedure or during follow-up. Complications related to the pacemaker pocket and leads and the recommended treatments are listed in Table 55.9.[63] The most common complications in relation to pacemaker implantation are pneumothorax and lead dislodgement.

Pneumothorax occurs as a complication of subclavian vein puncture and does not occur after cephalic vein cutdown. To minimize the risk of pneumothorax, fluoroscopic guidance of the subclavian puncture should be used together with careful technique, which also reduces risk of other potential complications (hemothorax, inadvertent arterial puncture, air embolism, thoracic duct injury, and brachial plexus injury). Pneumothorax requiring drainage occurs in 1% to 1.5% of implantations in which a subclavian approach is used.[64]

Lead dislodgement occurs during the immediate postoperative period in approximately 1% to 2% of implantations and in another 1% to 2% during the first 3 months of follow-up.[65] The use of screw-in leads in the atrium reduces atrial lead dislodgements to the same levels as for ventricular leads with passive fixation. Migration of a dislodged lead out of the heart may be associated with thromboembolic complications if it is not detected acutely.

In acute lead perforation, the lead must be withdrawn and repositioned. Most often, this is uncomplicated; however, careful monitoring for pericardial bleeding is necessary.

Inadvertent subclavian artery puncture occurs in 2% to 3% of attempts at subclavian vein puncture but is easy to recognize immediately and very rarely causes severe problems (hemothorax or arteriovenous fistula).[64] Inadvertent lead implantation in the left side of the heart should be corrected immediately.

Most pocket hematomas are small and do not need any treatment. Evacuation of the hematoma is very rarely needed (<0.5% of cases).[65] Needle aspiration increases risk of infection and should not be done. Careful hemostasis during operation and an INR not higher than 2 to 2.5 in anticoagulated patients are important to minimize the risk of hematoma, as is avoidance of giving heparin on the day of implantation.

Infections are severe complications of permanent pacing. The incidence of infection should be less than 0.5% to 1%.[65,66] Acute infections after initial implantation are rare; they are often associated with systemic symptoms and are often caused by *Staphylococcus aureus*. Later infections are more common and are often associated with *Staphylococcus epidermidis*. They are clinically more indolent than the early infections and often produce no systemic symptoms. Device replacement with insertion of a new device in an old chronic pocket increases the risk of such indolent *S. epidermidis* infections.

Endocarditis related to pacemaker lead infection is a rare but very serious complication that, if suspected, can be diagnosed by transesophageal echocardiography.[67]

Infections are prevented by a careful sterile technique during operation; moreover, we recommend antibiotic prophylaxis.[66,68] A temporary pacing lead increases the risk of later infection.[64] If infection occurs, the entire pacemaker system must be explanted, antibiotics administered, and a new pacemaker system implanted on the opposite side. Antibiotic therapy alone is not curative.

Pacemaker allergy due to contact sensitivity is very rare, but it has been described. This diagnosis should not be accepted until infection has been thoroughly ruled out.

Vein thrombosis occurs early or late after pacemaker implantation in 30% to 45% of patients. Most patients who have chronic venous thrombosis remain asymptomatic and do not need any treatment, but the venous occlusion may cause trouble in pacemaker reoperations. Acute venous thrombosis is likely to be symptomatic and may be complicated by pulmonary embolism. Diagnosis is obtained by venography. Management may include anticoagulation, thrombolysis, surgery, or percutaneous transluminal balloon venoplasty, depending on the duration, extent, and site of thrombosis as well as on the accompanying symptoms.[69]

Erosion of the skin by the pacemaker is uncommon and is often associated with implantation of the device outside the correct tissue plane. If the skin is intact and the pocket does not stick to the skin, reoperation with correct placement of the device is the treatment of choice. If the skin is broken or not freely moved over the pocket (i.e., the pocket sticks to skin), the entire system must be explanted as if it were infected.

PACEMAKER AND LEAD COMPLICATIONS AND APPROPRIATE TREATMENT

Complication	Treatment
Pocket complications	
Pocket hematoma	Observation; evacuation if large, not needle aspiration
Infection	Antibiotics, explantation of system, and implantation of a new system on opposite side when infection has resolved
Erosion	Relocation of pocket; if pacemaker pocket sticks to the skin or skin is broken, treat as infected
Migration of pacemaker	No treatment if no other complications
Twiddler's syndrome	Fixation of pacemaker and repositioning of lead
Lead complications	
Acute perforation	Repositioning; monitoring of pericardial bleeding, pericardiocentesis, or acute surgery if necessary
Dislodgement	Repositioning
Infection	Antibiotics, explantation of system, and implantation of a new system on opposite side when infection has resolved
Vein thrombosis	Anticoagulation, thrombolysis in case of superior vena cava syndrome
Migration	Lead extraction

Table 55.9 Pacemaker and lead complications and appropriate treatment.

Pacemaker Malfunction

Knowledge about the indication for pacemaker implantation, the type of pacemaker and leads implanted, and the previous functional status of the device is essential for the evaluation of pacemaker malfunction. A 12-lead surface electrocardiogram, equipment for fluoroscopy and echocardiography, and pacemaker programmers and manuals are necessary. In patients with suspected pacemaker malfunction, the history is obtained, the implantation site is inspected, and a physical examination is done. A 12-lead electrocardiogram is recorded with and without magnet application, which, in a device-specific manner, alters the pacing mode or rate. The pacemaker is interrogated by the programmer, and if they are available, the pacemaker event counters and intracardiac electrogram, including markers, are examined and printed. The pacemaker is tested as during routine follow-up (see Table 55.4), and the suspected malfunction is offered special attention.

Many suspected pacemaker malfunctions are caused by change in programming done by someone since the last evaluation. Lead failure is more common than device failure. Different pacemaker malfunctions and related causes are listed in Table 55.10.

Extracardiac stimulation may indicate an improper position of the lead or lead insulation failure. Pacemaker pocket stimulation is sometimes observed at unipolar output configuration and high output.

Changes in pacing mode and setting are usually caused by programming or battery depletion. Some dual-chamber devices change to a single-chamber mode to conserve power when the battery voltage drops below a certain value. Direct current conversion or other electromagnetic interference can cause mode change or polarity change or can trigger the elective replacement indicator in some pacemaker models. Automatic mode switching from DDD to VVI in case of atrial fibrillation and dropout of single ventricular complexes in DDD devices with algorithms promoting intrinsic ventricular conduction (see Fig. 55.4) are not pacemaker malfunctions but may be misinterpreted as such.

Change in pacing rate can occur because of different causes (see Table 55.10), of which the most common is programming. Battery depletion is associated with rate decline in some models.

In loss of pacing, there is no output, and no pacing artifact is present. Loss of pacing represents a potentially dangerous and lethal situation. It is important not to interpret bipolar pacing without visible pacing artifacts or automatic mode switching as loss of pacing. Temporary reprogramming of pacing polarity to unipolar and examination of the electrocardiogram and intracardiac electrograms should enable detection of those two "pseudomalfunctions." The actual programming of the AV delay, hysteresis, and sensor settings as well as activation of algorithms promoting intrinsic ventricular conduction and allowing dropout of single ventricular beats (see Fig. 55.4) should be considered before loss of pacing is diagnosed. Oversensing (see later) is a frequent cause of loss of pacing. Crosstalk is rare in new DDD devices because of ventricular blanking and ventricular safety pacing. Battery or circuit failure, lead fracture, and connection problems require reoperation.

In loss of capture, a pacing artifact is present, but there is no myocardial capture (Fig. 55.8). Undersensing with pacing in the myocardial refractory period is not loss of capture. In pacemaker-dependent patients, programming of the device to highest output may enable myocardial capture if there is threshold elevation. Threshold elevation within the first days of implantation indicates lead dislodgement, malposition, or perforation. Threshold may rise steadily over time until noncapture occurs, the so-called exit block, which is most commonly seen in some older leads, epicardial leads, and pediatric patients. Some antiarrhythmic agents (e.g., sotalol and propafenone) may increase the pacing threshold, as may metabolic factors (e.g., hyperkalemia and myxedema). Other causes are listed in Table 55.10.

In evaluation of undersensing (failure to detect normal intrinsic cardiac activity; see Fig. 55.8), it is important to know that the pacemaker may sense the intracardiac signal

PACEMAKER MALFUNCTION AND POSSIBLE CAUSES	
Malfunction	**Causes**
Extracardiac stimulation	Improper lead position, diaphragmatic stimulation, pacemaker pocket stimulation, lead insulation failure
Changes in mode and setting	Programming, battery depletion, automatic mode switching, special pacemaker algorithms, electrocautery, defibrillation, other electromagnetic interference
Rate change	Programming, battery depletion, circuit failure, magnet mode, atrial tracking, sensor-driven changes, oversensing, pacemaker-mediated tachycardia, crosstalk, runaway pacemaker, recording artifacts
Loss of pacing	Battery failure, circuitry failure, lead fracture, oversensing, crosstalk, automatic mode switching, hysteresis, lead and pacemaker not compatible or not connected properly
Loss of capture	Threshold elevation (lead maturation; later due to, for example, myocardial infarction, drugs or metabolic factors, or exit block), lead dislodgement, lead fracture, perforation, insulation failure, circuit or battery failure, cardioversion or defibrillation, electrocautery
Undersensing	Poor intracardiac signal, inappropriate sensitivity programming, atrial fibrillation or flutter, lead dislodgement, intrinsic beat falling in device refractory period, magnet application, myocardial infarction, device failure
Oversensing	Lead fracture, insulation failure, myopotential inhibition (unipolar systems), polarization current, far-field QRS sensing (AAI systems), T-wave sensing (VVI systems)
Pacemaker-mediated tachycardia	Sensor-driven tachycardia (programming of sensor parameters, inappropriate sensor activation), myopotential tracking, endless loop tachycardia, non–re-entrant ventriculoatrial synchrony

Table 55.10 Pacemaker malfunction and possible causes.

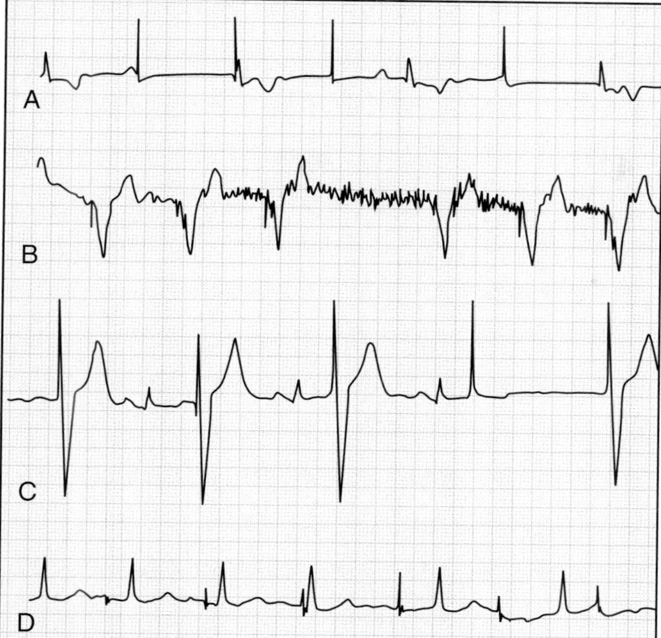

Figure 55.8 Electrocardiograms showing exit block, myopotential inhibition, and undersensing. Electrocardiograms showing VVI pacemaker with exit block **(A)**, VVI pacing with myopotential inhibition **(B)**, undersensing in patient with VVI pacemaker and normal intrinsic rhythm **(C)**, and undersensing in patient with AAI pacemaker and atrial fibrillation caused by the low-amplitude intra-atrial electrograms during atrial fibrillation **(D)**.

later than the start of the corresponding P wave or QRS complex on the surface electrocardiogram. Inappropriate setting of sensitivity or refractory periods is the most common reason for undersensing (see Table 55.10).

Oversensing (inappropriate sensing of electrical signals) is probably the most commonly encountered pacemaker malfunction. It may be indicated by rate change or loss of pacing. The most frequent cause of oversensing is myopotential inhibition, which occurs primarily in unipolar systems (see Fig. 55.8). Asking the patient to press the hands together firmly in front of the chest during electrocardiographic monitoring may be helpful in detecting oversensing. Far-field sensing of QRS complex (in AAI pacing) or the T wave (in VVI pacing) may be solved by reprogramming the sensitivity or refractory periods.

Sensor-driven pacemaker-mediated tachycardia most often is caused by inappropriate programming of sensor parameters, whereas external stimuli interacting with the specific sensor (e.g., use of a vibration-generating tool in a patient with a vibration sensor) is a rarer cause. Myopotential tracking is rare with a bipolar atrial lead. The classic endless loop tachycardia (in which sensing of a retrograde P wave initiates the AV interval, ending with a ventricular paced event and followed by a new retrograde P wave) is most often started by a ventricular premature beat but may be initiated by any situation that leads to a ventricular depolarization without a normal coupled atrial paced or sensed event. Endless loop tachycardia is prevented by appropriate programming of AV delay and PVARP and, in newer devices, by automatic algorithms to prevent endless loop tachycardia. Repetitive, non–re-entrant ventriculoatrial synchrony may result if the retrograde P wave falls in the PVARP.

Electromagnetic interference is caused by signals within the frequency spectrum that may be detected by the sensing circuit of the pacemaker. Electromagnetic interference can result in rate change, reprogramming, or sensing abnormalities. There are several potential sources of electromagnetic interference, including

- radiofrequency ablation;
- cardioversion or defibrillation;
- electrocautery;
- computed tomography or magnetic resonance imaging scanners;
- electroconvulsive therapy;
- transcutaneous electrical nerve stimulation; and
- cellular telephones, which should not be carried or held over or close to the pacemaker, although there is no health risk when they are placed over the ear.

SUMMARY

The clinical effect of pacing in patients who have Adams-Stokes syndrome and severe bradycardia is convincing, and permanent pacing is the treatment of choice with no acceptable alternatives in patients with symptomatic bradycardia. In recent years, large randomized trials have been conducted on the impact of different pacing modes on morbidity and mortality. Physiologic pacing should be the recommended standard. In patients who have AV block, DDDR pacing is optimal, single-lead VDD being an acceptable alternative. In patients who have sinus node dysfunction, AAIR pacing or DDDR pacing with the use of algorithms promoting intrinsic ventricular conduction is the optimal pacing mode. Patients who have chronic atrial fibrillation and bradycardia are the only patients for whom VVI pacing is the optimal pacing mode. Rate-adaptive pacemakers should be the standard.

Studies currently being performed are investigating the effect of cardiac resynchronization therapy in patients with bradycardia, need for ventricular pacing, and moderately reduced left ventricular function. The benefit of implanting the ventricular lead in positions other than the right ventricular apex—in the right ventricular septum or outflow tract or direct His bundle pacing—is also being investigated.

Technically, pacemakers have developed to small, multi-programmable devices. The latest innovations are pacemakers with self-adjusting sensors, semiautomatic devices that automatically adjust output and sensitivity, devices with extensive diagnostic abilities, and devices with features for remote monitoring. These newer advances probably will gain wider acceptance during the years to come. The evolution will continue, thereby improving the physiologic properties of pacing systems and making follow-up of patients easier.

chapter 56 Special Problems in Cardiac Pacing

a. Hemodynamic Sequelae of Right Ventricular Pacing

Mark A. Wood

DEFINITION OF PROBLEM

The right ventricle apex has been the target site for ventricular pacing for decades. However, in recent years, it is recognized that right ventricular pacing can result in serious sequelae. Right ventricular pacing produces a left bundle branch block electrical pattern of ventricular activation. As intrinsic left bundle branch block does, right ventricular pacing may result in deleterious patterns of wall strain in the left ventricle, ineffective contraction patterns, and detrimental ventricular remodeling. The result may be impaired left ventricular function and heart failure. The effects of right ventricular pacing on the development of heart failure are related to the frequency of ventricular pacing, the paced QRS duration, and the patient's underlying predisposition to heart failure. For both implantable cardioverter-defibrillator (ICD) and pacemaker patients, the risk of heart failure increases with the frequency of right ventricular pacing. In the DAVID trial, patients with low ejection fractions receiving ICDs were randomized to DDD pacing at 70 beats per minute or VVI pacing at 40 beats per minute (to minimize right ventricular pacing). The study was terminated prematurely because of higher combined incidence of death and hospitalization for heart failure in the DDD group with 58.9% ± 36.0% ventricular pacing compared with the VVI group with 3.5% ± 14.9% pacing. The MOST trial randomized sinus node dysfunction patients receiving pacemakers to DDDR or VVIR pacing. In a retrospective analysis, any amount of VVIR pacing or a cumulative percentage of DDDR pacing more than 40% of the time was associated with greater risk of heart failure than was a cumulative percentage of DDDR pacing 40% or less of the time. The risk of heart failure hospitalization was also increased proportionally with the paced QRS duration. Finally, the effects of right ventricular pacing on heart failure are heavily influenced by the underlying cardiac substrate and susceptibility to heart failure. In the MOST trial, the cumulative percentage of DDDR pacing more than 40% of the time essentially doubled the risk of heart failure in the pacemaker patients. Patients with normal ejection fraction, normal QRS duration, and no history of myocardial infarction or heart failure (typical of the pacemaker population) had low risk of heart failure (0.76% during 2 years) associated with infrequent ventricular pacing, which was doubled by frequent right ventricular pacing to about 1.4% during 2 years. Thus, many pacemaker patients tolerate right ventricular pacing with low risk of progression to heart failure. On the other hand, pacemaker patients with reduced ejection fraction, prolonged baseline QRS, and history of heart failure or myocardial infarction had a 32.4% risk of heart failure during 2 years with infrequent pacing that increased to 51.6% with frequent DDDR pacing. In contrast to the typical sinus node dysfunction patient, the presence of heart disease and heart failure is typical of the ICD population. Differences in myocardial substrate between these groups can explain the high incidence of heart failure in the DAVID trial (ICD patients) of 30% at 18 months versus 10% at 3 years for the pacemaker patients (MOST trial) with exposure to similar frequency of right ventricular pacing.

TYPICAL CASE

An active 72-year-old man undergoes DDDR pacemaker implantation for tachycardia-bradycardia syndrome. He is receiving amiodarone for paroxysmal atrial fibrillation. His intrinsic PR in sinus rhythm is 340 ms, and QRS duration is 95 ms (Fig. 56A.1). His left ventricular ejection fraction is 40% because of a prior myocardial infarction. He has class I-II heart failure symptoms. After 14 months of atrioventricular (AV) sequential pacing (see Fig. 56A.1), the patient develops new symptoms of class III congestive heart failure. Work-up reveals no ischemia, but his ejection fraction is now 28%. Marked ventricular dyssynchrony, mild left ventricular dilatation, and new mitral regurgitation are noted on echocardiography.

DIFFERENTIAL DIAGNOSIS

The late development of heart failure in this patient should incite a search for new myocardial ischemia, worsening hypertension, new valvular disease, medical noncompliance, atrial arrhythmias, or amiodarone-induced thyroid disease. In the absence of any of these conditions, the marked dyssynchrony and mitral regurgitation on echocardiography suggest right ventricular pacing–induced left ventricular dysfunction and remodeling. The delayed time course is typical,

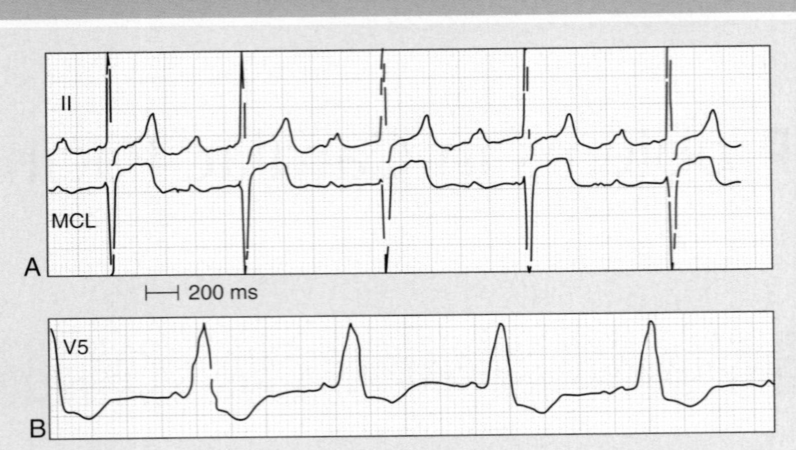

Figure 56A.1 Surface ECG with and without ventricular pacing. A, Surface electrocardiogram leads II and MCL showing sinus rhythm, P-P interval of 340 ms, and QRS duration of 95 ms. **B,** AV sequential pacing after pacemaker implantation with AV delay of 200 ms. Note the very wide paced QRS duration.

RISK FACTORS FOR RIGHT VENTRICULAR PACING–INDUCED HEART FAILURE
>40% cumulative right ventricular pacing in DDD mode
Any amount of cumulative right ventricular pacing in VVI mode
Prior myocardial infarction
Reduced left ventricular ejection fraction
Prior heart failure
Prolonged baseline QRS duration
Prolonged paced QRS duration

Table 56A.1 Risk factors for right ventricular pacing–induced heart failure.

METHODS TO REDUCE UNNECESSARY RIGHT VENTRICULAR PACING
AAI mode
Prolonged fixed AV delays
Program rate-responsive AV delay off
Program rate-responsive pacing off
Use AV search programs
Use minimal ventricular pacing algorithms
Program low lower rate limits, use hysteresis and low rate sleep functions
Other: direct His pacing or biventricular pacing at implant or revision

Table 56A.2 Methods to reduce unnecessary right ventricular pacing.

and the patient has risk factors for development of right ventricular pacing–induced heart failure, including prior ischemia, wide paced QRS, and history of reduced ejection fraction and heart failure (Table 56A.1).

TREATMENT OPTIONS

There are currently several strategies in use to minimize unnecessary right ventricular pacing in patients at risk for worsening heart failure (Table 56A.2).

For patients with sinus node dysfunction alone, AAI pacing can be considered. These patients have a low incidence of AV block (approximately 0.6% per year). For patients receiving dual-chamber systems at risk of AV block, ventricular pacing may sometimes be avoided by prolonging the AV delay. For patients with sinus node dysfunction, the intrinsic PR interval is usually less than 200 ms. In this patient, the intrinsic PR interval exceeded the maximal pacemaker AV delay, however. Inactivating rate response sensors or rate-responsive AV delays can prevent unnecessary ventricular pacing when intrinsic conduction is present.

Pacing algorithms specifically designed to minimize ventricular pacing from dual-chamber pacemakers are now available. AV search algorithms periodically prolong the AV delay during ventricular pacing, allowing intrinsic conduction to emerge if it is present (Fig. 56A.2). Failure to sense ventricular activity at the maximal AV delay results in reversion to ventricular pacing at a shorter AV delay. Some algorithms allow the device to function in AAI mode as long as a ventricular sensed event occurs within each consecutive P wave–to–P wave interval. Failure to sense ventricular activation results in ventricular pacing after the second atrial event (see Fig. 56A.2). The device reverts to DDD function if two of four consecutive cycles require ventricular pacing. Use of these algorithms can reduce ventricular pacing up to 94% and has been associated with outcomes similar to minimized VVI pacing at 40 beats per minute in the ICD patient population. These algorithms all compromise AV synchrony to reduce ventricular pacing. The relative benefits of these compromises need to be considered for each patient. For heart failure patients in whom ventricular pacing cannot be avoided or with prolonged baseline QRS durations, biventricular pacing may be a consideration. There is no consensus that any alternative site of right ventricular pacing attenuates the detrimental effects of right ventricular pacing. Finally, pure His pacing by specialized right ventricular lead positioning may result in normal paced QRS duration in the absence of distal

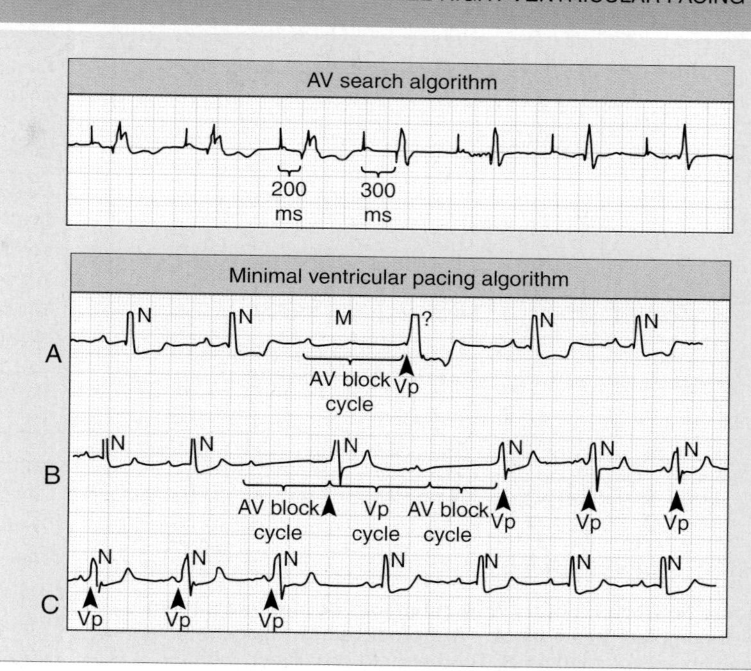

Figure 56A.2 Pacemaker algorithms to minimize right ventricular pacing. *Top panel,* AV search algorithm. On the surface electrocardiogram, the first three cardiac cycles show AV sequential pacing with AV delay of 200 ms. At a programmed interval, the AV delay is automatically extended to 300 ms for several cycles (fourth cardiac cycle). If intrinsic conduction is detected by the pacemaker, the extended AV delay is maintained. *Bottom panel,* Minimal ventricular pacing algorithm that allows switching between modified AAI and DDD modes if two of four consecutive P-P intervals do not contain a ventricular sensed event. **A,** On the surface electrocardiogram, there is sinus rhythm with a long intrinsic PR interval. The third P wave is nonconducted and results in ventricular pacing (V_P, *arrowhead*) at the end of the P-P interval without a QRS complex. **B,** Here, two of four cycles show AV block, and the device switches from AAI to DDD mode with ventricular pacing (V_P, *arrowheads*). **C,** In DDD mode, the device automatically switches back to AAI mode after the third cardiac cycle, and intrinsic conduction resumes.

conduction abnormalities. This technique has not gained widespread practice.

In this patient, echocardiography revealed resolution of ventricular dyssynchrony and mitral regurgitation during AAI pacing with intrinsic conduction. The device was reprogrammed to use a minimal ventricular pacing algorithm. After 6 months, the patient had significant improvement in heart failure symptoms, and the ejection fraction returned to 40%.

SUMMARY

Right ventricular pacing can induce ventricular dyssynchrony, abnormal left ventricular mechanical activation, and ventricular remodeling. Clinical heart failure may result, depending on the frequency of ventricular pacing, paced QRS duration, and underlying intrinsic risk of heart failure. Unnecessary right ventricular pacing can be greatly reduced by appropriate device selection and programming in most patients without advanced AV block.

b. Temporary Cardiac Pacing

Mark A. Wood

DEFINITION OF PROBLEM

Bradyarrhythmias are common in cardiac patients and the critically ill. The presentation of bradyarrhythmias is highly variable, ranging from asymptomatic to asystolic arrest. Temporary cardiac pacing may therefore be required on an elective or emergency basis. In addition, some clinical situations warrant prophylactic pacing owing to a high risk of severe bradycardia. The cardiologist must be knowledgeable about the indications for temporary cardiac pacing and possess the technical skills to initiate pacing when it is needed. In addition, from among several modalities of temporary pacing, the cardiologist must choose the one that is most appropriate for a given situation.

TYPICAL CASE

A frail 74-year-old woman with a history of hypertension presents to the emergency department with severe weakness and recurrent near-syncope for 1 week. The electrocardiogram shows complete heart block with left bundle branch escape at 42 beats per minute (Fig. 56B.1). Her blood pressure is 110/60 mm Hg, and she is without complaints while she is supine. She is scheduled for permanent pacemaker implantation later in the day and is transferred to the intensive care unit to wait. The cardiologist is consulted about the need for temporary cardiac pacing.

TREATMENT OPTIONS

Temporary cardiac pacing is indicated for sustained symptomatic or hemodynamically compromising bradyarrhythmias that are unresponsive to medical therapy. The indications for therapeutic and prophylactic temporary pacing are shown in Table 56B.1. Decisions about the mode of temporary pacing should take into consideration the urgency of the situation, the anticipated duration of temporary pacing, and the need to avoid specific complications (Table 56B.2).

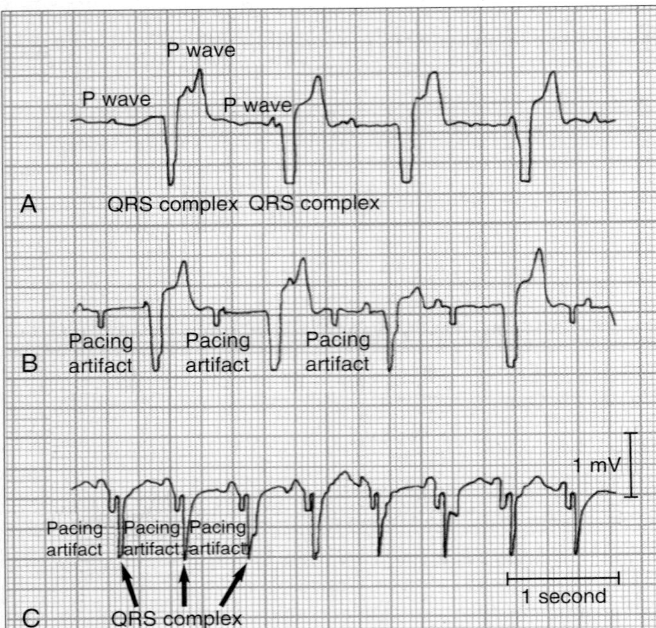

Figure 56B.1 Temporary transcutaneous pacing in a patient with complete heart block. A, Complete heart block with wide-complex escape rhythm. **B,** Subthreshold stimulation with a transcutaneous pacemaker fails to capture. **C,** A 1:1 ventricular capture with high current output. A QRS complex follows each pacing artifact. (With permission from Wood MA. Temporary cardiac pacing. In Ellenbogen KA, ed. Cardiac Pacing. © 1992, Oxford, Blackwell Scientific, 1992:162-210.)

Temporary transvenous pacing is the most robust method as it allows dual-chamber pacing and prolonged use. However, considerable operator experience is needed to initiate this mode safely. In urgent situations, temporary pacing wires can be passed blindly with balloon-tipped "floating" catheters or under electrocardiographic guidance. Fluoroscopic guidance is recommended whenever possible, however. Temporary pacemaker generators provide a full range of single-chamber (VVI, AAI) and dual-chamber (DDD, DVI) pacing modes. Contraindications to transvenous pacing include severe bleeding diathesis and mechanical tricuspid valve prosthesis. In the case of impassable tricuspid valve anatomy, ventricular capture may be achieved by pacing at high output from a lead placed in the coronary sinus. Stable temporary transvenous pacing can be achieved for periods of weeks with the use of an externalized active fixation permanent pacemaker lead connected to a permanent pacemaker generator affixed to the skin (Fig. 56B.2). Transvenous pacing through the femoral venous approach for more than 24 to 48 hours is associated with high rates of bacteremia and thrombotic phenomena even with anticoagulation.

Temporary epicardial pacing is frequently used in patients during the first few days after cardiac surgery. Pacing electrodes are fixed to the atrial and ventricular epicardial surfaces, and pacing wires are brought to the exterior through the skin. The electrodes will usually remain functional for several days. Placement of these electrodes is helpful during periods of bradycardia and for diagnosis and termination of some tachyarrhythmias that may occur during the postoperative period. Pacing thresholds usually rise by the fourth postoperative day.

INDICATIONS FOR TEMPORARY PACING
General
Medically refractory symptomatic bradyarrhythmia in the absence of contraindications
In the absence of acute myocardial infarction
Medically refractory sinus node dysfunction with symptomatic or hemodynamically compromising bradycardia
Medically refractory second- or third-degree AV block with symptoms
Third-degree AV block with wide QRS escape rhythm of ventricular response <50 bpm
In the setting of acute myocardial infarction
Medically refractory symptomatic sinus node dysfunction
Mobitz II second-degree AV block with anterior myocardial infarction
Third-degree AV block with anterior myocardial infarction
New bifascicular block
Alternating bundle branch block
Alternating Wenckebach block
New bundle branch block with anterior myocardial infarction
Bifascicular block of indeterminate age with anterior on indeterminate location
Bifascicular block and first-degree AV block
AV block (regardless of site of infarction) associated with marked bradycardia and symptoms (e.g., hypotension heart failure, low cardiac output)
Treatment of tachycardias
Termination of recurrent supraventricular tachycardias
Termination of recurrent ventricular tachycardia
Suppression of bradycardia-related ventricular tachycardia
Suppression of torsades de pointes
Prophylaxis
Swan–Ganz catheterization or right-sided heart biopsy in setting of left bundle branch block
Cardioversion in setting of sick sinus syndrome
New AV block or new bundle branch block in acute endocarditis (especially aortic valve endocarditis)
To allow pharmacologic treatment with agents that may exacerbate bradycardias (e.g., beta blockers in acute myocardial infarction or antiarrhythmic agents that suppress escape foci)

AV, atrioventricular.
From Wood MA. Temporary cardiac pacing. In Ellenbogen KA, Kay GN, Wilkoff BL, eds. Clinical Cardiac Pacing and ICDs, 4th ed. Philadelphia, WB Saunders, 2004:163-195.

Table 56B.1 Indications for temporary pacing.

Transcutaneous external pacing provides noninvasive cardiac stimulation by means of a specialized generator and self-adhesive patch electrodes adherent to the chest. This technique is extremely safe and rapid but produces ventricular capture in only about 60% to 80% of patients. Although it is very useful for prophylactic indications, the pain of

COMPARISON OF TEMPORARY PACING MODES				
Pacing mode	**Speed to Initiate**	**Advantages**	**Disadvantages**	**Uses**
Transcutaneous	Fastest	Fastest, simplest, and safest mode Minimal training required	Varaible capture Painful Ventricular pacing only	Cardiac arrest Prophylactic Long-term intermittent pacing
Transvenous	Slow	Most reliable Best long term Allows atrioventricular synchronous pacing	Invasive Slow to initiate Complications Most operator experience required	Cardiac arrest Prophylaxis Best for long-term continuous pacing
Epicardial (post–cardiac surgery)	Fast	Fast Allows atrioventricular synchronous pacing Does not require venous access	Thresholds deteriorate within days Available only postoperatively	Cardiac arrest Prophylactic Intermediate-term pacing (days)
Transesophageal	Slow	Safe Relatively simple Allows atrial pacing and recording	Ventricular capture rare Painful	Diagnostic recordings Atrial pacing (usually intraoperatively)

Table 56B.2 Comparison of temporary pacing modes.

transcutaneous stimulation makes it unsuitable for continuous pacing. Transcutaneous pacing can be initiated safely by personnel with a minimum of training while more definitive measures are awaited. Complications resulting from transcutaneous pacing are exceptionally rare. The large pacing artifact from transcutaneous pacing obscures ancillary electrocardiographic monitors. The electrocardiogram display of the pulse generator is heavily filtered and should be observed. Confirmation of capture by palpation of a peripheral pulse is also necessary.

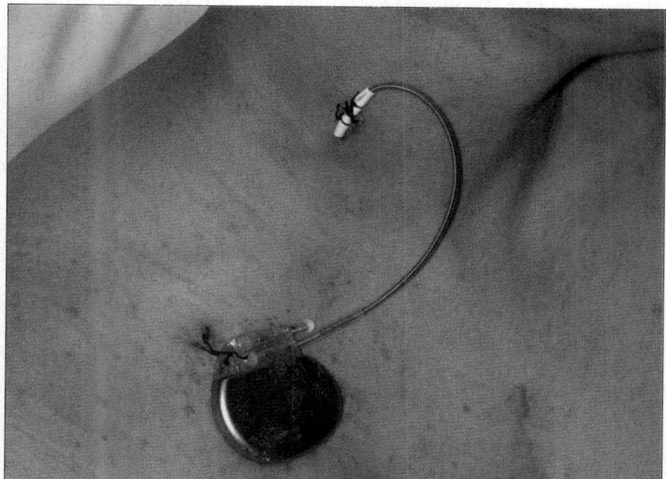

Figure 56B.2 Externalized "permanent" pacing system suitable for long-term temporary pacing. This system was used for 6 weeks during antibiotic therapy in a man with heart block after removal of an infected pacemaker system. The active fixation lead provides chronic stability.

Transesophageal pacing requires a specialized high-output generator and flexible dedicated transesophageal pacing catheter. This method consistently provides atrial pacing, but ventricular capture is rare. It is most commonly used to support atrial pacing or to terminate supraventricular tachycardias intraoperatively.

In this case, the patient was hemodynamically stable, and her advanced age made invasive procedures for short-term temporary pacing unattractive. Her slow wide-complex escape rhythm was an indication for temporary pacing, however. She had transcutaneous pacing patches applied prophylactically while awaiting permanent pacemaker implantation (see Fig. 56B.1). The temporary pacing rate was set below the patient's intrinsic rate of 42 beats per minute. This was done to protect the patient if her escape rhythm should abruptly deteriorate without subjecting her to the discomfort of transcutaneous pacing continuously. If continuous temporary pacing had been required, a transvenous electrode would have been preferred.

SUMMARY

The indications for temporary cardiac pacing are many but must be familiar to the practicing cardiologist. Both therapeutic and prophylactic indications exist. A variety of temporary pacing modes are available for use in different situations. Clinically, transvenous pacing and transcutaneous pacing have the greatest utility. Transcutaneous pacing is appropriate for prophylactic uses, given its safety and noninvasive implementation. Its speed makes it useful for emergency situations as well. Transvenous pacing can be used for any indication if the risk of bleeding complications and time for implementation are acceptable.

c. Diagnostic and Surgical Procedures in Patients with Pacemakers and Implantable Cardioverter-Defibrillators

Mark A. Wood

DEFINITION OF PROBLEM

The hospital setting can present a hostile electrical environment for permanent pacemakers and implantable cardioverter-defibrillators (ICDs). An assortment of medical equipment can interfere with device function and even cause permanent damage to the pacing system. Diagnostic and therapeutic equipment can affect implanted devices through electromagnetic interference (e.g., electrocautery, magnetic resonance imaging), high electrical current pulses (e.g., direct current cardioversion), or physical forces exerted on the generator (e.g., lithotripsy, radiation therapy). The recognition of potential procedure-related pacemaker problems falls to the cardiologist as part of the preoperative assessment.

TYPICAL CASE

A 64-year-old man with a permanent DDD pacemaker for high-grade heart block undergoes emergency surgical repair of a leaking abdominal aortic aneurysm. Preoperative pacemaker interrogation is not performed because of the urgency of the situation. During the surgery, asystole occurs repeatedly during electrosurgical cautery (Fig. 56C.1). In the recovery area, the pacemaker is noted to be pacing in VVI mode at a rate that is 10 beats per minute slower than the lower rate limit documented in clinic records. A consultation is requested for "pacemaker malfunction."

DIFFERENTIAL DIAGNOSIS

Figure 56C.1 demonstrates pacemaker inhibition by electromagnetic interference from the electrosurgical cautery. Pacemakers may sense the current of the cautery as QRS complexes and be inhibited. Sustained high-frequency electrical noise may trigger asynchronous pacing as a safety feature. Electromagnetic interference may also trigger inappropriate shocks in patients with implantable defibrillators. High-current exposure may cause reversion to a "reset" mode stored in nonvolatile electrical memory.

Reversion to reset mode was the reason for the slower pacing rate after surgery in this case. The features of the reset mode vary among different pacemaker models. Dual-chamber devices may revert to VVI or VOO modes. A change to unipolar output is a common safety feature. In most situations in which reset has occurred, normal pacemaker operation can be reprogrammed. However, in pacemakers with low battery voltages that are at or near elective replacement times, an attempt to revert to reset mode in response to electromagnetic interference may cause complete output failure from the device. Lithotripsy equipment, mechanical ventilation equipment, magnetic resonance imaging equipment, and dental equipment may trigger pacing at higher rates as a result of effects on rate-responsive pacemakers magnetic resonance imaging equipment may damage pacemaker/defibrilator generators and/or leads. All of these behaviors must be differentiated from preoperative pacer malfunction and intraprocedural damage to the pacing system.

TREATMENT OPTIONS

Periprocedural management of patients with pacemakers requires preoperative evaluation of the pacing system, appropriate intraoperative measures, and postoperative confirmation of the integrity of the pacing system.

Preoperatively, the pacemaker should be identified and interrogated, and a complete check of thresholds, battery status, and lead status should be performed. Before exposure to electrocautery, pacemaker-dependent patients should be reprogrammed to asynchronous (VOO) modes to prevent asystole. Pacemaker-dependent patients with pulse generators that are at or near the end of their battery life should receive temporary pacing wires. The use of triggered modes (VVT) can prevent pacemaker competition with the intrinsic rhythm in non–pacemaker-dependent patients.

Intraoperatively, a magnet can be applied to the pacemaker as needed to prevent inhibition during cautery. This maneuver would have been useful in this case because no time was available to reprogram the pacemaker preoperatively. Magnet application can inhibit antitachycardia therapies from ICDs but does not produce asynchronous (VOO or DOO) pacing. External surface electrodes for electrocautery should be placed as far from the pacemaker as possible. The use of bipolar cautery in short bursts can reduce the potential for interference. For defibrillation or direct current cardioversion in the patient with a pacemaker, the paddles (or patches) should be positioned more than 10 cm from the pulse generator (Fig. 56C.2). The device should be reinterrogated after conversion to exclude pacemaker reset or elevation in the pacing thresholds. Rate response functions should be inactivated before mechanical ventilation, external counterpulsation, and lithotripsy. Lithotripsy should be performed with caution in patients with abdominal pulse generators that will be submerged in a water tank. When the generator is submerged, the transmitted shock wave can damage components of the pulse generator.

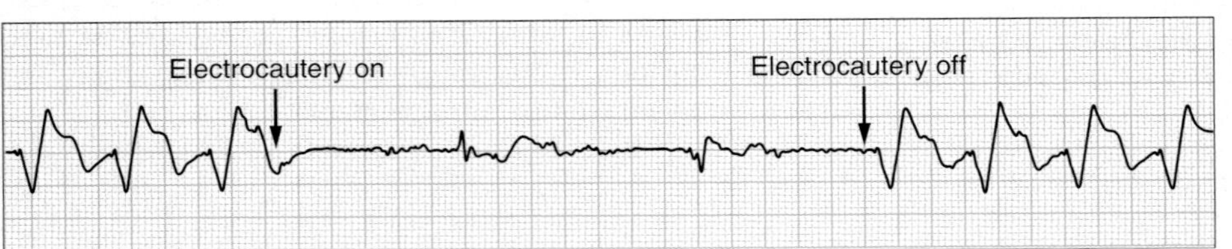

Figure 56C.1 Intraoperative electrocardiographic monitor tracing. This tracing shows ventricular tracking of sinus rhythm by a DDD pacemaker for the first three complexes. Electrocautery produces 4 seconds of asystole, after which pacing resumes.

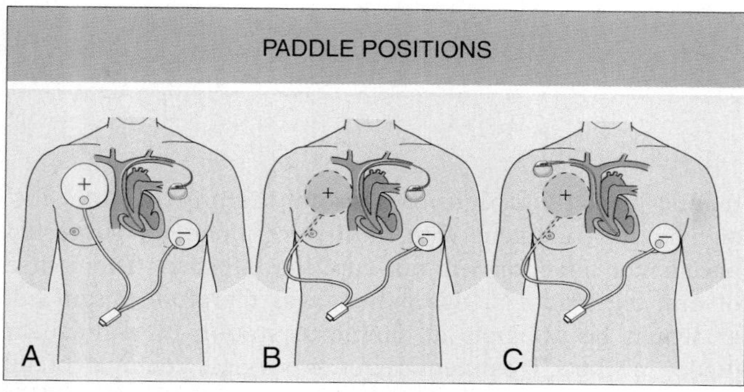

Figure 56C.2 Paddle positions for cardioversion of the pacemaker patient. **A,** For hand-held paddles, the apex-anterior position is used. **B,** For self-adhesive defibrillation patches, the apex-posterior position can be used. **C,** The apex-posterior position is preferred for patients with right-sided pacemaker implants. The defibrillation electrodes should always be more than 10 cm from the pacemaker.

Magnetic resonance imaging is generally avoided entirely in patients with pacemakers and ICDs, but this prohibition has been challenged by some centers studying highly selected patients, device systems, and scanning sequences. The safety of magnetic resonance imaging in device patients remains controversial, and no pacemaker or ICD system is approved for magnetic resonance imaging compatibility by the manufacturer or the Food and Drug Administration. Because magnetic resonance imaging can damage or reprogram pacemakers or cause current induction in the leads, reprogramming before the procedure does not preclude problems. Therapeutic irradiation for breast or lung cancer may damage pacemaker circuitry, and the device should be shielded if possible. Devices that cannot be excluded from the radiation field may need to be surgically relocated. Diathermy can cause pacemaker interference or even thermal damage if energy is applied over the pacemaker. Pacemaker interference from transcutaneous electrical nerve–stimulating units or electroconvulsive therapy is rare and does not routinely require protective measures.

SUMMARY

The vast arrays of therapeutic and diagnostic medical equipment in the modern hospital can cause transient or permanent pacemaker dysfunction. Physicians should be aware of the types of problems that may occur and of appropriate measures for prevention and correction (Table 56C.1). The most common interaction between pacemakers and equipment is inhibition from sources of electromagnetic interference, such as electrocautery. Fortunately, preprocedural reprogramming or judicious application of a magnet during the procedure can overcome most interactions with this source.

PERIPROCEDURAL DEVICE PROBLEMS AND SOLUTIONS

Procedure	Source of Interference	Effect on Pacemaker	Preventive Measures
Electrocautery	Electromagnetic interference	Inhibition	Reprogram to VOO or WT
	Electric current	Asynchronous pacing	Magnet application (VOO)
		Reset mode or reprogramming	Bipolar cautery in short bursts
		Circuitry and lead damage	Cautery at distance from pacemaker
Direct current cardioversion or defibrillation	Intense electric current	Reset mode	Paddle placement >10 cm from pacemaker
		Loss of capture	Anterior–posterior current path
		Circuitry or lead damage	
Magnetic responance imaging	Radiofrequency energy	Asynchronous pacing	Avoidance of magnetic resonance imaging
	Magnetic field	Reset mode	
	Current induction	Rapid pacing	
		Generator malfunction	
Lithotripsy	Hydraulic shock wave	Asynchronous pacing or inhibition	Shock synchronous to R wave
		Activation of rate response feature	Disable rate response
		Generator damage	Do not submerge generator in tank
Diathermy	Electromagnetic interference	Inhibition	Reprogram to VOO or WT
	Thermal energy	Loss of capture	Apply at distance from pacemaker
		Reset mode	
Radiofrequency catheter ablation	Electromagnetic interference	Inhibition	Deliver energy >4 cm from pacing lead electrodes
	Electric current	Loss of capture	Reprogram to VOO
		Reset mode	
Radiation therapy	Ionizing radiation	Generator component failure	Shield pacemaker
		Loss of capture	Follow dosimetry
			Frequent pacemaker follow-up

Table 56C.1 Periprocedural device problems and solutions.

d. Lead Extraction

Mark A. Wood

DEFINITION OF PROBLEM

Device- and lead-related complications may require removal (extraction) of pacing or defibrillator leads. The development of percutaneous lead extraction techniques with over-the-lead telescoping sheath systems has obviated the need for a surgical approach in most patients. This has reduced procedural morbidity and expanded the indications for extraction. The cardiologist should recognize situations that are appropriate for lead extraction and be aware of the potential risks of the procedure to make sound decisions about this procedure for the individual patient.

TYPICAL CASE

A 58-year-old woman with heart block, heart failure, and ventricular tachycardia undergoes an implantable cardioverter-defibrillator (ICD) generator change for battery depletion. She has atrial, right ventricular, and transcoronary sinus left ventricular leads associated with her biventricular ICD system as well as two abandoned leads from a previous pacemaker system. The leads range in age from 4 to 15 years (Fig. 56D.1). Two weeks after the generator change, she develops pain and inflammation at the pacemaker site. She is treated with oral antibiotics by her local physician but develops purulent drainage from the generator site. She is referred to the implanting physician. Blood cultures are negative.

DIFFERENTIAL DIAGNOSIS

The patient has an ICD pocket infection resulting from contamination at the time of her generator change. *Staphylococcus* species are the most common pathogens in surgically related pocket infections. Because of the presence of a foreign body, treatment with antibiotics alone for suspected pacemaker infection will not cure the infection. The course of oral antibiotics in this patient was therefore misguided, as would be attempts at simple aspiration of a fluctuant device pocket. Treatment requires surgical removal of all foreign bodies associated with the pacemaker system. This includes complete removal of all leads associated with the pocket because all must be considered contaminated. Simply cutting the leads in the pocket is associated with high rates of infection recurrence.

TREATMENT OPTIONS

The indications for pacemaker lead extraction are shown in Table 56D.1. Sepsis, endocarditis, and recurrent bacteremias involving ICD or pacemaker leads are life-threatening conditions and mandate lead removal. Extensive scarring of chronic leads to the vasculature and endocardium prevents lead removal by simple traction. Percutaneous lead removal by use of a telescoping laser or electrocautery sheath system over the lead is the treatment of choice (Fig. 56D.2). The end-firing laser or electrocautery energy emitted from the perimeter of the smaller inner sheath lyses adhesions along the course of the lead. A larger outer sheath passed over the inner sheath to the lead tip provides countertraction against the heart to prevent tearing of the myocardium by tension on the lead. A sheath system for snaring and removal of leads from the femoral approach is also available.

Before lead extraction, it is recommended that a transesophageal echocardiogram be obtained in bacteremic patients to exclude valvular endocarditis and large vegetations on the

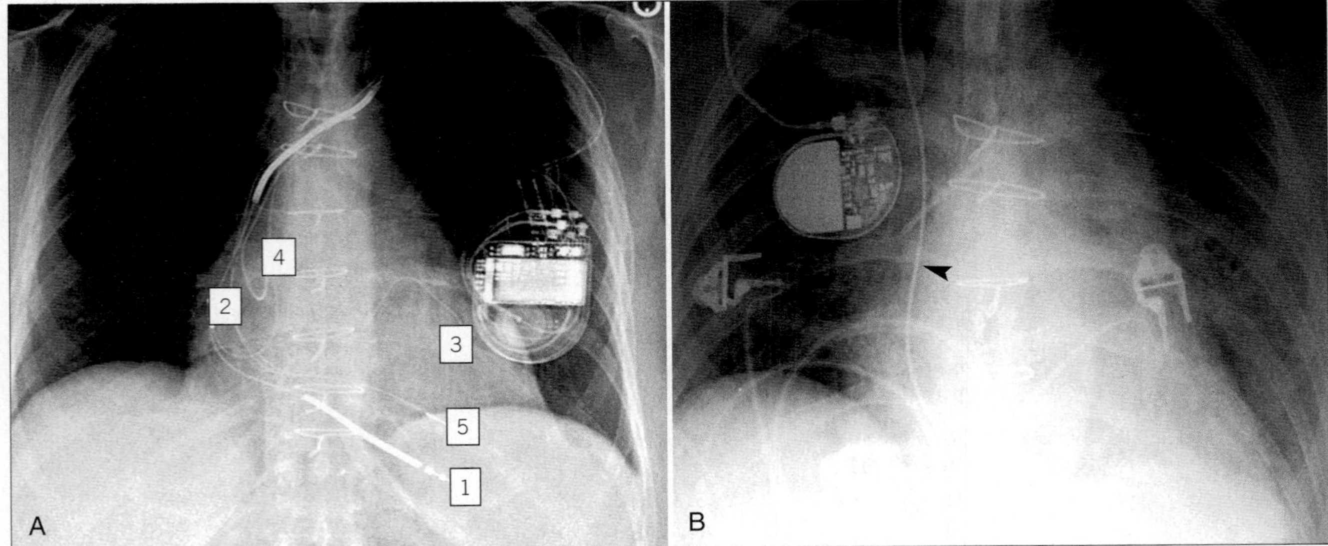

Figure 56D.1 **A,** Anteroposterior chest radiograph showing five leads before lead extraction: 1, right ventricular ICD lead; 2, right atrial lead; 3, left ventricular coronary sinus lead; 4, abandoned right atrial lead; 5, abandoned right ventricular lead. **B,** After extraction, a single transvenous temporary pacing lead is maintained through the right internal jugular vein connected to an externalized permanent pacemaker generator.

INDICATIONS FOR PACEMAKER AND IMPLANTABLE CARDIOVERTER-DEFIBRILLATOR LEAD EXTRACTION
Mandatory
Sepsis
Endocarditis
Lead migration with perforation or arrhythmias
Necessary
Pocket infection
Erosion
Device interaction
Lead replacement in thrombosed vein
Optional
Pain
Abandoned leads

Table 56D.1 Indications for pacemaker and implantable cardioverter-defibrillator lead extraction.

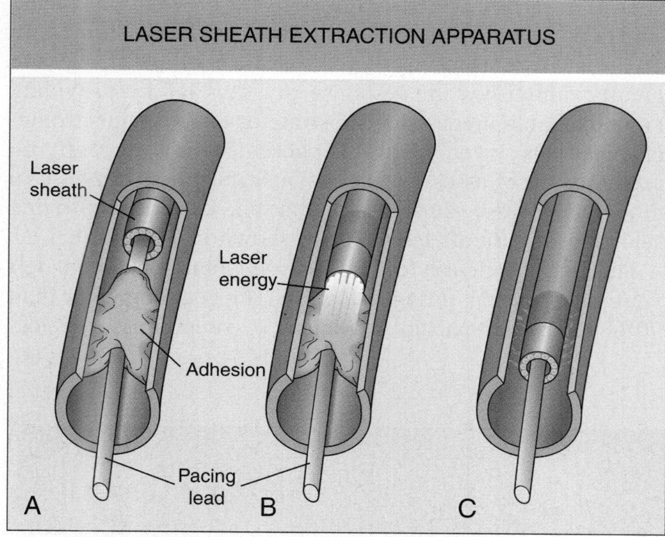

Figure 56D.2 Laser sheath extraction apparatus. A, The inner laser sheath of the telescoping sheath system is advanced over the lead until vascular adhesions are encountered. **B,** Laser energy emitted from the perimeter of the sheath lyses the fibrous tissue making up the adhesion. **C,** Once the adhesion is eliminated, the site of the adhesion is crossed. This process is repeated until the larger outer sheath can be advanced to the lead tip to apply countertraction against the myocardium. Without this countertraction, the wall of the heart could invert or tear under the pull of the lead that is required to dislodge the tip from the myocardium.

leads that might cause septic pulmonary emboli if they are dislodged by the sheaths. For infected leads that cannot be extracted with the sheath apparatus, surgical removal is necessary. The sheath systems can recanalize thrombosed veins and so provide venous access in an otherwise occluded vessel.

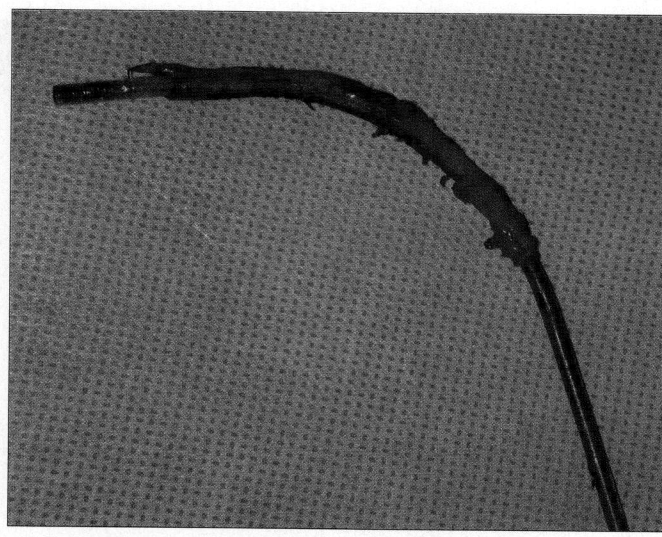

Figure 56D.3 Heavy fibrous ingrowth into the high-voltage coil of an extracted ICD lead.

The reduced morbidity of percutaneous lead extraction has led to elective indications for explantation, such as removal rather than abandonment of leads in young patients and lead removal to “debulk” the venous system.

Lead extraction is a potentially dangerous procedure that must be performed only by those experienced with this technique. Life-threatening complications occur in 2% of cases, including death in approximately 0.4%, hemopericardium, hemothorax, and pulmonary embolism.

The success rate for complete lead extraction is inversely related to the implant duration of the lead. Extraction is successful in 96% of cases when the leads are less than 1 year old but in only 72% of cases when the leads are older than 8 years. Success rates are also lower for ventricular leads, for passive fixation leads, and in the hands of inexperienced operators. Complications are more likely in women, in leads with longer implant duration, with inexperienced operators, and when calcification of the leads has occurred. Tissue ingrowth into the coils of ICD leads also renders these more prone than pacing leads to complications (Fig. 56D.3).

This patient underwent successful laser sheath extraction of all five leads (see Fig. 56D-1). A temporary externalized pacemaker system was used for 2 weeks during continued antibiotic therapy before a new device was implanted.

SUMMARY

Percutaneous extraction is the method of choice for removal of pacemaker or ICD leads. The indications for extraction include elective removal of abandoned leads and recanalization of thrombosed subclavian veins. Despite the technical advances with lead extraction, the possibility of life-threatening complications demands thoughtful consideration of the risks and benefits in each patient.

e. Failure of Resynchronization Therapy

Mark A. Wood

DEFINITION OF PROBLEM

Cardiac resynchronization therapy (CRT) is an established adjunct to medical therapy in selected patients with systolic heart failure. Benefits may include symptomatic relief, improved functional capacity, survival benefit, and beneficial cardiac structural remodeling. Nevertheless, up to 30% of patients may fail to respond. The causes of failure to respond to CRT are many and require a systematic approach to be remedied.

TYPICAL CASE

A 68-year-old woman with nonischemic cardiomyopathy (ejection fraction, 20%), QRS duration of 155 ms, and class III heart failure undergoes implantation of a CRT implantable cardioverter-defibrillator (ICD). Prehospital discharge evaluation shows satisfactory thresholds and a posterolateral coronary sinus lead position (Fig. 56E.1). During 3 months of follow-up, her ICD thresholds remain stable; however, she reports no clinical improvement in her condition. She is referred for further evaluation.

DIFFERENTIAL DIAGNOSIS

Failure to respond to CRT can be attributable to three general causes: shortcomings in selection of patients, problematic lead position, and failure to consistently pace the left ventricle. The therapeutic basis for CRT is the electrical and mechanical preexcitation of late activating left ventricular wall segments that, uncorrected, lead to inefficient ventricular contraction patterns. In the absence of ventricular dyssynchrony, CRT is not expected to be beneficial. Current guidelines include only QRS duration as a surrogate indicator for dyssynchrony; however, multiple studies have demonstrated this association to be weak. Those with QRS duration below 150 ms or with right bundle branch block appear to have lower response rates. The usefulness of echocardiographic measures to identify responders to CRT could not be confirmed under critical study.

After the best selection of patients, the next challenge to CRT is optimal left ventricular lead placement. Even among patients with typical left bundle branch block on electrocardiography, the sites of maximal electromechanical wall motion delays may vary widely, and current techniques empirically target the posterior-lateral left ventricle for lead placement. Problems arise when there are no coronary venous branches overlying this segment or when the pacing site does not correspond to the site of dyssynchrony. In addition, extensive myocardial scar at the pacing site greatly diminishes the response rate to CRT by providing an unexcitable myocardial substrate or one with electromechanical delay even when it is paced. There is currently no ready means of assessing the resynchronization response to any lead position during implantation. Criteria improving selection of patients for CRT are shown in Table 56E.1.

The final challenge to CRT is to maintain consistent left ventricular pacing during follow-up. The goal of greater than 90% ventricular pacing is frequently compromised by loss

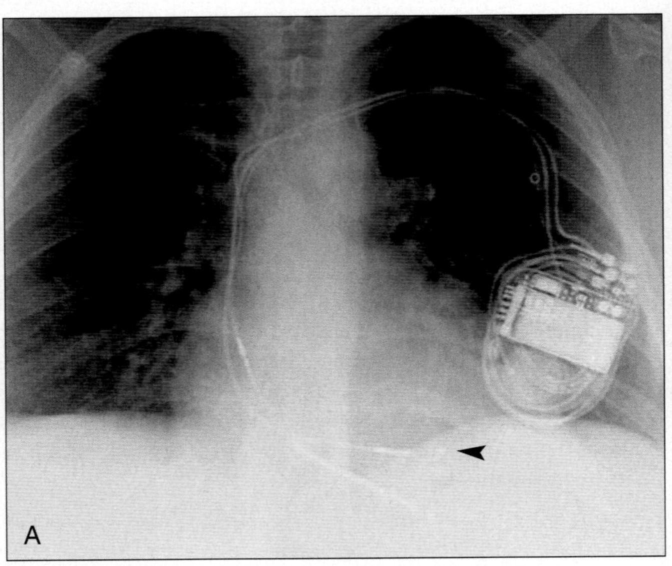

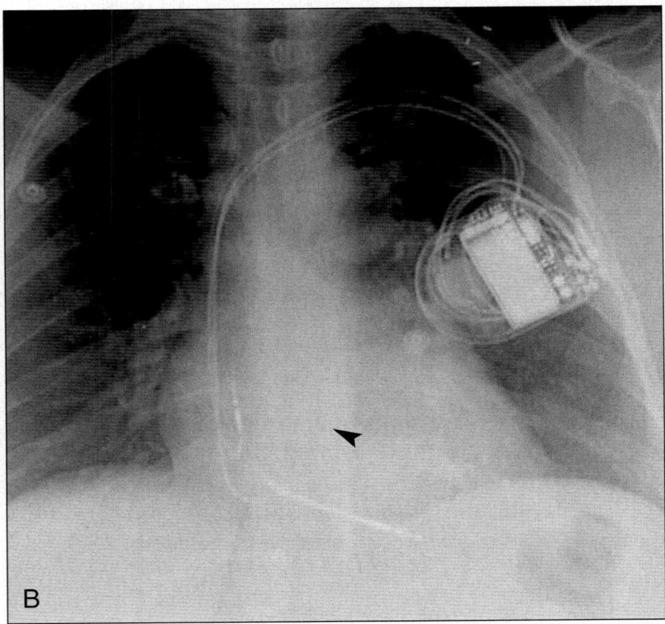

Figure 56E.1 A, Anteroposterior chest radiograph showing coronary sinus left ventricular lead position *(arrowhead)* after ICD implantation. **B,** Anteroposterior chest radiograph showing dislodgement of the coronary sinus lead to the base of the left ventricle *(arrowhead)* during follow-up.

PREDICTORS OF RESPONSE TO RESYNCHRONIZATION THERAPY		
	Response More Likely	**Response Less Likely**
QRS duration	>150 ms	<150 ms
Heart disease	Nonischemic	Ischemic
Functional class	III-IV	II
Interventricular conduction delay	Left bundle branch block	Right bundle branch block
Lead position	Posterior-lateral	Anterior or inferior
Scar burden (magnetic resonance imaging or perfusion imaging)	Low burden Nontransmural Posterolateral segments spared	High burden Transmural Posterolateral segments involved

Table 56E.1 Predictors of response to resynchronization therapy.

of ventricular capture, lead dislodgement, painful phrenic nerve stimulation, atrial fibrillation with rapid ventricular response, or issues related to device programming.

TREATMENT OPTIONS

A systematic approach to the failure to respond to CRT is given in Figure 56E.2. Not uncommonly after implantation, there is loss of ventricular pacing from elevated thresholds or lead dislodgement. Left ventricular capture can usually be accurately diagnosed by the presence of a Qr or qR complex in leads I and aVL and a prominent R wave in V_1 (Fig. 56E.3). Loss of the q or Q wave in lead I is highly predictive of loss of left ventricular capture. Capture can be confirmed by use of the device programmer and the data log interrogated for the percentage of paced and sensed ventricular complexes. Atrial fibrillation and loss of atrial tracking are common causes of loss of left ventricular pacing despite adequate thresholds. Once consistent left ventricular pacing is confirmed, assessment for non–device-related problems, such as hypervolemia or hypovolemia, ischemia, and medical noncompliance, is often warranted. If no medical issues are identified, optimization of the device programming is indicated. This involves programming the atrioventricular delay and timing of right and left ventricular stimulation (usually under echocardiographic guidance) to optimize ventricular filling patterns, to reduce mitral regurgitation, and to maximize cardiac output. Finally, failure to respond to all of these measures should lead to re-assessment of the left ventricular lead position. Lead revision may be necessary either by the transvenous approach or by surgical placement of an epicardial lead if transvenous pacing has failed.

In this case, the pacing thresholds remained stable, but chest radiography revealed dislodgement of the left ventricular lead to the base of the heart and presumably removed from the area of dyssynchrony (see Fig. 56E.1). The patient underwent revision of the lead to its original location with significant improvement in functional capacity.

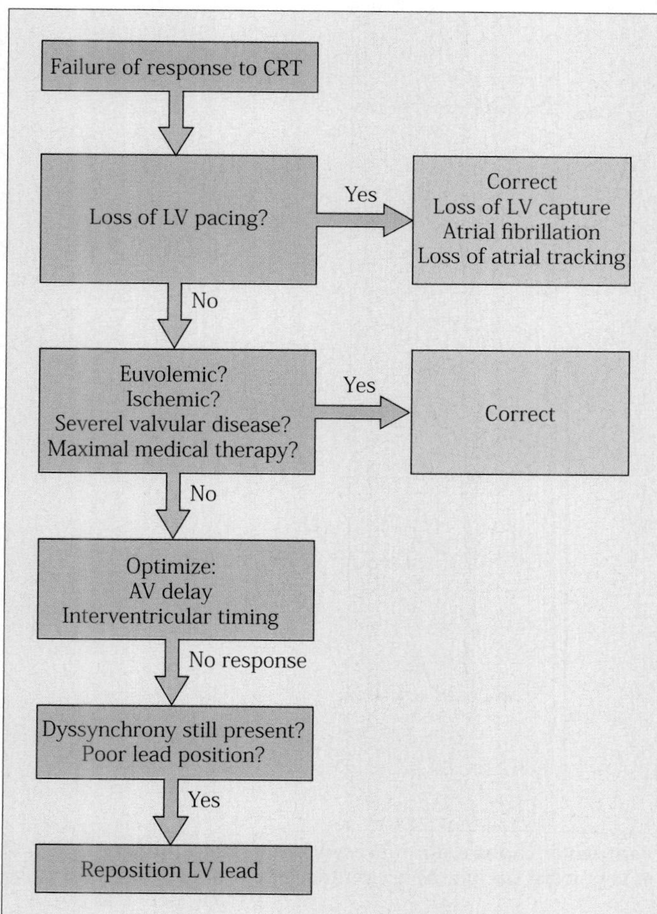

Figure 56E.2 Schematic for systematic evaluation of failure to respond to cardiac resynchronization therapy. AV, atrioventricular; LV, left ventricular.

SUMMARY

CRT is a valuable adjunctive therapy to select patients with congestive heart failure. Response to CRT requires appropriate selection of patients, appropriate lead placement, and attention to device programming.

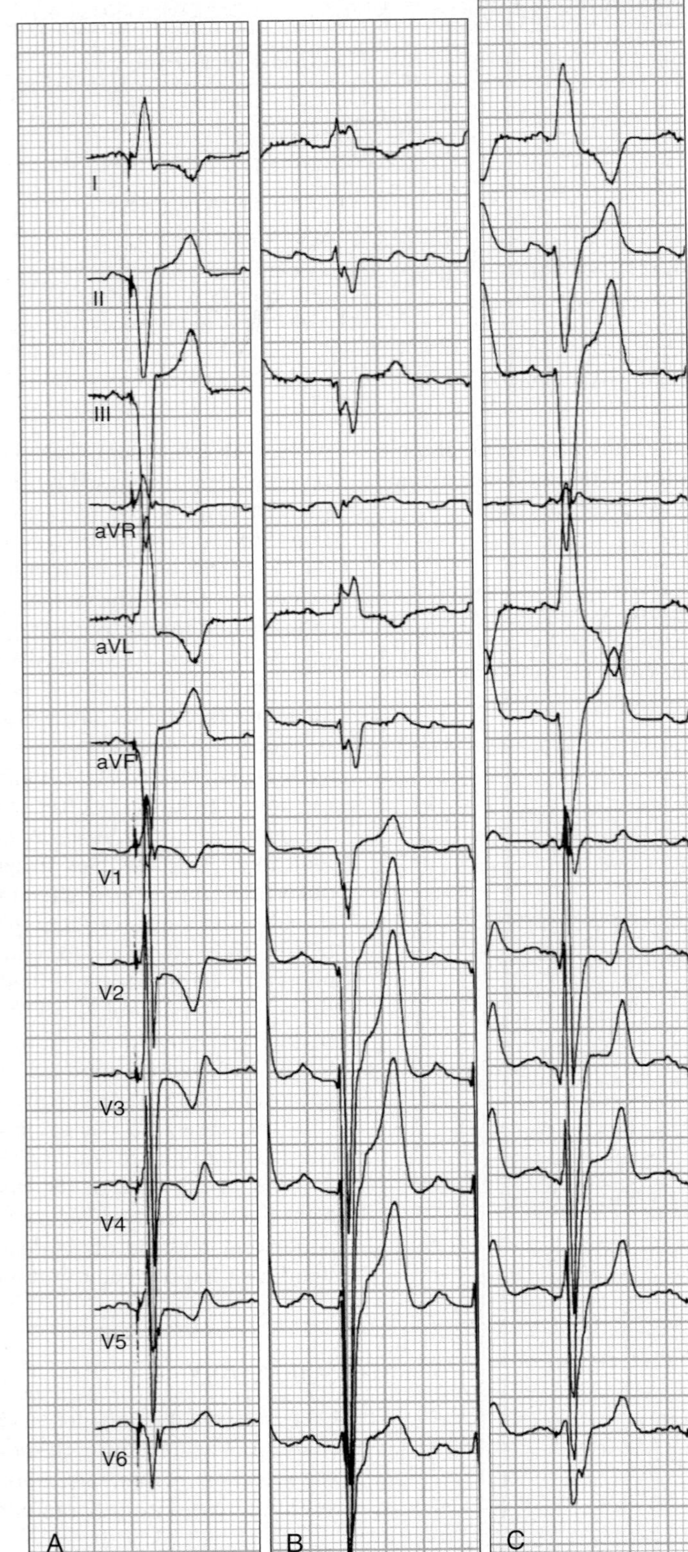

Figure 56E.3 Surface electrocardiogram leads useful to confirm left ventricular capture during resynchronization therapy. The absence of Q waves in leads I and aVL is very suggestive of loss of left ventricular pacing. **A,** left ventricular pacing; **B,** right ventricular pacing; **C,** intrinsic conduction.

chapter 57

Supraventricular Tachycardia

Carlos A. Morillo

Definition

- Supraventricular tachycardia is any tachycardia that originates in the atria or that uses the atrium or atrioventricular junction and that requires the participation of tissue above the bifurcation of the bundle of His for propagation as a critical component of the tachycardia circuit.

Key Features

- Atrioventricular nodal re-entrant tachycardia and atrioventricular reciprocating tachycardia are usually manifested in younger patients who do not have structural heart disease.
- Atrial tachycardias, atrial fibrillation, and atrial flutter are frequently associated with structural heart disease or pulmonary disease. Electrocardiographic features are helpful in establishing origin of tachycardia.

Therapy

- The severity and frequency of symptoms determine therapy of choice.
- Pharmacologic therapy is a good option, although recurrence rates may be high.
- Radiofrequency ablation has been proved to be a safe and a highly curative procedure, approaching success rates near 95% for most supraventricular tachycardias.

Supraventricular tachycardia (SVT) occurs in all age groups and is associated with varying causes, heart rates, and frequency and severity of heart disease. Recent population-based studies have reported a prevalence of 2.25 per 1000 persons and an incidence of 35 per 100,000 person-years. In the United States, there are approximately 89,000 new cases of SVT each year and 570,000 people with SVT at any time.[1] The potential for the development of tachycardia-induced cardiomyopathy resulting from uncontrolled SVT highlights the importance of prompt and appropriate therapy. Current management includes pharmacologic control and elimination of the arrhythmogenic substrate by catheter-guided radiofrequency ablation.

ANATOMY AND PATHOLOGY

The conduction system is composed of a fine network of modified cardiac cells that are related to the origin and transmission of the cardiac impulse. The anatomic substrate of the arrhythmia determines the type of tachycardia. SVT originating near the sinus node area, such as sinus node re-entry or inappropriate sinus tachycardia, is related to the anatomic structures near the sinus node and is influenced by autonomic tone modulation. The sinus node is located subepicardially in the terminal groove formed by the lateral junction of the superior vena cava and the right atrium. Experimental studies in canine and human atria have demonstrated that there are variable sites of origin of earliest activation, dependent largely on baseline heart rate and autonomic tone.[2] Appropriate balance between impulse formation and autonomic tone may be critical in the initiation and maintenance of rhythm disorders that originate near the sinus node, such as inappropriate sinus tachycardia (see Chapter 53).[3,4]

The role of the specialized conduction tissue within the atrial tissue between the sinus node and the atrioventricular (AV) node has been contested. It is clear that there are no insulated tracts in the atria that resemble structures such as the proximal His-Purkinje system. However, conduction preferentially proceeds through the major muscle bundles, namely, the crista terminalis, delimiting the junction between the smooth posterior wall and the trabeculated anterior wall, and the anterior lip of the fossa ovalis.[5,6]

The compact AV node is located in the lower part of the right atrium within the triangle of Koch (Fig. 57.1). The anatomic boundaries of the triangle of Koch are delineated by the tendon of Todaro (a fibrous extension of the eustachian valve), the septal leaflet of the tricuspid valve, and the coronary sinus ostium.

The bundle of His is the direct continuation of the AV node. It crosses through the central fibrous body into the posteroinferior portion of the membranous septum. Three distinct histologic cell types—atrionodal cells, nodal cells, and nodal-His cells—constitute the AV node. The exact anatomic correlates of dual AV nodal conduction are still under investigation. Anatomic, histologic, and electrophysiologic correlates have recently been documented in AV nodal re-entrant tachycardia (AVNRT).[7-10]

Since the early 1900s, several investigators have documented the existence of posterior inputs into the AV node. In the 1960s, James[11,12] and Truex and Smythe[13] provided the basis for the current understanding of the AV node. They suggested that the AV junctional area is divided into three regions:

- the compact AV node, located in the anterosuperior atrial septum; and
- two nodal pathways, the anterosuperior (fast) pathway, located in the anterior interatrial septum, and the posteroinferior (slow) pathway, originating near the ostium of the coronary sinus.

The mechanism and structural basis of AVNRT are depicted in Figure 57.2. Dual AV node physiology, characterized by longitudinal dissociation of AV node conduction, plays an

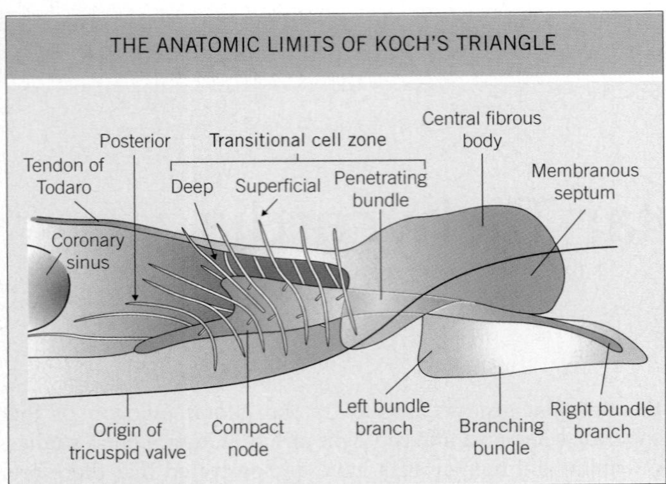

Figure 57.1 The anatomic limits of Koch's triangle. (From Becker AE, Anderson RH. Morphology of the human atrioventricular junctional area. In Wellens HH, Lie KL, Janse MJ, eds. The Conduction System of the Heart. Leiden, Stenfert Kroese, 1976:263-286. © 1976 Stenfert Kroese, Leiden.)

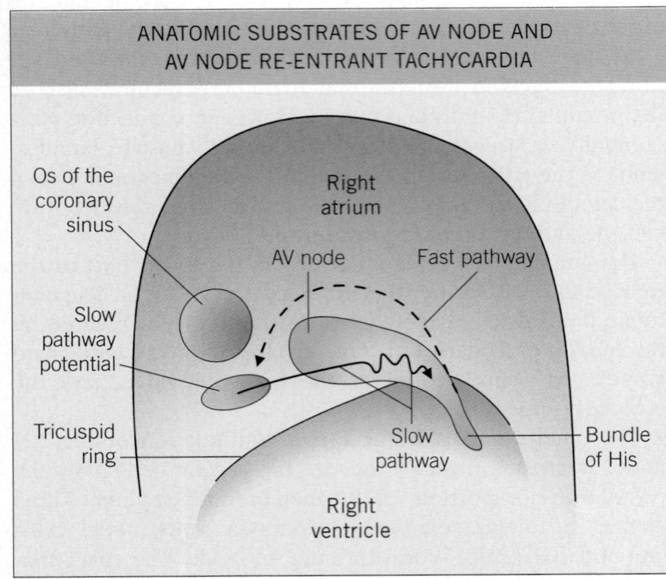

Figure 57.2 Anatomic substrates of AV node and AV node re-entrant tachycardia.

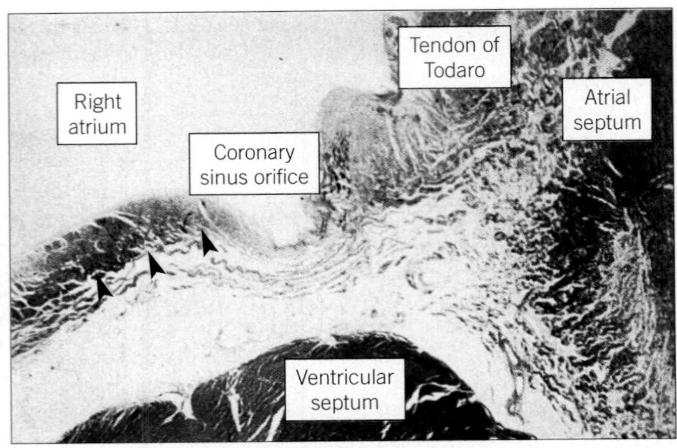

Figure 57.3 Right-sided posteroinferior connections to the coronary sinus. Arrowheads indicate intact right-sided posterior approaches to the AV node inferior to the coronary sinus orifice. Histologic evidence obtained from a canine experimental preparation. (From McGuire MA, Robotin M, Yip ASB, et al. Electrophysiologic and histologic effects of dissection of the connections between the atrium and posterior part of the atrioventricular node. J Am Coll Cardiol 1994;23:693-701. Reprinted with permission from the American College of Cardiology.)

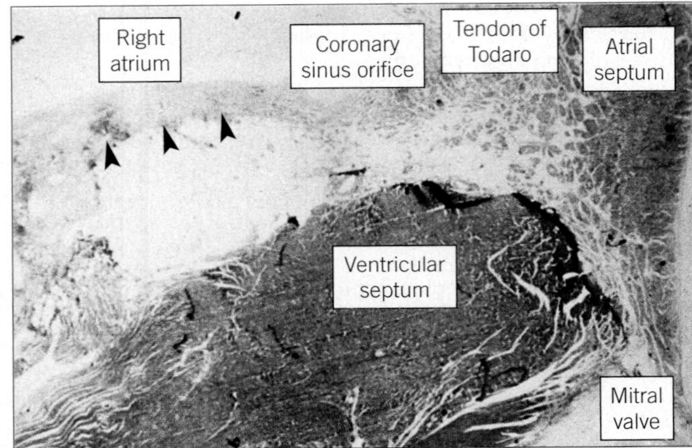

Figure 57.4 Fibrosis of the posteroinferior atrionodal connections. Histologic evidence after dissection of the area shown in Figure 57.3. The right-sided posterior connections to the AV node *(arrowheads)* have been replaced by fibrous tissue. (From McGuire MA, Robotin M, Yip ASB, et al. Electrophysiologic and histologic effects of dissection of the connections between the atrium and posterior part of the atrioventricular node. J Am Coll Cardiol 1994;23:693-701. Reprinted with permission from the American College of Cardiology.)

important role in the genesis of AVNRT. However, the lack of documented dual-pathway physiology does not preclude inducing AVNRT. The role of the slow and fast pathways is undisputed in the generation of AVNRT. However, the exact anatomic and electrophysiologic correlation of these pathways is controversial.[5] McGuire and colleagues[14-16] have clearly established the nature of the posterior and anterior inputs of the AV node in a series of elegant experimental preparations (Figs. 57.3 and 57.4). This gives rise to the typical or " common" type of AVNRT, which is characterized by anterograde conduction over the slow pathway with retrograde conduction over the fast pathway. It remains unclear whether these structures are actually single fibers or bundles of fibers that traverse the anterior and posterior inputs of the AV node. In contrast, the atypical or "uncommon" type of AVNRT uses the fast pathway for anterograde conduction and the slow pathway for retrograde conduction. Other varieties of AVNRT include retrograde conduction over the slow pathway in the so-called slow-slow type of AVNRT.[17-20]

SVTs associated with pre-excitation syndromes (e.g., Wolff-Parkinson-White syndrome) are related to the electrophysiologic properties of the AV node and the accessory pathway, and they depend on different refractory periods of the structures involved. This disorder is extensively reviewed in Chapter 60. Similarly, SVTs such as atrial fibrillation, atrial flutter, and atrial tachycardia are discussed in detail in Chapters 58 and 59.

CLASSIFICATION OF SUPRAVENTRICULAR TACHYCARDIA	
AV Node–Dependent Junctional Tachycardias	**AV Node–Independent Atrial Tachycardias**
AVNRT Typical ("common," slow-fast) Atypical ("uncommon," fast-slow)	Sinus tachycardia Physiologic Inappropriate Sinus node re-entry
AVRT Concealed accessory pathway Wolff-Parkinson-White syndrome	Atrial tachycardia Unifocal Multifocal
Junctional Junctional ectopic tachycardia	Atrial flutter Atrial fibrillation

AV, atrioventricular; AVNRT, atrioventricular nodal re-entrant tachycardia; AVRT, atrioventricular re-entrant tachycardia.

Table 57.1 Classification of supraventricular tachycardia.

Classification

Several classifications have been proposed for SVT. An approach that combines both anatomic substrate and mechanisms may be clinically applicable and useful. In principle, the term SVT by itself is an anatomic misnomer because half of the tachyarrhythmias classified as SVT involve the participation of an accessory pathway and nodal ventricular or atrial tissue for the maintenance of the re-entry circuit. An initial, useful, and practical approximation is to classify tachycardias as AV node–dependent junctional tachycardias and AV node–independent atrial tachycardias (Table 57.1). The advantage is that appropriate SVT diagnosis may be achieved in most cases without the need for intracardiac recordings.[21-24]

AV Node–Dependent Junctional Tachycardias

Junctional tachycardias are SVTs that either originate from or require the AV node as a critical component of the tachycardia circuit. The two most common are AVNRT and AV re-entrant tachycardia (AVRT) (Fig. 57.5). Another unusual AV node–dependent junctional tachycardia is the permanent form of junctional tachycardia. The permanent form of junctional tachycardia is frequently incessant, is predominantly diagnosed in young patients, and may lead to tachycardia-induced cardiomyopathy (Fig. 57.6).[25-27]

Automatic junctional tachycardia, also known as junctional ectopic tachycardia or nonparoxysmal junctional tachycardia, originates from the AV junction probably as a consequence of enhanced automaticity or triggered activity. This arrhythmia is rarely seen in adults and is usually triggered by AV node injury after operative repair of complex congenital heart disease in children.[28-30]

AV Node–Independent Atrial Tachycardias

Atrial tachycardias that originate and are maintained in the atria do not involve the AV node as a necessary part of the re-entrant circuit. The AV node acts as a "bystander" to the tachycardia. Sinus node tachycardia, both physiologic and inappropriate, and sinus node re-entry are in this category. Other atrial tachycardias may be either unifocal or multifocal, atrial flutter and atrial fibrillation (see Chapters 58 and 59).

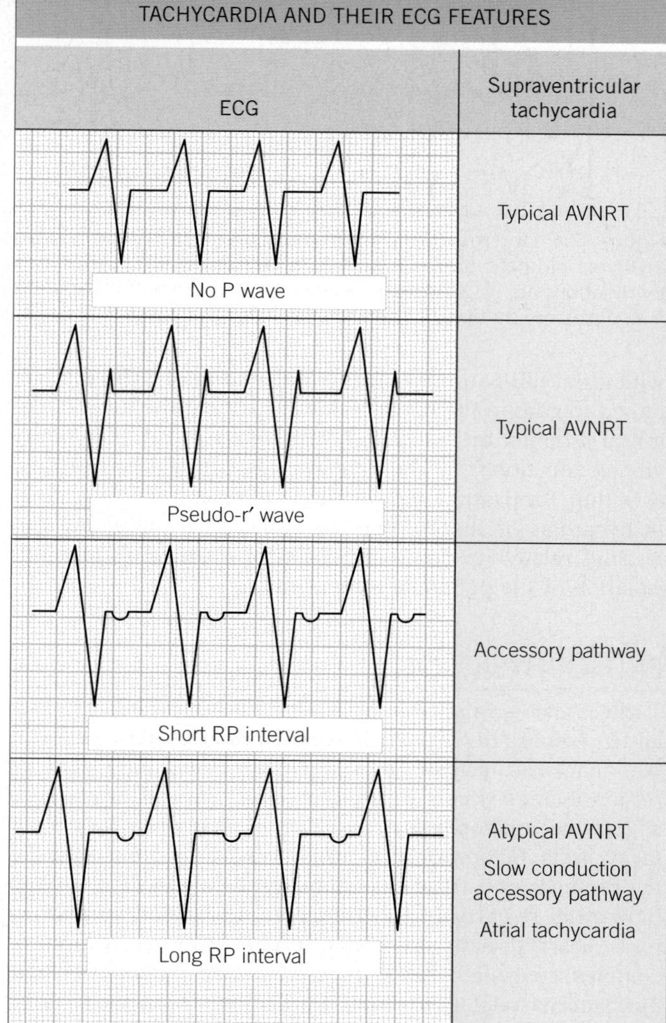

Figure 57.5 The most frequent types of supraventricular tachycardia and their electrocardiographic (ECG) features. AVNRT, atrioventricular nodal re-entrant tachycardia.

Differentiation of AV Node–Dependent and AV Node–Independent Atrial Tachycardias

A tachycardia can usually be classified as AV node dependent clinically by observing termination of tachycardia by blocking the AV node with a vagal maneuver such as carotid sinus massage or the use of an AV node–blocking drug such as adenosine; of course, adenosine may terminate tachycardia without necessarily causing block in the AV node. Once a tachycardia has been classified as either AV node dependent or AV node independent, further insight into the mechanism is warranted. Re-entrant mechanisms are usually observed in AV node–dependent junctional tachycardias and may be related to an anatomic obstacle. In contrast, AV node–independent atrial tachycardias are usually related to abnormal impulse formation. This approach may prove useful for the selection of pharmacologic therapy that targets the mechanisms of the atrial arrhythmia.[9,23,31]

The recent introduction of pulmonary vein isolation and wide area circumferential ablation associated with linear lesions in the left atrium as a treatment strategy in patients

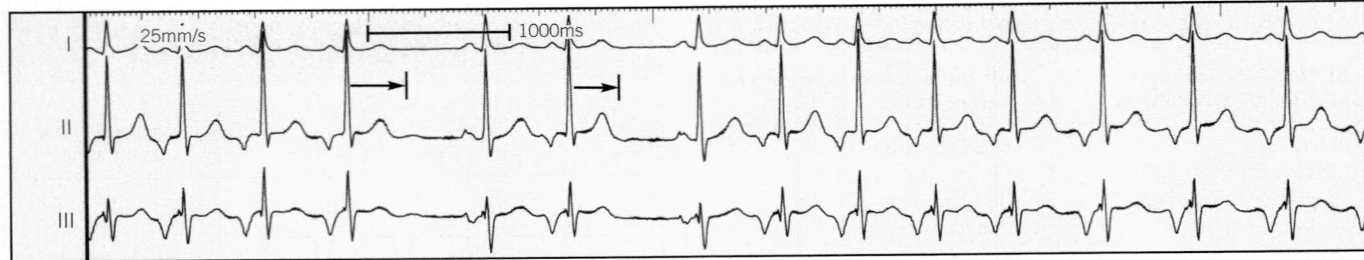

Figure 57.6 **Electrocardiogram in permanent junctional reciprocating tachycardia.** This electrocardiographic rhythm strip is from a 14-year-old patient. The P waves are inverted in the inferior leads, and the RP interval is longer than the PR interval. Spontaneous terminations are noted *(arrows)* without a retrograde P wave, indicating block in the retrograde limb of the re-entrant circuit (i.e., accessory pathway). The first cycle after the pause is sinus; it is followed by incessant tachycardia.

with atrial fibrillation has led to a new form of SVTs that are linked to gaps in the linear lesions usually at the level of the mitral isthmus or associated with recovery of pulmonary vein conduction.[32,33] These tachycardias should be classified as either focal atrial tachycardias or macroreentrant atrial tachycardias or flutters that are usually perimitral but can also be related to anatomic obstacles created by previous isolation of the pulmonary vein ostia.[34]

PATHOPHYSIOLOGY

Tachycardias arising from or around the sinus node are usually a response to physiologic stress, such as exercise or fever. An abnormal increase in sympathetic tone may also be responsible, as occurs in thyrotoxicosis. Several drugs, such as caffeine, aminophylline, and alcohol, may precipitate sinus tachycardia. Ectopic or focal atrial tachycardia often occurs in the presence of cardiac or pulmonary disease. SVT related to intra-atrial re-entry is also frequently associated with structural heart disease and often occurs after correction of complex congenital heart disease.[8,35] The pathophysiologic mechanisms related to atrial fibrillation, atrial tachycardia and atrial flutter, and pre-excitation syndromes are discussed in detail in Chapters 58, 59 and 60, respectively.

The mechanisms that lead to AVNRT have been described before. The role of dual pathways in AV node conduction is undisputed as a mechanism of tachycardia. However, alternative explanations have been proposed by Jalife,[36] who documented that re-entry may occur in a linear structure if conduction proceeds electrotonically along an area of block. Another pathophysiologic mechanism for AVNRT may be related to nonuniform anisotropy within the intricate anatomic structure of the AV node, leading to longitudinal dissociation and re-entry. Postmortem histologic evidence obtained from a patient with AVNRT who had successfully undergone radiofrequency ablation of the slow pathway revealed the presence of a right atrial lesion 1.15 cm from the compact AV node (Fig. 57.7).[37] Most investigators concur with the idea that at least two AV node inputs exist: a posteriorly located slow pathway, which usually has a short refractory period; and a fast pathway, which is anteriorly located, possibly in the anterior interatrial septum, and usually has a long refractory period.[5,14,19,20,28] It remains to be proven whether there is a lower common pathway and, if there is, whether this pathway is completely embedded in the compact AV node. Other mechanisms, such as atrial stretching, electrical remodeling, and autonomic modulation, are discussed in detail in Chapters 58 and 59. The effects of pulmonary

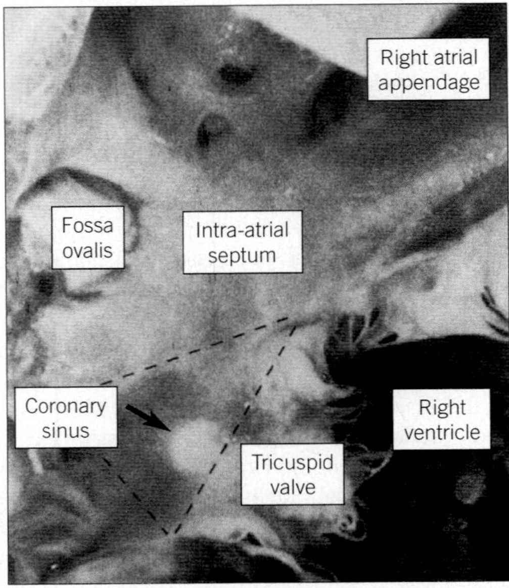

Figure 57.7 **Gross pathology of the right atrium after removal of the anterior wall of the right atrium.** Koch's triangle is depicted by the dashed lines from the os of the coronary sinus to the tricuspid annulus along the tendon of Todaro. The arrow indicates the lesion produced by radiofrequency ablation of the slow pathway. The border of the lesion is well delineated and lies 1.15 cm from the compact AV node. (From Olgin JE, Ursell P, Kao AK, Lesh MD. Pathological findings following slow pathway ablation for AV nodal reentrant tachycardia. J Cardiovasc Electrophysiol 1996;7:625-631. Reprinted with permission from the American College of Cardiology.)

disease and structural heart disease on the mechanisms of SVTs such as atrial flutter and fibrillation as well as ectopic atrial tachycardia are also discussed in Chapters 58 and 59.

CLINICAL PRESENTATIONS

A frequent finding in patients with SVT is recurrent palpitations with episodes of varying duration that may have first occurred in childhood. Palpitations, chest fullness, and "skipped" beats, associated with lightheadedness, presyncope, and occasionally syncope, are typical manifestations of SVT. Syncope during SVT is generally related to impaired vasomotor response to upright posture during tachycardia rather than to the fast heart rate.[38] Although characteristic clinical manifestations rarely identify a specific type of SVT, some clinical features may be helpful in distinguishing between the different forms of SVT in some circumstances. Heart rate is a feature, although a nonspecific finding because of marked overlap in the different types of SVT. Nevertheless, in AV node–dependent junctional tachycardias, the rate may range between 150 and 250 beats per minute. Neck pounding, caused by cannon waves, is an important diagnostic clue thought to be practically pathognomonic of AVNRT.[39]

It is difficult to distinguish between AVNRT and AVRT clinically, especially in patients without overt pre-excitation. Nonetheless, several electrocardiographic features may provide the diagnosis. AV node–dependent junctional SVTs are usually paroxysmal and associated with abrupt initiation and termination. In contrast, AV node–independent atrial tachycardias originating near or around the sinus node, such as sinoatrial re-entry and inappropriate sinus tachycardia, usually are nonparoxysmal with gradual onset and termination.

The association with structural heart disease is much greater in adults who have atrial tachycardia (80% to 90%) than in adults who have junctional tachycardia (5% to 10%). This is to be expected because most junctional tachycardias are related to a congenital substrate, whereas most atrial tachycardias are related to acquired structural heart disease.[40,41]

Reproducible termination of SVT with vagal maneuvers (e.g., carotid sinus massage, deep breathing, Valsalva maneuver) strongly suggests AV node–dependent tachycardias, although some atrial tachycardias, particularly sinus node re-entry, may be terminated by vagal maneuvers.

The age at onset may be helpful. Adolescents and young adults are more likely to have AVRT. In contrast, healthy middle-aged adults who have new symptoms and no evidence of structural heart disease are more likely to have AVNRT. Elderly patients who have a history of pulmonary or cardiac disorders usually have ectopic atrial tachycardia, atrial fibrillation, or atrial flutter.[8]

The clinical manifestations of SVT are usually nonspecific. However, precipitating factors (e.g., exercise, caffeine, cigarette consumption, relation to emotional upsets, and alcohol intake) should always be sought. Similarly, other features, such as regularity or irregularity of the rhythm and onset and termination of tachycardia, may be helpful. Incessant atrial tachycardia that is highly symptomatic and occasionally associated with acute heart failure is the characteristic clinical presentation of post–atrial fibrillation ablation atrial tachycardias.

Sinus Tachycardia

Sinus tachycardia may be either a physiologic response or an inappropriate response. Sinus tachycardia may be defined as heart rate of more than 100 beats per minute with normal P-wave axis and morphology. It is usually associated with hyperadrenergic states or triggered by hypovolemia, fever, pain, or hyperthyroidism. Initiation and termination are usually gradual (warm-up and cool-down). Correction of the precipitating cause usually restores normal sinus rhythm.

Inappropriate sinus tachycardia has been described in young, healthy adults. It predominantly affects women in their early 20s to mid-40s. Inappropriate sinus tachycardia is an ill-defined clinical syndrome with varied manifestations. It is characterized by an exaggerated heart rate response to physiologic demands or increased resting heart rate associated with myriad symptoms. Clinical manifestations range from mild palpitations to incapacitating incessant tachycardia associated with presyncope, syncope, and chronic fatigue.[39] It is unclear whether inappropriate sinus tachycardia is pathophysiologically related to postural orthostatic tachycardia syndrome or chronic orthostatic intolerance or whether it is a distinct syndrome. Clinically, there may be an overlap between these entities, and proper autonomic testing is recommended for appropriate classification and guidance of therapy.[42,43] Diagnostic criteria for inappropriate sinus tachycardia are summarized in Table 57.2. Pathophysiologic mechanisms include[3,4,44]

- enhanced sinus node automaticity;
- the presence of an automatic right atrial focus (near the sinus node); and
- impaired autonomic modulation (β receptor hypersensitivity or reduced vagal efferent modulation).

DIAGNOSTIC CRITERIA FOR INAPPROPRIATE SINUS TACHYCARDIA
P-wave axis and morphology during tachycardia similar or identical to sinus rhythm
Resting heart rate 100 bpm or heart rate 100 bpm induced by minimal exertion or postural changes
Exclusion of secondary cause
Exclusion of sinus node re-entry or right atrial tachycardia

Table 57.2 Diagnostic criteria for inappropriate sinus tachycardia.

Sinus Node Re-entrant Tachycardia

Sinus node re-entrant tachycardia presents with paroxysmal onset and sudden termination, usually precipitated by premature atrial cycles. Sinus node re-entry is rarely a clinical problem and is usually an incidental finding during Holter monitoring. The P wave is identical to that of sinus rhythm, and the rate is usually less than 150 beats per minute. During electrophysiologic testing, tachycardia is induced and terminated by critically timed atrial extrastimuli. The atrial activation sequence and intra-atrial conduction time are similar to those of sinus rhythm.[45,46]

DIAGNOSTIC TECHNIQUES

History and physical examination are fundamental to the diagnosis of SVT. Recording of heart rate and rhythm and other physical findings may be useful. Patients who have SVT generally have sustained episodes documented by 12-lead electrocardiography. The 12-lead electrocardiographic recording during an episode of SVT remains the cornerstone of the diagnosis. A stepwise approach to the surface electrocardiogram is fundamental for an appropriate diagnosis. Rate, rhythm (i.e., regular or irregular), P-wave polarity and relation with the QRS complex, QRS alternation, termination and initiation of the tachycardia, and effect of bundle branch block on tachycardia cycle length should be assessed.

Heart rate has poor specificity for the differentiation between SVTs, namely, AV node–dependent and AV node–independent tachycardias. Electrocardiographic characteristics of AV node–dependent tachycardias may help differentiate AVNRT from AVRT. The typical or common type of AVNRT is characterized by a heart rate that ranges between 100 and 250 beats per minute. The re-entrant circuit during typical (slow-fast) AVNRT conducts in an anterograde direction down the slow pathway and in a retrograde direction up the fast pathway, resulting in almost simultaneous activation of atria and ventricles. This activation pattern results in a retrograde P wave that is almost fully embedded in the QRS complex during tachycardia and may appear as a pseudo–S wave in lead II or pseudo–r′ wave in lead V_1 (Fig. 57.8). Initiation of typical AVNRT may be preceded by an atrial premature beat blocked in the fast pathway, allowing anterograde conduction over the slow pathway associated with lengthening of the PR interval (Fig. 57.9).

Atypical or uncommon AVNRT re-entrant circuit courses in the opposite direction (fast-slow) resulting in a delayed, negative retrograde P wave with a characteristic PR interval that is shorter than the RP interval during tachycardia. Examination of P waves and RP and PR intervals during narrow-complex tachycardia (in which the QRS complex is shorter than 0.12 second) is a useful initial approach for the patient with SVT. Polarity of the P wave may also be helpful. A positive P wave in lead V_1 has a sensitivity of 93% and a specificity of 88% in predicting a left atrial focus. On the other hand, a positive or biphasic P wave in lead aVL has a sensitivity of 88% and a specificity of 79% for a right atrial focus.[8] The differential diagnosis of short versus long RP tachycardias is summarized in Table 57.3. In essence, a narrow QRS tachycardia with a short RP and a long PR interval is primarily due to AV node–dependent junctional tachycardias such as AVNRT or AVRT. In contrast, a long RP interval and a short PR interval are

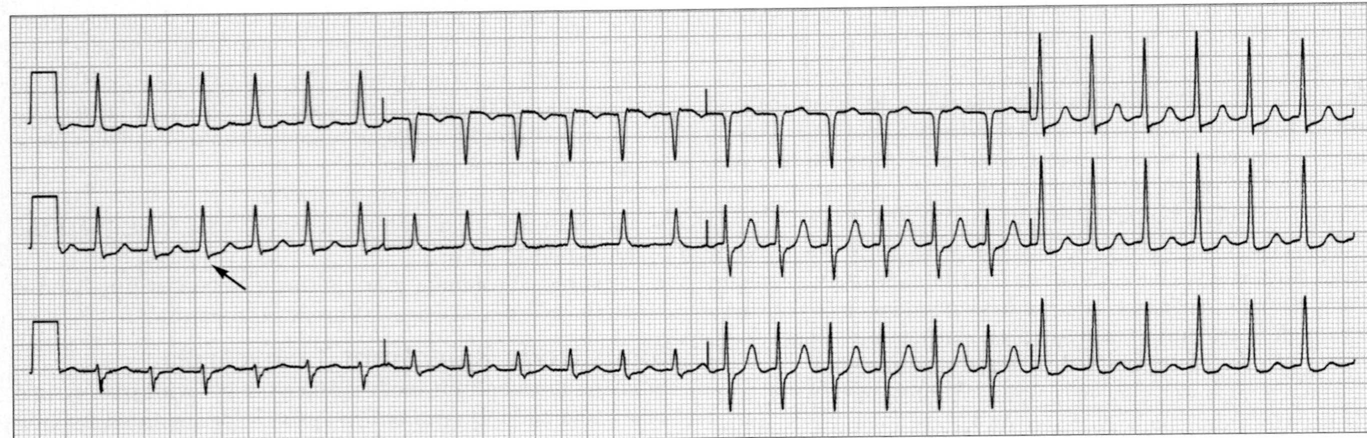

Figure 57.8 Twelve-lead electrocardiogram (ECG) showing a narrow-complex QRS tachycardia. This is characterized by a rate of 145 beats per minute. No P waves are clearly seen. A pseudo–S wave *(arrow)* can be seen in lead II, suggesting a retrograde P wave. Electrophysiologic study demonstrated the presence of dual pathways and induction of the same tachycardia, corresponding to typical AV nodal re-entrant tachycardia.

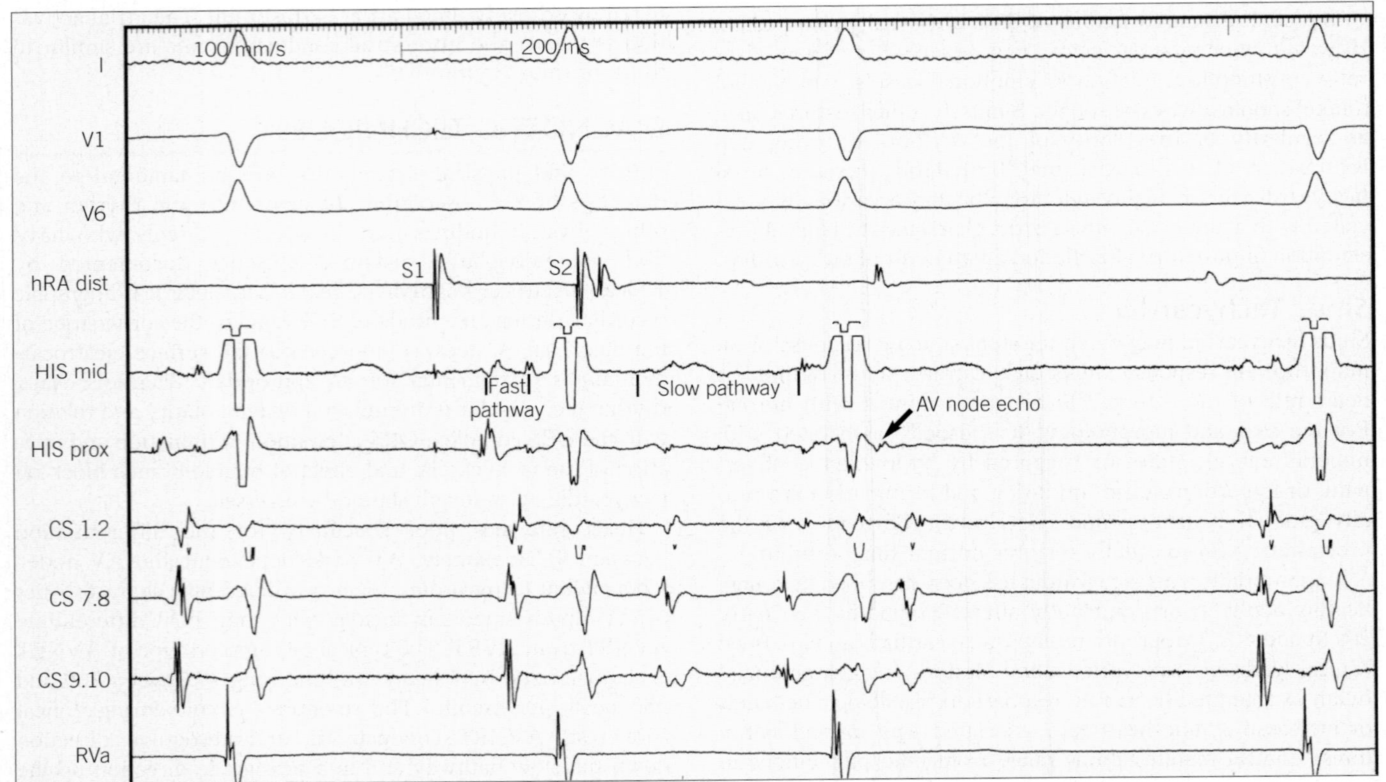

Figure 57.9 Electrophysiologic demonstration of dual AV nodal pathways. Introduction of an early coupled atrial premature beat (S2) blocks the fast pathway proceeding over the slow pathway with induction of an AV node echo beat. Surface leads I, V_1, and V_6 and intracardiac recordings are displayed. CS, coronary sinus; CS 1.2, distal; CS 9.10, proximal; HIS, bundle of his recording; hRA, high right atrium; RVA, right ventricular apex.

NARROW-COMPLEX QRS TACHYCARDIAS WITH SHORT VERSUS LONG RP INTERVAL	
Short RP Internal	**Long RP Interval**
Typical AVNRT	Atypical AVNRT
AVRT	AVRT (slow retrograde conduction) The permanent form of junctional tachycardia Atrial tachycardia Sinus node re-entry Inappropriate sinus tachycardia

AVNRT, atrioventricular nodal re-entrant tachycardia; AVRT, atrioventricular re-entrant tachycardia.

Table 57.3 Narrow-complex QRS tachycardias with short versus long RP interval.

related to both AV node–independent and AV node–dependent tachycardias, such as atrial tachycardia, sinus node re-entry, inappropriate sinus tachycardia, or atypical AVNRT and AVRT with slow retrograde conduction over an accessory pathway.[47] A simplified stepwise approach is shown in Fig. 57.10. More recently, other authors have proposed a more complex stepwise algorithm for the prediction of AVNRT and AVRT based on the analysis of the retrograde P wave during SVT (Fig. 57.11).[46,48] Another diagnostic clue derived from the 12-lead electrocardiogram is the effect of bundle branch block on the tachycardia cycle length. Prolongation of tachycardia cycle length during bundle branch block usually indicates the participation of an accessory pathway ipsilateral to the bundle branch morphology. QRS complex alternation has been ascribed to AVRT-mediated SVT. However, this appears to be related to tachycardia rate more than to mechanism.

In summary, several electrocardiographic features may be helpful in differentiating AVNRT and AVRT. These features include

- the presence of a delta wave during sinus rhythm, which supports AVRT being responsible for the tachycardia;
- the presence of a pseudo–S wave in lead II or a pseudo–r′ wave in lead V_1, which is highly suggestive of AVNRT; and
- prolongation of tachycardia cycle length associated with bundle branch block, which supports AVRT using an accessory pathway ipsilateral to the bundle branch block.

Patients who have infrequent episodes of palpitations or sustained SVT not documented by electrocardiography may have Holter monitoring or loop recorders. Exercise testing may be indicated when tachycardia is induced by exercise or other hyperadrenergic states. Under continuous electrocardiographic recording, vagal maneuvers may be helpful for the diagnosis and termination of SVT. Termination by vagal maneuvers (e.g., Valsalva maneuver, carotid sinus massage, gagging, cold face test) usually indicates that the tachycardia is AV node dependent. Slowing of the tachycardia rate may reveal blocked P waves or flutter waves.[49] Incessant atrial tachycardias manifesting after atrial fibrillation ablation are a diagnostic challenge. However, some electrocardiographic characteristics have been recently reported and are useful in determining the mechanism and origin of these focal or macroreentrant tachycardias[32,33]:

- cycle length shorter in mitral isthmus flutter compared with left focal atrial tachycardias;
- positive flutter waves in inferior and precordial leads and negative flutter waves in leads I and aVL suggests counterclockwise mitral isthmus–dependent flutter;
- negative flutter waves in inferior and precordial leads and positive flutter waves in leads I and aVL suggests clockwise mitral isthmus–dependent flutter;

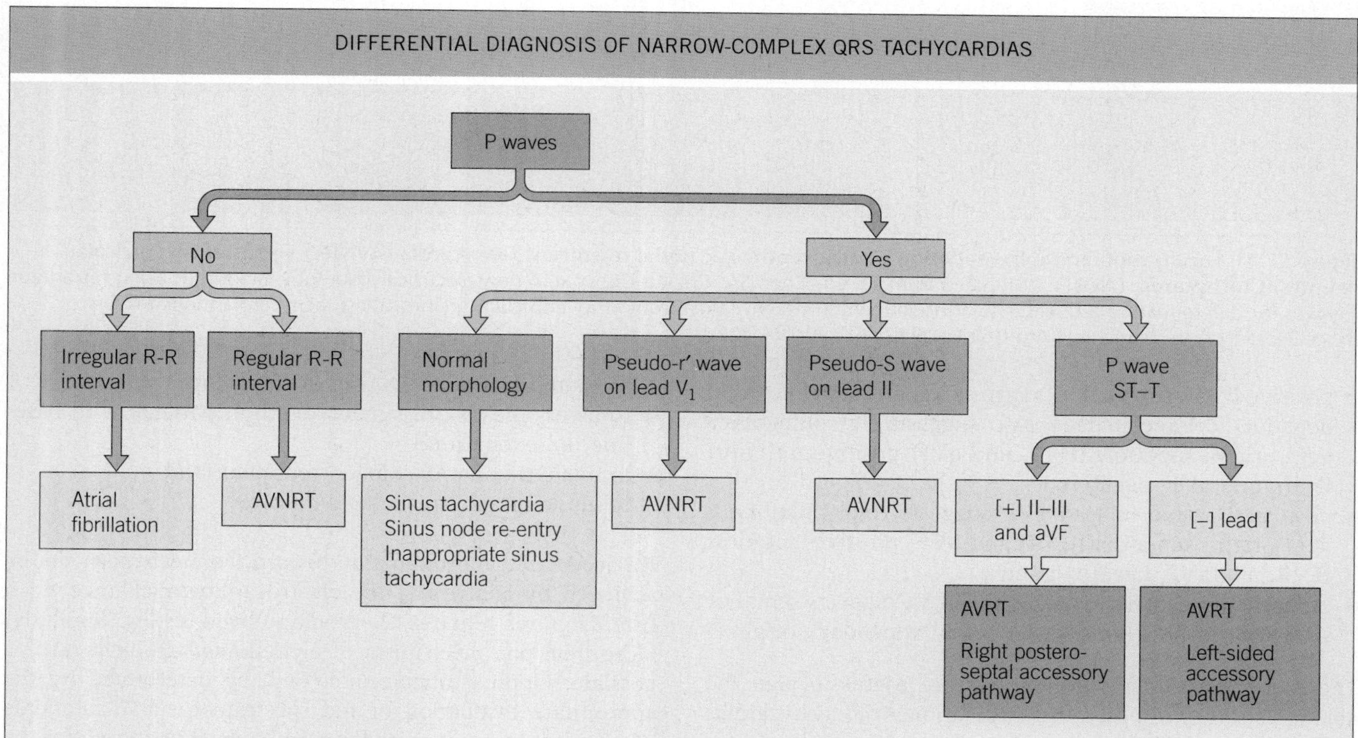

Figure 57.10 Differential diagnosis of narrow-complex QRS tachycardias. AVNRT, atrioventricular nodal re-entrant tachycardia; AVRT, atrioventricular re-entrant tachycardia.

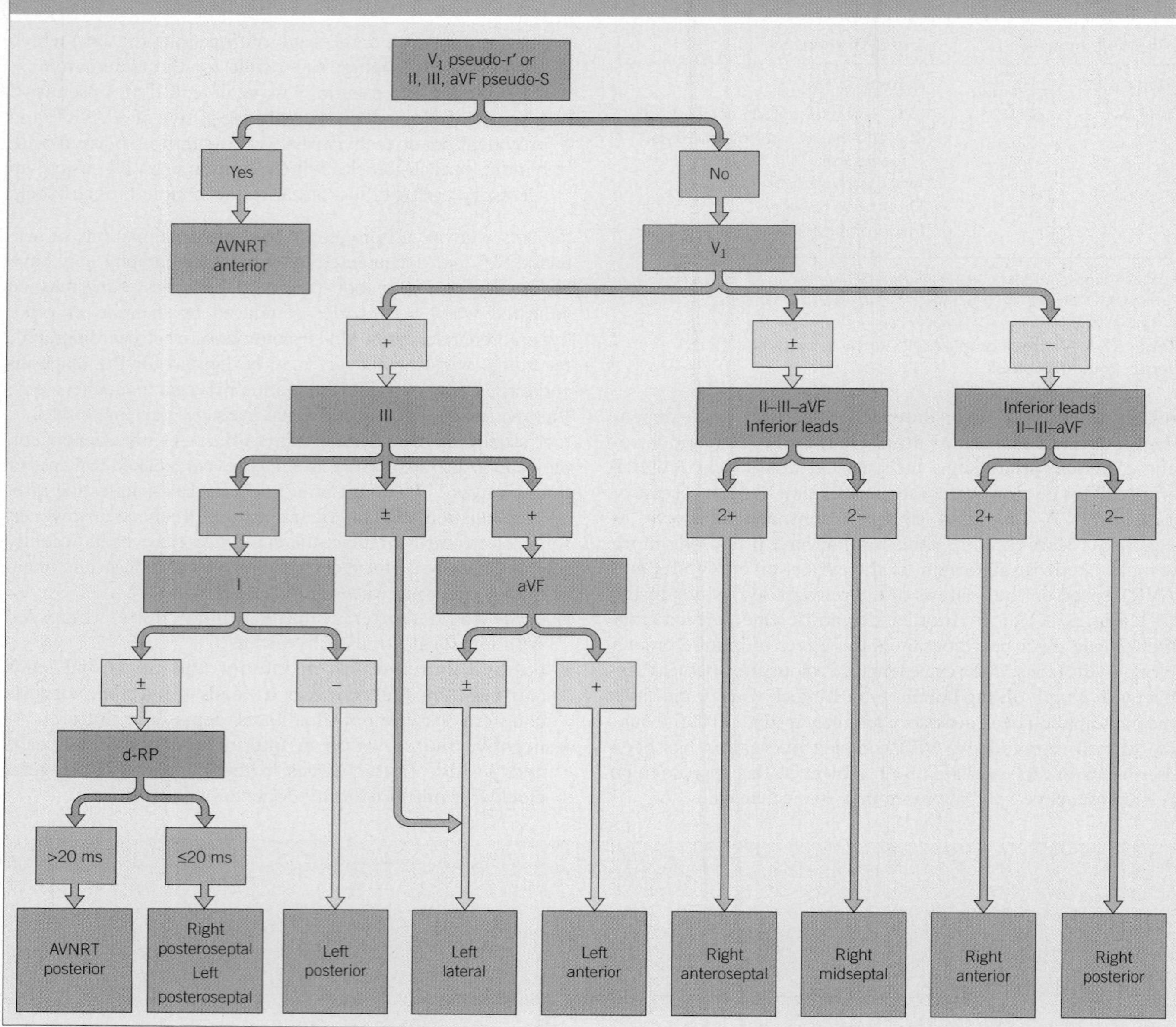

Figure 57.11 Localization and differentiation of atrioventricular nodal re-entrant tachycardia (AVNRT) versus atrioventricular re-entrant tachycardia (AVRT). (Modified from Tai CT, Chen SA, Chiang CE, et al. A new electrocardiographic algorithm using retrograde P waves for differentiating atrioventricular node reentrant tachycardia from atrioventricular reciprocating tachycardia mediated by concealed accessory pathway. J Am Coll Cardiol 1997;29:394-402.)

- positive P wave in lead V_1 suggests left atrial tachycardia;
- negative P wave in lead aVL suggests left pulmonary vein origin; superior: II, III, and aVF, positive; inferior: II, III, and aVF, negative;
- positive P wave in lead aVL suggests right pulmonary vein origin; superior: II, III, and aVF, positive; inferior: II, III, and aVF, negative; and
- biphasic or negative P wave in lead V_1 suggests septal or superior mitral isthmus or left atrial appendage origin.

These electrocardiographic features are useful to plan the ablation strategy of post–atrial fibrillation atrial tachycardias (Figs. 57.12 and 57.13 a-c).

Invasive electrophysiologic testing is indicated in patients with SVT for the following reasons:

- to establish the mechanism of the tachycardia;
- to assess the risk of sudden death in patients with baseline pre-excitation;
- to evaluate pharmacologic treatment; and
- to guide nonpharmacologic therapy.

An acceptable approximation toward the mechanism can be achieved by analysis of the electrocardiogram; however, a firm diagnosis requires electrophysiologic testing. Similarly, more than one mechanism of arrhythmia, although rare, is possible. Optimal management will be determined by the appropriate evaluation of the substrate for SVT. Patients who have infrequent episodes of SVT who do not wish to take daily therapy or to undergo catheter-guided radiofrequency ablation should not be studied invasively. Indications for

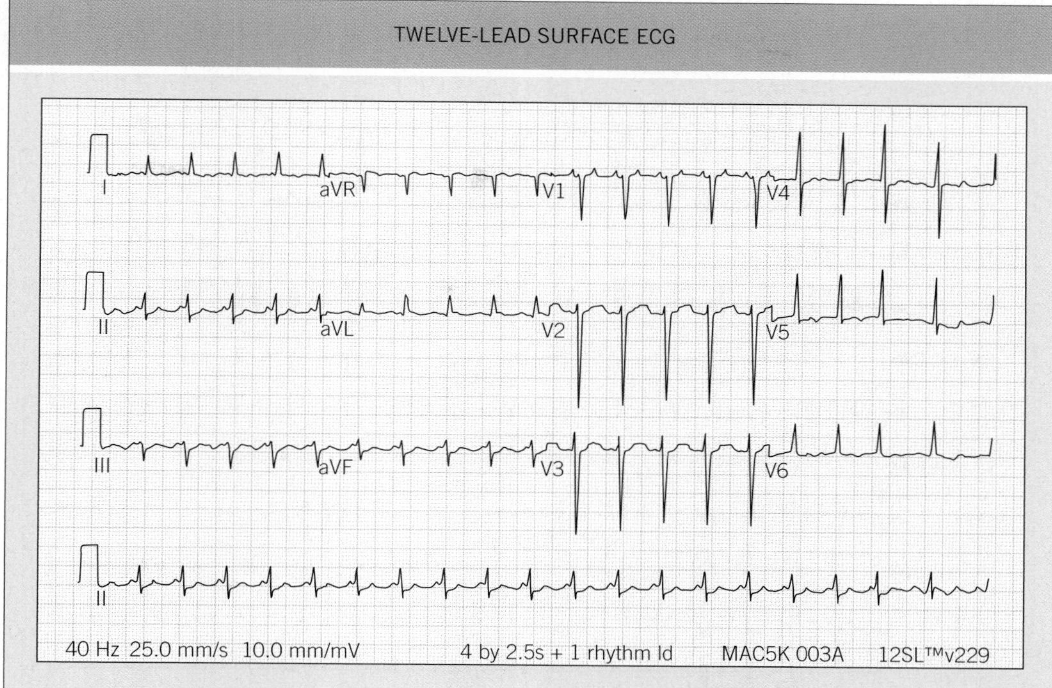

Figure 57.12 Twelve lead surface ECG from a patient presenting with incessant left atrial flutter 3 months post atrial fibrillation ablation. Flutter waves are positive in leads II, II and aVF and biphasic in lead I and aVL suggesting a counter-clockwise mitral annulus dependent flutter.

specific disorders, such as atrial fibrillation, atrial tachycardia and flutter, and the pre-excitation syndromes, are discussed in detail in Chapters 58, 59 and 60, respectively. Currently, most patients who undergo invasive electrophysiologic testing have radiofrequency ablation performed during the same session.[50]

Electrophysiologic study of the patient with SVT varies according to the suspected arrhythmia. Introduction of multipolar electrode catheters to the high right atrium, the bundle of His recording position, the right ventricular apex, and the coronary sinus is usually performed. Once the catheters are placed, programmed stimulation is performed. Studies in SVT usually begin with ventricular stimulation to determine the pattern of retrograde activation as well as the refractory periods of the right ventricle and the ventriculoatrial conducting system. Ventricular incremental pacing is then performed until ventriculoatrial block occurs or a cycle length of 250 ms is achieved. If baseline pre-excitation is present, atrial stimulation at different sites (right atrium and coronary sinus) and cycle lengths (600, 500, and 400 ms) is performed to enhance anterograde conduction over the accessory pathway, if it exists. Subsequently, atrial programmed stimulation is performed and incremental atrial pacing and introduction of single or multiple atrial extrastimuli are delivered until refractoriness of both the AV node and atrial tissue is achieved. The behavior of AV node conduction during atrial programmed stimulation clarifies the mechanism of AVNRT. Discontinuous AV node conduction was first described in humans in 1974 by Rosen and colleagues.[51] Progressively shorter coupled premature atrial extrastimuli result in an abrupt increase in AV nodal conduction. Critically timed earlier atrial extrastimuli block the fast pathway and conduct over the slow pathway, causing dissociation ("jump") in AV conduction, which results in the appearance of atrial echo beats or initiation of AVNRT (see Fig. 57.14). Dual-pathway physiology may not necessarily be associated with AVNRT. In fact, approximately 10% of adults and 35% to 46% of children have discontinuous AV node properties. In almost 80% of patients with AVNRT, dual-pathway physiology is documented at electrophysiologic testing.

Evidence of AV node dual-pathway conduction may also be obtained by rapid atrial or ventricular incremental pacing. An abrupt increase of 40 to 50 ms (jump), in response to a 10-ms decrement of atrial extrastimuli, indicates dual-pathway physiology. Diagnostic electrophysiologic features consistent with AVNRT include

- documentation of a critical atrium-His interval for initiation of tachycardia;
- atrial depolarization buried within the QRS complex during SVT;
- His-ventricle interval greater than or equal to conducted impulses; and
- evidence of AV node dual-pathway physiology.

Many patients do not present with AV node dual-pathway physiology. Atropine or isoproterenol infusion may reveal dual AV node conduction.[52] Diagnosis with AVRT may be achieved by introducing premature ventricular contractions during tachycardia. This technique consists of delivery of a ventricular extrastimulus at the time when the bundle of His is refractory and measurement of the effect on atrial cycle length. During typical AVNRT, ventricular extrastimuli do not usually advance the atrial cycle length, suggesting lack of participation of an accessory pathway (Fig. 57.14).[53]

A detailed description of electrophysiologic findings during AVRT and other AV node-independent SVTs is given in Chapter 60.

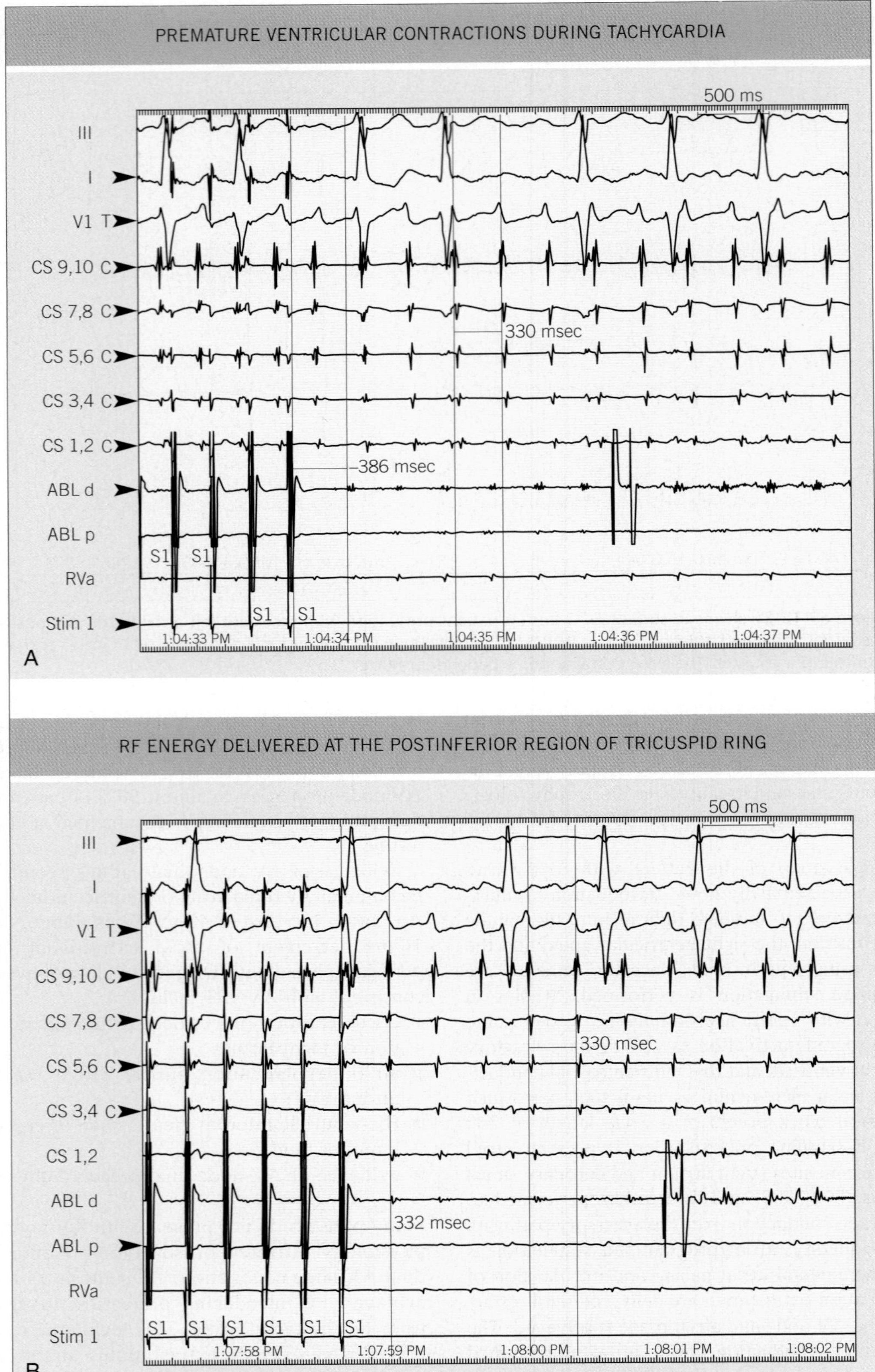

Figure 57.13 Same patient as in Figure 57.12 during entrainment maneuvers and RF ablation. **A,** Left atrial roof pacing entraining atrial flutter with a post pacing interval > 50 ms, **B,** left lateral coronary sinus entrainment with a PPI of < 20 ms demonstrating a macroreentrant counter-clockwise mitral annulus dependent flutter.

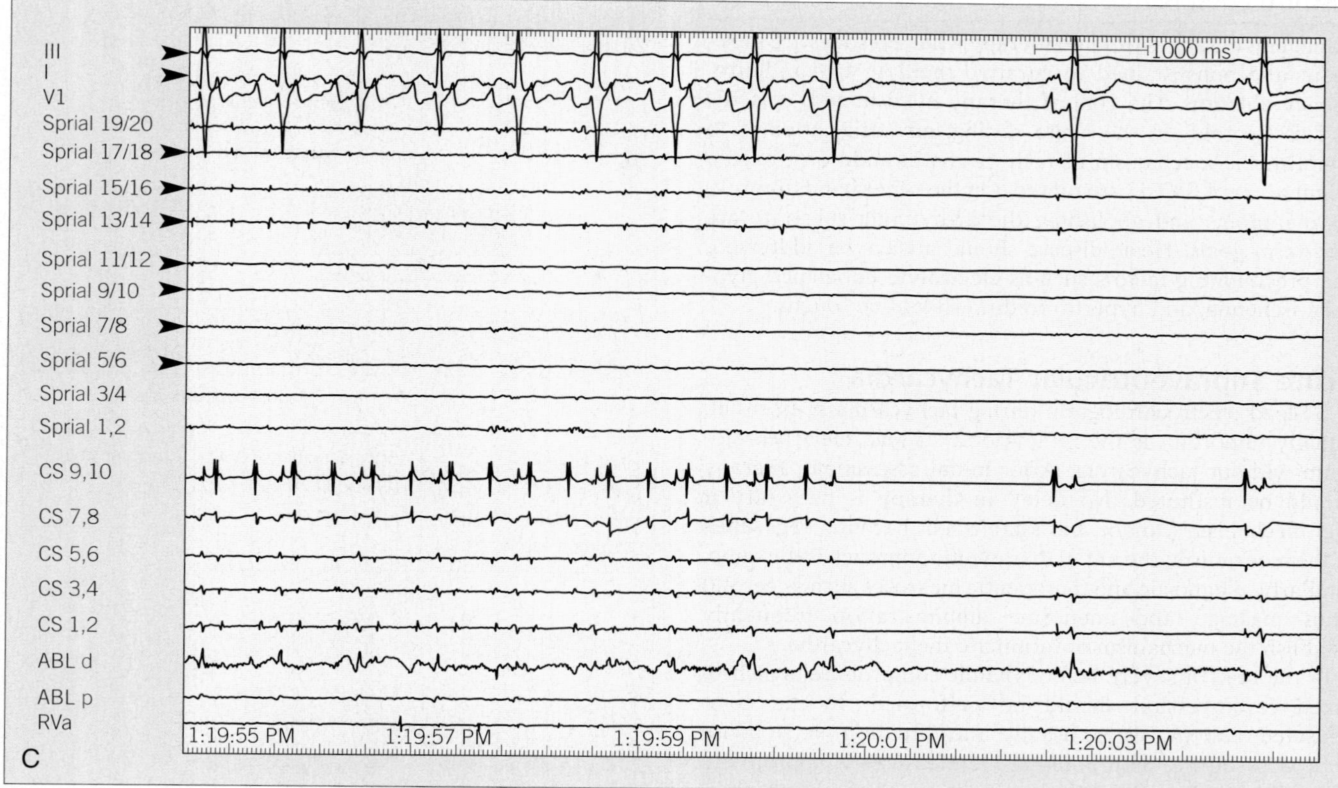

Figure 57.13 C, Radiofrequency ablation lesion delivered at the mitral isthmus area terminating left atrial flutter. Surface leads III, I and V1 and intracardiac recordings are displayed. Abl, ablation; CS, coronary sinus; CS 1,2, distal; CS 9,10, proximal (catheter was well imbedded in the coronary sinus); Rva, right ventricular apex; spiral; (circular catheter located in the left inferior pulmonary vein ostium).

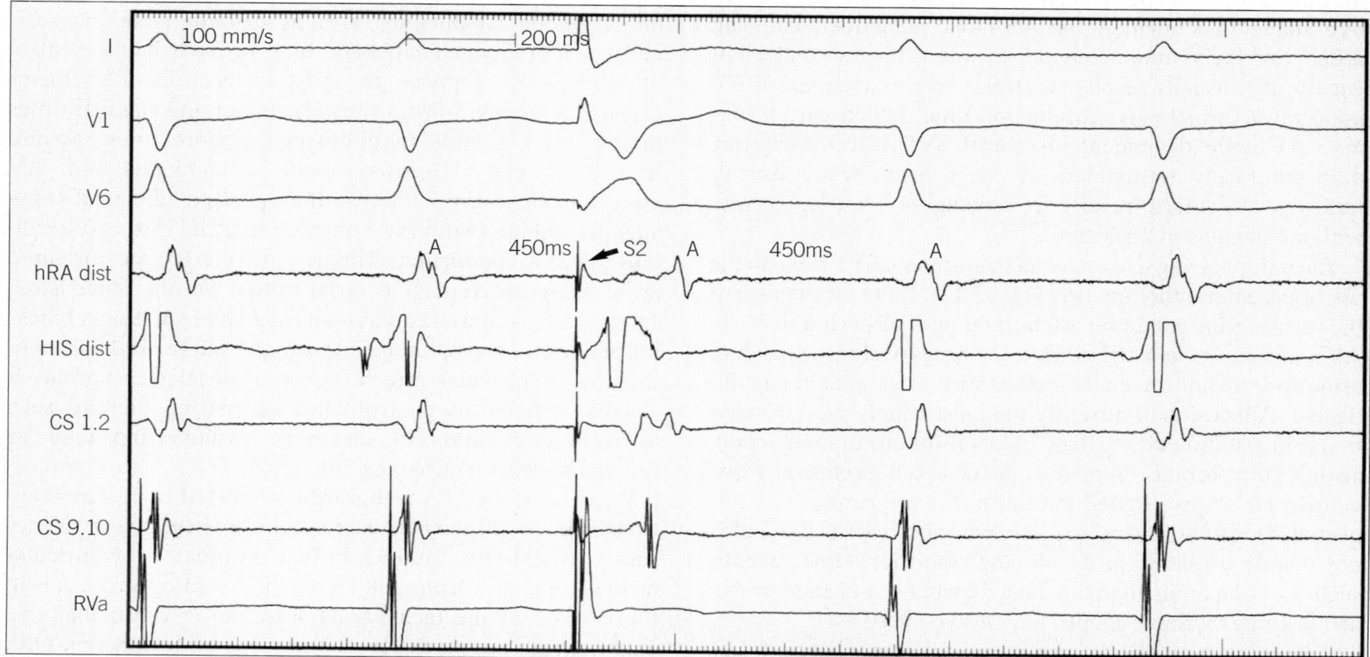

Figure 57.14 Introduction of premature ventricular contractions during tachycardia. This, if timed to coincide with the refractory period of the bundle of His bundle (S2), does not advance atrial activation, indicating that the tachycardia circuit is not mediated by an accessory pathway but by AV node re-entrant tachycardia. Surface leads I, V1 and V6, and intracardiac recordings are displayed. CS, coronary sinus; CS 1, 2 distal; CS 9, 10 proximal; HIS, bundle of His recording; hRA, high right atrium; RVa, right ventricular apex.

MANAGEMENT

Management ranges from no therapy when episodes are infrequent and nonsustained to curative therapy with radiofrequency ablation. The goal of therapy in sustained, episodic SVT is twofold. In the acute setting, an initial attempt to establish the mechanism of tachycardia in addition to acute termination of SVT is warranted. On the other hand, improving symptoms and abolishing the arrhythmia substrate are long-term goals. Heart disease should always be addressed, and precipitating factors such as electrolyte imbalance, hypoxia, ischemia, and hyperthyroidism should be sought.

Acute Supraventricular Tachycardia

A 12-lead electrocardiogram during tachycardia is essential. Equally important is the review of a 12-lead electrocardiogram without tachycardia. After initial assessment, therapy should be instituted. No delay in therapy is necessary if the mechanism cannot be established because regardless of the mechanism, the initial therapeutic approach is the same. Similarly, diagnostic and therapeutic measures such as carotid sinus massage and adenosine administration frequently establish the mechanism or terminate the tachycardia.

In the case of severe hemodynamic compromise, synchronized cardioversion should be performed. In the compensated patient, as is usually the situation, a stepwise approach starting with noninvasive measures is appropriate (Fig. 57.15). Maneuvers that increase vagal efferent output, such as the Valsalva maneuver or carotid sinus pressure, should be performed. Special care should be taken before carotid sinus massage to assess carotid artery disease. In the absence of bruits, gentle pressure is applied over the carotid sinus for 5 to 10 seconds. If there is no change in the tachycardia cycle and termination is not elicited, contralateral massage should be performed in the same fashion. Alternative maneuvers include the Valsalva maneuver, the gag reflex, and facial immersion in iced water. Increased efferent vagal traffic usually results in a transient prolongation of AV node refractoriness and conduction time, which may terminate AV node–dependent junctional SVT. Atrial tachycardias are rarely terminated by vagal maneuvers; usually transient AV block results in slowing of ventricular rate without changes in atrial rate.[54,55]

The failure of vagal maneuvers to terminate SVT leads to the use of parenteral therapy (see Fig. 57.15). If the mechanism of the tachycardia cannot be established or is suspected to be an AV node–dependent arrhythmia, the drugs of choice are adenosine and calcium channel blockers such as verapamil and diltiazem. Adenosine is currently the most widely used because of its almost immediate effect and its short duration of action, lasting only seconds. Similarly, adenosine is preferred when ventricular or pre-excited (antidromic) tachycardias are suspected. However, adenosine is much more expensive and is not readily available in developing countries. Other agents, such as verapamil, digoxin, beta blockers, and membrane-active antiarrhythmic agents, may also be used.[55,56]

Adenosine may also be useful for patients who have suspected AV node–independent tachycardias. Adenosine may occasionally terminate atrial tachycardia, but more frequently it blocks AV node conduction, allowing the clear identification of P waves. The same is true for atrial flutter.

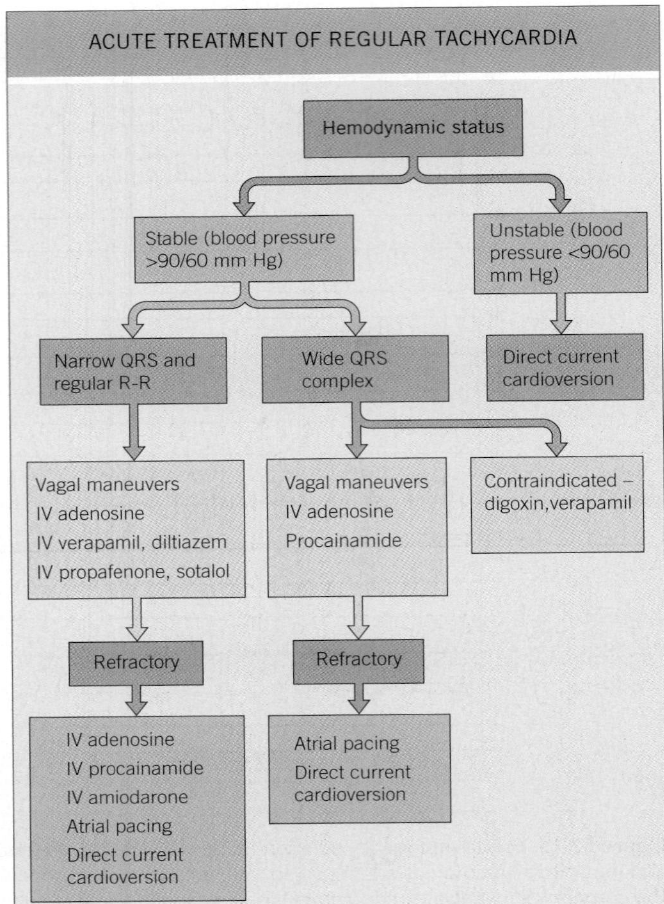

Figure 57.15 Acute treatment of regular tachycardia.

Administration of agents that have a more sustained effect on AV node conduction, such as digoxin, beta blockers, and calcium channel blockers, may provide better control of ventricular response to atrial tachycardia. The membrane-active class I drugs (procainamide) and class III drugs (amiodarone, sotalol, ibutilide) may restore sinus rhythm. In general, class I agents should be combined with AV node–blocking agents because the vagolytic effects of some agents combined with the reduction in atrial rate may facilitate 1:1 AV conduction. This is particularly true for rapid atrial tachycardias such as atrial flutter. On the other hand, agents such as sotalol and amiodarone have additional blocking actions on the AV node and may be safely used as monotherapy. Ventricular rate response in atrial tachycardias is usually difficult to control, and alternative therapy such as pace termination or electrical cardioversion may be preferred (see also Chapter 50).[31,51]

Wide-complex QRS tachycardia suspected to be supraventricular in origin may be successfully managed with adenosine. Adenosine infrequently terminates ventricular tachycardia, and transient effects are a safeguard even in the event that the tachycardia substrate is ventricular. An empiric, safe approach for undiagnosed wide-complex QRS tachycardias is to administer an antiarrhythmic agent that is effective at both the ventricular and supraventricular levels. Infusion of most class Ia, Ic, or III drugs[56] may be suitable in patients without structural heart disease.

Long-term Control of Supraventricular Tachycardia

The need for long-term control of SVT should be individualized. Factors that may influence the decision to initiate chronic therapy include frequency and severity of episodes. A patient who has had a single, mildly symptomatic episode may choose to defer therapy. This is acceptable in the absence of the Wolff-Parkinson-White syndrome, which merits further assessment (see Chapter 60). Other factors that influence the decision for therapy include age, left ventricular function, individual profession, and timely access to medical facilities. An aggressive position should be taken in patients who present with syncope, even if the syncopal episodes are infrequent. The need for therapy is undisputed in patients who have persistent pre-excitation and a potential risk for development of rapid atrial fibrillation and ventricular fibrillation. Detailed discussion of this issue can be found in Chapter 60.

The introduction of catheter-guided radiofrequency ablation has dramatically changed the approach to the patient with SVT.[57,58] Several studies have confirmed the cost benefits of radiofrequency ablation over pharmacologic therapy in patients who have refractory SVT. The current approach is to offer the patient with SVT who requires long-term therapy the option of radiofrequency catheter ablation as curative therapy. Long-term pharmacotherapy is chosen for those patients who decline catheter ablation or for whom catheter ablation has failed and for those in whom ablation is considered to carry a high risk of complications, such as inadvertent AV block. Ablation may also be deferred in infants, young children, and pregnant women. Pharmacologic therapy is preferred in patients who have arrhythmias not currently treatable by ablation, such as multifocal atrial tachycardia.

Selection of the pharmacologic agent is largely empiric and is based on trial and error, the main objectives being efficacy, safety, and tolerability. Electrophysiologically guided therapy has fallen into disuse because diagnosis and cure of the tachycardia during a single study has basically eliminated the need for electropharmacologic testing.

The empiric pharmacologic approach is usually based on the mechanism of tachycardia. In the case of AV node–dependent tachycardias, therapy may be directed at the AV node or the accessory pathway, or both. In the presence of pre-excitation, targeting of the accessory pathway is preferable unless a low-risk potential for sudden death has been documented. Class Ia, Ic, and III agents prolong the refractory period of the accessory pathway and potentially limit the ventricular rate response in the event of atrial fibrillation. In the absence of pre-excitation, AV node–blocking agents are preferred, possibly because of the lower potential of proarrhythmia. The initial choice is a matter of the physician's preference and his or her familiarity with the agent prescribed. Combination of AV node–blocking agents may be useful in patients who experience recurrences with monotherapy. However, the risk of adverse effects, such as transient AV block, may also be increased. The membrane-active Ia and Ic agents are useful in a broad range of patients, particularly younger patients, who tend to be more intolerant to AV node–blocking drugs. Class I agents should not be used in patients who have left ventricular function below 35% because of the high risk of proarrhythmia. However, class I agents may be safely and effectively used in patients who do not have significant heart disease (Table 57.4).[59,60] Detailed descriptions of the mechanisms of action, dosing, and adverse effects can be found in Chapter 50.

Catheter-Guided Radiofrequency Ablation

A detailed description of the principles and techniques involved in catheter-guided radiofrequency ablation can be found in Chapter 51. Briefly, several multipolar catheters are introduced, guided by fluoroscopy, and placed in the high right atrium, bundle of His position, right ventricular apex, and coronary sinus. Once the arrhythmia substrate

ACUTE PHARMACOLOGIC THERAPY FOR SUPRAVENTRICULAR TACHYCARDIA

Drug		Dose	Side Effects
AV node-blocking agents	Adenosine	6-12 mg bolus	Flushing, dyspnea, chest pain
	Verapamil	0.15 mg/kg during 2 minutes	Hypotension, bradycardia
	Diltiazem	0.25-0.35 mg/kg during 2 minutes	Hypotension, bradycardia
	Digoxin	0.5-1 mg during 2-10 minutes	Digoxin toxicity
	Propranolol	1-3 mg at 1 mg during 1 min	Hypotension, bradycardia
Class I antiarrhythmic agents: Use with caution in patients with congestive heart failure and an ejection fraction <40%	Quinidine	6-10 mg/kg at 10 mg/min	Hypotension
	Procainamide	10-15 mg/kg at 50 mg/min	Hypotension
	Disopyramide	1-2 mg/kg at 10 mg/min	Hypotension
	Propafenone	1-2 mg/kg at 10 mg/min	Bradycardia, gastrointestinal disturbance
	Flecainide	2 mg/kg at 10 mg/min	Bradycardia, dizziness
Class III antiarrhythmic agents	Sotalol	1-15 mg/kg at 10 mg/min	Hypotension, proarrhythmia
	Amiodarone	5 mg/kg during 5-10 minutes	Hypotension, bradycardia

Note that disopyramide, propafenone, flecainide, and sotalol are not available for parenteral use in the United States.

Table 57.4 Acute pharmacologic therapy for supraventricular tachycardia.

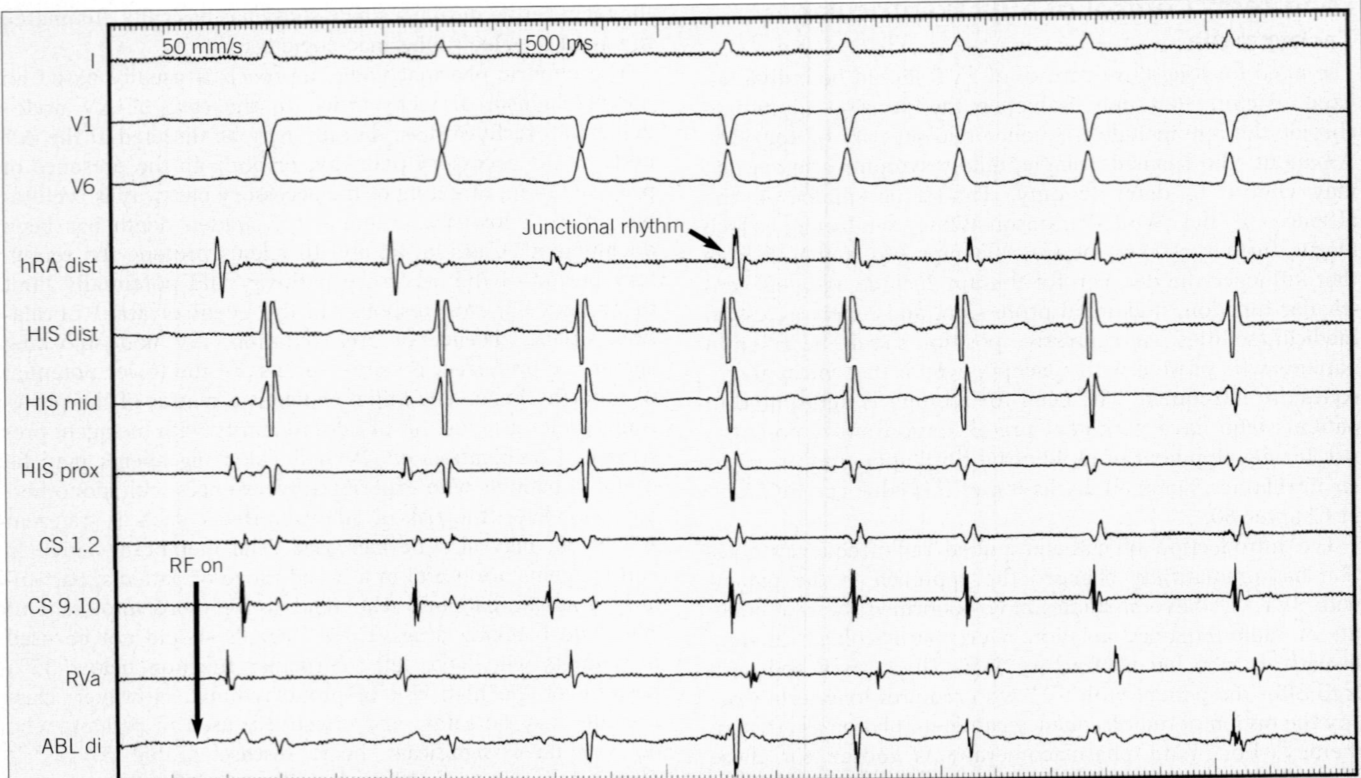

Figure 57.16 Radiofrequency (RF) energy delivered at the posteroinferior region of the tricuspid ring at the level of the coronary sinus os. Junctional rhythm is elicited almost immediately after initiation of radiofrequency energy delivery, indicating successful ablation of the slow pathway. Surface leads I, V_1, and V_6 and intracardiac recordings are displayed. CS, coronary sinus; CS 1,2, distal; CS 9,10, proximal; HIS, bundle of His recording; hRA, high right atrium; RVa, right ventricular apex.

has been reproduced and located, a steerable radiofrequency catheter is introduced for mapping of the area of interest (e.g., the mitral or tricuspid valve rings, the right or left atrial tissue, the cavotricuspid isthmus, or the AV node). Radiofrequency energy is delivered at the site of earliest activation or is anatomically guided, as in the case of slow pathway ablation (Fig. 57.16). Success is defined by elimination of the tachycardia or loss of pre-excitation, as in the case of the Wolff-Parkinson-White syndrome. Success rates vary according to the arrhythmia substrate and the operator's experience. In general, high success rates of 90% to 98% in patients with AV node–dependent tachycardias and 60% to 80% in patients with AV node–independent tachycardias such as atrial tachycardia and atrial flutter have been reported. Overall, the incidence of complications is low, with minimal morbidity and rare mortality during the procedure. A learning experience curve has been reported, but high rates of success are reported within 6 months of initiating the use of catheter ablation in individual centers.[8,17-19,37,52,54,57,58,61,62] Surgical management has been largely replaced by catheter-guided radiofrequency ablation. However, for patients in whom ablation has failed, surgery remains a viable option in centers with good surgical experience.

PROGNOSIS

The prognosis of SVT is generally benign, particularly in the absence of structural heart disease. In patients who have structural heart disease, the prognosis of SVT is strongly linked to the evolution of heart disease. Failure to ablate the arrhythmia substrate successfully is associated with a relatively high recurrence of SVT. However, success rates after initial failure approach 100% in experienced centers. In some special circumstances, such as incessant atrial tachycardias, the permanent form of junctional tachycardia, atrial fibrillation, and possibly atrial flutter, prognosis may be associated with the potential for development of tachycardia-induced cardiomyopathy. In these circumstances, restoration of sinus rhythm is imperative and has produced reversal of left ventricular dysfunction in some cases. Limitations of long-term pharmacologic therapy include frequent arrhythmia breakthroughs and the potential for proarrhythmia, especially in patients who have compromised left ventricular function.

SUMMARY

Supraventricular tachycardia is a common clinical problem that poses a challenge for the clinician. A systematic approach to the analysis of certain electrocardiographic features usually provides an acceptable approximation of the origin of the tachyarrhythmia. Currently, catheter-guided radiofrequency ablation is the standard of care for most SVTs, with high success rates. Prevention of incessant or recurrent episodes is warranted, particularly in patients who have the permanent form of junctional tachycardia, atrial fibrillation, and atrial flutter, because of the potential for development of tachycardia-induced cardiomyopathy and electrical remodeling.

chapter 58

Atrial Fibrillation

Gregory Y. H. Lip and John P. DiMarco

Definition

- Atrial fibrillation is characterized by disorganized electrical and mechanical atrial activity with an irregularly irregular ventricular response.

Key Features

- Atrial fibrillation is the most common sustained cardiac rhythm disorder, and its prevalence is increasing as the number of elderly people in the general population increases.
- The prognostic significance of atrial fibrillation depends on the severity of the patient's underlying condition, the response to therapy, and the risk for thromboembolic events.
- Atrial fibrillation is classified by temporal pattern into paroxysmal, persistent, and permanent forms.

Therapy

- Therapy is directed at control of symptoms and prevention of thromboembolic events.
- Strategies based on either rate control or maintenance of sinus rhythm may be appropriate.
- Catheter and surgical ablation may be effective in selected individuals.

Atrial fibrillation is the most common sustained cardiac rhythm disorder, with a high prevalence in an increasingly elderly population.[1-4]

Atrial fibrillation is the most common diagnosis for arrhythmia-related hospitalizations (Fig. 58.1).[5] Because atrial fibrillation is so common and is often highly symptomatic, many clinicians frequently face important therapeutic decisions concerning the need for antiarrhythmic and antithrombotic therapy.

The presence of atrial fibrillation confers significant mortality and morbidity, owing to an increased risk of stroke and thromboembolism and to potentially adverse hemodynamic effects that may result in heart failure and decreased exercise tolerance, as well as impaired quality of life.[6]

The diverse clinical presentations of atrial fibrillation make the development of a single, generalized strategy for its management difficult. Atrial fibrillation is usually associated with heart disease, but a significant proportion of patients with atrial fibrillation have no other clinically manifested heart disease. Investigation and management should be tailored and individualized to the specific clinical scenario associated with the atrial fibrillation in each patient. In the past decade, major advances have been made in the management of atrial fibrillation; these advances reflect not only innovations in technology, but also, perhaps more important, a better understanding of the pathophysiology responsible for this arrhythmia and its consequences.[7]

Epidemiology

In the Framingham study, the incidence of atrial fibrillation in subjects older than 22 years was 2%; it was slightly more common in men (with an incidence of 2.2%) than in women (1.7%).[1] The prevalence was 0.5% for subjects in the age range 50 to 59 years; this increased to 8.8% in subjects aged 80 to 89 years.

In the United Kingdom, the recent Screening for Atrial Fibrillation in the Elderly study[8] found the baseline prevalence of atrial fibrillation to be 7.2%, with a higher prevalence in men (7.8%) and the elderly (age >75 years, 10.3%). In the Renfrew-Paisley cohort, the prevalence of atrial fibrillation was 8 per 1000 in men and 5 per 1000 in women.[6] In the West Birmingham Atrial Fibrillation Project, the prevalence of atrial fibrillation was 2.4% in two general practices, in which the most common causes were hypertension (37%) and ischemic heart disease (29%); interestingly, only one third of the patients in the survey had ever presented to a hospital.[2]

The incidence of atrial fibrillation among older adults, studied during a 3-year follow-up period in the Cardiovascular Health Study population, was 19.2 per 1000 person-years among adults older than 65 years[3]; an increased incidence was associated with age, gender, and the presence of other cardiovascular disease at baseline. In the Renfrew-Paisley cohort, the incidence of atrial fibrillation was 0.9 new cases per 1000 patient-years in men and 0.2 new cases per 1000 patient-years in women.[9] In the Framingham study, secular trends in the prevalence of atrial fibrillation in subjects aged 65 to 84 years suggest an increase in the age-adjusted rates of atrial fibrillation. In men, the rate increased from 3.2% (1968 to 1970) to 9.1% (1987 to 1989); the change in women was not significant.[10] The incidence of atrial fibrillation is rising, increasing by 12.6% during the past 2 decades, and data from a 20-year study in Olmsted County, Minnesota, project that 15.9 million people in the United States will have atrial fibrillation by 2050.[11]

The lifetime risk for the development of atrial fibrillation was examined in the Framingham study,[12] which found that the lifetime risk at age 40 years was 26% for men and 23% for women; in those without previous or concurrent congestive heart failure or myocardial infarction, the lifetime risk for atrial fibrillation was approximately 16%. Similar estimates of the epidemiology and lifetime risk of the

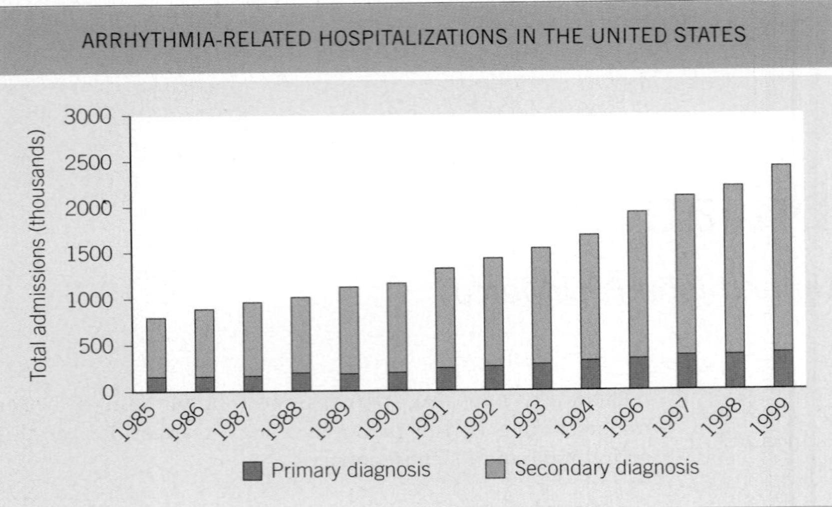

Figure 58.1 Arrhythmia-related hospitalizations in the United States. (Modified from Wattigney WA, Mensah GA, Croft JB. Increasing trends in hospitalization for atrial fibrillation in the United States, 1985-1999: implications for primary prevention. Circulation 2003;108:711-716.)

development of atrial fibrillation were reported by the Rotterdam study.[13] Thus, the lifetime risk for the development of atrial fibrillation is approximately 1 in 4 for subjects 40 years or older.

The Framingham study also examined the clinical characteristics and mortality of subjects 55 to 94 years of age who developed atrial fibrillation during 40 years of follow-up. Of the original 5209 subjects, 296 men and 325 women developed atrial fibrillation, and those who did so were more likely to have hypertension, left ventricular hypertrophy on an electrocardiogram (ECG), and histories of smoking, myocardial infarction, congestive heart failure, valvular heart disease, and cerebrovascular disease at baseline. Atrial fibrillation was associated with a relative risk (RR) for death of 1.5 in men and 1.9 in women, and this did not vary by age. Most of the excess of mortality attributed to atrial fibrillation occurred soon after diagnosis of atrial fibrillation.[1]

Up to one third of patients with atrial fibrillation may have idiopathic or "lone" atrial fibrillation; this is a diagnosis of exclusion, for cases in which no precipitating cause of the atrial fibrillation can be identified and in which no overt evidence of organic heart disease is seen.[3] Although previous data suggested that lone atrial fibrillation may be a benign condition, the Paris Prospective study reported that the relative risk associated with idiopathic atrial fibrillation for cardiovascular mortality was 4.22 (95% CI, 2.10-8.47) and that for total mortality, it was 1.97 (95% CI, 1.14-3.40).[14]

Much of the available clinical epidemiology of atrial fibrillation has been derived from predominantly Caucasian populations. The world literature on atrial fibrillation in non-Caucasian populations is extremely sparse and is limited to small series from Ethiopia, Hong Kong, China, Japan, and multiethnic communities in Europe. Among Afro-Caribbeans living in the United Kingdom, the most common underlying etiologic factor was hypertension, whereas among Indian Asians, ischemic heart disease was more common, in keeping with the more prevalent cardiovascular conditions among these ethnic groups in the United Kingdom.[15] More effective control of hypertension and prevention of ischemic and valvular heart disease are likely to shift the appearance of atrial fibrillation to more elderly age groups.

Causes

Atrial fibrillation may occur in both cardiac and noncardiac disease, or it may present in the absence of any overt condition (Table 58.1). In elderly patients who have atrial fibrillation, subclinical cardiac disease may be detected by rigorous testing,[3] but subclinical disease rarely affects treatment decisions.

Hypertension

In developed countries, hypertensive heart disease is currently the most common underlying disorder in patients with atrial fibrillation, accounting for approximately 50% of cases in several studies.[1-3,6] Atrial fibrillation may be secondary to left atrial dilatation, occurring in hypertensive patients as a

CONDITIONS RELATED TO ATRIAL FIBRILLATION

Cardiac Causes	Noncardiac Causes
Hypertensive heart disease	Autonomically mediated (sympathetic or parasympathetic)
Valvular disease	Toxin exposure
Coronary heart disease	Endocrinopathy (especially thyroid disease)
Cardiomyopathy (all forms)	Pulmonary disease
Pericardial disease	Neurologic disorders
Intracardiac masses	Idiopathic
Electrical disease	
Sinus node dysfunction	
Tachycardia induced	
Familial	
Cardiothoracic surgery	
Congenital heart disease	

Table 58.1 Conditions related to atrial fibrillation.

consequence of reduced left ventricular compliance. In addition, hypertension may be associated with underlying coronary artery disease, which in itself is a risk for atrial fibrillation and thromboembolism. Alcohol can cause both hypertension and atrial fibrillation. Atrial fibrillation is one of many manifestations of hypertensive heart disease, especially if associated hypertensive left ventricular hypertrophy is present.[16] Increasing pulse pressure is a strong predictor of subsequent atrial fibrillation.[17]

Not only does hypertension lead to more atrial fibrillation, uncontrolled hypertension is a major associate of stroke and systemic embolism, even in anticoagulated atrial fibrillation patients; this emphasizes the need for good blood pressure control.[18]

Valvular Disease

Valvular disease is a particularly important cause of atrial fibrillation because its presence substantially increases the thromboembolic risk of patients who have chronic atrial fibrillation. Up to 20% of patients who have mitral stenosis and atrial fibrillation develop embolic events, and these most commonly (in 60% to 75% of cases) affect the cerebral circulation. Among patients with mitral stenosis, the risk of stroke and thromboembolism for patients in atrial fibrillation is three to seven times that of those who remain in sinus rhythm.

Rheumatic heart disease is associated with a high prevalence of atrial fibrillation. In a study of the predictors for atrial fibrillation in approximately 1100 patients with rheumatic heart disease, the highest frequency of atrial fibrillation (70%) was found in those with mitral stenosis, mitral regurgitation, and tricuspid regurgitation.[19] Atrial fibrillation occurred in 29% of those with isolated mitral stenosis, 16% of those with isolated mitral regurgitation, and 52% of those with both conditions. However, when concurrent mitral valve disease is absent, atrial fibrillation is relatively infrequent in patients with aortic stenosis (about 1%) unless heart failure is present.

Coronary Heart Disease

A low proportion of patients who have coronary heart disease develop atrial fibrillation unless associated complicating factors are present, such as heart failure or hypertension. Atrial fibrillation may complicate the early phase of acute myocardial infarction in 10% to 15% of cases and is often a marker of extensive myocardial damage and a poor prognosis. In one study of 4108 patients with acute myocardial infarction admitted to 16 area hospitals, the overall incidence of new atrial fibrillation was 9.7%, with a 1.7-fold increase in mortality.[20] By multivariate analysis, atrial fibrillation was not found to be an independent risk factor for mortality, but rather was associated with older age and a higher prevalence of heart failure, shock, or serious ventricular arrhythmias. Atrial fibrillation with an acute myocardial infarction usually occurs during the initial 24 hours and is self-limited in the absence of heart failure or a previous history of atrial fibrillation. Transient atrial fibrillation after myocardial infarction may be a contributor to stroke.

Among patients who have chronic stable coronary heart disease, atrial fibrillation occurs fairly infrequently. For example, in the Coronary Artery Surgery Study,[21] the prevalence of chronic atrial fibrillation was 0.6%. Atrial fibrillation was usually associated with older age (older than 60 years), male gender, mitral regurgitation, and congestive heart failure. No association was seen between atrial fibrillation and the number of coronary arteries involved. Nevertheless, the presence of atrial fibrillation was an independent predictor of increased mortality, with a 7-year survival of 38% compared with 80% for those without atrial fibrillation (RR, 1.98).

Cardiac Surgery

Atrial fibrillation is a common complication of cardiac surgery and is associated with increased morbidity and mortality, a prolonged hospital stay, and increased costs. Postoperative atrial fibrillation occurs in 20% to 40% of patients undergoing coronary artery bypass surgery, usually between the second and eighth postoperative days.

The likelihood of developing atrial fibrillation after cardiac surgery is increased

- in the elderly;
- in those who have had previous episodes of atrial fibrillation;
- in those who have significant stenosis of the right coronary artery; and
- in those in whom beta blockers were discontinued preoperatively.[22]

A recent prospective study reported that left atrial volume is a strong and independent predictor of postoperative atrial fibrillation.[23] Thus, the risk of postoperative atrial fibrillation potentially could be predicted by left atrial volume and age.

Thyroid Disease

Atrial fibrillation occurs in about 20% to 25% of older patients who have overt thyrotoxicosis, but it is uncommon in patients younger than 30 years. The risk of atrial fibrillation is also increased up to threefold in patients with subclinical hyperthyroidism. In a population-based study of 5860 subjects aged 65 years, the biochemical finding of subclinical hyperthyroidism was associated with atrial fibrillation; even in euthyroid subjects with normal serum thyroid-stimulating hormone levels, serum free thyroxine concentrations were independently associated with atrial fibrillation.[24] One clinical clue to thyroid-associated atrial fibrillation may be the failure of digoxin to control the resting ventricular rate without the addition of beta blockers. Cardioversion should not be attempted while the patient is thyrotoxic because atrial fibrillation usually recurs in this setting.

Alcohol

Acute and chronic alcohol ingestion is a common cause of atrial fibrillation. Atrial fibrillation may be seen in up to 60% of binge drinkers, regardless of whether an underlying alcoholic cardiomyopathy is present. Episodes of atrial fibrillation frequently coincide with heavy alcohol consumption, giving rise to the term *holiday heart syndrome*. Alcohol-induced atrial fibrillation may occur even in healthy people who have otherwise normal hearts and who may be at no risk of atrial fibrillation if they abstain from alcohol. Chronic alcohol excess can cause hypertension or even a dilated cardiomyopathy, leading to the development of atrial fibrillation secondary to heart failure.

Cardiomyopathy

Atrial fibrillation is present in up to 28% of patients with hypertrophic cardiomyopathy and is associated with hemodynamic deterioration and increased mortality. These changes are reversible after cardioversion or effective control of ventricular rates. Atrial fibrillation is present in up to 20% of patients who have dilated cardiomyopathy, but the prognosis depends on the severity of myocardial dysfunction. In mild to moderate heart failure, atrial fibrillation is not associated with increased morbidity or mortality, but both total mortality and mortality from sudden death are increased in patients with advanced heart failure and atrial fibrillation.

Genetic Causes

During the past 10 years, a number of families with inherited patterns of atrial fibrillation have been investigated. Mutations associated with atrial fibrillation have been identified in four genes encoding various potassium channel subunits. These mutations result in shortening of the atrial action potential duration and the atrial effective refractory period. Other genes have been mapped to different loci, but the genes have not been identified. Patients with structural heart disease may also have an increased susceptibility to atrial fibrillation because of inherited DNA polymorphisms. This field is rapidly developing and should provide new insights into the pathogenesis of atrial fibrillation.[4,25]

ANATOMY AND PATHOLOGY

Aside from changes relating to underlying heart disease, anatomic structural changes including fibrosis, necrosis, fat and amyloid infiltration, and inflammation are present in patients who have atrial fibrillation.[26] Histologic examination of the atrial tissue of patients with atrial fibrillation has demonstrated patchy fibrosis, perhaps leading to the differences in atrial refractoriness and conduction velocity. Fibrosis may be a reaction to an inflammation or a degenerative process, and the sinus node may also be involved by fibrosis or fatty infiltration. In patients with mitral valve disease, severe atrial endocardial damage has been noted on scanning electron microscopy, contributing to thrombogenesis (Fig. 58.2).[27] Despite these data, a unique pathologic process responsible for atrial fibrillation has not yet been identified.

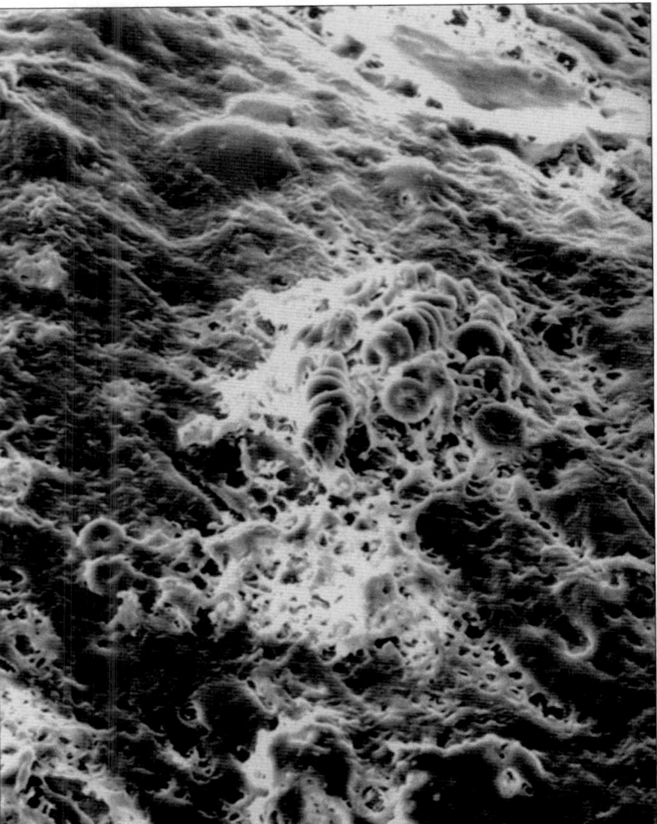

Figure 58.2 Severely damaged left atrial appendage with endocardial thrombotic mass. (From Goldsmith et al.[27])

PATHOPHYSIOLOGY

Hemodynamics

The clinical manifestations of atrial fibrillation relate to the loss of atrial systolic function and an irregular ventricular response, the rate of which typically is determined by the conduction and refractory properties of the atrioventricular (AV) node. The loss of atrial systolic function results in impaired hemodynamic function of the heart. Atrial fibrillation causes a fall in cardiac stroke output of approximately 10% in normal subjects, with a greater decrease seen at fast ventricular rates. This loss becomes more important clinically with increasing age and progressive impairment of left ventricular systolic or diastolic function because in these conditions, atrial systole makes a greater contribution (30% or more) to the overall stroke volume. In addition to the loss of AV synchrony, the irregular and often inappropriate ventricular rates seen in atrial fibrillation result in suboptimal ventricular filling and thus may further compromise cardiac output, an effect particularly important in patients with mitral stenosis. Cardioversion of atrial fibrillation with poorly controlled ventricular rates usually improves the left ventricular ejection fraction and exercise capacity, but the improvement occurs gradually after the procedure.

Loss of atrial systolic function results in stasis within the left atrium, leading to intra-atrial thrombus formation and an increased risk of stroke and thromboembolism. During episodes of atrial fibrillation, echocardiography can detect spontaneous echo contrast as a result of the formation of erythrocyte aggregations and thrombus in the atria. Stasis within the left atrium has been related to hemostatic abnormalities that are suggestive of a hypercoagulable state and that involve coagulation factors and abnormal endothelial and platelet function. These abnormalities of hemostasis have been related to changes in inflammatory indices and growth factors.[28,29] This hypercoagulable state is altered by antithrombotic therapy and by cardioversion of atrial fibrillation to sinus rhythm. Prothrombotic indices in atrial fibrillation have been shown to be prognostically relevant, being predictive of stroke and vascular events, and can be used to refine clinical stroke risk stratification.[7,30] Atrial natriuretic peptide levels are also increased in patients with atrial fibrillation and contribute to hemoconcentration and an increased risk for thrombus formation.

Atrial fibrillation is associated with heart failure in approximately 20% to 50% of patients. Atrial fibrillation and heart failure are related in several ways. Atrial fibrillation may lead to heart failure by loss of atrial transport. If diastolic dysfunction is present, as in left ventricular hypertrophy, a change in rhythm from sinus rhythm to atrial fibrillation, with loss of atrial "kick," may precipitate heart failure. In patients with mitral stenosis, atrial fibrillation contributes to heart failure both by loss of atrial contraction and by compromise of the diastolic filling time. Fast, uncontrolled heart rates, if prolonged, also produce functional, ultrastructural, and microscopic changes within the myocardium that may result in progressive left ventricular dilatation and reduction of left ventricular systolic function; this is referred to as tachycardia-induced cardiomyopathy. In a patient who has chronic heart failure and is in sinus rhythm, increased intracardiac pressures may lead to atrial stretch and dilatation, predisposing to both the development and recurrence of atrial fibrillation.

Electrophysiology

Several potential electrophysiologic mechanisms may be responsible for atrial fibrillation (Fig. 58.3).[4,31] One postulated mechanism is multiple wavelet re-entry, in which a critical number of wavefronts continuously sweep through the atria in random fashion. The multiple wavelet hypothesis requires the presence of a minimum number of wavefronts (more than five or six) and enough atrial tissue to permit their simultaneous propagation. An alternate hypothesis is that only one or two primary re-entrant circuits or rotors are constantly forming and disappearing, but the cycle lengths in these circuits are too short to allow the rest of the atria to follow in an organized fashion, resulting in "fibrillatory conduction."[31] It has been shown clinically that atrial fibrillation may be produced by rapid tachycardias from either focal sources, commonly found in the musculature of the pulmonary veins, or stable re-entrant circuits that drive the remaining atrial tissue until degeneration to atrial fibrillation occurs.[31,32] The pulmonary veins, which include muscular sleeves that may be electrically active, and the posterior left atrial wall are now considered the critical structures involved in the re-entrant excitation that leads to the initiation of atrial fibrillation. However, as the duration of atrial fibrillation increases, excitation frequency in other sites may become more important.

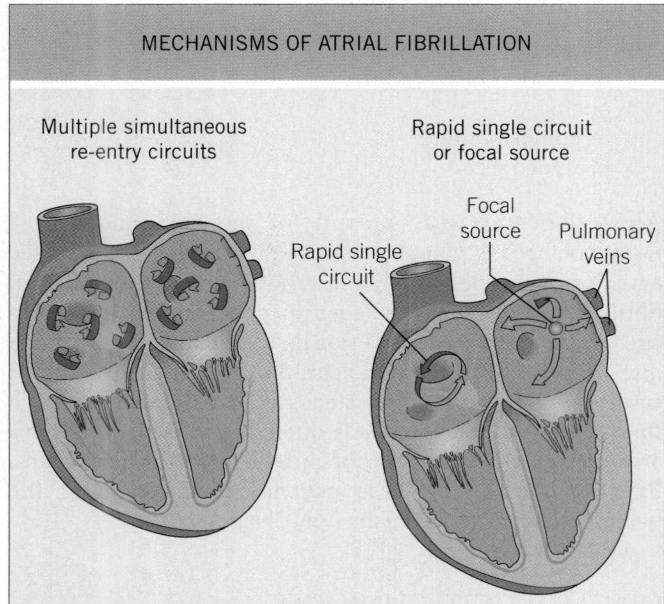

Figure 58.3 Mechanisms of atrial fibrillation. The mechanisms include multiple simultaneous and unstable re-entry circuits in both atria and a small, rapid re-entrant circuit or a source.

The cellular action potential changes seen in atrial fibrillation are a decrease in duration and a depression of plateau potential.[4,32] The action potential exhibits altered restitution; therefore, the response to rapid changes in rate is attenuated and vulnerability to the propagation of premature depolarizations is increased. Changes in calcium handling, reductions in I_{to}, I_{Kur}, and $I_{Ca\text{-}L}$, and increases in I_{K1} and $I_{K,ACh}$ are thought to be the responsible ionic mechanisms. Disorganization and fragmentation of gap junctions have been described. Metabolic factors arising from the rapid rate and genetic factors also play a role in modulating channel activity. These changes develop in a time-dependent fashion as a result of the rapid atrial rate. Thus, atrial fibrillation is a self-perpetuating phenomenon by means of what has been termed electrical remodeling.[32] Sinus node function is also depressed. All of these changes are reversible over time after restoration of sinus rhythm.

The electrophysiology of the AV node plays an important part in the clinical manifestations of atrial fibrillation. The atrial cycle length in atrial fibrillation is short (usually less than 160 ms), and multiple impulses bombard the AV node during its refractory period and are not conducted. Some impulses, although they are not fully conducted, partially penetrate the node and reset the refractory period for subsequent impulses. This process of "concealed conduction" is the key to achieving control of ventricular rates in atrial fibrillation. When atrial fibrillation occurs in patients with pre-excitation, extremely rapid ventricular rates may occur because the refractory period of the accessory connection, rather than that of the AV node, may be the chief determinant of AV conduction (see Chapter 60).

CLINICAL PRESENTATIONS

Clinical Classification

Several approaches for classifying atrial fibrillation have been devised.[4,7] In general, atrial fibrillation can be categorized as acute or chronic.

- *Acute atrial fibrillation* refers either to an episode of atrial fibrillation related to a transient, reversible cause, or to a patient's first episode of atrial fibrillation.
- *Chronic atrial fibrillation* implies recurrent, prolonged or continuing episodes.

Chronic atrial fibrillation can be subclassified as either

- paroxysmal (self-terminating) atrial fibrillation; or
- sustained atrial fibrillation.

Sustained atrial fibrillation can in turn be categorized as

- persistent atrial fibrillation, which is sustained atrial fibrillation that can be successfully cardioverted; and
- permanent atrial fibrillation, which is sustained atrial fibrillation that is resistant to or not appropriate for cardioversion.

Among patients who have chronic forms of atrial fibrillation, this temporally based clinical classification can assist management strategies, particularly in relation to rhythm control or rate control. Rhythm control is the approach for paroxysmal and persistent atrial fibrillation, whereas rate control is the strategy applied for permanent atrial fibrillation. In paroxysmal atrial fibrillation, the episodes are generally self-terminating; therefore, the goals of therapy are the prevention of paroxysms and long-term maintenance of sinus rhythm. In sustained atrial fibrillation, the therapeutic goal is either cardioversion to sinus rhythm (persistent atrial fibrillation) or heart rate control. Antithrombotic therapy for moderate or high-risk patients is an important component of both strategies. Figure 58.4 illustrates this approach.

Differentiation of these clinical categories depends on

- the history given by the patient;
- ECG documentation of the current episode; and
- the duration of the most recent previous episode of atrial fibrillation.

Although this classification is helpful, considerable variability exists, both among patients and in the same patient, in the temporal pattern of atrial fibrillation episodes, and approaches to therapy must be individualized, especially in relation to symptoms. Furthermore, paroxysmal atrial fibrillation may become permanent (8% at 1 year, 18% at 4 years), especially with increasing age.[33]

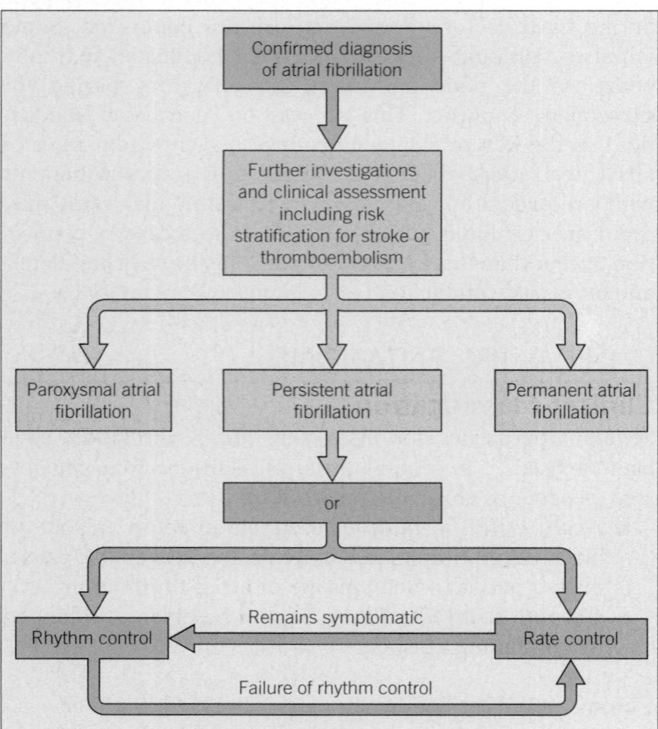

Figure 58.4 Treatment strategy decision tree in relation to clinical subtypes of atrial fibrillation.

Other classifications may also be helpful. Some patients have paroxysmal atrial fibrillation that is clearly mediated by changes in autonomic tone. Acetylcholine shortens the duration of the atrial action potential and facilitates induction of atrial fibrillation. The clinical syndrome of vagally induced atrial fibrillation occurs at night or after meals, especially in male patients who have organic heart disease. By contrast, some patients have atrial fibrillation that is adrenergically mediated and is seen only during exercise, emotion, and stress.

Symptoms

Atrial fibrillation is encountered in a wide variety of clinical settings. For example, it may be discovered incidentally in an asymptomatic patient; it may develop in a patient who merely has a fever or chest infection; or it may be found in a patient with a ventricular rate greater than 200 beats per minute who is too light-headed to stand up. Both symptomatic and asymptomatic episodes of atrial fibrillation can occur in the same patient.[34] Paroxysmal atrial fibrillation has a circadian pattern with decreased frequency and duration between 10 AM and 12 noon.

Asymptomatic atrial fibrillation is usually discovered incidentally by cardiac auscultation, a routine 12-lead ECG, or a 24-hour ECG recording undertaken for unrelated reasons. Asymptomatic atrial fibrillation has the same prognostic implications as symptomatic atrial fibrillation.[35] The duration of atrial fibrillation may be unknown in such patients. Other patients who have new-onset atrial fibrillation present with symptoms related to the arrhythmia.

Symptoms during atrial fibrillation vary, depending on the ventricular rate, the underlying functional status of the heart, and the duration of atrial fibrillation. Minor symptoms include

- palpitations;
- a sense of the heart racing;
- fatigue;
- light-headedness;
- increased urination; and
- mild shortness of breath.

More severe symptoms include

- congestive heart failure;
- angina;
- hypotension; and
- presyncope.

Atrial fibrillation may present for the first time with a thromboembolic complication (e.g., stroke or systemic embolus). Syncope is a rare but serious complication of atrial fibrillation, but it may be seen in patients who have preexcitation, enhanced AV nodal conduction, sinus node disease, or severe structural heart disease (e.g., hypertrophic cardiomyopathy) or aortic stenosis. In patients who have sinus node disease, syncope is often due to periods of sinus arrest when the paroxysm of atrial fibrillation terminates. Effective therapy of these patients usually requires the implantation of a pacemaker (see Chapter 53).

DIAGNOSTIC TECHNIQUES

An outline of the basic work-up for patients with atrial fibrillation is given in Table 58.2.[4] The investigation of atrial fibrillation requires a careful clinical history (including a past

INITIAL EVALUATION OF PATIENTS WITH ATRIAL FIBRILLATION
Minimum evaluation
History and physical examination
Electrocardiography
Chest radiography
Echocardiography
Laboratory studies (thyroid, renal function)
Optional studies
Exercise testing or ambulatory electrocardiography
Transesophageal echocardiography
Electrophysiologic study
Modified from Fuster V, Ryden LE, Cannom DS, et al. ACC/AHA/ESC 2006 guidelines for the management of patients with atrial fibrillation: a report of the American College of Cardiology/American Heart Association Task Force on Practice Guidelines and the European Society of Cardiology Committee for Practice Guidelines (Writing Committee to Revise the 2001 Guidelines for the Management of Patients with Atrial Fibrillation). J Am Coll Cardiol 2006;48:e149-e246.

Table 58.2 Initial evaluation of patients with atrial fibrillation.

medical history) with emphasis on certain clinical features. The history should cover whether the symptoms are sustained or intermittent and whether any complications are present, such as heart failure, stroke or thromboembolism). Other useful data include

- the date of the first episode;
- information about acute precipitating factors or chronic conditions linked to atrial fibrillation;
- how symptoms are relieved;
- the typical duration of episodes and the typical interval between them;
- the duration of the current or most recent episode; and
- current and past drug treatment.

Blood Tests

At the initial consultation, basic blood tests, including a full blood count, biochemistry (renal function, electrolytes), and thyroid function tests, are done. A full blood count is useful to exclude anemia because anticoagulation may be considered. Serum urea and electrolytes are relevant for consideration of drug therapy (e.g., the dose of digoxin is reduced with renal impairment). The risk of atrial fibrillation is increased by clinical and subclinical hyperthyroidism; therefore, the serum thyroid-stimulating hormone level should be measured in all patients with atrial fibrillation, even if no symptoms suggestive of thyrotoxicosis are seen.

Chest Radiography

A chest radiograph may occasionally be useful in patients with atrial fibrillation. For example, in young patients who have atrial fibrillation, a chest radiograph may provide a clue to congenital heart disease, such as an atrial septal defect. In older patients, the chest radiograph can give information on heart size and the presence of heart failure or coexisting intrathoracic pathology.

Documentation of the Arrhythmia

The arrhythmia should be documented, ideally with a standard 12-lead ECG. The characteristic ECG findings in atrial fibrillation include (Fig. 58.4)

- rapid baseline oscillations or fibrillatory waves that vary in size, shape, and timing;
- the absence of discrete P waves; and
- an irregularly irregular ventricular rate.

The ECG may also provide a clue to the etiology or electrophysiologic features that may have caused the atrial fibrillation (e.g., a previous myocardial infarction, left ventricular hypertrophy or pre-excitation). Often patients present with previous symptoms suggestive of atrial fibrillation but are in sinus rhythm at the time of their evaluation. If symptoms occur on a daily basis, a 24-hour ambulatory ECG should provide the diagnosis. If symptoms occur less frequently, a patient-activated event recorder or an implanted loop recorder is more likely to provide a diagnosis.

Echocardiography

An echocardiogram provides important information for the initial evaluation of most patients with atrial fibrillation.[4,36] Either transthoracic echocardiography or transesophageal echocardiography (TEE), or a combination of the two, may be appropriate. The initial goal of echocardiographic evaluation should be to establish the presence or absence of structural heart disease, including valvular abnormalities, congenital anomalies, chamber dimensions, pericardial thickening or effusions, and ventricular function.

Left atrial size is an important predictor of outcome in patients with atrial fibrillation because in most series, significant left atrial enlargement has been shown to reduce the chances of successful cardioversion and long-term maintenance of sinus rhythm. Left atrial enlargement may also increase the risk of stroke owing to a greater potential for stasis in the dilated chamber.

Although transthoracic echocardiography is adequate for assessing chamber size, detection of thrombi or assessment of the left atrial appendage anatomy and function requires the transesophageal approach. When TEE is used, up to 27% of patients with atrial fibrillation of longer than 3 days' duration may show detectable thrombi (Fig. 58.5). A

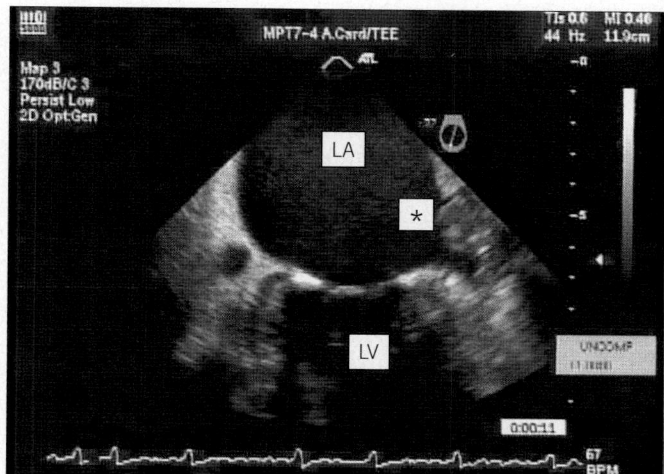

Figure 58.5 Transesophageal echocardiogram (TEE) of a thrombus *(asterisk)* in the left atrial appendage. A TEE was performed before a cardioversion attempt in a patient with atrial fibrillation, hypertrophic cardiomyopathy, and left atrial enlargement. LA, left atrium; LV, left ventricle. The TEE also demonstrates spontaneous echo contrast (SEC) in the left atrium.

prethrombotic finding, spontaneous echo contrast (also called smoke), is due to erythrocyte aggregation in the low-flow state and is even more common. Other TEE indices of high stroke risk include the presence of a left atrial thrombus, low left atrial appendage velocities, dense spontaneous echo contrast, and complex aortic plaque in the descending aorta.[36]

Any condition that leads to atrial hypertension, atrial stretch, or atrial fibrosis can result in atrial fibrillation. Mitral valve disease commonly leads to atrial fibrillation and may be clinically difficult to identify without echocardiography. Systolic and diastolic ventricular dysfunction can also lead to atrial hypertension and atrial fibrillation and, if present, should influence the choice of therapies for either rate control or maintenance of sinus rhythm.

Diastolic dysfunction is increasingly recognized as a predictor of subsequent atrial fibrillation. In an analysis from Olmsted County, Minnesota, the subsequent development of atrial fibrillation in patients without diastolic dysfunction was 1% versus approximately 12% in patients with moderate diastolic dysfunction and 20% in those with severe diastolic dysfunction (restrictive physiology).[37]

Other Investigations

If the patient complains of angina, the clinician should determine whether the angina occurs only during attacks of atrial fibrillation arising from an uncontrolled ventricular rate or whether it occurs independently of the arrhythmia. Exercise testing occasionally may be needed to clarify the severity of underlying cardiac ischemia. Exercise or ambulatory electrocardiography may also aid in assessment of the adequacy of drug treatment in heart rate control. Cardiac catheterization is usually required only if indicated by symptoms or if noninvasive test results suggest active ischemia.

Electrophysiologic Testing

Invasive electrophysiologic studies have only a limited role in the routine evaluation of patients with atrial fibrillation unless catheter ablation is planned. Electrophysiologic studies of atrial fibrillation should be reserved for the following situations:

- when another arrhythmia (e.g., atrial flutter or atrial or supraventricular tachycardia) is thought to be the cause of the atrial fibrillation;
- when other electrophysiologic abnormalities or symptoms (e.g., pre-excitation, sinus node dysfunction, syncope) require clarification or therapy;
- when catheter ablation is planned.

MANAGEMENT

Certain questions should be considered in the approach to management of a patient with atrial fibrillation:

- Is the diagnosis of atrial fibrillation certain, and are any other associated arrhythmias or conduction abnormalities present?
- Can any precipitating factors or predisposing conditions be identified, and are these factors reversible or preventable?
- Do the patient's symptoms warrant urgent intervention?
- Are restoration and maintenance of sinus rhythm of critical importance, or is effective rate control likely to be adequate?

Acute Atrial Fibrillation

Patients with acute atrial fibrillation are those with a recent onset of continuing atrial fibrillation that is seen within 48 hours after the onset.[38] This category therefore includes patients with a first or recurrent episode of persistent atrial fibrillation, as well as those with a continuing episode of paroxysmal atrial fibrillation. The approach to patients presenting with acute-onset atrial fibrillation depends on the initial assessment of the individual's hemodynamic status because patients who are hemodynamically compromised may require emergency direct current cardioversion (Fig. 58.6). On admission, while definitive therapy is planned, all patients should be administered intravenous unfractionated or subcutaneous low-molecular-weight heparin to minimize the risk for thromboembolism (Table 58.3). Patients with associated complications (e.g., heart failure, stroke, thromboembolism) should be managed accordingly. In patients with an inappropriately fast heart rate, rate control with beta blockers, rate-limiting calcium antagonists (verapamil, diltiazem), or digoxin may be considered. Pharmacologic conversion using either intravenous or oral therapy may be considered, as outlined in Table 58.4. If cardioversion is considered and the duration of atrial fibrillation is longer than 48 hours, a minimum of 4 weeks of anticoagulation after cardioversion is recommended (see Table 58.3).[4]

Paroxysmal Atrial Fibrillation

Paroxysmal atrial fibrillation commonly is defined as episodes that usually last less than 48 hours, and no longer than 7 days, before spontaneous termination. In patients with paroxysmal atrial fibrillation, the goals of therapy are to control symptoms caused by the episodes and to prevent thromboembolic complications.[4,39] Symptom control may be accomplished either with antiarrhythmic therapy for long-term maintenance of sinus rhythm or with AV nodal–blocking agents to control ventricular rates during paroxysms.

If a patient is experiencing only mild and infrequent symptoms, it may be possible to avoid chronic therapy with antiarrhythmic drugs and their potential for extracardiac and cardiac toxicity. General measures should always be considered (e.g., caffeine or alcohol withdrawal and stress counseling), as should atrial pacing for conditions that may benefit from it (e.g., sick sinus syndrome).

Effective rate control in patients with paroxysmal atrial fibrillation is often challenging. These patients are usually in sinus rhythm, and the effects of AV nodal–blocking agents on ventricular rates in a future atrial fibrillation episode are unpredictable. Digoxin should be avoided as monotherapy for rate control, inasmuch as evidence suggests that it makes paroxysmal atrial fibrillation worse. The major effect of digoxin on the AV node is to enhance vagal tone, and there should be little vagal influence on the ventricular rate during exercise or stress. Calcium channel blockers and beta blockers may help control the ventricular rate in paroxysmal atrial fibrillation, but they may not reduce the frequency of episodes. However, patients who have atrial fibrillation only during exercise or stress may respond well to beta blockers.

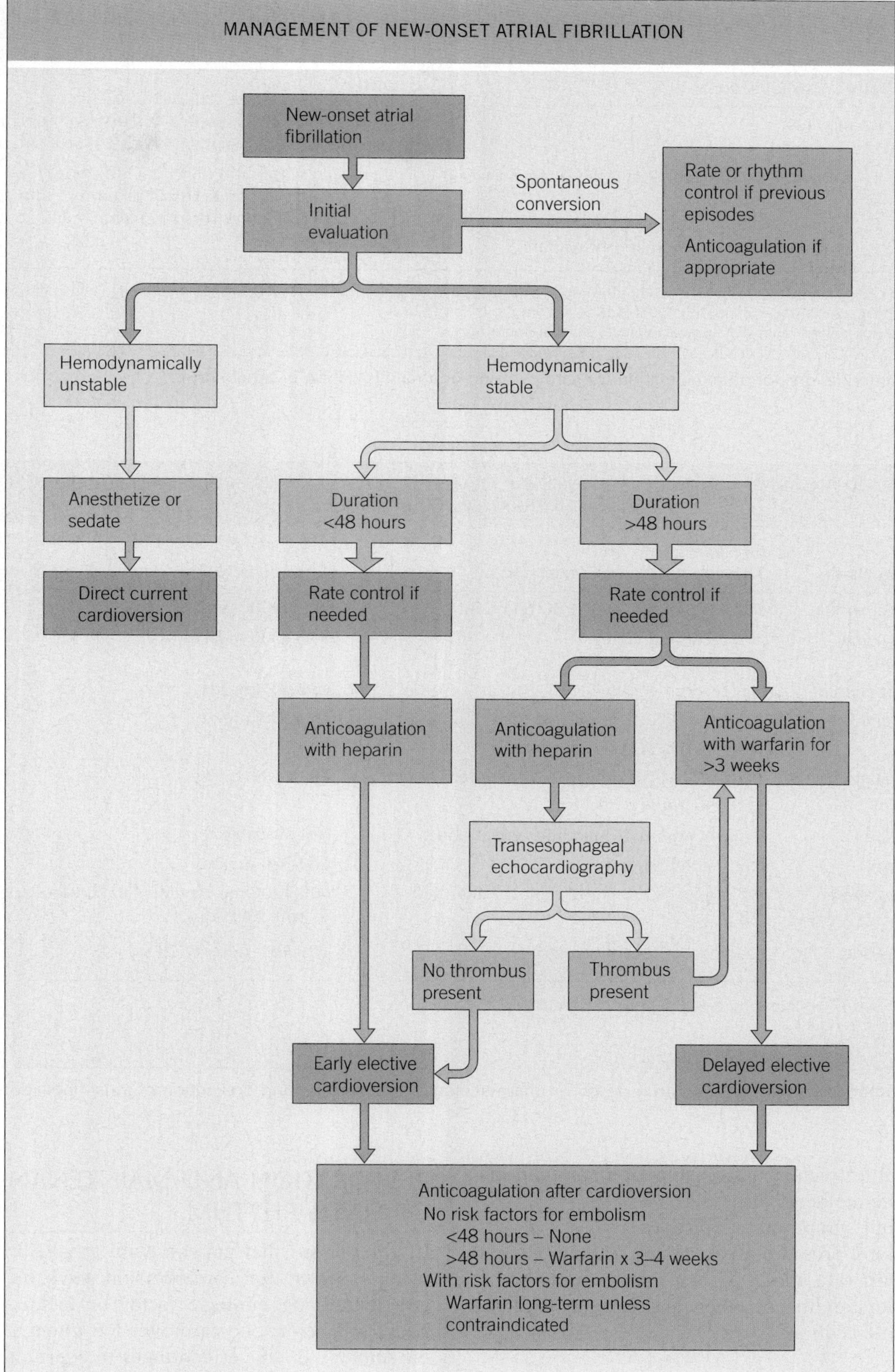

Figure 58.6 Management of new-onset atrial fibrillation.

The principles for use of class I and class III antiarrhythmic drugs in patients with paroxysmal atrial fibrillation are the same as for the use of these drugs to prevent recurrence in patients with persistent atrial fibrillation (discussed later in this chapter and in Chapter 50). In patients with minimal heart disease, oral loading doses of propafenone or flecainide may be used intermittently (the so-called pill in the pocket approach) to terminate acute episodes or shorten paroxysms.

In patients with paroxysmal atrial fibrillation, a "pill in the pocket" strategy can be considered in those who have

RECOMMENDATIONS FOR ANTICOAGULATION FOR CARDIOVERSION OF ATRIAL FIBRILLATION OR ATRIAL FLUTTER		
Duration of Arrhythmia	**Before Cardioversion**	**After Cardioversion**
<48 hours	Not required	Estimate risk of recurrence and assess chronic risk for stroke. If either is high, maintain INR at 2.0-3.0 with warfarin.
≥48 hours	1. Warfarin to maintain INR at 2.0-3.0 for 3-4 weeks *or* 2. TEE; if negative for thrombus, initiate and maintain anticoagulation (heparin and/or warfarin)	*All patients:* Warfarin (INR, 2.0-3.0) for at least 4 weeks. *After 4 weeks:* Estimate risk of recurrence and assess chronic risk for stroke. If either is high, maintain INR at 2.0-3.0 with warfarin.

Modified from Singer DE, Albers GW, Dalen JE, et al. Antithrombotic therapy in atrial fibrillation: the Seventh ACCP Conference on Antithrombotic and Thrombolytic Therapy. Chest 2004;126(Suppl 3):429S-456S.
INR, international normalized ratio; TEE, transesophageal echocardiogram.

Table 58.3 Recommendations for anticoagulation for cardioversion of atrial fibrillation or atrial flutter.

RECOMMENDED ANTIARRHYTHMIC DRUG DOSES FOR PHARMACOLOGIC CARDIOVERSION AND PREVENTION OF ATRIAL FIBRILLATION RECURRENCE			
Drug Class	**Drug Name**	**Intravenous or Oral Therapy for Rapid Conversion**	**Chronic Oral Drug Therapy to Prevent Recurrence***
Ia	Procainamide	500-1200 mg IV during 30-60 minutes	2000-4000 mg/day
	Quinidine sulfate	Not recommended	600-1200 mg/day
	Disopyramide	Not recommended	450-600 mg/day
Ic	Flecainide	1.5-3.0 mg/kg IV during 10 minutes† 200-400 mg PO	150-300 mg/day
	Propafenone	1.5-2 mg/kg IV during 10-20 minutes† 300-450 mg PO	400-600 mg/day
III	Ibutilide	1 mg IV during 10 minutes, repeat once	Not available
	Sotalol	Not recommended	160-320 mg/day
	Amiodarone	5-7 mg/kg IV during 30 minutes, then 1.2-1.8 g/day	400-1200 mg/day for 7 days, then taper to 100-300 mg/day
	Dofetilide	Loading not recommended	125-500 μg every 12 hours

*Initiation of oral therapy without loading may also result in conversion.
†Not available in North America.
IV, intravenously; PO, orally.

Table 58.4 Recommended antiarrhythmic drug doses for pharmacologic cardioversion and prevention of atrial fibrillation recurrence.

- no history of left ventricular dysfunction, valvular disease, or ischemic heart disease;
- infrequent but symptomatic episodes;
- a systolic blood pressure greater than 100 mm Hg and a resting heart rate above 70 beats per minute; and
- a good understanding of when and how to take the prescribed medications.

Antithrombotic therapy of paroxysmal atrial fibrillation should be considered because patients with paroxysmal atrial fibrillation have a stroke rate similar to that of patients with chronic atrial fibrillation.[40,41] Nevertheless, the range of thromboembolic risk in such patients is likely to be wide because a patient who has one short paroxysm once a year is likely to be at less risk than a patient who has long daily paroxysms.

RESTORATION AND MAINTENANCE OF SINUS RHYTHM

It is important that patients with atrial fibrillation who are being assessed for cardioversion have an assessment for any underlying etiologic factor or factors that should be addressed before the cardioversion attempt. If the underlying etiology or trigger continues to exert an effect, attempts at cardioversion may be unsuccessful. An algorithm for the management of new- or recent-onset atrial fibrillation is presented in Figure 58.6.

Not all patients can be successfully cardioverted. Predictors of refractoriness to cardioversion or unsuccessful maintenance of sinus rhythm include

- the age of the patient;
- the duration of the arrhythmia;

- the presence of uncontrolled hypertension;
- the severity of any structural heart disease; and
- the presence of other systemic diseases.

Left atrial size may also be an important predictor of outcome, but patients who have mild or moderate left atrial enlargement usually can be converted.

The duration of continuous arrhythmia before the conversion attempt is perhaps the most important factor. The probability of remaining in sinus rhythm after cardioversion increases twofold in patients who have had a short duration of atrial fibrillation (less than 3 months) compared with patients who have had atrial fibrillation for longer than 12 months. Few patients who have had persistent atrial fibrillation for longer than 2 years can be converted and then successfully maintained in sinus rhythm.[4]

If atrial fibrillation is secondary to hyperthyroidism, cardioversion should be delayed until thyroid function has returned to normal. Atrial fibrillation as a complication of cardiac surgery is common and tends to be self-limiting within 10 to 14 days after surgery; therefore, cardioversion may not be required if ventricular rates can be controlled. In atrial fibrillation in patients with myocardial infarction or a low ejection fraction, the optimal approach to antiarrhythmic therapy for restoration of sinus rhythm has yet to be ascertained. Patients who have sinus node dysfunction, as in the bradycardia-tachycardia syndrome, are also relatively unfavorable candidates for cardioversion unless back-up pacing support is provided.

The optimal time for a cardioversion attempt depends on the hemodynamic status of the patient and the duration of the episode. Patients with hemodynamic collapse or those who remain highly symptomatic require urgent or early cardioversion. In other patients, the duration of the arrhythmia influences management.

Thromboembolism is the most worrisome complication after cardioversion of persistent atrial fibrillation. It is infrequent in atrial fibrillation of less than 48 hours' duration, but it has been noted to occur after pharmacologic or electrical cardioversion in up to 7% of patients who have nonvalvular atrial fibrillation of more than 48 hours' duration without the use of anticoagulation. The incidence in patients who have mitral valve disease is even higher.

Several mechanisms and risk factors contribute to thromboembolism after cardioversion of atrial fibrillation. A mechanical explanation is that resumption of atrial systolic function results in the embolization of any preexisting clot within the left atrium. Recovery of atrial contraction is delayed and may take up to 3 weeks after cardioversion, and thrombi may form during this period. However, virtually all embolic events occur in the first week after conversion.[42]

A recently formed, poorly adherent thrombus is more likely to dislodge at the time of cardioversion; more chronic thrombi usually are firmly adherent as a result of fibroblastic infiltration. An estimate of the time required for the latter process is approximately 14 days. Adequate anticoagulation for this period might prevent new clot formation and allow the most recently formed thrombi to become sufficiently adherent. However, this interval cannot be precisely defined and is likely to vary according to the patient's hemodynamic status, atrial size and underlying atrial pathology, and the intensity of anticoagulation. Cardioversion itself may actually promote new thrombus formation owing to transient atrial dysfunction ("stunning") in the postcardioversion period.

Studies using TEE have demonstrated development of spontaneous echo contrast and thromboembolic complications after cardioversion, even in the absence of demonstrable left atrial thrombi before the procedure. Furthermore, atrial fibrillation is associated with abnormalities of hemostasis, blood rheology, and endothelial dysfunction, which confer a hypercoagulable state that is transiently more severe after cardioversion.[28,43] Atrial fibrillation is also associated with elevated levels of atrial natriuretic peptide, which may contribute to hemoconcentration, a raised hematocrit, and subsequent thromboembolism and stroke. Finally, cerebral blood flow appears to be increased after cardioversion from atrial fibrillation to normal sinus rhythm, and this may predispose to cerebral embolism in the distribution of the middle cerebral artery.

Recommendations have been published for anticoagulation to prevent thromboembolism after cardioversion of atrial fibrillation (see Table 58.3).[4,44] Anticoagulation must be continued in the presence of a high risk of recurrence after cardioversion or if the patient has risk factors for stroke and thromboembolism. Factors indicating a high risk for recurrence include a history of failed attempts at cardioversion, significant structural heart disease, a history of atrial fibrillation for longer than 12 months, and recurrence after a previous cardioversion.

TEE may be used to facilitate early cardioversion. TEE has a high sensitivity and specificity for detecting left atrial thrombi. Theoretically, if TEE shows an absence of thrombi before cardioversion and if anticoagulation is then maintained throughout the period of atrial recovery, the delay of several weeks before cardioversion may be avoided. In a TEE-guided approach to cardioversion, the patient is anticoagulated with heparin, and warfarin is initiated (target international normalized ratio [INR], 2.0-3.0). A multiplane TEE is performed to assess left atrial size and the presence of atrial thrombi. If a thrombus is seen, cardioversion is postponed. The patient is anticoagulated for a minimum of 4 weeks, and a follow-up TEE is performed to document thrombus resolution before cardioversion is attempted. Anticoagulation with warfarin should be continued for at least 4 weeks after atrial fibrillation cardioversion in all patients, regardless of the cardioversion method.

TEE-guided cardioversion is probably the best strategy for patients at increased risk of warfarin morbidity to decrease the duration of anticoagulation and also for patients with a short duration (2 to 30 days) of atrial fibrillation at presentation, in whom a delay might render the atrium more unstable. Recent studies indicate that the TEE-guided approach has a safety profile similar to that of conventional management and may be cost-effective in some situations.[44]

Electrical Cardioversion

Electrical cardioversion restores sinus rhythm in patients with atrial fibrillation by repolarizing the atrial myocardium, thereby restoring organized activity. After an initial asystolic period, the sinoatrial node should resume its role as cardiac pacemaker. The success rate of electrical cardioversion is highly influenced by the underlying etiology. The highest recorded success rates for cardioversion are seen in patients whose atrial fibrillation is secondary to hyperthyroidism (which has been corrected), and the lowest rates are seen in patients with severe mitral regurgitation. Attention to proper technique for external cardioversion greatly improves efficacy. R-wave synchronization is necessary to avoid shock-induced ventricular arrhythmias. Technical aspects that have to be considered include

- the electrode's size;
- the placement of the electrode (anteroapical or anteroposterior);
- the transthoracic impedance, a factor influenced by pressure on the electrodes;
- the efficacy of the dispersive gel and previous shocks;
- the defibrillation waveform (monophasic versus biphasic); and
- the amount of stored energy.

Biphasic shocks are more effective than monophasic shocks of equal energy. An initial energy of 125 J may be used for biphasic shocks, and 200 J is advised for monophasic shocks.

Limited evidence is available about the effect of antiarrhythmic agents on energy requirements and the success rate of cardioversion. Early failure may be due either to a high atrial defibrillation threshold or to immediate or early recurrence of atrial fibrillation. Ibutilide (1 to 2 mg intravenously) has been reported to lower the high atrial defibrillation threshold and prevent recurrence and may be given during the same procedure. When atrial fibrillation is difficult to convert and long-term therapy is indicated, loading with a class III antiarrhythmic drug (e.g., amiodarone, sotalol, or dofetilide) before the cardioversion attempt may result in success. Internal cardioversion using shocks from an intracardiac electrode and the use of up to 720 J of transthoracic shocks have been reported to be effective in resistant cases. The introduction of external defibrillators with biphasic waveforms and judicious use of antiarrhythmic drugs to facilitate defibrillation and prevent early recurrence have limited the need for these steps.

Nonembolic complications of external cardioversion are rare but include

- ventricular arrhythmia;
- sinus bradycardia;
- hypotension;
- pulmonary edema;
- skin burns; and
- transient ST segment and T-wave abnormalities.

Pharmacologic Cardioversion

An alternative to electrical cardioversion, especially for patients with recent-onset atrial fibrillation, is pharmacologic cardioversion. It should be noted that a high percentage of episodes of new-onset atrial fibrillation terminate spontaneously within 24 to 48 hours, even without specific therapy. Patients with long-standing atrial fibrillation rarely convert with drug therapy alone. Therefore, published studies on the efficacy of any antiarrhythmic drug may have different placebo-conversion rates, depending on the study's entry criteria. Only a few randomized trials that have compared drugs for conversion are available. Table 58.4 lists the agents that are effective for pharmacologic conversion of atrial fibrillation. Ibutilide is available only in an intravenous formulation and is most useful in acute settings, when long-term antiarrhythmic therapy is not planned. The other agents listed may be selected if chronic therapy will be used. Selected patients may be able to terminate episodes using oral loading doses of propafenone or flecainide on an outpatient basis. Only patients without important structural heart disease should be candidates for this "pill in the pocket" approach.

Antiarrhythmic Drugs to Prevent Recurrence

No antiarrhythmic drug is uniformly effective for preventing recurrent atrial fibrillation. Therefore, the algorithm for drug selection in the most recent guidelines established by the American College of Cardiology/American Heart Association/European Society of Cardiology (ACC/AHA/ESC) is based on a balance of safety and efficacy in patients with various cardiac diagnoses[45] (see Fig. 58.7). In randomized trials that have compared various antiarrhythmic agents, amiodarone has been shown to be superior to sotalol and to class I agents.[46-48] Comparisons of sotalol and class I agents typically have shown no significant difference in efficacy. Very little comparative data are available for more recently developed agents, such as dofetilide, dronedarone, or azimilide. In postoperative patients, β-adrenergic drugs have been shown to be helpful in preventing episodes in patients at risk.

It is difficult to eliminate all recurrences of atrial fibrillation with drug therapy. Therefore, in patients with paroxysmal atrial fibrillation, a decrease in the frequency or severity of episodes to a level that is acceptable to the patient is a practical goal. In patients with persistent atrial fibrillation, prolongation of the intervals between cardioversions is a reasonable target. Using this strategy, a single recurrent episode would not necessitate a change in therapy. If the frequency of episodes dictates a change, either higher doses of the current drug or another agent may be tried. Using this type of approach, many patients can be successfully maintained in sinus rhythm with a combination of drug therapy and periodic cardioversions.[49]

A particular concern with the use of antiarrhythmic drugs for treatment of atrial fibrillation is the risk of proarrhythmia. Virtually all antiarrhythmic drugs may cause sinus node dysfunction or AV block in susceptible individuals. Class Ia and class III antiarrhythmic drugs may lengthen the QT interval and produce polymorphic ventricular tachycardia, which can be fatal (Fig. 58.8). Class Ia and Ic drugs and amiodarone may organize atrial fibrillation to atrial flutter with a long cycle length. If AV nodal conduction is not blocked, 1:1 conduction may occur, with hemodynamic collapse (Fig. 58.9).

Permanent Atrial Fibrillation and Control of the Heart Rate

In permanent atrial fibrillation, the management strategy should be effective control of the heart rate and appropriate

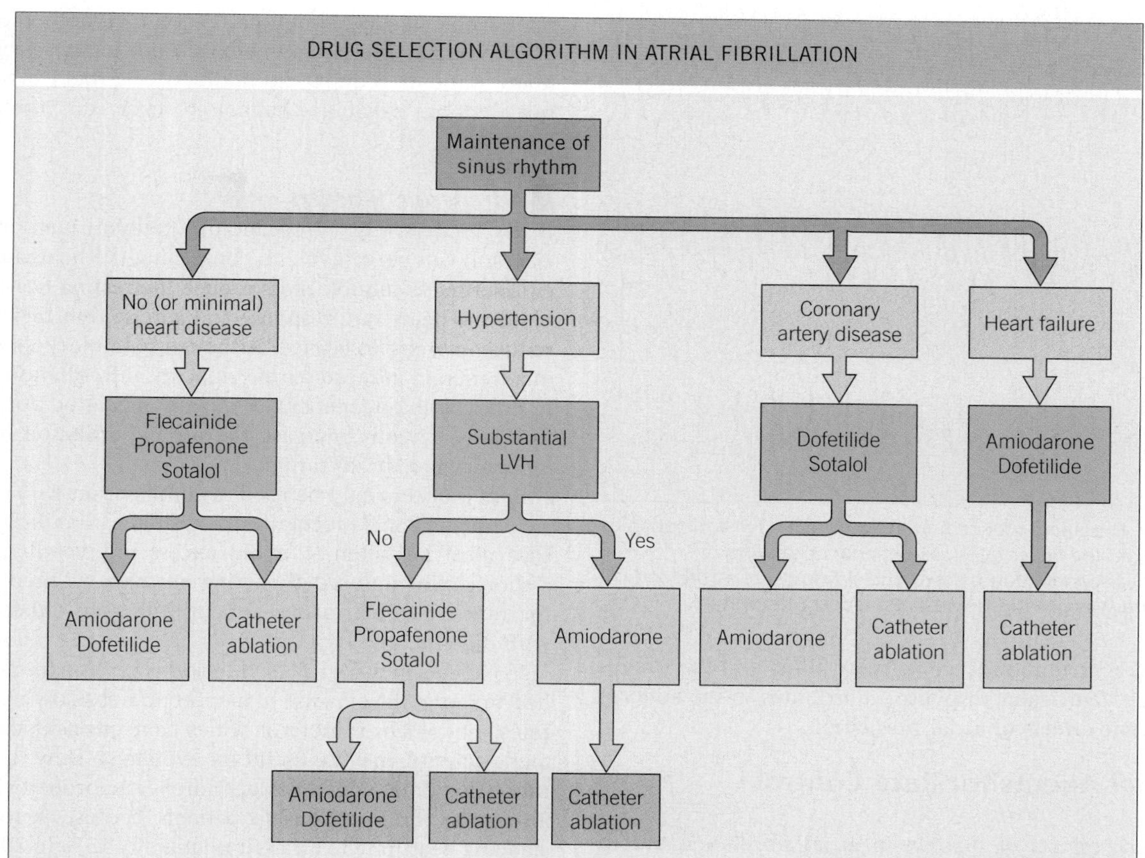

Figure 58.7 Drug selection algorithm in atrial fibrillation. LVH, left ventricular hypertrophy. (From Fuster V, Ryden LE, Cannom DS, et al. ACC/AHA/ESC 2006 guidelines for the management of patients with atrial fibrillation: a report of the American College of Cardiology/American Heart Association Task Force on Practice Guidelines and the European Society of Cardiology Committee for Practice Guidelines [Writing Committee to Revise the 2001 Guidelines for the Management of Patients with Atrial fibrillation]. J Am Coll Cardiol 2006;48:e149-e246.)

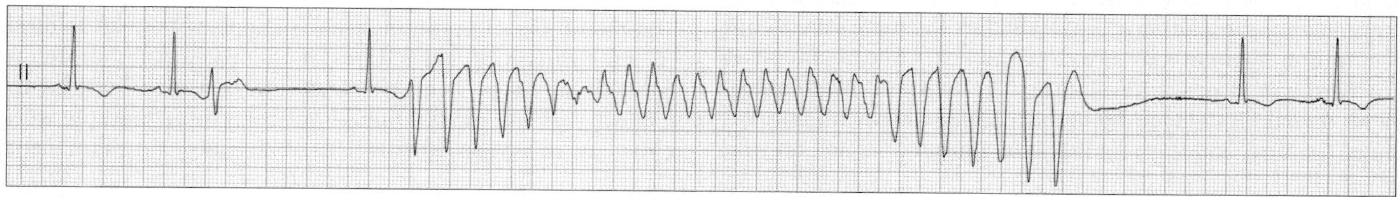

Figure 58.8 Torsades de pointes after conversion of atrial fibrillation. This patient had received intravenous ibutilide and converted to sinus rhythm. Shortly afterward, this episode of polymorphic ventricular tachycardia was recorded.

antithrombotic therapy. Strategies for heart rate control are often complex, and both pharmacologic (Table 58.5) and nonpharmacologic approaches may be appropriate. In patients with pre-excitation, agents that affect the AV node may actually worsen the heart rate in atrial fibrillation (see Chapter 60).

The definition of adequate rate control in atrial fibrillation is still controversial. Optimal control of the heart rate during atrial fibrillation is probably the heart rate that maximizes cardiac output. One definition of effective control of the heart rate is a ventricular rate that ranges between 60 and 80 beats per minute at rest and between 90 and 115 beats per minute during moderate exercise. A recent consensus conference stated that the ventricular rate should be under 90 beats per minute at rest and under 180 beats per minute during exercise.[50]

The heart rate response during a 6-minute walk test is a convenient way to assess heart rate control in many patients. Heart rate control in patients with paroxysmal atrial fibrillation is extremely challenging because the heart rate during sinus rhythm does not predict the atrial fibrillation heart rate, which may vary widely in the same individual during recurrent episodes. Even patients who present with highly symptomatic episodes probably have other spells that are asymptomatic.

Uncontrolled heart rates in atrial fibrillation may have an untoward effect on cardiac function, resulting in a tachycardia-induced cardiomyopathy. This factor, along with the loss

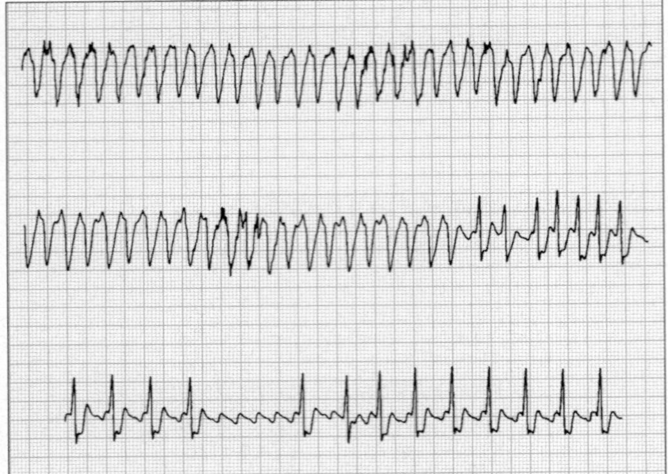

Figure 58.9 Flecainide-induced atrial flutter with 1:1 and variable conduction. At the faster rate, use-dependent slowing of intraventricular conduction is seen. The slowing rate at the end of the recording was produced with intravenous metoprolol.

of an atrial contribution to ventricular filling and the irregularity of the ventricular response, contributes to the adverse hemodynamic effects of atrial fibrillation.

Individual Agents for Rate Control

Digoxin

The primary effects of digoxin in atrial fibrillation are to enhance vagal tone and prolong AV node refractoriness. In heart failure, the increase in cardiac contractility and the improvement in hemodynamics with digoxin also reduce symptoms of low output and reflex sympathetic activation. However, digoxin is less likely to control the ventricular rate during fever, stress, or exercise (e.g., when vagal tone is low and sympathetic tone is high). It also has little or no ability to terminate the arrhythmia. Even with an adequate serum concentration, digoxin may not slow the heart rate at the onset of paroxysmal atrial fibrillation. The onset of rate control with digoxin is delayed for several hours, even with intravenous therapy, and this relatively slow onset of action may be undesirable in acute situations. Digoxin monotherapy is most effective in stable patients who do not exercise vigorously. Many patients require the addition of a beta blocker or a rate-limiting calcium channel blocker for optimal rate control.

β-Adrenergic Blockers

Beta blockers (e.g., propranolol, atenolol, metoprolol, and esmolol) can be valuable in controlling the heart rate in specific settings. Beta blockers reduce the resting heart rate and blunt the heart rate response to exercise, but they may also reduce exercise tolerance. Although beta blockers are useful in adrenergic-induced paroxysmal atrial fibrillation, their use in bradycardia-dependent or vagally mediated atrial fibrillation may actually increase the atrial fibrillation burden by inducing sinus bradycardia.

Beta blockers may be used in combination with digoxin or a calcium channel blocker for persistent atrial fibrillation, but care must be taken to avoid excess bradycardia. Esmolol, a short-acting and rapidly acting intravenous agent, is useful for rate control in acute atrial fibrillation, either alone or with digoxin.

In patients in whom a beta blocker controls exercise-induced heart rates at the expense of inappropriately slow resting heart rates, pindolol or xamoterol, which have intrinsic sympathomimetic activity, may be useful for avoiding a slow resting heart rate. Clonidine, which has antiadrenergic properties, may be an option for hypertensive patients because it reduces the standing heart rate in atrial fibrillation by 15% to 20%.

Calcium Channel Blockers

The calcium channel blockers verapamil and diltiazem increase refractoriness and slow conduction in the AV node and are often effective agents for heart rate control. They can be administered intravenously in the emergency setting, but their negative inotropic effects (particularly in the case of verapamil) require cautious use in patients with heart failure. In acute situations, bolus doses of either verapamil or diltiazem, followed by a maintenance infusion, can be used to control the ventricular rate. Long-term oral therapy with either agent is also effective for rate control in permanent

DRUG LOADING AND MAINTENANCE REGIMENS FOR CONTROL OF VENTRICULAR RATE IN ATRIAL FIBRILLATION

Drug Class	Drug Name	Acute Intravenous Therapy	Chronic Oral Therapy
Beta blockers*	Metoprolol	2.5-5 mg every 5 minutes up to 15 mg	50-200 mg/day
	Propranolol	0.15 mg/kg (1 mg every 2 minutes)	40-240 mg/day
	Esmolol	0.5-mg bolus, then 0.05-0.2 mg/kg per minute	NA
	Pindolol	NA	7.5-30 mg/day
	Atenolol	5 mg during 5 minutes, repeat in 10 minutes	25-100 mg/day
	Nadolol	NA	20-80 mg/day
Calcium channel blockers	Verapamil	0.075-0.15 mg/kg during 2 minutes; 0.005 mg/kg per minute	120-360 mg/day
	Diltiazem	0.25-0.35 mg/kg, followed by 5-15 mg/h	120-360 mg/day
Cardiac glycoside	Digoxin	0.75-1.5 mg in divided doses during 12-24 hours	0.125-0.375 mg/day

*Other beta blockers may also be useful.
NA, not available.

Table 58.5 Drug loading and maintenance regimens for control of ventricular rate in atrial fibrillation.

atrial fibrillation. Although they slow the ventricular rate, verapamil and diltiazem do not directly cardiovert atrial fibrillation to sinus rhythm. Exercise capacity should increase when verapamil or diltiazem is used to control the heart rate in atrial fibrillation.

Other Antiarrhythmic Agents for Rate Control

Class I antiarrhythmic agents are not usually advocated for the control of the heart rate in chronic atrial fibrillation. Indeed, class Ia agents (e.g., quinidine) may increase AV nodal conduction because of their anticholinergic effects. Propafenone may reduce the heart rate during paroxysms of atrial fibrillation owing to its limited beta-blocking activity. Amiodarone has sympatholytic and calcium channel blocking properties that depress AV nodal conduction, and this may be helpful for controlling the ventricular rate in atrial fibrillation and flutter. However, in view of its spectrum of side effects, amiodarone should not be used as the first-line agent for heart rate control. It therefore is useful only when other AV nodal–blocking agents fail to slow the ventricular rate adequately or are not well tolerated.

Nonpharmacologic Therapy in Atrial Fibrillation

If pharmacologic measures fail to prevent the recurrence of atrial fibrillation or to control the ventricular rate, nonpharmacologic strategies should be considered. These include pacemakers, atrial defibrillators, catheter ablation for either rate control or prevention of atrial fibrillation, and surgery. In patients with baseline left ventricular dysfunction, consideration should be given to the use of biventricular pacing for long-term support after AV junctional ablation.[51]

Pacemaker Therapy

The traditional indications for pacing in patients with atrial fibrillation are sinus node dysfunction with the bradycardia-tachycardia syndrome and AV block. Both sinus node dysfunction and AV block may be the result of necessary antiarrhythmic therapy. In patients with sick sinus syndrome, the incidence of atrial fibrillation declines significantly with atrial pacing. Atrial pacing may prevent the development of atrial fibrillation that occurs during bradycardia by reducing atrial premature beats, which may initiate atrial fibrillation, and by preventing long pauses, which can cause increased dispersion of repolarization.

VVIR pacing is the mode of choice in patients with permanent atrial fibrillation. Dual-chamber pacemakers, which can convert automatically to a VVIR or DDIR mode if an atrial arrhythmia is detected, should be considered in patients with paroxysmal atrial fibrillation. (See Chapter 55 for an explanation of pacing mode designations.) Pacing strategies that use higher than normal lower rate limits, prevention algorithms, and dual-site atrial pacing have been developed and may be effective in selected patients. Implantable atrial defibrillators have also been developed that can sense the onset of atrial fibrillation and deliver a shock or a burst of high-frequency stimulation to restore sinus rhythm.[52] These devices can be set to function either in an automatic mode or in a patient-activated mode, but poor patient tolerance for shocks has limited their use.

Catheter Ablation of AV Conduction

Catheter ablation of AV conduction with placement of a permanent pacemaker is an effective and highly reliable method of achieving ventricular rate control in patients who have atrial fibrillation. In patients who have permanent atrial fibrillation, a VVIR pacemaker is used. In patients with paroxysmal atrial fibrillation, a DDDR pacemaker may be used with mode switching during paroxysms. Standard rules for anticoagulation of patients with atrial fibrillation still apply. AV junctional ablation and VVIR pacemaker treatment were effective and superior to drug therapy in controlling symptoms in patients previously resistant to or intolerant of drug therapy, although cardiac performance was not modified by the treatment.[53] To prevent deleterious effects of right ventricular pacing in patients with left ventricular dysfunction, biventricular pacing should be considered.[51] Other procedures to modify the AV node and achieve better rate control without producing complete heart block have been described but are less reliable and not as frequently used.

Catheter and Surgical Ablation

Elimination of atrial fibrillation through catheter ablation has been a challenging goal. In some patients, atrial fibrillation is due to one or more rapidly firing atrial foci, which most commonly are located near the orifice or within the pulmonary veins. The strategy has been to isolate the pulmonary veins using lesions around their ostia in the left atrium. This blocks the exit and entrance of electrical impulses and has resulted in at least short-term elimination of arrhythmia in many patients, particularly those with paroxysmal atrial fibrillation and normal-sized atria.[4,54,55] Other patients may be more responsive to previously ineffective antiarrhythmic drugs.

Ablation in a pulmonary vein carries with it a risk of pulmonary vein stenosis and pulmonary hypertension, but this risk has been reduced by the placement of lesions in the pulmonary vein atrium rather than in the vein itself.[54] Other complications of catheter ablation procedures include esophageal injury with an atrioesophageal fistula, phrenic nerve injury, thromboembolism, left atrial tachycardias, and cardiac tamponade.

In patients with persistent atrial fibrillation, ablation maneuvers in addition to pulmonary vein isolation are often required. Linear ablation lines on the posterior left atrial wall, across the roof or along the mitral isthmus may be useful. Some electrophysiologists target regions with complex fractionated atrial electrograms or the vagal ganglionic plexuses around the atria. Most operators now use a stepwise ablation approach, recognizing that more than a single procedure may be required.[56]

Several surgical procedures have been described for atrial fibrillation.[4,54,57,58] In the maze operation, multiple linear incisions are made in the atria, excising both atrial appendages and isolating the pulmonary veins (Fig. 58.10). Theoretically, this should result in isolated regions of atrial tissue that are too small to sustain atrial fibrillation. In appropriate patients, the maze procedure eliminates atrial fibrillation and restores AV synchrony. Recent modifications of the maze technique have lowered the incidence of postoperative sinus node dysfunction. Adverse effects after the maze procedure include massive fluid retention (in approximately 5% of patients), which may be related to loss of atrial

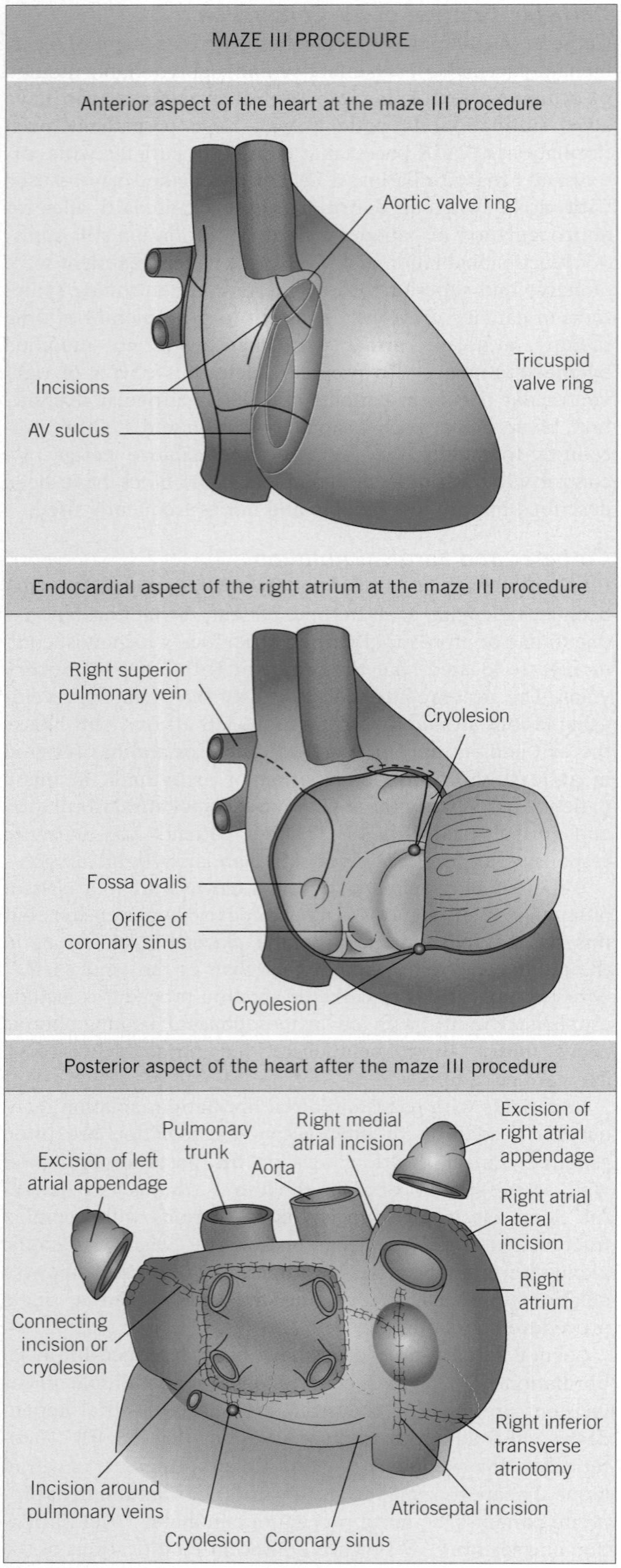

Figure 58.10 In the posterior aspect of the heart after the maze III procedure, note that the left atrial appendage has been amputated at its base. AV, atrioventricular.

natriuretic peptide, and frequent atrial arrhythmias in the early postoperative period. Recently it has been shown that a set of radiofrequency or cryoablation lesions that isolates the pulmonary veins may be useful as a separate procedure or in conjunction with another cardiac surgical procedure. These approaches appear promising and are now routinely recommended by many surgeons as an adjunct to mitral valve surgery in patients with or without previous atrial fibrillation.

Rate Control versus Rhythm Control

Traditionally, the initial strategy for most patients who present with any form of atrial fibrillation has been to restore and maintain sinus rhythm. The clinical impression was that by following a rhythm control strategy, symptoms would be relieved, the risk of stroke diminished, and quality of life and, perhaps, survival enhanced. Although widely accepted by clinicians, these assumptions had not been tested in clinical trials until recently. The Atrial Fibrillation Follow-up Investigation of Rhythm Management (AFFIRM) study[59] enrolled 4060 patients in North America and randomized them between strategies either for rhythm control or for rate control. Patients with both paroxysmal and persistent atrial fibrillation could be included, and only patients at substantial risk for stroke or death because of age or comorbidity were enrolled. Any clinically accepted therapy was allowed in both arms. After 3.5 ± 2 years, follow-up, a trend toward a lower mortality in the rate control arm was seen. The two groups showed equal changes in quality of life and functional status. No difference between the groups was seen in stroke rate or bleeding.

Four smaller trials, the Pharmacological Intervention in Atrial Fibrillation (PIAF) study,[60] the Rate Control versus Electrical Cardioversion (RACE) trial,[61] the Strategies in Atrial Fibrillation (STAF) trial,[62] and the How to Treat Chronic Atrial Fibrillation (HOT CAFE)[56] trial, have also failed to show reductions in stroke or mortality with a primary strategy of rhythm control. However, the recent Japanese Rhythm Management Trial in Atrial Fibrillation (J-RHYTHM)[63] showed that many patients with paroxysmal atrial fibrillation preferred a rhythm control strategy. Preliminary data from the Atrial Fibrillation–Congestive Heart Failure (AF-CHF) trial also failed to show improved survival with a rhythm control strategy in patients with systolic dysfunction and symptoms of heart failure.[64] Therefore, either a rhythm control or a rate control strategy may be chosen for a patient based on the individual's symptomatic response and personal preference (Fig. 58.11).

Antithrombotic Therapy for Atrial Fibrillation

Nonrheumatic atrial fibrillation has been associated with a fivefold increase in the risk of ischemic stroke compared with that of sinus rhythm. This translates into a 5% to 7% yearly risk in patients who are older than 65 years or who have other risk factors for stroke. Atrial fibrillation is usually present in about 15% to 20% of patients who present with stroke, and such patients are at higher risk of recurrent stroke, more severe strokes, greater disability, and a lower rate of discharge back to their own homes. These stroke events are associated with a 1.5 to 3 times higher mortality than that seen in patients in sinus rhythm.

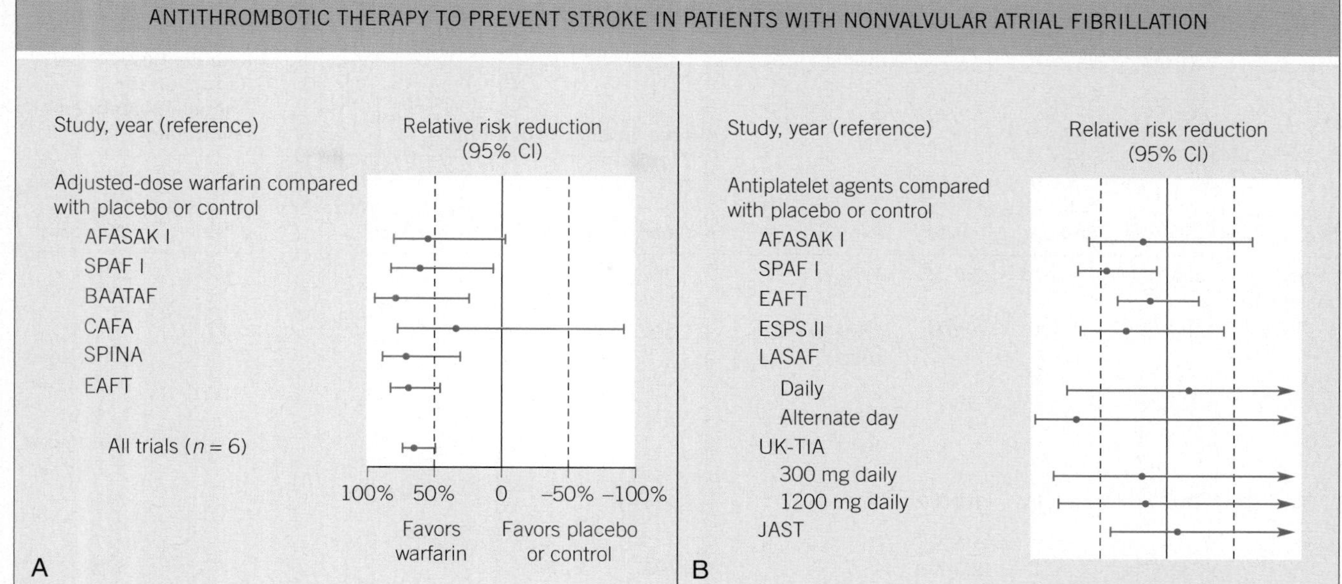

Figure 58.11 Antithrombotic therapy to prevent stroke in patients with nonvalvular atrial fibrillation. (Data from Hart RG, Pearce LA, Aguilar MI. Meta-analysis: antithrombotic therapy to prevent stroke in patients who have nonvalvular atrial fibrillation. Ann Intern Med 2007;146:857-867.)

In the mid-1980s, five randomized, prospective clinical trials were initiated independently to define the value of anticoagulant prophylaxis with warfarin in patients with atrial fibrillation.[65-69] Consistent results for the benefit of oral anticoagulation were seen in the five initial primary prevention studies, several subsequent studies,[70,71] and one secondary prevention trial in patients with nonrheumatic atrial fibrillation and a history of transient ischemic attack or minor stroke[72] (Table 58.6).

Anticoagulation Therapy

In the Atrial Fibrillation Investigators' pooled meta-analysis of the five initial primary prevention trials, a 4.5% annual rate of all strokes was found in the control group and a 1.4% rate in the warfarin group.[73] This difference represents an overall risk reduction of 68% (95% confidence interval [CI], 50%-79%). Warfarin prophylaxis resulted in a similar risk reduction in stroke with residual deficit, a decrease in mortality of 33%, and a 48% decrease in the combined adverse outcome (stroke, systemic embolism, or death). Warfarin was particularly beneficial as secondary prevention in the European Atrial Fibrillation Trial (EAFT),[72] in which the risk of stroke was reduced from 12% per year to 4% per year (hazard ratio, 0.34; 95% CI, 0.20-0.57).

The most recent meta-analysis[74] found that when compared with the control, adjusted-dose warfarin reduced stroke by 64% (95% CI, 49%-74%). Absolute increases in major extracranial hemorrhage were small (≤0.3% per year) on the basis of meta-analysis. Oral anticoagulation was also associated with reduced all-cause mortality compared to placebo, by about 30%.

Despite these impressive figures, the efficacy of warfarin prophylaxis is probably underestimated because most strokes in patients who were randomized to warfarin occurred while the patients were not, in fact, taking warfarin or were significantly under-anticoagulated at the time of the event.

In analyses of the optimal anticoagulation intensity for stroke prevention in atrial fibrillation, the stroke risk was substantially increased at an INR less than 2.0. In a study by Hylek and colleagues,[75] the INR was a powerful and independent determinant of the risk of stroke. For example, compared with patients with an INR of 2.0, patients with an INR of 1.7 had a twofold increase in the risk of stroke.

Antiplatelet Therapy

Analysis of the randomized trial data (see Table 58.6) has shown that aspirin is substantially less effective than warfarin. Aspirin had limited effects on severe strokes or mortality, although in the pooled analysis, aspirin did reduce strokes by 21% (95% CI, 0-37; $P = .05$) and the combined outcome of stroke, embolism, or death by 28%.[74] In the EAFT,[72] aspirin also was less effective than warfarin when used as secondary prophylaxis in patients who had had a previous stroke or transient ischemic attack (hazard ratio, 0.60; 95% CI, 0.41-0.87).

The apparent benefit of aspirin from the meta-analysis was driven largely by the data from the Stroke Prevention in Atrial Fibrillation (SPAF I) trial, which was the only trial to show a benefit for aspirin in stroke prevention in patients with atrial fibrillation (relative risk reduction [RRR], 42%). Nonetheless, in this trial a major inconsistency was seen between the results for the warfarin-eligible arm (RRR, 94%) and the warfarin-ineligible arm (RRR, 8%); these results were pooled to get the apparent RRR of 42%.[76]

Combination therapy with aspirin plus clopidogrel was inferior to therapeutic anticoagulation for stroke prevention in one large trial.[77] However, in this study, a subgroup comparison of subjects who were warfarin naïve compared to warfarin users at entry suggested that those who were warfarin naïve could derive less benefit from anticoagulation.

Among low-risk atrial fibrillation patients, the recent Japanese Atrial Fibrillation Stroke Trial showed no difference

RANDOMIZED TRIALS FOR PREVENTION OF THROMBOEMBOLIC EVENTS IN NONRHEUMATIC ATRIAL FIBRILLATION

				Annual Embolic Event Rate				Relative Risk Reduction for Annual Thromboembic Event Rate	
Trial		Follow-up (years)	INR	Aspirin	Warfarin	Placebo	Low-dose Warfarin and Aspirin	Aspirin	Adjusted-Dose Warfarin
Primary prevention	SPAF I[69]	1.3	2.0-3.5	3.6%	2.3%	6.3%-7.4%		42%	67%
	SPAF II[70]	2.3	2.0-3.5	1.9% in those aged < 75 years	1.3%				33% in those aged > 75 years
				4.8% in those aged > 75 years	3.6%				17% in those aged < 75 years*
	SPAF III[71]	1.1	1.8-3.2		1.9%				74%†
			1.2-1.5				7.9%		
	CAFA[67]	1.3	2.0-3.0		3.5%	5.2%			37%
	BAATAF[66]	2.2	1.5-2.7		0.41%	3%			86%
	AFASAK[65]	2.0	2.8-4.2	5.5%	2%	5.5%		14%	60%
	SPINAF[68]	1.8	1.5-2.5		0.9%	4.3%			73%
	MIWAF[82]	1.2	2.0-3.0 <1.5		0%‡ 3.7%‡				100%
Secondary prevention	EAFT[72]	2.3	2.5-4.0	10%	4%	12%		17%	66%

In the Stroke Prevention in Atrial Fibrillation (SPAF II) study, warfarin was compared with aspirin without an untreated control group; the study found that patients younger than 75 years who did not have risk factors (e.g., hypertension, recent heart failure, or a previous thromboembolic event) were at low risk and might not benefit from anticoagulation. Patients older than 75 years did benefit from anticoagulation. In the Boston Area Anticoagulation Trial in Atrial Fibrillation (BAATAF), aspirin was allowed in the control group. In the Atrial Fibrillation, Aspirin, Anticoagulation (AFASAK) study from Copenhagen, Denmark, the primary events included intracranial hemorrhage. CAFA, Canadian Atrial Fibrillation Anticoagulation study; EAFT, European Atrial Fibrillation Trial; INR, international normalized ratio; MWINAFS, Minidose Warfarin in Nonrheumatic Atrial Fibrillation study.

*The control group received aspirin at a dosage of 325 mg once a day.

†The comparison group was low-dose warfarin and aspirin.

‡Ischemic stroke only.

Table 58.6 Randomized trials for prevention of thromboembolic events in nonrheumatic atrial fibrillation.

between aspirin and placebo for stroke events; however, aspirin takers had more adverse effects (especially bleeding).[78]

Anticoagulant versus Antiplatelet Therapy

The Studio Italiano Fibrillazione Atriale (SIFA) study recently reported that a new antiplatelet agent, indobufen, at a dosage of 100 to 200 mg two times a day, was comparable to adjusted-dose warfarin in preventing stroke in 916 patients with chronic atrial fibrillation and a recent cerebrovascular event.[79] In this secondary prevention study, the 12-month primary event rate was 10% in the warfarin group and 12% in the indobufen group (P = NS).

The recent randomized Birmingham Atrial Fibrillation Treatment of the Aged (BAFTA) study[80] compared adjusted-dose warfarin (INR, 2.0-3.0) with aspirin (75 mg/day) in 973 elderly patients (>75 years) with atrial fibrillation (mean age, 81.5 years) in a U.K. general practitioner setting. This trial reported a primary event rate (defined as a fatal or disabling stroke, whether ischemic or hemorrhagic; intracranial hemorrhage; or clinically significant arterial embolism) of 1.8% per annum in the warfarin arm, compared with 3.8% per annum in the aspirin arm (RR, 0.48; 95% CI, 0.28-0.80; $P = .003$; number needed to treat (NNT) for 1 year to prevent one primary event, 50). For the endpoint of stroke per se, the annual risk was also significantly reduced for warfarin as compared with aspirin (1.6% versus 3.4%; RR, 0.46 [0.26-0.79]; $P = .003$), with the main benefit seen for severe or disabling stroke rather than fatal stroke. It is noteworthy that the risk of major hemorrhage was similar in the two treatment groups in the BAFTA trial.

Including the BAFTA data, the recent meta-analysis by Hart and coworkers[74] reported that the relative risk reduction by warfarin over aspirin is 39% (95% CI, 19%-53%).

Combined Warfarin and Aspirin Therapy

The SPAF III trial[71] compared the use of low-dose and fixed-dose warfarin (INR, 1.2-1.5) plus aspirin (325 mg/day) with standard dose-adjusted warfarin therapy (INR, 2.0-3.0) in 1044 patients with atrial fibrillation who were at high risk of stroke and thromboembolism. This study included women older than 75 years and patients with a systolic blood pressure above 160 mm Hg, poor left ventricular function, or a previous thromboembolic event. Compared with adjusted-dose warfarin therapy, low-dose warfarin plus aspirin was associated with significantly higher rates of

- ischemic stroke or systemic embolism (7.9% versus 1.9% per year; $P < .0001$);
- disabling stroke (5.6% versus 1.7% per year; $P = .0007$); and
- vascular death or a primary event (11.8% versus 6.4% per year, $P = .002$).

In the lowest risk patients (n = 892), a history of hypertension conferred a stroke risk approximately 3.5 times (approximately 3.5% per year; 95% CI, 2.5-5.2) that of the remaining "low risk" cohort (1% per year; 95% CI, 0.6-2.0), despite the addition of aspirin at 325 mg daily.

The Second Copenhagen Atrial Fibrillation Aspirin Anticoagulation (AFASAK-2) trial[81] compared daily treatment with warfarin (1.25 mg), warfarin (1.25 mg) plus aspirin (300 mg), and aspirin (300 mg) alone with adjusted-dose warfarin (INR, 2.0-3.0) in chronic atrial fibrillation. The trial included 677 subjects, but it terminated early after publication of SPAF III. The primary event rates at 3 years were 11.9%, 12.8%, 8.4% and 8.3% ($P = .67$), suggesting a trend toward superiority of adjusted-dose warfarin over low-intensity anticoagulation or aspirin-warfarin combination therapy.

A similar study by Pengo and associates[82] involving 303 patients who were randomized to low-intensity, fixed-minidose warfarin (INR, <1.5) or adjusted-dose therapy (INR, 2.0-3.0) reported an increased event rate in the fixed-minidose warfarin group (11.1% versus 6.1%), suggesting that this regimen was not useful.

What about adding antiplatelet therapy to adjusted-dose therapeutic anticoagulation? The Fluindione, Fibrillation Auriculaire, Aspirin et Contraste Spontané (FFAACS) investigators conducted a randomized trial of fluindione (an oral anticoagulant) versus fluindione plus aspirin.[83] This trial was stopped early because of poor recruitment, but it showed a substantially higher bleeding rate with combination therapy. A retrospective analysis of the combined dataset of two contemporary, randomized clinical trials of anticoagulation, the Stroke Prevention using an Oral Thrombin Inhibitor in Atrial Fibrillation (SPORTIF III and V) trials, compared aspirin users with nonusers.[84] This study found no additive effect of taking aspirin when a patient was anticoagulated (with either warfarin or ximelagatran) in preventing stroke or reducing vascular events (including death or myocardial infarction); however, it did find a significant increase in bleeding risk when aspirin was combined with anticoagulation. Of note, the rate of myocardial infarction with aspirin and warfarin (0.6% per year) was not significantly different from that with warfarin alone (1% per year).

This lack of benefit of aspirin may not apply to every antiplatelet agent. For example, one trial (n = 1209) randomized atrial fibrillation patients to triflusal (an antiplatelet drug that is a cyclooxygenase inhibitor), to acenocumarol (an anticoagulant), or to combination therapy.[85] The primary outcome was lower with combined triflusal-acenocumarol therapy than with anticoagulant therapy in both groups.

Two increasingly common situations in which anticoagulation therapy may require the addition of antiplatelet therapy (aspirin or clopidogrel) are percutaneous coronary intervention (with stenting) and presentation with an acute coronary syndrome.[86] A suggested management schema for such patients is presented in Table 58.7.

New Anticoagulant Drugs for Atrial Fibrillation

Much interest has arisen in the development of alternative anticoagulant drugs, given the many limitations associated with warfarin, including the requirement for regular monitoring and warfarin's interactions with other drugs, food, and alcohol.

The two main classes of anticoagulant drugs are the direct thrombin inhibitors and the oral factor Xa inhibitors. The first direct thrombin inhibitor, ximelagatran, was compared with warfarin in the SPORTIF III and V trials and was found to be noninferior to warfarin for stroke prevention, with potentially less bleeding.[84] However, the risk of liver toxicity led to the withdrawal of this drug. Ongoing large studies in atrial fibrillation involving other oral direct thrombin inhibitors (e.g., dabigatran) and oral factor Xa inhibitors (e.g., rivaroxaban and apixiban) may provide evidence for these drugs in the near future.

Risks of Antithrombotic Therapy for Atrial Fibrillation

The annual risk of intracranial hemorrhage increased from 0.1% in controls to 0.3% in warfarin groups in the pooled analysis, representing an excess of two episodes of intracranial bleeding per year per 1000 patients treated.[74] The risk

ANTICOAGULATION IN CHRONIC NONVALVULAR ATRIAL FIBRILLATION

Patient Group	Risk Factors	Estimated Risk	Recommendation
Age <65 years	Present	High	Warfarin
	Absent	Low	Aspirin or nothing
Age 65-75 years	Present	High	Warfarin
	Absent	Moderate	Warfarin or aspirin
Age > 75 years	Present	High	Warfarin
	Absent	Moderate to high	Warfarin

Risk factors are previous transient ischemic attack or stroke, hypertension, heart failure, diabetes mellitus, clinical coronary artery disease, thyrotoxicosis, and left ventricular dysfunction.

Table 58.7 Anticoagulation in chronic nonvalvular atrial fibrillation.

is increased as much as threefold in patients who have bled previously, and both bleeding and hemorrhagic stroke may be more common in patients aged 75 years or older. The risk of death from a major bleeding episode ranged from 13% to 33%, and the risk of morbidity in those who survived such an event was as high as 15%.

The bleeding risk with anticoagulation was particularly associated with an INR above 3.0, fluctuating INRs, and uncontrolled hypertension. An association with increasing age also has been found. In the SPAF II study,[70] for example, the benefits of warfarin were nearly counteracted by an increased risk of intracranial hemorrhage in the warfarin group, which was unexpectedly high in patients older than 75 years, at 1.8% per year. However, the rate of intracranial hemorrhage in this group was substantially higher than that reported in the original five trials (on average, 0.3% per year), which may reflect the higher intensity of anticoagulation in the SPAF II study (INR up to 4.5). Even low-dose aspirin may increase the risk of major hemorrhage by twofold, to 0.5% per year in elderly people.

A systematic review, done as part of the evidence-based U.K. National Institute for Health and Clinical Excellence guidelines on atrial fibrillation management, identified the following patient characteristics as risk factors for anticoagulation-related bleeding complications: advanced age, uncontrolled hypertension, a history of myocardial infarction or ischemic heart disease, cerebrovascular disease, anemia or a history of bleeding, and concomitant use of other drugs, such as antiplatelet agents.[87] The presence of diabetes mellitus, controlled hypertension, and gender were not identified as significant risk factors. What is evident is that many risk factors for anticoagulation-related bleeding are also indications for the use of anticoagulants in atrial fibrillation patients, as shown by the close correlation between bleeding risk and stroke risk calculated by the CHADS2 score.[89]

RISK STRATIFICATION FOR STROKE AND THROMBOEMBOLISM

The data from the studies discussed here provide the clinician with sufficient information on which to assess the risk of stroke and the need for anticoagulation (Table 58.8).

In a recent systematic review of seven studies (including six entirely independent cohorts) by the Stroke Risk in Atrial Fibrillation Working Group,[88] the most consistent independent risk factors for stroke in atrial fibrillation were a previous stroke or transient ischemic attack (RR, 2.5; 95% CI, 1.8-3.5), increasing age (RR, 1.5 per decade; 95% CI, 1.3-1.7), a history of hypertension (RR, 2.0; 95% CI, 1.6-2.5), and diabetes mellitus (RR, 1.7; 95% CI, 1.4-2.0). Female gender was inconsistently associated with stroke risk, and the evidence was inconclusive on whether heart failure or coronary artery disease was independently predictive of stroke. However, the risk of bleeding was high in many patients and must be considered when anticoagulation therapy is recommended.[89] Given that some stroke risk factors

SCHEMES FOR STROKE RISK ASSESSMENT IN PATIENTS WITH ATRIAL FIBRILLATION

	High	Intermediate	Low
Atrial Fibrillation Investigators (AFI; 1994)[73]	Age >65 years; history of hypertension, CAD, or diabetes mellitus		Age <65 years; no high-risk features
SPAF Investigators trial (1995)[69]	Women age >75 years; systolic blood pressure >160 mm Hg; LV dysfunction (on echocardiogram or clinically)	History of hypertension; no high-risk features	No history of hypertension; no high-risk features
$CHADS_2$ scheme (2001)[7]	Score 3-6	Score 1-2	Score 0
Framingham study (2003)[7]	Weighted point scoring system (low risk, 0-7; intermediate risk, 8-13; high risk, 14-31)—points given for following risk factors: old age (maximum score <10); gender (women = 6, men = 0); high blood pressure (<4); and diabetes (6). Total score (maximum 31 points) corresponds to predicted 5-year stroke risk		
ACCP guidelines (2004)[7]	Previous stroke, TIA, or systemic embolic event; age >75 years; moderately or severely impaired LV function with or without congestive cardiac failure; hypertension or diabetes	Age 65-75 years with no other risk factors	Age <65 years with no risk factors
NICE guidelines (2006)[7]	Previous ischemic stroke, TIA, or thromboembolic event; age ≥75 years with hypertension, diabetes, or vascular disease; clinical evidence of valvular disease or heart failure, or impaired LV function on echocardiography	Age ≥65 years with no high-risk factors; age <75 years with hypertension, diabetes, or vascular disease	Age <65 years with no history of embolism, hypertension, diabetes, or other clinical risk factors
ACC/AHA/ESC guidelines (2006)[4]	Previous thromboembolism (stroke, TIA, systemic embolism); valvular disease, more than one of the following: age ≥75 years, hypertension, heart failure, impaired LV systolic function, or diabetes mellitus	Age ≥75 years, hypertension, heart failure, impaired LV systolic function, or diabetes mellitus	Atrial fibrilation only (no other risk factors)

TIA, transient ischemic attack; CAD, coronary artery disease; LV, left ventricular.

Table 58.8 Schemes for stroke risk assessment in patients with atrial fibrillation.

were derived from the non-warfarin arms of trial cohorts, the review did not systematically look for some risk factors (e.g., coronary or peripheral artery disease).

These stroke risk factors have been used to inform the development of risk stratification schemas, to help identify patients at high risk of stroke, who would benefit most from anticoagulation therapy.

Decisions about anticoagulation should be based on the patient's age and the presence or absence of risk factors. All patients with rheumatic heart disease who have atrial fibrillation should receive warfarin. Patients who have nonvalvular atrial fibrillation may be stratified into low-, moderate-, and high-risk groups. High-risk patients should receive adjusted-dose warfarin with a target INR of 2.0 to 3.0. Low-risk patients should receive either nothing or aspirin. Therapy for moderate-risk patients is controversial, with some practitioners preferring warfarin and others preferring aspirin.

If contraindications to both warfarin and aspirin exist (particularly gastrointestinal bleeding or allergy), they should be carefully documented in the clinical notes; in cases of uncertainty, the patient should be referred to a specialist in cardiology.

As shown in Table 58.9, many guidelines are available, some based directly on event-rate analyses, others produced by expert consensus committees. A survey by Lip and colleagues[90] found that consensus is still lacking among consultant physicians on the question of anticoagulation for atrial fibrillation, and the varied perception of risk-benefit ratios in this survey suggests that much work is still needed for optimal risk stratification and the provision of suitable prophylaxis of stroke and systemic embolism for patients with chronic nonvalvular atrial fibrillation. Prescription of warfarin for low-risk patients who do not need it increases the risk of bleeding in these patients and imposes the inconvenience of regular attendance at anticoagulant clinics for monitoring.

For now, a clinically appropriate approach involves a strategy of careful clinical assessment in conjunction with risk stratification for atrial fibrillation (Fig. 58.12), in which the highest risk groups for stroke and thromboembolism are targeted for anticoagulation and low-risk subjects could be adequately treated with aspirin.

PROGNOSIS

Atrial fibrillation may adversely influence the prognosis both by increasing the risk of thromboembolic events and by aggravating or directly causing heart failure or ischemia. Lethal reactions to attempts at therapy (e.g., proarrhythmic responses to drug therapy or bleeding caused by anticoagulants) may also contribute to an increase in mortality in patients with atrial fibrillation. In the Framingham study, atrial fibrillation was associated with an odds ratio for death of 1.5 (95% CI, 1.2-1.8) among men and 1.9 (95% CI, 1.5-2.2) among women after adjustment for multiple clinical parameters.[1] The greatest absolute impact of atrial fibrillation on the prognosis is seen when it occurs in patients with advanced heart disease or other comorbid diseases.

ANTICOAGULATION IN HIGH-RISK SITUATIONS

	Usual Strategy Recommended	Perceived Potential Bleeding Risk	Presentation of Acute Coronary Syndrome	Management after Percutaneous Coronary Intervention
Patients at low risk for stroke	Aspirin	"	"	Bare metal stent: aspirin plus clopidogrel for 4 weeks, then aspirin DES: aspirin plus clopidogrel for 6-12 months, then aspirin
Patients at high risk for stroke	Warfarin	Low	No	Use bare metal stent if possible Bare metal stent: triple therapy with warfarin, aspirin, and clopidogrel for 2-4 weeks, then change to warfarin plus clopidogrel for up to month 12, then warfarin alone. DES: triple therapy with warfarin, aspirin, and clopidogrel for 3-6 (or more) months, then warfarin plus clopidogrel for up to month 12, then warfarin alone
		Low	Yes	Bare metal stent or DES: triple therapy with warfarin, aspirin, and clopidogrel for 3-6 (or more) months, then warfarin plus clopidogrel for up to month 12, then warfarin alone
		High*	No	Use bare metal stent if possible Bare metal stent: triple therapy with warfarin, aspirin, and clopidogrel for 4 weeks, then change to warfarin alone DES: triple therapy with warfarin, aspirin, and clopidogrel for 4 weeks, then warfarin plus clopidogrel for up to month 12, then warfarin alone
		High*	Yes	Bare metal stent or DES: triple therapy with warfarin, aspirin, and clopidogrel for 4 weeks, then warfarin plus clopidogrel for up to month 12, then warfarin alone

DES, drug-eluting stent. Doses: aspirin 75 mg/day, clopidogrel 75 mg/day, warfarin adjusted to target INR 2.0-2.5.

*Particular attention is paid to the following risk factors: age older than 75 years; antiplatelet drugs (e.g., aspirin or clopidogrel) or nonsteroidal anti-inflammatory drugs; more than one drug treatment (polyphamacy); uncontrolled hypertension; history of bleeding (e.g., pepticular or cerebral hemorrhage); and history of poorly controlled anticoagulation treatment.

Table 58.9 Anticoagulation in high-risk situations.

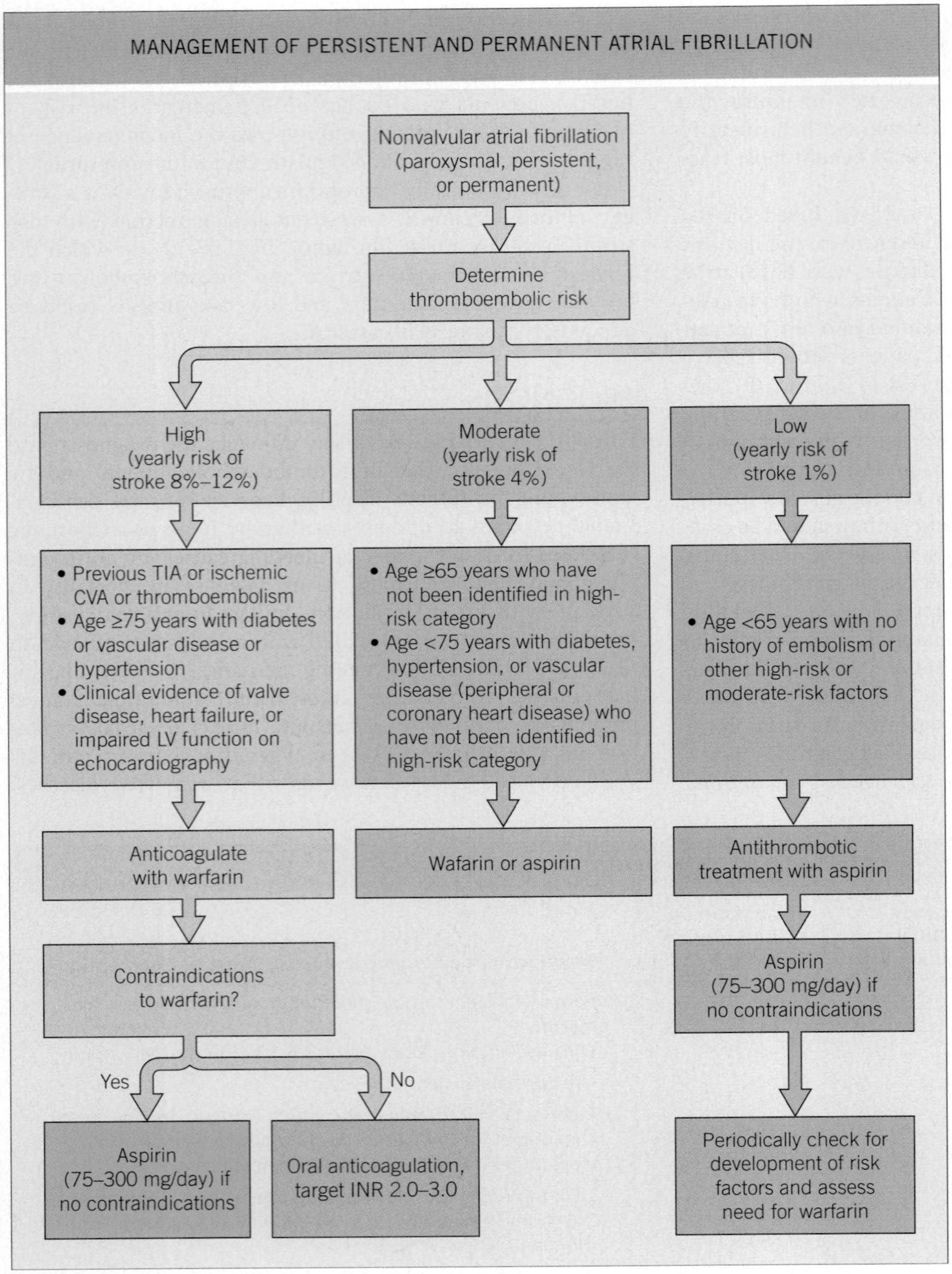

MANAGEMENT OF PERSISTENT AND PERMANENT ATRIAL FIBRILLATION

Figure 58.12 Management of persistent and permanent atrial fibrillation. TIA, transient ischemic attack; CVA, cerebrovascular accident; LV, left ventricular.

In patients who do not have significant heart disease, atrial fibrillation has a lesser effect on survival.

As strategies for appropriate anticoagulation, effective rate control, and heart failure management continue to evolve, it may be that the magnitude of the independent effect of atrial fibrillation will be lessened in the future.

SUMMARY

Atrial fibrillation is the most common sustained arrhythmia in adult populations. Although atrial fibrillation itself is usually not life-threatening, it leads to significant patient morbidity and economic costs and contributes to stroke and heart failure. Clinical decisions in patients who have atrial fibrillation are often difficult, and no uniformly effective and safe therapies are available. In some patients, ventricular rate control and anticoagulation may be preferable to aggressive attempts to maintain sinus rhythm with repeat cardioversions and antiarrhythmic drug therapy. Newer strategies, such as less toxic antiarrhythmic agents, catheter ablation, improved surgical approaches, and atrial defibrillators, offer promise for the future, but their efficacy and optimal use still need to be demonstrated. For now, a comprehensive approach that considers all therapeutic options is indicated (see Fig. 58.12).

chapter 59

Atrial Tachycardias and Atrial Flutter

Francis D. Murgatroyd

Definition

- Atrial tachycardias are tachycardias arising purely in the atrial tissue, that is, having a mechanism that does not depend on any part of the atrioventricular junction or ventricle.

Key Features

- Atrial tachycardias are seldom inherently dangerous but may be markers of serious underlying conditions.
- Sinus tachycardia is usually a physiologic response; true inappropriate sinus tachycardia is rare and difficult to treat.
- The recognition of an atrial arrhythmia is based on the demonstration that the arrhythmia is not dependent on 1:1 atrioventricular conduction.
- The exact diagnosis of an atrial arrhythmia is increasingly important now that many can be cured by catheter ablation.
- Atrial flutter carries a significant risk of thromboembolism.

Therapy

- Medical treatment of atrial arrhythmias may require both an atrioventricular node–blocking agent and an antiarrhythmic (membrane-active) drug.
- Atrial flutter responds less well than atrial fibrillation to antiarrhythmic drugs.
- Catheter ablation is effective in treating most types of atrial flutter and monomorphic atrial tachycardias.
- Anticoagulant therapy should be considered in patients with atrial flutter as with atrial fibrillation.

The firm diagnosis of an atrial arrhythmia depends on the demonstration that it is not dependent on conduction to the ventricles. Differentiation between atrial arrhythmias is usually possible by analysis of the P-wave rate and morphology. These arrhythmias can accompany structural cardiac disease and other conditions, but many are idiopathic. The severity of symptoms is highly variable, depending largely on the ventricular rate and the cardiac status of the patient.

Atrial arrhythmias are seldom inherently dangerous, but they may indirectly affect a patient's prognosis in three ways:

- the resulting tachycardia may precipitate acute heart failure, angina, or syncope in susceptible individuals;
- a chronically increased ventricular rate may lead to "tachycardia cardiomyopathy"; and
- atrial flutter may give rise to thromboembolism.

NOMENCLATURE OF ATRIAL ARRHYTHMIAS

In the last 2 decades, our understanding of the mechanisms and anatomic origins of all the common atrial and supraventricular arrhythmias has been greatly improved by invasive techniques. It is now recognized that some of the terms historically used to describe these arrhythmias and based solely on electrocardiographic findings occasionally give rise to confusion.[1] In this chapter, the following definitions are used (Fig. 59.1).

Sinus tachycardia (whether physiologic, re-entrant, or inappropriate) arises from the region of the sinus node. *Atrial tachycardia* (increasingly called ectopic or focal atrial tachycardia) arises from a circumscribed locus elsewhere in the atria. Whether the mechanism is automatic or microreentrant, the arrhythmia effectively arises from a point source.

Atrial flutter describes any macroreentrant circuit within the atria. Continuous activation occurs repeatedly over an anatomically determined path that measures centimeters in length.

Typical atrial flutter (also known as common atrial flutter) has a characteristic electrocardiographic appearance and is caused by counterclockwise activation of the right atrium, passing through the cavotricuspid isthmus (see later).

Atrial fibrillation consists of multiple irregular wavelets of atrial activation (see Chapter 58).

Supraventricular tachycardias (atrioventricular and atrioventricular nodal re-entrant tachycardia) depend on conduction over the atrioventricular node or an accessory atrioventricular pathway (see Chapters 57 and 60).

Atrial fibrillation and supraventricular tachycardias are dealt with elsewhere in this book.

ANATOMY AND PATHOLOGY

Gross Anatomy of the Atria

The anatomy of the atria is complex, reflecting the embryologic processes that gave rise to the chambers.[2] The right atrium has two parts, divided by the crista terminalis. The larger part has a smooth wall approximately 2 mm thick, derived from part of the embryologic sinus venosus. This includes the openings of the venae cavae, the posterior wall between these vessels, the posterior part of the right atrial appendage, and the fossa ovalis. The crista terminalis is a bundle of parallel myocardial fibers that can be several millimeters thick. It extends in a C shape from the inferolateral right atrium, in front of the orifice of the inferior vena cava, obliquely around the anterolateral right atrium to the roof of

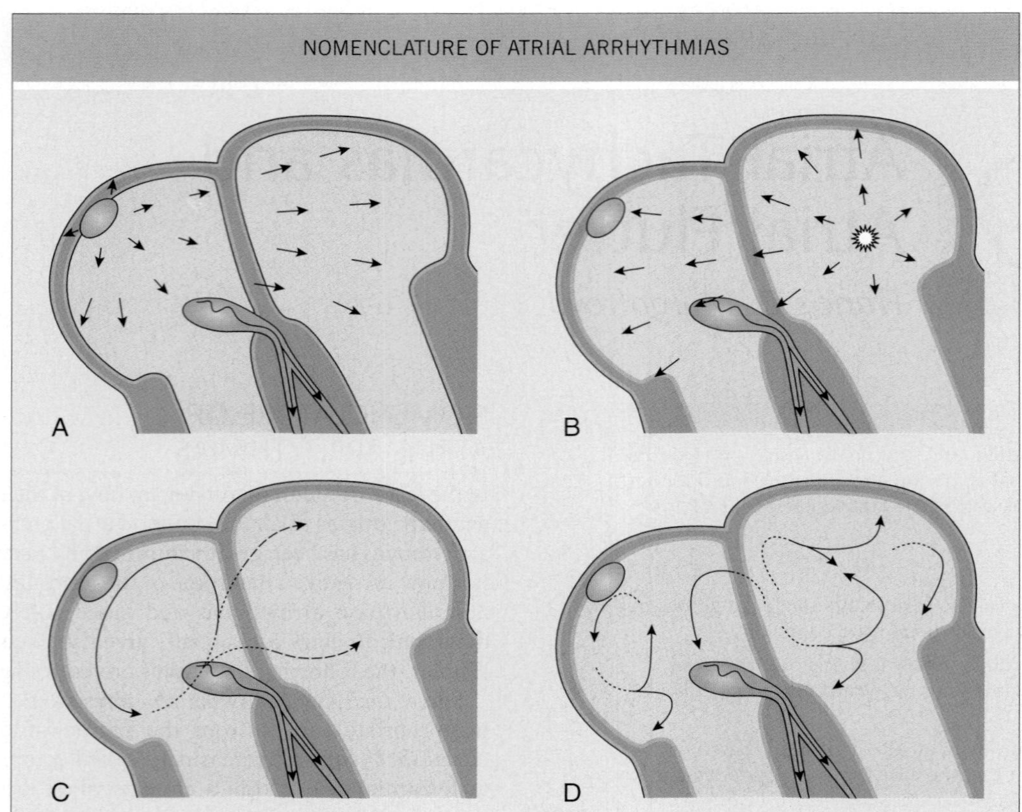

Figure 59.1 Nomenclature of atrial arrhythmias. A, Sinus tachycardia, whatever its mechanism, originates within the perisinus region. The P-wave morphology and endocardial atrial activation sequence are indistinguishable from those seen in sinus rhythm. Most sinus tachycardia (whether physiologic or pathologic) has an automatic mechanism, although sinus node re-entry is diagnosed when the tachycardia behavior suggests a re-entrant mechanism. **B,** Atrial tachycardia (often known as ectopic atrial tachycardia) arises from a site elsewhere within the atria. This may be an automatic focus or a microreentrant circuit. The P-wave morphology and endocardial atrial activation sequence differ from those seen in sinus rhythm. **C,** Atrial flutter is a regular macroreentrant tachycardia confined to one atrium, passively activating the other. As well as typical flutter (illustrated), various atypical forms have been described (see Fig. 59.3). **D,** Atrial fibrillation consists of multiple activation wavelets propagating chaotically in the atria. These may be self-sustaining or "driven" by a rapid focus or circuit.

the right atrium. Its fibers continue anterior to the fossa ovalis toward the atrioventricular junction. Pectinate muscles fan out perpendicular to the crista terminalis into the anterior section of the atrium, whose wall (paper-thin in places) they support. This anterior section includes the right atrial appendage and is the vestibule of the tricuspid valve.

The left atrium is considerably simpler. Most of it has a smooth wall approximately 3 mm thick, formed by the enlarged remnant of the embryologic common pulmonary vein, which becomes the confluence of the four pulmonary veins. A relatively small area of trabeculated muscle exists in and around the left atrial appendage, which varies greatly in both shape and volume. The anatomy of the pulmonary veins and their openings into the left atrium is also highly variable; a common orifice, branching into three or more veins, is frequently seen, especially on the left.[3] Myocardial sleeves may extend from the left atrium over the pulmonary veins for a distance of up to 3 to 4 cm; these are more commonly seen with the superior veins than the inferior veins.[4]

The true interatrial septum, where the left and right atria make contact, is fairly small. Most of its area is the floor of the fossa ovalis, derived from the embryologic septum primum, whose superior rim is the infolded groove between the right pulmonary veins and the superior vena cava (Waterston's groove to the cardiac surgeon). The inferior rim of the fossa ovalis is derived from the septum secundum and is continuous with other septal structures: the sinus septum, which separates the fossa ovalis and right atrium from the coronary sinus, and the muscular atrioventricular septum, which divides the right atrium from the left ventricle.

Specialized Tissue within the Atria

The sinus node lies on the crista terminalis superomedial to the opening of the superior vena cava. It is approximately 2 cm long and 0.5 cm wide. Its central compact zone surrounds the sinus node artery and is surrounded by a transitional cell zone, which is in contact with the atrial myocardium of the crista terminalis. The sinus node has dense parasympathetic and sympathetic innervation.

The atrioventricular node lies at the apex of the triangle of Koch in the low right atrium, adjacent to the anteroseptal portion of the tricuspid annulus. The compact portion of the atrioventricular node is a small bean-shaped structure lying on the atrial septal side of the central fibrous body. It is surrounded by a rim of transitional cells, derived from atrial myocytes, that approach the node from the posteroinferior, anterosuperior, and septal–left atrial directions. The atrioventricular node is also densely innervated.

The existence of specialized conducting pathways between the sinus and atrioventricular nodes has been proposed. However, it is now believed that preferred conduction routes are determined by anatomic and functional considerations rather than by distinct bundles of specialized fibers.

Atrial Structures Relevant to Arrhythmia in Health and Disease

A number of anatomic aspects of the atria, both gross and microscopic, may contribute to the substrate for arrhythmia. First, the orifices of the seven inlets and two outlets to the atria can act as anatomic boundaries for re-entrant circuits. Second, the complex arrangement of atrial fibers and gap junctions predisposes to anisotropic conduction.[5] Thus, the crista terminalis conducts rapidly along its length but can become a line of functional block in the perpendicular direction during typical atrial flutter (see later). Likewise, it is thought that anisotropic conduction due to fiber orientation may give rise to the zone of slow conduction in the inferoposterior right atrium that is part of the substrate for re-entry in typical atrial flutter. Third, in vitro studies of atrial tissue have shown that in addition to the classic "spike and dome" action potentials characteristic of nonspecialized myocytes, triangular action potentials characteristic of "pacemaker" cells can be recorded. Certain locations within the atria, particularly the crista terminalis, seem to be particularly common sites of automatic activity.[6] The musculature at the antrum and proximal segment of each pulmonary vein can give rise to rapid electrical firing based on a number of mechanisms, including automaticity, triggered activity, and microreentry, that may initiate or drive atrial arrhythmias.[7,8] Finally, a number of structural and functional changes are seen in diseased atria. These include increased excitability due to lowered diastolic potentials, extensive denervation, and degenerative change with adipose infiltration. Focal fibrosis of the atrial myocardium, which greatly affects conduction, is a normal age-related change in the elderly[9] and is increased in virtually all long-standing cardiac disease states.

PATHOPHYSIOLOGY

Sinus Tachycardia

Sinus tachycardia is almost always a physiologic response to exercise, pain or other psychological stress, or pathologic conditions such as dehydration. Pathologic sinus tachycardia is exceptionally rare.

The sinus rate is almost entirely determined by autonomic tone. Both vagal tone and adrenergic tone alter the pacemaker current (I_f) that determines the slope of phase 4 depolarization in sinus node cells. Idiopathic sinus tachycardia (see later) probably involves an alteration of this mechanism, as the tachycardia exhibits the electrophysiologic features of enhanced automaticity and is sensitive both to changes in autonomic tone and to beta blockade. The underlying cause appears to be a primary abnormality of the sinus node, causing increased β-adrenergic sensitivity. Efferent sympathovagal balance in the supine and erect positions appears to be normal, but the intrinsic heart rate (i.e., after autonomic blockade) is abnormally high, the diving reflex is depressed, and the dose-response curve of sinus rate to isoproterenol infusion is shifted to the left.[10] On the other hand, there appears to be some overlap of this condition with the postural orthostatic tachycardia syndrome, which is a primary autonomic abnormality characterized by an exaggerated heart rate response to erect posture in the absence of hypotension.

In contrast to idiopathic sinus tachycardia, sinus node re-entry (by definition) exhibits the characteristics of a re-entrant arrhythmia in the electrophysiology laboratory. A microreentrant circuit is assumed to be responsible.

Atrial Tachycardias

Atrial tachycardias encountered in clinical practice have been ascribed to a number of mechanisms on the basis of their onset and termination and the effects of various interventions (Table 59.1). Enhanced automaticity is the presumed mechanism when tachycardia cannot be initiated or terminated by pacing but is facilitated by isoproterenol. The tachycardia typically accelerates ("warms up") just after its initiation and slows just before termination. This is the most common mechanism of atrial tachycardia in young people with structurally normal hearts. It also accompanies chronic pulmonary disease and pneumonia, myocardial infarction, and metabolic disturbances including intoxication with alcohol and stimulant drugs.

Triggered activity can be induced or accelerated by rapid atrial pacing,[11] and the initial cycle length of the tachycardia and the time to its onset are directly related to the pacing cycle length but are not dependent on intra-atrial conduction delay. Like enhanced automaticity, this pattern is common in patients without structural heart disease. In one series, electrophysiologic study indicated triggered activity in 10 of 71 patients with atrial tachycardia, all consistently terminated by verapamil.[12] This type of ectopic atrial tachycardia is also sometimes terminated by adenosine.

Microreentry is presumed to be the mechanism of atrial tachycardia that is easily initiated and terminated in the electrophysiology laboratory. It is usually seen in patients with structural heart disease and atrial enlargement and especially in surgically repaired congenital heart disease. It is typically paroxysmal and may coexist with atrial flutter and fibrillation; indeed, microreentry in the vicinity of the pulmonary vein ostia is thought to be one of the mechanisms perpetuating atrial fibrillation.[8]

Typical Atrial Flutter

Typical atrial flutter was first described a century ago, but its mechanism and anatomic basis were established relatively recently.[13-18] The arrhythmia can be entrained, indicating a re-entrant circuit with an excitable gap. The circuit is confined to the right atrium, propagating in a counterclockwise direction around the tricuspid annulus (as viewed from the cardiac apex) (Fig. 59.2). Activation descends the free wall of the atrium and ascends through a zone of slow conduction adjacent to the tricuspid annulus before ascending the septum to the roof. Laterally, the crista terminalis forms a line of functional block contiguous with the inferior vena cava.

MECHANISMS AND DIAGNOSTIC FEATURES OF ATRIAL TACHYCARDIAS

	Sinus Node Re-Entry	Intra-Atrial Re-Entry	Atrial Automaticity	Triggered Activity
Initiation	Initiation by PACs, PVCs; atrial and ventricular pacing independent of IACD	Initiation by PACs only during atrial relative refractory period resulting in IACD	Cannot initiate with PACs Independent of IACD May "warm up"	Can initiate with PACs or atrial pacing, independent of IACD PCL and PAC coupling interval directly related to TCL and interval to onset
P wave; atrial activation sequence	Identical to sinus	Differs from sinus		
PR interval	Relates physiologically to atrial rate alone (unlike SVT)			
Effect of AV block	Does not usually affect atrial tachycardias (unlike SVT)			
Vagal maneuvers, adenosine	Slow then abruptly terminate tachycardia	May produce AV block, but arrhythmia itself not terminated	May produce AV block, but arrhythmia itself not terminated	May produce AV block, arrhythmia occasionally terminated
Effect of atrial pacing	Pacing and PACs may terminate tachycardia		May overdrive suppress, cannot terminate	May accelerate tachycardia

AV, atrioventricular; IACD, intra-atrial conduction delay; PAC, premature atrial complex; PCL, pacing cycle length; PVC, premature ventricular complex; SVT, supraventricular tachycardia; TCL, tachycardia cycle length.

Modified from Josephson ME. Supraventricular tachycardias. In Josephson ME, ed. Clinical Cardiac Electrophysiology. Techniques and Interpretations. Philadelphia, Lea & Febiger, 1993:181-274.

Table 59.1 Mechanisms and diagnostic features of atrial tachycardias.

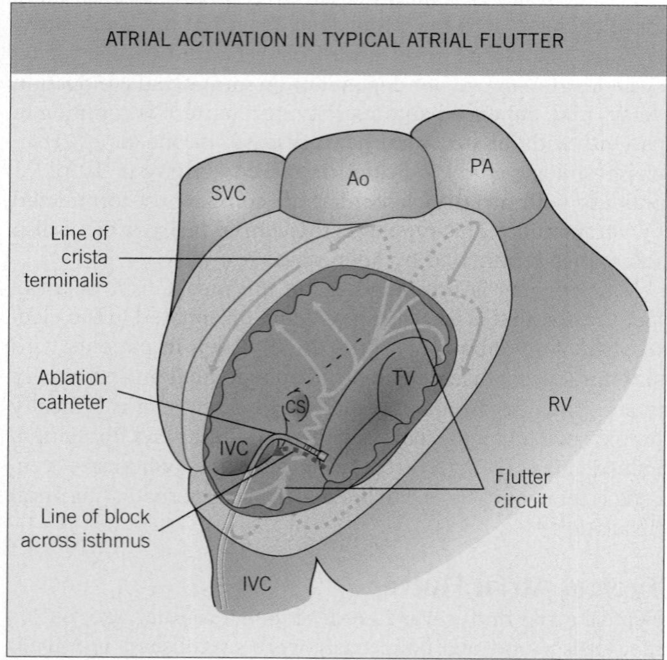

Figure 59.2 Diagram of atrial activation in typical atrial flutter. Typical atrial flutter. Activation travels rapidly down the free wall of the right atrium and passes through the isthmus between the openings of the inferior vena cava and the tricuspid valve, into an area of slow conduction along the tricuspid annulus. From there, activation ascends the interatrial septum, passively activating both the posterior portion of the right atrium and the left atrium. Ao, aortic root; CS, coronary sinus os; IVC, inferior vena cava; PA, pulmonary artery; RV, right ventricle; SVC, superior vena cava; TV, tricuspid valve.

Activation of the posterior right atrium and of the left atrium is passive. Passage through the isthmus between the inferior vena cava and the tricuspid annulus is obligatory, and this forms the basis for ablative treatment.

Atypical Atrial Flutter

Other atrial macroreentrant circuits have been described (Fig. 59.3). The most common is clockwise flutter, in which activation follows the same path as typical flutter (and is therefore also isthmus dependent) but in the opposite direction. Truly atypical atrial flutter is heterogeneous. It can be unstable, spontaneously terminating, or organizing into typical or clockwise flutter or into atrial fibrillation. The atrial rate is usually greater than with typical flutter. As the same morphology of atypical flutter tends to recur in an individual patient, it is likely that the pattern of activation is at least partly determined by fixed anatomic boundaries. In a study of 33 patients with atypical flutter, clockwise flutter was induced in 19 patients in the electrophysiology laboratory, and truly atypical flutter was induced in 20.[19] Scar-related atrial flutter after surgery for congenital heart disease and ablative procedures may be considered a distinct entity. The long oblique atriotomy required for the repair of septal defects, the baffles created in the Mustard and Senning procedures, and the conduit created in the Fontan procedure produce scars that frequently act as the substrate for macroreentrant circuits. After the Mustard and Senning procedures, the proportion of patients in sinus rhythm steadily declines and the incidence of flutter increases, despite modifications aimed at preserving sinus node functions.[20-23] Scar-related atrial flutter is increasingly seen as a complication of surgical and catheter ablation procedures for atrial

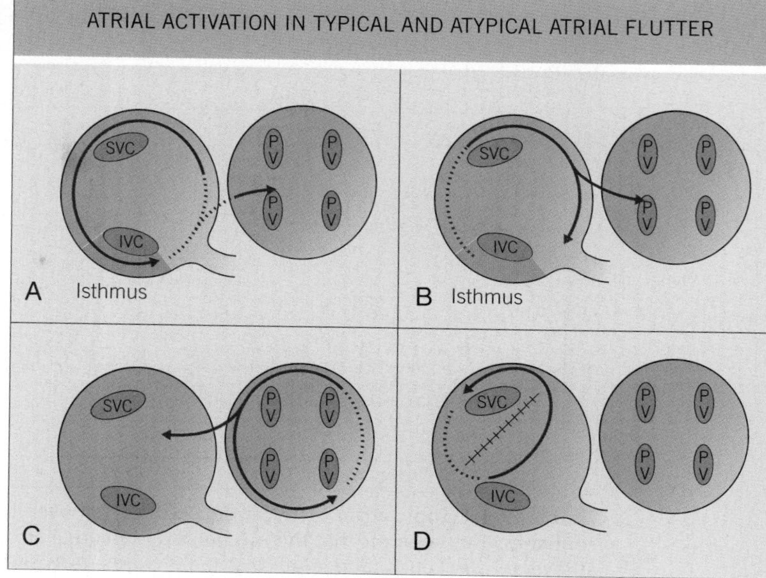

Figure 59.3 Atrial activation in typical and atypical flutters. Forms of atrial flutter. A, Typical atrial flutter as described in Figure 59.2. Right atrial activation travels around the tricuspid annulus in a counterclockwise direction as viewed from the cardiac apex. **B,** Clockwise flutter is essentially the same circuit in reverse. Passage through the cavotricuspid isthmus *(shaded)* is obligatory for both these circuits, and this forms the basis of curative catheter ablation. **C,** Truly atypical atrial flutter can have a variety of paths involving one or more fixed anatomic obstacles. Activation around the left atrium, bounded anteriorly by the mitral annulus and posteriorly by the pulmonary veins, is one of several flutter circuits seen as a complication of catheter ablation for atrial fibrillation. **D,** Scar-related atrial flutter is a common late complication of surgery for congenital heart disease. IVC, inferior vena cava; PV, pulmonary vein; SVC, superior vena cava.

fibrillation. In some cases, this is due to incomplete isolation of a pulmonary vein, allowing impulses to escape as if from a point source; in others, incomplete linear lesions can act as the substrate for macroreentrant circuits.[24-27]

CLINICAL PRESENTATIONS

Sinus Tachycardias

Physiologic Sinus Tachycardia

Sinus tachycardia, even though it may be a presenting feature, is usually an accompaniment to illness, physiologic stress, or anxiety. A full history and physical examination, accompanied by appropriate investigation (particularly to assess endocrine status and the possibilities of infection, heart failure, and dehydration), usually reveal an underlying cause. The context of the medical consultation (the "white coat" syndrome) may itself contribute, and ambulatory monitoring can be very useful to determine whether the tachycardia persists outside this environment.

Only if physiologic responses and psychological factors have been rigorously excluded can a sinus tachycardia be considered pathologic.

Inappropriate Sinus Tachycardia

Ambulatory monitoring and exercise testing show that inappropriate sinus tachycardia takes two forms.[28] In the typical form, sinus tachycardia is present both at rest (usually above 100 beats per minute) and on exertion. In the second form (which is either less common or perhaps less commonly recognized), the rate is nearly normal at rest but increases more than is appropriate on exertion.

Both forms are seen most commonly in young adults, with a preponderance of women. The condition is diagnosed with particular frequency among those working in the medical and allied professions; this may reflect an increased rate of detection and documentation in these groups.

Sinus Node Re-entrant Tachycardia

Sinus node re-entrant tachycardia is a common form of atrial microreentry. It is characterized by a paroxysmal nature (abrupt onset and termination), a P-wave morphology that is indistinguishable from that of sinus rhythm, and a PR interval that is normal for the heart rate. In the electrophysiology laboratory, the atrial activation sequence is identical to that in sinus rhythm, and the tachycardia can be initiated and terminated by critically timed premature atrial complexes, most easily near the sinus node. Although sinus node re-entry is frequently seen in the electrophysiology laboratory, it is rarely clinically relevant.[29]

Atrial Tachycardias

Atrial tachycardias account for approximately 10% of supraventricular tachycardias noted in the electrophysiology laboratory.[30,31] The P-wave morphology differs (although sometimes subtly) from that in sinus rhythm, and the tachycardia does not involve the atrioventricular node. Thus, the PR interval is related simply to the atrial rate; slight variations in the P-P interval are common, and atrioventricular block does not interrupt the tachycardia (Fig. 59.4). When episodes of tachycardia cease, the last beat is usually conducted to the ventricles, so that the last event inscribed on the electrocardiogram is a QRS complex. Conversely, termination of supraventricular tachycardia is usually caused by block in the atrioventricular node so that the last event is a nonconducted P wave.

Certain forms of atrial tachycardia deserve particular mention.

Benign Atrial Tachycardia of the Elderly

Ambulatory monitoring in apparently healthy elderly individuals frequently shows short-lived episodes of moderate atrial tachycardia (Fig. 59.5), which are usually asymptomatic and apparently have no prognostic significance.

Atrial Tachycardia with Block

Atrial tachycardia with coexistent atrioventricular block may be a hallmark of severe digitalis intoxication (Fig. 59.6), generally with plasma levels above 4.0 nmol/L. However, it is not a pathognomonic finding as was once thought. In one series from the 1960s, 22% of cases of atrial tachycardia

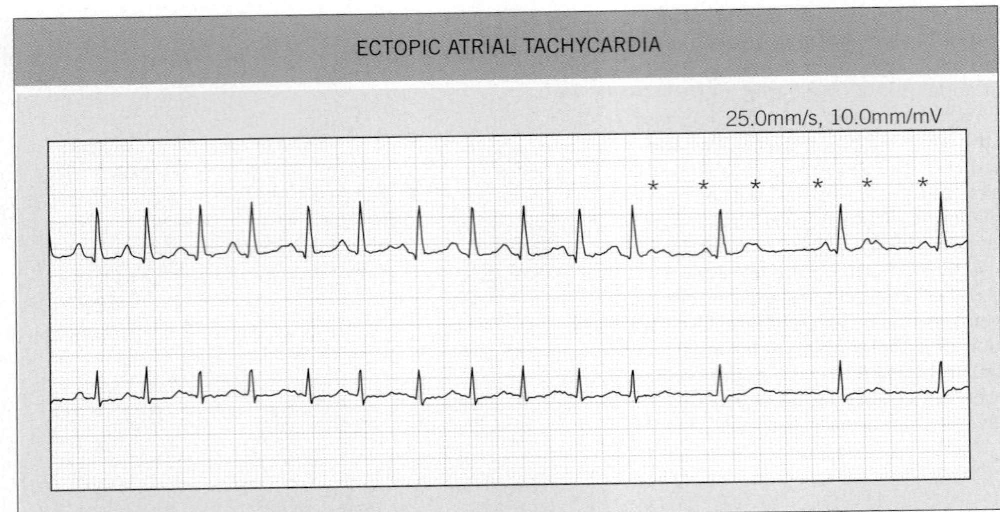

Figure 59.4 Ectopic atrial tachycardia. With 2:1 atrioventricular block *(right),* the arrhythmia continues. This confirms that the mechanism is an atrial arrhythmia and not dependent on atrioventricular conduction. Note that the P waves *(asterisks)* are slightly irregular.

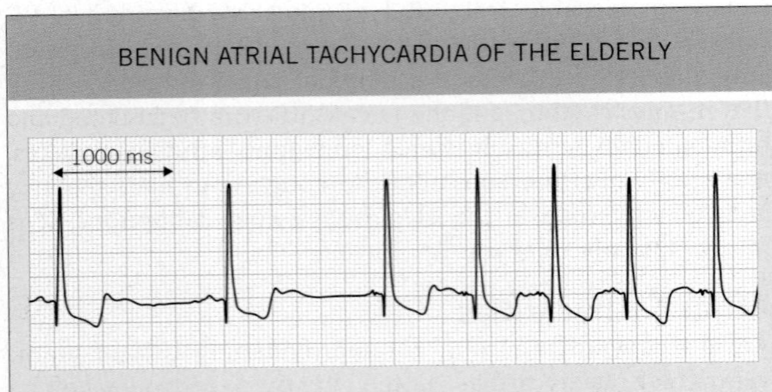

Figure 59.5 Benign atrial tachycardia of the elderly. This section of ambulatory monitoring was recorded at night. The tracing shows sinus bradycardia with a rate of approximately 40 beats per minute, followed by the abrupt onset of a relative tachycardia of more than 90 beats per minute, with a different P-wave morphology. (Reproduced with permission from Murgatroyd FD, Camm AJ. Atrial arrhythmias. Lancet 1993;341:1317-1322.)

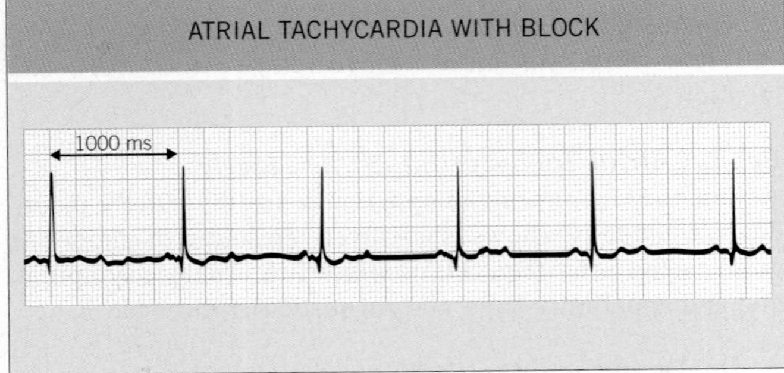

Figure 59.6 Atrial tachycardia with block. A moderate atrial tachycardia with 2:1 atrioventricular block is seen in this patient with digitalis intoxication. (From Naccarelli GV, Shih H-T, Jalal S. Sinus node reentry and atrial tachycardias. In Zipes DP, Jalife J, eds. Cardiac Electrophysiology. From Cell to Bedside, 2nd ed. Philadelphia, WB Saunders, 1995:607-619.)

with block were not caused by digitalis,[32] and now that digoxin intoxication is much rarer, this proportion is probably considerably lower. Digitalis toxicity may be exacerbated by hypokalemia. The atrial rate may be anywhere from 100 to 250 beats per minute, and second-degree atrioventricular block may be seen even at the lower end of this range.

Multifocal Atrial Tachycardia

Multifocal atrial tachycardia (as opposed to a "wandering atrial pacemaker," a type of bradycardia) is an uncommon arrhythmia typically seen in ill, elderly patients. The tachycardia is irregular and exhibits at least three P-wave shapes (Fig. 59.7). The ventricular response is usually between 100 and 160 beats per minute and appears irregularly irregular, so the arrhythmia can easily be mistaken for atrial fibrillation. Although multifocal atrial tachycardia can be found in healthy individuals, it is most commonly seen in the critically ill.[33] At least 60% of patients have significant pulmonary disease, and the arrhythmia accompanies exacerbations of obstructive pulmonary disease, respiratory or cardiac failure, infective episodes, surgery, and metabolic disturbances in the severely ill in whom hypoxia and acidosis are present.

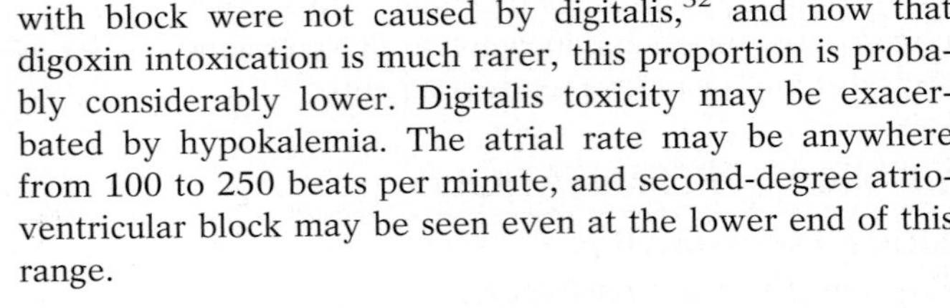

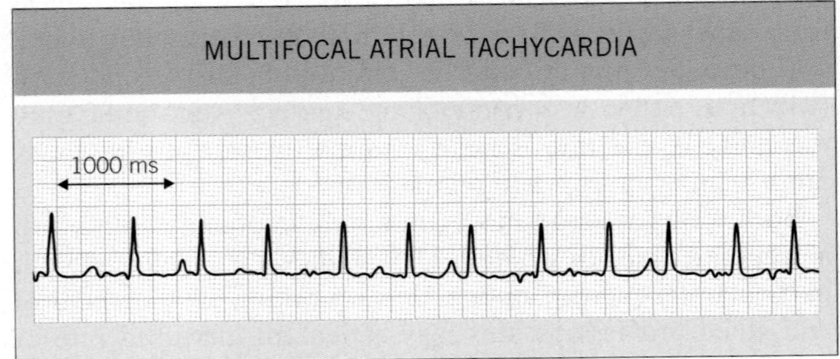

Figure 59.7 Multifocal atrial tachycardia. At least four distinct P-wave shapes can be discerned. The ventricular rhythm is irregular, and this arrhythmia can be confused with atrial fibrillation. (Reproduced with permission from Murgatroyd FD, Camm AJ. Atrial arrhythmias. Lancet 1993;341:1317-1322.)

Typical Atrial Flutter

Epidemiology

An early compilation showed an incidence of typical atrial flutter between 0.4% and 1.2% among hospital-reviewed electrocardiograms; the arrhythmia was almost five times more common in men than in women.[34] Atrial flutter and fibrillation commonly alternate in the same patient. Atrial flutter is also associated with mitral and tricuspid valve disease, chronic airflow obstruction, and other conditions that cause significant right atrial enlargement. The arrhythmia typically lasts for hours to weeks, and short-lived episodes are exceptional. Conversely, chronic atrial flutter lasting months or years is unusual (although not unknown) as atrial fibrillation generally supervenes in the long term. This is probably due to a tachycardia-induced electrical remodeling of the atrium.[35] The converse of this process occurs when atrial fibrillation is organized into atrial flutter by class I antiarrhythmic drugs that increase the refractory period.

Electrocardiographic Diagnosis

Typical atrial flutter is characterized on the surface electrocardiogram by regular atrial activity that has a cycle length of 175 to 250 ms (usually very close to 200 ms). There are discrete positive P waves separated by an isoelectric interval in lead V_1, and a sawtooth pattern, with a slow downstroke and rapid upstroke, is seen in the inferior leads (Fig. 59.8). The rapid upstroke is probably due to left atrial activation and may be absent when flutter occurs in patients who have undergone ablation for atrial fibrillation.[36]

The P-wave rate can be considerably slower when flutter occurs in the presence of class I and class III antiarrhythmic drugs. The ventricular response is usually regular as atrioventricular conduction tends to be unchanging at any one time. Most commonly, an atrioventricular ratio of 2:1 or 3:1 gives a ventricular rate around 150 or 100 beats per minute, respectively. Higher degrees of atrioventricular block may give rise to lower ventricular rates, and occasionally Wenckebach-type atrioventricular conduction can give rise to an apparently irregular ventricular rate.

The diagnosis of atrial flutter is rarely difficult when the atrioventricular ratio is 3:1 or greater, as flutter waves are easily visible. With 1:1 and 2:1 conduction, however, the flutter waves may be difficult to discern because of overlapping QRS and T waves. Atrial flutter should be suspected in the presence of a regular tachycardia with a ventricular rate around 300 or 150 beats per minute. The diagnosis can be confirmed by transiently increasing the level of atrioventricular block with use of vagal maneuvers or drugs such as adenosine.

A number of antiarrhythmic drugs used in the treatment of atrial fibrillation or flutter can predispose to 1:1 conduction of atrial flutter to the ventricles. Class Ia and Ic agents can slow the atrial rate sufficiently to allow 1:1 conduction over the atrioventricular node where previously only 2:1 conduction was possible. Because of the rapid ventricular rate and the effect of these drugs on the His-Purkinje system, conduction is usually aberrant, and the typical result is a wide-complex tachycardia that may resemble ventricular tachycardia (Fig. 59.9). Again, vagal maneuvers or adenosine can be used to aid differential diagnosis (Fig. 59.10). The 1:1 conduction of atrial flutter is most commonly seen now with flecainide and propafenone because of the frequency of their use and potent effect on atrial cycle length. Class Ia agents (quinidine, disopyramide, procainamide) can also cause 1:1 conduction of atrial flutter, and this may be aided by an anticholinergic effect on the atrioventricular node. Conversely, 1:1 conduction of atrial flutter is seldom seen with class III agents (sotalol, amiodarone) because of blocking action on the node.

Clinical Presentation

The clinical presentation of atrial flutter depends on the underlying cardiac status of the patient and especially on the ventricular response. If the ventricular rate is 75 or 100 beats per minute, patients are often asymptomatic. The 2:1 atrioventricular conduction (ventricular rate around 150 beats per minute) may present with palpitations and breathlessness or more severe symptoms in patients with angina or

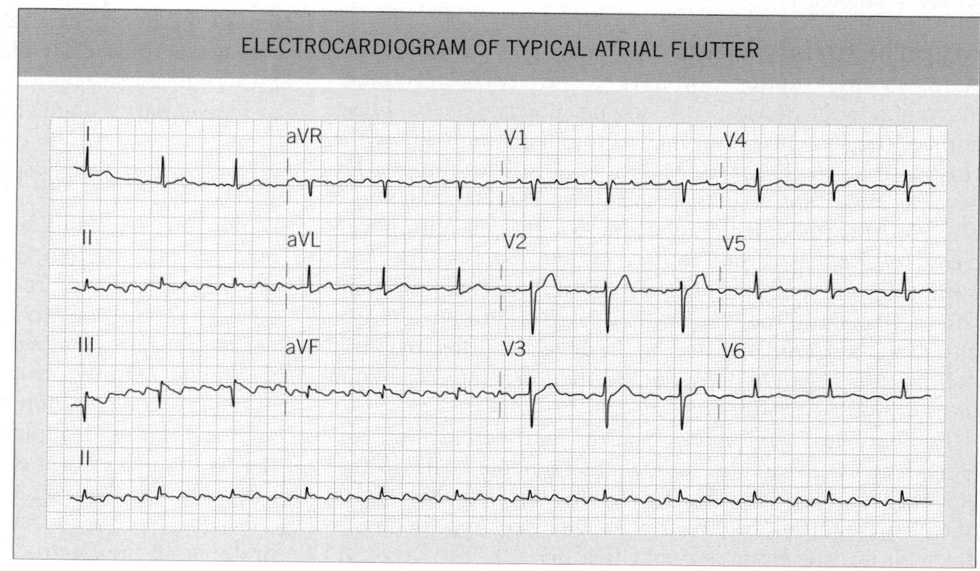

Figure 59.8 A 12-lead electrocardiogram of typical atrial flutter. Typical atrial flutter (counterclockwise, isthmus dependent). The atrial cycle length is 200 ms, and in V_1 there are discrete positive P waves separated by an isoelectric interval. In the inferior leads, there is a classic sawtooth pattern with a slow downstroke and a rapid upstroke.

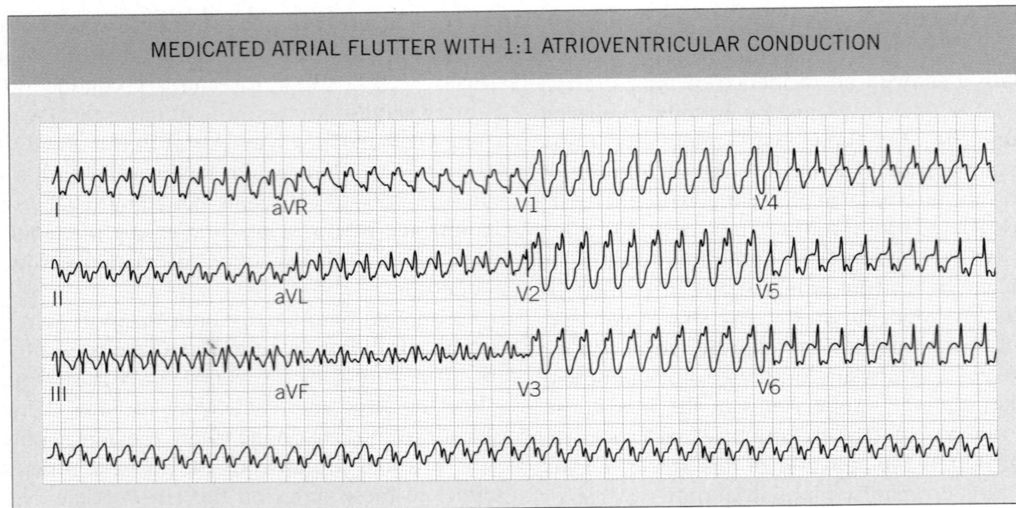

Figure 59.9 Medicated atrial flutter with 1:1 conduction. A 12-lead electrocardiogram from a patient treated with propafenone for paroxysmal atrial fibrillation and flutter. The drug has slowed the flutter cycle length to 250 ms. At this rate, 1:1 conduction over the atrioventricular node occurs with right bundle branch block. This can be mistaken for ventricular tachycardia.

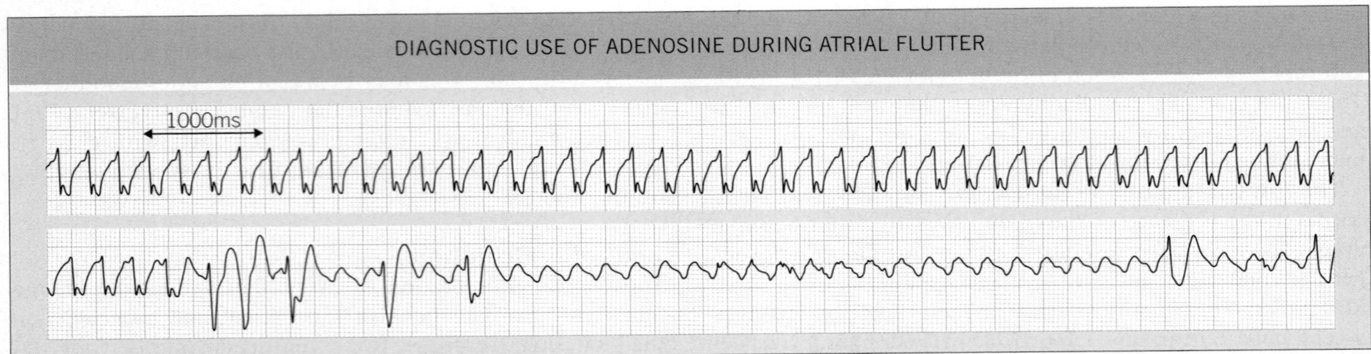

Figure 59.10 Diagnostic use of adenosine during atrial flutter. *Upper trace,* Wide QRS complex tachycardia with cycle length of 250 ms (in the same patient as in Fig. 59.9). The mechanism of tachycardia cannot be determined from this trace alone. *Lower trace,* The administration of intravenous adenosine causes transient atrioventricular block and reveals the underlying atrial flutter.

heart failure. Sustained 1:1 atrioventricular conduction is rare but usually causes extreme symptoms and, often, hemodynamic collapse.

Atypical Atrial Flutter

Atypical atrial flutter can have a variety of electrocardiographic appearances. The original description by Puech and colleagues[37] probably related to what is now known as clockwise atrial flutter. Recognition of this arrhythmia has become important as it is amenable to catheter ablation.[38] The electrocardiographic appearance, although not entirely characteristic, has certain fairly constant features. The atrial cycle length is similar to that of typical flutter; the predominant deflection in the inferior limb leads is positive and usually shows a degree of notching. In the chest leads, the atrial deflection is negative in V_1 and positive in V_6, but the point of transition is variable (Fig. 59.11).[19]

Truly atypical atrial flutter, such as that seen in adult congenital heart disease, is more heterogeneous. The surface electrocardiogram may bear a resemblance to that typical of clockwise flutter, or the atrial activity may appear sinusoidal with no isoelectric segment (Fig. 59.12). The "type II" atrial flutter originally described by Wells and colleagues[13] in postoperative patients may be initiated by attempts to terminate the typical form by use of rapid pacing but is itself unaffected by pacing. Atrial activity may be very rapid, and it is not entirely clear that this arrhythmia is indeed caused by a single macroreentrant circuit as opposed to a rapid focus or indeed partly organized propagation of atrial fibrillation.

DIAGNOSTIC TECHNIQUES

Deductions regarding arrhythmia mechanism can often be made from a rhythm strip, but invasive electrophysiologic study is occasionally required. However, in most cases, the 12-lead surface electrocardiogram of an arrhythmia is both necessary and sufficient for its diagnosis. The electrocardiographic features have been described for each arrhythmia in the preceding section of this chapter. The key to differentiation of atrial arrhythmias from supraventricular tachycardias is the demonstration that atrioventricular conduction is not critical to the maintenance of the arrhythmia.

When 1:1 or 2:1 atrioventricular conduction makes interpretation of the electrocardiogram difficult, vagal maneuvers

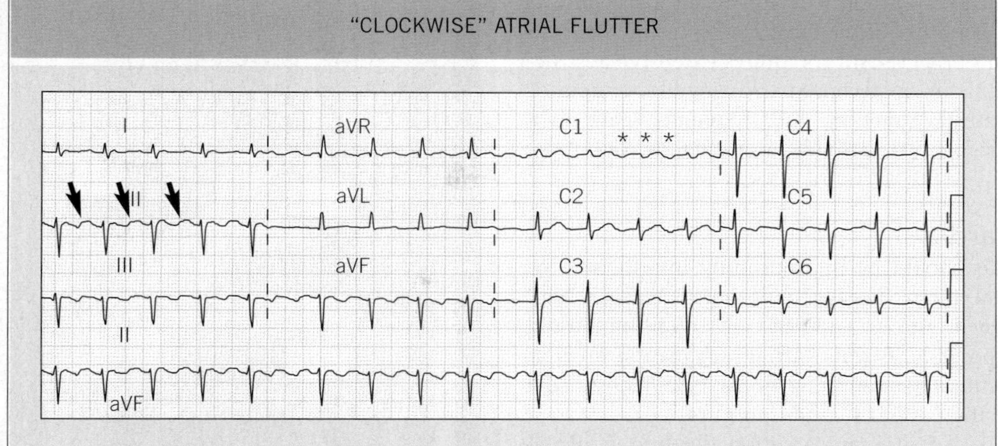

Figure 59.11 Clockwise atrial flutter. A 12-lead electrocardiogram of atypical flutter of the clockwise, isthmus-dependent type. Because of medication (sotalol), the atrial cycle length is slightly prolonged at 260 ms. Unlike in typical atrial flutter, the P waves in V_1 *(asterisks)* are negative and wide. In the inferior leads, the sawtooth pattern is less pronounced and more equiphasic, and there is slight notching *(arrows),* a common finding in clockwise flutter. The diagnosis was confirmed by entrainment mapping during electrophysiologic study, and conventional ablation of the cavotricuspid isthmus was curative.

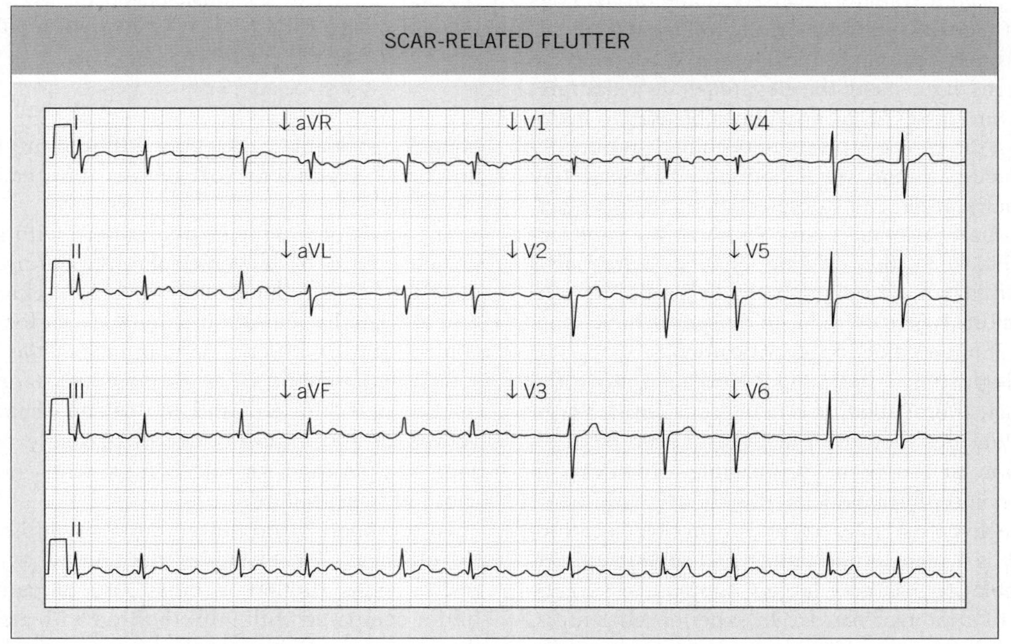

Figure 59.12 Scar-related flutter. A 12-lead electrocardiogram of atypical atrial flutter occurring 30 years after surgical repair of an atrial septal defect. The P wave is positive but wide in V_1, with little or no isoelectric interval. In the inferior leads, the negative sawtooth pattern of typical flutter is absent; if anything, P waves are positive. Mapping confirmed that the flutter circuit involved the right atriotomy scar.

or adenosine can be used to transiently increase atrioventricular block and reveal the underlying P-wave rate and morphology (see Fig. 59.10). An esophageal electrocardiogram is occasionally useful if atrial activity cannot be easily discerned from the surface. Electrophysiologic study yields the most information about atrial arrhythmias; the source of an ectopic rhythm can be deduced by standard multipolar electrodes and pinpointed with a mapping catheter. Much can be learned about the arrhythmia mechanism by use of pacing techniques and drugs (see Table 59.1).

MANAGEMENT

Sinus Tachycardia

The majority of sinus tachycardias are physiologic, and only the underlying condition needs treatment. Even if the tachycardia is clearly pathologic, specific treatment other than reassurance is seldom necessary. For patients with intractable symptoms, initial treatment is usually with a cardioselective beta blocker or verapamil, although other antiarrhythmic agents have been tried. In exceptional cases, catheter ablation of the sinus node can be performed. This is not a straightforward procedure. Abolition of inappropriate sinus tachycardia (as opposed to sinus node re-entry) requires extensive destruction of sinus nodal tissue, may cause narrowing of the superior vena cava–right atrium junction, and frequently leads to a pacemaker requirement to provide a normal chronotropic response.[39,40]

Atrial Tachycardia

Atrial tachycardias should be appropriately investigated to rule out structural heart disease, pulmonary disease, and metabolic imbalance, and any underlying condition should be treated when possible. Regular atrial tachycardia precipitated during an acute illness and multifocal atrial tachycardia tend to resolve if the patient's condition improves.

In the special case of digitalis intoxication, the drug should be withdrawn and serum potassium should be kept at the high end of the normal range (4.5 to 5.0 mmol/L if possible). Although the resulting atrial tachycardia may not itself cause decompensation, the clinician should be aware of the risk of malignant ventricular arrhythmias. Cardioversion should be performed only after insertion of temporary ventricular pacing because ventricular standstill may occur in the presence of digitalis toxicity. The toxicity can be rapidly reversed by the intravenous administration of digoxin-specific antibody fragment.

The antiarrhythmic treatment of atrial tachycardia may be directed at the arrhythmia itself, the elevated ventricular rate, or both. Drugs from classes Ia, Ic, and III can be used to maintain sinus rhythm; the choice is partly determined empirically and by patient factors. Drugs are seldom able to completely suppress atrial tachycardia, and a drug acting on the atrioventricular node is usually also necessary. To lower the ventricular rate, beta blockers, the calcium channel antagonists verapamil and diltiazem, and digoxin can be used. The efficacy of digoxin alone is greatly reduced by sympathetic tone; it is therefore of limited value in the critically ill.

Electrophysiologic study is indicated if the diagnosis of atrial tachycardia is unclear or if ablation is being considered. Surgical experience indicates that atrial tachycardia can be abolished by resection of the tissue responsible. However, in many cases, especially those associated with structural heart disease, atrial tachycardia may recur in another location; repeated surgery is a major undertaking and seldom considered. Catheter ablation has now largely supplanted surgery in the treatment of atrial tachycardia. In experienced centers, procedural success rates are high and complications rare. For patients with atrial tachycardia due to automatic foci and otherwise normal hearts, catheter ablation is usually curative (Fig. 59.13).[41] For others, the risk of recurrence at another site is greater, but repeated procedures can be undertaken.

In patients with intractable atrial tachycardia that is resistant to drug therapy and in whom curative catheter ablation is not possible, atrioventricular nodal ablation with implantation of a permanent ventricular pacemaker should be considered. This is particularly suitable in elderly patients and those in whom atrial tachycardia coexists with atrial fibrillation.

Atrial Flutter

As with atrial tachycardia, the presence of structural heart disease and other underlying pathologic processes must be assessed in patients with atrial flutter. This assessment may

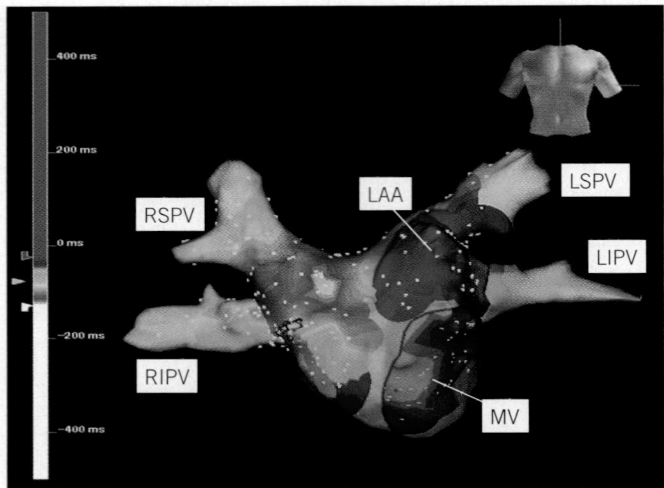

Figure 59.13 Ectopic atrial tachycardia in the left atrium. Representation of the left atrium in the anteroposterior view. A color map of electrical activation (white and red, earliest; blue and indigo, latest) is superimposed. Activation is demonstrated to arise from a focus on the roof, anterior to the antrum of the right superior pulmonary vein. This activation map was obtained with a nonfluoroscopic mapping system (NavX, Endocardial Solutions, Inc.). LAA, left atrial appendage; MV, mitral valve; LIPV, LSPV, RIPV, RSPV, left inferior and superior, right inferior and superior pulmonary veins.

identify reversible causes and will indicate the appropriateness and probability of success of available treatment modalities.

The goals of treatment in a patient with atrial flutter can include control of the ventricular rate during arrhythmia, termination of arrhythmia, and prevention of arrhythmia recurrence. Digitalis remains in common use for ventricular rate control, but its efficacy is marginal in the context of high sympathetic tone, such as during exercise or illness. For this reason, beta blockers and the calcium channel antagonists verapamil and diltiazem are increasingly preferred. Diltiazem may be used for rate control when high rates are the cause of heart failure.[42]

To terminate atrial flutter, antiarrhythmic drugs are of little efficacy. For example, flecainide has been found to restore sinus rhythm in only 20% of patients with atrial flutter compared with 90% of those with atrial fibrillation[43]; the efficacies of most other drugs are similar or lower. An exception to this rule is some of the newer class III agents. Intravenous ibutilide (up to 2 mg) and dofetilide (up to 8 μg/kg) have been reported to achieve pharmacologic cardioversion of atrial flutter in up to 70% of cases, although torsades de pointes is an occasional complication.[44,45] Electrical methods are generally preferred for the termination of atrial flutter. Overdrive pacing from the high right atrium is classically used, initially at a cycle length 10 ms shorter than that of the flutter, then decreasing in 10-ms steps, using either repeated bursts or progressive "ramp" pacing. Capture of the atria is confirmed when positive P waves are seen in lead II; pacing can then be abruptly terminated or gradually slowed to a normal rate. High pacing outputs (up to 20 mA) are frequently required to ensure atrial capture, and the procedure need not be abandoned until repeated attempts have been made at cycle lengths down to 150 ms. More often than not, successful termination of atrial flutter is accompanied by a transitional period of atrial fibrillation. The efficacy of overdrive pacing is improved, and the likelihood of producing atrial fibrillation reduced, if an antiarrhythmic drug such as procainamide or ibutilide has been given.[46] Synchronized direct current shocks are particularly effective in cardioverting atrial flutter; sinus rhythm can often be restored with energies as low as 25 J, and shocks of 100 J are virtually always effective.

There are few published data specifically relating to the prophylaxis of atrial flutter; but in general, antiarrhythmic drugs have only modest efficacy. Agents from classes Ia and Ic are often used, with some success. However, as complete arrhythmia suppression is rarely achieved, and accelerated ventricular rates are a common problem with these drugs (see earlier), the addition of an atrioventricular node–blocking drug is strongly recommended. The class III antiarrhythmic agents sotalol (usually 80 to 240 mg/day in divided doses) and amiodarone (usually 200 mg/day) are increasingly used for the prevention of atrial flutter. Again, there are few data specific to this arrhythmia regarding efficacy. Accelerated ventricular rates seem to be far less of a problem with these agents, presumably because of their additional effects on atrioventricular nodal conduction. Both amiodarone and sotalol have their drawbacks, however. Some patients, especially younger ones, may tolerate poorly the side effects of sotalol related to beta blockade, and the QT interval must be closely observed when the drug is initiated because of the appreciable risk of torsades de pointes. Proarrhythmia is rare with amiodarone, but because of its well-known potential for extracardiac toxicity, this drug is not normally the first choice.

A number of nonpharmacologic treatments for atrial flutter have been proposed. Success with overdrive pacing to terminate the arrhythmia acutely prompted the investigation of implanted atrial pacemakers with antitachycardia pacing capability. The long-term efficacy of these devices proved limited, and they are rarely used now. However, atrial flutter can often be terminated by overdriving in the clinic by use of the noninvasive programmed stimulation feature present in many pacemakers. Antitachycardia pacing has re-emerged recently as a capability in certain implantable defibrillators, which are able to distinguish atrial from ventricular arrhythmias and deliver both pacing and cardioversion therapies.[47] The place of such devices, and that of stand-alone atrial defibrillators, in the management of patients with atrial flutter is not yet clear.[48]

Catheter Ablation for Atrial Flutter

The greatest advances in the management of typical atrial flutter in recent years have been in the field of ablation. In the 1980s, intraoperative and catheter mapping confirmed the path of the re-entrant circuit and identified the region of the subeustachian isthmus as both the zone of slow conduction and the narrowest portion of the circuit (Fig. 59.14; see also Fig. 59.2).[49] Cryoablation in this region was effective in preventing atrial flutter, although not atrial fibrillation. Surgery has now been supplanted by catheter ablation for atrial flutter. Initial attempts at modifying the zone of slow conduction (identified by mapping or anatomically) were able to terminate flutter and to prevent its reinitiation acutely, but long-term success rates were disappointing. Catheter ablation is therefore instead directed at creation of a line of block across the subeustachian isthmus, usually by delivery of a series of

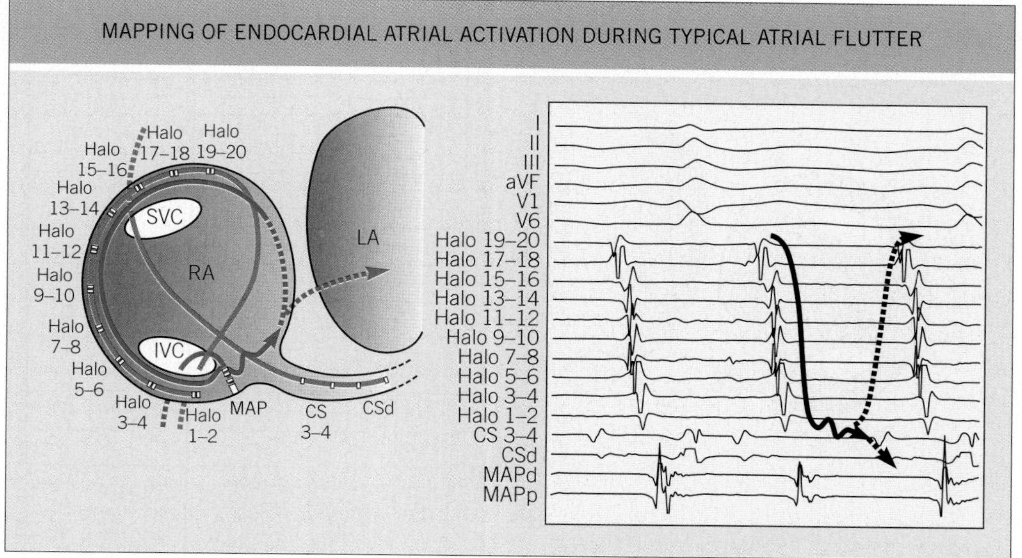

Figure 59.14 Mapping of endocardial atrial activation during typical atrial flutter. *Left,* A multipolar catheter (electrodes numbered Halo 1 to 20) has been advanced through the inferior vena cava (IVC) to record right atrial (RA) activation, parallel to the tricuspid annulus. Another catheter (numbered CS 3-4) has been advanced through the superior vena cava (SVC) to record left atrial (LA) activation through the coronary sinus, and a mapping catheter is positioned at the cavotricuspid isthmus (MAP). *Right, from top to bottom,* Surface electrocardiogram leads, bipolar endocardial electrograms recorded from the right atrial and coronary sinus electrodes and the mapping catheter. The flutter circuit *(arrowhead)* travels in a counterclockwise direction around the right atrium, activating the multipolar electrode from pole 20 to pole 1, followed by the mapping catheter. Activation then passes through the zone of slow conduction before passively activating the left atrium (recorded in the coronary sinus) and ascending the interatrial septum.

radiofrequency lesions between the tricuspid annulus and the orifice of the inferior vena cava but sometimes between the tricuspid annulus and the coronary sinus os.[17] When permanent bidirectional conduction block across the isthmus is achieved (Fig. 59.15), the long-term "cure" rate for atrial flutter approaches 100%.[50] In 10% to 20% of patients, difficulty is encountered in achieving this goal, largely because of the thickness and irregularity of pectinate muscle in the isthmus. Repeated ablation procedures and catheter designs yielding deeper lesions can largely circumvent this problem.[51]

Because of the high success rate and low complication rate now achievable, catheter ablation for typical atrial flutter should be considered at an early stage for symptomatic patients. Indeed, ablation may now be preferable to antiarrhythmic drugs as first-line therapy, although it must be borne in mind that atrial fibrillation occurs in at least 25% of patients during long-term follow-up after flutter ablation.[52,53] This is especially the case in those patients known to have a history of atrial fibrillation or impaired left ventricular function (the risk in one study being only 10% in those with neither of these risk factors), which responds better than atrial flutter

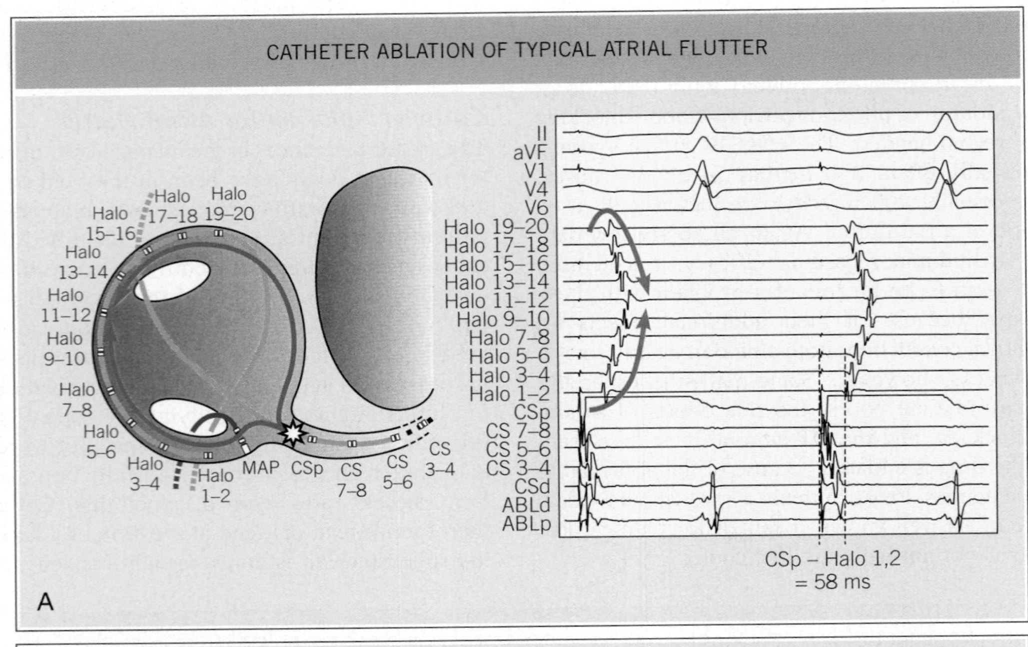

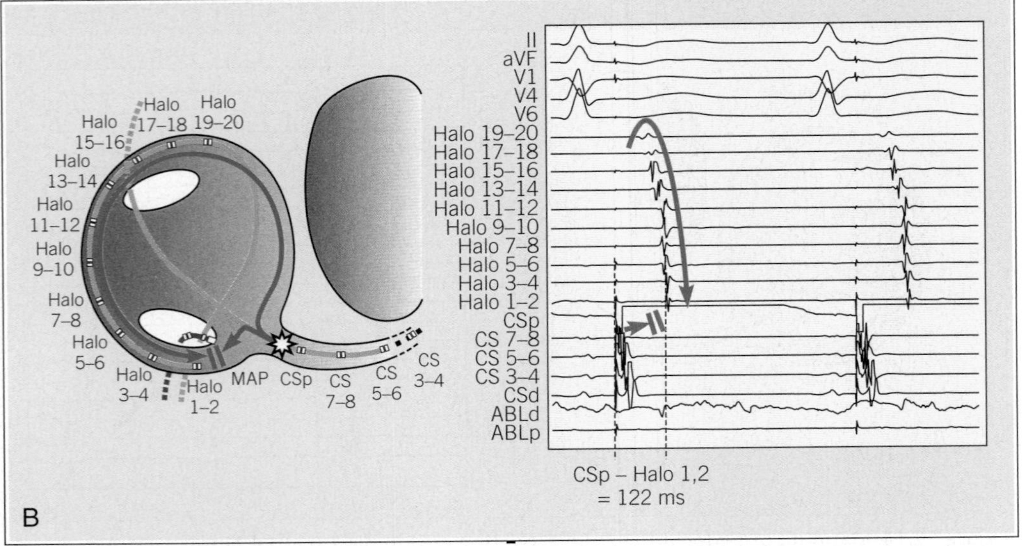

Figure 59.15 Catheter ablation of typical atrial flutter: validation of conduction block across cavotricuspid isthmus. A, When the proximal coronary sinus is paced before ablation, activation spreads around the right atrium in both clockwise and counterclockwise directions. Activation in the multipolar catheter is earliest at the proximal (Halo 19-20) and distal (Halo 1-2) ends and latest at the middle poles. **B,** After successful ablation, clockwise propagation of the impulse in the right atrium is not possible owing to block across the cavotricuspid isthmus. Activation spreads solely in the counterclockwise direction; the distal poles of the multipolar catheter (Halo 1-2) now record the latest electrogram, and the time taken for the impulse to reach these poles has greatly increased. Block of counterclockwise propagation across the isthmus can be similarly documented by pacing from Halo 1-2 (not shown).

to antiarrhythmic medication.[54] Finally, isthmus ablation appears to be successful in suppressing atrial flutter that complicates antiarrhythmic drug treatment for atrial fibrillation.[55]

Certain forms of atypical flutter are also amenable to catheter ablation. Clockwise flutter shares the same path as typical flutter with the direction reversed. The arrhythmia is dependent on conduction across the subeustachian isthmus, so ablation of this isthmus (as for typical flutter) is generally curative.[38,56] Unfortunately, clockwise flutter cannot be identified with certainty from the surface electrocardiogram. Intracardiac mapping and entrainment are necessary to confirm that the arrhythmia is isthmus dependent before ablation. Truly atypical flutter may resemble typical or clockwise flutter on the surface electrocardiogram but is not isthmus dependent. Mapping to identify the causative circuit is difficult with conventional techniques as the rhythm tends to be unstable, degenerating into atrial fibrillation or reorganizing into another form of atrial flutter. Newer mapping technologies, such as nonfluoroscopic mapping (Fig. 59.16), can assist in defining the flutter circuits and targeting ablation strategies.

Mapping and ablation of atrial flutter related to surgery for congenital heart disease present a spectrum of difficulty. The long atriotomy scars used for the closure of atrial and ventricular septal defects may constitute the anatomic obstacle around which the flutter circuit revolves. The circuit can be blocked by creating a line of ablation lesions between the scar and another fixed obstacle, typically the inferior vena cava or tricuspid annulus. In patients with atrial flutter complicating Mustard or Senning and Fontan procedures, catheter ablation is considerably more challenging and currently less successful. The identification of the flutter circuits is difficult because the atrial anatomy is complex and the circuits are caused by atrial stretching as well as by the surgical scars. Although identified flutter circuits can often be rendered noninducible acutely, long-term success is limited by the appearance of new flutter circuits; this is particularly the case with the Fontan procedure.[20,57] It is likely that improvements in atrial arrhythmias after surgery for congenital heart disease will come partly from newer mapping technologies[58] and partly from modifications to surgical technique that avoid creation of the arrhythmia substrate (see Chapter 128).

Despite the advances made in mapping and ablation of the various types of atrial flutter, there remain a few patients refractory both to these techniques and to conventional pharmacologic treatment. In such patients, catheter ablation of the atrioventricular node with permanent ventricular pacing remains a simple option for ventricular rate control. Although the arrhythmia (and therefore the possible need for anticoagulation) is unaffected, the need for antiarrhythmic medication is obviated, which can be a particular advantage in the elderly and those with impaired ventricular function. Consideration should be given to biventricular rather than right ventricular pacing to avoid left ventricular dyssynchrony.[59]

PROGNOSIS

In general, atrial tachycardias and flutters carry very little intrinsic risk. However, adverse consequences are related to the presence of underlying disease, the short- and long-term effects of increased ventricular rate, and the possibility

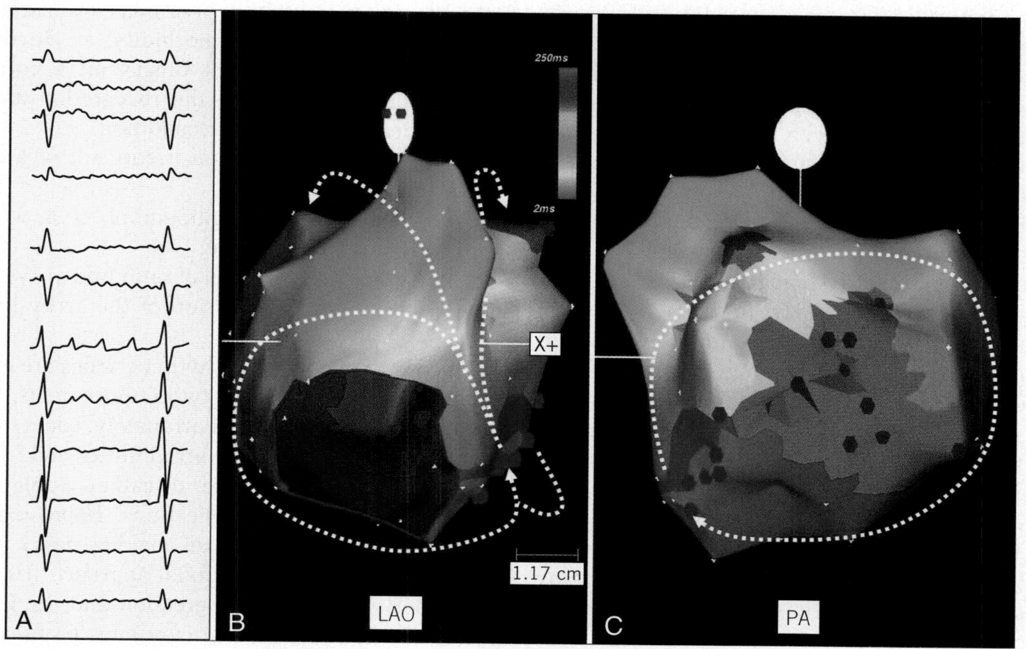

Figure 59.16 Left atrial flutter. Atypical atrial flutter in the left atrium. **A,** The 12-lead electrocardiogram (I, II, III, aVR, aVL, aVF, V_1 to V_6) showing atrial activity, the regularity of which is apparent only in the chest leads. **B** and **C,** Representations of the left atrium in the left anterior oblique (LAO) and posteroanterior (PA) projections. A color map of electrical activation (red, earliest; blue and indigo, latest) is superimposed. Activation is seen to rotate around two electrically silent zones: the mitral annulus (lower part of **B**, depicted as a cutout) and the posterior left atrium (gray area in **C**). A number of radiofrequency lesions (dark red dots) were made to create a line of block between these two silent zones and thus abolish this flutter circuit. The activation map was obtained by a nonfluoroscopic mapping system (Carto, Biosense Webster, Inc.), courtesy of Drs. P. Jais and M. Haïssaguerre.

of thromboembolic sequelae. The likelihood of arrhythmia recurrence appears to be high in untreated patients when no reversible cause is found; this includes those with idiopathic atrial flutter, coexistent cardiomyopathy, and corrected congenital heart disease.

Underlying Disease

The prognosis is generally excellent in patients with otherwise normal hearts, and short-lived episodes of slow atrial tachycardia are so common in the elderly that they can be considered normal.[60] At the other extreme, mortality may be as high as 60% when multifocal atrial tachycardia occurs in the critical care setting.[61] This, however, reflects the severity of the underlying disease rather than the arrhythmia itself.

Likewise, atrial flutter appears to confer very little intrinsic risk in patients with normal hearts, cardiomyopathy, or congenital heart disease. One large series of patients with flutter diagnosed before 25 years of age (81% of whom had surgically corrected or uncorrected congenital heart disease and only 8% of whom had structurally normal hearts) found 83% alive at mean follow-up of 6.5 years and 50% alive without atrial flutter.[62] After the Mustard or Senning and Fontan procedures, the late loss of normal sinus node function and the occurrence of atrial flutter are common and often reflect poor hemodynamic function and a risk of sudden death.[63]

Effects of Tachycardia

Very rapid ventricular rates caused by atrial arrhythmias with 1:1 atrioventricular conduction may cause angina, syncope, and hemodynamic collapse. A particularly common cause in adults is medicated atrial flutter (see earlier), which responds to the addition of an atrioventricular node–blocking drug. Theoretically, extreme ventricular rates in susceptible patients (critical coronary stenosis, Wolff-Parkinson-White syndrome, hypertrophic cardiomyopathy) could lead to ventricular fibrillation. However, this form of sudden death is probably an even rarer complication of atrial tachycardia and flutter than it is of atrial fibrillation.

Atrial arrhythmias that cause the ventricular rate to be persistently elevated can eventually lead to progressive ventricular dilatation and systolic dysfunction.[64] This tachycardia cardiomyopathy develops slowly (months or longer) and typically accompanies ventricular rates between 120 and 180 beats per minute; patients with persistently higher rates tend to present at an early stage. It has most often been described with atrial fibrillation but can also accompany incessant atrial tachycardia and atrial flutter.[65,66] The degree of ventricular dysfunction can be severe, and tachycardia cardiomyopathy can be difficult to distinguish at presentation from an idiopathic dilated cardiomyopathy *causing* atrial arrhythmia. However, tachycardia cardiomyopathy usually resolves to a striking extent with successful antiarrhythmic treatment or ventricular rate control.

Thromboembolic Risk

Atrial tachycardia has not been shown to carry a thromboembolic risk, presumably because the coordination of atrial mechanical activity is preserved. Atrial flutter was also thought to carry little or no risk of thromboembolic complications until recently. However, left atrial thrombus is detectable by transesophageal echocardiography in 11% of patients with atrial flutter, with spontaneous echo contrast in another 23%. In about a third of patients who are successfully cardioverted, atrial mechanical function is impaired and recovers only gradually.[67,68] In a series of 191 patients referred with atrial flutter, 11 patients gave a history of thromboembolism (four after cardioversion or catheter ablation), and nine more events occurred during 26 ± 18 months of follow-up. Risk factors for thromboembolism were hypertension (the only independent predictor), organic heart disease, left ventricular failure, and diabetes.[69] Retrospective analysis indicates that effective anticoagulation significantly reduces the incidence of thromboembolism in atrial flutter.[70] Randomized controlled studies have not been performed and are unlikely to be. In addition to this intrinsic thromboembolic risk, atrial flutter often coexists with atrial fibrillation, and atrial fibrillation frequently develops despite curative ablation of atrial flutter. For these reasons, anticoagulant prophylaxis is strongly recommended for patients with atrial flutter and risk factors for thromboembolism and around the time of cardioversion, as with atrial fibrillation. Even after successful catheter ablation of atrial flutter, high-risk patients should continue anticoagulation because of the ongoing risk of atrial fibrillation.

SUMMARY

Atrial arrhythmias constitute an increasing proportion of the workload of cardiologists in the developed world. This is probably due in part to an increasing prevalence in an aging population, in part to improved diagnostic methods, and in part to a switch in attention from supraventricular tachycardias as they are gradually eradicated by catheter ablation.

Although rarely putting the patient at immediate life-threatening risk, atrial arrhythmias are associated with considerable cardiovascular morbidity, as either a cause or an effect. Their management hinges on a correct electrocardiographic diagnosis and the recognition and treatment of any underlying pathologic condition.

As with atrial fibrillation, treatment of atrial tachycardia and flutter is focused on

- the reduction of thromboembolic risk with anticoagulation where appropriate;
- the control of ventricular rate; and
- the attempted suppression of the arrhythmia itself.

Anticoagulant and antiarrhythmic drugs are generally able to achieve the first of these two requirements, but the last has often proved frustrating. Fortunately, some of the most resistant arrhythmias—typical atrial flutter and focal atrial tachycardia—are now amenable to catheter ablation with a high cure rate and few complications. Improved understanding and technical advances are making many atypical flutters amenable to an interventional approach. However, because of underlying disease progression and the incidence of late atrial fibrillation, the term *cure* must be used with care.

Catheter ablation is clearly superior to antiarrhythmic drugs for the suppression of typical (and often atypical) atrial flutter and is increasingly useful for unifocal atrial tachycardia, although antiarrhythmic drugs still have a role. In patients with other associated risk factors, the need to consider anticoagulation cannot be overemphasized. Even after apparently successful flutter ablation, the possibility of asymptomatic arrhythmia recurrence and the development of atrial fibrillation means that this risk should not be forgotten.

chapter

60 Pre-excitation Syndromes

James W. Leitch and Malcolm Barlow

Definition

- Pre-excitation is activation of part of the ventricle by an anomalous connection before it is depolarized by the normal atrioventricular (AV) conducting system.

Key Features

- Most pathways connect the atrium and ventricle (AV, 97%), with rare variants such as atriofascicular (1% to 3%) connections.
- Presentation is usually in infancy or in young adults with supraventricular tachycardia (70%) or atrial fibrillation (30%).
- The spectrum of presentations is from asymptomatic (30% to 50%) to recurrent debilitating episodes of tachycardia and rarely to tachycardia-induced cardiomyopathy and sudden death.
- Sudden death results from rapid ventricular response to atrial fibrillation.

Therapy

- Symptomatic patients should undergo diagnostic electrophysiologic study.
- Catheter ablation is highly effective and is the preferred therapy.
- Asymptomatic patients with inducible supraventricular tachycardia and AV connections capable of rapid conduction may consider catheter ablation.

The history of pre-excitation has been summarized by Prystowsky.[1] As is usually the case with eponymously christened diseases, Wolff, Parkinson, and White[2,3] were not the first to describe pre-excitation, which had been reported by several investigators previously. The report by Wolff of the 11 cases collected by White and Parkinson clearly described the clinical syndrome of an electrocardiographic abnormality (short PR interval and wide QRS complex) in young patients with paroxysmal tachycardia and otherwise normal hearts. In any case, the abbreviated eponym WPW has a certain alliterative attractiveness, and it imparted a scientific air to a condition that in 1930 was completely unexplained. In fact, Wolff, Parkinson, and White thought that the electrocardiographic abnormality was a result of bundle branch block; it was only 2 years later that the correct interpretation of pre-excitation was postulated.[4] Key developments leading to our current understanding of pre-excitation include

- the development of a theory to explain the findings of pre-excitation[4];
- the histologic confirmation of this theory in patients with pre-excitation[5];
- the development of a technique to characterize pre-excitation and associated arrhythmias, namely, electrophysiologic studies;
- the demonstration that surgical division of accessory pathways cured the Wolff-Parkinson-White (WPW) syndrome[6,7]; and
- the refinement of accessory pathway localization and development of energy delivery systems that allowed catheter-based therapy for pre-excitation syndromes.[8,9]

EPIDEMIOLOGY

The prevalence of pre-excitation has been estimated to be about 0.1% to 0.2%,[10-12] but this figure may underestimate the true prevalence of the congenital abnormality at birth. Electrocardiograms are not collected routinely in healthy neonates, and the prevalence of pre-excitation decreases with age as some patients spontaneously lose accessory pathway conduction.[11,13] Most information about the fate of adults with pre-excitation is derived from Army and Air Force personnel,[11] and there are obvious problems with these sample populations. More recently, a population-based study found that the incidence of pre-excitation was around 4 per 100,000 of the population per year, with about half of the patients presenting with asymptomatic electrocardiographic abnormalities.[14] For reasons that are unexplained, pre-excitation is 1.5 to 2 times as common in males as in females. There is a bimodal distribution of age at presentation, with some patients presenting in infancy and the majority as young adults.

ANATOMY AND PATHOPHYSIOLOGY

A classification of pre-excitation is shown in Figure 60.1. Almost all patients who have symptomatic pre-excitation have an accessory atrioventricular (AV) connection. Accessory AV pathways can be conceptualized as a developmental "defect" in the insulation that separates the atrial and ventricular fibrous rings (see Fig. 60.1). At early stages of development of the heart, the atrium and the ventricle are continuous. The development of the AV sulcus and central fibrous body separates the atrium and ventricle into two syncytia connected only by the AV node and the bundle of His. Failure of this process could be considered to result in an accessory AV connection. This naive explanation for accessory pathways does not account for the anatomic location of accessory AV pathways, which are found far more commonly in the left side of the heart, or for the histologic observations of a well-formed fibrous annulus at the site of accessory AV

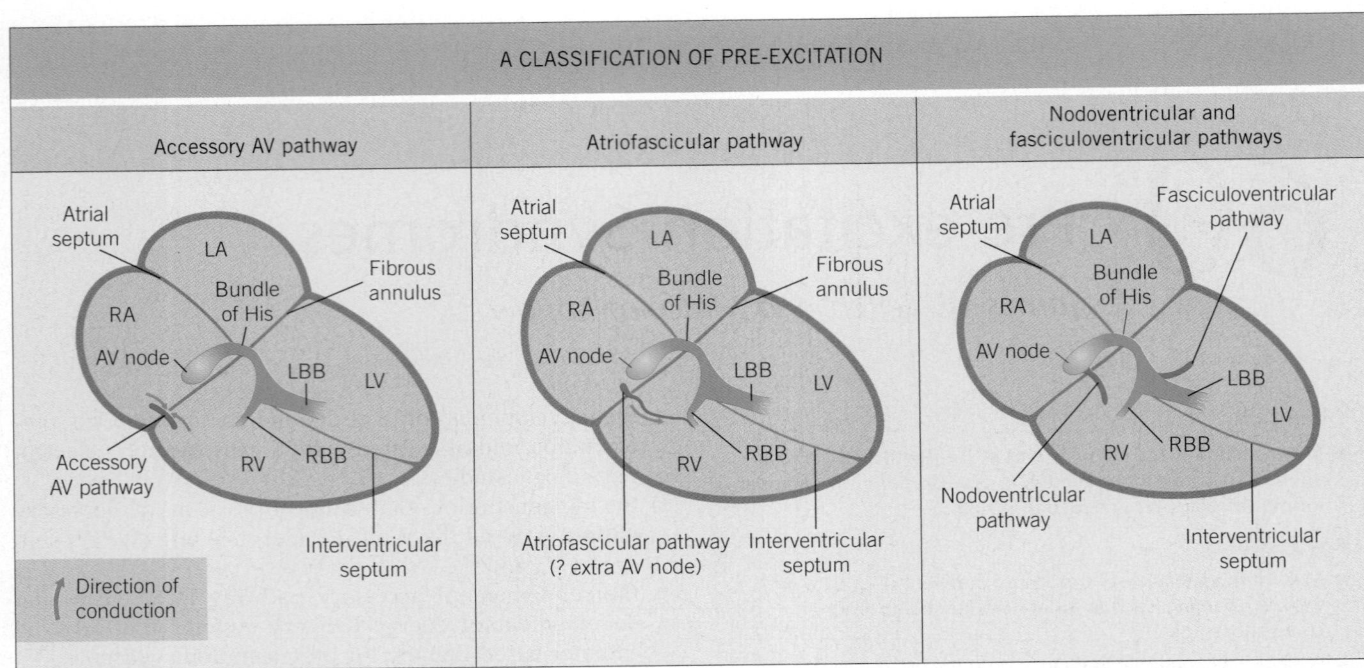

Figure 60.1 A classification of pre-excitation. AV, atrioventricular; LA, left atrium; LBB, left bundle branch; LV, left ventricle; RA, right atrium; RBB, right bundle branch; RV, right ventricle.

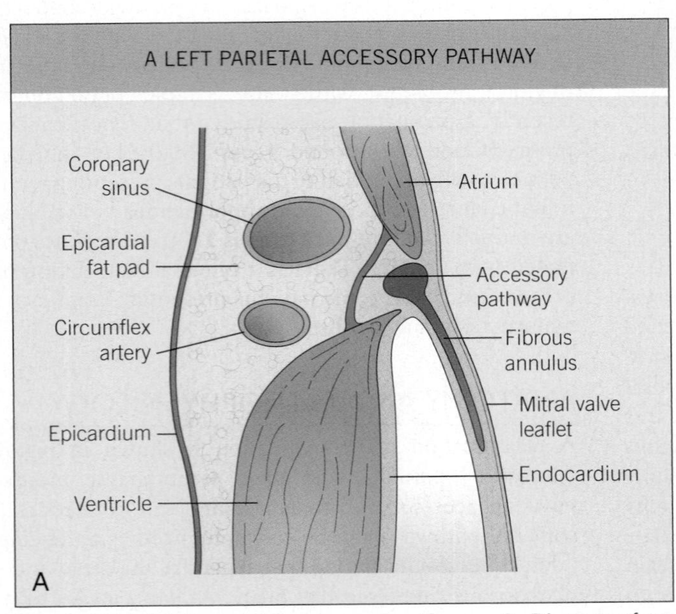

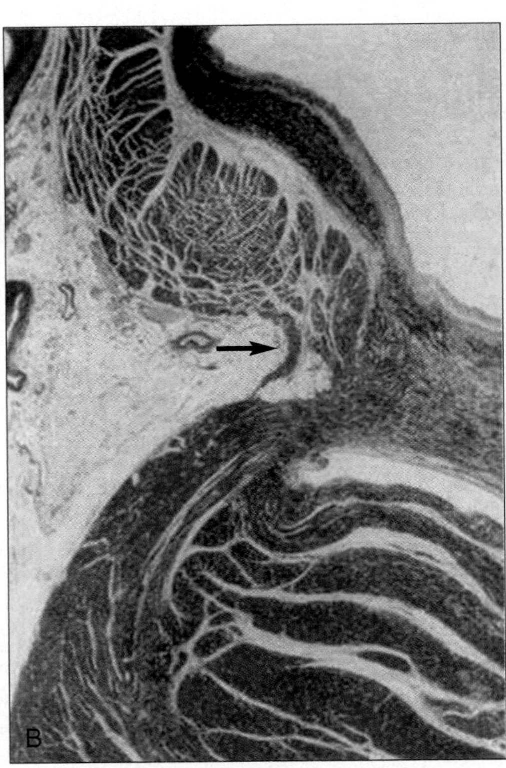

Figure 60.2 A left parietal accessory pathway. A, Diagram of an accessory pathway. **B,** A pathologic specimen from a patient who died suddenly with WPW syndrome. The arrow points to the left parietal accessory pathway. (From Basso C, Corrado D, Rossi L, Thiene G. Ventricular preexcitation in children and young adults. Atrial myocarditis as a possible trigger of sudden death. Circulation 2001;103:269-275. Reproduced with permission of the American Heart Association.)

connections.[15] In the reported pathologic cases of accessory AV pathways in the left AV annulus, the accessory connection runs in the epicardial fat pad, skirting a normally developed fibrous annulus (Fig. 60.2). Other structures close to the accessory pathway in the left epicardial fat pad are the coronary sinus and the circumflex coronary artery. Some posterior accessory AV pathways are related to diverticula of the coronary sinus that invaginate the ventricular muscle (Fig. 60.3).[16] This association suggests that the excess predominance of accessory AV connections in the left AV annulus may relate

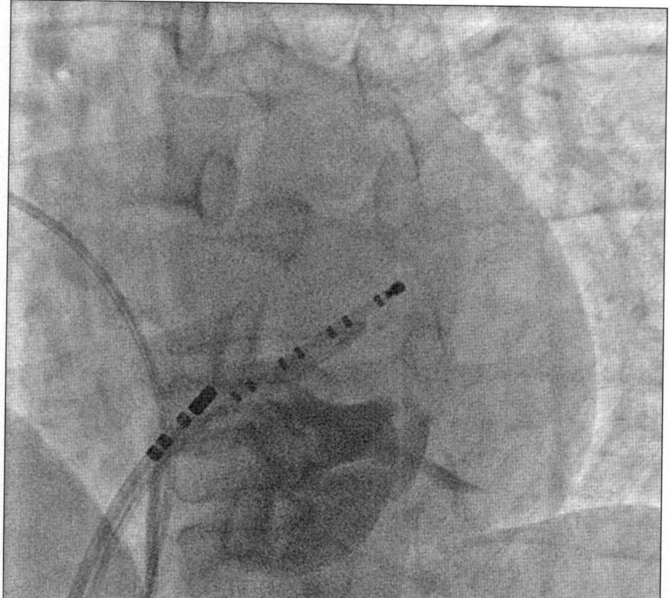

Figure 60.3 Left anterior oblique angiographic image of large coronary sinus diverticulum associated with WPW syndrome. The 8-pole electrode catheter lies in the body of the coronary sinus and the ablation catheter is positioned in the coronary sinus near the neck of the diverticulum. The large body of the diverticulum lies over the ventricle. The muscular fibers of the diverticulum serve as the accessory connection between the atrium and ventricle.

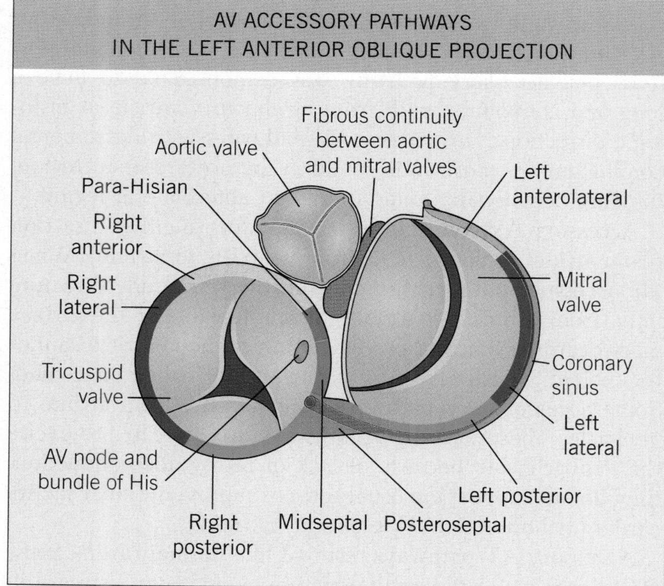

Figure 60.4 Location of atrioventricular (AV) accessory pathways in the left anterior oblique projection.

in some way to the development of the branches of the coronary sinus that pass from the sinus into the left ventricle.

Accessory AV pathways in the left AV annulus occur only in that part of the junction related to the mural leaflet of the mitral valve that occupies the posterior, lateral, and anterolateral aspects of the mitral circumference (Fig. 60.4). In the "anteromedial" portion of the left annulus, where the aortic leaflet of the mitral valve is in continuity with the aortic valve, it is not possible to have a direct AV connection because the left atrium attaches directly to the aortic root.[15] In the right AV annulus, AV connections can occur at any point in the circumference of the valve, but they are much less common than in the left AV annulus. Accessory AV pathways in the right annulus also skirt the fibrous annulus and run in the epicardial fat pad, which is generally larger and deeper than the epicardial fat pad in the left AV annulus. They may also travel to the ventricle along the endocardial aspect of the fibrous annulus.

The most common congenital abnormality associated with pre-excitation is Ebstein's anomaly. It is not surprising that a malformation involving the attachment of the tricuspid valve to the annulus should be associated with accessory AV connections. About 15% of patients with Ebstein's disease have an accessory AV connection, which is usually but not always located at the tricuspid annulus adjacent to the abnormal attachment of the tricuspid valve.[17] Multiple accessory connections are common in Ebstein's anomaly, sometimes with a combination of AV and atriofascicular connections.[17,18] Accessory AV pathways are rarely associated with other congenital anomalies, such as aortic stenosis, transposition of the great arteries, and left ventricular noncompaction.[19] Pre-excitation can also occur as a result of direct AV muscle connections unrelated to the fibrous annulus, such as between the atrial appendages and the underlying ventricular muscle, and in association with cardiac tumors and giant cardiac diverticula (see Fig. 60.3).

Genetics of Pre-excitation

In the great majority of cases, isolated WPW syndrome has no familial link. However, an inheritable form of the disease exists, expressing itself as isolated familial WPW syndrome, as a component of more extensive cardiac disease (e.g., hypertrophic cardiomyopathy), or as part of a multisystem syndrome (e.g., glycogen storage diseases). This topic has recently been summarized by Ehtisham and Watkins.[20]

To investigate the frequency of familial isolated WPW syndrome, one study examined the prevalence of pre-excitation in 2343 first-degree relatives of 383 patients with electrophysiologically proven accessory pathways.[21] Thirteen relatives (3.4%) had one or more accessory pathways, a prevalence of 0.55% compared with the usual prevalence of 0.1% to 0.2%. The affected families were more likely to have multiple accessory pathways, and the pattern of inheritance appeared to be autosomal dominant. This estimate of the proportion of familial WPW syndrome almost certainly underestimates the true situation as clinical information was obtained only for symptomatic relatives. In reality, the only sure way of determining the true prevalence of accessory AV connections in family members is through electrophysiologic testing of all individuals. Any assessment short of this will underestimate the prevalence.

The association between WPW syndrome and congenital heart disease has already been noted. The most common example is Ebstein's anomaly, the familial form of which is inherited in an autosomal dominant fashion with the abnormality mapped to chromosome 11q.[22] The association between hypertrophic cardiomyopathy and ventricular pre-excitation has been recognized for many years.[23] Although features suggestive of pre-excitation (shortened PR and abnormal QRS) may be seen in 5% to 10% of affected patients, electrophysiologic evidence of an accessory AV connection (often a fasciculoventricular connection) is found in only a subset.

Families with ventricular pre-excitation and supraventricular tachycardia, cardiac hypertrophy, cardiac conduction defects, and skeletal myopathy have recently been described.[24-26] Mutations affecting the gene *(PRKAG2)* encoding the γ_2 regulatory subunit of the AMP-activated protein kinase, located on chromosome 7q3, have been found to be responsible for this syndrome.[27] The defect is inherited in an autosomal dominant manner with a high degree of penetrance. Although original descriptions suggested that this was a form of hypertrophic cardiomyopathy, in contrast to typical hypertrophic cardiomyopathy, the gene defect does not involve the cardiac sarcomere, myofibrillar disarray is not evident, and the hypertrophy is characterized by glycogen accumulation. However, because of the prominent cardiac hypertrophy, some cases formerly identified as hypertrophic cardiomyopathy have in fact turned out to have *PRKAG2* mutations.[28] Transgenic mice models have been developed, and intriguingly, ventricular pre-excitation with electrophysiologic characteristics identical to human WPW syndrome appears to occur as a result of defects in the fibrous annulus, allowing direct contact between atria and ventricles, rather than to be due to muscle bridges around the outside of the annulus, as is the case in isolated WPW syndrome. It has been postulated that these defects may be secondary to the glycogen deposition and that this syndrome may explain the pre-excitation that can accompany other glycogen storage diseases such as Pompe's disease and Danon's disease.[29]

Finally, WPW syndrome may occur as part of a multisystem disorder. Mention has already been made of the glycogen storage diseases. In addition, mitochondrial diseases such as Leber's optic neuropathy and Leigh syndrome have been reported to be associated with WPW syndrome.[30]

Accessory Atrioventricular Connections

Anatomic Classification

Accessory AV connections were traditionally divided into four regions (left free wall, right free wall, posteroseptal, and anteroseptal) on the basis of the surgical anatomy.[31] As Anderson and Ho[15] have demonstrated, the "posteroseptal" region is not actually septal but rather is formed by the muscular floor of the coronary sinus overlying the posterior ventricular mass and abutting the right atrium. Similarly, the "anteroseptal" region as described by the surgeon represents the most medial aspect of the right parietal AV junction.

The classification of accessory AV connections is primarily useful as a way of communicating and aiding curative therapy with ablation. For this reason, electrophysiologists classify accessory pathways on the basis of the endocardial electrophysiologic and radiologic landmarks (see Fig. 60.4). In this classification

- accessory pathways located between the bundle of His recording position and the orifice of the coronary sinus are labeled midseptal;
- accessory pathways adjacent to the bundle of His (recognized by a recording of a potential from a Hisian pathway and an accessory pathway with the same catheter electrodes) are classified as anteroseptal or para-Hisian; and
- accessory pathways located within and posterior to the orifice of the coronary sinus, and not clearly in the right or left parietal AV junction, are labeled posteroseptal.

Accessory pathways in the left and right parietal AV annulus can be further subdivided into posterior, lateral, and anterior locations. Although the anatomist might disagree with this traditional, well-known terminology, it does have functional significance. For example, midseptal accessory pathways carry the highest risk of inadvertent AV block with catheter ablation because of the proximity of the AV node. Posteroseptal pathways may require detailed mapping of the left and right posterior annulus along with angiography and mapping of the coronary sinus because of the complex anatomy in this region and the possibility of coronary sinus anomalies.

Electrophysiologic Properties

Accessory AV pathways are usually composed of normal working muscle and have electrophysiologic properties similar to those of atrial and ventricular muscle. As the accessory pathway is stimulated at faster rates, it conducts at the same velocity until the refractory period of the pathway is reached and it abruptly "blocks." By contrast, the normal AV node demonstrates decremental conduction, with prolongation of the conduction time until block occurs (Wenckebach AV block). These differing properties of the AV node and the accessory connection explain a central feature of pre-excitation. With atrial ectopics or during an electrophysiologic study with increasing rates of atrial stimulation, pre-excitation becomes more pronounced. Examples of this behavior are shown in Figures 60.5 and 60.6.

On occasion, accessory AV pathways have pronounced decremental conduction like that of the AV node. Possible explanations for decremental accessory pathway (AP) conduction include the presence of specialized conducting tissue in the accessory pathway and unusual geometry of the accessory AV connection. For example, in one case, a decremental posteroseptal accessory pathway was demonstrated to have a long and convoluted path from atrium to ventricle at histologic dissection.[32] Accessory AV pathways with decremental conduction are most often found in the posteroseptal region; they are occasionally found in the left anterolateral region.[32]

Accessory AV connections may conduct in either direction (from atrium to ventricle or from ventricle to atrium). When the accessory pathway conducts in the retrograde direction only (from ventricle to atrium), it is not visible on the surface electrocardiogram, and pre-excitation of the ventricle cannot be elicited. These accessory pathways are called concealed. Some accessory AV pathways conduct only from atrium to ventricle. These accessory pathways are able to pre-excite the ventricle, but because of lack of retrograde conduction, they do not support the usual form of supraventricular tachycardia (orthodromic AV re-entry; Fig. 60.7).

Accessory AV pathways respond like normal cardiac muscle to changes in the autonomic milieu. With an increase in adrenergic tone, the refractory period decreases and the accessory pathway is able to conduct at faster stimulation rates. The opposite effect occurs with an increase in vagal tone. These responses, although in the same direction as the response of the AV node, are smaller in magnitude than the response of the AV node. This differential response may cause changing amounts of pre-excitation on the surface electrocardiogram, depending on the level of autonomic tone.[33] For example, during stress testing, the degree of pre-excitation may become less obvious as adrenergic tone increases and conduction time over the AV node shortens.[34]

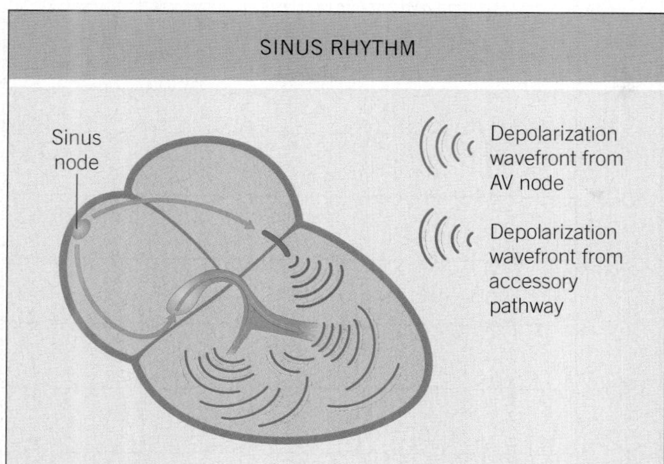

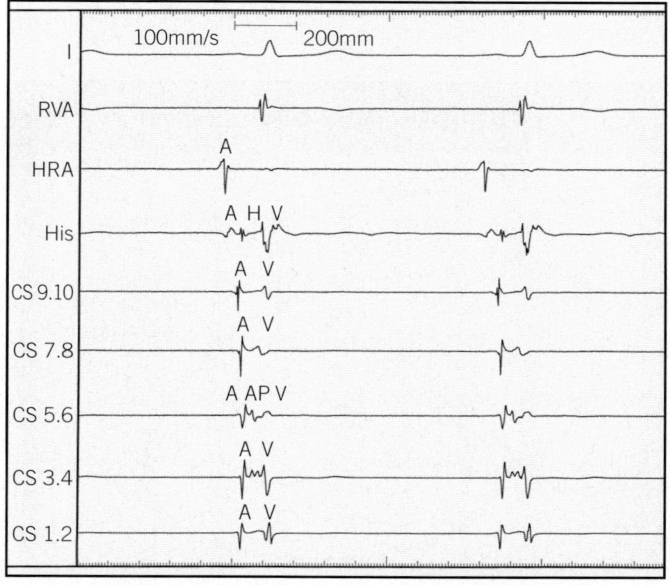

Figure 60.5 Pre-excitation in sinus rhythm. In sinus rhythm, only a small portion of the left ventricle adjacent to the accessory pathway is pre-excited. Tracings at electrophysiologic study show almost no pre-excitation in lead I and normal AH and HV intervals on the His bundle recording. However, early ventricular activation and an accessory pathway potential (AP) can be recorded from poles 5 and 6 of the coronary sinus (CS) catheter. A, atrium; HRA, high right atrium; RVA, right ventricular apex; V, ventricle.

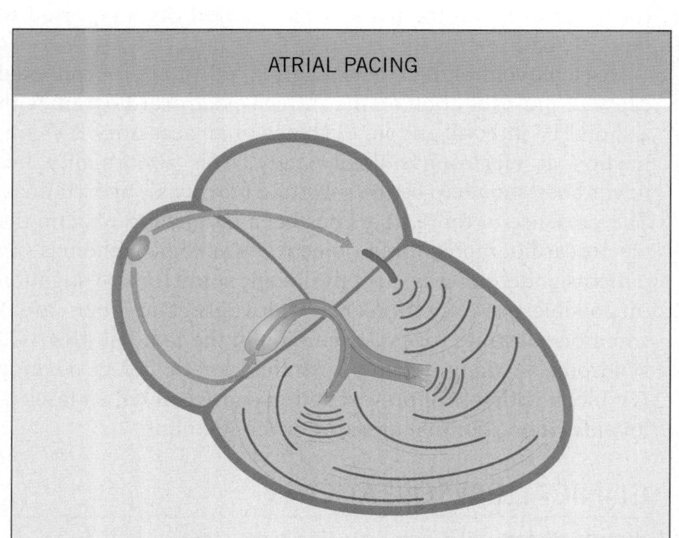

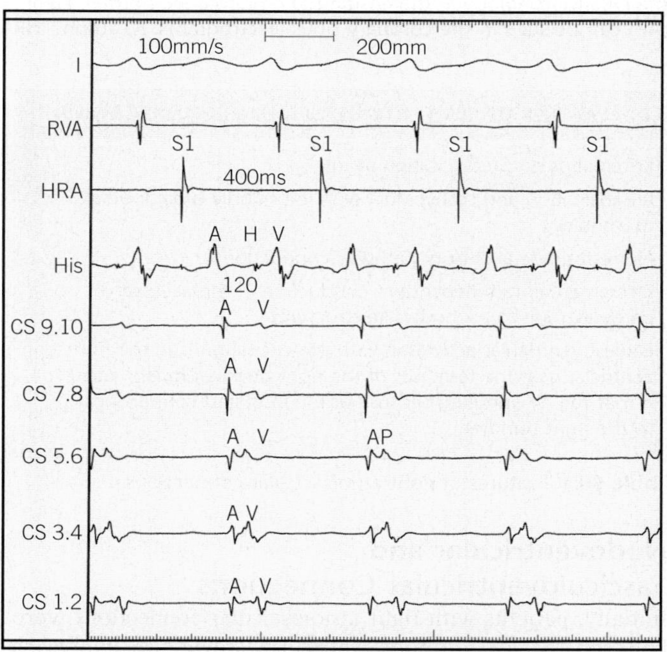

Figure 60.6 Increased pre-excitation with atrial pacing. During atrial pacing at a cycle length of 400 ms (150 beats per minute), AV nodal conduction time (AH interval) increases. Conduction time over the accessory pathway is unchanged from baseline, and consequently the degree of pre-excitation increases. A, atrium; AP, accessory pathway potential; HRA, high right atrium; RVA, right ventricular apex; V, ventricle.

Atriofascicular Connections

Atriofascicular connections account for about 1% to 3% of cases of pre-excitation. Atriofascicular pathways might represent a duplication of the normal conducting system (see Fig. 60.1). The proximal end of the atriofascicular connection probably consists of specialized conducting tissue that resembles the normal AV node.[15] These AV node remnants can be found in normal hearts in the right AV annulus, but they usually have no functional significance. They appear to be derived from the ring of specialized conducting tissue that surrounds the tricuspid annulus in the fetal heart.[15] In patients who have an atriofascicular connection, it is postulated that an AV node–like remnant is connected to the right bundle branch or to the distal right ventricle by a long, insulated connection that resembles a bundle of His. This anatomy results in a characteristic electrocardiographic and electrophysiologic profile (Table 60.1), which distinguishes these connections from the more common AV pathways.[35,36]

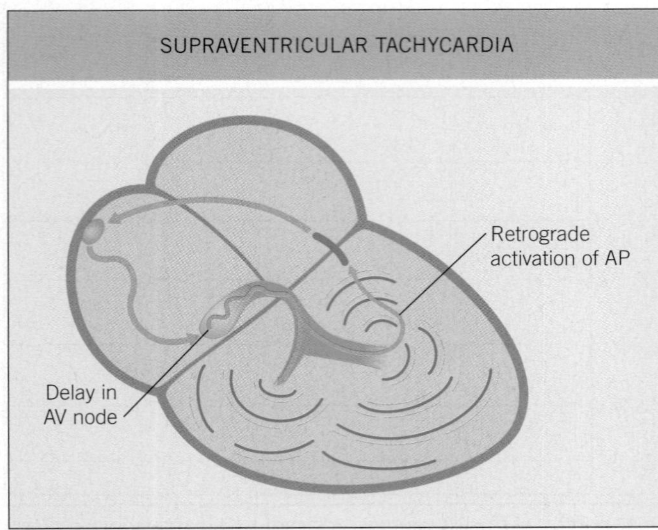

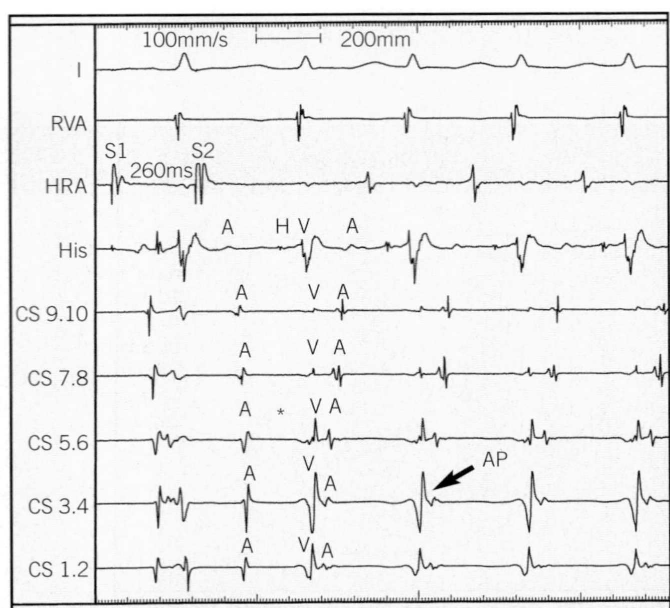

Figure 60.7 Induction of orthodromic AV re-entry. During tachycardia, the retrograde limb is the accessory pathway (AP) and the anterograde limb is the AV node. A premature atrial stimulus (S2) is delivered at a coupling interval of 260 ms. The refractory period of the accessory pathway is reached, and conduction of the premature stimulus shifts to the AV node with a longer conduction time and no pre-excitation. If the delay in AV nodal conduction is sufficient, re-entry using the accessory pathway will occur. The HV interval and the QRS morphology in the ensuing tachycardia are normal. Early eccentric retrograde atrial activation and an accessory pathway potential (AP) can be seen in the coronary sinus electrograms. A, atrium; HRA, high right atrium; RVA, right ventricular apex; V, ventricle.

FEATURES OF RIGHT ATRIOFASCICULAR CONNECTIONS
Minimal or no pre-excitation at rest
Pre-excitation and tachycardia with left bundle branch block morphology
No retrograde accessory pathway conduction
Decremental, rate-dependent conduction in the accessory pathway (due to AV node–like structure)
Earliest ventricular activation with pre-excitation is in the right ventricle, near the terminus of the right bundle branch, and not at the AV annulus (because of the insulated connection to the right bundle)

Table 60.1 Features of right atriofascicular connections.

Nodoventricular and Fasciculoventricular Connections

Initially, patients with right atriofascicular connections were believed to have a "nodoventricular" fiber also known as a Mahaim fiber. This misunderstanding arose because the electrophysiologic features of atriofascicular connections (see Table 60.1) are also theoretically compatible with a nodoventricular fiber (see Fig. 60.1). Surgical and catheter ablation has demonstrated that most patients with this electrophysiologic profile have an atriofascicular connection or, occasionally, a "conventional" right AV accessory pathway with decremental properties.[37]

As originally described by Mahaim, nodoventricular connections are normal variants of AV node histology and do not appear to have functional significance.[38,39] Although there are isolated reports of patients with tachycardia that could be attributed to a nodoventricular connection, definite proof of the participation of these fibers in a re-entry circuit is lacking. Nodoventricular connections are rarely a substrate for tachycardia on the basis of the isolated cases reported so far.

Fasciculoventricular fibers (see Fig. 60.1) are a postulated cause of pre-excitation on the surface electrocardiogram with a short HV interval and no evidence of an accessory AV connection at electrophysiologic study. This abnormality has never been shown to be the substrate for cardiac arrhythmias. The presence of these fibers has been invoked to explain the electrocardiographic and electrophysiologic findings in patients undergoing electrophysiologic study for investigation of possible pre-excitation. Fasciculoventricular fibers are a common substrate for pre-excitation in the familial *PRKAG2* syndrome.[25] Many patients with this genetic defect develop AV block with loss of pre-excitation consistent with a fasciculoventricular fiber that arises after the AV node.

CLINICAL PRESENTATIONS

Asymptomatic Pre-excitation

The relative frequency of asymptomatic pre-excitation is uncertain, but in one study, about half the presentations of pre-excitation were asymptomatic.[14] Most often, pre-excitation in an asymptomatic person is diagnosed when electrocardiography is performed incidentally, for instance, workplace screening.[40] In a young patient who is otherwise well, a diagnosis of the WPW syndrome, with its implication of potentially dangerous heart disease, can be quite overwhelming. Apart from the psychological aspects, certain safety-critical occupations and the armed forces have specific regulations that may preclude employment for people who have pre-excitation.

As is discussed later, current recommendations for investigation and therapy are strongly influenced by the presence or absence of symptomatic supraventricular tachycardia. Therefore, it is critical to carefully assess the nature of any symptoms to determine whether they are related to pre-excitation. It is possible both to incorrectly attribute symptoms to the underlying electrocardiographic abnormality and to overlook atypical symptoms and incorrectly describe the patient as asymptomatic. It is not uncommon for patients to become aware of ectopic beats and minor changes in heart rhythm after an incidental diagnosis of pre-excitation and to attribute these symptoms to the electrocardiographic abnormality. Although it is usually possible to diagnose ectopic beats from the history and to reassure the patient that this arrhythmia is incidental to pre-excitation, it can be more difficult to distinguish between paroxysmal supraventricular tachycardia and sinus tachycardia. Young children may not present with typical "palpitations" and may be thought to be asymptomatic when in fact they suffer from potentially serious tachyarrhythmias related to the accessory pathway. Therefore, in some patients, event monitoring may be required to determine whether the symptoms are genuinely related to pre-excitation.

Studies of asymptomatic patients indicate that about 70% do not have inducible AV re-entrant tachycardia at the time of electrophysiologic study, most often because the accessory pathway has poor or absent retrograde conduction.[40] The usual re-entrant circuit in patients who have pre-excitation and supraventricular tachycardia (orthodromic AV re-entry) requires retrograde conduction over the accessory pathway (see Fig. 60.7).

In the one third of asymptomatic patients who do have inducible orthodromic AV re-entry, tachycardia is often nonsustained and terminates spontaneously. It is likely that a proportion of these patients experience clinical episodes of supraventricular tachycardia that are relatively brief and therefore asymptomatic. The properties of the AV node and, to a lesser extent, the accessory pathway are dynamic and are influenced by autonomic function and the aging process. The frequency of premature beats—the usual triggers for arrhythmia—is also variable and tends to increase with age. Therefore, patients may develop symptoms only quite late in life or in special circumstances, such as competitive sport, that cause marked catecholamine stimulus. On occasion, the first manifestation of pre-excitation is with the occurrence of atrial fibrillation as a result of other heart disease. In general, however, accessory pathway and AV node function deteriorate with age, and it is uncommon for symptoms to develop after the age of 50 years.[14] Furthermore, loss of pre-excitation is a well-recognized phenomenon, occurring in 10% to 15% of asymptomatic patients observed for 5 years.[40,41]

Supraventricular Tachycardia

The symptoms of paroxysmal supraventricular tachycardia are described elsewhere in this book. AV re-entry is usually less dependent on autonomic tone than are other forms of supraventricular tachycardia, such as AV node re-entrant tachycardia and ectopic atrial tachycardia. Therefore, patients with AV re-entry are often unable to identify precipitating circumstances for their arrhythmia other than sudden body movement that may produce an ectopic trigger. It is not uncommon for AV re-entry to occur when the patient is completely at rest or during sleep. For the same reasons, AV re-entry is often a stable arrhythmia, lasting for hours at a time and requiring intervention such as intravenous administration of adenosine for termination. As with other forms of supraventricular tachycardia, it is easy to mistakenly attribute the symptoms of nonsustained AV re-entry to anxiety and panic attacks. In children and the elderly, typical symptoms of paroxysmal palpitations may not be reported. Instead, symptoms of breathlessness, dizziness, or even frank syncope may be the only clues to the presence of supraventricular tachycardia.

Orthodromic AV re-entry is the most common form of supraventricular tachycardia associated with pre-excitation. In this form of tachycardia, the accessory pathway is activated in the retrograde direction, and consequently the surface electrocardiogram is not pre-excited. Tachycardia is usually initiated by a critically timed ectopic beat that exploits the difference in the refractory periods of the accessory pathway and AV node and produces unidirectional block in one AV connection.

A less common form of accessory pathway–dependent tachycardia is antidromic AV re-entry, with anterograde conduction over the accessory pathway and retrograde conduction over the normal conducting system or over another accessory pathway. The ventricle is completely pre-excited during antidromic AV re-entry (Fig. 60.8). The reasons that antidromic tachycardia is inducible in only about 5% of patients with pre-excitation have been evaluated.[42,43] Antidromic tachycardia is usually initiated by an atrial premature beat that blocks in the AV node and conducts over the accessory pathway. Most patients do not develop sustained re-entry if this event occurs because, unlike in the AV node, there is no delay in conduction over the accessory pathway with a premature beat, and so the activation wavefront enters the ventricle and reaches the bundle of His and the AV node retrogradely before these structures have recovered excitability. For induction of antidromic tachycardia to occur, there must be

- a reasonable distance between the accessory pathway and the region of the bundle of His so that the activation wavefront does not arrive too rapidly at the His region (this means that it is very unusual to find antidromic tachycardia in patients who have single septal accessory pathways);
- a short anterograde accessory pathway refractory period; and
- a short retrograde refractory period of the bundle of His and the AV node to allow continued retrograde activation during tachycardia.

Pre-excited tachycardia is more likely to occur if there is a second accessory pathway that can act as the retrograde limb of the circuit. Antidromic tachycardia is the only form of AV re-entry that can occur in patients who have a single atriofascicular connection and no other accessory pathways because these pathways lack retrograde conduction. In addition, the AV node–like property of the atriofascicular connection facilitates induction of AV re-entry by allowing the requisite delay with a conducted atrial premature beat.

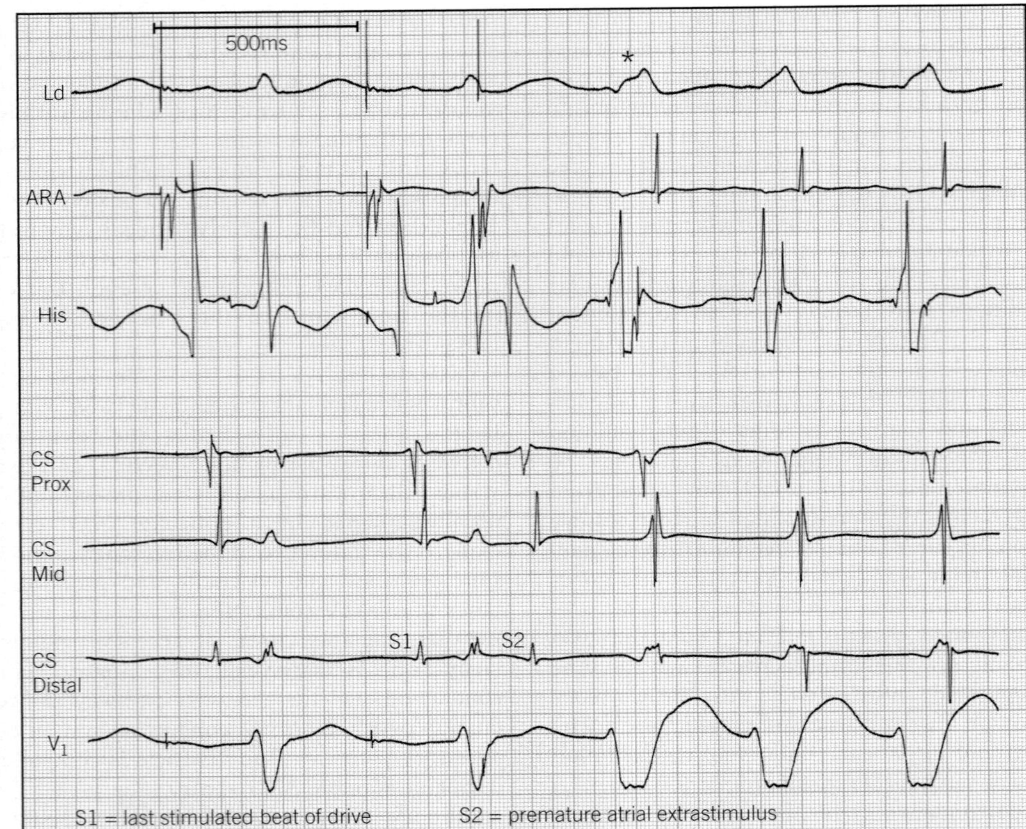

Figure 60.8 Induction of antidromic tachycardia in a patient with an atriofascicular accessory pathway. Note the prolongation of both AH conduction (over the AV node) and A delta conduction (over the accessory pathway) with atrial pacing. With tachycardia *(asterisk),* the ventricle is fully pre-excited, and the bundle of His potential is recorded at the onset of ventricular activation.

Incessant Supraventricular Tachycardia

Supraventricular tachycardia can occasionally be incessant, with continuous tachycardia during months and sometimes years. This type of presentation often occurs with accessory pathways that have slow conduction, so that there is a stable re-entrant tachycardia with a heart rate of 120 to 140 beats per minute.[44] This produces a characteristic electrocardiogram (Fig. 60.9). Because there is little change in the heart rhythm, patients may be unaware of palpitations and present only when tachycardia-induced cardiomyopathy develops or when the tachycardia is found incidentally. This form of AV re-entry tachycardia has been labeled permanent junctional reciprocating tachycardia.

Rapid incessant tachycardia, as demonstrated in animal models of pacing-induced heart failure,[45] inevitably leads to cardiac dysfunction. The speed with which heart failure develops is influenced primarily by the tachycardia rate, with heart failure developing within weeks with heart rates above 180 beats per minute and sometimes not at all with heart rates in the range of 120 to 140 beats per minute.

It is important to consider this diagnosis in a patient who has tachycardia and heart failure. Ablation of the accessory pathway usually results in complete resolution of cardiomyopathy.

Atrial Fibrillation

Atrial fibrillation was noted to be part of the spectrum of the WPW syndrome from the first descriptions of the clinical syndrome in 1930. Most series report occurrence of atrial fibrillation or atrial flutter (or both) in 15% to 35% of symptomatic patients who have pre-excitation, usually in addition to AV re-entry.[46-48] Atrial fibrillation is usually a secondary arrhythmia induced by AV re-entry.[49] During supraventricular tachycardia, atrial pressure and volume increase rapidly, and there is a marked increase in sympathetic tone. These factors produce acute electrophysiologic changes in the atria that favor induction of atrial arrhythmias.[50] Atrial myocarditis has also been found in some patients who die suddenly with WPW syndrome, and in these patients, the initiation of atrial fibrillation might be independent of the accessory pathway.[51]

Atrial fibrillation, once present, often sustains longer than AV re-entry because it is unresponsive to the Valsalva maneuver and other similar interventions and does not terminate with spontaneous ectopics. Therefore, even if there has been a long previous history of palpitations from nonsustained AV re-entry, the first presentation to the hospital may well be with atrial fibrillation (Figs. 60.10 and 60.11).

Sudden Death

The risk of dying suddenly of arrhythmias associated with pre-excitation is low but difficult to estimate precisely. Reasons for this include the following.

- Sudden cardiac death (SCD) is a rare outcome of an uncommon disease; therefore, for accurate information about this complication to be acquired, the screening and follow-up of hundreds of thousands of individuals for many years would be required, which has proved impossible to date.

- Much of the current information on the natural history of WPW syndrome comes from case series reports from tertiary referral centers or from selected individuals (such as Air Force recruits), which is consequently subject to significant selection bias.
- The natural history of symptomatic WPW syndrome has been inexorably altered with the advent of ablative therapies.
- Pre-excitation as a cause of sudden death is likely to be underdiagnosed because of the difficulty in making a pathologic diagnosis of WPW syndrome without a premorbid electrocardiogram to guide the dissection (one estimate suggests that pre-excitation accounts for about 10% of sudden unexpected deaths in young patients).[51]

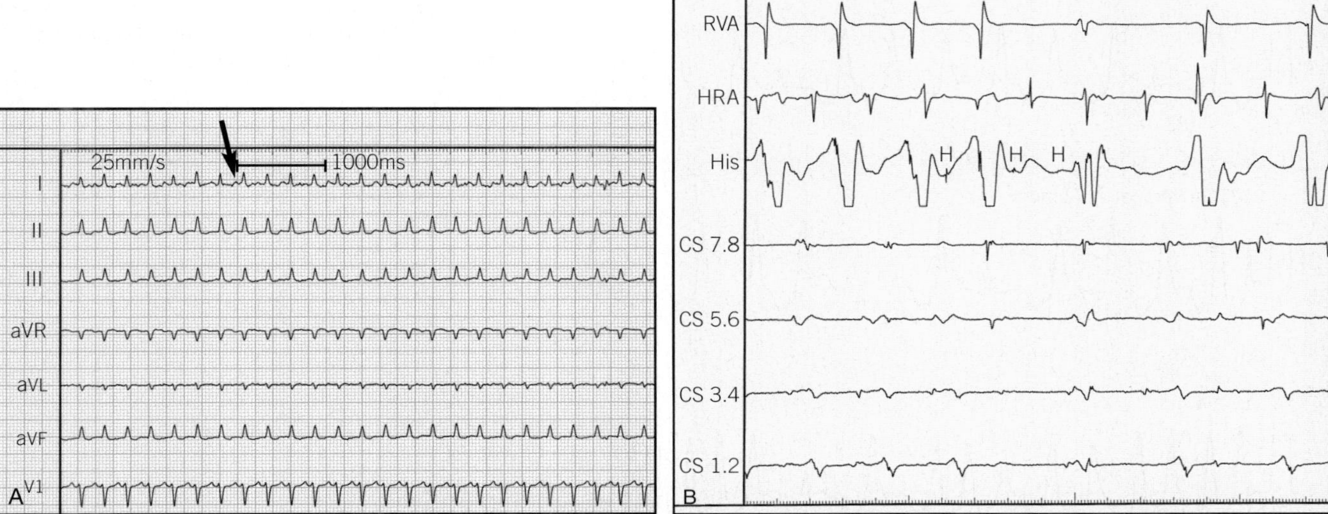

Figure 60.9 Incessant tachycardia with a decremental accessory pathway. A, Electrocardiogram obtained in a 20-year-old man with developmental delay who presented with heart failure and dilated cardiomyopathy (ejection fraction, 20%). Note the long VA interval with the P wave *(arrow)* just before the QRS complex. The patient was unaware of tachycardia. **B,** Intracardiac recordings of spontaneous onset of tachycardia. The retrograde limb of the tachycardia is a decremental accessory pathway that was localized to the left anterolateral region (CS 1.2), adjacent to the aortic valve. Note the long VA interval of 160 ms. Cardiac function returned to normal after catheter ablation of the accessory pathway. CS, coronary sinus electrograms; His, bundle of His; HRA, high right atrium; RVA, right ventricular apex.

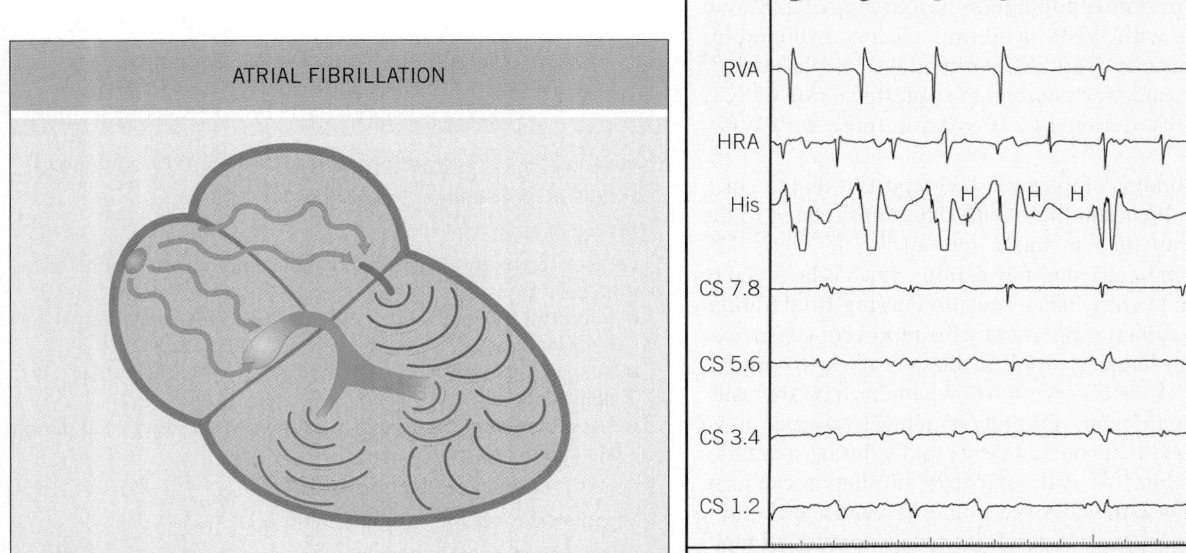

Figure 60.10 Pre-excited atrial fibrillation. In atrial fibrillation, conduction can occur both over the accessory pathway to give pre-excited beats and over the AV node to give normal QRS complex beats *(arrow)*. The proportion of pre-excited beats depends on the relative properties of the accessory pathway and the AV node, which may vary with changes in autonomic tone. HRA, high right atrium; RVA, right ventricular apex.

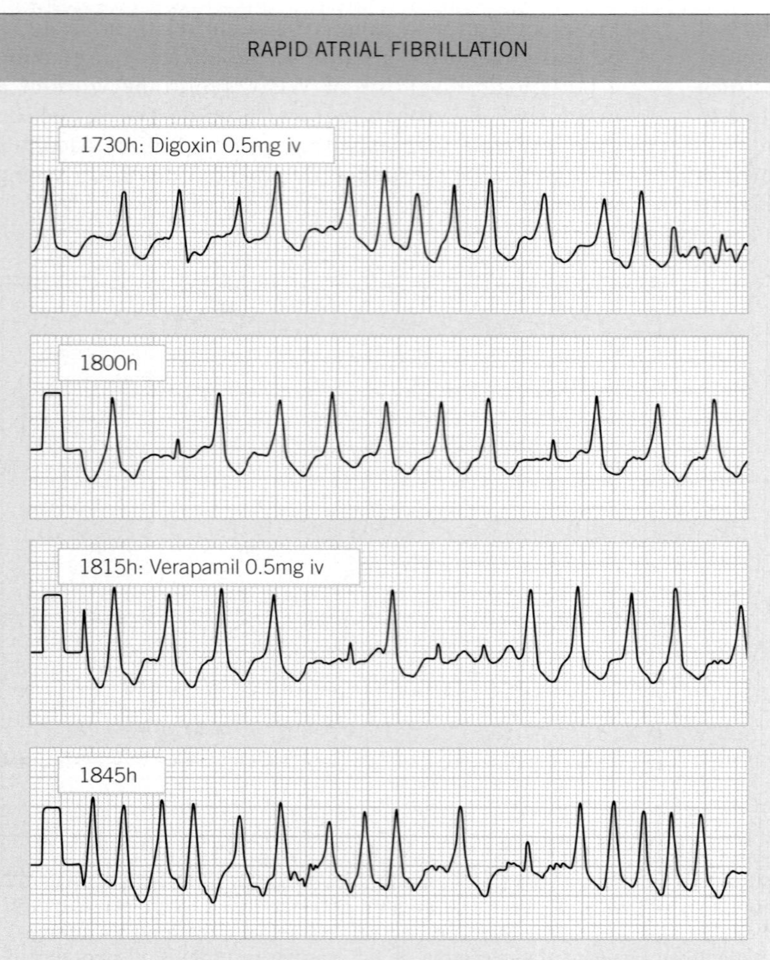

Figure 60.11 Rapid atrial fibrillation. These rhythm strips were recorded from a 35-year-old patient who presented with rapid atrial fibrillation. The patient had experienced palpitations for 5 years consistent with supraventricular tachycardia but had not sought medical attention. Pre-excitation was not recognized, and the initial treatment was 0.5 mg digoxin intravenously. Note that the shortest pre-excited R-R interval is about 200 ms (300 beats per minute), indicating a significant risk of ventricular fibrillation. At 1815, verapamil (0.5 mg) was given intravenously. As expected, there was no slowing in the ventricular response, which at 1845 is a little faster than before the digoxin and verapamil had been given. At 1900, the patient had a cardiac arrest with ventricular fibrillation and was defibrillated to sinus rhythm. The patient subsequently underwent catheter ablation.

Despite these limitations, the evidence suggests that sudden death is a rare event. For instance, one population-based study of 113 residents of all ages from Olmsted County with WPW syndrome (50% of whom were asymptomatic at the time of diagnosis) reported an incidence of SCD of 0.15% per year (two deaths).[14] In another population-based study of 228 adult military aviators with WPW syndrome electrocardiographic pattern, there was one death (SCD rate of 0.02% per year).[52] Finally, a recent guidelines statement suggested a rate of SCD of 0.15% to 0.39% during 3 to 10 years in those with WPW syndrome.[53]

One common finding of the published reports is that the incidence of death is higher in those with symptoms related to the accessory pathway than in those without.[13,14,40,41,47,52,54-58] Death results from ventricular fibrillation, which is believed to be a result of rapid ventricular stimulation during atrial fibrillation. This explanation is supported by the reports of ventricular fibrillation during induced atrial fibrillation at electrophysiologic studies and by the observation that patients who are resuscitated from ventricular fibrillation almost always have accessory pathways that conduct very rapidly during spontaneous atrial fibrillation.[46,47] Although atrial fibrillation can arise de novo in patients with WPW syndrome, as mentioned before, it is believed in most cases to result from degeneration of rapid AV re-entrant tachycardia. Therefore, it is understandable that patients with symptomatic WPW syndrome would be at higher risk for SCD than asymptomatic patients.

Studies reporting on cases of aborted SCD associated with pre-excitation have been consistent in identifying a number of high-risk markers (Table 60.2). In addition, many of the patients have been described to suffer this complication during heightened adrenergic states.[54] On

FACTORS ASSOCIATED WITH GREATER RISK OF SUDDEN CARDIAC DEATH IN PATIENTS WITH WOLFF-PARKINSON-WHITE SYNDROME
Male gender (85% of sudden cardiac death in WPW syndrome)
History of AV re-entrant tachycardia
History of atrial fibrillation
An accessory pathway capable of rapid anterograde conduction as evidenced by ■ a shortest R-R interval of <200 ms during pre-excited atrial fibrillation, or ■ a mean R-R interval of <250 ms during pre-excited atrial fibrillation, or ■ a short anterograde accessory pathway refractory period during electrophysiologic studies
Presence of multiple accessory pathways
Septal location of the accessory pathway
Age younger than 35 years

Table 60.2 Factors associated with greater risk of sudden cardiac death in patients with Wolff-Parkinson-White syndrome.

occasion, ventricular fibrillation is precipitated by inappropriate treatment of rapid atrial fibrillation by AV node–blocking agents, such as calcium channel blockers and digoxin (see Fig. 60.11).

DIAGNOSTIC TECHNIQUES

Electrocardiography

The electrocardiogram is the cornerstone of the diagnosis of pre-excitation, which is confirmed by the presence of a short PR interval and a delta wave. The delta wave obscures normal ventricular depolarization and also results in an abnormal pattern of repolarization. In the presence of pre-excitation, the electrocardiogram is uninformative about myocardial structure and the presence or absence of myocardial ischemia (Fig. 60.12).

The degree of pre-excitation on the resting electrocardiogram depends on the location of the accessory pathway and the conduction time over the AV node. Pre-excitation may be subtle if the accessory pathway is located far from the sinus node in the left lateral AV annulus because the accessory pathway is activated later than the AV node. For this reason, right-sided and septal accessory connections generally show more pre-excitation than left-sided connections do. Similarly, if the AV node conduction is accelerated by sympathetic stimulation, pre-excitation may be less obvious. If the diagnosis of pre-excitation is in doubt, it can be either confirmed or refuted by recording an electrocardiogram during an adenosine injection (Fig. 60.13).[59]

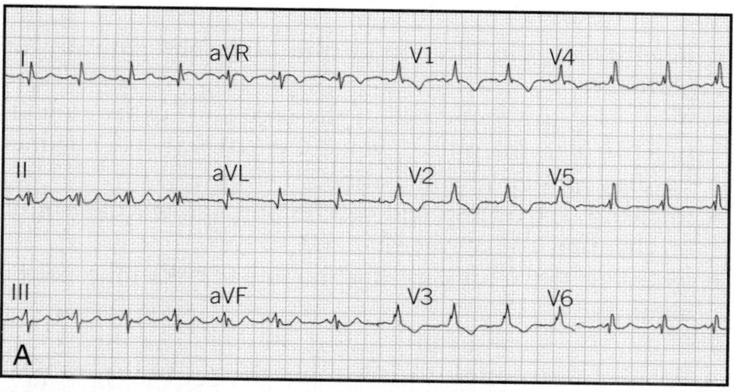

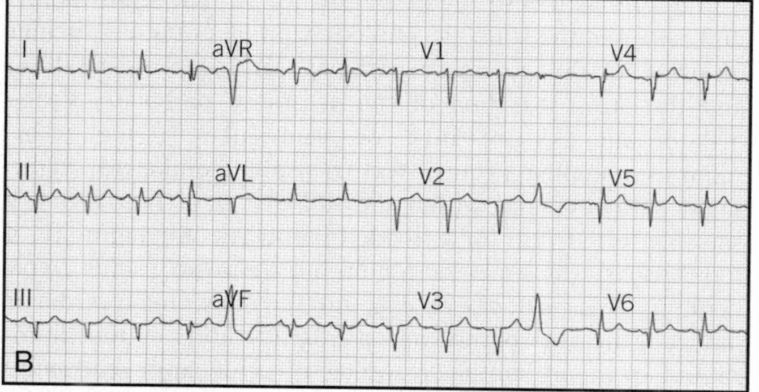

Figure 60.12 Pre-excitation with a left lateral accessory pathway. A, This electrocardiogram was recorded in a 60-year-old patient who presented with a large myocardial infarction. The electrocardiogram was interpreted as showing acute posterior myocardial infarction but in fact shows pre-excitation with a left lateral accessory pathway. There was also a history of recurrent palpitations consistent with supraventricular tachycardia. **B,** The electrocardiogram after catheter ablation of the accessory pathway. Note the Q waves in the inferior and anterior locations, which are indicative of previous myocardial infarctions that had been completely obscured by pre-excitation.

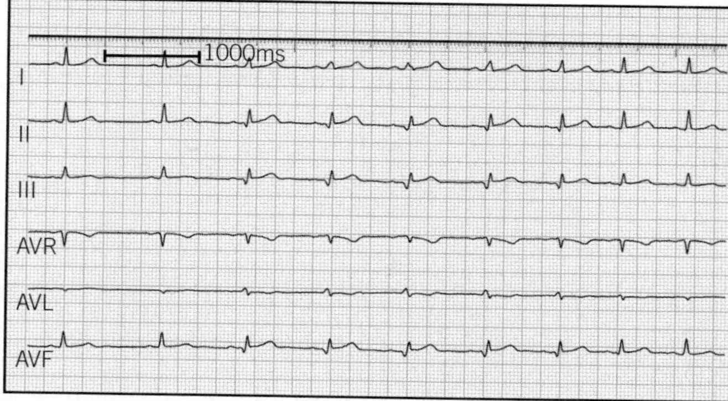

Figure 60.13 Use of adenosine to expose accessory pathway conduction. The baseline electrocardiogram shows no pre-excitation. With adenosine (12 mg), AV node conduction slows and pre-excitation from a posteriorseptal accessory pathway is exposed.

Many sophisticated algorithms to localize the accessory pathway from the characteristics of the delta wave have been proposed.[31,60] However, the general location of the accessory pathway (right parietal, left parietal, posteroseptal, or anteroseptal) can be estimated by a fairly simple process. The location in the left-to-right plane is determined by examining the delta wave in the chest leads. The pathway is almost always left-sided if the delta wave is positive in lead V_1. If the delta wave is negative or isoelectric in lead V_1 but strongly positive in leads V_2 and V_3, the pathway is usually located septally. Right-sided pathways generally have a precordial delta-wave progression, which is similar to the normal R-wave progression with a transition in leads V_3 and V_4. The location in the anterior-posterior plane is determined by the delta-wave vector in the limb leads. For instance, with respect to septal accessory pathways, posteroseptal pathways have a negative delta wave in leads II, III, and aVF. As the location becomes more anterior, lead II and then lead III becomes upright so that all three leads have a positive vector with anteroseptal pathways.

Intermittent pre-excitation recorded on a resting electrocardiogram is a valuable sign that the accessory pathway has poor anterograde conduction. Intermittent conduction over the accessory pathway at normal heart rates indicates that it cannot sustain a rapid rate during atrial fibrillation and that it therefore poses no risk of sudden death. Of course, as in concealed accessory pathways that have no anterograde conduction at all, an accessory pathway with intermittent pre-excitation may still have robust retrograde conduction and support supraventricular tachycardia.

Noninvasive Testing

In the presence of pre-excitation, routine stress testing for the assessment of myocardial ischemia is of little use because the repolarization abnormality obscures electrocardiographic evidence of ischemia. In this case, other techniques are necessary. Sudden loss of pre-excitation during a stress test indicates an accessory pathway with a long refractory period that generally will not conduct rapidly during atrial fibrillation. This must be interpreted with caution because

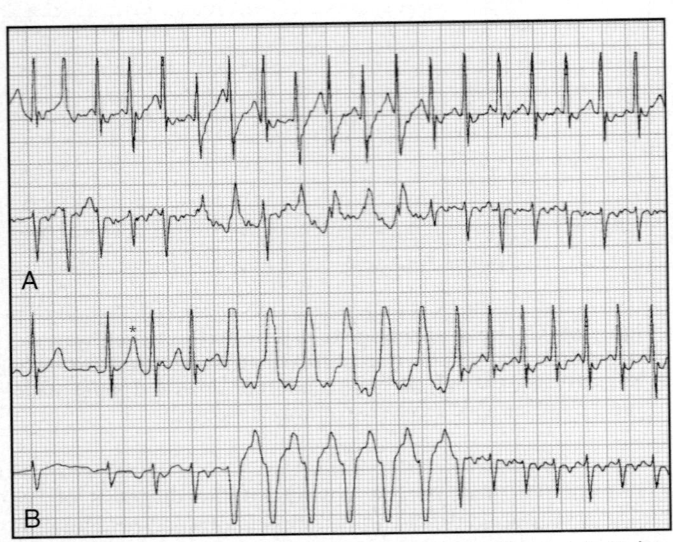

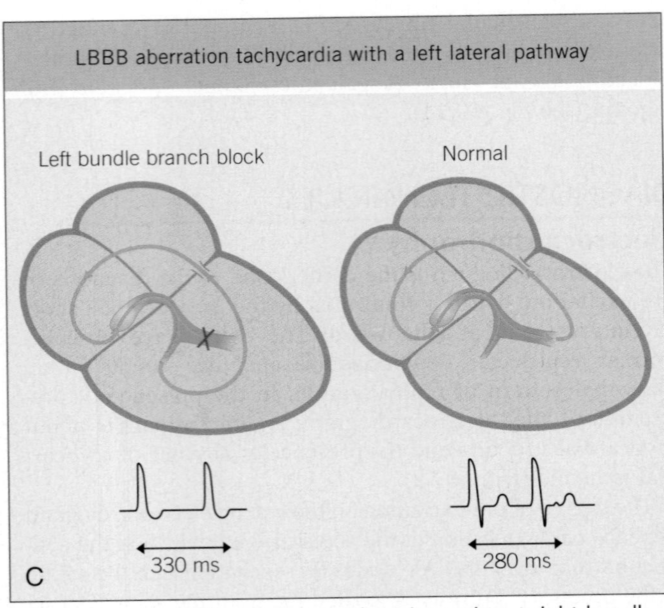

Figure 60.14 Concealed left lateral accessory pathway. A, Holter monitor recordings. The recordings show intermittent right bundle branch block aberration during supraventricular tachycardia. There is no change in cycle length of tachycardia with right bundle branch block. **B,** The tracings show initiation of supraventricular tachycardia by an atrial ectopic *(asterisk)*. The third to eighth beats of tachycardia have left bundle branch block aberration and a longer cycle length (330 ms) than the subsequent beats, which do not have left bundle branch block aberration (cycle length of 280 ms). This indicates that the retrograde limb of the tachycardia is a left lateral accessory pathway. **C,** Diagram showing why the tachycardia circuit is longer with bundle branch block ipsilateral to the site of the accessory pathway. LBBB, left bundle branch block.

enhancement of AV node conduction during stress testing may lead to the gradual reduction of pre-excitation, without actual loss of anterograde accessory pathway conduction. Routine echocardiography is worthwhile, especially in the case of right parietal accessory pathways, to determine whether there is any associated cardiac disease, such as Ebstein's anomaly. Premature activation of the pre-excited portion of the ventricle can be visualized at echocardiography, but this is a fairly crude approach to localization of the accessory pathway. Routine 24-hour Holter monitoring is generally of little value, and event monitoring is recommended if there is doubt about the nature of intermittent palpitations.[61] Any recordings of tachycardia should be carefully scrutinized for clues to the mechanism of tachycardia and the location of the accessory pathway (Fig. 60.14).

Electrophysiologic Study

Electrophysiologic study is indicated for assessment of risk of sudden death and as a prelude to catheter ablation for patients who wish to proceed to curative therapy. In general, electrophysiologic study is recommended for all symptomatic patients with pre-excitation.[53] Electrophysiologic study is also recommended for asymptomatic patients in high-risk occupations and professional athletes.[53] Electrophysiologic study not only provides an assessment of the risk of ventricular fibrillation but also demonstrates the location of the accessory pathway or pathways, the mechanism for tachycardia, and the presence of other types of arrhythmias. Therefore, electrophysiologic study has largely replaced noninvasive risk assessment of accessory pathway function.

The aims of electrophysiologic study in patients who have pre-excitation include

- determining the location of the accessory pathway or pathways;
- measuring the properties of the accessory pathway and, in particular, the rate at which the pathway will conduct during rapid atrial stimulation;
- inducing tachycardia and determining the mechanism or mechanisms of tachycardia; and
- assessing the feasibility and potential risks of catheter ablation.

A detailed description of electrophysiology testing in pre-excitation has been provided elsewhere.[62] The most important aspect of the study is detailed mapping of the ventricular insertion of the accessory pathway (during pre-excitation) and the atrial insertion of the accessory pathway (during orthodromic AV re-entry or ventricular pacing). This requires mapping around the tricuspid annulus for right-sided pathways and within the full extent of the coronary sinus or left atrium for left-sided pathways. Angiography of the coronary sinus may be required if a coronary sinus diverticulum is suspected (see Fig. 60.3). When tachycardia is induced, the anterograde and retrograde limbs of the circuit should be identified by mapping of atrial and ventricular activation and by the use of pacing interventions. If catheter ablation is indicated, it can be performed at the same time as the diagnostic study.

MANAGEMENT

Acute Arrhythmias

Orthodromic AV re-entry should be managed in the same way as other forms of supraventricular tachycardia: by vagal maneuvers and, if necessary, by injection of adenosine.

Intravenous administration of verapamil can also be used safely for orthodromic AV re-entry. If AV re-entry recurs repeatedly after temporary interruption with adenosine, intravenous verapamil, an intravenous class III antiarrhythmic agent such as sotalol or ibutilide, or a class I agent such as flecainide provides more sustained antiarrhythmic action than adenosine does.

Atrial fibrillation with a rapid ventricular response caused by pre-excitation requires urgent attention because of the small but definite risk of ventricular fibrillation. When there is hemodynamic embarrassment or a ventricular response of more than 250 beats per minute, cardioversion is the safest and most effective way of restoring sinus rhythm. If the arrhythmia is well tolerated and the ventricular response is less than 250 beats per minute, an intravenous class III agent such as sotalol has moderate efficacy and is safe. Class I agents, such as flecainide and procainamide, can also be used with similar efficacy. Digoxin and calcium channel blockers such as verapamil and diltiazem should be avoided (see Fig. 60.11) because they are completely ineffective and may increase the risk of cardiac arrest.

Long-term Management

The management of symptomatic pre-excitation has been revolutionized by the development of catheter ablation. Radiofrequency catheter ablation almost always eliminates accessory pathway conduction without the need for major surgery and with minimal risk of complications. Recent publications report success rates of close to (but not quite) 100%.[9,63,64] Ablation of the accessory pathway eliminates the symptoms of arrhythmias related to pre-excitation and any possibility of ventricular fibrillation as a result of rapid conduction over the accessory pathway.[65] Catheter ablation carries a small risk of significant complications, which occur in about 1% of cases. Complications of catheter ablation are discussed in Chapter 51. Ablation of accessory pathways in the midseptal and para-Hisian region may be associated with inadvertent damage to the AV node, with the need for pacemaker implantation. In skilled hands, the risk of AV block with pathways in this location is less than 1%. Rarely, embolic stroke may occur during or after left-sided ablation, and there are isolated reports of coronary artery damage. Mortality associated with the procedure has been estimated to be about 1 in 1000.[66-68]

These small risks need to be put into perspective by considering the alternatives of either long-term antiarrhythmic drug therapy or continued episodes of arrhythmia. In a young and otherwise healthy patient, long-term drug therapy is an unpalatable option and one that is rarely completely effective. Continued episodes of supraventricular tachycardia are inconvenient and often engender considerable anxiety even when the accessory pathway has been shown to be "safe." Therefore, in general, catheter ablation is the preferred solution to the problem of symptomatic arrhythmias with pre-excitation. When the accessory pathway is capable of rapid anterograde conduction, patients should be advised to undergo catheter ablation without reservation. Patients who have only brief and infrequent episodes of tachycardia and in whom electrophysiologic study demonstrates an accessory pathway with modest anterograde conduction properties may find the small risks of catheter ablation unacceptable in comparison to their minimal symptoms. These patients may prefer just to treat the episodes of tachycardia when they occur and consider catheter ablation at a later time if it proves necessary. As always, recommendations need to be tempered by individual circumstances, such as occupation, age, and the presence of comorbidity. For example, a patient who has minimal symptoms may elect to undergo catheter ablation if he or she is engaged in a safety-critical occupation in which even occasional episodes of tachycardia are unacceptable. The indications for catheter ablation in patients with pre-excitation are shown in Table 60.3.

INDICATIONS FOR CATHETER ABLATION	
Unequivocal recommendation for catheter ablation	Presentation with ventricular fibrillation
	Presentation with rapid atrial fibrillation (shortest pre-excited R-R interval <250 ms)
	Recurrent SVT with potentially dangerous accessory pathway (shortest pre-excited R-R interval during AF at EPS <250 ms)
	Incessant SVT with ventricular dysfunction
Catheter ablation strongly recommended	Recurrent SVT with significant impairment in quality of life from episodes of tachycardia
Catheter ablation optional	Infrequent, brief episodes of SVT without impairment in quality of life and with a "safe" accessory pathway (shortest pre-excited R-R interval at EPS during AF >250 ms)
Catheter ablation generally not recommended	Asymptomatic pre-excitation

AF, atrial fibrillation; EPS, electrophysiologic study; SVT, supraventricular tachycardia.

Table 60.3 Indications for catheter ablation.

Drug Therapy

Drug therapy may be a useful alternative in patients with symptomatic arrhythmias who do not wish to undergo catheter ablation or as a temporizing measure before definitive therapy. It is advisable to start with drugs that are safe and well tolerated, such as simple beta blockers like atenolol, even if the efficacy is less than that of more potent antiarrhythmic agents. If a simple beta blocker is ineffective, then sotalol, propafenone, and flecainide are reasonable options. The newer class III agents, such as dofetilide, should also prove to be moderately effective. Amiodarone is not generally recommended because of the potential for toxicity with long-term use.

It is important to explain that antiarrhythmic medication is rarely completely effective and that the aim of treatment is to decrease the frequency and severity of arrhythmia episodes. The individual risks of antiarrhythmic drugs should also be carefully explained before use.

No maintenance treatment may be appropriate in patients who have infrequent episodes of tachycardia, particularly when tachycardia is amenable to vagal maneuvers such as the Valsalva maneuver. All patients should be educated in the use of the Valsalva technique, which is usually most effective if applied immediately after the onset of tachycardia while the patient is lying supine. If tachycardia persists for more than 30 minutes or if there are persisting symptoms of pre-syncope or angina, the patient should be advised to come to the hospital for assessment and treatment.

Management of the Asymptomatic Patient

Approximately 25% to 50% of patients with WPW syndrome resuscitated from ventricular fibrillation have this as their initial presentation.[46,47,54] This type of statistic raises concern that sudden death may be a not uncommon initial manifestation of pre-excitation and that asymptomatic patients should therefore undergo risk stratification and ablation of potentially dangerous pathways. However, it is rare for ventricular fibrillation to be the initial symptom, and most patients have prior symptoms that are overlooked or ignored. From a population perspective, the risk of sudden death in an asymptomatic patient with pre-excitation is not known precisely, but it has been estimated to be less than 1 in 1000.[10,11,14,40,52,56-58] At this level of risk, it is difficult to aggressively advocate an intervention such as catheter ablation, which has a risk of about 1% of significant complications.

Pappone and colleagues[41,69,70] have published a series of reports addressing the role of electrophysiologic risk assessment and prophylactic catheter ablation in asymptomatic patients. They have shown that an ablation strategy based on the inducibility of AV re-entrant tachycardia or atrial fibrillation and the age of the patient is effective in reducing the occurrence of symptomatic arrhythmias and SCD with low risk of complications, in both children and adults with asymptomatic WPW syndrome. The significant findings in these reports are (1) the relatively high rate of SCD of 0.34% per year (7 of 477 patients), a rate much higher than seen in other studies; (2) the development of criteria (electrophysiologic and clinical) predictive of higher risk of SCD; and (3) the demonstration of an acceptably low rate of serious complications of the diagnostic electrophysiologic study and catheter ablation procedures.

Has the time arrived, therefore, to revisit the guidelines for diagnostic electrophysiologic study and catheter ablation in asymptomatic WPW syndrome? Certainly, these studies along with previous reports do lend credence to the development of criteria that may reasonably separate asymptomatic patients into lower and higher risk categories. However, even if the current complication rate of electrophysiologic study or catheter ablation has declined in comparison with the 1990s, it is debatable whether the low risk of complications achieved in these studies (no deaths, strokes, heart attacks, tamponade, or need for permanent pacing) is applicable to the general electrophysiology community. Finally, if the rate of SCD in asymptomatic patients is lower than reported by Pappone and colleagues, which is likely in light of the evidence from earlier studies, the impetus for investigation of asymptomatic patients will be less. Articles summarizing these and other issues related to this topic have been published.[71,72]

Certain special circumstances applicable to asymptomatic patients may reasonably be regarded as exceptions to the general recommendation that electrophysiologic study is unnecessary. These include certain occupations, such as the armed forces, police forces, and safety-critical occupations like airline pilots and train drivers, and those wishing to compete in professional high-energy sports. It may also be argued that children constitute a special group as the recognition of symptoms related to tachyarrhythmias can be challenging and because SCD can have such a devastating effect on the family and community. In the final analysis, the patient or family may elect to have electrophysiologic study and catheter ablation (if high risk) after having become familiar with the risks and benefits of this procedure relative to the risk of nonintervention.

PROGNOSIS AND SUMMARY

Initial descriptions of pre-excitation indicated that the prognosis, although generally good, was variable, with a significant proportion of patients suffering heart failure and sudden death as a result of uncontrolled tachycardia. With the advent of antiarrhythmic drugs, fatal events became uncommon, but many patients still suffered from debilitating episodes of tachycardia and the need for lifelong drug therapy. Surgical treatment of pre-excitation heralded a new era with the promise of cure, but it was never a universal treatment because of the morbidity of open heart surgery. In the current era, the prognosis of pre-excitation is excellent, and there are few patients who cannot be cured of pre-excitation and the associated arrhythmias by catheter ablation.

chapter

61 Special Problems in Supraventricular Arrhythmias

a. Coexisting Paroxysmal Supraventricular Tachycardias

Li-Wei Lo and Shih-Ann Chen

DEFINITION OF PROBLEM

The coexistence of double tachycardias has been reported in many patients. Double tachycardias may not be identified during noninvasive testing (such as with the 12-lead electrocardiogram, Holter monitor, cardiac event recorder, or exercise testing), and the patients may present with similar symptoms (palpitations, chest discomfort) during every attack. The incidence of double tachycardias in patients with paroxysmal supraventricular tachycardia (SVT) had been reported to be around 2% to 3%. Although the possibility is not high, an unrecognized switch from one tachycardia to another tachycardia creates confusion and can lead to a suboptimal clinical outcome. It had been reported that the transition between two SVTs could be due to a spontaneous atrial premature beat, conduction block in one limb of the tachycardia, or tachycardia-induced tachycardia. However, if there is a large difference between the two tachycardia cycle lengths, the two tachycardias may be induced under different circumstances. Therefore, a detailed electrophysiologic study plays an essential role in recognizing the second tachycardia in the patients with this problem.

TYPICAL CASE

A 20-year-old woman had been relatively well during the past until half a year ago, when frequent attacks of sudden-onset palpitations occurred. She visited the emergency department, where paroxysmal SVT was diagnosed. Adenosine was administered intravenously to terminate the tachycardia. Her resting electrocardiogram was normal sinus rhythm without any ventricular pre-excitation. The electrocardiogram of the clinically documented tachycardia exhibited a narrow QRS complex tachycardia without any obvious P waves. Transthoracic echocardiography revealed a structurally normal heart except for a mild mitral valve prolapse without any mitral regurgitation. Because the tachycardia occurred very frequently and the symptoms became more severe, the patient was referred for an electrophysiologic study and curative ablation therapy.

DIFFERENTIAL DIAGNOSIS

During the baseline electrophysiologic study, dual atrioventricular nodal pathways were found, and the tachycardia was induced by ventricular burst pacing under an isoproterenol infusion (2 μg/min). The atrial activation sequence during the SVT was identical to that during ventricular pacing, with a concentric activation pattern. Sudden prolongation of the AH interval was observed during the initiation of the SVT, with an HA interval shorter than the AH interval and a VA interval of less than 70 ms during the tachycardia, which favored the diagnosis of typical atrioventricular nodal reentrant tachycardia (AVNRT; Fig. 61A.1). While termination of the tachycardia was attempted by atrial pacing, there was a change in the atrial activation sequence to an eccentric pattern with the earliest activation in the high right atrium (Fig. 61A.2). Coexisting orthodromic reciprocating tachycardia or atrial tachycardia (AT) may have contributed to those findings. However, there was not an eccentric atrial activation pattern during baseline ventricular pacing, and the tachycardia could not be reset. In addition, a wide QRS complex tachycardia with a right bundle branch block pattern also developed during the tachycardia and exhibited the same tachycardia cycle length and VA interval. The tachycardia then accelerated (a change in the tachycardia cycle length from 350 ms to 325 ms) and returned to the previous concentric atrial activation pattern.

From this evidence, the coexistence of typical AVNRT and AT was considered in this patient. It had been reported that a spontaneous transition from one tachycardia to another is more likely if the two tachycardias have similar cycle lengths; the cutoff point of 25 ms had an 80% positive predictive value for a transition. The atrial stimulation from the retrograde atrial activation during the AVNRT reactivated the atrium. During burst atrial pacing, the AVNRT terminated and then was reinitiated with an upper common pathway block because of AT firing in the right atrium. Because the cycle length of the AT was slightly longer than that of the AVNRT, the AVNRT then conducted retrograde to the high right atrium after several beats, and the AT stopped. Therefore, we were able to observe the transition between the AT and AVNRT.

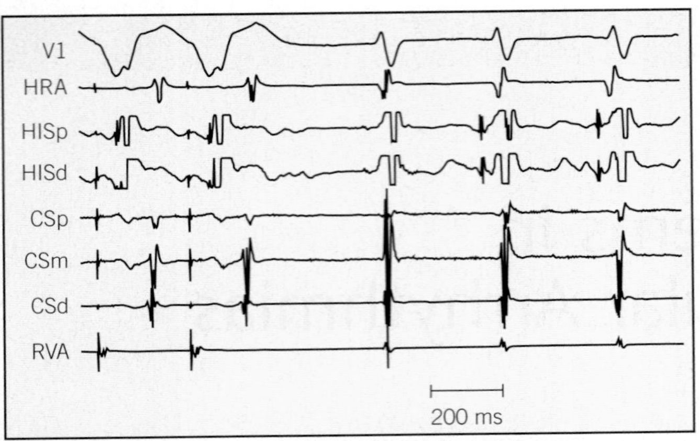

Figure 61A.1 Induction of typical AVNRT by ventricular pacing. Ventricular pacing at a cycle length of 260 ms is shown on the left with 1:1 conduction up the fast pathway. On cessation of the pacing after the retrograde conduction up the fast pathway, the conduction then went down the slow pathway, leading to typical AVNRT. HRA, high right atrial electrogram; HISp and HISd, proximal and distal His bundle electrograms; CSp, CSm, and CSd, proximal, middle, and distal coronary sinus electrograms; RVA, right ventricular apex electrogram.

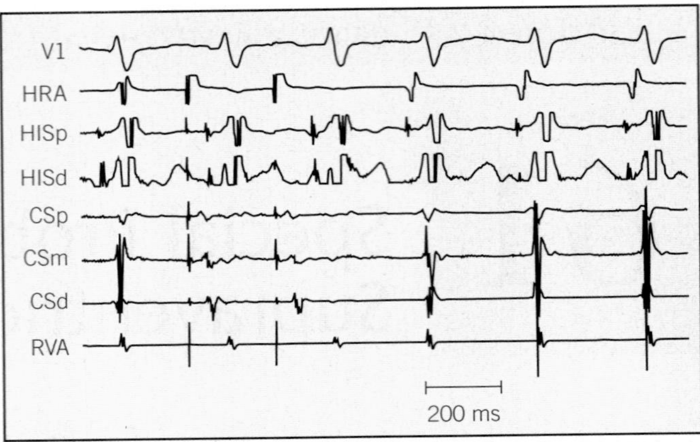

Figure 61A.2 Induction of atrial tachycardia by atrial pacing during typical AVNRT. Atrial tachycardia was initiated and recorded at the HRA after atrial pacing while the typical AVNRT still continued with an upper common pathway block. The atrial tachycardia slowed down, and then the HRA was activated by the retrograde fast pathway activation thereafter (not shown in this tracing). HRA, high right atrial electrogram; HISp and HISd, proximal and distal His bundle electrograms; CSp, CSm, and CSd, proximal, middle, and distal coronary sinus electrograms; RVA, right ventricular apex electrogram.

TREATMENT OPTIONS

In the case described here, manifested by an increasing frequency of the tachycardia and symptoms, the early initiation of an electrophysiologic study and curative catheter ablation was strongly indicated. A detailed diagnostic study before the therapeutic radiofrequency ablation to determine any factors that participated in the tachycardia was important to ensure that the ablation was not directed toward a clinically insignificant area. Because of the dual atrioventricular nodal physiology, inducibility of typical AVNRT, and easy transition of AT back to typical AVNRT, the ablation was first carried out at the anterograde slow pathway of the atrioventricular node in the lower part of Koch's triangle.

After the ablation, there was only anterograde fast atrioventricular nodal conduction and poor retrograde atrioventricular nodal conduction. It was therefore questioned as to how often a second tachycardia would be clinically relevant and whether it would require an additional ablation to control the symptoms. That issue still remained undetermined. However, the induction of sustained AT appeared to render the patient susceptible to subsequent tachycardia occurrences, and an additional catheter ablation of the AT focus was therefore warranted in an effort to prevent any tachycardia recurrence.

After the successful ablation of the anterograde slow atrioventricular nodal conduction, the AT was still inducible and was sustained under burst atrial and ventricular pacing without any preceding AVNRT. The patient then underwent three-dimensional electroanatomic mapping (with an EnSite array) for the AT ablation. The AT focus was located along the upper crista terminalis. After a careful mapping and ablation, the patient no longer had any episodes of the clinically documented tachycardia.

SUMMARY

Double tachycardias bring double troubles in the electrophysiology laboratory. A detailed electrophysiologic evaluation and careful assessment of the tachycardia cycle length and activation sequence may help in identifying a second tachycardia. The recognition of a second tachycardia can mean the difference between a successful outcome and an unsuccessful outcome. It is important to be alert to the possibility of double tachycardias during the ablation procedure as switching from one tachycardia to another creates confusion and can lead to a suboptimal outcome of the procedure.

b. Chronic Atrial Fibrillation

Li-Wei Lo and Shih-Ann Chen

DEFINITION OF PROBLEM

Atrial fibrillation (AF) is the most common arrhythmia and is associated with palpitations, cerebral and systemic embolization, aggravation of congestive heart failure, and possibly increased mortality. The prevalence of AF increases with age. Multiple random propagating wavelets, focal electrical discharges, and localized re-entrant activity with fibrillatory conduction are implicated in the mechanisms of AF. AF is believed to require a trigger for initiation and a substrate abnormality for perpetuation. The trigger plays a key role in the genesis of paroxysmal AF, whereas chronic AF depends also on atrial substrate abnormality. In the past decade, radiofrequency catheter ablation has become an effective treatment of patients with paroxysmal AF. In selected patients with chronic AF, it is possible to investigate the substrate properties with mapping, to ablate sources of the AF ectopy, and to modify the atrial substrate sufficiently to achieve restoration of sinus rhythm.

TYPICAL CASE

A 56-year-old man experienced frequent palpitations and chest pain during a 5-year period and was diagnosed with paroxysmal AF, initially treated with amiodarone. There was no history of hypertension, thyroid disorders, or alcohol abuse. Echocardiography revealed a structurally normal heart. The AF became persistent for the past 2 years while he was taking amiodarone, and he was referred for radiofrequency catheter ablation.

DIFFERENTIAL DIAGNOSIS

The electrocardiographic diagnosis of chronic AF is not generally challenging, and there are no other realistic diagnostic alternatives.

In this case, sustained AF was verified during the baseline electrophysiologic study. The bilateral pulmonary vein and coronary sinus recordings all demonstrated rapid disorganized fibrillatory activity (Fig. 61B.1). With use of a NavX electroanatomic system, biatrial geometries were constructed to facilitate the mapping and ablation procedures. Mapping of complex fractionated atrial electrograms (CFAEs) locates abnormal substrate potentially targeted for ablation (Fig. 61B.2), and linear ablation techniques are designed to prevent macroreentry. The CFAE sites over the anterior septum and left atrial appendage base were suspected to be potentially important for the perpetuation of the AF.

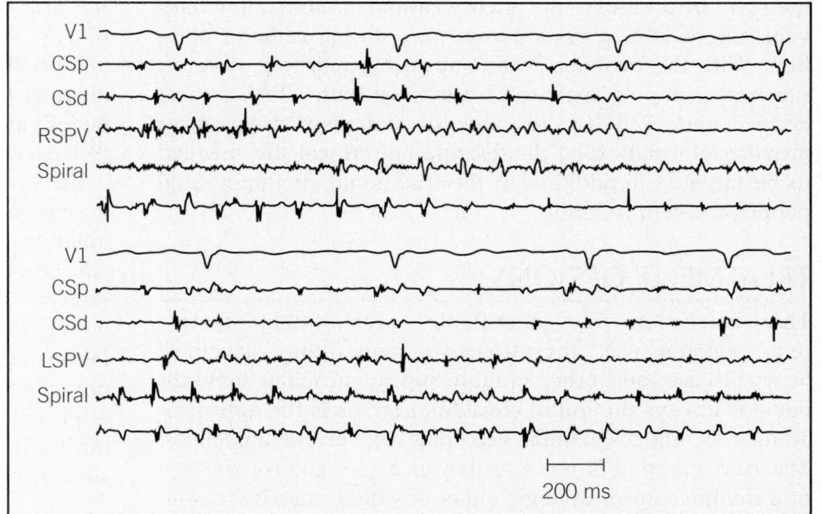

Figure 61B.1 Disorganized rapid electrical activity in the bilateral pulmonary veins before the catheter ablation. Intracardiac electrograms during atrial fibrillation in the coronary sinus and bilateral pulmonary vein recordings collected from the coronary sinus and spiral catheters. CSp and CSd, proximal and distal coronary sinus electrograms; RSPV and LSPV spiral, right superior and left superior pulmonary vein electrograms recorded by the spiral catheter.

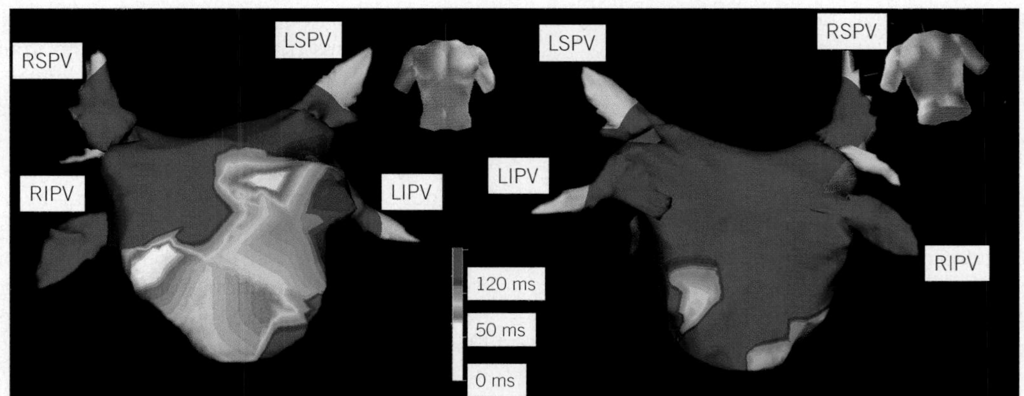

Figure 61B.2 Example of complex fractionated atrial electrogram (CFAE) maps. Shown are the anteroposterior and posteroanterior projections of the three-dimensional electroanatomic depictions of the left atrium in the left and right panels, respectively. In both panels, the color annotations show a range from white, with a mean CFAE cycle length of 50 ms or less, all the way through purple, with a mean CFAE cycle length of more than 120 ms. During the preablation CFAE map, most fractionated electrograms were located over the anterior septum and left atrial appendage base. Termination of AF developed during the ablation of the anterior septal CFAE site. RSPV, right superior pulmonary vein; RIPV, right inferior pulmonary vein; LSPV, left superior pulmonary vein; LIPV, left inferior pulmonary vein.

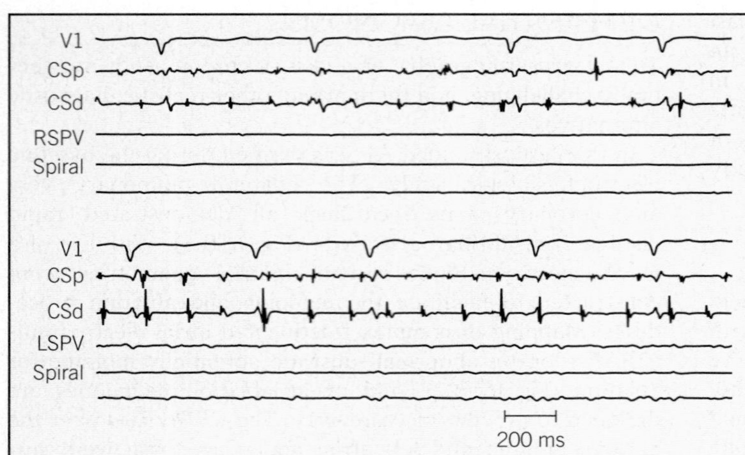

Figure 61B.3 Intracardiac electrograms after encircling the bilateral pulmonary veins. Although the AF still persisted after the circumferential pulmonary vein isolation, the electrical activity was silent within the bilateral pulmonary veins. CSp and CSd, proximal and distal coronary sinus electrograms; RSPV and LSPV spiral, right superior and left superior pulmonary vein electrograms recorded by the spiral catheter.

Recognition of pulmonary vein ectopy in the initiation and maintenance of AF still remains the first step during ablative therapy. In addition, the identification of non–pulmonary vein triggers also plays a pivotal role during catheter ablation. With the evolving techniques using mapping systems, substrate mapping tools to locate areas with CFAEs, short cycle length activity, or sites of dominant frequencies provide information on the discrete but critical sites needed to be targeted in addition to the traditional circumferential pulmonary vein isolation.

TREATMENT OPTIONS

The correction of identifiable precipitating factors (e.g., alcohol use, thyrotoxicosis, underlying structural heart disease, and other curable supraventricular arrhythmias) is always the initial consideration, as is the appropriateness of anticoagulation according to current guidelines. The next question is the selection of a rate control strategy or a rhythm control strategy, either of which could be reasonably selected for this individual. A sinus rhythm strategy was selected. Pharmacologic rhythm control can be attempted with class Ic drugs (propafenone, flecainide) or class III agents (amiodarone).

Pharmacologic rhythm control is generally indicated before nonpharmacologic therapy, but catheter ablation is being increasingly used in the event that pharmacologic rhythm control is not successful. The isolation of the pulmonary veins still remains the cornerstone of the procedure in nonparoxysmal AF. Atrial tissue at the "antrum" of the pulmonary vein is targeted rather than the pulmonary vein itself to dissociate the pulmonary veins from the left atrium and to create conduction block between the pulmonary veins and atria. Additional atrial ablation, usually including linear lesions at the roof and mitral isthmus (joining the left pulmonary veins from the mitral ring), is required to eliminate the arrhythmogenic substrate involved in the perpetuation of AF. Ablation of areas with fractionated atrial activity potentially arrhythmogenic (CFAEs) is becoming more prevalent in the procedure, although the precise mechanism of benefit and the identification of critical CFAEs remain active research questions.

Because this patient had symptomatic chronic AF for 2 years refractory to multiple drugs, he underwent catheter ablation. Rapid disorganized activity in the pulmonary veins was noted. After right and left pulmonary vein isolation, pulmonary vein electrical activity became silent without termination of the AF (Fig. 61B.3). Additional linear ablation lesions applied over the mitral isthmus and roof areas did not eliminate the AF. Finally, sinus rhythm was restored after ablation of identified CFAEs, especially in the left atrium in the anterior septal area. The patient remained in sinus rhythm after the ablation procedure.

SUMMARY

The management of chronic AF remains challenging and restoration of sinus rhythm potentially important. Antiarrhythmic drug therapy is the initial choice when a sinus rhythm strategy is elected, but "curative" catheter ablation is now feasible and emerging as an alternative. New ablative and mapping technologies to identify substrate are being refined and developed, and sinus rhythm can be achieved in the range of 70% in laboratories actively developing this procedure. The mechanism of success and the optimal ablation strategies are in evolution, but this therapy is emerging as a mainstream alternative in patients with persistent atrial fibrillation.

c. Pseudo–Atrial Fibrillation: An Infrequent Presentation of Paroxysmal Supraventricular Tachycardia

Li-Wei Lo and Shih-Ann Chen

DEFINITION OF PROBLEM

Atrial fibrillation (AF) generally presents as an irregularly irregular rhythm and is common in our daily practice. However, ventricular irregularity may also result from variable atrioventricular (AV) conduction in response to a rapid but regular atrial rate, as with supraventricular tachycardia (SVT). This phenomenon happens during the onset and termination of paroxysmal SVT and less so during a sustained period of the arrhythmia. In re-entrant arrhythmias, the tachycardia cycle length depends on the total conduction time of the entire tissue involved in the re-entrant circuit. Thus, oscillations in the conduction velocity and refractoriness within the re-entrant circuit are manifested by similar cycle length alternation. In patients with multiple AV conduction pathways or accessory pathways, an SVT may in particular be irregular for this reason and potentially be confused with AF. Careful analysis of the 12-lead electrocardiogram and electrophysiologic testing can provide the correct diagnosis. A high index of suspicion for this is especially appropriate in younger patients without risk factors for AF.

TYPICAL CASE

A 25-year-old man without structural heart disease had a 10-year history of frequent palpitations and chest discomfort, occurring at least twice a month. He visited a local emergency department, where a ventricular rate of up to 150 beats per minute was noted and AF was diagnosed. His resting electrocardiogram revealed sinus rhythm without ventricular pre-excitation. The electrocardiogram during tachycardia revealed irregular narrow-complex tachycardia without any apparent group beating (Fig. 61C.1). P waves could be seen only occasionally and were superimposed on the ST segment. Because he was young, without comorbidity, and experienced frequent attacks, he was referred to our clinic for further evaluation. An electrophysiologic study and possibly curative ablation therapy were arranged.

DIFFERENTIAL DIAGNOSIS

During baseline electrophysiologic study, atrial and ventricular extrastimulus testing revealed dual anterograde and retrograde AV nodal physiology. A fast-slow AV nodal re-entrant

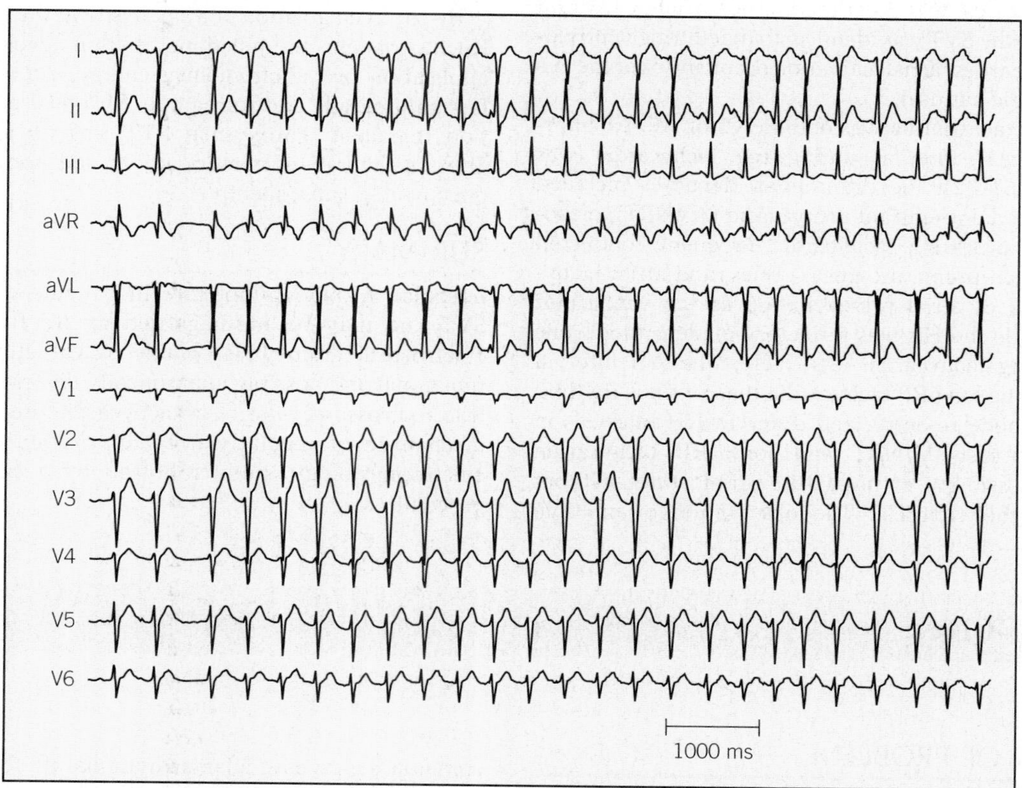

Figure 61C.1 The 12-lead electrocardiogram of the clinical tachycardia documented at presentation. The electrocardiogram mimics atrial fibrillation with an irregular narrow-complex tachycardia without group beating. P waves could be seen only occasionally and were superimposed on the ST segment intermittently.

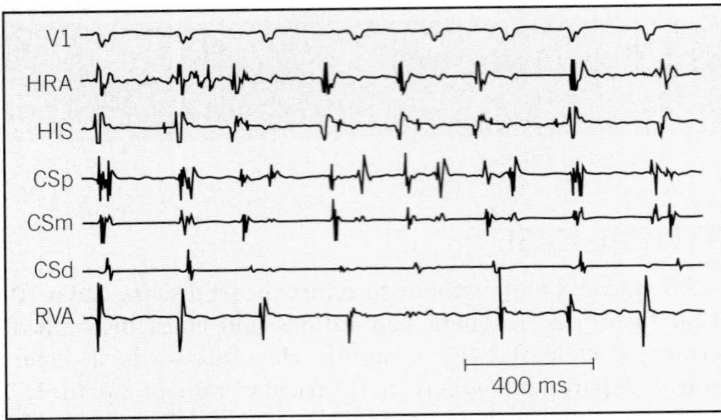

Figure 61C.2 Irregular atrioventricular nodal re-entrant tachycardia (AVNRT) related to dual anterograde and retrograde atrioventricular nodal properties. The first two beats represent a slow-fast AVNRT. The third beat is an atrial premature beat that is concealed in the atrioventricular node and terminates the slow-fast AVNRT, giving rise to a fast-slow AVNRT. The sixth beat develops a "1P2Q" response with any coexisting retrograde slow pathway block; the impulse is conducted through the node down both the anterograde fast and slow pathways, then the tachycardia returns to a slow-fast AVNRT. HRA, high right atrial electrogram; HIS, His bundle electrogram; CSp, CSm, and CSd, proximal, middle, and distal coronary sinus electrograms; RVA, right ventricular apex electrogram.

echo beat was identified during atrial extrastimulation. Intravenous infusion of isoproterenol (2 μg/min) was required to facilitate the induction and maintenance of the clinical tachycardia (see Fig. 61C.1). Although irregular, a "regularly irregular" pattern of the QRS complexes with intermittently discernible P waves was identified. The atrial activation sequence during the SVT was identical to that during ventricular pacing, with earliest atrial activation occurring over the His bundle (concentric pattern).

This irregular tachycardia was definitely not AF. An alternation in the AH interval during the tachycardia was observed (Fig. 61C.2); the differential diagnoses included multiform AV nodal re-entrant tachycardia (AVNRT), orthodromic AV reciprocating tachycardia, frequent conducted and nonconducted premature atrial cycles, and atrial tachycardia. The lack of atrial pre-excitation during ventricular extrastimuli while the His was refractory made orthodromic AV reciprocating tachycardia less likely. The AH interval was shorter during long RP tachycardia than in sinus rhythm, suggesting AV node re-entry, and different HH intervals in comparing slow-fast AVNRT and long RP tachycardia excluded the possibility of premature atrial cycles without conduction to the ventricle. The observation of multiple "jumps" in performance of atrial and ventricular pacing during the onset of the tachycardia and initiation of the tachycardia with a V-A-V sequence essentially excluded atrial tachycardia.

From this evidence, the regularly irregular narrow QRS complex tachycardia was diagnosed as irregular AVNRT. This variant can occur in up to 5% of patients with AVNRT. The irregularity may stem from anatomically different AV node pathways. However, studies have suggested that anisotropic conduction–induced functional pathways are responsible for this AV nodal physiology. Up to 42% of patients with multiple anterograde slow pathways experience the simultaneous elimination of all those pathways at a single ablation site.

TREATMENT OPTIONS

The patient had increasing frequency of attacks, and rapid AF was considered from the surface electrocardiogram. Under the circumstances, catheter ablation is a reasonable first-line option to further medical therapy. AF was not inducible after administration of isoproterenol, and consequently AV node re-entry was considered to be the only relevant clinical arrhythmia in this individual. It was observed that the fast pathway was anatomically distant from the multiple slow pathways, and most of the slow pathways could be successfully ablated after targeting of a single site or multiple sites, even though all may not have been clinically relevant. The immediate and long-term success rates of slow pathway ablation are excellent with minimal morbidity. Therefore, catheter ablation was offered to this patient.

He received ablation at a single site in the lower portion of Koch's triangle, and junctional rhythm developed during the application of radiofrequency energy. After ablation, only fast anterograde and retrograde AV nodal pathway conduction remained. Paroxysmal SVT was no longer inducible after the therapeutic intervention, and none was clinically documented subsequently.

SUMMARY

Irregular AVNRT is not rare in patients with paroxysmal SVT and may be misdiagnosed as AF from the surface electrocardiogram. It is curable by catheter ablation. The functional and possibly anatomically diverse slow pathways lead to gross irregularity of tachycardia. Recognition of this mechanism of regularly irregular rhythm can lead to an electrophysiologic study followed by a curative ablation procedure.

d. Atrial Flutter

Bruce D. Walker

DEFINITION OF PROBLEM

Atrial flutter, a common arrhythmia in the adult population (incidence between 0.4% and 1.2%), often coexists with atrial fibrillation. It is associated with valvular heart disease, congenital heart disease, and chronic airways disease and is a common supraventricular arrhythmia after open heart surgery. Typical atrial flutter is caused by macroreentry in the right atrium with conduction occurring in a counterclockwise direction, resulting in a typical sawtooth pattern in the inferior limb leads and positive flutter waves (F waves) in V_1.

Less commonly, flutter may conduct clockwise around the right atrium, producing F waves of the opposing polarity on the electrocardiogram. Other atypical forms of atrial flutter may occur in association with surgical scars, especially after congenital heart surgery. Typical atrial flutter may cause recurrent palpitations, dyspnea, or chest pain. It is generally less responsive to antiarrhythmic drugs, and the ventricular rate can be more difficult to control than atrial fibrillation. Inadequate rate control in the long term may predispose to tachycardia-induced cardiomyopathy. The risk of thromboembolism during atrial flutter is similar to that of atrial fibrillation; hence, antiplatelet and anticoagulant therapy should be considered in all patients.

TYPICAL CASE

A 54-year-old man presented with rapid, regular palpitations associated with dyspnea and mild dizziness on a background of documented paroxysmal atrial fibrillation and flutter. The episodes were usually several hours in duration and were not associated with chest pain, dyspnea, presyncope, or syncope. There was no history of coronary, valvular, or congenital heart disease. His relevant medical history included maturity-onset diabetes mellitus, obesity, hypertension, and previous tobacco use. He was treated with flecainide, 100 mg twice a day; ramipril, 10 mg daily; glyburide, 20 mg twice a day; metformin, 1 g twice a day; and aspirin, 81 mg daily. In the past, he had been treated with propafenone, 300 mg twice a day, but this was discontinued because of gastrointestinal upset. Sotalol, 120 mg twice a day, was not effective in suppressing his symptoms. He worked as a professional in a sedentary occupation, did not regularly exercise, and consumed 10 g of alcohol each day. Examination revealed a blood pressure of 150/80 mm Hg and no evidence of cardiac failure or pulmonary abnormalities.

DIFFERENTIAL DIAGNOSIS

A 12-lead electrocardiogram obtained on presentation shows atrial flutter with a 2:1 ventricular response (Fig. 61D.1). The diagnosis is based on the presence of a classic sawtooth pattern best seen in the inferior limb leads with no isoelectric interval and atrial rate of about 280 per minute. The F-wave axis is consistent with the presence of typical counterclockwise flutter in the right atrium (negative in leads II, III, and aVF; positive in V_1). The differential diagnosis is atrial tachycardia, which is unlikely given the rapid atrial rate, lack of isoelectric interval, and F-wave morphology.

A chest radiograph showed a normal cardiothoracic diameter and no evidence of pulmonary venous congestion. A transthoracic echocardiogram showed normal cardiac chambers and valves.

TREATMENT OPTIONS

Acute Treatment

There are two major alternatives for the initial treatment of this arrhythmia, restoration of sinus rhythm (by electrical cardioversion, atrial pace-termination, or antiarrhythmic drug therapy) and ventricular rate control. A decision between these options depends on whether the cardiac status is compromised as a direct result of the arrhythmia (e.g., hypotension, heart failure, ischemic chest pain). Cardioversion is the preferred option in this setting if rate control is not achievable. This carries a risk of thromboembolism similar to that of atrial fibrillation, particularly if atrial flutter has persisted for more than 48 hours and the patient has not been therapeutically anticoagulated for more than 1 month before cardioversion. Under such conditions, transesophageal echocardiography should be performed to exclude left atrial thrombus unless the patient is so compromised that the cardioversion is deemed urgent. The success rate for cardioversion of atrial flutter is 95% to 99% and can be

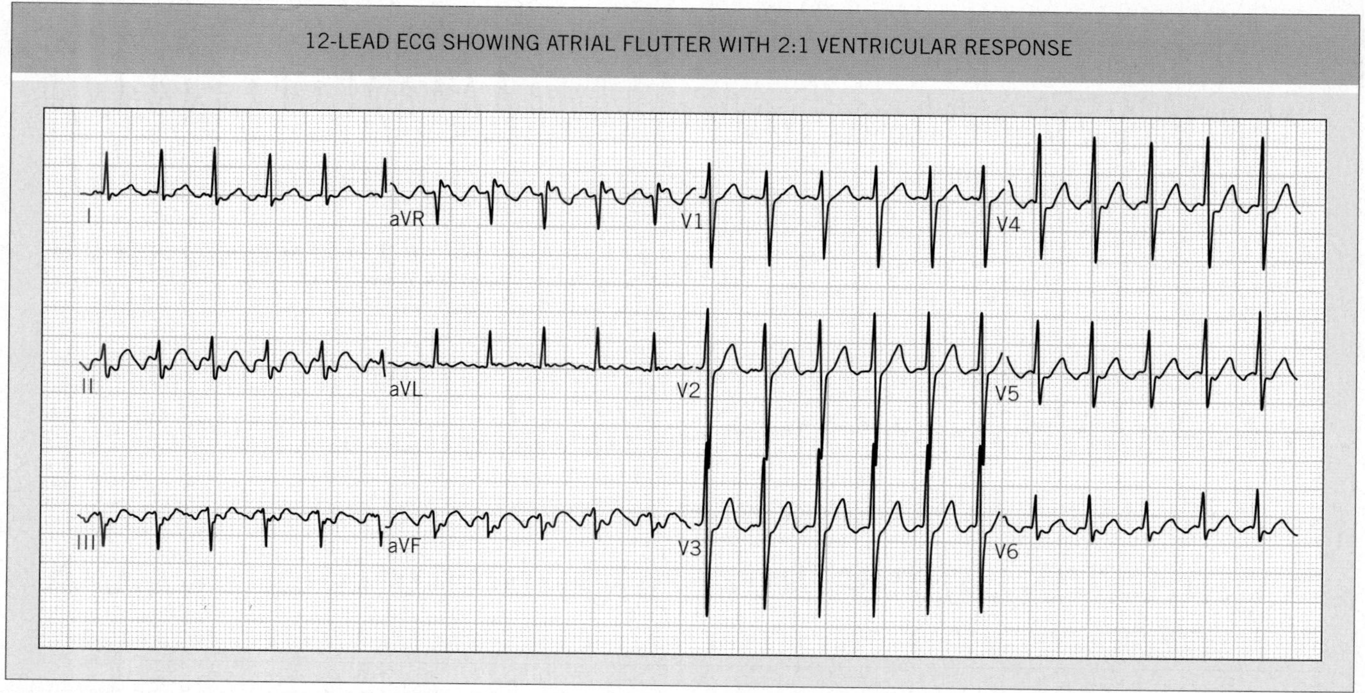

Figure 61D.1 The 12-lead electrocardiogram showing atrial flutter with 2:1 ventricular response. Flutter wave morphology suggests typical counterclockwise pattern of right atrial activation.

achieved with low energy (20 to 50 J) in many cases. In this case, cardioversion was not attempted because the patient was not compromised, there was uncertainty as to the duration of atrial flutter, and the patient was not anticoagulated.

Overdrive pace-termination confers the same risk of thromboembolism but can be performed without the need for general anesthesia or sedation. It is therefore useful for patients with a high anesthetic risk or in the nonfasted patient. The technique involves introduction of a single pacing wire into the high right atrium through a large peripheral vein. The atrium is paced 10% to 20% faster than the spontaneous flutter rate for 15 to 30 seconds to ensure adequate atrial capture. Sudden or gradual cessation of pacing results in termination of atrial flutter. If it is unsuccessful, the same maneuver can be attempted with a faster pacing rate, a new right atrial pacing site, or an increased stimulus strength (up to 20 mA). Alternatively, atrial pacing may be performed through temporary epicardial pacing wires in patients who have undergone cardiac surgery or with use of an esophageal electrode. Rapid atrial pacing can provoke atrial fibrillation, which may precede reversion to sinus rhythm. If atrial fibrillation persists, it is usually associated with a slower ventricular response.

Antiarrhythmic drug therapy is less effective than these strategies for acute reversion of atrial flutter. The success rates for termination vary between 40% and 70% for class Ia, class Ic, and class III agents. Ibutilide, a newer class III agent, appears to have greater efficacy than other antiarrhythmic drugs but is available only for intravenous use. Antiarrhythmic agents may also be commenced to facilitate electrical cardioversion and maintenance of sinus rhythm after cardioversion.

Acute ventricular rate control in atrial flutter can be achieved with use of drugs that preferentially slow conduction through the atrioventricular (AV) node, such as β-adrenoreceptor blockers, calcium channel antagonists, and digoxin. Intravenous loading with a beta blocker (e.g., esmolol, metoprolol) or calcium channel antagonist (e.g., diltiazem, verapamil) is the treatment of choice. Bolus doses can be given with blood pressure monitoring until adequate rate control is achieved (<100 beats per minute). In this case, rate control was initially achieved with intravenous diltiazem, then long-term treatment was initiated with atenolol.

Chronic Treatment

The alternatives for long-term treatment of paroxysmal atrial flutter also depend on whether the goal is maintenance of sinus rhythm or ventricular rate control. Antiplatelet and anticoagulation therapy must be considered in the context of either strategy. Rhythm control can be achieved with use of antiarrhythmic drugs or with a definitive procedure, such as catheter ablation of the tricuspid valve–inferior vena cava isthmus or surgery. AV node–blocking agents or AV node ablation followed by permanent pacemaker implantation is used for long-term rate control.

Long-term antiarrhythmic therapy with a class Ia, class Ic, or class III antiarrhythmic agent is variably effective for suppression of symptomatic paroxysmal atrial flutter. Class Ic and class III agents are better tolerated and more effective than class Ia drugs. Amiodarone is likely to be the most effective drug but carries the potential risk of serious adverse effects and is not generally used as first-line therapy. Caution should be exercised with class Ic agents because they may cause 1:1 ventricular conduction due to slowing of the atrial rate and a vagolytic effect on the AV node (Fig. 61D.2). This complication is best prevented by the coadministration of an AV node–blocking agent.

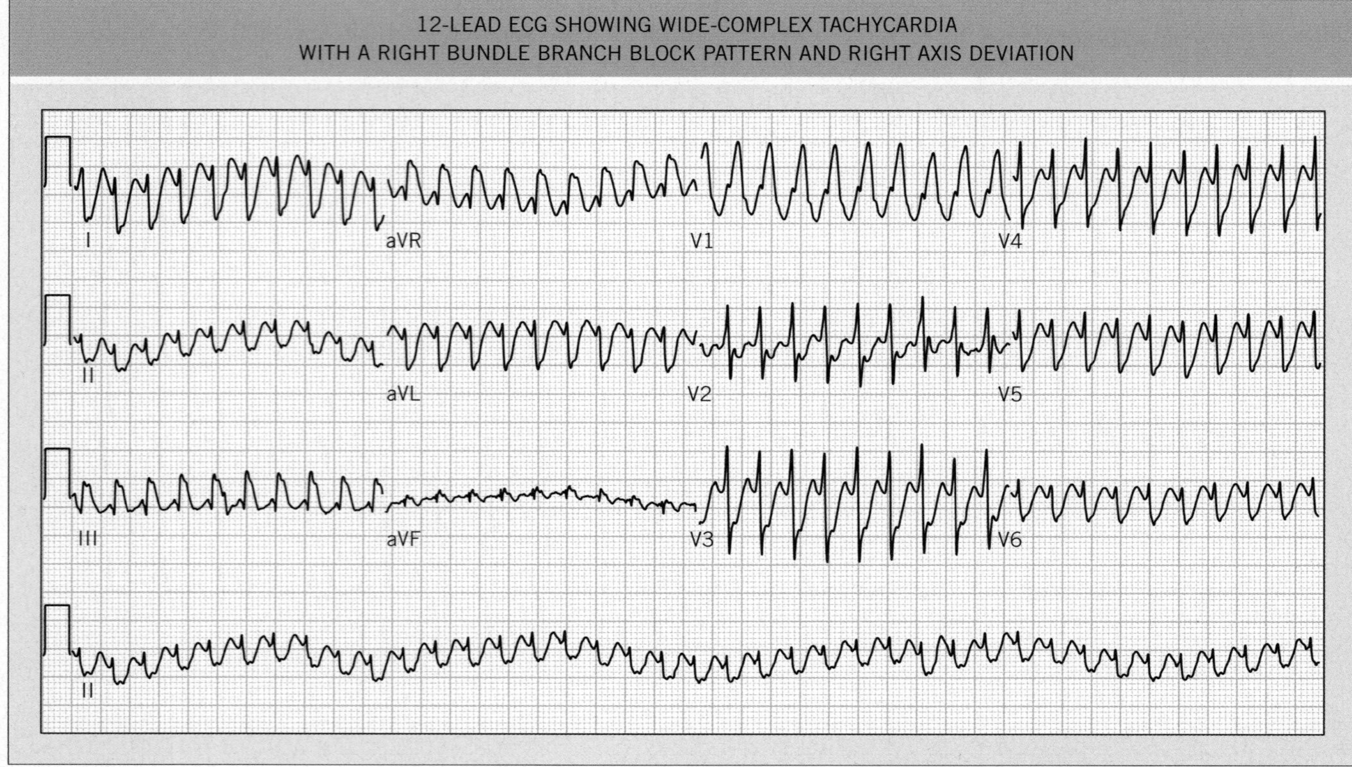

Figure 61D.2 The 12-lead electrocardiogram showing wide-complex tachycardia with a right bundle branch block pattern and right axis deviation. Administration of adenosine resulted in reversion to atrial flutter with a variable block, confirming a diagnosis of atrial flutter with 1:1 conduction.

Catheter ablation is indicated for patients with recurrent symptomatic paroxysmal, persistent, or chronic atrial flutter for whom antiarrhythmic therapy has failed or who have poor ventricular rate control. In this case, there was difficulty in achieving adequate rate control, so the patient underwent semiurgent catheter ablation. The subeustachian isthmus, a narrow zone of slow conduction, is the target of ablation. A line of block across the subeustachian isthmus is achieved by creating serial or continuous lesions from the tricuspid valve annulus to the inferior vena cava. The procedure has an 85% to 90% success rate in elimination of atrial flutter with a low risk of serious complication. It should be considered for early treatment of patients with poor ventricular rate control, tachycardia-induced cardiomyopathy, or a history of 1:1 ventricular conduction.

SUMMARY

Atrial flutter may be difficult to suppress with long-term antiarrhythmic treatment, and ventricular rate control is critical to the prevention of symptoms and maintenance of normal ventricular function. As illustrated in this case, catheter ablation for typical atrial flutter is a reasonable option for patients who become refractory to antiarrhythmic treatment or fail to achieve adequate rate control.

e. Atrial Fibrillation Complicated by Heart Failure

Bruce D. Walker

DEFINITION OF PROBLEM

Atrial fibrillation (AF) occurs in 10% to 20% of patients with mild to moderate heart failure but increases in frequency up to 50% in the setting of severe or advanced disease. AF is a major adverse prognostic factor in heart failure and is associated with a 1.3- to 3-fold increase in mortality. Impaired atrial contractile function, loss of atrioventricular synchrony, and irregular ventricular rhythm may contribute to a decrease in cardiac output. In patients with recent-onset heart failure, AF with a poorly controlled ventricular rate should be suspected as the possible underlying cause in the absence of other reversible factors, such as myocardial ischemia, valvular disease, and metabolic or infiltrative disorders.

TYPICAL CASE

A 50-year-old man presented with a 1-month history of increasing dyspnea on exertion, orthopnea, and intermittent palpitations (NYHA functional class II). He had no past history of viral illness, hypertension, or ischemic, valvular, or congenital heart disease and denied use of cardioactive medication or stimulants. There was no family history of cardiomyopathy or cardiac arrhythmias. Examination revealed an irregular pulse (110 beats per minute), blood pressure of 105/60 mm Hg, and signs of biventricular heart failure.

Differential Diagnosis

The 12-lead electrocardiogram revealed disorganized atrial activity consistent with AF and a ventricular rate of 140 beats per minute (Fig. 61E.1). There were no acute ST or T-wave changes, and the QT interval was within normal limits. The serum electrolyte values and renal, hepatic, and thyroid function test results were normal. Transthoracic echocardiography showed mild left ventricular dilatation with severe global impairment in systolic function (ejection fraction, 30%), mild biatrial dilatation, and normal cardiac valves.

TREATMENT OPTIONS

Management of AF is first targeted at achieving rate control and addressing the risk of thromboembolism. Whereas spontaneous reversion of AF occurs in 30% to 80% of patients within 24 hours of onset, the history suggests a more prolonged course, given the duration of symptoms.

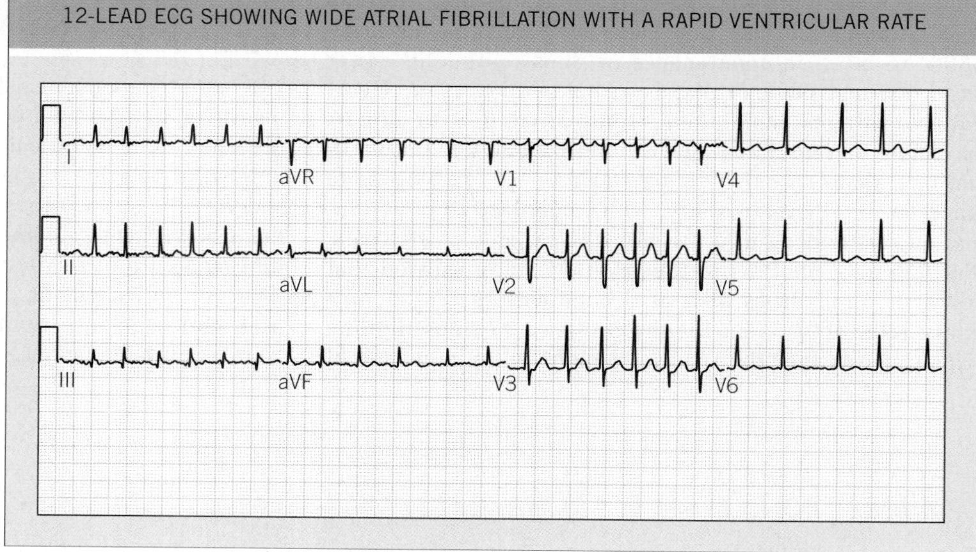

Figure 61E.1 The 12-lead electrocardiogram showing atrial fibrillation with a rapid ventricular rate.

Ventricular rate control in the context of heart failure could be achieved with amiodarone, digoxin, or low-dose β-adrenoreceptor blockade. Drugs with negative inotropic properties, such as verapamil, diltiazem, and high-dose beta blockers, should be avoided. The optimal target heart rate is not well established but should be in the range of 60 to 80 beats per minute at rest and up to 120 beats per minute during exertion. These measures alone may improve hemodynamics and blood pressure. The major predictors of stroke and systemic embolism in nonvalvular AF include previous stroke or transient ischemic attack, hypertension, left ventricular dysfunction, advanced age, diabetes mellitus, and coronary artery disease. Anticoagulation should therefore be considered with the use of standard intravenous heparin, subcutaneous low-molecular-weight heparin, or warfarin. Direct current cardioversion may be considered if there is marked hemodynamic instability and inadequate rate control and if transesophageal echocardiography is available.

In this case, a strategy of rhythm control was pursued as rate control proved difficult to achieve. Pharmacologic reversion with class I agents or sotalol is relatively contraindicated because of the increased risk of proarrhythmia and hemodynamic compromise in the setting of known left ventricular dysfunction. Direct current cardioversion was planned, the absence of left atrial thrombus having been confirmed on transesophageal echocardiography. In spite of biphasic shocks at 200 J, 300 J, and 360 J with electrodes in the anteroposterior position, AF persisted and the procedure was abandoned. The patient remained symptomatic with mild left ventricular failure on clinical examination. For this reason, treatment was continued with oral amiodarone (200 mg three times a day), digoxin (125 μg daily), carvedilol (3.125 mg twice daily), and furosemide (40 mg daily), with full anticoagulation with use of enoxaparin. Repeated cardioversion was performed successfully in 1 week by a single 200-J biphasic shock. The post-reversion electrocardiogram showed sinus rhythm with no abnormality in atrioventricular conduction, QRS axis, or bundle branch block.

Evidence from large clinical trials (e.g., AFFIRM, CHF-STAT, DIAMOND) and studies of catheter ablation for AF highlight the potential benefit of maintaining sinus rhythm in patients with AF and left ventricular dysfunction. Amiodarone and dofetilide have moderate efficacy (50% to 80%) in maintenance of sinus rhythm at 1 year after pharmacologic or direct current cardioversion. Heart failure patients maintaining sinus rhythm with antiarrhythmic therapy have lower mortality and less hospitalization than proarrhythmia (1.0% to 2.0%) and amiodarone-related toxicity, which may lead to discontinuation of the drug in up to 50% of patients at 10 years. Furthermore, analysis of the AFFIRM study showed that antiarrhythmic drugs were associated with increased mortality after adjustment for the presence of sinus rhythm. This suggests that the survival benefit in maintenance of sinus rhythm may be offset by the impact of adverse effects.

Catheter ablation of persistent AF in the setting of left ventricular dysfunction may be associated with 60% to 80% success in restoration and maintenance of sinus rhythm at 12 months with an improvement in left ventricular ejection fraction (up to 20%), exercise capacity, and quality of life. There remains a 1% to 5% risk of significant complication associated with this procedure, including cardiac perforation, tamponade, stroke, pulmonary vein stenosis, phrenic nerve paralysis, and atrioesophageal fistula. Furthermore, the long-term efficacy, the impact on left atrial mechanical function and autonomic function, and therefore the requirement for anticoagulation are unknown. In this case, the patient had recurrent AF within 3 months of cardioversion and catheter ablation was performed. Circumferential pulmonary vein isolation and linear ablation of the mitral isthmus and left atrial roof resulted in restoration of sinus rhythm during the procedure. Three months after the procedure, the patient was reassessed clinically with resting 12-lead electrocardiography and 24-hour Holter monitoring, which revealed maintenance of sinus rhythm. Repeated echocardiography showed mild left ventricular dilatation with normal systolic function (ejection fraction, 55%) and mild left atrial dilatation. Anticoagulation was continued for another 3 months and anti-failure medication for the next year.

If rhythm control could not be achieved in the long term, a rate control strategy with beta blockade (e.g., metoprolol, carvedilol, bisoprolol) and digoxin would be a reasonable option. Atrioventricular node ablation with implantation of a permanent pacemaker ("ablate and pace") is an alternative to pharmacologic rate control and is particularly beneficial in those with persistent symptoms, inadequate rate control, or adverse effects from medication. An ablate and pace strategy may be associated with a reduction in symptoms and improved quality of life, but there is no apparent mortality benefit versus medical therapy. Preliminary evidence suggests that a further benefit in left ventricular function may be achieved with implantation of a biventricular pacemaker in such patients, although larger randomized studies are pending (e.g., AVERT AF trial).

SUMMARY

AF is an independent risk factor for increased mortality in heart failure. Patients with AF and poor rate control may develop left ventricular dysfunction, which can be improved by achieving adequate rate control and then considering the option of restoration of sinus rhythm. This may be achieved with a combination of antiarrhythmic medication and cardioversion or catheter ablation. Although the issue of anticoagulant discontinuation remains controversial, anticoagulants should be continued in the absence of convincing and ongoing surveillance to exclude "silent" AF.

f. Atrial Fibrillation and Anticoagulation

Bruce D. Walker

DEFINITION OF PROBLEM

Atrial fibrillation (AF) is a major independent risk factor for stroke, with a prevalence of nearly 10% in patients older than 80 years. The estimated risk of stroke varies from 0.5% per year in young patients with lone AF to 12% per year in patients with AF and a previous stroke. The major predictors of stroke and systemic embolism in nonvalvular AF include previous stroke or transient ischemic attack, hypertension, left ventricular dysfunction, advanced age, diabetes mellitus, and coronary artery disease. Antiplatelet agents decrease the risk of stroke by 20% compared with placebo, whereas warfarin reduces stroke risk by 60% compared with placebo and 40% compared with aspirin. The choice of antithrombotic therapy is based on risk stratification by the use of these predictors and the presence of comorbidities that may contribute to risk of bleeding.

TYPICAL CASE

A 72-year-old man presented with a 1-month history of intermittent palpitations on a background of hypertension, type 2 diabetes, and prostate carcinoma treated with external beam radiation therapy. He had no past history of ischemic, valvular, or congenital heart disease. There was no history of gastrointestinal or genitourinary bleeding. His medications at presentation included ramipril (10 mg daily), metformin (500 mg twice daily), gliclazide (80 mg twice daily), and finasteride (5 mg daily). Examination revealed blood pressure of 160/85 mm Hg, an irregular pulse (100 beats per minute), normal heart sounds, and no signs of biventricular heart failure.

DIFFERENTIAL DIAGNOSIS

A 12-lead electrocardiogram showed AF and voltage criteria for left ventricular hypertrophy (Fig. 61F-1). Transthoracic echocardiography showed mild concentric left ventricular hypertrophy with normal systolic function, moderate left atrial dilatation, and normal cardiac valves. A 24-hour Holter monitoring showed AF with an average ventricular rate of 88 per minute, with a maximum rate of 195 per minute and no bradycardia or ventricular arrhythmias.

TREATMENT OPTIONS

The patient has two "moderate" risk factors, hypertension and diabetes, that place him at moderate risk for stroke. In the CHADS2 stratification scheme, this would yield a score of 2 with an expected stroke rate of 2.5% per year. Anticoagulation was commenced with warfarin because AF duration was longer than 48 hours, with a target international normalized ratio (INR) range of 2.0 to 3.0. This confers maximum protection against stroke without a significantly increased risk of major bleeding. Rate control was initiated with metoprolol, 50 mg twice daily, which eliminated his symptoms. The patient was unenthusiastic to pursue the option of rhythm control by antiarrhythmic therapy or direct current cardioversion.

Three months later, the patient presented with severe rectal bleeding with an INR of 2.6 requiring reversal of anticoagulation and 2-unit blood transfusion. Proctitis, confirmed on rectosigmoidoscopy, was most likely secondary to previous radiation therapy. Evaluation of potential thromboembolic risk included transesophageal echocardiography, which showed severe left atrial spontaneous echo contrast and poor left atrial appendage mechanical function without evidence of thrombus. As a result of these findings, the options included resumption of anticoagulation with a target INR of 2.0, antiplatelet therapy, catheter ablation of AF, operative left atrial appendage removal, left atrial appendage occlusion device, and no further treatment. Whether these interventions will replace more conventional

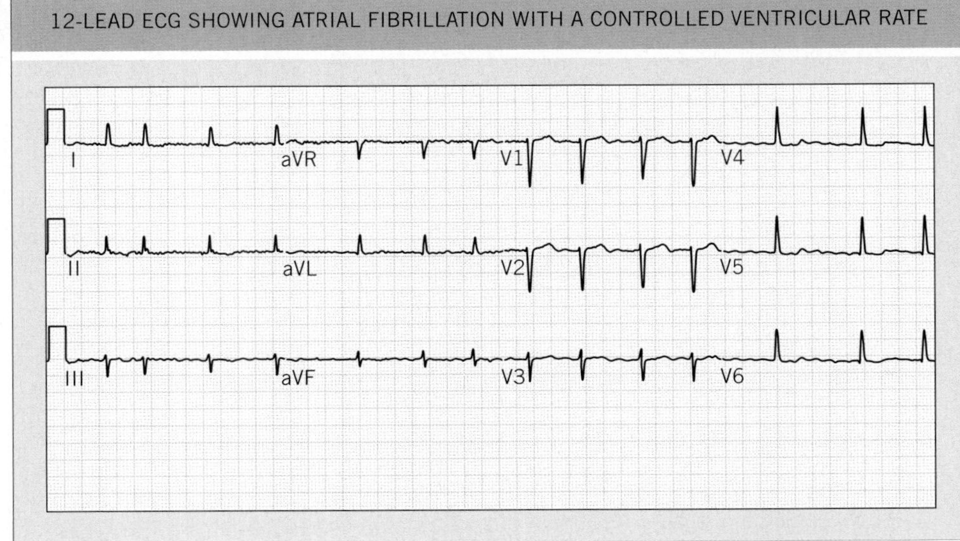

Figure 61F-1 The 12-lead electrocardiogram of atrial fibrillation with a controlled ventricular rate.

strategies for the reduction of thromboembolic risk in AF awaits confirmation from current clinical trials. The annual rate of major bleeding with warfarin is about 1% with major risk factors including age older than 65 years, history of gastrointestinal or other major hemorrhage, alcohol abuse, concomitant use of antiplatelet agents, uncontrolled hypertension, and renal or hepatic disease. The patient preferred to be treated with antiplatelet therapy alone (aspirin, 100 mg daily) and remained stable with only minor rectal bleeding.

SUMMARY

This case highlights one of the difficulties encountered with long-term anticoagulation for the prevention of stroke in AF. Although elderly patients are at higher risk of thromboembolism, there is also an increased risk of hemorrhage, particularly in those older than 80 years (annual rate, 3% to 4%). In low-risk AF patients (age <65 years, no heart disease or hypertension), aspirin alone is recommended for thromboembolism prophylaxis.

chapter 62

Ventricular Tachycardia

Glenn D. Young, Kurt C. Roberts-Thomson, Martin K. Stiles, and Prashanthan Sanders

Definition

- Ventricular tachycardia is a rapid rhythm (>100 beats per minute) arising from the ventricular tissue.

Key Features

- Most frequent cause of sudden cardiac death.
- Most often occurs in structurally abnormal hearts.
- Tachycardia mechanism is often re-entry involving diseased myocardium but can be due to triggered or enhanced automaticity.

Therapy

- Acute therapy involves a trial of drug therapy or cardioversion (in the hemodynamically compromised patient) and treatment of precipitants.
- Secondary prevention in patients with normal hearts usually involves drug therapy or ablation.
- Secondary prevention in patients with structural heart disease usually involves insertion of a defibrillator, with drug therapy and ablation reserved for frequent arrhythmias.

The diagnosis of ventricular tachycardia encompasses a range of conditions sharing the common feature of origin within the ventricular myocardium or the specialized conductive tissue distal to the atrioventricular node. Empirically, a rate of 100 beats per minute is used as a lower limit for the diagnosis of ventricular tachycardia, although practically, the rate is more often in excess of 150 or even 200 beats per minute. The cardinal diagnostic feature is the presence of broad and frequently atypical QRS complexes on the electrocardiogram during tachycardia. Although it occurs most often in patients with structural heart disease, there are forms that do occur in the absence of cardiac disease. Ventricular tachyarrhythmias are the most common cause of sudden cardiac death in our community. In the past, treatment has been primarily pharmacologic, although this has little impact on the prognosis of patients with ventricular tachycardia. More recently, the use of the implantable defibrillator and ablation therapy have improved the outlook for patients with ventricular arrhythmias.

ANATOMY AND PATHOPHYSIOLOGY

The importance of anatomic or structural changes in determining arrhythmia mechanism is recognized for most arrhythmias and holds true also for ventricular tachycardia. The most common substrate for ventricular tachycardia is ischemic heart disease. The likelihood of ventricular arrhythmia in patients with coronary artery disease relates directly to the extent of myocardial damage and scarring. Ejection fraction remains the cornerstone of predicting the risk of ventricular arrhythmia in the patient with coronary artery disease.[1] The mechanism for this monomorphic ventricular tachycardia is almost always re-entry maintained by the surviving myocytes within extensive areas of infarction.[2] The interdigitation of spared myocardium with scar tissue at the border zone of infarcted areas allows the development of an isthmus of slowed and anisotropic conduction in the border zones between scar and healed myocardium, and this forms the anatomic substrate that allows re-entry to be established (Figs. 62.1 and 62.2). Cell-to-cell propagation may also be affected by a variety of factors associated with myocardial infarction, further affecting the conduction and propagation of the electrical wavefront through the damaged tissue. In addition to changes in conduction velocity, abnormalities in repolarization frequently play a role in the genesis of re-entry arrhythmias. Refractory periods within regions of surviving muscle in the scarred tissue may also be prolonged and more variable than in the surrounding normal cardiac tissue. The electrophysiologic correlates of these abnormalities have been shown to be fractionated, low-amplitude, and prolonged signals.[3,4] These anatomic and electrophysiologic substrates form the basis of the fundamental requirements for re-entry (Fig. 62.3; see also Figs. 62.1 and 62.2).

The substrate for ventricular tachycardia during acute ischemia and infarction is likely quite different from that with a chronic infarct, and the precise mechanisms are less well understood. Although re-entry may still play an important role in the setting of acute myocardial infarction, perhaps with the involvement of the Purkinje network, the mechanisms early in an acute event are probably due to abnormal automaticity (Fig. 62.4).

The pathophysiologic mechanism of ventricular arrhythmias in hypertrophic and dilated cardiomyopathy is also not well characterized. Monomorphic ventricular arrhythmias are less common, as polymorphic ventricular tachycardia and ventricular fibrillation predominate. Nevertheless, the most likely electrophysiologic mechanism remains re-entry but with less well defined and delineated substrate than that seen in the postinfarction patient.

CLASSIFICATION OF VENTRICULAR TACHYCARDIA

Ventricular tachycardia may be classified according to a number of criteria. The morphology on the electrocardiogram (monomorphic or polymorphic), the duration of the

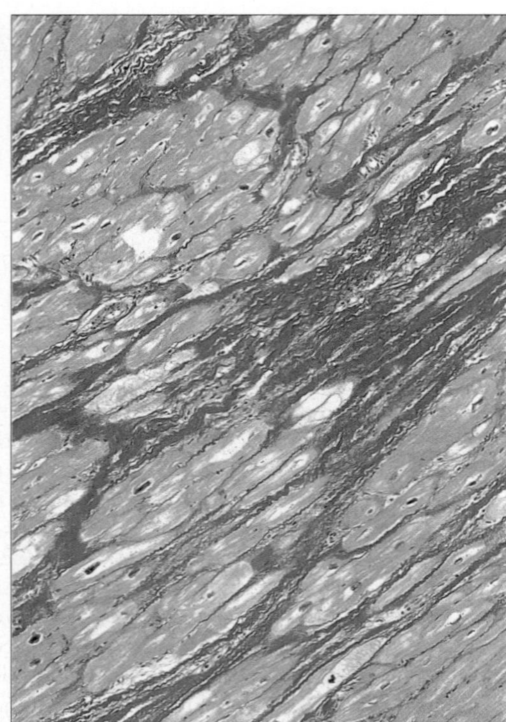

Figure 62.1 Patchy fibrosis in the border zone of healed myocardial infarction. This photomicrograph shows viable tissue interdigitating with regions of fibrosis, providing a substrate for ventricular tachycardia. Verhoeff–van Gieson stain. (Courtesy of Dr. Helen Cathro, University of Virginia, Charlottesville.)

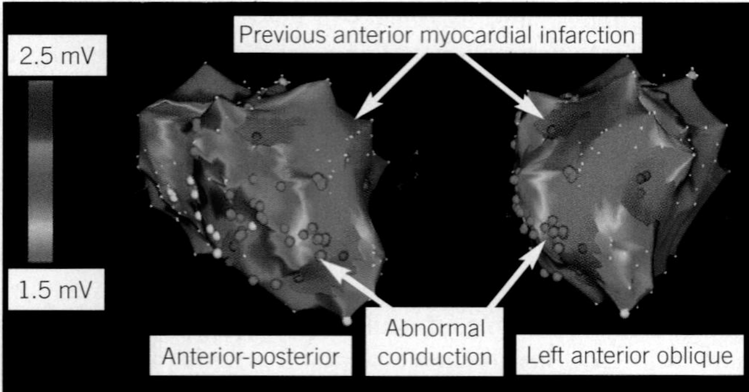

Figure 62.2 Electroanatomic three-dimensional map of the ventricle in a patient with an old anterior myocardial infarction and recurrent, hemodynamically compromising ventricular tachycardia. This map superimposes the bipolar voltage on the three-dimensional geometry of the ventricle to demonstrate the presence of scar. The area in red denotes the very low voltage region; gray represents areas of electrical silence. Together, these regions form the scar that resulted from the previous infarction. Healthy tissue is seen to produce large tissue voltages and is denoted in purple. In the border zone between the scar and healthy tissue, several electrograms are noted; fractionation or double potentials indicate areas of slowed conduction that could form an isthmus maintaining tachycardia (blue dots). In this case, pace mapping was performed around the border of the scar and compared with clinical tachycardia episodes. These sites were ablated by linear lesions within the scar border zone to eliminate inducible ventricular tachycardia.

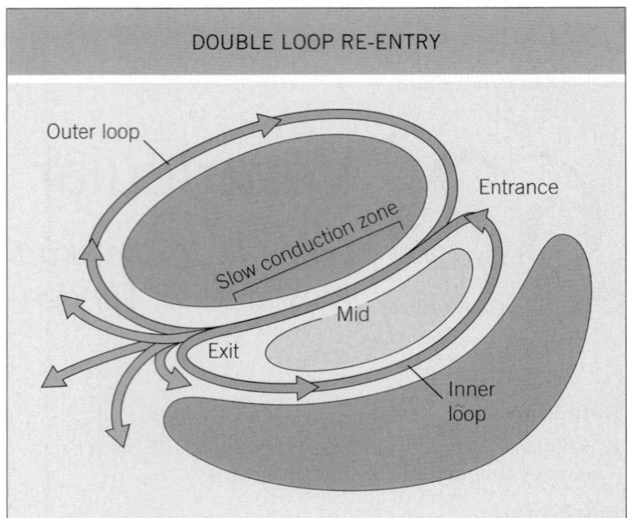

Figure 62.3 Double loop re-entry. This schematic diagram of a ventricular tachycardia circuit has an outer loop and an inner, protected loop that join in a central zone of slow conduction, the critical portion of the circuit. Pacing from within this slow conduction zone can be used to guide ablation.

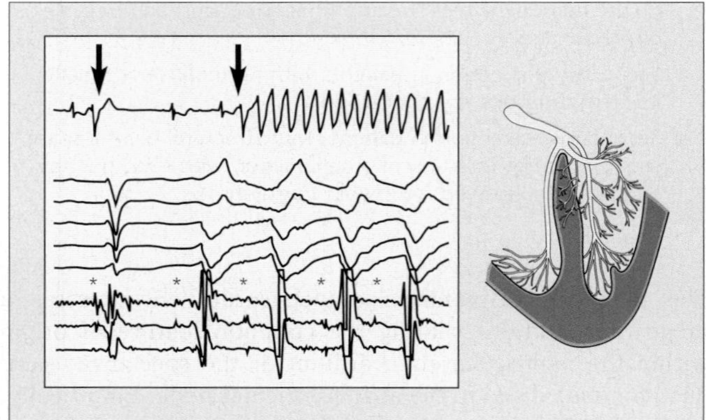

Figure 62.4 Ventricular tachycardia initiated from the Purkinje arborization in the setting of an acute myocardial infarction. Demonstrated is a schematic of the Purkinje arborization on the right. In the top panel, the rhythm strip is seen with an episode of rapid ventricular tachycardia and fibrillation initiated by an ectopic beat. Interestingly, the same ectopic beat is seen to occur in isolation, a few beats before the initiation of sustained arrhythmia *(arrows)*. The lower panel indicates the mapping of this initiating beat to a site at which a Purkinje potential precedes ventricular activation *(asterisks)*. In this example, repetitive firing from this Purkinje site initiates tachycardia. Ablation to eliminate the Purkinje triggers is effective in suppressing arrhythmia.

arrhythmia (sustained or nonsustained), and the underlying mechanism of the arrhythmia (re-entry, enhanced automaticity, or triggered automaticity) are some of the criteria by which ventricular tachycardias have been segregated. The clinical and electrocardiographic criteria used to classify ventricular tachycardia are listed in Tables 62.1 and 62.2, respectively. The electrocardiogram during ventricular tachycardia demonstrates a broad-

CLASSIFICATION OF VENTRICULAR TACHYCARDIA		
Rate	≥100 bpm	Ventricular tachycardia
	<100 bpm	Accelerated idioventricular rhythm
QRS pattern	Uniform QRS	Monomorphic
	Variable QRS	Polymorphic
QRS morphology	Positive in V_1	Right bundle type
	Negative in V_1	Left bundle type
	Positive in II, III, aVF	Inferior axis
	Negative in II, III, aVF	Superior axis
Duration	≥30 seconds	Sustained
	≥3 beats <30 seconds	Nonsustained
Frequency	Separate episodes	Sporadic
	Unable to maintain sinus rhythm	Incessant

Table 62.1 Classification of ventricular tachycardia.

DIFFERENTIAL DIAGNOSIS OF WIDE-COMPLEX TACHYCARDIA	
Favoring supraventricular tachycardia	Irregularly irregular intervals "Classic" RBBB or LBBB pattern QRS <140 ms (RBBB) or <160 ms (LBBB) History of SVT or pre-excitation QRS unchanged or just wider than in sinus rhythm
Favoring ventricular tachycardia	Atrioventricular dissociation Fusion or capture beats QRS >140 ms (RBBB) or >160 ms (LBBB) Positive chest lead QRS concordance QRS axis −60 to −180 degrees Heart disease, especially prior MI, present

LBBB, left right bundle branch block; MI, myocardial infarction; RBBB, right bundle branch block; SVT, supraventricular tachycardia.

Table 62.2 Differential diagnosis of wide-complex tachycardia.

complex rhythm with prolonged QRS duration (>120 ms) and usually abnormal QRS morphology, particularly compared with the electrocardiogram in sinus rhythm. On the basis of the morphology in lead V_1, ventricular tachycardia is usually defined as having either a right or left bundle branch block morphology, which may help predict its chamber of origin as left or right ventricle, respectively. This rule, however, is not infallible, particularly with tachycardia that has an exit site close to the interventricular septum. In addition, in the setting of previous left ventricular myocardial infarction, the ventricular tachycardia is almost always localized to the left ventricle irrespective of the electrocardiographic morphology.

PATHOPHYSIOLOGY: VENTRICULAR TACHYCARDIA ASSOCIATED WITH SPECIFIC DISEASES

Coronary Artery Disease

Coronary artery disease and in particular myocardial infarction offer the appropriate environment for the development of ventricular arrhythmias. The types of arrhythmia differ during the phases of evolution of myocardial infarction.[5] In the acute phase of myocardial infarction and during ischemia, polymorphic ventricular tachycardia and ventricular fibrillation predominate (see Fig. 62.4). Monomorphic ventricular tachycardia due to re-entry is the principal arrhythmia seen in the chronic phase after myocardial infarction. The intervening period between the index infarction and subsequent arrhythmia can be many years. The likelihood of ventricular tachycardia arising after myocardial infarction is related to the size of the infarct and overall left ventricular function. Larger infarcts offer more potential for re-entry because of the larger area of interface between damaged and normal myocardium. The left ventricular ejection fraction has been consistently shown to be a major determinant of the likelihood for development of ventricular arrhythmia.[6] Endocardial and intraoperative mapping supports the fact that these arrhythmias arise at the border zone between infarcted tissue and residual normal myocardium. All of the requirements for the establishment of re-entry, namely, parallel paths of conduction separated by anatomic or functional barriers, slowed conduction, and disturbed repolarization, exist in this border zone area. These factors probably contribute variably to the establishment and maintenance of sustained monomorphic ventricular tachycardia in different individuals. Endocardial mapping in sinus rhythm has demonstrated markedly fractionated and low-amplitude potentials in the peri-infarct regions of patients with recurrent ventricular tachycardia (Figs. 62.5 and 62.6).[7] These potentials not only represent the electrophysiologic markers for the areas of slowed conduction but may also signify a target site for catheter ablation therapy for these arrhythmias.

Dilated Cardiomyopathy

Patients with dilated cardiomyopathy, like those with ischemic left ventricular impairment, are at substantial risk for development of serious ventricular arrhythmia. The risk of malignant arrhythmia increases with heart failure severity.[8] The mechanism of arrhythmia in individuals with dilated cardiomyopathy is less well understood than in patients with ischemic heart disease. Monomorphic ventricular tachycardia is less common, and not infrequently, multiple morphologic patterns of ventricular tachycardia can occur. The substrate in dilated cardiomyopathy is more likely to be patchy myocardial cell death and fibrosis throughout the myocardium, producing fewer reproducible re-entry circuits than are found in chronic ischemic heart disease. This patchy scar can be perianular and epicardial in distribution. Risk assessment in patients with dilated cardiomyopathy and advanced left ventricular impairment is difficult as none of the currently available tests has sufficient specificity or sensitivity to be of real value.[9] Patients with dilated cardiomyopathy and ejection fraction below 35% who suffer sustained ventricular arrhythmia or syncope have a high risk of sudden cardiac death and need to be considered for aggressive therapy.

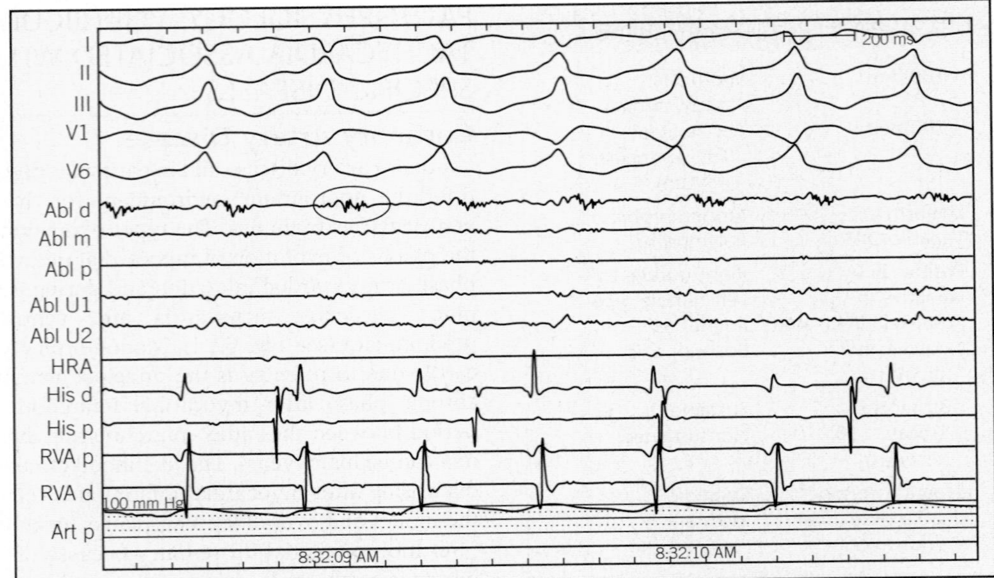

Figure 62.5 Electrograms during mapping in the border zone between scar and viable tissue. On the distal ablation signal (Abl d), a prolonged, low-amplitude, and delayed activation is seen during ventricular tachycardia. Abl d, Abl m, and Abl p refer to the ablation distal, mid, and proximal bipoles. Abl U1 and U2 denote the ablation unipoles. HRA, high right atrium; His, His electrogram; RVA, right ventricular apex; Art p, arterial pressure.

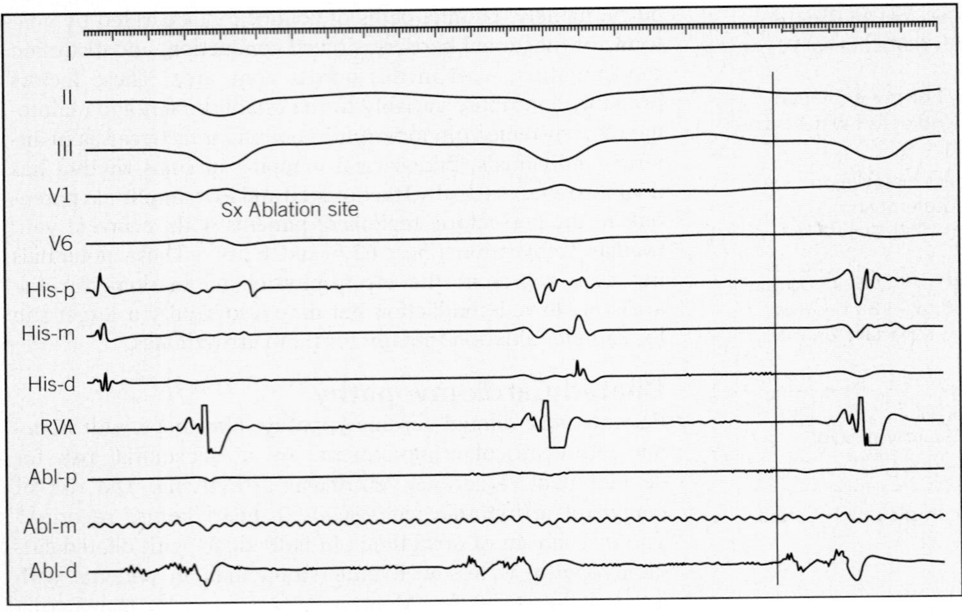

Figure 62.6 Another example of low-amplitude and prolonged activation in the isthmus of re-entry in the scar border zone. In this case, the fractionated low-amplitude electrogram on the distal ablation catheter (Abl-d) is seen to precede the surface electrocardiogram QRS complex in timing. Abl-d, Abl-m, and Abl-p refer to the ablation distal, mid, and proximal bipoles. His, His electrogram; RVA, right ventricular apex.

Sustained bundle branch re-entry is a specific form of ventricular tachycardia that occurs in patients with dilated cardiomyopathy. This arrhythmia, in its most frequently encountered form, uses the right bundle as the anterograde limb and the interventricular septum and the left bundle as the retrograde pathway. Characteristically, the surface QRS morphology demonstrates a left bundle branch pattern with a superiorly directed axis. Importantly, the arrhythmia mechanism requires disease within the conduction system, and the conduction system is critically involved in the tachycardia mechanism (Fig. 62.7). This form of ventricular tachycardia may account for 20% to 40% of presentations with monomorphic ventricular tachycardia in patients with dilated cardiomyopathy.[10] The recognition of this tachycardia is of particular clinical importance as recurrence can be prevented by ablation of the right bundle branch.

Hypertrophic Cardiomyopathy

The natural history of hypertrophic cardiomyopathy is variable, but most patients follow a relatively benign course. However, this condition is associated with an increased risk of sudden cardiac death, and ventricular arrhythmia is likely to account for a significant proportion of these sudden deaths. A number of factors, such as septal thickness, genotype, family history of malignant arrhythmia, syncope, and nonsustained arrhythmia, may help predict individuals at

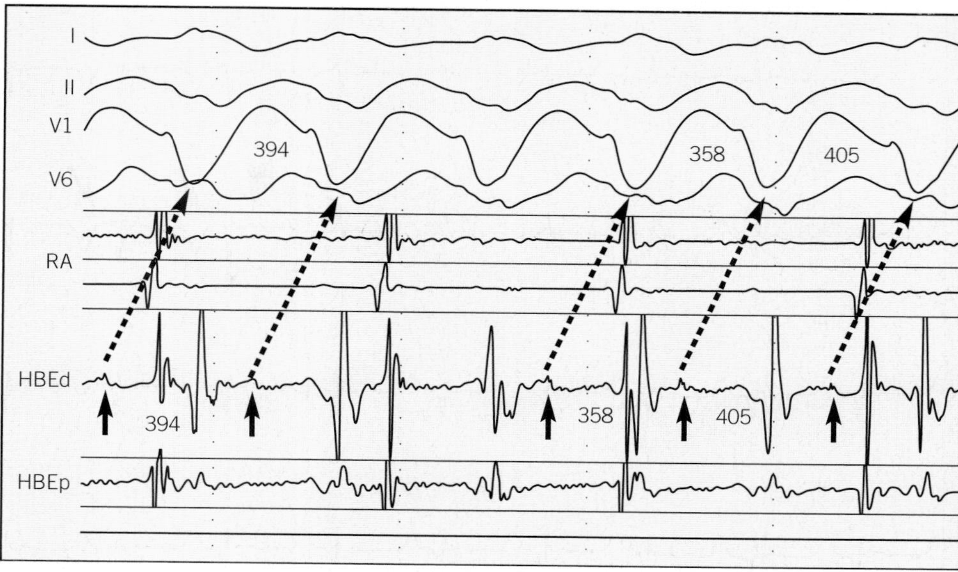

Figure 62.7 Intracardiac mapping during bundle branch re-entry tachycardia. Demonstrated are four electrocardiographic leads together with recordings from the right atrium (RA) and the proximal and distal electrode pairs at the His recording. The recording shows a broad complex on the surface electrocardiogram with a negative terminal component to V_1. The presence of VA dissociation is seen with an unrelated and slower atrial (RA recording). The involvement of the conduction system in the tachycardia circuit is confirmed by the presence of a His recording *(arrows)* before each ventricular complex and by the variation in the His-His activation preceding that observed in the ventricle. This arrhythmia was successfully eliminated by ablation of the right bundle.

higher risk of sudden death.[11] Although the risk of sudden cardiac death is low when it is considered across the spectrum of this condition, hypertrophic cardiomyopathy accounts for up to 50% of all cases of sudden cardiac death in competitive athletes.[12] Monomorphic ventricular tachycardia is much less frequent than in patients with ischemic heart disease. In long-term follow-up of high-risk patients with hypertrophic cardiomyopathy and an implantable defibrillator, ventricular fibrillation is responsible for at least 50% of appropriate defibrillator discharges.[13]

Arrhythmogenic Right Ventricular Cardiomyopathy/Dysplasia

This condition is an inherited disorder of cardiac muscle and presents most often with nonsustained or sustained ventricular arrhythmia. It accounts for up to 10% of cases of sudden cardiac death in individuals younger than 65 years.[14] The cardinal feature of this disease is patchy fatty and fibrous infiltration of the right ventricle (Fig. 62.8), with left ventricular involvement occurring rarely and usually only later in the disease process. Most often this condition presents in men before the age of 40 years. Traditionally, a definite diagnosis of arrhythmogenic right ventricular cardiomyopathy/dysplasia has required histologic finding of transmural fibrofatty replacement of the right ventricular myocardium at biopsy or necropsy. However, increasingly, there is acceptance of features on magnetic resonance imaging to allow premorbid diagnosis (see Fig. 62.8). Clinical diagnosis is based on a scoring system incorporating historical features and results of investigations.[15] The baseline electrocardiographic features are variable but include T-wave inversion across the anterior chest leads and the presence of an epsilon wave (Fig. 62.9). Monomorphic ventricular tachycardia with left bundle morphology occurs as the predominant

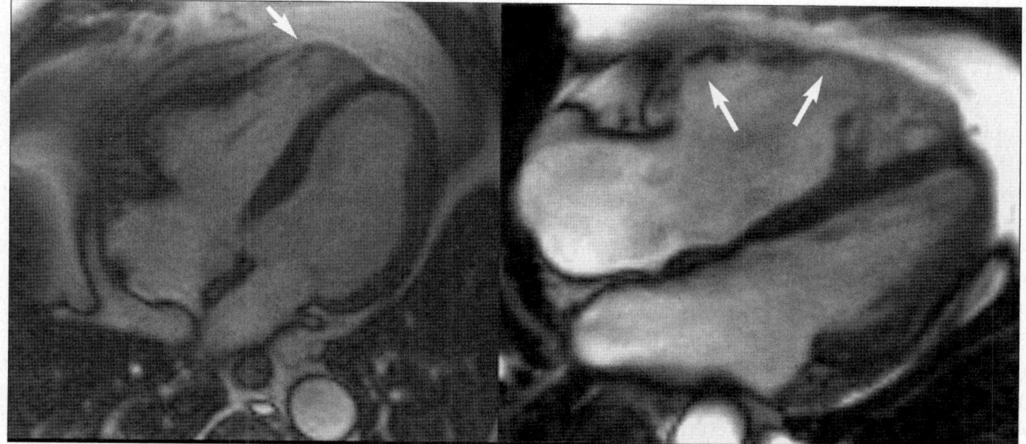

Figure 62.8 Magnetic resonance imaging in arrhythmogenic right ventricular cardiomyopathy/dysplasia. Two separate cases are demonstrated. The illustration on the left demonstrates thinning and dilatation of the right ventricular wall *(arrow)*. The one on the right demonstrates more advanced disease with right ventricular dilatation, systolic and aneurysmal bulging of the right ventricular wall, and fatty infiltration of the wall.

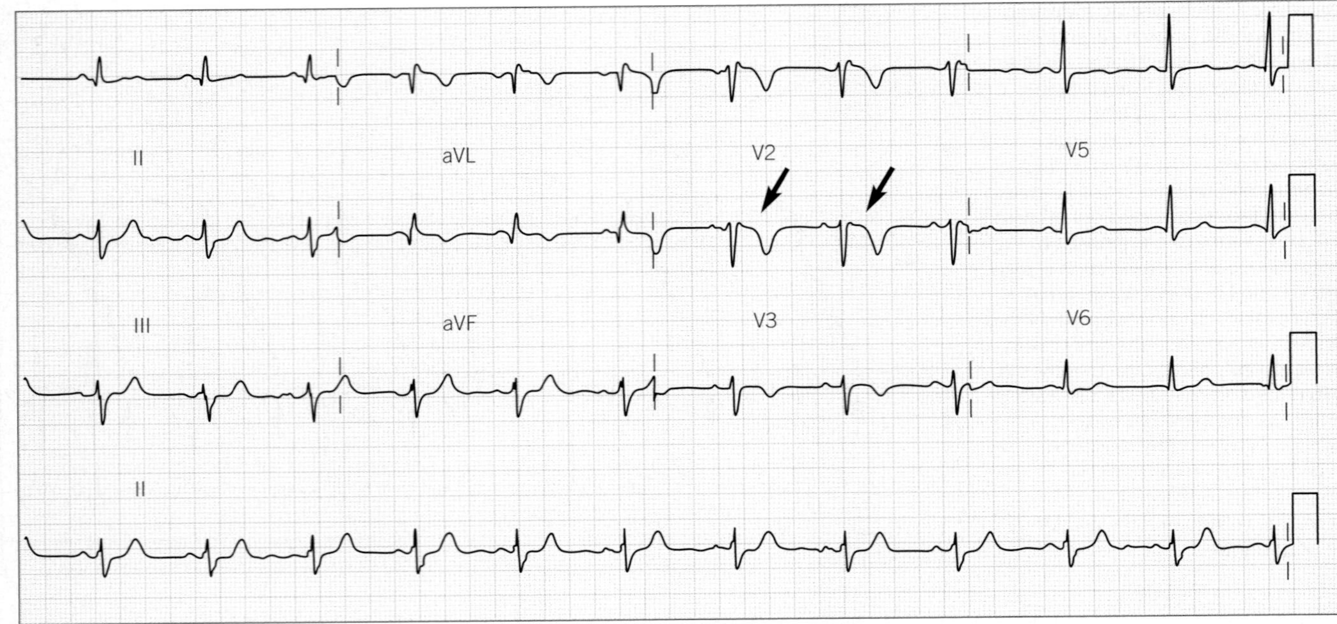

Figure 62.9 Electrocardiogram from a patient with a clinical diagnosis of arrhythmogenic right ventricular cardiomyopathy/ dysplasia. The electrocardiogram indicates T-wave inversion throughout the anterior chest leads and the suggestion of an epsilon wave *(indicated by arrows).*

arrhythmia. Affected individuals may have multiple morphologic forms of ventricular tachycardia because of the diffuse nature of the disease and the potential substrate for multiple re-entry circuits. It is imperative that this condition be differentiated from idiopathic right ventricular tachycardia, which also presents with left bundle ventricular tachycardia, but in contrast to arrhythmogenic right ventricular dysplasia usually has a benign prognosis. The natural history of subjects with arrhythmogenic right ventricular dysplasia is variable, but the presence of symptomatic heart failure and the occurrence of spontaneous ventricular tachycardia predict a poorer outcome.

Ventricular Tachycardia in the Normal Heart (Idiopathic Ventricular Tachycardia)

This group of conditions is characterized by recurrent ventricular tachycardia in the absence of structural heart disease. It often presents in young adults and may be associated with very frequent episodes of tachycardia. It accounts for approximately 10% of cases of ventricular tachycardia evaluated by electrophysiology laboratories in the United States.[16] Several distinct entities exist, and careful evaluation of the electrocardiogram can help elucidate the origin of the tachycardia. The most common form of idiopathic ventricular tachycardia is that which arises from the right ventricular outflow tract region. This ventricular tachycardia usually has left bundle morphology with an inferior axis (Fig. 62.10). Patients with this form of tachycardia frequently have premature ventricular contractions that have the same morphology as the sustained tachycardia. The mechanism of this tachycardia is catecholamine-mediated delayed after-depolarizations and triggered activity.[17] The implications of this mechanism are that episodes of tachycardia are frequently induced by exercise or other catecholaminergic stimuli. At electrophysiologic study, programmed extrastimuli rarely induce arrhythmia, but isoproterenol infusions and rapid burst pacing may provoke episodes. Even at very high rates, this tachycardia is usually well tolerated because the underlying ventricular function is usually normal. Less frequently, some of these outflow tract ventricular tachycardias have been localized to the left ventricular outflow tract or the aortic cusps.

Another form of idiopathic ventricular tachycardia that has a characteristic electrocardiographic appearance is left ventricular tachycardia involving the fascicles of the left ventricle. This was originally described by Zipes,[18] and the original electrocardiographic criteria were a right bundle branch appearance with a left axis deviation (Fig. 62.11). This ventricular tachycardia uses the left posterior fascicle as a critical part of the circuit. Subsequently, other forms using different parts of the conduction system have been described. Fascicular ventricular tachycardia has a number of characteristic features that include the typical electrocardiographic morphology, the ability to induce the tachycardia with atrial pacing, the termination of the ventricular tachycardia with intravenous verapamil (so-called verapamil-sensitive ventricular tachycardia), and the absence of other cardiac disease.[16] In contrast to outflow tract tachycardia, fascicular tachycardia fulfills many of the criteria required for the diagnosis of re-entry as an arrhythmia mechanism. As with outflow tract tachycardia, catheter ablation can be a highly effective form of therapy for this condition. Less frequently, other sites, such as the mitral annulus, have been described as a source of idiopathic ventricular tachycardia. Tachycardia-induced cardiomyopathy may occur in these patients, even without sustained ventricular tachycardia, and it can be difficult to determine whether the tachycardia or the cardiomyopathy is the primary condition.

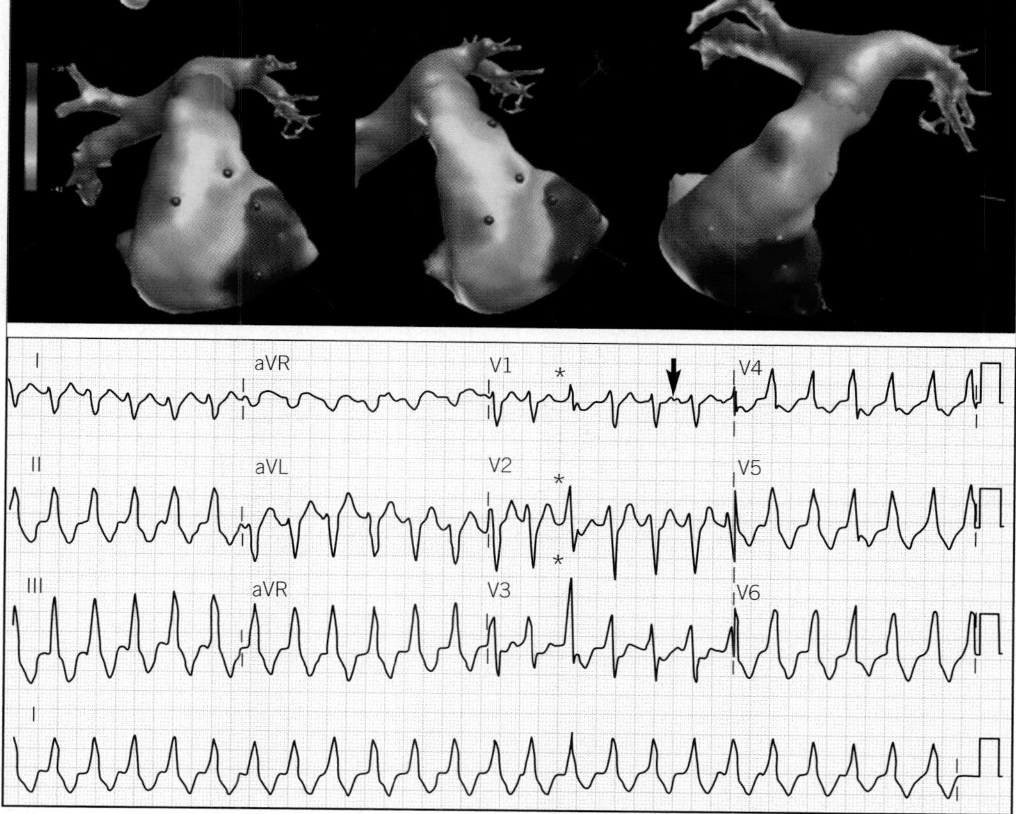

Figure 62.10 Electrocardiogram of right ventricular outflow tract ventricular tachycardia. It has the typical left bundle branch block morphology with an inferior axis. There are additional electrocardiographic features of ventricular tachycardia demonstrated in this electrocardiogram. First, there is a captured or fusion beat demonstrated as the second beat in the anterior chest leads *(asterisk)*. This beat clearly has a different morphology from that of tachycardia. Second, there is also evidence of ventricular-atrial dissociation with intermittent P waves *(arrow)*. The upper panel demonstrates progressive mapping to identify the site of earliest activity. The mapping progresses from right to left with more points being added to the activation map. Eventually in the rightmost panel, a single earliest point is identified for ablation. This tachycardia is localized to a typical site of the posterior septal right ventricular outflow tract.

CLINICAL PRESENTATIONS

The symptoms of ventricular tachycardia relate to the degree of hemodynamic compromise that the arrhythmia produces. In the case of profound hemodynamic disturbance, this can result in cardiac arrest. Recurrent self-terminating ventricular tachycardia can cause the clinical syndrome of recurrent presyncope and syncope. In a patient with left ventricular dysfunction, presyncope and syncope are associated with increased mortality,[19] and these symptoms need careful evaluation to exclude the possibility of recurrent ventricular tachycardia as the underlying cause.

In cases of less profound decompensation, the symptoms may be of more gradual onset and may reflect the effects of diminished cardiac output. This can include breathlessness due to pulmonary congestion, exacerbation of angina, reduced exercise capacity, or, if well tolerated, simply an awareness of palpitation. In some instances, slow and incessant arrhythmia may produce a tachycardia-associated cardiomyopathy, although this syndrome is more commonly associated with incessant atrial arrhythmia.

The extent to which ventricular tachycardia results in hypotension and cardiac decompensation is determined by the interplay of a number of factors. The tachycardia rate is clearly an important factor, with very rapid arrhythmias more likely to produce collapse and cardiac arrest. In addition to tachycardia rate, the degree of underlying ventricular dysfunction plays a critical role in the extent to which the arrhythmia is tolerated. The greater the severity of left ventricular dysfunction, the more likely tachycardia will be associated with more profound hemodynamic effects. Other factors, such as autonomic response, current drug therapy, and duration of the arrhythmia, will influence the presentation of ventricular tachycardia. In some cases, the atrioventricular dissociation that can occur in ventricular tachycardia can result in a vagal reflex that initiates vasodilatation and hypotension.

In instances of ventricular tachycardia in patients without other cardiac disease, the episodes may be associated with nonspecific symptoms or may be asymptomatic and detected serendipitously during investigation of other problems. The presence of ventricular tachycardia and complete heart block in a patient should raise suspicion of an infiltrative process.

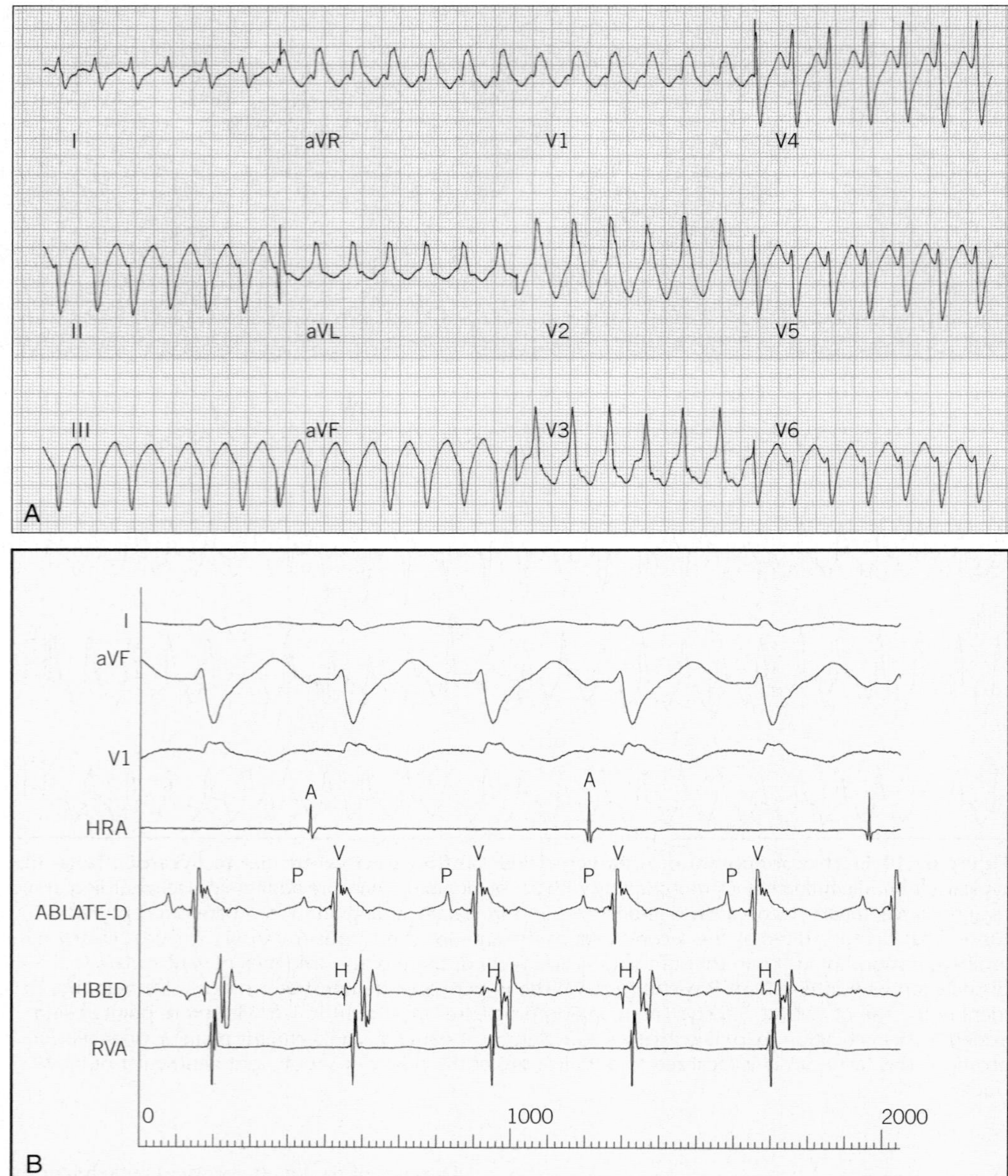

Figure 62.11 Verapamil-sensitive left ventricular tachycardia. A, The tachycardia has a right bundle branch block, left axis pattern. **B,** Intracardiac recordings with a catheter positioned at the ablation site (ABLATE-D) show a P potential. A, atrium; HRA, high right atrium; HBED, distal bundle of His; RVA, right ventricular apex; V, ventricle.

DIAGNOSTIC TESTS IN VENTRICULAR TACHYCARDIA

A diagnostic dilemma not infrequently encountered in clinical practice is the patient who presents with a broad-complex tachycardia (QRS duration $\geq$ 120 ms). The question that arises as a consequence of this presentation is whether this represents ventricular tachycardia or a supraventricular arrhythmia with aberrant conduction within the ventricle. In assessing an individual presenting with broad-complex tachycardia, the history, physical examination, and 12-lead electrocardiographic characteristics are all helpful.

A wide range of symptoms may be encountered with ventricular tachycardia as described previously in this chapter. Whereas hypotension and cardiovascular collapse are more common with ventricular arrhythmias, the extent of decompensation is not a reliable guide to the basis of the arrhythmia. The history of a prior myocardial infarction makes a broad-complex tachycardia highly likely (in excess of 90%) to be ventricular in origin.[20]

In the scenario of a broad-complex tachycardia, the clinical examination and electrocardiography provide complementary information. Both may provide features that are highly suggestive or diagnostic of ventricular tachycardia. The clinical signs and electrocardiographic features that indicate ventricular tachycardia reflect the atrioventricular dissociation that is usually present in this condition. The clinical signs that support ventricular tachycardia are variability of the first heart sound on cardiac auscultation, irregular cannon waves in the jugular venous waveform, and variable arterial pressure wave. These signs are most obvious at rapid ventricular rates.[21] The electrocardiographic features that are highly suggestive of a ventricular origin of a broad-complex tachycardia are dissociated P-wave activity and fusion or capture beats (see Fig. 62.10). In contrast to the clinical signs of atrioventricular dissociation, the electrocardiographic signs are more evident at slower ventricular rates. Table 62.2 presents the electrocardiographic characteristics that support ventricular tachycardia over supraventricular tachycardia with aberrant ventricular conduction.

If, after careful assessment, the diagnosis remains uncertain, ventricular tachycardia should be assumed. Therapy for supraventricular tachycardia inappropriately administered during ventricular tachycardia can have serious adverse consequences.[22]

Another diagnostic dilemma is the occurrence of single or multiple episodes of broad-complex tachycardia when a definitive diagnosis has not been made at the time of presentation or when the broad-complex tachycardia may be noted on telemetry or ambulatory monitoring and therefore is undiagnosed. Critical to the evaluation of these individuals is the assessment as to the presence or absence of other cardiac disease. In particular, ejection fraction is important in determining the likelihood that the episodes have been ventricular in origin and in determining subsequent prognosis. Echocardiography should be undertaken as a first-line investigation in the assessment of an individual with broad-complex tachycardia. It provides a range of information including left and right ventricular wall structure and function, presence of regional wall motion abnormalities suggesting coronary artery disease, presence of cardiac hypertrophy, and assessment of valvular function. Echocardiography can in most instances provide a formal assessment of left ventricular ejection fraction. Given the frequency of coronary artery disease as a cause of ventricular tachycardia, it is crucial to exclude this as a cause. Investigations that may be required are determined by the results of the initial clinical, electrocardiographic, and echocardiographic assessment. These may include exercise stress testing, particularly if the episodes are associated with situations of heightened catecholaminergic drive; coronary angiography if coronary artery disease or anomalous coronary anatomy is suspected; magnetic resonance imaging, particularly if arrhythmogenic right ventricular dysplasia or an infiltrative cardiomyopathy is suspected (see Fig. 62.8); cardiac biopsy; and cardiac electrophysiology studies. If an infiltrative cardiomyopathy is suspected, further investigations may be warranted on the basis of clinical suspicion.

Electrophysiology studies have several uses in patients with ventricular tachycardia. The primary role in the diagnosis of a broad-complex tachycardia is the inducibility of ventricular tachycardia and the exclusion of a supraventricular arrhythmia with aberrant or accessory conduction. In the case of ventricular tachycardia secondary to coronary artery disease, the electrophysiology study using programmed extrastimuli has a high likelihood of inducing the clinical arrhythmia with reasonable reproducibility. In other disease states, such as dilated and hypertrophic cardiomyopathy and in the case of idiopathic ventricular tachycardia, the ability to reproduce the clinical arrhythmia at electrophysiology study is much lower. Nevertheless, when it is inducible, it can allow confirmation of the mechanism of the tachycardia, which can have important treatment implications by identifying potential targets for ablation. Bundle branch re-entry tachycardia is reported to account for anywhere from 5% of all monomorphic ventricular tachycardia in patients with coronary artery disease[23] to 40% of ventricular tachycardia occurring in individuals with nonischemic cardiomyopathy.[24] In this particular form of ventricular tachycardia, catheter ablation can be highly effective (see Fig. 62.7). Additional information that electrophysiology study provides is in evaluating concurrent conduction system disease and in the assessment of hemodynamic tolerance and the effectiveness of antitachycardia pacing in terminating the arrhythmia, both being relevant for the choice of potential device therapy.

In using electrophysiology studies in evaluation of patients with ventricular tachycardia, it is important to compare the 12-lead electrocardiogram of any induced arrhythmia to the spontaneous event to ensure that you are dealing with the same arrhythmia. In the patient with confirmed ventricular tachycardia, a thorough assessment as to the substrate underlying the arrhythmia, the diagnosis of potentially reversible or contributing causes, and an assessment of likely prognosis are required.

There is considerable debate as to the utility of invasive electrophysiology testing in assessing the likelihood of spontaneous ventricular arrhythmia in high-risk individuals. More recent evidence has suggested that the presence or absence of inducible arrhythmia at invasive electrophysiology study does not predict subsequent events in either coronary artery disease patients[25] or those with dilated cardiomyopathy.[26] Other modalities that have been suggested in this setting, particularly in patients with coronary artery disease, have been signal averaged electrocardiography, heart rate variability, and microvolt T-wave alternans, with variable reports of sensitivity and specificity.

MANAGEMENT

Acute Management

The initial management of a patient who presents with ventricular tachycardia is determined by the nature of the symptoms and the hemodynamic state. If significant hypotension or other cardiovascular compromise (severe chest pain, pulmonary edema, or disturbed conscious state) is present, immediate direct current cardioversion should be considered. Although ideally the patient should be anesthetized before electrical cardioversion, it can be safely performed under sedation if the facilities for a general anesthetic are not available.

In the more stable patient, attempts at pharmacologic reversion can be attempted (Fig. 62.12). Although intravenous lignocaine has been traditionally used as the first-line agent, its efficacy is low, and procainamide may be a better choice.[27,28] The acute effects of intravenous amiodarone are primarily antiadrenergic and blockade of the atrioventricular node; the effects on myocardial conduction and refractoriness are of more gradual onset, making it less suitable for the acute termination of stable ventricular tachycardia.[29] Amiodarone has been proved to be valuable in patients with recurrent ventricular arrhythmias despite cardioversion or when other agents have failed.[30] Other intravenous agents that are

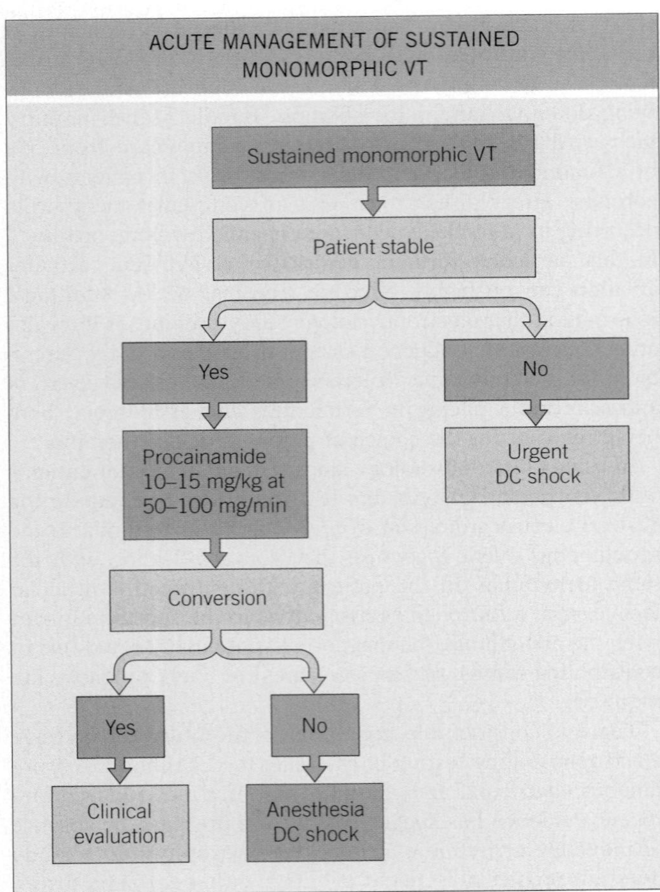

Figure 62.12 Acute management of sustained monomorphic ventricular tachycardia (VT).

available and may be considered when first-line drugs have proved ineffective include sotalol and flecainide. Both of these agents tend to have significant hypotensive effects, limiting their use in this situation.

In all instances, the effects of the intravenous drugs on the patient's blood pressure, QRS duration, and QT interval need to be continuously monitored. If drug therapy is proving ineffective or producing unacceptable hemodynamic or electrocardiographic changes, such as hypotension, marked QRS widening, or excessive QT prolongation, then progression to electrical cardioversion is appropriate.

Similarly, verapamil causes hypotension and should be reserved for cases highly likely to be verapamil-sensitive left fascicular ventricular tachycardia. Adenosine is of no value in most forms of ventricular tachycardia and should be used only in situations in which supraventricular tachycardia with aberrancy is likely. With all acute trials of drug therapy, the physician must be prepared to progress to electrical cardioversion if there is any evidence of compromise (as before).

In addition, acute precipitants such as electrolyte disturbances, drug intoxications, and acute myocardial infarction need to be identified and appropriate therapy initiated.

Secondary Prevention

Pharmacologic Therapy

After an episode of sustained ventricular tachycardia in the absence of therapy, recurrent arrhythmia is frequent and mortality rates are in the order of 20% at 12 months.[31] In patients with idiopathic ventricular tachycardia, it may be warranted to attempt a trial of drug therapy before ablation. In patients with structural heart disease, with the exception of beta blockers, empiric antiarrhythmic therapy has no role in the management; in most instances, this results in increased mortality. Even after class I antiarrhythmic drugs had been demonstrated to have adverse effects on mortality, empiric amiodarone has continued to be used in patients surviving an episode of ventricular tachycardia or out-of-hospital cardiac arrest.

In the past, either electrophysiology study or ambulatory monitoring–guided drug testing was suggested as a means of predicting the likely efficacy of antiarrhythmic drug therapy in preventing recurrence of ventricular arrhythmia. The role of electrophysiology study in predicting drug efficacy has been largely dismissed. Whereas empiric amiodarone has been shown to be superior to guided drug therapy with class I agents, it is not clear that it is superior to no antiarrhythmic therapy.[32] It is evident from the trials comparing implantable defibrillator therapy to amiodarone in patients with spontaneous sustained ventricular arrhythmias that despite amiodarone therapy, recurrence rates are significant and mortality is on the order of 10% to 20% at 12 months.[33,34] These trials have also demonstrated that implantable defibrillator therapy is superior to pharmacologic therapy with class III agents (see later).

Although antiarrhythmic therapy alone, be it empiric or guided by invasive or noninvasive means, has no role in the long-term management of ventricular tachycardia, it can have an important adjunctive role to implantable defibrillator therapy. In particular, beta blockers and amiodarone have been shown to reduce the incidence of defibrillator shocks in patients with implantable defibrillators.[35,36] A clear benefit for sotalol compared with conventional beta blockers in this role has not been established.

Catheter Ablation

Radiofrequency catheter ablation has been applied to the treatment of ventricular tachycardia occurring in association with structural heart disease and also that occurring in the absence of other cardiac disease (idiopathic ventricular tachycardia). The strategy used during an ablation procedure depends on the nature and underlying mechanism of the arrhythmia, its inducibility, the hemodynamic tolerance, and the equipment available to the operator.

Idiopathic ventricular tachycardia tends to occur in younger individuals, and episodes are often associated with exercise or emotion. Whereas there are a number of different causes, as a group, the risk of serious cardiovascular compromise and sudden death is very low. Although drug therapy with relatively simple agents such as beta or calcium channel blockers may be effective, many patients choose to have an ablation performed to obviate the need for long-term pharmacotherapy or when drug therapy is ineffective. The most common cause of idiopathic ventricular tachycardia is that arising in the outflow regions of the right and, to a lesser extent, the left ventricle. Whereas the 12-lead electrocardiogram during tachycardia may act as an initial guide to the location of the tachycardia, intracardiac mapping is used to determine the precise ablation site. Intracardiac mapping often uses both activation mapping (localizing the earliest site of endocardial activation during ventricular tachycardia; see Fig. 62.10) and pace mapping during sinus rhythm to find an endocardial site where pacing approximates the QRS morphology of the tachycardia.[16] Catheter ablation for outflow tract tachycardia has a success rate in excess of 90%, with little morbidity and mortality arising from the procedure.

The other common form of idiopathic ventricular tachycardia is that arising within the fascicular system of the left ventricle (see Fig. 62.11). Unlike in outflow tract ventricular tachycardia, pace mapping is of limited use in guiding ablation of this condition. Pacing in relatively large areas of the septum results in captures of the Purkinje system and nearly perfect pace maps, even though the captured area is not critical to the tachycardia circuit. Mapping of Purkinje potentials during ventricular tachycardia with ablation directed to the earliest recorded Purkinje potential can result in high success rates.[37]

The indications for ablation of ventricular tachycardia in the patient with underlying structural heart disease are less clear. In the majority of cases, ablation is reserved for those patients who have incessant ventricular tachycardia, that resulting in frequent discharges from an implantable defibrillator, or slow ventricular tachycardia that makes implantable defibrillator programming difficult because of the overlap with physiologic heart rates. In patients with underlying cardiac disease, and in particular those with reduced left ventricular ejection fraction, catheter ablation may be successful in treating the index tachycardia. However, there is no evidence to date to suggest any change in the overall prognosis. If it is available, the 12-lead electrocardiogram will give an indication as to the likely exit site for the tachycardia. A left bundle branch appearance suggests exit in the septum or right ventricle, whereas a dominant R wave in V_1 suggests a left ventricular origin. In the absence of an electrocardiogram during tachycardia, imaging of the heart to identify likely areas of interest is useful. In particular, in patients with ischemic heart disease, areas of prior infarction are likely to be the site of origin of monomorphic ventricular tachycardia. In catheter ablation of ventricular tachycardia in patients with underlying structural heart disease, two strategies are used. In the patient with inducible ventricular tachycardia that is hemodynamically tolerated, activation and entrainment mapping can be used to identify critical parts of the ventricular tachycardia circuit that would be amenable to focal ablation within the critical isthmus (Fig. 62.13; see also Figs. 62.5 and 62.6). With these techniques, high procedural success rates (suppression of the index ventricular tachycardia) are possible, but recurrence develops in at least one quarter of patients.[38] In patients who have unstable ventricular tachycardia, alternative techniques for catheter ablation have evolved. In these individuals, identification of the likely substrate for the ventricular tachycardia uses the 12-lead electrocardiogram morphology of the tachycardia, pace mapping (Fig. 62.14), and newer mapping systems to identify areas of scarring and in particular the border zone between scar and normal tissue that represents the usual site of origin for monomorphic ventricular tachycardia (see Fig. 62.2). This involves the ability to record an endocardial bipolar voltage with use of catheters that can annotate this on a three-dimensional anatomic shell created by the mapping system. In this way, the likely exit sites for ventricular tachycardia can be identified and linear ablation performed through the border zone area to connect dense scar to areas of normal myocardium or to anatomic boundaries such as the valve annulus. The targeting of channels within scar may also interrupt tachycardia circuits.

Ablation of ventricular tachycardia in disease states other than coronary artery disease is associated with lower success rates. In dilated and hypertrophic cardiomyopathy, monomorphic ventricular tachycardia represents a small percentage of all arrhythmias. When monomorphic ventricular tachycardia occurs, it may be due to focal myocardial scarring, but delineation of the boundaries of the scar and precise mapping of the ventricular tachycardia circuit and identification of a suitable ablation site are generally more difficult.[39] Importantly, the existence of intramyocardial and epicardial tissue that could maintain ventricular tachycardia is increasingly recognized.

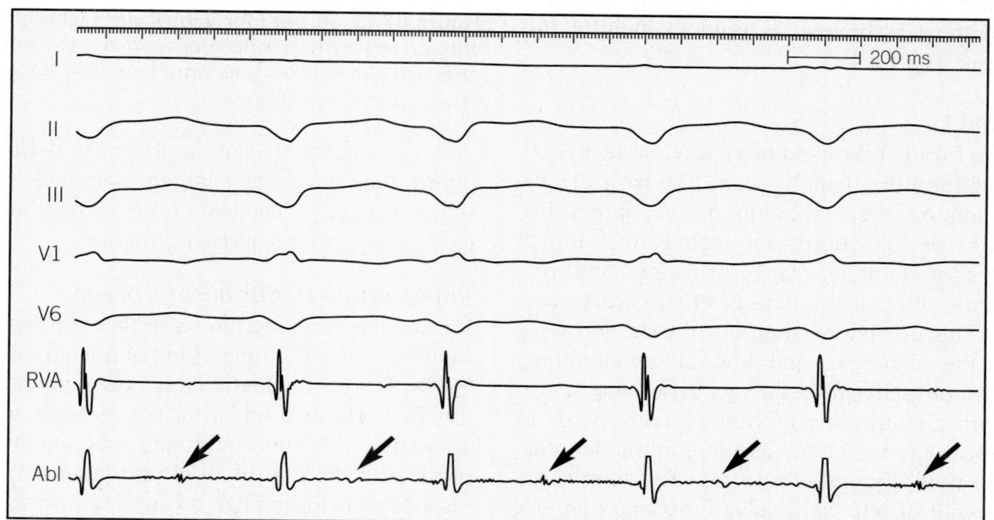

Figure 62.13 Mapping during ventricular tachycardia. In this case, a mid-diastolic potential *(arrows)* on the ablation catheter (Abl) indicates activity throughout the tachycardia cycle length suggestive of re-entry and implicates the position of the catheter within the isthmus of tachycardia, a suitable site for ablation.

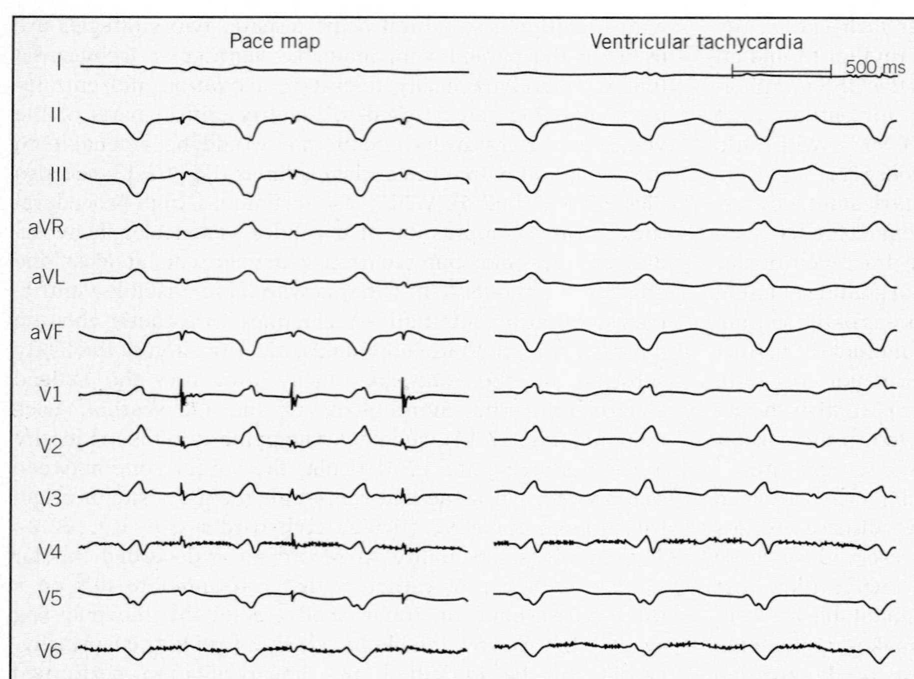

Figure 62.14 Pace mapping to identify the critical isthmus for ventricular tachycardia. In this case, in which tachycardia *(right panel)* resulted in hemodynamic compromise, pace mapping is used to identify the critical isthmus. The pacing artifact is seen, followed by a long stimulus to QRS, with identical activation of the ventricle as during tachycardia (as suggested by the identical morphology of the resultant QRS). These features are suggestive of pacing well within the critical isthmus as depicted in Figure 62.3 as the area of slowed conduction.

Percutaneous approaches are now used to perform intramyocardial needle ablation to target myocardial tissue or to access the pericardium for epicardial ablation when ventricular tachycardia cannot be eliminated by an endocardial approach.

There have been a limited number of reports of successful ablation for polymorphic ventricular tachycardia or ventricular fibrillation. Such procedures have been limited to patients with incessant arrhythmias who have required multiple cardioversions as a lifesaving measure with idiopathic ventricular fibrillation, acutely after myocardial infarction, with long QT syndrome, and with Brugada syndrome. Ablation in this situation has targeted the ventricular ectopic beat that initiates sustained arrhythmia. This has invariably arisen from the Purkinje arborization and less frequently the right ventricular outflow tract. A combination of activation and pace mapping techniques is used to identify the initiating trigger (see Fig. 62.4).

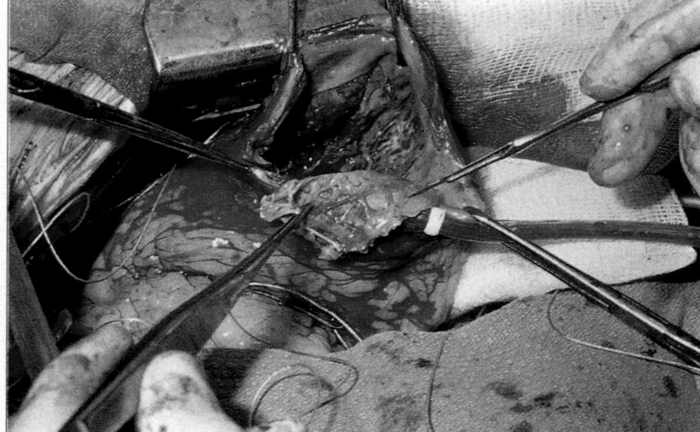

Figure 62.15 Surgery for ventricular tachycardia. A large anterior aneurysm has been opened and the subendocardium resected. The resected area would normally be left in place during a routine aneurysmectomy.

Surgical Therapy

Surgical techniques for the treatment of ventricular tachycardia have been used for more than 30 years. The basis of surgery is the excision or direct ablation of the underlying anatomic substrate for the ventricular tachycardia. Initial surgical approaches for ventricular tachycardia involved simple aneurysmectomy, often at the time of other cardiac surgery (Fig. 62.15). This procedure often left the border zone regions between the aneurysm and normal myocardium, where the majority of tachycardia circuits arise, and hence was associated with limited efficacy. Subsequently, various forms of subendocardial resection, either empiric or map guided, have been used. Extensive resection has been associated with worsening of left ventricular function, whereas less extensive procedures, even when they are map guided, have limited efficacy. The morbidity and mortality associated with these procedures are substantial, and with the improvements in percutaneous catheter-based techniques and the availability of implantable defibrillators, surgical approaches have been largely confined to patients having other surgical procedures and in centers with an established cardiac arrhythmia surgical program.

Implantable Defibrillator Therapy

Implantable cardioverter-defibrillator therapy has evolved substantially since the time of initial human implants in the early 1980s. Device implantation is now a percutaneous technique usually performed under local anesthesia and sedation and is associated with minor morbidity and minimal mortality. Much of the reduction in the risks associated with implantation has resulted from technologic advances allowing the use of transvenous lead systems and generators that can be sited in the subclavian fossa. Sophistication of the detection and treatment algorithms has reduced the incidence of inappropriate therapies (for supraventricular arrhythmias) and has allowed many episodes of arrhythmia to be treated with antitachycardia pacing rather than with defibrillation.[40] Parallel to advances in technology, there has been improved understanding of the role of this therapy both in individuals who have survived an episode of serious ventricular arrhythmia (secondary prevention) and in those at higher risk of this event (primary prevention).

A number of randomized trials have assessed the role of implantable defibrillator therapy in secondary prevention of ventricular arrhythmia. In particular, between 1997 and 2000, three trials demonstrating the superiority of defibrillator therapy over drug therapy (principally amiodarone) for survivors of cardiac arrest or hemodynamically unstable arrhythmia were published. The AVID, CIDS, and CASH trials all demonstrated a mortality reduction associated with defibrillator therapy. Although the magnitude of this benefit varied, a pooled analysis of these trials demonstrated an overall mortality reduction of 28% for implantable defibrillator therapy compared with amiodarone.[41]

More recently, the survival advantage seen for implantable defibrillator therapy in secondary prevention has also been documented in patients at high risk of ventricular arrhythmia but without documented events, termed primary prevention therapy. A number of factors have been postulated to predict increased risk for ventricular arrhythmia in patients after myocardial infarction or in those with heart failure. These include the presence of frequent ventricular ectopy or nonsustained ventricular tachycardia, the presence of late potentials on signal-averaged electrocardiography, inducibility at electrophysiology study, the presence of microvolt T-wave alternans, reduced heart rate variability, and reduced left ventricular ejection fraction (LVEF).[42] Of these, LVEF remains the primary measure used in assessing risk of ventricular arrhythmia. For more than 30 years, reduced LVEF has been recognized as a marker for increased risk of ventricular arrhythmia and indeed overall cardiac mortality in patients with ischemic heart disease and nonischemic cardiomyopathy. The role of tests for susceptibility to ventricular arrhythmia over and above LVEF remains to be established. The accumulated evidence supporting the role of LVEF in predicting sudden death and serious cardiac arrhythmia in patients with ischemic heart disease and cardiomyopathy spurred a series of trials in which the role of implantable defibrillator therapy in a primary prevention role in high-risk individuals was assessed. These studies have demonstrated a mortality benefit in patients with reduced LVEF but no documented sustained ventricular arrhythmia that is comparable to the benefit seen when implantable defibrillator therapy is used after resuscitated cardiac arrest or sustained ventricular tachycardia. Two trials in particular have reinforced the role of implantable defibrillator therapy for primary prevention. The Multicenter Automatic Defibrillator Implantation Trial II (MADIT II) prospectively randomized 1232 patients with prior myocardial infarction and LVEF below 30% without previous electrophysiologic testing to implantable defibrillator or conventional treatment.[43] This trial revealed a reduction in all-cause mortality in the defibrillator treatment arm by 31% at 20 months of follow-up compared with the conventional therapy. The Sudden Cardiac Death–Heart Failure Trial (SCD-HeFT) included patients with both ischemic and nonischemic cardiomyopathies and an ejection fraction of less than 30%.[44] At just under 4 years of follow-up, there was a 23% relative risk reduction (7% absolute) associated with defibrillator therapy. Although there is now a substantial body of evidence supporting the role of implantable defibrillator therapy for primary prevention of sudden cardiac death in individuals at increased risk, considerable work remains to establish the best methods for risk stratification over and above reduced ejection fraction.

PROGNOSIS

Ventricular tachycardia is a condition that has a number of causes and occurs in individuals with and without heart disease. The prognostic implications of the finding of nonsustained ventricular tachycardia are unclear. Previously, the finding of nonsustained ventricular tachycardia in individuals with ischemic disease and low ejection fraction and some patients with nonischemic cardiomyopathy has been thought to indicate an adverse outcome, in particular indicating a greater risk of sudden death. More recent evidence has shed doubt on the utility of nonsustained ventricular tachycardia as a marker of adverse outcome.[1]

In the situation of sustained ventricular tachycardia, the prognosis is determined by the nature and extent of the underlying cardiac condition more than by the arrhythmia itself. In individuals with ventricular tachycardia occurring in the otherwise normal heart, prognosis is excellent and the management is determined by the extent of symptoms and often by the patient's preference. Increasingly in these patients when frequent or sustained episodes exist, catheter ablation is chosen over long-term drug therapy.

The occurrence of sustained ventricular tachycardia in association with ischemic heart disease or cardiomyopathy is associated with high recurrence rates and a substantial risk of sudden cardiac death. In the secondary prevention trials examining implantable defibrillator therapy, the annual mortality in the medical treatment arm was between 10% and 15%, and approximately half of the deaths were likely to be due to recurrent arrhythmia.[41] Similarly, in patients with cardiomyopathy, mortality rates after an episode of sustained ventricular arrhythmia are substantial.[9,10] In all of these cohorts of patients, implantable defibrillator therapy has been shown to have a substantial benefit in reducing arrhythmic and total mortality.

SUMMARY

Ventricular tachycardia is a condition that has many modes of presentation ranging from fatal or near-fatal arrhythmic episodes to asymptomatic detection on clinical examination, electrocardiography, or cardiac monitoring. Likewise, it has a number of underlying electrophysiologic mechanisms. Critical to the evaluation of the individual with ventricular tachycardia is the determination of whether it reflects serious underlying cardiac disease or is idiopathic and occurring in the otherwise normal heart. Because of limited efficacy and limited effect on prognosis, drug therapy has in many instances been replaced with nonpharmacologic measures such as catheter ablation and implantable defibrillator therapy.

chapter 63

Inherited Arrhythmia Syndromes

Katherine T. Murray and Dan M. Roden

Definition

- The inherited arrhythmia syndromes are familial disorders characterized by an increased risk of sudden death in patients with a structurally normal heart, typically in association with electrocardiographic abnormalities.

Key Features

- In a young, otherwise healthy patient, the development of arrhythmias (e.g., ventricular tachycardia or atrial fibrillation) warrants evaluation for an inherited arrhythmia syndrome or cardiomyopathy.
- The long QT syndrome, a disorder of cardiac repolarization, is characterized by QT prolongation and enhanced susceptibility to polymorphic ventricular tachycardia, often triggered by physical or emotional stress.
- In the short QT syndrome, patients with a markedly abbreviated QT interval demonstrate both atrial and ventricular tachyarrhythmias as well as a high risk of sudden death.
- The Brugada syndrome is characterized by spontaneous or drug-induced right precordial ST elevation on the surface electrocardiogram and a high prevalence of serious ventricular arrhythmias.
- Patients with catecholaminergic polymorphic ventricular tachycardia have a normal electrocardiogram at rest but develop exercise- or emotion-induced polymorphic ventricular tachycardia, causing syncope or sudden death.

Therapy

- For patients with adrenergically mediated arrhythmias, β-adrenergic receptor blockers can reduce clinical events.
- After a cardiac arrest and in some cases syncope, an implantable cardioverter-defibrillator is the treatment of choice to improves survival.

LONG QT SYNDROME

The long QT syndrome (LQTS) is the most common inherited arrhythmia syndrome.[1] It is characterized by a prolonged QT interval on the baseline electrocardiogram and an increased risk of serious ventricular arrhythmias causing syncope or cardiac arrest, often in response to physical or emotional stress.[1-6] For many years, two forms of the LQTS were recognized on the basis of the pattern of inheritance: the more common Romano-Ward syndrome, displaying autosomal dominant transmission; and the Jervell and Lange-Nielsen syndrome, with autosomal recessive inheritance and a more severe clinical phenotype. Beginning in the 1990s,[7] there has been considerable progress in identification of genes harboring mutations that cause LQTS, and clinical features of the disorder vary according to the genetic defect. The LQTS is increasingly recognized as an important cause of sudden death in young, otherwise healthy persons.

ANATOMY AND PATHOLOGY

As patients with the LQTS have structurally normal hearts, the findings on physical examination and cardiac imaging (e.g., by echocardiography or magnetic resonance imaging) are typically normal. Similarly, autopsy findings are unremarkable. Recently, two subtypes have been identified having prominent extracardiac abnormalities, Andersen's and Timothy syndromes (see later).[8,9] For Timothy syndrome, various congenital heart defects (including patent ductus arteriosus, ventricular septal defect, and tetralogy of Fallot) have been described.

PATHOPHYSIOLOGY

To date, mutations in 10 genes have been causally linked to the LQTS (Table 63.1).[1,10] Most encode ion channel subunits; the remaining encode proteins that regulate ion channel function or expression (e.g., *ANK2*). In most cases, mutations cause loss of function. For K^+ channels that form the basis of repolarizing K^+ currents, this loss of function causes lengthening of the cardiac action potential and QT interval. For Na^+ and Ca^{2+} channels, mutations cause persistent inward current during the plateau phase of the action potential (often termed a gain of function), prolonging repolarization. Mutations in the first three genes identified (responsible for the clinical subtypes LQT1, LQT2, and LQT3) account for approximately 85% of cases.[10] For some ion channels, specific mutations that affect critical regions of the channel protein carry a worse prognosis. For some subtypes (LQT5, LQT6, LQT9, and LQT10), relatively few cases have been described to date linking the genetic abnormality to LQTS.[10]

CLINICAL PRESENTATIONS

LQTS is primarily a disorder of children and young adults; symptoms typically develop between the ages of 10 and 15 years (mean, 12 years).[11] However, the age for initial symptoms can range from the first to the sixth decade of life, and this may vary with the genetic subtype. LQTS is now recognized to contribute to the sudden infant death syndrome (SIDS).[12] The incidence of mutations is estimated to be at

LONG QT SYNDROME SUBTYPES

Subtype	Gene	Protein or Alias	Chromosomal Locus	Ionic Current Affected
LQT1	*KCNQ1*	KvLQT1	11p15.5	↓I_{Ks}
LQT2	*KCNH2*	HERG	7q35-q36	↓I_{Kr}
LQT3	*SCN5A*	Nav1.5	3p21	↑I_{Na}
LQT4	*ANK2*	Ankyrin-B	4q25-q27	Multiple
LQT5	*KCNE1*	MinK, Isk	21q22.1-q22.2*	↓I_{Ks}
LQT6	*KCNE2*	MiRP1	21q22.1*	↓I_{Kr}
LQT7	*KCNJ2*	Kir2.1, IRK1	17q23.1-q24.2	↓I_{K_1}
LQT8	*CACNA1C*	Cav1.2	12p13.3*	↑I_{Ca-L}
LQT9	*CAV3*	Caveolin-3	3p25*	↑I_{Na}
LQT10	*SCN4B*	Navβ.4	11q23*	↑I_{Na}
JLN1	*KCNQ1*	KvLQT1	11p15.5	↓I_{Ks}
JLN2	*KCNE1*	MinK, Isk	21q22.1-q22.2*	↓I_{Ks}

*Although mutations have been described in this gene in individuals with this disorder, formal genetic linkage to this locus has not yet been demonstrated.

I_{Ks}, slow component of the delayed rectifier K^+ current; I_{Kr}, rapid component of the delayed rectifier K^+ current; I_{Na}, Na^+ current; I_{K1}, inward rectifier K^+ current; I_{Ca-L}, L-type Ca^{2+} current.

Modified from Wilde AA, Tan HL. Inherited arrhythmia syndromes. Circ J 2007;71(Suppl A):A12-A19.

Table 63.1 Long QT syndrome subtypes.

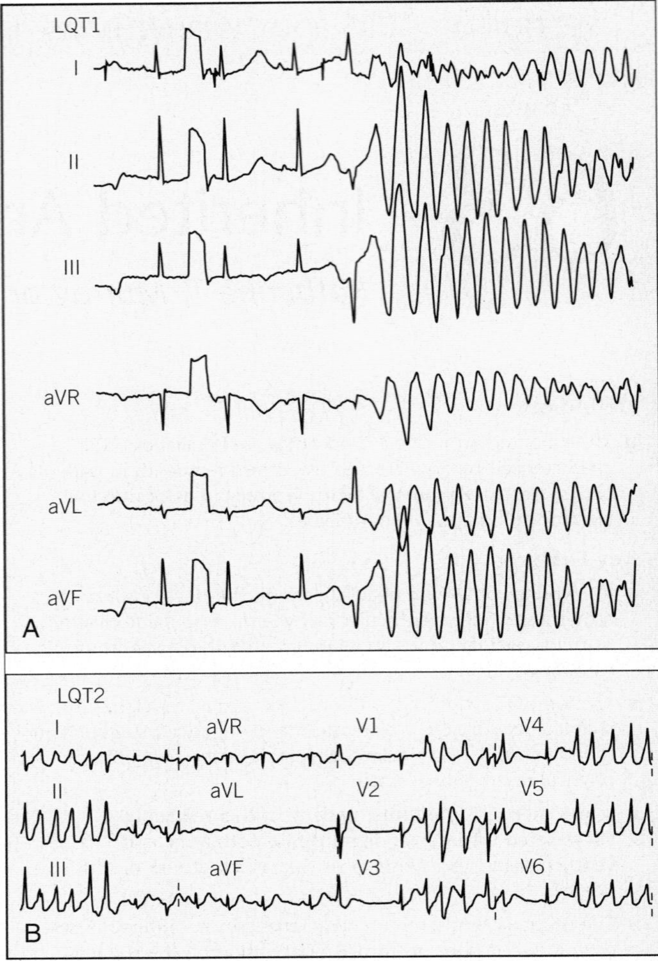

Figure 63.1 Torsades de pointes in the long QT syndrome. A, In a patient with the LQT1 subtype, torsades de pointes occur during an exercise test without a pause preceding the onset of the arrhythmia. **B,** In a patient with LTQ2, the arrhythmia follows a pause for multiple episodes shown in the example. (Modified from Wilde AA, Tan HL. Inherited arrhythmia syndromes. Circ J 2007;71 [Suppl A]:A12-A19.)

least 1 in 2000.[1] However, this is difficult to estimate, given that the prevalence of asymptomatic carriers has not been defined. A female predominance is apparent if detection of the LQTS is made purely on electrocardiographic and clinical grounds, as opposed to genotyping.[3] As most patients who have LQTS demonstrate autosomal dominant inheritance, it would be expected that the proportion of males and females should be equal. The female predominance as well as other nonmendelian features of the inheritance pattern suggests that other factors probably play a role in the phenotypic expression of this syndrome.[1]

Typically, symptomatic patients present with palpitations, presyncope, syncope, seizure-like activity, or cardiac arrest. Because they are young and otherwise healthy people, patients are often misdiagnosed as having a seizure disorder or vasovagal syncope. Syncope usually results from a form of polymorphic ventricular tachycardia (VT) known as torsades de pointes, which occurs in the setting of significant QT interval prolongation (Fig. 63.1). Available evidence indicates that the initiating event of this arrhythmia is an early after-depolarization or spontaneous depolarization during a prolonged action potential that interrupts phase 2-3. Early after-depolarizations probably trigger intramural re-entry because of the associated heterogeneity of repolarization also present (see later). Patients with LQT3 can have bradycardia, and this may contribute to symptoms. Degeneration to ventricular fibrillation is the usual mechanism for sudden death. Overall, the risk of syncope in patients with autosomal dominant LQTS averages 5% per year.[3] After the initial presentation of syncope, mortality can be greater than 20% in the first year and approaches 50% at 10 years. Symptoms tend to abate during pregnancy but are exacerbated in the postpartum state. Genetic testing has revealed that a number of patients harboring LQTS mutations are asymptomatic and have normal QT intervals, termed variable penetrance of the disease.[13] The explanation for this phenomenon is currently not known.

There is a strong genotype-phenotype correlation, with clinical features that are generally specific to the genetic subtype (Table 63.2).[1,10,11,14] This includes electrocardiographic patterns (Fig. 63.2), clinical triggers, and response to therapy, although in general overlap exists. The most common form is LQT1, in which mutations in *KCNQ1* cause loss of function for an adrenergic-sensitive K^+ current (the slowly activating delayed rectifier K^+ current, I_{Ks}).[15] Onset of symptoms is usually between the ages of 5 and 15 years, and arrhythmias are triggered by physical or emotional stress, especially swimming and diving. During exercise or epinephrine infusion, the QT interval fails to shorten

CLINICAL FEATURES OF THE COMMON LONG QT SUBTYPES			
	LQT1 *(KCNQ1)*	LQT2 (*KCNH2*)	LQT3 (*SCN5A*)
Incidence	30%-35%	25%-30%	5%-10%
Triggers	Emotional or physical stress, swimming, diving	Emotional or physical stress, sudden loud noise	Rest, sleep
Typical resting electrocardiogram	Broad T wave	Low-amplitude T wave with notching	Long isoelectric ST segment, narrow T wave
Arrhythmia onset	No pause	Pause	Not established
QT response to exercise	Does not shorten normally	Normal	Accentuated shortening
Response to beta blockers	Yes	Less than for LQT1	Uncertain

Modified from Roden DM. Clinical practice. Long-QT syndrome. N Engl J Med 2008;358:169-176.

Table 63.2 Clinical features of the common long QT subtypes.

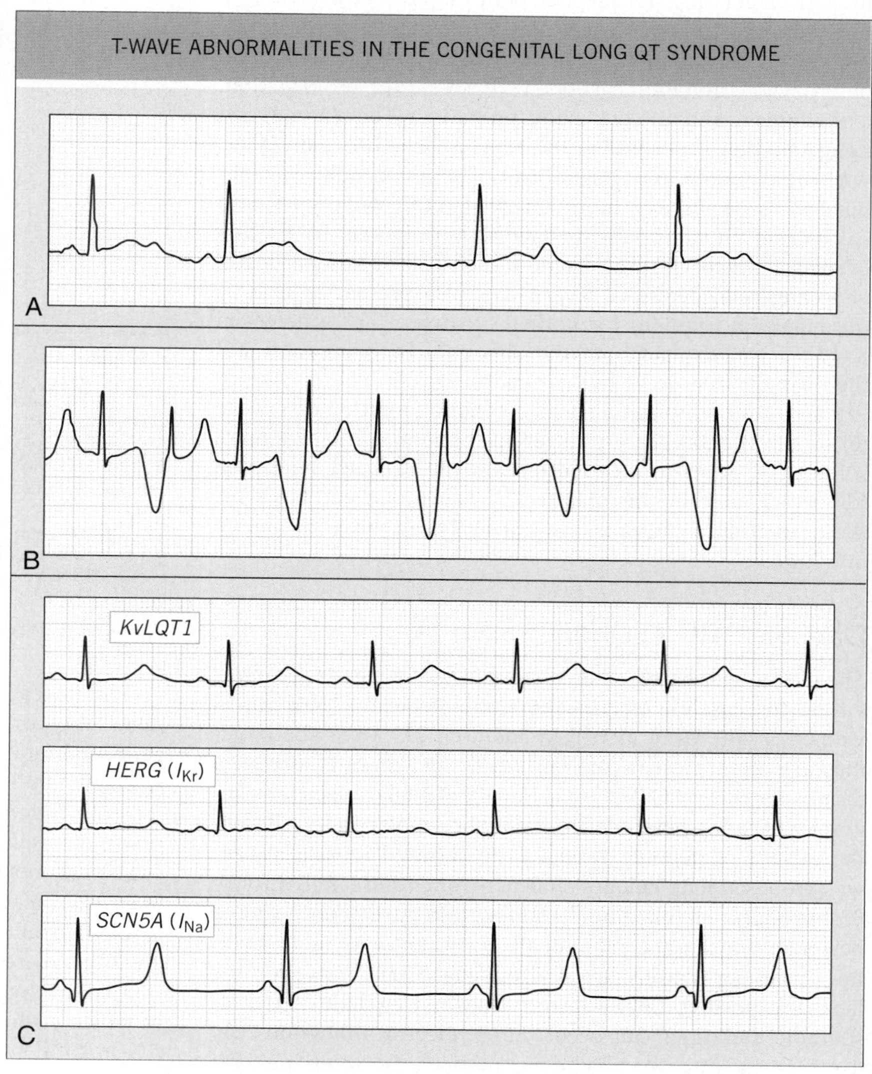

Figure 63.2 T-wave abnormalities in the long QT syndrome. A, An example of bifid T waves with T-wave lability. **B,** A rhythm strip from a patient with the long QT syndrome demonstrating T-wave alternans, with the T wave alternating between downward and upright configurations. **C,** Examples of the typical electrocardiographic pattern seen in patients with the LQT1, LQT2, and LQT3 subtypes are shown. (Modified from Roden DM, Lazzara R, Rosen M, et al. Multiple mechanisms in the long-QT syndrome. Current knowledge, gaps, and future directions. The SADS Foundation Task Force on LQTS. Circulation 1996;94:1996-2012.)

normally. Typically, the onset of torsades de pointes is tachycardia (not pause) dependent (see Fig. 63.1a).[16] In LQT2, mutations are present in *KCNH2* (or *HERG*, which encodes the rapidly activating component of the delayed rectifier K^+ current, I_{Kr}).[17] I_{Kr} is a target for many drugs that cause the acquired LQTS; thus, this discovery provided a mechanistic link between the congenital and acquired forms of LQTS. Age at onset of LQT2 is typically during puberty; arrhythmic events can occur with stress or at rest. A prominent trigger is loud auditory stimuli (such as an alarm clock). Episodes of VT are usually preceded by a pause (see Fig. 63.1b),[16] giving rise to the short-long-short initiating sequence often described for torsades. LQT3 results from mutations in *SCN5A* that disrupt inactivation of the cardiac

Na^+ channel.[18,19] Symptoms can start at puberty or later, and they commonly occur at rest or during sleep. Clinical evidence indicates that the prognosis with the LQT3 subtype is more ominous than for LQT1 or LQT2.

Two forms of the LQTS present with prominent extracardiac manifestations. In Andersen's syndrome[8] (LQT7), patients demonstrate facial and skeletal abnormalities, periodic paralysis, and ventricular arrhythmias, including bidirectional VT (in which the QRS morphology alternates by 180 degrees on a beat-to-beat basis). The baseline electrocardiogram can reveal prominent U waves in addition to QT prolongation. The prognosis appears to be more benign than for usual forms of LQTS, although sudden death has been reported. In Timothy syndrome[9] (LQT8), there is multiorgan dysfunction, with associated syndactyly of the hands or feet, congenital heart defects, immune deficiencies, intermittent hypoglycemia, and autism. For both of these disorders, it is likely that the involved genes play a role in embryonic development. Rarely, patients can be homozygous or compound heterozygote mutation carriers, with severe QT prolongation, arrhythmias, and a very poor prognosis. The Jervell and Lange-Nielsen syndrome is the term attached to individuals who carry mutations of both alleles of genes encoding I_{Ks} subunits. This results in a more severe clinical phenotype, with early onset (90% of patients have a clinical event by 8 years of age), marked QT prolongation, high risk of sudden death, and congenital deafness. KvLQT1 is also present in cells of the inner ear required for normal hearing. Thus, a defect in KvLQT1 can explain both the abnormal repolarization and the deafness that occur in this syndrome.

It is noteworthy that a specific genetic mutation can cause different phenotypes in different patients. For example, some LQT3 mutations can also cause the Brugada syndrome (discussed later in this chapter).[20] The molecular basis for these overlap syndromes is currently an area of active investigation.

DIAGNOSTIC TECHNIQUES

The diagnosis is based on an abnormally prolonged QTc interval on the baseline electrocardiogram (typically ≥460 ms in women, ≥440 ms in men[1]). In addition, TU wave abnormalities are often present (see Fig. 63.2), and there is increased dispersion of the QT interval on the 12-lead electrocardiogram, indicating heterogeneous cardiac repolarization. Before the advent of genetic testing, a point-based scoring system was proposed that includes clinical features and family history (Table 63.3).[21] In eliciting the family history, evidence should be sought for unanticipated death consistent with an arrhythmic event (e.g., cardiac arrest, drowning, SIDS). However, the lack of a positive family history does not exclude LQTS, as sporadic mutations can occur. Serial electrocardiograms can assist in making the diagnosis, particularly when patients initially fall into the uncertain category. Holter monitoring should be performed in all patients to look for asymptomatic arrhythmias, post-pause QT prolongation, and T-wave changes. Exercise testing is useful to observe the QT response to stress. Electrophysiologic testing is not useful because arrhythmias are not induced by programmed stimulation. An echocardiogram should be obtained to rule out structural heart disease. All first-degree relatives should be screened by electrocardiography in confirmed cases.

DIAGNOSTIC CRITERIA FOR THE LONG QT SYNDROME

			Points
Electrocardiographic findings*	Duration of QTc†	>480 ms{1/2}	3
		460-470 ms{1/2}	2
		450 ms (males){1/2}	1
	Torsades de pointes‡		2
	T-wave alternans		1
	Notched T wave in three leads		1
	Low heart rate for age§		0.5
Clinical history	Syncope‡	with stress	2
		without stress	1
	Congenital deafness		0.5
Family history‖	Family members with definite long QT syndromes¶		1
	Unexplained sudden cardiac death before the age of 30 years among immediate family members		0.5
Scoring	<1 point	Low probability of long QT syndrome	
	2-3 points	Intermediate probability of long QT syndrome	
	>4 points	High probability of long QT syndrome	

*In the absence of medications or disorders known to affect these electrocardiographic features.
†QTc calculated by Bazett's formula, where QTc = QT interval/√(RR interval).
‡Mutually exclusive.
§Resting heart rate below the second percentile for age.
‖The same family member cannot be counted in both aspects of the family history.
¶Definite long QT syndrome is defined by a long QT syndrome score >4.
From Schwartz PJ, Moss AJ, Vincent GM, et al. Diagnostic criteria for the long QT syndrome. An update. Circulation 1993;88:782-784.

Table 63.3 Diagnostic criteria for the long QT syndrome.

Genetic testing is now commercially available for the common subtypes. This is most useful to delineate the involved gene or mutation for therapeutic purposes and to identify affected family members. However, there is the potential for both false-negative and false-positive results, and appropriate counseling is an essential component of genotyping.

The differential diagnosis includes other causes of syncope (e.g., vasovagal; familial cardiomyopathies, such as hypertrophic cardiomyopathy; and other inherited arrhythmia syndromes) and other reasons for QT prolongation (e.g., medications, hypothyroidism, hypocalcemia). The incidence of LQTS mutations in patients who present with drug-induced LQTS ranges from 5% to 20%.[1,22]

MANAGEMENT

Although no placebo-controlled, randomized clinical trials have been performed in patients with LQTS, data from large registries indicate that beta blockers and the implantable cardioverter-defibrillator (ICD) afford the most effective therapy (Table 63.4).[11] Whereas an ICD is indicated after aborted cardiac arrest and persistent symptoms despite adequate beta blockade, its role in other situations is more

GUIDELINES FOR MANAGEMENT OF THE LONG QT SYNDROME*		
Recommendation	Level of Evidence†	Comment
No participation in competitive sports	I	Includes patients with the diagnosis established by means of genetic testing only
Beta blockers	I	For patients who have QTc interval prolongation (>460 ms in women and >440 ms in men)
	IIa	For patients with a normal QTc interval
Implantable cardioverter-defibrillator	I	For survivors of cardiac arrest
	IIa	For patients with syncope while receiving beta blockers
	IIb	For primary prevention in patients with characteristics that suggest high risk; these include LQT2, LQT3, and QTc interval >500 ms

*Data are from the American College of Cardiology, the American Heart Association, and the European Society of Cardiology, in collaboration with the European Heart Rhythm Association and the Heart Rhythm Society.[11]

†Levels of evidence are as follows: I, conditions for which there is evidence or general agreement, or both, that a given procedure or treatment is beneficial, useful, and effective; II, conditions for which there is conflicting evidence or divergence of opinion, or both, about the usefulness and efficacy of a procedure or treatment; IIa, conditions for which the weight of evidence or opinion is in favor of usefulness and efficacy; and IIb, conditions for which the usefulness and efficacy are less well established by evidence or opinion.

From Roden DM. Clinical practice. Long-QT syndrome. N Engl J Med 2008;358:169-176.

Table 63.4 Guidelines for management of the long QT syndrome.

controversial. Interestingly, a family history of sudden death is not predictive of cardiac arrest in other family members.

For risk stratification, the QTc interval is the most powerful parameter, with greatest risk for values of 500 ms or more.[11] For patients with LQT3, the risk is higher regardless of the QT interval, especially for males. Symptoms before puberty also indicate a worse prognosis.

For beta-blocker therapy, long-acting agents (e.g., nadolol) are usually recommended. Compliance with medication is essential as noncompliance can contribute to recurrent symptoms. Patients with LQT1 appear to have the best response; the drugs are less effective for LQT2 and LQT3 (see Table 63.2). For recurrent symptoms with beta blockers and other high-risk patients (early symptom onset, QTc ≥500 ms), an ICD may be indicated. Beta blockers should be used in conjunction with ICDs as the adrenergic stress of a shock can precipitate additional arrhythmias. More data are needed to assess the role of ICDs as first-line treatment in the absence of clinical events. Whereas Na^+ channel blockers preferentially block abnormal late Na^+ current and can shorten the QT interval in LQT3 patients,[23] there is a risk of exacerbating the Brugada syndrome, and their role in this situation is unclear.[1]

For asymptomatic mutation carriers at low risk (older, normal QT interval), therapy is not indicated. For younger patients, beta blockers are reasonable, especially in the setting of any QT prolongation. It is currently recommended that all patients with LQTS refrain from participation in competitive sports and that drugs that prolong QT interval or deplete K^+ or Mg^{2+} be avoided.[11] In addition, they should be cautioned to avoid K^+ depletion through diarrhea or excessive sweating by taking K^+ supplements during such periods.

PROGNOSIS

Both beta blockers and ICDs provide superior survival in patients with symptomatic LQTS, and mortality can be reduced to less than 3% to 4% in 5 years with standard therapy. Patients with the Jervell and Lange-Nielsen syndrome have a worse prognosis than that of other patients. A major challenge remains to identify asymptomatic patients at lower apparent risk of sudden death who should be aggressively treated.

SUMMARY

The LQTS is an important cause of sudden death in young, otherwise healthy patients. It should be considered when syncope or cardiac arrest occurs in patients with structurally normal hearts, especially when symptoms are adrenergically mediated.

SHORT QT SYNDROME

In the early 1990s, it was recognized that an abnormally short QT interval is also associated with an increased risk of sudden death.[24] Subsequently in 2000, the short QT syndrome (SQTS) was first described.[25] This very rare disorder may be highly lethal, and patients are susceptible to both atrial and ventricular arrhythmias.[26-29]

ANATOMY AND PATHOLOGY

Routine evaluation reveals that these patients have structurally normal hearts, with no detectable abnormalities by cardiac catheterization, echocardiography, or magnetic resonance imaging. Autopsy data in patients with the SQTS have been unremarkable.[26]

PATHOPHYSIOLOGY

To some extent, the SQTS represents a mirror image of the LQTS. Mutations have been described thus far in three genes that encode K^+ channel proteins[6,10] and are also associated with LQTS (including *KCNH2*, *KCNQ1*, and *KCNJ2*; Table 63.5). These mutations lead to functional defects that are opposite of those seen for LQTS, with a gain of function and increased K^+ current. This leads to more rapid repolarization, causing shortening of the cardiac action potential, the QT interval on the surface electrocardiogram, and refractoriness in both the atrium and ventricle during electrophysiologic testing. Recently, a group of patients with loss-of-function mutations in Ca^{2+} channel subunits causing the Brugada syndrome were noted to have abnormally short QTc intervals (330 to 370 ms) as well.[30]

CLINICAL PRESENTATIONS

This is a rare disorder with relatively few cases described thus far. In most families, inheritance appears to be autosomal dominant. The disease onset typically occurs at a young age,

SUBTYPES FOR OTHER INHERITED ARRHYTHMIA SYNDROMES					
	Subtype	**Gene**	**Protein or Alias**	**Chromosomal Locus**	**Ionic Current Affected**
Short QT syndrome	SQT1	*KCNH2*	HERG	7q35-q36*	↑I_{Kr}
	SQT2	*KCNQ1*	KvLQT1	11p15.5*	↑I_{Ks}
	SQT3	*KCNJ2*	Kir2.1, IRK1	17q23.1-q24.2*	↑I_{K1}
Brugada syndrome	BS1	*SCN5A*	Nav.15	3p21	↓I_{Na}
	BS2	*GPD1L*	Glycerol-3-phosphate dehydrogenase 1–like protein	3p22.3	↓I_{Na}
	BS3	*CACNA1c*	Cav1.2	12p13.3*	↓$I_{Ca\text{-}L}$
	BS4	*CACNB2b*	Cavβ2b	10p12	↓$I_{Ca\text{-}L}$
Catecholaminergic polymorphic ventricular tachycardia	CPVT1	*RYR2*	Ryanodine receptor	1q42.1-q43	↑SR Ca^{2+} release
	CPVT2	*CASQ2*	Calsequestrin	1p13.3-p11	↑SR Ca^{2+} release

*Although mutations have been described in this gene in individuals with this disorder, genetic linkage to this locus has not yet been demonstrated.
I_{Kr}, rapid component of the delayed rectifier K^+ current; I_{Ks}, slow component of the delayed rectifier K^+ current; I_{K1}, inward rectifier K^+ current; I_{Na}, Na^+ current; $I_{Ca\text{-}L}$, L-type Ca^{2+} current; SR, sarcoplasmic reticulum.
Modified from Wilde AA, Tan HL. Inherited arrhythmia syndromes. Circ J 2007;71(Suppl A):A12-A19.

Table 63.5 Subtypes for other inherited arrhythmia syndromes.

although sudden death has been reported in patients from 3 months to 70 years of age.[11,14] Patients can present with palpitations, syncope, or cardiac arrest, and a familial history of sudden death may be present. Supraventricular arrhythmias such as atrial fibrillation have been observed in addition to ventricular tachyarrhythmias. The disorder may be highly lethal, although with the small number of cases thus far, there may be a tendency to overestimate severity. In a recent series of 29 patients diagnosed with SQTS (by methods that included genetic testing), the mean age at diagnosis was 30 years (range, 4 to 80 years).[28] For the group, 67% were symptomatic, with cardiac arrest in 10 patients.

DIAGNOSTIC TECHNIQUES

The surface electrocardiogram is characterized by a persistently short QT interval over a wide range of heart rates, usually with tall, peaked T waves (Fig. 63.3).[14,26,29] For the patients initially described, the QTc was 300 ms or less. However, the exact cutoff for definition of the SQTS is

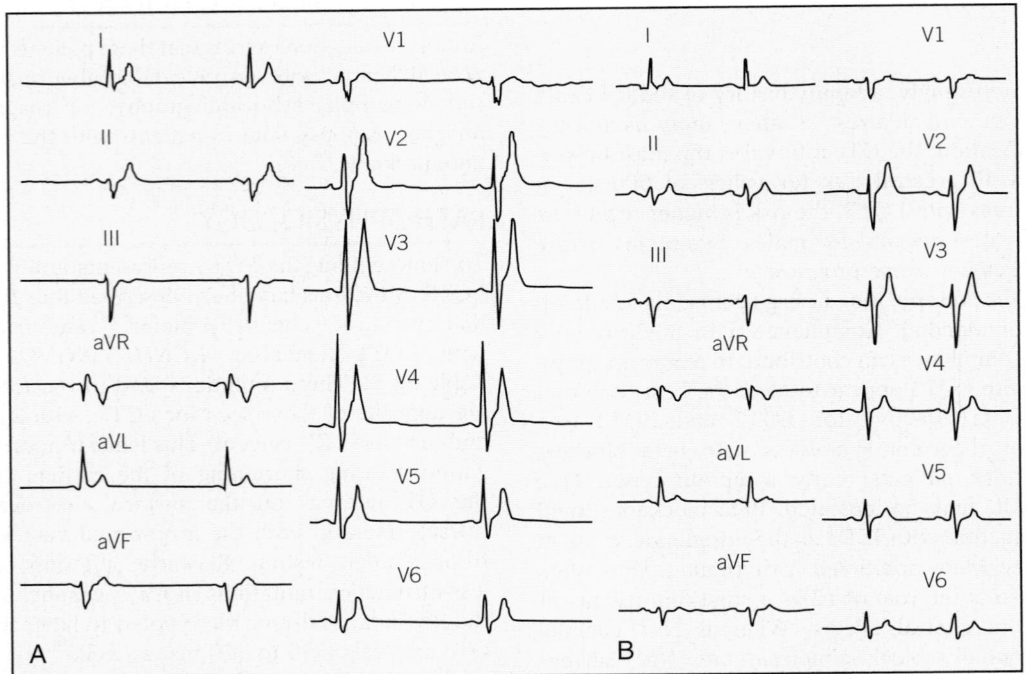

Figure 63.3 The electrocardiogram in the short QT syndrome. Examples of 12-lead electrocardiograms are shown for two patients with the short QT syndrome having a QT interval of 280 ms **(A)** and 220 ms **(B)**. (Modified from Gaita F, Giustetto C, Bianchi F, et al. Short QT syndrome: a familial cause of sudden death. Circulation 2003;108:965-970.)

currently not defined. No patients have been identified with a QTc above 340 ms. In a retrospective study of a random population of more than 10,000 middle-aged individuals, a QTc below 340 ms was seen in 0.4%, with a QTc below 320 ms in 0.1%.[31] Among individuals with such short QT intervals, cardiovascular and all-cause mortality was not increased. However, these findings are limited by a low event rate in the population, the retrospective nature of the study, and the exclusion of younger individuals, for whom the incidence of SQTS is likely to be increased. At electrophysiologic testing, atrial and ventricular refractory periods are shortened, and ventricular tachyarrhythmias are often induced by programmed stimulation. The differential diagnosis includes other entities that can cause a short QT interval (e.g., hypercalcemia and digoxin therapy) and tall T waves (e.g., hyperkalemia, ischemia). As for LQTS, family members should be screened to identify affected relatives.

MANAGEMENT

Given the small number of cases that have been described, management remains poorly defined. However, the only effective therapy to date is the ICD (Table 63.6).[10,11,14,28] Placement of an ICD is recommended for post-arrest and other high-risk patients (e.g., after syncope). Spurious shocks due to T-wave oversensing can occur, and devices should be programmed accordingly to minimize this risk. Quinidine may prolong the QT interval and suppress inducibility in some patients, but its value in long-term management is unknown.[10] It may also reduce T-wave amplitude and thus help prevent ICD oversensing.

PROGNOSIS

Because patients with this syndrome were identified less than a decade ago, the long-term prognosis for these individuals is not well defined. However, the ICD appears to be effective in reducing mortality. The risk of arrhythmic events in genetically affected individuals with a normal QT interval is not known.

SUMMARY

The SQTS is a recently described disorder consisting of abnormally short repolarization and increased susceptibility to atrial and ventricular arrhythmias. It should be considered in patients with a QTc of 340 ms or less if other factors suggestive of arrhythmia (e.g., syncope or positive family history) are present.

BRUGADA SYNDROME

The Brugada syndrome is characterized by spontaneous or drug-induced ST elevation in the right precordial leads, often associated with conduction delay, and a propensity for

GUIDELINES FOR MANAGEMENT OF OTHER INHERITED ARRHYTHMIA SYNDROMES

	Recommendation	Level of Evidence	Comment
Short QT syndrome	Implantable cardioverter-defibrillator	Not defined	For survivors of cardiac arrest
Brugada syndrome	Implantable cardioverter-defibrillator	I	For survivors of cardiac arrest
		IIa	For patients with syncope and spontaneous electrocardiographic pattern
		IIa	For patients with sustained VT
	Monitor the spontaneous electrocardiographic pattern	IIa	For patients with drug-induced electrocardiographic pattern
	Isoproterenol	IIa	For VT storm
	Quinidine	IIb	For VT storm
	Electrophysiologic testing	IIb	For risk stratification in patients with spontaneous electrocardiographic pattern
Catecholaminergic polymorphic VT	Beta blockers	I	For patients with spontaneous or stress-induced ventricular arrhythmias
		IIa	For children with the diagnosis established by means of genetic testing only
		IIb	For adults with the diagnosis established by means of genetic testing only
	Implantable cardioverter-defibrillator with beta blockers	I	For survivors of cardiac arrest
		IIa	For patients with syncope or sustained VT with beta blockers

VT, ventricular tachycardia.

Modified from Zipes DP, Camm AJ, Borggrefe M, et al. ACC/AHA/ESC 2006 guidelines for management of patients with ventricular arrhythmias and the prevention of sudden cardiac death: a report of the American College of Cardiology/American Heart Association Task Force and the European Society of Cardiology Committee for Practice Guidelines (Writing Committee to Develop Guidelines for Management of Patients With Ventricular Arrhythmias and the Prevention of Sudden Cardiac Death). J Am Coll Cardiol 2006;48:e247-e346.

Table 63.6 Guidelines for management of other inherited arrhythmia syndromes.

serious arrhythmias.[10,14,20,32-34] Although reportedly rare (except in Southeast Asia), it is increasingly recognized as a cause for sudden death in otherwise healthy individuals.

ANATOMY AND PATHOLOGY

Evaluation of patients with Brugada syndrome typically reveals no evidence of structural heart disease by standard imaging modalities. However, there is increasing evidence that abnormalities may be present at the microscopic level. Examination of an explanted heart from a patient with Brugada syndrome revealed fibrosis and fatty infiltration in the right ventricular outflow tract.[35] In a recent series of 18 Brugada syndrome patients, cardiac catheterization revealed ventricular microaneurysms; endomyocardial biopsy demonstrated histologic changes that included fibrofatty infiltration and lymphocytic inflammatory infiltrates (Fig. 63.4b).[36] At present, it is not clear whether myocarditis can stimulate Brugada syndrome or whether some Brugada syndrome patients in reality have subclinical heart disease.

PATHOPHYSIOLOGY

As for other inherited arrhythmia syndromes, mutations in multiple different genes are associated with the Brugada syndrome (see Table 63.5),[6,10] with autosomal dominant inheritance. In 1998, mutations in the cardiac Na^+ channel gene *SCN5A* were first described; more than 70 have been reported to date. However, *SCN5A* mutations are present in 20% or less of Brugada syndrome patients.[33] The overall functional effect is a reduction in cardiac Na^+ current.[10,20] In addition, more common DNA variants (or polymorphisms) can also influence Na^+ current magnitude. A promoter haplotype (group of cosegregating variants) associated with reduced Na^+ current was discovered in Asian persons,[37] although a connection with Brugada syndrome has not been reported. Currently, it is hypothesized that reduced Na^+ current causes slowed conduction or exaggeration of heterogeneous repolarization across the right ventricular myocardial wall to produce ST elevation and enhanced arrhythmia susceptibility. Mutations in *SCN5A* can cause LQTS, Brugada syndrome, conduction system disease, atrial fibrillation, and overlap syndromes.[10,20,33] In addition, multiple different phenotypes have been ascribed to the same mutation. The basis for these observations is currently an area of active investigation. A small number of Brugada syndrome patients demonstrate mutations in the gene encoding glycerol-3-phosphate dehydrogenase 1–like protein[38] (GPD1-L), which may regulate *SCN5A* expression. As noted before, mutations in Ca^{2+} channel subunit genes were recently identified in a disorder with features of both the Brugada and short QT syndromes.[30] Mutations in *SCN1B*, encoding a Na^+ channel modulatory subunit, have also been associated with Brugada syndrome.[39]

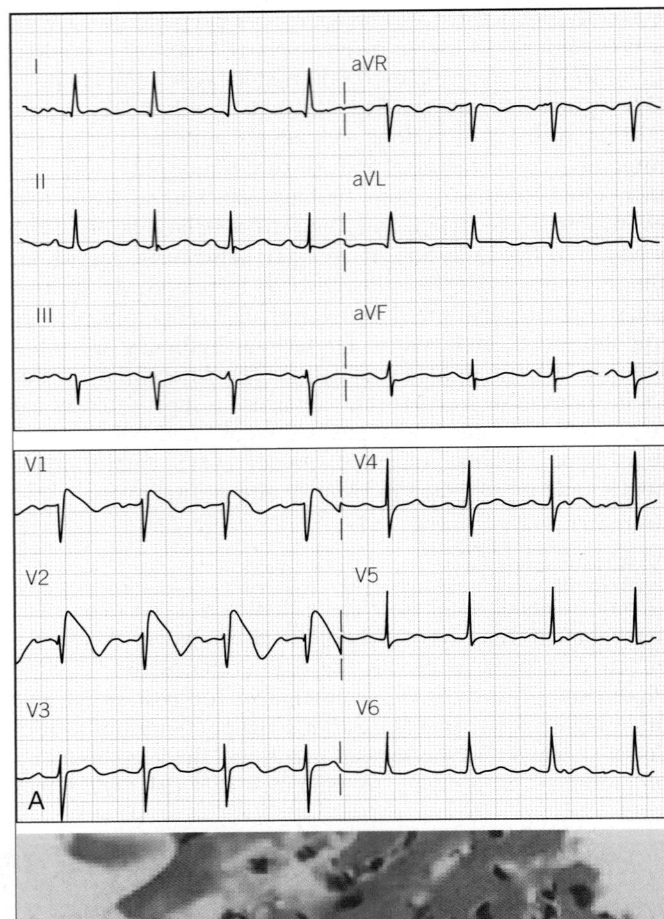

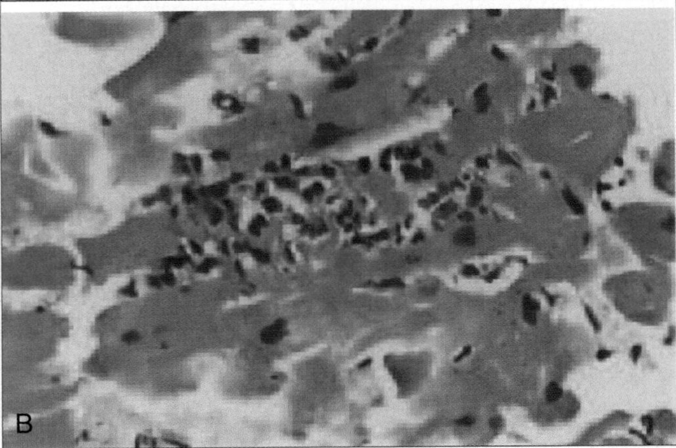

Figure 63.4 Electrocardiographic and microscopic abnormalities in the Brugada syndrome. A, The 12-lead electrocardiogram is shown for a patient with the Brugada syndrome, with ST elevation in leads V_1 and V_2. (From Brugada P, Brugada J. Right bundle branch block, persistent ST segment elevation and sudden cardiac death: a distinct clinical and electrocardiographic syndrome. A multicenter report. J Am Coll Cardiol 1992;20:1391-1396.) **B,** Right ventricular endomyocardial biopsy sample (hematoxylin and eosin stain) is shown from a patient with the Brugada syndrome, demonstrating a lymphocytic inflammatory infiltrate. (Modified from Frustaci A, Priori SG, Pieroni M, et al. Cardiac histological substrate in patients with clinical phenotype of Brugada syndrome. Circulation 2005;112:3680-3687.)

CLINICAL PRESENTATIONS

The overall incidence of Brugada syndrome is estimated to be 5 in 10,000 persons, although the true prevalence is unknown, given the intermittent nature of the electrocardiographic findings.[33] Higher rates have been noted in Japan (1 in 4000) and Southeast Asia (possibly 1%). Most patients are male, with an 8:1 male-to-female predominance for unknown reasons. The onset is typically in the third to fourth decade of life, but it can occur in infancy (causing SIDS).[10,14,32,33] Patients can present with syncope or cardiac arrest, with clinical events that often occur at rest or during sleep. Arrhythmias can also be triggered by fever and large meals. Unfortunately, sudden death is not infrequently the initial manifestation of the disease. The risk of cardiac arrest due to polymorphic VT or ventricular fibrillation is approximately 10% to 15% by the age of 60 years.[33] Up to 20% of patients can have supraventricular arrhythmias, usually atrial fibrillation.[32,33] A family history of sudden death may be present, but it does not predict risk of arrhythmic events.

DIAGNOSTIC TECHNIQUES

The electrocardiographic hallmark of the Brugada syndrome is ST elevation (at least 2 mm) in the right precordial leads (V_1 to V_3; Fig. 63.4a). The ST elevation is "coved," with a descending terminal portion of the ST segment. Incomplete or complete right bundle branch block may also be present. There is frequently evidence of diffuse conduction delay, with prolonged PR and QRS intervals. The ST elevation may occur spontaneously or after drug challenge with a Na^+ channel blocker (e.g., procainamide, ajmaline, or flecainide). The sensitivity of drug challenge is not clear, but for *SCN5A* mutations, it is estimated to be 77%.[33] There is evidence that moving the precordial leads to a higher intercostal space will increase detection of ST elevation. However, the false-positive rate of such electrocardiograms is not known. Inferior ST elevation has been reported. Evidence indicates that spontaneous ST elevation is typically intermittent, if enough recordings are obtained. The autonomic nervous system appears to play a role in the manifestation of the Brugada electrocardiographic pattern as right precordial ST elevation is suppressed by isoproterenol and aggravated by acetylcholine as well as by a full stomach.[33] The signal-averaged electrocardiogram is useful in Brugada syndrome as late potentials are detected in roughly half the patients. More data are needed to determine whether late potentials predict clinical events. At electrophysiologic testing, there is evidence of infra-Hisian conduction slowing (prolonged HV interval) and increased inducibility of ventricular arrhythmias. Family members should undergo electrocardiographic recordings or monitoring for screening purposes. The differential diagnosis includes acute ischemia, electrolyte disturbances, myocarditis, and arrhythmogenic right ventricular dysplasia.

MANAGEMENT

For patients with an aborted cardiac arrest or syncope, the ICD is the treatment of choice (see Table 63.6).[11] There is considerable debate about the management of asymptomatic patients with the Brugada electrocardiographic pattern.[11,32,33] The role of electrophysiologic testing for risk stratification of these patients has been controversial. Available evidence indicates that spontaneous ST elevation carries a greater risk than the drug-induced form. A recent meta-analysis of 30 prospective studies including more than 1500 patients indicated that the relative risk of clinical events is increased in patients with a spontaneous electrocardiographic pattern but not for a positive family history or inducibility at electrophysiologic testing.[40] At present, ICD implantation for asymptomatic patients with overt ST elevation may be reasonable. Drugs that exacerbate the electrocardiographic pattern (e.g., class I antiarrhythmics, tricyclic antidepressants, local anesthetics, cocaine, and beta blockers) should be avoided. During a febrile illness, attempts should be made to lower body temperature, and medical attention should be sought. For frequent ICD shocks or VT storm, recommended therapy includes isoproterenol or quinidine.[11] Whereas amiodarone has not proved useful, quinidine has been shown to prevent inducibility of ventricular arrhythmia in up to 76% of Brugada syndrome patients.[33]

PROGNOSIS

For symptomatic patients, the ICD is effective therapy to reduce mortality. It is currently not known whether patients with Brugada syndrome will develop evidence of overt cardiomyopathy over time.

SUMMARY

The Brugada syndrome represents an increasingly recognized cause of serious ventricular arrhythmias and sudden death in otherwise healthy patients. Prolonged monitoring and frequent electrocardiograms are often required for the diagnosis because the electrocardiographic pattern can be intermittent.

CATECHOLAMINERGIC POLYMORPHIC VENTRICULAR TACHYCARDIA

Initially described in 1987, catecholaminergic polymorphic ventricular tachycardia (CPVT) is a rare but highly lethal disorder characterized by adrenergically mediated syncope and sudden death.[10,11,41,42] The hallmark of this disease is stress-induced ventricular arrhythmias, including bidirectional VT, in the setting of a normal electrocardiogram at baseline.

ANATOMY AND PATHOLOGY

Imaging studies have revealed no evidence of overt structural heart disease in these patients. To date, there have been no reports of microscopic abnormalities during histologic studies of myocardium from patients with CPVT.

PATHOPHYSIOLOGY

The bidirectional VT seen in this disorder (Fig. 63.5) resembles that observed with digitalis toxicity. As for cardiac glycoside toxicity, evidence to date indicates a central role for impaired Ca^{2+} homeostasis and intracellular Ca^{2+} overload in CPVT.[10,41,42] Most cases are due to mutations in the gene encoding the cardiac ryanodine receptor (*RYR2;* see Table 63.5), which serves as the Ca^{2+} release channel in the sarcoplasmic reticulum, with autosomal dominant inheritance. These defects appear to cause diastolic Ca^{2+} leak through RyR2 channels. The resultant intracellular Ca^{2+} overload promotes triggered activity in the form of delayed after-depolarizations, causing VT. *RYR2* mutation knockin mice display delayed after-depolarizations at rest, which are aggravated by isoproterenol.[43] CPVT is also caused by mutations in the gene encoding the cardiac isoform of calsequestrin *(CASQ2),* the major sarcoplasmic reticulum Ca^{2+} buffering protein; the *CASQ2*-linked disease is autosomal recessive, that

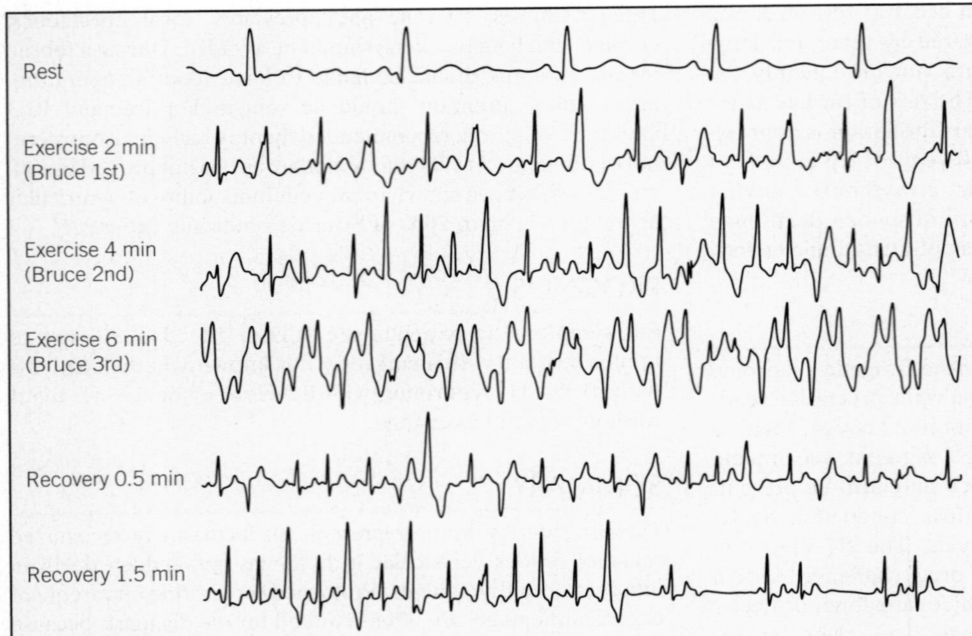

Figure 63.5 Exercise-induced arrhythmias in the catecholaminergic polymorphic ventricular tachycardia syndrome. During a treadmill test, ventricular arrhythmias are observed that worsen in a progressive manner. Bidirectional VT develops at 6 minutes of exercise, with gradual resolution of arrhythmias in recovery. (From Liu N, Colombi B, Raytcheva-Buono EV, et al. Catecholaminergic polymorphic ventricular tachycardia. Herz 2007;32:212-217.)

is, patients are homozygous for loss-of-function mutations. Together, these two genes account for up to 70% of patients with CPVT. The disorder is familial in about 30% of cases, with autosomal dominant inheritance for *RYR2* mutations and autosomal recessive transmission for *CASQ2*.

CLINICAL PRESENTATIONS

The mean age at onset is 8 years; most patients present by adolescence.[41] Death can occur in infancy, and like the other inherited arrhythmia syndromes, CPVT appears to contribute to SIDS. Patients present with exercise- or emotion-induced syncope or cardiac arrest. A particularly prominent trigger is swimming, which is also seen in LQT1. The risk of serious arrhythmias is high; approximately 20% of patients die suddenly by the age of 16 years, whereas mortality is 30% to 50% by the age of 40 years if it is left untreated.[41] Sudden death is the initial manifestation in about 10% of cases. There is a family history of stress-mediated arrhythmic symptoms in approximately 30%. The differential diagnosis includes LQTS, which also causes adrenergically mediated VT. Patients with Andersen's syndrome can also display bidirectional VT. However, the presence of periodic paralysis and dysmorphic features distinguishes these patients. Digoxin toxicity or poisoning should also be considered in cases of bidirectional VT.

DIAGNOSTIC TECHNIQUES

At baseline, the electrocardiogram is typically unremarkable (see Fig. 63.5). Resting bradycardia and prominent U waves have been reported. Treadmill testing is critical for the diagnosis. As exercise heart rate exceeds 110 to 130 beats per minute, ventricular premature depolarizations begin to occur. Arrhythmia complexity increases with continued exercise, with development of bigeminy, polymorphic or bidirectional VT (see Fig. 63.5), and occasionally ventricular fibrillation. Supraventricular arrhythmias can also occur. Long-term monitoring (e.g., with an implantable loop recorder) can be useful. Electrophysiologic testing is not warranted as ventricular arrhythmias are not inducible by programmed stimulation. Isoproterenol infusion can induce VT, but the role of this provocative challenge to predict subsequent clinical events is not clear.

MANAGEMENT

Beta blockers can reduce arrhythmias and clinical events (see Table 63.6).[10,11,41] Long-acting agents such as nadolol are typically used, and it is recommended to escalate to the highest tolerated dose. However, protection with beta blockers is only partial (up to 30% of patients will still have VT[14]), in at least some cases due to noncompliance or underdosing. For these patients and those suffering an aborted cardiac arrest, an ICD is recommended.[11] It is important to continue beta blockers after ICD placement; VT storm and death have occurred otherwise. For acute termination of VT, intravenous administration of beta blockers is recommended; amiodarone, lidocaine, and magnesium are not effective. Overall, verapamil is clearly less effective than beta blockers are. CPVT patients should avoid strenuous exercise.[10]

PROGNOSIS

Despite the frequency of severe ventricular arrhythmias, many patients do well with long-term survival by current management strategies. The prognosis for heterozygote carriers of *CASQ2* mutations remains to be clarified.

SUMMARY

In addition to LQTS, CPVT should be considered in the young patient with stress-mediated ventricular arrhythmias, a normal electrocardiogram, and a structurally normal heart. Identification of these patients is critical, given that beta blockers and the ICD usually provide effective therapy.

chapter 64

Sudden Cardiac Death

Paul LeLorier and John G. Carr

Definition

- Sudden cardiac death is unexpected total circulatory arrest within 1 hour of the onset of symptoms or without any warning.

Key Features

- Coronary artery disease is the most prevalent cause.
- Risk is increased in the presence of reduced left ventricular ejection fraction, congestive heart failure, and nonsustained ventricular tachycardia.
- The most common mechanism is ventricular tachyarrhythmia.

Therapy

- Defibrillator implantation is the treatment of choice for secondary prevention in the majority of survivors and for primary prevention in patients at high risk for sudden cardiac death.

Sudden cardiac death is defined as unexpected death, occurring within 1 hour from the onset of symptoms, that is not directly attributable to other factors. It is the leading cause of mortality in industrialized nations, accounting for 12% of all natural deaths and 50% of all deaths attributable to cardiovascular disease.[1] In the United States, approximately 300,000 people die suddenly each year. Recent advances in the care of acute coronary syndromes and heightened awareness of modifiable risk factors have led to an overall decrease in cardiovascular mortality, but the proportion of deaths that are sudden has remained constant during the past several decades. Although the greatest incidence occurs in cohorts with identifiable risk factors, most events occur in individuals without prior known risk factors (Fig. 64.1). Therefore, interventions aimed at reducing the incidence in the highest risk groups will have a modest effect on the number of sudden deaths in the population as a whole. The immediate cause leading to the final common pathway of total hemodynamic collapse is most frequently ventricular tachycardia (VT) and ventricular fibrillation (VF); asystole, pulseless electrical activity, aortic rupture, and cardiac tamponade account for the remainder (Fig. 64.2). The proximate events leading to these fatal ventricular arrhythmias result from a wide spectrum of underlying disease states, mediated by physiologic and environmental triggers.

PATHOPHYSIOLOGY

Underlying Disease Substrates

Structural Heart Disease

Coronary Artery Disease

Coronary artery disease and its sequelae remain the most important contributors to sudden cardiac death, accounting for 80% of sudden death in industrialized nations (Table 64.1). Paradoxically, within this group are both the most elusive and the most predictably high risk individuals at risk for sudden cardiac death. It is both ironic and sobering that more than half of those individuals who die suddenly of cardiovascular causes have no prior diagnosis of coronary artery disease.[2] In the general population, two thirds of these episodes are associated with rupture or erosion of an atherosclerotic plaque,[3] suggesting ischemia as being the major cause of sudden death in the general population. Extensive atherosclerosis is the most common finding in sudden death victims at autopsy, although a history of prior myocardial infarction is present in only 45%.[4] The importance of coronary disease in sudden cardiac death is further attested to in an autopsy series of 100 patients in which 44% of victims of sudden cardiac death had recent major coronary thrombi, 30% had minor thrombi, and 21% had plaque fissuring; only 5% had no acute changes.[5] Other data suggest that it is the presence of atherosclerosis, rather than its location or distribution, that is the critical feature in sudden cardiac death as there is no clear predilection for proximal versus distal disease or for left versus right. From these data, a significant portion of those dying of sudden cardiac death would be best served by improved identification of those nonobstructive coronary lesions at risk for acute thrombosis, an area of active research. Improved therapy for acute coronary syndromes that do not end in sudden cardiac death has led to an increase in post–myocardial infarction survival and in doing so has increased the proportion of individuals with identifiable risks and triggers for malignant ventricular arrhythmias.

After a myocardial infarction, the risk of sudden death is increased from baseline, peaking in the first 6 months. Heart failure and left ventricular function are the two most important predictors of higher risk of sudden death. In the setting of systolic dysfunction, ventricular ectopy gains importance as a predictor of sudden cardiac death. In the postinfarction population, the risk of sudden death is higher if complex ventricular ectopy is present, with the risk being 5% during a 3- to 5-year period.[6] If nonsustained VT is present, the risk

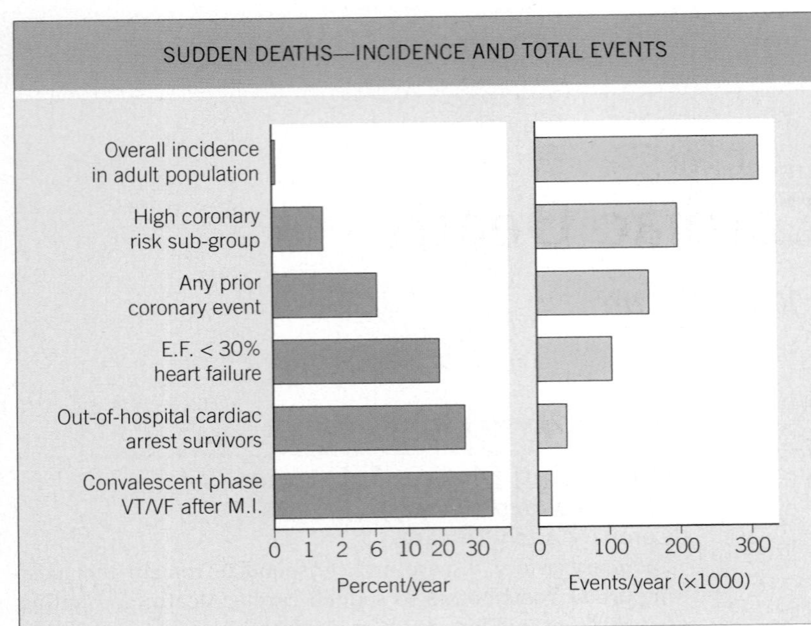

Figure 64.1 Sudden cardiac deaths among population subgroups. Estimates of incidence (percent/year) and total number of sudden cardiac deaths per year are shown for the overall adult population in the United States and for higher risk subgroups. The overall estimated incidence is 0.1% to 0.2% per year, totaling more than 300,000 deaths per year. Within subgroups identified by increasingly powerful risk factors, the increasing incidence is accompanied by progressively decreasing total numbers. The horizontal axis for the incidence figures is nonlinear. EF, ejection fraction; MI, myocardial infarction; VT/VF, ventricular tachycardia/fibrillation. (With permission from Myerburg RJ, Kessler KM, Castellanos A. Sudden cardiac death: structure, function, and time-dependence of risk. Circulation 1992;85[Suppl I]:I2-I10.)

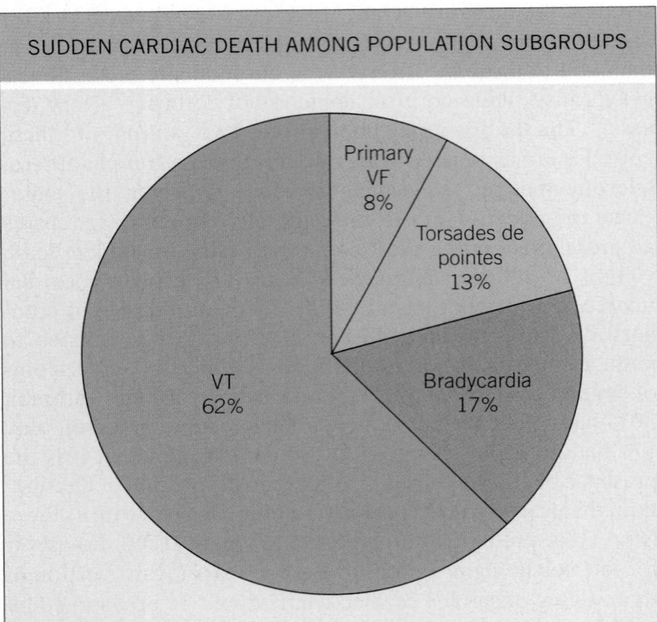

Figure 64.2 Sudden cardiac deaths among population subgroups. VT, ventricular tachycardia; VF, ventricular fibrillation (Modified from Bayés de Luna A, Coumel P, Leclercq JF. Ambulatory sudden cardiac death: mechanisms of production of fatal arrhythmia on the basis of data from 157 cases. Am Heart J 1989;117:151-159.)

CAUSES OF SUDDEN CARDIAC DEATH

Cause	Example
Structural heart disease	
Ischemic (70%-80%)	Myocardial ischemia or infarction Coronary plaque rupture, fissure, ulceration, or spasm Previous infarction Congenital: anomalous origin of coronary artery
Nonischemic (10%-15%)	Idiopathic dilated cardiomyopathy Hypertrophic cardiomyopathy Acute myocarditis Right ventricular dysplasia Infiltrative diseases Inflammatory diseases Congenital diseases and repairs
No structural heart disease (10%-15%)	
Channelopathies	Long QT syndrome Brugada syndrome Primary ventricular fibrillation
Accessory pathways	Wolff-Parkinson-White syndrome
Toxic or drug induced	Acquired long QT
Acute mechanical (5%)	Aortic rupture Ventricular rupture Commotio cordis

Table 64.1 Causes of sudden cardiac death.

increases further; rates up to 32% have been reported.[7,8] Because patients with decreased ejection fraction and poor functional class have a higher arrhythmia burden yet have a larger proportion of nonarrhythmic death, it is unclear whether the presence of such arrhythmias provides an independent predictor.[9] Uretzky and Sheahan[10] reported that patients assigned to New York Heart Association (NYHA) class II have an annual mortality of 5% to 15%, with sudden death accounting for 50% to 80%; patients assigned to NYHA class IV have a 30% to 70% annual mortality, with only 5% to 30% being caused by sudden death. Conversely, when there is no structural heart disease, the presence of monomorphic VT is not generally associated with a worse prognosis. Therefore, presence of ectopy or VT and functional classification or left ventricular ejection fraction are relatively crude predictors of individuals who are likely to have sudden death.

Structural abnormalities of the coronary arteries other than atherosclerotic disease are rare (<1%) and as such are an infrequent cause of sudden death in the general population. The risk of sudden death may be quite high for afflicted individuals, depending on the specific anomaly. Anomalous origin of the left coronary artery from the right aortic sinus of Valsalva with passage between the pulmonary trunk and the aorta is the most lethal of the coronary anomalies and has been linked to sudden death with exertion. It is believed that the proximal artery is kinked at its origin with exercise and compressed between the aorta and pulmonary trunk, resulting in ischemia. Anomalous origin of the left coronary artery from the right aortic sinus with subsequent passage anterior to the pulmonary trunk or posterior to the aorta and anomalous origin of the right coronary artery from the left sinus of Valsalva, despite its passage between the aorta and pulmonary trunk, have been reported to a lesser degree in association with sudden death. Other nonatherosclerotic primary coronary abnormalities include spontaneous dissection from connective tissue diseases, arteritis, and abnormal vasoreactivity. Coronary artery dissection as a sequela of proximal aortic dissection or during the prenatal period has been described. Further, coronary artery embolization resulting in sudden cardiac death can be due to left-sided endocarditis, thrombi on aortic or mitral valves, or mural thrombus. Sudden death in these cases results from the acute ischemia or reperfusion that ensues.

Nonischemic Dilated Cardiomyopathy

The causes of nonischemic dilated cardiomyopathies are varied, ranging from structural, to genetic, to metabolic and toxic myocardial insults that all ultimately lead to compromised systolic function. It is estimated that 10% of patients resuscitated from cardiac arrest have underlying nonischemic dilated cardiomyopathy.[11] As with the ischemic cardiomyopathies, sudden death is estimated to account for up to 40% to 50% of the overall mortality in these patients. Further, the overall incidence of dilated cardiomyopathy may be on the rise because of the impact of improved medical treatment strategies in reducing mortality due to congestive heart failure.

Mortality in this population is closely related to the degree of ventricular impairment and the duration of disease. As ejection fraction deteriorates and clinical heart failure progresses, mortality increases, but the proportion of sudden death to overall deaths is reduced. Sudden death accounts for approximately 60% of mortality in patients assigned to class II but only 30% in patients assigned to class IV.[12] This probably reflects the increase in the competing risk of pump failure over time. During end-stage heart failure, bradyarrhythmias may predominate over tachyarrhythmias as a cause of sudden death. In a series of 22 hospitalized patients awaiting transplantation, 62% of monitored cardiac arrests were a result of bradycardia or electromechanical dissociation.[13]

Nonsustained VT is commonly seen on ambulatory recordings with a frequency related to the degree of heart failure. Although it serves as an independent marker of increased mortality, the strength of its association with sudden death is controversial. Programmed stimulation is generally not helpful because of a low sensitivity and poor specificity in predicting arrhythmic events. The occurrence of syncope in the setting of idiopathic dilated cardiomyopathy has been shown to be predictive of a significantly higher risk of subsequent sudden death[14] and may serve as an indication for specific treatment.

Hypertrophic Cardiomyopathy

Hypertrophic cardiomyopathy results from genetically heterogeneous mutations in multiple genes encoding both sarcomeric and contractile proteins. It is marked by the presence of variable patterns of left ventricular hypertrophy in the absence of systemic cause and is strongly associated with myocardial disarray at the cellular level. Its prevalence is estimated at 1 in 500 of the general population. Initial studies of referred populations have demonstrated a risk of sudden death approaching 3% to 5% annually with increased vulnerability during adolescence.[15] A pooled longitudinal study from nonreferred populations suggests that the incidence of sudden death is significantly lower, approaching only 1% per year.[16] Hypertrophic cardiomyopathy is the leading cause of sudden death in athletes younger than 35 years and is exercise related in up to 40% of cases of sudden death.[17] Whereas large-scale echocardiographic screening for all athletes is not feasible, a screening physical examination and history may identify individuals at increased risk before participation in competitive athletics.

The mechanism of sudden death is most often fast VT that rapidly degenerates into VF. Although presentation with sustained monomorphic VT is rare, electrogram analysis from implantable cardioverter-defibrillator (ICD) discharges in those previously resuscitated from cardiac arrest reveals rapid VT at the onset of treated events in the majority of cases. These ventricular tachyarrhythmias are likely to result from altered conduction and inhomogeneous repolarization due to a combination of hypertrophy, myocyte disarray, interstitial fibrosis, and myocardial ischemia.

Risk stratification in this population is imprecise and complicated by the low positive predictive value of clinical variables. However, several markers have been linked to an increased risk, and the presence of multiple risk factors appears to confer additive risk. A family history of sudden death in affected relatives is an important prognostic feature. The presence of nonsustained VT and exercise-induced hypotension have been linked to an increased incidence of sudden death. Unexplained syncope during exertion in young patients may be a particularly ominous warning sign. The degree of hypertrophy has been correlated with outcome and found to be an independent marker with a linear and progressive association with increased risk; patients with a ventricular septum greater than 30 mm are at very high risk, especially when they present at a young age. Several gene mutations have been associated with a particularly high incidence of sudden death in selected kindreds[18]; however, the large and growing number of genetic alterations identified currently limits the application of genetic analysis as a widespread screening tool.

Arrhythmogenic Right Ventricular Dysplasia

Arrhythmogenic right ventricular dysplasia is a progressive autosomal dominantly inherited disease marked by various degrees of patchy replacement of the right ventricular myocardium with fatty or fibrofatty tissue. It is characterized clinically by ventricular arrhythmias and sudden death. On histologic examination, apoptosis and inflammation may be present (Fig. 64.3). Mutations have been linked to chromosomes 1, 2, 3, and 14, and in at least one form (type 2), the disorder appears to be related to abnormalities in intracellular calcium regulation.[19] Incomplete penetrance may account for a family history being recognized in approximately 30%

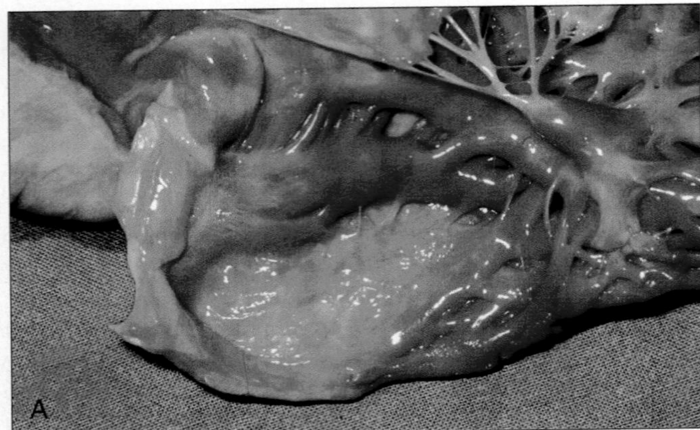

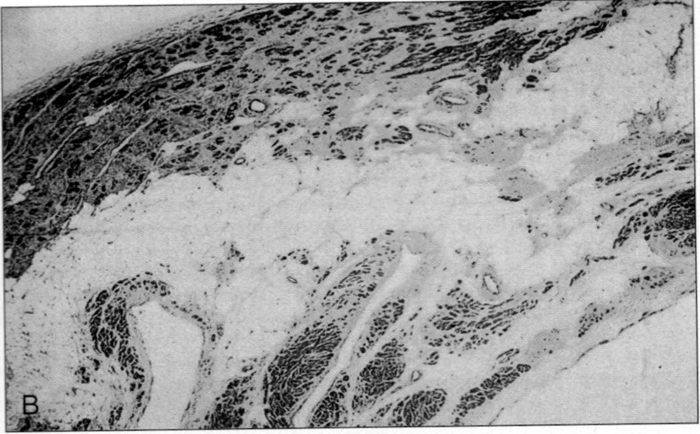

Figure 64.3 A, Pathology specimen of the right ventricle just inferior to the tricuspid valve demonstrating the typical fatty tissue infiltration of the right ventricular myocardium in arrhythmogenic right ventricular dysplasia. B, Photomicrograph of the right ventricular free wall. The specimen is a full-thickness sample with both pericardium (superior) and myocardium (inferior) demonstrated. (From Aziz S, McMahon RF, Garratt CJ. Sudden cardiac death in arrhythmogenic right ventricular dysplasia. Circulation 2000;101:825-827.)

to 50% of affected individuals. A disproportionate number of males are affected, and presentation is most common in adolescence or young adulthood.

Morbidity from ventricular arrhythmias is substantial. Patients often present with palpitations or syncope associated with left bundle branch block pattern VT arising from the right ventricle. The right ventricular inflow tract, outflow tract, and anterolateral free wall are most often involved, but left ventricular involvement may be present in up to 47% of cases.[20] The risk of sudden death in this disorder has not been well defined. Arrhythmogenic right ventricular dysplasia has been identified as the leading cause of sudden death in a cohort of young Italian athletes, lending support to the perception that sudden death is often the first manifestation of disease and that exercise may be a potent trigger. Among those presenting with palpitations or syncope, the rate of sudden death is estimated at 1% to 2% annually.

Inflammatory and Infiltrative Disease

Acute and chronic myocarditis has been associated with sudden death. In an autopsy series of 19 military recruits who died suddenly, evidence of myocarditis was detected in eight (five nonrheumatic, three rheumatic), with the majority of sudden deaths associated with exertion.[21] A single center in France has reported that in 5% of sudden deaths, evidence of acute or chronic lymphocytic myocarditis associated with fibrosis was seen on autopsy.[22] In a pooled series of 1961 patients who died suddenly before the age of 45 years, lymphocytic myocarditis was reported at autopsy in 97 (5%).[23]

Evidence of cardiac involvement in sarcoidosis is present in up to 20% of cases but is clinically manifested in only approximately 5%.[24] There appears to be a tropism for the septum and inferior wall, with a range of involvement from mild ventricular dysfunction to discrete aneurysms and severe global dilated myopathy. The incidence of ventricular arrhythmias is unknown but appears to be linked to the extent of myocardial involvement. Ventricular arrhythmias run the spectrum from premature ventricular contractions, through nonsustained and sustained VT, to VF and sudden death. One autopsy series documented that 67% of deaths from cardiac sarcoid occurred suddenly.[25] The contribution of bradycardia to sudden deaths is not known but may be significant, given the predilection of sarcoidosis to affect the conduction system.

Cardiac amyloidosis is frequently complicated by nonsustained VT, syncope, and sudden death. These patients are at risk for bradycardia from sinus node involvement, and His-Purkinje conduction delay is almost universally manifested. Syncope is frequently encountered because of chronotropic incompetence as well as inappropriate vascular responses due to dysautonomia. Sudden death represents the most common mode of death and can occur at any stage after diagnosis. In a cohort of patients prophylactically implanted with ICDs, sustained rapid VT and VF were common; however, successful defibrillation attempts often failed to resuscitate patients because of ensuing electromechanical dissociation.[26]

Primary Electrophysiologic Disease

In approximately 5% of patients resuscitated from cardiac arrest, no overt structural abnormality is apparent, and episodes of sudden death are attributable to functional abnormalities in ion channels that principally affect repolarization. Chief among these disorders are the long QT syndrome and Brugada syndrome.

The congenital long QT syndrome is caused by genetic mutations that alter the protein subunits of potassium or sodium channels, leading to changes in channel function and resulting in prolonged repolarization. Prolongation of repolarization provides a favorable environment for recurrent polymorphic VT (torsades de pointes). Mutations of the *KCNQ1 (KVLQT1)* gene (long QT syndrome 1) and *KCNH2 (HERG)* gene (long QT syndrome 2) lead to a decreased repolarizing potassium current; mutation of the *SCN5A* gene creates an alteration in the sodium channel resulting in an increased depolarizing sodium current. These genetic mutations account for approximately 90% of congenital long QT syndromes and are inherited in an autosomal dominant pattern. Diagnosis is typically made in childhood or adolescence, but presentation can be delayed for decades. Syncope with exertion and seizures in children are common presenting symptoms; a significant percentage of patients present with aborted sudden cardiac death. In long QT syndrome 1, heightened emotional states such as fright and anger as well as physical exertion (especially swimming) have been identified as potent triggers. In contrast, in long QT syndrome 3, episodes appear more common at rest or during sleep.

The Brugada syndrome is a more recently recognized repolarization disorder marked by incomplete right bundle branch block and persistent ST-segment elevation in the anterior precordial leads.[27] A mutation of *SCN5A* resulting in loss of sodium channel function and enhanced inactivation underly this disorder. Inheritance is autosomal. Shortened repolarization localized to epicardial layers of the myocardium may be responsible for persistent ST-segment elevation and create an environment favorable to re-entry and ultimately VF. The syndrome is manifested more often in males than in females. The risk of cardiac arrest has not been precisely defined but is considerable. Sudden death in an early cohort of 63 patients was 30% at 3 years[28]; however, a subsequent cohort of 200 had a substantially lower overall risk with the exception of a subgroup that experienced syncope.[29] The role of electrophysiologic study as a means of risk stratification is controversial.

Malignant ventricular arrhythmias induced by adrenergic stimulation in a structurally normal heart have been increasingly recognized since their initial description in 1978.[30] The potential molecular substrates for this entity have only recently been appreciated, however. Catecholaminergic polymorphic VT and familial polymorphic VT appear to arise from an abnormality of intracellular Ca^{2+} regulation secondary to mutations in two sarcoplasmic proteins. Missense mutations in the gene encoding the ryanodine receptor calcium channel *(RYR2)* appear to be inherited in an autosomal dominant fashion; a much rarer mutation in the gene encoding calsequestrin *(CASQ2)* is inherited in an autosomal recessive fashion. Recent evidence suggests that mutations in *RYR2* result in a "gain of function," with β-adrenergic stimulation leading to a 10-fold increase in sarcoplasmic calcium release and "after-depolarizations" that can precipitate ventricular arrhythmias.[31] These mutations appear to be particularly lethal; family history reveals one or more sudden cardiac deaths in 30% of cases, often occurring at a young age. Unfortunately, *RYR2* mutations appear to account for only about 50% of clinically diagnosed cases; thus, there are likely to be more unrecognized mutations. Interestingly, a form of arrhythmogenic right ventricular dysplasia (type 2) has recently been linked to mutations in the ryanodine receptor, suggesting a spectrum of disease in these catecholaminergically induced ventricular arrhythmias.

On rare occasions, sudden death is associated with Wolff-Parkinson-White syndrome with manifest pre-excitation over an atrioventricular bypass tract. The mechanism of sudden death is triggered by atrial fibrillation, with rapid and irregular ventricular activation over the bypass tract resulting in VF (Fig. 64.4). Mechanistically, the bypass tract must be capable of 1:1 conduction at rapid rates, that is, a short refractory period. Klein and associates[32] have noted that survivors of cardiac arrest universally demonstrate refractory periods shorter than 250 ms. This finding, however, suffers from low specificity and lacks positive predictive value for sudden death, which for the overall population of symptomatic Wolff-Parkinson-White patients is less than 1:1000 annually.

Finally, in a small percentage of cardiac arrest survivors, no structural or electrophysiologic abnormality is identified. Over time, it is likely that these patients will be found to be afflicted from a yet to be discovered channelopathy or extracardiac trigger. In any case, survival after a cardiac arrest in the absence of identifiable abnormality or clear precipitant is associated with a substantial rate of recurrence, estimated to be as high as 30% during the ensuing 3 years.[33]

Transient Risk Factors

Ischemia

It is well known that myocardial infarction can occasionally be complicated by VT or VF. However, clinical and autopsy series[34,35] have shown that only 20% of survivors of out-of-hospital cardiac arrest and cases of sudden death are associated with an acute transmural infarct. Because the results of the study by Taylor and colleagues[3] indicate plaque rupture in two thirds of individuals who succumbed to sudden death, this suggests that acute ischemia rather than infarct is responsible for the majority of these deaths. The finding of embolization and platelet aggregates in the distal coronary beds of more than 50% of sudden death survivors lends further weight to this theory. Transient occlusion and reperfusion with associated reperfusion arrhythmias may be responsible for many of these deaths in individuals without clinical evidence of infarction. Reperfusion may induce electrical instability by means of triggered activity mediated by sudden alterations in extracellular calcium[36] and by re-entry promoted by changes in gap junction conduction.[37] If there is presence of an additional substrate, such as scar from a previous myocardial dysfunction, hypertrophy, or fiber disarray from a cardiomyopathy, a lethal rhythm may then be maintained.

Activity

It is recognized that sudden death appears to occur at a higher frequency during or shortly after vigorous exertion. Between 6% and 17% of all sudden deaths occur in association with exertion[38]; the mechanism in most of these cases is believed to be due to plaque rupture. Examination of the Physicians' Health Study demonstrated a relative risk of sudden death during and within the 30 minutes after exercise to be 16.9, although the absolute risk during any given episode was extremely low (1 per 1.51 million),[39] and habitual exercise lowered this risk.

Smoking

The association between cigarette smoking and coronary artery disease is well established. The Framingham study shows a twofold to threefold increase in sudden death risk in each decade of life between 30 and 59 years.[40] In a study of 310 survivors of out-of-hospital cardiac arrest, a 27% incidence of recurrent cardiac arrest at 3 years was observed in individuals who continued to smoke compared with 19% in those who quit.[41] The mechanism by which smoking promotes sudden death may be in part related to its induction of coronary spasm with resulting ischemia-reperfusion arrhythmias and its effect on platelet function.

Acquired Long QT Syndrome

The acquired long QT syndrome can develop in response to several circumstances, such as electrolyte abnormalities, bradycardia, and drugs.[42,43] At least two thirds of those affected are women. The incidence is 0.5% to 8% for most antiarrhythmic

12-LEAD ELECTROCARDIOGRAPHIC PATTERN OF WOLFF-PARKINSON-WHITE SYNDROME

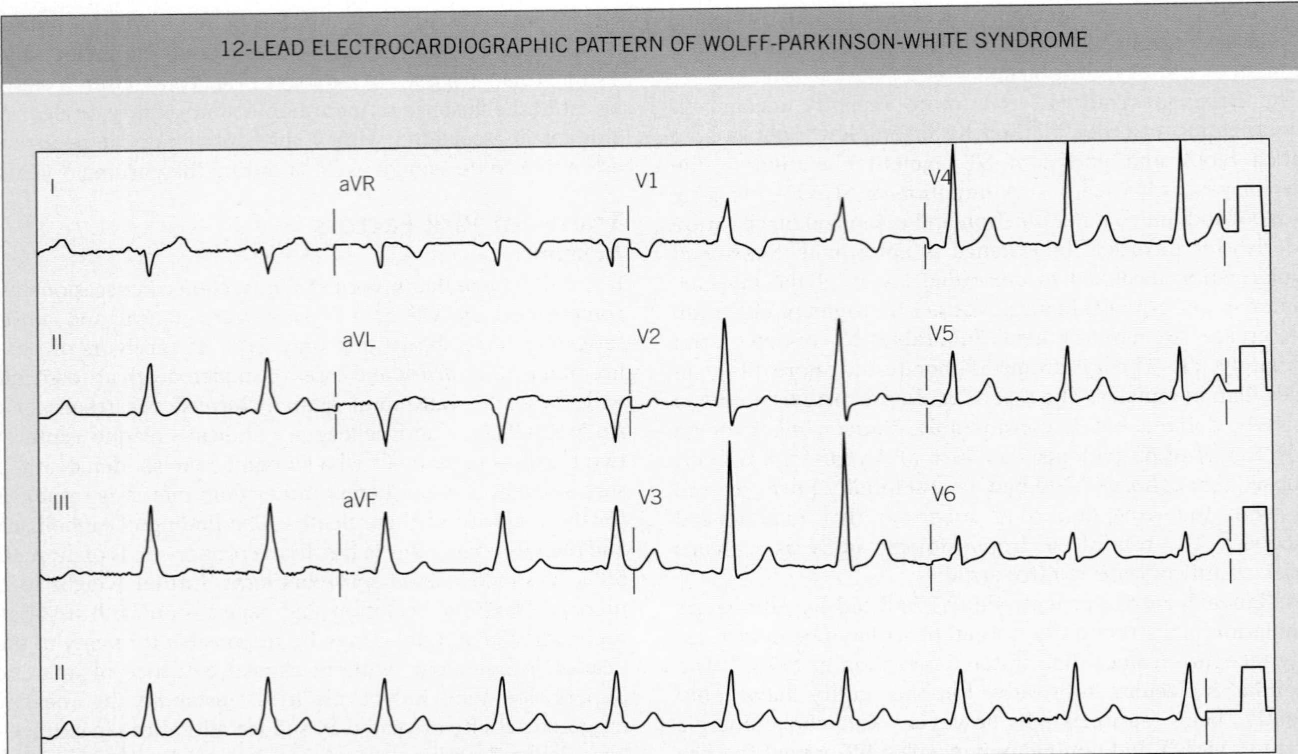

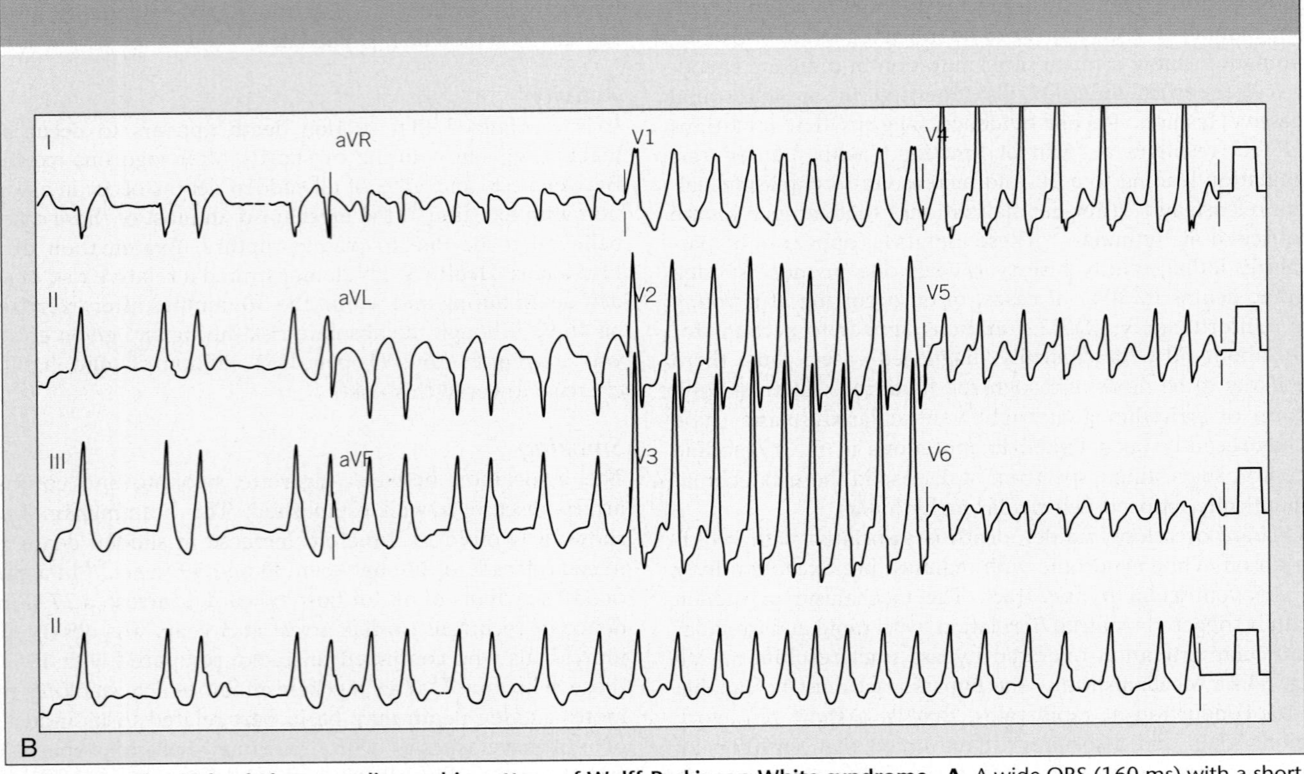

Figure 64.4 The 12-lead electrocardiographic pattern of Wolff-Parkinson-White syndrome. A, A wide QRS (160 ms) with a short PR interval and delta waves are evident. Positive QRS in V_1, II, III, and aVF and predominantly negative QRS in I and aVL suggest a left lateral location. **B,** During atrial fibrillation, extremely rapid conduction through the accessory pathway to the ventricle with cycle lengths as short as 240 ms (>250 beats per minute).

drugs, including quinidine, sotalol, and ibutilide.[42] However, it can clearly occur with drugs without primarily antiarrhythmic properties, such as tricyclic antidepressants, nonsedating antihistamines, phenothiazines, antimalarials, certain antibiotics, antifungals, and cisapride. A study by Siscovick and coworkers[44] demonstrated an increased risk of sudden death in patients taking thiazide diuretics when a potassium-sparing drug was not prescribed. However, the finding of low potassium concentration in sudden death survivors is very common, partly owing to the kaliuric action of high catecholamine states, and linking it to the etiology of the arrest should be done cautiously. Potassium depletion, magnesium depletion, and hypercalcemia may all prolong the QT in susceptible individuals. Myocardial hypertrophy and T-wave abnormalities also predispose to the acquired long QT syndrome.

In patients who have the acquired long QT syndrome, it is very important that the underlying cause be identified and reversed. Offending agents should be stopped, bradycardia should be corrected, and electrolytes should be repleted. Acutely, the preferred therapy for torsades de pointes in the setting of the acquired long QT syndrome is intravenous administration of magnesium. Magnesium therapy does not normalize the QT, however, so underlying causes should continue to be corrected.

Autonomic Tone

Studies documenting episodes of sudden death during Holter monitoring have demonstrated increases in sinus rate and frequency of ventricular extrasystoles before the onset of VF. These events have preponderance for the early morning hours, suggesting circadian variations in sympathetic tone as potential contributors to autonomic instability. In animal models of acute ischemia, either alone or in the setting of chronic infarction, there is good evidence linking the increase in sympathetic activity to VF. In these models, β-receptor blockade appears to be protective against ischemia-mediated VF.

A clear link between abnormal vagal input to the heart and the increased risk of sudden death has been described both in animal models of ischemia and in humans after an infarction. In a study of 78 postinfarction patients, baroreflex sensitivity, a reflection of parasympathetic inputs to the sinus node, was noted to be significantly lower in the individuals who subsequently died.[45] Overall, interactions between the sympathetic and parasympathetic nervous systems in the heart are incompletely understood, but their influence on the advent of sudden death remains compelling.

CLINICAL PRESENTATIONS

In the Seattle experience,[46] the typical sudden death survivor is a 64-year-old man (81%) with coronary artery disease and a remote history of myocardial infarction. Only 19% had evidence of new ST elevation myocardial infarction at the time of arrest and 38% had a diagnosis of myocardial infarction established by enzyme analysis. Prodromes such as chest pain, dyspnea, palpitations, and fatigue have been reported in some population studies, but a prospective study showed that only 12% of victims had consulted a physician in the preceding 6 months with complaints of new or worsening angina[47] compared with 33% with myocardial infarctions.

The initial rhythm in sudden death has been a matter of controversy. It has long been assumed to be VF because VT was rarely observed by paramedics on arrival at the scene. Recent trials have helped to elucidate this point. A study looking at the outcomes of rapid defibrillation by security officers in casinos,[48] in which the mean time from collapse to attachment of a defibrillator was 3.5 ± 2.9 minutes, showed that VF accounted for 71% of the initial rhythms. The remainder either had asystole or pulseless electrical activity. In sudden death survivors with a mean left ventricular ejection fraction of 42% ± 18% and a 70% prevalence of coronary artery disease receiving ICDs with electrogram storage ability, VT was the most common stored arrhythmia as an initial rhythm.[49] This conflicts with the findings of Raitt and associates,[50] in which VF was more commonly found. The reason for this discrepancy is not clear but may be due to different patient subsets and how the original rhythm is defined. Most believe that the original rhythm is an organized ventricular rhythm that within a few seconds degenerates into VF (Fig. 64.5).

The rhythm on arrival of the paramedics influences prognosis. In the Seattle experience, 40% of victims have VF as the initial recorded rhythm, and 26% of these (or 10% of the total) will be discharged from the hospital without neurologic sequelae with aptly timed cardiopulmonary resuscitation, paramedical arrival, and automatic external difibrillators.[46] In the study by Valenzuela and coworkers,[48] 56% were discharged from the hospital when the rhythm was VF compared with 0% for asystole or pulseless electrical activity.

The induction of hypothermia by endovascular cooling has been a great advance in the management of comatose survivors of out-of-hospital cardiac arrest. Cooling to 33°C for 24 hours has been proved safe, with improved survival and short-term neurologic recovery (53%) compared with standard treatment (34%).[51] (See Chapter 65).

DIAGNOSTIC TECHNIQUES

Diagnostic techniques have two main goals: determination of the cause of sudden death in survivors and identification of individuals at high risk for development of sudden death (primary prevention). Sudden death survivors merit a thorough investigation as to the cause of their arrest. Although the electrocardiogram is limited in predicting high risk for sudden death, it is very useful at establishing causality and prognosis if certain abnormalities are present in survivors. Such diagnoses as long QT syndrome, Brugada syndrome, arrhythmogenic right ventricular dysplasia, Wolff-Parkinson-White pattern, old myocardial infarctions, aneurysms, and left ventricular hypertrophy are hallmarks of high risk of recurrence if no intervention is done.

Further investigations should include a drug history with drug screen; family history; history of syncope or presyncope; cardiac enzyme analysis; cardiac imaging; determination of serum potassium, calcium, and magnesium levels; and continuous electrocardiographic monitoring. The presence or absence of significant coronary artery disease should be established early, preferably by coronary angiography, as should determination of left ventricular function. Metabolic derangement, acute ischemia or infarcts, and drug effects have

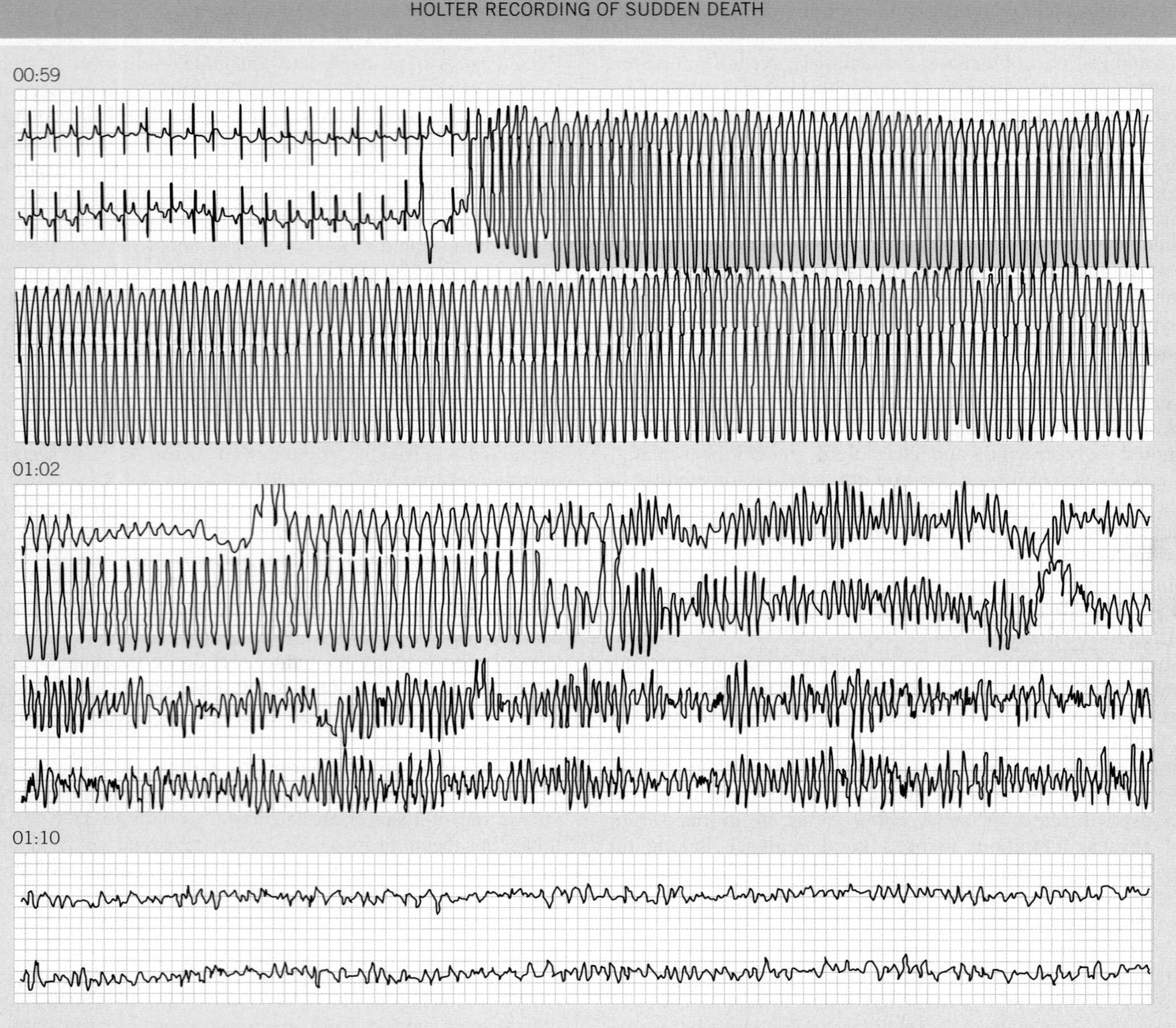

Figure 64.5 Holter recording of sudden death. The tracing shows an organized monomorphic ventricular tachycardia progressively degenerating into ventricular fibrillation. (From Aziz S, McMahon RF, Garratt CJ. Sudden cardiac death in arrhythmogenic right ventricular dysplasia. Circulation 2000;101:825-827.)

traditionally been considered to portend a good prognosis if the causative agent is avoided in the future. This has been put into question by an AVID substudy in which individuals with "correctable causes" remained at high risk for death, suggesting that further work is needed in terms of determining which causes of VF are truly reversible.[52] The term *primary VF* refers to sudden death in individuals without structural, electrical, or coronary abnormalities in whom no correctable cause can be identified.

Given the limitations of the 12-lead electrocardiogram and left ventricular function in determining which patients are at sufficiently high risk, other diagnostic modalities have evolved. The inducibility of sustained ventricular tachyarrhythmia by programmed electrical stimulation has been identified as a marker of heightened risk of arrhythmic death. Inducibility in patients who have had sustained VT or cardiac arrest survivors in whom no identifiable cause exists predicts a high risk of recurrent life-threatening arrhythmias. In individuals with prior myocardial infarction and documented VT, the sensitivity for induction of VT is 90%.[53] In patients without a prior infarct, the sensitivity is much less.[54] In very high risk patients, such as those with ischemic cardiomyopathies and syncope and sudden death survivors, a normal finding on electrophysiologic testing is often considered a false-negative result so that implantation of a defibrillator is often performed despite noninducibility.[55]

Given the false-negatives with electrophysiologic testing, its poor sensitivity in the absence of prior myocardial infarctions, and its invasive nature, other markers of high risk for arrhythmic death have been sought. Signal averaging of the electrocardiogram amplifies, filters, and improves the resolution of small potentials in the terminal portion of the QRS complex. These are thought to represent late potentials and prospective substrates for lethal tachyarrhythmias. Although the negative predictive value is excellent, its positive predictive value is low; thus, although it identifies a low-risk group, it is not sufficiently powerful to detect a high-risk individual.[56]

Two other markers of abnormal repolarization have been studied. QT dispersion represents the difference between the maximal and minimal QT intervals on a 12-lead electrocardiogram and has been advanced as a potential predictor of sudden death. However, the feasibility of obtaining any meaningful information from this method has been questioned because of several methodologic constraints.[57] T-wave alternans, defined as microvolt changes in T-wave amplitude from beat to beat, is the other measure of abnormal repolarization. Its presence in high-risk patients at specified heart rates identifies a high risk for arrhythmic deaths.[58] Until recently, this method of risk stratification had been validated only for individuals with ischemic cardiomyopathy. However, the ALPHA study showed that even in nonischemic individuals with NYHA class II or class III symptoms, an abnormal T-wave alternans test was associated with a fourfold higher risk of cardiac death and life-threatening arrhythmias.[59] Conversely, those in whom T-wave alternans tests were normal were found to have a very good prognosis at 18 months.

The role of the autonomic system in triggering sudden death has been well established. Heart rate variability looks at the relative influences of the sympathetic and parasympathetic systems on heart rate, both on a 12-lead electrocardiogram and during a 24-hour period. Reduced variability in R-R intervals during 24 hours translates into decreased parasympathetic tone. In combination with other risk factors, it has a relatively high accuracy for determining the risk of sudden death.[60]

MANAGEMENT

Data from the Trials on Prophylactic Implantable Cardioverter-Defibrillators

Secondary Prevention

The use of antiarrhythmic agents for the prevention of sudden death has been almost uniformly disappointing. The Cardiac Arrhythmia Suppression Trial (CAST)[61] examined the results of suppression of premature ventricular contractions after myocardial infarction with flecainide, encainide, and moricizine. The trial was prematurely stopped because of increased mortality in the treatment group and has led to the classification of group I agents as contraindicated in patients with structural heart disease. Amiodarone has shown more promise; two trials (EMIAT, CAMIAT)[62,63] showed no increase in mortality over placebo, and one (GESICA)[64] showed improved mortality compared with placebo. After several smaller studies showed a mortality benefit from ICD therapy, large randomized and prospective studies were designed to evaluate the role of ICDs in primary and secondary prevention of sudden death. The Antiarrhythmics Versus Implantable Defibrillators (AVID)[65] trial conducted a randomized comparison of ICD versus either amiodarone or sotalol in patients who had had life-threatening ventricular tachyarrhythmias (Fig. 64.6). These patients either had been resuscitated from VF (45%) or were cardioverted from hemodynamically significant sustained VT (55%). All patients with sustained VT had left ventricular ejection fractions of less than 40%; the average left ventricular ejection fraction of the group was about 31% in both arms. Although patients in the medication arm were randomized to either amiodarone (empirically dosed) or sotalol (dose guided by Holter or electrophysiologic testing), 96% were receiving amiodarone by the time of discharge. The overall survival at 1 year was 89% for the ICD group and 82% for the antiarrhythmic group. At 3 years, the survival was 75% for the ICD group and 64% for the medical treatment group, hence representing a 29% reduction in mortality at 3 years for the ICD. One major criticism leveled at the AVID study related to the disparity in beta-blocker use between the arms: 42% in ICD patients and 17% in the medication arm.

Two additional large trials addressed the issue. The Cardiac Arrest Study Hamburg (CASH)[66] randomized cardiac survivors with documented tachyarrhythmias to receive an ICD or amiodarone, propafenone, or metoprolol. The propafenone arm was subsequently discontinued because of higher mortality compared with ICD. The study found a 23% (nonsignificant) reduction in all-cause mortality in the ICD arm compared with amiodarone or metoprolol. Of note, no beta blockers were used in the ICD arm, and the mean ejection fraction in the study was about 45%. The Canadian Implantable Defibrillator Study (CIDS)[67] randomized patients who had been resuscitated from VF, VT, or unmonitored syncope with subsequently documented VT to receive either an ICD or amiodarone. The ICD group was found to have 20% (nonsignificant) relative risk reduction in all-cause mortality. The mean ejection fraction in this study was approximately 33%, and there was a significantly higher use of beta blockers in the ICD arm. A post hoc multivariate Cox analysis of the CIDS data determined that age 70 years or older, ejection fraction of 35% or less, and NYHA class III or class IV were predictors of individuals who were most likely to benefit from ICD therapy.[68] A meta-analysis of AVID, CASH, and CIDS found that ICD therapy had a 28% relative risk reduction in total mortality compared with amiodarone, which was due almost entirely to a 50% reduction in arrhythmic death.[69] On the basis of the data from these trials, one can conclude that ICD therapy is superior to amiodarone at improving survival after cardiac arrest.

Primary Prevention

As noted earlier, the largest social impact by the successful treatment of sudden cardiac death would be expected in the general population who are at lowest risk. Despite recent advances in automatic external defibrillators and the public health initiative that has made this lifesaving intervention widely available in certain settings, survival of a first arrhythmic event remains dismal both in mortality and in resulting morbidity. Because of the low survival associated with out-of-hospital cardiac arrest, some trials have aimed to examine the strategy of primary prevention, which is implantation of ICDs in high-risk groups to prevent a first occurrence of sudden death. The Multicenter Automatic Defibrillator Implantation Trial (MADIT)[70] was based on the knowledge that nonsustained VT in patients who had had a myocardial infarction and with reduced left ventricular

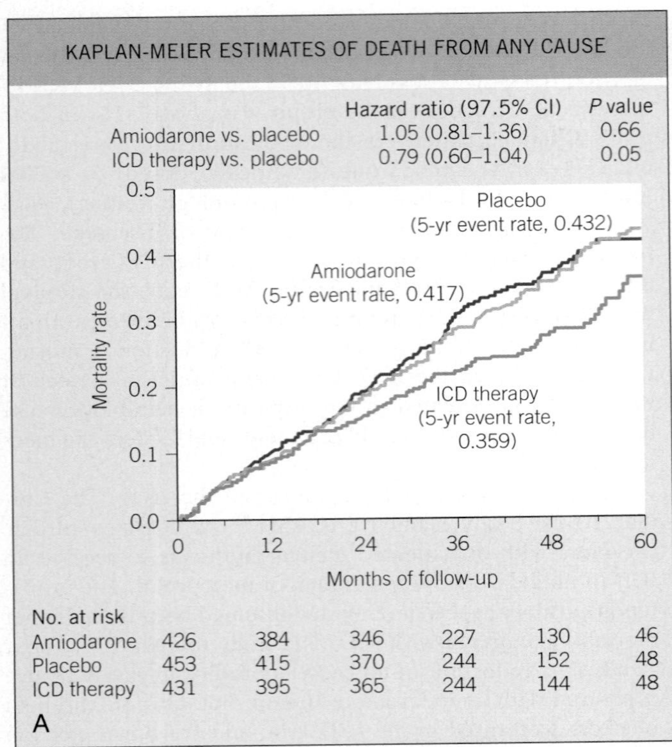

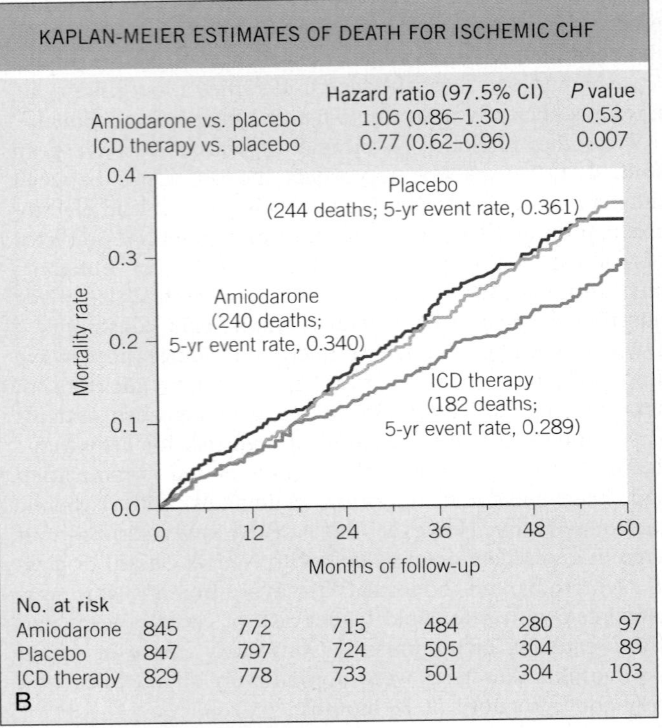

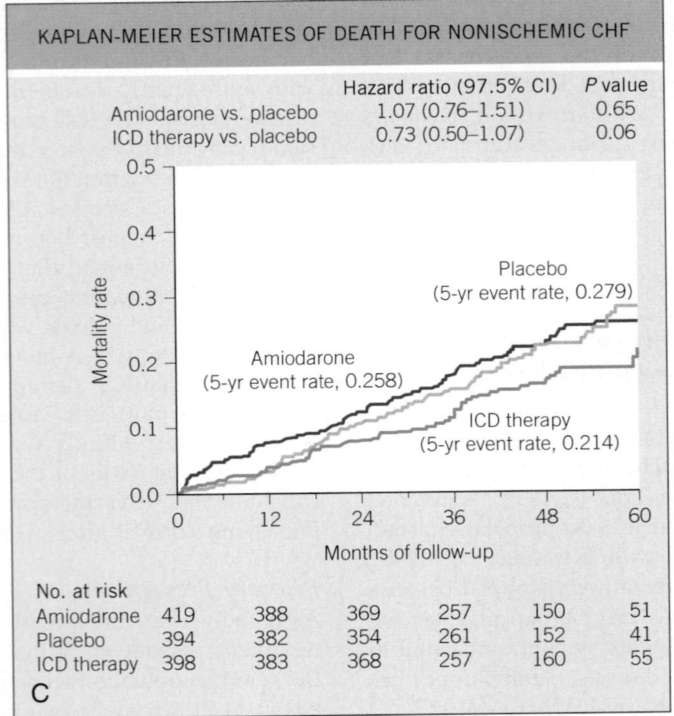

Figure 64.6 A, Kaplan-Meier estimates of death from any cause. B and **C,** Kaplan-Meier estimates of death from any cause for the prespecified subgroups of ischemic **(B)** and nonischemic **(C)** congestive heart failure (CHF). ICD, implantable cardioverter-defibrillator. (Data from Bardy GH, Lee KL, Mark DB, et al. Amiodarone or an implantable cardioverter-defibrillator for congestive heart failure. N Engl J Med 2005;352:225-237.)

function is associated with a 2-year mortality of 30%.[71] The study included patients with nonsustained asymptomatic VT, ejection fraction less than 35%, prior myocardial infarction, and inducible sustained VT that was not suppressible with procainamide. Patients were randomized to receive either an ICD or an antiarrhythmic drug, which in most cases (75%) was amiodarone. The trial was terminated early because of a 54% reduction in mortality rate in the ICD arm. Again, the use of beta blockers was higher in the ICD arm.

The Coronary Artery Bypass Graft (CABG) Patch Trial[72] used an abnormal signal-averaged electrocardiogram as a high-risk predictor in patients with a left ventricular ejection fraction of 35% or less undergoing coronary artery bypass surgery. Patients were randomized to ICD versus no therapy, and no survival advantage could be found for the ICD. The reason for the conflict in findings with those of MADIT I may be that revascularization is a potent prevention of VF or VT. Another may be that VT inducibility with invasive testing is more powerful than the signal-averaged electrocardiogram at identifying individuals in whom an ICD will be beneficial.

The role of the defibrillator in preventing sudden death in patients in whom VT is inducible at electrophysiologic study is supported by further studies. The Multicenter Unsustained Tachycardia Trial (MUSTT) investigators[73] sought to test the hypothesis that antiarrhythmic therapy guided by electrophysiologic testing can reduce the risks of sudden death and cardiac arrest among patients with coronary artery disease, left ventricular dysfunction (ejection fraction ≤40%), and spontaneous unsustained VT. Patients in whom VT could be induced were randomized to no antiarrhythmic therapy or antiarrhythmic therapy. Patients randomized to antiarrhythmic therapy received class I agents (26%), amiodarone (10%), sotalol (9%), or defibrillators (46%). The mean ejection fraction was 30%. It was found that the 5-year estimates of overall mortality were not significantly lower for the patients receiving electrophysiologically guided therapy (42%) than for those assigned to no antiarrhythmic therapy (48%). However, in looking at the benefit of defibrillators alone, there was a significant decrease in both arrhythmic death and overall mortality (see Fig. 64.6). A follow-up to the same study[74] examined the differences in outcome between inducible and noninducible patients and found a small but significant difference in both arrhythmic death (32% versus 24%) and overall mortality (48% versus 44%) at 5 years.

The MADIT II trial[75] investigated the role of the defibrillator in patients with very low ejection fraction (≤30%) and prior myocardial infarction. Patients were randomly assigned to a defibrillator or conventional medical therapy, and electrophysiologic testing was not required. During an average follow-up of 20 months, the mortality rates were 19.8% for the conventional therapy group and 14.2% for the defibrillator group. Documentation of nonsustained VT was not required.

The effectiveness of ICD therapy was once again confirmed and the indications broadened by the results of the Sudden Cardiac Death in Heart Failure Trial (SCD-HeFT).[76] More than 2500 patients were randomly assigned to receive either amiodarone or an implantable single-chamber ICD in addition to conventional therapy. This trial included patients who had NYHA class II or class III heart failure symptoms with an ejection fraction of 35% or less, regardless of whether the cause was ischemic or nonischemic. The ICD treatment group demonstrated a 23% reduction in all-cause mortality compared with placebo and no significant difference between amiodarone and placebo. The primary endpoint was death from any cause. Importantly, this was the first trial to demonstrate a mortality benefit in patients with nonischemic cardiomyopathy (see Fig. 64.6).

For patients with coronary artery disease, therapy aimed at decreasing ischemia and congestive heart failure is the cornerstone of prevention. The use of beta blockers after a myocardial infarction has been determined to decrease the incidence of sudden death, as have angiotensin-converting enzymes inhibitors.

In 1998, ICD placement became the therapy of choice for survivors of sudden death and for patients with coronary artery disease who present with sustained VT. In such a situation, even if revascularization is possible, the ICD remains the treatment of choice. This situation should not be confused with that in which an arrest accompanies acute ischemia or infarction, in which management of the coronary artery disease is the primary objective. VF occurring within 24 hours of acute myocardial infarction is usually attributed to ischemia and reperfusion and does not imply a worsened prognosis. On the other hand, sustained monomorphic VT cannot be ascribed to ischemia and warrants further electrophysiologic evaluation.

On the basis of the results of the MUSTT study and others, electrophysiologically guided drug testing has been replaced by ICD implantation in individuals with primary VF and VT. Patients in whom nonsustained VT is observed and revascularization is planned should be tested for inducibility after they have been revascularized. Likewise, if sustained VT occurred in the setting of ischemia, inducibility needs to be assessed after revascularization.

The ICD is the best option today for prevention of sudden cardiac death, with excellent efficacy and a very low complication rate. Therefore, the ICD is the treatment of choice for individuals who are at high risk for sudden cardiac death: survivors of sudden cardiac death, aborted sudden cardiac death, syncope with subsequent documented ventricular tachyarrhythmia (spontaneous or induced), and arguably even syncope in patients with severely decreased ejection fraction, regardless of whether any arrhythmias are documented.[55] Detailed guidelines for the use of ICDs for prevention of sudden death have been published jointly by the American College of Cardiology, the American Heart Association, European Society of Cardiology, and the Heart Rhythm Society (see Table 66.3 and Chapter 66).[78]

Because the benefit of ICDs in a large population is clear but relatively small, clinical judgment is currently considered necessary to select patients most likely to benefit from the potential increase in life expectancy. Furthering of our ability to foresee which individuals are most likely to derive benefit from this technology is still needed.

chapter 65

Cardiopulmonary Resuscitation: Evidence-Based Improvements in Basic Life Support

Jose A. Joglar and Richard L. Page

Definition

- Cardiopulmonary resuscitation includes all measures to provide assisted circulation to vital organs to prevent irreversible damage and to reestablish a stable cardiac rhythm and hemodynamics in victims of cardiac arrest.

Key Features

- Cardiac arrest remains a leading cause of death in the Western world.
- External chest compression provides a small but critical fraction of normal cardiac output and improves survival when it is administered early.
- For the majority of adults in cardiac arrest, defibrillation represents definitive treatment.

Clinical Implications

- Newer cardiopulmonary resuscitation techniques aimed at improving outcomes in cardiac arrest victims are under investigation, and recent guidelines with stronger emphasis on scientific evidence have been released.
- High-quality chest compressions should be provided, with interruption kept to an absolute minimum.
- The automated external defibrillator allows minimally trained operators to provide defibrillation to victims of cardiac arrest, with resultant improvement in survival when the shock is delivered promptly. For victims who have been unconscious for more than 4 to 5 minutes, 2 minutes of CPR should precede the first shock.
- Therapeutic hypothermia enhances outcome in comatose survivors of cardiac arrest.
- The postresuscitation period represents a fertile area for investigation.

Heart disease remains a leading cause of death in industrialized countries. For example, in the United States, heart disease was a primary cause of mortality in 2004, accounting for 654,092 cases or 27% of all deaths.[1] The proportion of these that are considered "sudden" varies, as vital statistics do not specifically define "cardiac arrest" or "sudden death." Nevertheless, on the basis of surrogate data, approximately 160,000 patients are treated for out-of-hospital cardiac arrest in North America every year, and 330,000 die of coronary artery disease either outside the hospital or in emergency departments.[2]

Unfortunately, survival from cardiac arrest remains poor; even in cities with advanced emergency medical systems, survival to discharge from the hospital without neurologic damage averages 6% or less. The poor survival statistics can be attributed to several factors, including delay in recognition of cardiac arrest, delay in activation of emergency medical systems, lack of widespread knowledge of cardiopulmonary resuscitation (CPR), and delay in arrival of trained professionals. In response to these difficulties in delivery of emergency care, guidelines on the sequence of events to be followed in the setting of a cardiac arrest have been developed, called the chain of survival. The four links of the chain are

- recognition of the event and activation of the emergency medical service;
- CPR;
- prompt defibrillation, if it is indicated; and
- administration of advanced cardiac life support, including advanced airway management and the administration of drugs.

In 2005, the American Heart Association published guidelines for CPR and emergency cardiovascular care.[2] These most recent guidelines are based on the most extensive evidence review of CPR yet published. Based on evidence from human and animal studies, the guidelines place emphasis on simplifying the information that rescuers need to learn and to remember. There is also emphasis on preventing interruption of chest compressions and avoiding detrimental interventions such as hyperventilation. The classification of recommendations based on the level of evidence is detailed in Table 65.1.

Time to defibrillation is considered the most important determinant of survival in cardiac arrest as most adults who suffer a witnessed cardiac arrest initially demonstrate ventricular arrhythmias. In recognition of this fact, the public access defibrillation initiative seeks to make early defibrillation "widespread" and to provide cardiac arrest victims with a better chance of survival.[3] Significant advances have been made in public access defibrillation thanks to the development of the modern automated external defibrillator (AED), which allows lay responders with modest training to deliver cardiac defibrillation. The AED incorporates advanced technology, such as a biphasic shock waveform, but is simple to use. Early experience in specific environments, such as in casinos and aboard commercial aircraft, confirmed that early defibrillation translates into improved survival. Consequently, guidelines have emphasized the importance of early defibrillation and include AED training in the course for basic life support.

The chance of survival is high when the cardiac arrest is witnessed, the initial rhythm is ventricular tachycardia or

APPLYING CLASSIFICATION OF RECOMMENDATIONS AND LEVEL OF EVIDENCE.			
Class I	**Class IIa**	**Class IIb**	**Class III**
Benefit >>> Risk	**Benefit >> Risk**	**Benefit ≥ Risk**	**Risk ≥ Benefit**
Procedure/treatment or diagnostic test/assessment should be performed/ administered.	It is reasonable to perform procedure/administer treatment or perform diagnostic test/ assessment.	Procedure/treatment or diagnostic test/ assessment may be considered.	Procedure/treatment or diagnostic test/ assessment should not be performed/ administered. It is not helpful and may be harmful.

Table 65.1 Applying classification of recommendations and level of evidence. (From International Liaison Committee on Resuscitation, 2005.[7]

fibrillation, and prompt CPR and defibrillation are provided. In contrast, when the initial rhythm is bradyasystole (ventricular rates below 60 beats per minute, periods of asystole, or both), the prognosis is grim. The only exception is when the arrest is witnessed and the bradycardia is due to easily correctable causes such as hypoxemia. When the cardiac arrest is unwitnessed and the initial rhythm is asystole, survival is nearly zero. In patients with pulseless electrical activity (the presence of an organized cardiac rhythm without a palpable pulse), the goal is to identify and to correct the cause, which may include pulmonary embolism, cardiac tamponade, myocardial infarction, and other factors. When the patient is believed to have been unconscious for more than 3 minutes, it is recommended that CPR for 2 minutes precede shock from the AED.

Unfortunately, in many cases after return of spontaneous circulation, neurologic dysfunction frequently occurs, probably as a result of reperfusion injury after blood flow is reestablished. This and other factors contribute to a period of postresuscitation dysfunction that is associated with substantial morbidity and mortality. For this reason, the second step in resuscitation, and one that is fertile for clinical investigation, is aimed at the treatment and prevention of postresuscitation injury and disease.

BASIC LIFE SUPPORT

Basic life support defines the sequence of actions taken during the first few minutes of a cardiac arrest and comprises the first three links in the chain of survival, including early activation of the emergency medical system, early CPR, and early defibrillation. As most adult victims of cardiac arrest will benefit from early defibrillation, an important component of basic life support is AED training and use.

Cardiopulmonary Resuscitation

The aim of basic CPR is to prolong viability until definitive treatment, usually a defibrillator, becomes available. Studies have shown that when CPR is administered promptly by bystanders, the odds of survival improve approximately twofold.[4] Furthermore, CPR plus defibrillation within 3 to 5 minutes of collapse can produce survival rates as high as 75%.

Mechanism of Action

Two basic mechanisms are believed to be operative for the production of forward blood flow during CPR:

- an increase in intrathoracic pressure during chest compression forces blood out of the chest (thoracic pump theory); and
- direct myocardial compression forces additional blood out of the heart (cardiac pump theory).[5]

During the decompression phase of CPR, a transient pressure gradient is generated between the aorta and right atrium, which allows myocardial perfusion.[6]

Description of Technique

The 2005 guidelines provide the sequence of steps for performing basic CPR (Fig. 65.1).[2] Initially, the rescuer checks for response by tapping on the victim and yelling, “Are you all right?” Once a rescuer confirms that the victim is unresponsive, the rescuer should immediately activate the local emergency medical system and get an AED if it is available. The next step is airway management. To relieve airway obstruction, the head is tilted back by applying backward pressure on the victim’s forehead, and the chin is lifted (the head tilt–chin lift maneuver). In suspected trauma to the neck, the jaw is thrust forward without head tilt (jaw thrust maneuver). The rescuer then looks, listens, and feels for ventilations. If the patient is not breathing, 2 breaths are administered either mouth to mouth or by use of a breathing mask. Breaths are given during 1 second with enough volume to cause the victim’s chest to rise with each breath. This recommended 1-second duration to make the chest rise applies to all forms of ventilation during CPR and is one important change compared with the prior 2000 guidelines.

Unless the rescuer is a health care professional, he or she should not palpate for a pulse but rather should initiate chest compressions without checking for a pulse if the patient is not breathing. Health care professionals should not spend more than 10 seconds searching for a pulse before initiating chest compressions as this effort can be unreliable even for trained professionals.[7]

Because effective chest compressions are essential for providing critical blood flow during CPR, the 2005 guidelines emphasize the quality of chest compressions, and algorithms were revised to minimize interruption in chest compressions. These changes are based on animal studies that have demonstrated improved coronary perfusion and survival rates when compressions are uninterrupted as well as on clinical studies demonstrating suboptimal compression technique in a high percentage of cases, even when CPR was provided by trained professionals. Therefore, the guidelines call for rescuers to “push hard and push fast.”[2] Chest compressions should be applied in a rhythmic fashion to the lower half of the sternum (between the nipples) to a depth of 4 to 5 cm, at a rate of approximately 100 compressions per minute. The chest must be allowed to recoil fully between compressions. The 2005 guidelines recommend that a ratio of 30 compressions to 2 ventilations be maintained, regardless of whether one or two rescuers are involved

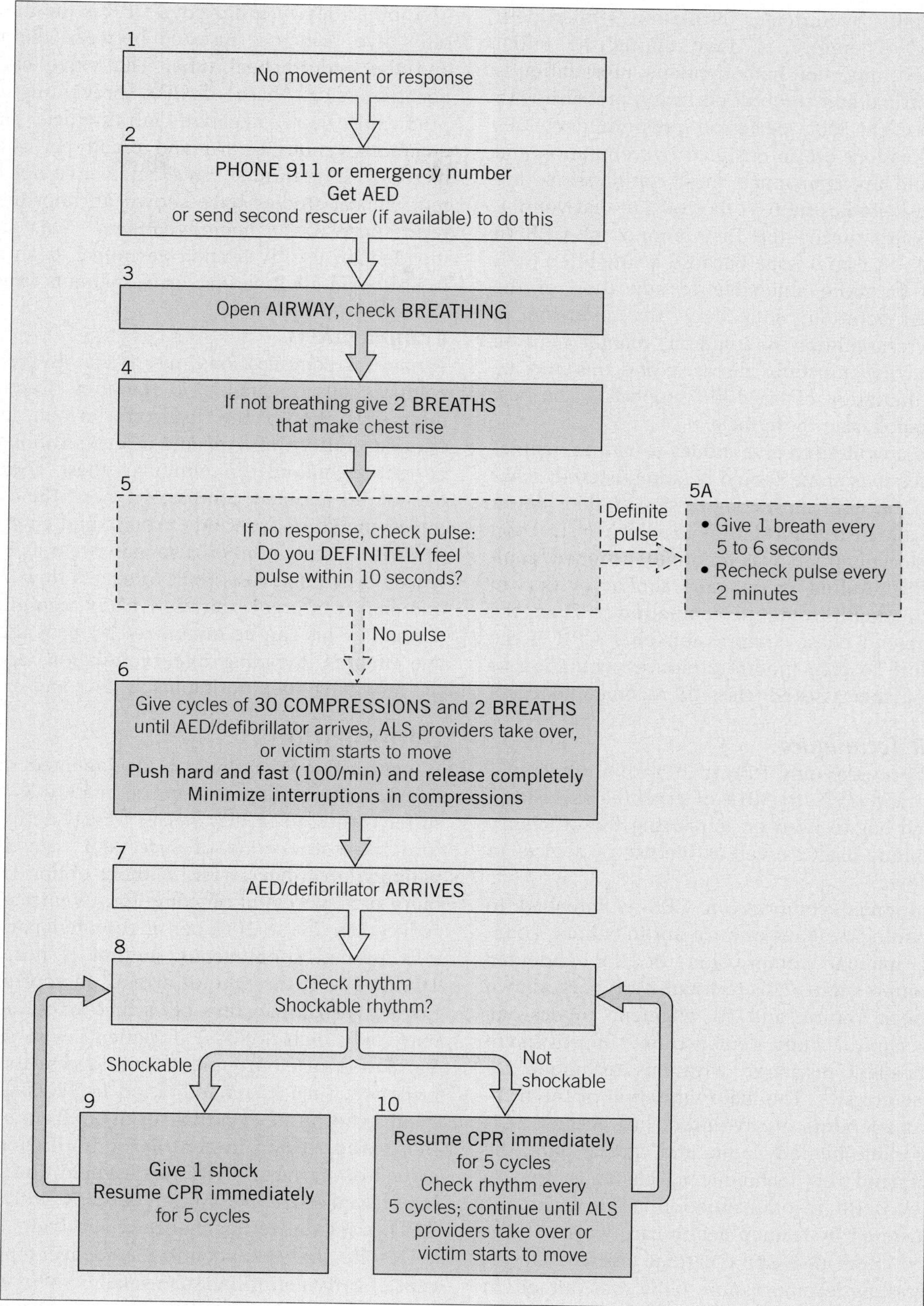

Figure 65.1 Algorithm for basic life support. AED, automated external defibrillator; ALS, advanced life support; CPR, cardiopulmonary resuscitation. (With permission from International Liaison Committee on Resuscitation. 2005 International Consensus on Cardiopulmonary Resuscitation and Emergency Cardiovascular Care Science with Treatment Recommendations. Circulation 2005;112:III1-III130. Copyright © 2005 American Heart Association.)

(in prior guidelines, the ratio was 15 to 2). This change aims not only to minimize interruptions of chest compressions but also to reduce the likelihood of hyperventilation, which can be detrimental. Once the airway is secured by endotracheal intubation, compressions may be continuous, with a ventilation rate of 8 to 10 breaths per minute.

Compression-only CPR

In adults who suffer cardiac arrest as a result of ventricular fibrillation, the value of mouth-to-mouth ventilation has been brought into question.[8] It has been demonstrated that spontaneous gasping can maintain adequate minute ventilation, Pa_{O_2}, and Pa_{CO_2}.[9] Furthermore, the arterial system of adults who succumb to ventricular fibrillation is filled with oxygenated blood. Therefore, at least during the initial 5 minutes, the most important hemodynamic intervention is to generate myocardial and cerebral perfusion pressure with chest compressions. In fact, perfusion pressure decreases when chest compressions are interrupted by ventilation and takes time to build up again once chest compressions are reinitiated.[8] Clinical studies support the concept that ventilation is not necessary during the first minutes of CPR in adults.[10] This is not a trivial issue because a simplified CPR technique would be more amenable to education of the general public. In addition, data show that aversion to mouth-to-mouth resuscitation is common, mainly because of fears of contracting infectious diseases, and this may be a disincentive to initiation of basic life support.[11] The new 2005 guidelines emphasize these facts.

If the rescuer is unwilling to give mouth-to-mouth ventilation, chest compressions alone should be administered; it has been shown that CPR with chest compression alone is better than no CPR at all. In a clinical trial in which instruction from dispatchers to volunteers was randomly assigned, compression-only CPR resulted in outcome similar to that of compressions plus mouth-to-mouth ventilation.[12] Thus, the guidelines recommend chest compression–only CPR if the rescuer is unwilling to give mouth-to-mouth ventilation or if the CPR is dispatcher assisted (class IIa recommendation).

Alternative CPR Techniques

As standard CPR provides only 15% to 20% of normal myocardial perfusion and 25% to 30% of cerebral perfusion,[5] extensive research has focused on improving the efficiency of the CPR technique itself as well as the use of devices to enhance blood flow.

Interposed abdominal compression CPR is intended to simulate the physiologic effects of intra-aortic balloon counterpulsation by manual compression of the abdomen between chest compressions. This technique has been shown to enhance venous return and to augment myocardial perfusion, and a clinical study demonstrated improvement in survival to hospital discharge with this technique for in-hospital cardiac arrest.[13] The main limitation of the technique is that two operators are required; but because it is safe and has favorable hemodynamic and clinical data, the guidelines recommend this technique as an alternative to standard CPR (class IIb recommendation). This technique should be administered by trained health care workers; it is not recommended in out-of-hospital cardiac arrest.

Active compression-decompression CPR was aimed at creation of negative pressure by use of a suctioning device on the sternum. This allows a decrease in the intrathoracic pressure during the decompression phase and increases the difference in intrathoracic pressure between the upstroke and downstroke phases of chest compression. Despite the theoretical potential of this technique, a randomized study failed to show clinical benefit.[14] A preliminary study demonstrated potential benefit of the use of a pneumatically cycled circumferential thoracic vest compared with manual CPR.[15] The study was limited by its small size, but greater aortic and coronary perfusion pressures were obtained with this device. Whether it will translate into important clinical benefits remains to be determined.

Another device to improve CPR is the impedance threshold valve, which is inserted between the ventilation bag and the endotracheal tube. The valve closes during the decompression phase of CPR, preventing inspiration and producing more negative intrathoracic pressure, which enhances venous return and organ perfusion.[16] Although increased long-term survival rates have not been documented, clinical studies have shown an improvement in short-term survival and hemodynamics.[17] This device is recommended for use by trained personnel as an adjunct to CPR in intubated adult cardiac arrest patients (class IIa).

Complications

Numerous complications may occur as the result of chest compressions, including rib fractures, fracture of the sternum, separation of the ribs from sternum, lung trauma, and even lacerations of liver and spleen. Although adherence to correct technique can minimize these complications, they cannot be avoided completely; nevertheless, concerns for injury should not preclude prompt and energetic application of CPR. Gastric inflation also may occur as a complication of rescue breathing, as a result of excess flow volume and rate, and may promote aspiration from regurgitation of gastric contents. This can be minimized by providing 1-second rescue breaths, avoiding hyperventilation, and ensuring that the airway is open during inspiration and expiration.

Defibrillation

A ventricular arrhythmia is documented during the initial minutes after collapse in approximately 85% of adults who suffer witnessed cardiac arrest.[18] Early defibrillation is therefore the cornerstone of successful resuscitation for most patients in cardiac arrest. Without defibrillation, the probability of a successful outcome from ventricular fibrillation is reduced by 7% to 10% per minute; few patients will survive if a normal spontaneous rhythm is not restored within 10 minutes of the time of arrest.[4] In contrast to the overall low survival for victims of cardiac arrest, survival rates are extremely high (>80%) in patients who suffer ventricular fibrillation in environments with access to immediate defibrillation, such as rehabilitation facilities. Furthermore, the great majority of eventual survivors from cardiac arrest are those who remain in ventricular fibrillation at the time of arrival of rescuers.[4] With this in mind, the new 2005 guidelines emphasize integration of CPR with the use of the AED to maximize the chance of survival.

Despite the overwhelming evidence supporting the concept of early defibrillation, a small body of evidence suggests that in those patients with "prolonged" ventricular fibrillation, defibrillation could do harm by converting to a resuscitation-refractory rhythm. Several animal studies have demonstrated that after prolonged cardiac arrest, the rate of return of spontaneous circulation was significantly improved when drugs and CPR were administered before defibrillation. Cobb and associates[19] conducted an observational study involving more than 1100 patients and demonstrated that 90 seconds of CPR before defibrillation resulted in improved survival (24% compared with 30%; $P = .04$). This benefit was predominantly seen in those who had been in arrest for more than 4 minutes (17% compared with 27%; $P = .01$).

Therefore, the new guidelines make a distinction in whether shock or CPR is to be provided first. Accordingly, when any rescuer witnesses either an out-of-hospital arrest or an in-hospital cardiac arrest and an AED is immediately available on-site, the rescuer should use the AED as soon as possible. In contrast, when an out-of-hospital cardiac arrest is not witnessed by emergency medical services personnel, the rescuer should give about 5 cycles of CPR (roughly 2 minutes) before checking the electrocardiogram rhythm and attempting defibrillation (class IIb).

Another important change in the new guidelines is the incorporation of the 1-shock protocol. In view of the high efficacy rate for the first shock with modern AED technology (>90% success) and to minimize interruption of chest compressions, the new recommendations are that when ventricular fibrillation or pulseless ventricular tachycardia is present, "the rescuer should deliver 1 shock and should then immediately resume CPR, beginning with chest compressions (class IIa). The rescuer should not delay resumption of chest compressions to recheck the rhythm or pulse. After 5 cycles (about 2 minutes) of CPR, the AED should then analyze the cardiac rhythm and deliver another shock if indicated (class IIB)."[2]

Mechanism of Defibrillation and Waveforms

Successful defibrillation depends on the administration of a shock to generate current flow through the heart that is sufficient to produce a strong, transient electrical field. This field interacts with myocardial cells that are characterized by a nonuniform and unpredictable distribution of refractoriness and partial refractoriness as a result of circulating ventricular fibrillation wavefronts. The mechanism of termination of cardiac arrhythmia by defibrillation remains unclear, but three different theories exist:

- The critical mass hypothesis suggests that a critical mass of myocardium is depolarized, with the remainder insufficient to sustain ventricular fibrillation.[20]
- The upper limit of vulnerability hypothesis argues that successful defibrillation requires a shock strength that exceeds the upper limit of vulnerability. Energies below this threshold reinitiate ventricular fibrillation by stimulating portions of the myocardium during the vulnerable period.[21]
- The progressive depolarization hypothesis, which integrates elements of the two preceding theories, states that stronger shocks depolarize more refractory myocardium, prolonging and synchronizing repolarization and refractoriness to decrease the probability of fibrillation after the shock.[22]

An important advance in the past decade has been the development of alternative waveforms for defibrillation. Specifically, newer defibrillators now use biphasic waveforms, which are superior to the traditional monophasic waveform because they require less energy for successful defibrillation. These waveforms have been of tremendous benefit for public access defibrillation because AEDs that incorporate biphasic waveforms can be built with smaller batteries and components, leading to an overall reduction in cost, size, and weight. Biphasic waveforms are now standard in implantable defibrillators as they have been shown to reduce energy requirements by 25% to 45%.[23]

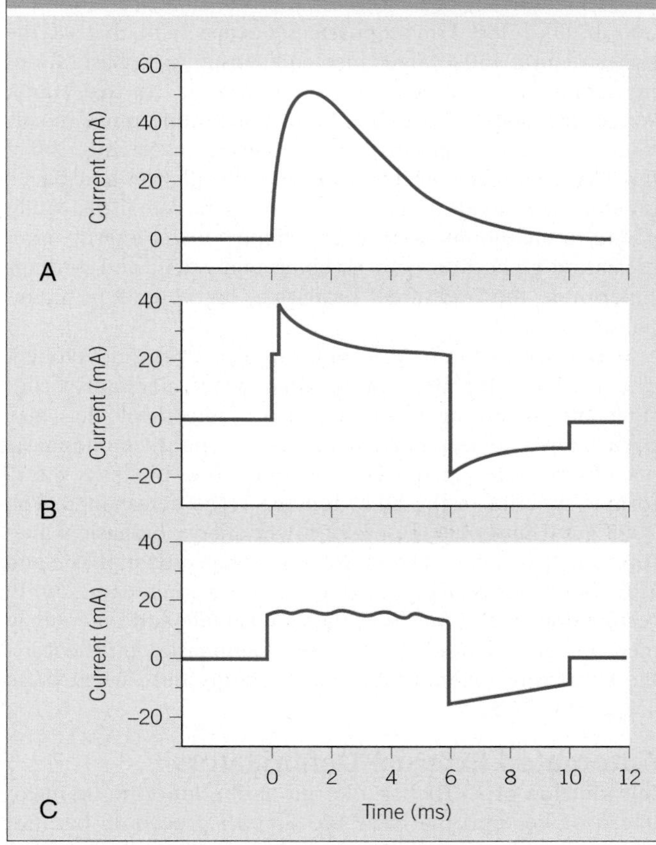

Figure 65.2 Different waveforms available for defibrillation. A, Damped sinusoidal monophasic. **B,** Truncated exponential biphasic. **C,** Rectilinear biphasic. (With permission from Takata TS, Page RL, Joglar JA. Automated external defibrillators: technical considerations and clinical promise. Ann Intern Med 2001;135:990-998.)

Monophasic waveforms deliver electrical energy in a single polarity—the current travels in a single direction. In contrast, with a biphasic waveform (Fig. 65.2), current reverses during the shock to travel in the opposite direction for a specific period (usually about 30% of the overall pulse duration). The advantage possessed by the biphasic waveform may derive from its ability to lower the defibrillation threshold by creating longer post-shock refractoriness in a greater percentage of cells than can be achieved with monophasic shocks.[24]

Traditionally, monophasic shocks were delivered as a progressive escalating sequence, usually 200 J, 300 J, and 360 J. This strategy attempted to minimize the amount of energy required for defibrillation, theoretically diminishing the potential for myocardial injury from the shock. By contrast, biphasic waveform devices can be equally successful or even superior with a series of three nonescalating shocks (150 J, 150 J, and 150 J). Impedance measurements during the delivered shock allow alterations to both the amount of current and the duration of current delivery (impedance compensating). Human studies conducted under controlled circumstances in the electrophysiology laboratory have shown equivalent defibrillation efficacy for 115 J and 130 J biphasic truncated shocks and 200 J damped monophasic shock.[25] A multicenter randomized prospective study compared the efficacy of defibrillation of the standard escalating 200 J/300 J/360 J monophasic sequence with that of the nonescalating 150 J impedance-compensating biphasic series in victims of out-of-hospital cardiac arrest.[26] In that study, which included 115 patients, there was no difference in survival in the two groups, but the group receiving 150 J biphasic treatment achieved faster defibrillation and had a greater likelihood of good cerebral function. This study added to the mounting data that support lower energy, nonescalating biphasic shocks as being equivalent and perhaps superior to the traditional escalating, higher energy monophasic shocks.

Variations of biphasic waveforms have been developed. The rectilinear biphasic, for example, which maintains a constant current during the first phase of the shock, has also been shown to be superior to higher energy monophasic waveforms (see Fig. 65.2).[27] Whether one biphasic waveform is superior to the other remains to be determined. The 2005 guidelines give the use of lower energy biphasic waveform for first shock (150 to 200 J for truncated biphasic and 120 J for rectilinear biphasic) a class IIa recommendation. In recognition of the fact that many hospitals and emergency medical services systems still use monophasic defibrillators, the consensus recommendation for energy dose when these are used is 360 J.

Automated External Defibrillators

Introduction of AEDs has allowed defibrillation to be introduced earlier into the basic life support procedure because the arrival of someone who is trained in the interpretation of arrhythmias is no longer required. These devices can analyze cardiac rhythm automatically and then deliver a commanded shock.

Most modern AEDs are designed in ways compatible with a public access defibrillation strategy: they are small, light, rugged, and inexpensive; they have the ability to self-test and to deter misuse; they provide data archiving and retrieval; and they require little maintenance. Furthermore, the lower energy requirement of biphasic waveforms is of great importance as it allows use of lithium batteries. Lithium batteries have a predictable life expectancy, do not require recharging or maintenance, and are energy dense; most types do not require special disposal.

With the use of sophisticated microprocessors, rhythm interpretation occurs through analysis of the surface electrocardiogram, measuring various components such as amplitude, frequency, slope, and wave morphology integration. The device also filters extraneous signals, such as motion artifact, loose electrodes, and nearby radio transmission, which could interfere with correct interpretation.

AEDs have performed extremely well in the interpretation of cardiac arrhythmias. The accurate detection of ventricular fibrillation with recommendations to shock range from 96% to 100%, whereas accurate withholding of defibrillation in appropriate rhythms (sinus tachycardia, asystole) approaches 100%.[28] The rare errors in electrocardiogram analysis have been those of omission, in which the device recommends no shock be given, typically in the presence of fine ventricular fibrillation. AEDs will also recommend shock for ventricular tachycardia as long as the rate exceeds the AED programmed value. The shocks are not synchronized; for this reason, the device is specified for use only in an unconscious victim without signs of circulation.

AEDs can malfunction occasionally, and safety advisories and recalls have been issued by the Food and Drug Administration mainly because of electrical or software problems.[29] One study reported 370 fatal AED malfunctions between 1996 and 2005. Yet, this number was just a very small fraction of the total number of lives saved by these devices each year.[29]

Operation of Automated External Defibrillators

AEDs are shock-advisory devices. That is, after interpreting the rhythm, the AED "advises" administration of a shock by a voice prompt and requires the operator to take the final step of pressing the "shock" button. There are four universal steps to operation of an AED:

1. The device is turned on, which initiates a series of voice prompts that guide the user through subsequent steps.
2. The electrode pads are attached. The operator is instructed by voice prompt and diagram to place electrode pads in an anterolateral position. If the victim is wet or diaphoretic, the chest should be dried with a cloth or towel.
3. The device automatically analyzes the rhythm. Instructions are given to stop CPR and any other possible motion artifact.
4. If the interpreted rhythm is ventricular fibrillation, the device will advise shock. For the shock to be delivered, the operator must manually depress the shock button.

Newer AED models are designed such that the instructions provided by visual and voice prompts meet the most recent resuscitation guidelines. Furthermore, some models provide the rescuer guidance through the entire CPR sequence.

Operation of the AED even by untrained lay persons is easy, as demonstrated by Grundy and colleagues.[30] They compared times to defibrillation achieved by sixth-grade elementary school children without prior AED training with those of trained emergency medical technicians during a mock cardiac arrest. The naive sixth graders defibrillated the mock victims in 90 seconds, only 23 seconds longer than the 67 seconds taken by the paramedics. The difference was considered to be of no clinical importance.

Field Experiences with the Automated External Defibrillator

During the past 15 years, extensive experience with the AED has been accumulated. Initially, the devices were made available to "nontraditional" first responders, such as firefighters and police officers in emergency medical systems, because it was recognized that police officers and firefighters often appear at the scene of a cardiac arrest before trained medical personnel in some communities. In a landmark trial, investigators in Seattle studied survival after firefighters were provided AEDs.[31] Survival rates for patients with ventricular fibrillation significantly improved when they were treated by firefighters using an AED compared with those receiving only basic life support until the arrival of paramedics (30% compared with 19%, respectively; $P < .01$). This improvement in survival resulted from shortening of the time to defibrillation by 5.1 ± 3.2 minutes.

Although some other reports of the use of AEDs by nontraditional responders have been favorable, improvement has not been universal; failure to show benefit apparently relates to a failure to decrease the time to defibrillation.[32] Moreover, results from a meta-analysis confirmed the importance of shortening the time to defibrillation to improve survival.[33]

Subsequently, the AED was tested in special environments, such as commercial airlines and casinos. People traveling aboard commercial airlines are exposed to factors that may precipitate sudden cardiac death, including the stress of flying, the exertion to reach the gate, the disruption of circadian rhythms, and the reduced oxygen in the cabin (equivalent to that at an altitude of about 8000 feet [2438 m] above sea level). Furthermore, when a cardiac arrest occurs during flight, it would take an airplane at least 20 minutes to reach ground-based assistance, eliminating all but the most remote chance of survival. Therefore, in 1997, American Airlines became the first U.S. airline to place AEDs aboard their aircraft; the experience with the first 200 AED uses was reported.[34] Ventricular fibrillation was documented in 14 individuals, and appropriate recommendation to shock was made in all 14. Survival to discharge from the hospital after shock was 40%; all the patients were discharged with good neurologic function. In the remaining cases, the AED appropriately identified nonshockable rhythms with 100% specificity. The sequence of electrograms for one of the first victims is demonstrated in Figure 65.3.

Further experience with the AED has been obtained in casinos, where patrons are exposed to a number of stresses (including lack of sleep, long travel, alcohol ingestion, and the anxiety and excitement associated with gaming). This environment, coupled with a population that is often older and sedentary, creates a situation in which cardiac arrest is not uncommon. The close security measures that are in place, with video surveillance, allow prompt recognition of cardiac arrest and measurement of the time to resuscitation. In 1997, a group of casinos in Nevada and Mississippi began placing AEDs on their premises and training their security personnel in their use. Data were published from 10 casinos in the first 30 months of the program, including cardiac arrest in 148 victims.[35] Ventricular fibrillation was documented in 105 cases; of these, 86% were witnessed. When the collapse was witnessed, the time to defibrillation was 4.4 ± 2.9 minutes, whereas it took paramedics 9.8 ± 4.3 minutes to arrive. Survival overall was 59%, but when defibrillation was performed in less than 3 minutes, survival was 74%. Historical models would have predicted a survival of 10% for patients defibrillated by standard paramedics.

Public Access Defibrillation

Public access defibrillation involves the deployment of AEDs in the community for immediate use by medically naive lay persons, with the aim of providing rapid defibrillation to cardiac arrest victims before the arrival of trained personnel.[3] The lay people expected to be the first to receive AED training include nontraditional responders such as police officers and ski patrol members, employees of corporations or public places with AED programs, and responders to persons at high risk, such as friends and family members.

In a large prospective randomized study, the Public Access Defibrillation Trial, deployment of lay volunteer–rescuer CPR plus AED programs in targeted public settings resulted in doubling of the number of survivors from out-of-hospital ventricular fibrillation sudden cardiac arrest compared with programs that provided early emergency medical services call and early CPR only.[36]

To optimize resources, it is recommended that AEDs be placed at public locations where the incidence of cardiac arrest is high, such that there is a reasonable possibility that the devices will be used. Studies have shown that there are a number of public venues that fulfill these criteria, including international airports, county jails, large shopping malls, public sports arenas, and large industrial sites (i.e., sites having more than 250 adults older than 50 years present for more than 16 hours per day).[37] Although this represents the most efficient use of the AED, placement in these locations alone would miss 75% of the cardiac arrests that occur in public places (where the risk in any one place is small but where, overall, most such arrests occur). AED deployment has also been recommended in places where call-to-shock time cannot be achieved in less than 5 minutes by conventional emergency systems. In some locations, such as in schools, cardiac arrest is rare; therefore, an AED program would not be cost-effective by traditional measures. Yet other important considerations can influence the decision to implement and to maintain an AED program, such as emotional and legal concerns. Furthermore, some authors argue that a school-based training in emergency activation and CPR is worthwhile because these skills provide potential benefit throughout the community and not just at school.[38]

One example of a successful public access defibrillation in high-risk locations is the Chicago Heart Save Program. In the program, implemented at Chicago's O'Hare and Midway airports, AEDs were deployed in a strategic location to allow 1-minute access within the airports.[39] The units were alarmed and well marked, and a high-profile education campaign was conducted at the airports. A total of 21 cardiac arrests were reported during the first 10 months; 18 patients had documented ventricular fibrillation, and 11 were resuscitated with intact neurologic function. Of note, the rescuers for 6 of the 11 resuscitated patients had no prior AED training.

AEDs continue to be deployed in diverse locations (such as high-rise buildings and golf courses), and public awareness continues to grow. It is likely that this will continue and widespread public access defibrillation will become a reality.

ADVANCED CARDIOVASCULAR LIFE SUPPORT

Despite the correct administration of basic life support, patients will frequently fail to achieve return of spontaneous circulation. This is when the fourth link in the chain of survival, early advanced care, is provided. Advanced cardiovascular life support includes

- definitive airway control with endotracheal intubation;
- establishment and maintenance of intravenous access; and
- administration of pharmacologic agents for resuscitation.

In addition, specific causes for the arrest should be considered and appropriate treatment administered if reversible factors are identified.

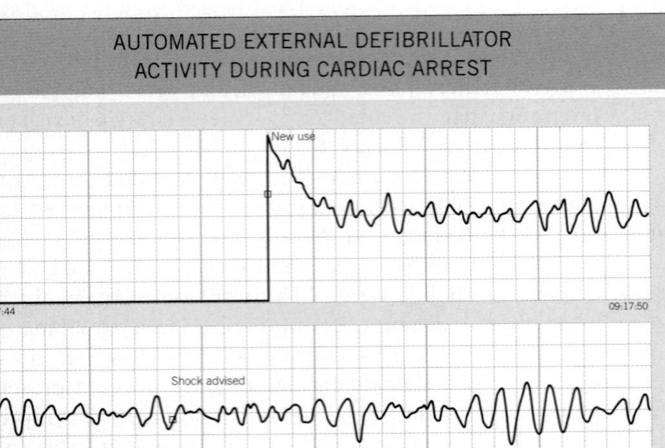

Figure 65.3 A playback of device activity as recorded on the memory card from an automated external defibrillator during a cardiac arrest aboard a commercial airliner. The actions of the device are recorded on the electrogram. Ventricular fibrillation is recognized and shocked successfully, resulting in sinus bradycardia with 2:1 conduction. The arrows point to P waves. The patient subsequently developed 1:1 conduction and later atrial fibrillation while the QRS slowly narrows. (With permission from Page RL, Hamdan MH, McKenas DK. Defibrillation aboard commercial aircraft. Circulation 1998;98:1429-1430.)

As opposed to CPR and early defibrillation, typical advanced cardiovascular life support therapies, such as insertion of advanced airways and pharmacologic support of the circulation, have not been shown to increase rate of survival to hospital discharge.[ref] Therefore, chest compressions should not be interrupted during drug administration.

The advanced cardiovascular life support algorithm for treatment of pulseless cardiac arrest is summarized in Figure 65.4.

Pharmacology

Epinephrine (Adrenaline)

Epinephrine (adrenaline) is the vasopressor of choice during resuscitation. Mediated by α-adrenergic receptor stimulation, it improves coronary and cerebral blood flow by increasing peripheral vasoconstriction. However, the benefit of increased myocardial blood flow is at least partially antagonized by the β-receptor–mediated increase in myocardial oxygen consumption, which may worsen postresuscitation myocardial dysfunction.

Despite widespread use of this drug, demonstration of its benefit in clinical arrest is scarce. The optimal dose of epinephrine has been controversial. The "traditional" 1-mg dose was derived from surgical experience, in which it was used for intracardiac administration to restart the arrested heart. Several clinical studies have been conducted to determine whether higher doses would be beneficial in humans.[40] These studies have shown occasional improvement in the rate of return of spontaneous circulation with higher dose epinephrine (0.07 to 20 mg/kg) but no improvement in

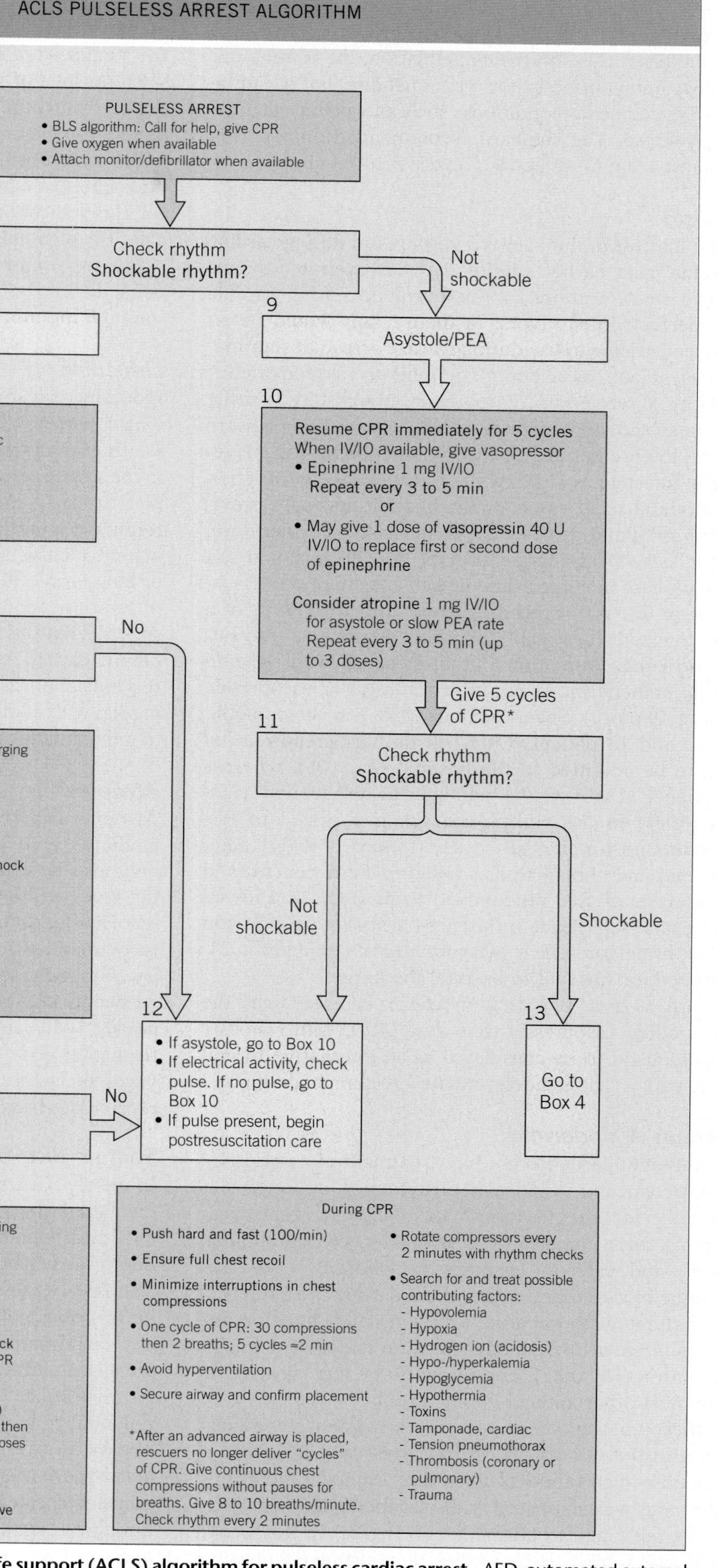

Figure 65.4 Advanced cardiovascular life support (ACLS) algorithm for pulseless cardiac arrest. AED, automated external defibrillator; BLS, basic life support; CPR, cardiopulmonary resuscitation; IO, intraosseous; IV, intravenous; PEA, pulseless electrical activity; VF, ventricular fibrillation; VT, ventricular tachycardia. (With permission from International Liaison Committee on Resuscitation. 2005 International Consensus on Cardiopulmonary Resuscitation and Emergency Cardiovascular Care Science with Treatment Recommendations. Circulation 2005;112:III1-III130. Copyright © 2005 American Heart Association.)

survival to discharge from the hospital. In view of these data, epinephrine has a class IIb recommendation; the routine use of high-dose epinephrine is not recommended, but it can be considered for specific conditions, such as calcium channel blocker overdose. The standard recommended epinephrine dose remains 1 mg intravenously every 3 to 5 minutes.

Vasopressin

The initial interest in the value of vasopressin during cardiac arrest stems from earlier studies that demonstrated supraphysiologic concentrations of this hormone during cardiac arrest, especially in survivors. In theory, this would be an ideal vasoconstrictor to use during cardiac arrest; at supranatural doses, it acts as a potent peripheral vasoconstrictor, mediated by V_1 receptors. Vasopressin administered during CPR has been shown to increase coronary perfusion pressure as it causes intense peripheral vasoconstriction of skin, skeletal muscle, intestine, and fat, with relatively less constriction of coronary and renal vasculatures. In addition, there is evidence for vasodilatation of the cerebral vessels. Furthermore, because it lacks β-adrenergic activity, the drug should not cause an increase in myocardial oxygen consumption.

Promise in the use of this drug grew after the results of a small randomized study were published; 40 patients who suffered ventricular fibrillation out of hospital were treated with either epinephrine (1 mg intravenously) or vasopressin (40 U intravenously). Seven patients (35%) in the epinephrine group and 14 patients (70%) in the vasopressin group survived to be admitted to the hospital ($P = .06$), whereas three patients (15%) in the epinephrine group and eight patients (40%) in the vasopressin group survived to discharge from the hospital ($P = .16$).[41] Subsequently, additional animal and human studies failed to show benefit, and a meta-analysis of five randomized trials (LOE 1) showed no statistically significant differences between vasopressin and epinephrine for return of spontaneous circulation, 24-hour survival, or survival to hospital discharge.

Therefore, as these two drugs appear to be equivalent, the guidelines allow vasopressin (one dose, 40 U intravenously or intraosseously) to be considered as an alternative to epinephrine, with a "class indeterminate" recommendation.

Intravenous Amiodarone

Intravenous amiodarone is used for treatment of a variety of supraventricular and ventricular arrhythmias, although it is labeled only for the treatment of malignant ventricular arrhythmias. It is a complex drug, with effects on the sodium, potassium, and calcium channels in addition to α- and β-adrenergic blocking properties. Amiodarone is a preferred agent in patients with impaired left ventricular function and atrial or ventricular arrhythmias because it does not impair cardiac contractility and is considered to be less proarrhythmic than most other antiarrhythmic agents.

The efficacy of amiodarone for shock-resistant ventricular fibrillation in out-of-hospital cardiac arrest was investigated in two double-blind randomized studies. Amiodarone (5 mg/kg or 300 mg) was compared with placebo in the first study (ARREST trial)[42] and to lidocaine (1.5 mg/kg) in the second study (ALIVE trial).[43] Both studies demonstrated improved survival to hospital admission with amiodarone. There was no difference in survival to discharge from the hospital, mainly because survival was very low in both groups, and the studies were not powered toward this endpoint.

The results of ARREST and ALIVE and accumulated evidence from other earlier studies indicate that intravenous amiodarone should be the drug of choice for shock-resistant ventricular fibrillation. Furthermore, previous studies with lidocaine have failed to demonstrate benefit from the drug for this indication. The 2005 guidelines give amiodarone a class IIb recommendation. The usual dose of amiodarone is a 300-mg rapid infusion with repeated 150-mg doses as needed, followed by an infusion of 1 mg/min for 6 hours, then 0.5 mg/min to a maximum daily dose of 2 g.

Lidocaine

Lidocaine is a sodium channel–blocking antiarrhythmic agent with a narrow therapeutic window used for the treatment of ventricular arrhythmias. The drug appears to be most effective in the setting of acute myocardial ischemia or infarction. In cardiac arrest, it has traditionally been the drug of choice for refractory ventricular fibrillation, despite a lack of proof of benefit for this indication as no study has proved short-term or long-term efficacy. In fact, some studies suggest lower rates of return of spontaneous circulation and a higher incidence of asystole, reasons for which it receives a class indeterminate recommendation. As stated previously, amiodarone is favored for this indication. The recommended dose for cardiac arrest is 1.5 mg/kg, with additional boluses of 0.5 to 0.75 mg/kg as needed to a maximum of 3 mg/kg during a 1-hour period.

Atropine

Atropine sulfate is most effective in reversing cholinergic-mediated bradycardia, hypotension, and vagal reactions. It may also be effective in reversing atrioventricular block at the level of the atrioventricular node but not at the level of the His-Purkinje system. During cardiac arrest, atropine is recommended for asystole or slow pulseless electrical activity, although no prospective study has shown this drug to be beneficial in this setting. The usual dose is 1 mg intravenously, with repeated doses every 3 to 5 minutes as needed, to a total dose of 3 mg; in most adults, this results in full vagal blockade. In view of the scant data, this drug also receives a class indeterminate recommendation.

Sodium Bicarbonate

In the past, administration of sodium bicarbonate was recommended during closed chest compression because of the belief that bicarbonate would buffer the hydrogen ions produced during anaerobic metabolism and therefore would improve acidosis. However, clinical data suggest that treatment with buffers does not improve outcome. In fact, this type of therapy could actually be detrimental by causing a paradoxical increase in intracellular carbon dioxide tension and a decrease in myocardial and cerebral tissue intracellular pH. Other potentially harmful effects include inhibition of oxygen release as a result of extracellular alkalosis, hyperosmolarity and hypernatremia, volume overload, and inhibition of administered catecholamines. Control of the acid-base balance during cardiac arrest is best achieved by adequate ventilation and rapid restoration of the circulation.

Alternative buffer agents do not appear to improve survival during cardiac resuscitation. A Norwegian study involving 502 adults who had asystole or ventricular fibrillation demonstrated no survival benefit after the use of a combination buffer agent (250 mL of a mixture of sodium bicarbonate, trometanol, and phosphate, with a buffering capacity of 500 mmol/L) compared with placebo, despite the fact that most patients were acidotic on arrival to the hospital.[44]

Management of Pulseless Electrical Activity

Pulseless electrical activity (PEA) is defined by the presence of an organized rhythm on the electrocardiogram in the absence of a palpable pulse. It is advisable to corroborate the absence of pulse in more than one location to avoid being misled by a preexisting carotid artery obstruction. The best hope for this group of patients is identification and treatment of a specific cause immediately, which may include pulmonary embolism, hypovolemia, pneumothorax, coronary thrombosis, and others. In addition, general resuscitation measures are mandatory, such as chest compressions, support of ventilation, and administration of epinephrine (adrenaline) and atropine as stated in the PEA algorithm (see Fig. 65.4).

In general, a fast narrow-complex rhythm with PEA indicates a relatively normal heart responding to a severe clinical condition, such as hypovolemia or cardiac tamponade, that would improve with a specific intervention. In contrast, PEA with a wide QRS complex and bradycardia may represent evidence of dying myocardium or may indicate a specific critical rhythm disturbance, such as in hyperkalemia or tricyclic toxicity. Great effort should be made to search for possible causes; the width and rate of the QRS provide important clues. Clues from the physical examination include distended neck veins, which would suggest pericardial tamponade, and unilateral absence of breath sounds, suggestive of tension pneumothorax.

Unfortunately, the prognosis for out-of-hospital PEA is poor; only 4% of affected individuals survive to discharge from the hospital.[45] A randomized study evaluated the effectiveness of routine administration of tissue plasminogen activator to patients with PEA under the theoretical reasoning that pulmonary embolism and coronary thrombosis are common causes and after smaller studies suggested a possible benefit. This study, which included 233 patients, demonstrated no benefit from tissue plasminogen activator and confirmed the grim prognosis associated with out-of-hospital PEA.[46] Nevertheless, certain limitations of this study must be mentioned. First, in this study, PEA was required to be present only for more than 1 minute during the arrest (it was not required to be the primary diagnosis). Second, patients with a clearly defined cause for PEA were excluded. It is therefore very likely that many of the patients in this study had PEA as a manifestation of terminal pump dysfunction and not as a result of a reversible cause. It is therefore important to stress that the results of this study should not be generalized to specific patients identified as having pulmonary embolism or myocardial infarction. Thus, thrombolytic should not be used routinely in cardiac arrest victims but may be considered on a case-by-case basis, such as when pulmonary embolus is suspected (class IIa recommendation). Ongoing CPR is not a contraindication to fibrinolysis.

Management of Bradyasystole

The term *bradyasystole* refers to rhythms below 60 beats per minute or periods of asystole, or both. In general, the prognosis for patients with bradyasystole is extremely poor. Engdahl and colleagues[47] reported an overall survival to discharge from the hospital of 2% for 1635 patients with out-of-hospital cardiac arrest in whom the initial rhythm was asystole, with no survivors among those with unwitnessed arrest who were older than 70 years. A possible exception to this poor prognosis is when patients with witnessed cardiac arrest develop bradyasystole as a result of a correctable situation such as hypoxemia.

Before accepting the diagnosis of asystole, one must switch electrocardiogram leads and maximize the electrocardiographic amplifier gain to check for possible fine ventricular fibrillation, as this rhythm is more amenable to treatment. Transcutaneous pacing has been advocated, but a large clinical study demonstrated no benefit, even when paramedics performed this intervention as early as possible.[48] The algorithm for management of asystole is demonstrated in Figure 65.4. This algorithm emphasizes the issue of "not starting" and "when to stop" resuscitation, as asystole is most often a confirmation of death and not a treatable rhythm.

POSTRESUSCITATION INJURY

Many patients who achieve return of spontaneous circulation after arrest subsequently succumb to later complications. Consequently, a second step in resuscitation care involves the treatment and prevention of the postresuscitation syndrome, which is a complex of serious abnormalities, including cardiogenic shock, hypovolemic shock, systemic inflammatory response syndrome, and multiorgan dysfunction. Postresuscitation care is now recognized as a critical component of advanced life support.

Several phases in the postresuscitation syndrome have been described:

- Initially, cardiovascular dysfunction is seen, which is usually reversible after 12 to 48 hours. This nonlethal myocardial injury, probably mediated by oxygen radicals, results in postresuscitation cardiac dysfunction and arrhythmias.[49]
- Global hypoxia leads to microvascular and cerebral dysfunction and damage.
- After the first 24 hours, the hemodynamic status improves, but increased intestinal permeability predisposes the victim to sepsis syndrome that can be manifested days later and often leads to rapid demise.
- Alternatively, multiple-organ dysfunction syndrome can be seen, resulting from continued deterioration of splanchnic organs.

Unfortunately, very few studies have been conducted to support the routine use of techniques aimed at targeted correction of the different systemic derangements mentioned, and other studies have failed to show positive results. Exceptions to this are published trials on the use of therapeutic hypothermia. Mild hypothermia (32°C to 34°C) is simple, safe, and effective, and the adverse effects observed with moderate hypothermia (28°C to 32°C), such as ventricular fibrillation, are avoided.

Two landmark randomized studies, one from Australia and one from Europe, demonstrated improved outcomes in comatose survivors of out-of-hospital cardiac arrest.[50,51] In the Australian study, which involved 77 patients, hypothermia to 32°C was induced by application of ice packs to head and torso of survivors of cardiac arrest and maintained for 12 hours. In this study, 49% of patients in the hypothermia group survived and had a good outcome, compared with 26% in the normothermia group. In the European study, involving 275 patients, hypothermia to 32°C to 34°C was induced with the use of an external cooling device and maintained for 24 hours. The results were similarly encouraging, with 55% of the hypothermia group showing a favorable neurologic outcome compared with 39% in the normothermia group. In addition, fewer of the hypothermia patients had died by 6 months (41% compared with 55%; $P = .02$). In both studies, temperature was monitored by tympanic or bladder thermometers, and sedative and paralyzing agents were given to prevent shivering.

In view of the positive results from these studies, induction of mild hypothermia (32°C to 34°C for 12 to 24 hours) is recommended in comatose and hemodynamically stable adult patients with return of spontaneous circulation after out-of-hospital cardiac arrest. When the initial rhythm is ventricular fibrillation, recommendation is class IIa; for non–ventricular fibrillation, it has a class IIb recommendation. This remains an area under extensive investigation, including clinical trials for other types of emergencies, such as stroke, as well as initiation of hypothermia in the prehospital setting.[52]

ETHICAL ISSUES

The issue of whether to initiate resuscitation efforts is complicated. Attempts at reversal of death might not be consistent with some patients' desires or their best interests, so provisions must be considered to avoid misunderstanding or the undertaking of futile resuscitative efforts. It is also important that health care professionals understand that they are not obligated to provide care that appears inappropriate or futile. The best way to avoid such events is to address the issues before they happen. The patient may have expressed a wish to forego resuscitation efforts through advanced directives or "do not resuscitate" orders. Family and friends should be made aware of advanced directives so that the emergency medical system is not activated in case of an emergency, and rescuers should look for emergency bracelets or any other objective documentation that would preclude resuscitation efforts. It is therefore recommended that all adults receive resuscitation unless they meet the following criteria delineated by the 2005 guidelines:

- The patient has a valid do not resuscitate order.
- The patient has signs of irreversible death, such as rigor mortis or decapitation.
- No physiologic benefit can be expected on the basis of the presence of deteriorating vital function despite maximal treatment, such as in terminal sepsis.

In addition, during out-of-hospital cardiac arrest, attempting CPR is not required if it would put the rescuer at risk of physical injury.

Another difficult decision is when to terminate resuscitation efforts. In adults, the chance of survival without severe neurologic impairment is essentially zero when CPR is administered for more than 25 minutes without return of spontaneous circulation, unless there is intermittent ventricular fibrillation or tachycardia or the arrest is associated with trauma, hypothermia, drug overdose, or respiratory etiology.[53] Furthermore, in the case of adults who do not respond to an adequate trial of advanced cardiovascular life support on the field, rapid transportation to the emergency department does not improve survival and is usually futile.[54] One study reported that for patients who suffer cardiac arrest while in the hospital, if the arrest is unwitnessed, the initial rhythm is not ventricular tachycardia or fibrillation, and the resuscitation lasts longer than 10 minutes, then the survival is zero.[55]

SUMMARY

CPR is a series of interventions intended to prevent irreversible damage to vital organs during cardiac arrest and ultimately to restore normal circulatory function. Initially, a basic sequence of resuscitation would involve emergency system activation, assisted ventilation, and closed chest compressions. During chest compression, emphasis is placed on good technique and minimal interruptions.

For the majority of adult patients in cardiac arrest, ventricular defibrillation represents definitive treatment and should be provided without delay. AEDs have developed into effective devices that allow people with modest training to deliver cardiac defibrillation effectively and safely. The modern AED is simple to use and incorporates advanced technology including biphasic waveform, sophisticated rhythm analysis, and advanced battery technology. On the basis of the recent studies and developments, widespread distribution of AEDs and further progress in the public access defibrillation strategy are expected.

For patients in pulseless electrical activity or asystole, the prognosis is poor, and the only hope is to find and to treat a potentially causative condition. The second step in resuscitation of victims who have achieved return of spontaneous circulation involves the treatment and prevention of the postresuscitation syndrome. For this group of patients, therapy with mild hypothermia has been shown to improve survival and to preserve neurologic function.

chapter

66 Implantable Defibrillators

Kathy L. Lee and Chu-Pak Lau

Definition

- The implantable cardioverter-defibrillator (ICD) is an electronic device used to treat ventricular tachyarrhythmias automatically with electrical shocks or pacing.

Key Features

- Most ICDs are implanted subcutaneously in the pectoral region and connected to endocardial lead systems.
- When the preset detection criteria of ventricular arrhythmias are met, the device automatically delivers programmed therapies for arrhythmia termination.
- ICD therapies include bradycardia pacing, antitachycardia pacing, cardioversion, and defibrillation.
- Apart from the single-chamber ICD, the dual-chamber ICD and the ICD with resynchronization therapy are used increasingly in patients with coexistent conditions such as atrial arrhythmia and heart failure.

Clinical Implications

- ICD therapy is indicated for patients with structural heart disease and life-threatening ventricular tachyarrhythmias.
- The ICD is used to prevent sudden death in patients with advanced structural heart disease and severe left ventricular dysfunction.

The first human implantation of an implantable cardioverter-defibrillator (ICD) was reported in 1980 by Mirowski.[1] He conceived the idea of an automatic defibrillator in the 1960s after the sudden death of his close friend and colleague. In 1985, the ICD was approved by the U.S. Food and Drug Administration. Throughout the years, the ICD has evolved from a sizable nonprogrammable shock-box with epicardial patches that required thoracotomy for implantation to a much smaller programmable device with tiered-therapy and an endocardial lead system suitable for subcutaneous pectoral implantation (Fig. 66.1). Furthermore, advancement in technology enables the ICD to offer electrical therapy for commonly coexistent conditions like atrial arrhythmias and congestive heart failure.

Throughout the past decade, large-scale randomized clinical trials have provided consistent evidence of the clinical efficacy of device therapy. The ICD is proven to be superior to antiarrhythmic drugs in patients with structural heart diseases who suffer from hemodynamically significant ventricular arrhythmias (see also Chapters 62 and 64).[2-4] In postinfarction patients at risk for arrhythmic death, prophylactic ICD implantation confers survival benefit.[5-7] Other randomized trials further expanded the role of the ICD in primary prevention of sudden death in patients with poor left ventricular function of both ischemic and nonischemic causes (Fig. 66.2).[8-10]

DESCRIPTION

Components

An ICD consists of the pulse generator and the lead system. The single-chamber ICD, dual-chamber ICD, and ICD incorporating cardiac resynchronization therapy are commercially available. ICD interrogation, follow-up, and programming are performed with an external programmer.

Pulse Generator

The pulse generator includes a titanium “can,” a battery, capacitors, sensing and amplification, pacing output, and high-voltage output circuits. The titanium can of an ICD may also function as an electrode for defibrillation.

Battery

The battery and capacitors constitute most of the pulse generator. Devices delivering higher energies and those with greater longevity tend to be larger. Most contemporary devices are smaller than 40 cc and weigh less than 100 g. The life spans of ICDs are 3 to 7 years on average, depending on the frequency of shocks and percentage of time pacing.

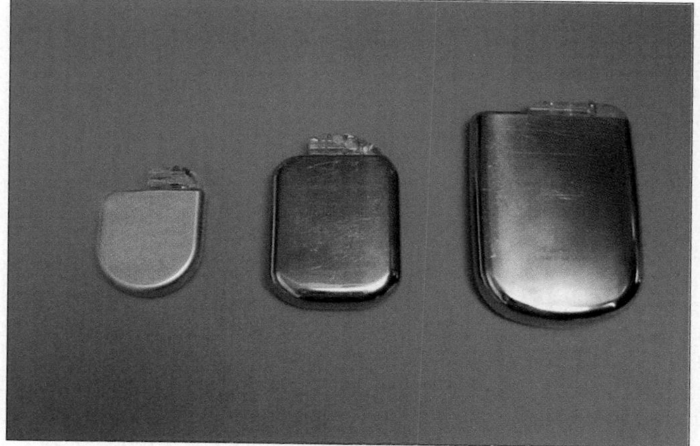

Figure 66.1 Evolution of the ICD. An abdominal ICD in the late 1980s *(right),* an ICD in the 1990s *(middle),* and a pectoral ICD in the 2000s *(left).*

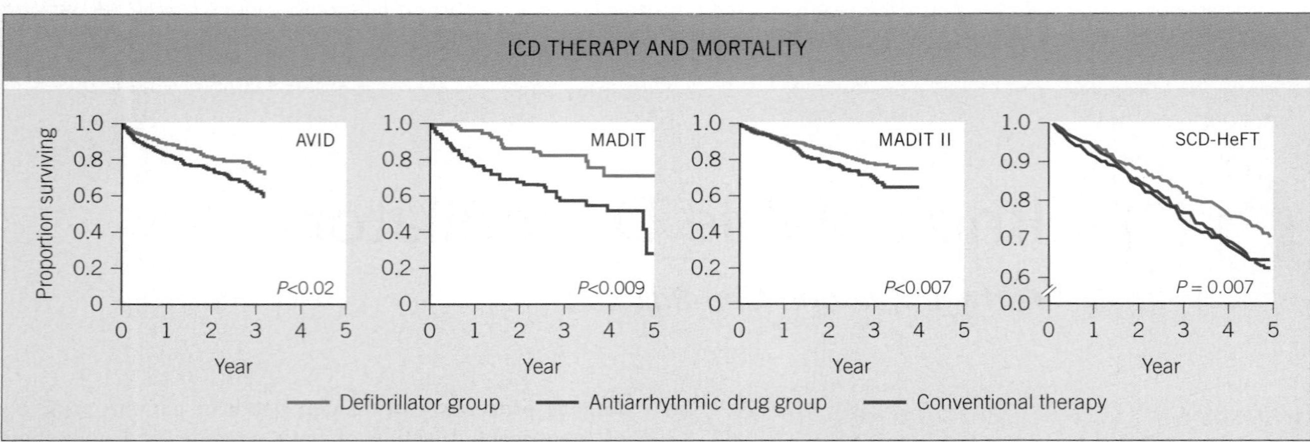

Figure 66.2 Plots of actuarial total survival in four multicenter randomized trials involving the use of implantable defibrillators. Antiarrhythmics Versus Implantable Defibrillator Trial (AVID) is a secondary prevention trial. Multicenter Automatic Defibrillator Implantation Trial (MADIT), MADIT II, and Sudden Cardiac Death in Heart Failure Trial (SCD-HeFT) are primary prevention trials. (From AVID Investigators,[2] Moss et al.,[5,7] and Bardy et al.[8])

Capacitors

Whereas the battery is the source of power, the capacitor transforms and temporarily stores the energy before discharge. The capacitors need to be reformed periodically for optimal function. Therefore, the capacitor automatically charges and then discharges without delivery of a shock to the patient every 1 to 6 months, depending on programming.

Sensing and Amplification System

The sensing and amplification system is for appropriate detection of QRS complexes even during ventricular fibrillation when the electrograms are minute, without sensing of artifacts that may cause inappropriate detection. High- and low-pass filters are used to suppress artifacts such as myopotentials. Adopting dynamic sensing in the ICD can eliminate T-wave sensing while preserving its capability to sense ventricular fibrillation. For instance, with auto-adjusting sensitivity, after a sensed event, the sensitivity is immediately decreased but falls back exponentially to the programmed value (Fig. 66.3). The defibrillator maintains its high sensitivity to electrical signal during most of the cardiac cycle except instantly after an intrinsic event such as the T wave.

Bradycardia Sensing and Pacing Circuits

When required, bradycardia pacing and antitachycardia pacing are delivered from the low-voltage pacing output circuit. The sensing parameters for bradycardia pacing are different from those used for sensing of tachycardia.

High-Voltage Output Circuits

The high-voltage circuit is used for charging of the capacitor and delivery of the charge to the myocardium through the lead system when ventricular arrhythmia detection criteria are satisfied.

Lead Systems

ICD leads convey electrical signals to the pulse generator for analysis and deliver pacing and shocking currents to the myocardium. Previously, defibrillation electrodes were epicardial patches, and thoracotomy was required for ICD implantation. Currently, endocardial lead systems with or without subcutaneous patches or arrays are used almost exclusively.

A dual-coil ICD lead consists of a pair of proximal and distal defibrillation coils (Fig. 66.4). The tip electrode functions as the cathode of the pace-sense lead; the anode may be the

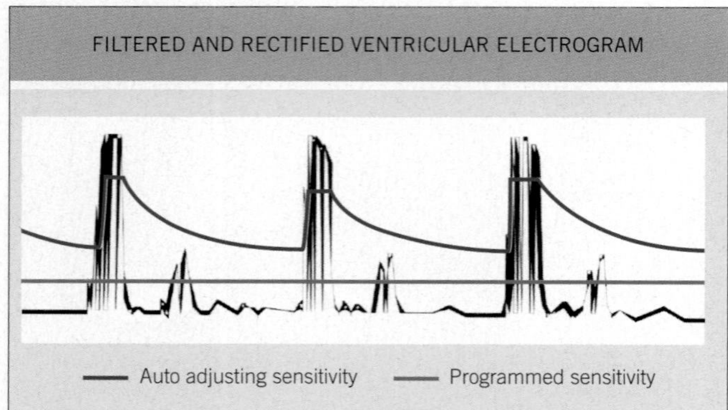

Figure 66.3 Auto-adjusting sensitivity in the ICD. The sensing threshold resets to a high value immediately after a sensed event but decreases progressively afterward. This helps eliminate oversensing of the T wave but avoids undersensing of the fine electrograms during ventricular fibrillation.

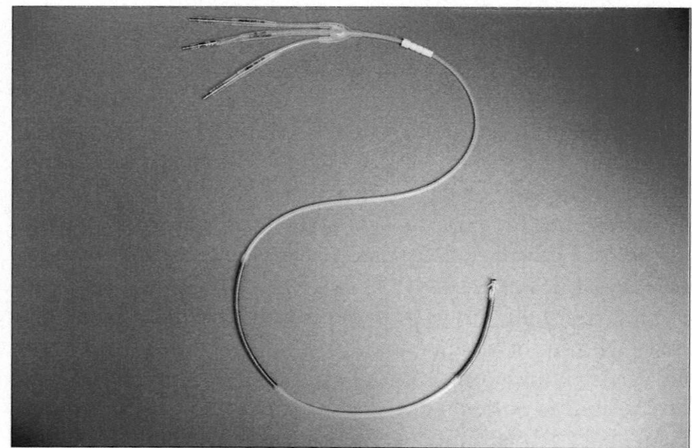

Figure 66.4 Dual-coil defibrillation lead.

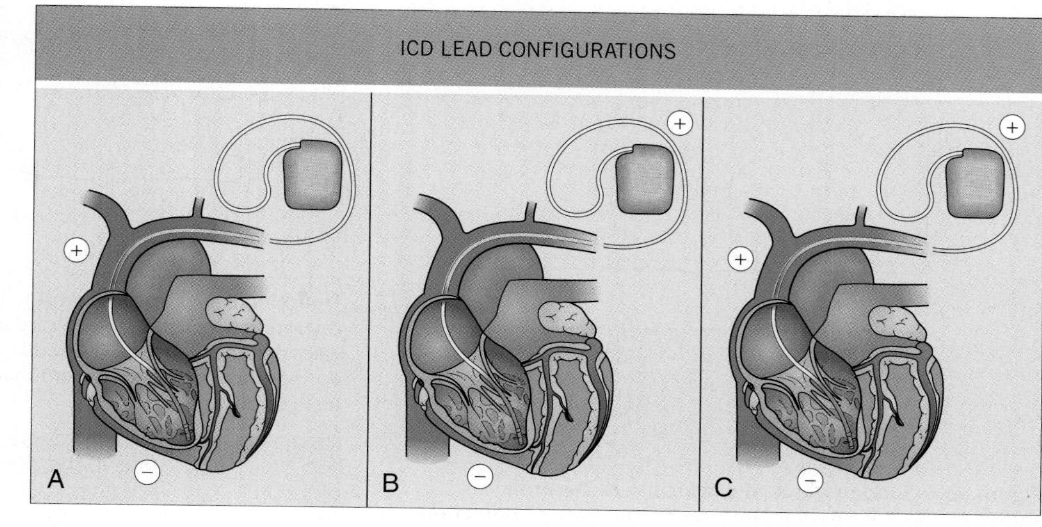

Figure 66.5 Endocardial defibrillation electrode configurations. A, Dual-coil configuration with the cathode in the distal coil at the right ventricle and the anode in the proximal coil at the superior vena cava–right atrium. **B,** Single-lead unipolar defibrillation system with the cathode in the right ventricle and the anode in the ICD can. **C,** Triad configuration with the cathode in the right ventricle and the anode in the proximal coil and the ICD can.

proximal spring electrode of the distal coil (integrated bipolar electrode) or a separate ring electrode located between the tip and the distal coil (dedicated bipolar electrode). Sensing in a dedicated bipolar defibrillation lead may be better than in an integrated bipolar lead during the immediate post-shock period. For a single-coil ICD lead, the defibrillation efficacy can be enhanced by an additional defibrillation lead placed in the superior vena cava or innominate vein. Most pectoral systems involve the ICD generator can as an active electrode (a "hot" or "active" can). As shown in Figure 66.5, different combinations of electrode configurations with a dual-coil lead and a generator can are possible.

A regular pace-sense lead is used in the right atrium for sensing and pacing in dual-chamber ICDs. A left ventricular lead is used in a coronary vein to achieve sensing and pacing of the left ventricle for cardiac resynchronization therapy.

ICD Programmer

ICD programmers are manufacturer-specific programming and display units. While the programmer wand is positioned near the ICD pocket, telemetry interface is established with the programmer. With radiofrequency technology, wireless communication between certain newer implantable devices and the programmer over a distance within several meters can be established. Device information including its operation, programmed parameters, and stored episode data can be obtained. Follow-up, testing, and programming of the ICD are also performed with the programmer. Remote monitoring of ICD parameters is also possible with wireless technology and data storage in an Internet server.

Principles of Operation

There are four fundamental functions in an ICD. They are bradycardia pacing, detection, therapy, and storage of arrhythmia episodes. Advanced features include rate-adaptive dual-chamber pacing, atrial therapies, and cardiac resynchronization therapy.

Bradycardia Pacing

In general, the pacing output, sensitivity, and other pacing parameters are programmed separately from those used for antitachycardia pacing. Advanced features such as rate-adaptive pacing and dual-chamber pacing are now widely available.

Detection

Recognition of arrhythmia primarily relies on rate sensing. When the rate of the sensed R waves falls into the rate-defined tachycardia zone, the detection algorithm is initiated and the counter is augmented.

When the counter reaches a critical value, therapy programmed for that tachycardia zone is delivered. In tiered-therapy devices, up to three rate-defined zones can be programmed to allow therapies of incremental aggressiveness (Table 66.1). Antitachycardia pacing or low-energy cardioversion may be tried initially and high-energy defibrillation deferred. Because the arrhythmia may terminate spontaneously during charging of the capacitor, a noncommitted device will reconfirm that the rate criterion is still satisfied before delivery of the shock.

In the ventricular fibrillation zone, highly sensitive detection criteria are applied, as prompt and aggressive therapy is warranted for ventricular fibrillation. In the ventricular tachycardia zones, various enhancement criteria are programmable to improve arrhythmia classification.[11] Inappropriate shocks due to supraventricular tachycardias such as sinus tachycardia or atrial arrhythmias are common when their R-R intervals fall within the rate zone. In single-chamber devices, algorithms such as "onset," "interval stability," and "electrogram width" help classify arrhythmias. In dual-chamber devices, atrial sensing is incorporated into the dual-chamber detection algorithms for arrhythmia classification.

HIERARCHY OF TIERED THERAPY

Zone	Brady	Normal	VT	FVT	VF
Rate (beats/minute)	<50	50-149	150-169	170-199	≥200
First device therapy	Pacing	None	ATP	ATP or CV	DeFib

VT, ventricular tachycardia; FVT, fast ventricular tachycardia; VF, ventricular fibrillation; ATP, antitachycardia pacing; CV, cardioversion; DeFib, defibrillation.

Table 66.1 Hierarchy of tiered therapy.

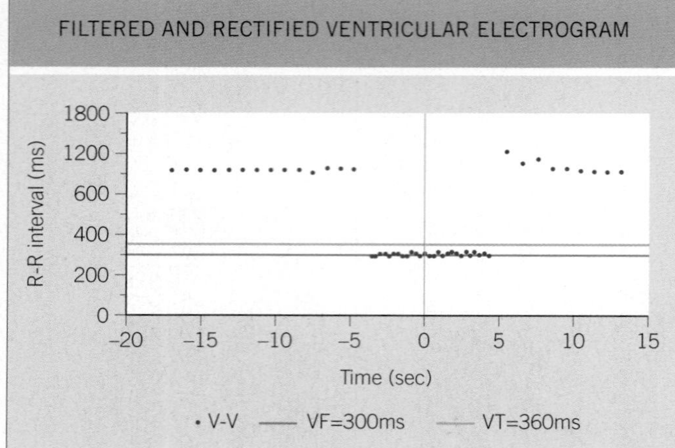

Figure 66.6 Sudden onset of ventricular tachycardia as shown in the R-R interval plot around the time of detection (time 0). The R-R interval changed from 900 to 300 ms abruptly at tachycardia onset. A 17.3-J shock terminated the tachycardia.

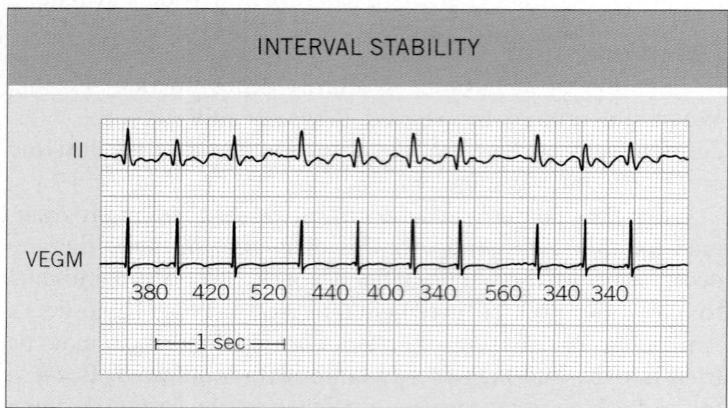

Figure 66.7 Interval stability in atrial fibrillation. The cycle length is grossly irregular during atrial fibrillation as shown in the electrogram strip. The upper panel shows surface electrocardiogram lead II (II), and the lower panel shows intracardiac electrograms (VEGM). The numbers are measurements of the R-R intervals in milliseconds.

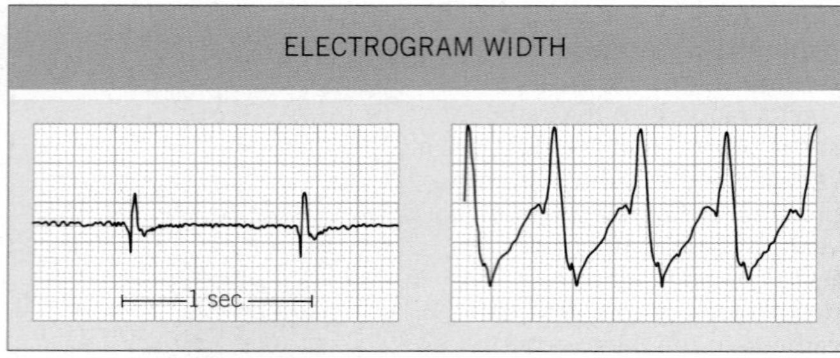

Figure 66.8 Electrogram width. Electrogram width in sinus rhythm and ventricular tachycardia as recorded in the far-field electrogram (see text). The width of the electrogram is 70 ms during sinus rhythm and more than 120 ms during ventricular tachycardia.

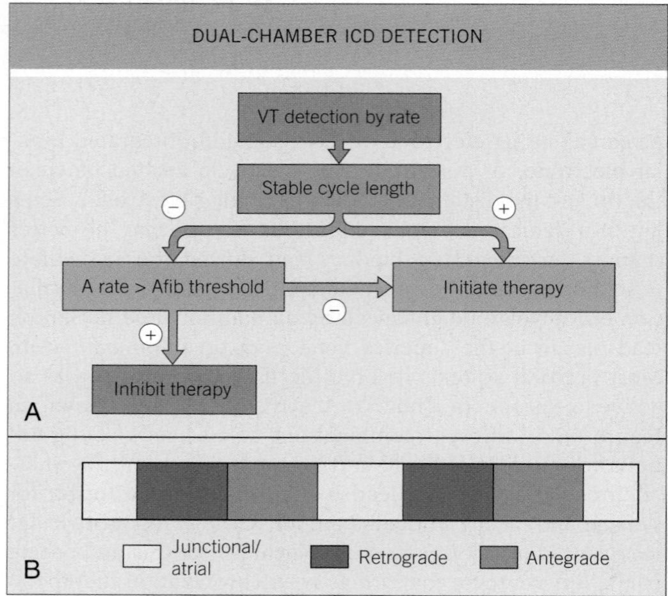

Figure 66.9 Two examples of dual-chamber algorithms. A, When the rate of a tachycardia falls into the detection zone and the tachycardia cycle length is regular, it will be classified as ventricular tachycardia, and therapy will be initiated. If the cycle length is not regular and the atrial rate exceeds the atrial fibrillation detection rate (Afib threshold), the tachycardia will be classified as atrial fibrillation, and therapy will be inhibited. **B,** When a tachycardia falls into the detection zone, the number and position of atrial events relative to ventricular events are determined. Common patterns of atrial and ventricular relationship in sinus, ventricular, and junctional tachycardias are matched to classify the arrhythmia.

The onset criterion may differentiate sinus tachycardia from ventricular tachycardia, as sinus tachycardia is usually gradual in onset, whereas ventricular tachycardia occurs abruptly. If programmed on, a sudden decrease in cycle length before detection is required to fulfill the onset criterion before therapy is delivered (Fig. 66.6). Interval stability may differentiate atrial fibrillation from ventricular tachycardia, as the cycle length tends to be irregular during atrial fibrillation (Fig. 66.7). When programmed on, the R-R cycle length must be relatively constant to initiate therapy. The electrogram width criterion is based on the measured duration of the intracardiac electrogram as recorded from the two defibrillation electrodes (far-field electrogram). Wide complexes are classified as ventricular in origin and narrow complexes as supraventricular (Fig. 66.8). Of note, detection error may occur in case of relatively narrow ventricular tachycardia or supraventricular tachycardia with bundle branch aberrancy. These criteria may increase the specificity of arrhythmia detection, but the sensitivity of ventricular tachycardia detection may be slightly compromised. These algorithms should be applied with caution, especially with poorly tolerated ventricular tachycardia.[12]

By incorporation of an atrial lead, dual-chamber ICDs can offer more diagnostic and therapeutic options for patients with frequent paroxysmal atrial arrhythmias.[13] Current dual-chamber algorithms are mostly constructed on the basis of the atrial rate and ventricular rate, with or without the timing relationship of their electrograms (Fig. 66.9).

Therapy

Tiered-therapy devices provide a hierarchy of increasingly aggressive electrical therapies for arrhythmias in ascending tachycardia zones. They include antitachycardia pacing, cardioversion, and defibrillation (see Table 66.1).

Antitachycardia Pacing

Rapid pacing can penetrate and interrupt re-entrant circuits. Antitachycardia pacing drains little energy and causes no

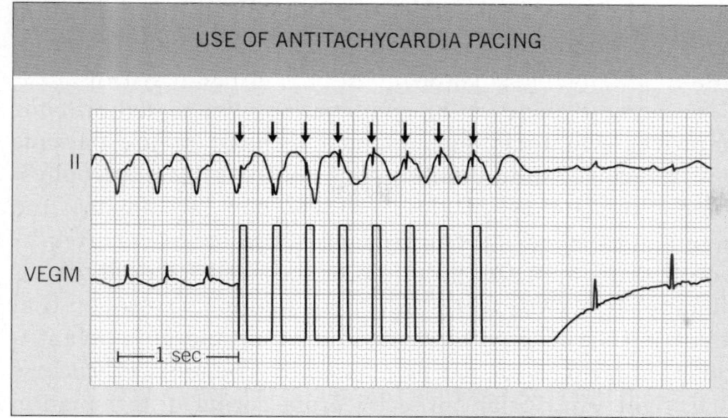

Figure 66.10 Antitachycardia pacing. Termination of ventricular tachycardia by burst pacing *(arrows)*. VEGM, intracardiac ventricular electrogram.

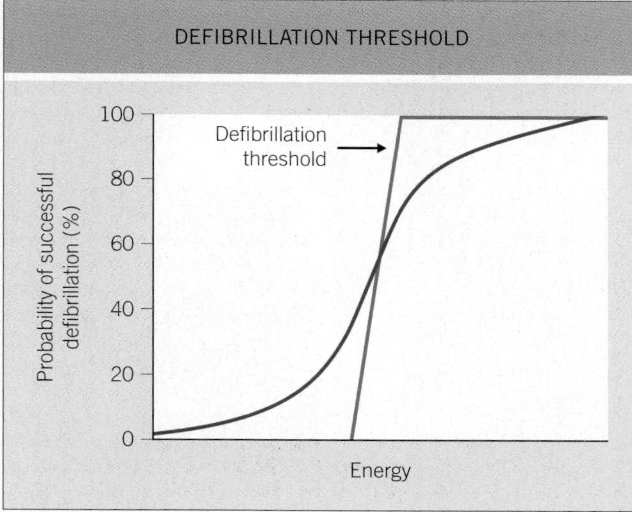

Figure 66.11 Dose-response curve of defibrillation. A defibrillation threshold implies that there is a cutoff between effective and ineffective energies. A defibrillation curve shows that a higher energy is associated with a greater chance of success in defibrillation. (Modified from Davy J, Fain ES, Dorian P, et al. The relationship between successful defibrillation and delivered energy in open-chest dogs: reappraisal of the "defibrillation threshold" concept. Am Heart J 1987;113:77-84.)

discomfort to the patient, although unsuccessful pacing trains may lead to tachycardia acceleration or degeneration.[14] Burst pacing is delivery of a train of pacing pulses at a fixed cycle length, usually as a certain percentage of the tachycardia cycle length (Fig. 66.10). Ramp pacing is delivery of a train of pacing pulses in which the coupling intervals shorten progressively. It is often safe and effective to program empiric antitachycardia pacing as initial therapy to terminate ventricular tachycardia.[15] Limiting the number of antitachycardia pacing trains may prevent undue delay in delivery of the next tier of effective therapy.

Cardioversion

Cardioversion attempts to terminate a tachycardia circuit by simultaneously depolarizing a large portion of the myocardium, rendering tissue refractory. Low-energy synchronized shock may be used to terminate a monomorphic ventricular tachycardia. However, even low-energy shocks at 1 to 2 J are painful and may cause degeneration of ventricular tachycardia into ventricular fibrillation.

Defibrillation

Ventricular fibrillation is a chaotic rhythm characterized by multiple circulating wavefronts in different stages of depolarization and repolarization. Defibrillation is termination of the fibrillation process by delivery of a nonsynchronized electrical current. Successful defibrillation is accomplished only when the electrical shock depolarizes a sufficient amount of tissue to stop the fibrillation wavefront from propagating. Defibrillation efficacy is best described by a sigmoidal dose-response curve that shows the probability of successful defibrillation for a shock of certain energy (Fig. 66.11). There is no single energy level above which all shocks are successful in termination of ventricular fibrillation.[16]

For successful defibrillation to be achieved, a strong electrical field is needed to synchronize all the cells. For monophasic shock, the ICD capacitor is discharged between the anode and the cathode to the heart. For biphasic shock, the polarity of the pulse is reversed during its delivery. The first phase of a biphasic pulse behaves like a monophasic pulse, but the second phase reduces the electrical requirements of the first phase. Reinitiation of the fibrillation wavefront may be prevented as the residual charge on the cells in a region that receives borderline stimulation with lower shock strength is removed during the second phase.[17] Biphasic pulses are in general more effective than monophasic pulses with similar pathways and reduce the defibrillation threshold significantly.[18]

Electrogram Storage

All episodes of tachycardia detection are registered in the device. After interrogation, the dates and times of occurrences of arrhythmias, cycle lengths, intracardiac electrograms, therapies delivered, and outcomes can be retrieved. This is useful for validation of device function and for retrospective arrhythmia classification.

Dual-Chamber ICD

Dual-chamber ICDs can be classified into two categories according to their functions. A dual-chamber ICD provides dual-chamber sensing and pacing and ventricular defibrillation (Fig. 66.12). Atrial therapies such as atrial burst pacing and atrial defibrillation are available in some dual-chamber ICDs.

A separate permanent pacemaker was historically needed in ICD patients with significant bradycardia.[19] However, there were risks of adverse device-device interactions, and vigorous testing was mandatory. Examples of such device-device interactions include sensing of the pacing artifact during ventricular fibrillation as an R wave, leading to inhibition of therapy; sensing of the pacing stimuli, causing double counting; and inappropriate detection and reset of the pacemaker to VOO mode after defibrillation.[20]

In the Antiarrhythmics Versus Implantable Defibrillators (AVID) trial, atrial fibrillation was shown to be an independent predictor of mortality in ICD patients.[2] Because of the high incidence of atrial arrhythmia in the ICD population, other than specific arrhythmia discrimination algorithms to reduce inappropriate shocks, prevention and termination of such arrhythmias are also important goals in the

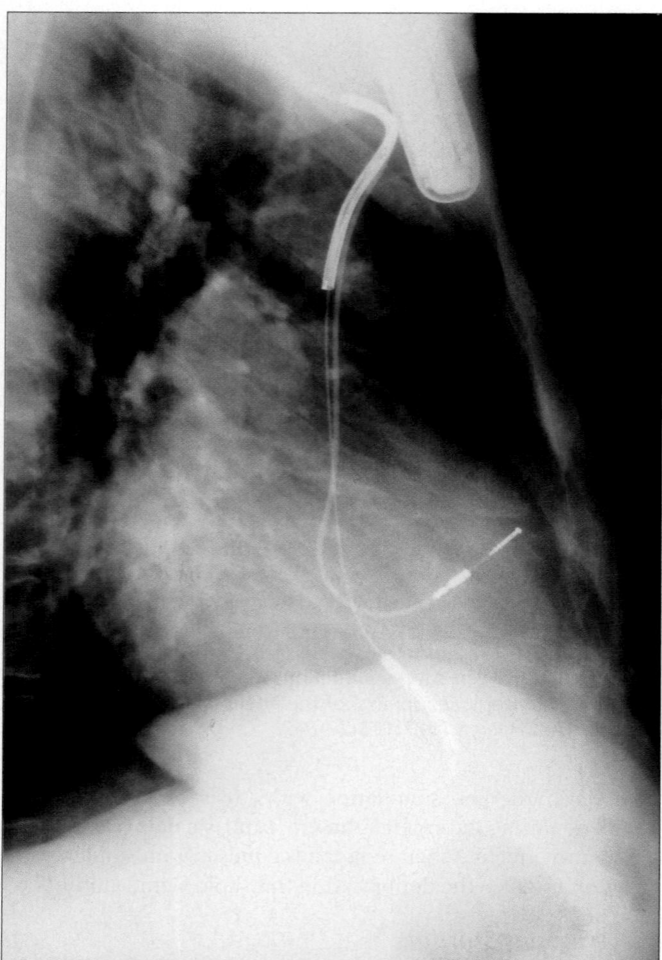

Figure 66.12 Lateral chest radiograph showing a dual-chamber ICD.

development of the newer generation dual-chamber ICD. The use of high-rate overdrive pacing in an ICD with atrial therapies has been shown to be effective in terminating half of all the spontaneous atrial episodes.[21] This suggests that many episodes of clinical atrial fibrillation begin with a more organized rhythm that can be pace terminated promptly. In patients with standard ICD indications and atrial arrhythmias, atrial pacing and shock therapies of a dual-chamber ICD significantly reduce the atrial fibrillation burden. It has been shown that repeated conversion of atrial fibrillation to restore sinus rhythm is associated with a reduction in the total arrhythmia duration and left atrial size. This reverse remodeling effect may be important in the ICD population because coexistent left ventricular dysfunction is common and maintenance of sinus rhythm desirable.[22] However, discomfort to the patient associated with atrial defibrillation is an important limitation of this therapy.

ICD with Cardiac Resynchronization Therapy

Biventricular pacing is an established therapy to improve survival and functional status of heart failure patients with low ejection fraction associated with intraventricular conduction delay. In a cardiac resynchronization pacing device, by optimization of the atrioventricular interval and correction of intraventricular as well as interventricular conduction delay, atrial-synchronized biventricular electrical stimulation improves ventricular diastolic filling, reduces mitral regurgitation, and increases cardiac output. Cardiac resynchronization therapy alone or in combination with a defibrillator improves symptoms and outcome in heart failure patients with prolonged QRS duration.[10,23] As favorable electrophysiologic remodeling of the ventricle may accompany the hemodynamic and structural changes, cardiac resynchronization therapy appeared to diminish the need for defibrillator therapy in a crossover study.[24] In another crossover trial involving the ICD with resynchronization therapy, biventricular antitachycardia pacing appeared to be more efficacious than right ventricular antitachycardia pacing in termination of ventricular tachycardia[25] (see Chapter 74).

Implantation Procedure and Technique

ICD implantation is usually carried out under local anesthesia and conscious sedation in the electrophysiology laboratory or operation room under fluoroscopic guidance. Electrophysiologists, sometimes with the help of surgeons, perform most procedures. With decreasing device volume, the surgical technique becomes similar to that of pacemaker implantation (see also Chapter 55).

Left-sided implantation is preferred to achieve better configuration for the defibrillation vector involving the defibrillator can. After skin disinfection and draping, a left pectoral skin incision is made. Venous access is obtained from cutdown of the left cephalic vein if possible. Left axillary or subclavian vein puncture may also achieve venous access, but it is better to avoid this approach, especially for the defibrillation lead, as it is associated with fracture due to "crush" damage between the clavicle and the first rib. Separate venous access is often required for implantation of multiple leads. The right ventricular defibrillation lead is advanced to the right ventricular apex or high septal region, with the distal end of the proximal coil positioned near the right atrium–superior vena cava junction. The distal coil should be apposing the septum to facilitate defibrillation. According to the critical mass hypothesis, successful defibrillation is accomplished by an electrical shock depolarizing a sufficient amount of the myocardium between the electrodes. In dual-chamber ICD implantation, the atrial pace-sense lead is advanced to the right atrial appendage. Apart from achieving satisfactory pacing and sensing parameters, it is important to avoid far-field R-wave sensing, which may cause double counting in the atrial channel and inhibition of therapy for ventricular tachycardia. For the ICD with resynchronization therapy, an additional left ventricular pace-sense lead is required (Fig. 66.13). Measurements of sensing and pacing parameters are obtained by use of a pacing system analyzer (see Chapter 55). Maximum output pacing with 10 V is recommended for detection of diaphragmatic capture.

After satisfactory lead positions and measurements are obtained, the leads should be sutured to the underlying muscle layer with anchoring stitches. A subcutaneous pocket with sufficient room for the ICD and its leads is created in the pectoral region. With the reduced volume of current devices, submuscular implantation is rarely required in adults. However, because an ICD is still significantly larger than a pacemaker, it is important to avoid a pocket that is too tight, too high, or too lateral. A bulky device in a tight

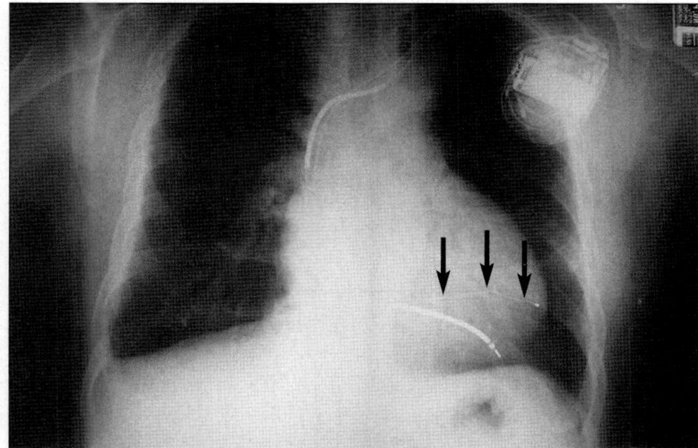

Figure 66.13 Chest radiograph showing an ICD with cardiac resynchronization therapy. The arrows show the left ventricular lead in the posterior coronary vein.

pocket may cause excessive stretch and subsequent pocket erosion. An ICD placed too high or too laterally may cause discomfort by friction on the clavicle or the shoulder joint with arm movement.

Defibrillation Threshold Testing

During ICD implantation, it is important to ensure that satisfactory ventricular fibrillation detection and defibrillation can be achieved. Previously, this was tested with an external cardioverter-defibrillator connected to the ICD lead. With the new advances in defibrillation waveform and technology, the rate of successful implantation is now close to 100%. Most manufacturers recommend performance of defibrillation testing with the implanted device. The defibrillation threshold is defined clinically as the lowest energy required to terminate ventricular fibrillation reproducibly.

Various protocols are used during an implantation procedure. A step-down to failure approach is usual. The programmed first shock energy requires a certain safety margin above the defibrillation threshold because successful defibrillation is a function of probability. It is usually programmed at twofold or 10 J above the defibrillation threshold. Most electrophysiologists start testing at 15 to 20 J and step down by 3 to 5 J. Repeated testing with an additional shock at the lowest energy with successful defibrillation is required to increase the accuracy and reproducibility, especially if the programmed energy is close to the maximum shock energy of the device.

To simplify the procedure and to minimize the number of ventricular fibrillation inductions and shocks delivered to high-risk patients, one can apply the "10 J margin" rule and assume that two consecutive successes at 20 J provide an adequate safety margin for implantation of a device with a maximum output of 30 J. If the implantation criteria cannot be met, one can consider reversing the electrode polarity, changing the lead position, or adding a subcutaneous patch or array.

During defibrillation testing, the patient should be monitored and connected to an external defibrillator with cutaneous defibrillation patches. The test should be performed with the patient adequately sedated and with the external defibrillator fully charged up. Delivery of a T-wave shock, high-rate ventricular burst pacing, or alternating current can induce ventricular defibrillation. If the first test energy fails to terminate ventricular fibrillation, a second shock programmed at maximum energy should follow. If both shocks fail to terminate the ventricular fibrillation, an external rescue shock should be delivered immediately (Fig. 66.14). To allow a safety margin on sensing, the device may be tested with the lowest sensitivity programmed for ventricular fibrillation detection. Depending on the clinical status of the patient, around 5 minutes of rest is usually allowed between each defibrillation test. The episode data and intracardiac electrograms are scrutinized for correct function.

After satisfactory defibrillation testing, the device pocket is closed in layers. A chest radiograph is required to verify lead position and to exclude pneumothorax. A predischarge device check is useful for detection of early lead migration. Predischarge defibrillation testing is indicated if the test was not performed during ICD implantation or if lead migration is suspected.

Device Programming

In general, ICD programming should be tailored to the patient's clinical presentation, results of defibrillation testing, and electrophysiology study. On the other hand, because not all ventricular tachycardias are inducible, and an induced arrhythmia may not be identical to the spontaneous arrhythmia, ICD programming is frequently empiric.

Detection and therapy are the most important programmable parameters to consider. For ventricular fibrillation

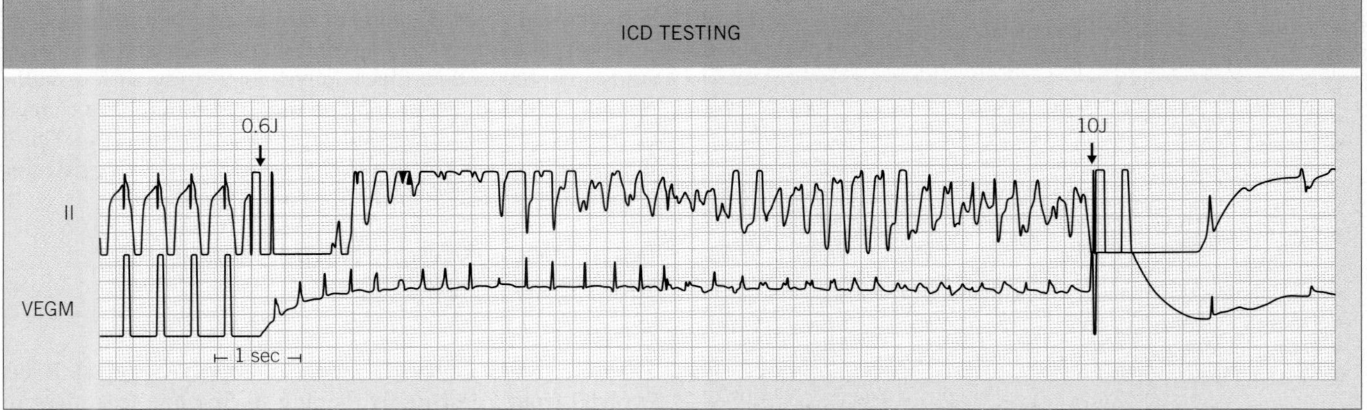

Figure 66.14 ICD testing. A T-wave shock at 0.6 J was delivered to induce ventricular fibrillation. Ventricular fibrillation was detected and successfully terminated by a 10-J shock from the ICD. VEGM, intracardiac ventricular electrogram.

detection, a nominal cycle length of 300 to 320 ms is often used. For ventricular tachycardia detection, the cycle length is usually programmed to 40 ms or more above that of the clinical tachycardia. Tiered-therapy devices allow different therapies to be delivered to arrhythmias, depending on cycle length. The first shock energy for ventricular fibrillation needs to be twice that of or 10 J above the defibrillation threshold, and subsequent shocks are usually programmed at the maximum shock energy. For hemodynamically stable ventricular tachycardia, one can attempt antitachycardia pacing before cardioversion.

Detection enhancement criteria may be programmed on if necessary. In case of slow ventricular tachycardia, especially after antiarrhythmic drugs, the cycle length may overlap with that during sinus tachycardia. The onset criterion may be programmed on to enhance arrhythmia classification. With coexistent atrial fibrillation, the interval stability criterion may be helpful to distinguish atrial fibrillation from ventricular tachycardia. The electrogram width criterion may be helpful in differentiating ventricular tachycardia from supraventricular tachycardia.

Patient Follow-up and Troubleshooting

Device follow-up is intended to check for the occurrence of any arrhythmia, therapy delivered, lead performance, and battery status (Table 66.2). The follow-up interval should preferably not exceed 4 months. Unscheduled follow-up is often required if patients report receiving ICD shocks, especially multiple or apparently inappropriate shocks.

After device interrogation, the episode log will indicate the arrhythmia count. Further details, such as the timing of occurrence, cycle length, arrhythmia classification, therapies delivered, and outcome, can also be obtained. The stored electrogram is retrieved to verify appropriate sensing. Noise detection, crosstalk, sensing of noncardiac signals, and T- or P-wave oversensing are sought. Real-time monitoring of the electrocardiogram with intracardiac electrograms and the marker channel may be helpful in identifying oversensing (Fig. 66.15). In case of suspected lead fracture, the patient

OVERVIEW OF ROUTINE ICD FOLLOW-UP
Review arrhythmia episodes
■ Date and time
■ Cycle length
■ Therapy
■ Outcome
■ Retrospective arrhythmia classification
Review programmed settings and device status
■ Brady pacing
■ Detection and enhancement criteria
■ Therapy
Assess battery status
■ Voltage
■ Charge time
Determine lead performance
■ Sensing, real-time electrogram, and marker channel
■ Pacing threshold
■ Pacing impedance
■ Shocking lead impedance

Table 66.2 Overview of routine ICD follow-up.

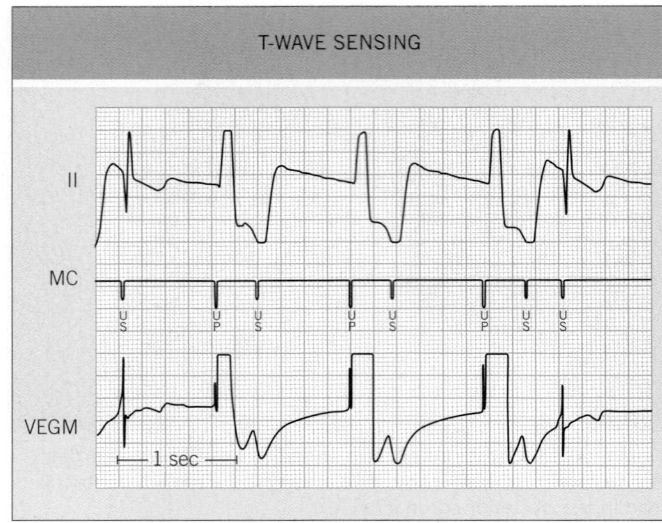

Figure 66.15 T-wave sensing as indicated by real-time marker. The upper panel shows surface electrocardiogram lead II, the middle panel shows the marker channel (MC), and the lower panel shows real-time intracardiac ventricular electrograms (VEGM). During ventricular pacing, the T wave was sensed as a ventricular signal, leading to double counting.

may move the arm around or perform the maneuver that provoked the ICD shock while ICD therapy is temporarily disabled (Fig. 66.16). The stored electrograms are useful for retrospective analysis and arrhythmia diagnosis. For instance, the onset, regularity, electrogram width, and relationship between atrial and ventricular electrograms in dual-chamber devices facilitate arrhythmia classification.

The voltage indicates the status of the battery. If the manufacturer-specified elective replacement index is reached, timely device replacement is required. The charge time is also an indicator of battery and capacitor performance. If the charge time exceeds the manufacturer-specified upper limit, a manual capacitor reform should be performed to see whether the charge time shortens. Subsequently, more frequent automatic capacitor reformation may be needed. If the charge time is still prolonged, the device may need to be replaced for safety reasons.

To check for lead performance, measurement of P- and R-wave amplitudes, T- or P-wave oversensing, pacing threshold, pacing impedance, and defibrillation lead impedance are obtained. These may indicate lead dislodgement or lead fracture. A chest radiograph should be obtained for comparison with the old films. In case of suspected malfunctioning or inappropriate programming of the ICD, electrophysiology study may be needed. Electrophysiology study with or without defibrillation testing may be required if there is a change in antiarrhythmic drugs and after ablation therapy. These may alter the cycle length and characteristics of the ventricular arrhythmia or change the defibrillation threshold.

INDICATIONS, CONTRAINDICATIONS, AND OBJECTIVES

Objectives

The objective of device therapy is to improve survival. It has evolved from a last-resort therapy to first-line treatment in cardiac arrest survivors. In patients with structural heart

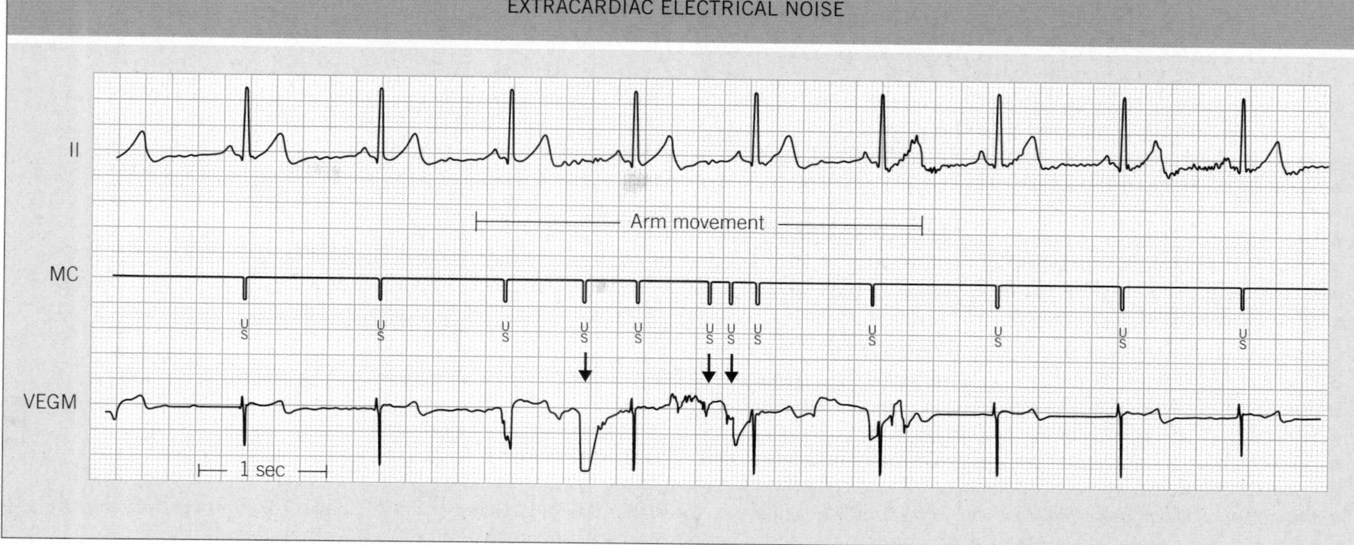

Figure 66.16 Intermittent electrical noise generated because of lead fracture. Extracardiac electrical noise reproduced during arm movement *(arrows)* was sensed as ventricular signal. MC, marker channel; VEGM, intracardiac ventricular electrogram.

disease who present with sudden cardiac arrest, spontaneous ventricular tachycardia, or syncope of undetermined cause with inducible ventricular arrhythmias at electrophysiology study, ICD is indicated.[26,27] For asymptomatic but high-risk patients, prophylactic ICD implantation has also been shown to improve overall survival.[28]

Indications

Secondary Prevention

The indications for ICD therapy are listed in Tables 66.3 and 66.4. For secondary prevention of sudden death, the ICD is indicated in treatment of ventricular tachyarrhythmias complicating structural heart diseases. In the Antiarrhythmics Versus Implantable Defibrillators (AVID) trial, the first large-scale randomized study to compare device therapy with conventional therapy in patients with left ventricular dysfunction and ventricular fibrillation or hemodynamically significant ventricular tachycardia, mortality in the device arm was reduced by 31% at 3 years ($P < .02$).[2] Of note, among the 1016 patients randomized, most patients in the conventional treatment arm were treated with amiodarone (see Fig. 66.2). In a post hoc subgroup analysis, it was found that the survival benefit in AVID was largely limited to patients with left ventricular ejection fraction of less than 35%.[29] Results of other studies like the Canadian Implantable Defibrillator Study (CIDS) and Cardiac Arrest Study Hamburg (CASH) also supported that the ICD is superior to medical therapy in secondary prevention of ventricular arrhythmias. In CIDS, 659 patients with ventricular fibrillation, symptomatic ventricular tachycardia, or syncope with either inducible ventricular tachycardia or spontaneous nonsustained ventricular tachycardia were randomized to receive an ICD or amiodarone. The ICD arm had 20% reduction in total mortality and 33% reduction in arrhythmic death after 5 years, although statistical significance was not reached ($P = .14$ and $P = .09$, respectively).[3] In CASH, 288 cardiac arrest survivors were randomized to receive an ICD, amiodarone, or metoprolol. After 57 months, there was 23% reduction in all-cause mortality in ICD patients, but statistical significance was also not reached ($P = .08$).[4] The use of thoracotomy systems among some patients in these trials might have resulted in higher perioperative mortality, and the survival benefit of ICD might have been understated.

The ICD is also indicated in patients with syncope of undetermined origin and clinically relevant inducible ventricular tachyarrhythmias at electrophysiology study. In the presence of ventricular dysfunction or prior myocardial infarction, the cause of syncope is likely to be ventricular tachyarrhythmias if other causes are excluded. It has been shown that in this situation, the subsequent rate of appropriate ICD discharge is high.[30-32]

Primary Prevention

The role of ICD in primary prevention of sudden death in patients with coronary artery disease and left ventricular dysfunction was established after the Multicenter Automatic Defibrillator Implantation Trial (MADIT), Multicenter Unsustained Tachycardia Trial (MUSTT), and MADIT II.

In MADIT, patients with previous myocardial infarction, depressed left ventricular function (ejection fraction of 35% or less), and nonsustained ventricular tachycardia underwent electrophysiology study. Among them, 196 patients with inducible sustained ventricular tachyarrhythmias but not suppressed by procainamide were randomized to receive an ICD or conventional therapy. The ICD group had a 54% reduction in mortality at 2 years ($P = .009$), and the benefit was greatest in patients with the lowest left ventricular ejection fraction (see Fig. 66.2).[5]

MUSTT was designed to compare electrophysiology-guided therapy and no active treatment in high-risk patients with asymptomatic nonsustained ventricular tachycardia. The 2202 patients with previous myocardial infarction and ejection fraction of 40% or less underwent electrophysiology study before randomization. The noninducible patients were followed up in the registry. The 704 inducible patients

MAJOR INDICATIONS FOR ICD THERAPY IN ADULTS
Class I (general agreement of benefit with ICD therapy)
■ Cardiac arrest due to ventricular fibrillation or hemodynamically unstable sustained VT after evaluation to define the cause of the event and to exclude any completely reversible causes.
■ Structural heart disease and spontaneous sustained VT, whether hemodynamically stable or unstable.
■ Syncope of undetermined origin with clinically relevant, hemodynamically significant sustained VT or VF induced at electrophysiological study.
■ LVEF less than 35% due to prior MI, at least 40 days post-MI with NYHA functional Class II or III.
■ Nonischemic dilated cardiomyopathy (DCM) with an LVEF less than or equal to 35% and NYHA functional Class II or III.
■ LV dysfunction due to prior MI, at least 40 days post-MI with an LVEF less than 30%, and NYHA functional Class I.
■ Nonsustained VT due to prior MI, LVEF less than 40%, and inducible VF or sustained VT at electrophysiological study.
Class II (ICD therapy reasonable or may be considered)
■ Unexplained syncope, significant LV dysfunction, and nonischemic DCM.
■ Sustained VT and normal or near-normal ventricular function.
■ HCM with 1 or more major risk factors for SCD.
■ Arrhythmogenic right ventricular dysplasia/cardiomyopathy (ARVD/C) and 1 or more risk factors for SCD.
■ Long-QT syndrome with syncope and/or VT while receiving beta blockers.
■ Miscellaneous high risk conditions including Brugada syndrome, catecholaminergic polymorphic VT, Chagas' disease, cardiac sarcoidosis, giant cell myocarditis, left ventricular noncompaction, and other familial cardiomyopathies associated with sudden death.
Class III (not indicated; risk of ICD therapy exceeds expected benefit)
■ No reasonable expectation of survival with an acceptable functional status for at least 1 year, even if they meet ICD implantation criteria specified in the Class I and II recommendations above.
■ Incessant VT or VF.
■ Significant psychiatric illnesses that may be aggravated by device implantation or that may preclude systematic follow-up.
■ NYHA Class IV drug-refractory congestive heart failure when cardiac transplantation or cardiac resynchronization therapy are not indicated.
All primary SCD prevention ICD recommendations apply only to patients who are receiving optimal medical therapy and have reasonable expectation of survival with good functional capacity for more than 1 year. (From Epstein AE, DiMarco JP, Ellenbogen KA, et al. ACC/AHA/HRS 2008 guidelines for device-based therapy of cardiac rhythm abnormalities: a report of the American College of Cardiology/American Heart Association Task Force on Practice Guidelines. Circulation 2008:117:e350-e408.)

Table 66.3 Major indications for ICD therapy in adults.

were randomized to receive conventional therapy with no antiarrhythmics or electrophysiologically guided treatment. Patients who remained inducible despite class Ia antiarrhythmics, propafenone, or sotalol were randomized to receive an ICD or further drug testing until all patients received either an ICD or an effective drug. At 5 years of follow-up, mortality was 9% in patients who received ICD, 34% in patients treated with an effective drug guided by electrophysiology study, and 32% in patients randomized to no antiarrhythmics ($P < .001$).[6]

In MADIT II, 1232 patients with prior myocardial infarction and left ventricular ejection fraction of 30% or less were randomized to ICD or conventional medical therapy in a 3:2 ratio. No nonsustained ventricular arrhythmias or electrophysiology study was required for enrollment. During an average follow-up of 20 months, the mortality in the ICD group was 14.2%, and that of the control group was 19.8% (31% risk reduction; $P = .02$).[7] This study demonstrated that prophylactic ICD implantation offered significant survival benefit in patients with advanced left ventricular dysfunction after myocardial infarction (see Fig. 66.2).

There were three primary prevention trials that failed to demonstrate any survival benefit of ICD implantation in certain subgroups of patients with coronary artery disease and left ventricular dysfunction. The Coronary Artery Bypass Graft (CABG) Patch Trial compared the ICD and usual care in 900 CABG candidates with ejection fraction of 35% or less and an abnormal signal-averaged electrocardiogram.[33] The Defibrillators in Acute Myocardial Infarction Trial (DINAMIT) compared the ICD with best medical therapy in 674 patients 6 to 40 days after acute myocardial infarction, in class I to III, with ejection fraction of 35% or less, and with abnormal autonomic tone manifested as depressed heart rate variability or elevated 24-hour heart rate.[34] The Beta-blocker Strategy plus ICD (BEST-ICD) compared the ICD with medical therapy in 138 patients within 1 month after an acute myocardial infarction.[35] Patients were randomized to medical therapy or invasive risk stratification by electrophysiology study if their ejection fraction was 30% or less and associated with frequent ventricular ectopics, abnormal signal-averaged electrocardiogram, or heart rate variability. Inducible patients were implanted with an ICD and noninducible patients received medical therapy. The lack of benefit of the ICD in these categories of patients may be due to the fact that ventricular arrhythmia is not a predominant cause of death or, because of ongoing ventricular remodeling early after acute myocardial infarction or CABG, that the substrate for ventricular arrhythmogenesis is still evolving.

The Sudden Cardiac Death in Heart Failure Trial (SCD-HeFT) compared the ICD plus conventional therapy to conventional therapy alone and conventional therapy plus empiric amiodarone in patients with class II and class III heart failure of more than 3 months and ejection fraction of 35% or less.[8] This is so far the largest trial of the ICD in primary prevention of sudden death in heart failure, with 2521 patients of both ischemic and nonischemic causes randomized. During 45.5 months of follow-up, patients randomized to the ICD had 23% lower mortality compared with conventional therapy ($P = .007$) with or without amiodarone (see Fig 66.2). The benefit of the ICD was consistent in patients with either ischemic or nonischemic cardiomyopathy.

In selected heart failure patients with widened QRS and regardless of etiology, the ICD offered significant survival benefit in addition to cardiac resynchronization therapy. The Comparison of Medical Therapy, Pacing, and Defibrillation in Heart Failure (COMPANION) study compared cardiac resynchronization therapy with or without an ICD to best medical therapy in 1520 class III/IV heart failure patients with QRS of 120 ms or more and ejection fraction of 35% or less. Cardiac resynchronization therapy in combination with an ICD resulted in 36% relative reduction in total mortality ($P = .003$), whereas cardiac resynchronization therapy alone was associated with a nonsignificant 24% relative reduction ($P = .059$) in total mortality after 12 months of follow-up.

There were three smaller primary prevention trials that were limited to patients with nonischemic dilated cardiomyopathy. The Cardiomyopathy Arrhythmia Trial (CAT) randomized 104 patients with nonischemic cardiomyopathy and ejection fraction of 30% or less to receive an ICD or no device.[36] The Amiodarone Versus Implantable Defibrillator Randomized Trial (AMIOVIRT) randomized 103 patients with nonischemic cardiomyopathy and nonsustained ventricular tachycardia to an ICD or amiodarone.[37] Both trials had a relatively low mortality (30% at 6 years in CAT and 20% at 3 years in AMIOVIRT) and failed to demonstrate any difference in survival between the ICD arm and the control arm. However, they are small trials that are grossly underpowered to assess survival benefit. In the Defibrillators in Nonischemic Cardiomyopathy Treatment Evaluation (DEFINITE), 458 patients with nonischemic dilated cardiomyopathy, class I to class III heart failure, ejection fraction of 35% or less, and ambient ventricular arrhythmias (frequent premature ventricular beats or nonsustained ventricular tachycardia) were randomized to receive an ICD or conventional therapy. After 29 months of follow-up, there was a nonsignificant 35% reduction in all-cause mortality ($P = .08$) and highly significant 80% reduction in arrhythmia death ($P = .006$).

Since 2002, when the latest guideline on ICD implantation was released from the American College of Cardiology/American Heart Association/North American Society for Pacing and Electrophysiology Committee (see Table 66.3), a number of important ICD trials have been published. The evolving guidelines are likely to incorporate alterations for primary prevention in high-risk patients (see Table 66.4). As clinical trials used slightly different cutoff values for ejection fraction, a range of values (e.g., ejection fraction of 30% to 35% or less) is therefore included on the basis of trials that enroll patients within that range of ejection fraction.[27]

Current evidence from multiple randomized trials shows that patients with significant left ventricular dysfunction of both ischemic and nonischemic causes benefit from ICD implantation; whether all patients who fulfill the criteria should receive an ICD is controversial. Additional risk assessment strategy is required for better identification of patients who need an ICD. Currently, there are some data to suggest that abnormal micro–T-wave alternans may identify heart failure patients at risk of sudden death. However, confirmatory results from additional prospective randomized studies are needed.

Some congenital or hereditary conditions are associated with a high risk for ventricular tachyarrhythmias and sudden cardiac death. Examples are congenital long QT syndrome, Brugada syndrome, arrhythmogenic right ventricular dysplasia, and hypertrophic cardiomyopathy (see Chapters 63 and 79). Because these diseases cause potentially lethal electrical disorder but infrequently affect the left ventricular systolic function, the prognosis should be good if fatal arrhythmias can be aborted promptly. Because there is no large randomized trial on most of these conditions, the selection criteria for prophylactic ICD implantation should be based on the best available contemporary evidence and results of comprehensive risk stratification.

Contraindications

The ICD is contraindicated if there is a transient reversible cause, such as myocardial infarction or electrolyte imbalance, to account for the ventricular arrhythmias. Incessant ventricular tachycardia or fibrillation is also considered a contraindication, as incessant arrhythmias will cause frequent device therapy and rapid battery drainage. Ablation therapy should be offered if the arrhythmia is amenable to surgical or catheter ablation.

Defibrillator therapy should not be prescribed in patients with New York Heart Association (NYHA) class IV drug-refractory heart failure, patients who are not candidates for cardiac transplantation and cardiac resynchronization therapy, and patients with terminal illnesses with projected life expectancy not more than 6 months. The ICD is also contraindicated in patients with significant psychiatric illnesses that may be aggravated by device implantation or may preclude follow-up.

Device therapy is not indicated in patients with recurrent syncope of undetermined cause but without inducible ventricular tachycardia or fibrillation at electrophysiology study.

COMPLICATIONS

Although there is evidence to support ICD therapy in patients at high risk for sudden death, this therapy is not entirely free of complications. Nearly half of ICD patients experience device-related adverse events within 1 year of implantation. The perioperative mortality of nonthoracotomy ICD implantation is below 1%; earlier series that involved thoracotomy procedures with or without concomitant surgical operations reported a much higher mortality. The morbidities associated with ICD implantation are related to the operative procedure or are complications related to the system itself.

Early surgical complications of ICD implantation include pocket hematoma, pneumothorax, hemothorax, lead perforation, and lead dislodgement. Pocket infection happens in around 1% of procedures and can be early or delayed. Like pacemaker pocket infection, it is usually related to the implantation procedure, and the organism is frequently *Staphylococcus aureus*. The clinical presentation includes general signs of infection such as redness, swelling, tenderness, fever, and leukocytosis. Intravenous antibiotics may be useful in controlling only the most superficial infection. In general, for ICD system infection, it is required to explant the generator and the leads to eradicate the organisms. Early ventricular defibrillation lead dislodgement is infrequent enough to preclude predischarge defibrillation testing in many centers.

Late complications of ICD implantation are mostly related to lead malfunction or frequent shocks. ICD lead fracture is a common late complication, and the failure rate at 10 years reaches 20%.[38] A fractured lead may generate electrical noise especially during arm movement. This may cause inappropriate ICD therapy. A high impedance of the pace-sense lead and reproduction of the noise signals with arm movement may help recognize this complication. Radiography may identify the fractured site, which is commonly located at the junction between the clavicle and the first rib. A loose connector may generate similar electrical noise and cause high impedance in the pace-sense circuit. Both conditions require surgical intervention for correction. If only the pace-sense function is lost, a pace-sense lead may be added in the right ventricle as a partial replacement procedure. Device and defibrillation lead malfunctions are increasingly reported as the number of devices implanted increases over time (see the section on special issues, device recalls).

Inappropriate therapy was identified as a major late complication of ICD implantation. The potential causes are shown in Table 66.4. The incidence of supraventricular arrhythmias causing device therapy is reported to be 20% to 30%. Despite the use of antiarrhythmic drugs and arrhythmia discrimination algorithms, the incidence of inappropriate ICD therapies remains high (Fig. 66.17). The availability of the dual-chamber ICD enables dual-chamber sensing, atrial electrogram storage, and development of dual-chamber algorithms for arrhythmia discrimination. Although these algorithms are reported to be highly sensitive and specific, controversies exist as to whether dual-chamber ICDs have an advantage over single-chamber devices in reduction of inappropriate therapies. Small clinical studies comparing single- and dual-chamber devices showed that the incidence of inappropriate ICD therapies was not reduced because of atrial undersensing or problems in the design of the algorithm.[39] Large trials are required to confirm this. Furthermore, accuracy in arrhythmia classification is likely to be algorithm specific. Continuous modification of the algorithm design and flexibility in programming are likely to result in improvement in the arrhythmia classification of dual-chamber ICDs.

CAUSES OF INAPPROPRIATE ICD THERAPY
Fractured pace-sense lead
Loose connector
External electromagnetic interference
T- or P-wave oversensing
Supraventricular arrhythmias including sinus tachycardia
Pacemaker-defibrillator interaction leading to sensing of the pacing artifacts and double counting

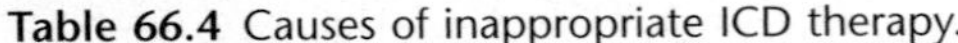

Table 66.4 Causes of inappropriate ICD therapy.

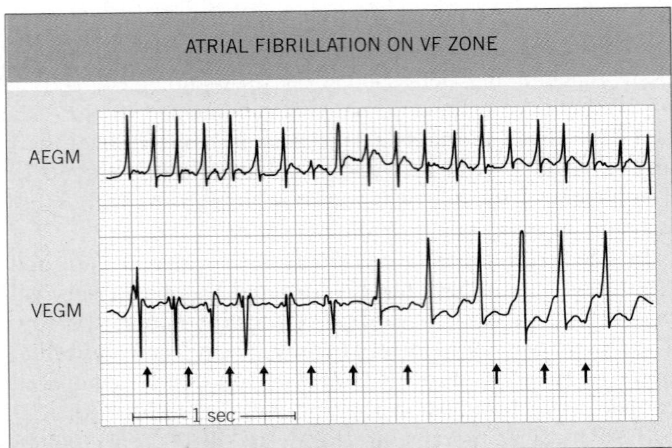

Figure 66.17 Rapid ventricular rate during atrial fibrillation. The upper panel shows atrial electrograms (AEGM) and the lower panel shows ventricular electrograms (VEGM). During this episode of atrial fibrillation, 10/11 R-R intervals fall into the ventricular fibrillation (VF) detection zone programmed at 320 ms. For safety purposes, dual-chamber algorithms do not apply in the zone of ventricular fibrillation. The arrow denotes an R-R interval equal to or less than 320 ms.

Inappropriate programming of dual-chamber pacing in ICD patients with impaired left ventricular function who do not require bradycardia pacing may increase heart failure hospitalization or death. It is recommended to encourage intrinsic conduction by programming pacing at a low backup rate or a long atrioventricular interval to minimize unnecessary right ventricular pacing.

Electrical storm, or frequent appropriate ICD shocks, may be associated with deteriorating heart failure, myocardial ischemia, electrolyte imbalance, or drug proarrhythmia. In addition to optimization of cardiovascular therapy, a salvage procedure such as catheter ablation of ventricular tachycardia may be needed to reduce arrhythmia episodes. Amiodarone is frequently used as an adjuvant antiarrhythmic agent in ICD recipients. Electrophysiology study and defibrillation testing may be required after initiation of antiarrhythmic drugs as the defibrillation threshold may change and the tachycardia cycle length may increase to above that originally programmed for tachycardia detection.

Sudden death occurs in ICD patients at 1% to 5% per year in different trials. The cause of death may be related to device malfunction or patient factors. Device-related causes include device inactivation, battery depletion, failure of sensing, failure of detection due to inappropriate programming of detection or enhancement criteria, and high defibrillation threshold. Patient-related causes include pulseless electrical activity, myocardial ischemia or infarction, and incessant ventricular arrhythmias.[40]

ICD-induced proarrhythmia is rare but potentially fatal. Possible causes are summarized in Table 66.5.

ICD-INDUCED PROARRHYTHMIAS
Acceleration or degeneration of ventricular tachycardia after antitachycardia pacing or low-energy cardioversion
Induction of atrial fibrillation by T-wave shock, low-energy cardioversion, or defibrillation
Induction of ventricular tachyarrhythmias by antitachycardia pacing initiated as inappropriate therapy for supraventricular tachyarrhythmias
Post-shock bradycardia
Post-shock increase in pacing threshold resulting in failure to capture
Pacemaker-mediated tachycardia in dual-chamber ICD
Pacemaker-ICD interaction leading to reset of a separate pacemaker after a shock

Table 66.5 ICD-induced proarrhythmias.

SPECIAL ISSUES

Device Selection

With the introduction of dual-chamber ICDs, incorporation of atrial therapies, and cardiac resynchronization therapy, device selection becomes a challenge to the implanting physicians. Apart from various functions and programmability, basic characteristics of these devices, such as size, longevity, complexity, and cost, should also be considered. Current evidence supports that a dual-chamber ICD is indicated in patients who have a concomitant indication for physiologic pacing, such as sinus node disease, atrioventricular nodal block, or drug-induced bradycardia. A dual-chamber ICD is also indicated in special conditions, such as congenital long QT syndrome, in which dual-chamber or atrial-based pacing may be beneficial. Furthermore, refined dual-chamber arrhythmia discrimination algorithms and enhanced atrial therapies are preferable for patients with frequent supraventricular arrhythmias. NYHA class III and class IV heart failure, low left ventricular ejection fraction, and prolonged QRS duration are indications for an ICD with cardiac resynchronization therapy.

Driving Restrictions

There is no legal restriction on noncommercial driving in ICD patients in the United States, Europe, or Asia. Physicians commonly advise their patients to refrain from driving for 6 months after device implantation to assess the frequency of arrhythmia and their reaction to device therapy.[41] Patients who receive an ICD for primary prevention, except for the first week after the procedure, are not restricted from driving in the absence of any symptom or appropriate device therapy for ventricular arrhythmia.[42] There is no evidence that the rate of serious traffic accidents involving ICD patients as drivers is increased compared with that of the general population.

Quality of Life

In most patients, the quality of life is improved after ICD implantation. In a minority of patients with undue worries about their health, psychological distress may develop after device implantation. Frequent ICD shocks may also cause anxiety and depression. It is important for physicians to understand the psychological impact of device therapy, and early referral to patient support groups, clinical psychologists, or counselors should be encouraged.

Cost-effectiveness

ICD therapy is perceived to be expensive because the initial cost is high. However, the available literature suggests that the ICD is a cost-effective therapy in secondary prevention of sudden death. In terms of cost per quality-adjusted life-year gained, device therapy is comparable to other well-accepted therapeutic interventions for cardiovascular diseases.[43] However, the number needed to treat for prevention of one sudden death at 36 months ranged between 3 and 39 according to various primary prevention trials.[44] In view of the enormous health care cost potentially involved, a solution in enhanced selection of patients is warranted. This provides the foundation for future research aimed at identification of patients most likely to benefit from an ICD.

Device Recalls

Reports of device malfunctions have increased as indications for the device have expanded and the volume of implantation has increased. As these reports gain media attention, patient anxiety and uncertainty in accepting device therapy also grow. Professional organizations, regulatory agencies, and the device industry are trying to manage this problem by encouraging vigilant postmarketing surveillance, standardization of terminology, and improvement of the system for physician notification and reporting of adverse events. Although ICD advisories are frequent and the number of devices affected is large, the actual number of device malfunctions is very low compared with the number of lives saved by ICDs implanted. The risk of device malfunction should be balanced against the risk of device replacement in the course of individual consideration regarding ICD recalls.

Provider of Device Therapy

In the United States, it has been reported that cardiologists without proper accreditation and training in ICD implantation have begun implantation and follow-up of ICDs. Although they may be able to master the surgical technique of device implantation, the proper management of device therapy, such as programming, troubleshooting, and treating complications, is beyond their capacity. This practice is doubtful on both professional and ethical grounds. As stated in guidelines of professional organizations, prescription, implantation, and follow-up of an ICD should be performed by accredited physicians.

SUMMARY

The ICD has evolved from an innovative idea to become a real device implanted by an electrophysiologist in the cardiac catheterization laboratory under local anesthesia. ICD technology continues to advance in the transvenous implantation procedure, generator size reduction, system longevity, arrhythmia discrimination, and programmable features such as rate-adaptive pacing, atrial therapies, and cardiac resynchronization therapy. The ICD is proven to be effective in preventing sudden death in various categories of high-risk patients as shown in both secondary and primary prevention trials. It is associated with modest complications. Device-based monitoring of hemodynamic status, myocardial ischemia, and autonomic changes of the patients may benefit patient management in addition to conventional clinical assessment. Furthermore, remote access of device information, monitoring signals, and safety alerts enable Internet-based follow-up as well as early detection of cardiac events and decompensation. Upcoming ICD trials will focus on evaluation of new technology, cost-effectiveness, and enhanced selection of patients at risk for sudden death.

chapter

67 Special Problems in Ventricular Arrhythmias

a. Multiple Shocks from an Implanted Cardioverter-Defibrillator—I

John M. Miller

DEFINITION OF PROBLEM

The implantable cardioverter-defibrillator (ICD) has revolutionized treatment of malignant ventricular tachyarrhythmias, such as ventricular tachycardia (VT) and ventricular fibrillation (VF). In some cases, though, these devices seem to go out of control, resulting in repeated shocks to the patient. This scenario has many possible causes, one of which is illustrated in the following case.

TYPICAL CASE

A 56-year-old man suffered an acute inferior wall myocardial infarction 5 years ago, complicated by mild congestive heart failure. One month ago, he had an episode of presyncope for which a rescue squad was summoned. On arrival, he was found to have a heart rate of 200 beats per minute and blood pressure of 90/60 mm Hg. The electrocardiogram showed VT that was cardioverted to sinus rhythm in the emergency department. Subsequent evaluation showed no new myocardial damage. An echocardiogram showed an ejection fraction of 35% and no evidence of a mural thrombus. He underwent placement of a single-chamber ICD and was discharged the following day. He did well for 3 weeks, at which time he began experiencing recurrent palpitations and lightheadedness. His ICD shocked him twice on one day and once the following day, but he never lost consciousness. Stored electrograms retrieved at ICD interrogation showed several VT episodes, some of which were terminated with antitachycardia pacing (Fig. 67A.1a), but others required shocks (Fig. 67A.1b).

DIFFERENTIAL DIAGNOSIS

Despite the sophistication of current ICDs, it is sometimes difficult to know whether shocks delivered in the absence of loss of consciousness are appropriate (for VT or VF) or inappropriate (e.g., for rapidly conducted atrial fibrillation, sinus tachycardia, artifact from lead fracture). Stored electrograms in ICDs allow the physician to "play back" a prior episode and to analyze whether the device functioned correctly (see Fig. 67A.1). In cases of multiple shocks, it is important to analyze each episode because not all of them may be identical. It is possible that one arrhythmia, such as atrial fibrillation, may trigger one ICD therapy (pacing) that may initiate another arrhythmia, such as VT or VF. In this case, it may be as important to control the initiating event as subsequent ones.

TREATMENT OPTIONS

In this case, a variety of options are available to prevent recurrence of this patient's situation (ICD shocks due to frequent VT recurrences that cannot always be pace terminated). These include

- reprogramming of the ICD to a more aggressive pacing strategy that might terminate VT more readily;
- administration of antiarrhythmic drugs either to decrease the frequency of VT episodes or to make VT more easily terminable by pacing; and
- radiofrequency catheter ablation to decrease the frequency of or entirely eliminate VT recurrences.

There are several factors to be considered in deciding which option to choose. In case of ICD reprogramming, can the ICD successfully terminate VT with more aggressive antitachycardia pacing algorithms without resulting in arrhythmia acceleration or VF requiring a shock? This is very often possible and can be tested in the electrophysiology laboratory by inducing VT with the ICD's noninvasive programmed stimulation feature (no temporary transvenous catheters are needed). If this strategy works, it prevents recurrent shocks—but not recurrent VT and subsequent ICD therapies, which may occasionally fail to terminate VT, resulting in shocks.

Administration of antiarrhythmic drugs may prevent some or all VT episodes or alter antitachycardia pacing effectiveness (either improving or worsening). Choices of drugs may be limited by the degree of heart failure and concern for ventricular proarrhythmia. Amiodarone is often used in this

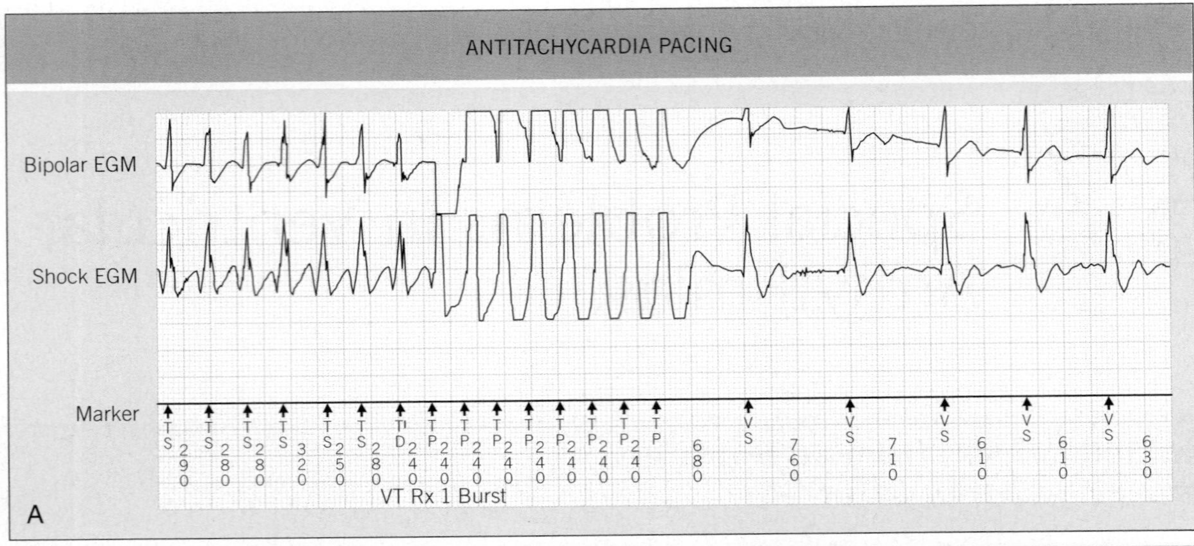

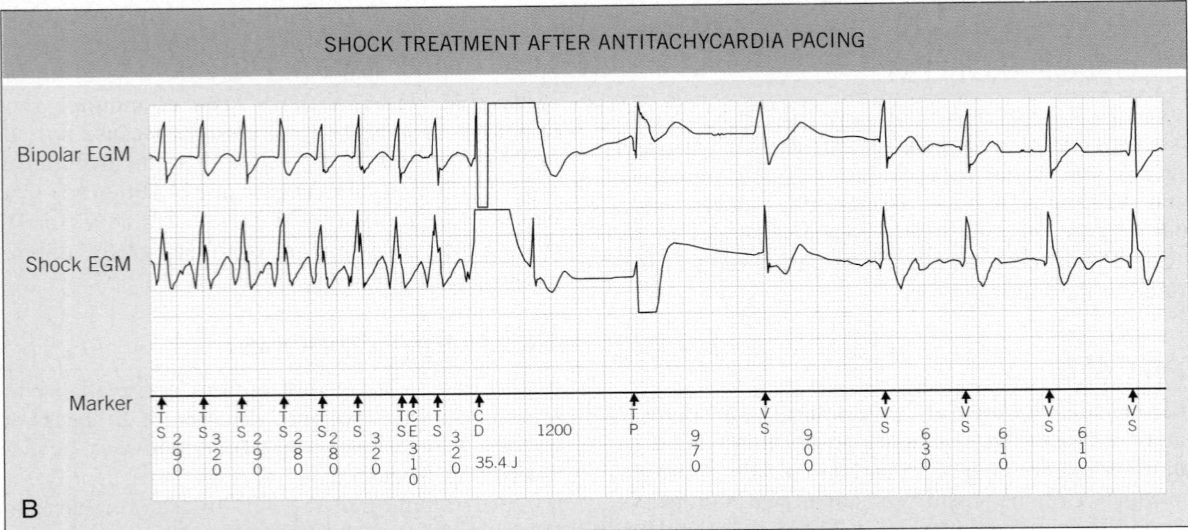

Figure 67A.1 Stored electrograms and marker channels from ICD interrogation. A, An episode of VT is successfully treated with antitachycardia pacing that results in sinus rhythm. **B,** Another episode of VT is successfully treated by a shock after several attempts at antitachycardia pacing had failed to terminate the episode.

situation because of its relatively better efficacy and side effect profiles, keeping in mind that some serious side effects, such as pulmonary toxicity, can rarely be lethal yet are difficult to predict. Drugs used in this setting can slow the VT rate during breakthrough recurrent episodes to such a degree that it no longer meets detection criteria and is thus not treated by the ICD. In addition, some antiarrhythmic drugs, such as amiodarone, may increase the defibrillation threshold. If a patient has a VF episode in this setting and the ICD is not able to terminate VF because of the presence of a drug that elevates defibrillation energy requirements beyond the device's capability, the patient will likely die. Thus, the ICD system must be thoroughly tested after initiation of antiarrhythmic medications to ensure proper functioning and may require reprogramming or modification.

Radiofrequency ablation has been used in this setting with good results. The advantages of this strategy are that if it is successful, the patient will have fewer or no episodes of recurrent VT, and it avoids the potential problems associated with use of antiarrhythmic medications. The major drawback of this procedure is that it is another catheterization with the attendant procedural risks, one of which is the possibility of systemic thromboembolism due to dislodgement of a left ventricular thrombus (present in some such cases). However, there are few other disadvantages to trying this option. Even if the procedure is completely unsuccessful (i.e., no VTs could be ablated), all the other treatment options are still available. Ablation is most readily applied in patients whose VT is hemodynamically tolerated (i.e., neither loss of consciousness nor severe angina or dyspnea is present during VT) because prolonged periods in VT are necessary to perform adequate left ventricular endocardial mapping for selection of target sites for radiofrequency delivery. A variety of mapping tools have been devised over the years that have increased the likelihood of a successful outcome for VT ablation (Fig. 67A.2, left). By use of these tools, the "culprit" VT (the morphology recorded during recurrent episodes) can be successfully ablated with radiofrequency energy in more than 80% of postinfarction

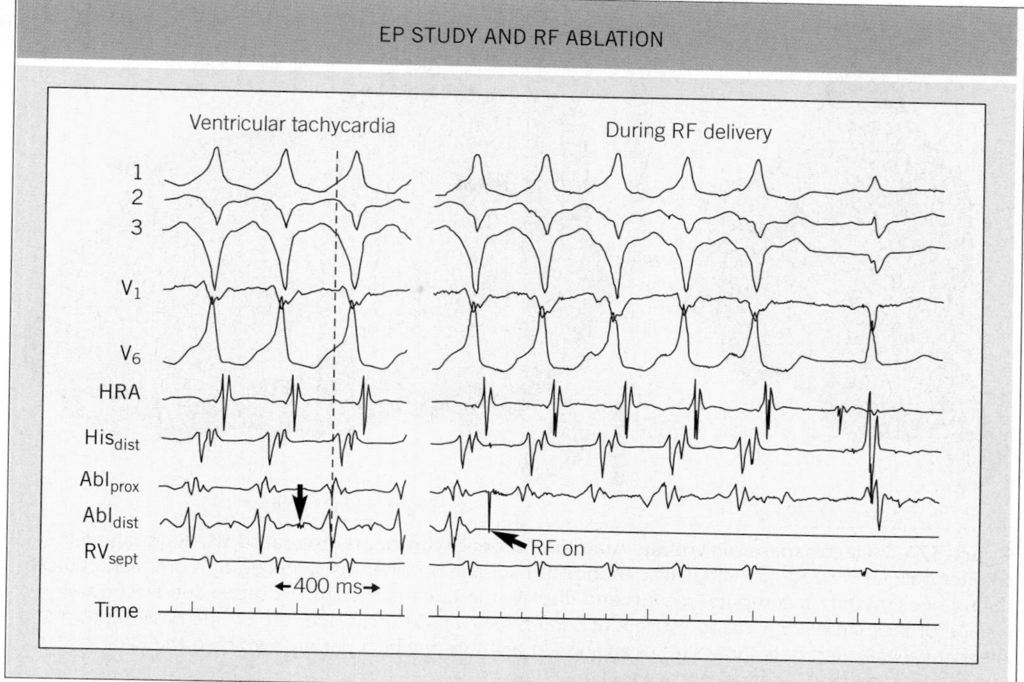

Figure 67A.2 Recordings during electrophysiology (EP) study and radiofrequency (RF) ablation in this patient. Shown are five surface electrocardiogram leads and intracardiac recordings from the high right atrium (HRA), the distal (dist) and proximal (prox) His bundle catheter electrodes, the ablation site (Abl), and the right ventricular septum (RV_{sept}). At left, an isolated mid-diastolic potential is seen *(vertical arrow)* that corresponds to electrical events in a critical part of the VT circuit. At right, delivery of radiofrequency energy *(diagonal arrow)* at this site results in nearly immediate termination of VT, resulting in sinus rhythm. This VT could not be reinitiated thereafter.

patients. However, most of these patients have multiple morphologies of VT inducible at electrophysiology study, and controversy remains about how aggressive one must be in attempting to ablate all VT morphologies. Most evidence suggests that if a VT morphology is induced at electrophysiology study and not ablated, it is likely to recur spontaneously at some future time. This is of obvious concern in a patient who does not have an ICD. In contrast, in the patient discussed here, the potential consequences of occasional recurrent VT episodes are much less serious. There is no evidence that VT ablation creates the possibility for additional ventricular arrhythmias. Finally, there is little likelihood of altering ICD performance or dislodging the lead because most mapping is carried out in the left ventricle. The patient was ideal for this treatment option because he tolerated his VT hemodynamically and echocardiography revealed no left ventricular thrombus. He preferred ablation to antiarrhythmic medications and underwent the ablation procedure without complications. At electrophysiology study, four morphologies of VT were induced and mapped. Two radiofrequency applications in the inferior basal region eliminated all inducible VT (Fig. 67A.2, right). He has not had any further ICD therapies during a follow-up period of 2 years.

Ablation therapy has recently been extended to patients whose VT is poorly tolerated hemodynamically. Several strategies have been employed:

- ablation of areas in the region of prior myocardial damage at which pacing closely mimics or replicates the QRS configuration during VT ("pace mapping");
- isolation of the region from which VT is likely to arise by making a continuous line of radiofrequency applications surrounding the infarct zone;
- ablation of selected portions of the border zone between prior infarction and more normal myocardium that have very low voltage signal amplitudes during sinus rhythm; and
- temporary use of circulatory support (intra-aortic balloon pump, percutaneous ventricular assist device) to offer hemodynamic stability during VT induction and mapping in a patient who otherwise would not tolerate sustained VT.

Results have been very encouraging with these strategies, reducing the frequency of recurrent device therapies dramatically. These new strategies require application of sophisticated mapping tools for proper selection of appropriate target sites for ablation, including electroanatomic contact mapping and noncontact mapping with multipolar electrode arrays that can correlate the electrical characteristics of a site in the heart (amplitude, timing) with its actual three-dimensional anatomic location (Fig. 67A.3).

It is reasonable—in fact essential in some cases—to employ several strategies, such as a combination of antiarrhythmic drugs and reprogramming of the device. As noted, the use of antiarrhythmic drugs alone may slow the VT rate so that it falls below the previously programmed detection rate or render VT more difficult to terminate with pacing therapies.

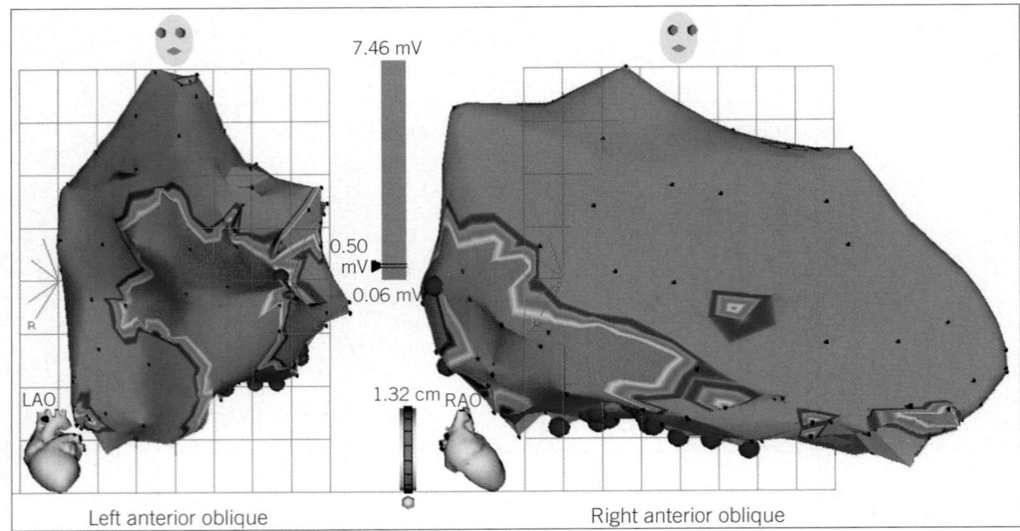

Figure 67A.3 Electroanatomic voltage map in a patient with poorly tolerated VT. Right and left anterior oblique views of left ventricular endocardial voltage obtained by sampling of more than 100 sites during sinus rhythm; a computer records and displays the three-dimensional location and electrogram voltage of sites sampled. A voltage scale is at center; low-voltage areas (red) are on the basal septum and inferolateral wall. Red dots show sites of ablation at areas from which pacing mimicked the QRS configuration during VT episodes (pace match).

SUMMARY

This case illustrates some of the difficulties in managing patients with ICDs. Fortunately, there are many good therapeutic options from which to choose. The combination of increasing sophistication of ICDs and success rates with catheter ablation will likely make this clinical problem less difficult to manage in the future.

b. Multiple Shocks from an Implanted Cardioverter-Defibrillator—II

John M. Miller

DEFINITION OF PROBLEM

The implantable cardioverter-defibrillator (ICD) is clearly successful at preventing sudden death from recurrent ventricular arrhythmias. The ICD's fundamental purpose is to ensure that no episodes of ventricular tachycardia or ventricular fibrillation escape detection and therapy. In achieving this goal, the device occasionally inappropriately delivers therapy when rapid signals are detected that are not of ventricular origin. Causes include rapidly conducted supraventricular arrhythmias, electrical "noise" from external electromagnetic power sources, and conductor fracture in the lead. This can pose difficult diagnostic and management problems, as illustrated in the following case.

TYPICAL CASE

A 63-year-old woman with moderate mitral regurgitation and reduced left ventricular systolic function had a cardiac arrest from which she was successfully resuscitated. Evaluation excluded all known reversible causes (infarction, metabolic disturbance, drug toxicity), and she underwent ICD implantation with a single-chamber (ventricular) device capable of antitachycardia pacing and shocks of up to 35 J. Testing during her implantation showed that the ICD reliably terminated ventricular tachycardia or ventricular fibrillation with 10 J shocks. The ICD was programmed to deliver the full 35 J output whenever ventricular tachycardia detection criteria were met (>160 beats per minute for 2 seconds). She did well for 8 months but while driving one day had a minor automobile accident; her seat/shoulder belt and air bag prevented significant injury. She was evaluated in the emergency department and released. Later that night, while sweeping her garage, she received five shocks in rapid sequence without premonitory symptoms. She asked for assistance, and while an ambulance was en route, she received two more shocks. In the emergency department, she was found to be in sinus rhythm at 90 beats per minute and had a blood pressure of 110/70 mm Hg. Examination showed no injury, and the murmur was unchanged. While sitting up to be examined, she had another shock during sinus rhythm. Interrogation of the device revealed the stored electrogram from the most recent shock (Fig. 67B.1). The lead impedance was normal and captured well at 1.0 V at 0.5 ms (normal values), and the chest radiograph showed no discontinuities in the lead. All other measurements were within normal limits, including shock lead impedance.

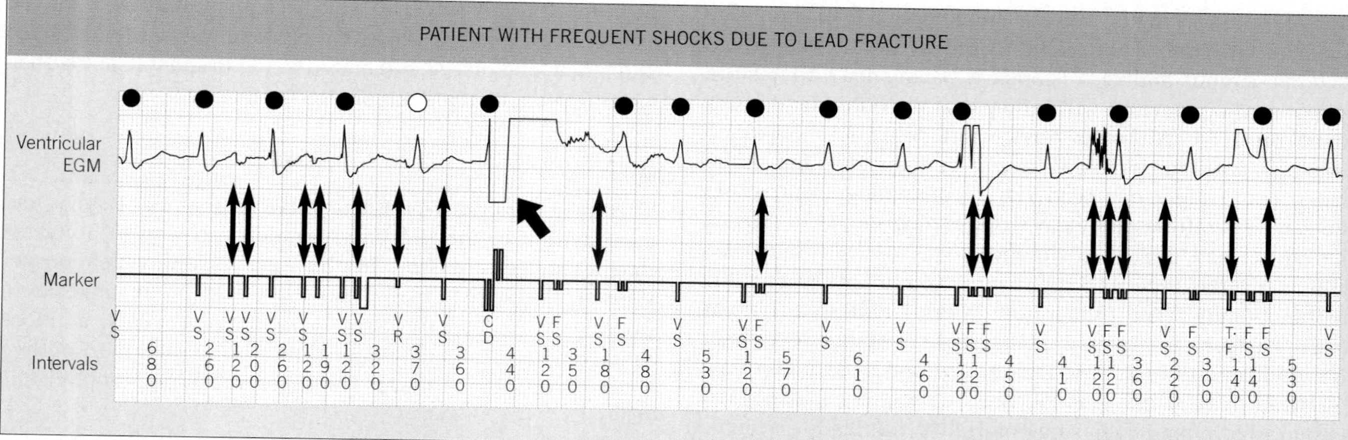

Figure 67B.1 Stored ICD electrogram from a patient with frequent shocks due to lead fracture. One shock is shown *(diagonal arrow)*. Dark circles at the top indicate appropriately sensed normal QRS complexes (denoted by VS in marker; FS denotes interval short enough to detect ventricular fibrillation); white circle shows a QRS that was not sensed. Double-ended arrows show falsely sensed events on the electrogram and marker channel.

DIFFERENTIAL DIAGNOSIS

When a previously stable patient begins having frequent ICD shocks, a careful, focused history should be obtained as to whether new myocardial events may have occurred (worsening heart failure, ischemic pain), new drugs have been added or old ones removed, symptoms have been experienced before shocks, or trauma has been sustained in the region of the device and leads. In this case, the patient's minor automobile accident resulted in damage to the ICD lead when the device's forward motion was suddenly stopped by the shoulder restraint. The sudden sharp motion whereby the lead was fixed beneath the clavicle resulted in a break in one conductor of the lead. Whereas the broken ends touch most of the time, establishing electrical continuity, they can separate and reappose, resulting in "make-break" noise simulating ventricular fibrillation. When the patient subsequently used adjacent muscles vigorously while sweeping, she inadvertently caused this make-break phenomenon. The lead was clearly malfunctioning despite an interrogation that showed no abnormal measurements (impedance, threshold). False shocks due to lead fracture should be distinguished from other causes of inappropriate shocks, such as T-wave oversensing (Fig. 67B.2), environmental noise, and supraventricular arrhythmias, which are all treated differently.

TREATMENT OPTIONS

Once the diagnosis is made, the only definitive therapy is replacement of the lead. Until that can be done, the device should be prevented from shocking the patient further by either programming arrhythmia detections off or taping a pacemaker magnet securely over the device (that "blinds" it from detecting and therefore treating any arrhythmia). Because the patient is thereby left without a working ICD,

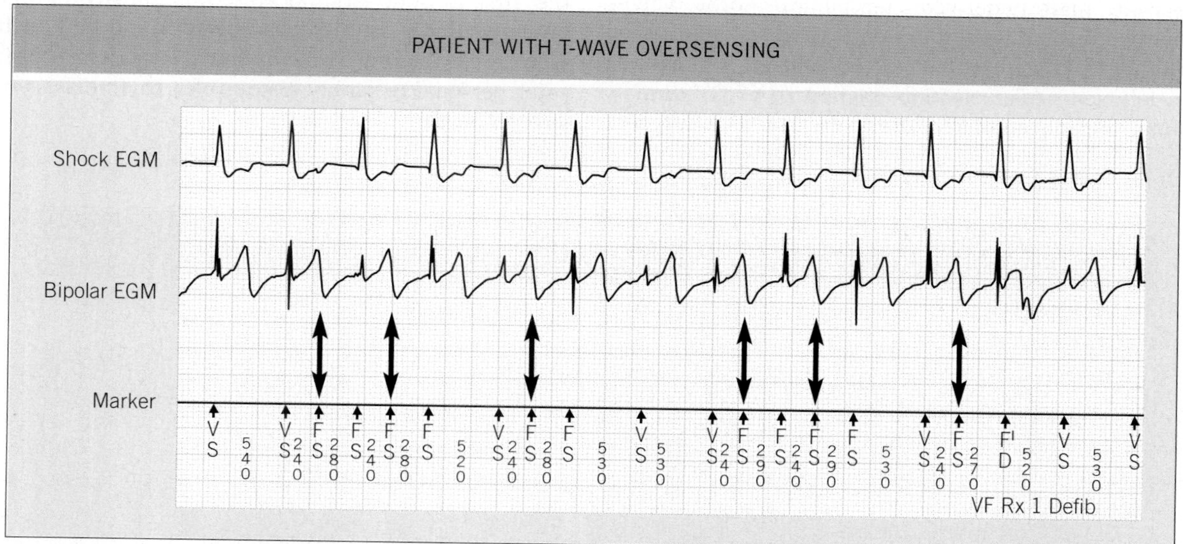

Figure 67B.2 Stored ICD electrogram from a patient with T-wave oversensing leading to an inappropriate shock. Double-ended arrows show T waves in bipolar sensing lead that are large enough to be detected, thus double counting on some beats. Ventricular fibrillation detection criteria were met at the right side of the strip, and a shock followed several seconds later.

inpatient monitoring is critical. The defective lead should be replaced as soon as feasible. Controversy exists as to whether simply adding a standard pacing lead to restore proper sensing function will suffice or if the entire lead needs to be replaced. Although device interrogation showed no problems with the shocking circuit components, the initial injury could have damaged other conducting elements in the lead. Therefore, many electrophysiologists opt to replace the entire lead in such a situation. This decision may also depend on the type and number of conductors within the malfunctioning lead (integrated versus dedicated bipolar lead). Further controversy exists about whether to extract the old lead and replace it with a new one or to add a new ICD lead next to the original. Lead extraction is associated with morbidity and even some mortality, but leads that have been in place for less than 1 year can generally be removed safely. In this patient's case, the old lead was easily extracted and a new one placed and mated to the original ICD that had several years of remaining battery capacity.

SUMMARY

This case illustrates how a carefully obtained history and examination of the ICD interrogation can lead to a correct diagnosis (lead fracture in this case), from which proper therapy flows. It is likely that there will be an increase in prevalence of lead fractures in the coming years, as more younger, physically active patients who are likely to outlive the service life of many leads are receiving prophylactic ICDs.

c. Recurrent Ventricular Fibrillation after Aortic Valve Surgery

John M. Miller

DEFINITION OF PROBLEM

Postoperative arrhythmias, most typically atrial fibrillation and flutter, are common. These prolong hospitalization and delay recovery but are usually self-limited. More serious ventricular arrhythmias are less common but can be far more difficult to manage. Causes include perioperative myocardial infarction, electrolyte imbalance, rewarming, and sometimes reperfusion of an area of myocardium (with coronary bypass surgery) that allows previously ischemic tissue to participate in arrhythmogenesis. The following case explores these possible causes as well as others.

TYPICAL CASE

A 64-year-old man underwent mechanical aortic valve replacement because of moderate stenosis and severe insufficiency (native bicuspid valve). Preoperative evaluation showed a left ventricular ejection fraction of 65%, normal wall motion, and no coronary artery disease. The surgery was uncomplicated, and he was easily weaned from bypass. His first postoperative day in the intensive care unit was likewise uncomplicated; but the following evening, he began having short bursts of ventricular tachycardia (VT), some of which deteriorated into ventricular fibrillation (VF). Frequent unifocal ventricular premature complexes (VPCs) seemed to precede each episode (Fig. 67C.1). He was shocked back to sinus rhythm, but episodes continued for the next 2 hours. Intravenous amiodarone, lidocaine, and metoprolol had little effect; temporary pacing with use of epicardial wires also was of no benefit. He remained hemodynamically stable when in sinus rhythm, without electrocardiographic evidence of ischemia or QT prolongation; electrolyte values were all normal, as was serum creatinine concentration. Troponin level was normal at the time of the first episode and increased minimally several hours after the first several shock episodes. No new medications were given before his arrhythmia episodes. There was no prior personal or family history of arrhythmias, syncope, or sudden death.

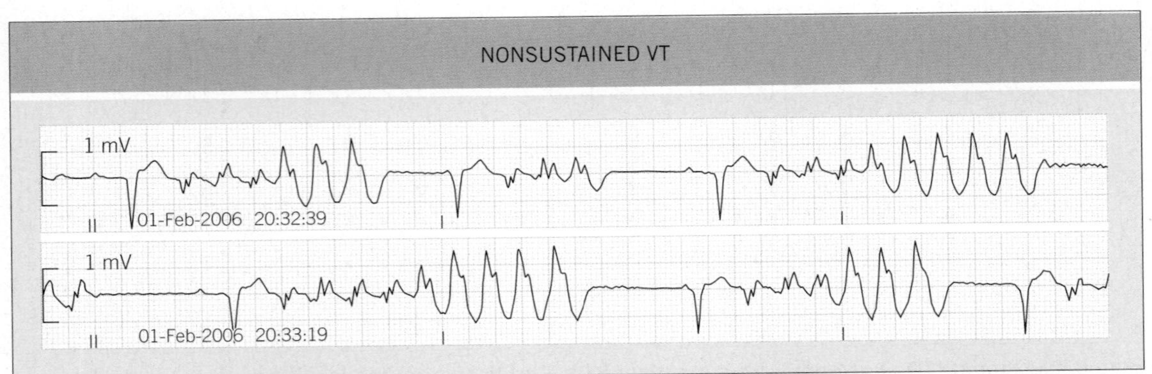

Figure 67C.1 Nonsustained VT. Rhythm strips from the intensive care unit showing bursts of nonsustained VT, each preceded by a VPC of the same morphology; the last episode on the strip degenerated to VF, requiring an external shock. The QT interval during sinus rhythm complexes is normal.

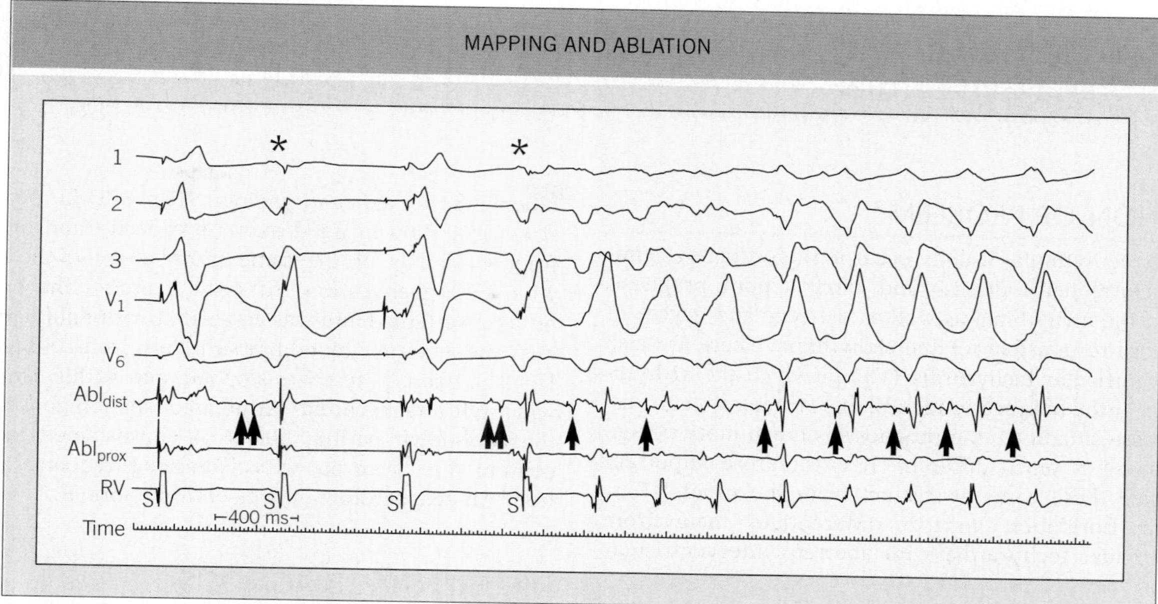

Figure 67C.2 Intracardiac recordings during mapping and ablation. During baseline right ventricular pacing (S, stimulus artifact), two of the initiating VPCs occur *(asterisk)*. The ablation catheter recordings show sharp, low-amplitude spikes occurring substantially earlier than the VPC QRS complexes *(arrows)*; these are also usually evident during the ensuing polymorphic arrhythmia.

DIFFERENTIAL DIAGNOSIS

Fortunately, this dramatic presentation is rare. Quick action must be taken to stabilize the patient and to exclude potential arrhythmia provocateurs, such as myocardial ischemia, physical irritants (e.g., a pulmonary artery catheter that is irritating the right ventricle), electrolyte abnormalities, and drug effects. In this case, all of these were quickly dismissed. This patient's recurrent ventricular arrhythmia had a stereotypical onset, initiated by the same morphology of VPC on almost every occasion. In such situations, these VPCs typically originate in or near the His-Purkinje system in cells that repetitively discharge so rapidly that ventricular activation cannot maintain a consistent pattern (hence, polymorphic VT or VF) or a burst of rapid discharges results, in turn initiating VF. In either case, the cells providing the trigger for this "focal VF" are the culprits. This disorder has been reported in individuals without obvious structural heart disease; in those with idiopathic as well as postinfarction or ischemic cardiomyopathy, acute myocardial infarction, Brugada syndrome, and long QT syndrome; and in patients after valve surgery. It can be a cause of VT "storm." Factors that cause these foci to suddenly become very active are not known. If it is untreated, death from intractable arrhythmia is certain.

TREATMENT OPTIONS

In this patient, after exclusion of known extrinsic promoters of ventricular arrhythmias, treatment quickly moved to high-dose amiodarone and beta blockade. In some cases, this is either effective by itself or gets the patient through a critical period, after which the focus appears to become less active or even dormant. In this patient, although this decreased the frequency of episodes to one every few hours, more aggressive therapy was clearly needed. The following day, the patient was taken to the electrophysiology laboratory for attempted mapping and ablation of a possible focus of the triggering VPC. Fortunately in this case, frequent monomorphic VPCs were still present (some of which initiated VT and VF episodes during the study). Right ventricular mapping showed no sites of likely origin; because of the recent aortic valve prosthesis, the left ventricle was mapped by use of an atrial transseptal approach. On the inferior aspect of the apical septum, characteristic narrow potentials were observed that were up to 90 ms before the QRS onset of triggering VPCs (Fig. 67C.2). Ablation at this site resulted in immediate cessation of the VPCs as well as of further VT and VF episodes. The patient continued recovering from his surgery and underwent ICD implantation the day before discharge. Whether this is necessary is unclear because there are relatively few cases in the literature. However, because the consequences of having even one episode of recurrent VT or VF without ICD backup are so severe, ICD therapy is used in almost all cases.

SUMMARY

VT and VF may occur in a variety of settings. When episodes recur in rapid sequence, one must make a diligent (and expedited) search for possible causes. In some cases, recurrent arrhythmias are dependent on stereotypical initiator VPCs that arise within or near the His-Purkinje system and can be mapped and successfully ablated, thereby eliminating further VT and VF episodes.

d. A Young Woman with Palpitations and Ventricular Tachycardia

John M. Miller

DEFINITION OF PROBLEM

Ventricular arrhythmias usually occur in the setting of significant structural heart disease and carry a poor prognosis because of the arrhythmia as well as the type and degree of heart disease responsible for the arrhythmia. There are also cases of ventricular tachycardia (VT) in which the arrhythmia occurs in the absence of identifiable structural heart disease. In these situations, the prognosis is much more benign and treatment is much different. It is therefore important to recognize these cases as distinct from the usual VT or ventricular fibrillation and to differentiate them from supraventricular tachycardia with aberrant interventricular conduction.

TYPICAL CASE

A 34-year-old mother was referred for evaluation of increasingly frequent palpitations and occasional lightheadedness. Her family physician obtained an ambulatory electrocardiogram (ECG) that showed several episodes of nonsustained VT, ranging in length from 3 to 30 beats at a rate of nearly 200 beats per minute (Fig. 67D.1). On further questioning, she said that she had been having these palpitations for several years, but she noted that they had increased in frequency and duration in the last few months. She recalled presyncope on one or two occasions but never syncope and was not sure that palpitations had been associated with the presyncope. She denied chest pain, viral illness, or shortness of breath and was in overall good health. Her palpitations were more frequent during her aerobics class. She had no family history of arrhythmias, but her father had undergone bypass surgery at the age of 43 years. She took no medications, consumed alcohol only socially, and never used tobacco. Her physical examination findings were entirely normal except for occasional skipped beats on cardiac examination. A resting ECG showed sinus rhythm with frequent ventricular premature complexes having a left bundle branch block inferior axis morphology (Fig. 67D.2). An exercise stress test showed good exercise capacity and increasingly frequent bursts of the same morphology of nonsustained wide QRS tachycardia. At peak exercise, the arrhythmia became sustained and was associated with mild lightheadedness and a systolic blood pressure drop from 140 to 100 mm Hg. The exercise test was stopped, and within 1 minute the wide QRS tachycardia terminated spontaneously. During the cool-down period, bursts of nonsustained tachycardia continued to occur but with decreasing frequency and duration. An echocardiogram was entirely normal.

DIFFERENTIAL DIAGNOSIS

Potential causes of wide-complex tachycardia include supraventricular tachycardia with aberration, supraventricular arrhythmia with conduction to the ventricles over an accessory atrioventricular pathway (Wolff-Parkinson-White syndrome), and VT. The first two diagnoses do not appear to be relevant in this woman's case because there is no atrial activity preceding the first beat of the tachycardia (see Fig. 67D.1), which should certainly be present in supraventricular arrhythmia. Thus, she has VT; but is it of a type that carries a poor prognosis or a good one? A list of VTs having a left bundle branch block configuration appears in Table 67D.1. It can be seen from this that most diagnoses carry a poor prognosis if they are untreated; only those occurring in the absence of structural heart disease have a good prognosis. It is thus important to determine the type and severity of any underlying heart disease. The sinus rhythm ECG often helps in making a distinction, as shown in Table 67D.1. Additional useful diagnostic tests are echocardiography and occasionally magnetic resonance imaging (especially useful if right ventricular dysplasia is being considered). It is important to distinguish right ventricular dysplasia from other forms because its clinical behavior is similar in many respects to VT in the absence of heart disease

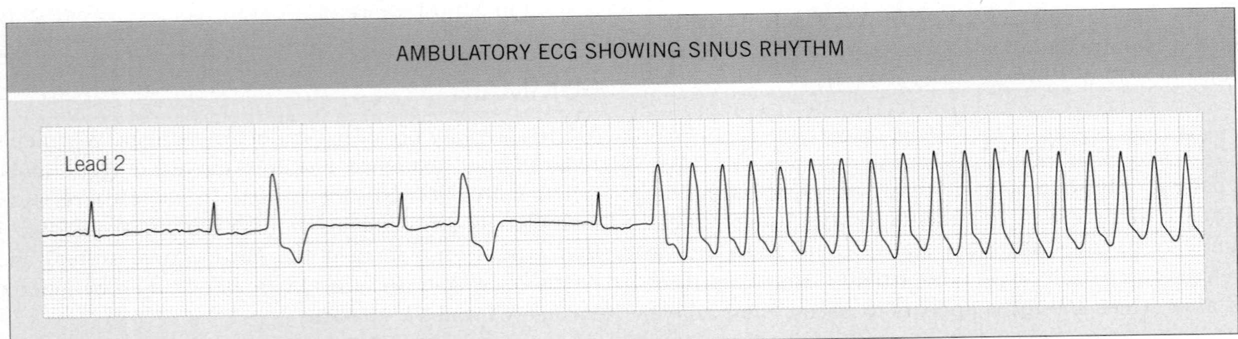

Figure 67D.1 Ambulatory ECG showing sinus rhythm. The ambulatory ECG strip shows sinus rhythm with ventricular premature complexes followed by a run of VT, all of a single morphology. This VT terminated 2 seconds later.

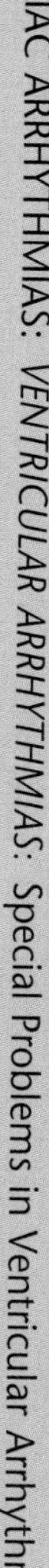

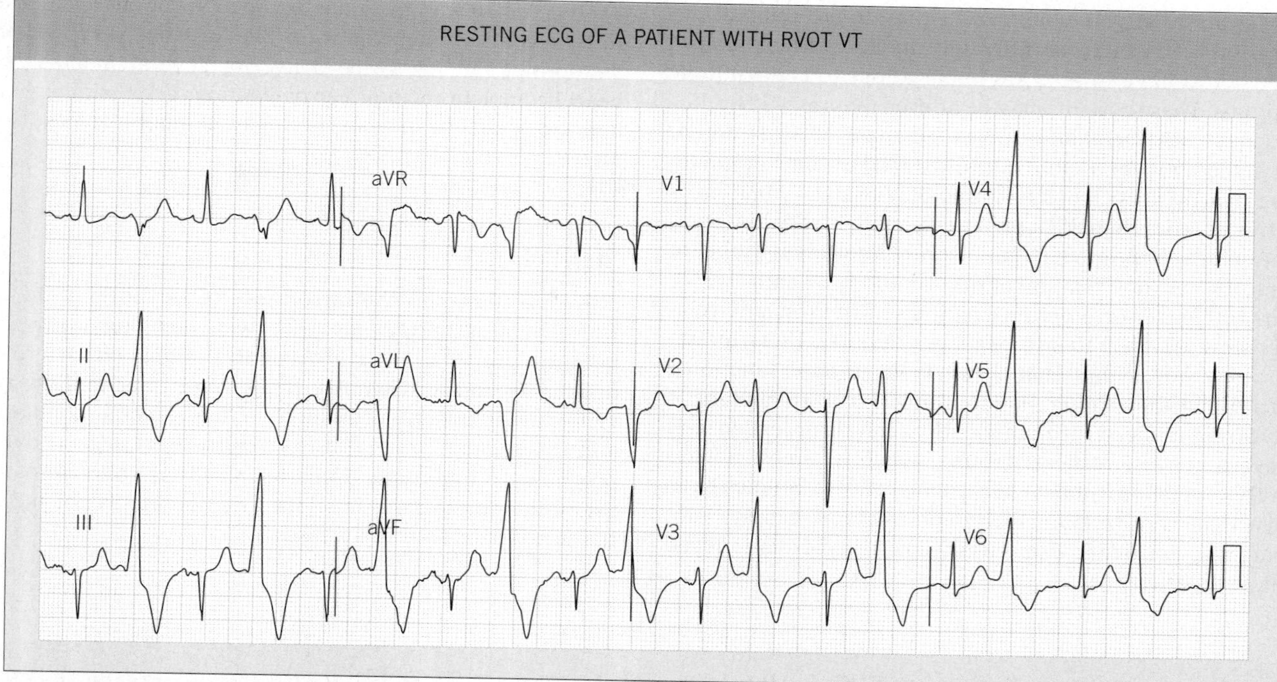

Figure 67D.2 Resting ECG of a patient with right ventricular outflow tract (RVOT) VT. Note isolated ventricular premature complexes in a bigeminal pattern having uniform morphology, rapid upstrokes of the QRS complex, and typical left bundle branch block, inferior axis configuration.

CAUSES OF VENTRICULAR TACHYCARDIA HAVING A LEFT BUNDLE BRANCH BLOCK CONFIGURATION

Diagnosis	Typical Sinus Rhythm ECG	Untreated Prognosis	Therapy
Postinfarction VT	Q-wave infarct common	Poor	AAD, ICD; RFA
Cardiomyopathic VT	Widened QRS	Poor	ICD, AAD; RFA
Bundle branch re-entry VT	Typical LBBB, left axis	Poor	RFA; ICD
Sarcoidosis	RBBB, left axis	Poor	AAD, ICD
Arrhythmogenic right ventricular dysplasia	Epsilon wave, IRBBB, inverted T wave in V_1-V_4	Poor	ICD, AAD; RFA
Normal heart			
Right ventricular outflow tract	Normal; VPCs	Good	Beta blocker; RFA
Aortic cusp–sinus of Valsalva	Normal; VPCs	Good	Beta blocker; RFA
Right ventricular inflow tract	Normal	Good	Beta blocker; RFA

AAD, antiarrhythmic drugs; ECG, electrocardiogram; ICD, implantable cardioverter-defibrillator; IRBBB, incomplete right bundle branch block configuration; LBBB, left bundle branch block configuration; RBBB, right bundle branch block configuration; RFA, radiofrequency ablation; VPCs, ventricular premature complexes; VT, ventricular tachycardia.

Table 67D.1 Causes of ventricular tachycardia having a left bundle branch block configuration.

(exercise provocation), it is inherited (and thus would have implications for this woman's siblings and children), and is associated with an increased incidence of sudden death. In contrast, this woman has no family history of arrhythmias or sudden death, her sinus rhythm ECG is normal except for ventricular premature complexes characteristic of a right ventricular outflow tract origin, and although her VT is exercise related, it occurs typically in frequent bursts of nonsustained VT rather than as strictly sustained episodes separated by days or weeks. Thus, her diagnosis is most consistent with right ventricular outflow tract VT in the absence of heart disease, and she has a good overall prognosis.

TREATMENT OPTIONS

In patients with right ventricular outflow tract VT, a variety of treatment options are available. Some patients require no treatment because of minimal symptoms and a benign prognosis (some patients are asymptomatic, and the diagnosis is made on routine electrocardiography). In patients who seek treatment for palpitations or presyncope, beta blockers have very good efficacy. The dose should be adequate for suppression of symptoms related to the arrhythmia, without causing typical beta-blocker side effects. Alternatively, calcium channel blockers such as verapamil and diltiazem may be used. Many patients with this disorder are relatively young and either do not tolerate the side effects of otherwise effective medications or simply prefer not to have to take any medications to control their symptoms. These patients may be offered therapy with radiofrequency catheter ablation; most of these VTs, as noted, arise in the right ventricular outflow tract, but some originate in the nearby aortic root's sinuses of Valsalva. Ablation is curative in more than 85% of patients, with a very low complication rate. Treatment in this disorder is purely for relief of symptoms and not for prevention of sudden death, which occurs rarely if ever. Very rare patients have incessant, relatively slow VT (120 to 140 beats per minute); these individuals may be asymptomatic and have normal functional capacity, but they should be monitored for development of tachycardia-induced cardiomyopathy. This disorder can lead to severe congestive heart failure, which is almost always entirely reversible if the tachycardia is treated. Studies have shown that even frequent ventricular ectopic activity (not actual VT episodes) can result in tachycardia-induced cardiomyopathy.

This woman was given the therapeutic options and decided to try a course of beta blockers. She has done very well with metoprolol (50 mg twice daily) for several months, with nearly complete relief of her palpitations even with exercise, and she is able to function normally without significant side effects.

SUMMARY

This case illustrates the importance of establishing the correct diagnosis in patients with wide-complex tachycardia because prognosis and treatment options differ greatly, depending on the diagnosis. Right ventricular outflow tract tachycardia is not uncommon in the general population, and its recognition as a distinct entity with a good overall prognosis is important. Catheter ablation, although a very useful therapy in cases in which drug therapy is not successful, is not necessary in all cases.

e. The Acquired Long QT Syndrome

Katherine T. Murray and Dan M. Roden

DEFINITION OF PROBLEM

The acquired form of the long QT syndrome (LQTS) is a disorder that usually occurs as a complication of therapy with drugs that prolong the QT interval. Another common presentation is syncope in a patient with new-onset atrioventricular block due to progressive conduction system disease. Patients typically demonstrate normal cardiac repolarization under drug-free or baseline conditions. However, on exposure to precipitating factors that include QT-prolonging drugs, electrolyte disturbances, and bradycardia, marked prolongation of the QT interval can occur in susceptible people. Symptoms can include palpitations, presyncope, syncope, seizure-like activity, and sudden death due to the occurrence of a polymorphic ventricular tachycardia that is associated with significant QT prolongation (≥500 ms), known as torsades de pointes. Recognition of this clinical syndrome is essential because therapy differs from that used for most forms of ventricular tachycardia, and removal of the offending agent or condition is critical.

CASE PRESENTATION

A 54-year-old woman with long-standing hypertension and recurrent palpitations presented to the emergency department because of persistent symptoms. She was found to be in atrial fibrillation with a ventricular rate of 107 beats per minute. After admission, her rhythm spontaneously converted overnight. At discharge, she was prescribed sotalol (80 mg orally twice a day), verapamil SR (240 mg orally once daily), and warfarin. Approximately 3 months later, she developed fever, diarrhea, and vomiting. After 24 hours, she suffered a syncopal episode and was admitted. The serum potassium concentration was 3.1 mEq/L. Continuous telemetry revealed nonsustained ventricular tachycardia and severe QT prolongation (Fig. 67E.1).

DIFFERENTIAL DIAGNOSIS

Other causes of reversible QT prolongation include hypothyroidism and hypocalcemia. In addition, mutations found in the congenital LQTS are detected in 5% to 20% of patients with the acquired form. For many of these patients, some degree of QT prolongation persists at baseline after recovery. During torsades de pointes, the morphology of the QRS complex changes over time (i.e., it is polymorphic), although periods of more monomorphic-appearing ventricular tachycardia can be interspersed (see Fig. 67E.1), especially if only a single electrocardiographic lead is available. The onset of the arrhythmia usually follows a premature beat and a pause, or a so-called short-long-short sequence. The beat that follows a pause often demonstrates the clearest evidence for QT interval prolongation. The initiating event of torsades de pointes is an early after-depolarization, or a spontaneous depolarization that interrupts phase 2 or 3 of an abnormally long action potential. Because dispersion of repolarization is often present with QT prolongation, it is likely that after-depolarizations trigger intramural re-entry to sustain the arrhythmia. Torsades de pointes should not be confused with polymorphic ventricular tachycardia seen in other clinical situations, especially unstable ischemic heart disease. Here, the tachycardia is usually (but not always) not pause dependent and is faster (often above 300 beats per minute), and QT prolongation is absent. The distinction is critical because the two conditions require different therapy.

Figure 67E.1 Marked QT prolongation. Telemetry strips are shown after admission to a monitored unit. For the nonsustained episode of torsades de pointes shown in the top strip, there is marked QT prolongation after a pause, leading to arrhythmia initiation (long-short sequence). The arrhythmia appears to be monomorphic in the bottom strip.

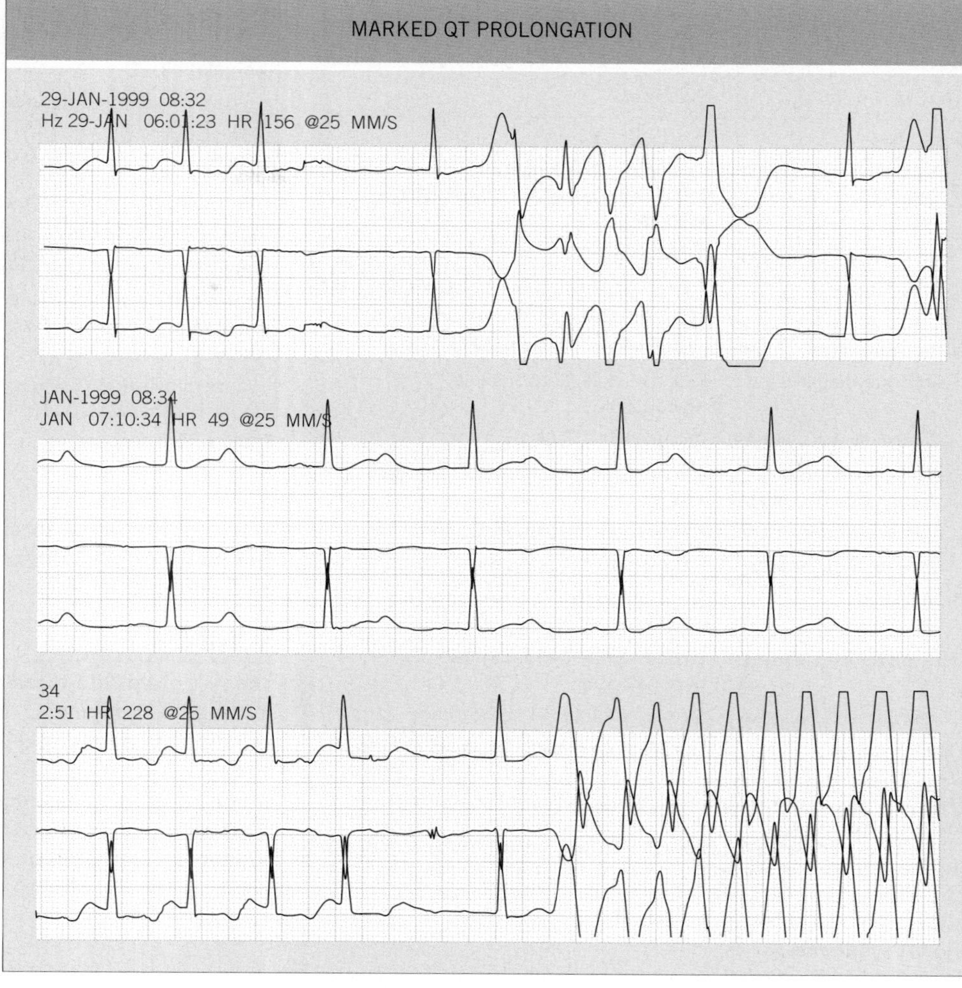

TREATMENT OPTIONS

An important aspect for clinicians is preventing the development of acquired LQTS in susceptible patients. This disorder occurs in a variety of conditions associated with QT prolongation, including exposure to antiarrhythmic agents, bradycardia, and electrolyte disturbances (Table 67E.1); in addition, a variety of commonly used, noncardiac medications have been implicated. Risk factors for the development of the acquired LQTS are shown in Table 67E.2. Excessive QT prolongation can occur early during the course of drug therapy (especially with quinidine), even after the first dose. For this reason, it is recommended that most QT-prolonging antiarrhythmics be started in the hospital with continuous monitoring. With most drugs, the incidence of acquired LQTS is dose related. Thus, the lowest effective dose should be sought. In some situations, excessive QT prolongation can develop during chronic therapy, particularly if bradycardia or new electrolyte disturbances develop, as in the case presented. Not all drugs that increase the QT interval confer the same risk. In particular, amiodarone can produce marked QT prolongation, even though the overall incidence of torsades de pointes is less than 1% during therapy. This low incidence almost certainly results from additional properties of amiodarone, such as its antiadrenergic features and block of the inward currents that underlie after-depolarizations.

In patients with the acquired LQTS, it is critical that the underlying cause be identified and eliminated. The offending pharmacologic agent should be stopped, and bradycardia and electrolyte depletion should be corrected. Acutely, the therapy of choice for torsades de pointes is intravenous magnesium sulfate, 1 to 2 g during 5 to 10 minutes. Additional magnesium may be needed and should be administered to achieve a serum level of at least 2.0 mg/dL. Magnesium therapy does not normalize the QT interval, even though it can suppress arrhythmias. Supplemental potassium should also be given if the serum potassium level is below 4.5 mEq/L. In some cases, ventricular arrhythmias may persist despite therapy directed at electrolyte depletion, especially if the patient is bradycardic. In this case, maneuvers that increase the heart rate to shorten the QT interval can be critical to terminate ventricular tachycardia. This can be accomplished either by temporary cardiac pacing or, in patients without evidence or significant risk of coronary artery disease, by an intravenous infusion of isoproterenol. For reasons that are not well understood, it can take a period of days for the QT to become normal and the arrhythmias to cease.

After resolution of the acquired LQTS, patients should be cautioned to avoid all QT-prolonging drugs. An exception to this may be amiodarone, which has been used successfully

CONDITIONS THAT CAUSE THE ACQUIRED LONG QT SYNDROME	
Type of Condition	**Examples**
Drug use	
Antiarrhythmic agents	Quinidine, procainamide, disopyramide, sotalol,* amiodarone, ibutilide*
Lipid-lowering agents	Probucol
Antibiotics	Trimethoprim-sulfamethoxazole, erythromycin,* pentamidine
Antihistamines	Terfenadine,*† astemizole*†
Antifungal agents	Ketoconazole,* fluconazole, itraconazole
Gastrointestinal agents	Cisapride†
Antidepressants (tetracyclic, tricyclic)	Amitriptyline, imipramine,* doxepin
Phenothiazines	Chlorpromazine, thioridazine*†
Antipsychotic agents	Haloperidol,* risperidone*
Bradycardia	Sinus bradycardia, atrioventricular block
Electrolyte disturbances	Hypokalemia, hypomagnesemia, hypocalcemia
Cerebrovascular diseases	Stroke, intracranial hemorrhage
Dietary status	Liquid protein diets, anorexia nervosa

*Known to be a potent blocker of the rapid component of the delayed rectifier K^+ current, I_{Kr}.
†Withdrawn or relabeled by the Food and Drug Administration because of the risk of torsades de pointes.

Table 67E.1 Conditions that cause the acquired long QT syndrome.

RISK FACTORS FOR THE ACQUIRED LONG QT SYNDROME
Female sex
Hypokalemia, hypomagnesemia
Bradycardia
Diuretic use
High drug doses or concentrations (except quinidine)
Recent conversion from atrial fibrillation
Rapid intravenous drug infusion
Baseline QT interval prolongation, T-wave lability (excessive QT interval prolongation, T-wave lability or changes during drug therapy)
Congenital long QT syndrome

Table 67E.2 Risk factors for the acquired long QT syndrome.

to treat arrhythmias in such patients. Nevertheless, amiodarone may rarely cause torsades de pointes, and it should be used with caution in such patients.

SUMMARY

The risk of this life-threatening disorder can be minimized by starting QT-prolonging drugs in a monitored setting and avoiding them in susceptible patients. Treatment requires prompt correction of the offending cause, intravenous administration of magnesium, and therapy to increase the heart rate and to shorten the QT interval. Identification of patients at very high or very low risk would be helpful.

SECTION 5

HEART FAILURE AND CARDIOMYOPATHY

chapter 68

Physiology of the Normal and Failing Heart

Helmut Drexler and Gerd Hasenfuss

Definition

- Heart failure can be defined as a clinical syndrome that is based on abnormal structure or function of the heart and clinical symptoms and signs of heart failure such as dyspnea, fatigue, and fluid retention.

Key Features

- Heart failure is characterized by abnormalities of left ventricular function and neurohumoral regulation and is accompanied by effort intolerance and reduced prognosis.
- The decrease in cardiac function is probably the consequence of alterations in specific signal events related to biomechanical stimuli and alterations in cytoskeletal proteins, myocyte survival pathways, and sarcoplasmic reticulum calcium cycling. It is followed by cardiac remodeling, neurohumoral and cytokine activation, and muscle wasting, resulting inevitably in progression of the disease.

Heart failure is a major health care problem and one of the most frequent reasons for patients to be admitted to the hospital. The incidence of heart failure is increasing rapidly (1% of the population in the Western world), particularly with the aging of the population around the world, including in developing countries. Despite significant advances in its treatment, the prognosis of heart failure remains poor. Heart failure is the final common pathway to death in cardiovascular disease, including pressure overload (i.e., hypertension), volume overload (i.e., mitral regurgitation), myocardial infarction, and inherited or acquired cardiomyopathies.

One attractive concept, which has been stressed for decades, is the crucial role of cardiac hypertrophy as an adaptive and maladaptive process, more recently extended by delineation of opposing (yet related) pathways that lead to cell death or affect regeneration processes. Major efforts have been made to understand basic processes that lead to hypertrophy, such as the response of the myocardium to physical stress (i.e., pressure overload) at a cellular and molecular level. From this viewpoint, heart failure may be considered a disorder of altered stress pathways or secondary to mutations in one or more genes.

However, heart failure is a clinical syndrome and, in this sense, receives attention primarily from physicians caring for patients whose clinical manifestations vary little despite the multiple causes that lead to this syndrome. Several definitions have been outlined over the years, although none has been generally satisfying. This reflects the complexity of this syndrome, which is characterized by reduced cardiac output and increased venous return accompanied by molecular abnormalities that cause progressive deterioration of the failing heart and, quite probably, premature myocyte cell death and suppress the ability of cardiac regeneration.[1]

PHYSIOLOGY OF CARDIAC CONTRACTION AND RELAXATION

Excitation-Contraction Coupling

The performance of the heart as a pump depends on the coronary circulation, the function of the myocytes, and the composition of the extracellular matrix. At the level of the myocyte, the contraction-relaxation cycle is controlled by excitation-contraction coupling.

Excitation-relaxation coupling comprises processes that are involved in calcium activation of contractile proteins and the subsequent removal of calcium, facilitating relaxation.[2] The initial event is activation of sodium channels, resulting in rapid sodium influx and depolarization of the membrane (Fig. 68.1). As a consequence, voltage-gated, dihydropyridine-sensitive sarcolemmal calcium channels (dihydropyridine receptors) are opened, allowing an influx of calcium into the myocyte. There is proximity between one or a few sarcolemmal calcium channels and one or a few calcium channels of the sarcoplasmic reticulum (ryanodine receptors [RyRs]). This may enable calcium influx through a single sarcolemmal calcium channel to increase a local pool of calcium sufficiently to open adjacent RyRs to release calcium. This local, punctate increase of calcium is termed calcium spark according to its visualization by confocal microscopy.[3] It is the sum of these local calcium releases that generates a global cytoplasmic increase in calcium, which causes activation of contractile proteins. The global increase in calcium is immediately followed by calcium removal, resulting in subsequent deactivation of the contractile machinery. Calcium removal from the cytosol occurs by activity of the sarcoplasmic reticulum (SR) calcium pump and by exchange of calcium for sodium by the sarcolemmal Na^{+}-Ca^{2+} exchanger.[2]

The contractile machinery is composed of the thick (myosin) and thin (actin) filaments, the thin filament regulatory systems, and the cytoskeleton components. The fundamental contractile unit in the myocardium is the sarcomere, which spans from Z line to Z line (Fig. 68.2). The Z lines appear to be the anchor proteins at which intermediate filaments of the cytoskeleton are connected to actin filaments. From the Z lines, the thin filaments project 1 μm from each end toward the center of the sarcomere. The thick filaments are 1.6 μm long and centered on the M line, where thick filaments are connected to each other.

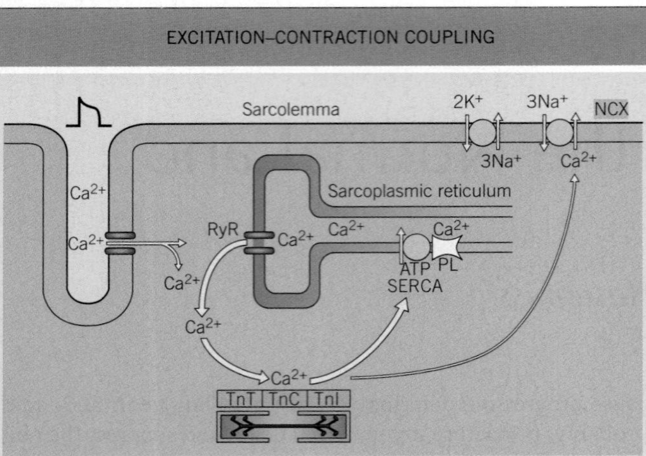

Figure 68.1 Excitation-contraction coupling processes of a myocyte. ATP, adenosine triphosphate; NCX, Na^+-Ca^{2+} exchanger; PL, phospholamban; RyR, ryanodine receptor; SERCA, sarcoplasmic reticulum Ca^{2+}-ATPase; Tn, troponin.

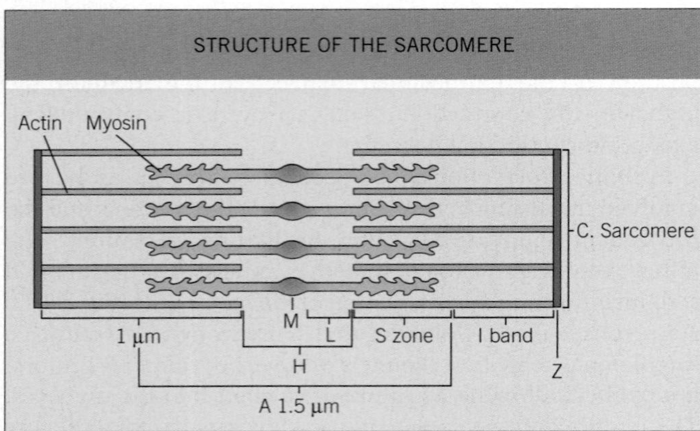

Figure 68.2 Structure of the sarcomere. Thick filaments, composed of myosin, are localized to the A band. In the I band, only thin C filaments are present.

The thick filament is composed largely of myosin, each molecule of which has a long α-helical tail and a globular head (Fig. 68.3). The heads form the cross-bridges, which interact with the thin filament, containing the site of ATP hydrolysis, and have two light chains associated with each head. The thin filament is composed of two chains of the globular protein G-actin, which form the helical, double-stranded actin polymer. In the groove between the actin strands, a long flexible protein, tropomyosin, is located. Furthermore, at every seventh actin, there is a troponin complex attached to tropomyosin. The tropomyosin-troponin system represents the regulatory unit of the contractile machinery. The troponin complex is made up of three subunits: troponin T (the tropomyosin-binding subunit), troponin C (the calcium-binding subunit), and troponin I (the inhibitory subunit).[4]

Under relaxed conditions (low cytoplasmic calcium concentration, ~0.1 μM Ca^{2+}), the actin–cross-bridge reaction is blocked or in a weak binding state because of the steric blocking position of tropomyosin. Troponin T is tightly bound to tropomyosin, and troponin I is tightly bound to actin. The interaction of troponin C and troponin I is weak.

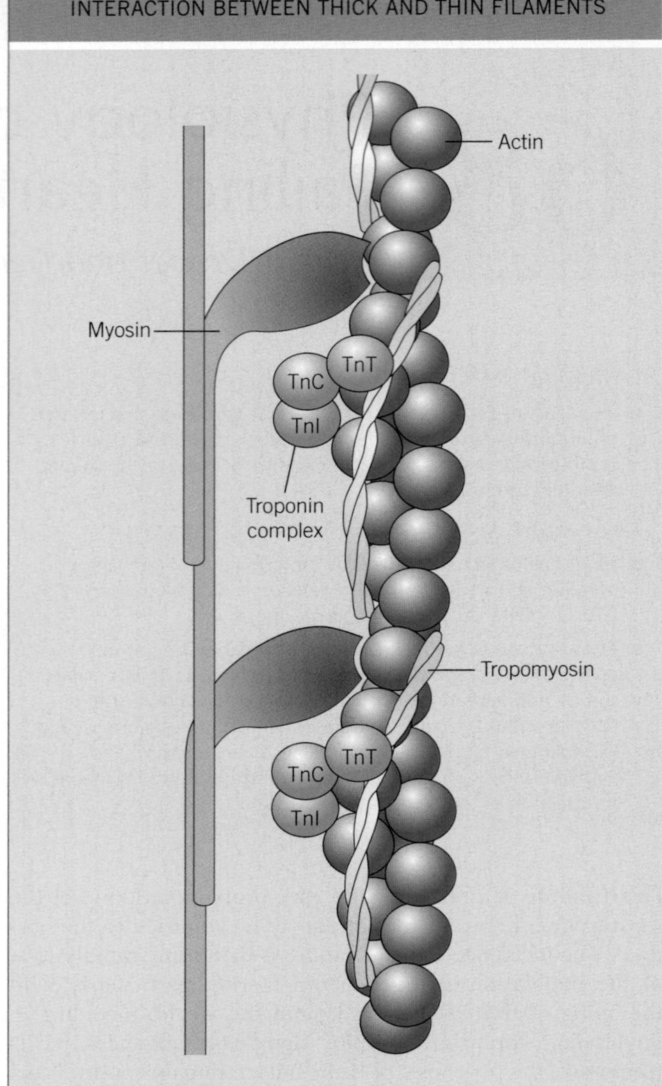

Figure 68.3 Interaction between thick (myosin) and thin (actin) filaments. Tn, troponin.

Activation occurs when calcium binds to the regulatory site of troponin C. This promotes a cascade of changes in protein-protein interactions that result in

- strong troponin C–troponin I interaction;
- weakened troponin I–actin interaction;
- weakened troponin T–tropomyosin interaction; and
- a movement of tropomyosin that finally promotes strong interaction between actin and the cross-bridge.[5]

Regulation of Contraction and Relaxation

The contractile force of the myocardium results from the number of actin-myosin cross-bridge interactions per unit of time. This number depends on the amount of calcium bound to troponin C, which is a function of calcium availability and the affinity of troponin C to calcium, as well as on the behavior of the individual cross-bridge cycle. Augmentation of calcium affinity to troponin C, increased recruitment of cross-bridges per number of calcium ions bound, and prolongation of the attachment period of the individual cross-bridge cycle are termed calcium sensitization or increased calcium sensitivity.

At the level of the myocyte, contractile performance is regulated mainly by four different mechanisms.

Alteration in Sarcomere Length

Alteration in sarcomere length (preload) is an important mechanism for regulation of myocardial performance. The underlying principle is that the maximum force depends on the degree of overlap between thick and thin filaments. However, it was shown that an increase in sarcomere length also increases SR calcium release as well as calcium sensitivity of the myofilaments. This relationship between sarcomere length and force underlies the Frank-Starling law, whereby increased diastolic volume leads to increased systolic contraction.

β-Adrenoceptor Stimulation

Under physiologic conditions, the sympathetic nervous system plays a central role in the response of the heart to acute stress.[6] Circulating or locally released catecholamines bind to myocardial β_1- and β_2-adrenoceptors. β-Adrenoceptors couple to adenylyl cyclase through stimulatory G proteins (G_s). Stimulation of adenylyl cyclase by G_s results in production of cyclic adenosine monophosphate (cAMP). Binding of cAMP to protein kinase A activates this enzyme, which subsequently results in phosphorylation of target proteins. In the myocardium, protein kinase A phosphorylates ion channels and proteins that are involved in calcium homeostasis, contractile proteins, and metabolic enzymes, and it may translocate to the nucleus to regulate gene transcription.

β-Adrenoceptor stimulation increases myocardial performance by the following effects. Increased calcium influx through L-type calcium channels after β-adrenoceptor stimulation results in increased calcium-triggered calcium release from the SR through SR calcium release channels (RyRs), the activity of which may also be regulated by protein kinase A–dependent phosphorylation.[7] Increased rate and degree of calcium activation of contractile proteins result in increased contractile force and rate of force development of the myocardium.[8] In addition, the rate of relaxation is considerably increased because of phosphorylation of the thin filament regulatory protein troponin I and phospholamban. Phosphorylation of troponin I decreases calcium affinity of the myofilaments and increases dissociation of calcium. The cAMP-dependent phosphorylation of phospholamban results in stimulation of the SR calcium pump.

Frequency-Dependent Regulation of Contractile Force

An increase in frequency of contraction increases contractile force by an increase in transsarcolemmal calcium influx and calcium release from the SR. This important regulatory mechanism is termed the force-frequency relation, strength-interval relation, or treppe (staircase) phenomenon and was first observed by Bowditch in the isolated frog heart.

Peptide Hormones

Peptide hormones such as angiotensin and endothelin as well as cytokines influence contraction and relaxation of the heart by different mechanisms.

PATHOPHYSIOLOGY OF HEART FAILURE

Traditionally, heart failure has been defined as a pathophysiologic state in which an abnormality of cardiac function is responsible for the inability of the heart to pump an adequate volume of blood to meet the requirements of the metabolizing tissues. This definition reflects the concept that impaired contractility and the reduced ability of the heart to eject blood are responsible for the clinical syndrome. However, many patients have structural cardiac alterations that impair systolic and diastolic function but do not have clinical signs of heart failure because compensatory mechanisms maintain cardiac output and peripheral perfusion. Therefore, heart failure is now considered a cardiocirculatory disorder more than simply a disease of the heart.

Historically, heart failure was considered to be a cardiorenal problem, leading to volume expansion and edema. On the basis of a better understanding of systolic and diastolic contraction and the observations of systolic dysfunction in experimental and clinical heart failure, the concept of mechanical pump failure dominated the 1960s and 1970s and prompted pharmacologic approaches to increase cardiac contractility. The presence of systemic vasoconstriction suggested that circulatory failure was an important component of the disease, and vasodilator treatment was consequently introduced. During the past 15 years, experimental and clinical studies have demonstrated that heart failure is also characterized by increased neurohumoral activation, particularly of the sympathetic nervous system and the renin-angiotensin-aldosterone system. Increased neurohumoral activity is now regarded as a major pathophysiologic component contributing to the symptoms and progression of heart failure. More recently, there is increasing evidence to implicate cytokine activation in heart failure, introducing the concept that heart failure involves an inflammatory component that may have both functional and structural consequences.

Conceptually but also from a clinical point of view, it is important to recognize that the clinical syndrome of heart failure emerges because of compensatory mechanisms that represent a beneficial short-term response to impaired cardiac function but that are associated with detrimental long-term consequences[9] (Table 68.1). However, the primary event that leads to heart failure appears to be the loss of a critical quantity of functioning cardiomyocytes—after an injury of the heart, such as acute myocardial infarction; as a result of infection, toxins, inflammation, or genetic causes; or in response to prolonged pressure-volume overload due to hypertension or valvular heart disease. This assumption includes the possibility that altered cardiac contractility represents the primary disturbance, which in turn is associated with adaptive mechanisms. However, alternatively, excessive cardiac overload and ventricular remodeling may represent the primary insult responsible for activation of compensatory mechanisms. This distinction has important implications because it would suggest different targets for therapeutic intervention. Although the primary disturbance may differ in the individual patient, attempts to improve cardiac contractility by positive inotropic agents failed to improve the course of the disease.[10] In contrast, interventions that limited ventricular remodeling and inhibited neurohumoral activation were associated with improved survival.[11] The incidence and progression of heart failure after an initial

SHORT-TERM AND LONG-TERM RESPONSES TO IMPAIRED CARDIAC PERFORMANCE		
Response	**Short-term Effects (mainly adaptive; hemorrhage, acute heart failure)**	**Long-term Effects (mainly deleterious; chronic heart failure)**
Salt and water retention	Augments preload	Pulmonary congestion, anasarca
Vasoconstriction	Maintains pressure for perfusion of vital organs (brain, heart)	Exacerbates pump dysfunction, increases cardiac energy expenditure
Sympathetic stimulation	Increases heart rate and ejection	Increases energy expenditure
Desensitization		Energy sparing
Cytokine activation	Vasodilatation, antiapoptotic (?)	Skeletal muscle catabolism, deterioration of endothelial function, impaired contraction, left ventricular remodeling
Hypertrophy	Unloads individual muscle fibers	Deterioration and death of cardiac cells: cardiomyopathy of overload
Capillary deficit		Energy starvation
Mitochondrial density	Increases; helps meet energy demands	Decreases; energy starvation
Appearance of slow myosin		Increases force integral, decreases shortening velocity and contractility; energy sparing
Prolonged action potential		Increases contractility and energy expenditure
Decreased density of sarcoplasmic reticulum calcium pump sites		Slows relaxation, possibly energy sparing
Increases collagen	May reduce dilatation	Impairs relaxation

Modified from Katz AM. The cardiomyopathy of overload: a major determinant of prognosis in congestive heart failure. N Engl J Med 1990;322:100-110.

Table 68.1 Short-term and long-term responses to impaired cardiac performance.

insult seem to vary considerably from patient to patient, depending on genetic factors. Identification of such genetic polymorphisms of candidate genes as susceptibility genes to develop heart failure and as modifier genes to determine the progression of the disease and therapeutic response will considerably influence prevention and treatment of heart failure in the future. In this respect, there is experimental evidence that disruption of the dystrophin-glycoprotein complex in virally infected myocytes is important to viral propagation in the heart, suggesting an interaction between an acquired and hereditary etiology of dilated cardiomyopathy.[12]

In response to as yet ill-defined signals, possibly including wall stress, baroreceptor activation, or tissue underperfusion, compensatory adjustments come into play. These include

- the Frank-Starling mechanism, which enhances cardiac contraction in response to increased preload (presumably by lengthening of the sarcomere);
- ventricular dilatation and myocardial hypertrophy, which are associated with altered cardiac gene expression; and
- activation of the sympathetic and renin-angiotensin systems (resulting in increased heart rate or contractility).

Although these adaptive mechanisms may be adequate in acute heart failure to maintain overall pumping performance of the heart, the long-term implications are less advantageous and are implicated in a variety of adverse long-term functional and structural changes. However, whereas stretch-induced expression of genes in the myocardium may exert only limited compensatory cardiovascular effects, some of these proteins (e.g., brain natriuretic peptides) may serve as useful clinical markers for diagnosis, response to treatment, and prognosis.[13]

MYOCARDIAL ALTERATIONS OF THE FAILING HEART

Functional Alterations

Human heart failure has many underlying causes, the frequencies of which have changed considerably over the years. At present, the leading cause is coronary heart disease, which accounted for 67% of heart failure cases during the 1980s according to the Framingham Heart Study.[14] Most of these patients also had a history of arterial hypertension (57%). Valvular heart disease underlies failure in about 10% of patients, and 20% of heart failure cases are attributable to primary myocardial diseases, of which dilated cardiomyopathy predominates. Regardless of the original cardiac abnormality, the advanced heart failure syndrome presents a complex picture, including disturbed myocardial function, ventricular remodeling, altered hemodynamics, neurohumoral activation, cytokine overexpression, and vascular and endothelial dysfunction.

At the level of the myocardium, characteristic functional, biochemical, and molecular alterations that occur in end-stage heart failure have been described.

Several clinical and experimental studies have indicated that alteration of the force-frequency relation represents a characteristic functional defect observed in the failing human heart (Fig. 68.4). As discussed before, the positive relation between rate of myocardial contraction and contractile force represents an important regulatory mechanism of the cardiovascular system. However, in failing human myocardium, the force-frequency relation is flattened or inverted.[15] The altered force-frequency behavior in failing human myocardium has also been observed in clinical studies showing depressed frequency potentiation of hemodynamic parameters of myocardial performance.[16]

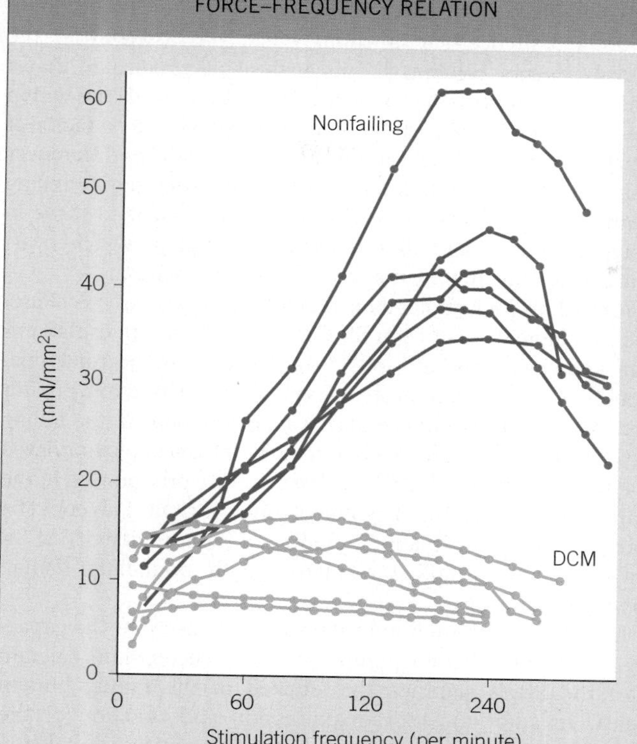

Figure 68.4 Force-frequency relation in failing (dilated cardiomyopathy [DCM]) and nonfailing human myocardium. Experiments were performed in isolated muscle strip preparation from human hearts. (From Mulieri LA, Hasenfuss G, Leavitt BJ, Allen PD, Alpert NR. Altered myocardial force-frequency relation in human heart failure. Circulation 1992;85:1743-1750.)

There is accumulating evidence that changes in the excitation-contraction coupling system underlie the alteration of myocardial function of the failing heart. Changes in excitation-contraction coupling may result from primary alterations of calcium cycling, from alterations in the β-adrenoceptor adenylyl cyclase system, and from alterations at the level of the contractile proteins.

Alteration of Calcium Cycling in Human Heart Failure

Several studies have indicated that altered calcium cycling may play a dominant role in the disturbed myocardial function of end-stage human heart failure. It was concluded that the total amount of calcium cycling and the rate of calcium removal are reduced in the failing human myocardium and that systolic free calcium is reduced and diastolic calcium increased.[17,18] It was further shown that alteration of calcium transients depends on the frequency of stimulation. With use of the photoprotein aequorin to evaluate calcium transients in isolated muscle strip preparations, it was observed that the frequency-dependent rise in the calcium transients is blunted and that even an inversion of the calcium-frequency relation occurs in most ventricular muscle strip preparations from end-stage failing human hearts.

Subcellular Alterations Underlying Altered Calcium Cycling

Transsarcolemmal Calcium Influx

Calcium entry through voltage-gated L-type calcium channels is the key event causing the transition from the resting state of the myocardium to contraction. Several studies have been performed to evaluate abundance of the L-type calcium channel α subunit in failing and nonfailing human myocardium, but data have not been consistent.[19]

Unaltered levels of the α_1 subunit of L-type calcium channels would be consistent with functional measurements indicating that calcium current densities measured during basal conditions are similar in isolated myocytes from failing hearts with dilated cardiomyopathy and from nonfailing hearts.[20] Interestingly, measurements suggested that the function of L-type calcium channels may be altered in human heart failure.[21] Piot and associates[21] observed that increasing frequencies augment calcium currents in myocytes from nonfailing hearts, whereas high-frequency up-regulation of calcium currents was attenuated or lost in myocytes from hearts with reduced left ventricular function. These findings may indicate that altered transsarcolemmal calcium influx and in particular lack of frequency-dependent up-regulation of transsarcolemmal calcium influx may contribute to altered excitation-contraction coupling in the failing human heart.

Sarcoplasmic Reticulum Function

Calcium release from the SR depends on the following components:

- the activation of RyRs by L-type calcium influx;
- the number of RyRs present in the SR membrane;
- the functional status of release processes, which includes calcium binding and diffusion within the SR as well as refractoriness of RyRs from previous activation; and
- the SR calcium load (i.e., the amount of calcium available for release).

Ryanodine Receptors and Sarcoplasmic Reticulum Calcium Release

The calcium-sensitive RyR, which is located in the immediate vicinity of the L-type calcium channel, is activated by a local increase in calcium subsequent to transsarcolemmal calcium influx. Once it is activated, the channel opens and releases calcium for activation of contractile proteins. This process is termed calcium-induced calcium release. Several groups have studied mRNA expression of the RyR in human heart failure, and results have not been consistent.[19] At the level of the protein, no change in RyR levels between failing and nonfailing hearts was consistently observed.[22,23] Whether function of RyRs is altered in human heart failure is currently unknown.

There is evidence that altered function of the RyR may be relevant for the pathophysiologic process of human heart failure. The RyR was shown to be a macromolecular complex including protein kinase A, the protein phosphatases PP1 and PP2A, an anchoring protein (mAKAP), sorcin, calmodulin, FKBP12 or FKBP12.6, and other proteins. FKBP12 and FKBP12.6 seem to play an important role for the regulation of the RyR.[24] Marx and colleagues[25] showed that protein kinase A–dependent phosphorylation of RyR regulates the binding of FKBP12.6 to the channel, both in vitro and in vivo. They postulated that protein kinase A hyperphosphorylation of the RyR channel is a contributing factor in the pathophysiologic mechanism and progression of heart failure. Protein kinase A phosphorylation of the RyR2 dissociates the regulatory subunit FKBP12.6 from the channel, resulting in pronounced altered channel function. As a consequence, destabilization of the channel and subconductance states as well as uncoupling of neighboring channels and diastolic calcium leak through the channel may result. Accordingly, it was shown that overexpression of FKBP12.6 in rabbit myocytes results in reduced spontaneous SR calcium leak, increased SR calcium content, and increased isotonic shortening of isolated myocytes.[26]

Calcium transport into the SR occurs by SR Ca^{2+}-ATPase, which transports two calcium ions per molecule of high-energy phosphate hydrolyzed against a high ion gradient from a free intracellular calcium concentration between 100 nmol/L and 10 µmol/L to a free calcium concentration in the SR of approximately 1 mmol/L.[2] The SR competes with the sarcolemmal Na^+-Ca^{2+} exchanger (Fig. 68.5). The SR Ca^{2+}-ATPase is regulated by phospholamban.[27,28] Dephosphorylated phospholamban is an inhibitor of SR Ca^{2+}-ATPase activity. The inhibition has been suggested to involve direct protein-protein interaction followed by conformational changes in SR Ca^{2+}-ATPase, resulting in a decrease in the affinity of the calcium pump for calcium. It has been recognized that phosphorylation of phospholamban by calcium/calmodulin-dependent protein kinase (CaM kinase; Thr17) and by protein kinase A (Ser16) results in stimulation of SR Ca^{2+}-ATPase.[28,29]

SR calcium uptake or SR Ca^{2+}-ATPase activity and mRNA are reduced in the failing human myocardium compared with the nonfailing human heart; however, observations at the level of the protein findings have been controversial. Importantly, a significant correlation exists between SR Ca^{2+}-ATPase protein levels and myocardial function, which was assessed by the force-frequency relation.[30] This analysis also indicated that a wide variation exists in protein levels of SR Ca^{2+}-ATPase within the group of failing hearts (protein levels differed by a factor of four) and that this variation in protein levels matches differences in myocardial function. In other words, in a subgroup of failing hearts, SR Ca^{2+}-ATPase protein levels are similar to those in nonfailing hearts, and this is associated with preserved myocardial systolic function by the force-frequency relation.

Regarding phospholamban regulation of SR Ca^{2+}-ATPase, the stoichiometry between SR Ca^{2+}-ATPase and phospholamban is crucial for SR Ca^{2+}-ATPase activity and myocardial function. SR Ca^{2+}-ATPase protein levels are decreased to a greater proportion than protein levels of phospholamban in the failing myocardium,[23] suggesting that in the basal low phosphorylated state, inhibition of SR Ca^{2+}-ATPase is more pronounced in the failing than in the nonfailing human myocardium. This could be one possibility to explain the finding of reduced activity of SR Ca^{2+}-ATPase in failing compared with nonfailing human myocardium.

In summary, there is considerable evidence that the capacity of the SR calcium pump system to accumulate calcium into the SR is significantly reduced in the failing human heart. In addition, altered expression and function of the Na^+-Ca^{2+} exchanger may further compromise SR calcium accumulation (see later).

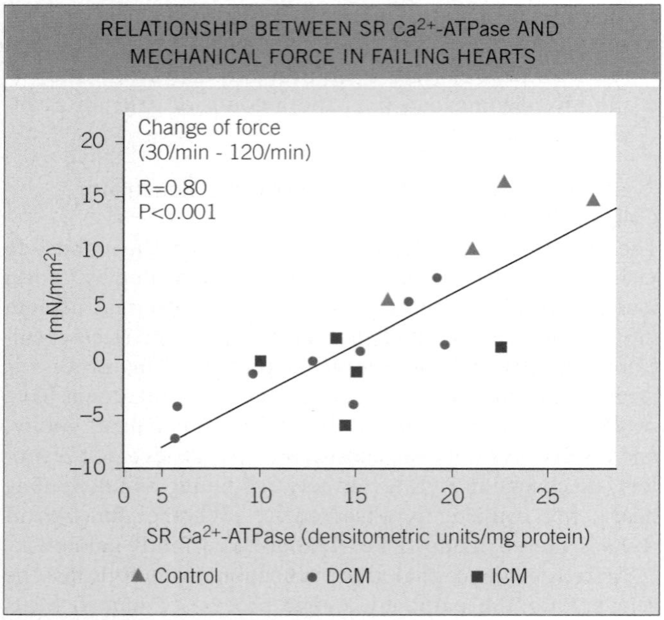

RELATIONSHIP BETWEEN SR Ca^{2+}-ATPase AND MECHANICAL FORCE IN FAILING HEARTS

Figure 68.5 Relationship between SR Ca^{2+}-ATPase and mechanical force in failing hearts. The graph shows the relationship between change in twitch tension after an increase of the stimulation frequency from 30/min to 120/min and protein levels of sarcoplasmic reticulum (SR) Ca^{2+}-ATPase normalized per total protein. DCM, dilated cardiomyopathy; ICM, ischemic cardiomyopathy. (From Hasenfuss G, Reinecke H, Studer R, et al. Relation between myocardial function and expression of sarcoplasmic reticulum Ca^{2+}-ATPase in failing and nonfailing human myocardium. Circ Res 1994;75:434-442.)

Transsarcolemmal Calcium Transport

Sarcolemmal calcium transport is dominated by activity of the Na^+-Ca^{2+} exchanger, whereas the sarcolemmal calcium pump is not considered to contribute quantitatively to beat-to-beat calcium elimination and myocardial relaxation.[31] The Na^+-Ca^{2+} exchanger extrudes one calcium ion for three sodium ions using the electrochemical sodium gradient.[32] In this mode, it produces a net movement of charge resulting in a net inward current. The Na^+-Ca^{2+} exchanger is also voltage dependent and can reverse its mode during the action potential. Under experimental conditions with high intracellular sodium levels, the Na^+-Ca^{2+} exchanger can promote calcium influx sufficiently to induce excitation-contraction coupling. Na^+-Ca^{2+} exchanger mRNA and protein levels and activity are significantly increased in the failing human heart,[33,34] and this appears to have functional relevance because the diastolic performance of failing human myocardium correlates inversely with the protein levels of the Na^+-Ca^{2+} exchanger (Fig. 68.6). Although increased Na^+-Ca^{2+} exchanger levels in failing hearts may compensate for reduced SR Ca^{2+}-ATPase levels to maintain low diastolic Ca^{2+} levels and to improve diastolic performance, these alterations may also promote systolic dysfunction by sarcolemmal calcium efflux and unloading of SR.[35,36]

Calcium Activation of Contractile Proteins

Disturbed function of the failing myocardium could also result from altered response of the contractile machinery to calcium or from altered function of the actin-myosin cross-bridge cycle itself. Several studies consistently indicated altered actin-myosin cross-bridge function in the failing human heart with

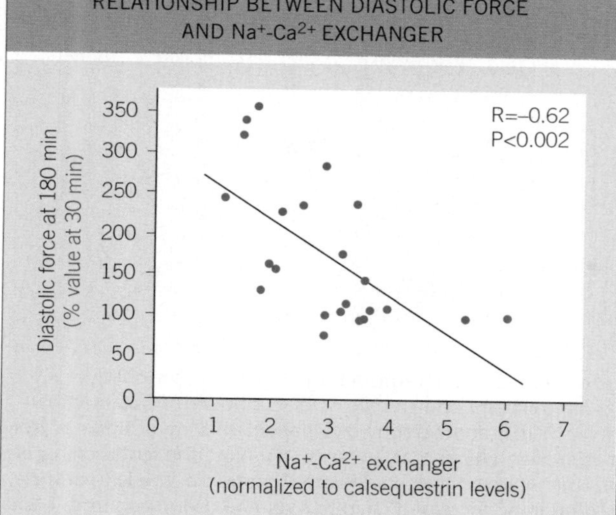

Figure 68.6 Relationship between diastolic force and Na^+-Ca^{2+} exchanger. The graph shows the relationship between the change in diastolic tension after an increase of the stimulation frequency from 30/min to 180/min, given as a percentage of the diastolic force value at 30/min, and protein levels of the Na^+-Ca^{2+} exchanger. Na^+-Ca^{2+} exchanger protein levels were normalized to calsequestrin protein levels. All data are from end-stage failing human hearts with dilated or ischemic cardiomyopathy.

decreased myosin and myofibrillar ATPase activity, decreased cross-bridge cycling rate, and increased cross-bridge force-time integral.[37] These alterations in cross-bridge function may contribute to altered power development and impaired relaxation of the failing human heart.

Similar alterations of cross-bridge function have been observed in rodent models of myocardial hypertrophy. However, previous studies suggested that unlike the situation in small mammals, alteration in cross-bridge function may not be related to myosin isoform shift because it was observed that the β-myosin heavy-chain isoform predominated in the left ventricle of nonfailing and failing human hearts.[38] This is in contrast to more recent studies showing that the α-myosin heavy-chain mRNA isoform was decreased in failing human hearts.[39,40] Alternative to a myosin isoform shift, the alteration in cross-bridge function may, however, be related to changes in troponin T isoforms or alterations in myosin light chains.[41,42]

Controversy also exists about myofilament calcium sensitivity, which was suggested to be unchanged[43] or decreased.[44] Wolff and colleagues[45] suggested that calcium sensitivity was increased in failing myocardium from hearts with dilated cardiomyopathy, which might be caused in part by reduction of protein kinase A–dependent phosphorylation of myofibrillar regulatory proteins. Although myosin content may be decreased by about 20% through replacement by connective tissue, maximum calcium-activated force was suggested to be similar in failing and nonfailing human myocardium.[46]

Preload-dependent regulation of myocardial force is an important regulatory mechanism (the Frank-Starling mechanism). Whether this fundamental mechanism is attenuated in the failing human heart is controversial[44,47]; however, a principal dependency of myocardial contractile force on sarcomere length has been demonstrated.[47]

Influence of the β-Adrenoceptor and cAMP System

Many studies have shown that the β-adrenergic signal transduction pathway is altered in the failing human heart. This results from a decrease in myocardial β_1-adrenoceptor density, which is partly due to decreased expression of the β_1-adrenoceptor gene demonstrated at both the mRNA and protein levels.[48] Both the β_1 and β_2 receptors are markedly uncoupled from G proteins in failing hearts—a process attributed to increased levels of myocardial β-adrenoceptor kinase (β-ARK) and increased $G\alpha_i$ mRNA and protein concentrations.[49] Alteration in the β-adrenoceptor adenylyl cyclase system may contribute to altered excitation-contraction coupling by decreased protein kinase A–dependent phosphorylation of proteins, such as L-type calcium channels, RyR, phospholamban, and troponin I.[45] This would be consistent with observations that forskolin, an activator of adenylyl cyclase, can partially normalize the inverse force-frequency relation in failing myocardium from human hearts with mitral regurgitation.[50] Moreover, inhibition of β-ARK is able to restore a pathologic phenotype and to improve survival.[51]

Critical Appraisal of Calcium Handling in the Failing Heart

At the level of the myocardium, disturbed SR function seems to play a central role in the altered systolic and diastolic performance of the failing human myocardium. Under physiologic conditions, calcium released from the SR is the dominant source for systolic activation of contractile proteins. Diastolic relaxation depends on calcium removal from the cytosol by the SR and the sarcolemmal Na^+-Ca^{2+} exchanger. There is considerable evidence that a major defect of excitation-contraction coupling is a decreased capacity of the SR to accumulate calcium. This may result from a decreased number of calcium pumps, an increased phospholamban inhibition of the pump, or a decreased activity of the pump by other mechanisms. In addition, because SR Ca^{2+}-ATPase competes with Na^+-Ca^{2+} exchanger for calcium, increased Na^+-Ca^{2+} exchanger activity may contribute to decreased SR calcium accumulation. Furthermore, disturbed regulation of RyRs by FKBP12 may be involved.

The decreased capacity of the SR to accumulate calcium may be of minor relevance at low heart rates. However, at higher heart rates—with a decreased time available for calcium transport—SR calcium accumulation may become inadequate, calcium release from the SR may decline, and systolic activation of contractile proteins may decrease. This is consistent with the findings of an altered force-frequency relation, a frequency-dependent decrease in calcium transients, and a decreased post–rest potentiation in the failing human heart. Altered transsarcolemmal calcium influx and, in particular, attenuation of frequency-dependent up-regulation of L-type calcium current may contribute to the reduced SR calcium load. Furthermore, alterations in the β-adrenoceptor adenylyl cyclase system with altered cAMP levels may be involved.

A second consequence of decreased SR function is diastolic calcium accumulation, which may result in diastolic activation of contractile proteins and disturbed diastolic function. Because SR Ca^{2+}-ATPase and Na^+-Ca^{2+} exchange work in concert to remove calcium from the cytosol, increased activity of the Na^+-Ca^{2+} exchanger may compensate for decreased SR calcium transport and preserve diastolic function. Accordingly, in failing human myocardium, diastolic function is correlated with protein levels of Na^+-Ca^{2+} exchanger. Of course, calcium eliminated across the sarcolemma by the Na^+-Ca^{2+} exchanger is no longer available for systolic activation of contractile proteins. Furthermore, the exchange of one calcium ion for three sodium ions results in an inward current, which may cause electrical instability. Therefore, alteration of calcium handling with increased activity of Na^+-Ca^{2+} exchanger relative to SR Ca^{2+}-ATPase may contribute to disturbed myocardial function as well as to the development of arrhythmias in patients with heart failure.

Studies in phospholamban knockout mice indicate that lack of phospholamban inhibition of the calcium pump increases SR calcium uptake and contractility of the myocardium. Interestingly, animals with dilated cardiomyopathy due to knockout of a cytoskeletal protein, the muscle-specific LIM protein, can be rescued from the left ventricular dilatation and failure by knockout of phospholamban.[52] These intriguing observations raise the possibility that overcoming the defect in calcium delivery to myofilaments by reducing the inhibitory action of phospholamban or reinstituting SR Ca^{2+}-ATPase (SERCA) activity[53] can prevent the disruption of the cytoskeletal network. Moreover, these observations point to a role of the cytoskeleton for Ca^{2+} signaling in the myocardium. Thus, a novel therapeutic approach to heart failure may involve gene therapy or small molecules that specifically interfere with the phospholamban-SERCA pump interaction or activity. In fact, chronic suppression of heart failure has been achieved in animal models of heart failure by cardiac gene delivery of phospholamban mutants.[54]

THE CARDIAC REMODELING PROCESS

Ventricular remodeling can be defined as any structural change of the left (or right) ventricle in response to a change in loading conditions, including alterations in ventricular mass and chamber size and shape. Ventricular remodeling develops in response to increases in afterload (pressure overload) or preload (volume overload), and it also may result from myocardial injury. Pressure overload results in concentric hypertrophy (i.e., thickened left ventricular walls by sarcomeres added in parallel), whereas eccentric hypertrophy results from sarcomeres added in series as seen in volume overload.

After myocardial infarction, the extent of left ventricular chamber enlargement, or remodeling, is directly related to infarct size. During the first several days after a moderate to large myocardial infarction, the left ventricular cavity enlarges because of infarct expansion (i.e., elongation and thinning of the infarcted segment; Fig. 68.7). Progressive left ventricular dilatation, however, may continue for months to years. This time-dependent process appears to result from elongation of noninfarcted wall segments. A large component of the chamber dilatation results from a structural change in the ventricular wall, partially related to elongation of myocytes generated by new sarcomeres organized in series, by myocyte slippage, by collagen reorganization, and possibly by myocyte apoptosis. Ventricular remodeling has a short-term benefit because stroke volume will be larger by the Frank-Starling mechanism; however, the long-term

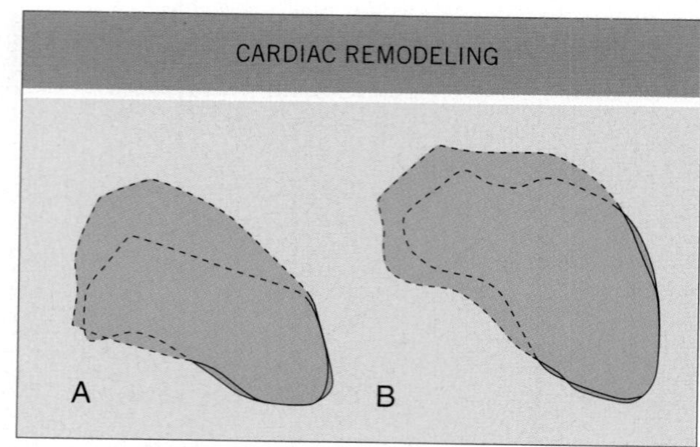

Figure 68.7 Cardiac remodeling. Right anterior oblique end-diastolic and end-systolic cardiac silhouettes obtained by left ventricular angiography of a patient with myocardial infarction on admission **(A)** and at 2 weeks **(B)**. Note the lengthening of both the infarcted and noninfarcted portion of the left ventricle, resulting in an increased chamber volume. (Modified from McKay RG, Pfeffer MA, Pasternak RC, et al. Left ventricular modeling after myocardial infarction: a corollary to infarct expansion. Circulation 1986;74:693-702.)

structural and biochemical adaptations are detrimental to the course of the disease (Fig. 68.8).[55,56]

The morphologic changes that take place in the noninfarcted myocardium or in response to pressure-volume overload are accompanied by microscopic evidence of eccentric myocyte hypertrophy and increased interstitial fibrosis. Progressive deterioration of global left ventricular pump performance after myocardial infarction appears to be attributable to emerging myocardial dysfunction of regions that showed normal wall motion initially (in the noninfarcted and nonischemic left ventricle). Quite probably, the transition to failure is related to profound changes in the expression of multiple genes that regulate the composition of contractile elements, cytoskeleton, and extracellular matrix; ion homeostasis; myocyte cell loss to both apoptosis and necrosis[57]; and ability of cell division of resident cardiac stem cells.[58] In fact, it is conceivable that the regenerative capacity of the myocardium may deteriorate with aging and cardiovascular diseases. Progressive chamber enlargement is associated with a poor

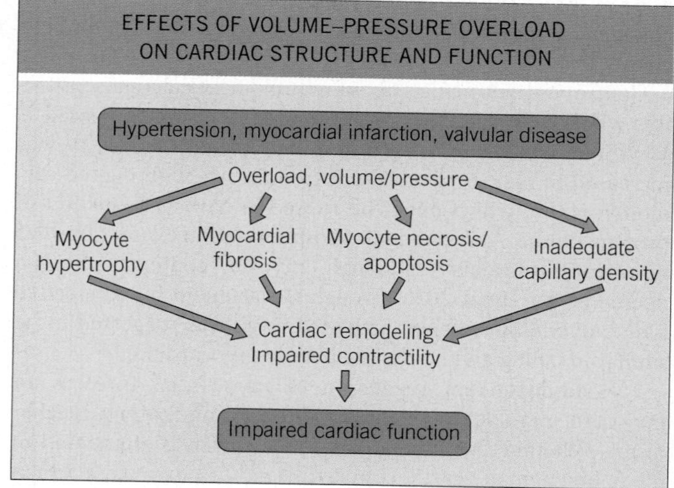

Figure 68.8 Proposed mechanisms by which volume-pressure overload affects cardiac structure and function.

prognosis; in other words, the extent of left ventricular remodeling is an important prognostic factor such that the greater the degree of left ventricular dilatation, the worse the outcome, supporting the notion that ventricular remodeling is a maladaptive process.

The remodeling process in both animal models and humans is associated with the development of eccentric hypertrophy (i.e., an increase in myocardial mass without or with only minimal increase in wall thickness, accomplished by an elongation in cardiac myocytes; Fig. 68.9).[59,60] Nonmyocytes, particularly fibroblasts, are also major contributors to remodeling. Both the production and degradation of the collagen network are regulated by fibroblasts, which in the presence of eccentric hypertrophy produce additional extracellular matrix to maintain structural integrity of the ventricular wall, resulting in increased interstitial fibrosis.[61] However, the presence of increased interstitial collagen is associated with reduced capillary density and increased oxygen diffusion distance, possibly facilitating ischemia. In addition to hypertrophy and fibrosis, the left ventricle shows a more spherical shape after injury such as myocardial infarction, which is associated with increased wall stress, abnormal distribution of fiber shortening, and dilatation of the mitral annulus with subsequent mitral regurgitation.

The molecular mechanisms that are involved in ventricular remodeling are still incompletely understood. However, both cardiomyocytes and nonmyocytes are sensors of pressure overload. In response to biomechanical stress, growth signals are generated by the release of growth factors and cytokines, including peptides that stimulate G protein–coupled receptors such as endothelin 1, angiotensin II, interleukin 6–related cytokines, tumor necrosis factor α, and growth factors that activate receptor tyrosine kinases such as insulin-like growth factor. Thus, the activation of cell surface receptors and their signaling targets, such as ras and $G\alpha_q$, by growth factors appears to represent the first step in the initiation of growth of cardiomyocytes and might also involve increases in intracellular calcium concentrations associated with calmodulin-dependent pathways, including calcineurin. There is some evidence that downstream effectors, including mitogen-activated protein kinases such as JNK and p38 (α versus β isoform), are important switches that modulate the balance between pathways to hypertrophy and apoptosis. In fact, biomechanical stress concomitantly activates hypertrophic and apoptotic programs. There is experimental evidence that activation of specific signaling pathways serves a survival pathway in cardiomyocytes,[62] that is, activation of gp130-dependent signaling or ERB2 provides a survival pathway favoring compensatory hypertrophy and blocking myocyte apoptosis.[63] Vice versa, lack of cardiac ERB2 receptors or its blockade by antibodies is associated with the development of dilated cardiomyopathy or may result in left ventricular dysfunction.[54,64,65] Signaling by these pathways appears to be severely altered in the failing human heart,[66] thus providing one explanation for the progression of heart failure.

There is also some evidence that cardiac hypertrophy and angiogenesis are coordinately regulated during physiologic or adaptive cardiac hypertrophy, and impairment of this interplay leads to transition of contractile dysfunction and heart failure, that is, loss of coordinated myocyte growth and angiogenesis can promote the progression from adaptive hypertrophy to heart failure.[67] Growth-promoting signals appear to simultaneously induce cardiac hypertrophy and angiogenesis; impaired expression of myocardial angiogenetic factors during pressure overload results in impaired angiogenesis and is associated with progression from adaptive to maladaptive hypertrophy and transition to cardiac failure.[68]

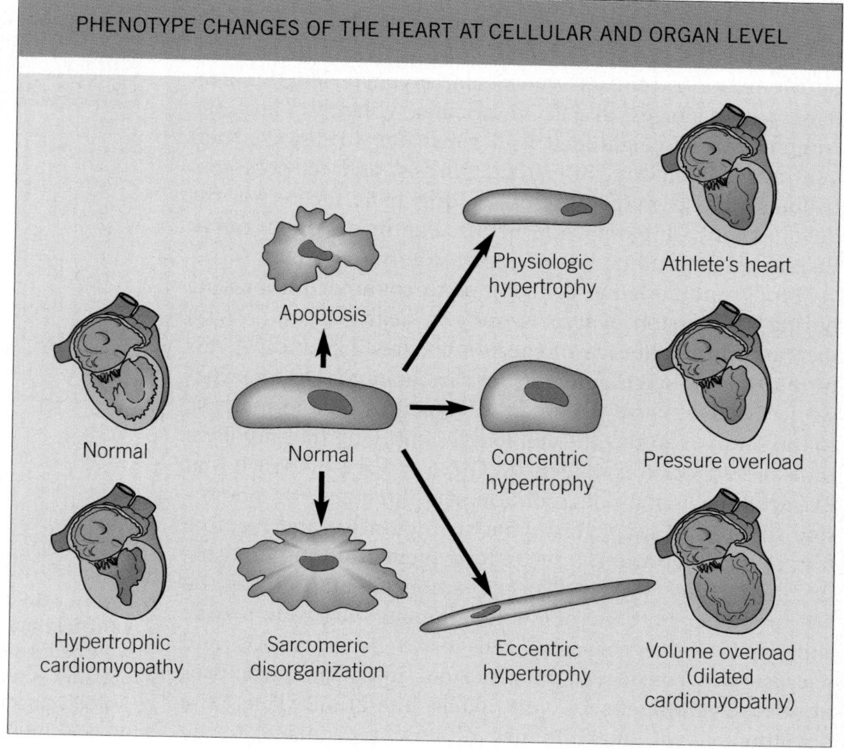

Figure 68.9 Phenotype changes of the heart at the cellular and organ level. Normal muscle cells can grow in a physiologic way, as typically seen in an athlete's heart; however, this can develop into concentric hypertrophy as a result of pressure overload, eccentric hypertrophy due to volume overload, or dilated cardiomyopathy. Mutations of sarcomeric proteins result in disorganization and in hypertrophic cardiomyopathy. In response to stimuli such as biomechanical stress or growth factors, both hypertrophic and apoptotic pathways are activated and may lead to apoptosis under ill-defined circumstances.

In contrast to pressure overload and concentric hypertrophy, the chamber dilatation in dilated cardiomyopathy has been associated with alterations in the cytoskeleton of the myocardium. The matrix proteins may represent an integrated component of the biomechanical sensor that links hemodynamic overload to intracellular signals. Indeed, the disruption of cytoskeletal proteins in knockout animals has resulted in dilated cardiomyopathy, and genetic defects in cytoskeletal components (i.e., the cardiac actin gene) have been noted to be involved in patients with familial dilated cardiomyopathy. In contrast, mutations in sarcomeric proteins cause hypertrophic cardiomyopathy (see Chapter 79).

As outlined before, activation of the renin-angiotensin system and adrenergic stimulation occur with pressure overload. Stretch of myocytes due to increased load results in paracrine-autocrine release of angiotensin II, resulting in early gene expression, which promotes the growth of cardiomyocytes. However, angiotensin II is also mitogenic for cardiac fibroblasts, stimulates collagen formation, and provides a positive feedback regulation by inducing the transforming growth factor β1 gene. Moreover, stretching of the cardiomyocytes activates the expression and release of multiple cytokines,[69,70] which appears to play a prominent role in balancing collagen degradation and synthesis (i.e., by regulating metalloproteinases).[71,72]

Isolated Myocyte Function and Changes in Myocyte Shape

The global alterations of left ventricular architecture that characterize postinfarction remodeling are accompanied by morphologic and intrinsic functional alterations in cardiomyocytes. However, the impairment of isolated myocyte contractile function in nonischemic myocytes may be minimal, with quite normal intracellular calcium transients at baseline and during inotropic stimulation and normal shortening-frequency relationship. However, myocytes from failing hearts demonstrate significant structural remodeling, in particular elongation, which is consistent with experimental observations that left ventricular myocyte length correlates with changes in left ventricular volume. Thus, the combination of heightened wall stress due to distorted left ventricular geometry, interstitial fibrosis, and cell loss contributes to and may represent a dominant factor for the development of global left ventricular dysfunction rather than simply a gradual loss of contractile function.

Myocyte remodeling contributes to chamber remodeling during progression of hypertrophy to heart failure.[69] With increased load, the size of cardiomyocytes increases. A disproportionate lengthening of the cardiac myocytes emerges while the transverse diameter of myocytes fails to increase to the same extent as the cell length, implying that myocyte transverse growth is defective. There is some evidence that extracellular matrix degradation sets the stage for side-to-side slippage of myocytes, whereas reparative and reactive fibrosis may represent a secondary event resulting in a stiffer myocardial wall.[73] Thus, chamber dilatation can be attributed to both myocyte lengthening and side-to-side slippage. In this scenario, cell losses by apoptosis and necrosis are considered to represent important processes in the development of ventricular dilatation. Thus, the development of heart failure is now recognized to be related not only to reduced contractility but also to a progressive structural disorder of left ventricular remodeling. However, intrinsic contractile dysfunction of cardiac myocytes and myocyte loss and remodeling are likely to be separate but related processes that act in concert; in other words, hypertrophy and increased myocyte length are associated with changes in gene expression that lead to intrinsic myocyte contractile dysfunction and contribute to ventricular dilatation and further activation of neurohumoral signals for growth.

Altered Left Ventricular Function

Altered left ventricular function and chamber remodeling result in characteristic alterations in left ventricular function that can be described in terms of an altered left ventricular pressure-volume relationship (Fig. 68.10). Left ventricular dilatation and reduced systolic function result in a rightward displacement of the pressure-volume curve with increased left ventricular end-diastolic volumes and pressure. Despite increased preload, stroke volume is reduced and end-systolic pressure to volume ratio (index of contractility) is depressed (curve B). Additional diastolic dysfunction due to incomplete relaxation after disturbed excitation-contraction coupling processes and increased stiffness due to altered extracellular matrix composition cause an additional upward shift of the pressure-volume relation (curve C). The integral of the pressure-volume relationship reflects left ventricular pressure-volume work or stroke work. The ratio of pressure-volume work to myocardial energy consumption reflects efficiency of the left ventricle as a pump. It is obvious from Figure 68.10 that pressure-volume work is reduced. Moreover, because myocardial oxygen consumption depends on volume and pressure (wall stress), it is obvious that the efficiency of contraction is considerably reduced in failing hearts with reduced systolic and diastolic performance.

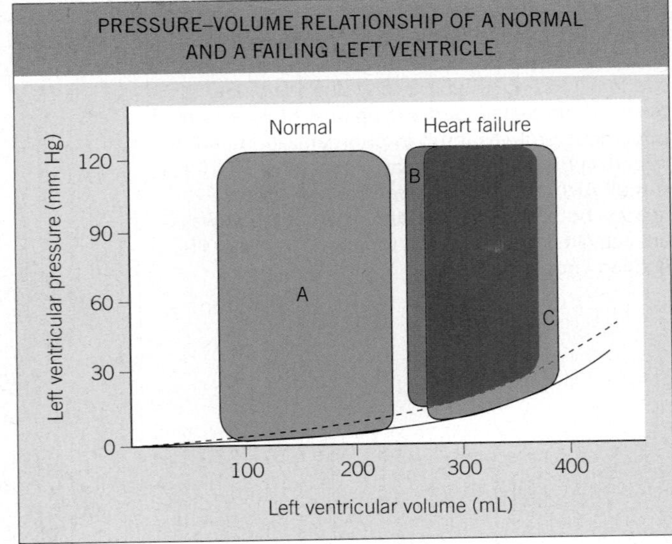

Figure 68.10 Pressure-volume relationship of a normal left ventricle and a failing left ventricle. In A, the normal pressure-volume relationship is shown. In B, the left ventricular end-diastolic pressure is increased because of chamber remodeling and reduced systolic ejection. In C, there is additional diastolic dysfunction with upward replacement of the diastolic pressure-volume relation.

NEUROHUMORAL ACTIVATION AND ITS FUNCTIONAL CONSEQUENCES

To compensate for myocardial cell dysfunction, both cardiac and neurohormonal mechanisms are activated to normalize cardiac function and output. Whereas the ventricle increases its contraction secondary to elevated diastolic tension (preload) and the Frank-Starling principle, the sympathetic nervous system is activated in response to decreased cardiac output; the resulting stimulation of β-adrenergic receptors in the noninjured myocardium increases both the force and frequency of contraction. These two compensatory mechanisms involve different but complementary, intracellular calcium–dependent inotropic pathways. Whereas sympathetic activation increases the delivery of calcium to myofilaments, ventricular dilatation enhances sensitivity of the myofilaments to calcium.

Although hemodynamic and neurohormonal mechanisms provide inotropic support, they are associated with an increased long-term burden and risk. Ventricular dilatation and the activation of the sympathetic nervous system and renin-aldosterone-angiotensin system (by peripheral vasoconstriction and increased afterload) enhance diastolic wall stress, which markedly affects its architecture and increases cardiac energy expenditure. Thus, the compensatory short-term adaptation by the activation of the neurohumoral axis is associated with detrimental long-term cardiac effects, representing a vicious circle (Fig. 68.11). The primary adaptive response to increased load of the ventricles is the development of cardiac hypertrophy, which includes both quantitative and qualitative changes of the myocardium (see earlier).

Consequences of Sustained Neurohormonal Activation

When cardiac output falls, systemic perfusion pressure is maintained mainly by peripheral vasoconstriction and sodium retention, which are both characteristic findings in patients with overt heart failure and are attributable to the interaction of hemodynamic and neurohormonal factors. Several neurohormonal systems are activated in patients with heart failure that cause peripheral vasoconstriction. The sympathetic nervous system is activated early in the disease process, whereas the renin-angiotensin system is usually triggered once symptoms develop, and vasopressin is released mainly in very advanced stages of the disease when systemic perfusion is threatened (Fig. 68.12). In addition to these circulating factors, heart failure is accompanied by an increased endothelial release of locally active vasoconstricting factors such as endothelin (Fig. 68.13).[74]

These endogenous vasoconstrictor factors are counterbalanced by endogenous vasodilators. In normal individuals, natriuretic peptides attenuate the release of norepinephrine (noradrenaline), renin, and vasopressin as well as their actions on peripheral blood vessels and within the kidneys. The release of endothelium-derived relaxing factor (nitric oxide) normally counteracts the vasoconstricting factors; in fact, a continuous basal release of nitric oxide keeps the vasculature in a dilated state. However, the effects of circulating and locally active vasodilators are attenuated in patients with heart failure. The release of atrial natriuretic peptide is blunted in chronic heart failure, and the effects of both atrial and brain natriuretic peptide lose their ability to suppress the release of renin or to dilate peripheral blood vessels.[75] Similarly, the vascular availability of nitric oxide is markedly reduced in patients with heart failure.[76] Thus, diminished vasodilator forces leave the actions of vasoconstrictors unopposed. The reduced bioavailability of nitric oxide may have functional consequences well beyond lack of vasodilatory capacity because nitric oxide is involved in several fundamental protective functions of the endothelium.[75] Importantly, the interaction of the sympathetic and renin-angiotensin systems amplifies their vasoconstricting effect (e.g., increased sympathetic activity increases release of renin and vice versa; angiotensin enhances the release of both norepinephrine and vasopressin).

In addition to neurohormonal activation, mechanical factors may contribute to increased peripheral resistance. Sodium retention may impair the vasodilator capacity of peripheral blood vessels, either because of an increase in the sodium content of peripheral vessels or because edema enhances the compressive forces of perivascular tissues. Long-term activation of vasoconstrictor systems is associated with structural alterations in both peripheral conduit and resistance vessels, which may limit the increase in blood flow during periods of increased demand, such as exercise.

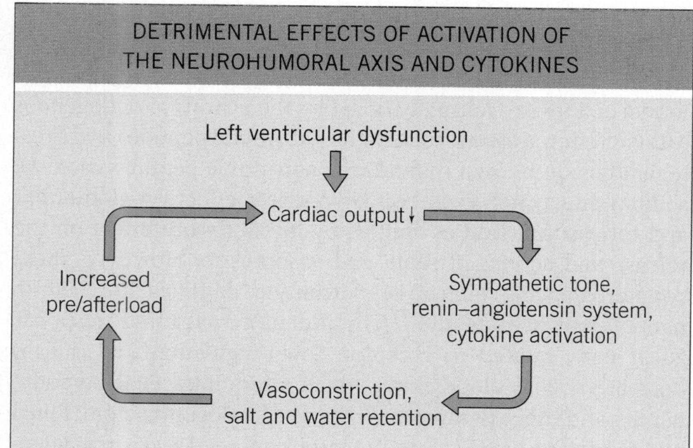

Figure 68.11 Vicious circle by which activation of the neurohumoral axis and cytokines exerts detrimental long-term cardiac effects. Impaired cardiac output activates the sympathetic nervous system, the renin-angiotensin system, cytokines, and other neurohumoral factors to maintain systemic blood pressure. However, increased systemic vascular resistance, sodium and water retention, and the direct cardiac effects of these factors have adverse long-term implications.

Sodium Retention

Neurohumoral activation leads to sodium and water retention in patients with heart failure. The alteration in fluid balance results to a large extent from the direct and indirect effects of the renin-angiotensin system on glomerular and tubular function. Angiotensin exerts constrictor effects on the efferent arteriole; the resulting increase in filtration fraction alters the peritubular balance of hydraulic and oncotic forces, such that proximal tubular sodium reabsorption is enhanced. In addition, angiotensin augments sodium reabsorption directly and indirectly by stimulating the release of aldosterone. Angiotensin causes water retention by two mechanisms: increasing water

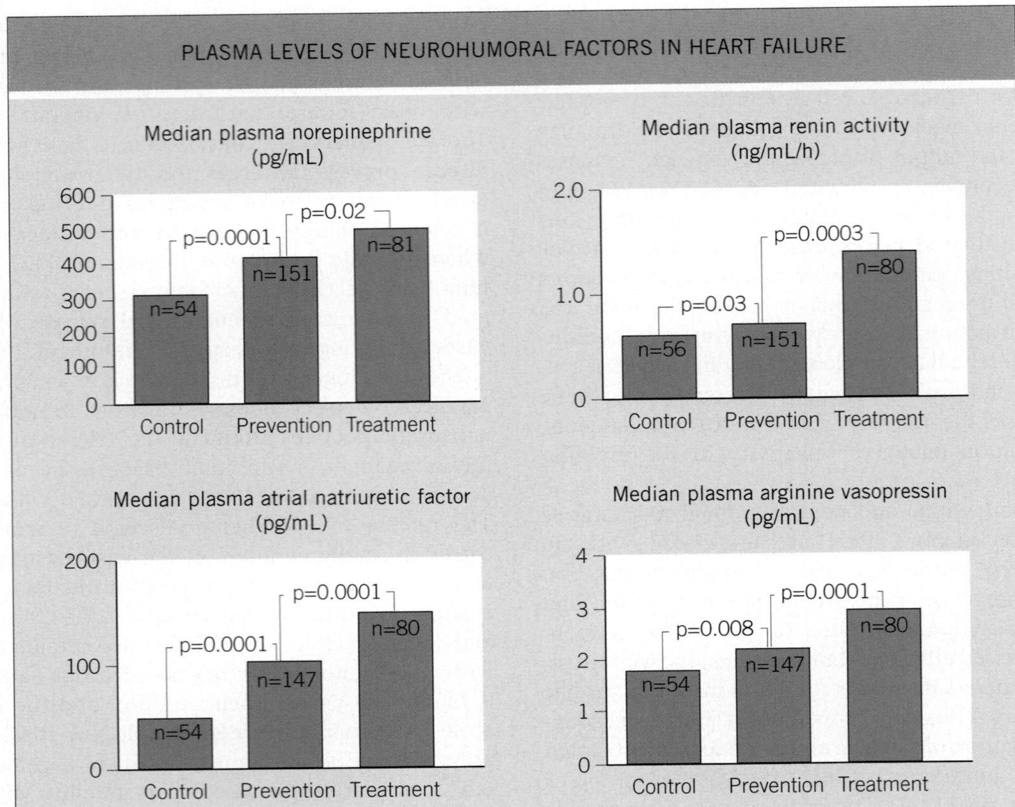

Figure 68.12 Plasma levels of neurohumoral factors in patients with heart failure. Plasma levels of norepinephrine (noradrenaline), renin activity, atrial natriuretic factor, and arginine vasopressin in normal individuals and in patients with asymptomatic left ventricular dysfunction (prevention) and patients with symptomatic overt congestive heart failure (treatment). (Modified from Francis GS, Benedict C, Johnstone DE, et al, for the SOLVD Investigators. Comparison of neuroendocrine activation in patients with left ventricular dysfunction with and without congestive heart failure. Circulation 1990;82:1724-1729.)

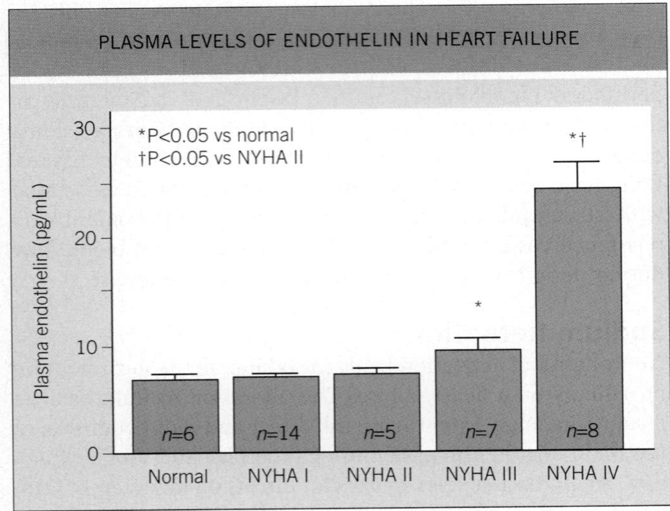

Figure 68.13 Plasma levels of endothelin in patients with heart failure. Plasma levels of endothelin of healthy subjects and patients with congestive heart failure at different New York Heart Association (NYHA) functional classes. (From Wei CM, Lerman A, Rodeheffer RJ, et al. Endothelin in human congestive heart failure. Circulation 1994;89:1580-1586.)

intake by stimulating the brain thirst center and reducing water excretion by enhancing the release of vasopressin. Sodium and water retention is potentiated by the stimulation of renal sympathetic nerves early in the course of heart failure and by a fall in renal blood flow in patients with reduced resting cardiac output at an advanced stage.

The effects of the renin-angiotensin system and related hormonal actions are normally offset by the actions of endogenous salt-excreting systems, such as the natriuretic peptides and prostaglandins. In normal individuals, natriuretic peptides increase sodium and water excretion by a direct effect on glomerular and tubular function as well as by an inhibitory effect on the release and actions of renin and vasopressin. However, these counterbalancing effects of natriuretic peptides are lost in patients with heart failure.[77] The attenuated natriuretic response is, in part, related to receptor down-regulation and due to decreased renal blood flow, which alters intrarenal hemodynamics and triggers intrarenal release of vasoconstrictors. Renal hypoperfusion also leads to the intrarenal release of prostaglandins, which exert some natriuretic and diuretic effects. However, these actions are limited by the inhibitory effect that renal hypoperfusion itself has on sodium and water excretion.

The development of peripheral vasoconstriction and sodium retention in heart failure represents an important shift in the priority of the cardiovascular system. Before the onset of heart failure, endogenous mechanisms are directed to the support of cardiac function. Once heart failure is established, the main goal is to maintain systemic perfusion pressure. Peripheral vasoconstriction and sodium retention result not only from excessive activation of endogenous vasoconstrictor systems but also from a loss of counterregulatory vasodilator influences, such as the impaired availability of endothelial nitric oxide. Thus, a disturbed balance of vasoconstricting and vasodilating forces contributes to a large extent to the hemodynamic burden of the failing heart, the function of which is already compromised by the loss of compensatory myocardial mechanisms.

Peripheral Adaptations and the Development of Clinical Symptoms

Impaired cardiac contractility and ventricular remodeling are not necessarily associated with clinical signs of heart failure but may be present in an asymptomatic patient. Thus, clinical symptoms appear to be related not to cardiac dysfunction as such but to compensatory mechanisms, such as an activated renin-angiotensin system and sympathetic nervous system, and possibly to activation of cytokines, such as tumor necrosis factor α and interleukin 6 (Fig. 68.14). However, the activation of the neurohumoral and cytokine axis and the extent of cardiac dysfunction and ventricular remodeling are important determinants of prognosis.

Traditionally, fatigue has been thought to arise from the impaired cardiac pumping capacity delivering inadequate amounts of oxygen, which leads to a buildup of products of anaerobic metabolism within the exercising muscle.[78] Dyspnea was thought to arise from the effects of impaired cardiac function, increasing left atrial pressure and thereby producing pulmonary congestion. However, there is evidence that persistent vasoconstrictor drive and endothelial dysfunction rather than cardiac output limitation impair effective muscle blood flow. A wide array of structural and functional abnormalities have been described in the muscle itself that can explain some of the fatigue of this condition even without impaired muscle blood flow.[79] Furthermore, even the differentiation between fatigue and dyspnea may be artificial in many patients as either symptom can occur with subtle alterations in the exercise testing procedure. There are few differences between patients who are limited by fatigue and those limited by dyspnea. In many patients, a sensation of exhaustion may have elements of both.

Finally, the cause of the perceptions of fatigue and dyspnea may arise from similar sensory afferents from the abnormal muscle of chronic heart failure patients. Fatigue appears to be related to peripheral adaptation, including impaired peripheral perfusion during exercise, reduced oxidative capacity of skeletal muscle, impaired muscle strength, and possibly reflex mechanisms associated with alterations in the metabolism of skeletal muscle (Fig. 68.15). Notably, however, in most cases of chronic heart failure, cardiac output remains close to normal during the early stages of exercise, and it is only near the peak of exercise that any perceptible reduction in cardiac output is seen. During the early phases of exercise, nevertheless, muscle blood flow is reduced compared with that in normal individuals because of diversion of blood flow away from the muscle in addition to a reduction in the size of the muscle and its vascular bed. These abnormal responses are associated with early muscle fatigue, but which factor is the most prominent precursor of fatigue is not clear.

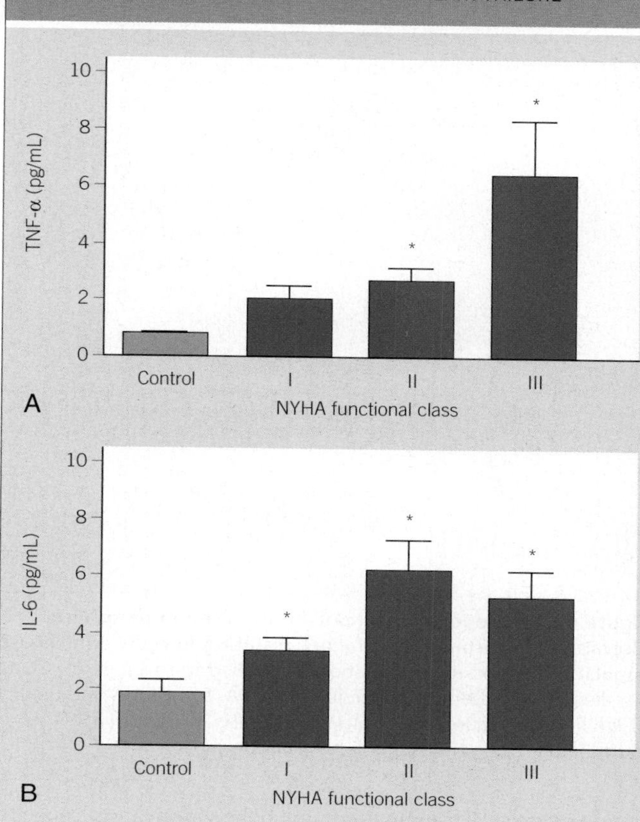

Figure 68.14 Plasma levels of cytokines in patients with heart failure. Plasma levels of tumor necrosis factor α (TNF-α) **(A)** and interleukin 6 (IL-6) **(B)** of healthy subjects and patients with congestive heart failure at different New York Heart Association (NYHA) functional classes. (From Torre-Amione G, Kapadia S, Benedict C, Oral H, Young JB, Mann DL. Proinflammatory cytokine levels in patients with depressed left ventricular ejection fraction: a report from the Studies of Left Ventricular Dysfunction [SOLVD]. J Am Coll Cardiol 1996;27:1201-1206. © American College of Cardiology.)

Attempts to augment muscle blood flow by increasing the pumping capacity of the heart during exercise have not produced increases in exercise tolerance or any reduction in fatigue. This may be either because the cardiac output was not the acutely limiting factor or because the augmented output was not perfusing the muscle but was passing through the skin circulation.

The metabolic abnormalities in patients with heart failure result not from inadequate oxygen delivery but from inadequate oxygen use by mitochondria (i.e., they are related to reduced mitochondrial content), which would decrease the rate of aerobic metabolism.[80] In many patients with chronic heart failure, the increase in blood flow to working muscle with exercise is attenuated for each given workload compared with that in normal persons.[81] Oxygen consumption at each level of work is lower in patients with chronic heart failure and is accompanied by an early increase in plasma lactate concentration. The reduced maximal blood flow to working muscle during exercise occurs predominantly in oxidative working muscle and is primarily caused by an abnormality of arteriolar vasodilatation

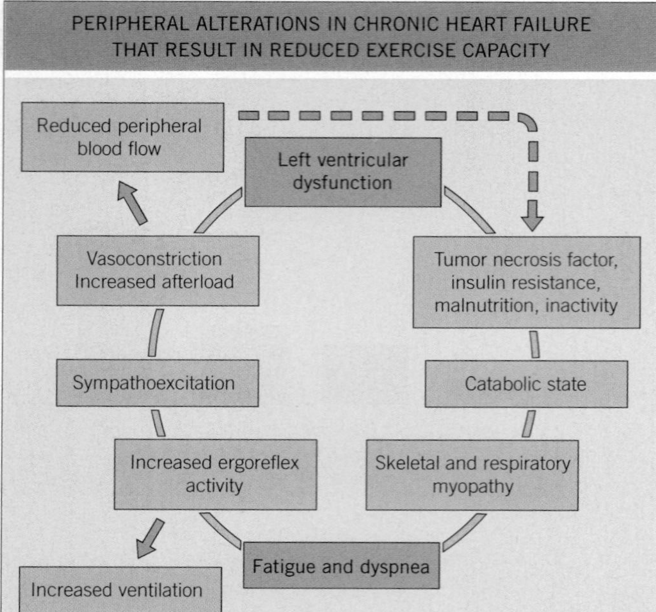

Figure 68.15 Proposed mechanisms involved in peripheral alterations in chronic heart failure resulting in reduced exercise capacity. See text for explanation. (Modified from Coats AJ, Clark AL, Piepoli M, Volterrani M, Poole-Wilson PA. Symptoms and quality of life in heart failure: the muscle hypothesis. Br Heart J 1994;72 [Suppl]:S36–S39. © BMJ Publishing Group.)

during exercise. This impaired metabolic vasodilatory capacity within skeletal muscle in patients with chronic heart failure during exercise is attributed to several factors,[76] including excessive sympathetically mediated vasoconstriction, activation of the plasma renin-angiotensin system, increased levels of endothelin, and impaired endothelium-dependent dilatation (i.e., reduced stimulated release of nitric oxide during exercise).[75]

Beyond skeletal muscle perfusion, intrinsic abnormalities of skeletal muscle metabolism and atrophy (reduced muscle mass) and biochemical alterations, including a shift in fiber-type distribution of skeletal muscle, emerge in patients with advanced heart failure.[79] These alterations in skeletal muscle result in reduced concentration of oxidative enzymes (Fig. 68.16) and, consequently, in impaired oxidative capacity of skeletal muscle as well as reduced maximal force production by large muscle groups. Thus, exercise capacity is, in part, determined by the condition of the working muscle. Changes similar to those seen in skeletal muscle are also seen in the respiratory muscles. Respiratory muscle endurance as assessed by maximal sustainable ventilatory capacity is reduced in patients with heart failure. There is early deoxygenation of respiratory muscles, alterations in diaphragmatic histology, and increased diaphragmatic work and deoxygenation of the accessory muscles of ventilation. These changes contribute to the sensation of breathlessness and fatigue in patients with heart failure. Whereas the alterations of skeletal muscle of chronic heart failure are, in part, due to deconditioning, other potential factors include malnutrition, increased insulin resistance, free radical activity, increased sympathetic tone, and increased plasma levels of tumor necrosis factor,[82] notably in patients with neurohormonal activation. Cytokines may contribute to the development of the anorexia and cachexia and adversely affect muscle metabolism and function, may enhance production of free radicals, and may contribute to the attenuated peripheral vascular response to endothelium-mediated vasodilators. In addition, cytokines such as tumor necrosis factor α and interleukin 6 affect myocyte growth, force of contraction, and extracellular matrix composition.[80]

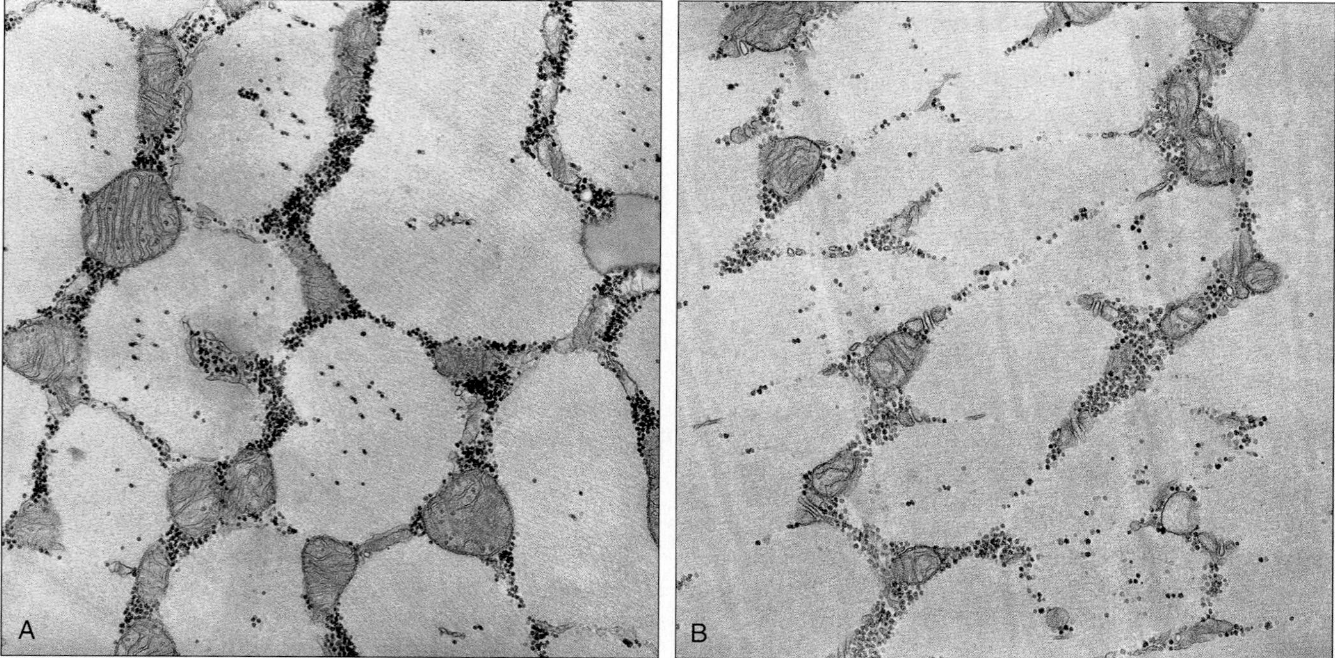

Figure 68.16 Electron microscopy of skeletal muscle from a healthy subject and a patient with severe chronic heart failure. Note the smaller cross-sectional area of the muscle fibers and the reduced size and staining (cytochrome-*c* oxidase) of the mitochondria in heart failure **(B)** than in healthy skeletal muscle **(A)**, reflecting the reduced oxidative capacity of the skeletal muscle.

CLINICAL IMPLICATIONS: PROGRESSION OF THE DISEASE

Although activation of the adrenergic and renin-angiotensin system is effective for short-term compensation, the sustained neurohumoral activation is associated with long-term adverse consequences, including progressive left ventricular dysfunction, remodeling, pump failure, and reduced survival (Fig. 68.17). Although the precise way in which hemodynamic and neurohormonal factors interact to cause progression of heart failure remains undefined, there is some evidence that several mechanisms are involved, including energy depletion, increased ventricular wall stress, altered cardiac gene expression, elevated oxidative stress, myocyte necrosis, and apoptosis (Fig 68.18).

Heart rate, contractile state, and wall stress are the three major determinants of myocardial oxygen consumption. Therefore, the failing heart has a much greater metabolic need compared with a normal (smaller) ventricle operating at a lower heart rate. Increases in cardiac pressure and volume may facilitate the occurrence of myocardial ischemia by augmenting energy expenditure while decreasing subendocardial perfusion, especially in patients with coronary artery disease. The hypertrophic response to stress increases energy demands while reducing energy supply by impairing oxygen diffusion in thickened ventricular walls. In addition, interstitial fibrosis and impaired coronary perfusion caused by functional (endothelial) and structural changes in coronary resistance vessels and capillary network of the coronary circulation result in increased diffusion distance for oxygenated blood, predisposing the failing ventricle to ischemia. High-energy phosphate reserves may be compromised and substrate use may be altered in the failing heart, resulting in an "energy-starved heart."[9] The state of energy deprivation is thought to have long-term detrimental effects on cellular processes and should contribute to progressive cardiac myocyte dysfunction.

Prolonged activation of the sympathetic nervous system and renin-angiotensin system exerts adverse effects on the heart independent of their hemodynamic action. High concentrations of norepinephrine and angiotensin exert direct toxic effects on myocardial cells, including calcium overload in the failing heart, increasing oxygen free radicals. In addition, increased activity of the sympathetic nervous system and renin-angiotensin system may exert adverse electrophysiologic effects and thereby provoke life-threatening ventricular arrhythmias. Sustained hemodynamic stress and neurohormonal activation can cause necrosis and apoptosis of myocardial cells in previously noninjured segments of the heart.

The activated renin-angiotensin system and cytokine activation have profound effects on extracellular matrix deposition. Discrete changes in the activity of enzymatic systems that are responsible for extracellular matrix degradation (matrix metalloproteinases and tissue inhibitors of metalloproteinases) contribute to changes in left ventricular geometry and thereby in the process of left ventricular remodeling in heart failure.[81] Ventricular remodeling increases wall stress, and this can cause irreversible structural remodeling of the heart because of slippage and elongation of myocardial fibers. In addition, progressive ventricular dilatation may cause dilatation of the mitral valve annulus, with subsequent mitral regurgitation. Finally, although the process of hypertrophy

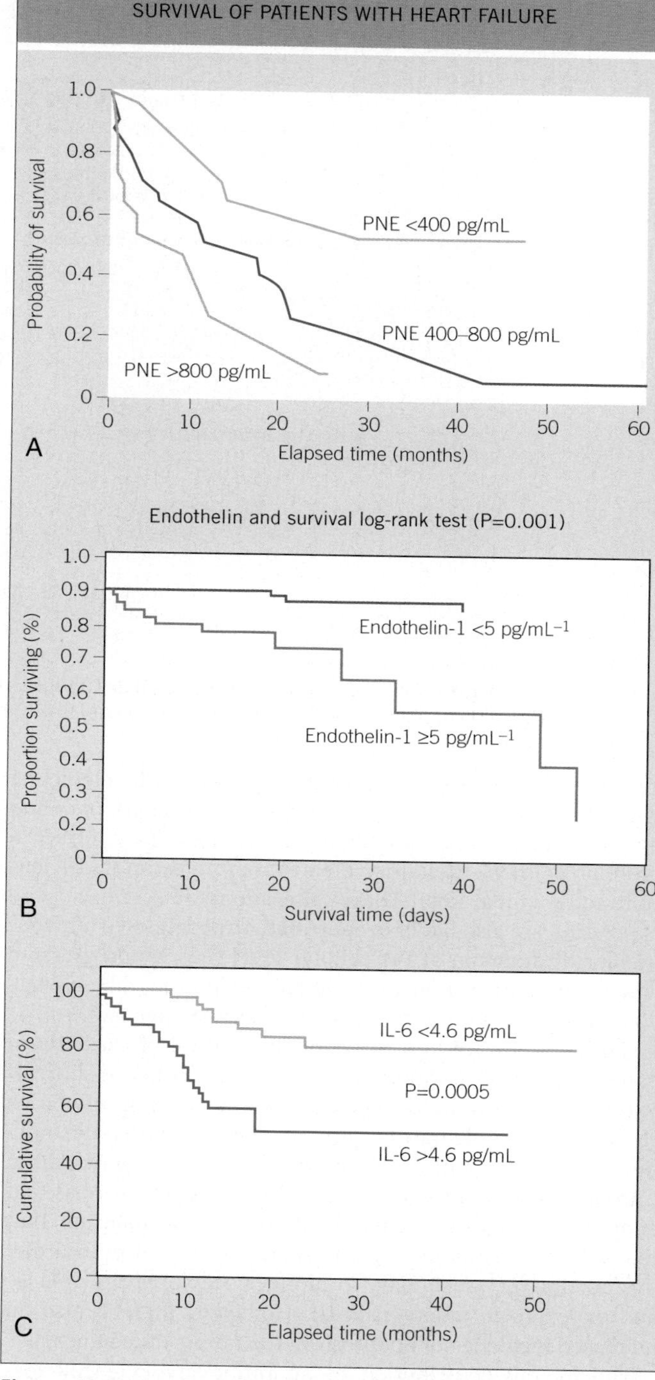

Figure 68.17 Survival of patients with heart failure. Survival is related to plasma levels of norepinephrine **(A)**, endothelin **(B)**, and interleukin 6 (IL-6) **(C)**. PNE, plasma norepinephrine. (**A** from Cohn JN, Levine TB, Olivari MT, et al. Plasma norepinephrine as a guide to prognosis in patients with chronic congestive heart failure. N Engl J Med 1984;311:819-823; © Massachusetts Medical Society. **B** from Pousset F, Isnard R, Lechat P, et al. Prognostic value of plasma endothelin-1 in patients with chronic heart failure. Eur Heart J 1997;18:254-258. **C** from Tsutamoto T, Hisanaga T, Wada A, et al. Interleukin-6 spillover in the peripheral circulation increases with the severity of heart failure and the high plasma level of interleukin-6 is an important prognostic predictor in patients with congestive heart failure. J Am Coll Cardiol 1998;31:391-398. © American College of Cardiology.)

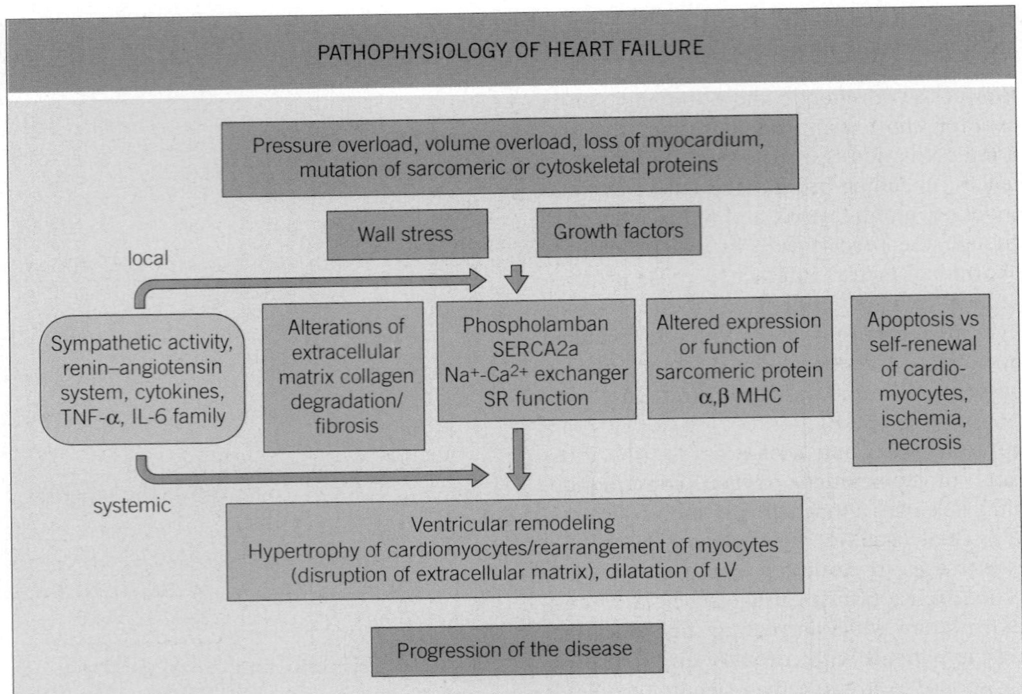

Figure 68.18 Pathophysiology of heart failure. IL, interleukin; LV, left ventricle; MHC, myosin heavy chain; SERCA, SR Ca^{2+}-ATPase; SR, sarcoplasmic reticulum; TNF, tumor necrosis factor.

increases the number of functioning contractile elements, alterations in gene expression that involve calcium handling by the sarcoplasmic reticulum and changes in contractile proteins or their regulatory elements produce an inefficient contractile apparatus. These alterations in cardiac gene expression are also likely to contribute to progressive left ventricular dysfunction at the cellular level (i.e., by progressive deterioration of systolic function and by limiting the myocardial reserve in times of stress, such as during exercise).

Cardiac myocyte loss is a common feature of cardiomyopathic processes. Although the degree of cell loss is difficult to quantify, loss of myocytes within viable portions of ventricles probably contributes to progressive myocardial dysfunction in patients with ischemic or dilated cardiomyopathy. Cardiac myocyte loss may occur through both necrosis and apoptosis. Necrosis occurs by cytotoxic mechanisms that may emerge in situations of both acute and chronic myocardial dysfunction (i.e., secondary to cardiac norepinephrine release and exposure to angiotensin II). However, there is also an increased incidence of apoptosis in the failing human heart.[83]

The overall contribution of apoptotic myocyte cell loss to progression of heart failure is far from established, but neurohumoral and cytokine activation has been shown to exert apoptosis of cardiac myocytes by several mechanisms. Apoptosis most probably occurs as a response to prolonged growth stimulation in the adult differentiated myocyte. However, although the adult myocyte may have lost the ability to divide (or with an insufficiently high cell division rate), there is growing evidence that resident cardiac stem cells and possibly engrafting circulating cells may provide some regenerative potential for the heart, in particular after cardiac injury.[83-85] The progressive loss of this limited self-renewing capability in aging and heart failure may shift the balance to progressive loss of cardiomyocytes and progression of the disease.

Conversely, neurohumoral/autocrine-paracrine signals that are activated or induced in the failing human heart can predispose to both necrosis and apoptosis. A loss of myocytes would further enhance the load on the remaining cardiomyocytes and thereby set in motion a vicious circle within the heart (Fig. 68.19).

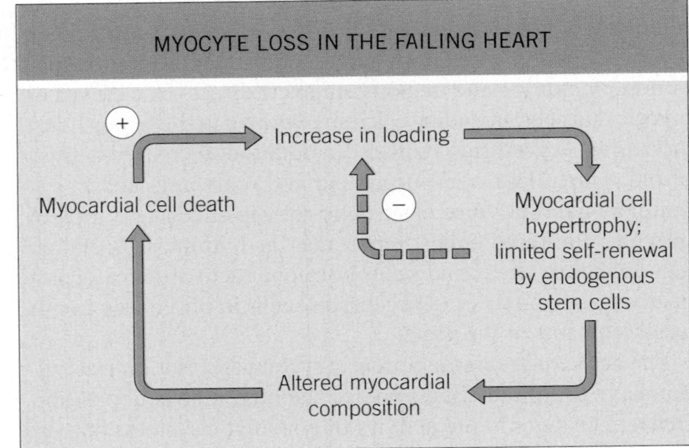

Figure 68.19 Vicious circle of myocyte loss in the failing heart. Hypertrophy, by increasing the number of contractile units in the overloaded heart, reduces the loading on each sarcomere and so is beneficial (−). However, hypertrophy also initiates myocardial changes that cause the cells of the failing heart to deteriorate and die, thereby establishing a vicious circle that by reducing the number of contractile units increases the load on each surviving cell (+). (From Katz AM. Changing strategies in the management of heart failure. J Am Coll Cardiol 1989;13:513-523. © American College of Cardiology.)

chapter 69

Assessment of the Patient with Heart Failure

Ayan R. Patel and Marvin A. Konstam

Definition

Heart failure is cardiac dysfunction resulting in an inability to achieve a cardiac output adequate to meet systemic metabolic demands, at rest or with exertion, at normal ventricular filling pressures.

Key Features

- Heart failure is the only common cardiovascular disease increasing in prevalence and incidence. Five-year mortality rates for this condition are as high as 50%, and it is the most frequent cause of hospitalization in patients older than 65 years.
- Evaluation of patients with suspected heart failure includes assessment of left ventricular function, identification of potentially reversible causes, and determination of prognosis.

Clinical Implications

- Because patients who have heart failure experience considerable morbidity and mortality, detection and specific treatment of reversible causes are critical. Patients who have coronary heart disease should be evaluated for the presence of ischemic viable myocardium and potential for revascularization. Left ventricular function should be characterized to guide medical therapy and to determine prognosis.

Heart failure is a common condition, both in the United States and worldwide, and it is a frequent cause of hospitalization. In the United States, more than 5 million people suffer from heart failure,[1] and global estimates of prevalence for those aged 65 years or older range from 30 to 130 per 1000 of this population.[2] The incidence of heart failure rises with age,[3] and in view of the burgeoning elderly population, the prevalence of this disease is likely to continue to increase.

Despite continued advances in the treatment of heart failure, mortality rates remain high. In recent clinical trials, the 1-year mortality for placebo groups has ranged from 8% to 13%, and mortality rates outside of clinical trials are likely to be higher.[4] Heart failure mortality rates in the community exceed 50% during 5 years.[3] In addition, this condition often results in frequent hospitalizations and limitations on quality of life. The relatively high prevalence of heart failure has economic implications as well because evaluation and management of this disease consume a significant amount of health care resources. It is estimated that in the United States, heart failure accounts for more than 1 million hospitalizations each year,[5] and the annual cost of heart failure management has been estimated at U.S. $20 billion to $40 billion.[1]

Heart failure is defined as cardiac dysfunction resulting in an inability to achieve a cardiac output adequate to meet systemic metabolic demands, at rest or with exertion, at normal ventricular filling pressures. In the United States, coronary artery disease and hypertension are major causes of heart failure; other important causes include idiopathic cardiomyopathy, valvular disease, and diabetes mellitus (Table 69.1).[3,6,7]

Although most cases of heart failure occur in the setting of systolic left ventricular dysfunction, a substantial proportion of patients have normal or nearly normal left ventricular ejection fractions but can exhibit signs and symptoms similar to those of patients with reduced ejection fractions. According to some estimates, up to 40% of cases of heart failure overall and even a higher proportion among the elderly may occur in patients with preserved ejection fractions.[8] Hypertension, left ventricular hypertrophy, and ischemia are common causes of this presentation as a result of impaired diastolic function, but diastolic dysfunction may also be due to restrictive cardiomyopathies. In addition, pericardial disease with constriction may result in heart failure despite normal systolic performance. High-output heart failure is rare and may occur in the setting of severe anemia, thyrotoxicosis, Paget's disease, or beriberi.

There are several objectives of the initial evaluation of a patient with possible or definite heart failure:

- the diagnosis must be confirmed;
- left ventricular function should be evaluated;
- specific reversible causes, including myocardial ischemia in some patients, should be identified and treated; and
- information that allows assessment of prognosis, particularly in patients who may be candidates for cardiac transplantation or investigational approaches, should be collected.

Patients with the classic symptoms and signs described here are easy to diagnose, but some patients, especially older patients, may present atypically with fatigue, abdominal discomfort, or altered mentation. Conversely, patients with typical signs, including dyspnea and edema, may have pulmonary disease, obesity, or venous insufficiency without an underlying cardiac abnormality.

Although most patients with heart failure have impaired left ventricular systolic function, many may not. Because most effective therapies have been studied only in patients with systolic dysfunction, information about left ventricular function is important in guiding therapy.

MAJOR CAUSES OF HEART FAILURE
Coronary artery disease
Hypertension
Idiopathic
Valvular disease
Infectious myocarditis (e.g., viral, protozoal, bacterial)
Toxins (e.g., anthracyclines, cyclophosphamide, alcohol, cocaine, cobalt, lead)
Tachycardia-related cardiomyopathy
Stress-induced cardiomyopathy
Endocrine disorders (e.g., diabetes, hyperthyroidism, hypothyroidism)
Infiltrative disease (e.g., sarcoidosis, amyloidosis, hemochromatosis)
Hypertrophic cardiomyopathy
Collagen vascular disease
Muscular dystrophies
Peripartum cardiomyopathy
Nutritional deficiencies

Table 69.1 Major causes of heart failure.

DESCRIPTION OF PROCEDURES

General Evaluation

History and Physical Examination

Symptoms consistent with heart failure (Table 69.2) may be categorized into those related to

- pulmonary congestion;
- systemic venous congestion; and
- low cardiac output.

However, a significant portion of patients who have marked left ventricular dysfunction do not present with symptoms of heart failure. Marantz and coworkers[9] reported that 20% of patients with left ventricular systolic dysfunction (ejection fraction of less than 40%) do not have clinical evidence of heart failure. Thus, although the presence of symptoms is diagnostically useful, a significant number of patients with left ventricular dysfunction are asymptomatic.

SYMPTOMS OF HEART FAILURE
Pulmonary congestion
Dyspnea on exertion
Orthopnea
Paroxysmal nocturnal dyspnea
Systemic venous congestion
Peripheral edema
Ascites
Abdominal pain or nausea
Low cardiac output
Decreased exercise tolerance or fatigue
Change in mental status or confusion

Table 69.2 Symptoms of heart failure.

The most common symptom related to pulmonary congestion is dyspnea on exertion. Orthopnea is a sensation of dyspnea that occurs when the patient is supine, and it may be present in patients who have severe heart failure. Paroxysmal nocturnal dyspnea is another symptom of severe heart failure and is characterized by shortness of breath that awakens the patient from sleep. Dyspnea on exertion has been demonstrated to be more sensitive for the presence of elevated filling pressures than orthopnea and paroxysmal nocturnal dyspnea, which are more specific symptoms.[10]

Patients who have right-sided heart failure may present with symptoms of systemic venous congestion. The most common symptom is peripheral edema, although its presence is relatively nonspecific. In severe right-sided heart failure, ascites and hepatic congestion may lead to gastrointestinal symptoms such as abdominal pain and nausea. Symptoms attributable to low cardiac output include fatigue, decreased exercise tolerance, and altered mental status. As these symptoms are nonspecific, it is important to consider the diagnosis of heart failure as well as potential noncardiac causes in patients who report them.

The New York Heart Association (NYHA) classification system is commonly used to categorize the severity of symptoms (Table 69.3).[11] Although it is subjective, the NYHA system is useful in classifying severity of heart failure and has been shown to correlate with prognosis.[12] In most cases, the degree of functional limitation can be ascertained from the history. In some patients, the degree of limitation is difficult to judge from the history, and consideration may be given to performing cardiopulmonary exercise testing to quantify functional impairment as a means of determining the degree to which additional treatment is needed. In addition, cardiopulmonary exercise testing is useful in assessing prognosis when cardiac transplantation is being contemplated (see evaluation of exercise capacity).

A careful review of the history is useful in determining the likelihood of heart failure as well as possible causes in a given patient. A history of coronary artery disease, hypertension, or diabetes mellitus increases the probability of heart failure. In addition, it is important to elicit a history of significant alcohol use or of cocaine use. A history of dietary noncompliance or exacerbating medications (such as nonsteroidal anti-inflammatory agents) can be helpful in determining the cause of decompensation in patients with existing heart failure.

NEW YORK HEART ASSOCIATION CLASSIFICATION SYSTEM	
Class I	No symptoms with ordinary activity
Class II	Mild limitation of physical activity; symptoms with ordinary physical activity
Class III	Marked limitation of physical activity; symptoms with less than ordinary physical activity
Class IV	Symptoms with any physical activity or at rest

From Criteria Committee, New York Heart Association. Diseases of the Heart and Blood Vessels. Nomenclature and Criteria for Diagnosis, 6th ed. Boston, Little, Brown, 1964.

Table 69.3 New York Heart Association classification system.

SIGNS OF HEART FAILURE ON PHYSICAL EXAMINATION
Left-sided heart failure and pulmonary venous congestion
Pulmonary rales
Decreased breath sounds
Dullness to percussion
Third heart sound
Displaced apical impulse
Right-sided heart failure and systemic venous congestion
Peripheral edema
Elevated jugular venous pressure, prominent *v* wave–*y* descent
Hepatojugular reflux
Hepatomegaly
Ascites
Right-sided third heart sound
Left parasternal heave
Low cardiac output
Tachycardia
Pulsus alternans
Decreased pulse pressure
Hypotension

Table 69.4 Signs of heart failure on physical examination.

Findings on physical examination can help to make the diagnosis of heart failure (Table 69.4). However, because most of these findings are not highly sensitive, their absence does not necessarily exclude the possibility of heart failure. Conversely, some of the signs associated with heart failure are relatively nonspecific and may occur in other, noncardiac conditions.

In pulmonary congestion, rales may be auscultated on lung examination. Wheezing may also occur in patients who have pulmonary edema, and decreased breath sounds or dullness to percussion may develop in the presence of pulmonary effusions. In severe cases of pulmonary congestion, the patient may be overtly tachypneic.

Signs of systemic venous congestion may predominate in patients who have right-sided heart failure, even when it results from chronic left ventricular dysfunction. Elevation of the jugular venous pressure reflects increased right-sided filling pressures and may therefore be helpful in monitoring volume status. In addition, the presence of an increased *v* wave and steep *y* descent of the jugular venous pulse is consistent with high right atrial pressures. Hepatojugular reflux should also be assessed to elicit evidence of elevated right-sided filling pressures. A left parasternal right ventricular heave indicates right ventricular enlargement or elevated right ventricular systolic pressure, and a right-sided third heart sound, which increases in intensity with inspiration, may develop in the presence of high right ventricular filling pressures. Ascites may be noted in patients who have severe right-sided heart failure, and hepatomegaly may develop as a result of hepatic congestion. A pulsatile liver is suggestive of severe tricuspid regurgitation. Peripheral edema is a common finding, but it is nonspecific in the absence of other signs of heart failure.[10] Several noncardiac conditions may cause peripheral edema; these conditions include venous stasis, lymphatic obstruction, and hypoalbuminemia. Although edema of the lower extremities caused by heart failure is usually bilateral, it may be asymmetric in some cases. Sacral edema may also be noted in patients with marked edema, particularly if they are recumbent much of the time.

Patients who have heart failure may also manifest signs and symptoms of low cardiac output. Tachycardia may ensue in low-output states, and pulsus alternans may be noted. A reduced pulse pressure may develop, and a proportional pulse pressure of less than 25% has been reported as correlating with a cardiac output of less than 2.2 L/min/m.[2,13] Patients with low-output states tend to maintain relatively low blood pressures, and orthostatic hypotension may occur, particularly in patients receiving diuretic or vasodilator therapy. The physical finding with the highest predictive value is the third heart sound, which reflects increased left ventricular filling pressures and is a marker of poor prognosis.[10,14] In addition, a displaced and diffuse apical impulse may be palpated in patients with a dilated left ventricle and systolic dysfunction. In the presence of severe pulmonary hypertension, a left parasternal right ventricular heave and loud pulmonary component of the second heart sound may be appreciated. Although there are no specific symptoms of low cardiac output, these patients often experience fatigue and activity intolerance and may exhibit altered mentation and renal dysfunction.

Routine Laboratory Studies

Many of the routine laboratory tests provide information about alternative or concomitant diagnoses and systemic dysfunction resulting from heart failure; alternatively, they may be necessary to guide and to monitor therapy. Relevant routine laboratory tests include complete blood count, electrolyte determinations, creatinine concentration, blood urea nitrogen concentration, liver function tests, fasting blood glucose concentration, and plasma lipid levels (Table 69.5).

Measurement of hemoglobin and hematocrit is useful to exclude anemia as a precipitating cause of heart failure or, if the anemia is severe, to suggest that it may be an alternative cause of many of the symptoms and signs of heart failure. Renal failure and nephrotic syndrome may mimic some of the presenting features of heart failure. In addition, renal dysfunction may result from hypoperfusion of the kidneys in heart failure and is a key parameter to be monitored during treatment with angiotensin-converting enzyme inhibitors. Electrolyte abnormalities are common and important in heart failure patients, especially during diuretic therapy. Hyponatremia may occur in severe heart failure as a result of activation of the renin-angiotensin system; it is associated with a worse prognosis. Liver function abnormalities, especially hypoalbuminemia, may indicate cirrhosis, which may mimic heart failure by causing fluid retention and dyspnea. Liver function may also be impaired as a result of right-sided congestion in heart failure.

In elderly patients or patients with atrial fibrillation, thyroid function tests should be performed to exclude the possibility of hyperthyroidism or hypothyroidism. Both of these conditions can be manifested with fluid retention and symptoms of dyspnea and fatigue, and both are easily treatable.

ROUTINE TESTING IN THE ASSESSMENT OF HEART FAILURE

Test	Abnormalities
Electrocardiography	Q waves ST-T wave abnormalities Left ventricular hypertrophy Right ventricular hypertrophy Low voltage (infiltrative cardiomyopathy, pericardial effusion, hypothyroidism) Intraventricular conduction disturbances Tachyarrhythmias
Chest radiography	Cardiomegaly Increased interstitial densities (including Kerley's B lines), diffuse alveolar densities Pleural effusions
Complete blood count	Anemia
Urinalysis	Proteinuria, casts
Blood urea nitrogen and creatinine concentration	Renal dysfunction
Electrolyte analysis	Hyponatremia, hyperkalemia, hypokalemia
Albumin concentration	Hypoalbuminemia
Thyroxine (T_4) concentration, thyroid-stimulating hormone level (atrial fibrillation or age > 65 years without obvious etiology)[5]	Hyperthyroidism or hypothyroidism

Table 69.5 Routine testing in the assessment of heart failure.

Diabetes mellitus is an important risk factor for heart failure, especially in women, and should be considered in the evaluation of patients with heart failure. Dyslipidemia is a risk factor for coronary artery disease and should be treated aggressively because recurrent ischemic events play an important role in the progression of heart failure.

Chest Radiography

A chest radiograph is generally obtained as part of the initial evaluation for heart failure. Cardiomegaly is the most common radiographic finding and is reported to be present in 46% of patients with left ventricular end-diastolic pressure of more than 15 mm Hg.[10] Radiographic manifestations of heart failure include cephalization of pulmonary venous vessels, increased interstitial markings, pleural effusions, and cardiomegaly. In severe heart failure, diffuse alveolar densities may be present. The chest radiograph may also be helpful in distinguishing between cardiac and pulmonary causes of dyspnea.

Electrocardiography

The electrocardiogram in heart failure is generally nonspecific, although evidence of the underlying etiology may be present. Typical electrocardiographic abnormalities are listed in Table 69.5. The electrocardiogram may provide evidence of ischemic heart disease, left ventricular hypertrophy, right ventricular hypertrophy, pericardial effusion, or infiltrative cardiomyopathy. Bundle branch block and intraventricular conduction delay are common in patients who have heart failure, and prolonged QRS duration is a predictor of poor prognosis.[15] Furthermore, intraventricular conduction abnormalities may be associated with discoordination of left and right ventricular contraction and relaxation, thereby contributing to impaired hemodynamics. The electrocardiographic finding of QRS prolongation is therefore clinically relevant because biventricular pacing for resynchronization therapy should be considered in patients with ventricular dyssynchrony who are symptomatic despite medical therapy.[16,17] Currently, prolonged QRS duration is the primary marker used to identify patients with heart failure who may benefit from resynchronization therapy, although echocardiographic methods of identifying ventricular dyssynchrony are also under investigation. Tachyarrhythmias and bradyarrhythmias should be noted; both can be associated with or precipitate heart failure. However, if these are suspected, more effective methods for detecting abnormal rhythms (ambulatory monitoring or event recorders) should be employed.

Pulmonary Testing

As noted before, patients who present with new onset of dyspnea or worsening dyspnea are often diagnosed as having chronic obstructive pulmonary disease. Evidence of cardiomegaly should strongly point to a cardiac origin, and echocardiography (see later) can confirm this judgment. Routine pulmonary function testing is not recommended and can be misleading because heart failure and pulmonary disease often coexist. Pulmonary function testing, however, is appropriate if left ventricular systolic function is not abnormal and the cardiac origin of symptoms remains in doubt.

Plasma Biomarkers of Heart Failure

Because of limitations in the reliability of clinical findings and routine tests in detecting heart failure, circulating neurohormonal levels have been investigated as potential markers for left ventricular dysfunction. In chronic heart failure, activation of compensatory mechanisms results in elevated levels of several neurohormonal factors. Multiple studies have established that levels of norepinephrine (noradrenaline) and natriuretic peptides are increased in left ventricular systolic dysfunction and that elevated levels of these neurohormones can provide prognostic information.[12,18-21]

Chronic heart failure results in activation of both the sympathetic nervous system and renin-angiotensin system. Increased plasma renin activity reflects activation of the renin-angiotensin system and is associated with poor prognosis in heart failure; however, because plasma renin activity tends to fluctuate, its utility as a prognostic marker may be limited.[18] Activation of the sympathetic nervous system in chronic heart failure results in increased levels of norepinephrine. High circulating norepinephrine levels have been observed even in early stages of left ventricular dysfunction, and a stepwise increase in norepinephrine levels has been observed as the degree of heart failure progresses.[19] In addition, norepinephrine levels have been found to be predictive of prognosis in both symptomatic and asymptomatic patients with left ventricular dysfunction.[12,18] It has been noted, however, that there is considerable variation in norepinephrine levels among heart failure patients, and cardiac natriuretic peptides have proved superior to norepinephrine in both diagnosis of heart failure and prediction of its prognosis.[20]

Atrial natriuretic peptide and brain natriuretic peptide (BNP) levels are usually increased in patients who have heart failure, particularly when they are symptomatic.[20,21] The cardiac natriuretic peptides have multiple hemodynamic and neurohormonal effects, such as arterial and venous vasodilator effects, natriuretic activity, and suppressive effects on the sympathetic nervous system and renin-angiotensin-aldosterone system. BNP is released by the left ventricle in response to increased myocardial stretch and therefore circulates at increased levels in patients with left ventricular dysfunction. It is a better predictor of ventricular function and prognosis than is atrial natriuretic peptide.[20] It is also more stable. N-terminal pro-BNP (NT-proBNP) is the inactive product released when pro-BNP is cleaved to form BNP. It has also emerged as a useful marker of cardiac function, volume overload, and prognosis and has the advantage of being even more stable than BNP, thereby reflecting myocardial events during a longer time frame. Both BNP and NT-proBNP may be assayed through commercially available kits as diagnostic tests for heart failure. Low levels of these peptides have a high negative predictive value for the presence of clinical heart failure.[21] However, falsely low levels may be seen in patients with right-sided heart failure, heart failure with preserved systolic function, or obesity. Very high levels of BNP indicate a poor prognosis, with higher subsequent mortality and readmission levels.

Clinical trials have demonstrated significant value for assays of both BNP and NT-proBNP in the emergency department diagnosis of patients presenting with dyspnea.[22,23] These tests should not be viewed as a replacement for clinical assessment. However, in conjunction with clinical assessment, they improve diagnostic accuracy and therefore may serve to improve the delivery of effective care to patients in this setting. Routine assays of BNP and NT-proBNP to facilitate clinical management of patients known to have heart failure, in both the inpatient and ambulatory settings, remain more controversial. Several small studies have suggested improved clinical outcomes from a strategy entailing medication dosing based on results of these tests.[24,25] Further work is needed to confirm these encouraging findings and to clarify that similar results would not be obtainable through more aggressive routine medication dosing.

Several other categories of circulating biomarkers have been shown to correlate with clinical outcomes in patients with heart failure. These include inflammatory markers, such as C-reactive protein, and markers of myocardial injury, such as troponin T and troponin I.[26,27] Cardiac troponin I is associated with impaired hemodynamics, progressive left ventricular dysfunction, and increased mortality rates in advanced heart failure.[28] At present, the role of assaying these biomarkers in facilitating diagnosis or patient management remains to be clarified. It is possible that future therapies may be personalized to specifically counter inflammatory or ischemic mechanisms in select patients on the basis of such measurements.

Evaluation of Left Ventricular Function

Assessment of left ventricular function is essential in all patients with suspected heart failure. Evaluation of the degree of systolic dysfunction is particularly important in view of the fact that angiotensin-converting enzyme inhibitors and beta blockers have been demonstrated to be beneficial in patients with moderate to severe left ventricular dysfunction, even in those who are asymptomatic. Furthermore, distinguishing patients with reduced ejection fractions from those with preserved systolic function is critical because the management of these conditions differs. In addition, multiple studies have demonstrated that the degree of left ventricular dysfunction is an important prognostic marker. Several noninvasive imaging techniques are available to evaluate left ventricular function.

Echocardiography

Echocardiography has the advantage of being a versatile imaging modality and is more widely available, is less costly compared with other imaging modalities, and avoids the modest radiation exposure associated with nuclear medicine testing. Two-dimensional echocardiography is the most commonly used method for assessing ventricular function, regional wall motion, and chamber size. This technique has been demonstrated to have good reproducibility when it is interpreted by experienced readers.[29] The primary disadvantage is that the echocardiographic window may be limited in some patients because of body habitus, obesity, or pulmonary disease, although technical advances in newer equipment have considerably reduced the number of unsatisfactory studies.

In addition to providing an assessment of biventricular function and chamber size, two-dimensional echocardiography may be useful in identifying many of the underlying causes of heart failure and associated disease. Echocardiography in conjunction with Doppler echocardiography can diagnose and quantify valvular abnormalities, which may often be correctable. Segmental wall motion abnormalities, particularly when they are severe and associated with segmental wall thinning (which is indicative of scarring), suggest an ischemic etiology, but nonischemic dilated cardiomyopathy may also display some degree of regional heterogeneity. Conversely, patients who have severe ischemic cardiomyopathy may develop global hypokinesis. In stress-induced (tako-tsubo) cardiomyopathy, characteristic wall motion abnormalities that do not correspond to a coronary territory are present; the distal ventricle and apex are typically involved, but other patterns of involvement have been reported. Other potential causes of heart failure, such as intracardiac shunts and other congenital abnormalities, can also be detected on echocardiography. Typical echocardiographic findings may suggest infiltrative and restrictive cardiomyopathies. Pericardial abnormalities may be detected, including sometimes unsuspected pericardial effusions. Complications of ventricular dysfunction, such as intracardiac thrombi (Fig. 69.1), may be identified.

Echocardiography may be helpful in determining whether diastolic function is abnormal. In hypertensive heart disease, left ventricular hypertrophy may be present. However, heart failure with preserved systolic function may occur in the absence of left ventricular hypertrophy.[8]

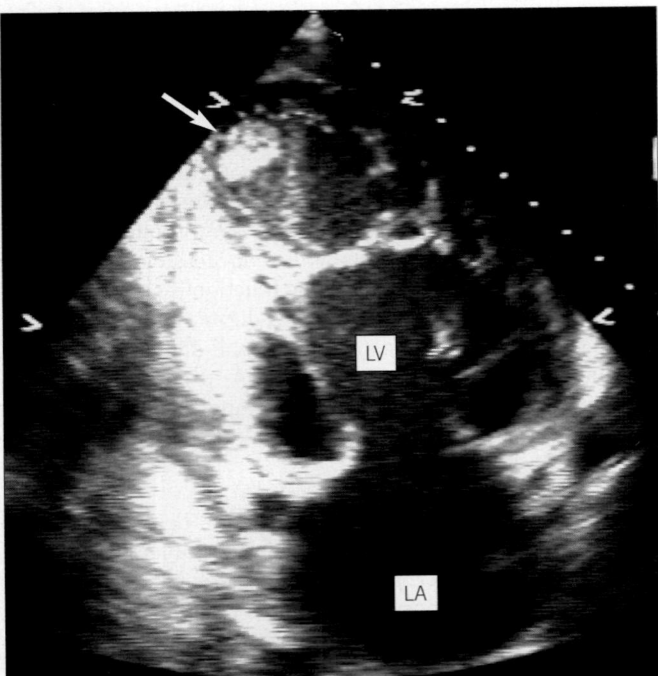

Figure 69.1 Apical thrombus. Two-dimensional echocardiographic image demonstrating left ventricular apical thrombus *(arrow)* in a patient with severe left ventricular dysfunction. LA, left atrium; LV, left ventricle.

Doppler echocardiography may be useful in detecting evidence of abnormal diastolic function (Fig. 69.2) in patients with heart failure. The typical finding in early diastolic dysfunction is an "abnormal relaxation" ventricular inflow pattern, which develops as relatively less filling occurs during early diastole because of increased ventricular stiffness, resulting in an increased reliance on atrial contraction for diastolic filling. A decrease in the ratio of the early diastolic filling (E) wave velocity to the atrial contraction (A) wave velocity and a prolonged E-wave deceleration time are observed in the mitral inflow Doppler examination. In late stages of diastolic dysfunction, a "restrictive" pattern develops. The restrictive filling pattern is characterized by a high ratio of the peak E-wave velocity to the peak A-wave velocity and a shortened E-wave deceleration time, which occur as a result of rapid early ventricular filling in the presence of high atrial and ventricular diastolic pressures. A restrictive filling pattern may occur in patients with systolic dysfunction who have advanced heart failure and high left atrial pressures and is an indicator of poor prognosis in such patients.[30]

Although these abnormal patterns are useful if they are present, they can be influenced by loading conditions, and the absence of an abnormal filling pattern does not exclude the possibility of diastolic abnormalities. In intermediate stages of disease, patients may exhibit a "pseudonormal" pattern as they evolve from the abnormal relaxation phase to the restrictive phase. Abnormalities of pulmonary venous flow (Fig. 69.3), such as blunting of the systolic venous component or a prominent atrial reversal wave, reflect increased left atrial pressures and may be helpful in distinguishing normal from pseudonormal mitral inflow patterns.[31]

Tissue Doppler imaging has emerged as an additional tool for assessing diastolic function (see Fig. 69.2). In patients with abnormal diastolic function, the tissue Doppler E′ wave may be blunted. The ratio of the mitral inflow E wave/tissue Doppler E′ wave has also been demonstrated to be indicative of left ventricular diastolic pressures. An E/E′ ratio of 15 or more has a high positive predictive value for elevated left ventricular diastolic pressure, whereas an E/E′ ratio of 8 or less has a high predictive value for normal left ventricular diastolic pressure.[32] However, E/E′ ratios between 8 and 15 represent a "gray zone," in which other parameters (such as left atrial enlargement and abnormal pulmonary venous flow pattern) may be helpful in determining whether elevated left atrial pressures are present.

Three-dimensional echocardiography is now available as a clinical tool for evaluation of cardiac anatomy as well as for quantification of chamber size and left and right ventricular ejection fraction (Fig. 69.4). Ventricular volumes and ejection fraction obtained by three-dimensional echocardiography correlate well with other methods, such as cardiac magnetic resonance imaging.[33,34] Three-dimensional echocardiography eliminates many of the potential technical sources of error that may occur in two-dimensional quantification but is still dependent on the underlying image quality.

Radionuclide Angiography

Radionuclide ventriculography can also be used to assess left and right ventricular functions and volumes, although the latter measurements are not routinely made in most laboratories. This technique is performed by labeling of red blood cells with radioactive isotope in vitro and injection of the tagged cells. The labeled cells reach equilibrium with the circulating volume, and images are obtained from many cardiac cycles and gated to the cardiac cycle. Radionuclide ventriculography offers the advantage of more precise quantitation of ejection fraction.

In an experienced laboratory, this method provides a quantitative assessment of biventricular function with reproducibility; adequate images can be obtained in most patients, although accuracy may be reduced in patients with very irregular rhythms. Information about diastolic function can be obtained from measurement of time to peak diastolic filling and peak filling rate. Regurgitant fraction may also be calculated, but this method provides only limited information about valve function.

Cardiac Magnetic Resonance Imaging

Cardiac magnetic resonance (CMR) imaging provides excellent spatial and contrast resolution for visualization of the myocardium and cardiac chambers. CMR provides three-dimensional quantitation of left and right ventricular volumes and ejection fraction, and a high degree of interstudy reproducibility has been reported.[35] Wall motion abnormalities, valvular lesions, pericardial abnormalities, and congenital cardiac abnormalities can also be visualized, although echocardiography is a better established method for the quantification of valvular disease. When gadolinium contrast imaging is used, myocardial scarring in a coronary distribution pattern on delayed enhancement images can indicate ischemic heart disease. In patients with nonischemic or infiltrative cardiomyopathies, delayed enhancement in noncoronary patterns may be seen. Because of rare reports

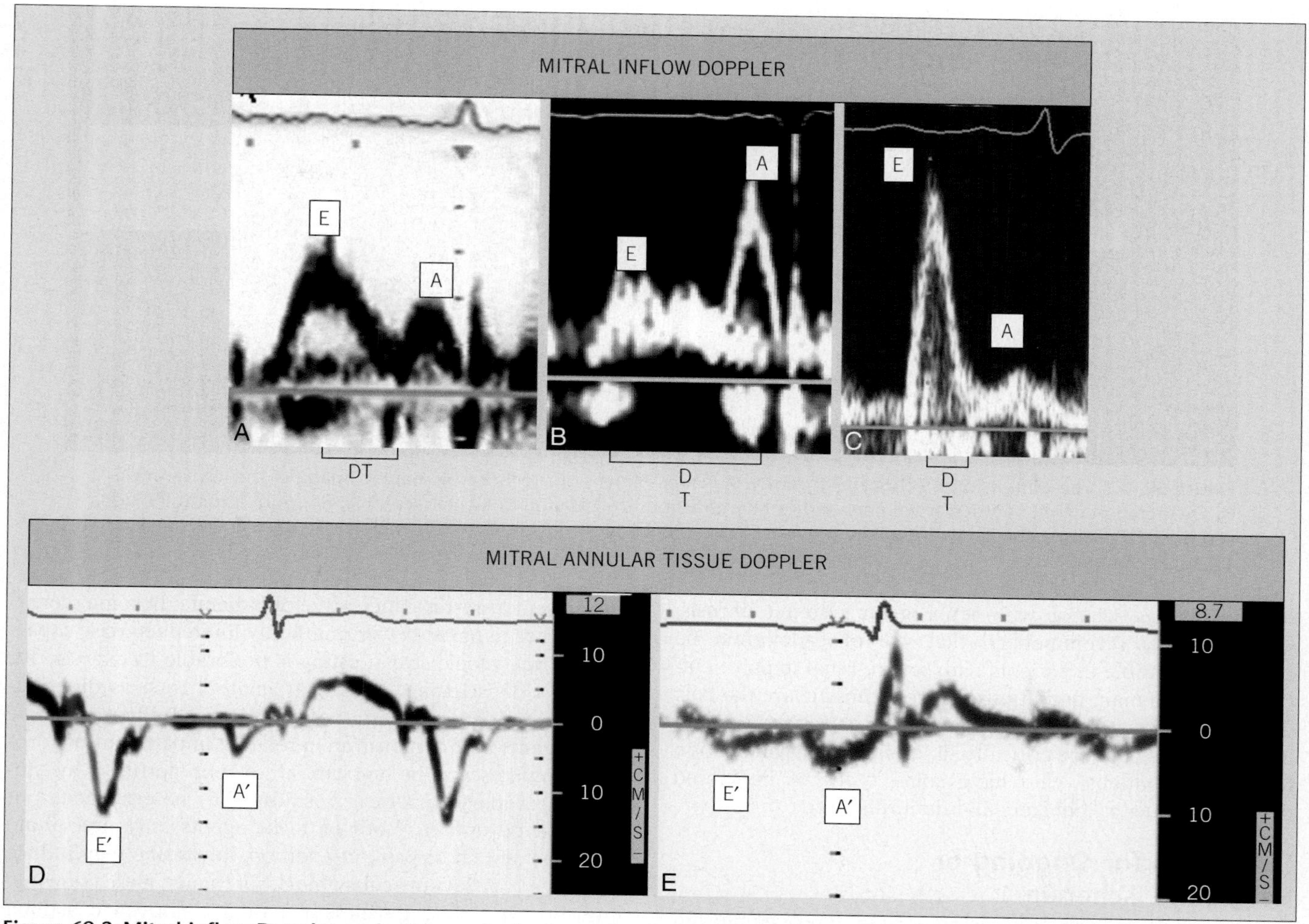

Figure 69.2 Mitral inflow Doppler evaluation and mitral annular tissue Doppler evaluation. A, Normal mitral inflow pattern. **B,** Abnormal relaxation pattern. **C,** Restrictive pattern. **D,** Normal tissue Doppler pattern. **E,** Abnormal tissue Doppler pattern. E, early ventricular filling wave; A, ventricular filling wave caused by atrial contraction; DT, deceleration time; E′, early diastolic tissue Doppler annular velocity; A′, late diastolic tissue Doppler annular velocity.

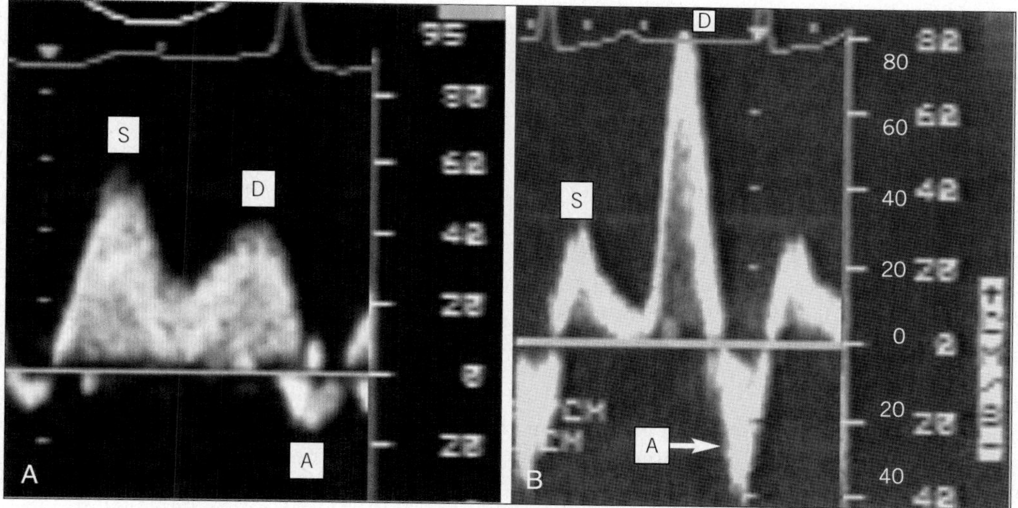

Figure 69.3 Doppler examination of pulmonary venous flow. A, Normal pulmonary venous flow. **B,** Abnormal pulmonary venous flow with blunting of the systolic component and prominent atrial reversal wave due to high left atrial pressures. S, systolic component; D, diastolic component; A, atrial reversal wave.

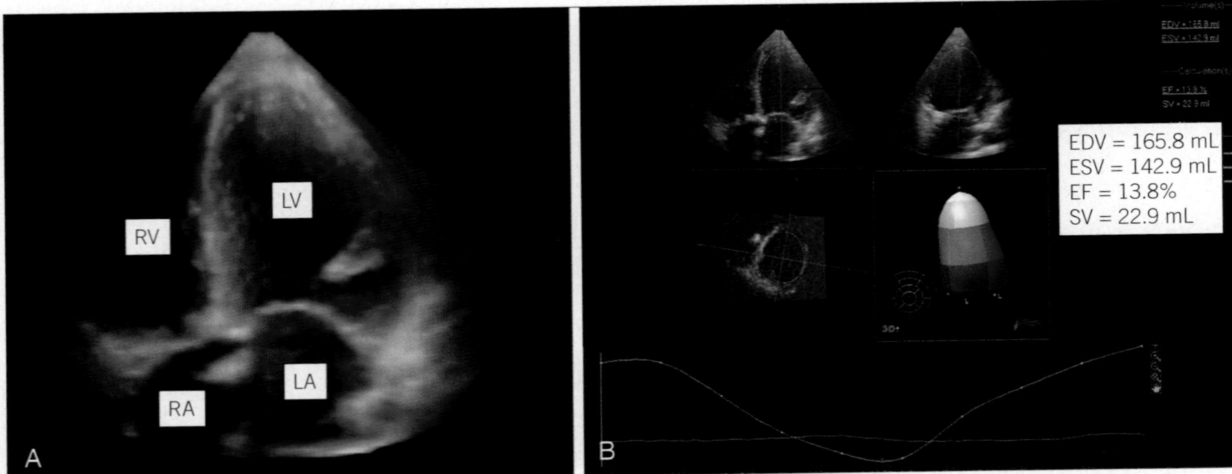

Figure 69.4 Three-dimensional echocardiography. A, Three-dimensional echocardiographic image of the left ventricle. **B,** Quantitation of left ventricular volumes and ejection fraction. LV, left atrium; LV, left ventricle; RA, right atrium; RV, right ventricle; EDV, left ventricular end-diastolic volume; ESV, left ventricular end-systolic volume; EF, left ventricular ejection fraction; SV, stroke volume.

of a possible association with nephrogenic systemic fibrosis, it is presently recommended that use of gadolinium be avoided if possible in patients with severe renal impairment. Currently, the main limitations of this technique are the lack of widespread availability, the inability to perform this imaging in patients who are critically ill, and the contraindication to CMR in patients who have some types of implanted devices (such as pacemakers and defibrillators).

Evaluation for Ongoing or Reversible Ischemia

Several cohort analyses have demonstrated improved mortality among patients who have heart failure and reduced ejection fraction and who are undergoing coronary artery bypass graft surgery compared with medically treated patients.[5] Although a randomized trial would be most valuable, these cohort data suggest a benefit of revascularization among patients who have viable but threatened myocardium. In patients with angina who are candidates for revascularization, coronary angiography is recommended; noninvasive testing may provide additional useful information in patients in whom the degree of ischemia or viability is uncertain. In heart failure patients who have a history of myocardial infarction but no symptoms of angina, noninvasive testing for myocardial ischemia and, if appropriate, myocardial viability is recommended (Fig. 69.5).[5] The beneficial yield of evaluation for ischemia in patients who do not have a history of myocardial infarction or angina is less clear, but noninvasive testing for ischemia should be considered in patients who may otherwise be good candidates for revascularization procedures.

Imaging Techniques

Several stress imaging techniques for detection of ischemia in patients with heart failure are available. Scintigraphic techniques include exercise and pharmacologic myocardial perfusion imaging. These methods use myocardial uptake of radionuclide tracers (agents labeled with either thallium Tl 201 or technetium Tc 99m) to determine myocardial perfusion. Perfusion defects that develop with stress but that are not present at rest are indicative of ischemia. In some scenarios, such as in patients with markedly limited exercise capacity, pharmacologic stress testing is preferable to exercise for diagnosis of ischemia. Arteriolar dilators such as dipyridamole and adenosine are commonly used pharmacologic stress agents that demonstrate a relative impairment of coronary flow reserve in myocardial regions perfused by stenosed coronary arteries, resulting in heterogeneity of radionuclide uptake. Both of these agents may precipitate headache and chest pain; in addition, adenosine may induce short-lived atrioventricular block or sinus node slowing. Bronchospasm may develop in patients who have asthma or very severe obstructive lung disease. The effects of adenosine are very short, lasting only 1 to 5 minutes. Intravenous administration of aminophylline can rapidly reverse the effects of dipyridamole. Exercise and dobutamine echocardiography are well-established methods for assessment of ischemia. Because the normal expected response to exercise or dobutamine is an increase in contractility, these methods use stress-induced wall motion abnormalities or worsening of baseline regional dysfunction to detect ischemia. Although the doses of dobutamine used for stress testing may be very high (up to 40 μg/kg per minute), complications are infrequent[36]; they include chest pain, arrhythmias, headache, nausea, tremor, and anxiety. Coronary computed tomographic angiography provides a noninvasive examination of coronary anatomy and may be useful when physiologic testing for ischemia is equivocal in patients presenting with new-onset heart failure. Computed tomographic angiography has a high negative predictive value for significant coronary disease.[37] The limitations of this method include technical difficulties with image interpretation in the presence of coronary stents or significant coronary calcification, potential risk of contrast nephrotoxicity, and associated radiation exposure.

In patients who have established coronary artery disease, noninvasive testing for viable or "hibernating" myocardium is useful for identification of those patients who are likely to have improvement in regional ventricular function after revascularization. Hibernating myocardium is defined as

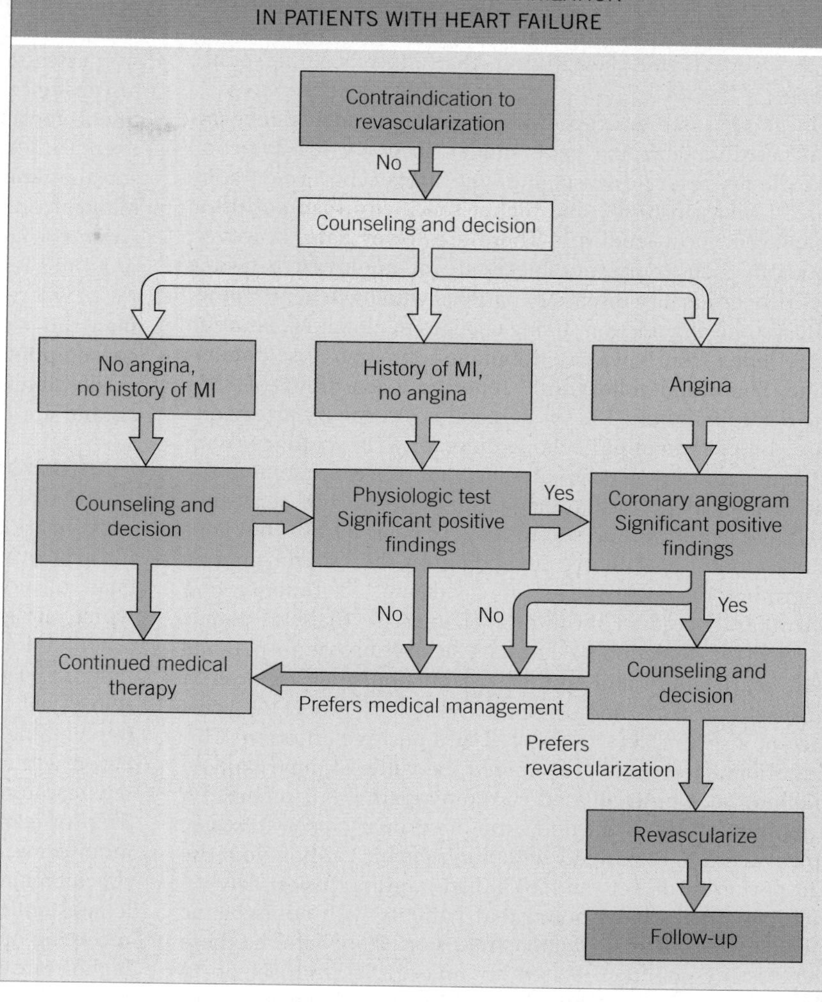

Figure 69.5 Evaluation of patients with heart failure for revascularization. MI, myocardial infarction. (From Konstam M, Dracup K, Baker D, et al. Heart Failure: Evaluation and Care of Patients with Left Ventricular Systolic Dysfunction. Clinical Practice Guideline No. 11. Rockville, Md, Agency for Health Care Policy and Research, Public Health Service, U.S. Department of Health and Human Services, 1994. AHCPR publication 94-0612.)

myocardium that is viable but asynergic due to chronic underperfusion. Positron emission tomography, ^{201}Tl perfusion single-photon emission computed tomography (SPECT) imaging, ^{99m}Tc-sestamibi SPECT imaging, dobutamine echocardiography, and delayed enhancement CMR have been demonstrated to be useful in identification of areas of viable but hypoperfused myocardium.[35,38-41]

Positron emission tomography (PET) has been considered the "gold standard" for identification of viable myocardium. PET imaging identifies viable myocardium by determining mismatch between metabolic activity and perfusion in a given region of myocardium. Regions of viable but ischemic myocardium demonstrate enhanced or preserved uptake of metabolic tracers such as [^{18}F]fluorodeoxyglucose, a glucose analogue commonly used to detect metabolic activity.[38] PET imaging with a perfusion tracer (most commonly [^{13}N] ammonia) is compared with [^{18}F]fluorodeoxyglucose imaging to determine mismatch of perfusion and metabolic activity. Although PET has the advantage of being able to detect metabolic activity, use of PET imaging has been limited because of its high cost and lack of widespread availability; SPECT imaging and low-dose dobutamine echocardiography are therefore commonly used to detect viability in patients who have heart failure.

Thallium 201 is a potassium analogue taken up only by viable cells, and its uptake by dysfunctional myocardium is therefore indicative of retained viability. Thallium 201 redistributes over time according to concentration gradients, and thallium imaging techniques use this redistribution property and delayed imaging to detect areas of myocardium that are viable but underperfused because of severe coronary artery disease. Perfusion defects that persist after delayed imaging are consistent with scarring, whereas the resolution of such defects after redistribution provides evidence of retained viability.

In contrast to thallium, ^{99m}Tc-sestamibi binds to mitochondria in myocardial cells and demonstrates minimal redistribution. However, because myocardial uptake of ^{99m}Tc-sestamibi occurs only in the presence of preserved cellular integrity, this agent may also be used to identify viable myocardium. Although ^{99m}Tc-sestamibi has not been studied as extensively as ^{201}Tl for detection of viability, there is evidence that both agents are comparable in predicting recovery of ventricular function.[40,41]

Dobutamine echocardiography can identify viable myocardium by detecting augmentation of regional contractility with administration of low-dose dobutamine. A biphasic response may also be observed, in which improved contractility with low-dose dobutamine is followed by a deterioration of function at high doses. Use of biphasic response as a marker of viability provides a higher specificity and lower sensitivity than low-dose response alone.[42]

In general, stress echocardiography and nuclear myocardial perfusion imaging have similar accuracy for detection of coronary artery disease, although stress echocardiography has a lower sensitivity and higher specificity than perfusion imaging in most studies.[43] There are fewer data, however, about the sensitivity and specificity of noninvasive testing for coronary artery disease in patients who have heart failure and systolic dysfunction. Using changes in global wall motion score index from low-dose dobutamine to high-dose dobutamine, Sharp and colleagues[44] reported a sensitivity of 83% and a specificity of 71% for detection of coronary artery disease by dobutamine echocardiography in patients with dilated cardiomyopathy. Studies that have examined the use of nuclear perfusion imaging in patients with heart failure have demonstrated sensitivities of nearly 100% but generally modest specificity, depending on the criteria used to determine the significance of a defect.[45,46] Tauberg and coworkers[45] studied the utility of exercise thallium planar imaging for detection of coronary artery disease in patients with heart failure and systolic dysfunction; they reported a sensitivity of 97% and a specificity of 75% when the presence of a severe defect was used as a positive criterion. Chikamori and associates[46] examined the value of dipyridamole thallium imaging in dilated cardiomyopathy and reported a sensitivity of 100% for detection of coronary artery disease; however, 73% of patients with nonischemic cardiomyopathy had perfusion defects and 38% had large perfusion defects. Multiple studies have noted that patients with nonischemic cardiomyopathy may demonstrate perfusion defects; these defects are possibly related to myocardial fibrosis or to abnormal myocardial blood flow reserve. However, these defects tend to be smaller and less severe than true ischemic defects.[46,47]

Dobutamine echocardiography appears to have higher specificity and lower sensitivity than SPECT imaging for predicting functional recovery after revascularization.[47] An analysis of several clinical studies that examined recovery of ventricular function reported positive predictive values of 69% for ^{201}Tl SPECT and 83% for dobutamine echocardiography and negative predictive values of 90% for ^{201}Tl SPECT and 81% for dobutamine echocardiography.[48] More recently, contrast-enhanced CMR imaging has emerged as an additional method for assessment of myocardial viability. On delayed CMR imaging, gadolinium contrast agents diffuse out of normal myocardium but accumulate in areas of scar or fibrosis. Several studies have indicated that this method predicts regional recovery of left ventricular function after revascularization.[49] Analyses of dobutamine echocardiography, SPECT imaging, and PET studies have demonstrated that the presence of myocardial viability on noninvasive testing is associated with a survival benefit after revascularization in patients with coronary artery disease and left ventricular dysfunction; conversely, if myocardial viability is absent, revascularization does not appear to confer a survival benefit compared with medical therapy.[50]

Evaluation of Exercise Capacity

In patients in whom exercise tolerance cannot be determined from the history, exercise testing can provide a more objective assessment of functional capacity. The 6-minute walk test distance may also be used as a means of assessing functional capacity in patients with heart failure. In addition, exercise testing with measurement of maximum oxygen consumption provides important prognostic information. Mancini and colleagues[51] demonstrated that heart failure patients with a maximum exercise peak oxygen consumption of 14 mL/kg per minute or less had a 1-year survival rate of 47%, whereas those with peak oxygen consumption of more than this had a 1-year survival rate of 94%. Peak oxygen consumption during maximum exercise is therefore useful in identifying heart failure patients who have a poor prognosis and are likely to benefit from cardiac transplantation.

Evaluation of Arrhythmias

Ventricular arrhythmias occur commonly in patients who have heart failure, and sudden cardiac death occurs in up to 50% of these patients.[52,53] However, although the presence of nonsustained ventricular tachycardia portends a worse prognosis, this increase in mortality is in part accounted for by an increase in death from congestive heart failure.[54] The Multicenter Automatic Defibrillator Implantation Trial (MADIT) reported improved mortality with implantable cardioverter-defibrillator (ICD) placement compared with conventional therapy in patients who had ischemic cardiomyopathy, left ventricular ejection fraction of 35% or less, nonsustained ventricular tachycardia on Holter monitoring, and inducible ventricular tachycardia despite procainamide during electrophysiologic testing.[55] However, a substantial number of patients in this study were not receiving optimal therapy for heart failure, and there was a higher rate of beta-blocker use in the group that was randomized to ICD placement. The MADIT II study randomized patients with ischemic cardiomyopathy (left ventricular ejection fraction $<30\%$) to ICD therapy versus no ICD therapy.[56] Patients enrolled in this study were not required to have evidence of ventricular arrhythmias. MADIT II demonstrated a significant improvement in mortality in the ICD group compared with the non-ICD group. Of some concern, however, is the observation that there was a trend toward a higher incidence of new or worsened heart failure in the defibrillator group in MADIT II; the reasons for this finding are not clear and warrant further evaluation. The Sudden Cardiac Death in Heart Failure Trial (SCD-HeFT) demonstrated that in patients with mild or moderately symptomatic ischemic or nonischemic cardiomyopathy and left ventricular ejection fraction of 35% or less, ICD implantation improved survivals.[57] Whereas there is growing evidence that ICD therapy improves mortality in patients with heart failure, the identification of which patients are most likely to benefit from prophylactic ICD placement remains a challenge, given the lack of reliable markers of sudden cardiac death within this population.

Evaluation of Intracardiac Hemodynamics

In patients with clear evidence of heart failure, clinical and noninvasive assessment of hemodynamics generally provides adequate information for management. In patients under consideration for cardiac transplantation, right-sided heart catheterization can determine whether pulmonary hypertension is present and, if so, whether it is reversible with administration of vasodilators. Irreversible severe pulmonary hypertension contraindicates cardiac transplantation and may necessitate consideration of heart-lung transplantation. In refractory patients, more aggressive therapy may be guided by hemodynamic measurements.

Tissue Characterization by Endomyocardial Biopsy

Endomyocardial biopsy is generally not indicated, but it may be useful in rare circumstances when cardiomyopathy caused by systemic disease (e.g., sarcoidosis or amyloidosis) is suspected. In addition, in cases of new-onset nonischemic heart failure that present with a fulminant course (such as cardiogenic shock or malignant arrhythmias), endomyocardial biopsy should be considered to evaluate for giant cell myocarditis. The prompt diagnosis of giant cell myocarditis has therapeutic implications because there is some evidence that immunosuppressive therapy is beneficial in such patients, although such an approach has never been subjected to randomized, controlled investigation of clinical outcomes. Endomyocardial biopsy has a low diagnostic yield for other forms of myocarditis, and as biopsy findings do not usually affect management, it is not generally advocated for detection of myocarditis. Endomyocardial biopsy is associated with a risk of arrhythmias and myocardial perforation, and it should therefore be performed only by experienced operators and only when the results are likely to influence management.

Combining Data to Assess Prognosis

A number of clinical, hemodynamic, and laboratory parameters have been identified as markers of poor prognosis in patients who have heart failure (Table 69.6). Clinical variables associated with decreased survival include NYHA functional class III or class IV, decreased exercise peak oxygen consumption, elevated jugular venous pressure, and presence of a third heart sound.[12,15] Electrocardiographic findings that predict a poor prognosis include intraventricular conduction disturbances, ventricular arrhythmias, and atrial fibrillation.[12,16,19] Left ventricular size and ejection fraction correlate inversely with survival, and several laboratory markers, including hyponatremia and increased neurohormonal levels, are predictive of poor outcome.[12,19,21] The presence of multiple adverse indicators should initiate consideration of transplantation in appropriate candidates.

PROGNOSTIC MARKERS IN HEART FAILURE
NYHA class
Third heart sound
Elevated jugular venous pulse
Cardiomegaly
Left ventricular ejection fraction
Right ventricular function
Left ventricular filling pressure
Right atrial pressure
Restrictive mitral inflow pattern on Doppler examination
Hyponatremia
Natriuretic peptide levels (brain natriuretic peptide, atrial natriuretic peptide)
Plasma renin activity
Norepinephrine level
Peak exercise oxygen consumption
Ventricular arrhythmias
Atrial fibrillation
Intraventricular conduction delay

Table 69.6 Prognostic markers in heart failure.

ACCURACY

In view of the high prevalence of heart failure, effective evaluation and management of this disease can have a significant impact on health care in terms of morbidity, mortality, and hospitalization. The clinical practice guidelines[5] produced by the Agency for Health Care Policy and Research in the United States identified several common errors that occur in the assessment of heart failure. Potential errors in diagnosis include

- lack of thorough evaluation for noncardiac causes of symptoms;
- misdiagnosis of heart failure as chronic obstructive lung disease;
- misdiagnosis of noncardiac peripheral edema as heart failure; and
- failure to identify and to treat reversible causes of heart failure.

Errors in management may occur if evaluation of left ventricular function is not performed or if evaluation of angina or other evidence of ischemia is not pursued. In addition, errors of overutilization, such as inappropriate use of invasive or noninvasive testing rather than of symptoms for routine monitoring, can occur. In most cases, patients can be adequately monitored by careful assessment of symptoms, weight, and level of activity. Although initial assessment of ventricular function is useful, routine monitoring of left ventricular ejection fraction is generally not helpful in guiding management.

DIAGNOSTIC STRATEGY

Heart failure is a common clinical syndrome, but its clinical presentation may be similar to that of other conditions that produce dyspnea, edema, fatigue, and exercise intolerance. This chapter reviews the various diagnostic modalities employed in the evaluation of patients presenting with symptoms or signs consistent with heart failure, and a stepwise approach to this evaluation is outlined in Figure 69.6. The history, physical examination, and routine laboratory studies are initially used to confirm the presence of heart failure and to exclude noncardiac conditions that can mimic the symptoms of heart failure. The next step usually involves an investigation of ventricular anatomy and function. This allows patients to be classified into groups with systolic dysfunction, diastolic function, primary valvular lesions, or transient factors that intermittently depress function. Additional testing, including selected use of angiography, biopsy,

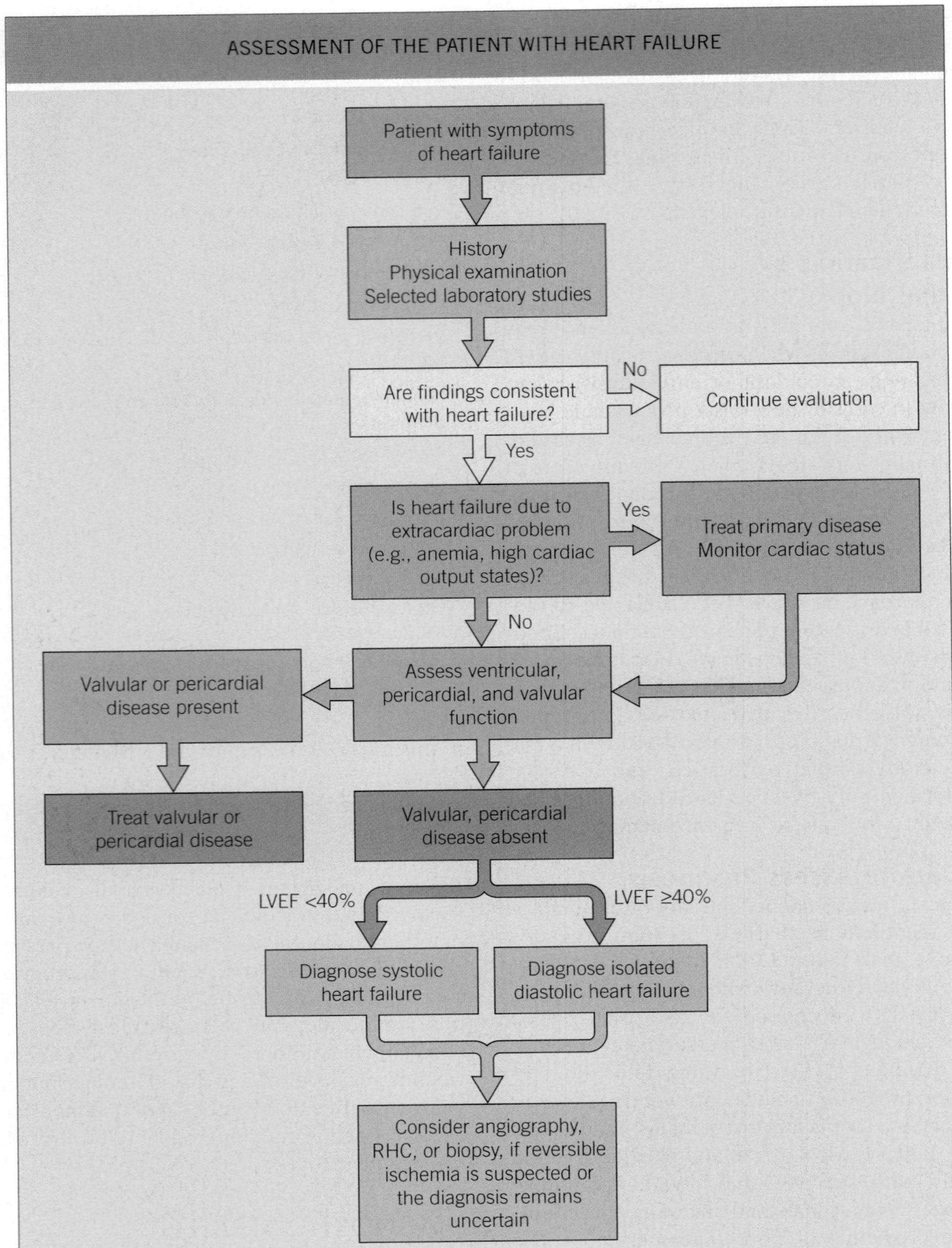

Figure 69.6 Strategy for assessment of the patient who has heart failure. LVEF, left ventricular ejection fraction; RHC, right-sided heart catheterization.

rhythm monitoring, and hemodynamic measurement, can then establish a specific cause, assess prognosis, and provide data on which treatment may be based.

SUMMARY

Initial assessment of patients with suspected heart failure should include determination of left ventricular function and evaluation for underlying etiology and potentially reversible causes. Additional testing may be indicated in some cases and must be individualized. A high index of suspicion must be maintained for reversible ischemic disease, with a low threshold for performing a noninvasive assessment for myocardial viability and inducible ischemia. Finally, in patients who have severely symptomatic heart failure, assessment of prognostic variables can provide useful information, particularly in patients in whom cardiac transplantation is a consideration.

chapter 70

Acute Heart Failure and Shock

Steven M. Hollenberg and Joseph E. Parrillo

Definition

- Acute heart failure is defined as the rapid onset of symptoms and signs secondary to abnormal cardiac function. It can occur as the first manifestation of a failing heart or on the background of chronic heart failure. Shock is a syndrome comprising an array of symptoms, signs, and laboratory abnormalities that result from systemic hypoperfusion. Ineffective tissue perfusion produces widespread organ dysfunction and cellular injury, and death will result if shock is not reversed rapidly.

Key Features

- The history, physical examination, and laboratory data offer critical insight into the underlying cause of acute heart failure and shock. Although coronary artery disease remains the most common etiology, other causes should be excluded by a careful review of all data.
- The clinical presentation of acute heart failure differs by syndrome.
- The clinical presentation of shock is similar regardless of the cause, with the constellation of hypotension, tachycardia, tachypnea, clouded sensorium, and oliguria.

Therapy

- Progress in management of cardiogenic shock has resulted from the interplay of increased understanding of pathogenesis, more rapid and aggressive application of supportive measures, and, most important, institution of a strategy of early revascularization therapy with angioplasty, stenting, or coronary bypass surgery.
- The pulmonary artery catheter remains an important tool for patients with shock and may be used to optimize hemodynamics.
- The use of intra-aortic balloon pumps and left ventricular assist devices continues to increase with emerging results of clinical trials and improved device design.

Acute heart failure is defined as the rapid onset of symptoms and signs secondary to abnormal cardiac function. It can occur as the first manifestation of a failing heart (acute "de novo" heart failure) or on the background of chronic heart failure, in which case the term *acute decompensation* is often applied. The cardiac dysfunction can be related to systolic or diastolic dysfunction, to abnormalities in cardiac rhythm, or to inadequate compensation for changes in preload or afterload. Acute heart failure is often life-threatening and requires urgent treatment.

Shock is a syndrome resulting from tissue oxygen delivery insufficient to meet metabolic demands. Its causes can be separated into cardiogenic, extracardiac obstructive, hypovolemic, and distributive forms of shock. Cardiogenic shock is a state of inadequate tissue perfusion resulting from the inability of the heart to deliver an adequate cardiac output.

Circulatory shock is diagnosed at the bedside by observing hypotension along with a combination of clinical signs indicative of poor tissue perfusion, including oliguria, clouded sensorium, and cool, mottled extremities. Cardiogenic shock is identified after documentation of myocardial dysfunction and exclusion or correction of factors such as hypovolemia, hypoxia, and acidosis. Hemodynamic criteria include sustained hypotension (systolic blood pressure <90 mm Hg for at least 30 minutes) and a reduced cardiac index (<2.2 L/min/m^2) in the presence of elevated pulmonary capillary occlusion pressure (>18 mm Hg). The pathophysiology and clinical presentations of shock are outlined in Figure 70.1.

PATHOPHYSIOLOGY

Acute Heart Failure

Acute coronary syndromes are the most frequent precipitants of acute de novo heart failure (42% in the EuroHeart Failure Survey), with three quarters of cases resulting from myocardial infarction rather than unstable angina.[1] Arrhythmias, particularly atrial fibrillation, are common precipitants of both de novo heart failure and acute decompensation. Extracardiac factors such as infection, anemia, thyroid disease, and renal dysfunction are important, particularly in the acute care setting. Noncompliance with medication, often resulting in suboptimal control of hypertension, is an important factor in acute decompensation of chronic heart failure, with or without concomitant dietary indiscretion.

Heart failure can be broken down into several different classifications: acute versus chronic, left sided versus right sided, systolic versus diastolic dysfunction. It is important for the clinician to distinguish between systolic and diastolic dysfunction as both the diagnostic work-up and therapeutic sequence differ. Although congestive heart failure results most commonly from decreased systolic performance, diastolic dysfunction, defined clinically as cardiogenic pulmonary congestion in the presence of normal systolic performance, is becoming more common as a cause of congestive heart failure, particularly in the elderly. Diastolic heart failure is more common in women than in men. The estimated prevalence of diastolic heart failure is 30% to 35% overall and more than 50% in patients older than 70 years.[2]

PATHOPHYSIOLOGY AND CLINICAL PRESENTATIONS OF SHOCK							
Type of shock		Forward cardiac output	CVP	PCWP	SVR	Clinical exam	Comments
Cardiogenic shock Pump failure	Left ventricular MI	⇓⇓⇓	⇑⇑	⇑⇑⇑	⇑⇑	+S$_3$, +S$_4$	Extensive infarct (>40% LV)
	Right ventricular MI	⇓⇓	⇑⇑⇑	⇔or⇓	⇑	Right sided +S$_3$,+S$_4$	Concomitant inferior wall MI common, consider if elevated right-sided filling pressures with normal/low PCWP or hypotension with clear lung fields
	Non-CAD cardiomyopathy	⇓⇓⇓	⇑⇑	⇑⇑⇑	⇑⇑	+S$_3$,+S$_4$	Includes myocarditis, idiopathic, inflammatory causes
	Allograft failure	⇓⇓⇓	⇑⇑	⇑⇑⇑	⇑⇑	+S$_3$,+S$_4$	Includes cellular and humoral rejection
	Infiltrative disease (late)	⇓⇓⇓	⇑⇑	⇑⇑⇑	⇑or⇔	+S$_4$ (early)	Characteristic echocardiographic appearance
	Trauma	⇓⇓	⇑or⇔	⇑⇑	⇑or⇔	Variable	Site involved: RA/RV > LA/LV May see combined shock (i.e., hypovolemic vs. obstructive with pump failure)
Mechanical causes	Acute aortic regurgitation Native or prosthetic	⇓⇓	⇔	⇑⇑ or ⇑⇑⇑	⇑⇑	EDM	Endocarditis most common cause; IABP contraindicated
	Acute mitral regurgitation Native or prosthetic	⇓⇓	⇑or⇔	⇑⇑⇑⇑	⇑⇑	ESM	Prominent PCWP *v* wave IABP very effective
	Aortic stenosis	⇔	⇑or⇔	⇑⇑	⇑⇑		Symptoms may become manifest with increased metabolic demand: e.g., pregnancy, exercise, thyrotoxicosis, sepsis
	Mitral stenosis	⇔	⇑or⇔	⇑⇑⇑	⇑⇑		
	VSD (acute post MI)	⇓or ⇓⇓	⇑or⇑⇑	⇑or⇑⇑	⇑⇑	HSM, thrill	May be 3–5 days s/p MI, uncommon event but high mortality
	Free wall rupture (post MI)	⇓or ⇓⇓	⇑or⇑⇑	⇑or⇑⇑	⇑⇑	Silent	Catastrophic presentation 1–3 days s/p MI, earlier presentation with lytics
Obstructive shock	Pericardial tamponade	⇓⇓ (LV)	⇑⇑⇑	⇑⇑	⇑⇑	Silent	Pressure equalization: RA mean, RV EDP, PA diastolic, PCWP within 5 mm Hg
	Pulmonary embolism	⇓⇓ (RV)	⇑⇑⇑	⇔	⇑or⇑⇑	RV S$_3$ or S$_4$, RV lift	RV dysfunction, moderate increase PA pressure (40–50 mm Hg)
Hypovolemic shock	Blood or volume loss	⇓	⇓⇓⇓	⇓⇓⇓	⇑or⇔	Silent	Look for source of blood or volume loss
Distributive shock	Septic shock	⇑or⇑⇑	Initial ⇓⇓	⇓⇓	⇓⇓⇓⇓	Hyperdynamic precordium	Early antibiotics, supportive care, identify occult source (e.g., abscess)
	Anaphylactic shock	⇔or⇑		⇓⇓	⇓⇓⇓⇓	None	Document antigen exposure, treatment is epinephrine
Combined shock (precise hemodynamics often difficult to predict)							
Septic and cardiogenic		⇓⇓	⇓or⇔	⇑⇑	⇓or⇓⇓	Variable	Common settings: sepsis-induced LV dysfunction Infection (e.g., pneumonia) after MI
Cardiogenic and hypovolemic		⇓⇓⇓	⇓or⇓⇓	⇑or⇑⇑	⇑⇑⇑	Variable	Free wall rupture after MI, gastrointestinal bleeding with thrombolytics after MI
Hypovolemic and obstructive		⇓⇓	⇓or⇔	⇓⇓	⇑⇑⇑	Quiet precordium	Ruptured aortic dissection with tamponade

Figure 70.1 *See legend on opposite page.*

Figure 70.1 Pathophysiology and clinical presentations of shock. CAD, coronary artery disease; CVP, central venous pressure; EDM, early diastolic murmur; ESM, early systolic murmur; EDP, end-diastolic pressure; HSM, holosystolic murmur; IABP, intra-aortic balloon pump; LA, left atrium; LV, left ventricle; PA, pulmonary artery; MI, myocardial infarction; PCWP, pulmonary capillary wedge pressure; PDM, pandiastolic murmur; RA, right atrium; RV, right ventricle; SEM, systolic ejection murmur; SVR, systemic vascular resistance; VSD, ventricular septal defect.

Cardiogenic Shock

Cardiac dysfunction in patients with cardiogenic shock is usually initiated by myocardial infarction or ischemia. The myocardial dysfunction resulting from ischemia worsens that ischemia, creating a downward spiral (Fig. 70.2).[3] When a critical mass of left ventricular myocardium (usually about 40%)[4] is ischemic or necrotic and fails to pump, stroke volume and cardiac output are decreased. Compensatory mechanisms include sympathetic stimulation to increase heart rate and contractility and renal fluid retention to increase preload. These mechanisms may become maladaptive and can actually worsen the situation when cardiogenic shock develops. Increased heart rate and contractility increase myocardial oxygen demand and exacerbate ischemia. Fluid retention and impaired diastolic filling caused by tachycardia and ischemia may result in pulmonary congestion and hypoxia. Vasoconstriction to maintain blood pressure increases myocardial afterload, further impairing cardiac performance and increasing myocardial oxygen demand. This increased demand, in the face of inadequate perfusion, worsens ischemia and begins a vicious circle that will end in death if it is uninterrupted.

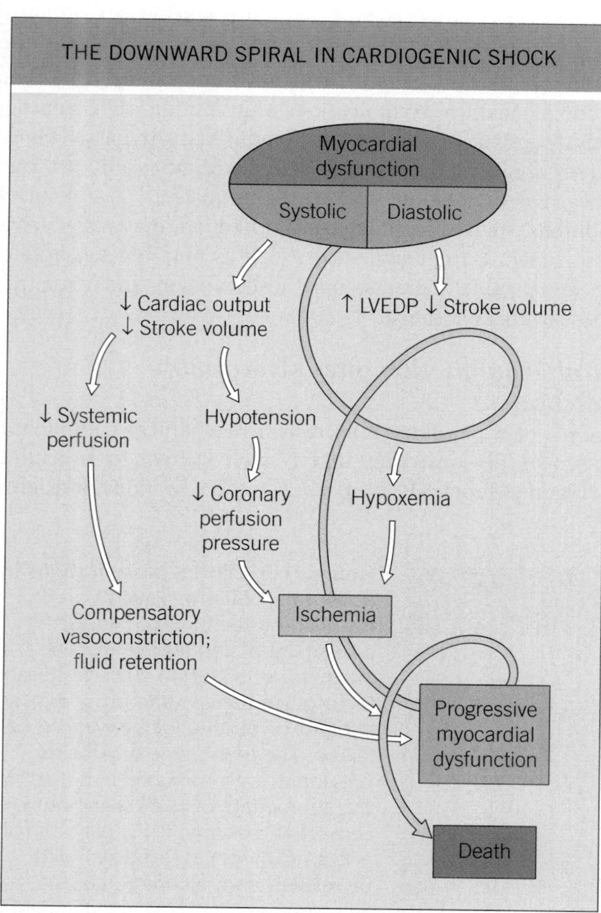

Figure 70.2 The downward spiral in cardiogenic shock. Stroke volume and cardiac output fall with left ventricular dysfunction, producing hypotension and tachycardia that reduce coronary blood flow. Increasing ventricular diastolic pressure reduces coronary blood flow, and increased wall stress elevates myocardial oxygen requirements. All of these factors combine to worsen ischemia. The falling cardiac output also compromises systemic perfusion. Compensatory mechanisms include sympathetic stimulation and fluid retention to increase preload. These mechanisms can actually worsen cardiogenic shock by increasing myocardial oxygen demand and afterload. Thus, a vicious circle can be established. LVEDP, left ventricular end-diastolic pressure. (Modified with permission from Hollenberg SM, Kavinsky CJ, Parrillo JE. Cardiogenic shock. Ann Intern Med 1999;131:47-59.)

Recent data suggest that not all patients fit into this classic paradigm. In the SHOCK trial, the average systemic vascular resistance was not elevated, and the range of values was wide, suggesting that compensatory vasoconstriction is not universal. Supporting this notion is the fact that the mean ejection fraction in the SHOCK trial was only moderately decreased (30%), indicating that mechanisms other than pump failure were operative.[5,6] In the SHOCK trial, some patients had fever and elevated white blood cell counts along with decreased systemic vascular resistance, suggesting a systemic inflammatory response syndrome.[7] Other studies have also shown elevations of white blood cell counts and cytokines in cardiogenic shock, confirming an inflammatory component in some of these patients. This has led to an expansion of the classic paradigm to include the possibility of the contribution of inflammatory responses to vasodilatation and myocardial stunning, leading clinically to persistence of shock.[8]

At the cellular level, tissue hypoperfusion and consequent cellular hypoxia lead to anaerobic glycolysis, with depletion of ATP, accumulation of lactic acid, and intracellular acidosis. Failure of energy-dependent ion transport pumps decreases transmembrane potential, causing accumulation of sodium and calcium, myocyte swelling, and activation of intracellular proteases.[9] If the ischemia is sufficiently severe and prolonged, myocardial cellular injury can become irreversible.[9] Although myocyte necrosis clearly predominates in acute ischemia, accumulating evidence indicates that apoptosis (programmed cell death) may also contribute to myocyte loss in myocardial infarction, especially in the border zone of infarcts.[10] Activation of inflammatory cascades, oxidative stress, and stretching of myocytes have been proposed as mechanisms that activate the apoptotic pathways. Apoptosis is a potential therapeutic target, and inhibitors of apoptosis have been found to attenuate myocardial injury in animal models of postischemic reperfusion.[11]

Another important concept is that dysfunctional ischemic myocardium may not be irretrievably lost. This reversible dysfunction can be described in two main categories: stunning and hibernation. Myocardial stunning represents postischemic dysfunction that persists despite restoration of normal blood flow; because normally perfused myocardium is viable, myocardial performance is expected to recover completely.[12] Stunning appears to result from a combination of oxidative stress with reperfusion, perturbation of calcium homeostasis, and decreased myofilament responsiveness to calcium.[13] Hibernating myocardium is a term originally coined to denote myocardial segments with persistently impaired function at rest due to severely reduced coronary blood flow; inherent in this definition of hibernating myocardium is the notion that function can be normalized by improving blood flow.[14,15] Hibernation can be seen as an adaptive response to restore equilibrium between flow and function.[14] Although hibernation is conceptually different from myocardial stunning, recent investigations have challenged the clear distinction between the two conditions. It is now clear that repetitive episodes of myocardial stunning can occur in areas of viable myocardium subtended by a critical coronary stenosis and that such episodes can recapitulate the hibernation phenotype, complicating the distinction between myocardial stunning and hibernation.[13,14,16]

Regardless of the degree of overlap, consideration of myocardial stunning and hibernation is vital in patients with cardiogenic shock because of their therapeutic implications. Contractile function of hibernating myocardium improves with revascularization, and stunned myocardium retains inotropic reserve and can respond to inotropic stimulation.[13] The notion that some myocardial tissue may recover function emphasizes the importance of measures to support hemodynamics and thus to minimize myocardial necrosis in patients with shock.

CLINICAL PRESENTATIONS

Acute Heart Failure

Acute heart failure has been classified clinically on the basis of observation of peripheral perfusion (warm or cold) and auscultation of the lungs (wet or dry). The patients can be classified as warm and dry, warm and wet, cold and dry, or cold and wet (Fig. 70.3). This classification, in addition to being readily applicable to guide therapy in the clinical setting, has been shown to have prognostic value to predict outcomes.[17]

Cardiogenic Shock

The predominant cause of cardiogenic shock is left ventricular failure in the setting of acute myocardial infarction.[18] Cardiogenic shock usually results from an extensive acute infarction, although a smaller infarction in a patient with previously compromised left ventricular function may also precipitate shock. Patients may have cardiogenic shock at initial presentation, but shock often evolves during several hours, suggesting that early treatment may potentially prevent shock.[18,19] Angiography most often demonstrates multivessel coronary disease.[18] This is important because development of compensatory hyperkinesis in myocardial segments not involved in an acute infarction is a normal response that helps maintain cardiac output. Failure to develop such a response, either because of previous infarction or because of high-grade coronary stenoses, is an important risk factor for cardiogenic shock and death.[20]

Other important causes of acute heart failure and shock include mechanical complications of infarction, right ventricular dysfunction, prolonged cardiopulmonary bypass, valvular disease, myocardial contusion, sepsis with unusually profound myocardial depression, and cardiomyopathy.[3,18] Concurrent conditions, such as hemorrhage or infection, may also contribute to shock. Iatrogenic factors, such as beta-blocker application in unstable patients, may also worsen and even may cause cardiogenic shock.

Mitral Regurgitation after Myocardial Infarction

Rupture of a papillary muscle is a mechanical complication of myocardial infarction that is well known to precipitate cardiogenic shock. It is more common in inferior than in

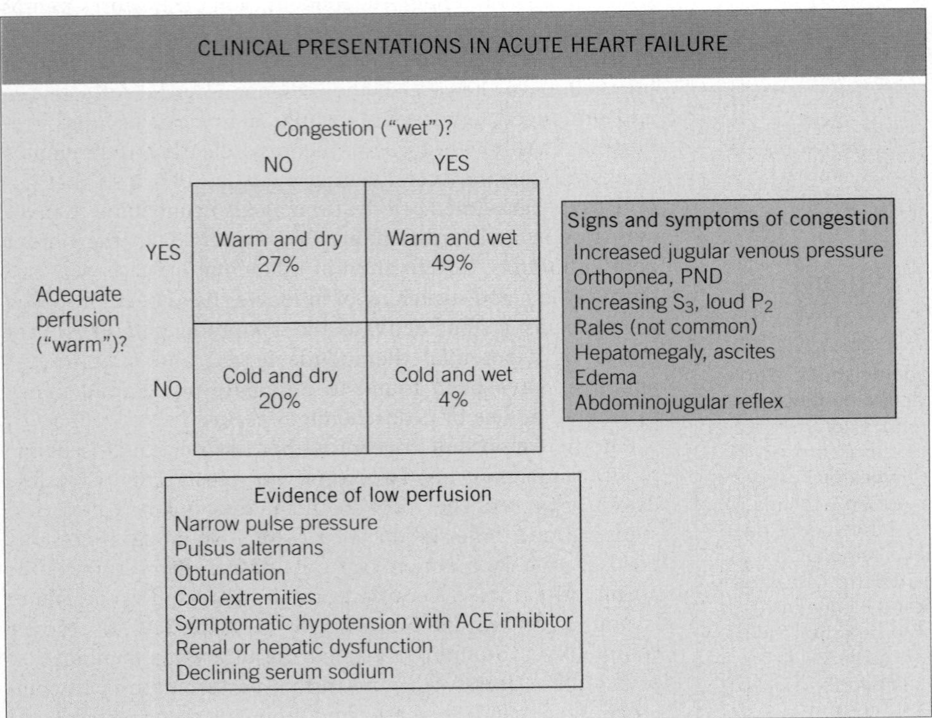

Figure 70.3 Clinical presentations in acute heart failure. Patients are classified on the basis of bedside assessment of congestion and the adequacy of perfusion. This classification helps guide therapy and prognosis for patients presenting with advanced heart failure. The percentage of patients presenting with each profile is listed in the appropriate box. ACE, angiotensin-converting enzyme; PND, paroxysmal nocturnal dyspnea. (Modified with permission from Nohria A, Lewis E, Stevenson LW. Medical management of advanced heart failure. JAMA 2002;287:628-640.)

anterior myocardial infarction because the posterior papillary muscle has a single blood supply in most patients, and it commonly presents dramatically, with rapid onset of pulmonary edema and shock. The clinical examination of patients with severe mitral regurgitation in this setting often reveals a hyperdynamic precordium with a prominent S_3 gallop and a holosystolic murmur, although the murmur may be soft or inaudible in many cases because cardiac output is reduced.

Papillary muscle rupture, however, is relatively uncommon. A much more common and more important contributor to myocardial dysfunction is ischemic mitral regurgitation. The classic view of ischemic mitral regurgitation is that it results from dysfunction of the papillary muscles. This view has been challenged by animal experiments demonstrating that reducing papillary muscle dysfunction does not cause either prolapse of the mitral valve leaflets or mitral regurgitation, and ischemic mitral regurgitation now appears to result primarily from changes in left ventricular geometry that cause displacement of the papillary muscles such that they no longer effectively close the mitral valve in systole.[21] As such, ischemic mitral regurgitation is a dynamic process that may change over time, which has implications for its correction.[21] With respect to the development of cardiogenic shock, postinfarction left ventricular remodeling may cause ischemic mitral regurgitation, precipitating the development of shock or contributing to its severity.

Postinfarction Ventricular Septal Defect

The frequency of acute rupture of the interventricular septum has decreased in the reperfusion era to an incidence of less than 1%,[22] but this complication still represents about 4% of patients with cardiogenic shock.[23] Hypertension, advanced age, and female gender are predisposing factors. The incidence is bimodal, either within 24 hours or 3 to 5 days after acute infarction. Early ruptures are due to intramural hematomas that dissect into tissue, and the later ruptures result from ongoing tissue necrosis.[22]

Patients with ventricular septal rupture have severe heart failure or cardiogenic shock, with a pansystolic murmur and a parasternal thrill, although both of these findings may be subtle in the presence of a low cardiac output. The hallmark finding is a left-to-right intracardiac shunt ("step-up" in oxygen saturation from right atrium to right ventricle) when right-sided heart catheterization is performed. The diagnosis is most easily made with echocardiography (Fig. 70.4).

Right Ventricular Infarction

Right ventricular infarction may occur after occlusion of the proximal right coronary artery, almost always in the setting of concomitant inferior left ventricular infarction. Clear lung fields in a patient with hypotension should suggest the possibility of right ventricular infarction or concomitant intravascular volume depletion; the presence or absence of jugular venous distention can be an important clue in differentiation.

Free Wall Rupture

Left ventricular free wall rupture occurs in less than 1% of acute myocardial infarctions but accounts for 7% of deaths. Like the other mechanical complications, its incidence is bimodal, with a peak within the first 24 hours and another at 3 to 5 days.[18] The classic patient is elderly, female, and hypertensive. The early use of fibrinolytic therapy reduces the incidence of cardiac rupture, but late use (>14 hours) may increase the risk. Most patients present with acute pericardial tamponade due to blood accumulation in the pericardial sac.

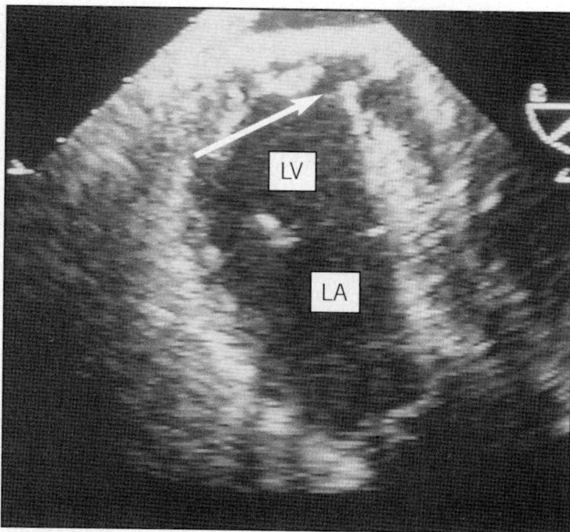

Figure 70.4 This patient developed a ventricular septal defect *(arrow)* along the distal aspect of the interventricular septum after an extensive Q-wave anterior wall myocardial infarction. This transesophageal echocardiographic image shows the disruption in the septum in the area of infarcted and thinned myocardium. LA, left atrium; LV, left ventricle.

Pseudoaneurysm with leakage may be heralded by chest pain, nausea, and restlessness, but frank free wall rupture presents as a catastrophic event with a pulseless rhythm.[18] A pericardial effusion may be visualized by echocardiography, sometimes with layered high acoustic echoes that suggest blood clots; a myocardial tear may be seen in up to 40% of cases.[24] Contrast ventriculography is not a sensitive way to detect a small rupture.

Cardiomyopathy and Other Causes

Cardiomyopathy can result from myocarditis, ischemia, or infiltration and may present with either acute heart failure or shock. Myocarditis is commonly associated with a viral infection, but there are a number of other causes, including autoimmune disorders (systemic lupus erythematosus, acute rheumatic fever, and rheumatoid arthritis), drugs (especially cocaine), and hypersensitivity. Clinical clues that suggest myocarditis include the diffuse nature of myocardial dysfunction, a recent history of a viral illness, and the absence of risk factors for coronary artery disease. Giant cell myocarditis is especially virulent and frequently results in a fatal outcome despite therapy.[25] Presentation with conduction system disease along with left ventricular dysfunction should raise the suspicion of giant cell myocarditis.

Acute myocarditis can be benign and self-limited; fulminant, with severe congestive heart failure or atrial and ventricular arrhythmias; or chronic, with typical symptoms of heart failure. Fulminant myocarditis commonly produces shock that requires pharmacologic or mechanical support, but cardiac function recovers in most cases, resulting in prolonged survival. Peripartum cardiomyopathy is a form of dilated cardiomyopathy that usually begins in the third trimester but may present after delivery. The clinical course

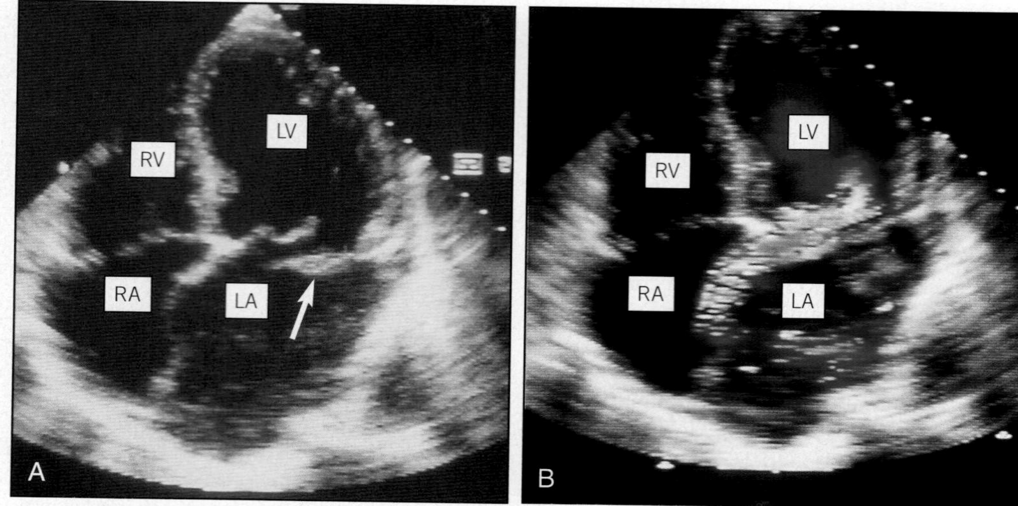

Figure 70.5 **A,** Two-dimensional apical four-chamber echocardiographic image showing flail posterior mitral valve leaflet *(arrow)* due to primary chordal rupture. **B,** Color flow imaging demonstrates severe mitral regurgitation with an eccentric jet. LA, left atrium; LV, left ventricle; RA, right atrium; RV, right ventricle.

is variable, with complete or nearly complete recovery of ventricular performance in 50% to 70% of patients, usually in the first 6 months, and persistent left ventricular dysfunction in others. Subsequent pregnancies in women who have recovered have been associated with relapses.

Infiltrative cardiomyopathies such as amyloidosis, sarcoidosis, and hemochromatosis usually present initially with diastolic dysfunction and manifestations of heart failure, but systolic dysfunction can be seen later in the course, sometimes resulting in progression to shock.

Shock due to cardiac trauma usually occurs from exsanguination after myocardial or aortic rupture or as a consequence of cardiac tamponade. Myocardial contusion may occur without evidence of bone injury to the thoracic cage. Left ventricular dysfunction is usually transient but may be severe enough to cause heart failure and even shock. Transient depression of ventricular contractility is common after cardiopulmonary bypass and is usually reversible within 24 to 48 hours; this probably represents myocardial stunning.[13] The depression of contractility can be severe enough to cause cardiogenic shock, and therapy with inotropic agents, vasodilators, and even mechanical support may be necessary.

Valvular Heart Disease

Acute Mitral Regurgitation

With acute mitral regurgitation, the large volume of regurgitant blood causes a significant elevation in left atrial pressure. This pressure is transmitted to the pulmonary veins, resulting in pulmonary edema and secondary right-sided heart failure as pulmonary pressure rises acutely. These increased pressures can be seen in the pulmonary capillary wedge pressure tracing as large v waves. Forward cardiac output falls dramatically with the large regurgitant fraction, producing hypotension and shock.

The most common causes outside of the setting of acute myocardial infarction are spontaneous chordal rupture ("primary rupture"), infective endocarditis, rheumatic fever, and trauma. Posterior leaflet chordae rupture more often than anterior chordae. Primary or secondary chordal rupture results in more severe mitral insufficiency than does rupture of the tertiary chords, and a flail leaflet may be identified on echocardiography (Fig. 70.5).

Patients present acutely with dyspnea, tachypnea, or frank pulmonary edema. Rales may be evident, and the left ventricular apical impulse is hyperdynamic. The murmur is best heard at the base but can radiate anywhere and can be soft or even absent as cardiac output falls. With secondary right-sided heart failure, central venous pressure rises and a prominent v wave may be evident on examination of the jugular venous pulse.

Acute Aortic Regurgitation

Acute aortic regurgitation most commonly results from infective endocarditis with leaflet destruction, but it may also be due to traumatic injury, acute aortic dissection, or, rarely, spontaneous rupture of a sinus of Valsalva aneurysm. Valvular incompetence produces a pandiastolic aortic–left ventricular gradient, and regurgitant fractions may exceed 50%. Forward cardiac output falls as left ventricular diastolic pressure and left atrial and pulmonary venous pressures rise, and pulmonary edema may ensue.

Patients appear ill with tachycardia, tachypnea, and restlessness. The pulse pressure is usually narrow, indicating decreased forward stroke volume, and the bounding pulsations seen with chronic aortic regurgitation are usually absent. S_1 is often soft or absent due to premature mitral valve closure. P_2 may predominate with a relatively soft A_2. An S_3 and S_4 are frequently heard with acute ventricular volume overload. The diastolic murmur of acute aortic regurgitation tends to be short, decrescendo, and blowing in quality and is best heard along the sternal border or at the apex. Patients with acute, severe aortic regurgitation have profound shock, and surgical intervention often provides the only chance for survival (see Chapter 94).

Aortic Valve Stenosis

Shock due to aortic stenosis may result from increasing metabolic demands or from concomitant left ventricular failure, which may be precipitated by atrial fibrillation. Examination typically reveals tachycardia with hypotension. S_1 may be normal or loud, and the S_2 may be soft or single due to loss of the aortic component. An S_4 is prominent in sinus rhythm, but the presence of an S_3 is variable.

The murmur is often soft or absent, as cardiac output is low. It is best heard at the base and may radiate to the right carotids. The carotid pulses demonstrate the characteristic delayed upstroke and diminished volume.

Occult critical aortic stenosis should be considered in patients presenting with unexplained shock as intervention can be lifesaving.

Mitral Stenosis

Chronic mitral stenosis rarely produces shock without atrial fibrillation, supraventricular tachycardia, thyrotoxicosis, or pregnancy. Patients with moderate to severe mitral stenosis (mitral valve area $\leq$1.3 cm^2) compensate with elevated left atrial and pulmonary venous pressure to maintain normal cardiac output. With critical mitral stenosis (mitral valve area $\leq$1.0 cm^2), a left atrial pressure of 25 mm Hg or more is common. The transmitral diastolic flow duration is inversely related to heart rate and directly related to stenosis severity, an important consideration when metabolic demands exceed the ability to augment cardiac output.

Patients present with pulmonary vascular congestion even though left ventricular function is normal. Right ventricular failure is more common because of secondary pulmonary hypertension.

Prosthetic Valve Dysfunction

Prosthetic valvular dysfunction, especially left sided, most often produces shock due to valvular regurgitation. Acute prosthetic valve regurgitation may result from sewing ring dehiscence, infective endocarditis, or catastrophic mechanical failure. The hemodynamic consequences are identical to those seen with native valves. Clinical presentations are dramatic, and associated mortality rates are high.

Acute prosthetic valve thrombosis may cause valvular stenosis. Tissue valves (porcine heterografts or preserved homografts) in the aortic and mitral position generally begin to degenerate during the fourth or fifth postoperative year, and the failure rate is 20% by 10 years; up to 50% of valves in the aortic position and 45% of valves in the mitral position fail by 15 years. Fortunately, tissue valves rarely fail abruptly; thus, shock due to acute tissue valve insufficiency is uncommon.

Extracardiac Obstructive Shock

Pericardial Tamponade

When pericardial fluid accumulates and the fibrous parietal pericardium reaches its elastic limit, pressure within the pericardial space increases rapidly. The right atrium is generally affected first, followed by the right ventricle, the left atrium, and finally the left ventricle (Fig. 70.6). One exception occurs after cardiac surgery, when loculated fluid collections can lead to regional tamponade involving specific chambers including the left ventricle.

This extracardiac obstruction to filling decreases ventricular preload and cardiac output. The major determinant of whether a pericardial effusion will cause shock is the rapidity with which the fluid accumulates. Patients at risk for shock due to tamponade are those with malignant disease, infection (such as tuberculosis), recent trauma, evolving aortic dissection, or severe pericarditis. Less commonly, patients with end-stage renal disease or hypothyroidism may develop tamponade.

Patients appear ill and uncomfortable and are usually unable to lie flat. Examination reveals distended neck veins with prominent *x* and blunted or absent *y* descents. Tachypnea is common, as is tachycardia, pulsus paradoxus, and hepatomegaly; diminished heart sounds are less common (34%). Hypotension is a late sign.

Pulmonary Embolism

When embolic material (e.g., thrombus, air, fat, or tumor) obstructs 30% or more of the pulmonary vasculature, the right ventricle often cannot generate adequate pressure to compensate for the increased resistance to flow. In the absence of preexisting pulmonary hypertension, it is uncommon for the right ventricle to be able to generate pressures exceeding 40 to 50 mm Hg after pulmonary embolism. The resulting right ventricular dilatation increases wall stress and provides a substrate for right ventricular ischemia. Right ventricular failure may ensue, with further dilatation and

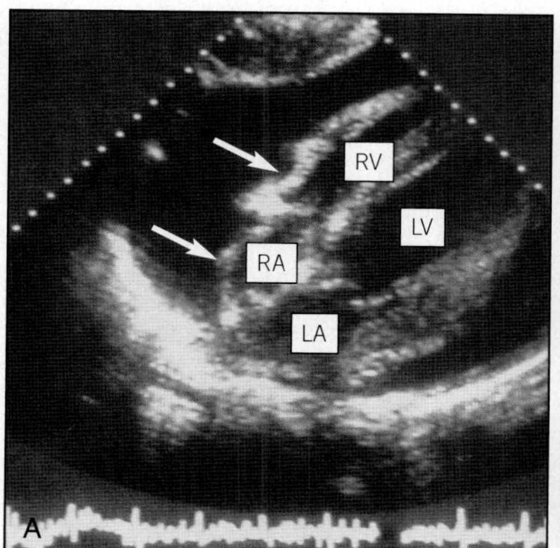

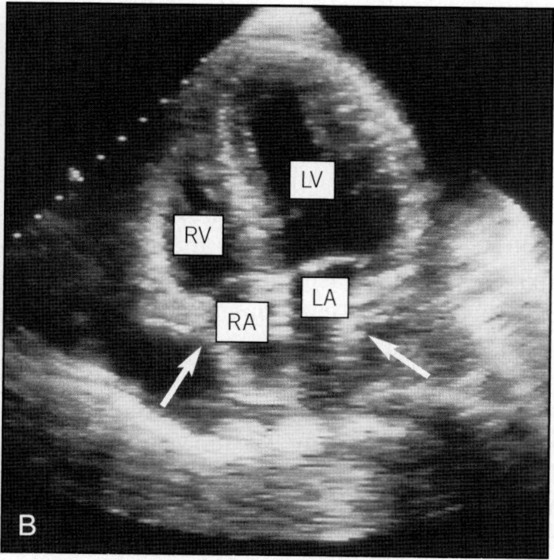

Figure 70.6 **A,** Tamponade may produce collapse of the right atrial and right ventricular free wall *(arrows)* during diastole. **B,** Left atrial collapse can also occur by the same mechanism *(arrows)*. LA, left atrium; LV, left ventricle; RA, right atrium; RV, right ventricle.

tricuspid insufficiency, increased right ventricular end-diastolic and right atrial pressure, and finally a fall in cardiac output and shock. Arrhythmias, especially bradyarrhythmias, are also common and may cause syncope. Patients may even present with syncope, severe dyspnea, or sudden death due to electromechanical dissociation.

The clinical diagnosis of massive pulmonary embolus is made by clinical suspicion more than by any specific findings on physical examination. Signs and symptoms of pulmonary embolism in general are nonspecific and include chest pain, pleuritic chest pain, dyspnea, apprehension, cough, hemoptysis, diaphoresis, and syncope.

Hypovolemic Shock

Hypovolemic shock, the most common type of shock, results from reduced circulating blood volume, preload, and thus stroke volume. When blood volume is reduced sufficiently (generally more than 20%) to overwhelm compensatory mechanisms, cardiac output and blood pressure fall. The clinical setting may be obvious (e.g., gastrointestinal bleeding, vomiting, dehydration, trauma, burns, or surgery) or occult (e.g., aortic dissection or aortic aneurysm rupture). Patients are typically hypotensive, are tachycardic with cool extremities, and may be pallid if they are anemic.

Distributive Shock

Distributive shock produces ineffective tissue oxygen delivery and extraction associated with inappropriate peripheral vasodilatation despite preserved or increased cardiac output. Blood may be shunted at the organ, tissue, or capillary level.[26] Shunting may be due to inappropriate vascular regulation or dysfunction of oxygen and nutrient utilization at the cellular level. The prototype of distributive shock is septic shock. Patients are hypotensive and tachycardic and may manifest fever, chills, rigors, or an obvious nidus of infection.

Myocardial systolic dysfunction is common in the setting of septic shock but may be unrecognized. Ventricular dysfunction is usually mild but may predominate and produce a low cardiac output in a minority (10% to 15%) of patients.

Other causes of distributive shock include the following:

- Anaphylactic shock follows exposure to a specific antigen in a sensitized individual. The allergic reaction that ensues produces large amounts of histamine, prostaglandins, leukotrienes, kinins, and other mediators, resulting in widespread microvascular leak and peripheral vasodilatation.
- Neurogenic shock occurs in patients with spinal cord injuries and other profound neurologic insults. Decreased sympathetic output may contribute to a fall in preload and afterload with resultant hypotension and shock.
- Endocrine catastrophes such as Addison's disease may result in shock because of inadequate corticosteroid release in response to a stressor; microvascular leakage plays a role as well. As with other conditions in which peripheral resistance is inappropriately low, organ perfusion pressure falls, and shock may ensue.

Combined Shock

Although shock can be categorized on the basis of underlying pathophysiologic changes, in the clinical setting, patients may demonstrate elements of more than one type of shock simultaneously. During septic shock, elements of distributive and hypovolemic shock can be complicated by myocardial impairment. Traumatic shock can also be complicated by elements of both hypovolemic and distributive shock. In a given patient, the nature of the circulatory disturbance may change with time and therapy. This can complicate management of patients as the treatment approaches may be disparate.

Multiple Organ Dysfunction Syndrome

The final product of tissue hypoperfusion is end-organ dysfunction, and although all organ systems may be affected to varying degrees, certain systems are most susceptible (Table 70-1).[3] Central nervous system autoregulation of blood flow fails when the mean blood pressure falls below 55 to 60 mm Hg. The generalized cerebral ischemia that may ensue can impair patients' levels of consciousness and may produce coma.

MULTIPLE ORGAN DYSFUNCTION SYNDROME

Organ System	Clinical Manifestations
Pulmonary	Ventilation-perfusion mismatch (shunt) CO_2 production rises with requisite increased ventilation and work of breathing Impaired gas exchange ⇒ fall in Po_2 and PH, increase in Pco_2 Pulmonary capillary leak ⇒ adult respiratory distress syndrome
Central nervous system	Altered level of consciousness (confusion ⇒ coma) Watershed infarct (MAP ≤50 mm Hg)
Cardiovascular	Catecholamine levels rise with secondary increase in heart rate and contractility Myocardial oxygen demands rise Systolic dysfunction: demands > supply, depressant factors Diastolic dysfunction Arrhythmias: supraventricular, ventricular
Kidney	Low MAP reduces GFR Renal ischemia produces acute tubular necrosis and renal failure Renal failure leads to rise in serum potassium concentration, metabolic acidosis, volume retention
Gastrointestinal	Ileus Gastritis, pancreatitis Gut ischemia leads to loss of mucosal barrier to organisms, increased lactate production, and lactic acidosis
Liver	Increased gluconeogenesis causes hyperglycemia, hypoglycemia, late hepatic failure Centrilobular necrosis increases serum transaminases and bilirubin ("shock liver") Intrahepatic cholestasis, acalculous cholecystitis
Hematologic	Reduced drug clearance Disseminated intravascular coagulation (10% of septic and hypovolemic shock patients) Coagulation abnormalities Thrombocytopenia
Immune	Cellular immunosuppression Humoral immunosuppression
Endocrine	Inadequate insulin secretion Adrenal insufficiency Impaired parathyroid function

GFR, glomerular filtration rate; MAP, mean arterial pressure.

Table 70.1 Multiple organ dysfunction syndrome.

Acute lung injury is common, with impaired gas exchange, hypoxemia, and decreased lung compliance, significantly increasing the work of breathing. Lung injury may also result in exudation of proteinaceous fluid into the alveolar space (adult respiratory distress syndrome).

Acute renal failure develops in about a third of patients with shock, usually due to acute tubular necrosis resulting from inadequate renal perfusion. The development of renal failure confers an adverse prognosis, with mortality ranging from 50% to 80%. Therapy is largely supportive, with some evidence suggesting that more intensive dialysis may improve outcomes.[27]

Hepatic dysfunction can be manifested by increased serum concentrations of transaminases, lactate dehydrogenase, and bilirubin and also by synthetic failure, with decreased concentrations of albumin and clotting factors. Splanchnic hypoperfusion can result in stress ulceration, ileus, and malabsorption. Hematologic dysfunction may cause thrombocytopenia and disseminated intravascular coagulation, and immune dysfunction may be present as well.

DIAGNOSIS

General Principles and Physical Examination

Shock is a syndrome comprising an array of symptoms, signs, and laboratory abnormalities that result from systemic hypoperfusion and consequent cellular and organ dysfunction. Because initiation of supportive therapy before shock causes irreversible damage to vital organs is important, evaluation and therapy must begin simultaneously. A practical approach is to make a rapid initial evaluation on the basis of a limited history, physical examination, and specific diagnostic procedures. Supportive therapy to maintain blood pressure, oxygenation, and tissue perfusion should be initiated concomitantly. Such support is crucial to stabilize the patient with shock to allow time for the institution of definitive interventions aimed at reversal of the underlying pathologic process.

Differentiation of low from high cardiac output is the first priority and can often be accomplished by bedside physical examination. Patients with inadequate perfusion are usually ashen or cyanotic and can have cool skin and mottled extremities. Cerebral hypoperfusion may cloud the sensorium. Pulses are rapid and faint and may be irregular in the presence of arrhythmias. In contrast, normal or high-output shock is often characterized by a widened pulse pressure with a low diastolic pressure and warm extremities.

Low-Output Failure

The first issue is to determine cardiac filling pressures. Patients with hypovolemic shock and low filling pressures have flat neck veins, have no evidence of pulmonary congestion, and generally lack cardiac gallops.

Patients with elevated filling pressures have jugular venous distention or signs of hepatic or peripheral venous congestion. The presence of a prominent right ventricular heave, jugular venous *v* waves, loud P_2, right-sided S_3 or S_4, or risk factors for deep venous thrombosis warrants consideration of pulmonary embolism. By comparison, the constellation of distended neck veins with a prominent *x* descent, distant heart sounds, and an exaggerated pulsus paradoxus (>10 mm Hg) suggests pericardial tamponade. In both of these scenarios, signs of left-sided heart failure should be absent.

A laterally displaced and sustained left ventricular apical impulse, soft heart sounds, and S_3 suggest left ventricular dysfunction. Clinical signs of congestive heart failure should be sought as well. Jugular venous distention and pulmonary rales are usually present, although their absence does not exclude the diagnosis. Left ventricular dysfunction resulting from noncoronary myopathies is suggested by antecedent viral illness, fever, and younger age. Patients with valvular heart disease can present with characteristic murmurs, although these murmurs can change when low cardiac output and shock are present.

Normal or High Cardiac Output Failure

Patients with distributive shock have clinical findings suggestive of high or normal output. Septic shock is recognized in the presence of infection and is the most common form of distributive shock. Anaphylaxis is suspected in the presence of angioedema or threatened laryngeal closure. Neurogenic insults causing shock are typically severe, including hemispheric stroke, subarachnoid hemorrhage, and trauma.

Addisonian crisis should be a consideration in the setting of known adrenal or pituitary insufficiency or recent steroid taper. Shock from liver failure is seen with fulminant hepatic dysfunction due to hepatitis (infectious or chemical), ischemic injury, or end-stage liver disease. Likewise, severe pancreatitis resulting in shock is recognized in the setting of severe abdominal pain, nausea or vomiting, and elevated amylase or lipase.

DIAGNOSTIC TECHNIQUES

Laboratory Testing

Initial diagnostic tests should include measurement of arterial blood gases, electrolyte determinations, blood urea nitrogen and creatinine concentrations, complete blood count, liver function studies, coagulation parameters, and cardiac enzyme analysis. Serum calcium, phosphorus, and magnesium concentrations should be checked as well. With organ hypoperfusion, it is common to observe increased lactic acid levels due to tissue hypoxia and anaerobic metabolism.

Measurement of enzymes released into the serum from necrotic myocardial cells after infarction can aid in the diagnosis of myocardial infarction. The classic biochemical marker of acute myocardial infarction is elevation of the creatine kinase MB isoenzyme; but troponin T and troponin I, constituents of the contractile protein apparatus of cardiac muscle, are both more sensitive and specific for the detection of myocardial damage, and troponin measurement has superseded creatine kinase MB isoenzyme analysis in most settings. Troponin elevation identifies a subpopulation at increased risk for complications.[28]

B-type natriuretic peptide (BNP) is produced by ventricular myocytes in response to increased wall stress (i.e., increased filling pressures and stretch). Circulating concentrations of BNP and the amino-terminal fragment (NT-proBNP) of its prohormone (proBNP) are increased in congestive heart failure in proportion to the severity of symptoms, the degree of left ventricular dysfunction, and the cardiac filling pressures. Following the introduction of rapid, automated assays for determination of BNP and NT-proBNP, measurement of BNP has been used to distinguish between heart failure and pulmonary causes of dyspnea.[29] In addition, in patients presenting with acute dyspnea, elevations of both BNP and

NT-proBNP provide prognostic information above and beyond conventional risk markers.[28] Increased plasma levels of BNP and NT-proBNP, however, are not entirely specific for heart failure and may be influenced by a variety of cardiac and noncardiac conditions.

Chest Radiography

Chest radiography may suggest a specific diagnosis (e.g., aortic dissection or sepsis due to pneumonia). Cardiomegaly may result from ventricular failure or tamponade (in which case the heart may appear flask shaped). Prominent pulmonary arteries may be seen with pulmonary emboli (loss of peripheral vasculature) as well as with pulmonary hypertension. Severe mitral or aortic valvular calcification suggests stenosis in the right clinical setting.

Electrocardiography

A 12-lead electrocardiogram should be performed immediately on presentation. This may reveal evidence of infarction or arrhythmias. Conversely, an entirely normal electrocardiogram makes it unlikely that myocardial ischemia is the cause of cardiogenic shock. Whereas the electrocardiogram can be diagnostic in the setting of myocardial infarction, it is most often nonspecific in other settings. Most patients with shock are tachycardic and many have nonspecific ST and T-wave changes. Other important findings may include low QRS voltage or electrical alternans in tamponade, $S_1Q_3T_3$ pattern in pulmonary embolus (15%), and new-onset heart block in endocarditis with perivalvular abscess. In patients with inferior infarction, electrocardiography with right-sided leads should be done to look for right ventricular infarction.

Echocardiography

To the physician confronted with a critically ill patient, echocardiography can be a key element in successful differential diagnosis.[30] This is particularly true in the evaluation of patients with acute heart failure or suspected cardiogenic shock, and early echocardiography should be routine.[9] Expeditious evaluation of global and regional left ventricular performance is crucial for management of congestive heart failure, with or without suspected myocardial ischemia. Echocardiography is simple and safe; it permits systemic interrogation of cardiac chamber size, left and right ventricular function, valvular structure and motion, atrial size, and anatomy of the pericardial space. Doppler interrogation can be used for noninvasive assessment of right and left ventricular filling pressures, pulmonary artery pressures, stroke volume, and cardiac output.

Echocardiography is extremely useful for the rapid diagnosis of mechanical causes of shock after myocardial infarction, such as papillary muscle rupture and acute mitral regurgitation, acute ventricular septal defect, and free wall rupture and tamponade.[31] In some cases, echocardiography may reveal findings compatible with right ventricular infarction. Echocardiography can also reveal alternative diagnoses, such as valvular abnormalities, pericardial tamponade, and hypertrophic cardiomyopathy. Acute right-sided heart failure, manifested by a dilated and hypokinetic right ventricle without hypertrophy suggestive of chronic pulmonary hypertension, can suggest pulmonary embolism.[32]

Transthoracic echocardiographic images may be suboptimal because of poor acoustic windows in critically ill patients, particularly those who are obese, have chronic lung disease, or are on positive-pressure ventilation. Contrast echocardiography may be used to improve image quality.[33] Transesophageal echocardiography can also provide better visualization, particularly of valvular structures, and can be performed safely at the bedside.

Pulmonary Artery Catheterization

Pulmonary artery catheterization provides simultaneous assessment of filling pressures and cardiac output and can be quite useful for initiation and monitoring of therapy. Hemodynamic profiles of patients with different forms of shock are shown in Figure 70.1. The hemodynamic profile of cardiogenic shock includes a pulmonary capillary wedge pressure greater than 18 mm Hg and a cardiac index less than 2.2 L/min/m^2.[34] Invasive hemodynamic monitoring can reveal unrecognized volume depletion in patients with suspected cardiogenic shock.[3,9] Hemodynamic monitoring can also be useful in the diagnosis of mechanical complications of infarction. Right-sided heart catheterization may reveal an oxygen step-up diagnostic of ventricular septal rupture or a large *v* wave that suggests severe mitral regurgitation (Fig. 70.7), although *v* waves may be present in acute ventricular septal defect as well. Equalization of diastolic

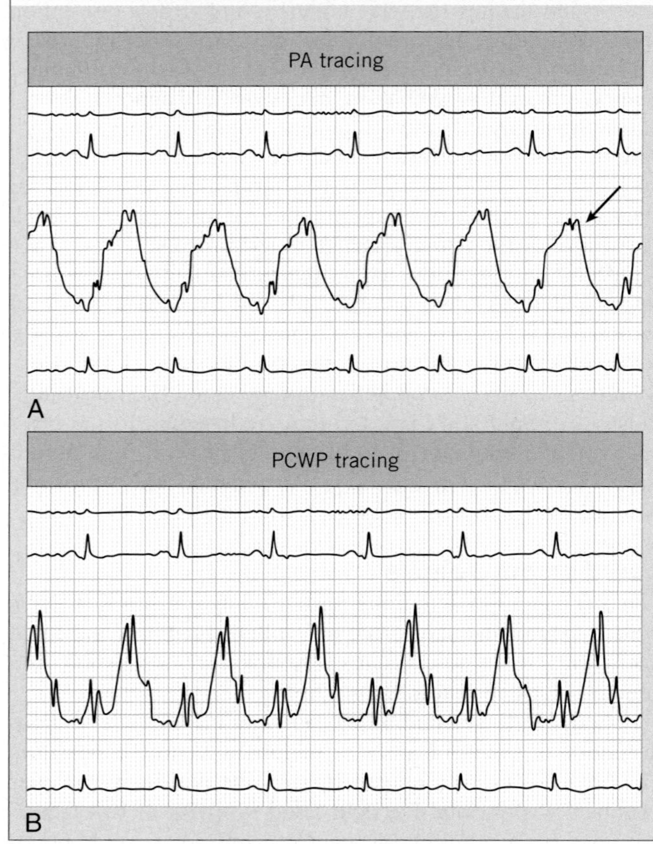

Figure 70.7 Right-sided heart catheter tracings from a patient with severe, acute mitral regurgitation (MR). The pulmonary capillary wedge pressure (PCWP) tracing **(B)** shows a large *v* wave with an overall waveform that might be confused for a pulmonary artery (PA) pressure waveform **(A)**. The peak of the *v* wave can be seen, embedded in the PCWP tracing *(arrow)*.

filling pressures may suggest pericardial tamponade. The hemodynamic profile of right ventricular infarction includes high right-sided filling pressures in the presence of normal or low occlusion pressures.[35]

Pulmonary artery catheterization can also be used to assess the adequacy of global perfusion. Mixed venous oxygen saturation is an indicator of the balance between oxygen delivery and consumption. In an otherwise stable patient, desaturation of hemoglobin in mixed venous blood can reflect decreased cardiac output.[36] Mixed venous oxygen saturation can be measured by withdrawal of a blood sample from the pulmonary artery or continuously by employment of an oximetric pulmonary artery catheter.

The pulmonary artery catheter provides hemodynamic data not easily inferred from physical examination or laboratory evaluation. Although prospective trials may never be able to demonstrate conclusively that acquisition of hemodynamic data leads to decreases in mortality, the benefits of more rapid diagnosis seem clear, and optimization of supportive therapy is often best guided by hemodynamic assessment.[36] Severe hypotension (defined as systolic blood pressure of less than 80 mm Hg), therapy with vasopressor or inotropic agents, and cardiogenic shock represent class I indications for pulmonary artery catheter hemodynamic monitoring in the latest American College of Cardiology/American Heart Association guidelines.[37]

MANAGEMENT

Acute Heart Failure

The initial step in the management of acute heart failure is to establish the clinical diagnosis and to define the patient's clinical scenario by presentation characteristics as described before. Noninvasive monitoring of blood pressure, respiratory rate, electrocardiogram, and oxygen saturation should be initiated.

Symptomatic improvement is the focus of treatment during the first few hours after acute heart failure presentation. In patients with severe dyspnea or respiratory distress, noninvasive respiratory support, usually by providing continuous positive airway pressure but sometimes wth both inspiratory and expiratory support (bilevel ventilation), can be very helpful. Noninvasive respiratory support has a number of theoretical advantages, making it an attractive therapy for the early treatment of acute heart failure syndromes. It augments cardiac output, decreases left ventricular afterload, and increases functional residual capacity and respiratory mechanics, and it can reduce the work of breathing. Noninvasive respiratory support has been shown in recent meta-analyses to reduce the need for mechanical ventilation, and there was a reduction in mortality that was significant for use of continuous positive airway pressure (but not for bilevel ventilation).[37a,37b] Initial therapy consists of a positive pressure of 5 to 7.5 cm H_2O, with titration to clinical response. Noninvasive respiratory support should not, however, be used when there is the need for emergent intubation, and if patients do not manifest rapid clinical improvement with noninvasive respiratory support, the strategy should be reconsidered.

The three main goals are to stabilize the patient clinically, to normalize filling pressures, and to optimize perfusion to vital organs. Therapy is thus targeted to physiologic endpoints. The pathophysiologic rationale for reducing filling pressures in acute heart failure is fairly straightforward. Loop diuretics are the most common first-line agent around the world for the treatment of patients with acute heart failure, but there is surprisingly little clinical trial evidence for their use as monotherapy, and one small study suggests that vasodilators may be superior.[38] Acute therapy with vasodilators is recommended to improve both hemodynamics and symptoms; diuretics can be added, with care not to cause overdiuresis and thus compromise renal function. Patients receiving diuretics should be reevaluated in 30 minutes to 1 hour for improvement in symptoms, physical findings, and hemodynamics. Gradual diuresis is the goal, not sudden production of large volumes of urine. Electrolytes should be monitored closely. In patients with limited response to diuretics, early use of ultrafiltration is an option to effectively reduce congestion and to improve symptoms. Ultrafiltration can reduce length of stay in the hospital and may lead to a decrease in readmissions for acute heart failure.[38a]

Currently available vasodilators include nitrates, nitroprusside, and nesiritide. Nitrates include nitroglycerin, isosorbide mononitrate, and isosorbide dinitrate. Nitrates relieve pulmonary congestion primarily through direct venodilatation and may decrease ischemia, an effect that is often desirable given the high incidence of coronary artery disease in heart failure patients. In severely decompensated heart failure, intravenous nitroglycerin, started at low doses, is preferred because of questionable absorption of oral and transdermal preparations and for ease of titration. Doses may need to be increased if tolerance develops. Nitroprusside is a balanced arterial and venous vasodilator with a very short half-life, facilitating rapid titration. Nitroprusside is particularly useful in settings in which acute afterload reduction is needed. Coronary steal is a concern in patients with ischemia, and nitroglycerin is preferred in these patients. Nesiritide, a recombinant form of human B-type natriuretic peptide, is a venous and arterial vasodilator that may also potentiate the effect of diuretics. Nesiritide has been shown to lower wedge pressures significantly more than either intravenous nitroglycerin or placebo in early heart failure,[39] but meta-analyses have suggested that nesiritide may worsen renal function and decrease survival at 30 days compared with conventional therapies.[40] The degree to which these issues are applicable to use in patients with acute heart failure and hemodynamic decompensation is controversial, but the potential adverse effect on long-term outcome is a significant concern, resolution of which awaits completion of appropriately powered prospective clinical trials.

Initial Approach to Patients with Shock

A management algorithm for shock is shown in Figure 70.8. Patients with shock should be treated in an intensive care unit. Continuous electrocardiographic monitoring and pulse oximetry should be performed. Bladder catheterization is routine and central venous access usual, although the diagnostic work-up should not be delayed to insert a central line.

In shock states, measurement of blood pressure by use of an arterial cannula provides the most appropriate and reproducible measurement of arterial pressure. Noninvasive monitoring by auscultation or oscillometric methods is commonly inaccurate in hypotensive patients, and these methods

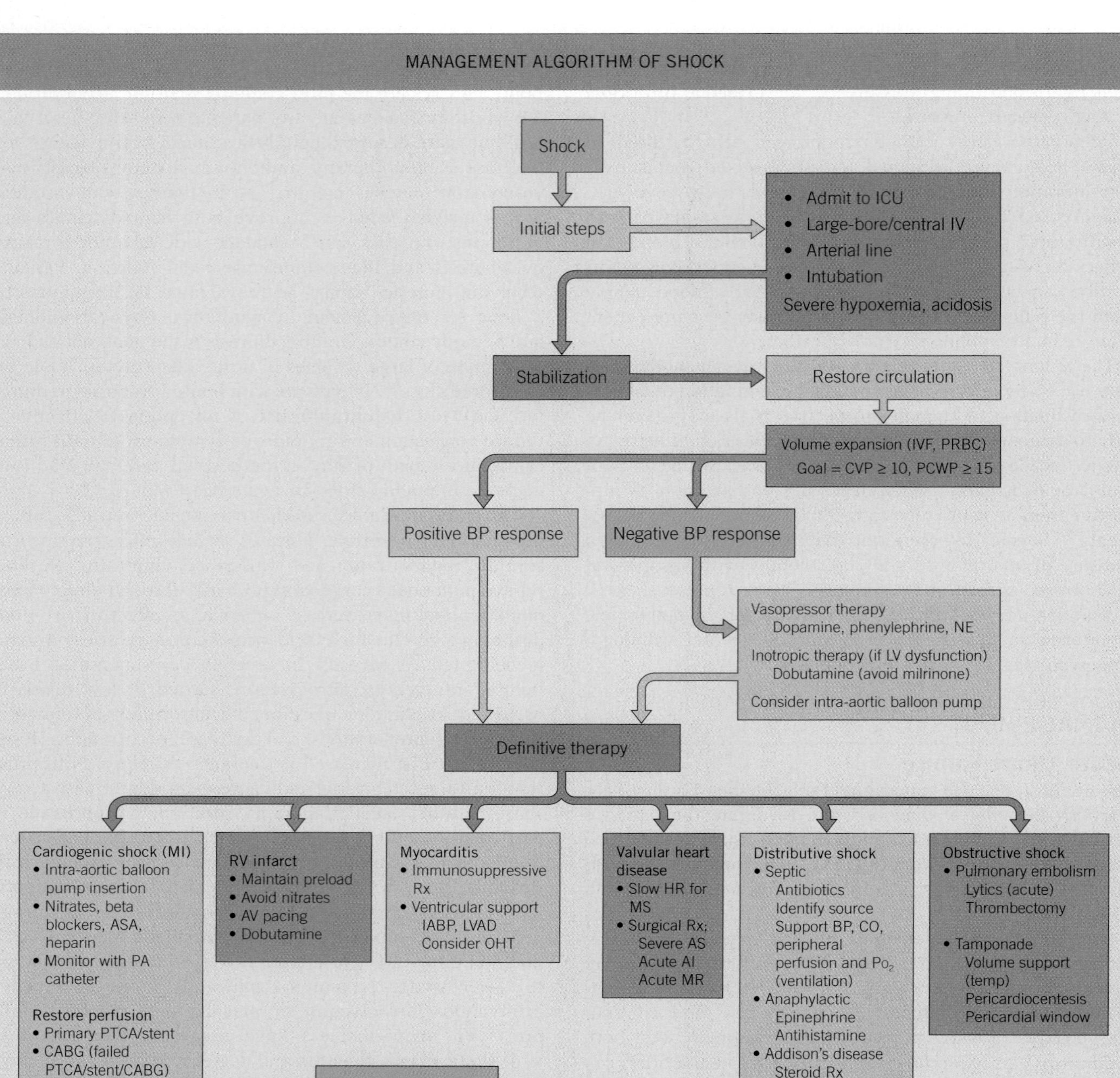

Figure 70.8 Management strategy for shock based on three critical steps: initial management, stabilization, and definitive therapy. AI, aortic insufficiency; AS, aortic stenosis; ASA, aspirin; AV, atrioventricular; BP, blood pressure; CABG, coronary artery bypass grafting; CO, cardiac output; CVP, central venous pressure; HR, heart rate; IABP, intra-aortic balloon pump; ICU, intensive care unit; IVF, intravenous fluids; LV, left ventricle; LVAD, left ventricular assist device; MI, myocardial infarction; MR, mitral regurgitation; MS, mitral stenosis; NE, norepinephrine; OHT, orthotopic heart transplantation; PA, pulmonary artery; PCWP, pulmonary capillary wedge pressure; PRBC, packed red blood cells; PTCA, percutaneous transluminal coronary angioplasty; RV, right ventricle; Rx, therapy; VSD, ventricular septal defect.

measure arterial pressure only intermittently. Arterial cannulation allows beat-to-beat analysis so that decisions about therapy can be based on immediate and reproducible blood pressure information.[36]

Maintenance of adequate oxygenation and ventilation is critical. Many patients require intubation and mechanical ventilation, if only to reduce the work of breathing and to facilitate sedation and stabilization before cardiac catheterization.

Electrolyte abnormalities should be corrected because hypokalemia and hypomagnesemia predispose to ventricular arrhythmias. Relief of pain and anxiety with morphine sulfate (or fentanyl if systolic pressure is compromised) can reduce excessive sympathetic activity and decrease oxygen demand, preload, and afterload. Arrhythmias and heart block should be corrected promptly with antiarrhythmic drugs, cardioversion, or pacing.

Fluid Resuscitation

The initial approach to the hypotensive patient should include fluid resuscitation unless frank pulmonary edema is present. Patients are commonly diaphoretic, and relative hypovolemia may be present in as many as 20% of patients with cardiogenic shock.[41] Patients with myocardial infarction and low cardiac index and low pulmonary capillary wedge pressure, most of whom have reduced stroke volume and compensatory tachycardia,[34] would be expected to respond to fluid infusion with an increase in stroke volume, although the magnitude of such a response depends on the degree of ischemia and cardiac reserve.

Fluid infusion is best initiated with predetermined boluses titrated to clinical endpoints of heart rate, urine output, and blood pressure. Ischemia produces diastolic as well as systolic dysfunction, and thus elevated filling pressures may be necessary to maintain stroke volume in patients with cardiogenic shock. Patients who do not respond rapidly to initial fluid boluses or those with poor physiologic reserve should be considered for invasive hemodynamic monitoring. Optimal filling pressures vary from patient to patient but usually range from 12 to 20 mm Hg; hemodynamic monitoring can be used to construct a Starling ventricular function curve at the bedside, identifying the filling pressure at which cardiac output is maximized. Maintenance of adequate preload is particularly important in patients with right ventricular infarction.

Vasopressors

When arterial pressure remains inadequate, therapy with vasopressor agents may be required to maintain coronary perfusion pressure. Maintenance of adequate blood pressure is essential to break the vicious circle of progressive hypotension with further myocardial ischemia. The choice of a particular vasoactive agent depends on the clinical setting and goals (Table 70-2).[42]

Dopamine, which acts directly on myocardial β_1-adrenergic receptors and acts indirectly by releasing norepinephrine, has both inotropic and vasopressor effects. Dopamine also dilates specific dopamine receptors in the renal and splanchnic circulation. The net effect of dopamine administration is dependent on the dosage; effects on contractility predominate at doses below 10 μg/kg per minute, and α-adrenergic effects predominate above 20 μg/kg per minute. Dopamine is usually preferable as the initial choice in patients with systolic pressures below 80 mm Hg because it increases both blood pressure and cardiac output.[3,43]

When hypotension remains refractory, norepinephrine, a natural catecholamine with potent α-adrenergic and less pronounced β_1-adrenergic effects, may be necessary to maintain organ perfusion pressure. Its predominant effect is vasoconstriction, with little change in cardiac output. Norepinephrine is more potent than dopamine and may be more effective at reversing hypotension in patients with shock. Norepinephrine is usually started at 0.02 to 0.04 μg/kg per minute and titrated to effect.

Both dopamine and norepinephrine can cause tachycardia and increased peripheral resistance, which may exacerbate myocardial ischemia, and are arrhythmogenic. Phenylephrine, a selective α_1-adrenergic agonist, may be a good choice when tachyarrhythmias limit therapy with other vasopressors; doses start at 0.75 μg/kg per minute and range to 4 μg/kg per minute.

Vasopressin infusion at 0.01 to 0.03 U/min produces peripheral vascular vasoconstriction, and this may be a useful adjunct in septic shock and other forms of shock that are unresponsive to norepinephrine or dopamine. There is some concern that vasopressin infusion may either decrease splanchnic perfusion or redistribute blood flow away from the splanchnic mucosa, and, in sepsis at least, it is conceptualized as replacement therapy for relative deficiency rather than as a vasopressor agent to be titrated to effect. A randomized clinical trial recently reported that vasopressin added to norepinephrine appears to be as safe and effective as norepinephrine in fluid-resuscitated patients with septic shock.[44]

Vasopressor infusions need to be titrated carefully in patients with cardiogenic shock to maximize coronary perfusion pressure with the least possible increase in myocardial oxygen demand. It is also mandatory to ensure that filling pressures are optimal. Hemodynamic monitoring is useful in this regard.

Inotropic Agents

In patients with inadequate tissue perfusion and adequate intravascular volume, cardiovascular support with inotropic agents should be initiated. Dobutamine, a selective β_1-adrenergic receptor agonist, can improve myocardial contractility and increase cardiac output; dosage starts at 2.5 μg/kg per minute and is titrated to 20 μg/kg per minute as needed.[3] Dobutamine may exacerbate hypotension in some patients and can precipitate tachyarrhythmias.[3,43]

Phosphodiesterase inhibitors such as milrinone increase intracellular cyclic adenosine monophosphate by mechanisms not involving adrenergic receptors, producing both positive inotropic and vasodilatory actions. This effect may be important in patients with chronic heart failure, in whom chronic elevation of circulating catecholamine levels can produce down-regulation of β-adrenergic receptors.[45] Milrinone has fewer chronotropic and arrhythmogenic effects than catecholamines do, but it has the potential to cause hypotension due to vasodilatation and has a long half-life; in patients with tenuous clinical status, its use is often reserved for situations in which other agents have proved ineffective.[46] Standard administration of milrinone calls for a bolus loading dose of 50 μg/kg followed by an infusion of 0.5 μg/kg per minute, but many clinicians eschew the loading dose (or halve it) in patients with marginal blood pressure.

Levosimendan is a novel agent that increases cardiac myocyte calcium responsiveness and also opens ATP-dependent potassium channels, giving the drug both inotropic and vasodilatory properties. Levosimendan, unlike catecholamines, does not increase myocardial oxygen consumption. The SURVIVE study compared levosimendan with dobutamine in patients with acute heart failure and ejection fraction of less than 30% who had symptoms and clinical signs of low cardiac output despite intravenous

VASOPRESSORS AND INOTROPES USED IN SHOCK

				Order of Use			
				Cardiogenic Shock		Distributive Shock	
Agent	**Dose**	**HR/ Contractility**	**Vasoconstrict/ Vasodilate**	**Restore BP**	**Cardiac Output**	**Restore BP**	**Comments**
Dopamine	5-10 μg/kg/min	++/++	Variable	NA	++	NA	
	10-20 μg/kg/min	+++/ +++++	++–+++/0	+	+++	+	First-line agent to restore BP
Dobutamine	2.5-20 μg/kg/min	++/++++	0/++	NA	+	NA	First-line agent to improve cardiac output but arrhythmogenic
Norepinephrine	2-20 μg/kg/min	+/++	++++/0	++	NA	++	Purer vasoconstrictor than dopamine
Epinephrine	1-20 μg/kg/min	++++/ ++++	++++/+++	Avoid	Avoid	++++	Potent inotrope; significant increase in myocardial oxygen requirements; equipotent vasoconstrictor and vasodilator
Phenylephrine	20-200 μg/kg/min	0/0	+++/0	+++	NA	+++	Purest vasoconstrictor; least arrhythmogenic
Isoproterenol	1-5 μg/kg/min	++++/ ++++	0/++++	Avoid	+(if OHT)	NA	Ideal for HR response in heart transplantation; arrhythmogenic and vasodilator properties limit use elsewhere
Milrinone	0.375-0.75 μg/kg/ min	+/+++	0/++	NA	++	NA	Inotrope of choice if pulmonary HTN or failed dobutamine trial; generally avoid bolus

Relative potency on scale of 0 to ++++. BP, blood pressure; HR, heart rate; HTN, hypertension; NA, not applicable; OHT, orthotopic heart transplantation.

Table 70.2 Vasopressors and inotropes used in shock.

diuretics and vasodilators. Although levosimendan showed some early benefit, with a reduction in worsening heart failure, the primary outcome, all-cause mortality at 6 months, was not different (26.0% versus 27.9%; HR = 0.91; CI, 0.74-1.13).[47] Levosimendan is not currently available in the United States but has been approved for use in some countries in Europe and South America. Levosimendan has the potential to cause hypotension and thus should be used with some caution in patients with cardiogenic shock.

Intra-aortic Balloon Counterpulsation

Intra-aortic balloon pump (IABP) counterpulsation reduces systolic afterload and myocardial oxygen consumption and augments diastolic perfusion pressure, increasing cardiac output, coronary perfusion, and systemic blood pressure.[48] Inflation and deflation of the IABP are timed (by electrocardiography or arterial pressure) to augment aortic pressure in early diastole and to reduce aortic pressure at end-diastole, just before the onset of ventricular ejection (Fig. 70.9).

The effects of IABP, in contrast to those of inotropic or vasopressor agents, occur without an increase in oxygen demand, and decreased afterload is accomplished without lowering of blood pressure. In patients with cardiogenic shock and compromised tissue perfusion, IABP can be an essential support mechanism to stabilize patients and to allow time for definitive therapeutic measures to be undertaken.[49] Contraindications and complications of the IABP are discussed in Chapter 75.

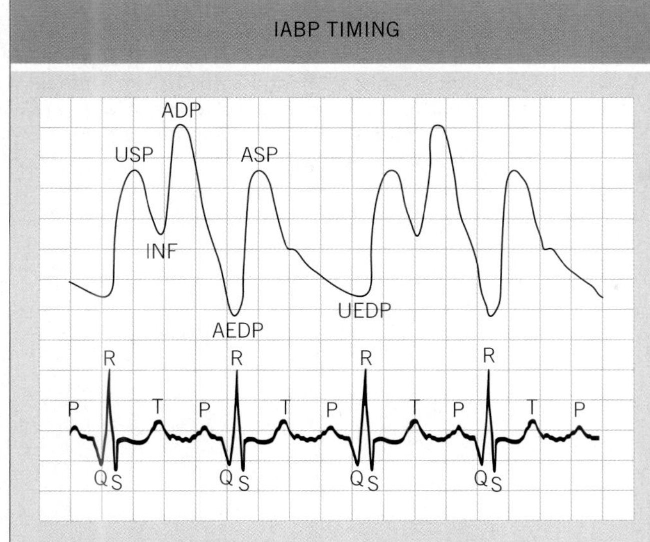

Figure 70.9 Optimal timing of an intra-aortic balloon pump (IABP). Arterial pressure tracing from a patient with an intra-aortic balloon pump. The balloon was set at 2:1 to evaluate timing. Inflation (INF) was timed to the dicrotic notch to follow aortic valve closure. There is augmentation of diastolic pressure (ADP) and lowering of the end-diastolic pressure with augmented beats (AEDP) compared with the unaugmented end-diastolic pressure (UEDP). The augmented systolic pressure (ASP) is often lower than the unaugmented systolic pressure (USP) as well.

Left Ventricular Assist Devices

A growing body of evidence supports the use of ventricular assist devices for acute heart failure and shock (see Chapter 75). The decision to support the left ventricle, the right ventricle, or both ventricles is clinical. Most patients receive isolated left ventricular support systems. Preexisting pulmonary hypertension and right ventricular dysfunction increase the likelihood of requiring right ventricular support after left ventricular support is initiated. Isolated right ventricular support is more common after orthotopic heart transplantation to temporarily support the right ventricle in the face of elevated pretransplantation pulmonary pressures.[50]

Cardiogenic Shock due to Myocardial Infarction

Stabilization

The initial treatment of cardiogenic shock in the setting of acute myocardial infarction management is outlined earlier. The initial goals of improved cardiac output and oxygen delivery have been shown to improve whole-body oxygen consumption[51] and may prevent or reverse multisystem organ failure. Measures routinely employed and proven to improve outcome after myocardial infarction, such as nitrates, beta blockers, and angiotensin-converting enzyme inhibitors,[52] have the potential to exacerbate hypotension in cardiogenic shock and should be withheld until the patient stabilizes.

After initial stabilization and restoration of adequate blood pressure, tissue perfusion should be assessed by a combination of clinical, laboratory, and hemodynamic parameters.[53] If tissue perfusion remains inadequate, inotropic support or intra-aortic balloon pumping should be initiated. If tissue perfusion is adequate but significant pulmonary congestion remains, diuretics may be employed. Vasodilators can be considered as well, depending on the blood pressure. If tissue perfusion is adequate and no pulmonary congestion is present, then no further resuscitative measures are needed (Fig. 70.10). In each of these situations, however, expeditious cardiac catheterization should be performed and the patient assessed for revascularization; prompt reperfusion is the key to achieving a good outcome in patients with cardiogenic shock. Patients who show clinical improvement after thrombolytic therapy and IABP should also eventually undergo cardiac catheterization.

Primary Angioplasty and Stenting

An extensive body of observational and registry studies has shown consistent benefits from revascularization for patients with cardiogenic shock, but such retrospective studies cannot be regarded as definitive. Two randomized controlled trials of revascularization for patients with myocardial infarction have now been published. The Should We Emergently Revascularize Occluded Coronaries for Cardiogenic Shock (SHOCK) study[5,54] was a randomized, multicenter trial that assigned patients with cardiogenic shock to receive optimal medical management—including IABP and thrombolytic therapy—or to cardiac catheterization with revascularization by percutaneous transluminal coronary angioplasty or coronary artery bypass grafting. Survival with invasive treatment was improved from 47% to 56% at 30 days, but this difference did not quite reach statistical significance ($P = .11$).[5] At 6 months, the absolute risk reduction was 13% (50% compared with 63%; $P = .027$), and this risk reduction was maintained at 12 months (mortality, 53% versus 66%; $P < .03$).[54] Subgroup analysis showed a substantial improvement in mortality rates in patients younger than 75 years.[5] The SMASH (Swiss Multicenter trial of Angioplasty SHock) trial[55] had a very similar design but was terminated early because of difficulties in recruitment of patients. In SMASH, a reduction in 30-day mortality to that in the SHOCK trial of 9% was observed (31% in the invasive group versus 22% in the medically managed group; RR = 0.88; 95% CI = 0.6-1.2; P = NS).[55] This benefit was also maintained at 1 year.

When the results of both the SHOCK and SMASH trials are put into perspective with results from other randomized controlled trials of patients with acute myocardial infarction, an important point emerges: despite the moderate *relative* risk reduction (for SHOCK, 0.72; for SMASH, 0.88), the *absolute* benefit is important, with 9 lives saved for 100 patients treated at 30 days in both trials and 13 saved per 100 patients treated at 1 year in the SHOCK trial. This latter figure corresponds to a number needed to treat of 7.6.

Coronary artery stenting is becoming routine, both in elective cases and as a component of primary angioplasty for acute myocardial infarction; normal coronary flow is restored in more than 90% of patients, and short-term outcome is good.[56] Data in patients with cardiogenic shock are more sparse, but success rates with direct percutaneous transluminal coronary angioplasty have been good.[57,58] Adjunctive glycoprotein IIb/IIIa inhibition is also becoming more routine in high-risk patients undergoing percutaneous coronary intervention. Recent data indicate that abciximab

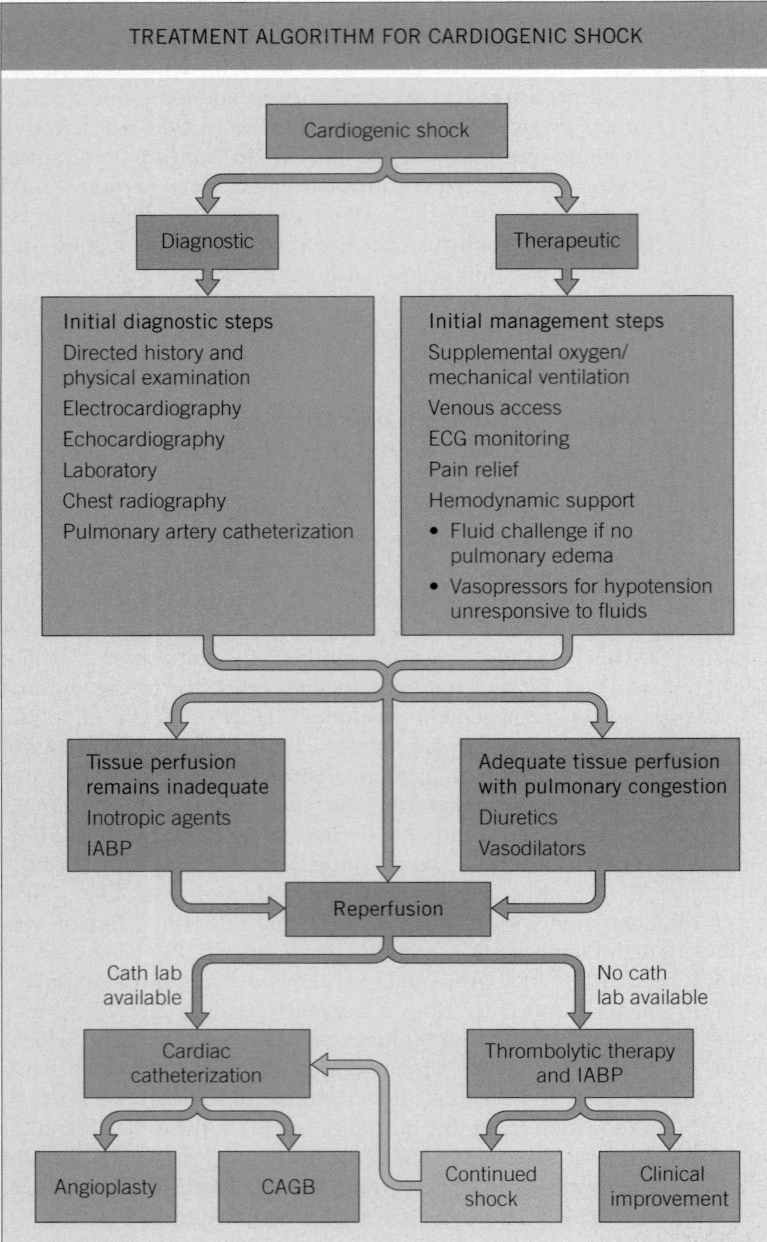

Figure 70.10 An approach to the diagnosis and treatment of cardiogenic shock caused by myocardial infarction. CABG, coronary artery bypass grafting; ECG, electrocardiographic; IABP, intra-aortic balloon pumping. (Modified with permission from Hollenberg SM, Kavinsky CJ, Parrillo JE. Cardiogenic shock. Ann Intern Med 1999;131:47-59.)

added to stenting improves outcomes in patients with myocardial infarction undergoing coronary stenting.[59]

Stabilization with IABP and thrombolysis followed by transfer for cardiac catheterization may be used if percutaneous transluminal coronary angioplasty is not immediately available. IABP may be a useful adjunct to thrombolysis in this setting by increasing drug delivery to the thrombus, improving coronary flow to other regions, preventing hypotensive events, or supporting blood pressure and ventricular function until areas of stunned myocardium can recover. Data from two large registries have shown improved mortality in patients treated with fibrinolytic therapy when IABP was also employed.[60,61] Although selection bias is clearly a confounding factor in these studies, two retrospective studies[62,63] showed improved in-hospital survival and outcomes in patients with cardiogenic shock treated with IABP followed by thrombolysis and subsequently transferred for revascularization.

Coronary Artery Bypass Grafting

Coronary artery bypass grafting can be performed on patients with shock, even during cardiopulmonary resuscitation. One-year and 10-year survival rates of 77% and 60%, respectively, have been reported for patients undergoing emergency coronary artery bypass grafting for cardiogenic shock due to acute myocardial infarction.

Transplantation

Emergency transplantation is rarely feasible, but appropriate patients may undergo left ventricular assist device insertion as a bridge to transplantation. Five-year survival rates in the range of 45% to 76% have been reported.

Surgical or Invasive Options

Definitive therapy for mechanical complications of acute myocardial infarction is surgical. Partial or complete papillary muscle disruption is a surgical emergency. Afterload reduction and IABP are used for initial stabilization but are temporizing measures; surgical valve repair or replacement should be undertaken as soon as possible because clinical deterioration can be sudden.[64]

The timing of repair for ventricular septal rupture has been more controversial, but most authorities now suggest that repair should be undertaken early, within 48 hours of the rupture. Concomitant right ventricular infarction confers a negative prognosis in this setting, and inferior ventricular septal defect has a worse prognosis than anterior. Important considerations include conservative trimming of right ventricular muscle and repair of papillary muscle if rupture is present. More recently, a technique of infarct–ventricular septal defect exclusion has been advocated.

Left ventricular free wall rupture, presenting as tamponade, may require immediate pericardiocentesis to restore blood pressure, followed by prompt operative repair. Such patients are at high risk of cardiac arrest at the time of anesthesia induction. Rarely, left ventricular free wall rupture can seal spontaneously. Such patients can be treated conservatively with bed rest and beta blockers, and long-term survival is possible.[65]

Right Ventricular Infarction Management

In patients with right ventricular infarction, right ventricular preload should be maintained with fluid administration. In some cases, however, fluid resuscitation may increase pulmonary capillary wedge pressure but may not increase cardiac output, and overdilatation of the right ventricle can compromise left ventricular filling and cardiac output.[66] Inotropic therapy with dobutamine may be more effective in increasing cardiac output in some patients, and monitoring with serial echocardiograms may also be useful to detect right ventricular overdistention.[66] Maintenance of atrioventricular synchrony is also important to optimize right ventricular filling, and some patients may benefit from atrioventricular sequential pacing.[35] For patients with continued hemodynamic instability, IABP may be useful, particularly because elevated right ventricular pressures and volumes increase wall stress and oxygen consumption and decrease right coronary perfusion pressure, exacerbating right ventricular ischemia.

Reperfusion of the occluded coronary artery is also crucial. A study using direct angioplasty[67] demonstrated that restoration of normal flow resulted in dramatic recovery of right ventricular function and mortality of only 2%, whereas unsuccessful reperfusion was associated with persistent hemodynamic compromise and 58% mortality.

Valvular Heart Disease

Emergency surgery should be considered for cases of shock resulting from acute aortic regurgitation or aortic dissection involving the ascending aorta.[68] In cases of severe mitral stenosis, cardiac output can be improved with use of agents to slow the heart rate to facilitate diastolic filling. In addition, mitral orifice enlargement can be achieved by catheter-based or surgical mitral valvuloplasty.

Extracardiac Obstructive Shock

Pericardial Tamponade

Initial therapy involves fluid administration to help maintain right-sided transmural filling pressures in the face of pericardial compression. Vasopressors may be used to maintain blood pressure as well, but these are temporizing measures in patients with cardiac tamponade; definitive therapy requires removal of pericardial fluid. The heart is maximally stimulated by sympathetic drive, and exogenous inotropic agents add little.

Patients with tamponade physiology should be considered for emergent pericardiocentesis. Because of the steepness of the pericardial compliance curve, prompt relief can be obtained with removal of only a small amount of fluid. For patients requiring prolonged drainage, a multihole pigtail drainage catheter can be left in place until drainage is decreased to less than 50 mL/day.[69] The fluid can also be removed by surgical creation of a pericardial window. This is preferred when biopsy specimens are required, the fluid is loculated, the fluid has reaccumulated, or the patient is coagulopathic.

Pulmonary Embolism

The use of thrombolytic therapy has been advocated for patients with hemodynamic compromise after pulmonary embolism[70] and, recently, for patients without shock but with right ventricular dysfunction or evidence of pulmonary hypertension by echocardiography.[71] Thrombolytics (recombinant tissue plasminogen activator, streptokinase, and urokinase) are more effective than heparin in relieving acute pulmonary arterial occlusion.[71-73] Few differences have been noted between the various thrombolytic regimens; however, the use of recombinant tissue plasminogen activator is associated with more rapid resolution of right-sided pressures.[71-73]

Distributive Shock

In septic shock, therapy is largely supportive, with an emphasis on a vigorous search for an infectious source, early administration of appropriately broad-spectrum antibiotic coverage, aggressive fluid resuscitation, and early institution of hemodynamic support.[74] Despite supportive care, septic shock is still associated with mortality rates of 35% to 60%. Combinations of clinical and physiologic variables, the source of infection, circulating levels of cytokines, and the number of organ systems affected have all been shown to predict outcomes in septic shock. A multicenter trial reported a significant reduction in 30-day mortality (from 31% to 25%) with recombinant activated protein C in patients with severe sepsis and more than one organ failure.[75]

Anaphylactic shock is corrected with subcutaneous or infused epinephrine. Addisonian crisis–related shock is stabilized with stress doses of intravenous corticosteroids.

chapter 71

Heart Failure due to Systolic Dysfunction

Gary S. Francis and W. H. Wilson Tang

Definition

- Heart failure is a clinical syndrome characterized by a constellation of signs and symptoms (including shortness of breath and fatigue) due to structural or functional impairment of the heart to fill with or to eject blood. Any form of heart disease can ultimately lead to heart failure.

Key Features

- Heart failure due to systolic dysfunction typically culminates in a progressively dilated heart with reduced ejection phase indices (often described by a low left ventricular ejection fraction).
- There is frequently associated mitral and tricuspid insufficiency, pulmonary hypertension, and diastolic dysfunction, particularly in the late stages.
- Fluid retention is a frequent although not invariable accompaniment of heart failure.

Therapy

- Outpatient medical treatment consists of sodium restriction, angiotensin-converting enzyme inhibitors or angiotensin II receptor blockers, and β-adrenergic blockers. In some patients, aldosterone receptor antagonists, fixed-dose hydralazine and isosorbide dinitrate, and digoxin may be helpful.
- Chronic diuretics and electrolyte replacement are often needed to maintain euvolemia.
- Device therapy includes the implantable cardioverter-defibrillator and cardiac resynchronization therapy (or biventricular pacemaker).
- Advanced surgical therapy consists of coronary artery bypass grafting or valve repair or replacement, ventricular reconstructive surgery, mechanical assist devices, and cardiac transplantation.

Heart failure is an extremely complex clinical syndrome that can be caused by virtually any form of heart disease. There is always some underlying abnormality of cardiac structure or function.[1] The syndrome of heart failure is accompanied by symptoms of shortness of breath and fatigue at rest or with exertion, although recent guidelines have also highlighted the need to recognize those patients without symptoms who are at risk for development of heart failure (such as patients with diabetes or prior myocardial infarction).[2] Heart failure should be distinguished from "circulatory congestion" in symptomatic patients with no underlying cardiac dysfunction (e.g., patients who have severe anemia, arteriovenous shunting, or acute renal failure),[3] although controversy about how to define heart failure remains.[4]

The term "congestive" heart failure has been abandoned because patients with heart failure frequently manifest no evidence of edema or tissue congestion, particularly when they are treated aggressively.[5] The widespread use of potent loop diuretics and combination diuretic therapy often results in patients having clear lungs and no edema.[6] Although such patients may still complain of severe exercise intolerance and manifest severe impairment of cardiac systolic dysfunction, they exhibit no manifestations of "congestion" (some even do not require the routine use of diuretic therapy). Therefore, the term *heart failure* may be a more appropriate description.

Heart failure has both acute and chronic manifestations regardless of whether the left ventricular (LV) systolic function is compromised or preserved. The acute and chronic presentations are quite different. Acute heart failure is often referred to as acute pulmonary edema, and this has an entirely different management strategy from that for chronic heart failure.[7,8] In general, the onset of acute heart failure is accompanied by severe shortness of breath, orthopnea, and diaphoresis. It requires immediate attention, with the primary goal being relief of pulmonary congestion.[9] Although there is an association between altered hemodynamics and symptoms of acute heart failure, a favorable hemodynamic response does not necessarily translate into a favorable long-term outcome, especially when there is evidence of organ dysfunction.[10,11] Chronic heart failure can also be manifested as acute decompensation (or exacerbation) with acute pulmonary edema that is otherwise indistinguishable from new-onset acute heart failure. However, many patients with chronic heart failure are ambulatory and can function reasonably well. Although limited by breathlessness and fatigue, patients who have chronic heart failure are usually able to conduct their ordinary daily affairs without the need for prompt therapeutic intervention.

Patients who have heart failure can be grouped into those with dominant abnormalities of systolic function and those who have abnormalities mainly of diastolic function (so-called diastolic heart failure or heart failure with preserved systolic function).[12] The distinction between heart failure due to systolic dysfunction and diastolic dysfunction is complicated by the fact that diastolic dysfunction nearly always coexists with systolic dysfunction, and the degree of severity may vary widely.[13,14] Systolic ejection is coupled physiologically to myocardial relaxation, which makes it difficult to separate out pure systolic and diastolic heart failure. Furthermore, there is no universally accepted, single diagnostic criterion to precisely define diastolic heart failure. The diagnosis and management of diastolic heart failure are discussed in detail in Chapter 73. The primary focus of this chapter is on those patients who present with heart failure and LV dilatation with reduced LV ejection fraction.

ANATOMY AND PATHOLOGY

The anatomic hallmark of heart failure due to systolic dysfunction is remodeling, usually in the form of LV dilatation or hypertrophy.[15] Heart failure from any cause appears to perpetuate a change in the shape and structure of the heart, termed cardiac remodeling, which culminates in an increase in LV end-diastolic and end-systolic volumes, a more spheroid LV shape, and an obligatory increase in LV wall stress. In certain types of heart failure, the right ventricle may be dominantly affected (i.e., cor pulmonale; see Chapter 84). However, in patients who have coronary artery disease and other forms of cardiomyopathy, it is usually the left ventricle that predominantly dilates. The right ventricle may later dilate in response to elevated LV filling pressures and chronic pulmonary hypertension. Biventricular failure may occur in sequence or in parallel. The increase in LV wall stress leads to an increase in myocardial oxygen requirements. There is a close inverse relationship between increased wall stress and decline of LV systolic performance.[16]

It was pointed out in 1960 by Linzbach[17] that heart failure is accompanied by major morphometric and anatomic changes in the cardiac myocytes, including hypertrophy. To this day, it remains unclear exactly how and when the transition from adaptive hypertrophy to heart failure occurs.[18] Although there is no major increase in the length of the sarcomeres as the left ventricle progressively dilates, there is an increase in the size of the cardiac cells. Normal LV filling results in a change in sarcomere length from 1.4 to 2.0 μm. The maximum lengthening of sarcomeres, even in severe heart failure, is only slightly beyond 2 μm. This would suggest that the cardiac muscle fibers are unable to adapt to any great extent by intrinsic sarcomere stretch. Rather, there must be an increase in the size of the cells (i.e., an increase in the number of sarcomeres) to accommodate the marked chamber dilatation that occurs. To some extent, the increase in LV chamber dimension and wall stress is offset by an increase in wall thickness (i.e., hypertrophy). The hypertrophy "adapts" the chamber to heightened preload and afterload conditions, thereby maintaining its performance characteristics. Overall, LV mass is increased in heart failure. However, the dominant anatomic change in both experimental and human heart failure is an increase in cardiac cell length rather than an increase in myocyte cross-sectional area.[19,20]

During normal postnatal growth of the heart, the cardiac myocytes become both wider and longer, maintaining a fixed length-width ratio. When heart failure ensues from either coronary disease or dilated cardiomyopathy, there is an alteration in the cardiac myocyte length-width ratio.[21] There is a disproportionate increase in cell length compared with cell width. This is one of the most consistent changes that occurs as part of the remodeling process in chronic heart failure. Some of the longest cells observed in human hearts are from the failing left ventricle.[20] They are larger than cells seen in physiologic hypertrophy. Human cardiac myocytes normally tend to be binucleated. The increase in the size of the cardiac myocytes is usually unaccompanied by nuclear ploidy or an increase in the number of nuclei. Although not proved, there is now a growing recognition that remodeling at the cellular level may contribute importantly to chamber enlargement in human heart failure.[20]

The increase in cardiac chamber size in heart failure is largely a structural problem, and a low LV ejection fraction is to some extent obligated by the increase in LV chamber size.[22] For example, maintenance of a normal ejection fraction of 62% in a left ventricle with an end-diastolic volume of 350 to 400 mL would deliver an enormous stroke volume, perhaps one that might even cause disruption of the normal homeostatic coupling between the heart and the periphery. In a sense, the low LV ejection fraction may be adaptive in the context of such a large LV end-diastolic volume, thus protecting the peripheral circulation from an unusually high pulse pressure. One could argue that a large chamber volume "obligates" a reduced ejection fraction to maintain normal homeostatic coupling.

Today's working model of heart failure represents a probable transition from an index event of a susceptible individual, beginning with a genetic mutation or acute injury due to myocardial infarction or inflammation, passing through a progressive remodeling phase, and finally arriving at the clinical syndrome of heart failure (Table 71.1).[23-26] The known responses to acute or chronic myocardial injury include myocyte growth with deposition and replacement of interstitial collagen. Additional factors that probably

TRANSITION MODEL OF SYSTOLIC HEART FAILURE

Index Event	Structural Remodeling and Heart Failure	Clinical Syndrome of Progression of Disease
Acute myocardial infarction	Myocyte hypertrophy	Salt and water retention
Gene mutations	Fibrosis, chamber dilatation	Congestion, edema
Acute inflammation	Collagen strut dissolution	Low cardiac output
Onset of hypertension	Cell dropout (apoptosis)	Diastolic dysfunction
Valvular heart disease	Cell necrosis	Increasing symptoms
	Neuroendocrine activation	
	Cytokine release	
	Increased wall stress	
	Chamber dysfunction	

This model states that there is an index event, such as a myocardial injury or expression of mutation. This progresses to a remodeling phase and ultimately to the full expression of the clinical syndrome of heart failure. There is plasticity of the phenotype, with variation in pace of development of progression.

From Francis GS. Changing the remodeling process in heart failure: basic mechanisms and laboratory results. Curr Opin Cardiol 1998;13:156-161.

Table 71.1 Transition model of systolic heart failure.

contribute to LV remodeling include myocyte slippage, perhaps caused by dissolution of collagen struts that normally hold the cells together, and increased cell loss caused by the process of apoptosis. Many of the processes are present in all patients, but the quantitative contributions of myocyte slippage and apoptosis to the cardiac remodeling process are not entirely clear. Moreover, there are some who believe that there is an overall increase in the number of cardiac myocytes during the development of hypertrophy and remodeling of heart failure,[27-29] although the classic teaching up to now has been that cardiac cells, being highly differentiated, are unlikely to enter into the cell cycle.[30] Eventually, the remodeling process and its hemodynamic burden, aggravated by activation of multiple neurohormones and cytokines, causes a further change in the size and the shape of the heart, leading to cardiomegaly and reduced LV systolic function.[23] The process is extraordinarily complex, with activation of multiple, redundant signaling pathways and crosstalk between signal transduction pathways. There is a highly complex interaction between mechanical signals, such as stretch of cell membranes, and various neurohormones and cytokines, making a single "silver bullet" therapy an unrealistic concept.

As the heart progressively enlarges, there may be secondary dilatation of both the mitral and the tricuspid valve annuli and support structures, leading to mitral and tricuspid insufficiency. The added hemodynamic burden of volume overload contributes to further LV remodeling and a more spheroid shape to the heart. Both atria as well as the right ventricle may also show substantial enlargement, which is noticeable on the electrocardiogram, echocardiogram, and chest radiograph.

In summary, the anatomic and pathologic changes that occur during heart failure are multifactorial and highly complex. They are a result of a confluence of hemodynamic and neuroendocrine forces, always initiated by an index event. Despite intensive research during the past 2 decades into LV remodeling, the process remains incompletely understood. There is now a firm belief that hypertrophy occurs early in the syndrome of heart failure, probably in response to hemodynamic perturbations and neurohumoral forces, and it may initially be adaptive to a perceived threat or injury to the myocardium itself. The index event can be due to any number of causes, including acute myocardial infarction, acute myocarditis, acute or chronic volume overload, genetic mutations, toxic drug therapy, and even the gradual development of pheochromocytoma. There is then a transition from "adaptive" hypertrophy to "maladaptive" overt heart failure, but what drives the pace and nature of this transition has remained elusive. How much of the problem is actually structural and how much is functional is not always clear. Undoubtedly, various growth factors, neurohormones, and cytokines are involved, with the ultimate phenotypic expression being that of an earlier fetal program associated with myocyte growth, increased apoptosis, and altered "growth" of the interstitium.[31]

When acute myocardial infarction is the inciting index event, loss of contractile tissue and replacement fibrosis in the heart contribute in a substantial manner to cardiac dysfunction.[32] Patients with dilated cardiomyopathy also have increased deposition of interstitial collagen. In some patients, a disparity between up-regulated expression of some matrix metalloproteinases and a lack of corresponding increase in tissue inhibitors of the matrix metalloproteinases favors a persistent matrix metalloproteinase activation state within the myocardium and is likely to contribute to the progressive LV remodeling process.[33] Despite the uncertainties about the mechanisms of LV remodeling, an improved understanding of this process has led to the development of new therapies such as angiotensin-converting enzyme inhibitors,[34,35] angiotensin II receptor blockers,[36,37] aldosterone antagonists,[38] and β-adrenergic blockers.[39,40] These treatments appear to manifest their benefit primarily through the inhibition of progressive LV remodeling. Rather than primarily affording acute hemodynamic relief, they appear to retard the slow progression of heart failure by abrogating or even reversing the LV remodeling process.[41-43]

PATHOPHYSIOLOGY

Despite decades of study, the pathogenesis of heart failure remains a subject of much debate. Investigators have gradually observed an evolution from a simple hemodynamic model to a complex neurohumoral model, largely based on evidence that inhibition of neurohormones rather than stimulation of an inotropic state leads to improvement in survival (Table 71.2). Although it is clear that the syndrome of heart failure is often characterized by abnormal loading conditions, including an increased impedance to LV ejection and elevated LV filling pressures, the mechanism by which the development of reduced force occurs has remained elusive and continues to be debated. Clearly, there is no single molecular abnormality that underlies heart failure; rather, there is a host of findings that are largely model dependent.[44] Many of the molecular abnormalities observed in experimental models, such as alteration in phospholamban messenger RNA and protein levels, are model dependent and variably observed in failing human hearts. Some investigators have demonstrated a significant reduction of the sarcoplasmic reticulum–specific calcium uptake and calcium adenosine triphosphatase activities in preparations from failing myocardium, suggesting a diminished amount of sarcoplasmic reticulum calcium adenosine triphosphatase per cell.[44] The findings are complicated by the fact that decreased functional capacity of the sarcoplasmic reticulum to recycle calcium in the failing myocardium is at least in part compensated by other cellular mechanisms, such as increased activity of the sodium-calcium exchanger. Although abnormal calcium cycling is clearly part of the pathogenesis of heart failure, it is not always clear whether such observations are driving reduced contractility or secondary epiphenomena.

There is clear evidence of cardiac myosin isoform switching in experimental heart failure.[44] There may also be myosin gene switching in human cardiac hypertrophy and failure. In human heart failure, there is a diminishment in the α-myosin heavy chain with an increase in the β-myosin heavy chain.[45] This alteration in gene expression of myosin heavy chain isoforms, if translated into protein expression, would lead to a decrease in myosin adenosine triphosphatase enzyme velocity and a slower speed of contraction. However, alterations in cardiac contractile protein isoforms have uncertain functional consequences.[46,47] Could such molecular abnormalities

FACTORS THAT LEAD TO THE PROGRESSIVE REMODELING OF THE LEFT VENTRICLE

Progressive Remodeling and Heart Failure			Counter-regulatory Factors
Cell Growth	**Fibrosis**	**Apoptosis**	
Angiotensin II	Angiotensin II	TNF-α	Natriuretic peptides (ANP, BNP)
Catecholamines	Endothelin	Fas ligand	Bradykinin
Endothelin	Aldosterone		Nitric oxide
TNF-α	TGF-β		
Growth hormone	Matrix metalloproteinases		
Insulin-like growth factor			
Leukemia inhibitory factor			
Cardiotrophin 1			
Mechanical stretch			

Growth of cardiac myocytes is a primary feature and is due to a host of growth factors, including neurohormones and cytokines. Mechanical stretch also seems to be important and may directly stimulate growth and indirectly promote cell growth by releasing intracellular angiotensin II. Fibrosis is promoted by activation of the renin-angiotensin-aldosterone axis and through activation of endothelin and transforming growth factor β (TGF-β). Apoptosis regulation is altered through changes in the expression of p53, Bcl-2, and Bax genes, perhaps as a consequence of increases in tumor necrosis factor α (TNF-α) acting to stimulate the Fas ligand. Programmed cell death is enhanced, producing cell dropout. Counterregulatory forces, including atrial natriuretic factor or atrial natriuretic peptide (ANP) and B-type natriuretic peptide (BNP), are activated. Nitric oxide, driven by bradykinin and ANP, may have antigrowth properties and hold uncontrolled growth in check to some extent; however, on balance, cardiac myocytes elongate, which contributes to left ventricular remodeling.

Modified from Francis GS. Changing the remodeling process in heart failure: basic mechanisms and laboratory results. Curr Opin Cardiol 1998;13:156-161.

Table 71.2 Factors that lead to the progressive remodeling of the left ventricle.

explain reduced force development in human heart failure? Perhaps, but it seems more likely that there is a convergence of many diverse factors, some of them functional and some of them structural. It is seemingly the convergence of these many factors that ultimately leads to diminished cardiac function, cardiomegaly, and the clinical syndrome of systolic heart failure.

There are other cellular abnormalities that may contribute importantly to the pathophysiologic process of heart failure. Heart failure is characterized by a reduction in β-adrenergic signal transduction. This possibly protective "adaptation" results from a reduced density of membrane β-adrenergic receptors[48,49] as well as alterations in G coupling proteins.[50,51] There is now general agreement that $G\alpha_i$ messenger RNA and protein concentrations are increased in heart failure, and this could conceivably inhibit adenylyl cyclase activity in the failing heart,[52] further protecting the heart from excessive β-adrenergic stimulation.

There are additional functional disturbances related to loss of adrenergic control in the syndrome of heart failure. For example, under normal conditions, an increase in the frequency of the heartbeat augments LV contractile force. This is known as the positive force-frequency relationship. The failing heart, assessed by various measures of myocardial contractility, typically demonstrates a marked reduction in the positive inotropic force-frequency effect.[53] This abnormality of the force-frequency relationship could play some role in the impairment of cardiac function during exercise in patients who have heart failure.

Heart failure is also characterized by important peripheral abnormalities. Reflex control mechanisms are altered, contributing in part to excessive sympathetic nervous system activity. Blunted responses to endothelium-dependent vasodilatation in patients who have heart failure have also been described.[54] The role that this abnormality plays in reduced exercise tolerance is not entirely clear, but it may contribute to impaired blood flow to skeletal muscles. There are also primary abnormalities of skeletal muscle that appear to play a role in the exercise limitation of heart failure patients, including muscle atrophy, impaired muscle function, and altered muscle metabolism.[55-57]

Insulin resistance is also prevalent in patients with heart failure[58,59] and relates to the severity and etiology of heart failure.[60] Some of these changes result from diminished muscle activity and deconditioning, but others may represent manifestations of the activation of neurohormones and cytokines so commonly observed in patients with chronic heart failure. Increased adrenergic drive in heart failure itself has also been shown to raise free fatty acid oxidation and insulin resistance and has been suggested as a cause of impaired peripheral vasodilatation and vascular activity resulting from diminished nitric oxide production, increased LV afterload, and increased atherogenicity.[61]

In summary, a host of molecular, physiologic, and structural abnormalities in heart failure undoubtedly converge and contribute to LV remodeling and diminished myocardial contractile function. There is no single underlying mechanism of systolic dysfunction in heart failure. Importantly, the progression of heart failure to very advanced stages is a dynamic process that usually occurs during months to years. Although drugs such as digitalis and diuretics can reduce the signs and symptoms of heart failure to some extent, the cornerstone of therapy remains drugs such as angiotensin-converting enzyme inhibitors and β-adrenergic blockers, which are designed to slow the progression of the syndrome rather than to provide immediate hemodynamic benefit. Neurohormone and cytokine augmentation is common in heart failure (see Table 71.2). The neurohormones, cytokines, and other peptides probably contribute to the remodeling process as well as to endothelial and skeletal muscle dysfunction and provide a rationale for multiple pharmacologic interdictions. There is even recent evidence to suggest that myocardial gene expression may be restored after neurohormonal antagonism.[62]

CLINICAL PRESENTATION

Patients who have chronic heart failure often pass through a phase of asymptomatic LV dysfunction followed by the gradual development of exercise intolerance, shortness of breath, fatigue, edema, ascites, and, ultimately, a state of skeletal muscle wasting or cachexia. The clinical presentation can be dominated by any of these manifestations, and all signs

EXACERBATING FACTORS AND COMMON CAUSES OF ACUTE AND CHRONIC SYSTOLIC HEART FAILURE
Exacerbating factors for acute heart failure
Acute myocardial infarction
Uncorrected high blood pressure
Atrial fibrillation and other arrhythmias
Negative inotropic drugs (e.g., verapamil, nifedipine, diltiazem, beta blockers)
Other drugs (e.g., thiazolidinediones, nonsteroidal anti-inflammatory drugs)
Excessive alcohol
Endocrine abnormalities (e.g., diabetes mellitus, hyperthyroidism, hypothyroidism)
Drug and sodium noncompliance or lack of information given to patient about diet and medications
Concurrent infections (e.g., pneumonia, viral illnesses)
Common causes of chronic heart failure
Coronary artery disease
Hypertensive cardiovascular disease
Diabetes mellitus
Valvular heart disease
Dilated cardiomyopathy (20%-30% are familial)
Infiltrative cardiomyopathy
Hypertrophic cardiomyopathy

Table 71.3 Exacerbating factors and common causes of acute and chronic systolic heart failure.

and symptoms may occur simultaneously in patients who have very advanced heart failure. Heart failure is a dynamic process, waxing and waning as the function of the heart and its interaction with the kidneys, neurohormones, and peripheral circulation vary with time. Patients may reach a steady-state condition for a time, but acute exacerbations occur frequently, leading to an undulating process of spontaneous improvement and relapse. The causes of acute clinical decompensation are numerous (Table 71.3).

Patients with a large, dilated heart and reduced LV ejection fractions may occasionally demonstrate no signs or symptoms of heart failure. Such patients can be identified by echocardiographic population screening.[63] Such patients may also be identified by mass population screening of plasma B-type natriuretic peptide (BNP), which appears to increase even before the onset of symptoms.[64] Echocardiography or measurement of plasma BNP levels may provide an effective method of screening for LV systolic dysfunction in a general population, especially if it is targeted to those at high risk. However, rigid definitions of normal LV chamber size and LV dysfunction in epidemiologic studies are, to some extent, arbitrary. The same applies to plasma BNP levels. There is a distribution of ventricular size in the population at large, with some normal people in the extreme ranges. For example, highly trained athletes can have LV internal diastolic chambers by M-mode echocardiography of up to 70 mm, which in other subjects would be considered severe chamber dilatation.[65] Dilated cardiomyopathy is defined by some as an enlarged LV internal end-diastolic dimension of 2.7 cm/m^2 and an ejection fraction of less than 45%.[66,67] Even patients who have so-called asymptomatic dilated cardiomyopathy and LV dysfunction commonly demonstrate a reduction in exercise tolerance, although young patients who have severe LV dysfunction may have striking preservation of exercise capacity. Likewise, the plasma BNP level may be elevated in elderly women without obvious heart failure, and it can be less than 100 pg/mL in patients with well-compensated but obvious cardiomyopathy (unpublished observations). More research will be required before these screening tools can be thoroughly verified.

Chronic heart failure, like fever or renal failure, is not a diagnosis that can stand alone. It is a clinical syndrome, and it frequently has an identifiable cause (see Table 71.3). The heart is usually enlarged in systolic LV dysfunction, and it becomes more spherical over time. As left atrial pressure rises, the left atrium also dilates, and this dilatation is often made worse by chronic mitral insufficiency. However, the symptoms of dyspnea that are so common in patients with chronic, ambulatory heart failure are not closely related to left atrial pressure.[68,69] Although it was long taught that dyspnea resulted primarily from "backward" heart failure (i.e., increased left atrial pressure), more current evidence argues strongly against this theory. The two cardinal symptoms of chronic heart failure are dyspnea and fatigue, but neither is completely understood. For example, the limiting symptoms of dyspnea and fatigue can be manipulated in an individual patient during progressive exercise testing by altering the details of the exercise test.[70] A rapidly induced incremental exercise load leads more commonly to dyspnea, whereas a more slowly induced workload more often leads to fatigue. The limiting symptom varies regardless of the pulmonary capillary wedge pressure achieved.[71] Moreover, symptoms of dyspnea during exercise do not relate to pulmonary artery pressure during studies of 24-hour ambulatory pressure monitoring in patients who have chronic heart failure.[72]

Dyspnea is poorly understood, even in normal subjects. Its mechanism in chronic obstructive lung disease is also in doubt. What is known is that patients with chronic heart failure demonstrate a relative hyperventilation even during mild exercise, as manifested by an increase in minute ventilation ($\dot{V}_E$) relative to carbon dioxide production ($\dot{V}CO_2$), resulting in an abnormally steep $\dot{V}_E$-$\dot{V}CO_2$ slope. One theory is that ergoreflex systems[73] and central carbon dioxide chemosensitivity sensors[74] have increased gain in patients who have heart failure, leading to an exaggerated ventilatory response to exercise and marked activation of the sympathetic nervous system.

Fatigue, particularly during exercise, is also a common presenting complaint of chronic heart failure. Often, patients cannot easily distinguish between dyspnea and fatigue, and they frequently coexist. The mechanism of fatigue is highly complex and includes[75]

- impaired muscle blood flow;
- skeletal muscle wasting;
- deficient endothelial function; and
- disordered skeletal muscle structure and function.

Objective measures of LV function, such as ejection fraction, bear little relation to the fatigue experienced by patients who have heart failure. Rather, structural and metabolic abnormalities in the skeletal muscles and their impaired coupling to the peripheral circulation correlate more strongly with exercise intolerance.[75] This concept is supported by the observation that even heart transplantation fails to “normalize” exercise tolerance in patients who have long-standing heart failure.[76] Patients who have advanced muscle wasting demonstrate reduced vascular conductance to skeletal muscles, which leads to an increase in vascular resistance; this observation highlights the importance of skeletal muscle abnormalities in chronic heart failure.

Peripheral edema, ascites, and anasarca occur later, usually in advanced heart failure. This is despite the fact that retention of sodium occurs very early in the setting of LV dysfunction, before edema ensues or there is any change in renal blood flow.[75] The mechanism of sodium and water retention in heart failure is multifactorial and still incompletely understood. However, it occurs in experimental heart failure before there is a reduction in renal blood flow.[77,78] Eventually, in advanced heart failure, renal blood flow is reduced, even though glomerular filtration is maintained until quite late in the syndrome. Glomerular filtration rate is maintained as a result of vasoconstriction of the efferent glomerular arterioles by angiotensin II and norepinephrine (noradrenaline). This mechanism tends to maintain intraglomerular hydraulic pressure, at least temporarily. The transmural plasma oncotic pressure gradient also increases over the length of the peritubular capillaries, which favors increased resorption of sodium and water by the proximal tubules. The renin-angiotensin-aldosterone axis is activated early in the syndrome of heart failure and progressively strengthens its grip during acute exacerbations; this further aggravates salt and water retention.[79] Circulatory congestion, edema, ascites, and anasarca are the natural end consequences of these events, particularly if dietary sodium is not restricted or loop diuretics are not properly employed.

Although salt and water retention can contribute to the clinical manifestations of chronic heart failure, the kidneys themselves are usually intrinsically normal. When the kidneys of a patient who has had heart failure are transplanted into a normal environment, they usually function normally. It appears as though the kidneys in the setting of heart failure “sense” a decrease in blood volume, despite what is apparently an increased blood volume. How the kidney senses the “effective circulating volume” is not well defined.[80] It is possible that the unifying drive to develop heart failure is a perceived threat to organ perfusion or to reduced blood pressure in the face of impaired cardiac function.[80-82] Whatever the signals are, the kidney responds by unleashing a multitude of mechanisms basically designed to expand blood volume and to protect blood pressure. These observations are consistent with the hypothesis that neurohormonal activation is a central force in the pathogenesis of heart failure.[83]

Cachexia is a severe complication of many chronic illnesses, including acquired immunodeficiency syndrome, cancer, and heart failure. Patients who have heart failure usually do not develop cachexia until very advanced stages, but it has long been recognized as a terminal manifestation of the syndrome.[84] Cachexia is defined as a documented, unintentional, nonedematous weight loss of 5 kg or more and a body mass index of less than 24 kg/m^2. Patients who have heart failure have increased plasma levels of tumor necrosis factor α (TNF-α).[85] This has now been confirmed by several other laboratories.[86,87] TNF-α, interleukin 1, and interleukin 6 are cytokines known to be important in tissue catabolism. As well as being linked to cachexia, these cytokines are increased in heart failure, and they probably contribute to LV remodeling and may have negative inotropic effects on cardiac myocytes. The detection of cardiac cachexia in patients who have heart failure implies highly advanced disease and a poor prognosis. Biventricular failure is often evident by the time cachexia is present. Bone mass may also be reduced. Although plasma levels of TNF-α correlate with the amount of documented weight loss, the relevance of serial assessment of TNF-α is not yet established. Clinical trials of drugs designed to inhibit cytokine activity in heart failure are ongoing, but at least one large trial using etanercept (a fusion protein that inactivates TNF-α activity) failed to improve survival.[88,89] A similar trial with a monoclonal antibody to TNF-α (infliximab) was also unsuccessful, thus leaving some questions about the role of cytokines in the pathogenesis of heart failure.

During the past few years, through the interrogation of large databases and careful observation, it has become apparent that about 20% of patients with chronic heart failure are anemic, depending on how one defines anemia.[90] Multiple mechanisms appear to be operative, including iron deficiency, dilutional factors, and the anemia of chronic disease. There may also be an inability to process erythropoietin signals, as erythropoietin levels are usually increased in patients with heart failure and tend to mirror the severity of heart failure. A trial of darbepoetin alfa is now under way (Reduction of Events with Darbepoetin in Heart Failure [RED-HF]) to test the hypothesis that increasing the hemoglobin levels by darbepoetin in patients with heart failure will improve survival of patients. Patients receiving this form of therapy need to be monitored carefully; there is clear risk of thrombotic complications that can occur as the hemoglobin level rises.[91] The ideal hemoglobin target for patients with heart failure is still not fully understood.

DIAGNOSIS

Perhaps the most important diagnostic approach in the management of systolic heart failure is performance of the clinical history and physical examination. With use of the information gained at the bedside, an attempt can be made to define the etiology of the heart failure and the duration of symptoms and to elucidate factors that might be contributing to acute exacerbation, such as dietary indiscretion or medical noncompliance. It is usually possible, although not always, to determine at what point in the natural history of the syndrome a patient might be by a thorough and comprehensive history and physical examination. The presence or absence of circulatory congestion, valvular insufficiency, and cardiac cachexia as well as other signs of advanced heart failure can be evaluated at the time of initial contact with the patient. This allows an assessment of prognosis and the implementation of appropriate treatment strategies. An assessment of the patient’s functional disability is also important. Diagnostic techniques important in the evaluation of patients with heart failure include an assessment of cardiac structure and function by echocardiography. In selected cases, candidates for coronary revascularization should be sought by stress testing or coronary arteriography, or both. BNP is usually elevated in patients with heart failure, and a normal plasma BNP level is strong evidence against the diagnosis of overt heart failure in symptomatic patients. These issues are covered in more detail in Chapter 69.

MANAGEMENT

The goals of treatment in patients with heart failure due to systolic dysfunction are to relieve symptoms, to prolong survival, and to prevent or to delay progression to more severe cardiac dysfunction. Pharmacologic therapy has evolved greatly during the past 2 decades. All patients who have chronic, ambulatory heart failure due to systolic dysfunction should be considered for treatment with angiotensin-converting enzyme inhibitors and beta blockers because both classes of drug prolong survival and prevent progressive dysfunction and remodeling. Although experience is more limited in patients with systolic dysfunction who have no apparent symptoms, angiotensin-converting enzyme inhibitors prevent progression to clinical heart failure in this group, and beta blockers are likely to be similarly or even more effective (based on limited data in patients who have asymptomatic low ejection fractions and earlier postinfarction trials).[34,35,39,40] Diuretics and digoxin are often indicated in those who have evidence of fluid retention and persistent symptoms. The further addition of spironolactone has an important role in the treatment of patients with advanced heart failure.[38] Angiotensin receptor blockers are useful in patients found to be intolerant of angiotensin-converting enzyme inhibitors, and their role has been expanded with the publication of new clinical trials in patients with systolic heart failure.[92] Fixed-dose hydralazine and isosorbide dinitrate combination has also been shown to provide morbidity and mortality benefits in African American patients with systolic heart failure as an add-on therapy to standard neurohormonal antagonists.[93] These recommendations are based on evidence from a large number of randomized, controlled clinical trials and are covered in more detail in Chapter 72.

PROGNOSIS

It is important to determine the prognosis of patients who have systolic heart failure because

- the patients and their families want to know the natural history of the disorder so that they can plan their lives;
- knowing the prognosis is critical in considering the timing of heart transplantation; and
- understanding the prognosis helps the physician to plan long-term management strategies, including newer surgical interventions.

Numerous factors have been suggested as predictive of survival in patients with heart failure (Table 71.4). Moreover, the prognosis of patients who have heart failure appears to be changing, as evidenced by longitudinal experiences in several centers. One program has reported a 33% improved survival since 1989 for patients who have advanced heart failure,[94] and the Framingham group has reported an incremental improvement in survival in patients treated with contemporary therapy during the past 2 to 3 decades. This large reduction in mortality, particularly in sudden death, may reflect the use of new therapeutic advances, including improved arrhythmia management by implantable cardioverter-defibrillators (ICDs).[95] Being able to make better predictions of how patients will fare clearly helps the patient to plan for the future and may identify subgroups of patients for whom different approaches to treatment may be preferred. Predictive information tends to be most useful when the data can be used to influence an immediate solution for an individual patient rather than just to provide general prognostic information. Among the many factors that have been used to predict prognosis in heart failure, only peak $\dot{V}O_2$ has been routinely used as a selection criterion for heart transplantation.[96] Reliance on a single physiologic prognostic factor seems imprudent, however. The peak $\dot{V}O_2$ is somewhat dependent on the patient's age. For example, $\dot{V}O_2$ of less than 50% predicted for age and size in a young patient implies that the patient should be listed for heart transplantation even if the peak $\dot{V}O_2$ exceeds 14 mL/kg per minute. Peak exercise systolic blood pressure,[97] maximal exercise, heart rate, heart rate recovery after exercise, and increased ventilatory response ($\dot{V}E/\dot{V}CO_2$ ratio) are also useful predictors of prognosis in patients with heart failure.[98]

The development of the physician's impression about an individual patient's prognosis is also important. In clinical terms, physicians often develop their own mortality estimates in bayesian terms, which should then be modified on the basis of formal data. The cause of the heart failure is important. It now seems clear that the extent of underlying coronary artery disease contributes more prognostic information than the clinical diagnosis of ischemic or nonischemic cardiomyopathy.[99] The New York Heart Association (NYHA) functional classification, although subjective, carries important prognostic information. A third heart sound gallop rhythm, a low cardiac output, a reduced ejection fraction, a low blood pressure, and a high pulmonary capillary wedge pressure all relate to prognosis in an independent manner, but none can be used as a single variable to predict prognosis in an individual patient. Previous attempts to quantify risk prediction used many of these parameters.[100] The Seattle Heart Failure Model (SHFM) has been developed by a consortium of investigators to better understand the factors that predict mortality in patients with chronic heart failure.[101] This model incorporated patients enrolled in six randomized trials or registries, a total of 10,538 patients with predominantly systolic dysfunction. The SHFM score provides information about the likely mode of death among ambulatory patients with heart failure. Scores from models should not replace informed, compassionate clinician-patient conversations and do not predict with accuracy what may happen to an individual patient. Rather, they are an exercise in probability based on a large experience.

We now know that risk assessment based on single factors has limited accuracy and reproducibility. Individual predictors often conflict and are only weakly correlated. Only by combining individual clinical characteristics into a multivariable predictive index can the analysis be made coherent. The ability to predict which patients are at increased risk of sudden death remains poor. This is a serious deficiency in our

PREDICTORS OF WORSENING SURVIVAL IN CHRONIC SYSTOLIC HEART FAILURE				
Clinical and Functional Assessment	**Structural Assessment**	**Electrophysiologic Assessment**	**Hemodynamic Assessment**	**Laboratory Assessment**
Ischemic etiology	LV end-diastolic diameter (LVIDd >65 mm)	Tachycardia	Low cardiac index (<2.0 L/min/m^2)	Hyponatremia
Long disease duration	Reduced LV ejection fraction (LVEF <35%)	Presence of atrial fibrillation	Elevated filling pressures (pulmonary artery pressure, PCWP, or LV end-diastolic pressure)	Renal insufficiency
Clinical instability	Lack of LVIDd/LVEF response after therapy	Wide QRS duration		Elevated natriuretic peptides (ANP, BNP)
History of syncope	Concomitant diastolic dysfunction	Presence of nonsustained or sustained ventricular tachycardia		Elevated renin, catecholamines (NE >600-900 pg/mL)
High NYHA class	Concomitant pulmonary hypertension and/or RV dysfunction	Abnormal signal-averaged ECG		Elevated cytokines or endothelin levels (research)
Peak $\dot{V}O_2$ ≤14 mL/kg/min	Concomitant valvular dysfunction	Abnormal T-wave alternans		
Increased $\dot{V}E/\dot{V}CO_2$ slope				
Abnormal heart rate recovery				
Short distance on 6-minute walk				

$\dot{V}E/\dot{V}CO_2$, ventilation with respect to carbon dioxide production; $\dot{V}O_2$, oxygen consumption; ANP, atrial natriuretic peptide; BNP, B-type natriuretic peptide; ECG, electrocardiography; LV, left ventricle; LVEF, left ventricular ejection fraction; LVIDd, left ventricular end-diastolic internal dimension; NE, norepinephrine; NYHA, New York Heart Association; PCWP, pulmonary capillary wedge pressure; RV, right ventricle.

Table 71.4 Predictors of worsening survival in chronic systolic heart failure.

ability to manage heart failure because sudden death often occurs unexpectedly and most often in seemingly stable patients. ICDs cannot be placed in all patients who are at risk because the cost would be prohibitive. Rather, the risk of sudden death must somehow be gauged, and selected patients who would derive a more robust benefit need to be identified. Those patients receiving class I antiarrhythmic agents and those patients who have less severe forms of heart failure appear to be at greater risk of sudden death, but more research in this area is needed. Use of microvoltage T-wave alternans during exercise may be as useful as provocative electrophysiologic testing,[102] but more experience is necessary as the data about its utility continue to be conflicting. Meanwhile, the Sudden Cardiac Death in Heart Failure Trial (SCD-HeFT) indicated that in patients assigned to NYHA class II or class III with an ejection fraction of 35% or less on good background therapy, simple shock-only ICDs decreased mortality by 23%.[103] The second Multicenter Automatic Defibrillator Implantation Trial (MADIT II) suggests that patients with a history of myocardial infarction and LV ejection fraction of less than 30% may be protected from sudden death by ICD implantation,[104] but the cost-effectiveness of this approach needs close scrutiny.

Two important advances in the care of advanced systolic heart failure patients during the past years have been cardiac resynchronization therapy and ventricular assist devices as destination therapy. In patients with conduction delays (QRS >130 ms), cardiac resynchronization therapy has demonstrated significant benefit in reducing both morbidity and mortality in symptomatic patients with an ejection fraction of 35% or less.[105] Meanwhile, for end-stage heart failure patients, ventricular assist device support can provide the last-resort option with better survival over medical therapy,[106] and it may even have the ability to provide an opportunity for the reversal of ventricular remodeling in some patients.[107] Other advanced cardiothoracic surgical options include coronary artery bypass surgery and valvular surgeries, ventricular remodeling surgery, and cardiac transplantation.

Last, controversy about the use of long-term anticoagulation in heart failure persists. There are no data from randomized, controlled clinical trials to guide us in this regard. There is still considerable controversy about who should receive anticoagulation in the setting of heart failure. Even aspirin is controversial. A randomized, controlled trial is seemingly unrealistic; the event rate is so low as to mandate a very large sample size with prolonged follow-up. For now, patients with a previously documented systemic embolism, patients with atrial fibrillation, patients with large anterior myocardial infarction and very low ejection fraction, and patients with noncompaction cardiomyopathy should be considered for anticoagulation. A retrospective analysis of the Studies of Left Ventricular Dysfunction

(SOLVD) database indicated that patients receiving either aspirin or warfarin derive an additional survival advantage over patients who are not anticoagulated.[108]

SUMMARY

Patients who have heart failure represent a growing epidemic. Whereas morbidity, mortality, and age-adjusted incidence and prevalence of coronary heart disease are all declining, heart failure and atrial fibrillation are becoming more common. These two conditions are largely diseases of older patients, and we can expect further incremental growth as the population continues to age. Therapy is improving, but there is still much room for the development of innovative technologic and pharmacologic interventions. We are now in an era of consensus guidelines, evidence-based medicine, and cost controls. It is contingent on physicians to keep abreast of developments, particularly with regard to randomized controlled trials, which, in combination with skillful judgment, are most likely to advance the overall best interest of our patients.

chapter 72

Management of the Patient with Chronic Heart Failure

Barry M. Massie

Definition

- Chronic heart failure is a common condition that is responsible for a large number of deaths and considerable morbidity and cost.

Key Features

- Management of the patient with chronic heart failure must be multifaceted, including both pharmacologic therapy and nonpharmacologic approaches, such as dietary and activity counseling, patient and family education, and close follow-up.
- The goals of pharmacologic therapy are first to prevent heart failure and, once it is present, to improve symptoms, to prevent progression of left ventricular dysfunction, and to prolong survival.

Therapy

- Appropriate use of diuretics is critical to symptom management, but treatment with neurohormonal antagonists, including angiotensin-converting enzyme inhibitors, beta blockers, and spironolactone, is the key to preventing progression and prolonging survival.
- In patients who are in sinus rhythm, digoxin is primarily used as an adjunct in patients who remain symptomatic despite optimal treatment with diuretics and these neurohormonal antagonists.
- The roles of implantable cardioverter-defibrillators and cardiac resynchronization with biventricular pacemakers are evolving.

Chronic heart failure (CHF) is a common condition that is growing in both incidence and prevalence.[1] The pathophysiology and diagnosis of CHF are covered in Chapters 68, 69, 71, and 73. Despite major advances in the pharmacologic treatment of patients with CHF, mortality rates often exceed 10% per year and range from 20% to 50% in the most severely affected patients.[1] CHF also remains a major cause of morbidity and a major user of health care resources, primarily because it is one of the most frequent causes of disability and admission to the hospital in older individuals.[1]

UNDERLYING ABNORMALITIES

Although CHF may be caused by abnormalities of the heart valves, congenital conditions, or excessive systemic metabolic or flow requirements, there is underlying myocardial damage or dysfunction in the large majority of cases. The symptoms and signs of CHF primarily reflect the severity of underlying myocardial dysfunction and the resulting hemodynamic derangements.[2] These may result from impaired systolic (contractile) function caused by the loss of myocardium (from myocardial infarction or progressive cardiomyopathy) or dysfunction of still viable myocardium (ischemia, tachycardia, or exposure to excessive endogenous hormonal stimulation or exogenous toxins). Alternatively or concomitantly, the dysfunction may be primarily diastolic as a result of reduced myocardial compliance or impaired myocardial relaxation, usually due to myocardial fibrosis or hypertrophy.

IDENTIFICATION OF REVERSIBLE CONDITIONS

Relatively few of the causes of CHF are reversible or amenable to specific treatment, but these should be assiduously sought and addressed (see Chapters 69 and 81).[3-5] The most important of these are valvular abnormalities and myocardial ischemia resulting from coronary artery disease. These conditions can usually be recognized or suspected from the patient's history and physical examination, with confirmation by echocardiography for valvular abnormalities and stress testing or coronary angiography in the case of myocardial ischemia. Other relatively common reversible conditions (as a result of avoidance, treatment, or spontaneous remission) include alcohol, thyroid dysfunction, myocarditis, tachyarrhythmias, and bradyarrhythmias.

GOALS OF THERAPY

In most patients with CHF, there is no specific treatment; nonetheless, a growing number of nonpharmacologic and drug treatments are available that substantially improve symptoms and outcomes. Table 72.1 lists the goals of CHF treatment and some of the approaches that have proved effective in achieving them.

Prevention

The importance of measures for the prevention of heart failure has only recently been adequately emphasized. The American College of Cardiology/American Heart Association CHF guidelines adopted a new approach to the classification of heart failure that emphasizes both the evolution and the progression of the disease (Table 72.2).[3] Four stages are defined, the first two of which identify patients in whom prevention is the key goal:

- Stage A consists of patients who are at high risk for the future development of CHF but have no identifiable structural abnormality of the heart.
- Stage B refers to patients who have structural abnormalities that are known to predispose to CHF but have never experienced symptoms of heart failure.

GOALS OF TREATMENT IN CHRONIC HEART FAILURE	
Goal	**Examples**
Prevention	Blood pressure control (especially systolic blood pressure) Treatment of dyslipidemia Secondary prevention in postinfarction patients Beta blockers Angiotensin-converting enzyme inhibitors Antithrombotic therapy Treatment of dyslipidemia Treatment of asymptomatic left ventricular dysfunction Angiotensin-converting enzyme inhibitors Beta blockers
Symptom reduction and improved activity tolerance	Exercise training Diuretics Angiotensin-converting enzyme inhibitors Digoxin Beta blockers
Prevent progression (remodeling)	Angiotensin-converting enzyme inhibitors Beta blockers Spironolactone* Angiotensin receptor blockers† Cardiac resynchronization (biventricular pacing)
Prolong survival	Angiotensin-converting enzyme inhibitors Beta blockers Spironolactone Angiotensin receptor blockers*† Implantable cardioverter-defibrillators*
Reduce resource use	Disease management Diuretics Angiotensin-converting enzyme inhibitors Beta blockers Digoxin Spironolactone Cardiac resynchronization

*Treatment that has not been definitively demonstrated to accomplish a goal but is likely to do so on the basis of other results and the known mechanisms of action.
†For use in patients intolerant of angiotensin-converting enzyme inhibitors.

Table 72.1 Goals of treatment in chronic heart failure.

- Stage C includes patients with current or prior symptoms of CHF.
- Stage D identifies patients with end-stage disease who require specialized treatment strategies.

Figure 72.1 schematically indicates the progression of heart failure and the appropriate interventions at each stage.

Key interventions to prevent heart failure in stage A are the rigorous control of hypertension (especially systolic hypertension in older patients),[6] lipid-lowering treatment in those at risk for myocardial infarction,[7] and use of angiotensin-converting enzyme (ACE) inhibitors in patients at high risk for vascular events.[8] The primary preventive measures in stage B are interventions in postinfarction patients to prevent recurrent infarction or left ventricular remodeling or dysfunction (ACE inhibitors, beta blockers, antithrombotic agents, and lipid-decreasing treatments)[9-11] and in patients with asymptomatic left ventricular dysfunction of other causes (ACE inhibitors, beta blockers).[10,12]

Amelioration of Symptoms

For patients with clinical CHF, the first objective of treatment is to reduce symptoms and improve quality of life. To a significant degree, the symptoms are caused by volume retention and the underlying hemodynamic abnormalities. Thus, salt restriction, diuretics, and other agents that reduce ventricular filling pressures and improve cardiac output (digoxin, direct-acting vasodilators, and ACE inhibitors) are effective. However, the origin of the most frequent symptoms, exercise intolerance and dyspnea, is complex and multifactorial, reflecting in part abnormalities of skeletal muscle and ventilation.[13] Exercise training has emerged as one of the most effective interventions for relief of symptoms.[14]

Prevent Progression

The greatest advance in the management of CHF during the past 2 decades has been the recognition that several medications can prevent progressive left ventricular dysfunction and dilatation, a process often termed remodeling. Although the initial abnormalities in CHF result in hemodynamic dysfunction, the deleterious effects of excessive neurohormonal responses to these derangements are responsible for progression of this syndrome.[15,16] Excessive circulating and myocardial concentrations of angiotensin II, aldosterone, catecholamines, endothelin, and proinflammatory cytokines appear to induce or to exacerbate myocyte loss and dysfunction and interstitial fibrosis. This leads to progressive myocardial dilatation, pathologic hypertrophy, and further dysfunction. Inhibitors of the renin-angiotensin-aldosterone system and beta blockers prevent or even reverse this remodeling process, thereby preventing further deterioration of left ventricular function.

Prolong Survival

Medications that prevent or slow the progression of left ventricular dysfunction would be expected to prolong survival, and this has proved to be the case with ACE inhibitors,[17,18] beta blockers,[19-22] and spironolactone.[23] However, 40% to 50% of deaths in patients with CHF are sudden, and therefore the goal of prolonging survival entails prevention of sudden death. Although sudden death is often believed to be caused by ventricular fibrillation, there are a number of potential underlying mechanisms in the setting of heart failure, including myocardial infarction and bradyarrhythmias resulting from sinus node or conduction abnormalities and reflex-mediated responses to severe hemodynamic abnormalities.[24] Beta blockers, in particular, have reduced the incidence of sudden death by 40% to 50%, probably by affecting each of these mechanisms.[25]

STAGES OF HEART FAILURE FROM THE AMERICAN COLLEGE OF CARDIOLOGY/AMERICAN HEART ASSOCIATION GUIDELINES		
Stage	**Description**	**Examples**
A	Patients at high risk of developing HF because of the presence of conditions that are strongly associated with the development of HF. Such patients have no identified structural or functional abnormalities of the pericardium, myocardium, or cardiac valves and have never shown signs or symptoms of HF	Systemic hypertension; coronary artery disease; diabetes mellitus; history of cardiotoxic drug therapy or alcohol abuse; personal history of rheumatic fever; family history of cardiomyopathy
B	Patients who have developed structural heart disease that is strongly associated with the development of HF but who have never shown signs or symptoms of HF	Left ventricular hypertrophy or fibrosis; left ventricular dilatation or hypocontractility; asymptomatic valvular heart disease; previous myocardial infarction
C	Patients who have current or prior symptoms of HF associated with underlying structural heart disease	Dyspnea or fatigue due to left ventricular systolic dysfunction; asymptomatic patients who are undergoing treatment for prior symptoms of HF
D	Patients with advanced structural heart disease and marked symptoms of HF at rest despite maximal medical therapy and who require specialized interventions	Patients who are frequently hospitalized for HF or cannot be safely discharged from the hospital; patients in the hospital awaiting heart transplantation; patients at home receiving continuous intravenous support for symptom relief or being supported with a mechanical circulatory assist device; patients in a hospice setting for the management of HF

HF, heart failure.

Table 72.2 Stages of heart failure from the American College of Cardiology/American Heart Association guidelines.[3,4]

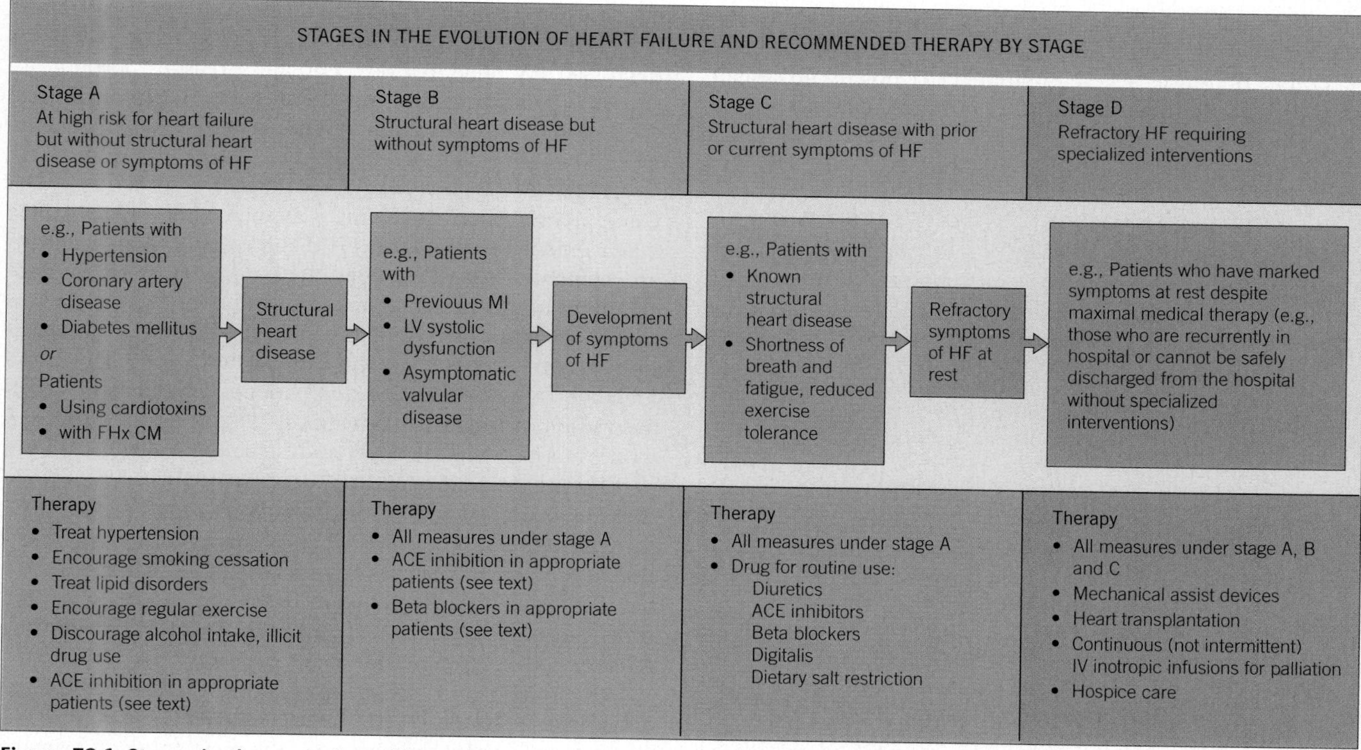

Figure 72.1 Stages in the evolution of heart failure and recommended therapy by stage. ACE, angiotensin-converting enzyme; FHx CM, family history of cardiomyopathy; HF, heart failure; IV, intravenous; LV, left ventricular; MI, myocardial infarction. (With permission from Hunt SA. ACC/AHA 2005 guideline update for the diagnosis and management of chronic heart failure in the adult. J Am Coll Cardiol 2005;46:e1-e82.)

Although antiarrhythmic drugs have appeared to have more adverse than beneficial effects in this setting, there is growing evidence supporting wider use of implantable cardioverter-defibrillators (see Chapter 66).[26] Coronary revascularization and cardiac transplantation are appropriate approaches in selected individuals (see Chapter 75).

Reduce Use of Resources

A final goal of CHF management is to reduce use of resources. The key to this is the optimal use of effective medications and dietary modification. Any intervention that accomplishes the first three objectives should also prevent admission to the hospital and reduce the cost of managing CHF.

However, prescription of medications does not appear to be sufficient in many patients. Specific strategies have been designed to prevent heart failure readmissions by use of nurse case managers, heart failure clinics, home visits, and home monitoring.[27,28]

NONPHARMACOLOGIC INTERVENTIONS

Although drug treatment of CHF has advanced markedly during the past 2 decades, nonpharmacologic interventions continue to have an important and sometimes critical role. These are often neglected by physicians because it is thought that patients are unlikely to follow their recommendations, but for many patients, compliance with these approaches is no worse than that with medication use. Table 72.3 lists nonpharmacologic approaches that have an important role in the effective management of patients with CHF.

Dietary Recommendations

Sodium and Fluid Restriction

As a result of activation of the renin-angiotensin-aldosterone system and changes in glomerular hemodynamics that favor proximal sodium reabsorption, CHF is a salt-retaining state. Therefore, salt restriction is an important component of the management of all symptomatic patients. With the advent of potent diuretics, severe sodium restriction is no longer essential in mild to moderate CHF, but these patients should not use added salt and should avoid excessively salty food, limiting their daily sodium intake to 2 to 2.5 g (about 5 to 6 g of salt). High salt intake in patients taking diuretics increases potassium loss and exacerbates hypokalemia. Only with more severe symptoms and high diuretic requirements does it become essential to restrict daily sodium consumption further, to 1.2 to 1.8 g (3 to 4.5 g of salt). As important as limiting overall salt intake is the need to minimize fluctuations in sodium intake so that the diuretic requirements can be matched to the sodium intake.

Fluid restriction is not a necessary component of CHF management, except in the minority of patients with refractory fluid retention, significant hyponatremia, or severely impaired renal function. Hyponatremia is typically a result of excessive activation of the renin-angiotensin and arginine-vasopressin systems, both of which stimulate thirst and the latter of which causes retention of free water. Severe hyponatremia (serum sodium concentration <130 mmol/L) is associated with a poor prognosis but importantly usually occurs in the setting of increased total body sodium concentration, so effective treatment requires limitation of free water intake to 1 to 1.5 L/day, usually with concomitant diuretic therapy.

Alcohol Intake

Alcohol is an important cause of dilated cardiomyopathy, and alcohol can further impair left ventricular function when it is depressed for other reasons. For these reasons, alcohol use should be discouraged in most CHF patients, although there are no well-controlled studies to support this recommendation.

NONPHARMACOLOGIC APPROACHES FOR THE MANAGEMENT OF CHRONIC HEART FAILURE

Approach	Recommendations
Dietary advice	Sodium restriction of 2.5 g (2.0 g in more severe heart failure) Fluid restriction, primarily for hyponatremia Low-fat diet and calorie restriction when indicated Abstention from alcohol or restriction to one drink per day
Activity and exercise counseling	Encourage regular activity in all patients Exercise training and cardiac rehabilitation in stable, motivated patients
Patient and family education	Explanation of heart failure and its common symptoms Reasons for salt restriction Medications and importance of compliance Need for daily weight measurements Recognition and management of worsening heart failure
Disease management approaches	Home visits by nurse or pharmacist Telephone monitoring and counseling by nurse Automated transfer of weight and vital sign data Comprehensive heart failure clinics

Table 72.3 Nonpharmacologic approaches for the management of chronic heart failure.

General Nutritional Measures

General nutritional counseling is an important aspect of CHF management because obesity, diabetes, and atherosclerosis are common associated conditions. Obesity itself is associated with hypervolemia and fluid retention, so weight loss can be an important adjunctive goal. Conversely, malnutrition is not uncommon in patients with severe CHF. Basal metabolic rates are increased in patients with CHF, and malabsorption may occur in advanced CHF. Muscle loss is common even in moderate CHF, and cachexia, contributed to in part by negative nitrogen balance, may occur in 3% to 15% of patients, depending on the definition used.[29]

Many patients with CHF take vitamins and other nutritional supplements, such as antioxidants. Coenzyme Q10 has been particularly popular. However, when controlled trials have been performed, they have not been positive, although adverse effects have not been reported.

Exercise and Activity Counseling

Exercise or activity intolerance is the most common primary complaint of most patients with CHF. For many years, it was believed that exercise was limited by high left ventricular filling pressures, resulting in dyspnea or impaired cardiac output reserve, leading to reduced peripheral blood flow to the exercising muscles. It is now apparent that the mechanisms responsible for exercise intolerance are more complex.[13] Peripheral blood flow is limited not just by central hemodynamic abnormalities but also by impaired vasodilatation and endothelial dysfunction. Skeletal muscle abnormalities, including atrophy, selective loss of oxidative fibers and oxidative capacity, increased dependence on glycolytic metabolism, and increased muscle fatigue, have been observed and appear to explain, in part, the dissociation between the severity of cardiac dysfunction and exercise intolerance. Excessive ventilation and ventilatory muscle fatigue may partially explain the symptoms of dyspnea. Inactivity may play a part in these changes, but they are in some ways dissimilar to those associated with deconditioning and, in animal models, are not explained by decreased activity. However, nearly all of these abnormalities can be improved, if not reversed, by exercise training, in the absence of significant improvements in central hemodynamics.[14]

These findings together with the favorable experience of cardiac rehabilitation programs in patients with coronary heart disease have led many authorities to recommend exercise training for patients with heart failure. Although many patients are older and have significant comorbidities that may make it difficult to participate in or may interfere with exercise, small randomized studies have consistently shown that aerobic and resistive training, performed either in a supervised setting or at home after counseling, at levels of 40% to 75% of peak oxygen consumption, results in increased exercise capacity, improved quality of life, and reduced sympathetic nervous system activity. The last finding raises the possibility of a beneficial effect on prognosis. To date, there is inadequate information with which to assess the effect of exercise training on the natural history of CHF, but the symptomatic and psychological benefits are evident. Importantly, exercise has been well tolerated in patients with stable New York Heart Association (NYHA) class I to class III symptoms, without evidence of increased risk of either life-threatening arrhythmias or clinical deterioration.

Thus, a progressive exercise program should be recommended to appropriate stable candidates.[4,5] In general, this should be initiated after a maximal or submaximal monitored exercise test has been performed. In patients with severe CHF or associated symptomatic coronary disease, it is prudent for the initial sessions to be supervised. However, most patients can be counseled to carry on a gradually progressive program of walking or stationary cycling. In any case, the often-made recommendation for patients with heart failure to remain sedentary and avoid unnecessary activity should be eliminated.

Disease Management

Despite the tremendous efficacy of current medical management, patients with CHF are frequently admitted to the hospital.[1] Particularly troublesome is the 30% to 50% rate of readmission to the hospital within 3 to 6 months of discharge. There are many contributing factors, including suboptimal in-hospital treatment, inadequate follow-up early after discharge, lack of understanding of the condition and its treatment on the part of the patient, noncompliance with dietary recommendations or medicines, and inadequate procedures to detect and to enable early intervention during subsequent episodes of deterioration. A number of approaches to improve the management of CHF have been evaluated and implemented.[27] Measures that appear effective include education of the patient and family, evaluation early after discharge (at home or in the office), close tracking of weight changes, and systems that facilitate close communication between patients and providers. Specially trained nurses or pharmacists can have an important role.[28] Nonetheless, those groups of patients who benefit most from these potentially costly programs and the optimal interventions have not been determined.

PHARMACOLOGIC THERAPY

Table 72.4 lists the classes of agents that can be used in the management of CHF resulting from systolic dysfunction (see Chapter 73 for discussion of treatment of CHF with intact systolic function). Overviews of pharmacologic treatment are provided in recently updated guidelines.[4,5]

Diuretics

Mechanism of Action and Pharmacology

Although the kidneys are structurally relatively normal in most patients with CHF, hemodynamic and neurohormonal abnormalities produce marked alterations in renal function.[30] Reduced cardiac output and blood pressure diminish renal perfusion pressure and flow. Systemic and local activation of the renin-angiotensin-aldosterone and sympathetic nervous systems induces compensatory intrarenal hemodynamic and tubular responses. Although both afferent and efferent arterioles are constricted, the latter predominate, with a resulting increase in filtration fraction and preservation of glomerular filtration rate. However, the consequent increase in proximal tubule hydrostatic pressure relative to the peritubular capillaries leads to increased sodium and water reabsorption in the proximal tubule. Chronic increases in sodium delivery also

CLASSES OF DRUGS USED IN THE MANAGEMENT OF PATIENTS WITH CHRONIC HEART FAILURE

Drug Class	Examples
Diuretics	Thiazide and thiazide-like agents Loop diureticzs Potassium-sparing agents
Inhibitors of the renin-angiotensin-aldosterone system	Angiotensin-converting enzyme inhibitors Angiotensin receptor blockers Aldosterone antagonists
β-Adrenoceptor blockers	β_1 Selective (metoprolol, bisoprolol) Nonselective with alpha-blocking activity (carvedilol)
Digitalis glycosides	Digoxin
Direct-acting vasodilators	Inorganic nitrates Nesiritide Hydralazine Calcium antagonists
Intravenous positive inotropic agents	Dobutamine Phosphodiesterase inhibitors Dopamine Levosimendan*
Ancillary therapies	Antithrombotic agents Antiarrhythmic drugs

*Not available in the United States and many other countries.

Table 72.4 Classes of drugs used in the management of patients with chronic heart failure.

lead to an increase in the capacity of the distal tubules to reabsorb sodium. Increased circulating aldosterone concentrations also stimulate sodium-potassium exchange in the collecting ducts, and increased vasopressin concentrations enhance free water reabsorption and stimulate thirst.

The role of diuretics is to overcome these maladaptive responses and to stimulate sodium excretion.[31,32] Table 72.5 lists the diuretics most frequently used in CHF, their sites of action, and information about their dosing and use. There are several classes of diuretics, with different primary mechanisms and sites of action along the renal tubules. However, with the exception of the aldosterone receptor antagonists, the activity of diuretics is dependent on their tubular concentration. Thus, they must be filtered or secreted into the urine, with the latter process predominating because most are highly protein bound.

The loop diuretics inhibit the Na^+-K^+-$2Cl^-$ cotransporter in the epithelial cells of the thick ascending portion of the loop of Henle, markedly increasing Na^+ and Cl^- excretion.[30] They can increase Na^+ excretion to 20% to 25% of the filtered load while at the same time maintaining free water clearance. Because the loop diuretics are actively secreted, they maintain their efficacy down to very low glomerular filtration rates (creatinine clearances <5 mL/min). These properties make the loop diuretics the preferred agents for patients with more than mild propensity for sodium retention. Loop diuretics are active as long as a threshold tubular concentration is achieved. This usually occurs after a 20- to 80-mg dose of furosemide (frusemide), 1 to 4 mg of bumetanide, or 10 to 40 mg of torsemide, unless gastrointestinal absorption is impaired or renal function is severely abnormal. Higher doses may modestly prolong the diuretic response, but if a greater diuresis is desired, several daily doses will be much more effective.

The thiazide and thiazide-like diuretics inhibit Na^+-Cl^- transport in the distal convoluted tubule.[30] At this point in the nephron, there is less potential to reabsorb Na^+, and these diuretics increase Na^+ excretion by only 5% to 10%. In addition, they tend to reduce the clearance of free water, which may lead to hyponatremia. The thiazides are more weakly secreted than the loop diuretics and lose their activity when the creatinine clearance decreases to 25 to 30 mL/min. However, the thiazides do have weak carbonic anhydrase–inhibiting properties, which may enhance proximal tubular Na^+ excretion.

DIURETICS USED FOR CHRONIC HEART FAILURE

Diuretic	Site and Mechanism of Action	Usual Dose Range	Adverse Effects	Comment
Thiazides and thiazide-like agents				
Hydrochlorothiazide	Inhibit Na^+-Cl^- transport in the distal tubule	25-100 mg/day	↓K^+, ↓Mg^{2+}, hyponatremia, ↑uric acid, glucose intolerance	Preferable for blood pressure control
Bendroflumethiazide		2.5-20 mg/day		Inadequate for severe fluid retention
Metolazone		2.5-10 mg/day		Useful in combination with loop diuretics for refractory edema
Chlorthalidone		25-100 mg/day		
Indapamide		2.5-5 mg/day		
Loop diuretics				
Furosemide	Inhibition of Na^+-K^+-$2Cl^-$ cotransport in the thick ascending loop of Henle	20-640 mg/day	↓K^+, ↓Mg^{2+}, hyponatremia, ↑uric acid	For hypertension, must be given in divided doses
Bumetanide		0.5-20 mg/day		For severe fluid retention, effective dose should be given 2-3 times daily
Torsemide		20-400 mg/day		
Ethacrynic acid		25-400 mg/day		At higher doses, combination with thiazide-type agent may be more effective. Ethacrynic acid primarily for patients with sulfur allergy
Potassium-sparing agents				
Triamterene	Inhibition of Na^+ reabsorption and Na^+-K^+ exchange in distal convoluted tubule and cortical collecting duct	50-200 mg/day	↑K^+	Follow potassium concentration closely when used with angiotensin-converting enzyme inhibitor
Amiloride		5-20 mg/day	Gastrointestinal side effects	
Aldosterone antagonists				
Spironolactone Eplerenone	Competitive aldosterone antagonist in the distal convoluted tubule and cortical collecting duct	12.5-50 mg/day 25-100 mg/day	↑K^+ Breast enlargement and tenderness with spironolactone	Follow potassium concentration and renal function closely

Table 72.5 Diuretics used for chronic heart failure.

Both loop and thiazide diuretics increase Na^+ delivery to the distal nephron and therefore enhance Na^+-K^+ exchange, with resulting kaliuresis and potential hyponatremia. The potassium-sparing agents inhibit the Na^+ channels of the distal convoluted tubule and cortical collecting duct and diminish this exchange but have little net effect on Na^+ or water excretion. Mineralocorticoid antagonists accomplish the same objective by a different mechanism of action but with additional beneficial effects (see later discussion of aldosterone antagonists).

Indications and Recommendations for Use

Because most patients with symptomatic heart failure have some degree of Na^+ and fluid retention, most will require treatment with diuretics.[33] Patients have fewer symptoms, better exercise tolerance, and fewer exacerbations of heart failure when they are maintained at or near "dry weight," which can be defined as the absence of edema and a jugular venous pressure of less than 8 cm H_2O.[34] When the propensity to fluid retention is mild, thiazides may be the preferred agents because they have a less abrupt onset and longer duration of action. They are also more effective antihypertensive agents than the loop diuretics, unless the loop diuretics are given in multiple daily doses or the glomerular filtration rate is severely impaired. However, most patients with moderate to severe CHF will require treatment with loop diuretics.

Management of Diuretic Resistance

Most patients with CHF can be maintained at the desired volume status with twice-daily doses of a loop diuretic. However, some 10% to 20% will not respond to doses of furosemide up to 160 mg twice daily (or the equivalent with other agents); these may be termed diuretic resistant.[31] There are two general explanations for this phenomenon: inadequate delivery of the diuretic to the tubular lumen and inadequate diuretic response to adequate intratubular concentrations of the diuretic (Table 72.6). The most common cause of perceived diuretic resistance is the use of doses below this threshold or large single daily doses. In some cases, diuretic doses are reduced to allow the introduction of ACE inhibitors or beta blockers, but these agents do not reduce and may even exacerbate fluid retention. Patients with severe renal dysfunction may require much greater doses because glomerular blood flow and diuretic secretion may be impaired. Similarly, patients with very low albumin concentrations may not deliver adequate doses of diuretic to the glomerulus because these agents are highly protein bound. Another factor is the relatively poor bioavailability of some loop diuretics, especially furosemide.[35] Substitution with more bioavailable agents may improve response and clinical outcome, as demonstrated by a study that compared torsemide with furosemide.[36] If a diuretic response is observed after dosing, the appropriate strategy may be to decrease the interdose intervals. Continuous infusions of furosemide (10 to 40 mg/h) may be markedly effective in many "resistant" patients.

Two other mechanisms for diuretic resistance have been recognized.[31] One, termed braking, is a short-term reduction in response, particularly after a marked diuresis, resulting in volume contraction. More important is the occurrence of enhanced distal tubular Na^+ reabsorption during chronic treatment, resulting from hypertrophy of the distal tubular epithelial cells and increased capacity for distal Na^+ reabsorption. A markedly effective approach to this form of resistance is the use of combinations of loop and thiazide or thiazide-like agents because the latter will inhibit distal Na^+ reabsorption.[37] Metolazone (2.5 to 10 mg) is often used because it may be secreted more actively than other thiazides. However, the magnitude of the response is unpredictable, and there is potential for very large diuretic and kaliuretic responses that may be life-threatening, so this must be approached with great caution and under close monitoring.

MECHANISMS AND MANAGEMENT OF DIURETIC RESISTANCE IN HEART FAILURE

Mechanism	Management
Inadequate delivery of diuretic to active site (renal tubules)	
Patient noncompliance	Patient education; observe dosing
Inadequate gastrointestinal absorption	Intravenous administration; use more bioavailable agent (torsemide)
Hypoalbuminemia (reduced protein binding)	High-dose intravenous therapy; coadminister albumin
Impaired renal blood flow	Use loop diuretics; coadminister inotropic agent or low-dose dopamine
Impaired tubular diuretic secretion (with renal dysfunction)	Use loop diuretics; administer high doses
Inadequate response to diuretic	
Short period of tubular exposure to threshold concentrations	Increase frequency of dosing; use intravenous infusion
Braking (temporary resistance due to intravascular contraction)	More gradual diuresis; replace intravascular volume
Diuretic tolerance (increased Na^+ reabsorption)	Combination of loop and distal agent to overcome distal hypertrophy
Concomitant sodium retention	Minimize sodium intake (dietary, intravenous fluids); avoid nonsteroidal anti-inflammatory drugs

Table 72.6 Mechanisms and management of diuretic resistance in heart failure.

The final and most difficult cause of diuretic resistance is poor renal perfusion because of low cardiac output, the so-called cardiorenal syndrome. Inotropic support or even left ventricular assist devices may be the only effective approach to this condition (see later).

Adverse Effects

Treatment with diuretics, although essential, is not without its downside.[31] The major problems are those that may be anticipated by the underlying physiology—electrolyte imbalance and neurohormonal activation. Hypokalemia and the often concomitant hypomagnesemia are the most frequent and have the potential to induce life-threatening arrhythmias and digitalis toxicity. Careful monitoring of electrolytes after initiating or increasing diuretic doses is critical, especially when combinations of loop and thiazide diuretics are used. Maintenance of serum potassium concentrations between 4 and 5 mmol/L is preferable to provide a cushion against changes in diuretic response. Consideration should be given to the use of potassium-sparing agents rather than potassium replacement because these also prevent magnesium loss. Aldosterone antagonists have additional desirable myocardial effects and reduce mortality and morbidity in advanced heart failure.

Diuretics also stimulate the activity of the renin-angiotensin-aldosterone system and the sympathetic nervous system, with potential deleterious effects on the progression of myocardial dysfunction and the natural history of CHF. Thus, diuretics should not be used without concomitant treatment with inhibitors of these systems, in particular ACE inhibitors and, in advanced CHF or with high doses of diuretics, spironolactone.

Inhibitors of the Renin-Angiotensin-Aldosterone System

Mechanisms of Action

The response of the renin-angiotensin-aldosterone system in CHF and the rationale for its inhibition are discussed in Chapter 71 and extensively reviewed elsewhere.[38,39] However, the early notion of the renin-angiotensin system as a predominantly intravascular system serving to regulate arterial pressure, renal function, and adrenal mineralocorticoid secretion is now known to have been simplistic. Important newer concepts that are relevant to CHF include the presence of a tissue renin-angiotensin system in the heart, kidneys, and blood vessels; the presence of non–ACE-mediated pathways for angiotensin II generation; and the more widespread role of aldosterone as a mediator of the myocardial fibrosis and remodeling. Furthermore, the interactions between the renin-angiotensin system and the activity of the sympathetic nervous system, bradykinin, prostaglandins, and nitric oxide are now recognized to have potentially important roles in the adverse effects of its activation and beneficial responses to its inhibition.[38-41]

Some of these aspects of the renin-angiotensin system are illustrated schematically in Figure 72.2. From this, it can be appreciated that an ACE inhibitor will diminish but not fully prevent the generation of angiotensin II and aldosterone. It will also increase concentrations of bradykinin and prostaglandins, which will have a variety of actions on the blood vessels and the heart. There are increasing data indicating that bradykinin may play a part in many of the beneficial effects of ACE inhibitors on myocardial remodeling and endothelial and vascular function. Similarly, studies have shown that inhibition of prostaglandin synthesis reduces the hemodynamic response and perhaps the clinical benefit of ACE inhibitors. Angiotensin receptor blockers (ARBs) should inhibit angiotensin II–mediated actions more completely than do ACE inhibitors, assuming comparable tissue penetration and activity. However, an ARB may not share in the beneficial effects mediated by bradykinin and prostaglandins. Finally, neither an ACE inhibitor nor an ARB fully blocks the production of aldosterone, which is also regulated by serum potassium concentrations and adrenocorticotropic hormone. Some of these concepts have been validated by the demonstration of "breakthrough" (e.g., initial reduction but subsequent restoration) in the concentrations of angiotensin II and aldosterone during chronic ACE inhibitor and ARB treatment and by the results of clinical trials.[42,43]

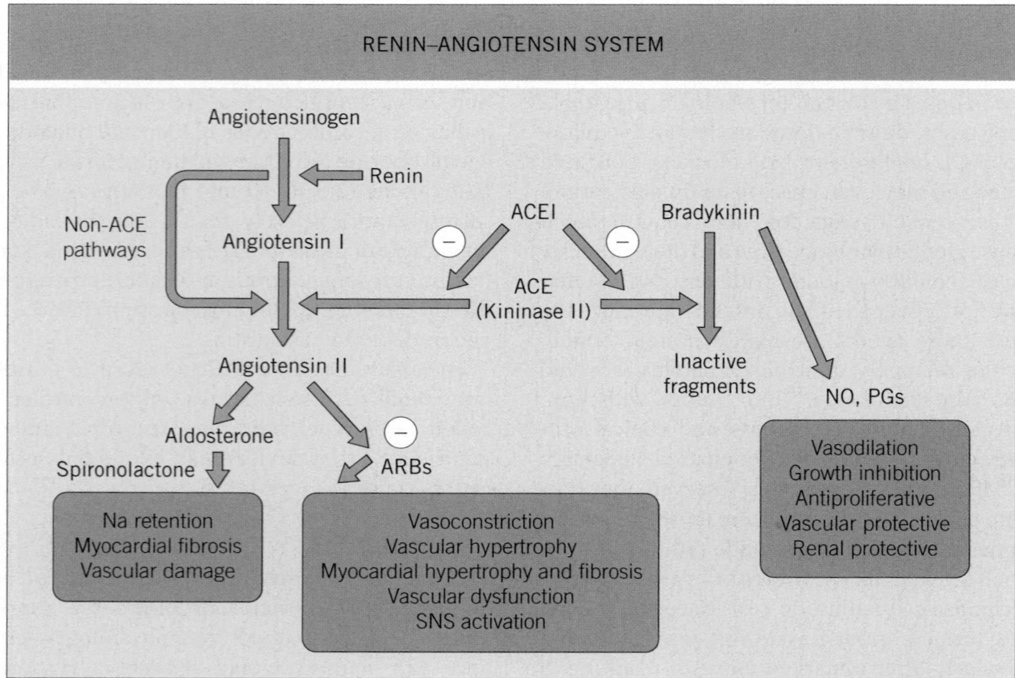

Figure 72.2 Renin-angiotensin system. ACE, angiotensin-converting enzyme; ACEI, ACE inhibitor; ARBs, angiotensin receptor blockers; NO, nitric oxide; PGs, prostaglandins; SNS, sympathetic nervous system.

Indications

There is compelling evidence that inhibition of the renin-angiotensin-aldosterone system results in symptomatic and prognostic improvement in patients with CHF and prevents progressive deterioration of left ventricular function in patients with asymptomatic systolic dysfunction.[4,5,18,31,39,44] This has been demonstrated both early after large myocardial infarction and in patients with chronically reduced ejection fractions. Three classes of agents are available that inhibit some components of the renin-angiotensin-aldosterone system: ACE inhibitors, ARBs, and aldosterone antagonists. However, the more frequent and severe occurrence of angioedema with vasopeptidase inhibitors without counterbalancing evidence of greater benefit may prevent their approval. Table 72.7 lists the most commonly used inhibitors of the renin-angiotensin-aldosterone system, with their mechanisms of action, doses, and major clinical results in patients with CHF and left ventricular systolic dysfunction. These are discussed in greater detail in the following.

Angiotensin-Converting Enzyme Inhibitors

Results of Clinical Trials

The clinical experience with ACE inhibitors is now enormous. These agents have been shown to improve symptoms and exercise tolerance and to prolong survival in patients with severe and mild to moderate CHF and in asymptomatic chronic and post–myocardial infarction left ventricular systolic dysfunction.[4,5,18,31,39,44] A meta-analysis of the results of most of the major trials reported a total mortality reduction of 23% (95% confidence interval [CI], 12% to 33%) and a reduction in the composite of total mortality plus CHF-related admissions to the hospital of 35% (95% CI, 26% to 43%).[18]

Indications and Recommendations for Use

On the basis of these results, there is widespread consensus that patients with symptomatic CHF or asymptomatic left ventricular ejection fractions of less than 40% should be treated with an

INHIBITORS OF THE RENIN-ANGIOTENSIN-ALDOSTERONE SYSTEM IN CHRONIC HEART FAILURE			
Class and Drug	**Usual Starting Dose**	**Usual Target Dose**	**Results of Major Trials**
Angiotensin-converting enzyme inhibitors			
Captopril	12.5 mg q8h	50 mg q8h	Multicenter trial[45]: ↑exercise tolerance, ↓symptoms in moderate CHF SAVE[9]: ↑survival, ↓CHF in post–myocardial infarction left ventricular dysfunction
Enalapril	2.5 mg q12h	10 mg q12h	CONSENSUS[46]: ↑survival in severe CHF SOLVD treatment[17]: ↑survival, ↓hospitalizations in mild-moderate CHF SOLVD prevention[10]: ↓new-onset CHF in asymptomatic left ventricular dysfunction V-HeFT II[46]: ↑survival compared with hydralazine-nitrates in moderate CHF
Lisinopril	5 mg q24h	20 mg q24h	Multicenter trials: ↑exercise tolerance, ↓symptoms in mild to moderate CHF ATLAS[47]: ↓mortality and morbidity with high-dose (35 mg) versus low dose (5 mg) in moderate to severe CHF
Ramipril	2.5 mg q12h	5 mg q12h	AIRE[48]: ↓mortality, ↓worsening CHF in post–myocardial infarction heart failure
Angiotensin receptor blockers			
Losartan	25 mg q24h	50 mg q24h or q12h	ELITE I[49]: effects on renal function and sex similar to those of captopril in elderly CHF patients ELITE II[50]: trend toward ↓survival versus captopril in elderly CHF patients OPTIMAAL[51]: trend toward ↓survival versus captopril in post–myocardial infarction patients
Valsartan	80 mg q24h	160-320 mg q24h	Val-HeFT[52,53]: large trial of valsartan versus placebo added to ACE inhibitor, showing no difference in survival but a small reduction in survival plus hospitalizations for heart failure. An impressive reduction in mortality and morbidity was seen in patients who were not receiving ACE inhibitors at baseline.
Candesartan	4-8 mg q24h	16-32 mg q24h	CHARM[54]: large program evaluating candesartan versus placebo added to ACE and versus placebo in ACE-intolerant patients in patients with ejection fraction >40%; results pending
Irbesartan	75 mg	150-300 mg	I-Preserve: 3600-patient trial in patients with heart failure and preserved ejection fraction (≥45%)
Aldosterone antagonists			
Spironolactone	25 mg q24h	25 mg q24h	RALES[23]: ↑survival, ↓hospitalizations in severe CHF
Eplerenone	50 mg q24h	50-100 mg q24h	EPHESUS[55]: 17% reduction in mortality in post–myocardial infarction patients with ejection fraction ≤40% and heart failure

Table 72.7 Inhibitors of the renin-angiotensin-aldosterone system in chronic heart failure.

ACE inhibitor unless it is not tolerated or is contraindicated. Although physicians have been very cautious in prescribing these agents, there are few contraindications to their use. These include pregnancy, history of angioedema, known severe bilateral renal artery stenosis, and uncorrected hyperkalemia (potassium concentration >5.5 mmol/L). Although ACE inhibitors may cause significant and sometimes symptomatic hypotension and worsening renal function when they are initiated, even systolic blood pressures below 80 mm Hg (if asymptomatic) and serum creatinine concentrations above 3.0 mmol/L are not absolute contraindications to their use if appropriate caution and monitoring are used. Patients with increased risk of early hypotension, renal dysfunction, or hyperkalemia include those with preceding low blood pressures (systolic <100 mm Hg), preexisting renal dysfunction or prerenal azotemia, or hyponatremia (a marker of activation of the renin-angiotensin system) and diabetic individuals with nephropathy or preexisting hyperkalemia.

In patients who do not fall into these high-risk groups, the starting doses should be as follows: captopril, 12.5 mg every 8 hours; enalapril, 2.5 mg every 12 hours; lisinopril, 5 mg every 24 hours; ramipril, 2.5 mg every 24 hours; or the equivalent with other agents. Patients should be instructed to report symptoms of hypotension, and blood pressure, renal function, and serum potassium concentrations should be measured after 1 to 2 weeks. Doses may be incremented at 1- to 2-week intervals. Patients in the aforementioned higher risk groups should have their treatment initiated at half these doses; they also need to be monitored more closely. In these patients, it is advisable to initiate treatment with captopril because the peak hypotensive response occurs at 30 to 60 minutes, allowing monitoring in the clinic. Telephone contact after 24 to 72 hours is advisable, and laboratory testing should be performed no later than 1 week after initiation of treatment. Longer acting, more convenient agents may be substituted after dose titration.

Two important unresolved issues are whether one ACE inhibitor is preferred to another and what the target dose should be. Because there are favorable clinical outcome data for at least six ACE inhibitors in CHF or related settings, it is likely that the benefits are class effects. Most trials have used higher target doses than are used in clinical practice (150 to 300 mg of captopril, 20 to 40 mg of enalapril, or the equivalent) and have achieved relatively high maintenance doses (captopril >100 mg/day, enalapril >15 mg/day), even in patients with severe CHF. The Assessment of Treatment with Lisinopril and Survival (ATLAS) trial showed a beneficial trend in survival and a significant 25% reduction in the composite of mortality plus admissions to the hospital for heart failure in patients treated with doses of lisinopril close to 30 mg compared with doses of 5 mg.[47] Thus, it is recommended that doses for patients be titrated to the target doses used in the major trials, if these are tolerated. Asymptomatic hypotension, increases in serum creatinine concentration that stabilize, and potassium concentrations of 5.0 to 5.4 mmol/L should not be considered contraindications to further up-titration if appropriate caution is used.

Adverse Effects

Apart from the adverse effects discussed before, ACE inhibitors are generally safe and well tolerated. The most common side effect is dizziness, which is often unrelated to blood pressure changes and occurs in 5% to 15% of patients. This often resolves spontaneously or with adjustment in concomitant medication (by avoiding simultaneous administration of several vasodilating or hypotensive agents). A chronic nonproductive cough occurs in 5% to 10% of patients (more frequently in women) and usually requires discontinuation if it recurs after rechallenge. Rashes occur in 1% to 3% of patients (most commonly with captopril), and angioedema occurs in less than 0.3% (more frequently in African Americans).

Angiotensin Receptor Blockers

Results of Clinical Trials

The rationale for and theoretical limitations to the use of ARBs are discussed earlier and have recently been reviewed.[39] These agents have been shown to improve hemodynamic measurements in patients, without or with concomitant ACE inhibitor therapy.[56,57] The Evaluation of Losartan in the Elderly (ELITE) trial tested the hypothesis that the ARB losartan would cause less renal dysfunction than the ACE inhibitor captopril. No difference was observed,[49] but an unexpectedly lower number of deaths was observed in the losartan group, although the number of events was very small. The much larger ELITE II trial was designed to test the hypothesis that losartan is superior to captopril in prolonging survival in patients with CHF.[50] This trial not only did not confirm the earlier result but demonstrated a trend to a greater mortality rate with losartan (hazard ratio, 1.13; CI, 0.9-1.35; $P = .16$). The occurrence of the secondary endpoint of sudden death plus resuscitated cardiac arrest was also greater with losartan (hazard ratio, 1.25; CI, 0.98-1.60; $P = .08$). A subsequent post–myocardial infarction trial, the Optimal Trial in Myocardial Infarction with Angiotensin II Antagonist Losartan (OPTIMAAL), comparing captopril and losartan, also exhibited a trend toward poorer survival with losartan than with captopril (relative risk, 1.13; 95% CI, 0.99-1.28; $P = .07$).[51] Whether these results are specific to losartan or to the relatively low dose used (50 mg once daily) or reflect a general advantage of ACE inhibitors over ARBs in these patients is uncertain. Trials soon to be completed that are using more potent doses of candesartan and valsartan in patients with heart failure and after myocardial infarction will address this question.[54,58] The Valsartan Heart Failure Trial (Val-HeFT) evaluated the effect of adding the ARB valsartan to optimally treated patients, of whom 85% were receiving ACE inhibitors and 34% were receiving beta blockers.[52] There was no difference in survival but a 13% lower incidence of the coprimary endpoint of mortality and heart failure morbidity (primarily admissions to the hospital for worsening CHF). The most impressive finding in this study was the highly significant reductions in mortality and combined mortality and morbidity in the 366 patients who were not taking ACE inhibitors.[53] This trial provides the first evidence that ARBs share the beneficial effects on prognosis observed with ACE inhibitors.

Indications and Recommendations for Use

Although confirmation is awaited from current trials, it is reasonable to recommend an ARB for patients with heart failure who do not tolerate an ACE inhibitor because of cough and, possibly, angioedema. However, the relative efficacy of these two classes is not clear, and the results with losartan raise the possibility that they are not equivalent.

Aldosterone Antagonists

Clinical Trial Results

In the past, it was assumed that ACE inhibitors would suppress aldosterone concentrations, and therefore spironolactone was not considered for treatment of CHF. Indeed, because of the potential risk of hyperkalemia with the two agents together, spironolactone was generally considered to be contraindicated. However, the observation that aldosterone concentrations remain increased in CHF despite chronic treatment with ACE inhibitors and experimental data indicating that spironolactone prevents myocardial fibrosis in models of hypertension and left ventricular hypertrophy led to a reconsideration of its role.[43] To this end, the Randomized Aldactone Evaluation Study (RALES) trial—a survival study in 1663 patients with severe CHF defined by NYHA class IV symptoms at entry or within the previous 30 days and ejection fractions of less than 35%—was undertaken, comparing spironolactone (25 mg/day) with placebo.[59] To the surprise of most physicians and many investigators, spironolactone was associated with a 30% reduction in mortality (95% CI, 18%-40%; $P < .001$) and a 35% lower occurrence of death plus admission to the hospital because of CHF (95% CI, 23%-46%). Serious hyperkalemia was uncommon, but patients were observed carefully, with frequent laboratory testing. In practice, spironolactone has been used in less severe heart failure, sometimes in place of or in the absence of concomitant diuretic treatment, raising important safety concerns.[60]

A new, more selective aldosterone antagonist, eplerenone, should become available shortly. This agent has been investigated in hypertensive patients and appears to be as effective as spironolactone. Eplerenone has not been studied in CHF, but a large trial of post–myocardial infarction patients with heart failure or left ventricular dysfunction, EPHESUS (EPlerenone's neuroHormonal Efficacy and SUrvival Study),[55] demonstrated a 17% reduction in death, with the main impact being on sudden death, and a significant decrease in heart failure hospitalizations. Importantly, these benefits were observed on top of ACE inhibitors and beta blockers in most patients.

Indications and Recommendations for Use

Although the RALES results are striking, they should not be extrapolated to very different groups of patients. Thus, spironolactone should be given to patients with NYHA class IV CHF who are receiving ACE inhibitors or those with advanced class III symptoms who are receiving substantial doses of loop diuretics. Although routine use of spironolactone in patients with milder CHF is not recommended, it may be reasonable to use this agent in place of potassium replacement in those with diuretic-induced hypokalemia. It should not be substituted for an ACE inhibitor and probably should not be used in place of standard diuretics in patients with fluid retention. Additional information is required before recommendations can be made concerning eplerenone.

Adverse Effects

The main concern with aldosterone antagonists is hyperkalemia, and close monitoring is required. In RALES, potassium concentrations were measured every 4 weeks for 12 weeks and then at 3-month intervals, but an earlier measurement 7 to 14 days after initiation is prudent. Breast enlargement or pain was observed in 10% of men. Eplerenone, which has a lower affinity for androgen and progesterone receptors, may minimize this side effect, but a relatively high risk of hyperkalemia has been noted in hypertension studies, especially in diabetic patients.

Beta Blockers

Mechanisms of Action

Activation of the sympathetic nervous system in CHF and its adverse prognostic significance have been recognized for many years.[61] However, it has been uncertain whether sympathetic activation is an adaptive response that serves as a marker for severe CHF, whether it has a mechanistic role in the progression of myocardial dysfunction, or whether it exerts both roles at different stages of the disease. High concentrations of catecholamines are known to cause acute and chronic myocardial damage in humans (e.g., with pheochromocytomas) and in experimental models, but whether this process occurs in CHF and how it occurs are unclear.

Potential mechanisms by which excessive catecholamine stimulation may cause myocardial damage include energetic imbalance (oxygen requirements exceeding supply), stimulation of pathologic myocardial hypertrophy, down-regulation and uncoupling of adrenergic receptors, desensitization of contractile proteins, increased oxidative stress, and induction of apoptosis.[16,61-63] In addition, sympathetic activation and catecholamines can provoke arrhythmias by a variety of mechanisms. However, the conclusive evidence for the deleterious effects of sympathetic nervous system activation has come not from the laboratory but from the clinic, as treatment with beta blockers has proved not dangerous but rather protective and beneficial.

Results of Clinical Trials

More than 14,000 patients with CHF have now been studied in randomized, placebo-controlled trials of beta blockers with mortality or mortality and morbidity endpoints.[25,63] This experience substantially exceeds that with ACE inhibitors in CHF. Of the large-scale trials, three have used the β_1-selective agents bisoprolol and metoprolol: the Cardiac Insufficiency Bisoprolol (CIBIS I) study,[64] the CIBIS II trial,[20] and the Metoprolol Randomized Intervention Trial in Heart Failure (MERIT-HF).[21] Three have used the nonselective agents carvedilol and bucindolol: the U.S. carvedilol trials,[19] the Carvedilol Prospective Randomized Cumulative Survival Study (COPERNICUS),[65] and the Beta-blocker Evaluation of Survival Trial (BEST).[66] Carvedilol also has alpha-blocking activity, and bucindolol produces mild vasodilatation by a mechanism that is not clearly defined but may be intrinsic sympathomimetic activity. In all these studies, the beta blocker was added to background treatment that included diuretics and ACE inhibitors in the great majority and digoxin in many of the participants. Most of the patients had NYHA class II or class III symptoms, with a smaller number having class IV symptoms. The patients in COPERNICUS had severe class III or class IV symptoms but were required to be stable at the time of entry to the study. The upper limit for ejection fraction was generally 35% or 40%, but it was 25% in COPERNICUS.

Table 72.8 summarizes the results from these trials. With the important exception of BEST, in each of the trials with more than 1000 participants, beta-blocker therapy produced substantial and highly significant reductions in mortality, exceeding 30%. In BEST, the 10% lower mortality rate with bucindolol was not statistically significant and differed substantially from that observed with the other agents.[66] Whether

MAJOR BETA-BLOCKER HEART FAILURE TRIALS				
Drug and Trial	**Starting Dose**	**Target Dose**	**Population**	**Main Results**
Metoprolol (β_1 selective) MERIT-HF[21]	12.5-25 mg q24h (SR)	200 mg q24h	Class II-IV*	34% ↓ mortality, 41% ↓ sudden death, ↓hospitalizations
Bisoprolol (β_1 selective) CIBIS I[64] CIBIS II[20]	1.25 mg q24h	5 mg q24h	Class II-III	Trend toward ↓ mortality, ↓hospitalizations
	1.25 mg q24h	10 mg q24h	Class III-IV*	34% ↓ mortality, 44% ↓ sudden death, ↓hospitalizations
Carvedilol (nonselective, weak alpha blockade)	3.125 mg q12h	25-50 mg q12h	Class II-III	38% ↓ death + cardiovascular hospitalizations
U.S. trials program[19] COPERNICUS[65]	3.125 mg q24h	25 mg q12h	Class III-IV	35% ↓ death, 24% ↓ death or hospitalization
Bucindolol (nonselective, weak vasodilator) BEST[66]	3 mg q12h	50-100 mg q12h	Class III-IV	Nonsignificant 10% ↓ in mortality, ↓hospitalizations
Carvedilol vs. metoprolol IR COMET[67]	Carvedilol, 3.125 mg bid	Carvedilol, 25 mg bid	Class II-IV*	17% ↓ in mortality with carvedilol compared with metoprolol IR
	Metoprolol IR, 5 mg bid	Metoprolol IR, 50 mg bid		

*Class IV patients in MERIT-HF and CIBIS II had relatively low mortality rates and probably did not have very severe CHF.

Table 72.8 Major beta-blocker heart failure trials.

this can be attributed to differences in characteristics of the patients (BEST included sicker patients and a substantial proportion of blacks, neither of which groups benefited), differences in the pharmacology of the study drug (possible intrinsic sympathomimetic activity), or chance is unclear. However, COPERNICUS enrolled patients with equally severe or more severe CHF and had a strikingly positive result with carvedilol, which is a nonselective beta blocker.[65] Sudden cardiac death was also reduced by 40% to 50%.[25] When assessed in these trials, symptoms consistently improved, but exercise capacity did not increase. Importantly, in all of these large studies, there were significant reductions in CHF hospitalizations. Although early deterioration was observed in some patients treated with beta blockers, during long-term therapy, withdrawals for worsening heart failure were generally less frequent in the beta blocker–treated patients.

Indications and Recommendations for Use

This large favorable clinical trial experience supports a recommendation that beta blockers be used in all patients with CHF who have stable class II or class III symptoms attributable to left ventricular systolic dysfunction unless contraindicated.[4,5] On the basis of the results of COPERNICUS and the small numbers of patients with severe heart failure in CIBIS II and MERIT, patients with current or recent class IV symptoms should also be treated if they are clinically stable and free of volume overload and the treating physician is experienced in management of these patients.

The role of beta blockers in asymptomatic left ventricular dysfunction is less well established, but the favorable results from a group of 366 patients within the U.S. carvedilol trials and the extensive experience with beta blockers in postinfarction patients suggest that beta blockers should be considered in these patients also. Evidence for the use of beta blockers in postinfarction patients with reduced systolic function has been strengthened by the findings of the Carvedilol Post-Infarct Survival Control in Left Ventricular Dysfunction (CAPRICORN) study,[11] in which 1959 patients with recent myocardial infarction and ejection fraction no greater than 40% were treated with carvedilol titrated to 25 mg twice daily or placebo. Mortality was lower in the carvedilol group (hazard ratio, 0.77; CI, 0.60-0.98; P =.03), as was the composite of death or recurrent nonfatal infarction (hazard ratio, 0.71; CI, 0.57-0.89; P =.002).

The keys to the successful use of beta blockers are the selection of appropriate candidates, initiation of treatment at very low doses, and gradual up-titration with close monitoring (Table 72.9). In general, patients should be stable and free of significant volume overload when beta blockers are initiated because early deterioration may occur. Diuretics and ACE inhibitors should be initiated, and their doses should be stabilized. However, recent trials have demonstrated that once they are stabilized, patients with advanced heart failure and patients in whom treatment with beta blockers is initiated at the end of hospital admissions may actually exhibit the greatest benefit, although some of them will not tolerate these drugs. Contraindications to the use of beta blockers include asthma or severe chronic obstructive pulmonary disease with bronchospasm, symptomatic bradycardia or atrioventricular block, and insulin-requiring diabetes with frequent hypoglycemic episodes. Most patients with chronic obstructive pulmonary disease, however, tolerate at least low-dose beta-blocker treatment well, although use of a β_1-selective agent is preferable. Patients with heart rates below 60 beats per minute need to be monitored closely and may benefit less than those with resting tachycardia. Asymptomatic hypotension (systolic blood pressure <80 to 90 mm Hg) is not a contraindication but may make carvedilol, with its alpha-blocking activity, a less favorable choice.

The usual starting doses of beta blockers are carvedilol, 3.125 mg every 12 hours; metoprolol tartrate (immediate release), 6.25 mg or 12.5 mg every 12 hours (or every

RECOMMENDATIONS FOR ADMINISTRATION OF BETA BLOCKERS IN CHRONIC HEART FAILURE
Candidates
Stable class II or class III symptoms and left ventricular ejection fraction <40%-45%
Stable class IV patients without fluid retention
Asymptomatic patients with reduced ejection fraction
No clinical evidence of fluid retention (rales, edema, significantly increased jugular venous pressure)
Receiving stable doses of ACE inhibitors and diuretics
Heart rate >60 beats per minute and absence of more than first-degree atrioventricular block
No noncardiac contraindications to beta blockade
Starting doses
Carvedilol, 3.125 mg q12h
Metoprolol tartrate, 6.25-12.5 mg q12h or q24h in severe heart failure
Metoprolol succinate (extended release), 12.5-25 mg q24h
Bisoprolol, 1.25 mg q24h
Monitoring
If pretreatment systolic blood pressure <100 mm Hg, observe blood pressure during 1-2 hours for carvedilol
Patient to report change in weight, edema, or dyspnea immediately
Telephone contact after 3-5 days for more symptomatic patients
Examination or telephone contact within 2 weeks in all patients
Titration
Up-titration (dose doubling) at intervals of at least 2 weeks
Target doses are carvedilol, 25 mg q12h; metoprolol tartrate, 50-75 mg q12h; metoprolol succinate, 200 mg q24h; bisoprolol, 10 mg q24h
Management of adverse effects
Dizziness, hypotension (most common with carvedilol, usually early and transient)
No intervention necessary if mild
Stagger other hypotensive medications
If necessary, temporarily reduce vasodilators (nitrates, ACE inhibitors)
Fluid retention, worsening dyspnea
Increase diuretics if mild and continue same dose of beta blocker
If more than mild, reduce beta-blocker dose and increase diuretics
When stable, try to increase beta-blocker dose at more gradual rate
Bradycardia
Obtain electrocardiogram to exclude atrioventricular block or sinus node dysfunction
May continue beta blocker if asymptomatic and heart rate >50 beats per minute
Consider pacemaker if indication for beta blocker is strong
Management of decompensation
Diuretics are first line of therapy
Try to avoid abrupt discontinuation of beta blocker, but may reduce by 50% and taper gradually if necessary
Inotropic support with dobutamine or milrinone (milrinone may be more effective with beta blocker)

Table 72.9 Recommendations for administration of beta blockers in chronic heart failure.

24 hours in patients with more severe CHF); metoprolol succinate (extended release), 12.5 to 25 mg every 24 hours; and bisoprolol, 1.25 mg every 24 hours. Patients should be counseled to weigh themselves daily and promptly report weight gains of 3 pounds (1.5 kg), edema, or increased dyspnea. Telephone contact within a few days is advisable in patients with more severe symptoms, any degree of prior fluid retention, and low blood pressure or heart rate before treatment. Titration should occur in intervals of no less than 2 weeks and may be performed at routine visits at longer intervals. Approximately 10% of stable patients will experience some degree of worsening heart failure, usually several days after the first or second titration step. This can generally be managed by increasing the doses of diuretics while maintaining or dropping back one step on the dose of beta blocker. The other relatively frequent side effects during

titration are dizziness and postural hypotension. These are more common with carvedilol but usually resolve spontaneously or by staggering the doses of concomitant hypotensive medications. In some cases, doses of other vasodilators, such as nitrates or ACE inhibitors, need to be temporarily reduced. In the clinical trials, most patients tolerated titration to the target doses (carvedilol, 25 mg every 12 hours; bisoprolol, 10 mg every 24 hours; metoprolol tartrate, 50 to 75 mg every 12 hours; and extended-release metoprolol, 200 mg every 24 hours). Therefore, titration to these doses is recommended, although there is evidence that patients who do not attain them still sustain benefit.

The dramatic, approximately 35% reduction in mortality achieved in trials with carvedilol, metoprolol (extended release), and bisoprolol emphasizes the importance of administering a beta blocker to all patients with systolic heart failure unless they have contraindications or intolerance. Because the 3029-patient Carvedilol or Metoprolol European Trial (COMET) demonstrated a 17% reduction (hazard ratio, 0.83; 95% CI, 0.74-0.93; P =.0017) in mortality with carvedilol (target dose, 25 mg twice daily; mean total daily dose, 42 mg) compared with immediate-release metoprolol (target dose, 50 mg twice daily; mean daily dose, 85 mg),[67] the question of whether there is a preferred beta blocker for heart failure patients arises. It is unclear and controversial whether the COMET result reflects insufficient magnitude or duration of $beta_1$ blockade with immediate-release metoprolol or additional benefits of the $beta_2$ and alpha blockade afforded by carvedilol.

Adverse Effects

The side effects of beta blockers are well known. The primary additional concern in heart failure is the potential for early deterioration in patients who are relying on adrenergic activity for compensation. How to avoid or to deal with this possibility is discussed in the preceding section. However, in the major trials, treatment with beta blockers was exceedingly well tolerated, with adverse events and withdrawals occurring no more frequently in the active treatment group than in the placebo group.

Digitalis Glycosides (Digoxin)

The initiating abnormality in most patients with CHF is failure of the pumping performance of the left ventricle. This is a result of impaired myocardial contractile function or loss of contractile units. Therefore, use of drugs that increase myocardial contractility is a logical approach to treatment. Indeed, digitalis glycosides are the oldest pharmacologic treatment for CHF, and one, digoxin, remains in widespread use. However, more potent positive inotropic agents that work by different mechanisms of action (β-adrenoreceptor stimulation or phosphodiesterase inhibition) have been repeatedly found to accelerate the progression of CHF and to reduce survival, so digitalis remains the only commonly used positive inotropic agent for long-term treatment.

Mechanisms of Action

The digitalis glycosides bind to and competitively inhibit the Na^+,K^+-ATPase on the cardiac myocyte cell membrane and in other tissues.[68] Inhibition of this energy-dependent pump results in increased concentrations of intracellular Na^+, which favor Na^+-Ca^{2+} exchange. The greater cytosolic Ca^{2+} concentrations then increase contractile protein cross-bridge formation and myocyte shortening. In recent years, it has become clear that the digitalis glycosides have additional noncardiac effects.[69] These agents sensitize carotid and cardiac baroreceptors, which results in reduced central nervous system sympathetic outflow and a decrease in circulating concentrations of norepinephrine. Other data indicate a direct or indirect suppression of renal renin release. To what extent these actions play a part in the clinical response to digitalis is unknown, but they may distinguish these agents from drugs with more powerful positive inotropic effects.

Results of Clinical Trials

The digitalis glycosides have long been the subject of controversy; both experts and practitioners hold markedly divergent views on their efficacy and safety. Much of this disagreement resulted from poorly designed, often very short duration studies that included patients whose degree of left ventricular dysfunction was unknown and used surrogate endpoints. Studies during the past 2 decades have clarified this picture. Several moderate-sized placebo-controlled studies examined the effect of digoxin on symptoms, exercise tolerance, and clinical status in patients with low ejection fractions and moderate to severe CHF symptoms.[70-73] Each showed a clear benefit with regard to these endpoints. The Prospective Randomized Study of Ventricular Function and Efficacy of Digoxin (PROVED) and Randomized Assessment of Digoxin and Inhibitors of Angiotensin-Converting Enzyme (RADIANCE) were withdrawal trials in patients without and with ACE inhibitor background treatment, respectively.[72,73] Figure 72.3 illustrates the primary results—the incidence of death or deterioration during the 90-day period of observation. These results indicate that digoxin prevented worsening of CHF in patients with or without concomitant ACE inhibitor treatment but that the lowest rate of deterioration occurred in patients maintained with a diuretic, ACE inhibitor, and digoxin.

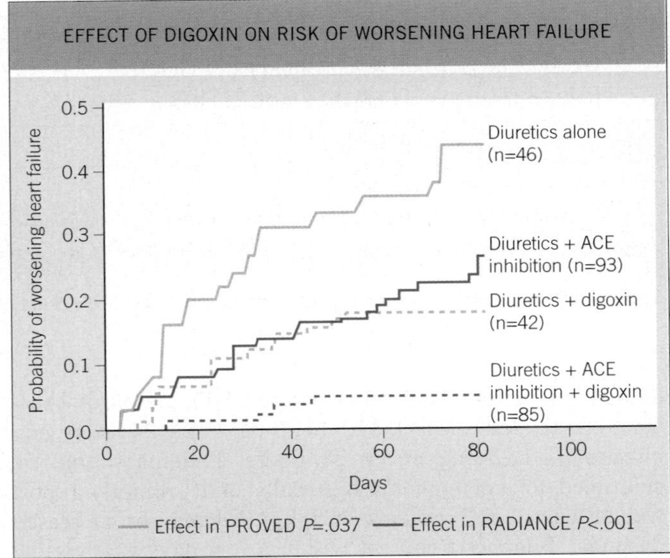

Figure 72.3 Effect of digoxin on risk of worsening heart failure. ACE, angiotensin-converting enzyme.

The Digitalis Investigation Group (DIG) trial evaluated the effect of digitalis on survival in 6800 patients with NYHA class II and class III CHF in sinus rhythm with ejection fractions of less than 45%.[74] During a mean follow-up period of 37 months, no difference was noted between patients randomly assigned to receive digoxin or placebo. There were fewer deaths from worsening CHF in those receiving digoxin, but these were balanced by a greater number from myocardial infarction or sudden death. Digoxin reduced the occurrence of admissions to the hospital for worsening heart failure by 28%. The greatest benefit was seen in patients with more severe symptoms, lower ejection fractions, and greater left ventricular dilatation. This result together with those of the earlier studies indicates that digoxin improves the symptoms of CHF and prevents its deterioration, particularly in patients with more severe left ventricular dysfunction, but neither increases nor decreases survival.

Indications and Recommendations for Use

On the basis of the aforementioned trial results, digoxin can be recommended primarily for patients with CHF and reduced ejection fractions who remain symptomatic despite optimal treatment with diuretics and ACE inhibitors. Because it appears to be more effective in patients with more severe symptoms and systolic dysfunction, it may be preferable to initiate digoxin before the use of beta blockers in this subgroup, but because of the beneficial prognostic effect of beta blockers, they are a more appropriate third agent for patients with mild to moderate CHF. In patients who are in atrial fibrillation or have episodic supraventricular tachyarrhythmias, digoxin may be an appropriate first-line agent. There are no data to support the use of digoxin in patients with asymptomatic left ventricular dysfunction.

Digoxin is cleared by the kidney, and downward adjustments of the dose are necessary for patients with renal dysfunction and low lean body mass (both of which are frequent in the elderly). Nomograms are available with which to estimate the appropriate starting dose of digoxin,[74] but as a rule, doses of 0.25 mg/day are appropriate for normal-sized patients with normal serum creatinine concentration who are younger than 70 years. Doses of 0.125 mg/day are appropriate for smaller and older individuals, and lower doses should be used with more severe renal dysfunction. A number of drugs will increase serum digoxin concentrations, including quinidine, amiodarone, verapamil, propafenone, flecainide, and spironolactone. Downward adjustments of the dose by about 50% are required with the first four of these. Several drugs, including erythromycin, tetracycline and related antibiotics, and proton pump inhibitors, may increase the gastrointestinal absorption of digoxin. Routine monitoring of digoxin concentrations is not recommended, but measurement after 7 to 10 days is indicated in patients with renal dysfunction or after the initiation of agents that interact with digoxin. The relationship between serum concentrations of digoxin and efficacy is not known, but in general, concentrations between 0.5 and 1.2 ng/mL are considered appropriate. Digoxin toxicity is infrequent with concentrations less than 2 ng/mL and rare at those less than 1.6 ng/mL. Retrospective analyses from several trials have suggested a greater mortality rate in patients with concentrations greater than 1.2 ng/mL, but it is unclear whether this is an effect of excess digoxin or a marker of more severe CHF.

Adverse Effects

Although digoxin toxicity is much feared, it has become relatively uncommon with the improvement in understanding of its pharmacology and the ability to monitor drug concentrations. The most important forms of toxicity are arrhythmias. Digoxin can both stimulate automaticity of junctional and ventricular myocytes and increase atrioventricular block. Common manifestations of increased automaticity are ectopic beats, accelerated junctional rhythms, paroxysmal atrial tachycardia, and ventricular tachycardia. These can often be corrected by administration of potassium, even when potassium concentrations are normal. Lidocaine (lignocaine) or phenytoin may be useful for ventricular tachyarrhythmias. Overdrive pacing is often effective, but electrical cardioversion should be avoided if possible because it may exacerbate ventricular arrhythmias. Conduction abnormalities include sinus bradycardia, sinus arrest, sinoatrial exit block, and atrioventricular block. Often these are asymptomatic and can simply be observed, but if necessary, atropine is usually effective. Rarely is temporary pacing required.

Administration of digoxin-specific Fab fragments can rapidly reverse the effect of digoxin, but this is indicated only in life-threatening situations (generally recurrent ventricular tachycardia or fibrillation, usually after intentional overdosage). The half-life of digoxin Fab fragments is substantially less than that of digoxin itself, so digoxin concentrations may increase and toxicity may recur 24 to 48 hours after its administration.

Other less serious but more common adverse effects of digoxin include nausea and visual disturbances, often described as yellow vision or blurring.

Direct-Acting Vasodilators

The modern era of heart failure management was ushered in by the recognition that alteration of the loading conditions of the left ventricle could modulate cardiac function. This was initially accomplished by agents such as sodium nitroprusside and phentolamine but subsequently with oral or nonparenteral administration of direct-acting vasodilators, such as the inorganic nitrates and hydralazine, which were convenient for chronic treatment. However, with the advent of ACE inhibitors, which achieve the same hemodynamic effects but also prevent the progression of CHF and improve its prognosis, the use of direct-acting vasodilators for CHF has been relegated to adjunctive therapy in special situations. However, organic nitrates and the novel vasodilator nesiritide are useful in the management of acute decompensated heart failure, although this topic is beyond the scope of this chapter.

Mechanisms of Action

Agents that dilate the arteriolar resistance vessels can reduce left ventricular afterload, defined as the impedance to left ventricular ejection but reflected by systemic vascular resistance and left ventricular systolic wall stress. This can facilitate increases in cardiac output as effectively as positive inotropic drugs. Agents that dilate the venous bed reduce left or right ventricular preload, defined as end-diastolic volume or pressure. This results in reduction of left and right atrial pressures, with resultant improvements in dyspnea and edema. Agents or combinations of agents that have both actions can produce marked hemodynamic benefits. These short-term hemodynamic effects occur with many classes of drug, such as the nitrates, hydralazine, minoxidil, alpha blockers, and calcium channel blockers, as well as with inhibitors of the renin-angiotensin system. However, the clinical responses depend on other actions of these drugs, such as whether they stimulate or interfere with neurohormonal systems, whether tolerance to their effects developed, whether they have direct or indirect positive or negative inotropic actions, and whether they produce generalized vasodilatation or differentially affect specific beds.

Results of Clinical Trials

Although many of the aforementioned drugs produced hemodynamic improvement, very few studies showed sustained clinical improvement. However, by current standards, these trials were underpowered to detect meaningful benefit. The Vasodilator Heart Failure (V-HeFT I) trial was the first large-scale trial to evaluate the clinical efficacy of vasodilator therapy and was the first to address the question of whether drug treatment could improve the prognosis of patients with CHF.[75] This study randomly allocated 642 patients with mild to moderate symptoms to groups to receive placebo, prazosin (5 mg every 6 hours), or the combination of hydralazine (50 mg) and isosorbide dinitrate (40 mg every 6 hours). Although prazosin had no effect on survival, the hydralazine–isosorbide dinitrate combination reduced mortality by 34% (95% CI, 4%-54%). However, when the subsequent V-HeFT II trial compared this combination with enalapril, the 2-year mortality rate was 25% lower with the ACE inhibitor as a result of a 38% lower incidence of sudden death.[46]

Subsequent interest centered on the calcium channel blockers, which are potent and better tolerated arteriolar dilators, although they all possess negative inotropic properties in vitro. Anecdotal reports and subsequent retrospective analyses of trials in postinfarction patients indicated that nifedipine, diltiazem, and verapamil could precipitate worsening heart failure. Several trials have evaluated newer dihydropyridine calcium channel blockers, which are relatively more vascular selective. The largest, Prospective Randomized Amlodipine Survival Evaluation (PRAISE), randomly assigned 1153 patients with severe (NYHA class IIIb or class IV) CHF and ejection fractions of less than 30% to amlodipine (10 mg/day) or placebo.[76] There were no significant differences either in the primary endpoint of death from any cause or admission to the hospital for major cardiovascular events or in total mortality. These results confirmed for the first time that a calcium channel blocker could be administered safely to patients with severe CHF. Interestingly, the subset of patients believed to have CHF of a nonischemic etiology exhibited a 31% reduction in the primary endpoint with amlodipine. However, this result was not corroborated in the much larger PRAISE-2 trial, which failed to show any benefit from amlodipine in patients with nonischemic cardiomyopathy.

Despite the apparent safety of amlodipine in patients with CHF, studies with this drug and other vasoselective calcium channel blockers such as felodipine have failed to demonstrate any improvement in symptoms. The relatively small studies with felodipine are also not sufficiently robust to confirm the safety of this agent, and a tendency to more frequent early deterioration was observed.[77,78] Thus, the use of calcium channel blockers should be limited to the treatment of ancillary conditions, such as angina and hypertension, rather than the treatment of CHF itself, and amlodipine should be the preferred agent because it is the only calcium agonist for which safety in patients with CHF has been confirmed.

The Flolan International Randomized Survival Trial (FIRST), which randomly assigned 471 patients with severe CHF to a chronic intravenous infusion of prostacyclin, a potent arterial dilator, or placebo, was terminated prematurely because of a strong trend toward increased mortality without any evidence of symptomatic benefit.[79] More recently, some physicians have begun to administer intermittent infusions of nesiritide, or recombinant B-type natriuretic peptide, to patients with severe heart failure, but there are no data supporting the efficacy of this approach.

Indications and Recommendations for Use

Despite the favorable results of V-HeFT I, the role of direct-acting vasodilators is limited. Although the combination of hydralazine and isosorbide dinitrate is probably safe and may be effective, ACE inhibitors are preferred. In intolerant patients, ARBs are preferable to hydralazine–isosorbide dinitrate because of their greater convenience and tolerability and the accumulating data supporting their beneficial effects on prognosis.[53] The nitrates are effective and safe for the treatment of angina in the CHF population, and hydralazine may be helpful in diminishing mitral regurgitation when this is severe.[80] Calcium channel blockers are not indicated for the treatment of CHF, but amlodipine may be considered for the management of concomitant angina refractory to nitrates or persistent hypertension. However, beta blockers should be considered first because they have a well-demonstrated beneficial effect on prognosis.

Adverse Effects

The side effects of the available vasodilators are well known. Nitrates produce headache and gastrointestinal side effects, and hydralazine induces nausea and, rarely, the drug-induced lupus syndrome. Approximately 20% of patients will not tolerate one or both agents, and a larger number will not achieve the recommended doses. Amlodipine, although safe overall, causes fluid retention in some patients with CHF and may be associated with a greater incidence of pulmonary edema.[76]

Chronic or Intermittent Use of Positive Inotropic Drugs

Digoxin is the only oral agent with positive inotropic actions that is available in the United States, but many others have been investigated.[81] These have included β-adrenoreceptor agonists (xamoterol, pirbuterol, and sustained infusions of dobutamine) and phosphodiesterase inhibitors (including milrinone, amrinone, enoximone, pimobendan, and flosequinan). Both of these classes of drug increase intracellular cyclic adenosine monophosphate, with resultant increases in cytosolic Ca^{2+}, which mediates the enhanced contractile response. All the agents studied thus far have significantly increased mortality or have been associated with a trend toward increased mortality, primarily as a result of markedly more occurrences of sudden death.[82-84] Indeed, this may be the disadvantage that goes with the reduction in sudden death observed with beta blockers. Furthermore, although acute hemodynamic improvement with these agents is often dramatic, evidence of sustained clinical benefit is lacking.

Nonetheless, enthusiasm for chronic positive inotropic treatment persists. Some practitioners use inotropic infusions in the routine management of acute decompensated heart failure. However, a trial in 951 patients, in which newly admitted patients were allocated randomly to either a 48-hour infusion with milrinone or placebo, found a significantly greater incidence of treatment failures and serious adverse effects (sustained hypotension and new-onset atrial fibrillation and ventricular tachycardia or fibrillation) in the milrinone group and no evidence of short- or long-term benefit.[85] Whether this negative result reflects on positive inotropic agents in general or is specific to beta agonists and phosphodiesterase inhibitors is unclear, although a trial demonstrating better outcomes with the calcium sensitizer levosimendan than with dobutamine suggests that there may be important differences among agents.[86]

Another application of positive inotropic therapy has been administration of short-term infusions to outpatients on a recurring basis. Although there is no doubt that inotropic infusions are highly effective in some patients admitted to the hospital with severely decompensated heart failure, particularly those with the cardiorenal syndrome, in which sufficient diuresis cannot be obtained without progressive deterioration of renal function, there are no controlled studies to support the benefit of intermittent infusions to outpatients. Indeed, the two small studies with control groups suggest that this approach may also increase mortality.[87,88]

Antithrombotic Therapy

Many physicians routinely anticoagulate patients with dilated cardiomyopathy, with the goal of preventing systemic arterial emboli from intracardiac thrombi. Although anticoagulation is definitely indicated in appropriate patients with chronic or intermittent atrial fibrillation or flutter, who are at very high risk for embolic events, there are few data to support routine anticoagulation in patients with sinus rhythm.[89] Indeed, in recent trials, the annual incidence of embolic events has been 1% to 3%, which is relatively low compared with the annual mortality rates and far lower than the embolic rate in patients with atrial fibrillation. In prospective studies, it is not even clear that patients with chronic left ventricular thrombi (detected more than 3 to 4 months after myocardial infarction) are at increased risk for embolic events. Therefore, chronic anticoagulation can be recommended only for those patients with CHF with atrial fibrillation or flutter, for those patients with prior embolic events, and perhaps for those with mobile or protruding thrombi.

In contrast, retrospective analyses of nonrandomized subsets of patients enrolled in the Studies of Left Ventricular Dysfunction (SOLVD) trials have reported that patients with CHF who are receiving warfarin may have a lower risk of death, sudden death, and coronary events.[90] Whether these findings are confounded by differences in the characteristics of patients who are treated with warfarin is unclear, and identical analyses from the same trials showed a similar potential benefit from aspirin.[91] However, patients receiving aspirin did not appear to benefit from treatment with ACE inhibitors, raising the possibility of an interaction in which aspirin, by virtue of inhibiting ACE inhibitor–induced increases in prostaglandin production, may diminish the efficacy of ACE inhibition.[92] This hypothesis will be tested in the current Warfarin and Antiplatelet Therapy in Chronic Heart Failure (WATCH) trial, which is comparing warfarin, aspirin, and clopidogrel (an antiplatelet agent that acts through a mechanism that is not cyclooxygenase dependent) in patients with CHF and sinus rhythm.

Until WATCH is completed, physicians should treat patients with CHF and underlying coronary or atherosclerotic vascular disease with an antithrombotic agent (warfarin, aspirin, or possibly clopidogrel), but aspirin should be avoided in those with primary cardiomyopathy.

Antiarrhythmic Treatment

Sudden death is responsible for 40% to 50% of the fatal events in patients with CHF and is particularly devastating in patients with mild symptoms. It has often been assumed that these events are caused by ventricular tachyarrhythmias because ventricular arrhythmias are ubiquitous in patients with CHF, and most episodes of sudden death in patients without CHF are caused by ventricular arrhythmias. However, there is growing evidence that several underlying mechanisms operate. In advanced heart failure, a surprising number of these episodes represent bradyarrhythmias and conduction disturbances, most probably precipitated by worsening pump failure with resultant activation of ventricular baroreceptors and consequent vagal stimulation.[24] A substantial number of episodes of sudden death are induced by acute coronary events, which would explain the lower incidence of sudden death in patients receiving antithrombotic agents, discussed in the previous section.[93]

The most important new observation, however, is that treatment with beta blockers can prevent 40% to 50% of the episodes of sudden death.[25] Therefore, these agents should be the first line of treatment to prevent this outcome. Unfortunately, beyond routine treatment with beta blockers, there are no proven approaches for the identification of patients who are at particularly high risk for sudden death as opposed to death from any cause. Sudden death is most frequent in patients with more severe symptoms, more severe left ventricular dysfunction, and underlying coronary artery disease, but these are the same patients who have the greatest overall mortality. The presence of asymptomatic ventricular arrhythmias adds little to the identification of patients who are candidates for sudden death.[94]

Therefore, the role of treatment with antiarrhythmic agents and devices in the population of patients with heart failure remains controversial and in flux. These topics are discussed in detail in Chapters 66 and 74.

FUTURE APPROACHES TO THE TREATMENT OF CHRONIC HEART FAILURE

Although enormous advances have occurred in the treatment of patients with CHF, mortality rates remain high, and the affected population continues to grow. Therefore, development of new agents that will improve on or supplement existing treatments continues. However, several promising pharmacologic agents for the treatment of CHF have recently failed to show benefit in large clinical trials. These include the vasopeptidase inhibitor omapatrilat, several endothelin antagonists, and two antagonists of tumor necrosis factor α. Although there is now evidence that an ARB is effective in patients who do not tolerate ACE inhibitors, it is disappointing that these two classes are not additive. There are a number of reasons that may explain these failures. One obvious factor is the markedly improved prognosis of patients participating in clinical trials. This in part reflects the vigorous treatment that these individuals receive, making it more difficult to show additive benefits. This may particularly be the case with additional neurohormonal antagonists in patients already receiving effective doses of ACE inhibitors, beta blockers, and, in some cases, spironolactone. These failures may also reflect the choice of the wrong targets or the administration of incorrect dosages. Nevertheless, investigations with promising agents and new approaches continue.[95,96]

The greatest current excitement lies with encouraging results with new devices, including wider use of implantable cardioverter-defibrillators in patients with heart failure,[26] cardiac resynchronization with biventricular pacemakers,[97] and use of left ventricular assist devices as long-term (destination) therapy.[98] These devices are discussed in Chapters 66, 74 and 75, respectively. The appropriate use of these approaches remains to be defined, and economic considerations are likely to play a part. Other novel approaches, such as the use of stem cells and gene therapy, are also under active investigation.

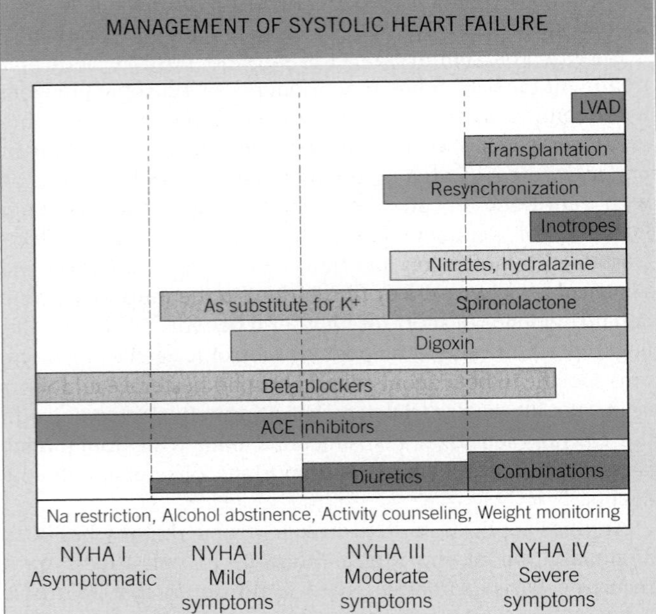

Figure 72.4 Management of systolic heart failure. ACE, angiotensin-converting enzyme; LVAD, left ventricular assist device; NYHA, New York Heart Association.

SUMMARY

From the foregoing, it should be clear that CHF is a serious condition that requires a multifaceted approach for optimal management. Important nonpharmacologic approaches include dietary counseling, recommendations for activity and exercise, and sufficient education of the patient and the patient's family to allow the patients to participate in their own management. Additional programs to improve compliance with medication and monitoring of clinical status have a role, at least in patients with more advanced symptoms.

There are a growing number of effective drugs for the treatment of CHF, and virtually all patients with symptomatic or asymptomatic left ventricular systolic dysfunction require polypharmacy. The art of managing heart failure is to use these agents in the appropriate patients, in the appropriate sequence, and in the appropriate manner. Figure 72.4 illustrates how the various classes of medication should be used in relation to the severity of the patient's symptoms.

Diuretics are the mainstay of management in symptomatic patients but have no role (other than the management of hypertension) in asymptomatic individuals. As symptoms and fluid retention become more severe, doses of diuretics should be increased, and diuretic combinations are often indicated. Optimal use of diuretics is the key to the successful management of advanced heart failure.

ACE inhibitors are indicated in all patients with asymptomatic or symptomatic left ventricular systolic dysfunction. Contraindications to and adverse effects of ACE inhibitors are few, and neither asymptomatic hypotension nor moderate to severe renal dysfunction should dissuade physicians from using them. Doses should be titrated to concentrations that have proved to be effective in clinical trials. On the basis of the results of recent trials, ARBs appear to be effective alternatives to ACE inhibitors in patients intolerant of them.

Beta blockers have proved to be strikingly effective and are indicated for much more widespread use. They are indicated in patients with stable NYHA class II, class III, and class IV CHF and are likely to be effective in patients with asymptomatic left ventricular systolic dysfunction. Despite the appropriate concern of physicians about using agents that have, until recently, been contraindicated in patients with CHF, they are generally well tolerated. The key is appropriate selection of the patient, use of low initial doses, and slow, careful up-titration. Particular care must be taken in the selection and initiation of beta blockers in patients with class IV CHF, and their use in this group of patients should be reserved for those whose physicians have considerable experience in managing severe heart failure.

The role of digoxin has evolved. With the exception of patients in atrial fibrillation, it is now a third- or fourth-line agent. However, digoxin is effective in reducing the symptoms of heart failure and is generally safe when it is dosed appropriately. Digoxin is recommended primarily for patients who remain symptomatic despite optimal treatment with diuretics and ACE inhibitors. It may be used before or after beta blockers in patients with mild to moderate symptoms but not instead of them.

Spironolactone is an old drug with a new role in CHF. Its efficacy has been demonstrated in patients with advanced heart failure, in whom it should be added to diuretics, ACE inhibitors, and, in most cases, digoxin. Some of these patients may be receiving beta blockers, but others may be too unstable for them. Whether spironolactone is effective in patients with milder symptoms is uncertain, but it is probably appropriate in patients receiving high doses of diuretics who require potassium replacement. Eplerenone, a more selective aldosterone receptor antagonist, is an alternative to spironolactone, especially in patients with side effects related to spironolactone-induced estrogenic activity.

The role of direct-acting vasodilators in this potpourri of drugs is less clear. By and large, they are most useful as ancillary agents for the management of angina and, rarely, persistent hypertension. However, as has been shown in this chapter, nitrates and hydralazine may provide additive benefit in patients who remain symptomatic despite other approaches.

At the far end of the pharmacologic spectrum are the intravenous inotropes. Their use in advanced heart failure is largely based on anecdotal experience; but in a very limited number of patients, they may have a beneficial role. Cardiac resynchronization is a promising and probably more attractive approach to patients with advanced symptoms. Implantable cardioverter-defibrillators will have a growing role in a broad range of heart failure, but defining that role will be difficult. Left ventricular assist devices have proved to be an effective bridge to cardiac transplantation, but technologic improvements and reductions in cost will be essential if they are going to have more than a niche role in long-term management.

chapter 73

Diastolic Heart Failure

Walter J. Paulus, William H. Gaasch, and Michael R. Zile

Definition

- The diagnosis of diastolic heart failure requires three conditions to be simultaneously satisfied: (1) signs or symptoms of congestive heart failure, (2) left ventricular (LV) ejection fraction above 50%, and (3) objective evidence of diastolic LV dysfunction derived from either invasively measured LV filling pressures or echocardiographic/tissue Doppler imaging indices of abnormal diastolic function.

Key Features

- Patients with diastolic heart failure are usually older, more often are women, and frequently have comorbidities such as arterial hypertension, obesity, and diabetes.
- Patients with diastolic heart failure have a concentrically remodeled left ventricle with high LV mass-volume ratio, prominent cardiomyocyte hypertrophy, and alterations in the extracellular matrix.
- Diastolic LV dysfunction is the mechanism responsible for diastolic heart failure, and other coincident hemodynamic abnormalities, such as a high arterial stiffness, exert their effect through worsening of diastolic LV dysfunction.

Management

- Control of arterial hypertension, volume overload, and myocardial ischemia with antihypertensives, diuretics, and revascularization.
- Angiotensin-converting enzyme inhibitors, angiotensin receptor blockers, and beta blockers have a symptomatic but as yet no clearly proven prognostic benefit in diastolic heart failure.

The diagnosis of diastolic heart failure is based on the presence of a triad consisting of signs or symptoms of congestive heart failure, normal or slightly impaired (>50%) left ventricular ejection fraction (LVEF), and objective evidence of diastolic left ventricular (LV) dysfunction. Objective evidence of diastolic LV dysfunction can be obtained by invasive techniques or noninvasive imaging and consists of evidence of abnormal LV relaxation, filling, or diastolic distensibility. Diastolic heart failure currently accounts for more than 50% of all heart failure cases in Western societies. Although prognosis (both mortality and morbidity) of patients with diastolic heart failure was initially perceived to be better than prognosis of patients with systolic heart failure, recent evidence shows prognosis to be equally poor in both conditions.[1] Furthermore, whereas the prognosis of patients with systolic heart failure has improved during the last 2 decennia as a result of modern heart failure therapy, the prognosis of patients with diastolic heart failure has not improved significantly during the same time.[2]

ETIOLOGY AND PATHOLOGIC ANATOMY

In patients with signs or symptoms of congestive heart failure and a normal or slightly impaired LVEF, diastolic LV dysfunction can arise from epicardial fibrosis or calcification, endocardial fibrosis, myocardial fibrosis, myocardial deposits, myocardial hypertrophy, and myocardial ischemia. Specific causes (Table 73.1) include constrictive pericarditis (see Chapter 82); endomyocardial fibrosis (see Chapter 81); radiation-induced myocardial fibrosis; hypertrophic cardiomyopathy (see Chapter 79); hypertensive heart disease; ischemic heart disease; and infiltrative cardiomyopathy (see Chapter 81) with myocardial deposition of amyloid (amyloidosis), iron (hemochromatosis), or glycosphingolipids (Fabry's disease; Fig. 73.1). Myocardial hypertrophy and myocardial fibrosis are usually prominent pathologic features. As a result of myocardial hypertrophy, there frequently is electrocardiographic or echocardiographic evidence of LV hypertrophy.[3-5] In diastolic heart failure, the LV hypertrophy leads to concentric LV remodeling evident from a high LV wall mass-volume ratio and a high relative wall thickness (septal + posterior wall thickness/LV internal diameter; Fig. 73.2). This pattern of LV remodeling contrasts with the LV remodeling observed in patients with systolic heart failure, who frequently present with a lower than normal LV wall mass-volume ratio and a low relative wall thickness.[6] Myocardial ultrastructure also differs between diastolic and systolic heart failure:

- Patients with diastolic heart failure have a cardiomyocyte diameter that on average is 50% larger than the cardiomyocyte diameter observed in patients with systolic heart failure (Fig. 73.3).[6]
- Although it is elevated in both patient groups, patients with diastolic heart failure have lower collagen volume fraction (11%) than that of patients with systolic heart failure (16%).[7]
- On electron microscopic images, patients with diastolic heart failure have higher myofibrillar density than do patients with systolic heart failure,[8] who frequently have loss of myofilaments (Fig. 73.4).

Furthermore, on both electron microscopic and immunofluorescent images stained for α-actinin, patients with diastolic

SPECIFIC CAUSES OF DIASTOLIC HEART FAILURE	
Epicardial fibrosis	Constrictive pericarditis
Endocardial fibrosis	Endomyocardial fibrosis
Myocardial fibrosis	Radiation induced
Myocardial deposits	Amyloidosis
	Hemochromatosis
	Fabry's disease
Myocardial hypertrophy	Hypertrophic cardiomyopathy Hypertensive heart disease
Myocardial ischemia	Ischemic heart disease

Table 73.1 Specific causes of diastolic heart failure.

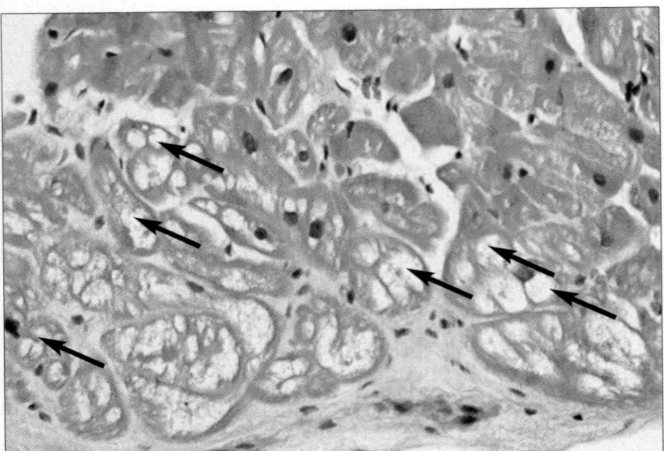

Figure 73.1 Myocardial glycosphingolipid deposition *(arrows)* related to Fabry's disease and observed in a patient with diastolic heart failure.

heart failure have significant widening of the Z disk (Fig. 73.5).[7] Increased myocardial collagen deposition in patients with diastolic heart failure results from altered expression patterns of matrix metalloproteinases and of tissue inhibitors of matrix metalloproteinases. The shift in the balance between matrix metalloproteinases and tissue inhibitors of matrix metalloproteinases is also obvious in plasma; hypertensive patients with LV hypertrophy have decreased expression of matrix metalloproteinases 2 and 13, and hypertensive patients with LV hypertrophy and diastolic heart failure have both decreased expression of matrix metalloproteinases 2 and 13 and increased expression of tissue inhibitors of matrix metalloproteinases 1 and 4.[8] One third of the patients presenting with diastolic heart failure have a normal value of collagen volume fraction in their endomyocardial biopsy samples.[9] Their LV end-diastolic pressure and LV stiffness modulus are, however, comparable to those of patients with a high value of collagen volume fraction in the endomyocardial biopsy tissue. This finding suggests that factors in addition to collagen deposition also contribute to the high in vivo LV stiffness observed in these patients. Intrinsic cardiomyocyte stiffness is one of these factors. Intrinsic cardiomyocyte stiffness is elevated in patients with diastolic heart failure,[9] and this finding could be related to modified expression of the cytoskeletal protein titin. Titin functions as a bidirectional spring responsible for early diastolic LV recoil and late diastolic LV stretch. In patients with systolic heart failure, titin isoform expression shifts toward the more compliant isoform, whereas in patients with diastolic heart failure, such a shift is absent.[6]

PATHOPHYSIOLOGY

Although diastolic heart failure is now widely recognized as an important cause of cardiac morbidity and mortality, it remains uncertain if diastolic heart failure is indeed a distinct heart failure phenotype or a mere precursor stage of systolic heart failure.[10,11] Because of possible continuity of diastolic and systolic heart failure and because diastolic LV dysfunction is not unique to diastolic heart failure but also occurs in patients with systolic heart failure, diastolic heart failure is often referred to as heart failure with normal LVEF or heart failure with preserved LVEF.[12]

Does Diastolic Heart Failure Evolve to Systolic Heart Failure?

Although global LV systolic performance is normal in patients with diastolic heart failure,[13] they have a reduced tissue Doppler LV long-axis shortening velocity.[14] LV long-axis shortening velocity is produced by longitudinal muscle fibers that originate from the mitral annulus, wrap around the apex, and reinsert on the mitral annulus at a location that is opposite to the one from which they depart. Systolic contraction of these fibers results not only in LV long-axis shortening but also in LV twisting, which in contrast to LV long-axis shortening is preserved in patients with diastolic heart failure.[15] This divergence suggests that in patients with diastolic heart failure, the reduced LV long-axis shortening velocity results not from a contractile deficit of these longitudinal muscle fibers but from the LV shape change and a concomitant reduction in long-axis length. Additional reasons for the heart failure syndrome in diastolic heart failure not to arise from disturbed LV long-axis function are the following[16]: as many as 50% of the diastolic heart failure patients in published studies did not exhibit depressed LV long-axis shortening velocity; depressed LV long-axis shortening was also observed in patients with LV hypertrophy and no heart failure; LV long-axis shortening has little impact on LV stroke volume, which is mainly produced by shortening of the LV minor axis; and reported LV long-axis shortening velocity was never normalized for LV or body size.

Continuity between diastolic and systolic heart failure is also inferred from the unimodal distribution of LVEF in registries such as the EuroHeart Failure Survey[17] and in large heart failure trials, such as the CHARM study, which recruited patients with both normal and reduced LVEF.[18] In the EuroHeart Failure Survey, however, the respective distributions of LVEF for both genders clearly differed from one another, with LVEF peaking at 35% in the male heart failure population and at 55% in the female heart failure population (Fig. 73.6)[17]; the unimodal distribution observed in the global population therefore derives from an inappropriate summation of LVEF data of both genders. A median value of 55% observed in the LVEF distribution of the female gender illustrates the high prevalence of diastolic heart failure in women.

Figure 73.2 Contrasting patterns of LV remodeling in systolic and diastolic heart failure.

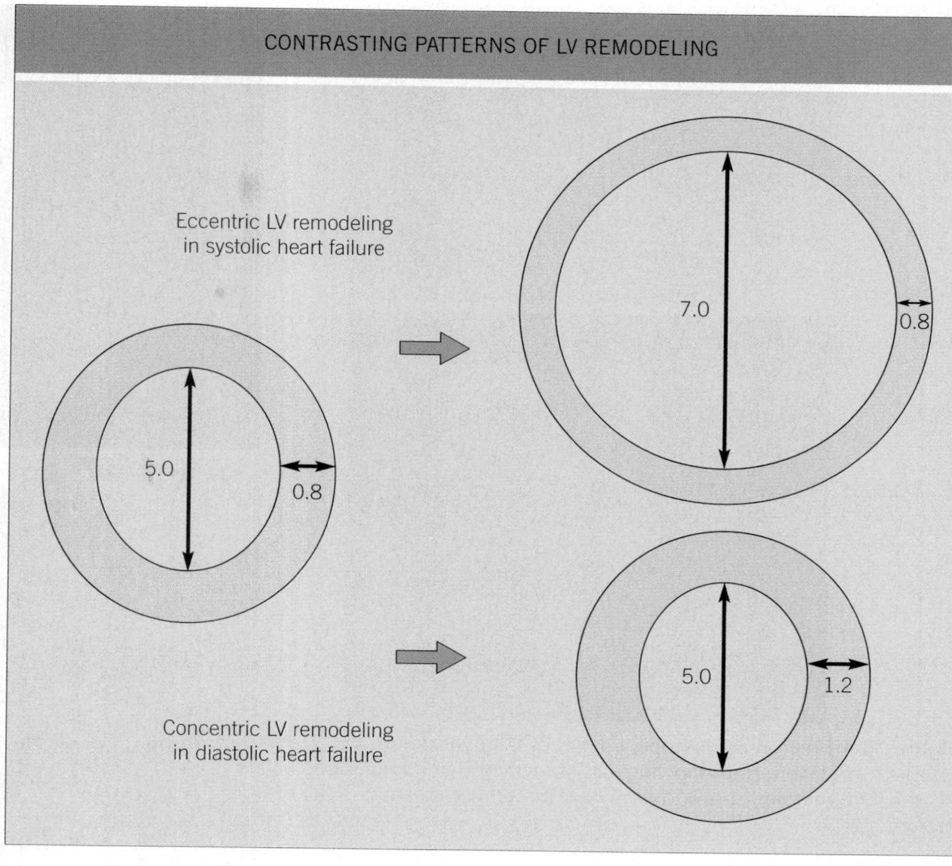

Figure 73.3 Patients with diastolic heart failure (DHF; *right-hand panels*) have larger cardiomyocyte diameters than do patients with systolic heart failure (SHF) irrespective of collagen volume fraction (CVF).

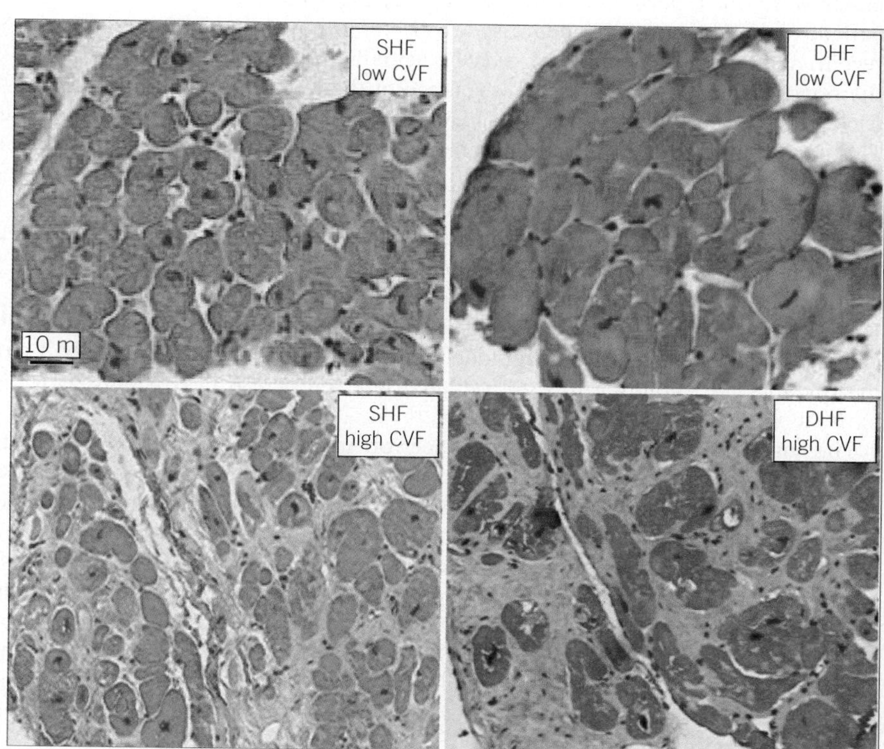

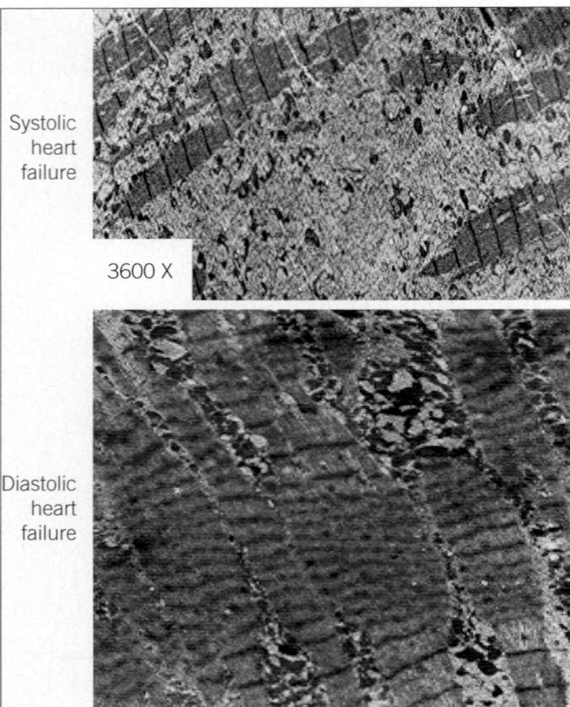

Figure 73.4 Electron microscopic images of LV myocardium in systolic heart failure *(top)* showing loss of myofibrils and in diastolic heart failure *(bottom)* showing preserved sarcomeric striation pattern.

Another frequently cited argument for diastolic heart failure evolving to systolic heart failure is the evolution toward a dilated phenotype in hypertensive heart disease[19] and in hypertrophic cardiomyopathy.[20] In many of the previous studies observing such an evolution, interval coronary events either were not reported or were significantly higher in the patients who developed a depressed LVEF. Moreover, a recent and large epidemiologic survey actually observed the opposite, namely, progressive shrinkage of the left ventricle in hypertensive heart disease as LV failure develops.[21] This study obtained LV echocardiograms in controls, hypertensives, and hypertensives with heart failure and found a progressive reduction of LV end-diastolic volume index from control (62 mL/m^2) to hypertensives (60 mL/m^2) and to hypertensives with heart failure (56 mL/m^2). This study also confirmed the findings of a number of earlier studies.[8,13,22] Furthermore, in hypertrophic cardiomyopathy, a disease also characterized by concentric LV remodeling and diastolic LV dysfunction, the evolution toward a dilated left ventricle is extremely low (3.5%).[20]

The macroscopic, microscopic, and electron microscopic differences observed in myocardium procured from patients with diastolic and systolic heart failure are illustrated in the previous section and support that diastolic heart failure is a distinct heart failure phenotype characterized by concentric LV hypertrophy, cardiomyocyte hypertrophy, and preserved myofilamentary density. These anatomic differences are paralleled by functional differences, such as a higher cardiomyocyte resting tension in diastolic heart failure, and by unequal expression of matrix metalloproteinases, tissue inhibitors of matrix metalloproteinases, or titin isoforms. Finally, in many

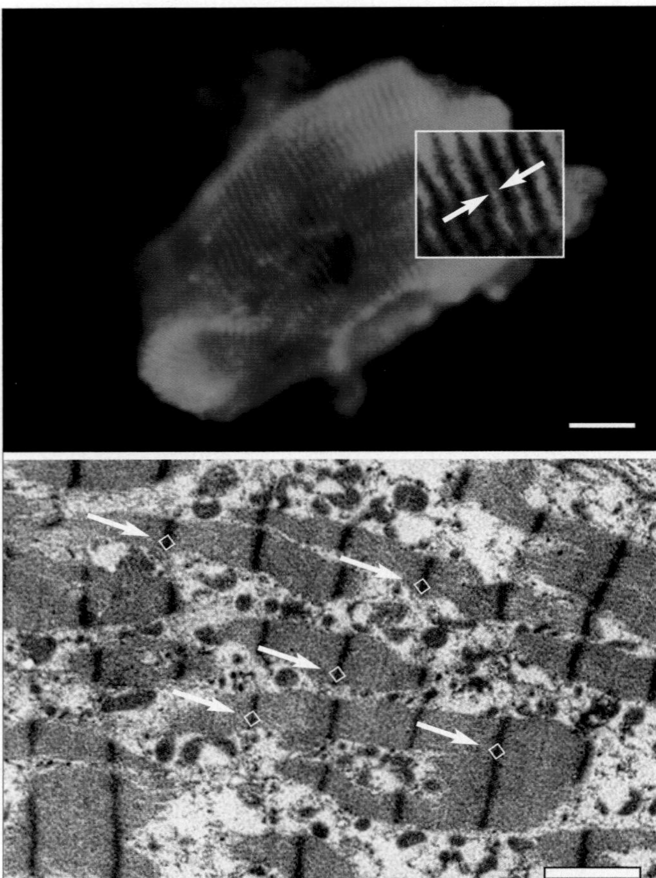

Figure 73.5 Widening of the sarcomeric Z disks observed in α-actinin–stained immunofluorescent image *(top)* and electron microscopic image *(bottom)* of LV myocardium of a patient with diastolic heart failure (arrows indicate Z disks).

therapeutic trials, patients with diastolic heart failure have failed to respond, in contrast to patients with systolic heart failure. As a result of this poor response to modern heart failure therapy, the prognosis of patients with diastolic heart failure has remained unchanged during the last 2 decennia.[2]

Therefore, these data overwhelmingly support the conclusion that diastolic heart failure is indeed a distinct heart failure phenotype and not a mere precursor stage of systolic heart failure.

Does Diastolic Heart Failure Result from Diastolic Left Ventricular Dysfunction?

Patients with diastolic heart failure have manifest diastolic LV dysfunction evident from slow LV relaxation and high diastolic LV stiffness.[22] Apart from diastolic LV dysfunction, patients with diastolic heart failure also have a high LV end-systolic stiffness (slope of the end-systolic pressure-volume relation; Fig. 73.7, right-hand panel).[23] This combined LV diastolic and systolic stiffening turns the left ventricle into a fixed stroke volume pump with hypotension during arterial vasodilatation and an amplified hypertensive response to exercise. The latter not only induces an inappropriate rise in myocardial energy demand but also exacerbates diastolic LV dysfunction. Other mechanisms that eventually could contribute to diastolic heart failure include LV volume

Figure 73.6 Unequal distributions of LVEF in both genders, with LVEF peaking at 35% in the male heart failure population and at 55% in the female heart failure population. A median value of 55% observed in the LVEF distribution of the female gender illustrates the high prevalence of diastolic heart failure in women.

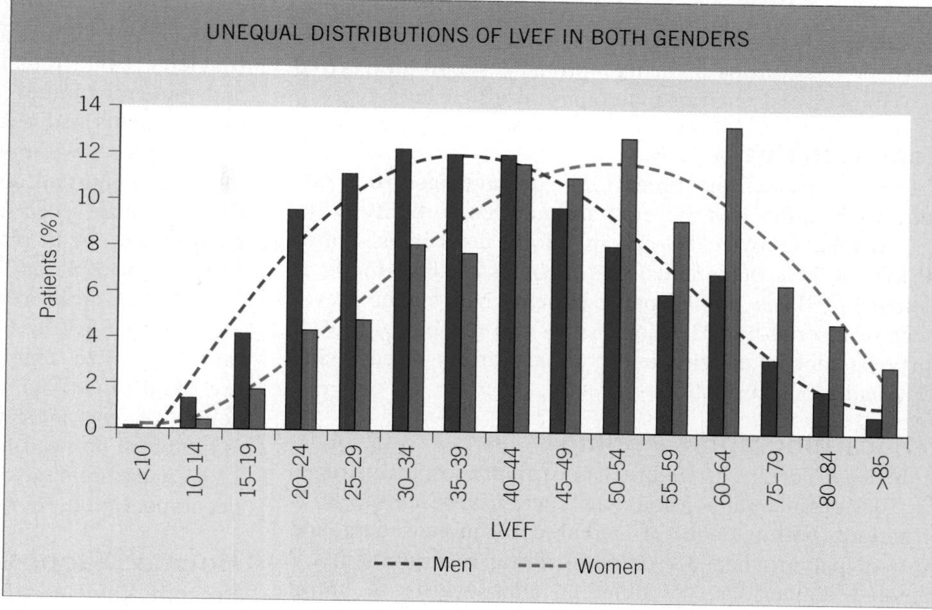

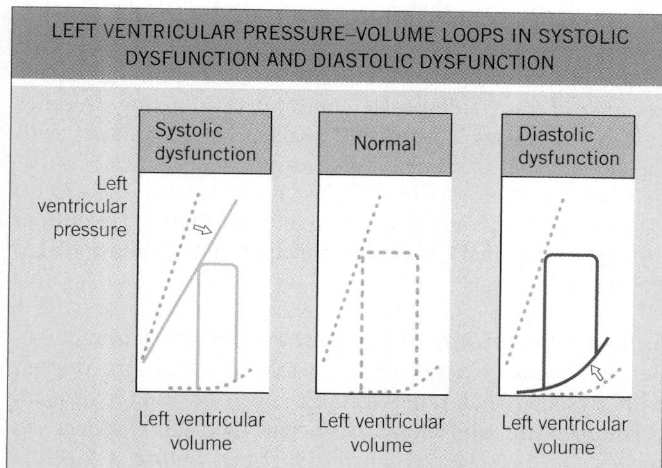

Figure 73.7 Left ventricular pressure-volume loops in systolic and diastolic heart failure. In systolic heart failure, contractility is depressed and the end-systolic pressure-volume relation is displaced down and to the right; the diastolic LV pressure-volume relation is either unchanged or displaced to the right. In diastolic heart failure, LV diastolic stiffness is increased and the diastolic LV pressure-volume relation is displaced up and to the left. Furthermore, the end-systolic LV pressure-volume relation is also displaced up and to the left. Because of steep diastolic and end-systolic LV pressure-volume relations, the left ventricle functions as a fixed stroke volume pump, which is not influenced by changes in preload or afterload.

overload[24] because of anemia, renal failure, or obesity; atrial remodeling and dilatation,[25] which again reflects underlying diastolic LV dysfunction; and impaired chronotropic or vasomotor responses,[26] although this remains debated.[27]

Therefore, in conclusion, diastolic LV dysfunction manifested as slow LV relaxation and high diastolic LV stiffness is the mechanism responsible for diastolic heart failure. Other coincident hemodynamic abnormalities observed in these patients either exert their effect through diastolic LV dysfunction or result from diastolic LV dysfunction.

CLINICAL PRESENTATION

Case Report

A 77-year-old woman with a history of arterial hypertension and diabetes was admitted to the hospital because of pulmonary edema. She was treated by a general practitioner with spironolactone (50 mg once daily) and insulin. She reacted promptly to intravenous administration of furosemide and nitroglycerin. Her electrocardiogram showed regular sinus rhythm at 74 beats per minute and LV hypertrophy. On admission, blood pressure was 210/95 mm Hg, and NT-proBNP was elevated (1860 pg/mL; normal value, <120 pg/mL). After recompensation, a transthoracic echocardiogram was obtained, which ruled out significant valvular heart disease and showed LV end-diastolic dimension of 41 mm, LVEF of 77%, and E/E′ ratio of 15 (E, early mitral valve flow velocity; E′, tissue Doppler early diastolic lengthening velocity). Cardiac catheterization showed no significant coronary artery disease and LV pressure of 185/30 mm Hg, pulmonary capillary wedge pressure of 22 mm Hg, pulmonary artery pressure of 48/21/33 (systolic/diastolic/mean), LVEF of 79%, and LV end-diastolic volume index of 49 mL/m^2. Hospital course was uneventful, and the patient was discharged with antihypertensive medications and insulin.

Clinical Characteristics

The New York Heart Failure Consortium completed a prospective multicenter registry of patients hospitalized for diastolic heart failure.[28] Diastolic heart failure patients were usually women (75%). The women included in the registry were on average 4 years older than the men (72 versus 68 years). Black non-Hispanic patients presented on average 8 years earlier than did patients of other racial background. Preexisting chronic symptoms of dyspnea were present in 75% of cases. A precipitating event leading to the episode of pulmonary edema and the hospitalization could be identified in only 50% of cases and consisted in decreasing frequency of uncontrolled arterial hypertension (>200 mm Hg), nonadherence to prescribed medications, valvular heart disease, acute coronary syndromes, atrial arrhythmias, and renal or pulmonary insufficiency.

Comorbidities

Arterial hypertension preexisting on average 10 years before admission was the most frequent comorbidity (75% of patients), followed by obesity (body mass index above 30 kg/m^2; 50% of patients) and diabetes mellitus (50% of patients).[29] Black non-Hispanic patients had higher prevalence of arterial hypertension (85%) and of obesity (60%). Forty percent of patients had coronary artery disease, and 25% had atrial fibrillation.

Echocardiographic Findings

In the New York Heart Failure Consortium prospective registry,[28] LV chamber dimensions and function were normal, 80% of patients had evidence of increased LV muscle mass, and 10% of patients had 3+ or more mitral regurgitation. LV chamber dimensions, LV function, and severity of mitral regurgitation were identical when data obtained at the time of acute decompensation were compared with data obtained a couple of days later after recompensation.[29] The increased LV muscle mass with normal LV chamber dimensions was consistent with concentric LV remodeling, a prominent anatomic LV feature in diastolic heart failure.[3,6] When hypertensive patients have diastolic LV dysfunction without diastolic heart failure, prevalence of LV hypertrophy is much lower, as evident from both the WHO MONICA project, which observed a 15% prevalence of LV hypertrophy,[30] and the VALIDD trial,[31] which observed a remarkably low (3%) prevalence of LV hypertrophy. This finding implies that diastolic LV dysfunction may precede LV hypertrophy and suggests that increased myocardial stiffness might be a stimulus to and not a consequence of LV hypertrophy.

DIAGNOSTIC STRATEGY

In contrast to systolic heart failure, which can be diagnosed by signs or symptoms of fluid overload in the presence of a reduced LVEF (<40%), the diagnosis of diastolic heart failure is often more challenging. Obvious signs of fluid overload, such as lung crepitations, distended neck veins, or pedal edema, are usually evident if the patient presents in an emergency department with acute decompensated heart failure and pulmonary edema, but these physical examination signs can be absent if the patient presents in an outpatient clinic with exercise-related dyspnea. Because diastolic heart failure patients are older and because comorbidities such as obesity are frequent, it can be unclear if breathlessness on exertion results from pulmonary congestion or physical deconditioning. If, as a corollary to systolic heart failure, the diagnosis of diastolic heart failure is based on presence of symptoms and a normal or only mildly reduced LVEF (i.e., LVEF >50%), physical deconditioning because of old age and obesity could be erroneously diagnosed as diastolic heart failure. The high risk for a false-positive diagnosis of diastolic heart failure was illustrated by the CHARM-Preserved trial,[32] which recruited patients suffering from dyspnea (NYHA classes II to IV) and who had a history of hospitalization for a cardiac reason and LVEF above 40%. An echocardiographic substudy of this trial later revealed that less than half of the recruited patients had moderate to severe LV diastolic dysfunction and that these patients had a significantly poorer outcome than that of the patients without diastolic LV dysfunction.[33] Measurements of abnormal diastolic LV function, of abnormal cardiac structure such as LV hypertrophy[5] and left atrial enlargement, or of plasma levels of natriuretic peptides are therefore considered necessary for the diagnosis of diastolic heart failure apart from signs or symptoms of fluid overload and a normal LVEF. For the evaluation of LVEF, it is important to realize that LVEF and LV chamber dimensions are identical at the time of acute decompensation and a couple of days later after recompensation[29] and that there is therefore no need to assign more diagnostic weight to the LVEF measurement obtained within 72 hours of the acute decompensation episode.[34]

How to Diagnose Diastolic Heart Failure

Recently, the Heart Failure and Echocardiography Associations of the European Society of Cardiology jointly published an updated set of criteria for the diagnosis of diastolic heart failure, which includes measures of LVEF, LV volumes, LV diastolic function, LV hypertrophy, left atrial size, and heart failure biomarkers.[35] Such an update had become necessary because of the widespread clinical use of tissue Doppler evaluation and of NT-proBNP analysis. In accordance with this updated set of criteria, three conditions need to be satisfied for the diagnosis of diastolic heart failure (Fig. 73.8): (1) signs or symptoms of congestive heart failure, (2) normal or mildly abnormal LV systolic function, and (3) diastolic LV dysfunction.

Signs or Symptoms of Congestive Heart Failure

Because many patients with diastolic heart failure present with dyspnea and no detectable signs of fluid overload, symptoms are considered sufficient clinical evidence to suggest the presence of congestive heart failure. Objective evidence of reduced exercise performance is optional and can be provided by exercise testing with measurements of peak exercise oxygen consumption (marked limitation, $\dot{V}O_2max$ <14 mL/kg per minute) or by the 6-minute walking test (marked limitation, <300 m).

Normal or Mildly Abnormal LV Systolic Function

The proposed cutoff values are LVEF above 50%, which excludes patients with abnormal LV systolic function, and LV end-diastolic volume index below 97 mL/m^2, which excludes patients with LV enlargement. LVEF and LV end-diastolic volume index should be measured in accordance with the recent recommendations of the American Society of Echocardiography and the European Association of Echocardiography.[36]

Evidence of Diastolic LV Dysfunction

Invasive diagnostic evidence of diastolic LV dysfunction can be obtained by measurement of the mean pulmonary capillary wedge pressure (>12 mm Hg), the LV end-diastolic pressure (>16 mm Hg), the time constant of LV relaxation

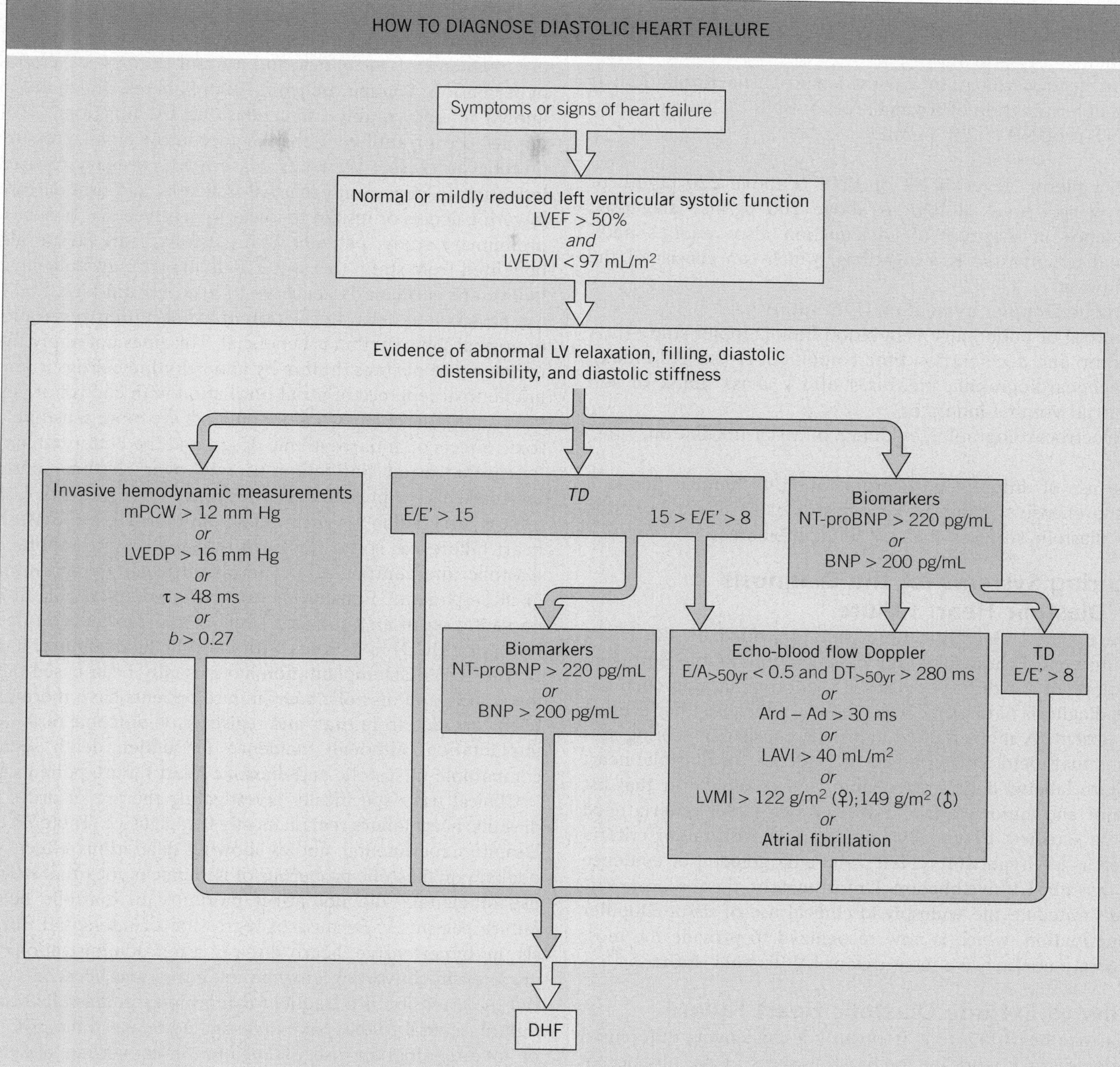

Figure 73.8 Diagnostic flow chart to diagnose diastolic heart failure in a patient suspected of having diastolic heart failure. Ad, duration of mitral valve atrial wave flow; Ard, duration of reverse pulmonary vein atrial systole flow; *b*, constant of left ventricular chamber stiffness; BNP, brain natriuretic peptide; DHF, diastolic heart failure; DT, deceleration time; E, early mitral valve flow velocity; E′, early TD lengthening velocity; E/A, ratio of early (E) to late (A) mitral valve flow velocity; LAVI, left atrial volume index; LVEDP, left ventricular end-diastolic pressure; LVEDVI, left ventricular end-diastolic volume index; LVEF, left ventricular ejection fraction; LVMI, left ventricular mass index; mPCW, mean pulmonary capillary wedge pressure; NT-proBNP, N-terminal pro brain natriuretic peptide; TD, tissue Doppler; τ, time constant of left ventricular relaxation.

($\tau > 48$ ms), or the LV stiffness modulus ($b > 0.27$). Noninvasive diagnostic evidence of diastolic LV dysfunction is preferably derived from myocardial tissue Doppler examination ($E/E' > 15$; E, early mitral valve flow velocity; E′, tissue Doppler early diastolic lengthening velocity). If myocardial tissue Doppler examination yields values suggestive of but nondiagnostic for diastolic LV dysfunction ($15 > E/E' > 8$), tissue Doppler examination needs to be implemented with other noninvasive investigations to provide diagnostic evidence of diastolic LV dysfunction. These noninvasive investigations can consist of the following:

- a blood flow Doppler study of mitral valve flow velocity (E/A ratio < 0.5 and deceleration time > 280 ms combined, for patients older than 50 years; A, atrial mitral valve flow velocity) eventually combined with pulmonary vein flow velocity ($Ard - Ad > 30$ ms; Ard, duration of atrial reverse pulmonary vein flow velocity; Ad, duration of atrial mitral valve flow velocity);

- an echocardiographic measure of left atrial volume index (>40 mL/m^2) or of LV mass index (women, >122 g/m^2; men, >149 g/m^2);
- an electrocardiogram with evidence of atrial fibrillation; or
- a determination of plasma level of BNP (>200 pg/mL) or NT-proBNP (>220 pg/mL).

If the plasma level of NT-proBNP is above 220 pg/mL or the plasma level of BNP is above 200 pg/mL, diagnostic evidence of diastolic LV dysfunction also requires additional noninvasive investigations, which can consist of the following:

- tissue Doppler evaluation (E/E′ ratio);
- mitral or pulmonary vein blood flow Doppler study (E/A ratio and deceleration time combined; Ard − Ad index);
- echocardiographic measures of LV mass index or left atrial volume index; or
- electrocardiographic evidence of atrial fibrillation.

The use of different echocardiographic techniques allows a comprehensive noninvasive assessment of LV relaxation, LV diastolic stiffness, and LV filling pressures.[37]

Scoring Systems for the Diagnosis of Diastolic Heart Failure

The updated diagnostic flow chart provided by the Heart Failure and Echocardiography Associations of the European Society of Cardiology[35] uses a dichotomous approach for the diagnosis of diastolic heart failure, which is either present or absent. A more refined approach consists of scoring systems that yield distinct levels of evidence for diastolic heart failure labeled definite, probable, and possible[34] or that list major and minor criteria[38]; at least two major criteria need to be satisfied, eventually implemented with minor criteria such as LV hypertrophy, left atrial enlargement, or evidence of diastolic LV dysfunction. Unfortunately, these scoring systems antedate the widespread clinical use of tissue Doppler examination, which is now recognized to provide the most accurate noninvasive measures of LV diastolic stiffness.[39]

How to Exclude Diastolic Heart Failure

Diastolic heart failure is frequently a challenging differential diagnosis in a work-up for breathlessness in the absence of detectable signs of fluid overload. The Heart Failure and Echocardiography Associations of the European Society of Cardiology therefore also proposed a set of criteria for the exclusion of diastolic heart failure (Fig. 73.9).[35] If a patient with breathlessness and no signs of fluid overload has an NT-proBNP level of less than 120 pg/mL or a BNP level of less than 100 pg/mL, any form of heart failure is virtually ruled out because of the high negative predictive value of plasma natriuretic peptides, and pulmonary disease becomes the most likely cause of breathlessness. If an echocardiogram confirms the absence of valvular or pericardial disease, LVEF and LV volumes should be measured. If the LVEF exceeds 50%, if the LV end-diastolic volume index is below 76 mL/m^2, and if the patient has no atrial fibrillation, atrial dilatation (left atrial volume index < 29 mL/m^2), LV hypertrophy (LV mass index: women, <96 g/m^2; men, <116 g/m^2), low tissue Doppler shortening velocity (>6.5 cm/s), or high tissue Doppler E/E′ (E/E′ < 8), the diagnosis of heart failure with normal LVEF is ruled out.

MANAGEMENT

Current guidelines for the management of diastolic heart failure recommend fastidious and careful control of arterial hypertension, volume, ischemia, and diabetes, which are all known to unfavorably affect diastolic LV function.[40] This implies use of antihypertensives to control blood pressure, diuretics to correct LV volume overload, coronary revascularization to prevent myocardial ischemia, and oral glucose-lowering agents or insulin to lower hyperglycemia. In a small preliminary study, patients with diastolic heart failure also benefited from statin therapy.[41] Patients with diastolic heart failure are particularly sensitive to loss of atrial kick, and in the presence of atrial fibrillation or atrial flutter, restoration of normal sinus rhythm is beneficial. This does not imply that maintenance of sinus rhythm by antiarrhythmic drugs is preferable to acceptance of atrial fibrillation with control of ventricular response. Heart failure patients are more sensitive to toxic effects of antiarrhythmic drugs, and the better outcome in chronic atrial fibrillation of rate over rhythm control therefore also applies to diastolic heart failure patients. Usefulness of cardiac resynchronization therapy for diastolic heart failure has so far not been assessed despite reports of diastolic interventricular and intraventricular dyssynchrony in these patients. Equally unclear is the potential benefit of implantation of an automatic implantable cardioverter-defibrillator (AICD) in patients with diastolic heart failure. Indications for AICD implantation have usually been based on a low LVEF, and diastolic heart failure patients have therefore been excluded from trials and registries on outcome of AICD implantation, although incidence of sudden death seems comparable in systolic and diastolic heart failure patients.[1]

Clinical trials specifically investigating the use of drugs in diastolic heart failure remain mostly inconclusive (Table 73.2). Despite experimental studies showing deleterious effects of ouabain on diastolic properties of ischemic myocardial strips, use of digitalis did not affect mortality in diastolic heart failure patients.[42] Because of regression of interstitial fibrosis in hypertensive heart disease after administration of angiotensin-converting enzyme inhibitors and because arterial hypertension is a frequent comorbidity in diastolic heart failure, several studies have investigated or are in the process of investigating the use of angiotensin-converting enzyme inhibitors, angiotensin receptor blockers, and spironolactone in patients with diastolic heart failure. In patients with preserved LVEF after myocardial infarction, enalapril[43] and perindopril[44] (PREAMI) had favorable effects, respectively, on symptoms or on LV dilatation but not on cardiovascular death or need for hospitalizations. PREAMI specifically addressed the use of angiotensin-converting enzyme inhibitors for the prevention of eccentric LV remodeling after small myocardial infarctions[44] and did not provide evidence that perindopril modifies the concentric LV remodeling observed in diastolic heart failure patients. The PEP-CHF trial specifically enrolled elderly heart failure patients with echocardiographic evidence of diastolic dysfunction but no systolic LV dysfunction. In this trial, perindopril improved exercise tolerance, reduced the need for heart failure hospitalizations, but failed to alter all-cause mortality.[45] Remarkably similar results have been observed with angiotensin receptor blockers in diastolic heart failure. In patients with

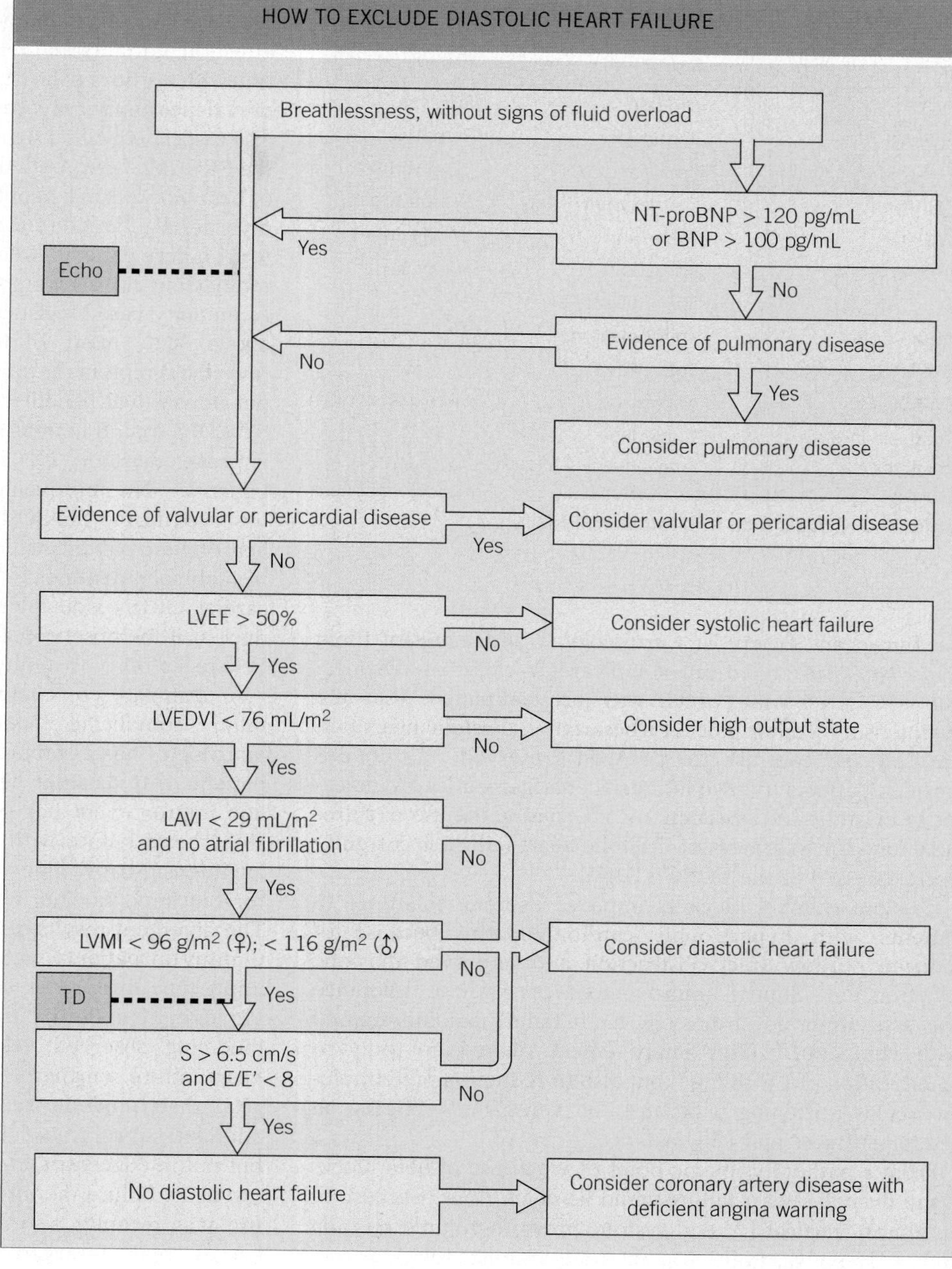

Figure 73.9 Diagnostic flow chart to exclude diastolic heart failure in a patient presenting with breathlessness and no signs of fluid overload. LAVI, left atrial volume index; LVEDVI, left ventricular end-diastolic volume index; LVEF, left ventricular ejection fraction; LVMI, left ventricular mass index; S, TD shortening velocity; TD, tissue Doppler.

a hypertensive response to exercise and diastolic LV dysfunction, losartan significantly improved exercise tolerance compared with either placebo[46] or hydrochlorothiazide.[47] The VALIDD trial studied the same population of hypertensive patients with diastolic LV dysfunction and reported an improvement of diastolic LV relaxation velocity after valsartan.[31] A similar improvement, however, was also observed with blood pressure–lowering agents, which did not specifically target interstitial myocardial fibrosis. This nonsuperiority of valsartan suggests other mechanisms, such as cardiomyocyte resting tension, to be more important. This suggestion is supported by the lower myocardial collagen volume fraction[7] and the higher cardiomyocyte resting tension[6] observed in patients with diastolic heart failure compared with systolic heart failure. A large randomized trial looking at the effects of candesartan in patients with diastolic heart failure (CHARM-Preserved)[32] resulted, like PEP-CHF, in a reduction of heart failure hospitalizations but no survival benefit. These results were clearly inferior to the results obtained with the same drug in patients with systolic heart failure. Patient recruitment in CHARM-Preserved did not require objective evidence of diastolic LV dysfunction as evident from an echocardiographic substudy of CHARM-Preserved, in which only 44% of patients had moderate to severe evidence of diastolic LV dysfunction. The majority of patients in CHARM-Preserved therefore did not satisfy the criteria for diastolic heart failure recently proposed by the Heart Failure and Echocardiography Associations of

CLINICAL TRIALS IN DIASTOLIC HEART FAILURE		
Trial	**Drug**	**Result**
DIG	Digoxin	Survival =
PREAMI	Perindopril	Remodeling ↓
PEP-CHF	Perindopril	Symptoms ↓
CHARM-Preserved	Candesartan	Symptoms ↓
VALIDD	Valsartan	LV relaxation =
I-Preserve	Irbesartan	Survival =
TOPCAT	Spironolactone	?
ALDO-DHF	Spironolactone	?
PREDICT	Eplerenone	?
SWEDIC	Carvedilol	LV relaxation =
Japanese-DHF	Carvedilol	?
SENIORS	Nebivolol	Survival ↑

Table 73.2 Clinical trials in diastolic heart failure.

the European Society of Cardiology,[35] and many of them could have suffered from a noncardiac cause of dyspnea. The I-Preserve trial, which was just completed, uses the angiotensin receptor blocker irbesartan in diastolic heart failure, but in contrast to CHARM-Preserved, it requires enrolled patients to have left atrial enlargement as an indicator of diastolic LV dysfunction.[48,49] Finally, the use of spironolactone for treatment of diastolic heart failure is currently being assessed in the TOPCAT trial.

Calcium channel blockers improve exercise tolerance in patients with hypertrophic cardiomyopathy because of reduced outflow tract obstruction and improved diastolic LV function. Similar improvement of exercise tolerance was also observed in diastolic heart failure patients treated with verapamil.[50] This improvement related not only to amelioration of LV filling[50] but also to reduction of ventriculovascular stiffening[51] because of verapamil's effects on arterial stiffness and LV elastance.

From a pathophysiologic point of view, use of beta blockers in diastolic heart failure could be deleterious. Because of an almost vertical LV end-systolic pressure-volume relation and a steep diastolic LV pressure-volume relation (see Fig. 73.7, right-hand panel), the left ventricle of patients with diastolic heart failure functions as a fixed stroke volume pump, which is exclusively dependent on heart rate to increase its output. A blunted heart rate response to exercise because of administration of beta blockers could therefore unfavorably affect exercise tolerance in these patients. Furthermore, isolated cardiomyocytes procured from patients with diastolic heart failure have a high in vitro diastolic stiffness, which significantly contributes to the high in vivo LV diastolic stiffness.[9] Administration of protein kinase A corrects this high in vitro cardiomyocyte stiffness.[9] Use of beta blockers lowers myocardial protein kinase A activity and could theoretically worsen diastolic LV stiffness in diastolic heart failure. Clinical observations on the use of beta blockers in diastolic heart failure seem to confirm these pathophysiologic drawbacks, and trials with beta blockers in diastolic heart failure have been less convincing than in systolic heart failure. In elderly postinfarction patients with a preserved LVEF, propranolol had a favorable and significant effect on mortality and reinfarction rate.[52] In a similar population with a history of heart failure, a preserved LVEF, and a high prevalence of prior myocardial infarction, beta-blocker use was also associated with a significant reduction in mortality.[53] Like the PREAMI study, both these studies addressed the usefulness of beta blockers in a population of patients with a limited prior myocardial infarction and not in a typical population of diastolic heart failure patients, who are characterized by concentric LV remodeling and a high prevalence of arterial hypertension. A community-based registry of heart failure patients with LVEF above 40%, many of them elderly hypertensive women, revealed symptomatic improvement and fewer hospitalizations but no survival benefit during carvedilol treatment.[54] In the SWEDIC trial, 6 months of carvedilol treatment also failed to improve diastolic LV function in diastolic heart failure patients.[55] No improvement in diastolic LV function was also observed in the SENIORS trial despite improved survival in heart failure patients with a preserved or a reduced LVEF during nebivolol treatment.[56] The beta blocker nebivolol has myocardial nitric oxide–releasing properties, and it is therefore unclear if the observed survival benefit relates to blockade of beta receptors or to antihypertrophic properties of nitric oxide.

In summary, in contrast to patients with systolic heart failure, convincing evidence is still lacking that modern pharmacologic heart failure therapy improves prognosis in patients with diastolic heart failure. So far, mostly symptomatic improvement has been observed in patients with diastolic heart failure with use of a variety of drugs, including angiotensin-converting enzyme inhibitors, angiotensin receptor blockers, calcium channel blockers, and beta blockers. The divergent results of modern pharmacologic heart failure therapy in patients with systolic and diastolic heart failure imply that different myocardial signal transduction pathways are operative during the eccentric and concentric LV remodeling observed, respectively, in systolic and diastolic heart failure. Furthermore, these divergent results also suggest that modern heart failure therapy predominantly addresses signal transduction pathways activated in eccentric but not in concentric LV remodeling. The inefficacy of modern heart failure therapy in patients with diastolic heart failure was recently also illustrated by a large epidemiologic survey that observed improved prognosis over time in patients with systolic heart failure but not in patients with diastolic heart failure.[2]

PROGNOSIS

Earlier data on prognosis of patients with diastolic heart failure suggested better prognosis in diastolic heart failure than in systolic heart failure. Most of these data were derived from ambulatory populations, with relatively less information on hospitalized patients. Moreover, similar to therapeutic trials in diastolic heart failure, inclusion criteria for diastolic heart failure varied widely. A large population-derived cohort study overcame most of these inadequacies and demonstrated similar 1-year mortality rates in patients with systolic and diastolic heart failure of 26% and 22%, respectively.[1] This study also revealed similar rehospitalization rates and heart failure–related rehospitalization rates in both groups.

SUMMARY

Diastolic heart failure currently accounts for more than 50% of all heart failure patients in Western societies. Specific causes of diastolic heart failure include constrictive pericarditis, endomyocardial fibrosis, hypertrophic cardiomyopathy, infiltrative cardiomyopathy, and ischemic and hypertensive heart disease. Diastolic heart failure patients frequently are elderly and more commonly women. They often have multiple comorbidities, such as arterial hypertension, obesity, and diabetes mellitus, and a concentrically hypertrophied left ventricle with a high LV wall mass-volume ratio, prominent cardiomyocyte hypertrophy, and abnormal extracellular matrix. The diagnosis of diastolic heart failure rests on a triad consisting of signs or symptoms of congestive heart failure, normal LVEF (>50%), and objective evidence of diastolic LV dysfunction. Objective evidence of diastolic LV dysfunction is preferably derived from invasive measurements of LV filling pressures or from noninvasive tissue Doppler indices of abnormal diastolic function. Current guidelines for the management of diastolic heart failure recommend control of arterial hypertension, volume overload, ischemia, and diabetes. Modern heart failure therapy with angiotensin-converting enzyme inhibitors, angiotensin receptor blockers, and beta blockers provides a symptomatic benefit but no prognostic benefit in patients with diastolic heart failure. One-year mortality of patients with diastolic heart failure approaches 22%, and prognosis in diastolic heart failure is therefore comparable to prognosis in systolic heart failure.

chapter 74

Cardiac Resynchronization Therapy

John G. F. Cleland, Ahmed Tageldien Abdellah, Nidal Maarouf, and Neil Hobson

The basic premise of cardiac resynchronization therapy (CRT) is that cardiac dyssynchrony complicates or causes heart failure and that retiming of the sequence of contraction can improve cardiac function, thereby improving symptoms and reducing cardiovascular morbidity and mortality (Fig. 74.1). There is no doubt that atriobiventricular pacing is clinically effective, but the reasons that it is effective are far from certain.[1] Ultimately, it may be that cardiac dyssynchrony is the basis for the effects of CRT but that cardiac dyssynchrony is so poorly understood, so difficult to measure, or so ubiquitous that it is clinically irrelevant to select patients for this therapy on this basis.[2] This chapter reviews the existing data, focusing on substantial randomized controlled trials and existing guidelines, and attempts to interpret them for current clinical practice and future research.

PATHOPHYSIOLOGY OF CARDIAC DYSSYNCHRONY

Conceptually, cardiac dyssynchrony means that the orderly sequence of cardiac contraction and relaxation is disturbed, leading to a decline in cardiac efficiency (Fig. 74.2).[3] Cardiac dyssynchrony can take many forms, which commonly coexist. Atrioventricular (AV) dyssynchrony is caused by delayed ventricular contraction. Atrial relaxation leads to a fall in atrial pressure and the backward flow of blood through the AV valves during late diastole that leads, in turn, to a decline in diastolic ventricular pressures and volume that impairs ventricular contractile performance. Intraventricular dyssynchrony refers to late activation of parts of the left ventricular (LV) myocardium, usually the posterolateral wall. It may affect circumferential or longitudinal contraction. Late activation of some segments leads to a slower rise in systolic pressure and delayed LV ejection and also to slower relaxation and delayed LV filling. The left ventricle expends energy changing shape as regions that are contracting deform regions that either have not yet started to contract or have already started to relax. Blood is thus moved around the LV chamber rather than ejected from it. If the interventricular septum—which forms part of both ventricles—is activated before the LV free wall (i.e., left intraventricular mechanical delay), this will result in right ventricular (RV) ejection greatly preceding LV ejection and interventricular dyssynchrony, unless the right ventricle is also severely diseased, which is a poor prognostic sign. Delayed activation of papillary muscles leading to mitral regurgitation during systole is another important aspect of dyssynchrony. Whether interatrial dyssynchrony or dyssynchronous contraction within the thickness of the myocardial wall has an important effect on cardiac function is uncertain.[1-3] Which aspect of dyssynchrony is most important overall is uncertain, and it is likely that the most important aspect of dyssynchrony varies from patient to patient and over time.[4]

THE EPIDEMIOLOGY OF HEART FAILURE AND CARDIAC DYSSYNCHRONY

Heart failure is common but complex and the final expression of many different cardiac diseases and pathophysiologic processes. Ischemic heart disease, hypertension, and atrial fibrillation, alone or in combination, are common causes. The prevalence of heart failure is maintained at relatively low levels because most patients die within a few years of diagnosis. Heart failure is better described by its incidence.[5] About one person in every five will develop heart failure, and most of these patients will die as a complication of it. Indeed, recent reports show that 80% of people who die as a consequence of myocardial infarction will first develop heart failure.[6]

The prevalence and incidence of dyssynchrony are essentially unknown because no robust definition exists. It is exceedingly unlikely that dyssynchrony is an all-or-nothing problem, and so any definition would have to choose an arbitrary number to define dyssynchrony.[7] This is further complicated by the fact that there are many more than a dozen different measures of dyssynchrony assessing widely varying aspects of its pathophysiology. No one is sure which are relevant. Different types of dyssynchrony may have additive adverse effects on cardiac function. Dyssynchrony may vary over time and with stress, and its nature will vary from patient to patient.[8]

Historically, a QRS duration of more than 120 ms has been taken as supportive evidence of ventricular dyssynchrony. Surveys suggest that about one quarter of patients with heart failure have a QRS width of 120 ms or more but that among patients with LV systolic dysfunction (LVSD), it may be nearer 40%.[9] In the EuroHeart Failure Survey, of 5934 hospital deaths and discharges with an electrocardiogram and assessment of LV function, 2107 (36%) had LV ejection fraction (LVEF) of 35% or less, and of these, 42% had QRS of 120 ms or more (Fig. 74.3).[9] However, QRS duration is only a rough guide to the prevalence of intraventricular and interventricular dyssynchrony at rest and may better reflect the severity of LVSD rather than dyssynchrony.[9] There are no detailed echocardiographic studies in large populations. One of the largest included just 158 patients with LVEF of 35% or less. The prevalence of both inter-dyssynchrony (>40 ms difference in onset of aortic and pulmonary flow) and

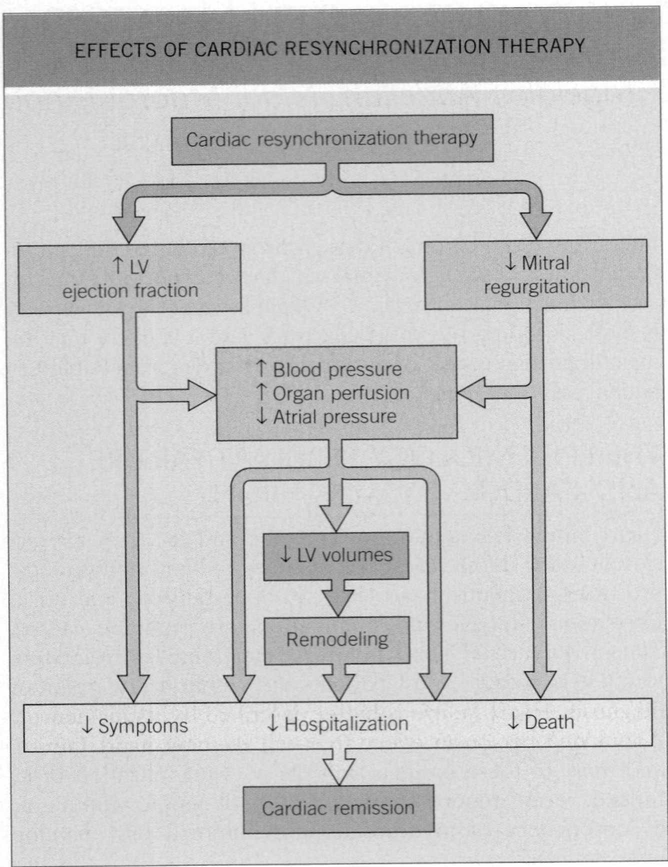

Figure 74.1 Effects of cardiac resynchronization therapy.

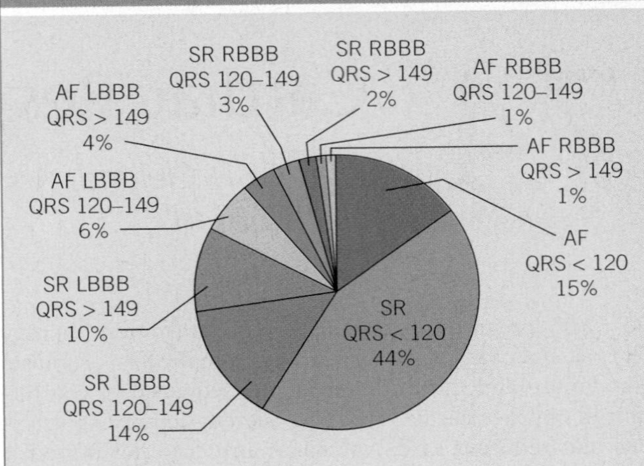

Figure 74.3 The prevalence of QRS prolongation in patients with left ventricular systolic dysfunction. AF, atrial fibrillation; LBBB, left bundle branch block; RBBB, right bundle brunch block; SR, sinus rhythm.

intraventricular dyssynchrony (>50 ms in an eight-segment model using tissue Doppler imaging) was more than 70% in patients with QRS of more than 150 ms, around 55% in those with QRS of 120 to 150 ms, and, for intraventricular dyssynchrony, about 30% in those with QRS duration of less than 120 ms.[10]

The incidence of dyssynchrony and whether it can resolve are unknown. The incidence of new-onset bundle branch block is about 10% per annum. Patients with LVSD and left bundle branch block have an adverse prognosis, and patients with new-onset left bundle branch block have an even worse outcome (Fig. 74.4).[11]

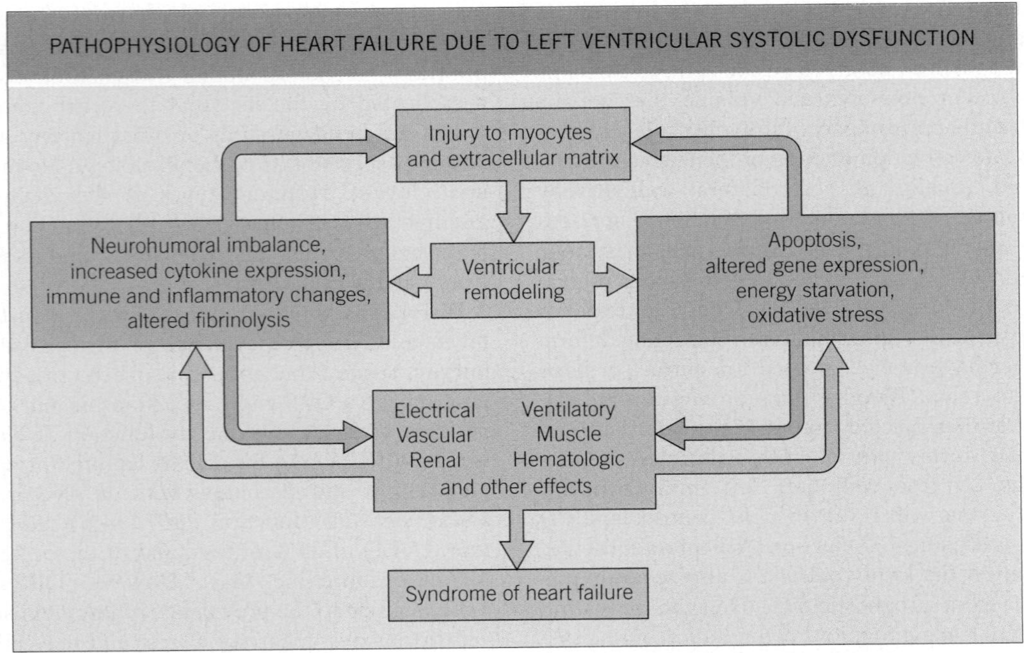

Figure 74.2 Pathophysiology of heart failure due to left ventricular systolic dysfunction. (From McMurray JJ, Pfeffer MA. Heart failure. Lancet 2005;365:1877-1889.)

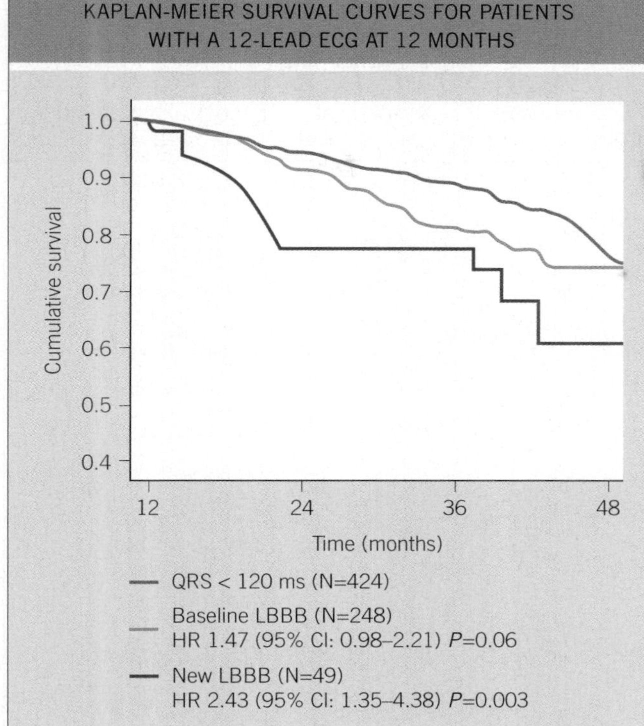

Figure 74.4 Kaplan-Meier survival curves for patients with a 12-lead electrocardiogram (ECG) at 12 months. Patients are split by QRS duration. Shown are those patients with a QRS of less than 120 ms at baseline and follow-up, those with left bundle branch block (LBBB) at baseline, and those developing new left bundle branch block during the first year's follow-up.[11]

It may be that increased QRS duration just signifies worse ventricular function and that ventricles with worse function are more likely to show dyssynchrony. Many studies show that QRS duration predicts prognosis in patients with heart failure, but the majority of the evidence shows that dyssynchrony, after correction for the severity of ventricular dysfunction, predicts a better outcome.[12] This probably reflects the fact that for a given severity of ventricular dysfunction, there is more surviving myocardium in a dyssynchronous rather than in a synchronous ventricle. In other words, an ejection fraction of 30% is true in a patient without dyssynchrony but is an underestimate of the "true" synchronous ejection fraction when dyssynchrony is present.

A SHORT REVIEW OF CLINICAL TRIALS

There is powerful evidence from a series of randomized controlled trials that CRT is an effective treatment of patients with heart failure who fulfilled their entry criteria (Table 74.1), which universally included patients with LV dilatation and systolic dysfunction, predominantly with wide QRS and in sinus rhythm.[1,13] Patients with a broad range of symptoms were included. Echocardiographic evidence of dyssynchrony was generally not required.

MUSTIC TRIALS

These trials were conducted single blind, that is, the investigator but not the patient knew whether the CRT device was switched on. Patients who had a successful implantation and survived the run-in period were randomly assigned to periods of pacing switched on or off. These trials included 48 assessable patients in sinus rhythm[14] and 41 assessable patients with slow atrial fibrillation.[15] Patients with slow atrial fibrillation had a ventricular demand rate-responsive (VVIR) pacemaker set to pace at 70 beats per minute during the control period. The primary endpoint was meters walked in 6 minutes. Important secondary endpoints were quality of life by use of the Minnesota Living With Heart Failure (MLWHF) questionnaire and patient preference. The study showed clear benefits with CRT switched on for patients in sinus rhythm but less clear benefits for those in atrial fibrillation, perhaps because of the high ventricular pacing rate or the lack of atrial activity.

CONTAK

This study started as a double-blind crossover study in patients with a successful device implantation but evolved into a parallel-arm study lasting 6 months and including 490 patients.[16] At least 257 patients (52%) were in New York Heart Association (NYHA) class II and at least 209 (43%) were in NYHA class III-IV at the time of randomization. The primary endpoint of the study was initially peak exercise oxygen consumption but was changed to worsening heart failure events. The trial failed to meet its revised primary endpoint but did show that patients assigned to CRT-on had a greater improvement in exercise capacity and LV function. Clinical benefit at 6 months was greater in more symptomatic patients, but recovery of LV function was similar regardless of symptom severity.

MIRACLE

This was a double-blind study (Fig. 74.5). All patients had a device implanted. Patients who survived a postimplantation run-in period were randomly assigned to atriobiventricular pacing switched on or off for 6 months. The primary endpoints of this study were NYHA class, quality of life score on the MLWHF scale, and distance walked in 6 minutes, all of which improved significantly (P =.005 or better).[17] This study established CRT as an effective treatment of symptoms. Hospitalization for heart failure was also reduced (P <.05).

MIRACLE ICD

This was a double-blind study, similar in concept and design to the MIRACLE study but conducted in patients for whom an implantable cardioverter-defibrillator (ICD) was indicated because of cardiac arrest or symptomatic ventricular arrhythmia.[18] The primary endpoints were the same as in the MIRACLE trial. Improvements in symptoms and quality of life but not in exercise capacity were observed. Mortality and hospitalization for heart failure were not reduced. Overall, this study suggested that the benefits of CRT might be less in the presence of an ICD. This may reflect the inclusion of patients less likely to benefit symptomatically because they were receiving a device mainly on prognostic criteria.

MIRACLE ICD II

The design and inclusion criteria were identical to those of MIRACLE ICD except that it included only NYHA class II patients.[19] The study suggested that cardiac function improved with CRT to a similar extent as in patients assigned to NYHA class III-IV. Most assessments of symptom

ENTRY CRITERIA FOR RANDOMIZED CONTROLLED TRIALS OF CARDIAC RESYNCHRONIZATION THERAPY										
					Entry Criteria					
Study	N	Design	Follow-up (months)	Pacing Mode	ICD	Sinus Rhythm	NYHA Class	EF (%)	LVEDD (mm)	QRS Duration (ms)
MUSTIC[14]	48	Single-blind crossover	3	CRT on vs. off	No	Yes	III	<35	>60	>150
MUSTIC AF[15]	41	Single-blind	3	CRT on vs. off VVI backup 70 bpm	No	No	III	<35	>60	>200 (RV paced)
CONTAK CD[16]	490	Double-blind crossover	3-6	CRT on vs. off	Yes	Yes	II-IV	≤35	Median 71	≥120
MIRACLE[17]	453	Double-blind parallel-arm	6	CRT on vs. off	No	Yes	III-IV	≤35	≥55	≥130
MIRACLE ICD[18]	369	Double-blind parallel-arm	6	CRT on vs. off	Yes	Yes	III-IV	≤35	≥55	≥130
MIRACLE ICD II[19]	186	Double-blind parallel-arm	6	CRT on vs. off	Yes	Yes	II	≤35	≥55	≥130
COMPANION[20]	1520	Unblinded parallel-arm	12 (for control group)	CRT-D vs. CRT vs. control	No	Yes	III-IV	≤35	Median 67	≥120
CARE-HF and extension[21,22]	813	Unblinded parallel-arm	30 (38 for extension)	CRT vs. control	No	Yes	III-IV	≤35	>30 mm/m (height)	120-149 + interventricular dyssynchrony or ≥150
REVERSE	610	Double-blind parallel-arm	12 (24 in Europe)	CRT on vs. off	Optional	Yes	I-II	≤40	≥55	≥120

EF, ejection fraction; ICD, implantable cardioverter-defibrillator; LVEDD, left ventricular end-diastolic diameter; NYHA, New York Heart Association

Table 74.1 Entry criteria for randomized controlled trials of cardiac resynchronization therapy.

response were not improved. This may reflect the difficulty in showing improvement in patients with mild symptoms and the need for longer follow-up to show differences in the rate of deterioration.

COMPANION

This trial (Fig. 74.6) compared the effects of CRT (n = 617), CRT-D (cardiac resynchronization therapy pacemaker plus backup defibrillation; n = 595), and pharmacologic management alone (n = 308) on morbidity and mortality[20] in patients who had been hospitalized for heart failure in the previous year and satisfied standard entry criteria (see Table 74.1). The primary outcome was a composite of all-cause hospitalization or all-cause mortality and was dominated by the former. It is likely that many hospitalizations were for minor problems. Although the prestated intention was to compare each intervention with control, because two patients were allocated to each intervention for every control patient and because numerically more events occurred in the intervention groups, it was better powered to show differences between devices. At 6-month follow-up, CRT and CRT-D had improved symptoms, quality of life, and exercise capacity by a similar amount. The study was stopped early because there was a highly significant reduction in the primary endpoint in both groups and in all-cause mortality in the CRT-D group and because of a high rate of implants in the control group. Trials that stop early overestimate the benefit in the arm of the trial that drove the decision. Overall, this trial showed that CRT and CRT-D could improve morbidity and mortality to a similar extent. As CRT is less expensive and associated with fewer complications, it suggests that CRT is the preferred treatment for most patients with heart failure. It also shows that the benefits of CRT are not diminished in the presence of an ICD, which was a concern raised by MIRACLE ICD.

CARE-HF

This trial (Fig. 74.7) compared the effects of CRT (n = 409) with pharmacologic management alone (n = 404).[21,22] In addition to the criteria shown in Table 74.1, patients with QRS of 120 to 149 ms also had to have an echocardiographic measure of dyssynchrony. The primary outcome was

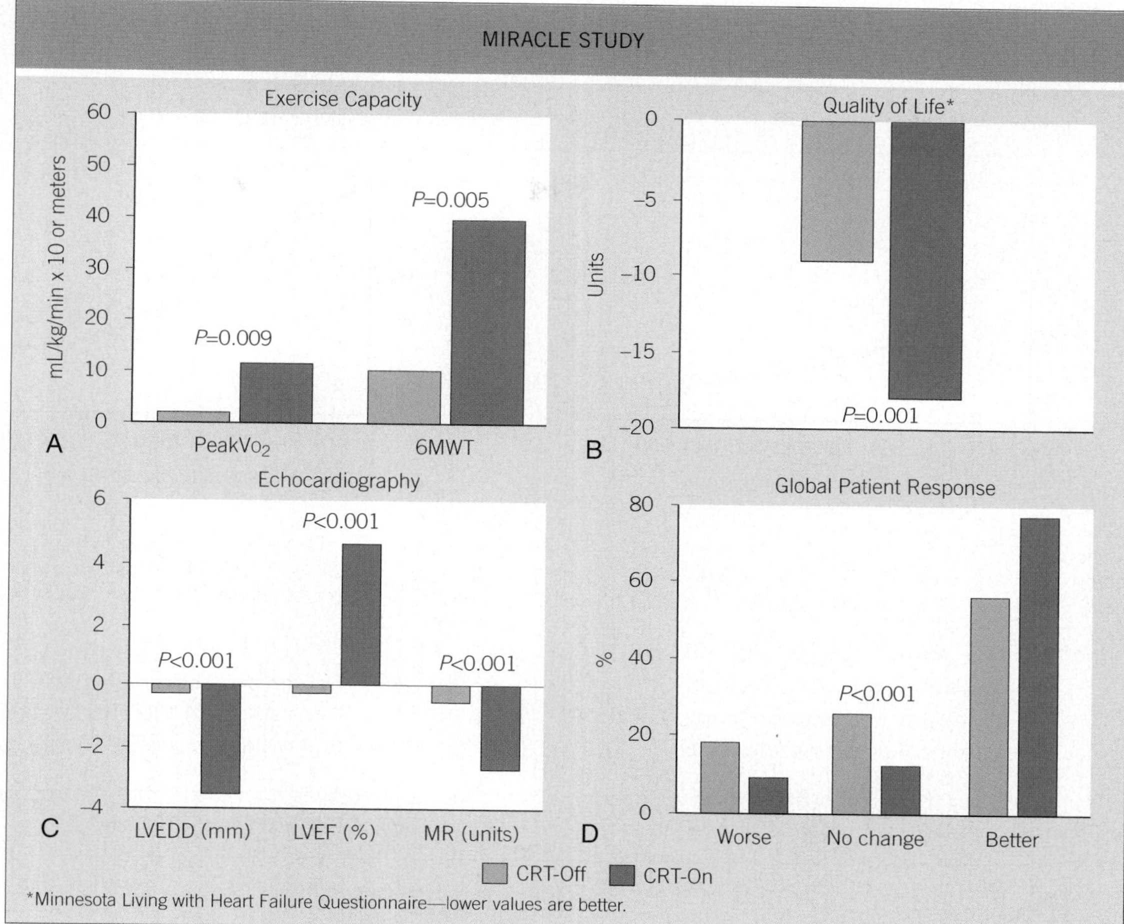

Figure 74.5 MIRACLE study. LVEDD, left ventricular end-diastolic diameter; LVEF, left ventricular ejection fraction; 6MWT, 6-minute walk test; MR, mitral regurgitation.

unplanned hospitalization for a major cardiovascular event or all-cause mortality. The study was completed according to plan (median follow-up, 29.4 months) and included an extension phase to allow analysis and presentation of results (median follow-up, 37.6 months). Because of the long follow-up, the larger control group, and the low crossover rate, CARE-HF was better powered than COMPANION to show the effects of CRT. CRT improved cardiac function, symptoms, and quality of life. Effects were evident within 3 months and persisted for at least 18 months. There were highly significant reductions in the primary endpoint (by 37%), all-cause mortality (by 40% in the extension phase), death due to worsening heart failure (by 45%), and sudden death (by 46%). The risk of death or urgent hospitalization for worsening CHF was reduced by 52%. These results established CRT as part of the routine management of heart failure.

Meta-analysis

A meta-analysis of trials shows that the benefits of CRT are consistent across trials (Fig. 74.8).[13]

RETHINQ

This was a 6-month double-blind study of only 172 patients designed to investigate the effects of CRT in patients who needed an ICD and who had a QRS of less than 130 ms, NYHA class III symptoms, and echocardiographic dyssynchrony.[23] The study showed that CRT improved symptoms (P =.006) regardless of QRS duration but had no effect on exercise capacity or quality of life. Inappropriate statistical analysis suggested that peak exercise oxygen consumption may have improved in the subset with QRS of 120 to 130 ms. A test for heterogeneity in response according to QRS duration would probably have been neutral. The study provides no evidence that selection of patients on the basis of echocardiographic dyssynchrony is valuable.

REVERSE

This was a double-blind study conducted predominantly in patients with mild symptoms of heart failure and permitted inclusion of LVEF up to 40%, although the mean LVEF was similar to that in CARE-HF.[24] CRT improved cardiac function, appeared to improve symptoms or to prevent their worsening, and reduced morbidity after only 1 year of follow-up. Many of the patients continue in an extension phase. Interim reports from the extension phase indicate a lower morbidity and mortality in patients assigned to CRT-on.

RHYTHM II ICD and DECREASE-HF

These randomized trials compared simultaneous biventricular pacing with echocardiographically "optimized" VV programming.[25,26] They suggested little difference between these interventions. By inference, these studies suggest that VV interval timing plays little role in the effects of CRT and that interventricular and perhaps intraventricular dyssynchrony are not the primary target of therapy.

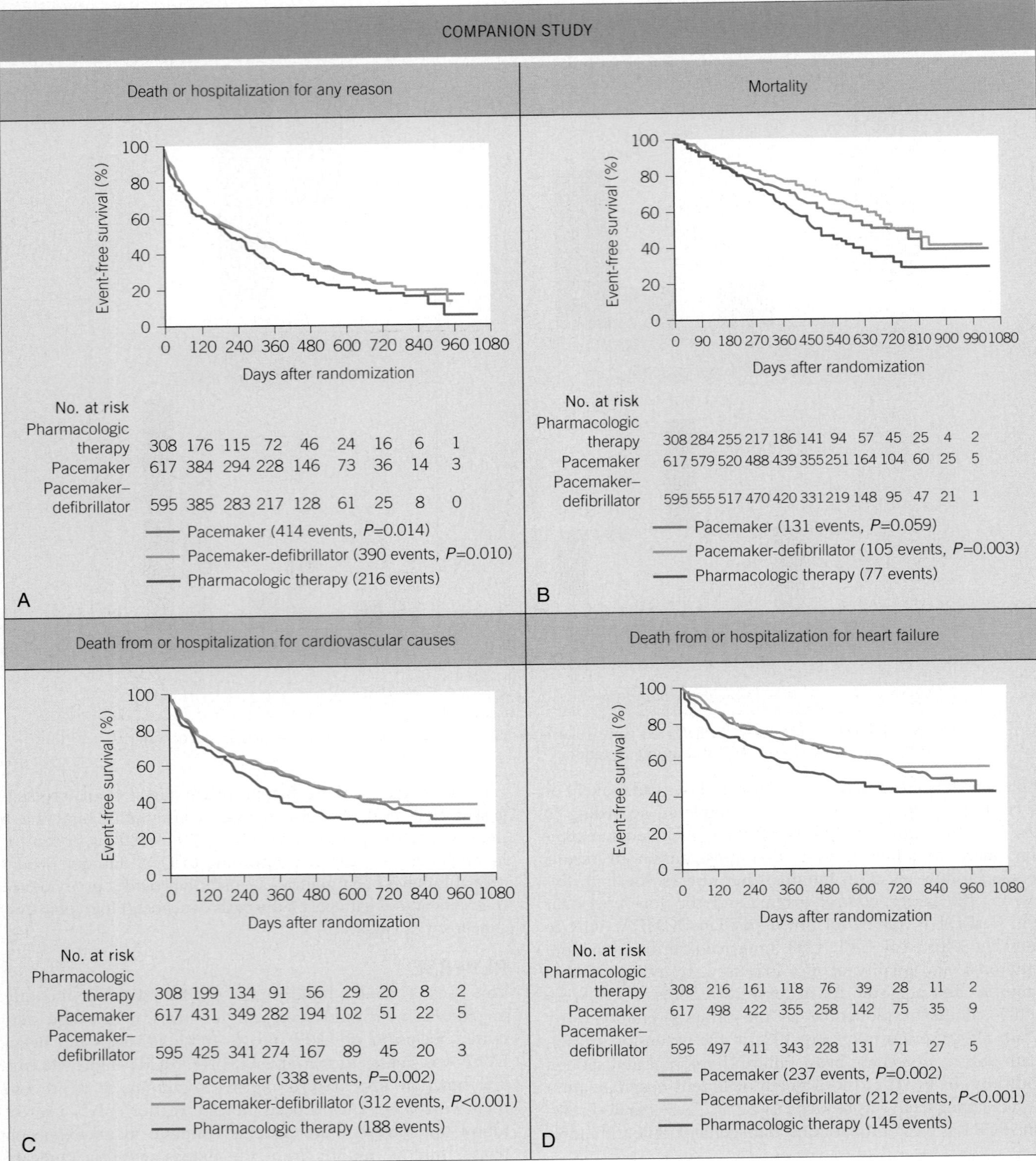

Figure 74.6 COMPANION study.

Smaller Randomized, Controlled Studies

Small trials suggest that in patients with LVSD and heart failure, upgrading right to biventricular pacing improves cardiac function.[27] Stimulation of the left ventricle at multiple sites may be superior to stimulation of only one.[28] In patients with atrial fibrillation and cardiac dysfunction, AV ablation followed by biventricular pacing is superior to RV pacing in terms of symptoms, exercise capacity, ventricular function, and perhaps morbidity and mortality.[29]

CRT or CRT-D

There is a substantial cost difference between CRT and CRT-D. CRT-D may prevent more sudden deaths but also carries the risk of increased morbidity from inappropriate

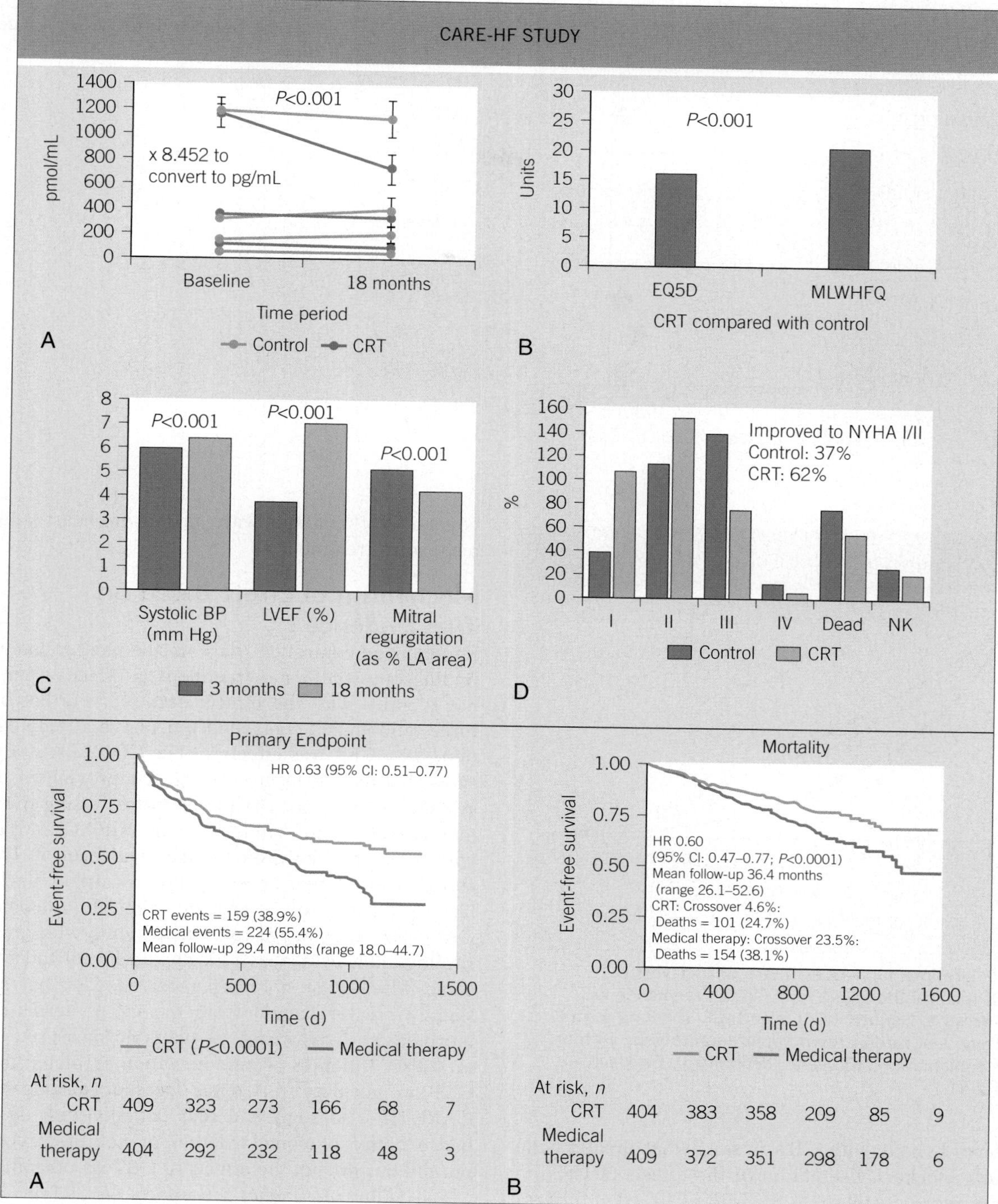

Figure 74.7 CARE-HF study.

(i.e., in the absence of ventricular tachycardia) or unnecessary (i.e., for ventricular tachycardia that would have self-terminated) shocks. However, a projected lifetime analysis of CARE-HF[30] (Fig. 74.9), assuming that a CRT-D device would prevent about two thirds of sudden deaths that occurred with CRT, suggests that CRT-D rather than CRT might be cost-effective and affordable for patients who are expected to survive more than about 7 years if death from heart failure or arrhythmias is prevented. Age is one of the best predictors of such risk. On the other hand, given that most patients with LVSD who require an ICD have or will develop dyssynchrony, it seems unwise and uneconomical to implant an ICD rather than CRT-D.[31]

IMPACT OF CARDIAC RESYNCHRONIZATION THERAPY ON SYMPTOMS

The effect of CRT on morbidity and mortality is substantial and similar to the effects of beta blockers during 12 months of follow-up. No substantial placebo-controlled trial of beta blockers continued much beyond 1 year, and so the evidence

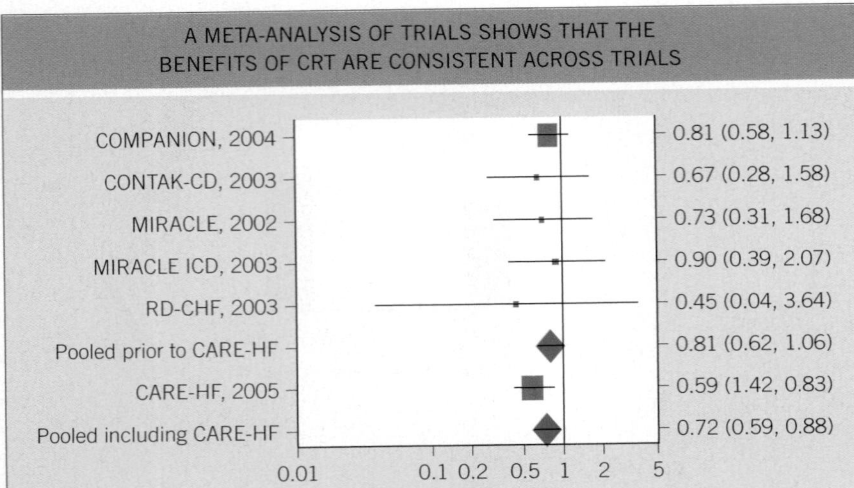

Figure 74.8 A meta-analysis of trials shows that the benefits of CRT are consistent across trials.

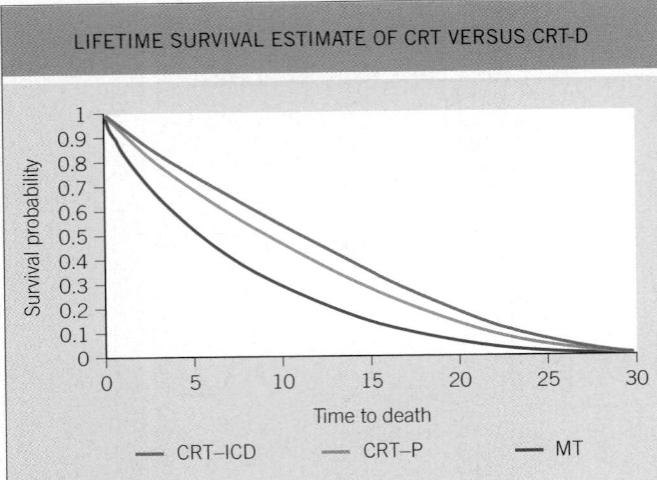

Figure 74.9 Lifetime survival estimate of CRT versus CRT-D. MT, medical therapy. (From Yao G, Freemantle N, Calvert M, Bryan S, Daubert J-C, Cleland JGF. The long-term cost-effectiveness of cardiac resynchronization therapy with or without an implantable cardioverter-defibrillator. Eur Heart J 2007;28:42-51.)

for long-term benefit with CRT is somewhat greater than that for beta blockers. Estimation of the effects of CRT on symptoms is more complex. In the MIRACLE trial, 59% of CRT recipients versus 37% of controls improved by at least one NYHA class. Quality of life, measured with the MLWHF questionnaire, is widely used and provides a means of comparing trials and different treatments. The effects of CRT on MLWHF are summarized in Table 74.2 and compared with other interventions.[2] The effect of CRT appears more substantial than that of many other interventions. Recent reports show that the benefit persists for at least 18 months and probably much longer.[32] However, the magnitude of the symptom response is highly variable. Some patients obtain a dramatic improvement and others deteriorate. Change is, of course, highly dependent on the starting point because patients with few symptoms have less room for improvement, and presumably there is a point of no return beyond which patients with very severe heart failure cannot respond to treatment.

Mechanism of Effect Based on Trial Evidence

Randomized controlled trials are the most robust method of finding out whether a treatment is effective but often do not identify why the effects occurred. Further analysis of three randomized controlled trials have attempted to determine why CRT was effective. The CONTAK study failed to show that dyssynchrony predicted improvement in LV end-systolic volume, but the method of assessing dyssynchrony may have been too crude.[33] In the MIRACLE trial, patients with greater echocardiographic evidence of LV dyssynchrony had a larger improvement in cardiac function, but it lacked power to investigate clinical outcomes.[34] The CARE-HF study suggested that patients with greater echocardiographic evidence of LV dyssynchrony had a better outcome whether or not they received CRT but also had a slightly greater benefit from therapy in terms of reduced morbidity.[35,36] However, no variable measured at baseline or within 3 months of randomization predicted the effect of CRT on mortality.[35] A tissue Doppler imaging substudy of CARE-HF also suggested that patients with dyssynchrony had a better outcome whether or not they received CRT but did not predict the effects of CRT on outcome.[37]

The failure to predict the effects of CRT in randomized controlled trials contrasts starkly with the numerous reports of small observational trials mostly from single centers.[2] These generally suggest that patients with dyssynchrony have a better outcome after CRT implantation. However, the investigators failed to distinguish between outcome and treatment effect, a fatal error.

Patients with greater dyssynchrony are more likely to have dilated cardiomyopathy. Patients with dilated cardiomyopathy are more likely to improve their ventricular function in response to all sorts of interventions and also have a better prognosis. As noted before, the dyssynchronous ventricle, for a given LVEF, is intrinsically less sick. It is not surprising that patients with dyssynchrony do better with CRT in observational studies because they were going to

EFFECT OF GUIDELINE-INDICATED THERAPIES ON QUALITY OF LIFE OR SYMPTOMS IN HEART FAILURE				
Study (and number in QoL analysis)	**Intervention**	**Baseline Minnesota Score (higher is worse)**	**Duration**	**Change compared to control group**
SOLVD-treatment (N = 77)	Enalapril vs placebo	30		Improved 5 points $P<0.01$
DIG study (N = 589)	Digoxin vs placebo	30	12 mo	No difference
Beta-Blocker Review	Beta-blockers vs placebo	Variable	6-12 mo	Generally no difference observed
Val-HeFT (N = 3010)	Valsartan vs placebo (added to ACE inhibitors)	32	~24 mo	Improved 1.75 points $P=0.005$
MIRACLE (N = 453)	CRT on vs off	59	6 mo	Improved 9 points $P<0.001$
MIRACLE-ICD (N = 319)	CRT on vs off In ICD patients	56	6 mo	Improved 6.5 points $P=0.02$
MIRACLE-ICD-II (N = 177)	CRT on vs off In ICD patients	40	6 mo	No difference
COMPANION (N = 1267)	CRT or CRT-D vs neither	NA	6 mo	Improved 14 points $P<0.001$
CARE-HF (N = 813)	CRT vs no CRT	44	3 mo	Improved 10.6 points $P<0.001$
CARE-HF (N =813)	CRT vs no CRT	44	18 mo	Improved 10.7 points $P<0.001$
REVERSE	CRT on vs off	28	12 mo	No difference

QoL, quality of life; SOLVD, Studies of Left Ventricular Dysfunction; DIG, Digitalis Investigation Group; Val-HeFT, Valsartan Heart Failure Trial.

Table 74.2 Effect of guideline-indicated therapies on quality of life or symptoms in heart failure.

have a better outcome anyway. Larger multicenter observational studies show that measures of dyssynchrony are poorly reproducible and are weak predictors of outcome, confirming the observations from randomized trials.[38] Observational trials are also difficult to interpret because they use surrogate outcomes, such as improved LV function. The CARE-HF trial shows that patients with ischemic heart disease have less improvement in LV function but as great or greater reduction in mortality.[7,21] In other words, changes in LV function with CRT are a poor surrogate for its effect on mortality.

Two other considerations suggest that selection of patients on the basis of dyssynchrony is futile. First, investigations suggest that most dilated, poorly functioning ventricles become dyssynchronous when stressed.[39] Second, QRS becomes progressively wider in patients with heart failure, with about 10% of patients with LVSD developing new-onset left bundle branch block each year.[11] This suggests that many patients who do not have obvious dyssynchrony initially will develop it later. In other words, the long-term effects of CRT cannot be predicted because the substrate for the effect of CRT is absent at the time of implantation. Whether a policy of careful repetitive dyssynchrony monitoring would be superior to prophylactic implantation is not clear. If dyssynchrony is a highly mutable state, then routine rather than selective implantation would be the better policy.

Two potential mechanisms of CRT effect that have received insufficient attention are AV dyssynchrony and mitral regurgitation. There were no substantial randomized controlled trials of AV dyssynchrony, but the small trials that were done had mixed results.[13,14] It is possible that the major benefit of CRT is reduction in AV dyssynchrony while ensuring that interventricular dyssynchrony does not get worse. Studies of CRT programming suggest that in contrast to VV programming, AV programming can make a profound difference. In the CARE-HF study, the two most powerful predictors of prognosis were NT-proBNP and the severity of mitral regurgitation.[35] When these were reassessed 3 months after randomization, they were even more powerful predictors of outcome, although they explained only about 25% of the overall benefit of CRT on prognosis. Correction of mitral regurgitation could be an important mechanism of benefit. Indeed, in our experience, patients with moderately severe mitral regurgitation that is corrected by CRT are likely to be super-responders.

HEALTH ECONOMIC ASPECTS OF CARDIAC RESYNCHRONIZATION THERAPY

Health economics is about spending money wisely, not about cutting costs. Prolonging life will usually incur additional health care costs. The simplest way to reduce costs is to let patients die quickly by medical neglect, if you can avoid the legal bill! This is clearly unethical and not a view supported by any health care administration. Unlike with pharmacologic therapy, most of the costs of CRT and CRT-D are incurred at the time of implantation rather than spread evenly throughout the course of therapy. There is a large difference in costs between CRT and CRT-D that needs to be justified by superior outcomes. CRT is highly cost-effective when it is applied in most clinical scenarios (Fig. 74.10).[30,40] However, CRT-D is cost-effective only when it is applied to patients with a relatively good life expectancy, taking into account the expected

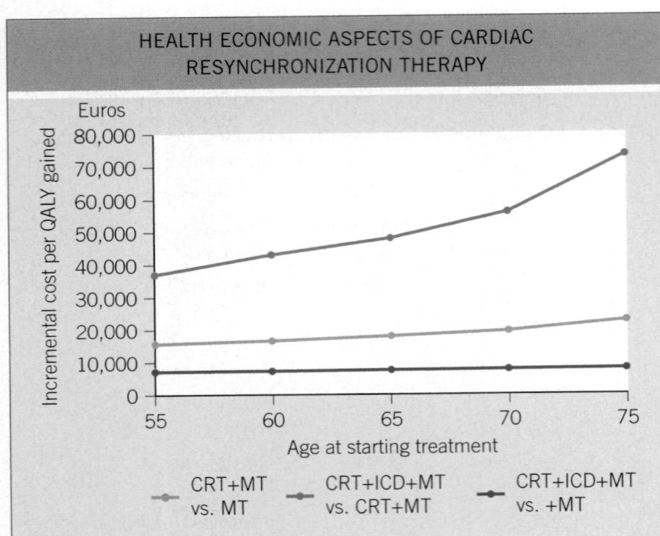

Figure 74.10 Health economic aspects of cardiac resynchronization therapy (CRT). ICD, implantable cardioverter-defibrillator; MT, medical therapy; QALY, quality-adjusted life-years.

benefits of CRT-D. A life expectancy of about 7 years after device implantation is a reasonable threshold from a health economic viewpoint.

Selection of Patients

To understand how investigation might help in the selection of patients, it is first necessary to consider existing guidelines on selection of patients and how they came about. Guidelines from the U.S. National Institute for Health and Clinical Excellence and the European Society of Cardiology differ little.[41,42] They suggest that CRT should be used in patients with chronic heart failure who have prolonged QRS duration, LVEF of 35% or less, and moderate or severe symptoms in sinus rhythm despite standard pharmacologic therapy. Evidence of cardiac dyssynchrony should be sought, according to some guidelines, when the QRS duration is between 120 and 149 ms. Why has this guidance come about? No one has ever shown that CRT does not work in patients excluded from treatment by this guidance. These criteria were developed by scientific committees on the basis of educated guesswork to conduct a clinical trial to show a treatment effect. They were not designed to show which patients did not benefit. Absence of evidence should not be confused with evidence of absence of an effect. CRT probably works equally well in many patients currently excluded by guidelines from receiving CRT. Jumping to premature conclusions about what does or does not work does not help patients. Of course, absence of evidence cannot be construed as evidence of effect either. An open mind, clinical judgment, and logical deduction all need to be employed in selecting an appropriate patient for CRT.

Should Symptoms Be Used to Select Patients for Therapy?

CRT can improve symptoms only if the patient has severe enough symptoms in the first place so that a benefit can be noticed when the treatment is effective. However, many patients with heart failure do not remain stable for long periods but have periodic worsening in response to change in the underlying disease, diet, therapy, or intercurrent events. CRT might retard the development[19,43,44] or recurrence[17,20] of symptoms. On the other hand, there is little evidence that symptoms predict the effect of CRT on prognosis.[43] More symptomatic patients tend to have a worse prognosis, but the results of simple tests, such as brain natriuretic peptide level, are a far better guide to outcome than symptoms are.[45] Also, it is not clear that the sickest patients benefit the most from CRT. As with any treatment, there are those too well to benefit and those too sick.

Recent data from CARE-HF showed that about 20% of patients reported that they had no or only mild symptoms of heart failure at the time of randomization.[43] These patients had a slightly better prognosis than that of other patients but the same relative benefit in terms of morbidity and mortality as that of more symptomatic patients. The REVERSE study enrolled patients with no or only mild stable symptoms and showed substantial improvement in LV function and a reduction in hospitalization for worsening heart failure within 1 year.[24]

QRS Duration

Patients with a broad QRS have a worse prognosis and more evidence of ventricular dyssynchrony on imaging. People have subsequently drawn sweeping but unjustified conclusions about this relationship.[2] QRS is an indicator of a more dilated, more poorly functioning left ventricle.[9] Dyssynchrony is more common in more dilated ventricles. QRS prolongation and dyssynchrony probably occur together because they are both associated with sick ventricles. Whereas QRS duration has repeatedly predicted a poor outcome,[46] dyssynchrony on imaging has not.[35-37] Indeed, dyssynchrony may be associated with a more favorable prognosis after adjusting for the severity of ventricular dysfunction.[2] It is likely that the adverse prognostic significance of increased QRS duration reflects its association with the severity of LV dilatation and dysfunction rather than the degree of dyssynchrony. Recently, the RETHINQ study reported that CRT did not improve treadmill exercise capacity after 6 months in patients with QRS duration of less than 130 ms and dyssynchrony on echocardiography.[27] The study was not highly powered and not long enough to show effects on clinical outcomes. However, CRT did improve symptoms, regardless of QRS duration. This study provides no support to the concept that either dyssynchrony on imaging or QRS duration is important for selection of patients. However, few patients with QRS duration of less than 130 ms have been recruited in clinical trials of CRT so far.

Heart Rhythm

Studies have so far focused on patients in sinus rhythm. There is little evidence on which to base arguments for or against CRT in patients with atrial fibrillation (AF). The two most substantial studies used AV ablation to control ventricular rate and then compared RV versus biventricular pacing.[2,15] The apparent benefit of CRT may owe more to a deleterious effect of RV pacing than to CRT and constitutes a poor argument for use of CRT in patients with AF. CRT does not appear to alter the risk for development of AF.[47] Patients who developed AF after device implantation in

CARE-HF did worse than other patients but not as poorly as patients who developed AF in the control group. Perhaps the most worrying piece of evidence that CRT might not work in AF comes from studies of device programming. These suggest that moderate alterations in VV interval make little difference to cardiac function[2,26] but that programming of the AV interval can make a large difference.[2] If AV dyssynchrony rather than ventricular dyssynchrony is the key to the success of CRT, benefit in patients with AF might be less or absent, and all efforts to select patients by ventricular dyssynchrony imaging are futile. Studies conducted more than a decade ago suggested that pacing with a shortened AV delay might be beneficial for patients with heart failure. The randomized controlled trials conducted were small and lacked sufficient power to show an effect one way or the other.[2,48] The reason that CRT seems to work better than pacing with a short AV delay may just reflect either adequately powered studies or the fact that CRT improves AV synchrony without making interventricular dyssynchrony worse.

Blood Pressure

Low systolic blood pressure predicts a poor outcome in patients with heart failure.[46] CRT is a unique intervention for heart failure as it is the only treatment, so far, that increases blood pressure and improves outcome. A rise in blood pressure is often one of the immediate responses to CRT and is used by some to select the site for LV pacing.[2] Interestingly, low systolic blood pressure is one of the few variables that independently predicts a greater benefit from CRT.[36]

Imaging

Echocardiography may be a major barrier to the appropriate deployment of CRT, but it is still necessary. We cannot be sure that a dilated, poorly functioning left ventricle is an absolutely necessary substrate for CRT to be effective, but unlike for ventricular dyssynchrony and QRS, there is no evidence yet to challenge this assumption. Patients with severe aortic valve disease are unlikely to respond. Research in "diastolic" heart failure has only recently become possible with the development of reliable indicators of diastolic heart failure, such as amino-terminal brain natriuretic peptide.[49]

Severity of Left Ventricular Dysfunction

Most of the landmark studies of CRT chose LVEF of 35% or less as an entry criterion, but the REVERSE study recently raised the threshold to 40% and showed that benefit in terms of recovery of LV function and in morbidity and mortality was similar to that observed in CARE-HF.[24] About 75% of patients in studies of CRT had LVEF below 30%, and trials usually required patients to also have marked LV dilatation. However, these are echocardiographic measurements and therefore prone to substantial measurement error. Patients with LVEF well above 40% will undoubtedly have been recruited in these studies. There is no evidence that the severity of LVEF predicts benefit from CRT.[35,36]

Ventricular Dyssynchrony

Unfortunately, studies have not attempted to select patients on the basis of AV dyssynchrony. A huge amount of energy has been expended on investigating the ability of a great variety of echocardiographic measures of ventricular dyssynchrony to predict the benefit of CRT, with little success.[2] As noted before, dyssynchrony is a marker of a better prognosis, probably because it indicates the existence of a larger amount of viable myocardium for a given LVEF. This confounds observational studies because patients with dyssynchrony will do better whether or not they receive CRT. Randomized trials have failed to show that intraventricular dyssynchrony predicts benefit,[34,35] although this could reflect the inadequacy of the techniques used rather than a problem with the concept. In CARE-HF and MIRACLE, greater echocardiographic evidence of LV dyssynchrony did predict a slightly greater reduction in death or heart failure hospitalization, but the effect was modest,[35] and intraventricular mechanical delay was associated with a better outcome even in the control group (Fig. 74.11).

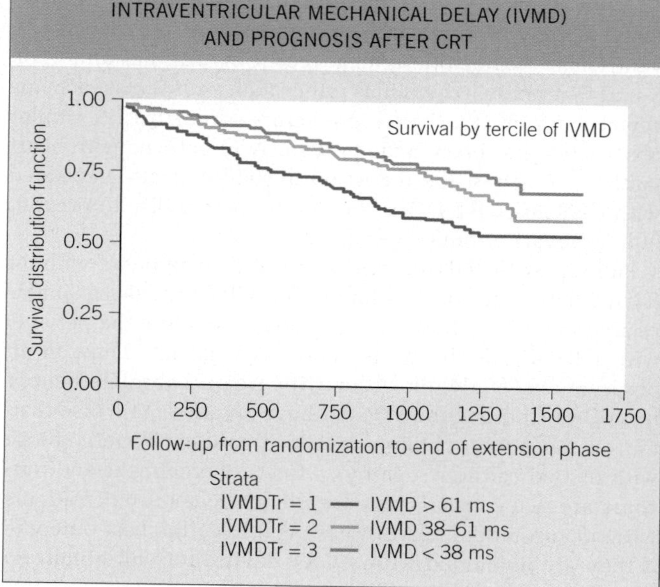

Figure 74.11 Intraventricular mechanical delay (IVMD) and prognosis after CRT.

Left Ventricular Scar

Clearly, a heavily scarred ventricle cannot recover as much contractile function despite stimulation. Patients with ischemic heart disease (IHD) are more likely to have substantial myocardial scar. Scar probably accounts for why patients with LV dysfunction due to IHD have a worse prognosis and gain a smaller improvement in LV function with CRT[35] than do patients who do not have IHD. However, IHD is not a determinant of the relative or absolute benefits of CRT on symptoms, quality of life, or prognosis in randomized studies. Indeed, because the prognosis of patients with IHD is worse, the absolute benefit of CRT quality is greater in this group. Whether scar predicts clinical benefit from CRT is uncertain.[2]

This paradox between the effects of CRT on LV function and outcome in patients with IHD suggests that only some of the benefit of CRT is mediated by improving ventricular function. CRT reduces the risk of sudden cardiac death,[21] and it is possible that CRT suppresses arrhythmias directly or by even small improvements in cardiac function. Interestingly, a study of implantable loop recorders in patients with ventricular dysfunction after a recent myocardial infarction found that bradyarrhythmias rather than ventricular tachyarrhythmias were the better predictors of death.[24] A similar observation has been made previously in patients with heart failure.[50] Much of the reduction in sudden death associated with CRT and CRT-D may be due to their ability to prevent fatal bradyarrhythmic events.

Patients with IHD do not do as well as patients without IHD, whether or not they have CRT. CRT provides a similar relative benefit to both but not enough to allow the patients with IHD to "catch up" to those who do not. Thus, in an observational study, the group with greatest absolute benefit from CRT (those with IHD) still have an outcome worse than that of those who obtain a smaller treatment benefit (those with dilated cardiomyopathy). Effects of treatment and outcome are two concepts that should not be confused. Patients without substantial heart disease will have the best outcome if they are implanted with a CRT device but will obtain no benefit from it and may be harmed.

Mitral Regurgitation

Reduction of mitral regurgitation is, along with a rise in systolic blood pressure, one of the most immediate and often substantial effects of CRT, and reduction in mitral regurgitation by CRT is associated with an improved outcome.[36] However, whereas mitral regurgitation, at least when it is functional, may form part of the basis for response to CRT, it has not been shown to predict benefit.

This discussion highlights the fact that no preimplantation measurement predicts response to CRT in a clinically useful way. A clinician who knows that the left ventricle is dilated and contracts poorly can judge by use of clinical skills alone which patients are most likely to derive benefit from CRT.

Does the Early Response to CRT Predict Long-term Benefit?

Another approach to trying to understand the relationship between dyssynchrony and CRT is to investigate the early response to CRT. There are many reasons why CRT might fail to improve ventricular function, including failure of the device to capture the ventricles (due to either high stimulation thresholds or the onset of atrial fibrillation with a rapid intrinsic ventricular response), lack of a myocardial substrate that can respond to CRT (for instance, scar), and progression of the underlying disease. The initial echocardiographic response to CRT is the sum of the ability of the left ventricle to respond and the adequacy of intervention.[35] If resynchronization of baseline dyssynchrony accounts for the response to CRT, the early response should predict the benefit that the patient will acquire in the long term.

Again, unfortunately, this is not the case.[6] Whereas reduction in mitral regurgitation, rise in blood pressure, and improved LV function all predict a better prognosis after intervention, altogether they explain only about 25% of the long-term benefit of CRT.[35] Some other factors are at play. It may be that small improvements in LV function have striking benefits on arrhythmia risk in some patients with heart failure. However, ultimately, it may be our lack of understanding of the nature of cardiac dyssynchrony that is the problem. Dyssynchrony may be a nearly universal problem of the diseased left ventricle, in which case there is no need to try to detect it. Still more problematic is the possibility that dyssynchrony at rest waxes and wanes over time.[1] Faced with trying to select patients by serial stress echocardiography on a regular basis, maybe it is just cheaper and more effective to implant.

TECHNIQUE OF IMPLANTATION

The extra, technically demanding step in CRT implantation is the transvenous insertion of the LV lead into one of the tributary veins draining into the coronary sinus. The coronary sinus is initially cannulated with a specially designed, preshaped sheath that has many shapes and sizes to accommodate the variable anatomy of the coronary sinus and retrograde venography to visualize cardiac venous anatomy (Fig. 74.12). The LV lead is inserted into the target marginal, posterior, or posterolateral veins, and a stable position is found that does not pace the phrenic nerve. Monitoring of arterial pressure may help optimize the pacing site as there is some evidence that the rise in systolic blood pressure associated with CRT predicts a better response. However, this is not a well-established fact. Sometimes, a target vein is unavailable, and a surgical implantation should be considered through mini-thoracotomy.

SAFETY AND COMPLICATIONS OF CARDIAC RESYNCHRONIZATION THERAPY

CRT implantation is a relatively safe procedure. Randomized controlled trials show that CRT implantation is successful in approximately 93% of patients. Procedure-related risks include death (0.3%, although there were none in CARE-HF) and a 4% to 5% chance of problems such as coronary vein dissection and perforation and pneumothorax. The most common early problems are hematoma around the generator, displacement of one or more leads (usually the LV lead), and infection (1% to 2%). Late complications are loss of capture and, especially with CRT-D, malfunction of the RV lead and inappropriate or unnecessary shocks.

OPTIMIZATION AND MAXIMIZING RESPONSE

As noted, so far, there has been little success in selecting patients likely to have a substantial response to CRT. The same may be said for the selection of patients for most other cardiovascular treatments, including coronary bypass surgery, angioplasty, implantable defibrillators, and pharmacologic therapy. It is not clear why the clinical community has become obsessed about this aspect of CRT. Enlightened cardiologists put more effort into optimizing the treatment response to CRT than in the technical details of patient selection. A good clinician, knowing that the patient has heart failure associated with LV dilatation, can select patients suitable for CRT with bedside skills alone.

Trials show that programming of the VV interval has little clinical effect, supporting the notion that ventricular dyssynchrony is not the basis for the effect of CRT.[25,26] However,

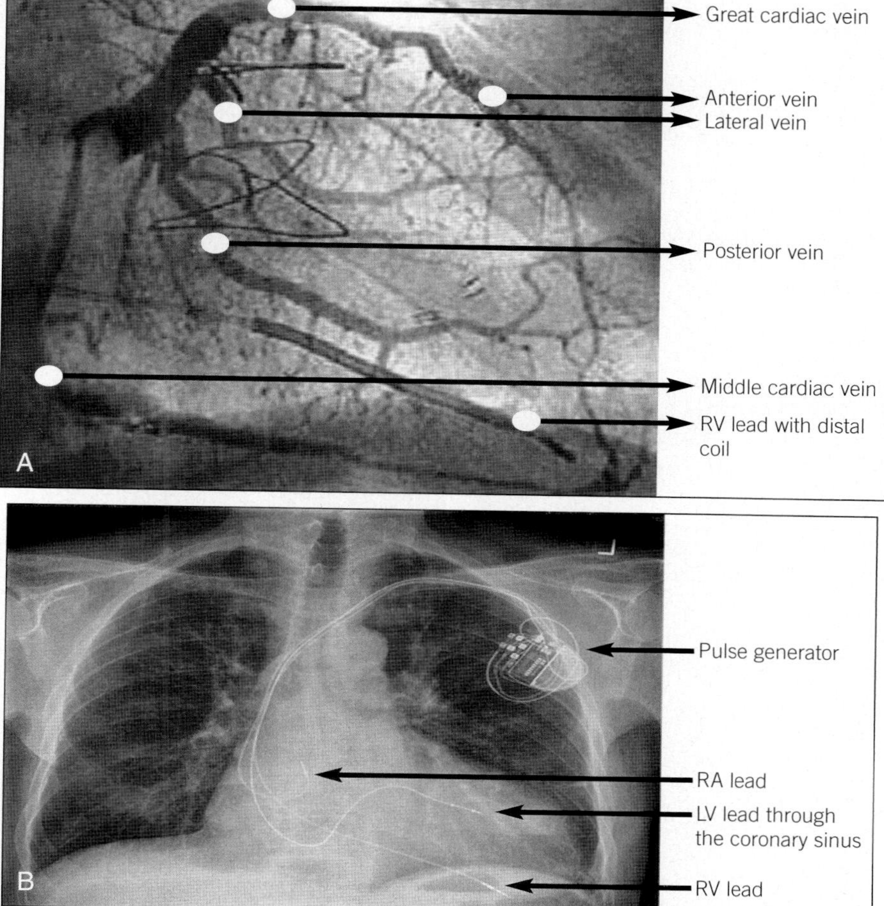

Figure 74.12 A, Retrograde coronary venogram (right anterior oblique view) in a patient undergoing a biventricular ICD implantation. The occlusive balloon is placed in the coronary sinus. The lateral vein is the most commonly used vein for placement of the LV lead, but posterior-lateral, posterior, and anterior veins could be suitable targets to achieve satisfactory pacing. **B,** Chest radiograph showing a biventricular pacemaker with three leads: RA lead, LV lead, and RV lead. (From Albouaini K, Egred M, Rao A, Alahmar A, Wright DJ. Cardiac resynchronization therapy: evidence based benefits and patient selection. Eur J Intern Med 2008;19:165-172.)

AV programming, which has been much less well studied, may have a large effect, suggesting that atriobiventricular pacing works mainly by enhancing AV synchrony, reducing mitral regurgitation, and not making VV dyssynchrony worse. Echocardiography probably has a valuable role in the optimization of the AV interval. Optimization should probably be done before the patient leaves the hospital and repeated after 3 and 12 months and perhaps annually thereafter.

SUMMARY

CRT is a highly effective treatment for patients selected according to current guidelines. Symptomatic patients in sinus rhythm, with LVEF of 35% or less and QRS of more than 150 ms, clearly benefit. However, patients with few or perhaps none of these characteristics may benefit as much if not more. Patients who are unlikely to die of anything else other than an arrhythmia or heart failure within the next 5 to 7 years should have a CRT-D device. On the other hand, it may be wise to implant CRT-D rather than an ICD in patients who require an ICD who have LVSD. Perhaps the biggest problem with CRT is its success. The benefits are so dramatic and immediate in some patients that the more modest and delayed benefit observed in most may cause disappointment. Although sicker patients provide more immediate gratification in terms of symptom response, gains in longevity are often measured in months. In contrast, patients with few symptoms who already have a moderately good prognosis may gain extra years of life. The physician and the patient need to be clear what they are using CRT for.

chapter 75

Surgery, Mechanical Circulatory Assist Devices, and Cardiac Transplantation for Heart Failure

James B. Young

Definition

- Surgical interventions in patients who have heart failure can correct specific problems that cause heart failure (e.g., coronary and valvular heart disease) and support the circulation (ventricular assist devices) or entirely replace the heart (cardiac transplantation and total artificial heart implantation).
- Some surgical procedures are designed to counter detrimental cardiac remodeling by eliminating valvular regurgitation (e.g., mitral valve repair), by restoring more normal left ventricular geometry (e.g., aneurysmectomy, infarct exclusion, or partial left ventricular resection), or by replacing cardiac pump function virtually (mechanical circulatory assist devices) or entirely (cardiac transplantation and the total artificial heart).
- Determination of which heart failure patients might benefit with surgical therapies requires careful assessment of patients by a joint cardiology and cardiovascular surgery team.

Key Features

- Proper selection of patients and tailoring of surgical options to specific clinical situations are critical.
- Surgical procedures must be coupled to appropriate heart failure pharmacotherapy and devices such as biventricular pacers and defibrillators.

Clinical Implications

- The surgical armamentarium for heart failure is large and should be coupled to medical and electrophysiologic treatments.
- Gratifying results with surgery in carefully selected patients can be anticipated.
- Some surgical interventions seemingly ameliorate pathophysiologic processes of detrimental cardiac remodeling, whereas others aim to establish more normal intracardiac pressures and circulatory flow by correcting anatomic abnormalities.

During the past decade, a great deal of insight has been gained into surgical strategies that might ameliorate heart failure. Interestingly, aside from cardiac transplantation or mechanical circulatory assist device insertion, cardiac surgery in advanced heart failure was previously often contraindicated. New knowledge and evolving surgical techniques are now showing significant promise, at least in part because of the use of state-of-the-art pharmacotherapy before and after surgical intervention. With this combination strategy, specialized heart failure treatment centers have evolved, with resultant improvements in outcomes. Many surgical procedures ameliorate specific cardiac difficulties that lead to heart failure. Some attenuate detrimental cardiac remodeling (the key to the progressive pathophysiologic changes of this syndrome), and others are designed to improve circulatory flow directly.

Table 75.1 details operations that are, perhaps, helpful in select heart failure patients. Both acute and chronic ischemic heart disease can be addressed with coronary revascularization. Mitral valve repair or replacement for papillary muscle rupture or dysfunction in a setting of acute myocardial infarction or chronic ventricular ischemia can ameliorate profound hemodynamic compromise, as can closure of a ventricular septal defect that develops after a myocardial infarction. In patients who have ischemic cardiomyopathy and long-term complications of myocardial infarction, repair of a left ventricular pseudoaneurysm with aneurysmorrhaphy or aneurysmectomy has proved helpful. More recently, operations designed to remove akinetic segments of the left ventricle, so-called infarct exclusion (the Dor procedure), have been performed.

Valvular heart disease produces abnormal preload and afterload that are detrimental in settings of ventricular dysfunction. Aortic, mitral, and tricuspid valve replacement or repair for primary stenotic or regurgitant lesions is also important. Ventricular remodeling procedures are designed to normalize ventricular shape and, subsequently, function. The premise behind these operations is that a reduction in ventricular radius will translate into a decrease in ventricular volume and, thus, ventricular wall stress. Wall stress is one of the primary stimulants of abnormal ventricular hypertrophy and cardiac remodeling that leads to further heart failure. These procedures include aneurysmorrhaphy and aneurysmectomy procedures and the infarct resection operation (Dor procedure). Mitral valve repair or replacement will also reduce the volume overload of mitral regurgitation and cause the ventricle to decrease its size. Two procedures, now for the most part abandoned, that addressed cardiac remodeling in creative and unique fashion are partial left ventriculectomy (the Batista procedure) and dynamic cardiomyoplasty (rotating the latissimus dorsi into the thorax and wrapping the heart with it). Mechanical circulatory support procedures, such as intra-aortic balloon pump placement, extracorporeal oxygenation system implantation, ventricular assist device insertion, and total artificial heart, benefit patients who have cardiogenic shock and more profound end-stage heart failure syndromes. These procedures can be

SURGICAL PROCEDURES THAT MAY BE HELPFUL IN HEART FAILURE	
For ischemic heart disease	Coronary artery bypass graft surgery (for both acute and chronic ischemic heart failure syndromes) Mitral valve repair or replacement for papillary muscle rupture Closure of post–myocardial infarction ventricular septal defect Ventricular pseudoaneurysm repair Aneurysmorrhaphy or aneurysmectomy Infarct exclusion procedure (Dor operation)
For valvular heart disease	Aortic valve repair or replacement for primary aortic stenosis or aortic incompetence Mitral valve repair or replacement for primary mitral stenosis or mitral incompetence Tricuspid valve repair or replacement for primary tricuspid stenosis or tricuspid incompetence
Ventricular remodeling procedures	Partial left ventriculectomy (Batista operation)—largely abandoned Infarct exclusion procedure (Dor operation) Aneurysmorrhaphy or aneurysmectomy Mitral valve repair for secondary mitral regurgitation Dynamic cardiomyoplasty—largely abandoned
Circulatory support procedures	Intra-aortic balloon pump placement Use of extracorporeal membrane oxygenator Ventricular assist device insertion Total artificial heart implantation
Cardiac replacement	Ventricular assist device insertion (virtual heart replacement) Artificial heart implantation (total heart replacement) Cardiac transplantation

Table 75.1 Surgical procedures that may be helpful in heart failure.

done to "bridge" patients to recovery enough to allow device removal, to other more permanent devices, or to transplantation. Cardiac replacement can be the ultimate surgical procedure in individuals with advanced heart failure. Virtual replacement is noted with ventricular assist device insertion, whereas total replacement is the goal of the artificial heart and cardiac transplantation. Obviously, these procedures completely remove the diseased heart.

The rationale for surgical procedures in heart failure is summarized in Table 75.2. Coronary revascularization operations are designed to improve heart perfusion and to resuscitate ischemic or hibernating myocardium. Reduction of cardiac preload and afterload perturbation by repair of valvular or other structural abnormalities leads to improved ventricular geometry with improved metabolic function. Indeed, aneurysmectomy, aneurysmorrhaphy, and infarct exclusion all focus on creation of a more appropriate ventricular geometry and left ventricular mass to volume ratio, which decreases left ventricular wall tension and, then,

RATIONALE FOR SURGICAL PROCEDURES IN HEART FAILURE
Myocardial perfusion to resuscitate viable myocardium that might recover function and decrease angina
Correction of preload or afterload abnormalities
Increase forward stroke volume
Normalize ventricular geometry
Increase left ventricular mass-volume ratio
Decrease left ventricular wall tension
Reduce myocardial oxygen demand
Alter pathologic molecular and cellular responses

Table 75.2 Rationale for surgical procedures in heart failure.

myocardial oxygen demand. Elimination of mitral regurgitation should increase forward stroke volume in addition to beneficial left ventricular cavity shape changes. All of these changes are likely to attenuate or to reverse detrimental molecular and cellular responses to increased wall stress.

This chapter considers operations performed for ischemic heart disease, procedures for valvular heart disease (both primary and secondary), ventricular remodeling procedures, and mechanical circulatory support tactics, including ventricular assist device insertion and cardiac replacement with the total artificial heart and heart transplant.

OPERATIONS FOR HEART FAILURE IN THE SETTING OF ISCHEMIC HEART DISEASE

Description of Procedures

Coronary artery bypass graft (CABG) surgery is the most commonly performed operation in heart failure patients. Growing experience with coronary revascularization strategies, such as off-pump coronary procedures (beating heart surgery), may be decreasing the operative risk in the heart failure subset. New strategies for cardioplegia and compulsive operative techniques have made mortality rates for most patients acceptable. The use of arterial conduits has resulted in more durable benefits. Unfortunately, many patients who require coronary revascularization for heart failure have had multiple previous sternotomies or additional valvular lesions that need to be addressed, and this makes many operations a special challenge.

Indications, Contraindications, and Objectives

Patients who have asymptomatic left ventricular dysfunction, compensated congestive heart failure, overt congestive heart failure, chronic end-stage heart failure, or acute cardiogenic shock (particularly in the setting of myocardial infarction or unstable angina pectoris) may benefit from CABG surgery. Relief of active ischemia is generally associated with clinical improvement and decreased heart failure morbidity and mortality. Patients who have coronary artery disease predominate in most heart failure populations, particularly those that have been studied in large, randomized clinical trials. In the Studies of Left Ventricular Dysfunction (SOLVD) trials,

38% of patients had angina pectoris and 66% had a previous myocardial infarction.[1] In patients who have asymptomatic left ventricular dysfunction, the risk for development of symptomatic congestive heart failure was increased twofold to threefold in patients with angina pectoris and fourfold to sixfold in patients with previous myocardial infarction. In the Framingham study, coronary heart disease alone or in combination with hypertension was the most common problem causing heart failure.[2]

Because of the prevalence of coronary heart disease and the ability of coronary artery revascularization procedures to prevent some pathophysiologic sequelae, many consensus guidelines for heart failure diagnosis and treatment have been developed.[3-5] A consensus has emerged among many that three groups of heart failure patients might be amenable to revascularization and should be searched for:

- patients who have angina;
- patients who have a history of previous myocardial infarction and no current angina but demonstrate large areas of so-called viable myocardium (that is, "stunned" or "hibernating" myocardium that does not properly contract and, if it is satisfactorily perfused, is likely to have recovery of function); and
- patients who have neither angina nor a past history of myocardial infarction but who belong to a high-risk subset of coronary heart disease.

Many clinical trials have addressed the utility of surgical coronary revascularization in heart failure patients.[6] Both ischemic and hibernating myocardium should be addressed. Hibernating myocardium describes nonfunctional segments of the myocardial wall that are hypoperfused and noncontractile but still viable; hibernating myocardium is distinct from ventricular scar or ischemic zones. Patients who do not have ischemia or hibernation and who demonstrate only postinfarction scar seem less likely to benefit from revascularization procedures but may be suitable candidates for some left ventricular remodeling operations, particularly the infarct exclusion or Dor procedure.[6] However, no randomized clinical trials have specifically evaluated the outcome of CABG surgery in heart failure patients, and most published studies preceded the era of aggressive multidimensional pharmacologic therapy. The three large randomized clinical trials of CABG surgery versus medical management actually excluded patients with clinically significant congestive heart failure and left ventricular dysfunction, particularly severely reduced left ventricular ejection fraction (LVEF) of less than 35%.[7-9] Nonetheless, cohort studies that have evaluated the effect of CABG surgery on survival in patients who have heart failure and severe angina have shown generally positive results.[6] Many patients who have diabetes mellitus exhibit silent myocardial ischemia,[10] but the amount of ischemia required to justify intervention when symptoms are absent is not well characterized. We are fortunate to have a large-scale, international, multicenter randomized surgical trial for revascularization in patients with heart failure about to conclude. Results from this study will, undoubtedly, influence how the existing heart failure treatment consensus guidelines change in the next few years. The Surgical Treatment of Ischemic Heart Failure (STICH) trial[11] is designed to test two primary hypotheses of surgical therapeutic strategies in patients with left ventricular systolic dysfunction and obstructive coronary artery disease suitable for bypass surgery. The first hypothesis is that improvement in myocardial perfusion by CABG combined with intensive medical therapy improves long-term survival compared with medications alone. The second hypothesis is that left ventricular reconstruction (surgical optimization of ventricular shape and size) in patients with anterior left ventricular akinesia combined with medical therapy and CABG improves long-term survival free of cardiac hospitalization compared with CABG and medical therapy. Secondary endpoints of this trial include cardiac mortality and morbidity, health resource utilization, cost and effectiveness, quality of life, and exercise capacity as well as treatment-specific prediction of primary trial endpoints by baseline measurements of myocardial ischemia and viability and by baseline and post-treatment measurements of ventricular size and function and neurohormonal and proinflammatory cytokine levels. This will be a landmark study that drives into the very core of controversy about medical versus surgical therapy for ischemic heart disease. Several thousand patients have been enrolled into this study, and follow-up should be completed shortly.

At present, however, heart failure treatment guidelines generally suggest that patients with heart failure and no substantive contraindications to surgery or percutaneous interventions who have activity-limiting angina pectoris, angina that occurs frequently at rest, or recurrent episodes of acute pulmonary edema in a setting of diminished LVEF should undergo coronary angiography as an initial diagnostic test to determine whether suitable targets for CABG (Table 75.3) or angioplasty are present. Some patients may need subsequent physiologic testing to quantify and to localize ischemic myocardium or to determine myocardial viability.[3-5]

One must take into consideration the overall severity of the heart failure syndrome, particularly the degree of hemodynamic disturbance. This will, in large part, be related to the extent of left ventricular akinesia and dyskinesia and to the extent of ischemia or hibernation. One must judge the degree of viability versus scar tissue. Importantly, there must be adequate revascularization targets. Concomitant cardiac abnormalities, such as mitral regurgitation, may make one more inclined toward operative

HIERARCHY OF CONSIDERATIONS FOR CORONARY ARTERY BYPASS GRAFT SURGERY IN HEART FAILURE
Severity of heart failure syndrome (hemodynamic disturbance militates against success)
Extent of left ventricular akinesia or dyskinesia (scar)
Extent of left ventricular ischemia or hibernation (viability)
Revascularization targets (coronary anatomy)
Accompanying cardiac abnormalities (e.g., mitral regurgitation)
Comorbid conditions (e.g., diabetes, renal dysfunction, chronic obstructive pulmonary disease, peripheral vascular disease)
Long-term goals (reduction in symptoms, morbidity, and mortality)
Alternative strategies (medications, percutaneous transluminal coronary angioplasty, transmyocardial laser revascularization, heart transplantation)

Table 75.3 Hierarchy of considerations for coronary artery bypass graft surgery in heart failure.

intervention because this problem could also be addressed at the time of surgery. However, concomitant mitral valve repair or replacement in this setting is still controversial. The size and location of left ventricular scar is important as one might consider combining surgical revascularization with infarct resection and left ventricular remodeling, as the STICH trial is addressing. Comorbid conditions that might limit success (e.g., severe diabetes mellitus, renal dysfunction, chronic obstructive pulmonary disease, or troublesome peripheral vascular disease) must be put into perspective and may limit one's enthusiasm for an operation.

When patients who have heart failure and coronary artery disease present without significant angina pectoris, physiologic stress testing can be performed to determine the degree of myocardial ischemia, hibernation, and scarred or nonviable myocardium. Several approaches are available, including perfusion scintigraphy with use of thallium Tl 201 or technetium Tc99m sestamibi in conjunction with exercise or coronary vasodilators, dobutamine stress echocardiography, and positron emission tomography (see Chapter 20).

Surgical considerations in the setting of coronary heart disease and heart failure are presented in Figure 75.1. In cases of cardiomyopathy and substantive congestive heart failure caused by ischemic heart disease when there are no adequate coronary targets for revascularization, one can consider only remodeling operations designed to address akinetic or dyskinetic left ventricular scar and couple this approach with mitral valve repair designed to eliminate mitral regurgitation. If no significant akinesia or dyskinesia or severe mitral regurgitation is present, transmyocardial laser revascularization has been reported to be beneficial if active ischemia is present. The only alternative, however, is often cardiac transplantation. Certainly, patients who undergo infarct exclusion or mitral valve repair but who have unsatisfactory results could also be considered for heart transplantation. Among patients who have adequate coronary revascularization targets, one might differentiate between those who have only moderate or moderately severe left ventricular systolic dysfunction manifested by an LVEF of 25% to 50% and those who have more profound systolic left ventricular dysfunction and symptomatic heart failure (such as patients whose LVEF is less than 25%).

In mild to moderate heart failure, patients who have three-vessel coronary artery disease would probably do best with CABG surgery. The choice of procedure is more difficult in patients who have two-vessel disease. Patients who do not

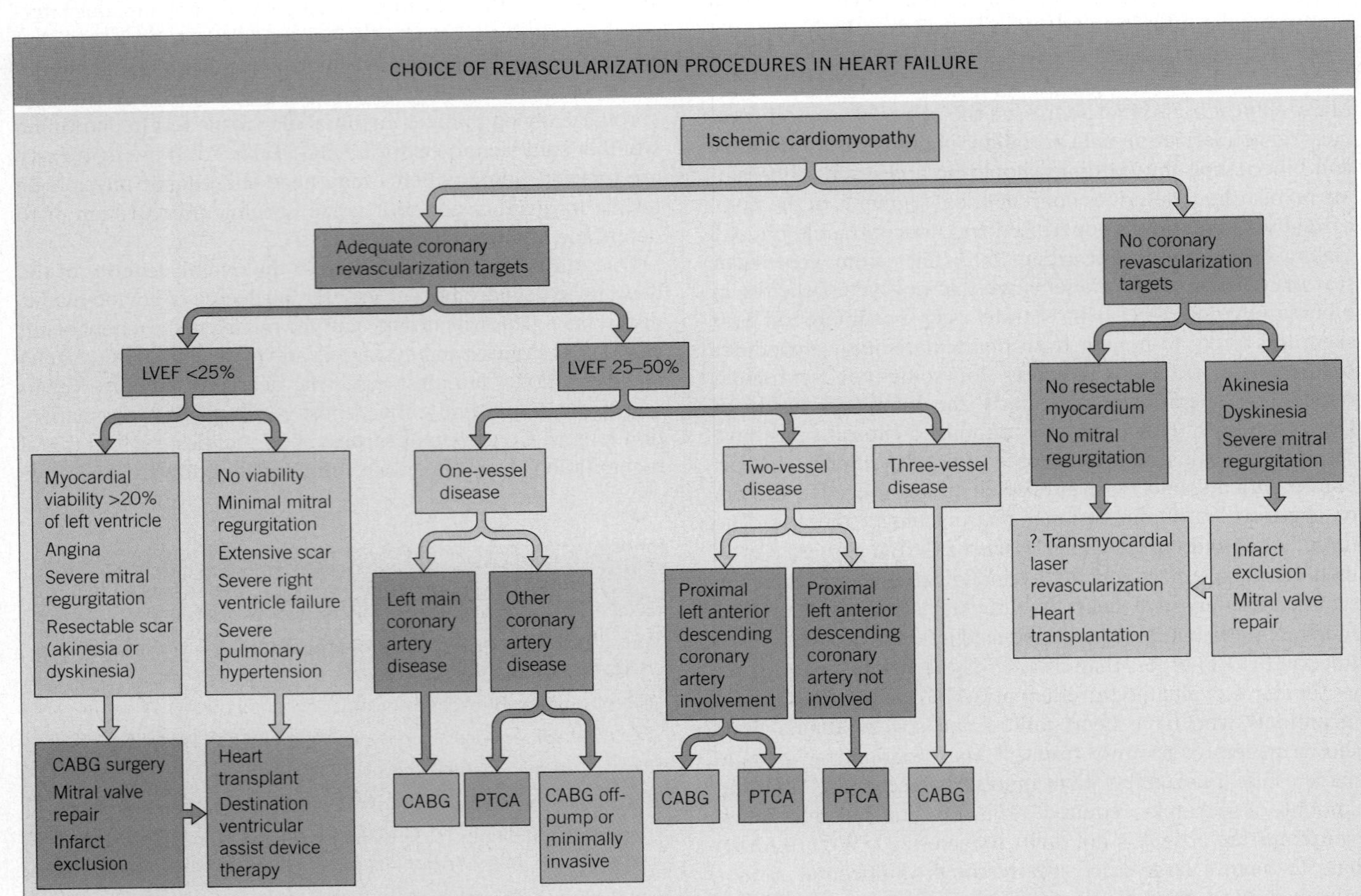

Figure 75.1 Choice of revascularization procedures in heart failure. Approaches should be dictated by the degree of left ventricular dysfunction, the presence of significant amounts of viable myocardium, the severity of valvular regurgitation, the amount of resectable myocardial scar, and the suitability for ventricular assist device or heart transplantation "bailout." Targets for revascularization must also be present. These considerations will dictate, in large part, which patients may be candidates for percutaneous revascularization strategies as well. All patients, regardless of procedure, require appropriate medication treatments and atherosclerotic cardiovascular risk factor prevention. CABG, coronary artery bypass graft; LVEF, left ventricular ejection fraction; PTCA, percutaneous transluminal coronary angioplasty.

have involvement of the proximal left anterior descending coronary artery might be best served by percutaneous coronary revascularization procedures, if these can be done. On the other hand, those who have proximal left anterior descending coronary artery disease coupled to other lesions might be better served by CABG surgery. Nonetheless, many in this cohort could be candidates for percutaneous transluminal coronary angioplasty. Patients who have mild to moderate left ventricular systolic dysfunction in the face of one-vessel coronary disease also represent a challenge. Clearly, patients who have left main coronary artery disease should have surgery, but other one-vessel lesions should be addressed according to lesion location and suitability for percutaneous intervention. Coronary artery bypass grafting off cardiopulmonary bypass and minimally invasive procedures make surgical intervention in one-vessel disease more attractive.

The main challenge appears to be in patients who have an LVEF of less than 25% and coronary revascularization targets (see Fig. 75.1). In this group of patients, myocardial viability should be assessed; if the total quantity of ischemic and hibernating myocardium together is greater than 20% of the left ventricle, revascularization procedures should be considered because greater benefit is anticipated. Furthermore, if there is severe mitral regurgitation or resectable scar as manifested by ventricular wall akinesia or dyskinesia, CABG surgery coupled to mitral valve repair and infarct exclusion could be recommended (Fig. 75.2). In patients who are undergoing these procedures but who fail to be weaned from cardiopulmonary bypass support, ventricular assist device insertion as a bridge to cardiac transplantation should be considered. Patients who have limited viable myocardium, minimal mitral regurgitation, extensive scar, or severe right ventricular failure with severe pulmonary hypertension should also be considered for ventricular assist device implantation as a bridge to cardiac transplantation. Again, many of these issues will be better clarified when the results of the STICH trial are available.

Risks of Coronary Artery Bypass Graft Surgery

Although patients who have heart failure benefit from revascularization, LVEF still remains an important predictor of operative mortality.[12,13] However, reports suggest that LVEF has fallen from being the most important predictor of adverse outcome to become the fourth most important (after repeated CABG surgery, emergency operations, and age).[13] Compared with patients who have an LVEF above 40%, those who have an LVEF below 20% have a threefold to fourfold higher chance of dying perioperatively.[12] Early postoperative mortality of about 12% has been reported in patients who have an LVEF below 20%,[12,13] although this experience is now somewhat dated. Elefteriades and colleagues[13] more recently summarized a single-center experience in patients who have an LVEF of less than 30% and suggested that hospital mortality should be closer to 5%.

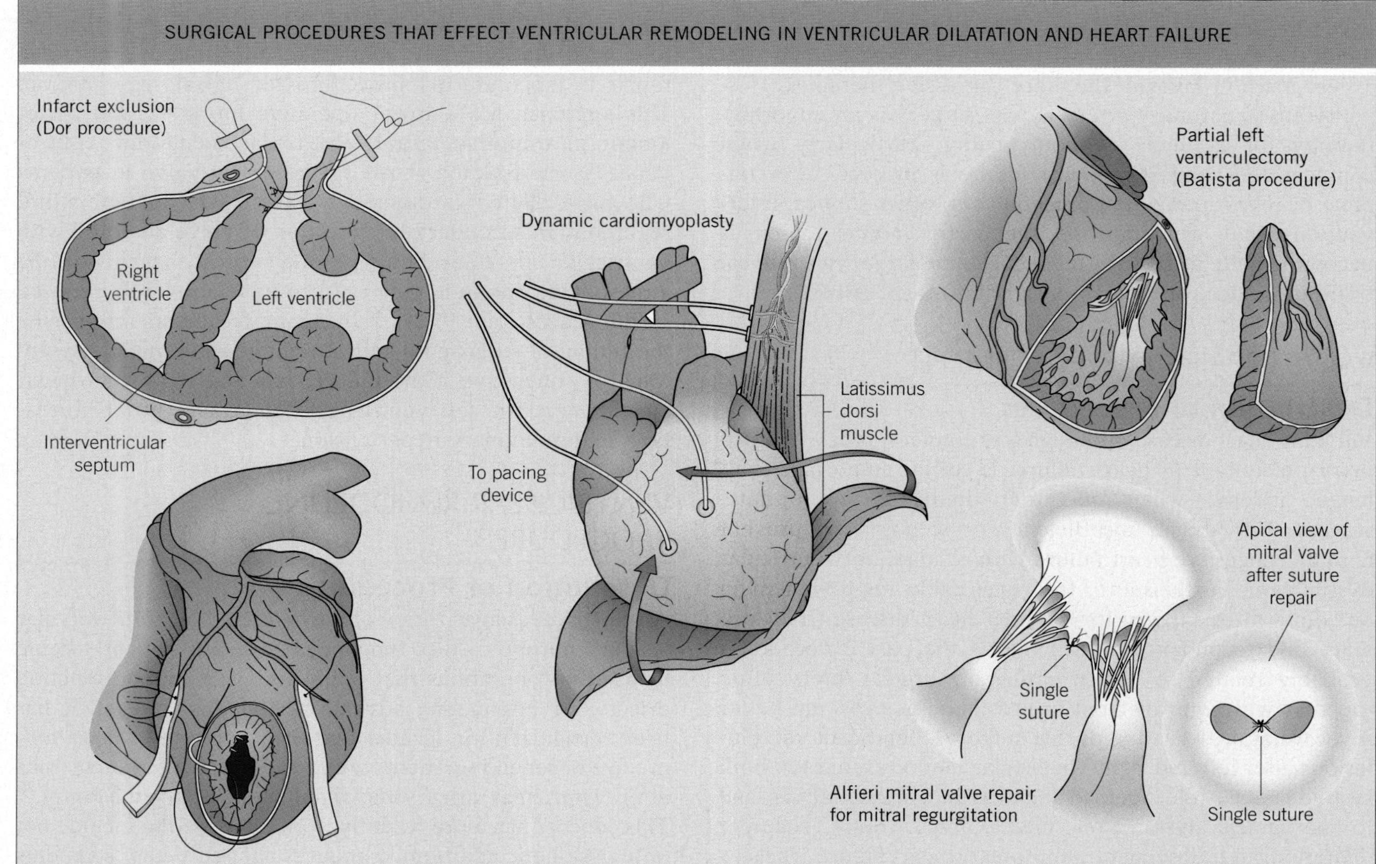

Figure 75.2 Surgical procedures that effect ventricular remodeling in ventricular dilatation and heart failure. These procedures are designed to alter myocardial geometry and to decrease excessive myocardial loading states. It is hoped that this might prevent detrimental cardiac remodeling and even induce regression of hypertrophy.

Important determinants of mortality after CABG surgery include

- age, with a 0.5% increase in risk per year after 60 years;
- diabetes mellitus;
- significant renal dysfunction;
- significant hepatic dysfunction;
- significant obstructive pulmonary disease;
- significant cerebrovascular disease; and
- female sex.

In addition, previous cardiothoracic surgery, the need for emergency CABG surgery (usually in the setting of a failed percutaneous transluminal coronary angioplasty attempt or acute myocardial infarction), or concomitant valve heart surgery increases operative mortality.[12]

One group of patients with ischemic heart disease that deserves particular attention are those presenting with an acute ischemic event and cardiogenic shock. Such patients were recently studied in the SHOCK trial (Should We Revascularize Occluded Coronaries in Cardiovascular Shock).[14-16] In this multicenter randomized study, surgical or percutaneous revascularization strategies were studied compared with medical therapies when patients presented with an acute ischemic event. Patients who underwent CABG had 30-day and 1-year mortalities of 42% and 56%, respectively. Although the results are seemingly worse than the results of CABG in compensated congestive heart failure patients, those randomized to the medical therapy arm had worse outcomes (56% 30-day and 75% 1-year mortality). The difference in mortality between the revascularization and medical treatment groups was statistically significant at the 1-year mark in favor of the more aggressive therapies.

Presently, coronary artery bypass surgery is an important therapy for ischemic cardiomyopathy, particularly when compensated congestive heart failure is present. The coupling of revascularization procedures to other surgical interventions that can improve the heart failure milieu is becoming quite attractive. Indeed, several large-scale clinical trials are under way to gain insight into these issues.

VALVE REPAIR OR REPLACEMENT

Description of Procedures

Valvular heart disease, although less common today as a primary precipitant of heart failure, is still an important challenge. Indeed, when operative timing is appropriate, surgery for valvular insufficiency or stenosis can prevent chronic congestive heart failure with residual left ventricular dysfunction. Furthermore, the remarkable improvement in outcomes after surgery for valvular heart disease (both primary and secondary disease) during the past 2 decades is probably related to better timing of surgical intervention together with improvement in prosthetic devices and better myocardial preservation during surgery. Significant valvular lesions alter left and right ventricular hemodynamics in both systole and diastole. Preload and afterload abnormalities lead to mechanical dysfunction, muscle hypertrophy, chamber dilatation, and subsequent symptomatic heart failure. The surgical approach to primary valvular disease is discussed in Chapters 99 and 100. Because mitral regurgitation associated with left ventricular dilatation and heart failure constitutes a problem different from that expressed by those patients with primary valvular heart disease, this chapter discusses surgery to correct mitral regurgitation due to heart failure.

Chronic mitral regurgitation may be associated with cardiac remodeling characterized by ventricular hypertrophy, ventricular dilatation, and atrial enlargement. Unless mitral regurgitation is acute and massive, the lesion usually progresses in an insidious fashion and causes ventricular dysfunction before symptoms of heart failure are noted. One particularly challenging issue is whether mitral regurgitation caused by ventricular dilatation associated with cardiomyopathy is a significant contributor to adverse ventricular remodeling with subsequent dysfunction. Patients who present with asymptomatic left ventricular systolic dysfunction believed to be caused by mitral regurgitation should have the lesion corrected. Once LVEF has fallen below 60% in a setting of significant mitral regurgitation, the long-term prognosis is poor. Similarly, when the end-systolic dimension of the left ventricle exceeds 4.5 cm, the prognosis of mitral regurgitation is not good. Another adverse prognostic indicator is right ventricular dysfunction associated with pulmonary hypertension. Patients who have a right ventricular ejection fraction of less than 30% are also believed to be at significant risk for an adverse event. As with aortic stenosis, concomitant coronary heart disease complicates the situation, and the relative contribution of valvular regurgitation in coronary heart disease, particularly when heart failure is present, needs to be clarified.

Because the submitral apparatus (including the chordae tendineae and papillary muscles) plays a critical part in systolic and diastolic left ventricular function, mitral valve repair is the preferred procedure for mitral regurgitation. This approach has a lower operative mortality and better long-term result than mitral valve replacement. More controversial is the isolated repair of the mitral valve in patients who have dilated cardiomyopathy and concomitant mitral regurgitation secondary to distortion of valve anatomy with ventricular dilatation. Some reports suggest that this can be a reasonable option in patients who have a severely reduced LVEF (see Chapter 99).[17-22] In summary, factors influencing the timing of surgery for mitral regurgitation include symptoms of congestive heart failure, left and right ventricular ejection fraction, left ventricular dimensions, atrial fibrillation, and pulmonary hypertension.

VENTRICULAR REMODELING PROCEDURES

Description of Procedures

Although revascularization of the heart and repair of valvular lesions improve cardiac function, efforts are currently being focused on operations that might improve cardiac function directly by attenuating adverse remodeling. Indeed, it has been recognized for decades that the symptoms of heart failure are lessened in patients who have ventricular aneurysms after ventricular aneurysmorrhaphy or aneurysmectomy.[23] This concept has more recently been expanded to include not only dyskinetic and frankly aneurysmal ventricular segments but also large akinetic regions of scar (particularly scar that involves the anterior left ventricular wall).[24-27] It used to be thought that resection of such akinetic regions did not improve outcome in ischemic cardiomyopathy. With experience, this type of ventricular reconstruction has evolved from a linear aneurysm repair, which involved removal of the free wall of the anterior left ventricle, to a more complicated repair that excludes the infarcted septum and free wall (see Fig. 75.2). Current experience with infarct exclusion operations has evolved from the experience of Jatene,[28] Dor,[25,26] Dor and colleagues,[27] Cooley and associates,[23] and David.[21] The Dor procedure (see Fig. 75.2) as well as ventricular aneurysm resection improves ventricular muscle function primarily because of amelioration of perturbed wall tension and ventricular shape. According to the law of Laplace, wall tension = $P \times r/2h$, where P is intraventricular pressure, r is the left ventricular radius, and h is the wall thickness. The Laplace surgical concept was expanded by Batista to include idiopathic dilated cardiomyopathy and some cases of valvular heart disease and Chagas' disease.[24,29,30]

All of the geometric and physiologic factors that are characteristic of advanced heart failure (increased left ventricular chamber dimension, elevated left ventricular end-diastolic pressure, mitral regurgitation, and eccentric hypertrophy) contribute to increased circumferential and meridional wall stress.[31] In addition, myocyte elongation without any equivalent increase in myocyte diameter leads to an increased length-width ratio, which has been observed in humans and other species.[32] Importantly, survival has been shown to correlate with left ventricular size in dilated cardiomyopathy[33] after acute myocardial infarction.[34] It has been speculated that sudden cardiac death in the setting of marked chamber dilatation is precipitated by subendocardial ischemia and arrhythmias that are in turn precipitated by increased wall stress in a setting of a dilated hypertrophied ventricle.

Partial left ventriculectomy, also known as heart reduction surgery or the Batista procedure, was used to ameliorate difficulties engendered by cardiac dilatation and remodeling.[35-40] The operation, as originally described, involved removal of a triangular wedge of the lateral wall of the left ventricle, with amputated segments weighing more than 100 g (see Fig. 75.2). Obviously, this is a prototypic operation for changing the shape of the ventricle to a more normal configuration and should be studied from that perspective.[40] In general, the mitral valve repair involves apposition of the anterior and posterior mitral leaflets with a single suture, thus creating a double-orifice mitral valve that yields a characteristic figure-of-eight appearance when the mitral valve is viewed in the short-axis echocardiographic configuration (see Fig. 75.2).

Although initial experience with this procedure was encouraging, longer term follow-up of these patients has been disappointing, and the operation has fallen out of favor in a number of circles. At the Cleveland Clinic Foundation, 62 procedures were performed between 1996 and 1998. Patients had dilated cardiomyopathy, and 59 of 62 were on the heart transplant waiting list (with about half of these supported by inotropic infusions and awaiting heart transplantation in the hospital). Before surgery, the mean LVEF was 13.5%, and mean peak oxygen consumption at exercise was 10.8 mL/kg per minute; at the time of the operation, 61% were assigned to New York Heart Association (NYHA) class IV. The perioperative mortality was 3.2%, and 1- and 2-year mortality rates were 68% and 78%, respectively. Importantly, 16% required postoperative left ventricular assist device placement for perioperative cardiogenic shock. At 1 year, in survivors, NYHA class improved from 3.7 to 2.2. Survivors had improved LVEF and decreased left ventricular volumes at 3 months. By 1 year, survivors who had an initial increase in ejection fraction, hemodynamics, and exercise tolerance subsequently worsened to a plateau level, with ejection fraction going from 13% preoperatively to 32% postoperatively and 24% at 1-year ($P < .0001$).[39,40]

Dynamic cardiomyoplasty is another operation that has been performed intermittently during the past decades but is no longer performed with any frequency.[41,42] Theoretically, the procedure should boost left ventricular systolic performance by wrapping the left or right latissimus dorsi muscle circumferentially around the heart (see Fig. 75.2). The muscle is dissected out from the posterior thorax and rotated carefully from the normal anatomic position into the chest, with great attention paid to preservation of the neurovascular pedicle. Critical to success of this operation is conversion of skeletal muscle performance from fatigable to fatigue-resistant fibers with appropriate repetitive electrical stimulation. Although early clinical studies of this operation suggested that contractile performance is marginally improved, possibly more important was the diastolic buttressing of the heart that appeared to limit further cardiac dilatation. Despite more than 600 cardiomyoplasty procedures being performed and reported worldwide, the benefits of operation did not seem to justify risks.[43] Although initially it seemed that quality of life and functional class were improved at the 6-month observation points, benefits were largely lost in the long term. This operation has largely been abandoned, and commercial efforts to develop the muscle stimulating-pacing device have been halted, but observations of some seemingly beneficial left ventricular remodeling after this girdling surgery spawned development of new approaches to surgical remodeling with devices. Possibly similar to the restraining effects of dynamic cardiomyoplasty, these newer approaches attempt to maintain more normal left ventricular shape and diameter, which theoretically leads to decreased left ventricular wall stress and decreased myocardial oxygen demand and consumption, improves contractile function and efficiency, and inhibits further detrimental remodeling. The Acorn CorCap Cardiac Support Device (Acorn Cardiovascular, Minneapolis, Minn) is an elastic mesh "sock" that is wrapped and pulled up over the heart and snugged up to gently girdle the entire left and right ventricular surface. In animal models of heart failure, at the 3- to 6-month follow-up point, LVEF was increased and ventricular volumes and wall stress were reduced.[44,45] In an intriguing investigation, Sabbah and coworkers[46] demonstrated that after CorCap placement, associated with left ventricular volume reduction, animals had altered gene expression (down-regulation of stretch-mediated p21-ras and sarcoplasmic reticulum adenosine triphosphatase), indicative of early reverse remodeling. In exploratory human studies, patients with idiopathic dilated cardiomyopathy who had wrap replacement at the time of coronary artery bypass grafting had decreased left ventricular end-diastolic diameter after 3 months (63 mm versus 53 mm;

$P = .025$). No patient demonstrated problems with the coronary graft after the procedure.[47] Clinical trial data are presently under review, with some concerns generated by regulatory authorities about pivotal trial design but a belief expressed that there might be utility to the procedure eventually demonstrated. This is yet to be determined.

Another creative device, the Myosplint (Myocor, Minneapolis, Minn), was designed to prevent detrimental left ventricular remodeling and to reduce ventricular volumes by use of a transventricular splint. Several devices are placed across the ventricular cavity from the lateral left ventricle through the posterior interventricular septum. After the splints are tightened, the ventricle has a bilobed configuration that, mathematically, is associated with reduced left ventricular wall stress. In a canine model of pacing tachycardia–induced heart failure, Myosplint placement had an acute and chronic increase in LVEF (27% to 37%), decreased end-systolic and end-diastolic left ventricular volumes, and diminished wall stress compared with sham-operated controls.[48] In humans undergoing heart transplantation, immediately before amputation of the native heart, Myosplint insertion effected acute left ventricular volume changes similar to those seen in the animal studies.[49] Clinical trials with this device have yet to clarify their best precise use, and some have suggested that they are best used to reduce mitral regurgitation. Neither the CorCap nor the Myosplint device is clinically available, but they demonstrate the concepts of ventricular remodeling surgery that have evolved. It is anticipated that other methods of changing ventricular shape will follow similar principles, and their effectiveness will be demonstrated or refuted by properly controlled clinical trials.

MECHANICAL CIRCULATORY SUPPORT DEVICES

Description of Devices

Several circulatory support systems are available, including

- the intra-aortic balloon pump, which is the oldest device and the simplest to insert;
- extracorporeal systems that are similar to cardiopulmonary bypass devices or extracorporeal pumps;
- a variety of intracorporeal devices, some of which have been used for sustained periods; and
- total artificial hearts.

Mechanical circulatory assist devices that are useful in patients who are in cardiogenic shock or advanced and end-stage heart failure range widely in their concepts and sophistication.[50-53] Intra-aortic balloon counterpulsation devices inserted percutaneously were first proposed in the early 1960s as a way of augmenting failing circulatory systems. Although this approach is not focused, in the strict sense, on direct mechanical flow augmentation, it remains the most commonly used form of mechanical assistance in left ventricular failure. Its advantage lies in the fact that it is relatively simple to insert, and it carries a low risk. It is used most commonly in patients who have severe heart failure or who are in cardiogenic shock after a myocardial infarction or cardiac surgery. Unfortunately, the device can be left in place only for several days or at most a few weeks, and it requires patients to be immobilized because the usual access site is a femoral artery.

Temporary mechanical cardiac assistance can also be accomplished for short times by use of extracorporeal non-pulsatile centrifugal flow pumps that are integral components of cardiopulmonary bypass circuits. When an oxygenating device (membrane) is inserted, this is referred to as extracorporeal membrane oxygenation (ECMO). Although adequate flow and oxygenation can be accomplished satisfactorily with ECMO, it is rarely successful for more than a few days. Blood component trauma, thromboembolism, and infection are troubling limiting factors that occur with ECMO. As with the intra-aortic balloon counterpulsation device, use of ECMO is usually limited to those patients who are in cardiogenic shock and are believed to have reversible left ventricular dysfunction. Some patients may have this device inserted as a bridge to other operations, such as cardiac transplantation or a permanent ventricular assist device system.

Some ventricular assist systems are designed to function for sustained periods ranging from days to months or years. The pump itself must have appropriate inflow and outflow conduits with directional valve or impeller systems to generate proper flow direction. The pump chamber is the essential volumetric portion of the machine with, of course, a blood-device interface that ideally does not cause blood component trauma and is not thrombogenic or immunologically active. The controller system of any device regulates the circulatory pressure, heart rhythm, and pump interface system. Ultimately, the controller is responsible for modulating "cardiac" output. The pump driver is the activator system that creates flow; it is generally an electric motor component, or it operates by pneumatic displacement. The driver power source (whether a pneumatic or electric motor system is used) is derived from either wall socket alternating current or a battery pack. Interestingly, transcutaneous battery pack energy delivery systems have been developed. Finally, for pulsatile systems, an air displacement chamber or an external venting line is necessary to handle displaced air volume as the pump sac fills and empties.

A number of important parameters must be considered when long-term mechanical circulatory support systems are created (Table 75.4). Obviously, the pump must develop effective pressure and flow support. Whether pulsatile configurations are important during long-term circulatory support has not been clarified. The device should have the potential for easy removal so that rapid repair or replacement can be effected for pump malfunction. Ideally, the device should be able to be simply explanted or turned off and safely left in place if ventricular recovery occurs. The device should be small and use an efficient power source; it should be completely implantable, and it should not have percutaneous connections. It should also be quiet and produce little motion of its own. Obviously, the device should be reliable, be durable, and have a low infection risk (i.e., it should be completely implantable); it should not produce thrombus (which could embolize), and it should cause minimal blood component trauma and be nonimmunogenic. That is a very demanding list for any mechanical system implanted into a biologic environment.

IMPORTANT PARAMETERS FOR AN IDEAL LONG-TERM MECHANICAL CIRCULATORY SUPPORT SYSTEM
Effective pressure-flow support
Potential for easy removal
Rapid repair or replacement for pump malfunction
Ability to explant or to shut off if ventricle recovers
Small device
Efficient power source
Completely implantable
No percutaneous connections
Quiet
Little movement
Reliability
Durability
Low infection risk
Minimal blood component trauma
Nonimmunogenic

Table 75.4 Important parameters for an ideal long-term mechanical circulatory support system.

Indications, Contraindications, and Objectives

The objectives of mechanical device insertion are, obviously, to ameliorate circulatory pressure and flow perturbation. Today, devices are inserted when it is believed that cardiac recovery is likely to occur to the extent that the device can be removed.[54] This is, however, a relatively rare occurrence. Most often, a mechanical circulatory system is inserted as a bridge to heart transplantation. Mancini and associates[55] retrospectively reviewed their experience at Columbia Presbyterian Hospital, New York, to determine which patients were likely to tolerate left ventricular assist device explantation. During a retrospective case review, only 5 of 111 left ventricular assist device recipients were identified as potential explant patients. Prospectively, 18 of 29 patients were studied, with 15 patients exercised during maximal device support. However, only one of these patients had the device explanted successfully. Observations were that significant myocardial recovery after left ventricular assist device therapy in heart failure patients occurs in only a small percentage of patients. This is in contrast to a more successful experience reported by Müller and coworkers[54] in Berlin. This group has successfully removed devices from more than 20 patients. An interesting characteristic of successful device weaning in the Berlin experience was the presence of antibodies directed at myocardial β receptors. A correlation existed between the disappearance of these antibodies and the ability to wean patients from ventricular assist device therapy. Left ventricular assist device bridging to "recovery" is an emerging concept that must be carefully explored, but it does have a theoretical rationale.[49] Delineation of successful candidates for this procedure and clarification of intervention strategies must occur before widespread implementation of this practice occurs.

Factors to consider in evaluating patients for ventricular assist device insertion are related to

- severity of circulatory impairment;
- likelihood of cardiac function recovery;
- presence of comorbid conditions or irreversible hepatic or renal dysfunction; and
- suitability of the patient for heart transplantation.

General and relative contraindications to ventricular assist device insertion are detailed in Table 75.5. Both very small

GENERAL AND RELATIVE CONTRAINDICATIONS TO THE INSERTION OF A VENTRICULAR ASSIST DEVICE	
Contraindications	**Examples**
Technical	Body surface area <1.5 m² or >2.5 m² Weight >150% ideal Highly calcified aorta Substantive aortic insufficiency Mechanical aortic valve prosthesis Inability to anticoagulate Some pacing or automatic implantable cardioverter devices create electrical interference
Hemodynamic	Right atrial pressure >20 mm Hg despite intense diuresis and vasodilatation Pulmonary capillary wedge pressure generally <15 mm Hg with therapy Cardiac index generally >2.0-2.5 L/min per m² without parenteral inotropes
Pulmonary	Chronic ventilator dependence Recent pulmonary embolism Severely impaired pulmonary function (forced expiratory volume in 1 second <50% predicted) Fixed pulmonary hypertension (pulmonary artery pressure >60 mm Hg), transpulmonary gradient >17 mm Hg, pulmonary vascular resistance >5 Wood units while receiving intense pulmonary vasodilator therapy
Peripheral vascular	Significant aortic aneurysm (>5 cm) Peripheral vascular disease with limb claudication Significant cerebrovascular disease (previous stroke or transient ischemic attacks in the presence of internal carotid artery plaque or lesion)
Irreversible end-organ dysfunction	Cirrhosis Liver enzymes more than three times normal or bilirubin concentration 3.0 mg/dL (51 μmol/L) Primary coagulopathy International normalized ratio >1.8 or partial thromboplastin time more than twice control time in the absence of anticoagulation Serum creatinine concentration >3.0 mg/dL (250 μmol/L) or creatinine clearance <30 mL/min (0.5 mL/s)
Active infection	Particularly sepsis syndrome
Psychosocial issues that have an impact on compliance	Alcohol dependence or abuse Major psychiatric illness Inadequate social support systems
Endpoint of support unclear	Patient is not a candidate for heart transplantation

Table 75.5 General and relative contraindications to the insertion of a ventricular assist device.

and very large patients can be problematic. Individuals with a highly calcified aorta or significant aortic regurgitation will have problems related to outflow graft insertion and left ventricular emptying. A mechanical aortic valve prosthesis is likely to remain closed during complete or relatively complete ventricular unloading and therefore is predisposed to thrombus formation. Some devices require intense anticoagulation; patients for whom this is impossible are not suitable candidates for such devices. Furthermore, pacing and automated internal cardioverter-defibrillator devices can be problematic because of electronic interference. Hemodynamic contraindications generally include right atrial pressure above 20 mm Hg despite intense diuresis and vasodilatation. Insertion of a right ventricular assist device may support circulatory function in these circumstances, but this adds another dimension of complexity. Systolic pulmonary artery pressure above 60 mm Hg or a transpulmonary gradient of more than 17 mm Hg or a pulmonary vascular resistance of more than 5 Wood units (if the patient is receiving intense pulmonary vasodilator therapy) portends trouble when left ventricular assist devices are used alone. Furthermore, patients who are chronically ventilator dependent or have substantively impaired pulmonary function from obstructive pulmonary or restrictive lung disease that is not due to congestive heart failure and patients who have had recent pulmonary embolism with infarction do poorly after left ventricular assist device insertion.

Other general or relative contraindications to device insertion include an aortic aneurysm of more than 5 cm, peripheral vascular disease with limb claudication, and significant cerebrovascular disease (such as a previous stroke or transient ischemic attack in the presence of significant internal carotid artery lesions). Irreversible end-organ dysfunction (as manifested by hepatic cirrhosis or severe congestive hepatopathy with liver enzymes more than three times normal or a bilirubin concentration above 3 mg/dL) has been associated with poor outcome. A platelet count of less than 50,000 cells, primary coagulopathy, an international normalized ratio above 1.8 and a prothrombin time longer than twice the control time in patients who are not anticoagulated, a serum creatinine level above 3 mg/dL, and a creatinine clearance of less than 30 mL/min have also been associated with a poor outcome. Active infection is a contraindication to device insertion, particularly when sepsis syndrome is present. Postoperative device infection can be a disaster. Psychosocial issues that may have an impact on long-term compliance with treatment, such as alcohol dependence or abuse, major psychiatric illness, and inadequate social support systems, lead to substantial difficulties after device insertion. Finally, devices should not be inserted when the endpoint of support is unclear (generally meaning that cardiac transplantation is not an option).

Several devices that are available now or are being studied are shown in Figures 75.3 to 75.6. The extracorporeal Abiomed ventricular assist system (see Fig. 75.3) is a pneumatically driven device that is essentially built from plastic components. This pump is used for relatively short-term support and is extracorporeal. It is attached to the patient's bedside, and it can be set up in right and left ventricular support format (see Fig. 75.3).

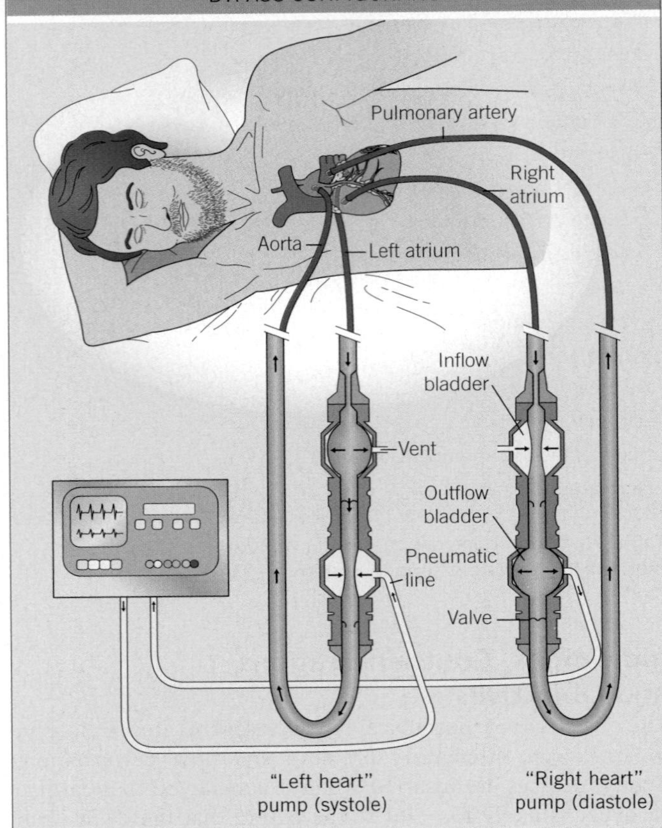

Figure 75.3 Abiomed bedside extracorporeal pneumatic ventricular assist system in biventricular bypass configuration.

The Thoratec extracorporeal pneumatically driven ventricular assist device (see Fig. 75.4) is also extracorporeal, but it is more portable than the Abiomed system and can support the circulation for longer times. Various patterns of left ventricular and combined right and left ventricular support can be used.

Figure 75.5 demonstrates the general configuration for intra-abdominal implantation of the Novacor and HeartMate "wearable" electric left ventricular assist device systems. The remarkable miniaturization of the controller systems and battery pack power sources can be appreciated.

Figure 75.6 details the DeBakey-MicroMed/NASA ventricular assist device, which is much smaller than any of the other available pulsatile implantable systems and is designed to be placed subdiaphragmatically. It is driven by a small controller system that can also be operated by battery power. The pump is a continuous-flow system with rapidly spinning impellers that are driven by a magnetic motor. Another example of this sort of pump is the Jarvik 2000, which has the advantage of being inserted directly into the left ventricular apex. Obviously, these devices have many theoretical advantages, including simplicity, ease of insertion, small size, potential for fewer infections (smaller drivelines), and less cost. Unknown is the potential for adverse effects of chronic nonpulsatile blood flow. Furthermore, these devices do not flow at levels that will, in general,

Figure 75.4 Thoratec extracorporeal pneumatic ventricular assist device. The device is shown in left ventricular assist configuration, in two biventricular assist setups, and in cross section. Ao, aorta; RA, right atrium; PA, pulmonary artery; LVAD, left ventricular assist device; RVAD, right ventricular assist device.

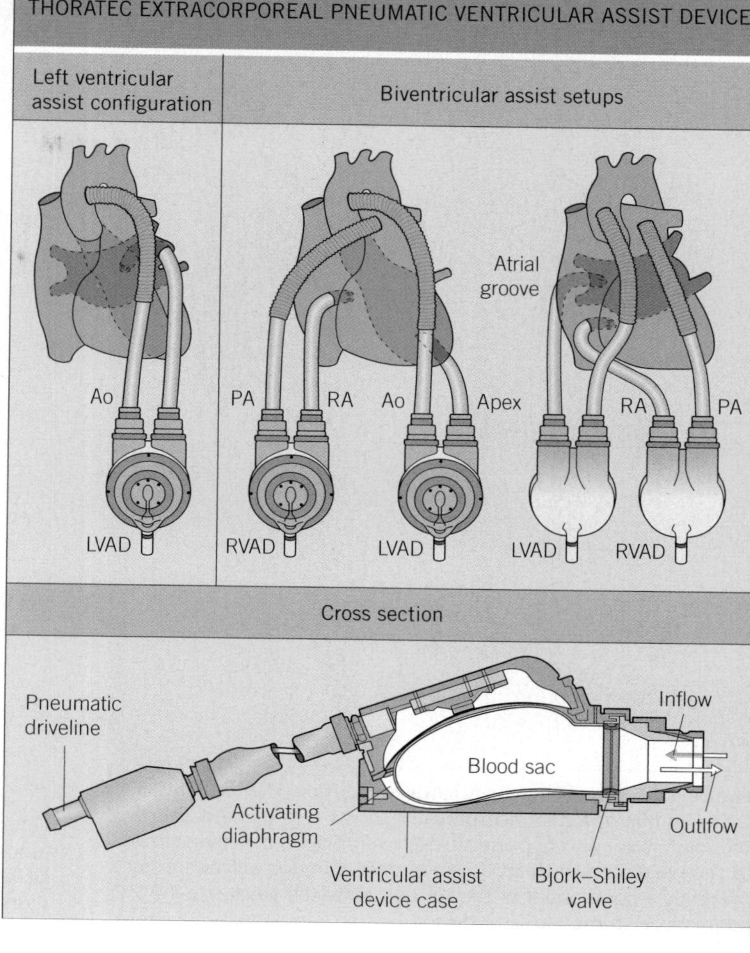

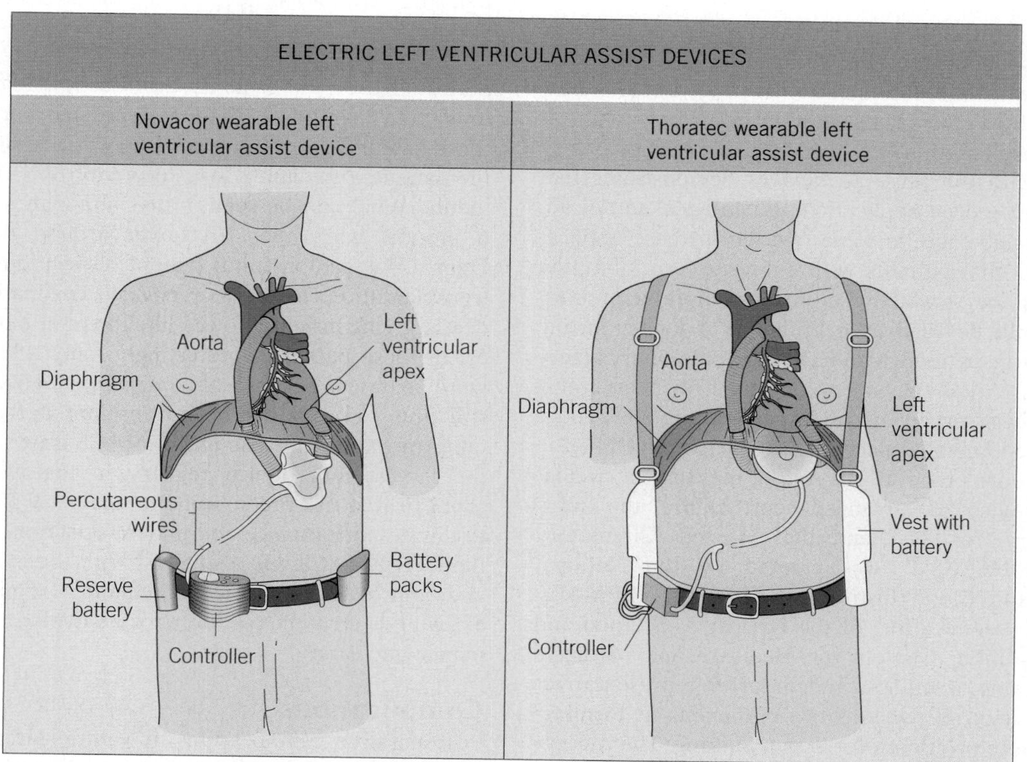

Figure 75.5 Electric left ventricular assist devices. These two devices are subdiaphragmatic, sump from the left ventricular apex, and have the outflow cannula anastomosed to the ascending aorta. Both devices have portable power and controller systems that allow remarkable mobility and activity of the patient.

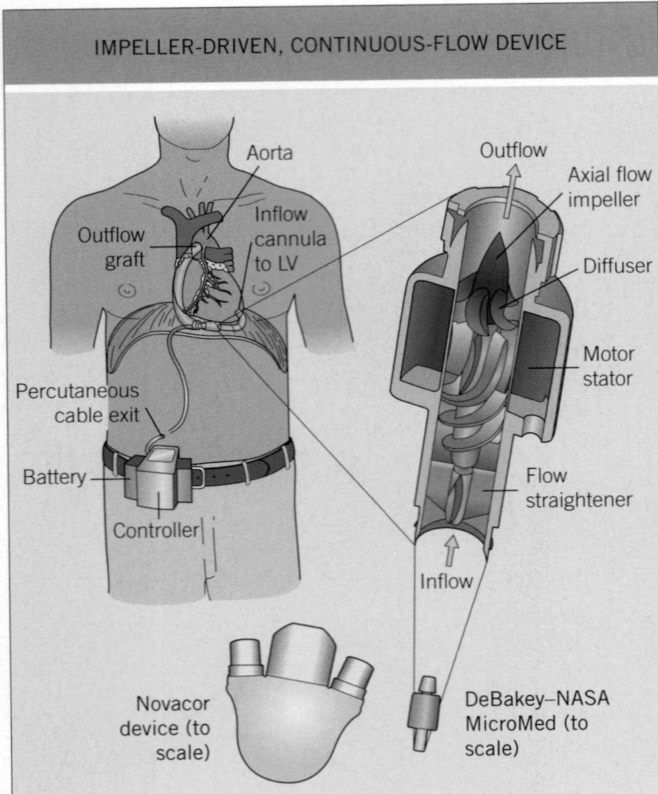

Figure 75.6 Impeller-driven, continuous-flow device. This DeBakey-MicroMed intracorporeal machine is implanted below the diaphragm and bypasses the left ventricle in a fashion similar to the Novacor and HeartMate systems, although valves are not presently a component of the system. Note the small size in comparison to the Novacor device.

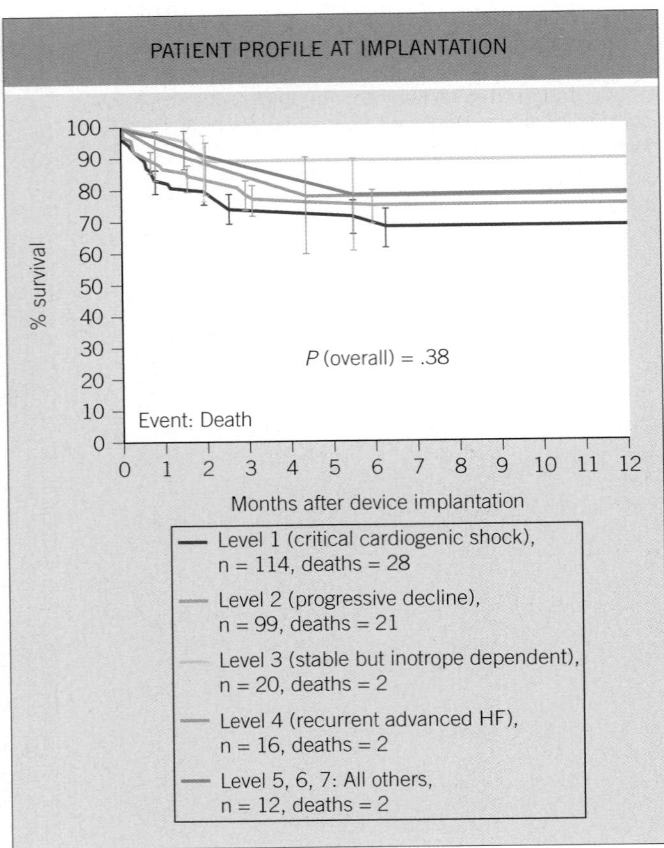

Figure 75.7 Patient profile at implantation. The hazard function analysis of devices implanted in different patient types, all very ill, but from those having acute cardiogenic shock to the slightly more stable patient with simply long-term inotropic support requirements. What can be seen is that although survival rates at 6 months vary, they all hover around the 80% mark. HF, heart failure.

completely support the circulation. Ongoing clinical trials are evaluating these pumps in bridge-to-transplant protocols. Indeed, the HeartMate II impeller-driven continuous-flow pump was recently given regulatory approbation for use as a bridge to transplantation.

Experience with the pulsatile devices demonstrates that each has its own special application, advantages, and disadvantages. Although there is some overlap in these applications, it appears that patients with extensive postinfarction shock may best be served by a smaller, more temporary device that could be used as a bridge to a longer lasting one, whereas large patients who have high pulmonary artery pressures and are likely to wait a long time for heart transplantation are best served by the larger and arguably more durable intra-abdominally placed pulsatile flow machines.

To describe more precisely the role of mechanical circulatory support devices in advanced heart failure, the Interagency Registry for Mechanically Assisted Circulatory Support (INTERMACS)[56] was created by the National Heart, Lung, and Blood Institute (NHLBI). INTERMACS was devised as a joint effort of the NHLBI, U.S. Food and Drug Administration, Centers for Medicare and Medicaid Services, clinicians, scientists, and industry representatives in conjunction with the University of Alabama at Birmingham and the United Network for Organ Sharing. The registry is approaching 1000 patients, and 93 sites are participating with an anticipated total to well above 100 in the United States. Figure 75.7 is the hazard function analysis of devices implanted in different patient types, all very ill, but from those having acute cardiogenic shock to the slightly more stable patient with simply long-term inotropic support requirements. What can be seen is that although survival rates at 6 months vary, they all hover around the 80% mark. Figure 75.8 demonstrates patient disposition with regard to transplantation, bridge to recovery, destination therapy, or death, giving insight into the likelihood of outcomes of interest in these patients. Interestingly, only 4% of the devices were removed because of "recovery," whereas 42% were still alive and 31% had been transplanted; the 6-month mortality rate was 23%. As INTERMACS grows, it will become the largest multidevice registry in the world and allow sophisticated risk prediction of outcomes while giving clarity to device performance and patient selection. It is hoped that the INTERMACS will also assist with the evaluation of new and improved mechanical circulatory support devices by allowing a creative platform for analyzing machine performance and safety.

Complications

Postoperative complications of ventricular device insertion vary widely and are also to be quantitated in INTERMACS, but today's data suggest that the most important ones include

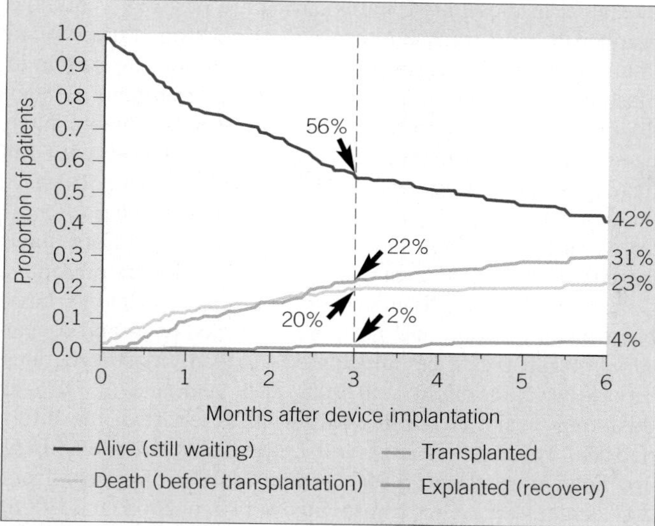

Figure 75.8 Patient disposition with regard to transplantation, bridge to recovery, destination therapy, or death, giving insight into the likelihood of outcomes of interest in these patients. Interestingly, only 4% of the devices were removed because of "recovery," whereas 42% were still alive and 31% had been transplanted; the 6-month mortality rate was 23%.

bleeding associated with device implantation and coagulopathies that develop as a consequence of cardiopulmonary bypass and major open heart surgical intervention. One of the more frightening and challenging complications after left ventricular assist device insertion is right-sided circulatory failure. Approximately 20% of patients who require left ventricular assist device implantation have right ventricular dysfunction, which can be severe. Factors that predispose to this complication include

- air embolism through pulmonary circuits;
- poor intrinsic right ventricular contractility;
- myocardial stunning;
- pulmonary hypertension;
- cardiac arrhythmias; and
- volume status.

Naturally, the right ventricle must supply an adequate output through the lungs to the left ventricle to allow proper oxygenation and ventricular assist device filling. Pulmonary hypertension exacerbates intrinsic right-sided heart failure and must be avoided if possible. Unfortunately, pulmonary hypertension is exacerbated by transfusion-induced cytokine storm during therapy for excessive bleeding. Insertion of biventricular mechanical support is sometimes necessary.

Thromboembolic complications are another nemesis. Bleeding is more common than thromboembolism and is generally perioperative. In view of the risk of long-term thromboembolism, most patients receive continuous anticoagulation therapy after perioperative coagulation parameters have normalized. Because of the textured blood-contacting surface of the HeartMate pulsatile device, thromboembolism with this device seems to be less of a problem, and long-term maintenance with platelet-inhibiting drugs alone is generally possible.

Because ventricular assist devices violate the integrity of natural barriers to infection (as none now available for routine use is completely implantable), pump pocket infection, driveline infection, and device "endocarditis" are problematic and sometimes devastating. All patients undergoing left ventricular assist device insertion receive antimicrobial prophylaxis before the operation, and clinicians should have a low threshold for treating clinical signs of infection during support.

The use of left ventricular assist device insertion as a permanent alternative to heart transplantation has recently been studied in the randomized evaluation of mechanical assistance for the treatment of congestive heart failure (so-called REMATCH protocol).[57-59] This trial involved patients with more advanced end-stage heart failure than in those participating in any previous congestive heart failure randomized study. Baseline characteristics of the patients included a mean LVEF of 17% and serum creatinine levels of 1.8 mg/dL (mean). The trial results in these patients with terminal heart failure were compelling in terms of survival and quality of life. One-year survival rates were nearly doubled for the left ventricular assist device insertion group (the implantable HeartMate pulsatile device was used in this study). Absolute reduction in the mortality rate of 24% at 1 year was noted, and survival nearly tripled at 2 years, with the median survival of 408 days for the left ventricular assist device patients versus 150 days for those in the optimal medical treatment group. The trial also demonstrated rapid and extended improvement in NYHA class in many ventricular assist device–supported patients. Quality of life, measured by mobility, functionality, and mental status, was equal to or superior to that of those being treated medically. At baseline, 97% of the ventricular assist device patients and 98% of the medically managed patients were in NYHA class IV. At 1 month, 52% of the HeartMate patients were in NYHA class I or class II, compared with none of the medically managed patients. At 1 year, 72% of the surviving HeartMate patients were in class I or class II versus 18% of the medically managed patients. The successes, however, were attenuated by the fact that multiple device-related complications were apparent, including device failure from mechanical malfunction, infection, and embolic events. Nonetheless, this was the first trial to suggest that ventricular assist device insertion as "destination therapy" holds promise for terribly advanced end-stage heart failure patients. Devices that are less complicated, totally implantable, and more durable will likely generate much interest in their use in patients who have this degree of heart failure and are not candidates for alternative surgical procedures or cardiac transplantation. INTERMACS is vitally interested in this use of devices and will supplement the data presently available from the trials done for registration. As with bridging indications, selection of patients is critical to success, and we do not yet have complete clarification of the best populations in which to use these devices.

CARDIAC TRANSPLANTATION

Description of Procedure

Cardiac transplantation is truly a miraculous operation for patients with advanced and end-stage heart failure, who have a high likelihood of premature death and who suffer greatly from congestive and low cardiac output syndromes.[60,61] Orthotopic or heterotopic implantation configuration can be used for cardiac transplantation (Fig. 75.9); heterotopic (or "piggyback") transplantation is now done rarely. Procurement of donor hearts is usually done during multiorgan retrieval in suitable organ donors. Unfortunately, only a limited supply of heart-beating brain-dead cadavers is available; in the United States during the past few years, the number of heart transplant procedures performed has leveled out at around 2500 cases per year. Furthermore, to sustain in reasonable fashion this number of heart transplants, older donors and donors formerly thought less acceptable have been used. For example, the proportion of donors used for heart transplantation who have been older than 50 years increased from 2.1% to almost 10%. Patients dying of cerebrovascular accidents and becoming heart donors have increased from 20% to almost one third of donors presently. Despite this, and although heart transplant recipients have been much more ill and unstable, remarkable 1- and 5-year survival rates can be anticipated. Indeed, most programs report survivals of 80% to 90% at 1 year and of 70% to 80% at 5 years. According to the 2008 report of the International Society for Heart and Lung Transplantation, there are now more than 75,000 patients in their registry from 203 centers reporting transplants between 2005 and 2006. Although falling from a peak of close to 4500 heart transplantations done in 1995 to about 3000 done in 2005, the numbers have remained around 3000 yearly for the last half-decade or so.

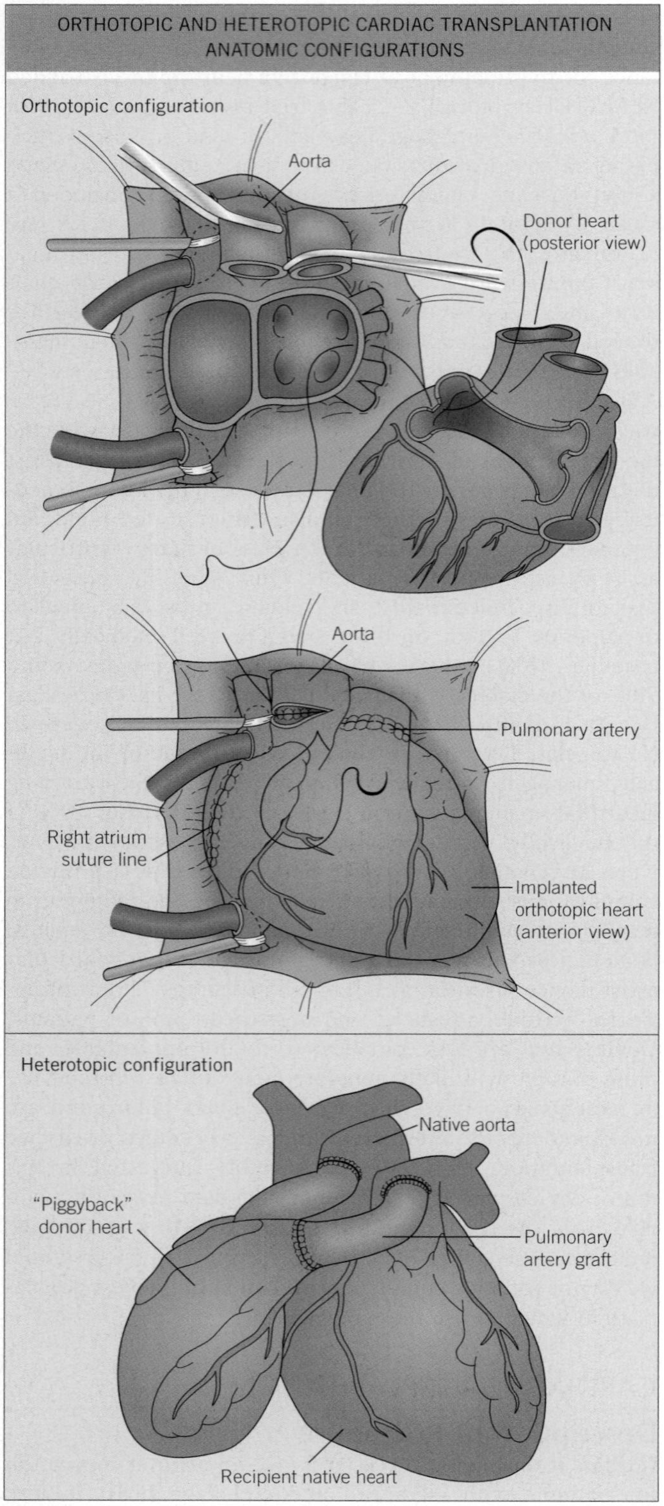

Figure 75.9 Orthotopic and heterotopic cardiac transplantation anatomic configurations.

Indications, Contraindications, and Objectives

When to consider cardiac transplantation and the decision process are shown in Table 75.6 and Figure 75.10. Because replacing the heart requires major operative intervention and chronic immunosuppressive therapy, the risk-benefit ratio must be carefully weighed in each individual patient. Furthermore, the likelihood of success must be considered carefully when the few donor hearts available are balanced against the many patients with advanced end-stage heart failure who might benefit from transplantation. Clearly, irreversible heart disease is a requirement, and potential candidates should be receiving optimal medical therapy. Furthermore, the patient should not be a candidate for

REASONS TO CONSIDER HEART TRANSPLANTATION
Irreversible and progressive heart disease
Maximally tolerated and appropriate pharmacotherapy in place
Not candidate for alternative surgical procedures
6- to 12-month survival estimated to be <50%
Unacceptable functional status and quality of life
Maximal oxygen consumption with exercise <14 mL/kg per minute or <55% of predicted for age and sex (while respiratory exchange ratio >1.10 and anaerobic threshold surpassed)
Patient depends on parenteral inotropes to avoid hemodynamic compromise
Patient likely to survive heart transplantation surgery
Patient likely to tolerate rigors of chronic immunosuppressive therapies
Patient not allosensitized
Patient candidate for mechanical circulatory support, if necessary, as bridge to transplantation
Patient willing to undergo radical surgery

Table 75.6 Reasons to consider heart transplantation.

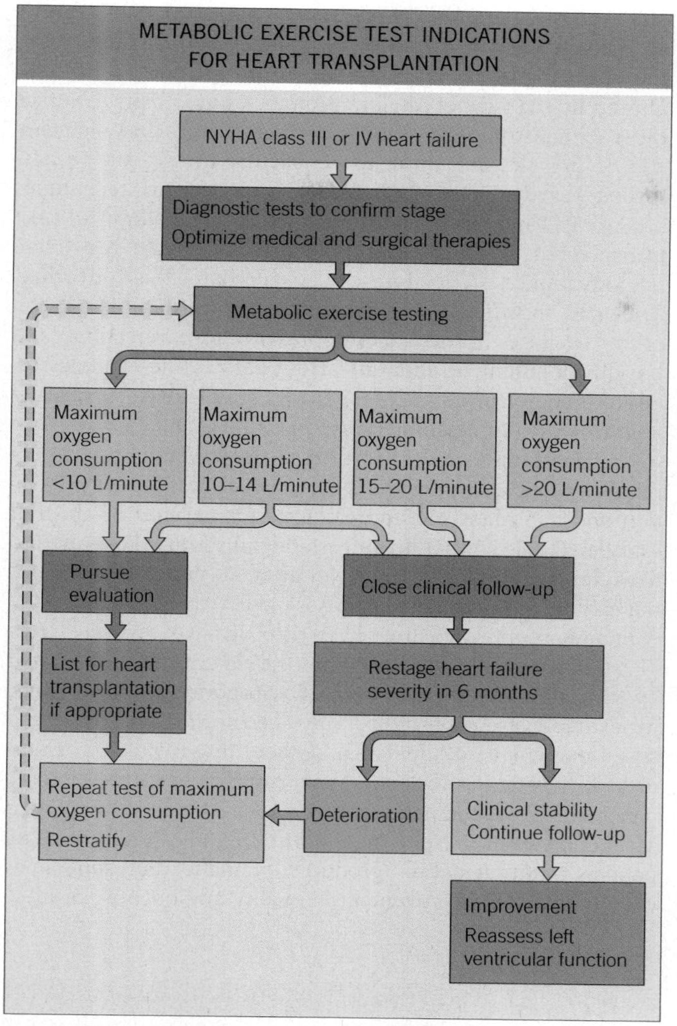

Figure 75.10 Metabolic exercise test indications for heart transplantation. NYHA, New York Heart Association.

alternative surgical procedures that might ameliorate the situation, even if only partially, and so obviate need for cardiac transplantation. Six- to 12-month survival without transplantation and with maximal medical therapy should be estimated at less than 50%. Furthermore, the patient should have unacceptable functional status and quality of life because of the heart failure. Recent consensus guidelines generated by the American Society of Transplantation[61] suggest that maximum oxygen consumption with exercise should be less than 14 mL/kg per minute or less than 55% of the predicted maximum for age and sex (after a respiratory exchange ratio above 1.10 has been achieved and the anaerobic threshold has been surpassed). Further indications include patients who require parenteral inotropic therapy to maintain a reasonable hemodynamic state. Candidates should also be likely to survive transplantation surgery and to tolerate chronic, immunosuppressive therapy. They should not have significant comorbid conditions that limit this likelihood. Patients should also be candidates for mechanical circulatory support, if necessary, as a bridge to transplantation. Finally, the patient must be willing to undergo the rigors of this radical surgical intervention and understand the commitment necessary for long-term care.

PERCEIVED CONTRAINDICATIONS TO HEART TRANSPLANTATION
Coexistent systemic illness (comorbid conditions) that portends a poor long-term prognosis
Irreversible renal dysfunction
Irreversible hepatic dysfunction
Severe or significant peripheral and cerebrovascular disease (claudication, transient ischemic attack, or cerebrovascular accident)
Diabetes mellitus with substantive end-organ damage
Active infection (particularly sepsis)
Coexisting malignant neoplasm
Acute pulmonary embolism or infarction
Active peptic ulcer disease
Active diverticulosis or diverticulitis
Certain myocardial infiltrative diseases (amyloidosis, hemochromatosis)
Severely elevated, "fixed" pulmonary artery pressures
Morbid obesity
Profound osteoporosis
Psychosocial instability or substance abuse (including nicotine use)

Table 75.7 Perceived contraindications to heart transplantation.

Contraindications to cardiac transplantation must be considered as well (Table 75.7).[61] Coexistent systemic illness that portends poor long-term prognosis militates against success after transplantation. Irreversible renal or hepatic dysfunction creates problematic issues with drug administration. Immunosuppressive agents have substantial toxicity that will predispose to worsening renal insufficiency and renal failure and can even induce hepatic coma. Severe and significant peripheral and cerebrovascular disease that causes claudication, transient ischemic attacks, or nonembolic cerebrovascular accidents should probably preclude a patient from being a serious candidate for transplantation. Diabetic patients who have substantive end-organ damage such as proliferative retinopathy, nephropathy, or peripheral vascular disease often deteriorate after heart transplantation. Because patients will be receiving intense immunosuppressive protocols, active infection, particularly sepsis, at the time of transplantation is a contraindication, as is active coexistent neoplasm. Acute pulmonary embolism and infarction predispose to complications, as do active peptic ulcer disease, diverticulosis, and diverticulitis. These issues generally should be resolved before transplantation is seriously considered. Certain myocardial infiltrative diseases that cause heart failure, such as amyloidosis and hemochromatosis, can recur in the allograft. Such patients are generally not well served by transplantation. Severely elevated and "fixed" pulmonary artery pressures produce postoperative right-sided heart failure and have been associated with adverse outcome. If pulmonary artery pressures cannot be diminished with aggressive therapeutics, patients will suffer from right-sided heart failure after heart transplantation. Morbid obesity, interestingly, is a significant independent risk factor for poor outcome after transplantation. Profound osteoporosis is made worse by post-transplantation immunosuppressive therapy and represents a relative contraindication. Finally, psychosocial instability and, in particular, substance abuse (including persistent nicotine use) must be carefully considered and weighed during determination of the patient's suitability for transplantation.

Complications

Although transplanted hearts work remarkably well, cardiac allografts do not function totally normally, and exercise tolerance in transplant recipients is somewhat less than might be expected (Table 75.8). The transplanted heart is a denervated preparation (from both an afferent and efferent perspective). This creates altered reflex control of peripheral vasoconstriction and dilatation, which leads to altered salt and water regulation. Vagus nerve control of heart rate is absent, and there is a blunted heart rate response to exercise. Rapid resting heart rates are the norm. Hemodynamics are altered by the type of implantation technique (biatrial versus bicaval anastomosis). Donor-recipient atrial asynchrony can be present, and atrial to ventricular transit can be perturbed (particularly when bicaval anastomosis techniques are used). There is an early restrictive physiology in most transplanted hearts as well as long-term, occult, restrictive hemodynamics. Rejection can exacerbate this difficulty. Tricuspid insufficiency is common. Myocardial injury can occur because of inadequate preservation, rejection, and the development of allograft arteriopathy. These processes, either alone or often in combination, may lead to substantial abnormalities of diastolic or systolic function.

Complications noted after cardiac transplantation generally relate to a suppressed immune system, which predisposes to infection and malignant transformation or the ravages of allograft rejection (Table 75.9). Allograft arteriopathy, sometimes referred to as chronic rejection, accounts for most late graft losses. Indeed, the half-life of transplanted hearts is only 10 to 12 years.

Immunosuppressive drugs have their own toxicities and complications, which are distinct from the risk of infection caused by the immunosuppression itself. Cyclosporine and tacrolimus, for example, are nephrotoxic, cause seizures, induce hypertension, and create dyslipidemia. Other drug-related problems include hepatic insufficiency, renal insufficiency, osteoporosis, pancreatitis, and nuisance problems such as gingival hyperplasia and hirsutism. Despite these difficulties, in carefully selected patients, transplantation produces dramatic and sometimes even miraculous improvement in quality and quantity of life.

ISSUES RELATED TO OBSERVATIONS OF CARDIAC ALLOGRAFT FUNCTION	
Hemodynamics	Donor-recipient atrial asynchrony Bicaval versus biatrial anastomosis Early myocardial restrictive physiology Late occult myocardial restrictive physiology
Allograft denervation	Altered reflex neuroendocrine control of peripheral vasoconstriction and vasodilatation Altered sodium- and water-regulated secretion of vasopressin, renin, angiotensin, and aldosterone Absence of anginal syndrome during ischemia Absent vagus nerve control Blunted heart rate response to exercise Loss of diurnal blood pressure fluctuation Hypersensitivity to circulating catecholamines Exaggerated response to acetylcholine
Altered humoral homeostatic feedback loops	Atrial natriuretic peptide secretion enhanced Elevated circulating catecholamines Increased paracrine peptides (endothelin) Elevated exercise circulating catecholamines
Myocardial injury or maladaptation	Organ preservation or recovery injury Operative complications Allograft rejection Cardiac allograft vasculopathy Hypertensive heart disease Ventricular hypertrophy
Donor-related issues	Effect of brain death on cardiac function Donor-recipient size mismatch Age-related diastolic dysfunction Preexisting atherosclerosis Preexisting ventricular hypertrophy Preexisting cardiomyopathy Preexisting structural heart disease (e.g., atrial septal defect, anomalous coronary artery anatomy)

Table 75.8 Issues related to observations of cardiac allograft function.

COMPLICATIONS AFTER HEART TRANSPLANTATION	
Allograft rejection	Humoral rejection Vascular rejection Cell-mediated rejection
Infection	Bacterial Viral Cytomegalovirus Hepatitis Herpesvirus
Allograft arteriopathy	Obstructive coronary artery disease
Malignant transformation	Skin cancers Solid organ malignant neoplasms Post-transplantation lymphoproliferative disorder
Immunosuppressive drug-related difficulties	Nephrotoxicity Seizures Meningitis and encephalitis Hypertension Dyslipidemia Osteoporosis Obesity Cholelithiasis Cholestasis Pancreatitis Hirsutism Gingival hyperplasia

Table 75.9 Complications after heart transplantation.

SUMMARY

Multiple surgical strategies are available to help manage heart failure. These options should be tailored to individual circumstances and never pursued in a vacuum. Concomitant medical therapeutics are mandatory and should be coupled to these surgical procedures in an attempt to optimize the patient's outcome. Electrophysiologic procedures such as arrhythmia ablation, cardiac resynchronization pacers, and defibrillator implantation are critical in appropriate patients as well. Individuals with established heart failure who have been aggressively treated with medications and observed for extended periods but who have progressive symptoms should be considered for surgical therapies when appropriate. Cardiac transplantation is available to only a minority of the diseased population, and therefore other alternatives should always be kept in mind. Newer surgical modalities focus on decreasing myocardial wall stress and, theoretically, reducing subsequent molecular and circulatory pathophysiologic derangements. In heart failure, ventricular performance is clearly reduced; however, individual myocyte contractile function may remain at reasonable levels. If contractile function is intact, performance might be improved by altering myocyte load. In the future, more sophisticated quantification of the degree of apoptosis and fibrosis in the cardiac system may help guide decisions about which patients would benefit from the diverse therapies, including operative interventions.

chapter 76

Special Problems in Chronic Heart Failure

a. Mechanisms of Exercise Intolerance and Exercise Training

Kai C. Wollert and Helmut Drexler

DEFINITION OF PROBLEM

In acute heart failure, the symptoms suffered by the patient usually reflect inadequate cardiac output or pulmonary congestion and can be adequately treated by interventions that correct hemodynamic status. In stable chronic heart failure, a discrepancy often exists between measurements of left ventricular function and the severity of symptoms. Against this background, it is more difficult for the treating physician to know how to modify therapy for a noncongested patient with heart failure who remains symptomatic and desires an improved exercise capacity.

TYPICAL CASE

A 62-year-old man presented with the insidious onset of fatigue and exertional dyspnea, leading eventually to a presentation with acute dyspnea and swollen ankles. He was diagnosed with heart failure and treated with intravenous and oral diuretics. The patient was stabilized, and angiotensin-converting enzyme inhibitor and beta-blocker therapy was commenced. Cardiac catheterization revealed an enlarged, poorly contracting ventricle with normal coronary arteries. Ventricular biopsy uncovered features of a dilated cardiomyopathy. During a 2-year period, he required one admission when he had omitted his medication, but he was easily stabilized again. At this stage, he was markedly limited even when taking his medication. He was experiencing New York Heart Association (NYHA) class III symptoms, and he was being limited by dyspnea on mild exertion and generalized muscle fatigue. He was encouraged by his cardiologist to start a supervised exercise training program. During the next year, his left ventricular function was still poor, with an ejection fraction of 32%; however, his exercise tolerance had gradually improved.

DIFFERENTIAL DIAGNOSIS

Factors affecting exercise tolerance in heart failure are summarized in Table 76A.1. Peripheral vascular and skeletal muscle alterations can lead to more marked exercise intolerance than would be expected for an individual patient on the basis of measurements of ejection fraction alone. Marked skeletal muscle fatigue during exercise testing is indicative of chronic muscle deconditioning in heart failure patients. More detailed testing may reveal a loss of peripheral muscle bulk and reduced maximal leg or arm blood flow. A cardiopulmonary exercise test is the key investigation in most cases. In patients with nonedematous heart failure, the development of arterial oxygen desaturation during exercise suggests the presence of important concomitant lung disease, which needs to be diagnosed and treated.

TREATMENT OPTIONS

Current practice guidelines recommend endurance exercise training in stable patients with chronic heart failure. Before a training program is started, the cause of heart failure needs to be clarified, and severe stenotic or regurgitant valvular disease needs to be treated. Myocardial revascularization and implantable cardioverter-defibrillator implantation should be performed according to current guideline recommendations. Because agreements on a universal exercise prescription do not exist, an individualized approach is recommended. Gas exchange measurements offer an objective assessment of functional capacity (peak oxygen consumption) and should be used to derive an individual exercise prescription and to monitor changes in functional status. Heart rate–derived exercise prescriptions may be inaccurate in the current era of beta blockers. Endurance training should be initiated in a supervised setting at low intensity (e.g., 50% of peak oxygen consumption for 10 minutes three or four times a day). Home training should follow the early supervised period. Usually 20 to 30 minutes of exercise 3 to 5 days a week at 60% of peak oxygen consumption is initially recommended. Frequent follow-up is advised to assess the benefits of the home exercise program, to determine any unforeseen problems, and to advance to higher levels of exertion if lower levels of work are well tolerated.

Exercise training can lead to improvements in peak exercise capacity, exercise duration, and heart failure–related

FACTORS AFFECTING EXERCISE TOLERANCE IN HEART FAILURE
Blunted ability to increase cardiac output during exercise due to
■ impaired intrinsic cardiac contractility
■ blunted heart rate reserve
■ reduced β-adrenergic responsiveness
■ exercise-induced myocardial ischemia, mitral regurgitation, arrhythmias
Impaired peripheral vasodilatory capacity due to
■ endothelial dysfunction
■ vascular deconditioning related to disuse
■ excessive sympathetic stimulation
■ activation of the renin-angiotensin system
Skeletal muscle alterations due to
■ hypoperfusion of exercising muscle
■ deconditioning related to disuse
■ reduced mitochondrial volume density
■ reduced oxidative and increased glycolytic metabolism

Table 76A.1 Factors affecting exercise tolerance in heart failure.

symptoms. In general, quality of life improves in parallel to the improvements in exercise capacity. Moreover, impressive physiologic gains can be achieved by exercise training. These include an increase in peak oxygen consumption; an improvement in the autonomic control of the circulation, with a reduction in sympathetic nervous system activity and an enhancement in vagal activity; and improvements in endothelial function and in skeletal muscle biochemical and histologic characteristics. The results of training in heart failure, however, are not uniform. Some patients either are unable to complete an exercise program or achieve no increase in exercise capacity from so doing. These patients seem to be those with limiting cardiac output rather than those limited by secondary changes in the periphery. This distinction is quite plausible as training appears to achieve the majority of its beneficial effects through peripheral mechanisms with little or no effect on resting left ventricular function.

SUMMARY

Exercise intolerance is inextricably linked to the diagnosis of heart failure. However, there is often a marked discrepancy between left ventricular function and symptomatic limitation. Impaired peripheral vasodilatory capacity, endothelial dysfunction, and skeletal muscle deconditioning may all contribute to the symptoms and exercise intolerance in heart failure patients. Significant symptomatic improvements can be achieved by supervised exercise training programs in selected patients with stable heart failure, with no evidence of exercise-induced ventricular arrhythmias and ischemia or severe valvular disease.

b. Cardiac Cachexia

Stefan D. Anker and Piotr Ponikowski

DEFINITION OF PROBLEM

During the natural course of chronic heart failure (CHF), significant weight loss (often termed cardiac cachexia) may occur in some patients. This should be viewed as a serious complication of the CHF syndrome as it adversely affects morbidity and mortality of patients.

The development of cachexia is not a unique feature of CHF. It has several similarities to cachexias complicating other chronic illnesses, including malignant cancer, chronic obstructive pulmonary disease, chronic kidney disease, rheumatoid arthritis, and AIDS.

Cardiac cachexia affects 10% to 15% of patients with CHF and is always an ominous sign. Survival of cachectic heart failure patients is extremely poor, worse than in many malignant diseases, as nearly half of these subjects are dead within 18 months. Unfortunately, the predictors of weight loss development in CHF remain largely unknown. In clinical practice, cachectic CHF patients tend to be somewhat older than noncachectic patients, have longer duration of heart failure, and have more advanced disease, often with biventricular heart failure or predominant right ventricular component. However, the presence and severity of cachexia are not necessarily associated with the traditional measures of CHF severity. The transition from clinically and body weight stable disease to a stage in which weight loss and body wasting occur is poorly understood, and the time lines vary widely between patients.

Cardiac cachexia complicating CHF is a generalized process that encompasses loss in all body compartments: skeletal musculature, fat tissue (energy reserves), and bone tissue (osteoporosis).

The pathophysiologic mechanism of cardiac cachexia is complex. What exactly initiates the process of weight loss and body wasting in CHF still remains unknown; there is probably not a single cause as a number of processes occur simultaneously (Fig. 76B.1). It has already been established that numerous mechanisms are able to trigger tissue wasting and that most of these are found to be activated early in the development of CHF. Many of these pathways are initially activated as compensatory mechanisms to protect the heart and the circulation from damage and to compensate for impaired myocardial function. Mediators that have been implicated in this process include proinflammatory cytokines, catecholamines, angiotensin II, aldosterone, cortisol, and natriuretic peptides, to name a few. Nutritional factors also contribute to cachexia; they include alterations in food intake and appetite in some cases, imbalance between anabolic and catabolic factors, and increased bowel wall permeability and impaired absorption of nutrients from the gut. In addition, bowel wall edema may yield translocation of bacteria or endotoxin, which is the responsible stimulus that triggers the release of proinflammatory cytokines, which further contributes to cachexia in a vicious circle mechanism.

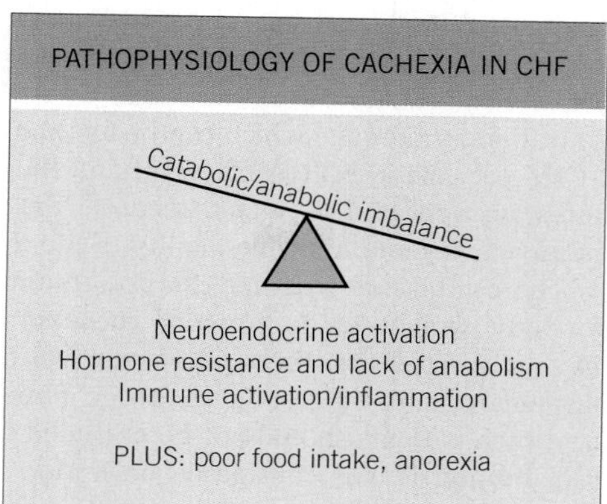

Figure 76B.1 Pathophysiology of cachexia in CHF.

TYPICAL CASE

A 70-year-old man with a 6-year history of CHF (etiology: coronary artery disease, acute myocardial infarction 8 years ago, coronary artery bypass grafting) presented with complaints of increasing fatigue, weakness, and exertional dyspnea. His medication consisted of angiotensin-converting enzyme inhibitor (enalapril, 10 mg twice daily), beta blocker (carvedilol, 12.5 mg twice daily), diuretic (furosemide, 40 mg daily), aspirin, and statin (atorvastatin, 20 mg daily). He reported that he was quite well until 1 to 2 months ago. At that time, he had started feeling more weakness during everyday activities, being predominantly limited by generalized muscle fatigue (in NYHA class III). He also noticed that he had started losing weight about 8 months ago. This observation was triggered because relatives commented on the loose fit of his trousers. For the last 10 years, weight loss had always been his aim and his physician's advice; this was based on presence of overweight with a body mass index (BMI) of 28 kg/m^2 (calculated from patient's comments). In the last 8 months, he lost about 12 kg (current BMI, 24 kg/m^2), although he did not notice any significant change in his appetite and food intake. On physical examination, there was neither pulmonary congestion (confirmed by radiography) nor peripheral edema. Echocardiography assessment did not reveal any significant changes from the last evaluation (enlarged left ventricular cavity; left ventricular ejection fraction, 36%). His biochemistry results revealed elevated BNP level, low serum cholesterol level (total cholesterol, 3.3 mmol/L), normal serum albumin level (4.1 g/dL), and mild anemia (hemoglobin level, 11.8 g/dL). This case illustrates the case of a patient with long-lasting history of mild CHF who developed significant weight loss with concomitant symptoms of weakness and deterioration in exercise capacity, despite optimal therapy and without any clear triggering factor.

DIFFERENTIAL DIAGNOSIS AND CLINICAL IMPLICATIONS

Recently, a consensus definition of cachexia in chronic illness has been published.[27] According to this definition, cachexia can be diagnosed when weight loss >5% in 12 months or less is in evidence and when 3 or 5 diagnostic criteria (including presence of anorexia, fatigue, and reduced muscle strength, low fat-free mass and biochemical abnormalities) are fulfilled. The following need to be excluded: starvation, malabsorption, primary depression, hyperthyroidism, and age-related muscle loss.

To assess for presence of cachexia and alterations in body composition, the following approaches are used in clinical practice: history of voluntary or involuntary weight loss; changes in body mass index; calculations of percentage of predicted ideal mass matched for sex, age, and height (by Metropolitan Life Insurance reference tables); anthropometric measurements (skinfold thickness, arm muscle circumference); and scores including biochemical assessments like serum albumin concentration. To verify the clinical term cachexia or muscle wasting more objectively, the assessment of body composition with dual-energy x-ray absorptiometry (called DEXA and allowing simultaneous measurement of lean muscle, fat, and bone tissue), computed tomographic scanning, and magnetic resonance imaging of leg musculature have been applied in recent years.

Clinical Definition of Cardiac Cachexia

In patients with CHF without signs of other primary cachectic states (such as cancer, chronic obstructive pulmonary disease, severe renal dysfunction, thyroid disease, AIDS), cardiac cachexia can be best defined as nonedematous weight loss of 6% or more of total body weight within the last 6 to 24 months. This definition was validated by the SOLVD and V-HeFT II databases on the basis of the assumption that a "best" definition should provide the highest sensitivity-specificity product to predict subsequent mortality. In this context, the average weight before the onset of heart disease should be used as the previous normal weight. From the practical point of view in heart failure patients, the presence of edema may further complicate the assessment of weight loss, which highlights the importance of assessment of changes in body weight in the nonedematous state. If weight change data are not available, a BMI of 21 kg/m^2 or less for men or a BMI of 20 kg/m^2 or less for women is considered sufficient to establish a diagnosis of cachexia.

Some authors argue that in addition to weight, a BMI criterion should be added (for instance, BMI less than 24.0 kg/m^2) to exclude previously obese patients who could have lost weight intentionally. Very few patients are able to lose weight when they want to lose weight. When weight loss is thought to be intentional (this can only be a subjective statement by the patient) but is achieved only after many years of trying and in the presence of a significant cachexia-associated chronic illness, presence of cachexia is many times more likely than successful dieting.

An important issue is to differentiate cardiac cachexia occurring in the natural course of CHF from "lack of food." In contrast to cachexia, the latter is reversible once food is supplied. The diagnostic process should focus on assessing important cachexia-associated symptoms. Development of cachexia in the natural course of CHF syndrome usually coincides with severe symptoms of dyspnea and weakness, which further result in poor quality of life. Weight loss in CHF is related to very poor outcome, independently of the other established prognosticators in CHF. Hence, presence of cachexia should be included in efforts to prognosticate heart failure patients.

The differential diagnosis of weight loss and weakness or fatigue in CHF is complex as it includes virtually all important chronic and malignant illnesses. Most important may be that recent onset of significant weight loss can also be a sign of malignant cancer. The complexity of the differential diagnosis of cardiac cachexia prohibits a detailed description in this setting but should always remind us to think beyond cardiology.

TREATMENT OPTIONS

Treatment of cardiac cachexia should be viewed in the context of prevention of weight loss and therapy for cachexia.

Angiotensin-converting enzyme inhibitors and beta blockers, which constitute a core of pharmacologic therapy in heart failure, both decrease the risk of weight loss. In addition, patients treated with beta blockers may ultimately experience a significant increase in body weight related to better outcome. Recent investigations have shown that approximately two thirds of the weight gain caused by beta blockers is in the form of fat tissue. This may indicate increased energy conservation (storage).

Intervention studies suggest that multiple micronutrient supplementation is potentially beneficial for cachectic patients, and it should contain antioxidant supplements and B-group vitamins. These studies have not yet been performed in CHF patients with cachexia.

Some therapeutic approaches are currently pursued to reverse weight loss in patients with cachexia. Cardiac cachexia has not specifically been targeted yet. None of the following treatments is currently approved for the treatment of cachexia in CHF or any other chronic illness (with the exception for use in AIDS-associated weight loss). The therapeutic concepts comprise interventions with appetite stimulants, anabolic steroids, and growth hormone and other novel anabolics (like myostatin antibodies, ghrelin, selective androgen receptor modulators, and anti-inflammatory therapies).

Exercise training programs, which can be applied to stable cachectic CHF patients in NYHA classes II and III, may also be an interesting option. This would increase the levels of daily physical activity and improve quality of life. However, it has not been established whether exercise training is able to restore body weight or to prevent cachexia in CHF. Reports have suggested that the relative survival benefit of heart transplantation is biggest in cachectic patients with CHF; hence, such patients should not be excluded from possible transplantation if it is considered an option at all. In contrast, it appears that left ventricular assist device therapy is not particularly helpful in CHF patients with low BMI.

SUMMARY

During the natural course of CHF in some patients, significant weight loss (often termed cardiac cachexia) may occur. Cardiac cachexia affects 10% to 15% of patients with CHF and is always an ominous sign for morbidity and mortality. In patients with CHF without signs of other primary cachectic states, cardiac cachexia can be diagnosed when nonedematous weight loss of 6% or more of total body weight within the last 6 to 24 months is present. The differential diagnosis of weight loss and weakness or fatigue in CHF is complex as it includes virtually all important chronic and malignant illnesses.

c. The "Cardiorenal Syndrome": Clinical Presentation, Pathophysiology, and Treatment

Marco Metra, Livio Dei Cas and Barry M. Massie

CASE PRESENTATION

A. P. is a 67-year-old man with severe cardiac dysfunction. Despite aggressive and appropriate medical therapy and implantation of a CRT-D device, he remained clinically symptomatic and had been admitted multiple times for heart failure.

On this admission, he presented a 13-kg weight gain, dyspnea at rest, massive peripheral edema and probable ascites, elevated jugular venous pressure, pleural effusion, and hepatomegaly. His blood pressure was 90/60 mm Hg. Laboratory studies showed moderate impairment in renal function with serum creatinine concentration of 1.5 mg/dL, estimated glomerular filtration rate (GFR) of 50 mL/min/1.73 m^2, serum hemoglobin level of 11.5 g/dL, and serum sodium concentration of 135 mEq/L. His echocardiogram showed severe left ventricular dysfunction with a left ventricular ejection fraction of 18%, severe left ventricular dilatation, severe mitral regurgitation and secondary tricuspid regurgitation, restrictive filling pattern, and inferior vena cava congestion. He was taking warfarin, digoxin (0.125 mg), furosemide (250 mg twice daily), spironolactone (50 mg), valsartan (40 mg), and carvedilol (6.125 mg twice daily).

He was started on intravenous furosemide (100-mg bolus followed by infusion of 500 mg/day). There was a moderate diuretic response (1800 to 2000 mL/day); but on the third day after admission, he became oliguric and gained 2 kg of body weight, and serum creatinine and blood urea nitrogen concentrations rose from 1.5 to 2.6 mg/dL and 74 to 145 mg/dL, respectively. He failed to respond to low-dose dopamine or treatment with positive inotropes. Although he experienced a transient increase in diuresis with the addition of metolazone (10 mg), this was attended by a further increase in serum creatinine concentration to 4.3 mg/dL and a further decline in serum sodium concentration to 128 mEq/L. Continuous arteriovenous hemofiltration was then initiated, with subsequent negative fluid balances and progressive improvement in renal function. After 6 days of continuous arteriovenous hemofiltration, the patient was free of congestion, and serum creatinine concentration declined to 2.34 mg/dL. He was discharged 3 days later with oral therapy similar to that before admission. Weight gain developed again after 6 weeks, with another readmission to the hospital in the following week.

DEFINITION, PREVALENCE, AND PROGNOSTIC IMPLICATIONS

Many definitions of "cardiorenal syndrome" have been proposed, but this term is generally used to describe the presence or development of renal dysfunction in patients with

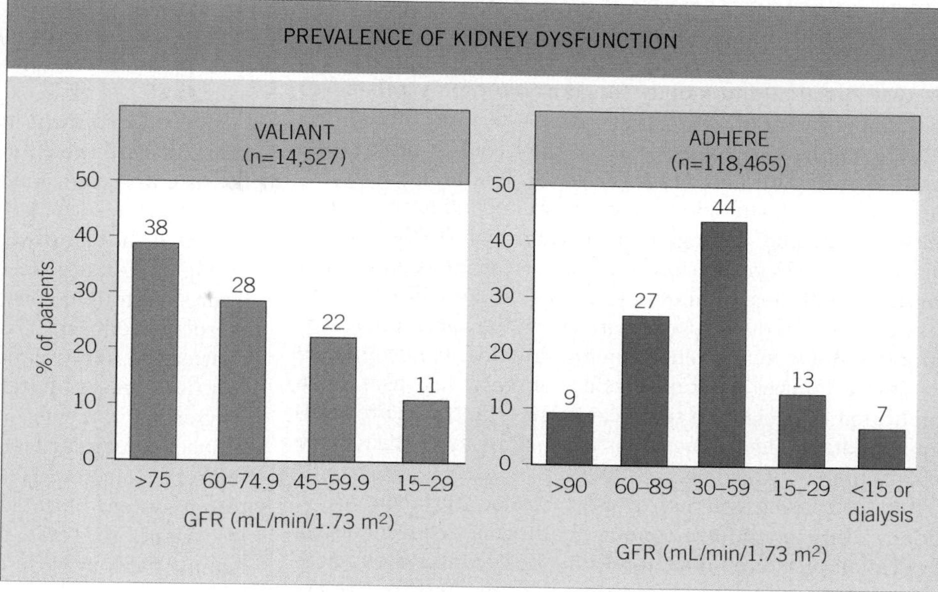

Figure 76C.1 Prevalence of kidney dysfunction. Prevalence of kidney dysfunction among patients with recent myocardial infarction (VALIANT trial) and patients hospitalized for acute decompensated heart failure (ADHERE). GFR, glomerular filtration rate. (Data from Anavekar NS, McMurray JJ, Velazquez EJ, et al. Relation between renal dysfunction and cardiovascular outcomes after myocardial infarction. N Engl J Med 2004;351:1285-1295; and Heywood JT, Fonarow GC, Costanzo MR, Mathur VS, Wigneswaran JR, Wynne J; ADHERE Scientific Advisory Committee and Investigators. High prevalence of renal dysfunction and its impact on outcome in patients hospitalized with acute decompensated heart failure: a report from the ADHERE database. J Card Fail 2007;13:422-430.)

cardiac dysfunction.[1,2] Although most patients with this presentation are volume overloaded, some patients may not be congested but suffer from low cardiac output. Excessive diuresis should also be considered in these cases.

Cardiorenal syndrome is common, with an estimated GFR of less than 60 mL/min/1.73 m^2 present in 33% of the patients with a recent myocardial infarction and left ventricular dysfunction or heart failure[3] and in up to 64% of the patients admitted for acute decompensated heart failure (Fig. 76C.1).[4] Furthermore, 30% to 45% of patients hospitalized for acute decompensated heart failure develop worsening renal function, defined by a serum creatinine concentration of 0.3 mg/dL or more and an increase in serum creatinine concentration of more than 25% from initial values.[1,5] Milder increases in serum creatinine concentration (e.g., >0.1 mg/dL) are even more frequent and are also associated with worse prognosis (Fig. 76C.2).[6] An increase in serum creatinine concentration generally occurs during the first 3 days of hospitalization, and then values remain high or even continue to rise in the following 2 weeks because it may take 5 to 7 days for serum creatinine concentration to achieve steady state after a change in GFR.

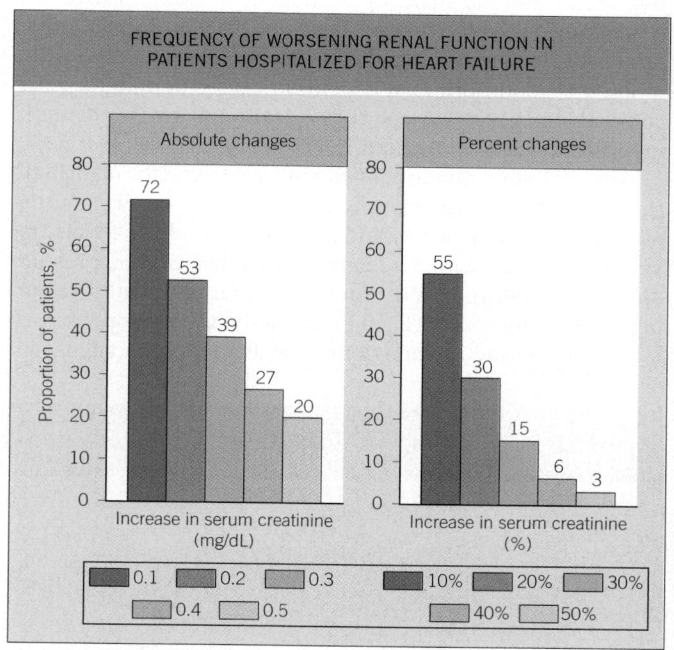

Figure 76C.2 Frequency of worsening renal function in patients hospitalized for heart failure. (Data from Gottlieb SS, Abraham W, Butler J, et al. The prognostic importance of different definitions of worsening renal function in congestive heart failure. J Card Fail 2002;8:136-141.)

Renal dysfunction is one of the most powerful independent adverse prognostic predictors in heart failure patients. Studies in ambulatory patients have shown that even a serum creatinine level above 1.3 mg/dL and an estimated GFR of less than 60 mL/min are associated with an increased risk of death. The relation between renal function and outcomes is stronger than that of most traditional clinical indicators, including NYHA class and left ventricular ejection fraction.[7] A recent meta-analysis has shown a more than 60% increase in the risk of death in patients developing worsening renal function (hazard ratio, 95%; confidence intervals, 1.62, 1.45-1.82 for ambulatory patients and 1.61, 1.35-1.93 for in-hospital patients).[8]

However, the finding of a relation with prognosis, even if it is confirmed by multivariate analysis, does not prove a mechanistic role of cardiorenal syndrome in the progression of the disease. There are, however, other reasons that this syndrome may be important for a patient's clinical course in addition to disease progression. These include increased length of hospital stay, need for increased diuretic doses, and lower tolerance and less use of lifesaving therapies (including angiotensin-converting enzyme inhibitors, aldosterone antagonists, and even beta blockers) in the patients with cardiorenal syndrome.

MECHANISMS: KIDNEYS AGAINST THE HEART AND VICE VERSA

Cardiac function and kidney function are tightly related so that impairment of one organ causes dysfunction of the other, creating a vicious circle that may lead to progressive multiorgan failure and death (Fig. 76C.3). Cardiac dysfunction and renal dysfunction often occur concomitantly as they share causes and pathogenetic mechanisms (Table 76C.1). Diabetes and hypertension are among the most important causes of both heart failure and chronic kidney disease, and thus they are frequently associated with the cardiorenal syndrome and worsening renal function in patients hospitalized for heart failure.[9,10] Renovascular disease has also been implicated, especially in some case series, but there are inadequate data to determine its prevalence or mechanistic role in cardiorenal syndrome.[11]

Besides sharing common causes, cardiac dysfunction and kidney dysfunction have common pathogenetic mechanisms. Activation of the renin-angiotensin-aldosterone system, activation of the sympathetic nervous system, impaired organ perfusion and ischemia, inflammation, and increased oxidative stress are the main determinants of both cardiac and renal damage. Activation of these mechanisms by one organ may cause or exacerbate the dysfunction or damage of the other.[1,12] Neurohormonal activation causes peripheral vasoconstriction, tissue hypoperfusion, salt and water retention, myocardial remodeling, and renal damage.

Hemodynamic abnormalities may also directly contribute to renal dysfunction. Hypotension and low cardiac output may impair renal perfusion. Furthermore, elevated central venous pressure with associated high renal venous pressure diminishes transrenal perfusion pressure, potentially resulting in tissue hypoxia. This, in turn, activates a compensatory mechanism termed tubuloglomerular feedback, an adenosine A_1 receptor–mediated process that down-regulates renal energy use by inducing afferent arteriolar vasoconstriction and reducing energy-requiring proximal tubular sodium excretion.

Medical treatment may itself play a contributory role as a cause of cardiorenal syndrome. High doses of diuretics are consistently associated with more frequent worsening of renal function.[5,10] An increase in sodium load to the distal tubule, as after furosemide administration, is sensed by the juxtaglomerular cells, causing adenosine release, glomerular afferent arteriole constriction, and reduced GFR (tubuloglomerular feedback). However, it is difficult to dissect the cause-and-effect relationship because underlying renal dysfunction causes diuretic resistance. Similarly, angiotensin-converting enzyme inhibitors and receptor blockers can reduce glomerular blood flow, also causing transient worsening renal function. However, both diuretics and renin-angiotensin system blockers are critical elements of heart failure treatment, so these short-term effects must be balanced against the long-term benefits.

TREATMENT

Preservation of renal function has become a major endpoint of treatment of heart failure patients. This is primarily based on studies showing the independent prognostic value of renal dysfunction and worsening renal function as well as on data suggesting that worsening renal function may be related to worse outcomes after drug treatment.[12]

Diuretics

Diuretics are a mainstay of treatment of patients with acute decompensated heart failure as they relieve fluid retention and congestion. However, high doses or excessive use of diuretics can be associated with worsening renal function,

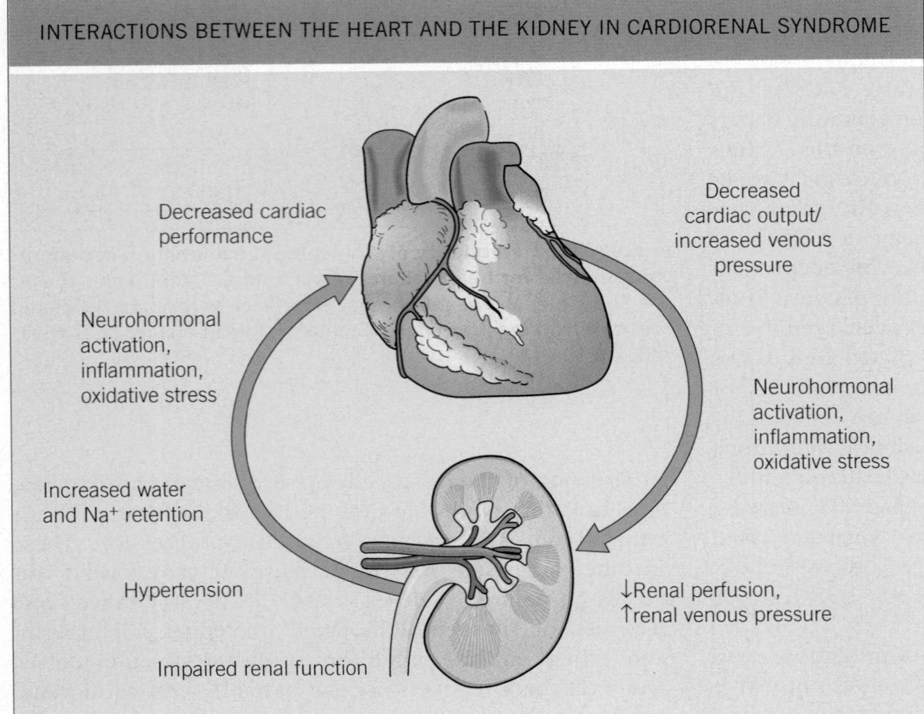

Figure 76C.3 Interactions between the heart and the kidney in cardiorenal syndrome.

CAUSES OF AND PATHOGENETIC MECHANISMS IN CARDIORENAL SYNDROME
Concomitant cause of cardiac and renal disease
Hypertension
Diabetes
Atherosclerotic vascular disease (coronary artery disease, renal vascular disease)
Concomitant mechanisms of cardiac and renal dysfunction
Activation of the renin-angiotensin-aldosterone system
Activation of the sympathetic nervous system
Inflammation
Increased oxidative stress
Hemodynamic impairment and fluid retention (specific of cardiac dysfunction)
Low cardiac output–renal hypoperfusion
Increased central venous pressure–renal venous pressure
Increased intra-abdominal pressure
Medical treatment
Diuretics
Loop diuretics
Thiazide diuretics
Combination diuretic therapy
Aldosterone antagonists
Angiotensin-converting enzyme inhibitors and angiotensin receptor blockers
Discontinuation of nonsteroidal anti-inflammatory drugs
Specific of chronic kidney dysfunction
Accelerated calcifying atherosclerosis–vascular stiffening
Increased asymmetric dimethylarginine

Table 76C.1 Causes of and pathogenetic mechanisms in cardiorenal syndrome.

at least in part by activating tubuloglomerular feedback and neurohormonal activation. Diuretic resistance is a hallmark of advanced heart failure and cardiorenal syndrome. Patients with substantial volume overload and elevated central venous pressure may show an improvement in renal function with diuresis. Diuretics are generally necessary but should be used cautiously and with close monitoring.

Vasodilators

Nitrates, sodium nitroprusside, and, in the United States, nesiritide are often used to decrease preload and afterload and thus to relieve congestion and to increase forward cardiac output in patients with acute decompensated heart failure and normal or high blood pressure. However, there is little evidence that these agents improve renal blood flow, and if they cause hypotension, they may actually have the opposite effect. Natriuretic peptides evoked considerable enthusiasm initially because in normal subjects and some animal models of heart failure, they improve natriuresis and GFR; but this has not proved to be the case in the patients with heart failure, perhaps because of the associated hypotension they may induce.[12]

Inotropic Agents

Inotropic agents are indicated in patients with acute decompensated heart failure and signs of low cardiac output and peripheral hypoperfusion. As renal impairment may be a sign of peripheral hypoperfusion, they are frequently used in patients with cardiorenal syndrome. Dopamine, administered at small doses, increases renal blood flow in normal subjects; but in heart failure patients, no consistent effect on renal function and outcomes has been observed, at least when accompanying hypotension is not present. Similarly, the use of β-adrenergic agonists (dobutamine) and phosphodiesterase inhibitors (milrinone, enoximone) has not had a significant effect on renal function or outcomes in patients with cardiorenal syndrome.

Newer and Investigational Treatments

Several newer agents have become available or are being actively investigated that may have a potential role in the management of patients with cardiorenal syndrome.

Vasopressin V_2 Receptor Antagonists

These agents are selective inhibitors of V_2 receptors in the distal nephron that regulate aquaresis (free water excretion). Accordingly, they are effective for the treatment of hyponatremia, especially when it is caused by inappropriate vasopressin release and excessive water retention. Their effects in an unselected study group of patients hospitalized for acute decompensated heart failure have been studied in the Efficacy of Vasopressin Antagonism in Heart Failure Outcome Study with Tolvaptan (EVEREST) trial. Administration of tolvaptan was associated with a greater decline in body weight and with a transient improvement in symptoms and signs of congestion in the first days of hospitalization. Notably, changes in renal function in the tolvaptan and placebo groups did not differ despite the higher doses of diuretics in the latter group.[13] Chronic treatment with tolvaptan also was associated with slightly less diuretic use but no difference in death or readmission for worsening heart failure compared with placebo.

Adenosine A_1 Receptor Antagonists

Adenosine is an important regulator of renal blood flow, salt excretion, and function. A_1-selective blockers inhibit renal counterregulatory actions of adenosine resulting from increased adenosine in the setting of heart failure and diuretic-induced natriuresis. Several such agents, for both intravenous and oral use, are under active investigation. Thus far, the one agent studied in the clinical setting of acute decompensated heart failure, rolofylline, appears to produce dose-dependent increases in diuresis and natriuresis associated with lesser need for loop diuretics and with preservation of renal function compared with placebo-treated patients.[14]

Ultrafiltration

New devices using venovenous ultrafiltration provide a relatively simple approach to mechanical fluid removal, making this approach available in a variety of clinical settings. Compared with diuretic treatment, ultrafiltration is not associated with as much neurohormonal activation. It also facilitates greater and more rapid removal of fluid and, especially, of salt than aggressive diuresis does. Although ultrafiltration was not associated with either greater symptom improvement or better renal function in a prospective randomized trial compared with furosemide, there was an apparent reduction in readmissions for heart failure between 30 and 90 days after discharge—a potentially important finding but one that requires replication.[15]

SUMMARY

Cardiorenal syndrome is a term connoting the intersection between cardiac dysfunction and renal dysfunction, most frequently in patients with heart failure. Although the underlying mechanisms have not been fully characterized, this presentation in the setting of acute decompensated heart failure and in chronic heart failure is associated with poor short- and long-term outcomes. At present, there is no therapeutic intervention with proven benefit in outcomes in this setting, but reasonable treatment objectives include maintaining renal perfusion by maintaining arterial pressure, decongesting the patient to lessen central venous pressure, avoiding excessive diuresis, and maintaining as much as possible treatment with neurohormonal antagonists that are known to prolong survival and to prevent readmissions. Novel approaches are undergoing investigation and are greatly needed.

d. Anemia in Heart Failure

Peter van der Meer and Dirk J. Van Veldhuisen

DEFINITION OF PROBLEM

Anemia is commonly observed in patients with chronic heart failure (CHF). The prevalence of anemia depends on both the severity of heart failure and the diagnostic criteria. It has been shown that the percentage of patients with hemoglobin levels below 12 g/dL increased from 9% in NYHA class I to 79% in NYHA class IV heart failure. In a large meta-analysis, it has been shown that one third of the CHF patients are considered anemic.[1]

PATHOPHYSIOLOGY AND CLINICAL IMPLICATIONS

Although anemia is common in patients with CHF, only a few studies have investigated the origin of anemia in CHF. Several potential mechanisms may be involved. Chronic renal failure is likely to be an important contributor. Reduced kidney function and anemia frequently occur in patients with CHF; half of the CHF population has an estimated glomerular filtration rate below 60 mL/min, indicating an impaired renal function. In turn, CHF can cause renal failure because of a decreased cardiac output and relative renal vasoconstriction, leading to chronic renal ischemia, subsequent lowering of erythropoietin levels, and ultimately anemia. On the other hand, anemia can also provoke or worsen CHF. Once anemia has developed, the increased cardiac workload results in left ventricular hypertrophy and ultimately worsens cardiac function, which in turn impairs renal function, resulting in a vicious circle, the so-called cardiorenal anemia syndrome.

Because many patients with CHF have a normal or only slightly impaired renal function, other factors probably play a role in the presence of anemia in CHF.[2] Hematinic deficiencies may be implicated in the anemia observed in CHF patients. There may be reduced levels of iron, folate, and vitamin B_{12} related to poor nutrition, malabsorption, and cardiac cachexia. Furthermore, the use of aspirin and oral anticoagulation can lead to microscopic amounts of gastrointestinal blood loss, contributing to the anemia. Lower hemoglobin levels are also frequently observed in inflammatory conditions. It has been shown that patients with CHF express elevated levels of cytokines, which in turn may reduce the hematopoietic proliferation. Anemia can also originate from increased plasma volume (hemodilution). In addition, treatment of CHF might induce anemia. It has been shown that inhibition of the renin-angiotensin system reduces hematopoietic activity.

Several studies have linked the presence of anemia to an impaired outcome. In one of the largest cohorts studied so far, comprising more than 50,000 CHF patients, lower hemoglobin levels were associated with a gradual increase in mortality. Mortality risk increased from 50% in patients with hemoglobin levels between 11.0 and 12.0 g/dL to 300% in patients with hemoglobin levels below 9.0 g/dL compared with nonanemic patients, independent of other known predictors of mortality in CHF.

TREATMENT OPTIONS

Intervention studies have assessed the efficacy of erythropoietin in a limited number of patients with CHF. Erythropoietin and the intravenous administration of iron corrected anemia and were associated with a significant increase in left ventricular ejection fraction and decrease in NYHA class, which was reflected by almost 90% reduction in the number of hospitalizations. Moreover, erythropoietin treatment significantly increased peak oxygen consumption ($\dot{V}O_2$) and exercise duration in patients with moderate to severe CHF. In principle, the first clinical studies have all shown that erythropoietin can correct anemia and that oral iron resulted in an improvement in NYHA status and exercise endurance. Moreover, renal function improved, and there was a significant decrease in plasma B-type natriuretic peptide levels as well as reduced need for hospitalization in patients treated with erythropoietin. Although these trials showed beneficial effects, the sample sizes of these studies were relatively small, preventing far-reaching conclusions. A middle-sized multicenter phase II study evaluated the effects of darbepoetin (a long-acting erythropoietin analogue) on surrogate cardiovascular endpoints in 165 patients with CHF. Treatment with darbepoetin was safe and effectively raised hemoglobin level. Moreover, it significantly improved the clinical status as measured by the Kansas City Cardiomyopathy Questionnaire; however, no significant improvement in exercise tolerance could be observed. Larger randomized studies are clearly needed to determine the impact on morbidity and mortality. Therefore, a large-scale trial to assess the effect of anemia correction on cardiovascular mortality in patients with CHF was designed.[3] This large phase III morbidity and mortality trial, the Reduction of Events with Darbepoetin alfa in Heart Failure (RED-HF), will provide more data to answer the question of whether erythropoietin in anemic heart failure patients is beneficial.

SUMMARY

Anemia is common in patients with CHF and related to an impaired outcome independent of other known prognosticators. The origin of anemia in CHF is diverse and related to several factors, including renal failure, resistance of the bone marrow to erythropoietin due to cytokines, hematinic deficiencies, and medication use. Small-scale clinical trials in CHF have shown some improvement on surrogate endpoints. Currently, a large morbidity and mortality study evaluating the effect of erythropoietin treatment in anemic CHF patients is being conducted. At present, the current guidelines do not recommend erythropoiesis-stimulating agents in anemic CHF patients, and such use should be assessed only in an investigational setting, notwithstanding the promising results of small-scale clinical trials.

e. Depression in Heart Failure

Christiane E. Angermann

DEFINITION OF PROBLEM

A major depressive episode is diagnosed on the basis of several well-defined criteria as the presence of depressed mood and loss of interest. Major depression is four to five times more common in patients with chronic heart failure (CHF) than in the general population. In a recent meta-analysis, the overall prevalence of clinically significant (major) depression was reported to be 21.5% in patients with CHF.[1] Significantly higher short- and long-term morbidity and mortality rates have been demonstrated in patients with CHF suffering from major (but not minor) depression as a comorbidity[2,3] (Fig. 76E.1); worse outcome in terms of health-related quality of life and higher costs for hospitalizations have also been reported. Possible mechanisms mediating this relationship include biologic (e.g., severity of CHF, autonomic and immunologic dysregulation, systemic inflammation, multiple comorbidities), behavioral (health behavior, impaired compliance with pharmacologic and nonpharmacologic therapy), and psychosocial factors as well as gender, with higher estimated prevalence rates in women. There is growing evidence that major depressive disorder and cardiovascular disease may also share genetic susceptibilities.[4]

DIAGNOSIS OF DEPRESSION

The diagnosis of depression requires distinct changes of mood characterized by

- sadness;
- loss of interest and pleasure, energy, and self-esteem; and
- in addition, at least two of the following psychophysiologic changes: sleeping disorders, loss of appetite, feeling

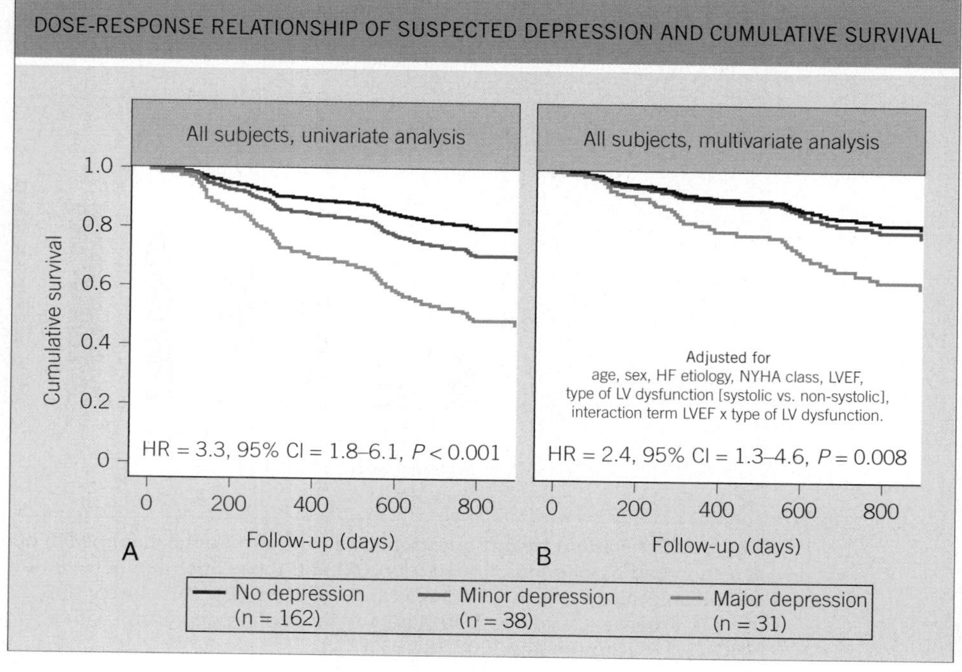

Figure 76E.1 Dose-response relationship of suspected depression according to PHQ-9 and cumulative survival. After multivariable adjustment, only major depression remains predictive of increased all-cause mortality. (Modified from Faller H, Störk S, Schowalter M, et al. Depression and survival in chronic heart failure: does gender play a role? Eur J Heart Fail 2007;9:1018-1023. Epub 2007 Jul 30.)

of guilt, decreased sexual desire, decreased working ability, crying, and suicidal tendencies.

These changes must last for at least 2 weeks and interfere significantly with the patient's professional situation or family relations. Thus, the diagnosis is based on operational criteria without taking into consideration etiologic factors. As in other mental disorders, no biologic tests that would allow the diagnosis to be verified are presently available.

Standardized and validated physician- or patient-administered questionnaires, some of which are listed in Table 76E.1, may alternatively be used as screening tools for assessment of suspected depressive symptoms in heart failure patients. Cutoff scores are then used to classify the severity as absent, mild, moderate, or severe. The short form of the two-item Patient Health Questionnaire (PHQ-2) has been established as a brief multipurpose measure adequate for the detection, grading, and monitoring of depression and associated impairments, such as work disability (Fig. 76E.2).[5] It consists of only two questions that might easily be integrated in the patient's interview during routine cardiologic check-up. The PHQ diagnosis of depression compares favorably with the National Institute of Mental Health Diagnostic Interview Schedule (DIS) and the Structured Clinical Interview for Depression (SCID), which are administered by mental health specialists to establish the diagnosis of a major depressive disorder according to the *Diagnostic and Statistical Manual of Mental Disorders* (DSM-IV) and are employed as reference standards.

More recently, additional evaluation of anxiety, cognitive function, and quality of life has been recommended in CHF patients as anxiety and cognitive impairment are frequent in this population of elderly patients and may require

COMMON STANDARDIZED AND VALIDATED INSTRUMENTS FOR DEPRESSION SCREENING AND FOR THE ASSESSMENT OF ANXIETY, COGNITIVE FUNCTION, AND QUALITY OF LIFE
Depression screening and monitoring
Beck Depression Inventory (BDI)
Hamilton Rating Scale for Depression (HAM-D)
Patient Health Questionnaire (PHQ) 2 and 9
Montgomery-Asberg Depression Rating Scale (MADRS)
Depression diagnosis
National Institute of Mental Health Diagnostic Interview Schedule (DIS)
Structured Clinical Interview for Depression (SCID)
Anxiety assessment
Patient Health Questionnaire on General Anxiety Disorder (PHQ-GAD)
Cognitive function
Mini-Mental State Examination (MMSE)
Quality of life
Generic
Short Form Health Survey-36
Disease specific
Kansas City Cardiomyopathy Questionnaire (KCCQ)
Minnesota Living with Heart Failure Questionnaire (MLHFQ)

Table 76E.1 Common standardized and validated instruments for depression screening and for the assessment of anxiety, cognitive function, and quality of life.

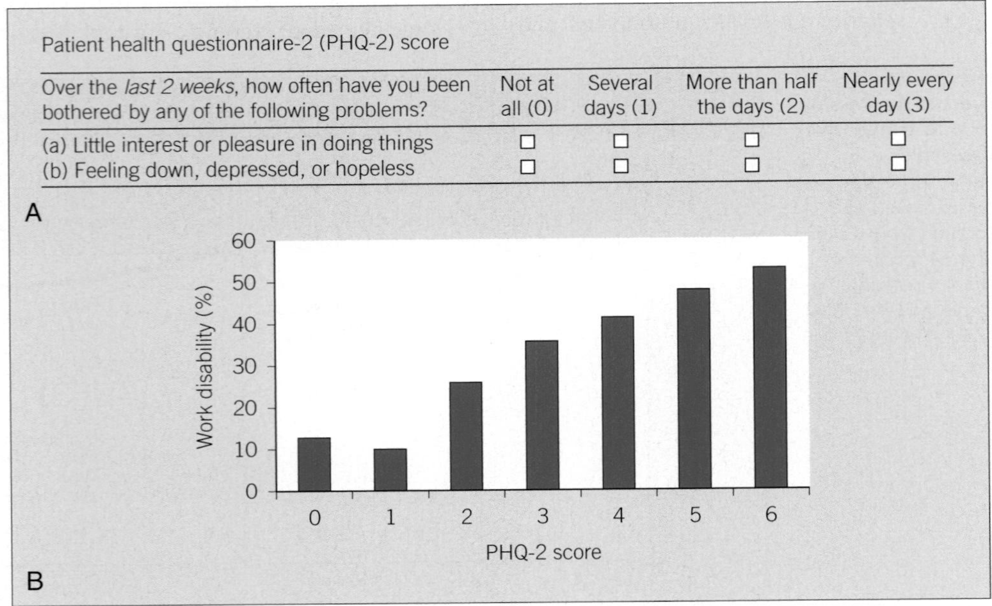

Figure 76E.2 Patient health questionnaire. The two-item patient health questionnaire (PHQ-2) for detection and monitoring of depression **(A)** and the relationship between the rate of work disability and mean PHQ-2 score in 1619 medical outpatients **(B)**. (**A** courtesy of B. Löwe. **B** modified from Löwe B, Kroenke K, Gräfe K. Detecting and monitoring depression with a two-item questionnaire [PHQ-2]. J Psychosom Res 2005;58:163-171.)

additional therapeutic consideration. Also, depression has emerged as the main determinant of generic as well as disease-specific quality of life, which from the point of view of the patients represents a particularly important treatment goal and may thus influence the choice of management strategies in the individual subject. Table 76E.1 lists a selection of appropriate respective instruments.

PATHOPHYSIOLOGIC CONSIDERATIONS

Figure 76E.3 illustrates possible pathophysiologic links between affective disorders such as depression, psychosocial stressors such as chronic severe illness, and cardiovascular disease.[6] Dysregulation of autonomic nervous control represents one plausible mechanism that may mediate the adverse effects of depression in CHF. Reduced parasympathetic and increased sympathetic tone lowers the threshold for myocardial ischemia and cardiac events. High levels of circulating catecholamines may contribute to recurrent endothelial injury. Most studies investigating the role of sympathetic nervous system dysregulation in depression found a higher resting heart rate, decreased heart rate variability, and increased norepinephrine excretion, all serious risk factors even in the general population. Elevated catecholamines may promote procoagulant processes by potentiating platelet activation and may also enhance platelet activation through direct agonist effects. Further, increased sympathetic tone is associated with increased levels of plasma cortisol, serotonin, renin, aldosterone, angiotensin, and free radicals. Several studies implicate involvement of the immune system in the relationship of depression and cardiovascular disease.[7] Depression may also have an adverse impact on behavioral factors, such as smoking, diet, physical activity, and compliance with treatment recommendations.

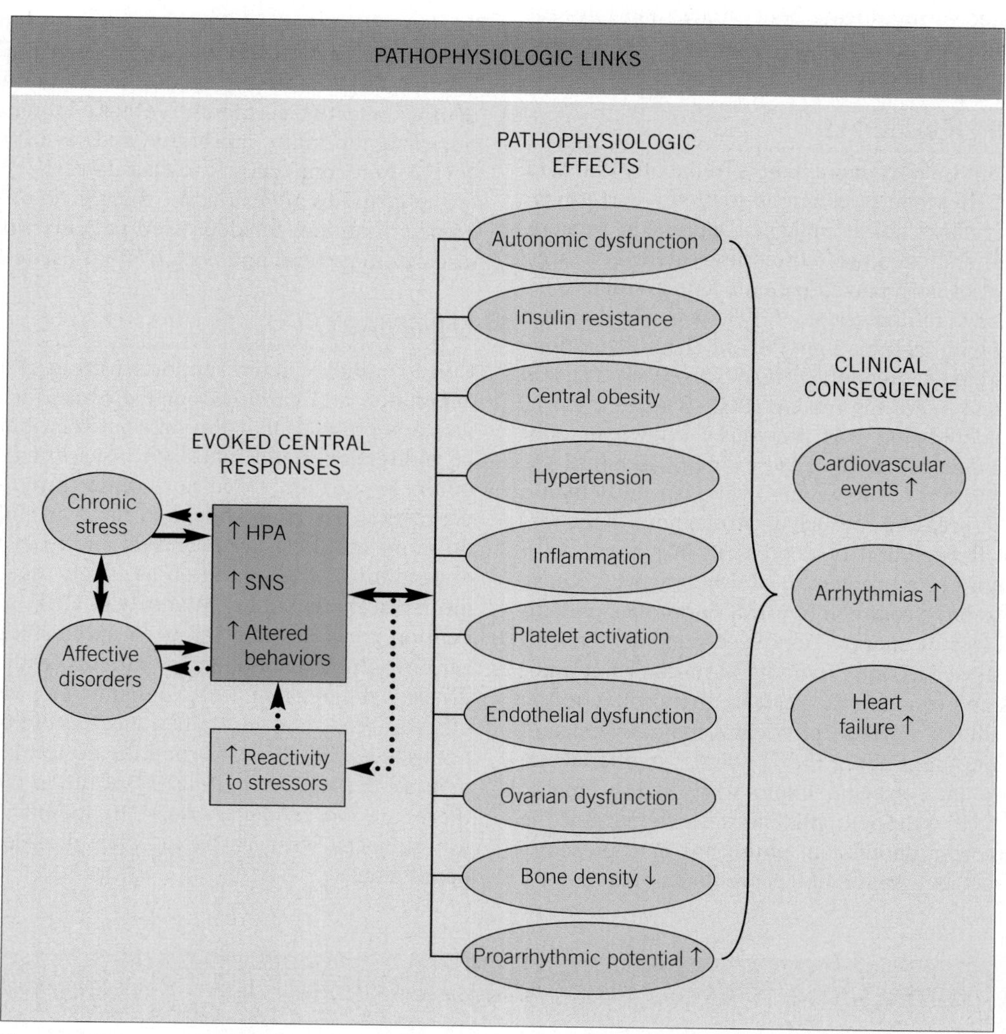

Figure 76E.3 Possible pathophysiologic links between affective disorders (e.g., depression), psychosocial stressors, and cardiovascular disease. The stressors activate the sympathetic nervous system (SNS) and the hypothalamus-pituitary-adrenal axis (HPA) and modify behavior. This results in pathophysiologic effects that are likely to increase the cardiovascular risk, with the consequence of a higher clinical event rate. Vice versa, risk factors and comorbidities in cardiovascular disease may potentially evoke central responses and increase the risk of depression. (Modified from Rozanski A, Blumenthal JA, Davidson KW, Saab PG, Kubzansky L. The epidemiology, pathophysiology, and management of psychosocial risk factors in cardiac practice: the emerging field of behavioral cardiology. J Am Coll Cardiol 2005;45:637-651.)

Bidirectional mediators have been implicated in the association of depression and cardiovascular risk. In addition to efferent effects of the sympathetic nervous system on the immune system, a reverse relationship has also been documented such that inflammatory processes cause central nervous system responses through both humoral and neural pathways.[7] It is still uncertain how depression and inflammation are causally related in CHF. It has been postulated, however, that elevated plasma levels of proinflammatory cytokines induce production of cytokines in the brain, which then activates the hypothalamus-pituitary axis, elicits a stress response, and inhibits serotonin activity.[8] Depression is also a risk factor for an incident cardiac event among initially healthy individuals; on the basis of meta-analysis, people with clinically significant depression have, compared with the general population, a more than 2.5-fold risk of myocardial infarction or cardiac death.[9] To further elucidate these complex pathophysiologic pathways, prospective studies, such as the ongoing MOOD-HF multicenter trial, are needed to investigate both clinical and relevant biochemical parameters of potential relevance and to test interventions likely to have an impact on these factors.[10]

CLINICAL IMPLICATIONS

Clinically significant (major) depression is frequently detected in patients with CHF when screening is routinely performed. However, in everyday clinical practice, depression remains often undiagnosed and even more often untreated. In a large consecutive cohort of hospitalized patients with systolic CHF, an overall prevalence of depression of 39% was found on the basis of screening with the nine-item Patient Health Questionnaire (PHQ-9). Minor depression (PHQ-9 score 9 to 11) was present in 15% and major depression (PHQ-9 score >11) in 24%. However, depression was previously known in only 16% (12% of the men and 26% of the women), and only 8% (6% of the men and 8% of the women) were currently taking antidepressants. The reasons for such underdiagnosis of depression are several. Recognition of depression in patients with CHF may sometimes be a problem in clinical practice because the two conditions have common physical symptoms, particularly fatigue and loss of energy. Depressed patients, but also their attending physicians, may in addition misinterpret emotional symptoms and erroneously attribute them solely to the chronic somatic illness. Further, physicians may be reluctant to explicitly ask questions about their patients' emotional status because they lack specific exploratory skills. Finally, because current CHF treatment guidelines do not suggest the treatment of comorbid depression, physicians may presently not perceive correct recognition of this problem as mandatory.

TREATMENT OPTIONS

Recognition of the prognostic importance of depression in cardiovascular disease has increased the demand for evidence-based treatment guidelines in this population. However, robust clinical pathways for the management of psychosocial risk factors are lacking, and current guidelines for the treatment of CHF do not provide specific handling directives. Although several previous outcome trials in depressed patients with cardiovascular disease proved the safety and antidepressant efficacy of selective serotonin reuptake inhibitors (reviewed in reference 10), there is no evidence that beyond improvement of depression these strategies favorably affect morbidity and mortality. So far, no larger randomized treatment trials to evaluate either antidepressant efficacy or long-term effects on somatic endpoints of antidepressants in CHF patients have been published. The ongoing SADHART-CHF study, which compares pharmacotherapy with either the selective serotonin reuptake inhibitor sertraline or placebo tablets, includes CHF patients in NYHA functional class II. The MOOD-HF study will be the first to generate results on the safety and efficacy of yet another selective serotonin reuptake inhibitor, escitalopram, regarding mortality, morbidity, and severity of depression in NYHA functional class II to class IV CHF.[10] Until the results of these studies are available, there is no evidence-based reference treatment for depressed patients with cardiovascular diseases in general and with CHF in particular.

SUMMARY

Considerable evidence supports a strong association between depression and cardiovascular disease, including CHF. Evidence is growing that the link between both disorders may be bidirectional and that each disease may give rise to the other or further enhance disease progression. Although depression has been shown to have an unfavorable impact on short- and long-term survival and to increase health care expenditures, the condition is rarely diagnosed and even more rarely treated in patients with CHF. No secondary prevention trials have so far been successful in reducing hard cardiovascular endpoints in patients with coronary artery disease, whereas in CHF patients, no data on treatment efficacy regarding mortality and morbidity have yet been published at all. Thus, beyond the desirable goal of improvement of depression and quality of life in individual patients, there are no evidence-based treatment recommendations for subjects with cardiovascular diseases and comorbid depression.

f. Disease Management Programs in Heart Failure

Christiane E. Angermann

SCOPE OF PROBLEM

Chronic heart failure (CHF) is a disease of the elderly and one of the most prevalent medical disorders; it is associated with serious impairment of quality of life and carries a poor prognosis comparable to that of common malignant neoplasms. With the introduction of more effective medical and interventional treatment strategies in coronary artery disease and the progressive aging of the industrial societies, both the incidence and prevalence of CHF and the annual number of CHF-related hospitalizations have increased, and affected patients are major consumers of health care resources. CHF has emerged as the most costly cardiovascular problem in developed countries, and 1% to 2% of total health care expenditures are related to this condition.

In this situation, appropriate actions to improve health care strategies would have the potential to dramatically improve health care results. To date, underutilization of available therapies has remained a common problem of the CHF population. Barriers precluding state-of-the-art medical care are complex and relate to characteristics of the "real world" patients, who differ from those enrolled in pharmacologic treatment trials, as well as to physician-related factors and to various administrative and financial obstacles within the different health care systems. Unless innovative management strategies are developed and implemented on a large scale, the situation will undoubtedly continue to deteriorate as the prevalence of CHF continues to increase.

The term *disease management* typically refers to multidisciplinary efforts to improve the quality and cost-effectiveness for selective patients suffering from chronic conditions. These programs involve interventions designed to enhance adherence to scientific guidelines and treatment plans.[1] Compared with traditional sectoral approaches, the superior effectiveness of multidisciplinary disease management, which integrates the endeavors of different health care providers (Fig. 76F.1), has been demonstrated in numerous randomized trials and has been confirmed by meta-analysis in CHF patients.[2,3] Consequently, a recommendation to use such programs has been included in the most recent American and European Society of Cardiology treatment guidelines for CHF.[4] The success of disease management has, however, not been consistent throughout (details in references 2, 3, and 5). Although components of successful health care delivery models in CHF have been published,[6] it has still remained uncertain which elements entail the efficacy of a specific intervention. To date, this constitutes a major obstacle to more general application and funding of such programs and therefore represents a major goal for future health care research.

COMPONENTS AND GOALS OF DISEASE MANAGEMENT

The components of patient care and monitoring that are recommended in the European treatment guidelines for CHF are listed in Table 76F.1.[4] Their superordinate goal is the physiologic and psychosocial stability of the patient.[6] The degree of instability is the main determinant of the required intensity of disease management and thus the quantity of personnel time to be devoted to an individual subject. Further, decisions about the patient's medical therapy, such as changes in the dosages of drugs and referral to another health care provider, such as a cardiologist or other specialist (e.g., psychiatrist, geriatric specialist, nephrologist, or endocrinologist) or to a transplant center, are usually triggered by changes in the patient's stability. Although the intervals between contacts of patient and caregiver usually increase with time and improving self-management abilities on the patient's side, it is important to establish and to maintain a schedule of telephone communication and office visits to ascertain compliance on a long-term basis; further, easy access to a team member should always be available in case of emergencies. Important criteria of clinical stability and implications of these monitoring goals for the strategies to be applied during disease management are detailed elsewhere.[6] Table 76F.2 lists major topics to be addressed during regular communication with CHF patients. If it is successful, this approach is supposed to improve patient outcome, including decreased symptoms, improved quality of life, reduced rates of hospital admissions and mortality, and decreased health care costs.[6]

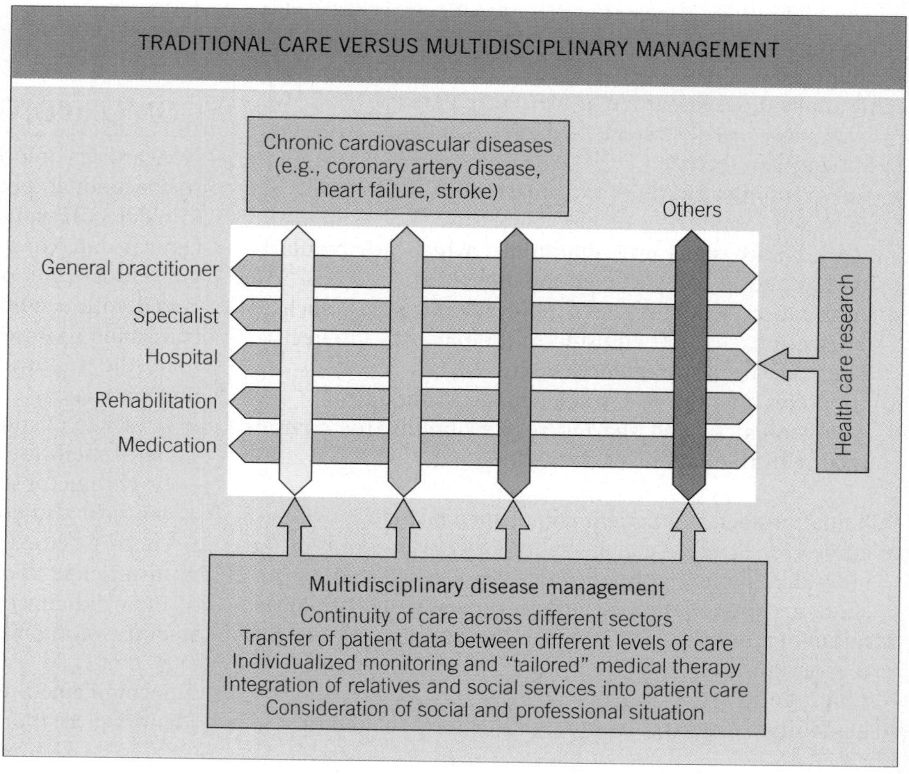

Figure 76F.1 Schematic diagram comparing traditional, sectorally organized care *(horizontal gray arrows)* and multidisciplinary disease management across different levels of care *(vertical colored arrows)* in patients with chronic cardiovascular diseases. Health care research accompanying the process is essential to better clarify which components of disease management are essential to produce positive outcomes in terms of decreased mortality and hospitalization rates, improved quality of life, and reduced costs.

RECOMMENDED COMPONENTS OF CARE AND FOLLOW-UP PROGRAMS AS INDICATED IN THE MOST RECENT UPDATE OF THE GUIDELINES ON THE DIAGNOSIS AND TREATMENT OF CHRONIC HEART FAILURE
Use a multidisciplinary team approach
Vigilant follow-up, first follow-up within 10 days of discharge
Discharge planning
Increased access to health care
Optimizing medical therapy with guidelines
Early attention to signs and symptoms (e.g., telemonitoring)
Flexible diuretic regimen
Intense education and counseling
Integration of inpatient and outpatient care
Attention to behavioral strategies
Address barriers to compliance
Modified from Swedberg K, Cleland J, Dargie H, et al; Task Force for the Diagnosis and Treatment of Chronic Heart Failure of the European Society of Cardiology. Guidelines for the diagnosis and treatment of chronic heart failure: executive summary (update 2005): the Task Force for the Diagnosis and Treatment of Chronic Heart Failure of the European Society of Cardiology. Eur Heart J 2005;26:1115-1140.

Table 76F.1 Recommended components of care and follow-up programs as indicated in the most recent update of the guidelines on the diagnosis and treatment of chronic heart failure.

COMPLIANCE WITH TREATMENT

The success of endeavors to implement state-of-the-art pharmacologic and nonpharmacologic treatment according to guidelines depends on the patient's commitment and adherence to the recommended therapeutic regimen. Strategies to ensure compliance of patients must therefore clearly define the roles of patients and their relatives, physicians, nurses, and other caregivers in the overall management plan. Noncompliance with CHF medical treatment and diet plans is common and has been identified as the major cause of rehospitalization, in particular in elderly persons.[6]

Commonly used strategies to assist patients with their treatment plan include

- daily reminder routines and clearly laid out forms to aid daily self-monitoring of blood pressure, heart rate, and heart failure signs and symptoms, which are regularly paid attention to by a team member;
- information brochures on CHF-relevant issues, such as medication, that are adjusted to the patient's intellectual level and are also regularly discussed;
- pill boxes containing 1 week's medication; and
- involvement of and sharing responsibilities for compliance with the patient's relatives.

Potential obstacles to patient compliance include

- advice for lifestyle changes without consideration of the individual patient's circumstances in life, which may preclude accommodation of certain recommended changes;
- failure to extend education and counseling to persons responsible for providing food or administration of drugs; and
- inadequate discharge planning after hospitalization.

MAJOR TOPICS OF IMPORTANCE FOR EDUCATION AND COUNSELING OF PATIENTS SUFFERING FROM CHRONIC HEART FAILURE
Coping strategies for a life with CHF
Explanation of clinical course and prognosis of CHF
Symptoms of worsening CHF
Action plan in case of worsening CHF
Self-monitoring of blood pressure, heart rate, and CHF symptoms and signs
Social services and community support
Patient preferences and end-of-life decisions
Pharmacotherapeutic regimen
Nature and mode of action of each drug (CHF and noncardiac)
Dosages of drugs, potential side effects
Importance of compliance
Individualized compliance strategies
Financial issues (if a problem)
Physical activities and working ability
Explanation of the role of regular physical activity for CHF therapy
Individualized exercise and training program
Compliance strategies
Sexual life
Work and leisure activities
Dietary issues
Sodium intake
Fluid restriction and consideration of renal function
Understanding alcohol restriction
Nutritional value and calorie content of food

Table 76F.2 Major topics of importance for education and counseling of patients suffering from chronic heart failure.

COMORBIDITIES—A KEY ISSUE

Noncardiac comorbidities including psychiatric disorders and socioeconomic problems are highly prevalent, in particular in older CHF patients, and strongly associated with adverse clinical outcomes. Data from the literature indicate that a large proportion of deaths and discharges for CHF are associated with conditions other than CHF that may precipitate, contribute to, or complicate hospital admission.[7] In this context, the following factors indicate an increased risk of noncompliance:

- presence of multiple comorbidities, such as anemia, diabetes mellitus, renal impairment, cerebrovascular insult, or chronic obstructive airway disease;
- physical and cognitive limitations;
- social isolation;
- insufficient social support mechanisms;
- financial concerns; and
- depression and anxiety.

Noncompliance in the context of multimorbidity has been identified as the most important determinant of increased hospitalization rates and health care costs.[8] Another problem related to multiple comorbidities is polypharmacy, which increases not only the risk of noncompliance by itself but also the possibility of drug-drug interactions; moreover, the presence of several concurrent diseases may lead to under-prescription of evidence-based CHF pharmacotherapy on the side of attending physicians because of safety concerns (e.g., diminished use of aldosterone antagonists in patients with renal dysfunction or of beta blockers in patients with asthma). In summary, comorbidities are a critical yet frequently neglected determinant of both clinical management requirements and compliance.

HOSPITAL DISCHARGE AND OUTPATIENT HEART FAILURE MANAGEMENT

If discharge management is inadequate, patients may be unable or lack insight into the necessity to comply with complex treatment regimens that not uncommonly are introduced during hospitalization. A successful transition into the outpatient setting needs to be prepared with a comprehensive, multidisciplinary discharge schedule, which needs to take into consideration sociodemographic factors and involve patients, relatives, the patient's general practitioner, and social services and other ancillary support as necessary. Discharge planning also includes an assessment of the need for outpatient follow-up by a specialist. Patients at high risk for readmission, such as elderly, multimorbid subjects living alone, should be monitored more closely in the home setting, if such a service is available.

Regarding outpatient disease management programs for patients with CHF, there are considerable discrepancies between different countries. In the CHF clinic model, care is provided in a specialized medical outpatient facility usually attached to a hospital or alternatively by a cardiologist in private practice or by general practitioners with special experience and interest in CHF. Visits by nurses or physicians responsible for future outpatient care while the patient is still in the hospital are desirable but—at least in Germany—still an exception. In nurse-based care, specialized CHF nurses assist the cardiologist in coordinating and delivering care. We have encouraging experiences with nurses delivering education and counseling by telephone according to a structured schedule with an intensity tailored to the needs of the individual patient and the severity of CHF; in this case, nurses are supervised by a CHF specialist. In nurse-directed care, a nurse, usually an advanced practice nurse, has primary responsibility for the day-to-day care of CHF patients. Although this model of disease management has been used successfully for years in some countries (e.g., Great Britain, The Netherlands), legal barriers in other countries (e.g., Germany) still preclude self-responsible care including prescription and up-titration of CHF medication to be delivered by nurses.

In the implementation phase of a specific CHF disease management program, the characteristics of the target population must be taken into account. The guidelines clearly state that it is likely that "the optimal model will depend on local circumstances and resources and whether the model is designed for specific sub-groups of patients or the whole CHF population."[4] As studies comparing the relative effectiveness of different disease management strategies are scarce and have not been conclusive,[5] further health care research accompanying the application of disease management and the success of specific components is needed.

PALLIATIVE CARE

In general, modern medicine aims to prevent illness and to engineer rescues from injury or other disease by appropriate means. "High-tech" medicine as practiced in the developed countries has been slow to adapt to the new challenges of chronic illness in old age, in which palliative care may be more appropriate. There is a growing need for continuity of care across settings and across the changing challenges of worsening illness that cannot be met by a sectorally organized type of care. In this respect, the integrated multidisciplinary approach of disease management may contribute to better coping with the shortcomings of modern medicine because it shares many goals of palliative care as defined by the World Health Organization.[9] According to the World Health Organization, palliative care "is applicable early in the course of illness, in conjunction with other therapies that are intended to prolong life, and includes those investigations needed to better understand and manage distressing clinical complications."[9] If required in conjunction with palliative care specialists, the disease management team might also take responsibility for many of these aspects of palliative care. The service needs of their patients may change during the course of illness from a more disease-modifying "curative" approach in the earlier stages to more palliative symptom management in advanced CHF.

Further, the patient's preferences and end-of-life decisions should be discussed with the family of elderly patients who are difficult to stabilize, and patients should be encouraged to provide some form of advance directive. The inclusion of counseling about cardiopulmonary resuscitation training may assist family members to better understand the risks of sudden death and to better cope with their family member's illness.

SUMMARY

Incidence and prevalence of CHF are increasing. Current treatment guidelines for the diagnosis and treatment of CHF[4] provide the rationale for the implementation of disease management programs in the management of this large population of patients. The success of disease management depends critically on the development of multidisciplinary strategies that integrate different health care providers in the inpatient and outpatient setting and generate networks across different levels of care. This includes discharge planning and monitoring as well as education and counseling in the outpatient setting tailored to individual needs. Such an integrated approach is likely to contribute to better patient compliance and improved outcomes, which include alleviation of symptoms and better functional status, superior quality of life, reduced morbidity and lower rates of readmission to the hospital, possibly reduced health care expenses, and prolonged survival.

g. Stem Cell Therapy after Myocardial Infarction

Kai C. Wollert and Helmut Drexler

DEFINITION OF PROBLEM

Modern reperfusion strategies and advances in pharmacologic management of acute myocardial infarction have resulted in an increasing proportion of patients surviving the acute event. Some of these patients develop adverse left ventricular remodeling and heart failure. None of our current therapies addresses the underlying cause of the remodeling process, that is, the loss of cardiomyocytes in the infarcted area. It has been shown experimentally that adult stem and progenitor cells may reduce infarct size, enhance neovascularization, and improve functional recovery when they are transplanted into an infarcted heart. The mechanisms of these effects are incompletely understood but may involve secretion of paracrine factors from the transplanted cells. In the meantime, initial clinical trials have been performed to test this new therapeutic concept in patients after myocardial infarction.

TYPICAL CASE

A 63-year-old man was admitted with a first anterior ST-segment elevation myocardial infarction. The patient presented 8.5 hours after chest pain onset. He underwent immediate coronary angiography, percutaneous transluminal coronary angioplasty, and stenting of his proximally occluded left anterior descending coronary artery. Magnetic resonance imaging 4 days after coronary reperfusion revealed extensive anteroseptal akinesia and a left ventricular ejection fraction of 37%. The patient was offered participation in an ongoing clinical trial of intracoronary bone marrow cell transfer after acute myocardial infarction. After informed consent was provided, 120 mL of bone marrow was harvested under a brief general anesthesia. The bone marrow was processed by density gradient sedimentation according to current good medical practice regulations to reduce the volume of the preparation and to deplete erythrocytes and platelets. Six days after coronary reperfusion, bone marrow cells were infused into the infarct-related artery through the central lumen of an over-the-wire balloon catheter. The patient was discharged the next day with standard medical therapy. Six months later, left ventricular ejection fraction had improved to 43% as shown by repeated magnetic resonance imaging.

TREATMENT OPTIONS

Conceptually, a variety of stem and progenitor cells could be used for cardiac cell therapy after myocardial infarction. Each cell type has its own profile of advantages, limitations, and practicability issues and may (or may not) have an impact on cardiac structure or function through distinct mechanisms. Most investigators have chosen a pragmatic approach by using unfractionated bone marrow cells, which contain different stem and progenitor cell populations, including endothelial progenitor cells, mesenchymal stem cells, and, possibly, multipotent progenitor cells. One recent trial has investigated the impact of skeletal myoblast transplantation after myocardial infarction. Table 76G.1 provides an overview of the randomized controlled clinical trials that have been published to date.

Bone Marrow Cell Trials

Bone marrow cells have been delivered by intracoronary infusion in all randomized studies. In four trials, cells were delivered within a few days after coronary reperfusion; in one trial, bone marrow cells were transplanted months and years after myocardial infarction. The combined experience from these studies indicates that intracoronary delivery of unselected bone marrow cells is feasible and safe in the short and mid term. Improvements in regional and global left ventricular ejection fraction were observed after cell therapy in the Bone Marrow Transfer to Enhance ST-Elevation Infarct Regeneration (BOOST) trial, the Reinfusion of Enriched Progenitor Cells and Infarct Remodeling in Acute Myocardial Infarction (REPAIR-AMI) trial, and the Transplantation of Progenitor Cells and Recovery of Left Ventricular Function in Patients with Chronic Ischemic Heart Disease (TOPCARE-CHD) trial. In the Leuven-AMI trial, significant improvements in regional contractility were observed; however, no significant increase in left ventricular ejection fraction was reported. The Autologous Stem Cell Transplantation in Acute Myocardial Infarction (ASTAMI) trial was the only study that did not report a beneficial effect on left ventricular functional parameters. Although the reasons for these somewhat heterogeneous results are not clear, it has been argued that differences in the timing of cell transfer and the cell preparation methods may have been critical.

Initial Experience with Skeletal Myoblasts

The recently completed Myoblast Autologous Grafting in Ischemic Cardiomyopathy (MAGIC) trial was the first randomized, placebo-controlled study of myoblast transplantation after myocardial infarction. Patients were treated with culture-expanded, autologous skeletal myoblasts or placebo at least 4 weeks after myocardial infarction. Cells were injected into the infarct border zone during bypass surgery. Myoblast transplantation did not improve regional or global left ventricular function, the primary endpoints of the trial. Notably, a significant decrease in left ventricular volumes was noted after cell therapy. A higher number of arrhythmias was noted in the myoblast-treated patients, but this did not translate into differences in major adverse cardiac events after 6 months.

SUMMARY

It appears that bone marrow cell transfer has the potential to improve left ventricular ejection fraction recovery after myocardial infarction, if the right cell type and timing of cell delivery are employed. Recent meta-analyses support this

Study	Design	N	Cell Type	Dose	Time of Cell Delivery (after AMI)	Outcome	
						Improved	No Change
Leuven-AMI	Placebo controlled	32 treated 34 controls	Mononucleated BMCs	130 mL	1 day	Regional contractility	Global LVEF LVEDV
REPAIR-AMI	Placebo controlled	95 treated 92 controls	Mononucleated BMCs	50 mL	3-6 days	Global LVEF	LVEDV
BOOST	Open, controlled	30 treated 30 controls	Nucleated BMCs	128 mL	6 ± 1 days	Regional contractility Global LVEF	LVEDV
ASTAMI	Open, controlled	47 treated 50 controls	Lymphocytic BMCs	50 mL	6 ± 1 days	—	Global LVEF LVEDV
TOPCARE-CHD	Open, controlled	23 controls 35 treated	Mononucleated BMCs	50 mL	81 ± 72 months	Global LVEF	LVEDV
MAGIC	Placebo controlled	30 controls 67 treated	Skeletal myoblasts	400 or 800 $\times 10^6$	>4 weeks	LVEDV LVESV	Regional contractility Global LVEF

In BOOST, cells were prepared by gelatin-polysuccinate density gradient sedimentation, which retrieves all nucleated cell types from the bone marrow; REPAIR-AMI, TOPCARE-CHD, and Leuven-AMI employed a Ficoll gradient, which recovers the mononuclear cell fraction. Although a similar cell isolation protocol was used in ASTAMI, the cell yield was lower compared with REPAIR-AMI. Dose refers to the average amount of bone marrow that was harvested or the numbers of myoblasts injected. Only patients with complete imaging studies are considered here.

AMI, acute myocardial infarction; BMCs, bone marrow cells; LVEF, left ventricular ejection fraction; LVEDV, left ventricular end-diastolic volume; LVESV, left ventricular end-systolic volume.

Table 76G.1 Randomized cell therapy trials in patients with acute myocardial infarction and ischemic heart failure.

conclusion. At the present stage, little is known about the long-term effects of bone marrow cell therapy after myocardial infarction. Moreover, the impact of bone marrow cell transfer on clinical endpoints is currently unknown, and patients should not be treated outside well-designed clinical trials. On the basis of our current knowledge, skeletal myoblasts do not appear to represent a suitable cell source. Possibly, modification of the cells, for example, to enhance their capacities for survival and integration after intramyocardial delivery, will yield more successful results in the future.

h. Role of Biomarkers as Prognostic Markers in Patients with Chronic Heart Failure

Kalkidan G. Bishu and Inder S. Anand

During the last 2 decades, use of rational therapies with neurohormonal blockers has led to a remarkable improvement in survival of patients with heart failure. In spite of this, the prognosis of heart failure remains dismal in many subgroups, with the annual mortality varying from less than 8%[1] to 75%.[2] Health care providers need to know about long-term prognosis not only to counsel patients and their families but also to help make informed decisions about medications, devices, transplantation, and end-of-life care. A large number of clinical, hemodynamic, echocardiographic, exercise, and biomarker variables have been shown to predict adverse outcomes in patients with heart failure in small clinical studies.[3] These results have generally not been validated in large, prospectively designed studies. More recently, several models have used some of the previously identified prognostic markers to predict survival, with variable results and accuracy.[4-7] The Seattle Heart Failure Model used several traditional clinical, echocardiographic, and biochemical parameters and medication use to predict survival.[6] The accuracy of the model was excellent, with predicted versus actual 1-year survival rates of 73.4% versus 74.3% in the derivation cohort and 90.5% versus 88.5%, 86.5% versus 86.5%, 83.8% versus 83.3%, 90.9% versus 91.0%, and 89.6% versus 86.7% in the five validation cohorts from different heart failure clinical trials. In this model, none of the new novel biomarkers, discussed later in this subchapter, was used. Whether use of biomarkers in the construction of newer models would help improve our ability to predict outcomes in heart failure patients is unclear. Unfortunately, there are only a few large heart failure studies that have measured some of the newer biomarkers at baseline and during follow-up. The Valsartan in Heart Failure Trial (Val-HeFT) has perhaps the largest such database and provides a unique insight into the potential role of biomarkers for risk stratification of heart failure patients.[8] In this subchapter, we summarize some of the findings from the Val-HeFT database. Some of the biomarkers measured in Val-HeFT were investigational but may become available as commercial assays are developed.

Val-HeFT was a randomized, placebo-controlled, double-blind, multicenter trial in 5010 men and women with symptomatic heart failure that evaluated the efficacy of the angiotensin receptor blocker valsartan.[8] Patients in stable NYHA class II to class IV heart failure with left ventricular ejection fraction below 40% and left ventricular internal dimension in diastole indexed to body surface area above 2.9 cm/m^2 on echocardiography were eligible. All patients had to be receiving stable pharmacologic treatment for heart failure, which could include angiotensin-converting enzyme inhibitors, beta blockers, digoxin, diuretics, hydralazine, or nitrates. The study had two primary endpoints: mortality and the first morbid event, which was defined as death, sudden death with resuscitation, hospitalization for heart failure, or administration of intravenous inotropic or vasodilator drugs for 4 hours or more without hospitalization. Hospitalization for heart failure was a secondary endpoint. Several clinical, echocardiographic, and routine biochemical measurements and a number of neurohormonal and other biomarkers including brain natriuretic peptide (BNP), NT-proBNP, norepinephrine, aldosterone, endothelin, high-sensitivity C-reactive protein (hs-CRP), growth differentiation factor 15 (GDF-15), troponin T (TnT), and high-sensitivity troponin T (hs-TnT) were measured.

It is likely that different biomarkers provide prognostic information about diverse pathophysiologic aspects of the syndrome. Plasma levels of BNP and NT-proBNP are considered to indicate ventricular dysfunction and wall stretch[9]; CRP and uric acid are markers of inflammation and oxidative stress[10,11]; norepinephrine, endothelin 1, and renin are markers of hemodynamic stress, and endothelin 1 may also be an indicator of vascular endothelium-induced peripheral vasoconstriction.[12] Troponin elevation indicates myocardial injury. Use of a battery of biomarkers related to different mechanisms of disease may therefore be a surrogate of disease progression.

NATRIURETIC PEPTIDES AND NOREPINEPHRINE

There are three peptides in the natriuretic peptide family, atrial natriuretic peptide, BNP, and C-type natriuretic peptide. The natriuretic peptides are produced in response to ventricular wall stretch that is closely linked to the pathophysiologic process of heart failure,[9] and several studies have documented the importance of BNP as a predictor of outcomes. In Val-HeFT, baseline levels of BNP, NT-proBNP, and norepinephrine as well as changes over time in these neurohormones predicted mortality and first morbid events.[13,14] Figure 76H.1a shows that BNP is a stronger predictor of outcomes than norepinephrine is. More important, compared with patients who did not have a change in BNP or norepinephrine over time, patients with the greatest percentage decrease in BNP or norepinephrine had the lowest mortality, whereas patients with the greatest percentage increase in BNP or norepinephrine had the highest mortality (Fig. 76H.1b). In a direct comparison, NT-proBNP was found to be superior to BNP in predicting the first morbid event but not mortality.[15] Interestingly, increase or decrease in BNP was also associated with a similar directional change in left ventricular internal dimension in diastole, suggesting a pathologic link between left ventricular structure and BNP.[14]

Serial measurements of BNP have also been shown to have prognostic value in patients with acute decompensated heart failure. In a cohort of 114 admissions for acute decompensated heart failure, Logeart and colleagues[16] found that a discharge BNP level of less than 350 ng/L was associated with 16% mortality or hospitalization for heart failure compared with an event rate of 93% in the group with BNP levels of more than 700 ng/L. A high predischarge BNP level may suggest residual volume overload and therefore predict higher hospital readmission rates. However, "dry" BNP level varies considerably and is unique to individual patients. Although the strategy of BNP-guided therapy was found to

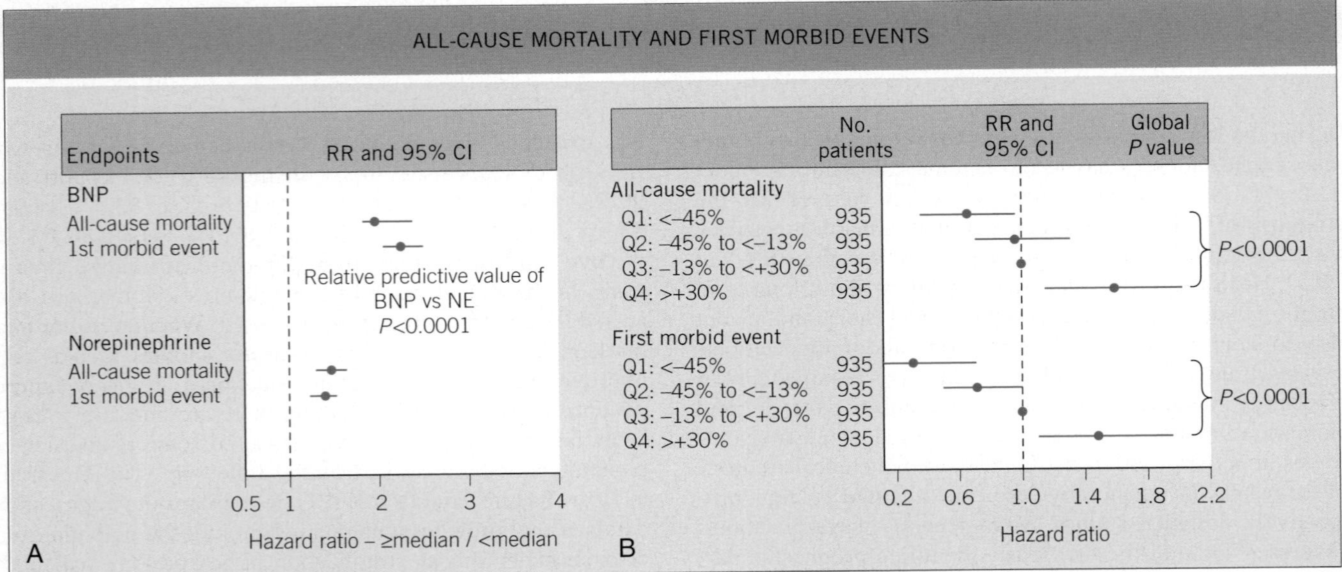

Figure 76H.1 All-cause mortality and first morbid events. **A,** All-cause mortality and first morbid events with brain natriuretic peptide (BNP) and norepinephrine (NE) levels above and below median. **B,** All-cause mortality and first morbid events for quartiles of change in BNP level from baseline to 4 months. (**A** and **B** from Anand IS, Fisher LD, Chiang YT, et al. Changes in brain natriuretic peptide and norepinephrine over time and mortality and morbidity in the Valsartan Heart Failure Trial [Val-HeFT]. Circulation 2003;107:1278-1283.)

be helpful in a few studies,[17,18] further work is required before this approach can be recommended for routine practice.

INFLAMMATORY MARKERS

CRP is an inflammatory cytokine produced in the liver. It has emerged as an important risk factor for systemic atherosclerosis and in particular for coronary artery disease.[10] Few studies have investigated the role of CRP in heart failure. In Val-HeFT patients, plasma concentration of hs-CRP was higher than in the general population, and patients with higher hs-CRP concentration had features of more severe heart failure than did those with lower hs-CRP concentration.[19] The cumulative likelihood of death increased with increasing quartiles of hs-CRP concentration. Relative to the lowest hs-CRP quartile, the risk of mortality was increased in the highest hs-CRP quartile in multivariable models (hazard ratio [HR], 1.51; 95% CI, 1.2-1.9; $P < .001$). Moreover, hs-CRP concentration was an independent predictor of mortality and added incremental prognostic information to that provided by BNP level alone (Fig. 76H.2a). Levels of both BNP and hs-CRP above the median were indicative of a particularly high relative risk compared with levels below the median values (HR, 2.08; 95% CI, 1.64-2.63; $P < .001$).

Uric acid, a product of xanthine oxidase metabolism, is another marker of chronic inflammation. There has been considerable interest in uric acid as a prognostic marker of poor outcomes in heart failure.[20] In one study, uric acid levels above the median more than doubled the risk of 1-year mortality (>484.5 μmol/L; relative risk, 2.6; 95% CI, 1.6-4.3; $P < .0001$).[20] However, the strategy to lower uric acid levels with oxypurinol was not shown to be associated with improved outcomes in the OPT-CHF trial.[21]

MARKERS OF MYOCARDIAL NECROSIS

Troponins T and I are protein components of thin myofilaments released with myocyte damage and may be modestly elevated in heart failure patients even in the absence of myocardial ischemia. With use of a conventional assay, TnT was found to be elevated in 10% of patients in the Val-HeFT population, and de novo release of TnT was detected in 3.6% of patients at the 4-month follow-up. Both the presence of TnT at baseline (HR = 1.6; 95% CI, 1.3-2.0; $P < .001$) and new detection of TnT during follow-up (HR = 3.2; 95% CI, 2.3-4.5; $P < .001$) were found to be independent predictors of mortality.[22] A high-sensitivity TnT (hs-TnT) assay, that is, 10 times more sensitive than the conventional assay, was developed recently. By use of

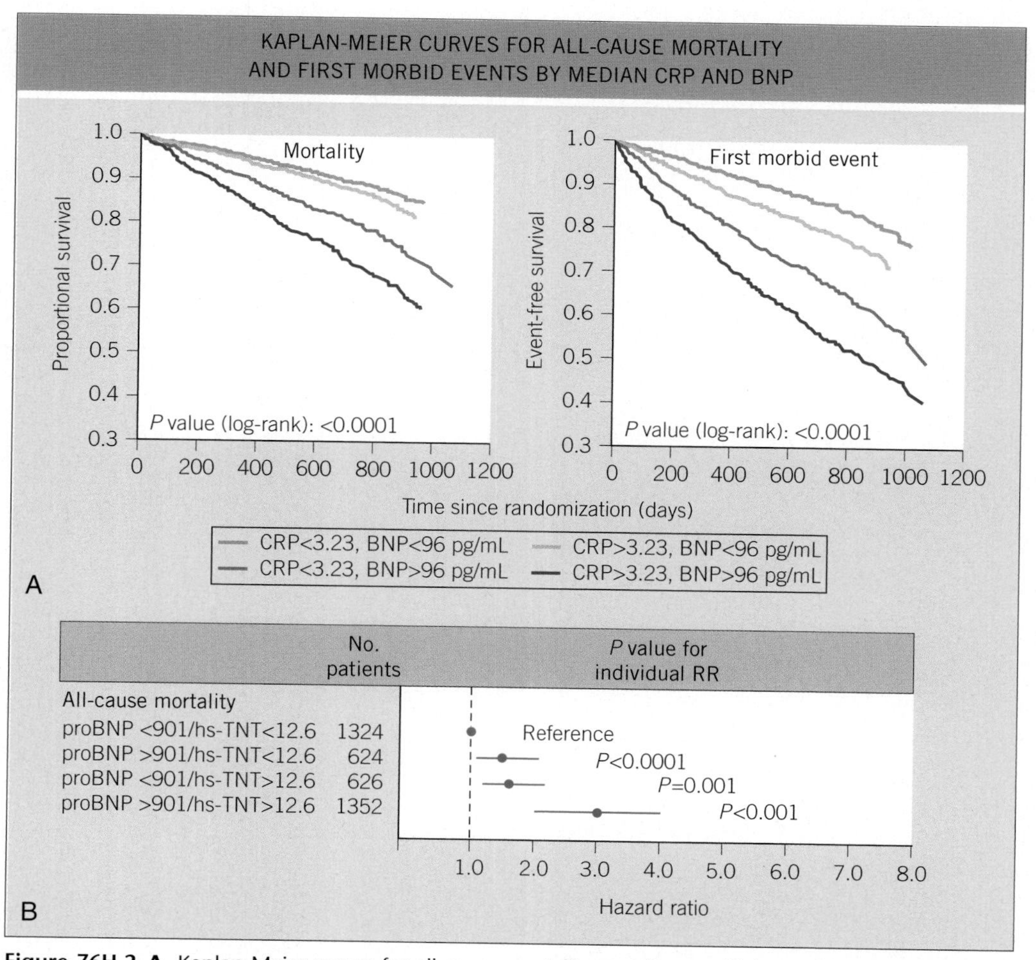

Figure 76H.2 **A,** Kaplan-Meier curves for all-cause mortality and first morbid events by median CRP and BNP levels. (From Anand IS, Latini R, Florea VG, et al. C-reactive protein in heart failure: prognostic value and the effect of valsartan. Circulation 2005;112:1428-1434.) **B,** All-cause mortality with NT-proBNP and hs-TNT levels above and below median.)

this assay, 92% of Val-HeFT patients were found to have hs-TnT present, suggesting ongoing necrotic or apoptotic myocyte death in the majority of patients with chronic stable heart failure. The presence of hs-TnT was also a strong independent predictor of mortality and provided prognostic information in heart failure patients incremental to that provided by other powerful predictors of outcome like BNP (Fig. 76H.2b).[23]

ENDOTHELIN

Peptides of the endothelin family are synthesized by the vascular endothelium and mediate vasoconstriction. Endothelin 1 (ET-1) and its precursor (big ET-1) are elevated in heart failure; a big ET-1 level above 0.83 pmol/L was an independent predictor of all-cause mortality in Val-HeFT (HR, 1.49; 95% CI, 1.20-1.84; *P* =.0003).[24]

GROWTH DIFFERENTIATION FACTOR 15

GDF-15 is a stress-responsive member of the transforming growth factor β cytokine superfamily. Its expression is upregulated in the presence of various myocardial stressors including reactive oxygen species, inflammation, and experimental pressure overload in animals.[25] In a cohort of 455 chronic heart failure patients, Kempf and associates[25] found GDF-15 quartile-related increase in mortality of 10.0%, 9.4%, 33.4%, and 56.2% (*P* <.001). GDF-15 was also shown to be a strong independent predictor of outcomes in Val-HeFT.[26] A baseline GDF-15 level above the median level of 2027 ng/L was a significant independent predictor of death (HR, 1.5; 95% CI, 1.06-2.14), first morbid event (HR, 1.56; 95% CI, 1.19-2.04), and hospitalizations for heart failure (HR, 1.93; 95% CI, 1.33-2.80) compared with a GDF-15 level below the median.[26]

SUMMARY

It is clear from this discussion that numerous biomarkers reflecting different pathophysiologic aspects of the disease are elevated in heart failure and independently predict poor outcomes. Incorporation of these biomarkers into multimarker risk stratification models for chronic heart failure may help improve our ability to predict adverse outcomes, enhance our understanding of the pathogenesis of heart failure, and help guide treatment.

chapter 77

Myocarditis and Inflammatory Cardiomyopathy

Heinz-Peter Schultheiss and Uwe Kühl

Definition

- Myocarditis is an inflammatory disease of the myocardium caused by infectious and noninfectious agents.

Key Features

- Progressive damage of the myocardium and the development of heart failure may be caused by either chronic viral infection or chronic inflammation.
- The host's immune response after viral infection influences the further clinical course of myocarditis and inflammatory cardiomyopathy.

Therapy

- Treatment of heart failure remains primarily supportive. Preliminary results from ongoing treatment trials, however, suggest that specific antiviral or anti-inflammatory treatment strategies are successful in patients who are carefully selected and characterized according to biopsy-based diagnostic criteria.

DEFINITION AND CLASSIFICATION

Myocarditis is an inflammatory disease of the cardiac muscle caused by intramyocardial infiltration by immunocompetent cells after any kind of cardiac injury. However, classic myocarditis mainly occurs by the host's immune response against organisms that cause common infectious illnesses, as a manifestation of hypersensitivity, or as a toxic reaction to drug administration. Chronic inflammatory events may survive successful clearance of initial cardiotoxic agents, be triggered or amplified by autoimmunologic processes, or develop in the context of systemic diseases. In many cases, however, the cause of inflammatory changes, which may spread from a focus or be diffused throughout the cardiac muscle, remains unclear. The extensive use of myocardial biopsy led to an agreement on the histomorphologic classification of myocarditis at a conference of leading cardiovascular pathologists in Dallas in 1987.[1] According to these so-called Dallas criteria, active myocarditis is typically characterized by a mononuclear cellular infiltrate with myocytolysis or degeneration of adjacent myocytes, whereas cellular infiltrates without myocyte necrosis are defined as borderline myocarditis (Table 77.1). Although these criteria can define acute or active myocarditis unequivocally, the diagnosis of borderline myocarditis is consistent with the existence of a myocardial inflammatory process, although it constitutes no definite proof. Histologic classification can result only from a follow-up biopsy carried out after some time has elapsed. If lymphocytic infiltrates persist in this biopsy sample, the findings correspond to ongoing myocarditis. If the infiltrates have decreased significantly in number or are no longer detectable at the time of biopsy, the diagnosis is healing myocarditis or healed myocarditis, respectively. Focal myocardial cell necrosis characteristic of active myocarditis is detectable only during the first 7 to 14 days of the early phase of the disease. As a result of this focal distribution of myocyte necrosis or the reduced numbers of inflammatory cells in the later stages of chronic inflammation, the findings on histologic examination are of only limited use because the sensitivity and specificity are methodologically reduced.[2,3] The World Health Organization Task Force on the definition and classification of cardiomyopathies has developed updated recommendations for the classification and diagnosis of cardiomyopathies. This definition introduces inflammatory cardiomyopathy—chronic myocarditis with impaired ventricular function—as a new entity among secondary or specific cardiomyopathies (Table 77.2).[4] Because clinical and histologic classification criteria alone are unsuitable for a clinically useful classification of inflammatory cardiac muscle disease, only the combination of clinical and histologic diagnosis with the results of new diagnostic examination procedures, such as immunohistochemical analysis of the inflammatory process and molecular biology virus detection, ensures a reliable diagnosis and a clinically relevant classification of inflammatory heart disease.[5]

OCCURRENCE AND FREQUENCY

The incidence of myocarditis is difficult to establish, given the varying severity of the symptoms. Evidence of myocarditis may be found in 1% to 9% of routine autopsy cases and in 17% to 19% of those performed for unexplained sudden cardiac death in young people, emphasizing the importance of myocarditis as a cause of sudden cardiac death.[6,7] The prevalence of histologic inflammation in recent-onset idiopathic dilated cardiomyopathy varies widely and has been estimated in approximately 10% to 40% of analyzed endomyocardial biopsy specimens.[8-12] An inflammatory process that involves cardiac muscle can have various causes (Table 77.3). Intramyocardial

DEFINITION OF MYOCARDITIS	
Active myocarditis	Inflammatory infiltration of the myocardium with necrosis and/or degeneration of adjacent myocytes
Borderline myocarditis	Inflammatory infiltration without myocytolysis; does not prove myocarditis unless follow-up biopsy demonstrates persistence of myocardial inflammation
No myocarditis	Normal myocardium or pathologic tissue without inflammation
Histologic definitions from the Dallas criteria.[1]	

Table 77.1 Definition of myocarditis.

DEFINITION OF CHRONIC MYOCARDITIS AND INFLAMMATORY CARDIOMYOPATHY	
Chronic myocarditis	
With viral persistence	Chronic myocardial inflammation
Autoimmune type	Normal left ventricular contractility *or* Regional wall motion abnormalities (EF > 55%)
Inflammatory cardiomyopathy	
With viral persistence	Chronic myocardial inflammation
Autoimmune type	Impaired ventricular contractility (EF < 55%) Ventricular dilatation
EF, ejection fraction. Data from Richardson et al.,[4] Kühl et al.,[70] and Kereiakes and Parmley.[13]	

Table 77.2 Definition of chronic myocarditis and inflammatory cardiomyopathy.

CAUSES OF MYOCARDITIS	
RNA viruses	Picornaviruses (coxsackieviruses A, B; echovirus; poliovirus) Orthomyxoviruses (influenza viruses A, B, C) Paramyxoviruses (rubella, mumps) Hepatitis C virus Togavirus (dengue fever, yellow fever, rubella)
DNA viruses	Adenoviruses Parvovirus B19 Herpesviruses (herpesvirus 6, cytomegalovirus, Epstein-Barr virus, varicella) Human immunodeficiency virus
Bacteria	Diphtheria Salmonella Corynebacteria
Spirochetes	*Chlamydia pneumoniae* *Borrelia burgdorferi*
Rickettsia	*Rickettsia rickettsii* *Coxiella burnetii*
Protozoa	*Trypanosoma cruzi* (Chagas' disease) *Toxoplasma gondii* Malaria Amebiasis Leishmaniasis
Parasites	Trichinella Echinococcus Ascaridae
Others	*Mycoplasma* *Legionella*
Fungi	*Aspergillus* *Candida* *Cryptococcus* *Histoplasma*
Toxic substances	Alcohol Anthracyclines Catecholamines Interleukin 2 Interferon alfa

Table 77.3 Causes of myocarditis.

inflammation frequently accompanies an episode of various septic illnesses and bacterial endocarditis. Among the protozoan diseases, Chagas' disease often affects the heart. Among the noninfectious entities, inflammation of the heart complicates about 20% of cases of sarcoidosis, and intramyocardial inflammation may affect up to 70% of patients suffering from collagen diseases, especially rheumatic fever.

Although virtually any bacterial agent can cause myocardial dysfunction, viral forms are the most common cause now. Most have a subclinical course. Meta-analysis of polymerase chain reaction (PCR) studies in patients who had heart biopsies with clinically suspected myocarditis or dilated cardiomyopathy demonstrated an odds ratio of 3.8 for viral presence compared with control patients. The overall incidence of myocarditis in viral infections is estimated at 3% to 6%.[13] Ten percent to 15% of virus-related myocarditis is caused by enteroviruses (Table 77.4). Apart from enteroviruses, analysis of endomyocardial biopsy specimens employing molecular biology techniques has also identified, with geographic differences and varying degrees of frequency, erythrovirus genotypes 1 and 2, human herpesvirus type 6, adenoviruses, human immunodeficiency virus, cytomegalovirus, herpes simplex virus type 2, and hepatitis C virus in the myocardium,[14-20] which are detected in 40% to 60% of patients with clinically suspected myocarditis and dilated cardiomyopathy. If the substantial number of cases involving a clinically suspected diagnosis (recent onset of arrhythmia, contraction disorders, cardiac enlargement) is included, however, the figures are likely to be even higher. Nevertheless, because of the low mortality of acute virus-induced myocarditis in adults, there are only a few autopsy findings relating to this stage of the disease. Mortality is often due to arrhythmia-related sudden death after fulminant myocarditis. Although these are far from being representative of all cases of myocarditis, they do constitute an important clinical entity.

DETECTION OF ENTEROVIRAL RNA IN ENDOMYOCARDIAL BIOPSY SPECIMENS OF PATIENTS WITH MYOCARDITIS AND DILATED CARDIOMYOPATHY			
Authors	**Method**	**Myocarditis**	**DCM**
Bowles et al. (1986)	Slot blot	4/8	5/11
Archard et al. (1991)	Slot blot	23/9	8/47
Wiegand et al. (1990)	Dot blot	—	1/6
Easton et al. (1988)	In situ hybridization	6/12	—
Iracy et al. (1990)	In situ hybridization	2/7	—
Kandolf et al. (1991)	In situ hybridization	23/95	8/47
Jin et al. (1990)	PCR	2/28	3/20
Weiss et al. (1991)	PCR	1/5	0/11
Zoll et al. (1992)	PCR	—	1/5
Grasso et al. (1992)	PCR	—	0/21
Koide et al. (1992)	PCR	3/9	8/25
Towbin et al. (1996)	PCR	90/191	26/132
Pauschinger et al. (1999)	PCR	24/102	44/149
Total		178/553 (32%)	99/463 (21%)

PCR, polymerase chain reaction.

Table 77.4 Detection of enteroviral RNA in endomyocardial biopsy specimens of patients with myocarditis and dilated cardiomyopathy.

PATHOPHYSIOLOGY

Acute Myocarditis

The inflammatory infiltrate, which may be mild, moderate, or severe, is typically lymphocytic but may also include eosinophilic, neutrophilic, or a mixed type of cells. In rare cases, multinucleated giant cells (giant cell myocarditis) or eosinophils dominate the active inflammatory process. Giant cell myocarditis is associated with autoimmune diseases (20%) but may also occur as a manifestation of drug hypersensitivity. Poorly formed granulomas and myocyte necrosis in association with mixed lymphocytic infiltrates composed of lymphocytes, plasma cells, histiocytes, and eosinophils are common. Overt myocyte necrosis is also found in the idiopathic hypereosinophilic syndrome but less frequently in allergic or parasite-induced eosinophilic myocarditis, in which direct drug-related toxicity and necrotizing vasculitis contribute to the pathogenesis. The infiltrates are composed of lymphocytes, histiocytes, and eosinophils but no giant cells.

In the United States and western Europe, viral infection and postinfectious autoimmune processes are thought to be the most common causes of this histologically defined diagnosis. Viral genomes have been detected in various frequencies, with or without inflammation. Virus-induced myocarditis in humans is assumed to develop through three phases. The early phase is the viral phase, followed by innate and acquired immune reactions and subsequently cardiac remodeling.[19]

The early phase, in the context of the general viral infection, is initiated by infection of cardiac myocytes, fibroblasts, or endothelial cells through receptor-mediated endocytosis.[16,21-24] Viral proteins are translated, and virus replication occurs in the myocardial cells.[25] The direct virus-related cytolysis of cardiomyocytes is already detected before any inflammatory infiltrate develops and appears to be decisive in rare, fulminating cases of myocarditis accompanied by rapidly developing cardiac failure and early death of the host. The unusual pathogenicity of the viruses and the resulting myocytolysis, causing a significant loss of contractile tissue, account for a clinical picture that is consistent with a rapidly progressive and often irreversible dilated cardiomyopathy.[26] Cytokines released by macrophages activate natural killer (NK) cells, which directly kill virus-infected heart cells through perforin- and granzyme-mediated lysis.[27-29]

The activation of antigen-specific cell-mediated immunity initiates the second phase of viral clearing. Myocardial damage is directly caused by the innate and acquired immune responses that are triggered by the ubiquitous Toll-like receptors and specific humoral and cellular responses to foreign molecular antigens.[30-33] Numerous in vivo and in vitro studies have revealed that the ability of the host to eradicate an invading organism effectively depends on the class of the effector-specific immune response generated. In general, T_H1 lymphocytes, which are characterized by the production of proinflammatory cytokines, including type I and type II interferons, are important for protection against intracellular pathogens such as viruses.[34-37] Usually, the virus is eliminated effectively by the emerging inflammatory response because of direct cell-mediated cytotoxicity and the increased formation of antiviral interferons accompanying this inflammatory process.[38]

A pronounced myocardial inflammatory process is not necessarily associated with all viral infections with rapidly progressive viral heart disease, indicating impaired or delayed antiviral immune control.[16] Some patients show insufficient activation of the cellular immune response and the corresponding specific and nonspecific defense mechanisms mediated by NK cells and cytotoxic effector T lymphocytes. The immune response is often dampened by the invading virus, which subsequently escapes the host's immune surveillance. This condition favors the development of viral persistence (Fig. 77.1), which in turn leads to ventricular dysfunction resulting either from direct lytic infection of cardiomyocytes, endothelial cell damage, and cytoskeletal remodeling or from an interaction between the virus or viral proteins and the cellular protein and RNA synthesis. The cytotoxic effect of the virus, the virus-associated chronic inflammation, and the interruption of the synthesis of vitally important cellular components may initially damage some individual cells but may ultimately affect the whole myocardium, finally resulting in heart failure.[39,40]

In a significant proportion of patients with acute myocarditis, the inflammatory reaction heals spontaneously within a few weeks of successful virus elimination. Unspecific intercellular fibrosis of various degrees may constitute the sole tangible histomorphologic correlate of the inflammatory process. In the long run, matrix remodeling may constitute the substrate for postinfectious or postinflammatory progression of heart failure or arrhythmias in patients lacking other comprehensible causes of their disease.

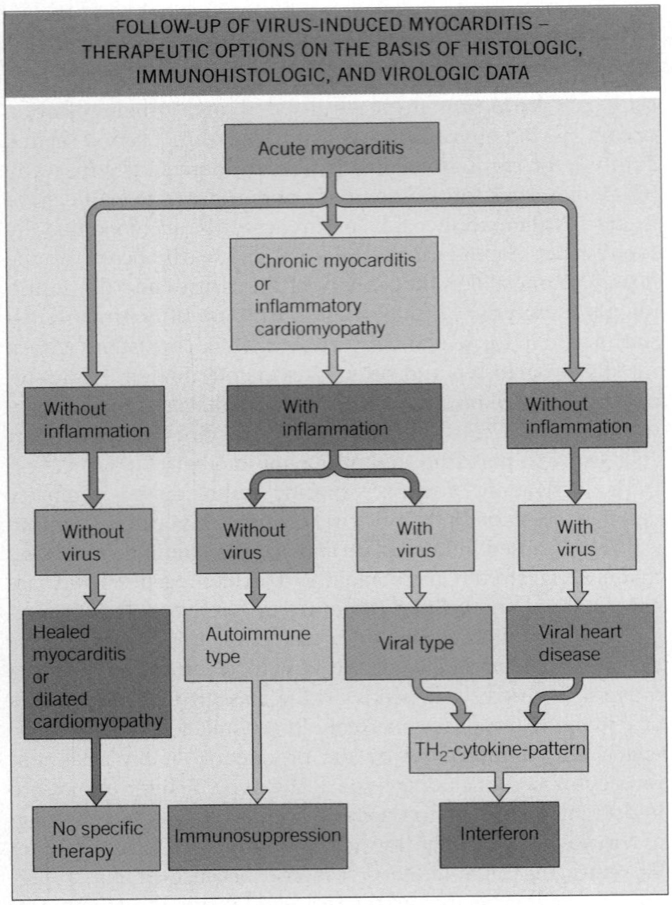

FOLLOW-UP OF VIRUS-INDUCED MYOCARDITIS – THERAPEUTIC OPTIONS ON THE BASIS OF HISTOLOGIC, IMMUNOHISTOLOGIC, AND VIROLOGIC DATA

Acute myocarditis
Chronic myocarditis or inflammatory cardiomyopathy
Without inflammation
With inflammation
Without inflammation
Without virus
Without virus
With virus
With virus
Healed myocarditis or dilated cardiomyopathy
Autoimmune type
Viral type
Viral heart disease
TH_2-cytokine-pattern
No specific therapy
Immunosuppression
Interferon

Figure 77.1 Follow-up of virus-induced myocarditis. Therapeutic options on the basis of histologic, immunohistologic, and virologic data.

Chronic Myocarditis

The pathophysiologic mechanisms of this chronic phase are less well defined than the acute and subacute phases of myocarditis. The inflammatory process may not resolve spontaneously either because of persistence of the viral genome or because of the initiation of an autoimmune response, and this process may be responsible for persisting symptoms and progressively impair cardiac function (see Fig. 77.1).[39,41] Activated T lymphocytes that react with viral as well as with myocardial antigens predominate in this chronic phase of intramyocardial inflammation. The myocardial tissue continues to be interspersed with diffuse, mild to moderate lymphocytic infiltrates. Active myocytolysis is no longer present at this time. The contingents of myocytes destroyed as a result of the elimination of virus or immune-mediated injury are replaced by reparative fibrosis. The left ventricle is not often enlarged at this stage of the disease. During this stage of the disease, a transition from the initial infection-triggered response to a chronic autoimmune response has occurred, constituting a chronification of the disease (chronic myocarditis; see Fig. 77.1).[42]

Inflammatory Cardiomyopathy

The antiviral effect of the interferons produced in the context of the immune response is only partly due to inhibition of virus replication. Most important, virus elimination is a result of the destruction of virus-infected myocardial cells by specific and nonspecific cellular defense mechanisms (NK cells, cytotoxic T lymphocytes, macrophages). The healing process therefore results primarily from a partial destruction of myocardial tissue that is not capable of regeneration. The ensuing myocardial damage depends on the scale of the cellular virus infection and increases with growing virus dispersion. Under clinical conditions, this myocardial damage is frequently not detectable during the early stage of the disease when virus infection is low because the myocardium can compensate sufficiently for a partial loss of tissue (chronic myocarditis). The ongoing loss of myocardial tissue and its replacement during many years by connective tissue may lead to the clinical manifestation of dilated cardiomyopathy through remodeling (see Fig.77.1). Independently of the myocardial damage caused by the demise of cardiomyocytes, chronic intramyocardial inflammation or viral persistence can continue to damage the myocardial tissue. Viral persistence, especially persistence of enteroviral replication in the myocardium, is associated with increased mortality.[43-45]

Spontaneous improvement of ventricular function after virus clearance and partial reversibility of ventricular dysfunction after antiviral treatment with interferons suggest that ventricular dysfunction in patients with chronic viral heart disease is not solely caused by an irreversible loss of cardiomyocytes but often is a reversible process[46,47] that may in part be due to interference of virus-encoded proteins or mRNA with myocyte function and matrix integrity.[40,48,49] Because similar humoral and cellular immune phenomena that point toward a virus-induced, active autoimmune process have been reported in both myocarditis and dilated cardiomyopathy patients, it was postulated that these two conditions in fact constituted different stages of the same disease.[19,50] In other words, chronic myocarditis might convert into inflammatory cardiomyopathy.[51] The cases documented so far indicate that 12% of clinically suspected myocarditis patients and 40% of biopsy-proven myocarditis cases manifest dilated cardiomyopathy (Table 77.5). However, detailed epidemiologic data with respect to inflammatory cardiomyopathy are not yet available.

DEVELOPMENT OF DILATED CARDIOMYOPATHY IN PATIENTS WITH CLINICALLY SUSPECTED MYOCARDITIS

Authors	Year	N	DCM	Follow-up (years)
Levander-Lindgren	1965	154	13 (8%)	7
Berigtsson/Lamberger	1966	90	17 (19%)	5
Sianani	1968	22	5 (23%)	Not given
Bergström	1970	15	0 (0%)	4
Smith	1970	22	6 (27%)	6
Gerzen	1972	45	16 (36%)	5
Das	1980	6	3 (50%)	2
Hayakawa	1983	20	3 (30%)	4
Levi	1988	68	10 (15%)	15
Remes	1990	18	5 (28%)	23
Total		**460**	**78 (17%)**	

DCM, dilated cardiomyopathy.

Table 77.5 Development of dilated cardiomyopathy in patients with clinically suspected myocarditis.

DIAGNOSTIC TECHNIQUES

Clinical Presentation

The majority of patients with acute myocarditis have a clinically inapparent course, and cardiovascular symptoms may be minimal. Because of the often asymptomatic course, many patients with myocarditis will not be aware that they are affected and will not seek medical attention. A typical characteristic of myocarditis is the emergence of cardiac complaints a few days or weeks after a viral infection in a formerly healthy patient. However, as experience has shown, such a correlation is traceable in only about 30% to 50% of patients. The patient with subacute myocarditis often presents with subtle changes in exercise tolerance, with easy fatigability and malaise. Shortness of breath may occur, with relatively low exercise tolerance (Table 77.6). Atypical chest pain is common, particularly if there is associated pericarditis or endothelial dysfunction. Complaints of palpitations may be caused by rhythm abnormalities. Many patients with this presentation will experience resolution within 4 to 12 weeks. In others, the uncharacteristic symptoms described will persist or symptoms and ventricular dysfunction will progress over time. Such patients may develop a chronic disease.

Frequently, only temporary electrocardiographic changes or an incidental echocardiographic diagnosis of ventricular wall motion dysfunction points to a myocardial disease in otherwise barely affected patients. In this setting, myocarditis may easily be overlooked. The pathologic findings usually recede completely within a few days or weeks. It is unclear whether the resulting, usually minimal myocardial damage has any significance for the future course of the disease.

CLINICAL PRESENTATION AND SYMPTOMS OF PATIENTS WITH MYOCARDITIS AND INFLAMMATORY CARDIOMYOPATHY

Symptoms	Acute Myocarditis	Chronic Myocarditis	Inflammatory Cardiomyopathy
History of viral infection	+	+	(+)
Reduced physical efficiency	++	+	+
Atypical angina pectoris	−/+	−/+	−/+
Angina pectoris on exertion	−/+	−/+	−/+
Palpitations	++	++	+
Arrhythmias	++	+	+
Dyspnea at rest	(+)	−/(+)	(+)/+
Dyspnea on exertion	+/(+)	+/(+)	++

− unusual; (+) rare; + common, ++ typical.

Table 77.6 Clinical presentation and symptoms of patients with myocarditis and inflammatory cardiomyopathy.

If the disease begins with an acute onset and severe thoracic pain, it is not clinically distinguishable from acute myocardial infarction (Fig. 77.2). Other patients may develop rapidly progressive dyspnea, which can progress to cardiac

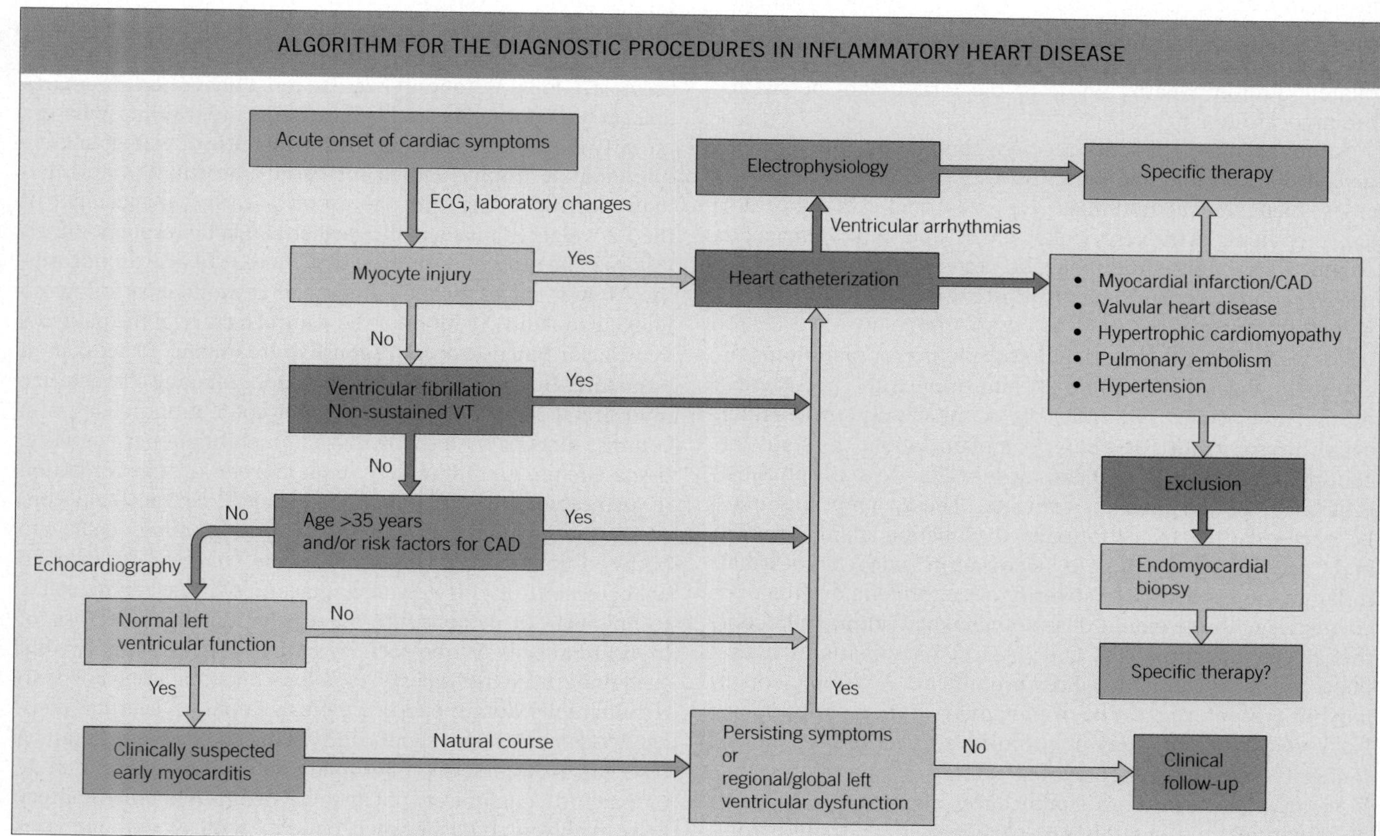

Figure 77.2 Algorithm for the diagnostic procedures in inflammatory heart disease. CAD, coronary artery disease; ECG, electrocardiography; VT, ventricular tachycardia.

decompensation. Rapid onset of symptoms and hemodynamic compromise often requires high-dose vasopressor support and ventricular assist device for appropriate stabilization. This fulminant acute myocarditis is a clinically rare event, often taking a dramatic course in particular cases. Early mortality is high (up to 42%) in patients who require mechanical circulatory support in the management of heart failure. These fulminant inflammatory processes are, however, associated with a long-term outcome (11-year mortality <10%) better than that of a nonfulminant presentation of myocarditis patients (mortality >50%), if patients survive the initial critical phase.[52-54] This may indicate that local intramyocardial inflammation is not detrimental and, moreover, that inflammation may reflect an attempt of the immune system to eliminate cardiotropic viruses.

In patients with nonfulminant lymphocytic myocarditis, spontaneous improvement occurs in 40% to 57%, and clinical improvement is more common in those with chest pain or arrhythmias at the onset.[26,55] Long-term prognosis of lymphocytic myocarditis is poor, particularly in patients with heart failure at presentation. During a mean period of 3 years, 20% of patients develop dilated cardiomyopathy, and a 20% to 56% mortality has been reported within 5 to 10 years.[26,53,56,57] Corresponding data of patients with documented chronic myocarditis or inflammatory cardiomyopathy do not yet exist. A lack of spontaneous short-term improvement and adverse long-term prognosis have been reported for patients with myocarditis and virus persistence.[43,45,47] Because different virus infections have been detected in patients with acute myocarditis, dilated cardiomyopathy, and end-stage dilated cardiomyopathy (explanted hearts), it is suggested that persistence of the virus after viral myocarditis might predispose to the later development of dilated cardiomyopathy and that the virus might persist in the myocardium.[8,14,18,26,44,55,58-60]

Although many patients recover completely, progressive myocardial cell loss and death have been reported. In other cases, malignant arrhythmias (e.g., ventricular tachycardia) are prevalent. Atrioventricular block and intraventricular conduction abnormalities may be associated with infection with certain viruses, such as Epstein-Barr virus, or with myocarditis caused by *Borrelia burgdorferi*.

There is no characteristic clinical picture of symptoms of chronic myocarditis.[57] The only hint often is the persistence of the nonspecific symptoms of a subacutely progressing active myocarditis. Patients complain about a state of continual physical weariness, nonspecific loss of physical efficiency, or dyspnea on exertion. These symptoms may be partly caused by endothelial dysfunction of myocardial and peripheral arteries in association with myocardial inflammation because the severity of endothelial dysfunction correlates with the extent of endothelial activation and endothelial cell infection.[61-63] On physical examination, tachypnea and tachycardia are most prominent. A chronic cough may be present, suggestive of pulmonary venous congestion. Neck vein distention may be prominent, together with hepatomegaly secondary to elevated systemic venous pressure. If ventricular function is significantly affected, the picture of symptoms and signs is not clearly distinguishable from that of a dilated cardiomyopathy.

Noninvasive Diagnostic Techniques

If the symptoms are so pronounced that the patient visits the physician during the first days of myocarditis, sinus tachycardia that is out of proportion to fever or other clinical events, arrhythmias, and electrocardiographic abnormalities that range from T-wave inversion to frank ST-segment elevation and bundle branch block, depending on the region and extent of inflammatory damage, can be documented. Creatine kinase (CK) and CK-MB, frequently raised by a factor of 2 to 5, and raised troponin T levels also suggest myocardial cell damage. It is not possible to distinguish these cases from acute myocardial infarction, either electrocardiographically or chemically in the laboratory (see Fig. 77.2). Other laboratory parameters, such as erythrocyte sedimentation rate and transaminase levels, are often increased, but this is rather an effect of the underlying infection and does not allow one to draw conclusions about myocardial involvement (Table 77.7). Ventricular contractility might be unaffected during the early stage, but regional or, less frequently, global wall motion abnormalities can be proved echocardiographically in about 50% to 60% of all cases.

After a period of about 1 to 2 weeks, the acute laboratory chemical and echocardiographic changes characteristic of the early phase of the disease have receded. Myocardial contractile dysfunction recedes at a significantly slower pace, although it does normalize in many cases. Noticeable electrocardiographic findings for this follow-up phase (14 days after appearance of the cardiac symptoms) include nonspecific changes in ST segments or T inversion, sinus tachycardia or a slow normalization of the pulse after stress, supraventricular and ventricular premature beats, and conduction system abnormalities (see Table 77.7).

On echocardiographic examination, regional left ventricular wall motion abnormalities of varying scope are particularly discernible. Global systolic myocardial function is often unremarkable, at least during the early phase of the myocarditis, whereas an early diastolic dysfunction exists. Increase of wall diameters (pseudohypertrophy due to increased interstitial water content), corresponding with the proof of early enhancement of the T2-weighted image in the cardiac magnetic resonance analysis, may be present during the first 2 weeks of acute myocarditis. At later stages, echocardiography is useful as a follow-up imaging modality to monitor the natural history of the patient's ventricular function or in response to treatment. T2 relaxation parameters in cardiac magnetic resonance imaging characterize myocardial tissue according to water content and changes in contrast kinetics by local changes in membrane permeability, tissue edema, and ultimately tissue fibrosis or scar formation in association with inflammatory events.[64] Extracellular contrast agents such as gadolinium-DTPA differentially distribute between inflamed and scarred tissue, leading to delayed enhancement on T1-weighted images.[65,66] Nuclear medicine techniques can demonstrate myocardial damage. Necrosis of myocardial cells can be seen by antimyosin scintigraphy, but such findings are not specific to myocarditis. Radionuclide ventriculography during exertion reveals latent myocardial damage by demonstrating significantly reduced or absent pumping reserves. However, an abnormality detected by nuclear study or imaging technique cannot distinguish different inflammatory cells or differentiate between patients with or without virus infection.

DIAGNOSTIC VALUE OF NONINVASIVE CLINICAL FINDINGS FOR THE DIAGNOSIS OF MYOCARDITIS AND INFLAMMATORY CARDIOMYOPATHY

Clinical Findings		Active Myocarditis	Chronic Myocarditis	Inflammatory Cardiomyopathy	Diagnostic Accuracy	Comments
Laboratory parameters	CK-MB	+	–	–	Low	Only acute stage and after exclusion of other cardiac diseases
	Troponin T	+	(+)	(+)	Low	No differentiation from other cardiac diseases (e.g., AMI); indicates myocyte necrosis
	C-reactive protein	(+)	–	–	None	
	ESR	+	–	–	None	
	Virus serology	(+)	–	–	None	Low sensitivity, no correlation with organ involvement
ECG	ST elevation	+	–	–	Low	Only acute stage and after exclusion of AMI
	ST deviation	+	–	–	None	Indication for myocyte necrosis
	T inversion	(+)	(+)	(+)	None	No differentiation from other cardiac diseases
Holter ECG	Sinus tachycardia	++	(+)	(+)	Low	Only acute stage
	SVES, VES	+	+	+	None	No differentiation from other cardiac diseases (e.g., ischemic heart disease or cardiomyopathies)
	Atrial fibrillation	+	+	+	None	
	Supraventricular tachycardia	(+)	(+)	(+)	None	
	Bundle branch block	(+)	(+)	+	None	
Echocardiography	Wall edema	+	–	–	Low	After exclusion of cardiac diseases caused by or associated with myocardial hypertrophy
	Pericardial effusion	++	–	–	Good	
	Cardiomegaly	(+)	(+)	+	None	
	Impaired systolic contractility:					
	Local or regional	+	+	+	Good	Only after exclusion of other cardiac diseases
	Global	(+)	(+)	++	Good	Only after exclusion of other cardiac diseases
	Impaired diastolic function	(+)	+	+	None	
Chest radiography	Cardiomegaly	(+)	(+)	+	None	Low sensitivity
	Pericardial effusion	(+)	–	–	None	Low sensitivity
	Pulmonary edema	(+)	(+)	(+)	None	Seen after cardiac decompensation

– unusual; (+) possible; + common; ++ typical. AMI, acute myocardial infarction; CK, creatine kinase; ECG, electrocardiography; ESR, erythrocyte sedimentation rate; SVES, supraventricular extra beats; VES, ventricular extra beats.

Table 77.7 Diagnostic value of noninvasive clinical findings for the diagnosis of myocarditis and inflammatory cardiomyopathy.

Invasive Diagnostic Techniques

Differentiation from other cardiac diseases that evoke similar clinical symptoms is important. Valvular heart disease can be identified by echocardiography. The differentiation of inflammatory cardiomyopathy from ischemic cardiomyopathy is not possible noninvasively, even with the aid of stress echocardiography, because stress-induced regional dysfunction in ventricular walls can also occur in myocarditis. After exclusion of other causes of heart failure, cardiomyopathy or myocarditis may be assumed. None of the noninvasively obtained diagnostic parameters (see Table 77.7) allows an unequivocal diagnosis of myocardial inflammation (myocarditis or inflammatory cardiomyopathy) or viral infection. Because of the low specificity of noninvasive examination methods, subsequent invasive approaches are indicated, especially in patients with overt heart failure (see Fig. 77.2).[57,67] The diagnosis of intramyocardial inflammation or viral infection is confirmed only by the analysis of endomyocardial biopsy tissue. Viral genomes or a myocardial inflammatory response frequently constitutes the only tangible pathologic finding in patients without clear ventricular dysfunction or arrhythmias of uncertain etiology.

Histology

The diagnosis of myocarditis is still largely based on histomorphologic criteria according to the Dallas classification (see Table 77.1).

Essential pitfalls that have contributed to the greatly divergent findings of different studies on the prevalence of intramyocardial inflammation in suspected myocarditis and dilated cardiomyopathy are many. Given the patchy nature of the myocardial lesions, the sample size, or the number of biopsy specimens obtained and the fact that the strongly subjective component inherent in the histologic assessment of myocardial tissue causes substantial interobserver variability, it is not surprising that substantial sampling error exists.[3,10,68,69] Furthermore, because the majority of patients—because the course of the disease is usually subacute—do not undergo invasive diagnostic techniques and biopsy until reparative processes have already taken place in the myocardial tissue, histologic diagnosis of myocarditis based on the Dallas criteria is usually no longer possible at this stage of the disease. Comparative analyses of biopsy samples and myocardial tissue obtained at autopsy have revealed that even in cases of proven myocardial inflammation with the sampling of at least five myocardial biopsy specimens, the cellular infiltrates that exist are histologically recorded in only about 60% of patients. It follows that a purely histologic work-up of myocardial biopsy specimens is not sufficient for the detection of chronic myocardial inflammation.[19]

Immunohistochemistry

Apart from its low sensitivity and specificity, the main disadvantage of histologic assessment of myocardial biopsy specimens is the absence of sensitive markers for an active immunologic process. In contrast, immunohistochemical diagnostic techniques offer an enormous diagnostic potential stemming from the multitude of disposable monoclonal antibodies; this potential surpasses by far the possibilities of a purely histologic analysis of the inflammatory reaction.[70,71] The differentiation, characterization, and quantification of the activated interstitial cells or invading immune cells (e.g., leukocytes, B cells, macrophages, NK cells, endothelial cells) account for a specific assessment of the myocardial inflammatory process (Table 77.8 and Fig. 77.3). Moreover, the homogeneous distribution of endothelial cell adhesion molecules within the myocardium, irrespective of focal infiltrates, substantially reduces the sampling error (see Fig. 77.3).[72]

The higher sensitivity and specificity of immunohistologic examination compared with histology as well as the enormous amount of extra information acquired became obvious during the course of a prospective study of 658 patients who underwent endomyocardial biopsy for clinically suspected myocarditis or dilated cardiomyopathy. On histologic evaluation, about 97% of the examined tissue exhibited no evidence of inflammation. On immunohistologic evaluation, however, a persisting inflammatory process with increased lymphocytic infiltrates and simultaneously intensified expression of cell adhesion molecules was demonstrated in about 49% of the endomyocardial biopsy specimens examined (Figs. 77.4 and 77.5).[72]

CURRENT STATUS OF DIAGNOSTIC PROCEDURES	
Histology	Diagnosis of acute myocardial inflammation with cell necrosis (according to the Dallas criteria)
	Histomorphologic analysis of cardiac tissue
Immunohistology	Diagnosis of chronic myocardial inflammation
	Quantification of inflammatory cells
	Differentiation of inflammatory cells
	Detection of activated infiltrating lymphocytes or macrophages
	Analysis of cell-independent markers of inflammation (adhesion molecules)
Viral diagnostic techniques	Detection of viral RNA or DNA
	Analysis of viral replication

Acute myocarditis and pathologic histomorphologic changes of cardiac tissue are best analyzed by routine histology staining methods, although sensitivity for the detection of tissue inflammation and cell necrosis is low. For analysis of chronic inflammation, only immunohistology can be recommended. Detection of viral RNA and DNA requires molecular biologic methods, such as the polymerase chain reaction or in situ hybridization.

Table 77.8 Current status of diagnostic procedures.

Virology

Even positive serologic test results cannot prove virus infection of the myocardium. A positive diagnosis of viral infection of the myocardium is confirmed only by analysis of endomyocardial biopsy specimens by molecular biology methods, such as in situ hybridization or PCR. These methods enable the detection of viral RNA and DNA even if only a few copies of the infective genome are present (see Table 77.4). Furthermore, when group-specific primers and sequencing of amplified genomes are employed, homology screening for different virus strains can be conducted with PCR.[20] Finally, an actively replicating virus can be differentiated from a nonreplicating, resting viral genome by molecular biology techniques.[25]

Biopsy-Guided Classification of Inflammatory Heart Muscle Disease

With regard to the pathophysiology of chronic myocarditis, it is currently unresolved whether cardiotropic viral infection or persistence constitutes the sole significant factor in the genesis and progression of the disease or whether it is feasible that autoimmune mechanisms are induced during the viral infection that then secondarily account for the continuing damage to the myocardium and progression of the disease. Because pathologic-anatomic and especially clinical diagnosis is fraught with numerous problems, an etiologic classification based on histology, immunohistochemistry, and molecular biology is obviously preferable in view of the improvements in techniques that have been made in recent years. These techniques not only may contribute to a thorough understanding of the underlying pathologic mechanisms but may also ultimately be decisive as to the choice of a specific immunomodulatory treatment. The current standard of diagnostic procedures should suggest a routine histologic staining technique that allows the analysis of histomorphologic changes and might depict myocytolysis (active myocarditis). For the analysis of chronic inflammatory processes, however, immunohistologic methods are

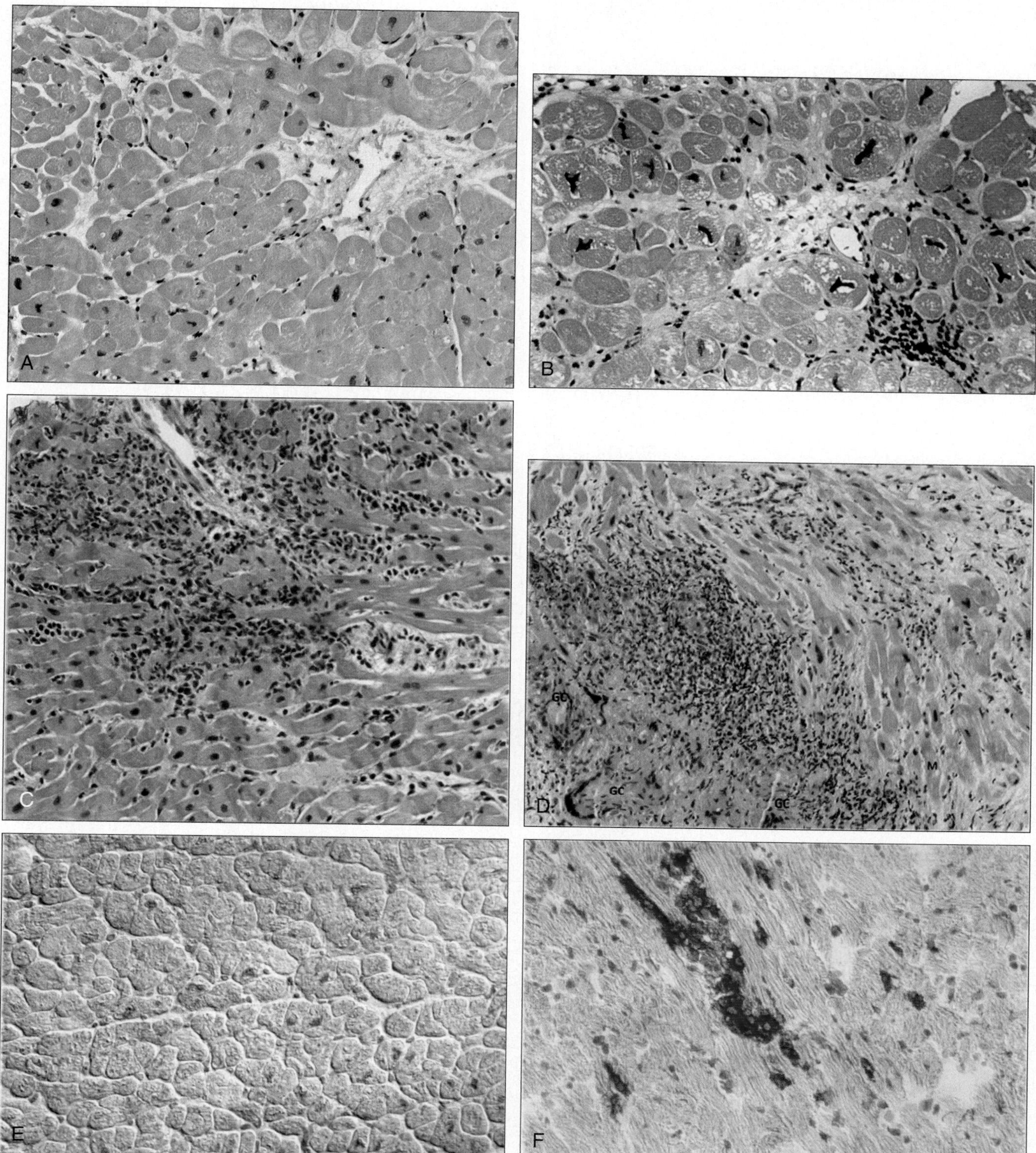

Figure 77.3 Histologic staining of endomyocardial biopsy specimens. **A,** Normal myocardial tissue. **B,** Borderline myocarditis with sparse interstitial lymphocytes; one focal lymphocytic infiltrate is seen without myocyte damage. **C,** Lymphocytic myocarditis with prominent lymphocytic infiltration and myocyte damage. **D,** Giant cell myocarditis with dense inflammatory infiltrate composed of lymphocytes, macrophages, few plasma cells, few eosinophils, multinucleated giant cells, and myocyte necrosis. **E** to **I,** Immunohistologic staining of endomyocardial biopsy specimens. **E,** No evidence of intramyocardial infiltration (magnification $\times$ 400). **F,** focal $CD3^{+}$ infiltrate suggestive of myocytolysis (magnification $\times$ 400).

(*Continued*)

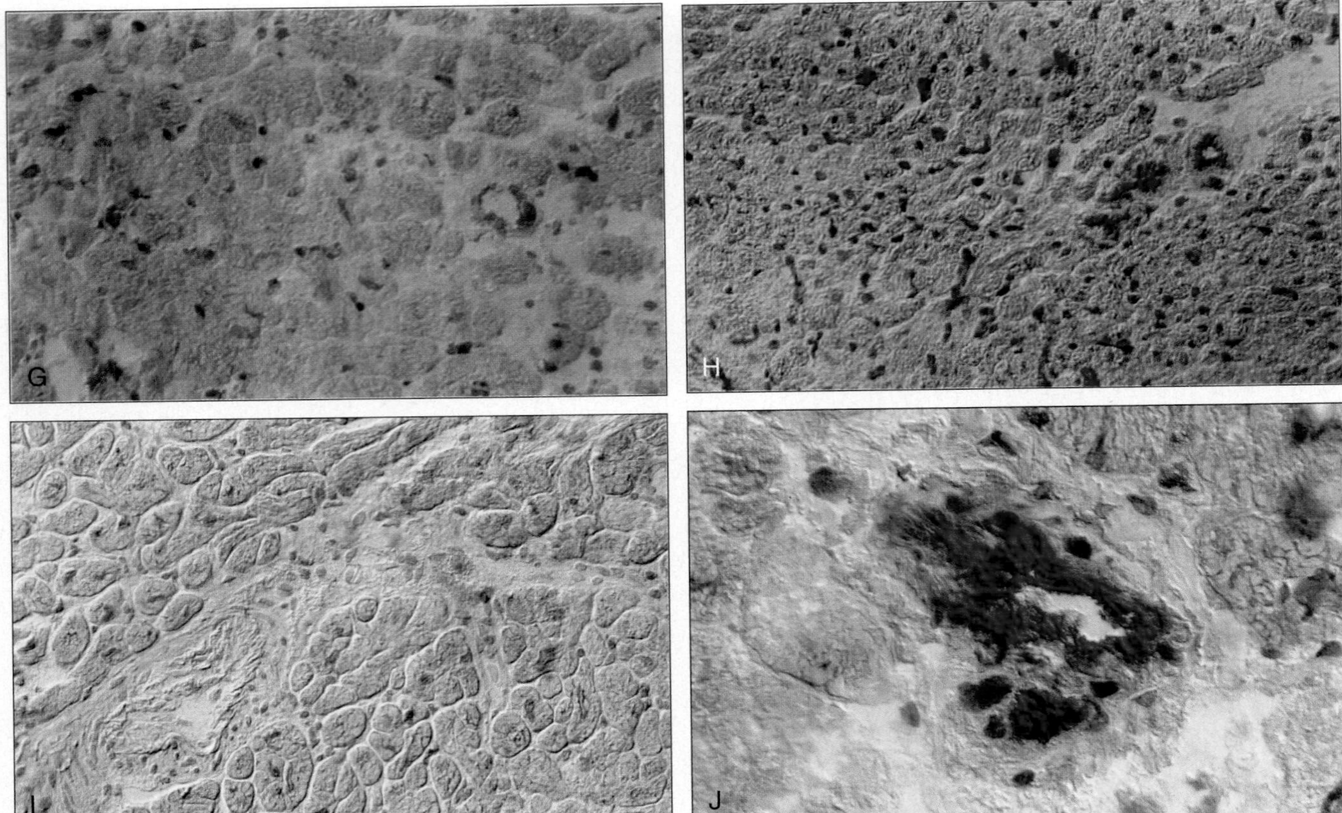

Figure 77.3—cont'd Histologic staining of endomyocardial biopsy specimens. G, Baseline expression of intercellular adhesion molecule (ICAM) 1 in a biopsy specimen without evidence of intramyocardial inflammation (magnification × 100). **H,** Abundant ICAM-1 expression in a specimen positive for inflammatory cardiomyopathy (magnification × 100). Note the homogeneous distribution of ICAM-1 immunoreactivity within the section (compare with **G**). **I,** Absence of vascular cell adhesion molecule (VCAM) 1 immunoreactivity in a cross-sectioned vessel of a specimen without evidence of intramyocardial infiltration (magnification × 400). **J,** Enhanced VCAM-1 expression in a biopsy specimen positive for inflammatory cardiomyopathy (magnification × 400).

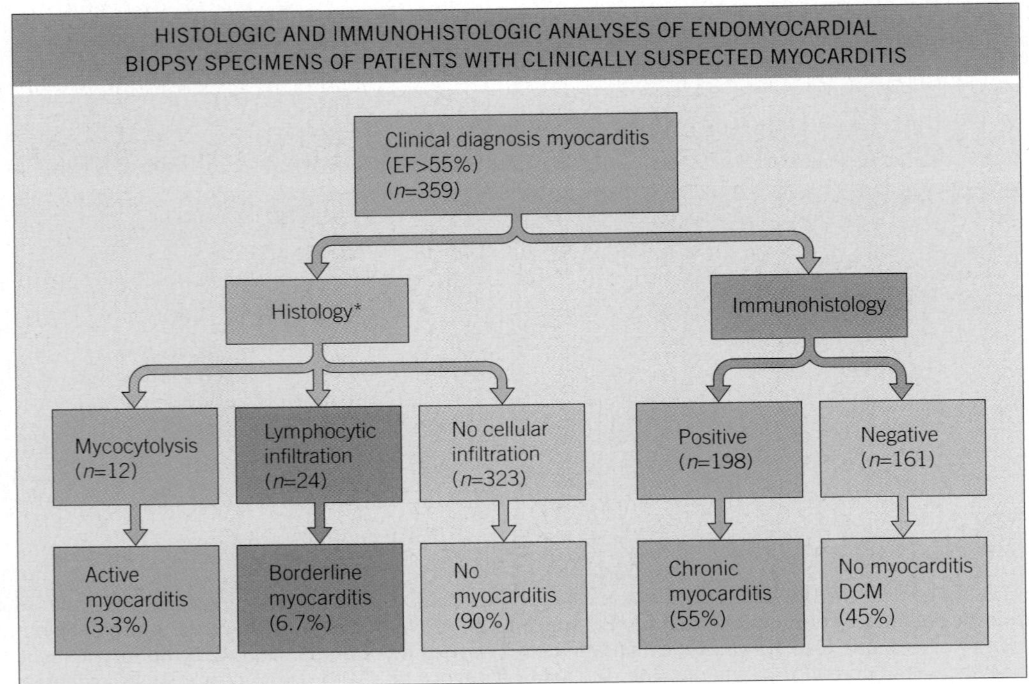

Figure 77.4 Histologic and immunohistologic analyses of endomyocardial biopsy specimens of patients with clinically suspected myocarditis. *According to the Dallas criteria.[1] DCM, dilated cardiomyopathy; EF, ejection fraction.

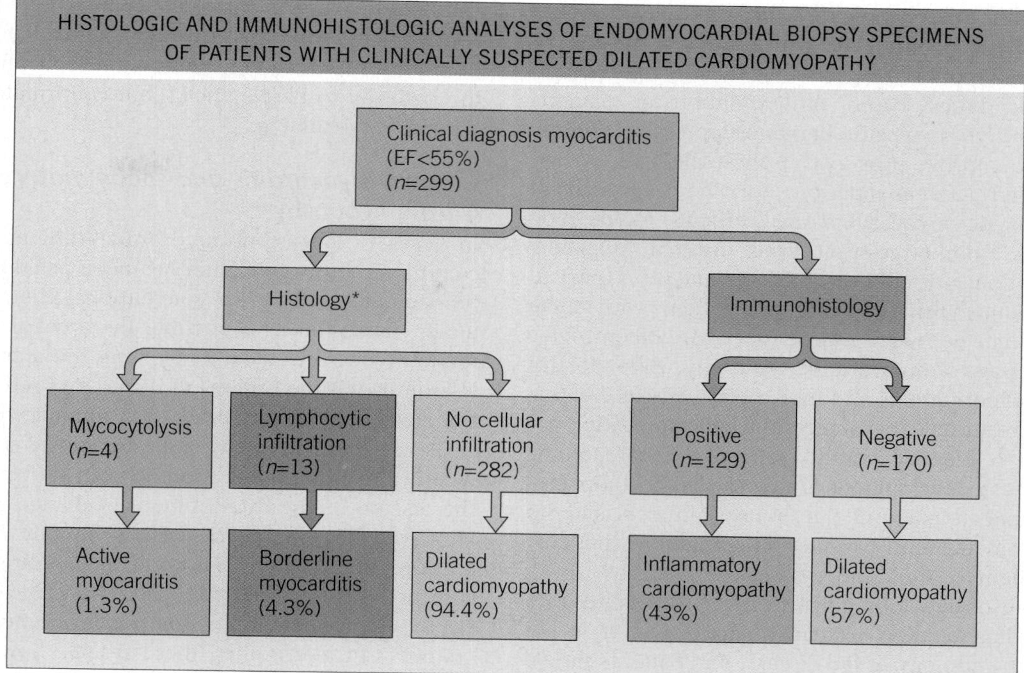

Figure 77.5 Histologic and immunohistologic analyses of endomyocardial biopsy specimens of patients with clinically suspected dilated cardiomyopathy.[70] *According to the Dallas criteria.[1] EF, ejection fraction.

recommended. Detection of viral genome, viral replication, and virus subtypes requires molecular biologic techniques such as PCR or in situ hybridization and sequence analysis of the genome products. On the basis of the data obtained by these methods, patients with a clinically suspected diagnosis of myocarditis or dilated cardiomyopathy can be subclassified to different entities (see Fig. 77.1).

In healed myocarditis and dilated cardiomyopathy, no evidence can be documented either for intramyocardial inflammation or for viral infection. The persisting cardiac symptoms are presumably due to irreversible sequelae after complete elimination of the virus. Viral heart disease is characterized by intramyocardial virus persistence without evidence for inflammation. Chronic myocarditis and inflammatory cardiomyopathy, on the other hand, are both characterized by the immunohistologic proof of an active inflammatory process within the myocardium. A virus may persist in the myocardium (viral type) but is not necessarily present at this stage of the disease (autoimmune type).

MANAGEMENT

The prognosis for patients with severe left ventricular dysfunction is poor, and dilated cardiomyopathy represents the primary indication for heart transplantation worldwide. In general, the progression of dilated cardiomyopathy cannot be halted by symptomatic therapy with digitalis, diuretics, angiotensin-converting enzyme inhibitors, and beta-blocking agents, particularly because the possible triggering causes, such as inflammation and cardiotropic viruses, remain untreated.

The interdisciplinary combination of histologic, immunohistochemical, and molecular biology analyses has introduced a new era of classifying dilated cardiomyopathy on the basis of the prevailing etiopathogenesis. These insights may ultimately improve the treatment options for dilated cardiomyopathy patients (see Fig. 77.1).[19] The current American College of Cardiology/American Heart Association (ACC/AHA) guidelines for the treatment of heart failure and a recent scientific statement from the AHA/ACC and the European Society of Cardiology on the role of endomyocardial biopsy in the management of cardiovascular disease consider endomyocardial biopsy for patients with rapid progressive cardiomyopathy refractory to conventional therapeutic management, for patients with an unexplained cardiomyopathy that is associated with progressive conduction system disease or severe arrhythmias, or if cardiovascular symptoms develop in systemic disease known to cause left ventricular dysfunction.[67,73] At present, the optimal time frame for starting therapy is speculative because of the lack of data. However, therapy should certainly begin as early as possible and before the development of serious ventricular dysfunction because complete normalization of ventricular function is unlikely to be achieved once severe myocardial damage has occurred. Because of the progressive nature of the disease, the option of specific antiviral or anti-inflammatory treatment should be considered even in more long-standing disease.

General Aspects of Therapeutic Management

Active Myocarditis

More than 50% of patients with advanced cardiac dysfunction accompanying lymphocytic myocarditis will develop residual ventricular dysfunction or may progress to transplantation or death within 4 to 6 years from onset.[10,11,19]

The outcome of untreated patients with giant cell or eosinophilic myocarditis is even worse, with a median survival of less than 6 and 12 months, respectively.[74] These figures indicate that rapid biopsy-based differentiation of patients requiring supportive or specific immunosuppressive therapy is mandatory to improve prognosis in these patients.

Evidence-based recommendations for the treatment of active lymphocytic myocarditis are difficult to develop because results from large-scale trials are not available. If clinical symptoms are mild or moderate and left ventricular function remains virtually unaffected, patients with active myocarditis do not necessarily need special treatment. During the initial phase of myocarditis, especially while electrocardiographic abnormalities and increased levels of creatine kinase can be recorded, hospitalization and monitoring are recommended to identify and to prevent life-threatening arrhythmias or the development of myocardial decompensation. In the subacute stage of the disease, physical activity should be avoided until cardiac inflammation (possibly verified by endomyocardial biopsy) has resolved.

The treatment of developing heart failure in patients with active myocarditis remains primarily supportive. It is not dependent on the etiology of the disease, and patients should be treated according to the guidelines proposed by the ACC/AHA Task Force on Practice Guidelines, including angiotensin-converting enzyme inhibitors, diuretics, digitalis, and beta blockers (see also the later section on Lyme disease).[73] Heart transplantation is at present the only possible curative therapy for end-stage heart failure. Implantation of a mechanical cardiac support system in patients with rapidly progressive heart failure may improve cardiac function and stabilize acute cardiac decompensation. Preliminary results have shown that mechanical assist devices can gain several months before transplantation becomes essential (see Chapter 75).

Ventricular arrhythmia is common in patients with active myocarditis, but it does not require specific therapy in most cases. If patients present with severe refractory ventricular arrhythmias, antiarrhythmic treatment with amiodarone or implantable cardioverter-defibrillators is necessary. Similarly, patients with atrioventricular block may require insertion of a temporary pacemaker. Because myocarditis may result in spontaneous remission, long-term antiarrhythmic therapy should be given only after all methods of controlling arrhythmia have proved to be unsuccessful.

Giant cell myocarditis and eosinophilic myocarditis usually respond to immunosuppressive therapy, and rapid treatment improves prognosis.[74] Such specific treatment is, however, not indicated for histologically confirmed active lymphocytic myocarditis (Dallas criteria) in view of the negative effects of specific treatment in animal experiments and the high rate of spontaneous healing in active myocarditis. The pooled data from a meta-analysis showed that spontaneous healing varied widely and that 57% of all patients analyzed achieved clinical and hemodynamic improvement through physical rest combined with conventional cardiac heart failure therapy. Immunosuppression is also not indicated in patients with virus infections because adverse prognosis has been reported.[44] In patients with recent onset of cardiomyopathy or myocarditis, high-dose intravenous immune globulin treatment does not augment the improvement of left ventricular ejection fraction compared with the natural course of the disease. Virustatic therapy at this early stage of the disease, with detectable viral replication, would seem theoretically to be beneficial, but confirmatory clinical data are not yet available.

Chronic Myocarditis and Inflammatory Cardiomyopathy

In cases of persistent myocardial inflammation in which continuing viral replication has been excluded, immunosuppression, in addition to conventional therapy, is currently under discussion as a possible therapy for chronic autoimmune myocarditis. The aim of the therapeutic intervention is to interrupt the process of disordered self/foreign recognition and the resultant anticardiac immune response.

As yet, there have been no randomized studies confirming whether this treatment approach can prevent progression of the disease or the development of dilated cardiomyopathy. However, the short-term results of a few smaller studies and one randomized trial point in this direction.[9,44,75,76] In contrast, the American Myocarditis Study could not demonstrate improvement in ventricular function or clinical course.[77] In interpreting these results, however, it must be borne in mind that this randomized investigation included only patients with histologically confirmed active myocarditis. This and other studies, moreover, failed to make an appropriate immunologic or molecular biologic characterization of the patients or to investigate possible viral persistence, and it also failed to consider the high spontaneous healing rate of active myocarditis. Therefore, the negative treatment results of this trial and similarly designed studies are not surprising. The extremely variable spontaneous course of myocarditis and the impossibility of adequately assessing the clinical course through a single observation mean that it is necessary to follow up the clinical findings and the myocardial inflammatory process after 4 to 6 months to evaluate the natural course. If chronic persistent inflammation is then found without evidence of improved myocardial function, we recommend immunosuppressive therapy. Currently, randomized studies using a variety of diagnostic protocols are exploring a range of different treatment strategies. Until these studies yield results, immunosuppressive and antiviral treatment should continue to be limited to special centers.

Viral Heart Disease

The effectiveness of antiviral treatment for myocardial enteroviral infection has mainly been demonstrated in animal myocarditis models.[78] The precondition for successful antiviral therapy is molecular biologic proof of viral genome in the myocardium with or without inflammation.[44] According to the preceding classification (see Fig. 77.1), patients with chronic viral cardiac disease or chronic virus-induced myocarditis and a T_H2 cytokine profile (indicating insufficient production of antiviral interferons) are potential candidates for antiviral therapy—using, for example, interferon.

Specific Treatment

Interferon Therapy

When interferon alfa was introduced into clinical practice, first observations in four patients did not demonstrate a beneficial effect with respect to virus clearance or left ventricular contractility in patients treated with a protocol using 9 million units of interferon alfa per week for 6 months.[79] In a second study, patients with clinical evidence of myocarditis or dilated cardiomyopathy were treated with interferon alfa or thymomodulin.[46,80] Left ventricular contractility improved after 6 months of therapy, but virus infection of the myocardium before and after treatment was not documented in this study. Data from an open, uncontrolled interferon beta treatment study have provided first evidence that antiviral interferon beta therapy effectively clears enteroviral and adenoviral infections of the myocardium in patients with chronic heart failure when it is given subcutaneously every other day in addition to constant heart failure medication. The treatment was administered subcutaneously three times a week, using 6 million units of interferon beta per injection. This dosage was well tolerated, and no patient deteriorated.[46] Because this favorable treatment response of enteroviruses and adenoviruses has been confirmed in subsequent studies including one randomized trial (BICC study),[87] interferon beta may be considered a realistic treatment option for these two infectious agents. Treatment data of other cardiotropic viruses (e.g., parvovirus B19) are still lacking, however, and these viruses or virus subtypes may demand different treatment modalities, some of which are currently tested in different phase I and phase II studies. At present, immunomodulatory treatment of virus-associated heart disease still remains an option for expert centers and clinical trials.

Immunosuppressive Therapy

Giant cell myocarditis is a heterogeneous disorder with variable rates of recurrence and severity that may need multiple drug regimens, including cyclosporine (trough level of 100 to 150 μg) and initial high-dose methylprednisolone tapered from 1 mg/kg to 10 mg/day within 6 to 8 weeks or more slowly. Immunosuppression is maintained for 1 year but should be continued in case of recurrence. Some patients may need lifelong therapy (L. Cooper, personal communication). Eosinophilic myocarditis and myocarditis caused by autoimmune or hypersensitivity reactions may well respond to standard immunosuppression.

The immunosuppressive treatment regimens in chronic myocarditis or inflammatory cardiomyopathy and autoimmune disorders involve corticosteroids, azathioprine, or cyclosporine. α-Methylprednisolone is generally given at a rate of 1 mg/kg body weight (for children, 1 to 2 mg) initially for 4 weeks, tapering the dosage biweekly in increments of 10 mg until a maintenance dose of 10 mg is reached. The treatment should last for 6 months. In cases of persisting inflammation (35% to 40% of patients are affected by this), azathioprine may be administered in addition to low-dose corticosteroid. This appears to be effective, however, only if a sufficient level of immunosuppression is achieved, which is signaled by a reduction in peripheral lymphocytes to levels of around 1000/μL. Provided an adequate molecular biology and immunohistochemical characterization of the patients is performed, both clinical and hemodynamic improvement can be achieved in 65% to 70% of cases with immunosuppressive treatment, thus significantly exceeding the rates of hemodynamic change due to spontaneous remission.[44,75,76]

Hyperimmune Sera and Immune Adsorption

Several attempts have been made to inhibit virus replication by means of passive immunization with hyperimmune sera or to improve hemodynamic dysfunction by eliminating autoantibodies or antigens from the serum by performing immune adsorption. Uncontrolled studies suggested a potential benefit from intravenous immune globulins.[81] Later randomized trials, however, showed no specific benefit of intravenous immune globulins on improvement of left ventricular ejection fraction because patients improved spontaneously with or without immune globulin treatment in the patient cohort with acute-onset dilated cardiomyopathy.[82] Significant improvement of left ventricular dysfunction and clinical symptoms was reported after immune adsorption, in parallel with the elimination of circulating cardiodepressant immunoglobulin subclass G3 autoantibodies.[83,84] Immune adsorption has been performed in one to five courses at 1-month intervals. During each course, patients underwent one immune adsorption session daily on 3 to 5 consecutive days. With use of protein A columns, a 40% reduction of total immunoglobulin G and a reduction of more than 85% of immunoglobulin G3 were achieved during each session. After the final immune adsorption session, the patients received 0.5 g/kg polyclonal immunoglobulin G during a period of 6 hours to restore the immunoglobulin G plasma levels. Hemodynamic improvement at 6 months was found to be comparable between single-course and repeated-course immune adsorption treatment strategies.[83,85] Recent data indicate that the negative inotropic effects of immunoglobulin G may be triggered by an Fcγ receptor located at the cardiomyocyte surface.[86] These observations suggest that activation of the humoral immune response could play a functional role in cardiac dysfunction of patients with inflammatory cardiomyopathy. Influencing the humoral immune system by immune adsorption may thus provide a therapeutic option for patients with immune-mediated heart failure. This treatment regimen is currently being tested in a randomized clinical trial.

OTHER CAUSES OF MYOCARDITIS

Cytomegalovirus

The endemic rate of cytomegalovirus is high (>50%), and the prevalence of chronic infection accounts for about 25%. Cytomegalovirus-related mononucleosis, the most common manifestation of cytomegalovirus infection, can be manifested in the myocardium as pericarditis and less frequently as myocarditis. The infection is more significant in immunosuppressed patients.

Hepatitis C Virus

Hepatitis C virus appears to be a new etiologic agent mainly seen in Asian countries such as Japan. Higher prevalence of hepatitis C infections in those countries may account for the higher detection rates of hepatitis C virus genomes in cardiomyopathy patients. Symptomatic myocarditis is generally observed in the first month after onset of hepatitis C. In contrast to other forms of myocarditis, a hypertrophied myocardium is more frequent than myocardial dilatation. Although progressive heart failure and fatal outcome have been reported in some patients with persisting virus infection, virus clearance is generally associated with recovery of myocardial function and morphology.

Human Immunodeficiency Virus

Even though cardiac anomalies have been described in 25% to 70% of autopsy examinations, cardiac complaints are rare in human immunodeficiency virus (HIV) infection. Cardiac manifestations of HIV infection often appear as a result of opportunistic infections. About 30% of all cases show cardiovascular involvement; manifest cardiac disease occurs in 2% to 8% of HIV-infected patients. The prevalence of myocardial damage is about 15%, and that of clinically symptomatic myocardial dysfunction is about 6%. Heart failure is likely to occur only in the late stages of AIDS. The average survival after the onset of HIV-related severe heart failure is 1 to 3 months (see Chapter 131).

The etiology of HIV-related cardiomyopathy is not precisely understood. It can be induced by the HIV infection itself, by an accompanying opportunistic infection (including enteroviruses), by toxins, or by malnutrition (e.g., selenium deficiency in the late stage). Furthermore, therapeutic drugs such as virustatic agents (interleukin 2, azidothymidine), antibiotics (pentamidine, amphotericin B), and chemotherapeutic agents (doxorubicin, interferon alfa) used to treat HIV-associated malignant neoplasms may also be implicated. In addition, drug abuse may contribute to heart failure. Although myocardial infarctions are more frequent in connection with cocaine abuse, cardiomyopathies and arrhythmia also occur. Pentamidine, which is used for the treatment of *Pneumocystis carinii* infections, may have an effect similar to that of ganciclovir, inducing sustained ventricular arrhythmias and torsades de pointes tachycardias. The significance of myocarditis is not clear, however. The detectable cardiomyocyte necrosis may be caused either by the cytotoxicity of HIV or by accompanying virus infections (e.g., cytomegalovirus or enteroviruses). The HIV genome can be detected by in situ hybridization and PCR in myocytes and lymphocytes of the myocardium of symptomatic patients who still have normal myocardial function. Replicating HIV has not yet been demonstrated. Other infections may also have cardiotoxic effects because of the severe immune defect. In heart tissue obtained at autopsy, cytomegalovirus is detectable by molecular biology in 50% of cases involving cardiac dysfunction. Fungi, especially *Cryptococcus neoformans, Aspergillus, Histoplasma,* and *Candida* species, have also been reported to be causal for HIV-related myocarditis. Even though cardiac toxoplasmosis is more common (12%), it rarely leads to myocardial inflammation. As in the case of ordinary myocarditis, autoimmune mechanisms have also been postulated.

Chlamydia

Chlamydiae are ubiquitously present gram-negative bacteria. The distinctive types are *Chlamydia psittaci, Chlamydia trachomatis,* and *Chlamydia pneumoniae;* the last is reportedly the cause of pericarditis, endocarditis, and myocarditis. Although the majority of these cases of myocarditis run a subclinical course, lethal outcomes have also been documented.

Diphtheria

Diphtheritic myocarditis has rarely been seen since the immunization-related decrease in prevalence of the disease. However, diphtheria continues to be of some importance in developing countries, primarily among children. The toxin of *Corynebacterium diphtheriae* affects predominantly nerves and the myocardium, resulting in polyneuropathies, cardiomegaly, and severe congestive heart failure. Cardiac involvement is typically seen in 20% to 30% of patients and develops 5 to 7 days after the onset of the disease, as demonstrated by electrocardiography. Serious cardiac dysfunction is less common, but these cases have a high mortality rate, accounting for more than 60%. The cardiac-related overall mortality of this disease is about 30%. The long-term prognosis is generally good, once the patient has survived the acute illness, although cardiomyopathy and conduction blocks may persist in isolated cases. Severe cases are treated with diphtheria antitoxins and intravenous penicillin.

Rickettsia

Rocky Mountain spotted fever, caused by *Rickettsia rickettsii,* is characterized by a generalized vasculitis due to endothelial cell infection and is frequently associated with endocarditis. Tachycardia, hypotension, and symptoms of shock can occur. Involvement of coronary vessels, resulting in thrombotic occlusions and pericarditis, has been described; primary myocardial involvement is unusual. Mortality ranges between 5% and 10%, especially connected with symptoms of shock.

Lyme Disease

Lyme disease (borreliosis) is caused by *Borrelia burgdorferi.* This systemic disease is characterized by erythema chronicum migrans, fever, arthralgia, and myalgia. Cardiac manifestations may occur in 4% to 10%, especially in the absence of appropriate antibiotic therapy. The predominant feature is primarily atrioventricular conduction abnormalities, which can rapidly progress to bradycardia, requiring a pacemaker. Acute myocarditis with left ventricular decompensation is rare. The diagnostic procedure is based on the history (tick bite, presence in endemic areas) and serologic test results, which may be negative during the first 4 to 8 weeks. A negative serology result during this period does not therefore preclude an infection. Intravenous antibiotics (20 million units of penicillin G daily for 2 weeks or, in mild cases, a 3-week course of oral doxycycline or ceftriaxone) are recommended. Complete recovery is usual, and the development of cardiomyopathy is rare.

Malaria

Cardiac involvement in malaria infections is rare and almost exclusively limited to infection with *Plasmodium falciparum.* Unspecific electrocardiographic changes occur in about 37% of all cases. Coronary capillary occlusion by parasites has been described in isolated cases.

Chagas' Disease

Chagas' disease is the most frequent nonviral myocardial infection. It is caused by *Trypanosoma cruzi* and is limited to Central and South America, particularly Brazil and Argentina. Some 20 million people are assumed to be infected. Infection can also occur through contaminated blood products, which can therefore lead to isolated cases outside the endemic area. Acute myocarditis with marked interstitial cellular infiltrates around damaged cardiomyocytes occurs only rarely in the acute phase of Chagas' infection, when parasites infiltrate cardiac fibers. Involvement of the endocardium or pericardium may result in thrombus formation or pericardial effusion, respectively. Chronic infection with cardiac and gastrointestinal manifestations affects about 10% to 30% of all primarily infected persons, years or often decades later. This disease constitutes the major cause of cardiomyopathy and cardiac death within the endemic areas. The characteristic presentation includes muscle hypertrophy, ventricular dilatation with ventricular thrombi, and thinned walls. Right ventricular involvement is common. On histologic examination, autoimmune phenomena similar to those of virus-induced myocarditis are seen. In most cases, there is extensive fibrosis. Drug therapy is problematic and has little influence on the chronic course of the disease. After successful heart transplantation, recurrence of the disease has been seen during immunosuppressive treatment even after intensive preoperative antibiotic treatment of the parasites.

SUMMARY

Myocarditis is caused by a wide variety of pathologic conditions, in particular by viral infections, and often precedes the development of dilated cardiomyopathy. The infecting virus initiates the disease process and then may persist as an insidious molecular pathogen, causing ongoing cardiac damage (viral heart disease). If the host's immune system can effectively clear the viral infection, cardiac inflammation often resolves. Dysregulation of the immune response, however, may result in a persisting pathologic autoimmune process (chronic myocarditis, inflammatory cardiomyopathy), causing progression of left ventricular dysfunction. Cytokines play a critical role in the development of virus persistence and chronic inflammation.

Because pathologic-anatomic and especially clinical diagnosis is fraught with numerous problems, the current standard of the biopsy-based diagnostic procedures means that routine histologic staining, which allows the analysis of histomorphologic changes and may demonstrate myocytolysis (active myocarditis), is quite appropriate. For the analysis of chronic inflammatory processes, immunohistologic methods are recommended. Detection of viral genome and viral replication requires molecular biology techniques, such as PCR or in situ hybridization. The etiologic classification thus obtained not only contributes to a thorough understanding of the underlying pathomechanisms but may also be ultimately decisive as to the choice of a specific immunomodulatory treatment.

Preliminary results from ongoing treatment trials suggest that specific antiviral or anti-inflammatory treatment strategies are successful in patients who have been carefully selected and characterized according to biopsy-based diagnostic criteria. At present, the optimal time frame for starting antiviral or immunosuppressive therapy is speculative because of the lack of data. However, treatment should certainly begin as early as possible and before the emergence of serious ventricular dysfunction because complete normalization of ventricular function is unlikely to be achieved once serious myocardial damage has occurred.

chapter 78

Dilated Cardiomyopathy

a. Dilated Cardiomyopathy

Priya Kansal, Michelle C. Montpetit and John B. O'Connell

The umbrella term *dilated cardiomyopathy* includes a heterogeneous group of heart muscle diseases characterized by ventricular chamber enlargement and systolic dysfunction[1] with normal left ventricular wall thickness.[2] Diverse causes like genetic mutations, infections, autoimmune triggers, and toxins can lead to the final common pathway of ventricular dilatation and compromised systolic function. It is a common cause of heart failure and the most frequent cause of heart transplantation.[2]

EPIDEMIOLOGY

The actual incidence of dilated cardiomyopathy is not precisely known. Population-based studies estimate that the incidence varies from 3.9 to 7.9 per 100,000 person-years. The prevalence of dilated cardiomyopathy in persons younger than 55 years is 17.9 per 100,000.[3] Statistically significant associations have been observed between dilated cardiomyopathy and low annual income, history of asthma, and black race, which are independent of other risk factors.[4] The incidence in Asian populations is reported to be between 1.3 and 3.6 per 100,000 person-years.[5,6] The incidence in Hispanic and other minority populations is unknown.

NATURAL HISTORY

The clinical course is highly variable and difficult to predict. Some patients are asymptomatic and may have left ventricular dilatation for months to years.[7] In a retrospective analysis, it has been estimated that up to 14% of patients with dilated cardiomyopathy may present in this fashion.[8] The mean time between initial symptoms and presentation to a physician has been observed to be 1.3 years.[7] Most patients come to the attention of the health care system with a syndrome of volume overload. Death is due to progressive pump failure or arrhythmias.[7] Population-based studies estimate overall survival rates of 95% at 1 year and 80% at 5 years.[9]

PATHOPHYSIOLOGY

The primary abnormality in dilated cardiomyopathy is contractile dysfunction. There is four-chamber enlargement with proportionately thin cardiac walls that increases myocardial wall stress, compromising subendocardial blood flow and worsening myocardial function.[10]

Histologic examination demonstrates extensive areas of interstitial and perivascular fibrosis. Loss of contractile proteins, such as titin and α-actinin, may be the first and decisive event initiating an adaptive change in cytoskeleton- and membrane-associated components. Necrosis, cellular infiltrates, and ultrastructural degeneration with an altered nucleus-cytoplasm relationship are noted. Contractile proteins are down-regulated; cytoskeletal proteins desmin and tubulin and membrane-associated proteins such as vinculin and dystrophin are up-regulated, and those of the intercalated disk are irregularly arranged. Abnormal cytoskeletal proteins correlate with diastolic and contractile dysfunction in these patients. The enlarged interstitial space contains accumulations of fibroblasts, extracellular matrix components, macrophages, and microvascular elements consistent with fibrosis.[11] Whether these pathologic processes are a consequence of toxic, viral, or immunologic insults or are due to a genetic predisposition has not yet been conclusively established. It is thought that many of the cases of dilated cardiomyopathy may actually be myocarditis that went undetected and therefore are infectious in etiology. Many investigators have described detection of virus in the myocardium by polymerase chain reaction testing.[12]

ETIOLOGY

There are a multitude of causative agents implicated in the generation of dilated cardiomyopathy. The most clinically relevant ones are listed in Table 78A.1.

CLINICAL FEATURES

A small number of patients with dilated cardiomyopathy are asymptomatic and are discovered during routine clinical testing.[3] Although the course of disease can be highly variable and unpredictable, most patients present with symptoms of left ventricular dysfunction; 80% to 90% of patients are in New York Heart Association (NYHA) class III to class IV heart failure by the time they come to attention.[13] Dyspnea on exertion, orthopnea, paroxysmal nocturnal dyspnea, and occasionally chest discomfort similar to typical angina can be seen.[10] Fatigue and effort limitation can be profound and may be the only

ETIOLOGY OF DILATED CARDIOMYOPATHY
Idiopathic
Inherited syndromes
Familial autosomal dominant
X-linked
Mitochondrial
Toxins
Ethanol, cocaine
Chemotherapeutic agents (anthracycline, trastuzumab [Herceptin])
Antiretroviral agents (zidovudine, didanosine)
Lead, cobalt, mercury
Endocrine abnormalities
Hypothyroidism
Thyrotoxicosis
Pheochromocytoma
Cushing's disease
Diabetes mellitus
Nutritional deficiencies
Thiamine (beriberi)
Selenium
Carnitine
Electrolyte abnormalities
Hypocalcemia
Hypophosphatemia
Uremia
Infectious causes
Viral (human immunodeficiency virus, coxsackieviruses A and B, cytomegalovirus, adenovirus)
Rickettsial (Q fever, typhus)
Bacterial (meningococcal, diphtheria, mycobacteria)
Spirochetal (Lyme disease)
Parasitic (Chagas' disease, *Toxoplasma*)
Fungal *(Histoplasma, Aspergillus, Candida)*
Inflammatory
Collagen vascular disorders (systemic lupus erythematosus, scleroderma, dermatomyositis)
Hypersensitivity myocarditis
Sarcoidosis
Neuromuscular diseases
Duchenne's and Becker's muscular dystrophies
Emery-Dreifuss muscular dystrophy
Erb's limb-girdle dystrophy
Myotonic dystrophy
Friedreich's ataxia
Other
Hypertension
Obesity
Sleep apnea
Stress induced (tako-tsubo)
Left ventricular noncompaction
Peripartum cardiomyopathy
Arrhythmogenic right ventricular dysplasia
Tachycardia-mediated cardiomyopathy
Mitochondrial myopathies
Giant cell myocarditis

Table 78A.1 Etiology of dilated cardiomyopathy.

symptoms manifested. Abdominal distention, early satiety, right upper quadrant pain, nausea, and anorexia attributable to right-sided heart failure may occur.[14] This may lead to the mistaken diagnosis of biliary or hepatic disease, especially in young people. Patients may present with the onset of atrial or ventricular arrhythmias and pulmonary or systemic embolization. On occasion, the initial presentation may be a stroke, transient ischemic attack, syncope, or sudden death.

The findings at physical examination depend on the stage of the disease process. Early on, there may be few abnormal physical signs. Systemic blood pressure may be normal or low with a narrow pulse pressure. Hypertensive patients may present with elevated blood pressure. Pulsus alternans is common in severe left ventricular failure. Signs of right-sided heart failure and tricuspid regurgitation are common. Enlargement of the liver may be noted together with raised jugular venous pressure, peripheral edema, and ascites in advanced right-sided failure. The degree of jugular venous pressure elevation can provide an estimate of central venous pressure. A laterally displaced diffuse apical impulse reflects left ventricular dilatation. A left parasternal lift may be noted. There may be paradoxical splitting of the second heart sound (if there is left bundle branch block) or an accentuated pulmonary component of the second heart sound in the presence of pulmonary hypertension. Systolic murmurs of mitral and tricuspid regurgitation are common, caused by the dilatation of the valvular rings and structural remodeling.[15] Once cardiac decompensation occurs, ventricular gallop sounds (S_3) and tachycardia can be expected. At this time, dullness to percussion of the lung bases and lung crackles may be heard, signifying pleural effusion and interstitial pulmonary edema. Cool peripheral extremities with hypotension suggest the development of cardiogenic shock.

HISTORY

The goal of initial evaluation of a patient presenting with a dilated cardiomyopathy is to determine the etiology and to identify potentially reversible causes. The importance of obtaining history and performing a physical examination focused on identification of cardiac and noncardiac disorders or behaviors that might cause or accelerate the development or progression of heart failure is emphasized.[16] A history of current and past use of alcohol, illicit drugs, current or past standard or "alternative therapies," and chemotherapy drugs should be obtained.[16] A detailed family history should be obtained to identify patients with familial syndromes. Assessment should be made of the patient's ability to perform routine and desired activities of daily living. Calculation of body mass index along with documentation of initial heart rate, blood pressure, and weight is pertinent. The recommendations of the American College of Cardiology/American Heart Association (ACC/AHA) for evaluation of patients with heart failure (Table 78A.2) are applicable to those with dilated cardiomyopathy.

LABORATORY INVESTIGATIONS

Initial laboratory evaluation should include complete blood count, urinalysis, serum electrolyte determinations (including calcium and magnesium), blood urea nitrogen concentration, serum creatinine concentration, fasting blood glucose level (glycohemoglobin), lipid profile, liver function tests, and thyroid-stimulating

RECOMMENDATIONS FOR THE INITIAL CLINICAL ASSESSMENT OF PATIENTS PRESENTING WITH HEART FAILURE: ACC/AHA PRACTICE GUIDELINES.16
1. A thorough history and physical examination should be obtained/performed in patients presenting with HF to identify cardiac and non-cardiac disorders or behaviors that might cause or accelerate the development or progression of HF (Level of Evidence: C).
2. A careful history of current and past use of alcohol, illicit drugs, current or past standard or "alternative therapies," and chemotherapy drugs should be obtained from patients presenting with HF (Level of Evidence: C).
3. In patients presenting with HF, initial assessment should be made of the patient's ability to perform routine and desired activities of daily living (Level of Evidence: C).
4. Initial examination of patients presenting with HF should include assessment of the patient's volume status, orthostatic blood pressure changes, measurement of weight and height, and calculation of body mass index (Level of Evidence: C).
5. Initial laboratory evaluation of patients presenting with HF should include complete blood count, urinalysis, serum electrolytes (including calcium and magnesium), blood urea nitrogen, serum creatinine, fasting blood glucose (glycohemoglobin), lipid profile, liver function tests, and thyroid-stimulating hormone (Level of Evidence: C).
6. Twelve-lead electrocardiogram and chest radiograph (PA and lateral) should be performed initially in all patients presenting with HF (Level of Evidence: C).
7. Two-dimensional echocardiography with Doppler should be performed during initial evaluation of patients presenting with HF to assess LVEF, LV size, wall thickness, and valve function. Radionuclide ventriculography can be performed to assess LVEF and volumes (Level of Evidence: C).
8. Coronary arteriography should be performed in patients presenting with HF who have angina or significant ischemia unless the patient is not eligible for revascularization of any kind (Level of Evidence: B).

Table 78A.2 Recommendations for the initial clinical assessment of patients presenting with heart failure: ACC/AHA practice guidelines.[16]

hormone concentration.[16] Screening for hemochromatosis or human immunodeficiency virus infection is reasonable in selected patients. Diagnostic tests for rheumatologic diseases, amyloidosis, or pheochromocytoma are reasonable in patients in whom there is a clinical suspicion of these diseases.[16] A chest radiograph (posteroanterior and lateral) should be obtained. Screening for sleep-disordered breathing is appropriate as it is an independent risk factor for development of dilated cardiomyopathy.[16]

ELECTROCARDIOGRAPHY

A twelve-lead electrocardiogram should be obtained in all patients with suspected dilated cardiomyopathy. Sinus tachycardia is a common finding, as are nonspecific ST-T wave abnormalities and left bundle branch block. Atrial or ventricular arrhythmias may be noted.[15]

IMAGING

Two-dimensional echocardiography with Doppler study should be performed to assess left ventricular ejection fraction, left ventricular size, wall thickness, and valve function.[16] Dilated cardiomyopathy is characterized by reduced left ventricular function and increased end-diastolic volumes or dimensions. Ejection fraction is the most widely used index of left ventricular systolic function and is a powerful prognostic indicator. A value of less than 45% is considered abnormal.[17] End-diastolic dimension above 3.2 cm/m^2 indexed to body surface area represents a dilated left ventricle. End-diastolic volume of greater than 75 mL/m^2 is the partition value used for abnormal ventricular parameters.[17] Calculated left ventricular mass greater than 88 g/m^2 in women and 102 g/m^2 in men is considered to be increased. Diastolic function, a reflection of left ventricular filling pressures, has also been correlated with prognosis. Patients with evidence of restrictive filling have significantly worse outcomes than those of patients with normal filling pressures for any given degree of systolic dysfunction.[18] Augmentation in ejection fraction and left ventricular sphericity with dobutamine on stress studies helps identify patients who are most likely to demonstrate improvement in left ventricular function over time.[19]

Radionuclide ventriculography can also be performed to assess left ventricular ejection fraction and volumes in patients in whom a poor acoustic window precludes accurate quantifications as described before. It is of limited use in determining etiology because it fails to provide information about valvular disease or hypertrophy.

Significant reduction in myocardial blood flow on positron emission tomography is associated with an increased risk of death or progression of heart failure.[20] Uptake of radiolabeled *m*-iodobenzylguanidine (MIBG) has been used to predict risk of sudden cardiac death in advanced heart failure by assessing the extent of sympathetic activation in the myocardium.[21]

Cardiac magnetic resonance imaging can be used to assess irreversible myocardial injury, which is detected as late gadolinium hyperenhancement of the myocardium. Cardiac magnetic resonance imaging can be used to evaluate the underlying cause of a newly diagnosed cardiomyopathy by differentiating between ischemic and nonischemic causes.[22] In addition, specific patterns of hyperenhancement may be helpful in differentiating causes such as myocarditis, dilated cardiomyopathy, cardiac amyloidosis, sarcoidosis, and vasculitis.[23]

INVASIVE TESTING

Cardiac catheterization with coronary arteriography should be considered in all patients presenting with heart failure who have angina or significant ischemia, if they are candidates for revascularization. Noninvasive imaging to detect myocardial ischemia and viability is reasonable in patients with known coronary artery disease without angina. Right-sided heart catheterization is used as a valuable aid in guiding optimal medical therapy in severely symptomatic hospitalized patients who are refractory to standard therapy.

Endomyocardial biopsy can be useful in patients presenting with heart failure when a specific diagnosis is suspected that would influence therapy but is not recommended as routine work-up.[16] Current recommendations for biopsy are reserved for (1) patients with new-onset heart failure of less than 2 weeks' duration associated with hemodynamic compromise and (2) new-onset heart failure of 2 weeks' to 3 months' duration associated with a dilated left ventricle and new ventricular arrhythmias, advanced heart block, or failure to respond to usual care within 1 to 2 weeks. This strategy is focused on identification of patients with giant cell myocarditis, which carries a grim prognosis.[24] Biopsy can also be considered in a patient with chronic heart failure if an infiltrative disease is suspected.[24] There have been several attempts to determine if identifying and quantifying the presence of virus in the myocardium of individuals with dilated cardiomyopathy have clinical relevance, but there is not consensus, and testing in a clinical setting is currently not recommended.[25]

EXERCISE TESTING

Maximal exercise testing with or without measurement of respiratory gas exchange or blood oxygen saturation is reasonable in patients presenting with exertional dyspnea to help determine the cause of exercise limitation when the etiology of symptoms is uncertain. Metabolic testing is also used to identify high-risk patients who are candidates for cardiac transplantation or other advanced treatments.[16] A simple, inexpensive, reproducible alternative to metabolic testing is the 6-minute walk test. The test reproduces the activity of daily life, allows objective evaluation of exercise tolerance, provides prognostic evaluation, and permits evaluation of response to medical treatment.[26] T-wave alternans testing may also be a valuable adjunct in determining the risk of sudden death in dilated cardiomyopathy patients, although it has been shown in favorable light in only one study.[27]

TREATMENT

Management of patients with dilated cardiomyopathy is multifaceted and needs to be dynamic, given the unpredictable course of the disease. Education of patients is vital and needs to be tailored to the stage of disease. Knowledge of basis for symptoms, identification of precipitating factors, ability to monitor self for signs of volume overload, and awareness of a protocol for contacting a provider have been shown to markedly reduce hospitalizations. Patients should be educated about treatment goals for blood pressure and heart rate. A flexible diuretic regimen minimizes the deleterious effects of this therapy and should be instituted if possible.[28] Education about dietary sodium restriction is necessary for all patients, whereas fluid restriction is indicated only for patients with advanced systolic dysfunction and persistent hypervolemia.

The pharmacologic treatment of acute and chronic heart failure is discussed in other chapters and is applicable to the management of dilated cardiomyopathy. ACC/AHA and Heart Failure Society of America guidelines-driven pharmacologic therapy is recommended on the basis of ACC/AHA stages of heart failure.[16] The life-prolonging pharmacologic therapies for chronic heart failure are angiotensin-converting enzyme inhibitors or angiotensin receptor blockers, beta blockers, and aldosterone antagonists.[29-36] These drugs have also been shown to reduce hospitalizations and to improve quality of life. Statins have not been studied prospectively but have been shown to reduce mortality in retrospective analyses. However, this therapy is not currently recommended for treatment of heart failure without coronary disease or other risk factors.[37,38] The possible interaction of aspirin with angiotensin-converting enzyme inhibitors has also been studied in retrospective analyses and found not to meet statistical significance.[39] Aspirin has been shown to reduce the risk of major ischemic events in patients without heart failure, and even though this benefit has not been established in patients with heart failure, current recommendations are in favor of aspirin administration in patients who have risk factors for such events.[16] Anticoagulation with warfarin is most justified in patients who have experienced a previous embolic event or who have paroxysmal or persistent atrial fibrillation. Anticoagulation should also be considered in patients with underlying disorders that may be associated with an increased thromboembolic risk, like amyloidosis or left ventricular noncompaction in patients with familial dilated cardiomyopathy and a history of thromboembolism in first-degree relatives.[16]

Assessment of the risk of sudden cardiac death is important not just for prognosis but also for therapeutic decision making. Implantable cardiac defibrillator therapy is indicated in patients who have a left ventricular ejection fraction of 35% or less and who are in NYHA functional class II or class III. Patients should not have a reversible cause of transient left ventricular dysfunction and be optimized on medical therapy.[40] Those with evidence for ventricular dyssynchrony as manifested by prolongation of QRS duration receive additional symptomatic improvement from biventricular pacing.[41] Studies are under way to assess and to define dyssynchrony on imaging, which may identify further subsets of patients who can benefit from this intervention.

There are several surgical therapies for severe dilated cardiomyopathy, including mitral valve and tricuspid valve surgery, ventricular reduction surgery, ventricular assist devices, and heart transplantation. Mitral valve annuloplasty is offered to ischemic and nonischemic cardiomyopathy patients with severe mitral regurgitation due to annular dilatation. The ACORN trial evaluated the CorCap device primarily in patients with nonischemic cardiomyopathy. A substudy of the trial randomized patients to receive mitral valve annuloplasty versus mitral valve annuloplasty plus the CorCap cardiac support device. The results suggested improved left ventricular dimensions and improved NYHA class in patients with surgical elimination of mitral regurgitation with low mortality.[42] Because of a lack of randomized trials and lack of long-term benefit, mitral valve annuloplasty in dilated cardiomyopathy patients is currently not recommended in ACC/AHA or other heart failure guidelines. Other types of ventricular reduction surgeries include the Dor procedure and the SAVER procedure, but these are more frequently offered to patients also undergoing coronary revascularization. Dilated cardiomyopathy is a common indication for ventricular assist device implantation and for cardiac transplantation in appropriate patients. The HARPS trial is currently evaluating the potential for ventricular recovery in dilated cardiomyopathy patients with ventricular assist devices, neurohormonal antagonists, and the β-agonist clenbuterol.[43]

PROGNOSIS

Survival in patients with dilated cardiomyopathy varies on the basis of clinical, structural, hemodynamic, and biochemical factors. Historically, 5-year overall mortality rates have been reported ranging from 50% to 60%.[44] More recently, observed mortality in patients has ranged from 10% to 15% at 2.5 years.[45] Clinical features associated with a worse prognosis are hypotension, presence of S_3, elevated jugular venous pressure, and poor effort tolerance as reflected in NYHA class.[46] Maximal oxygen consumption on exercise testing integrated with functional class has shown a mortality of 20% per year in patients with NYHA class III and $\dot{V}O_2$max of 10 to 15 mL/kg per minute, and this rises to 60% in patients in class IV with $\dot{V}O_2$max of less than 10 mL/kg per minute.[46] Structural abnormalities such as increased left ventricular volumes or mass, mitral or tricuspid regurgitation, and left atrial enlargement portend worse outcomes.[47] Echocardiographic demonstration of restrictive filling pattern confers a poorer prognosis.[48] Elevated levels of serum norepinephrine, B-type natriuretic peptides, and endothelin 1 are associated with limitation of survival.[46] Hyponatremia and elevation in serum urea nitrogen or creatinine concentration have also been correlated with poorer outcomes. On the basis of a recent study, the patients more likely to improve are younger patients; those with higher systolic blood pressure, lower serum creatinine level, shorter mean QRS interval, and lower prevalence of diabetes; and female patients.[49]

Several risk models have been proposed to predict survival based on the variables discussed. The most widely used estimate for in-hospital mortality in acute decompensated heart failure is based on the ADHERE Registry data. Blood urea nitrogen level of 43 mg/dL or higher (≥15.35 mmol/L), serum creatinine level of 2.75 mg/dL or higher (≥243.1 μmol/L), and systolic blood pressure of less than 115 mm Hg were independent predictors of high risk for in-hospital mortality in the analysis. Patients were stratified into low-, intermediate-, and high-risk groups by use of a CART analysis showing mortality risks ranging from 2.1% to 21.9%.[50] A similar prediction model in use for stable outpatients is the Seattle Heart Failure Model. This resource is available on-line and provides an accurate estimate of mean, 1-, 2-, and 3-year survival as well as cumulative effects of adding medications or devices to a patient's regimen.[51]

SUMMARY

As research progresses and the etiologic agents of dilated cardiomyopathy are revealed—whether they are genetic, infectious, or inflammatory—this particular chapter will get shorter. Although we currently apply testing and therapy similarly in all patients with heart failure, further research should allow us to better prevent, to predict, and to treat the specific disease that afflicts patients with dilated cardiomyopathy.

b. Genetics

Philippe Charron and Michel Komajda

The role of genetics in dilated cardiomyopathy (DCM) has been underestimated for a long time, but it is now recognized that familial DCM accounts for approximately 20% to 35% of all cases of DCM.[1]

INHERITANCE AND PENETRANCE

The mode of inheritance is variable, but the most common is autosomal dominant with therefore a 50% risk for transmission to first-degree relatives. The other patterns of inheritance, autosomal recessive, X-linked, and mitochondrial, are obviously less frequent. In addition, an autosomal dominant disease may be manifested by an atypical presentation—an isolated case with a de novo mutation; in this particular case, the heterozygous mutation is not transmitted by one of the two parents as the mutation is absent in the parents, and paternity had been confirmed. The penetrance of a mutation is the percentage of mutation carriers who express the phenotype, that is, have developed or will develop the disease (with or without symptoms). Penetrance of DCM gene mutations is estimated to be age related (with progressively increased risk of cardiac expression with age, even in adults) and may be incomplete in some cases (no cardiac expression at advanced age), but data are still limited.

GENES AND MUTATIONS

More than 20 different causal genes have been identified in DCM (Table 78B.1 and Fig. 78B.1),[1-3] each with a low prevalence (ranging from less than 1% to 10%), and all together are supposed to be involved in less than one third of DCM families. There are therefore other, yet unknown genes responsible for familial DCM. A first group of genes involved in DCM is related to cytoskeletal proteins (dystrophin, sarcoglycan, desmin, metavinculin), leading to the hypothesis that DCM could result from impaired cytoskeletal force transmission and mechanotransduction. However, other groups of genes, with different underlying signaling pathways, were subsequently related to DCM: sarcomeric (such as β-myosin heavy chain) and Z band–related genes (such as myopalladin), nuclear membrane genes (lamins A and C), calcium cycling genes (phospholamban), and cytoplasmic membrane channels (*SCN5A*). The pathophysiologic mechanism of the disease remains largely unknown, especially regarding a possible common final pathway.

GENOTYPE-PHENOTYPE RELATIONS

Some gene mutations are associated with a specific phenotype. Mutations of genes encoding intermediate filaments or cytoskeletal proteins (dystrophin, dystrophin-sarcoglycan

Chromosomal locus	Gene	Protein	Inheritance	Phenotype and Associated Abnormality
DCM autosomal dominant inheritance				
1p1-q21	*LMNA*	Lamins A and C	AD	DCM + conduction system disease ± skeletal myopathy (AD Emery-Dreifuss or limb-girdle muscular dystrophies)
1q32	*TNNT2*	Cardiac troponin T	AD	Pure DCM
1q42-43	*RYR2*	Ryanodine receptor 2	AD	DCM + sinus node dysfunction, ventricular arrhythmia
2q14-q22	?	?	AD	DCM + conduction system disease
2q31	*TTN*	Titin	AD	Pure DCM
2q35	*DES*	Desmin	AD	Pure DCM
3p21	*SCN5A*	Sodium channel type V, α subunit	AD	DCM + conduction defect and arrhythmia
3p22-p25	?	?	AD	DCM + conduction system disease
5q33	*SGCD*	δ-Sarcoglycan	AD	Pure DCM
6q12-q16	?	?	AD	Pure DCM
6q21	*LAMA4*	laminin α4	AD	Pure DCM
6q22	*PLN*	Phospholamban	AD	Pure DCM
6q23	?	?	AD	DCM + skeletal myopathy (limb-girdle muscular dystrophy) ± conduction system disease
6q23-q24	*EYA4*	Eya4	AD	DCM + sensorineural deafness
9q13-q22	?	?	AD	Pure DCM
9q22-q31	?	?	AD	Pure DCM
10q21.1	*MYPN*	Myopalladin	AD	Pure DCM
10q22-q23	*VCL*	Metavinculin	AD	Pure DCM
11p11	*MYBPC3*	Cardiac myosin-binding protein C	AD	Pure DCM
12p12.1	*ABCC9*	ATP-sensitive K channel	AD	Pure DCM
14q12	*MYH7*	β-Myosin heavy chain	AD	Pure DCM
15q14	*ACTC*	α–Cardiac actin	AD	Pure DCM
15q22	*TPM1*	α-Tropomyosin	AD	Pure DCM
DCM autosomal recessive inheritance				
3p13	*ALMS1*	Alms1 protein	AR	DCM in Alström syndrome
4q12	*SCGB*	β-Sarcoglycan	AR	Limb-girdle muscular dystrophy + severe DCM
6p24	*DSP*	Desmoplakin	AR	DCM + woolly hair and keratoderma
19q13.4	*TNNI3*	Cardiac troponin I	AR	Pure DCM
DCM X-linked inheritance				
Xp21	*DMD*	Dystrophin	X-linked	X-linked DCM, Duchenne's and Becker's muscular dystrophies
Xq28	*G4.5*	Tafazzin	X-linked	X-linked infantile DCM, Barth syndrome, hypertrophic DCM, endocardial fibroelastosis, and left ventricular noncompaction
Xq28	*EMD*	Emerin	X-linked	X-linked Emery-Dreifuss muscular dystrophy

AD, autosomal dominant; AR, autosomal recessive; DCM, dilated cardiomyopathy.

Table 78B.1 Genes and mutations.

complex, desmin) can be responsible for DCM associated with skeletal myopathy, either clinical or subclinical with an increased plasma level of creatine kinase. Lamin A/C gene mutations can cause DCM with early conduction disorders (atrioventricular block of variable degree, sinus node dysfunction), early supraventricular or ventricular arrhythmia, and sometimes skeletal myopathy.[4,5] Considering common and isolated forms of DCM, and due to the fact that most mutations described so far are private or observed in few families, little information is available on genotype-phenotype relationship and prognostic stratification. However, it has been suggested that β-myosin heavy chain gene *(MYH7)* mutations were associated with late onset, incomplete penetrance, and delayed major cardiac events compared with cardiac troponin T *(TNNT2)* mutations.

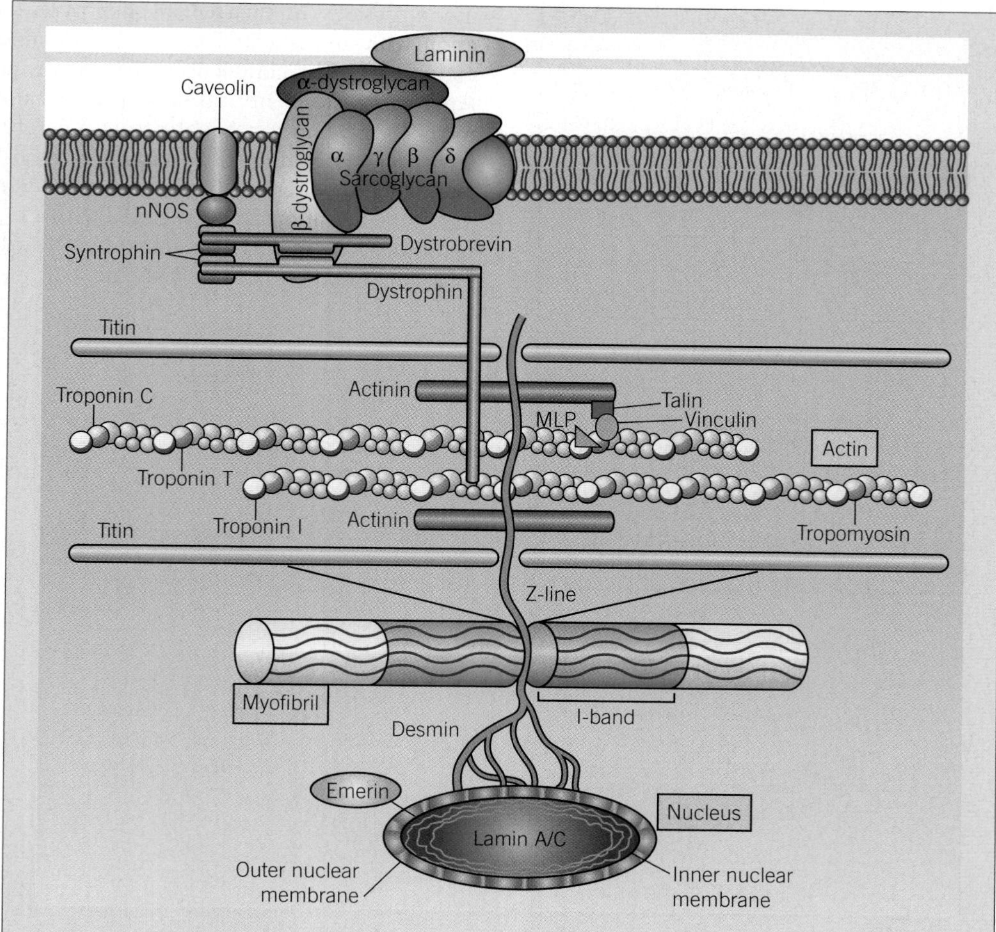

Figure 78B.1 Proteins involved in the development of dilated cardiomyopathy. Identified genes that result in dilated cardiomyopathy include the cytoskeletal protein-encoding genes β- and δ-sarcoglycan in the sarcolemma; dystrophin and the intermediate filament protein-encoding genes desmin and lamin A/C; and sarcomeric protein-encoding genes actin, β-myosin heavy chain, and cardiac troponin T. MLP, muscle LIM protein; nNOS, neuronal nitric oxide synthase. (From Towbin JA, Bowles NE. The failing heart. Nature 2002;415:225-233.)

NON-MONOGENIC FORMS OF DILATED CARDIOMYOPATHY

About two thirds of DCM cases are related to a sporadic disease that is considered to be of multifactorial origin with a genetic component. Some studies have observed the association of genetic polymorphisms with the risk for development of the disease (susceptibility genes) or with the risk of a severe prognosis (modifier genes) or with a differential response to pharmacologic treatment (pharmacogenetic interactions).[6] However, analysis of these factors in clinical practice cannot be recommended because the observed odds ratio is usually low and because the results are based on populations of limited size and have to be confirmed in separate and large populations.

PRACTICAL ISSUES

Because DCM is a genetic disease with mendelian inheritance in at least one third of all cases, routine echocardiographic evaluation can be recommended in all first-degree relatives of a patient with a diagnosis of DCM.[7] The aim is to identify asymptomatic affected relatives who could benefit from early management and treatment, namely, angiotensin-converting enzyme inhibitors (Fig. 78B.2). This strategy could also identify relatives with minor abnormalities (such as isolated left ventricular enlargement or mild depressed systolic function) who could benefit from a serial echocardiographic follow-up, as these individuals are at high risk for development of the disease within a family with a documented affected member.[8]

Genetic testing and genetic counseling may also be offered to patients and families with DCM to improve medical management through preclinical diagnosis and sometimes a better prognostic stratification.[7,9] At present, and in the context of common and pure forms of familial DCM, genetic testing can be proposed but cannot be systematically recommended in routine practice because of the low rate of mutation identification and the high cost of the molecular analyses. A possible exception concerns the β-myosin heavy chain mutations, which could be involved in up to 10% of these families. In contrast, the yield of genetic testing is high

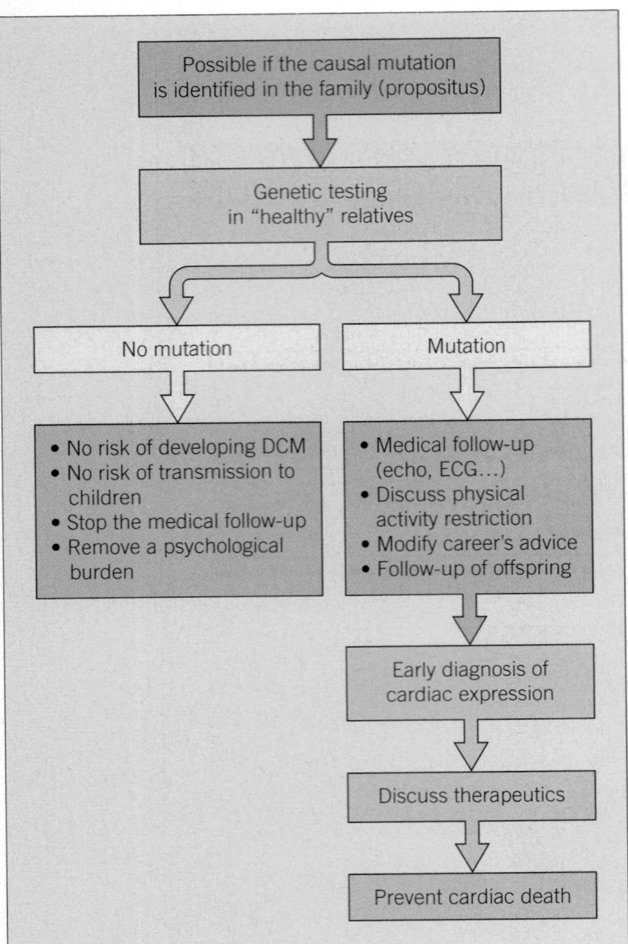

Figure 78B.2 Main outcomes of predictive genetic testing in autosomal dominant dilated cardiomyopathy (DCM).

in the presence of a particular phenotype, such as the association with mild skeletal myopathy, isolated creatine kinase elevation, early conduction defects, or early arrhythmia. Apart from the identification of preclinical mutation carriers in relatives, who can benefit from a careful cardiac follow-up, the identification of a particular gene in a family may lead to better therapeutic management. For example, lamin A/C gene mutations are associated with a high rate of sudden death, leading to early pacemaker and cardioverter-defibrillator implantation in these patients.[5]

chapter 79

Hypertrophic Cardiomyopathy

Perry M. Elliott, Andrew S. Flett, and William J. McKenna

Definition

- Hypertrophic cardiomyopathy is defined by the presence of increased ventricular wall thickness or mass in the absence of loading conditions sufficient to cause the observed abnormality. The most common etiology is an autosomal dominant disorder caused by mutations in genes that encode cardiac sarcomeric proteins.

Key Features

- The disease is the most common inherited cardiovascular disorder, affecting up to 1 in 500 of the general population.
- The pathologic hallmarks of the disease are myocardial hypertrophy, myocyte disarray (usually in association with myocardial fibrosis), and small-vessel disease.

Clinical Implications

- Clinical manifestations include systolic and diastolic dysfunction, myocardial ischemia, arrhythmia, abnormal vascular responses, and skeletal muscle dysfunction.
- Serious complications include ventricular arrhythmia, sudden death, thromboembolism, heart failure, and infective endocarditis.
- Treatment is designed to abolish or to alleviate symptoms when possible and to prevent disease-related deaths.

Hypertrophic cardiomyopathy is defined by the presence of myocardial hypertrophy in the absence of loading conditions (e.g., hypertension or valve disease) sufficient to cause the observed abnormality.[1] Cases of unexplained left ventricular hypertrophy have been described for more than 100 years, but it was not until the 1950s that hypertrophic cardiomyopathy was established as a diagnostic entity, after the publication of Sir Russell Brock's paper "Functional Obstruction of the Left Ventricle"[2] and Donald Teare's description of asymmetric myocardial hypertrophy.[3]

Since then, the concept of hypertrophic cardiomyopathy has evolved from one of a disorder defined solely by the presence of asymmetric septal hypertrophy and left ventricular outflow obstruction to a syndrome encompassing a range of conditions that cause myocardial hypertrophy, the most common of which is a genetically determined disorder of the cardiac sarcomere.[4] The pathophysiologic process and clinical presentation of the disease are heterogeneous, ranging from asymptomatic gene carriers who have very minor electrocardiographic and echocardiographic abnormalities to patients who have severe hypertrophy, diastolic dysfunction, arrhythmias, and disabling symptoms.

ANATOMY

Macroscopic Anatomy

Sixty percent to 70% of patients with hypertrophic cardiomyopathy have an asymmetric distribution of myocardial hypertrophy that affects the interventricular septum more than the lateral or posterior walls (Fig. 79.1). In the remainder of patients, myocardial hypertrophy is concentric or affects one or more myocardial segments elsewhere in the ventricle. Hypertrophy that affects only the left ventricular apex is uncommon, except possibly in Japanese patients.[5] Isolated right ventricular hypertrophy is unreported, but right ventricular involvement is present in approximately 30% of patients who have left ventricular disease. In patients who have left ventricular outflow tract obstruction (see later), there may be a patch of subendocardial thickening on the septum, caused by repeated contact with the anterior leaflet of the mitral valve.[6] The mitral valve itself is also frequently abnormal, with elongation of one or both leaflets or anomalous insertion of the papillary muscles into the main body of the leaflet.[7,8]

Fibrosis is common and often extensive. A small proportion of patients develop a "burnt-out" phase that is characterized by wall thinning and cavity dilatation.[9]

Microscopic Anatomy

The most prominent microscopic feature of hypertrophic cardiomyopathy is myocyte disarray (Fig. 79.2).[10] This consists of

- loss of the normal parallel arrangement of myocytes;
- abnormal intercellular connections; and
- variation in the diameter and length of individual myocytes.

Within cells, there is variation in nuclear size and disruption of myofibrillar architecture. The abnormal myocytes sometimes form circles around areas of increased connective tissue and are often associated with areas of myocardial fibrosis. Myocyte disarray is reported in congenital heart disease, hypertension, and aortic stenosis, but it is more extensive in hypertrophic cardiomyopathy, in which it affects 5% to 40% of the total myocardium.

Many patients have abnormal, small intramural arteries (with an external diameter of less than 15 mm) that are characterized by medial hypertrophy and apparent narrowing of their lumens.[11] This "small-vessel disease" and the apparent mismatch between myocardial mass and coronary circulation in hypertrophic cardiomyopathy probably contribute to the impaired coronary vasodilator reserve and regional myocardial ischemia and consecutive myocardial scarring.

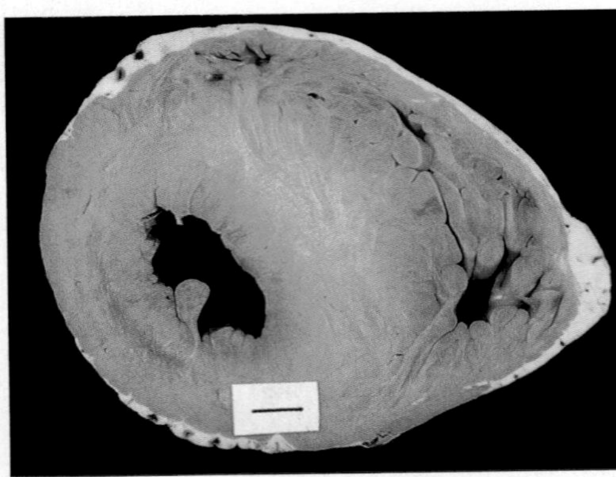

Figure 79.1 Severe asymmetric hypertrophy of the interventricular septum and a disordered pattern of large muscle bundles in hypertrophic cardiomyopathy. (Courtesy of Professor M. Davies, St. George's Hospital Medical School, London.)

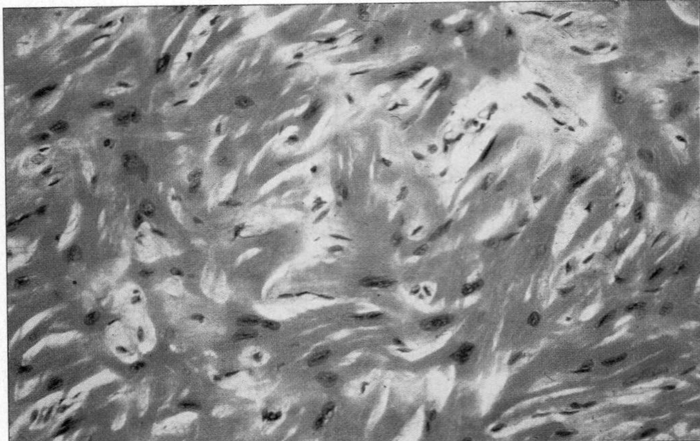

Figure 79.2 Myocyte disarray. Myocardial section (hematoxylin and eosin stain) demonstrating myocyte disarray. Individual myocytes vary in length and diameter and contain abnormal nuclei. There are abnormal intercellular connections, and cells form circles around areas of increased connective tissue. (Courtesy of Professor M. Davies, St. George's Hospital Medical School, London.)

BIOCHEMISTRY

Calcium Homeostasis

Limited studies of isolated muscle preparations have demonstrated abnormal calcium homeostasis during muscle contraction. In particular, hypertrophic cardiomyopathy muscle fibers show two calcium transients[12,13]:

- an early and short-lived calcium current, which is believed to be caused by release of stored calcium from sarcoplasmic reticulum; and
- a second, more prolonged phase of calcium current, which is believed to be caused by increased uptake of calcium through membrane channels.

These abnormalities are associated with slow and dyssynchronous left ventricular relaxation that impairs early ventricular filling and may be associated with delayed afterdepolarizations.

Natriuretic Peptides

The natriuretic peptides are a group of circulating hormones with actions that include natriuresis and vasodilatation. In normal hearts, atrial natriuretic peptide (ANP) is secreted from the atria in response to an increase in atrial volume. There is usually negligible expression of ANP in the ventricles. In patients who have hypertrophic cardiomyopathy, several studies have shown that ANP plasma concentrations are fourfold or fivefold greater than normal and that ANP gene expression occurs in the ventricle.[14]

Brain natriuretic peptide (BNP) is structurally similar to ANP, but in mammalian hearts, it is mainly secreted from the ventricles. Plasma concentrations of BNP are strikingly increased in patients with hypertrophic cardiomyopathy, with the greatest concentrations (85 times normal) in patients who have left ventricular outflow tract obstruction.[15] More recently, studies have shown that BNP concentrations in children are strongly correlated with degree of left ventricular hypertrophy, outflow tract gradient, transmitral flows, and exercise capacity. In addition, levels were higher in children with implantable cardioverter-defibrillators than without.[16]

The ratio of BNP to ANP in hypertrophic cardiomyopathy is much higher than that in other myocardial diseases (e.g., congestive cardiac failure), which suggests that the underlying stimulus to BNP secretion is much greater in hypertrophic cardiomyopathy. Studies indicate that increased BNP concentrations at rest may be a predictor of silent myocardial ischemia in hypertrophic cardiomyopathy.[17]

Fatty Acid Metabolism

Several studies using radiolabeled fatty acid analogues have demonstrated abnormal fatty acid metabolism in some patients who have hypertrophic cardiomyopathy.[18] Investigations in a Japanese population have linked abnormal myocardial fatty acid uptake—measured by iodine 123–labeled 15-(*p*-iodophenyl)-3-*R*,*S*-methylpentadecanoic acid single-photon emission computed tomography—to reduced CD36 antigen expression on platelets or point mutations in CD36 cDNA.[19] It is suggested that CD36 is associated with long-chain fatty acid transport across cell membranes.

GENETICS

The estimated prevalence of familial hypertrophic cardiomyopathy derived from a large echocardiographic study is approximately 1 per 500 of the general population.[20] Molecular genetic studies have shown that familial hypertrophic cardiomyopathy is a disease with autosomal dominant inheritance caused by mutations in any one of 11 different genes, each encoding proteins of the cardiac sarcomere (Fig. 79.3)[21-23]:

- β-myosin heavy chain (chromosome 14q11);
- α-myosin heavy chain (chromosome 14q11);
- β–cardiac troponin T (chromosome 1q32);
- cardiac myosin–binding protein C (chromosome 11p11);
- α-tropomyosin (chromosome 15q22);
- cardiac troponin I (chromosome 19p13.2-q13.2);
- the essential myosin light chain (chromosome 3p21);
- the regulatory myosin light chain (chromosome12q23-p21);

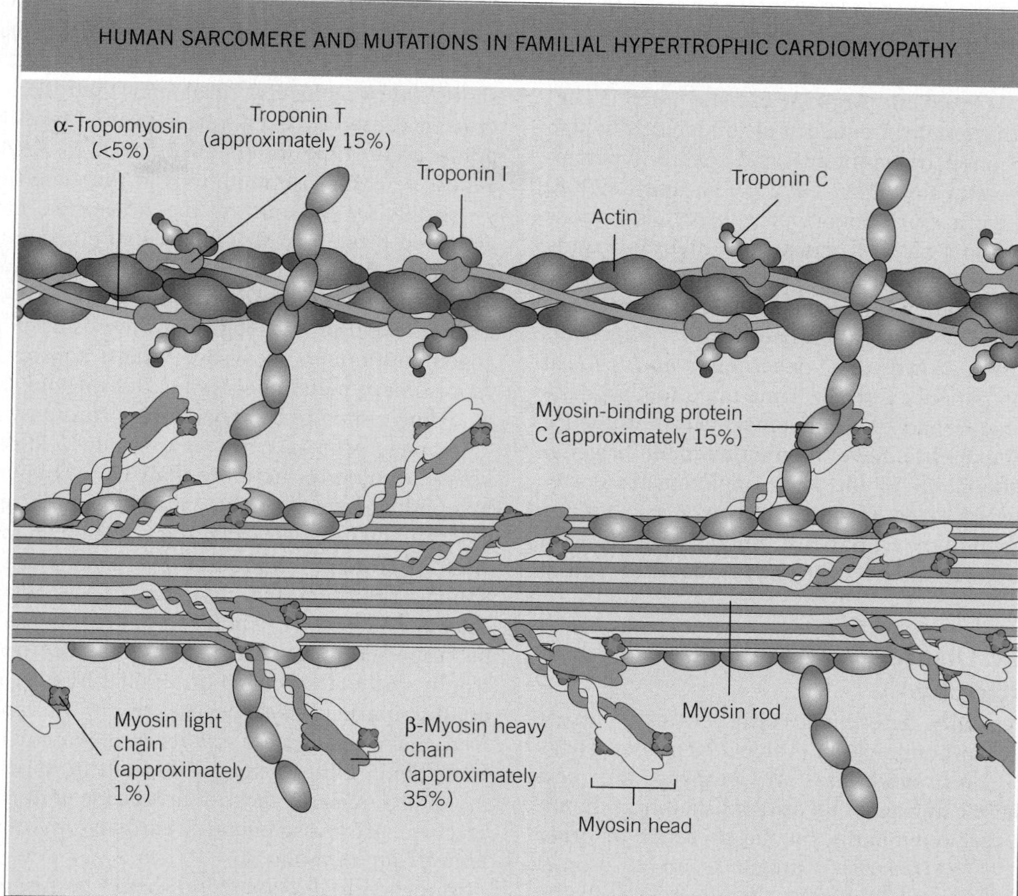

Figure 79.3 Human sarcomere and mutations in familial hypertrophic cardiomyopathy. All the mutations that have been described in familial hypertrophic cardiomyopathy occur in genes that encode cardiac sarcomeric proteins. The most frequent mutations occur in the head or head-rod region of the gene that encodes the β-myosin heavy chain. The estimated frequencies of these mutations and of mutations in other sarcomeric protein genes are shown.

- cardiac troponin C;
- cardiac α-actin (chromosome 15q14); and
- titin (chromosome 2p31).

Current estimates suggest that up to 60% of hypertrophic cardiomyopathy is caused by mutations in one of these genes. The most commonly affected genes are β-myosin heavy chain, cardiac myosin–binding protein C, and cardiac troponins T and I. The genetic diversity is compounded by intragenetic heterogeneity, with more than 150 mutations in β-myosin heavy chain alone. Many families have their own "private" mutation.

The majority of hypertrophic cardiomyopathy mutations are missense mutations or minor truncations caused by a single amino acid substitution. All β-myosin heavy chain point mutations produce missense codons and occur in the head or the head-rod region of the β-myosin heavy chain protein,[24] which suggests that they may disturb the function of critical domains of β-myosin heavy chain that are involved in contractility. Some mutations also cause a change in the charge of the substituted amino acid and may produce conformational changes in the protein structure.

Variable Penetrance and Expression

Clinical penetrance varies between individuals with the same sarcomeric protein mutation. Clinical penetrance varies with age, in that hypertrophy can develop during the teenage growth spurt. Gene carriers who do not have overt disease by their mid-20s can go on to develop it in later life, although the proportion that have so-called late-onset disease remains to be determined. Studies in individuals who have mutations in the gene encoding cardiac myosin–binding protein C have suggested that this gene is particularly prone to a delayed onset, after the second and third decades.[25-27] Some studies have also shown that although death before the age of 40 years is uncommon in patients with cardiac myosin–binding protein C mutations, cumulative survival decreases from more than 80% in the fourth decade to less than 50% in patients older than 50 years, suggesting that once disease is expressed, disease-related complications such as arrhythmia, heart failure, and thromboembolism are just as common as they are in some other sarcomeric protein mutations.[25]

Preliminary data suggest that some of the observed clinical heterogeneity in hypertrophic cardiomyopathy may reflect the genetic heterogeneity of the disease. For example, cardiac troponin T mutations can be associated with mild hypertrophy but extensive myocyte disarray and a high incidence of premature death.[28,29] Some β-myosin heavy chain mutations (e.g., Arg403Gln, Arg453Cys, and Arg719Gln) are associated with a greater frequency of sudden death, high penetrance, early onset of symptoms, and severe hypertrophy, whereas others (Val606Met, Gly256Gln, and Leu908-Val) appear to have a more benign prognosis.[22] Mutations in the α-tropomyosin (<5% of cases) and myosin-binding protein C mutations (15% to 20% of cases) have variable morphologic expression, with a generally good prognosis and a low incidence of sudden cardiac death.[24] However, many studies have shown that penetrance and clinical expression vary in patients with the same mutation, suggesting that other genetic and environmental factors influence development of the disease. Several potential modifier genes encoding the components of the renin-angiotensin-aldosterone system have emerged recently and may account for the significant phenotypic variability among patients with hypertrophic cardiomyopathy who have identical causal mutations.[30,31]

Other Genetic Disorders That Cause Hypertrophy

Many other genetically determined disorders can present with hypertrophic cardiomyopathy (Table 79.1). Friedreich's ataxia and Noonan's syndrome are perhaps the best described, and these can usually be distinguished from familial hypertrophic cardiomyopathy by the presence of other clinical features.[32,33] Friedreich's ataxia is an autosomal recessive condition caused by a trinucleotide repeat in the gene that encodes a protein called frataxin, which is involved in mitochondrial iron metabolism.[34] Noonan's syndrome (which can cause ventricular hypertrophy and is characterized by unusual facial characteristics, eye abnormalities, short stature, bleeding problems, and skeletal malformations) is caused by mutations in protein tyrosine phosphatase nonreceptor type II *(PTPN2)*, *SOS1*, *KRAS*, and *RAF1* genes.[35-38] Missense mutations in the gene that encodes the γ_2 regulatory subunit of the adenosine monophosphate–activated protein (AMP) kinase cause a syndrome of Wolff-Parkinson-White in association with conduction abnormalities and left ventricular hypertrophy. In contrast to hypertrophic cardiomyopathy, histologically there is accumulation of glycogen within myocytes, so it is most appropriately regarded as a primary metabolic storage disease and should therefore be distinguished from hypertrophic cardiomyopathy in terms of management and risk assessment.[39] Mutations in AMP kinase account for no more than 1% of hypertrophic cardiomyopathy cases.[40] Other nonsarcomeric gene mutations associated with myocardial hypertrophy include human muscle LIM protein[41] (a promoter of myogenesis) and phospholamban promoter (an inhibitor of sarcoplasmic reticulum calcium ATPase).[42] Anderson-Fabry disease should always be suspected in case of late-onset concentric cardiac hypertrophy without evidence of familial hypertrophic cardiomyopathy, particularly because recent therapeutic advances have made this disease and its cardiovascular manifestations treatable.[43] Other genes implicated in hypertrophic cardiomyopathy include those that encode mitochondria: tRNA-glycine, tRNA-isoleucine, cardiac myosin light-peptide kinase, and caveolin 3.

Mitochondrial dysfunction should be suspected in patients who have

- exclusively maternal inheritance;
- disproportionate exercise limitation and severe acidosis on exercise; or
- other clinical features, such as subclinical skeletal muscle disease, retinitis pigmentosa, or deafness.

GENETICALLY DETERMINED DISORDERS THAT CAN PRESENT WITH HYPERTROPHIC CARDIOMYOPATHY IN CHILDHOOD OR ADULTHOOD	
Syndromes	Noonan's syndrome
	Friedreich's ataxia
	Lentiginosis
	Swyer's syndrome (gonadal dysgenesis)
Metabolic disorders	Acyl-coenzyme A dehydrogenase deficiency
	Carnitine deficiency
	Glycogen storage diseases (Pompe's disease, Forbes' disease)
	Hurler's syndrome
	Hunter's syndrome
	Anderson-Fabry disease
	Phosphorylase b kinase deficiency
	Debrancher enzyme deficiency
	Mitochondrial cytopathies

Hypertrophic cardiomyopathy has been described in a large number of often rare metabolic disorders, only some of which are listed here. Most present in infancy and childhood, but others, such as Fabry's disease and mitochondrial DNA mutations, can present in adulthood.

Table 79.1 Genetically determined disorders that can present with hypertrophic cardiomyopathy in childhood or adulthood.

PATHOPHYSIOLOGY

Systolic Function

Patients with hypertrophic cardiomyopathy typically have small left ventricular cavity dimensions with normal or increased ejection fraction. Regional systolic function may be abnormal, particularly in the interventricular septum, where both longitudinal and circumferential shortening are often reduced. Cardiac output is also reduced on exercise or during pharmacologic stress.[44] Development of left ventricular dilatation and systolic impairment is associated with a poor prognosis.[45]

Left Ventricular Outflow Tract Obstruction

Twenty-five percent of patients with hypertrophic cardiomyopathy have a resting pressure gradient between the left ventricular outflow tract and aorta. Other patients may develop a gradient only during physical or pharmacologic maneuvers that reduce afterload or preload or increase ventricular contractility.[46] In fact, recent evidence suggests it may be more common than previously estimated, with one

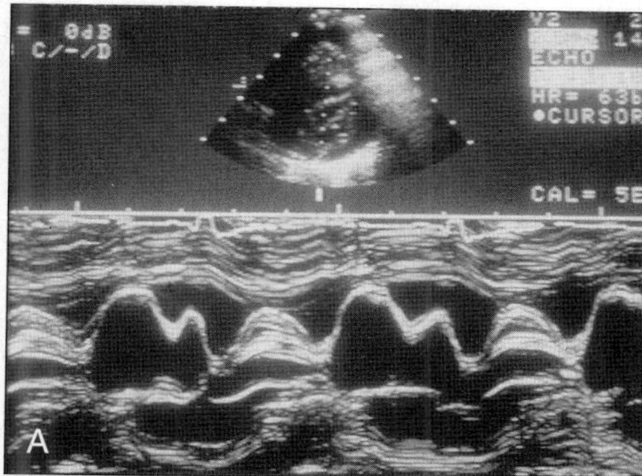

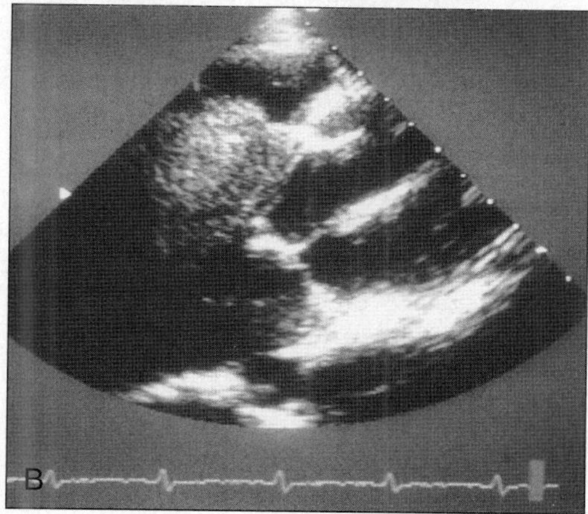

Figure 79.4 Left ventricular outflow tract obstruction. **A,** M-mode echocardiogram in a patient with asymmetric septal hypertrophy and left ventricular outflow tract obstruction demonstrating asymmetric septal hypertrophy and systolic anterior motion of the mitral valve. The timing and duration of contact caused by anterior motion between the mitral valve and the septum can be used to estimate the severity of the outflow gradient. **B,** Two-dimensional echocardiogram in a patient with left ventricular outflow tract obstruction demonstrating the characteristic anterior motion of the anterior mitral valve leaflet. As the distal portion of the leaflet bends toward the septum, it makes contact with the septum and causes obstruction.

series identifying outflow obstruction in 70% of hypertrophic cardiomyopathy patients on exercise echocardiography.[47] Left ventricular outflow tract gradients are nearly always associated with an abrupt forward movement—systolic anterior motion—of the anterior mitral valve leaflet (Fig. 79.4). Less commonly, the posterior leaflet makes contact with the septum. For a long time, it had been suggested that systolic anterior motion develops because septal hypertrophy and outflow tract narrowing produce a high-velocity stream above the mitral valve that causes the tip of the anterior mitral valve leaflet to be "sucked" against the septum by the Venturi effect.[40] Another hypothesis has been that abnormal anterior positioning of the mitral leaflets results in drag forces on the undersurface of the anterior leaflet during ventricular ejection. This theory is supported by the onset of systolic anterior motion before aortic valve opening, the presence of systolic anterior motion only in the center of the anterior leaflet, and the occurrence of systolic anterior motion in the absence of septal hypertrophy.[48] Additional factors that predispose to systolic anterior motion include abnormalities in the primary mitral valve apparatus, such as leaflet elongation and anomalous insertion of papillary muscles into the valve.[7,8]

For many years, there was continuing debate about the significance of left ventricular outflow gradients. The hypothesis that the outflow gradient represents true obstruction to left ventricular ejection is based on several observations[41]:

- the subaortic gradient develops simultaneously with contact caused by systolic anterior motion between the mitral valve and the septum;
- its severity correlates with the time at onset and the duration of the apposition between the mitral valve and septum;
- a significant proportion of ventricular ejection occurs in the presence of the subaortic gradient;
- left ventricular ejection time is prolonged; and
- aortic flow profiles in patients with severe gradients demonstrate a characteristic midsystolic deceleration that coincides with mitral valve–septal contact.

Perhaps the most persuasive evidence is the clinical improvement that is observed after successful surgical or pharmacologic relief of outflow tract obstruction. Mitral regurgitation occurs in almost all patients who have obstructive hypertrophic cardiomyopathy as a consequence of systolic anterior motion and abnormal mitral leaflet coaptation (Fig. 79.5) and in approximately 30% of patients who have nonobstructive hypertrophic cardiomyopathy.

Recent data suggest that left ventricular outflow tract obstruction is an independent predictor of sudden death that is related to the severity of obstruction, along with the usual risk markers for sudden death (Table 79.2). However, in patients who are asymptomatic even with left ventricular outflow tract obstruction, the absolute risk of sudden death remains low (<0.5% per annum).[49,50]

Diastolic Function

In patients who have hypertrophic cardiomyopathy, left ventricular relaxation is altered by myocyte hypertrophy, myocyte disarray, abnormal intracellular calcium flux, distorted ventricular geometry, and myocardial ischemia. Left ventricular

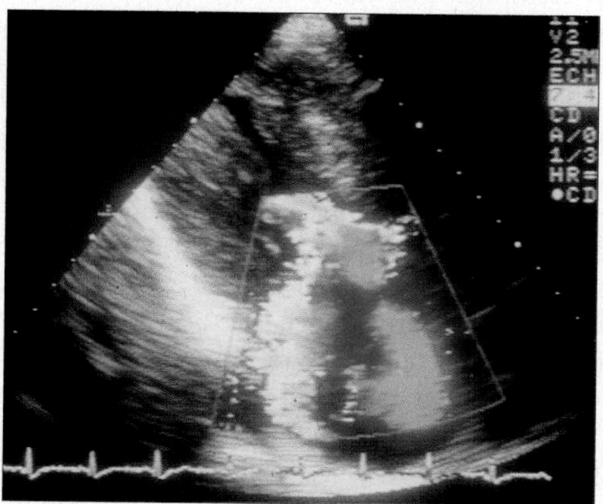

Figure 79.5 Color-flow Doppler study from apical two-chamber view. There is increased velocity in the left ventricular outflow tract caused by anterior motion of the mitral valve and systolic contact between the anterior leaflet and the septum. The anterior motion of the mitral valve causes failure of mitral leaflet coaptation and mitral regurgitation.

RISK FACTORS FOR SUDDEN CARDIAC DEATH IN HYPERTROPHIC CARDIOMYOPATHY: SENSITIVITY, SPECIFICITY, AND PREDICTIVE ACCURACY OF SELECTED FACTORS

Risk Factor	Sensitivity (%)	Specificity (%)	Positive Predictive Accuracy (%)	Negative Predictive Accuracy (%)
Blood pressure (in patients younger than 40 years)[72]	75	66	15	97
Nonsustained ventricular tachycardia during Holter monitoring[19]	69	80	22	97
Syncope[59]				
Overall	29	83	25	86
In those younger than 45 years	42	82	29	89
Family history of sudden cardiac death	42	79	28	88
Left ventricular hypertrophy ≥30 mm[95]	26	88	13	95

Table 79.2 Risk factors for sudden cardiac death in hypertrophic cardiomyopathy: sensitivity, specificity, and predictive accuracy of selected factors.

compliance is reduced by altered ventricular geometry, fibrosis, and increased diastolic ventricular interaction.

Studies using echocardiography, ventriculography, and radionuclide angiography have demonstrated a spectrum of diastolic abnormalities that includes[42]

- prolonged time to peak filling;
- reduced relative volume during rapid filling;
- prolonged isovolumic relaxation time;
- increased atrial contribution; and
- reduced rates of posterior wall thinning.

It is clear that no single pattern is typical of the disease; abnormal relaxation is the predominant abnormality in some patients, reduced left ventricular compliance in others. Diastolic dysfunction causes dyspnea and exercise limitation; in a small subset of patients, it may cause severe biatrial enlargement, pulmonary hypertension, and severe right-sided heart failure with edema, ascites, and hepatomegaly.

Arrhythmia

Arrhythmias are common. Paroxysmal episodes of atrial fibrillation occur in approximately 20% to 25% of patients with hypertrophic cardiomyopathy, with an age-related increase in incidence. Predisposing factors include left atrial enlargement, severe left ventricular hypertrophy, and left ventricular outflow tract obstruction.[51,52] Chronic atrial fibrillation is present in 5% of patients at initial presentation, and it develops in another 10% in the first 5 years after diagnosis.[45] Despite being usually well tolerated and self-limited, atrial fibrillation is a major determinant of embolic stroke and other peripheral vascular events, with an annual incidence of 0.8% and a prevalence rate of 6%, leading to death and disability most commonly in the elderly.[53]

Isolated ventricular ectopic beats and nonsustained ventricular tachycardia are common; nonsustained ventricular tachycardia occurs in up to 25% of adults during ambulatory electrocardiography.[45] Documented sustained monomorphic ventricular tachycardia is uncommon and is often associated with apical left ventricular aneurysms in patients with mid-cavity obliteration.[54] Possible contributory factors include myocyte disarray, abnormal intercellular connections, myocardial fibrosis, and myocardial ischemia.

Abnormal atrioventricular nodal or His-Purkinje conduction is a relatively frequent finding at electrophysiologic testing, but the incidence of clinically significant conduction block in hypertrophic cardiomyopathy is uncertain. The presence of familial conduction disease should prompt consideration of disease caused by mutations in the AMP kinase gene or mitochondrial DNA.

Abnormalities of Skeletal Muscle Function

Many patients with hypertrophic cardiomyopathy complain of muscle fatigue during exercise. Several studies have demonstrated a range of abnormalities in skeletal muscle structure and function, including abnormal electromyographic recordings, selective type 1 fiber atrophy, focal myofibrillar loss, lipid vacuoles, and abnormal mitochondrial ultrastructure. Some of these features may be secondary phenomena, but mutations in genes such as β-myosin are expressed in both skeletal and cardiac muscle fibers. Some preliminary data suggest that the severity of skeletal muscle fiber dysfunction may vary between different mutations.[55]

Autonomic Dysfunction

A number of studies have suggested that autonomic function is abnormal in patients who have hypertrophic cardiomyopathy, but findings in published studies have been contradictory. Some studies have demonstrated selective reduction in cardiac parasympathetic activity (reduced heart rate variability during respiration and Valsalva maneuver), whereas others have shown reduced sympathetic tone (reduced low-frequency component of heart rate variability).[56] This variability in reported abnormalities probably reflects the effects of patient selection and drug treatment and the various and complex mechanisms of autonomic dysfunction in hypertrophic cardiomyopathy.

In different subgroups of patients, a number of stimuli may be important, including

- left atrial dilatation;
- hyperdynamic left ventricular systolic function;
- activation of ventricular mechanoreceptors; and
- myocardial ischemia.

These different mechanisms of autonomic disturbance are reflected in the reported associations between different components of heart rate variability and left atrial size, left ventricular cavity dimensions, and left ventricular wall thickness.

Abnormal Vascular Responses

Twenty-five percent of all patients who have hypertrophic cardiomyopathy have an abnormal blood pressure response during upright exercise. This is manifested as a failure of the blood pressure to increase from baseline or as a decrease in blood pressure during exercise. In a minority of these patients, this can be explained by the development of a substantial left ventricular outflow gradient during exercise, but abnormal responses also occur in patients who have nonobstructive disease. Abnormal blood pressure responses are associated with small left ventricular cavity dimensions[57] and, in some individuals, inappropriate vasodilatation in nonexercising muscles. In addition, reflex dilatation of venous capacitance beds is described in patients with syncope and exercise-induced hypotension.[58] The trigger for these abnormal peripheral vascular responses may be the activation of left ventricular baroreceptors by increased wall stress or, possibly, myocardial ischemia. The presence of a vasodepressor response in patients who have hypertrophic cardiomyopathy may also explain the poor tolerance of paroxysmal atrial arrhythmia or sinus tachycardia in some patients. In some patients, ejection fraction and stroke volume fall during exercise and may contribute to the abnormal blood pressure response.[46] The mechanism for the fall in stroke volume may be myocardial ischemia.

Myocardial Ischemia

Several pathophysiologic mechanisms may cause microvascular angina in hypertrophic cardiomyopathy. Left ventricular hypertrophy increases myocardial oxygen demand and extravascular compressive forces and may decrease the density of coronary arterioles. Myocyte disarray results in inefficient myocardial contraction and thereby contributes to increased oxygen demand.

Several studies have described medial thickening and apparent narrowing of small intramural vessels in the hearts of patients with hypertrophic cardiomyopathy, particularly in regions of myocardial scarring and in hearts affected by "end-stage" dilatation. Systolic compression of larger septal perforator vessels and epicardial coronary vessels is well recognized and may explain the sometimes dramatic systolic flow reversal seen in proximal coronary vessels. Positron emission tomographic studies have demonstrated a significant impairment of microvascular flow in hypertrophic cardiomyopathy compared with normal controls. Reduction in flow is seen in hypertrophic cardiomyopathy with mild or even no symptoms and may be associated with an adverse outcome including progression of heart failure symptoms, arrhythmia, and death.[59]

CLINICAL IMPLICATIONS

Clinical Presentation

The majority of patients who have hypertrophic cardiomyopathy have few or no cardiac symptoms, but in hospital-based populations, dyspnea, chest pain, unexplained syncope, and palpitation are common. Fatigue is also common and can be the major limiting symptom. Chest pain may be exertional and may occur at rest, and it is frequently precipitated by eating. Syncope and presyncope can be caused by paroxysmal arrhythmia, conduction system disease, and abnormal vascular responses during exercise; but in many cases, no underlying cause is identified, even after extensive investigations. Palpitations are often associated with symptomatic cardiac contractions and ventricular ectopy, but supraventricular arrhythmias are the most frequent cause of sustained palpitations.

Although there are many classic descriptions of the physical findings in hypertrophic cardiomyopathy, physical examination is unremarkable in the majority of patients. Some patients may have a rapid upstroke to the arterial pulse, a sustained left ventricular impulse, and a palpable left atrial beat. A prominent *a* wave in the jugular venous pressure wave, caused by reduced right ventricular compliance, may be observed in a minority of patients. Auscultation may reveal a fourth heart sound, reflecting atrial systole into a "stiff" left ventricle, in patients who are in sinus rhythm. Left ventricular outflow tract obstruction causes a systolic murmur at the left sternal edge that radiates to the aortic and mitral areas but usually not into the neck or axilla. Severe left ventricular outflow obstruction may be associated with reverse splitting of the second heart sound. A characteristic feature of the outflow tract murmur is its dependence on ventricular volume, such that physiologic and pharmacologic interventions that reduce afterload and venous return (e.g., standing, Valsalva maneuver, or amyl nitrate) increase its intensity, whereas interventions that increase afterload and venous return (e.g., squatting or phenylephrine) reduce it. Most patients who have left ventricular outflow gradients also have mitral regurgitation.

Electrocardiography

Although the majority of patients who have hypertrophic cardiomyopathy have an abnormal electrocardiogram, there are no patterns that are specific to the disease. A normal electrocardiogram is present in 6% of hypertrophic cardiomyopathy patients, and 35% do not meet voltage criteria for hypertrophy. In those with voltage criteria for left ventricular hypertrophy, repolarization abnormalities are usual, but isolated increases in voltage without ST-segment and T-wave changes are rare. Pathologic Q waves also occur frequently, most commonly in the inferolateral leads, and criteria for left and right atrial enlargement are also commonly seen. Giant negative T waves in the mid-precordial leads are said to be characteristic of Japanese patients with apical involvement,[5] but they are also seen in Western patients who have more extensive hypertrophy. Some patients have a short PR interval with a slurred QRS upstroke that can be difficult to distinguish from preexcitation.[60]

A study of patients with hypertrophic cardiomyopathy relating electrocardiographic changes to findings on cardiovascular magnetic resonance imaging has shown that abnormal Q waves are related to upper anterior septal thickness and that the depth of negative T waves is related to distal hypertrophy.[61] The presence of wide Q waves and the absence of normal septal Q waves are associated with fibrosis.

Echocardiography

Echocardiography remains the mainstay investigation for the diagnosis of hypertrophic cardiomyopathy in individual patients. The classic M-mode echocardiographic abnormalities in hypertrophic cardiomyopathy include

- asymmetric hypertrophy of the interventricular septum;
- systolic anterior motion of the mitral valve;
- small left ventricular cavity;
- septal immobility; and
- premature closure of the aortic valve.

The routine use of two-dimensional echocardiography has confirmed that asymmetric hypertrophy is the most common abnormality, but it has also shown that virtually any pattern of hypertrophy is consistent with a diagnosis of hypertrophic cardiomyopathy (Fig. 79.6).[62]

When a ratio of the thickness of the septum to the thickness of the free wall of 1.3:1 is used to define asymmetry, concentric hypertrophy accounts for only 1% to 2% of all cases, but this proportion increases to approximately 31% when a ratio of 1.5:1 is used. Several scoring systems for the severity of hypertrophy can be used. The Wigle index uses the degree of septal thickness and the extension of hypertrophy to the left ventricular apex[41] (measured from the apical four-chamber view to determine the extent of septal involvement and the parasternal short-axis view at the level of the mitral valve leaflet tips to assess anterolateral wall involvement).

The mechanisms of systolic anterior motion and outflow gradients have been reviewed. True systolic anterior motion occurs before peak anterior movement of the posterior left ventricular wall. Pseudo–systolic anterior motion is an exaggeration of the normal anterior movement of the mitral valve in systole that reaches its peak at the end of systole, when the posterior left ventricular wall has fully contracted. The time at onset and the duration of the contact between the mitral leaflet and the septum in systole correlate with the magnitude of the outflow tract pressure gradient.

Commonly, gradients are measured by use of continuous-wave Doppler echocardiography and the modified Bernoulli equation:

$$\text{Peak gradient} = 4V_{max}^2$$

where V_{max} is the maximum velocity across the left ventricular outflow tract.

The typical continuous-wave recording shows a late-peaking velocity profile, but when left ventricular outflow tract obstruction is severe, the Doppler envelope may become holosystolic. This can make differentiation from the mitral regurgitation that frequently accompanies systolic anterior motion difficult.

The broad spectrum of diastolic abnormalities in patients who have hypertrophic cardiomyopathy results in an equally diverse range of echo-derived indices of diastolic function. In addition to the classic impaired relaxation and restrictive patterns of left ventricular filling, ventricular asynchrony often results in abnormal intracavity flows during isovolumetric contraction and relaxation. In particular, patients with apical hypertrophy may have flow from the apex toward the outflow tract in diastole.

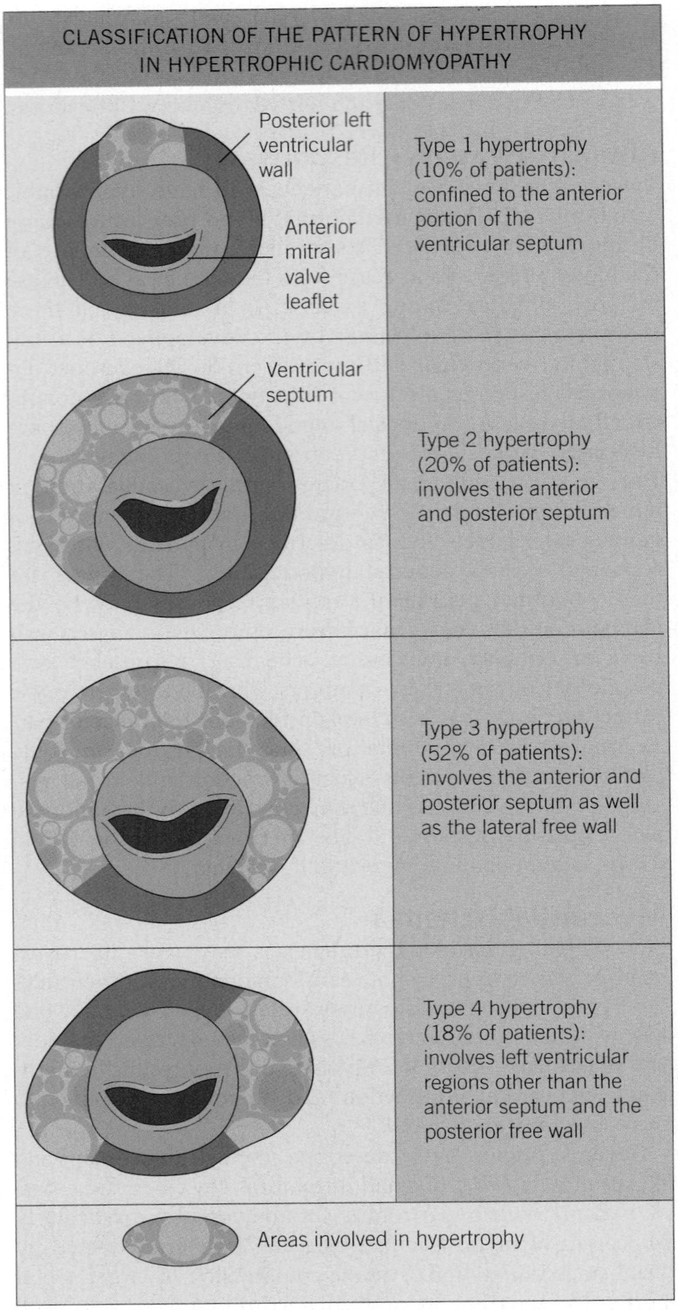

CLASSIFICATION OF THE PATTERN OF HYPERTROPHY IN HYPERTROPHIC CARDIOMYOPATHY

Figure 79.6 Classification of the pattern of hypertrophy in hypertrophic cardiomyopathy. The Maron classification of the different patterns of hypertrophy with their approximate frequency in patients with hypertrophic cardiomyopathy is summarized. With the discovery of the underlying genetic basis of familial hypertrophic cardiomyopathy, it is now clear that many patients do not fulfill conventional diagnostic criteria. Some patients have only very mild hypertrophy that can be associated with severe diastolic dysfunction. (Modified with permission from Maron BJ, Gottdiener JS, Epstein SE. Patterns and significance of the distribution of left ventricular hypertrophy in hypertrophic cardiomyopathy: a wide angle, two-dimensional echocardiographic study of 125 patients. Am J Cardiol 1981;48:418-428. © 1981, Elsevier Science Ltd.)

As in other cardiac diseases, interrogation of pulmonary vein velocities with pulsed Doppler study may be a useful aid for the interpretation of transmitral velocities. Increasingly, tissue Doppler examination is being used to measure myocardial velocities in a variety of diseases, and studies in patients who have hypertrophic cardiomyopathy have demonstrated reduced myocardial contraction and relaxation velocities. Tissue Doppler examination has demonstrated a significantly lower systolic and diastolic mitral annular velocity in genotypically positive patients without left ventricular hypertrophy compared with individuals without gene defects.[63]

Cardiovascular Magnetic Resonance

Cardiovascular magnetic resonance is particularly useful if diagnostic doubt remains after routine clinical evaluation (including echocardiography). For example, echocardiographic views of the left ventricular apex are frequently technically challenging because of near-field artifact, so in patients thought to have apical hypertrophy (unexplained repolarization abnormalities on electrocardiography), cardiovascular magnetic resonance imaging may be helpful.[64] Also, apical cavity obliteration, microaneurysms, thrombus, and left ventricular noncompaction can be easily identified. Cardiovascular magnetic resonance is able to detect hypertrophy in other areas of myocardium not easily seen on echocardiography, in particular the basal anterior-anteroseptal and anterolateral left ventricular free wall.[65] In addition, cardiovascular magnetic resonance can be helpful when there are anatomic variations: right ventricular structures, false tendons or trabeculae, membranes, and complex multilevel obstruction.

With the use of gadolinium-DTPA–based contrast agents, focal areas of fibrosis can be identified.[66] Gadolinium is an extracellular contrast agent and accumulates in areas of scar, making the area brighter or hyperenhanced on magnetic resonance imaging (termed late gadolinium enhancement). One limitation of the technique is when there is diffuse infiltration or fibrosis (e.g., amyloid), which will potentially be missed by cardiovascular magnetic resonance as only regional differences can be easily detected.

Late gadolinium enhancement is common in hypertrophic cardiomyopathy, occurring in up to 80% of individuals in one series.[67] Although the significance is not fully defined, the extent of late gadolinium enhancement and hence scarring is correlated with clinical risk markers for sudden death and progression to heart failure and is predictive of nonsustained ventricular tachycardia.[68,69] Clinically, extensive late gadolinium enhancement in young patients appears to be particularly adverse, and such a finding, particularly in individuals with one conventional risk factor for sudden death, may help with the difficult clinical decisions surrounding implantable cardioverter-defibrillator implantation.

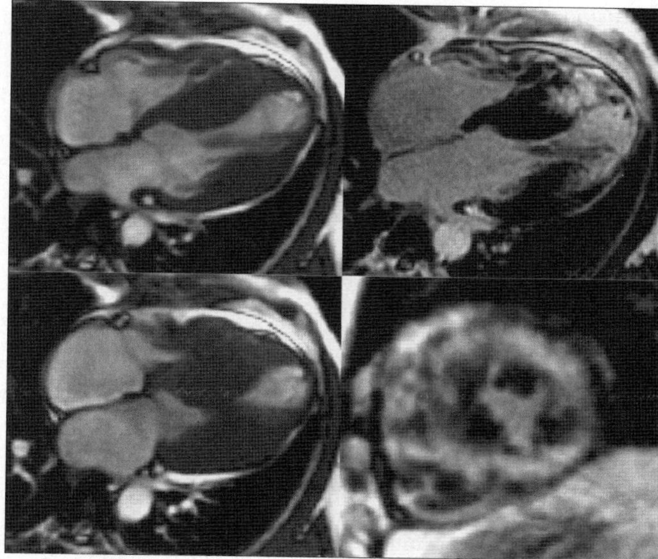

Figure 79.7 Cardiovascular magnetic resonance images. *Top left,* Diastolic four-chamber frame demonstrating left ventricular hypertrophy. *Bottom left,* Systolic view showing apical aneurysm. *Top right,* Late gadolinium four-chamber view. Normal myocardium (black) is seen in the basal nonhypertrophied areas; compare with the extensive late gadolinium enhancement (bright) in the hypertrophied ventricle and surrounding the apical aneurysm. *Bottom right,* Short-axis slice through the apical left ventricle with extensive late gadolinium enhancement.

Cardiac Catheterization

Cardiac catheterization has been superseded by echocardiography for the diagnosis of hypertrophic cardiomyopathy. The major use of cardiac catheterization is the exclusion of coronary atherosclerosis in older patients who have chest pain. In patients with left ventricular outflow tract obstruction, outflow pressure gradients can be measured by performing careful pressure monitoring during pullback across the aortic valve (Fig. 79.7) or by measuring simultaneous aortic and left ventricular inflow pressures through a transseptal puncture. Substantial outflow gradients may be associated with an early initial spike in the aortic pressure wave, followed by a secondary dome-shaped tidal wave before the dicrotic notch. In addition, the pulse pressure may be reduced in amplitude after an extrasystole, which reflects an increase in the outflow gradient during the potentiated post-extrasystolic beat (the Brockenbrough sign). Pulmonary capillary wedge pressure and left ventricular end-diastolic pressure are often increased in patients with and without outflow obstruction, but right atrial and right ventricular pressures are typically normal, except in patients with significant right ventricular outflow gradients or severe restrictive physiology. Resting cardiac output is usually normal or increased, except in patients who have advanced disease and systolic impairment.

In patients who have obstructive hypertrophic cardiomyopathy, left ventricular angiography may show a septal bulge encroaching on the left ventricular outflow tract during systole, together with systolic anterior motion of the anterior mitral valve leaflet and mitral regurgitation. In patients who have hypertrophy that is confined to the left ventricular apex, the ventricular angiogram may show a characteristic spade-shaped appearance in the right anterior oblique projection.

Radionuclide Studies

A number of studies using both planar and single-photon emission computed tomography thallium Tl 201 myocardial perfusion imaging have demonstrated a high prevalence of perfusion abnormalities in patients with hypertrophic cardiomyopathy.[70] Fixed perfusion defects are associated with increased left ventricular cavity dimensions, reduced shortening fraction, and lower peak exercise oxygen consumption, suggesting that they represent areas of myocardial fibrosis. The disparity between mild clinical symptoms and reversible perfusion defects may reflect some of the intrinsic limitations of single-photon imaging. Thallium 201 perfusion defects represent relative differences in myocardial uptake of ^{201}Tl, and it is possible for a relatively homogeneous reduction in coronary vasodilator reserve to remain undetected by qualitative analysis of ^{201}Tl perfusion images.

Positron emission tomography is theoretically superior to conventional single-photon imaging because of its greater resolution and its ability to quantify myocardial blood flow. Studies using nitrogen 13–labeled ammonia have demonstrated reduced coronary flow reserve during pharmacologic coronary vasodilatation in both hypertrophied and nonhypertrophied myocardium,[71] and some data indicate that symptomatic patients have lower mean coronary flow reserve than do patients without chest pain.

The relationship of myocardial blood flow abnormalities to myocardial metabolism has been investigated with use of fluorine 18–labeled deoxyglucose.[72] Areas of mismatch between blood flow and [^{18}F]deoxyglucose are believed to indicate the presence of ischemic myocardium; such areas have been described at rest and during exercise in some patients.

Cardiopulmonary Exercise Testing

Cardiopulmonary gas exchange responses during exercise can be used to provide an objective measure of functional capacity and to discriminate between respiratory and circulatory causes of exercise intolerance. Exercise testing in patients who have hypertrophic cardiomyopathy provides useful clinical data on symptoms, myocardial ischemia, vascular responses, and potential mechanisms of exercise intolerance. It may also be useful in the detection of rare metabolic causes of left ventricular hypertrophy. Studies in patients who have hypertrophic cardiomyopathy have demonstrated that most have reduced peak oxygen uptake and anaerobic threshold.[73]

Some patients have indirect evidence for impaired stroke volume response, the mechanism of which includes diastolic dysfunction, left ventricular outflow tract obstruction, and possibly chronotropic incompetence. A substantial number of patients have an as yet unexplained increased ventilatory equivalent for carbon dioxide during exercise. A similar response is observed in patients who have congestive cardiac failure; possible explanations include increased physiologic dead space, abnormal microvascular function, and abnormal respiratory stimulation. In addition to these "central" mechanisms for exercise limitation, there are data that suggest a role for abnormal peripheral oxygen kinetics in hypertrophic cardiomyopathy patients.

DIAGNOSTIC CRITERIA

Unexplained left ventricular hypertrophy that exceeds two standard deviations from the normal (typically more than 15 mm in adults) is usually sufficient for a diagnosis of hypertrophic cardiomyopathy to be made. In children and adolescents, the diagnosis can be more difficult because the complete phenotype may not be manifested in young "gene carriers." Even in adults, it is increasingly recognized that many have very mild clinical expression of the disease. Diagnostic criteria based on the principle of major and minor criteria have been proposed.[74] They are intended to apply only to relatives of patients who have unequivocal (clinically or genetically proven) hypertrophic cardiomyopathy, not to isolated cases of nondiagnostic electrocardiographic or echocardiographic abnormalities (Table 79.3).

Differentiation from Hypertensive Heart Disease

In the absence of a family history, the differentiation between hypertensive heart disease and hypertrophic cardiomyopathy can be problematic. Patients who have hypertrophic cardiomyopathy tend to have more severe hypertrophy than hypertensive patients do, and a maximal wall thickness of more than 20 mm in a white patient should always raise the suspicion of hypertrophic cardiomyopathy. Concentric hypertrophy is more frequent in hypertension, whereas asymmetric septal hypertrophy is more frequent in hypertrophic cardiomyopathy, but both of these patterns have low specificity. Systolic anterior motion of the mitral valve occurs in both diseases, but the combination of complete systolic anterior motion with a substantial left ventricular outflow gradient and asymmetric septal hypertrophy is highly suggestive of hypertrophic cardiomyopathy.

Athlete's Heart

The normal cardiovascular adaptation to regular physical training can make differentiation of "athlete's heart" from hypertrophic cardiomyopathy difficult. Although differentiation between this condition and hypertrophic cardiomyopathy may require a period of detraining for 3 to 6 months, there are a number of clinical features that can be used to separate pathologic hypertrophy from normal physiologic adaptation. A diagnosis of hypertrophic cardiomyopathy is favored by cardiovascular symptoms and a family history of hypertrophic cardiomyopathy and premature sudden death. The typical "athletic" electrocardiogram demonstrates voltage criteria for left ventricular hypertrophy, sinus bradycardia, and sinus arrhythmia, but Q waves, ST-segment depression, and deep T-wave inversion are rare and more suggestive of cardiomyopathy. Even the most intense athletic training is associated with only a modest increase in myocardial mass, with less than 2% of elite athletes having a wall thickness of more than 13 mm,[75] but as a substantial minority of patients with familial hypertrophic cardiomyopathy present with a wall thickness in the same range, objective differentiation between physiologic and pathologic left ventricular hypertrophy, solely based on echocardiographic or electrocardiographic criteria, may be problematic. In this situation, metabolic exercise testing may indicate the diagnosis through a significantly greater peak oxygen uptake and anaerobic threshold in athletes compared with individuals with familial hypertrophic cardiomyopathy.[76] Athletic hypertrophy is greatest in endurance sports such as rowing and cycling. Isometric activities alone do not appear to cause a substantial hypertrophic response. An increase in left ventricular cavity dimension with preserved systolic function is

PROPOSED DIAGNOSTIC CRITERIA FOR HYPERTROPHIC CARDIOMYOPATHY IN FIRST-DEGREE RELATIVES OF PATIENTS WITH UNEQUIVOCAL DISEASE	
Major Criteria	**Minor Criteria**
Echocardiography	
Left ventricular wall thickness ≥13 mm in the anterior septum or posterior wall or ≥15 mm in the posterior septum or free wall Severe systolic anterior motion of the mitral valve	Left ventricular wall thickness of 12 mm in the anterior septum or posterior wall or 14 mm in the posterior septum or free wall Moderate systolic anterior motion of the mitral valve (no leaflet-septum contact) Redundant mitral valve leaflets
Electrocardiography	
Left ventricular hypertrophy and repolarization changes	Complete bundle branch block or (minor) interventricular conduction defects (in left ventricular leads)
T-wave inversion in leads I and aVL (≥3 mm with QRS-T axis discordance ≥30 degrees), in leads V_3-V_6 (≥3 mm), or in leads II, III, and aVF (≥5 mm)	Minor repolarization changes in left ventricular leads
Abnormal Q waves (>40 ms or >25% of R wave) in at least two leads of II, III, aVF (in the absence of left anterior hemiblock), V_1-V_4, or in leads I, aVL, V_5, and V_6	Deep S wave (>25 mm) in lead V_2 Unexplained syncope, chest pain, or dyspnea

Some patients with hypertrophic cardiomyopathy do not fulfill "conventional" diagnostic criteria for the disease. In this scheme, a diagnosis of hypertrophic cardiomyopathy in first-degree relatives of patients with the disease could be made in the presence of one major criterion, or two minor echocardiographic criteria, or one minor echocardiographic plus two minor electrocardiographic criteria.
With permission from McKenna WJ, Spirito P, Desnos M, Dubourg O, Komajda M. Experience from clinical genetics in hypertrophic cardiomyopathy: proposal for new diagnostic criteria in adult members of affected families. Heart 1997;77:130-132.© BMJ Publishing Group.

Table 79.3 Proposed diagnostic criteria for hypertrophic cardiomyopathy in first-degree relatives of patients with unequivocal disease.

more typical of an athlete, in contrast to the small, hyperdynamic ventricles seen in hypertrophic cardiomyopathy. Left atrial enlargement can occur in some athletes, but this reflects an increase in preload and is not associated with diastolic dysfunction.

Hypertrophic Cardiomyopathy in the Elderly

Idiopathic left ventricular hypertrophy similar to that seen in familial hypertrophic cardiomyopathy may present in middle-aged patients.[77] Compared with younger patients, such individuals tend to have milder hypertrophy localized to the anterior interventricular septum and a more ovoid or ellipsoid left ventricular cavity than the more typical crescentic shape seen in younger patients.

Several hypotheses have been proposed to explain hypertrophic cardiomyopathy in the elderly. Hypertension is more frequent in the elderly population, but the lack of any major differences in left ventricular morphology in hypertensive and nonhypertensive patients with hypertrophic cardiomyopathy suggests that it is not an important factor. A characteristic feature in elderly patients is the increased angulation of the aorta with respect to the long axis of the left ventricle. It is suggested that this, together with some shrinkage of the heart, results in the upper septal bulge and in narrowing of the outflow tract sufficient to cause obstruction.

Systematic pedigree analysis is limited in most series of elderly patients, but the available data suggest that less than 13% of patients have a family history of hypertrophic cardiomyopathy, compared with more than 50% of younger patients. As discussed earlier, a proportion of patients with late-onset disease have mutations in cardiac myosin–binding protein C.[78]

COMPLICATIONS

The most important complication of hypertrophic cardiomyopathy is sudden death or death after heart failure or stroke. The reported incidence of sudden death varies from less than 1% in "nonreferral" annual populations to more than 4% in some early tertiary referral center studies. The risk of sudden death is greatest in patients who present in childhood or adolescence. It is believed that the major mechanism of sudden death is ventricular arrhythmia. However, sudden death from conduction disease is also recognized, although its precise frequency is uncertain. Untreated atrial fibrillation is associated with a 4% annual risk of systemic emboli, particularly in patients with left atrial enlargement. Patients with outflow tract obstruction or mitral regurgitation are at increased risk for infective endocarditis and should receive conventional antibiotic prophylaxis before surgical and dental procedures.

SYMPTOMATIC THERAPY

Figure 79.8 shows a working algorithm for the treatment of symptomatic patients. In general, treatment is more successful in patients who have symptoms attributable to left ventricular outflow tract obstruction than it is in patients who have the nonobstructive form of the disease. The essential principle of treatment is that therapy should be targeted, when possible, to the likely mechanism of symptoms.

Left Ventricular Outflow Tract Obstruction

The medical treatment of obstructive hypertrophic cardiomyopathy is largely empirical, mostly depending on the patient's subjective perception of symptomatic benefit.

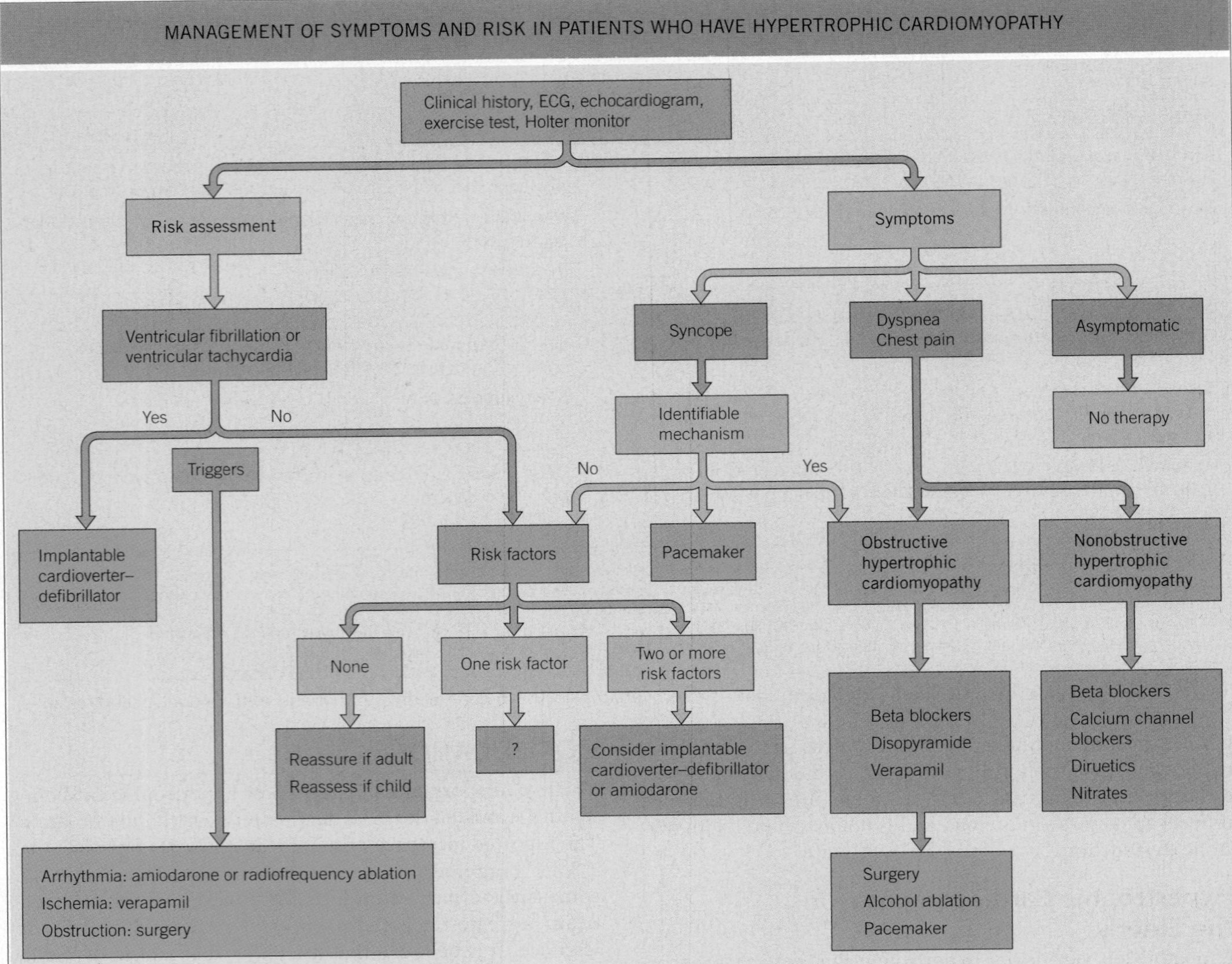

Figure 79.8 Suggested management of symptoms and risk in patients who have hypertrophic cardiomyopathy.

Despite the lack of controlled data, beta blockers are the first-line treatment in symptomatic patients with hypertrophic cardiomyopathy, particularly if they have provocable outflow gradients. Verapamil can also be an effective treatment of outflow obstruction, but it occasionally precipitates dramatic worsening of symptoms and hemodynamic compromise. If verapamil is used, it should always be commenced at low doses under medical supervision. Disopyramide has been evaluated more systematically and is effective in gradient reduction and symptom relief because of its negative inotropic properties, but its anticholinergic side effects may be limiting in elderly patients and its beneficial effects may not persist.[79] However, it is best used in combination with a beta blocker because disopyramide alone may accelerate atrioventricular node conduction, with the potential risk of rapid ventricular rates occurring. Cibenzoline, another class I antiarrhythmic agent with fewer anticholinergic effects, has been shown to be effective in reducing gradients and improving symptoms.[80] When medical treatment fails to relieve obstructive symptoms, there are three treatment options:

- surgery;
- dual-chamber atrioventricular sequential pacing; and
- injection of alcohol into the septal perforator branches of the left anterior descending artery.

Surgery

Surgery has been throughout the past 40 years and still remains the "gold standard" for patients with hypertrophic cardiomyopathy who have refractory symptoms and outflow tract gradients greater than 50 mm Hg. Numerous studies have demonstrated that correctly performed myotomy or myectomy (Morrow procedure) of the interventricular septum relieves symptoms and improves exercise capacity in more than 70% of cases.[81] In addition, long-term survival is returned to that of the general population and is improved compared with obstructive hypertrophic cardiomyopathy without operation.[82] Most modern series suggest that the mortality risk of the procedure is 1% or less, and preoperative transesophageal echocardiography has made complications of the procedure, such as ventricular septal defects and complete heart block, increasingly rare. Postoperative left bundle branch block is common, and many patients develop trivial aortic regurgitation. The traditional myectomy has been adapted to include more extensive mobilization of the papillary muscles.[83] A study of myectomy patients with postoperative echocardiography has demonstrated a significant reduction in septal and free wall thickness, a reduction in systolic anterior motion of the mitral valve, and an increase in left ventricular end-diastolic dimensions.[84]

Mitral valve replacement also relieves outflow obstruction, but it does so at the cost of increased operative and long-term complications. Mitral valve replacement should be considered only if patients have other intrinsic abnormalities of the mitral valve.

Dual-Chamber Atrioventricular Sequential Pacing

In some patients, dual-chamber pacing results in a reduction in the peak gradient, possibly by altering the activation sequence of the interventricular septum. Data on its clinical efficacy are contradictory, but several randomized crossover clinical trials have demonstrated that subjective symptomatic benefit and reduction of outflow gradient during pacing were not accompanied by objective evidence of improved exercise capacity. There was also evidence for a substantial placebo effect.[85,86] However, there was a subset of elderly patients (older than 65 years) who experienced objective clinical benefit with pacing, so that this treatment modality might at least be a therapeutic alternative for this subgroup, particularly as these patients may not be candidates for surgery because of their frequent comorbidities.[79] For pacing to work at all, the ventricle must be maximally preexcited, and it is argued that some pacing failures relate to the presence of short native atrioventricular delays that preclude physiologically beneficial programmed atrioventricular delays because of their detrimental effect on left ventricular filling. This may be overcome by pharmacologic slowing of intrinsic atrioventricular node conduction with beta blockers and calcium channel blockers or by radiofrequency ablation of the atrioventricular node.

Percutaneous Transluminal Septal Myocardial Ablation

Another approach to obstructive hypertrophic cardiomyopathy is to create a localized septal infarction by selective injection of alcohol into one or more of the septal perforator branches of the left anterior descending artery (Fig. 79.9). The main effects of this procedure are necrosis and thereby a thinning of the basal septal wall thickness, an enlargement of left ventricular outflow tract, and an elimination of systolic anterior motion and outflow obstruction.

Subsequent complications relate to inadvertent leakage of alcohol into the left anterior descending artery, extensive myocardial infarction, and occurrence of greater degrees of atrioventricular block that persist in up to 10% to 22%, requiring permanent pacemaker implantation. These limitations can be minimized by the peri-interventional use of contrast echocardiography. This ensures accurate delivery of the alcohol to the correct area of myocardium.[87] In contrast to surgery, alcohol ablation is associated with the development of right bundle branch block in most patients. Published data suggest that the technique is generally safe and that it can relieve outflow tract obstruction and improve symptoms to a similar degree as myotomy-myectomy, although a study demonstrated surgery to be superior in gradient reduction.[88] Initial long-term follow-up data indicate that reduction of septal thickness and outflow gradient reduction are continuous processes during the first 3 to 6 months.[89] Hence, reablation or alternative treatments should not be considered until at least 3 months after the initial procedure.

As yet, progressive ventricular dilatation and late arrhythmic complications have not been described. However, lack of long-term follow-up has led most authorities to suggest avoidance of alcohol in young patients.

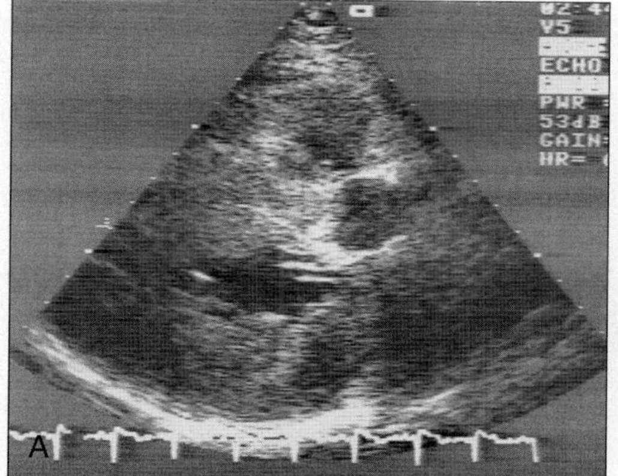

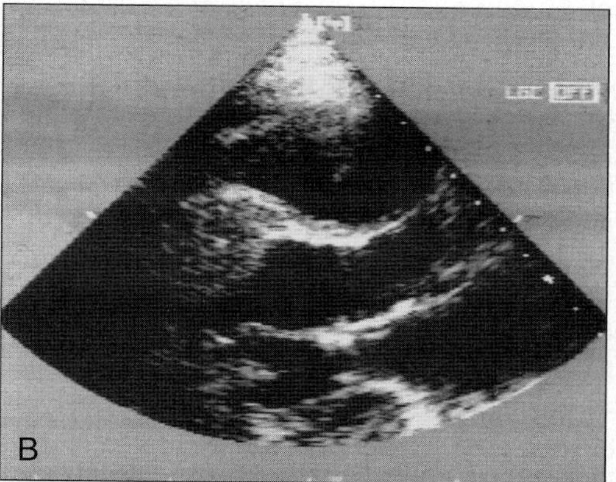

Figure 79.9 Selective coronary injection of alcohol in hypertrophic cardiomyopathy. A, Parasternal, long-axis, two-dimensional echocardiogram demonstrating severe concentric left ventricular hypertrophy and systolic anterior motion of the mitral valve in a severely symptomatic patient with hypertrophic cardiomyopathy and an outflow tract gradient of 120 mm Hg. **B,** Parasternal, long-axis, two-dimensional echocardiogram from the same patient 3 months after selective coronary injection of alcohol. There is dramatic localized thinning of the anterior septum, similar to that seen after septal myectomy. This was associated with a reduction in outflow gradient to less than 30 mm Hg, a reduction in left atrial size, and an improvement in symptoms.

Nonobstructive Hypertrophic Cardiomyopathy

There are few prospective data on medical treatment of patients who do not have left ventricular outflow tract obstruction. Calcium channel blockers and beta blockers may be effective in relieving chest pain and dyspnea, and in patients with high filling pressures, judicious diuretic treatment may also relieve congestive symptoms. Nitrates have not been extensively evaluated in patients who have hypertrophic cardiomyopathy, and they are contraindicated in patients with obstruction. Nevertheless, they can be effective in patients who have troublesome angina and breathlessness. Patients who go on to develop ventricular dilatation and wall thinning should be treated with conventional vasodilator-diuretic combinations.

Cardiac transplantation should be considered only in patients who have end-stage congestive cardiac failure or severe refractory restrictive physiology.

Supraventricular Arrhythmia

In some patients who have hypertrophic cardiomyopathy, rapid atrial fibrillation can provoke hemodynamic deterioration and even sudden death. It is also associated with a significant risk of thromboembolism. When atrial fibrillation provokes severe clinical deterioration, urgent direct current cardioversion is required. Cardioversion is also the treatment of choice in patients who have new-onset atrial fibrillation without hemodynamic deterioration.

Persistent atrial fibrillation can be tolerated in the long term if the ventricular response is controlled, but because it is associated with an increased risk of systemic thromboembolism in all patients with persistent or paroxysmal atrial fibrillation, anticoagulation should be initiated.[47] Amiodarone is effective in preventing recurrences, and beta blockers with or without class III activity and calcium channel blockers may also be useful for controlling the rate. The role of class I agents in preventing atrial fibrillation in hypertrophic cardiomyopathy has not been studied in any systematic manner. In some very rare circumstances, rate control may be achieved only by atrioventricular nodal ablation and pacemaker treatment.

PREVENTION OF SUDDEN DEATH AND RISK FACTOR STRATIFICATION

The identification and treatment of patients with hypertrophic cardiomyopathy who are at risk of sudden death remain a clinical challenge; the diverse disease phenotype has meant that the experience of sudden death and the views on its prevention can vary between centers. There is general agreement that patients who have already experienced sustained ventricular arrhythmia are at significant risk of sudden death, with a greater than 30% chance of recurrence in the 7 years after their initial event.[90] In some patients, it may be possible to identify a potentially treatable trigger for ventricular arrhythmia, such as supraventricular arrhythmia or myocardial ischemia. However, the more typical situation is one in which no obvious trigger can be identified. Evidence indicates that the medium-term outlook for patients who have a history of cardiac arrest or syncopal ventricular tachycardia and who are treated with an implantable cardioverter-defibrillator is good, and this should now be the treatment of choice.[91] The management of patients who do not have a history of sustained ventricular arrhythmia is more controversial. All patients should undergo a noninvasive risk stratification assessment, including clinical history, two-dimensional echocardiography, Holter monitoring, and maximal exercise testing.[92-94] Several clinical features are established as markers of an increased risk of premature sudden cardiac death (see Table 79.3).[19,50,66,95]

Recent evidence suggests that patients with two or more risk factors are at sufficiently high risk to warrant consideration of prophylactic antiarrhythmic therapy. In patients with only a single risk factor, clinical decision making is more difficult as most risk markers have only a modest positive predictive accuracy when they occur in isolation. Until more data are available, treatment in this group is determined largely by the strength of the given risk factor.

At present, there are only two options for treatment, namely, amiodarone and implantation of a cardioverter-defibrillator. However, neither has been prospectively evaluated in a randomized fashion in patients who have the disease. In a study of two consecutive age- and sex-matched populations with nonsustained ventricular tachycardia,[96] patients who were treated with low-dose amiodarone had a significantly lower rate of sudden death than did patients treated with "conventional" antiarrhythmic drugs (predominantly disopyramide) (Fig. 79.10). In the case of implantable cardioverter-defibrillators, a study has reported appropriate discharge rates of 11% per annum in patients with a history of sustained ventricular arrhythmia and 5% in patients with risk factors for sudden cardiac death but no history of sustained ventricular tachycardia and fibrillation.[74] Given the superior effect of the implantable cardioverter-defibrillator compared with amiodarone in multicenter studies in patients with ischemic heart disease and heart failure, most authorities

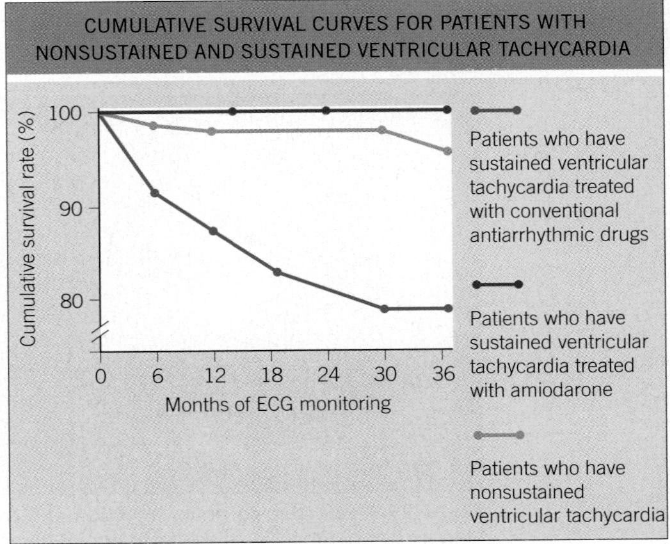

Figure 79.10 Cumulative survival curves for patients with nonsustained and sustained ventricular tachycardia. (Modified with permission from McKenna WJ, Oakley CM, Krikler DM, et al. Improved survival with amiodarone in patients with hypertrophic cardiomyopathy and ventricular tachycardia. Br Heart J 1985;53:412-416.)

generally agree that patients with several clinical risk factors should be considered for implantable cardioverter-defibrillator therapy. In the absence of prospective randomized trials, the choice of treatment in patients with only a single risk factor is determined by the clinical context and by the opinions of the patient and the physician.

Pregnancy

The hemodynamic adaptations associated with pregnancy might be assumed to pose increased risk. In fact, serious complications and mortality are rare.[97] However, caution should be applied in use of drugs with cardioactive properties during pregnancy and labor. In addition, conventional epidural anesthesia causes peripheral vasodilatation with a theoretical risk, especially in the presence of left ventricular outflow tract obstruction.

SUMMARY

In the past few decades, the concept of hypertrophic cardiomyopathy as a disease typified by asymmetric hypertrophy and outflow tract obstruction has evolved to that of a family of predominantly genetically determined disorders. The genetic heterogeneity of the disease is matched by a remarkable spectrum of pathophysiologic and clinical manifestations that make hypertrophic cardiomyopathy one of the most capricious of all cardiac disorders. In spite of this, certain basic principles can be used to guide treatment in patients who have the disease, and although the clinical algorithms available at present are far from perfect, the pace of current work in this fascinating field augurs well for the future.

chapter

80 Special Problems in Myocarditis and Cardiomyopathy

a. Peripartum Cardiomyopathy

Afshan Hameed and Uri Elkayam

DEFINITION OF PROBLEM

Peripartum cardiomyopathy (PPCM) is a rare form of cardiomyopathy of uncertain etiology with potential life-threatening consequences in women of childbearing age. Criteria for the diagnosis of PPCM are listed in Table 80A.1. Although the majority of patients with PPCM are diagnosed during the last month of pregnancy or the first postpartum month, a significant number of cases are diagnosed as early as the third month of gestation (Fig. 80A.1). The incidence of PPCM varies among geographic regions and has recently been estimated to be about 1:3000 to 4000 in the United States, 1:1000 in South Africa, and as high as 1:300 in Haiti.

TYPICAL CASE

A 25-year-old primigravida presented at 38 weeks of gestation with a 1-month history of shortness of breath and dyspnea on exertion after walking a few steps. She was found to be in pulmonary edema. The patient did not have a previous history of cardiac disease. An echocardiogram revealed left ventricular (LV) dilatation and dysfunction with an ejection fraction of 24%. After optimization of medical therapy, she underwent a cesarean delivery of a female infant weighing 2915 g with Apgar scores of 8 and 9 without complications.

After delivery, the patient underwent a complete work-up, including cardiac catheterization and right ventricular endomyocardial biopsy. Cardiac catheterization revealed normal coronary arteries with moderate LV dysfunction, and the biopsy results were inconclusive. A repeated evaluation of LV function 1 month later by multiple gated acquisition scan revealed normal LV size and function and an ejection fraction of 62%.

ETIOLOGY

The cause of PPCM remains unknown. Risk factors include advancing age, multiparity, African descent, multiple gestation, hypertension, and use of tocolytic therapy.

An unusual form of prolactin (16 kDa) in the maternal circulation has recently been linked to the development of cardiomyopathy in mice. Other studies suggest an immunologic basis to the disease, and high titers of autoantibodies against select cardiac tissue proteins have been described in these patients. In addition, elevated levels of inflammatory cytokines, such as C-reactive protein, tumor necrosis factor α, interleukin 6, and soluble Fas receptors (an apoptosis signaling receptor), are thought to play a role in the pathogenesis of PPCM. Abnormalities of the hormone relaxin leading to excessive relaxation of cardiac muscle with resultant myocardial dysfunction have also been implicated.

PATHOLOGY

Specimens from patients with PPCM usually demonstrate dilatation of the heart and myocardial pallor. Ventricular thrombi are often seen. Endocardial thickening and pericardial fluid have been noted occasionally. Biopsy specimens have demonstrated interstitial edema and occasionally lymphocytic infiltration. The role of endocardial biopsy in PPCM for diagnosis and treatment is limited.

CLINICAL PRESENTATION

The signs and symptoms of PPCM are typical for a patient with heart failure. Commonly described symptoms include dyspnea, which is nearly a universal finding. In addition, orthopnea, decreased exercise tolerance, cough, hemoptysis, and leg edema are frequently encountered. Nonspecific fatigue, palpitations, chest pain, and abdominal pain are common and usually tend to confuse the initial clinical presentation. On occasion, thromboembolism may be the only presenting feature.

Physical examination often reveals tachycardia, increased jugular venous pressure, cardiomegaly, right ventricular heave, and third heart sound in addition to mitral and tricuspid regurgitation, pulmonary rales, and peripheral edema.

Routine evaluation includes 12-lead electrocardiography, chest radiography, and M-mode and two-dimensional Doppler echocardiography. The electrocardiogram usually demonstrates sinus tachycardia with nonspecific ST-segment and T-wave abnormalities. The PR and QRS intervals may be prolonged, suggesting intraventricular conduction delay and occasionally bundle branch block.

CRITERIA FOR DIAGNOSIS OF PERIPARTUM CARDIOMYOPATHY
Development of cardiac failure during pregnancy or within 6 months of delivery
Absence of determinable cause of cardiac failure
Demonstrable impairment of left ventricular ejection fraction <45%

Table 80A. 1 Criteria for diagnosis of peripartum cardiomyopathy.

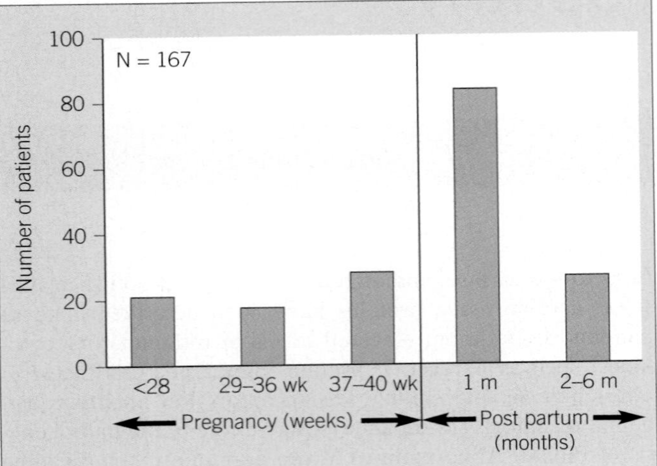

Figure 80A.1 Time at presentation of peripartum cardiomyopathy in 167 women. (Modified from Elkayam U, Akhter MW, Singh H, et al. Pregnancy-associated cardiomyopathy. Clinical characteristics and a comparison between early and late presentation. Circulation 2005;111:2050-2055; and Elkayam U, Tummala PP, Rao K, et al. Maternal and fetal outcomes of subsequent pregnancies in women with peripartum cardiomyopathy. N Engl J Med 2001;344:1567-1571.)

Chest radiography invariably shows cardiomegaly. In addition, pulmonary venous congestion, bilateral basilar infiltrates, and small pleural effusions are commonly seen.

Echocardiography usually shows LV dilatation and impairment of systolic performance. Right ventricular and bilateral atrial enlargements as well as mitral and tricuspid regurgitation are often found.

Characteristic hemodynamic abnormalities include markedly elevated right and left ventricular filling pressures, moderate pulmonary hypertension, increased systemic and pulmonary vascular resistance, and decreased stroke volume and cardiac output.

THERAPY

Medical therapy for PPCM is similar to that for other forms of congestive heart failure and includes sodium restriction and the use of diuretics, beta blockers, vasodilators, and digoxin. Angiotensin-converting enzyme inhibitors are contraindicated in pregnancy because of the fetal risks of renal failure, oligohydramnios, pulmonary hypoplasia, and demise. These agents, however, should be used after delivery until LV function normalizes. Whenever vasodilator therapy is required, hydralazine and organic nitrates are the combination of choice. Beta blockers have been shown to improve survival in cardiomyopathy patients, and it is reasonable to consider beta-blocker therapy in patients with PPCM after initial treatment of volume overload. Digoxin is beneficial for its inotropic effects and rate control in cases of atrial fibrillation and is considered safe during pregnancy and lactation. Because of the high incidence of thromboembolic events, anticoagulants should be strongly considered at the time of diagnosis and may be continued until normalization of LV function. There is emerging evidence of the benefit of bromocriptine therapy in patients with PPCM. This therapy remains experimental, however. The benefit of immunosuppressive therapy is questionable and is not recommended. As PPCM is often reversible, the temporary use of an intra-aortic balloon pump or LV assist device may aid in stabilizing patients until recovery of LV function. Cardiac transplantation has been performed successfully. This procedure should be considered in patients who continue to deteriorate or remain severely symptomatic beyond a few months post partum.

PROGNOSIS

Approximately 50% of patients have marked improvement in LV function and clinical symptoms. Recovery usually occurs within 6 months from the time of initial diagnosis. Death or heart transplantation has been reported in approximately 20% of patients with PPCM. Prognosis seems to be related to the severity of LV dilatation and dysfunction and evidence of myocardial damage at the time of diagnosis, lack of recovery at 2 to 6 months post partum, and African race.

EFFECT OF SUBSEQUENT PREGNANCY

Subsequent pregnancy in patients who have a history of PPCM may result in recurrence of LV dysfunction (Fig. 80A.2) and symptomatic heart failure even if there

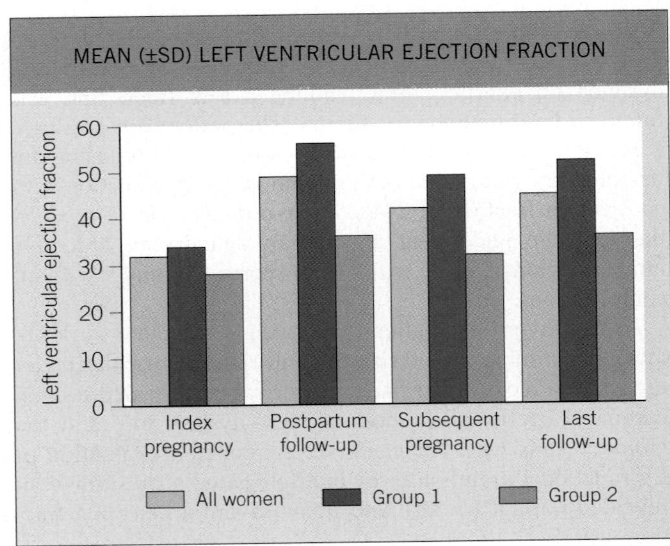

Figure 80A.2 Toxic cardiomyopathy, cancer drugs, and Herceptin mean (+SD) left ventricular ejection fraction. Left ventricular ejection fractions in 44 women at the time of the diagnosis of peripartum cardiomyopathy (index pregnancy), at postpartum follow-up, during the first subsequent pregnancy, and at the last follow-up a mean of 72 months after the subsequent pregnancy. (With permission from Elkayam U, Tummala PP, Rao K, et al. Maternal and fetal outcomes of subsequent pregnancies in women with peripartum cardiomyopathy. N Engl J Med 2001;344:1567-1571.)

has been normalization of cardiac function after the initial cardiomyopathic episode. An additional pregnancy is especially risky in patients who have persistent LV dysfunction. More than 50% of such patients have been reported to have heart failure during their subsequent pregnancy, with a mortality rate of up to 25%. In addition, there is a significantly higher risk of premature deliveries and therapeutic abortions. This group of patients should therefore be strongly counseled against future pregnancies.

b. Chagas' Heart Disease

Harry Acquatella

DEFINITION OF PROBLEM

Chagas' heart disease affects approximately 18 million people in Latin America, where it causes approximately 45,000 deaths annually.[1] Cases in the United States and in Europe usually occur in individuals who have lived in or emigrated from Latin America.[2] Most of these people are of low socioeconomic status and had lived in poor housing conditions in which Triatomine bugs (from the family Reduviidae) transmit the protozoan flagellate *Trypanosoma cruzi* to animals or humans. Trypanosomes present in bug feces penetrate through the skin into the bloodstream to invade the heart and other tissues. The infection is unrecognized in most patients, but it may also occur after blood transfusion, with transplantation, by congenital transmission, or by oral ingestion.[3] Chagas' disease has an acute and chronic form.[3-5] The acute form is rare and may present as an acute myopericarditis.[5] Chronic cardiac manifestations may appear after a long period of several decades (latent or undifferentiated form); the majority remain asymptomatic, whereas about one quarter become symptomatic.[2,4,6,7]

TYPICAL CASE

A 45-year-old man consults his physician because of irregular heartbeats. Physical examination findings are normal. On electrocardiography, premature ventricular contractions, right bundle branch block, and abnormal ST-T segment elevation on left precordial leads can be seen (Fig. 80B.1). The patient had lived during his infancy in a country in which Chagas' disease is highly endemic in rural areas. Routine laboratory test results were within normal limits. Serologic test results were positive for Chagas' disease. Two-dimensional echocardiography disclosed mild left ventricular dilatation, a small left ventricular apical aneurysm, and a slightly diminished ejection fraction (Fig. 80B.2). Holter monitoring for 24 hours disclosed intermittent first-degree atrioventricular block, multifocal premature ventricular contractions, and short runs of ventricular tachycardia. Coronary angiography was normal.

DIFFERENTIAL DIAGNOSIS

The acute form may be expressed clinically after 1 to 4 weeks of the infection, usually in childhood. Symptoms include fever, malaise, edema, lymph node enlargement, sweating, tachycardia, extrasystoles, and hepatosplenomegaly. In those having cardiac involvement, pericardial effusion appears in more than half of the cases,[5] occasionally leading to tamponade. By echocardiography, ventricular dimensions and systolic function are normal in most.[7] In those developing cardiomegaly and systolic dysfunction, the prognosis is ominous. Most patients recover spontaneously without the infection's being recognized.[4] After several decades, the chronic form of Chagas' disease may be expressed clinically; the described case is an example of such a usual presentation.[2,4,6,8]

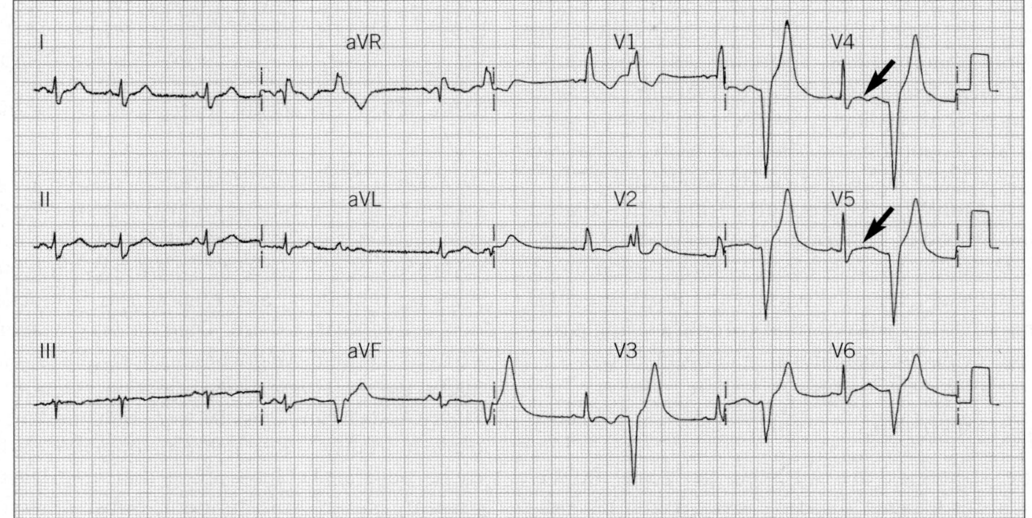

Figure 80B.1 Electrocardiogram in Chagas' disease. Note right bundle branch block, ventricular bigeminy, and convex upward ST-T segment elevation in leads V_3 to V_5, suggestive of a left ventricular aneurysm.

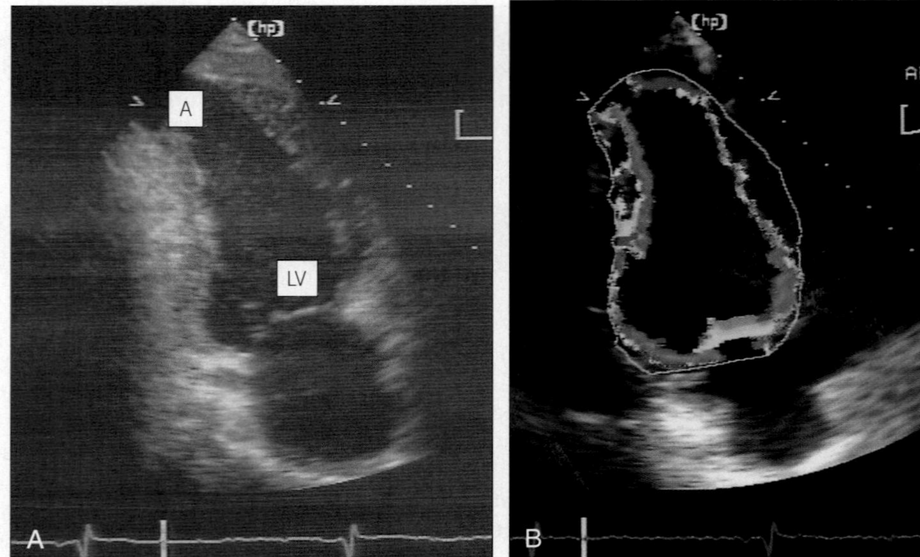

Figure 80B.2 End-systolic two-chamber left ventricular apical echocardiogram in Chagas' disease. A, A narrow-necked left ventricular apical aneurysm can be seen. A, apical aneurysm; LV, left ventricle. **B,** The same view with color kinesis. The normal inward systolic motion of the left ventricular wall is displayed in blue-green, and the apical dyskinesis is displayed in red.

The diagnosis of Chagas' disease rests on epidemiologic features, serologic test results, and clinical findings. Symptoms occur in about 30% of seropositive persons. Cardiac manifestations predominate, but in southern countries of South America, digestive symptoms (megaorgans) may also appear.[2] Complaints are of arrhythmias, fatigue, heart failure, chest pain, and systemic or pulmonary embolic phenomena. Although many patients present with evidence of ventricular arrhythmias and atrioventricular and intraventricular conduction defects, as did the patient described, others may present with a picture of dilated cardiomyopathy with biventricular heart failure. A combination of electrocardiographic findings highly suggestive of Chagas' disease includes right bundle branch block or left anterior hemiblock (each seen in about 40% of cases), or both; ventricular arrhythmias (seen in more than 80%); abnormal ST-segment elevation and T-wave inversion on precordial electrocardiographic leads (seen in 30%); and various degrees of atrioventricular block. Left ventricular apical contraction abnormalities, including left ventricular aneurysms and dilated, poorly contracting ventricles, are seen on two-dimensional echocardiography.[7] Nearly 70% of seropositive people are asymptomatic, and half of these have a normal electrocardiogram and a normal life expectancy.[2,4,6,8]

Chagas' disease should be differentiated from other dilated cardiomyopathic processes of hypertensive, ischemic, or primary origin. Left bundle branch block is more common in these disorders. Because Chagas' disease may cause segmental wall motion abnormalities with normal coronaries, angiography should be performed when clinical uncertainty exists.

TREATMENT OPTIONS

The therapeutic strategies are outlined in Table 80B.1. Specific treatment for Chagas' disease (benznidazole) is indicated in acute Chagas' disease with or without cardiac manifestations.[2] The role of treatment in the latent phase and once clinical cardiac involvement exists is at present under discussion. It appears to diminish disease progression without significantly affecting mortality.[9] Treatment of the chronic cardiac disease is palliative and is directed to the individual manifestations of the disease.[10] Diuretics, angiotensin-converting enzyme inhibitors, and angiotensin II blockers can improve congestive heart failure. Digoxin may exacerbate ventricular arrhythmias and conduction abnormalities. Lack of β-blocking agent use, left ventricular ejection fraction, and New York Heart Association Class IV were independent predictors of all-cause mortality.[11] Resynchronization devices have been shown to be beneficial. Once severe left ventricular dysfunction is present, the prognosis is poor. Substantial survival improvement has been obtained by cardiac transplantation. Parasiticidal treatment in the host before and frequently after the graft is necessary to avoid acute myocarditis.

THERAPEUTIC STRATEGIES IN CHAGAS' HEART DISEASE	
Antiparasitic drugs: benznidazole or nifurtimox	Acute Chagas' disease Disease reactivation in immune suppressed patients (transplantation, cancer chemotherapy, AIDS)
Symptomatic ventricular arrhythmias	Empiric amiodarone or drug selection by programmed electrical stimulation
Atrial fibrillation	Amiodarone, electric cardioversion Surgical or catheter ablation
Heart failure symptoms	Angiotensin-converting enzyme inhibitors, angiotensin II blockers, spironolactone, beta blockers Low salt, diuretics, warfarin Heart transplantation Pacemaker in symptomatic bradyarrhythmias and conduction abnormalities Resynchronization, automatic-internal-cardioverter-defibrillator

Table 80B. 1 Therapeutic strategies in Chagas' heart disease.

Arrhythmias and sudden death are common. Low-dose amiodarone is the agent of choice, often resulting in a high and sustained rate of suppression of ventricular couplets and tachycardia. Class I antiarrhythmic drugs may induce proarrhythmic effects (including torsades de pointes) and depress contractility. Implantable cardioverter-defibrillator, ablation, or aneurysmectomy may be considered when malignant ventricular arrhythmias become drug resistant. Pacemaker implantation for symptomatic conduction disturbances is associated with improved survival except in subjects with low left ventricular function.[10]

SUMMARY

This patient had typical clinical, electrocardiographic, and echocardiographic findings of chronic Chagas' heart disease as well as the common difficulties encountered in treatment before development of heart failure or sudden death.

c. Diabetic Cardiomyopathy

Thomas H. Marwick

DEFINITION OF PROBLEM

Diabetic cardiomyopathy is the term used to describe patients with diabetes mellitus who have established heart failure with normal coronary arteries and without other known causes. However, this picture represents end-stage disease, is indistinguishable from any other nonischemic cardiomyopathy, and has the same treatment implications with inhibitors of the renin-angiotensin and sympathetic systems.

It seems likely that effective prevention of end-stage diabetic cardiomyopathy will require identification and treatment of the subclinical stage (American College of Cardiology/American Heart Association stage B). Typically, patients with early diabetic primary myocardial disease are described as being asymptomatic, but in fact many patients have exercise intolerance (usually dyspnea). The clinical challenge relates to the attribution of this exercise intolerance in a patient with type 2 diabetes to primary myocardial disease because these patients have multiple comorbid conditions that may in part explain their symptoms. These include obesity as well as concerns about the possibility of coronary artery disease leading to dyspnea as an angina equivalent.

TYPICAL CASE

The typical presentation is in a middle-aged to elderly patient, more commonly female, with obesity (body mass index >30) and type 2 diabetes, often with poor glycemic control. Typically, the patient complains of exertional dyspnea, usually functional class 2, perhaps with some orthopnea, but it would be unusual to present with acute pulmonary edema at this early stage in the disease. The patient may complain of chest tightness associated with dyspnea, but the symptoms are inconsistent with typical angina. The physical examination shows the patient to be overweight or obese, with a borderline blood pressure (e.g., 150/90 mm Hg), a pulse rate of 72, and no clinical signs of heart failure. The resting electrocardiogram is normal.

DIFFERENTIAL DIAGNOSIS

The differential diagnosis of diabetic myocardial dysfunction in this situation includes hypertensive heart disease, coronary artery disease, obesity, and chronic lung disease. The investigation of choice is echocardiography, often with exercise echocardiography.

The typical resting echocardiographic findings are shown in Figure 80C.1. The patient could be expected to have a normal ejection fraction, no regional wall motion abnormalities, perhaps borderline left ventricular hypertrophy with normal left ventricular mass due to a small left ventricular cavity, and no evidence of valve disease. The diastolic measurements show delayed relaxation and may have evidence of increased filling pressure (e.g., mild left atrial enlargement and increased ratio of early transmitral velocity [E] to tissue diastolic velocity [E′]). Often, only E′ is reduced, consistent with abnormal myocardial diastolic performance.

Disturbances of diastolic function in diabetic subjects are common; some reports document their presence in 50% to 75% of apparently healthy patients. Abnormalities of myocardial performance, measured by tissue velocity and deformation (Fig. 80C.2), have been documented in 25% to 30% of patients. It is unclear whether these are more specific for patients who deteriorate or respond to medical therapy.

Whereas an ordinary treadmill exercise test offers the benefit of documenting the reduction of exercise capacity, the performance of exercise echocardiography adds useful information to the evaluation of these patients, despite the absence of angina. There are two reasons for this. First, the test excludes the presence and contribution of ischemia. Dyspnea is a frequent presenting symptom of coronary artery disease and should be considered an angina equivalent for the purpose of assessing pretest probability of coronary artery disease and suitability for noninvasive testing. Second, the calculation of exercise E/E′ can be used to document an increment of filling pressure with exercise, reflecting an increase in left atrial pressure without an increment in myocardial diastolic velocity. Although the resting echocardiographic parameters may identify left ventricular filling problems and abnormal myocardial properties, evidence of raised filling pressure with exercise makes it likely that the diastolic findings are a cause of exercise intolerance rather than a coincidental finding (Fig. 80C.3).

TREATMENT OPTIONS

The treatment steps for advanced diabetic cardiomyopathy are the same as those for patients with heart failure of any other etiology.

For early diabetic heart disease, probably the most important general step is to improve glycemic control. Although

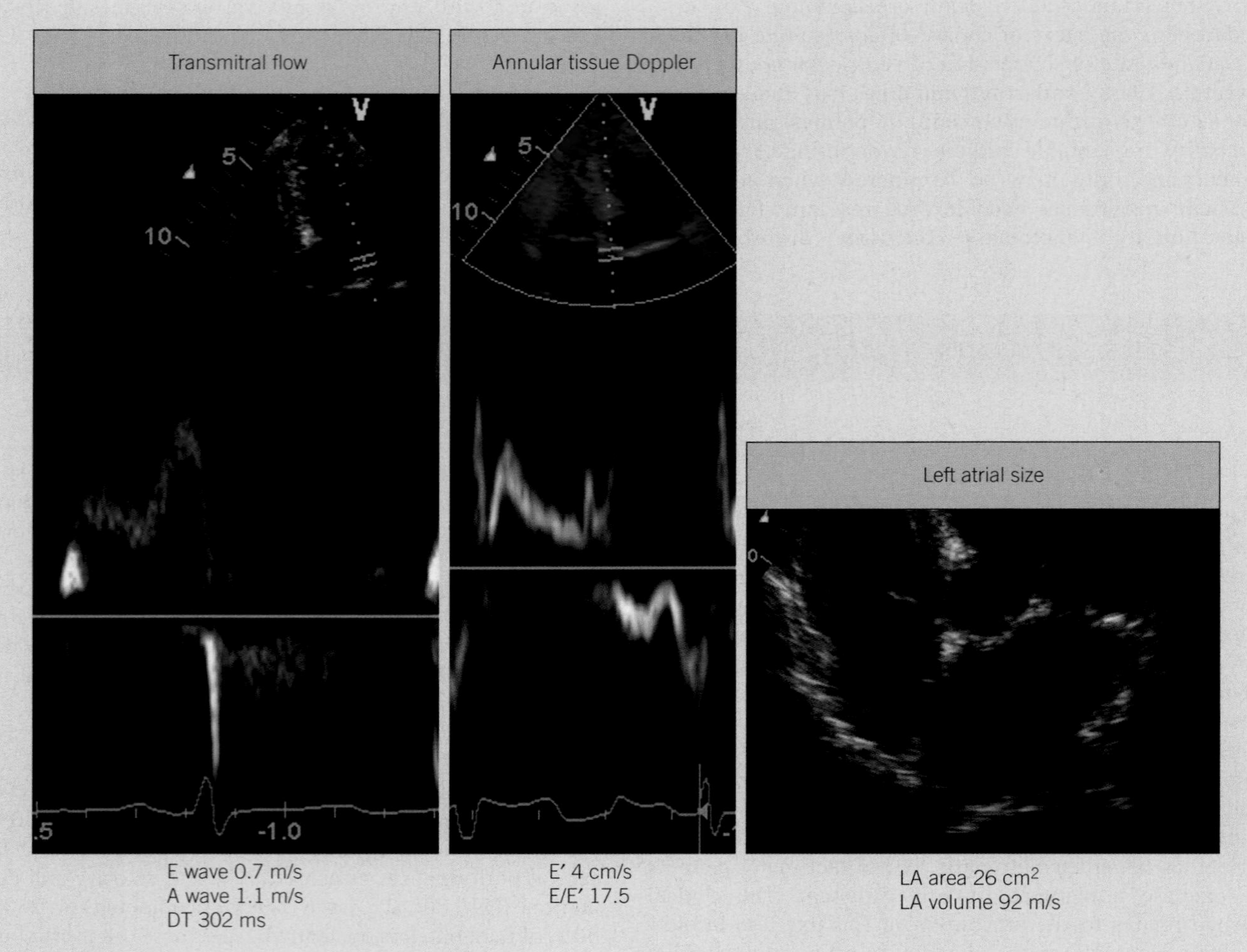

Figure 80C.1 Left ventricular filling. Transmitral flow shows an E:A ratio of 0.63 and deceleration time of more than 300 ms, demonstrating delayed relaxation. Increased filling pressure is evident from reduced annular diastolic velocity (E′) with an increased E/E′ ratio of 17.5 and is supported by increased left atrial size.

the impact of this on global diastolic indices is ambiguous, studies of myocardial dysfunction show improved glycemic control to be beneficial. Insulin sensitizers may be considered on theoretical grounds because insulin resistance is an important contributor to myocardial dysfunction, but there is no evidence to support the use of biguanides, for example, in preference to insulin. Thiazolidinediones may not be a good choice because of their propensity to provoke heart failure and the association of some members of the class with coronary events. Exercise training has been shown to benefit glycemic control and improves insulin sensitivity, and there is limited evidence to suggest that it may improve primary myocardial disease among poorly controlled diabetic subjects with this condition.

Weight loss is central in the management of diastolic dysfunction. Clearly, a number of mechanisms may be responsible for improving the well-being of overweight patients. Relatively minor degrees of weight reduction offer significant metabolic benefits, and there is evidence of improved myocardial function in response to weight reduction in obese individuals.

Good blood pressure control is a cornerstone of the management of patients with diastolic dysfunction, although it is unclear whether this is of benefit in the normotensive diabetic subject. There is evidence to support the presence of myocardial fibrosis in diabetic myocardial disease. As this is likely to be mediated by aldosterone, there may be benefits of specific drug therapy in these subjects, particularly angiotensin-converting enzyme inhibitors, angiotensin receptor blockers, and aldosterone blockade. Other antifibrotic therapies include inhibitors of transforming growth factor β as well as agents to break cross-links caused by protein glycation.

SUMMARY

Atherosclerosis is often considered the major cause of diabetic heart disease, but left ventricular dysfunction is rapidly emerging as an important consequence of diabetes. Diabetes and heart failure are strongly linked, and not just through comorbidities such as hypertension, obesity, and coronary artery disease because diabetes alone may cause left ventricular dysfunction. The current epidemics of type 2 diabetes and obesity are likely to feed the growth of heart failure in both the developed and developing worlds.

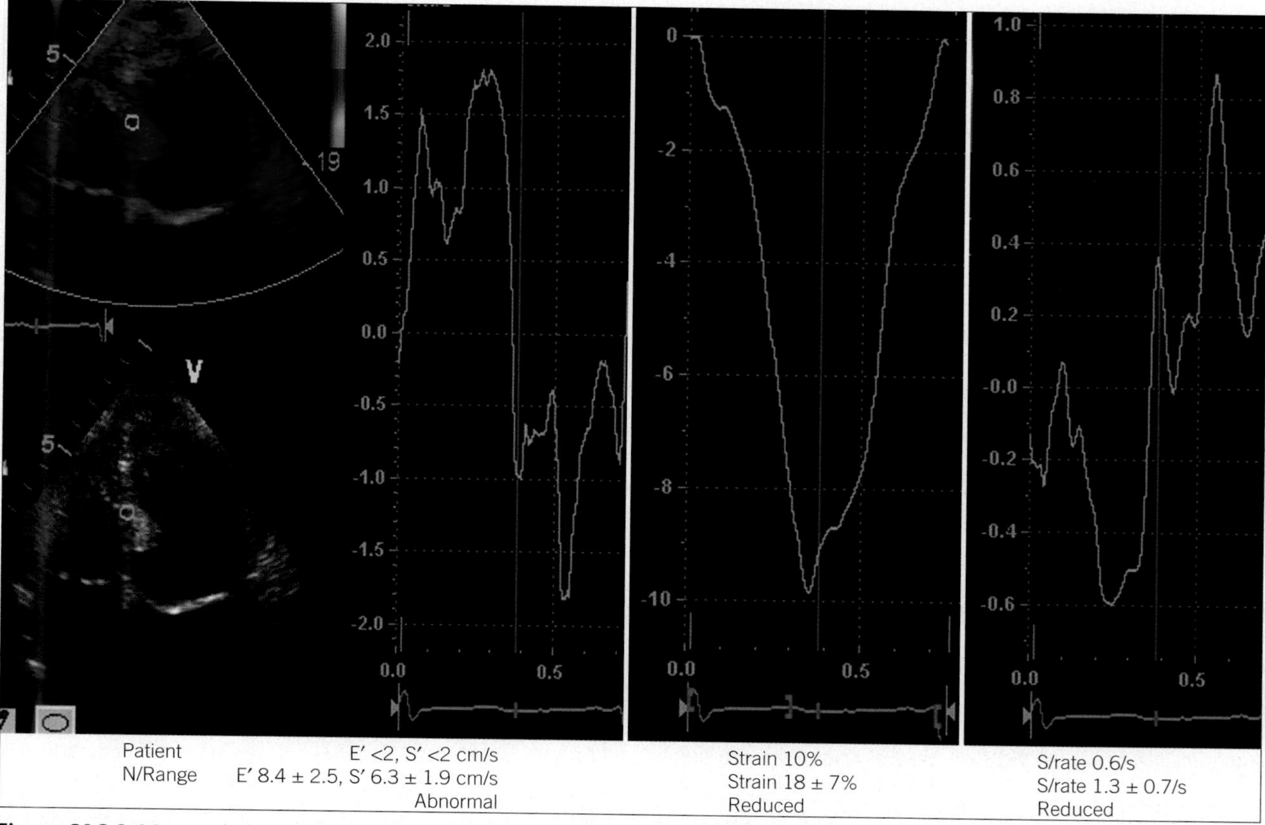

Figure 80C.2 Myocardial properties. Systolic and diastolic myocardial tissue velocities are reduced, as are strain and strain rate.

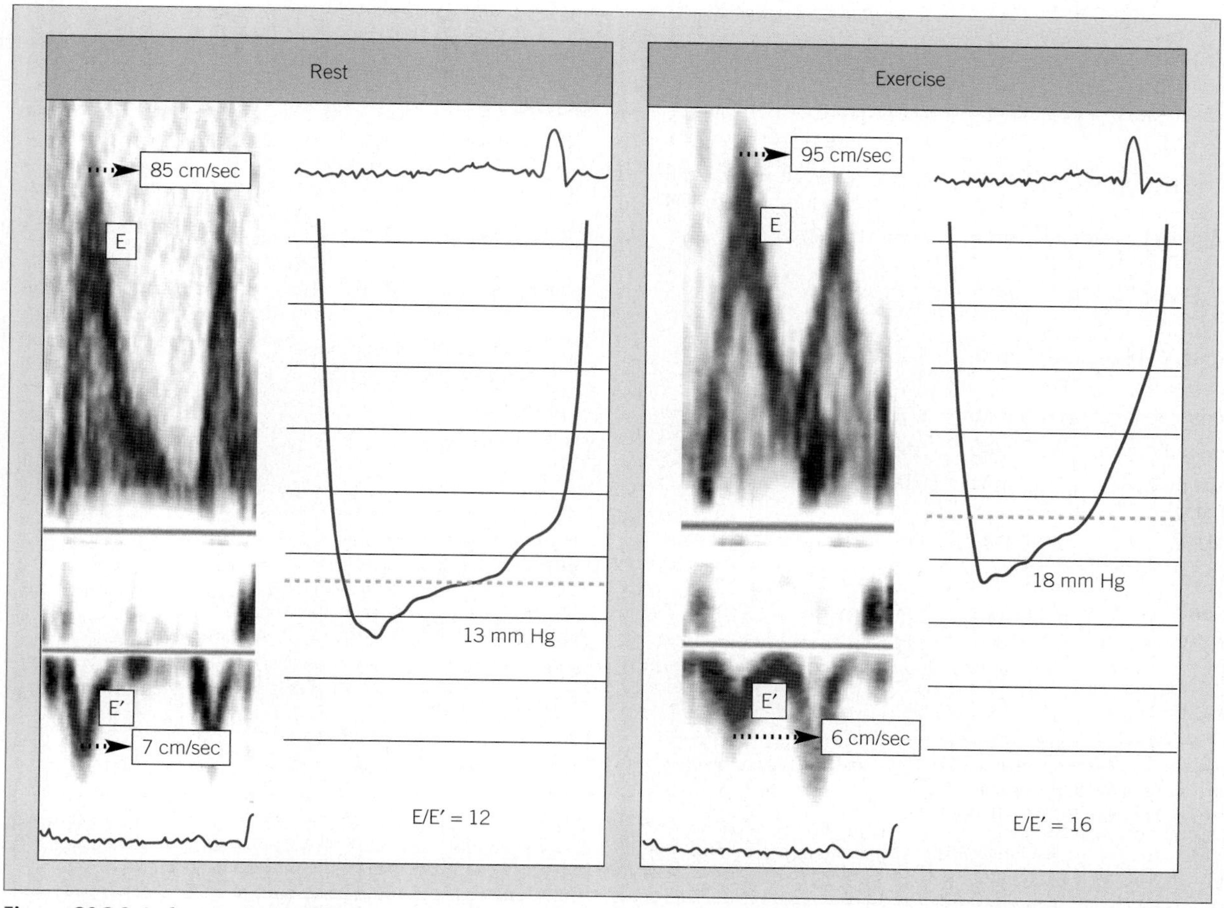

Rest
85 cm/sec
E
13 mm Hg
E′
7 cm/sec
E/E′ = 12
Exercise
95 cm/sec
E
18 mm Hg
E′
6 cm/sec
E/E′ = 16

Figure 80C.3 Left ventricular filling response to exercise. In another patient, left ventricular diastolic pressure is measured invasively at rest and during supine exercise. The increment of measured end-diastolic pressure from 13 to 18 mm Hg is matched by an increase of E/E′ from 12 to 16.

d. Toxic Cardiomyopathy, Cancer Drugs, and Herceptin

Gilles de Keulenauer and Thomas Force

DEFINITION OF PROBLEM

Drugs that target protein kinases (enzymes that regulate multiple processes in all cells, including cell proliferation, cell death, and motility) have become a mainstay of cancer therapeutics. The agents are of two types, monoclonal antibodies and small-molecule tyrosine kinase inhibitors. They can be recognized because the generic names for monoclonal antibodies end in -mab, and those for tyrosine kinase inhibitors typically end in either -inib or -enib (Table 80D.1).[1,2] These drugs target kinases, mutations in which or gene amplifications of which drive cancer progression (see (Table 80D.1). Some have radically altered prognosis of specific cancers. For example, trastuzumab (Herceptin), which targets the human epidermal growth factor receptor 2 (Her2, also known as ErbB2), has markedly increased

TYROSINE KINASE INHIBITORS AND MONOCLONAL ANTIBODIES IN CANCER

Agent	Class	Tyrosine Kinase Targets	Malignant Neoplasms	Cardiotoxicity/(rate)/Other
Imatinib (Gleevec)	TKI	ABL1/2, PDGFRα/β, KIT	CML, Ph+ B-ALL, CMML, HES, GIST	Yes/(low)*
Dasatinib (Sprycel)	TKI	ABL1/2, PDGFRα/β, KIT, SRC family	CML	Yes/(low to moderate)*/QT prolongation
Nilotinib (Tasigna)	TKI	ABL1/2, PDGFRα/β, KIT	CML	Unknown
Sunitinib (Sutent)	TKI	VEGFR1/2/3, KIT, PDGFRα/β, RET, CSF-1R, FLT3	RCC, GIST	Yes/(moderate)/hypertension, hypothyroidism
Lapatinib (Tykerb)	TKI	EGFR (ErbB1), HER2 (ErbB2)	HER2† breast cancer	No
Sorafenib (Nexavar)	TKI	c-/B-Raf, VEGFR2/3, PDGFRα/β, KIT, FLT3	RCC, melanoma	Yes/(low?)*/ACS, hypertension
Gefitinib (Iressa)	TKI	EGFR (ErbB1)	NSCLC	No*
Erlotinib (Tarceva)	TKI	EGFR (ErbB1)	NSCLC, pancreatic cancer	No*
Temsirolimus (Torisel)	Novel	mTOR (indirect; binds to FKBP12 and complex inhibits mTOR)	RCC	No*
Trastuzumab (Herceptin)	mAb	HER2 (ErbB2)	HER2† breast cancer	Yes/(moderate, especially in metastasized setting)
Bevacizumab (Avastin)	mAb	VEGF-A	Colorectal cancer, NSCLC	Yes/(low to moderate)*/ arterial thrombosis
Cetuximab (Erbitux)	mAb	EGFR (ErbB1)	Colorectal cancer, squamous cell carcinoma of head and neck	No*
Panitumumab (Vectibix)	mAb	EGFR (ErbB1)	Colorectal	No*
Rituximab (Rituxan)	mAb	CD20	B-cell lymphoma	Unknown
Alemtuzumab (Campath)	mAb	CD52	B-cell CLL	Yes (in patients with mycosis fungoides, Sézary syndrome)
Lestaurtinib†	TKI	JAK2/FLT3		Unknown
Pazopanib†	TKI	Multitargeted	RCC	Unknown
Vandetanib†	TKI	VEGFR/EGFR	NSCLC	Unknown
Cediranib‡	TKI	VEGFR	NSCLC	Unknown
Alvocidib‡	TKI	CDK	CLL	Unknown
Enzastaurin‡	TKI	PKCβ	B-cell lymphoma	Unknown

*Effect on left ventricular function has not been determined and therefore these represent best guesses.
†New Drug Applications expected 2008.
‡New Drug Applications expected 2010.
ACS, acute coronary syndrome; CLL, chronic lymphocytic leukemia; CML, chronic myelogenous leukemia; CMML, chronic myelomonocytic leukemia; GIST, gastrointestinal stromal tumor; HES, hypereosinophilic syndrome; mAb, humanized monoclonal antibody; NSCLC, non–small cell lung cancer; Ph+ B-ALL, Philadelphia chromosome–positive B-cell acute lymphocytic leukemia; RCC, renal cell carcinoma; TKI, tyrosine kinase inhibitor.

Table 80D. 1 Tyrosine kinase inhibitors and monoclonal antibodies in cancer.

survival in patients with Her2-positive breast cancer, and imatinib (Gleevec), which targets the Bcr-Abl fusion protein created by the translocation that produces the Philadelphia chromosome, has done the same for patients with chronic myeloid leukemia. However, cardiotoxicity of some of these agents has become apparent (see Table 80D.1).[3] Because prospective evaluations of left ventricular function have not generally been included in pre–Food and Drug Administration (FDA) approval clinical trials of these agents, the magnitude of the problem is not clear for most of these agents. For example, of the eight approved tyrosine kinase inhibitors, only two have been studied prospectively with determinations of left ventricular ejection fraction (LVEF). For one, lapatinib (Tykerb), which also targets Her2, none was identified, although this study was biased by selection of patients already treated with trastuzumab and therefore patients who had not developed congestive heart failure (CHF) in the setting of Her2/ErbB2 inhibition in the past.[4,5] For another, sunitinib (Sutent), significant cardiotoxicity was seen.[6] The reasons for the toxicity are complex; but in some cases (as with trastuzumab and imatinib), a target of the drug serves an important role not only in driving cancer progression but also in maintaining cardiomyocyte "health."[7-10] Thus, inhibition of that target can stall or even cure cancer progression but can also lead to cardiotoxicity.

There are currently 21 FDA-approved monoclonal antibodies; and although there are only eight approved tyrosine kinase inhibitors, six more are expected to file New Drug Applications in the next two years (see Table 80D.1).[11] Furthermore, an additional approximately 150 tyrosine kinase inhibitors are currently in or are planned to be in clinical trials. Thus going forward, cardiotoxicity of these agents is an issue with which cardiologists will need to be familiar.

Herein, we examine cardiotoxicity of two agents, trastuzumab and sunitinib, because these are, at this point, the best documented inducers of cardiotoxicity by agents targeting protein kinases. We also use these as examples of why agents targeting tyrosine kinases in cancer can lead to cardiotoxicity.

TYPICAL CASE

Trastuzumab

Trastuzumab is a humanized monoclonal antibody directed to the extracellular domain of the Her2/ErbB2 tyrosine kinase receptor. This receptor is overexpressed in 20% to 25% of human breast cancers, but it is also expressed on cardiomyocytes, where it heterodimerizes with ErbB4 to initiate a cell-protective signaling program.[7,10,12] Trastuzumab is associated with an increased risk of cardiac dysfunction, which is greatest in patients receiving concurrent anthracyclines such as doxorubicin (Adriamycin) (CREC analysis, overall rate of cardiac dysfunction 27%, severe heart failure in 16%). When it is used as adjuvant therapy after completion of anthracycline therapy, cardiac dysfunction is less frequent (NSABP B-31 trial, discontinuation of trastuzumab due to cardiac reasons in 19%, the majority of which were asymptomatic declines of LVEF), and CHF symptoms are usually milder. Risk for cardiac dysfunction is associated with the patient's age, hypertension, cumulative anthracycline dose, and body mass index.

The patient was a 65-year-old woman with body mass index of 31, mild diabetes, and essential hypertension controlled with a thiazide diuretic. She was diagnosed with lymph node–positive and Her2 protein–overexpressing breast cancer. After surgery and four cycles of doxorubicin and cyclophosphamide, she received weekly trastuzumab. Six months later, she experienced mild but increasing exertional dyspnea and peripheral edema. LVEF by radionuclide ventriculography had dropped from 63% before trastuzumab therapy to 49%.

Sunitinib

Sunitinib is one of the first multitargeted tyrosine kinase inhibitors. Typically, this means that a drug inhibits kinases regulating both cancer cell growth and tumor vascularization (see Table 80D.1). Of the small-molecule inhibitors, sunitinib appears to be the one most commonly associated with cardiotoxicity. For example, in one series of 75 patients treated with the agent, 8% of patients developed CHF, and 19% experienced declines in LVEF of at least 15 points. An additional series of six cases of sunitinib-associated CHF have also been reported.[13]

The patient was a 37-year-old woman with a metastatic gastrointestinal stromal tumor. Imatinib therapy had recently failed, and the patient was enrolled in a clinical trial assessing the efficacy of sunitinib in imatinib-resistant gastrointestinal stromal tumor. There was no history of cardiovascular disease and no risk factors for it. The patient was treated with the FDA-approved dose (50 mg/day on a 4-week on/2-week off schedule). At week 71 of treatment, the patient presented with chest pain, shortness of breath, and fatigue. On physical examination, elevated jugular venous pressure, basilar rales, and bipedal edema were noted. Blood pressure had risen from her baseline of 120/76 mm Hg to 156/88 mm Hg. B-type natriuretic peptide concentration was 1400 pg/mL. Troponin I level was normal. Chest radiography showed pulmonary edema. Because this was one of the first patients to present with CHF while receiving sunitinib, the patient underwent cardiac catheterization, which showed no coronary artery disease. LVEF by radionuclide ventriculography had declined from 57% at baseline to 38%.

DIFFERENTIAL DIAGNOSIS

Diagnosis of heart failure in cancer patients can be quite challenging because these patients typically have multiple reasons for having shortness of breath, fatigue, and peripheral edema, and the symptoms can be attributed to causes other than CHF. Furthermore, many cancer patients have multiple comorbidities, including cardiovascular comorbidities. Thus, one must consider other causes of CHF, including myocarditis. There are specific additional issues to consider in this population of complex patients—most important, prior anticancer therapies including radiation and anthracyclines. The hypertension that was seen in the patient treated with sunitinib is typical of agents that inhibit activity of the vascular endothelial cell growth factor (VEGF)/VEGF receptor system including the small-molecule inhibitor sorafenib (Nexavar) and the monoclonal antibody that "traps" VEGF, bevacizumab (Avastin).[14] The latter has also been associated with arterial thromboses, especially in older patients. Mild elevations of troponin I can be seen in these patients even without other evidence of myocardial injury, and the significance of this is not clear. These modest increases in troponin I did not appear to predict adverse events or deterioration in LVEF in patients taking sunitinib.[6]

For agents other than sunitinib and trastuzumab, especially the monoclonal antibodies and tyrosine kinase inhibitors directed at the EGF receptor antagonists (e.g., cetuximab, panitumumab, erlotinib, and gefitinib), CHF appears to be rare, and therefore alternative explanations should be sought. The imatinib group (including dasatinib and nilotinib) is not as clear (again, LVEF determinations have never been done with any of these agents).

TREATMENT OPTIONS

At present, the most prudent course is to discontinue treatment with the agent and, depending on the severity of the CHF, to institute standard heart failure management. On the basis of limited experience, it does appear that the deterioration in LVEF improves or even returns to normal, sometimes simply with stopping of the drug and in other cases with stopping of the drug and addition of a heart failure regimen.[6] For most if not all of these drugs, however, the long-term cardiac outcome is unknown, and given the progressive nature of CHF, possible late declines in cardiac function must be kept in mind. If LVEF recovers, even if not fully, the question then becomes whether to resume therapy. These patients need to be receiving the drug or the cancer will inexorably progress. This is a situation that requires close cooperation with the oncology service. First one must determine if there are viable treatment options other than resuming therapy with the offending agent. If not, then on the basis of limited experience, it may be reasonable, in light of the alternative of cancer progression, to treat the patient with an angiotensin-converting enzyme inhibitor or receptor antagonist, with or without a beta blocker, and carefully reinstitute therapy, but only after any hypertension, if it is present, has been tightly controlled. Of course, the patient must be fully apprised of the "experimental" nature of this approach. Serial assessment of left ventricular function should be undertaken. In the two cases presented, both patients were started on heart failure regimens; LVEF improved significantly to within the normal range (although not fully back to baseline), and cancer therapy was resumed without further major declines in LVEF. Again, in patients who need to continue the drug indefinitely, LVEF must be monitored closely. Perhaps more sensitive ventricular parameters, such as those derived from tissue Doppler imaging, will increase sensitivity of detection of ventricular dysfunction in the future.

SUMMARY

Although the kinase inhibitors used in cancer treatment are a class of agents, they are distinct in that targets are often quite different.[3] If a specific target plays a critical role in cardiomyocyte function or "health," then cardiotoxicity can be expected. The problem is that in most cases, this is not known. Therefore, the clinician must keep an open mind, consider the possibility that the agent may be at fault, but aggressively search for other explanations because if they are found, cancer therapy may be able to be continued as the other cause is addressed. Finally, aggressive management of heart failure and hypertension is the cornerstone of therapy and may allow patients to continue treatment, which is ultimately the goal.

chapter 81

Restrictive and Infiltrative Cardiomyopathies

Naveen L. Pereira and G. William Dec

Definition

- Restrictive and infiltrative cardiomyopathies are rare diseases of the heart muscle characterized by elevated filling pressures, normal left ventricular volumes, and usually preserved LVEF.

Key Features

- Common causes include amyloidosis, sarcoidosis, endomyocardial fibrosis, and idiopathic restrictive cardiomyopathy.
- Congestive heart failure with predominantly right-sided physical findings is the most common form of presentation.

Therapy

- Treatment is usually disease specific, but symptomatic relief may be attempted with diuretics and preload-reducing agents.

RESTRICTIVE CARDIOMYOPATHIES

Restrictive cardiomyopathies are the least commonly encountered forms of heart muscle disease.[1] Compliance is abnormal, resulting in rapid early diastolic filling but diminished or absent atrial filling. Restrictive cardiomyopathy can be classified according to etiology as primary or secondary. Primary restrictive cardiomyopathy includes idiopathic restrictive cardiomyopathy and endomyocardial fibrosis. Common secondary causes include infiltrative cardiomyopathies such as amyloidosis, sarcoidosis, hemochromatosis, storage disorders such as Fabry's disease, and metastatic cancers. A classification based on frequency of occurrence is outlined in Table 81.1. Unlike in dilated and hypertrophic disease, a familial component is rare in restrictive cardiomyopathy.

CLINICAL PRESENTATION

Congestive heart failure is the most frequent initial manifestation, and common symptoms include dyspnea on exertion, fatigue, and lower extremity edema. Chest pain occurs infrequently. Physical examination typically reveals prominent right-sided findings with jugular venous distention and prominent x and y descent without respiratory variation (Kussmaul's sign). Hepatomegaly, ascites, and pedal edema are seen in advanced cases. The apical impulse may or may not be displaced but is usually palpable. The first and second heart sounds are normal; a third heart sound is occasionally audible. Functional mitral and tricuspid murmurs are frequently present.

DIAGNOSTIC TECHNIQUES

Electrocardiography and Chest Radiography

The electrocardiogram often demonstrates nonspecific repolarization changes. Low voltage, pseudoinfarction pattern, left or right bundle branch blocks, and atrioventricular conduction delays are common findings and should suggest an infiltrative process. Cardiomegaly is mild or absent; prominent atrial enlargement may be seen with increased interstitial markings and pleural effusions.

Echocardiography

Normal right and left ventricular systolic function and normal chamber dimensions with biatrial enlargement on echocardiography in the presence of congestive heart failure should suggest restrictive cardiomyopathy. Increased left ventricular wall mass may represent an infiltrative process. Abnormal diastolic ventricular compliance is reflected by the following Doppler echocardiographic findings (Fig. 81.1): increased early diastolic filling velocity (E) due to elevated atrial pressures, decreased atrial filling velocity (A) due to elevated ventricular diastolic pressures, E/A ratio of 1.5 or more, decreased deceleration time (<125 ms), and decreased isovolumic relaxation time.[2] A marked decrease in systolic/diastolic pulmonary venous flow ratio due to high atrial pressures and an augmented atrial reversal velocity due to decreased ventricular compliance are also frequently seen.

Hemodynamics

Right- and left-sided filling pressures are elevated, and cardiac index is depressed. Right atrial pressure is elevated with prominent x and y descents and lacks respiratory variation. The classic square root sign (i.e., a prominent, early decrease in ventricular diastolic pressure followed by a rapid rise to a plateau, which facilitates early diastolic filling) characterizes restrictive physiology. Right ventricular systolic pressures can be 50 mm Hg or higher, whereas right ventricular diastolic pressures are usually less than one third of the systolic pressures. Left ventricular diastolic pressures are typically 5 mm Hg or higher than right ventricular diastolic pressures, but it is not uncommon for both to be nearly identical.

Endomyocardial Biopsy

Endomyocardial biopsy plays an important role in the diagnostic management of patients with restrictive cardiomyopathy. Cardiac involvement in systemic diseases such as

CLASSIFICATION OF RESTRICTIVE CARDIOMYOPATHY
Common causes
Amyloidosis
Idiopathic restrictive cardiomyopathy
Tropical endomyocardial fibrosis (in equatorial countries)
Uncommon causes
Sarcoidosis
Hemochromatosis
Hypereosinophilic endomyocardial fibrosis (in temperate countries)
Rare causes
Scleroderma
Storage diseases
■ Fabry's disease
■ Gaucher's disease
■ Hurler's disease
■ Glycogen storage diseases
Radiation
Metastatic malignant neoplasms (e.g., melanomas, lymphomas)

Table 81.1 Classification of restrictive cardiomyopathy.

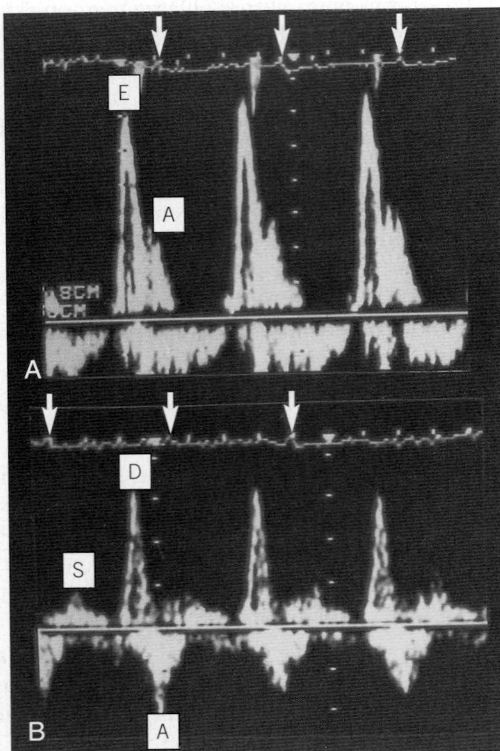

Figure 81.1 Doppler echocardiography in restrictive cardiomyopathy. A, Transmitral inflow pattern by Doppler echocardiography demonstrating prominent restrictive physiology. There is evidence for increased early diastolic filling velocity (E) and markedly decreased atrial filling velocity (A). **B,** Pulmonary venous flow pattern showing decreased systolic (S)/diastolic (D) pulmonary venous flow ratio and a prominent atrial reversal velocity (A). (Courtesy of Mary E. King, MD, Cardiac Ultrasound Laboratory, Massachusetts General Hospital, Boston, Mass.)

amyloidosis and hemochromatosis can be definitively established with endomyocardial biopsy. Biopsy is also useful in differentiating restrictive cardiomyopathy from constrictive pericarditis.[3]

MANAGEMENT

Therapy should be directed toward the specific underlying cardiomyopathy (see later). Judicious use of diuretics can control pulmonary congestion, peripheral edema, and ascites. Even mild hypovolemia in the presence of a nondilated, stiff ventricle can further decrease stroke volume and cause dizziness, prerenal azotemia, and low-output state. Supraventricular arrhythmias, particularly atrial fibrillation, are common and should be treated aggressively to maintain atrial contractility and diastolic filling. Bradyarrhythmias are not uncommon in infiltrative diseases and often necessitate permanent pacemaker implantation.

DIFFERENTIATION OF RESTRICTIVE CARDIOMYOPATHY FROM CONSTRICTIVE PERICARDITIS

Restrictive cardiomyopathy and constrictive pericarditis have similar physiology, and differentiation of the two conditions may be difficult (Fig. 81.2). Constrictive pericarditis is more likely if pericardial thickening (≥10 mm) is demonstrated on computed tomographic or magnetic resonance imaging. A decrease in mitral transvalvular velocities during inspiration as measured by Doppler echocardiography in constrictive pericarditis helps distinguish this condition from restrictive cardiomyopathy. Newer techniques, such as Doppler tissue imaging, have shown ventricular diastolic expansion to be reduced in restrictive cardiomyopathy. The most common hemodynamic criterion employed to differentiate the two conditions is equalization of right and left ventricular diastolic pressures.[4] This finding has a 92% positive predictive value for constrictive pericarditis and 70% for restrictive cardiomyopathy. The poor specificity of this sign for constrictive pericarditis improves if hemodynamic equalization persists during a volume challenge. Discordance in right and left ventricular pressures in constrictive pericarditis as evidenced by an inspiratory increase in right ventricular systolic pressures and decrease in left ventricular systolic pressures, which demonstrates ventricular interdependence, has been reported to be the most sensitive and specific hemodynamic criterion for differentiation of constrictive pericardial disease.[5] Coronary phasic flow characteristics have also been used to help make the distinction between the two conditions. Ultimately, if there are discordant imaging and hemodynamic data, endomyocardial biopsy may be indicated to rule out a specific restrictive cardiomyopathy.

AMYLOID HEART DISEASE

Cardiac amyloidosis is characterized by the deposition of twisted β-pleated sheet fibrils of various precursor proteins and accounts for approximately 10% of all nonischemic cardiomyopathies. Amyloidosis may be primary, secondary, familial, senile, or dialysis associated. Primary amyloidosis

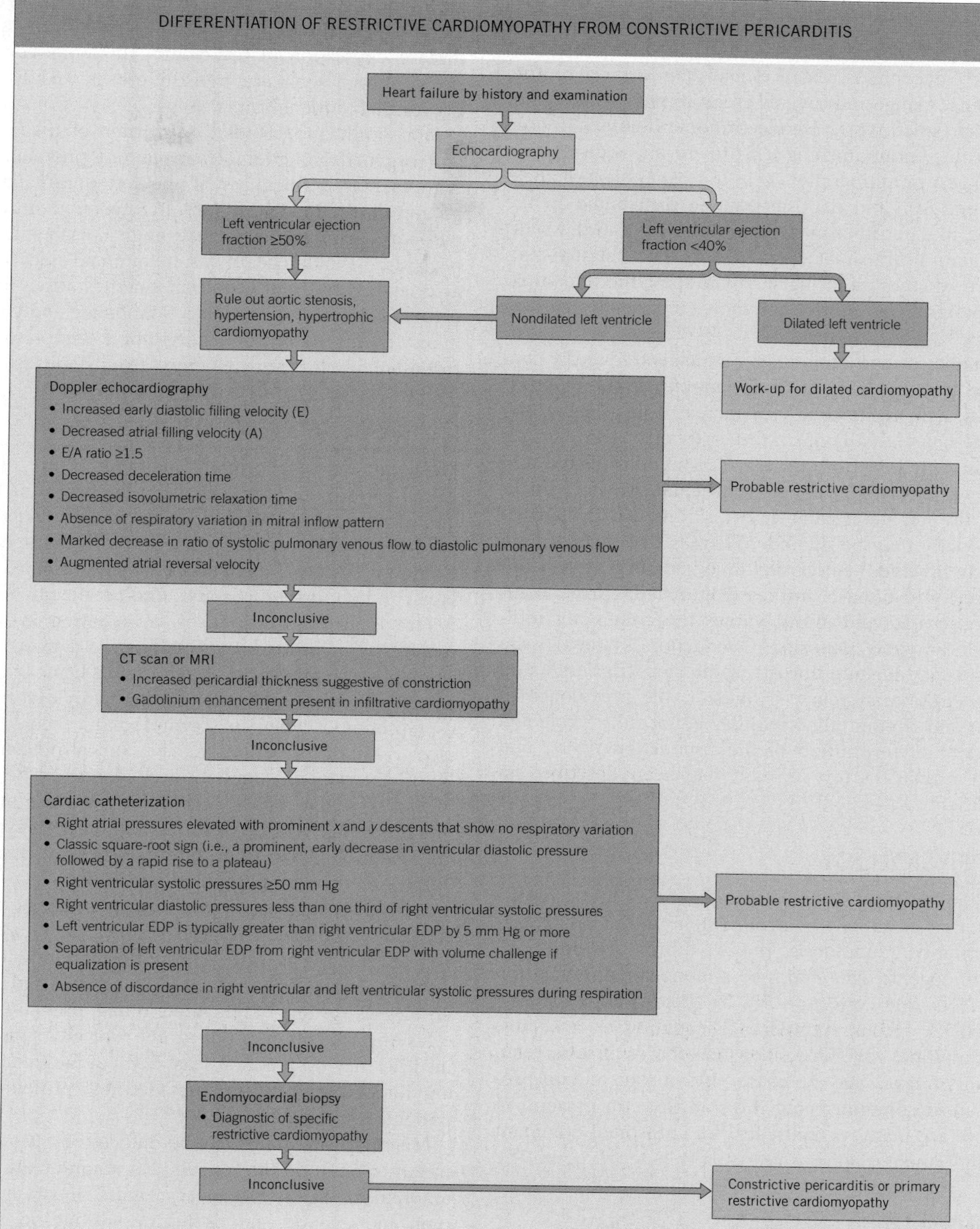

Figure 81.2 Differentiation of restrictive cardiomyopathy from constrictive pericarditis. CT, computed tomography; MRI, magnetic resonance imaging; EDP, end-diastolic pressure.

(AL) accounts for 85% of cases in the United States and is associated with plasma cell dyscrasias resulting in deposition of fibrils composed of monoclonal κ or λ immunoglobulin light chains.[6,7] Secondary amyloidosis (AA), characterized by tissue deposition of protein A, is associated with chronic inflammatory diseases such as rheumatoid arthritis, inflammatory bowel disease, osteomyelitis, tuberculosis, and leprosy. Renal involvement is typical, but cardiac involvement is rare. Familial amyloidosis is usually an autosomal dominant disorder commonly caused by mutations in the transthyretin (prealbumin) gene. More than 100 such mutations of transthyretin have been reported and account for approximately 10% to 20% of amyloid cases. Senile systemic amyloidosis is found in up to 25% of patients older than 80 years but is an uncommon cause of clinically significant cardiac amyloidosis.[8] Dialysis-related amyloidosis is characterized by β_2-microglobulin amyloid deposits predominantly found in osteoarticular structures but that can be detected in the hearts of patients who have undergone hemodialysis for a prolonged time.[9]

ANATOMY AND PATHOLOGY

On microscopic examination, amyloid deposits appear as eosinophilic, amorphous, extracellular deposits on routine tissue staining. Congo red reveals green birefringence under polarized light microscopy. By electron microscopy, amyloid appears as fine, nonbranching 7.5- to 10-nm-wide protein fibrils arranged in antiparallel or in a cross β-pleated sheet configuration. Amyloid deposits can be distributed in the interstitium, in a perifiber or nodular pattern, or in the walls of the intramural arterioles (Fig. 81.3).[10] The vascular pattern is more common in primary amyloidosis; the interstitial nodular pattern is more common in senile cardiac amyloidosis.

Unlike senile cardiac amyloidosis, which is frequently confined to the heart, AL amyloidosis commonly involves extracardiac sites, such as the kidneys, pancreas, spleen, liver, and rectum. The heart usually has a firm, rubbery texture and is increased in weight.[11] Both atria are commonly dilated and infiltrated with amyloid. The left ventricular walls are thickened, and the left ventricular cavity size is usually normal but occasionally may be dilated. Whereas the endocardium is frequently involved, pericardial involvement is dependent on the severity of disease. Intracardiac thrombi are uncommon. The tricuspid and mitral valves are commonly infiltrated with amyloid deposits. Conduction system tissue involvement may include fibrosis of the sinoatrial node and of the His-Purkinje system.[12] However, the prevalence of conduction and rhythm abnormalities is not fully explained by the extent of infiltration of the conduction tissue, and epicardial coronary artery disease has been described in 15% of patients.

PATHOPHYSIOLOGY

In familial and primary amyloidosis, genetic mutation results in formation of unstable precursor proteins and fibril deposition. In primary amyloidosis, the AL fibrils are produced from amyloidogenic light chains by a monoclonal population of plasma cells that constitute 5% to 10% of bone marrow plasma cells; λ chains are twice as common as κ chains, except in multiple myeloma, in which the reverse is seen. Familial amyloidosis may be caused by various mutant proteins, the most common being the transthyretin protein, of which there are many variants. It is an autosomal dominant disease, and affected persons are usually heterozygous. The methionine 30 variant is the most prevalent variant worldwide. Certain unidentified age-related factors result in phenotypic disease expression in the elderly. In senile cardiac amyloidosis, normal sequence transthyretin is usually detected by myocardial immunohistochemistry.

Fibril infiltration leads to distortion of tissue architecture and organ dysfunction. Heart failure prevalence increases with increased thickness of the left ventricular walls and greater deposition of amyloid. Involvement of the intramural coronary arteries may cause angina, ischemic myocardial necrosis, or sudden death despite minimal epicardial coronary arterial involvement. Unusual manifestations include pericardial effusion and cardiac tamponade, valvular involvement leading to mitral regurgitation, and systemic arterial thromboemboli that result from atrial standstill.

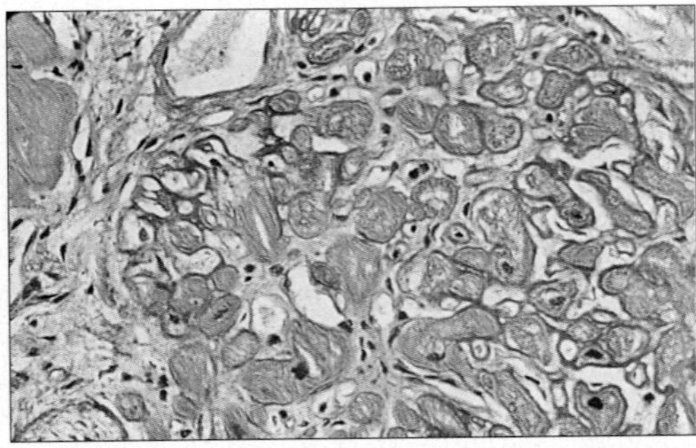

Figure 81.3 Endomyocardial biopsy specimen from a patient who has cardiac amyloidosis. Photomicrograph of a myocardial specimen stained with Congo red shows marked congophilia (red) of the amyloid deposits in the interstitium.

CLINICAL PRESENTATION

Most patients with primary amyloidosis are older than 40 years. Syndromes at presentation in decreasing order of frequency include renal failure, heart failure, carpal tunnel syndrome, peripheral neuropathy, and orthostatic hypotension.[6] Common systemic complaints include fatigue, weight loss, facial and periorbital purpura, and bone pain. Whereas heart failure is an initial mode of presentation in only 17% of patients with primary amyloidosis, its prevalence increases as the disease progresses. The onset of heart failure portends a poor prognosis. Senile cardiac amyloidosis is usually asymptomatic; when it is symptomatic, heart failure is the most common presentation. The clinical presentation of the Ile 122 variant in familial amyloidosis can be very similar to that of senile cardiac amyloidosis because of the absence of light chains in urine or serum and onset of symptoms after the age of 60 years. Heart failure, however, is not a common initial presentation in familial amyloidosis.

Syncope is a common symptom and may be due to orthostatic hypotension, bradyarrhythmias, or tachyarrhythmias; angina pectoris is rare. Atrial fibrillation will develop in 20% to 30% of patients as a result of atrial enlargement, atrial infiltration, or elevated filling pressures. Pericardial effusions are common but rarely clinically significant. Renal insufficiency occurs in at least 50% of patients with primary amyloidosis and is accompanied by proteinuria in most patients.

Macroglossia, which can be detected by prominent indentation of teeth on the tongue, is a unique feature of primary amyloidosis in the advanced stages. Hepatomegaly is common, but splenomegaly is an unusual finding. Waxy cutaneous papules, alopecia, and scleroderma-like skin infiltration may also be seen. Polyarthropathy, which is usually bilateral and symmetric, may also occur. Hemorrhagic complications due to factor 10 deficiency may rarely be seen.

DIAGNOSTIC TECHNIQUES

Electrocardiography and Chest Radiography

The two most common and diagnostically useful electrocardiographic patterns in AL amyloidosis are a pseudoinfarction pattern and low QRS voltage. Unlike in AL amyloidosis, the electrocardiographic voltage is well preserved in familial amyloidosis. Atrial tachyarrhythmias (especially atrial fibrillation), premature ventricular complexes, and heart block are commonly observed. Abnormal signal-averaged electrocardiography has been described in one third of patients with primary amyloidosis, and echocardiographic evidence of cardiac amyloid appears predictive of sudden death. The cardiac silhouette is usually normal; pleural effusions and interstitial edema are common. Pulmonary involvement rarely may present as a solitary nodule or interstitial infiltration.

Echocardiography

M-mode echocardiography typically shows a nondilated left ventricle and thickening of the interventricular septum, posterior wall, and right ventricular free wall.[13] Decreased electrocardiographic voltage to echocardiographic left ventricular cross-sectional area ratio suggests amyloid heart disease.[14] Left atrial enlargement and small pericardial effusions are common. Left ventricular systolic function is normal except in advanced states. A characteristic "speckled" pattern of increased myocardial echogenicity may be seen, particularly in the interventricular septum (Fig. 81.4). Interatrial septal thickening is less common but more specific for amyloid heart disease. Diastolic function is impaired early in the course of the disease as seen by an E/A ratio reversal and a prolonged deceleration time by Doppler echocardiography. Early systolic dysfunction is reflected by a prolonged isovolumic contraction time. As the disease progresses and symptoms become more prominent, pseudonormalization of the E/A ratio occurs and then a more typical restrictive filling pattern emerges.[15] Echocardiographic variables have been shown to correlate with symptoms and survival. Left ventricular wall thickness correlates directly with the occurrence of heart failure and inversely with survival. Shortened deceleration time and an increased early diastolic filling velocity to atrial filling velocity ratio are also strong predictors of survival. Familial amyloidosis cannot be distinguished from primary amyloidosis by echocardiographic features.

Magnetic Resonance Imaging

Magnetic resonance imaging has been used in a small number of patients with cardiac amyloidosis and has the capability of detecting amyloid protein as low-intensity signals by tissue characterization in addition to high-resolution imaging of the atrial and ventricular myocardium. Late subendocardial contrast enhancement occurs in more than 40% of AL amyloid patients and correlates with increased amyloid load.[6,16] Magnetic resonance imaging may have the potential to monitor progress as far as response to therapy is concerned in these patients.

Tissue Biopsy

Common sites of tissue biopsy for detection of systemic amyloidosis include rectal mucosa, abdominal fat, skin, bone marrow, kidney, and myocardium. The demonstration of amyloidosis on the abdominal fat aspirate in conjunction with an abnormal echocardiogram can be indirectly used to diagnose cardiac amyloid. However, if noninvasive test results are abnormal but not typical, definitive diagnosis of cardiac involvement can be established only by endomyocardial biopsy.

Diagnostic Approach to Determine the Type of Amyloid

The sensitivities of the various tests used to diagnose the presence of amyloid are outlined in Table 81.2. Once the diagnosis of amyloid has been established, it is important to determine the type of amyloid deposition for further therapeutic considerations (Fig. 81.5). AL amyloidosis is usually confirmed by evidence of plasma cell dyscrasia manifested in the urine, serum, or bone marrow. Conversely, patients who have light chains in urine or serum do not necessarily have amyloidosis. Routine serum protein electrophoresis in AL amyloidosis may show an M-band spike in only 50% of cases. Immunofixation electrophoresis of the serum and urine is far more sensitive in detection of abnormal light chains like κ or λ. Bone marrow biopsy allows detection of

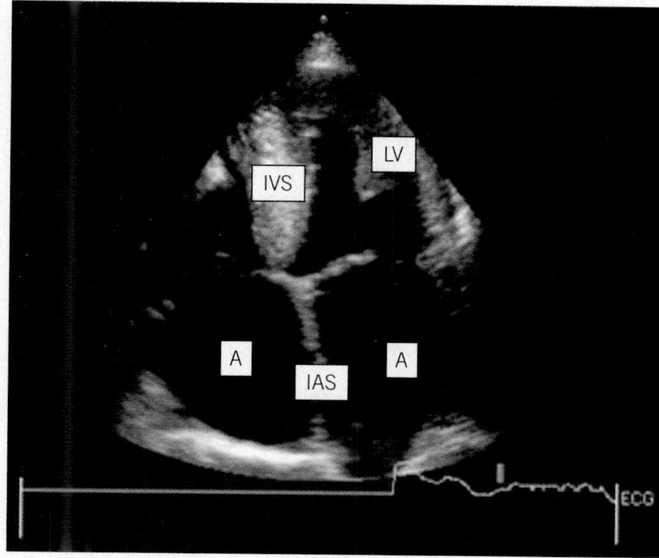

Figure 81.4 Two-dimensional echocardiography in cardiac amyloidosis. Apical four-chamber view demonstrates increased septal (IVS) and lateral wall (LV) thickness with a "speckled" pattern, enlarged atria (A), and thickened interatrial septum (IAS).

SENSITIVITIES OF DIAGNOSTIC TESTS IN CARDIAC AMYLOIDOSIS

Diagnostic test		Sensitivity (%)
Electrocardiography	Low voltage	63–80
	Q waves	60–93
Echocardiography	Speckled appearance	45–87
	Interatrial septum thickening	60
Tissue biopsy	Abdominal fat pad aspiration	80
	Rectal biopsy	70–85
	Bone marrow biopsy	50–56
	Skin biopsy	50–90
	Endomyocardial biopsy	100
Radionuclide imaging	Technetium Tc 99m pyrophosphate scintigraphy	23

Table 81.2 Sensitivities of diagnostic tests in cardiac amyloidosis.

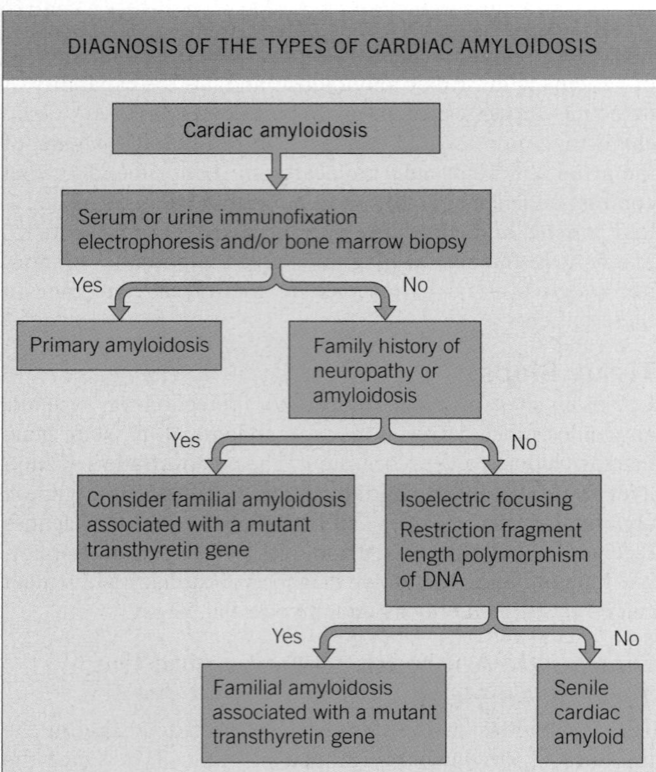

Figure 81.5 Diagnosis of the types of cardiac amyloidosis. The diagnosis of senile cardiac amyloid is confirmed by positive staining of myocardial tissue with antibody to prealbumin. (Modified from Falk RH, Comenzo RL, Skinner M. The systemic amyloidoses. N Engl J Med 1997;337:898-909.)

monoclonal proliferation of plasma cells, which confirms the diagnosis when routine serum or urine test results are nondiagnostic, and it also helps detect the presence of multiple myeloma. Familial amyloidosis is diagnosed by demonstration of an abnormal transthyretin mutant by genetic testing. Myocardial tissue staining for prealbumin usually confirms the diagnosis of senile cardiac amyloidosis.

MANAGEMENT

Patients with cardiac amyloidosis are unusually sensitive to digoxin and calcium channel blockers, probably because of their direct binding to the amyloid fibril, and these agents should be avoided.

Specific treatment options aimed at reducing protein deposition remain limited in primary amyloidosis. A randomized prospective trial has demonstrated that treatment with melphalan and prednisone resulted in a median survival of 18 months, whereas median survival was 8 months in the colchicine-treated patients.[17] The benefit was most evident in those patients who had a decreased concentration of serum or urine monoclonal protein, circulating immunoglobulin light chains, or NT-proBNP with treatment.[18] Recurrent amyloid deposition can occur in the cardiac allograft in solitary heart transplantation histologically in approximately 60% of patients, and actuarial survival rates are approximately 60% at 1 year and 30% at 5 years. High-dose intravenous melphalan with autologous peripheral blood stem cell transplantation has been used to treat patients with primary amyloidosis, resulting in clinical response and improved survival, especially in patients with good functional status and minimal cardiac and other organ involvement.[18,19] Carefully selected patients with heart failure and AL amyloidosis have been treated with sequential cardiac and stem cell transplantation, with initial promising results.[20] In patients who have amyloidosis associated with a mutant transthyretin gene, liver transplantation may be curative; survival at 5 years is comparable to that with liver transplantation performed for other reasons. Although initial reports indicated amyloid regression and clinical improvement after liver transplantation due to elimination of variant transthyretin production, studies indicate that cardiac and other organ progression can occur from continued deposition of wild-type transthyretin.[21,22]

PROGNOSIS

In patients with primary amyloidosis, the median duration of survival is approximately 1 year after diagnosis but only 6 months after the onset of heart failure. Common causes of death include progressive heart failure, arrhythmias, and renal failure. Almost 25% to 30% of deaths are sudden and may be due to bradyarrhythmias or tachyarrhythmias. Clinical variables associated with a poor prognosis include advanced New York Heart Association (NYHA) functional class, cachexia, heart failure, hepatomegaly, and stress-associated syncope. Biomarkers associated with a poor prognosis included persistent elevation of circulating free light chains, troponin, and NT-proBNP. Reported survival averages 8 months when troponin T is elevated compared with 21 months when it is not.[23] Similarly, NT-proBNP can fall rapidly during chemotherapy; a 30% reduction in NT-proBNP has been associated with improved event-free survial.[18] Finally, a 50% reduction in free immunoglobulin light chains can occur after chemotherapy and parallels a reduction in biomarkers and clinical improvement.[18] Echocardiographic features that predict decreased survival include increased left ventricular wall thickness, reduced systolic function, and right ventricular dilatation.[22,24] Doppler study predictors of poor outcome include a shortened deceleration time and an increased E/A ratio.[25] The extent of interstitial amyloid deposition determined by endomyocardial biopsy may also correlate with survival. The present modalities of treatment in primary amyloidosis have not had a significant impact on the survival rate, except cardiac transplantation in selected patients with high-dose chemotherapy and stem cell transplantation may improve survival.[26] Familial amyloidosis patients have a better prognosis, with a median survival of approximately 2 years after diagnosis.

ENDOMYOCARDIAL FIBROSIS

Endomyocardial fibrosis (EMF) can be classified as tropical, hypereosinophilic, or iatrogenic in origin. Tropical EMF is a disease entity commonly seen in equatorial countries such as Uganda, Nigeria, India, and Brazil; it accounts for approximately 20% of heart failure cases and 15% of cardiac deaths in equatorial Africa.[27] Hypereosinophilic EMF or late Löffler's endomyocardial disease is more commonly seen in temperate zones. The heart is involved in 75% of patients with hypereosinophilic syndrome. Iatrogenic factors producing EMF include methysergide, large doses of anabolic steroids, and, rarely, doxorubicin (Adriamycin).

ANATOMY AND PATHOLOGY

The heart size can be normal or small with characteristic fibrous encasing of the right ventricle, left ventricle, or both ventricles. Fibrosis typically involves the atrioventricular canal, papillary muscles, and cardiac apex, which can be obliterated by fibrous tissue or thrombus. Histopathologic examination reveals a layer of fibrin, collagen, and elastin fibrils, accounting for the endocardial thickening with fibrous septa extending into the myocardium. The interstitium has predominantly lymphocytic infiltrates. Eosinophil granule proteins are evident in cardiac tissues of patients with hypereosinophilic EMF but are uncommon in tropical EMF. Marked eosinophilia (>1500 eosinophils/mm^2) of any cause can produce endomyocardial disease.

PATHOPHYSIOLOGY

Nutritional factors (such as roots of cassava and plantains), environmental factors (such as thorium, cerium, and parasitic infections), and drugs (such as methysergide, anabolic steroids, and doxorubicin) have been implicated in the pathogenesis of EMF. Dietary and environmental factors probably play an important role in tropical EMF. The intracytoplasmic granular content of the eosinophil is thought to be responsible for causing toxic endomyocardial damage in hypereosinophilic EMF.

CLINICAL PRESENTATION

EMF commonly affects children and younger adults; the mean age at presentation is 35 years. In equatorial countries, there is a male preponderance; in European countries, women are more commonly affected. The illness has an insidious onset; a common initial manifestation is either left- or right-sided heart failure. A characteristic feature of right-sided heart failure in EMF is prominent, predominantly exudative ascites with little peripheral edema, especially in end-stage EMF. Mitral regurgitation and tricuspid regurgitation are commonly associated valvular abnormalities. Clinical features of hypereosinophilic EMF include weight loss, persistent unexplained fever, cough, rash, and biventricular heart failure.

DIAGNOSTIC TECHNIQUES

Electrocardiography and Chest Radiography

The electrocardiogram is usually unhelpful and may show sinus rhythm, nonspecific ST-T changes, atrial fibrillation, chamber enlargement, and intraventricular conduction delays. Likewise, the chest film is usually normal.

Echocardiography

Echocardiographic features include myocardial calcification, intracavitary thrombi, thickening of the anterior right ventricular wall, and small pericardial effusion. The right or left ventricular apical cavity is typically obliterated by thrombus or fibrous tissue.[28] Severe biatrial enlargement is the norm. Left ventricular systolic function is preserved, and diastolic chamber dimensions are reduced. Varying degrees of mitral and tricuspid regurgitation are evident on Doppler echocardiographic study.

Computed Tomography

EMF may be visualized as a linear calcification or low-attenuation band on electron beam computed tomographic imaging. This finding may be useful in differentiating this condition from constrictive pericarditis.

Endomyocardial Biopsy

Biopsy may be useful in identifying hypereosinophilic EMF in the early stages but is usually not required when marked peripheral eosinophilia is evident.

MANAGEMENT

Medical treatment usually consists of sodium and fluid restriction and diuretics. Corticosteroids are useful in the early phase of Löffler's endocarditis. Surgical treatment involves resection of the fibrous endocardium and replacement of the mitral and tricuspid valves. It provides symptomatic relief, decreases left ventricular end-diastolic pressures and left ventricular end-diastolic volumes, and may improve survival.[29] Operative mortality of 10% to 30% has been reported, but a more recent series found no perioperative deaths. Patients with NYHA class III or class IV symptoms derive most benefit from surgical treatment.

PROGNOSIS

Adverse prognostic indicators include moderate to severe biventricular fibrosis, presence of valvular regurgitation, and severity of heart failure at initial presentation.[30] Survival rates in a series of 145 patients were 76% at 1 year and 36% at 5 years. Surgically treated patients have a better 5-year survival at 60% to 70%. Mortality rates are high, up to 75% at 2 years after the onset of symptoms in tropical EMF because of poor response to medical therapy. Common causes of death include progressive heart failure, embolic phenomena, and pneumonia.

CARDIAC SARCOIDOSIS

More than 30% of patients with systemic sarcoidosis without cardiac complaints have subclinical cardiac involvement as manifested by thallium perfusion defects.[31] The relatively high prevalence is reflected in autopsy studies, in which pathologic cardiac involvement is seen in 20% to 25% of patients. However, only 5% of patients have symptomatic cardiac disease.

ANATOMY AND PATHOLOGY

The pathognomonic lesion in sarcoidosis is a noncaseating epithelioid cell granuloma (Fig. 81.6a). The extent and type of myocardial involvement are variable and can range from active granuloma to scar formation, sometimes resulting in formation of ventricular aneurysms. Granulomas are classically found

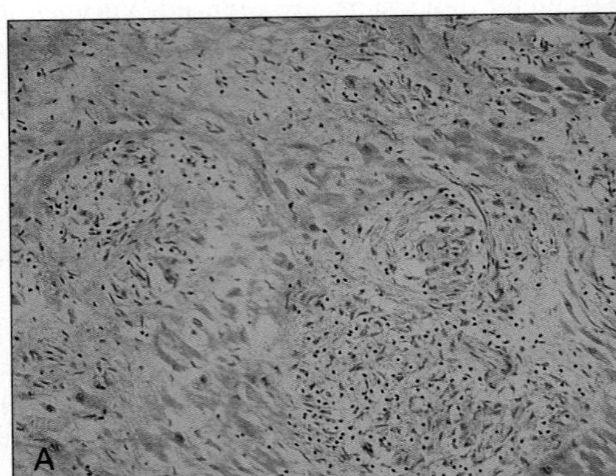

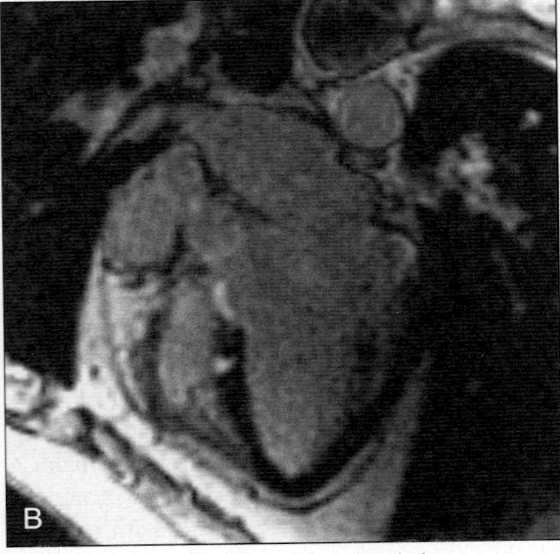

Figure 81.6 **A,** Histopathology of cardiac sarcoidosis. Photomicrograph shows characteristic noncaseating granulomas within the myocardium in association with lymphocytes and fibrosis. (Courtesy of H. Thomas Aretz, MD, Department of Pathology, Massachusetts General Hospital, Boston, Mass.) **B,** Delayed gadolinium enhancement on cardiac magnetic resonance imaging. Patchy focal enhancement in the basal septum and lateral walls is consistent with cardiac sarcoidosis. (Courtesy of James Glockner, MD, Department of Radiology, Mayo Clinic, Rochester, Minn.)

in the proximal portions of the left ventricle, basal septum, and conduction tissue, particularly the atrioventricular node. Infiltration of small coronary vessels is not uncommon.

PATHOPHYSIOLOGY

Granulomatous infiltration of the myocardium and subsequent healing with scar formation result in increased ventricular stiffness and diastolic dysfunction. Systolic dysfunction may develop later as the disease progresses. Infiltration of the atrioventricular node can cause heart block, and myocardial granulomas or scar can also serve as an automatic focus or facilitate re-entry for ventricular arrhythmias.[32] Small-vessel involvement may result in ischemia and sudden death. Papillary muscle infiltration may cause substantial mitral or tricuspid regurgitation. Genetic susceptibility has been implicated in the pathogenesis of the disease, with certain gene loci being linked to cardiac and renal involvement.

CLINICAL PRESENTATION

Myocardial sarcoidosis typically affects young or middle-aged adults and is typically associated with systemic sarcoidosis. A common clinical manifestation of cardiac sarcoidosis is complete heart block.[33] Sudden death due to high-degree atrioventricular block may be the initial presentation. Ventricular arrhythmias including ventricular premature complexes and ventricular tachycardia are also common. Heart failure may be present in 20% to 30% of patients and portends a poor outcome. Rarely, myocardial sarcoid may simulate a myocardial infarction or present as myocarditis or cardiac tamponade. Pulmonary hypertension occurs frequently in advanced sarcoidosis.

DIAGNOSTIC TECHNIQUES

Diagnostic Guidelines

The Japanese Ministry of Health and Welfare has published guidelines for the diagnosis of cardiac sarcoidosis.[34]

Electrocardiography and Chest Radiography

Typical electrocardiographic abnormalities include varying degrees of atrioventricular block (0.9% to 11.3% of patients), right or left bundle branch blocks (0.6% to 5.8%), ventricular ectopic activity (1.3% to 4.7%), and ST-T wave abnormalities (7.3% to 36.3%). A QS pattern mimicking myocardial infarction is occasionally seen, and increased QT dispersion has been reported. A normal chest radiograph is the rule and does not exclude cardiac involvement.

Serologic and Kveim-Siltzbach Skin Testing

Angiotensin-converting enzyme levels in serum or bronchoalveolar lavage fluid are insensitive for establishing the diagnosis but can be helpful for monitoring level of activity. A heat-treated suspension of a sarcoidosis spleen extract is injected intradermally, which on biopsy 4 to 6 weeks later yields sarcoid-like lesions in 70% to 80% of individuals with sarcoidosis. The test has less than 5% false-positive results but is not widely available.

Radionuclide Imaging

Myocardial perfusion imaging reveals reversible or fixed defects that correspond to abnormalities of the coronary microvasculature and the presence of scar or granulomas, respectively. A combination of thallium Tl 201 and gallium Ga 67 scintigraphy can be used to diagnose and to evaluate severity of cardiac sarcoidosis and to assess response to therapy.[35]

Echocardiography

The echocardiogram is usually normal in the early course of the disease but may be useful in diagnosis of advanced myocardial sarcoidosis. Features include systolic dysfunction with or without regional wall motion abnormalities particularly involving the basal portion of the septum, left ventricular cavity dilatation, mitral or tricuspid regurgitation, ventricular aneurysms, and, in a small proportion of cases, pericardial effusions.[36] Increased thickness of the interventricular septum, asymmetric septal hypertrophy, and apical hypertrophy have been rarely described. Ultrasonic tissue characterization by myocardial integrated backscatter analysis is more sensitive than two-dimensional echocardiography in detecting early cardiac involvement, especially in the basal septum.

Magnetic Resonance Imaging and Positron Emission Tomography

Gadolinium contrast–enhanced magnetic resonance (cardiac magnetic resonance) imaging demonstrates interstitial edema by enhancement of signal intensity in the affected myocardium, indicating granulomatous inflammation (Fig. 81.6b). The sensitivity and specificity of cardiac magnetic resonance imaging have been reported to be 100% and 78%, respectively, although histologic correlation is lacking.[37] Active sarcoid involvement of the heart on positron emission tomography can appear as a flow-metabolic mismatch. These techniques may therefore be useful in monitoring the effects of various treatment regimens on disease activity in the myocardium and may be more sensitive than ^{67}Ga and ^{201}Tl imaging in detection of cardiac sarcoidosis.[38]

Endomyocardial Biopsy

Endomyocardial biopsy is useful in detecting active myocardial sarcoid disease, but findings are positive in only 50% of patients because of the inhomogeneous distribution of granulomas. Myocardial biopsy does not always differentiate cardiac sarcoidosis from giant cell myocarditis, which has a worse prognosis.

Electrophysiologic Studies

Nonsustained ventricular tachycardia is common in sarcoid heart disease, but the prognosis of these patients is unclear. Ventricular tachycardia in these patients may not be associated with active disease and may be secondary to re-entry. Electrophysiologic studies have a high sensitivity for detection of inducible ventricular tachycardia in cardiac sarcoidosis and can aid in arrhythmia management,[39] but they should be reserved for patients with a history of recurrent palpitations, syncope, sudden death, or sustained or nonsustained ventricular tachycardia.

MANAGEMENT

Corticosteroids are generally used in the management of cardiac sarcoidosis, although most of the data are based on case series and case reports.[40] Steroids have been shown to improve myocardial perfusion imaging abnormalities with ^{201}Tl, ^{67}Ga, and positron emission tomography imaging as well as electrocardiographic abnormalities in a small proportion of patients. Left ventricular function has also been shown to improve with prednisone but is unlikely to improve in the presence of significant fibrosis, especially in advanced cases with left ventricular ejection fraction of less than 30%. Methotrexate has also been used in patients requiring long-term steroid therapy. Cyclophosphamide and infliximab have been used successfully in a few cases unresponsive to steroid therapy.

Implantation of a permanent pacemaker in advanced atrioventricular block and implantable cardioverter-defibrillator in cases of sustained ventricular tachycardia or electrophysiologically inducible ventricular tachycardia is indicated. Steroids may decrease the severity and frequency of ventricular arrhythmias, but their effect on sudden death prevention remains unproven.

Cardiac transplantation is a therapeutic option for end-stage cardiomyopathy or refractory arrhythmias in sarcoid heart disease; 1-year post-transplantation survival rates are reported at approximately 88%.[41] Recurrent sarcoid in the allograft can occur but is usually responsive to enhanced immunosuppression and does not affect long-term prognosis.[42]

PROGNOSIS

Survival ranges from 2 years to more than 10 years from the time of diagnosis and is highly dependent on the extent of myocardial involvement. Patients with pulmonary sarcoidosis who present with cardiac symptoms have a poorer prognosis than that of those who are asymptomatic. Sudden death and progressive heart failure are the two most common causes of death. Patients with dilated cardiomyopathy due to cardiac sarcoidosis compared with patients with idiopathic dilated cardiomyopathy have a worse prognosis. However, 5-year transplant-free survival rate in biopsy-proven sarcoidosis is much better than that of idiopathic giant cell myocarditis and has been reported at 70%.[43] A large series of Japanese patients with cardiac sarcoidosis treated with prednisone had a 5-year survival rate of 75%.[44] NYHA functional class, left ventricular end-diastolic diameter, and presence of sustained ventricular tachycardia were independent predictors of mortality. Patients receiving corticosteroids before the onset of significant left ventricular systolic dysfunction had a better clinical outcome than did those with established congestive heart failure.

IDIOPATHIC RESTRICTIVE CARDIOMYOPATHY

The criteria proposed to define idiopathic restrictive cardiomyopathy are elevated ventricular filling pressures, normal left ventricular internal dimensions, and absence of pericardial or endomyocardial disease and infiltrative cardiomyopathy.[45] Idiopathic restrictive cardiomyopathy is a rare disorder described in younger adults and children.

ANATOMY AND PATHOLOGY

The ventricular cavity size is usually normal, and biatrial enlargement may be present. Ventricular wall thickness is usually normal but may be mildly increased. Pathologic examination of the heart reveals three different forms: pure restrictive disease, hypertrophic-restrictive form, and mildly dilated restrictive form. On microscopic examination, there is marked interstitial fibrosis and myocyte hypertrophy.

PATHOPHYSIOLOGY

The pathogenesis of this disorder is not clear, but marked diastolic dysfunction is the rule. A familial form exists and suggests that there may be a genetic abnormality with a phenotypic expression of interstitial fibrosis and myocyte hypertrophy. Most familial cases suggest autosomal dominant inheritance with variable penetrance. Some cases are sporadic in occurrence. Desmin, a granulofilamentous material, has been identified on ultrastructural examination in myocardium and skeletal muscle in approximately 40% of cases.[46] Desmin-related myopathy is associated with mutations in desmin, αB-crystallin, and selenoproteins.

CLINICAL PRESENTATION

Heart failure is the usual mode of presentation. The mean age at presentation is generally between 20 and 30 years. Complete heart block has also been described in patients and kindreds. Atrial fibrillation is a frequent, late finding. Both proximal and distal skeletal myopathy may also be present, especially in the familial forms.

DIAGNOSTIC TECHNIQUES

Electrocardiography and Chest Radiography

Biatrial enlargement, atrial fibrillation, complete heart block, intraventricular conduction delays, and biventricular hypertrophy are frequent electrocardiographic findings. The chest radiograph is often normal, but increased cardiothoracic ratios and mild interstitial edema are not uncommon findings.

Echocardiography

Moderate left atrial enlargement is often observed, but left ventricular dimensions are usually normal.

Endomyocardial Biopsy

Endomyocardial biopsy is helpful to rule out specific causes of infiltrative and restrictive cardiomyopathy. The diagnosis of idiopathic restrictive cardiomyopathy is one of exclusion.

MANAGEMENT

Medical management consists of diuretics to control diastolic heart failure, management of supraventricular arrhythmias, and insertion of a permanent pacemaker for high-grade atrioventricular block. Cardiac transplantation is often necessary as patients respond poorly to medical management, and it often results in excellent survival despite the presence of significant pulmonary hypertension.[47]

PROGNOSIS

Prognosis in children is substantially worse than that in adults, with a mean survival of approximately 1 year after diagnosis.[48] One case series reported a mean duration to transplantation or death of 117 ± 57 months; however, another report described a 5-year survival rate of greater than 95%. Multivariate analysis has identified male sex, left atrial dimension above 60 mm, age older than 70 years, and higher NYHA functional class as predictors of poorer survival in adults.[49]

HEMOCHROMATOSIS

Primary or hereditary hemochromatosis is an autosomal recessive iron storage disease characterized by a disturbance in regulation of iron absorption. The secondary type is seen as a result of excessive exogenous iron overload, especially in patients with congenital anemias who receive chronic blood transfusions. Cardiac involvement in hemochromatosis has been reported in 15% of patients but appears less prevalent in recent years because of earlier detection and advances in therapy.

ANATOMY AND PATHOLOGY

Excessive deposition of iron occurs in a variety of tissues, including heart, liver, testis, and pancreas.[50] In advanced cases, the iron deposits can be grossly visualized, and these patients invariably have cardiac dysfunction. Microscopic iron deposition is identified by a positive Prussian blue reaction and occurs predominantly in the subepicardial myocardium. Iron deposits are usually sarcoplasmic in location but occasionally may involve the interstitium.

PATHOPHYSIOLOGY

Primary hereditary hemochromatosis is commonly caused by mutations in the *HFE* gene linked to chromosome 6p. The most common genetic mutations are C282Y and H63D. Juvenile hemochromatosis may be linked to mutations in chromosome 1q. Cardiac involvement leads to a combined restrictive and dilated pattern with evidence of both diastolic and systolic dysfunction. The extent of myocardial iron deposition correlates well with the extent of left ventricular dysfunction. Fibrosis within the ventricle is scanty and does not entirely account for the extent of cardiac dysfunction. Iron distribution in early disease is usually perinuclear; in later stages, the entire cytoplasm is involved, possibly resulting in mitochondrial damage and systolic dysfunction (Fig. 81.7). Atrial iron deposition correlates with the presence of supraventricular arrhythmias.

CLINICAL PRESENTATION

Hepatomegaly, abnormal liver function test results, and arthritis are common initial clinical features in systemic hemochromatosis.[51] However, the classic triad of skin pigmentation, hepatomegaly, and diabetes mellitus was present in only 8% of patients in one series. Dyspnea occurs in less than 15% of patients. The most common cardiac manifestation is heart failure; when it is present, right-sided failure findings such as ascites and edema predominate. Patients with juvenile hemochromatosis may primarily present with dilated cardiomyopathy and may have accompanying

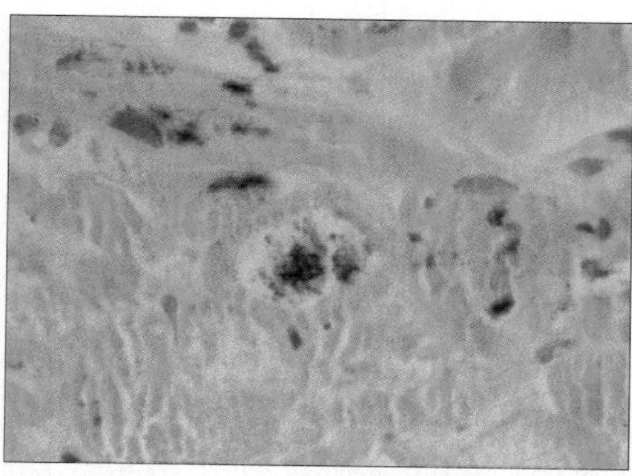

Figure 81.7 Endomyocardial biopsy specimen in a patient with hemochromatosis. Photomicrograph shows intracellular iron deposits (blue) in a myocardial biopsy specimen stained with Perls' iron stain. (Courtesy of H. Thomas Aretz, MD, Department of Pathology, Massachusetts General Hospital, Boston, Mass.)

hypogonadotropic hypogonadism, hepatomegaly, or hyperpigmentation typically before the age of 30 years.[52] Supraventricular arrhythmias, principally atrial fibrillation, can occur, but ventricular arrhythmias are infrequent.

DIAGNOSTIC TECHNIQUES

Serologic Testing

A fasting transferrin saturation of greater than 50% to 60% has been shown to be a highly sensitive screening test, especially for affected homozygotes. Serum ferritin (900 to 6000 μg/L) is a relatively sensitive but nonspecific test in detecting total body iron overload. Serum iron (180 to 300 μg/dL) is unreliable, and levels depend on nutritional status and blood loss.

Electrocardiography and Chest Radiography

Electrocardiographic abnormalities occur in 22% to 65% of patients with cardiac hemochromatosis. Common electrocardiographic findings include nonspecific repolarization abnormalities, low QRS voltage, intraventricular conduction delay, atrial fibrillation, and first-degree atrioventricular block. Cardiomegaly and pleural effusions are common chest radiographic findings.

Echocardiography

Unlike in most infiltrative cardiomyopathies, left ventricular thickening is not a characteristic feature of primary hemochromatosis. Mild thickening of left ventricular walls has been observed in some patients with normal left ventricular systolic function and may indicate early myocardial involvement because this thickening may resolve with therapy. Increased septal echogenicity similar to that of cardiac amyloidosis may be seen. As disease advances, cardiac findings include abnormal left ventricular systolic function, cavity dilatation, and biatrial enlargement.

Magnetic Resonance Imaging

Cardiac iron deposition is detected on magnetic resonance imaging by a reduction of myocardial signal intensity. Magnetic resonance imaging could be a valuable diagnostic aid in the early detection and management of these patients, although the sensitivity or specificity of this test in cardiac hemochromatosis is unknown.

Endomyocardial Biopsy

Biopsy is seldom necessary but can confirm the diagnosis when clinical features are equivocal. However, biopsy may yield false-negative results because of the predominant epicardial involvement of the myocardium.

Genetic Testing

Testing for common gene mutations in patients with hereditary hemochromatosis is important, especially for family screening and genetic counseling purposes.

MANAGEMENT

Therapy consists of phlebotomies and iron chelating therapy with chronic subcutaneous desferrioxamine. Periodic phlebotomies can reduce left ventricular diameter, left ventricular mass, and left atrial diameter and increase ejection fraction by echocardiography. Chelation therapy with desferrioxamine has also been reported to reverse cardiomyopathy.[53] Treatment may or may not result in actual depletion of iron deposits at the cellular level. Echocardiography and magnetic resonance imaging can monitor response to therapy. Improvement in symptoms and ejection fraction is variable and may occur within 6 to 12 months. Cardiac transplantation alone or with liver transplantation has been reported, without disease recurrence in the allograft, in patients with advanced cardiomyopathy for whom medical management has failed.[54]

PROGNOSIS

In an early series of 1098 patients with hemochromatosis, heart failure accounted for 31% of all deaths.[55] Cirrhosis of the liver, lack of response to venesection, and diabetes mellitus adversely affect long-term prognosis in primary hemochromatosis. Patients who do not have cirrhosis or diabetes mellitus and are treated with phlebotomies have a life expectancy comparable to that of the normal population.[56] Common causes of death in these patients include liver cirrhosis, hepatocellular carcinoma, and, rarely, cardiomyopathy. Heart failure is an important cause of mortality in patients with untreated hereditary and transfusion-related hemochromatosis. Although chelation therapy and repeated phlebotomy are most beneficial when they are instituted early, they can provide clinical improvement even when cardiomyopathy has developed.

STORAGE DISEASES OF THE MYOCARDIUM

A variety of myocardial storage diseases produce infiltrative cardiomyopathies. All are extremely rare and are summarized in Table 81.3.

STORAGE DISEASES OF THE MYOCARDIUM			
Type	**Metabolic Abnormality**	**Diagnostic Tests**	**Features**
Fabry's disease (X-linked recessive deficiency of α-galactosidase A)	Glycosphingolipid deposition	Low α-galactosidase activity in leukocytes, increased thickness of left ventricular walls by echocardiography, lamellar inclusion bodies in myocardial biopsy specimen	Mitral valve prolapse, infiltrative cardiomyopathy in the form of left ventricular hypertrophy that may regress with enzyme replacement therapy, arrhythmias, aortic stenosis, myocardial ischemia or infarction, mitral regurgitation
Hurler's syndrome (deficiency of α-L iduronidase, β-galactosidase)	Mucopolysaccharide deposition	Clear and granular cells in myocardial biopsy speciman, ultrastructural demonstration of abnormal cytoplasmic organelles	Mitral stenosis, mitral or aortic regurgitation, coronary arteriosclerosis, congestive heart failure
Glycogen storage diseases	Liver and muscle debranching enzyme, cardiac-specific phosphorylase kinase, lysosomal acid α-glucosidase	Enzyme deficiency in leukocytes, skeletal muscle or endomyocardial biopsy specimen; demonstration of glycogen by periodic acid–Schiff base staining of cells or glycogen granules by electron microscopy	Skeletal myopathy with or without cardiomyopathy in the form of left ventricular hypertrophy
Gaucher's disease (reduced β-glucocerebrosidase activity)	Glucocerebroside deposition	Decreased leukocyte glucocerebrosidase levels, thickened walls on echocardiography, histologic presence of myocardial interstitial Gaucher's cells	Restrictive cardiomyopathy, pericardial disease, valvular calcifications

Table 81.3 Storage diseases of the myocardium.

SUMMARY

Restrictive cardiomyopathy is the least commonly encountered cardiomyopathy but should always be considered when a patient presents with congestive heart failure and normal left ventricular systolic function. An important differential diagnosis is constrictive pericarditis, which is surgically treatable. Whereas hemodynamic features obtained at cardiac catheterization help make the diagnosis of restrictive cardiomyopathy, endomyocardial biopsy and imaging studies of the pericardium are not infrequently required. Treatment is usually disease specific and supportive with diuretics and preload-reducing agents.

chapter 82

Pericardial Disease

Yasmin Masood and Martin M. LeWinter

Definition

- Pericardial disease has numerous causes, mainly inflammatory and infectious, and multiple clinical presentations related to acute inflammation, hemodynamic effects on the heart, and acute and chronic complications.

Key Features

- A thorough history, physical examination, and electrocardiography in conjunction with hemodynamic and properly selected imaging modalities lead to accurate diagnosis and appropriate treatment strategies.

Therapy

- Therapy for pericardial disease is directed toward treatment of both the primary cause and the hemodynamic complications.

Numerous cardiac as well as systemic disease processes can affect the pericardium. The disease process may be transient and self-limited, as in acute pericarditis; chronic and progressive, as in constrictive pericarditis; or relatively sudden and life-threatening, as in cardiac tamponade. Infection, inflammation, fibrosis, and infiltration of tumors may cause changes in the thickness and fluid content of the pericardial sac, resulting in pericardial space constraints. Depending on the acuteness of these changes, there may be severe hemodynamic compromise, especially with pericardial fluid accumulation and cardiac tamponade. This chapter reviews the anatomy and physiology of the pericardium and the etiology, clinical presentation, electrocardiographic features, hemodynamics, imaging study findings, management, and treatment of these disease processes.

ANATOMY AND PHYSIOLOGY

The pericardium is composed of a fibrous parietal outer layer and an inner serous visceral membrane. The parietal membrane, composed of collagen and elastin fibers, allows the heart to sustain its position within the cardiothoracic cavity regardless of body position or respiration. This fibrous layer has ligamentous attachments to the sternum, xiphoid process, vertebral column, and diaphragm and tube-like extensions that enclose the origins of the great vessels.[1] The serous visceral membrane, composed of a monolayer of mesothelial cells, lines the epicardial surface of the heart. The mesothelial cells contain numerous microvilli and cilia that increase the surface area for fluid transport and provide a friction-bearing surface.[2] The visceral membrane reflects back on itself to line the parietal membrane from the inside (Fig. 82.1) at two points, proximal to the entry of the superior and inferior venae cavae in the right atrium and the oblique sinus of the pericardium, posterior to the left atrium. The parietal pericardium surrounds both ventricles, the entire right atrium, and portions of the caval vessels as mentioned. The left atrium is only partially enclosed within the parietal pericardium. The internal thoracic arteries constitute the main blood supply to the parietal pericardium. Blood from the pericardium drains into the azygos system. Pericardial lymphatic drainage occurs through anterior mediastinal nodes. The innervation of the pericardium is mainly from the phrenic nerves.[3,4]

The pericardium normally contains up to 50 mL of serous fluid, which is an ultrafiltrate of plasma. The visceral pericardium is believed to be the source of pericardial fluid in both normal and diseased states. Total protein concentration is lower than that in plasma, but there is a higher proportion of albumin. The pericardial fluid also contains phospholipids that serve as a lubricant in the pericardial cavity. A number of prostaglandins are found in the pericardial fluid and are believed to modulate cardiac electrophysiologic properties.[5]

The normal pericardium is elastic (compliant) up to cardiac volumes that correspond to about the upper limit of the operating volume of the normal heart. Above this volume, the pericardium relatively abruptly becomes noncompliant, that is, it has a small reserve volume. This behavior is ascribable to the collagen fibers in the parietal pericardium, which straighten as the pericardial sac becomes noncompliant. As a result, under normal conditions, physiologic changes in cardiac volume cause no more than modest changes in intrapericardial pressure (Fig. 82.2).[6,7] However, with acute, pathologic cardiac dilatation (e.g., due to regurgitant valvular disease or right ventricular myocardial infarction), the pericardium can exert an important restraining effect on increases in cardiac volume (Fig. 82.3).[8] In both of these conditions, the chambers of the heart dilate to a degree, placing constraints on the pericardial space. This increase in pericardial restraint (i.e., an increased contact force on the surface of the heart) increases the intracavitary filling pressures in the cardiac chambers, most prominently on the right side of the heart.

The pericardium also modulates direct diastolic ventricular interaction through the septum. Ventricular interaction (the capacity of one ventricle to influence the behavior of the contralateral ventricle) can be demonstrated under normal conditions. In diastole, this is manifested as a measurable,

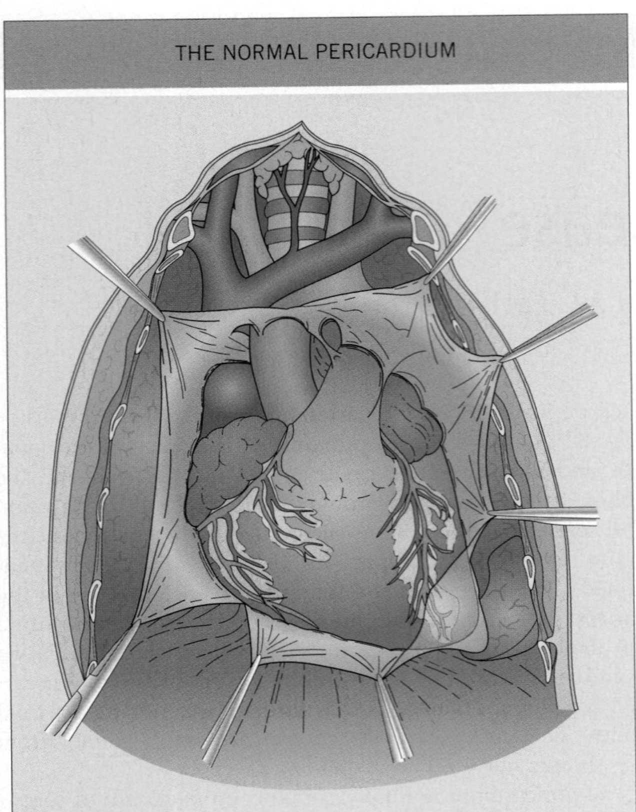

Figure 82.1 **The normal pericardium.** The parietal pericardium is lifted, showing extension enclosing the origin of great vessels. (From Spodick, DH. The Pericardium. New York, Marcel Dekker, 1997.)

modest contribution of the filling pressure of the left to the right ventricle and vice versa. Ventricular interaction is markedly exaggerated when the volume in the pericardial sac reaches the steep, noncompliant portion of the pericardial

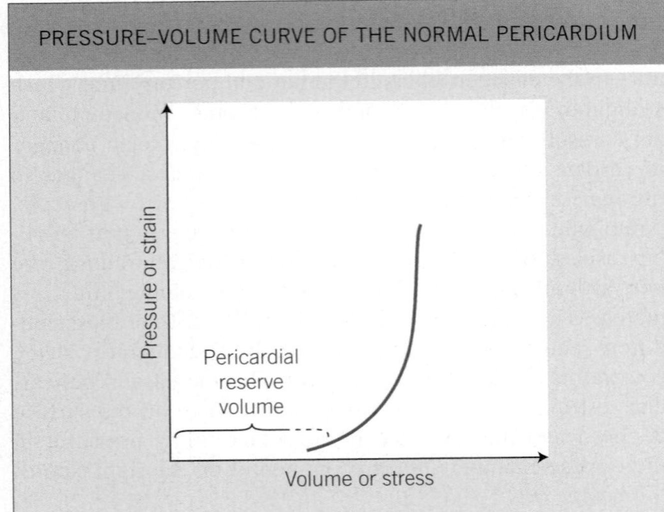

Figure 82.2 **Pressure-volume curve of the normal pericardium.** As volume is added to the pericardial space, a minimal change in intrapericardial pressure occurs. When the pericardial reserve volume is exceeded, a small further increment of added volume increases the pressure exponentially. (From Spodick, DH. The Pericardium. New York, Marcel Dekker, 1997.)

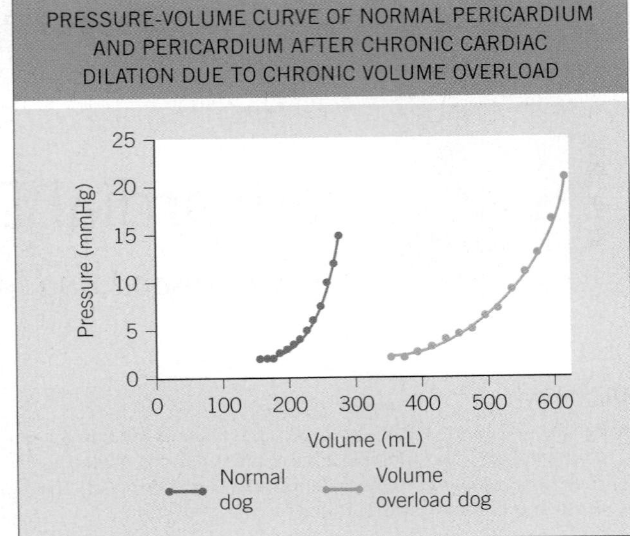

Figure 82.3 **Pressure-volume curve of normal pericardium and pericardium after chronic cardiac dilatation due to chronic volume overload.** The pressure-volume curve shifts to the right; as a result, the pericardium can accommodate a larger volume before the restraining effect on the heart occurs. (From Freeman G, LeWinter M. Pericardial adaptations during chronic cardiac dilation in dogs. Circ Res 1984;54:294-300.)

pressure-volume relation. At this point, the pericardium markedly influences filling pressure both directly and by augmenting diastolic interaction.[9] In effect, the cardiac chambers are constrained to function at a relatively fixed total volume within the pericardial sac. As a result, when the pericardial volume is abnormally large, an increase in filling of one chamber occurs at the expense of filling of the contralateral chamber. Thus, ventricular interaction also influences systolic function. Exaggerated ventricular interaction is a key pathophysiologic mechanism underlying pulsus paradoxus in cardiac tamponade.[10]

Similar pressure-volume relationships apply to increases in the fluid in the pericardial sac. As indicated earlier, the pericardial space has only a small reserve volume. Initial increases in pericardial fluid volume cause slight increases in intrapericardial pressure until the pericardial pressure-volume relation becomes very steep (noncompliant). At this point, additional increases in pericardial fluid volume cause an exponential increase in pericardial pressure. This in turn is transmitted to the inside of the cardiac chambers, causing markedly increased intracardiac pressures but reduced volumes with secondary effects on stroke volume and cardiac output. Conversely, removal of small amounts of pericardial fluid in cardiac tamponade can dramatically reduce intracardiac pressures.

In chronic cardiac diseases in which the total cardiac volume enlarges gradually (e.g., regurgitant valvular disease), the pressure-volume curve of the pericardium gradually shifts to the right, minimizing the restraining effects observed acutely. Thus, the pericardium stretches and can accommodate much larger cardiac volumes than it can acutely. A similar response occurs with a slowly accumulating pericardial effusion, which can be extremely large without causing cardiac tamponade.

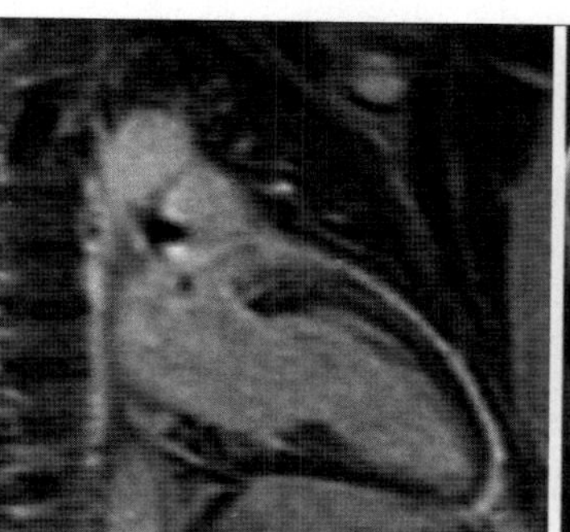
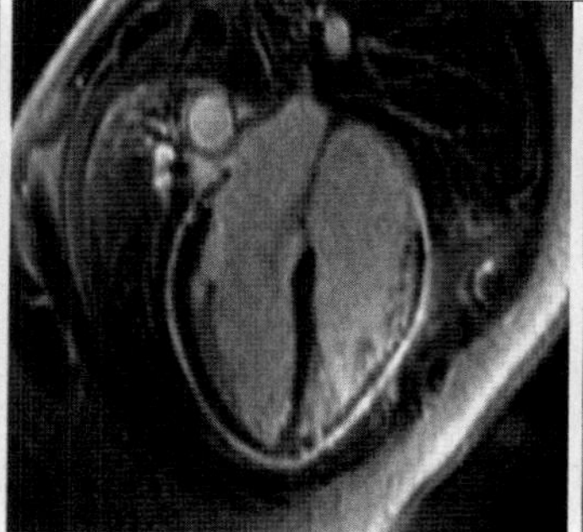
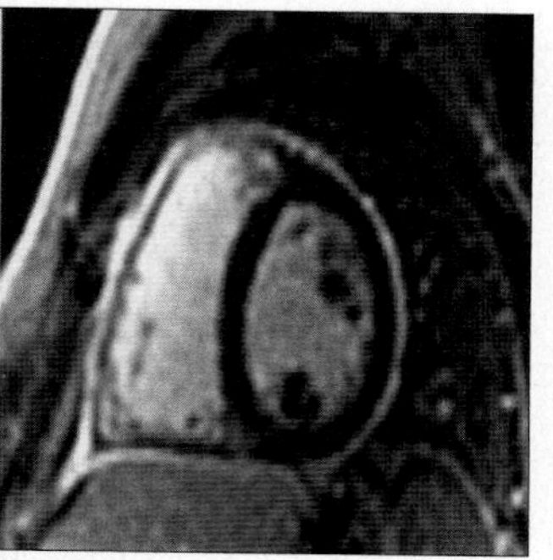

Figure 82.4 Inversion-recovery sequences showing diffuse hyperenhancement around the heart after gadolinium administration indicative of pericarditis.

ACUTE PERICARDITIS

The clinical syndrome of chest pain, pericardial friction rub, and serial electrocardiographic abnormalities defines acute pericarditis, an inflammatory response of the pericardial tissue typically characterized by increased vascularity, infiltration with polymorphonuclear leukocytes, and deposition of fibrin (Fig. 82.4). This syndrome can be the result of a variety of infectious and noninfectious causes (Table 82.1). However, the most common cause is viral. Because a specific virus is rarely implicated in individual cases, this category is usually termed idiopathic. In an uncertain number of cases, myocarditis accompanies a syndrome characteristic of pericarditis. The reverse may also occur, and a truly mixed picture of myopericarditis is occasionally present (Fig. 82.5).

CLINICAL PRESENTATIONS

Chest pain is the most common presenting symptom, although it may be absent, especially with more subacute or chronic causes, such as rheumatoid disease or tuberculosis. The pain often begins relatively abruptly; it is typically sharp in quality and pleuritic. It is exacerbated by coughing and recumbency and relieved by sitting up and leaning forward. Pericardial pain may radiate to the trapezius ridge; if it is present, this radiation is nearly specific for pericarditis.

MAJOR CAUSES OF ACUTE PERICARDITIS WITH ESTIMATED PERCENTAGES	
Idiopathic or viral	
Coxsackie A, coxsackie B, echovirus, adenovirus	78%
Neoplasms	
Lung carcinoma, breast carcinoma, leukemia, lymphoma	7%
Tuberculosis	5%
Infectious	
Bacterial, fungal, toxoplasmosis	4%
Collagen vascular diseases	
Rheumatoid, systemic lupus erythematosus, scleroderma	3%
Other	
Uremia, post–myocardial infarction, postcardiac surgery, radiation induced, drugs	3%

Table 82.1 Major causes of acute pericarditis with estimated percentages.

However, it may also radiate in a fashion similar to the discomfort of myocardial ischemia. Systemic manifestations including low-grade fever and influenza-like symptoms may accompany or precede the chest pain. High fevers are unusual and suggest bacterial pericarditis.

The pericardial friction rub is pathognomonic of pericarditis, although its absence does not exclude pericardial inflammation. It is best heard with the diaphragm of the stethoscope at the left mid to lower sternal edge with the patient sitting up and leaning forward. The pericardial friction rub classically consists of three components corresponding to atrial systole, ventricular systole (loudest), and early ventricular diastole (Fig. 82.6).[11] In about one third of patients, the rub is biphasic; in about 10%, it is monophasic. The friction rub is believed to be generated by contact between the inflamed pericardial surfaces. However, it can be heard even in the presence of a large effusion.[12] The rub can be remarkably transitory. When a rub is not heard initially in a suspected case of pericarditis, frequent auscultation can be rewarding in establishing the diagnosis.

DIAGNOSTIC TECHNIQUES

Electrocardiography is the most useful diagnostic test in patients presenting with chest pain; electrocardiographic abnormalities appear in about 90% of patients with acute pericarditis.[13] These have been classically divided into four stages.[14] Stage I is characterized by ST-segment elevation in all leads except aVR and V_1, with a normal T-wave axis. Unlike in acute myocardial infarction, the ST segment is usually concave upward, and the leads in which elevation is observed do not correspond to usual infarction lead distributions (Fig. 82.7). In stage II, the ST segment returns to baseline and flattening of T waves occurs, typically during several days. T-wave inversion occurs in stage III, sometimes with ST-segment depression. In stage IV, ST segments and T waves return to normal. Complete normalization may require weeks to months. There is considerable variability in the ST-T abnormalities of pericarditis, and they need not go through each of these phases in an individual case. In addition to ST-segment and T-wave changes, PR-segment depression has been reported in about 80% of patients.[13] PR-segment depression is one of the earliest electrocardiographic manifestations of pericarditis, occurring in the first few hours of presentation and often preceding ST-segment elevation.[15]

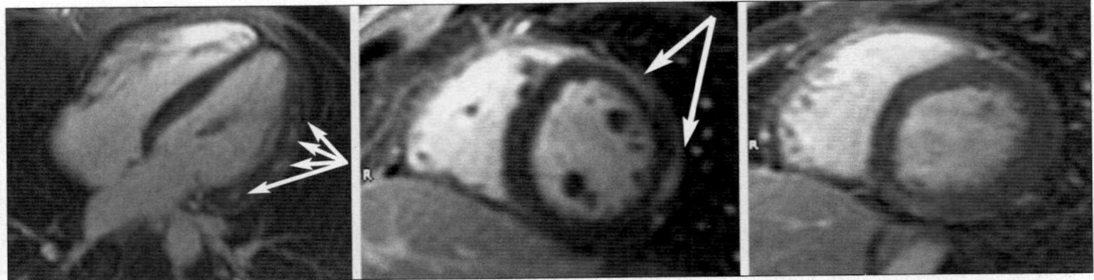

Figure 82.5 Gradient echo inversion-recovery sequence in a case of myopericarditis. There is patchy delayed hyperenhancement after administration of gadolinium *(arrows)* indicative of myocarditis in the four-chamber long-axis view, thickened pericardium indicative of pericarditis in the mid short-axis view, and normal myocardium in the basal short-axis view slice (no delayed hyperenhancement).

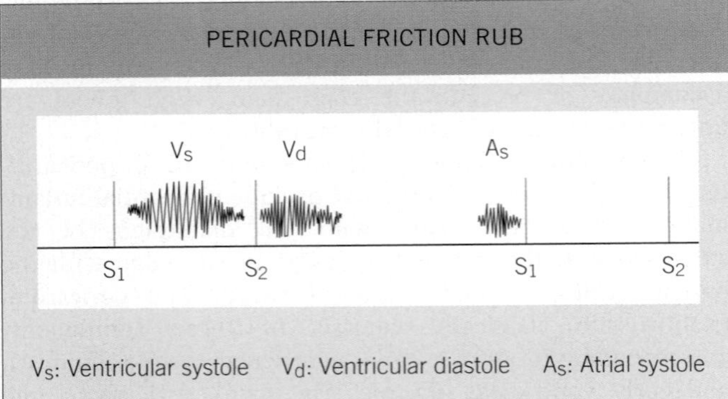

Figure 82.6 Schematic representation of a phonogram of pericardial friction rub with its three components: ventricular systole (V_s), ventricular diastole (V_d), and atrial systole (A_s). S_1, first heart sound; S_2, second heart sound.

The ST-segment elevation of pericarditis can be differentiated from the normal variant of early repolarization if the ratio of ST to T wave in V_6 is greater than 0.25. Furthermore, evolutionary ST- and T-wave changes as described before are not observed with early repolarization. Sinus tachycardia is common in patients with acute pericarditis. Ventricular tachycardia and conduction abnormalities are suggestive of myocardial involvement with ischemia, inflammation, or fibrosis and should not be considered a manifestation of acute pericarditis.

Nonspecific inflammatory responses are evident in several laboratory test abnormalities. Mild leukocytosis and elevation in erythrocyte sedimentation rate are often found. Biomarker changes characteristic of myocardial necrosis are usually absent but can occur in the presence of associated myocarditis. Moreover, troponin I can be significantly elevated in 20% of patients with acute pericarditis.[16] Specific diagnostic laboratory tests should be tailored to the clinical presentation. Blood cultures, fungal serology, human immunodeficiency virus (HIV) testing, and tuberculin skin testing should be obtained if a nonviral infectious agent is suspected (in cases of routine "idiopathic" pericarditis, viral titers are not ordinarily indicated). The measurement of blood urea nitrogen, creatinine, thyroid-stimulating hormone, thyroxine, antinuclear antibodies, and rheumatoid factor is also indicated in situations in which the presentation suggests a specific etiology.

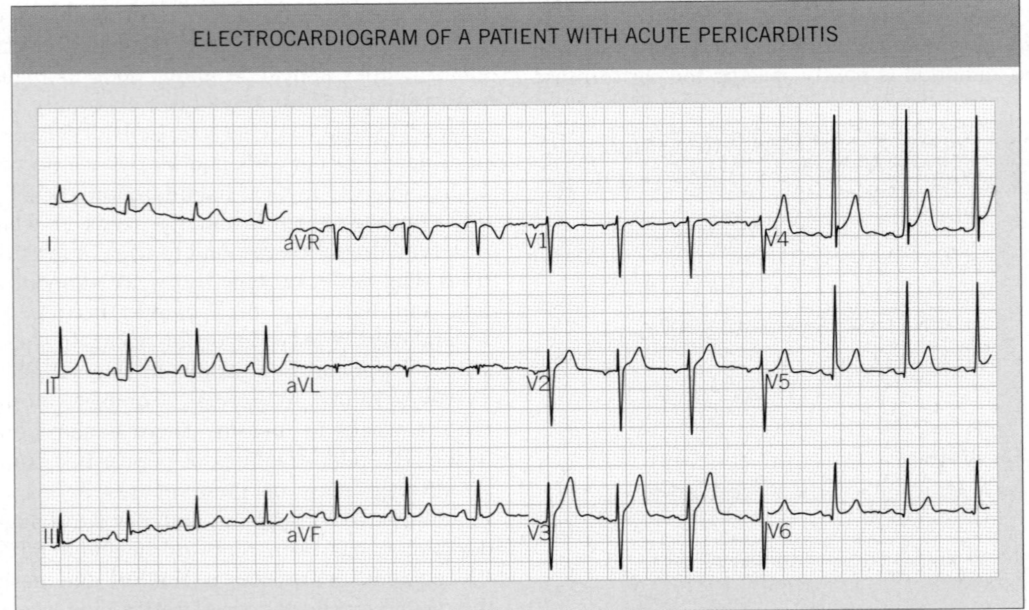

Figure 82.7 Electrocardiogram of a patient with acute pericarditis. Note the diffuse ST elevation and PR depression.

A chest radiograph should be obtained in all cases. It is normal in uncomplicated acute, idiopathic pericarditis. However, the cause of the pericarditis may be clarified if an adjacent pneumonic process or lung neoplasm is identified. Enlargement of the cardiac silhouette may be observed if a significant pericardial effusion complicates acute pericarditis.

Echocardiography is a very sensitive test for the detection of pericardial effusion or tamponade. However, the diagnosis of acute pericarditis is made by documenting the clinical syndrome of chest pain, pericardial friction rub, and characteristic electrocardiographic abnormalities, not by the presence of a pericardial effusion. At the same time, small effusions are fairly common and support the diagnosis of pericarditis if there is uncertainty. Moderate or larger effusions are unusual in acute, idiopathic pericarditis.

The utility of additional diagnostic testing in acute pericarditis, including pericardiocentesis and pericardial biopsy (if more than a small effusion is present), has been addressed in prospective studies.[17] Noninvasive testing was performed as an initial step, followed by fluid analysis or pericardial biopsy. These studies revealed that the diagnostic yield of pericardiocentesis with fluid analysis or a pericardial biopsy has a much higher positive predictive value in sicker patients and those with a complicated presentation but is of little use in typical patients who respond to initial, conservative therapy.

MANAGEMENT

In 70% to 90% of the patients with acute pericarditis, the course is self-limited without complications. Treatment of acute pericarditis (idiopathic or viral) is aimed at alleviation of symptoms and prevention of recurrences and complications. Treatment of other causes of pericarditis is aimed at the primary disease causing pericardial inflammation, as discussed later. Hospitalization is not always required. Reliable patients with presentations typical of idiopathic or viral pericarditis and no evidence of a significant effusion by echocardiography, whose discomfort can be relieved effectively with initial treatment as outlined later, can be managed as outpatients. Acute pericarditis responds well and frequently dramatically to nonsteroidal anti-inflammatory drugs (NSAIDs). Although indomethacin is often recommended as the NSAID of choice, we prefer ibuprofen (600 to 800 mg every 6 hours) as initial treatment because it is effective and less toxic. Although aspirin is currently rarely used for acute, uncomplicated pericarditis, it is an acceptable alternative at doses of 650 mg every 6 to 8 hours if it is well tolerated. For acute attacks, colchicine can also be considered an alternative or supplement to NSAIDs. If symptoms are severe and persist for more than 48 hours despite NSAID treatment, colchicine should be strongly considered. Colchicine is administered at a dose of 1 mg daily for 10 to 14 days after a 2- to 3-mg oral loading dose.[18] Corticosteroids should be avoided in patients with acute pericarditis if at all possible because their use may be associated with an increased incidence of recurrences. If corticosteroids cannot be avoided, the recommended course is prednisone, 60 mg daily for 2 days with tapering during 7 days. Studies indicate that concomitant use of rosuvastatin with an NSAID (indomethacin) may accelerate the reduction of inflammation and recovery. This interesting finding deserves additional study to more definitively delineate the role of statins in pericarditis.[19]

Antibiotics should not be administered unless purulent pericarditis is documented. Anticoagulation (heparin or warfarin) should be avoided if possible during the acute phase of pericarditis of any cause. However, in ischemic syndromes and myocardial infarction, the indications for anticoagulation outweigh the exceedingly small risk of intrapericardial bleeding. The risk of intrapericardial bleeding in ischemic syndromes does not appear to be increased by platelet glycoprotein IIb/IIIa receptor antagonists. Patients with pericarditis who must receive drugs that interfere with hemostasis should be observed carefully and frequently for signs of effusion or tamponade by physical examination and echocardiography.

Recurrent episodes of pericarditis after successful initial treatment occur in about 15% to 30% of patients. Occasional patients with what is initially thought to be idiopathic pericarditis manifest evidence of a specific etiology as they develop recurrences (e.g., systemic lupus erythematosus). Recurrences usually respond to a repeated course of the initially successful treatment. A small number of patients develop multiple bouts of recurrent chest discomfort, which can be debilitating. Some have surprisingly little in the way of objective evidence of pericardial inflammation with these episodes. These patients often present difficult management problems. Repeated courses of NSAIDs or colchicine appear to be equally effective. Once a recurrent acute episode has passed, colchicine is generally effective as prophylaxis for recurrent symptoms. We currently recommend its routine use in patients with multiple bouts of recurrent pericardial pain. The most common side effects of colchicine are nausea and diarrhea, which leads to dose reduction or cessation of treatment in 10% to 15% of the patients. Again, corticosteroids should be avoided if possible for recurrent episodes.[20] Among patients with recurrent pericarditis, that is, more than two relapses, the aggregate of published and unpublished studies has shown corticosteroid use to be an independent risk factor for recurrence after colchicine therapy.[21] If there is no response to other treatments, short courses of corticosteroids may be initiated. In these difficult cases, combined use of NSAIDs or even immunosuppressive drugs such as cyclosporine or azathioprine may aid in minimizing corticosteroid dosage. There are also few case reports of benefit from use of intravenous immune globulins in patients with chronic idiopathic pericarditis.[22] Pericardiectomy has also occasionally been employed for treatment of recurrent pericarditis. Results have in general been disappointing, probably because it is impossible to remove the entire pericardium, and the underlying inflammatory processes may also involve the pleura. Nonetheless, we have encountered occasional patients with impressive responses to pericardiectomy.

Pericardial effusion is not unusual in patients with acute pericarditis but usually rarely produces adverse hemodynamic consequences. Constrictive pericarditis is a complication of chronic pericardial inflammation and is discussed later. The proportion of cases of idiopathic or viral pericarditis that go on to pericardial constriction is very small.

PERICARDIAL EFFUSION

Pericardial effusion not infrequently is an incidental finding on echocardiography. Most are small and probably represent extremes within the normal distribution of pericardial fluid volume. Rarely, however, incidental effusions can be moderate to remarkably large. The natural history of large, incidental effusions is unclear. Most effusions of moderate size or greater, and virtually all that result in cardiac tamponade, are caused by pericardial injury or inflammation. Thus, the etiology and differential diagnosis of pericardial effusion are essentially those of pericarditis (see Table 82.1), with exceptions being processes such as congestive heart failure, nephrotic syndrome, and hypothyroidism that can produce effusion without pericardial inflammation.

CLINICAL PRESENTATIONS

Pericardial effusions are rarely symptomatic unless they are complicated by cardiac compression. Associated symptoms are usually related to pericardial inflammation or the underlying disease causing the effusion. Pericardial effusions that accumulate slowly can exceed 2 liters in volume without hemodynamic compromise. However, rapid increases in intrapericardial fluid of as little as 150 to 200 mL can raise the intrapericardial pressure to a level sufficient to cause cardiac compression. In practice, most effusions that cause tamponade in medical patients are intermediate between these two extremes. Rarely, large pericardial effusions can compress adjacent structures and cause symptoms. Thus, compression of bronchi or the trachea can lead to cough, compression of the vagus nerve can cause hiccups, and compression of lung parenchyma can cause crackles. If a large pericardial effusion is present, the heart sounds are usually muffled. Pulsus paradoxus and abnormal jugular venous pressure do not occur unless there is significant elevation in the intrapericardial pressure.

DIAGNOSTIC TECHNIQUES

In the presence of a large pericardial effusion, the electrocardiogram often demonstrates low QRS voltage. Electrical alternans is virtually pathognomonic of a large pericardial effusion, usually with cardiac tamponade. It is caused by the curious phenomenon of the heart's swinging in the pericardial fluid with a frequency equal to half the heart rate (Fig. 82.8).

With a large effusion, the chest radiograph demonstrates enlargement of the cardiac silhouette with a "water bottle"–shaped heart (Fig. 82.9). Enlargement does not occur with effusions of less than approximately 250 mL; an important implication of this is that a rapidly accumulating, hemodynamically significant effusion need not enlarge the cardiac silhouette.

Echocardiography is the most sensitive and practical method for detection of pericardial effusion (Fig. 82.10). Pericardial effusion can be posterior (this is where nonloculated effusions first accumulate), circumferential (Fig. 82.11), or loculated. The best echocardiographic views are the parasternal short-axis view and the apical four-chamber view for posterior and circumferential effusions, respectively. Subcostal views are best for loculated fluid overlying the right atrium. It is important to differentiate pericardial from pleural effusion. Left pleural effusions are seen in the parasternal long-axis view posterior to the descending aorta, whereas pericardial fluid is situated anterior to the descending aorta.

Pericardial effusions can also be detected with magnetic resonance imaging (MRI) and computed tomography (CT).

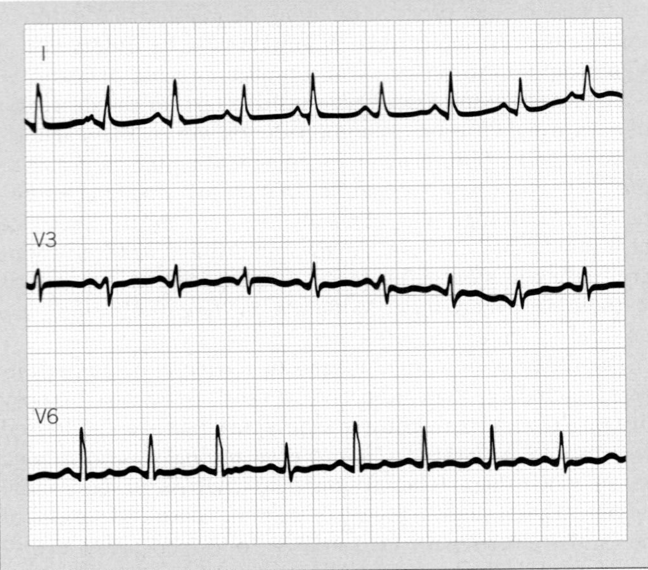

Figure 82.8 Electrocardiogram of a patient with cardiac tamponade showing electrical alternans. (From Shabetai R. The Pericardium. New York, Grune & Stratton, 1981:279-324.)

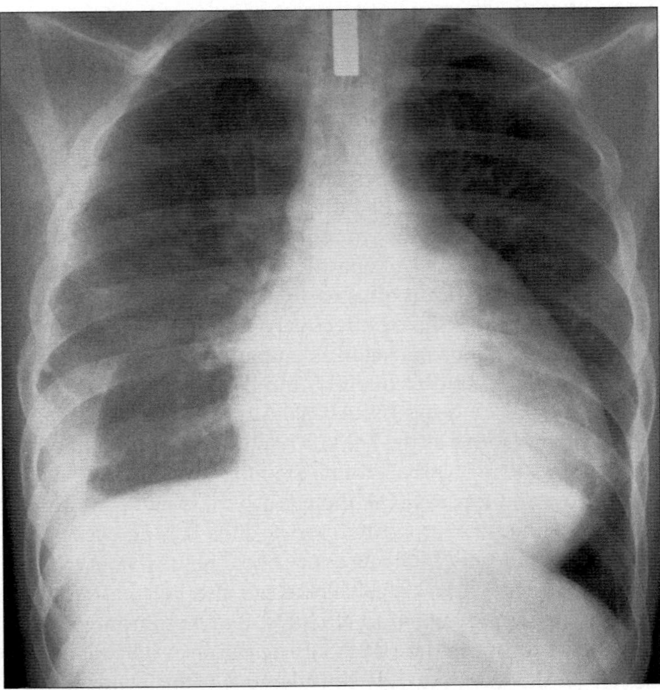

Figure 82.9 Chest radiograph from a patient with a pericardial effusion showing typical "water bottle" heart.

For routine assessment of the size and location of pericardial effusions, echocardiography is the most accessible and convenient method and is often less costly than MRI or CT. However, CT and MRI are valuable in patients in whom echocardiographic views are technically inadequate. CT and MRI are also useful to assess loculated pericardial effusion, to differentiate hemorrhagic from nonhemorrhagic effusion, to measure pericardial thickness, and to detect

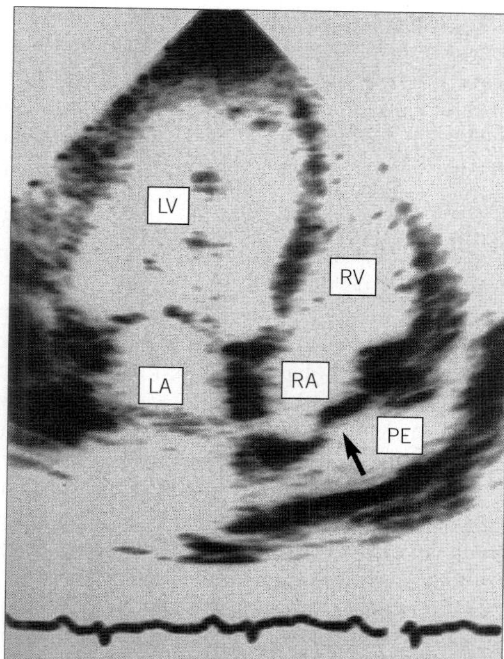

Figure 82.10 Echocardiograph of a patient with a large circumferential pericardial effusion. LA, left atrium; RA, right atrium; RV, right ventricle; LV, left ventricle; PE, pericardial effusion.

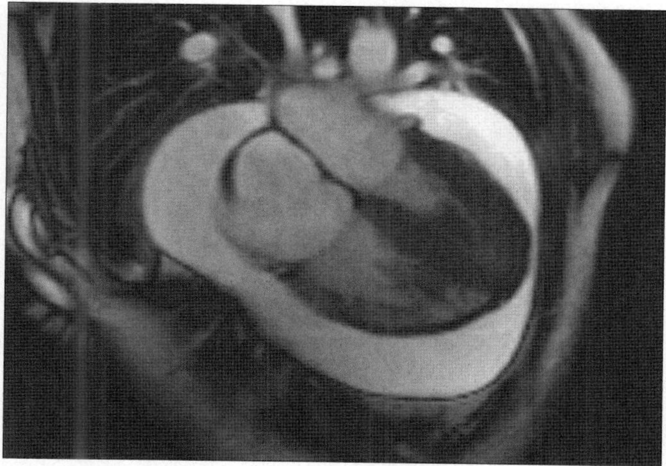

Figure 82.11 Gradient echo image showing hyperdense signal on T1 weighting illustrates severe circumferential pericardial effusion in a patient with systemic lupus erythematosus.

enhancement of the pericardium when constrictive pericarditis is suspected. For differentiation of small pericardial effusion from thickened pericardium, cine MRI with gradient echo or steady-state free precession is superior to CT or echocardiography because it can demonstrate ventricular sliding over the pericardium. Typically, pericardial effusions are visualized on MRI turbo spin echo as a hyperintense signal on T2-weighted images and a hypointense signal on T1-weighted images. As previously noted, a high signal intensity is also seen on MRI T2 cine gradient echo and steady-state free precession sequences. Chest CT by use of Hounsfield units and cardiac MRI by use of T1 and T2 weighting may be helpful in distinguishing the type of pericardial effusion (i.e., hemorrhagic versus nonhemorrhagic; Fig. 82.12).

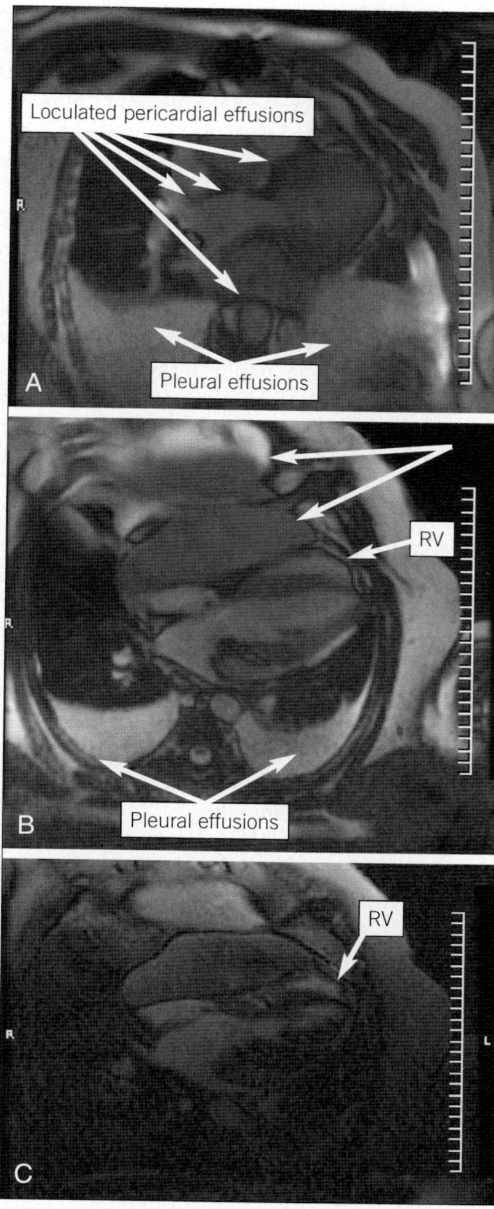

Figure 82.12 Patient with pericardial effusion and pleural effusion. T1-weighted gradient echo images show multiple areas of loculated hemorrhagic pericardial effusion and bilateral pleural effusions (**A** and **B**). Low (dark) and high (bright) signal in the pericardial effusion indicates subacute bleeding compressing the right ventricle (*arrows,* **B**), and high signal is seen within the bilateral pleural effusions (**A** and **B**). Inversion-recovery sequence shows heterogeneity of signal within the pericardial effusion indicative of subacute bleeding **(C)**. RV, right ventricle.

MANAGEMENT

In patients with small, incidentally detected pericardial effusions, we do not ordinarily recommend any further evaluation. The appropriate management of moderate to large effusions without evidence of cardiac compression that are detected incidentally in asymptomatic individuals is uncertain. We recommend a chest radiograph (if one has not been obtained previously), routine blood testing to look for hematologic and thyroid abnormalities and rheumatologic disease, and skin testing for tuberculosis. An unanswered question is when such effusions should be drained, if at all. We usually recommend draining them electively by closed pericardiocentesis because cardiac tamponade can occur in about 30% of patients with large idiopathic chronic pericardial effusion.[23] However, it is also perfectly reasonable to alert these patients to symptoms of increasing effusion and to manage them conservatively by performing serial echocardiography.

In the case of effusions not detected incidentally, drainage is mandatory only if cardiac compression (or compression of other structures) is present or purulent pericarditis is suspected. Thus, chronic (>6 months), moderate to large effusions considered secondary to known systemic diseases such as hypothyroidism, malignant neoplasia, uremia, nephrotic syndrome, and chronic heart failure need not necessarily be drained. With effusions that are not chronic or are of unknown duration, drainage is often indicated on an individualized basis. In patients without cardiac tamponade, a trial of NSAIDs or colchicine can be administered to reduce the effusion before drainage is considered. In effusions for which an autoimmune disorder is the etiology, corticosteroids can be administered in addition to other anti-inflammatory medications. We particularly favor draining such effusions in patients with cancer or immunocompromise, in whom delineation of sometimes unusual infectious causes is critical. Pericardial effusion in patients with cancer is not necessarily due to metastatic implants. Infections have already been mentioned. Another occasional cause of effusion in cancer patients is obstruction of the pericardial lymphatic drainage due to mediastinal lymphadenopathy.

Whether drainage is undertaken or not, appropriate attempts to delineate the etiology of pericardial effusions are critical. It is important to search carefully for nonviral causes, especially systemic diseases, infections, and malignant neoplasms, as outlined in Table 82.1. Pericardial fluid should routinely be stained and cultured for detection of bacteria (including tuberculosis) and fungi. As much fluid as possible should be submitted for detection of malignant cells as there is a reasonably high yield for diagnosis of malignant disease in patients with pericardial involvement. In tuberculous pericardial disease, several tests other than culture of fluid and examination of biopsy specimens are useful. These include adenosine deaminase, interferon γ, and polymerase chain reaction to detect viral RNA. Unless some other cause is evident, we believe that a relatively rapid test for tuberculosis (adenosine deaminase, polymerase chain reaction) is usually warranted because of the general difficulty of diagnosing tuberculous pericarditis and the delays involved in making a diagnosis by culture. There may also be a role for routine measurement of selected tumor markers as a general screen for malignant effusion and an adjunct to direct detection of malignant cells.

CARDIAC TAMPONADE

Accumulation of fluid in the pericardial space causing an increase in intrapericardial pressure and cardiac compression defines cardiac tamponade. It is usually a life-threatening situation and should be managed aggressively and promptly.

PATHOPHYSIOLOGY

Tamponade results in a spectrum of hemodynamic alterations. The condition is a pathophysiologic continuum ranging from mild to critical compression with marked reduction in cardiac output and cardiovascular collapse.[24] Critical tamponade can occur from as little as 150 mL of blood acutely introduced into the pericardial space or may require substantially more than 1 liter of slowly accumulating fluid. Clinically significant cardiac compression depends on several related factors. As noted before, the pericardial pressure-volume curve has a flat portion followed by a steep portion (see Fig. 82.2). As fluid is infused into the pericardial space, it initially fills the numerous recesses and sinuses of the parietal pericardium,[25] and the pressure rises slowly over the flat portion of the curve. As volume is added, the steep portion of the pressure-volume curve is eventually engaged, probably at total pericardial volumes just above the upper limits of the physiologic range of total cardiac volumes. At this point, additional increments of added volume increase intrapericardial pressure exponentially. The rise in the intrapericardial pressure defines a compressive force on the surface of the cardiac chambers that results in decreased transmural distending pressures and hence impaired filling.[26] The compressive force initially and most prominently affects the lower pressure, thinner walled right heart chambers. The intrapericardial portions of the caval vessels may actually be most sensitive to compression. Correspondingly, collapse of the right atrium, right ventricle, and caval vessels is a relatively early echocardiographic sign of cardiac tamponade. Effects on the left side of the heart are likely to be related as much to underfilling secondary to impaired right-sided heart output as to direct compression. The earliest hemodynamic effects of cardiac compression consist of mild elevations in the intracavitary cardiac filling pressures, with right-sided heart pressures rising more rapidly than left-sided heart pressures, and a modest reduction in stroke volume without overt hemodynamic deterioration.[27]

The reduction in stroke volume initiates compensatory mechanisms, chiefly reflex and neurohumorally mediated increases in adrenergic tone. Tachycardia helps maintain cardiac output. The increase in sympathetic outflow activates α-adrenergic peripheral receptors, which maintain blood pressure by peripheral vasoconstriction.[28] Activation of the renin-angiotensin-aldosterone system occurs relatively late. This contributes to decreased urinary sodium excretion and water retention in an effort to maintain blood pressure. Untreated tamponade leads to a progressive decline in cardiac output, with failure of compensatory mechanisms to maintain adequate perfusion pressure. Terminally, severe hypotension is followed by sinus bradycardia, cardiovascular collapse, and death.

CLINICAL PRESENTATION

Dyspnea and tachypnea are the most common presenting symptoms of slowly developing cardiac tamponade.[29] Patients with tamponade almost invariably are more comfortable sitting upright as opposed to supine. Anorexia, profound weakness, and lower extremity edema can occur but are less common presenting symptoms. As hemodynamic compromise progresses, patients become anxious and diaphoretic, with tachycardia and diminishing pulse pressure preceding cardiovascular collapse. In the terminal stages of tamponade, regardless of the speed of development, patients become stuporous or restless, with cold, clammy extremities, all of which are manifestations of shock.

Jugular venous distention is the most common physical finding in patients with cardiac tamponade. A single descent as a result of loss of the normal *y* descent may be appreciated at the bedside. Tachypnea, tachycardia, and arterial hypotension are also common physical findings. Patients may present with Beck's triad consisting of muffled heart sounds, hypotension, and increased jugular venous pressures. Pulsus paradoxus, defined as an inspiratory decline in systolic blood pressure by more than 10 mm Hg, is present in most patients. In severe tamponade, the paradoxical pulse is easily palpated. Pulsus paradoxus is an exaggeration of the normal, very small inspiratory decline in left ventricular stroke volume and systemic arterial pressure. During inspiration, the intrathoracic pressure decreases, with a resultant decrease in the elevated intrapericardial and intracavitary right atrial and ventricular pressures. As in normal subjects, the decrease in right-sided pressures causes an increase in venous return to the right side of the heart, with an accompanying increase in right ventricular volume. In cardiac tamponade, however, the cardiac chambers may be considered to operate at a fixed total volume dictated by the intrapericardial pressure. Accordingly, the increase in right ventricular volume during inspiration occurs at the expense of the already reduced left ventricular volume by shifting the interventricular septum to the left side. Loss of left ventricular preload thus causes the decrease in aortic flow and systolic arterial pressure during inspiration (Fig. 82.13).[30] Patients with preexisting ventricular dilatation who develop cardiac tamponade may not have a pulsus paradoxus. Examples are patients with atrial septal defect and, importantly, patients with aortic dissection and aortic valve disruption with acute regurgitation, in whom retrograde bleeding in the pericardial space is a common cause of death.[31] Loss of the normal *y* descent in the jugular venous pulse also results from the inability of the right atrium to empty during diastole because total cardiac volume is constrained.

DIAGNOSTIC TECHNIQUES

The electrocardiographic findings in cardiac tamponade are nonspecific. Those described previously in acute pericarditis and effusion may be seen. Electrical alternans of the QRS complex in a patient known to have pericardial effusion is highly suggestive of cardiac tamponade (see Fig. 82.8).[32] The chest radiograph does not differentiate pericardial effusion from cardiac tamponade, but it may demonstrate related pulmonary disease.

Echocardiography is the most sensitive and specific test for the diagnosis of cardiac tamponade. As discussed before, it provides information about the location and the extent of pericardial fluid. Moreover, in conjunction with Doppler flow velocity measurements, it also provides information about the hemodynamic significance of the effusion.[33] A hemodynamically significant effusion causes all of the cardiac chamber volumes to be relatively or absolutely small unless there is other cardiac disease. However, the most classic signs of cardiac tamponade are diastolic right atrial and right ventricular compression or "collapse."[34,35] Right ventricular diastolic collapse is a particularly good predictor of hemodynamically significant pericardial fluid. Doppler recordings of mitral and tricuspid inflow demonstrate abnormal respiratory variations in patients with cardiac tamponade. The mitral E wave decreases by more than 25% during inspiration compared with the expiratory phase (Fig. 82.14). In contrast, the tricuspid E wave demonstrates a greater than 50% increase during inspiration compared with the expiratory phase.[33,36] Thus, echocardiographic findings of pericardial effusion with right atrial and right ventricular collapse and an inspiratory decrease in transmitral E-wave velocity are diagnostic of cardiac tamponade. At present, there is no demonstrated advantage to the use of methods such as tissue and color-flow Doppler study in the diagnosis of cardiac tamponade.

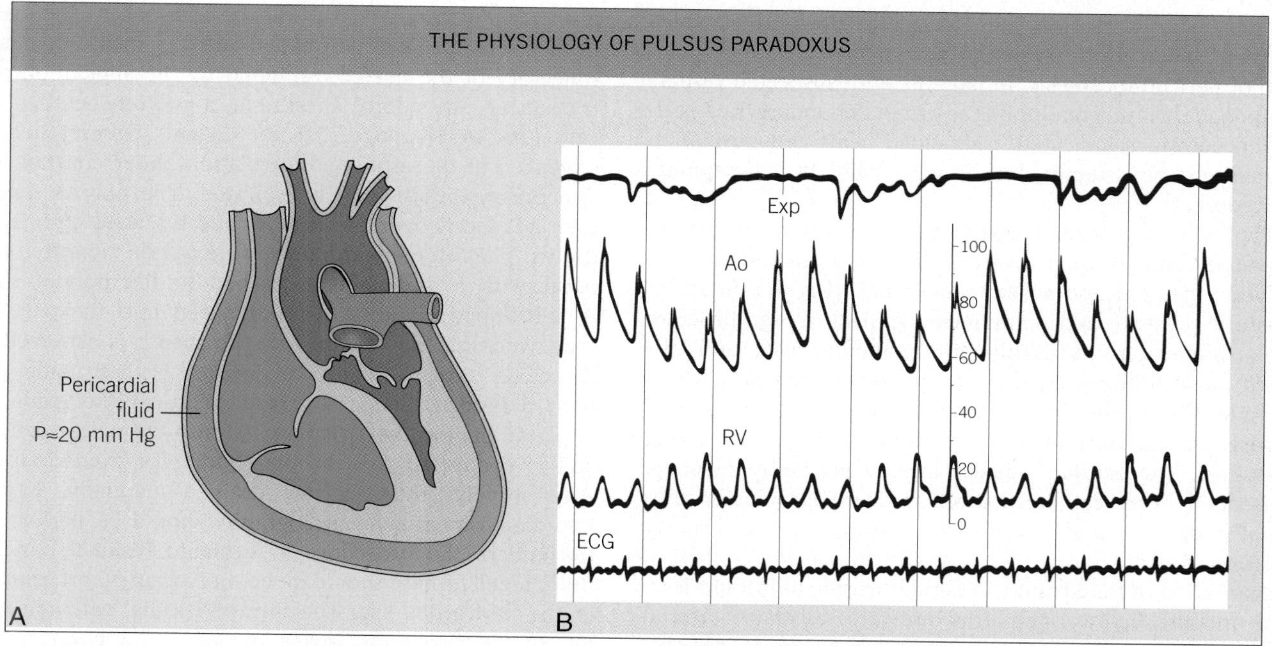

Figure 82.13 The physiology of pulsus paradoxus. A, During inspiration, the drop in intrathoracic pressure causes an increase in right-sided filling. The increase in right-sided volume occurs at the expense of left-sided filling with septal shift to the left. **B,** The reduced left-sided volume causes a reduced stroke volume and lower aortic pressure during inspiration. Exp, expiration; Ao, aorta; RV, right ventricle; ECG, electrocardiogram. (Modified from Shabetai R. The Pericardium. New York, Grune & Stratton, 1981:279-324.)

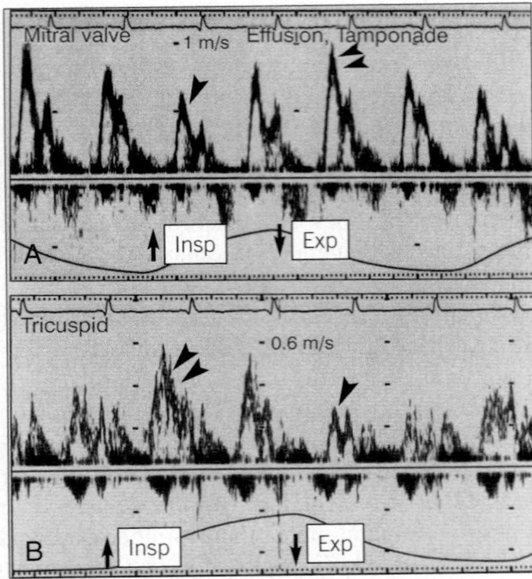

Figure 82.14 Doppler tracing of mitral **(A)** and tricuspid **(B)** inflow velocities in a patient with cardiac tamponade. Note the marked respiratory variation from inspiration (Insp) to expiration (Exp). (From Schutzman JJ, Obarski TP, Pearce GL, Klein AL. Comparison of Doppler and two-dimensional echocardiography for assessment of pericardial effusion. Am J Cardiol 1992;70:1353-1357. © 1992 American Journal of Cardiology.)

Echocardiography (along with the bedside examination) is usually reliable in delineating the hemodynamic significance of a pericardial effusion. Right-sided heart catheterization is primarily indicated when the echocardiogram is technically inadequate or borderline or hemodynamic findings may be obscured because of coexistent problems such as hypovolemia and overload states. It may also be useful to monitor hemodynamics as a guide during pericardiocentesis and to detect conditions such as effusive-constrictive pericarditis, pulmonary hypertension, and left ventricular failure, which may be evident from pressure tracings recorded on completion of pericardiocentesis. In patients with suspected cardiac tamponade whose condition is so grave that emergency pericardiocentesis is indicated, right-sided heart catheterization should not be attempted if it will delay the therapeutic procedure.

Typically, right-sided heart catheterization reveals an elevated right atrial pressure with the characteristic preserved *x* descent and absent *y* descent.[37] Right ventricular diastolic pressure and pulmonary capillary wedge pressure are also elevated. In full-blown tamponade, right- and left-sided heart filling pressures are equal and typically 15 to 20 mm Hg; if the intrapericardial pressure is measured before removal of fluid, it is equal to the intracardiac filling pressures. The cardiac index is usually markedly reduced. Left-sided heart catheterization and angiographic studies usually do not add useful information and are rarely performed.

Aspiration of fluid results in rapid lowering of intrapericardial pressure below right atrial pressure. Systemic arterial pressure and cardiac output improve pari passu. In straightforward tamponade, when the pericardial fluid is fully drained, intrapericardial pressure should drop to about 0 mm Hg and fluctuate with changes in intrathoracic pressure (Fig. 82.15). If filling pressures remain elevated despite removal of most or all of the effusion, the diagnosis of effusive-constrictive disease (see later) should be strongly considered. Hemodynamic alterations consistent with left-sided heart failure or pulmonary hypertension may also be evident after pericardiocentesis in patients with additional, coexistent disease.

MANAGEMENT

Drainage is the only effective treatment and should ordinarily be performed urgently or emergently, depending on individual circumstances. Removal of modest amounts of fluid (even 50 to 100 mL) usually results in substantial lowering in intrapericardial pressure and hemodynamic improvement. Echocardiographically guided, transcutaneous pericardiocentesis is usually the procedure of choice. In experienced hands, this is safe when the effusion is large. Pericardiotomy through a subxiphoid incision may also be used to evacuate pericardial fluid under pressure. This is sometimes the preferred method if there is question as to the size or loculation of fluid or if it is thought that pericardial biopsy is required. However, the advantage of direct pericardial visualization must be balanced against the risk of anesthesia in patients who are often very sick. Except in the most emergent of circumstances, blind percutaneous pericardiocentesis is unacceptable because of its high rate of mortality and morbidity.[38] Hemodynamic support with intravenous fluids and inotropic agents should be considered while preparing for pericardiocentesis, but these are temporizing measures only.

We recommend the following techniques for echocardiographically guided, closed pericardiocentesis. Two-dimensional echocardiography should be used to localize the pericardial effusion and to select the ideal entry site. The site should be the point on the body surface where the largest fluid accumulation is closest to the transducer. The distance from the skin to the pericardial space is measured and the trajectory of the needle estimated by the angulation of the transducer. After local anesthesia, a polytef-sheathed intracath (16- to 18-gauge, 5.1 to 8.3 cm) Deseret needle is advanced at the estimated angulation under constant negative pressure until fluid is aspirated. The polytef sheath is then advanced over the needle, and the steel core is withdrawn. The intrapericardial pressure can be measured at this point with a manometer attached to the polytef sheath. A soft-tipped guide wire is advanced into the pericardial space through the sheath, and the sheath is removed over the guide wire. A small skin incision is then made, and a 6 to 8 French dilator is introduced over the guide wire. A pigtail angiocatheter is inserted into the pericardial space and is connected to a suction bottle for fluid drainage.[39] Alternatively, fluid can be drained manually. Repeated two-dimensional echocardiography should be performed at the end of the procedure to evaluate residual pericardial fluid. Ideally, there should be no more than 50 mL remaining in the pericardial sac. The intrapericardial catheter can be left in the pericardial space for 24 to 72 hours to allow further drainage, with heparinized saline used as a flush.

Closed balloon pericardiotomy is a relatively new procedure that can be performed in conjunction with percutaneous pericardiocentesis after draining of a portion of the fluid.

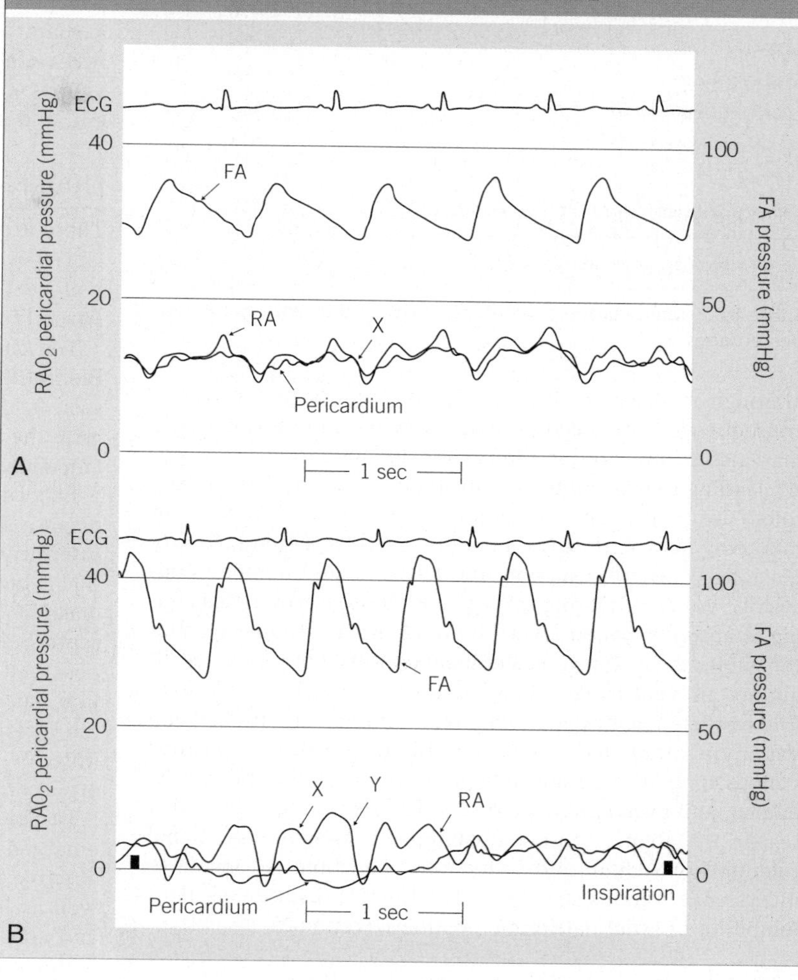

Figure 82.15 Simultaneous right atrial and intrapericardial pressure and femoral artery pressure before (A) and after (B) pericardiocentesis in a patient with cardiac tamponade. A, Reduced femoral artery (FA) pressure (scale, 0 to 100) with equalization of right atrial (RA) and pericardial pressure (scale, 0 to 40). Note the loss of diastolic *y* descent. **B,** Improvement of femoral artery pressure and restoration of pericardial pressure to 0. Note the reappearance of diastolic *y* descent. (Modified from Lorell BH, Grossman W. Profiles in constrictive pericarditis, restrictive cardiomyopathy, and cardiac tamponade. In Baim DS, Grossman W, eds. Cardiac Catheterization, Angiography and Intervention. Baltimore, Williams & Wilkins, 1996:801-857.)

A 20-mm-diameter, 3-cm balloon is inflated and drawn through the parietal pericardium to create a tear (i.e., a pleuropericardial window)[40] for drainage into the left hemithorax. The long-term efficacy of this procedure compared with conventional surgical pericardiotomy has not been evaluated.

Surgical pericardiotomy, or creation of a pericardial window, is usually the procedure of choice for recurrent effusions and is always the procedure of choice if there is no physician available with experience in closed pericardiocentesis (with the exception of dire emergencies). A subxiphoid pericardial window can be created under local or general anesthesia. A small longitudinal incision is made below the xiphoid process, the diaphragm is dissected away from the sternum, and the pericardium is opened under direct vision. A small section of the pericardium is resected, a tube is placed in the pericardial space for drainage, and the wound is closed. The tube is usually removed in several days after drainage ceases.[40] Although surgical pericardial windows have a significant failure rate, they remain the most reliable method to drain chronic effusions. This opinion may change if more data about balloon pericardiotomy become available.

CONSTRICTIVE PERICARDITIS

Constrictive pericarditis is the end stage of an inflammatory process that involves the pericardium, usually infectious, after surgery, or after radiation therapy. The end-result is dense fibrosis, often calcification, and adhesions of the parietal and visceral pericardium. Functionally, the heart becomes rigidly encased, with profound restriction of diastolic filling. In the past, tuberculosis was by far the most important cause of constrictive pericarditis, but the incidence of tuberculosis has become markedly reduced in developed countries. Correspondingly, the etiology of pericardial constriction is now much more diverse (Table 82.2). Some degree of transient pericardial constriction is not at all uncommon in the weeks or months after cardiac surgical procedures, despite the fact that most surgeons do not reapproximate the pericardium. In most cases, this is not clinically significant, but it does occasionally require treatment.

PATHOPHYSIOLOGY

The pathophysiologic consequence of constrictive pericarditis is markedly restricted filling of all chambers. In "pure" constriction, myocardial contractile function is preserved,

MAIN CAUSES OF CONSTRICTIVE PERICARDITIS WITH ESTIMATED PERCENTAGES	
Idiopathic pericarditis	40%
Post-CABG	30%
Tuberculosis	10%
Radiation induced	5%
Collagen vascular diseases	5%
Other	
Malignant neoplasm, uremia, purulent	5%

CABG, coronary artery bypass graft.

Table 82.2 Main causes of constrictive pericarditis with estimated percentages.

although ventricular ejection fraction may be reduced as a consequence of reduced preload. However, the myocardium may also be involved in the chronic inflammation and fibrosis, leading to true contractile dysfunction. During early diastole, the ventricles fill abnormally rapidly because of markedly elevated atrial pressures and accentuated early diastolic ventricular suction, the latter related to small end-systolic volumes. During early to mid diastole, ventricular filling is abruptly halted when the intracardiac volume reaches the limit set by the noncompliant pericardium. As a result, almost all ventricular filling occurs very early in diastole. The restricted ventricular filling is associated with marked elevation in atrial and ventricular filling pressures. Systemic venous congestion results in hepatomegaly, ascites, peripheral edema, and even cardiac cirrhosis. The reduced cardiac index results in fatigue, muscle wasting, and weight loss. Renal retention of sodium and water also contributes to increases in systemic venous and left-sided filling pressures, as does inhibition of atrial natriuretic peptide secretion.[41]

CLINICAL PRESENTATIONS

The usual presentation consists of signs and symptoms of predominantly right-sided heart failure with normal or nearly normal ventricular systolic function, as assessed by echocardiography. Thus, patients present with lower extremity edema, abdominal swelling, and often vague abdominal symptoms. Exertional dyspnea and orthopnea are also common. Generalized fatigue, muscle wasting, and weight loss are advanced symptoms that are usually secondary to chronically low cardiac output. Classic physical findings include marked elevation in jugular venous pressure with a prominent, rapidly collapsing *y* descent. Because the *x* descent is normal or perhaps somewhat exaggerated itself, the resulting jugular venous waveform has the appearance of an M or W shape. Kussmaul's sign, an inspiratory increase in systemic venous pressure, is usually present.[42] On occasion, the venous pressure will simply fail to decrease on inspiration rather than actually increase. These abnormalities of the venous waveform are in marked contrast to those observed in cardiac tamponade. About one third of patients have a pulsus paradoxus. Examination of the heart is most notable for the presence of a pericardial knock, corresponding to the early, abrupt cessation in ventricular filling. The pericardial knock is a relatively low frequency, early diastolic sound best heard at the left sternal border or the cardiac apex. Experienced examiners often recognize it as an "early" third heart sound. A significant number of patients with constrictive pericarditis have secondary tricuspid regurgitation and a characteristic murmur. Abdominal examination typically reveals hepatomegaly with or without ascites and hepatic venous pulsations. Lower extremity edema is usually present, and anasarca occurs in some cases.

DIAGNOSTIC TECHNIQUES

There are no specific electrocardiographic findings. Nonspecific T-wave abnormalities are often observed, with low-voltage QRS. Left atrial abnormality may also be present. Atrial fibrillation is present in a minority of patients.

The chest radiograph may show right atrial enlargement. Pleural effusions are not unusual. Pericardial calcification is seen in a small number of patients (Fig. 82.16) and should raise the suspicion of tuberculous pericarditis. However, calcification is not diagnostic of constrictive physiology.

Echocardiography can provide some important clues to the diagnosis; however, they are nonspecific and somewhat insensitive. Findings include pericardial thickening (although this is better visualized by MRI or CT) and prominent early diastolic filling. Abrupt displacement of the interventricular septum during early diastole (septal "bounce") may be observed (Fig. 82.17).[43,44] Signs of systemic venous congestion, such as dilatation of hepatic veins and distention of the inferior vena cava with blunted respiratory fluctuation (inferior vena cava plethora), are almost always seen but are also nonspecific.

Doppler echocardiographic flow velocity measurement has emerged as a useful tool to establish the diagnosis of constrictive pericarditis, with high sensitivity and specificity, as well as to differentiate between restrictive cardiomyopathy and constrictive pericarditis,[45-47] entities that share several features of pathophysiology and clinical presentation. Doppler findings in constrictive physiology are characterized by an exaggerated inspiratory decrease in left ventricular filling and retention of the normal inspiratory increase in right

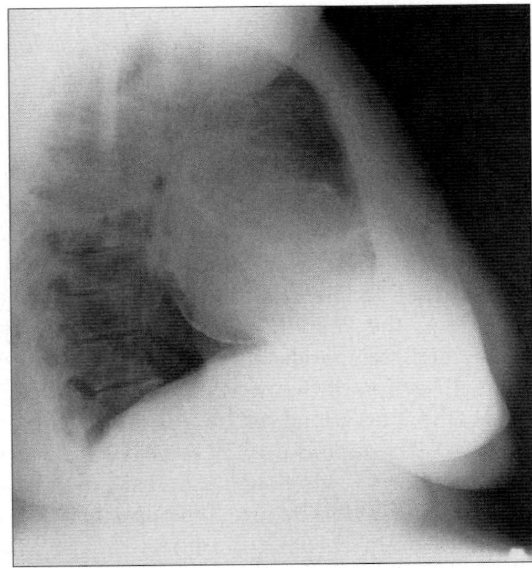

Figure 82.16 Chest radiograph showing marked pericardial calcifications in a patient with constrictive pericarditis.

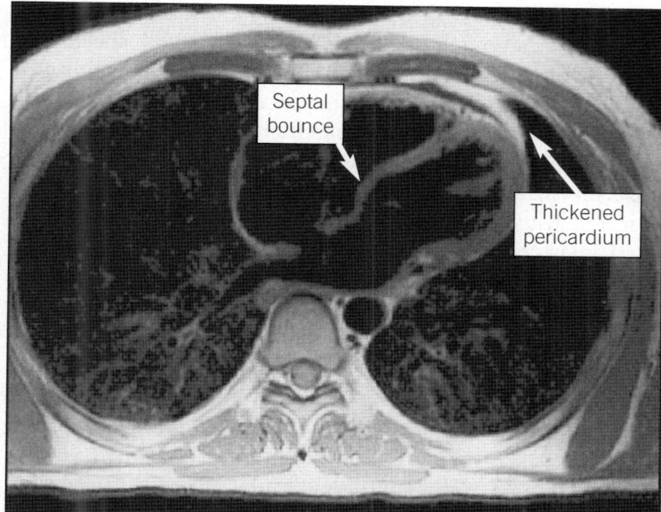

Figure 82.17 Turbo spin-echo images showing thickened pericardium and septal bounce, indicative of constrictive pericarditis.

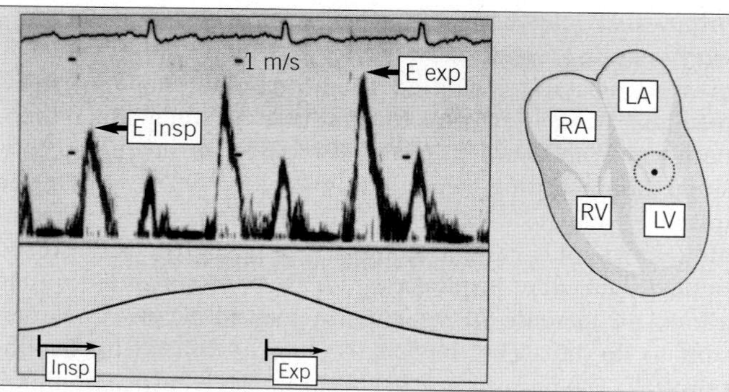

Figure 82.18 Mitral and tricuspid Doppler velocities in a patient with constrictive pericarditis. Upper panel shows mitral inflow velocities of E and A waves, with an approximate 50% increase in E velocity from inspiration (Insp) to expiration (Exp). LA, left atrium; LV, left ventricle; RA, right atrium; RV, right ventricle. (From Oh JK, Hatle LK, Seward JB, et al. Diagnostic role of Doppler echocardiography in constrictive pericarditis. J Am Coll Cardiol 1994;23:154-162. Reprinted with permission from the American College of Cardiology.)

ventricular filling (this despite the fact that caval flow is reduced or unchanged during inspiration). Typically, patients with pericardial constriction demonstrate a 25% or more increase in mitral E velocity during expiration compared with inspiration. Mitral E deceleration time is usually but not always less than 160 ms (Fig. 82.18).[48] In the minority of patients who do not have exaggerated mitral flow variation, maneuvers that decrease preload (head-up tilt, sitting) can unmask characteristic respiratory variation in mitral E velocity. When mitral inflow velocities by transthoracic echocardiography are technically inadequate or equivocal, measurement of pulmonary venous velocities with transesophageal echocardiography demonstrates pronounced respiratory variation, even larger than in the mitral inflow tract.[49] Tissue Doppler examination reveals increased E′ velocity of the mitral annulus as well as septal abnormalities corresponding to the bounce. Tissue Doppler examination appears to be at least as sensitive as conventional echocardiography and Doppler investigation for diagnosis of constriction.

The proposed mechanism of respiratory variation in left ventricular filling is related to the dissociation between intrathoracic and intracardiac pressures. The thickened, fibrotic pericardium isolates the cardiac chambers from the change in intrathoracic pressure with respiration (Fig. 82.19). During

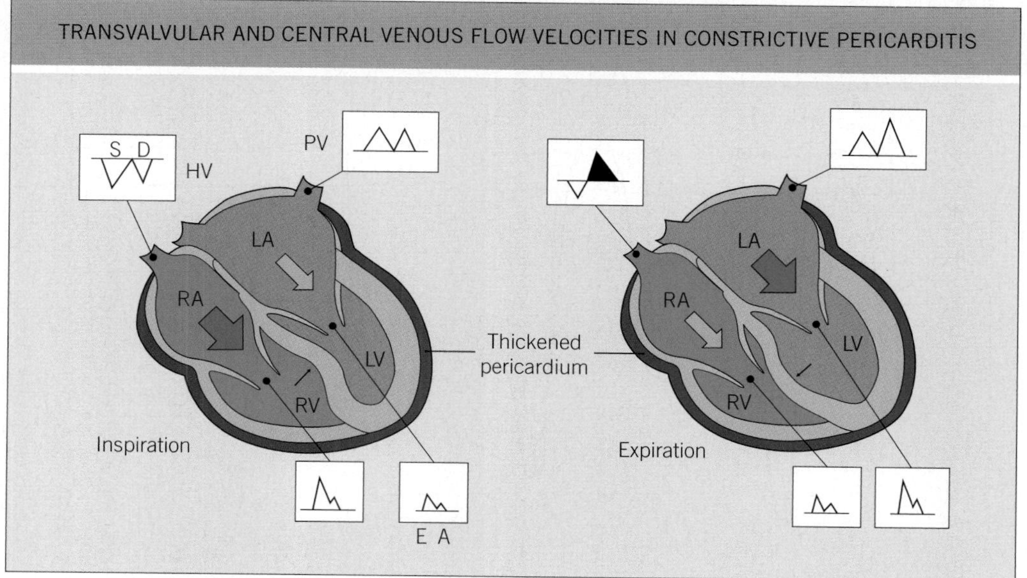

Figure 82.19 Schematic representation of transvalvular and central venous flow velocities in constrictive pericarditis. During inspiration, the decrease in left ventricular filling results in a leftward septal shift, allowing augmented flow in the right ventricle. The opposite change occurs during expiration. This is a result of the fixed cardiac volume dictated by the thickened pericardium. EA, mitral inflow; HV, hepatic vein; LA, left atrium; LV, left ventricle; PV, pulmonary venous flow; RA, right atrium; RV, right ventricle. (From Oh JK, Hatle LK, Seward JB, et al. Diagnostic role of Doppler echocardiography in constrictive pericarditis. J Am Coll Cardiol 1994;23:154-162. Reprinted with permission from the American College of Cardiology.)

inspiration, intrathoracic pressure drops and hence pulmonary venous pressure falls. However, the fall in intrathoracic pressure is not transmitted to the cardiac chambers. This resultant decreased pressure gradient between the pulmonary veins and cardiac chambers results in decreased left-sided filling during inspiration, with the variation in the mitral E velocity described before. Because of the presumably fixed total cardiac volume secondary to the fibrosed pericardium, the inspiratory decrease in left-sided filling allows an increase in right ventricular filling with a septal shift to the left. The opposite sequence occurs with expiration.[45,46] The inspiratory decrease in left ventricular filling presumably also accounts for the occurrence of a paradoxical pulse in constrictive pericarditis. These Doppler echocardiographic findings have an 88% sensitivity for the diagnosis of constrictive pericarditis.[48]

Echocardiography with Doppler flow measurements may be useful in differentiating constrictive from restrictive physiology. Patients with restrictive cardiomyopathy often have thick-walled ventricles due to infiltrative processes. Biatrial enlargement is also common in restriction. Enhanced respiratory variation in mitral inflow velocity of 25% or more with expiration compared with inspiration is seen in constriction but not in restriction. In restriction, there is markedly blunted pulmonary venous systolic flow with greater diastolic forward flow; in constriction, both systolic flow and diastolic flow are present. Hepatic vein flow demonstrates an enhanced flow reversal in expiration with constriction, whereas there is increased inspiratory flow reversal in restriction.[46,48] Interrogation of the mitral annulus by tissue Doppler examination often will show higher E′ values in constriction versus restrictive cardiomyopathy.[49,50] This has a higher sensitivity for making the distinction than mitral inflow parameters[51,52] and approximately 100% specificity. There is also incremental improvement in the sensitivity of distinguishing the two disease processes by combining E′ with systolic mitral annular velocity (S′) and the time difference between onset of mitral inflow (E) and E′ ($T_{E' - E}$).[53]

Cardiac catheterization is an important tool in the evaluation of constrictive physiology. Simultaneous right- and left-sided heart catheterization should be performed in most if not all patients who are suspected of having constrictive pericarditis. Typically, atrial, right ventricular diastolic, pulmonary capillary wedge, and left ventricular diastolic pressures are equal and elevated in the range of 15 to 25 mm Hg. Right atrial pressure demonstrates a preserved *x* descent with a prominent early *y* descent and roughly equal *a* and *v* wave heights, with the resultant M or W shape evident in the jugular veins as well.[37] Intraventricular pressure recordings reveal an early, marked diastolic dip followed by a plateau (dip-and-plateau or square root sign), corresponding to the early and rapid ventricular filling pattern (Fig. 82.20).

Hemodynamic differentiation between constrictive pericarditis and restrictive cardiomyopathy is often difficult. However, careful attention to the hemodynamic profile can identify some clues. In both conditions, right and left ventricular diastolic pressures are elevated. In restriction, however, diastolic pressure in the left ventricle is higher than in the right ventricle at rest or during exercise, usually by at least 3 to 5 mm Hg.[52] Simultaneous recording of right and left pressure waveforms that are not congruent favors restriction. Pulmonary hypertension is common with restrictive cardiomyopathy but rare in constrictive pericarditis. In addition, marked right ventricular systolic hypertension (>60 mm Hg)

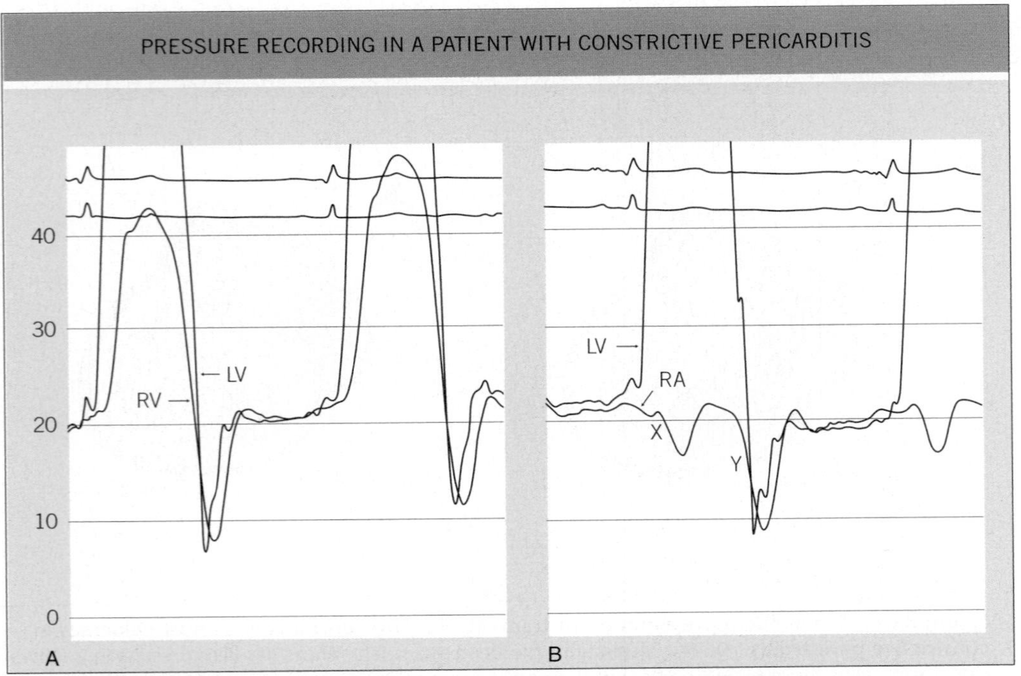

Figure 82.20 Pressure recording in a patient with constrictive pericarditis. A, Simultaneous right ventricular (RV) and left ventricular (LV) pressure tracings with equalization of diastolic pressure as well as dip-and-plateau morphology. **B,** Simultaneous right atrial (RA) and LV pressure with equalization of RA and LV diastolic pressure. Note the prominent *y* descent. (From Vaitkus PT, Cooper KA, Shuman WP. Constrictive pericarditis. Circulation 1996;93:834-835.)

is usually indicative of restrictive cardiomyopathy. The absolute level of atrial or ventricular diastolic pressure elevation is also sometimes useful in distinguishing the two conditions, with extremely high pressures (>25 mm Hg) much more common in restrictive cardiomyopathy.

CT and MRI are the best modalities for imaging of the pericardium itself and measurement of thickness, which is almost always increased in constriction.[54,55] However, pericardial thickening is not diagnostic of constrictive physiology and should always be accompanied by hemodynamic evaluation. Whereas CT tends to overestimate thickness of the pericardium in the presence of isodense effusions, the thickness of the normal pericardium measured by CT and MRI is less than 2 mm. A thickness of more than 4 mm is considered abnormal. The main disadvantages of CT are the use of iodinated contrast material and ionizing radiation. MRI provides a detailed and comprehensive examination of the pericardium without the need for iodinated contrast media or ionizing radiation. The "normal" pericardium visualized by MRI has been reported to be up to 4 mm in thickness. This measurement most likely reflects the entire pericardial "complex," with physiologic fluid representing a significant component of the measured thickness. The accuracy of diagnosis of constrictive pericarditis by MRI is 93% based on clinical suspicion and greater than 4-mm thickness. Calcification within the thickened pericardium may indicate acute or chronic pericarditis and is best detected by CT. Delayed enhancement with gadolinium may also reveal a pericardial inflammation. MRI can also provide real-time cine imaging during inspiration, providing anatomic and hemodynamic information that can aid in distinguishing constrictive pericarditis from restrictive cardiomyopathy. In patients with constrictive pericarditis, septal flattening or bounce is seen by gradient echo imaging (see Fig. 82.17). By use of velocity-encoded sequences, mitral and tricuspid valve inflows and pressures can be calculated. The diagnosis of constriction can be confidently made if there is clinical evidence of impaired diastolic filling and pericardial thickening, especially if calcification is present. Absence of pericardial thickening argues against the diagnosis of constriction but does not completely rule it out. Focal as well as diffuse thickening of the pericardium may be seen to cause compression of the heart, much more commonly on the right than on the left side. Detailed description of pericardial thickening may guide surgical treatment planning for pericardiectomy. Disadvantages of MRI include the need for long breath-holds, claustrophobia, and prolonged imaging time.

MANAGEMENT

Constrictive pericarditis is a progressive disease. Medical management with diuretics and salt restriction is useful for symptomatic relief of fluid overload and peripheral edema, but patients ultimately become refractory. Efforts should be made to slow the ventricular rate in patients with atrial fibrillation and rapid rates. However, excessive slowing should be avoided as these patients often have a fixed stroke volume. Digitalis is recommended as the initial treatment of choice. β-Adrenergic blockers and calcium channel blockers can also be employed for this purpose but must be used with great care.

Surgical pericardiectomy is the only definitive treatment. This is often an extensive and difficult procedure that may entail use of cardiopulmonary bypass. Pericardiectomy is associated with a 5% to 15% operative mortality. Perioperative mortality has decreased in the modern era from 14% to 4%, but late survival has not. This is probably because the frequency of elderly patients with constrictive pericarditis secondary to cardiac surgery and mediastinal irradiation is increasing.[56,57] Early mortality arises primarily as a result of low cardiac output, often in debilitated patients with prolonged pump runs caused by difficult dissections. The highest mortality occurs in patients with class III and class IV preoperative symptoms. Symptomatic improvement occurs in more than 90% of patients who survive the operation. Five-year survival is in the range of 75% to 85%. Pericardiectomy should be performed early in the disease process, before marked clinical deterioration and myocardial damage occur.

EFFUSIVE-CONSTRICTIVE PERICARDITIS

A significant number of patients with pericarditis present with a syndrome that combines elements of effusion-tamponade and constriction, with a subacute or more chronic course. It is not unusual for an inflammatory effusion to dominate the picture initially, with constrictive findings prominent later. Hemodynamics do not fully normalize after pericardiocentesis in these patients and may more closely resemble constriction after fluid removal. Causes are diverse, but most common are malignant disease, radiation therapy, and tuberculosis. Physical, hemodynamic, and echocardiographic abnormalities are often mixtures of those associated with effusion and constriction and may vary considerably with time as the syndrome progresses. Diagnosis may require acquisition of intrapericardial fluid and biopsy samples if the etiology is not obvious. It is important to be cautious in performing closed pericardiocentesis in these patients when they do not have large effusions. Management is tailored to the specific cause if it is known. In our experience, it is not at all unusual for these patients to ultimately require pericardiectomy.

SPECIFIC CAUSES OF PERICARDIAL DISEASE

Bacterial Pericarditis

A wide variety of organisms can cause bacterial pericarditis.[58] Direct extension from pneumonia or empyema accounts for the majority of cases. In these cases, the most common agents are staphylococci, pneumococci, and streptococci. Hematogenous spread during bacteremia and contiguous spread after thoracic surgery or trauma are also important mechanisms of bacterial pericarditis. The incidence of hospital-acquired, methicillin-resistant staphylococcal pericarditis after thoracic surgery has increased during the past decade. Anaerobic organisms are usually the cause in patients with infections of the mediastinum and head and neck.

The clinical presentation is usually high-grade fever with shaking chills. Patients may complain of dyspnea and chest pain. A pericardial friction rub is present in about half of cases. The disease may be unsuspected secondary to the nature of underlying or associated illnesses, such as severe pneumonia or mediastinitis after thoracic surgery. Laboratory findings include leukocytosis with left shift, and there may be widening of the cardiac silhouette on chest radiography. The electrocardiogram shows typical ST-segment and T-wave changes of acute pericarditis along with low voltage if there is a large effusion. Two-dimensional echocardiography is very helpful in this setting. It almost always demonstrates a significant pericardial effusion with or without adhesions. CT and MRI may be used to differentiate exudative from transudative pericardial effusion in patients with suspected bacterial pericarditis. On CT, fluid density and heterogeneity suggest the presence of exudate. On MRI, intermediate signal intensity on spin-echo T1-weighted images suggests exudate.

Cardiac tamponade is often the cause of hemodynamic deterioration in patients with bacterial pericarditis and can be confused with septic shock. Suspected or proven bacterial pericarditis should be considered a medical emergency and prompt surgical drainage or percutaneous pericardiocentesis with long-term catheter drainage performed if exudative fluid is obtained. High specific gravity, leukocytosis, low glucose concentration, and elevated protein levels are characteristic of pericardial fluid in bacterial pericarditis. Intravenous antibiotics should be selected according to the Gram stain and culture results.

The prognosis of bacterial pericarditis is generally poor, with mortality rates up to 70%.[59] This probably reflects delays in diagnosis, disease severity, and comorbidities. Early drainage of the pericardial fluid or pericardiotomy may help prevent the late complication of constrictive pericarditis. Intrapericardial streptokinase has been administered to selected patients with purulent or loculated effusions and may obviate the need for a window.

Pericardial Disease and Human Immunodeficiency Virus

A wide variety of causes of pericardial disease have been reported in patients infected with HIV. It is estimated that 21% of patients infected with HIV have pericardial involvement.[60] In industrialized countries, pericarditis is typically idiopathic; in Africa, it is usually caused by a variety of microorganisms. Pericardial disease is the most common cardiac manifestation of HIV disease, and the most common abnormality is an effusion.[61] Moderate to large effusions are indicative of more advanced stages of infection and are associated with Kaposi's sarcoma, tuberculosis, pulmonary infections, and heart failure. The HIV virus itself may be the cause in some cases.

Symptomatic patients usually present with dyspnea or chest pain. Symptoms are secondary to pericardial inflammation or a large pericardial effusion. Symptomatic pericardial effusion or cardiac tamponade is often caused by infection or a neoplasm. Tuberculosis is the most common infectious cause of symptomatic pericardial effusion, being present in 86% to 100% of such patients in Africa infected with HIV.[62] In contrast, in the general population of HIV-infected patients, the majority of effusions are small, asymptomatic, and without an identifiable cause. The most common infectious agents identified are *Mycobacterium tuberculosis* and *Mycobacterium avium-intracellulare*. However, a wide variety of organisms, often unusual, have been implicated. Lymphomas and Kaposi's sarcoma are the most common neoplasms associated with effusion.[60]

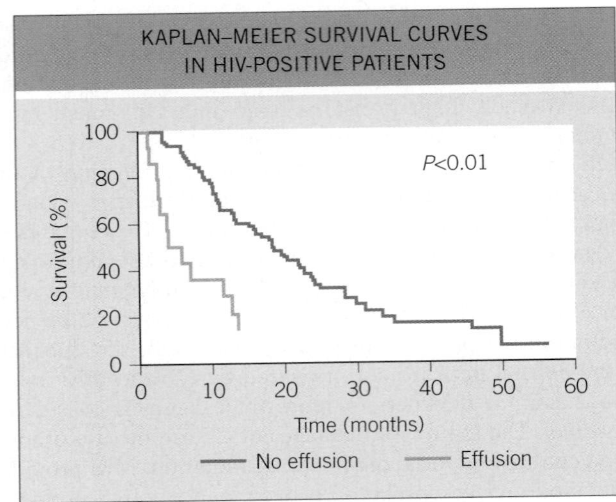

Figure 82.21 Kaplan-Meier survival curves in HIV-positive patients with and without pericardial effusion. (From Heidenreich P, Eisenberg M, Keel L, et al. Pericardial effusion in AIDS: incidence and survival. Circulation 1995;92:3229-3234.)

Asymptomatic patients with pericardial effusion do not require pericardiocentesis. Symptomatic pericardial effusions should be drained and an identifiable cause sought. Constrictive pericarditis is rare in patients with HIV infections. When it occurs, it is usually secondary to *M. tuberculosis* infection. A study by Heidenreich and colleagues[63] demonstrated that pericardial effusions in HIV disease, even when small, usually occur in the context of full-blown AIDS and are strongly associated with a shortened survival. This was independent of the CD4 count. The mortality at 6 months for patients with effusion was ninefold greater than in subjects without effusion (Fig. 82.21). There is little published information about the effect of highly active antiretroviral drugs on the natural history and etiology of HIV-associated pericardial disease.

Tuberculous Pericarditis

The incidence of tuberculosis has decreased in the industrialized world and, along with it, tuberculous pericardial disease. However, it is still a major problem in the immunocompromised host.[64] Thus, in patients infected with HIV, the most common cause of symptomatic pericardial effusion is tuberculosis. Pericardial involvement is usually secondary to retrograde spread from peribronchial or mediastinal lymph nodes or hematogenous spread from the primary focus.

The clinical presentation of tuberculous pericarditis is usually subacute to chronic, with systemic symptoms of fever, malaise, and dyspnea in association with a pericardial effusion. Later in the disease process, patients may present with hemodynamic compromise secondary to tamponade.[65] Many patients are properly classified as having a subacute, effusive-constrictive syndrome, and a number develop late constrictive pericarditis even with antituberculous treatment.[65,66] Clinical evidence of pulmonary tuberculosis may be absent or subtle. This is one of the chief reasons that the diagnosis is sometimes unsuspected.

Making the diagnosis of tuberculous pericardial disease has been notoriously difficult. A definitive diagnosis is made by isolation of the organism from pericardial fluid or biopsy tissue. However, the yield for isolation of the organism from pericardial fluid is low. The probability is increased if both pericardial fluid and a biopsy specimen are examined early in the effusive stage of the disease. Thus, there is a definite role for biopsy in selected patients. The finding of granulomas without viable bacilli is helpful but not diagnostic of tuberculous pericarditis because granulomas can be found in rheumatoid and sarcoid pericardial disease. A positive tuberculin skin test response certainly increases suspicion, but it is often not useful in immunocompromised hosts. Measurement of adenosine deaminase, an enzyme produced by white blood cells in pericardial fluid, markedly improves diagnostic capabilities. In a prospective study of patients with pericardial effusion, a level of adenosine deaminase in excess of 40 U/L had a sensitivity of 93% and a specificity of 97% for the diagnosis of tuberculous pericarditis.[67] Adenosine deaminase should be routinely measured whenever tuberculous pericardial involvement is suspected. Finally, use of polymerase chain reaction performed on pericardial fluid specimens has the potential to revolutionize the accuracy and timeliness of the diagnosis of tuberculous pericardial disease.

The treatment of tuberculous pericarditis should start with a four-drug regimen (isoniazid, rifampicin, pyrazinamide, and ethambutol), and treatment should be maintained for at least 6 months. The addition of corticosteroid treatment may decrease mortality and lower the incidence of repeated pericardial drainage or need for pericardiectomy.[68] The use of corticosteroids has not been resolved in HIV-infected patients and does not appear to have any effect once patients develop constriction. In comparison to closed pericardiotomy and pericardiocentesis, patients with tuberculous effusions who undergo open drainage are less likely to require repeated pericardiocentesis and may have reduced development of constriction. We recommend pericardiectomy for most patients with tuberculous effusive-constrictive pericarditis. Pericardiectomy performed late in the disease, when calcification is present, has an increased mortality.

Fungal Pericarditis

Fungal infections are rare causes of pericarditis. Patients who are immunocompromised or receiving corticosteroids and intravenous drug abusers are at increased risk for opportunistic fungal pericarditis. Histoplasmosis is the most common. Typically, a patient living in or having traveled through an endemic area presents with signs and symptoms of acute pericarditis. Treatment is symptomatic and does not require amphotericin B except for disseminated disease. However, patients need to be observed in the hospital because about half can develop a rapidly accumulating pericardial effusion that can lead to tamponade. Other fungal organisms implicated in pericarditis include *Coccidioides, Aspergillus,* and *Candida* species.

Uremic Pericarditis and Dialysis-Associated Pericardial Disease

The incidence of classic uremic pericarditis has decreased markedly since the introduction of widespread dialysis. The etiology of uremic pericarditis is unclear. Toxic metabolites, hypercalcemia, and hyperuricemia and hemorrhagic, viral, and autoimmune mechanisms have all been implicated.[69,70] The clinical presentation is sometimes that of acute pericarditis with chest pain, fever, leukocytosis, and pericardial friction rub. Alternatively, patients may present with a large, asymptomatic pericardial effusion that can cause hypotension during or after dialysis (so-called low-pressure cardiac tamponade). Conventional cardiac tamponade with hemodynamic compromise can also occur.

The management of uremic pericarditis is intensive hemodialysis (along with drainage in patients with hemodynamic compromise). This has been shown to reduce both symptoms and the size of pericardial effusion.[70] Heparin should be used cautiously during hemodialysis because this can lead to hemorrhagic pericarditis with tamponade or chronic constriction. Subxiphoid surgical pericardiotomy with instillation of steroids in the pericardial space has also been advocated. Recurrent, symptomatic pericardial effusions are best treated with pericardiectomy.

Pericardial disease and symptoms can appear de novo in patients undergoing chronic hemodialysis, despite the fact that blood urea nitrogen and creatinine concentrations are normal or only mildly elevated. Some of these patients have painful pericarditis without significant effusion, whereas others develop effusions of varying size, which once again may be manifested as hypotensive episodes during or after dialysis. Because classic uremic pericarditis is clearly associated with markedly elevated blood urea nitrogen and creatinine concentrations, it is likely that the mechanism of pericardial involvement in chronic dialysis patients differs. Accordingly, we prefer to consider these patients as having dialysis-related pericardial disease. Treatment is empiric, depending on the presentation. In our experience, intensifying dialysis is marginally beneficial at best, presumably because these patients are already receiving regular dialysis. Corticosteroids should be avoided in this group of patients.

Acute Post–Myocardial Infarction Pericarditis and Dressler's Syndrome

Acute post–myocardial infarction pericarditis occurs during the first several days to about a week after a Q-wave myocardial infarction and is due to transmural necrosis with inflammation affecting the adjacent visceral and parietal pericardium. On the basis of autopsy studies, around 40% of patients with large Q-wave infarctions have pericardial inflammation.[71] Most commonly, pericarditis is asymptomatic and identified by auscultation of a rub. When it is symptomatic, patients develop pleuritic chest pain within the same time frame. It is important to distinguish pericardial pain from ischemic discomfort. Ordinarily, this is not difficult on clinical grounds. The typical electrocardiographic changes of acute pericarditis are uncommon after infarction. Pericardial inflammation is localized to the infarct area; hence, the electrocardiographic changes will not reflect a diffuse abnormality. Re-elevation of the ST segment in the infarcted area, often subtle, may be present. An atypical T-wave evolution has also been described after postinfarction pericarditis. This consists of persistent upright T waves or early normalization of inverted T waves. The latter T-wave changes have been shown to be highly sensitive for postinfarction pericarditis.[72]

Postinfarction pericarditis is a benign process and does not cause hemodynamically significant effusion. However, it is associated with relatively large transmural infarctions. The treatment is entirely symptomatic. We recommend augmentation of the usual low-dose aspirin administered to these patients (to 650 mg three or four times per day) or acetaminophen (paracetamol) for symptomatic relief. There is evidence of a higher incidence of early postinfarction myocardial rupture in patients receiving corticosteroids and possibly nonaspirin NSAIDs after Q-wave acute myocardial infarction, probably due to inhibition of scar formation.[73] Thus, these drugs should be avoided, although low-dose NSAIDs are not likely to be harmful. We do not recommend modifying heparin administration when postinfarction pericarditis is detected.

Dressler's syndrome is a pleuropericarditis that occurs weeks to months after an acute myocardial infarction. The incidence has been considered to be about 4% of all patients presenting with acute myocardial infarction, but there is a general impression that the incidence has been decreasing for some time. Dressler's syndrome is believed to have an autoimmune etiology due to sensitization to myocardial cells at the time of necrosis. Antimyocardial antibodies have been demonstrated in patients with Dressler's syndrome.[74] However, these antibodies are nonspecific. The inflammation involves the pleura and the pericardium. In contrast to early postinfarction pericarditis, the pericardial inflammation in this syndrome is diffuse and not localized to the myocardial injury site. Physical examination may reveal pleural or pericardial friction rubs. The chest radiograph may show a pleural effusion or enlargement of the cardiac silhouette. The electrocardiogram may demonstrate ST-segment elevation and T-wave changes typical of acute pericarditis. Although Dressler's syndrome is ultimately a self-limited disorder, admission to the hospital for observation and possible hemodynamic monitoring should be considered. Aspirin, NSAIDs, and colchicine are often effective for symptomatic relief. A short course of prednisone (40 to 60 mg/day) can be used in patients who do not respond to treatment or for recurrent symptoms.[75]

Post–Cardiothoracic Surgery and Postpericardiotomy Pericarditis

Trauma and blunt injury to the chest cavity and heart or cardiothoracic surgery with direct injury to the pericardium can cause pleuropericardial inflammation. The clinical presentation is usually pleuritic chest pain or dyspnea associated with fever and leukocytosis occurring days to months after the insult. The pathophysiologic process is thought to involve a systemic immunologic response after cardiac injury. The electrocardiogram may show nonspecific ST-T wave changes, and the chest radiograph may reveal pleural effusions. Small to moderate pericardial effusion may be evident on echocardiography, but cardiac tamponade is rare. Treatment with NSAIDs usually results in an excellent response within 48 hours. There have been numerous case reports of use of colchicine for refractory cases, and clinical trials are under way to evaluate the use of colchicine for primary prevention of postpericardiotomy syndrome.[76] Corticosteroid therapy is reserved for patients with unresponsive, severe, or recurrent symptoms.

Pericardial Involvement in Autoimmune Diseases

Rheumatoid Arthritis

Pericardial involvement is common in rheumatoid arthritis. Autopsy studies have shown pericardial inflammation in about 50% of patients.[76] This is evident clinically in up to 25%. Patients often present with chest pain, fever, and dyspnea. Acute pericarditis usually occurs in association with exacerbations of the underlying disease. Asymptomatic large pericardial effusion and cardiac tamponade can also be presenting manifestations of pericardial involvement in rheumatoid arthritis. Constrictive pericarditis can result from long-standing pericardial inflammation. In patients with disease exacerbation, the management of associated acute pericarditis or pericardial effusion without tamponade is first and foremost the same as that employed to treat the exacerbation. Pericardial manifestations seem to respond well to high-dose aspirin or NSAIDs. Pericardial effusions causing cardiac tamponade should of course be drained. Recurrent tamponade is a good indication for a pericardial window. Suppressive therapy with colchicine has also been shown to be effective for recurrent symptoms.[77]

Systemic Lupus Erythematosus

Pericarditis is the most common cardiovascular manifestation of systemic lupus erythematosus.[78,79] It is not at all unusual for pericarditis to be the first manifestation of the disease. About 40% of patients with systemic lupus erythematosus develop pericarditis at some time, usually in conjunction with flares of the disease and involvement of other serosal surfaces. Typical patients present with pleuritic chest pain, low-grade fever, and symptoms related to serosal inflammation elsewhere. The electrocardiogram often shows typical findings of acute pericarditis. The chest radiograph may show enlargement of the cardiac silhouette if effusion is present, along with pleural effusions and often parenchymal infiltrates. Pericardial effusions have high protein and low glucose content and a white cell count below $10,000/mL^3$ (see Fig. 82.11). It is important to exclude purulent, fungal, or tuberculous pericarditis because the majority of these patients are being treated with immunosuppressive medications. Most patients respond to corticosteroids or immunosuppressive therapy used to treat the disease flare. Hemodynamic compromise secondary to cardiac tamponade is estimated to occur in 10% of patients with systemic lupus erythematosus.[78,79] Accordingly, we recommend hospitalization of these patients for monitoring of hemodynamic complications until clinical stability is achieved.

Scleroderma

Patients can present with large pericardial effusion or acute pericarditis. The incidence of clinical pericarditis with chest pain and pericardial friction rub is about 10%. Late constrictive pericarditis has been described and carries a poor prognosis.[80,81] Treatment of pericarditis in scleroderma patients is often unrewarding. The response to aspirin and NSAIDs is unpredictable. It is important to perform right-sided heart catheterization in patients presenting with dyspnea or right-sided heart failure to evaluate pulmonary vascular disease, which is relatively common.

Post-Irradiation Pericarditis

Mediastinal and thoracic irradiation is currently standard treatment of a variety of neoplasms. Hodgkin's disease, non-Hodgkin's lymphoma, and breast carcinoma are the most common neoplasms associated with radiation-induced pericarditis. Factors that influence the degree of injury to the pericardium include total dose delivered, amount of cardiac silhouette exposed, nature of the radiation source, and duration and fractionation of therapy. Recent series have reported a 2.2% incidence of clinically evident pericarditis in conjunction with modern techniques of radiation delivery. However, the incidence can be as high as 20% when the entire pericardium is exposed.[82]

The clinical presentation takes one of two forms: acute pericarditis with chest pain, fever, and malaise; or a delayed form of pericardial injury that can occur months to years after treatment. Asymptomatic effusions are also common with radiation injury. Late manifestations of pericardial injury occur from about 1 year to up to 20 years after radiation treatment.[83] Patients can present with symptomatic pericarditis and effusion with or without cardiac compression or circulatory congestion due to constrictive pericarditis. Effusions can evolve into constriction (i.e., effusive-constrictive pericardial disease).

Radiation-induced pericarditis and pericardial effusion can be confused with malignant effusions. Malignant effusions are usually associated with other evidence of disease recurrence and metastases. Hypothyroidism induced by mediastinal irradiation can also contribute to a large pericardial effusion. Pericardiocentesis with fluid analysis for malignant cells and thyroid function tests can differentiate radiation-induced effusion from other causes. Large, symptomatic pericardial effusions should be drained either percutaneously or surgically. Recurrent pericardial effusions are often treated with pericardiectomy. Surgical pericardiectomy should also be performed in patients with constrictive physiology. However, the mortality in this group of patients appears to be relatively high.

Neoplastic Pericarditis

Primary benign or malignant tumors of the pericardium are very rare. They include lipomas, hemangiomas, lymphangiomas, teratomas, neurofibromas, fibrosarcomas, and mesotheliomas. Mesotheliomas and fibrosarcomas are lethal. With the advent of HIV infection, Kaposi's sarcoma and lymphomatous involvement of the pericardium have been widely described. Pericardial tumor implants are the usual cause of effusion in patients with known malignant neoplasms, although obstruction of lymphatic drainage by mediastinal lymph nodes is occasionally observed. The leading cause of cardiac tamponade in developed countries is malignant disease. Lung (40%) and breast (22%) carcinoma and lymphomas (15%) are the most common causes of malignant effusion. Gastrointestinal carcinoma, melanoma, and sarcomas are less common.[84,85]

An asymptomatic, incidental pericardial effusion may be the presenting sign of pericardial involvement in patients with malignant neoplasms, although many present with large, symptomatic effusions or tamponade. The electrocardiogram is variable but usually shows nonspecific T-wave abnormalities with low-voltage QRS. ST-segment elevation is somewhat unusual but can occur. In addition to echocardiography, MRI and CT scanning can be useful to evaluate metastatic disease in the pericardium and adjacent structures. On MRI, most neoplasms have medium signal intensity on T1-weighted spin-echo images and high signal intensity on T2-weighted images.

It is important to evaluate the life expectancy of patients before choosing a treatment modality. Terminally ill patients require palliative measures with drainage of effusions primarily to aid in relief of symptoms. However, patients with an overall good prognosis deserve a more aggressive approach, which can be gratifying in a surprisingly large number.[86] In some cases, a single drainage of fluid will provide prolonged relief. Instillation of tetracycline or chemotherapeutic agents has been advocated to encourage pericardial sclerosis. External beam radiation therapy is an option in patients with radiation-sensitive tumors. A pericardial window or even complete surgical pericardiectomy should be considered in patients with recurrent symptoms not responding to these measures who continue to have a good prognosis otherwise.

Congenital Anomalies of the Pericardium

Pericardial cysts are rare congenital malformations. They are usually fluid filled, located at the right costophrenic angle, and identified as an incidental finding on a chest radiograph. The diagnosis is usually confirmed by echocardiography. No treatment is required.

Congenital Absence of the Pericardium

Congenital absence of the pericardium is rare and can be complete or partial. Partial absence is usually associated with other cardiac anomalies, including atrial septal defect, bicuspid aortic valve, and pulmonary malformations. Total absence of the pericardium is usually asymptomatic, However, it can cause apparent cardiac dilatation. Partial absence of the pericardium is usually symptomatic and may allow herniation of portions of the heart through the defect. Patients may present with chest pain, syncope, or even sudden death. Echocardiography and MRI are the diagnostic tools that are most informative. Appropriate surgical correction should be performed to prevent cardiac strangulation.

SUMMARY

Pericardial disease has multiple clinical presentations and both acute and chronic complications. Acute or idiopathic pericarditis is the most common and benign form of pericardial disease. It is usually self-limited and rarely leads to complications. Asymptomatic, incidental pericardial effusions are occasionally detected on routine chest radiography or during echocardiography. These are often related to an identifiable, underlying disease but are typically idiopathic when they are moderate in size or larger. Cardiac tamponade is an emergency that should be treated promptly; otherwise, cardiovascular collapse and death can ensue. Constrictive pericarditis is a chronic complication of pericardial disease leading to restricted diastolic filling of the cardiac chambers with circulatory congestion. Surgical pericardiectomy is usually curative for this disease. In the future, improved technology and refinement of noninvasive imaging should allow better understanding and earlier diagnosis of pericardial disease as well as easier differentiation from other cardiac pathologic processes.

chapter 83

Pulmonary Arterial Hypertension

Richard Krasuski

Definition

- Pulmonary arterial hypertension is defined by a mean pulmonary artery pressure greater than 25 mm Hg, a pulmonary capillary wedge pressure less than 15 mm Hg, and a pulmonary vascular resistance greater than 3 Wood units.
- Pulmonary arterial hypertension is an alteration in the histologic architecture and function of pulmonary arterioles.

Key Features

- Pulmonary arterial hypertension results from endothelial proliferation and dysfunction.
- Right ventricular function is the main determinant of survival in pulmonary arterial hypertension.
- Echocardiography is an extremely valuable diagnostic tool for evaluation of the patient with suspected pulmonary arterial hypertension.
- Heart catheterization is required to establish the diagnosis, to guide appropriate therapy, and to determine prognosis.

Therapy

- Several pulmonary arterial hypertension–specific therapeutic classes have been developed, and multiple clinical trials have been performed to demonstrate the efficacy of these agents in patients with pulmonary arterial hypertension.
- Evidence-based guidelines have been published to assist in clinical management of pulmonary arterial hypertension.
- Continuous intravenous epoprostenol therapy improves symptoms, exercise tolerance, hemodynamics, and survival in patients with advanced pulmonary arterial hypertension.
- Prostacyclin analogues allow novel administration techniques to avoid some of the shortcomings of epoprostenol, and clinical outcomes with these agents are being actively examined.
- Oral endothelin antagonists improve exercise tolerance in patients with pulmonary arterial hypertension, and open-label, uncontrolled data also suggest improved long-term outcomes with bosentan.
- Phosphodiesterase type 5 inhibitors improve exercise tolerance and hemodynamics in patients with pulmonary arterial hypertension.

The pulmonary vasculature is normally a low-pressure, low-resistance system, and consequently the right ventricle is designed as a volume pump, not a pressure pump. A multitude of diseases may increase pulmonary artery pressure and result in right ventricular dysfunction. The classification of pulmonary hypertension has been revised by the World Health Organization (WHO) and is displayed in Table 83.1.[1] Category 1, pulmonary arterial hypertension (PAH), is the focus of this chapter. Diseases of the left side of the heart, such as left ventricular dysfunction, hypertensive heart disease, and aortic or mitral valve disease, can elevate pulmonary artery pressure by raising left atrial pressure. This represents pulmonary venous hypertension, and treatment in such cases should be directed at the underlying left-sided heart disease. Diseases of lung parenchyma, such as emphysema and pulmonary fibrosis, may cause mild to moderate pulmonary hypertension and represent WHO category 3. Chronic thromboembolic pulmonary hypertension may be manifested with symptoms and hemodynamic findings similar to those of idiopathic pulmonary hypertension and is further discussed in Chapter 85. Disorders directly affecting the pulmonary vasculature, such as schistosomiasis and sarcoidosis, may also result in pulmonary hypertension.

Idiopathic pulmonary arterial hypertension (IPAH), previously referred to as primary pulmonary hypertension, was first described hemodynamically by Dresdale in 1951. It is what is left unexplained after the known causes of PAH have been excluded. The pulmonary vessel histopathology of IPAH is indistinguishable from that of a number of known causes of pulmonary hypertension, such as congenital heart disease, anorexigen use, human immunodeficiency virus infection, portopulmonary hypertension, and collagen vascular disease. These entities also fall in WHO category 1, PAH. The identical endothelial pathologic process strongly suggests that the changes in the pulmonary vessels are a final, common pathway for endothelial injury that can be precipitated by a variety of causes, some of which are known and others of which are not.

ANATOMY AND PATHOLOGY

The pathologic process of the pulmonary vessels in PAH is complex and poorly understood. Endothelial cell proliferation is a hallmark of the disease, but it is not known at what stage of the disease this process occurs. The reduction in endogenous vasodilators (nitric oxide and prostacyclin) and the increase in endogenous vasoconstrictors (endothelin and thromboxane) are integral to the pathogenesis of the disease and represent the basis of currently available therapies.

Classically, PAH has been characterized by the presence of the plexiform lesion, which is a mass of disorganized vessels with proliferating endothelial cells, smooth muscle cells, myofibroblasts, and macrophages (Fig. 83.1). The role of the smooth muscle cell in PAH is also complex. Interconversion can occur between fibroblasts, smooth muscle cells, and endothelium, and new vessel formation may also be possible.

WORLD HEALTH ORGANIZATION (WHO) NOMENCLATURE AND CLASSIFICATION OF PULMONARY HYPERTENSION
Diagnostic classification
1. Pulmonary arterial hypertension
1.1. Primary pulmonary hypertension (a) Sporadic (b) Familial 1.2. Related to (a) Collagen vascular disease (b) Congenital systemic to pulmonary shunts (c) Portal hypertension (d) HIV infection (e) Drugs/toxins (1) Anorexigens (2) Other (f) Persistent pulmonary hypertension of the newborn (g) Other
2. Pulmonary venous hypertension
2.1. Left-sided atrial or ventricular heart disease 2.2. Left-sided valvular heart disease 2.3. Extrinsic compression of central pulmonary veins (a) Fibrosing mediastinitis (b) Adenopathy/tumors 2.4. Pulmonary veno-occlusive disease 2.5. Other
3. Pulmonary hypertension association with disorders of the respiratory system and/or hypoxemia
3.1. Chronic obstructive pulmonary disease 3.2. Interstitial lung disease 3.3. Sleep-disordered breathing 3.4. Alveolar hypoventilation disorders 3.5. Chronic exposure to high altitude 3.6. Neonatal lung disease 3.7. Alveolar–capillary dysplasia 3.8. Other
4. Pulmonary hypertension due to chronic thrombotic and/or embotic disease
4.1. Thromboembolic obstruction of proximal pulmonary arteries 4.2. Obstruction of distal pulmonary arteries (a) Pulmonary embolism (thrombus, tumor, ova and/or parasites, foreign material) (b) In situ thrombosis (c) Sickle cell disease
5. Pulmonary hypertension due to disorders directly affecting the pulmonary vasculature
5.1. Inflammatory (a) Schistosomiasis (b) Sarcoidosis (c) Other 5.2. Pulmonary capillary hemangiomatosis
Modified from Rich S, ed. Primary Pulmonary Hypertension: Executive Summary from the World Symposium–Primary Pulmonary Hypertension 1998. Available at http://www.who.int/ncd/cvd/pph.html.

Table 83.1 World Health Organization (WHO) nomenclature and classification of pulmonary hypertension.

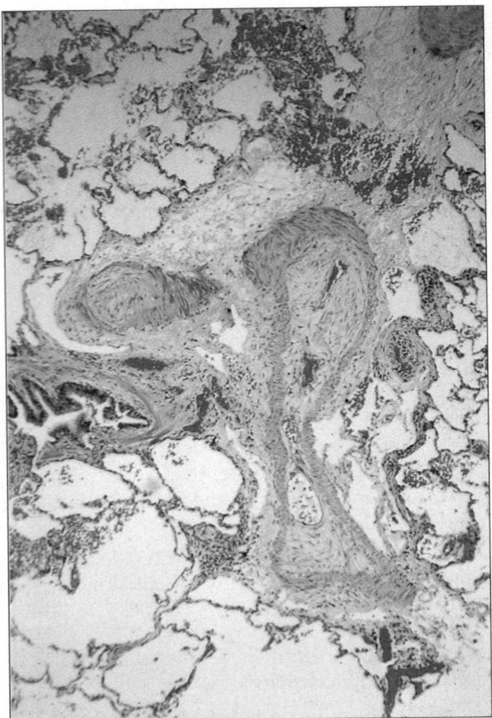

Figure 83.1 The cross-sectional area of the pulmonary vessels is markedly reduced because of endothelial proliferation in this patient with pulmonary arterial hypertension.

Furthermore, different types of smooth muscle cells may exist in the different layers of the vessel wall and may play different roles in the pathogenesis of the disease. In the large muscular and elastic arteries, smooth muscle cell hypertrophy occurs, and dissolution of the elastic lamina is a common finding. Smooth muscle cells may also contribute to intimal thickening. Precursor smooth muscle cells, similar to pericytes, may also contribute to the thickening process. A number of matrix-degrading enzymes, including elastase, metalloproteinases, and tenascin, appear to be involved in these pathologic changes and may also stimulate smooth muscle cell proliferation and migration.

PATHOPHYSIOLOGY

Basic research has provided insights into the causes of PAH. The voltage-regulated (Kv) potassium channel in smooth muscle has been demonstrated to be abnormal in the pulmonary arteries of patients with IPAH, resulting in vasoconstriction.[2] Researchers have demonstrated a loss of prostacyclin synthase enzyme and gene expression in the pulmonary vessels of patients with IPAH, and it has been demonstrated that patients with IPAH have decreased prostacyclin production.[3] It is not clear whether this is a cause or consequence. Endothelial cell products of nitric oxide synthase production are also reduced and correlate inversely with the extent and severity of the histologic lesions.[4] Similarly, endothelin 1 expression is inversely related to nitric oxide synthase.[5]

In situ small-vessel thrombosis may be an additional contributing factor to the cause or propagation of PAH. Abnormalities in platelet activation and function occur, and biochemical markers of a procoagulant environment are present. Thrombosis may play an important role involving growth factors, platelets, and the vessel wall in many of the proposed processes in the cause or progression of the disease. Increased shear stress caused by elevated pressure or flow can be an initiator of PAH, as seen in congenital cardiovascular shunts. It may also enhance progression of the disease when it is stimulated by other factors. Increased shear forces on the endothelial cell probably cause the release of mediators that induce vascular smooth muscle growth, which results in remodeling of the pulmonary arteries.

CLINICAL PRESENTATIONS

Pulmonary hypertension is an insidious killer. By the time symptoms occur, the disease is often very advanced; without treatment, death can occur in less than 3 years. Even when symptoms appear, they are often nonspecific, such as breathlessness and chest pain, and because the patients are often young and otherwise healthy, they are discounted by both patient and physician.

A prospective study, the Primary Pulmonary Hypertension Patient Registry, recorded presenting symptoms in 187 patients diagnosed with IPAH (Table 83.2).[6] Dyspnea was by far the most common presenting symptom, occurring in 60% of patients, and virtually all of the patients developed this symptom during the course of the disease. Fatigue, chest pain, and syncope were other common presenting symptoms. Peripheral edema and fatigue were present in patients who had advanced disease and were experiencing right-sided heart failure. Also, chest pain, syncope, and palpitations became more frequent as the disease progressed.

The physical findings in early pulmonary hypertension are subtle, such as increased intensity in P_2 and a right ventricular lift (Table 83.3). As the disease advances, nearly all patients develop the murmur of tricuspid regurgitation. Pulmonary regurgitation is less common. A right-sided, fourth heart sound is common, and a prominent *a* wave in the jugular venous pulse may also be recognizable. Once right ventricular failure ensues, peripheral edema is common, as is distention of the neck veins with prominent *a* and *v* waves in the jugular pulse. Late in the disease, a prominent right-sided third heart sound develops, and sometimes ascites occurs.

The natural history of IPAH is generally one of progressive decline. Historically, predictors of survival include functional class, hemodynamics, and exercise tolerance. Once right-sided heart failure occurs, death usually follows within months to years (Fig. 83.2).[7]

PRESENTING SYMPTOMS IN PULMONARY HYPERTENSION: U.S. NATIONAL INSTITUTES OF HEALTH PATIENT REGISTRY

Symptom	Initial (%)	Eventual (%)
Dyspnea	60	98
Fatigue	18	75
Chest pain	7	48
Near syncope	5	38
Edema	3	38
Palpitations	5	33

Modified from Rich S, Dantzker DR, Ayres SM, et al. Primary pulmonary hypertension. A national prospective study. Ann Intern Med 1987;107:216-223.

Table 83.2 Presenting symptoms in pulmonary hypertension: U.S. National Institutes of Health patient registry.

PHYSICAL FINDINGS IN PULMONARY HYPERTENSION

Accentuated P_2	93%
Tricuspid regurgitation murmur	40%
Right-sided S_4	38%
Peripheral edema	32%
Right-sided S_3	23%
Cyanosis	20%
Pulmonary insufficiency murmur	13%

Modified from Rich S, Dantzker DR, Ayres SM, et al. Primary pulmonary hypertension. A national prospective study. Ann Intern Med 1987;107:216-223.

Table 83.3 Physical findings in pulmonary hypertension.

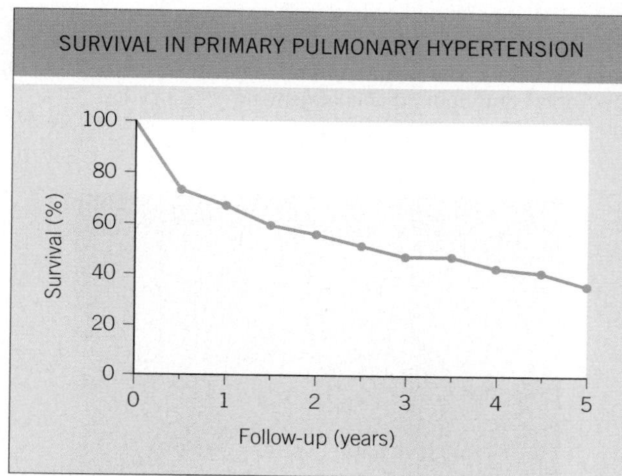

Figure 83.2 Survival in primary pulmonary hypertension. The survival curve from the National Institutes of Health national registry for primary pulmonary hypertension demonstrates the poor prognosis in patients. (Modified from D'Alonzo GE, Barst RJ, Ayres SM, et al. Survival in patients with primary pulmonary hypertension. Results from a national prospective registry. Ann Intern Med 1991;115:343-349.)

DIAGNOSTIC TECHNIQUES

A number of diagnostic modalities provide useful information about patients with PAH. Early in the disease process, the electrocardiogram may be normal; but by the time the patient is symptomatic, the QRS complex usually demonstrates right ventricular enlargement (Fig. 83.3). As the disease progresses, right axis deviation and right atrial enlargement are common. Arrhythmias are uncommon in this disease, but supraventricular tachycardias are occasionally encountered.

When PAH is mild (pulmonary artery mean pressure, 35 mm Hg), the chest radiograph is often normal. Moderate pulmonary hypertension (pulmonary artery mean pressure, 40 to 45 mm Hg) usually produces some enlargement of main and proximal pulmonary arteries. When the pulmonary hypertension is advanced, in addition to pulmonary artery dilatation, the right atrium and ventricle are also enlarged,

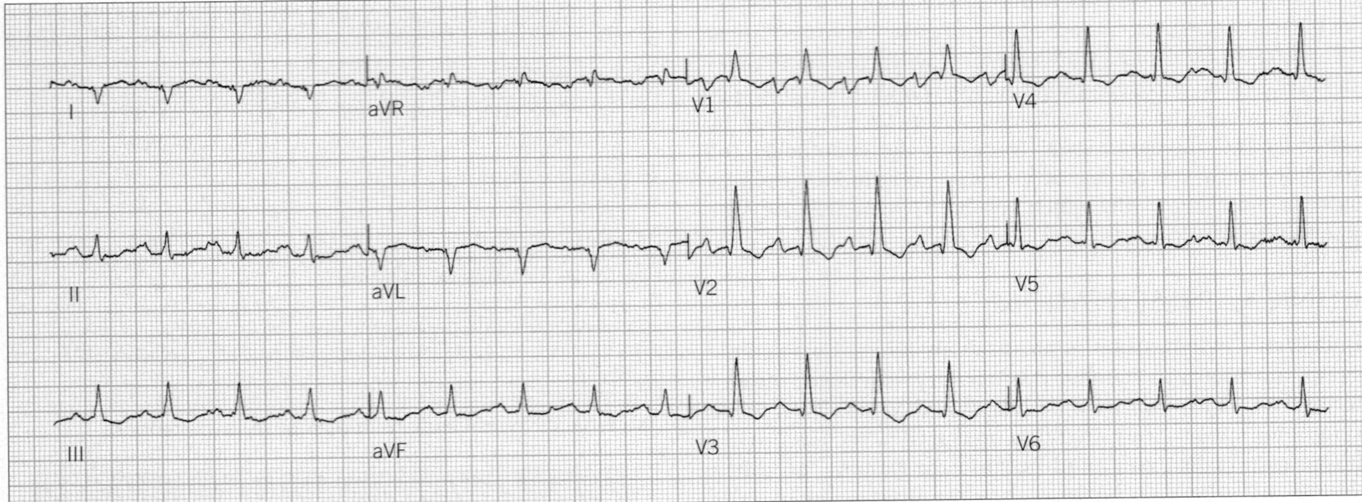

Figure 83.3 Electrocardiogram from a patient with advanced pulmonary hypertension demonstrating right axis deviation, right ventricular hypertrophy, and right atrial enlargement.

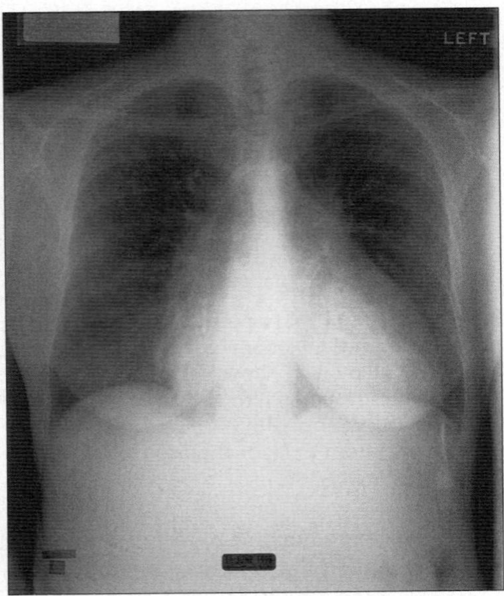

Figure 83.4 Chest radiograph of a patient with severe intrinsic pulmonary vascular disease demonstrating enlargement of the main pulmonary artery, right ventricle, and right atrium.

producing cardiomegaly (Fig. 83.4). Extensive parenchymal lung disease, especially fibrosis, indicates that it is the likely cause of the pulmonary hypertension. Massively enlarged pulmonary arteries may be associated with PAH related to a congenital systemic-to-pulmonary shunt.

Evaluation of exercise performance is useful for objective determination of the effect of pharmacologic therapy and prognosis. The 6-minute walk is most commonly employed because of its ease of performance and lack of need for specialized equipment. Modified treadmill protocols may also be useful. Formal exercise testing with continuous measure of lung and arterial oxygen and carbon dioxide concentrations may also be useful and correlates with survival.[8]

Echocardiography is an extremely valuable diagnostic tool for evaluation of the patient with suspected PAH. If there is significant elevation in pulmonary pressure, the right atrium and right ventricle are usually dilated. The more severe the elevation of pressure or the longer it is present, the greater the dilatation. Once pulmonary pressure is elevated, tricuspid regurgitation is nearly always present and allows calculation of the right ventricular systolic pressure (Fig. 83.5). The echocardiogram is also useful for excluding left-sided heart causes of the pulmonary hypertension, such as left ventricular dysfunction or mitral valve disease. Subtle findings of left-sided heart disease include left atrial enlargement and abnormal diastolic filling parameters (>stage I dysfunction). Echocardiography, through the use of color Doppler imaging or through injection of intravenous agitated saline, may also detect congenital cardiovascular shunts that may provoke PAH. Isolated partial anomalous pulmonary venous return can be missed as the source of PAH because the agitated saline contrast study will be normal in these cases (shunt is left to right only in this anatomic defect).

Radioisotope ventilation-perfusion scanning is the preferred method by which to exclude chronic pulmonary thromboembolism as a cause of pulmonary hypertension in a patient with unexplained dyspnea. Symptomatic pulmonary hypertension due to chronic thromboembolic disease is virtually always associated with a very abnormal lung scan, showing large areas of hypoperfusion. Minor perfusion abnormalities are common in PAH but are rarely confused with the large defects caused by thromboembolic disease.[9] Although it is excellent to exclude acute pulmonary embolism in the appropriate clinical setting, spiral computed tomography may underestimate clot burden in smaller pulmonary vessels.

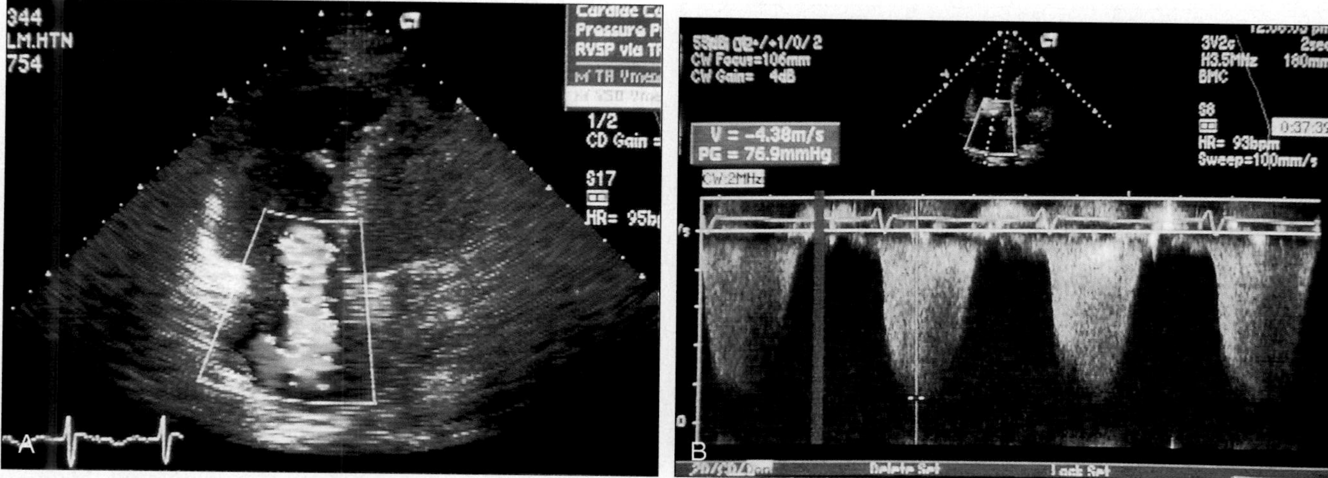

Figure 83.5 Echocardiography in primary hypertension. A, Color-flow Doppler study depicts the tricuspid regurgitant jet in a patient with primary pulmonary hypertension. **B,** Continuous-wave Doppler study measures the velocity of the tricuspid jet, which exceeds 4 m/s in this patient.

Pulmonary function testing should be performed as part of the initial evaluation of the patient with newly diagnosed pulmonary hypertension to exclude parenchymal lung disease as the cause. Pulmonary function test results are usually normal in patients with IPAH. Some patients may demonstrate mild to moderate reduction in diffusion capacity.[6] Oxygen saturation is usually normal in patients with IPAH. Significant desaturation suggests intracardiac shunting due to either congenital heart disease or a patent foramen ovale.

Cardiac catheterization remains the cornerstone for making the diagnosis of PAH. Right-sided heart catheterization documents the pulmonary artery pressure, cardiac output, and pulmonary vascular resistance. Right atrial pressure is also measured; along with cardiac output, it is the most important hemodynamic determinant of prognosis.[7] The National Institutes of Health patient registry demonstrated that cardiac indices of less than 2.0 L/min per m^2 and right atrial pressures of 20 mm Hg or greater are associated with an extremely shortened life expectancy (Fig. 83.6). Cardiac catheterization also identifies any intracardiac shunts and evidence of other structural abnormalities. A simple shunt run should be performed in all patients with a measurement of the superior and inferior vena cava saturations and the pulmonary artery saturation. The pulmonary artery saturation should normally approximate the mixed venous saturation (estimated by adding 3 times the superior vena cava saturation to the inferior vena cava saturation and dividing by 4).[10] If the pulmonary artery saturation is more than 7% higher than the mixed venous saturation, a shunt is likely to be present.

It is crucial to obtain an adequate pulmonary capillary wedge pressure or, if necessary, a left ventricular end-diastolic pressure. If it is elevated (>15 mm Hg), the diagnosis is likely to be pulmonary venous hypertension, and the patient should be treated accordingly. An elegant way to differentiate pulmonary arterial from pulmonary venous hypertension is continuous recording of the capillary wedge pressure and then pulmonary artery pressure during deflation and careful, slight withdrawal of the balloon catheter (Fig. 83.7).

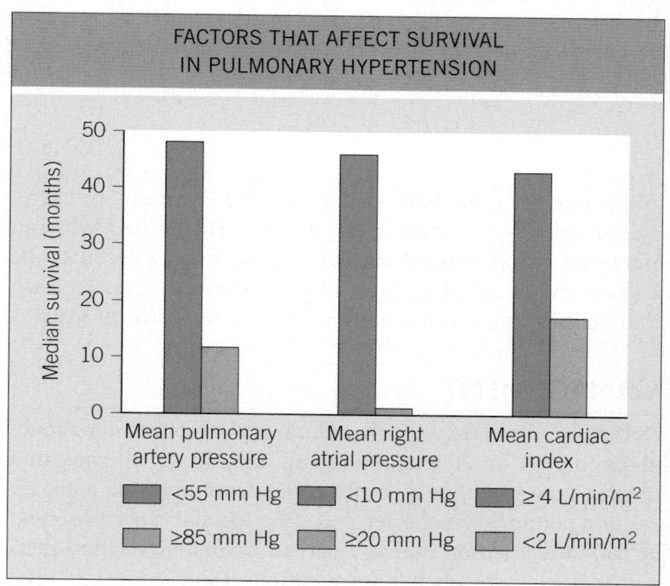

Figure 83.6 Factors that affect survival in pulmonary hypertension. The median survival in patients with pulmonary hypertension is related to the degree of right atrial and pulmonary artery pressure elevation and to how severely the cardiac index is suppressed. (Modified from D'Alonzo GE, Barst RJ, Ayres SM, et al. Survival in patients with primary pulmonary hypertension. Results from a national prospective registry. Ann Intern Med 1991;115:343-349.)

At the time of diagnostic catheterization, it is important also to test the pulmonary vascular reactivity because it is very useful in determining the best treatment strategy.[11] Hemodynamic measurements are made at baseline and during prostacyclin or adenosine infusion or nitric oxide

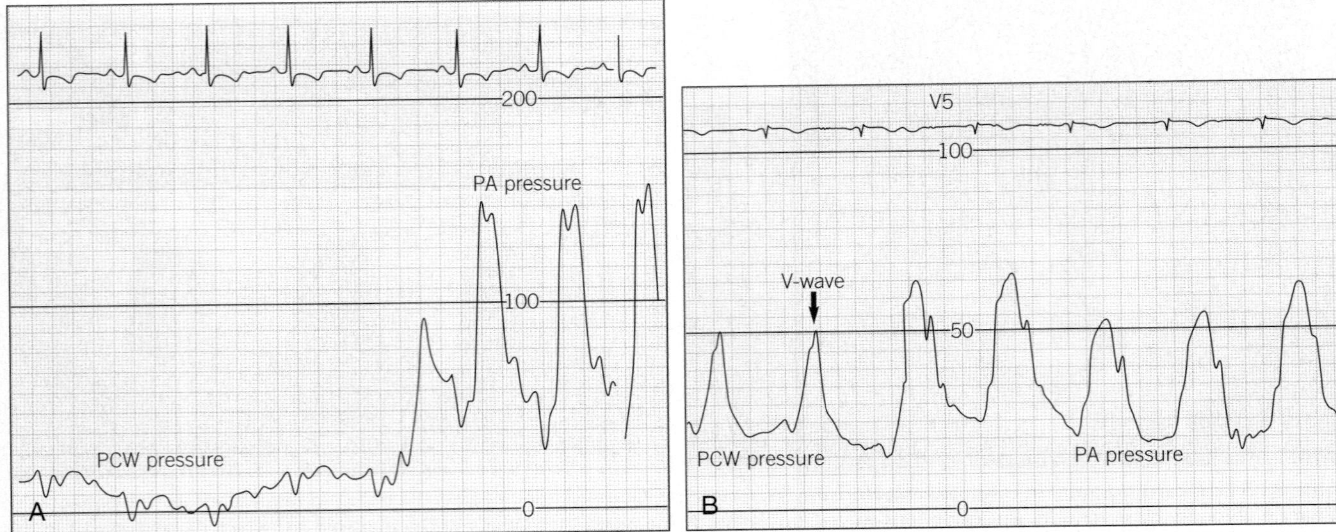

Figure 83.7 Hemodynamic tracings from cardiac catheterizations performed in patients with pulmonary arterial hypertension (A) and pulmonary venous hypertension (B). In pulmonary arterial hypertension **(A),** the left atrial pressure (estimated by the pulmonary capillary wedge pressure) is low, and there is a significant "step-up" in pressure going back into the pulmonary artery from the wedge position after balloon deflation. In pulmonary venous hypertension **(B),** although the pulmonary artery pressure is elevated, it is not disproportionately elevated compared with the left atrial pressure. Also note the large *v* waves on the tracing suggestive of either a stiff left atrium or significant mitral regurgitation, both suggestive of left-sided heart dysfunction as the cause of elevated right-sided heart pressures. Numbers on the *y* axis are pressures in millimeters of mercury. PA, pulmonary arterial; PCW, pulmonary capillary wedge.

inhalation. A reduction of 10 mm Hg or more in mean pulmonary artery pressure to 40 mm Hg or less with an increased or unchanged cardiac output is considered to be a good indicator of a favorable response to oral calcium channel blocker therapy and improved long-term survival.

MANAGEMENT

Optimally, all patients with pulmonary hypertension should undergo their initial evaluation and initiation of therapy in a medical center with a specialty clinic devoted to the management of pulmonary hypertension.[12] Functional capacity should be formally assessed in every patient as guideline-based therapy is dependent on this information (Table 83.4).[13,14] The proliferation of new therapies has resulted in frequent updates to these guidelines, although evidence-based therapy remains a novel approach to this disease entity.

Patients should be encouraged to participate in some form of regular exercise to promote physical fitness. Studies have suggested a significant benefit from formalized pulmonary and cardiovascular rehabilitation programs in pulmonary hypertension that may even exceed the benefits of adding a typical pharmacologic agent.[15,16] Activities should be aerobic in nature, and patients should be advised to avoid activities that abruptly increase intrathoracic pressures, such as lifting weights. Patients should limit themselves on the basis of the development of chest pain, excessive shortness of breath, or dizziness and should be encouraged to start their routines slowly and to build their intensity during the course of several weeks to months.

Female patients should be counseled about the critical importance of avoiding pregnancy because of the extremely high reported risk of maternal and fetal morbidity and mortality.[17] Ideally, women should be offered two forms of contraception including a barrier form and a low estrogen pill or injection, the latter to avoid induction of a hypercoagulable state with estrogen. Should patients become pregnant, they should be counseled to consider elective termination. Care for these patients should involve obstetricians with experience in management of complex patients.

Patients with hypoxemia (oxygen saturation <90%), either at rest or with exercise, should receive supplemental oxygen. Studies have suggested that nocturnal desaturation can occur in pulmonary hypertension, even in the absence of exercise-induced hypoxia, and therefore nocturnal oximetric evaluation is advised for most patients.[18]

Conventional Pharmacologic Therapies

Diuretics (typically furosemide) are frequently used to reduce excessive edema in patients with right-sided heart failure. They are particularly useful when hepatic congestion, ascites, and edema are present. In refractory cases, a switch to a better absorbed loop diuretic such as torsemide or the addition of a potassium-sparing diuretic such as aldactone can be helpful. For the latter, doses in excess of 50 mg may be necessary to achieve the intrinsic diuretic effect. The use of concurrent thiazide diuretics, such as metolazone (Zaroxolyn), can be particularly effective but requires careful monitoring of electrolytes. In some instances, patients may require temporary treatment with intravenous diuretics.

Digoxin, a cardiac glycoside, increases cardiac output and reduces circulating neurohormones.[19] No long-term efficacy or safety data regarding the use of glycosides in pulmonary hypertension exist, however, and in patients with fluctuating renal clearance, dosing should be closely monitored to prevent toxicity. Digoxin may also have utility as a rate-controlling

OVERVIEW OF THE AMERICAN COLLEGE OF CHEST PHYSICIANS GUIDELINES ON MEDICAL THERAPY FOR PULMONARY ARTERIAL HYPERTENSION			
Recommendation	**Level of Evidence**	**Net Benefit**	**Grade of Recommendation**
Calcium channel blockers			
Acute responders to vasoreactivity testing and an absence of right-sided heart failure may be treated with oral CCB, with careful reassessment:			
1. IPAH	Low	Substantial	B
2. Secondary PAH from underlying conditions	Expert opinion	Intermediate	E/B
Sildenafil			
Patients who are not candidates for or who have failed CCB therapy can initiate long-term therapy for the following function class:			
1. II or III	Good	Substantial	A
2. IV	Low	Indeterminate	C
Intravenous epoprostenol			
Patients who are not candidates for or who have failed CCB therapy can initiate long-term therapy for the following function class:			
III or IV	Good	Substantial	A
Treprostinil			
Patients who are not candidates for or who have failed CCB therapy can initiate long-term therapy for the following function class:			
1. II			
SC or IV	Low	Small/weak	C
2. III or IV			
a. SC	Fair	Intermediate	B (III), C (IV)
b. IV	Low	Intermediate	C (III and IV)
Inhaled iloprost			
Patients who are not candidates for or who have failed CCB therapy can initiate long-term therapy for the following function class:			
1. III	Good	Intermediate	A
2. IV	Fair	Intermediate	B
Bosentan			
Patients who are not candidates for or who have failed CCB therapy can initiate long-term therapy for the following function class:			
1. III	Good	Substantial	A
2. IV	Fair	Intermediate	B

Strength of recommendation scale: A, strong; B, moderate; C, weak; D, negative; E, expert opinion only followed by strength of expert opinion consensus. CCB, calcium channel blocker; IPAH, idiopathic pulmonary arterial hypertension; IV, intravenous; PAH, pulmonary arterial hypertension; SC, subcutaneous.

Table 83.4 Overview of the American College of Chest Physicians guidelines on medical therapy for pulmonary arterial hypertension.

agent in patients who develop atrial fibrillation as it avoids the negative inotropic effects associated with beta-blocker and calcium channel blocker administration.

Anticoagulant therapy has been associated with an improved survival in one prospective and two retrospective studies.[20-22] In patients who were nonresponders to calcium channel blockers, a significant improvement in survival was noted in those treated with anticoagulants, with a survival of 91%, 62%, and 47% after 1, 2, and 3 years compared with 52%, 31%, and 31% in patients who did not receive anticoagulants.[21] Although the effectiveness of warfarin anticoagulation in patients with PAH has never been tested in a prospective randomized long-term trial, on the basis of the known pathogenesis of PAH and the available data, the use of low-dose warfarin to maintain an international normalized ratio of 2.0 to 2.5 times control is recommended. The only subgroup in whom this strategy may not apply is in the Eisenmenger population, in which a significant risk for hemoptysis exists; the risks and benefits in these patients need to be carefully weighed before anticoagulation is initiated.

Calcium Channel Blockers

Calcium channel blockers were among the first vasodilators to be used in the setting of IPAH, and early studies suggested that up to 25% of IPAH patients acutely respond to calcium channel blockers. This number was probably grossly overestimated, and response to calcium channel blockers appears to occur even less frequently in patients with other types of PAH. Favorable response is usually predicted by the pulmonary vasodilator challenge at the time of cardiac catheterization. Of a group of 17 patients who acutely responded to high-dose calcium channel blockers, Rich and colleagues[21] reported a 94% 5-year survival rate with therapy compared with a 36% survival rate among patients who did not respond to therapy. Sitbon and associates[23] retrospectively evaluated 557 consecutive patients with IPAH who underwent acute vasodilator testing with inhaled nitric oxide or intravenous epoprostenol. Acute responders were defined by a decrease of more than 20% in mean pulmonary artery pressure and pulmonary vascular resistance. Acute responders were prescribed a calcium channel blocker and observed every 3 to 6 months. Patients were classified as long-term responders if their function class was I or II after 1 year of therapy without the need for additional PAH medications. Of the 70 acute responders to vasoreactivity testing, 38 patients remained responsive to calcium channel blockers after 1 year; this represented less than 7% of the total cohort. Survival was improved in the calcium channel blocker responder group compared with the calcium channel blocker failure group, although the study was not powered to detect such differences. The long-term responders had a mean pulmonary artery pressure at the time of acute vasodilator testing of 33 ± 8 mm Hg at baseline compared with 46 ± 10 mm Hg for the calcium channel blocker failure group. This important study suggests that only a small subset of patients will benefit from calcium channel blockers and should be identified by vasoreactivity testing.

Empiric calcium channel blocker therapy should be discouraged, and calcium channel blockers with negative inotropic effects, such as verapamil, should generally be avoided. When they are used without the benefit of hemodynamic monitoring, calcium channel blockers may worsen right ventricular failure and potentially result in premature death. Depending on the patient's stability, one may consider starting calcium channel blockers under invasive hemodynamic guidance to monitor the safety and efficacy of treatment. An increase in right atrial pressure, a decline in cardiac output, or an obvious clinical deterioration warrants discontinuation of therapy.

Prostacyclin (Epoprostenol) and Prostacyclin Analogues

Prostacyclin is a metabolite of arachidonic acid that is produced primarily in the vascular endothelium, and patients with PAH have deficiencies in prostacyclin and prostacyclin synthase.[24] The major pharmacologic actions of prostacyclin include potent vasodilatation of the pulmonary and systemic arterial and venous beds and inhibition of platelet aggregation. Prostacyclin analogues include treprostinil, iloprost, and beraprost, which are typically administered by subcutaneous, inhalational, and oral routes, respectively.

Intravenous Prostacyclin

Intravenous prostacyclin (epoprostenol, Flolan), a potent, short-acting vasodilator with a half-life of 3 to 6 minutes, has been well studied in PAH. A seminal open-label trial randomized 81 patients with IPAH assigned to function class III or class IV to continuous intravenous epoprostenol and conventional therapy or conventional therapy alone for 12 weeks.[25] The 6-minute walk distance, mean pulmonary artery pressure, and pulmonary vascular resistance improved in the epoprostenol group but worsened under conventional therapy, and all eight patients who died in the study were receiving only conventional therapy. In a randomized trial conducted in 111 patients with function class III and class IV PAH associated with scleroderma, 6-minute walk distance, mean pulmonary artery pressure, and pulmonary vascular resistance improved in the epoprostenol group compared with conventional therapy alone, although no survival difference was found.[26]

The long-term efficacy of intravenous epoprostenol has been evaluated in several observational studies.[27-29] The first study observed 162 consecutive patients with function class III or class IV IPAH for a mean of 36 months.[11] In addition to improvements in exercise endurance, mean pulmonary artery pressure, and pulmonary vascular resistance, survival at 1, 2, and 3 years was significantly improved (88%, 76%, and 63%) compared with predicted survival (59%, 46%, and 35%). The second study found similar results for 178 patients with function class III or class IV IPAH.[29] In addition to 6-minute walk distance and pulmonary artery pressure improvements, survival at 1, 2, and 3 years was significantly improved. For the 55% of patients reassigned to function class I or class II at 3 months, survival was 100%, 93%, and 88% at 1, 2, and 3 years. Another observational study observed 91 patients with function class III or class IV PAH (49 with IPAH).[27] At 1 year, 6-minute walk distance, mean pulmonary artery pressure, and pulmonary vascular resistance remained better in the IPAH patients, and survival was improved (85%, 76%, and 65% compared with predicted survival of 62%, 49%, and 39%). Intravenous epoprostenol therefore appears to benefit survival in function class III and class IV IPAH and has been approved by the Food and Drug Administration (FDA) for use in patients with IPAH and PAH secondary to the scleroderma spectrum of disease.

Epoprostenol is administered through a permanent intravenous catheter and delivered by an ambulatory infusion system. The delivery system is complex and requires that patients learn the techniques of sterile preparation of the medication, operation of the ambulatory infusion pump, and care of the permanent intravenous catheter. Side effects related to epoprostenol therapy are common and include headache, flushing, nausea, diarrhea, and an unusual type of jaw discomfort that occurs with the first bite or two of a meal. Other chronic side effects include thrombocytopenia, weight loss, foot pain, gastropathy, and ascites. In most patients, the symptoms are minimal and well tolerated. Other complications related to epoprostenol therapy include infection of the central venous catheter and unintended interruptions of therapy. The expected local central line infection rate is in the range of 0.22 to 0.68 per patient per year, and the rate of bacteremia is 0.14 to 0.39 per patient per year.[25,26,28-30] Because of the very short half-life, even a brief interruption in therapy can result in rebound pulmonary hypertension and has been fatal in some instances. Catheter thrombosis is fortunately a rare event. In addition, as with nearly every therapeutic option with the exception of calcium channel blockers, epoprostenol is very expensive.

Dosing of epoprostenol is somewhat problematic. Early on, it was noted that tolerance to the beneficial effects of epoprostenol seemed to occur. This led clinicians to the practice of progressively increasing the dose in anticipation of symptoms. Unfortunately, patients treated with chronic epoprostenol therapy may suffer adverse effects related to high cardiac output states.[31] In such cases, patients can undergo successful reduction in the dose of epoprostenol without a change in pulmonary artery pressure but with substantially fewer side effects related to epoprostenol.

Subcutaneous and Intravenous Treprostinil

Because of the complexities of epoprostenol administration and the associated infections and other potentially severe adverse events, an alternative mode of delivery of prostaglandins has been desired. Treprostinil (Remodulin), a prostacyclin analogue, has a longer half-life (4.5 hours) than prostacyclin and is stable at room temperature, thereby obviating the need for refrigeration. It was initially designated for subcutaneous administration to prevent the need for central access and to reduce the risks of infection. In a 12-week double-blind, placebo-controlled trial, 470 patients with functional class II to class IV IPAH or PAH associated with congenital systemic-to-pulmonary shunts or connective tissue disease on conventional therapy were randomized to continuous subcutaneous treprostinil or placebo.[32] The 6-minute walk distance and mean pulmonary artery pressure improved with treprostinil but worsened with placebo. No difference in death, transplantation, or clinical deterioration was seen. The most common adverse event was infusion site pain (85% in the treprostinil group and 27% of placebo patients). An open-label extension of this study observed 860 patients for 4 years to evaluate long-term safety and efficacy.[33] Of the 15% of patients who continued to receive subcutaneous treprostinil alone, survival at 1, 2, 3, and 4 years was 88%, 79%, 73%, and 70%. For the 332 patients with IPAH, survival at 1, 2, 3, and 4 years was improved (91%, 82%, 76%, and 72% compared with predicted survival of 69%, 56%, 46%, and 38%). Site pain was the most common adverse event (92% of patients), and a significant number of patients discontinued therapy because of this during the first year of treatment.

Most patients experience pain or erythema at the site of subcutaneous treprostinil infusion. In some patients, these symptoms are severe enough to limit dose escalation. Numerous remedies have been used in an attempt to control this infusion site reaction. No therapy has emerged as uniformly successful to treat this problem; however, current recommendations include local therapies such as warm and cold packs and nonsteroidal anti-inflammatory agents. Narcotic opioids should not be used to control pain.

Because of the high frequency of site pain with subcutaneous administration, intravenously administered treprostinil has been studied in a 12-week open-label prospective trial of 16 patients with function class III and class IV IPAH and PAH due to connective tissue disease or congenital heart disease.[34] In the 14 patients who completed the trial, 6-minute walk distance, mean pulmonary artery pressure, and pulmonary vascular resistance improved from baseline. Similar results were found in an open-label trial transitioning 31 patients in function class II and class III from epoprostenol to intravenous treprostinil.[35] The effects on quality of life are currently being evaluated in patients rapidly switched from epoprostenol to intravenous treprostinil and observed for 8 weeks.[36] The long-term efficacy of intravenous treprostinil in patients in function class II to class IV is still being evaluated. The strength of evidence in the updated treatment guidelines does not exceed epoprostenol for patients in function class III or class IV, and the subcutaneous form of treprostinil has been given a higher evidence grade than the intravenous form.[14] A new, inhaled form of treprostinil is currently being investigated, and initial results appear promising.[37]

Inhaled Iloprost

Iloprost (Ventavis) is a prostacyclin analogue with a half-life of 25 minutes available in intravenous, subcutaneous, and inhaled forms. The inhaled form has been studied the most extensively. Aerosolized particles of inhaled iloprost are deposited as alveolar particles and selectively vasodilate the pulmonary vasculature. A 12-week trial randomized 203 patients with function class III or class IV IPAH or PAH secondary to appetite suppressants, chronic thromboembolic disease, or connective tissue disease to inhaled iloprost or placebo on a background of conventional therapy.[38] The primary endpoint was defined as an improvement of 10% or more in 6-minute walk distance and at least a one–function class improvement. At 12 weeks, the primary endpoint was reached by 16.8% of patients in the iloprost group compared with 4.9% of patients in the placebo group ($P < .007$). Marked improvements in 6-minute walk distance, mean pulmonary artery pressure, and pulmonary vascular resistance were also seen.

In a prospective open-label study of 76 patients with function class II to class IV IPAH treated with inhaled iloprost for 535 ± 62 days, freedom from death, transplantation, change to intravenous prostanoid therapy, or change to or addition of other oral PAH therapy occurred in 81%, 53%, 29%, 20%, 17%, and 13% of patients at 3 months and at 1, 2, 3, 4, and 5 years.[39] No significant improvement in expected survival was seen with therapy. In general, therefore, inhaled iloprost appears to be an effective treatment of patients with function class III and class IV PAH, but effects on long-term survival remain unclear. The short half-life of iloprost requires inhalation six to eight times daily and somewhat limits the practicality of its use.

Oral Beraprost

Beraprost is an orally active epoprostenol analogue that has been used primarily in Japan for the treatment of pulmonary hypertension. Beraprost has a short half-life and must be given three or four times per day, preferably with food. A retrospective analysis suggested an improved survival in 24 patients treated with beraprost compared with 34 patients treated with conventional therapy in Japan.[40] A double-blind, randomized, controlled European trial evaluated beraprost in

130 patients with function class II or class III PAH.[41] From baseline to week 12, a slight improvement in 6-minute walk distance was seen. There were also favorable trends in hemodynamic parameters. In a similarly designed trial performed in the United States, beraprost or placebo was administered to 116 patients with class II or class III PAH.[42] Although results looked promising at 6 months, including less disease progression and improvement in 6-minute walk distance, these findings were not sustained during longer follow-up time (9 and 12 months). Beraprost is not commercially available in the United States at this time.

Endothelin Receptor Antagonists

Endothelin 1 is a potent vasoconstrictor and smooth muscle mitogen. Patients with PAH have increased expression of endothelin 1, and its level has been correlated with disease severity.[43] Endothelin receptor antagonists are designed to halt the effects of endothelin 1 and offer another pharmacologic class for the treatment of PAH. Bosentan (Tracleer) was the first oral endothelin receptor antagonist studied in PAH. A double-blind, placebo-controlled study of 32 patients with function class III or class IV IPAH or PAH secondary to scleroderma demonstrated significant improvements in 6-minute walk distance, pulmonary artery pressure, and pulmonary vascular resistance at 12 weeks.[44] Clinical worsening occurred in three patients, all of whom were receiving placebo. An open-label study involving 29 of the original 32 patients continued for 15.3 ± 3.2 months and demonstrated persistent 6-minute walk distance improvements at 6 months.[45] In 11 patients who underwent right-sided heart catheterization, pulmonary vascular resistance was improved, although pulmonary artery pressure was unchanged. Function class improved in 41.4% of patients at 6 months and remained stable at 1 year.

The Bosentan Randomized Trial of Endothelin Antagonist Therapy (BREATHE-1) randomized 213 patients with function class III or class IV IPAH or PAH secondary to connective tissue disease to placebo or bosentan.[46] At 16 weeks, 6-minute walk distance improved with bosentan but declined with placebo, with the greatest improvement seen in patients receiving 250 mg daily. Function class improved to class II in 38% and 34% of patients receiving 250 mg and 125 mg compared with 28% receiving placebo; 4% in the combined bosentan group improved to class I compared with no patients receiving placebo. Bosentan also improved the secondary endpoint of time to clinical worsening.

The long-term efficacy of bosentan has been examined in patients receiving bosentan during the two placebo-controlled trials and their extension studies. A total of 169 patients with function class III or class IV IPAH were observed for 2.1 ± 0.5 years.[47] During the study, 19 patients died, 3 had transplantation, and 12% received alternative or additional PAH therapy. Survival at 1 and 2 years was 96.4% and 88.5% compared with predicted survival of 69.2% and 57.3%. Of the patients who were alive at 1 and 2 years, 78% and 55% were receiving bosentan monotherapy. The most common adverse effect was elevated hepatic transaminases (more than three times the upper limit of normal), seen in 14.9% of patients. Baseline function class and 6-minute walk distance were the most powerful predictors of survival.

A retrospective analysis of 103 consecutive patients with function class III or class IV IPAH showed improvements in 6-minute walk distance and pulmonary artery pressure at 16 weeks in patients treated with bosentan.[48] After 24 ± 15 months, prostanoid therapy had been initiated in 44% of patients. Survival at 1 and 2 years was 90% and 87% compared with predicted survival of 63% and 45%. Bosentan was stopped because of elevated liver enzymes in three patients, in whom levels returned to normal within 12 weeks of discontinuation. Long-term survival was assessed in a cohort of 139 patients with function class III IPAH treated with bosentan therapy and compared with 346 historical controls treated with intravenous epoprostenol.[49] Survival for the bosentan cohort was 97% and 91% at 1 and 2 years compared with 91% and 84% in the epoprostenol cohort.

At the 2007 European Society of Cardiology Congress, the Endothelin Antagonist Trial in Mildly Symptomatic PAH (EARLY) was presented.[50] This study randomized 185 patients in function class II to bosentan or placebo for 6 months. A significant 23% reduction in pulmonary vascular resistance was seen as well as a trend toward improvement in 6-minute walk distance. Death, hospitalization, or symptomatic progression was significantly delayed with bosentan (3% versus 11% with placebo; $P = .01$). Although these results suggest that bosentan could be beneficial in symptomatic patients in function class II, the study has yet to be formally subjected to peer review.

Ambrisentan (Letairis) is a second endothelin receptor antagonist approved for treatment of PAH. In a trial of 64 patients with function class II or class III IPAH or PAH associated with connective tissue disease, anorexigen use, or human immunodeficiency virus infection, the 6-minute walk distance, mean pulmonary artery pressure, and pulmonary vascular resistance improved after 12 weeks of therapy, although no dose relationship to clinical effect was seen.[51] Function improved by at least one class in 36.2% and was maintained in patients with open-label drug until at least 24 weeks. Clinical worsening was reported in 20.3% of patients.

The ARIES-1 and ARIES-2 trials were 12-week placebo-controlled trials that demonstrated improvements in exercise capacity and symptoms in patients with PAH.[52] The long-term efficacy of ambrisentan has been examined in a continuation study of these two phase III placebo-controlled trials.[53] A total of 383 patients with PAH were treated with ambrisentan for approximately 1.4 years. At 24 and 48 weeks, 99% and 84% of patients continued to receive ambrisentan monotherapy. The 6-minute walk distance and function class improvements were maintained through 48 weeks in all dosage groups. Survival at 1 year ranged from 94% to 97%, and the long-term incidence of elevated liver function test results did not appreciably change from the 12-week incidence. Further studies, particularly randomized trials, are needed to more fully evaluate the long-term efficacy and safety of ambrisentan. Ambrisentan was listed as an investigational agent in the latest treatment guidelines[14] but was recently approved by the FDA for treatment of PAH. On the basis of available trial data, it should be considered an alternative endothelin receptor antagonist for patients with function class II and class III PAH.

Sitaxsentan is an endothelin receptor antagonist that has not yet been approved for treatment of PAH in the United States. The Sitaxsentan to Relieve Impaired Exercise 1

(STRIDE-1) study randomized 178 patients with function class II and class III IPAH or PAH associated with connective tissue disease or congenital heart disease to 12 weeks of placebo or sitaxsentan and demonstrated improvement in 6-minute walk distance and pulmonary vascular resistance.[54] In STRIDE-2, 247 patients with function class II to class IV IPAH or PAH associated with connective tissue disease or congenital heart disease were randomized to placebo, two different sitaxsentan doses, or open-label bosentan.[55] At 18 weeks, 6-minute walk distance worsened in the placebo group but improved in all the treatment groups. Function class improved or was unchanged in 98% of patients receiving high-dose (100 mg) sitaxsentan compared with 87% of patients receiving placebo ($P = .04$), yet no difference was seen with lower dose (50 mg) sitaxsentan or open-label bosentan compared with placebo. Time to clinical worsening did not differ between groups. Sitaxsentan has a well-described interaction with warfarin, and patients require a decrease in warfarin dose to maintain a therapeutic international normalized ratio when sitaxsentan is added.[56] Long-term outcomes with sitaxsentan are unknown, and it remains unapproved by the FDA.

Overall, the endothelin receptor antagonists are a promising therapeutic class for treatment of PAH and are an oral therapeutic option. The most common adverse effect is hepatotoxicity, which may limit their use in certain populations of patients. Liver function test results must be monitored monthly on therapy. Also, because of the risk for teratogenicity, pregnancy is contraindicated with therapy.

Phosphodiesterase Inhibitors

Nitric oxide stimulation of vascular endothelium increases cyclic guanosine 3′,5′-monophosphate (cGMP) levels and results in vasorelaxation. Phosphodiesterase type 5 inhibitors rapidly break down cGMP and attenuate the effect. In the pulmonary vasculature, phosphodiesterase type 5 is highly expressed, and its inhibition can sustain the vasodilatory effect of nitric oxide. Inhibitors of phosphodiesterase type 5 (such as sildenafil and tadalafil), initially developed as antianginals and more recently marketed for erectile dysfunction, appear to have potent vasodilatory effects in the pulmonary vasculature of patients with PAH.

Sildenafil (Revatio) has been reported to improve functional class and exercise tolerance in both observational and small, randomized clinical studies.[57,58] The Sildenafil Use in Pulmonary Arterial Hypertension (SUPER) study randomized 278 patients with function class II to class IV IPAH or PAH associated with connective tissue disease or previously repaired congenital shunts to 12 weeks of either placebo or sildenafil (20, 40, or 80 mg three times daily).[59] The sildenafil group had improvements in 6-minute walk distance, functional class, and mean pulmonary artery pressure with all three dosages compared with placebo. Death, hospitalization, or initiation of an alternative PAH therapy was similar between placebo and sildenafil-treated patients. The majority of patients in the SUPER trial were assigned to function class II or class III, and these patients now have the strongest evidence for benefit with sildenafil therapy.[59] The FDA has approved sildenafil for treatment of PAH at a dose of 20 mg three times daily.[13,14] In an open-label extension of sildenafil therapy to 1 year, 86% of patients continued sildenafil monotherapy (although most with a dose of 80 mg three times daily) and had stable improvements in 6-minute walk distance.

Tadalafil is another phosphodiesterase type 5 inhibitor with a substantially longer half-life than sildenafil. The current evidence on the efficacy of tadalafil for treatment of PAH is limited. An interesting prospective observational study of 16 consecutive symptomatic Eisenmenger syndrome patients with PAH treated with 12 weeks of tadalafil showed marked improvements in function class and 6-minute walk distance.[60] A phase III clinical trial recently finished enrollment of 406 patients with PAH randomized to receive various dosages of tadalafil versus placebo for 16 weeks, with eligibility to extend therapy to 52 weeks.[61] Clinical outcomes, including 6-minute walk distance and function class, will be measured, and results of this study could establish tadalafil as an efficacious alternative to sildenafil for treatment of PAH. Currently, tadalafil is not approved for PAH.[14]

Future Directions in the Medical Management of PAH

The recently updated guidelines on the medical management of PAH are largely based on trials that studied the various agents as monotherapies,[14] which appears to be quite different from what is practiced worldwide. The guidelines are most important in determining which pharmacologic class is the best option for initial therapy, yet a large proportion of patients may need additional therapies to halt the progressive nature of PAH. Combination therapy for PAH is therefore an important and exciting area of current research for the management of PAH.

Because of the multiple mechanisms involved in the pathogenesis of PAH, it seems reasonable to hypothesize that combining therapeutic classes could improve treatment efficacy and prevent the toxicity seen with higher dose monotherapy. Recently published trials using combination therapy for PAH are summarized in Table 83.5. These generally small trials have shown short-term benefits in exercise capacity or hemodynamics with certain combinations, but long-term survival has not been examined. A number of larger trials are currently ongoing and should provide further insight into the efficacy and safety of combination therapy. Although combination therapy may prove to be the future of PAH management, its cost-effectiveness will also need to be weighed carefully.

In Figure 83.8, a treatment algorithm for PAH is proposed on the basis of the updated American College of Chest Physicians guidelines and current clinical practices. Medical management in PAH is shifting toward initiation of therapy in less symptomatic patients and being more aggressive (i.e., combination therapy). Use of a structured format by which patients are assessed for response to treatment and initiation of combination therapy when certain parameters are not met may become the paradigm by which PAH is approached in the future. Hoeper and colleagues[62] have shown that use of a goal-oriented approach in 123 consecutive PAH patients significantly improved survival at 1, 2, and 3 years compared with both historical controls and the predicted survival. In this study, 43% of patients required two drugs and 16% required three drugs to reach the prespecified treatment goals.

OVERVIEW OF COMPLETED COMBINATION THERAPY TRIALS IN PAH				
Study	**Length**	**No. of Patients**	**Therapeutic Agents**	**Results**
Prostanoids + endothelin receptor antagonists				
BREATHE-2[66]	16 weeks	33	Epoprostenol + bosentan or placebo	Nonsignificant trend toward improvement in hemodynamics with combination therapy No change in 6MW distance or FC
Hoeper et al.[67]	12 weeks	40	Iloprost alone or iloprost + bosentan	No change between the two groups Study terminated prematurely
STEP[68]	12 weeks	67	Bosentan + iloprost or placebo	Improved 6MW distance, FC, and hemodynamics
Seyfarth et al.[69]	13.5 ± 5 months	16	Bosentan added to existing iloprost	Sustained improvements in 6MW distance and FC
Channick et al.[70]	12 weeks	12	Inhaled treprostinil to existing bosentan	Improved 6MW distance, FC, and hemodynamics
Prostanoids + phosphodiesterase inhibitors				
Wilkens et al.[71]	2 hours	5	Sildenafil or iloprost or combination	Improved hemodynamics with combination therapy
Ghofrani et al.[72]	3 hours	30	Sildenafil or iloprost or combination	Improved hemodynamics with combination therapy
Gomberg-Maitland et al.[73]	12 weeks	9	Sildenafil added to existing treprostinil	6MW distance improved compared with baseline
PACES[74]	16 weeks	267	Epoprostenol + sildenafil or placebo	6MW distance, survival, and time to clinical worsening improved with combination therapy
Phosphodiesterase inhibitors + endothelin receptor antagonists				
Hoeper et al.[75]	9 months	9	Sildenafil added to existing bosentan	Sustained improvement in 6MW distance
Minai et al.[76]	19 months	3	Sildenafil added to existing bosentan	Sustained improvement in FC
COMPASS-I[77]	60 months	45	Sildenafil added to existing bosentan	Improvement in hemodynamics from baseline

6MW, 6-minute walk; FC, function class; PAH, pulmonary arterial hypertension.

Table 83.5 Overview of completed combination therapy trials in PAH.

Percutaneous and Surgical Options

A palliative form of therapy, graded atrial balloon septostomy, is an option for patients refractory to medical therapy. Sandoval and colleagues[63] have demonstrated that graded or stepwise balloon dilatation of the atrial septum can be done safely. Systemic saturations are monitored during the procedure, and further dilatation is not performed when arterial saturation falls to 75% or the left ventricular diastolic pressure reaches 18 mm Hg. Interestingly, peripheral oxygen delivery is found to be improved because the increased cardiac output more than compensates for the fall in hemoglobin saturation. Currently, in the United States, balloon septostomy is reserved for those patients who are deteriorating in spite of continuous intravenous prostacyclin and are candidates for lung transplantation. The procedure is not recommended for patients in the terminal stages of the disease (late class IV with advanced right-sided heart failure) because of the high procedural mortality. More recently, an expandable stent technique has been developed that may allow more precise control over the size of the defect that is created.[64]

Lung transplantation has been performed successfully in patients with IPAH for more than a decade.[65] Because these patients have severe right ventricular dysfunction, it was originally believed that heart-lung transplantation was the only transplantation option. More recently, bilateral lung transplantation and single-lung transplantation have been performed successfully in patients with IPAH. The immediate reduction in pulmonary artery pressure and pulmonary vascular resistance is associated with an improvement in right ventricular function. Bilateral lung transplantation is preferred at most centers because there is greater pulmonary vascular reserve should the patient sustain rejection or infection. Single-lung transplantation may be preferred in some situations because the operation is technically less challenging and the wait time is shorter. As with any type of organ transplantation, the major long-term morbidity and mortality are related to the high incidence of rejection and

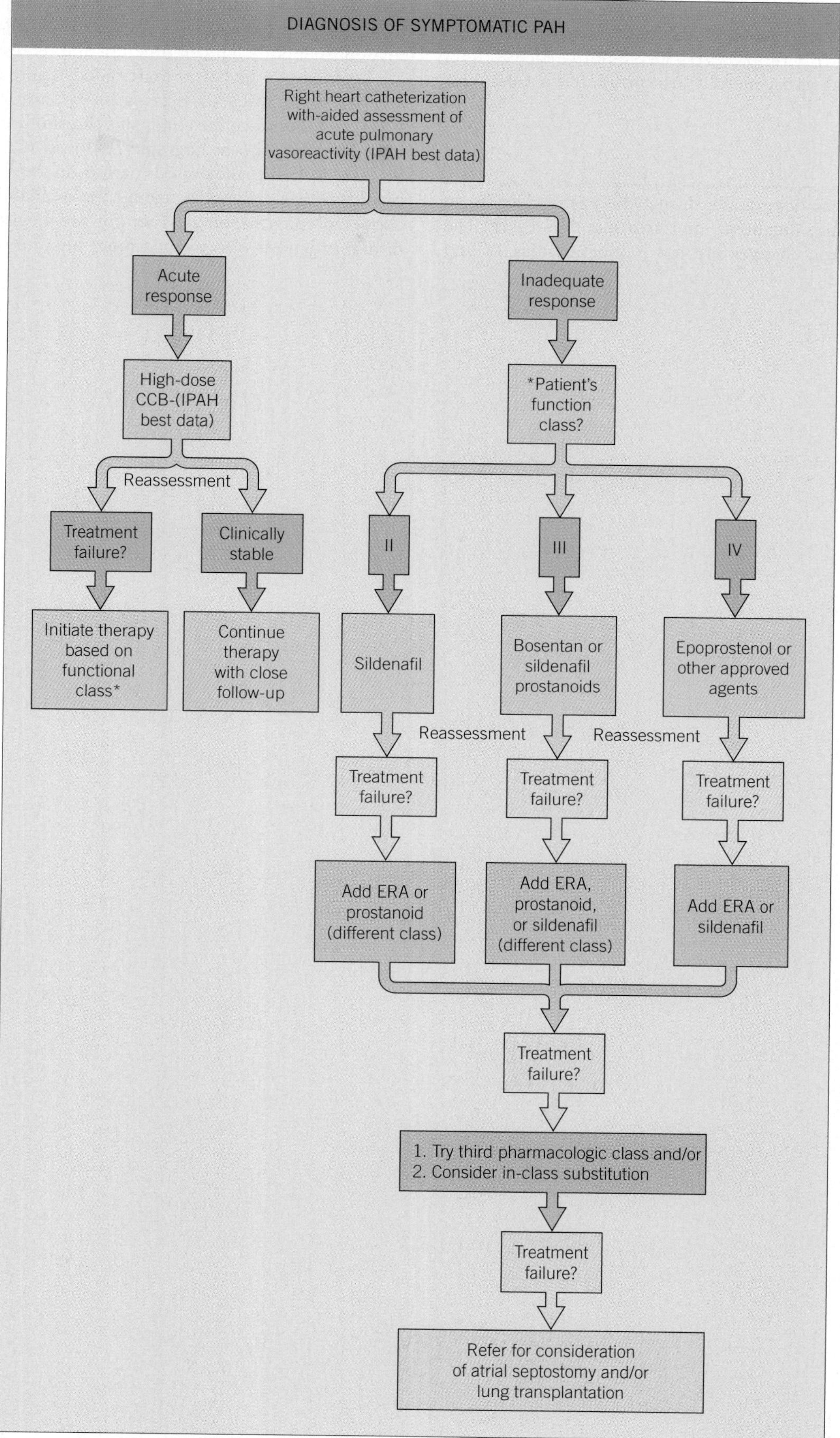

Figure 83.8 Algorithm for the medical management of PAH based on American College of Chest Physicians guidelines. CCB, calcium channel blocker; ERA, endothelin receptor antagonist; IPAH, idiopathic pulmonary arterial hypertension; PAH, pulmonary arterial hypertension.

opportunistic infections. In addition, lung transplantation carries a high risk for the development of bronchiolitis obliterans. In the era of multiple PAH-specific drug classes, lung transplantation should generally be considered a treatment of last resort.

SUMMARY

Great progress has been made during the past 2 decades in our understanding, diagnosis, and treatment of PAH. The anatomic-histologic changes are not pathognomonic of any specific etiology but represent the final common pathway in response to endothelial injury. Molecular mechanisms related to endothelial cell function and its response to injury are beginning to be better understood. There is much greater awareness of diseases that cause or are associated with PAH, and therefore the clinician's threshold to use diagnostic tools, such as echocardiography, is lower. Consequently, the disease is being diagnosed earlier in its course. Finally, breakthroughs in treatment and the availability of multiple classes of pharmacologic therapy are beginning to turn a dismal prognosis into a much more hopeful one.

chapter 84

Right-Sided Heart Failure in Chronic Lung Diseases and Pulmonary Arterial Hypertension

Harm Jan Bogaard, Anton Vonk Noordegraaf, and Norbert F. Voelkel

Definition

- Right-sided heart failure and cor pulmonale relate to altered structure and function of the right ventricle as a result of pulmonary hypertension associated with chronic obstructive pulmonary disease (COPD) or other lung diseases with chronic hypoxia.

Key Features

- The right ventricular response to pulmonary hypertension is highly variable and related not only to mechanical overload but also to right ventricular ischemia, oxidative stress, inflammation, and biventricular interaction.
- Clinical features of right ventricular failure result from low cardiac output, elevated right atrial pressure, and neurohormonal activation.

Therapy

- There is no proven benefit of pulmonary vasodilators in COPD-associated pulmonary hypertension.
- Long-term oxygen therapy benefits hypoxemic patients, and sodium restriction or diuresis minimizes fluid retention.

Historically, the right ventricle (RV) of the heart has been attributed a rather insignificant role in normal physiology and cardiovascular disease. In the first half of the 20th century, destruction of the RV in dogs with an open pericardium was shown not to affect resting cardiac output.[1] The relative resistance of the RV to ischemia led to the belief that in coronary artery disease, infarction of the RV is of much less importance than infarction of the left ventricle (LV). Absence of successful treatments for pulmonary arterial hypertension (PAH) and pulmonary hypertension associated with chronic obstructive pulmonary disease (COPD) and absence of methods to reliably assess RV function contributed to a further neglect of the right side of the heart. However, several developments have led to a renewed interest in the RV. Pulmonary hypertension was shown to contribute significantly to the mortality of patients with left-sided heart failure[2] and COPD.[3] A better understanding of the mechanisms underlying pulmonary vasoconstriction and vascular remodeling in PAH has led to moderately successful new therapies. New diagnostic methods have emerged to assess RV function, starting with the development of the pulmonary artery catheter and proceeding to modern imaging techniques like magnetic resonance imaging, three-dimensional echocardiography, and positron emission tomography.

The clinical hallmarks of right-sided heart failure are a reduced cardiac output and retention of fluid in interstitial spaces (edema) and body cavities (ascites, pleural effusion, pericardial effusion). Right-sided heart dysfunction and failure contribute to the pathophysiologic process and outcome of many diseases that are covered elsewhere in this book: ischemic heart disease, valvular heart disease, congenital heart disease (e.g., tetralogy of Fallot, transposition of the great arteries, Ebstein's anomaly, Eisenmenger's syndrome), and dilated cardiomyopathy, to name just a few. This chapter focuses on the development of right-sided heart failure associated with lung diseases or hypoxemia (cor pulmonale) and right-sided heart failure associated with PAH. An increase in pressure in the pulmonary circulation is the primary but not the only reason for adaptive responses in the RV in these conditions. The cellular and molecular mechanisms that govern the transition from adaptive RV hypertrophy to dilatation and failure have not been studied, nor do we understand the development of RV failure in response to LV pressure overload. To assume that we just have to study the LV to understand RV failure may be ill-advised, in particular because there are various structural, functional, and even developmental differences between the right and left ventricles.

DIFFERENCES BETWEEN THE RIGHT AND LEFT VENTRICLES

The RV is thinner than the LV and has a different shape. This is associated with a low pressure in the pulmonary circulation. The thin-walled RV facilitates quick adaptation to changes in preload. Because an increase in wall stress not only increases myocardial oxygen demand but also decreases myocardial perfusion, an important adaptation of the LV to the high-pressure systemic circulation is an increase in wall thickness and the change to a more rounded shape (as opposed to the RV tetrahedron; Fig. 84.1). It follows from the Laplace relationship that in a thin-walled sphere, an increase in intraluminal pressure results in an increase in wall stress, unless the thickness of the chamber walls is augmented or the internal radius of the chamber is reduced. The fact that the RV cannot develop or sustain similar configurational changes in the setting of pulmonary hypertension might indicate that the RV is inherently different from the LV. This notion is supported by evidence for differences in developmental origin. LV and atrial myocytes in the linear heart tube are derived from the primary heart field, whereas cells of the RV and outflow tract have their origin in the anterior heart field and are added to the linear heart tube later in development.[4,5] Perhaps reflective of the different

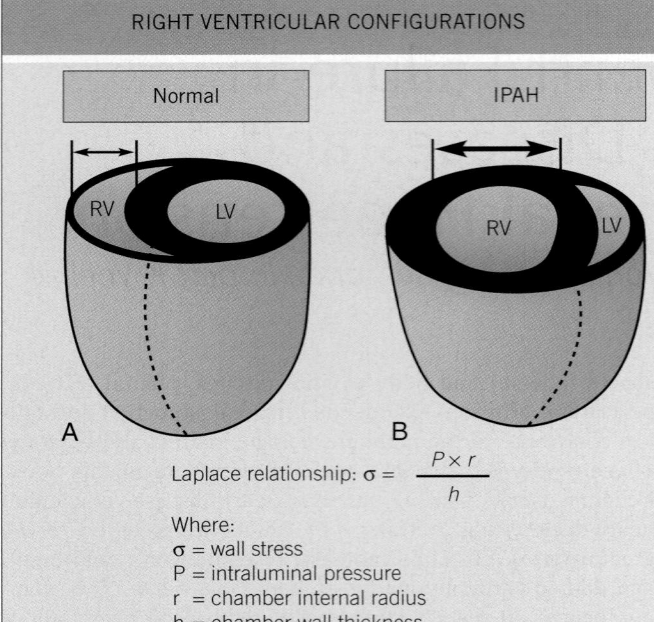

Figure 84.1 Right ventricular configurations in health and pulmonary hypertension. According to the Laplace relationship, pulmonary hypertension is characterized by an increased right ventricular wall stress (σ) due to an elevated intraluminal pressure (P) and a larger chamber radius (r), unless right ventricular wall thickness (h) is augmented by hypertrophy. IPAH, idiopathic pulmonary arterial hypertension.

sites of cellular origin, during embryonic development, gene expression patterns in the two ventricles are different. The *TBX5* gene, encoding a T-box transcription factor, is initially expressed throughout the linear heart tube with subsequent expression predominantly in the LV and atria but not in the RV myocytes that are added.[6] Examples of transcription factors that are specifically important for RV morphogenesis are myocyte enhancer factor 2C,[7] GATA-4,[8] and Bop.[9] At specific time points during cardiac development, the basic helix-loop-helix transcription factors Hand1 and Hand2 show restricted patterns of expression in the RV and LV, respectively.[10] Whether differences in the embryonic development have implications for how the RV and LV respond to hypoxia and pressure overload is unknown.

PULMONARY HYPERTENSION ASSOCIATED WITH CHRONIC LUNG DISEASES OR HYPOXEMIA

The following paradox pertains to the associations between pulmonary hypertension, right-sided heart failure, and chronic lung diseases. Chronic lung disease (in particular COPD, one focus in this chapter) is the second most important cause of pulmonary hypertension and right-sided heart failure, after left-sided heart failure. Severe pulmonary hypertension and right-sided heart failure are uncommon in COPD and are usually mere markers of hypoxemia and disease severity (and, therefore, prognosis) rather than direct causes of mortality. The very high prevalence of COPD (which is still increasing, especially in women) translates into significant morbidity and mortality of right-sided heart failure in COPD. A better understanding of the mechanisms determining the transition from RV adaptation to failure would benefit both these patients and patients with PAH.

In dealing with right-sided heart failure in chronic lung disease, it is important to consider the large heterogeneities between patients in (1) the susceptibility to development of pulmonary hypertension and (2) the susceptibility to development of right-sided heart failure in the context of established pulmonary hypertension. In general, the definition of pulmonary hypertension in the context of chronic lung disease incorporates a different mean pulmonary arterial pressure (mPAP) threshold to separate normal from abnormal (>20 mm Hg instead of the usual >25 mm Hg in PAH). The prevalence of COPD-associated pulmonary hypertension in the general population is unknown. The population at risk is large, however; a study conducted in the early 1980s in the United Kingdom showed that 0.3% of the Sheffield population older than 45 years had a partial oxygen pressure of less than 55 mm Hg in combination with a forced expiratory volume in 1 second of less than 50% of predicted.[11] This would translate into 60,000 subjects at risk for COPD-associated pulmonary hypertension in the United Kingdom and 300,000 patients in the United States. Even taking into account the fact that this study was conducted in an area with a large coal mining industry, the considerable increase in COPD prevalence in the last 2 decades probably indicates that the problem has become much larger still. For comparison, the yearly incidence of idiopathic PAH is about 5 to 25 cases per 1 million adult inhabitants.[12] In severe COPD, the mPAP increases by approximately 0.5 to 3 mm Hg per year, and elevated mPAP is an acknowledged predictor of poor prognosis in COPD patients.[13]

Although mPAP between 20 and 35 mm Hg is clearly abnormal, we doubt whether this degree of pulmonary hypertension is of clinical significance in COPD. Because the progression of pulmonary hypertension in COPD is usually slow, these patients are unlikely to develop severe pulmonary hypertension later in the course of the disease. COPD patients with mild pulmonary hypertension at rest may develop more pronounced—even severe—pulmonary hypertension during exercise, and if so, it may contribute to their reduced exercise tolerance. Figure 84.2 shows the wide variability in hemodynamic responses (both mPAP and cardiac output) between COPD patients.[14] An attenuated pulmonary pressure response with phosphodiesterase type 5 inhibition (see later) does not translate into an increased exercise capacity in COPD.[15,16] Increases in mPAP in COPD may also occur during episodes of oxygen desaturation during sleep.[17] Again, the overall significance of these hypertensive episodes is unclear. The prevention of nocturnal hypoxia by oxygen supplementation has no survival benefit in COPD patients who are normoxic at daytime, even though this treatment reduces nocturnal pulmonary hypertension.[18]

The prevalence of a moderately elevated mPAP (between 35 and 45 mm Hg) was about 10% in a group of 205 French COPD patients who underwent a right-sided heart catheterization in the work-up for lung reduction surgery or transplantation.[19] Another 3.7% of these patients had a severely elevated mPAP (>45 mm Hg). The degree of airflow obstruction in some of

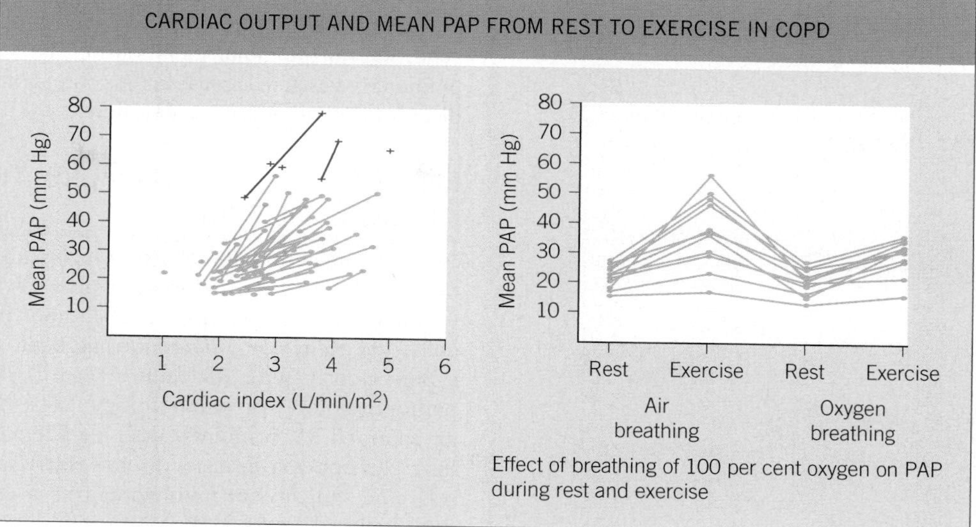

Figure 84.2 Increase in cardiac output and mean pulmonary artery pressure (PAP) from rest to exercise in chronic obstructive pulmonary disease (COPD). There is a large heterogeneity in the initial values but also in the responses *(left)*. The right panel shows the attenuated increase in pulmonary artery pressure with supplemental oxygen breathing, which is partly but not fully explained by a relief of hypoxic pulmonary vasoconstriction. (Reproduced from Burrows B, Kettel LJ, Niden AH, et al. Patterns of cardiovascular dysfunction in chronic obstructive lung disease. N Engl J Med 1972;286:912-918.)

these patients was not as severe as would be expected from their degree of hypoxemia. This led the authors to speculate that they had identified a subgroup of atypical patients in whom pulmonary vascular disease is more important than chronic airway disease.[19] An alternative explanation would be the coincidence of COPD (which is, after all, very common) with a second disease, such as idiopathic pulmonary fibrosis (also smoking related) or idiopathic PAH. There may be a genetic predisposition to development of pulmonary hypertension in COPD because a polymorphism in the gene encoding the serotonin transporter was shown to predict the severity of pulmonary hypertension in COPD.[20] Even though it occurs in only a minority of COPD patients, severe pulmonary hypertension is an indicator of a worse prognosis.[21]

Pathophysiology of Pulmonary Hypertension Associated with Chronic Lung Disease or Hypoxia

The usual suspect accused of the development of pulmonary hypertension in COPD is hypoxia, which is undoubtedly, both acutely and chronically, associated with an increase in pulmonary vascular resistance (PVR). A negative correlation exists in COPD between arterial oxygen saturation and the pulmonary artery pressure. Pulmonary vasoconstriction in response to acute alveolar hypoxia is an important physiologic control mechanism to optimize ventilation-perfusion matching and to prevent hypoxemia, at the expense of an increase in PVR. Both in normal subjects and in COPD patients, a considerable variability exists in the degree of hypoxic pulmonary vasoconstriction.[22] Although the acute effects of hypoxia on pulmonary vascular smooth muscle cell function may explain the increase in PVR during acute exacerbations and in patients with nocturnal desaturations and sleep apnea, the pulmonary vascular structural changes (vascular remodeling) that are associated with chronic hypoxia are of equal or greater importance to explain the increased PVR in COPD. Chronic hypoxia is associated with hypertrophy of the muscular media of small pulmonary arteries and muscularization of pulmonary arterioles, which are normally nonmuscular. These changes may come about by the direct action of hypoxia on smooth muscle cells and endothelial cells and from activation of signaling pathways in response to the increased intravascular pressure that follows hypoxic pulmonary vasoconstriction, thus creating a positive feedback loop (Fig. 84.3). Hypoxia also leads to increased expression of erythropoietin, and the resulting polycythemia increases blood viscosity and, hence, PVR. However, and importantly, mechanisms unrelated to hypoxia can lead to pulmonary hypertension in COPD in specific circumstances. It has been recognized for some time that pulmonary vascular remodeling is not fully reversed by long-term oxygen therapy[23] and may even occur in nonhypoxemic COPD patients[24] or smokers without airflow obstruction.[25] The vascular changes seen in the last two instances may be due to cigarette smoke–induced endothelial dysfunction, but because they are not associated with an increase in mPAP, their significance remains unexplained. Destruction of alveolar septa (emphysema) with a concomitant destruction of pulmonary vessels will lead to an increase in resting PVR only if it is very severe (>60% destruction) because the pulmonary vascular bed has a considerable reserve capacity. An increase in left atrial pressure during acute exacerbations of COPD and a hyperdynamic circulation due to hypercapnia can increase mPAP without an increase in PVR but are likely of importance in few patients. Pulmonary vascular in situ thrombosis[26] or undiagnosed pulmonary embolism[27] and intracardiac shunts may contribute to pulmonary hypertension in some COPD patients. Last,

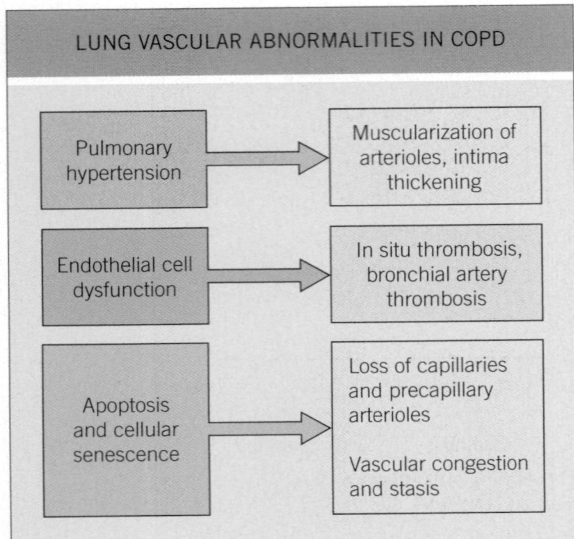

Figure 84.3 Lung vascular abnormalities in COPD. The increase in pulmonary artery pressure induced by hypoxic pulmonary vasoconstriction leads to muscularization of arterioles and intima thickening, which creates a positive feedback loop, further elevating pulmonary vascular resistance. Direct effects of cigarette smoke are endothelial cell dysfunction, apoptosis, and hypercoagulability, which lead to a decrease in pulmonary vascular reserve by destruction and obstruction of capillaries. (Reproduced from Voelkel NF, Cool CD. Pulmonary vascular involvement in chronic obstructive pulmonary disease. Eur Respir J Suppl 2003;46:28s-32s.)

the increase in mPAP with exercise is related not only to pulmonary vascular disease and dysfunction but also to compression of alveolar capillaries due to air trapping and increases in positive end-expiratory pressures.

Pulmonary Hypertension in Other Conditions Associated with Chronic Hypoxia

The current opinion on the prevalence of pulmonary hypertension in diffuse parenchymal lung disease (in particular idiopathic pulmonary fibrosis) very much resonates what is known about pulmonary hypertension in COPD: pulmonary hypertension does occur, but there are no large-cohort epidemiologic data (numbers on prevalence vary between 8% and 84%[28]). Pulmonary hypertension is usually not severe, barring perhaps some "atypical" patients, and pulmonary hypertension is associated with but is not necessarily causally related to prognosis. It sometimes leads to right-sided heart failure, but it is difficult to predict in which patients. Treatment with supplemental oxygen and diuretics has been advised, but the place of vasodilators in the treatment regimen is uncertain. Similarly, little is known about the importance of pulmonary hypertension in disorders that are associated with hypoxemia due to alveolar hypoventilation (e.g., kyphoscoliosis, neuromuscular disease, and the obesity-hypoventilation syndrome). It can be safely assumed that these conditions very rarely lead to severe pulmonary hypertension. When severe pulmonary hypertension occurs in any patient with chronic lung disease or hypoxia, the diagnostic process has not ended. In these patients, an additional explanation for the increase in pulmonary artery pressure should be considered. Frequently, an additional explanation will be left-sided heart failure (e.g., LV diastolic dysfunction due to systemic hypertension in the obesity-hypoventilation syndrome) or pulmonary embolism. The idiopathic PAH-like pulmonary vascular disease in the context of a connective tissue disorder also requires consideration.

RIGHT-SIDED HEART FAILURE: THE BIG CLINICAL PICTURE

We recognize that there are categorically three pathways that will lead to RV failure and that RV failure subsequent to left-sided heart disease carries a poor prognosis. For decades, the term *cor pulmonale* has been used by clinicians synonymously with RV failure regardless of the dominant pathophysiology or pathobiology. Here we point out that an enlarged RV combined with leg edema can be caused by lung parenchyma disease, disease restricted to the lung vessels, and lung vessel involvement as a consequence of LV dysfunction (Fig. 84.4). It is rather intuitive that as the entry criteria and pathobiologic features are different in each category, treatment will need to be tailored to the underlying mechanism. How can this be? The likely answer is that there is more to RV failure than afterload and that the etiology of cor pulmonale is not understood. The larger question then becomes, Why does the RV fail, and what is the difference between "good" and "bad" RV hypertrophy?

In the context of exclusive pulmonary precapillary vascular disease as in idiopathic PAH, a progression of the angiogenic vaso-obliteration has been thought to be the etiologic explanation for the terminal RV failure; we suggest that this in itself is not a sufficient explanation. Even more incomplete is our understanding of the pulmonary venous hypertension component in patients with an initial LV problem. It appears that more patients with the combination of LV disease and pulmonary hypertension are now being diagnosed and that mPAP is an important predictor of mortality in these patients (Fig. 84.5).[29] Whether this is due to frequent echocardiographic monitoring of patients with LV disease or a longer survival of heart failure patients, or both, is unknown.

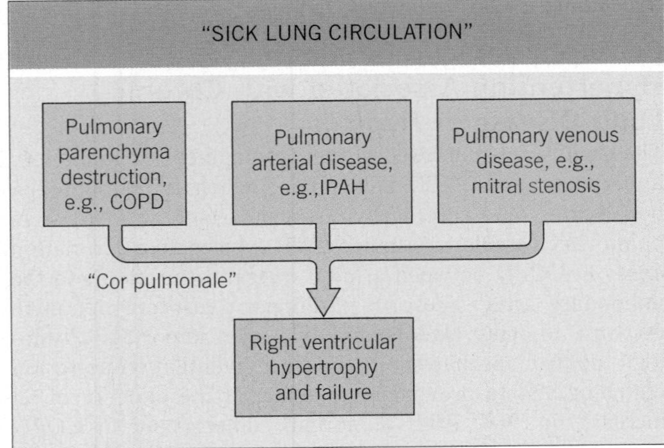

Figure 84.4 Three categories of diseases leading to an elevated pressure in the pulmonary circulation, right ventricular hypertrophy, and right ventricular failure. The common denominator is a "sick lung circulation." COPD, chronic obstructive pulmonary disease; IPAH, idiopathic pulmonary arterial hypertension.

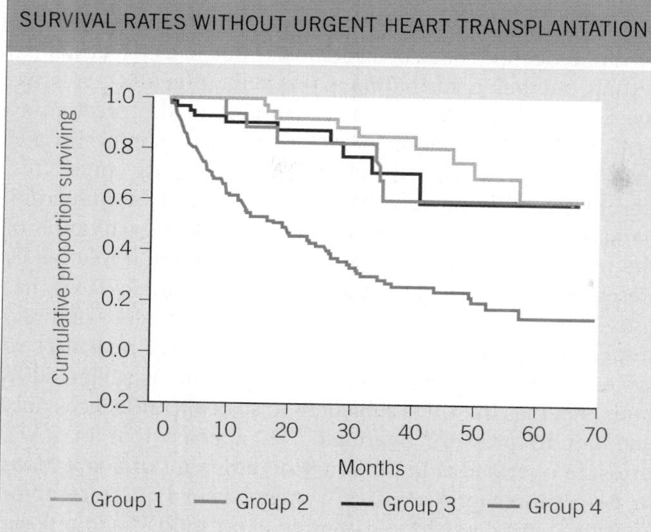

Figure 84.5 Survival rates without urgent heart transplantation in patients grouped according to the coupling between mean pulmonary artery pressure (mPAP) and right ventricular ejection fraction (RVEF). Group 1: normal PAP, preserved RVEF (n = 73); group 2: normal PAP, low RVEF (n = 68); group 3: high PAP, preserved RVEF (n = 21); and group 4: high PAP, low RVEF (n = 215). (Reproduced from Ghio S, Gavazzi A, Campana C, et al. Independent and additive prognostic value of right ventricular systolic function and pulmonary artery pressure in patients with chronic heart failure. J Am Coll Cardiol 2001;37:183-188.)

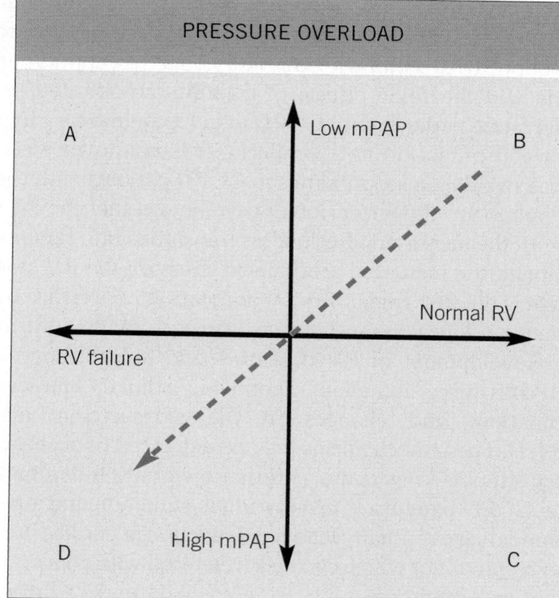

Figure 84.6 Pressure overload. Pressure overload eventually leads to right-sided heart failure, but the relationship is not always linear (as depicted by the dashed line). Some patients present with right-sided heart failure despite a relatively normal pulmonary artery pressure (panel A). Others have preserved right-sided heart function despite considerable elevation of right ventricular afterload. mPAP, mean pulmonary artery pressure; RV, right ventricle.

What we begin to appreciate is that the survival of patients with a relatively maintained LV ejection fraction and pulmonary hypertension is poor and that vasodilator drugs are relatively contraindicated. The reader is reminded of the fact that prostacyclin treatment of patients with heart failure increased the mortality of this group of patients.[30] As in mitral stenosis with fixed pulmonary hypertension, we have no clearly effective treatment options. Until we have learned how to reverse the structural (venous, but not only!) lung vessel disease, we may focus on a strategy that intends to preserve RV contractile function as the pulmonary artery pressure will likely remain high and vasodilator refractory.

This view as depicted in Figure 84.4 acknowledges that the common denominator or link between the three categories is the "sick lung circulation" but that the form or degree of the lung vessel involvement is different. It matters greatly when it comes to designing treatment whether the lung vessel abnormalities are precapillary, postcapillary, or both (as in pulmonary veno-occlusive disease and in some patients with eosinophilic granulomatosis or scleroderma) or whether a large disease component is due to vessel and capillary loss (as in severe emphysema). We also need to emphasize that the still very popular pathogenetic concept of pulmonary hypertension → RV hypertrophy = cor pulmonale is most certainly ill-conceived and in need of revision. This traditional linear concept is problematic because it attempts a strict causal connection between pulmonary artery pressure and cor pulmonale (Fig. 84.6, dashed line). As we will point out (see later), many patients apparently have cor pulmonale without severe pulmonary hypertension, and in a large number of patients with severe pulmonary hypertension, the pulmonary artery pressure alone is not a sufficient explanation for the RV failure. Thus, the clinical spectrum of RV function has more the appearance of a compass, with pulmonary artery pressure and RV function as the x and y coordinates that describe the position of a patient in this spectrum.

THE RIGHT VENTRICLE UNDER PRESSURE: FROM ADAPTIVE HYPERTROPHY TO DILATATION AND FAILURE

Classic teaching has it that the first response of the RV to an elevated afterload is to increase its muscle mass. Because the heart is considered a terminally differentiated organ, the increase can result only from cellular hypertrophy. When the right-sided heart cannot sustain this adaptation, contractile dysfunction and dilatation follow. Although this course of events may be essentially true (whereas the notion of terminal differentiation is pertinently wrong),[31] there are no detailed reports in the literature on the natural course of right-sided heart morphologic changes associated with pressure overload and chronic smoke exposure. In clinical practice, patients frequently present with a dilated heart without prior documentation of cardiac hypertrophy. We have yet to begin to probe the mechanisms that underlie the transition from RV hypertrophy to dilatation in right-sided heart failure associated with PAH or chronic lung diseases. Moreover, it is not understood which mechanisms guide the generally excellent recovery of the heart after lung transplantation and pulmonary endarterectomy for chronic thromboembolic pulmonary hypertension.[32,33] Although it is well recognized that disease-specific myocardial involvement contributes to cardiac dysfunction in sarcoidosis, systemic sclerosis, and amyloidosis,[34-36] it has not been explored whether the cellular and molecular determinants of pulmonary vascular remodeling in idiopathic or familial PAH—or in COPD for that matter—can also cause myocardial dysfunction. It is unknown how individual susceptibilities to hypoxia and the toxic effects of cigarette smoke determine whether some patients with COPD develop pulmonary hypertension and others do not. Similarly, it is unknown whether the same or other susceptibilities in COPD patients with established pulmonary hypertension determine whether the RV can cope with the increased afterload or transitions into failure.

Although the increased mechanical stress on the RV cardiomyocyte is the first trigger for RV adaptation in pressure overload, many additional mechanisms are expected to contribute to the development of RV dilatation and failure: neurohormonal activation, ischemia, apoptosis, cellular senescence, inflammation, and changes in the extracellular matrix (Fig. 84.7). These mechanisms may be enhanced or accelerated by cigarette smoking and a chronic low-grade inflammatory state in COPD patients.[37] Contractile dysfunction and adverse RV remodeling eventually lead to a reduction in cardiac output, the development of which can be accelerated with concomitant tricuspid regurgitation (due to RV dilatation), ventricular interdependence, and arrhythmias.

Cellular and Molecular Mechanisms Involved in the Transition from Hypertrophy to Dilatation

The increase in ventricular mass induced by an increase in afterload is predominantly hypertrophy and the result of protein synthesis and an increase in cell size through the addition of sarcomeres. Recently, the existence of proliferating cardiac progenitor cells[31] and the influx of bone marrow–derived progenitor cells developing into cardiomyocytes[38] have been demonstrated in an experimental setting, but their contribution to the adaptation to RV pressure overload is unknown. Protein synthesis in the cardiomyocytes is directly induced by stretch sensed by integrins and stretch-activated ion channels in cardiac cells (myocytes, fibroblasts, endothelial cells)[39] and enhanced by autocrine, paracrine, and neurohormonal influences (e.g., activation of the renin-angiotensin and sympathetic systems; Table 84-1). Research on hearts of patients with idiopathic PAH has provided some insight into the relative contributions of direct responses to pressure overload and additional responses to systemic influences; the RV of PAH patients is subjected to both, whereas the LV is subjected to systemic influences only and not to pressure overload.[40] It appears that in PAH, pressure overload is the primary determinant of adaptations in β-adrenoreceptor density,[41] angiotensin type 1 receptor density,[42] atrial natriuretic peptide expression,[43] and myosin heavy chain (MHC) and α-actin contents.[43,44] In contrast, the increase in angiotensin-converting enzyme expression is likely a response to systemic influences because it is increased in both ventricles in PAH.[42]

Theoretically, RV dilatation can result from a change in preload or afterload, the loss of cardiomyocyte contractile force (due to functional, structural, or numerical changes in cardiomyocytes), or a change in the connective tissue surrounding the cardiac myocytes. It is generally believed that the same signaling mechanisms that lead to adaptive hypertrophy eventually contribute to ventricular dysfunction and

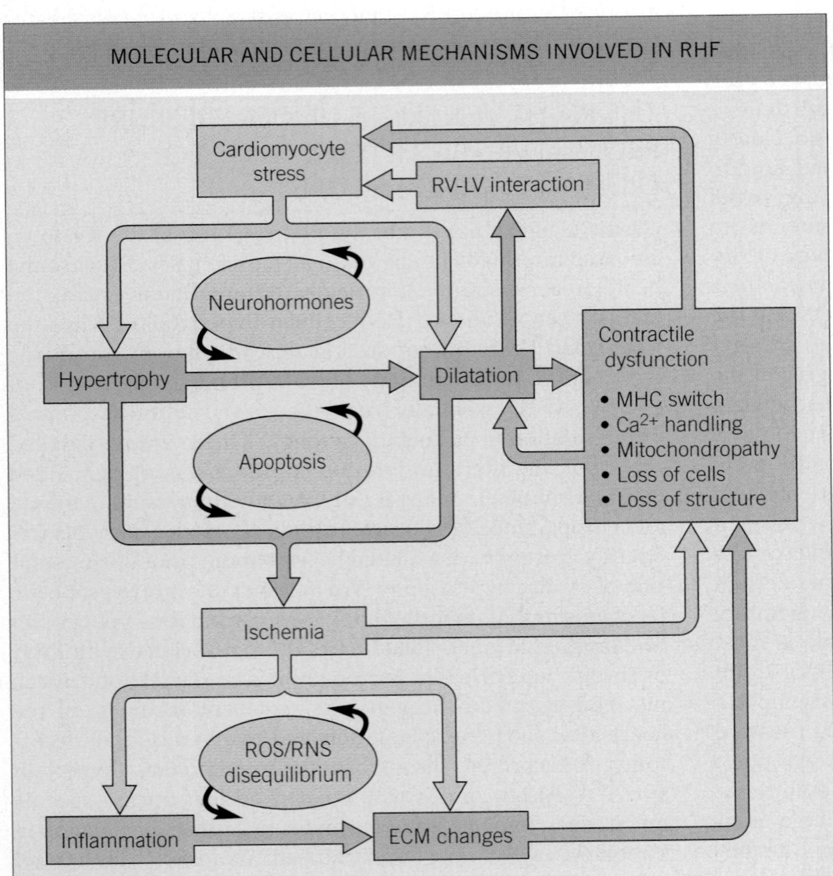

Figure 84.7 Hypothetical molecular and cellular mechanisms involved in the development of right-sided heart failure (RHF) in pulmonary hypertension. Cardiomyocyte stress in the setting of pulmonary hypertension may be predominantly caused by the increased pulmonary resistance. Different amplifying and modifying loops lead to contractile dysfunction, imposing further stress on remaining cardiomyocytes. ECM, extracellular matrix; MHC, myosin heavy chain; RNS, reactive nitrogen species; ROS, reactive oxygen species.

NEUROHORMONES AND AUTOCRINE AND PARACRINE FACTORS POSSIBLY INVOLVED IN RIGHT-SIDED HEART FAILURE		
	Known Direct Cardiac Effects	**Evidence for Involvement in Right-Sided Heart Failure Associated with Pulmonary Hypertension**
Angiotensin II	Hypertrophy, inflammation, fibrosis, contractile dysfunction	Increased AT1R density after PAH in rabbits; genetic variation in ACE expression affects PAH survival
Catecholamines	Contractile dysfunction with sustained activation	Sympathetic hyperinnervation in MCT model
Endothelin 1	Hypertrophy; inhibition of apoptosis; effects on contractility depending on duration of stimulation	Unknown long-term effects on RV adaptation to pressure overload
Prostaglandins	Unknown whether prostacyclin increases cardiac output by vascular or cardiac effects	Improved RV contractility and capillary-to-myocyte ratio in a flow-associated PAH model
Aldosterone	Mediates effects of angiotensin II	No data
Transforming growth factor β1	Mediates effects of angiotensin II	No data
Natriuretic peptides	Attenuate hypertrophy; antiapoptotic, antifibrotic	Up-regulated in experimental and human PAH; importance for RV adaptation unclear
Nitric oxide	Complex effects, through cGMP related and unrelated pathways	cGMP may acutely increase RV contractility in experimental and human PAH
Adrenomedullin	Inhibits endothelin 1, Ras, and sympathetic signaling; long-term effects unclear	No data
Growth hormones	Hypertrophy, antiapoptotic	No data
Platelet-derived growth factor	Antiapoptotic, anti-inflammatory	No data

ACE, angiotensin-converting enzyme; AT1R, angiotensin type 1 receptor; cGMP, cyclic guanosine monophosphate; PAH, pulmonary arterial hypertension; RV, right ventricle.

Table 84.1 Neurohormones and autocrine and paracrine factors possibly involved in right-sided heart failure.

dilatation. One of the hallmarks of maladaptive cardiac growth is the switch in isotype of the major thick filament protein MHC (α-MHC/β-MHC switch) in cardiomyocytes. In the normal adult human RV, the α-MHC isotype makes up about 23% to 34% of total MHC, β-MHC the remainder. The reduction in α-MHC content (down to ±5%) that is encountered in PAH-associated right-sided heart failure[43] can have important functional consequences. β-MHC has lower ATPase activity than α-MHC; the disappearance of the latter results in a significant decrease in systolic function.[45] Stressed hearts not only exhibit thick filament changes but also show increased expression of the thin filaments α-skeletal actin and α-smooth muscle actin at the cost of α-cardiac actin.[46] Because α-skeletal actin is up-regulated in the RV of newborn calves with hypoxic pulmonary hypertension, whereas LV α-skeletal actin remains unchanged, it seems that pressure overload is a stimulus for this response.[44] Contractile dysfunction in LV failure is associated with alterations in enzymes and ion channels involved in myocyte excitation-contraction coupling, with mitochondrial abnormalities, with depletion of myocardial ATP and high-energy phosphate metabolites (creatine and phosphocreatine), and with modifications of myocardial substrate use (from fatty acids to glucose). The extent to which these mechanisms play a role in RV failure has received little attention.

Right Ventricular Myocardial Ischemia in Pulmonary Hypertension

Smoking leads to both coronary artery disease and COPD. It is therefore likely that myocardial ischemia plays a role in a substantial proportion of patients with COPD and right-sided heart failure; but even with a normal coronary arterial anatomy, patients with severe pulmonary hypertension may present with chest pain and RV ischemia.[47] By use of magnetic resonance imaging in PAH patients, an impaired systolic flow could be demonstrated in the right coronary artery and a reduction in mean blood flow in those patients with severe RV hypertrophy.[48] This reduction in coronary blood flow was attributed to systemic hypotension and enhanced systolic compression of the coronary vessels due to hypertrophy. Both ventricular dilatation and an elevated systolic pressure increase RV wall stress, thus enhancing myocardial oxygen consumption and contributing to an imbalance between oxygen supply and demand. Pressure overload is associated with loss of myocardial microvessels, and this capillary loss may contribute to tissue hypoxia.[49,50] Attempts to increase coronary driving pressures in PAH with phenylephrine were associated with a decline in RV performance and cardiac output, possibly because of vasoconstriction of the right coronary artery or pulmonary arteries.[51]

In pulmonary hypertension, myocardial hypoxia can be worsened by several additional mechanisms, including decreased nitric oxide–mediated vasodilatation of RV small arteries,[52] changes in cardiac myoglobin content and mitochondrial distribution, chronic hypoxemia due to disturbances in pulmonary gas exchange (particularly in COPD), right-to-left shunting through a patent foramen ovale, and (in severe output failure) increased peripheral oxygen extraction. In very rare instances, extreme dilatation of the pulmonary trunk can lead to compression of the left anterior descending artery, which supplies parts of the anterior wall of the RV.

Involvement of Apoptosis in the Development of Right Ventricular Dilatation

Cardiomyocyte apoptosis (programmed cell death, an energy-dependent process) is rare in the normal heart, with 1 apoptotic cardiomyocyte in 10^4 to 10^5 cells.[53] However, apoptosis rates increase to 1 in 400 in human heart failure.[54,55] In animal models, apoptosis rates vary widely, with rates as high as 14% in ischemia-reperfusion and lower than 1% in chronic pressure overload.[56] The rate of RV cardiomyocyte apoptosis is elevated after pulmonary artery banding in rats.[57,58] Even very low rates of apoptosis (one fifth of that seen in human heart failure) have been shown to cause lethal dilated cardiomyopathy in a mouse model.[59]

Oxidative and Nitrosative Stress

Heart failure is associated with increased generation of reactive oxygen and nitrogen species and reduced activity of cytoprotective enzymes. Excessive production of reactive oxygen species (ROS) and reactive nitrogen species (RNS) induces contractile dysfunction through suppression of enzymes involved in excitation-contraction coupling and through polynitrosylation of the ryanodine receptor. ROS and RNS favor cardiac remodeling through enzyme inactivation and induction of cell damage, apoptosis, and inflammation. One of the few exceptions to the literature in which studies on the LV predominate is a report on transgenic deletion of the cytoprotective ("antioxidant") enzyme heme oxygenase 1 (HO-1). In mice subjected to hypoxia, HO-1 deletion led to severe RV dilatation and failure, unrelated to pulmonary vascular vasoconstriction or remodeling but associated with myocardial infarction, inflammation, fibrosis, and cardiomyocyte apoptosis.[60] HO-1 is induced in vascular smooth muscle cells and cardiomyocytes by many stressors, such as stretch, shear stress, ROS, hypoxia, cytokines, heme, and heavy metals. HO-1 catalyzes the oxidation of heme to carbon monoxide and biliverdin, which is subsequently reduced to bilirubin.[61] Carbon monoxide stimulates soluble guanylate cyclase and induces vasodilatation.[62] HO-1 has antioxidant properties by degrading the pro-oxidant heme and generating the antioxidant bilirubin.[63]

Inflammation and Immune Activation in Right Ventricular Failure

RV ischemia may lead to inflammation and immune activation by accumulation of hypoxia-inducible factor 1α and ROS/RNS formation.[64,65] Furthermore, Rho kinase (ROCK) activation associated with RV hypertrophy may exacerbate cardiac inflammation by leading to ineffective clearance of apoptotic cells (efferocytosis).[66] Patients with chronic heart failure have increased serum levels and myocyte expression of the proinflammatory cytokines tumor necrosis factor α, interleukin 1, and interleukin 6, with elevated levels correlating with disease severity reflected in clinical and hemodynamic parameters.[67] Elevations of serum sST2, which is the soluble isoform of the interleukin 1 receptor family member ST2 (ST2L is the other, transmembrane, isoform), also predict worse prognosis in patients with chronic heart failure.[68]

Changes in the Extracellular Matrix

The heart's matrix scaffold is predominantly collagen with relatively small amounts of fibronectin, laminin, and elastin. The collagen is organized as an intricate network of fibers that surround, group, and interconnect individual myocytes, myofibrils, muscle fibers, and muscle bundles. Its proximity to the contractile apparatus implies that the extracellular matrix likely influences diastolic and systolic function as well as ventricular size and shape.[69,70] Moreover, the extracellular matrix determines the milieu for electrical propagation, and when the matrix is inhomogeneous, it predisposes to conduction abnormalities and arrhythmia.[71] Both increased collagen content of the heart (fibrosis), which is tightly linked to transforming growth factor β1 signaling, and excessive degradation of the matrix by matrix metalloproteinases will adversely affect myocardial systolic and diastolic function.[69,71,72] Transforming growth factor β1and matrix metalloproteinase signaling are linked in a complex fashion.[71] RV endomyocardial biopsy specimens of patients with PAH show increased levels of fibrosis,[43] confirming earlier findings in rats after pulmonary artery banding.[73] Because scar formation and fibrosis are very common responses to tissue hypoxia, it is possible that these findings are related to microcirculatory insufficiency. Degradation of the extracellular matrix may contribute to decompensated heart failure and ventricular dilatation in PAH because failing hearts have an increased density of mast cells capable of activating matrix metalloproteinases by secreting tumor necrosis factor α, tryptase, and chymase.[69] The only observation of myocardial mast cell infiltration in pulmonary hypertension has been in a very specific animal model (nude rats treated with the vascular endothelial growth factor receptor blocker SU5416),[74] and it is unclear whether such mast cell infiltration also exists in other animal models or human PAH.

RIGHT-SIDED HEART FAILURE IN PATIENTS WITH CHRONIC LUNG DISEASE ASSOCIATED WITH PULMONARY HYPERTENSION

The clinical features of right-sided heart failure result from low cardiac output, increased right atrial pressure, and secondary neurohormonal activation, which all have been discussed in detail in other chapters. A low cardiac output is associated with dyspnea on exertion, decreased exercise tolerance, and, in more advanced stages, renal failure. Pooling of venous blood and activation of the renin-angiotensin system leads to edema in the extremities, ascites, and pericardial and pleural effusions. In very severe cases, elevated venous pressures in the splanchnic circulation can lead to protein-losing enteropathy and immune deficiency. Dilatation of the right atrium and sympathetic activation are associated with atrial tachyarrhythmias and sudden death.

It is unknown what proportion of COPD patients with associated pulmonary hypertension develop right-sided heart failure. Data are lacking. Even a very small proportion of all COPD patients would still translate into a large number (probably larger than patients with PAH-associated right-sided heart failure) because of the ever-increasing prevalence of COPD in general. Evidently, the prevalence would depend on the definition used for right-sided heart failure. Cor pulmonale customarily has been diagnosed when fluid retention exists, but it has become clear that fluid retention in COPD may occur without severe right-sided heart dysfunction. Hypoxia and hypercapnia enhance sodium retention, which is associated with a reduced renal plasma flow and an activated renin-aldosterone system.[75] In a small group of 20 hypoxic COPD patients with pulmonary hypertension and varying degrees of hypercapnia, pressure-volume relationships in the RV suggested relatively well preserved RV contractility.[76] RV hypertrophy can be demonstrated in normoxic patients with moderate airflow obstruction, without a clear effect on RV or LV function at rest.[77] COPD patients have a reduced exercise stroke volume response,[15,78] but this finding may just as well be explained by deconditioning. As already stated, the term *cor pulmonale* is now more obscure than 2 or 3 decades ago. We believe we know it when we see it, but we do not understand what it is.

Ventricular Interdependence

Under normal physiologic conditions, the effect of LV function on RV function and vice versa can be neglected; but when RV afterload is increased, the complex interaction of both ventricles may influence RV adaptation. Two mechanisms of ventricular interaction have been proposed: (1) direct ventricular interaction mediated by the pericardium and (2) interventricular asynchrony. At present, the role of the pericardium in the adaptive process of the RV in PAH is not clear. Because both ventricles share the same pericardial space, dilatation of the RV will be accompanied by increased pericardial stretch. This inward-directed force may hamper RV dilatation and, mediated by the interventricular septum, impair LV filling. The effects of pericardial constraint on LV filling have been demonstrated in an acute model of RV pressure overload in dogs.[79] Opening of the canine pericardium facilitated LV filling and consequently improved cardiac output.[79,80] The consequences of pericardial constraint in chronic pressure overload are less clear.[81]

A more important mechanism of ventricular interaction in PAH is interventricular asynchrony. Synchronous RV and LV pressure measurements in PAH patients showed that a significant right-to-left transseptal pressure gradient is present at the time of maximal leftward septal displacement measured by magnetic resonance imaging (Fig. 84.8).[82] The mechanism behind this asynchrony is that RV pressure overload leads to prolonged contraction of the RV free wall.[83] At the time that the LV has entered its early diastolic phase, RV pressure exceeds LV pressure. As a result, a transseptal pressure gradient leads to paradoxical septum movement.[84] The consequence of this leftward septal bowing is not only ineffective RV end-systolic contraction but also impaired LV early diastolic filling.[85] A decreased LV end-diastolic volume (i.e., preload) directly impairs LV output according to the Frank-Starling mechanism.[85,86] Both pericardial constraint and impaired LV filling may influence the perfusion of the right coronary artery and thus oxygen supply to the LV.

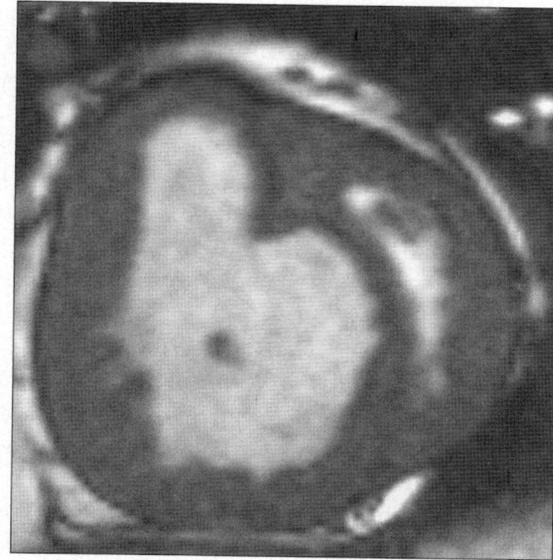

Figure 84.8 Magnetic resonance image of right ventricular hypertrophy and dilatation in severe pulmonary hypertension. Right ventricular pressure overload leads to prolonged contraction of the right ventricular free wall. At the time that the left ventricle has entered its early diastolic phase, right ventricular pressure exceeds left ventricular pressure. As a result, a transseptal pressure gradient leads to paradoxical septum movement. The consequence of this leftward septal bowing is not only ineffective right ventricular end-systolic contraction but also impaired left ventricular early diastolic filling (ventricular interdependence).

ASSESSMENT OF RIGHT VENTRICULAR FUNCTION

Assessment of RV function and pulmonary arterial pressure requires invasive methods and modern imaging techniques, although suspicions may be raised by abnormalities on the chest radiograph (globular appearance of the heart, encroachment of the retrosternal airspace) and electrocardiogram (e.g., right axis deviation, right atrial enlargement, R or R′ > S in V_1). A COPD patient with a low oxygen saturation of the arterial blood is evidently at risk of pulmonary hypertension, and elevated serum levels of the neurohormone NT-proBNP indicate the presence of heart failure of any cause.

Right-Sided Heart Catheterization

A firm diagnosis of PAH cannot be made without right-sided heart catheterization. When an elevated mPAP is established, measurements of cardiac output (CO) and pulmonary artery occlusion pressures (PAOP) and calculation of the PVR = (mPAP − PAOP)/CO allow distinction between PAH (elevated PVR), a hyperdynamic circulation (high CO, normal PVR), and pulmonary venous hypertension (normal PVR, normal CO, high PAOP). Significant prognostic information is obtained when the right atrial pressure and cardiac output are measured.[87] Because mPAP may decline in severe right-sided heart failure owing to a decrease in cardiac output, this variable is a less firm predictor of mortality.

Echocardiography

Air is a poor transmitter of sound waves, and therefore pulmonary hyperinflation complicates echocardiography in COPD. An adequate examination has been reported in 44% to 85% of COPD patients.[88,89] A higher percentage may be achieved by a transesophageal approach, but the required sedation is unattractive in patients with respiratory failure. Two-dimensional echocardiography (preferably in the parasternal axis in COPD) can be used to measure RV wall thickness, to assess RV dilatation, and to determine the presence of important indicators of RV failure (e.g., pericardial effusion, paradoxical movement of the interventricular septum). In a substantial number of COPD patients, accurate estimation of the systolic pulmonary artery pressure is impossible.[89]

Magnetic Resonance Imaging

The crescent shape of the RV prohibits accurate estimations of RV dimensions and cavity volumes by echocardiography. Magnetic resonance imaging is therefore probably the "gold standard" to noninvasively estimate cardiac output.[90] Cardiac output has more prognostic significance than RV ejection fraction in pulmonary hypertension, which is the reason that radionuclide assessments of RV ejection fraction are not commonly used. Disadvantages of magnetic resonance imaging are its high cost and limited availability.

Exercise Testing

The 6-minute walk distance is used as a prognostic predictor in pulmonary hypertension and as a guide toward treatment adjustments. More sophisticated cardiopulmonary exercise testing allows assessment of gas exchange abnormalities that are characteristic of pulmonary hypertension: low anaerobic threshold, low oxygen pulse, low peak oxygen uptake, and exaggerated ventilatory response. However, these characteristics are not sensitive enough to distinguish COPD patients with associated pulmonary hypertension from those patients without.[91]

MANAGEMENT OF PULMONARY HYPERTENSION AND RIGHT-SIDED HEART FAILURE ASSOCIATED WITH CHRONIC LUNG DISEASE OR HYPOXIA

The treatment of PAH is discussed in Chapter 83. There is no proven benefit of (and, in fact, not much rationale for) treatment of mild pulmonary hypertension in COPD. Long-term oxygen therapy benefits hypoxemic patients (see later) and may partly do so by reducing pulmonary artery pressure. There is no proven benefit of pulmonary vasodilators in severe COPD-associated pulmonary hypertension. In patients with right-sided heart failure, sodium restriction and diuretics are used to minimize fluid retention. Atrial fibrillation and high-grade atrioventricular block may have profound hemodynamic consequences in right-sided heart failure, and therefore an effort should be made to maintain sinus rhythm. COPD patients benefit from exercise rehabilitation, and the presence of pulmonary hypertension should not be considered a contraindication. On the contrary, exercise training is also of benefit to PAH patients.[92]

Oxygen Therapy

Two large trials evaluated the benefit of long-term oxygen therapy in hypoxemic COPD patients. Both the Nocturnal Oxygen Therapy Trial and the Medical Research Council trial showed that long-term oxygen therapy significantly improves survival in COPD patients with a PaO_2 of less than 55 mm Hg, and a considerable proportion of these patients had established pulmonary hypertension.[93,94] In the latter study, mPAP was shown to remain stable with long-term oxygen therapy, whereas it increased in untreated patients.[94] The best hemodynamic results can be achieved with longer durations ($>$16 hours/day) of oxygen supplementation.[93,95] Despite the fact that oxygen desaturation is a predictor of worse prognosis in idiopathic pulmonary fibrosis, the only randomized trial evaluating long-term oxygen therapy in these patients failed to show a beneficial effect.[96]

Pulmonary Vasodilators

The main concern with pulmonary vasodilator therapy in hypoxemic lung disease is a worsening of the hypoxemia. After all, hypoxic pulmonary vasoconstriction is a physiologic response that protects the organism from ventilation-perfusion mismatch. It has been suggested that the phosphodiesterase type 5 inhibitor sildenafil very specifically dilates pulmonary vessels in well-ventilated lung areas,[97-100] which would make this drug safe in COPD. It was recently shown in a group of 15 patients with moderate to severe COPD (nine had pulmonary hypertension at rest) that 3 months of sildenafil treatment lowered mPAP but had no effect on exercise capacity or exercise stroke volume. Surprisingly, there are no reports of larger studies evaluating sildenafil in COPD.

Lung Transplantation

Patients with severe COPD and moderate or severe associated pulmonary hypertension are usually not considered candidates for lung volume reduction surgery but should be evaluated for lung transplantation.[101] Even single-lung transplantation can normalize pulmonary artery pressures in COPD patients with associated pulmonary hypertension, and this result is maintained 2 years after surgery. However, the survival benefit of double-lung transplantation may be superior to that of single-lung transplantation.[102]

SUMMARY

When pulmonary hypertension occurs in patients with chronic lung disease or hypoxemia, it is usually not severe. It is associated with but not necessarily causally related to prognosis. However, pulmonary hypertension is severe in some COPD patients, in whom it can lead to right-sided heart failure and death. It should be treated with supplemental oxygen and diuretics when necessary, but the place of vasodilators is uncertain. When severe pulmonary hypertension occurs in any patient with chronic lung disease or hypoxia, the diagnostic process has not ended. In these patients, an additional explanation for the increase in pulmonary artery pressure should be considered. The cellular and molecular mechanisms behind the transition from adaptive hypertrophy to RV dilatation and failure are not well understood. Decreased cardiomyocyte contractility (related to reexpression of fetal-type contractile proteins and disturbances in calcium handling and energy generation) and loss of cardiomyocyte numbers due to apoptosis enhance the stress imposed on remaining cardiomyocytes and trigger autocrine, paracrine, and neuroendocrine signaling pathways that can either compensate the diminished force generation or lead to further deterioration. RV ischemia (due to increased oxygen demand, decreased coronary perfusion, and microcirculatory insufficiency), ROS/RNS disequilibrium, inflammation, changes in the extracellular matrix, and RV-LV interaction contribute to the creation of a vicious circle that finally results in right-sided heart failure. That the heart failure is potentially reversible is a lesson learned from patients who have received a lung transplant. An understanding of the repair program of the recuperating RV may provide important clues directed toward strategies to induce cellular myocardial repair in view of persistent hemodynamic stress.

chapter 85

Pulmonary Embolism

Stavros Konstantinides and Wolfgang Kasper

Definition

- Pulmonary embolism (PE) and deep venous thrombosis are two clinical presentations of venous thromboembolism and share the same risk factors and predisposing conditions. In most cases, PE is a consequence of deep venous thrombosis of the lower extremities. Nonthromboembolic causes of PE are rare.

Pathophysiology and Risk Assessment

- Several acquired and hereditary disorders predispose to venous thromboembolism. Pathogenesis involves venous stasis, vessel wall injury, and systemic thrombophilia.
- Right ventricular dysfunction is an important determinant of prognosis in the acute phase of PE. It can be clinically diagnosed, when it is associated with persistent hypotension or shock, or detected by imaging tests or biomarkers.
- On the basis of clinical presentation and the detection of right ventricular dysfunction, PE can be classified as high risk (clinically massive), intermediate risk (submassive), and low risk.

Diagnosis

- In the hemodynamically stable patient, diagnostic work-up should start with the assessment of clinical (pretest) probability, preferably based on explicit, validated scores.
- Measurement of D-dimer levels is the second step in patients with low or intermediate clinical probability for PE.
- Former algorithms required the combination of single-detector computed tomography or ventilation-perfusion scintigraphy with venous ultrasonography and, occasionally, pulmonary angiography to confirm or to exclude PE safely.
- At present, multidetector-row computed tomography used as the only imaging modality permits the diagnosis or exclusion of PE in most cases.

Therapy

- Low-molecular-weight heparins are the mainstay of initial anticoagulation for low-risk and intermediate-risk PE.
- Thrombolysis or, alternatively, surgical or catheter-based recanalization should be reserved for high-risk PE.
- Selected patients with intermediate-risk PE may also benefit from thrombolysis.
- Secondary prophylaxis (oral anticoagulation) should be given for at least 3 to 6 months to patients with a first, unprovoked episode of venous thromboembolism. The optimal duration of treatment should weigh the bleeding risk of vitamin K antagonists against the lifelong elevation in the risk of PE recurrence.

Morbidity and mortality associated with pulmonary embolism (PE) remain high despite important advances in cardiovascular diagnosis and treatment. The annual incidence rate of venous thromboembolism has been estimated at 100 to 150 cases per 100,000 population per year; approximately one third of these patients present with acute PE and two thirds with deep venous thrombosis.[1] Case fatality rates vary widely, depending on the clinical severity of the thromboembolic episode,[2-5] but it is generally estimated that 10% of all patients with acute PE die during the acute phase of the disease. Overall, 1% of patients admitted to the hospital die of acute PE, and 10% of all hospital deaths are PE related.[6-8] These epidemiologic data indicate that our current wealth of information about PE is yet to be translated into an effective approach to the disease in clinical practice. The importance of deep venous thrombosis of the lower extremities in the pathogenesis of PE is now well understood, and several acquired or hereditary conditions that predispose to venous thrombosis have been identified. Beyond recommendations to maintain a high index of clinical suspicion, standardized scores of clinical probability, laboratory screening tests, and noninvasive imaging diagnostic procedures have been developed. Prospective accuracy and outcome trials have recently documented the usefulness and safety of novel diagnostic strategies when they are applied in the appropriate setting. Nevertheless, underdiagnosis and overdiagnosis of PE still occur frequently. The treatment of hemodynamically stable patients with confirmed PE has been simplified thanks to the widespread use of low-molecular-weight heparins; patients with persistent arterial hypotension and shock benefit from emergency pharmaceutical (thrombolysis) or surgical recanalization. On the other hand, uncertainty persists about the optimal treatment of normotensive patients with subclinical right ventricular dysfunction. This chapter reviews our current state of knowledge of venous thromboembolism, placing particular emphasis on the integration of traditional and novel diagnostic and therapeutic options into an effective, safe, and practicable management concept.

ANATOMY AND PATHOLOGY

Early surgical and postmortem studies demonstrated that almost 90% of pulmonary emboli originate in the leg veins. Recently, the importance of upper extremity venous thrombosis has been increasing as a result of intravenous drug abuse and the frequent use of central venous catheters in medicine. Thromboemboli from the veins appear as long, thin, friable structures with a smooth surface and a roughly cylindrical V or Y shape corresponding to the lumen of the vessel or vessel ramification in which they originated. Pale layers of platelets and fibrin alternating with dark red erythrocyte layers can be seen on their surface.[9] In vivo, venous thrombi in transit can occasionally be detected by echocardiography. They appear as highly mobile, relatively large serpentine masses floating in the right side of the heart (or, infrequently, caught in a patent foramen ovale before causing paradoxical embolism). Small, round or oval thrombi originating in the right atrium or ventricle are rarely found as a cause of PE.

As they follow the distribution of flow in the pulmonary circulation, detached venous or cardiac thrombi embolize more frequently into the lower lobes and prefer the right lung to the left lung. In contrast, disseminated peripheral thrombosis within the small muscular pulmonary arteries is encountered in idiopathic pulmonary arterial hypertension. It is believed to develop in situ as a secondary phenomenon rather than as the result of chronic thromboembolic disease. Most affected patients have had no history of PE or deep venous thrombosis. However, there are no specific histologic characteristics to allow unequivocal differentiation between the two entities.

The endogenous fibrinolytic mechanisms of the lung are capable of dissolving most thromboemboli, regardless of their size, if the patient survives the acute event. Progression to chronic thrombotic arteriopathy and chronic thromboembolic pulmonary hypertension is infrequent although not as rare as previously thought.[10,11] This process involves fibrous organization of the clot and neoangiogenesis, leading to partial recanalization.[12] Pulmonary infarction is also an uncommon complication of PE in the absence of preexisting heart failure or terminal illness because the lung normally receives a collateral blood supply from the bronchial arteries.

PATHOGENESIS AND PATHOPHYSIOLOGY

A variety of acquired and hereditary disorders have been implicated in the pathogenesis of venous thromboembolism. Their prothrombotic effect involves one or more of the mechanisms that make up the classic Virchow's triad (Fig. 85.1):

- venous stasis;
- increased blood coagulability;
- injury to the vessel wall.

Thrombi have been shown to originate in the venous sinuses and valve cusp pockets of the calf, that is, in areas of slow or turbulent flow. Locally disturbed flow clearly predisposes to and amplifies thrombosis by impairing the clearance of coagulation factors. Venous stasis caused by external compression, prolonged immobilization, or incompetent venous valves may substantially enhance this effect. In addition, several acquired disorders, including cancer and the antiphospholipid antibody syndrome, are associated with a systemic prothrombotic tendency. Temporary conditions associated with acquired thrombophilia include pregnancy and the use of oral contraceptives or postmenopausal hormone replacement therapy.

Genetic abnormalities related to thrombophilia (see Fig. 85.1) can now be identified in up to 30% of unselected patients who have venous thromboembolism and at least 50% of those with familial thrombosis. Most of them involve steps of the activated protein C pathway, the most potent endogenous anticoagulant mechanism (Fig. 85.2).[13] Resistance to activated protein C is almost exclusively caused by a single point mutation in the factor V gene, which has a prevalence of 3% to 5% in whites; in patients who have deep venous thrombosis, its prevalence is 20%. Risk of thromboembolism is increased between 5- and 10-fold in heterozygotes. Nevertheless, most carriers remain unaffected, and the need for

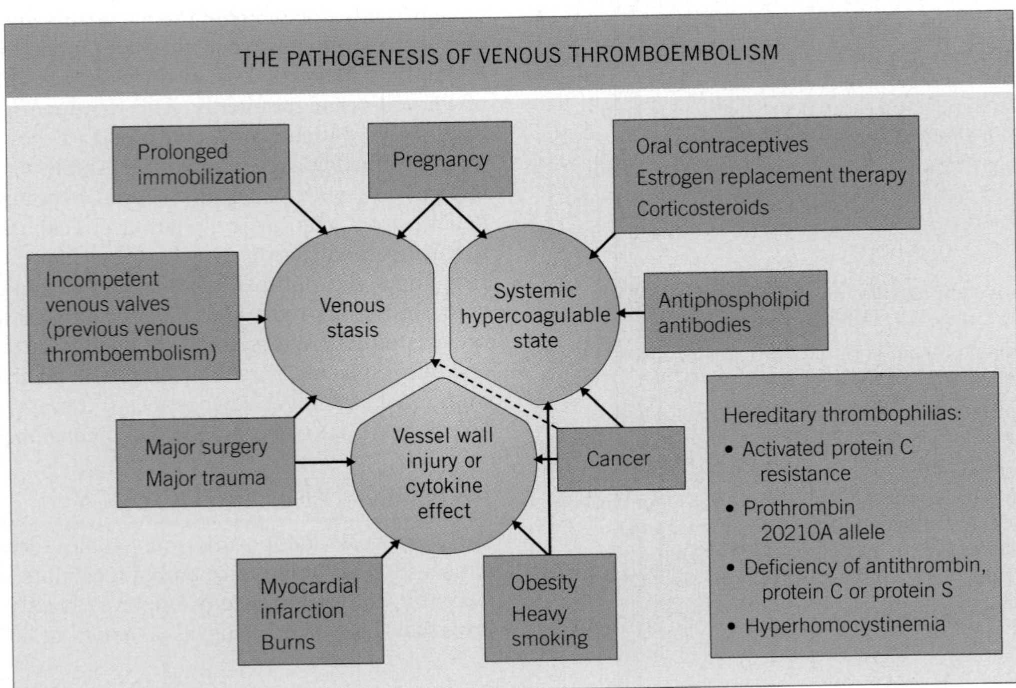

Figure 85.1 Pathogenesis of venous thromboembolism.

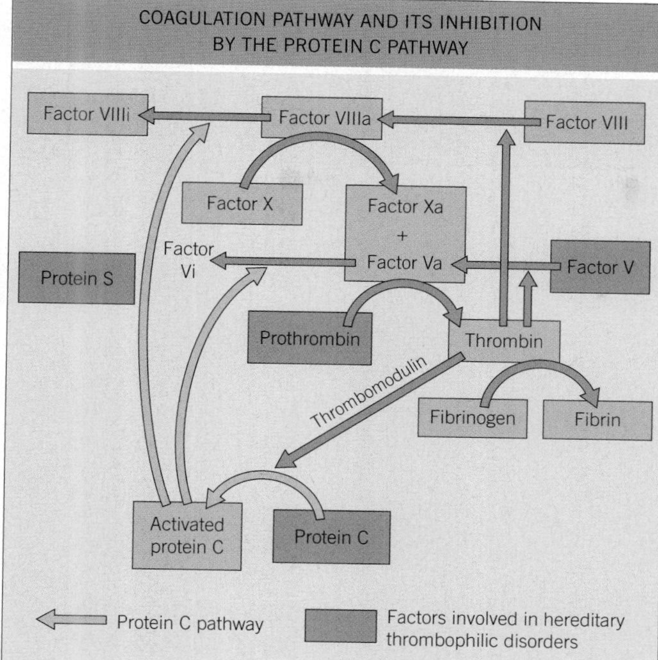

Figure 85.2 Coagulation pathway and its inhibition by the protein C pathway. Factors Va, VIIIa, Xa, activated coagulation factors V, VIII, and X; Vi, inactivated factor V; VIIIi, inactivated factor VIII. (Modified from Murin S, Marelich GP, Arroliga AC, Matthay RA. Hereditary thrombophilia and venous thromboembolism. Am J Respir Crit Care Med 1998;158:1369-1373.)

recurrent PE prophylaxis in the absence of other risk factors is controversial. Prothrombin 20210A mutation has also recently been shown to be a frequent but mild thrombophilic disorder. Deficiencies of protein C, protein S, or antithrombin are more infrequent, and they are characterized by genotypic and phenotypic variability. Antithrombin deficiency is associated with a high incidence of thrombosis. Importantly, hereditary abnormalities tend to coexist and potentiate one another in patients who have venous thromboembolism. Thus, recurrent thrombosis before the age of 40 years or a family history of venous thromboembolism may require testing for all known defects. On the other hand, routine screening of unselected patients after the first episode of deep venous thrombosis or PE does not currently appear to be a cost-effective approach.

Local injury to the vessel wall or cytokines released from tumors or from injured or infarcted tissue are required to trigger thrombus formation. Inflammatory cytokines and platelet products stabilize thrombi by stimulating the synthesis of antifibrinolytic factors (plasminogen activator inhibitors) by the cells of the vessel wall. At the same time, however, up-regulated plasminogen activators control and contain the thrombotic response, facilitating clot dissolution or organization. Therefore, the formation of vascular thrombi and their fate are determined by the continuous and complex interplay between thrombogenic and fibrinolytic mechanisms both at the local level and in the systemic circulation.

Increased pulmonary artery pressure occurs in 60% to 70% of patients who have PE and roughly correlates with the anatomic severity of thromboembolic obstruction. In addition, vasoconstrictive factors released from the thrombus and reaction to hypoxia contribute to the increase in pulmonary vascular resistance. Moreover, preexisting cardiac or pulmonary disease may enhance the hemodynamic impact of an acute thromboembolic event. Right ventricular dilatation and hypokinesis result from the interplay of these factors and may initiate a vicious circle of increased myocardial oxygen demand, myocardial ischemia or infarction, and left ventricular preload reduction. Ultimately, inability to maintain the cardiac index and arterial pressure leads to cardiogenic shock. Thus, right ventricular dysfunction is the critical hemodynamic event and an important determinant of the clinical presentation, course, and prognosis of PE.

Classification of Clinical Severity

Acute PE covers a wide spectrum of clinical severity, and the mortality rates during the acute, in-hospital phase ranged between less than 1% and well above 50% in different studies.[2-5,14] The principal clinical factor that determines disease severity, and thus the diagnostic and therapeutic approach to a patient with suspected acute PE, is the presence or absence of hemodynamic instability at presentation due to acute right ventricular dysfunction. High-risk, clinically massive PE indicates overt right ventricular failure that results in refractory arterial hypotension and shock (commonly defined as systolic blood pressure $<$90 mm Hg or a pressure drop $\geq$40 mm Hg for at least 15 minutes). This condition accounts for almost 5% of all cases of acute PE and is associated with a high risk of in-hospital death, particularly during the first few hours after admission. On the other hand, the absence of overt hemodynamic instability indicates non–high-risk PE, which is generally associated with a favorable outcome, provided the disease is diagnosed correctly and anticoagulation can be instituted without delay.

CLINICAL PRESENTATIONS AND DIFFERENTIAL DIAGNOSIS

Numerous clinical symptoms and signs, some of which are listed in Table 85.1, may be associated with acute PE.[15,16] However, their low specificity rarely permits prompt clinical differentiation of PE from other major cardiovascular syndromes. Thus, earlier studies indicated that massive PE was diagnosed during life in only 15% to 30% of cases, whereas pulmonary angiography was reported to be normal in as many as 80% of patients with clinically suspected PE. In the past years, research focused on standardizing the clinical probability (pretest likelihood) of the disease and optimizing the subsequent use of diagnostic imaging procedures to confirm or to exclude PE. This resulted in the development and validation of explicit scores based on clinical symptoms, signs, and predisposing factors. The scores shown in Table 85.2 assist the clinician in classifying the clinical suspicion of PE as low, intermediate, or high.[17,18] Their use is strongly recommended in current guidelines.

Clinically massive, high-risk PE should always be considered in patients who are admitted with unexplained acute systemic hypotension or cardiogenic shock (Fig. 85.3). History taking, if it is feasible, can strengthen this suspicion by providing one or more predisposing factors for PE (see Fig. 85.1). Clinical signs of leg vein thrombosis should be sought, but their absence does not exclude PE. In specific

REPORTED INCIDENCE OF CLINICAL, LABORATORY, RADIOLOGIC, AND ELECTROCARDIOGRAPHIC FINDINGS IN PATIENTS WITH SUBSEQUENTLY CONFIRMED PULMONARY EMBOLISM AS OPPOSED TO THOSE IN WHOM THE DIAGNOSIS WAS REJECTED

		PE Present (%)	PE Absent (%)
		n = 219	n = 546
Symptoms	Dyspnea	80	59
	Pleuritic chest pain	52	43
	Substernal chest pain	12	8
	Cough	20	25
	Hemoptysis	11	7
	Syncope	19	11
Signs	Tachypnea (≥20/min)	70	68
	Tachycardia (≥100/min)	26	23
	Signs of deep venous thrombosis	15	10
	Fever (>38.5°C)	7	17
	Cyanosis	11	9
Chest radiography	Atelectasis, parenchymal abnormalities	49	45
	Pleural effusion	46	33
	Pleura-based opacity	23	10
	Elevated diaphragm	36	25
	Prominent central pulmonary artery with decreased pulmonary vascularity (Westermark's sign)	36	6
Blood gas analysis	Arterial hypoxemia	75	81
Electrocardiography	Right-sided heart strain	50	12

Modified from Miniati et al.[15] and Stein et al.[16]

Table 85.1 Reported incidence of clinical, laboratory, radiologic, and electrocardiographic findings in patients with subsequently confirmed pulmonary embolism as opposed to those in whom the diagnosis was rejected.

circumstances, other sources of embolism have to be considered (e.g., amniotic fluid embolism during parturition, fat embolism in major trauma, and air embolism in patients who have an unprotected central venous catheter). Symptoms and signs of distress, including dyspnea and tachypnea, tachycardia, and diaphoresis, are present in up to 95% of patients with massive PE, but they are not particularly helpful with regard to differential diagnosis. Cyanosis indicates arterial hypoxemia, which results from ventilation-perfusion mismatch in the lung and a concurrent decrease in mixed venous partial oxygen pressure to values below normal. However, cyanosis may accompany any condition that causes cardiovascular insufficiency and peripheral tissue hypoxia. Conversely, profound cyanosis that does not respond to the administration of oxygen may be due to an intracardiac right-to-left shunt through a patent foramen ovale.[19] Of greater specificity are indications of right-sided heart failure, including neck vein distention with prominent *v* waves, palpable right ventricular impulse, right-sided gallop rhythm with a third heart sound, and tricuspid regurgitation (see Fig. 85.3). Although these signs may also be encountered in pericardial tamponade or right ventricular myocardial infarction, an accentuated pulmonary component of the second heart sound or a systolic murmur over the pulmonary valve points toward pulmonary hypertension and increased right ventricular afterload. At this stage, postcapillary pulmonary hypertension caused by mitral valve dysfunction or decompensated left ventricular failure also comes into the differential diagnosis. Apart from the auscultatory findings of mitral or aortic valve disease and left-sided gallop rhythms with third or fourth heart sounds, the presence of pulmonary edema generally characterizes these conditions.

PE may also cause injury to the pulmonary parenchyma, with alveolar flooding and hemorrhage. Patients suffering acute PE occasionally present with cough or hemoptysis, and respiratory examination may reveal reduced breath sounds or crackles. However, frank pulmonary edema, particularly if it is bilateral, rules out PE in most cases. In addition, the diagnostic value of auscultation and percussion of the lungs lies in the exclusion of tension pneumothorax, which may otherwise be manifested with symptoms and signs that are identical to those of massive PE.

Clinical diagnosis of acute PE becomes extremely difficult and unreliable in the presence of right ventricular infarction or cardiomyopathy. The same is true for chronic cor pulmonale caused by congenital cardiac defects (particularly atrial septal defect) or severe chronic pulmonary disease, including primary pulmonary hypertension. Unfortunately, these conditions also obscure most of the diagnostic tests.

Diffuse neurologic impairment is not an uncommon finding in hemodynamically compromised patients and may also accompany massive PE. However, a focal neurologic deficit (transient ischemic attack or stroke) or peripheral arterial ischemia in combination with cyanosis and signs of right-sided heart failure

VALIDATED SCORES FOR CLINICAL (PRETEST) PREDICTION OF PULMONARY EMBOLISM PROBABILITY

Revised Geneva Score		Wells Score	
Risk factors	**Points**	**Risk factors**	**Points**
Age >65 years	+1		
Previous DVT or PE	+3	Previous DVT or PE	+1.5
Surgery or fracture within 1 month	+2	Recent surgery or immobilization	+1.5
Active cancer	+2	Active cancer	+1
Symptoms		**Symptoms**	
Unilateral lower limb pain	+3		
Hemoptysis	+2	Hemoptysis	+1
Clinical signs		**Clinical signs**	
Heart rate		Heart rate >100/min	+1.5
75-94/min	+3		
≥95/min	+5		
Pain on lower limb, deep venous palpation, and unilateral edema	+4	Clinical signs of DVT	+3
		Clinical judgment	
		Alternative diagnosis less likely than PE	+3
Clinical probability	**Total**	**Clinical probability**	**Total**
Low	0-3	Low	0-1
Intermediate	4-10	Intermediate	2-6
High	≥11	High	≥7
		Clinical probability (dichotomized)	
		PE unlikely	0-4
		PE likely	>4

DVT, deep venous thrombosis; PE, pulmonary embolism.
Modified from Wells et al.[17] and Le Gal et al.[18]

Table 85.2 Validated scores for clinical (pretest) prediction of pulmonary embolism probability.

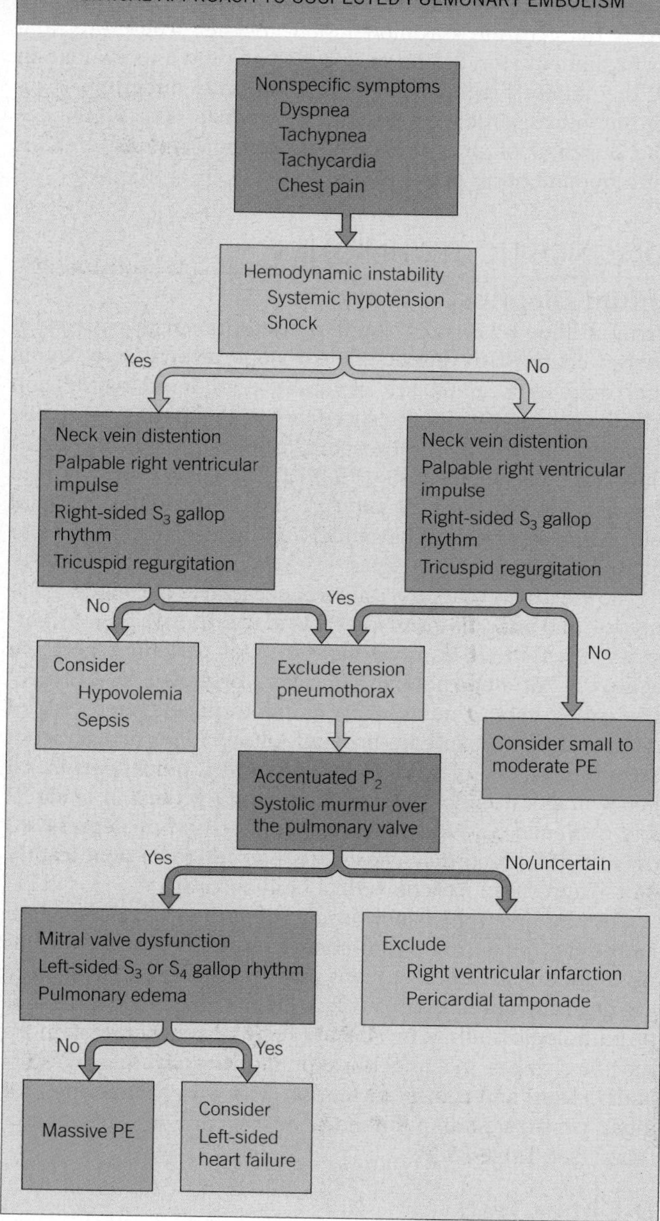

Figure 85.3 Clinical approach to suspected pulmonary embolism. PE, pulmonary embolism; P_2, pulmonary component of the second heart sound; S_3, third heart sound; S_4, fourth heart sound.

should raise the suspicion of paradoxical embolism because increased right atrial pressure facilitates passage of thrombi through a patent foramen ovale. The cardiovascular risk in patients with massive PE and a patent foramen ovale is particularly high, but the therapeutic implications of this unfavorable combination remain to be determined.

In patients who present without systemic hypotension (see Fig. 85.3), suspicion of clinically nonmassive (non–high-risk) PE is usually based on the presence of dyspnea, chest pain, or hemoptysis of recent onset together with evidence of deep venous thrombosis or the presence of one or more risk factors for thrombosis (see Tables 85.1 and 85.2). Pleuritic chest pain is often associated with peripheral (subpleural) emboli and is generally not difficult to differentiate from the pain of acute pericarditis or myocardial ischemia when it is present in its typical form. Together with hemoptysis, pleural rub, or auscultatory findings of pulmonary consolidation, it suggests that pulmonary infarction has probably occurred. A moderate increase in temperature is common in pulmonary infarction, but temperature above 100.4°F (38°C) is usually a sign of superimposed infection with pneumonia. With regard to differential diagnosis, in drug addicts or patients with central venous catheters, a febrile syndrome that includes symptoms of PE may result from tricuspid or (rarely) pulmonary valve endocarditis.

Non–high-risk PE is not a clinical emergency, but it may become one if significant residual deep venous thrombosis leads to recurrent thromboembolic events. Therefore, and as explained later, attention needs to be drawn to evaluation of the patient's leg vein status in addition to underlying prothrombotic disorders because these two factors will influence the duration of oral anticoagulation for secondary venous thromboembolism prevention.

DIAGNOSTIC TECHNIQUES

Initial Diagnostic Work-up

Arterial blood gases are routinely determined in patients in whom acute PE is suspected. Although arterial hypoxemia and mild hypocapnia are generally considered to indicate PE, the sensitivity and the specificity of this finding were disappointingly low in the Prospective Investigation of Pulmonary Embolism Diagnosis (PIOPED).[20] The same was true for the alveolar-arterial oxygen difference. Thus, arterial blood gas determinations cannot, by themselves, be used to guide management strategies.

The electrocardiogram is always necessary to exclude acute myocardial infarction and may reveal transitory signs of right-sided heart strain in more than 75% of patients who have acute PE. Although not by themselves diagnostic for PE, electrocardiographic findings may point to an elevated risk of death during the acute (in-hospital) phase. In particular, atrial arrhythmias, complete right bundle branch block, peripheral low voltage, pseudoinfarction pattern (Q waves) in leads III and aVF, and ST-segment changes (elevation or depression) over the left precordial leads were reported to be significantly more frequent in patients with a fatal outcome.[21]

Chest radiography is performed primarily to exclude pneumothorax. It may reveal pulmonary infiltrates, basal atelectasis, or pleural effusion—findings that occasionally accompany PE. Overall, more than 70% of patients with PE may have subtle pathologic findings on chest radiographs. In contrast, more specific changes, including focal pulmonary oligemia (Westermark's sign) and central distention with abrupt tapering of a lobar or segmental pulmonary artery, are less frequently found (see Table 85.1).

D-Dimer Test

Plasma D-dimer assay is a valuable laboratory test for screening of patients with suspected PE. D-dimers result from endogenous fibrinolysis, which is almost invariably present in PE. The enzyme-linked immunosorbent assay (ELISA) has a 97% sensitivity in detecting plasma D-dimer concentrations of more than 500 mg/L, and the negative predictive value approaches 99%. Conversely, D-dimers are also detectable in acute myocardial infarction, pneumonia, and a variety of systemic diseases, especially in older patients or those who have been admitted to the hospital several days before the index event. Thus, a positive assay yields no specific diagnostic information. It is nevertheless useful, serving as an indication for further (imaging) tests in a patient with low or intermediate clinical probability of PE as part of contemporary diagnostic strategies that are presented later.

D-dimer levels are negative in only 10% of patients with a high clinical probability, who in turn represent only 10% of all patients with suspected PE. Thus, as the absolute number of patients with the combination of a high probability and a negative D-dimer test result is very small, testing for D-dimers is not recommended in patients with a high clinical probability for PE. On the other hand, a negative D-dimer test result has been established as a reliable rule-out criterion in patients with low or intermediate clinical probability for PE. This is particularly true when a highly sensitive (ELISA) D-dimer assay is used. In this case, a negative test result permits PE to be ruled out, and thus therapeutic anticoagulation to be safely withheld, without further testing in around 30% of patients in the emergency department.[22-24] In comparison, quantitative latex-derived assays and whole-blood agglutination assays have a lower sensitivity in the range of 85% to 90%.[25] With the most extensively studied assays (Tinaquant, SimpliRED), the 3-month thromboembolic risk in patients with a low clinical probability is less than 1% when they are left untreated. However, their safety for ruling out PE has not been established in the moderate clinical probability group.

Imaging Modalities

In most cases, PE originates from deep venous thrombosis of the lower limbs. Thus, diagnosis of deep venous thrombosis in a patient clinically suspected of having acute PE is sufficient to set the indication for anticoagulant treatment without further testing.

Lower limb compression ultrasonography has largely replaced venography for diagnosis of deep venous thrombosis. Compression ultrasonography, which has a sensitivity of more than 90% and a specificity of approximately 95% for proximal vein thrombosis, detects abnormality in 30% to 50% of all patients with PE and more often if clinical signs of deep venous thrombosis are also present.[26,27] The diagnostic yield of compression ultrasonography in suspected PE can be raised to more than 40% by performing complete ultrasonography, which includes the distal veins, although this may be accompanied by a decrease in specificity to 85% or less. More recently, computed tomographic (CT) venography, combined with CT pulmonary angiography in a single procedure, was proposed as a "simple" alternative to compression ultrasonography for diagnosis of deep venous thrombosis in patients with suspected PE. Although this approach increased the diagnostic sensitivity of CT pulmonary angiography for diagnosis of venous thromboembolism from 83% to 90% in the PIOPED II study, the increase in negative predictive value was marginal,[28] and it is therefore debatable whether CT venography as a routine procedure justifies the risks of irradiation to the pelvis, especially in younger adults.

The ventilation-perfusion lung scan is an established diagnostic test for suspected PE. The criteria for interpretation and classification of the results have been revised since their initial description in the PIOPED study (Table 85.3).[29-32] Several earlier prospective clinical outcome studies demonstrated that it is safe to withhold anticoagulant therapy in patients with a normal lung scan.[33,34] These results were recently confirmed by a randomized trial comparing ventilation-perfusion scan with computed tomography.[35] In this large series, only 2 of 247 patients (0.8%) with exclusion of PE on the basis of a normal lung scan were treated with

REVISED PIOPED CRITERIA FOR THE DIAGNOSIS OF ACUTE PULMONARY EMBOLISM BY VENTILATION-PERFUSION LUNG SCAN	
	Post-Test Probability of PE
Normal	<2%
No perfusion abnormalities	
Very low probability	<10%
Nonsegmental perfusion defects Perfusion defect smaller than radiographic finding Stripe sign Triple match mid-upper lung <3 small segmental defects	
Low probability	<15%
Multiple matched defects >3 small segmental defects Nonsegmental defects	
Intermediate probability	33%
1 moderate or <2 large defects Corresponding lower lung zone and radiographic abnormality Ventilation-perfusion defects and lung effusion Difficult to categorize as high or low probability	
High probability	>85%
2 large segmental defects without ventilation or radiographic abnormality 1 large and 2 moderate perfusion defects 4 moderate perfusion defects	
Modified from Freitas et al.[31] and Stein and Gottschalk.[32]	

Table 85.3 Revised PIOPED criteria for the diagnosis of acute pulmonary embolism by ventilation-perfusion lung scan.

anticoagulants. These patients were found to have proximal deep venous thrombosis on ultrasound examination. The remaining 245 patients were left untreated, and none of them suffered a recurrent thromboembolic event during follow-up.

Although a normal lung scan is a reliable test to rule out PE, the high frequency of nondiagnostic "intermediate probability" scans is often considered a practical limitation of the method, as these necessitate further diagnostic testing to exclude or to confirm PE. In the past decade, multistep diagnostic algorithms were developed and validated on the basis of the lung scan assisted by the clinical probability, D-dimer testing, and compression venous ultrasonography.[36,37] Such algorithms permitted the diagnosis or exclusion of PE in more than 80% of patients and were recommended in previous guidelines,[38] but they proved difficult to implement correctly in clinical practice because of their complexity and the relatively frequent need for invasive pulmonary angiography. More recent studies have suggested that data acquisition in a tomographic mode, such as single-photon emission computed tomography (SPECT), increases diagnostic accuracy and reduces the frequency of nondiagnostic lung scans. SPECT imaging may also allow the application of automated detection algorithms for PE.[39,40]

The value and the use of CT pulmonary angiography for diagnosis and clinical decision making in suspected PE have increased dramatically with recent improvements in CT technology. Studies using "first-generation," single-detector spiral computed tomography in suspected PE reported a diagnostic sensitivity of 70% and a specificity of 90%.[41,42] It follows that a normal single-detector CT study appears, by itself, insufficient for ruling out PE. On the other hand, the combination of a normal single-detector CT study and the absence of proximal deep venous thrombosis on lower limb venous ultrasonography in patients with non–high clinical probability was associated with a very low (1%) 3-month thromboembolic risk as demonstrated by outcome studies.[43,44]

Since the introduction of multidetector-row computed tomography (MDCT) with a high speed of acquisition along with high spatial and temporal resolution, CT angiography has become the method of choice for imaging the pulmonary vasculature for suspected PE in routine clinical practice (Fig. 85.4). The recent PIOPED II study observed an overall diagnostic sensitivity of 83% and a specificity of 96%.[45] More specifically, in patients with a low or intermediate clinical probability of PE as assessed by the Wells score, a normal MDCT study had a high negative predictive value for PE, reaching 96% and 89%, respectively. This, however, decreased to only 60% in those with discordant, that is, high clinical (pretest), probability. Conversely, the positive predictive value of an abnormal CT scan was high (92% to 96%) in patients with an intermediate or high clinical probability but much lower (58%) in patients with discordant (low) pretest likelihood of PE. Thus, the findings of PIOPED II demonstrate how important it remains to correctly assess the clinical probability of PE before performing and interpreting imaging procedures. In a prospective management study including 756 consecutive patients referred to an emergency department with clinical suspicion of PE, all patients with high clinical probability and those with a non–high clinical probability and a positive ELISA D-dimer test result underwent lower limb ultrasound and MDCT examinations.[22] The proportion of patients in whom a proximal deep venous thrombosis was found on ultrasound examination despite a normal MDCT scan was only 0.9%. In another outcome study, all patients classified as PE likely on the basis of the dichotomized Wells score (see Table 85.2) and those with a positive D-dimer test result underwent MDCT. The 3-month thromboembolic risk in the patients left untreated because of a normal CT scan was 1.1%, confirming the high negative predictive value of the method.[46] A more recent randomized controlled trial reached similar conclusions.[35]

On the basis of current evidence, a normal MDCT scan appears adequate for exclusion of PE in patients with non-high (i.e., intermediate or low) clinical probability of the disease, whereas it remains, at present, controversial whether patients with a normal CT scan despite a high clinical probability should undergo further diagnostic testing by compression lower limb ultrasonography, lung scan, or even pulmonary

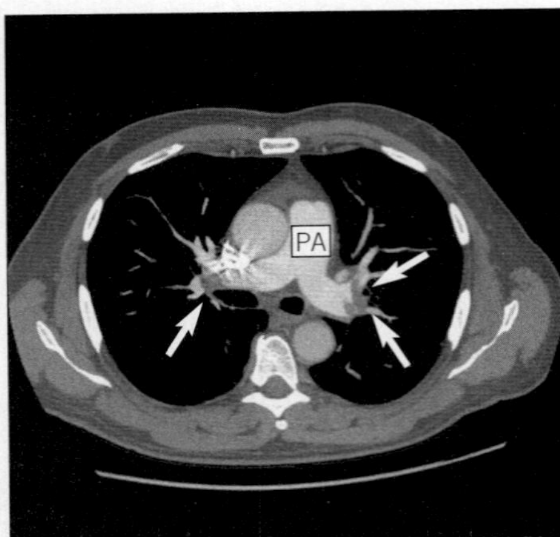

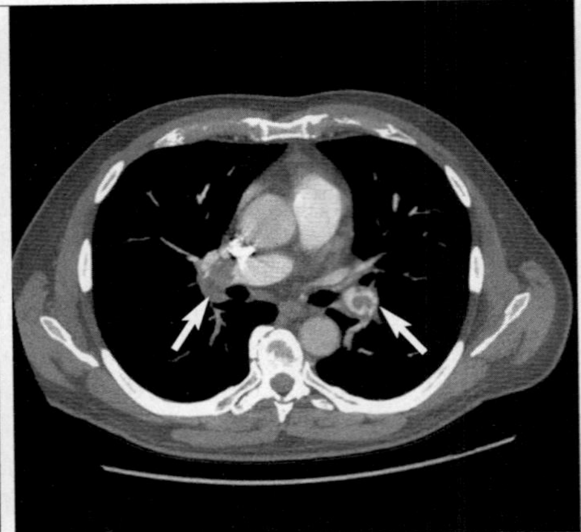
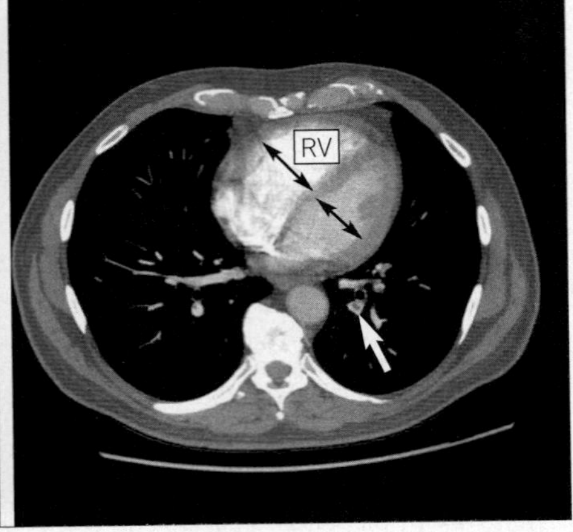

Figure 85.4 Demonstration of pulmonary artery emboli on multidetector (16-row) CT pulmonary angiography. Thrombi are seen as filling defects *(arrows)* in the right and left pulmonary arteries (PA, *left panel*) and in their lobar branches *(middle panel)*. In this patient, thrombi were traced down to the subsegmental level and were accompanied by an enlargement of the right ventricle (RV, *right panel;* right-to-left ventricular dimension ratio >0.9).

angiography. On the other hand, an abnormal MDCT scan at the segmental (or a more proximal) level is adequate proof of PE in patients with high or intermediate clinical probability, whereas further testing may be considered to exclude a false-positive result in patients with low clinical probability.

For decades, selective pulmonary angiography was the "gold standard" for unequivocal confirmation of PE. Because of its (presumed) high specificity and its ability to visualize thrombi down to the subsegmental level, it was used in all major trials that evaluated novel diagnostic and therapeutic regimens for PE. Complete or partial intraluminal filling defects are considered to be typical signs of PE, but vessel tapering or "cutoff" may occasionally be the principal finding. Several scoring systems were introduced for quantitative assessment of pulmonary vascular occlusion. However, angiographic indices of severity correlate only roughly with clinically important predictors of outcome and, in particular, with the impact of the thromboembolic event on right ventricular function. Moreover, pulmonary angiography carries all the known risks of an invasive procedure, including injury to the right ventricle and hemorrhagic complications, particularly in patients who are candidates for thrombolytic treatment.[47] The results of studies that evaluated the accuracy of contemporary diagnostic modalities, particularly that of MDCT, and the impact of noninvasive diagnostic strategies on the patient's outcome have shown that confirmation or exclusion of PE and therapeutic decisions are currently possible without the use of pulmonary angiography in most patients.[22,28,35,46]

The role of echocardiography in the diagnosis of PE is to assess the pressure overload imposed on the right ventricle by the thromboembolic event and the resulting increase in pulmonary artery pressure.[14,48-51] The sensitivity of echocardiography in detecting these changes was shown in several studies to range from 80% to 100%. In particular, right ventricular enlargement (defined as a right ventricle that appears larger than the left ventricle in the apical or subcostal four-chamber view or as a right ventricular end-diastolic diameter of more than 30 mm in the left precordial view at the level of the mitral valve apparatus) appears to be a simple and sensitive diagnostic finding in this regard. In addition, Doppler ultrasonography permits a reliable assessment of pulmonary artery pressure and its response to treatment. In some of the patients, diagnosis of right ventricular hypertrophy or excessive pulmonary hypertension may identify chronic cor pulmonale due to recurrent PE (chronic thromboembolic pulmonary hypertension).[52] Finally, contrast echocardiography is capable of diagnosing a right-to-left shunt through a patent foramen ovale in up to 35% of patients who have massive PE, indicating a particularly high risk of profound arterial hypoxemia or paradoxical embolism.[19]

In contrast to other imaging procedures, imaging of the pulmonary embolus itself is not the primary scope of cardiac ultrasonography. However, mobile thrombi can be detected in the right-sided heart chambers or the central pulmonary artery segments in up to 11% of PE patients if they are carefully sought (Fig. 85.5). Transesophageal imaging offers superior resolution and greater sensitivity in visualizing thrombotic material (see Fig. 85.5). However, it is poorly tolerated by patients with PE, who are often dyspneic and agitated, and it should be reserved for intubated patients or those in whom transthoracic imaging is of poor quality.

In summary, echocardiography is primarily a risk stratification and not a diagnostic tool in acute PE,[53] with the exception of patients presenting with hemodynamic instability (see later).

Contemporary Diagnostic Strategies and Algorithms

Suspected High-Risk Pulmonary Embolism in a Patient with Hypotension or Shock

Management of the unstable patient with suspected high-risk (massive) PE should always direct the focus on rapid institution of recanalization treatment to reverse right ventricular failure and to save the patient's life. The assessment of clinical probability, preferably by use of one of the scores mentioned before, is mandatory as a first step, whereas there is no rationale for performing a D-dimer test in such an emergency situation.

According to the algorithm proposed in Figure 85.6, bedside echocardiography is the fastest and thus most appropriate initial test to confirm acute right ventricular failure. Additional information that can be obtained from ultrasound imaging includes the presence of large floating intracardiac thrombi, which indicate an imminent threat of recurrent

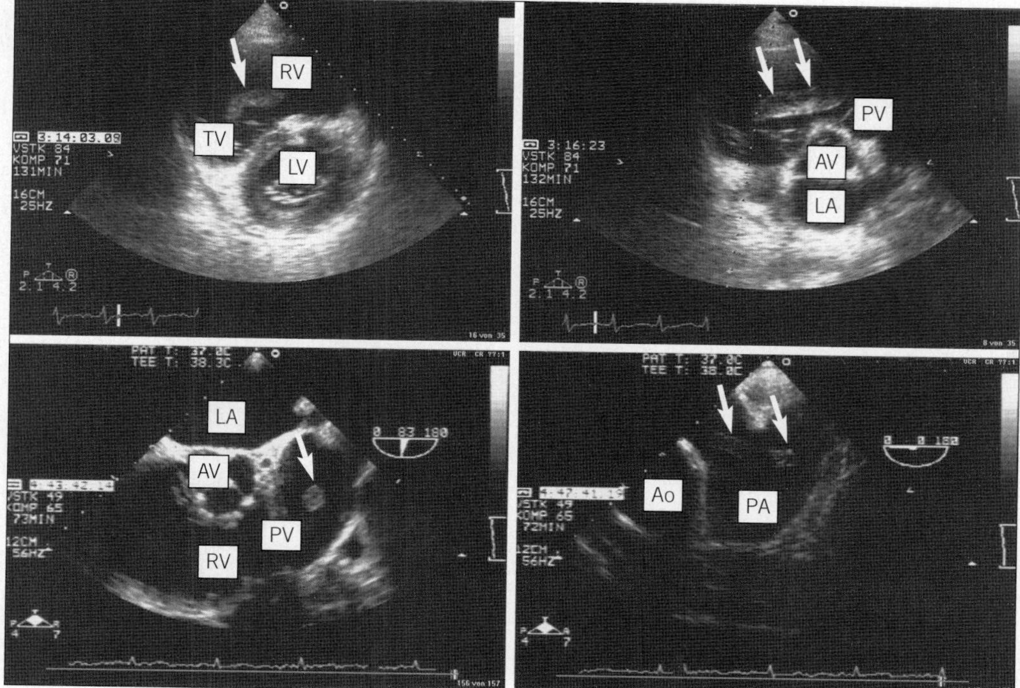

Figure 85.5 *Upper panels,* In this short-axis parasternal transthoracic view, a long mobile thrombus *(arrows)* can be seen protruding through the tricuspid valve into the right ventricle *(left)* and from there through the pulmonic valve into the pulmonary artery *(right)*. *Lower panels,* During this transesophageal examination, a mobile thrombus *(arrows)* was observed in the pulmonary artery distal to the right ventricle and the pulmonic valve *(left)*; in the transverse plane, the thrombus was found to have a typical serpentine form and to override the bifurcation of the pulmonary artery *(right)*. Ao, ascending thoracic aorta; AV, aortic valve; LA, left atrium; LV, left ventricle; PA, pulmonary artery; PV, pulmonic valve; RV, right ventricle; TV, tricuspid valve.

massive PE. Finally, and importantly, echocardiography may provide alternative explanations for the patient's hypotension and shock, such as left ventricular failure due to cardiomyopathy or large myocardial infarction, critical valvular disease, pericardial tamponade, or aortic dissection. In mechanically ventilated patients, transesophageal echocardiography is a useful alternative to transthoracic imaging, permitting direct visualization of possible thrombi in the right atrium, foramen ovale, right ventricle, or proximal segments of the common and right pulmonary artery.

If bedside echocardiography is not available on an emergency basis or its findings are nondiagnostic, CT pulmonary angiography is the fastest and most reliable diagnostic method. Selective invasive pulmonary angiography is rarely necessary unless the patient is already in the catheterization laboratory because of suspected myocardial infarction or if catheter-based aspiration of the pulmonary thrombus is a treatment option.

Suspected Non–High-Risk Pulmonary Embolism in a Normotensive Patient

Numerous multistep algorithms have been proposed and prospectively validated for the diagnostic work-up of normotensive patients with suspected nonmassive PE. According to established algorithms that were recommended in previous guidelines[38] and are still valid today,[54] lower limb venous compression ultrasonography is the initial imaging method in patients with an elevated D-dimer level and in those with a high clinical probability for PE. It will detect deep venous thrombosis in about 10% of the patients and can thus help establish a definite diagnosis in approximately 15% of the entire initial cohort. Single-detector CT scan has, as already mentioned, a relatively low diagnostic sensitivity, but the combination of a normal CT scan, a normal lower limb ultrasound examination, and a low or intermediate clinical probability can safely rule out PE. In hospitals in which ventilation-perfusion lung scan is the preferred imaging modality, the combination of a low-probability scan and a low clinical probability of PE can be used to safely exclude PE. At the other end of the spectrum, a high-probability ventilation-perfusion scan generally establishes the diagnosis of PE, although further tests may be necessary in patients with low clinical probability because of the low positive predictive value of the lung scan in this setting. In all other combinations of lung scan findings and clinical probability, further tests, such as spiral computed tomography or even selective pulmonary angiography, are necessary.

More recent algorithms, such as the one shown in Figure 85.7, are based on the superior sensitivity of MDCT and its ability to confirm or to exclude PE without the need for venous ultrasonography as an intermediate step. As previously mentioned, false-negative results of MDCT have been reported in patients with a high clinical probability of PE.[28] This fact underlines the importance of assessing clinical (pretest) probability before interpreting the results of imaging studies, including MDCT. However, such discrepancies appear to be infrequent in clinical practice, and their implications regarding the need for further testing to exclude PE remain controversial in light of the reassuring results of outcome trials.[46]

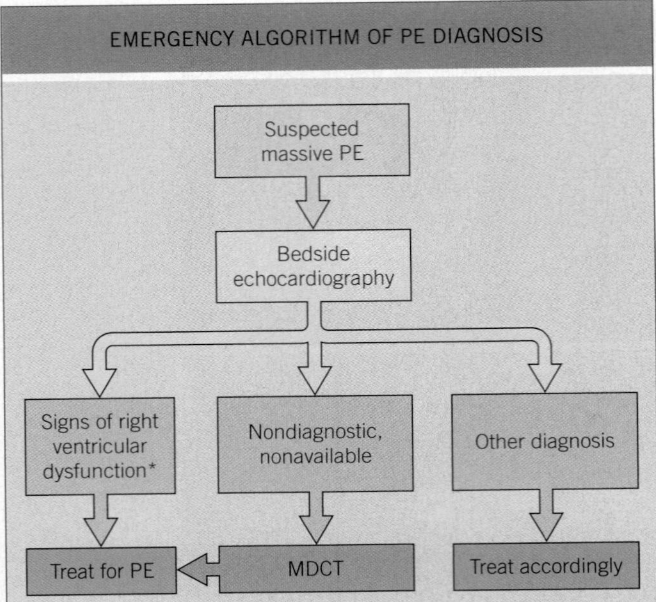

Figure 85.6 Emergency algorithm of PE diagnosis in the high-risk patient presenting with persistent hypotension or shock. *Signs of right ventricular dysfunction include the following: right ventricular diastolic diameter of more than 30 mm (parasternal view) or right-to-left ventricular dimension ratio greater than 1 (apical or subcostal view); systolic flattening of the interventricular septum; tricuspid insufficiency pressure gradient of more than 30 mm Hg in the absence of right ventricular hypertrophy; and presence of the McConnell sign, that is, normokinesia or hyperkinesia of the apical segment of the right ventricle free wall combined with hypokinesia of the remaining parts of the right ventricle free wall. MDCT, multidetector-row computed tomographic pulmonary angiography. (Modified from Konstantinides SV. Acute pulmonary embolism revisited: thromboembolic venous disease. Heart 2008;94:795-802.)

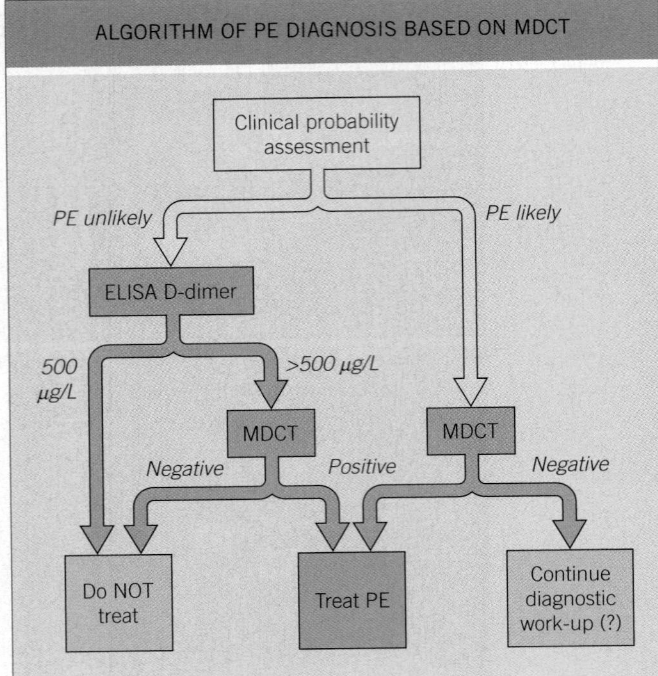

Figure 85.7 Prospectively validated algorithm of PE diagnosis based on multidetector-row computed tomographic (MDCT) pulmonary angiography. ELISA, enzyme-linked immunosorbent assay; PE, pulmonary embolism.

INITIAL TREATMENT

In acute PE, cardiovascular mortality is highest during the first few hours. In patients who survive the early phase, the risk is determined by the potential for recurrent thromboembolic events. Thus, management of PE must focus on two major goals:

- the early reversal of right-sided heart dysfunction, if present; and
- the prevention of recurrent thromboembolism.

Anticoagulation

Anticoagulant treatment should be administered to all patients on clinical suspicion of acute PE, that is, without awaiting definitive confirmation by imaging procedures.[38] Intravenous unfractionated heparin is still the preferred mode of initial anticoagulation

- for patients with severe renal impairment (creatinine clearance <30 mL/min);
- for patients at high risk of bleeding;
- for high-risk, hypotensive patients with clinically massive PE; and, as a rule,
- for extremely overweight, underweight, or old patients.

A weight-adjusted bolus injection of 80 U/kg is followed by an infusion rate of 18 U/kg per hour. Subsequent infusion rates are adjusted by use of activated partial thromboplastin time (aPTT)–based nomograms to achieve and to maintain therapeutic aPTT prolongation.[55] The aPTT should be measured 4 to 6 hours after the bolus injection and subsequently 3 hours after each dose adjustment or once daily when the target dose has been reached.

With the exception of these circumstances, unfractionated heparin has largely been replaced by low-molecular-weight heparin given subcutaneously at weight-adjusted doses. A meta-analysis of 12 trials confirmed that low-molecular-weight heparins are at least as efficacious and at least as safe as unfractionated heparin.[56] Currently approved low-molecular-weight heparins include

- enoxaparin, 1 mg/kg every 12 hours (1.5 mg/kg once daily is also approved in some countries);
- tinzaparin, 175 U/kg once daily; and
- the pentasaccharide fondaparinux, 5 mg (for body weight <50 kg), 7.5 mg (for body weight of 50 to 100 kg), or 10 mg (for body weight >100 kg) once daily.

Routine anticoagulation monitoring (i.e., measurement of anti–factor Xa levels) is not necessary in patients receiving low-molecular-weight heparin, but it should be considered during pregnancy. In this case, anti-Xa levels should be determined 4 hours after the morning injection; the proposed target range is 0.6 to 1.0 IU/mL for twice-daily and 1.0 to 2.0 IU/mL for once-daily administration. Because of the risk of heparin-induced thrombocytopenia, monitoring of the platelet count is recommended during treatment with either unfractionated or low-molecular-weight heparin with the exception of fondaparinux.

Anticoagulation with unfractionated heparin, low-molecular-weight heparin or fondaparinux should be continued for at least 5 days. Oral anticoagulants (vitamin K antagonists) should be initiated as soon as possible in all hemodynamically stable patients, preferably on the same day as heparin. Parenteral anticoagulation can be stopped as soon as the international normalized ratio has been in the therapeutic range (between 2.0 and 3.0) on 2 consecutive days.

Benefits and Risks of Thrombolysis

Randomized trials performed during a 30-year period[57] have consistently shown that thrombolytic therapy for PE effectively resolves thromboembolic obstruction and promptly reduces pulmonary artery pressure and resistance with a concomitant increase in cardiac output. One of the largest trials also demonstrated a significant improvement in right ventricular function as assessed by echocardiography 3 hours after treatment with recombinant tissue plasminogen activator.[51] In the only randomized thrombolysis trial with clinical endpoints, early thrombolytic treatment given to normotensive patients with evidence of right ventricular dysfunction significantly reduced the need for emergency escalation of therapy during the hospital stay.[58]

Overall, up to 92% of patients with PE appear to respond favorably to thrombolysis as indicated by clinical and echocardiographic improvement within the first 36 hours.[59] The greatest benefit is observed when treatment is initiated within 48 hours of symptom onset, but thrombolysis can still be useful in patients who have had symptoms for 6 to 14 days.[60] On the other hand, the hemodynamic benefits of thrombolysis over heparin alone appear to be confined to the first few days. In patients who are alive 1 week after treatment, the improvement in the severity of vascular obstruction and right ventricular dysfunction appears to be similar in thrombolysis-treated and heparin-treated patients.[61] Moreover, thrombolysis also carries a significant bleeding risk. According to the data derived from thrombolysis trials in acute PE, a cumulative rate of major bleeding of up to 13% and a rate of intracranial or fatal hemorrhage reaching 2% should be anticipated,[62,63] although the risk of major or life-threatening bleeding may be lower if noninvasive imaging methods are used in the diagnostic work-up of PE.[51,58] Thus, taken together, the available data suggest that thrombolysis should be reserved for those patients in whom a high risk of *early* PE-related death is anticipated.

Currently approved thrombolytic regimens for PE include

- streptokinase, 250,000 IU as a loading dose during 30 minutes, followed by an infusion of 100,000 IU/h during 12 to 24 hours;
- urokinase, 4400 IU/kg as a loading dose during 10 minutes, followed by 4400 IU/kg per hour during 12 to 24 hours; and
- alteplase (recombinant tissue plasminogen activator), 100-mg infusion during 2 hours, with the first 10 mg usually given as bolus injection.

A short (during 15 minutes) infusion regimen of alteplase at the dosage of 0.6 mg/kg (maximum dosage, 50 mg) can be used in emergency situations (e.g., during cardiopulmonary resuscitation). Satisfactory hemodynamic results also have been obtained with double-bolus reteplase, two injections (10 U) 30 minutes apart, although this drug is not officially approved for PE. Preliminary uncontrolled data appear to support the efficacy and safety of tenecteplase in acute PE.

Surgical or Catheter-Based Embolectomy

Pulmonary embolectomy remained a rarely performed rescue operation for several decades, and limited data existed about its efficacy and safety. Recent technical advances in transportable extracorporeal assist systems, and particularly the timely involvement of the cardiac surgeon as part of an interdisciplinary approach to high-risk PE, may contribute to better postoperative outcomes.[64] Currently, pulmonary embolectomy is a recommended therapeutic option in patients with high-risk PE in whom there are absolute contraindications to thrombolysis or if thrombolysis has failed. The same recommendations apply to catheter embolectomy or fragmentation of proximal pulmonary arterial clots.

Inferior Vena Cava Filters

Cava filters may be used as a means of primary or secondary PE prevention. However, the data about their relative safety and efficacy remain inconclusive. Comparison with therapeutic anticoagulation has to take into account the fact that anticoagulation is very effective in preventing recurrent thromboembolism in patients treated for symptomatic PE. For example, recurrence rates under effective anticoagulation are in the range of 3% even in the presence of free-floating thrombi in the proximal leg veins,[65] and fatal PE occurs in 0.4% to 1.5% of patients during treatment with heparin or warfarin.[66] In one study, inferior vena cava filter placement increased the risk of recurrent leg vein thrombosis during the long term.[67] At present, temporary inferior vena cava filters have a role in the prevention of PE only if anticoagulation is absolutely contraindicated or in cases of recurrence in spite of adequate medical treatment.

DIFFERENTIAL THERAPY BASED ON RISK STRATIFICATION

High-Risk Patients

In view of the high early mortality and complication risk associated with clinically massive PE,[3,68,69] existing guidelines[38,70,71] and most clinicians agree that patients who present with persistent arterial hypotension or shock are in need of immediate recanalization of the occluded pulmonary arteries with thrombolytic agents or, alternatively, surgical or catheter-based procedures. In fact, pooled data from five trials that included hemodynamically unstable patients appear to suggest a significant reduction of death or PE recurrence after thrombolysis in this high-risk group.[57]

Non–High-Risk Patients: Distinction Between Low and Intermediate Risk

A meta-analysis of randomized trials that excluded hypotensive patients with high-risk PE suggested that heparin anticoagulation is sufficient as the initial treatment of PE and that thrombolysis may have no clinical benefits in this setting.[57] Nevertheless, several years ago, registry data generated the hypothesis that the detection of subclinical right ventricular dysfunction in a normotensive patient with acute nonmassive PE may help define an elevated death risk in the acute phase.[2,3] It was further postulated that these patients may benefit from early thrombolytic treatment.[72]

Imaging of the Right Ventricle

As discussed before, echocardiography is capable of detecting the morphologic and functional changes of the right ventricle as a result of acute pressure overload. A number of parameters permit the noninvasive diagnosis of right ventricular dysfunction at the bedside. Several registries and cohort studies could demonstrate an association between these parameters and a poor in-hospital outcome in terms of PE-related death and complications.[14,48-51] Nevertheless, the potential therapeutic implications of cardiac ultrasonography, particularly with regard to thrombolysis, in normotensive patients with PE remain the subject of debate. The persisting uncertainty may partly be due to the lack of standardization of the echocardiographic criteria and the absence of adequately powered, controlled studies focusing on normotensive patients with PE.[73] Furthermore, differential diagnosis between acute PE and chronic thromboembolic pulmonary hypertension may be difficult, although some echocardiographic criteria have been proposed to distinguish between acute and chronic cor pulmonale.[52]

The largest randomized thrombolysis trial to date, which included 256 normotensive patients with right ventricular dysfunction (mainly) detected by echocardiography, reported a significantly reduced incidence of the primary endpoint (30-day mortality or need for treatment escalation) in patients who underwent early thrombolysis as opposed to those treated with heparin alone. However, there was no significant influence of the type of treatment on mortality rates during the acute phase of PE.[58] It is thus likely that further information (beyond echocardiographic findings) is needed before the decision can be made to perform thrombolysis in a normotensive patient with acute PE.

Four-chamber views of the heart on MDCT, which is currently the preferred method for diagnosis of PE in most institutions, may detect right ventricular enlargement due to acute cor pulmonale and possibly predict early death. In a large retrospective series, 30-day mortality was twice as high in patients with right ventricular enlargement, defined as right-to-left ventricular dimension ratio greater than 0.9, compared with those without this finding (15.6% versus 7.7%).[74] Another retrospective study evaluated the prognostic value of a predefined diameter ratio of 1.0 (axial four-chamber views without post-processing of the CT images) during 3-month follow-up.[75] The negative predictive value of a small right ventricle reached 100%, whereas the positive predictive value of a right-to-left ventricular dimension ratio greater than 1.0 for PE-related mortality was rather low (10.1%).

Biomarkers

Elevated cardiac troponin I or T levels, which are a sensitive indicator of myocardial cell damage and microscopic myocardial necrosis, are found in 11% to 50% of patients with acute PE. A large number of studies that were included in a meta-analysis[76] could show that cardiac troponin elevation correlates with the presence of right ventricular dysfunction on echocardiography and possesses a high (97% to 100%) negative predictive value with regard to death or complication risk in the acute phase. Thus, normal troponin levels may rule out an adverse outcome in patients with PE. However, the positive predictive value of these biomarkers is probably low. Consequently, troponin elevation alone does not suffice to predict early death or complications in patients with acute PE, and it is unlikely that it could, by itself, identify intermediate-risk patients as potential candidates for thrombolytic treatment. The natriuretic peptides BNP and NT-proBNP are characterized by extreme prognostic sensitivity and a negative prognostic value that is probably higher than that of the cardiac troponins. On the other hand, they exhibit a very low specificity and positive prognostic value in the range of 12% to 25%.[77] Furthermore, appropriate cut-off levels for distinguishing between a "positive" and a "negative" BNP or NT-proBNP test result have not yet been prospectively validated. Heart-type fatty acid–binding protein is a small cytoplasmic protein that is abundant in the heart. After myocardial cell damage, it diffuses rapidly through the interstitial space and appears in the circulation as early as 90 minutes after symptom onset, reaching its peak within 6 hours. It might provide prognostic information superior to that of cardiac troponins in acute PE.[78]

At present, the existing evidence appears to support the rationale for risk stratification algorithms for normotensive patients with confirmed acute PE (Fig. 85.8). These algorithms combine the information provided by an imaging procedure (echocardiography or computed tomography) and a biomarker test, preferably troponin I or T. The therapeutic implications of identifying an intermediate-risk patient group are currently being evaluated in a large multinational trial that plans to randomize more than 1000 normotensive patients with acute PE. It is expected that this study will be able to resolve the long-lasting debate on the possible indications for thrombolytic treatment in selected normotensive patients with acute PE.

RECURRENCE OF PULMONARY EMBOLISM AND LONG-TERM SECONDARY PROPHYLAXIS

PE, particularly idiopathic, unprovoked PE, is considered a life-long disease, and chronic secondary prophylaxis is necessary. Without continuing anticoagulation, as many as 50% of patients with symptomatic proximal deep venous thrombosis or PE will suffer a recurrent episode within the first 3 months.[79] The frequency of recurrence appears to be independent of the initial clinical manifestation of venous thromboembolism, but recurrent venous thromboembolism is three times more likely to be manifested as PE if the initial clinical event was PE than if it was deep venous thrombosis.[80] This fact emphasizes the need for effective secondary prophylaxis in patients who have suffered PE. To date, most of the studies addressing recurrence prophylaxis for venous thromboembolism have included patients with deep venous thrombosis rather than focusing on PE alone. The available data indicate that the long-term recurrence rate may be 30% or even higher after 8 to 10 years,[81-83] and it was found that indefinite treatment might be capable of reducing the risk for recurrent thromboembolism by up to 90%.[84] Thus, oral anticoagulants (vitamin K antagonists) are highly effective in preventing recurrent thromboembolism, but they do not eliminate the risk of subsequent recurrence after their discontinuation, regardless of the duration of treatment.[85,86] On the other hand, the benefits of chronic oral anticoagulation are partly offset by the increased risk of major bleeding.[84,87]

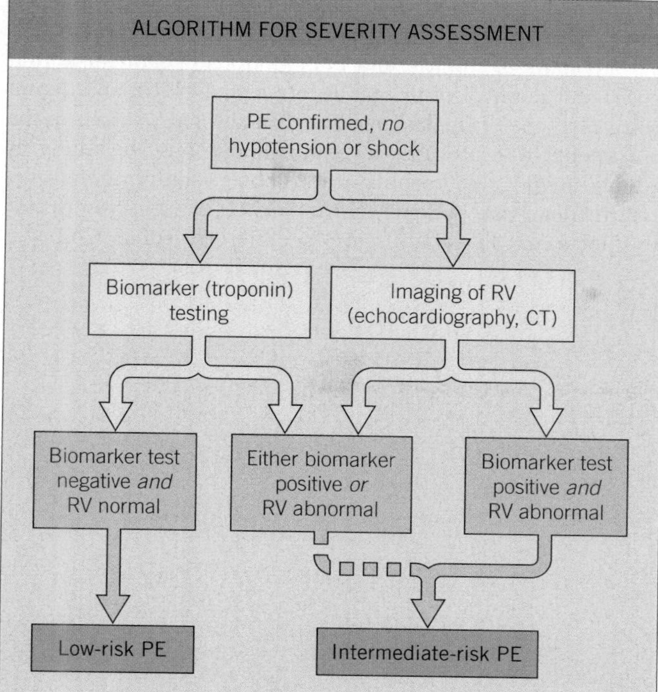

Figure 85.8 Risk stratification of PE: contemporary algorithm for severity assessment. CT, computed tomography; PE, pulmonary embolism; RV, right ventricle.

The recommended duration of oral anticoagulation after an episode of acute PE has been reviewed in recent guidelines and is based on these considerations (Table 85.4).[71] As a rule, treatment with vitamin K antagonists should be continued for 3 months after a first episode of PE triggered by a transient risk factor (trauma, surgery, immobilization, pregnancy, contraceptive use, or hormonal replacement therapy) and for longer periods (preferably 6 to 12 months) for patients with unprovoked PE. Indefinite oral anticoagulation should be considered and discussed on an individual basis for patients with a first manifestation of unprovoked PE and a low risk of bleeding, and it is clearly recommended for most patients with a second unprovoked episode of venous thromboembolism. Patients with high-risk thrombophilia or active cancer are also candidates for long-term oral anticoagulation. On the other hand, it is at present unclear whether and to what extent the severity of the initial event and possibly other clinical and hemodynamic factors, such as persistent pulmonary hypertension on echocardiography, may determine recurrence-related fatality rates and affect long-term therapeutic decisions. It also remains to be confirmed whether D-dimer testing 1 month after discontinuation of vitamin K antagonists may be used to resume or definitely to terminate therapy in patients who have received oral anticoagulants for 3 months after the first episode of idiopathic vein thrombosis or PE.[88]

Novel, vitamin K–independent oral anticoagulants are currently under investigation for primary and secondary prophylaxis of venous thromboembolism. In particular, the selective oral thrombin inhibitor dabigatran and the oral factor Xa inhibitor rivaroxaban have already yielded promising data in phase III clinical trials. If they are eventually approved for the treatment and long-term secondary prophylaxis of venous thromboembolism, these drugs may increase the safety of chronic oral anticoagulation and compliance of patients.

SUMMARY

Until recently, the diagnosis and management of acute PE were characterized by a high degree of complexity along with a lack of both efficacy and efficiency. The clinical symptoms and signs of acute PE are known to be nonspecific, and the same limitation applies to the findings of bedside tests such as electrocardiography, chest radiography, and clinical chemistry. In the past, the limitations of individual diagnostic tests led to the development of complex multistep diagnostic algorithms, which were successfully validated in prospective management studies but have proved extremely difficult to implement in clinical practice. As a result, the diagnosis of potentially life-threatening PE was frequently missed in many patients who subsequently died of the disease without receiving appropriate treatment, whereas other patients unnecessarily underwent potentially hazardous, time-consuming, and costly procedures because of poorly documented clinical suspicion. The recent development of structured models for assessment of clinical pretest probability, the widespread use of D-dimer testing in patients with intermediate or low clinical probability, and the enormous technical advances of MDCT have begun to change the approach to patients with suspected PE. These modalities form the basis for contemporary noninvasive diagnostic

RECOMMENDED DURATION OF ANTICOAGULATION FOR SECONDARY PREVENTION OF VENOUS THROMBOEMBOLISM	
First episode with transient risk factor (trauma, surgery, immobilization, pregnancy, contraceptive use, or hormonal replacement therapy)	3 months
First episode, unprovoked (no transient risk factor), or with low-risk thrombophilia (e.g., heterozygous activated protein C resistance, G20210A prothrombin mutation)	At least 3 months, preferably 6-12 months; consider indefinite treatment in selected patients with low bleeding risk
First episode with homozygous or combined thrombophilia, antiphospholipid syndrome	At least 12 months
Recurrent venous thromboembolism, active cancer	Indefinite anticoagulation

Modified from Kearon et al.[71] and Torbicki et al.[89]

Table 85.4 Recommended duration of anticoagulation for secondary prevention of venous thromboembolism.

algorithms that are reliable, fast, and easy to follow and to implement by clinicians. Overt right ventricular failure with hemodynamic instability at diagnosis clearly indicates high-risk PE. In the remaining patients, the prognostic importance of right ventricular dysfunction has also been demonstrated, and a number of studies confirmed the value of echocardiography, computed tomography, and laboratory biomarkers for risk stratification of normotensive patients with PE into a low-risk and an intermediate-risk group. Current treatment regimens for hemodynamically stable patients with PE are based on low-molecular-weight heparins; early thrombolysis and technical advances in surgical and interventional treatment permit successful removal of thrombus in massive PE. In an attempt to resolve one of the last persisting major controversies in the treatment of acute PE, a multinational ongoing study is testing the possible benefits of thrombolysis in normotensive, intermediate-risk patients with evidence of right ventricular dysfunction. (ClinicalTrials.gov Identifier: NCT00639743).

VALVULAR HEART DISEASE

SECTION

6

chapter 86

Noninvasive Assessment of Valvular Function

Otto A. Smiseth, Reidar Bjørnerheim, and Sigurd Nitter-Hauge

Definition

- Two-dimensional echocardiography and Doppler study provide data on both valvular structure and function and are frequently superior to invasive studies for the diagnosis of valvular heart disease.

Key Findings

- Valvular structure and left ventricular performance are best appreciated by two-dimensional and M-mode echocardiography.
- Doppler study assesses the severity of valvular stenosis through the calculation of pressure gradient and valve area.
- Two-dimensional color Doppler study confirms the diagnosis of valvular regurgitation by showing a regurgitant jet.
- Transesophageal echocardiography is more sensitive than transthoracic echocardiography for the detection of valvular vegetations.

Clinical Implications

- Serial Doppler measurements of transvalvular velocities are important for follow-up of prosthetic cardiac valves.

In most cases, the diagnosis of valvular heart disease is made by a combination of the patient's history, clinical findings, and echocardiography. Some additional diagnostic information is provided by electrocardiography and chest radiography. Two-dimensional echocardiography in combination with Doppler study provides information about valve structure and allows assessment of the severity of the lesion.[1] In many ways, echocardiography is superior to invasive studies because it provides more comprehensive data on structure as well as on function. These include quantitative data on ventricular and valvular function and pulmonary artery pressures. Echocardiography should include a comprehensive evaluation of all heart valves, searching for associated valve diseases. In patients with aortic valve disease, evaluation and dimension measurements of the ascending aorta should also be performed. In interpreting dimensions of the left ventricle and other cavities, it is important to take into account the patient's body size, and for some measurements, it is preferable to index dimensions to body surface area. Transesophageal echocardiography should be considered when transthoracic examination is suboptimal and when valve thrombosis, prosthetic valve dysfunction, and endocarditis are suspected. Three-dimensional echocardiography is undergoing promising developments, but its added value in routine clinical work is not yet clear. Stress testing with exercise electrocardiography is useful to unmask symptoms in patients who claim they are asymptomatic. Magnetic resonance imaging and radioisotope methods still have limited application, and in most centers they are not used for the evaluation of patients who have valvular heart disease, even if magnetic resonance imaging is a promising diagnostic tool with increasing availability.[2,3] Fluoroscopy is useful to assess leaflet motion in mechanical valves and to evaluate prosthesis stability.

MITRAL STENOSIS

Mitral stenosis continues to be an important cause of cardiac disease, particularly in the nonindustrialized parts of the world. Rheumatic heart disease is by far the most common cause of mitral stenosis and accounts for about 90% of cases. In some patients, mitral stenosis is caused by mitral annular calcification that extends into the leaflets. There also are rare cases of congenital mitral stenosis. In mitral stenosis secondary to rheumatic heart disease, there is typically diffuse thickening of the leaflets, fusion of the commissures, and fusion and shortening of the chordae tendineae. This leads to restricted opening of the valve and obstruction of flow into the left ventricle. The disease progresses slowly. There is often combined mitral stenosis and mitral regurgitation, and the aortic valve is often affected as well.

DIAGNOSTIC PROCEDURES AND TECHNIQUES

Echocardiography

Mitral stenosis is easily diagnosed by two-dimensional echocardiography, which shows thickening of the valve leaflets with commissural fusion and diminished leaflet separation in diastole (Fig. 86.1). The leaflet thickening is most marked along the margins. A most characteristic finding is diastolic doming of the valve, with wider separation of the basal portions than of the leaflet tips. In typical cases, the anterior leaflet has the appearance of a hockey stick in the parasternal long-axis view (see Fig. 86.1). This pattern is the result of relative sparing of the basal portions of the valve, which are separated widely by the elevated left atrial pressure. If the valve is extensively calcified, the doming may disappear. The parasternal short-axis view shows a small valve orifice with fish-mouth appearance. When the disease progresses, the thickening and calcification of the valve expand toward the annulus. This is in contrast to mitral annular calcifications, which start at the annulus and may expand toward the mitral tips.

Because of thickening of the valve, the M-mode echocardiogram shows multiple echoes originating from the leaflets

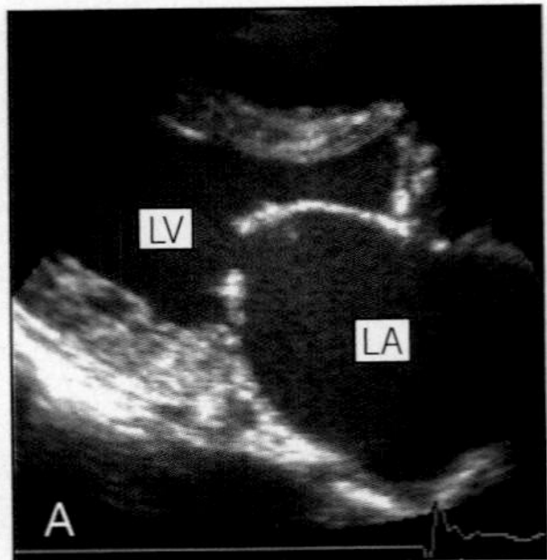

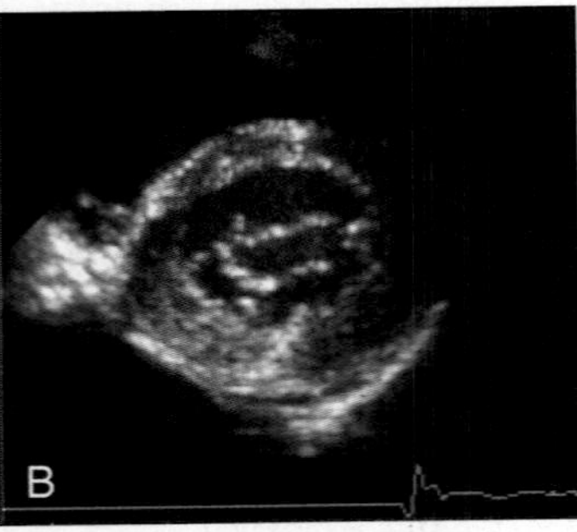

Figure 86.1 Two-dimensional echocardiography in mitral stenosis. A, Parasternal long-axis view through a stenotic mitral valve demonstrating typical diastolic doming of the anterior leaflet. **B,** The short-axis view shows the fish-mouth appearance of the stenotic valve. LA, left atrium; LV, left ventricle.

(Fig. 86.2). Furthermore, the M-mode echocardiogram typically shows decrease or loss of the initial diastolic closure motion of the anterior leaflet. This results from persistence of transmitral flow throughout diastole, which is caused by the elevated transmitral pressure gradient. This sign is not specific for mitral stenosis. A more specific sign is diastolic anterior motion of the posterior leaflet. This is in contrast to the normal valve, for which the M-mode trace of the posterior leaflet is an approximate mirror image of that of the anterior leaflet (i.e., at onset of filling, when the anterior leaflet moves anteriorly, the posterior leaflet moves posteriorly). Because of fusion of the commissures, the larger and more mobile anterior leaflet pulls both leaflets anteriorly in early diastole. In mild mitral stenosis, however, this sign may be absent. Another finding in mitral stenosis is a slight leftward motion of the interventricular septum at onset of diastole.

A mobile atrial myxoma or another atrial tumor may obstruct the mitral valve and may mimic the clinical findings as well as some of the M-mode echocardiographic findings in mitral stenosis. Two-dimensional echocardiography, however, demonstrates the tumor.

The mitral valve area is calculated on a parasternal, short-axis, two-dimensional image after the plane has been adjusted to obtain the smallest possible valve orifice. In most patients, this method gives an accurate measure of the anatomic area, which compares well with the area determined during cardiac surgery.[4] However, dense fibrosis and calcification broaden the echo from the edges of the orifice and may lead to underestimation of the area, whereas echo dropouts may lead to overestimation. Improper gain setting can either enlarge or reduce the measured area. The area should be measured in early diastole when the valve is maximally distended. In most cases, however, reliable estimation of severity is obtained by Doppler studies, and planimetry of the valve area is a supplementary method.

Doppler Studies

Transmitral Pressure Gradient as Measured by Doppler Study

The instantaneous pressure gradient is derived from the simplified Bernoulli equation, where V is the velocity of flow:

$$\Delta P = 4V^2$$

The use of this equation has proved to be an accurate method for calculation of the pressure gradient in mitral stenosis.[5-7] From the apical view, the jet is easily localized by two-dimensional color Doppler study, and continuous-wave Doppler examination is used to obtain maximum velocities (Figs. 86.3 and 86.4). It is important to minimize the angle between the direction of the jet and the sampling beam. The mean transmitral pressure gradient by Doppler interrogation correlates well with the invasive mean gradient.

The transmitral gradient is influenced by the flow across the valve. During tachycardia (e.g., atrial fibrillation with rapid ventricular rate), there is shortening of diastole, and the stroke volume therefore needs to cross the valve in a shorter time. This leads to a higher gradient, although the stenosis is unchanged. Similarly, in mitral regurgitation, there will be increased diastolic flow across the valve and

Figure 86.2 Parasternal M-mode registration in mitral stenosis. This is the same mitral valve as in Figure 86.1.

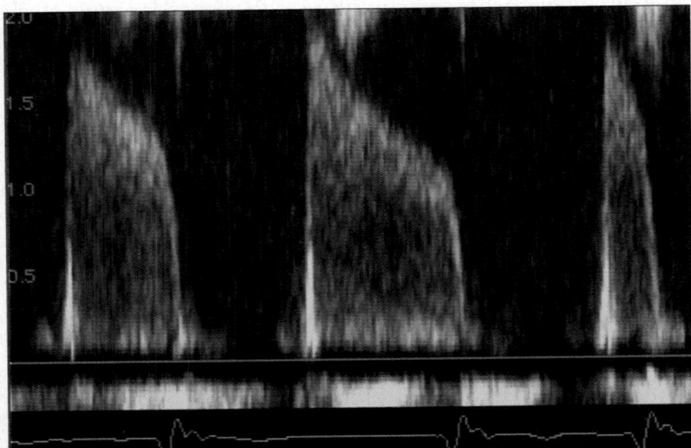

Figure 86.3 Pulsed Doppler study of mitral inflow in a patient with mitral stenosis and atrial fibrillation. By tracing of the flow profile, the gradient can be determined. During prolonged R-R intervals, the pressure half-time gives an excellent estimate of the stenotic valve area.

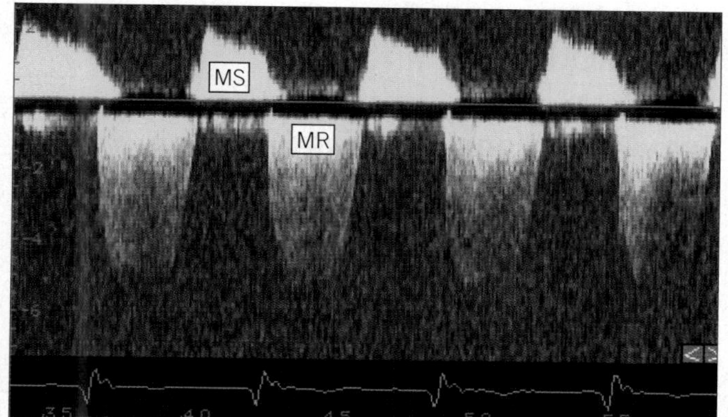

Figure 86.4 Continuous-wave Doppler study through the mitral valve in combined mitral stenosis (MS) and mitral regurgitation (MR). The study demonstrates that the regurgitation starts immediately after inflow has finished. This is in contrast to aortic flow, which is slightly delayed during isovolumetric contraction.

therefore an increased gradient. None of these factors, however, reduces the accuracy of the Doppler-derived gradient.

When there is discrepancy between symptoms and a modest gradient, the patient should be reexamined during exercise (e.g., actively lifting the legs or pedaling against moderate resistance). When the valve is severely stenotic, even a small increase in flow causes a marked increase in gradient. In some cases, even passive leg elevation will markedly increase the transmitral pressure gradient. One should also try to estimate systolic pulmonary artery pressure from the tricuspid regurgitation velocity.

Pressure Half-time Method

In mitral stenosis, the transvalvular pressure gradient remains elevated throughout diastole. The more severe the stenosis is, the less steep the decrease in the gradient.[8] The pressure half-time is the time that it takes for the gradient to decrease to half of its initial value, and this can be calculated by Doppler study with use of the simplified Bernoulli equation. On the Doppler velocity trace, the pressure half-time is measured directly from the monitor. In normal subjects, the mitral pressure half-time is less than 60 ms; during mitral stenosis, it ranges from 100 to 400 ms or longer.[7] Sometimes the slope of the transmitral velocity curve is not linear. Then the dominant slope is measured, ignoring the early spike and the last part of the curvature. Pressure half-times longer than 220 ms usually indicate valve areas below 1.0 cm^2, and the mitral valve area can be approximated as 220 divided by the pressure half-time in milliseconds.[8] Mitral valve area is normally between 4 and 6 cm^2. Severe mitral stenosis is present when the area is 1 cm^2 or less; moderate stenosis is present when the area is 1.1 to 1.5 cm^2; and mild stenosis is present when the area is 1.6 to 2 cm^2. In most cases, mitral stenosis does not give symptoms until the orifice area is less than 1.5 cm^2.

Patients who do not have mitral stenosis but who do have impaired left ventricular relaxation may also have prolonged pressure half-times. In these patients, however, the peak transmitral E (early) velocity is not elevated.

The pressure half-time is affected by changes in left atrial or left ventricular compliance and by the presence of aortic regurgitation. Left ventricular compliance determines how much left ventricular pressure increases for a given volume increment. In patients who have reduced left ventricular diastolic compliance, caused, for example, by left ventricular hypertrophy, the blood that enters the left ventricle causes a marked increase in left ventricular pressure, and the transmitral gradient decreases rapidly. Similarly, aortic regurgitation causes a more rapid rise in left ventricular diastolic pressure and thus shortens the pressure half-time. In spite of these limitations, the pressure half-time is a very useful measure of the degree of mitral stenosis. Because the pressure gradient varies with flow, it is essential to estimate valve area as well as pressure gradient.

Other Methods to Determine Mitral Orifice Area

As with the calculation of the area of a stenotic aortic valve, the continuity equation can be used to calculate mitral orifice area. The calculation is based on the principle of similar flow volume across the mitral valve and the aortic or pulmonary valve. The method for calculation of stroke volume in aortic stenosis is described elsewhere. Mitral orifice area is calculated as stroke volume divided by mitral velocity-time integral. In the presence of aortic regurgitation, flow across the pulmonary valve can be used instead, although the accuracy of calculations of the pulmonary valve area is not very good, and aortic flow measurements are preferred. Mitral regurgitation introduces an error in the calculation.

The proximal isovelocity surface area or flow convergence method may also be used to determine mitral orifice area.[9]

CHOICE OF THERAPY

Echocardiography provides important information about the choice of therapy, which may be surgical commissurotomy, balloon valvuloplasty, or valve replacement. Mitral leaflet mobility, valvular and subvalvular thickening, and degree of calcification are important factors to be considered. A high degree of valve mobility favors balloon valvuloplasty. Limited mobility of the leaflets, marked thickening, extensive calcification, and subvalvular changes with extensive thickening and shortening of the chordal structures are associated with poor outcome from balloon valvuloplasty. The presence of significant mitral regurgitation favors surgical treatment. The ideal case for balloon valvuloplasty is a patient who has a pliable valve with little calcification and no or only mild mitral regurgitation.

Patients with mild mitral stenosis (valve area >1.5 cm^2) usually do not have symptoms at rest. However, symptoms may be precipitated by exercise, fever, or atrial fibrillation. This is due to tachycardia, which reduces the diastolic filling time and leads to compensatory elevation of left atrial pressure. Symptoms may also be precipitated by pregnancy because of increased transmitral flow rate. When there is doubt about symptoms, stress testing may be useful as it may unmask symptoms and provide an objective evaluation of functional status. In asymptomatic patients, yearly clinical evaluation is recommended, and echocardiography is needed only when there is a change in clinical status. Patients who develop symptoms are potential candidates for balloon valvuloplasty or surgery. Patients with severe mitral stenosis and New York Heart Association (NYHA) functional class III or class IV heart failure have a poor prognosis if left untreated, and balloon valvuloplasty or surgery is indicated unless there is complicating comorbidity. When in doubt, Doppler examination is recommended to assess transmitral pressure gradient and pulmonary artery pressure during or immediately after exercise. If the mean transmitral pressure gradient rises above 15 mm Hg and pulmonary artery systolic pressure exceeds 60 mm Hg, it means a hemodynamically significant mitral stenosis.

SUMMARY

The diagnosis of mitral stenosis is confirmed by

- two-dimensional echocardiography showing leaflet thickening and diastolic doming (hockey-stick appearance) in the parasternal long-axis view and a fish-mouth orifice in the short-axis view;
- M-mode echocardiography showing a decrease in the initial diastolic closure motion of the anterior leaflet and diastolic anterior motion of the posterior leaflet; and
- the finding of a distended left atrium.

In most patients, the severity of mitral stenosis is adequately determined from the mean pressure gradient and area by the pressure half-time method. When in doubt, the results should be confirmed by direct measurement of the area of the orifice by planimetry of the two-dimensional image. Pulmonary artery pressure should be determined from the tricuspid regurgitation velocity.

MITRAL REGURGITATION

Mitral regurgitation is the second most frequent valve disease after aortic stenosis. The causes of mitral regurgitation include primary disease in the valve apparatus and regurgitation, which is due to left ventricular disease. Mitral regurgitation is suspected during clinical examination by a systolic murmur and presence of the third heart sound. Echocardiography is the principal examination and should include assessment of severity of regurgitation, underlying mechanisms, and reparability. In most cases, transthoracic echocardiography provides sufficient diagnostic information. Before mitral valve surgery and in particular in considering mitral valve repair, transesophageal echocardiography should be done to assess feasibility of repair. The results of mitral valve repair should be evaluated intraoperatively by transesophageal echocardiography to enable immediate surgical correction if necessary. Acute mitral regurgitation due to papillary muscle rupture may be difficult to detect clinically and should be suspected in patients with shock during myocardial infarction. Importantly, the murmur may be of low intensity or may be absent.

Mitral regurgitation may be secondary to abnormalities of

- the valve leaflets;
- the mitral annulus;
- the chordae tendineae; or
- the papillary muscles and their adjacent musculature.

It can result from

- rheumatic heart disease;
- annular dilatation and calcification;
- degenerative disease;
- endocarditis; or
- myocardial ischemia or infarction.

DIAGNOSTIC PROCEDURES AND TECHNIQUES

Echocardiography and Two-Dimensional Color and Continuous-Wave Doppler Studies

Mitral regurgitation is easily detected by two-dimensional color Doppler study, which shows retrograde flow across the mitral valve in systole (Fig. 86.5). The best views for two-dimensional color-flow study are the parasternal long-axis view and the apical view. The sensitivity of Doppler echocardiography for detection of mitral regurgitation approaches 100%. The specificity for significant regurgitation is excellent. In a large number of patients, however, Doppler study shows small regurgitations that are considered to have little or no clinical significance. Regurgitant jets that are small and are seen only in early systole appear to be part of normal leaflet closure.

Determination of the cause of mitral regurgitation is possible in most cases.[10] When the cause is rheumatic heart disease, there is thickening and reduced mobility of the leaflets. In mitral valve prolapse, there is systolic ballooning of the affected leaflet into the left atrium, and the regurgitant jet is typically eccentric (see Fig. 86.5). Because of the saddle shape of the mitral annulus, even a normal valve may appear to prolapse on the apical four-chamber view,[11] and one should look for consistent findings in other views. The parasternal long-axis view should be used, and the diagnosis should not be made unless leaflet displacement is more than 2 mm behind a line connecting the anterior and posterior

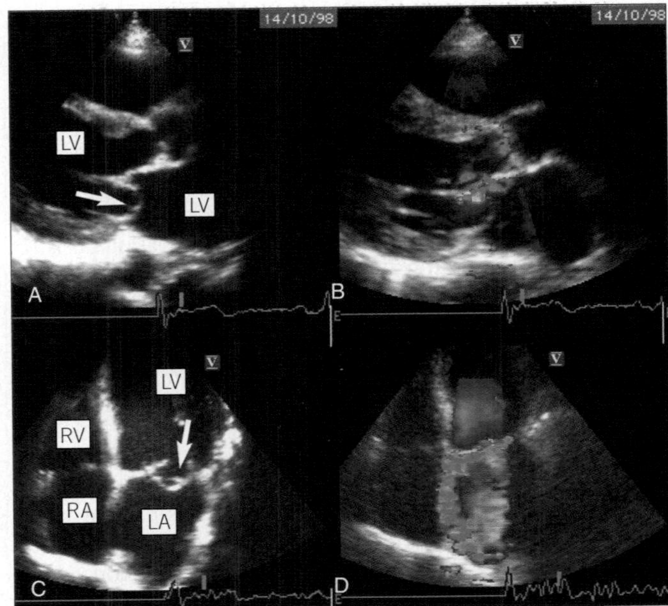

Figure 86.5 Echocardiographic studies in mitral regurgitation. Parasternal long-axis views show prolapse of the posterior mitral leaflet (**A**, *arrow*) with corresponding flow directed along the anterior mitral leaflet toward the atrial septum **(B)**. Apical four-chamber views show the prolapse more clearly (**C**, *arrow*), and the extension of the regurgitation is better visualized **(D)**. The jet is spoon shaped, broad, and thin along the wall, and it is therefore easily underestimated. LA, left atrium; LV, left ventricle; RA, right atrium; RV, right ventricle.

margins of the annulus. The diagnosis of mitral prolapse is supported by the findings of a late systolic eccentric jet, mid to late systolic posterior displacement of leaflet tissue on the M-mode echocardiogram, and thickened leaflets. In mitral regurgitation caused by infective endocarditis, vegetations may be identified.

In mitral regurgitation caused by papillary muscle dysfunction, there is myocardial dysfunction consistent with coronary artery disease. In some cases, the dysfunction is due to scarring and shrinkage of the papillary muscle, which limits leaflet motion, and the retracted leaflet does not close all the way to the level of the mitral annulus.[12] The echocardiographic signs of papillary muscle dysfunction are not reliable, however, and the echocardiographic findings are suggestive rather than conclusive.

Objective assessment of severity of the regurgitation is done by echocardiography and requires the combined use of a number of echo Doppler modalities. The following should be assessed in each patient:

- extension of the regurgitant jet into the left atrium;
- signal intensity of the regurgitant jet;
- transmitral early filling velocity;
- pattern of flow in the pulmonary veins;
- systolic pulmonary artery pressure; and
- impact on the left atrium and the left ventricle.

Although each of these approaches has a number of limitations, in combination they are very useful for clinical decision making.[13,14] In addition to these methods (which are only semiquantitative), there are quantitive methods that have proved to be useful in some laboratories. These include the continuity equation and the proximal flow convergence method. Furthermore, the width of the vena contracta represents a semiquantitative measure of the regurgitation.

Extension of the Regurgitant Jet into the Left Atrium

Determination of jet extension in the left atrium by pulsed Doppler examination was previously the most widely used method to estimate the severity of mitral regurgitation. The method is time-consuming and has been replaced by color-flow mapping. Maximum jet area is calculated in absolute terms or as a fraction of left atrial cross-sectional area. With consistent use of instrument settings in a given laboratory, the jet area method is useful in grading mitral regurgitation.[15] However, the jet area is dependent on a number of factors, which include gain setting, pulse repetition frequency, field depth, direction of the jet, and loading conditions. Importantly, for a given regurgitant volume, a jet along the atrial wall appears smaller than a free jet, the Coanda effect.[16]

Signal Intensity of the Regurgitant Jet

The strength of the continuous-wave Doppler signal of the regurgitant jet relative to that of anterograde transmitral flow provides some information about the severity of the regurgitation (Fig. 86.6). This method, however, has many limitations.

Transmitral Early Filling Velocity

When the mitral regurgitation is severe, the elevated left atrial pressure causes increased peak early transmitral filling velocities (>1.2 m/s).

Pattern of Flow in the Pulmonary Veins

In severe mitral regurgitation, the marked systolic elevation of left atrial pressure causes reversal of systolic pulmonary venous flow (see Fig. 86.6).[17] This can be measured as peak negative velocity or as a systolic velocity-time integral. Reversal of systolic pulmonary venous flow has 96% specificity and 52% sensitivity for diagnosis of severe mitral regurgitation.[18] A blunted systolic flow wave and a systolic-to-diastolic velocity ratio of less than 1 may be seen in

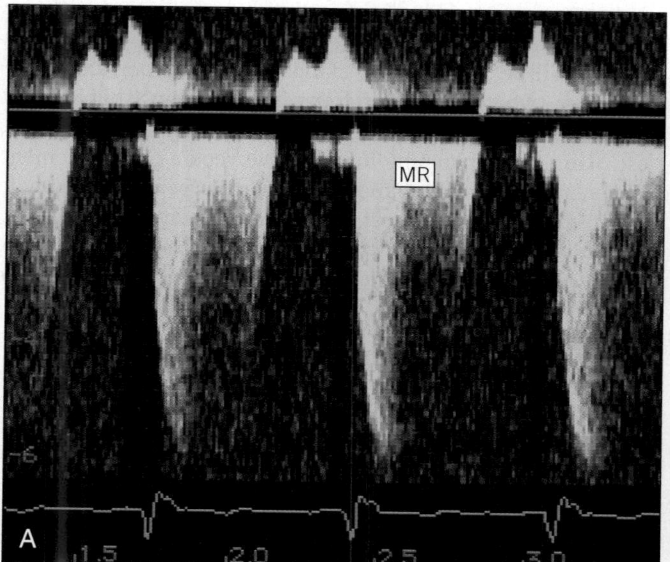

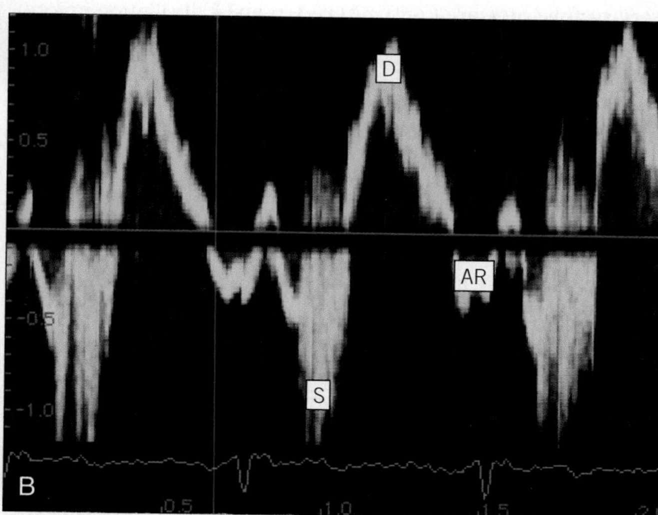

Figure 86.6 Signal intensity of the mitral regurgitant jet and reversal of pulmonary venous systolic flow. A, Continuous-wave Doppler study through severe mitral regurgitation (MR) demonstrating early maximal flow. The intensity is less than expected from the severe regurgitation owing to oblique direction of the flow. **B,** The pulsed Doppler study of the pulmonary vein shows reversed systolic flow (S), high diastolic wave (D), and broad reversed atrial contraction wave (AR). The S wave is partly disturbed by the regurgitant jet entering the vein directly, giving a broadened and less clean appearance than the rest of the tracing.

moderate mitral regurgitation. However, systolic-to-diastolic velocity ratios of less than 1 are seen normally in young adults as well as in patients who have left ventricular systolic dysfunction and elevated left ventricular filling pressure. Therefore, a blunted systolic velocity has little diagnostic value.

In most patients, adequate Doppler signals can be obtained by transthoracic echocardiography, placing the pulsed Doppler sample volume about 1 cm into a pulmonary vein. Most often, the right upper pulmonary vein gives the best recordings. High-quality images can easily be obtained by transesophageal echocardiography in nearly every patient.

Pulmonary Artery Systolic Pressure

Severe mitral regurgitation leads to elevated left atrial pressure and in turn to elevated pulmonary artery systolic pressure. Systolic pulmonary artery pressure can be estimated from a tricuspid regurgitation jet.[19]

Impact on the Left Atrium and the Left Ventricle

In chronic mitral regurgitation, an atrial diameter of more than 5.5 cm supports the diagnosis of severe regurgitation. A dilated left ventricle with an end-diastolic diameter above 7.0 cm is also consistent with severe regurgitation. A reduction in the left ventricular ejection fraction and a progressive increase in end-systolic diameter and volume are important criteria in deciding on the timing of mitral valve surgery.

Mitral valve surgery is indicated in patients who have symptoms due to chronic mitral regurgitation but no contraindication to surgery. In general, mitral valve surgery is indicated in asymptomatic patients when the regurgitation is severe and there is reduced left ventricular function (i.e., left ventricular ejection fraction $\leq$0.60 or left ventricular end-systolic diameter $\geq$4.5 cm). In severe mitral regurgitation, a substantial fraction of the left ventricular stroke volume is ejected into a low-pressure chamber, and therefore the lower limit for normal ejection fraction is higher than the conventional limit of 0.50. In patients with preserved left ventricular systolic function, the finding of markedly elevated pulmonary artery systolic pressure (>50 mm Hg) or atrial fibrillation favors surgical treatment. In patients with markedly reduced left ventricular function (ejection fraction <0.30), surgical treatment is associated with a very high risk. In such patients, feasibility of valve repair and low comorbidity may justify surgery.[20]

Quantitative Methods

The proximal isovelocity surface area (PISA) method can be useful in laboratories with sufficient experience with the method. The PISA method is based on the principles of conservation of flow and the continuity equation.[21] The acceleration of flow toward the regurgitant orifice on the left ventricular side of the mitral valve can be visualized with color flow. All flow that passes through the regurgitant orifice must also pass through the zone of flow convergence. Because the flow convergence zone is approximately hemispheric, there are isovelocity hemispheres of diminishing radius but increasing velocity as one approaches the regurgitant orifice. Because all flow that passes through the regurgitant orifice must first pass through each of the isovelocity hemispheres, it is possible to calculate regurgitant volume as the product of the velocity in one of the hemispheric shells and the surface area of the hemisphere (i.e., $2\pi r^2$).[21] By use of the aliased velocities, it is possible to read the velocity directly off the monitor, and the radius is measured on the same image as the distance from the blue-red aliasing interface to the level of the mitral leaflets. Near the orifice, the shells tend to become flatter and lose their hemispheric shape, and it is recommended that either the first or the second aliasing zone be used. If the first aliasing zone is close to the regurgitant orifice, it may be too flat to allow this calculation to work. This problem can be reduced by lowering the pulse repetition rate or by zero shifting, thus extending the first aliasing zone. The PISA method is time-consuming in clinical practice. Simplifications have been proposed, for instance, a nomogram in which the radius of the proximal isovelocity surface area is entered together with the aliasing velocity, which is given by the ultrasound machine.[22]

Serial Testing

Asymptomatic patients with moderate mitral regurgitation and preserved left ventricular function can usually be evaluated annually with clinical examination and with echocardiography performed every 2 years. Asymptomatic patients with severe mitral regurgitation and preserved left ventricular function need more frequent controls, and the time intervals should be individualized. When there is uncertainty about the duration of the mitral regurgitation, a second visit should be scheduled relatively soon to make sure that the condition is stable. When there are borderline values of left ventricular dimensions or ejection fraction, the patients need closer monitoring. In general, patients with severe mitral regurgitation and preserved left ventricular function should be seen every 6 months for clinical evaluation, and echocardiography should be performed every year. The patients should be instructed to report promptly any change in functional status and should be followed up accordingly.

Mitral Annulus Dimension

Figures 86.7 through 86.10 illustrate how mitral annulus diameters are measured. The mitral valve is elliptical and may be distorted by disease. Therefore, a minimum of measurements will be in the three standard planes (long-axis/three-chamber, two-chamber, and four-chamber views), but it is wise to scan the whole mitral ring from the apex to detect the greatest diameter in planning mitral valve repair or replacement. In general, the window giving the most perpendicular view to the structure gives the most exact measurement because of better radial resolution compared with the lateral resolution of ultrasonography. These measures are useful in evaluating the cause of regurgitation and in planning mitral valve surgery.

SUMMARY

Mitral regurgitation is suspected by typical murmur and is confirmed by color Doppler study. The cause of the regurgitation can in most instances be determined by echocardiography. The severity of mitral regurgitation is determined by taking into account clinical symptoms and signs and by using multiple echocardiographic criteria. Severe regurgitation is indicated by

- a large color-flow area (aliased velocities);
- an increased transmitral early filling velocity;
- a dense continuous-wave Doppler signal;
- the reversal of pulmonary vein systolic flow; and
- an elevated pulmonary artery systolic pressure.

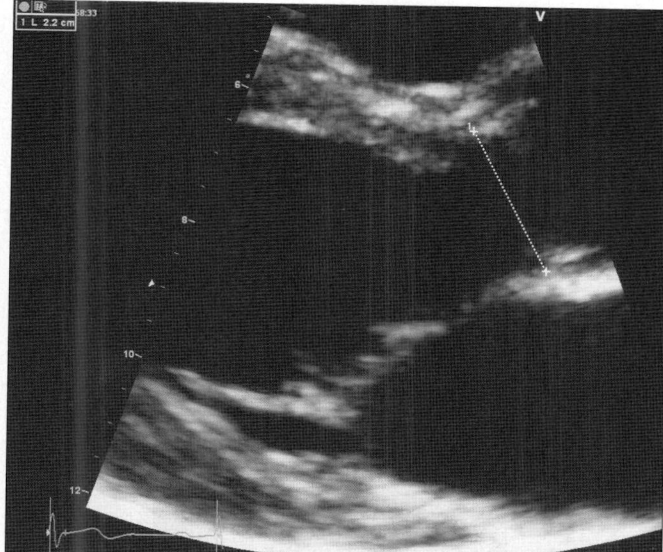

Figure 86.7 The left ventricular outflow tract diameter is measured between the hinge points of the aortic valve leaflets at its greatest diameter in parasternal or apical long-axis views. Here, the left ventricular outflow tract is approximately circular. Measurements are taken from inner edge to inner edge. Color flow may be useful to better define tissue-blood interfaces.

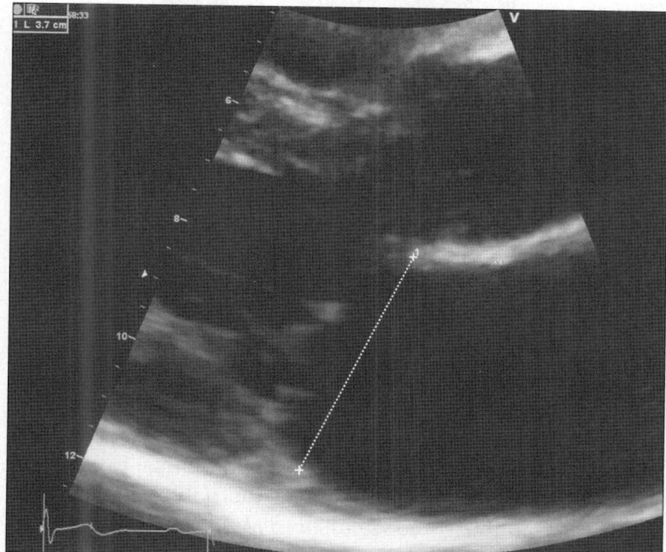

Figure 86.8 Measurement of mitral annulus diameter. Measurement of the anterior and posterior hinge points of the leaflets is usually possible from the parasternal long-axis view, in this case best determined in systole. One has to scan the whole cardiac cycle for the best delineation of the measuring points.

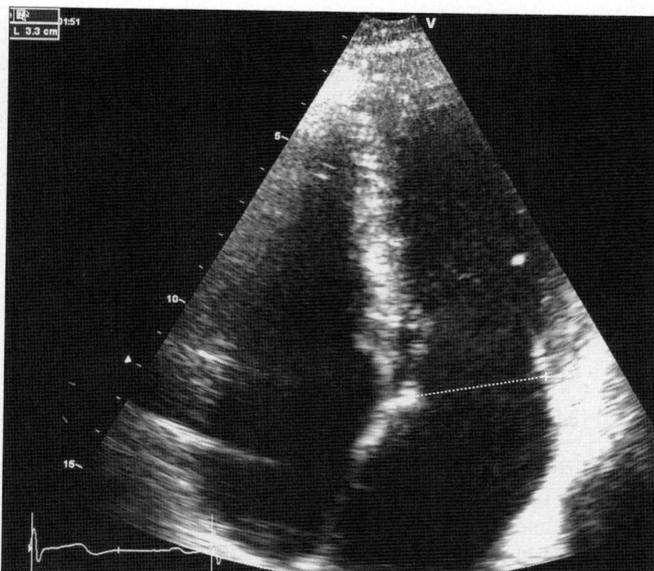

Figure 86.9 Measurement of mitral annulus diameter. Four-chamber view. The scan plane should not be placed too anteriorly to avoid the outflow tract.

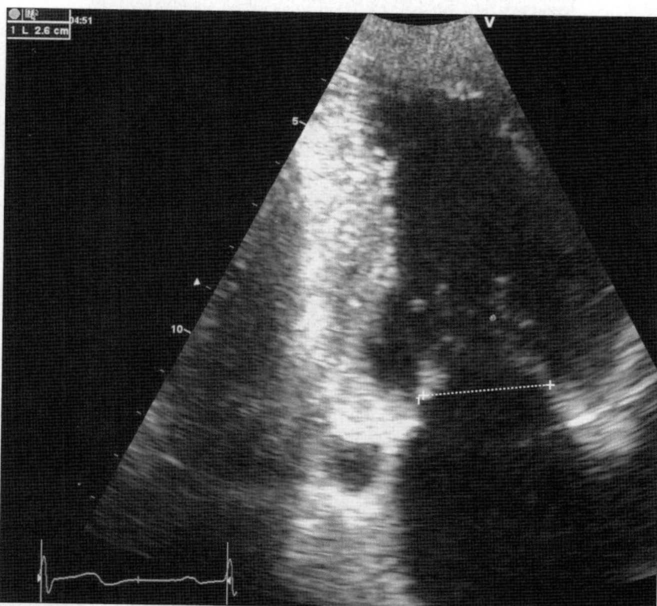

Figure 86.10 Measurement of mitral annulus diameter. Two-chamber view. Even if there often may be difficulties in observing the free wall of the left ventricle in the two-chamber view, the mitral annulus is most often clearly seen and can be measured.

In chronic mitral regurgitation, markedly dilated left atrium and dilated left ventricle support the presence of severe regurgitation.

AORTIC STENOSIS

There are three major causes of adult aortic valve stenosis:

- rheumatic heart disease;
- senile-calcific degeneration; and
- congenital bicuspid aortic valve with secondary calcification.

In the Western world, senile-calcific aortic stenosis accounts for almost half of the cases. In other parts of the world, rheumatic etiology still dominates. Aortic stenosis due to rheumatic heart disease is characterized by commissural fusion and fibrosis as well as by calcification of the cusps. Furthermore, rheumatic aortic stenosis is invariably accompanied by mitral valve disease.

Senile-calcific aortic stenosis is characterized morphologically by nodular excrescences within the valve pockets that restrict motion. The bicuspid aortic valve is characterized by leaflets of unequal size, the larger of which often contains a fibrous ridge (raphe) at the site of congenital fusion. When there is marked calcification of the valve pockets, this produces a narrowed orifice that is shaped like an ellipse. When there is little calcification, systolic doming of the stenotic valve is often seen; this is most common in young patients who have congenital or rheumatic disease.

Aortic sclerosis, which is defined as valve thickening without obstruction to left ventricular outflow, is a condition that may be prognostic for development of aortic stenosis. Aortic sclerosis is present in about 25% of adults older than 65 years and has been associated with adverse clinical outcome related to valve hemodynamics.[23-25]

DIAGNOSTIC PROCEDURES AND TECHNIQUES

Echocardiography

From the parasternal long- and short-axis views, two-dimensional echocardiography reveals thickening and reduced motion of the leaflets, and M-mode echocardiography shows reduced cusp separation and often multiple echo lines in the aortic root (Figs. 86.11 and 86.12). Normal aortic valve area in the adult is 3 to 4 cm^2, and normal opening produces about 2 cm of leaflet separation. Cusp separation smaller than 1.2 cm suggests significant aortic stenosis. The M-mode echocardiogram, however, is inaccurate and cannot be used to grade the severity of aortic stenosis. In patients who have noncalcific aortic stenosis with systolic doming (as in bicuspid aortic valve), the restriction of the valve opening may occur distal to the M-mode cursor, and the M-mode echocardiogram may therefore appear normal. Two-dimensional echocardiography is helpful in sorting out this problem by showing the bicuspid valve, and Doppler studies show increased velocities across the valve. Two-dimensional echocardiography is a highly sensitive method for detection of aortic stenosis and for separation of aortic stenosis from aortic sclerosis. It is necessary, however, to perform Doppler echocardiography to determine the severity of the aortic stenosis. As a result of the stenosis, the velocity across the valve is increased, indicating increased transvalvular pressure gradient.

Owing to increased wall stress, there is usually left ventricular hypertrophy. The transmitral filling velocities may show signs of impaired relaxation with a relative shift in filling toward end-diastole. At a late stage in the disease, the left ventricle may decompensate, with progressive dilatation and reduction in ejection fraction.

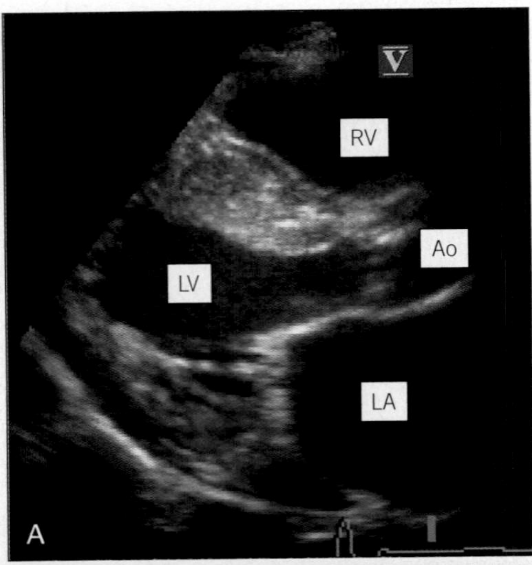

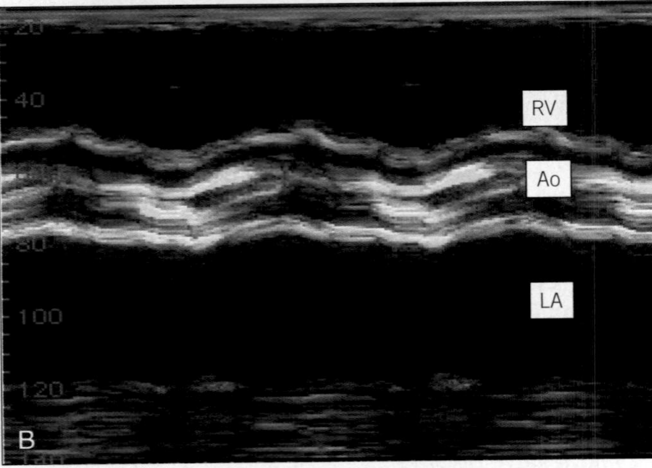

Figure 86.11 Echocardiography of aortic stenosis. A, Parasternal long-axis view of a stenotic aortic valve in systole. The valve is thickened, with reduced opening. The walls, in particular the interventricular septum, are hypertrophic. **B,** Corresponding M-mode study through the stenotic valve. Ao, aorta; LA, left atrium; LV, left ventricle; RV, right ventricle.

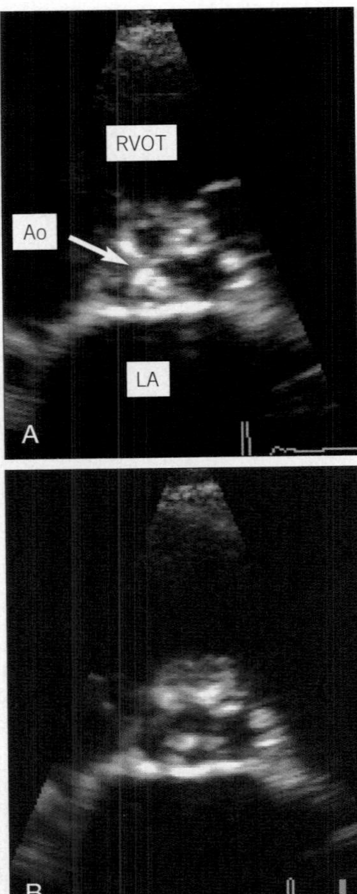

Figure 86.12 Calcified aortic valve. Parasternal short-axis view in diastole **(A)** and systole **(B)** shows high echo density and limited opening. Ao, aortic valve; LA, left atrium; RVOT, right ventricular outflow tract.

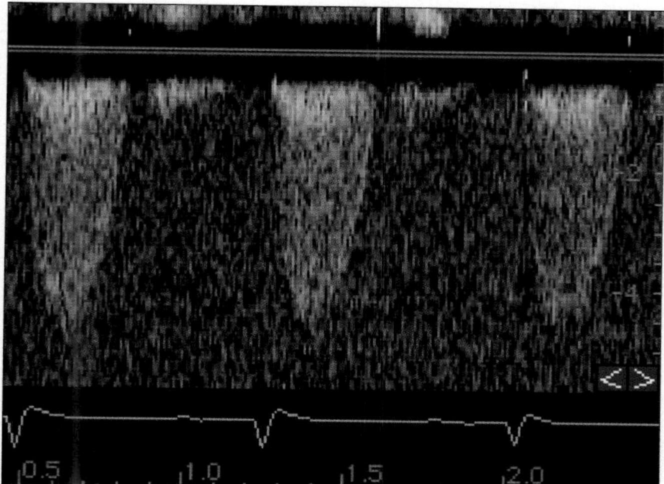

Figure 86.13 Continuous-wave Doppler study through a stenotic aortic valve. The maximum pressure gradient was 74 mm Hg, and the mean gradient was 47 mm Hg. The calculated stenotic area was 0.7 cm^2.

Degree of valvular calcification, size of the aortic annulus, and secondary dilatation in the ascending aorta should be assessed. These factors are important for the surgeon.

Aortic stenosis is graded in terms of pressure gradient and valve area. The pressure gradient is calculated from the continuous-wave Doppler signal (Fig. 86.13).[7,26-28] From the additional measurement of left ventricular outflow tract (LVOT) velocity by pulsed-wave Doppler study and LVOT diameter, it is possible to calculate aortic valve area.[29-31]

Pressure Gradient

The most critical step in the ultrasound evaluation of aortic stenosis is the careful search for maximum velocity across the valve by continuous-wave Doppler study. It is recommended that one start from the apical position, with the patient in the left lateral decubitus position, and use the two-dimensional image as a guide. The patient should then be turned to the right lateral decubitus position and measurements made from the right intercostal spaces. Velocities should also be recorded from the suprasternal position; in some patients, the subcostal position gives the best signal. A nonimaging continuous-wave Doppler transducer is recommended as it is smaller and fits better between the ribs. The highest obtained velocities should be used.

The velocities are related to the pressure difference across the valve as described by the Bernoulli equation. By use of the simplified Bernoulli equation, which ignores the viscous term and the flow acceleration term, the pressure difference across the valve can be calculated with good accuracy.[28,30]

The mean gradient and the maximum gradient are calculated from the velocity curve. In a clinical context, the mean gradient is more important than the maximum gradient because the mean gradient is a better measure of the systolic load on the left ventricle and approximates the peak-to-peak gradient obtained from invasive studies. In general, a mean pressure gradient of more than 40 mm Hg indicates severe aortic stenosis with a small valve area, whereas a mean gradient of less than 10 mm Hg indicates no aortic stenosis. Mean gradients in the range of 10 to 25 mm Hg suggest mild stenosis, and mean gradients in the range of 25 to 40 mm Hg suggest moderate stenosis. However, in patients who have reduced systolic function, a gradient in the range of 20 to 50 mm Hg may reflect severe stenosis with a small area due to the flow dependency of transvalvular gradients.

The flow dependency is the most important limitation when gradient determinations are used to quantify aortic stenosis. When stroke volume is reduced, there is reduced flow across the valve, and this leads to a smaller gradient. On the other hand, a mildly stenotic valve may have a high gradient if stroke volume is markedly increased, as in aortic regurgitation. Therefore, one should always try to obtain aortic valve area in patients with aortic stenosis. When the gradient is less than 50 mm Hg, the determination of area becomes increasingly important. Stress echocardiography with low-dose dobutamine may be useful as a means to differentiate between true severe aortic stenosis and reduced valve area due to reduced flow. The dobutamine stress testing, however, should be performed only in centers with significant experience in dobutamine stress testing, and appropriate interpretation of the test requires significant experience with this specific procedure during aortic stenosis.

Ideally, the Doppler gradient should be calculated as $4(V_2^2-V_1^2)$, where V_2 is peak velocity and V_1 is velocity proximal to the stenosis. When V_1 is small relative to V_2, the error is small when V_1 is ignored. However, when the aortic stenosis is mild or when the prestenotic velocity is high (more than 1 m/s), as in aortic regurgitation, the contribution from V_1^2 becomes important, and the transvalvular gradient is overestimated by assuming that $\Delta P = 4V^2$. In general, however, this limitation is not of great importance in the presence of severe stenosis.

Pitfalls

A mitral regurgitant jet can be misinterpreted as an aortic stenosis jet, particularly when the mitral regurgitant jet is directed against the posterior aortic wall, as in prolapse of the posterior mitral leaflet. This problem is solved by examining the timing of the jet in relation to the opening and closing of the two valves, by obtaining consistent signals from more than one window, and by confirming a typical aortic stenosis shape of the Doppler spectral display.

The findings on two-dimensional echocardiography should also be consistent with the Doppler data.

In patients who have variations in stroke volume as a result of arrhythmias, the gradient may vary markedly from beat to beat, and an average of multiple consecutive beats should be used.

Valve Area

Because flow in the distal LVOT is equal to flow across the aortic valve, the continuity equation can be used to calculate valve area (Fig. 86.14).[29,30,32] Valve area is equal to stroke volume divided by the time-velocity integral of peak velocities across the valve:

$$\text{Stroke volume} = A_{LVOT} \times VTI_{LVOT}$$

The continuity principle anticipates that $A_{LVOT} \times VTI_{LVOT} = A_{ao} \times VTI_{ao}$. Consequently, $A_{ao} = A_{LVOT} \times VTI_{LVOT}/VTI_{ao}$.

In other words, stroke volume is calculated as the product of LVOT area (A_{LVOT}) and LVOT velocity-time integral

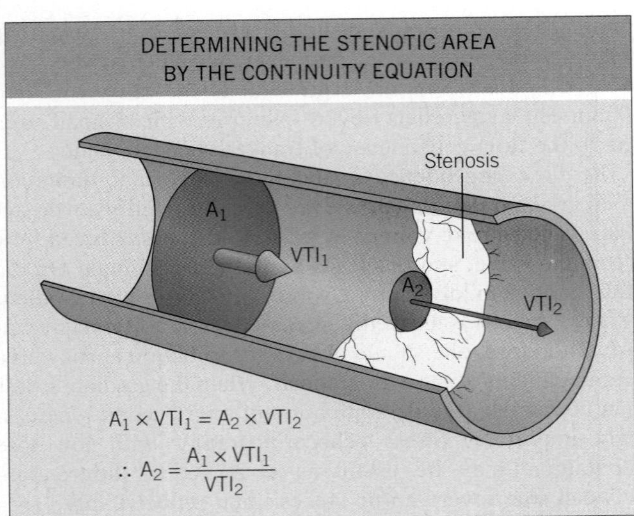

Figure 86.14 Determination of the stenotic area by the continuity equation. A_1 is calculated from the diameter in the left ventricular outflow tract (LVOT), assuming a nearly circular distal part of the LVOT. A_2 is the area within the stenosis. VTI_1 is measured by pulsed Doppler study, and VTI_2 is measured by continuous-wave Doppler study.

(VTI_{LVOT}). Outflow tract area is calculated from its diameter measured just proximal to the stenosis, using a two-dimensional parasternal long-axis view and assuming that the LVOT is circular (see Fig. 86.7). The diameter should be measured in midsystole at the annulus, from the trailing edge of the anterior echo to the leading edge of the posterior echo. The measurement of LVOT diameter represents the largest source of error in the calculation of valve area. In general, an area of 1.0 cm^2 or less means severe aortic stenosis. In a large patient, however, an area of 1 cm^2 may indicate severe stenosis; in a small patient, an area as low as 0.7 cm^2 may be adequate. Areas between 1.0 and 1.5 cm^2 mean moderate aortic stenosis, and areas above 1.5 cm^2 mean mild aortic stenosis.[33]

Because of the potential inaccuracies in its calculation, valve area alone cannot be relied on for clinical decision making. It should always be considered in combination with pressure gradient, left ventricular function, and clinical status.

The LVOT velocity-time integral is measured from an apical window by pulsed-wave Doppler study. The sampling position is moved stepwise toward the valve, and measurements are taken proximal to the site at which the velocities accelerate more abruptly. The area with flow acceleration may not be well defined, however, and this represents a source of error in the calculation. Figure 86.7 illustrates how to measure LVOT diameter. Septal hypertrophy or other outflow tract obstruction may preclude the calculation of left ventricular stroke volume. One should attempt to measure diameter and velocities from the same anatomic site. The velocity-time integral of the aortic stenosis jet (VTI_{ao}) is measured from the window that gives the highest velocities.

Peak velocities may be used in the continuity equation instead of the velocity-time integral. One advantage of measuring velocity-time integrals rather than peak velocities is that the calculation of stroke volume and cardiac output serves as a control that the measurements are not too far off.

Because aortic stenosis can be associated with dilatation of the ascending aorta, one should always measure aortic root dimension. For the anatomy of the thoracic aorta to be fully delineated, supplementary studies with computed tomography or magnetic resonance are often needed.

When in doubt, transesophageal echocardiography should be performed and valve area should also be determined by planimetry to ascertain whether the data are consistent. Determination of aortic valve area by transesophageal echocardiography is not an accepted quantitative method, but it can be useful in identifying patients with severe aortic stenosis.

Unless there is complicating comorbidity, nearly all symptomatic patients with severe aortic stenosis are candidates for aortic valve replacement. In asymptomatic patients, there is disagreement about indications for surgery. Sudden death in aortic stenosis is rare in asymptomatic patients. However, after onset of symptoms, annual mortality is high. Therefore, the patients should be monitored closely for development of symptoms. Echocardiographic signs of reduced left ventricular systolic function and hypertrophy are markers of high risk, and their presence supports the need for surgical treatment.

Exercise Testing

Exercise testing is contraindicated in symptomatic patients with aortic stenosis because of the high risk of complications. However, exercise testing may be useful for unmasking of symptoms and for risk stratification in asymptomatic patients with severe aortic stenosis.[20,23] Electrocardiographic ST depression during exercise occurs in about 80% of adults with asymptomatic aortic stenosis and has no known prognostic value. Exercise testing, however, can unmask symptoms and show limited exercise capacity or abnormal blood pressure response. The interpretation of the exercise test is important in relation to choice of therapy. Breathlessness on exercise, however, may be difficult to interpret in physically inactive patients, particularly in the elderly, and decision making with regard to surgery may still be difficult. In physically active patients, an abnormal exercise test is a strong indication for surgery in asymptomatic severe aortic stenosis. Exercise testing in asymptomatic patients should be done under the supervision of an experienced physician and with close monitoring of blood pressure and electrocardiogram.

SUMMARY

The major causes of aortic stenosis are rheumatic heart disease, senile-calcific degeneration, and bicuspid aortic valve. Aortic stenosis is suspected from the history and clinical findings and is confirmed by the combined use of two-dimensional and M-mode echocardiography and Doppler study. Severity of aortic stenosis is determined by measuring maximum velocity across the valve and calculating mean pressure gradient. As the gradient is flow dependent, it is also essential to calculate orifice area.

AORTIC REGURGITATION

Aortic regurgitation is caused by

- diseases that affect the aortic valve, such as endocarditis, rheumatic heart disease, and degenerative changes in a bicuspid or tricuspid valve; and

- conditions that lead to dilatation of the aortic root, such as various connective tissue diseases and the so-called idiopathic dilatation of the aortic root (or annuloaortic ectasia).

DIAGNOSTIC PROCEDURES AND TECHNIQUES

The most important clinical signs in chronic aortic regurgitation are a diastolic murmur and exaggerated arterial pulsations with low diastolic pressure. In acute aortic regurgitation, however, peripheral signs are less marked. Pulse pressure may not be increased because systolic pressure is reduced, and the diastolic murmur may be short and soft due to rapid pressure equalization between the aorta and the left ventricle.

Echocardiography and Two-Dimensional Color and Continuous-Wave Doppler Studies

Aortic regurgitation can be easily visualized by two-dimensional color Doppler study as reversed flow through the valve in diastole (Figs. 86.15 and 86.16). In addition, continuous-wave Doppler study gives jet velocities and the timing of reversed flow. Any associated or causal lesion in the valve itself or in the aortic root can often be identified by tissue echo. In some patients, there may be fine diastolic fluttering of the anterior mitral leaflet, which vibrates between the two jets. In some patients, there may be premature closure of the mitral valve and short deceleration time of early mitral velocity (<150 ms) due to marked elevation in left ventricular diastolic pressure. About 30% of people older than 75 years are found to have some degree of aortic regurgitation (usually minimal) when studied by Doppler echocardiography.[34]

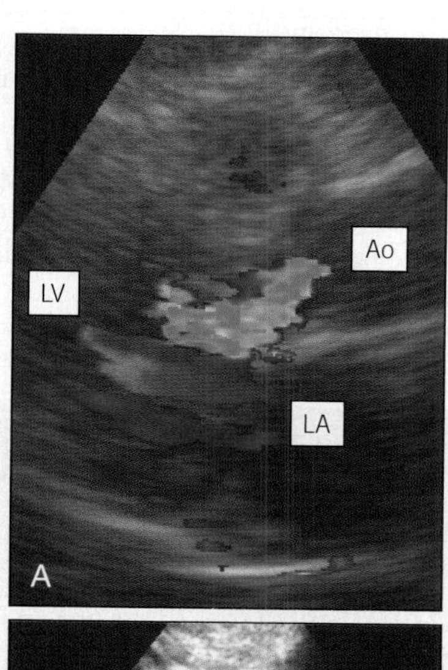

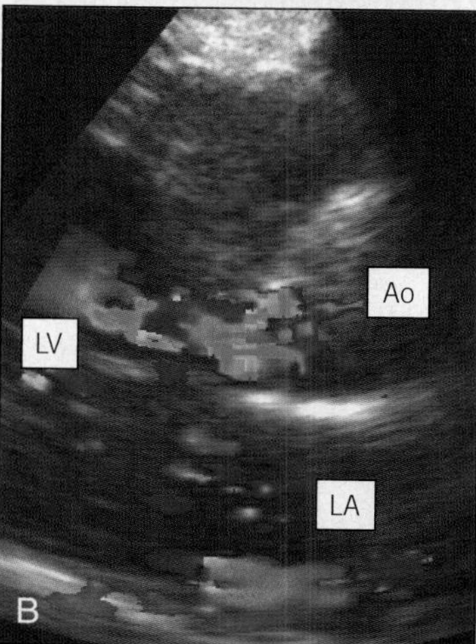

Figure 86.15 Parasternal long-axis view with color Doppler study in aortic regurgitation. A, Patient with a narrow origin of the regurgitant jet, indicating a small regurgitation. **B,** Another patient with a wide origin of the regurgitant jet, indicating a severe regurgitation. Ao, aorta; LA, left atrium; LV, left ventricle.

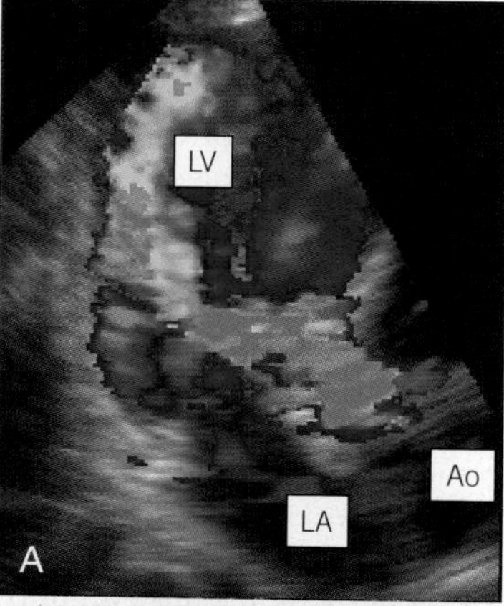

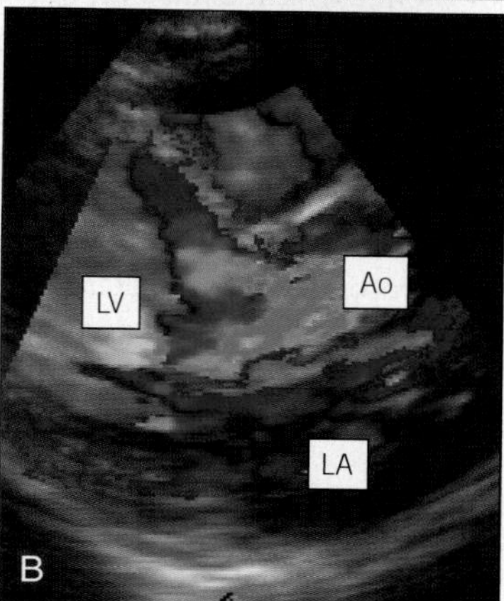

Figure 86.16 Severe aortic regurgitation. A, Apical view showing a wide jet reaching to the apex. **B,** Parasternal long-axis view showing a wide origin of the jet, although this view does not demonstrate that the jet extends far into the ventricle. Ao, aorta; LA, left atrium; LV, left ventricle.

Determination of the severity of aortic regurgitation by echocardiography requires the combined use of a number of echo-Doppler modalities. In each patient, it is recommended that the following be assessed:

- proximal regurgitant jet dimension in the LVOT;
- decay rate of the regurgitant velocity (pressure half-time);
- diastolic flow reversal in the descending aorta or peripheral arteries;
- intensity of the regurgitant flow signal compared with anterograde flow; and
- left ventricular stroke volume, which is increased when there is a large regurgitant volume.

In experienced laboratories, quantitative measurement of regurgitant volume and regurgitant surface area can be performed.

For timing of surgery, it is important to determine the impact of the regurgitation on left ventricular function. One should attempt to define the mechanism of regurgitation and to determine the feasibility of valve repair. For the latter issue to be resolved, transesophageal echocardiography may be required.

Proximal Jet Area and Diameter in the Left Ventricular Outflow Tract by Color Doppler Study

Extension of the regurgitant jet in terms of color-flow area correlates poorly with angiographic grading of aortic regurgitation,[35] and this reflects the difficulty of separating the contributions from aortic regurgitation and mitral inflow. Measurement of the jet length is also an unreliable method as patients with mild aortic regurgitation may have a narrow jet that extends far into the left ventricular cavity. The diameter or cross-sectional area of the jet at its origin is the best color Doppler index of severity of aortic regurgitation.[35] The area of the jet measured at the level of the aortic valve should in principle reflect the size of the defect. For optimal spatial resolution, a parasternal view should be used. The maximum diameter or cross-sectional area of the jet is measured at the junction of the LVOT and the aortic annulus and is expressed in percentage of LVOT diameter or area in the same location. As an approximation, jet diameter ratios of less than 25% indicate mild aortic regurgitation, ratios between 25% and 50% indicate moderate regurgitation, and ratios of more than 50% indicate severe regurgitation. There are several limitations to this approach, including dependency on jet direction and shape as well as spatial resolution and settings of the Doppler instrument.

Decay Rate of the Regurgitant Velocity by Continuous-Wave Doppler Study

As aortic regurgitation causes blood to flow from the aorta into the left ventricle during diastole, aortic pressure decreases faster and left ventricular pressure rises faster than normally. Therefore, the decay rate of the diastolic aortic to left ventricular pressure gradient is increased and reflects the severity of the aortic regurgitation.[36-38]

A measure of the decay rate is the pressure half-time (i.e., the time required to reach half of the initial gradient as estimated by continuous-wave Doppler study; Fig. 86.17). In general, a pressure half-time of 400 ms has been reported as separating mild from hemodynamically significant aortic regurgitation, and a half-time of 250 to 300 ms separates moderate from severe aortic regurgitation.

The pressure half-time, however, is determined not only by the regurgitant orifice area but also by the compliance of the aorta and the rate of volume losses to the peripheral circulation and to the left ventricle. In patients who have a dilated aorta and increased aortic compliance, a large volume can leave the aorta with a small decrease in aortic pressure, and therefore the pressure half-time is prolonged. An increase in peripheral resistance tends to prolong the half-time, as this reduces runoff to the periphery. Reduced left ventricular diastolic compliance tends to shorten the half-time, as left ventricular pressure rises markedly with small increments in left ventricular volume.

Diastolic Flow Reversal in the Descending Aorta and Peripheral Arteries by Pulsed-Wave Doppler Study

With severe aortic regurgitation, there is diastolic flow reversal in peripheral arteries. This can be measured in the subclavian and the carotid arteries. Most often, flow reversal is

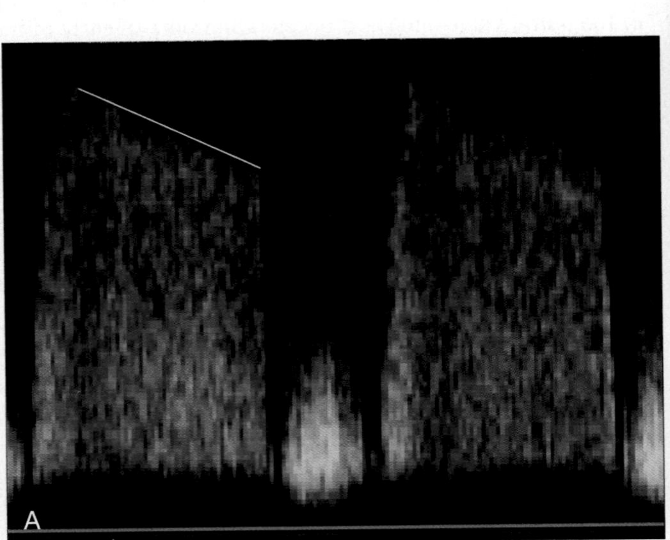

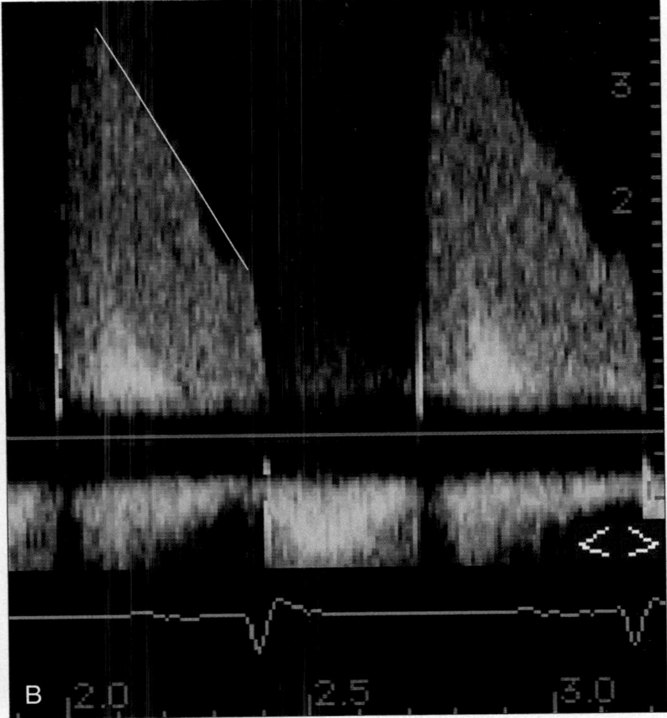

Figure 86.17 Continuous-wave Doppler study through aortic regurgitant jets. A, Small regurgitant jet (pressure half-time is 900 ms). **B,** Large regurgitant jet (pressure half-time is 175 ms). The added lines indicate the tracing for calculation of pressure half-time.

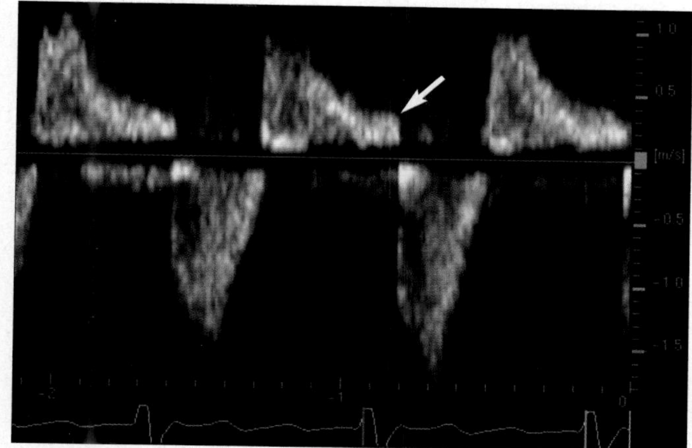

Figure 86.18 Pulsed Doppler study in the descending limb of the aortic arch. This study was recorded from the suprasternal notch. Diastolic regurgitant flow can be seen, with increased end-diastolic velocity, 0.40 m/s *(arrow)*, which indicates a severe aortic regurgitation.

measured in the descending thoracic aorta (Fig. 86.18) and can be assessed as the ratio between end-diastolic flow velocity and peak systolic flow velocity[39] or as an absolute reversed velocity. There are no established velocity criteria for grading of regurgitation. It has been proposed that a reversed velocity of 0.25 m/s or more at end-diastole indicates severe aortic regurgitation.

In patients who have marked dilatation of the ascending aorta, however, this method tends to underestimate aortic regurgitation severity, as a large volume pendulates between the left ventricle and the ascending aorta. Furthermore, it can be predicted that diastolic flow reversal is dependent on the heart rate (i.e., bradycardia reduces end-diastolic flow reversal, and tachycardia leads to higher end-diastolic reverse velocities). Another problem in the aortic arch is a flow pattern at the inner curvature different from that at the outer curvature. In general, however, holodiastolic flow reversal in the descending aorta and peripheral arteries indicates moderate or severe aortic regurgitation. The more peripherally the reversed flow is observed, the more severe the regurgitation.

Intensity of the Regurgitant Flow Signal

High regurgitant jet signal intensity relative to intensity of forward flow supports hemodynamically significant aortic regurgitation. The grading by this method, however, is subjective.

Stroke Volume

A large stroke volume calculated from diameter and velocity in the LVOT is consistent with significant aortic regurgitation. Direct calculation of the regurgitant volume is feasible, but the methods are not suitable for routine clinical use.

Aortic Dimensions

It is recommended that diameter of the ascending aorta be measured at four different levels (annulus, sinuses of Valsalva, sinotubular junction, and maximum diameter of the ascending aorta), and indexing for body surface area can be recommended especially in patients of small body size and women.[20] The indications for combined valve and aortic root surgery are outlined in recent guidelines.[20]

Impact on Left Ventricular Function

Aortic regurgitation imposes additional volume load on the left ventricle. As an adaptive response, the left ventricle dilates to accommodate the regurgitant volume, and in early stages of the disease, it may show exaggerated wall motion. With severe aortic regurgitation, the ventricle continues to dilate and may eventually fail. For the sake of a good long-term prognosis, it is essential to perform valve surgery before there is irreversible injury of the ventricle. Left ventricular size and ejection fraction are important markers of disease progression, and marked changes may indicate irreversible injury.

In patients with severe aortic regurgitation and symptoms (NYHA class II to class IV or angina), surgical treatment is usually recommended even if ejection fraction is normal. In patients with no symptoms, surgery is generally recommended if left ventricular ejection fraction is below normal ($\leq$0.50). Valve replacement is also recommended in asymptomatic patients with normal ejection fraction if there is marked left ventricular dilatation (end-diastolic diameter >7.0 to 7.5 cm or end-systolic diameter >5.5 cm).[20,23] When left ventricular diameter approaches these values, the patient should be monitored closely with frequent echocardiograms (every 4 to 6 months). Body size should be taken into account when these numbers are used, but there is lack of agreement as to whether normalization to body surface area should be done.[23] It is also important to remember that the variability of diameter measurement is about 0.5 cm. Therefore, one should look for trends in the measurements and not put too much emphasis on a small change between two sets of measurements. In patients with long-standing arterial hypertension and reduced left ventricular compliance and in patients with concomitant mitral stenosis, there may be less left ventricular dilatation, and the dimension criteria referred to before do not strictly apply. In such patients, it is more important to monitor left ventricular ejection fraction. Pulmonary artery pressures should be estimated by Doppler study, and the finding of pulmonary hypertension is another sign that the ventricle has begun to fail. In acute aortic regurgitation, the criteria for when to operate are different, and early surgical intervention is important.

Serial Testing

Most patients with mild or moderate aortic regurgitation can be seen by a cardiologist on a yearly basis, and it is usually sufficient with echocardiography every 2 years. Patients with severe aortic regurgitation and normal left ventricular function should be seen a few months after the first visit to make sure that the condition is stable. If measurements and clinical condition are stable, follow-up can be done annually; but in some patients, more frequent visits are needed, depending on clinical status. In patients with dilated aortic root and especially in patients with Marfan's syndrome or bicuspid aortic valve, examination of the aorta should be performed on a yearly basis and with closer intervals if there are signs of progressive aortic enlargement.

SUMMARY

Aortic regurgitation is suspected from clinical findings and is confirmed by two-dimensional color Doppler study as reversed flow through the valve in diastole. Severity of the regurgitation is best determined by taking into account the clinical condition and by using several echocardiographic parameters, which include assessment of proximal jet dimension in the LVOT, decay rate of the regurgitant velocity (pressure half-time), and diastolic flow reversal in the descending aorta or peripheral arteries. It is also essential to determine the impact of the regurgitation on left ventricular function. Surgery should be performed before there are signs of irreversible damage of left ventricular function.

TRICUSPID VALVE DISEASE

Acquired tricuspid stenosis is rare and is most often caused by rheumatic heart disease. The mitral lesion is typically more severe and usually dominates. Tricuspid stenosis may also occur with carcinoid and endomyocardial fibrosis. Two-dimensional echocardiography shows doming, thickening, and restricted motion of the leaflets. The M-mode findings resemble those in mitral stenosis.

The pressure half-time method has never been validated for the tricuspid valve, and planimetry of the valve area is difficult for technical reasons. A mean pressure gradient of more than 5 mm Hg is considered indicative of clinically significant tricuspid stenosis.[20,40]

Tricuspid regurgitation is common and is most often due to right ventricular dilatation. Other causes are rheumatic heart disease, prolapse, carcinoid, and endocarditis. Quantification is not easy as there is no good reference method. Systolic flow reversal into the inferior vena cava and hepatic veins supports severe regurgitation. A large jet by color-flow imaging also supports severe regurgitation (Fig. 86.19). The Doppler technique for detection of tricuspid regurgitation is highly sensitive, and a minor degree of incompetence is common even in people who have no known heart disease.

PULMONARY VALVE DISEASE

The most common pulmonary valve problem is congenital pulmonary stenosis. Acquired pulmonary stenosis is most commonly caused by carcinoid disease; the next most common causes are rheumatic disease and endocarditis. Pulmonary stenosis may also be seen in association with other congenital lesions. Echocardiography may show systolic doming, and Doppler examination shows increased transvalvular velocities.

A small degree of pulmonary regurgitation is often detected by pulsed and color Doppler studies, even in normal subjects. Significant pulmonary regurgitation is most often due to pulmonary hypertension, either primary or secondary to other cardiac disorders. Pulmonary regurgitation may also be seen in endocarditis and in carcinoid. Pulmonary regurgitation in general has a benign course, and the clinical outcome is determined by the associated heart disease.

ENDOCARDITIS

The echocardiographic criterion for diagnosis of endocarditis is the finding of vegetations on one of the valve leaflets. The mitral valve is most frequently involved. Aortic valve endocarditis may seed and infect the anterior mitral leaflet and the chordae. Vegetations may arise in the LVOT immediately below the valve. Tricuspid endocarditis is suggested by the triad of narcotic addiction, fever, and multiple lung lesions (septic emboli).

Vegetations can be demonstrated by two-dimensional echocardiography as well as on M-mode echocardiography. They are seen as an echogenic mass (Figs. 86.20 to 86.22). It is important to look for complications of the endocarditis, including

- abscess formation, which in some cases can be seen as a structure with an echo-free center;
- perforation of the leaflet with regurgitation; and
- fistulas.

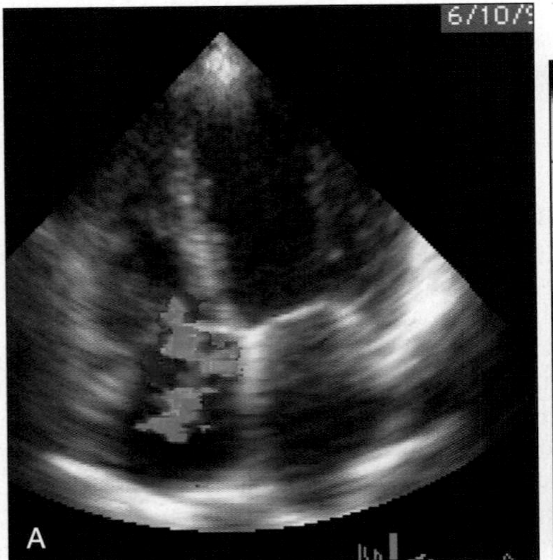

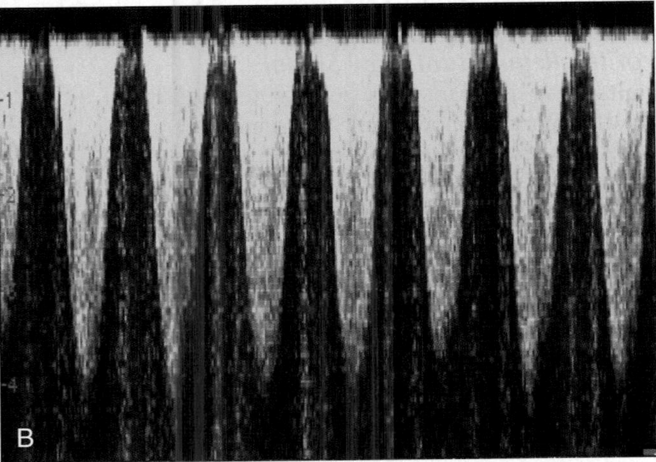

Figure 86.19 Echocardiography of tricuspid regurgitation. A, Apical four-chamber view with color Doppler study through a tricuspid valve with a medium to severe regurgitation. **B,** Corresponding continuous Doppler recording through the jet demonstrating a peak velocity of 4 m/s, which indicates a systolic pressure in the right ventricle of at least 64 mm Hg (plus the pressure in the right atrium).

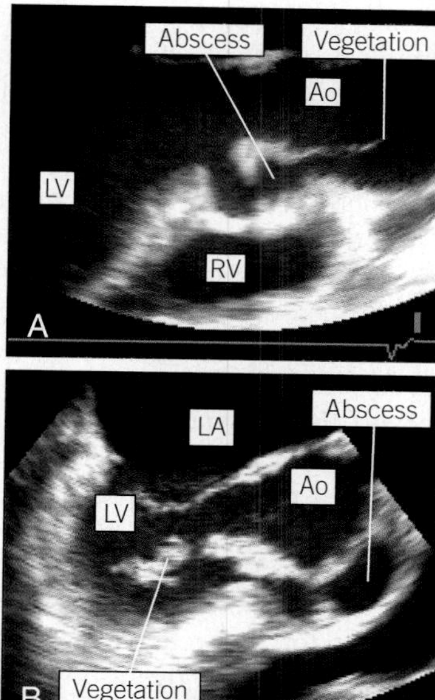

Figure 86.20 Transesophageal long-axis views in systole (A) and diastole (B) through an infected aortic valve. A, A long, slim vegetation stretches from the anterior part of the aortic valve in systole. **B,** In diastole, the same vegetation is pendulating into the left ventricle, where it looks more bulky because it is cut differently. In addition, there are abscesses between the aorta and the right ventricular outflow tract. Ao, aorta; LV, left ventricle; RV, right ventricle.

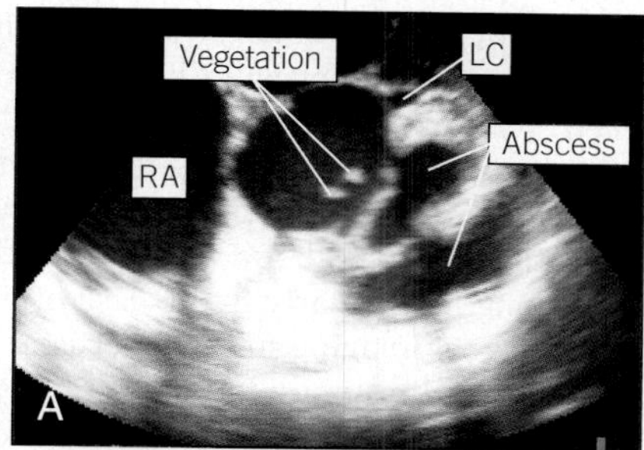

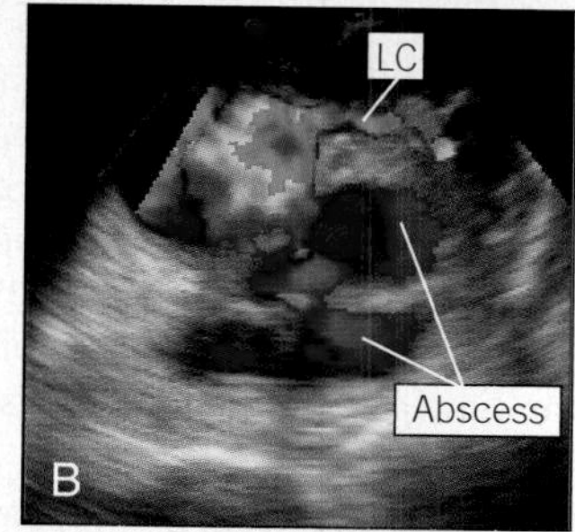

Figure 86.21 Transesophageal short-axis views through the aortic bulb in a patient with an infected aortic valve. These studies are from the same patient as in Figure 86.20. **A,** Vegetations in the aorta can be seen, as can abscesses between the aorta and the right ventricular outflow tract. **B,** The scan is positioned at the level of the main stem of the left coronary artery (LC), where flow is demonstrated. RA, right atrium.

Transesophageal echocardiography is far more sensitive than transthoracic echocardiography in detecting vegetations and complications from endocarditis; the sensitivities are approximately 60% and 90%, respectively.

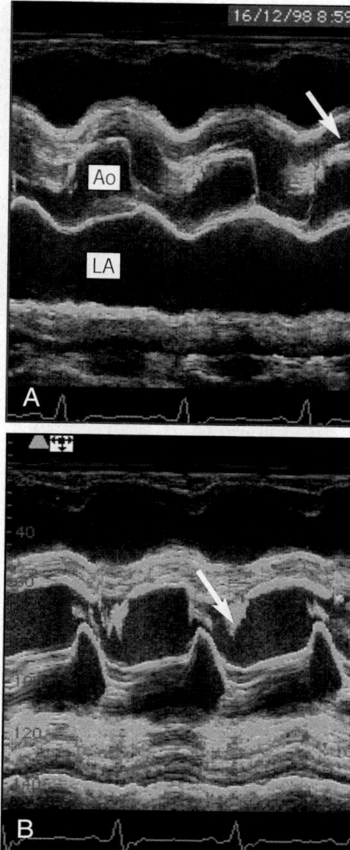

Figure 86.22 Vegetations in patients with infected valves. These transthoracic studies are from the same patient as in Figures 86.20 and 86.21. **A,** M-mode recording through the aortic valve showing vegetations during systole *(arrow)*. **B,** M-mode recording through the mitral valve. Thick vegetations appear in late diastole *(arrow)*. Ao, aorta; LA, left atrium.

Vegetations can be seen for several months to years after the endocarditis has been cured. In acute endocarditis, the vegetations appear soft and with variable degrees of independent motion, whereas chronic or healed vegetations are more echo dense and fixed.

PROSTHETIC CARDIAC VALVES

ASSESSMENT OF PROSTHETIC VALVE FUNCTION

The mechanical prostheses normally produce different sounds related to valve opening and closure, and it is difficult in most cases to tell from a clinical examination whether valve function is normal. Echocardiography is the main tool for assessment of prosthetic valve function. The difference in physical characteristics and hemodynamic profiles of the various prostheses complicates the assessment. Furthermore, most of the prostheses cause acoustic shadowing and reverberations, which obscure structural echoes and Doppler signals from behind the valve. These problems can be reduced by adjusting the gain and by using multiple views. In many cases, transesophageal echocardiography is necessary, particularly for evaluation of a mitral prosthesis.

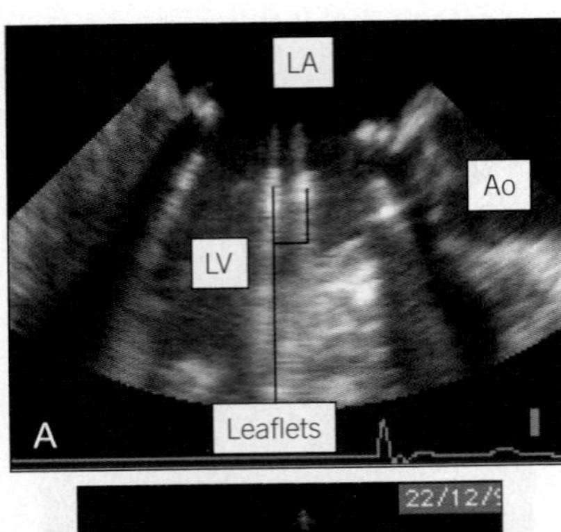

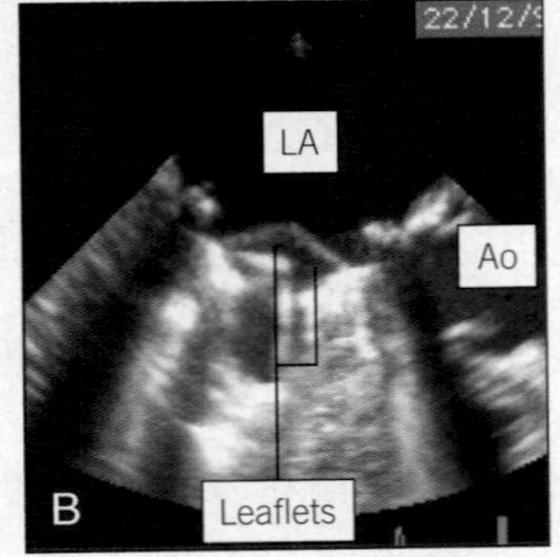

Figure 86.23 Transesophageal echocardiograms of a normal bileaflet mechanical prosthesis in the mitral position. The valve during diastole **(A)**, with the leaflets open, and systole **(B)**, with the leaflets closed. Observe the dense echo shadowing into the left ventricle from both the valvular annulus and the two leaflets. Ao, aorta; LA, left atrium; LV, left ventricle.

The ball-cage prosthesis produces very bright echoes on two-dimensional echocardiograms. The M-mode echocardiogram shows characteristic changes as the ball moves between closed and open position. In patients who have a single disk prosthesis, it is often possible to see the motion of the disk from an apical view. With the bileaflet tilting disk, it may be possible to see both disks open and become parallel (Fig. 86.23). During imaging of a bioprosthesis, the stents can be seen protruding from the valve. The motion of the tissue leaflets may be difficult to visualize, but it is similar to that of the native valve.

Doppler echocardiography provides reliable information about flow velocities across the various types of prostheses.[7,41] The normal prosthetic valve is slightly stenotic compared with a native valve, and therefore velocities across the valve are somewhat higher than normal. The degree of stenosis varies, depending on the type, size, and position of the prosthetic valve. Table 86.1 shows expected normal velocities and calculated pressure gradients from some of the most common prostheses. To determine whether a valve is stenotic, it is essential to compare the measured values with the expected values for that particular prosthesis at comparable size. It is also important to take into account the flow across the valve. Therefore, calculation of valve area by the continuity equation is useful (see Fig. 86.14).[42-44] The continuity principle assumes similar flow across the two measurement sites. For an aortic prosthesis, the use of subvalvular velocity-time integral and area is valid even with aortic regurgitation. For a mitral prosthesis, however, the presence of either aortic or mitral regurgitation makes aortic flow invalid as a reference flow. For calculation of area of a mitral prosthesis, the Doppler pressure half-time has been used.[9] Because the pressure half-time method was derived from patients with rheumatic mitral stenosis, the use of the empiric constant 220 may not give true valve areas for different valve types. The mitral prosthesis area may be grossly overestimated. For a given patient, however, the pressure half-time method is useful in long-term follow-up.

In some patients, the size of the prosthesis is too small relative to the flow rate. Such valve-heart mismatch results in a high gradient in a normally functioning valve.

The pressure gradients derived from Doppler velocities, however, are influenced by pressure recovery,[45] more so than in patients who have stenotic native valves. Therefore, the Doppler-derived pressure gradients are somewhat higher than the invasive gradients. The clinical impact of pressure recovery in prosthetic valves remains to be determined.

All tilting disk prostheses normally have some regurgitation (Fig. 86.24).[46] It is important to distinguish this physiologic leak from paravalvular regurgitation that occurs between the sewing ring and the annulus. The quantitation of regurgitation through prosthetic valves is difficult with transthoracic imaging, particularly in the case of mitral prostheses. Transesophageal imaging may be necessary to determine the exact site of the regurgitation. Paravalvular leaks are difficult to quantify because they adhere to the wall (Coanda effect), and the regurgitation may be underestimated. Some paravalvular leak is common immediately after valve replacement and may decrease over time. The clinical significance depends on the size of the regurgitation. Aortic and mitral prosthesis regurgitations should be quantified by the same methods as described for native valves.

It is important that every patient have a baseline echocardiographic study some time after surgery to be used as reference

EXPECTED DOPPLER MEAN PRESSURE GRADIENTS FOR BILEAFLET PROSTHESES OF VARIOUS SIZES

Valve size (mm)	19	21	23	25	27	29	31	33
Aortic valve (mm Hg ± SD)	N = 8 17.1 ± 5.6	N = 14 12.1 ± 3.6	N = 12 9.4 ± 4.0	N = 22 9.1 ± 3.0	N = 17 6.8 ± 2.5			
Mitral valve (mm Hg ± SD)					N = 13 3.5 ± 1.0	N = 17 3.4 ± 1.0	N = 10 3.5 ± 0.9	N = 4 4.8 ± 2.5

From Ihlen H, Mølstad P, Simonsen S, et al. Hemodynamic evaluation of the CarboMedics prosthetic heart valve in the aortic position: comparison of noninvasive and invasive techniques. Am Heart J 1992;123:151-159; and Bjørnerheim R, Ihlen H, Simonsen S, Sire S, Svennevig J. Hemodynamic characterization of the CarboMedics mitral valve prosthesis. J Heart Valve Dis 1997;6:115-122.

Table 86.1 Expected Doppler mean pressure gradients for bileaflet prostheses of various sizes.

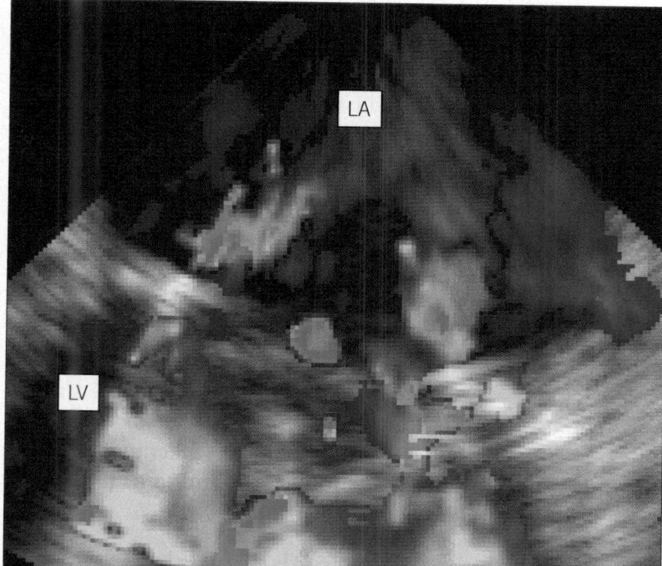

Figure 86.24 Transesophageal echocardiogram during systole of normal bileaflet mechanical prosthesis in the mitral position. Observe the normal intravalvular regurgitation (the small central jet between the leaflets and the corresponding two jets between the leaflets and the annulus on either side). These jets are generally easy to discriminate from paravalvular jets, which have higher velocities and are brighter on color Doppler evaluation. LA, left atrium; LV, left ventricle.

for later follow-up studies.[47] Owing to the wide range of normal velocities, a given set of values are less important than a series of measurements that show changes over time.

A complete baseline assessment with clinical examination, electrocardiography, chest radiography, routine blood tests, and transthoracic echocardiography should be done at the first postoperative outpatient evaluation within 12 weeks after surgery, ideally 2 to 4 weeks after discharge. Alternatively, the baseline echocardiogram can be done before discharge at the end of the postoperative stay; but the clinical evaluation with electrocardiography, chest radiography, and blood tests is still needed within 12 weeks. All patients who have undergone valve surgery require lifelong follow-up by a cardiologist.[20] Clinical examination should be done annually and whenever new cardiac symptoms occur. In the latter case, echocardiography should be done promptly to assess valve function. Routine chest radiography is not indicated. In patients with mechanical valves who are stable and have no symptoms or clinical evidence of left ventricular dysfunction, further routine echocardiographic testing is not needed.[23] In patients with significant regurgitation or whenever there is a question about prosthesis function, echocardiography should be done as indicated. Echocardiography is indicated in every patient with a prosthetic valve whenever there is a new murmur or a change in clinical status.

For bioprostheses, annual echocardiography is recommended after the fifth year and more frequently when there are signs of significant degeneration. Transprosthesis pressure gradient should be interpreted in relation to baseline values in the individual patient rather than in comparison with theoretical values. Fluoroscopy is useful to evaluate leaflet motion in mechanical valves when valve thrombosis or pannus is suspected and to demonstrate rocking of a dehiscing prosthesis.

The postoperative blood tests should include international normalized ratio, complete blood count, blood creatinine concentration, and lactate dehydrogenase concentration. The last is a useful marker of hemolysis.

When echocardiography does not provide an adequate answer, cardiac magnetic resonance imaging can be done and is safe for all commercially available prosthetic heart valves.[23]

ASSESSMENT OF PROSTHETIC VALVE MALFUNCTION

In a patient with a prosthetic valve, all new cardiac symptoms or signs of infection should raise suspicion of valve malfunction or endocarditis. The different valve types generate different clicking sounds, which correspond to opening and closure of the prosthesis. Auscultation may provide important information. Decreased intensity of one or both sounds or a malposition within the cardiac cycle (delayed opening or closure) should raise suspicion of malfunction from thrombus formation. Echocardiography is of major importance in sorting out valve problems, and transesophageal echocardiography is superior to conventional transthoracic imaging.

Thrombus Formation

Thrombus formation on the prosthesis may prevent valve closure and lead to regurgitation, or it may restrict opening and cause stenosis (Fig. 86.25). The impairment of leaflet motion may be partial and intermittent, and a careful echocardiographic examination is required. Increased echo

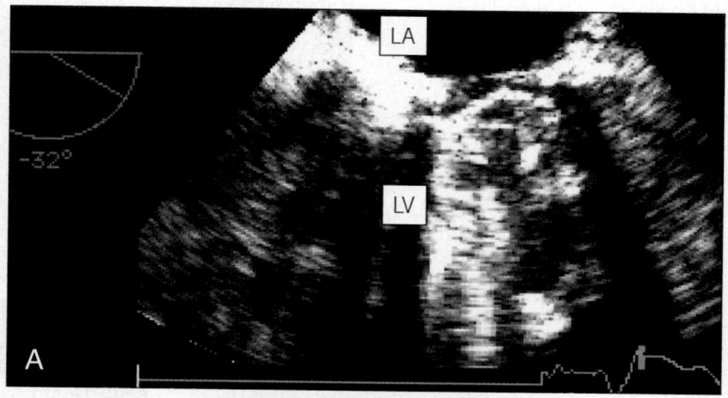

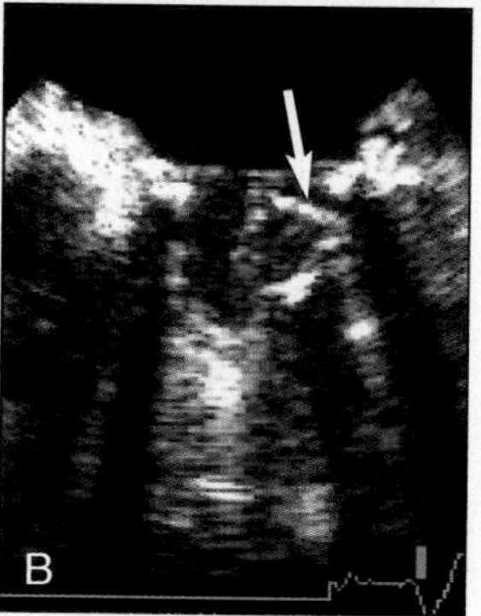

Figure 86.25 Transesophageal echocardiograms of a pathologic bileaflet mechanical prosthesis in the mitral position. A, Normal systolic closure is demonstrated. **B,** In late diastole, the posterior leaflet is fully open, whereas the anterior leaflet is still closed *(arrow)*. Whether this was caused by thrombus or pannus could not be diagnosed by echocardiography. LA, left atrium; LV, left ventricle.

densities within the valve suggest thrombus formation or vegetations. Tissue ingrowth or pannus formation sometimes interferes with valve function.

Bacterial Endocarditis

Because prosthetic valves are foreign bodies, they are associated with a high risk of bacterial endocarditis. As with thrombus formation, the formation of vegetations may interfere with leaflet closure or opening and cause valvular stenosis or regurgitation. Vegetations may be identified on two-dimensional echocardiograms as well as on M-mode echocardiograms. However, transthoracic echocardiography has limited sensitivity for detection of vegetations, and transesophageal echocardiography has much higher sensitivity and is essential to determine whether the infection has invaded the surrounding tissues and whether more than one valve is involved.

Prosthetic valve endocarditis has a high incidence of abscess formation (Fig. 86.26). On the two-dimensional echocardiogram, the abscess is seen as an echo-dense structure, which often has an echo-free center. The abscesses may not respond to antibiotics. They may lead to paravalvular fistulas, may perforate to the cardiac chambers, and may cause valve dehiscence.

Valve Dehiscence

Dehiscence is caused by rupture of one or more of the sutures that attach the sewing ring to the annulus of the excised native valve. It is most often accompanied by paravalvular regurgitation. Underlying endocarditis should be ruled out. The dehiscence is characterized echocardiographically by abnormal rocking of the valve and sewing ring relative to the annulus.

Paravalvular Leaks and Hemolysis

Blood tests for hemolysis should be part of routine follow-up in valve patients. Lactate dehydrogenase is the most useful biochemical marker of hemolysis. In patients with hemolytic anemia, there is need for closer assessment of the valve by transesophageal echocardiography. There is consensus to recommend reoperation if the paravalvular leak is related to endocarditis or if it causes hemolysis needing repeated blood transfusions or leading to severe symptoms (European Society of Cardiology guidelines).

Degeneration of Bioprosthetic Valves

Bioprosthetic valves undergo progressive calcification and degeneration. This leads to leaflet thickening, which interferes with valve function. After 5 to 10 years, it is common to see significant regurgitation; in some cases, stenosis is seen as well.

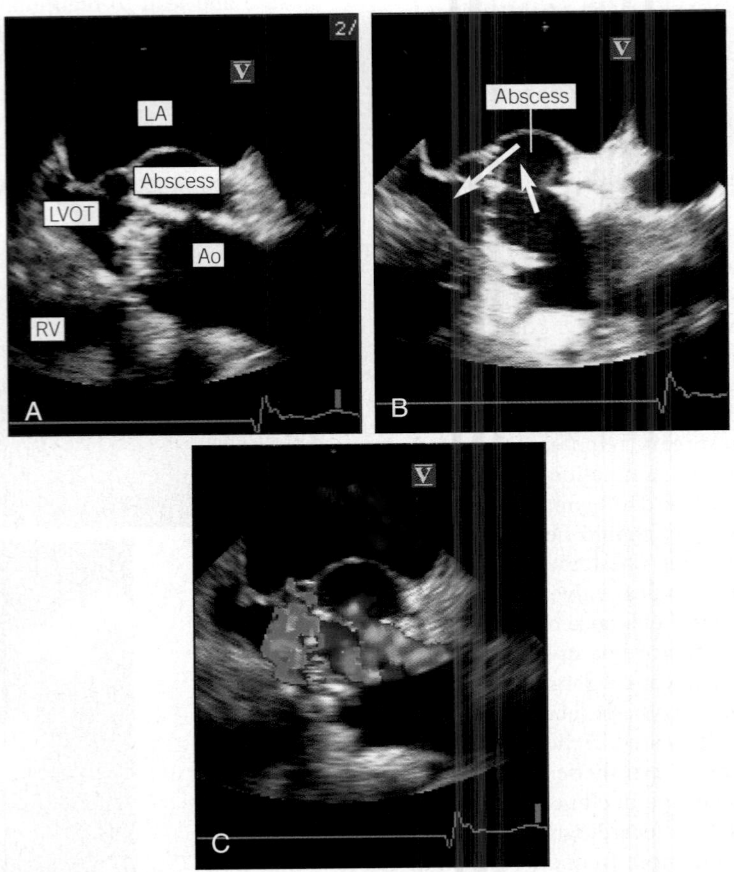

Figure 86.26 Transesophageal echocardiograms of an aortic valve with a two-compartment perforated abscess. The abscess can be seen in slightly different views on the left atrial side of the prosthesis (**A** and **B**), resulting in paravalvular fistula from the aorta through the abscess to the left ventricular outflow tract (**B**, *arrows*). The flow is shown in **C** by color Doppler study. Ao, aorta; LA, left atrium; LVOT, left ventricular outflow tract; RV, right ventricle.

chapter 87

Invasive Assessment of Valvular Function

Peter Wenaweser, Stephan Windecker, and Otto M. Hess

Definition

- Valvular dysfunction is characterized by the interplay of valve leaflets, the subvalvular apparatus, annular morphology, and stroke volume.

Key Features

- The accuracy of noninvasive assessment of valvular function by echocardiography has become comparable to that of invasive assessment in many cases.
- Limitations of noninvasive assessment, such as poor echocardiographic quality, and the presence or absence of coronary artery disease still render an indication for the performance of cardiac catheterization.
- In patients with anginal symptoms, invasive evaluation may be necessary to distinguish between symptomatic coronary artery disease and symptoms caused by valvular dysfunction itself.

Clinical Implications

- Preoperative evaluation of coronary anatomy is necessary in older patients to make a decision about combined surgery.
- Cardiac catheterization offers the possibility of performing balloon valvuloplasty and, in elderly patients (>75 years) with multiple comorbidities, of performing percutaneous valve replacement.
- The indication for invasive assessment of valvular function should be decided carefully, when clinical symptoms and laboratory findings suggest surgical correction of valve lesions.

To assess uncomplicated valvular heart disease, it is usually sufficient to carry out serial echocardiographic evaluations. Even in the preoperative assessment, fewer and fewer invasive examinations are performed. However, they remain necessary whenever coronary artery disease must be excluded, the echocardiographic assessment is of poor quality, there are discrepancies between clinical symptoms and echocardiographically derived data, or exact hemodynamic values are required.

DESCRIPTION OF PROCEDURE

A catheter protocol for most valvular diseases includes right-sided heart catheterization for assessment of right-sided heart pressure, cardiac output, and, when necessary, pulmonary vascular resistance. Left-sided heart catheterization aims to determine the transvalvular pressure gradient and left ventricular end-diastolic pressure in aortic stenosis. Retrograde passage of severe aortic stenosis may prove to be difficult, so transseptal puncture with anterograde entry into the left ventricle may be necessary in some cases.

In aortic regurgitation, determination of the central aortic and left ventricular end-diastolic pressure is essential. Angiography, including ventriculography and aortography to determine the regurgitant fraction and left ventricular volumes, is mandatory.

In mitral stenosis, left ventricular end-diastolic pressure, left atrial pressure (transseptally), or, alternatively, pulmonary capillary pressure during right-sided heart catheterization is measured. As a nonoperative measure for the treatment of severe mitral stenosis, mitral valvuloplasty has gained increasing popularity in recent years by use of transseptal catheterization.

In mitral regurgitation, left-sided heart catheterization includes the determination of left ventricular end-diastolic pressure. Left atrial pressures are assessed from pulmonary capillary wedge pressure. Angiography of the left ventricle is carried out to evaluate total left ventricular volume and the regurgitant fraction.

Coronary angiography is carried out when it is indicated to exclude coronary artery disease preoperatively.

INDICATIONS AND OBJECTIVES

Aortic Stenosis

It is routine practice to perform cardiac catheterization in patients of middle age or older to evaluate coronary artery status before surgery.[1] Younger patients without significant risk factors may be assessed noninvasively. Despite the remarkable difficulty in proving that concomitant revascularization of diseased coronary vessels at the time of aortic valve replacement enhances survival beyond that expected for aortic valve replacement alone,[2] it is currently recommended that combined aortic valve replacement and aorto-coronary bypass surgery be performed even when the degree of aortic stenosis is only moderate.

Cardiac catheterization should include both left- and right-sided heart catheterization. Usually, the gradient across the aortic valve is obtained by pullback of the pigtail catheter. Most patients with aortic stenosis will have a normal cardiac output, normal right ventricular and pulmonary capillary pressure, and normal ejection fraction. Left ventricular end-diastolic pressure is increased as an expression of left ventricular hypertrophy with increased chamber stiffness (diastolic dysfunction). A prominent *a* wave is seen in the pulmonary capillary, left atrial, and left ventricular pressure curves. The aortic pressure contour shows a characteristic delay and an anacrotic notch in the upstroke (Fig. 87.1). When the catheter is removed in patients with severe aortic stenosis (valve area

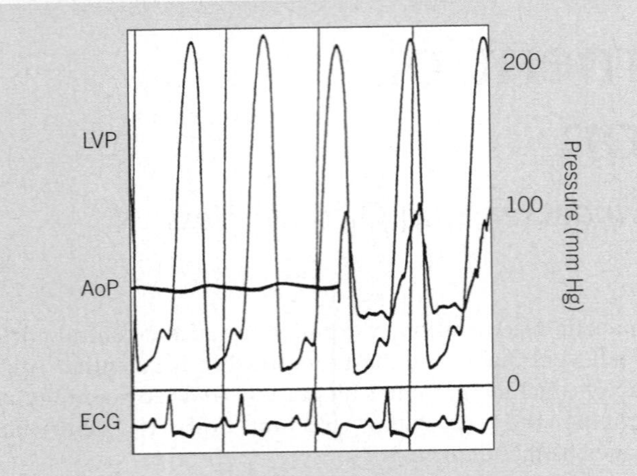

Figure 87.1 Left ventricular–aortic pressure (LVP-AoP) gradient in a patient with severe aortic stenosis. The high *a* wave in the left ventricular pressure (LVP) curve is an expression of the reduced left ventricular compliance. The aortic pressure (AoP) curve shows the typical delay and an anacrotic notch in the upstroke.

<0.6 cm^2), systemic arterial pressure may increase (Carabello's sign), which is another indicator of the severity of the stenosis. The pathophysiologic mechanism is probably based on the additional obstruction of the already significantly restricted valve opening by the removal of the retrogradely inserted catheter.

The severity of aortic stenosis is judged more reliably by calculation of the aortic valve area, which is determined invasively by relating the mean transvalvular gradient to the patient's cardiac output with simultaneous measurement. It is usually calculated by the Gorlin formula, which takes into account the aortic flow and the transvalvular pressure gradient.[3]

According to Torricelli's law

$$F = A \times V \times C_c$$

where F is the flow volume during the valve opening time (mL/s), A is the valve area (cm^2), and C_c is the flow velocity coefficient. Except during the complete opening of a heart valve, the flow through the opening is always less than the flow through the true valve area. This physical phenomenon is expressed by the constant C_c.

Gorlin set the pressure gradient in relation to the flow velocity:

$$V^2 = (C_v)^2 \times 2gh \text{ or } V = (C_v)\sqrt{2gh}$$

where V is the flow velocity (cm/s), C_v is the flow velocity coefficient (takes into account the loss of energy when pressure is changed to velocity), g is the gravitational acceleration (980 cm/s^2), and h is the transvalvular pressure gradient (cm H_2O). Hence, it follows that

$$A = F/C_c \times C_v\sqrt{2gh} \text{ or } A = F/C_c \times 44.3\sqrt{(P_1 - P_2)}$$

where C is a correction factor derived from the comparison between calculated and empirically measured valve areas during autopsies and includes C_c, C_v, a conversion factor from millimeters of mercury to centimeters of water, and other unknown factors; it equals 1 for aortic, pulmonary, and tricuspid valves as well as for a patent ductus arteriosus, whereas it is 0.85 for the mitral valve. The correction factor 44.3 is derived from $\sqrt{2g} = \sqrt{1960}$; the pressure gradient h is derived from $P_1 - P_2 = P$, where P_1 is equivalent to the pressure before the aortic valve and P_2 is equivalent to the pressure after the valve.

The pressure gradient is dependent not only on the flow velocity but also on the duration of flow (i.e., from the time during which the blood passes the stenosed valve). The duration of flow is given in seconds and is multiplied by the heart rate. The flow volume is calculated from cardiac output (CO) divided by the duration of flow. Hence, it follows that

$$A = CO/t \times 44.3 \times C\sqrt{\Delta P}$$

For the aortic and the pulmonary arteries, the systolic duration of flow is used; and for the mitral and tricuspid valves, the diastolic. The peak-to-peak systolic pressure gradient is often used, and the resulting valve area agrees well with the planimetric mean gradient when the stenosis is significant.

As an additional indicator of stenosis severity, aortic valve resistance (AVR) can be determined as

$$\text{AVR} = G \times \text{SEP} \times \text{HR} \times 1330/\text{CO}$$

where CO is the cardiac output (mL/min), SEP is the systolic ejection period (s), HR is the heart rate (bpm), and G is the mean transvalvular gradient (mm Hg).

Aortic valve resistance is simply the mean gradient divided by the cardiac output and involves no discharge coefficients or empiric constant.[4] It seems helpful in low-flow states for distinguishing patients who have truly stenotic valves from patients who have small calculated areas but in whom severe aortic stenosis is not present.[5]

A low-gradient, low-flow situation[6] has recently been described in patients with severe aortic stenosis and normal ejection fraction. These patients have been traditionally deferred from valve replacement, but outcome data have shown a worse prognosis in these patients.[6] Our data have indicated that this low-flow, low-gradient situation in severe aortic stenosis with maintained left ventricular function is rare, being around 5% of all patients with severe aortic stenosis.

Aortic valve areas of less than 0.8 cm^2 are generally considered to represent severe valvular aortic stenosis. In the presence of good left ventricular function, the resting systolic pressure gradient may exceed 100 mm Hg without symptoms at rest or with exercise. In the presence of normal left ventricular function, there is an increase in cardiac output with exercise, which may be normal in severe aortic stenosis owing to a disproportionately prolonged ejection period and, in part, to a stretching of the valve at higher systolic pressures.

Although echocardiographic assessment may be sufficient, angiography of the left ventricle has generally been included in the examination. Patients with left ventricular heart failure and high filling pressures may tolerate the additional volume load of the contrast agent poorly, but the use of nonionic or low osmolar contrast agents has reduced these risks considerably. Information derived from angiography includes the evaluation of left ventricular function, regional wall motion abnormalities, and the mitral valve. In addition, left ventricular wall thickness and muscle mass may be calculated. An aortogram gives information about the size of the annulus and the aorta ascendens, the number of cusps, and the presence of aortic regurgitation.

Aortic Regurgitation

Invasive assessment is indicated when the regurgitation is severe, the patient becomes symptomatic, the left ventricular ejection fraction is below 50%, and the echocardiographically determined end-systolic diameter is more than 55 mm or the end-diastolic diameter is more than 70 mm.[7]

The aortic pressure curve shows a typical high amplitude between systolic peak pressure and diastolic pressure, corresponding to the water-hammer pulse (Fig. 87.2). This is created by the very large stroke volume ejected into the aorta, which compensates for the volume regurgitated into the left ventricle during diastole. In acute aortic regurgitation, before eccentric hypertrophy has had time to occur, total stroke volume and pulse pressure will not be increased, and thus most of the physical signs will be absent (see Chapter 94). Another hemodynamic clue to the severity of aortic regurgitation is the rapid rise in diastolic left ventricular pressure (see Fig. 87.2). In aortic regurgitation, left ventricular filling is rapid because it occurs both as blood enters the ventricle from the left atrium and as blood is regurgitated through the incompetent aortic valve into the left ventricle.

With acute severe aortic regurgitation, there may be a premature closure of the mitral valve induced by the very high left ventricular filling pressure through the double filling of the left ventricle (see Fig. 87.2). This is an ominous sign in acute aortic regurgitation and usually indicates that aortic valve replacement will be necessary. In these patients, there is no or little left ventricular dilatation, and acute aortic regurgitation is associated with a massive increase in left ventricular diastolic pressure. In contrast to the chronic form, the blood pressure is not increased. Early mitral closure is detected on physical examination as a soft S_1 and can be confirmed visually during echocardiography or hemodynamically as left ventricular pressure rises above simultaneously recorded left atrial or wedge pressure in mid-diastole (see Fig. 87.2).

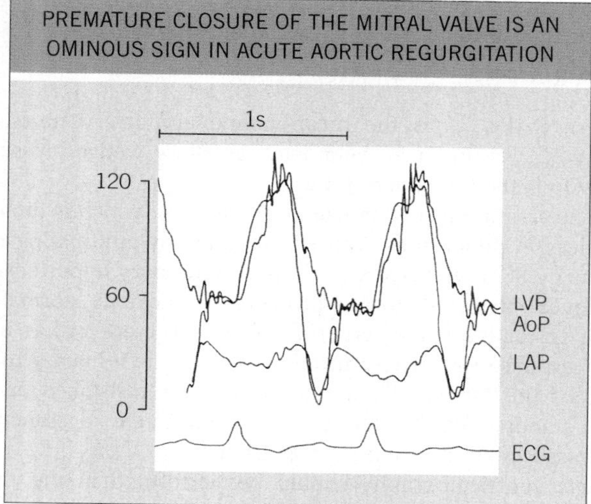

Figure 87.2 Aortic pressure curve in a patient with severe aortic regurgitation. There is a typical high amplitude between systolic peak pressure and diastolic filling pressure corresponding to the water-hammer pulse. AoP, aortic pressure; LAP, left atrial pressure; LVP, left ventricular pressure.

Right-sided heart catheterization is used to measure the left atrial (wedge) pressure. Supra-aortic angiography serves to demonstrate the severity and dynamics of aortic regurgitation. The morphologic features of the ascending aorta will help distinguish aortic regurgitation due to valvular or aortic disease. In the presence of a bicuspid valve, the characteristic poststenotic dilatation of the ascending aorta, as in aortic stenosis, is seen; in cystic medial disease, especially Marfan's syndrome, there is a balloon-like dilatation of the ascending aorta that involves the entire aortic root.

The most helpful information obtained during invasive assessment of the severity of aortic regurgitation is provided by qualitative and quantitative angiography. During qualitative angiography, a catheter is placed in the aorta, and the severity of regurgitation is judged by opacification of the left ventricle. Moderate aortic regurgitation is present when the regurgitant fraction amounts to 30% to 50%. When it is higher than 50%, aortic regurgitation is severe. Semiquantitative assessment of the severity of aortic regurgitation is based on a visual estimate of the concentration of contrast medium in the left ventricle:

- first degree: confinement of the jet to the left ventricular outflow tract and disappearance with each systole;
- second degree: the contrast jet remains in the left ventricle during more than one systolic contraction;
- third degree: there is no actual jet but a continuous filling with opacification of the left ventricle during two or three heart cycles; and
- fourth degree: the whole left ventricle is opacified within one beat, and the contrast agent is washed out slowly during several heartbeats.

Quantitative assessment of the regurgitant fraction (fao) may be done through a combination of angiographic volumetry and the calculation of the cardiac output by Fick's principle:

$$\text{fao} = \text{TSV}_{(\text{angio})} - \text{FSV}_{(\text{Fick})}/\text{TSV}_{(\text{angio})}$$

where $\text{TSV}_{(\text{angio})}$ is the total angiographic stroke volume and $\text{FSV}_{(\text{Fick})}$ is the forward stroke volume (Fick's principle).

Quantitative left ventricular angiography serves to assess ventricular function and dilatation. The left ventricular end-diastolic volume is increased twofold to threefold in chronic aortic regurgitation and ranges usually between 170 and 220 mL/m^2 (Fig. 87.3). As a consequence of ventricular dilatation, the ejection fraction is usually decreased. The incidence of coronary artery disease is lower than in patients with aortic stenosis and amounts to approximately 20% to 30%. Nevertheless, preoperative invasive evaluation of the coronary arteries is recommended for patients older than 40 years.

Mixed Aortic Stenosis and Regurgitation

Calculation of the valve area is not possible with more than mild aortic regurgitation. Judgment of the severity of mixed aortic valve disease must rely on the systolic gradient, regurgitant volume, and left ventricular function.

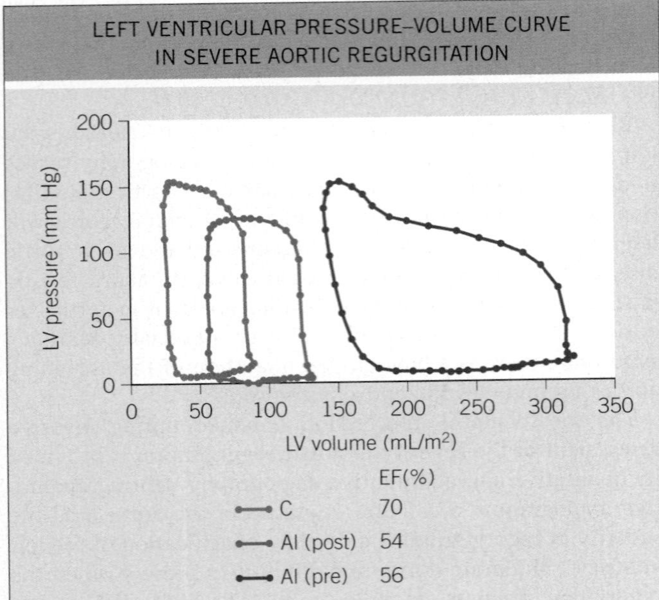

Figure 87.3 Left ventricular pressure-volume curve of a patient with severe aortic regurgitation before and 25 months after successful aortic valve replacement in comparison with a control patient. Before surgery, there is a massive dilatation of the left ventricle. Left ventricular (LV) ejection fraction (EF) is decreased mildly. The regurgitant fraction amounts to 67%. After surgery, there is a substantial decrease but not normalization of LV volume. Left ventricular ejection fraction remains unchanged. AI, aortic insufficiency; C, control; post, post surgery; pre, presurgery.

Mitral Stenosis

The normal mitral valve opening amounts to 4 to 6 cm^2. Moderate stenosis is present if it is 1 to 1.5 cm^2; severe mitral stenosis has a mitral valve opening of less than 1 cm^2. The key measurements during cardiac catheterization are simultaneous pressures in the left atrium (or the pulmonary capillary wedge pressure) together with the left ventricle and a long pressure tracing to determine the diastolic filling period. This is especially the case if the patient is in atrial fibrillation with widely varying diastolic filling periods. Pulmonary capillary wedge pressure closely approximates the left atrial pressure, but this requires that great care be taken to ensure that the pulmonary capillary wedge pressure is indeed a true wedge pressure. The pulmonary capillary wedge pressure contour shows a prominent *a* wave of atrial systole and a slow *y* descent due to delayed emptying of the left atrium with mitral obstruction (Fig. 87.4). With atrial fibrillation, there will be no *a* wave. The *a* wave in the left ventricle is either absent or markedly attenuated in mitral stenosis. Gorlin's original formulation for calculation of valve areas[3,8] is described in the section on aortic stenosis (see earlier). In mitral stenosis, the validity of this calculation depends on the accuracy of pulmonary capillary wedge pressure and left atrial pressure. If there is doubt, a direct left atrial pressure by the transseptal technique should be used, and the correction factor is 0.9 rather than 0.85.[9]

A detailed description of the transseptal technique is given later. The diastolic filling period is measured from the simultaneous wedge and left ventricular diastolic tracings, but in practice, it can be taken from an ascending aortic tracing;

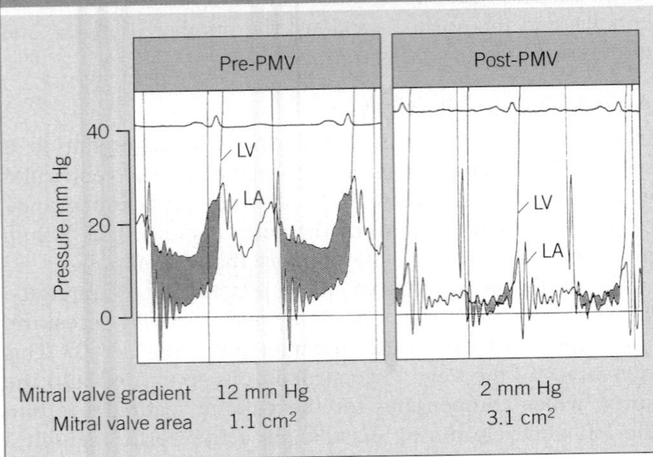

Figure 87.4 Simultaneous registration of the pressure curve in the left atrium (LA) and the left ventricle (LV) shaded in a patient with severe mitral stenosis before *(left)* and after *(right)* valvuloplasty. The area corresponds to the pressure gradient over the mitral valve. PMV, percutaneous mitral valvuloplasty.

ΔP is the mean diastolic gradient, measured as the difference in pressure between the left atrial (pulmonary wedge) and the left ventricular pressure over time and is best assessed planimetrically.

The relationship of the mean diastolic gradient to diastolic flow in mitral stenosis is an exponential rather than a linear one. Furthermore, it is evident that the pressure gradient across the valve is a function of heart rate as well as of flow because diastole is proportionally shortened more than systole during higher heart rates; tachycardia will increase the pressure gradient.

Pulmonary hypertension in mitral stenosis results mainly from passive rise due to an elevated pulmonary artery wedge pressure, but it may be caused by pulmonary arteriolar vasoconstriction and sometimes by tissue changes associated with long-standing pulmonary hypertension.[10] The pulmonary vascular resistance (PVR) is estimated by the formula

$$PVR = PAP_{(mean)} - PAW_{(mean)}/Qp$$

where $PAP_{(mean)}$ is the mean pulmonary artery pressure, $PAW_{(mean)}$ is the mean pulmonary capillary wedge pressure, and Qp is the pulmonary flow.

The simple ratio is known as Wood unit, which is dimensionless. A dimensional value is obtained by multiplying this value by 80 to yield dynes × s/cm^5. Pulmonary hypertension in severe mitral stenosis will decrease and may normalize with corrective valve surgery.[11] The decreased cardiac output response to exercise in mitral stenosis is in part a function of the increased pulmonary vascular resistance or, in long-standing cases, due to right ventricular dysfunction and associated tricuspid regurgitation.

Left ventriculography should be performed in the right and left anterior oblique views. Pure or predominant mitral stenosis should show little or no mitral regurgitation. An enlarged right ventricle will displace the left ventricle posteriorly. The left ventricle is usually of normal size. Mitral stenosis is sometimes associated with left ventricular dysfunction in the presence of mitral regurgitation or aortic valve disease or as a result of postrheumatic myocarditis. Therefore, the left ventricle must be evaluated for dilatation, ejection fraction, and regional wall motion abnormalities. Although angiography may yield important information on the pliability of the valve and the subvalvular mitral apparatus, these are better evaluated by echocardiography.

Contrast material injected into the pulmonary artery may visualize the left atrium well during the levophase. Left atrial angiography has been largely replaced by echocardiography for assessment of valve mobility and the presence of thrombi.

Mitral Regurgitation

The evaluation of mitral regurgitation today is a domain of echocardiography because invasive evaluation does not appear to be more accurate than the noninvasively acquired data.

Angiographic quantification of regurgitant flow is not entirely satisfactory. Left ventriculography is commonly used to assess the magnitude of regurgitant flow with the right and left anterior oblique views. A commonly used grading is I to IV, in analogy to that described in the section on aortic regurgitation (see earlier). Grade I is trivial to mild insufficiency, in which a bolus of contrast material enters the left atrium without completely opacifying the chamber; grade IV is massive regurgitation into the left atrium, in which the left atrium is more densely opacified than the left ventricle. There is often regurgitation of contrast material into the pulmonary veins. Grade II and grade III are in between: grade II is mild to moderate, with the left atrium completely but faintly opacified and left atrial opacification that is less dense than left ventricular opacification; grade III is moderately severe, with early opacification of the left atrium, in density equal to that of the left ventricle. Although grade I and grade II are probably not capable of causing symptoms or muscle dysfunction in most circumstances, grade III and grade IV may cause symptoms, severe hemodynamic overload, and left ventricular dysfunction. Unfortunately, this semiquantitative system is often ambiguous. Frequently, the diagnosis is grade III,[12] and the proper management for patients in this range of severity is unclear. The regurgitant volume may be calculated from forward stroke volume by hemodynamic studies (i.e., Fick's principle; see earlier) and total stroke volume by angiography (difference between end-diastolic and end-systolic volumes). The regurgitant fraction is formulated as before (see equation under aortic regurgitation).

This method has a large margin of error and must be carried out with simultaneous measurements. Furthermore, it is probably invalid in atrial fibrillation. The exact regurgitant fraction that imposes a load on the heart severe enough to cause symptoms and eventually muscle dysfunction is unknown. However, most patients with mitral regurgitation requiring mitral valve surgery have regurgitant fraction values of greater than 0.5 (= 50%), which suggests that at least this amount of regurgitation is required to precipitate enough decompensation to warrant surgical correction. Furthermore, there is evidence that left ventricular function does not return to normal after surgery, probably because the valve prosthesis leads to a sudden increase in afterload when the low impedance leak is closed.[13] Thus, a regurgitant fraction in the range of 40% to 50% or greater is probably the severity required to cause symptoms and decompensation.

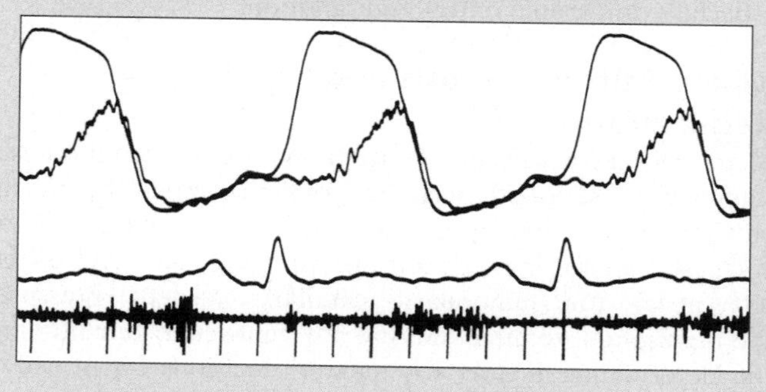

Figure 87.5 Left ventricular and left atrial pressure in a patient with chronic mitral regurgitation. Because of regurgitation of blood into a dilated atrium with a reduced compliance, the *v* wave is increased. The electrocardiogram demonstrates the timing of the *v* wave that peaks during late systole. Left ventricular end-diastolic pressure is elevated.

In acute mitral regurgitation, the ventriculogram will demonstrate a relatively normal ventricular size and massive regurgitant flow into the left atrium.

For hemodynamic evaluation of mitral regurgitation, right-sided heart catheterization should be performed to measure pulmonary capillary wedge pressure (Fig. 87.5). In symptomatic patients with mitral regurgitation, the left atrial pressure is usually elevated because pulmonary congestion is responsible for the patient's symptoms. Failure of the pulmonary capillary wedge pressure to increase suggests that the patient is well compensated or that mitral regurgitation is mild and symptoms may be coming from another source. However, it might be that the patient is well compensated at rest but that left atrial pressure rises during exercise, producing the symptom of dyspnea on exertion. Simple elevation of the patient's legs, which introduces sudden volume loading, allows us to distinguish which of these mechanisms is operative.

The wedge pressure tracing classically shows a steep rise in the v wave, with a rapid y descent as the unobstructed valve opens, because during systole, the left atrium fills both with blood returning from the pulmonary veins and with blood regurgitated across the incompetent mitral valve. The presence of a v wave twice the mean pulmonary capillary wedge pressure is usually consistent with severe mitral regurgitation (see Fig. 87.5). In pure mitral insufficiency, there should be little or no end-diastolic gradient across the mitral valve. However, the magnitude of the v wave is dependent on both the magnitude of regurgitant flow and the compliance of the left atrium.[14] The v waves are therefore impressively tall in acute mitral regurgitation in which there is a large regurgitant volume and a relatively noncompliant left atrium. In chronic mitral regurgitation, a large v wave may or may not be present because progressive dilatation of the left atrium may be associated with markedly increased compliance, so that even a large regurgitant volume may not elicit characteristic pressure contour changes in the left atrium.[15] Although the *v* wave is of clinical interest, few therapeutic decisions are made on the basis of its presence, especially in chronic mitral regurgitation.

Mixed Mitral Stenosis and Regurgitation

Mixed mitral stenosis and regurgitation occur when there is a significantly elevated diastolic gradient across the mitral valve as well as angiographically significant regurgitation of contrast material into the left atrium. Here, the level of the left atrial (or pulmonary capillary wedge) pressure, the regurgitant volume, and the left ventricular function are the determining factors for making decisions about valve dilatation or replacement.

Pulmonary, Tricuspid, and Prosthetic Valves

Pulmonary stenosis is a congenital disease usually diagnosed and treated in childhood. In adults, the severity has traditionally been inferred from pressure gradient measurements in the pulmonary artery and the right ventricle, with assessment of simultaneous cardiac output.[16] The pressures can be taken simultaneously or during withdrawal. The pulmonary valve area can be calculated by the Gorlin formula[3] and the mean systolic gradient. There has been substantial immediate and long-term success in the treatment of adults and children with balloon valvuloplasty.[17]

Tricuspid Valve Disease

Hemodynamic evaluation of tricuspid stenosis includes simultaneous pressure recordings in the right atrium and right ventricle, simultaneous measurement of cardiac output and heart rate, and determination of the diastolic filling period. The valve area can be calculated by the Gorlin formula,[3] provided the regurgitation is mild. However, as with aortic stenosis, discharge coefficients for the estimation of valve area from the Gorlin formula have never been developed. In general, relatively small tricuspid valve gradients (approximately 5 to 6 mm Hg) may be consistent with severe tricuspid stenosis. As with mitral stenosis, if the resting hemodynamics leave some doubt about the severity of the stenosis, exercise hemodynamics should be obtained.

The right atrial tracing in tricuspid stenosis will show sustained elevation of right atrial pressure. The rhythm is usually atrial fibrillation, and an *a* wave is seldom seen. The presence of a consistent end-diastolic gradient establishes the diagnosis because functional tricuspid regurgitation alone should not be associated with an end-diastolic gradient.

Tricuspid insufficiency is a diagnosis best made by a skilled clinician. The hallmark of tricuspid insufficiency is a large *v* wave in the right atrial pressure tracing that gives rise to deep jugular pulsations readily apparent on inspection of the neck veins. As tricuspid regurgitation worsens, the right atrial pressure tracing begins to resemble the right ventricular pressure tracing (Fig. 87.6).

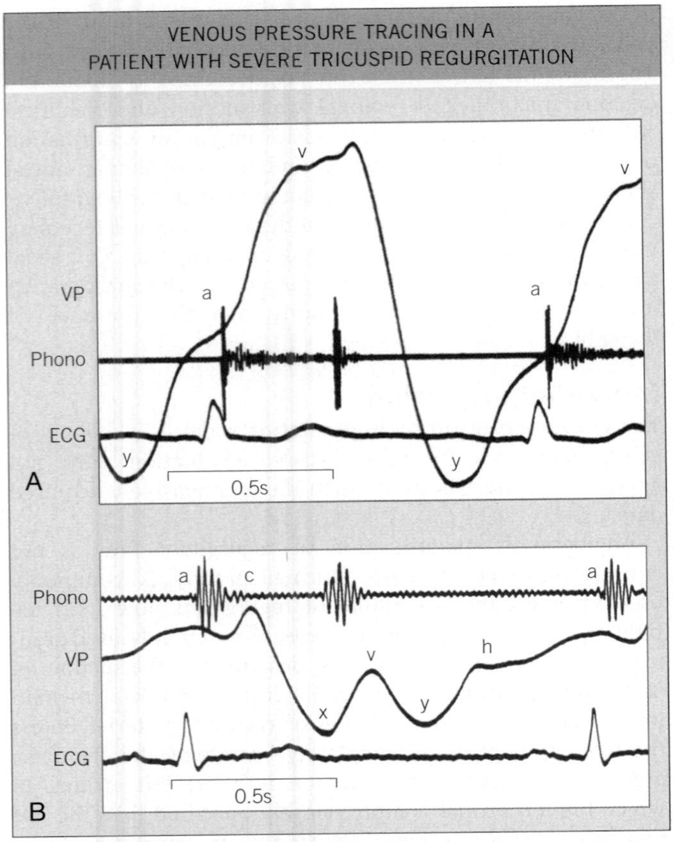

Valve Prostheses

Valve prostheses are evaluated hemodynamically by methods identical to those for native valves. However, unlike native valves, mechanical prostheses cannot be crossed with a catheter without causing acute regurgitation, thereby invalidating any measurement. A mitral prosthesis can be evaluated with the pulmonary capillary wedge and left ventricular pressures. A prominent *v* wave is commonly seen in the wedge pressure in the presence of a mitral prosthesis without regurgitation. The prominent *v* wave may be due to decreased atrial compliance in the presence of the prosthesis. With a mechanical aortic prosthesis, transseptal access to the left ventricle is necessary. Ball valves may be crossed with a small straight catheter without interfering excessively with ball motion. However, retrograde passage of a catheter across a single tilting disk valve must pass through the major orifice. A catheter passed into the minor orifice can become entrapped, resulting in a catastrophe. In the case of the double-leaflet valves, retrograde passage is avoided because of potential catheter entrapment.

Bioprostheses pose no technical difficulties for cardiac catheterization. They can be crossed readily without significantly altering hemodynamics. Tricuspid valve prostheses are commonly bioprosthetic, but tilting disk valves can be cautiously traversed in this low-pressure system.

Invasive evaluation of regurgitant prosthetic valves in the aortic and mitral position is performed identically as for native valves. Both qualitative and quantitative angiography are employed, but retrograde passage should be avoided.

VENOUS PRESSURE TRACING IN A PATIENT WITH SEVERE TRICUSPID REGURGITATION

Figure 87.6 Venous pressure tracing in a patient with severe tricuspid regurgitation. A, The tracing resembles the right ventricular pressure tracing with a high *v* wave. **B,** The tracing is from a control patient.

Transseptal Puncture

It is usually not recommended to enter the left ventricle retrogradely across a mechanical aortic valve prosthesis because the catheter itself may get stuck on the valve prosthesis and may alter the hemodynamics. In addition, it is sometimes impossible to cross a stenotic aortic valve. Here, the transseptal technique is useful.[18,19] Furthermore, it is the route used for balloon dilatation of mitral stenosis. Briefly, a venous catheter with a preshaped distal curve and tapered tip is introduced over a guide wire through the right femoral vein to the superior vena cava. With an aortic prosthesis or aortic valve calcification, the level of the aortic valve is readily identified. Otherwise, a pigtail catheter should be advanced into the aortic cusps to mark the level of the valve. The venous catheter is then exchanged for a 7 French or 6 French Brockenbrough catheter, which is positioned with its tip in the superior vena cava. A preshaped steel needle with a curved tip and an arrow at its end to indicate the direction of the curve at the tip is advanced through the catheter to within 1 cm of its tip. The entire assembly is gently pulled down until the tip of the catheter is in the upper right atrium. At this juncture, it is important to ensure that the tip of the catheter is pointing posteromedially (toward the left shoulder) to avoid the aorta. The lumen of the needle is connected to pressure, and the assembly is slowly drawn down until the tip jumps slightly. If this is at the level of the aortic valve, this usually represents the upper limbus of the fossa ovalis. The needle is then extended through the catheter so that approximately 1 cm of needle is exposed. The patient is then instructed to report any chest or throat pain. The operator gently pushes the needle posteromedially until it moves across the septum with a sudden jump when it enters the left atrium. If the patient experiences chest pain, the needle is not in the fossa but rather in the muscular part of the septum and must be repositioned. When the needle enters the left atrium, a pressure change will be obvious. The chamber can be confirmed by drawing of a blood sample, which should be fully saturated. The catheter can be smoothly pushed over the needle into the left atrium, and the needle is withdrawn. The tip of the catheter can then be maneuvered into the left ventricle. From a technical standpoint, there are at least three contraindications to transseptal puncture:

- left atrial myxoma (which is commonly attached to the rim of the fossa ovalis);
- cystic media disease with massive dilatation of the aorta; and
- significant thrombi in the left atrium, especially in the presence of long-standing atrial fibrillation.

Significant thrombi can be excluded with reasonable confidence by transesophageal echocardiography.

Balloon Valvuloplasty

Originally introduced for the treatment of (and now the standard treatment for) pulmonary stenosis by Brock,[19] the technique has been used increasingly for mitral valvuloplasty.

Up until 1990, a double-balloon technique was used most frequently, whereas later the Inoue technique with a single balloon was used to dilate the stenosis. For mitral stenosis, transseptal catheterization is done after routine hemodynamic measurements and coronary angiography. Before mitral valvuloplasty, the left atrial pressure and the transvalvular pressure gradient are measured. An 8 French valvuloplasty catheter is then passed over the guide wire to the level of the interatrial septum, and the septal opening is dilated. After its removal, a 12 French balloon catheter is passed through the septum and into the mitral annulus. The balloon is inflated for 10 to 15 seconds with a mixture of normal saline and contrast medium under radiographic control until the waist of the balloon is no longer visible and the balloon falls back into the left atrium (Fig. 87.7). Several dilatations are sometimes necessary. A fractioned procedure is also recommended by several authors to reduce the risk of sudden valvular rupture with consequent severe mitral

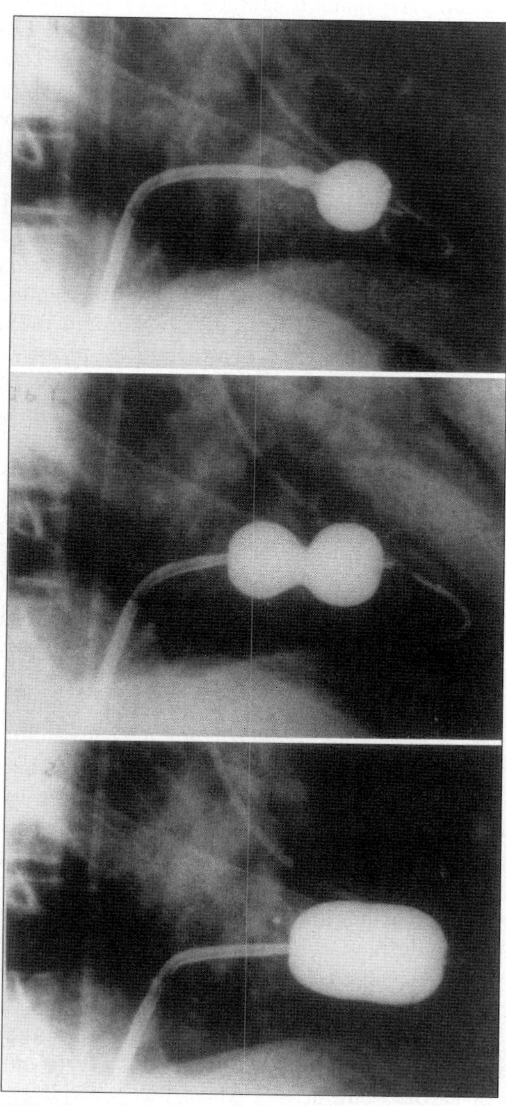

Figure 87.7 Mitral valvuloplasty performed by the Inoue technique. The catheter is placed in the mitral valve and the distal part of the Inoue balloon inflated *(top)*. The balloon is then pulled back in the mitral valve and inflated for 10 to 15 seconds under fluoroscopic control *(middle)* until the waist of the balloon is no longer visible *(bottom)* and the balloon falls back into the left atrium.

regurgitation. Immediately after the valvuloplasty, the transvalvular pressure is again determined. At the end of the procedure, left ventricular angiography is carried out to document the degree of an eventually newly developed regurgitation.

Percutaneous Aortic Valve Replacement

Percutaneous treatment of aortic stenosis has been increasingly used in elderly patients considered inoperable because of severe comorbidities. Currently, two different systems are used for retrograde implantation of the aortic valve prosthesis in high-risk patients with severe aortic stenosis, namely, the Edwards-Sapien valve and the CoreValve self-expanding prosthesis.[20,21] With both systems, the aortic valve is retrogradely crossed with a stiff guide wire, and the stenosed valve is predilated with a 22- or 24-mm balloon under rapid pacing with 160 to 200 beats per minute (reduces valve motion). The balloon catheter is then replaced by the valve prosthesis, which is balloon expanded for the Edwards-Sapien valve or self-expanded for the CoreValve (Fig. 87.8). Both valve prostheses press the native valve toward the wall, allowing the bovine or porcine stented valve to expand. The pressure gradient immediately disappears, and aortic pressure increases. The size of the introducer sheath varies between 18 and 24 French and limits this intervention to patients with appropriately sized femoral and iliac arteries without severe tortuosity. In elderly patients with small vessels, the Edwards-Sapien valve can also be implanted transapically through a small incision of the skin and the apex.[22] First results with these valve prostheses are promising, but long-term outcome is not known, and procedural complications are still rather high. There is a considerable learning curve for the operators.

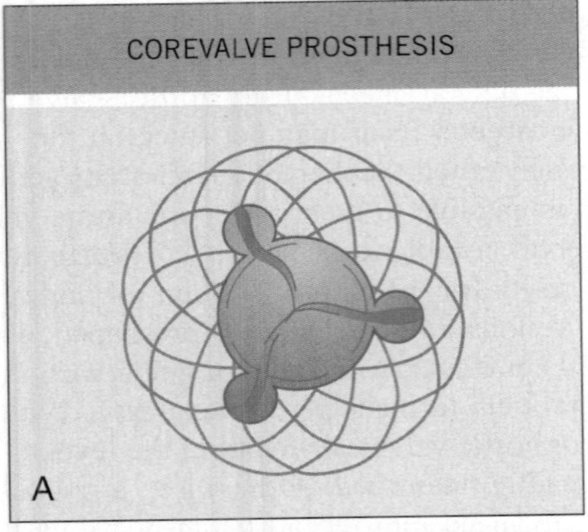

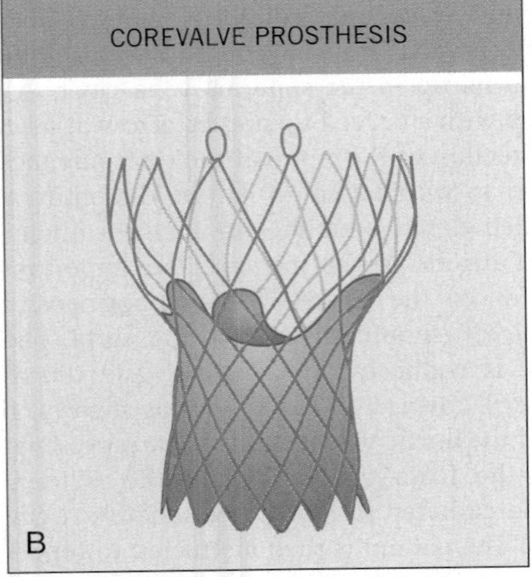

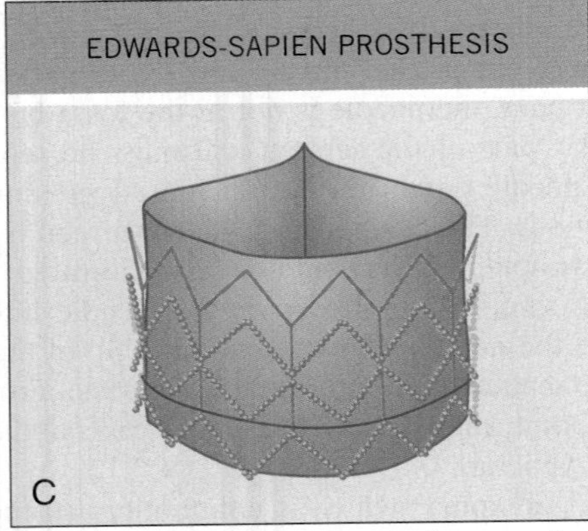

Figure 87.8 Photographs of the CoreValve prosthesis (A, view from the top; B, front view) and the Edwards-Sapien prosthesis (C) for percutaneous aortic valve replacement. The CoreValve is self-expanding and is implanted through an 18 French delivery sheath. The Edwards-Sapien valve is mounted on a balloon and implanted through balloon inflation. The size of the introducer sheath is 24 French.

ACCURACY

Cardiac Output

The techniques available for measurement of cardiac output include the Fick method, the thermodilution technique, the dye dilution technique, and the angiographic technique as mentioned before. The Fick method, which uses carefully measured oxygen consumption and arteriovenous oxygen difference, is the "gold standard" for measurement of cardiac output but has its own inherent problems. A longer period of steady state is needed to allow the time to collect the expired air, and respirations must be regular and uniform (the most extreme example in which the Fick principle cannot be applied is Cheyne-Stokes respiration). However, the Fick principle has the virtue of being usable in severe right or left ventricular failure, severe valve regurgitation, and intracardiac shunts. Because of the inconvenience of measuring oxygen consumption, some laboratories use algorithms that generate assumed oxygen consumption. Such assumptions may produce as much as a 20% error in the estimation of cardiac output.[23,24] Thus, this practice should be used with caution in the assessment of severity of aortic valve stenosis.

The thermodilution technique for determination of cardiac output is less accurate at low cardiac outputs. The technique also tends to underestimate cardiac output when tricuspid regurgitation is present.

The dye dilution technique may underestimate cardiac output if concomitant aortic or mitral regurgitation is present. The angiographic technique requires the accurate calculation of end-diastolic and end-systolic volumes. This condition can be met by paying careful attention to detail, especially in measuring the angiographic correction factor.

Aortic Valve Area

The Gorlin formula is usually accurate in assessing the true aortic valve area when valve flow exceeds 150 mL/s, which is approximately equivalent to a cardiac output of 4.5 L/min. At lower flows, the formula is less accurate because calculated aortic valve area varies directly with flow. Thus, as flow falls, calculated aortic valve area becomes smaller, regardless of the true severity of the aortic stenosis. Flow dependence at lower flows probably occurs because the empiric constant for the aortic valve was never developed[3] and has been assumed erroneously to be 1.0. It is also likely that at lower flows, there is less mechanical force present to separate the aortic valve cusps. Thus, the functional valve orifice is actually smaller at lower flows.

Transvalvular Gradient

Measurement of the transvalvular gradient is also fraught with difficulty. A serious source of error in gradient measurement arises from improper placement of the catheter, which should be well into the body of the left ventricle, as this position represents most accurately the pressure overload. Because there is a substantial gradient between the body of the left ventricle and the aortic outflow tract in most patients with aortic stenosis, positioning of the catheter in the outflow tract will produce inaccurate data, although in both cases the recordings are typical left ventricular pressure tracings.[25]

Mitral Valve Area

The calculated mitral valve area is subject to many errors.[26] The pulmonary capillary wedge pressure is used for left atrial pressure, the constant may be variable,[8] and a significant mitral regurgitation may coexist. Cardiac output measurements also may have a margin of errors, as mentioned before. However, unlike the calculated valve area in aortic stenosis, the calculated valve area in mitral stenosis is usually a more accurate reflection of the true severity of mitral stenosis.[3] The difference in accuracy of the valve area calculations for the two different valves probably arises from the fact that the Gorlin formula was validated for aortic stenosis and that an empiric constant was determined for the mitral valve.

Aortic and Mitral Regurgitation

In most cases, the severity of aortic or mitral regurgitation can be established only after all diagnostic modalities, including qualitative and quantitative ventriculography, are taken into consideration.[27]

Percutaneous Aortic Valve Replacement

The most common complications of percutaneous aortic valve replacement are device related: perivalvular aortic regurgitation, which is usually mild to moderate; obliteration of the coronary ostia, which is rare; or misplacement of the valve prosthesis with embolization in the aorta or ventricle. Periprocedural adverse events are cardiac death with disruption of the native valve, perforations with pericardial tamponade, severe arrhythmias, aortic dissection, and hemodynamic instability. Procedural mortality ranges between 8% and 12% in most studies. Other complications are cerebral embolization, bleeding and dissection at the vascular puncture site, renal dysfunction, and multiorgan failure.

COMPLICATIONS

Complications of invasive assessment of valvular function are basically similar to those of cardiac catheterization. Specific complications in the invasive assessment of valvular function include the following conditions.

Transseptal Puncture

When it is performed correctly, complications should be infrequent. Perforation of the atrial free wall may occur and may lead to tamponade. If the needle is pointing anteriorly, the aorta may be entered. If the needle is too low, one may mistake the coronary sinus for the fossa ovalis, but this can be avoided by noting the level of the aortic valve. Because of the possibility of perforation of the atrial free wall, the patient should not be heparinized until after completion of transseptal puncture. An atrial septal defect is detected angiographically or oxymetrically in approximately 15% of patients, and a patent foramen ovale can be found in up to 30% of all patients.

Balloon Valvuloplasty

The most common complication of balloon valvuloplasty is the development of valvular regurgitation, which occurs in approximately 10% to 20% of patients. However, newly developed valvular regurgitation leading to immediate surgery occurs in approximately 0.5% to 1% of patients. Other complications include arrhythmias, air or thrombi embolism, and ventricular perforation in approximately 1% to 2% of patients.

DIAGNOSTIC STRATEGY

Pressure Gradient Measurement

Damping will underestimate the peak systolic pressure; conversely, if overshoots are not recognized, the peak pressure will be overestimated. Optimally, the aortic pressure should be measured in the ascending aorta because systolic pressure in the femoral artery is amplified and peaks later than the pressure in the ascending aorta.

Determination of Pulmonary Capillary Wedge Pressure

Pulmonary capillary wedge pressure approximates closely left atrial pressure when great care is taken to ensure that the right-sided heart catheter is properly wedged. There should be a significant and abrupt change in pressure compared with the pulmonary artery, and the pressure contour should be of venous configuration with a large *a* wave if the patient is in sinus rhythm; but with atrial fibrillation, it may be fairly nondescript. For verification, a blood sample drawn from the wedge position can be taken, which should be fully saturated. To confirm that the catheter is properly wedged, it is important to note that the *v* wave of the pulmonary capillary wedge tracing follows the T wave of the electrocardiogram. Furthermore, the pulmonary artery pressure should be greater than the mean pulmonary capillary wedge pressure. If there is uncertainty about the validity of the wedge pressure after observing these precautions and wedging at several sites, direct measurement of the left atrial pressure may be necessary.

Technical Difficulties in Aortic Stenosis

The stenotic aortic valve is often calcified and distorted. Manipulation of the pigtail angiographic catheter through the stenotic valve into the left ventricle requires considerable skill. This is related in part to the small and distorted orifice and in part to the somewhat downward and leftward displacement of the valve itself by the poststenotic dilatation of the ascending aorta. A straight-tipped guide wire should be used to straighten out the pigtail curvature. Systematic probing of the aortic valve is undertaken, making use of the curvature in the catheter itself to alter the angle of the probing wire. Should the pigtail catheter be unsuccessful in entering the left ventricle, one will often be successful with the use of the Amplatz left coronary catheter with a straight guide wire. Then, with use of an exchange wire, the Amplatz catheter can be exchanged for a pigtail catheter. Rarely, it is impossible to cross the aortic valve retrogradely, and one must perform transseptal puncture to gain access to the left ventricle.

Valve Area Calculation

As noted before, valve area calculated by the Gorlin formula is flow dependent, which represents a particular problem when a low gradient is measured at a cardiac output of less than 4.5 L/min. Many patients with low transvalvular gradients and low cardiac output do not have truly severe aortic stenosis despite the small calculated valve area[5] but may rather suffer from cardiomyopathy coexisting with mild aortic stenosis. Those patients will probably not exhibit marked improvement after aortic valve replacement. For identification of patients with low cardiac output and severe aortic stenosis, infusion of nitroprusside or of dobutamine (dobutamine stress echocardiography) to increase cardiac output has been suggested.[5]

Mitral Regurgitation

During left ventriculography, ventricular ectopy, which causes artifactual mitral regurgitation, must be avoided. A second error that must be avoided is injection of an amount of contrast material that is inadequate to opacify the enlarged left atrium and ventricle. This flaw in technique can cause serious underestimation of the degree of regurgitation. As a rule, 45 mL of contrast material should be injected during 3 or 4 seconds.

SUMMARY

Despite the accuracy of assessing the severity of valvular function noninvasively, invasive evaluation is still performed for two major reasons: to assess coronary anatomy in patients who are usually at risk for having coronary disease because of their age and to add further hemodynamic information in cases in which severity of the disease is still in doubt after noninvasive testing.

chapter 88

Rheumatic Fever

Mohammed R. Essop and Tanvier Omar

Definition

- Rheumatic fever represents a multisystem disorder due to an abnormal immune response to a preceding streptococcal pharyngitis and is characterized by a proliferative inflammatory reaction involving connective tissue.

Key Features

- Carditis, polyarthritis, subcutaneous nodules, chorea, and erythema marginatum are the major manifestations.
- Carditis is by far of greatest significance and may lead to chronic rheumatic heart disease.

Therapy

- Appropriate antibiotics to eradicate the streptococcal infection and to prevent further episodes.
- Salicylates for relief of arthralgia.
- Bed rest and surgical intervention for hemodynamically severe valvular regurgitation.
- The use of corticosteroids is controversial.

There is a tremendous regional variation in the epidemiology of rheumatic fever. Whereas coronary artery disease is the major cardiovascular affliction in industrialized countries, acute rheumatic fever and its progression to chronic rheumatic heart disease constitute the major burden of cardiac disease in developing nations. Worldwide, rheumatic fever is the most common cause of cardiac disease in children and young adults. The incidence of rheumatic fever in many developing countries exceeds 100 per 100,000.[1] In the United States, the incidence of rheumatic fever has progressively declined from more than 100 per 100,000 population at the turn of the century to current estimates of 2 per 100,000. The reasons for the declining incidence of rheumatic fever are not entirely clear but in part probably relate to less overcrowding and better sanitation and general living conditions, all of which result in a reduction in infectious diseases in general and streptococcal infections in particular. The impact of antimicrobial therapy is uncertain because there was a notable decline in the incidence of rheumatic fever even before the advent of antibiotics. Furthermore, the marked reduction in incidence of acute rheumatic fever has occurred despite an unchanged incidence of streptococcal pharyngitis. Of great interest is the recent resurgence of rheumatic fever in geographically distinct areas of the United States, with the first outbreak being reported in 1987.[2] These outbreaks were usually associated with mucoid strains of group A streptococci belonging to M types 1, 3, 6, and 18. These strains were previously rarely recovered, suggesting that the incidence of rheumatic fever may be related to outbreaks of rheumatogenic strains of streptococci. The reduction in rheumatic fever has been too rapid for changes in host susceptibility to be postulated as a cause of this.[3]

IMMUNOPATHOGENESIS

Several lines of evidence suggest that rheumatic fever occurs as a result of a group A streptococcal pharyngitis. Outbreaks of rheumatic fever usually accompany epidemics of rheumatogenic streptococcal pharyngitis, and both the primary and secondary attacks can be prevented with specific antimicrobial therapy. Several theories have been advanced concerning the mechanism by which group A streptococci induce rheumatic fever. The most tenable theory is that M proteins from rheumatogenic strains (Fig. 88.1) share certain epitopes with cardiac myosin and sarcolemmal membrane protein.[4,5] Antibodies produced in the host against these epitopes of streptococci cross-react with cardiac tissue, resulting in an inflammatory response in pericardium, myocardium, and endocardium. In addition to the humoral response, there is mounting evidence that a heightened cellular response may be intimately involved in the disease process.[6-8] Implicit in this concept is that the observed host immune response is abnormal.[9] Whether this abnormal immune response is genetically programmed or represents an acquired alteration in host defense or immunologic mechanisms is unclear.[10]

ANATOMY AND PATHOLOGY

The acute phase of rheumatic fever is characterized pathologically by a diffuse exudative and proliferative inflammatory reaction involving connective tissue and collagen. The inflammatory infiltrate comprises lymphocytes, polymorphonuclear leukocytes, histiocytes, and eosinophils. Aggregation of multinucleated giant cells gives rise to the characteristic Aschoff nodule of rheumatic fever (Fig. 88.2). On histologic examination, there is edema and fibrinous degeneration of collagen with fragmentation and disintegration.

Although the inflammatory changes may be diffuse, affecting the heart, joints, brain, and cutaneous and subcutaneous tissues, Aschoff nodules are seen only in cardiac tissue. Furthermore, long-term sequelae of the inflammatory response are seen only in the heart.

From a gross anatomic point of view, there is a pancarditis involving the endocardium, myocardium, and pericardium. However, it is involvement of the endocardium, including

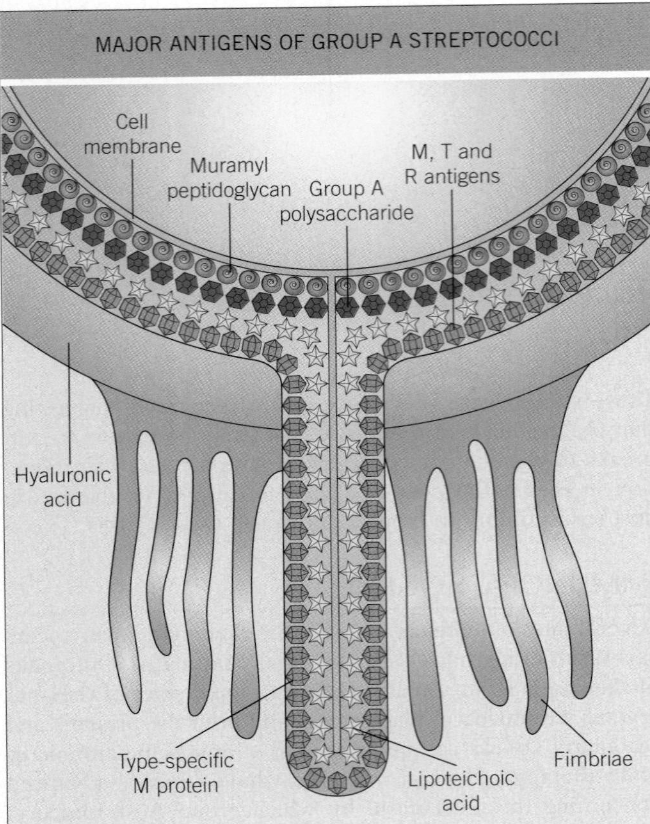

Figure 88.1 Schematic of the major antigens of group A streptococci.

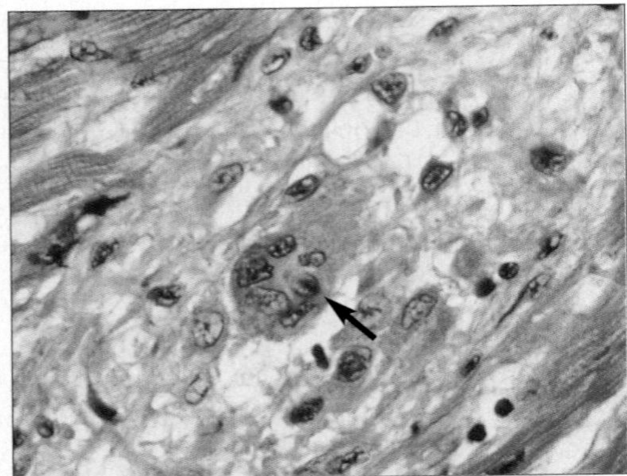

Figure 88.2 Aschoff nodule in the myocardium. The Aschoff nodule is characteristic of rheumatic fever, and the nodule consists of multinucleated giant cells *(arrow)* surrounded by macrophages and T lymphocytes. The adjacent myocardial fibers appear intact.

the valvular and subvalvular apparatus, that gives rise not only to the acute manifestations of the disease but, most important, to the development of chronic rheumatic valvular disease with all its varied manifestations. For reasons that are not clear, the mitral valve is most commonly affected, followed by the aortic, tricuspid, and pulmonary valves. On macroscopic examination, the valves may appear remarkably normal or may show some thickening and small verrucous vegetations measuring 1 to 3 mm at the leaflet

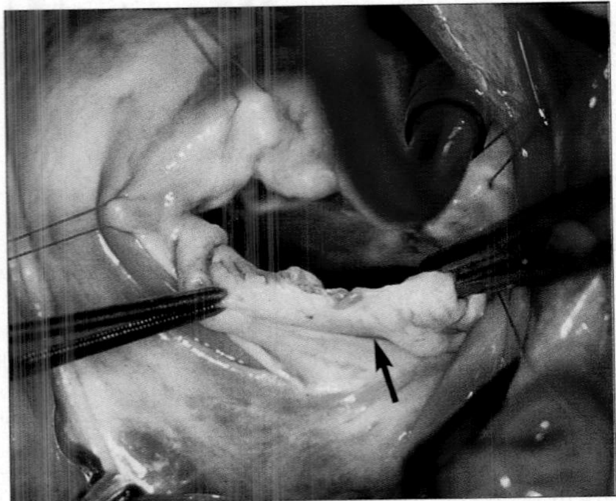

Figure 88.3 View from the left atrium of the mitral valve in a patient with acute rheumatic fever. The leaflets show evidence of rheumatic activity with edematous thickening and verrucous vegetations at the leaflet margins *(arrow)*.

margins (Fig. 88.3). Histologic examination, however, frequently reveals edema, inflammatory cell infiltration, and capillary proliferation. Gross and Friedberg[11] noted a predilection for the atrioventricular valve rings and emphasized that involvement here frequently preceded the appearance of interstitial valvulitis. This is consonant with our echocardiographic and surgical observations that among others, dilatation of the posterior mitral annulus is the predominant mechanism in the pathogenesis of acute rheumatic mitral regurgitation.[12-14] A similar mechanism, although less well documented, has been observed by us in the case of acute rheumatic fever with aortic regurgitation.[13,15]

Although acute inflammatory cell infiltrates and Aschoff nodules are frequently seen in the myocardium of patients with acute rheumatic fever, there is generally scanty histologic evidence of injury or loss of myocardial fibers.[16] An arteritis of the intramyocardial branches of coronary arteries occasionally occurs, but we have never observed clinical myocardial infarction in these patients.

A serofibrinous pericarditis is common, especially in patients with severe episodes of carditis, but it usually resolves completely, leaving normal pericardium. Adhesions may occur, but these are never sufficiently severe to cause pericardial constriction. Small pericardial effusions are common, but cardiac tamponade does not occur.

PATHOPHYSIOLOGY

The pathophysiology of acute rheumatic fever, as it pertains to the heart, essentially relates to the mechanism and consequences of valvular regurgitation and the issue of left ventricular contractile function.

Variable severity of mitral regurgitation is the most common abnormality, and elaboration of the mechanism has an important bearing on the principles of echocardiographic diagnosis and surgical management of this condition. Severe mitral regurgitation has been documented by us[13,14,17] and others[18,19] to be almost invariably caused by prolapse of the anterior mitral leaflet. Prolapse occurs mainly as the result of dilatation of the posterior mitral annulus, but several additional anatomic and geometric factors play a role. These include hamstringing or shortening of the posterior

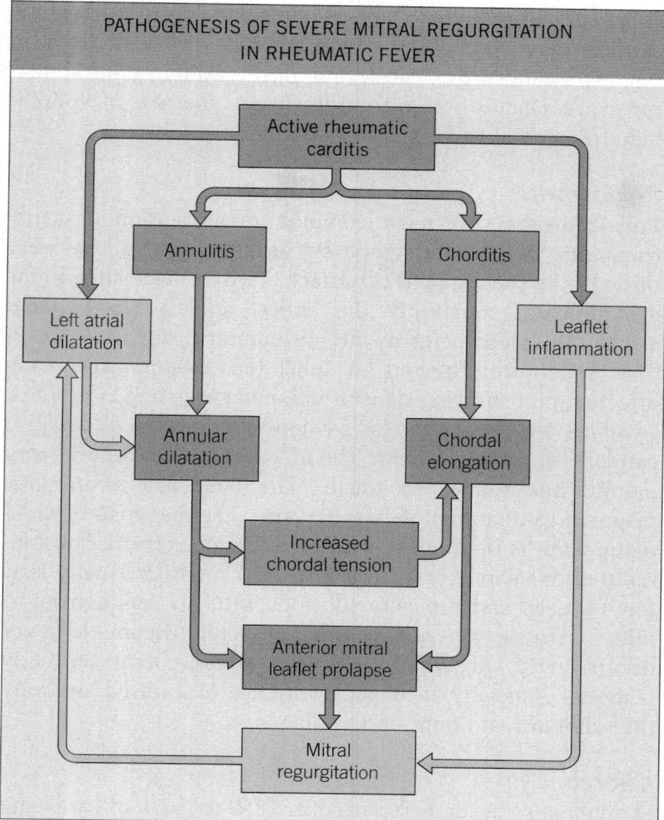

Figure 88.4 Pathogenesis of severe mitral regurgitation in rheumatic fever.

leaflet, retraction of the anterior leaflet, loss of the keystone mechanism of mitral valve closure, chordal elongation, and abnormal spatial relationship between the papillary muscle and valve as a consequence of left ventricular and atrial dilatation (Fig. 88.4). If the resulting mitral regurgitation is severe, there is progressive volume overloading of the left ventricle with a rise in pressure in the left ventricle at end-diastole, left atrium, and pulmonary artery. The left ventricle at presentation in severe cases is almost always dilated, suggesting that the progression of mitral regurgitation has not been rapid.[20] Severe pulmonary hypertension, as seen in patients with chronic rheumatic valvular disease, is unusual.

Aortic regurgitation is the second most frequent abnormality in patients with acute rheumatic fever. We have previously shown the mechanism to be similar to that of mitral regurgitation.[15] Because the aortic annulus is much smaller than the mitral annulus, even mild increases in its dimension may significantly impair leaflet coaptation and result in severe regurgitation. Like that of mitral regurgitation, the development of aortic regurgitation is probably subacute, occurring after several clinically apparent or occult episodes of acute carditis. Thus, the left ventricle is almost always significantly dilated, and the echocardiographic or hemodynamic findings of acute severe aortic regurgitation are absent.

Combined severe mitral and aortic regurgitation is frequent and in our experience occurs in about one third of patients.[21] This combination imposes a severe volume overload and results in significant left ventricular enlargement.

Although histologic evidence of myocarditis is present in 32% to 95% of autopsy cases[22] and was reported in every patient undergoing endomyocardial biopsy during the active phase of the disease, it is not clear that these features are related to abnormalities of left ventricular contractile function. It is both our experience[20] and that of others[23] that left ventricular dilatation and heart failure rarely occur in the absence of hemodynamically significant mitral regurgitation with or without accompanying aortic regurgitation. In patients with active rheumatic carditis presenting with overt heart failure, functionally severe mitral regurgitation with its anatomic correlate of annular dilatation, chordal elongation, and prolapse of the anterior mitral leaflet has been observed sufficiently frequently by us[14] to be regarded as a pathoanatomic hallmark of the disease. To clarify the relative contribution of volume overload induced by valvular regurgitation and myocardial dysfunction due to rheumatic myocarditis to the overall degree of left ventricular dilatation, we analyzed left ventricular dimensions and function noninvasively in a group of young patients with documented active rheumatic carditis before and after successful isolated mitral or combined mitral and aortic valve replacement.[20] Prompt reduction in left ventricular dimensions and preservation of fractional shortening after isolated mitral or combined mitral and aortic valve replacement provided good evidence that rheumatic carditis is not accompanied by myocardial contractile dysfunction to any significant degree. Distinction between left ventricular dilatation and congestive heart failure arising as a consequence of contractile dysfunction due to rheumatic myocarditis or volume overloading associated with valvular regurgitation has important clinical implications because the definitive treatment of severe regurgitant lesions is prompt surgery.

CLINICAL PRESENTATION

Because there is no specific clinical or laboratory test for the diagnosis of rheumatic fever, diagnosis rests on an evaluation of the various clinical and laboratory manifestations of the disease. Early diagnosis and treatment may diminish or eliminate the rheumatic activity, highlighting the importance of an accurate and prompt clinical assessment in these patients. If it is untreated, the initial rheumatic attack is self-limited, and the vast majority subside spontaneously within a period of 12 to 15 weeks.[23]

The most common signs of the disease are carditis, polyarthritis, and chorea; subcutaneous nodules and erythema marginatum are less frequent but no less characteristic. In 1944, T. Duckett Jones formulated criteria for the diagnosis of rheumatic fever.[24] The usefulness of these criteria was reaffirmed in 1992 by the American Heart Association's expert committee.[25] The criteria serve as a useful diagnostic framework but, as also emphasized by the expert committee, are not a substitute for mature clinical judgment. The clinical and laboratory findings are divided into major and minor manifestations on the basis of the diagnostic importance of a particular finding (Table 88.1). If it is supported by evidence of a preceding group A streptococcal infection, the presence of two major or of one major and two minor criteria indicates a high probability of the disease.

MODIFIED JONES CRITERIA FOR THE DIAGNOSIS OF RHEUMATIC FEVER	
Major manifestations	Carditis Polyarthritis Chorea Erythema marginatum Subcutaneous nodules
Minor manifestations	Clinical findings Arthralgia Fever Laboratory findings Elevated acute-phase reactants Elevated erythrocyte sedimentation rate Elevated C-reactive protein level Prolonged PR interval on electrocardiography
Supporting evidence of antecedent group A streptococcal infection	Positive throat culture or rapid streptococcal antigen test result Elevated or rising streptococcal antibody titer
Rheumatic fever may be diagnosed in the presence of two major or one major and two minor criteria with evidence of streptococcal infection.	

Table 88.1 Modified Jones criteria for the diagnosis of rheumatic fever.

Major Manifestations

Carditis

The endocardium, myocardium, and pericardium are involved in varying degrees. However, clinically, rheumatic carditis is almost always associated with a murmur of valvulitis, and in the absence of a murmur, the diagnosis should be made with great caution. Mitral regurgitation is the most common abnormality and results in an apical pansystolic murmur radiating toward the axilla. The apical mid-diastolic or Carey-Coombs murmur is much less frequent and is caused either by increased diastolic flow associated with mitral regurgitation or by structural abnormality of the mitral valve and papillary muscles. Concomitant aortic regurgitation can be detected in approximately 50% of the cases, but isolated aortic insufficiency is less frequent. The tricuspid and pulmonic valves are rarely involved in the acute phase. These murmurs must all be differentiated from murmurs that are functional or flow related or those arising as a result of congenital or chronic rheumatic valvular disease. Myocarditis is diagnosed clinically by the presence of tachycardia, cardiac enlargement, and features of heart failure, although all of these may reflect significant valvular incompetence. Pericarditis is associated with chest pain, and severe tenderness on sternal pressure applied with the heel of the hand is a sign that we have found characteristic and useful. Auscultation may reveal distant heart sounds due to effusion or a pericardial friction rub. Pericardial effusions only rarely result in tamponade, and pericardial constriction almost never occurs. Pericarditis occurs in approximately 6% to 12% of the patients and is generally a sign of fairly severe active rheumatic carditis. Pericarditis in the absence of a murmur should cast doubt on the diagnosis and prompt a search for alternative causes, such as collagen vascular disorders or viral infections. Rheumatic carditis may sometimes be difficult to differentiate from infective endocarditis. Relevant distinguishing clinical features are negative blood cultures and absence of splinter hemorrhages or other signs of systemic embolism.

Polyarthritis

Polyarthritis is the most common manifestation of acute rheumatic fever. The symptoms usually begin at the very onset of the rheumatic fever attack. Two or more large joints are affected, commonly the knees, ankles, elbows, and wrists. It is characteristically asymmetric and migratory. The joints are affected in quick succession, with each affected joint showing signs of inflammation such as redness, swelling, and local heat for 24 hours to 1 week, although it can last for up to 3 weeks. The affected joint is usually very painful and tender to touch. The pain has a dramatic response to treatment with salicylates. The diagnosis of rheumatic fever is in doubt if arthritis does not improve substantially after salicylates. If it is untreated, arthritis usually lasts for 4 weeks and typically subsides with no residual deformity. Because the polyarthritis of acute rheumatic fever occurs early, at which time the streptococcal antibody response is usually at its peak, absence of a raised antibody titer should cast doubt on the diagnosis.

Chorea

Sydenham's chorea is reported in 13% to 34% of cases and is more frequent in female patients. Although the frequency is relatively low, it is one of the most specific signs of rheumatic fever. It is a late manifestation and usually occurs at least 3 months after the onset of the episode of acute rheumatic fever. Thus, when chorea is manifested, all the other clinical signs of rheumatic fever may have disappeared. Emotional lability and irritability are usually the earliest manifestations. This is followed by the appearance of purposeless, rapid, nonrepetitive involuntary movements. It may affect any muscle, but typically those of the extremities and face are involved. The involuntary movements are more evident when the patient is awake, are worsened by stress and fatigue, and disappear during sleep. These movements must be differentiated from tics, athetosis, conversion reactions, and hyperkinesia. Speech may be affected, being explosive and halting. The symptoms of Sydenham's chorea usually resolve in 1 to 2 months but in some cases may persist for more than 2 years. Roughly a quarter of all patients presenting with pure Sydenham's chorea will in the long term be found to have rheumatic mitral valve disease. Whether this represents recurrent attacks of rheumatic fever or recrudescence of mild carditis that was present from the beginning is unknown.

Erythema Marginatum

Erythema marginatum is seen in less than 10% of patients. It is an evanescent, pink or faintly red, nonpruritic rash that occurs mainly on the trunk and proximal extremities but never on the face. The lesions are variable in size, are usually macular, but may be slightly papular. The margins are thin and colored, with a pale rounded center. They appear as enlarging rings, or when they fuse, they may take a serpiginous pattern. The rash may be elicited or accentuated by application of heat and blanches on pressure. Although an infrequent sign, its presence is an important confirmatory sign of rheumatic fever.

Subcutaneous Nodules

Subcutaneous nodules are detected in 10% to 16% of patients with an initial attack of rheumatic fever. They are discrete, firm, painless, and mobile, measuring 0.5 to 2.0 cm. They are usually located over the extensor surfaces of the joints or over bone prominences such as the occipital scalp and spinous processes of vertebrae. The overlying skin is freely movable and is not inflamed. Nodules are a relatively late manifestation. They often appear more than 3 weeks after the onset of the other manifestations, and therefore the early diagnosis of rheumatic fever does not rely on the detection of subcutaneous nodules, but their presence is rather a confirmatory sign. Multiple nodules are almost invariably associated with signs of rheumatic carditis. They usually disappear in 1 to 2 weeks.

Minor Clinical Manifestations

Arthralgia, defined as pain in one or more joints without objective evidence of inflammation, and fever are common but nonspecific manifestations of rheumatic fever. Arthralgia must not be considered a minor manifestation when arthritis is present. Fever with no specific pattern is almost always present at the onset of rheumatic fever, but temperature rarely exceeds 104°F (40°C). Low-grade fever may persist for 1 to 2 weeks.

Other Manifestations

Several features not included in the Jones criteria are sometimes seen in patients with rheumatic fever. These include epistaxis, abdominal pain, splenomegaly, and digital clubbing.[13]

Exceptions to the Jones Criteria

There are three instances when rheumatic fever can be diagnosed without strictly adhering to the Jones criteria. Chorea may be the only manifestation of rheumatic fever. In the absence of any other cause and especially in the appropriate age group, rheumatic fever may be diagnosed by this finding alone. Similarly, indolent carditis at a time by which other features of rheumatic fever have waned may be the only manifestation of the disease. Finally, patients with recurrent attacks may not meet the specified criteria. Rheumatic fever may be diagnosed in these patients, provided the prior episodes have been reliably documented and there is sufficient supporting evidence of a recent group A streptococcal infection.

DIAGNOSTIC TECHNIQUES

Nonspecific Laboratory Findings

The acute-phase reactants including erythrocyte sedimentation rate and C-reactive protein constitute minor criteria for the diagnosis of rheumatic fever. They are sensitive but nonspecific markers of inflammation and are almost always increased in patients with polyarthritis or acute carditis except when salicylates or steroids have been administered. In patients with isolated chorea, they are usually normal. Anemia may result in a more rapid sedimentation rate, and the opposite occurs in the presence of severe congestive heart failure. C-reactive protein levels are less sensitive to external factors and may be a more useful test to follow disease activity. A normochromic normocytic anemia is common.

Supporting Evidence of Preceding Group A Streptococcal Infection

With the exceptions mentioned, laboratory evidence of an antecedent group A streptococcal infection is a specified requirement for the diagnosis of rheumatic fever. The criteria require either demonstration of group A streptococci in the throat or an elevated or rising titer of streptococcal antibodies.

At the time of diagnosis of rheumatic fever, only about 25% of patients have a positive throat culture for group A streptococci. The low isolation rate is due to several factors, including

- the 10- to 14-day latent period between infection and development of rheumatic fever;
- the failure to consider the diagnosis, causing inappropriate delay in obtaining culture specimens; and
- the prior exposure to antibiotics.

Several rapid group A streptococcal antigen detection kits are available. These tests are specific but lack sensitivity. For this reason, a negative test result should be confirmed by a conventional throat culture. Interpretation of throat cultures or the antigen test result is further complicated by the fact that group A streptococci may colonize the normal pharynx, their presence being unrelated to the clinical illness under investigation. Because streptococci found in the pharynx may not represent active infection, elevated or rising serum antibody titers provide more definitive evidence of a recent streptococcal infection.

Serologic evidence of a group A streptococcal infection is predicated on an elevated or rising streptococcal antibody titer. Antibody determination is especially useful because the onset of the clinical manifestations of rheumatic fever coincides with the peak antibody response. A negative test result therefore has a high predictive value in excluding the diagnosis. A significant antibody response is defined as a rise in titer of two or more dilution increments between the acute- and convalescent-phase specimens, irrespective of the absolute antibody level. Antibody responses to several streptococcal extracellular antigens may be measured, including streptolysin O, streptolysin S, hyaluronidase, streptokinase, deoxyribonucleases A to D, and nicotinamide adenine dinucleotidase. Of these, the anti–streptolysin O (ASO) and anti–deoxyribonuclease B (anti–DNase B) assays are used most commonly. ASO titers are elevated in about 80% of patients with rheumatic fever but in only 20% of those with chorea as the only manifestation. The definition of an elevated ASO titer may be difficult because the range is variable and dependent on several factors, including age, geographic location, and season of the year. Arbitrarily, an elevated ASO titer is defined as that value that is exceeded by less than 20% of the population being studied. By use of this definition, an ASO titer is considered to be increased if it exceeds 240 Todd units in adults or 320 Todd units in children. Titers of ASO may be measured by a commercially available slide agglutination test. This test should be used for screening purposes only, and if the result is negative, a definitive titration should still be done. Low to normal levels of ASO when the clinical suspicion is high should be followed by measures of other antibodies, including anti–DNase B and, if necessary, antihyaluronidase titer. Titers of anti–DNase B exceeding 120 Todd units in adults or 240 Todd units in children are regarded as being elevated. With use of three different antibody tests, an elevated titer for at least one test can be demonstrated in about 95% of patients with rheumatic fever and 80% of patients with isolated Sydenham's chorea.

Electrocardiographic Features

First-degree heart block constitutes a minor Jones criterion for the diagnosis of rheumatic fever and occurs frequently. However, it may occur in any post-streptococcal infection and is not specific for rheumatic carditis or the later development of rheumatic valvular disease. Other features include tachycardia and repolarization abnormalities, but these are not considered minor criteria.

Chest Radiography

This is not specific for rheumatic fever. The size of the heart and presence of pulmonary venous congestion are dependent on the severity of the underlying valve lesions. A normal chest film appearance should not therefore exclude the diagnosis.

Echocardiography

Although valvular regurgitation is frequently the hallmark of rheumatic fever with carditis and is the forerunner of the long-term complications of this disease, until recently little has been known about the mechanism of valvular dysfunction. Furthermore, an appreciation of the pathology and pathophysiology of valvular regurgitation is germane to any surgical endeavor to restore competence of the mitral and aortic valves. Neither postmortem analysis nor observations made intraoperatively in a flaccid nonbeating heart are able to appreciate the dimensions and spatial relationships of the valvular and subvalvular components of the mitral valve.

Echocardiography is an easily applied, noninvasive technique with excellent resolution and has made a unique contribution to our understanding of the pathogenesis of valvular regurgitation in rheumatic carditis. In a detailed echocardiographic analysis of 73 young patients (mean age, 13 years) with acute carditis and severe mitral regurgitation, we have demonstrated[14] varying degrees of prolapse of the anterior mitral leaflet in 94% (Figs. 88.5 and 88.6). Echocardiographically detected prolapse, defined as failure of leaflet edge coaptation during systole, was confirmed in every patient at the time of surgery. An increase in the mitral annular diameter, mainly of the posterior annulus, is the primary cause of leaflet prolapse (Fig. 88.7). The mean mitral annular diameter in our patients was 37 mm compared with a diameter of 23 mm in a control group matched for age and sex. To validate the hypothesis that mitral annular dilatation is the primary abnormality in rheumatic fever and not secondary to severe mitral

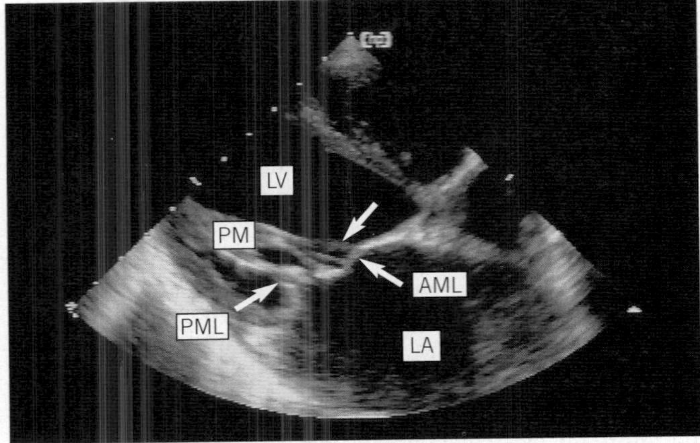

Figure 88.5 Transthoracic echocardiogram in a 14-year-old patient with rheumatic fever and severe mitral regurgitation. This parasternal, long-axis, end-systolic echocardiogram shows characteristic prolapse of the anterior mitral leaflet. The marginal chordae to the anterior leaflet are mildly thickened and elongated *(arrows)*. Note that the leaflets themselves appear relatively normal. AML, anterior mitral leaflet; LA, left atrium; LV, left ventricle; PM, papillary muscle; PML, posterior mitral leaflet.

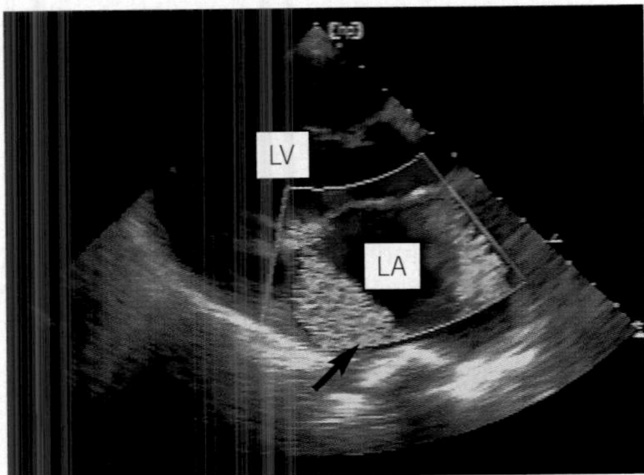

Figure 88.6 Color Doppler study in a patient with rheumatic fever and severe mitral regurgitation. Note the typical posteriorly directed jet *(arrow)* due to prolapse of the anterior leaflet. LA, left atrium; LV, left ventricle.

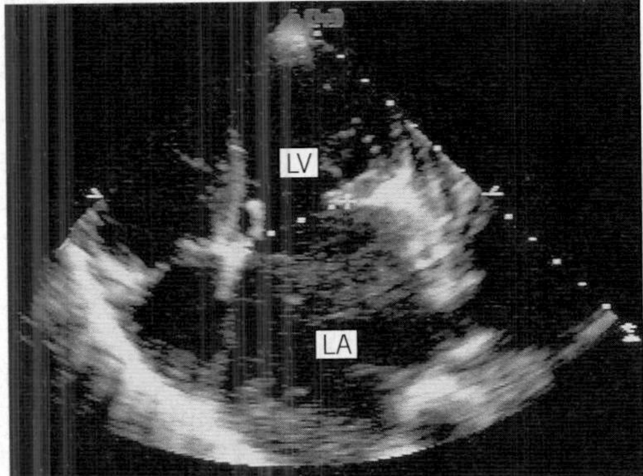

Figure 88.7 Transthoracic apical four-chamber view in a 12-year-old patient with rheumatic fever and severe mitral regurgitation. The mitral annulus is dilated at 39 mm. The left atrium is markedly enlarged. LA, left atrium; LV, left ventricle.

regurgitation with left ventricular dilatation, we measured annular diameter in a group of patients with mild mitral regurgitation and a matched control group with normal hearts.[26] Although the annular diameter was smaller than that measured in patients with severe mitral regurgitation, even patients with mild mitral regurgitation had larger annuli compared with controls. The occurrence of annular dilatation in children in whom mitral regurgitation was mild and in whom neither left atrial nor left ventricular enlargement was advanced lends further proof to the hypothesis that mitral annular dilatation is a primary event in the pathogenesis of rheumatic mitral regurgitation. Further proof for this hypothesis is the fact that despite the young age of this group of patients, relatively large diameter annuloplasty rings or mechanical prostheses can be inserted in the mitral position.[17]

Another feature of severe mitral regurgitation in rheumatic fever is elongated chordae to the anterior mitral leaflet, but without rupture (see Fig. 88.5). It is probable that both primary involvement by the rheumatic process and secondary exposure to increased tensile stresses during ventricular systole contribute to elongation of the chordae.[14] Apart from some shortening of the posterior mitral leaflet due to stretching of the annulus, the morphologic appearance of the leaflet is remarkably normal. Thus, severe mitral regurgitation in rheumatic fever is the result of annular dilatation and chordal elongation with resultant prolapse and is not, at least in the early stages, due to abnormalities of the leaflets themselves.

Color Doppler study is useful in quantifying the severity of mitral regurgitation and almost invariably shows a posteriorly directed jet, confirming anterior leaflet prolapse. The abnormalities of the mitral valve that have been described are characteristic of patients with rheumatic fever and severe mitral regurgitation. In an unselected group of patients presenting with rheumatic fever and carditis, Vasan and colleagues[27] were able to document mitral valve prolapse in only 9% of patients with a first attack of carditis and in 16% with recurrent carditis. The severity of mitral regurgitation in these patients is unfortunately not documented. In their series, the most frequent echocardiographic abnormality was leaflet thickening and nodules possibly representing verrucous vegetations. Other series have noted a higher incidence of mitral valve prolapse. Wu and coworkers[28] noted mitral valve prolapse in 30% of their patients with rheumatic fever and mitral regurgitation. Mitral valve prolapse also correlated with a larger cardiac size and a less favorable long-term outcome. In a series of patients receiving rheumatic fever prophylaxis with less than moderate mitral regurgitation, Lembo and colleagues[19] found an 80% incidence of echocardiographically detected mitral valve prolapse.

Differentiation of rheumatic mitral valve prolapse from degenerative or myxomatous mitral valve disease is important.[17] Rheumatic prolapse always involves the anterior leaflet, whereas myxomatous prolapse has a predilection for the posterior leaflet. Myxomatous leaflets are thickened, voluminous, and redundant, with significant systolic bulging or billow toward the left atrium. In contrast, the leaflets in rheumatic carditis with mitral regurgitation show minimal thickening, redundancy, or billow.

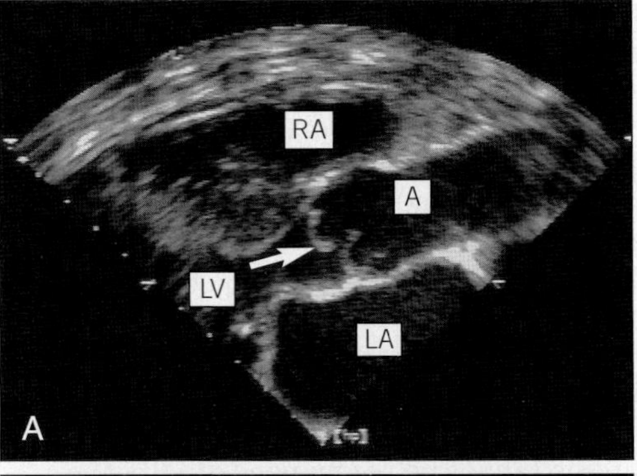

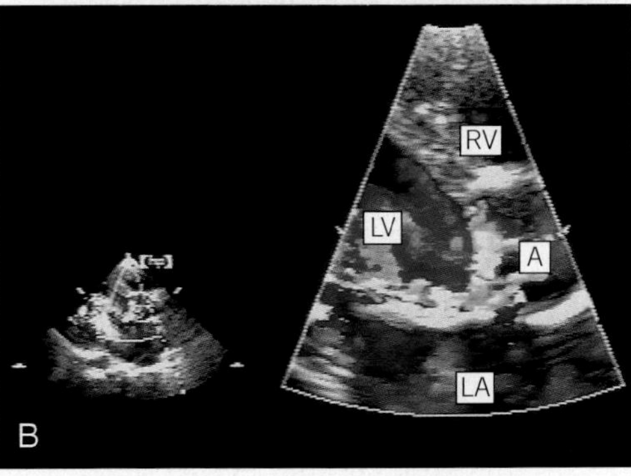

Figures 88.8 Transesophageal long-axis view in a patient with rheumatic fever and severe aortic regurgitation. There is a prolapse of the right coronary cusp. Color Doppler study **(B)** confirms a posteriorly directed jet. A, aorta; LA, left atrium; LV, left ventricle; RV, right ventricle.

We have also had the opportunity to evaluate the mechanism of severe aortic regurgitation in rheumatic fever.[15] As in the case of the mitral valve, annular dilatation with leaflet prolapse appears to be the predominant mechanism (Fig. 88.8). Because the aortic annulus is much smaller than the mitral annulus, even minor changes in its diameter may result in significant prolapse and regurgitation.

Despite careful auscultation, valvular regurgitation may sometimes be inaudible with the stethoscope. In these cases, echocardiography may play a useful role in enhancing the detection of carditis. Thus, Doppler echocardiography was the sole means for the diagnosis of carditis in 25% of the patients in one series[2] and increased the diagnosis of carditis based on the Jones criteria from 72% to 91% in another.[29] Furthermore, functional murmurs in young, febrile, and anemic patients are quite common. By differentiating these from the murmur of mitral regurgitation, Doppler echocardiography could potentially reduce the rate of false-positive diagnoses. The American Heart Association guidelines for the diagnosis of rheumatic fever published in 1992[25] do not encourage the use of echocardiography as the sole criterion for the diagnosis of carditis. Whereas there is some justification for this, including the possibility of overdiagnosis and the lack of prospective studies evaluating the role of echocardiography, there is an emerging body of evidence emphasizing the utility of Doppler echocardiography for the diagnosis of rheumatic carditis.[30] We would concur with Veasy[30] that echocardiography has the potential of becoming a useful diagnostic tool and should be incorporated in the future into the Jones criteria.

Endomyocardial Biopsy

On histologic examination, the only pathognomonic feature of rheumatic carditis is the Aschoff nodule. A series evaluating the utility of endomyocardial biopsy found Aschoff nodules in only 27% of the patients with clinically documented carditis according to the revised Jones criteria.[31] Whether the Aschoff nodules were truly absent or not seen because of sampling error is not known. Nonspecific myocyte or interstitial alterations occurred in most patients with clinically definite rheumatic carditis and were absent in those with clinically inactive disease. On the basis of these data, routine endomyocardial biopsy for the diagnosis of rheumatic carditis cannot be recommended.

MANAGEMENT

Several aspects of management need to be considered, including primary prevention, secondary prevention, treatment of the acute attack, and bacterial endocarditis prophylaxis.

Primary Prevention

Prevention of the first attack of rheumatic fever requires the prompt recognition and treatment of a group A streptococcal pharyngitis. Pharyngitis has a multifactorial etiology, with only about 30% of sore throats being of streptococcal etiology. The vigor with which a group A streptococcal etiology is sought depends on local circumstances. In an affluent setting where the prevalence of rheumatic fever is low, throat swabs or a rapid antigen assay to confirm group A streptococcus should be obtained before initiation of specific antibiotic therapy. However, in areas where rheumatic fever is endemic and financial resources are limited, antibiotic treatment of all sore throats without microbiologic confirmation is not an unreasonable approach. Despite optimal treatment of all patients presenting with a sore throat, rheumatic fever may not be entirely preventable for two reasons:

- many episodes of streptococcal pharyngitis are asymptomatic; and
- despite their in vitro susceptibility, streptococci are not always eradicated from the pharynx after appropriate antibiotic therapy.[10]

Most streptococci, however, remain extremely sensitive to penicillin, which can be administered either as a single intramuscular injection of benzathine penicillin (1.2 million units) or a 10-day course of oral phenoxymethyl penicillin (250 mg every 6 hours). Erythromycin (250 mg every 6 hours for 10 days) is appropriate for patients allergic to penicillin. Up to 30% of patients who receive appropriate antibiotic therapy become carriers of group A streptococci despite clinical recovery. However, chronic pharyngeal carriage does not appear to pose a threat in populations with a low prevalence of rheumatic fever.[32] As pointed out by Stollerman,[32] in areas where rheumatic fever has a high prevalence, continuous microbiologic surveillance is particularly important to identify known and new rheumatogenic M serotypes but especially if multivalent vaccines are to be developed in the future.

Secondary Prevention

Much of the morbidity of rheumatic fever is due to repeated flares of disease activity initiated by recurrent episodes of group A streptococcal pharyngitis. Because asymptomatic pharyngitis can also trigger episodes of acute rheumatic fever, and even optimal treatment of symptomatic infections may fail to prevent recurrences, continuous prophylactic antibiotic therapy is the only way to prevent recurrent attacks of rheumatic fever and should be instituted promptly in any patient with documented rheumatic fever or rheumatic heart disease. Monthly intramuscular injection of 1.2 million units of benzathine penicillin is the most effective, although oral penicillin (125 to 250 mg every 12 hours) is also acceptable. Erythromycin (250 mg every 12 hours) is appropriate for those allergic to penicillin.

The duration for which prophylactic antibiotic therapy should be continued is controversial, bearing in mind that the risk of recurrent rheumatic fever decreases with advancing age and increasing intervals since the last episode. We have rarely encountered rheumatic fever beyond adolescence, even in a high-prevalence area for rheumatic disease. Prophylactic therapy beyond the age of 21 years, we therefore believe, is rarely necessary, but judgment for each patient should be individualized. Thus, individuals who have had an attack within the preceding 5 years and those at high risk of exposure to streptococcal infections, such as children and adolescents, parents with young children, teachers, military recruits, and health care personnel, should probably be treated for longer if not for a lifetime.

There is some evidence that patients with isolated chorea are more likely in the long term to develop mitral stenosis than are those presenting with isolated polyarthritis. These patients should therefore receive rheumatic fever prophylaxis even in the absence of documented heart disease or rheumatic fever.

Treatment of the Acute Attack of Rheumatic Fever

Irrespective of the result of throat cultures, which at the time of clinical presentation are likely to be negative anyway, all patients should be treated immediately for a presumed group A streptococcal pharyngitis as outlined earlier. Bed rest is important because it lessens joint pain and reduces the cardiac workload in patients with carditis. The duration of bed rest should be guided by symptoms and serum activity markers, but it should be enforced for a minimum of 8 to 12 weeks in patients with documented carditis. Most patients are able to return to unrestricted activity without residual cardiac disease.

The use of specific anti-inflammatory agents, including aspirin and glucocorticoids, is subject to controversy. Aspirin is effective for the relief of joint pain and should be used in high doses (100 mg/kg per day given every 4 to 6 hours), with further dosage guided by serum levels. Tinnitus, nausea, or vomiting requires a reduction in dose. Although corticosteroids are also effective in reducing inflammatory activity, there is little objective evidence that they alter the natural history of the disease. The U.K. and U.S. cooperative trial of adrenocorticotropic hormone, cortisone, and aspirin failed to show any advantage of corticosteroids in preventing cardiac damage at 1, 5, and 10 years.[33] Patients with mild carditis are likely to improve anyway, and most physicians currently limit the use of steroids to patients with cardiomegaly or heart failure. However, because heart failure in these patients is invariably due to hemodynamically significant valvular regurgitation, it is our belief that appropriate therapy is valve repair or replacement.[20] We are therefore in agreement with Stollerman[32] that corticosteroids are not appropriate for the routine treatment of rheumatic fever. Furthermore, corticosteroids are associated with serious side effects, among which fluid retention and hypertension are particularly undesirable in a patient with heart failure.

Although it is diminishing in frequency, in South Africa we continue to encounter a severe form of fulminant rheumatic carditis that afflicts patients in early adolescence. These patients present most commonly with severe mitral regurgitation but not infrequently with concomitant severe aortic regurgitation. Heart failure in these patients rarely responds to the usual measures, including intravenous diuretics, digitalis, and supportive inotropic therapy. Furthermore, as long as these patients remain in a hemodynamically compromised state, there is little success in attenuating rheumatic inflammatory activity despite bed rest and antibiotic therapy. Despite the disadvantages of prosthetic valve implantation in this young group of patients, it has been our experience[12,13,17,34,35] and that of others[36,37] that this treatment may be lifesaving and can be performed with a low mortality in experienced centers. Valve replacement is accompanied by a dramatic decline in rheumatic activity, suggesting that the rheumatic activity is perpetuated by the hemodynamic burden. Although mitral valve repair is desirable in these young patients, we have found the results disappointing, with a 5-year event-free survival of only 66% and a valve failure rate of 47%.[38]

A multivariate analysis identified active rheumatic carditis at the time of surgery as the only predictor of reoperation. Valve failure in these patients is not due to poor operative technique because the failure usually occurs late; rather, it is a reflection of the natural history of rheumatic valve disease with progressive fibrosis and scarring of the valve. Although externally the leaflet in rheumatic disease may appear beguilingly normal, histologic examination invariably demonstrates inflammatory cell activity, and it is therefore inevitable that this will adversely affect the long-term results of valve repair. It is our policy to recommend a valve repair in women of childbearing age, in patients in whom monitoring of warfarin anticoagulation is likely to be difficult, and in those patients who either at presentation or after a period of bed rest and penicillin treatment show some reduction in serum activity markers. Patients with gross rheumatic activity, often evident intraoperatively, do poorly after repair, and mitral valve replacement remains the most suitable option.

The technique of mitral valve repair is guided by the observed pathoanatomy and most often includes annular reconstruction with an annuloplasty ring and chordal shortening.[35] Prolonged bed rest and antibiotic prophylaxis against recurrent episodes of rheumatic fever are particularly important to prevent early breakdown of the repair.

Infective Endocarditis Prophylaxis

Patients with rheumatic fever and valvular regurgitation require endocarditis prophylaxis (see Chapter 99). It is often not appreciated that rheumatic fever prophylaxis does not offer protection against endocarditis and that appropriate measures need to be taken in this regard.

PROGNOSIS

During an epidemic of pharyngitis with rheumatogenic group A streptococci, rheumatic fever follows at an attack rate ranging between 1% and 5%. The magnitude of the immune response and duration of carriage of the organism are the major determinants of the attack rate. Appropriate antibiotic therapy for group A streptococcal pharyngitis reduces the attack rate to almost negligible levels. The attack rate for rheumatic fever in nonepidemic outbreaks of group A streptococcal pharyngitis may be much lower.

Even after the first episode of rheumatic fever, long-term sequelae of chronic rheumatic heart disease are manifested in only about half of the patients. The remaining half either recover completely or demonstrate some other noncardiac manifestation of the disease. The incidence of carditis, characterized by regurgitant murmurs, shows a diminishing frequency with age, ranging from 90% at age 3 years to about 30% in adolescence. The prognosis for patients who either escape carditis or have a very mild episode is excellent, with almost no development of late chronic rheumatic heart disease, provided recurrences of rheumatic fever are prevented. With increasing severity of carditis, the chances of escaping progression to chronic rheumatic heart disease are less; only 40% of patients presenting with heart failure are free of disease at 10 years, provided further recurrences of rheumatic fever are prevented. These data highlight the extreme importance of secondary antibiotic prophylaxis in the patient with rheumatic fever.

We believe that once there is significant scarring of the valve and commissural fusion, rheumatic disease is progressive even in the absence of recurrent episodes of acute carditis. This may in part be related to the adverse effects of turbulent blood flow with progressive leaflet rigidity, thickening, and calcification.

SUMMARY

Rheumatic fever remains a significant health issue in developing countries, with sporadic and unexplained outbreaks even in more advanced countries. The drain on global economic resources is considerable, and only an improvement in the general standards of living, coupled with early diagnosis and effective treatment of both group A streptococcal pharyngitis and acute rheumatic fever, offers any reasonable prospect of diminishing the ravages of this disease. Whereas the revised Jones criteria remain a useful tool for the diagnosis of rheumatic fever, there are inherent limitations, and they should by no means be applied in a rigid fashion. Apart from delineating the mechanisms of valvular regurgitation and providing an insight into left ventricular contractile function, echocardiography may make a useful contribution to the diagnosis of rheumatic fever with carditis and may possibly in the future be incorporated into the Jones criteria, in a manner similar to the new paradigm for the diagnosis of infective endocarditis. The limited availability of this technology may be the only impediment. The development of a vaccine against rheumatic fever represents a novel and exciting strategy for the control of this disease. The M protein molecule of rheumatogenic group A streptococci has already been completely characterized, extracted, modified, and tested in several studies that suggest a potential for an oral vaccine.[39] Armed with an effective vaccine and penicillin, we may yet succeed in eradicating the scourge of rheumatic fever.

chapter
89 Mitral Stenosis

Michael S. Kim and John D. Carroll

Definition

- Mitral stenosis is abnormal diastolic blood flow from the left atrium to the left ventricle.

Key Features

- Mitral stenosis is predominantly caused by rheumatic fever and continues to result in significant morbidity and mortality worldwide.
- Commissural fusion produces hemodynamic obstruction, with the development of increased pulmonary capillary pressures and limitation of cardiac output.
- The pathophysiologic process of mitral stenosis is generally logical and well understood, although the predilection of the disease for women and the variable occurrence of severe pulmonary hypertension remain unclarified.
- Atrial fibrillation is a common arrhythmia that precipitates hemodynamic decompensation and further increases the risk of thromboembolism as a result of left atrial enlargement, blood stagnation, and increased concentrations of prothrombotic markers.
- The clinical presentation varies according to the patient's age, symptoms (e.g., asymptomatic or critically ill), and presence or absence of concomitant valve abnormalities and during pregnancy.
- Diagnosis and characterization are possible by various forms of echocardiography with Doppler study, but the physical examination remains important, especially for initial detection before life-threatening complications occur.

Treatment

- Medical management includes pharmacologic reduction of the hemodynamic impact of obstruction, control of atrial fibrillation, reduction of thromboembolic risk, and prevention of endocarditis and recurrent acute rheumatic fever.
- Percutaneous mitral balloon valvuloplasty provides mechanical relief from moderate to severe stenosis early in the natural history of mitral stenosis and has replaced surgical commissurotomy as the initial intervention for those with suitable valve morphology. Advanced echocardiographic techniques, including real-time three-dimensional echocardiography, may improve selection of patients in the future.
- Surgical valve replacement remains the treatment of choice in symptomatic patients with more deformed valves.
- Whereas the natural history of mitral stenosis has been dramatically altered by advancements in medicine, the eradication of rheumatic fever remains the ultimate cure.

Mitral stenosis (MS) is a valvular lesion typically seen in adults and is most commonly a consequence of childhood rheumatic carditis. If it is left unrecognized or untreated, MS may result in serious and potentially fatal complications, such as pulmonary edema, systemic embolism, severe pulmonary hypertension, and endocarditis. Although the incidence of MS is greatest in countries where rheumatic fever is either uncontrolled or insufficiently contained, it nonetheless remains the cause of significant morbidity and mortality worldwide. Whereas many patients with MS in developing countries are young, in other areas of the world where rheumatic fever was eradicated decades ago, patients are often elderly. Immigration, however, has brought with it a resurgence of younger patients with this disorder to both the United States and other industrialized countries.[1]

ANATOMY AND PATHOLOGY

Rheumatic fever remains the predominant (i.e., >99% of cases) cause of MS.[2] In contrast, congenital MS, the predominant cause of the disease in children, is rarely seen in the adult population. In addition, mitral annular calcification may involve the valve leaflets and produce obstruction through functional leaflet immobility, although this finding remains relatively rare. Other rare causes of the disorder include carcinoid tumor, methysergide therapy, Fabry's disease, Whipple's disease, systemic lupus erythematosus, and mucopolysaccharidosis.

Rheumatic Heart Disease

Although rheumatic disease may affect several sites within the heart, the most common manifestation is valvulitis involving the edges of the mitral leaflets, which produces verrucae. These anatomic anomalies slowly progress during decades, are likely driven by abnormal flow dynamics caused by the initial injury, and lead to various anatomic and functional consequences (Fig. 89.1).

The mitral valve is involved in two thirds of patients with chronic rheumatic disease.[2] Unlike mitral regurgitation, MS is rarely observed during acute rheumatic fever but rather occurs later in the disease course and is denoted by its distinctive anatomic features. Hemodynamic obstruction typically occurs at the level of the mitral orifice and is predominantly caused by commissural fusion.[3] Over time and in cases of advanced MS, increased hemodynamic resistance commonly develops at the pulmonary vascular level, reflected by thickening of the arterial wall and obliteration

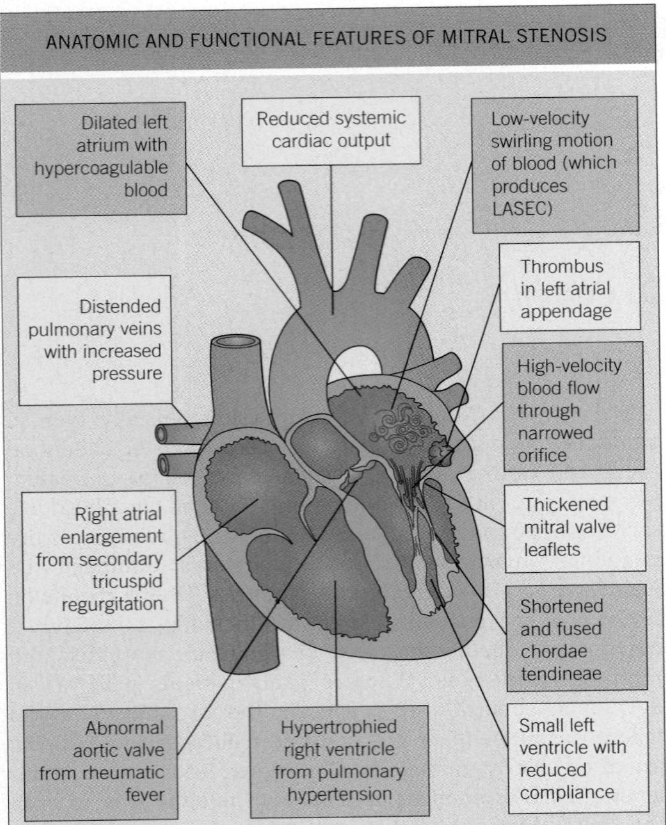

Figure 89.1 Anatomic and functional features of mitral stenosis. The heart undergoes a variety of anatomic and physiologic modifications from the initial rheumatic insult and the subsequent development of hemodynamically important mitral stenosis. LASEC, left atrial spontaneous echo contrast.

of small vessels. Significant obstruction at the subvalvular level is uncommon, although when it is present, it results from extensive chordal fusion coexistent with advanced obstruction at the level of the mitral orifice.

The normal mitral valve opens to an area of 4 to 6 cm^2 and involves the harmonious coordination of the delicate anterior and posterior leaflets, subvalvular apparatus, and mitral annulus.[3] In contrast, a narrowed mitral valve with an orifice of less than 1.5 cm^2 demonstrates an abrupt, plate-like narrowing of the valve orifice. In rheumatic MS in which commissural fusion is present, however, the valve orifice assumes the characteristic shape of a fish mouth. Although the leaflets may be thickened and resist opening, significant upstream and downstream tapering of the flow field is not traditionally present. Furthermore, during periods of enhanced cardiac output, such as occurs with exercise, the augmented magnitude of opening forces may result in a slightly larger orifice area than is present during resting conditions. All of these features are important anatomic features of rheumatic MS and play significant roles in the physiologic manifestations of obstruction.

Mitral Annular Calcification

Mitral annular calcification is commonly found on routine echocardiography, particularly in the elderly.[4] Mitral annular calcification is generally regarded as a benign process, although it may result in significant mitral regurgitation because of increased rigidity of the mitral annulus.[5] MS, however, remains a relatively rare complication of mitral annular calcification[6] and is seen in approximately 0.5% of outpatient echocardiograms.[7] Unlike rheumatic disease, which most commonly reduces valve opening by commissural fusion, calcific MS distinguishes itself by thin and mobile mitral leaflet tips with calcification of the interannular fibrosa extending down onto the mitral leaflets. This annular thickening directly results in reduced valve mobility and subsequent narrowing of the diastolic flow area. Studies indicate that reduced anterior mitral leaflet mobility is a key determinant in elevated resting mitral valve gradients (i.e., >5 mm Hg) and that reduced anterior mitral leaflet mobility is more important in producing a significant mitral valve gradient than the actual severity of mitral annular calcification.[7]

Although the severity of stenosis in most patients with mitral annular calcification will be relatively minor at rest, situations in which the heart rate rises and cardiac output is augmented (e.g., exercise, atrial fibrillation, anemia, severe systemic illnesses) may increase the mitral valve gradient enough to cause or to contribute to symptoms of dyspnea and fatigue (i.e., functional MS).

PATHOPHYSIOLOGY OF MITRAL STENOSIS

The pathophysiology of MS is characterized not only by classic hemodynamic findings but also by arrhythmias (especially atrial fibrillation), alterations in neurohumoral activation, development of thromboembolism, and irregularities in ventricular function. The effect of MS on circulatory pressures and blood flow has four clinically relevant aspects:

- increased transmitral pressure gradient in diastole;
- increased transmitral blood velocity with the formation of a flow jet;
- reduced total flow (i.e., cardiac output); and
- left atrial hypertension.[3]

The transvalvular pressure gradient is directly assessed by comparing a pressure waveform upstream from the obstruction (i.e., pulmonary capillary wedge or left atrial pressure) with the downstream left ventricular pressure waveform (Fig. 89.2). The degree of the diastolic gradient is a marker of stenosis severity. Clinically significant MS usually produces resting diastolic mean gradients of 10 to 20 mm Hg that dramatically increase during minimal exercise. With worsening of MS severity, the transvalvular gradient may eventually plateau because of an inherent decrease in transvalvular flow resulting from decreased cardiac output. A central concept in determining the clinical and hemodynamic significance of MS is that the transvalvular gradient is a marker of both obstruction severity and absolute flow across the narrowed valve.

MS can also be characterized by changes in the transvalvular velocity of blood flow. This property forms the basis of noninvasively derived measurements of transvalvular gradients by Doppler echocardiography.[8] Acceleration of blood flow below the orifice occurs in the discrete anatomic region of stenosis and produces a high-velocity laminar jet of blood emerging from the valve orifice. The velocity of the laminar

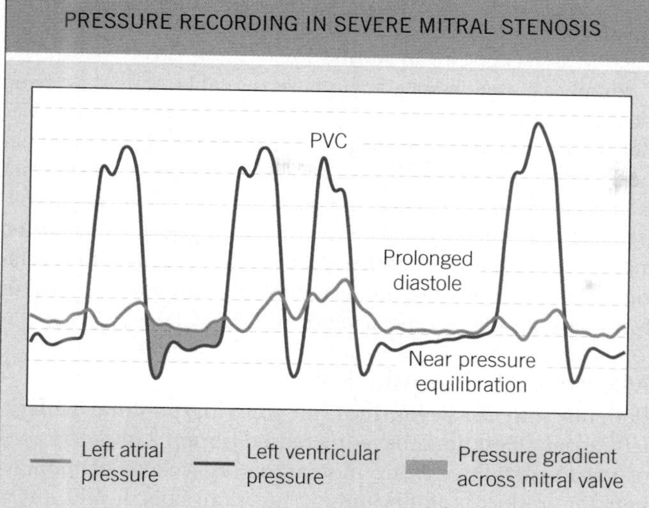

Figure 89.2 Pressure recording in severe mitral stenosis. Left atrial pressure and left ventricular pressures were measured by use of standard, fluid-filled catheters with an external pressure transducer. Two sinus beats are followed by a premature ventricular contraction (PVC) with a post-PVC prolongation of diastole. The pressure tracings demonstrate the transmitral gradient across the mitral valve and an increased left atrial pressure of 28 mm Hg caused by the obstruction of the mitral valve. The reduced gradient at the end of the prolonged diastole, with near pressure equilibration, is due to the decompression of the left atrium that is permitted by the additional time for blood to enter the left ventricle before the next contraction. This demonstration is relevant to the management strategy of slowing the heart rate with beta blockers.

jet can be noninvasively measured by echocardiography, resulting in a representative assessment of the transvalvular gradient.

The reduction in cardiac output often seen in MS is related to disease severity as well as to whether the measurement of cardiac output is made at rest or during states of increased flow (e.g., exercise, anemia, pregnancy, thyrotoxicosis, and systemic infection). Noticeable decreases in cardiac output may be apparent only during exercise in patients with moderate MS. In contrast, resting cardiac output in severe MS with pulmonary hypertension is often very low (on the order of 3.0 L/min) and is associated with mixed venous oxygen saturations of approximately 50%.[3]

The duration of the diastolic filling period also plays a vital role in determining the clinical impact of a given degree of MS. When heart rate is increased, the hemodynamic influence of MS dramatically worsens. Exercise-induced symptoms are related to marked increases in left atrial pressure resulting from an abbreviated diastolic filling period during periods of tachycardia, coupled with an increase in cardiac output. Similar increases in both the transvalvular gradient and left atrial pressure are also observed in the presence of atrial fibrillation with rapid ventricular response. The importance of diastolic filling time in MS forms the basis for the management strategy of promoting sinus bradycardia and optimal rate control in atrial fibrillation. Specifically, bradycardia results in a prolonged diastolic filling period and allows complete decompression of the engorged left atrium, thereby minimizing the transvalvular pressure gradient in the setting of markedly reduced left atrial pressure (see Fig. 89.2).

The increase in left atrial pressure is the final manifestation of MS and leads to a variety of clinical effects. Left atrial hypertension leads directly to increased pulmonary capillary pressure, which is manifested as increases in dyspnea, pulmonary edema, hemoptysis, pulmonary hypertension, and detrimental effects on the right-sided chambers (i.e., right ventricular enlargement and failure). Left atrial hypertension also leads to progressive left atrial dilatation, thereby increasing the risk of atrial fibrillation or thromboembolic complications. The normal left atrial pressure is less than 12 mm Hg, but in patients with moderate MS, left atrial pressure is often increased to 20 mm Hg at rest. With severe obstruction, left atrial pressure may range between 20 and 50 mm Hg, although the absolute value often varies according to the degree of effective medical therapy.

The slowly progressive nature of MS may mute the impact of increased left atrial, pulmonary venous, and capillary pressures. Thickening of the capillary vessel walls in advanced MS decreases the tendency for alveolar edema and instead promotes rupture and resultant hemoptysis in the setting of increased pressure. Thus, the oft-quoted pressure value of 25 to 28 mm Hg in the pulmonary capillary system commonly responsible for producing alveolar edema is often not applicable to patients with chronic MS. The protection against alveolar edema is not complete, however, and surges of pressure augmentation such as those that occur during exercise or in the setting of atrial fibrillation with a rapid ventricular response may produce acute and sometimes life-threatening symptoms of pulmonary edema.

Pulmonary Hypertension

Pulmonary hypertension frequently develops in patients with long-standing MS.[9] When pulmonary hypertension is present, several anatomic changes can be identified, including dilatation of the pulmonary arteries, reactive narrowing of the lumen, and intimal hyperplasia in smaller arterial vessels. Furthermore, the right ventricle may become hypertrophied in response to an increased hemodynamic load. Although varying degrees of right ventricular dysfunction often coexist with MS, the right ventricle responds favorably to commissurotomy or valvuloplasty by immediate augmentation of function. This observation suggests that the detrimental impact of MS on right ventricular function is primarily a manifestation of increased afterload and is often partially if not totally reversible if it is treated in a timely fashion. Right ventricular dilatation and failure may develop in long-standing MS, however, and are often accompanied by tricuspid regurgitation, increased right atrial pressures, and peripheral edema.

Left Ventricular Ejection Fraction

A reduced left ventricular ejection fraction in the setting of MS is relatively common, with a prevalence of approximately 30%.[10-12] The etiology of impaired left ventricular function remains debatable, but most likely it is patient specific and multifactorial in nature. Proposed causes include impaired diastolic filling, impaired myocardial contractility, reduced passive compliance of the posterobasal left ventricular myocardium from scarring or inflammation, and neurohumoral activation leading to vasoconstriction and increased afterload.[13] Interestingly, however, a reduced ejection fraction does not appear to alter long-term surgical or percutaneous outcomes.[9,14]

Neurohumoral Axis

Abnormal hemodynamic states evoke activation of the neurohumoral axis. Neurohumoral activation in MS can be demonstrated by microneurographically measured muscle sympathetic nerve activity and increased serum concentrations of various transmitters and metabolites.[13] In addition, neurohumorally mediated vasoconstriction may further increase afterload. This increase in sympathetic activity, however, has been shown to be completely reversed within 1 week after valvuloplasty.[13]

Exercise

The exercise limitation commonly felt by and objectively demonstrated in patients with MS is multifactorial and may not be solely attributed to the resting or exercise left atrial pressure or resting mitral valve area. For example, exercise limitation has also been related to both an inadequate augmentation in cardiac output and increases in peak pulmonary artery pressure during activity.[15]

Atrial Fibrillation

In patients with MS, atrial fibrillation often begins with paroxysmal episodes and eventually becomes persistent in nature. Development of atrial fibrillation in MS is a multifactorial process. Possible causes include dilatation of the atria from persistent increases in atrial pressure and prolonged valvular obstruction[16] and fibrosis of the atria, internodal tracts, and sinoatrial node (a possible complication of the initial rheumatic inflammatory process), resulting in abnormalities in conduction velocities and refractory periods and promoting various atrial arrhythmias. Finally, both systemic hypertension and coronary artery disease, if present with MS, are potential contributing factors.

Thromboembolism

The morbidity associated with MS is tightly associated with the presence of left atrial thrombus and systemic embolization (see Fig. 89.1). Thrombus formation in MS typically occurs in the left atrial appendage, although free-floating and intermittently obstructing large left atrial thrombi have been observed. Of patients with newly diagnosed MS not treated with anticoagulant therapy, nearly 20% will have a left atrial thrombus at the time of diagnosis.[17] As expected, left atrial thrombus is commonly associated with atrial fibrillation; more than 90% of patients with a detectable thrombus have coexistent atrial fibrillation.[18]

Left atrial enlargement is an independent risk factor for left atrial thrombi. The reduced velocity of blood motion within the dilated left atrium is suggested by left atrial spontaneous echo contrast (LASEC) or "smoke" on transesophageal echocardiography. LASEC represents the swirling pattern of echogenic blood, is an independent predictor of thrombus formation,[19] and is more prevalent in patients with a history of prior embolism (approximately 80%) than without (approximately 48%).[20] LASEC may be reversible, especially in patients with sinus rhythm after successful balloon valvuloplasty. However, LASEC may frequently persist even after successful valvuloplasty, especially in the presence of persistent atrial fibrillation.[21]

Finally, a region-specific hypercoagulable state has been postulated to exist in the left atrium of patients with MS, despite normal systemic coagulation activity.[22] This phenomenon is observed almost exclusively in patients with coexistent LASEC, but the mechanism for such regional hypercoagulability remains unknown. The increased regional coagulation activity, however, is counteracted by treatment with warfarin,[23] thereby reducing the incidence of subsequent thrombus formation despite the persistence of LASEC.[19]

Markers of Coagulation

Patients with MS, even those in sinus rhythm and without left atrial dilatation, have increased serum concentrations of various prothrombotic biomarkers as well as of biomarkers that reflect hypofibrinolytic function. Specifically, these patients have increased concentrations of tissue-type plasminogen activator, plasminogen activator inhibitor 1, D-dimer, and antithrombin III. Increases in biomarkers such as D-dimer and antithrombin III suggest high intravascular fibrin turnover, indicating enhanced coagulation activation and thrombogenesis.[24] In one study comparing 46 patients with MS in either sinus rhythm or atrial fibrillation, it was shown that in the presence of LASEC, coagulation activation, platelet activation, and endothelial dysfunction were comparable in patients with sinus rhythm and atrial fibrillation, suggesting that chronic anticoagulation should be considered in all patients with LASEC, regardless of their rhythm.[25] Although abnormal levels of coagulation biomarkers may contribute to an increased risk of stroke even in the absence of atrial fibrillation, before anticoagulation therapy can be broadly recommended for patients with MS who are in sinus rhythm or lack a dilated left atrium, larger prospective studies are needed to assess both the predictive value of biomarkers and the risk-benefit ratio of treatment based on their values.

CLINICAL PRESENTATION

Because MS occurs throughout the world, across cultures and age groups, and is manifested at various stages in the disease process, clinicians must appreciate this variability in disease presentation. Streptococcal pharyngitis and acute rheumatic fever generally occur in children between the ages of 5 and 15 years (median age of 9 and 11 years).[1] The age at which patients present with symptomatic MS after their initial rheumatic insult potentially depends on several mitigating factors. Presumably, younger patients presenting with symptomatic MS most likely represent a subgroup who suffered a more severe initial rheumatic insult. In addition, recurrent acute streptococcal infection and subsequent recurrent rheumatic carditis clearly accelerate the process of commissural fusion and deformation of different portions of the mitral valve apparatus.[1] Finally, later onset of symptoms may reflect a milder initial rheumatic insult, with slow progression of further valve deformity mediated by nonrheumatic processes.

Severe MS may emerge within 5 years of an episode of acute rheumatic fever. This so-called juvenile MS, however, is currently seen only in countries where acute rheumatic fever and repeated recurrences of the disease are common.[1] In countries where successful prevention of rheumatic fever has been achieved, MS generally afflicts the adult population, although the mean age at presentation remains highly variable. For example, in the United States, Canada, and Japan, the mean age at presentation of patients with symptomatic MS is 50 to 60 years; in China, Saudi Arabia, India, Korea, and South Africa, the mean age at presentation is 20 to 30 years.[1] Further complicating the issue of age demographics, immigration has made the demographic characterization of MS substantially less uniform.

The clinical and anatomic features of MS are somewhat age dependent. For example, older patients presenting with symptomatic MS have a higher incidence of atrial fibrillation, more severe functional limitation, and lower cardiac output compared with younger patients with similar degrees of calculated valve area reduction.[1] In addition, coronary artery disease coexists in 30% of patients older than 40 years with symptomatic MS, but it remains clinically silent in most cases. Furthermore, larger amounts of calcium are present in the valve apparatus in older patients, resulting in a lesser chance of the valve's being amenable to commissurotomy.[26] Last, it is not uncommon for the diagnosis of MS in the elderly to be made only after echocardiography, a phenomenon that may be related to more subtle auscultative findings (e.g., less pronounced S_1 or opening snap) secondary to valve calcification and subsequent deformation.

Finally, it is not unusual for a patient to present with severe, previously undetected MS even in societies with advanced medical care. The reason for this observation is likely to be related to the slow, progressive nature of the disease process, the adaptation toward more sedentary lifestyles, and the misinterpretation of symptoms by both patients and physicians with failure to recognize the disease in its early stages.

Major Symptoms

The most common symptoms of MS are dyspnea and fatigue, particularly in older patients. Because of their nonspecific nature, symptoms of MS are often attributed to other causes, further leading to delays in disease recognition. The evolution of atrial fibrillation, which is common in MS, however, often precipitates sudden clinical deterioration necessitating medical attention.

Cough, another common symptom, may be caused by either left atrial hypertension or compression of the left main bronchus or left recurrent laryngeal nerve secondary to left atrial enlargement. In addition, hemoptysis may occur from a variety of causes, including pulmonary embolism or infarction, pulmonary edema, paroxysmal nocturnal dyspnea, bronchitis, and pulmonary apoplexy with profuse hemorrhage.[27]

Syncope and sudden death are not nearly as common in severe MS as they are in aortic stenosis. These clinical symptoms may occur in the context of digitalis toxicity, massive pulmonary embolism, or coronary embolism.

Most patients with MS do not manifest true angina. Rather, transient increases in left atrial and pulmonary pressures often produce short-lived sensations of chest fullness or discomfort. The sudden onset of crushing chest pain, however, may represent an embolic acute myocardial infarction or severe pulmonary embolus.

The development of pulmonary hypertension in patients with MS is not apparent by history alone. Its presence, however, may contribute to complaints of dyspnea, fatigue, and angina. In addition, the subsequent development of right ventricular hypertrophy, dilatation, and decompensation along with tricuspid regurgitation may produce peripheral edema.

Presentation with a cerebral or cerebellar infarction is relatively common and is often a devastating manifestation of underlying MS. Transient or sustained focal neurologic symptoms or deficits may represent an embolic cerebral vascular event. In addition, peripheral embolisms to the lower extremity and the renal, coronary, and mesenteric arteries have been described in patients with MS. Embolic phenomena are most common in patients with coexisting left atrial enlargement, LASEC, or atrial fibrillation. Finally, transesophageal echocardiography or surgical inspection of the left atrium after the initial embolic event may reveal no residual thrombus. If possible, however, pathologic examination of a removed embolus is recommended to exclude the diagnosis of atrial myxoma.

Physical Examination

MS exhibits several distinct findings on physical examination (Table 89.1). Clinicians should maximize the yield from the cardiac assessment by examining patients with a careful, systematic approach in a quiet room and using maneuvers such as auscultation with the patient in the left lateral position and immediately after exercise. In fact, the diagnosis of MS by physical examination alone remains a defining skill in practitioners to whom patients with the disease may initially present.[28] Because the initial presentation of MS may involve a large disabling stroke or life-threatening pulmonary edema in the setting of atrial fibrillation, detection of the disease before such events occur has major clinical importance. Sadly, however, modern medicine tends to deemphasize the importance of the physical examination. The lost art of cardiac auscultation, excessive reliance on advanced technology, increased reliance on physician performance measures emphasizing efficiency, and shortening of time spent examining patients are all setting the stage for an increased likelihood of missing the diagnosis of MS.

Clinical Presentations in Subsets of Patients with Mitral Stenosis

Mitral Stenosis during Pregnancy

Cardiac decompensation in the pregnant patient with MS is a well-known syndrome that exposes both the mother and fetus to significant risk. Previously asymptomatic, well-compensated patients with MS may develop sudden, life-threatening symptoms of congestive heart failure during pregnancy.[29] Symptoms occur during pregnancy in as many as 25% of patients with MS. Clinical deterioration frequently occurs by the middle of the second trimester, which incidentally coincides with the time of maximal hemodynamic changes during normal pregnancy.[29-31] Further complicating the diagnosis, symptoms related to MS need to be considered in the context of the fatigue, mild breathlessness, and peripheral edema common during normal pregnancy. On physical

MAJOR PHYSICAL FINDINGS IN MITRAL STENOSIS	
Physical Finding	**Comments**
Increased loudness of S_1	The auscultatory finding that is usually easiest to detect, but it is not specific for mitral stenosis. Listen at the apex and compare S_1 with S_2; normally, S_1 is slightly louder at the apex than S_2.
	May be palpated
	Loudness directly related to preserved flexibility of leaflets
	Variable intensity with atrial fibrillation
	Intensity decreases with prolongation of PR interval
Opening snap	High-pitched and snapping in character. Search between the left lateral sternal border and apex using the diaphragm of the stethoscope. Do not confuse with P_2.
	Correlates with abrupt deceleration of the opening mitral leaflets and requires their mobility
	May become inaudible when leaflets become immobile and extensively scarred
Timing of opening snap	Interval between S_2 and opening snap shortens with progression of obstruction
Diastolic rumbling murmur at apex	A low-pitched sound best heard at apex with the bell of the stethoscope. When in doubt, listen immediately after limited exercise and with patient in left lateral decubitus position.
	Starts with opening snap
	Decrescendo nature of murmur is typically followed by presystolic accentuation in those with preserved atrial contraction
Increased loudness of P_2	Associated with pulmonary hypertension
Right ventricular heave	Associated with pulmonary hypertension in the presence of tricuspid regurgitation
Malar flush	Not common
Cardiac cachexia	Advanced, untreated disease
Peripheral cyanosis	Advanced, untreated disease; consider complicating condition
Peripheral edema	Advanced, untreated disease, usually in the presence of severe pulmonary hypertension and tricuspid regurgitation

P_2, pulmonary component of second heart sound; S_1, first heart sound; S_2, second heart sound.

Table 89.1 Major physical findings in mitral stenosis.

examination, the augmented cardiac output and young age of these patients usually produce more pronounced auscultative findings, including a loud S_1 and opening snap and an easily appreciated diastolic rumble.

Mitral Stenosis in the Setting of Left Ventricular Systolic or Diastolic Dysfunction

In patients with significant left ventricular systolic dysfunction, the transmitral gradient may not be as high as expected because of the depressed cardiac output. On physical examination, these patients may have a reduction in both the intensity of S_1 and the diastolic murmur.

In patients with diastolic dysfunction and preserved systolic function, the magnitude of increase in left atrial pressure may be out of proportion to the underlying severity of MS, thereby increasing symptom severity. Early in the disease process, early left ventricular diastolic pressures are often negative, representing the generation of diastolic suction created by the normal left ventricle.[3] This mechanism is lost when there is diastolic dysfunction due to an increase in late diastolic pressure from the noncompliant left ventricle.

Decompensated, End-Stage Mitral Stenosis

Patients with severe, end-stage MS are often cachectic and edematous. In addition, they may have gross hepatomegaly and advanced pulmonary hemosiderosis. In contrast, acute decompensation secondary to MS often presents with intractable pulmonary edema, severe pulmonary hypertension with right-sided heart failure, and low cardiac output syndrome.[32]

Mitral Stenosis with Multivalvular Involvement

MS often presents in the setting of concomitant valvular lesions. For example, given that rheumatic disease is the most common cause of MS, coexistent aortic stenosis is common. In these cases, the aortic stenosis may be more or less pronounced on physical examination, and progressive dyspnea often remains the chief complaint. In addition, combined MS and aortic insufficiency is fairly common. In these cases, the MS is typically advanced while the insufficiency remains mild to moderate in severity. Mitral balloon valvuloplasty is often an effective means to delay double valve replacement surgery, potentially for many years.

MS with mitral regurgitation, so-called mixed mitral valve disease, presents with symptoms typical to one or both disease states (i.e., fatigue, dyspnea). The physical examination, however, usually reflects the combined nature of the valve abnormality with a loud apical systolic murmur and a hyperdynamic precordium reflective of a volume-overloaded left ventricle.

MS with tricuspid stenosis is a rare occurrence, although tricuspid stenosis must always be excluded whenever MS is present. MS with tricuspid regurgitation, however, is a common valve combination and is most common in the setting of moderate to severe pulmonary hypertension. Four findings on physical examination indicative of clinically significant tricuspid regurgitation include peripheral edema, pulsatile hepatomegaly, pansystolic murmur along the left lateral sternal border that increases with inspiration, and regurgitant wave in the distended jugular veins.

DIAGNOSTIC TECHNIQUES

Electrocardiography

The standard 12-lead electrocardiogram not only documents the rhythm (i.e., atrial fibrillation) but often reveals information suggestive of MS or pulmonary hypertension (i.e., vertical or rightward axis deviation, R > S wave in V_1). Sinus rhythm may be accompanied by findings of left atrial conduction delay (a notched P wave in lead II and a broad P wave in lead V_1 with a negative terminal deflection). Although P-wave abnormalities correlate poorly with absolute left atrial pressure, they may normalize in shape after successful valvuloplasty.

Chest Radiography

A chest radiograph often reveals left atrial enlargement with elevation of the left main stem bronchus, straightening of the left-sided heart border, and presence of a double density.[33] Pulmonary artery enlargement and "fullness" in the retrosternal space secondary to right ventricular enlargement may also be present. Right atrial enlargement suggests the development of tricuspid regurgitation. Finally, variable degrees of pulmonary congestion are seen in the setting of clinical decompensation.

Echocardiography

Echocardiography with Doppler Study

Echocardiography with Doppler study provides an excellent means of confirming the diagnosis of MS, characterizing the severity of obstruction and both detecting and quantifying associated abnormalities in the pulmonary circulation and the right-sided heart structures. Noninvasive measurements of mitral valve area (MVA) correlate well with direct anatomic measurements. In addition, transthoracic echocardiography is frequently able to provide a semiquantitative representation of the size and shape of the orifice (Fig. 89.3). When a patient is considered for balloon valvuloplasty, an echocardiographic scoring system that assigns a score of 1 to 4 (1 = minimal, 4 = severe) to the morphologic features of valve thickening, mobility, calcification, and subvalvular fusion may be used to guide therapy.[1] A sum echocardiographic score of less than 8 identifies the traditional candidate for commissurotomy or valvuloplasty. A more complete assessment of the degree and symmetry of the commissural fusion is also routinely performed to identify those patients at greater risk for development of severe mitral regurgitation and less relief of obstruction from balloon valvuloplasty.

The peak and mean Doppler-derived diastolic gradients with continuous-wave velocity curves are comparable to gradient determination by direct measurement of left atrial and left ventricular pressures.[8] In fact, Doppler gradients are more accurate than invasively determined gradients calculated from pulmonary capillary wedge pressure (versus direct measurement) to assess left atrial pressure. Although the Doppler diastolic half-time may be complementary, traditional echocardiographic measurements should not be relied on immediately after commissurotomy or valvuloplasty or when significant left ventricular abnormalities coexist.

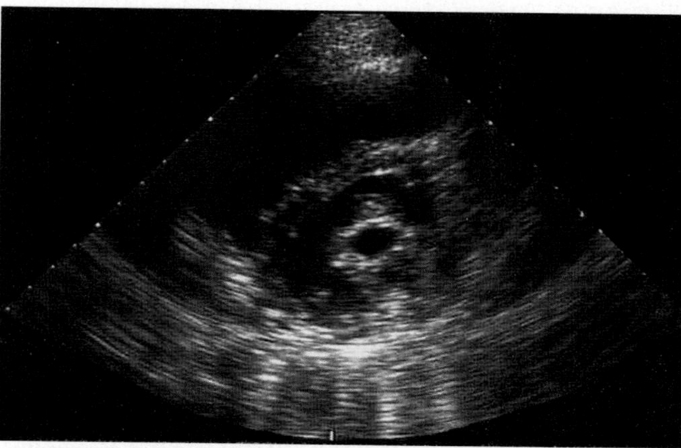

Figure 89.3 Anatomic substrate for balloon valvotomy. Short-axis, two-dimensional echocardiographic visualization of the fused commissures is important in determining the severity of obstruction and the potential benefit from balloon valvotomy. In this echocardiogram, both commissures are fused, the echogenicity is fairly uniform around the orifice (which is shaped like the mouth of a fish), and the stenosis appears severe. Therefore, it is likely that a balloon valvotomy will successfully open the fused commissures and reduce the severity of obstruction.

Finally, transmitral Doppler gradients and echocardiographic analysis of mitral annular motion velocity by pulsed Doppler tissue imaging are potentially valuable in the assessment of functional MS due to mitral annular calcification.[34] Severe calcification of the mitral annulus interferes with the active mitral annular motion necessary for normal valvular function. By echocardiography, this phenomenon is demonstrated as a reduction in the E′ velocity as determined by pulsed Doppler tissue imaging (Fig. 89.4). In addition, mitral annular calcification also results in a reduction in the normal annular dilatation during diastole, which by Doppler echocardiography is reflected in an increased mitral peak E velocity (see Fig. 89.4). Interestingly, this increased peak E velocity is present regardless of the underlying severity of mitral annular calcification (i.e., mild versus severe).[34] The combination of a high peak E velocity and reduced E′ velocity by Doppler echocardiography results in an elevated E/E′ ratio, reflecting an overall increase in left atrial pressure.

Dobutamine and Exercise Stress Echocardiography

Dobutamine and exercise stress echocardiography may be useful when the patient's symptoms are either ambiguous or out of proportion to the apparent severity of MS.[35] A low transmitral gradient is common in the setting of moderate MS with bradycardia and a reduced cardiac output, such as occurs in patients treated with beta blockers.[3] Doppler measurements of transmitral gradients and estimated pulmonary artery systolic pressure at rest and immediately after exercise may drastically differ, however, aiding in clinical decision making and determination of the need for additional therapeutic intervention.

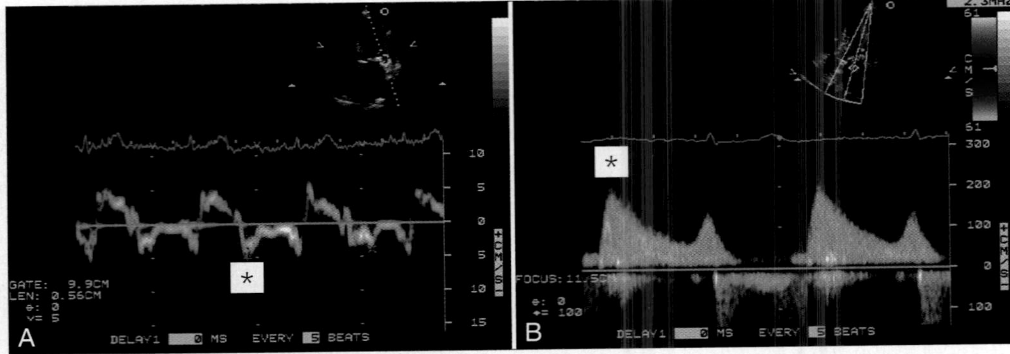

Figure 89.4 Doppler echocardiography evaluation of mitral annular calcification. A, Pulsed Doppler tissue imaging of the mitral annulus demonstrating a reduced E′ velocity *(asterisk)* of 5 cm/s. **B,** Continuous-wave Doppler recording of mitral inflow demonstrating an increased peak E velocity *(asterisk)* of 200 cm/s with a prolonged deceleration time, consistent with a transmitral gradient which does not equilibrate. The E/E′ is 40, indicative of markedly elevated left-sided filling pressure. However, while the LA pressure is likely elevated in this instance, the E/E′ data should be interpreted cautiously, as mitral annular calcification will be, by itself, associated with a reduced E′.

Transesophageal Echocardiography

Transesophageal echocardiography has proved to be a valuable tool in the screening of patients for intracavitary thrombus, especially in the left atrial appendage. Thrombi are found in approximately 20% of patients, most of whom are in atrial fibrillation. The positive predictive value of transesophageal echocardiography for detection of thrombi is 100%, with a negative predictive value of 98.9%.[36] Transesophageal echocardiography, however, does not usually add to information already provided by standard transthoracic echocardiography in the morphologic characterization of MS.

Real-Time Three-Dimensional Echocardiography

Significant technologic advancements in cardiac imaging made during the last decade have led to recent exposure to the next frontier in echocardiography, real-time three-dimensional (RT3D) echocardiography. RT3D echocardiography is unique in that the modality has a remarkable ability to clarify the unique spatial orientations of cardiac structures that are generally not adequately represented by standard two-dimensional echocardiography. RT3D echocardiography is ideally suited for assessment of the mitral valve because of the inherent complex, spatial interrelationships of the valve leaflets, chordae, papillary muscles, and myocardial walls (Fig. 89.5).[37,38] Studies of both transthoracic and transesophageal RT3D echocardiography demonstrate that calculation of MVA is more accurate, reproducible, and less variable by RT3D echocardiography compared with conventional two-dimensional methods.[39-43] In addition, two new indices for the evaluation of MS, mitral valve doming volume and mitral valve volume, have been introduced and proposed to predict both a propensity for atrial fibrillation and the success after therapeutic procedures such as balloon valvuloplasty.[44]

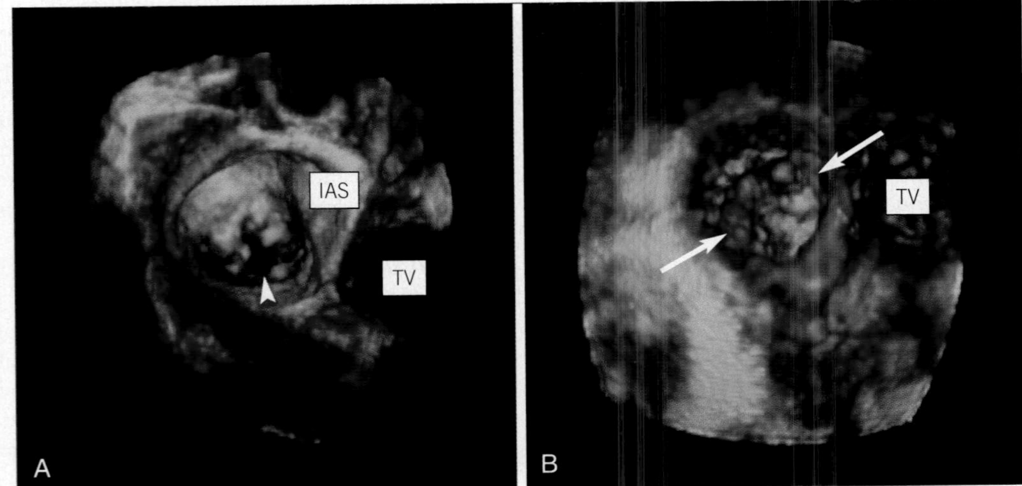

Figure 89.5 Real-time three-dimensional transesophageal echocardiography in the evaluation of mitral stenosis. A, Short-axis three-dimensional view from the left atrium illustrating a markedly reduced valve area *(arrowhead)*. **B,** Short-axis three-dimensional view from the left ventricle illustrating location and morphology of the papillary muscles and subvalvular apparatus *(arrows)*. IAS, interatrial septum; TV, tricuspid valve.

Although currently available evidence suggests that RT3D echocardiography is superior to traditional two-dimensional techniques in the diagnostic evaluation of MS (particularly in the determination of MVA), its use is not currently recommended in the most recent American College of Cardiology/American Heart Association practice guidelines for the management of valvular heart disease.[45] As more evidence mounts and as the use of RT3D echocardiography becomes more widespread, it is anticipated that this exciting new ultrasound modality will emerge as a standard diagnostic tool in the evaluation of patients with MS.

Cardiac Catheterization

The role of cardiac catheterization in the management of MS has evolved because of advances in noninvasive imaging modalities and the emergence of percutaneous mitral balloon valvuloplasty (PMBV) as a major therapeutic tool. In addition, invasive preoperative evaluation of patients with valvular stenosis undergoing surgery has changed during the past decade in that although 96% of these patients still undergo cardiac catheterization, only 18% (compared with 63% a decade ago) undergo invasive hemodynamic assessment of MS severity.[46]

In contrast, invasive hemodynamic assessment of MS is commonly performed in the setting of PMBV and typically involves catheterization of both the right and left sides of the heart. Compared with pulmonary capillary wedge pressure, which typically overestimates the true transmitral pressure gradient by up to 43% because of transmitted artifacts in pressure waveforms, direct pressure recordings of the left atrium through transseptal catheterization provide a much more accurate and reproducible assessment of transmitral gradients (see Fig. 89.2). In addition, coronary angiography is typically performed when atherosclerosis is suspected clinically or several risk factors are present for it. Finally, left ventriculography is often performed to quantify mitral regurgitation, especially when the noninvasive assessment is indeterminate, given that management decisions are heavily dependent on quantification of regurgitation.

MANAGEMENT

The fundamental aspects in the management of patients with MS include performing an initial clinical evaluation, addressing issues surrounding medical management, and deciding the need, timing, and criteria for PMBV or mitral valve surgery. The American College of Cardiology/American Heart Association guidelines for the management of patients with valvular heart disease[45] provide a comprehensive, practical, and well-referenced approach to management of patients with MS.

The initial evaluation of a patient with known or suspected MS should include history, physical examination, surface electrocardiogram, chest radiograph, initial blood testing, and two-dimensional echocardiogram with Doppler study. On the basis of this evaluation, consideration is then given to the medical management options outlined in Table 89.2.

Medications focused on reducing the clinical impact of mitral valve obstruction are typically instituted either when symptoms are present or evidence suggesting a hemodynamically significant obstruction exists. In patients with underlying sinus

MEDICAL MANAGEMENT OF MITRAL STENOSIS

Goal	Strategies
Minimize the hemodynamic impact of obstruction	Limitation of exercise
	Beta blocker or calcium channel blocker with negative chronotropic properties
	Dietary salt restriction and diuretics
Treat atrial fibrillation	**Acute episode**
	Anticoagulation with assessment of thromboembolic risk before subsequent cardioversion
	Pharmacologic control of heart rate with digoxin, beta blocker, or calcium channel blocker that slows AV nodal conduction
	Cardioversion—immediate electrical conversion with hemodynamic or clinical instability
	Recurrent episodes
	Long-term anticoagulation with warfarin
	Pharmacologic control of heart rate with digoxin, beta blocker, or calcium channel blocker
	Antiarrhythmic drugs—group 1C drugs, group 1A drugs, or amiodarone
	Sustained episode
	Long-term anticoagulation with warfarin
	Pharmacologic rate control with digoxin, beta blocker, or calcium channel blocker
Prevent development of atrial thrombus	Long-term anticoagulation with warfarin
	Percutaneous balloon valvuloplasty (controversial)
	Prevent or treat atrial fibrillation
Prevent recurrent rheumatic fever	Antibiotic prophylaxis as outlined in AHA guidelines addressing the issues of agent and duration[45]
Prevent endocarditis	Guidelines issued by AHA[45]

AHA, American Heart Association; AV, atrioventricular.

Table 89.2 Medical management of mitral stenosis.

rhythm, medical therapy usually begins with beta blockade, although conflicting evidence and ongoing debate remain surrounding the efficacy of beta blockade in improving clinical outcomes.[47] Although beta blockade may reduce resting and peak exercise heart rate, studies suggest that it has no beneficial impact on treadmill exercise time, aerobic capacity, and ventilatory performance.[48] Furthermore, although pulmonary capillary wedge pressures during exercise are reduced in patients with severe MS treated with beta-blocker therapy, overall exercise performance is not enhanced, probably because of a blunted augmentation in cardiac output during activity.[49] In addition, in patients with severe pulmonary hypertension in the setting of MS, the disproportionate impact of beta-blocker therapy on cardiac output versus pulmonary capillary wedge pressure during exercise is often marked enough to cause significant increases in pulmonary vascular resistance.

In regard to noninvasive evaluation of valve morphology, the patient's underlying clinical status and the severity of the MS dictate the frequency of testing. Yearly echocardiographic examinations are rarely justifiable in clinically stable patients with mild to moderate disease. Although the rate of progression is not predictable across patients, the average reduction in MVA is generally slow, with a mean rate of 0.09 cm^2 per year.[50,51] However, changes in right ventricular dimensions and severity of tricuspid regurgitation may progress independently of changes in MVA.[51]

The timing of intervention, either percutaneous or surgical, in a patient with MS is based on clinical status, anatomic severity, risks of continued medical treatment, and determination of the risk-benefit ratio of intervention.[1] In the setting of MVA less than 1.5 cm^2, consideration should be given to PMBV. This MVA value is by no means absolute, however, and appropriate adjustments should be made in correlating lesion severity to overall body size.[3] In addition, anatomic estimates of stenosis severity should be combined with assessments of both symptoms and lifestyle limitations as well as the needs of the individual patient. The decision to intervene should also incorporate an assessment of any special needs or risks (e.g., desire for childbearing, planned major noncardiac surgery, reduction of risk for systemic embolization).

Percutaneous Mitral Balloon Valvuloplasty for Mitral Stenosis

In the last 2 decades, the treatment of MS has undergone an evolution, first with the worldwide introduction of PMBV in the late 1980s and subsequently intensifying since the approval by the Food and Drug Administration of PMBV with the Inoue balloon catheter in 1994. PMBV has proved to be a safe and cost-effective means by which to provide both short- and long-term improvements in symptoms and hemodynamic status in a broader spectrum of patients than those traditionally considered for surgical commissurotomy. In fact, this technique is associated with significantly less morbidity and improved long-term results compared with historic surgical data. The early (immediate) results of PMBV are incredibly gratifying; most investigators report that the valve area typically doubles (i.e., 1.0 cm^2 to 2.0 cm^2) after PMBV of a critically stenotic valve. Although the post-PMBV valve area is still smaller than the normal MVA of 3 to 5 cm^2, it is nonetheless sufficient to produce substantial hemodynamic benefits, including decreases in left atrial pressure and transmitral pressure gradient, reductions in pulmonary artery pressure, and increases in cardiac output. In addition, an added benefit after PMBV is a noticeable reduction in left atrial stiffness, which results in either enhanced left atrial function in patients with sinus rhythm or improved left atrial reservoir function in those with atrial fibrillation.[52] Finally, the hemodynamic impact of PMBV may be exaggerated in high-output states, such as pregnancy (Table 89.3) and morbid obesity.

The long-term results of PMBV rely heavily on several factors, including the patient's baseline characteristics, echocardiographic estimation of mitral apparatus deformity (i.e., echocardiographic score), history of prior commissurotomy, pre-PMBV and post-PMBV scores, and New York Heart Association (NYHA) functional class.[53] Reported outcomes of PMBV in studies of patients in developing countries, which typically involve younger patients with lower echocardiographic scores, may not truly reflect outcomes for the population of patients typically seen in the United States and other industrialized nations where rheumatic disease has long been controlled. For example, in one large study investigating the long-term results of PMBV in developing countries, the mean age of enrolled patients was 33 years. In this younger population, the survival rates were 98% at 5 years and 97% at 10 years, with event-free survival rates of 85% and 72%, respectively.[54] In contrast, a study examining the long-term results of PMBV in a large North American population enrolled patients with a mean age of 55 years.[55] In this population, the overall survival and event-free survival rates during the follow-up period were 87% and 53%, respectively. Patients

EXAMPLE OF THE HEMODYNAMIC IMPACT OF MITRAL BALLOON VALVOTOMY PERFORMED DURING PREGNANCY

	Before Balloon Valvotomy	Immediately after Balloon Valvotomy
Left atrial pressure	36 mm Hg	18 mm Hg
Mitral valve pressure gradient	25 mm Hg	14 mm Hg
Cardiac output	6.8 L/min	10.2 L/min
Calculated mitral valve area	1.3 cm^2	2.8 cm^2
Pulmonary arterial pressure	61/32 mm Hg (mean, 46 mm Hg)	41/19 mm Hg (mean, 28 mm Hg)
Right atrial pressure	12 mm Hg	6 mm Hg
Degree of mitral regurgitation	Trivial by color-flow Doppler study	Mild by color-flow Doppler study

Table 89.3 Example of the hemodynamic impact of mitral balloon valvotomy performed during pregnancy.

with baseline echocardiographic scores of less than 8, however, demonstrated significantly improved survival (82% versus 57%) and event-free survival (38% versus 22%) at 12-year follow-up compared with patients with scores of more than 8. This finding can be explained by the fact that patients with echocardiographic scores of more than 8 were generally older, more likely to have atrial fibrillation, and often assigned to NYHA class IV immediately before PMBV.

PMBV may be performed by several techniques, but the most common and extensively studied approach has been with the Inoue catheter.[56,57] During cardiac catheterization, a transseptal puncture is used to gain access to the mitral valve from the left atrium. A special balloon catheter (i.e., Inoue catheter) is advanced from the right femoral vein into the right atrium, through the transseptal puncture into the left atrium, and across the stenotic mitral valve. Inflation and rapid deflation of the balloon opens the stenotic valve by separation of the fused commissures as well as by fracture of calcific deposits in the leaflet tissue (Fig. 89.6).

The immediate technical failure rate of PMBV ranges from 0.8% to 2.3%.[1] Inability either to perform a successful transseptal puncture or to cross the stenotic valve with the Inoue balloon catheter occurs most commonly in the early experience of the operator and in elderly patients. Suboptimal short- and long-term hemodynamic results are a function of preprocedural factors, most of which revolve around readily identifiable valve and patient characteristics, as described before.

Major complications of death, systemic embolization, and cardiac perforation are rare. Procedure-related deaths occur in less than 1% of patients and typically result from cardiac perforation or occur in the context of a critically ill, moribund patient with end-stage MS. Rare cases of catastrophic emboli to the coronary arteries immediately after PMBV have been reported.[58]

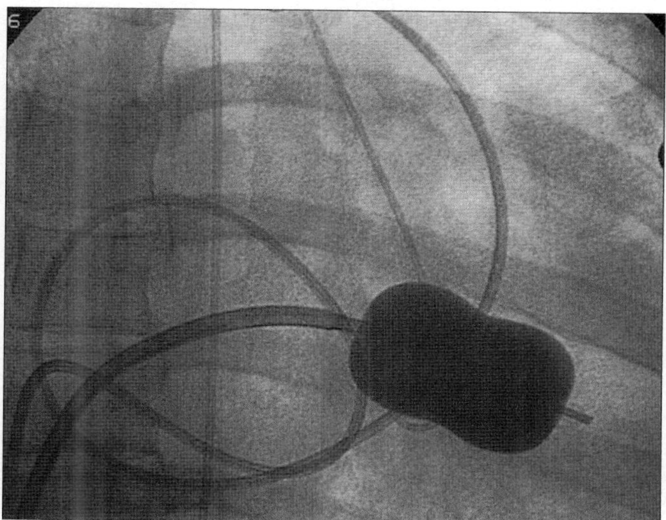

Figure 89.6 Inoue catheter for mitral balloon valvotomy. The balloon-tipped catheter is positioned across the stenotic valve and inflated. The narrowed orifice is subjected to the force from the transiently inflated balloon. When the procedure is successful, these forces break the scar tissue and allow greater opening of the mitral valve leaflets. This technique is a balloon commissurotomy that has evolved from the earlier extensive experience with closed and open commissurotomy.

The major complication of PMBV is mitral regurgitation. The incidence of worsening mitral regurgitation after PMBV, including trivial worsening, ranges between 14% and 37%.[1,59] The complication of severe mitral regurgitation occurs in approximately 5% of patients and is often attributed to tearing of a valve leaflet or chordae tendineae, although a central regurgitant jet with no obvious structural abnormality occurs in up to 26% of cases.[60] Emergency surgery for severe, hemodynamically significant mitral regurgitation is required in approximately 2% of cases, and it may be related to unfavorable mitral valve morphology before PMBV.[60] Residual moderate mitral regurgitation after PMBV is associated with both failure to improve symptomatically and persistent pulmonary hypertension. In these cases, elective mitral valve surgery is usually performed.

After removal of the Inoue catheter, a small atrial septal defect is commonly detected. Between 1% and 2% of patients will have a hemodynamically important left-to-right shunt with a Qp/Qs ratio above 1.5.[1] Few of these patients will require any therapy (i.e., percutaneous defect closure), given that the shunt resolves within 6 months in 67% of cases.

Use of Real-Time Three-Dimensional Echocardiography in Percutaneous Mitral Balloon Valvuloplasty

Traditional methods of assessing MVA after PMBV remain severely limited. Specifically, during the immediate post-PMBV period, hemodynamic factors (heart rate, cardiac index, cardiac rhythm, ventricular and atrial compliance) rapidly change, which can result in significant discrepancies in pressure half-time–derived MVA. In addition, determination of MVA by planimetry of the valve orifice in the short-axis view is similarly prone to substantial variation, given that after PMBV, the commissural fusion can split in an asymmetric fashion, making the planimetry tracing of the valve orifice less reproducible across observers. RT3D echocardiography, however, has been shown to overcome many of the limitations of traditional two-dimensional echocardiography in determining MVA after PMBV (Fig. 89.7). Specifically, RT3D echocardiography has been shown to be an effective technique to monitor the efficacy of PMBV, with improved accuracy and agreement with the Gorlin-derived MVA.[41,61] Finally, RT3D echocardiography has demonstrated remarkable utility during PMBV by enabling the detailed visualization of commissural splitting and leaflet tears previously not appreciated on traditional two-dimensional echocardiography.[62] As a result, RT3D echocardiography may potentially be used to guide and to optimize results of valvuloplasty procedures so that a maximal MVA can be obtained in the safest fashion.

Selection of Patients for Percutaneous Mitral Balloon Valvuloplasty and Surgery

During the last decade, the question of which treatment, PMBV or surgical repair or replacement, is preferred in MS has been extensively studied. The immediate clinical and

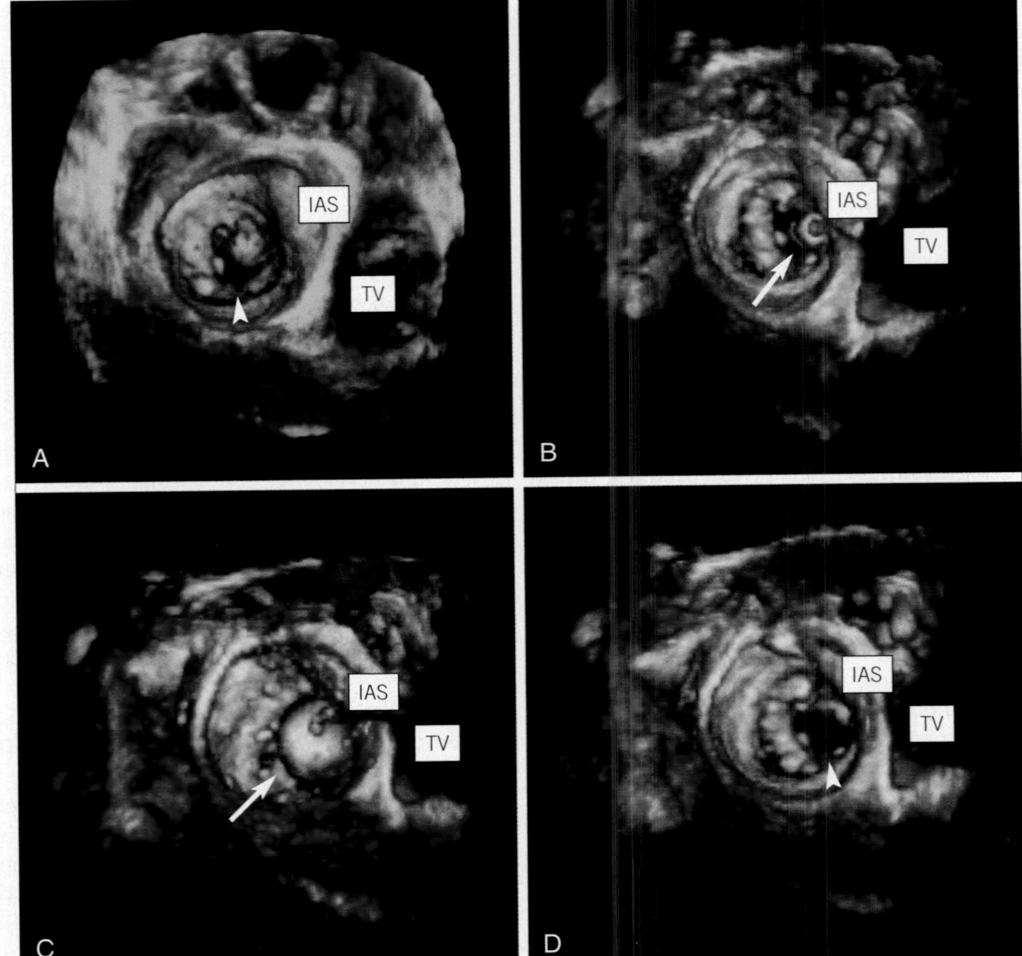

Figure 89.7 Real-time three-dimensional transesophageal echocardiography used during percutaneous mitral balloon valvuloplasty. A, Baseline image illustrating a markedly reduced mitral valve area *(arrowhead)*. **B,** Inoue balloon catheter *(arrow)* placed across the stenotic mitral valve. **C,** Inoue balloon catheter during maximal inflation *(arrow)*. **D,** Image illustrating a significantly larger mitral valve area *(arrowhead)* after percutaneous mitral balloon valvuloplasty. IAS, interatrial septum; TV, tricuspid valve.

hemodynamic results of PMBV compared with closed or open surgical commissurotomy were studied in three prospective randomized trials of young to middle-aged patients in South Africa, Tunisia, and India.[63-65] In these studies, no deaths or thromboembolic complications occurred in either group, and the incidence of increased mitral regurgitation was similar between the two groups. Open commissurotomy and PMBV resulted in equivalent clinical outcomes, and both methods were superior to closed commissurotomy in a 7-year follow-up period.[64] In addition, patients with favorable mitral valve anatomy who underwent PMBV demonstrated superior hemodynamic results and improved function class compared with surgical patients (72% of patients in the PMBV group demonstrated NYHA functional class I versus 57% of patients in the open commissurotomy group).[63,65] In the United States, PMBV has also demonstrated an economic benefit, with reductions in total hospital cost and shorter times of return of patients to increased productivity compared with surgical commissurotomy or valve replacement.[1] The economic benefit is not a universal finding, however, given that in some countries, the cost of surgical commissurotomy remains significantly lower than the cost of specialized equipment such as cardiac catheterization suites and Inoue balloon catheters.[56]

The decision to refer patients for PMBV or surgical valve replacement is heavily influenced by the expected long-term benefits of each treatment option, the inherent risks of surgery, and the individual patient's goals of treatment. A significant proportion of patients in the United States and other developed countries, however, tend to fall into a category demonstrating a 5-year event-free survival after PMBV of roughly 50%, although this value varies somewhat according to the degree of valve deformity as determined by the echocardiographic score (Fig. 89.8). The reason for this observed suboptimal event-free survival is likely to be explained by the inherently older population of patients with multiple comorbidities. The obvious lack of significant precision in predicting outcome after PMBV, however, introduces greater uncertainty than with many

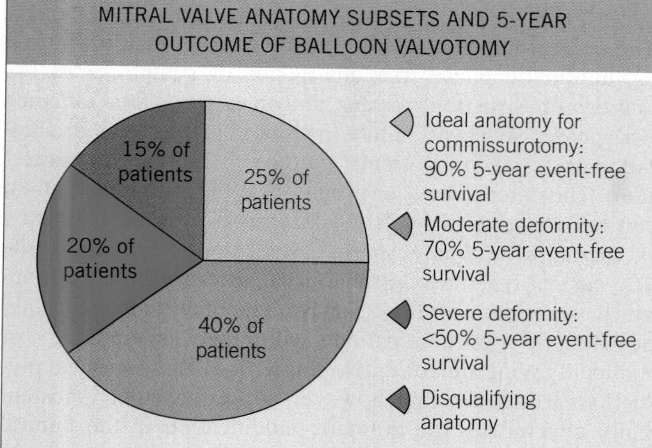

Figure 89.8 Mitral valve anatomy subsets and 5-year outcome of balloon valvotomy. The potential candidacy for balloon valvotomy is presented as a function of the frequency of all patients who have isolated mitral stenosis seen in clinical practice. Patients with valves that are not ideal for traditional surgical commissurotomy have undergone balloon valvotomy and have had 5-year event-free survivals that vary widely. Those with severe deformity should not undergo balloon valvotomy unless surgical valve replacement cannot be performed, and the acute and long-term expectations should be adjusted. The large "gray area" of patients with moderate deformities of the mitral valve apparatus remains clinically challenging, and it is controversial whether balloon valvotomy should be used as an alternative to surgical valve replacement. Patients with a disqualifying anatomy for balloon valvotomy may have minimal commissural fusion, extensive subvalvular obstruction, or marked asymmetry of commissural fusion.

other medical decisions. Thus, a careful preprocedural consultation and open discussion with the patient and family about treatment options and goals are paramount. Although the eventual need for surgical valve replacement remains a central reality for many patients, others derive sustained benefits from PMBV alone. For others still, PMBV is approached as a palliative procedure when surgery is not possible or desirable.

Surgery for Mitral Stenosis

The traditional surgical approaches to MS are open and closed commissurotomy and mitral valve replacement. The insight of manually enlarging the small opening in MS guided attempts by Cutler in the 1920s to physically enlarge the mitral opening.[66] In the 1950s, Bailey and Harken succeeded in developing a surgical procedure that served as the foundation for future closed mitral commissurotomy. Both open and closed commissurotomy have resulted in long-term survival and effective palliation in the vast majority of treated patients, especially in those younger than 40 years.

The surgical approach in treating patients with MS may also involve procedures treating structures beyond the valve leaflets. Such procedures include plication of an extremely large left atrium to improve hemodynamics, plication of the left atrial appendage to reduce the risk of thromboembolism, replacement of chordae to improve the function of the mitral apparatus, and variations on the maze procedure to treat atrial fibrillation. Finally, less invasive techniques for mitral valve surgery, although more technically challenging, may reduce bleeding, postoperative pain, and risk of infection and are a continued area of investigation.[67,68]

Mitral valve replacement is the treatment of choice in patients with severe MS who are not candidates for surgical commissurotomy or PMBV as well as in those with combined MS and mitral regurgitation. Although mitral valve replacement can be performed with a risk of less than 5% in young, healthy patients, in older patients with concomitant medical problems, the perioperative mortality may approach 20%.[69] Continued refinement of the surgical approach to mitral valve surgery, however, has improved perioperative risk and postoperative recovery time in those who are suitable for mini-thoracotomy and other approaches.

Management of Mitral Stenosis in Special Situations

Mitral Stenosis and Pregnancy

Hemodynamically significant MS should be corrected before pregnancy whenever possible. Medical management of the pregnant patient with mild to moderate MS requires careful attention to volume status, use of beta blockers and diuretics, and avoidance of warfarin.[29] If clinically important MS is discovered after pregnancy has begun, medical treatment may fail, and consideration of valve intervention is strongly recommended. Before the introduction of PMBV in 1984, surgery was the only treatment available for pregnant patients with severe MS and refractory symptoms of heart failure. Although surgical commissurotomy does not expose the mother to significant risk, the risk to the fetus is dramatic, with a reported fetal mortality of 6% to 33%. The increase in fetal mortality may be attributed to the effects of general anesthesia, thoracotomy, or need for extracorporeal circulation. In contrast, PMBV has been shown to be associated with significantly fewer fetal complications and reductions in both fetal and neonatal mortality.[70] Thus, PMBV is the preferable treatment approach and is usually performed in the late second trimester of pregnancy when radiation exposure to the fetus is of lesser concern. Successful PMBV performed during pregnancy for medically refractory MS results in symptomatic and hemodynamic improvement, improved likelihood of delivery of the fetus at full term, and rare reports of fetal loss (see Table 89.3).[30,31]

Decompensated, End-Stage Mitral Stenosis

Patients with severe end-stage MS may present with intractable pulmonary edema, severe pulmonary hypertension with right-sided heart failure, and low cardiac output syndrome. Thoracotomy for valve replacement or commissurotomy is often not entertained as a therapeutic option in these patients because of the extremely high perioperative risk. PMBV may be performed in these patients either as the sole intervention or as a therapeutic bridge to nonemergent, lower risk surgical valve replacement. The risks of PMBV in these patients are inherently greater, and the immediate hemodynamic effects are often not as marked as those seen in stable patients undergoing elective PMBV.[32]

Patients with Previous Surgical Commissurotomy

PMBV can be safely performed in patients who have undergone previous surgical commissurotomy. Compared with similarly aged patients who have not had prior surgical commissurotomy, however, patients with a previous surgical commissurotomy are more likely to have atrial fibrillation (19% versus 6%), mitral valve calcification (50% versus 36%), and total echocardiographic score above 8 (55% versus 24%), making them an inherently less favorable population for PMBV intervention.[71] Nonetheless, although the 5-year event-free survival is somewhat less in this subset of patients, the overall acute and intermediate efficacies of PMBV are comparable to those in patients without previous surgical commissurotomy.

Mitral Stenosis with Advanced Pulmonary Hypertension

Surgical decompression of the left atrium through mitral commissurotomy or mitral valve replacement often yields immediate regression of pulmonary hypertension in the postoperative period. After successful PMBV, severe pulmonary hypertension may also improve substantially; the effect is seen immediately, with a second phase of lowered pressures during weeks to months.[9] Studies suggest, however, that early PMBV (i.e., before the development of severe pulmonary hypertension) is both valuable and often indicated as it may yield a more optimal symptomatic and hemodynamic benefit.[72]

Mitral Stenosis with Concomitant Severe Tricuspid Regurgitation

It has been suggested for decades that tricuspid regurgitation, especially in the presence of pulmonary hypertension, may decrease after relief of MS. In patients with severe MS, tricuspid regurgitation is usually functional in etiology and results from right ventricular and tricuspid annular dilatation caused by long-standing pulmonary hypertension. Although some studies reported that baseline moderate to severe tricuspid regurgitation remains unchanged in 88% of patients after PMBV,[73] more contemporary studies demonstrate a substantial regression in significant tricuspid regurgitation after successful PMBV.[74] The impact of PMBV on reducing tricuspid regurgitation appears to depend heavily on the underlying severity of pulmonary hypertension.[75]

PROGNOSIS

The natural history of MS typically consists of a prolonged asymptomatic phase, the emergence of symptoms as the degree of obstruction worsens, and an eventual fatal outcome with progressive heart failure (embolism in the systemic circulation and, in some patients, pulmonary embolism or infection). The determinants of prognosis in the individual patient can be summarized by 10-year survival rates as a function of current symptomatic state.[76] With severe symptoms, the 10-year survival rate is less than 15%, whereas the asymptomatic patient demonstrates a survival rate of more than 80%. In addition, 60% of these patients will remain asymptomatic or minimally symptomatic during this period. These survival predictions are not absolute, however, as they have been substantially affected by the dramatic modification in the natural history of MS by the advent of PMBV.[77]

SUMMARY

Mitral stenosis is a valvular disorder requiring diagnostic acumen for its recognition and up-to-date medical knowledge for its management. Recognition of the disease process leads to a series of important management decisions. Although mitral stenosis remains a classic rheumatic valvular lesion, there has been a recent surge in knowledge surrounding both its underlying pathophysiology and management. This surge in contemporary information has been largely propelled by the emergence of percutaneous mitral balloon valvuloplasty as an important and widely used therapeutic option. Despite the efficacy of current therapies, however, the continued worldwide presence of mitral stenosis emphasizes the need both to pursue more effective methods of eradicating acute rheumatic fever, especially in nonindustrialized countries, and to develop more refined approaches for management of the disorder in those already afflicted.

chapter 90

Mitral Regurgitation

Blase A. Carabello

Definition

- Mitral regurgitation is abnormal systolic blood flow from the left ventricle to the left atrium.

Key Features

- Mitral regurgitation produces a potentially damaging volume overload on the left ventricle.
- Mitral regurgitation results in eccentric cardiac hypertrophy that is both adaptive and maladaptive.
- Echocardiography is the mainstay for surveillance against left ventricular dysfunction.

Therapy

- There is no proven medical therapy for chronic disease.
- Valve repair or replacement should occur before left ventricular ejection fraction falls below 60%, when end-systolic dimension approaches 45 mm, or when symptoms occur.

Mitral regurgitation is the second most common valve lesion (next to aortic stenosis) in the United States and is prevalent throughout the world. Severe mitral regurgitation causes a hemodynamic burden that ultimately injures the left ventricle if it is left untreated.[1,2] Fortunately, timely diagnosis of and therapy for the disease now return many patients with this valvular abnormality to a normal quality of life and life span.[3] The physician's recognition of the disease, its stages, and its proper therapy is at the apex of a successful outcome for the patient and is the focus of this chapter.

ANATOMY AND PATHOLOGY

The mitral valve and its apparatus are composed of the annulus, the anterior and posterior leaflets, the chordae tendineae, and the papillary muscles (Fig. 90.1). Abnormalities of any of these structures, which interact dynamically to maintain mitral valve competence, can lead to mitral regurgitation. When a lesion in part of the valve apparatus causes mitral regurgitation, the disease is termed primary (i.e., it is an abnormality of the mitral valve structure itself that has caused mitral regurgitation). When abnormalities in left ventricular function, shape, or contractile function cause malposition of the papillary muscles with or without dilatation of the annulus, the mitral regurgitation that results is said to be secondary to the abnormalities in ventricular geometry that have developed.

The mitral valve apparatus is a dynamic structure that not only maintains mitral valve competence during systole but is also an integral part of the left ventricle. At the beginning of left ventricular contraction, pressure in the left ventricle rapidly exceeds that of the left atrium and the pressure gradient between the two chambers closes the valve leaflets, which coapt, preventing mitral regurgitation. Contraction of the papillary muscles against the chordae tendineae helps prevent the leaflets from going beyond their coaptation point, thus maintaining valve competence. However, it is unclear whether papillary muscle contraction is necessary to prevent mitral regurgitation.[4] Papillary muscle contraction may not be necessary as long as the papillary muscles and chordae do not become elongated and the ventricle does not dilate. Thus, acute papillary muscle ischemia in isolation does not usually result in mitral regurgitation in experimental models.[5] On the other hand, papillary muscle elongation, leaflet elongation, chordal elongation, and chordal rupture can all lead to severe mitral regurgitation.

In addition to the tethering action of the papillary muscles on the chordae tendineae and mitral leaflets, the annulus itself is dynamic and contracts in size during systole. This sphincter-like effect further supports the valve and maintains leaflet coaptation.[6]

Chordae tendineae are classified as primary, secondary, or tertiary. Primary chordae insert on the edges of the mitral leaflets, preventing their eversion. Secondary chordae are attached to the ventricular side of the leaflets and prevent leaflet prolapse. Tertiary chordae arise directly from the left ventricle and attach only to the posterior leaflets. Rupture of a strategically placed primary or secondary chorda may cause immediate severe mitral regurgitation. Other chordae may rupture, causing little mitral regurgitation; however, any chordal rupture places more stress on the remaining chords. Thus, mitral regurgitation tends to beget mitral regurgitation, a process further reinforced by ventricular dilatation.

The incidence of the various pathologic processes that cause mitral regurgitation varies throughout the world. In developed countries, the most common cause of mitral regurgitation is myxomatous degeneration of the valve, which leads to thickened and redundant leaflets and elongated chordae tendineae. In this condition, the leaflets extend past their systolic coaptation point, allowing mitral regurgitation to occur. The second most common cause is ischemic heart disease. As noted before, papillary muscle ischemia by itself is usually not sufficient to cause mitral regurgitation. However, infarction or ischemia-mediated changes in the papillary muscles

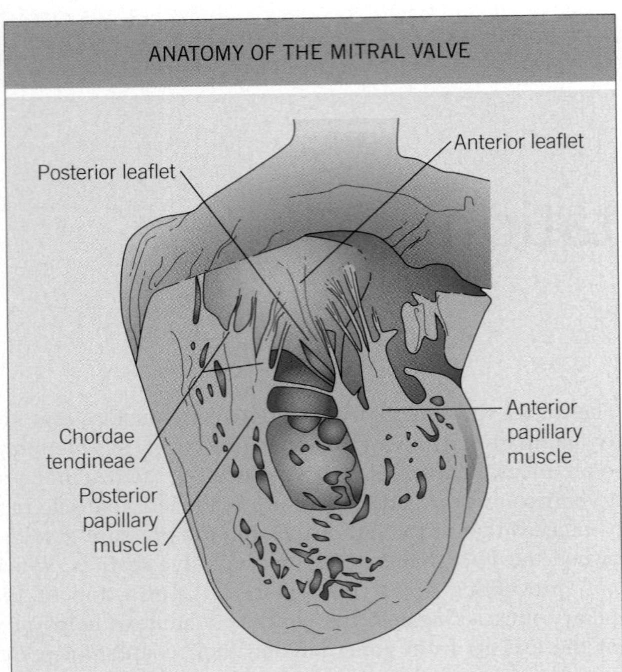

Figure 90.1 Anatomy of the mitral valve apparatus.

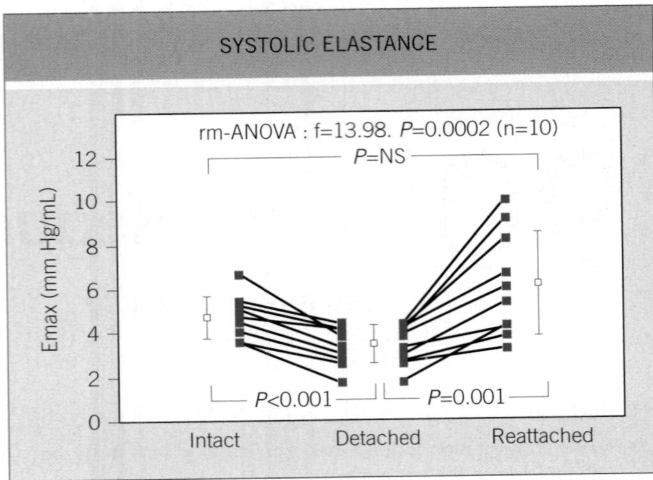

Figure 90.2 Systolic elastance (E_{max}), a measure of ventricular performance, is demonstrated at baseline, immediately after chordal disruption, and again after chordal reattachment. It is clear that the absence of chordal-ventricular interaction impairs ventricular performance, which is immediately restored when the apparatus is reintegrated. (From Sarris GE, Cahill PD, Hansen DE, et al. Restoration of left ventricular systolic performance after reattachment of the mitral chordae tendineae. The importance of valvular-ventricular interaction. J Thorac Cardiovasc Surg 1988;95:969-979.)

that result in their lengthening or regional wall motion abnormalities of the left ventricle that discoordinate left ventricular contraction lead to ischemic mitral regurgitation.

Other causes include infective endocarditis that destroys leaflets or chordae, collagen vascular disease, and rheumatic heart disease. In developing nations, rheumatic disease is still the main cause of mitral regurgitation. Unlike other causes of the disease that result in mitral regurgitation by allowing the leaflets to extend beyond their coaptation point, rheumatic disease leads to shortening of the chordae, preventing the valve leaflets from reaching their coaptation point. Recently, prolonged use of the anorectic drugs fenfluramine and dexfenfluramine has been shown to cause mitral leaflet thickening and regurgitation.[7] The mechanism and incidence of this disease are still in debate. In any case, the agents have been removed from the market and are no longer available.

Apart from the well-recognized function that the mitral valve apparatus has in maintaining mitral valve competence, the apparatus also has a major role in maintaining ventricular function.[8,9] The exact mechanism by which the mitral apparatus augments contraction is not clear, but it is certain that transection of the chordae causes a dramatic fall in left ventricular function (Fig. 90.2). In one scheme, shown in Figure 90.3, the shortening of the chordae early in isovolumetric systole reduces the apex-to-base length, in turn elongating the short axis of the heart. This might increase preload of the short-axis fibers just before contraction, in turn augmenting their function. Alternatively, the apparatus may play its role in maintaining left ventricular function by helping to maintain the prolate ellipsoid shape of the ventricle and by augmenting the fibrous skeleton that helps maintain ventricular stiffness. In many instances, ischemic or functional mitral regurgitation is the result of geometric changes in the left ventricle that lead to leaflet malcoaptation (Fig. 90.4).

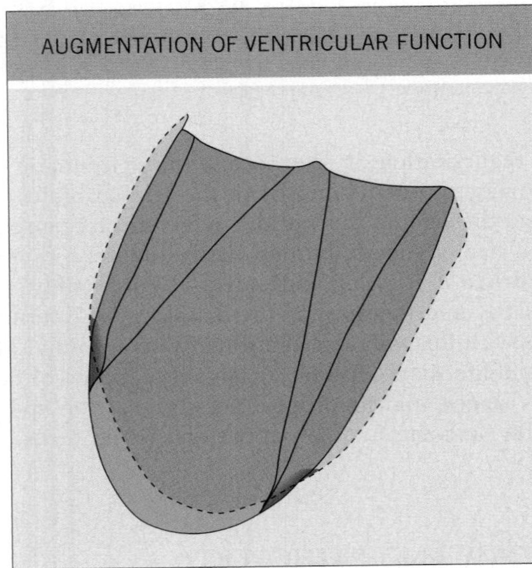

Figure 90.3 One mechanism by which the mitral valve apparatus might augment ventricular function. The solid line represents end-diastole. At the very beginning of systole, papillary muscle contraction shortens the long axis of the heart, in turn lengthening the short axis of the heart, causing sarcomere stretch and preload augmentation in the short axis, which is primarily responsible for left ventricular ejection.

PATHOPHYSIOLOGY

The pathophysiology of mitral regurgitation may be divided into three stages: acute, chronic compensated, and chronic decompensated (Fig. 90.5). Acute mitral regurgitation, such as might occur in chordal rupture, suddenly creates a new pathway for ejection of blood from the left ventricle into the left atrium, resulting in several hemodynamic alterations.

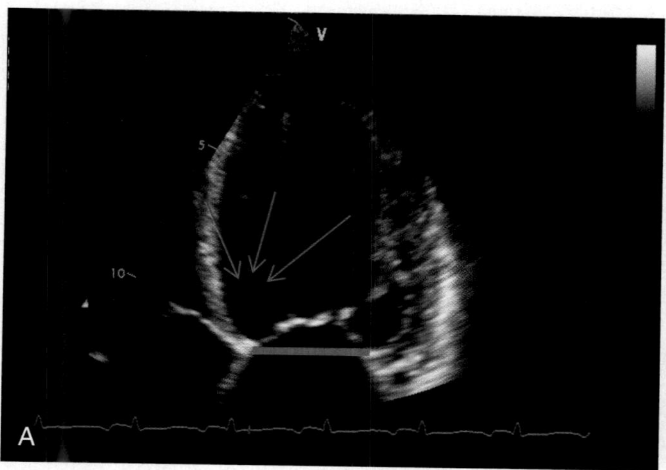

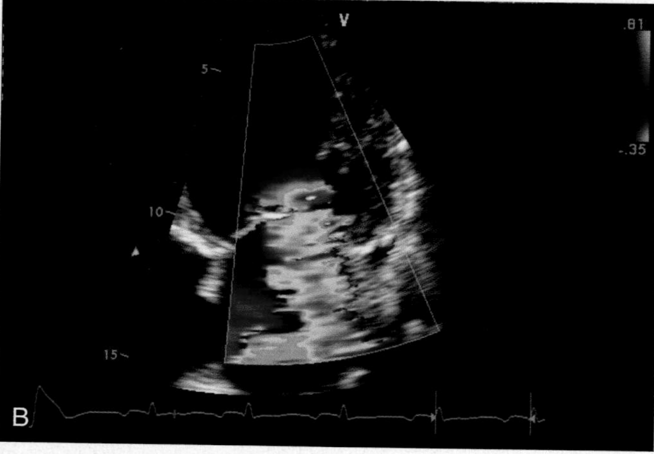

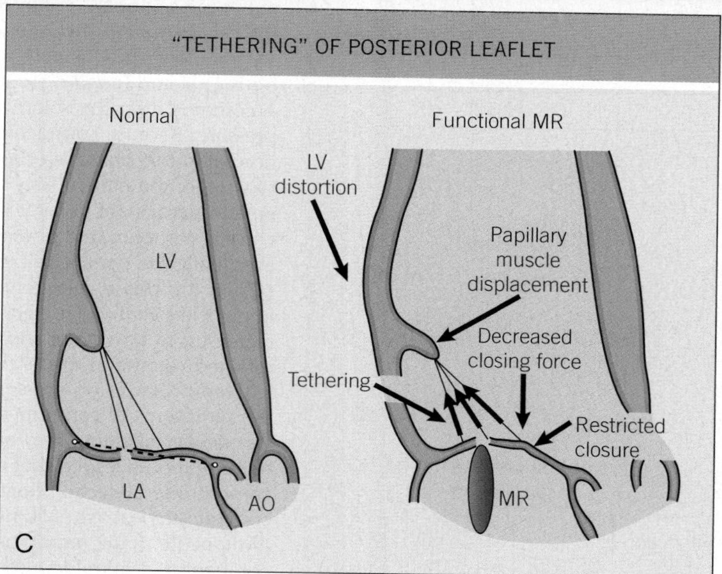

Figure 90.4 Leaflet malcoaptation. In functional or ischemic mitral regurgitation, the mitral leaflets and coaptation point *(arrows)* are displaced toward the apex **(A)**. Normal closure occurs at the annular line *(solid line)*. This malcoaptation is associated with severe mitral regurgitation, as is seen in the accompanying color Doppler still frame **(B)**. In this instance, the mechanism of mitral regurgitation is related to the dilated and dysfunctional left ventricle, resulting in distortion of the mitral valve apparatus. The mitral leaflets are morphologically normal, as described in the schematic diagram **(C)**. The left ventricular shape distortion is associated with apical displacement of the mitral apparatus and reduced leaflet closing force or restricted leaflet closure. The posterior leaflet, in this instance, is "tethered" with restricted motion, caused by the apical displacement of the papillary muscle. AO, aorta; LA, left atrium; LV, left ventricle; MR, mitral regurgitation.

First, because two pathways are now available for ejection, afterload decreases, facilitating more complete emptying, thereby reducing end-systolic volume. Filling of the left ventricle is augmented both from the volume returning from the pulmonary veins and from the regurgitated volume, resulting in increased diastolic volume. Concurrently, sarcomeres are stretched toward their maximum, increasing preload and augmenting the ability of the left ventricle to perform work through the Frank-Starling mechanism. These loading changes act in concert to increase total stroke volume. However, because a large portion of this total stroke volume is regurgitated into the left atrium, where it is ineffective, forward stroke volume is reduced and cardiac output falls. At the same time, augmented filling of the left ventricle increases end-diastolic pressure, which in turn increases left atrial pressure, causing pulmonary venous hypertension, pulmonary congestion, and dyspnea. At this point, the hemodynamics of congestive heart failure are manifested (a fall in cardiac output together with a rise in filling pressure), but ventricular muscle function is completely normal.

In many instances, the hemodynamic decompensation from acute mitral regurgitation is severe enough to warrant urgent surgery. However, if this acute phase can be tolerated, the patient may enter the chronic compensated phase. Compensation is provided by eccentric left ventricular hypertrophy. Individual myocytes lengthened by the addition of sarcomeres in series cause the chamber to dilate. Because left ventricular contractile function remains normal or nearly so in this phase, ejection performance remains supranormal. Thus, a large ejection fraction of an increased diastolic volume results in an increase in total stroke volume. In turn, forward stroke

STAGES OF MITRAL REGURGITATION

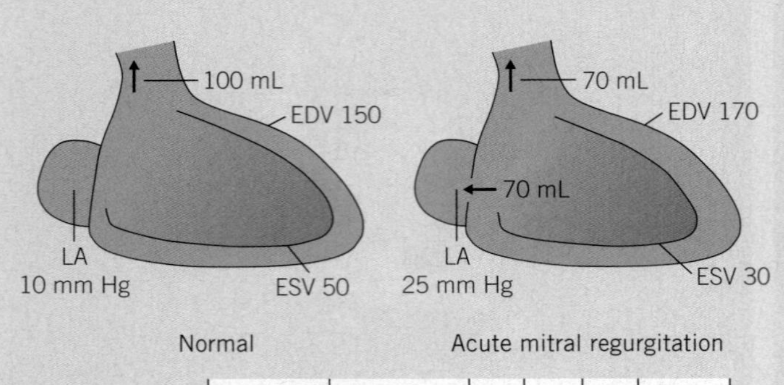

Normal

Acute mitral regurgitation

	Preload SL (μm)	Afterload ESS (kdyn/cm²)	CF	EF	RF	FSV (mL)
Normal	2.07	90	N	0.67	0.0	100
AMR	2.25	60	N	0.82	0.50	70

A

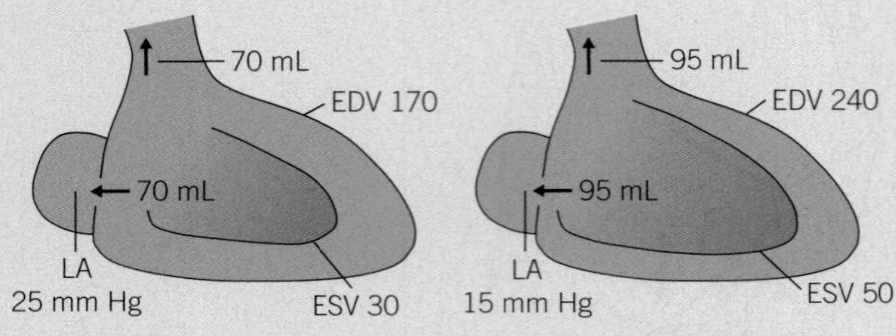

Acute mitral regurgitation

Chronic compensated mitral regurgitation

	Preload SL (μm)	Afterload ESS (kdyn/cm²)	CF	EF	RF	FSV (mL)
AMR	2.25	60	N	0.82	0.5	70
CCMR	2.19	90	N	0.79	0.5	95

B

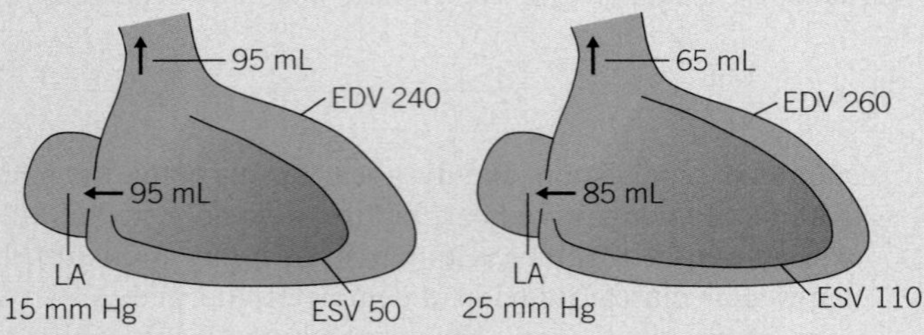

Chronic compensated mitral regurgitation

Chronic decompensated mitral regurgitation

	Preload SL (μm)	Afterload ESS (kdyn/cm²)	CF	EF	RF	FSV (mL)
CCMR	2.19	90	N	0.79	0.50	95
CDMR	2.19	120	↓	0.58	0.57	65

C

Figure 90.5 Stages of mitral regurgitation. In acute mitral regurgitation **(A)**, such as might occur after the rupture from major chordae tendineae, there is the sudden opening of an extra pathway for ejection of blood from the left ventricle. The regurgitant volume combined with the returning blood flow from the pulmonary vein increases left ventricular filling, in turn increasing sarcomere stretch and end-diastolic volume. The new pathway itself facilitates left ventricular ejection by reducing afterload, in turn reducing end-systolic volume. The volume overload must be contained in a small unprepared left atrium and left ventricle, in turn increasing left ventricular filling pressure. At this point, although left ventricular contractile function is normal, the patient experiences the physiology of congestive heart failure (increased filling pressure and decreased cardiac output). Although many patients with severe acute mitral regurgitation require immediate surgery, others may go on to enter the chronic compensated phase **(B)**. In this stage of mitral regurgitation, eccentric cardiac hypertrophy provides the compensation that allows substantial left ventricular enlargement. The increase in left ventricular volume permits both total and forward stroke volume to increase while accommodating the volume overload at a lower filling pressure. Because contractile function is normal or nearly normal in this phase, ejection fraction remains elevated. In this stage, the patient may be entirely asymptomatic and able to participate in fairly vigorous activity. Although the chronic compensated phase may be maintained for years, eventually the patient will enter the decompensated phase **(C)**. In this phase, left ventricular contractile dysfunction impairs left ventricular ejection, and end-systolic volume increases. In turn, total and forward stroke volume fall. The retained volume in the left ventricle again causes increased left ventricular filling pressure, and the patient may develop the symptoms of congestive heart failure in this phase. Ventricular dilatation may also worsen the mitral regurgitation. Despite that contractile function is now compromised, ejection fraction, although reduced from the compensated phase, still may be within "normal" range. AMR, acute mitral regurgitation; CCMR, chronic compensated mitral regurgitation; CDMR, chronic decompensated mitral regurgitation; CF, contractile function; EDV, end-diastolic volume; EF, ejection fraction; ESS, end-systolic stress; ESV, end-systolic volume; FSV, forward stroke volume; LA, left atrium; N, normal; RF, regurgitant fraction; SL, sarcomere length. (From Carabello BA. Mitral regurgitation, part 1: basic pathophysiologic principles. Mod Concepts Cardiovasc Dis 1988;57:53-58.)

volume is also increased, helping to normalize cardiac output. At the same time, enlargement of the left ventricle and left atrium allows the increased diastolic volume to be accommodated at a lower filling pressure, which is accomplished in part by increased chamber compliance and normal muscle compliance.[10,11] Thus, mitral regurgitation stands apart in cardiology as a situation in which pathologic change leads to improved rather than abnormal diastolic function. Enhanced chamber compliance develops from thinning of the left ventricular wall; it allows the ventricle to fill to a supernormal volume while permitting diastolic pressure to remain in the range in which pulmonary congestion does not develop. In this phase of mitral regurgitation, the patient may be entirely asymptomatic and able to engage in fairly vigorous activity without difficulty.

The patient may remain in the compensated phase for months or years. Eventually, however, left ventricular contractility diminishes. Because the left ventricle is now weakened, ejection is impaired and end-systolic volume increases. In turn, total stroke volume and forward stroke volume decline. The retained left ventricular volume increases end-diastolic volume and end-diastolic pressure. Usually, when the patient enters this stage, symptoms develop. However, some patients remain asymptomatic. Although ejection fraction is now diminished from both the acute and chronic compensated phases, ejection fraction still may remain in the "normal" range, even when the patient enters the decompensated phase.

Development of Eccentric Hypertrophy

The major compensatory mechanism for mitral regurgitation is the development of eccentric cardiac hypertrophy. The lengthening of individual cardiocytes increases chamber volume (and mass), allowing the ventricle to increase its total stroke volume. Thus, a ventricle with an ejection fraction of 70% and an end-diastolic volume of 100 mL produces stroke volume of 70 mL. If ejection performance is maintained and diastolic volume increases to 200 mL, total stroke volume doubles from 70 mL to 140 mL.

Some 30 years ago, Grossman and colleagues hypothesized that volume overload increased ventricular diastolic stress, which provided the signal for turning on the biochemical machinery that created new muscle mass. Recently, two studies have found that at least in experimental mitral regurgitation, this concept needs to be modified.[12,13] A sudden increase in end-diastolic stress caused by severe mitral regurgitation does not detectably increase protein synthesis rate. Conversely (and as a positive control), acute pressure overload increases protein synthesis rate by 35% within 6 hours after the increase in pressure (Fig. 90.6).[12] In fact, the hypertrophic process in mitral regurgitation was observed during the 3 months after creation of mitral regurgitation, and an increase in protein synthesis rate was never found.[13] Because the myocardial proteins are in constant flux, with synthesis and degradation occurring continually, an increase in mass in the absence of an increase in synthesis rate must by definition result from a decrease in degradation rate. Thus, it appears that the concentric hypertrophy that develops in experimental mitral regurgitation is "passive" and occurs

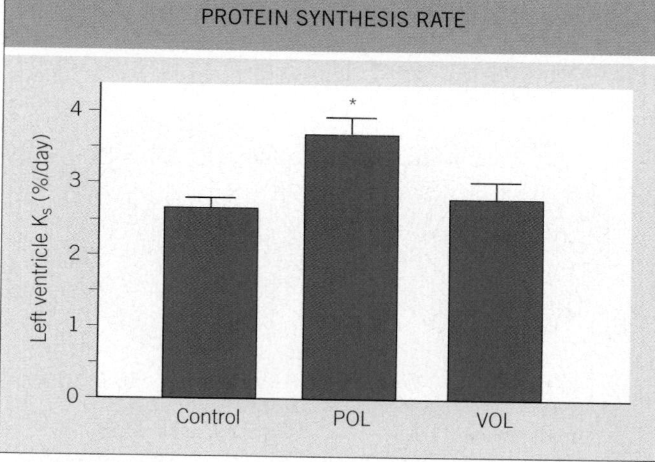

Figure 90.6 Protein synthesis rate. Myosin heavy chain synthesis rate (K_s) is demonstrated for controls, for dogs with the acute volume overload of mitral regurgitation (VOL), and for dogs with the acute pressure overload of aortic stenosis (POL). Within 6 hours after a pressure overload, there is a substantial increase in myosin protein synthesis rate, an increase that is not seen in mitral regurgitation. (From Imamura T, McDermott PJ, Kent RL, et al. Acute changes in myosin heavy chain synthesis rate in pressure versus volume overload. Circ Res 1994;75:418-425.)

from a slowing of degradation rather than from an increase in synthesis. How this process relates to the eventual development of contractile dysfunction is currently unclear. It may be that diminished degradation results in older cardiac proteins, which in some way impairs the ventricle's responses to adaptation, leading in turn to left ventricular dysfunction.

As noted before, the eccentric hypertrophy of mitral regurgitation enhances volume pumping. However, according to the law of Laplace, the stress or force on any given part of the myocardium is calculated as follows: (pressure × radius) ÷ thickness. For stress to remain normal when the radius term increases, as it does in eccentric hypertrophy, there must be a concomitant increase in wall thickness to offset radial lengthening. However, the opposite occurs in mitral regurgitation. The left ventricular wall is slightly thinner than normal, so that the ratio of radius to thickness becomes enlarged (Fig. 90.7).[14] Therefore, although the extra pathway for ejection of blood into the left atrium tends to reduce left ventricular afterload, afterload may be paradoxically normal or even increased because of the large radius-to-thickness ratio, which increases systolic stress (afterload).[15]

Thus, the changes in left ventricular geometry that occur in mitral regurgitation are both adaptive and maladaptive. The increase in radius is adaptive because it allows the ventricle to increase its overall volume-pumping capability. On the other hand, the discordance between the increase in radius and the decrease in thickness increases both systolic and diastolic stress. The increase in systolic stress (afterload) impairs left ventricular shortening. If Laplacian stress is in fact the signal for hypertrophy, the signal that is transmitted in mitral regurgitation is an incomplete or imperfect one in which eccentric hypertrophy occurs in the absence of enough concentric hypertrophy to normalize stress.

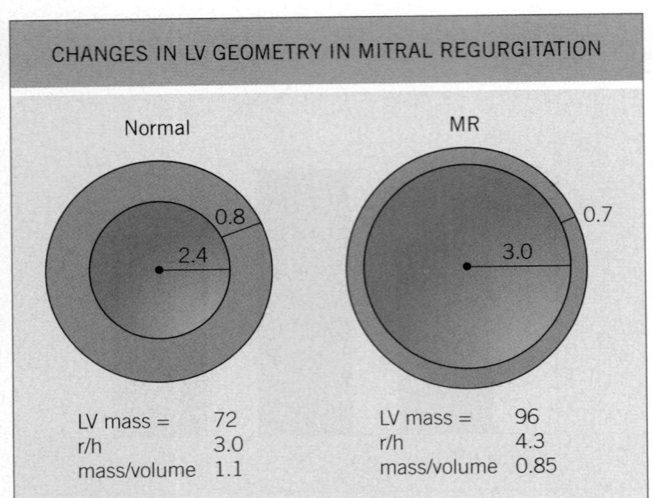

Figure 90.7 Changes in left ventricular (LV) geometry that occur in mitral regurgitation. The schematic shows the changes in left ventricular geometry that occur in mitral regurgitation (MR). The chamber radius increases while wall thickness decreases, in turn increasing the ratio of radius to thickness. This geometry change tends to increase wall stress.

Mechanisms of Left Ventricular Systolic Dysfunction

Patients with chronic severe mitral regurgitation may remain in the chronic compensated phase for years. However, left ventricular dysfunction eventually develops. Its causes are multifactorial.

Myofibrillar Loss

In the papillary muscles both from humans with mitral regurgitation and in whole hearts taken from dogs with experimental mitral regurgitation, there is substantial loss of contractile elements.[16,17] The 35% reduction in myosin found in dogs can almost entirely account for the amount of contractile dysfunction that is seen. In the few reports in humans, this degree of myofibrillar dropout has been seen primarily in the papillary muscles. Presumably, in this situation, myofibrillar loss contributes to papillary muscle dysfunction and potential worsening of mitral regurgitation, especially during stress.

Abnormal Calcium Handling

In the endocardium and epicardium in humans, Mulieri and coworkers[2] found a reduction in the force-frequency relationship. In normal subjects, as heart rate increases, myocardial contractility increases, presumably because of a net increase in calcium flux. Conversely, in heart failure (both in cardiomyopathy and in mitral regurgitation), the force-frequency relationship is blunted and has an early descending limb. Thus, as heart rate increases past a modest point, force generation diminishes rather than increases. This abnormal relationship can be returned to normal by the addition of forskolin, which serves to increase cyclic adenosine monophosphate development, in turn resulting in increased calcium transients and increased calcium-triggered calcium release. Thus, reduced density of the contractile proteins as well as abnormalities in calcium handling results in the left ventricular dysfunction of mitral regurgitation. We hypothesize that because of the decrease in the mass-to-volume ratio, there is insufficient myocardial mass to deliver the necessary volume to maintain compensation. In the absence of hypertrophic compensation, there is greater reliance on deleterious neurohumoral activation, especially on activation of the sympathetic nervous system.[18] In fact, in both naturally occurring and experimental mitral regurgitation, catecholamines are increased when decompensation occurs. Excess catecholamines may cause the loss of contractile elements.[19] Accordingly, when beta blockers are used or when mitral regurgitation is corrected, myofibrillar density may return to normal.[18,20]

Importantly, and irrespective of whether it is investigated in humans or in experimental animals, contractility can improve or return to normal after a timely correction of mitral regurgitation.[20,21] Unlike the contractile abnormalities that develop in dilated cardiomyopathy, the abnormalities in contractile function seen here are reversible, at least in the early stages of decompensation. In the dog model, reversal is predicated on renormalization of the number of contractile elements in the individual cardiocytes.[20] The mechanism of restoration of normal function in humans has not yet been studied.

Summary

Mitral regurgitation is compensated by the development of eccentric hypertrophy, which may accrue by a reduction in the degradation rate of myocardial proteins rather than by an increase in synthesis rate. Although the extra pathway for ejection into the left atrium tends to decrease afterload, the manner in which the ventricle remodels is a negative counterbalance to unloading and results in afterload returning to normal or even becoming greater than normal. In turn, the relative lack of hypertrophic compensation "forces" the ventricle to rely more heavily on neurohumoral mechanisms of compensation, many of which are deleterious. Activation of the adrenergic nervous system has been noted to be maladaptive in many chronic cases of cardiac decompensation, and excess catecholamine levels may in themselves be cardiotoxic. Persistently elevated catecholamines may be the cause of myofibrillar dropout and a further reduction in contractile function. In addition, abnormalities in calcium handling reduce the force-frequency relationship of the mitral heart. Fortunately, both in experimental animals and in humans, these abnormalities can be reversed by timely mitral valve replacement (or by beta blockers in the dog model).

CLINICAL PRESENTATIONS

Mild to Moderate Mitral Regurgitation

Mild to moderate mitral regurgitation causes no symptoms and is not typically noticed by the patient. It is usually detected initially by the health care provider as a holosystolic apical murmur during physical examination. Evidence of cardiac enlargement is usually absent, and a third heart sound is not heard. Mild to moderate mitral regurgitation does not require therapy but should be evaluated at baseline; the evaluation should include echocardiography to establish baseline ventricular function, lesion severity, and valve morphology. This examination will serve as a reference for the future surveillance of the disease.

Acute Severe Mitral Regurgitation

In acute mitral regurgitation, such as might occur with chordal rupture or bacterial destruction of the valve, a severe volume overload is placed on the otherwise unprepared left ventricle and left atrium. The result is a fall in cardiac output and an increase in left ventricular, left atrial, and pulmonary venous pressures, in turn leading to pulmonary congestion. Almost all such patients present with the symptoms that are typical of congestive heart failure (i.e., orthopnea, fatigue, and dyspnea on exertion). Because pressure in the small, noncompliant left atrium rises rapidly in systole, the pressure gradient between left ventricle and left atrium rapidly diminishes, reducing the driving force for blood to cross the regurgitant orifice, shortening the murmur of mitral regurgitation. Thus, the murmur in acute mitral regurgitation may be relatively short and unimpressive. However, a third heart sound is usually heard, which attests to the severity of the disease. Because cardiac dilatation has not had time to occur in acute mitral regurgitation, the apical impulse is not displaced and may not be hyperdynamic. The first heart sound is soft, and the second is usually split.

Chronic Severe Mitral Regurgitation

Even chronic severe mitral regurgitation may be tolerated for years without symptoms. Thus, physical examination rather than a complaint by the patient often brings the disease to the attention of the physician. During examination, an enlarged heart is noted as the apical impulse is displaced downward and to the left. An apical holosystolic murmur is heard, usually radiating to the axilla, and is usually accompanied by a third heart sound. In chronic compensated mitral regurgitation, the third heart sound reflects the filling of the left ventricle by the large volume stored in the left atrium and does not necessarily indicate heart failure.

Chronic Decompensated Mitral Regurgitation

As left ventricular contractile dysfunction develops, cardiac output falls and left atrial pressure increases, usually causing the symptoms that are typical of congestive heart failure, including dyspnea on exertion, orthopnea, and paroxysmal nocturnal dyspnea. However, some patients enter this decompensated phase without the development of symptoms. Because there are no reliable physical examination signs that decompensation has developed, asymptomatic transition into this stage can be detected only by objective changes in cardiac performance during echocardiography (see later).

Ischemic Mitral Regurgitation

Ischemic mitral regurgitation must be distinguished from organic mitral valve disease that develops in patients who happen to have coronary disease. The term *ischemic mitral regurgitation* implies that it is ischemia that has caused the mitral regurgitation. Typically, ischemic mitral regurgitation occurs in patients with known coronary disease who have had subsequent coronary events. Because, as noted before, transient ischemia by itself is usually not enough to cause mitral regurgitation by way of papillary muscle dysfunction,[5,6,22] it is unusual for mitral regurgitation to come and go as angina comes and goes in the absence of any other manifestation of coronary disease. Usually, there has been a previous myocardial infarction that has led to abnormalities in left ventricular wall motion. Ischemic mitral regurgitation often develops close to a myocardial infarction. Even when mild mitral regurgitation develops at the time of infarction, prognosis worsens, presumably because the presence of mitral regurgitation indicates severe ventricular damage.[23] The worse the ischemic mitral regurgitation is after myocardial infarction, the worse the prognosis. Despite the advances and improvement in prognosis that have occurred in nonischemic mitral regurgitation, the prognosis for severe ischemic mitral regurgitation still remains reduced compared with that of nonischemic mitral regurgitation.[24] However, recent reports suggest improving survival as surgical techniques have improved.[25,26]

DIAGNOSTIC TECHNIQUES

Electrocardiography

Once the diagnosis of mitral regurgitation has been made from physical examination, electrocardiography should be performed. This examination is useful as a later reference point should the patient develop atrial fibrillation (a common complication of mitral regurgitation) and in detecting myocardial infarction as one of the potential causes of the disease.

Chest Radiography

There is probably no need for chest radiography in patients with mild to moderate mitral regurgitation because it is likely to be normal, and if mitral regurgitation worsens with time, changes in heart size are more accurately quantified during echocardiography than by chest radiography. With severe disease, when there may be a question of whether the patient is compensated, chest radiography may be useful to objectively assess the presence of pulmonary congestion.

Echocardiography

Currently, echocardiography forms the basis for establishment of the diagnosis of mitral regurgitation, helping establish the cause, gauge severity, and assess progression of disease and of ventricular dysfunction.

Etiology

The most common cause of mitral regurgitation in developed countries is degeneration of the valve, causing mitral valve prolapse. During echocardiography, this abnormality is detected by finding thickened redundant mitral leaflets and elongated chordae tendineae so that one or both leaflets prolapse past the annular plane into the left atrium, moving past the point of coaptation and causing mitral regurgitation. The mitral annulus has a saddleback shape and is not uniplanar.[27] Thus, whether the leaflets have prolapsed above the annular plane must be judged with caution and should be seen in both the four-chamber and parasternal long-axis views.

If rupture of a chorda tendinea has led to mitral regurgitation, the ruptured chorda itself as well as a flail leaflet may be seen.

If endocarditis is the cause, vegetations on the leaflets or the chordae help confirm the diagnosis. In rheumatic disease, the typical hockey-stick rheumatic deformity of the valve is seen. There is restricted travel of the leaflets, so that they cannot extend to the point of coaptation, leading to regurgitation.

Assessment of Lesion Severity

Although color-flow Doppler examination of the valve is primarily used to assess severity, it cannot be overemphasized that this analysis must be performed in the context of left atrial and left ventricular size. If by history the disease is chronic and by Doppler examination the lesion is severe but left atrial size and left ventricular size are normal, there is incongruity in the data. The lack of cardiac dilatation suggests either that the disease is acute or that the color-flow study is overestimating the severity of the disease. Many cases of overestimation of mitral regurgitation occur in this situation.

Several techniques employ color-flow Doppler interrogation of the mitral valve to assess severity of the lesion. In most cases, the color-flow examination does provide good estimation of mitral regurgitation, but there are many exceptions that cause the diagnostician to be unsure in any given patient whether color flow is accurately reflecting disease severity.

Visual Estimation of the Color-Flow Signal

As the regurgitant jet passes from the left ventricle through the regurgitant orifice into the left atrium, flow accelerates, and it is this increase in red cell velocity that is detected by the ultrasound interrogation of the jet. In general, the more "disturbed" the flow detected in the left atrium, the greater the degree of mitral regurgitation.[28] However, it must be understood that the examiner is not viewing true flow but rather flow velocity, a concept that, if overlooked, can lead to misinterpretation. On the one hand, a small, high-velocity jet can entrain a large area of disturbed flow, causing an overestimation of the severity of mitral regurgitation. On the other hand, a jet that is directed laterally becomes confined and looks relatively small, which may lead to underestimation of the severity of mitral regurgitation.[29] The apparent degree of severity can further be affected by machine settings and the type of equipment used.[30]

Color-Flow Mapping

In an effort to provide a more quantitative estimation of mitral regurgitation, mapping of the jet in terms of its actual size or its size relative to left atrial size has been attempted. Although this process was initially viewed with enthusiasm, it has become clear that this technique is limited by the same factors that limit visual estimation. Thus, the time necessary to perform mapping probably is not justified by any real increase in the accuracy of severity estimation.

Proximal Isovelocity Surface Area

As the regurgitant jet on the ventricular side of the mitral valve approaches the orifice, it tends to develop a hemispheric shape. By the principle of the conservation of momentum, at the outside of the convergence zone, the area is large and the velocity is low; but as the jet approaches the regurgitant orifice, it becomes smaller in size but higher in velocity.[31] Regurgitant flow in the convergent jet can be calculated as the jet area × jet velocity. Velocity of flow at a given point in the jet can be determined by the machine settings. By calculating the area of the jet at the point of aliasing, where velocity is known, flow can be calculated. The area of a hemisphere is given as $2\pi r^2$, where r is the distance from the point of aliasing to the mitral valve plane. In turn, by dividing peak flow by peak velocity, the instantaneous area of the mitral valve orifice itself can be calculated. Areas of more than 0.4 cm^2 indicate a large mitral regurgitant orifice and therefore severe mitral regurgitation.[32] In fact, in one report, measured regurgitant orifice area was directly related to prognosis.[33]

When the proximal isovelocity surface area method works effectively, it provides increased accuracy in the assessment of the mitral regurgitant orifice and of the severity of the lesion. Unfortunately, this method also has several limitations. First, it is often impossible to detect the zone of convergence because the hemispheric pattern has simply not materialized. Second, it may be difficult to judge the radius length if the mitral plane is difficult to locate exactly. Third, although flow should be the same throughout the jet, the flow calculation in reality varies according to where in the jet the area and the velocity are measured.[34]

Vena Contracta Method

The vena contracta is the narrowest part of the regurgitant orifice on the atrial side of the valve before the jet begins to spread out. At this point, the jet size should accurately reflect the regurgitant orifice itself, and it can be obtained by measuring the jet there rather than using the extensive calculations shown before. In fact, there is good correlation between the vena contracta area and other measures of mitral regurgitation.[35] However, this method also has its limitations because it is affected unpredictably by changes in left ventricular afterload.[36]

Quantitative Echocardiography

Perhaps the most accurate (and most time-consuming) method of estimating the severity of mitral regurgitation is to calculate regurgitant flow and regurgitant fraction.[37] The total flow pumped by the left ventricle is the flow crossing the mitral valve during diastole; total flow can be calculated by multiplying the mitral valve orifice area by the time-velocity integral of flow across the valve. Forward flow is that flow determined at a nonregurgitant orifice (either the pulmonary, aortic, or tricuspid valve) and is equal to the area of that valve orifice multiplied by its time-velocity integral. By subtracting forward flow from total flow, regurgitant flow is calculated. Regurgitant fraction is equal to regurgitant flow divided by total flow. Typically, regurgitant fractions of more than 60% indicate severe mitral regurgitation, regurgitant fractions of less than 40% indicate moderate to mild mitral regurgitation, and regurgitant fractions in the range of 40% to 60% indicate moderate to moderately severe mitral regurgitation. Unfortunately, the time and labor necessary to perform this technique are considerable, which has caused it not to be widely applied in clinical practice.

Three-Dimensional Echocardiography

More recently, real-time three-dimensional echocardiography has been developed as an imaging technique complementary to two-dimensional echocardiography. This technique presents the clinician with a more anatomic view of the mitral valve akin to what the operating surgeon will see when the left atrium is opened during mitral valve surgery. Its exact role in the armamentarium of diagnosis is unclear, but the technique is likely to help in making the preoperative decision about whether the valve can be repaired.[38,39]

Summary

Echocardiography is indispensable in the assessment of mitral regurgitation. It helps establish the etiology, assess the impact of the lesion on left ventricular and left atrial size and function, and quantify the severity of the lesion. However, because color-flow estimation of mitral regurgitation severity can both underestimate and overestimate severity, no echocardiographic parameter should be allowed to stand by itself; rather, all must be taken in the context of the patient's history, physical examination, and chamber geometry.

Cardiac Catheterization

In cases in which all aspects of the clinical presentation and the noninvasive examination are consistent, cardiac catheterization may not be necessary to arrive at a diagnosis. However, in patients with risk factors for coronary disease (including age), catheterization is usually performed before surgery to accomplish coronary arteriography. If at this time the diagnosis of mitral regurgitation and its severity are uncertain, both hemodynamic studies and left ventriculography may be helpful in resolving the issue. In the symptomatic patient with mitral regurgitation, wedge pressure and pulmonary artery pressure should be elevated to confirm a hemodynamic cause of pulmonary congestion and the patient's symptoms. In acute mitral regurgitation, a large *v* wave is usually demonstrable in the pulmonary capillary wedge tracing. However, the presence or absence of a large *v* wave correlates only roughly with the severity of mitral regurgitation and is often not an important diagnostic benchmark unless the amplitude of the *v* wave is twice that of the mean pulmonary capillary wedge pressure.

If resting hemodynamics are relatively normal in the symptomatic patient, the cause of the symptoms is not apparent. Often, handgrip exercise that raises afterload causes a striking increase in the amount of mitral regurgitation, demonstrated by a marked increase in wedge pressure and its *v* wave, now uncovering the cause of the patient's symptoms.

During left ventriculography, the actual flow of radiopaque contrast material from left ventricle to left atrium is visualized (Fig. 90.8) and graded on a semiquantitative scale shown in Table 90.1. Like echocardiography, quantitative angiography can be performed in which total stroke volume is calculated as angiographic end-diastolic volume minus end-systolic volume, and forward stroke volume is the cardiac output determined by either the Fick or thermodilution method divided by heart rate. As with echocardiography, the time-intensive nature of calculating regurgitant volume and regurgitant fraction in this manner and error caused by lack of attention to the details of volume calculation in many busy catheterization laboratories prevent widespread use of this technique. However, semiquantitative ventriculography

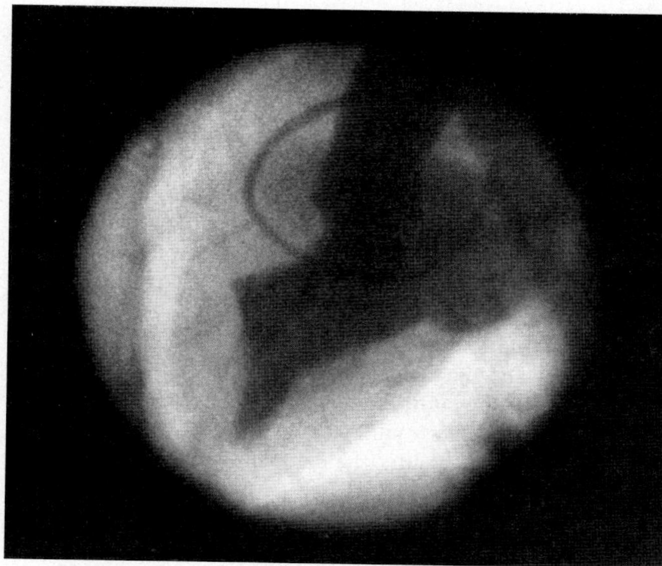

Figure 90.8 The left ventriculogram of a patient with mitral regurgitation. Contrast material is seen densely opacifying the left atrium.

SEMIQUANTITATIVE ANGIOGRAPHIC ASSESSMENT OF MITRAL REGURGITATION	
Grade	**Features**
1	Only a puff of contrast material enters the left atrium during systole
2	The left atrium becomes completely but faintly opacified with contrast material after several heartbeats
3	Equal opacification of left atrium and left ventricle
4	Greater opacification of the left atrium than the left ventricle

Table 90.1 Semiquantitative angiographic assessment of mitral regurgitation.

(see Table 90.1) can be quite useful in assessing the severity of mitral regurgitation, provided adequate contrast material is used. A common mistake is to use too little contrast material, which causes an underestimation of the severity of mitral regurgitation when a small amount of contrast material is diluted into both the enlarged left atrium and the enlarged left ventricle, making opacification appear unimpressive. In assessing the severity of mitral regurgitation, at least 50 to 60 mL of contrast material should be used to accurately estimate the degree of mitral regurgitation.

MANAGEMENT

Medical Therapy

Acute Mitral Regurgitation

The goal of therapy in acute mitral regurgitation is to lower left ventricular and left atrial filling pressure while increasing cardiac output. In the normotensive patient, this can be accomplished by the use of potent vasodilators such as nitroprusside. By lowering total peripheral resistance, nitroprusside causes a preferential increase in flow toward the aorta and away from the left atrium, in turn increasing forward cardiac output and decreasing regurgitant flow.[40] By reduction of regurgitant flow, filling pressure diminishes and the symptoms of pulmonary congestion may be relieved. If mitral regurgitation is so severe that hypotension has developed, vasodilators cannot be used because they lower blood pressure further. In such cases, intra-aortic balloon counterpulsation is initiated. Counterpulsation diminishes left ventricular afterload, in turn increasing forward flow while maintaining or even augmenting diastolic blood pressure. In cases severe enough to require either nitroprusside or intra-aortic balloon pumping, surgical correction of the mitral regurgitation should follow soon after medical stabilization has been accomplished. In less severe cases, diuretic therapy alone may be sufficient to relieve pulmonary congestion while "buying time" until eccentric cardiac hypertrophy allows the patient to enter the compensated phase.

Chronic Mitral Regurgitation

Because vasodilators are effective in the treatment of acute mitral regurgitation, it seems intuitive that vasodilators would be useful in the treatment of chronic mitral regurgitation. However, there are several theoretical and practical limitations why this may not be so. First, in mitral regurgitation, load is normal. Thus, the use of vasodilators to further lower afterload creates a situation of subnormal afterload with which there is very little clinical experience, and the outcome is unpredictable. Furthermore, afterload reduction decreases left ventricular force development, diminishing the force closing the mitral valve, potentially worsening rather than improving the condition.[41]

From a practical standpoint, there is simply no conclusive evidence that vasodilators are efficacious in the treatment of chronic mitral regurgitation, and their use is therefore problematic. Wisenbaugh and colleagues[42] found that in asymptomatic patients with mitral regurgitation, captopril (25 mg every 8 hours) did little to change cardiac volume status or performance. In a smaller group of symptomatic patients[43] (who presumably already manifested left ventricular dysfunction), vasodilators were effective in reducing cardiac size and mass, but it could be argued that surgery is preferable to medical therapy in such patients. However, many studies in humans and in dogs[44-48] have failed to show any important effect of angiotensin-converting enzyme inhibitors or angiotensin receptor blockers on mitral regurgitation. To be sure, these agents are not simple vasodilators, and other drugs may be more effective. However, until a large trial of vasodilators in mitral regurgitation is performed, the use of vasodilators in the treatment of chronic asymptomatic mitral regurgitation should be viewed as experimental and of uncertain efficacy.

Beta blockers have been successful in treating experimental mitral regurgitation[18,49] and also in treating mitral regurgitation secondary to cardiomyopathy[50] in humans. However, results of the treatment in humans of chronic severe primary regurgitation with beta blockers have yet to be reported.

Surgery

Mitral regurgitation is a mechanical lesion that requires mechanical correction provided by surgery. The ultimate goals of surgery are to prevent or to relieve symptoms, to maintain and to restore left ventricular function, and to allow a normal lifestyle and life span. Dramatic changes in our understanding of mitral regurgitation and the surgical practice to correct it have allowed important advances toward these goals, which are now usually attainable. Although 15 years ago there was only a 50% 10-year survival after mitral valve surgery, patients may now enjoy normal longevity after a properly timed and properly performed mitral valve operation.[3] The factors involved in the timing of surgery are

- the presence or absence of symptoms;
- the presence or absence of left ventricular dysfunction;
- the type of valve surgery performed;
- age; and
- whether the mitral regurgitation is primary or functional in origin. In primary mitral regurgitation, the regurgitation has caused a volume overload on the left ventricle, and restoration of valve competence "cures" the disease. In secondary mitral regurgitation, cardiomyopathy, either ischemic or idiopathic, has led to mitral regurgitation. Because removal of the mitral regurgitation does not cure the underlying muscle disease, the outcome is much less favorable.

Symptomatic Status

The presence or absence of symptoms alone affects outcome after surgery.[51] The development of symptoms is a negative statement about the patient's overall cardiovascular physiology and thus worsens prognosis. Whether the symptoms have developed because the regurgitation has worsened, because left ventricular dysfunction has begun to develop, because pulmonary pressure is increasing, or because of some combination of these events, the new onset of symptoms is an indication for surgery. Thus, the clinician should not be reassured because symptoms have developed in the absence of objective changes in left ventricular function or pulmonary artery pressure. Rather, the symptoms should be taken as a more complex measure of physiology that is not detectable by the simpler objective markers. The usual symptoms of mitral regurgitation are considered to be dyspnea and orthopnea. Although it is not truly a symptom, the onset of atrial fibrillation has a negative impact on prognosis.[52] Thus, recurrent or persistent atrial fibrillation probably should be considered a change in symptomatic status. Unless advanced age or other comorbid factors prevent surgery, most patients should undergo mitral valve repair or replacement at the time symptoms develop. In the future, assessment of brain natriuretic peptide may prove a useful adjunct to history alone in determining cardiovascular status.

Onset of Left Ventricular Dysfunction

Although the onset of symptoms in some cases heralds left ventricular dysfunction, silent left ventricular dysfunction without symptoms develops in other patients. Fortunately, there are now relatively reliable markers of left or right ventricular dysfunction that are helpful in the timing of surgery. As noted before, the favorable loading conditions of mitral regurgitation augment ejection fraction.[1] "Normal" ejection fraction in mitral regurgitation is about 65% to 70%.[3,53,54] There is substantial evidence that once left ventricular ejection fraction falls below 60%, outcome worsens (Fig. 90.9),

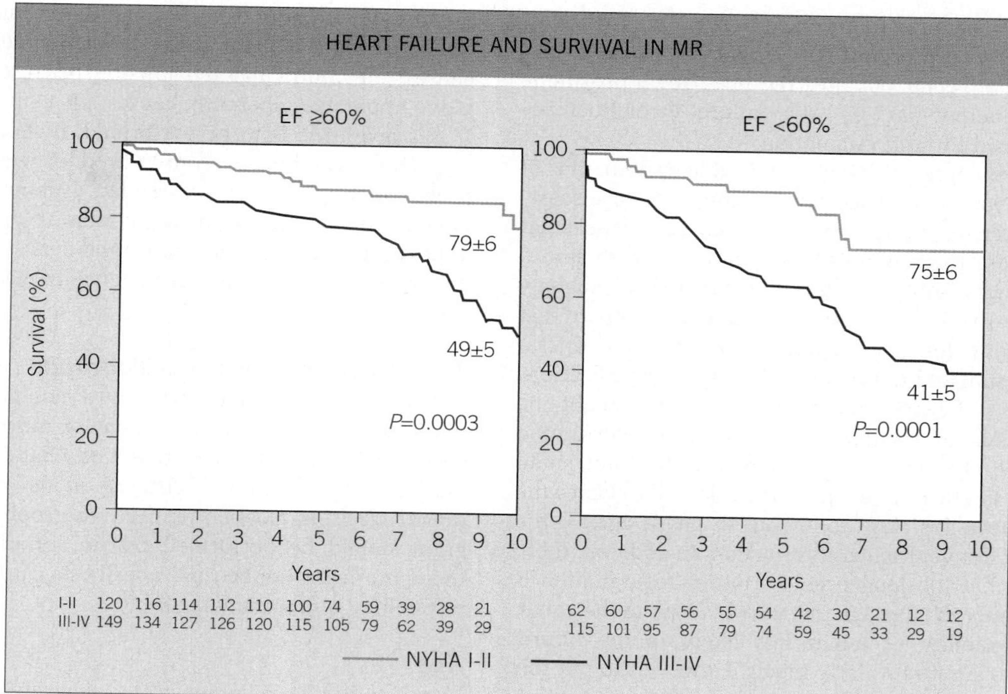

Figure 90.9 The impact of the presence or absence of the symptoms of heart failure on survivorship in patients with mitral regurgitation (MR). Even patients with normal left ventricular function had a poorer outcome if symptoms were present. EF, ejection fraction; NYHA, New York Heart Association class. (From Tribouilloy CM, Enriquez-Sarano M, Schaff HB, et al. Impact of preoperative symptoms on survival after surgical correction of organic mitral regurgitation: rationale for optimizing surgical indications. Circulation 1999;99:400-405.)

implying that left ventricular dysfunction is present at the time this threshold is crossed.[3,55,56] Thus, in general, patients with mitral regurgitation should be operated on before the ejection fraction falls below 60%.

Because the volume overload of mitral regurgitation augments preload, in turn augmenting ejection fraction, end-systolic dimension, which is relatively preload independent, has also been used to gauge left ventricular function.[56,57] Several studies indicate that when end-systolic dimension exceeds 45 mm or end-systolic volume exceeds 50 mL/m^2 (roughly equivalent to a 45-mm end-systolic dimension at echocardiography),[56,57] prognosis worsens (Fig. 90.10). Some studies indicate that for ejection fraction to return to normal postoperatively, end-systolic dimension should exceed 40 mm.[58] Thus, patients should also have surgery when repeated echocardiographic examinations demonstrate that end-systolic dimension is approaching 40 to 45 mm.

Although the effect of mitral regurgitation on left ventricular function has been correctly emphasized, it must be recognized that a consequence of mitral regurgitation is pulmonary artery hypertension, in turn impairing right ventricular function. When pulmonary artery pressure exceeds 50 mm Hg or when right ventricular ejection fraction falls below 35%, outcome is poor[56,59]; pulmonary hypertension is therefore also an indication for surgery.

Type of Mitral Surgery

Three types of mitral surgery are performed to correct mitral regurgitation: mitral valve repair, mitral valve replacement with conservation of the native mitral valve apparatus, and "standard" mitral valve replacement. Mitral valve repair is

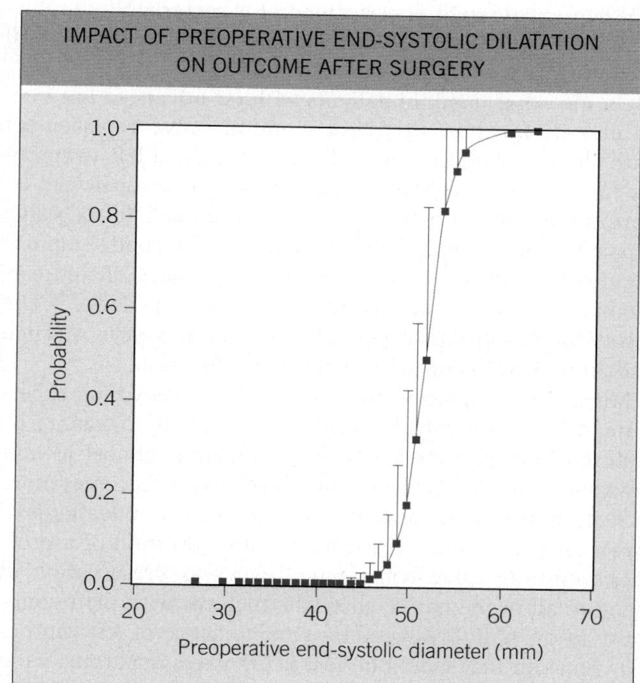

Figure 90.10 Probability of a poor outcome after surgery increases dramatically when preoperative end-systolic diameter exceeds 45 mm. Thus, surgery should be undertaken before end-systolic dilatation of this magnitude.[57]

preferable. Results after mitral valve repair are superior to those of a standard mitral valve replacement, in which the mitral apparatus is destroyed.[60] The better outcome probably derives from the importance of retaining the mitral valve apparatus in preserving left ventricular function and from the fact that repair obviates the need for a prosthetic valve and its inherent risks of valve failure, thromboembolism, and the need for anticoagulation.

Mitral valve repair is potentially applicable at both ends of the ventricular functional spectrum in mitral valve disease. In the asymptomatic patient with normal left ventricular function in whom there is no obvious indication for mitral surgery, one might apply an "atrial septal defect" analogy to mitral valve repair. In atrial septal defect, a repair that avoids a prosthetic device is performed at a very low operative risk to forestall and to prevent subsequent complications of the defect. Likewise, mitral valve repair might be practiced in a similar fashion because it can be performed at approximately 1% to 2% operative risk, does not entail the use of a prosthetic device, and is durable and obviates the postoperative need for close follow-up to guard against the development of left ventricular dysfunction. In addition, there is the concern that the longer severe mitral regurgitation is present, the greater the damage that may be done to the valve, making the possibility of repair less likely in the future; this concept also argues for early repair. However, to put this concept into practice, a repair must almost be guaranteed. If an unanticipated prosthesis is inserted, the atrial septal defect analogy is abrogated. In this circumstance, insertion of a prosthesis would be considered a complication of surgery. The concept must be taken in light of the fact that only about half of mitral valves are currently repaired in the United States.

When valve repair is performed, it is remarkably durable. In Carpentier's series of 162 patients, there were only 10 reoperations to 20 years of follow-up.[61]

On the other hand, in patients with far-advanced left ventricular dysfunction in whom a mitral valve replacement with chordal disruption would cause worsened left ventricular function and probably death, an adequate repair can be performed where a replacement cannot. Indeed, mitral valve repair has been employed in patients with secondary mitral regurgitation in the presence of severe primary dilated cardiomyopathy and ejection fractions as low as 15%.[62] The results in this group of patients were 70% 1-year survival and an improvement in left ventricular function.

Mitral valve replacement with chordal preservation is performed in cases in which mitral valve competence cannot be restored by repair itself. Although repair is almost always possible in simple posterior leaflet prolapse, it becomes more difficult in rheumatic disease,[63] in patients with bileaflet prolapse, and in patients with endocarditis. Insertion of a prosthesis ensures valve competence, whereas preservation of some or all of the native chordal structures with their continuity to the native valve allows maintenance of left ventricular function that would be lost if the valve apparatus were destroyed.[64,65] The disadvantage of this procedure is that it uses a prosthesis, subjecting the patients to all the risks of an artificial valve.

Finally, a standard mitral valve operation, in which the valve apparatus is removed and a prosthesis is inserted, should be avoided whenever possible, and it is now performed in only a minority of patients. The procedure should be reserved for those cases in which the valve and apparatus are already so badly distorted that they cannot be preserved. This operation, while ensuring valve competence, inevitably causes left ventricular dysfunction because removal of the valve apparatus inherently causes left ventricular damage.[66] If this operation is to be performed, it should be done only in patients who have well-preserved left ventricular function preoperatively. If left ventricular dysfunction has already developed and the mitral apparatus is removed, this will almost certainly result in a large and persistent fall in postoperative ejection fraction, persistence of heart failure, and a shortened life span.

Transesophageal Echocardiography

Transesophageal echocardiography can be used preoperatively to gain a better assessment of mitral valve anatomy and therefore a better assessment of what operation will ultimately be performed.[67] Because of its importance in the overall decision to operate, the transesophageal echocardiogram should be performed before surgery rather than in the operating room because anesthesia can alter the patient's physiology quite dramatically.[68]

Age

Many studies have demonstrated that advanced age (>70 to 75 years) is a greater risk factor for mitral surgery than it is for aortic surgery, and the outcome for elderly patients with mitral regurgitation is relatively poor.[60] Poorer prognosis applies especially if there is a need for a concomitant procedure such as coronary revascularization and if mitral valve replacement rather than repair must be performed.[60] However, recent reports are more encouraging with regard to surgical outcome in the elderly.[69-71] Although patients with symptoms should not be denied surgery simply because they are elderly, operation in elderly asymptomatic patients must be weighed very carefully and should probably not be performed if there is any question that a mitral valve replacement rather than a repair will be performed.

Secondary (Functional) Mitral Regurgitation

The prognosis for secondary mitral regurgitation remains poor despite the advances made in the treatment of nonischemic mitral regurgitation. The poor prognosis stems in part from the fact that a second potentially fatal heart disease is now automatically present and that even if the mitral regurgitation is repaired successfully, the coronary disease or primary myocardial disease may continue to progress. Furthermore, when secondary mitral regurgitation is present, severe left ventricular dysfunction almost always accompanies it. Nonetheless, this area is receiving intense interest. Led by Bach and Bolling,[62] several studies have demonstrated satisfactory operative mortality and reverse remodeling after mitral surgery for such patients.[72,73] On the other hand, there has been no evidence as yet of a survival benefit,[74] and some have questioned the utility of mitral surgery in such patients.[75,76] It seems clear that this issue will have to be settled from the results of randomized trials.

Catheter-Based Therapies

Percutaneous intervention for mitral regurgitation has recently engendered much excitement.[77] A variety of devices use two similar catheter-based approaches to therapy for mitral regurgitation. In one approach, a clip or suture is used to appose the two leaflets of the valve, producing a double-barrel mitral valve. This approach mimics the surgical approach of Alfieri[78] and has been successful in decreasing the amount of mitral regurgitation present at least in the short term.[79] The second approach uses the proximity of the coronary sinus to the mitral annulus in many patients. A variety of maneuvers are being used to change the shape of the coronary sinus, in turn altering the mitral annulus, reducing the mitral regurgitation present.[79] Still in their infancy, percutaneous interventions for mitral regurgitation await long-term data for judging their success.

SUMMARY

Severe mitral regurgitation places a volume overload on the left ventricle that is compensated by the development of eccentric left ventricular hypertrophy. Although this mechanism may allow patients to remain compensated for a variable length of time, eventually prolonged and severe hemodynamic overload leads to left ventricular dysfunction. A careful history and physical examination, together with echocardiography, are indispensable in assessing the severity of the disease and whether left ventricular dysfunction has begun to develop. When disparity exists between clinical presentation and echocardiography or between left ventricular geometry and the Doppler assessment of mitral regurgitation, hemodynamic evaluation, including left ventriculography, is essential.

The goal of therapy is to restore mitral valve competence early in the decompensation phase of the illness. Thus, when mild symptoms develop, when pulmonary artery pressure increases, or when left ventricular ejection fraction falls below 60% or end-systolic dimension exceeds 40 mm, surgery should be performed. In primary mitral regurgitation, mitral valve repair is the preferred operation because it carries a lower operative mortality and preserves postoperative left ventricular function. If competence cannot be restored by repair alone, apparatus conservation together with insertion of a prosthetic valve should be entertained. With proper surgical timing and technique, it is now possible to restore prognosis postoperatively to that of an age-matched unaffected population.

The favorable outcome now possible for primary mitral regurgitation is unfortunately not always applicable to secondary (functional) mitral regurgitation, in which the presence of two different heart diseases substantially worsens prognosis. In the case of secondary mitral regurgitation, the optimum timing of surgery and the most beneficial operation have still not been clarified.

chapter 91

Mitral Valve Prolapse

Richard B. Devereux

Definitions

- Mitral valve prolapse represents abnormal systolic displacement of the mitral valve leaflets into the left atrium.

Key Features

- Mitral valve prolapse is a dominantly inherited disorder of connective tissue with more consistent gene expression in women.
- Mitral valve prolapse may be diagnosed by a characteristic midsystolic click and late systolic murmur and by echocardiographic findings.
- Although most patients remain asymptomatic, complications can include heart failure, endocarditis, autonomic nervous system dysfunction, and arrhythmias.

Therapy

- Antibiotic prophylaxis is indicated if there is moderate or severe mitral regurgitation or if a patient has had previous endocarditis.
- Valve repair is indicated if heart failure or left ventricular dysfunction develops.

Mitral valve prolapse (MVP) is the most common structural abnormality of heart valves in industrialized countries, affecting 2% to 3% of adults.[1,2] By definition, MVP represents abnormal systolic displacement of the mitral valve leaflets superiorly from their normal position into the left atrium. This usually occurs because connective tissue components of the mitral valve (leaflets, chordae, and annulus) are enlarged in relation to the size of the supporting left ventricle (Fig. 91.1); but in some instances, it may occur because of the exaggerated distensibility of the mitral annulus.[3]

Most instances of MVP occur as a primary condition, which is usually passed from mothers or fathers to children of either gender in a pattern indicative of autosomal dominant inheritance.[4,5] Family studies show that the age at onset is usually between 10 and 16 years, that women more consistently demonstrate typical valvular findings, and that some mild cases become undetectable after the age of 50 to 60 years.[4,5] A small proportion of cases of MVP occur because of valvular deformity secondary to other heritable disorders of connective tissue, such as the Marfan and Ehlers-Danlos syndromes,[6] or on a dynamic basis because of disproportion between normal mitral valves and small left ventricles in such conditions as anorexia nervosa and atrial septal defect.

ANATOMY AND PATHOLOGY

Initial knowledge of the anatomy of MVP came from examination of specimens removed during surgery to replace severely regurgitant mitral valves. These studies showed enlargement, thickening, and distortion of mitral leaflets, often involving all three scallops of the posterior mitral leaflet and portions of the anterior leaflet, with elongation or rupture of chordae tendineae and dilatation of the mitral annulus.[7,8] Typically, thickening of the mitral leaflets reflected both increase in the fibrous layers on their atrial and ventricular surfaces and proliferation of loose, myxomatous connective tissue in the middle of the leaflets. The collagen bundles in this layer, which provide the valve's tensile strength, are commonly fragmented, providing a structural basis for the segmental stretching or "hooding" of mitral leaflet segments that occurs commonly in prolapsed mitral valves.

A study by Davies and colleagues,[9] based on 1984 consecutive autopsies in which the left ventricle was distended by water perfusion, revealed MVP as manifested by expansion of more than one third of the posterior leaflet or more than half of the anterior leaflet in 5% of women and more than 3% of men. In the approximately 25% of instances of MVP with more severe valvular abnormalities (e.g., chordal rupture or fusion of mitral leaflet segments to the free wall of the left ventricle), the mitral valve abnormality was considered to be the cause of death in about 40%. In this series, approximately 65% of those with MVP had involvement only of the posterior leaflet, about 10% had involvement only of the anterior leaflet, and 25% had involvement of both leaflets. Of note, in view of the current approach to use of two-dimensional echocardiography for diagnosis of mitral prolapse, 10% to 20% of individuals with MVP at necropsy or by angiography have involvement of the posterior leaflet's medial or lateral scallop (P1 and P3) but not its central scallop (P2), the one visualized in the echocardiographic long-axis view (see later). As noted by Davies and colleagues,[9] most prolapsed mitral valves are thickened, but "in some instances the valve appeared translucent and gelatinous." More recent echocardiographic studies show thickening of mitral leaflets, above the 97th percentile of normal (2 mm), in at least 60% of individuals with uncomplicated MVP and in even higher proportions of those with hemodynamically important mitral regurgitation or other complications.[10,11]

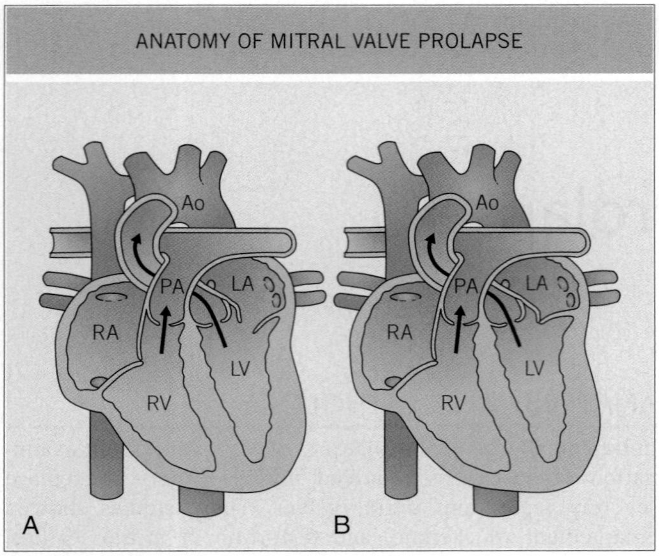

ANATOMY OF MITRAL VALVE PROLAPSE

Figure 91.1 Anatomy of mitral valve prolapse. Enlargement of mitral leaflets, annulus, and chordae in patients with mitral valve prolapse **(A)** compared with findings in healthy persons **(B)**. Ao, aorta; LA, left atrium; LV, left ventricle; PA, pulmonary artery; RA, right atrium; RV, right ventricle.

PATHOPHYSIOLOGY

Three lines of evidence indicate that most instances of MVP represent a heritable disorder of connective tissue. The first, discussed before, is the demonstration of abnormalities of collagen and other connective tissue components in prolapsed mitral valves studied at necropsy or after surgical excision. The observation of fragmentation of collagen bundles in prolapsed mitral leaflets[9] led to the attractive hypothesis that MVP might constitute a disorder of collagen; however, family studies have refuted linkage of MVP to the major fibrillar collagen genes.[12] Initial reports of loci for alternative candidates as the cause of MVP have not yet been confirmed.[13-16]

The second line of evidence, derived from family studies, is the demonstration that most individuals with MVP have other affected relatives, with MVP detectable by echocardiography in about 30% of adult parents, siblings, or children of index cases with MVP (Fig. 91.2).[4,5] Visual inspection of Figure 91.2 shows frequent transmission of MVP from mother to son or from father to daughter, forming the basis for formal genetic analyses showing autosomal dominant inheritance.[4] Examination of pedigrees in family studies demonstrates a reduced frequency of gene expression in children, adult men, and older women.

The third line of evidence derives from the demonstration of extravalvular connective tissue abnormalities associated with MVP. These include several-fold higher prevalences in individuals with MVP than in unaffected individuals of skeletal abnormalities, including mild scoliosis, pectus excavatum, and arachnodactyly, and of relatively low body weight[17-19] and documentation of connective tissue anomalies affecting the cardiac conduction system in MVP patients who had suffered sudden death.[20]

The etiologic abnormalities in connective tissue, the gene or genes for which have not yet been defined, cause the cardiac manifestations of MVP by producing a structural or dynamic disproportion between the size of the mitral valve's connective tissue elements and its muscular supports (papillary muscles and underlying ventricular walls).[3] In an elegant piece of clinical investigation, Fontana and coworkers[21] performed contrast angiography and phonocardiography in MVP patients in the supine and head-up tilt positions, demonstrating that reduction in left ventricular cavity size caused by diminished venous return allowed earlier billowing into the left atrium of the mitral leaflets and production of characteristic clicks and murmurs earlier in systole.

CLINICAL PRESENTATIONS

Although MVP was first recognized by its auscultatory features and by abnormal mitral valve motion revealed by angiography and echocardiography, reports soon appeared of a high prevalence of nonanginal chest pain, dyspnea, and anxiety-related symptoms in patients with MVP. The concept of an inclusive "MVP syndrome" proved clinically useful because it provided an explanation for common, troublesome, and otherwise confusing cardiovascular and psychological symptoms that is acceptable to patients and physicians alike. However, controlled studies have documented similar prevalences of chest pain and dyspnea as well as prolongation of the electrocardiographic QT interval among prolapse patients and cardiovascularly normal individuals evaluated in the same clinical or epidemiologic setting. MVP also appears to be no more common among patients with panic and anxiety disorders than among matched control subjects.

Our studies compared affected relatives (relatively unselected individuals with MVP) with unaffected relatives and spouses in more than 100 families of patients with MVP (who constitute genetically related and unrelated control groups).[17] Affected relatives were more likely than control subjects to have thoracic bone abnormalities (pectus excavatum, scoliosis, and "straight back"), low body weight and systolic blood pressure, and palpitations (Table 91.1). In contrast, we found no difference between MVP and control subjects in the prevalence of nonanginal chest pain, dyspnea, panic attacks, high anxiety, or electrocardiographic repolarization abnormalities (Table 91.2). We also found that MVP and panic attacks were associated with contrasting patterns of autonomic dysfunction.[22] More MVP than control subjects exhibited orthostatic hypotension and syncope, possibly related to reduced blood volume, whereas the group with panic attacks exhibited hyperreactive heart rate and blood pressure responses to orthostatic stress. Thus, MVP and panic disorders are biologically distinct as well as statistically unassociated.

In a separate, population-based sample, we confirmed the association of MVP with lower body weight and blood pressure and identified links with lower prevalence of diabetes, more favorable metabolic profile and left ventricular geometry, and better myocardial and renal function.[1] Thus, controlled studies—assessing families with multiple affected members, matched clinical patients, or members of a population-based sample—show a relatively narrow spectrum of adverse clinical features and also reveal potentially

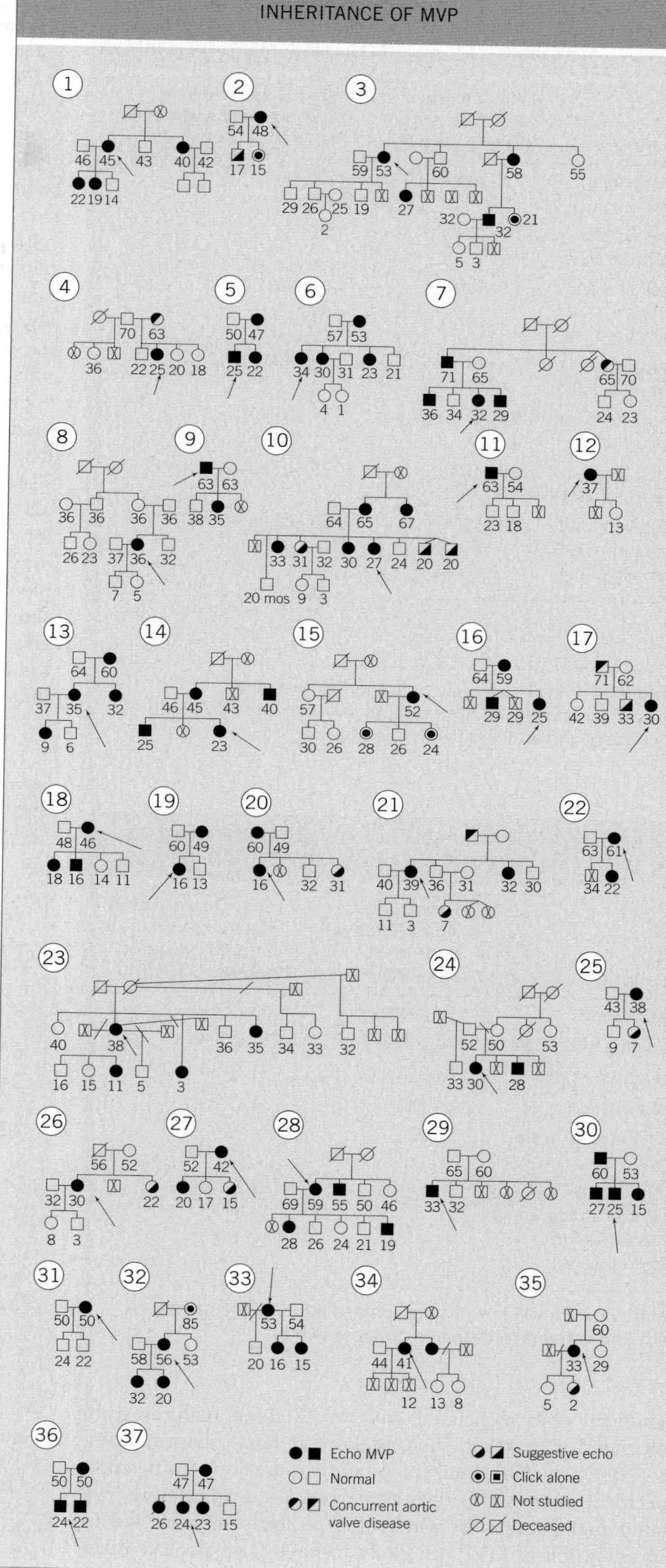

Figure 91.2 Inheritance of mitral valve prolapse (MVP). Pedigrees of families ascertained by an index case *(arrows)* with MVP and other affected *(filled)* female *(circles)* and male *(squares)* relatives. Ages of subjects are indicated beneath their symbols. (From Devereux RB, Brown WT, Kramer-Fox R, et al. Inheritance of mitral valve prolapse. Effect of age and sex on gene expression. Ann Intern Med 1982;97:826-832, with permission from the American College of Physicians.)

PREVALENCE OF AUSCULTATORY FEATURES AND EXTRACARDIAC MANIFESTATIONS OF MITRAL VALVE PROLAPSE (MVP) IN INDEX CASES AND AFFECTED FAMILY MEMBERS		
Feature	**First-Degree Relatives with MVP (n = 81)**	**First-Degree Relatives and Spouses without MVP (n = 232)**
Midsystolic click only	27 (33%)*	7 (3%)
Late systolic murmur only	14 (17%)†	8 (4%)
Click and late systolic murmur	13 (16%)*	1 (<1%)
Holosystolic murmur only	1 (1%)*	0 (0%)
Thoracic bone abnormalities	33 (41%)*	34 (15%)*
Body weight <90% of ideal	26 (32%)*	29 (13%)*
Systolic blood pressure <120 mm Hg	43 (53%)*	65 (28%)*

*P <.01.
†P <.001

Table 91.1 Prevalence of auscultatory features and extracardiac manifestations of mitral valve prolapse (MVP) in index cases and affected family members.

PREVALENCE OF SYMPTOMS IN ADULT FAMILY MEMBERS WITH AND WITHOUT MITRAL VALVE PROLAPSE (MVP)		
Symptom	**First-Degree Adult Relatives with MVP (n = 81)**	**First-Degree Adult Relatives and Spouses without MVP (n = 232)**
Palpitations	32 (40%)	53 (23%)
Atypical chest pain	14 (17%)	37 (16%)
Dyspnea	5 (6%)	21 (9%)
Panic attacks	6 (7%)	11 (5%)
Trait anxiety score >50	5 (6%)	14 (6%)
Inferior lead electrocardiographic repolarization abnormalities	9 (11%)	23 (10%)

Table 91.2 Prevalence of symptoms in adult family members with and without mitral valve prolapse (MVP).

beneficial ones associated with MVP. Even features truly associated with MVP, such as thoracic bone abnormalities, low body weight, and palpitations, are not sufficiently specific to be useful diagnostic features. Furthermore, we found that patients in whom nonspecific symptoms led to consideration of MVP are likely to have false-positive diagnoses resulting from misattribution to MVP of panic attacks and midsystolic murmurs.[23]

DIAGNOSTIC TECHNIQUES

In clinical practice, MVP is most commonly first recognized by auscultation. Typical auscultatory features are a midsystolic click and late systolic murmur, which is separated from the first heart sound by a silent interval but continues to or through the second heart sound. These sounds are best heard by listening over the left ventricular impulse and medial to it, with the patient in the supine, left decubitus, and sitting positions. Because systolic clicks may have other causes and mitral annular calcification may produce a late systolic murmur in older persons, it is important to perform physical maneuvers during auscultation that take advantage of the key role of valvular-ventricular disproportion in producing the manifestations of MVP (Fig. 91.3). When both a midsystolic click and late systolic murmur are present and vary appropriately in timing and intensity with maneuvers, or a loud midsystolic click exhibits appropriate mobility, the diagnosis is definitive.

As Figure 91.3 shows, maneuvers that reduce left ventricular chamber size will cause the click and onset of the murmur to move closer to the first heart sound, whereas the loudness of the click and murmur is affected by changes in blood pressure independent of changes in timing. Figure 91.3 shows how standard maneuvers during physical examination affect the click and murmur. It is especially important to time the onset after the first sound and continuation until the second sound of the late systolic murmur, as miscategorization

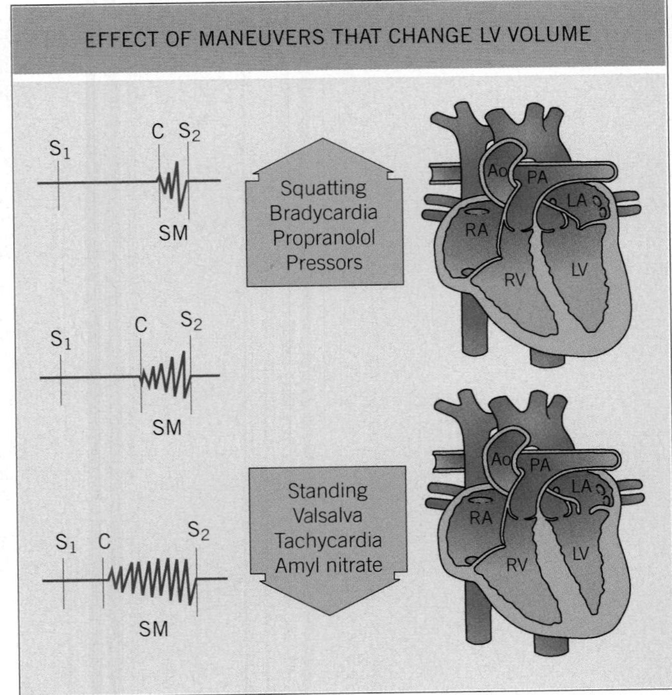

Figure 91.3 Effect of maneuvers that change left ventricular (LV) volume on the timing of the click (C) and murmur (SM) of mitral valve prolapse. The onset of the murmur and occurrence of the click move closer to the first heart sound (S_1) when left ventricular volume is reduced and farther from it when left ventricular volume is increased. Ao, aorta; LA, left atrium; PA, pulmonary artery; RA, right atrium; RV, right ventricle; S_2, second heart sound.

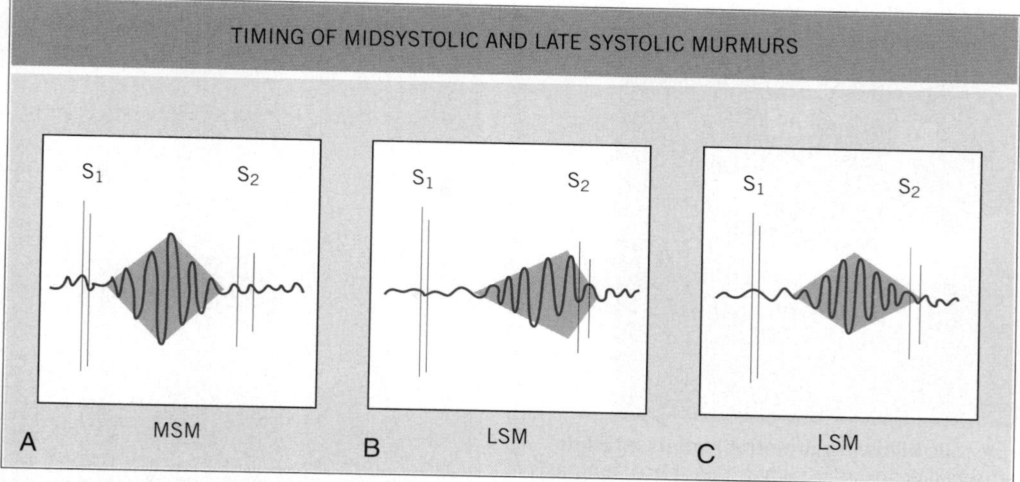

Figure 91.4 Timing of midsystolic and late systolic murmurs. A, A midsystolic murmur (MSM) begins after the first heart sound (S_1). **B** and **C,** Late systolic murmurs (LSM) begin after S_1 but continue to or through the second heart sound (S_2). Note that both types of murmur may have a crescendo-decrescendo configuration.

of midsystolic murmurs caused by normal blood flow in thin-chested persons or aortic sclerosis in older patients commonly causes false-positive diagnoses of MVP (Fig. 91.4). When both a midsystolic click and a late systolic murmur are present and respond appropriately to maneuvers, MVP can be diagnosed confidently by physical examination. If there are less specific auscultatory features, such as a soft or immobile midsystolic click or a late systolic murmur in a middle-aged or older individual, echocardiographic confirmation of MVP is desirable.

Echocardiography

Because of its ability to visualize the anatomy and function of the mitral valve, echocardiography is a nearly ideal method to detect and to characterize MVP.[24,25] The initial mainstay of echocardiographic diagnosis of MVP was demonstration on M-mode recordings of late systolic posterior motion, by more than 2 mm, of continuous mitral leaflet interfaces posterior to the valve's C-D line in late systole (Fig. 91.5). Late systolic buckling of mitral leaflets on M-mode tracings occurs simultaneously with the midsystolic click and onset of the late systolic murmur (see Fig. 91.5).

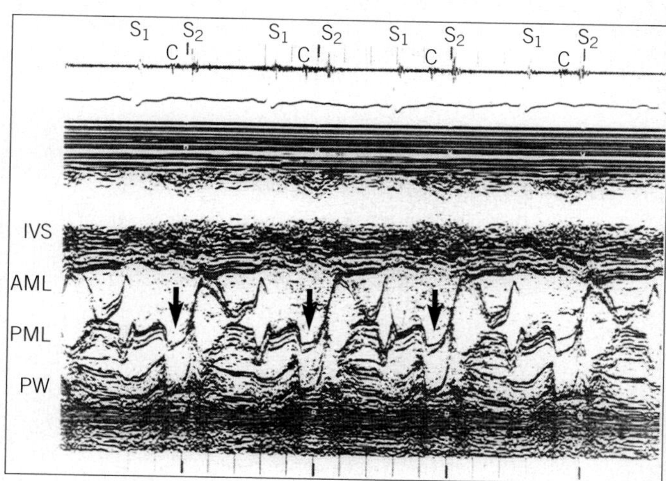

Figure 91.5 Late systolic prolapse. M-mode echocardiographic recording of the mitral valve demonstrating late systolic prolapse *(arrows)*. The simultaneous phonocardiogram shows a midsystolic click (C) and late systolic murmur. AML, anterior mitral leaflet; IVS, interventricular septum; PML, posterior mitral leaflet; PW, posterior wall; S_1, first heart sound; S_2, second heart sound.

Two-dimensional echocardiography has enhanced recognition and assessment of the severity of MVP. The condition can be accurately diagnosed by two-dimensional echocardiography when one or both mitral leaflets are seen to protrude or "billow" into the left atrium in systole in the parasternal or apical long-axis view (Fig. 91.6).[24,25] As noted before, however, this view principally visualizes the central scallops of the mitral leaflets (P2 and A2), potentially missing instances of prolapse localized to medial or lateral posterior leaflet scallops. Quantification of mitral leaflet motion on two-dimensional echocardiograms has shown that posterior motion of MVP on M-mode recordings may be produced either by leaflet billowing into the left atrium or, in some individuals, by posterior motion of the mitral leaflets due to exaggerated systolic distention of the mitral annulus.[26] It is important not to diagnose MVP on the basis of apparent protrusion of the mitral leaflets into the left atrium that is seen only in the apical four-chamber two-dimensional view, as this is a common consequence of the saddle shape of the mitral annulus (Fig. 91.7). Diagnosis of MVP by echocardiography should be based on either unequivocal systolic billowing of one or both mitral leaflets across the mitral annulus in two-dimensional parasternal or apical long-axis views or more than 2 mm of late systolic posterior displacement of continuous mitral leaflet interfaces in high-quality two-dimensional targeted M-mode recordings (which have the advantage, when a transverse scan is performed by sweeping the beam from near the interventricular septum to the lateral left ventricular wall, of visualizing the medial and lateral scallops of the posterior mitral leaflet).

Two-dimensional echocardiography is especially useful for identification of mitral valve abnormalities associated with severe forms of MVP. These include elongation of mitral

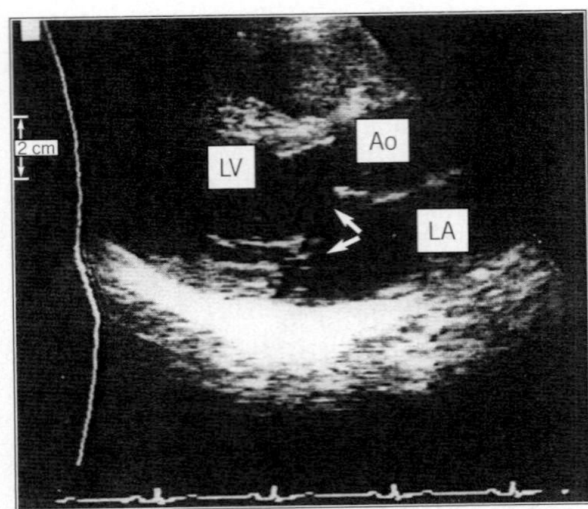

Figure 91.6 Late systolic billowing of mitral leaflets into left atrium. Two-dimensional echocardiogram in parasternal long-axis view showing late systolic billowing of both mitral leaflets *(arrows)* into the left atrium. Ao, aorta; LA, left atrium; LV, left ventricle.

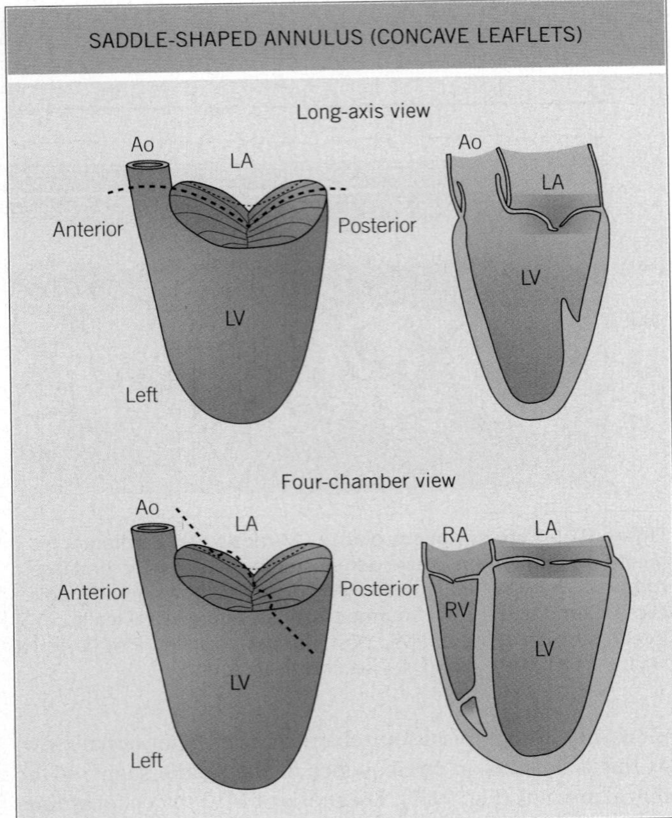

Figure 91.7 Artifactual mitral valve prolapse in the apical four-chamber view resulting from the saddle shape of the mitral annulus. Ao, aorta; LA, left atrium; LV, left ventricle; RA, right atrium; RV, right ventricle.

leaflets and annulus[27] and prominent leaflet thickening,[28] both of which are associated with severe mitral regurgitation. Billowing of one mitral leaflet segment that is so prominent that it loses apposition with the matching portion of the other mitral leaflet is an anatomic cause of severe regurgitation that can be readily visualized on two-dimensional echocardiography (Fig. 91.8).[29]

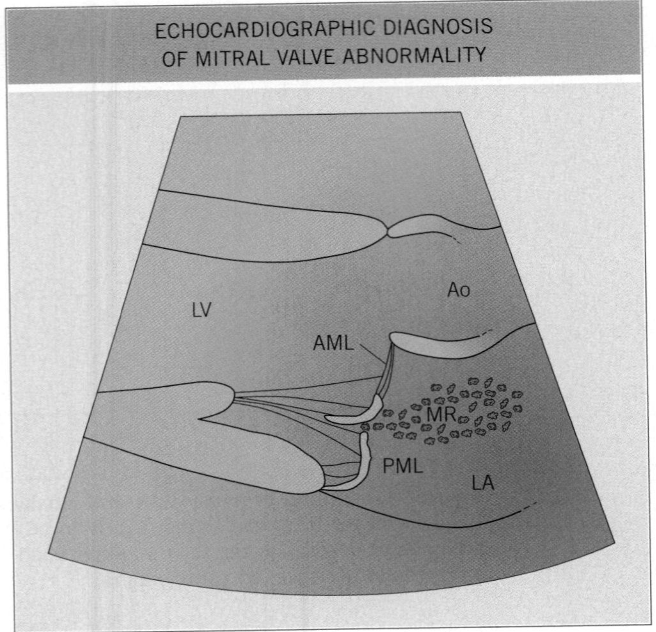

Figure 91.8 Echocardiographic diagnosis of mitral valve abnormality. Severe posterior mitral leaflet (PML) prolapse into the left atrium (LA) producing loss of coaptation with the anterior mitral leaflet (AML) and allowing severe mitral regurgitation (MR). Ao, aorta; LV, left ventricle.

Although conventional echocardiography and color-flow Doppler echocardiography are not useful for diagnosis of MVP, as there are many causes of mitral regurgitation, they are of great value for grading the severity of regurgitation, which in turn is the most important factor in determining the risk of major complications. Assessment of severity of mitral regurgitation is commonly performed by several sets of criteria. Despite their limitations, initial criteria based on jet length (<1.5 cm = 1+; 1.5 to 3 cm = 2+; 3 to 4.5 cm = 3+; >4.5 cm or to roof of the left atrium = 4+)[30] and jet/left atrial area ratios (e.g., <20% = 1+; 20% to 40% = 2+; 40% to 60% = 3+; >60% = 4+)[31] remain useful and easy to apply. More refined methods, including measurement of proximal jet width (the vena contracta),[32] proximal isovelocity surface area (PISA), actual jet volume by three-dimensional color Doppler study,[33] and calculated regurgitant volume and fraction, give even more precise estimates of the severity of regurgitation.

When color Doppler study is used to evaluate the severity of mitral regurgitation due to MVP, special attention is needed for the correct assessment of potential

- underestimation of the severity of wall-hugging jets;
- overestimation or underestimation of the regurgitant volume calculated by PISA as a result of asymmetric jet origin;
- underestimation or overestimation of the severity of regurgitation by regurgitant jet or left atrial area criteria if the atrium is dilated through the effects of chronic regurgitation or, conversely, if the atrium is relatively small; and
- overestimation or underestimation of the severity of regurgitation by jet length criteria in the presence of systemic hypertension or relatively low arterial pressure.

Three-dimensional echocardiography may be the ideal method to identify prolapse of all scallops of the posterior leaflet as well as of the more centrally situated anterior leaflet. With improved image quality and new approaches to image acquisition, real-time or rapidly reconstructed three-dimensional echocardiographic volume imaging is becoming feasible and may improve clinical assessment of the location and severity of prolapse of different portions of the mitral valve.[34]

MANAGEMENT

Appropriate care of an individual who has MVP depends on accurate diagnosis and on matching the intensiveness of evaluation and treatment to the level of risk (Table 91.3).[35] When the diagnosis is in doubt, echocardiography may be useful as an objective means to expunge a dubious diagnosis of MVP and to free a patient from unfounded concerns about heart disease and unwarranted treatment. Echocardiographic screening for MVP in unselected populations is not cost-effective; however, evaluation of adolescent and adult first-degree relatives of patients with unequivocal MVP is cost-effective because about 30% of such individuals have MVP. MVP is too rare before the age of 10 years to warrant screening.

Uncomplicated Mitral Valve Prolapse

The starting point of management for most patients with MVP is reassurance that they have a condition that is generally benign and may even be beneficial if they have inherited the tendencies, mentioned before, to low body weight and low blood pressure.[1,19] Management of patients with MVP should be matched to the risks of infective endocarditis and progressive mitral regurgitation. Because these risks are related to the presence of at least mild mitral regurgitation,[36,37] no specific treatment is needed for individuals with MVP, particularly women younger than 45 years without a mitral regurgitant murmur on any of several examinations with auscultation in multiple positions and isometric handgrip exercise or evidence of no more than 1+ mitral regurgitation by Doppler echocardiography. We reassure such individuals that the outlook is benign and may even be enhanced if they have low body weight and blood pressure. Antibiotic prophylaxis is not recommended unless the individual wishes maximum protection against even remote risks; reevaluation by auscultation and echocardiography is recommended at moderate intervals (perhaps every 5 years) to be certain that the patient has not passed into a higher risk group.

On the basis of present evidence, patients with echocardiographic MVP who even intermittently or with simple maneuvers such as sitting or handgrip exercise have soft late systolic murmurs of mitral regurgitation or who have Doppler echocardiographic evidence of trace or mild mitral regurgitation appear to be at modestly increased risk for endocarditis or progressive mitral regurgitation. In accord with the 2007 American Heart Association recommendations, we do not recommend infective endocarditis prophylaxis to such patients.[38] We have obtained evidence that endocarditis prophylaxis is cost-effective in MVP patients with obvious mitral regurgitation, documented by prior recognition of heart murmurs that are likely to have reflected moderate or severe regurgitation.[39] In view of suggestive evidence that elevated blood pressure may predispose to chordal rupture and progressive mitral regurgitation in patients with MVP,[40] we recommend antihypertensive treatment of all MVP patients with mild mitral regurgitation with even borderline systemic hypertension. Doppler echocardiography is important to define precisely the extent of mitral regurgitation, and this evaluation as well as auscultatory examination is warranted at more frequent intervals (every 2 to 3 years) to assess possible progression of regurgitation.

MATCHING RISK AND MANAGEMENT IN MITRAL VALVE PROLAPSE	
Level of Risk	**Definition and Management**
Lowest	Subjects without mitral regurgitant murmurs or Doppler regurgitation; especially women younger than 45 years **Management:** reassurance; no clear need for antibiotics; reevaluation and echocardiography at moderate intervals (5 years)
Moderate	Subjects with intermittent or persistent mital murmurs, mild Doppler regurgitation, and/or thickened valves **Management:** antibiotic prophylaxis with amoxicillin or clindamycin; treat even mild established hypertension; reevaluation and echocardiography more frequently (2–3 years)
High	Subjects with moderate or severe mitral regurgitation **Management:** antibiotic prophylaxis with amoxicillin (unless allergic); optimize afterload (arterial pressure); reevaluate with Doppler echocardiography and other tests if needed annually Consider valve repair or replacement for exertional dyspnea or decline of left ventricular function into low-normal range.

Table 91.3 Matching risk and management in mitral valve prolapse.

Mitral Valve Prolapse with Hemodynamically Important Mitral Regurgitation

Patients with MVP who have hemodynamically important mitral regurgitation are at greatest risk for endocarditis, sudden death, and need for mitral valve surgery. This group constitutes approximately 4% of adults with MVP. Severe mitral regurgitation in a patient with MVP can be identified on physical examination by a holosystolic or nearly holosystolic mitral regurgitant murmur associated with an audible third heart sound and leftward displacement of an enlarged, dynamic left ventricular impulse (Fig. 91.9). Objective confirmation of this complication can be obtained by demonstration of a large mitral regurgitant jet by color-flow Doppler echocardiography (Fig. 91.10). Echocardiography usually reveals left ventricular and left atrial enlargement, and it demonstrates a spectrum of morphologic valvular abnormalities, including leaflet and annular enlargement, distortion and thickening of leaflet segments, and redundancy or rupture of chordae tendineae.[10,27-29]

Because MVP patients with moderate or severe mitral regurgitation are likely to progress to cardiac decompensation if they suffer additional valve damage from endocarditis, which may include leaflet perforations that would render the prolapsed valve nonrepairable, we recommend antibiotic prophylaxis to such patients with amoxicillin

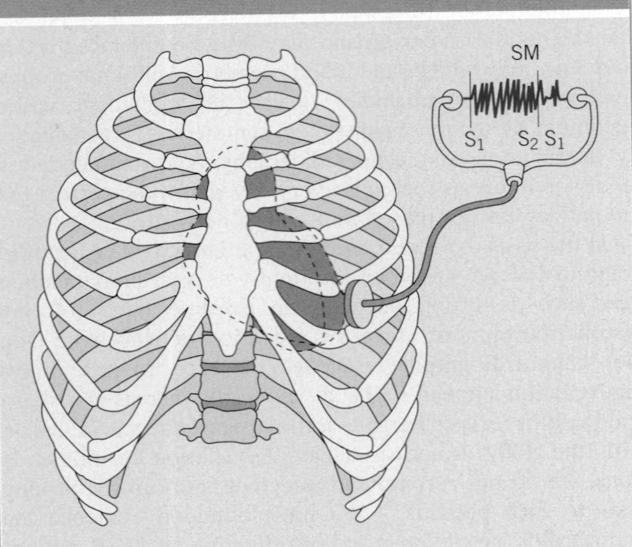

Figure 91.9 Diagnosis of severe mitral regurgitation in a patient with mitral valve prolapse (MVP). There is a nearly holosystolic mitral regurgitant murmur, with a third heart sound and leftward displacement of an enlarged left ventricular impulse, which is felt to the left of the midclavicular line in the fifth and sixth intercostal spaces, instead of being smaller than 2.5 cm in diameter and limited to one interspace, as it would be in a normal heart. S_1, first heart sound; S_2, second heart sound; SM, systolic murmur.

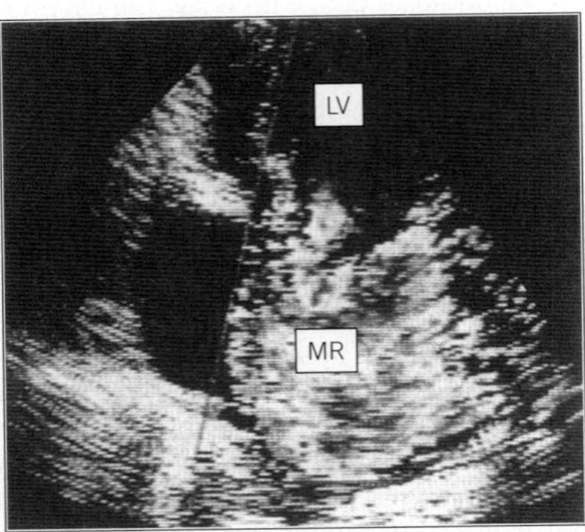

Figure 91.10 Severe mitral regurgitation demonstrated by color-flow Doppler echocardiography. The mitral regurgitation (MR) jet fills almost the entire left atrium, which is nearly 10 cm in diameter. LV, left ventricle.

(2 g) or clindamycin (600 mg) orally within 1 hour before dental procedures (see Table 91.3).[38] It is also theoretically attractive, although not of proven value, to treat even borderline systemic hypertension with antihypertensive drugs in such patients. Regular follow-up is required, with annual echocardiography, optimally with exercise stress.

Corrective valvular surgery, by valve repair rather than by valve replacement in most patients, is recommended either when patients develop dyspnea of more than New York Heart Association class II severity or when left ventricular systolic performance falls into the lower part of the normal range in the absence of symptoms. A simple partition value for recognition of the latter is left ventricular minor axis shortening of less than 31%, which has been reported to predict a suboptimal outcome after mitral valve surgery for severe mitral regurgitation. Frankly subnormal ventricular performance, with ejection fractions of 30% to 50%, should not preclude corrective valvular surgery, which may improve the poor survival associated with medical management of patients with severe mitral regurgitation and ventricular dysfunction.

It has been suggested but not yet proved that early repair of prolapsed mitral valves, before any of the preceding criteria are met, may yield better long-term results; however, this could also accelerate by many years the morbidity associated with valve surgery in some patients who would otherwise have had a stable long-term course. The excellent initial success, approaching 90%, with long-term durability of repair by experienced cardiac surgeons of severely regurgitant prolapsed mitral valves[41] makes repair rather than replacement the procedure of choice when surgery is needed in patients with MVP. Ongoing clinical trials indicate that substantial reduction of regurgitation due to severe prolapse of central mitral valve scallops (P2 and A2) can be achieved by transcatheter placement of a clip that anchors the mitral leaflets to each other,[42,43] suggesting that this may become an attractive option both for early repair of severely regurgitant mitral valves and for repair of such valves in individuals at exceptionally high operative risk because of advanced age or severe comorbidities.

Treatment of Arrhythmias

Arrhythmias in MVP may require treatment to relieve symptoms or to reduce risk of sudden death.[44] Palpitations, salvos of atrial premature complexes, and brief bursts of atrial tachycardia are found slightly more commonly in subjects with MVP than in normal individuals. Suggested mechanisms of arrhythmogenesis include stimulation of atrial pacemakers by the impact of prolapsing leaflets or mitral regurgitant jets and origin of impulses from electrically active cells, shown to have β-adrenoreceptors, in the mitral leaflets. However, many episodes of palpitation reflect awareness of forceful heart beating during sinus rhythm in thin individuals, and many episodes of atrial arrhythmia are asymptomatic. Awareness of palpitation in other prolapse subjects may coincide with simple ventricular premature complexes, but the prevalence of ventricular arrhythmias in controlled studies of MVP is not strikingly higher than that in normal subjects.

In our experience, many cases of atrial arrhythmia and some instances of ventricular premature contractions will respond to treatment with beta-blocking drugs (e.g., nadolol, beginning at a dose of 40 mg/day). However, periods of remission and exacerbation of symptoms may continue, as often occurs in the absence of treatment. Some patients with atrial arrhythmias respond favorably to verapamil (240 to 480 g/day of long-acting formulations). Episodes of supraventricular tachycardia in MVP patients are usually caused by re-entry in the atrioventricular node. If episodes are recurrent and disruptive to the patient, we offer electrophysiologic study and potentially corrective ablation of the extra electrical pathway, with a success rate of more than 90%. Because of their frequent side effects and occasional proarrhythmic activity, type I agents (such as flecainide and propafenone) or other agents with appreciable toxicity (e.g., sotalol and amiodarone) are used only when simpler regimens have failed in highly symptomatic subjects.

Whether to use antiarrhythmic drugs to prevent sudden death in patients with MVP and when to use them remain controversial. Sudden death is strongly concentrated in the minority of MVP patients with hemodynamically severe regurgitation; but even in this high-risk group, there is no evidence of benefit from antiarrhythmic drug treatment. Individuals with MVP with sustained ventricular tachycardia or resuscitation from near sudden death should be evaluated with electrophysiologic testing followed by use, when appropriate, of an implantable antitachycardia device. The rate of arrhythmic death among the larger population of subjects with otherwise uncomplicated MVP is too low for either potentially toxic antiarrhythmic agents or expensive antitachycardia devices to be cost-effective management strategies.

Treatment of Nonspecific Cardiovascular Symptoms

Management of patients with MVP and symptoms other than palpitations or dyspnea related to mitral regurgitation may require varied approaches. Chest pain, palpitations, and dyspnea may occur concurrently with severe anxiety and other symptoms, including tremor, dizziness, and diaphoresis, in repeated episodes termed panic attacks. If panic attacks occur spontaneously ("out of the blue") or in response to emotionally stressful situations such as elevators or crowded places, treatment with either pharmacologic or behavioral therapy for panic disorder guided by an experienced psychiatrist is often effective. Patients with these complaints do not generally respond well to cardiac medications such as beta blockers. Meticulous attention to details of clinical history is important because in some anxiety-prone individuals, the sudden onset of rapid palpitations due to paroxysmal atrial tachycardia or fibrillation may lead to other cardiovascular symptoms and secondary panic; this situation often responds well to appropriate medications (digoxin, beta blockers) and reassurance. Both panic disorder and repeated paroxysms of atrial arrhythmia may remit spontaneously or recur after a period of quiescence. Other chest pain syndromes with features suggestive of angina, esophageal disorders, or a musculoskeletal origin should not be attributed to MVP but rather should lead to appropriate further evaluation and specific treatment if it is clinically indicated.

Management of Autonomic Dysfunction

A variety of autonomic dysfunction syndromes may occur in patients diagnosed with or considered to have MVP. The most common of these in our experience consists of recurring episodes ranging from dizziness through presyncope, requiring the individual to sit or to lie down, to even frank syncope, which occurs most commonly with variably prolonged standing or with exercise on a hot day. These episodic symptoms may be associated with physical fatigue and a sense of being emotionally drained but occur in the absence of evidence of generalized autonomic failure or specific metabolic defects. In such patients, orthostatic hypotension (a fall in diastolic blood pressure of more than 10 mm Hg) or tachycardia (an increase in heart rate of more than 10 beats per minute) is usually provoked by 5 minutes of quiet standing.[19] Nausea, mild chest constriction, and bradycardia may precede actual syncope.

Detailed investigation commonly reveals a depressor response to head-up tilt testing and a deficit in blood volume; most such patients respond favorably to dietary salt supplementation or addition of sodium chloride tablets (1 g one to four times per day). Fludrocortisone acetate (0.05 to 0.1 mg/day) or clonidine hydrochloride (0.1 to 0.2 mg/day) may be added if necessary, with careful monitoring of blood pressure responses; individuals with features of neurocardiogenic syncope may benefit from treatment with atenolol, beginning at a dose of 25 mg/day. In some of our female MVP patients, orthostatic hypotension has remitted during the natural volume expansion of pregnancy.

A variety of other syndromes of autonomic dysfunction, characterized by evidence of sympathetic or parasympathetic overactivity, appear to occur with nearly equal frequency in individuals with and without MVP. Their evaluation commonly requires specialized testing.

PROGNOSIS

In general, MVP is a benign condition, and most patients will never have an important complication. However, a minority of affected persons develop severe mitral regurgitation, infective endocarditis, or sudden death. Because of the high population prevalence of MVP, an appreciable number of adults have these complications.

MVP has been found more commonly among patients with these complications than is expected for its prevalence of about 2% to 3% in unselected populations. Among patients with severe mitral regurgitation in industrialized countries, 38% to 64% have MVP as the underlying cause, whereas the proportion ranges from 11% to 29% among patients with infective endocarditis.[45] The data for neurologic ischemic episodes have been variable, and recent population-based data cast doubt on whether this is a true association.[46,47] Sudden death occurs with discernible frequency only among MVP patients with severe mitral regurgitation, although MVP has been found in a disproportionate number of the small minority of sudden death patients without obstructive coronary artery disease in some studies.[21] Prospective studies by our group indicated that complications of MVP occur at rates of about 1% annually in unselected individuals with this condition and about 3% per year in selected MVP patients referred to tertiary care hospitals.[37,48] A cross-sectional study of the Framingham offspring cohort found that prevalent mitral regurgitation, generally of mild degree, was associated with MVP, but other reported complications were not in a relatively healthy population free of referral bias.[3]

Identification of Patients with Mitral Valve Prolapse at Risk of Complications

By comparing characteristics of MVP patients with infective endocarditis and a control group of adults found to have MVP in our family studies, we were able to show that male gender, age older than 45 years, and history of a preexisting heart murmur were independently associated with infective endocarditis.[37] Compared with an average incidence of

1:20,000 per year in the general population, we estimated that infective endocarditis occurs annually in 1:1920 MVP patients with late or holosystolic mitral regurgitant murmurs versus 1:21,950 without a mitral systolic murmur. Similar calculations suggest annual incidences of infective endocarditis of 1:3540 among affected men and 1:2930 among individuals older than 45 years with MVP. The facts that major morbidity occurred in one third of our MVP patients with endocarditis during short-term follow-up (three deaths, four valve replacements) and that endocarditis appeared to be of dental origin in one third[49] suggest that infective endocarditis complicating MVP with moderate or severe mitral regurgitation is dangerous and may be partially preventable.

In long-term follow-up studies, we found the risk of complications of MVP, principally mitral valve repair or replacement but also including infective endocarditis, heart failure, and sudden death, to be increased by male gender, age older than 45 years, and especially a holosystolic murmur and left ventricular or left atrial dilatation. These findings result in overall complication rates that range from well below 0.5% annually in MVP subjects with a midsystolic click and normal heart size to about 7% per year among MVP patients (principally men) with clinical and echocardiographic evidence of moderate or severe mitral regurgitation.[37,48] Among all patients with MVP, the lifetime risk of needing mitral valve surgery is up to 5% among men and about 2% among women.[40,50,51] Initially mild regurgitation may become severe during prolonged follow-up.[52] In addition to irreversible risk factors of age and gender, high blood pressure may promote progressive regurgitation.

For sudden, presumably arrhythmic death, the annual risk may be as high as 1% among patients with severe regurgitation but less than 1:5000 in those with little or no mitral regurgitation.[53]

Infective endocarditis occurs in approximately one-quarter as many patients with MVP as develop severe regurgitation (Table 91-4), implying a cumulative risk of less than 1% by 75 years of age. The risk of endocarditis is increased about threefold in men compared with women, in persons older than 45 years compared with younger persons, and in MVP patients with a mitral regurgitant murmur.[30] In our studies,[54] mitral annular dilatation and leaflet elongation were more closely associated than leaflet thickening with the occurrence of infective endocarditis. About one third of endocarditis cases are of dental origin, similar to the experience with other predisposing valvular lesions; however, the importance of dental work in predisposing to infective endocarditis in MVP patients remains controversial.[55] During long-term follow-up, we have shown that a majority of patients with MVP who develop endocarditis require valve surgery or suffer cardiac death.[49]

Sudden death is the most feared, least understood, and perhaps rarest major complication of MVP. An increased risk of sudden death is well established in patients with severe mitral regurgitation, but this appears to relate to the degree of regurgitation rather than to MVP.[51] Instances of sudden death in patients without severe mitral regurgitation are often associated with prominent valvular deformity and increased heart weight, suggesting that unrecognized regurgitation or hypertension may have been present.[20,56] To date, neither specific arrhythmias nor electrocardiographic features such as repolarization abnormalities have been documented to identify patients with MVP who are at increased risk of sudden death.

ANNUAL OCCURRENCE IN THE USA OF COMPLICATIONS ASSOCIATED WITH MVP

Complication	Patients per Year (n)	Patients with Mitral Valve Prolapse (n)	Annual Events Attributable to Mitral Valve Prolapse (n)
Mitral valve surgery	16,000	25	4000
Infective endocarditis	9,000	13	1150
Sudden death	400,000	1	4000

Table 91.4 Annual occurrence in the USA of complications associated with MVP.

SUMMARY

Mitral valve prolapse occurs commonly, affecting 2% to 3% of adults, with family aggregation documenting predominantly autosomal dominant but also X-linked inheritance due to as yet undefined underlying gene defects. Enlargement, thickening, and in some instances heightened distensibility of the mitral valve's connective tissue elements (leaflets, chordae, and annulus) result in valvular-ventricular disproportion. This can be exploited at the bedside for the use of maneuvers that reduce left ventricular volume (e.g., sitting or standing) to make characteristic midsystolic clicks and late systolic murmurs move closer to the first heart sound. Echocardiographic demonstration of abnormal leaflet motion is the mainstay of objective diagnosis of MVP; auscultatory and Doppler echocardiographic assessment of the presence and degree of mitral regurgitation is the most effective means of stratifying risk of complications of MVP. Prevention of exacerbating moderate or severe mitral regurgitation by infective endocarditis, minimization of the stress imposed on regurgitant prolapsed valves, and surgical correction of severely regurgitant valves by mitral valve repair rather than by replacement when possible are the mainstays of therapy for MVP. With current management, complication rates range from about 0.5% per year in low-risk individuals without mitral regurgitation (a rate that may be more than offset by the benefits of low body weight and blood pressure) to nearly 7% per year in those with evidence at baseline of severe mitral regurgitation.

chapter 92

Special Problems in Mitral Valve Disease

a. Endoscopic Mitral Valve Repair

Filip P. Casselman, Oren Lev-Ran, Hugo Vanermen, and Frank Van Praet

DEFINITION OF PROBLEM

Asymptomatic patients with degenerative mitral valve regurgitation are usually treated conservatively. Because no cardiac surgical procedure has zero mortality, it is not evident to refer an asymptomatic patient to surgery. Furthermore, although it is desirable, mitral valve repair for degenerative mitral valve disease is not uniformly feasible. The database of the Society of Thoracic Surgeons indicates that currently in the United States, mitral valve repair for degenerative disease is performed in only 50% of operations.[1] The remainder of the patients undergo valve replacement and are exposed to the early and long-term complications of either a mechanical or bioprosthetic valve. Moreover, mitral valve repair is in most cases performed through a classic median sternotomy, resulting in a 20- to 30-cm midline scar.

Recent data have suggested an improved operative outcome in asymptomatic versus symptomatic patients with mitral valve regurgitation.[2] Experienced centers also report higher success rates in the repairability of degenerative mitral valve regurgitation.[3] Both of these findings have lowered the threshold to operate on asymptomatic or slightly symptomatic patients with degenerative mitral regurgitation. To overcome the invasiveness and postoperative aesthetic appearance of the standard procedure through median sternotomy, endoscopic mitral valve surgery has recently been introduced. Despite the fact that endoscopic mitral valve surgery has been available for more than 10 years[4] and robotic mitral valve surgery for more than 5 years,[5] both techniques have been practiced in only a limited number of centers, mainly because of the operator learning curve and the high additional cost. The feasibility, reproducibility, and durability of endoscopic mitral valve surgery in primary and reoperative procedures have now clearly been established.[6,7] Endoscopic mitral valve surgery also leads to an accelerated rehabilitation and high patient satisfaction.

TYPICAL CASE

A 69-year-old woman is known to have had mitral valve regurgitation for 5 years. The mitral regurgitation was graded 3/4, and the patient was asymptomatic. The mechanism of regurgitation was a combined leaflet prolapse; there was a slight prolapse of the A2 segment, a huge prolapse of P2, and a partial prolapse of P3 with uniform presence of excessive tissue (so-called Barlow's disease). Left atrial and ventricular dimensions as well as left ventricular function were normal. Given the asymptomatic status, the absence of repercussions on the heart, and the complexity of the pathologic process (which made a successful valve repair uncertain), the patient was treated conservatively. Six months ago, the patient experienced a brief period of palpitations, for which sotalol, 80 mg twice daily, was given. Afterward, the patient was still judged to be "asymptomatic," although there was decreased exercise tolerance on exercise testing (100 watts; 62% of predicted value), which was attributed to aging and sotalol therapy. Holter monitoring demonstrated a continuous sinus rhythm and echocardiography a grade 4/4 mitral valve regurgitation. The mechanism of the mitral valve regurgitation remained unchanged, with upper normal left atrial and ventricular dimensions and normal function.

TREATMENT OPTIONS

Despite worsening of the mitral valve regurgitation, the patient has remained asymptomatic, and cardiac repercussions of the mitral regurgitation are borderline. Furthermore, the patient's regurgitation pathophysiology remains complex, questioning the surgical repairability of the valve. A conservative approach could therefore be proposed while awaiting further cardiac deterioration or symptoms. Another approach is surgical intervention. Arguments in favor of surgical intervention include the improved outcome in asymptomatic patients versus symptomatic patients and the poor outcome of patients with reduced ventricular function or dilated cardiac chambers as a result of the volume load of mitral valve regurgitation.[2] The patient's condition can only worsen during conservative follow-up; the mitral valve cannot be cured without surgical intervention, and complications (e.g., ventricular function deterioration, cardiac chamber dilatation, or atrial fibrillation) may become irreversible.

Surgery becomes acceptable if the likelihood of valve repair is high. Although valve pathology is complex in this patient, an experienced valve repair team still has a high chance of performing an adequate valve reconstruction, thereby avoiding permanent postoperative anticoagulation. Another prerequisite to propose a surgical intervention is a low surgical mortality. Currently, the overall reported mortality for mitral valve repair procedures in the Society of Thoracic Surgeons database is 2%.[8] It is obvious that surgical mortality should not exceed this reported value in proposing surgery for asymptomatic patients. The surgical team should also aim to provide an appealing aesthetic result without compromising the valve repair.

SURGICAL PROCEDURE

The patient underwent a thoracoscopic mitral valve repair according to a previously described technique performed since February 1997 in more than 1000 procedures.[4,6] With use of a 6-cm right inframammary incision, the chest is entered (Fig. 92A.1). The whole procedure is performed with video assistance. The endocardiopulmonary bypass system is connected through the femoral vessels, and the heart is arrested by cardioplegia administered through an endoaortic balloon.

The preoperative pathology was confirmed at endoscopic operation; there was a prolapsing A2 segment (Fig. 92A.2) as well as prolapse of the P2 and P3 segments of the posterior leaflet (Fig. 92A.3). Accordingly, the patient first underwent a major quadrangular resection of P2 with sliding plasty of the P1 and P3 segments to fill the gap and to lower the height of the posterior mitral valve leaflet. This was done to avoid systolic anterior motion of the anterior valve leaflet after the repair. The prolapsing segment of A2 was corrected with two neochordae (Gore-Tex, W. L. Gore, Phoenix, Ariz), and the repair was stabilized with a mitral valve Carpentier-Edwards Physio 34 (Edwards Lifesciences, Irvine, Calif) annuloplasty ring (Fig. 92A.4 shows the final result). There was no residual mitral valve regurgitation postoperatively, and the patient made an uneventful recovery. The postoperative aesthetic result at 6 weeks is shown in Figure 92A.5.

By this technique, successful mitral valve repair for degenerative mitral valve disease was achieved in 83.5% of cases with an overall mortality of 1.8%. The endoscopic technique allows any type of mitral and tricuspid valve repair. This therapeutic strategy is also appreciated by the patient as evident from a high patient satisfaction rate: 93.5% of the patients report no or only mild postoperative pain; 98.4% of the patients are pleased with the cosmetic result; and 60% of the patients have resumed work or other daily activities within 8 weeks.[6]

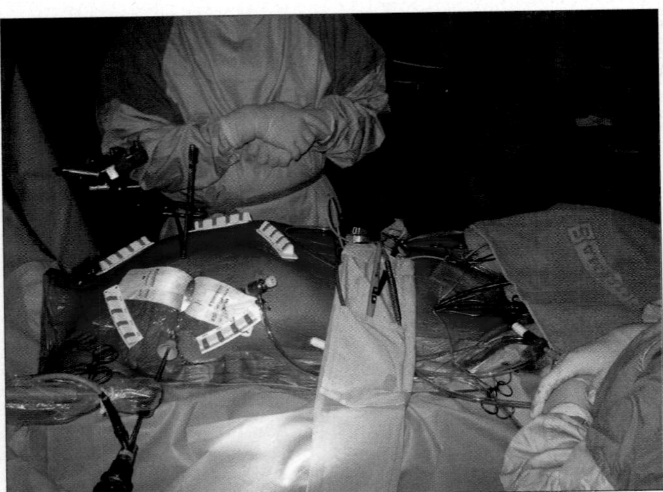

Figure 92A.1 Operative setup for an endoscopic procedure. The heart-lung machine is connected through the femoral vessels. The approach is performed by a small inframammary incision. A camera is introduced *(left lower corner)*, which enables the surgeon to follow the intrathoracic manipulations on a screen (video assistance).

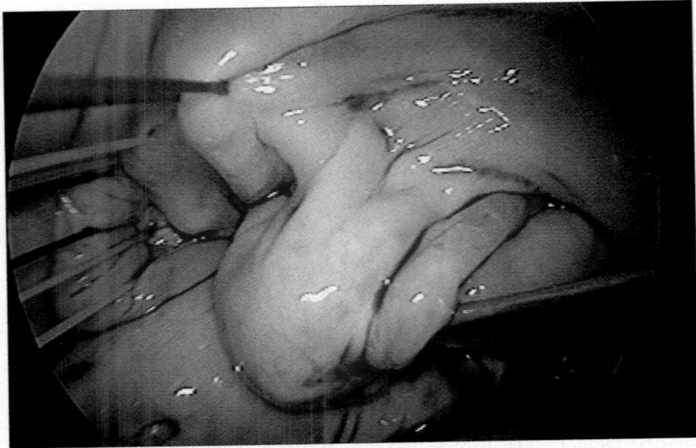

Figure 92A.2 Perioperative endoscopic view demonstrating prolapse of the middle segment of the anterior mitral valve leaflet (segment A2).

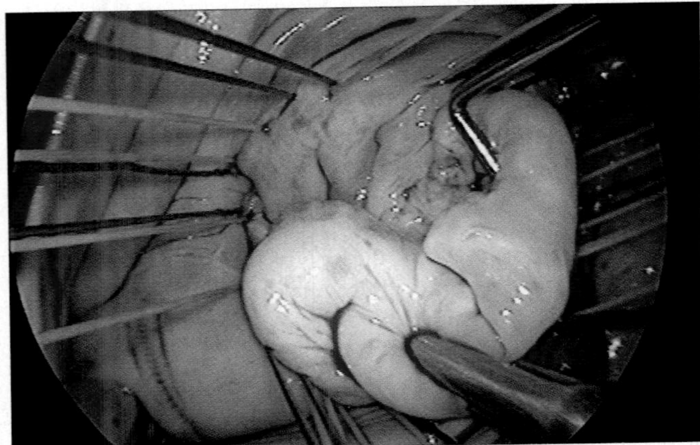

Figure 92A.3 Perioperative endoscopic view demonstrating prolapse of the middle and posteromedial segments of the posterior mitral valve leaflet (segments P2 and P3).

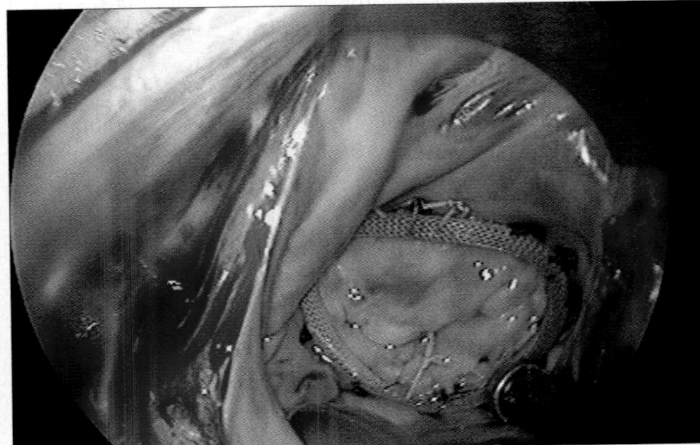

Figure 92A.4 Final result after fluid injection in the left ventricle to pressurize and to test the mitral valve competence (note the neochordae on A2 and the ring annuloplasty).

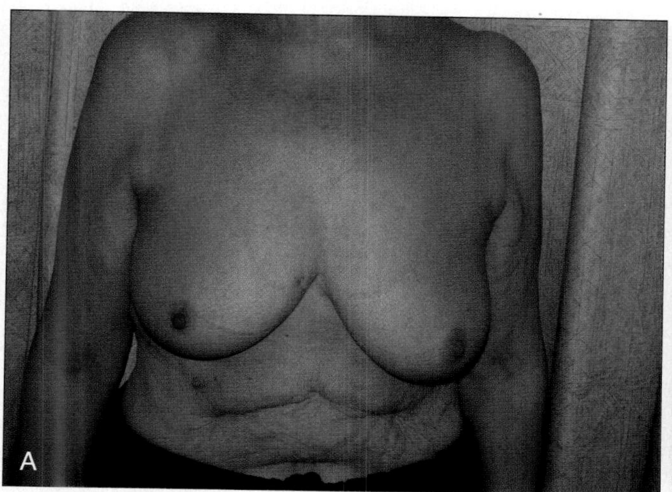

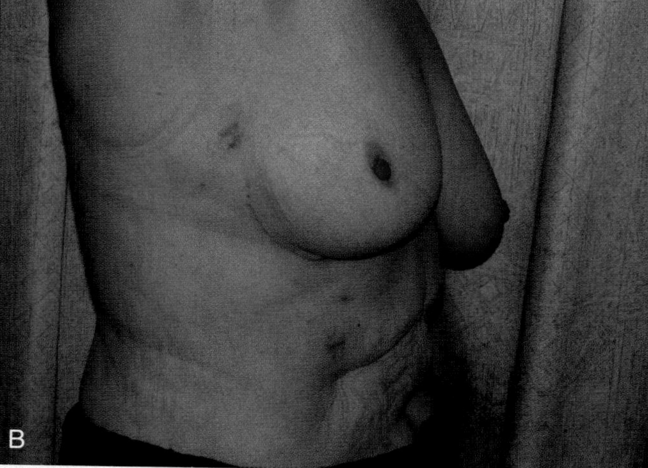

Figure 92A.5 Postoperative aesthetic result. A, Frontal view. **B,** Lateral view.

SUMMARY

Outcome of mitral valve repair in asymptomatic patients is superior to that in symptomatic patients. This finding, associated with a vast experience in endoscopic mitral valve repair, resulting in a high percentage of success (83.5%) and a low operative mortality (1.8%), has allowed earlier intervention in mitral valve regurgitation whereby an endoscopic mitral valve repair procedure is performed in asymptomatic patients, as soon as a grade 3/4 mitral valve regurgitation is observed.

b. Antiarrhythmic Surgery for Atrial Fibrillation

Filip P. Casselman, Frank Van Praet, Hugo Vanermen, and Peter Geelen

DEFINITION OF PROBLEM

Patients with organic mitral valve disease frequently develop atrial fibrillation as part of the pathologic process. In these patients, the mitral valve disease develops first and atrial fibrillation develops later as a secondary phenomenon.[1] When surgery is indicated, the primary goal is to correct the mitral valve disease with addition of an antiarrhythmic procedure to prevent persistence or recurrence of atrial fibrillation.[2-4]

In another group of patients, atrial fibrillation develops first. Initially paroxysmal, atrial fibrillation later becomes persistent or permanent. The fibrillating atria as well as the mitral valve annulus dilate, and mitral valve regurgitation occurs. This mitral valve regurgitation is initially mild and centrally located. As the mitral annular dilatation progresses, it becomes difficult to determine which came first, atrial fibrillation or mitral valve regurgitation. If surgery becomes indicated for either symptomatic, therapy-resistant atrial fibrillation or mitral valve regurgitation, the goal of the intervention will be twofold: abolishment of atrial fibrillation and restoration of a competent mitral valve.

TYPICAL CASE

A 50-year-old man has a 5-year history of atrial fibrillation. Initially, he experienced short but symptomatic episodes of paroxysmal atrial fibrillation. An echocardiographic evaluation at that time revealed grade 2 central mitral valve regurgitation with normal cardiac dimensions. The patient was treated conservatively with antiarrhythmic therapy, which decreased the incidence of atrial fibrillation paroxysms. During the following years, the patient progressed from paroxysmal to persistent and finally to permanent atrial fibrillation, which was poorly tolerated. His blood pressure remained borderline (100/60 mm Hg), and exercise tolerance was limited. A new echocardiographic evaluation confirmed a grade 2 mitral valve regurgitation and a dilated left atrium (52 mm). The left ventricular function remained normal. Despite adequate oral anticoagulation, the patient experienced a transient ischemic attack with detection of clot in the left atrial appendage on transesophageal echocardiography.

The patient underwent an endoscopic left atrial cryo-maze procedure with endoraphie of the left atrial appendage and mitral valve annuloplasty. During this minimally invasive procedure (Fig. 92B.1), a pulmonary vein box lesion is created with cryotherapy (Fig. 92B.2). In addition, the left isthmus is ablated and the left atrial appendage obliterated (Fig. 92B.3). Finally, a mitral valve annuloplasty is performed with a Carpentier-Edwards Physio 32 (Edwards Lifesciences, Irvine, Calif) annuloplasty ring (Fig. 92B.4).

The postoperative course was uneventful apart from one short episode of atrial fibrillation on the fourth postoperative day. The patient received antiarrhythmic and anticoagulant treatment for 6 months postoperatively. This therapy was subsequently discontinued, and the patient has remained free of atrial fibrillation recurrence for 2 years. At follow-up, an echocardiographic examination revealed absence of mitral valve regurgitation.

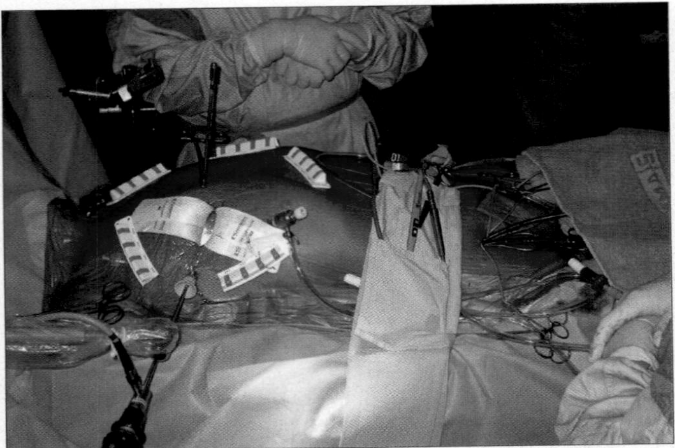

Figure 92B.1 The endoscopic procedure is performed as in endoscopic mitral valve surgery. A 2-inch submammary incision is used to introduce the cryocatheter and the mitral valve annuloplasty ring. The heart-lung machine is connected through the femoral vessels. A camera is introduced *(left lower corner)*, which enables the surgeon to follow the intrathoracic manipulations on a screen (video assistance).

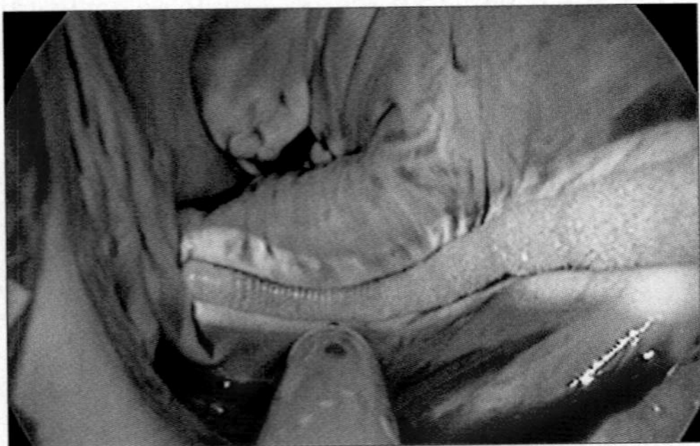

Figure 92B.2 The lower ablation line is drawn, connecting right and left inferior pulmonary veins. Note the large ablation zone.

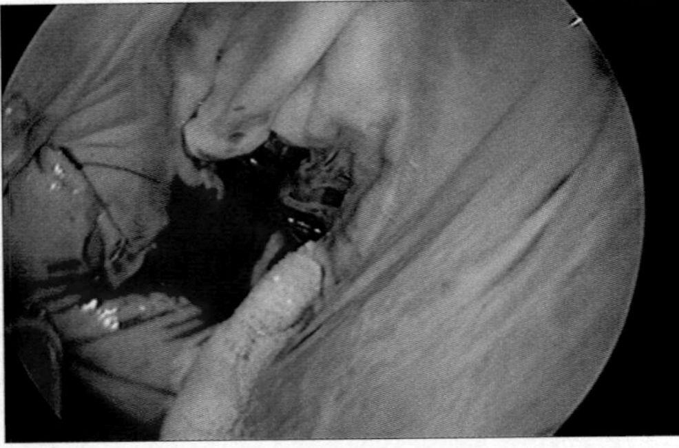

Figure 92B.3 Ablation of the left isthmus, connecting the box lesion to the mitral valve annulus. Note also the obliterated (closed) left atrial appendage (see surgical suture in left upper corner).

DIFFERENTIAL DIAGNOSIS

It is frequently unclear whether the patient first had atrial fibrillation and developed secondary mitral valve regurgitation or if the mitral valve regurgitation was the initial insult. To distinguish between both conditions, stress echocardiography can be helpful. Some patients develop a marked increase in severity of mitral regurgitation during exertion as initially described in ischemic heart disease.[5] If stress echocardiography yields an abnormal result, the mitral valve regurgitation at rest underestimates the severity of the mitral valve disease. The atrial fibrillation then complicates severe mitral valve regurgitation, which prompts earlier surgery.

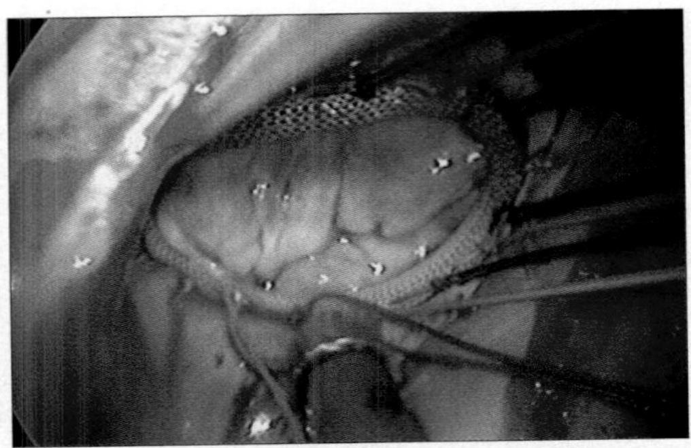

Figure 92B.4 A mitral annuloplasty ring completes the procedure.

TREATMENT OPTIONS

Two choices of intervention are available: transvascular atrial fibrillation ablation and left atrial appendage exclusion; and surgical intervention dealing with the rhythm disturbance, the left atrial appendage, and the mitral valve regurgitation.

Despite the fact that successful catheter ablation of permanent atrial fibrillation has been reported, the success ratio is lower than in paroxysmal atrial fibrillation, and multiple sessions are often required.[6] Furthermore, catheter-based left atrial appendage exclusion[7] is still in a preliminary phase. Therefore, a surgical procedure was preferred in the described patient. The procedure was performed thoracoscopically and consisted of three components: left atrial cryo-maze procedure, left atrial appendage obliteration, and mitral valve annuloplasty (see Figs. 92B.2 to 92B.4).

If the patient had presented with paroxysmal atrial fibrillation without left atrial appendage clot, a transvascular catheter-based procedure would have been preferable. Catheter ablation for paroxysmal atrial fibrillation provides a 1-year freedom from atrial fibrillation of 77%.[8] With use of a surgical strategy, 3-month freedom from atrial fibrillation is 86%.[9] In patients with mitral valve disease, two studies[3,4] have demonstrated less sinus rhythm restoration in patients undergoing only mitral valve surgery than in patients undergoing additional antiarrhythmic surgery. Both procedures are therefore usually combined. In addition, the left atrial appendage needs to be ligated in all cases with a history of neurologic events or demonstrated clot.

SUMMARY

In mitral valve disease, persistence of atrial fibrillation increases postoperative morbidity and mortality and negatively influences long-term outcome. Patients undergoing mitral valve surgery with a history of atrial fibrillation should therefore undergo an additional antiarrhythmic procedure to restore sinus rhythm and to improve postoperative outcome. Additional antiarrhythmic procedures can be performed with minimally invasive techniques. They do not add much operative time and provide a high success rate even in patients undergoing surgical ablation of permanent atrial fibrillation.

c. Percutaneous Mitral Valve Repair

David McCarty and Judy Hung

DEFINITION OF PROBLEM

Mitral regurgitation (MR) is a common valvular disorder and can be broadly classified as primary or secondary. Primary, or organic, MR results from valvular disease, such as mitral valve prolapse, rheumatic mitral disease, or endocarditis. Primary MR can progress to left ventricular failure in many patients if it is not surgically corrected. Definitive correction of the valvular structural abnormalities at present offers the only potential for improved survival and morbidity.[1] Current guidelines recommend mitral valve repair for chronic primary MR if the condition is severe and associated with symptoms or in asymptomatic patients if evidence of left ventricular dysfunction exists (left ventricular ejection fraction, 0.30 to 0.60; left ventricular end-systolic diameter >40 mm). Valve repair is preferred to replacement, and approximately 100,000 mitral valve procedures are performed worldwide per year.[1,2]

Secondary MR results from tethering of the mitral leaflets and hence restricted leaflet closure due to ventricular dilatation from ischemic heart disease or cardiomyopathy. Secondary MR is also referred to as functional or ischemic MR. The presence of MR secondary to global left ventricular dilatation or chronic ischemic disease confers a poor prognosis.[3,4] The therapy for ischemic MR remains unclear as there has been no survival benefit shown with ring annuloplasty for ischemic MR, and it should be performed on an individual basis.

The surgical approach to disease of the mitral valve has developed during several decades. It is now recognized that valve-sparing repair procedures in general have superior outcomes to valve replacement for the majority of patients. Techniques for surgical mitral valve repair are numerous and continue to be refined. Most operators combine insertion of an annuloplasty ring to correct annular dilatation with a leaflet repair procedure.

Many patients, however, are unsuitable for cardiac surgery, most often because of multiple medical comorbidities. Risks of a surgical approach include operative morbidity, complications of postoperative recovery, anticoagulation, prosthetic failure, and endocarditis.[5] Individuals who have cardiac decompensation are also at increased risk for surgical intervention. This can create a paradox if the reason for heart failure is due to decompensated MR but the patient is too sick to undergo repair of the mitral valve. Percutaneous treatments for MR are emerging and show promise for patients who are at high risk for surgery.

TYPICAL CASE

An 81-year-old man presented with increasing fatigue and shortness of breath on exertion during several months. There was an associated cough. He described paroxysmal nocturnal dyspnea and had noticed ankle swelling in the evenings.

Past medical history included treated systemic hypertension for many years, chronic liver disease, and metastatic prostatic carcinoma that was stable with hormone therapy.

On examination, his pulse was 72 beats per minute and regular. Blood pressure was 136/84 mm Hg. Peripheral pulses were symmetric. Jugular venous distention was noted, with the pulse visible at the root of the neck. The apical impulse was displaced laterally and located in the sixth intercostal space, anterior axillary line. Cardiac auscultation revealed a soft mitral component of the first heart sound, followed by a loud (grade 3/6) holosystolic murmur over the cardiac apex, radiating to the axilla. A third heart sound was also noted. There were fine bibasal end-inspiratory crackles audible at the lung bases. Ankle edema was noted.

Investigations revealed an enlarged cardiac silhouette on chest radiography with pulmonary vascular congestion. A 12-lead electrocardiogram showed sinus rhythm, with left ventricular hypertrophy and a lateral strain pattern. Transthoracic echocardiography was performed. The left atrium was enlarged. The left ventricle measured 61 mm at end-diastole, and the ejection fraction measured by the biplane method of disks was 45%. The mitral valve was noted to be myxomatously degenerated with thickening of the leaflets and chordae tendineae. During systole, both mitral leaflets prolapsed above the plane of the mitral annulus. Color Doppler examination across the valve revealed a large, centrally directed jet of MR filling 50% of the left atrium. The vena contracta measured 7 mm in the parasternal long-axis view. A large area of proximal flow convergence was present. On continuous-wave Doppler study, a dense jet was seen. Pulsed Doppler study of the pulmonary veins showed reversal of systolic flow consistent with severe MR. Quantitative analysis of mitral regurgitant flow revealed an effective regurgitant orifice area of 0.8 mm^2, with an estimated regurgitant fraction of 50%. The right ventricle was mildly dilated with preserved global function. The transtricuspid gradient was 65 mm Hg.

Cardiac catheterization confirmed severe MR with complete opacification of the left atrium within three cardiac cycles after injection of angiographic contrast material into the left ventricle. The mitral leaflets were noted to billow into the left atrium during systole. The mean pulmonary capillary wedge pressure was 15 mm Hg, with a v wave of 33 mm Hg. The cardiac output was estimated by the Fick calculation as 3.5 L/min. Right ventricular systolic pressure was 80 mm Hg. There was no major obstructive coronary artery disease.

The patient was presented to the cardiac surgical team for consideration of mitral valve repair or replacement. He was deemed to be at prohibitively high risk for cardiopulmonary bypass, given his preexisting comorbidities. After further consultation with the patient and his family, a decision was made to proceed with a percutaneous technique to repair the mitral valve.

PERCUTANEOUS OPTIONS

The two main approaches to percutaneous mitral valve repair are based on modifications of surgical mitral repair techniques: edge-to-edge technique and percutaneous mitral annuloplasty.

Edge-to-Edge Repair

The technique currently at the most advanced stage of development is the double orifice technique produced by snaring, approximating, and subsequently clipping together the middle scallops of the posterior and anterior mitral leaflets. This procedure seeks to emulate the edge-to-edge surgical approach initially described by Ottavio Alfieri.[6]

Preclinical Evaluation

Proof of concept, feasibility of percutaneous device deployment, and device safety were demonstrated in preclinical testing. St. Goar and coworkers[7] deployed a mitral clip percutaneously in 14 animals without MR in a porcine model. Examination confirmed successful device delivery with creation of a mitral double orifice. Fann and colleagues,[8] in a similar porcine model (n = 21), evaluated acute and long-term outcomes after device placement (up to 1 year). No acute deterioration in cardiovascular hemodynamics was observed after deployment. Sequential histopathologic surveillance confirmed that the device was incorporated into the surrounding valvular tissue, with complete endothelialization noted on scanning electron microscopy. Persistence of a mitral double orifice without the interim development of mitral stenosis was demonstrated. Two animals developed endocarditis during follow-up. A suture-based percutaneous device for edge-to-edge approximation is also undergoing evaluation in preclinical trials.[9]

Clinical Experience

The device was investigated in patients with MR in the Food and Drug Administration–approved phase I clinical trial EVEREST (Endovascular Valve Edge-to-Edge Repair Study).[2,10] This trial established criteria for selection of patients for percutaneous repair with the Evalve MitraClip system (Evalve Inc., Menlo Park, Calif) and a technical protocol for device delivery under transesophageal echocardiographic and fluoroscopic guidance. The MitraClip is a 4-mm-wide polyester-covered mechanical device with two clip arms that may be opened and closed by control mechanisms on the clip delivery system (Fig. 92C.1). The integral clip delivery system has coaxial steering control at the operator end and is inserted over a guide wire to the left atrium through a transseptal approach. Percutaneous introduction of the clip to the left atrium is followed by careful positioning across the mitral valve under transesophageal echocardiographic guidance. When optimal alignment perpendicular to the coaptation line is achieved, the operator first grasps the mitral leaflets to evaluate leaflet immobilization and reduction of regurgitation before subsequently capturing both leaflets within the arms of the clip and releasing the device.

Initial 6-month outcomes for 27 patients were reported by Feldman and coworkers.[10] The majority of patients had degenerative valve disease with posterior or bileaflet prolapse (93%). A significant proportion had indicators of advanced disease with documented congestive heart failure (59%), New York Heart Association class III or class IV (44%), and atrial fibrillation (41%). Patients were candidates for cardiac surgery if it was required. Among the exclusion criteria were quantitative evidence of severe left ventricular impairment (ejection fraction <0.30) and dilatation (left ventricular end-systolic diameter >55 mm). Successful clip implantation was achieved in 24 patients (Fig. 92C.2). Reduction in MR to 2+ MR or less by 1 month was achieved in 14 patients. Six of these patients subsequently required elective mitral valve surgery, three for partial clip detachment and three for persisting severe MR. One patient experienced a nonembolic cerebrovascular accident. Thirteen patients with satisfactory reduction in MR at 1 month continued to have 2+ MR or less at 6-month follow-up. The investigators concluded that the device was safe, and satisfactory reduction of MR was achieved in many patients.

Silvestry and associates[2] reported outcomes on the complete study cohort of 47 patients, incorporating further description of device delivery protocol and transesophageal

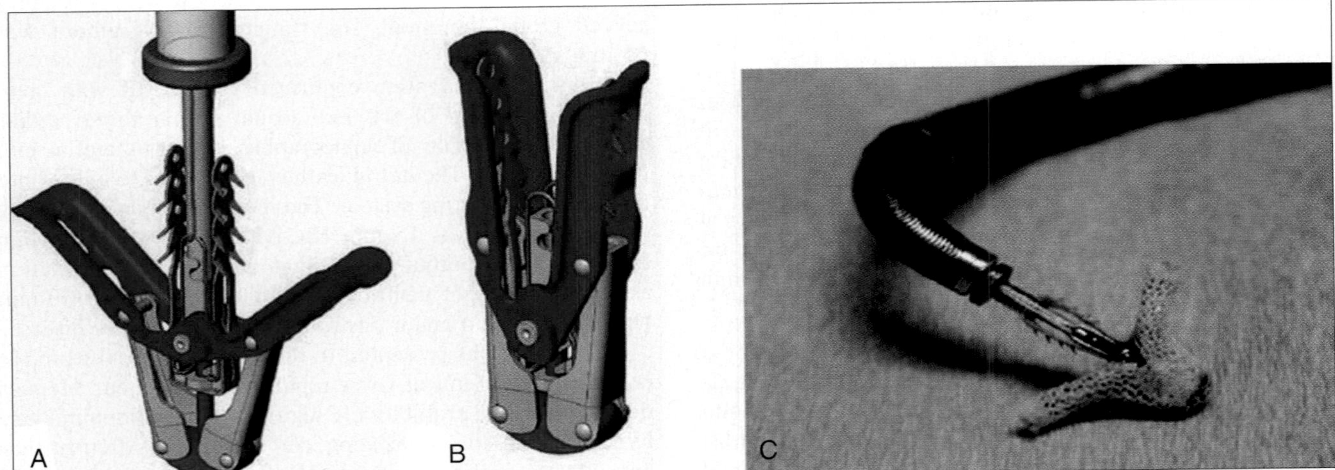

Figure 92C.1 A schematic of the Evalve MitraClip with the clip arms in the open **(A)** and closed **(B)** positions. The clip attached to the delivery system is shown in **C**. (From Feldman T, Wasserman HS, Herrmann HC, et al. Percutaneous mitral valve repair using the edge-to-edge technique: six-month results of the EVEREST Phase I Clinical Trial. J Am Coll Cardiol 2005;46:2134-2140.)

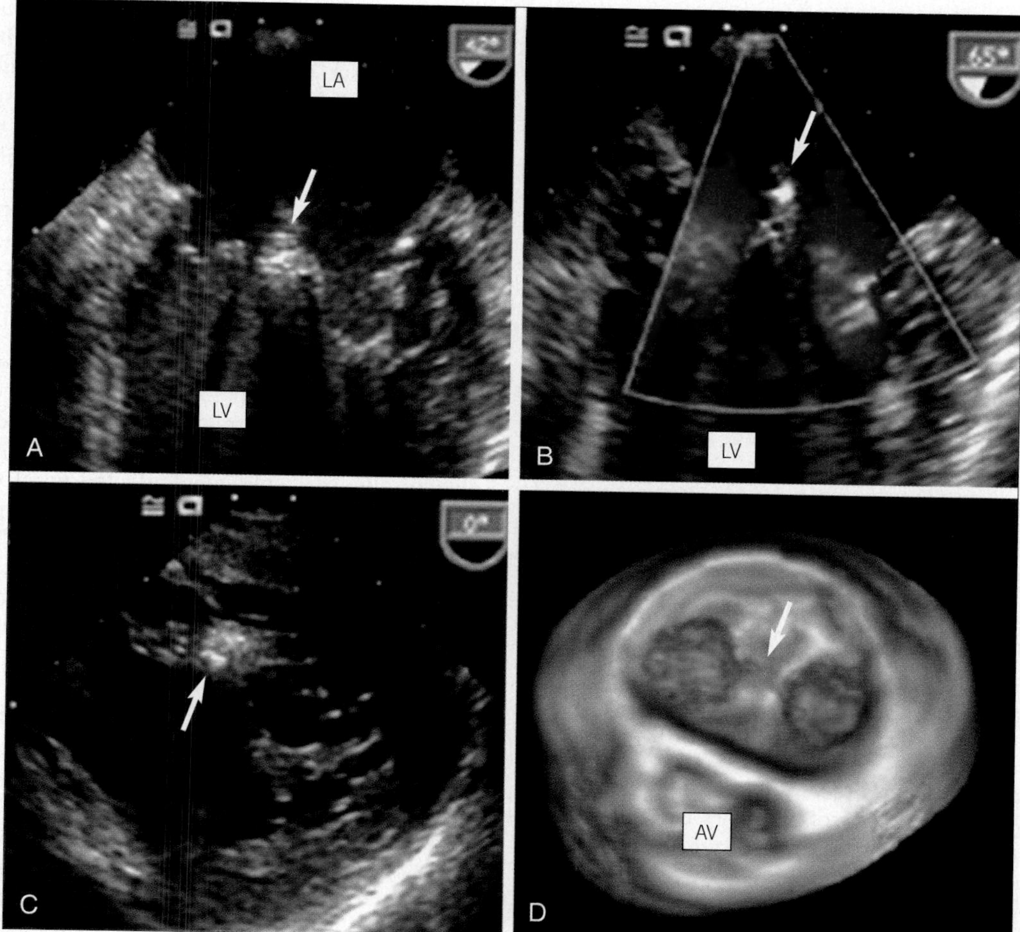

Figure 92C.2 The deployed MitraClip *(arrows)* is shown from a commissural transesophageal view **(A)** and a gastric short-axis view **(C)**. The double orifices are apparent on imaging by color Doppler two-dimensional echocardiography **(B)** and real-time three-dimensional transesophageal echocardiography **(D)**. AV, aortic valve; LA, left atrium; LV, left ventricle. (From Silvestry FE, Rodriguez LL, Herrmann HC, et al. Echocardiographic guidance and assessment of percutaneous repair for mitral regurgitation with the Evalve MitraClip: lessons learned from EVEREST 1. J Am Soc Echocardiogr 2007;20:1131-1140.)

echocardiographic guidance. In total, 87% had degenerative disease, with 13% functional MR. Forty-two patients received at least one clip, with five patients who had insufficient reduction of MR proceeding to uneventful valvular surgery. Two patients receiving clips required surgery before discharge (one partial detachment, one catheter malfunction). Thirty-four patients had acute procedural success with successful clip placement and MR of 2+ or less at discharge. The authors commented on the value of a standardized transesophageal echocardiography–guided device deployment protocol in decreasing exposure time, achieving uniformity of delivery technique, and achieving technical success. Collaboration between imaging, interventional, and surgical operators was encouraged.

Whereas the EVEREST study primarily included patients with degenerative MR, the investigators proposed that this technique could also be used in patients with other causes of regurgitation, such as ischemic disease. Comparison of outcomes after percutaneous versus surgical repair is currently being evaluated in the EVEREST II study.

Limitations of Edge-to-Edge Devices

Concerns surrounding this procedure include its widespread applicability to patients with MR of varying causes. The value of simple edge-to-edge approximation is debated in the surgical literature as this will not address other structural abnormalities often present in MR, such as papillary muscle displacement and annular dilatation.[11] Incomplete correction of MR is also a concern; the endpoint of mild (≤2+) MR is seen as too lax by some commentators. Initial concern about the subsequent development of mitral stenosis has not been substantiated, with reports excluding this after both surgical and percutaneous edge-to-edge repair.[2,7]

Percutaneous Mitral Annuloplasty

An alternative percutaneous approach under development seeks to achieve reduction in mitral annular dimensions by the percutaneous insertion of an annuloplasty device into the coronary sinus (Fig. 92C.3). This venous confluence in most individuals closely approximates the mitral annulus, lying within the left atrioventricular groove. In addition,

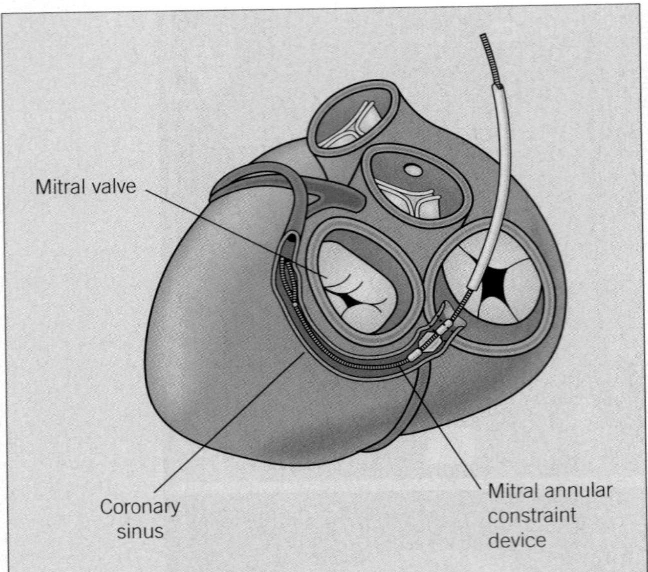

Figure 92C.3 A schematic illustrating the relationship of the coronary sinus to the mitral valve. An annuloplasty device is shown in the coronary sinus. (From Kaye DM, Byrne M, Alferness C, Power J. Feasibility and short-term efficacy of percutaneous mitral annular reduction for the therapy of heart failure–induced mitral regurgitation. Circulation 2003;108:1795-1797.)

percutaneous coronary sinus access is increasingly performed by cardiologists during ablation of accessory cardiac conduction pathways and for biventricular pacing.

Preclinical Evaluation

Kaye and associates[4] initially described delivery of a mitral annular constraint device in nine sheep with MR as a consequence of cardiomyopathy induced by rapid atrial pacing. The device consisted of a nitinol wire with proximal and distal anchor points and an intervening cable. Once it is positioned, tension may be gradually applied to the cable, effecting annular constraint. The incremental effect of annular modification on MR may be observed by echocardiographic or fluoroscopic imaging before the device is finally locked and released. After device delivery, the investigators confirmed reduced MR and pulmonary capillary wedge pressure, concluding that this occurred secondary to the observed decrease in the septal-lateral dimension of the mitral annulus. Hemodynamic monitoring demonstrated acute benefit with increased cardiac output. No coronary sinus injury was observed. In a separate experiment, the same group of investigators demonstrated continued reduction of MR with associated improvement in hemodynamic and neurohumoral status during 30 days of follow-up after device placement.[12]

Maniu and coworkers[13] described delivery of a similar annuloplasty device in a canine model. Eighteen animals with MR secondary to pacing-induced cardiomyopathy received devices. Coronary sinus venography was used before deployment to gauge anatomy and to size the device and after insertion to exclude coronary sinus dissection or disruption. After delivery of the device to the coronary sinus, tension was applied with direct visualization of MR reduction and to exclude compression of the neighboring left circumflex artery, coursing beside the sinus in the atrioventricular groove. Imaging can precisely define the optimal site for anchor placement, anchor size, device length, and degree of tension required. Deployment resulted in a decrease in mitral annular diameter and MR, determined by jet area. No significant changes in left ventricular pressures and systolic or diastolic function were observed. Initial reduction in the degree of MR was maintained to 4 weeks of follow-up. Compromise of the left circumflex was noted in two animals.

In addition to efficacy for reduction of MR in the dilated cardiomyopathy models described, percutaneous annuloplasty has also been shown to be effective in models of acute and chronic myocardial ischemia.

Liddicoat and colleagues[14] deployed a nitinol–stainless steel annuloplasty device coated in Teflon and polyethylene plastic (Viacor, Wilmington, Mass) in six sheep with MR secondary to acute posterolateral ischemia. Reduction or elimination of the resultant severe MR was initially observed after device delivery. Deployment effected a profound reduction in septal to lateral annular diameter, with improved mitral leaflet coaptation noted on epicardial echocardiography. Acute ischemia resulted in reduction in ejection fraction and increase in left ventricular volumes, which were partially reversed after device insertion. No harmful effects on systemic blood pressure were observed. After device retrieval, severe MR returned.

Daimon and coworkers,[15] using an ovine model of chronic ischemic MR, demonstrated decreased MR after percutaneous annuloplasty. The decrease resulted from an observed reduction in mitral annular anteroposterior diameter and leaflet tenting area measured by real-time three-dimensional echocardiography. No deleterious change in hemodynamics was noted acutely. No circumflex injury was observed (although it is unclear if ischemic models generated by prior ligation of the main circumflex artery or its branches permit meaningful assessment of this endpoint).

Clinical Experience

Three coronary sinus annuloplasty devices have been implanted in patients, with early reports of outcomes recently published.

The Viking device (Edwards Lifesciences Inc., Irvine, Calif) comprises proximal and distal stent anchors with an intervening nitinol bridge (Fig. 92C.4).[16] The distal anchor is placed in the great cardiac vein and the proximal anchor in the proximal coronary sinus. Application of tension to the bridge

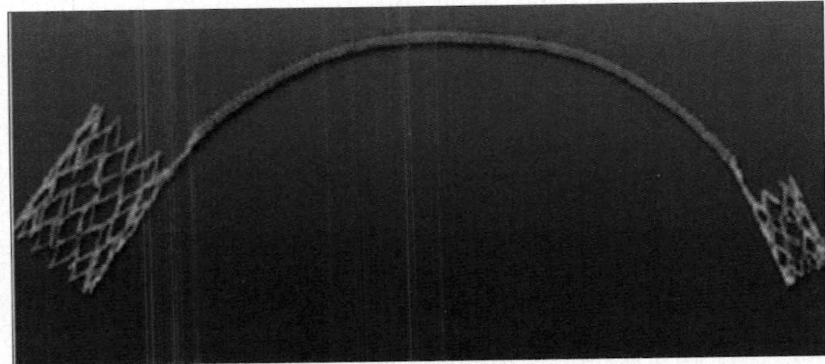

Figure 92C.4 The Edwards Viking coronary sinus annuloplasty device is shown with the smaller distal and larger proximal stent anchors. (From Webb JG, Harnek J, Munt BI, et al. Percutaneous transvenous mitral annuloplasty. Initial human experience with device implantation in the coronary sinus. Circulation 2006;113:851-855.)

segment results in constraint of the mitral annulus, the effect of which may be observed before final release of the system. The device was evaluated in five patients with chronic ischemic MR. Deployment was successful in four patients.[17] MR was reduced acutely in three patients. During follow-up, however, fracture of the connecting bridge from the anchors was noted in three patients. After device separation, the grade of MR increased.

The manufacturers subsequently modified the design of the device, reinforcing the bridge segment to produce the second-generation MONARC system. This device is currently undergoing evaluation in the EVOLUTION phase I clinical trial, recruiting patients with functional MR secondary to dilated cardiomyopathy or chronic ischemia. Preliminary results are available.[16] Of 55 enrolled patients, 49 underwent successful device delivery, with reduction of MR by one grade or more in 48.5% at day 30 of follow-up. There was continued remodeling after placement, and 92.3% of patients demonstrated this degree of reduction of MR by day 180. Three of nine patients experiencing major adverse cardiac events at day 30 were deemed to have device-related complications (two procedure-related cardiac tamponade after possible guide wire perforation of the coronary sinus, one myocardial infarction secondary to compression of a coronary artery). No bridge separations were reported. A subsequent larger multicenter registry, the EVOLUTION II trial, is planned.

The Viacor percutaneous mitral annuloplasty device (PTMA) consists of a multilumen retrievable catheter placed through the coronary sinus in the anterior interventricular cardiac vein.[16] Insertion of up to three rods of varying length and stiffness into the lumen effects conformational changes in the mitral annulus. This device is similar to that used by Daimon and Liddicoat in the preclinical experiments described before. Temporary placement of the device was evaluated by Dubreuil and coworkers[18] in four patients with ischemic MR. Transesophageal echocardiographic guidance was used to ensure optimal configuration of the device and reduction of MR. Placement was successful in three patients, in whom reduced mitral annular dimensions, improved leaflet coaptation, and decreased MR were then observed. No acute complications occurred in this small study. Whereas this technique offers flexibility in customizing the device to individual anatomy, a potential limitation is the number and combination of rod insertions to be evaluated to determine this. Human trials of a permanent device are currently under way.

The third coronary sinus annuloplasty device currently available is the CARILLON Mitral Contour System (Cardiac Dimensions, Kirkland, Wash). Of nitinol construction, this device was evaluated by Kaye, Byrne, and Maniu in the preclinical work described before. Proximal and distal mirror-image double-helix anchors are connected by an intervening nitinol bridge. Initial use in patients with functional MR and heart failure was reported by Duffy and coworkers.[19] Temporary placement of the device was undertaken in patients during a clinically indicated coronary angiography and left ventricular catheterization procedure. As the study was intended to evaluate the effects of only temporary annular plication, devices without a proximal anchor were placed and retrieved after observation of MR. The device could be anchored in four of five patients. Septal-lateral mitral annular diameter was reduced significantly by the system, with a trend to reduction in MR. The small sample size and slippage of two of the devices due to undersizing may have led to statistical significance not being achieved. No patients experienced complications or obstruction to coronary blood flow during device placement.

The AMADEUS trial is currently evaluating this device in European patients with heart failure and functional MR. Preliminary results are available.[16] Implantation has been successful in 70% of patients, of whom 80% have had documented reduction of MR. Two patients required device recapture after documentation of coronary artery compression that followed initial placement. A similar study (COMPETENT) is recruiting patients in the United States.

Limitations of Coronary Sinus Annuloplasty Devices

Concerns with this procedure include the variable anatomic relationship of the coronary sinus to both the mitral annulus and the circumflex artery.[20] Some have expressed concern that the procedure lacks essential elements inherent in surgical annuloplasty and is merely a "commissure-to-commissure" annuloplasty.[21] In addition, annuloplasty alone has been shown to be insufficient by itself to correct MR for some patients without concurrent leaflet repair. Reduction of the annulus in patients without severe dilatation of this structure may in fact interfere with leaflet coaptation and indeed worsen MR.

Other Techniques

Percutaneous septal sinus shortening has been proposed as a technique to reduce the septal-lateral diameter of the mitral annulus.[22] The system consists of a bridge element positioned between two anchors, placed in the interatrial septum and the great cardiac veins. Increasing tension in the bridge element effects a reduction in annular dimensions. Preclinical study in an ovine model of pacing-induced cardiomyopathy demonstrated proof of concept and technical feasibility. The device was efficacious in reducing the septal-lateral annular diameter and thereby functional MR. Longer term follow-up was associated with increased cardiac output, decreased pulmonary capillary wedge pressure, and improvement in biochemical indices of cardiac function. An early report of clinical use confirmed reduction in annular dimensions and MR before scheduled explantation of the device during elective cardiac surgery.[23]

Another technique under development is the application of radiofrequency energy to the mitral annulus to cause tissue heating, scarring, and annulus fibrosis. Initial preclinical work in an ovine model without generation of MR conducted by Heuser and associates[24] confirmed feasibility of this technique. Radiofrequency energy application to the mitral annulus delivered from a malleable probe positioned in the coronary sinus resulted in modification of MR by reduction of annular dimensions. The initial results persisted through 30 days of follow-up.

SUMMARY

Mitral regurgitation confers an adverse prognosis in many forms of cardiac disease. Many patients, however, are not candidates for surgical correction. The recent development of percutaneous valvular repair techniques offers potentially attractive alternative treatment options for these patients.

d. Radiation-Associated Valvular Heart Disease

Theo E. Meyer

DEFINITION OF PROBLEM

The improved long-term survival of many cancer patients treated with mediastinal irradiation has resulted in a higher likelihood of secondary cardiac disease presenting years after the initial treatment. Mediastinal irradiation can affect all the structures of the heart and is associated with a wide spectrum of acute and chronic cardiac disease, including pericarditis, accelerated atherosclerosis, myocardial fibrosis, valvular dysfunction, and conduction disturbances.[1-8] The pericardium is most often involved, and the conduction system is the least frequently affected. The overall incidence of clinically detectable radiation-induced heart disease varies from 5% to 30%, depending on the method of diagnosis.[9] Mediastinal irradiation is commonly used to treat patients with Hodgkin's disease, non-Hodgkin's lymphoma, seminoma, carcinoma of the breast, carcinoma of the lung, and carcinoma of the esophagus. Factors predictive of the risk of subsequent damage to the heart include total radiation dose to the mediastinum, use of radiation-blocking modalities, and age of the patient. Younger patients are more likely than older patients to present later in life with radiation-induced heart disease. Most of the patients received total doses of more than 3500 cGy delivered at 1000 to 1100 cGy per week.

Clinically significant radiation-associated valvular heart disease is not commonly encountered. However, postmortem analysis found fibrous thickening of the valvular endocardium in about 70% to 80% of patients who received more than 3500 cGy to the heart.[8,10] Left-sided valves seem to be more frequently involved than are right-sided valves.[8,10]

There is still uncertainty about which elements of the heart (blood capillaries, mesothelial cells) are the main targets of radiation, but some investigators have implicated the fibroblasts.[11] This may explain, in part, why the fibrous skeleton of the heart may be more prone to thickening and fibrosis after irradiation.

TYPICAL CASE

A 48-year-old woman is evaluated for dyspnea and chest tightness. She has a prior history of Hodgkin's disease, diagnosed during her teenage years. This was treated with mantle irradiation, with a total dose of 4500 cGy administered. Her echocardiogram showed normal left ventricular and right ventricular chamber size but severe calcification of the aortic-mitral curtain. Severe aortic regurgitation and moderate mitral regurgitation were detected by color-flow Doppler examination. She subsequently underwent coronary arteriography, which demonstrated critical stenoses of both the proximal left main and proximal right coronary arteries. She underwent successful multivessel coronary artery bypass surgery and replacement of the mitral and aortic valves.

DIFFERENTIAL DIAGNOSIS

In general, the symptoms and physical findings of significant radiation-associated valvular heart disease are not distinct from the symptoms and signs of valvular heart disease due to other causes. However, coexistent radiation-induced coronary or pericardial disease may alter the clinical presentation.

The diagnosis of radiation-associated valvular heart disease is based on a history of prior mediastinal irradiation and echocardiographic evidence of valvular thickening. The increased fibrous content of the left-sided valves after mediastinal irradiation correlates with the two-dimensional echocardiographic findings of variable aortic, mitral, and tricuspid valve thickening.[5,12-15] These echocardiographic findings are nonspecific for radiation-associated valvular heart disease because other conditions, such as rheumatic heart disease, are associated with similar findings. However, echocardiographic demonstration of thickening of the structures that define the aortic-mitral curtain (noncoronary aortic sinus, annular attachment and body of the noncoronary aortic leaflet, and annular attachment and body of the anterior mitral leaflet) may be highly suggestive of radiation-associated valvular heart disease after therapy for Hodgkin's disease (Fig. 92D.1).[15]

Preoperative coronary angiography and hemodynamic assessment are indicated to exclude underlying radiation-induced coronary and pericardial disease when surgical treatment is considered for significant valve disease.

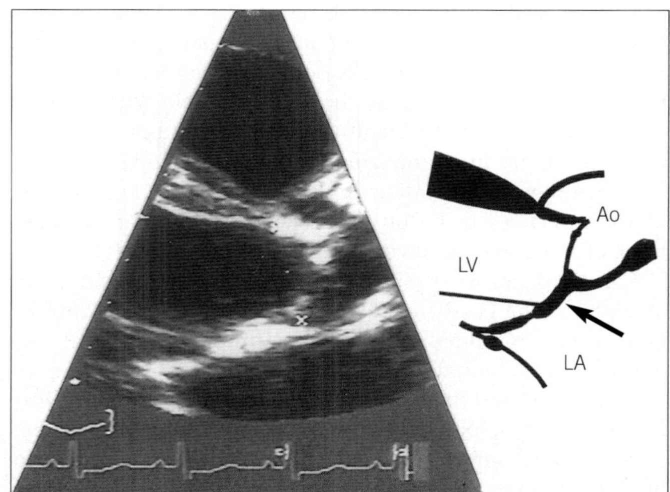

Figure 92D.1 A representative echocardiogram of a patient with radiation-associated mitral and aortic valve disease after mediastinal irradiation for Hodgkin's disease. *Left,* Parasternal long-axis two-dimensional echocardiographic image of the aorta and mitral valves and adjacent structures. *Right,* A diagrammatic representation of these structures. Thick lines denote thickening of the anatomic regions. Note the thickening of the aortic-mitral curtain *(arrow)*. Ao, aorta; LA, left atrium; LV, left ventricle.

TREATMENT OPTIONS

The medical and surgical management of patients with radiation-associated valvular heart disease is similar to that of all patients with valvular heart disease. The mortality after surgical intervention for radiation-induced valvular lesions is not prohibitive.[9] Because myocardial damage and fibrosis affect chiefly the right ventricle, particular attention should be given to right ventricular protection during cardiopulmonary bypass, and right ventricular dysfunction should be anticipated in the perioperative period.[9]

SUMMARY

Mediastinal irradiation affects all the structures of the heart and is associated with a wide spectrum of acute and chronic cardiac disease, including pericarditis, accelerated atherosclerosis, myocardial fibrosis, valvular dysfunction, and conduction disturbances.

Whereas clinically significant radiation-associated valvular heart disease is rare, fibrous thickening of the valvular endocardium is found in about 70% to 80% of patients who received more than 3500 cGy to the heart. Left-sided valves seem to be more frequently involved than right-sided valves are. The diagnosis of radiation-associated valvular heart disease is based on a history of prior mediastinal irradiation and echocardiographic evidence of valvular thickening.

Thickening of the aortic-mitral curtain appears to be a common finding in radiation-associated valvular heart disease. The medical and surgical management of patients with radiation-associated valvular heart disease is similar to that of all patients with valvular heart disease.

e. Vasodilator Therapy in Asymptomatic Mitral Regurgitation

William H. Gaasch

DEFINITION OF PROBLEM

Patients with chronic severe mitral regurgitation (MR) and symptoms of heart failure or left ventricular (LV) dysfunction are candidates for mitral valve repair or replacement.[1] However, the indications for such surgery in asymptomatic patients, especially those with normal LV function, remain controversial and depend on a variety of factors, such as valve repairability and atrial fibrillation. Many clinicians argue that because there are no symptoms to improve, not only does early surgery expose the patient to perioperative morbidity and mortality, but if repair of the native diseased valve cannot be achieved, the patient will also be exposed to the long-term complications of a prosthetic valve. Thus, many clinicians are reluctant to consider surgical correction of chronic MR in an asymptomatic patient. Medical therapy with a vasoactive drug, were it able to obviate or safely delay the need for surgery, would obviously be desirable. However, because of potential untoward effects and unproven long-term benefit, there is a persistent uncertainty about the utility of vasodilator therapy in asymptomatic patients with chronic MR.[2]

TYPICAL CASE

An asymptomatic 55-year-old man is found to have a holosystolic murmur, and his physician orders an echocardiogram. This study shows a mildly dilated left ventricle (end-diastolic dimension, 58 mm) with normal systolic function (ejection fraction, 65%), a left atrium of normal size, and a mitral valve prolapse with MR judged to be severe by color-flow Doppler criteria.

PATHOPHYSIOLOGY

MR burdens the left ventricle with a volume load that leads to a series of compensatory myocardial and circulatory adjustments.[3] With acute regurgitation and volume overload, the ventricle draws on preload reserve, and the total stroke volume increases by the Frank-Starling mechanism. In addition, the low-resistance runoff into the left atrium contributes to an increased ejection fraction and a decrease in systolic volume; according to the law of Laplace, systolic load (i.e., afterload) declines. Thus, in acute MR, an increased ejection fraction and increased total stroke volume occur as a result of an increase in LV preload and a decrease in afterload.

The major change that occurs during the evolution from acute to chronic MR is an enlargement of the ventricle. As this new state develops, the small hyperkinetic chamber of acute MR is converted to a large compliant chamber well suited to deliver a large stroke volume. This comes about through a dissolution of collagen weave and remodeling of the extracellular matrix with a rearrangement of myocardial fibers, in association with the addition of new sarcomeres and the development of eccentric LV hypertrophy. As a result, cardiomyocytes are longer, but preload at the sarcomere level (i.e., sarcomere length) returns toward normal. Moreover, the systolic unloading characteristic of acute MR is gradually replaced by normal systolic wall stresses.[4] Thus, the enhanced total stroke volume, seen in chronic compensated MR, is "mediated through a normal performance of each unit of an enlarged circumference."[3] At this time, LV contractility and ejection fraction are normal and total stroke volume is high as a result of the large end-diastolic volume. During this compensated phase of the disease, most patients remain asymptomatic. This would seem to be an ideal time for the use of vasodilator therapy—if such treatment could reliably reduce the volume overload and thereby protect the ventricle from progressive enlargement and decompensation.

The most elusive and poorly understood aspect of the pathophysiologic process of MR is the nature of the transition from the compensated to a decompensated state. This may occur as a consequence of progressive increments in the regurgitant volume, a gradual depression of myocardial contractility, or both. The decompensated state is characterized by substantial and progressive ventricular enlargement, high LV diastolic pressure and wall stress, increased systolic wall stress, and decline in the ejection fraction. The fall in ejection fraction is a consequence of both depressed LV contractile state and afterload excess. Progressive atrial enlargement and atrial arrhythmias are seen, pulmonary hypertension develops, and the patient becomes symptomatic. At this late (i.e., decompensated) stage, there may be irreversible depression of ventricular and atrial function, and although some patients may benefit from vasodilator therapy or surgery, an optimal surgical result is unlikely.

Hydraulic Determinants of Regurgitant Flow

The determinants of mitral regurgitant volume are best understood in the context of the orifice equation. This equation, based on the Torricelli principle, states that flow through an orifice varies by the square root of the pressure gradient across that orifice:

$$\text{MRV} = \text{MROA} \times C \times T_s \times \sqrt{\text{LVP} - \text{LAP}}$$

where MRV is mitral regurgitant volume, MROA is mitral regurgitant orifice area, C is constant, T_s is time or duration of systole, LVP is LV mean systolic pressure, and LAP is left atrial mean systolic pressure. In many patients with MR, the regurgitant orifice area is dynamic with variations that are dependent on LV geometry. The systolic pressure gradient across the valve also can vary dramatically. These two determinants of regurgitant volume are the primary therapeutic targets in patients with MR, and vasodilators have the potential to affect both. However, a reduction in the systolic pressure gradient between the ventricle and the atrium would be expected to have minimal impact on regurgitant flow if the regurgitant orifice area remains constant. Thus, a 10% to 15% decrease in the pressure gradient would produce only a 7% reduction in regurgitant volume.[2] Such a small change is unlikely to be detected with currently available techniques. Therefore, the goal of vasodilator therapy should be to reduce both the pressure gradient and the orifice size. This can often be accomplished in myopathic ventricles and secondary MR and in decompensated hearts with degenerative disease of the mitral leaflets. By contrast, a beneficial effect in asymptomatic patients with normal ventricular function and little or no LV enlargement is unlikely. Systemic vascular resistance, LV systolic wall stress (i.e., afterload), and contractile or inotropic state are not direct determinants of the regurgitant volume.

The Severity of Regurgitation

LV cineangiography and Doppler echocardiography are widely used to evaluate the severity of MR, but these methods are only semiquantitative. Calculations of the regurgitant volume or regurgitant fraction with catheterization or echocardiographic techniques can be more accurate, but the methods require careful attention to detail and until recently had not been widely applied. Moderate MR is said to be present when the regurgitant fraction is in the range of 30% to 50%; severe MR is defined as a regurgitant fraction of more than 50%. However, the regurgitant fraction varies inversely with the total stroke volume, and an increase in the LV end-diastolic volume or ejection fraction might reduce the regurgitant fraction—despite a constant regurgitant volume.

CLINICAL VASODILATOR STUDIES

The short-term effects of vasodilator therapy in patients with chronic MR have been variable and dependent, among other factors, on the agent employed.[5] For example, nitroprusside has produced a consistent decrease in the regurgitant volume and an increase in forward stroke volume, generally accompanied by a reduction in end-diastolic pressure and volume. Nitroglycerin tends to produce a reduction in end-diastolic volume with little effect on regurgitant volume or forward stroke volume. The short-term effects of angiotensin-converting enzyme (ACE) inhibitors appear to be less consistent, but there is a tendency for regurgitant flow to decrease during such treatment.

The long-term use of vasodilator therapy in chronic MR has virtually been limited to ACE inhibitors and AT_1 receptor blockers.[6-11] These agents tend to produce a decrease in the regurgitant volume, but the average changes are relatively small, and there are substantial individual variations in the magnitude of the effect.[9,10] A decrease in end-diastolic volume is not uniformly seen,[9] and exercise tolerance is not improved.[9,10] In one blinded study, therapy was withdrawn from one third of the patients because of side effects.[9] In another study, small changes in regurgitant orifice area and regurgitant volume were seen during angiotensin blockade, but neither LV size and function nor clinical outcomes were reported.[12] Most important, however, is that no published studies report a beneficial effect on clinical outcomes, such as a delay in the hemodynamic progression or the development of symptoms or, most important, a delay or decrease in the need for corrective surgery. Thus, "in the absence of systemic hypertension, there is no known indication for the use of vasodilating drugs or ACE inhibitors in asymptomatic patients."[1]

SUMMARY

Although no one would argue against the use of ACE inhibitors or perhaps AT_1 receptor blockers in myopathic hearts with secondary MR or in decompensated hearts with primary (valvular) MR, the available data do not provide strong support for the use of these agents in asymptomatic patients with valvular MR and normal LV size and function. Thus, a beneficial effect should not necessarily be expected in asymptomatic patients with normal LV size and function. By contrast, hemodynamic benefit might be expected in patients with severe MR and LV enlargement, especially those with early or mild symptoms or those with borderline LV function. When a compelling indication (e.g., hypertension, diabetes) exists for the use of ACE inhibitors or AT_1 receptor blockers in a patient with coexisting MR, these drugs should obviously be used. However, a long-term beneficial effect on the regurgitant lesion and long-term outcomes should not necessarily be expected, and most important, such therapy should not replace careful clinical follow-up, including periodic evaluation of the mitral structure, severity of regurgitation, and LV size and function.[1]

chapter 93

Aortic Stenosis

David M. Shavelle and Catherine M. Otto

Definition

- Aortic stenosis occurs when there is obstruction to the ejection of blood from the left ventricle, most commonly at the valvular level in adults.

Key Features

- Symptoms include angina, syncope, and congestive heart failure.
- Physical findings with hemodynamically significant aortic stenosis include sustained apical impulse, crescendo-decrescendo systolic murmur, single second heart sound, and abnormal carotid pulse contour.
- Echocardiography allows assessment of valve anatomy, severity of obstruction, and left ventricular geometry and function.

Therapy

- Aortic valve replacement is the only effective treatment of symptomatic patients.
- Asymptomatic patients should receive endocarditis prophylaxis, risk factor modification, and education about symptoms and disease progression.

For quality of life to be preserved as the population ages, it is important to identify and to treat appropriately diseases commonly encountered in the elderly. It is estimated that approximately 1% to 4% of adults older than 65 years have aortic valve stenosis, and many of these patients will develop severe obstruction requiring valve replacement surgery.[1,2] With improving access to health care, wide availability of noninvasive diagnostic tests, and evolving operative and endovascular techniques with low mortality, the primary care physician and cardiologist will both be faced with issues of establishing the diagnosis and determining the appropriate treatment of patients with aortic stenosis.

Degenerative disease of the aortic valve (aortic sclerosis) most likely represents an early stage in a disease process that eventually results in aortic stenosis. The degree of aortic valve calcification as detected by echocardiography increases with age; aortic sclerosis (valve calcification and a peak transaortic velocity by Doppler study of less than 2 m/s) occurs in 20% of patients aged 65 to 74 years and 48% of patients older than 84 years.[1,2] Similarly, aortic stenosis also increases in prevalence with age and is present in 1.3% of patients aged 65 to 74 years and 4% of patients older than 85 years. Physicians should therefore have a relatively low threshold for obtaining an echocardiogram in an elderly patient with a systolic murmur. In addition to age, several other risk factors have been associated with aortic sclerosis, including male gender, lipoprotein(a) level, height, hypertension, smoking, low-density lipoprotein cholesterol level, and diabetes mellitus.[2-5] In addition, metabolic syndrome is associated with an increased risk of aortic valve calcification.[6] Genetic factors may play a role on the basis of family studies and genome-wide linkage analysis.[7,8]

ANATOMY AND PATHOLOGY

The aortic valve serves a critical function in the heart by maintaining the anterograde flow of blood to the aorta when it is opened and preventing retrograde flow into the left ventricle when it is closed. The normal aortic valve consists of three thin, mobile fibrous cusps that are covered by a layer of endothelium and attach to the aortic wall in a crescentic or semilunar manner (Fig. 93.1). Each cusp is named according to its relationship to the coronary ostia, with adjacent cusps separated by one of three commissures.

The disease processes that result in stenosis of the aortic valve can be classified as congenital, rheumatic, degenerative (calcific), and rare causes (Table 93.1). Among congenital anomalies, a bicuspid valve is the most common, occurring in approximately 2% of the population. The frequency of bicuspid valves is greater in men (the male-to-female ratio is 2:1), and it is associated with coarctation of the aorta and aortic dissection. In adults undergoing valve replacement for severe aortic stenosis, more than 50% have a bicuspid aortic valve.[9] Bicuspid aortic valve disease is also associated with aortic root dilatation and an increased risk of aortic dissection.[10] The cusps are usually of unequal size and develop progressive thickening and calcification with age, resulting in reduced leaflet flexibility.

Rheumatic aortic valve disease is characterized by commissural fusion with leaflet thickening and fibrosis that produce a triangular valve orifice, and it is uniformly accompanied by mitral valve involvement. The valve may acquire calcium, but the degree is often less than with a bicuspid valve.

Degenerative disease (more recently referred to as calcific disease) occurs when a normal trileaflet aortic valve progressively acquires calcium in an active process that has many similarities to atherosclerosis.[11] The valvular lesions are characterized by intracellular and extracellular lipid accumulation and inflammatory cells, fibroblasts, and mineralization (Fig. 93.2). Valve calcification is an active process with expression of osteopontin, matrix metalloproteinase 2, and

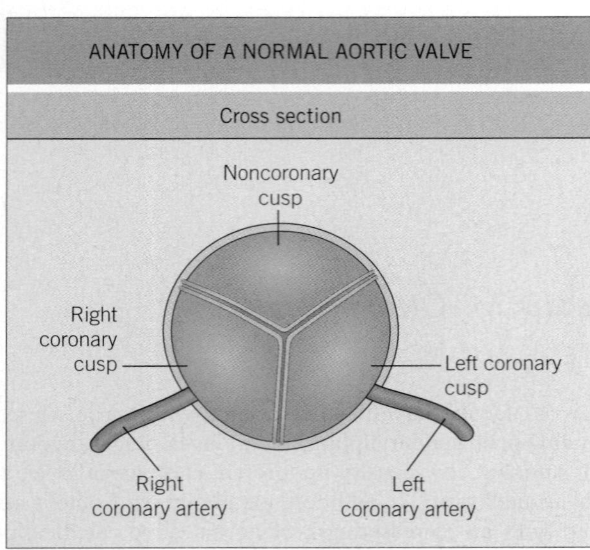

Figure 93.1 Anatomy of a normal aortic valve. Three cusps are named according to their relationship with the coronary ostia, and adjacent cusps are separated by one of three commissures.

CAUSES OF VALVULAR AORTIC STENOSIS
Congenital
Unicuspid valve
Bicuspid valve
Rheumatic
Degenerative (calcific)
Degenerative disease of three-cusped valve
Superimposed calcification of a bicuspid valve
Other rare causes
Homozygous type II hypercholesterolemia
Paget's disease of bone
Renal failure
Radiation exposure

Table 93.1 Causes of valvular aortic stenosis.

tenascin-C.[12-14] Hydroxyapatite crystal formation occurs early in the disease process and eventually leads to frank bone formation within the valve leaflets in end-stage disease.[15] Calcification begins at the base of the cusps and progresses toward the edges, with the commissures remaining open (Fig. 93.3). Accelerated valve calcification is seen in patients with homozygous type II hypercholesterolemia, Paget's disease of bone, renal failure, and radiation exposure.

Although each disease process that results in aortic stenosis causes specific changes to the normal valve tissue, it may be difficult to distinguish a bicuspid from a trileaflet valve once severe calcific changes are present. Therapeutic options are the same for symptomatic patients with aortic stenosis regardless of the underlying cause. However, establishment of the etiology may have clinical implications:

- degenerative (calcific) disease can be associated with calcification of the conduction system, resulting in heart block;

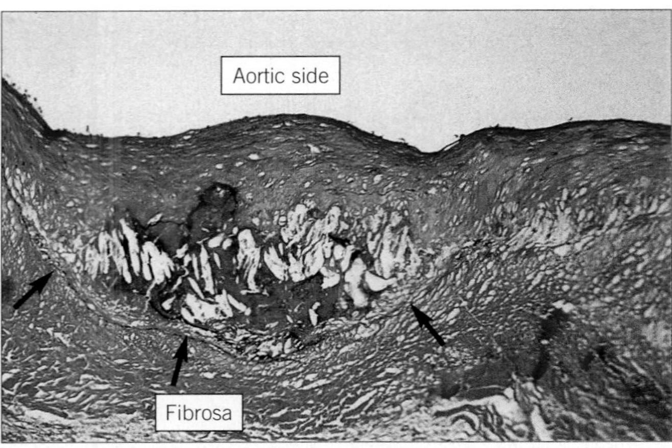

Figure 93.2 Histology of a typical lesion of degenerative (calcific) aortic stenosis. The lesion is on the aortic side of the valve leaflet with displacement of the elastic lamina *(arrows)* that normally lies adjacent to the endothelium. The lesion consists of an inflammatory cell infiltrate (macrophages and T lymphocytes), lipids (low-density lipoprotein, lipoprotein(a), oxidized low-density lipoprotein), microscopic calcification, and protein. Proteins involved in calcification, such as osteopontin, are also produced by a subset of lesion macrophages.

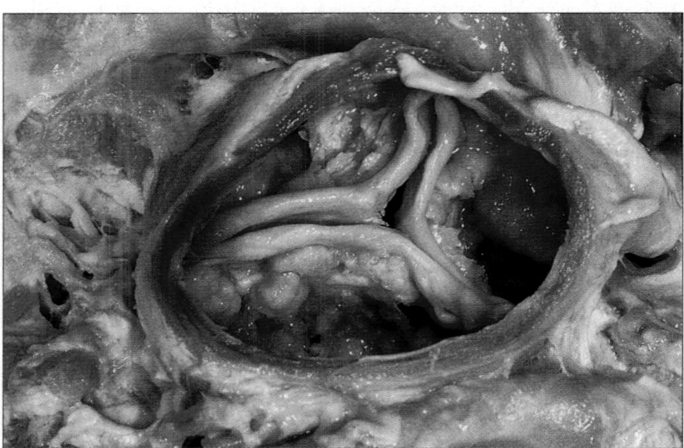

Figure 93.3 Gross pathology of degenerative (calcific) aortic stenosis. Large deposits of calcium are present on the aortic side of all three valve leaflets. Also note the absence of commissural fusion.

- a bicuspid valve is associated with aortic coarctation and aortic dissection; and
- mitral valve involvement is uniformly present with rheumatic aortic disease, and mitral stenosis may mask the symptoms of aortic stenosis as it reduces left ventricular preload and cardiac output.

PATHOPHYSIOLOGY

Resistance to flow by the narrowed aortic valve imposes a pressure overload on the left ventricle. In response, the left ventricle generates progressively higher pressures as stenosis worsens, with the development of an aortic transvalvular gradient. Several mechanisms attempt to compensate for this chronic pressure overload, according to the law of Laplace. The thickness of the left ventricular walls increases (hypertrophy) so that the ratio of pressure to thickness remains constant, thereby minimizing wall stress and left ventricular work. The law of Laplace states that

$$\text{Stress} = (\text{pressure} \times \text{radius})/(2 \times \text{thickness})$$

The costs of these compensatory mechanisms include

- reduced left ventricular compliance;
- increased myocardial oxygen demand;
- decreased coronary blood flow; and
- eventual left ventricular systolic dysfunction.

Hypertrophy results in a thick-walled and noncompliant left ventricular chamber. Reduced compliance impairs the ability to adequately fill the left ventricle under normal pressures, and left ventricular diastolic pressure increases. The left ventricle becomes more dependent on the atrial contribution to diastolic filling, and hemodynamic impairment can therefore result from the loss of atrial contraction (as in atrial fibrillation). Of note, there are substantial gender differences in the pattern of left ventricular hypertrophy in adults with aortic stenosis. Although left ventricular mass is increased in both men and women, women tend to have a small, thick-walled, hyperdynamic left ventricle, whereas men tend to have a dilated, hypokinetic left ventricle with relatively normal wall thickness.[16,17]

In addition to reduced compliance, the hypertrophied ventricle requires increased oxygen to meet its metabolic demands. The ability to perfuse the coronary vessels (coronary perfusion pressure) is the difference between the aortic diastolic and left ventricular diastolic pressures. Elevated left ventricular diastolic pressure reduces this gradient, limits coronary perfusion pressure, and may induce angina in the absence of obstructive coronary artery disease.[18,19]

Despite significant hypertrophy, the left ventricle maintains normal contractility until late in the disease course. Eventually, however, the increased pressure load overwhelms left ventricular contractile reserve, leading to left ventricular systolic dysfunction and chamber dilatation.

CLINICAL PRESENTATION

Valvular aortic stenosis is a gradually progressive disease, so that patients may remain asymptomatic for years. Not infrequently, the diagnosis is initially considered during a routine physical examination when a systolic murmur is heard. Because the prognosis of symptomatic patients is poor without surgical treatment, it is of paramount importance to identify the onset of symptoms, which marks a turn in the disease course.

Symptoms

The initial symptom of severe aortic stenosis in adults typically is decreased exercise tolerance or dyspnea on exertion. The "classic" symptoms of angina, syncope, and heart failure occur only late in the disease course and are rarely seen in patients with a known diagnosis who are observed prospectively.

Dyspnea occurring during exertion may reflect a limited ability to augment stroke volume adequately to meet the metabolic demand of exercise. However, dyspnea can reflect other processes, including coronary artery disease, left ventricular hypertrophy and diastolic dysfunction, chronic lung disease, and hypertension. Because valve obstruction develops slowly, many patients gradually reduce their activity level in an unconscious manner to avoid dyspnea and therefore are unaware of their current limitation unless they are specifically questioned or objectively evaluated.

Approximately 50% of patients with aortic stenosis have coexisting coronary artery disease to explain the development of angina.[19] Conversely, the absence of chest pain does not exclude the presence of significant coronary artery disease. In patients who experience angina in the absence of coronary disease, an imbalance between myocardial oxygen supply and demand is the proposed explanation. Increased demand occurs secondary to elevated left ventricular cavity pressure, prolonged left ventricular ejection time, and increased muscle mass, and various mechanisms have been described that impair coronary blood flow and limit supply.[18,20,21]

Syncope or presyncope is usually temporally related to exertion and occurs when elevated left ventricular cavity pressure stimulates baroreceptors that induce arterial hypotension, decreased venous return, and occasionally bradycardia.[22] Syncope at rest is more commonly the result of ventricular arrhythmias.

Physical Examination

The principal findings on physical examination in patients with significant aortic stenosis include a sustained apical impulse, a slow-rising and weak carotid pulse, and a crescendo-decrescendo systolic murmur (Fig. 93.4). The carotid pulse contour provides a more accurate measure of stenosis severity than do peripheral pulses (radial or brachial) because of its proximity to the left ventricle. Prolonged left ventricular ejection through the narrowed aortic valve yields a slow-rising pulse (pulsus tardus), and reduced stroke volume results in a weak or small-amplitude pulse (pulsus parvus). Elderly patients and those with long-standing hypertension may have a normal carotid pulse contour despite severe aortic stenosis because of reduced arterial wall compliance.

The apical impulse is typically nondisplaced and sustained, reflecting prolonged left ventricular ejection. A presystolic thrust may occasionally be palpated at the apex and coincides with the fourth heart sound generated by forceful atrial contraction into the noncompliant left ventricle. If the aortic valve leaflets are mobile, as in congenital as opposed to degenerative aortic stenosis, an ejection click may be heard at the base after the first heart sound. The second heart sound may be single as the aortic component is diminished because of calcification and stiffening of the valve leaflets. The finding of a normal second heart sound implies normal valve closure and the absence of severe stenosis.[23]

Turbulent flow across the narrowed aortic valve produces a crescendo-decrescendo systolic murmur that is best heard immediately downstream from the lesion over the ascending aorta in the second right intercostal space. The murmur is frequently well transmitted to the base of the neck and carotid arteries. On occasion, the murmur appears to radiate toward the apex as the high-pitched musical components are preferentially transmitted through solid tissue (chest wall and myocardium), simulating mitral regurgitation (the Gallavardin phenomenon). The murmur begins after isovolumetric

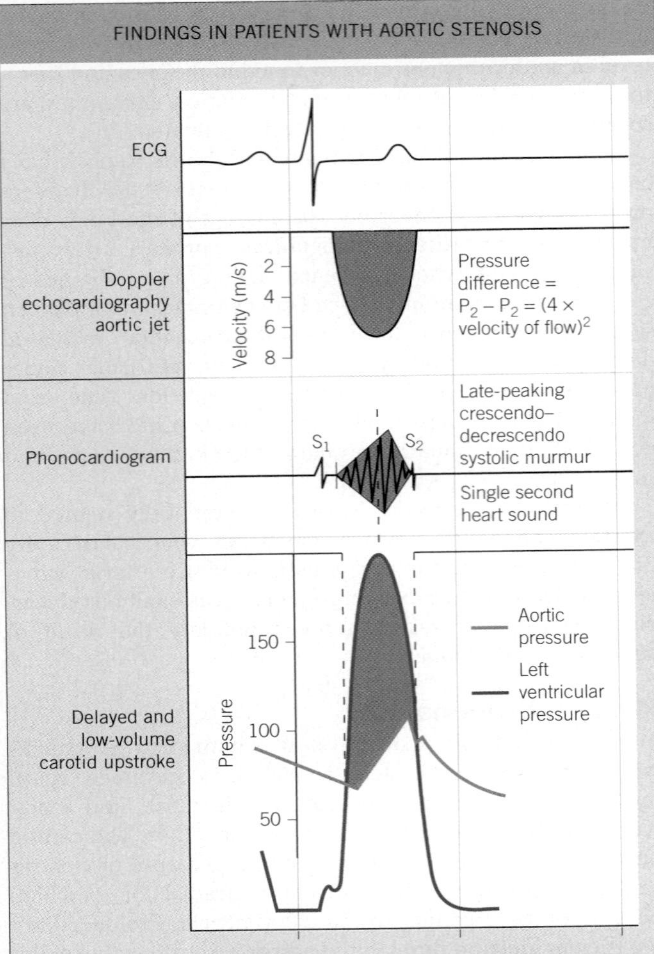

Figure 93.4 Findings from Doppler echocardiography, physical examination (phonocardiogram), and cardiac catheterization in a patient with aortic stenosis. Note that the Doppler maximum aortic jet velocity corresponds to the maximum instantaneous pressure gradient recorded at cardiac catheterization. As stenosis becomes more severe, the maximum gradient occurs later in systole so that the murmur peak on auscultation (phonocardiogram) is delayed. With severe aortic stenosis, the second heart sound is single because of the absence of the aortic component of the second heart sound.

contraction (approximately 0.06 second after the first heart sound) and ends before the second heart sound. This time interval is useful in distinguishing the murmur of mitral regurgitation, which begins immediately after the first heart sound and extends into and frequently obscures the second heart sound.

The rise and fall of the transaortic pressure gradient in systole is the basis for the shape and time to the peak intensity of the murmur. As stenosis severity increases, the time to peak intensity of the murmur is further delayed in the systolic ejection period. A late-peaking murmur therefore indicates more severe stenosis, but it often takes an experienced observer to appreciate this, and it may be absent if severe aortic stenosis coexists with conditions that increase the transaortic volume flow rate, such as aortic regurgitation.

The grade of the murmur may help quantify the severity of stenosis. A grade 4 murmur is highly specific for severe obstruction; conversely, severe stenosis is uncommon with a grade 1 murmur.[23] Intermediate grade murmurs (grade 2 and grade 3) may be present with varying degrees of stenosis and are therefore not as useful in determining the severity of stenosis. The murmur grade is dependent not only on the transaortic pressure gradient but also on the transaortic volume flow rate, transmission of the murmur to the chest wall, and orientation of the turbulent jet. Conditions that affect the transaortic volume flow rate (e.g., a low cardiac output), transmission of the murmur to the chest wall (e.g., obesity, emphysema), and orientation of the turbulent jet can also alter the grade of the murmur.

A number of other valvular and nonvalvular conditions can mimic the symptoms and physical findings of aortic stenosis (Table 93.2). Patients with hypertrophic cardiomyopathy may also present with a history of syncope, chest pain, and dyspnea and a systolic murmur. Although the apical impulse can be sustained and preceded by a presystolic thrust (fourth heart sound) as in aortic stenosis, the carotid upstroke and characteristics of the systolic murmur are distinctly different. In hypertrophic cardiomyopathy, the carotid upstroke is rapid and often displays a "spike-and-dome" configuration, in contrast to the slow-rising pulse of aortic stenosis. The systolic murmur is usually longer, harsher, and often best heard along the left sternal border with minimal radiation to the carotid arteries, and the murmur changes in intensity with various maneuvers. Squatting-to-standing action and the strain phase of the Valsalva maneuver increase murmur intensity because of a reduction in left ventricular preload; the murmur of aortic stenosis remains unchanged or decreases with these maneuvers. Both mitral regurgitation and ventricular septal defects also produce systolic murmurs. These lesions should not be confused with aortic stenosis as the murmurs are holosystolic, usually best heard along the left sternal border or cardiac apex, and accompanied by a normal carotid upstroke. Coarctation of the aorta may occasionally coexist with a bicuspid aortic valve and is identified by a brachial-femoral pulse delay and hypertension of the upper relative to the lower extremities.

DIAGNOSTIC TECHNIQUES

Pertinent findings from the history and physical examination are supplemented with information from the chest radiograph and electrocardiogram to suggest the diagnosis of aortic stenosis. The diagnosis is then confirmed by echocardiography; cardiac catheterization is reserved for situations in which the echocardiographic data are inconclusive or inconsistent with the clinical findings or the patient is at risk for coronary artery disease and requires coronary angiography before surgical valve replacement (Fig. 93.5).

Chest Radiography

Left ventricular hypertrophy may be seen as rounding of the cardiac apex. Overall cardiac size and left atrial size are normal and pulmonary venous hypertension is absent unless cardiac decompensation is present. Poststenotic dilatation of the proximal aorta suggests stenosis at the valvular level. Aortic valve calcification occurs in the majority of

DIFFERENTIAL DIAGNOSIS OF A SYSTOLIC MURMUR						
Condition	**Apical Impulse**	**Carotid Pulse Contour**	**Murmur Location (Radiation)**	**Effect of Maneuvers on Murmur Intensity**	**Murmur Duration**	**Additional Findings**
Aortic stenosis	Sustained, nondisplaced	Delayed upstroke, low volume	Second right intercostal space (carotid arteries)	No characteristic changes; increase after premature ventricular contracture	Midsystolic	Ejection sound; single or paradoxically split second heart sound; third and fourth sounds
Mitral regurgitation	Nonsustained, displaced	Normal	Apex (axillae)	Increase with handgrip; no change after premature ventricular contraction	Holosystolic	Third heart sound
Ventricular septal defect	Normal	Normal	Fourth left intercostal space (none)	No diagnostic changes	Holosystolic	Murmur often associated with thrill
Hypertrophic cardiomyopathy	Sustained, nondisplaced	Rapid upstroke, full volume	Fourth left intercostal space (none)	Increase with strain phase of Valsalva maneuver, on moving from squatting to standing position, and after premature ventricular contractions	Midsystolic	Third and fourth heart sounds; no ejection sound

Table 93.2 Differential diagnosis of a systolic murmur.

patients with significant stenosis and can be apparent on the lateral view, confirming that stenosis is located at the valvular level.

Electrocardiography

The electrocardiogram often shows left ventricular hypertrophy with or without repolarization abnormalities (strain pattern) in patients with significant aortic stenosis. However, severe aortic stenosis can be present without electrocardiographic evidence of left ventricular hypertrophy, and its absence should not mislead the clinician from the diagnosis.[24] Left bundle branch block may occasionally be present, and extensive calcification of the conduction system may result in first-degree atrioventricular block and rarely complete heart block.[21] The majority of patients are usually in normal sinus rhythm, and a normal electrocardiogram can be seen in 10% to 20% of patients with significant aortic stenosis. The presence of atrial fibrillation suggests coexisting rheumatic mitral valve disease or coronary artery disease.

Echocardiography

Echocardiography has emerged as the principal method of establishing the diagnosis of aortic stenosis.[25] The echocardiographic study should focus on

- defining the valve anatomy;
- determining the severity of stenosis;
- identifying other valvular or nonvalvular conditions; and
- assessing the left ventricular response to the pressure overload.

Valve characteristics of degenerative (calcific) disease include increased echogenicity and reduced systolic opening, frequently with increased echogenicity of the valve annulus. A trileaflet valve may be difficult to distinguish from a bicuspid valve when extensive fibrocalcific changes are present. Commissural fusion and coexisting mitral valve involvement are the distinguishing features of rheumatic aortic valve disease.

The severity of stenosis is reflected by

- aortic jet velocity;
- maximal and mean transaortic pressure gradients; and
- aortic valve area.

The aortic jet velocity is measured by Doppler echocardiographic methods as the maximal velocity across the aortic valve and has been shown to be predictive of symptom onset and clinical outcome in asymptomatic patients and to be accurate for clinical decision making in patients with symptomatic disease.[24,26] The pressure difference (gradient) between two chambers can be estimated by a modification of the Bernoulli equation:

$$\text{Pressure difference (gradient)} = 4(V)^2$$

The maximal gradient can be determined from the maximal velocity and the mean gradient by integrating the instantaneous pressure gradients over the systolic ejection period (Fig. 93.6). The velocity of a moving column of fluid increases through areas of narrowing but the volume of blood remains constant, according to a basic principle of fluid mechanics known as the continuity equation. This principle can be applied to determine the area of the aortic valve as shown in Figure 93.7.[27-29]

Echocardiography also allows evaluation of other potential causes of a systolic murmur, such as mitral regurgitation, hypertrophic cardiomyopathy, coarctation of the aorta, and ventricular septal defect. A large number (approximately 80%) of patients with aortic stenosis will have some degree of aortic regurgitation that should be quantified and may have implications for the timing of surgery. Other common coexisting valvular lesions include mitral annular calcification with mitral regurgitation in degenerative disease and mitral stenosis or regurgitation in rheumatic disease.

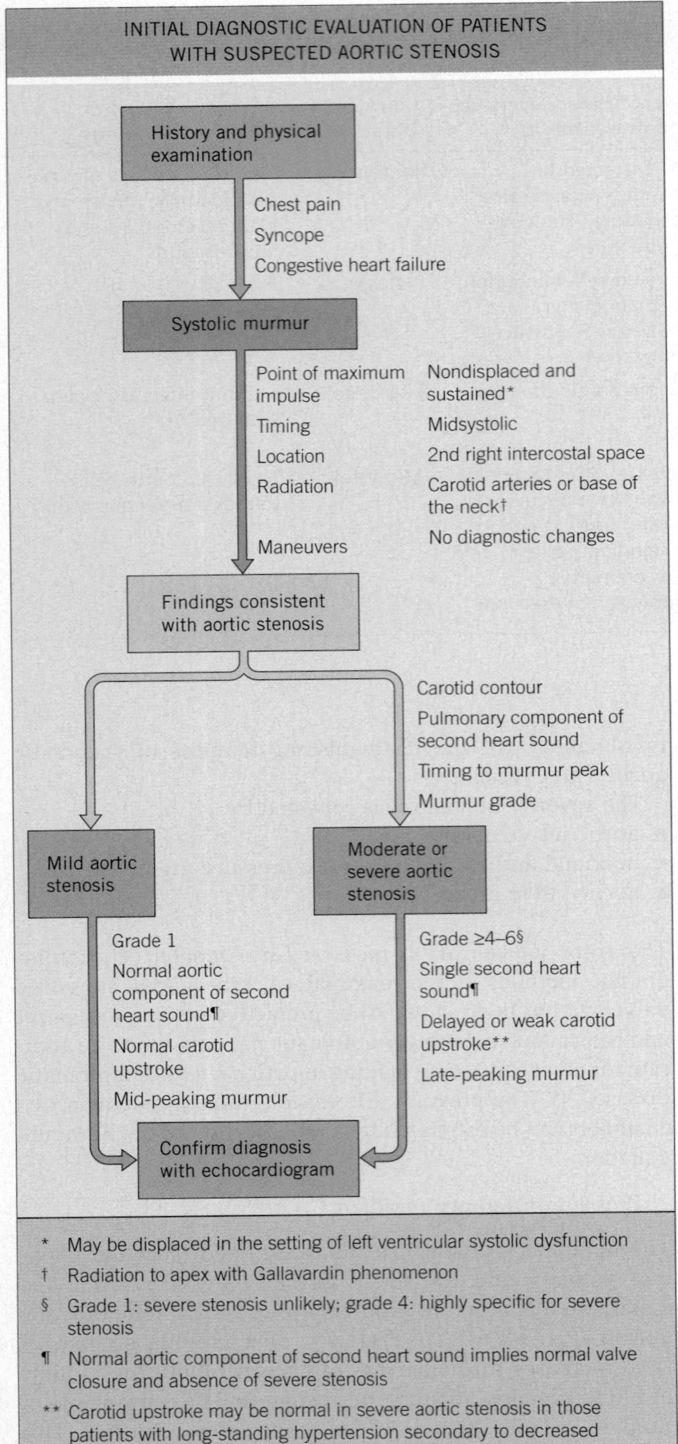

Figure 93.5 Diagnostic evaluation of patients with suspected aortic stenosis.

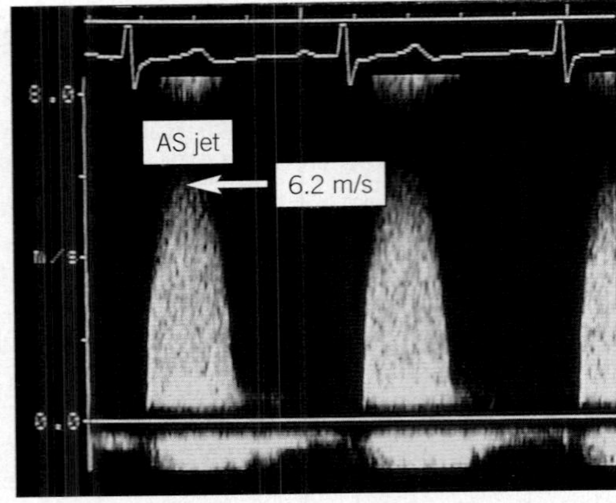

Figure 93.6 Doppler echocardiography recording of an aortic stenosis jet. The recording shows a maximum aortic jet velocity of 6.2 m/s corresponding to a maximum gradient of 154 mm Hg and a mean gradient of 92 mm Hg. AS jet, aortic stenosis jet.

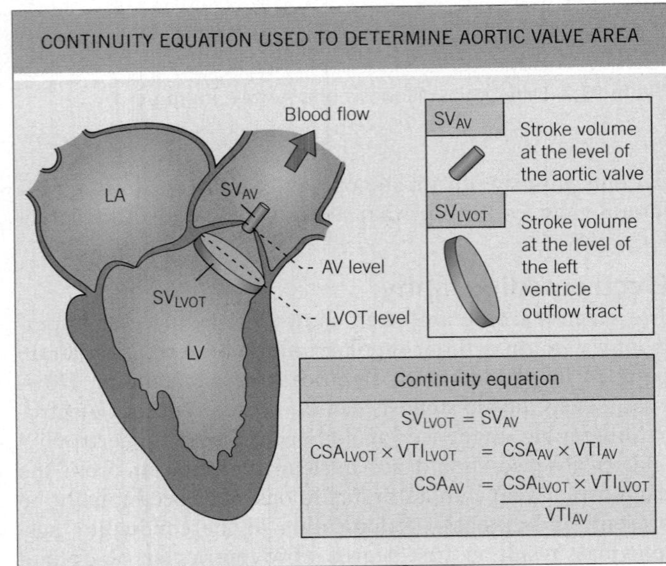

Figure 93.7 Diagram of the continuity equation that is used to determine the aortic valve area. The stroke volume at the aortic valve level (SV_{AV}) equals the stroke volume at the left ventricle outflow tract level (SV_{LVOT}) based on the principle of continuity of flow. The velocity-time integral (VTI) is measured with pulsed Doppler echocardiography in the left ventricular outflow tract and with continuous-wave Doppler echocardiography in the narrowed aortic valve orifice. The cross-sectional area (CSA) at the left ventricular outflow tract is measured on two-dimensional echocardiography, and the equation is solved for the cross-sectional area of the aortic valve (e.g., aortic valve area). AV, aortic valve; LA, left atrium, LV, left ventricle.

The left ventricle responds to the chronic pressure overload by developing left ventricular hypertrophy, which can be accurately identified by echocardiography. However, some patients have severe aortic stenosis without significant left ventricular hypertrophy. Typically, left ventricular systolic function remains well preserved until late in the disease course. Therefore, significant left ventricular systolic dysfunction suggests coexisting coronary artery disease or a cardiomyopathy. Coexistent diastolic dysfunction is common and is usually due to left ventricular hypertrophy, coronary artery disease, or a combination of both.

Other noninvasive approaches for the evaluation of aortic stenosis severity include three-dimensional echocardiography, which allows planimetry of valve area, and cardiac magnetic resonance imaging, which allows measurement of pressure gradient and valve area, but neither of these approaches is widely used.

Cardiac Catheterization

Invasive measurements of the transaortic valve gradient and calculation of the aortic valve area by the Gorlin formula are rarely needed when good-quality echocardiographic data are available. When the clinical and echocardiographic data yield conflicting results or the echocardiographic data are inconclusive, invasive measurements may be helpful. Patients at risk for coronary artery disease require coronary angiography so that bypass grafting can be performed at the time of valve replacement.

Accurate measurement of pressure gradients can be achieved by a single arterial puncture with a small-caliber (6 French) double-lumen catheter. The transaortic valve gradient is represented by three invasive measurements: the peak-to-peak gradient, the peak instantaneous gradient, and the mean gradient (Fig. 93.8). The peak-to-peak gradient is the difference between the peak left ventricular and peak aortic pressures and is usually less than the peak instantaneous gradient. The peak instantaneous gradient corresponds to the maximum gradient measured by Doppler echocardiographic methods. The mean gradient is average transaortic gradient during the systolic ejection period and is used in the Gorlin formula to calculate aortic valve area. Transaortic volume flow rate is measured by the thermodilution method, Fick method, or left ventricular angiography and is required in the Gorlin formula to calculate the aortic valve area. The Gorlin formula is flow dependent and in the setting of a low cardiac output may falsely overestimate the severity of stenosis. Measurements obtained during dobutamine infusion can augment cardiac output and may resolve this issue.[30]

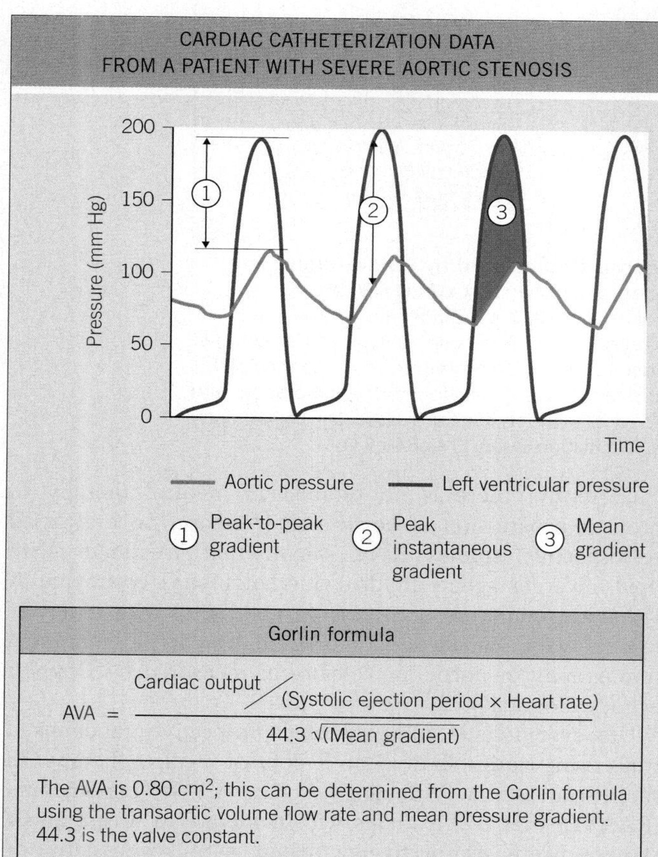

Figure 93.8 Cardiac catheterization data from a patient with severe aortic stenosis. The severity of stenosis is represented by the peak-to-peak gradient (75 mm Hg), the peak instantaneous gradient (105 mm Hg), and the mean gradient (55 mm Hg). With use of the cardiac output, systolic ejection period, heart rate, and mean gradient, the aortic valve area (AVA) is calculated by the Gorlin formula.

Stress Testing

Exercise treadmill testing is not routinely performed in the evaluation of patients with presumed aortic stenosis. Stress testing is contraindicated in symptomatic patients with aortic stenosis because of the risk of exercise-induced angina, syncope, congestive heart failure, or arrhythmias. Even asymptomatic patients with aortic stenosis often develop exercise-induced electrocardiographic changes despite normal coronary arteries, thus limiting the utility of treadmill testing for the detection of coronary artery disease. Exercise testing can be useful when it is unclear whether the patient is truly asymptomatic, when patients with moderate disease wish to increase their physical activity level, or when symptoms appear to be out of proportion to the severity of stenosis. The onset of symptoms during the exercise test or the failure of blood pressure to rise appropriately with exercise indicates hemodynamically significant aortic stenosis.[31,32]

Noninvasive nuclear imaging to detect coronary artery disease has been proposed as an alternative to coronary angiography.[33] Studies with exercise thallium Tl 201 show a reasonable accuracy for the detection of coronary artery disease but are further complicated by the risks of exercise-induced complications.[34] Pharmacologic stress testing with adenosine or dipyridamole has potential advantages over exercise because of a low incidence of precipitating myocardial ischemia and improved accuracy for identification of coronary artery disease.[33,35,36] Cardiac computed tomographic angiography and cardiac magnetic resonance imaging also provide diagnostic images of the proximal coronary arteries. When noninvasive coronary angiography is normal in a younger patient without cardiac risk factors, some clinicians would defer preoperative coronary angiography. However, most clinicians continue to perform coronary angiography before aortic valve surgery because of the importance of performing concurrent coronary artery bypass grafting if disease is present.

Valve Calcification Score

Cardiac computed tomography has been used to quantify the amount of aortic valve calcium with protocols similar to those used with coronary artery calcium scanning.[37] The amount of aortic valve calcium is related to the severity of aortic valve disease, with higher calcium scores associated with more severe aortic stenosis.[38] Several studies have used aortic valve calcium as measured by cardiac computed tomography as a clinical endpoint for therapeutic treatment trials.

MANAGEMENT

Asymptomatic Aortic Stenosis

The treatment of patients with aortic stenosis is dictated by the presence or absence of symptoms (Fig. 93.9). Asymptomatic patients should be educated about expected symptoms (exertional dyspnea, decreased exercise tolerance, chest pain, syncope, and congestive heart failure) and the time

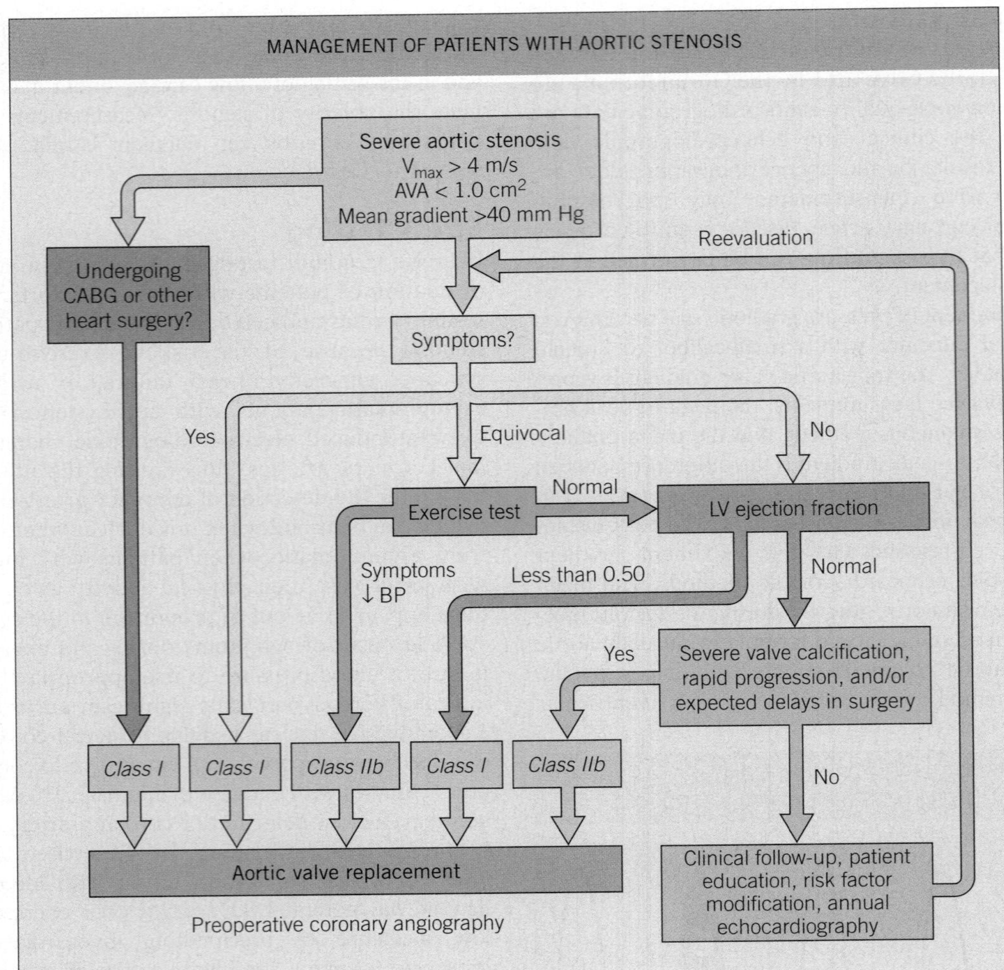

Figure 93.9 Management of patients with aortic stenosis documented by echocardiography. AVA, aortic valve area; BP, blood pressure; CABG, coronary artery bypass grafting; LV, left ventricle. (From Bonow RO, Carabello BA, Kanu C, et al. ACC/AHA 2006 guidelines for the management of patients with valvular heart disease: a report of the American College of Cardiology/American Heart Association Task Force on Practice Guidelines [writing committee to revise the 1998 Guidelines for the Management of Patients with Valvular Heart Disease]: developed in collaboration with the Society of Cardiovascular Anesthesiologists: endorsed by the Society for Cardiovascular Angiography and Interventions and the Society of Thoracic Surgeons. Circulation 2006;114:e84-e231.)

course for disease progression. Because patients with degenerative aortic valve disease share many of the same risk factors for coronary artery disease, modification of these factors should also be a major focus of treatment to prevent future cardiovascular events.

Given that the rate of progression in an individual patient is difficult to predict, it is prudent to perform periodic echocardiography even in asymptomatic patients. In patients who remain asymptomatic, echocardiography should be repeated as follows:

- mild stenosis (aortic jet velocity <3.0 m/s): every 3 to 5 years;
- moderate stenosis (aortic jet velocity 3.0-4.0 m/s): every 1 to 2 years; and
- severe stenosis (aortic jet velocity >4.0 m/s): every year.

Echocardiography is also indicated when symptoms develop, for any change in clinical status, and before any noncardiac procedure, including noncardiac surgery and childbirth.[39]

Currently, there is no established medical therapy to prevent progression of aortic valve disease. Several small retrospective studies have shown that treatment with lipid-lowering agents (hydroxymethylglutaryl–coenzyme A reductase inhibitors or statins) is associated with a slower rate of valve calcification measured by cardiac computed tomography or aortic jet velocity as measured by Doppler echocardiography.[40-42]

However, two recently reported prospective, randomized trials using statins showed no benefit of medical therapy. In the Rosuvastatin Affecting Aortic Valve Endothelium (RAAVE) trial, 121 patients with moderate to severe aortic stenosis were prospectively treated with rosuvastatin or placebo.[43] The study endpoint was change in aortic valve area and aortic jet velocity as measured by echocardiography. Those treated with rosuvastatin had a smaller decrease in aortic valve area and a smaller increase in aortic jet velocity compared with the placebo group. In the Scottish Aortic Stenosis and Lipid Lowering Trial, Impact on Regression (SALTIRE), 156 patients with an aortic jet velocity of more than 2.5 m/s were randomized to either atorvastatin or placebo.[44] The endpoint of the study was the change in aortic jet velocity as measured by echocardiography and the change in aortic valve calcium as assessed by cardiac computed tomography. Whereas low-density lipoprotein cholesterol was reduced to 63 mg/dL in those receiving atorvastatin, there was no difference in the aortic jet velocity or aortic valve calcium score between those receiving atorvastatin and those receiving placebo.

In the prospective randomized double blind study (SEAS) of simvastatin and ezitimide compared to placebo in 1873 adults with mild to moderate aortic stenosis, there was no difference between treatment groups in the composite outcome of aortic valve events and ischemic events, despite effective lowering of serum lipid levels.[45] There also was no effect of treatment on the rate of hemodynamic progression of valve obstruction, assessed by echocardiography jet velocity, mean gradient or valve area. Although there were fewer ischemic events in the treatment group, this difference was largely due to fewer coronary bypass procedures at the time of aortic valve replacement. The Aortic Stenosis Progression Observation: Measuring Effects of Rosuvastatin (ASTRONOMER) is still in progress.[46]

Symptomatic Aortic Stenosis

The prognosis of symptomatic patients is extremely poor without surgical treatment, with an average 2-year survival of approximately 50%.[47,48] Once patients develop symptoms, prompt surgical intervention is needed. The preoperative evaluation should focus on

- confirming the severity of stenosis;
- identifying any comorbid conditions that may have an impact on the surgical approach;
- performing angiography to evaluate coronary anatomy; and
- optimizing hemodynamics before surgery.

The primary options for valve replacement in adults are a bioprosthetic valve and a mechanical valve. In adults, aortic valve débridement techniques and balloon valvuloplasty have no role in the long-term management. The pulmonic autograft procedure is considered only infrequently in young adults. Operative mortality for aortic valve replacement averages 5.6%, with relative survival rates of 94.6% at 5 years, 84.7% at 10 years, and 74.9% at 15 years after valve replacement. Independent risk factors for postoperative mortality include the preoperative severity of symptoms and atrial fibrillation.[49]

After aortic valve replacement, symptoms resolve, left ventricular hypertrophy regresses, and systolic function improves.[50,51] Despite the improvement in left ventricular systolic function in the majority of patients after valve replacement, diastolic dysfunction can persist for 6 to 7 years after surgery.[52] Difficult problems in the management of adults with symptomatic aortic stenosis include evaluation of the patient with aortic stenosis and concurrent left ventricular systolic dysfunction (see Chapter 96A) and whether aortic valve replacement should be performed at the time of coronary artery bypass grafting in patients with moderate aortic stenosis (see Chapter 96B).

Ongoing research is evaluating the feasibility of percutaneously placed valves and alternative operative approaches. Cribier and coworkers[53] described the first case of a percutaneously placed aortic valve in a patient with critical aortic stenosis who was not an operative candidate in 2002. The percutaneous valve was made of three bovine pericardial leaflets mounted within a balloon-expandable stent. A subsequent series of 50 patients with severe, inoperable aortic stenosis showed that this approach is feasible, with sustained hemodynamic and clinical benefit.[54]

An alternative operative approach involves placement of a prosthetic valve through the left ventricular apex by a minithoracotomy without the need for cardiopulmonary bypass. Although long-term data are not available, clinical outcome at 6 months is acceptable.[55]

PROGNOSIS

Symptomatic Aortic Stenosis

The prognosis of patients with aortic stenosis depends on the presence or absence of symptoms.[47,56] Asymptomatic patients have a clinical outcome similar to that of age-matched controls without aortic stenosis, and there have been no reports of sudden death as the initial presentation of disease in adults.[24,56] Symptomatic patients with uncorrected aortic stenosis have survival rates of only 15% to 50% at 5 years.[56,57] Once symptoms occur, the risk of sudden death increases dramatically, so valve replacement surgery needs to be performed promptly at symptom onset. In patients who refuse surgery or have severe comorbid conditions making surgery very high risk, the expected clinical course is recurrent hospitalizations for heart failure symptoms or the occurrence of sudden death within a relatively short time.

Disease Progression in Asymptomatic Aortic Stenosis

The etiology of aortic stenosis can be useful in estimating the approximate age at symptom onset. Patients with secondary calcification of a congenitally bicuspid valve become symptomatic at 50 to 60 years; those with degenerative calcification of a trileaflet valve, at 70 to 80 years; and patients with rheumatic aortic disease, at 20 to 50 years.[58,59]

Prospective studies using Doppler echocardiography have further clarified the natural history of asymptomatic patients and made possible the estimation of time to symptom onset based on the Doppler aortic jet velocity. For patients with a baseline aortic jet velocity of greater than 4.0 m/s, 40% develop symptoms of aortic stenosis annually, with a higher rate of symptom onset in patients older than 50 years and those with moderate to severe valve calcification (Figs. 93.10 and 93.11).[24,60] The annual rate of symptom onset is only 8% in patients with an aortic jet velocity of less than 3.0 m/s. Those with an aortic jet velocity between 3 and 4 m/s have an intermediate likelihood of symptom onset; but even in this group, by 4 years, approximately 50% have developed symptoms warranting valve replacement.

Prospective studies evaluating the rate of hemodynamic progression in asymptomatic patients have shown that the average rate of increase in the maximal aortic jet velocity is 0.3 ± 0.3 m/s per year, with an increase in mean gradient of 7 ± 7 mm Hg per year and a decrease in aortic valve area of 0.12 ± 0.19 cm^2 per year.[24,61-63] However, the rate of hemodynamic progression in an individual patient may be more variable, and factors other than the Doppler velocity and aortic valve calcification to predict the rate of progression in an individual patient have not been identified.

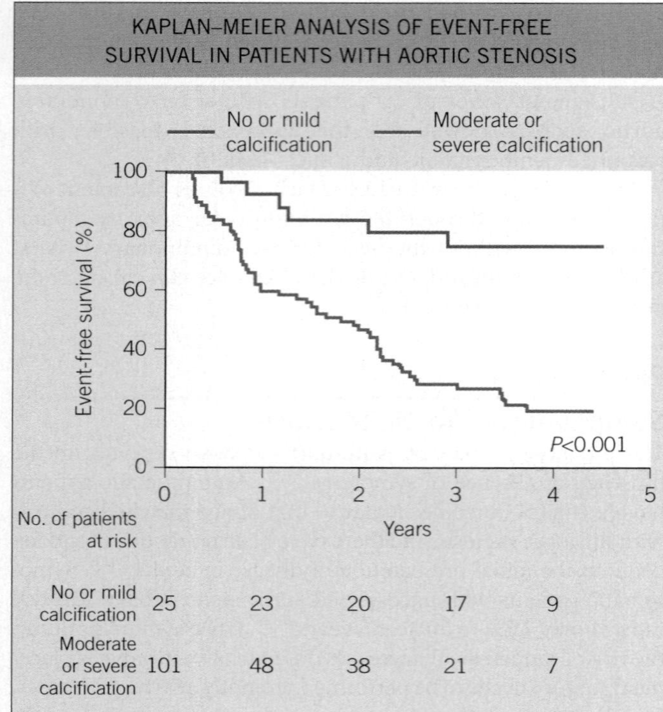

Figure 93.10 Kaplan-Meier analysis of event-free survival in patients with calcification. Kaplan-Meier analysis of event-free survival among 25 patients with mild or no aortic valve calcification compared with 101 patients with moderate or severe calcification. At study entry, all patients were asymptomatic and had a Doppler aortic jet velocity of at least 4 m/s. (From Rosenhek R, Binder T, Porenta G, et al. Predictors of outcome in severe, asymptomatic aortic stenosis. N Engl J Med 2000;343:611-617.)

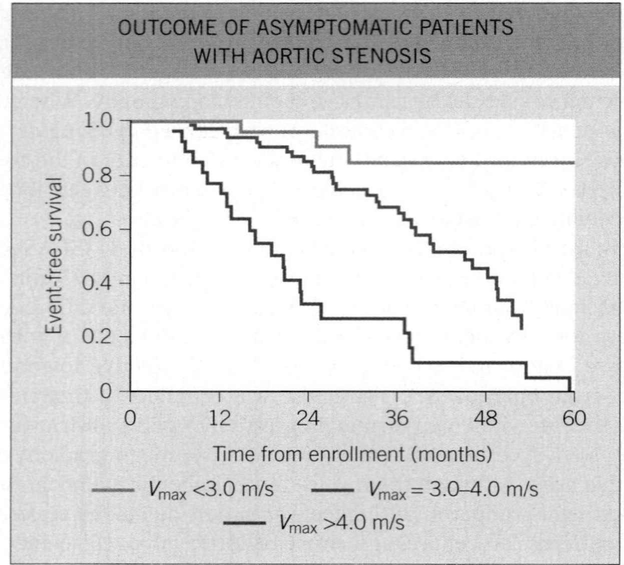

Figure 93.11 Outcome of asymptomatic patients with aortic stenosis as predicted by the aortic jet velocity with Cox regression analysis. (From Otto CM, Burwash IG, Legget ME, et al. Prospective study of asymptomatic valvular aortic stenosis. Clinical, echocardiographic, and exercise predictors of outcome. Circulation 1997;95:2262-2270.)

SUMMARY

Aortic stenosis occurs when there is obstruction to the ejection of blood from the left ventricle. In adults, the obstruction is commonly located at the aortic valve and is caused by degenerative or calcific disease. Aortic stenosis is a slowly progressive disease, with patients remaining asymptomatic for many years. The development of symptoms, including angina, syncope, and congestive heart failure, marks a turn in the disease course characterized by increased mortality without surgical intervention. Physical examination findings that indicate significant aortic stenosis include sustained apical impulse, crescendo-decrescendo systolic murmur, single second heart sound, and abnormal carotid pulse contour. Echocardiography has emerged as the principal method to establish the diagnosis and allows assessment of aortic valve anatomy, severity of valvular obstruction, and left ventricular response to pressure overload.

Aortic valve replacement is the only effective treatment of symptomatic patients. Asymptomatic patients should receive endocarditis prophylaxis, coronary risk factor modification, and education about expected symptoms and disease progression. The potential for medical therapy to slow or to prevent the disease process in the valve leaflets remains unclear.

chapter 94

Acute Aortic Regurgitation

Gerard P. Aurigemma and Theo E. Meyer

Definition

- Acute anatomic disruption of the aortic valve with sudden imposition of a large regurgitant volume on a normal or noncompliant left ventricle.

Key Features

- Causes include infective endocarditis, aortic dissection, and blunt chest trauma.
- Clinical recognition is by pulmonary edema and signs of low output; diastolic murmur of aortic regurgitation may be unimpressive.
- Clinical diagnosis is suggested by radiographic findings of pulmonary edema and normal heart size.
- Definitive diagnosis is usually made by echocardiography.

Therapy

- Urgent surgical management is required; short-term medical stabilization may be helpful in some instances.
- For patients who have bacterial endocarditis, an abbreviated course of antibiotics may be necessary because surgery should not be delayed.

Acute, severe aortic regurgitation is usually a catastrophic medical condition because of the sudden imposition of a large volume load on the left ventricle. Urgent surgical correction is necessary to avoid refractory pulmonary edema or cardiogenic shock. The clinician is most likely to encounter acute, severe aortic regurgitation in patients who have bacterial endocarditis, aortic dissection, or severe blunt chest trauma. This chapter reviews the principal causes of acute aortic regurgitation, its salient diagnostic features, and what, in our judgment, comprises the appropriate management approach for this condition.

ANATOMY AND PATHOLOGY

The causes of acute, severe aortic regurgitation are relatively few (Table 94.1). The most common causes include bacterial endocarditis, acute dissection of the ascending aorta, and blunt chest trauma.[1-6] The frequency with which acute, severe aortic regurgitation complicates bacterial endocarditis is not established, but it is not common. Similarly, aortic regurgitation of varying severity is believed to occur in at least 50% of cases of proximal aortic dissection,[7] but severe aortic regurgitation is not a frequent finding. When severe aortic regurgitation does complicate aortic dissection, it is the result of either disruption of the aortic valve apparatus by the dissecting hematoma or, possibly, interference with normal coaptation of the aortic valve by a prolapsing intimal flap. In instances of severe aortic regurgitation induced by blunt trauma, it has been hypothesized that a sudden increase in intrathoracic pressure, occurring in ventricular diastole, leads to rupture of the aortic valve leaflet or supporting apparatus.[6]

Other, less common causes of acute aortic regurgitation include balloon aortic valvuloplasty,[8] laceration of the aorta,[9] percutaneous balloon dilatation of aortic coarctation,[10] and nonbacterial endocarditis.[11] The aortic valve is also frequently involved in the syndrome of valvulopathy that results from anorectic drugs, a recently described disorder[12]; however, it is as yet unclear to what extent this entity produces acute, severe aortic regurgitation.

PATHOPHYSIOLOGY

The amount of regurgitant flow per beat through an incompetent aortic valve is largely determined by[2,13]

- the area of the regurgitant orifice;
- the diastolic pressure gradient between the aorta and the left ventricle; and
- the duration of diastole.

The hemodynamic consequences of severe aortic regurgitation, in turn, depend on[2,14-16]

- its severity;
- the rapidity with which the regurgitation develops;
- the compliance of the left ventricle; and
- peripheral vascular resistance.

In chronic aortic regurgitation, forward cardiac output and hemodynamics are not altered, despite a regurgitant volume that is similar to that encountered in acute aortic regurgitation. In chronic aortic regurgitation, the left ventricle has time to adapt to the hemodynamic burden, usually through the development of eccentric hypertrophy.[17] In recent-onset aortic regurgitation, however, the unadapted ventricle is subjected to a sudden increase in volume. This increase in volume leads to a precipitous increase in left ventricular diastolic pressure because the ventricle now operates, unlike in chronic aortic regurgitation, on the steep portion of the diastolic pressure-volume curve (Fig. 94.1). The pressure may exceed that of the left atrium, prematurely closing the mitral valve,[18-21] and it may then increase to equilibrate with aortic diastolic pressures, limiting further regurgitation and opening the aortic valve in diastole.

CAUSES OF ACUTE, SEVERE AORTIC REGURGITATION
Infective endocarditis
Aortic dissection
Blunt chest trauma
Miscellaneous
Balloon valvuloplasty
Nonbacterial endocarditis
Valvulopathy caused by anorectic drugs

Table 94.1 Causes of acute, severe aortic regurgitation.

Premature closure of the mitral valve protects the pulmonary vascular bed from markedly increased left ventricular diastolic pressures but limits or prevents effective atrial emptying.[16] Atrial contraction against a closed mitral valve leads to an increase in pulmonary venous pressure. However, when heart rate is increased to such an extent that atrial emptying occurs earlier in diastole (at the time when the mitral valve is still open), left atrial pressure decreases.[20] A competent mitral valve appears to be essential to the effectiveness of premature mitral closure in protecting the pulmonary vascular bed from the direct transmission of the significantly increased left ventricular diastolic pressures. If mitral regurgitation supervenes, this protection is lost, leading to marked increase in left atrial pressures and to a decrease in cardiac output.[2,14,16,20]

The forward stroke volume decreases and cardiac output is maintained through compensatory tachycardia. Pulmonary edema and circulatory collapse may occur because of the reduced stroke volume and the dramatic increase in left ventricular diastolic pressure. The situation is probably exacerbated in patients who have preexisting conditions that are associated with reduced left ventricular compliance (e.g.,

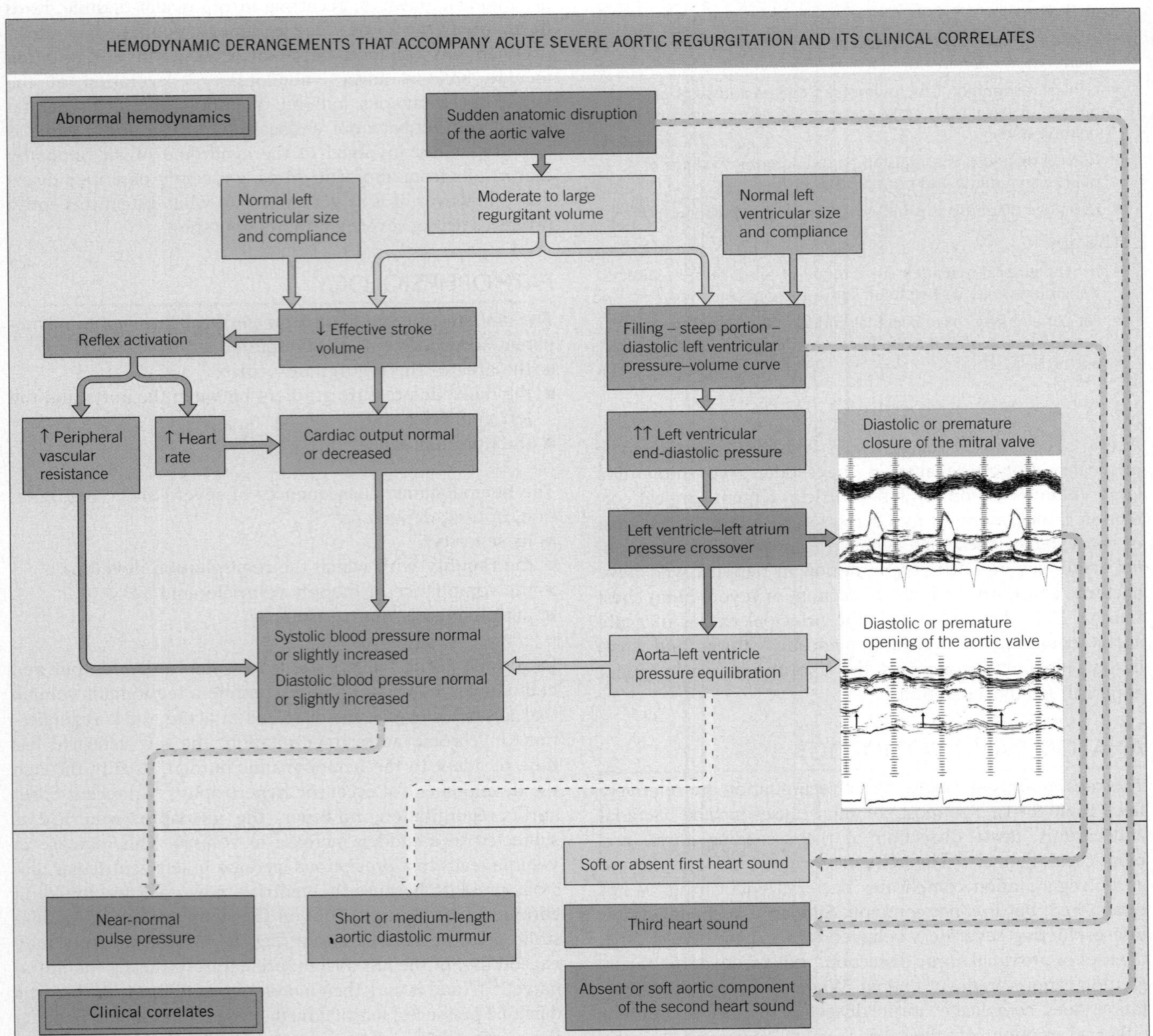

Figure 94.1 Hemodynamic derangements that accompany acute, severe aortic regurgitation and its clinical correlates.

hypertensive heart disease or coronary heart disease) because these people may have an even higher increase in left ventricular filling pressures.

CLINICAL PRESENTATIONS

Common Scenarios

Acute, severe aortic regurgitation should be considered in the differential diagnosis of all patients who suffer sudden unexplained hemodynamic collapse and respiratory failure. In our experience, these patients generally fit into one of three clinical categories:

- established aortic valve endocarditis with acute worsening of heart failure;
- acute aortic dissection; and
- blunt chest trauma with pulmonary congestion.

Perhaps the most common scenario in which acute, severe aortic regurgitation is encountered is in the patient with established aortic valve endocarditis who manifests acute worsening of heart failure. Variations of this situation, in which the bedside diagnosis may be difficult, may also occur. For example, patients who do not have an established diagnosis of endocarditis may present with fever, cardiorespiratory failure, and positive blood cultures. The murmur of acute, severe aortic regurgitation—which, even under ideal circumstances, may be unimpressive for the reasons cited later—may not be appreciated or may be obscured by noise associated with mechanical ventilation or loud rhonchi. A chest radiograph that shows pulmonary edema and a normal heart size may be the only clue to alert the clinician to the diagnosis in this setting.

The second scenario in which acute, severe aortic regurgitation is encountered is the patient with acute aortic dissection. In this instance, there is usually a history of sudden, severe back pain coupled with neurologic signs or absent pulses. When aortic regurgitation is present, it is likely to result in pulmonary edema and a compromised respiratory status.

Finally, acute, severe aortic regurgitation may complicate blunt chest trauma (e.g., striking the steering wheel in the course of a motor vehicle accident) and should be considered if the patient presents with pulmonary congestion. A new diastolic murmur, particularly if it is accompanied by chest radiographic signs of pulmonary edema, should alert the clinician to the diagnosis. However, as noted before, even if the murmur is not appreciated, the constellation of blunt chest trauma and pulmonary congestion should also raise suspicion of traumatic disruption of the aortic valve.

Auscultation

Many of the physical findings that are characteristic of chronic, severe aortic regurgitation are absent in acute aortic regurgitation. This is because most of the classic findings in chronic, severe aortic regurgitation depend on a widened pulse pressure (see Chapter 95). In acute aortic regurgitation, the pulse pressure is usually reduced owing to a reduced stroke volume and increased peripheral vascular resistance (see Fig. 94.1). Similarly, the diastolic murmur of aortic regurgitation may be abbreviated because the aortic pressure and the left ventricular diastolic pressure equilibrate rapidly. Tachycardia is usually present, and the first heart sound may be soft or absent as a result of premature closure of the mitral valve. A diastolic gallop (third heart sound) and Duroziez's sign[21] (see Chapter 95) are likely to be present.

DIAGNOSTIC TECHNIQUES

The diagnosis of acute, severe aortic regurgitation may not be considered unless the clinician pays attention to clues provided by the history, physical examination, and chest radiograph. Once the diagnosis is considered, in most instances, a comprehensive two-dimensional echocardiographic study, with transesophageal echocardiography if the transthoracic study is suboptimal, will usually provide the diagnosis. In most instances, echocardiography will also provide definition of the anatomic abnormality and characterization of the hemodynamic severity of aortic regurgitation.

The noninvasive assessment of aortic regurgitation includes an indirect assessment of the hemodynamic burden of the regurgitant volume load. The most straightforward method is to assess the timing of mitral valve closure. Premature closure of the mitral valve, indicating significantly increased left ventricular filling pressures, can be easily demonstrated by M-mode echocardiography (see Fig. 94.1). A caveat is that this echocardiographic sign may not be apparent when the heart rate is increased. Early closure of the mitral valve has been used to identify patients who require semiurgent surgery (Fig. 94.2).

Recent developments in two-dimensional echocardiography together with the advent of transesophageal echocardiography permit detailed anatomic examination of the incompetent aortic valve (Fig. 94.3). Echocardiographic examination of the aortic valve in bacterial endocarditis generally shows evidence of infection and may show evidence of extravalvular extension. In acute aortic regurgitation caused by acute dissection, the echocardiogram may disclose the mechanism of aortic regurgitation (Figs. 94.4 and 94.5).

Spectral and color-flow Doppler techniques are used to obtain a semiquantitative estimate of the severity of aortic regurgitation. According to the widely quoted color-flow grading scheme published by Perry and colleagues,[22] the width of the regurgitant stream at its origin relative to the size of the left ventricular outflow tract gives the best agreement with semiquantitative grading from contrast aortography. A ratio of the height of the aortic regurgitation jet to the height of the left ventricular outflow tract that exceeds 0.65 was found to be almost always associated with severe aortic regurgitation as assessed by contrast angiography.

Spectral Doppler (pulsed and continuous wave) techniques are also used to quantify the severity of aortic regurgitation. These techniques are particularly important when two-dimensional imaging is suboptimal. With the continuous-wave Doppler technique, signs of severe aortic regurgitation include a rapid deceleration of the spectral envelope of aortic regurgitation, with a pressure half-time of less than 300 ms.[21] Alternatively, the actual deceleration slope of the aortic regurgitation spectral display may be used, and a deceleration slope of more than 3.5 m/s^2 will separate severe aortic regurgitation from milder grades.[22] In addition, the mitral deceleration time may also be short (<150 ms), reflecting the rapid increase in diastolic pressures in the left ventricle.

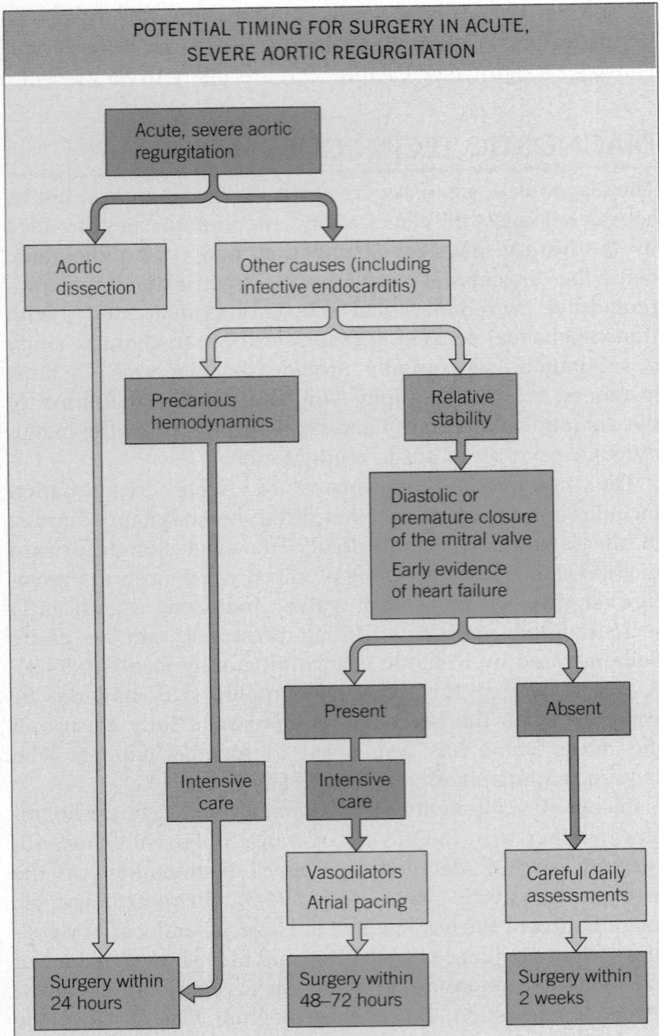

Figure 94.2 Potential timing for surgery in acute, severe aortic regurgitation.

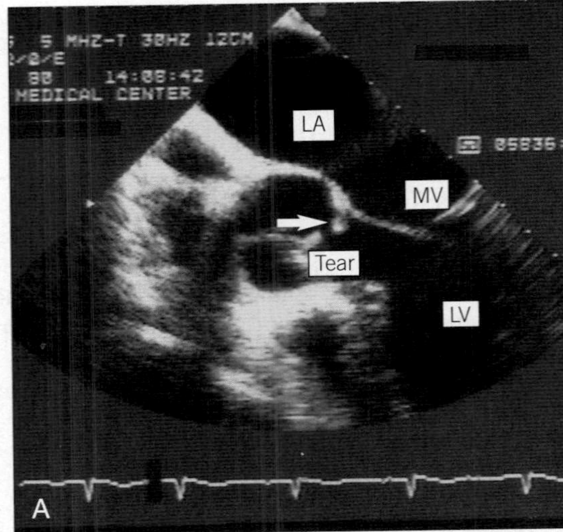

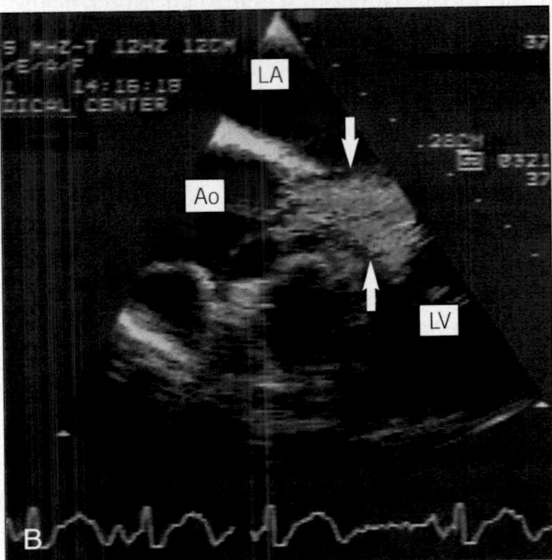

Figure 94.3 Acute, severe aortic regurgitation resulting from trauma. Transesophageal echocardiographic studies from a 68-year-old man who was involved in a motor vehicle accident in which he sustained severe thoracic and flank trauma. The physical examination on admission revealed evidence of pulmonary congestion and aortic regurgitation. The chest radiograph showed a normal heart size and pulmonary edema. The transesophageal echocardiographic study was performed to give a better idea of the cause of the aortic regurgitation. **A,** The aortic valve shows a tear in its noncoronary cusp *(arrow)*. The probe is in the esophagus. **B,** Color-flow mapping, in an orientation similar to that in **A**, demonstrates diastolic turbulence that encompasses the entire left ventricular outflow tract *(arrows)*. This finding is compatible with severe aortic regurgitation. Ao, aorta; LA, left atrium; LV, left ventricle; MV, mitral valve.

As a practical matter, much of the diagnostic evaluation that was provided in the past by invasive hemodynamics is now furnished by a complete echocardiographic examination. In our medical center, when the diagnosis of acute, severe aortic regurgitation is made on clinical grounds and supported by echocardiographic findings, invasive study serves mostly to confirm the hemodynamic findings provided by Doppler echocardiography. There are instances when valve surgery is undertaken on the basis of the clinical and echocardiographic findings alone. However, catheterization may be necessary to document the extent of coronary artery disease.

MANAGEMENT

Almost all patients with acute aortic regurgitation are hemodynamically compromised, even if at first glance they appear to be stable. The burden of sudden, severe volume overload inevitably leads to pulmonary edema and early death. There is, therefore, consensus that acute, severe aortic regurgitation frequently constitutes a surgical emergency.[2,23] As noted before, the early recognition of this clinical syndrome and its correct management are essential to ensure a good outcome for the patient. Earlier (rather than later) surgical intervention generally improves results and prevents the long-term complications of delayed operations in anatomically complex patients, once an accurate preoperative diagnosis is made and initial stabilization with medical therapy has been achieved. The inherent operative risk is far greater for this group of patients than for those who have chronic, severe aortic regurgitation because they are seriously ill at the time of the operation and have coexisting pathologic abnormalities, such as infective endocarditis or aortic dissection, that add to the complexity of the operation.

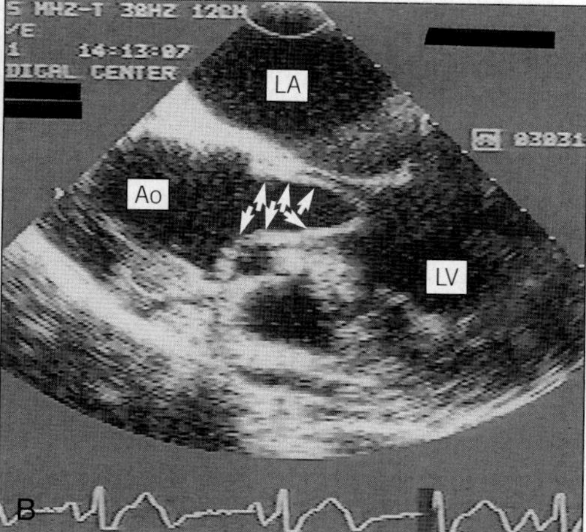

Figure 94.4 Acute, severe aortic regurgitation resulting from aortic dissection. Transesophageal echocardiographic images showing an intimal flap in a 79-year-old woman with acute aortic dissection. **A,** Systolic frame shows dilated aortic root and intimal flap *(arrows)*. **B,** In diastole, the intimal flap *(arrows)* prolapses across the aortic valve, contributing to aortic regurgitation. Ao, aorta; LA, left atrium; LV, left ventricle.

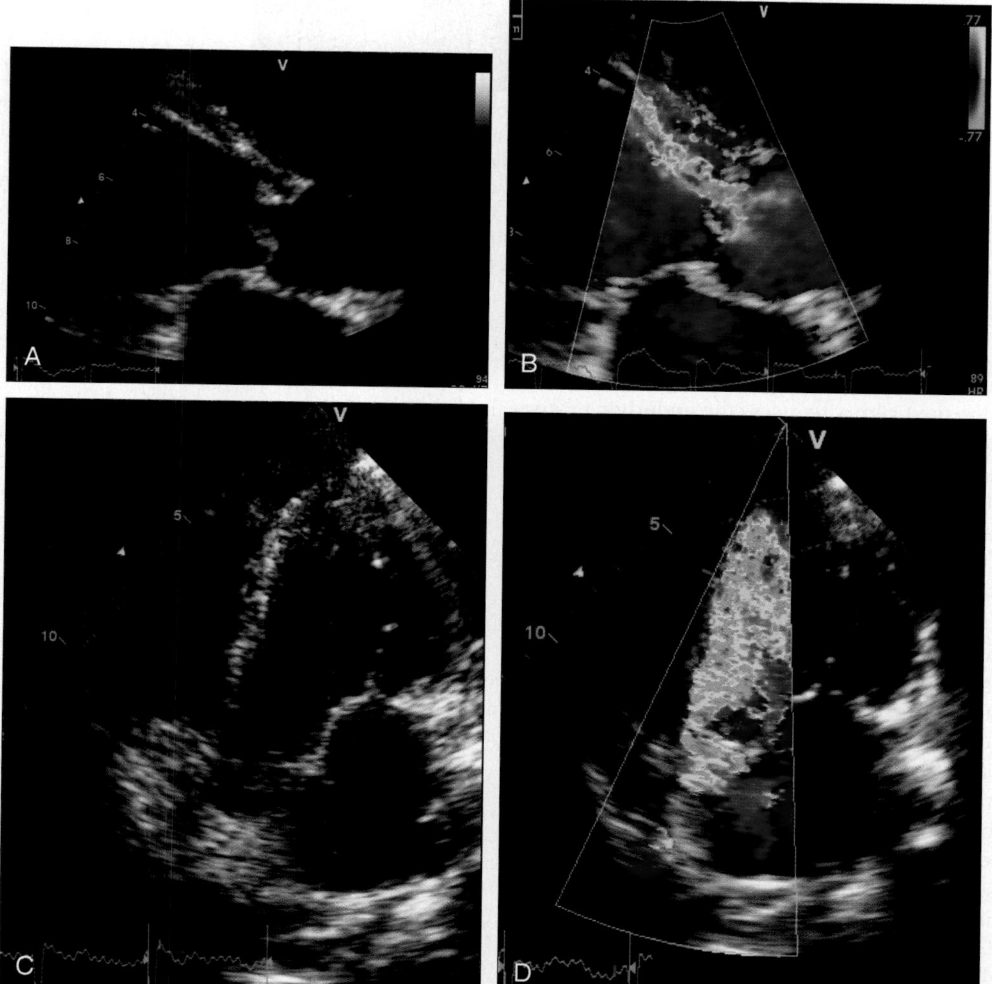

Figure 94.5 Images from the study of a 46-year-old man with aortic valve endocarditis caused by *Staphylococcus aureus*. **A,** Multiple vegetations affect both the right and noncoronary cusps, leading to complete leaflet malcoaptation. **B,** Image taken at a similar phase of the cardiac cycle shows the jet of aortic regurgitation, directed toward the interventricular septum. **C** and **D,** Apical five-chamber views with and without color-flow mapping of the regurgitant jet. Note that the spatial extent of the jet of aortic regurgitation is such that the entire left ventricular outflow tract is encompassed by color, and the turbulent flow extends to the apical region of the left ventricle.

(Continued)

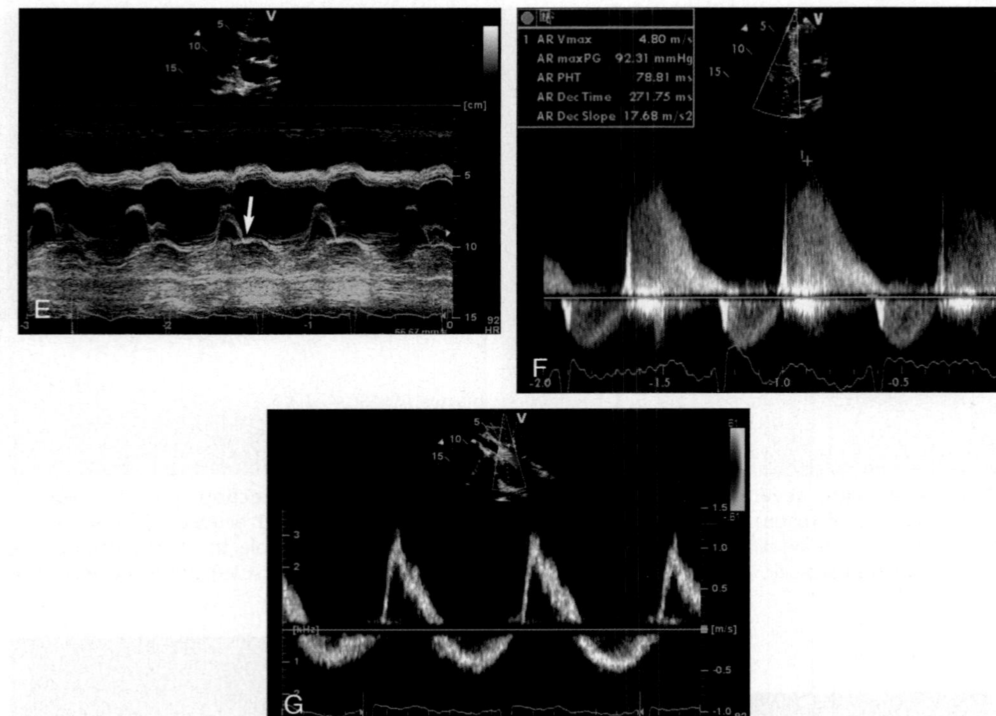

Figure 94.5—cont'd E, M-mode echocardiogram of the mitral valve in the same patient. There is early closure of the mitral valve *(arrow),* consistent with equalization of diastolic pressures in the left ventricle. **F** and **G,** Transaortic valve **(F)** and descending aortic **(G)** continuous-wave Doppler study in the same patient. The continuous-wave Doppler study shows extremely rapid equilibration of flow across the aortic valve. The deceleration slope of this signal is 1.7 m/s^2, and the pressure half-time is 78 ms. Values greater than 3.5 m/s^2 for the slope of this signal and less than 200 ms for the pressure half-time are indicative of severe aortic regurgitation. Also note that the regurgitation signal is extremely bright, an important indirect sign of severe aortic regurgitation.

Once the diagnosis of acute, severe aortic regurgitation has been established, the next step is to assess the underlying cause and hemodynamic state of the patient. Because these patients are usually hemodynamically unstable and in respiratory distress, initial stabilization is required in the intensive care unit before the diagnostic work-up for the underlying cause is commenced. Medical treatment is directed at reducing pulmonary venous congestion and maximizing cardiac output in an attempt to stabilize the hemodynamics before surgery.

Intravenous vasodilator therapy with nitroprusside can be effective in this regard. Increasing the heart rate by atrial pacing has also been shown to decrease regurgitant volume, left ventricular end-diastolic pressure, and pulmonary venous pressure in patients who have severe aortic regurgitation.[24] The principal aim of medical treatment is to optimize the patient's preoperative clinical status rather than to provide definitive treatment, which may potentially delay surgery.

The timing of surgery should be based on the hemodynamic status of the patient and the underlying cause. For example, when acute aortic regurgitation is secondary to aortic dissection, surgery within 24 hours should be contemplated. Similarly, surgery is also indicated within 24 hours if attempts at stabilizing the patient are unsuccessful. The echocardiographic finding of early closure of the mitral valve and the presence of pulmonary edema, which are clinical indicators of markedly increased left ventricular diastolic pressures, also mandate relatively early surgical intervention (within 48 to 72 hours). In the absence of early closure of the mitral valve or heart failure, careful daily assessments for hemodynamic deterioration or progression of disease are essential. These patients will require surgery, and it is best performed sooner rather than later (within 2 weeks of the onset of acute aortic regurgitation). Figure 94.2 summarizes the timing and treatment plan for acute regurgitation.

Severe aortic regurgitation secondary to infective endocarditis deserves special mention. In the past, there has been a reluctance among surgeons to operate early on patients who have infective endocarditis because of the presence of infected, friable tissue and hemodynamic instability. It was believed that implantation of a prosthesis in an infected area may lead to prosthetic endocarditis. These concerns have been shown to be unfounded, as judged by the results from several centers.[25,26] The overall operative mortality (<8%) and the incidence of prosthetic endocarditis (<10%) are low,[25,26] which reaffirms that procrastination in referral for surgery is not justified.

PROGNOSIS

Mortality with medical treatment is high (75%).[2] Early surgical intervention is therefore necessary. Because of the coexisting pathologic abnormalities, such as infective endocarditis and aortic dissection, mortality and morbidity in the first year after surgery amount to 25%.

SUMMARY

The clinician is most likely to encounter acute, severe aortic regurgitation, a life-threatening cardiovascular emergency, in the setting of aortic dissection, infective endocarditis, or blunt chest trauma. In these settings, severe increases in left ventricular filling pressures are occasioned by the marked increase in diastolic volume, in either a normal left ventricle or a noncompliant left ventricle (e.g., if there is a previous history of coronary or hypertensive heart disease). Therefore, patients who have acute, severe aortic regurgitation are likely to present with signs of pulmonary congestion and a low cardiac output but with a normal-sized heart on chest radiography. The physical examination, which can be rendered suboptimal in the setting of acute respiratory failure and mechanical ventilation, is remarkable for signs of hemodynamic compromise and pulmonary edema. The characteristic features of chronic, severe aortic regurgitation that relate to a widened pulse pressure and a long diastolic murmur are often absent with recent-onset aortic regurgitation.

The diagnosis is usually made by echocardiography, with use of the transesophageal approach when necessary. Urgent surgical management is the definitive treatment, after an initial period of medical stabilization.

chapter 95

Chronic Aortic Regurgitation

Walter J. Paulus

Definition

- Chronic aortic regurgitation implies the presence of chronic diastolic reflux of blood from the aorta into the left ventricle.

Key Features

- The most frequent causes of chronic aortic regurgitation are connective tissue disorders with dilatation of the aortic root, congenital heart disease, infective endocarditis, and rheumatic fever.
- It is frequently well tolerated, and during this asymptomatic period, the left ventricle progressively enlarges.

Treatment

- Surgical correction with aortic valve replacement is indicated in the presence of symptoms (dyspnea or angina) or with evidence of left ventricular dysfunction (left ventricular ejection fraction of less than 55% or left ventricular end-systolic internal dimension of more than 55 mm).

Chronic aortic regurgitation is characterized by chronic diastolic reflux of blood from the aortic root into the left ventricle because of malcoaptation of the cusps of the aortic valve as a result of

- shortening and retraction of the cusps, as occurs during rheumatic fever–induced valvular fibrosis; or
- dilatation of the aortic annulus, as occurs in certain connective tissue disorders.

ETIOLOGY AND PATHOLOGIC ANATOMY

Rheumatic Fever

Rheumatic fever is an important cause of aortic regurgitation. After the acute inflammation, valve leaflets become thickened and rigid, which leads to commissural retraction and fusion. Depending on the relative importance of aortic cusp retraction or fusion, regurgitation, stenosis, or mixed disease will dominate the clinical picture.

Syphilis

Aortic regurgitation accompanying syphilitic aortitis is rare. Leaflet retraction, cusp prolapse, and annular dilatation all appear to be involved. Other features of syphilitic aortitis include coronary osteal stenoses, linear calcifications of the ascending aorta on chest radiography, and saccular aneurysm of the ascending aorta.

Infective Endocarditis

Infective endocarditis usually results in massive and acute aortic regurgitation because of commissural vegetation, leaflet destruction, and leaflet perforation. Some forms of endocarditis, however, follow a chronic course (endocarditis lenta) that is characterized by more prominent tissue granulation and formation of valvular vegetations. Aortic infective endocarditis can occur on an apparently normal valve, but more frequently it occurs on a congenitally or rheumatically deformed valve or as a result of infection spreading from neighboring structures.

Aortic Sclerocalcific Disease

Calcium deposits of aortic sclerocalcific disease deform the aortic valve. This most frequently results in leaflet rigidity and aortic stenosis, but leaflet malcoaptation and aortic regurgitation may also occur.[1] Both clinical and experimental studies suggest that aortic sclerocalcific disease is a valvular manifestation of an active inflammatory process, similar to atherosclerosis.[2] Inflammatory injury induces production of matrix metalloproteinase 9 and tissue inhibitor of matrix metalloproteinase 1. Inflammatory response is more severe in aortic stenosis than in aortic regurgitation. In 27% of centenarian hearts, aortic regurgitation is present.[3]

Aortic Dissection

Aortic regurgitation in the presence of dissection of the ascending aorta is usually acute and results from prolapse and loss of attachment to the aortic wall of a sinus of Valsalva. In Marfan's syndrome, aortic regurgitation in the presence of dissection of the ascending aorta can sometimes be unrelated to the dissection process but caused by annular dilatation.

Trauma

Aortic regurgitation is the most common traumatic cardiac valvulopathy. It results from a direct thoracic impact or from sudden deceleration. The mechanism appears to be that the column of blood in the ascending aorta hits the closed aortic valve and causes rupture of one of the leaflets.

Connective Tissue Disorders

In patients who have aortic cystic medial necrosis (either isolated or associated with classic Marfan's syndrome), Ehlers-Danlos syndrome, or osteogenesis imperfecta, aortic regurgitation is the result of dilatation of the aortic annulus, which accompanies dilatation of the proximal portion of the ascending aorta. In patients who have ankylosing spondylitis, rheumatoid or psoriatic arthritis, or Reiter's syndrome, both annular dilatation and valvular inflammation-fibrosis contribute to the aortic insufficiency.

Congenital Heart Disease

Chronic aortic regurgitation can be present in patients who have congenital cardiac or aortic malformations, such as

- bicuspid or quadricuspid aortic valves;
- aortic valvular fenestrations;
- supravalvular aortic stenosis;
- membranous or tunnel-type subaortic stenosis;
- aneurysm of the sinus of Valsalva;
- coarctation of the aorta;
- subpulmonary and membranous ventricular septal defect; and
- congenital aneurysm of the membranous interventricular septum.

Reduced aortic elasticity and aortic root dilatation are frequently present in bicuspid aortic valves.[4] In coarctation of the aorta, arterial hypertension contributes to aortic annular dilatation. In subpulmonary or membranous ventricular septal defect and aneurysm of the interventricular septum, prolapse of the right or noncoronary aortic valve cusp because of lack of ventricular supporting structures hinders aortic leaflet coaptation. Chronic aortic regurgitation can also occur as a sequela of balloon valvuloplasty for congenital aortic stenosis.

Appetite-Suppressant Drugs

Multivalvular heart disease involving aortic, mitral, and tricuspid valves was first described in obese women who had been treated with the appetite-suppressant combination of fenfluramine and phentermine.[5] In patients who had undergone valve replacement, the pathologic findings resembled those of carcinoid heart disease, with proliferation of myofibroblastic cells with myxoid stroma. Subsequently, valvular insufficiency and, especially, aortic regurgitation were also demonstrated after use of fenfluramine alone or after use of dexfenfluramine either alone or in combination with phentermine.[6-8] The risk of significant valvular heart disease varies from 5% to 15% and depends on both dose and duration (>6 months) of the treatment with appetite-suppressant drug.[9]

Ergot-Derived Dopamine Receptor Agonists

Ergot-derived dopamine receptor agonists (pergolide, cabergoline) are often used in the treatment of Parkinson's disease and are associated with an increased risk of mitral regurgitation (six times the risk), aortic regurgitation (four times the risk), and tricuspid regurgitation (five times the risk). A higher risk is associated with higher cumulative dose.[10,11] High affinity of pergolide and of cabergoline for 5-hydroxytryptamine type 2B serotonin receptors is again involved.

Antiphospholipid Syndrome

Antiphospholipid syndrome is characterized by increased concentrations of antiphospholipid antibodies, venous or arterial thromboses, obstetric complications with recurrent fetal loss, and thrombocytopenia. Antiphospholipid syndrome is termed secondary in the context of an autoimmune disease such as systemic lupus erythematosus, a malignant neoplasm, or a drug-induced condition; it is termed primary in the absence of such an underlying disorder. The antiphospholipid antibodies contribute to the development of valvular lesions, as is evident from subendothelial deposits of immunoglobulins and complement in the deformed valves of patients who have antiphospholipid syndrome.[12] The morphologic alterations of the valvular lesions observed in patients who have antiphospholipid syndrome include sterile verrucose vegetations, as originally described by Libman and Sacks,[13] and valvular thickening. These two morphologic types of valvular lesion probably represent different stages of the same pathologic process.

Mediastinal Irradiation

Mediastinal irradiation can lead to fibrosis, thickening, and calcification of the aortic valve leaflets, sometimes necessitating aortic valve surgery.[14,15]

Prevalence and Relative Frequency of Causes of Chronic Aortic Regurgitation

Among a sample group of middle-aged to older adults, mild aortic regurgitation occurred in 7.3%, moderate in 2.4%, and severe in 0.3%.[16] In a study[17] of predictors for valve replacement in a large cohort (n = 104) of patients with chronic aortic regurgitation, the different causes of chronic aortic regurgitation were distributed as follows:

- connective tissue disorders with dilatation of the aortic root: 25%;
- congenital heart disease: 13%;
- rheumatic fever: 12%;
- infective endocarditis: 10%;
- aortic sclerocalcific disease: 7%; and
- unknown etiology: 35%.

A similar distribution of causes was recently also reported in patients undergoing aortic valve replacement in a tertiary referral center.[18]

PATHOPHYSIOLOGY

Assessment of the Severity of Aortic Regurgitation

Quantification of the severity of aortic regurgitation has been a challenge to clinicians since its original description. In his treatise on aortic regurgitation, Corrigan[19] noted that "the quantity of blood that regurgitates will be largely in proportion to the degree of inadequacy of the valves and to the length of the pause between contractions of the ventricle during which blood can be pouring back."

Quantitative Assessment of the Severity of Aortic Regurgitation

The following methods are used for quantitative assessment of the severity of aortic regurgitation:

- qualitative grading (grade 1 to grade 4) of regurgitant volume by supravalvular aortography;

- calculation of the regurgitant volume and regurgitant fraction;
- measurement of aortoventricular pressure half-time;
- measurement of the width of the regurgitant jet or of the vena contracta;
- mapping of the regurgitant jet within the left ventricle; and
- measurement of the effective aortic regurgitant orifice area.

Qualitative Grading of Regurgitant Volume by Supravalvular Aortography

The subjective observation of aortic incompetence during supravalvular aortography is usually expressed in four degrees of severity (grade 1 to grade 4) as illustrated in Figure 95.1.[20]

Such qualitative grading of regurgitant volume by supravalvular aortography correlates poorly with regurgitant volume, especially in the presence of left ventricular (LV) enlargement, which dilutes LV opacification by the regurgitant aortic flow.[21]

Calculation of the Regurgitant Volume and Regurgitant Fraction

In the cardiac catheterization laboratory, regurgitant volume is derived from the difference between the angiographic LV stroke volume and the Fick or thermodilution stroke volume.[22] Dividing the regurgitant volume by the body surface area produces the regurgitant volume index (Table 95.1). The regurgitant fraction corresponds to the regurgitant volume divided by the angiographic stroke volume (see Table 95.1).

These measurements are subject to several sources of error resulting from determination of cardiac output and quantification of LV volumes.

Measurement of Aortoventricular Pressure Half-time

Diastolic flow velocities can be obtained from the LV outflow tract by continuous-wave Doppler studies. These diastolic flow velocities correspond to the diastolic LV-aortic pressure gradient; the more rapid the downslope of the diastolic flow velocity, the more severe the aortic regurgitation (see Chapter 86).

Measurement of the Width of the Regurgitant Jet

By use of color Doppler echocardiography, the width of the regurgitant jet can be determined,[23] and the ratio of regurgitant jet diameter to LV outflow tract diameter can be calculated.

Mapping of the Regurgitant Jet within the Left Ventricle

Numerous studies suggest that the area of the regurgitant flow on two-dimensional color-flow mapping corresponds to the angiographic grade of valvular insufficiency and with the regurgitant volume.[24] Pitfalls in extrapolating the regurgitant flow area to the degree of valvular insufficiency include the visualization of a turbulent zone of blood that is being moved or pushed by the regurgitant volume and that is not part of the regurgitant volume itself and the high dependency of the size of the regurgitant jet on velocity of flow or arterial afterload. Indeed, increasing afterload has a significant effect on the regurgitant flow area beyond what would be expected for the change in regurgitant volume.

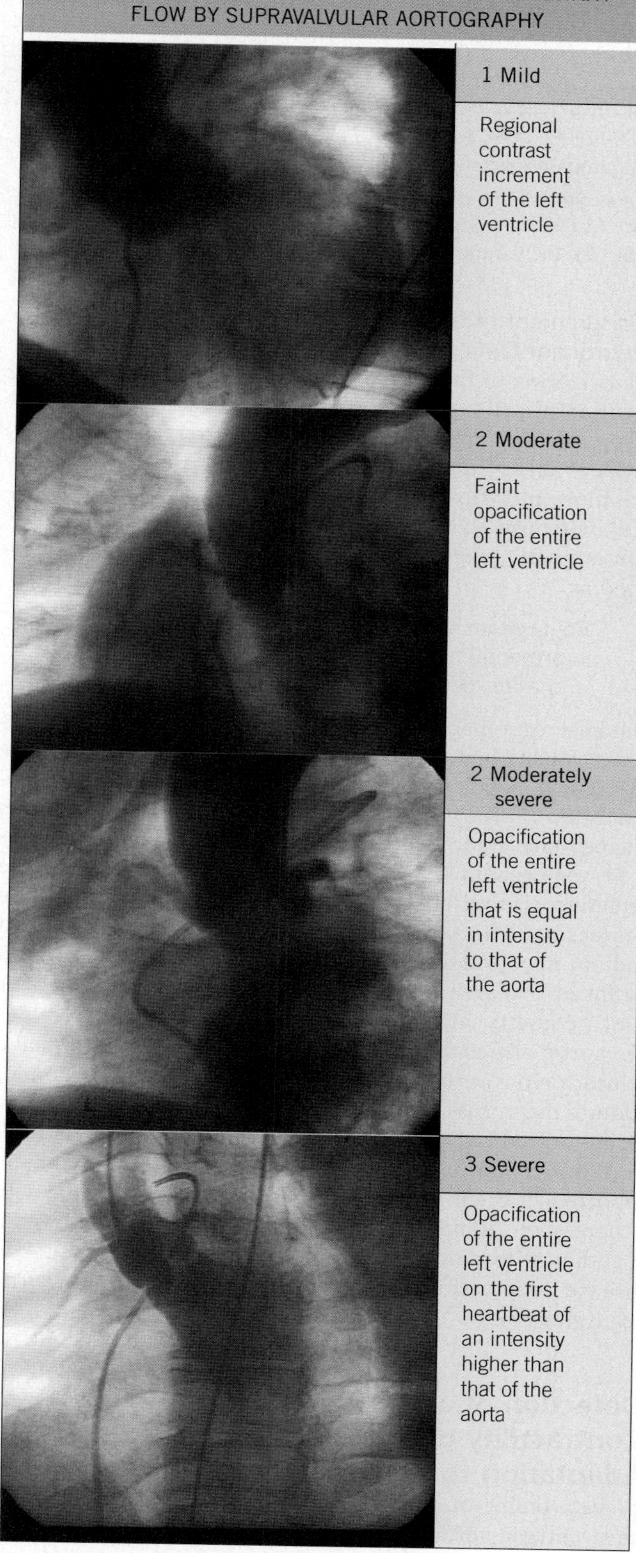

Figure 95.1 Qualitative grading of aortic valve regurgitant flow by supravalvular aortography.

QUANTITATIVE INDEXES OF AORTIC REGURGITATION				
	Aortic Regurgitation Grade			
Measure	**1 (mild)**	**2 (moderate)**	**3 (moderately severe)**	**4 (severe)**
Regurgitant volume index (mL/min per m^2)	<700	700-1700	1700-3000	>3000
Regurgitant fraction (%)	0-20	20-40	40-60	>60
Regurgitant aortic orifice area (cm^2)	<0.1	0.1-0.5	0.5-1.0	>1.0

Table 95.1 Quantitative indexes of aortic regurgitation.

Measurement of the Effective Aortic Regurgitant Orifice Area

Visualization of the acceleration flow area proximal to the regurgitant orifice can be obtained by Doppler color-flow mapping. This method calculates a proximal isovelocity surface area from the display of an aliasing velocity Doppler color-flow map proximal to the regurgitant orifice, with use of a hemispheric or hemielliptic model.[25] Subsequently, regurgitant volume flow rate can be calculated as

$$\text{Regurgitant volume flow rate (in L/min)} \\ = \text{proximal isovelocity surface area (in cm}^2) \\ \times \text{ aliasing velocity (in cm/s)} \times 0.06$$

Maximal regurgitant orifice area can be calculated as the regurgitant volume flow rate divided by maximal continuous-wave regurgitant Doppler flow velocity recorded within the regurgitant orifice.[26] The regurgitant aortic orifice area increases with angiographic grade (see Table 95.1).[27]

In experimental models of aortic regurgitation, the effective regurgitant aortic orifice area was reduced by decreasing arterial blood pressure during infusion of sodium nitroprusside.[28] This dynamic nature of the regurgitant orifice area may be secondary to a change in aortic root geometry at lower arterial pressure and resembles the aortic orifice variability observed in patients who have sclerocalcific aortic valvular stenosis during infusion of sodium nitroprusside.[29] In patients who have chronic aortic regurgitation, progressive enlargement of the regurgitant orifice during several years of follow-up has been reported.[30] Such enlargement is probably secondary to progressive dilatation of the aortic root[31] and could, together with deterioration of LV function, contribute to disease progression in patients who have chronic aortic regurgitation.

Detection of a Decline in Myocardial Contractility during Left Ventricular Adaptation to Volume Overload

Correct timing of aortic valve replacement in patients who have chronic aortic regurgitation and minimal or no symptoms implies early detection of a decline in myocardial contractility during the process of LV adaptation to the chronic volume overload of aortic regurgitation. Once myocardial contractility has become depressed, it will remain impaired even after valve replacement, and the patient will progress to congestive heart failure and premature death despite valve replacement.

Markers that have been proposed for the detection of declining myocardial contractility during LV volume overload of chronic aortic regurgitation are

- measures of the LV end-systolic pressure-volume (LVESP-LVESV) relationship;
- tissue Doppler LV long-axis shortening velocity;
- hemodynamic changes during exercise;
- elevated heart failure biomarkers; and
- alterations in myocardial gene expression.

Measures of the LV End-Systolic Pressure-Volume Relationship

The slope of the LVESP-LVESV relationship is a sensitive measure of LV contractility and is relatively independent of LV preload and afterload (Fig. 95.2). Determination of this slope is cumbersome and requires construction of at least two LV pressure-volume loops, one at rest and one after a pharmacologic intervention such as an intravenous infusion of sodium nitroprusside or phenylephrine. Numerous investigators have therefore tried to obtain similar information about LV performance from a single measurement of LV end-systolic performance. These measurements include

- LV end-systolic short-axis internal dimension (LVESID) and LVESV;
- the ratio of LVESP to LVESV and the ratio of LV peak systolic pressure (LVPSP) to LVESV; and
- the ratio of LV end-systolic wall stress (LVESWS) to LVESV and the ratio of LVESWS to LV ejection fraction (LVEF).

LV End-Systolic Short-Axis Internal Dimension and Volume

LV dimensions and volume at end-systole are independent of preload and vary only with afterload. End-systolic LV dimensions and volume have therefore been proposed as indexes of LV myocardial contractility in patients who have LV volume overload of chronic aortic regurgitation and as predictors of surgical outcome.[32-35] The use of end-systolic LV dimensions and volume as indexes of contractility assumes no derangement of LV afterload. This assumption is open to criticism because LV afterload measured as LV end-systolic myocardial wall stress (LVESWS) is greater in patients with chronic aortic regurgitation than it is in normal individuals and in patients with chronic mitral regurgitation.[36,37] This characteristic "afterload mismatch"[38] of chronic aortic regurgitation should be taken into account when LV end-systolic dimensions and volume are used as a guide to postoperative prognosis. This is because correction of the afterload mismatch by valve replacement could induce a larger improvement in LV end-systolic dimensions or volume than is predicted by preoperative measurements.

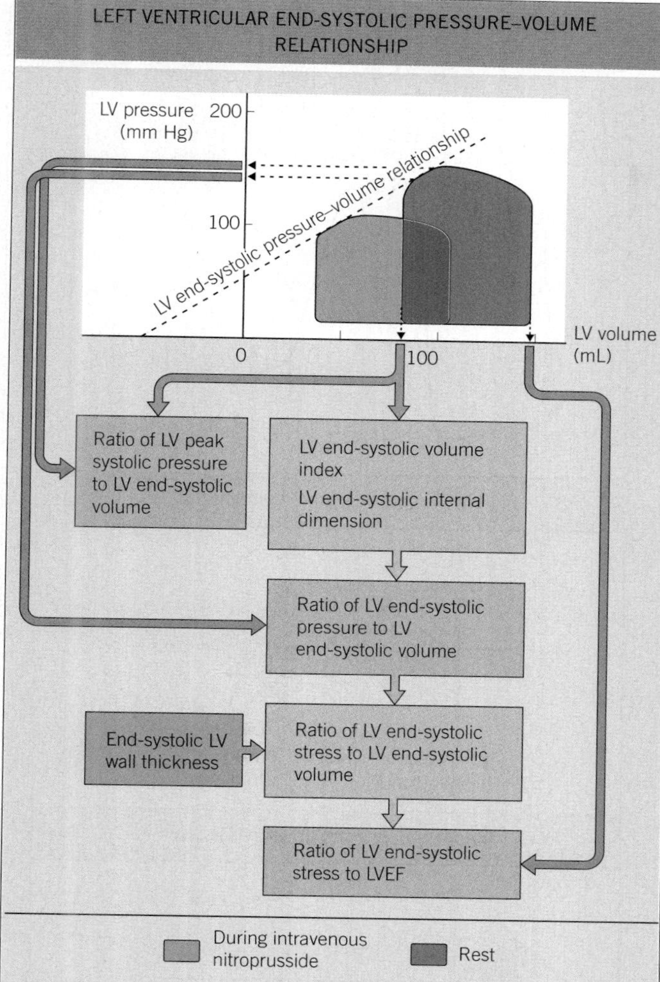

Figure 95.2 Use of the left ventricular end-systolic pressure-volume relationship for detection of left ventricular dysfunction in chronic aortic regurgitation. LVEF, left ventricular ejection fraction.

LV End-Systolic Pressure/Volume and LV Peak Systolic Pressure/End-Systolic Volume Ratios

In an attempt to correct for afterload variability, investigators used the ratio of LVESP to LVESV and the ratio of LVPSP to LVESV as measures of the LVESP-LVESV relationship.[39] For the ratio generated by a single point measurement to reflect the slope of a linear relation, the linear relation has to pass through the origin of the pressure-volume axes. This condition is not satisfied in clinical practice, in which the intercept of the LVESP-LVESV relation with the volume axis is variable, certainly in a dilated left ventricle. Moreover, replacement of LVESP with LVPSP is open to criticism because of the widened arterial pulse pressure in chronic aortic regurgitation.

LV End-Systolic Wall Stress/End-Systolic Volume and LV End-Systolic Wall Stress/LVEF Ratios

To include the degree of compensatory LV hypertrophy in the assessment, LVESP was replaced by LVESWS in several studies. LVESWS is indeed directly related to LVESP and LVESV and inversely related to LV end-systolic wall thickness. The ratio between LVESWS and LVESV was the only independent predictor of surgical outcome in patients with LV volume overload caused by chronic mitral regurgitation.[40] In patients with chronic aortic regurgitation, the ratio between LVEF and LVESWS[37] was a predictor of unfavorable outcome.[17]

Tissue Doppler LV Long-Axis Shortening Velocity

When tissue Doppler LV long-axis shortening velocity measured at the lateral mitral annulus drops below 9 cm/s, there is an increased need for aortic valve replacement in asymptomatic aortic regurgitation.[41]

Hemodynamic Changes during Exercise

Inability of LVEF to augment during exercise has been proposed as a marker of LV dysfunction in patients who have LV volume overload of chronic aortic regurgitation.[42] To account for altered loading conditions during exercise, the change in LVEF from rest to exercise has been normalized for the change in LVESWS from rest to exercise.[17] In a long-term (18-year) prospective study,[17] this ratio allowed prediction of the need for valve replacement and the occurrence of sudden cardiac death in asymptomatic patients with chronic aortic regurgitation.

Elevated Heart Failure Biomarkers

Both brain natriuretic peptide (BNP) and N-terminal pro-BNP (NT-proBNP) have diagnostic and prognostic value in patients with aortic valvular disease as they reflect LV hemodynamic stress related to LV pressure or volume overload. An NT-proBNP value of 600 pg/mL has been proposed as a cutoff value for patients with aortic regurgitation likely to experience an adverse event on follow-up.[43]

Alterations in Myocardial Gene Expression

A prolonged imposition of LV volume overload results in eccentric myocardial hypertrophy as an adaptive response. Eccentric myocardial hypertrophy is consistent with an increase in both LV volume and mass.[44]

Limited information has so far been obtained on myocardial gene expression during LV volume overload of chronic aortic regurgitation. In a rabbit aortic regurgitation model, cardiac fibroblasts reacted to the cyclical strain of the LV volume overload with an increase in fibronectin synthesis and little change in collagen content[45]; but in human aortic valve disease, high LV wall stress activated the myocardial renin-angiotensin system and led to an increase in both fibronectin and collagen.[46] In patients who have chronic aortic regurgitation, surgical procurement of LV endomyocardial biopsy specimens at the time of valve replacement revealed a positive correlation between expression of c-Myc oncoprotein and LVEF or reversibility of LV dysfunction and negative correlations between expression of c-Myc oncoprotein and LV end-systolic volume index, cell diameter, and fibrous content.[47] From these studies, it would appear that failure of proto-oncogene expression could serve as a marker of myocardial contractile dysfunction in patients who have chronic aortic regurgitation.

CLINICAL PRESENTATIONS

History

Chronic aortic regurgitation is often very well tolerated and discovered only at a routine physical examination. During this asymptomatic period, the left ventricle progressively enlarges. When symptoms of dyspnea or angina occur, cardiomegaly is usually considerable and LV dilatation has frequently progressed to the stage of myocardial dysfunction.[48] This emphasizes the importance of eventual surgical correction of the valvular abnormality of chronic aortic regurgitation in patients who have no or minimal symptoms.

When chronic aortic regurgitation has progressed to the symptomatic stage, symptoms of exertional dyspnea or angina are common. Angina results from a decline in coronary flow reserve, with a shift from predominantly diastolic to predominantly systolic epicardial blood flow.[49] Nocturnal angina can occur because of the decrease in heart rate at night, which prolongs the diastolic time interval of the cardiac cycle, increases the regurgitant volume, and decreases the coronary diastolic perfusion pressure. Syncope is a rare complaint and is more characteristic of stenotic valvular lesions, but it warrants further electrophysiologic investigation to exclude ventricular tachycardia.[50]

Physical Signs

Chronic aortic regurgitation produces many characteristic signs on physical examination; often, these are named after the physician who first described them.

Exaggerated arterial pulse (reflecting large LV stroke volume) and collapsing arterial pulse (reflecting LV runoff because of the regurgitant aortic valve) occur synchronously with each cardiac contraction. These signs are known as water-hammer pulse, Corrigan's pulse, or Vieussens' pulse. Exaggerated arterial pulsations are, however, not pathognomonic and are also observed in other conditions, such as patent ductus arteriosus, arteriovenous fistulas, and aging-related loss of arterial distensibility.

Arterial cuff blood pressure measurement reveals increased systolic arterial pressure and Korotkoff sounds sometimes persisting to "zero arterial pressure" (despite a diastolic arterial pressure that is rarely lower than 30 mm Hg) because of the presence of arterial sounds and murmurs. Auscultation of the femoral artery may reveal "pistol-shot" sounds, with a systolic and diastolic sound set up by vibrations of the arterial wall (Traube's sign) and a systolic murmur followed by a soft diastolic murmur of the aortic regurgitant flow (Duroziez's sign).

Capillary pulsations (Quincke's sign) can be observed and consist of alternating systolic redness and diastolic paleness of the fingernails or the lower lip during slight compression with a glass slide. Mechanocardiographic registration of the carotid pulse reveals a bisferiens pulse, especially in patients who have mixed aortic regurgitation and stenosis (Fig. 95.3). The "bite" taken out of the systolic portion of the carotid pulse in bisferiens pulse is attributed to a Venturi effect created in the aorta by the high-velocity jet of the ejected blood.[51]

The cardiac apical impulse is displaced inferiorly to the sixth or seventh intercostal space. It is hyperdynamic and felt over a wider than normal area of the thoracic wall. A mechanical recording of the apical impulse (apexcardiogram) reveals a fast-rising rapid filling wave without a slow filling wave and a prominent *a* wave because of continuous LV filling by aortic regurgitant flow (Fig. 95.4).

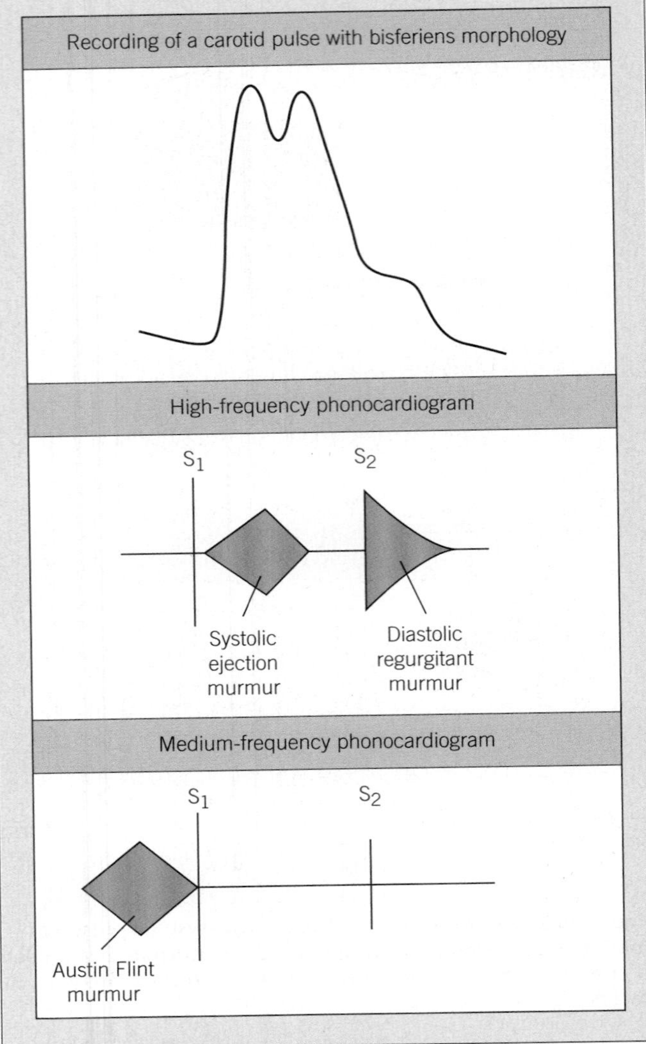

Figure 95.3 Carotid pulse recording and phonocardiography in chronic aortic regurgitation. S_1, first heart sound; S_2, second heart sound.

Auscultation

First, Second, and Third Heart Sounds

The first heart sound is usually soft because of increased LV filling pressures, which reduce the closing motion of the mitral valve, and because of frequent prolongation of the PR interval. The aortic component of the second heart sound is soft or absent, especially when aortic regurgitation is important. The pulmonary component of the second heart sound is obscured because of the early diastolic regurgitant murmur, which starts immediately after the aortic component. Therefore, the second heart sound can either be a single sound or have narrow or paradoxical splitting. Because of exaggerated rapid LV filling, from both the aorta and the left atrium, a third heart sound is often present.

Protosystolic Ejection Click

In mild and moderate aortic regurgitation, a protosystolic ejection click can be recorded from the apical area. It corresponds

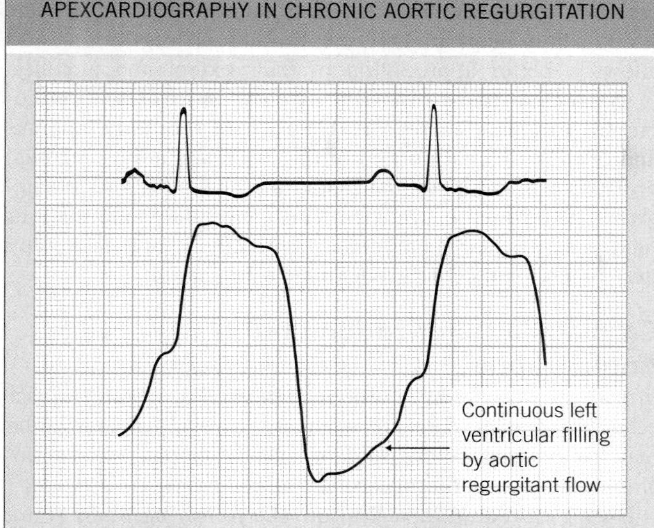

Figure 95.4 Apexcardiography in chronic aortic regurgitation.

to the rise in the carotid pulse recording and results from the deceleration of the opening motion of the stiffened aortic leaflets.

Midsystolic Ejection Sound

A pistol-shot sound can be heard over the right infraclavicular region because of abrupt cessation of the aortic distention. It corresponds to the first peak of the bisferiens pulse on the carotid pulse recording.

Systolic Ejection Murmur

A functional systolic ejection murmur, which results from the increase in ejection rate and stroke volume, is best heard in the second right intercostal space. It immediately follows the protosystolic ejection click, is of higher pitch than the ejection murmur of aortic stenosis, and ends well before the second heart sound (see Fig. 95.3).

Diastolic Regurgitant Murmur

A high-frequency diastolic murmur is the most important sign of aortic regurgitation (see Fig. 95.3). It starts immediately after the aortic component of the second heart sound and is loudest over the third or fourth intercostal space along the left sternal border or sometimes over the second or third right intercostal space. It radiates to the xiphoid and to the apex and is best heard while the patient is sitting up with the breath held in deep expiration. A high intensity usually corresponds to severe aortic regurgitation, but when cardiac output is low, severe aortic regurgitation can be present despite low intensity of the regurgitant murmur. In moderate to severe aortic regurgitation, the regurgitant murmur is holodiastolic. In mild aortic regurgitation, the murmur is decrescendo, usually of higher pitch and limited to the first part of diastole. In severe acute aortic regurgitation or in severe chronic aortic regurgitation with LV failure, the murmur shows a peak in early diastole rather than a progressive decline and attenuates abruptly thereafter because of equilibration of late LV diastolic and late aortic diastolic pressures. The diastolic regurgitant murmur of aortic regurgitation is accentuated by interventions that increase arterial pressure, such as exercise, and is reduced by interventions that decrease arterial pressure, such as inhalation of amyl nitrite. The murmur must be distinguished from the diastolic regurgitant murmur of pulmonary regurgitation, which starts after the pulmonary component of the second heart sound, is not accompanied by a widened arterial pulse pressure, and increases after amyl nitrite inhalation.

Protodiastolic Apical Rumble

A protodiastolic apical rumble is rare but sometimes occurs in moderate to severe aortic regurgitation, either because of an aortic regurgitant jet's directly hitting the superior portion of the mitral valve or because of superposition of the diastolic aortic regurgitant murmur and a loud third heart sound caused by simultaneous filling of the left ventricle from both the aorta and the left atrium.

Mid and Late Diastolic Apical Rumble (Austin Flint Murmur)

In contrast to a protodiastolic rumble, a mid and late diastolic rumble is more frequent in chronic aortic regurgitation (see Fig. 95.3). It can mimic mitral stenosis, and the absence of a loud first heart sound or an opening snap is helpful for differentiation between the two conditions. It varies in intensity from one diastole to another, which is also helpful to exclude organic mitral disease. The murmur is set up by vibrations of the mitral valve because of rapid inflow from the left atrium, especially at the time of left atrial contraction, because of partial closure of the mitral leaflets by the regurgitant aortic flow, and because of the increase in the LV diastolic pressures.[52] It is most frequently observed in severe chronic aortic regurgitation, but it can also occur in moderate chronic aortic regurgitation. It is absent in acute aortic regurgitation and in chronic aortic regurgitation accompanied by severe LV failure, when end-diastolic LV pressures exceed end-diastolic left atrial pressures and render forward transmitral flow impossible.

When LV filling pressures decrease because of LV dilatation and remodeling after the onset of acute aortic regurgitation, an Austin Flint murmur can appear. When filling pressures decrease further, the timing of the Austin Flint murmur during the cardiac cycle progressively shifts toward end-diastole. As with the diastolic regurgitant murmur, the intensity of the Austin Flint murmur augments when blood pressure increases during exercise and decreases when blood pressure decreases after inhalation of amyl nitrite. The Austin Flint murmur is of higher frequency than a presystolic fourth heart sound.

DIAGNOSTIC TECHNIQUES

Electrocardiography

The electrocardiogram is usually normal in patients who have minimal or moderate aortic regurgitation. In patients who have severe aortic regurgitation, LV hypertrophy will develop, and the amplitude of the QRS complex will increase. Initially, the T waves are upright and tall, consistent with LV hypertrophy of the diastolic overload type. As the disease progresses, inverted T waves and ST-segment depression appear. Incomplete left bundle branch block is observed in 30% of patients who have chronic aortic regurgitation and has been ascribed to the impact of the regurgitant jet on the proximal portions of the left bundle branch. Complete left or right bundle branch block is rare and is usually associated with mixed aortic valve disease. A first-degree atrioventricular block is common.

Chest Radiography

In chronic aortic regurgitation, marked LV enlargement occurs. This is especially obvious on the posteroanterior chest radiograph. Calcification of the aortic valve is present in aortic regurgitation of rheumatic or sclerocalcific etiology. Dilatation of the ascending aorta is usually present and shows up as prominence of the aortic knuckle on the left of the mediastinum and of the ascending aorta on the right of the mediastinum in the posteroanterior view. Enlargement of the left atrial silhouette suggests accompanying mitral valve disease or LV failure.

Echocardiography

Echocardiography has proved to be a useful tool for establishing the diagnosis and the etiology of chronic aortic regurgitation and for quantifying the severity of the chronic aortic regurgitation and the LV volume overload (see Chapter 86).[53]

Diagnosis

Before the advent of two-dimensional echocardiography, high-frequency diastolic fluttering of the anterior leaflet of the mitral valve was the most important feature of aortic regurgitation on M-mode echocardiographic examination. This results from the aortic regurgitant jet's hitting the anterior mitral valve leaflet. These high-frequency vibrations are not visible on two-dimensional examination because of insufficient temporal resolution, and they are not seen in mild aortic regurgitation, in the presence of a thickened and calcified mitral valve, or when the regurgitant jet is directed toward the interventricular septum (in which case high-frequency diastolic fluttering can be observed on the septal endocardium).

The diagnosis of aortic regurgitation is usually made through the use of Doppler investigations. Color Doppler imaging allows visualization of the aortic regurgitant jet in the LV cavity. The aortic regurgitant jet is composed of a zone of flow convergence that is proximal to the regurgitant orifice, a central cone of laminar flow through the regurgitant orifice, and a turbulent zone that is distal to the regurgitant orifice. The origin of the regurgitant flow can be visualized either centrally (if there is leaflet malcoaptation) or eccentrically (if there is cusp retraction, prolapse, or tear). Localization of the origin of the jet is especially important for establishing the paravalvular origin of aortic regurgitant flow in the presence of a valve prosthesis. Pulsed-wave Doppler study confirms the presence of aortic regurgitant flow when the Doppler sample volume is placed in the LV outflow tract, and continuous-wave Doppler study allows assessment of maximal regurgitant flow velocity.

Etiology

Echocardiographic examination also allows identification of the cause of chronic aortic regurgitation in the majority of cases. In rheumatic heart disease and in sclerocalcific disease, valve leaflets appear thickened and calcified and have limited mobility. In endocarditis, two-dimensional echocardiographic examination helps in the visualization of vegetations and allows a better appreciation of their extent and mobility. In connective tissue disorders, two-dimensional echocardiographic examination reveals dilatation of the aortic annulus and of the proximal portion of the ascending aorta, eventual prolapse of a cusp, and malcoaptation of the leaflets. In congenital heart disease, accompanying congenital malformations such as ventricular septal defect can easily be appreciated on two-dimensional echocardiographic examination.

Cardiac Catheterization and Angiography

In patients with chronic aortic regurgitation in whom Doppler echocardiographic data are adequate, cardiac catheterization may be omitted before surgery unless Doppler echocardiographic indexes conflict or coronary artery disease is suspected.[54]

During cardiac catheterization, the following findings are helpful in establishing the presence of aortic regurgitation or in quantifying it:

- widening of the aortic pulse pressure;
- approximation and eventual equilibration of aortic end-diastolic and LV end-diastolic pressures;
- qualitative grading of aortic regurgitation by supravalvular aortography;
- calculation of regurgitant volume and regurgitant fraction;
- visualization of the proximal portion of the ascending aorta by supravalvular aortography; and
- quantitative LV angiography to evaluate the severity of the LV volume overload.

Widening of the Aortic Pulse Pressure

Widening of aortic pulse pressure (Fig. 95.5) with a rapidly rising upstroke and significant peripheral arterial pressure amplification, with peak femoral artery systolic pressure exceeding central aortic pressure by 20 mm Hg, is helpful in establishing the presence of aortic regurgitation. Increased peak femoral artery systolic pressure results from modified arterial pressure wave reflections caused by high LV ejection velocity, increased systolic arterial pressure, and low diastolic arterial pressure.

Approximation and Eventual Equilibration of Aortic End-Diastolic and LV End-Diastolic Pressures

The end-diastolic aortic-LV pressure difference is inversely related to the severity of the aortic regurgitation and proportionally related to the chronicity of the aortic regurgitation and to the LV distensibility (see Fig. 95.5).

Qualitative Grading of Aortic Regurgitation by Supravalvular Aortography

Qualitative grading of aortic regurgitation by supravalvular aortography is usually expressed in four degrees of severity (grade 1 to grade 4; see Fig. 95.1).

Calculation of Regurgitant Volume and Regurgitant Fraction

The use of quantitative angiography to measure total LV stroke volume and the use of the Fick method or the thermodilution

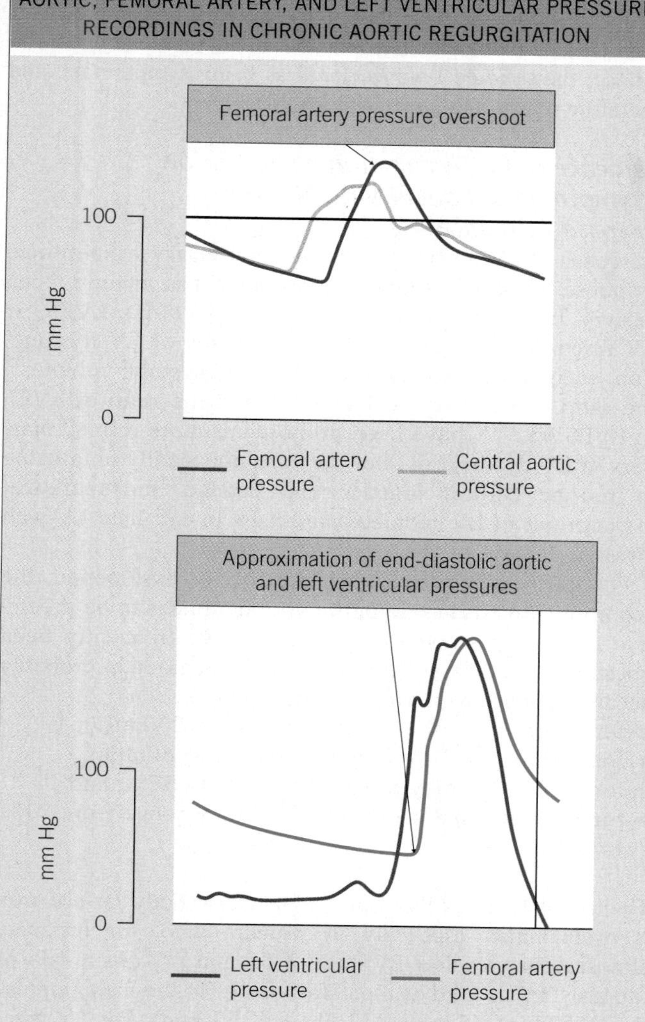

Figure 95.5 Aortic, femoral artery, and left ventricular pressure recordings in chronic aortic regurgitation.

cardiac output method to measure net forward stroke volume yield regurgitant volume as the difference between angiographic stroke volume and cardiac output stroke volume.[15] The regurgitant fraction corresponds to the regurgitant volume divided by the angiographic LV stroke volume.

Visualization of the Proximal Portion of the Ascending Aorta by Supravalvular Aortography

In patients who have connective tissue disorders, visualization of the proximal portion of the ascending aorta by supravalvular aortography is especially useful to appreciate the magnitude of dilatation of the aortic root and to give an indication of aortic root replacement at the time of aortic valve surgery (see Chapter 99).

Quantitative LV Angiography

Quantitative LV angiography can evaluate the severity of the LV volume overload. The magnitude of the LV volume overload that results from the chronic aortic regurgitation and the eventual LV dysfunction caused by "volume-overload cardiomyopathy" can be appreciated from quantitative angiographic measurement of LV end-diastolic and end-systolic volumes and from measurement of LVEF.

Computed Tomographic Scanning and Cine Nuclear Magnetic Resonance Imaging

Cine magnetic resonance imaging can be helpful in the diagnosis of chronic aortic regurgitation through quantification of regurgitant volumes and regurgitant orifice and through visualization of retrograde blood flow in the thoracic aorta. Both computed tomographic scanning and nuclear magnetic resonance imaging are powerful techniques for visualization of the ascending aorta. This is of special importance in connective tissue disorders, in which dilatation of the proximal portion of the ascending aorta (internal diameter $\geq$55 mm) necessitates replacement of the aortic root at the time of aortic valvular replacement. Computed tomography also has high diagnostic accuracy for the diagnosis of significant coronary artery disease in patients with chronic aortic regurgitation.[55]

MANAGEMENT

Optimal Timing of Aortic Valve Replacement

Choosing the optimal time for surgical correction of chronic aortic regurgitation remains a tough clinical challenge.[56] The goals of surgery for chronic aortic regurgitation are

- relief of symptoms; and
- prevention of irreversible LV dysfunction, which jeopardizes survival of the patient.

An optimal outcome for the patient after surgery is characterized by an early decline in LV volumes and an early increase in LVEF during the first 6 months after operation, with an additional late increase in LVEF during the first 3 to 7 years.[57] Despite advances in surgical technique, intraoperative myocardial preservation, and design of valvular prostheses, 20% to 30% of patients have suboptimal postoperative outcome because surgery is performed too late in the course of the disease, at a time when irreversible LV dysfunction has already occurred.[58]

Optimal timing of aortic valve replacement in chronic aortic regurgitation therefore implies early detection of a decline in myocardial contractility during the process of LV adaptation to the chronic volume overload. As discussed before, several markers have been proposed for early detection of a decline in myocardial contractility. The most frequently used markers are measures of LV contractility at rest by the LVESP-LVESV relationship and hemodynamic changes during exercise. Figure 95.6 sets out a proposed method to determine the optimal timing of aortic valve replacement in patients who have chronic aortic regurgitation.

Symptoms of Angina or Dyspnea

When a patient who has chronic aortic regurgitation has symptoms on initial evaluation, aortic valve replacement should be performed. The presence of preoperative functional

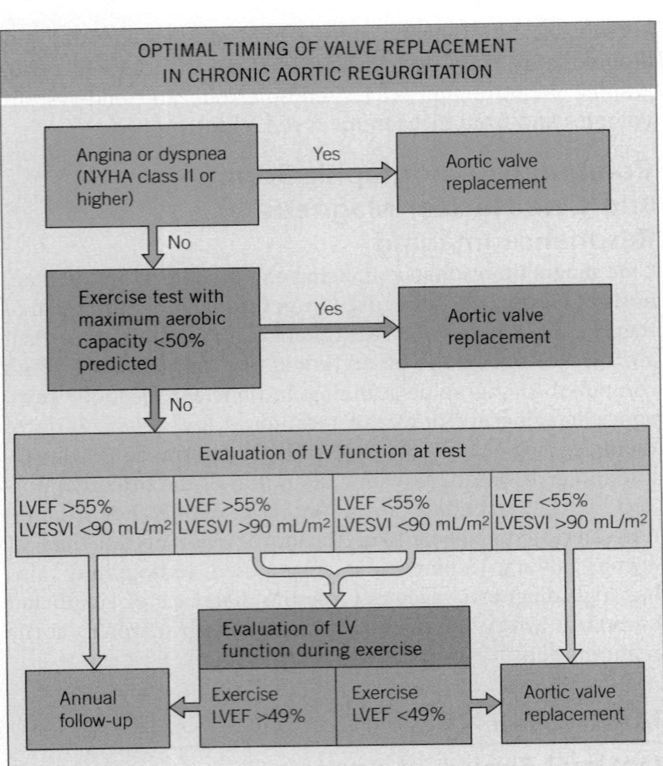

Figure 95.6 Optimal timing of valve replacement in chronic aortic regurgitation. LV, left ventricular; LVEF, left ventricular ejection fraction; LVESVI, left ventricular end-systolic volume index; NYHA, New York Heart Association.

New York Heart Association (NYHA) class III or class IV symptoms of dyspnea or angina is an independent determinant of excess postoperative immediate and long-term mortality,[59] especially in women.[60] In contrast, NYHA class II symptoms are associated with low operative mortality and excellent long-term postoperative survival.[59]

In symptomatic patients, measures of LV performance and of exercise tolerance are relevant to postoperative outcome. If a patient is symptomatic on initial evaluation and has an LVEF of more than 50%, postoperative prognosis is excellent. If a patient is symptomatic on initial evaluation and has an LVEF of less than 45%, prognosis is significantly poorer. If a symptomatic patient has poor exercise capacity on the treadmill, prognosis is also significantly poorer. In a group of initially asymptomatic patients with chronic aortic regurgitation,[17] development of symptoms (in 72% of patients) preceded the development of LV dysfunction (in 18% of patients) as the most common indication for aortic valve replacement. In this group of patients, the rate of progression to sudden death, symptoms (NYHA functional class II or above), or LV dysfunction averaged 6.2% per year.[17]

Objective Evidence of Reduced Exercise Tolerance in an Asymptomatic Patient

A patient with chronic aortic regurgitation who claims to have no or minimal symptoms should undergo an exercise treadmill or bicycle stress test.[61] A patient who cannot achieve 50% of his or her predicted aerobic capacity should be classified as having exercise intolerance, which is associated with poor postoperative prognosis and poor recovery of LV function.[57] In the course of their chronic illness, these patients have gradually restricted their physical activities and so become unaware of their exercise intolerance; they should be considered as being symptomatic and therefore referred for aortic valve replacement.

Evidence of LV Dysfunction at Rest in an Asymptomatic Patient with Normal Exercise Tolerance

Evidence of LV dysfunction at rest that marks a suboptimal response to aortic valve replacement has mainly been derived from measurement of LVESV, LVESID, LVEF, or LV fractional shortening. Other measures of LV dysfunction, such as the ratio of LVPSP to end-systolic volume,[39] the ratio of LVESWS to LVESV,[40] and the ratio of LVEF to LVESWS,[17,37] have been proposed as more refined markers of LV dysfunction, but they are not readily obtainable in routine clinical practice and depend on theoretical assumptions of LV geometry and mass to calculate LV wall stress.

For the routinely used measures of LV dysfunction, the reported cutoff values found in various studies to be predictive of poor postoperative outcome have frequently been questioned and have gradually been upgraded, probably because of improved surgical techniques:

- for LVESV,[33,35] they range from 60 to 200 mL/m^2;
- for LVESID,[32,34] they range from 55 to 60 mm;
- for LVEF,[28,62] they range from 35% to 55%; and
- for LV fractional shortening,[32,63] they range from 21% to 30%.

The use of an index that is not adjusted for body surface area is problematic, especially in women, who, for instance, almost never reach a LVESID of 55 mm.[60,64] As a rule of thumb, "55" is used as the cutoff value for the male population (LVEF of 55% and LVESID of 55 mm). For LV fractional shortening and for LV end-systolic volume index, the approximate values corresponding to 55 are 25% and 90 mL/m^2, respectively.

In an asymptomatic patient with normal exercise tolerance, LVESV or LVESID of less than 90 mL/m^2 or 55 mm and LVEF or fractional shortening of more than 55% or 25% are evidence of absence of LV dysfunction and justify postponement of valve replacement and annual reassessment. In an asymptomatic patient with normal exercise tolerance, LV volumes or dimensions of more than 90 mL/m^2 or 55 mm and LVEF or LV fractional shortening of less than 55% or 25% are evidence of LV dysfunction, and the patient should undergo aortic valve replacement. In an asymptomatic patient with normal exercise tolerance and conflicting values of LV dimensions and LV performance, LV imaging with another technique (e.g., angiography, cine nuclear magnetic resonance imaging) or the calculation of more refined indexes (e.g., the ratio of LVPSP to LVESV[39]) can be performed. If the outcome of additional imaging again yields an equivocal result, or if the ratio of LVPSP to LVESV is less than 1.72 mm Hg/mL per m^2, assessment of the LV hemodynamic response to exercise becomes desirable. Inability to improve LVEF during exercise might reflect an early stage of impairment of LV function and argue in favor of aortic valve replacement.[65]

Treatment

Medical Treatment

Medical treatment of patients who have asymptomatic chronic aortic insufficiency consists of vasodilator therapy to prevent LV dilatation. By reducing systemic vascular resistance, vasodilator drugs can increase forward cardiac output, reduce regurgitant flow, and decrease the LV volume overload.

The first drug to be used as vasodilator therapy for chronic aortic regurgitation was hydralazine. In a double-blind, placebo-controlled trial, patients receiving oral hydralazine (average daily dose, 216 ± 64 mg) had a significant reduction in both LV end-diastolic volume (18%) and end-systolic volume (24%) after 2 years of treatment.[66] Indications for surgery (i.e., development of symptoms or a significant decrease in LVEF) developed in 17% of patients in the placebo group and in 2% of the hydralazine-treated patients. In this study, a favorable response to vasodilator therapy with hydralazine was more likely if the initial LVESWS was low.

This raises the possibility that patients who have a high LVESWS are at risk for an unfavorable course, not only after aortic valve replacement but also during vasodilator therapy, probably because of the irreversibility of the LV myocardial damage. The usefulness of hydralazine is limited by frequent side effects, such as gastrointestinal symptoms, headache, flushing, and, in 9% of patients, development of a lupus-like syndrome. Alternative choices for vasodilator therapy in asymptomatic chronic aortic regurgitation are nifedipine,[67] enalapril,[68] and felodipine.[69]

After 6 years of follow-up, 34% of patients in the placebo group underwent aortic valve replacement, compared with 15% of the nifedipine-treated group.[56] In the placebo group, indications for valve replacement were development of symptoms or progression of LV dysfunction; whereas in the nifedipine-treated group, the only indication was progression of LV dysfunction. Furthermore, LV unloading with nifedipine resulted in normalization of LVEF, which was not observed in the placebo group.[70] Patients with asymptomatic aortic regurgitation who were randomly assigned to enalapril[68] experienced a significant reduction in LV end-diastolic and end-systolic volumes compared with those patients assigned to hydralazine. These positive results with nifedipine and enalapril were recently challenged; after 7 years of follow-up, need for surgery in asymptomatic patients with severe aortic regurgitation was similar in controls, enalapril-treated patients, or nifedipine-treated patients.[71] Beta blockade appears to limit aortic dilatation during childhood in children affected by Marfan's syndrome, thereby reducing aortic regurgitation and the need for aortic valve replacement.[72]

In symptomatic patients with chronic aortic regurgitation, aortic valve replacement is mandatory. In these patients, medical treatment is temporary and is intended to alleviate symptoms of dyspnea and angina. It can consist of digitalis, diuretics, and nitrates. Vasodilator drugs are also effective in decompensated chronic aortic regurgitation, but there is no information on their long-term effects. Bradycardia and atrial fibrillation are poorly tolerated and require immediate treatment. A history of sustained ventricular tachycardia, ventricular fibrillation, or syncope requires an electrophysiologic study and eventual implantation of a cardioverter-defibrillator.[50]

Surgical Treatment

Aortic valve substitutes implanted during surgery for chronic aortic regurgitation include mechanical valves, porcine heterograft tissue valves, stentless porcine heterograft tissue valves, aortic allografts, and pulmonary autografts. In patients who have chronic aortic insufficiency because of annuloaortic ectasia with a transverse diameter of the proximal portion of the ascending aorta exceeding 55 mm,[73] composite surgical replacement of the aortic valve and the ascending aorta is performed with use of a valved conduit or an allograft total root. In women in particular, aortic replacement at the time of aortic valve surgery should be considered because of the greater incidence of coexisting aortic disease and subsequent aortic rupture. In some patients who have significant aortic root dilatation and normal aortic valve leaflets on multiplane transesophageal echocardiography, reconstruction of the aortic root can be performed with preservation of the aortic leaflets (aortic valve–sparing operation). In these patients, correction of the aortic regurgitation will result from readjustment of the diameter of the ascending aorta at the sinotubular junction. The overall operative mortality rate for isolated aortic valve replacement has decreased over time and is now down to approximately 2%. Furthermore, operative mortality of patients with severe LV dysfunction also improved dramatically, such that aortic valve surgery in patients with severe LV dysfunction is no longer a high-risk procedure for which cardiac transplantation is a better option.[74] Among patients with rheumatic heart disease, a considerable number have mild aortic regurgitation at the time of mitral valve surgery, yet most do not progress to severe aortic regurgitation, and prophylactic aortic valve replacement at the time of mitral valve surgery does not seem to be indicated.[75]

The use of mechanical valves for aortic valve replacement offers the advantage of long-term valve durability but carries an increased risk of thromboembolism (0.5% to 3%/patient-year) and of bleeding secondary to anticoagulation (morbidity, 1.3% to 2.7%/patient-year; mortality, 0.1% to 0.5%/patient-year). In patients who have mechanical prostheses, the target international normalized ratio for anticoagulant management should be within the range of 3.0 to 4.5, as complication rates increase sharply above a ratio of 4.9 and below a ratio of 2.5.[76] The use of tissue valves eliminates the need for chronic anticoagulation and is accompanied by a reduced risk of thromboembolism, but it carries an increased risk of structural failure, which usually results in progressive valvular regurgitation and less frequently in valve stenosis. Structural degeneration of bioprosthetic valves is accelerated in the presence of metabolic syndrome.[77] A time-related risk for development of aortic regurgitation is also present for cryopreserved aortic allografts, with 25% of patients developing aortic regurgitation of NYHA functional class II during a 2-year follow-up,[78] but it remains minimal for the pulmonary autograft.[79]

The selection of a valve prosthesis depends on surgery-related factors and on patient-related factors:

- for a narrow aortic root, a low-profile mechanical valve is used;
- for a dilated aortic root, a valved conduit or a homograft total root replacement is preferred;

- for patients older than 65 years and in regular sinus rhythm, porcine heterograft tissue valves are recommended; and
- for women of childbearing age, an aortic allograft or pulmonary autograft is desirable.

The use of the pulmonary autograft for patients who have Marfan's disease and aortic insufficiency is questionable because of the diffuse nature of the connective tissue abnormality and the postoperative dilatation of the pulmonary autograft.[80]

PROGNOSIS

Prognosis in patients who have chronic aortic regurgitation depends on the symptomatic status of the patients. If a patient who has chronic aortic regurgitation presents on initial evaluation with symptoms (NYHA functional class II or above) of dyspnea or angina, or if such symptoms develop during follow-up, aortic valve replacement should be performed without delay. This is because once it is symptomatic, the condition can deteriorate rapidly, with death occurring within 4 years if the presenting symptom was angina and within 2 years if the presenting symptom was dyspnea. In asymptomatic patients, the annual rate of progression to sudden death, to symptoms that necessitate valve replacement, or to LV dysfunction that necessitates valve replacement is about 5%.

SUMMARY

Chronic aortic regurgitation results from chronic diastolic reflux of blood from the aortic root to the left ventricle because of malcoaptation of the aortic valve leaflets. Such malcoaptation can result from dilatation of the aortic annulus or from retraction of the aortic cusps. The most frequent causes are connective tissue disorders with dilatation of the aortic root, congenital heart disease, rheumatic fever, and infective endocarditis.

Chronic aortic regurgitation is often very well tolerated, with a prolonged asymptomatic period during which the left ventricle progressively enlarges. When symptoms of dyspnea or angina occur, cardiomegaly is usually considerable. Important physical signs are exaggerated and collapsing arterial pulsations and a high-frequency diastolic regurgitant murmur.

Doppler echocardiographic examination confirms the diagnosis and frequently establishes the severity and etiology of the valvular lesion and the extent of LV dysfunction. Cardiac catheterization and angiography are required if Doppler echocardiographic indexes are conflicting or when coronary artery disease is suspected.

Aortic valve replacement is indicated in the presence of symptoms or evidence of LV dysfunction (LVEF <55% or LVESID >55 mm). In asymptomatic patients, the annual rate of progression to sudden death, symptoms, or significant LV dysfunction is about 5%.

chapter

96 Special Problems in Aortic Valve Disease

a. Low-Gradient, Low-Output Aortic Stenosis

Paul A. Grayburn

DEFINITION OF PROBLEM

Aortic valve replacement is recommended in patients with severe, symptomatic aortic stenosis (AS) because it improves symptoms and life expectancy, even in the setting of left ventricular (LV) dysfunction. LV dysfunction in severe AS is usually due to afterload mismatch, such that valve replacement relieves the afterload excess imposed by the stenotic valve and improves LV performance. However, a small subset of patients with severe AS and LV dysfunction have a low transvalvular gradient and a low cardiac output. Operative mortality is high in these patients, and the clinician is faced with the difficult dilemma of how to predict which of these patients will benefit from valve replacement.

TYPICAL CASE

A 52-year-old man with New York Heart Association (NYHA) class IV heart failure was referred for cardiac transplantation. Two years previously, he presented with mild heart failure symptoms and was diagnosed with severe AS and mildly depressed LV systolic function (left ventricular ejection fraction [LVEF] of 40%). He refused aortic valve surgery. After that time, his heart failure symptoms progressively worsened, and his LVEF declined to 17%. His blood pressure was 92/60 mm Hg; heart rate, 101 beats per minute; and respiratory rate, 30 breaths/minute. He was afebrile. His neck veins were distended to the angle of the mandible, and the carotid pulses were diminished with a delayed upstroke. Auscultation of the chest revealed bilateral rales, a summation gallop, and a late-peaking grade 2/6 systolic ejection murmur. The electrocardiogram was notable for the absence of LV hypertrophy and the presence of nonspecific ST-T changes. Chest radiography showed an enlarged cardiac silhouette and pulmonary edema. A repeated echocardiogram showed a thickened aortic valve with a mean gradient of 17 mm Hg, calculated valve area of 0.7 cm^2, LV end-diastolic dimension of 7.4 cm, LVEF below 20%, and estimated right ventricular systolic pressure of 50 mm Hg. Cardiac catheterization demonstrated normal coronary arteries, mean transvalvular gradient of 17 mm Hg, and valve area of 0.7 cm^2.

A dobutamine echocardiogram was performed; the results are shown in Figure 96A.1. At baseline, the mean gradient was 17 mm Hg with a stroke volume of 35 mL and a valve area of 0.7 cm^2. At peak dose, stroke volume had increased to 45 mL, indicating that the dobutamine had significantly improved LV function. Mean gradient increased significantly to 29 mm Hg, and valve area remained at 0.7 cm^2.

DIFFERENTIAL DIAGNOSIS

This patient has AS associated with a low cardiac output and low transvalvular gradient. Such patients are at increased risk for operative mortality and morbidity. Because of this concern, he was referred to us for cardiac transplantation rather than for valve replacement. In evaluating such patients, it is important to consider the differential diagnosis in terms of pathophysiology. Critical to this consideration is the fact that aortic valve area may be underestimated in low-flow conditions because both the Gorlin formula and the continuity equation measure the effective valve area. During low-flow states, the aortic valve may not open to its full extent because of inadequate forward flow. Accordingly, a patient with a calculated valve area of 0.7 cm^2 in the setting of a low cardiac output and low gradient could have an aortic valve that is only moderately diseased but unable to open fully because of an underlying cardiomyopathy. Such a patient would not benefit from aortic valve replacement. On the other hand, it is clear that some patients have LV dysfunction secondary to anatomically severe AS. These patients often have inadequate LV hypertrophy, which allows wall stress to increase dramatically such that LV function declines. Relief of the afterload mismatch by valve replacement may improve LV function and result in a good clinical outcome.

The classic descriptor of the severity of AS is aortic valve area. Unfortunately, aortic valve area is least helpful in low-flow states. It is also dependent on body habitus and should be indexed for body surface area. Valve resistance has been proposed as a useful descriptor of the severity of AS and may be particularly useful in low-flow, low-gradient AS because it is less flow dependent than valve area.

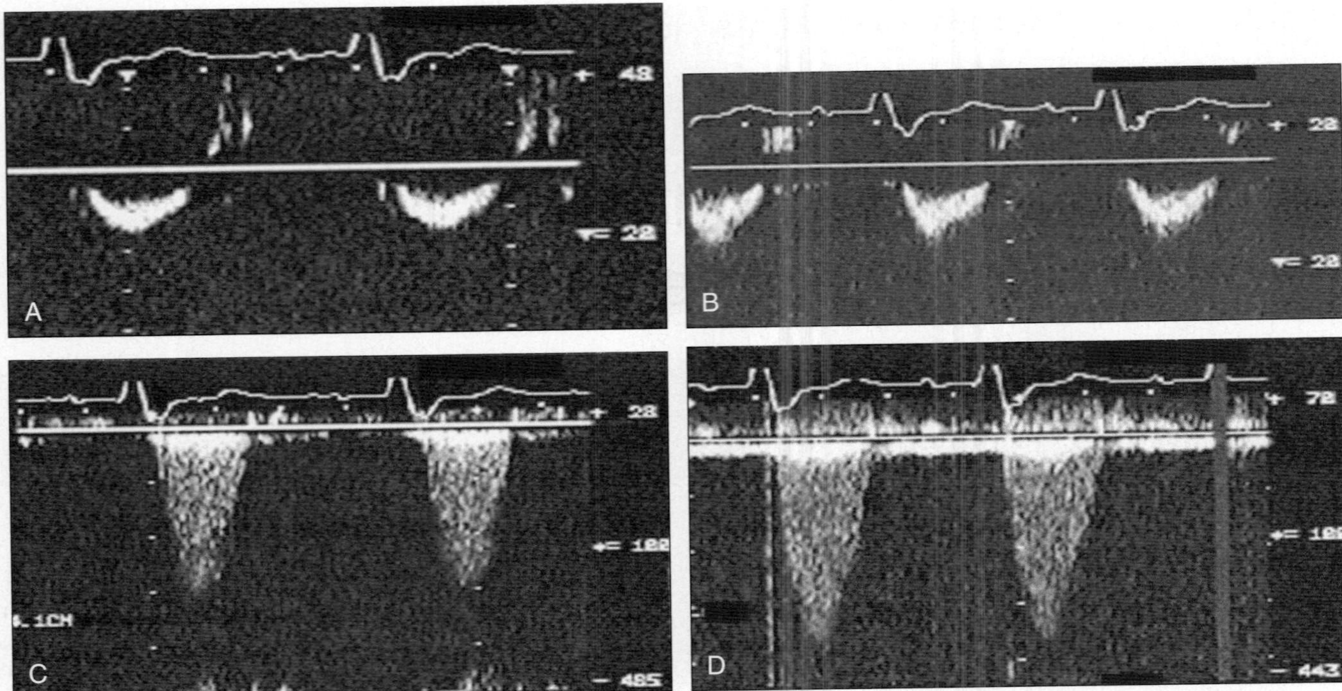

Figure 96A.1 Dobutamine echocardiograms. A, Baseline left ventricular outflow tract pulsed Doppler study showing a velocity-time integral of 6.6 cm and a stroke volume of 35 mL. **B,** At peak dobutamine dose, left ventricular outflow tract velocity-time integral increased to 8.4 cm, and stroke volume increased to 45 mL. **C,** Baseline continuous-wave Doppler study shows a peak velocity of 3.0 m/s and a mean gradient of 17 mm Hg. Aortic valve area by the continuity equation was 0.7 cm^2. **D,** At peak dobutamine dose, the peak aortic velocity increased to 3.6 m/s and the mean gradient to 29 mm Hg; the aortic valve area remained at 0.7 cm^2.

Resistance can be calculated from either catheterization or echocardiographic data as

$$1.33 \times \text{MPG} \times \text{SEP}/\text{SV}$$

where MPG is the mean pressure gradient in millimeters of mercury, SEP is the systolic ejection period in milliseconds, and SV is the stroke volume in milliliters. A valve resistance above 250 dynes • s/cm^5 is indicative of severe AS. A valve resistance below 200 dynes • s/cm^5 is probably not severe AS.

Dobutamine echocardiography is very helpful in determining the physiology of low-gradient, low-flow AS. Dobutamine should be infused at a starting dose of 5 g/kg per minute and increased every 3 to 5 minutes to no more than 20 mcg/kg/min. The goals are to increase forward flow across the aortic valve and to assess the effect of this maneuver on the mean gradient and valve area. Forward flow can be monitored by the velocity-time integral of the pulsed Doppler signal in the LV outflow tract. In our experience, there are three subsets of patients (Table 96A.1). First, mean gradient increases by at least 10 mm Hg without a significant change in valve area. These patients have physiology that is consistent with "fixed" AS and may benefit from valve replacement. Second, mean gradient may increase only slightly with a significant increase in valve area. These patients have only moderate AS in which the low-flow state fails to fully open the abnormal leaflets and results in a calculated valve area that overestimates the severity of AS. Such patients may be considered to have AS that is "relative" to the amount of forward flow. Third, patients in whom the LV dysfunction is characterized by severe fibrosis or necrosis may not have significantly increased LV stroke volume during dobutamine infusion. In such patients, it is not possible to determine the severity of the AS, although failure of the left ventricle to respond to dobutamine is generally thought to be a very poor prognostic indicator. Such patients may require transplantation rather than valve replacement.

HEMODYNAMIC RESPONSES TO DOBUTAMINE IN LOW-FLOW, LOW-GRADIENT AORTIC STENOSIS

	Fixed AS Group		Relative AS Group	
Variable	**Baseline**	**Dobutamine**	**Baseline**	**Dobutamine**
Aortic valve area (cm^2)	0.7 ± 0.1	0.7 ± 0.1	0.8 ± 0.1	1.1 ± 0.1*
Mean gradient (mm Hg)	23 ± 6	41 ± 11*	18 ± 2	22 ± 4
Valve resistance (dynes • s/cm^5)	190 ± 49	261 ± 71*	144 ± 15	115 ± 10

AS, aortic stenosis
*$P < .05$ compared with baseline value.

Table 96A.1 Hemodynamic responses to dobutamine in low-flow, low-gradient aortic stenosis.

TREATMENT OPTIONS

In this patient, the results of the dobutamine echocardiogram indicated reversible LV dysfunction due to severe AS. As a result, the patient underwent aortic valve replacement with an uneventful postoperative course. One month later, his LVEF was 40% and he was back to work with no heart failure symptoms. In our experience, patients with low-flow, low-gradient AS can be sent to valve surgery if the dobutamine echocardiogram and valve resistance indicate fixed AS. If it shows relative AS, we may elect to treat the patients medically for heart failure and are comfortable using angiotensin-converting enzyme inhibitors because they do not have fixed AS. If heart failure is severe, heart transplantation may be indicated. In patients in whom the LV dysfunction does not improve with dobutamine, transplantation may be the only alternative.

SUMMARY

Low-flow, low-gradient AS is associated with increased operative mortality. Decisions about management of such patients depend on accurate determination of whether the AS is causing LV dysfunction or whether severe LV dysfunction is preventing a moderately diseased aortic valve from opening fully. Dobutamine echocardiography is useful in clarifying the pathophysiology and in predicting which patients will benefit from aortic valve replacement.

b. Mild to Moderate Aortic Stenosis in Patients Undergoing Bypass Surgery

Paul A. Grayburn

DEFINITION OF PROBLEM

Because patients who are referred for coronary artery bypass grafting (CABG) are often older and have generalized atherosclerosis, it is not uncommon for them to have concomitant aortic stenosis (AS). In patients with severe AS, CABG is combined with aortic valve replacement (AVR). However, when the AS is of mild or moderate severity, it is not clear whether to perform AVR at the time of CABG or to wait until severe, symptomatic AS develops. On the one hand, it can be argued that the AVR should be performed at the time of CABG to avoid a reoperation a few years later. On the other hand, combined CABG and AVR increases the mortality of the operation and exposes the patient to the complications of an aortic valve prosthesis. Unfortunately, there are no randomized, controlled clinical trials to provide a definitive answer to this dilemma. Therefore, the clinical decision must be based on thoughtful clinical judgment and consideration of a number of important variables.

TYPICAL CASE

A 53-year-old man was referred for cardiac catheterization for evaluation of progressively increasing exertional angina during the past 3 months. He had no prior history of myocardial infarction, hypertension, or diabetes. He had never smoked. His low-density lipoprotein cholesterol level was 234 mg/dL, and his high-density lipoprotein cholesterol level was 25 mg/dL. His brother and two uncles had myocardial infarctions in their 50s. His blood pressure was 136/84 mm Hg, with a pulse rate of 76 beats per minute. Physical examination was remarkable for a grade 2/6 mid-peaking systolic ejection murmur that radiated to the carotids. His carotid upstrokes were brisk and not delayed. There was an S_4 gallop. His electrocardiogram showed minor nonspecific ST-T wave changes. An echocardiogram showed a moderately calcified aortic valve with decreased excursion, a peak aortic velocity of 3.2 m/s, a mean gradient of 24 mm Hg, and an aortic valve area of 1.2 cm^2.

At cardiac catheterization, he was found to have an 80% stenosis of the left main coronary artery with good distal targets and normal left ventricular function. The mean aortic valve gradient at catheterization was 23 mm Hg, with a valve area of 1.3 cm^2. He was scheduled for CABG, and the surgeons asked for an opinion as to whether to perform AVR.

DIFFERENTIAL DIAGNOSIS

The diagnosis in this case is not in question. The patient clearly has progressive angina and left main coronary disease, for which surgery is indicated. He also has mild to moderate AS. It is important in such cases to be certain that an accurate assessment of aortic valve area is made. In this case, the concordance between echocardiographic and catheterization data provides a high level of confidence in the hemodynamic assessment of the severity of AS. It is also useful to evaluate the degree of valve thickening and mobility by echocardiography and the amount of calcification by fluoroscopy. Transesophageal echocardiography can also be helpful in assessing valve morphology if the transthoracic echocardiogram is inadequate (Fig. 96B.1).

TREATMENT OPTIONS

There are three treatment options available in this case: first, isolated CABG can be performed without addressing the aortic valve; second, AVR can be combined with CABG; third, the aortic valve can be inspected and débrided at the time of CABG. There is no clear consensus about which of these options is optimal, and the decision will rest on clinical judgment in individual cases.

Several factors must be considered in making this judgment. In favor of replacing the valve at the time of surgery is the possibility that the patient may require reoperation within a few years if the valve is left alone. The natural history of progression of AS in a general population is a decrease in valve area of about 0.1 cm^2 per year. Thus, a typical patient with a valve area of 1.2 cm^2 might be expected to require AVR anyway in 4 to 5 years. Some

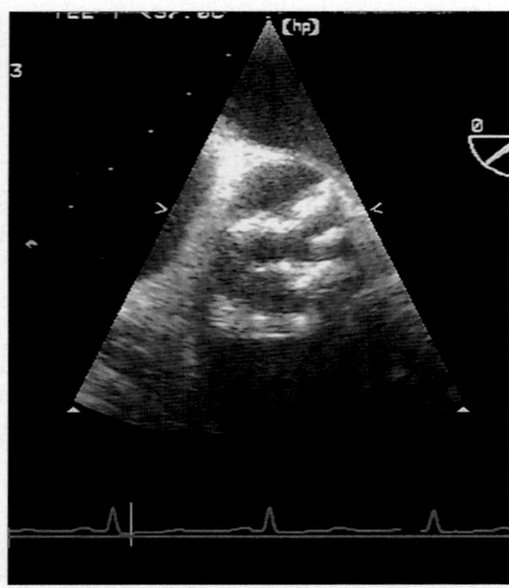

Figure 96B.1 Transesophageal short-axis view showing a moderately thickened aortic valve with reduced excursion.

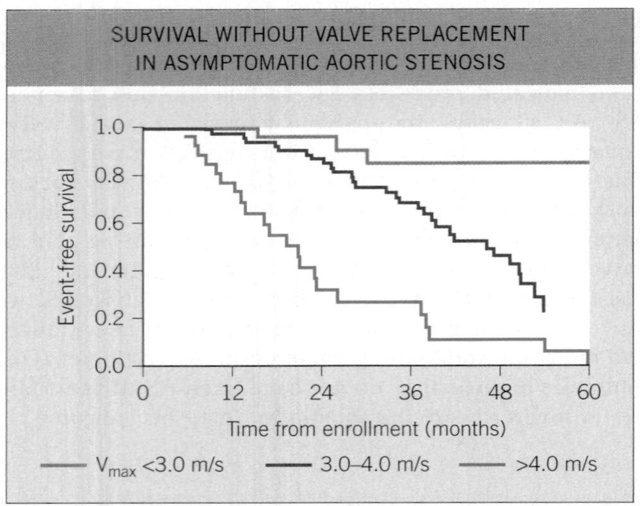

Figure 96B.2 Survival without valve replacement in 123 patients with asymptomatic aortic stenosis (AS). Patients are grouped according to peak aortic velocity on entry into the study. V_{max}, peak velocity. (From Otto CM, Burwash IG, Legget ME, et al. Prospective study of asymptomatic valvular aortic stenosis. Clinical, echocardiographic, and exercise predictors of outcome. Circulation 1997;95:2262-2270.)

patients have a faster rate of progression, and some patients demonstrate little progression; unfortunately, the rate of progression cannot be reliably predicted by baseline hemodynamic or clinical factors. However, Otto and colleagues (1997), in a prospective study of 123 patients with asymptomatic AS, showed that patients with a peak velocity below 3 m/s have an excellent 5-year event-free survival (Fig. 96B.2). Such patients would not be expected to benefit from prophylactic AVR. On the other hand, patients with a peak velocity above 3 m/s have a significant decrease in 5-year event-free survival and should be considered for AVR when CABG is indicated. An important advantage of peak velocity is that it is noninvasive, easy to measure, and, unlike aortic valve area, does not need to be indexed for body surface area.

The arguments against prophylactic AVR are that it increases the operative risk and exposes the patient to the risk of prosthetic valve endocarditis, thromboembolism, and anticoagulation. The risk of long-term anticoagulation can be avoided by use of a bioprosthesis. However, bioprosthetic valves have small effective orifice areas (1.0 to 1.6 cm^2, depending on annulus size) and therefore may not be optimal for prophylactic AVR in patients with mild to moderate AS undergoing bypass surgery because of patient-prosthesis mismatch. We prefer to use bileaflet mechanical valves because of their larger orifice areas and favorable hemodynamics. Newer generation bioprosthetic valves may be acceptable for prophylactic use, provided the annulus is large enough to accept a large enough valve to avoid patient-prosthesis mismatch. Finally, there is little experience with débridement of the valve in such cases. It is not clear whether this procedure would reduce the rate of progression of AS in the long term, although it does avoid the risks of prosthetic valve complications and anticoagulation.

SUMMARY

The most recent American College of Cardiology/American Heart Association guidelines consider AVR for moderate AS to be clinically indicated (class IIa). However, the decision of whether to perform prophylactic AVR in patients with mild to moderate AS undergoing CABG is a difficult one. Each case should be carefully considered on an individual basis. Factors in favor of AVR include a peak velocity of more than 3 m/s and rapid progression of AS on the basis of serial echocardiograms. On the other hand, if the patient has a small aortic annulus, patient-prosthesis mismatch may occur, such that a significant gradient persists across the prosthesis. In such cases, there may be no advantage to prophylactic AVR.

c. The Clinical Significance of Pressure Recovery in Aortic Stenosis

Philippe Pibarot and Jean G. Dumesnil

DEFINITION OF PRESSURE RECOVERY

The accurate assessment of the hemodynamic severity of the valvular stenosis is crucial for clinical decision making in patients with aortic stenosis (AS).[1] The severity of AS is generally determined by measurement of the pressure gradient across the valve or preferably, because it is less flow dependent, the effective orifice area (EOA) of the valve (Fig. 96C.1). When flow passes through the stenotic valve, there is a contraction and acceleration of the flow, and the area where the flow jet is the smallest is called the vena contracta. The EOA of the valve corresponds to the cross-sectional area of the vena contracta. In the clinical

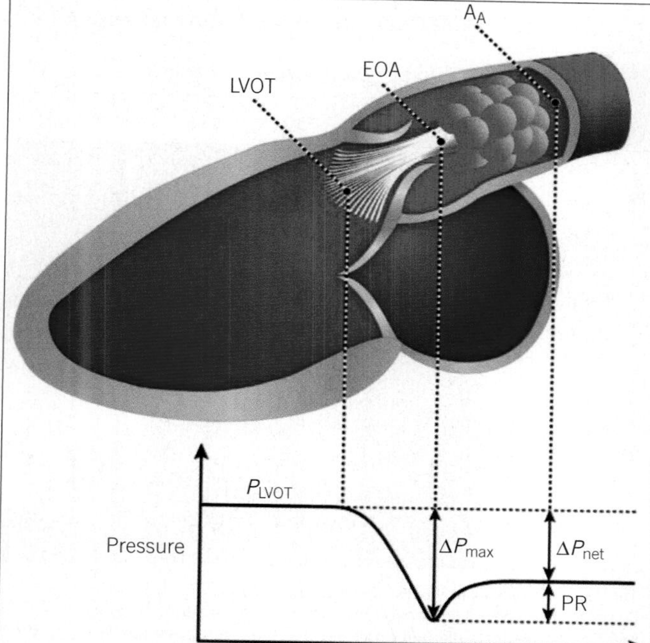

Figure 96C.1 Schematic representation of the flow and blood pressure across the left ventricular outflow tract, aortic valve, and ascending aorta during systole. A_A, cross-sectional area of the aorta at the level of the sinotubular junction; EOA, valve effective orifice area, that is, the cross-sectional area of the vena contracta of the transvalvular flow jet; LVOT, left ventricular outflow tract; P_{LVOT}, pressure in the left ventricular outflow tract; ΔP_{max}, maximum transvalvular pressure gradient recorded at the level of the vena contracta (gradient measured by Doppler echocardiography); ΔP_{net}, net transvalvular pressure gradient recorded after pressure recovery (gradient measured by catheter); PR, pressure recovery.

SUMMARY OF THE ECHOCARDIOGRAPHIC AND CATHETERIZATION DATA OF A 32-YEAR-OLD WOMAN WITH A HISTORY OF BICUSPID AORTIC STENOSIS		
	Doppler Echocardiography	Catheterization
Mean gradient (mm Hg)	40	27
EOA (cm^2)	0.87	1.0
Indexed EOA (cm^2/m^2)	0.57	0.66
Aortic diameter (mm)	25	—
Estimated pressure recovery[1] (mm Hg)	11	—
Estimated net mean gradient[2] (mm Hg)	29	—
Energy loss coefficient[3] (cm^2)	1.06	—
Energy loss index (cm^2/m^2)	0.7	—

EOA, effective orifice area.
[1,2,3]Calculated with the use of Equations 1, 2, and 3, respectively.

Table 96C.1 Summary of the echocardiographic and catheterization data of a 32-year-old woman with a history of bicuspid aortic stenosis.

setting, the EOA can be measured either by Doppler echocardiography with the use of the continuity equation or by left-sided heart catheterization with the Gorlin formula. Unfortunately, there are often discrepancies between Doppler echocardiographic and catheter measurements of EOA, which may result in divergent estimation of AS severity and bring some uncertainties in clinical decision making. Studies have demonstrated that these discrepancies between Doppler echocardiographic and catheter measurements are in large part due to the pressure recovery phenomenon.[2-4]

When the blood flow contracts to pass through a stenotic orifice, a portion of the potential energy of the blood (i.e., pressure) is converted into kinetic energy (i.e., velocity), thus resulting in a pressure drop and acceleration of flow (see Fig. 96C.1).[5] Downstream of the vena contracta, the flow jet re-expands and decelerates. Given that the total energy must remain constant, the kinetic energy is converted back into potential energy (i.e., blood velocity decreases, whereas blood pressure increases). Unfortunately, this energy conversion is not complete in the context of an abrupt obstruction, such as an aortic valve stenosis, because the sudden expansion of the flow jet downstream of the vena contracta generates flow turbulences. As a result of these turbulences, a large part of the kinetic energy is irreversibly dissipated as heat. The remaining portion of the kinetic energy that is reconverted to potential energy is called the pressure recovery (see Fig. 96C.1). The extent of this pressure recovery essentially depends on the relationship between the size of the valve orifice and the size of the aorta (see Fig. 96C.1).[2-8] The smaller the valve EOA relative to the size of the aorta, the more flow turbulences will occur and the less energy will be available to be recovered as pressure. Hence, the extent of pressure recovery generally becomes clinically relevant in patients with smaller aortas (i.e., with an aorta diameter at the sinotubular junction ≤30 mm) and especially in those with mild, moderate, or moderate to severe AS.[2-4,6,7,9] In this regard, Gjertsson and colleagues[9] reported that approximately 50% of the AS population have an aorta diameter of 30 mm or less. These findings suggest that a relatively high proportion of the patients with AS may have a substantial pressure recovery downstream of the aortic valve.

Patients with a large aneurysm of the ascending aorta have no pressure recovery and therefore a more important energy loss for a given valve EOA. Congenital bicuspid AS is often associated with dilatation of the ascending aorta, which may reduce the extent of pressure recovery and thereby increase the energy loss at the level of the aortic valve or root.

TYPICAL CASE

This is the case of a 32-year-old woman with a history of bicuspid AS. She recently had a few episodes of mild chest pain. The Doppler echocardiographic examination (Table 96C.1) revealed a mean gradient of 40 mm Hg and an aortic valve EOA of 0.87 cm^2 (indexed EOA: 0.57 cm^2/m^2), which is consistent with severe AS according to the American College of Cardiology/American Heart Association guidelines. She underwent a maximum bicycle exercise test with respiratory gas analysis. She reached 105% of her age- and gender-predicted maximum oxygen consumption. The reason for stopping exercise was fatigue; there was a

2-mm ST-segment depression but no chest pain during exercise. Cardiac catheterization was performed to determine the presence of coronary artery disease and to corroborate the severity of AS. Coronary angiography showed no evidence of coronary artery stenosis. However, the mean gradient measured by catheterization (27 mm Hg) was substantially lower than that measured by echocardiography, and the EOA was higher (1.0 cm^2) (see Table 96C.1). There is thus an important discrepancy between the echocardiographic and catheter assessments of stenosis severity.

RECONCILING ECHOCARDIOGRAPHIC AND CATHETER DATA

Doppler measurements rely on the maximum velocity or gradient measured across the aortic valve at the level of the vena contracta (see Fig. 96C.1). On the other hand, catheterization measurements are generally performed at a few centimeters downstream of the valve, where the pressure is fully recovered. As a result, the pressure gradient recorded by catheterization, which corresponds to the "recovered" or "net" pressure gradient, is generally lower than the Doppler gradient, which corresponds to the maximum gradient recorded at the level of the vena contracta. Likewise, EOA by the Gorlin formula is derived from recovered pressures, such that its value is higher than EOA derived by the continuity equation, which measures the actual area occupied by flow at the valvular level.

In this context, it should be emphasized that the guidelines were first established on the basis of data obtained from catheter measurements. The same cutpoint values (e.g., mean gradient >40 mm Hg or EOA <1.0 cm^2 for severe AS) were then extended to echocardiographic data on the assumption that Doppler and catheter measurements are equivalent. To this effect, the guidelines make no distinction between catheterization and echocardiographic measurements as if values for gradients and EOA measured by either technique are interchangeable. However, as demonstrated in several studies, these measurements are not equivalent, and differences in results of up to 50% may be observed between the two techniques, depending on the size of the aorta and the severity of the stenosis (Table 96C.2).[4,5,7,10] The extent of pressure recovery and thus the discrepancies between Doppler and catheter measurements are more important in patients with smaller aortas or with mild, moderate, or moderate to severe AS. Nonetheless, these discrepancies can in large part be reconciled by taking into account the pressure recovery phenomenon.

In patients with an aortic diameter of less than 30 mm, it becomes appropriate to account for pressure recovery by use of the formula proposed by Baumgartner and coworkers[2,3] to estimate the net gradient from Doppler measurements:

$$PR = \Delta P_{mean} \times 2 \times (EOA/A_A) \times (1 - EOA/A_A) \qquad \text{Equation 1}$$

$$\text{Net } \Delta P_{mean} = \Delta P_{mean} - PR \qquad \text{Equation 2}$$

where PR is the pressure recovery, A_A is the cross-sectional area of the aorta measured at the sinotubular junction, ΔP_{mean} is the mean pressure gradient measured by Doppler echocardiography, and net ΔP_{mean} is the net pressure gradient (i.e., the Doppler pressure gradient corrected for pressure recovery).

One can also calculate the energy loss coefficient (ELCo), a new parameter proposed by Garcia and associates,[5] that adjusts the Doppler EOA for the size of the aorta to take into account the pressure recovery:

$$ELCo = (EOA \times A_A)/(A_A - EOA) \qquad \text{Equation 3}$$

This energy loss coefficient is easily measurable by Doppler echocardiography and is more or less equivalent to the catheter EOA calculated with the use of the Gorlin formula.[4,10] Like the EOA, the energy loss coefficient should be indexed for body surface area to take into account cardiac output requirements in a given patient. A value of the energy loss index of 0.50-0.55 cm^2/m^2 or less is an indicator of severe AS.[5,11]

Physiologically, the net or recovered indexes (i.e., the catheter EOA and gradients or the energy loss coefficient and net gradients estimated by Doppler echocardiography) are more representative of the actual energy loss caused by the stenosis and thus of the increased burden imposed on the ventricle than the maximum gradient or EOA measured by Doppler echocardiography, and as such, they should be more closely related to symptoms. Accordingly, previous

CORRELATION BETWEEN DOPPLER AND GORLIN EOA

Doppler EOA (cm^2)	Aorta Diameter (mm)					
	20	25	30	35	40	45
0.4	0.5	0.4	0.4		0.4	0.4
0.5	0.6	0.6	0.5	0.5	0.5	0.5
0.6	0.7	0.7	0.7	0.6	0.6	0.6
0.7	0.9	0.8	0.8	0.8	0.7	0.7
0.8	1.1	1.0	0.9	0.9	0.9	0.8
0.9	1.3	1.1	1.0	1.0	1.0	1.0
1	1.5	1.3	1.2	1.1	1.1	1.1
1.1	1.7	1.4	1.3	1.2	1.2	1.2
1.2	1.9	1.6	1.4	1.4	1.3	1.3
1.3	2.2	1.8	1.6	1.5	1.5	1.4
1.4	2.5	2.0	1.7	1.6	1.6	1.5
1.5	2.9	2.2	1.9	1.8	1.7	1.7

This table provides the values of the energy loss coefficient, that is, the Doppler effective orifice area (EOA) corrected for pressure recovery, as a function of the aorta diameter measured at the sinotubular junction and the Doppler EOA. The energy loss coefficient is equivalent to the catheter EOA measured by the Golin Formula. The green area indicates the situations in which the pressure recovery is absent or negligible. In these situations, it is not relevant to calculate the net (i.e., recovered) indexes of stenosis severity. The yellow area represents the situations in which there is significant pressure recovery, but the differences between Doppler EOA and energy loss coefficient (or catheter EOA) are generally not clinically relevant. The red area indicates important pressure recovery that may result in misclassification of stenosis severity based on Doppler EOA. In these situations, it is important to calculate the net pressure gradient (Equation 2) and the energy loss coefficient (Equation 3).

Table 96C.2 Correlation between Doppler and Gorlin EOA

studies have demonstrated that the energy loss coefficient is superior to the Doppler EOA in predicting the actual energy loss and the occurrence of left ventricular dysfunction and adverse outcomes in patients with AS.[5,11] Not accounting for pressure recovery in patients with small aortas may lead to a discrepancy in the estimation of severity between Doppler echocardiography and invasive cardiac catheterization (see Table 96C.2).

In the case presented, the aortic diameter measured at the sinotubular junction was 25 mm, the pressure recovery estimated from the echocardiographic data by Equation 1 was 11 mm Hg, and the net mean gradient estimated by Equation 2 was 29 mm Hg, which is consistent with the gradient measured by catheter (see Table 96C.1). Consistently, the energy loss coefficient or "recovered EOA" calculated with Equation 3 (1.06 cm^2) was similar to the EOA determined by catheter with the use of the Gorlin formula. Hence, the discrepancy between the echocardiographic and catheter data observed in this patient with a small aorta is essentially due to the occurrence of an important pressure recovery downstream of the stenosis. In conclusion, this patient has a moderate AS and should be managed conservatively.

SUMMARY

Pressure recovery is a clinically relevant issue in patients with smaller aortas (diameter <30 mm) or with mild, moderate, or moderate to severe AS, whereby echocardiography tends to overestimate AS severity relative to American College of Cardiology/American Heart Association guidelines (see Table 96C.2). In these patients, the consideration of the net or recovered indexes of stenosis severity, such as the net pressure gradient (Equations 1 and 2) or the energy loss coefficient (Equation 3), allows the clinician to obtain a more accurate estimate of the actual energy loss caused by the stenotic valve, to reconcile the discrepancies between catheter and Doppler indexes of stenosis severity, and to achieve a more accurate assessment of stenosis severity and risk stratification.

d. Transcatheter Aortic Valve Replacement

Alain Cribier, Alan Zajarias, Helene Eltchaninoff, and Christophe Tron

Aortic stenosis is the most common form of adult acquired valvular heart disease in developed countries, increasing in prevalence with age.[1] The management of aortic stenosis in elderly patients, particularly when it is associated with comorbidities, is becoming an important issue for geriatricians and cardiologists. The only proven therapy for definitive relief of symptoms and improved survival is surgical valve replacement. The operative mortality and frequency of postoperative morbidity increase with age and become significantly higher when preexistent comorbidities, such as coronary artery disease, poor left ventricular function, renal insufficiency, pulmonary disease, and diabetes, are present.[2] Whereas the operative mortality rate for aortic valve replacement is below 4% in the general population, it may become prohibitive in this subset of patients (20% or greater). It is remarkable that approximately one third of patients with symptomatic aortic stenosis do not undergo surgical treatment, mainly because of old age, left ventricular dysfunction, and underlying cardiac and extracardiac comorbidities.[3] However, with medical treatment aimed at symptom palliation, the survival rate is known to be as low as 20% at 2 years.[4]

Since 2002, transcatheter aortic valve implantation has been a possible alternative treatment for this population at high risk for surgical valve replacement.

CASE PRESENTATION

An 84-year-old man with aortic stenosis began experiencing episodes of dyspnea on exertion during the last 2 years. His symptoms have recently progressed with dyspnea at rest, orthopnea, and increasing lower extremity edema. His past medical history is significant for coronary artery disease with surgical revascularization, hypertension, diabetes mellitus, dyslipidemia, chronic renal insufficiency (estimated glomerular filtration rate of 33 mL/min/m^2), and pulmonary hypertension. His physical examination is remarkable for marked fluid overload and pulmonary congestion, absence of the second heart sound, and harsh systolic murmur at the upper sternal border. His transthoracic echocardiogram shows a heavily calcified trileaflet aortic valve, decreased left ventricular systolic function with an ejection fraction of 32%, pulmonary systolic pressure of 60 mm Hg, mean aortic valve gradient of 42 mm Hg, and estimated valve area of 0.65 cm^2. Coronary angiography shows severe multivessel disease with patent left internal mammary graft to the left anterior descending coronary artery. With an estimated operative mortality risk (Society of Thoracic Surgeons score) of 17.8%, he was declined for surgery by two independent surgeons. Because of his age, baseline renal impairment, and other comorbidities, his risk of requiring dialysis after surgery is not trivial either. Few treatment options are available for him. Medical titration will improve his degree of congestion, but the underlying problem will remain. Percutaneous balloon aortic valvuloplasty may be attempted, but its success is accompanied by a high recurrence rate. Thus, he was referred for percutaneous aortic valve implantation.

PERCUTANEOUS PLATFORMS

Currently, there are two different percutaneous platforms that have been tested extensively in humans and have obtained the European CE mark: the Edwards Sapien valve (Edwards Lifesciences, Irvine, Calif) and the CoreValve ReValving System (CoreValve Inc., Irvine, Calif). At this time, patients with severe aortic valve stenosis

($\leq$0.7cm^2) associated with symptoms that are expected to benefit from isolated valve replacement, who have a high surgical risk, and who have been refused standard aortic valve replacement are exclusively considered for transcatheter aortic valve implantation.

Edwards Balloon-Expandable Valve

Since the first transcatheter aortic valve implantation in humans performed in Rouen, France, in April 2002,[5] more than 500 patients have been treated worldwide with the balloon-expandable valve. The current model used (Edwards Sapien valve) is a trileaflet bioprosthesis made of bovine pericardium mounted on a stainless steel balloon-expandable stent (Fig. 96D.1). The valve is placed in the subcoronary position with use of the calcified aortic annulus and native leaflets to anchor it in place. It is available in two sizes, 23 mm and 26 mm in diameter at full expansion, which require a 22 French and 24 French sheath for insertion, respectively.

Initial valve placement was done by the anterograde (transvenous) approach.[5,6] This route had the advantages of being completely percutaneous, avoiding arterial access complications, and crossing the native aortic valve through its smooth ventricular surface. However, it was technically challenging. The current retrograde approach[7] uses a catheter with a deflectable tip (RetroFlex catheter) that allows easier passage through arterial tortuosities and the aortic arch. The route's major advantages include the familiarity of the technique, as it resembles balloon aortic valvuloplasty, and its simplicity because the transseptal puncture is avoided. However, its limitation is vascular access; because of the size of the sheaths required for valve delivery, patient candidacy is limited by arterial diameter. The transapical approach is truly a mini-invasive surgical technique that requires an anterolateral thoracotomy, direct ventricular puncture, and sheath insertion.[8] The bioprosthesis is then introduced through the left ventricle under echocardiographic and fluoroscopic guidance. This avoids concerns of vascular access and potentially limits the risk of stroke as it avoids the passage of a large device across the aorta.

Currently, both surgeons and cardiologists determine the placement route after thoroughly assessing the diameter, tortuosity, and calcification of the aorta and the iliac and femoral arteries (Fig. 96D.2).

Transcatheter aortic valve implantation follows the same steps regardless of the route used. First, the aortic valve is crossed and dilated by a regular balloon valvuloplasty technique to increase the orifice area and to aid in traversing the native aortic valve and positioning the crimped stent-valve. The bioprosthesis is then implanted. Both the balloon aortic valvuloplasty and the valve deployment are performed under rapid ventricular pacing. Rapid ventricular pacing consists of stimulating the right ventricle at a rate of 180 to 220 beats per minute, dropping the systolic blood pressure to less than 60 mm Hg, reducing the cardiac output, and creating virtual cardiac standstill. This stabilizes the balloon during inflation, ensuring appropriate valve positioning and preventing the stent from being dragged by the balloon.

This technology provides remarkable hemodynamic improvement. Femoral insertion is accompanied by an increase in aortic valve area (0.6 to 1.7 cm^2), a fall in mean transvalvular gradient (46 to 11 mm Hg), and an improved left ventricular ejection fraction.[6,7] Perivalvular aortic insufficiency is seen in some of the patients; however, it is hemodynamically significant in a minority. The observed procedural mortality rate is dramatically lower than the predicted one (7.8% to 12% versus 30% to 34%), and the 1-year survival is 81%.[7] The transapical approach is associated with similar hemodynamic improvements. Its procedural and 30-day mortality rates are reported to be 13.6%, and actuarial survival at 110 days is 76%.[8]

CoreValve

The CoreValve ReValving System is a self-expanding nitinol-framed porcine pericardium prosthesis that has been developed for the treatment of native aortic stenosis and aortic regurgitation and to replace failing bioprostheses. The multilevel frame is placed retrograde across the left ventricular outflow tract and extends to the aortic root. It has three functional levels: (1) the lower portion with high radial strength to anchor the device in the annulus; (2) the middle portion, which provides high hoop strength where the bioprosthesis lies in a supra-annular position; and (3) the superior portion, with low radial strength, which flares into the ascending aorta, ensuring optimal orientation in relation to blood flow (Fig. 96D.3). The device, which has been used since 2004, was initially available on a 25 French catheter platform that

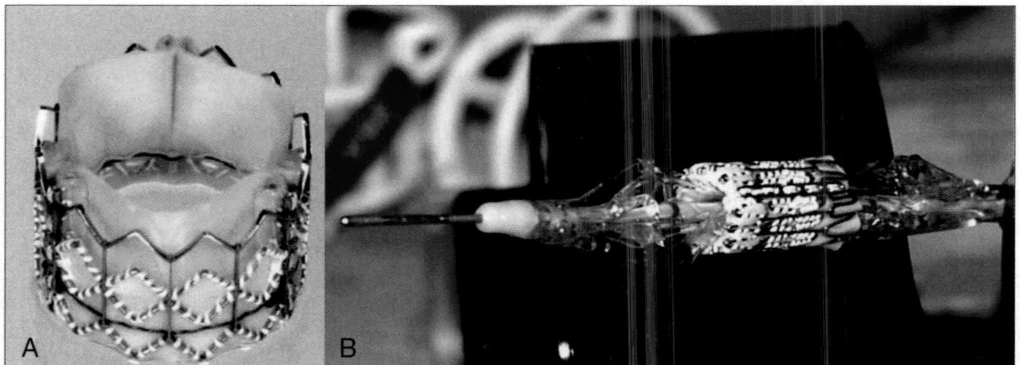

Figure 96D.1 A, Profile of the Edwards Sapien percutaneous valve. The valve is trileaflet, made of bovine pericardium, and mounted on a stainless steel stent partially covered on its distal half by a polyethylene terephthalate skirt. **B,** It is symmetrically crimped over a balloon to allow its insertion.

Figure 96D.2 Algorithm for selection of patients for transcatheter aortic valve implantation with the Edwards-Sapien valve.

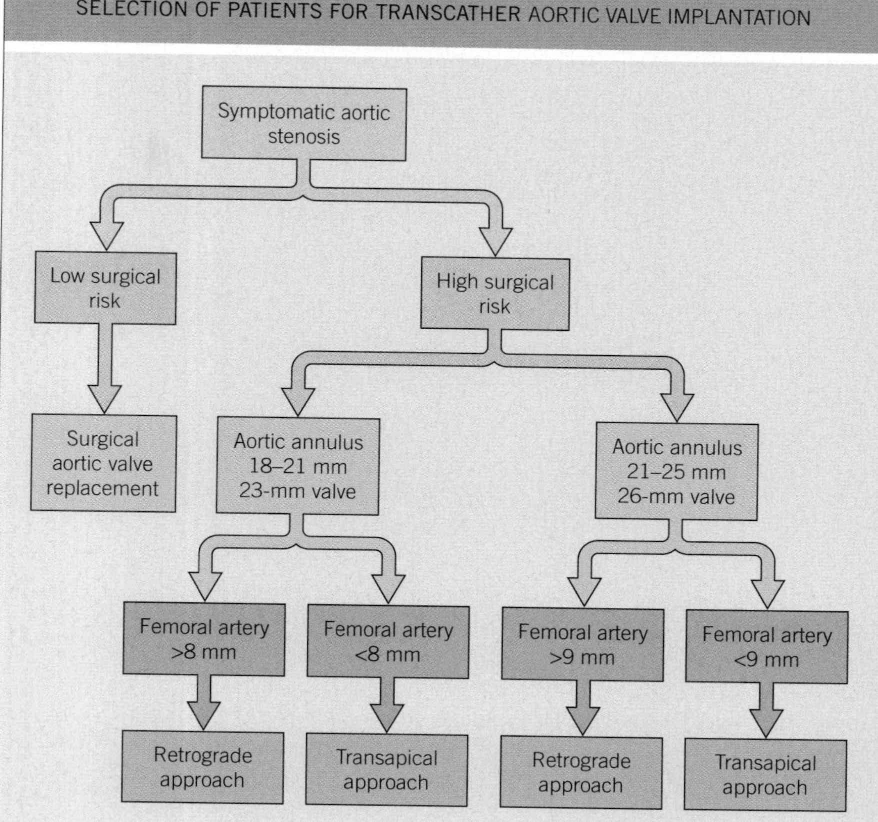

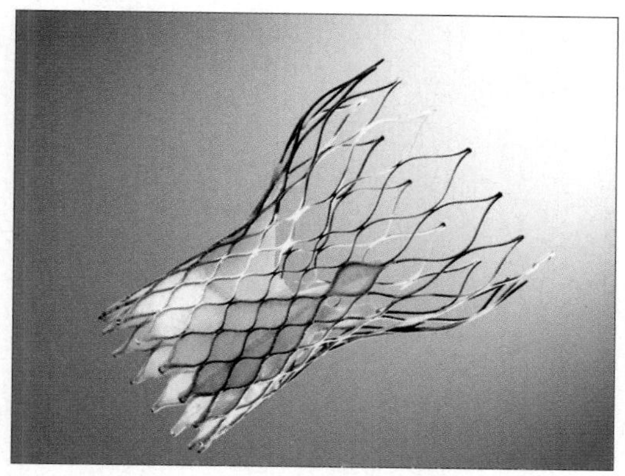

Figure 96D.3 The CoreValve ReValving System is composed of a 55-mm nitinol frame that allows anchoring at the level of the aortic annulus and aortic root and a porcine pericardium trileaflet valve that is delivered percutaneously.

required extracorporeal circulation support. This was replaced by second-generation (21 French) and third-generation (18 French) devices. The current 18 French device has evolved to a truly percutaneous procedure performed under local anesthesia, without circulatory assistance or rapid ventricular pacing. The results obtained with the two last generation devices are promising.[9] In a population of elderly patients at high surgical risk, the acute success rate was 88%. Valve implantation resulted in a marked reduction of the transvalvular gradient from 44 to 9 mm Hg with unchanged aortic regurgitation grade. Acute procedural success was 74%, and procedural and 30-day mortality rates were 6% and 12%, respectively. The major advantages of the Core-Valve prosthesis include a smaller sheath size and the ability to reposition the valve when it is partially deployed. This provides liberty to the operator to optimize the valve position during deployment. To date, more than 400 patients have been treated with this technology (E. Grube and M. Buchbinder, oral presentation, Transcatheter Cardiovascular Therapeutics, Washington, DC, October 2007).

SUMMARY

Percutaneous aortic valve replacement is a new and feasible therapeutic option for the high-risk surgical patient with symptomatic aortic stenosis and offers promising short- and mid-term results. Longer follow-up is needed to assess in vivo long-term valve durability. The next generation of valves will likely decrease sheath size, correct perivalvular leaks, allow valve repositioning, and improve the crossing profile of the valve catheter, making transcatheter aortic valve implantation a safer procedure and affecting its success. Unconditional cooperation between cardiologists, surgeons, anesthesiologists, and clinicians is required to ensure a prosperous future for transcatheter aortic valve implantation.

chapter 97

Tricuspid and Pulmonic Valve Disease

Theo E. Meyer and Dennis A. Tighe

Definition

- Stenosis of the valves and obstruction to flow or regurgitation of the tricuspid and pulmonic valves.

Key Features

- Tricuspid regurgitation has several primary and secondary causes. The most common primary cause is infective endocarditis; the most common secondary cause is pulmonary hypertension.
- Tricuspid stenosis is uncommon and usually well tolerated. It occurs in rheumatic heart disease or the carcinoid syndrome.
- Pulmonic stenosis is a congenital abnormality that may be manifested in adulthood.
- The primary diagnostic tool for these valve lesions is echocardiography.

Therapy

- Tricuspid valve disease is managed medically with diuresis and surgically by valve repair or replacement.
- Pulmonic stenosis can often be corrected by balloon valvotomy.

TRICUSPID VALVE DISEASE

TRICUSPID REGURGITATION

The clinical spectrum of patients with tricuspid regurgitation (TR) varies greatly and is largely determined by the cause of regurgitation and associated comorbid conditions. TR is detected frequently in normal subjects by color-flow Doppler echocardiography; if it is present, it is graded as trace, mild, moderate, or severe. The prevalence of trace TR is between 52% and 77%; mild TR is found in 13% to 26% of subjects in the Framingham study.[1] The high prevalence of trace TR by color-flow study suggests that this is a normal finding associated with tricuspid valve closure. The prevalence of more than mild grades of TR increases with age.[1] Moderate or more severe TR is found less commonly and may be a finding associated with minimal symptoms in some patients; but in others, it may be associated with a marked increase in morbidity and mortality when it coexists with left-sided valvular heart disease,[2-4] pulmonary hypertension, or right ventricular dysfunction or follows cardiac surgery.[5]

Functional Anatomy and Etiologic Considerations

The tricuspid valve has three leaflets that are supported by papillary muscles of varying size. The septal and the anterosuperior leaflets are the most prominent. The inferior leaflet is less constant than the other two. The tricuspid annulus is not a distinct collagenous structure like the mitral annulus, and as such, it is more prone to dilate in response to pressure and volume overload conditions of the right ventricle. In fact, tricuspid annular dilatation is the most common mechanism of severe TR. Whereas primary TR refers to a tricuspid valve lesion in the absence of elevated pulmonary pressures or dilating conditions of the right ventricle, secondary or functional TR refers to a right-sided valve lesion in the presence of these conditions (Table 97.1).

Pathophysiology

The hemodynamic consequences of TR depend on its severity, rapidity of onset, compliance of the right atrium and ventricle, and pulmonary vascular resistance (Fig. 97.1). The right ventricle is both volume and pressure overloaded when severe TR is secondary to pulmonary hypertension; but in primary ("low-pressure") TR, the right ventricle is predominantly volume overloaded. Both these overload conditions are associated with right ventricular and atrial dilatation, which in turn leads to further tricuspid annular dilatation and worsening regurgitation. Volume overload in the setting of a noncompliant right ventricle and atrium is associated with marked increases in right-sided filling pressures. Right atrial pressures may become "ventricularized" when a large regurgitant volume enters a fairly volume-loaded and noncompliant right atrium. Severe TR is also associated with a decreased right-sided forward stroke volume, which may cause exercise intolerance.[6] Thus, TR is relatively well tolerated in patients with compliant right ventricles and normal pulmonary artery pressures, whereas patients with significant TR and elevated pulmonary artery pressures usually develop marked right-sided heart failure.

Clinical Presentation

The symptoms and physical signs of TR are to a large extent dependent on coexistent cardiac conditions. In general, the symptoms are not distinct from the symptoms of right-sided congestion. However, symptoms such as anorexia, weight loss, right upper quadrant abdominal tenderness, abdominal discomfort, and leg swelling may be more pronounced when severe TR complicates right-sided heart failure. Patients who develop TR late after successful left-sided valve replacement often complain of a considerable reduction in their exercise capacity.[6]

Patients with severe TR often have poor peripheral perfusion as reflected by cold and cyanotic extremities and

ETIOLOGIC CONSIDERATIONS OF TRICUSPID REGURGITATION		
Functional Anatomy	**Etiology**	**Prevalence**
Primary TR		
Abnormal TV leaflets		
Scarred or retracted leaflets	Rheumatic heart disease[7]	Rare
	Carcinoid disease[8]	Rare
	Anorectic drugs[9]	Rare
	Radiation-associated valve disease[10]	Rare
Myxomatous leaflets	Myxomatous degeneration of TV	Rare
Destruction of leaflet tissue	Infective endocarditis	Most common cause of primary TR
	Pacing wires[19]	Increasing prevalence
	Right ventricular biopsies	Increasing prevalence
Abnormal position of TV annulus	Ebstein's anomaly	Rare
Abnormal right atrial geometry	Giant isolated right atrium	Rare
	Cardiac transplantation[20]	Increasing prevalence
Ruptured or retracted chordae tendineae of TV	Infective endocarditis	Common cause of primary TR
	Trauma	Rare
	Myxomatous chords	Rare
	Right ventricular biopsies	Increasing prevalence
	Rheumatic disease	Rare
	Endomyocardial fibrosis	Rare
Abnormalities of the papillary muscles	Trauma	Rare
	Right ventricular infarction	Rare
	Endomyocardial fibrosis	Rare
Unknown	After cardiac surgery	Not known
Secondary TR		
Tricuspid annular dilatation	Elevated pulmonary artery pressures	Most common cause of TR
	Left-sided valve lesions	Common
	Left ventricular dysfunction	Common
	Primary pulmonary hypertension	Rare
	Cor pulmonale	Common
	Intracardiac shunts	Rare
	Right ventricular dilating conditions in the absence of elevated pulmonary artery pressures	
	Atrial septal defect	Rare
	Right ventricular infarction	Rare

TR, tricuspid regurgitation; TV, tricuspid valve.

Table 97.1 Etiologic considerations of tricuspid regurgitation.

purplish discoloration of the cheeks. The hallmark physical finding of significant TR, distention and systolic pulsation of the neck veins, is accompanied invariably by an enlarged and pulsatile liver. Auscultation may reveal the typical systolic murmur of TR, which is predominantly localized over the left lower sternal area and increases with inspiration. The murmur may also be detected at the apex in patients with marked right ventricular dilatation. Failure to demonstrate an inspiratory increase in murmur intensity does not necessarily exclude severe TR; in some patients with flail leaflet or leaflet coaptation failure, the murmur may be soft or even absent because there is minimal flow turbulence. Frequently, a diastolic flow rumble is heard because of the increased diastolic flow across the tricuspid valve. Careful attention should be accorded to the underlying causes of functional or secondary TR, such as mitral stenosis, pulmonary hypertension, and causes of left ventricular failure.

Diagnostic Techniques

The diagnostic work-up of a patient with suspected TR should include an assessment of the

- presence and severity of the tricuspid regurgitant lesion
- functional anatomy of the tricuspid valve
- pulmonary artery pressures
- right and left ventricular systolic function
- left-sided valves

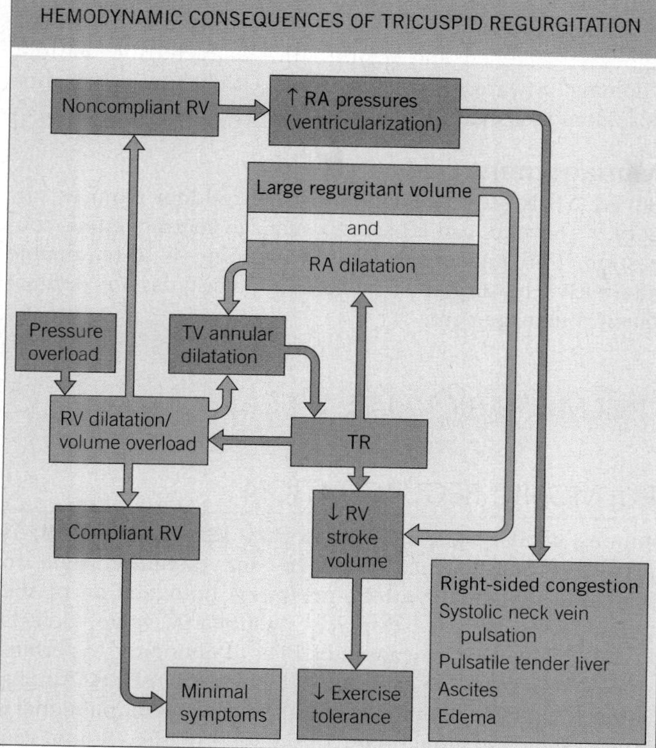

Figure 97.1 Hemodynamic derangements that accompany tricuspid regurgitation and its clinical correlates. RA, right atrium; RV, right ventricle; TR, tricuspid regurgitation; TV, tricuspid valve.

Electrocardiography

The electrocardiographic changes associated with TR are not specific and often reflect abnormalities associated with left-sided disease or pulmonary hypertension. Atrial fibrillation, right bundle branch block, and right precordial Q waves (V_1 and V_2) are the most suggestive electrocardiographic findings of significant TR.

Chest Radiography

The chest radiograph is not particularly helpful in diagnosis of TR. In general, cardiomegaly is evident in nearly all patients with severe TR, and there may be disproportionate enlargement of the right atrium and right ventricle. In patients with primary TR, the lung fields are usually fairly avascular. Patients with infective endocarditis of the tricuspid valve, however, often have multiple areas of cavitation in the lung fields due to septic emboli.

Echocardiography

Doppler echocardiography is generally the only imaging modality necessary to assess the functional anatomy of the tricuspid valve and to quantify the severity of TR. Moreover, this technique permits estimation of pulmonary artery pressures, assessment of right and left ventricular systolic function, and evaluation of the aortic or mitral valves.

Certain echocardiographic findings are specific and may help identify the primary disease involving the tricuspid valve. Certainly, the presence of mobile vegetations provides strong evidence that infective endocarditis is the primary process. The differential diagnosis of the echocardiographic finding of excessive thickening and retraction of the tricuspid leaflets includes rheumatic disease,[7] carcinoid disease,[8] anorectic drugs,[9] and radiation-associated valve disease (see Table 97.1 and Chapter 86).[10] The most common echocardiographic findings, however, are markedly dilated tricuspid annulus, right ventricular and atrial dilatation, and elevated pulmonary artery pressures.

Several Doppler echocardiographic findings have been used to quantify the severity of TR.[11,12] All of the currently available Doppler echocardiographic indexes of severity are largely qualitative and, at best, semiquantitative. The most commonly used are the color Doppler regurgitant jet area and the jet area as percentage of the right atrial area.[12] The finding of systolic flow reversal of vena cava and hepatic veins provides strong indirect evidence of severe TR. The vena contracta width of the tricuspid regurgitant jet as measured by Doppler color-flow study appears to correlate the most closely with severity of TR.[11] A vena contracta width of 6.5 mm or more is a very specific (93.3%) and fairly sensitive (88.5%) finding of severe TR.[11] However, the best approach to the quantification of TR severity is to integrate all these echocardiographic indexes of severity in conjunction with right atrial and ventricular size and systolic expansion of the right atrium. The color Doppler flow parameters of severity may not be accurate when severe TR is due to either a flail leaflet or tricuspid valvectomy for infective endocarditis. In this scenario, the low-pressure gradient between right ventricle and right atrium is likely to produce regurgitant flow with less turbulence and, hence, a less impressive area of disturbed flow in the right atrium.

Cardiac Catheterization

In the current era, invasive hemodynamic assessment of TR is unnecessary in most patients, although cardiac catheterization is often performed in patients with TR to evaluate coronary anatomy when surgery is planned for aortic or mitral valve disease. In milder forms of TR, right atrial and diastolic right ventricular pressures may be only mildly elevated; in more severe TR, the right atrial pressure tracings show a large *v* wave and progressive "ventricularization" of the right atrial pressure. In some cases of severe TR, the right ventricular and left ventricular diastolic pressure tracings appear to have the usual characteristics of patients with restrictive or constrictive physiology. This has led to the mistaken diagnosis of coexistent constrictive pericarditis.

Management

Primary Tricuspid Regurgitation

Diuretics are effective in alleviating the symptoms of right-sided congestion, such as abdominal fullness and leg edema. Severe TR due to infective endocarditis is usually well tolerated, and surgery is not indicated unless there is evidence of antibiotic failure. Surgery for primary TR could be considered when there is persistent and intractable right-sided heart failure. Tricuspid valve repair, if it is feasible, is preferred to valve replacement. When the valve leaflets themselves are diseased, abnormal, or destroyed, valve replacement with a low-profile mechanical valve or bioprosthesis is often necessary. A biologic prosthesis is preferred because of the high rate of thromboembolic complications with mechanical prostheses in the tricuspid position.

Functional Tricuspid Regurgitation

Medical treatment in patients with functional TR is directed toward treating and addressing the cause of right ventricular dilatation. In patients with severe TR secondary to cor pulmonale, for example, treatment should include measures that improve oxygenation, which may reduce pulmonary artery pressures. Similarly, aggressive medical management of left ventricular failure with consequent reduction in reactive pulmonary hypertension is likely to improve functional TR by providing systolic unloading of the right ventricle. Diuretics remain the mainstay for treatment of congestion in patients with functional TR.

In recent years, the indications for surgical repair of the regurgitant tricuspid valve at the time of surgery for left-sided valve lesions have become more liberal.[2] The reasons for this change in attitude are twofold: first, the recognition that tricuspid annuloplasty adds little additional morbidity and mortality to left-sided valve surgery; and second, the evidence that functional TR may lead to increased long-term mortality and morbidity.[5] The need for tricuspid valve repair at the time of surgery for left-sided valvular heart lesions depends on the tricuspid annular size and the presence of significant TR. Some investigators have recommended a tricuspid annular diameter of more than 30 mm as an indication for tricuspid valve surgery.[13] Others recommend repair when the ratio of the tricuspid regurgitant jet area to the right atrial area is 34% or more and the diastolic tricuspid annular size is more than 21 mm/m^2.[12,14]

The American College of Cardiology/American Heart Association guidelines for the management of patients with valvular heart disease recommend that tricuspid annuloplasty be considered for less than severe TR in patients undergoing mitral valve surgery when there is pulmonary hypertension or tricuspid annular dilatation.[15]

TRICUSPID STENOSIS

Pure tricuspid stenosis (TS) is a rare condition and is usually caused by rheumatic disease. TS occurs in about 5% of patients with rheumatic mitral valve disease and is almost always associated with mitral stenosis. Mild to moderate TS has also been documented in patients with carcinoid syndrome.[8] Other forms of TS are unusual and include congenital tricuspid atresia, pacemaker lead–related injury with leaflet fibrosis,[16] and right atrial tumors such as an atrial myxoma. Patients who had a bioprosthetic tricuspid valve may also present years later with clinical signs of TS due to marked degeneration and calcification of the bioprosthetic valve.[17] The symptoms of TS are usually similar to those of the concomitant mitral stenosis or mitral regurgitation.

Pathophysiology

The hemodynamic hallmark of TS is a mean diastolic pressure gradient of 2 mm Hg or more across the tricuspid valve. The gradient increases with inspiration and volume loading, and when the gradient is more than 5 mm Hg, systemic venous congestion is usually evident.

Diagnosis

The hallmark auscultatory finding of TS is a soft diastolic rumble that increases with inspiration, best heard along the left sternal border. This finding may be obscured by the murmur of coexisting mitral stenosis. Similar to TR, TS is confirmed by echocardiography. The tricuspid valve usually appears thickened and features the characteristic diastolic "doming" toward the right ventricle. Cardiac catheterization is seldom indicated for diagnosis of TS.

Management

Severe TS is often well tolerated and seldom requires surgery.[18] Diuretics can effectively manage central venous congestion. Percutaneous balloon valvotomy is a reasonable alternative to surgery if symptoms persist despite optimal medical management.

PULMONARY VALVE DISEASE

PULMONIC REGURGITATION

Among adults, significant pulmonary regurgitation (PR) is usually a consequence of valve ring dilatation (due to increased pulmonary artery pressures) or dilatation of the pulmonary artery.[21] Primary pulmonary valve defects (Table 97.2) are rare causes of PR.[21] Pulmonary hypertension of any cause can exacerbate the severity of PR. Among patients with congenital heart disease, peripheral pulmonary artery stenosis should be considered as this lesion can increase the degree of PR. The hemodynamic consequence of PR is right ventricular volume overload, which is most pronounced with concomitant pulmonary hypertension. A mild degree of PR is found commonly on routine echocardiography.

Clinical Presentation

Isolated PR can be tolerated for long periods. When it is accompanied by pulmonary hypertension and tricuspid valve disease, symptoms and signs of right ventricular failure can dominate the clinical picture. Among patients with repaired tetralogy of Fallot, atrial or ventricular arrhythmias and sudden death may be a consequence of right ventricular dilatation and systolic dysfunction due to long-standing, severe PR.[22]

Physical Examination

In the setting of pulmonary hypertension, significant PR can cause a sustained parasternal right ventricular impulse, palpable systolic pulsations due to pulmonary artery enlargement, and a tap indicative of pulmonary valve closure at

PRIMARY CAUSES OF PULMONARY REGURGITATION
Infective endocarditis
Iatrogenic valve injury
Catheter related
Surgical or balloon valvuloplasty
Congenital valve defects
Carcinoid syndrome
Traumatic valve injury
Rheumatic heart disease

Table 97.2 Primary causes of pulmonary regurgitation.

the second left intercostal space. An ejection sound and accentuation of the pulmonic component of the second heart sound (P_2) are also often present with coexisting pulmonary hypertension. The character of the diastolic murmur of PR depends on pulmonary artery systolic pressures. The murmur is brief and low pitched with pressures of 60 mm Hg or less and may be high pitched and blowing when pulmonary pressures exceed 60 mm Hg. Murmur intensity, regardless of pulmonary pressures, increases with inspiration.

Diagnostic Techniques

Electrocardiography

Incomplete or complete right bundle branch block is found commonly. Right ventricular hypertrophy is evident when there is pulmonary hypertension. A QRS duration of 180 ms or longer has been associated with ventricular tachycardia and sudden death among patients with repaired tetralogy of Fallot.[23]

Chest Radiography

Hemodynamically significant PR is often associated with dilatation of the pulmonary arteries and enlargement of the right ventricle on chest radiography.

Echocardiography

Right ventricular enlargement and signs of diastolic overload (paradoxical septal motion, septal flattening) are common with severe PR.[23] Right ventricular hypertrophy often accompanies pulmonary hypertension. Color-flow mapping can detect PR, but a formal grading system is not established. The end-diastolic velocity of the PR spectral profile can be used to estimate the pulmonary artery diastolic pressure.

Cardiac Magnetic Resonance Imaging

Cardiac magnetic resonance imaging can be used to assess right ventricular size and systolic function and is often more accurate than echocardiography for this purpose.[22] It also permits assessment of the right ventricular outflow region for areas that are aneurysmal or akinetic. Important parameters, such as right ventricular ejection fraction, pulmonary regurgitant fraction, and right ventricular end-systolic and end-diastolic volumes, can be obtained readily from cardiac magnetic resonance imaging.

Management

Therapy is often directed at the underlying cause. In isolation, PR seldom requires specific therapy. Right ventricular failure can be treated with diuretics. In some cases, such as with prior tetralogy of Fallot repair, surgical repair,[24] or among selected patients, percutaneous valve replacement[25] may be required, although the optimal timing is not certain.[22]

PULMONIC STENOSIS

Pulmonic stenosis (PS) is most often congenital in origin. Rarely, PS may be an acquired lesion. PS causes obstruction to right ventricular outflow with a consequent right ventricular pressure overload. In 80% to 90% of cases, the obstruction occurs at the valve level.[21] On pathologic examination, the pulmonic valve most often has three pliant leaflets with commissural fusion. In some cases, the valve can be bicuspid or dysmorphic (Noonan's syndrome). Secondary hypertrophy of the infundibulum accompanies valvular PS commonly. In the minority of cases, right ventricular outflow obstruction occurs at subvalvular, supravalvular, or pulmonary artery locations.

Clinical Presentation

Among adults, valvular PS is typically an isolated finding, but it may exist with other congenital defects. Mild PS is often asymptomatic. Patients with moderate or severe PS may present with fatigue, exertional dyspnea, angina, syncope, or sudden death due to decreased pulmonary blood flow.

Physical Examination

Significant PS is characterized by a prominent jugular venous *a* wave and a right ventricular lift. The first heart sound is normal and P_2 is diminished. If the valve is pliant, a systolic ejection click is often heard. The murmur of PS is of the systolic ejection type and best heard at the second left intercostal space. Cyanosis may occur with right-to-left shunting at the atrial level as with a patent foramen ovale or septal defect.

Diagnostic Techniques

Electrocardiography

With moderate or severe PS, right ventricular hypertrophy and right axis deviation can be found.

Chest Radiography

The heart appears normal in size, and pulmonary artery dilatation is often found with mild to moderate PS. Cardiomegaly and decreased vascular markings may be observed with severe PS.

Echocardiography

The size and function of the right ventricle (and right atrium) and thickness of the right ventricular free wall can be assessed.[26] Significant PS is associated with both systolic and diastolic interventricular septal flattening and right ventricular free wall hypertrophy. Right ventricular dilatation and systolic dysfunction are often observed. The location of stenosis can be determined by pulsed-wave and color-flow Doppler study. The severity of the stenosis is assessed by the modified Bernoulli equation to calculate the peak systolic gradient.

Cardiac Catheterization

Catheterization is required rarely for diagnosis of PS. When echocardiography fails to adequately assess PS, cardiac catheterization is indicated. Cardiac catheterization is also recommended when the peak systolic gradient is more than 36 mm Hg and the valve is amenable to balloon dilatation.[15]

Management

The most recent American College of Cardiology/American Heart Association guidelines[26] define mild PS as a peak systolic gradient of less than 36 mm Hg, moderate stenosis as peak gradients ranging from 36 to 60 mm Hg, and severe stenosis as a peak gradient of more than 60 mm Hg. Mild PS rarely exhibits significant hemodynamic progression and is generally characterized by a benign clinical course.[27]

Patients with severe disease are often symptomatic and will require intervention.[27] The procedure of choice is percutaneous balloon valvotomy.[28,29] Current class I indications for balloon valvotomy include symptomatic status with peak gradients above 30 mm Hg and asymptomatic patients with peak gradients above 40 mm Hg.[15] Long-term results are excellent, and infundibular stenosis regresses with time.[28,29] Valve surgery is reserved for those with dysmorphic or heavily calcified valves, subvalvular PS, and significant PR. Similar to balloon valvotomy, long-term results with surgery are quite good. After valvuloplasty, surveillance for the development of significant PR is required. Moderate PS can be managed medically, with intervention reserved for the development of symptoms.[27]

chapter 98

Infective Endocarditis

Jean Acar and Pierre-Louis Michel

Definition

- Infective endocarditis is an infection of the endocardium caused by microorganisms.

Key Features

- As a general rule, valvular endocardium is involved.
- Prompt diagnosis is essential for successful management and is now easier because of ultrasound techniques.

Therapy

- Appropriate antibiotic therapy is required.
- Cardiac surgery is often mandatory to improve the prognosis.
- Recommendations for prevention have changed.

EPIDEMIOLOGY

Infective endocarditis (IE) is not a rare disease. The precise incidence of the disease is unknown, but it is higher than evaluated from clinical series. The widespread use of echocardiography and particularly transesophageal echocardiography has enabled most cases, but not all, to be diagnosed. The yearly incidence reported in developed countries usually ranges between 1.7 and 6.2 per 100,000 of the population.[1-11]

Men are more frequently affected than women are, with a male-to-female ratio ranging between 1.6:1 and 2.5:1. The incidence of the disease increases after 30 years of age and exceeds 10 cases per 100,000 for people older than 50 years. Over time, a higher mean age of the patients with IE has been reported in most series. Cherubin and Neu[5] reported a mean age of 31 years in 1938 and 52 years in 1966. In the series of Delahaye and coworkers[2] and of Hoen and colleagues,[7] which included only cases of IE that were diagnosed in 1991 and in 1999, the mean age was 56 years and 59 years, respectively. In the series of Heiro and colleagues,[6] during 24 years (1980-2004), the mean age of patients increased significantly from 47.2 to 54.5 years.

During the past few decades, the incidence of the disease has been either stable or increasing.[4,7,8] For example, per 100,000 patient-years, it was

- 1.8 in 1983, 2.4 in 1991, and 3.0 in 1999 in France[2,7];
- 3.2 in 1945 and 6.8 in 1990 in Dusseldorf (Germany)[3]; and
- 3.6 in the review of contemporary case series encompassing a total of 3784 episodes of IE between 1993 and 2003.[4]

The stability and, in some countries, the increase in the rate of IE over time, in spite of the decrease in rheumatic valvular disease in industrialized countries, seem to be related to several factors:

- the increase in predisposing conditions, such as degenerative heart valve disease and prosthetic heart valves;
- the increase in nosocomial endocarditis, mainly in the elderly population, resulting from invasive procedures such as endovascular investigations, hemodialysis, and implanted endovascular or intracardiac devices;
- the increase in IE due to intravenous drug abuse;
- the improved diagnosis of endocarditis since the introduction of ultrasonography.

The microbiologic profile of IE also has changed. Staphylococci and oral streptococci account for most cases of disease, and staphylococci tend to prevail in some recent series.[4,6,7]

IE remains a major cause of severe valvular lesions. In autopsy studies in the 1960s, it was the cause of 15% of valvular diseases with predominant or pure valvular regurgitation. Recent data show that it is responsible for 10% to 25% of the cases of mitral and aortic regurgitation at surgery.[8] The prognosis has definitely improved during the past 10 years, but in spite of medical and surgical therapies, the mortality rate is still about 20%.

ANATOMY AND PATHOLOGY

The valvular apparatus is usually involved. The left-sided heart chambers, which are infected in more than 85% of cases of IE, are the most commonly involved. Isolated aortic lesions are observed in 55% to 60% of cases, isolated mitral lesions in 25% to 30% of cases, and associated mitral and aortic lesions in around 15% of cases. However, in some series, mitral IE has increased with time, whereas the proportions of aortic IE have decreased.[6] In right-sided IE (which accounts for 10% to 15% of the total cases), the tricuspid valve is more often involved than the pulmonary valve.[8,12]

The lesions consist of vegetations and valvular mutilations (Fig. 98.1). Thrombi are sometimes associated with vegetations. Vegetations are located on the valves and sometimes extend to the ventricular or atrial endocardium. They start along the valve closure line. At first, they form as small outgrowths that become a pinkish, red, or grayish mass, which is sessile or pedunculated and is a source of emboli. The size ranges from 0.2 to 4 cm. On histologic examination, they are composed of a mixture of fibrin and platelets; they contain a large inoculum of bacteria and are often enclosed in a layer of exopolysaccharides that hampers antibiotic penetration (Fig. 98.2). After sterilization, they decrease and disappear or, rarely, calcify.

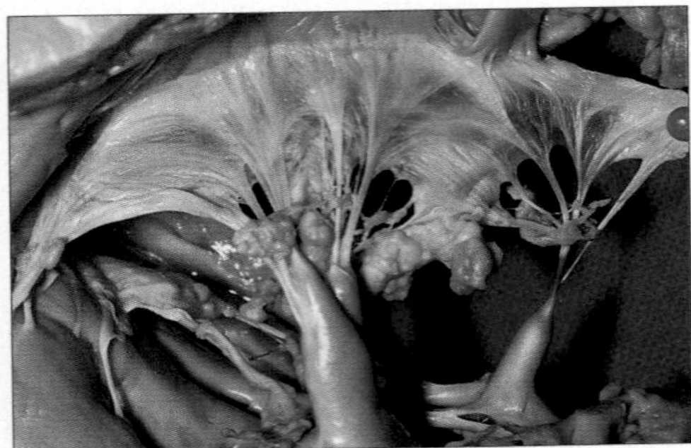

Figure 98.1 Tricuspid valve endocarditis. There are large vegetations on the leaflets and the chordae tendineae.

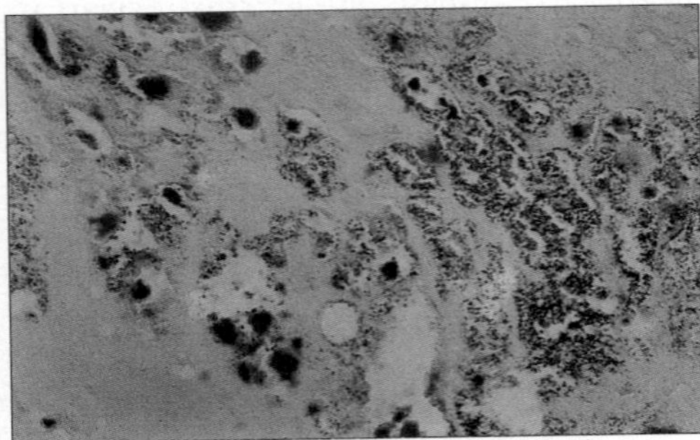

Figure 98.2 Mitral valve endocarditis. Microscopic section of vegetation (Gram coloration) showing clumps of bacteria. (Courtesy of R. Loire, Hospital Lyon, France.)

The degree of valvular mutilation depends on the type of IE, its duration, and its anatomic site. Mutilation consists of ulceration, tear, perforation, and rupture of mitral or tricuspid chordae tendineae. When the tear affects the insertion ring, either the cusp or the leaflet prolapses. This causes a sudden onset of valvular regurgitation. Perforation of cusps has been found at autopsy in two thirds of patients who had aortic valve IE (Fig. 98.3). Perforation of the anterior mitral leaflet usually results from contamination by a regurgitating aortic jet. A mitral valvular aneurysm may be the

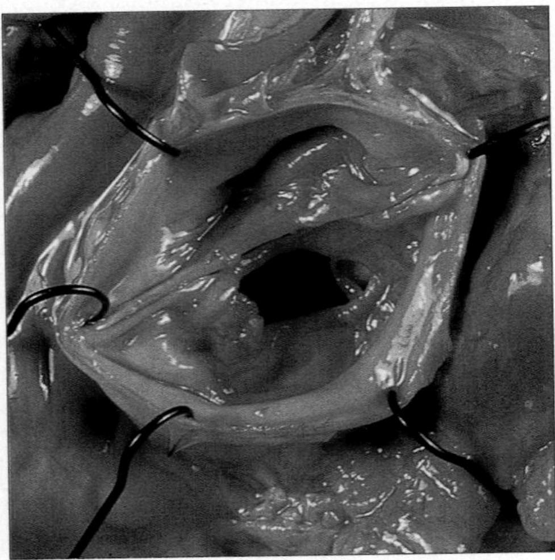

Figure 98.3 Aortic valve endocarditis. Note the bicuspid valve and the perforation of a cusp. (Courtesy of R. Loire, Hospital Lyon, France.)

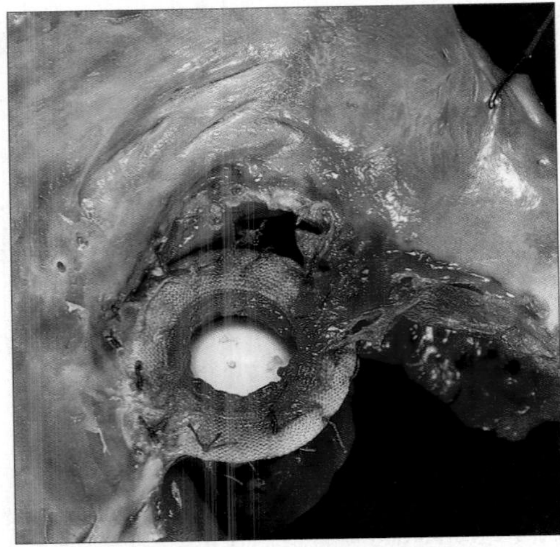

Figure 98.4 Anatomic finding in a patient who died of prosthetic valve endocarditis. There is dehiscence of the annulus ring with vegetations. The prosthetic valve was a mitral Starr-Edwards valve.

first step toward perforation. Rupture of mitral chordae tendineae is often multiple, involving the two leaflets.

Abscesses of the heart are observed in 20% to 40% of cases, mainly in the aortic valvular ring. They can spread to the surrounding structures, such as the aorta, the anterior mitral valve, and the interventricular septum, and they can cause a fistula between the two ventricles or between the left ventricle and the right atrium or connect the aorta and the right-sided heart chambers.

Myocardial lesions are usually the consequence of acute valvular regurgitation. They consist rarely of a diffuse myocarditis with minute disseminated abscesses, an isolated abscess, or a myocardial infarction secondary to coronary embolism.

An inflammatory or septic pericardial effusion is mainly observed in IE that is localized to the aortic valve.

Most extracardiac lesions result from arterial emboli in the kidneys, the spleen, the liver, the central nervous system, and the coronary arteries. Mycotic aneurysms involve mainly the sinuses of Valsalva, the cerebral arteries, the branches of the abdominal aorta (the mesenteric arteries), and, more rarely, the limb arteries and coronary arteries.

Prosthetic Valve Endocarditis

When mechanical valves are affected by IE, abscesses are particularly frequent, extending beyond the prosthetic ring into the annulus and periannular tissue. Ring abscess, septal abscess, fistulous track, and dehiscence of the prosthesis are frequent autopsy findings (Fig. 98.4). In cases of bioprosthetic valves, the anatomic lesions are more heterogeneous, varying from perivalvular extension to limited leaflet infection.

PATHOGENESIS AND PATHOPHYSIOLOGY

Pathogenesis

Endocarditis results from the colonization of the endocardium by microorganisms during episodes of bacteremia. A cause of bacteremia may be found in 50% to 70% of cases of IE. Table 98.1 specifies the predominant pathogens in IE

PREDOMINANT PATHOGENS IN INFECTIVE ENDOCARDITIS ACCORDING TO THE CAUSE OF BACTEREMIA

Portal of Entry	Predominant Pathogens*
Dental procedures and routine daily activities (e.g., tooth brushing, chewing food)†	Penicillin-sensitive streptococci‡
Infection of the respiratory tract Surgery of the oropharynx Surgery of the respiratory tract	Viridans group streptococci
Digestive tract infectious diseases Gastrointestinal tumors Therapeutic interventions in the gastrointestinal tract	Enterococci *Streptococcus bovis* Gram-negative bacilli Staphylococci
Urosepsis Urologic interventions	Enterococci Gram-negative bacilli *Staphylococcus aureus*
Gynecologic infections Gynecologic interventions	Streptococci Enterococci
Other Wound infections Skin injuries Osteomyelitis Indwelling catheters Chronic hemodialysis Intravenous drug abuse Cardiac catheterization Cardiac surgery	*Staphylococcus aureus* *Staphylococcus epidermidis* Gram-negative bacilli Fungi

*No cause of bacteremia is found in 30% to 50% of cases.

†The most frequent portal of entry. However, bacteremia causing infective endocarditis is probably more often related to a daily transfer of bacteria from mouth to blood than to occasional oral or dental procedures (see section on prevention).

‡Viridans group streptococci are usually penicillin sensitive, but in the past 2 decades, the percentage of resistant strains to penicillin, macrolides, and cephalosporin has been increasing.

Data from references 2, 3, and 7.

Table 98.1 Predominant pathogens in infective endocarditis according to the cause of bacteremia.

according to the cause of bacteremia. Mucosal surfaces are populated by a dense endogenous microflora. Trauma to a mucosal surface, particularly the gingival crevice around teeth, oropharynx, gastrointestinal tract, urethra, and vagina, releases many different microbial species transiently into the bloodstream. However, an undamaged endocardium is resistant to infection. Two factors therefore intervene to create endocarditis:

- aseptic fibrinoplatelet thrombus; and
- microorganisms.

Aseptic Fibrinoplatelet Thrombus

An aseptic fibrinoplatelet thrombus called nonbacterial thrombotic endocarditis is the prerequisite for the development of an infection. It develops on contact with a damaged endothelium and has been found in 1.3% of patients at autopsy in various diseases. Within the framework of IE, the usual cause of nonbacterial thrombotic endocarditis is a predisposing cardiac defect. Endothelial lesions are determined by the initial disease, such as rheumatic fever, and later by the rheologic conditions related to the valvular disease (e.g., the impact of a high-velocity jet, flow from a high-pressure chamber to a low-pressure chamber, and flow across a narrow orifice at high velocity). The site of endocardial lesions and nonbacterial thrombotic endocarditis corresponds closely with that of infected vegetations in patients who have IE. They are usually immediately beyond a valvular or subvalvular obstruction, on the atrial side of the valve in mitral or tricuspid regurgitation, on the right ventricular endocardium around a ventricular septal defect, and on the pulmonary artery wall opposite a patent ductus arteriosus.

Preexisting heart disease is found in 40% to 75% of cases of left-sided IE but is rarer in right-sided disease. Table 98.2 lists the cardiac conditions that carry a risk for the development of IE. In the absence of preexisting heart disease, it is supposed that the damage to the endothelium is the result of bacterial toxins. In some cases that are classified as primary endocarditis, minor degenerative cardiac lesions could not be detected but probably served as a nidus for initiation of endocarditis. Diabetes mellitus and infection with human immunodeficiency virus (HIV) may also increase the IE risk.

Microorganisms

An acute course of IE is, as a rule, caused by virulent pathogenic agents, and preexisting valve disease can be minimal or absent in such cases. Subacute IE usually affects patients who have major preexisting heart valve defects and is caused by less virulent pathogens, such as viridans streptococci.

Before colonization of the thrombus and the damaged endocardium by microorganisms can occur, several conditions must be satisfied (Fig. 98.5)[3,4]:

- resistance to serum bactericidal factors;
- formation of clusters of microorganisms, facilitating endocardial penetration and resulting from serum aggregating antibodies;
- reduced clearance capacity of the reticulohistiocyte system with respect to the infective agent; some conditions that cause complement consumption, reduced cellular immune reactivity, and immunosuppressive serum factors are associated with a reduced clearance capacity (e.g., AIDS, terminal renal insufficiency, alcoholism, and drug abuse); and
- adhesive power of microorganisms, which is promoted by multiple mechanisms, such as the ability of pathogens to produce dextran (in the case of streptococci), glycocalyx, or slime *(Staphylococcus epidermidis)* or to have receptors for fibronectin (*Staphylococcus aureus;* viridans streptococci; groups A, C, and G streptococci; enterococci; and *Candida* albicans); fibronectin can facilitate adherence of bacteria to the site of injury of the valve.

Figure 98.6 shows early steps in bacterial valve colonization.[4]

After the infection of the vegetation, the poor vascularization of the endocardium limits the effectiveness of the humoral defense mechanism. Fibrin deposits are also an effective barrier against phagocytes. Therefore, the vegetation grows from the multiplication of pathogens and the accumulation of cell detritus, platelets, and fibrin. The vegetation is not a totally sheltered site, however. It has been shown in experimental endocarditis that platelets produce a potent microbicidal material that kills some strains of streptococci and *S. aureus* in the vegetations.[16]

CARDIAC DISEASE AND THE RISK OF INFECTIVE ENDOCARDITIS		
Group A: Cardiac diseases with the highest risk		
Prosthetic valves	Mechanical, bioprosthetic, or homograft valves	Risk 5-10 times higher than in patients with native valve disease
Congenital heart disease causing cyanosis, uncorrected or with pulmonary-systemic shunts	Tetralogy of Fallot	Incidence of 2-3/1000 patient-years; risk is higher after a palliative pulmonary-systemic arterial anastomosis and lower after total correction
	Other	Incidence of 8/1000 patient-years
Previous IE	Promoting factors include drug addiction, poor dental hygiene, and underlying cardiac disease	
Group B: Cardiac diseases with moderate risk		
Valvular heart diseases	Aortic regurgitation	Underlying in 17%-36% of IE; incidence 0.4/1000 patient-years
	Aortic stenosis	Underlying in 10%-20% of IE
	Mitral regurgitation	Underlying in 20%-35% of IE
	Mitral valve prolapse with murmur	Risk 6-14 times higher than in control population
Congenital heart diseases	Ventricular septal defect	Incidence of 2-3/1000 patient-years; risk does not depend on the size of the defect; risk is higher in association with aortic regurgitation; risk is decreased by corrective surgery
	Bicuspid aortic valve	Important promoting factor for IE; found in 20%-25% of aortic IE
	Patent ductus arteriosus and coarctation of aorta	Previously high bacterial risk has greatly decreased as a result of correction during infancy or childhood
Hypertrophic obstructive cardiomyopathy	Incidence has not been exactly evaluated; severe obstruction is a promoting factor; mitral and aortic valves and endocardium of the left ventricle outflow tract are the sites of infection	
Group C: Cardiac diseases with low risk or no risk		
Mitral stenosis	Low risk when it is pure and isolated; incidence of 0.17/1000 patient-years	
Pulmonary stenosis	Incidence of 0.09/1000 patient-years	
Mitral annular calcification	Low risk	
Marfan's syndrome		
Cardiac pacemakers and implantable defibrillators		
Corrected left-to-right shunts		
Coronary artery bypass grafts	No risk	
Mitral valve prolapse without mitral regurgitation		
Interatrial communication (except atrioventricular septal defect)		

Note: In developing countries, rheumatic heart disease is the first predisposing factor for infective endocarditis (IE).
Group A includes cardiac diseases for which not only the incidence but also the morbidity and mortality of infective endocarditis are high. Guidelines from the American Heart Association[43] also include the following conditions in this group for which prophylaxis with dental procedures is recommended: completely repaired congenital heart defect with prosthetic material or device, whether it is placed by surgery or by catheter intervention, during the first 6 months after the procedure; repaired congenital heart diseases with residual defects at the site or adjacent to the site of a prosthetic patch or prosthetic device; and cardiac transplantation recipients who develop cardiac valvulopathy.
Data from references 8, 13 to 15, and 18 to 21.

Table 98.2 Cardiac disease and the risk of infective endocarditis.

Pathophysiology

Clinical manifestations of IE (Fig. 98.7) result from

- local intracardiac infection;
- embolization of vegetations and thrombi;
- metastatic infection;
- stimulation of the immune system; and
- activation of the coagulation system.

Local Intracardiac Infection

The consequences of intracardiac infection are highly variable. In some cases, antibiotic therapy allows a rapid sterilization of infected vegetations and avoids major damage to the valves and surrounding tissue. In many cases, cardiac infection leads to severe lesions. At first, valvular destruction is responsible for an acute regurgitation. Subsequently,

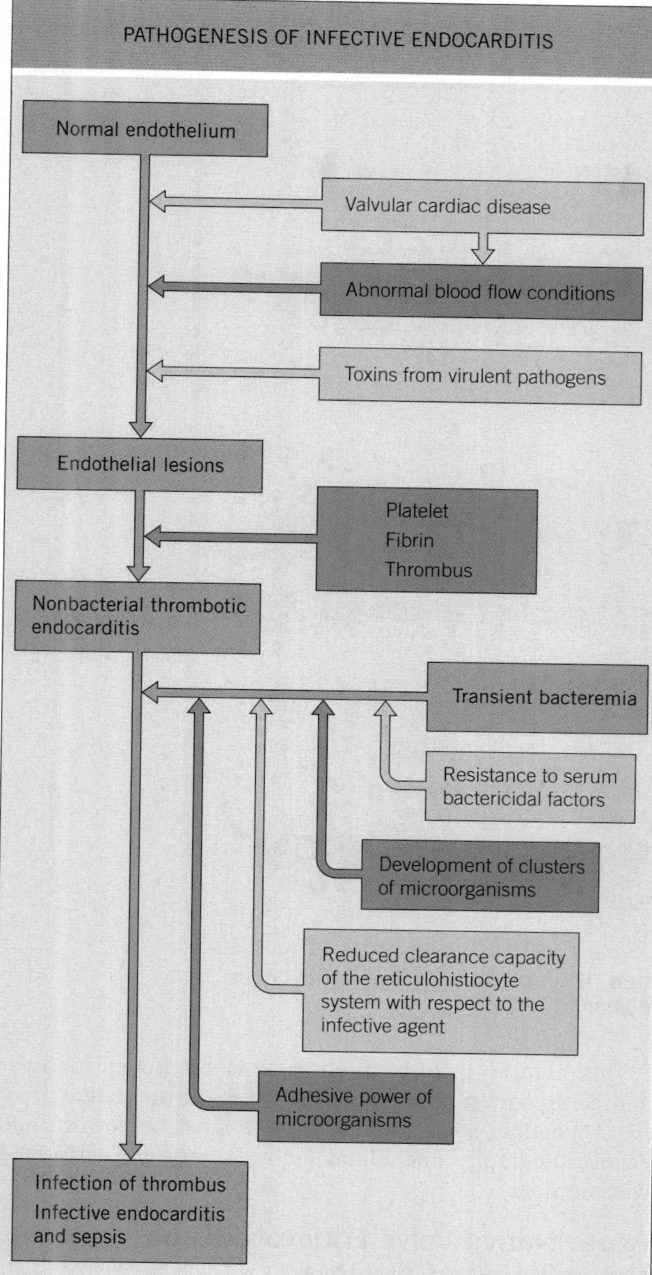

Figure 98.5 Pathogenesis of infective endocarditis.

aneurysms of the sinuses of Valsalva, intracardiac fistulas, conduction abnormalities, and septic pericarditis can result from spreading of valve ring abscesses in the paravalvular tissue.

Embolization of Vegetations and Thrombi

Embolization of vegetations may involve virtually any organ. It affects the systemic or pulmonary circulation according to the site of IE, and it can cause sterile or septic infarction. The highest risk of emboli occurs in infections that produce large, mobile vegetations, including infection due to *Candida* species, *S. aureus*, and HACEK and abiotrophic organisms.

Intracardiac thrombi may also be the source of embolism.

Metastatic Infection

Metastatic infection results from embolization or seeding of bacteria to remote sites. It may be obvious, with local signs, or more difficult to diagnose, presenting as a persistent fever in spite of antibiotic therapy. Mycotic aneurysms are produced by septic embolization to the vasa vasorum or by direct bacterial invasion of the arterial wall.

Stimulation of the Immune System

IE stimulates both the humoral and the cell-mediated immune systems. Activated circulating macrophages and splenomegaly express the cellular responses. Humoral stimulation is evident from circulating immune complexes, which is common in patients who have positive blood cultures and is seen in about half of the patients who have negative blood cultures. High titers of immune complexes have been found in IE of long duration, in the presence of extravascular manifestations, and in right-sided IE. Immune complex titers decrease and can disappear with effective antibiotic therapy and rise again with failure of treatment.

Deposits of immune complexes with complement along the glomerular basement membrane may entail a focal or diffuse glomerulonephritis and may be detected by kidney biopsy with appropriate staining of glomeruli. Arthritis and some peripheral cutaneous manifestations of IE (Osler's nodes) have been attributed to the local deposit of immune complexes.

Activation of the Coagulation System

The levels of circulating membrane activation molecules, such as E-selectin and P-selectin, have been found to be increased in patients with IE and significantly correlated to the risk of thromboembolic events.[17]

CLINICAL PRESENTATIONS

Clinical presentations of IE are variable.

Subacute Native Valve Endocarditis of the Left Side of the Heart

Subacute native valve endocarditis (NVE) of the left side of the heart is the most common clinical picture in IE. Symptoms occur within 2 weeks of bacteremia in more than 80% of patients.

Fever is the dominant symptom. It is often moderate, with a temperature lower than 102°F (39°C), and remitting. In patients who have known valvular heart disease, any unexplained fever for 5 days must lead to consideration of IE. However, fever is absent in about 5% of patients, particularly in cases of previous antibiotic therapy, in elderly people, in severe debility, and in chronic renal failure. In practice, the absence of fever does not allow the diagnosis of IE to be dismissed.

Nonspecific symptoms, such as sweating, shivering, fatigue, nausea, arthralgias, myalgias, and weight loss, are sometimes present.

Pathologic murmurs occur both as a result of preexisting heart disease and as a result of IE. Diastolic murmurs from aortic regurgitation and apical holosystolic murmurs from mitral regurgitation are common abnormalities. If the previous cardiac auscultatory findings are known, the discovery of a new murmur or a change in the intensity of a mitral or aortic murmur has a significant value for the diagnosis of IE; this occurs in 30% to 50% of patients.

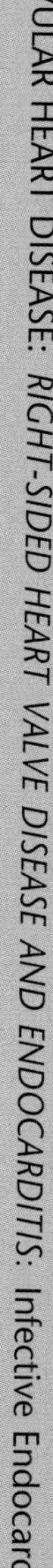

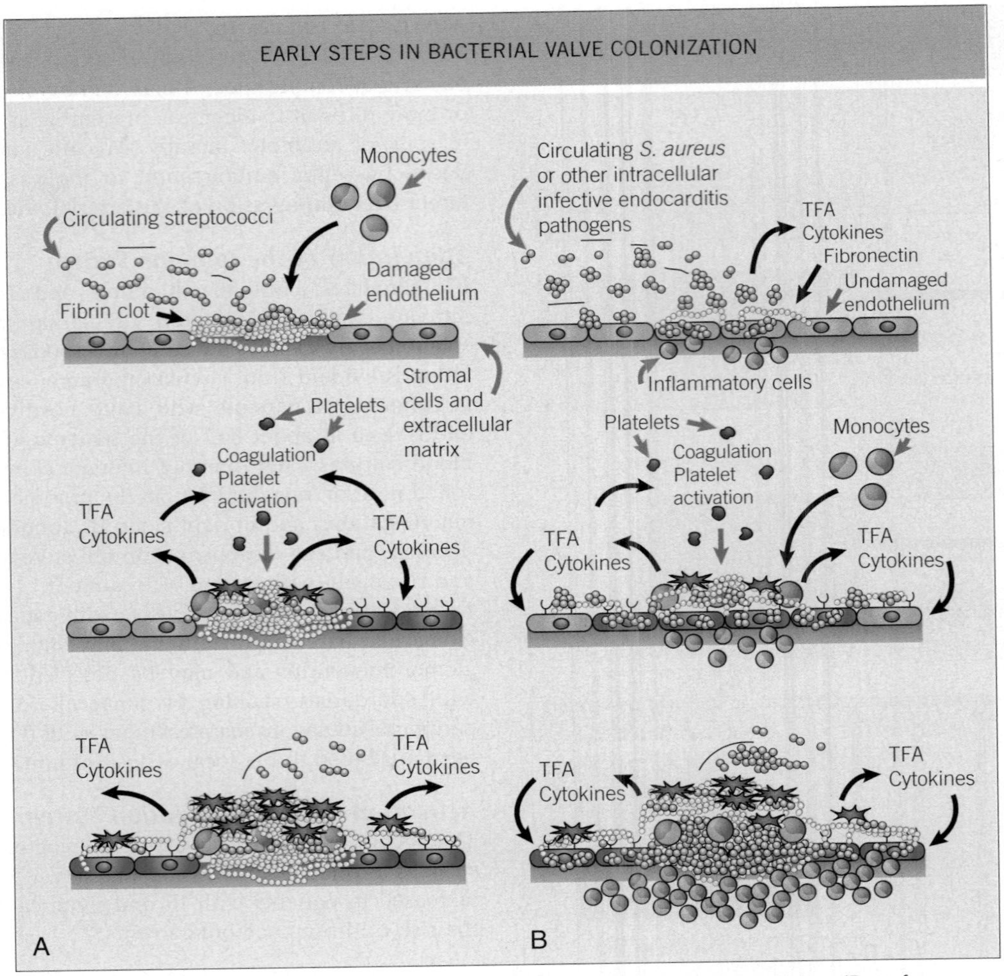

Figure 98.6 Early steps in bacterial valve colonization. TFA, tissue factor activity. (Data from Moreillon P, Que YA. Infective endocarditis. Lancet 2004;363:139-149.)

Peripheral signs are related either to sepsis or to vascular manifestations. These signs include

- splenomegaly, which is observed in 30% to 50% of cases;
- renal signs, such as microscopic hematuria and proteinuria, which occur commonly; and
- anemia-related pallor, which affects one quarter of patients.

Cutaneous manifestations are not specific for IE and are rarer than in the past because of earlier antibiotic therapy. Clubbing occurs late and is seen in 10% to 20% of patients. Between 10% and 40% of patients have petechiae, which are found on the extremities, above the clavicles, on the buccal and palatal mucosa, or on the palpebral conjunctiva. Splinter or subungual hemorrhages, which occur in 5% to 15% of cases, are dark red, linear, or sometimes flame-shaped streaks.

Osler's nodes, which are found in 10% to 20% of cases, are bluish red tumefactions that are pinhead to pea sized, painful on pressure, and located on the finger or toe pads. They disappear after a few days and without suppuration either spontaneously or after antibiotic therapy. Janeway's lesions are erythematous, irregularly defined, nontender, small (1 to 5 mm) areas that are located chiefly on the palms and soles. Roth's spots appear as oval retinal hemorrhages with a pale center and are found in 5% to 10% of cases.

This clinical picture, even if it is restricted to fever and cardiac murmurs, must bring to mind the diagnosis of IE. A possible source of bacteremia must be sought, and echocardiography and blood cultures must be performed without delay.

Acute Native Valve Endocarditis of the Left Side of the Heart

Acute NVE of the left side of the heart represents 5% to 10% of cases. The onset of infection is usually explosive; the clinical picture consists of severe sepsis and a high fever with temperature of 102°F to 104°F (39°C to 40°C), shivering, splenomegaly, and sometimes necrotic purpura. In many cases, there is no preexisting heart disease at the initial examination. Cardiac murmurs are often absent at the first examination but quickly appear as the result of valvular destruction. It should also be observed that acute IE evolves too quickly for the development of immunologic vascular phenomena.

As a rule, such occurrences of acute IE are caused by virulent pathogens, particularly *S. aureus,* but also by *Pseudomonas aeruginosa* and beta-hemolytic streptococci. The prognosis, if untreated, is poor. The two most frequent complications are left-sided heart failure and uncontrolled sepsis with metastatic infection.

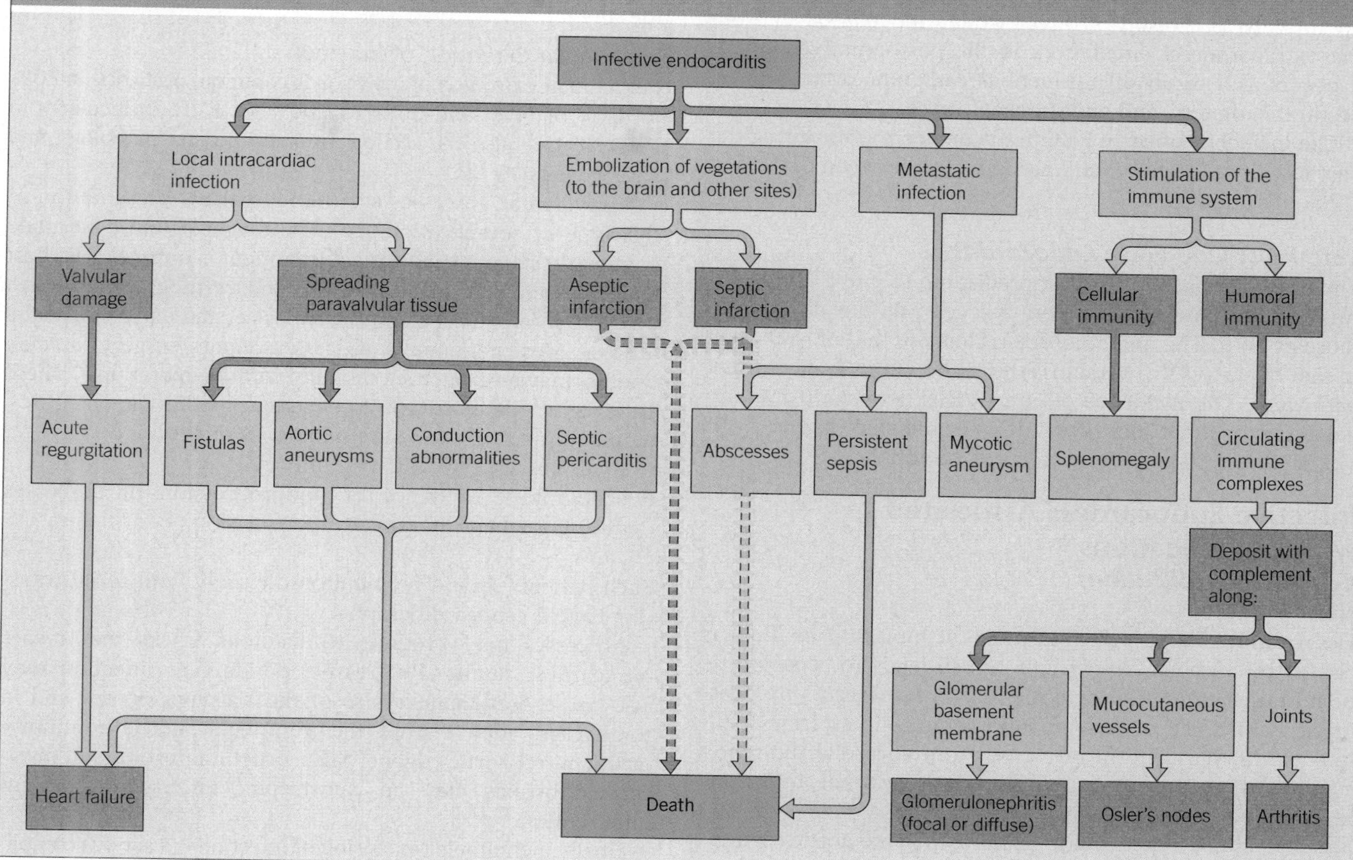

Figure 98.7 Pathophysiology of infective endocarditis.

Right-Sided Heart Valve Endocarditis

Right-sided heart valve endocarditis occurs in 5% to 10% of cases of IE.[3,18-20] The main cause is intravenous drug abuse. The valve most frequently damaged is the tricuspid valve (>70% of cases). Other sources of infection are rarer and include pacemakers,[20] central lines, skin or gynecologic infections, and bacteremia in patients who have congenital cardiac lesions (such as left-to-right shunts).

The clinical presentation is an acute endocarditis or, more often, pulmonary septic emboli, which occur in 75% of cases of IE due to intravenous drug abuse. Cardiac signs are not evident. A murmur of tricuspid regurgitation is heard in less than half of the patients. In the past, the diagnosis was often missed, but echocardiography and awareness of predisposing factors have now led to diagnosis of the disease in most patients.

The principal responsible pathogen is *S. aureus* (mainly in intravenous drug abuse). *S. epidermidis* (mainly in pacemaker IE), *P. aeruginosa*, streptococci, fungi, or polypathogens may also be responsible.

In intravenous drug abuse, the mortality rate of right-sided endocarditis is between 5% and 10%,[18] but recurrences are frequent, occurring in 30% of cases. The usual causes of death are respiratory insufficiency, left ventricular endocarditis, and complications of AIDS. In pacemaker IE, pacemaker removal is usually required, and the prognosis is more serious.

Prosthetic Valve Endocarditis

The frequency of prosthetic valve endocarditis (PVE) is between 10% and 25% of IE in developed countries. In early PVE, symptoms appear within 60 days after valve implantation; in late PVE, they occur later. Nevertheless, many cases appearing between 2 months and 1 year after surgery are likely to be nosocomial.

In recent studies, the cumulative risk of PVE was about 1% at 12 months and 2% to 3% at 60 months.[11] In most series, PVE is more frequent with aortic prosthetic valves or multiple valves and in patients who had been operated on for an infected native valve. The usual clinical presentation is that of an acute or subacute endocarditis with sepsis and prosthesis dysfunction that gives rise to signs of poorly tolerated regurgitation. An unexplained fever in a patient with a prosthetic valve should prompt careful evaluation for PVE. Color Doppler study and transesophageal echocardiography provide crucial contributions to the diagnosis. The echocardiogram may show vegetations, ring abscess, or dehiscence of the valve, and it can evaluate the degree and the exact site of the regurgitant flow. The prognosis has been improved by medical and often earlier surgical therapy, but it remains serious.

Early Prosthetic Valve Endocarditis

The microbiology of early PVE and of that occurring within the first postoperative year is distinctive. Staphylococci such as *S. aureus* and coagulase-negative species are predominant (around 50%), followed by gram-negative bacilli, fungi, streptococci, and enterococci. Contamination occurs intraoperatively as a result of direct wound inoculation or from the extracorporeal circulation; in the postoperative period, it occurs as a result of intravenous catheters, arterial lines, urethral catheters, and endotracheal tubes.

The incidence of early PVE has been decreasing during the past few decades, but it still accounts for between 0.4% and 1.2% of patients.[21]

Late Prosthetic Valve Endocarditis

The causes of bacteremia that predispose to late PVE, occurring beyond the first postoperative year, do not differ from those of NVE. The microbiology is closer to that of NVE than to that of early PVE. Viridans streptococci are the most usual pathogens. The incidence of late PVE is between 0.2% and 0.4% per patient per year; it is somewhat higher with bioprostheses than with mechanical valves.[21]

Infective Endocarditis Associated with Complications

Cardiac Complications

Heart Failure

Heart failure is the principal cause of mortality in IE. It is caused by valvular destruction, which leads to acute aortic or mitral regurgitation or both, and in some cases by prosthetic dehiscence or sudden intracardiac shunts from fistulous tracks. It is due in rare cases to myocardial infarction caused by coronary emboli or to myocardial infectious lesions.

Heart failure may develop acutely. In acute aortic regurgitation, clinical features appear early and are immediately severe. They include dyspnea, pulmonary edema, and sometimes angina pectoris. The physical signs differ from those observed in chronic aortic regurgitation. Tachycardia is the rule, and the pulse pressure is only slightly increased or normal. The arterial peripheral signs are less clear-cut, and the diastolic murmur is shortened. A soft first heart sound is often heard because the rapid ventricular filling that occurs in aortic regurgitation closes the mitral valve before the onset of systole. The chest radiograph shows pulmonary edema and a normal cardiac silhouette. Septic complications and cardiac failure lead to a mortality of 50% to 75% in the absence of cardiac surgery. Acute mitral regurgitation may cause pulmonary edema. There is no significant myocardial dysfunction, and recompensation is often successful with medical therapy that allows continuation of the antibiotic treatment and the postponement of surgery.

Heart failure may also develop insidiously, despite administration of appropriate antibiotics, as a result of a progressive worsening of valvular insufficiency and ventricular dysfunction. Echographic evaluation delineates the causes and severity of congestive heart failure. Progressive chamber enlargement, elevation of pulmonary artery pressures, and increasing valve insufficiency on serial evaluation indicate a trend toward decompensation. Surgical decision can be guided by echocardiographic detection of abscesses, fistulas, prosthetic dehiscence, or flail leaflets.

Heart failure in IE, irrespective of the course or mechanism, portends a severe prognosis with medical therapy alone and is usually an indication for rapid surgery. In practice, patients with IE and congestive heart failure, irrespective of the mechanism, should be immediately evaluated for surgery.

Periannular Extension of Infection

Periannular extension of infection is common, occurring in 10% to 40% of NVE and 56% to 100% of PVE, particularly in aortic IE (see also the section on anatomy and pathology and pathogenesis).

Paravalvular abscesses are the most usual presentation of this type of complication.[22-24] The diagnosis must be made at an early stage when surgical treatment is optimal. The best examination is transesophageal echocardiography, which provides information about the site, size, and extension of the abscess. Most periannular abscesses require surgery; a small number may be treated successfully without operation.[24] These patients include those who meet certain conditions:

- uncomplicated, non-staphylococcal infection;
- small abscesses (<2 cm^2); and
- echographic evidence of nonprogression of abscesses during medical therapy.

Such patients should be monitored closely with serial transesophageal echocardiography.

Abscesses may progress to fistulous tracks that create intracardiac shunts. Progressive periannular infection may also cause pseudoaneurysms of the Valsalva sinuses and in some cases may disrupt the ventricular aortic continuity or the mitral aortic trigone. Such structural lesions and intracardiac fistulas may be catastrophic and require urgent intervention.[23,25]

Finally, periannular extension of infection is a serious complication of IE, predicting a higher mortality rate, more frequent development of heart failure, and more frequent cardiac surgery.

Extracardiac Complications

Systemic arterial embolisms make up the majority of extracardiac complications. They are observed in 20% to 50% cases of IE. Up to 65% of emboli involve the central nervous system, and more than 90% of these emboli lodge in the distribution of the middle cerebral artery. Less often, emboli affect lower limbs, kidney, spleen, liver, coronary arteries, and bone. They may be multiple and recurrent, occurring principally within the month after the first episode (50% of cases in some series).[3] The first episode of emboli often occurs early, before hospital admission and before or within the first 2 weeks of antimicrobial therapy; of note, the rate of embolic events drops dramatically during the first 2 weeks of successful antibiotic therapy from 13 to less than 1.2 embolic events per 1000 patient-days.[11,26] Predisposing factors are the type of pathogens and the characteristics of the vegetations on echocardiography (see earlier). Emboli may be symptomatic or silent (e.g., in the kidneys or spleen). They are detected by ultrasound examination, computed tomographic scanning, or magnetic resonance imaging. In a recent series, the incidence of splenic involvement was evaluated by computed tomographic scanning in around 35% of cases of endocarditis.[27]

Extracardiac abscesses result from septic infarction or seeding of bacteria. They frequently involve the spleen (5% to 10% in autopsy series) and the kidneys and, rarely, the brain. It is estimated that only 5% of the patients with splenic infarction, which is a common complication of left-sided IE, will develop splenic abscess. Persistent or recurrent bacteremia, persistent fever, or other signs of sepsis are suggestive of splenic abscess. Abdominal computed tomography and magnetic resonance imaging are the best tests for diagnosis, with sensitivity and specificity of 90% to 95%. Definitive treatment is splenectomy, which is also required in rare cases of splenic rupture.[22,27]

Mycotic aneurysms may involve different arteries (see the section on anatomy and pathology). They have been reported in 2% to 15% of cases,[3] chiefly late in the course of IE.

Intracranial mycotic aneurysms (which are observed in 25% of mycotic aneurysms) account for 2.5% to 6.2% of all intracranial aneurysms. The distal middle cerebral artery branches are most often involved, especially the bifurcations. Intracranial mycotic aneurysms are multiple in 20% of cases. Streptococci and *S. aureus* account for approximately 50% and 10% of cases, respectively, and are seen with increased frequency among intravenous drug abusers with IE. They can cause severe localized headache or focal neurologic deficits but are often asymptomatic until the occurrence of a sudden hemorrhage. Some intracranial mycotic aneurysms leak slowly before rupture and produce mild meningeal irritation that is detected by lumbar puncture; the spinal fluid is sterile but contains erythrocytes, leukocytes, and elevated protein levels. Rupture may happen during the active period of IE or several months or years later. Intracranial mycotic aneurysms, in many cases, may also heal with effective antibiotic therapy.[28] Decisions concerning medical versus surgical therapy must be individualized according to the patient's age, underlying comorbid conditions, location of intracranial mycotic aneurysms, and results of frequent monitoring of imaging procedures. Intervention should be strongly considered if signs of enlargement or leakage develop.[22,28] Recently, endovascular treatment has been used successfully as an alternative to surgery.[29]

Extracranial mycotic aneurysms[22] may be intrathoracic, intra-abdominal, or located on limbs. Intrathoracic or intra-abdominal mycotic aneurysms are often asymptomatic until leakage or rupture occurs. Hematemesis, hematobilia, and jaundice suggest rupture of a hepatic mycotic aneurysm; arterial hypertension and hematuria suggest rupture of a renal mycotic aneurysm; and massive bloody diarrhea suggests the rupture of a mycotic aneurysm in the small or large bowel. Whatever the risks, surgery represents an improved chance of survival.

The diagnosis of limb mycotic aneurysm is easier. The appearance of a pulsatile mass in a patient with IE should suggest extracranial mycotic aneurysm. Surgery should be envisaged, despite the risks of reinfection and rupture of interposed vascular grafts, to avoid spontaneous rupture.

Neurologic complications occur in 30% to 40% of patients. They are caused by emboli, hemorrhages, and more rarely diffuse vasculitis and metastatic infection. Ischemic cerebral infarction is the most frequent pathologic lesion, occurring in more than 50% of patients with neurologic complications; intracranial hemorrhage is noticed in around 30% of cases. It may be secondary to hemorrhagic transformation of an ischemic cerebral infarction, or it may be caused by the rupture of a mycotic aneurysm.

More rarely, brain abscess, meningitis, and meningoencephalitis are observed. Focal neurologic symptoms such as hemiplegia and hemianopsia are frequent manifestations, usually caused by embolic strokes. They are the reason for hospital admission in 3% to 5% of patients subsequently proven to suffer from IE.[3] Therefore, any vascular accident associated with fever, particularly in a young patient, must bring to mind IE. Nonfocal neurologic symptoms such as severe headache must also draw attention to IE. The exact diagnosis of these complications is provided by neurologic tests (computed tomographic scanning, nuclear magnetic resonance imaging, or lumbar puncture). Computed tomographic scanning and magnetic resonance imaging have 90% to 95% sensitivity for intracerebral bleeding and may identify the location of an aneurysm. Magnetic resonance imaging is a promising new technique for the detection of intracranial mycotic aneurysm, but conventional four-vessel cerebral angiography remains the standard for evaluation of small aneurysms (<5 mm). In patients who have neurologic complications, the mortality rate of IE is high, around 40%.

Renal complications include immune-mediated glomerulonephritis, but renal problems may also be triggered by emboli, low cardiac output, and toxic antibiotic therapy. Nephrotic syndrome is rare. Acute renal insufficiency, which occurs in less than 15% of cases, carries a poor prognosis whatever its cause and frequently necessitates surgical treatment of IE.

Articular complications such as septic arthritis and spondylitis are rare.

Infective Endocarditis in Children

The incidence of IE in infancy and childhood is low, about 0.34 per 100,000 per year.[30] Predisposing cardiac lesions are found in 75% of cases after the neonatal period. Congenital heart disease, previously operated on in 50% of cases, is usual. Rheumatic aortic or mitral valve disease is rarer. Microbiology and clinical presentation are the same as in adults. Surgical therapy for congenital heart disease is a contributing factor to the increase in the survival rate, the aging of patients, and the risk of IE after operations with prosthetic material or residual high-velocity shunts. On the other hand, surgery reduces the risk of IE in a wide range of patients.[15]

Nosocomial Endocarditis

In community hospitals, 14% to 25% of all cases of endocarditis seen during the last decade were nosocomial, with important regional variations.[9,11,31,32] This type of IE often affects elderly patients and is the result of bacteremia associated with a hospital procedure. Infected intravascular devices give rise to at least half of these cases. Other sources include genitourinary or gastrointestinal tract procedures and surgical wound infection.[11]

Particular risk groups include the immunosuppressed with central venous catheters and those undergoing hemodialysis.[33] Predominant pathogens are staphylococci and enterococci. Nosocomial endocarditis is important because its case fatality rate is greater than 50%.[32]

Endocarditis in Intravenous Drug Users

The incidence of IE in intravenous drug users is estimated to be between 1.5 and 3.3 cases per 1000 person-years.[34] IE incidence is higher among HIV-seropositive intravenous drug users than among HIV-seronegative intravenous drug users. In HIV-1–positive intravenous drug users, both the risk and mortality from IE rise inversely with the CD4 count. Intravenous cocaine use has been associated with a particularly high risk.[19]

The IE of intravenous drug users usually concerns young men (mean age of 30 to 40 years, with a ratio of men to women of 4 to 6:1). The pathogens usually originate from the skin, explaining the predominance of *S. aureus*. In some cases, unusual pathogens are responsible for IE: gram-negative bacilli, polymicrobial infections, fungi, group B streptococci, and *Streptococcus mitis*.[18,22,34] The tricuspid valve is infected in more than 50% of cases, followed by the aortic valve and the mitral valve (10% to 25%, each one). Recent analyses have demonstrated that although *S. aureus* species predominate in intravenous drug users, cases of left-sided IE in this population are due equally to viridans group streptococci and *S. aureus*.[22] Biventricular and multiple valve infections may occur, particularly in *Pseudomonas* endocarditis; 60% to 80% of patients have no known preexistent valvular lesions.

Repeated injections of impure material could probably encourage cytokine production, valvular inflammation, and fibronectin deposition on previously healthy valve tissue, thereby predisposing to infection. The most frequent clinical presentation is right-sided heart valve endocarditis (for this topic and the prognosis, see the section on right-sided heart valve endocarditis).

DIAGNOSTIC TECHNIQUES

Diagnostic Criteria

IE is a highly variable disease. Decisions concerning clinical management are directly related to an accurate diagnosis. Diagnostic criteria are important to help distinguish endocarditis from other bacteremic syndromes. Furthermore, clinical research on the natural history, epidemiology, complications, and treatment outcomes of IE depends on the accurate identification of patients with this disease.[22] Following Pelletier and Petersdorf (1977) and Von Reyn and colleagues (1981), Durack and coworkers[35] in 1994 developed a new diagnostic scheme, namely, the Duke criteria. These criteria integrate the factors predisposing patients to IE, the blood culture isolate and persistence of bacteremia, and the echocardiographic findings with other clinical and laboratory information. Many studies have validated the Duke criteria; sensitivity is estimated at more than 80%, and specificity is high (≥95%). Nevertheless, clear deficiencies remain, and sensitivity is diminished in patients whose blood cultures are negative, in those with infections affecting a prosthetic valve or pacemaker lead, and in those with IE affecting the right side of the heart (particularly drug-misusing patients). Some modifications have been proposed to improve sensitivity (Table 98.3).[36,37]

Laboratory Diagnosis

A bacterial cause of IE is established by recovery of the infective agent from the blood or from surgically removed vegetations or embolic material. The bacteriologic diagnosis of IE is facilitated by the relative constancy of bacteremia. Three separate sets of blood cultures, obtained during 24 hours, are recommended to evaluate patients suspected of having endocarditis. Each set should include two flasks, one containing an aerobic medium and the other an anaerobic medium, into which at least 10 mL of blood should be placed. Each set of cultures should be obtained from separate

MODIFIED DUKE CRITERIA FOR THE DIAGNOSIS OF INFECTIVE ENDOCARDITIS

Criteria
Major criteria
■ Blood culture positive for IE
Typical microorganisms consistent with IE from two separate blood cultures: viridans streptococci, *Streptococcus bovis,* HACEK group, *Staphylococcus aureus,* or community-acquired enterococci, in the absence of a primary focus; or
Microorganisms consistent with IE from persistently positive blood cultures: at least 2 positive cultures of blood samples drawn >12 hours apart; or all of 3 or a majority of ≥4 separate cultures of blood (with first and last samples drawn at least 1 hour apart)
Single positive blood culture for *Coxiella burnetii* (which is rare in most clinical microbiology laboratories) or antiphase I IgG antibody titer >1:800
■ Evidence of endocardial involvement
New valvular regurgitation (increase or change in preexisting murmur not sufficient)
Abnormality on echocardiographic examination (transesophageal echocardiography is recommended in patients who have a prosthetic valve, who are rated as having at least possible IE by clinical criteria, or who have complicated IE), defined as follows: an oscillating intracardiac mass on a site of endocardial injury, a periannular abscess, and a new dehiscence of a prosthetic valve
Minor criteria
■ Predisposing cardiac condition or injection drug use
■ Fever: temperature >38°C (100.4°F)
■ Vascular phenomena: emboli, mycotic aneurysms, intracranial hemorrhage, conjunctival hemorrhages, and Janeway's lesions
■ Immunologic phenomena: glomerulonephritis, Osler's nodes, Roth's spots, rheumatoid factor
■ Microbiologic findings: positive blood cultures not meeting major criteria, serologic evidence of active infection with organism consistent with IE
■ Echocardiogram consistent with IE but not meeting major criteria
Diagnosis
Definite
■ Pathologic criteria
Microorganisms demonstrated by culture or histologic examination of a vegetation, a vegetation that has embolized, or an intracardiac abscess specimen; or
Pathologic lesions: vegetation or intracardiac abscess confirmed by histologic examination showing active IE
■ Clinical criteria
2 major criteria or 1 major criterion and 3 minor criteria or 5 minor criteria
Possible infective endocarditis
■ 1 major and 1 minor criteria
■ 3 minor criteria
Rejected
■ Firm alternative diagnosis
■ Resolution of IE syndrome with ≤4 days of antibiotics
■ No pathologic evidence of IE at surgery or autopsy with antibiotic therapy for ≤4 days

Modified Duke criteria[35] for the diagnosis of infective endocarditis. Criteria modified from Fournier et al.[36] and Li et al.[37]

Table 98.3 Modified Duke criteria for the diagnosis of infective endocarditis.

venipuncture sites to minimize the risk of false-positive results. The constancy of bacteremia in patients with IE makes it unnecessary to await the arrival of a fever spike or chills to obtain blood culture specimens. The most common pathogens responsible for IE are specified in Table 98.4. The need for sampling before antibiotic administration is self-evident, although surveys of contemporary practice show consistent failure in this respect.[10,38]

In 85% to 90% of cases of IE, blood cultures on routine media are positive; in 10% to 15% of cases, usual blood cultures are negative. Prior antibiotic therapy is the major cause of blood culture–negative IE, and it has been found in 50%

MICROBIOLOGIC FEATURES OF INFECTIVE ENDOCARDITIS

Organism	Frequency (%)	Comments
Streptococcus species	50-60	
Viridans streptococci	25-25	Most common: *S. sanguis, S. salivarius, S. mitis, S. mutans*
Group D streptococci	20-25	
S. bovis		The most common of group D streptococci in IE; prevalent among the elderly and associated with colonic lesion
Enterococcus species		Frequently implicated in nosocomial bacteremia and IE resistant to medical therapy
Groups A, B, C, G	5	Responsible for severe IE
S. pneumoniae	1-2	
Abiotrophic species	2-4	Difficult growth; growth in thioglycolate medium of blood culture or on medium supplemented with pyridoxal hydrochloride or L-cysteine
Staphylococcus species	15-40	
Coagulase positive *(S. aureus)*	15-30	The most common pathogen in early PVE and in IE associated with injection drug use and long-term indwelling intravenous catheter
Coagulase negative	3-8	Observed in PVE and rarely in NVE *(Staphylococcus lugdunensis)*
HACEK organisms		
Fastidious gram-negative bacilli: *Haemophilus, Actinobacillus, Cardiobacterium, Eikenella corrodens,* and *Kingella kingae*	2-3	Slow growth; occasionally require prolonged incubation and subculturing
Bacteria with an obligatory or predominant intracellular growth	5-8	Serologic tests; lysis-centrifugation system for blood cultures
Bartonella species (usually *B. henselae* or *B. quintana*)	3	PCR of valve or embolized vegetations; special culture techniques available, but organisms are slow growing and may require a month or more for isolation
Coxiella burnetii (Q fever)	2-5	Serologic tests; PCR, Giemsa stain, or immunohistologic techniques on operative specimens
Chlamydia species	Very rare	Serologic tests; direct staining of tissue with use of fluorescent monoclonal antibody
Tropheryma whipplei	Very rare	Histologic examination (silver and periodic acid–Schiff stains) of excised heart valve; PCR or culture of vegetation
Enterobacteriaceae and	1-1.5	
nonfermenting bacilli: *Pseudomonas, Acinetobacter, Alcaligenes*	1	
Fungi	0.5-1	Regular blood cultures often positive for *Candida* species; lysis-centrifugation system with specific fungal medium can increase yield; testing of urine for *Histoplasma capsulatum* antigen or of serum for *Cryptococcus neoformans* polysaccharide capsular antigen can be helpful
Aspergillus species *Candida* species		Accessible lesions (such as emboli) should be cultured and examined histologically for fungi
Heterogeneous group of bacteria	4	
Brucella	(1)	Serologic tests; slow growth; prolonged incubation
Corynebacteria, Peptococcus, Neisseria, Listeria	(3)	

Frequency: approximate percentage of cases. IE, infective endocarditis; NVE, native valve endocarditis; PCR, polymerase chain reaction; PVE, prosthetic valve endocarditis.

Modified from Delahaye et al.[8] and Mylonakis and Calderwood.[11]

Table 98.4 Microbiologic features of infective endocarditis.

of cases.[39] Suppression of bacteremia often persists for longer than the antibiotic is present in the blood. In patients who have not received antibiotic therapy, pathogens responsible for blood culture–negative IE are primarily *Coxiella burnetii*, then abiotrophic species, HACEK microorganisms, *Brucella* species, *Legionella* species, *Bartonella* species, *Chlamydia* species, *Tropheryma whipplei*, and fungi.[37,39] Laboratory diagnosis requires, depending on the pathogens, prolonged incubation (up to 3 to 4 weeks), special cultures, molecular techniques such as polymerase chain reaction to identify organisms in excised vegetations or systemic emboli, and serologic tests (see Table 98.4). Finally, because of modern bacteriologic and serologic techniques, the incidence of authentic blood culture–negative IE has decreased and is estimated to be about 5%.[22,39]

The use of other laboratory tests in the diagnosis of IE is limited. Erythrocyte sedimentation rate is usually elevated, as is the level of C-reactive protein, but these findings have little specific diagnostic value. A normochromic normocytic anemia is present in the majority of patients who have IE, but this finding is equally nonspecific. The white blood cell count may be normal or moderately elevated in patients who have subacute presentations, whereas patients who have staphylococcal IE usually have leukocytosis. Elevated levels of serum globulins, the presence of cryoglobulin and circulating immune complexes, and hypocomplementemia may also occur in some patients, but none of these findings is diagnostic. However, an elevated level of rheumatoid factor may occasionally be useful in diagnosis. When it is present in patients without a known previous rheumatologic disorder, this finding is considered to be one of the six minor criteria in the Duke criteria.[35]

The urine analysis is often abnormal. Microscopic hematuria and mild proteinuria are often found in the absence of other renal complications. The presence of red blood cell casts and a low serum complement level may be an indication of immune-mediated glomerular disease, which is a minor diagnostic criterion.[35]

Electrocardiography

An electrocardiogram should be part of the initial evaluation of all patients suspected of having IE. Besides the presence of ischemia or infarction, the electrocardiogram may also reveal the presence or the appearance of atrioventricular block. New atrioventricular, fascicular, or bundle branch block, particularly in the setting of aortic valve endocarditis, suggests a perivalvular extension of infection. A new atrioventricular block has an 88% positive predictive value for abscess formation but a low sensitivity (45%).[40]

Echocardiography

Echocardiography is essential to the diagnosis and management of patients who have IE. Echocardiographic evaluation should be performed in all patients clinically suspected of having IE, including those with negative blood cultures. Many patients who have NVE that involves the aortic or mitral valve can be imaged adequately by transthoracic echocardiography (TTE). Transesophageal echocardiography (TEE) has superior sensitivity and is recommended when clinical suspicion is high and a transthoracic examination is normal. It is also useful in all cases of PVE and when complications are suspected or before surgery.[41]

The superiority of TEE in the detection of prosthetic endocarditis is even greater than for native valve disease. Vegetations on the tricuspid valve are detected with equal frequency by TEE and TTE. However, endocarditis of the pulmonary valve and endocarditis at unusual sites, such as pacemaker wires, are more often recognized by TEE than by TTE. TEE can more readily detect complications of endocarditis, such as abscesses and fistula formation, than TTE can. The sensitivity of TEE in the detection of abscesses or infected pseudoaneurysms has been reported to be 87% to 100%, whereas that of TTE has varied from 28% to 43%. Therefore, TEE is considered the modality of choice for initial assessment of any patient at risk for perivalvular extension of IE.

TEE is also useful in assessing the mechanisms of mitral regurgitation, which is most often caused by leaflet perforation or rupture of the chordae. It is also a particularly sensitive method for the detection of mitral regurgitation in the presence of a prosthetic mitral valve.

Echocardiography cannot always differentiate between vegetations resulting from active IE and abnormalities caused by other noninfectious valvular lesions, such as those that occur in patients who have malignant neoplasms or in valvular lesions associated with lupus erythematosus or the antiphospholipid syndrome. In addition, valvular thickening, valvular calcification, rupture of chordae, benign leaflet nodules, suture material around a sewing ring (especially after mitral valve replacement), valvular thrombus, or pannus formation on valve structures may mimic vegetations. Similarly, it is not usually possible to distinguish active from healed vegetation. TEE and TTE may produce false-negative results if vegetations are small or have already embolized.

Echocardiography may also provide important physiologic information about ventricular function and an estimate of the severity of regurgitation. Mitral valve preclosure in the setting of acute aortic regurgitation implies a marked rise in left ventricular diastolic pressure and the likely need for more urgent intervention.

Controversy remains as to whether the echocardiographic characteristics of vegetations are of use in predicting embolization. Although it is not demonstrated in all studies, it is likely that patients who have larger vegetations (>10 or 15 mm in diameter[42]; Fig. 98.8) are at increased risk for embolic complications, especially if vegetations are attached to the anterior mitral leaflet. Embolic events do appear also to be predicted by an increase in vegetation size by TEE during 4 to 8 weeks of therapy.

The use of harmonic imaging has improved study quality without altering sensitivity in the detection of vegetations. The role of three-dimensional echocardiography has yet to be evaluated.

Other Diagnostic Techniques

Other imaging modalities, such as computed tomographic scanning and magnetic resonance imaging, have been used to assess the presence of para-aortic complications such as ring abscess. However, their utility compared with that of echocardiography has not yet been established.

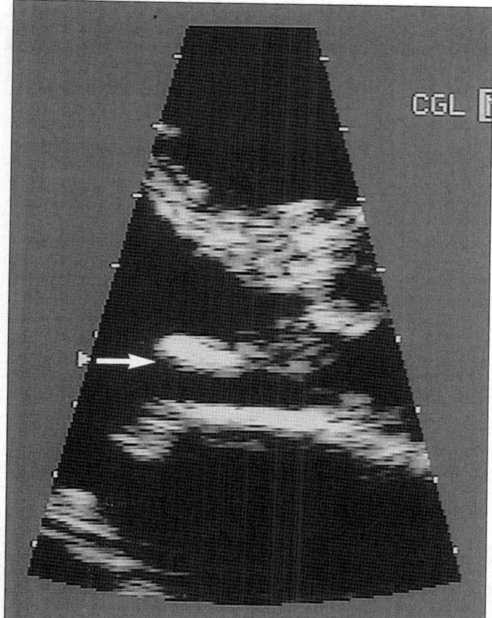

Figure 98.8 Parasternal long-axis echocardiographic view during diastole. There is a large vegetation *(arrow)* attached to the anterior mitral leaflet.

The role of cardiac catheterization in the evaluation of patients who have IE remains controversial. Doppler echocardiography allows a precise assessment of the hemodynamic and pathologic consequences of infection in most cases. The use of invasive techniques is usually limited to coronary angiography in some patients at high risk for coronary disease on the basis of their coronary risk factors.

MANAGEMENT

Prevention of Infective Endocarditis

For more than 50 years, recommendations have been made for the prevention of IE by expert groups both in the United States and in Europe. The guidelines of the European consensus (1995) and of the American Heart Association (1997) proposed a wide use of antibiotic prophylaxis in patients who underwent dental, gastrointestinal tract, or genitourinary tract procedures.

Recently, several national societies have released new guidelines that reduce greatly the indications of antibiotic prophylaxis in IE. The primary reasons for this revision are the following.

1. The responsibility of dental procedures as a cause of IE has been overestimated. Many clinical case reports and reviews implicating a dental procedure in the development of IE are debatable, either poorly documented or including cases with a remote preceding dental procedure.[43]

Some control studies have failed to prove a statistically significant link between dental procedures and IE.[44-46] The assertion that "bacteremia with organisms known to cause IE may occur in association with dental procedures," however, remains valid and has been supported by a recent French study [47]; yet the risk of IE resulting from a dental procedure appears very low .[43,45,47] The majority (95% to 98%) of patients with IE have not had, in recent series, a dental procedure within 2 weeks before the onset of symptoms of IE.

On the other hand, dental procedures are common in industrialized countries. The estimated risk of IE in adults with predisposing cardiac conditions undergoing dental unprotected procedures was 1 in 10,700 and 1 in 54,000, respectively, for patients with prosthetic valves and native valves in a recent French series.[47] The risk is evaluated as still lower in reports in the United States.[43] Therefore, a huge number of antibiotic prophylaxis treatments would be necessary to prevent a very low number of IE cases.

2. Antibiotic prophylaxis prevents viridans group streptococcal or enterococcal endocarditis in animals, but it is hazardous to extrapolate experimental data to human data. Indeed, the rabbit model requires high bacterial challenge, and the magnitude of bacteremia is much higher than that resulting from a dental procedure or from routine daily activities in humans.
3. IE is much more likely to result from frequent exposure to random bacteremias associated with daily activities than from bacteremia caused by a dental, gastrointestinal tract, or genitourinary tract procedure. Transient bacteremia is common with manipulation of the teeth and periodontal tissues, but there is a wide variation in reported frequencies[43] (e.g., tooth extraction, 10% to 100%, mean ratio around 50%; periodontal surgery, 36% to 88%). Indeed, transient bacteremia occurs frequently during routine daily activities unrelated to dental procedures: tooth brushing and flossing (20% to 68%), use of wooden toothpicks (20% to 40%), and chewing food (7% to 51%).

Finally, the cumulative risk over time of bacteremia, depending on the frequency and duration of exposure to bacteremia, is much higher from routine daily activities than from dental, gastrointestinal tract, or genitourinary tract procedures.[48]

4. The efficacy of antibiotic prophylaxis in the prevention of IE has not been absolutely proved in small retrospective studies.[44,46,49,50] The efficacy appears as probable in the survey of Duval and coworkers,[47] with an estimated protective efficacy of 70%.
5. The antibiotic prophylaxis is not risk free, and these risks must be compared with benefits of the prevention of IE.[43] Fatal anaphylactic reactions have been estimated to occur in 15 to 25 individuals per 1 million patients who receive a dose of penicillin and 1 case per 1 million patients from cephalosporin. Fatal reactions to a single dose of macrolides or clindamycin are extremely rare.

In addition, the widespread use of antibiotic prophylaxis promotes the emergence of resistant microorganisms most likely to cause endocarditis, such as viridans group streptococci and enterococci. The frequency of multidrug-resistant pathogens of these species has increased dramatically during the past decades.[43]

Four sets of revised guidelines have been published recently by the European Society of Cardiology (2004),[31] the British Cardiac Society/Royal College of Physicians (2004 and 2006),[51,52] the American Heart Association (2007),[43] and the French

Society of Cardiology (2002-2004).[53,54] These new guidelines on prophylaxis of IE take into account the considerations mentioned and agree about main issues with, nevertheless, some key exceptions.[55]

The following recommendations, however, cannot substitute for the physician's evaluation of the individual risk in a given patient.

Recommendation 1: Definition of the Groups at Risk

Group A is defined as high risk, for which the incidence but also the morbidity and mortality of IE are high. Group B has a moderate risk (lower incidence and severity). These two groups are detailed in Table 98.2.

In the other cardiac conditions, there is either no increased risk of IE or low risk (group C in Table 98.2).

Recommendation 2: Importance of Hygiene Measures

General hygiene measures are of major importance. The aim is to decrease the risk of bacteremia. These measures include oral dental and skin hygiene, disinfection of wounds, curative antibiotic treatment of infection, and strict compliance with asepsis in performing procedures at risk for infection.

A systematic surveillance of the oral and dental state is mandatory, at least twice a year for patients with heart diseases. In these patients, any procedure leading to a mucosal or skin wound must be avoided (acupuncture, skin piercing). Infusion catheters on patients at risk should be peripheral rather than central, and peripheral catheters should be replaced every 3 or 4 days.

Recommendation 3: Oral and Dental Care

In patients in group A and group B, it is recommended by the French Society of Cardiology that local chlorhexidine-based antiseptics be used as mouthwash for 30 seconds before dental procedures. However, the efficacy of topical antiseptics in reducing the frequency of bacteremia after dental procedures remains debated.

Indications for Systemic Antibiotic Prophylaxis

- Group A: antibiotic prophylaxis is recommended in patients with the highest lifetime risk of acquisition of IE and the highest risk of adverse outcome from IE (see Table 98.2) and undergoing dental procedures associated with a risk of IE (Table 98.5).
- Group B: in patients undergoing dental procedures with a risk of IE, antibiotic prophylaxis is not recommended by the American Heart Association; antibiotic prophylaxis is recommended by the European Society of Cardiology; and antibiotic prophylaxis is optional for the French Society of Cardiology.

Antibiotic prophylaxis should be chosen by health care professionals, taking into account the nature of the procedure and the patient's general condition. Table 98.6 lists factors that can influence this choice. Whatever the choice, it must be made after the patient is informed and his or her consent to the proposed strategy is obtained.

- For other cardiac conditions, antibiotic prophylaxis is not recommended.

DENTAL PROCEDURES FOR WHICH ENDOCARDITIS PROPHYLAXIS IS RECOMMENDED (FOR PARTICULAR CARDIAC DISEASES)
All dental procedures that involve manipulation of gingival tissue or the periapical region of teeth or perforation of oral mucosa
Some procedures are contraindicated, such as prostheses on teeth to be pulpectomized, inserting implants, and periodontal surgery. Pulp diseases, periodontal diseases, and trauma require extraction.
From Wilson W, Taubert KA, Gewitz M, et al. Prevention of infective endocarditis. Guidelines from the American Heart Association. Circulation 2007;116:1736-1754.

Table 98.5 Dental procedures for which endocarditis prophylaxis is recommended (for particular cardiac diseases).

FACTORS THAT MAY HELP IN CHOOSING WHETHER ANTIBIOTIC PROPHYLAXIS WILL BE PRESCRIBED WHEN PROPHYLAXIS IS OPTIONAL.[53,54]
Arguments for prescription
Age >65 years
Associated conditions
Cardiac, renal, respiratory, and hepatic insufficiency
Diabetes mellitus
Acquired, constitutional, or therapeutic (corticosteroids, immunosuppressive agents) immunodepression
Oral or dental condition
Inadequate oral or especially dental hygiene
Procedure
Important bleeding (intensity, duration)
Technically difficult procedure (prolonged procedure)
Patient's opinion after receiving information
Arguments against prescription
Allergy to several antibiotics
Patient's opinion after receiving information
Data from Danchin N, Duval X, Leport C. Prophylaxis of infective endocarditis: French recommendations 2002. Heart 2005;91:715-718.

Table 98.6 Factors that may help in choosing whether antibiotic prophylaxis will be prescribed when prophylaxis is optional.[53,54]

Before valve surgery, antibiotic prophylaxis is indicated as for patients assigned to group A. A complete radiologic dental assessment must be made; only pulped teeth or teeth that have had a perfect endodontic treatment (more than a year before) without periodontal enlargement and with a healthy periodontium are kept. Pulpectomized teeth with incomplete endodontic treatment and teeth presenting with periodontal lesions and persisting roots and apex are extracted at least 15 days before cardiac surgery.

Recommendation 4: Other Procedures at Risk

These recommendations are based on professional consensus in the absence of scientific data and cannot replace the clinician's judgment. Antibiotic prophylaxis is not recommended by the guidelines of the American Heart Association except for patients assigned to group A who undergo an invasive procedure of the respiratory tract, such as biopsy of the respiratory mucosa, tonsillectomy, and adenoidectomy. The European Society of Cardiology, British Cardiac Society/ Royal College of Physicians, and French Society of Cardiology propose antibiotic prophylaxis for some patients who undergo procedures at risk for IE. Table 98.7 details diagnostic and therapeutic interventions, other than dental procedures, associated with a risk of IE.

INTERVENTIONS OTHER THAN ORAL OR DENTAL PROCEDURES ASSOCIATED WITH A RISK OF INFECTIVE ENDOCARDITIS AND PROPHYLAXIS RECOMMENDATIONS

	Prophylaxis Recommendations			
Procedures	ESC[50]	BCS[51,52]	SFC[53,54]	AHA[43]
Tonsillectomy and adenoidectomy	+	+	+ group A	+
			Optional group B	
Esophageal dilatation or sclerotherapy	+	+	+	–
Instrumentation of obstructed biliary tracts	+	+	+	–
Transurethral prostatic resection*	+	+	+ group A	–
			Optional group B	
Biopsy of urinary tract or prostate	+	+	+ group A	–
			Optional group B	
Urethral dilatation or instrumentation	+	+	+ group A	–
			Optional group B	
Cystoscopy*	+	+	+ group A	–
			Optional group B	
Cesarean section	–	+	–	–
Vaginal delivery	–	–	Optional group A	–
			– group B	
Lithotripsy	+	–	Optional group A	–
			– group B	

*Contraindication in the presence of bacteriuria (SFC).
ESC, European Society of Cardiology; BCS, British Cardiac Society; SFC, Société Française de Cardiologie; AHA, American Heart Association.
+ antibiotic prophylaxis recommended; – antibiotic prophylaxis not recommended.

Table 98.7 Interventions other than oral or dental procedures associated with a risk of infective endocarditis and prophylaxis recommendations.

Recommendation 5: Antibiotic Prophylaxis Prescriptions

In general, antibiotic prophylaxis is initiated in the hour before the procedure (Tables 98.8 and 98.9). Nevertheless, if problems possibly leading to a specific infectious risk arise during or immediately after an intervention without prior antibiotic prophylaxis (important bleeding, long or difficult procedures), initiation of antibiotic prophylaxis as soon as possible after the procedure may be indicated.

Medical Therapy

General Principles

After the initial diagnosis is established, a search should be undertaken for the source of the valvular infection. The extent and nature of this search depend on the causative organism. If a source of the endocarditis can be found, its treatment or eradication should be carried out.

Antithrombotic Therapy

Anticoagulant therapy does not prevent embolization in IE and increases the risk of intracerebral hemorrhage; thereby, it is contraindicated in NVE, except in cases with a clear indication separate from IE. In the presence of intracranial hemorrhage or mycotic aneurysm, anticoagulant therapy should be suspended until the complications have resolved. In patients with PVE requiring anticoagulation, anticoagulant therapy should be cautiously continued. For some authors, heparin is a good alternative to oral anticoagulation. In *S. aureus* PVE, the hemorrhagic neurologic risk seems particularly high in patients receiving anticoagulant therapy, and it has been suggested that anticoagulation be suspended during the acute phase of illness.[56] If cardiac surgery is planned, warfarin should be discontinued and replaced with heparin. Despite experimental evidence to suggest a beneficial role of aspirin in reducing embolic complications and attenuating microbial virulence, a recent randomized trial in left-sided IE found no significant benefits and increased risk of bleeding.[57]

Antimicrobial Therapy

Once a diagnosis of IE has been established, antimicrobial therapy should be administered in a dose designed to give sustained bactericidal serum concentration. The intravenous route for antibiotic administration is the best because it provides maximal bioavailability. Most antibiotics are administered as short infusions (30 minutes). There are some exceptions. Penicillin G is usually administered continuously because of the risk of seizures secondary to the high serum concentrations achieved with intermittent infusion. One- to 2-hour infusions of vancomycin improve the tolerability of the drug. For antibiotics with concentration-dependent effects (β-lactams), the interval between infusions must be adjusted to take the elimination half-life into account. For antibiotics with time-dependent effects (aminoglycosides), administration is recommended two or three times daily. There are, however, clinical data in favor of once-daily administration of gentamicin in IE caused by penicillin-sensitive streptococci.[58] The duration of therapy has to be long enough to eradicate microorganisms growing in the valvular vegetation, where bacterial concentrations may be as high as 10^9 to 10^{10} organisms per gram of tissue.

ANTIBIOTIC PROPHYLAXIS FOR INFECTIVE ENDOCARDITIS IN DENTAL CARE AND UPPER RESPIRATORY TRACT PROCEDURES: ADMINISTRATION OF ANTIBIOTICS RESPECTING CONTRAINDICATIONS AND USUAL CONDITIONS OF USE AND SURVEILLANCE[43,50–54]			
	Antibiotic	**Dosage and Route of Administration**	
Ambulatory care*		**Single dose in the hour before the procedure**	
No allergy to β-lactams	Amoxicillin	3 g orally	
Allergy to β-lactams	Pristinamycin *or* clindamycin†	1 g orally 600 mg orally	
General anesthesia‡		**Before (in the hour before the procedure)**	**After (6 hours later)**
No allergy to β-lactams	Amoxicillin	2 g IV (infusion 30 min)	1 g orally
Allergy to β-lactams	Vancomycin *or* teicoplanin	1 g IV (infusion ≥60 min) 400 mg IV (bolus)	No second dose

*Oral pediatric dosage: amoxicillin, 75 mg/kg; clindamycin, 15 mg/kg; pristinamycin, 25 mg/kg, 2 g orally if the patient's weight is <60 kg.
†The respective percentage of streptococci strains with a decreased susceptibility to these two antibiotics must be taken into account for the choice.
‡Pediatric dosage: amoxicillin, 50 mg/kg intravenously before, 25 mg/kg orally 6 hours later; vancomycin, 20 mg/kg (maximum, 1 g); teicoplanin, no official approval for antibiotic prophylaxis in children.
Data from Danchin[53].

Table 98.8 Antibiotic prophylaxis for infective endocarditis in dental care and upper respiratory tract procedures: administration of antibiotics respecting contraindications and usual conditions of use and surveillance.

ANTIBIOTIC PROPHYLAXIS FOR INFECTIVE ENDOCARDITIS DURING UROLOGIC AND DIGESTIVE PROCEDURES: ADMINISTRATION OF ANTIBIOTICS RESPECTING CONTRAINDICATIONS AND USUAL CONDITIONS OF USE AND SURVEILLANCE[43,50-54]			
	Antibiotic	**Dosage and Route of Administration**	
		Before (in the hour of procedure)	**After (6 hours later)**
No allergy to β-lactams	Amoxicillin *then* gentamicin	2 g IV (infusion 30 min) 1.5 mg/kg IV (infusion 30 min) or IM	1 g orally No second dose
Allergy to β-lactams	Vancomycin *or* teicoplanin *then* gentamicin	1 g IV (infusion ≥60 min) 400 mg IV (bolus) 1.5 mg/kg IV (infusion 30 min) or IM	No second dose

Pediatric dosage: amoxicillin, 50 mg/kg intravenously before, 25 mg/kg orally 6 hours later; gentamicin, 2 mg/kg (maximum, 80 mg); vancomycin, 20 mg/kg (maximum, 1 g); teicoplanin, no official approval for antibiotic prophylaxis in children.
If antibiotic prophylaxis concerns a procedure for which the microorganism is a staphylococcus, pristinamycin should be used unless it is contraindicated.
Data from Danchin[53].

Table 98.9 Antibiotic prophylaxis for infective endocarditis during urologic and digestive procedures: administration of antibiotics respecting contraindications and usual conditions of use and surveillance.

Until recently, most patients who have IE received the entire duration of their antimicrobial therapy in the hospital. Technical advances allowing the safe administration of antibiotics at home combined with well-developed home care systems make it feasible to treat patients with IE on an outpatient basis. Patients should be selected for outpatient therapy only if they have responded clinically to inpatient therapy and if they have shown no evidence of complications. In addition, they should be hemodynamically stable, compliant, and capable of managing the technical aspect of intravenous therapy.[22]

Immediate initiation of antimicrobial therapy after blood culture samples have been obtained is appropriate in the management of patients with acute IE and of patients with hemodynamic decompensation requiring urgent surgical intervention. On the other hand, in hemodynamically stable patients suspected of having subacute IE, it is prudent to delay antibiotic therapy pending the results of initial blood cultures. Repeated blood cultures should be performed during the initial days of therapy to determine whether the bacteremia has been controlled. Fever associated with IE often resolves within 3 days after the start of appropriate antimicrobial treatment in patients with less virulent pathogens; defervescence occurs in 90% of patients before the end of the second week of treatment. The most common causes of persistent fever (>14 days) are the extension of infection beyond the valve (often with myocardial abscess), focal metastatic infection, drug hypersensitivity, and nosocomial infection or other complication of hospitalization such as pulmonary embolism. Both the efficacy and the tolerance of the treatment need to be carefully monitored. In terms of efficacy, apart from the absence of relapse at the end of the treatment, there is no totally reliable clinical or biologic criterion. This emphasizes the importance of clinical and biologic surveillance (disappearance of fever, sterilization of blood culture specimens, and normalization of inflammation markers) during treatment and in the subsequent 4 weeks.

Relapse of IE usually occurs within 2 months of the discontinuation of antimicrobial therapy. The relapse rate for patients with NVE caused by penicillin-susceptible viridans streptococci who have been treated with the recommended courses of therapy is generally less than 2%, and it is 8% to 20% for NVE due to enterococcal species. Among patients with IE caused by *S. aureus,* Enterobacteriaceae, or fungi, treatment failure often occurs during the primary course of therapy. A positive bacterial culture at the time of valve replacement surgery, particularly in patients with *S. aureus* infection, is a risk factor for subsequent relapse. The relapse rate in PVE is about 10% to 15%.

Endocarditis Caused by Viridans Streptococci and Streptococcus bovis

Most viridans streptococci and strains of *Streptococcus bovis* are highly susceptible to penicillin (minimum inhibitory concentration [MIC] of ≤0.1 μg/mL; Table 98.10). Treatment for 4 weeks with parenteral penicillin in doses of 12 to 18 million units/day or with 2 g of ceftriaxone sodium in a single

USUAL ANTIMICROBIAL THERAPY FOR ENDOCARDITIS CAUSED BY STREPTOCOCCI AND HACEK ORGANISMS

Pathogens	Antimicrobial Therapy: Antibiotic	Dosage and Route (for a day)	Duration (weeks)	Comments
Penicillin-susceptible viridans streptococci, *Streptococcus bovis,* and other streptococci with MIC of penicillin ≤0.1 μg/mL	Penicillin G *or*	200,000-300,000 U/kg IV	4	Preferred in most patients older than 65 years or with impairment of renal function
	amoxicillin *or*	100 mg/kg IV	4	If the streptococcus is very penicillin susceptible, the oral route of amoxicillin may replace the intravenous route for the last 2 weeks.
	ceftriaxone	2 g IV or IM	4	This type of monotherapy is used only in NVE.
	Penicillin G *or*	200,000-300,000 U/kg IV	2-6	A 2-week regimen of penicillin G or amoxicillin with gentamicin is appropriate for NVE without complications.
	amoxicillin +	100 mg/kg IV	2-6	
	gentamicin	3 mg/kg IV or IM	2	A 6-week regimen of penicillin G with gentamicin (2 weeks) is advised in PVE.
	Ceftriaxone +	2 g IV or IM	2	This regimen may be used in NVE.
	netilmicin	5 mg/kg IV	2	Alternative to netilmicin: gentamicin not to exceed 2 g/24 hours unless serum levels are monitored
	Vancomycin	30 mg/kg IV	4	Recommended for β-lactam–allergic patients
Relatively penicillin-resistant streptococci: MIC of penicillin >0.1 to 0.5 μg/mL	Penicillin G *or*	300,000-400,000 U/kg IV	4-6	A 4-week regimen of penicillin G (or amoxicillin) with gentamicin (2 weeks) is advised in NVE without complications.
	Amoxicillin +	200 mg/kg IV	4-6	
	gentamicin	3 mg/kg IV or IM	2	A 6-week regimen of penicillin or amoxicillin with gentamicin (2 weeks) is advised in PVE and NVE with complications.
Streptococcus species with MIC of penicillin >0.5 μg/mL, *Enterococcus* species, or abiotrophic species	Penicillin G *or*	300,000-400,000 U/kg IV	4-6	6 weeks of therapy is recommended for patients with symptoms >3 months, myocardial abscess, or selected other complications or with PVE.
	amoxicillin *or*	200 mg/kg IV	4-6	
	ampicillin +	200 mg/kg IV	4-6	

(Continued)

Pathogens	Antimicrobial Therapy			Comments
	Antibiotic	Dosage and Route (for a day)	Duration (weeks)	
	gentamicin	3 mg/kg IV or IM	4-6	
	Vancomycin + gentamicin	30 mg/kg IV 3 mg/kg IV or IM	4-6 4-6	Vancomycin with gentamicin is used for β-lactam–allergic patients or in patients with *Enterococcus* species resistant to penicillin. Monitor drug serum levels and renal function.
HACEK organisms	Ceftriaxone *or*	2 g IV or IM	4-6	A duration of 4 weeks is advised in NVE. A longer duration (6 weeks) is required in PVE.
	Ampicillin + gentamicin	200 mg/kg IV 3 mg/kg IV or IM	4-6 4-6	Alternative regimen to ceftriaxone, but some isolates that produce β-lactamase may be resistant to this regimen.

Penicillin G IV is given either continuously or in six equally divided doses.
Ceftriaxone IV may be used once daily. This regimen is particularly suited for outpatient therapy.
Amoxicillin and ampicillin IV are given in six doses.
Gentamicin IM or IV is given usually in three equally divided doses; some studies suggest that gentamicin once daily might be adequate.
Netilmicin IV is given in two doses.
Vancomycin is used in two equally divided doses and infused during at least 1 hour.
Teicoplanin may be an alternative to vancomycin.
MIC, minimum inhibitory concentration; NVE, native valve endocarditis; PVE, prosthetic valve endocarditis.
Data from references 11, 22, and 31.

Table 98.10 Usual antimicrobial therapy for endocarditis caused by streptococci and HACEK organisms.

daily dose can be expected to achieve a bacteriologic cure in up to 98% of patients. Selected patients with NVE who do not have evidence of complications can be treated with shorter courses (2 weeks) of combination therapy (penicillin G, or amoxicillin or ceftriaxone with gentamicin or netilmicin).[58] In patients who have prosthetic valves, a 6-week regimen of penicillin is recommended together with gentamicin for at least the first 2 weeks. Vancomycin is an effective alternative and is the drug of choice in patients who have a history of penicillin allergy.[52]

Patients who have IE caused by viridans streptococci with reduced susceptibility to penicillin ($0.1 < MIC < 0.5$) should receive penicillin G for a total of 4 to 6 weeks. Ampicillin and amoxicillin (200 mg/kg per day in six infusions) are alternatives to penicillin. Gentamicin should be added to this regimen for the first 2 weeks. For patients who are allergic to β-lactams, vancomycin is an acceptable alternative. Other streptococcal species (e.g., groups A, B, C, and G streptococci and *S. pneumoniae*) are occasional causes of IE. Therapy should be based on the results of susceptibility tests. With minimum inhibitory concentrations above 0.5 mg/mL, treatment is the same as for enterococcal endocarditis (see Table 98.10).

Endocarditis Caused by Enterococci

Enterococcus faecalis, Enterococcus faecium, and to a lesser extent *Enterococcus durans* are most commonly responsible for IE. Treatment of enterococcal endocarditis is complicated because the organisms are relatively resistant to penicillin, expanded-spectrum penicillin, and vancomycin (see Table 98.10). The degree of resistance to aminoglycosides is highly variable. It is found in about 10% of endocarditis strains of *E. faecalis*.

Standard therapy consists of a combination of intravenous penicillin G or ampicillin or amoxicillin combined with gentamicin for 4 to 6 weeks. Patients who have symptoms of less than 3 months' duration can usually be treated with 4 weeks of therapy. Patients with symptoms of more than 3 months' duration before initiation of therapy, those with a relapse of infection, and those with prosthetic valve infection should receive a 6-week course of therapy. Gentamicin therapy should be given at doses designed to achieve peak serum levels of approximately 3 μg/mL and trough serum concentrations of less than 1 μg/mL.

Patients who have a history of penicillin allergy should be treated with a combination of vancomycin and gentamicin for 4 to 6 weeks. Enterococcal IE caused by strains with an intrinsically high level of penicillin resistance (MIC >6 μg/mL) should be treated with a combination of vancomycin and gentamicin. When endocarditis is due to enterococci that are highly resistant to all aminoglycosides, monotherapy with amoxicillin or vancomycin is advised and should be continued for 8 weeks or more. Glycopeptide-resistant enterococci are often multidrug resistant. Newer agents, such as quinupristin-dalfopristin and linezolid, appear to be preferable options in this setting.[59] Surgical resection of the affected valve may be necessary.

Staphylococcal Endocarditis

The success of therapy for staphylococcal endocarditis is dependent on numerous factors (Table 98.11). These include whether the right- or left-sided valvular structures are involved, whether the staphylococci are susceptible or resistant to methicillin, and whether the infection is on a native or a prosthetic valve.

Native valve infection caused by methicillin-susceptible staphylococci is best treated by a semisynthetic penicillinase-resistant penicillin, such as cloxacillin or oxacillin sodium, for 4 to 6 weeks. Many authorities recommend the addition of gentamicin for the first 3 to 5 days of therapy. Patients who have a history of penicillin allergy can be treated either with a cephalosporin such as cefamandole or with vancomycin.

Selected patients who have NVE involving the right-sided heart valves can be successfully treated by a 2-week regimen with the combination therapy of nafcillin and gentamicin.

The only effective therapy for patients who have endocarditis caused by methicillin-resistant staphylococci is vancomycin. Monotherapy for 4 to 6 weeks is usually adequate. Teicoplanin may be an alternative, provided an adequate dosage is given.

SUGGESTED TREATMENT OF NATIVE VALVE ENDOCARDITIS AND PROSTHETIC VALVE INFECTIVE ENDOCARDITIS CAUSED BY STAPHYLOCOCCI

	Antimicrobial Therapy			
Pathogens	**Antibiotic**	**Dosage and Route (for a day)**	**Duration**	**Comments**
Native valve endocarditis				
Methicillin-susceptible staphylococci	Oxacillin *or* nafcillin	150 mg/kg IV	4-6 weeks	First choice of treatment Oxacillin and nafcillin are given IV in 6 doses. Cloxacillin is an alternative.
	+ gentamicin	3 mg/kg IV or IM	3-5 days	Gentamicin is optional for the first days of therapy.
	Cefamandole	75-100 mg/kg IV	4-6 weeks	Given in 6 doses Alternative for patients allergic to penicillin if hypersensitivity is not of the immediate type
	+ gentamicin	3 mg/kg IV or IM		
	or netilmicin	5-6 mg/kg IV	5-7 days	
Methicillin-resistant staphylococci	Vancomycin	30 mg/kg IV	4-6 weeks	Recommended for β-lactam–allergic patients
	Vancomycin	30 mg/kg IV	4-6 weeks	Alternative: teicoplanin Gentamicin optional
	± gentamicin	3 mg/kg IV or IM	3-5 days	
Prosthetic valve endocarditis				
Methicillin-susceptible staphylococci	Oxacillin *or* cloxacillin *or* nafcillin	150 mg/kg IV	≥6 weeks	Rifampin is optional; it increases the hepatic metabolism of numerous drugs, including warfarin.
	+ gentamicin	3 mg/kg IV or IM	2 weeks	
	+ rifampin	20-30 mg/kg PO	≥6 weeks	
	Vancomycin	30 mg/kg IV	≥6 weeks	Recommended for β-lactam–allergic patients
	+ gentamicin	3 mg/kg IV or IM	2 weeks	
	+ rifampin	20-30 mg/kg PO	≥6 weeks	
Methicillin-resistant staphylococci	Vancomycin	30 mg/kg IV	≥6 weeks	If the staphylococcus is resistant to gentamicin, an alternative third agent should be chosen on the basis of in vitro susceptibility testing.
	+ gentamicin	3 mg/kg IV or IM	2 weeks	
	+ rifampin	20-30 mg/kg PO	≥6 weeks	

Data from references 11, 22, and 31.

Table 98.11 Suggested treatment of native valve endocarditis and prosthetic valve infective endocarditis caused by staphylococci.

Patients who have PVE due to methicillin-sensitive *S. aureus* should be treated with nafcillin or an equivalent β-lactamase–resistant β-lactam antibiotic for at least 6 weeks. Many experts recommend simultaneous treatment with oral rifampin (rifampicin) and the addition of gentamicin for the first 2 weeks. In cases of infection due to methicillin-resistant staphylococci, combination therapy with intravenous vancomycin and oral rifampin is given for 6 to 8 weeks. The addition of gentamicin is recommended for the first 2 weeks.

Early surgical intervention should always be considered.

Endocarditis Caused by HACEK Organisms

All these organisms grow slowly in blood culture media. This delayed growth makes standard antibiotic susceptibility testing difficult. Although most HACEK organisms were sensitive to ampicillin in the past, this is no longer true. However, virtually all of these organisms are highly susceptible to third-generation cephalosporins, such as ceftriaxone and cefotaxime (see Table 98.10). Either agent is usually effective when it is given for 4 weeks to patients with NVE. Patients who have PVE should be treated for 6 weeks.[22]

Endocarditis from Unusually Encountered Organisms

The optimal therapy is still not adequately defined.[11,22] In all cases, most patients require valve surgery.

In a Q fever endocarditis, doxycycline with a second antimicrobial agent is the advised treatment, often given for 3 to 4 years until immunoglobulin G antibody titers drop below 1:400. The combination of doxycycline and hydroxychloroquine is associated with the lowest rate of relapse.[60]

In *Bartonella* endocarditis, most patients have been treated with a β-lactam antibiotic and an aminoglycoside. Fluoroquinolones are also bactericidal for these species.

In *Brucella* endocarditis, few patients have been cured only with antimicrobial agents (combination of doxycycline and rifampin for at least 8 weeks and up to 10 months after valve replacement).

In *Candida* and *Aspergillus* endocarditis, cure usually requires valve surgery in addition to amphotericin B.

IE caused by *Legionella* is rare and occurs mainly in patients with prosthetic valves. The usual treatment consists of a combination of a fluoroquinolone and rifampin. The duration of treatment should be at least 2 months, and valve surgery is almost always required.

In *Pseudomonas* IE, most cases are caused by *P. aeruginosa* and occur in the setting of intravenous drug abuse. Isolated right-sided IE is generally managed with antibiotic therapy (large doses of an antipseudomonal penicillin with an aminoglycoside). In left-sided disease, valve replacement is mandatory.

Culture-Negative Endocarditis

In patients with NVE, therapy includes penicillin or ampicillin, or ceftriaxone or vancomycin, often in combination with an aminoglycoside. In patients with PVE, within the initial 12 months after surgery, therapy often includes vancomycin and gentamicin. For patients with endocarditis that begins 12 months or more after valve surgery, ceftriaxone or cefotaxime could be added to cover HACEK organisms. If fever due to IE persists after empirical therapy, valve replacement should be considered.

Surgical Therapy

Cardiac surgery plays an important role in the treatment of complications of IE.

Indications for Surgery in Patients Who Have Active Infective Endocarditis

The indications for valve surgery in IE have not been evaluated in randomized controlled trials. Some recent studies have suggested that the benefits of surgical therapy have been overestimated.[61] However, many complications of NVE or PVE require, beyond all question, surgery. They are specified in Tables 98.12 and 98.13 from recommendations of the European Society of Cardiology,[31] the American College of Cardiology/American Heart Association,[62] and the French Society of Cardiology.[63]

SURGERY FOR NATIVE VALVE ENDOCARDITIS
1. Heart failure due to valve dysfunction (stenosis or regurgitation) 2. Evidence of perivalvular extension of infection (e.g., heart block; annular or aortic abscess; destructive penetrating lesions: sinus of Valsalva to right atrium, right ventricle, or left atrium fistula; mitral leaflet perforation with aortic valve endocarditis) 3. Aortic regurgitation or mitral regurgitation with hemodynamic evidence of elevated left ventricular end-diastolic or left atrial pressure, or moderate or severe pulmonary hypertension 4. Persistent infection after 7 to 10 days of adequate antibiotic therapy; infection due to fungal or other resistant organisms with a poor response to antibiotic treatment 5. Recurrent embolism and persistent vegetation despite appropriate antibiotic therapy
Indications 1 to 4 are in class I and indication 5 is in class IIa according to the guidelines of the American College of Cardiology/American Heart Association.[62]
A debated indication: mobile vegetation in excess of 10 mm. Indication depends on existence of previous emboli, site of valvular vegetations (mitral or aortic), and feasibility of conservative valve surgery.

Table 98.12 Surgery for native valve endocarditis.

SURGERY FOR PROSTHETIC VALVE ENDOCARDITIS
1. Heart failure due to prosthetic dysfunction 2. Evidence of periprosthetic extension of infection (see indication 2 for native valve endocarditis surgery in Table 98.11) 3. Prosthetic valve with evidence of increasing obstruction or worsening regurgitation 4. Prosthetic valve with dehiscence evident by cinefluoroscopy or echocardiography 5. Persistent infection after 7 to 10 days of adequate antibiotic therapy (see indication 4 for native valve endocarditis surgery in Table 98.11) 6. Recurrent emboli despite appropriate antibiotic treatment 7. Prosthetic valve with relapsing infection
Indications 1 to 5 are in class I and indications 6 and 7 are in class IIa according to the guidelines of the American College of Cardiology/American Heart Association.[62]

Table 98.13 Surgery for prosthetic valve endocarditis.

Surgery appears mandatory in at least 30% of cases with active IE and in another 20% to 40% after healing.[31] Early surgery in acute IE is frequently performed in one of two surgical patients. Surgery should be envisaged every time that a severe, surgically treatable complication of IE intervenes, if the patient has reasonable prospects of recovery with satisfactory quality of life after the operation. Surgery is not indicated if complications (severe embolic cerebral damage) or comorbid conditions make the prospect of recovery unlikely. Decisions about surgical intervention in patients with IE should be individualized with input from both the cardiologist and the cardiovascular surgeon.

Heart failure resulting from new or worsening valvular dysfunction is the most common indication for surgery. There is widespread consensus that surgical intervention has been shown to improve survival in most cases in which heart failure complicates endocarditis. The degree of hemodynamic instability of the individual patient is the major determinant of the timing of surgery; surgery should not be delayed in the setting of life-threatening congestive heart failure or cardiogenic shock due to surgically treatable valvular heart disease with IE. In these patients, urgent surgery is often mandatory. Heart failure caused by IE-induced aortic regurgitation has a worse prognosis than that of IE-induced mitral regurgitation. For patients who have severe, acute aortic regurgitation and progressive pulmonary edema, urgent surgery is mandatory. In the case of regression of heart failure and stable hemodynamics, the optimal timing remains controversial. In our view, early surgery should be performed after 2 weeks of antibiotherapy.[64,65]

Failure to achieve an adequate bactericidal response to therapy and to control infection remains an indication for surgical intervention. Certain organisms, such as methicillin-resistant staphylococci and vancomycin-resistant enterococci, cannot be effectively treated only with antibiotics. Fungal endocarditis is also notoriously difficult to cure with medical therapy alone. Most patients who have *Candida* endocarditis and virtually all patients who have endocarditis due to *Aspergillus* require surgery for control of the infection. Similarly, IE due to some unusual organisms is often an indication for combined medical and surgical therapy. A bacteriologic cure may also be difficult to achieve in patients who have PVE. PVE caused by organisms other than viridans streptococci and the HACEK group of microorganisms is difficult to cure with medical therapy. Most such patients require surgery. In addition, when PVE relapses after a course of medical therapy, a perivalvular infection is usually present.

However, not all patients with PVE require a surgical therapy. Around 20% of PVE may be cured only by medical therapy:

- noncomplicated PVE without abscesses or dehiscence evidenced by cinefluoroscopy or echocardiography;
- nonstaphylococcal PVE; and
- late endocarditis sited on bioprosthetic valves.

Nevertheless, the follow-up of these patients must be particularly strict during the months that follow the end of antibiotherapy.

In practice:

1. Consultation with a cardiovascular surgeon is recommended for every patient with complicated endocarditis so that the surgical team is aware of the patient who may suddenly need surgery.
2. Patients with PVE who receive warfarin anticoagulation and develop complicated endocarditis should have warfarin discontinued and replaced with heparin. This recommendation is less related to the possibility of hemorrhagic complication of endocarditis than to the possibility of urgent surgery. Likewise, aspirin, if it is part of the medical regimen, should also be discontinued.

Although a relationship may exist between vegetation characteristics (size, mobility, number) and the risk of embolism, the implication for surgical intervention remains controversial. Data on vegetations should be weighed in the context of the overall clinical picture to assess the benefits of surgery. Surgery should be considered in principle if there have been two episodes or more of embolization or one episode with a residual large (>10 mm) vegetation in the anterior mitral leaflet or if vegetation size increases after 4 weeks of antimicrobial therapy. However, these criteria for surgery are somewhat arbitrary because there are no data from prospective controlled trials. Indications for surgery should account for several points:

- Criteria based on embolic events should exclude cutaneous embolization, which is common, or embolism occurring before the institution of therapy.
- Because of the known decrease in embolic risk during the first weeks of antibiotic therapy, the benefit of surgery is greatest in the early phase of IE.
- Surgery is the more indicated as valve repair may be foreseen from echocardiographic evaluation rather than valve replacement. Therefore, patients with mitral IE are the best candidates.
- Surgery is also the more indicated as other predictors of complicated course are present (heart failure, annular abscess, antibiotic-resistant organisms).

Finally, the strategy for surgical intervention to avoid systemic embolization in IE remains specific to the individual patient. The optimal timing of surgery after a cerebral embolism is controversial because full heparinization and hypotension during open heart surgery potentially aggravate the neurologic injury. For some authors, a delay in operation for IE results in a lower complication rate.[66,67] If cardiac function permits, surgery should be delayed for 2 to 3 weeks for patients who have had a prior cerebral infarct. On the other hand, other series suggest that the timing of surgical intervention after stroke in patients with ischemic events does not appear to significantly affect outcome.[68,69] In patients who have sustained an intracranial hemorrhage or a hemorrhagic transformation of a cerebral infarction, surgery should be delayed until at least 3 weeks have elapsed.

Intracardiac abscess is another usual indication for surgery.

Type of Surgery

When surgery is performed for aortic valve endocarditis, valve replacement is mandatory. Patients who have extensive damage of the aortic root may require placement of a homograft.[70] Homografts have a constant but low risk for the development of sewing ring infections and IE, possibly related to improved penetration of antibiotics. In the absence of paravalvular lesions, the choice of valve substitute should be made by the usual criteria (i.e., age and the ability to take long-term anticoagulant therapy). For mitral and tricuspid valve endocarditis, valve repair appears to be the procedure of choice. Feasibility of valve repair in patients with active IE has been reported to be 80% or higher.[71-74] Some specific techniques are sometimes used. Autologous pericardial patching is used for leaflet perforation. Posterior chordal transposition to the anterior leaflet is mandatory if there is rupture of the anterior leaflet chordae. If the extent of the lesions is too great, the use of a partial homograft may be considered.[75]

Antimicrobial therapy should be continued after surgical intervention. The duration of postoperative antimicrobial therapy depends on the duration of preoperative therapy, the susceptibility of the organisms to antibiotics, the presence of paravalvular lesions, and the culture status of the vegetation.

In general, for IE with negative cultures of operative specimens, preoperative plus postoperative antimicrobial therapy should at least equal a full course of recommended therapy. For those patients who have a positive intraoperative culture, a full course of therapy should be given postoperatively.

Results

The operative mortality rate for surgery in active IE has varied over time and according to the different series. In most large series, it is between 5% and 25%.[61,64,65,69-81] The major determinants of operative mortality are

- hemodynamic status at operation, which is the principal factor of operative risk;
- increased age;
- type of IE: PVE involves a higher operative risk than NVE does; mortality rate is between 10% and 25% in PVE; in NVE without perivalvular infection, it is around 5% but higher in cases with abscesses;
- type of valve surgery: in patients with mitral valve endocarditis, the mortality rate of valve repair is lower than that of valve replacement.

The late results are satisfactory. Survival rates at 5 and 10 years after surgery range, respectively, from 70% to 80% and 60% to 70% in NVE, but actuarial survival rates are lower in PVE.[76-79] Endocarditis recurs in about 1% of patients per year and reaches 3% in IE with annular abscesses. Paravalvular leakage after valve replacement is seen in 5% to 15% of cases. Reintervention for reinfection or other valve complication is required in 2% to 3% of patients per year. The rates of patients free from reoperation at 10 years are usually between 70% and 90%. From multivariate analysis, PVE, preoperative neurologic complications, coagulase-negative staphylococcal IE, and annular infective invasion are the critical adverse determinants of late outcome.

Results after conservative surgery for infected mitral valve are noteworthy. Since the first report in 1990, several series have confirmed the advantages of mitral repair compared with valve replacement.[71,73,74,80,81]

PROGNOSIS

Prognosis of IE has greatly changed since effective antibiotherapy. Before the antibiotic era, the disease led to death within a few days to 2 years. At present, cure of IE occurs in a majority of cases. However, the mortality rate is still between 15% and 25%.

Several factors worsen the prognosis of IE and may require urgent cardiac surgery.

Clinical Factors

IE has a worse prognosis

- in the elderly;
- in cases with associated conditions: renal, respiratory, and hepatic insufficiency; diabetes mellitus; acquired immunodepression;
- in the presence of heart failure, which is the first determinant of mortality;
- in the presence of systemic embolization and neurologic symptoms; and
- in nosocomial endocarditis.

Bacteriologic Factors

IE is more severe when it is due to certain pathogens. Mortality rate has been estimated at 4% to 16% for viridans streptococci and *S. bovis;* 15% to 25% for enterococci; 25% to 47% for *S. aureus;* 5% to 37% for Q fever; and more than 50% for *P. aeruginosa,* Enterobacteriaceae, or fungi.[11]

Anatomic Factors

In NVE, disease that is localized to the aortic valve is more severe than mitral or tricuspid disease. PVE carries a worse prognosis because of prosthetic leakage, septic embolism, and persistent sepsis. Ring abscesses may be responsible for uncontrolled infection. They usually require surgery and increase the morbidity and mortality rates of cardiac intervention. Right-sided IE often shows a good response to antibiotics.

Delay in the Diagnosis and in Effective Medical and Surgical Treatment

Delay in diagnosis partly explains the persistent high mortality rate of IE. All patients who have unexplained fever and a cardiac murmur should be suspected of having IE. Echocardiography and blood cultures should be performed quickly and repeated if necessary.

SUMMARY

The incidence of IE is between 1.7 and 6.2 new cases per 100,000 people every year. This incidence has not decreased during the past few decades. The clinical presentations are variable: subacute or acute native valve endocarditis of the left side of the heart, right-sided heart valve endocarditis, prosthetic valve endocarditis, or a clinical picture associated with complications.

Diagnosis is often difficult. The mean period between the first symptom and the diagnosis exceeds 1 month in many series. An early diagnosis is a key factor for successful management. Physicians should be aware of the first signs of IE. Any unexplained and persistent fever in a patient at risk for IE requires echocardiography and blood cultures. Since 1980, diagnostic criteria have been proposed for the diagnosis of IE. The criteria most used are those of Duke University, which take into account specific echocardiographic findings.

Transthoracic echocardiography and transesophageal echocardiography with color Doppler study provide a crucial contribution to the diagnosis. Echocardiography is particularly useful for the detection and characterization of valvular vegetations, valvular regurgitation, ventricular dysfunction, and associated lesions (such as abscesses, shunts, and ruptured chordae). Echocardiography may be useful in the case of culture-negative IE or of persistent bacteremia whose source remains unidentified after appropriate evaluation.

Microbiologic methods have improved in recent years. At present, the rate of culture-negative endocarditis should be less than 10% of cases. Most frequently (in 50% of such cases), it results from prior antibiotic treatment. Among identified microorganisms, *Streptococcus* species are responsible for 50% to 60% of IE, and *S. bovis* endocarditis appears more frequent; staphylococci are identified in about a third of cases and are the predominant pathogens in early prosthetic valve endocarditis.

Since the introduction of effective antibiotherapy, many cases can be cured, but mortality rate is still about 20%. An improvement in the prognosis requires early diagnosis and adequate management based on appropriate antibiotic therapy and, in many cases, cardiac surgery.

chapter 99

Surgery for Valvular Heart Disease

Christophe Acar and Pierre Théodore

Definition

- In patients with valvular heart disease, cardiac surgery aims to restore normal valve function through either repair or replacement of the diseased valve.

Key Features

- Reconstructive valvular surgery is the preferred surgical procedure, especially for the diseased mitral valve.
- Valve replacement is the standard procedure for the diseased aortic valve.
- Age and cardiac rhythm are the main determinants for choosing between a mechanical and a biologic artificial valve.

Clinical Implications

- Valvular surgery restores normal valve function with excellent long-term results, especially after valve repair.

Surgical management of valvular heart disease started more than 50 years ago and has since gone through a phase of exponential growth. Although techniques became standardized for most types of repair and replacement procedures, surgical management of valvular heart disease still continues to evolve to respond to the changing profile of patients.

OPERATIVE APPROACH

A median sternotomy is the operative approach of choice for most valvular procedures. Use of this approach implies division of the sternum from suprasternal notch to xiphoid process. After opening of the pericardium, the entire heart becomes accessible, and a safe and excellent exposure of all cardiac valves can be obtained. This approach does not alter the respiratory function and allows a rapid healing with a very low rate of scar infection (1%). Other incisions are occasionally employed for particular indications. When a significant cosmetic concern exists, modifications such as the mini-sternotomy or a thoracotomy may confer aesthetic advantages. In case of reoperation, sternal re-entry raises a risk of traumatic injury to the enlarged heart. A right or a left thoracotomy can then be preferred to approach the tricuspid or the mitral valve on rare occasions in which the midline approach seems excessively dangerous.

EXTRACORPOREAL CIRCULATION AND MYOCARDIAL PROTECTION

Establishment of an extracorporeal circulation is a prerequisite for open heart interventions because it permits arrest of the heart and cessation of ventilation. Venous blood is drained through cannulas placed in the right atrium or in the venae cavae. Blood is oxygenated by a membrane oxygenator and returned to the patient with the aid of a roller pump through a cannula in the ascending aorta. The femoral artery is sometimes chosen as the site of arterial perfusion, especially for procedures involving ascending aorta or aortic arch or for redo interventions. During extracorporeal circulation, flow and mean arterial pressure are maintained within their physiologic ranges. The extracorporeal circuit contains a heat exchange system, allowing the temperature of the blood and hence the temperature of the patient to be closely regulated. Although some surgeons prefer a slight systemic hypothermia, which lowers the patient's core temperature to 28°C, the current trend is to maintain normothermia. Extracorporeal circulation requires anticoagulation with heparin, which is neutralized after separation from cardiopulmonary bypass with an appropriate dose of protamine.

Myocardial protection during the period of arrest is accomplished by injection of a cold (4°C) cardioplegic solution, derived from the extracorporeal circuit and cooled by the heat exchange system. Diastolic arrest of the heart occurs as a result of the drop in temperature and the addition of potassium chloride (20 mmol/L) to the cardioplegic solution. If the aortic valve is competent, the cardioplegic solution is usually delivered to the heart in an anterograde fashion through puncture of the ascending aorta. In case of aortic valve incompetence, selective cannulation of the coronary arteries is used to deliver the cardioplegic solution to the heart. Cardioplegia can also be achieved in a retrograde fashion by selective cannulation of the coronary sinus. The duration of cardiac arrest is variable, usually between 30 minutes and 4 hours, depending on the complexity of the procedure and operative technique. For optimal cardioprotection to be maintained, repeated doses of cardioplegia are administered at 30-minute intervals. The presence of aortic insufficiency, coronary artery stenoses, left ventricular hypertrophy, or severe left ventricular dysfunction requires particularly close attention to myocardial protection.

VALVULAR RECONSTRUCTIVE SURGERY

Valvular reconstruction is especially relevant for procedures involving the mitral and the tricuspid valves.

Mitral Valve Repair

Functional Classification

Three types of mitral insufficiency are described according to the Carpentier functional classification (Fig. 99.1)[1]:

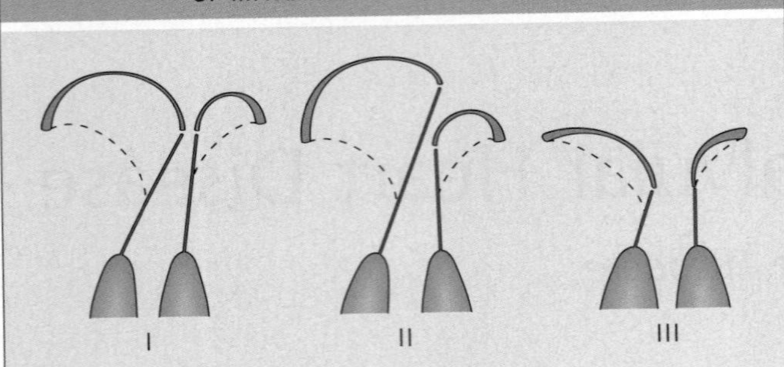

Figure 99.1 Carpentier functional classification of mitral valve insufficiency. Type I: normal leaflet motion. Type II: prolapse. Type III: restriction.

- type I, normal leaflet motion: regurgitation secondary to a dilated annulus or perforation of a leaflet;
- type II, excessive leaflet motion (prolapse): regurgitation secondary to a flail leaflet rising above the plane of the annulus in systole; and
- type III, reduced leaflet motion (restriction): regurgitation secondary to failure of coaptation, with the leaflet edge remaining below the plane of the annulus in systole.

The posterior leaflet is divided into three segments from the anterolateral commissure to the posteromedial commissure: P1, P2, and P3.[2] The mechanisms responsible for valvular dysfunction are appreciated preoperatively by echocardiography. Intraoperative inspection allows a more precise identification of valve lesions.

Analysis of Valvular Lesions

Degenerative Disease

Myxomatous degeneration of the mitral valve, so-called Barlow's disease, is the most common cause of acquired mitral insufficiency in Western society. The valve apparatus is thickened and yellowish with redundant leaflets characterized by an excessive tissue. The chordae tendineae are either elongated or ruptured, producing prolapse (functional type II). The myxomatous changes have a predilection for the median segment of the posterior leaflet (P2). Bileaflet prolapse is less frequent and is related to a diffuse myxomatous involvement of the valve; this is often the case in patients with Marfan's syndrome whose mitral valve is regurgitant.

Fibroelastic deficiency is another nosologic entity defined by isolated chordal rupture without myxoid degeneration. The leaflet tissue appears normal or pellucid. It is a senescence process localized to the mitral valve observed in elderly patients.

Annulus dilatation is a constant finding in both forms of degenerative mitral insufficiency. It is usually more pronounced in cases of Barlow's disease. Calcifications of the mitral annulus can be observed more often in elderly patients and in those with renal insufficiency, chronic hypertension, or severe myxomatous valvular degeneration. Both dilatation and calcification, when present, predominate in the posterior part of the mitral annulus.

Rheumatic Valve Disease

Mitral valve dysfunction is related to a slowly evolving fibrotic reaction secondary to the acute inflammatory phase of rheumatic fever. This process is characterized by a progressive thickening with leaflet retraction and chordae shortening, preventing coaptation in systole. The lesions of the valvular apparatus induce a restrictive-type mitral valve insufficiency (see Fig. 99.1, Carpentier type III). In addition, the mitral annulus is dilated to a variable extent. In children and adolescents with rheumatic mitral valve disease, because of the predominant restriction of the posterior leaflet, a relative prolapse of the anterior leaflet is often observed.

Rheumatic mitral disease is always associated with some degree of stenosis due to commissure and chordae fusion together with leaflet rigidity. Ultimately, calcification occurs and predominates on the leaflets at the level of chordal insertions; the annulus usually remains free of calcium.

Infectious Endocarditis

Acute endocarditis is responsible for characteristic lesions: abscess formation, perforation, vegetations, and chordal rupture. At the site of a valvular abscess, the endocardial surface is eroded and the surrounding leaflets appear thickened and infiltrated. The abscess is generally localized to the leaflets but can occasionally also involve the annulus. The natural progression of a valve abscess leads to leaflet perforation. When infection involves the leaflet edges or the chordae, it can result in chordal rupture and valve prolapse. Mitral vegetations that are made from fibrin deposits containing microorganisms carry a high risk of migration, particularly when they exceed 20 mm in size.

Ischemic Mitral Insufficiency

Ischemic mitral valve regurgitation is one of the rare causes of mitral dysfunction in which both valve prolapse and restriction can coexist (Fig. 99.2). Restriction is uniformly present in ischemic mitral insufficiency because of excessive systolic traction on the chordae due to a dysfunctional left ventricular segment. If an akinetic or dyskinetic myocardial segment involves the base of the papillary muscles, the

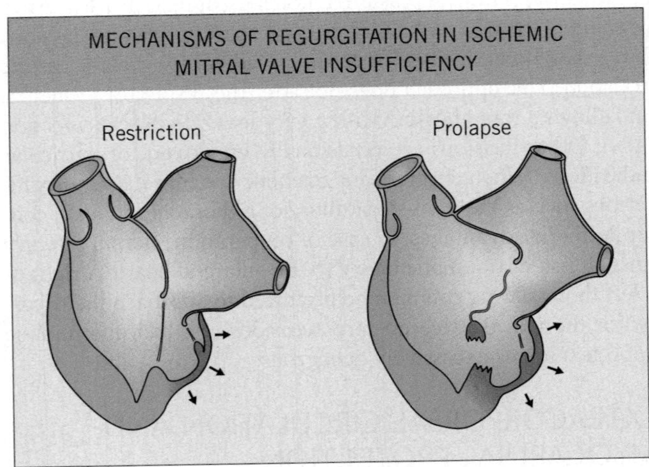

Figure 99.2 Mechanisms of regurgitation in ischemic mitral valve insufficiency. Restriction: excess traction on chordae inserted on the ischemic papillary muscle prevents leaflet coaptation. Prolapse: papillary muscle rupture.

distance separating the base of the papillary muscle from the mitral annulus will increase during systole, and the leaflets will be subjected to a tethering that prevents normal coaptation. In some cases, a segmental prolapse of the leaflet can be associated with the restrictive type of valvular dysfunction. Its mechanisms are multiple and depend on the anatomy of the ischemic papillary muscle. Rupture of the papillary muscle can be partial (detachment of a single head) or total. Rarely, prolapse is related to papillary muscle elongation.[3]

In 85% of cases, ischemic miral insufficiency involves the posterior papillary muscle because its blood supply is more precarious, being perfused either exclusively from the right coronary artery or from branches of the circumflex coronary artery. In contrast, the anterior papillary muscle receives its blood supply from both the left anterior descending coronary artery and its diagonal branches. Mitral annular dilatation is usually moderate in ischemic mitral regurgitation. In ischemic mitral insufficiency, the degree of regurgitation is variable with time and dependent on preload conditions.

Other Causes of Mitral Insufficiency

End-stage dilated cardiomyopathy can result in a restrictive pattern of mitral valve insufficiency (see Fig. 99.1). Similar to the mechanism described in ischemic mitral regurgitation, the failing left ventricle exerts excessive traction on the chordae tendineae during systole, which results in poor leaflet coaptation.[4] The other causes of mitral insufficiency concern a lesser number of patients: congenital abnormalities, such as the anterior leaflet cleft in atrioventricular canal; autoimmune disorders, in particular systemic lupus, producing fine vegetations adherent to retracted leaflets with shortened chordae; and endomyocardial fibrosis, resulting in an embedded posterior leaflet associated with a left ventricular apical thrombus.

Correction of Posterior Leaflet Prolapse

Posterior leaflet prolapse resulting from rupture or elongation of the chordae tendineae can be treated with quadrangular resection of the prolapsed segment (Fig. 99.3a).[5,6] When excess tissue is present on the posterior leaflet (i.e., myxomatous degeneration), it is additionally necessary to excise the leaflet and to perform a sliding leaflet plasty as described by Carpentier (Fig. 99.3b). Furthermore, in the event of annular calcification, decalcification followed by reconstruction with use of the sliding leaflet technique occasionally permits valve preservation.[7]

TREATMENT OF POSTERIOR LEAFLET PROLAPSE

A

B

Figure 99.3 Treatment of posterior leaflet prolapse.
A, Quadrangular resection of the posterior leaflet. **B,** Posterior leaflet resection with sliding plasty.

Correction of Anterior Leaflet Prolapse

A number of techniques have been described for correction of prolapse of the anterior leaflet. Chordal transfer from the posterior leaflet to the anterior leaflet is reliable and efficient regardless of the mechanism of the anterior leaflet prolapse (Fig. 99.4). A segment of posterior leaflet with its chordae tendineae is harvested and sutured to the anterior leaflet at the level of the prolapse. This technique has been the subject of several studies demonstrating excellent long-term results.[8,9] Other techniques include use of artificial chordae,[10,11] chordal shortening,[5] and closure of the central orifice of the mitral valve with creation of a double orifice (bow-tie repair) as described by Alfieri.[12]

Correction of Valve Restriction

Commissurotomy

The commissure is incised with preservation of a few millimeters of leaflet tissue at the annulus to regain the normal anatomic configuration. On occasion, the underlying chordae tendineae and papillary muscle are divided or even fenestrated.[5]

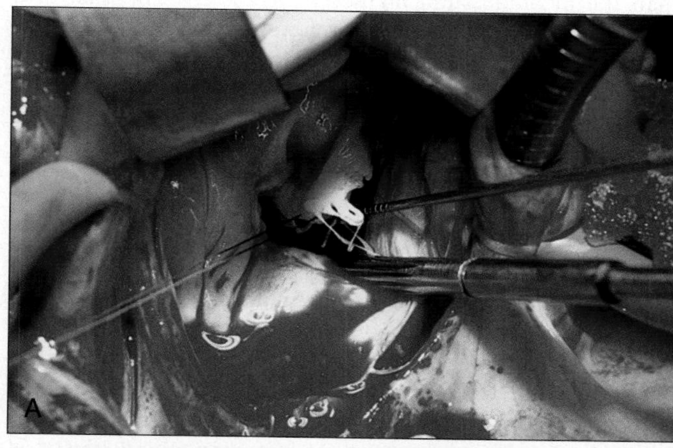

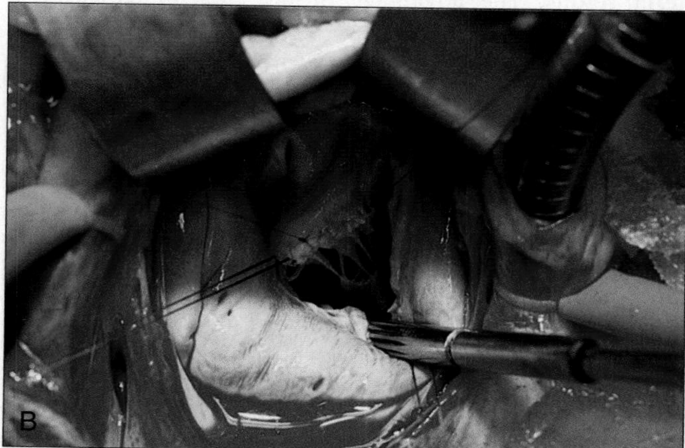

Figure 99.4 Chordal transfer from posterior leaflet to anterior leaflet. A, Ruptured chordae on the anterior leaflet.
B, Transposition of chordae from posterior to anterior leaflet.

Leaflet Augmentation with a Pericardial Patch

In the presence of frank retraction of the leaflets, the only technique that permits true mobilization of the mitral valve is leaflet augmentation with pericardium.[13] Autologous pericardium briefly treated with glutaraldehyde is an excellent material for leaflet enlargement. This technique can be applied to both anterior and posterior leaflets.

Principles of Prosthetic Ring Annuloplasty

The mitral annulus is a dynamic structure that changes both shape and size throughout the course of the cardiac cycle. The surface area of the mitral orifice decreases by a third during ventricular systole compared with its area during diastole. Contraction of the annulus occurs mainly in its posterior region because of direct insertion of myocardial fibers in this region of the annulus. The mitral orifice's shape is almost circular in systole and becomes oval in diastole. Although previously considered to be a flat structure, the annulus of the mitral valve is in fact saddle shaped, slightly concave in its short axis (anteroposterior) and convex in its long axis (bicommissural) because of the impression of the protruding aortic root.[2]

The mitral annulus is often dilated in the setting of mitral regurgitation. This dilatation is not homogeneous and occurs mostly in the posterior portion of the annulus with its sparse fibrous skeleton. The remodeling ring annuloplasty, as first described by Carpentier, aims to restore the normal proportions of the annulus with an anteroposterior diameter smaller than the bicommissural diameter (Fig. 99.5). The goal of a remodeling ring annuloplasty is not only to correct annular dilatation but also, especially in cases of degenerative valve disease, to augment the durability of the valve repair by reinforcing the valve sutures and by increasing the surface area of leaflet coaptation. The latter effect reduces tension exerted on the suture lines and on the dystrophic chordae tendineae. In the setting of mitral regurgitation due to restriction (i.e., ischemic, rheumatic, or cardiomyopathic etiology), the annulus is often only mildly dilated if at all. In these cases, reduction of the annular dimensions with an undersized ring annuloplasty compensates for the restrictive process through reinforcement of leaflet coaptation.

Mitral valve reconstruction without ring annuloplasty (Wooler repair) generally provides less favorable long-term results. The advantage of the ring annuloplasty is achievement of a reduction of the annulus precisely calibrated to the mitral orifice. Whereas some prosthetic rings are made of rigid materials meant to reshape the mitral orifice (Carpentier[1]), others are flexible, allowing slight changes in shape of the orifice during the cardiac cycle (Duran[14]). Some authors (Cosgrove[15]) use an incomplete prosthetic ring in an attempt to specifically reduce the most dilated segments of the annulus (commissural and posterior regions). In daily practice, a prosthetic ring is placed in most mitral repairs. Some exceptions are repair in very young children because of the risk of stenosis with growth, repair of a rheumatic mitral stenosis because of risk of residual stenosis related to leaflet rigidity, recurrent acute bacterial endocarditis because of risk of prosthesis infection, and severe hypertrophic cardiomyopathy because of risk of worsening the systolic anterior motion of the mitral valve.

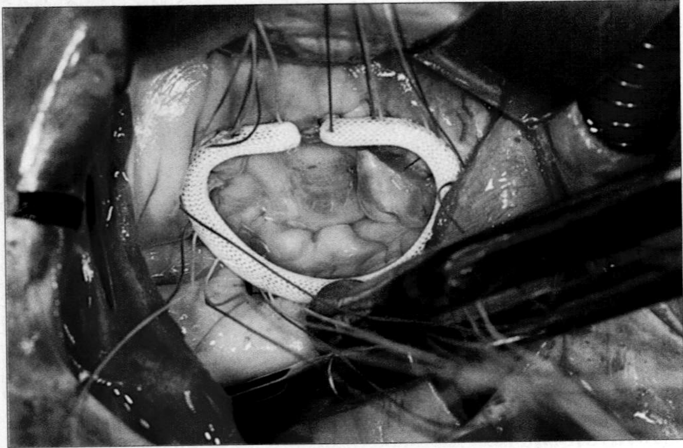

Figure 99.5 Carpentier mitral prosthetic ring.

Intraoperative Transesophageal Echography

All patients undergoing a valve repair undergo intraoperative assessment of the result by transesophageal echography. This test has significantly decreased the risk of early reoperation due to valve failure. Any persistent mitral dysfunction is immediately treated during an additional time of extracorporeal circulation; most frequently, a conservative treatment is possible, and valve replacement is rarely required.

Systolic anterior motion is a rare complication of mitral repair (2% in our experience). It is manifested by hemodynamic collapse on weaning from cardiopulmonary bypass and is detected by intraoperative transesophageal echocardiography. Excess tissue of the posterior mitral leaflet pushes the anterior mitral leaflet into the left ventricular outflow tract toward the interventricular septum, thus creating an obstruction to the ejecting bloodstream, a ventriculoaortic pressure gradient, and severe mitral regurgitation.[16] Systolic anterior motion results from an error in sizing of the prosthetic annular ring, thereby creating a neoannulus, which becomes too narrow to accommodate the excess valve tissue. Systolic anterior motion is primarily encountered in repair of Barlow's disease or in cases of hypertrophy of the interventricular septum. The treatment[16] of systolic anterior motion consists of upsizing of the prosthetic ring, more extensive resection of the posterior leaflet by a sliding leaflet plasty, or valve replacement if an adequate repair is not feasible.

Results

The results of mitral valve repair depend on the cause of valvular disease and on the operative technique.

Operative Mortality

In our experience of 514 cases from 1995 to 1998, the operative mortality was directly correlated to etiology. It was approximately 3% in degenerative mitral insufficiency. The risk was significantly higher in the elderly and in cases of severe annulus calcification. Because of younger age, the operative mortality of repair in rheumatic cases was low (1%). Conversely, the operative risk was much higher in patients suffering from acute endocarditis and ischemic cardiomyopathy (8%). Moreover, irrespective of the etiology, several studies have demonstrated higher mortality with mitral valve replacement compared with mitral valve repair.[17,18]

Long-term Results

It is now established that mitral valve repair, when it is technically feasible, offers better long-term results than mitral valve replacement with either bioprosthetic or mechanical prostheses. These superior results apply to long-term survival, to thromboembolic complications, and to need for reintervention.[17,18] The superiority of repair over replacement is obvious at 5 years after surgery and becomes even more evident after longer periods of follow-up.[19] Carpentier and associates[2] reported on a series of 206 consecutive patients and observed an actuarial survival rate of 83% at 10 years and 72% at 15 years. If only valve-related mortality is considered, survival is 83% at 15 years. Moreover, after 15 years of follow-up, nearly all patients were free of thromboembolic complications (94%) or of hemorrhagic complications (96%) related to use of anticoagulants. Finally, 87% of patients had no need for reintervention (actuarial rate of reoperation: 1% per patient-year).[2]

The cause of the valvular disease has a major influence on long-term results after mitral valve repair (Fig. 99.6). Degenerative mitral insufficiency is least likely to require reoperation, with 93% of patients free of reintervention at 15 years.[20,21] The portions of the valve affected by degenerative changes also affect outcome (Fig. 99.7). Isolated posterior leaflet repair rarely requires reintervention. In contrast, an anterior leaflet prolapse or prolapse of both leaflets carries a higher risk of reoperation.[15]

Repair of rheumatic mitral valve disease is associated with less favorable long-term outcome compared with repair of degenerative mitral valve disease.[2,19,22] For rheumatic patients, freedom from reintervention drops to 76% 15 years after surgery.[2] Among rheumatic patients, the age of the patient at the time of repair determines the risk of deterioration of the repair; the highest risk occurs in children and adolescents younger than 20 years.[22,23] Despite this higher risk of reoperation, mitral valve repair still offers a better short- and long-term outcome than mitral valve replacement in patients with rheumatic mitral valve disease. This superior outcome justifies the use of mitral valve repair whenever possible, even in patients with rheumatic heart disease.[23]

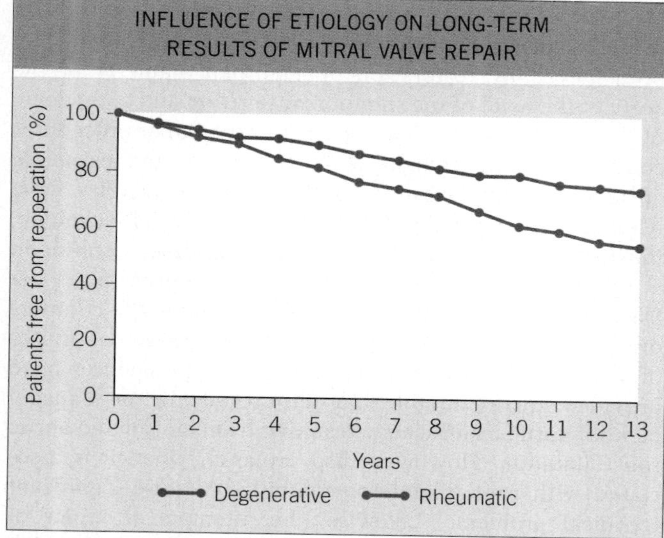

Figure 99.6 Influence of etiology on long-term results of mitral valve repair. The rate of reoperation is higher in rheumatic disease compared with degenerative disease.

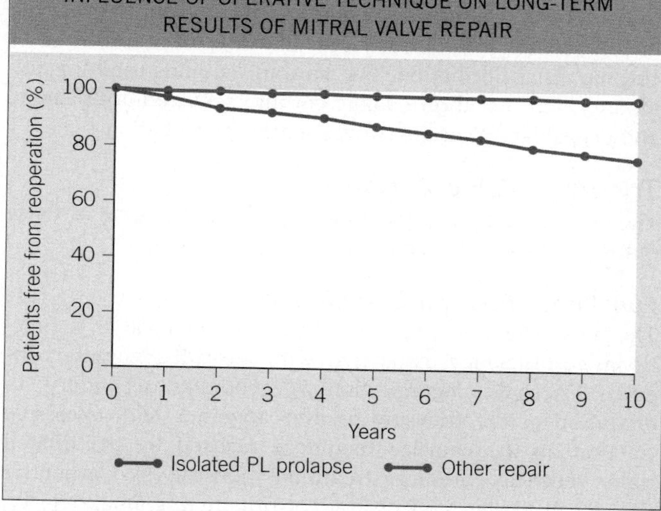

Figure 99.7 Influence of the operative technique on long-term results of mitral valve repair. The best results are observed in cases of an isolated procedure on the posterior leaflet (PL).

Mitral valve repair also offers durable results in acute infective mitral endocarditis, with almost 80% of patients free from events at 7 years,[24] and it is preferred to valve replacement in any case whenever it is technically possible. Long-term results of annuloplasty for ischemic mitral insufficiency have not yet reached such excellence; the risk of late death has remained relatively high, with only 58% survival at 5 years.[25]

Mitral Repair and Atrial Fibrillation

About 20% to 30% of patients presenting for mitral repair are in atrial fibrillation.[26,27] Compared with patients in sinus rhythm, patients with atrial fibrillation are usually older.[28] They present with more severe cardiac disease, such as ventricular and atrial dilatation and pulmonary hypertension. When atrial fibrillation has persisted for more than 1 year preoperatively, one rarely observes a return to sinus rhythm after mitral valve repair. Usually, only patients presenting with intermittent atrial fibrillation of recent onset (<3 months in duration) and a moderately dilated left atrium (<60 mm) are likely to reestablish sinus rhythm after mitral valve repair.[26,28] Restoration of sinus rhythm presents several advantages, including relief of palpitations and improved hemodynamics because of restored atrial kick. Above all, the presence of atrial fibrillation greatly increases the risk of thromboembolic complications and of hemorrhagic complications related to use of anticoagulants. The Cox procedure consists of creation of an atrial maze to eliminate re-entrant circuits thought to be responsible for atrial fibrillation.[29] At the Mayo Clinic, 78% of patients treated with mitral valve repair and the Cox procedure had returned to sinus rhythm versus 12% treated with mitral valve repair alone at follow-up 2 years postoperatively.[26] Because of its complexity, the Cox procedure has not been uniformly applied worldwide in patients with atrial fibrillation requiring mitral valve surgery. Pulmonary vein isolation, a simplification of the full maze procedure, has been proven to be almost as efficient. Nowadays, it is currently practiced in conjunction with mitral surgery in cases of intermittent or chronic atrial fibrillation. The various methods used for pulmonary vein isolation (classic cut and sew, radiofrequency, and cryoablation) are currently under investigation.

Tricuspid Valve Repair

The principles guiding tricuspid repair are the same as those outlined for mitral repair.

Functional Tricuspid Insufficiency

The most common problem of the tricuspid valve is functional insufficiency associated with left-sided valvular disease. Tricuspid regurgitation is generally secondary to dilatation of the tricuspid annulus together with excessive traction on the chordae tendineae exerted by the dilated right ventricle. Surgical treatment consists of Carpentier (Fig. 99.8), Duran, or Cosgrove prosthetic ring annuloplasty. The De Vega repair annuloplasty,[26] with a tacking running suture on the tricuspid annulus, is another option. The anterior and posterior sections of the valve are most commonly dilated in tricuspid insufficiency, whereas the septal leaflet is spared.[30,31] Tricuspid annuloplasties therefore primarily aim to reduce these two regions.

Progression of an overlooked tricuspid insufficiency has been shown to carry a poor prognosis with a high mortality at reoperation. Therefore, identification of the determinants of tricuspid leak worsening is critical before any left-sided valve procedure. Even if the amount of regurgitation is only mild to moderate, tricuspid annuloplasty is indicated in the following situations:

- evidence of permanent or transient right ventricular failure symptoms;
- valve disease secondary to rheumatic fever: besides the annulus dilatation, the tricuspid valve is frequently the site of organic lesions that have a potential for progression;
- elevated pulmonary pressure (systolic pressure >50 mm Hg);
- pronounced annulus distention (anteroposterior diameter >40 mm); and
- endocavitary pacemaker or defibrillator wire that somehow impairs leaflet motion.

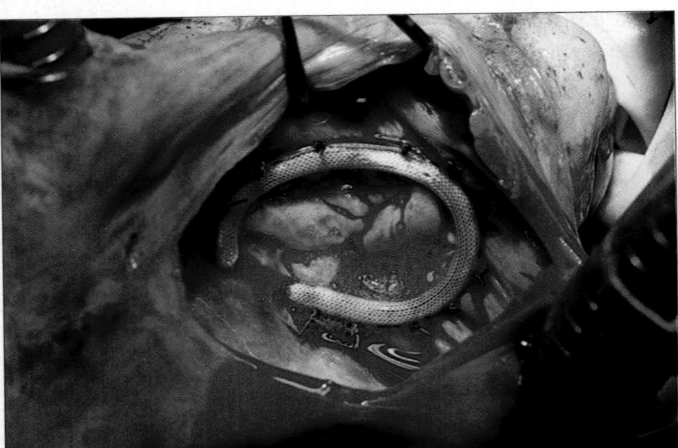

Figure 99.8 Carpentier tricuspid prosthetic ring.

Organic Tricuspid Insufficiency

Acute rheumatic fever produces a fibrotic involvement of the tricuspid valve that is frequently underestimated by echography. In typical cases, it results in regurgitation secondary to leaflet retraction together with some stenosis due to commissural fusion. Repair of the tricuspid valve comprises commissurotomy and ring annuloplasty.

Infectious endocarditis of the tricuspid valve occurs mainly in intravenous drug users or in cases of infection of endocavitary pacemaker leads. A medical management of these patients with antibiotics and removal of all prosthetic material is recommended in most cases. Surgery is rarely required in acute situations (threatening and monstrous vegetations, obstruction of the pulmonary trunk or of its proximal branches). Ultimately, surgical repair of a severely leaking tricuspid valve can occasionally be indicated.

In carcinoid syndrome, the extent of the valve fibrosis requires tricuspid valve replacement and also occasionally involves the pulmonary valve. Finally, traumatic papillary muscle or chordal rupture as well as tricuspid leaflet tearing is occasionally encountered after blunt trauma to the chest; in these uncommon cases, surgical repair should be postponed for several weeks after the accident.

Aortic Valve Repair

Replacement is the standard treatment of a diseased aortic valve. On occasion, reconstructive surgery of the aortic valve can be performed.

Dystrophic Aneurysm of the Ascending Aorta

The standard treatment of aneurysm of the ascending aorta with aortic insufficiency is the Bentall procedure,[32] which includes both replacement of the aortic root with a Dacron tube prosthesis with coronary artery reimplantation and replacement of the aortic valve (Fig. 99.9). Aortic insufficiency that accompanies ascending aortic aneurysms usually results from restricted motion of the valve cusps due to excess traction by the dilated aortic root. This results in incomplete central coaptation and aortic regurgitation. Most often, the aortic cusps are structurally normal. It has recently been shown that aortic valvular competency can be achieved by restoration of a normal diameter of the aorta at the level of the sinotubular junction and at the level of the aortic annulus. Two sparing aortic valve procedures consisting of replacement of the aortic root and ascending aorta with reimplantation of the coronary arteries have been described (see Fig. 99.9).[33,34] In the David technique, the aortic valve is included in the Dacron tube, resulting in a tubular aortic root[33]; in the Yacoub procedure, the Dacron tube is fashioned proximally to follow the contours of the crown-shaped aortic annulus to reproduce neosinuses of Valsalva.[34] These sparing aortic valve procedures have provided equally durable long-term results for the management of aortic insufficiency resulting from an isolated aortic root dilatation. However, cusp prolapse, when it is associated with root dilatation, continues to raise significant technical problems. Likewise, the attempts at repair of bicuspid aortic valves have been responsible for a high reoperation rate. In these instances, aortic valve replacement remains preferable.

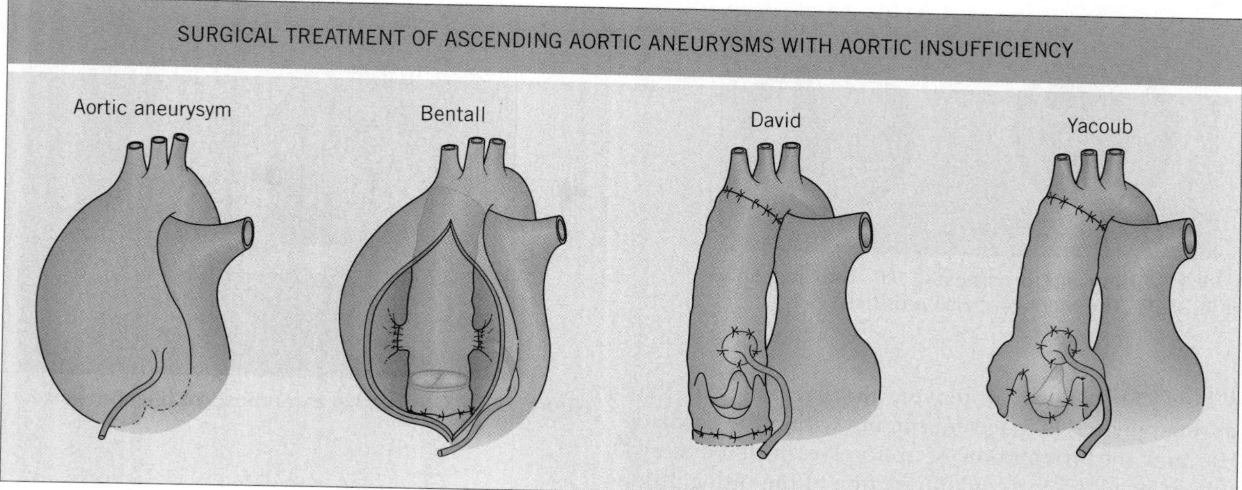

Figure 99.9 Surgical treatment of ascending aortic aneurysms with aortic insufficiency.

Other Aortic Valve Repairs

In the setting of acute aortic dissection, it is common to encounter aortic insufficiency related to extension of the dissection into the commissures. Treatment consists of suspending the three commissures on a felt strip. The long-term result of this approach is excellent, with a very low rate of reoperation.[35] Because of the satisfactory performance of modern prostheses, in particular in the aortic position, and the possibilities offered by homograft or autograft replacement, the indications for repair of other aortic valvular disease (such as endocarditis, rheumatic or congenital disorders) have remained anecdotal.

VALVE REPLACEMENT

Access to the aortic valve is obtained through a transverse aortotomy at the base of the ascending aorta. The incision is extended vertically in the direction of the noncoronary sinus. Access to the mitral valve is obtained by opening of the left atrium with an incision parallel to the interatrial groove. The diseased valve is removed together with eventual fragments of calcium adherent to the annulus. In an effort to preserve left ventricular structural architecture, the mitral valve is excised, if possible with preservation of the posterior leaflet and its chordae tendineae.

Any prosthetic valve consists of two elements: a sewing ring for fixation to the valvular orifice, generally made of Dacron and occasionally reinforced with silicone; and a mobile section that allows opening and closure of the orifice during the cardiac cycle. According to the nature of the mobile component, artificial valves are divided into two categories, mechanical and biologic. Age and cardiac rhythm are among the main determinants for choosing a specific artificial valve.

Mechanical Prosthetic Valves

There are various types of mechanical valves: the ball-cage prosthesis, the tilting disk prosthesis, and the bileaflet prosthesis.

Ball-Cage Prostheses

Constructed as a ball enclosed in a metallic cage, these prostheses were the first to be used in humans. The prototype of this valve is the Starr-Edwards valve first used in 1961 (Fig. 99.10).

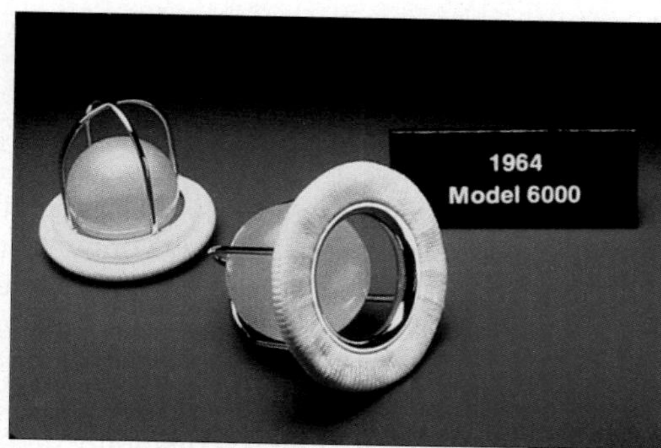

Figure 99.10 Ball-cage prosthesis. The Starr-Edwards prosthesis.

The most common Starr valve consisted of a Silastic ball surrounded by a cage of metal bars (model 6120 for the mitral position, model 3160 for the aortic position). The ball prosthesis partially obstructs blood flow, and flow through the prosthesis is turbulent.[36] As a consequence, a transvalvular pressure gradient can persist, particularly in a small prosthesis placed in the aortic position. Cellular elements of blood are traumatized when the ball makes contact with the cage, and hemolytic anemia can therefore occur. In addition, a ball-cage prosthesis is bulky, occupying a lot of space within the cardiac chambers. For these reasons, the number of ball-cage prostheses implanted today has remained small.

Tilting Disk Prostheses

The mobile element of these valves is a tilting disk held in place by two welded struts. The prototype of this prosthesis is the Bjork-Shiley introduced in 1969 (Fig. 99.11). A Bjork valve introduced in 1985 (the so-called convexo-concave) was plagued by several structural failures, mainly fracture of a strut resulting from the repetitive stresses of opening and closure. This model was withdrawn from the market. The hemodynamic characteristics of the tilting disk prosthesis are better than those of the ball-cage prosthesis. Nevertheless, because of a leaflet opening that amounts to only 60 degrees in certain models, a degree of obstruction to

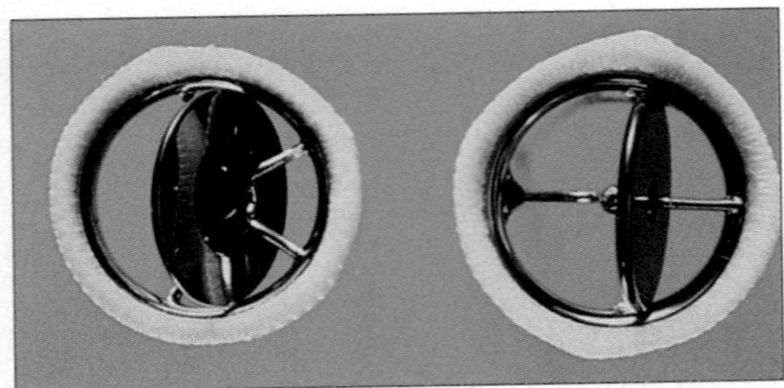

Figure 99.11 Tilting disk prostheses. *Left,* The Bjork-Shiley prosthesis. *Right,* The Medtronic-Hall prosthesis.

blood flow can persist. Moreover, the excursion of the disk during opening is space consuming within the cardiac cavities, and the orientation of the valve must be very carefully determined to avoid interaction of the tilting disk with the side walls of the cardiac chambers. A newer model of tilting disk prosthesis with proven durability, improved angle of disk opening, and reduced transvalvular gradient is the Medtronic-Hall Omnicarbon prosthesis (see Fig. 99.11).[37]

Bileaflet Prostheses

The clinical introduction of a bileaflet prosthesis in 1977 was a major breakthrough in the field of mechanical prosthetic valves. These valves are made of two semicircular pivoting disks. The leaflets of the prosthesis are made of pyrolytic carbons, a material considered to be less thrombogenic. This prosthesis possesses an excellent hemodynamic profile, with some degree of obstruction to blood flow observed only in prostheses of smaller size. The prototype is the St. Jude valve, which currently is the most commonly implanted mechanical prosthetic valve in the world. Since its introduction, the results obtained with this valve have been excellent. Newer prostheses resembling the St. Jude valve have become available, such as the CarboMedics (Fig. 99.12), Sorin Bicarbon, ATS, and Mira Edwards prostheses.

Limitations of Mechanical Prosthetic Valves

The most important risk linked to the use of a mechanical valve is valvular thrombosis. The risk of thrombosis is greatest in the first months after surgery. A thrombotic complication can be manifested as a systemic embolus with preserved function of the valve (nonobstructive thrombosis). Emboli can arise from fibrin deposits attached to the sewing ring of the prosthesis and sometimes show up as small abnormal echo signals. Valvular thrombosis can also interfere with the mechanical function of the valve (Fig. 99.13) and can

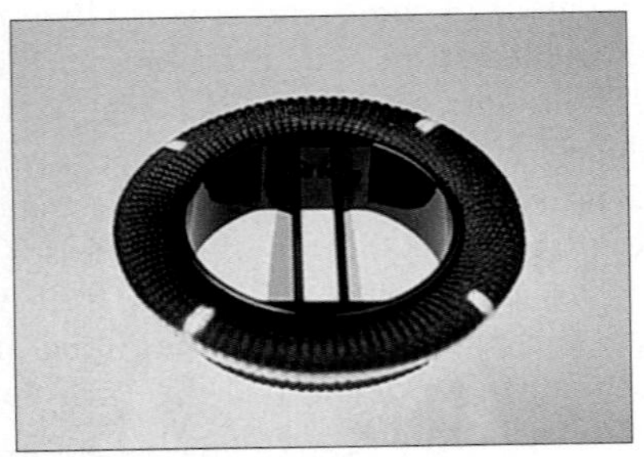

Figure 99.12 CarboMedics prosthesis.

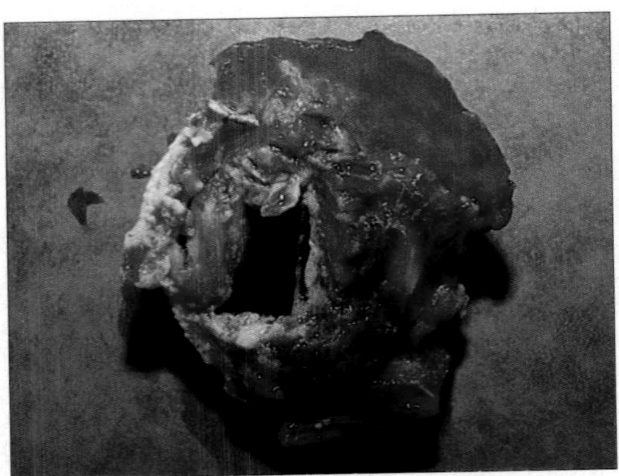

Figure 99.13 Obstructive thrombosis of bileaflet valve.

produce symptoms of acute valvular stenosis. In such a case, the thrombus usually arises from the struts and eventually progresses to the entire prosthetic apparatus to interfere with valvular mechanical function. Whatever mechanical valve is chosen, the thromboembolic risk persists throughout the life of the patient, with a linearized rate of 2% to 2.5% per patient-year.[38] As shown in the AREVA study,[39] a lower level of anticoagulation can be used for bileaflet prostheses in the aortic position (international normalized ratio of 2 to 3). For mechanical valves in the mitral position, a more aggressive anticoagulation regimen is warranted (international normalized ratio of 3 to 4.5). The risk of a hemorrhagic complication related to the use of anticoagulants is also 2% per patient-year.[39,40]

Biologic Valves

Biologic valves are separated into three groups on the basis of the origin of the biologic material: heterografts (animal origin), homografts (human donor), and autografts (tissues derived from the patient).

Bioprostheses (or Heterografts)

The use of valvular tissue, derived from animals after fixation in glutaraldehyde, was first reported by Carpentier in 1969.[41] Porcine bioprosthetic valves are fabricated from pig aortic leaflets mounted on metal-coated stents. Depending on the model, the noncoronary cusp, which in pigs is embedded in muscle and whose mobility is decreased, is either included (Hancock) or excluded (Carpentier-Edwards, Mosaic).

Pericardial bioprostheses are fabricated with bovine pericardium, a concept introduced by Ionescu. Ionescu valves were prone to cusp tearing along the rigid struts.[42] This problem was resolved by the Carpentier pericardial bioprostheses, which modified the fixation of the pericardium inside the rigid stent with a clipping system (Carpentier-Perimount; Fig. 99.14). Other models of pericardial valves have attempted to optimize the flow by mounting the pericardium outside the struts (Mitroflow). To fit the aortic annulus, the sewing ring of recent bioprostheses has been scalloped, allowing a slight upsizing compared with the plane configuration of the old models and that of mechanical valves.

Regardless of their type, bioprosthetic valves are subjected to degeneration. This process ultimately leads to tears and

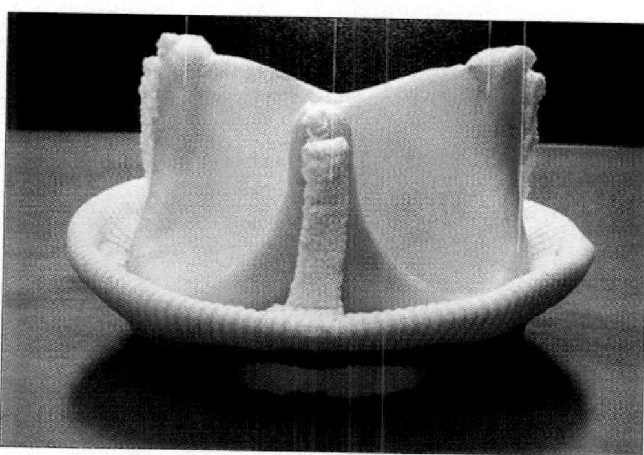

Figure 99.14 Pericardial Carpentier-Perimount bioprosthesis.

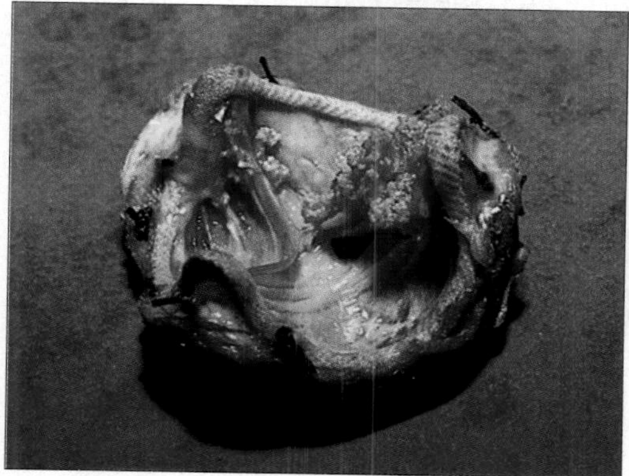

Figure 99.15 Bioprosthesis degeneration with leaflet tears and calcifications.

calcifications of the cusps (Fig. 99.15). The time course of valve failure is a function of the age of the patient because bioprostheses in children and young adults show faster degradation. Because of lower transvalvular pressures and brisker valve opening and closing, bioprostheses in the mitral position deteriorate faster than do bioprostheses in the aortic or tricuspid position. With the Carpentier-Perimount, the rate of freedom from reoperation after 15 years is 94% for the aortic valve and 78% for the mitral valve.[43] Bioprosthetic degradation usually is manifested as a valvular leak caused by a torn and prolapsed cusp or by commissural detachment. On occasion, bioprostheses may become purely stenotic because of calcification at the base of the cusps (most commonly pericardial bioprostheses).

The classic bioprosthesis consisted of animal tissue mounted on peaked metal stents surrounded by a sewing ring for fixation. In an effort to optimize the flow and to decrease the transvalvular gradient, stentless aortic bioprostheses have been developed. These substitutes consist of either a porcine valve including its attachment to the aortic wall (Freestyle, CryoLife-O'Brien) or a bovine pericardial valve sewn inside a pericardial tube. The lack of any rigid support allows the implantation of larger diameter valves whose hemodynamic profile is excellent. However, the technique of insertion is slightly more difficult than for a stented valve. It was hypothesized that reducing the constraints of the biologic tissue attached directly to the patient's aortic wall rather than to a rigid stent might improve the longevity of the prosthesis. Unfortunately, long-term studies have shown that stentless bioprostheses undergo degradation at the same speed as their stented counterparts do.[44]

Homograft Valves

Homografts have been used since the earliest days of cardiac surgery and are aortic, pulmonary, or mitral valves harvested from humans. These valves are obtained from transplant donors whose hearts had been refused, persons deceased from noncardiac causes, and explanted hearts of transplant recipients. Each country's legislation regulates the harvesting procedure for such valves.

The preservation method of the homografts has changed with time. In the 1960s, once harvested, the valves were dipped in a culture medium containing antibiotics at 4° C and had to be implanted within a 3-week time lapse. Since then, cryopreservation has become the routine technique. The homografts are stored at the tissue bank in liquid nitrogen at −160° C and are kept in a solution containing a cryopreservative agent (dimethyl sulfoxide), which prevents tissue fracture related to ice crystal formation. This method allows unlimited preservation of the valve.

Similar to stentless bioprostheses, homograft valves are not mounted on a rigid support and require a specific implantation technique. Two possibilities exist for placement of a homograft in the aortic position: implantation of the valve alone with a small sewing ring of homograft aortic wall (freehand) and replacement of the aortic root (Fig. 99.16). The freehand technique or subcoronary implantation carries a slight risk of distortion of the valve. Therefore, replacement of the whole aortic root is the most common procedure. Homografts are particularly useful in the management of infectious endocarditis as they are considered to be more resistant to infection because of absence of prosthetic material. More important, homograft replacement of the aortic root allows an easy treatment of any annular abscess cavities.

Homografts have an excellent hemodynamic profile but undergo a degenerative deterioration responsible for cusp tear or calcification and leading to reoperation. In several series, 80% of patients managed with aortic homografts were free of reoperation at 15 years.[45-47] The mitral homograft has been used for partial or complete valve replacement in very limited series.[48] However, the overall longevity of homografts does not appear to be far superior to that of bioprostheses.

Autograft Valves

The use of autograft valves is limited to transfer of the pulmonary valve to the aortic position, known as the Ross procedure (Fig. 99.17). In theory, the transposed pulmonary valve is viable and of unlimited durability. A pulmonary homograft is subsequently implanted into the vacated position on the right outflow tract. The Ross procedure is especially attractive if there is a component of subvalvular stenosis because of the possibility of performing an additional Konno-type outflow tract enlargement. Furthermore, because of its potential to grow, the Ross procedure is the preferable option in a developing child. Since the introduction by Ross of pulmonary valve autografting in 1967, excellent long-term results have been demonstrated, with 85% of

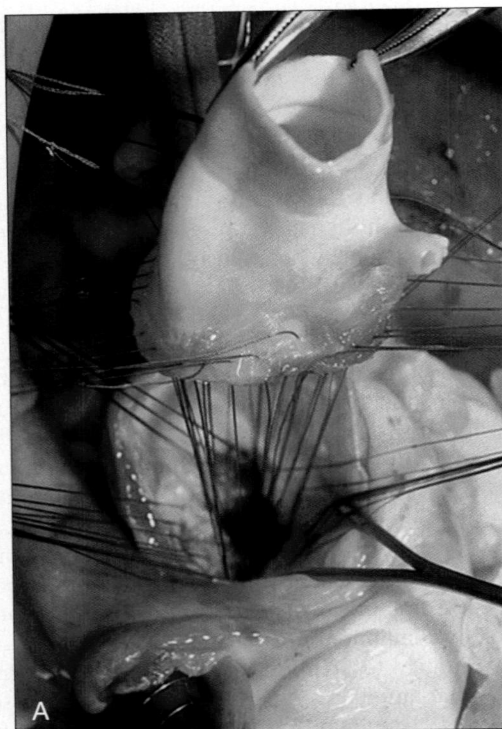

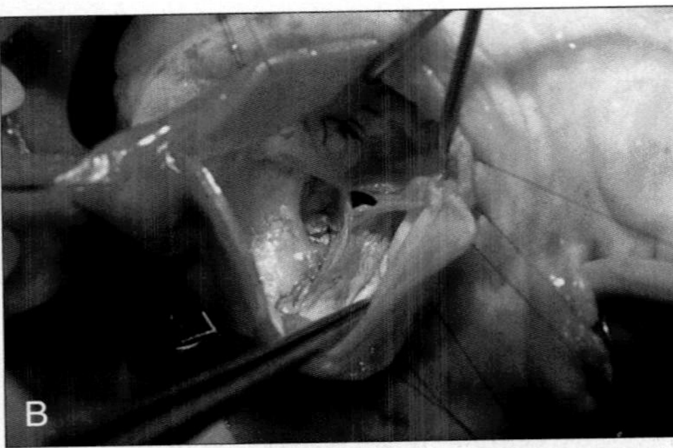

Figure 99.16 Placement of homograft in aortic position. A, Aortic root replacement with homograft. **B,** Freehand aortic homograft.

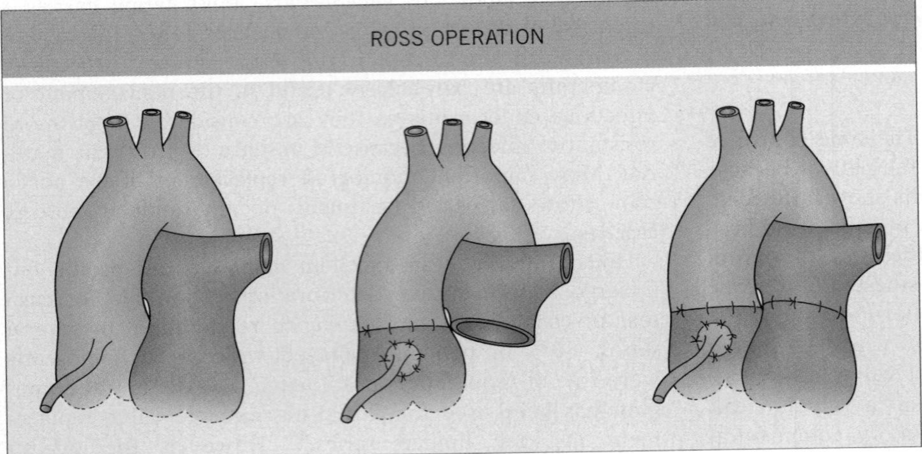

Figure 99.17 Ross operation.

patients free of reoperation after 20 years of follow-up.[49] Satisfactory results of the Ross operation have also been reported in the setting of complicated infective endocarditis.[50]

Long term, degradation of the homograft in the pulmonary position was thought to be the main and only cause for reoperation. Unfortunately, recent studies have shown occasional progressive dilatation of the pulmonary artery when it is subjected to a systemic pressure.[51] Beyond a certain extent, enlargement of the root leads to an excess traction on the commissures, resulting in autograft regurgitation. The risk of reoperation for autograft insufficiency appeared to be at least equal to that of pulmonary homograft failure.[51] This raised a serious concern as to the place of the Ross procedure in an adult population in which other simpler and reliable alternatives exist for aortic valve replacement.

Which Is the Preferred Valvular Substitute?

The choice of an artificial valve must first take into account the age of the patient.[52]

In Children

The Ross procedure is the operation of choice for aortic valve replacement. Pulmonary autografting provides a valve substitute capable of growth, and systemic anticoagulation in the developing child is avoided. A mechanical prosthesis is a potential option, keeping in mind lifelong anticoagulation therapy and monitoring. Because of their rapid rate of degradation in children, bioprosthetic valves are generally contraindicated in this age group. Homografts also undergo rapid deterioration. This limits their use in children to replacement of the pulmonary valve as part of a Ross procedure because eventual dysfunction is usually well tolerated in the pulmonary position.

In Adults Younger than 70 Years

In general, the preferred valve substitute in adults younger than 70 years is a mechanical prosthesis, particularly in patients who are already taking anticoagulants (e.g., for atrial fibrillation). On occasion, in younger patients with strong reasons for anticoagulation therapy to be avoided, a bioprosthesis or a homograft is a suitable alternative. These reasons include the desire for pregnancy, living in impoverished areas where anticoagulation monitoring is impossible, and engaging in sports with a high risk of traumatic injury. Furthermore, in cases of infective endocarditis, particularly those with aortic ring abscesses, a homograft is very useful. If life expectancy does not exceed 10 years (advanced congestive heart failure, severe coronary artery disease, cancer, or other significant comorbidity), a bioprosthesis is to be preferred.

For patients in the age range between 65 and 70 years, the choice of a valvular prosthesis remains controversial. A mechanical prosthesis is preferred in the absence of significant comorbidity (e.g., a woman with aortic stenosis without clinical coronary artery disease). Sometimes it is preferable to choose a bioprosthesis (e.g., a man with mitral valvular disease in the presence of significant coronary artery disease). A bioprosthesis is also preferable when there are associated diseases in which anticoagulation is contraindicated (e.g., osteoarthritis, gastrointestinal ulcer, or urologic disease).

In Patients Older than 70 Years

As a rule, these patients are offered a bioprosthesis. The presence of atrial fibrillation does not alter this preference.

chapter 100

Management of the Postsurgical Valve Disease Patient

John Kern and Bret Mettler

Many acceptable substitutes exist for the replacement of diseased heart valves. The ideal valvular prosthesis, as described by Harken,[1] remains the benchmark that all prosthetic valves attempt to achieve. Whereas prosthetic heart valves have continued to evolve, their inherent deficits and treatment requirements may result in postoperative complications requiring complex treatment algorithms. As the average age of the population increases, clinicians of all specialties are seeing more patients with prosthetic heart valves. Caring for these patients requires an understanding of the various valve types and the principles of postoperative management. It also requires an understanding of the pathophysiology and management of prosthetic valve dysfunction. In this chapter, the diagnosis and management of common problems in patients with valve replacement and repair are reviewed.

IMMEDIATE POSTOPERATIVE PERIOD

CLINICAL PRESENTATION

Cardiopulmonary bypass induces many physiologic changes that become apparent in the postoperative patient, and its duration is a determinant of the speed of recovery. Optimal management involves treatment of untoward trends early while avoiding overtreatment of acute hemodynamic changes associated with a physiologic dynamic state. Monitoring is aided by use of an arterial line that provides beat-to-beat blood pressure measurement and allows ease of access for blood gas determination.

Atrioventricular conduction abnormalities more commonly present after valvular heart surgery because of local edema and trauma to the conduction system. In anticipation of these potential problems, all patients undergoing valve replacement or repair should have epicardial pacing wires placed at the time of surgery and an electrocardiogram in the immediate postoperative period. Patients should be monitored for signs of malperfusion, which include a persistent or worsening acidosis, cool extremities, and low urine output. Whereas cardiac output and blood pressure are easily measured indexes of effective circulation, there are no absolute values that must be achieved. The markers of adequate end-organ perfusion, as demonstrated by the resolution of acidosis, an adequate urine output, and the awakening from anesthesia, are used to guide postoperative care. As anticoagulation is necessary for cardiopulmonary bypass, there is routinely some degree of postoperative bleeding. Mediastinal and pleural tube outputs are observed closely to ensure that this effect resolves. Postoperatively, a heparin-induced coagulopathy may persist as evidenced by an elevated partial thromboplastin time and bleeding. Treatment includes warming of the patient to normal body temperature and protamine reversal. If bleeding persists, re-exploration may be necessary.

DIAGNOSTIC TECHNIQUES

After valve replacement or repair, heart function and vasomotor tone are labile and may exhibit wide fluctuation in measured values. As a result, isolated hemodynamic measurements are less important than are trends in the same measurements over time. The alterations in normal physiology caused by cardiopulmonary bypass and cardioplegia-induced cardiac arrest require time to be corrected fully. In addition, ventricles damaged by years of native valve dysfunction do not "normalize" immediately after a successful valve operation. As patients warm and re-equilibrate after surgery, cardiac function should gradually improve and vasomotor tone should stabilize. These changes are marked by less variability in blood pressure and the ability to slowly wean the patient from any medications used to assist in separation from cardiopulmonary bypass.

Persistent hemodynamic lability or ongoing evidence of inadequate end-organ perfusion mandates additional investigation starting with a thorough physical examination. After cardiopulmonary bypass, failure to awaken from general anesthesia or signs of a focal deficit should prompt additional neurologic evaluation. Patients with impending tamponade will have diminished heart sounds, jugular venous distention, and equalization of right- and left-sided heart pressure. An undrained hemothorax may present with decreased breath sounds, hypotension, and difficulty in being weaned from the ventilator. It cannot be overstated that a complete physical examination in the management of the postsurgical valve disease patient will often give clues to additional investigative studies to be obtained to confirm the physician's suspicions.

A pulmonary artery catheter may be invaluable in sorting out problems and can aid the management of postoperative cardiac dysfunction by monitoring myocardial preload and afterload as well as pulmonary artery pressures. Frequently, a simple determination of the patient's volume status can be obtained by the pulmonary capillary wedge pressure. As rewarming and its attendant vasodilatation take place, patients may become relatively hypovolemic, resulting in a low pulmonary capillary wedge pressure; volume replacement may be required to improve cardiac output and tissue perfusion. This problem may be particularly pronounced in patients who have been treated for aortic stenosis, as their ventricles tend to be noncompliant and preload sensitive. In these patients, restoration of intravascular volume may be enough to restore adequate perfusion. When the pulmonary capillary wedge pressure is high and favors an intravascularly replete state, the addition of inotropic medications or afterload reduction may be indicated. A pulmonary artery catheter with mixed venous pulmonary oximetry provides additional information about oxygenation and can help guide further therapy.

Not infrequently, echocardiography is needed to supplement hemodynamic information. Diagnostic applications in the postoperative period include anatomic definition and physiologic interrogation of cardiac and vascular structures as well as real-time visualization of myocardial and valvular function. Transthoracic echocardiography is usually performed first as it is readily available and least invasive, but it may be difficult to interpret immediately after surgery because mediastinal air often obscures acoustic access to the heart. Because of this limitation, transesophageal echocardiography is often the study of choice in the postoperative patient. Transesophageal echocardiography is more accurate than transthoracic echocardiographic imaging for identification of valvular vegetations and complications of endocarditis, diagnosis of aortic dissection, evaluation of mitral valve prostheses, and intraoperative evaluation of mitral valve repair. Transesophageal echocardiography is also used to identify left atrial thrombus as a potential cardiac source of emboli and to exclude thrombus before elective cardioversion for atrial fibrillation. In the intensive care setting, transesophageal echocardiography has been used to determine the cause of unexplained hypotension and is particularly helpful after cardiac surgery in patients who are at increased risk for ischemia, hypovolemia, and pericardial tamponade; it may be useful to help optimize ventricular function and volume status.

Hemodynamic assessment by left- and right-sided heart catheterization may occasionally be required as an adjunct to echocardiography. Cardiac chamber pressures as well as transvalvular gradients are directly measured; valve surface area may be calculated by the Gorlin formula. Ventricular function can be directly evaluated with ventriculography, and coronary anatomy may be defined if there is evidence of postoperative ischemia. In patients who have lateral and posterior wall motion abnormalities after mitral valve surgery, a cardiac catheterization may be required to evaluate the circumflex coronary artery, as it runs parallel with the mitral orifice and may be injured during mitral valve surgery.

MANAGEMENT

Despite meticulous adherence to the principles of myocardial protection, perioperative myocardial damage related to ischemia-reperfusion injury may occur after cardiac operations that have been performed in an otherwise technically adequate manner. Recovery after surgically induced ischemia involves the resumption of normal oxidative metabolism, the restoration of myocardial energy reserves, and the repair of the ischemia-induced cellular changes. As myocardial recovery takes time, postoperative care should consist of supportive measures until this period resolves. Many surgeons advocate the use of a flow-directed pulmonary artery catheter for measurement and therapeutic manipulation of both the cardiac output and the central filling pressures. A cardiac index of at least 2.0 L/min/m^2 during the immediate postoperative period is required for normal recovery, and lower cardiac outputs have been shown to correlate with worse outcomes. At the tissue level, lower cardiac output leads to decreased end-organ perfusion and is manifested as a persistent lactic acidosis. Inotropic agents are often required for a short duration as myocardial function recovers. In the setting of severe myocardial dysfunction with evidence of end-organ ischemia, a balloon pump may be required. Pulmonary artery wedge pressure and central venous pressure can be measured and used as surrogates for left and right ventricular volume. Low central venous pressures can be treated with volume administration. Following valve replacement, afterload may be elevated in 10% of patients postoperatively and is shown by an elevated systemic vascular resistance. In this setting, afterload reduction may be beneficial, although the degree to which hemodynamic improvement can be obtained with afterload reduction is difficult to predict. Nitroglycerin, esmolol, and nitroprusside are the most commonly used agents in the immediate postoperative period. The control of postoperative heart rate and rhythm is important, and prudence dictates that temporary epicardial pacing leads be placed on the right atrium and ventricle in the event that pacing becomes necessary. In all valve replacement patients, optimal cardiac output often depends on appropriate atrial function leading to complete ventricular filling, higher cardiac output, and better tissue perfusion. Changes in heart rhythm after cardiac surgery are common and usually temporary, allowing early treatment with externally placed epicardial pacing wires. Patients with mitral valve disease are more likely than are patients with aortic valve disease to be in preoperative atrial fibrillation. Chronic atrial fibrillation is unlikely to revert to sinus rhythm postoperatively without a concomitant maze procedure. Atrioventricular conduction pathways are particularly at risk during mitral valve surgery, and conduction abnormalities may be seen in patients who would otherwise be in sinus rhythm. Infrequently, a permanent pacemaker may be required if symptoms persist.

The hemodynamic management of postoperative valve replacement patients has been described in a clear and concise manner.[2] Several general principles can be applied to patients with specific valve disease. Patients with aortic stenosis who have undergone valve replacement have hypertrophied, noncompliant left ventricles. As a result, most postoperative problems are related to inadequate preload. Adequate volume loading and judicious use of positive inotropic agents are required to achieve optimal cardiac output and end-organ perfusion. In addition, a low preoperative cardiac output may result in vasoconstriction that persists postoperatively. These patients are prone to persistent hypertension, and judicious afterload reduction is important to optimize peripheral perfusion. Aortic valve replacement rarely results in conduction abnormalities. Patients who have had surgery for mitral stenosis tend to have normal left ventricular compliance and are not prone to the same left ventricular dysfunction as are patients with aortic stenosis. However, these patients frequently have elevated pulmonary artery pressures and chronically pressure- and volume-overloaded right ventricles. Chronic pulmonary hypertension may not be immediately reversible after mitral valve replacement. These patients are at risk for right ventricular failure during the perioperative period. Treatment of pulmonary hypertension and isolated right-sided heart failure is not dissimilar to the management of a low cardiac output state and left ventricular failure. The preload as measured by central venous pressure may need to be increased to more than 20 mm Hg. β-Adrenergic agonists may be helpful at lower doses. At higher doses, they may further increase pulmonary artery pressure and worsen right-sided heart failure. Milrinone is beneficial for its inotropic effect as well as reduction of pulmonary vascular resistance. Targeted therapy for pulmonary hypertension includes prostacyclin-derived medications and nitric oxide. Inhaled prostacyclin is an excellent pulmonary vasodilator and is more easily administered than nitric oxide, and a transition may be made to sildenafil for use in the outpatient setting.

Other early problems encountered postoperatively include cardiac tamponade, bleeding, and poor ventricular function. Patients with low cardiac output and equivalent central venous and pulmonary artery pressure who experience a sudden drop in mediastinal tube output have tamponade until proven otherwise. If there is any question about the diagnosis, echocardiography is often useful and shows local hematoma compressing the right or left atrium. If the patient is stable, cardiac tamponade may occasionally be treated by manual evacuation of clots from the mediastinal tubes. If the patient is unstable or if evacuation is not immediately effective, the tamponade must be treated surgically with operative exploration. In all patients, there will be some degree of postoperative bleeding. Patients who have excessive bleeding are treated by correction of hypothermia and replacement of required clotting factors. Blood bank products required in the postoperative state may include fresh frozen plasma, cryoprecipitate, and platelets. If the patient is in renal failure before surgery, desmopressin is used to treat uremia-associated platelet dysfunction. If these interventions fail to control bleeding and the patient is warm with normal coagulation profiles and the surgeon's suspicion does not favor a surgically correctable source of bleeding, recombinant factor VII may be used. Historically, a surgical cause of bleeding must be entertained in a setting of normothermia and corrected coagulation parameters when mediastinal drainage tube output is more than 500 to 600 mL for 1 hour or 200 mL/h for 4 hours. In this setting, surgical exploration is most often indicated.

Poor intraoperative cardiac protection may result in decreased myocardial contractility in the immediate postoperative period. Although uncommon, this should be considered in patients with normal prosthetic valve function and who had normal preoperative ventricular function. Poor cardiac protection should be rare with the proper use of anterograde and retrograde cardioplegia, but when it occurs, it can be disastrous. The administration of inotropic medications is the first line of therapy, but temporary mechanical support (intra-aortic balloon pump, ventricular assist device) may be required in these patients while ventricular function recovers.

PROGNOSIS

Despite the advances in cardiac surgery, the results of surgical therapy for aortic and mitral valve replacement have not changed dramatically during the last quarter century. Many research efforts have attempted to identify specific patient cohorts and risk factors that will alter outcome for those patients requiring prosthetic valve replacement. For aortic valve replacement, the 30-day mortality has been reported between 2% and 5%. Mortality is increased to 6% to 15% by a prior median sternotomy, increased to 6% by the addition of concurrent coronary artery bypass grafting, and increased to 10% by the addition of mitral valve replacement. The most common complications after aortic valve operation include stroke in 1% to 2%, mediastinal bleeding requiring reoperation in 5% to 11%, wound infection in 1% to 2%, heart block requiring pacemaker placement in less than 1%, and renal failure requiring dialysis in 0.7%.[3]

The pathophysiology of mitral valve disease and the surgical options for treatment are complex and are explored in other chapters. The 30-day operative mortality with mitral valve replacement ranges from 4% to 7%.[4] The increased effort to preserve ventriculoannular continuity is the major factor associated with preservation of postoperative ventricular function and improved operative outcomes. In a review of the Society of Thoracic Surgeons database of 14,000 patients undergoing mitral valve replacement, the operative mortality was 6.4%. Predictors of operative mortality include age, urgency of the operation, renal failure, functional classification, requirement for reoperative surgery, and history of previous myocardial infarction with decreased cardiac function.[5]

The 10-year survival is 73.2% after aortic valve replacement with a mechanical prosthesis and 74.1% after replacement with a bioprosthetic valve. The 10-year survival after mitral valve replacement is 74.1% and 77.9% with respect to mechanical and bioprosthetic valves. The 10-year reoperation rate after bioprosthetic aortic valve replacement is 35.4%, whereas it is 21.3% after bioprosthetic replacement in the mitral position. Major bleeding and thromboembolic events are more common after mechanical mitral valve replacement.[6]

ANTICOAGULATION

CLINICAL PRESENTATION

The American College of Cardiology with the American Heart Association and the American College of Chest Physicians have published recommendations for the management of anticoagulation in valve replacement patients.[7,8] Whereas anticoagulation is undertaken at the discretion of the practitioner and must be tailored to the circumstances of the individual patient, it is an important adjunct for any patient undergoing valve replacement surgery. According to the guidelines, all patients undergoing valve replacement should be anticoagulated initially. The duration and intensity of anticoagulation then depend on the type of valve used, the length of time implanted, and the location of placement. The risk of thromboembolic events is greatest early after prosthetic valve insertion. As a result, many surgeons advocate the concomitant use of heparin and warfarin in the immediate postoperative period until a therapeutic international normalized ratio (INR) is reached. The need for heparin is controversial, and its benefit must be weighed against the risk of postoperative bleeding. As a result, the use of heparin varies widely and must be individualized. It has been our practice to begin heparin in patients with mechanical valves within 48 hours after surgery. The first dose of warfarin is administered the evening of the first postoperative day. The heparin is continued with the partial thromboplastin time maintained in the range of 60 to 80 seconds until the INR is near therapeutic values. Early anticoagulation is particularly critical for patients receiving a mechanical mitral valve and in those with identified risk factors for thromboembolic events. These additional risk factors include atrial fibrillation, history of previous thromboembolism, left ventricular dysfunction, and hypercoagulable conditions. At our institution, patients receiving a biologic prosthesis are treated with aspirin and warfarin and are not given heparin unless an additional risk factor is present. Patients who have had a mitral valve repair are treated in the same fashion. For those who have an increased risk of bleeding in the postoperative period, aspirin may be used solely after replacement with a biologic valve or after mitral valve repair.

As part of long-term health maintenance surveillance in valve replacement patients, physical examination should look for signs of valve dysfunction and complications related to chronic anticoagulation. New murmurs found during auscultation of the chest should be evaluated echocardiographically. An often asymptomatic complication of subtherapeutic anticoagulation is nonobstructive valve thrombosis. This is most commonly diagnosed when routine echocardiography is performed in the postoperative period.[9] Patients who are noncompliant with their anticoagulation medication may rarely present with catastrophic acute valvular thrombosis and symptoms of heart failure, syncope, and dyspnea. More often, they present after an arterial embolism from thrombus present on a valve leaflet with the constellation of symptoms predicted by the lack of circulation to the affected arterial bed (brain, mesentery, extremities). Alternatively, patients who present with neurologic changes and a supratherapeutic INR should be evaluated for a hemorrhagic stroke. Some patients may present with complaints of chronic fatigue, dyspnea on exertion, and melanotic stools and be found to have chronic anemia on their hematologic profile. On physical examination, they will have pallor of the skin; on rectal examination, they may have heme-positive stools. Any evidence of chronic anemia should be evaluated; likely sources are gastrointestinal bleeding and hemolysis.

DIAGNOSTIC TECHNIQUES

Patients suspected of having a thromboembolic event are initially evaluated with a thorough history and physical examination. Laboratory evaluation includes a hematologic and coagulation profile. For patients who have a history of previous thromboembolism or deep venous thrombosis, work-up for a hypercoagulable state is also completed. Echocardiography is performed to look for leaflet and flow abnormalities, to assess the presence of a transvalvular gradient, and to look for a thrombus attached to the prosthetic valve or within the cardiac chambers. Although transesophageal echocardiography is more sensitive in detecting partial valvular thrombosis and subtle changes in valve hemodynamics, transthoracic echocardiography remains the initial diagnostic tool for the detection of valvular thrombosis. In the setting of mitral valve replacement with a mechanical valve, transesophageal echocardiography is usually necessary, as acoustic shadowing from the prosthesis prevents complete evaluation of the left atrium. Evaluation of leaflet motion is also impaired in this position by transthoracic echocardiography.[10,11] The role of fluoroscopy as a first-line diagnostic tool has declined since the introduction of transesophageal echocardiography. A prerequisite for performance of a fluoroscopic study is the presence of a radiopaque prosthesis.[12] Fluoroscopy is currently used as an adjunct to transesophageal echocardiography when the diagnosis of subclinical valvular dysfunction is suspected but is unable to be confirmed.[13]

The initial management of the postsurgical valve replacement patient who presents with neurologic changes is illustrated in Figure 100.1. Patients with a neurologic deficit are promptly evaluated with computed tomography of the

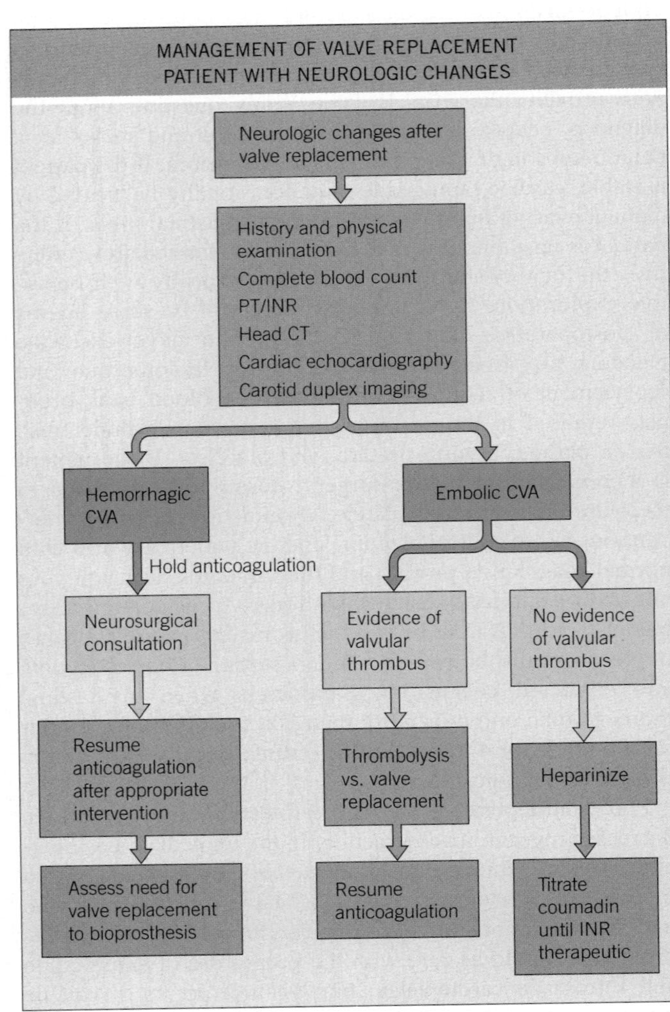

Figure 100.1 Algorithm for the management of the valve replacement patient with neurologic changes. CVA, cerebrovascular accident; INR, international normalized ratio; PT, prothrombin time. CT, computed tomography.

head. If there is evidence of an ischemic infarct, additional evaluation includes carotid duplex imaging and echocardiography to look for the source of embolism. If valve thrombosis is identified, either the patient is immediately heparinized with thrombolysis or valve replacement is performed. If the computed tomogram shows evidence of a hemorrhagic cerebrovascular accident, a neurosurgical consultation is obtained and anticoagulation is reversed until the INR is normal.

Patients who present with anemia or gastrointestinal bleeding should be evaluated for the source of blood loss. A stool guaiac test is done, and the patient is further examined with upper and lower endoscopy. Patients with a gastrointestinal source of bleeding not localized with endoscopy are further evaluated with a tagged red blood cell scan. Bleeding is rarely brisk enough to be localized with arteriography. In the setting of anemia not associated with blood loss, hemolysis should be suspected. This is particularly true in patients with mechanical valves. Laboratory profile would show an elevated lactate dehydrogenase level and a decreased haptoglobin level. A liver profile may show a conjugated hyperbilirubinemia. These patients have a higher incidence of pigmented gallstones.

MANAGEMENT

Anticoagulation management is determined by the type of prosthesis (mechanical or biologic), the position of implantation (aortic or mitral), and the presence of risk factors associated with thromboembolic complications. These risk factors include atrial fibrillation or thrombus, previous thromboembolism, and hypercoagulable state. Many would also include patients with severe left ventricular dysfunction, defined by an ejection fraction of less than 30%, in the higher risk group.

All patients with mechanical valves require warfarin therapy, with anticoagulation usually begun in the early postoperative period. We begin intravenous administration of heparin within the first 48 hours after surgery. The first dose of warfarin is administered the evening of the first or second postoperative day. Heparin use may be optional in the mechanical aortic valve patient, with warfarin therapy alone adequate. It has been our practice, however, to administer heparin to all patients with mechanical valves while the INR becomes therapeutic. The warfarin dose is titrated to maintain the INR between 2.5 and 3.5 for patients with mechanical mitral prostheses. In patients with a mechanical prosthesis of an older type (Starr-Edwards or mechanical disk valves, other than Medtronic-Hall prostheses) in the aortic position, the INR should be maintained between 2.5 and 3.5. In patients who do not have any risk factors for thromboembolism and who have undergone aortic valve replacement with a bileaflet mechanical valve or a Medtronic-Hall valve, warfarin therapy is indicated to achieve an INR of 2.0 to 3.0. In the subset of patients who have associated risk factors for thromboembolism, warfarin is indicated to achieve an INR of 2.5 to 3.5.[7,8]

At this time, the consensus opinion on which cardiovascular surgeons anticoagulate their patients after valve replacement with a biologic prosthesis is ambiguous. Although the current American College of Cardiology/American Heart Association guidelines state that the omission of warfarin therapy does slightly increase the early thromboembolic event rate, there are data to support withholding of anticoagulation.[14] At this time, all current national and international guidelines support the use of warfarin for 3 months after bioprosthetic valve replacement in the mitral position. In contrast, patients who receive bioprosthetic valves in the aortic position without identified risk factors for thromboembolic complications are routinely treated with antiplatelet therapy alone. A CTSNet survey with 726 respondents in 2004 found that 60% of surgeons did not routinely anticoagulate their patients after bioprosthetic aortic valve replacement. In this survey, 60% of surgeons thought that warfarin was no longer the standard of care.[15] A similar study performed in the United Kingdom found that 53% of surgeons never use warfarin after bioprosthetic aortic valve replacement and 33% do not anticoagulate tissue valve replacements.[16]

According to the published guidelines, all patients with a valve replacement, regardless of anatomic location or prosthetic valve type, should receive lifelong aspirin therapy of 75 to 100 mg/day. This is especially true in patients who have associated risk factors for thromboembolism. In high-risk patients with prosthetic heart valves in whom aspirin cannot be used, a growing population of literature supports the use of daily clopidogrel (75 mg/day) or increased warfarin therapy to achieve an INR of 3.5 to 4.5.[7,8] Recent trials evaluating the need for antiplatelet therapy after bioprosthetic aortic valve replacement in patients without thromboembolic risk factors showed that the addition of postoperative aspirin therapy conferred no advantage compared with no antiplatelet therapy.[17] At this time, opinion about the type and use of an antiplatelet agent is equivocal, with further investigation needed.

Despite adequate anticoagulation, valvular thrombosis will occasionally develop. Our management of patients with prosthetic valve thrombosis is initially based on the burden of thrombus and the patient's hemodynamic status. Patients whose prosthetic valve dysfunction is a result of pannus ingrowth must be distinguished from those with clot formation. Often, this can be a diagnostic dilemma best deciphered with echocardiography. If pannus formation is determined to be the cause of valvular obstruction, a second valve replacement is often required. Valve obstruction secondary to pannus formation is addressed later in this chapter. Patients who present with thrombosis and are hemodynamically stable may undergo attempted thrombolysis. Thrombolytic therapy, specifically recombinant tissue plasminogen activator, when it is used to treat stable patients with acute valvular thrombosis, has been shown to restore normal prosthetic valve function in approximately 80%.[18,19] Thrombolysis has also been shown to be superior to heparin treatment in patients with nonobstructive valve thrombosis.[9] If it is successful, anticoagulation is resumed, with increased frequency of anticoagulation and echocardiographic surveillance. If the patient is hemodynamically challenged or attempted thrombolysis is unsuccessful, surgical treatment is pursued. At the time of exploration, either operative thrombectomy or valve replacement is performed. We attempt to salvage the thrombosed valve if possible; however, when the valve is thought to be unstable or deteriorated, valve replacement is necessary. An algorithm for the evaluation and management of

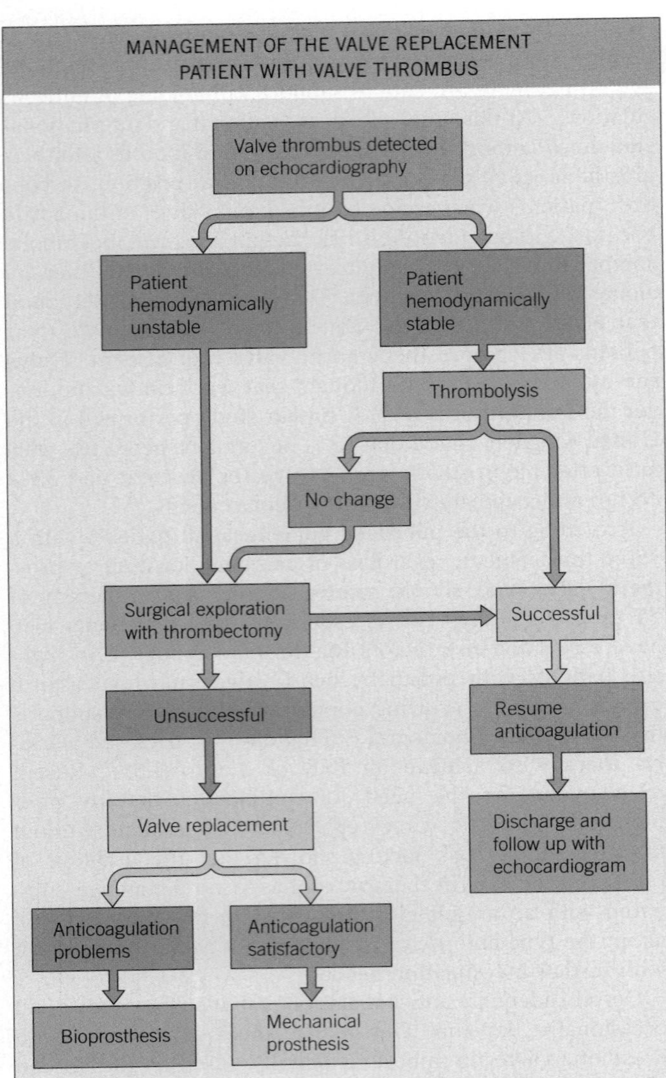

Figure 100.2 Algorithm for the management of the valve replacement patient with valve thrombus. (Modified from Cohn L, Doty D, McElvein R. Decision Making in Cardiothoracic Surgery. St. Louis, Decker/Mosby–Year Book, 1993.)

patients with valvular thrombosis as previously described is summarized in Figure 100.2.[20] Medication noncompliance may result in thromboembolic complications. If this is found to be the case, warfarin is resumed to the previous goal INR without additional increase required. In some cases, thromboemboli may be due to a hypercoagulable state. Patients who are hypercoagulable should have warfarin adjusted to maintain an INR of 3.0 to 4.0. In extreme circumstances in which anticoagulation is difficult to maintain or valve thrombosis is detected despite maintenance of an elevated INR, surgical replacement of the initial mechanical valve with a bioprosthetic valve may be indicated.

Patients with bleeding complications due to excessive anticoagulation are first stabilized with appropriate transfusions and cessation of anticoagulation therapy. After appropriate therapy for the hemorrhagic complication, these patients are restarted on heparin, and warfarin is carefully titrated until the INR is therapeutic. Often, patients with hemorrhagic complications are found to have a high INR that could be due to dietary changes or interactions with other medications. These patients should be counseled about appropriate diet and medicine interactions and should have an increased frequency of INR evaluation while warfarin is restarted. When patients present with a hemorrhagic cerebrovascular accident, anticoagulation is reversed and held until adequate evaluation and treatment of the neurologic event can be performed. After appropriate intervention, heparin and warfarin are restarted unless there is a contraindication to this therapy. If there is a high risk for recurrent hemorrhagic events, the patient is evaluated for a reoperation with implantation of a bioprosthesis.

Patients with valvular prostheses may require noncardiac invasive procedures. The key issue is to minimize the risk of thromboembolism while anticoagulation is held, minimizing the risk of procedure-related bleeding. Most surgical operations can safely be performed with an INR of 1.5 or less, which may be achieved by withholding of warfarin for 4 days. Neurosurgical operations are an exception and usually require a nearly normal INR to be performed safely. If warfarin is withheld for 4 days before an invasive procedure and is resumed soon after, the duration of time in which a patient's clot-forming ability is normal is brief.

Concerns are frequently raised about a "rebound" hypercoagulable state after warfarin therapy is restarted. Surgical procedures may cause hemostatic changes that may increase the risk of thromboembolism. Although this effect has been well documented with regard to venous thromboembolism, there is no evidence that surgery increases the risk of embolism in patients with prosthetic heart valves. The average rate of major thromboembolism in patients with mechanical heart valves who are not given anticoagulant therapy is estimated at 8% per year.[21] Anticoagulation reduces this rate by about 75%.[22] As a result, the risk of a significant thromboembolic event during a 4-day window of subtherapeutic INR levels is 0.09%. This risk may be lowered by use of intravenous heparin to decrease the duration of the subtherapeutic window. This may be appropriate in patients with additional risk factors or in whom the risk of bleeding is low. This risk must be weighed against the 11% reported risk of postprocedural bleeding in patients treated with intravenous heparin for 5 days after major surgery.[23] Patients with mechanical valves do not demonstrate a clear preoperative or postoperative benefit with the use of the traditional heparin window, and clinical thoughtfulness is required. A subset of patients who would be candidates for perioperative heparinization includes those with significant additional risk factors, such as a recent embolic event or a history of thromboembolism. In cases in which there is high risk for a thromboembolic event, preoperative heparin may be warranted, but the postoperative administration of heparin should still be approached with trepidation.

PROGNOSIS

The risk of thromboembolic complications is most prevalent in the first month after valve replacement. Meticulous management of anticoagulation is imperative during this critical time. In general, the risks of thromboembolic and hemorrhagic events in patients receiving anticoagulation therapy are 0.6% and 1.6% per year, respectively.[22] Almost all studies have shown that the risk of thromboembolism is greatest with a mechanical mitral valve prosthesis. The incidence of thromboembolic events in patients with mechanical valves and adequate anticoagulation ranged from 0.5% to 3% per patient-year; bleeding complications related to the anticoagulation therapy ranged from 0.7% to 6.3% per patient-year.[24] Patients with bioprosthetic valves, whether porcine or pericardial, have a long-term risk for thromboemboli of 0.2% to 3.3% per year.[25] The incidence of thromboembolism for bioprosthetic valves in the aortic position is 0.2% to 1.3% per patient-year; it increases to 1.5% to 2.0% for mechanical valves.[2]

Once a bleeding or thrombotic complication occurs, patients must be observed closely for recurrent episodes. Repeated episodes of bleeding in a patient with a mechanical valve and appropriate warfarin therapy may be an indication for valve replacement with a biologic valve.

ENDOCARDITIS

CLINICAL PRESENTATION

The postsurgical valve disease patient can present with endocarditis at any time. In most large series, the incidence of prosthetic valve endocarditis is reported between 2% and 4%.[26] By definition, early valvular endocarditis presents within 60 days postoperatively. Early prosthetic valve endocarditis results from contamination either during the operation or in the immediate postoperative period; the usual pathogens are *Staphylococcus epidermidis*, diphtheroids, fungi, and gram-negative bacteria. Risk factors identified for patients undergoing prosthetic valve replacement include initial valve replacement for native valve endocarditis, black race, male gender, and prolonged cardiopulmonary bypass time.[27]

Late prosthetic valve endocarditis occurs more than 60 days postoperatively and is believed to arise either from infection acquired after the perioperative period or from insidious infection acquired during the operation that has remained clinically quiescent. Late valve endocarditis occurring more than 1 year after valve replacement has been associated with sources of contamination including dental procedures, surgical procedures, gastrointestinal endoscopy, de novo infections, and drug abuse. The pathogens associated with late valvular endocarditis include streptococci, enterococci, and *Staphylococcus aureus; S. epidermidis* infection portends the best prognosis.

Prosthetic valve endocarditis, particularly early prosthetic valve endocarditis, may be difficult to diagnose. Fever is the most common clinical finding and is virtually always present.[28] However, in the postoperative period, there are many potential sources of fever, making this a nonspecific finding. Another physical finding is a new regurgitant murmur, frequently caused by valve dehiscence. Splenomegaly is present in 25% of early and 44% of late prosthetic valve endocarditis patients.[29] Other physical signs that are classically associated with native valve endocarditis, such as petechiae, Roth's spots, Osler's nodes, and Janeway's lesions, are found only rarely with prosthetic valve endocarditis. Patients with late valve endocarditis often have a more insidious course and may present with a fever of unknown origin. Cardiac conduction abnormalities are common in patients with endocarditis and have been associated with 47% of patients who present with prosthetic valve endocarditis.[30] A conduction aberration strongly suggests the formation of a paravalvular abscess and has been associated with a twofold higher mortality rate.[31]

Endocarditis of a prosthetic aortic valve can cause left-sided heart failure as a result of stenotic disease; endocarditis of a prosthetic mitral valve can cause pulmonary hypertension and right ventricular overload if the infection results in a mitral stenosis. Overall, the incidence of prosthetic valve endocarditis is remarkably low, and one recent review of patients with prosthetic aortic valves revealed that only 3.7% of these patients developed prosthetic valve endocarditis during their postoperative course. The risk for development of prosthetic valve endocarditis is 0.5% per patient-year for mechanical mitral valves versus 1.0% per patient-year for other types of valvular replacement.[32]

DIAGNOSTIC TECHNIQUES

When postsurgical valve replacement patients are febrile during the postoperative period, they are evaluated in the standard manner, including a thorough physical examination with attention paid to all surgical incisions and indwelling catheter sites. It is important to examine the extremities for evidence of thrombophlebitis. Chest radiography is performed, and urine, sputum, and indwelling catheter culture specimens are obtained to rule out a potential source of infection.

Initial evaluation for suspected prosthetic valve endocarditis includes blood cultures and echocardiography, which should be performed on all patients. Patients with positive blood cultures and an identifiable source of infection are treated with microbe-specific antibiotic therapy. Patients with persistently positive blood cultures, positive cultures without an identifiable source, or untoward septic decompensation require evaluation with echocardiography to rule out valvular abnormalities. Echocardiographic features consistent with prosthetic valve endocarditis include vegetations of the valve, a paravalvular leak, and a paravalvular abscess. Transthoracic echocardiography is readily available, but the image quality is operator dependent. Sonographic windows may be obscured by lung parenchyma, chest wall deformities, and pericardial adipose tissue. For prosthetic valve endocarditis, transthoracic echocardiography has been shown to be 50% sensitive and 90% specific.[33] In contrast, transesophageal echocardiography is nearly 100% sensitive and specific, making this the diagnostic modality of choice for prosthetic valve endocarditis. It is particularly valuable in visualization of a paravalvular abscess or an intracardiac fistula as a result of the infection.

If the patient is an operative candidate, coronary angiography is usually limited to patients older than 40 years or patients who have symptoms of coronary insufficiency. Preoperative computed tomography of the head cannot be overemphasized in the unconscious or focally impaired patient. Liberal use of abdominal computed tomography is encouraged to identify embolic abscesses to abdominal organs, such as the spleen or liver, because these infections potentially may reinfect the newly replaced valve.

MANAGEMENT

Prosthetic valve endocarditis is one of the most devastating complications of valve replacement and demands an aggressive management strategy and optimal timing of surgical reoperation. The decision to reoperate is complex and influenced by the valve involved, the extent of infection, the organism involved, and the confounding comorbidities of the patient. Timing of surgery is affected by the same factors and the patient's concurrent clinical course. Several series have reported a mortality rate of 60% in the medical treatment of prosthetic valve endocarditis.[34,35] Historically, prosthetic valve endocarditis has been considered an indication for surgery, but some patients may be able to be treated with medical management alone.

Patients in whom endocarditis develops early are likely to have had valve infection intraoperatively (from native valve endocarditis) or in the immediate perioperative period. When they are diagnosed with prosthetic valve endocarditis, patients should initially be treated with culture-specific antibiotics. Patients with streptococcal prosthetic valve endocarditis without evidence of significant left-sided heart failure, without echocardiographic evidence of annular abscess or pedunculated vegetations larger than 1 cm, and in whom blood cultures are aseptic within 72 hours may be managed with antibiotics alone. This is particularly true if the involved valve is an infected bioprosthesis. Initially, these patients need weekly surveillance echocardiography to identify early extension of the disease process. Dedication to a prolonged course of medical treatment in the clinical status of deterioration is ill advised.

Surgery is indicated in patients with life-threatening congestive heart failure or cardiogenic shock due to surgically treatable valvular heart disease if the patient has a reasonable prospect of recovery with satisfactory quality of life. Surgery should not be delayed once the patient has been clinically stabilized in the setting of congestive heart failure. Surgery is not indicated if complications or comorbid conditions make the prospect of recovery remote.

Surgery for prosthetic valve endocarditis in patients with stable hemodynamics is less clear. When antibiotic therapy is unsuccessful and infection persists, patients are evaluated for valve replacement. In addition, patients with endocarditis secondary to *S. aureus,* gram-negative organisms, or fungal species have little chance of sterilization with medical therapy. In this setting, we proceed early to surgical débridement and replacement of the infected valve.

The mortality rates associated with the surgical treatment of prosthetic valve endocarditis have fallen during the past decade. Perhaps the most important contribution to improved outcomes is an understanding of the need to radically excise infected cardiac tissue and the ability of surgeons to reconstruct it. Surgical modalities used for the treatment of prosthetic valve endocarditis depend on the severity and extent of the infectious process. The preoperative assessment of the extent of endocarditis helps in planning the operation, but the ultimate surgical procedure depends on the intraoperative findings. The patient is maintained with appropriate antimicrobial therapy through the surgical intervention and postoperative period. The pathologic manifestations of prosthetic valve endocarditis are manifold, and the most commonly involved area is the valve seat. This can cause abscess formation and extension into the adjacent cardiac structures, often resulting in paravalvular leak, dehiscence, conduction abnormalities, intracardiac fistula formation, or mycotic aneurysms.[36] Depending on the operative findings and the extent of infection, some patients can be treated with débridement of the infectious process and valve replacement with another prosthetic valve. Patients noted to have more extensive involvement of the aortic root need valvular replacement with reconstruction of the involved aorta. The valvular prosthesis used for replacement in situations of prosthetic valve endocarditis is a subject of debate. We tend to use homografts whenever possible. For patients with extensive aortic root abscesses, we favor an aortic homograft with reimplantation of the coronary ostia because aortic homografts are remarkable for their resistance to reinfection. In addition, the extra tissue that comes with an aortic homograft is useful for repair of defects caused by abscess formation or by débridement of infected structures. Series reports have shown the resistance of homografts to reinfection.[37] Options for replacement of an infected mitral valve are more limited. At this time, we do not recommend replacement of an infected mitral prosthesis with a homograft. We débride all infected tissue, reconstruct the annulus with autologous or bovine pericardium, and implant a new mechanical or biologic valve.[38]

Invasive procedures involving the respiratory tract, oropharynx, gastrointestinal tract, and genitourinary system may cause transient bacteremia that can seed prosthetic valves and result in prosthetic valve endocarditis. Guidelines for appropriate antimicrobial prophylaxis have been published.[39] A simplified algorithm for the evaluation and treatment of prosthetic valve endocarditis is illustrated in Figure 100.3.

PROGNOSIS

Approximately 10% of endocarditis cases occur in patients with prosthetic valves. Although most cases of prosthetic valve endocarditis involve the aortic valve, all prosthetic valves are susceptible. Patients who present with prosthetic valve endocarditis require expeditious diagnosis and management because of the prohibitively high mortality rate with delayed treatment. With a delay in care, the outcomes of prosthetic valve endocarditis are worse than those of native valve endocarditis.[40]

Not only is prosthetic valve endocarditis associated with higher operative mortality, it also adversely affects long-term survival relative to native valve endocarditis. Whereas the mortality in published series has varied, a recent large-center study reported the operative mortality for prosthetic valve endocarditis to be 18%.[41] In a report from the United Kingdom Heart Valve Registry on 322 cases of prosthetic valve endocarditis, the 30-day mortality was 20% and the 5- and 10-year survivals were 55% and 37%, respectively.[42] Investigators from the Cleveland Clinic reported an operative mortality of 13% among 146 patients with prosthetic valve endocarditis; among those who survived surgery, the 5-year survival was 82%.[43] In another report from the same institution on prosthetic aortic valve endocarditis treated exclusively with aortic valve homograft, the operative

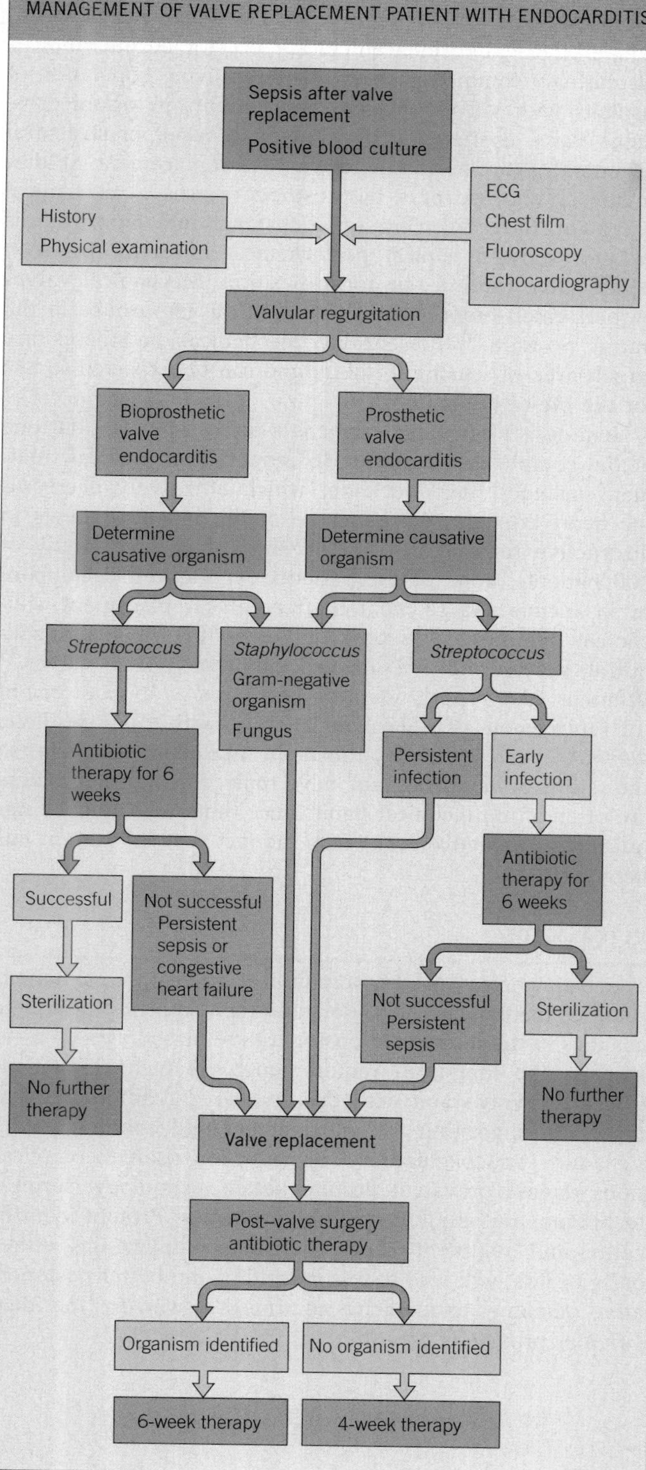

Figure 100.3 Management of valve replacement patient with endocarditis. (Modified from Cohn L, Doty D, McElvein R. Decision Making in Cardiothoracic Surgery. St. Louis, Decker/Mosby–Year Book, 1993.)

mortality was only 3.9% and the 5- and 10-year survivals were 73% and 56%, respectively.[44]

The main reason that the operative mortality for prosthetic valve endocarditis is higher than that for native valve endocarditis is the complexity of the operation and the fact that it is often associated with paravalvular abscess. Resection of aortic root abscess is indeed a complex operation, but resection of mitral annulus abscess can be even worse. Although aortic valve homografts are believed to be the best valve for aortic root abscess, they are not a substitute for radical débridement and implantation of the new valve in healthy tissue. Persistent or early recurrent endocarditis is probably related more to the surgeon's recognition of and ability to extirpate all infected tissues than to the type of valve used for replacement.[45] Resection of an abscess in the mitral valve annulus is a formidable operative procedure associated with high operative mortality, but we believe that it is the only way to eradicate the infection and to provide satisfactory long-term results.[46] Throughout this decade, in-hospital mortality for patients with prosthetic valve endocarditis has decreased from 20% to 10%.[26] The improved results that have been achieved in the surgical treatment of prosthetic valve endocarditis are partially a result of aggressive débridement of perivalvular abscesses and improved techniques of annular reconstruction with autologous or homologous tissue.[45]

OTHER PROBLEMS: VALVULAR OBSTRUCTION, DEGENERATION, AND HEMOLYSIS

CLINICAL PRESENTATION

Postsurgical valve disease patients can present with disorders related to the functional and physiologic deterioration of the prosthetic valve, including orifice obstruction secondary to pannus formation, leaflet degeneration of tissue valves, and hemolysis. The duration of time from the initial operation to clinically relevant valve-related dysfunction may be years, leading to initial diagnostic uncertainty.

Patients with a biologic prosthesis are prone to development of leaflet calcification. The thickened, immobile leaflets cause decreased outflow surface area and may be a nidus for calcific embolism. From the repetitive wear of the cardiac cycle, the tissue-preserved bioprosthetic leaflets are also prone to degeneratation.[47]

Pannus ingrowth from the surrounding paravalvular tissue results in an obstructive pathologic process and is seen in both bioprosthetic and mechanical prosthetic valves. Patients who present with symptoms of heart failure, abnormal or additional heart sounds, changing physical examination findings, or differing electrocardiographic features should be evaluated for prosthetic valve dysfunction. All patients with prosthetic valves, particularly those with bioprostheses, should be monitored for signs of valve leaflet degeneration with echocardiography. Patients who present with chronic anemia and no evidence of gastrointestinal bleeding should be evaluated for hemolysis.

DIAGNOSTIC TECHNIQUES

Patients who have undergone valve replacement should be evaluated by a cardiologist yearly. All patients with new symptoms of heart failure, dyspnea on exertion, and shortness of breath should undergo chest radiography and transthoracic echocardiography. Transesophageal echocardiography is reserved for situations in which transthoracic echocardiographic findings are ambiguous. In the rare situation in which the transesophageal echocardiographic data are also equivocal, we selectively use angiography to aid in the diagnostic process. Mechanical valve leaflet motion can be evaluated with fluoroscopy if a frozen leaflet is suspected and is not able to be visualized on echocardiography.

Diagnosis of pannus formation is best done with echocardiography. Patients suspected of having prosthetic valve–induced hemolysis are evaluated with serum haptoglobin and lactate dehydrogenase levels in addition to echocardiography. These patients have decreased haptoglobin levels and elevated lactate dehydrogenase levels secondary to red blood cell destruction. Echocardiography will often show a paravalvular leak, with regurgitant jets causing turbulent flow of blood elements that collide with the valve annulus, leading to hemolysis.

MANAGEMENT

In the evaluation of patients with prosthetic valve obstruction, an important distinction to be made is whether the obstruction is secondary to pannus ingrowth or thrombus formation. In contrast to patients with pannus ingrowth, patients with thrombus formation usually present earlier in the postoperative course and often have a shorter duration of symptoms.[11] Depending on the degree of symptoms, treatment varies from a strategy of increased anticoagulation to emergent valvular replacement. For patients with obstruction secondary to pannus formation, surgical therapy includes either pannus débridement or valve replacement. The exact mechanism of pannus formation is unknown, but most consider it to be long-term, chronic inflammation. Large series document complications secondary to pannus formation at 2.4%; identifiable risk factors are the use of a mechanical valve with a small orifice surface area, the use of a tilting disk valve, and the presence of a region of turbulent flow near the prosthetic valve annulus.[48]

The choice of the appropriate prosthesis at the initial surgery has long-term implications in minimizing complications related to prosthetic valve degeneration. Elderly patients with limited survival and patients with contraindications to anticoagulation are thought to be best treated with a biologic prosthesis, although no long-term increase in survival has been identified.[49] Elderly patients without contraindications to anticoagulation may be good candidates for mechanical prostheses in this era of improved patient survival and thus avoid the need for reoperation from valvular degeneration. Reoperative valve replacement surgery for degeneration is increasingly common, in view of the growing population of patients with valve replacements. Patients in whom prosthetic valve dysfunction develops as a result of structural degeneration are evaluated for valve re-replacement. Studies reviewing the use of a bioprosthetic versus a mechanical valve for re-replacement of a dysfunctional bioprosthesis did not show a clinical performance difference between either valve type in the aortic position. Mechanical valves outperformed bioprosthetic valves in all age groups in the mitral position.[50] Present-day mechanical prostheses are largely free of structural failure and can be expected to last for the life of the patient.

Hemolysis after valve repair is a rare occurrence but one of the complications leading to reoperation. Medical treatment includes beta blockade, which effectively decreases the heart rate and the exposure of the blood elements to destructive regurgitant forces.[51] In a prospective study of 300 patients, none of the patients experienced decompensated anemia. At 12 months after valve replacement, subclinical hemolysis was detected in 26% of patients with mitral valves and 5% of patients with aortic valves.[39] Whereas case reports identify hemolysis as a requirement for replacement of a mechanical valve with a bioprosthetic valve, in our experience, this is an infrequent necessity. In the setting of hemolysis and valve replacement, other factors are often of more clinical significance (hemodynamically significant paravalvular leak) than the fact that the patient has hemolysis.

SUMMARY

The management of the postsurgical valve disease patient requires the clinician to understand the complex physiologic changes in the immediate postoperative period as well as to manage the long-term requirements. As technology continues to evolve and with the diversity of different valve types, the algorithm for management will continue to be dynamic. Anticoagulation- and infection-related complications remain prevalent despite better technology, surgical technique, and modern imaging modalities. Prompt identification and treatment of postoperative complications, either early or late, will lead to less morbidity and better postoperative outcomes as medicine continues to wait for the ideal valvular prosthesis.[1,52]

chapter 101

Special Problems in the Surgically Treated Valve Disease Patient

a. How to Treat Perivalvular Leaks

Sandro Betocchi, Maria Angela Losi, and Massimo Chiariello

DEFINITION OF PROBLEM

Perivalvular leak indicates a regurgitation between the ring of a prosthesis and the native valvular annulus. Although perivalvular leaks may have an asymptomatic course and remain hemodynamically stable for a long time, the recognition of such a condition alerts surgeons and cardiologists (as the condition may be rapidly progressive) and leads to early redo operation. Symptoms of decreased cardiac output, such as fatigue, are usually present in patients with a large perivalvular leak. The flow disturbance caused by the prosthetic regurgitant lesion and the resultant increase in shear stress may produce clinical hemolysis. Moreover, patients who contract endocarditis in prosthetic heart valves are at high risk for development of perivalvular leak.

It is important to know how to recognize and to treat this condition so that irreversible heart or organ dysfunction is prevented, but redo operation is not necessarily proposed in all types of periprosthetic lesions.

TYPICAL CASES

Case 1

A 25-year-old man developed fatigue and a new systolic murmur 3 years after mitral valve replacement with a Starr-Edwards prosthesis for severe calcified mitral stenosis. At admission, the patient presented with a mild elevation in body temperature in the evening for the previous 3 weeks, but this had been overlooked by the patient. White blood cell count was increased. The hematocrit value was low, and there was evidence of elevated levels of lactate dehydrogenase and bilirubin as well as of hemoglobinuria.

The patient started antibiotic therapy. Transthoracic echocardiography was performed; this revealed prosthetic regurgitation. Subsequently, transesophageal echocardiography showed a perivalvular leak with severe regurgitation (Fig. 101A.1).

Case 2

A 50-year-old woman developed a systolic murmur in the early postoperative period after mitral valve replacement with a St. Jude valve for bioprosthesis malfunction. Transesophageal echocardiography was pivotal in establishing the diagnosis of perivalvular leakage; regurgitation appeared to be mild (Fig. 101A.2). The patient had no evidence of endocarditis or hemolysis.

DIFFERENTIAL DIAGNOSIS

In a patient with one or more prosthetic valves, prosthesis malfunction may be suggested by

- a new murmur;
- deterioration in the clinical condition;
- embolic episodes; or
- hemolysis.

Prosthesis malfunction may stem from intraprosthetic or extraprosthetic problems. Intraprosthetic malfunction includes defect of the ball or disk movement and structural degeneration. In the majority of patients with bioprostheses, the cause of malfunction is degeneration of the leaflets, leading to valve stenosis, regurgitation, and hemolysis. Prosthesis malfunction may be due to endocarditis, thrombus, or pannus formation. Each of these complications can be misdiagnosed as perivalvular leak.

Endocarditis

Endocarditis has been reported in 3% to 6% of patients with prosthetic heart valves. The incidence of this complication peaks at 5 weeks after surgery and reaches a plateau at 9 months. This condition carries a very high mortality rate, particularly in patients who have early endocarditis (i.e., during the first 60 days after heart surgery). Endocarditis may result in malfunction of bioprostheses due to leaflet infection and of mechanical prostheses due to defects in ball or disk movements caused by the presence of vegetations. Late endocarditis is the major cause of perivalvular dehiscence at late follow-up. Diagnosis can be reached by careful interrogation of patients (asking about, for example, fever and previous dental or genitourinary procedures known to be associated with a high risk for endocarditis) and the usual laboratory tests; these, however, may have little diagnostic value if they are performed long after the beginning of infection. Transthoracic and transesophageal echocardiography permit diagnosis (see Fig. 101A.1).

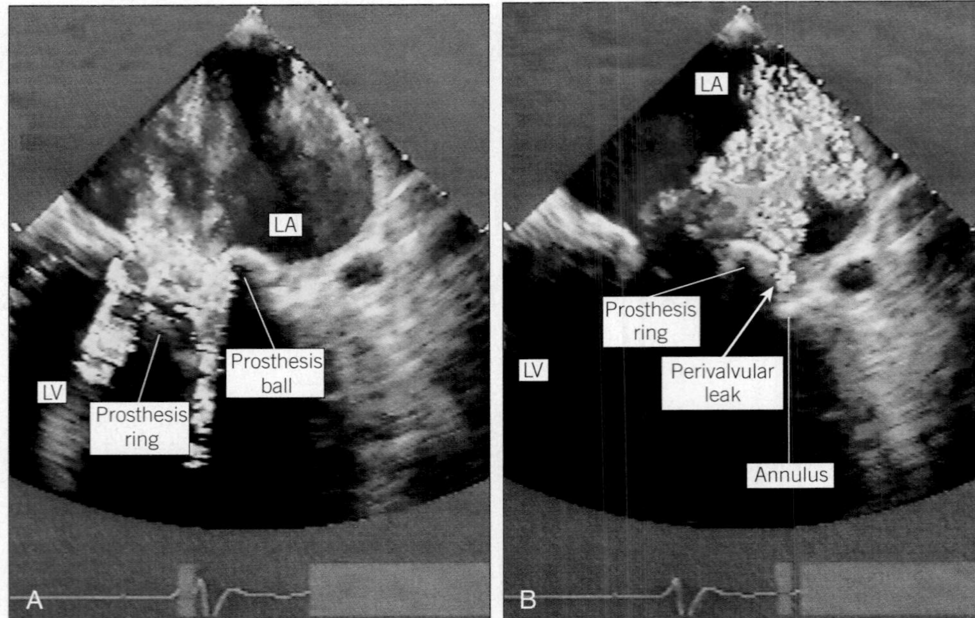

Figure 101A.1 Severe perivalvular leak. Transesophageal color Doppler echocardiographic images of the two-chamber view (90 degrees) in a patient with a Starr-Edwards valve in the mitral position. **A,** Image in diastole. Notice the filling flow around the ball. **B,** Image in systole. Notice the severe regurgitation going from the left ventricle (LV) into the left atrium (LA) between the prosthesis ring and the annulus; this is the perivalvular leak.

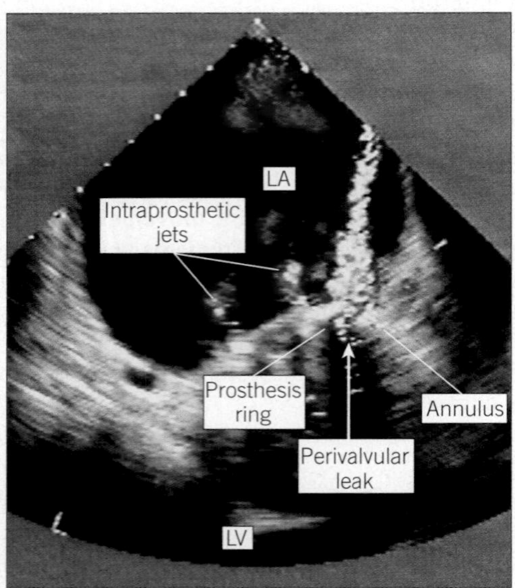

Figure 101A.2 Mild perivalvular leak. Transesophageal color Doppler echocardiographic image of the two-chamber view (90 degrees) during systole in a patient with a St. Jude valve in the mitral position. There are small, intraprosthetic, regurgitant jets (normal phenomenon). There is also mild regurgitation going from the left ventricle (LV) into the left atrium (LA) between the prosthesis ring and the annulus; this is the perivalvular leak.

Prosthetic Obstruction

The incidence of prosthetic valve obstruction has been estimated at 0.1% to 4% per year; in the majority of cases, it depends on thrombus formation resulting from inadequate anticoagulation. In almost 20% of patients, prosthetic obstruction is caused by pannus formation, either in isolation or in combination with thrombus. The onset of symptoms may be insidious or, more commonly, abrupt, presenting with cardiovascular collapse. In some cases, prosthetic thrombus causes an embolic event; rarely, it is totally asymptomatic, and in such cases it is occasionally detected by echocardiography. Thrombosis may induce prosthetic regurgitation because of lack of closure of prosthetic elements; this leads to an erroneous diagnosis of perivalvular leak. The decreased or absent opening or closing sounds help in the differential diagnosis. Transthoracic echocardiography shows increased transprosthetic pressure gradients. Transesophageal echocardiography usually clarifies the cause of malfunction.

Prosthetic Degeneration

Structural prosthetic degeneration or strut failure, resulting in stenosis or regurgitation, can occur in the early and late postoperative periods, although degeneration is uncommon during the first decade after implantation of mechanical valves. Ball degeneration in Starr-Edwards prostheses was common in models manufactured before 1965. In patients who have a new murmur and who had a ball-cage prosthesis implanted at least 20 years earlier, ball degeneration, so-called ball variance, should be suspected. In contrast, degeneration of the occluding disk in tilting prostheses is uncommon. So many cases of strut fracture have been reported in Bjork-Shiley convexo-concave valves, which were introduced in 1978, that the valve was withdrawn from the market in 1987. However, there are still almost 41,000 patients carrying these valves worldwide, and they may present with acute pulmonary edema, syncope, shock, neurologic deficits, or embolic episodes; these symptoms should suggest a strut prosthetic failure. High-resolution cineradiography is helpful for early diagnosis of strut failure.

Hemolysis

Hemolysis is frequent in patients with mechanical prostheses. Traumatic red blood cell destruction is revealed by a low hematocrit and an increased level of lactate dehydrogenase. Serious hemolysis may induce jaundice and hemoglobinuria and is therefore easily detected clinically, whereas compensated significant hemolysis is not, resulting in long-term complications such as renal hemosiderosis, cardiomyopathy, and gallstones.

Several mechanisms may contribute to the development of hemolytic anemia with normal and malfunctioning prosthetic valves, including shear stress, turbulence, pressure fluctuations, intrinsic abnormalities of the erythrocyte membrane, and interaction with foreign surfaces. Perivalvular leaks may induce hemolysis not only because of the flow disturbance in the regurgitation jet but also because of the exposure of the prosthetic ring surface. In fact, perivalvular leak is the major cause of hemolysis, which occurs in almost 40% of patients with this complication. However, hemolysis can be found even in patients with normally functioning prostheses. In patients with first-generation ball-cage prostheses, the incidence of hemolysis has been reported at between 6% and 15%; with the introduction of tilting disk valves and bioprostheses, the incidence of hemolysis in normally functioning valves has been significantly reduced, although it has not disappeared. Thus, although hemolysis does not always indicate the presence of perivalvular leak, its detection should prompt the physician to clarify the underlying cause.

Echocardiography

Perivalvular leak may be diagnosed noninvasively by echocardiography. Transthoracic echocardiography is the first diagnostic approach; for mitral prostheses, however, transthoracic echocardiography shows prosthetic regurgitation but does not allow identification of the type and extent of regurgitation owing to acoustic shadowing in the left atrium created by nonbiologic material. Because the esophagus lies adjacent to the posterior left atrium, with transesophageal echocardiography, the acoustic shadowing phenomenon is created in the left ventricle, leading to good visualization of the mitral prosthesis. For aortic prostheses, transthoracic echocardiography allows quantification of regurgitation, but transesophageal echocardiography is needed to identify its site of origin. Thus, transesophageal echocardiography is always necessary when a perivalvular leak is suspected.

TREATMENT OPTIONS

In patients with perivalvular leak, severe regurgitation or severe hemolysis warrants a redo operation (Fig. 101A.3). Because the most powerful predictor of survival in a redo operation is the New York Heart Association functional class, it is very important that surgery be performed before the patient deteriorates to class IV. In patients with endocarditis, surgery must be performed promptly (see Fig. 101A.3).

The patient described in case 1 underwent an urgent redo operation. Intraoperatively, vegetations were found on the mitral annulus that had not been seen by transesophageal echocardiography (see Fig. 101A.1). Unfortunately, the patient died in the early postoperative period because of refractory heart failure.

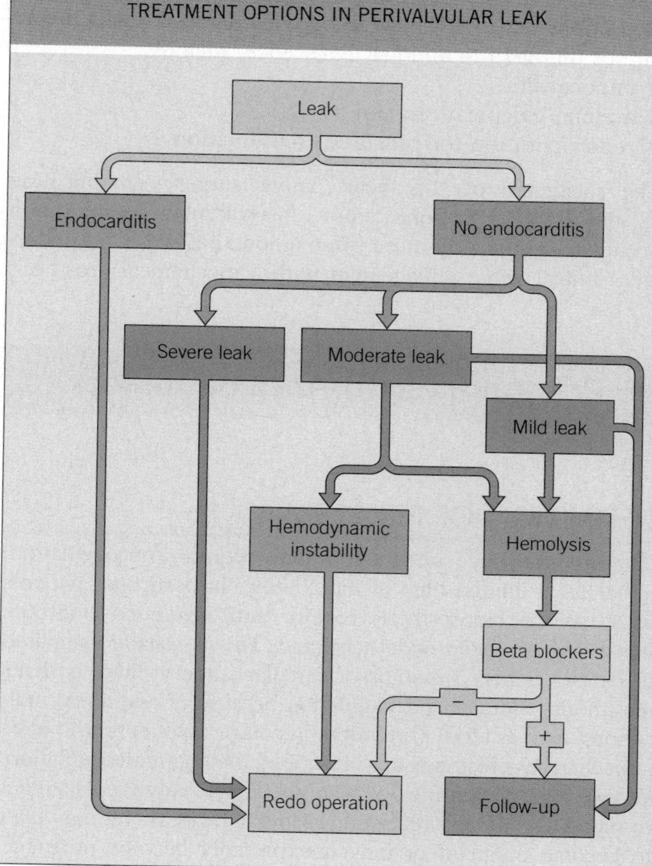

Figure 101A.3 Treatment options in perivalvular leak. + indicates favorable response to treatment with beta blockers; − indicates unfavorable response to treatment with beta blockers.

In patients who are believed to be poor operative candidates, a transcatheter umbrella may be an alternative treatment. The procedure, performed in the catheterization laboratory, involves the use of a new clamshell double umbrella, which is positioned on the defect after a determination of its size by a balloon-tipped catheter inflated in the defect itself.

In patients with a normally functioning prosthesis and hemolysis, medical treatment with beta blockers such as propranolol has been proposed. Although the exact mechanism of this therapy on hemolysis is unclear, beta blockers are thought to reduce the shear stress between erythrocytes and the foreign material by slowing the velocity of the blood. It may be postulated that this treatment is useful even in patients who have a small perivalvular leak and hemolysis. If this therapy is not effective, the perivalvular leak has to be surgically corrected to avoid chronic complications of hemolysis (see Fig. 101A.3).

Patients who have evidence of a mild perivalvular leak (see Fig. 101A.2) in the absence of endocarditis or hemolysis, like the patient presented in case 2, do not need a redo operation and should only be followed up (see Fig. 101A.3). The patient described in case 2 was followed up every 6 months. Three years later, she was clinically stable and showed a degree of perivalvular leak similar to that previously detected.

SUMMARY

Conditions that predispose to perivalvular leak include conditions that lead to annular dehiscence, such as
- endocarditis;
- annular calcification; and
- redo operation for prosthesis malfunction.

The incidence of this heart valve surgery complication is almost 4%. In one study, perivalvular regurgitation occurred significantly more often among patients who underwent mitral valve replacement with a mechanical prosthesis than among those who received a bioprosthesis. Perivalvular leak may be the first indicator of endocarditis in the late postoperative period. Surgical strategies have been described for the prevention of early postoperative leak.

However, the persistence of this complication in the early and late postoperative periods suggests that the use of the stethoscope in patients with heart prostheses, by revealing a new prosthetic murmur suggestive of prosthesis malfunction, continues to have a pivotal role, despite the introduction of new sophisticated diagnostic tools.

b. Pregnancy and Anticoagulants

Sandro Betocchi, Maria Angela Losi, and Massimo Chiariello

DEFINITION OF PROBLEM

Patients who have prosthetic valves require anticoagulation, either for a limited time or indefinitely. In particular, patients who have a bioprosthesis require anticoagulation until the valve ring has been endothelialized. This is usually estimated to happen within 3 months of valvular surgery; these patients may require longer anticoagulation because of additional indications, such as atrial fibrillation. In contrast, patients who have a mechanical prosthesis are prescribed lifelong anticoagulation. Women of childbearing age who need heart valve replacement or who have already received prosthetic heart valves may plan to become pregnant or may unexpectedly become pregnant. Pregnancy in women who have prosthetic heart valves is considered by the American College of Cardiology/American Heart Association guidelines for the management of patients with valvular heart disease to be associated with a high maternal and fetal risk. Potential complications are related to

- increased blood volume and hemodynamic load, leading to heart failure; and
- hypercoagulable state of pregnancy, leading to increased incidence of thromboembolic events.

In addition, problems associated with fetal exposure to anticoagulants and other cardiovascular drugs that the mother may need are to be carefully weighed.

A cardiologist is often faced with the problems associated with pregnancy in a woman with a prosthetic heart valve who needs anticoagulation. Although most patients in New York Heart Association functional class I or class II who have a functioning prosthesis can tolerate the load of pregnancy, discontinuation of treatment with drugs that are potentially harmful to the fetus (except oral anticoagulants) should be considered. In problem cases, exercise testing before conception may be used to evaluate whether the increased cardiac load of pregnancy can be tolerated. Gestation should be discouraged in patients in New York Heart Association functional class III or class IV because the additional burden imposed by pregnancy could further impair hemodynamics and pose an increased risk of death for both mother and fetus. The approach to pregnancy in women who have a valvular prosthesis that requires anticoagulation is twofold and concerns the balance of problems posed to the mother and the fetus.

EFFECTS OF ANTICOAGULATION ON THE MOTHER

Valve Thrombosis

Warfarin derivatives are effective in preventing thromboembolic events during pregnancy in patients with mechanical valves. Several studies of oral anticoagulants have been carried out in pregnant women who have mechanical valve prostheses. Although the number of patients included in each of them is understandably small, the reported incidence of valve thrombosis is rather low, ranging from 0% to as much as 14%. When a high complication rate was found, inadequate anticoagulation was identified as a cause.

These findings outline the need for careful monitoring of coagulation indexes during pregnancy because dosages of oral anticoagulants that warranted a satisfactory degree of anticoagulation before pregnancy may no longer be effective owing to the increase in coagulation factors during pregnancy. In contrast, work from one group suggests that the coagulation state is not much affected by pregnancy; hence, the dosage of anticoagulant drugs may be predicted beforehand. However, widespread intersubject dosing differences of warfarin are well recognized. Variants in two genes (two in *CYP2C9,* one in *VKORC1*), together with age and weight, explain approximately half of this variability. Indeed, the U.S. Food and Drug Administration (FDA) recently revised the product label of warfarin to recognize the potential effect of genetic makeup on drug dosing. However, pharmacogenetic-guided dosing has not been adequately tested in prospective trials. A study of 206 patients being initiated on warfarin, randomized to pharmacogenetic-guided or standard dosing and observed for up to 3 months, showed that the pharmacogenetic-guided algorithm selected an initial dose more closely predictive of the stable maintenance dose, led to fewer and smaller dose adjustments, and required fewer international normalized ratio (INR) assessments. Despite this, percentage out-of-range INR, the primary endpoint, did not differ significantly between arms. In subset analyses, pharmacogenetic guidance seemed promising for patients without mutations in either of the two genes (who required greater than average doses) and those with mutations in both genes (who had much lower requirements). These findings are important for better design of future randomized trials.

The incidence of thromboembolic events in patients who have prosthetic heart valves and who are correctly treated with oral anticoagulants during pregnancy is probably similar to that in the nonpregnant population. However, the use of warfarin during pregnancy is associated with an increased risk of spontaneous abortion, fetal hemorrhage, and teratogenesis, especially when it is taken between weeks 6 and 12 of gestation, and the risk appears to be dose related. Thus, many studies have been undertaken to reduce the dosage and the time of exposure to warfarin derivatives during pregnancy. Heparin as a replacement anticoagulation therapy has been used because it does not cross the placenta owing to its large molecular size and because women with venous thrombosis who received heparin during pregnancy have shown normal fetal and neonatal outcome without an increase in maternal bleeding complications. Long-term treatment with heparin has been associated with osteoporosis; however, the reduction in bone density as a consequence of long-term heparin therapy during pregnancy is usually reversible, the risk of symptomatic fracture is small, and the overall duration of heparin administration is relatively short. The point that needs to be clarified about the use of heparin as an anticoagulant during pregnancy is whether it is effective in preventing prosthetic valve thrombosis; an additional issue is whether the intravenous administration route is mandatory or whether the more practical subcutaneous route can be safely used. A high incidence of valve thrombosis (up to 25%) has been reported in women treated with heparin for the first trimester or throughout pregnancy. This high incidence is probably the consequence of an inadequate therapeutic target of activated partial thromboplastin time (aPTT). A target aPTT of 1.5 times the control value appears to be associated with high rates of valve thrombosis and arterial embolism. There is evidence that the clinical efficacy of heparin is optimized if the anticoagulant effect is maintained above a defined minimal level; an aPTT ratio of two or three times the control value is probably an appropriate target. It is relevant, however, that two deaths due to prosthetic thrombosis have been reported in a population of 37 pregnant women despite the fact that they had strictly followed their heparin treatment with a target aPTT of 2.5 times the control level.

Low-molecular-weight heparin (LMWH) derivatives may represent an interesting alternative to subcutaneous heparin as they have a better clinical profile, such as the potential for once-daily administration and no need for anticoagulation monitoring. However, as the pregnancy progresses, the volume of distribution for LMWH will change. Thus, in pregnant women, it is necessary to measure plasma anti-Xa levels 4 to 6 hours after the monitoring dose and to adjust the dose of LMWH to achieve an anti-Xa level of approximately 0.7 to 1.2 units/mL. At present (March 2009), although the effectiveness of LMWH derivatives as a substitute for warfarin in the prevention of thrombosis and pulmonary thromboembolism during pregnancy has been established, their role in preventing valve thrombosis or thromboembolic events in patients with artificial valves has yet to be assessed. Although the number of physicians prescribing LMWH during pregnancy in women with artificial valves is increasing, treatment failures are continually reported in the literature. Moreover, FDA-approved labeling indicated specifically that use of LMWH has not been studied sufficiently for prevention of cardiac valve prosthesis thrombosis in pregnant women. Nevertheless, the American College of Cardiology/American Heart Association guidelines for the management of patients with valvular heart disease suggest that dose-adjusted subcutaneous LMWH can be used during the first and the last weeks of pregnancy. In contrast with this statement, in the same guidelines, LMWH is not recommended in patients with mechanical valves who require interruption of warfarin therapy, in whom unfractionated heparin is mandated. Thus, the inclusion of LMWH in the prevention of cardiac valve thrombosis during pregnancy is still, in our opinion, to be debated.

Additional confounding factors are that prostheses in the aortic position pose less thrombotic risk than those in the mitral position and that older mechanical valves, such as Starr-Edwards and Bjork-Shiley valves, are more thrombogenic than newer valves, such as Medtronic-Hall, St. Jude Medical, and CarboMedics valves.

Second-generation prosthetic valves require anticoagulation therapy with warfarin at a lower prothrombin INR value. In one study, patients were treated with warfarin during the first two trimesters of gestation and with heparin during the last trimester. The target INR while receiving warfarin was 2.0 to 2.5, whereas the target aPTT while receiving heparin was 1.5 to 2.5 times the control value. Although anticoagulation was found to be within the therapeutic range in only about 40% of patients, the incidence of thromboembolism was low. These data may indicate a lower likelihood of thromboembolic events during pregnancy in patients with newer generation prosthetic heart valves.

Aspirin has been suggested as an addition to warfarin to reduce the dosage of warfarin that is required and the risk of valve thrombosis in nonpregnant patients; this strategy yielded a reduction in mortality and systemic embolism, but at the expense of an increased risk of minor bleeding (but not major bleeding). To date, there are no data on the association between warfarin derivatives and aspirin during pregnancy. The use of dipyridamole to the same effect is not recommended because of high fetal loss demonstrated in one study.

Bleeding

The reported incidence of serious bleeding during pregnancy with long-term heparin therapy varies from 2% to 12%. Abnormal peripartum bleeding or hematoma formation at the site of cesarean delivery has been observed in 13% of women who were receiving heparin or warfarin at the time of delivery. These complications were reported as benign.

EFFECTS OF ANTICOAGULATION ON THE EMBRYO OR FETUS

Spontaneous Abortion

Several reports have shown that the use of warfarin derivatives during the first trimester of pregnancy results in an increased incidence of spontaneous abortion, ranging between 16% and 44%. A lower rate of abortion seems to occur in women who are treated with heparin during the first trimester and the last 2 weeks of pregnancy. An incidence of abortions of about 35% was seen in women who were treated with warfarin derivatives in the first trimester of gestation, and the abortion rate fell to less than 10% in women who were treated with intravenous heparin during the same period.

However, conflicting data exist. A spontaneous abortion rate between 40% and 50% was seen in patients treated with subcutaneous heparin during the first trimester of pregnancy. Because patients were receiving warfarin at the beginning of the pregnancy, it has been postulated that this drug may be the key factor in early abortion and thus that warfarin replacement before or immediately after conception might be the answer. This hypothesis has not been supported by data. One group suggests that a warfarin dosage of 5 mg or less throughout pregnancy is associated with a low risk of spontaneous abortion, and they claim that if a sufficient anticoagulation is achieved at such dosages, no further caution is needed.

The mechanism of abortion during anticoagulation is not yet clear. It may occur during effective anticoagulation with either warfarin or heparin, probably as a result of placental hemorrhage.

Stillbirth and Neonatal Deaths

The fetus is susceptible to the risk of hemorrhage because of several interrelated factors that are centered on fetal vitamin K metabolism. In normal midgestation fetuses, the level of vitamin K_1 is only 20% of that in adults. Even in subtherapeutic doses, warfarin reduces fetal vitamin K further, to the point at which normal hemostasis is jeopardized. This results in intraventricular cerebral hemorrhage and consequent stillbirth or neonatal death. Stillbirth may also be due to placental hemorrhage and extreme prematurity. The incidence of stillbirths and neonatal deaths is markedly reduced if the mother is switched to heparin shortly before delivery. These data suggest that warfarin should be avoided at least during the last 2 weeks of pregnancy. It has been suggested that for the safety of both mother and fetus, heparin should be administered intravenously to hospitalized patients to obtain a rapid and adequate anticoagulant effect.

Embryopathy

The use of warfarin derivatives during pregnancy has been associated with the so-called warfarin embryopathy and with central nervous system abnormalities. The syndrome includes nasal bone hypoplasia and epiphyseal stippling (chondrodysplasia punctata). The mechanism of the warfarin embryopathy is not completely understood. Probably, the placental gradient maintains the fetus in a vitamin K–deficient state. Because the vitamin K–dependent proteins are necessary for tyrosine kinase activity, which controls growth regulation, depletion of vitamin K–dependent proteins abolishes the required stimuli for normal embryogenesis. To date, there is convincing evidence that warfarin causes an embryopathy when it is administered between weeks 6 and 12 of gestation, although it has been suggested that a warfarin dosage of 5 mg or less is relatively safe.

The incidence of reported warfarin embryopathy varies enormously, from less than 5% to as much as 67%. The American College of Cardiology/American Heart Association guidelines for the management of patients with valvular heart disease suggest that 4% to 10% is a reasonable estimate of the incidence of warfarin embryopathy.

TREATMENT OPTIONS

Management of women of childbearing age in need of cardiac valve replacement poses myriad problems in terms of prosthetic valve selection, clinical evaluation of the patient to assess whether hemodynamics will allow her to bear a child with an acceptable risk, and if so, the anticoagulation strategy if anticoagulation is needed. At present, no guidelines can be given that allow pregnancy in women who have prosthetic heart valves without additional risk to the mother or the child. Because none of the options that a cardiologist can offer is completely safe, it is highly recommended that the woman and possibly her partner be made aware of all the possibilities of treatment and the associated risks.

At the Time of Valve Replacement

If the woman is already pregnant, every effort should be made to delay surgery until after the delivery or until a planned cesarean delivery can be performed (Fig. 101B.1). If the woman is not pregnant, she should be made aware that a mechanical valve prosthesis implies the lifelong need of anticoagulation and that no anticoagulant treatment is totally safe for both the mother and the child. Oral anticoagulants of the warfarin type are safer for the mother but are associated with embryopathy and a high risk of spontaneous abortion and stillbirth. Heparin poses a high risk of prosthetic valve thrombosis, which can be lethal and can occur even if the targeted anticoagulation has been reached. Both anticoagulant agents carry some risk of bleeding, especially at the time of delivery.

If the patient opts for a mechanical valve, new, less thrombogenic valves (e.g., Medtronic-Hall, St. Jude, or CarboMedics valve) should be used because they allow a lower target INR and lower warfarin dosage (which seems to carry lower

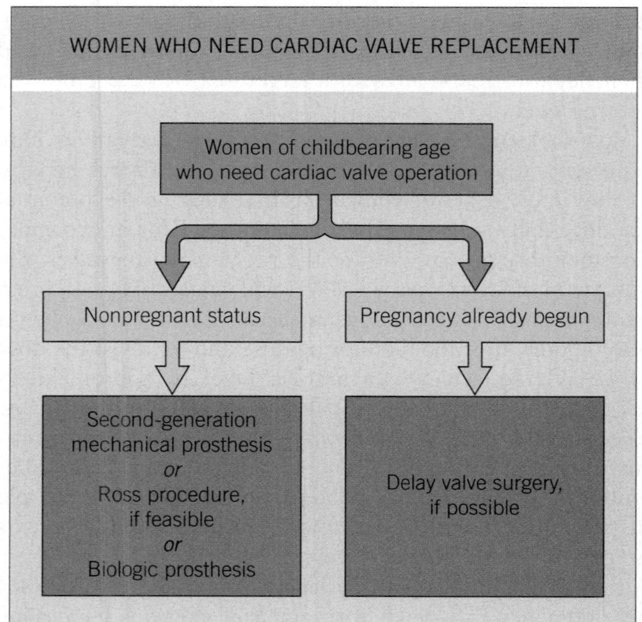

Figure 101B.1 Management of woman of childbearing age who need cardiac valve replacement.

risk to the fetus). Bioprostheses have the advantage of not requiring anticoagulation after the first 3 postsurgical months; their major disadvantage, however, is structural deterioration and shorter expected life span, more so for porcine than for pericardial prostheses. In addition, there is some evidence of an increased incidence of pregnancy-related bioprosthetic structural deterioration, which may require redo operation, during or soon after gestation. Therefore, biologic prostheses are not recommended for the general population younger than 50 years.

Women who plan to become pregnant after valve replacement, however, may consider the risks of receiving a mechanical valve too high and should be given the option of receiving a bioprosthesis, but they should be informed about the increased risk of bioprosthetic failure 6 to 8 years after implantation. If an isolated aortic valve replacement is needed, the Ross procedure (pulmonary autograft in the aortic position) could be offered as an option because it seems to have a better clinical profile than bioprostheses do. Because patients who have bioprostheses do not require anticoagulation unless they have additional indications or they have received the bioprosthesis within the previous 3 months, the following recommendations apply only to patients with mechanical valves.

Planned Pregnancy

After valve replacement, a woman and possibly her partner should be advised to plan pregnancies together with her cardiologist and her gynecologist and to take effective contraceptive measures at all other times (Fig. 101B.2). Patients with mechanical valves should be evaluated clinically and by echocardiography; if overt or subclinical heart failure or prosthetic valve malfunction is detected, pregnancy should be discouraged. The same applies to patients who must take drugs that are known to carry unwanted effects on the fetus (e.g., amiodarone, diuretics, calcium channel blocking agents). Because of the high risk when the fetus is exposed to warfarin from weeks 6 to 12 of gestation, the mother should be switched to heparin throughout the first trimester of pregnancy (see Fig. 101B.2). It has been hypothesized by Lee and colleagues (1986) that the use of warfarin increases the risk of abortion even before week 6 of gestation, and the use of heparin

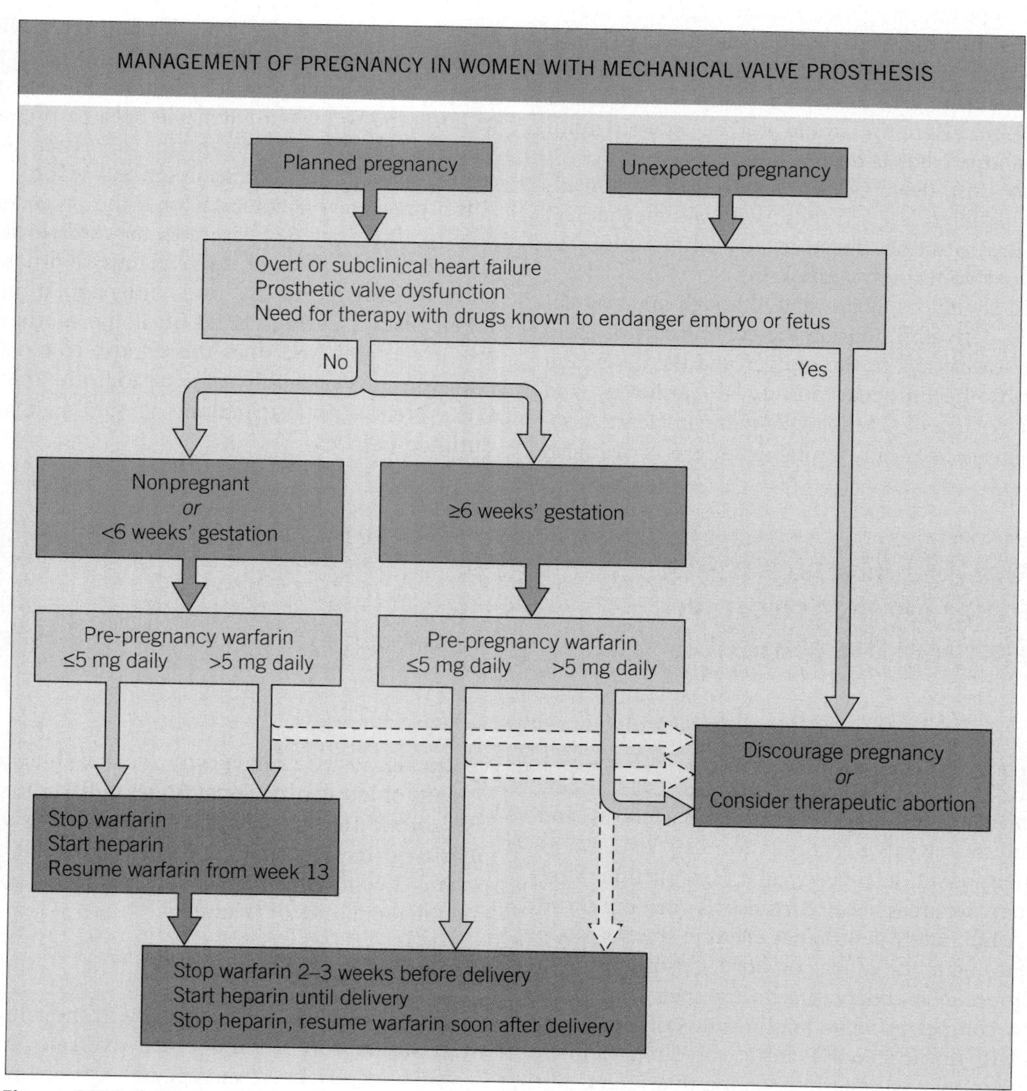

Figure 101B.2 Management of pregnancy in women with mechanical valve prosthesis.

before pregnancy and throughout the first trimester has been advocated. It has been suggested that the outcome of pregnancy is better with low warfarin dosage and that women taking 5 mg or less of warfarin daily before pregnancy can be reassured. Attractive as they are, these suggestions are hampered by the small number of patients and by the lack of a control group, and heparin still remains the safest treatment during the first trimester of pregnancy.

No further data on this topic exist. Because anticoagulation with heparin poses an increased risk of valve thrombosis, it is therefore reasonable to monitor signs of pregnancy carefully (such as frequent assessment of β-human chorionic gonadotropin levels) and to initiate treatment with heparin before week 6 and as soon as pregnancy is detected. Patients should be switched from warfarin to heparin while in the hospital so that aPTT can be carefully monitored and early signs of valve thrombosis can be detected. Heparin should be given subcutaneously twice a day, with a target aPTT (measured 6 hours after the last administration) of two to three times the baseline value. Dosage is usually 17,500 to 20,000 units every 12 hours. If LMWH is chosen, anti-Xa levels should be monitored at the same interval after administration, and levels of 0.7 to 1.2 units/mL should be sought.

After week 12 of gestation, patients should again be hospitalized to switch from heparin to warfarin (see Fig. 101B.2). Target INR will vary according to the type and position of the valve; it ranges from 2 to 3 to 3.5 if there is a high risk of thromboembolism. Heparin should not be stopped until an INR level of about 2 has been reached.

Addition of low-dose (80 mg daily) aspirin can be considered in high-risk patients (e.g., in those with old mechanical valves in the mitral position, those in atrial fibrillation, or those with a history of thromboembolism).

The cardiologist should be aware that although anticoagulation with warfarin derivatives during the central part of pregnancy carries the lowest risk to the mother and the fetus (and is recommended by the European Society of Cardiology and by the American College of Cardiology/American Heart Association), manufacturers explicitly prohibit the use of warfarin derivatives during pregnancy. This could pose legal problems if this point is not clarified to the mother, and possibly her partner or family relatives, and if written consent is not obtained.

In the final 2 or 3 weeks of gestation, patients should stop oral anticoagulants and initiate intravenous infusion of heparin while in the hospital. The target aPTT is two to three times the baseline value.

There is no evidence that a cesarean delivery has advantages over vaginal delivery, and therefore the option can be left to the mother. Heparin should be stopped at the onset of labor and resumed 6 to 12 hours after delivery. Oral anticoagulation should be resumed soon thereafter (see Fig. 101B.2). There appear to be no contraindications to breastfeeding because little warfarin is found in maternal milk.

Unexpected Pregnancy

A therapeutic abortion might be proposed to patients who have overt or subclinical heart failure or valve malfunction and to those who might not tolerate the hemodynamic burden of pregnancy or who might require a redo operation (see Fig. 101B.2). If a pregnancy is detected before week 6 of gestation, the woman should be made aware that the chance of a spontaneous abortion could be high (see Fig. 101B.2), especially at high warfarin dosages. In addition, she should receive the same kind of counseling as outlined before. Because the patient might not have been aware of the increased risks posed by anticoagulation to the embryo or fetus and to herself when she became pregnant, she might want to consider a therapeutic abortion. Anticoagulation strategy should proceed as described before.

If a pregnancy is detected (or if the pregnant woman seeks advice) after week 6 of gestation, the cardiologist should clearly state that the risks of spontaneous abortion and warfarin embryopathy posed by oral anticoagulation have already taken place (see Fig. 101B.2). If the mother considers the risk acceptable and does not choose to have a therapeutic abortion, it is probably safer to continue therapy with warfarin. Near delivery, patients should switch to heparin as outlined before.

c. Postoperative Management of Myocardial Dysfunction in Valvular Surgical Treatment

Sandro Betocchi, Maria Angela Losi, and Massimo Chiariello

DEFINITION OF PROBLEM

Patients who have aortic valve disease (both stenosis and regurgitation) and mitral valve regurgitation may experience temporary or permanent left ventricular dysfunction after valve replacement, whereas its occurrence is uncommon in mitral stenosis. A fall in left ventricular ejection fraction soon after valve replacement for mitral or aortic insufficiency is common and represents an adaptation to the increased afterload that the new competent valve imposes; it is often reversible. In patients with aortic stenosis, aortic valve replacement is followed by complex anatomic remodeling that affects left ventricular systolic and, mostly, diastolic function. If symptoms or signs of left ventricular systolic or diastolic dysfunction persist beyond the first few weeks after valve replacement, the physician may become concerned about the persistence and possible evolution of such dysfunction, its impact on prognosis, and the modalities of treatment.

TYPICAL CASE

A 48-year-old man with a history of shortness of breath and chest discomfort on moderate exercise for the previous 2 years experienced an episode of severe dizziness. On physical examination and on echocardiography, signs of predominant aortic stenosis with mild insufficiency were found. Owing to a poor acoustic window, echocardiography did not allow an estimate of left ventricular function and mass; equilibrium radionuclide angiography at rest showed a slightly reduced ejection fraction and a markedly abnormal peak filling rate (Fig. 101C.1). With exercise, a drop in ejection fraction by as much as 15 percentage points was seen (see Fig. 101C.1); this may be caused by severe coronary artery disease or by afterload mismatch resulting from aortic stenosis.

The patient underwent cardiac catheterization, which showed severe aortic stenosis (peak-to-peak gradient, 91 mm Hg) with increased left ventricular end-diastolic pressure (22 mm Hg) and pulmonary wedge pressure (mean, 17 mm Hg). Cardiac output was normal, and left ventricular volume was also normal at 88 mL/m^2. Coronary arteries were normal, whereas aortic angiography showed moderate valve regurgitation.

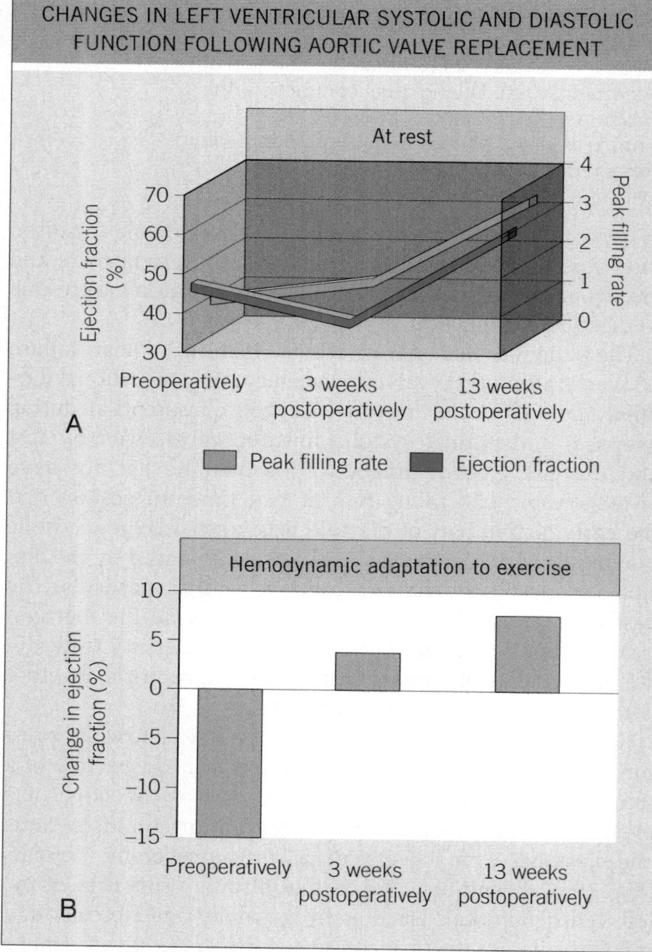

Figure 101C.1 Changes in left ventricular systolic and diastolic function following aortic valve replacement. A, Ejection fraction and peak filling rate as measured at rest by radionuclide angiography in the patient in the typical case who underwent aortic valve replacement for aortic stenosis. **B,** Exercise-induced changes in ejection fraction. Measurements were performed preoperatively, 3 weeks postoperatively, and 13 weeks postoperatively.

The patient underwent aortic valve replacement with a CarboMedics 23 prosthesis; his perioperative course was uneventful. He was discharged with warfarin, low-dose diuretics, and angiotensin-converting enzyme inhibitors, but he kept experiencing shortness of breath on moderate exercise. Therefore, 3 weeks after surgery, he was reevaluated. His resting ejection fraction was slightly lower than it had been preoperatively, but it rose with exercise by 4 percentage points (see Fig. 101C.1). Peak filling rate had increased but was still subnormal (see Fig. 101C.1).

Treatment was not changed and the patient was reevaluated at 13 weeks. At this time, he still complained of shortness of breath on moderate exercise and reported no substantial benefit from the operation in terms of exercise tolerance. His resting ejection fraction had strikingly risen by 23 percentage points and was within normal limits and further increased with exercise; peak filling rate had also increased remarkably and was normal (see Fig. 101C.1). Pulmonary vein Doppler echocardiography (Fig. 101C.2) showed increased velocity and duration of the reverse A pulmonary wave, which lasted longer than the mitral A wave. Left atrial fractional shortening (Fig. 101C.3) was also subnormal (14%; normal >16%). His maximum oxygen consumption during exercise was below normal (18 mL/kg per minute).

DIFFERENTIAL DIAGNOSIS

Left ventricular dysfunction after valve replacement carries a higher risk of early and late morbidity and mortality. Preoperative left ventricular dysfunction is the major predictor of the risk of having left ventricular dysfunction postoperatively. In a study of 257 patients who had preoperative subnormal left ventricular systolic function (ejection fraction of 40%) and who underwent valve replacement, an in-hospital mortality of 12.5% was found (19.4% for mitral valve replacement and 9.0% for aortic valve replacement). Perioperative mortality appears to be particularly elevated in patients with left ventricular dysfunction and low aortic valve gradients (<30 mm Hg) because low gradients may result from severe left ventricular dysfunction.

In another study, higher risk of early and late postoperative death was due independently to either systolic or diastolic dysfunction, and their association carried an additive risk. Symptoms of congestive heart failure are caused by isolated left ventricular diastolic dysfunction in about half of the patients with aortic stenosis; left ventricular hypertrophy affects both active relaxation and passive filling, and the increased fibrosis typically found in these patients alters distensibility. This highlights the need for identification of isolated diastolic dysfunction and for its diagnosis when it is associated with systolic dysfunction.

According to the guidelines of the European Study Group on Diastolic Heart Failure, the diagnosis of primary diastolic heart failure requires three obligatory conditions to be simultaneously satisfied:

- presence of signs or symptoms of congestive heart failure;
- presence of normal or only mildly abnormal left ventricular systolic function; and
- evidence of abnormal left ventricular relaxation, filling, diastolic distensibility, or diastolic stiffness.

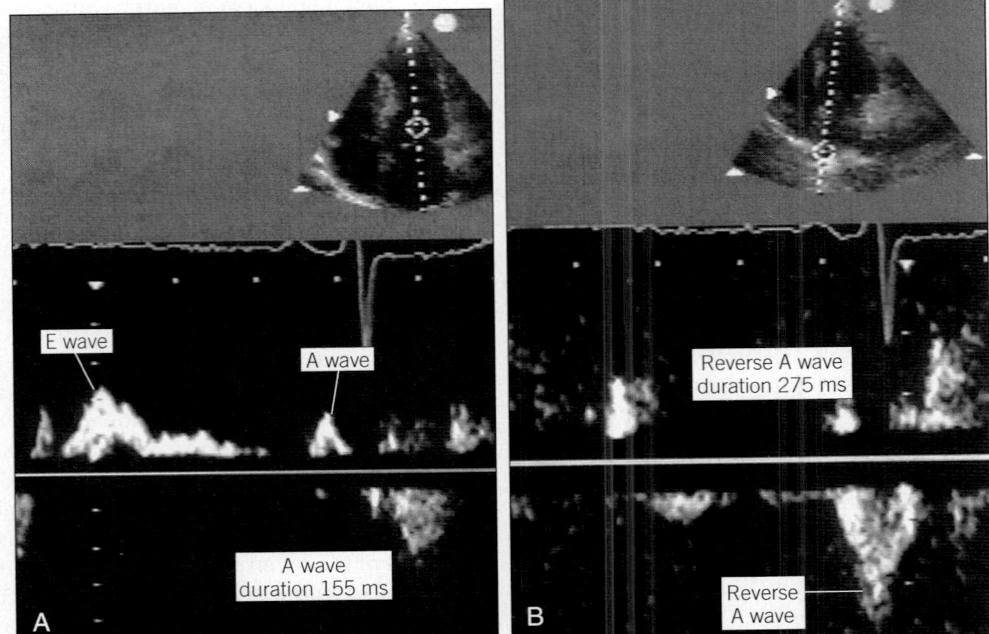

Figure 101C.2 Detection of altered left ventricular distensibility by Doppler echocardiography. Mitral inflow velocity **(A)** and pulmonary vein velocity **(B)** assessed by pulsed Doppler echocardiography. The duration of the A wave at the mitral level is much shorter than the duration of the reverse A wave at the pulmonary vein level (*thick horizontal lines*). During atrial contraction, the increase in left ventricular volume leads to a marked increase in left ventricular pressure, which exceeds the atrial pressure and further impedes left ventricular filling. As a consequence, retrograde flow into the pulmonary vein is increased. This indicates a reduced left ventricular distensibility.

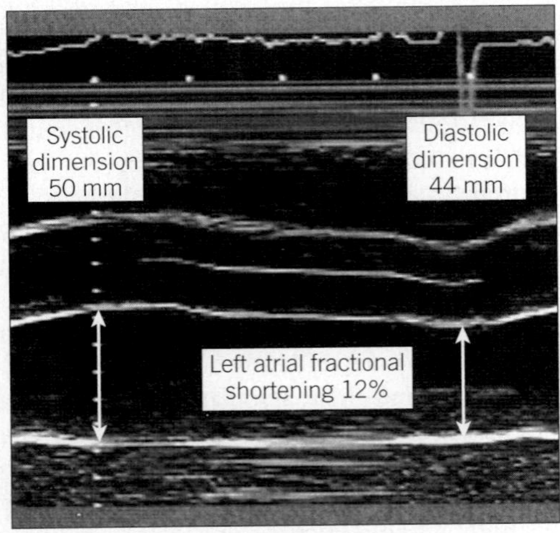

Figure 101C.3 Detection of altered left ventricular distensibility by M-mode echocardiography of the left atrium. During atrial emptying, left atrial dimension changes little, and hence the left atrial fractional shortening is reduced (normal value >16%). The increase in left ventricular pressure, which exceeds the atrial pressure, further impedes left atrial emptying. This indicates a reduced left ventricular distensibility.

An important issue has recently been raised that left ventricular systolic function has to be normal or mildly abnormal at the time of acute symptoms of congestive heart failure (such as pulmonary edema) for it to be positively concluded that such symptoms are due to isolated diastolic dysfunction. In fact, ischemia affecting a large portion of the left ventricle can cause left ventricular systolic dysfunction and symptoms of heart failure. If left ventricular systolic function is assessed after resolution of ischemia, it may be entirely normal, and one would be misled into thinking that symptoms were due to diastolic dysfunction.

The patient in this typical case had features of heart failure 13 weeks after aortic valve replacement (e.g., exertional dyspnea and subnormal maximal oxygen consumption during exercise) and normal systolic function as assessed by rest and exercise ejection fraction. However, he did not have an abnormal peak filling rate at that time, suggesting that the early, active part of diastole was normal. When systolic function is normal, exercise capacity is influenced by the diastolic properties of the left ventricle and, in particular, by passive distensibility; therefore, to understand the mechanisms of impaired exercise tolerance, it is necessary to evaluate passive diastolic properties of the left ventricle together with systolic function and early filling.

Reduced distensibility means that the left ventricular pressure-volume relationship is shifted upward, irrespective of a simultaneous change in stiffness. Stiffness is the slope of a pressure-volume curve obtained by plotting multiple static end-diastolic left ventricular pressure-volume points (Fig. 101C.4) and depends on the intrinsic properties of the left ventricular wall (such as hypertrophy and fibrosis) that influence its ability to increase volume for a given change in pressure.

Noninvasive assessment of stiffness is not possible, as diastolic left ventricular pressures cannot be measured noninvasively; only estimates of distensibility can be obtained. Decreased left ventricular end-diastolic distensibility can be inferred from a shortened Doppler mitral early filling wave

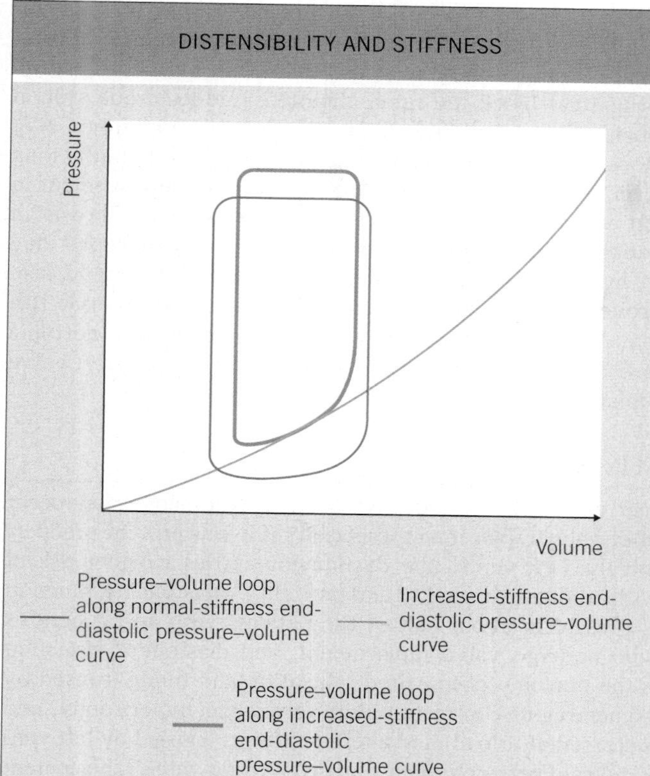

Figure 101C.4 Distensibility and stiffness. Pressure-volume loops along normal-stiffness and increased-stiffness end-diastolic pressure-volume curve. The red pressure-volume loop represents a loop at normal volume, whereas the green pressure-volume loop indicates the effect of volume load. The increase in volume is associated with a large increase in diastolic pressure. The pressure-volume loop along the normal-stiffness end-diastolic pressure-volume curve has the same diastolic pressure as the loop at high stiffness, but it accommodates a much larger volume.

(E) deceleration time or from a Doppler pulmonary vein flow tracing that shows reverse pulmonary venous atrial contraction (A) wave flow velocity of more than 350 mm/s or that exceeds in duration the mitral A wave. To understand these parameters, one has to keep in mind that a reduced left ventricular distensibility implies an impaired left atrial contraction, which results in an increased and prolonged retrograde flow toward the pulmonary veins and a shortened left ventricular filling during atrial contraction (a small increase in left ventricular volume caused by atrial emptying results in a large increase in end-diastolic pressure that exceeds left atrial pressure and interrupts filling). If the duration of pulmonary venous A wave exceeds the duration of mitral A wave by at least 30 ms, a left ventricular end-diastolic pressure of more than 15 mm Hg occurs with a sensitivity of 85% and a specificity of 79%.

An additional estimate of reduced distensibility is provided by the so-called restriction to inflow, a transmitral Doppler pattern consisting of an increased E/A ratio (more than 3.2) or a shortened E wave deceleration time (<140 ms). Although the presence of this pattern is very specific for a severely reduced distensibility, its sensitivity is low.

Another way of looking at distensibility is provided by an invasive study, in which the M-mode–derived left atrial fractional shortening yields a reliable estimate of left ventricular end-diastolic pressure. (Again, the decrease in left ventricular distensibility leads to an increase in end-diastolic pressure, which hampers left atrial emptying.) The patient in this example had Doppler and left atrial signs of reduced left ventricular distensibility (see Figs. 101C.2 and 101C.3).

TREATMENT OPTIONS

Diastolic dysfunction after aortic valve replacement for aortic stenosis is frequent and is the outcome of a complex rearrangement of the left ventricle. The reduction in intraventricular pressure leads to a decrease in left ventricular mass that begins soon after surgery, is significant after a few months, and becomes nearly normal by 1 to 2 years (Fig. 101C.5). The mass decrease is associated with favorable

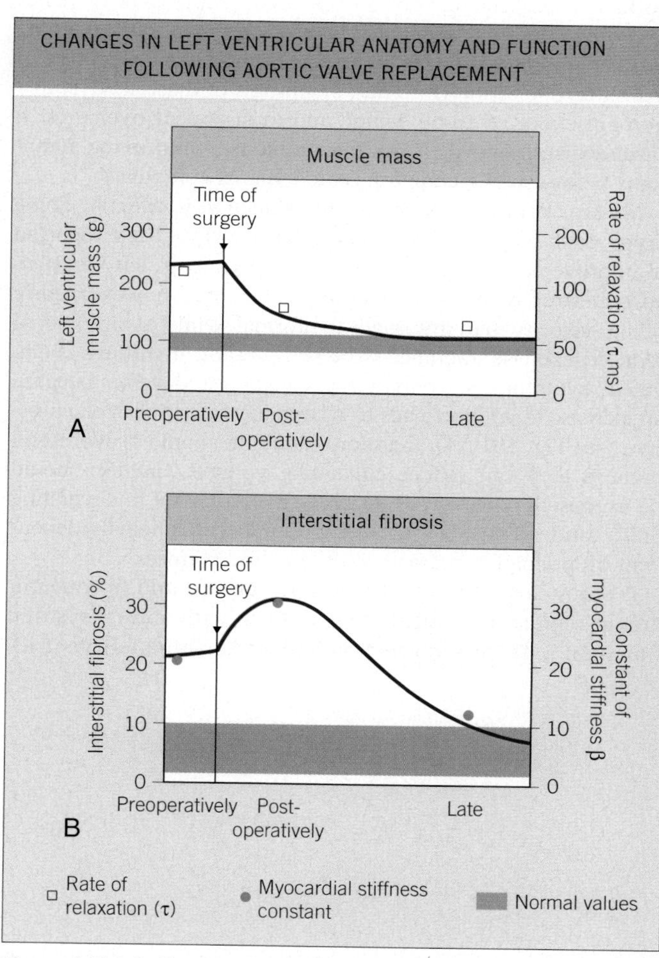

Figure 101C.5 Changes in left ventricular anatomy and function following aortic valve replacement. Left ventricular anatomy and indexes of diastolic function before (preoperatively), early (postoperatively), and late after aortic valve replacement (late) for aortic stenosis. **A,** Schematic changes in left ventricular muscle mass and, at given time points, in the rate of relaxation (τ). Muscle mass decreases early after aortic valve replacement, and such a decrease is paralleled by an improvement in τ, a measure of active diastolic function. **B,** Schematic changes in interstitial fibrosis and, at given time points, in the myocardial stiffness constant. In contrast to muscle mass, interstitial fibrosis rises after aortic valve replacement and declines much later; this is accompanied by an early worsening and a later decline in the myocardial stiffness constant, a measure of passive diastolic function.

effects on systolic and active diastolic mechanics: a decrease in the time constant of isovolumetric relaxation (τ). In the patient in this example, the ejection fraction, its change during exercise, and the peak filling rate were normal 13 weeks after aortic valve replacement (see Fig. 101C.1).

Unlike the changes in mass, interstitial fibrosis does not decrease in the short term, and in the setting of a mass decrease, the percentage fibrosis indeed increases (see Fig. 101C.5). As a consequence, myocardial stiffness increases. Therefore, soon after valve replacement for aortic stenosis, passive diastolic function worsens.

Fibrosis eventually decreases and returns to normal, but this process may take several years; normalization of interstitial fibrosis is associated with normalization in myocardial stiffness (see Fig. 101C.5). In an animal study, the development of left ventricular hypertrophy after banding of the ascending aorta was associated with an enhanced expression of genes encoding the extracellular matrix; removal of banding resulted in regression of hypertrophy and normalization of the extracellular matrix. Thus, symptoms of diastolic dysfunction are expected to be benign and to disappear over time; a cardiologist, however, faces the problem of improving symptoms before such a complex remodeling is completed.

Medical treatment of diastolic dysfunction is difficult. Some drugs, such as calcium channel blockers, have been reported to improve active diastolic function, especially in left ventricular hypertrophy. In the patient in this example, however, early filling velocity had returned to normal while symptoms of reduced exercise tolerance were still present. If stiffness is elevated, symptoms of pulmonary congestion develop because an increase in volume leads to a large increase in diastolic pressure (see Fig. 101C.4); therefore, diuretics should prove useful because they can reduce circulating volume. Caution should be exercised, however, as an excessive reduction in circulating fluids can lead to a fall in cardiac output that is heavily dependent on preload in patients with impaired stiffness.

A study has shown that collagen I and III and fibronectin are up-regulated in aortic stenosis even with normal systolic function; a depressed function and an elevated left ventricular end-diastolic pressure further contribute to such up-regulation. The activation of the renin-angiotensin-aldosterone system was held responsible for this matrix activation. Drugs that block the renin-angiotensin-aldosterone system (such as angiotensin-converting enzyme inhibitors, AT_1 blockers, and spironolactone) could prove useful in the long term, as they have been associated with an improvement in left ventricular remodeling and a decrease in fibrosis in patients with secondary left ventricular hypertrophy due to hypertension. Drugs that reduce heart rate could also prove useful, as they prolong filling time and increase filling. Beta blockers, however, have a negative inotropic and lusitropic effect that is unwanted soon after valve replacement.

SUMMARY

Left ventricular systolic and diastolic dysfunction may occur after valve replacement, especially if it was present preoperatively. Left ventricular dysfunction carries a higher risk of early and late morbidity and mortality. Diastolic dysfunction is present in about half of the patients with aortic stenosis who undergo valve replacement, and diastolic dysfunction is the outcome of impaired relaxation and filling (caused by asynchronous contraction, left ventricular hypertrophy, and increased afterload) and altered stiffness (caused by left ventricular hypertrophy and fibrosis). Aortic valve replacement leads to a prompt decrease and even normalization in left ventricular mass and active diastolic function. Fibrosis is also reversible, but the process takes much longer. Thus, signs and symptoms of impaired passive diastolic function may persist after an otherwise successful aortic valve replacement. Treatment of symptoms is largely empirical and includes reduction of the circulating volume and of heart rate. A possible role for drugs blocking the renin-angiotensin-aldosterone system has to be sought in aortic stenosis, as it has been in other forms of secondary left ventricular hypertrophy.

SECTION 7

CONGENITAL HEART DISEASE

chapter 102

Epidemiology of Congenital Heart Disease

Cynthia D. Morris

Issues/Problems

- Despite a reported recent increase in the prevalence at birth of some defects, it is likely that this is due to a technologic improvement in the ability to detect small, subclinical defects, such as muscular ventricular septal defects.
- Current knowledge of the environmental risk factors explains only a small component of the occurrence of heart defects.

Key Findings

- Congenital heart defects are defined as structural anomalies of the heart or great vessels present at birth.
- The prevalence of congenital heart defects is approximately 8 to 10 per 1000 live births, commonly cited as 1% of all births.
- The prevalence of complex and severe heart defects is greater in males than in females.
- Expansion of knowledge of chromosomal anomalies associated with the syndromic occurrence of congenital heart disease has yielded advancements in the understanding of developmental classifications, such as conotruncal defects.

Clinical Implications

- The natural history of congenital heart disease has changed with an improvement in survival from surgical repair.
- The recurrence rate of heart defect in offspring with one affected parent is 4% to 10%.

In the mid 20th century, an infant born with a congenital heart defect faced a life drastically altered both in duration and in quality. However, with the rapid evolution of medical and surgical therapeutic interventions, morbidity and mortality have radically decreased, and with these changes, the burden placed upon the families of patients has lessened. As the majority of children born with congenital heart disease now reach adolescence and adulthood, greater emphasis has been placed on understanding the etiology of the disorder with an eye to prevention and the demands placed on the health care system by this problem.

DIAGNOSTIC CRITERIA

Definition of Congenital Heart Disease

Congenital heart disease is defined as a structural anomaly of the heart or great vessels that is or could be of functional significance. It is present at birth even though diagnosis may come years, even decades, later. In common usage, this term does not include arrhythmias, even if they are noted at birth. Three other anomalies are often not included when considering the prevalence of congenital heart disease: mitral valve prolapse, bicuspid aortic valve, and patent ductus arteriosus associated with prematurity. Mitral valve prolapse has a prevalence later in life up to five times that of all congenital heart defects combined, and the proportion present at birth as opposed to the proportion developing later is unknown. Bicuspid aortic stenosis is often without sign or symptom and is often detected only with echocardiography, and thus is rarely included in studies of the occurrence of congenital heart disease. Patent ductus arteriosus in premature infants is difficult to document because it can close spontaneously with maturation or with pharmacologic management.

PREVALENCE AND INCIDENCE

Prevalence of Congenital Heart Disease

Accurate assessment of the prevalence at birth of congenital heart defects is critical to understanding the demands placed on the health care system, and the social and economic burdens placed on patients and their families. Knowledge of prevalence can assist in coordination of pediatric cardiology services as well as advanced diagnostic and treatment facilities within a region or a group of insured patients. As the population with congenital heart disease ages, an estimate of the number of children surviving to adulthood underscores the need to plan for adult cardiology services. Analyzing differences among populations may reflect the influence of genetic or environmental teratogens within an area or between countries. A higher than expected prevalence within a region or a change in prevalence over time may provide insight into the etiology. An accurate, ongoing assessment of prevalence at birth over time through birth defect monitoring programs could help detect changes that might be due to a new teratogen or an increase in a risk factor and could alert public health authorities.

Most surveys in the past decade have identified a birth prevalence of congenital heart defects of 4 to 12 children per 1000 live births, and a rate of 10 per 1000 (or 1% of all live births) is often cited.[1] Because the intensity and duration of case finding is reflected in the accuracy of the prevalence estimate, the best estimates of birth prevalence come from studies with an established birth cohort with repeated examinations through childhood. Richards and colleagues[2] gathered data from a comprehensive study of pregnancy in New York with frequent postnatal examinations and found a prevalence of 8.3 per 1000 live births.

The Collaborative Perinatal Program used the largest sample—more than 56,000 births occurring from 1957 to 1967[3]; children in the study were examined up to the age of 7 years. The rate of congenital heart disease was similar, at 8.1 per 1000 live births. At the Kaiser Foundation in Oakland, California, Hoffman and Christianson[4] followed pregnancies that resulted in 19,044 live births, with intensive follow-up until the youngest child in the study reached 5 years of age. Definite congenital heart disease was found in 8.8 per 1000 live births; when this figure was combined with possible heart defects, the resulting incidence was 10.4 per 1000 live births. (This study began in 1959 and ended in 1971, before the routine use of echocardiography.) In a more current era, the Metropolitan Atlanta Congenital Defects Program reported an occurrence of congenital heart disease of 9 per 1000 births from 1995 to 1997. This estimate is not clearly prevalence at birth or incidence as it includes some stillbirths and pregnancy terminations as well as all live births [5] (Table 102.1).

If one considers all the reports of the occurrence of heart defects, it would appear that the prevalence varies greatly over time and among populations. However, this is probably due to the duration and intensity of case finding, and sensitivity of diagnostic methods and of identifying all congenital heart defects in studies of population prevalence. It should be obvious that studies that rely on vital records, either birth or death certificates, significantly under-report prevalence. Birth certificates are a notoriously poor source of information, with only a small percentage of known malformations noted. As an example, a study that used heart defects recorded within the first week of life noted a prevalence at birth of only 2.8 per 1000.[6] Many congenital heart defects become apparent only later in infancy or in childhood rather than at birth. Only about 40% to 50% of heart defects are diagnosed within 1 week of birth, 80% to 90% are diagnosed within the first year of life, and perhaps 95% are diagnosed by 5 years of age. Two studies have used seemingly complete ascertainment but have followed children only up to the age of 1 year; in one the prevalence was 4.05 per 1000 live births,[7] and in the other it was 5.54 per 1000 live births.[8] This prevalence is considerably lower than that found in other studies that have followed subjects into later childhood.

The studies that have reported the highest birth prevalence have included a registry that follows a defined population or a combined effort of all pediatric heart referral centers in a region and have made an intensive effort to examine all children for heart defects through early childhood. Echocardiographic screening of a population can identify heart defects of minor significance and unlikely to be identified clinically. Although it is unlikely that these studies overestimate prevalence, given the multitude of difficulties in assessment, the smaller estimates may represent the prevalence of significant heart defects. With more complete case ascertainment, heart defects that may be asymptomatic are more likely to be diagnosed, such as mild pulmonary stenosis and small VSDs or atrial septal defects (ASDs). It should not be surprising that surveys that follow children only up to the age of 1 month or even 1 year show the lowest prevalence of heart defects. Ideally, to gain a true estimate of prevalence at birth, a large, diverse, population-based cohort from birth through infancy and childhood and perhaps up to the age of 18 years should be followed, with routine assessment by echocardiography and extensive autopsy evaluation of every death to eliminate referral bias.

The widespread use of two-dimensional echocardiography, which was introduced during the 1980s, has also affected prevalence estimates. With the ability to detect very small VSDs and ASDs as well as mild degrees of valvular stenosis, prevalence estimates have risen as diagnosis has been enhanced. The inclusion of these less severe defects will have an obvious impact when prevalences between regions or over time are compared, and their inclusion is important in studies of the etiology of congenital heart disease. However, this is less significant when the impact on the health care system is considered, because tiny VSDs and mild pulmonary stenosis require few health care resources.

Estimates of the Incidence of Congenital Heart Disease

The term prevalence is often used in connection with congenital heart disease because it constitutes incidence and duration. Incidence connotes the new occurrence of a disease or disorder (Table 102.2), and in the case of congenital heart defects, as with all birth defects, it comprises the occurrence of a defect at the time of cardiogenesis (or postnatally in the case of patent ductus arteriosus). Prevalence at the time of birth may be considerably less than incidence, given elective pregnancy termination, spontaneous abortion, and stillbirth.[9] In order to provide the best estimate of the occurrence of heart defects in studies of risk, it is important to understand the prenatal and postnatal occurrence of structural heart defects.

DETERMINING THE PREVALENCE AT BIRTH OF CONGENITAL HEART DEFECTS	
Determining the numerator	Examine all children by using optimal diagnostic methods
	Follow children beyond infancy and, if possible, through childhood
	Examine the hearts of children who die from any cause if possible
	Establish diagnostic criteria for congenital heart disease
Determining the denominator	Define the population base
	Only live births should be included

Table 102.1 Determining the prevalence at birth of congenital heart defects.

INCIDENCE VERSUS PREVALENCE	
Incidence	The rate or proportion of all pregnancies in which the fetus has a structurally abnormal heart at the time of cardiogenesis
Prevalence	The rate or proportion of the population affected by a heart defect at any given point in time
Prevalence at birth	The number of children born with a heart defect as a rate or proportion of the number of live births
Definition of the term incidence, prevalence, and prevalence at birth in the context of congenital heart disease.	

Table 102.2 Incidence versus prevalence.

Comparatively little information is known about the occurrence of heart defects in abortuses owing to the difficulty in observation, although these defects are more readily detectable in stillborn children and in fetuses that have been electively aborted. Most congenital malformations, including heart defects, have a higher rate of occurrence in stillbirths than in live births, particularly in fetuses lost early in gestation; such losses may be due in part to chromosomal anomalies. In the case of malformations that can be discovered only on examination of the heart, autopsy of the stillborn child is required for diagnosis. This is infrequently done because of a failure of health professionals to request and obtain permission for fetopsy, and because examination is often impossible owing to maceration. The increasing use of fetal echocardiography may lead to an observable increase in measured incidence but to a decrease in the prevalence at birth, particularly in pregnancies complicated by severe and complex defects, such as hypoplastic left heart syndrome and single ventricle and complete ASD, which some parents may choose to terminate.

Hoffman[10] estimated that the true incidence of congenital heart disease may be as high as 53 per 1000 pregnancies (Fig. 102.1).

The proportion of spontaneous abortions before 28 weeks of gestation may be as high as 40% and decline to 6% for fetal deaths after 28 weeks.[11] Although prevalence rates that include spontaneous abortions and stillbirths may have little relevance to the economic burden of congenital heart disease, these have great importance in the study of etiology.

Prevalence at Birth of Specific Heart Defects

The prevalence of specific heart defects may vary considerably among geographic regions, owing to small sample size, ascertainment bias, maternal age and risks, and possibly genetic variation. Hoffman[1] has tabulated the median proportion of congenital heart disease attributable to each specific defect from major population studies worldwide (Fig. 102.2).[5] As shown, ventricular septal defects are the most common of all heart defects at birth and account for about one in every three defects.

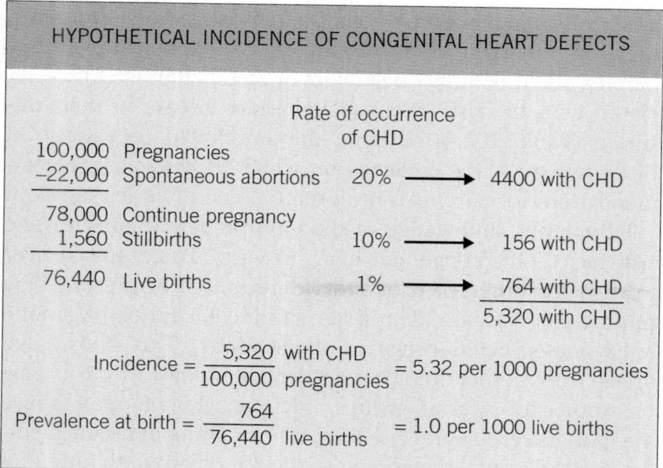

Figure 102.1 Hypothetical incidence of congenital heart defects. CHD, congenital heart defects.

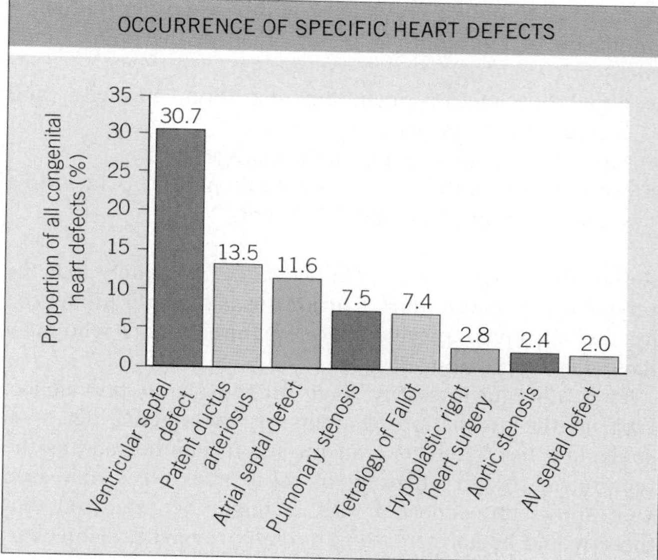

Figure 102.2 Occurrence of specific heart defects as a function of total prevalence at birth. AV, atrioventricular.

Secular Effects on Prevalence at Birth

Is it possible that the prevalence of specific congenital heart defects is increasing over time? In the Metropolitan Atlanta Congenital Defect Program, the prevalence of heart defects increased from 6.2 per 1000 to 9.0 per 1000 between 1995 and 1997.[5] VSD, tetralogy of Fallot, AV septal defects, and pulmonic stenosis all increased while the prevalence of D-transposition of the great arteries decreased. Although selective pregnancy termination with identification early in gestation can explain a decrease in serious or complex defects, improvement in diagnostic technology can explain an increase in less significant defects. An increase in VSDs was first noted in Sweden in the 1950s, and a birth defects monitoring project in the United States reported that the prevalence at birth of VSD had increased from 0.4 per 1000 births in 1970 to 0.8 per 1000 births in 1975.[11] Many subsequent reports demonstrated no change or a small increase in prevalence during this period. The combined evidence, however, indicates a lack of any compelling reason to suspect a true increase in the occurrence of VSD. Despite an apparent increase in detected VSDs, the rate of spontaneous closure by 1 year of age is reported to be unchanged over time, and the prevalence of defects requiring therapeutic intervention, particularly moderate to large defects, has also remained constant over time.[12]

In the case of patent ductus arteriosus, a nationwide monitoring project in the United States reported an increase from 0.4 per 1000 births in 1970 to 1.1 per 1000 births in 1975, and in metropolitan Atlanta, Georgia, an increase from 0.7 per 1000 live births in 1968 to 3.2 per 1000 live births in 1975 has been reported.[13] With an increase in the survivability of low-birth-weight premature infants within this same time period, perhaps this secular trend should not be surprising, given the association between patent ductus arteriosus and prematurity. Even comparing the birth prevalence within a defined region, a multitude of confounding factors may change over time, such as

- population factors, including migration, ethnicity, and socioeconomic factors;
- reproductive history and maternal age; and
- community and tertiary medical practice, including screening, diagnosis, and treatment.[14]

Rather than a true increase in incidence, it is likely that the prevalence of patent ductus arteriosus is strongly influenced by the improved survival of premature infants who may have died in previous decades.

Two other factors may have an impact on prevalence. First, as the population of adults of reproductive age with congenital heart defects is increasing in number and as the recurrence risk in offspring of those affected is increased well above the expected rate, it might be predicted that there would be an increase in overall prevalence. However, widespread use of fetal echocardiographic screening may reduce the birth prevalence through pregnancy termination of fetuses with severe cardiac malformations. In the United Kingdom, if the rate of implementation of fetal cardiac screening would increase to 54%, and if the rate of pregnancy termination was 50%, then 218 fewer children might be born with severe heart defects, approximately one of every eight children so affected.

Prevalence by Race and Ethnicity

Comparison of the regional prevalence of congenital heart disease throughout the world is impossible because of the paucity of data from Australia, Asia, and Africa in particular, as well as from the underassessment of heart defects in many populations.[1] Moreover, given the methodologic intensity necessary to make valid comparisons of prevalence among populations and the little additional information that this would provide, it is unlikely that such studies would be performed worldwide. The data that do exist, however, give no important reason to suspect a difference in the overall prevalence within Europe and the United States. However, examining differences in race and ethnicity within a population may provide insights.

Within the United States, there are indications of an important difference in the prevalence of congenital heart disease between black infants and white infants. In one report, the prevalence of coarctation of the aorta, aortic stenosis, Ebstein's anomaly, pulmonary atresia, and D-transposition of the great arteries within the first year of life was significantly higher in white children than in black children, yet the prevalence of pulmonary stenosis and heterotaxy was significantly higher in black children.[15] In a separate cohort, the rate of congenital heart defects in non-Hispanic whites was significantly higher than that for Mexican Americans or blacks; however, the rate of more severe heart disease requiring cardiac catheterization or surgery was similar between the groups.[16]

Although the timing of referral to a pediatric cardiologist was not related to ethnicity, income, or education, this does not exclude underascertainment of less severe heart defects in economically or medically disadvantaged populations.

DOMINANT HEART DEFECTS IN MALES AND FEMALES	
Males	**Females**
Hypoplastic left heart syndrome	Atrial septal defect
Double-outlet right ventricle	Patent ductus arteriosus
Coarctation of the aorta	Atrioventricular septal defects
Aortic stenosis	
D-transposition of the great arteries	
Pulmonary atresia	
Tricuspid atresia	
L-transposition of the great arteries	

Table 102.3 Dominant heart defects in males and females.

Prevalence at Birth by Sex

There are pronounced differences by sex in the distribution of heart defects (Table 102.3). In general, the prevalence of cyanotic and complex defects is significantly greater in males than in females. In a population study in Czechoslovakia, severe defects predominated, with higher ratios of males to females for double-outlet right ventricle, hypoplastic left heart syndrome, D-transposition of the great arteries, aortic stenosis, pulmonary atresia, tricuspid atresia, and congenitally corrected transposition.[17] All left heart defects, in particular hypoplastic left heart syndrome, aortic stenosis, and coarctation, show uniformly higher rates of occurrence in males than in females. Less severe defects, including ASD, patent ductus arteriosus, and atrioventricular (AV) septal defects, dominate in females. Ventricular septal defects and perhaps pulmonary stenosis appear to be evenly distributed by sex. Overall, there is a dominance of defects of greater complexity and higher mortality in males as compared to females. This may provide a clue to differential teratogenicity by the gender of the fetus, or more possibly to greater fetal wastage in males as compared to females.

RISK FACTORS

A scientific statement from the American Heart Association Council on Cardiovascular Disease in the Young[18] provides an excellent summary on noninherited risk factors. From this, there are emerging clues for clinicians to counsel prospective parents about potential behaviors or factors that may be associated with the risk of congenital heart disease in their offspring (Table 102.4). Despite the substantial prevalence at birth, however, the evidence on which to base these recommendations for parents is insubstantial and often inconsistent.

Ultimately, knowledge of the environmental and lifestyle risk factors for congenital heart disease (Table 102.5) may lead to the prevention of some defects, but at present, few teratogenic risks are identified, with the exception of genetic risks and selected drugs or medications. This knowledge arises from epidemiologic case-control studies in particular, or studies of special groups, such as women who abuse alcohol, have diabetes mellitus, or use anticonvulsant medications. This type of study, in particular, is prone to potential biased recall by mothers of case children; this plus failure to adequately control confounding factors can sometimes lead

COUNSELING PARENTS WHO HAVE AN INFANT WITH A CONGENITAL HEART DEFECT
■ Recurrence risk in offspring may approach 4%–10%. ■ Risk may be higher if more than one relative is affected with congenital heart disease. ■ Recurrent heart defects in offspring are often similar to that of the parent. ■ If the mother has compromised cardiac status, she should be referred to a cardiologist for management of pregnancy and delivery, optimally before she conceives. ■ Fetal echocardiography is recommended in the second trimester. ■ Genetic karyotyping may be warranted if fetal echocardiography demonstrates a heart defect.

Table 102.4 Counseling parents who have an infant with a congenital heart defect.

KNOWN OR SUSPECTED RISK FACTORS FOR CONGENITAL HEART DISEASE		
Maternal drug and medication use	Alcohol abuse	Thalidomide
	Cocaine abuse	Lithium
	Vitamin A congeners	Valproic acid
	Warfarin	Estrogens (possibly)
Maternal medical disorders	Insulin-dependent diabetes mellitus	
	Phenylketonuria	
	Coagulopathies, spherocytosis	
	Rubella, toxoplasmosis, other infections	
Environmental risks	Drinking water contamination by trichloroethylene, dichloroethylene	
Maternal nutrition	Low intake of folate	

Table 102.5 Known or suspected risk factors for congenital heart disease.

to spurious results. There are no published prospective cohort studies of the pathogenesis of congenital heart defects in the larger population. Because of the complications of studying the incidence of heart defects to include early termination of pregnancy, the specific effect of teratogens in pathogenesis can be difficult to assess.

Maternal Risk Factors

Maternal pregestational diabetes mellitus significantly increases the risk of cardiac defects in offspring, although gestational diabetes is not thought to increase this risk.[19,20] In the Baltimore-Washington study, maternal diabetes was responsible for a 3.2-fold increased risk of all structural heart defects; the increase was even more for double-outlet right ventricle, tetralogy of Fallot, and VSD.[21] Fetal malformations overall are clearly linked to glycemic control; if before conception and during pregnancy the mother is not hyperglycemic, then risk is equivalent to the general population.[22] This risk may take on increasing importance as the prevalence of obesity in young women increases globally, given that a sizable proportion of pregnancies are unplanned and may therefore involve inadequate glycemic control.

Maternal overweight and obesity (body mass index >26 kg/m) has been reported to be associated with increased risk of congenital heart defect in offspring.[23] While this may be independent of any effect of maternal diabetes, a similar pathway may be involved. Similarly, this may not be independent of nutritional intake nor an association with socioeconomic status.

Maternal infections associated with heart defects include rubella, toxoplasmosis, coxsackie B virus, Epstein-Barr virus, influenza, and mumps, but not Lyme disease. The broad spectrum of infections involved may indicate that maternal febrile illness in the first trimester may be associated with this risk.[24] Children exposed to human immunodeficiency virus type 1 in utero have been reported to have a rate of congenital cardiac defects some 5 to 10 times that expected; however, when compared to cohorts of children of uninfected women similarly screened, there is likely no real increase in risk.

Maternal phenylketonuria is associated with a sixfold increase in risk of congenital heart defect, particularly tetralogy of Fallot, VSD, patent ductus arteriosus, and single ventricle. Dietary control of phenylketonuria can significantly reduce that risk. In addition, maternal coagulopathies and spherocytosis have also been linked to congenital heart defects.

Nutrition

The epidemiologic observation that maternal supplemental folic acid in pregnancy is protective against neural tube defects has been extended through epidemiologic evidence of associations with orofacial clefts, conotruncal heart defects, midline abdominal defects, and urogenital malformations. Of five prior case-control studies, three demonstrated that use of a folic acid–containing supplement conferred significant magnitude of protection from conotruncal heart defects (OR ~0.50). In two studies, however, there was no association between folate supplementation and outcome. Although a recent Cochrane review[25] of the case-control studies of congenital heart defects concluded there was no significant risk reduction by folic acid supplementation for conotruncal defects (RR, 0.74; 95% CI, 0.14-3.32), in contrast, a prospective population-based study in Denmark[26] found significantly fewer malformations when folic acid supplementation began before 7 weeks' gestation. Evidence from a randomized trial of primary prevention of neural tube defects with folate supplementation in Hungary indicated fewer VSD in offspring, although not statistically significant.[27] Additional measurements of dietary intake and biologic markers of folate will be important, because a traditional placebo-controlled clinical trial of folate is not ethically possible.

Retinol intake from foods and supplements of more than 10,000 IU per day in the year before gestation has been reported to dramatically increase the risk of D-transposition of the great arteries but not other conotruncal defects with normally related vessels.[28] For lesser intake through diet or supplements, the data are inconsistent.

Many medications have been investigated as cardiac teratogens; many of these drugs appear to have no effect on cardiogenesis when taken during pregnancy, and others have been strongly associated with cardiac defects in infants. Drugs that are known cardiac teratogens include thalidomide, vitamin A congeners, and warfarins. Thalidomide has been associated with conotruncal defects, particularly truncus arteriosus and tetralogy of Fallot, and vitamin A congeners, such as isotretinoin and etretinate, have been associated with transposition of the great arteries and aortic hypoplasia. Other reports have linked the use of lithium, valproic acid, ibuprofen, angiotensin-converting enzyme inhibitors, some antiemetic agents, and some antineoplastic agents with heart defects.[18] Many antiepileptic drugs, such as valproate, carbamazepine, benzodiazepines and phenobarbital, in combination with caffeine have been associated in general with heart defects, and folic acid antagonists with conotruncal defects. Medications that appear to have no effect on the developing heart include penicillin, ampicillin, vaginal metronidazole, antivirals and antiretrovirals, corticosteroids, buproprion, serotonin reuptake inhibitors, and oral contraceptives. More uncertainty exists for diazepam, antiasthmatic drugs, and sympathomimetics. It should be noted, however, that some of these medications, as with serotonin reuptake inhibitors, may be associated with other congenital malformations.

Abuse of Illegal Drugs, Alcohol, and Tobacco

The overall incidence of fetal alcohol syndrome is 1.95 per 1000 births; among women who are heavy drinkers it is 49 per 1000 births.[29] Heart defects, particularly VSD, occur in perhaps half of all children with this syndrome; these defects include isolated defects and those in association with aortic regurgitation, coarctation, and subaortic stenosis. Tetralogy of Fallot and secundum ASD occur less commonly. A nonspecific teratogenic effect of alcohol on the developing heart is suggested because of the lack of one mechanistic classification of defect. At levels of alcohol consumption of one to two drinks per day in the first trimester, there is likely no associated increased risk of congenital heart defect. Although greater consumption of alcohol, more than two drinks a day, may be associated with increased risk, the precise relationship is unknown, as are the effects of binge drinking (more than five drinks on one occasion).[30]

Maternal cocaine use in pregnancy alters the maternal fetal-placental unit, and these alterations lead to changes in fetal blood flow and to hypoxemia. These changes have been demonstrated to have an effect on the developing chick heart, but the effect in humans is more uncertain. In a meta-analysis of six epidemiologic studies, cocaine use during pregnancy was not significantly associated with congenital heart malformations.[31] Subsequent to this, however, an association of cocaine use and congenital heart defects has been identified in two studies.

A meta-analysis of cigarette smoking discovered no strong relationship to the occurrence of congenital heart defects overall. However, for specific defects such as truncus arteriosus, ASD, and patent ductus arteriosus, maternal cigarette use has been reported to be associated with risk.

Caffeine likewise is not associated with congenital heart defects in risk groups of those who drink as much as four to eight cups per day.[32]

Environmental Risks

Environmental exposure can be difficult to assess in case-control studies, because exposure to precise products can be uncertain and at best is subject to recall bias. Nonetheless, there are suggestions that maternal exposure to organic solvents, paints, dyes, and lacquers may be associated with specific heart defects. Similarly, there is a higher risk of congenital heart defects in offspring of mothers who work in the agricultural industry. Pesticides and herbicides have been associated with conotruncal heart defects in at least one study.[18]

A higher incidence of congenital heart defects has been noted for parents who live in an area where the drinking water is contaminated by trichloroethylene, dichloroethylene, or chromium. Actual exposure of individuals was not assessed, and therefore a causal relationship cannot be established, although animal models have provided some corroborative evidence. Living near national priority list cleanup sites for hazardous waste also appears to somewhat increase risk of heart defects. There is some indication that maternal exposure in early gestation to air pollution through particulate matter and carbon monoxide may be associated with congenital heart defects. One indication of an effect of air pollution may be seasonality of the occurrence of heart defects. Only pulmonary valve stenosis has been noted to exhibit seasonality, however.

Birth Weight

The relationship between low birth weight and cardiac malformations is well described. In the Baltimore-Washington Infant Study, infants with tetralogy of Fallot, AV septal defects, hypoplastic left heart syndrome, pulmonary stenosis, coarctation of the aorta, VSD, and ASD were significantly more likely than controls to have low birth weight for gestational age after adjustment for important confounders.[33] In one study, infants with a congenital heart defect were about twice as likely to be small for gestational age as compared to controls. The broad spectrum of defects associated with low birth weight argues against a specific mechanism, such as reduced aortic blood flow, which would lead to growth retardation. In fact, embryonic growth retardation may increase the risk of congenital malformation; this has been noted very early in gestation in maternal diabetes. Disturbance of embryonic blood flow may accompany such growth retardation or may be causal.

Similarly, the risk of a cardiovascular malformation is significantly increased in infants born prematurely. In a cohort of more than 52,000 births in England, a cardiovascular malformation was identified in 5.1 per 1000 term infants and in 12.5 per 1000 premature infants, with an odds ratio of 2.4 (95% CI, 2.2-2.7).[34] This was particularly apparent with tetralogy of Fallot, pulmonary stenosis, aortic stenosis, coarctation of the aorta, complete atrioventricular septal defect, and ventricular septal defect. Approximately 16% of all infants with a heart defect were born preterm. Late stillbirths were also reported to be common with more severe and complex malformations, such as coarctation of the aorta, hypoplastic left heart, truncus arteriosus, double-outlet right ventricle, and double-inlet left ventricle.

Inheritance of Congenital Heart Defects

Knowledge of the genetic etiology of the origins of congenital heart disease has exploded in the last decade. Whereas multifactorial transmission had always been posited, it is now apparent that distinct genetic causes likely operate independently as well as in conjunction with other risks, such as lifestyle and environment. A scientific statement from the

American Heart Association, Congenital Cardiac Defects Committee, Council on Cardiovascular Disease in the Young has summarized current information in this field.[35]

In past decades, the recurrence rate of congenital heart defects in offspring of an affected parent was cited as 4% to 8%. Because previous reports were from the era before the recent expansion of genetic knowledge of congenital heart disease, it is now apparent that these proportions may include a substantial number of subjects or families with chromosomal anomalies, and the calculated recurrence may change depending on the composition of the population studied.

An increase in the population frequency of congenital heart defect could be anticipated if recurrence risk is increased in the offspring of parents who have a heart defect. Understanding of genetic mechanisms assumes increasing importance as the population of adults with congenital heart defects grows in number as a result of therapeutic improvements. Given the improving quality of life for this group, it is likely that with opportunities for reproduction, the birth prevalence of congenital heart defect, particularly more severe defects, may increase in subsequent generations.

Knowledge of the genetic basis of a heart defect may provide essential information for counseling prospective parents. This may yield benefit as well to increase understanding of the pathobiologic nature of the heart defect and to provide information to families, including siblings. This will help refine the risk of recurrence from a population perspective to individual risk. Knowledge of the genetic basis may indicate that the heart defect is part of a syndrome with the possibility of involvement of systems other than the heart, thereby improving care. It may also provide an indication of the long-term clinical outcome as well. Given that syndromes and extracardiac malformations are thought to occur in perhaps a quarter of all children, investigating etiology is particularly important.

Genetic testing should be part of the assessment plan for many families facing a heart defect during a pregnancy. Fetal echocardiography in the second trimester should be offered to all parents to allow planning for the remainder of the pregnancy and for the delivery. Amniocentesis or chorionic villus sampling may be offered to the parents to karyotype an affected pregnancy. Management may require the teamwork of a cardiologist and perinatologist for the mother and a pediatric cardiologist for the child.

Genetic Syndromes and Congenital Heart Defects

The recent rapid increase in the number of genetic anomalies associated with congenital heart defects (Table 102.6) has made multifactorial inheritance less likely. Given the specific nature of the heart defects associated with most syndromes, discovery of the chromosomal origins of a syndrome has been extremely important in advancing the understanding of the origins of disordered cardiogenesis. This is apparent in the association of chromosome 22q11 deletion with DiGeorge syndrome and microdeletion at 7q11.23 with Williams syndrome. The rapid increase in genetic knowledge may radically change our understanding of the etiology of congenital heart defects in the next decade (Table 102.7).

Microdeletions of chromosomal region 22q11 were first described in 1992 as a cause of conotruncal defects. Deletions at this same locus are responsible for 70% to 90% of cases of DiGeorge syndrome, which is associated with truncus arteriosus, interrupted aortic arch, tetralogy of Fallot and isolated VSD, and for velocardiofacial syndrome, which is associated with tetralogy of Fallot and VSD. In children who have isolated conotruncal defects, a 20% to 30% occurrence of 22q11 deletions has been noted.[36] This has a wide variation with the deletion noted rarely with transposition of the great arteries, in 8% to 35% of tetralogy of Fallot, and in 34% to 41% of truncus arteriosus.[35] The microdeletion 22q11 is inherited in an autosomal dominant manner in 6% to 28% of children. Sufficient evidence exists to warrant genetic testing for the 22q11 deletion in all patients who have truncus arteriosus, interrupted aortic arch, absent pulmonary valve syndrome, tetralogy of Fallot, anomalous origin of the pulmonary artery from the aorta, and any congenital heart defect associated with absence of the thymus. This defect is also associated with cleft

GENETIC AND HERITABLE SYNDROMES COMMONLY ASSOCIATED WITH CONGENITAL HEART DISEASE

- Down's syndrome
- Williams syndrome
- DiGeorge syndrome
- Holt–Oram syndrome
- Noonan's syndrome
- Turner's syndrome
- Velocardiofacial syndrome
- Goldenhar syndrome
- Alagille syndrome
- Smith–Lemli–Opitz syndrome
- Cri du chat syndrome
- Pierre–Robin syndrome
- Ellis–van Creveld syndrome
- Trisomy 13
- Trisomy 18
- Thrombocytopenia–absent radius syndrome
- Heart–hand syndromes
- CHARGE association
- VATERR/VACTERL association

CHARGE, coloboma, heart defects, atresia of the choanae, retarded growth and development, genital hypoplasia, ear anomalies or deafness; VACTERL, vertebral, anal, cardiac, tracheal, esophageal, renal, and limb anomalies; VATERR, vertebral defects, anal atresia, tracheoesophageal fistula, esophageal atresia, radial and renal anomalies.

Table 102.6 Genetic and heritable syndromes commonly associated with congenital heart disease.

ONGOING INVESTIGATIONS OF SYNDROMES, CONGENITAL HEART DEFECT, AND CHROMOSOMAL ANOMALY

Syndrome	Congenital Heart Defect	Chromosomal Anomaly
DiGeorge syndrome	Conotruncal defects	Chr 22q11 microdeletion
Williams syndrome and familial autosomal-dominant supravalvular aortic stenosis	Supravalvular aortic stenosis	Chr 7q11.23 hemizygosity or disruption
Familial total anomalous pulmonary venous return	Total anomalous pulmonary venous return	4p (possibly)
Holt–Oram syndrome	Atrial septal defect	Chr 12 (possibly)

Chr, chromosome.

Table 102.7 Ongoing investigations of syndromes, congenital heart defect, and chromosomal anomaly.

palate, hypocalcemia, hypernasal speech, learning disability, attention deficit disorder, and psychiatric disorders in older children and adults.

Because of the anatomic similarity between supravalvular aortic stenosis in Williams syndrome and that of an autosomal dominant defect, a common chromosomal origin was postulated. Disruption of the elastin gene localized to 7q11.23 may explain the autosomal dominant form of isolated supravalvular aortic stenosis apart from Williams syndrome.[37] Molecular genetic studies have demonstrated that hemizygosity at this elastin locus explains the occurrence of cardiac defects with Williams syndrome as well. The accompanying syndrome is associated with distinct facial features, mental retardation or cognitive disability, short stature, infant hypercalcemia, adult diabetes mellitus, and skeletal and renal anomalies.

Although Alagille syndrome is thought of as a primary liver and biliary disorder, it is associated with cardiovascular anomalies in more than 90% of children. This includes such anomalies as pulmonary valvular stenosis, peripheral pulmonary hypoplasia, and tetralogy of Fallot. This syndrome has been associated with a JAG1 mutation and 20p12 rearrangement or deletion.[35] This may be particularly relevant in some families, because other members may be asymptomatic yet affected by liver disease.

Down syndrome occurs in 9.2 per 10,000 live-born infants and is the most commonly identified syndrome associated with a heart defect, making up approximately three quarters of the syndromic occurrence. Cardiac defects occur in about 20% to 30% of all affected infants. In a large survey of three registries, AV septal defects occurred most frequently (in 39% of children), VSDs in 28%, and ASDs in 7%. Tetralogy of Fallot and patent ductus arteriosus each occurred in less than 5% of children.[38] Down syndrome occurs in approximately 75% of children who have an AV septal defect. Surgical intervention dramatically improves survival, and most children with Down syndrome are not at higher operative or postoperative risk; repair of AV septal defects or other heart defects has contributed greatly to the increasing life span.

Holt-Oram syndrome is the best recognized of a family of heart-hand syndromes; this autosomal dominant condition occurs in about 1 per 100,000 individuals. Diagnosis depends on skeletal preaxial radial ray anomalies, which may range from subclinical findings to phocomelia. Cardiac defects occur in perhaps 95% of all affected people. Structural cardiac anomalies (particularly ASDs and occasionally VSDs) are present in the majority, although conduction defects are noted in the absence of a heart defect. The Holt-Oram syndrome is caused by a mutation in the TBX5 transcription factor gene, chromosome 12q24.1.[35] Other types of heart-hand syndromes are rarer and, accordingly, are less well studied, but they are thought to be genetically distinct. Again, further study of these disorders may lead to a better understanding of the development of the atrial septum. Likewise, a single-gene defect for nonsyndromic ASD has been identified at NKX2.5 using linkage analysis; this same mutation may be associated with other heart and conduction defects.[39]

Noonan's syndrome is estimated to occur in 1 per 1000 to 2500 births. Although autosomal inheritance has been described, the syndrome can also occur sporadically. At present, no consistent chromosomal anomaly has been identified. Diagnosis is often based on characteristic facies, including broad and sloping forehead, ocular hypertelorism, and a deep philtrum. Cardiac defects involvement occurs in 80% to 90% of those affected with Noonan's syndrome, with a dysplastic, stenotic pulmonary valve and hypertrophic cardiomyopathy being the most characteristic. In a recent study of children undergoing pulmonary valvotomy, about 7% had Noonan's syndrome. However, the full range of cardiac defects has been reported, including ASD, VSD, and tetralogy of Fallot. To date, there are three known Noonan's syndrome disease genes, *PTPN11*, the most prevalent occurring in 40% to 50% of cases, as well as *SOS1* and *KRAS*.[35] A disease gene on chromosome 12 has been identified.

Other known chromosomal anomalies and syndromes commonly associated with congenital heart defects include cri du chat (monosomy 5p), Turner's syndrome (monosomy X), trisomy 13, trisomy 18, Goldenhar's syndrome, Smith-Lemli-Opitz syndrome, thrombocytopenia–absent radius syndrome, VATERR (vertebral defects, anal atresia, tracheoesophageal fistula, esophageal atresia, radial and renal anomalies), and VACTERL (vertebral, anal, cardiac, tracheal, esophageal, renal, and limb anomalies) associations, CHARGE (coloboma, heart defects, atresia of the choanae, retarded growth and development, genital hypoplasia, ear anomolies or deafness) association, and a large number of trisomy duplication syndromes.

PROGNOSIS

Natural History

One of the most dramatic events in pediatrics over the past three decades has been the development of surgical techniques that provide the chance of cure for some children who have congenital heart disease and dramatic improvements in survival and quality of life for others. For all major heart defects that have been studied, surgery improves prognosis, particularly in the case of those that carry a high infant mortality rate. Even when studied over time, given the decreasing operative mortality rate apparent over the previous 30 years, survival is consistently better with surgery, even in the earliest era of operative repair.

Advances in the past 30 years in pediatric cardiology have included

- a widespread use of interventional cardiac catheterization techniques, such as balloon valvotomy and noninvasive closure of ASD and patent ductus arteriosus;
- atrial septostomy;
- prostaglandin E_1 therapy and indomethacin for pharmacologic control of ductus;
- echocardiography for diagnosis; and
- surgical palliation of complex, cyanotic defects, such as truncus arteriosus and pulmonary atresia.

As a result of these changes, the number of children who survive to adulthood has increased dramatically; with this has come a need to monitor clinical results. Medical problems in adult survivors of congenital heart defects include

- arrhythmias, both supraventricular and ventricular, and a higher risk of sudden cardiac death;
- recurrent or residual lesions that may be of considerable physiologic consequence, including recurrent valvular stenosis or coarctation;
- sequelae of surgery, with the need to replace a cardiac valve, baffle, or conduit because of limited durability, patient growth, thrombogenesis, or endocarditis;

NEEDS OF ADOLESCENTS AND ADULTS AND SEQUELAE AFTER SURGICAL REPAIR OF CONGENITAL HEART DEFECT
Late complications of heart disease
Arrhythmias
Pulmonary hypertension
Endocarditis
Ventricular dysfunction
Late surgical complications
Recurrent or residual heart defect
Sequelae of surgery
Reproduction and family planning
Recurrence of heart defect in offspring
Functional status and quality of life
Insurability, employability

Table 102.8 Needs of adolescents and adults and sequelae after surgical repair of congenital heart defect.

- ventricular dysfunction from chronic hemodynamic overload or pulmonary hypertension or as a complication of surgery; and
- endocarditis, particularly with left-sided defects, a left-to-right shunt, and the presence of a valve or conduit.

The needs of these children and adults are summarized in Table 102.8.

Outcome Studies of Congenital Heart Defect

At no time in history has the number of children and adults with congenital heart disease been as large as it is at present. To assess the needs of this growing population, it is important to estimate the number of adults who have surgically corrected and uncorrected heart defects. This statistic is dependent on the birth prevalence of congenital heart defect, the frequency of successful intervention, and the mortality rate. An estimate of the pediatric population in 2000 indicated that 623,000 children had congenital heart disease in the United States; this includes 320,000 with simple heart defects, 165,000 with moderately complex defects, and 138,000 with highly complex heart defects.[40] Now that survival to adulthood is commonplace, this population is now aging. At the time of the Bethesda conference in 2000, there was an estimated 787,000 adults with heart defects. This includes 368,800 adults with simple heart defects, 302,500 with moderately complex defects, and 117,000 with highly complex heart defects.[41] In a separate study, the prevalence of congenital heart disease in the general population was 4.09 per 1000 adults and 0.38 per 1000 for severe heart defects, such as tetralogy of Fallot, transposition of the great arteries, truncus arteriosus, atrioventricular septal defects, and univentricular heart.[42] In the previous two decades, the proportion with severe defects increased particularly in adults. Females accounted for 57% of this adult population. Given the vagaries of estimating this population, this may be an underestimate. In fact, more than 1 million adults are now thought to have congenital heart defects. It is clear that, whereas in the past 50 years the overwhelming majority of the population with congenital heart defects were children, the adult population will outnumber the pediatric population and health resources will need to be modified to reflect this change. This indicates a true shift in the demographic profile of congenital heart defects that will have an impact on the provider and system needs of these individuals.

To date, sources of morbidity and mortality information on the long-term outcome after surgery for congenital heart defects are limited. The Natural History Study[43] provided important information about follow-up after surgery for VSD, aortic stenosis, and pulmonary valve stenosis, but the limited duration of follow-up and the limited diversity of congenital heart defects that were included restrict the impact of these data. Two medical centers that pioneered pediatric open heart surgery have compiled long-term outcomes of surgery. These include 30 years of follow-up after surgery for secundum ASD, VSD, or tetralogy of Fallot at the Mayo Clinic,[44,45] and 26- to 32-year follow-up after surgery for congenital heart defect in 1000 consecutive cases at the University of Minnesota.[46] The Society of Thoracic Surgeons has formed a national congenital heart surgery database, but this analyzes operative mortality only and does not evaluate long-term outcome. Lastly, the Oregon Registry of Congenital Heart Defect Surgery is a population-based registry that has followed a large cohort of patients who have undergone surgery for any of 14 different heart defects from 1958 up to the 1990s to determine long-term outcomes.[47]

Most importantly, none of the previously mentioned studies of natural history is ongoing, except for the two last-mentioned databases, and only the Oregon population registry has evaluated the changing nature of surgery over the past three to four decades. Moller and Anderson[46] have stated that "the management of children with a cardiac malformation is hampered by a paucity of information about the long-term clinical course" and that the ideal study of this would follow an entire cohort of children from birth to adulthood. Given the difficulties of such a study, information for clinical management of adults must depend on reports from individual series as well as on the larger population-based databases.

SUMMARY

Primary prevention of congenital heart defects is not possible at this time except for measures to eliminate alcohol and cocaine abuse in pregnancy. With greater knowledge of the genetic causes of heart defects, however, it may be possible to develop screening tests and to inform women who are at high risk.

Secondary prevention is possible with the use of fetal echocardiography, which can be used in women at high risk because of medical factors, familial risk, or exposure to teratogens. On identification of a heart defect, pregnancy termination can be offered to the mother if this is indicated. Genetic counseling can also be given. Neither preventive method is likely to have a marked impact on the incidence without population screening, which may not be warranted at present without additional understanding of the natural history of heart defects in utero, as well as the sensitivity and specificity of fetal echocardiography. Moreover, the impact of gene-nutrient and gene-environment interactions needs to be explored, given the burgeoning knowledge of chromosomal anomalies in congenital heart disease.

chapter 103

Embryology of Congenital Heart Disease

Adriana C. Gittenberger-de Groot, Monique R. M. Jongbloed, Marco C. DeRuiter, Margot M. Bartelings, and Robert E. Poelmann

Definition

- Normal and abnormal development of the heart are discussed in the context of their study in the era of molecular biology.

Key Features

- The myocardial heart tube, developing from a first and a second heart field, shows segments and transitional zones that, after looping and septation, result in a four-chambered organ with pulmonary and systemic circulations containing valves that direct blood flow, a conduction system for impulse generation, and a coronary vascular system for nutritional support.
- These developmental events are regulated by genes with complete interrelationships that cannot be regarded as isolated entities.

Clinical Implications

- Genetic therapy for the prevention or treatment of congenital heart disease is unlikely for some time, because of the complexities of gene interactions in these conditions.

Study of both normal and abnormal heart development benefits greatly from our evolving knowledge of developmental biology and the genes that have regulating roles. In this chapter, studies that use molecular biological approaches are referred to when they are considered to reveal basic mechanisms for normal or abnormal development. However, our expectations need to be modulated, because interactions in heart development involve gene complexes located on more than one chromosome. In this regard, most congenital heart abnormalities fall within the category of a multifactorial background, implying involvement of both genetic and environmental factors. This explains the variable expression of the severity of the malformations encountered within families with the same genetic background. To understand the pathogenesis of congenital heart disease, it is convenient to group the malformations in clusters that might involve common mechanisms, although regrouping might be necessary in the light of increasing knowledge gained from molecular biology research.

EMBRYONIC ORIGIN OF CARDIAC TISSUE

The heart is derived from two parallel cardiogenic zones that develop within the splanchnic mesoderm at the anterior part of the embryo. These zones, which at an early stage express cardiac-specific genes such as *Nkx2.5* and *GATA4-6*, will fuse in the midline to form the substrate for the cardiomyocytes of the primary heart tube. As early as the cardiogenic plate stage, gene patterns reveal that there is a future atrial (posterior) and ventricular (anterior) region.

This cardiogenic tissue envelops the precursors of the endocardium, which are for the greater part derived from a similar source as the remaining endothelial cells of the embryo that are recruited for vascular development (Fig. 103.1).[1] The resulting heart tube is connected to the developing pharyngeal arch arteries cranially and the omphalomesenteric veins caudally.

LOOPING OF THE HEART TUBE

The human cardiac tube grows and starts to pulsate by peristaltic movements at about the third week of development. These combined events modulate the looping process (Figs. 103.2 and 103.4). They also regulate the disappearance of the central part of the dorsal mesocardium that connects the heart tube to the dorsal wall of the embryo. The resulting opening allows a left-right connection in the pericardial cavity that will persist as the inner curvature (or sinus transversus) of the fully developed heart.

The looping program is regulated by a cascade of genes that are basic for the left-right programming of the embryo. These genes include, among others, *dynein*, *inversion*, *nodal*, *sonic hedgehog*, *bone morphogenetic protein*, *activin*, and *Pitx2*. The exact interactions are still unclear, but are based on an intricate system in which inhibition of active genes plays an important part.[2] Experiments in which these genes are manipulated reveal disorganization of the looping process.[3] The normal program leads to a rightward looping of the heart. Disturbance of these regulatory genes is followed by random looping and, in a number of cases, reversed looping to the left. Such abnormal looping does not primarily lead to dextrocardia, for example, but falls within the category of ventricular inversion. We are referring here to primary looping, in which the heart tube bends to either the right or the left. The fine tuning of this looping process, in which the cardiac outflow tract is brought in front of the atria with eventual wedging of the aorta in between the atrioventricular orifices, requires other mechanisms, among which is remodeling of the inner curvature (see Figs. 103.2 and 103.4).

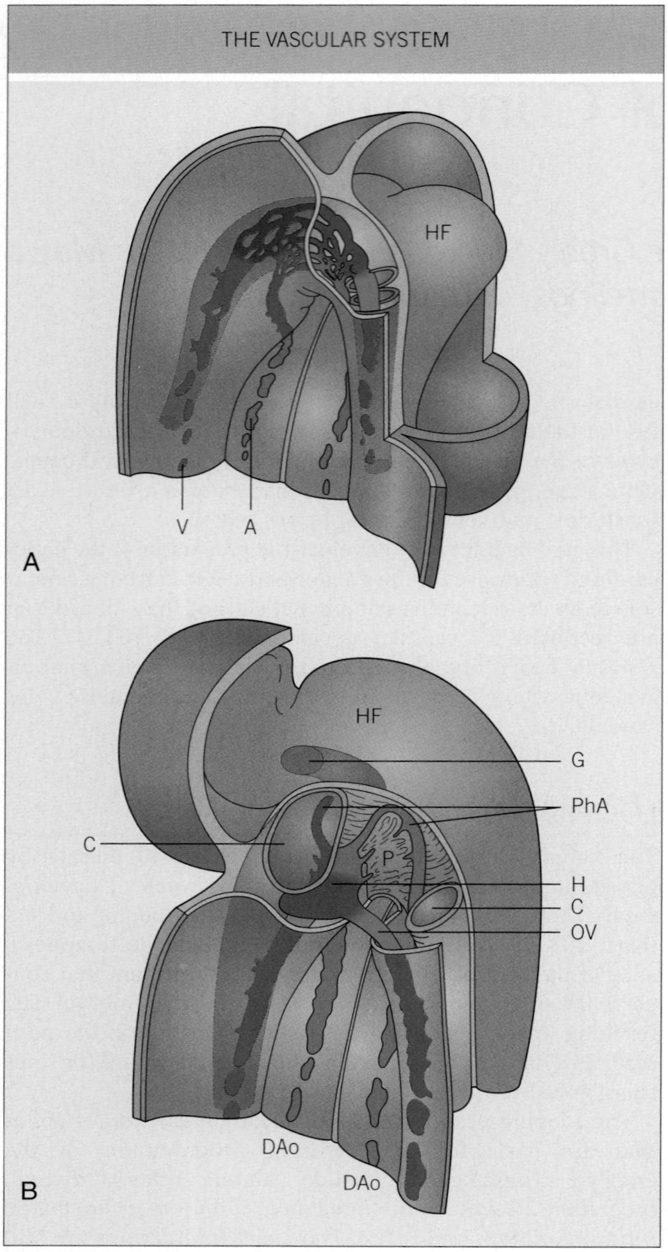

Figure 103.1 The vascular system, consisting of endothelium-lined blood vessels and the cardiac precursor, develops in the splanchnic mesoderm. A, The endothelial precursors merge to form a venous (V) and an arterial (A) network. **B,** After folding of the embryo, the heart region (H) becomes ventrally positioned. The endothelial network in this H (endocardium) becomes incorporated within the myocardium of the cardiac mesoderm. The omphalomesenteric veins (OV) enter the venous pole of the heart, while at the arterial pole the symmetric pharyngeal arch arteries (PhA) connect to the bilateral dorsal aortae (DAo) that run alongside the gut (G). C, coelomic cavity; HF, head fold.

FIRST AND SECOND HEART FIELD AND DEVELOPMENT OF THE SEGMENTS AND TRANSITIONAL ZONES WITHIN THE HEART TUBE

Recent data are consistent in that the primary heart tube, derived from the first heart field, consists of a small atrial part, an atrioventricular canal, and a primitive left ventricle (see Figs. 103.2 to 103.4). Both molecular data[4] and cell-tracing studies[5] have confirmed that a second heart field, located in the splanchnic mesoderm dorsal of the primary heart tube, is responsible for secondary lengthening of the heart tube at both the arterial (outflow) and sinus venosus (inflow) ends (see Fig. 103.2). Fig. 103.3 shows the still confusing nomenclature. At the outflow tract the terms *anterior heart field* and *secondary heart field* are used,[6] whereas at the inflow tract the term *posterior heart field* was introduced[7] to describe the sinus venosus myocardium precursors in the dorsal mesocardium connecting to the venous pole of the heart. The emerging data are highly relevant for the understanding of timing and development of outflow tract and inflow tract malformations.

Initially, the primary myocardial tube is lined by cardiac jelly on the inside, over its full length. During growth this cardiac jelly disappears or is remodeled into endocardial cushions (atrioventricular canal and outflow tract). In the heart tube we distinguish segments and transitional zones. The segments are the developing ballooning atria and ventricles, whereas the transitional zones are discerned in those parts that bear endocardial cushions (atrioventricular ring and ventriculo-arterial ring) and in those parts that are devoid of cushion tissue, such as the primary fold between the primitive left and right ventricle and the sinoatrial ring between the sinus venosus and the developing atrial segment (see Fig. 103.4).

It is essential to appreciate that, after looping, the transitional zones coalesce in the inner curvature of the heart tube. The cushion-bearing transitional zones will take part in septation and valve formation. The primary fold and the sinoatrial ring are essential for the development of the cardiac conduction system.

SEPTATION OF THE HEART

Adequate septation requires an intricate adjustment and alignment of segments and transitional zones.

Atrial Septation and Sinus Venosus Contribution

On the basis of recent data on the contribution of the posterior heart field to the sinus venosus (see Figs. 103.3 and 103.4), we have come to the conclusion that the dorsal wall of both right and left atrium including the primary atrial septum are derived from sinus venosus myocardium. The lower rim of the primary septum, which will form the valve of the foramen ovale, has a cushion-like structure, the so-called mesenchymal cap, that continues dorsally into the inferior atrioventricular cushion and the mesenchyme of the dorsal mesocardium, also called the spina vestibuli. This tissue of the mesenchymal cap fuses with the atrioventricular cushions and with components of the sinus venosus to close off the primary interatrial foramen. The primary septum develops fenestrations that coalesce to form the ostium secundum. The ostium secundum is bordered on the right side by the limbus. The limbus forms the free rim of the muscular septum secundum, which consists of two components.

- The superior and anterior extension are produced by infolding of the right-sided dorsal atrial wall. Immunohistochemical data point toward the fused left and right venous valves as being the free rim of this fold, which runs to the anterior part of the tricuspid orifice.

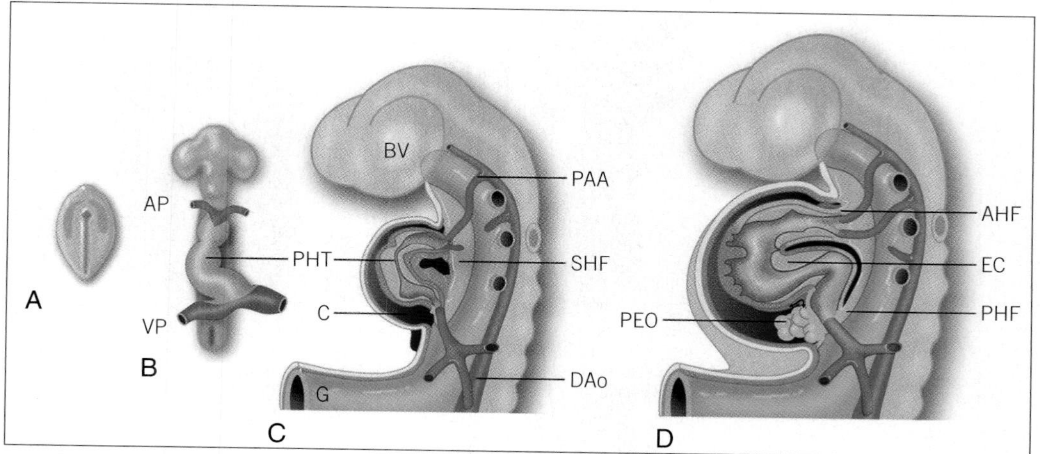

Figure 103.2 A, Schematic representation of the bilateral cardiogenic plates, which are derived from the splanchnic mesoderm. The plates fuse and form a primary heart tube (PHT) (**B**) that starts looping to the right. **C,** The PHT (brown) is lined on the inside by cardiac jelly (blue). The yellow area behind the PHT depicts the second heart field (SHF) that in later stages contributes myocardium to both the arterial and venous poles of the heart (yellow myocardium in **D**). **D,** The SHF can be divided into the anterior and posterior heart fields (AHF and PHF, respectively). The yellow lobulated structure that protrudes into the pericardial cavity at the venous pole of the heart is the proepicardial organ (PEO). AP, arterial pole; BV, brain ventricles; C, coelomic cavity; DAo, dorsal aorta; EC, endocardial cushion; G, gut; PAA, pharyngeal arch artery; VP, venous pole.

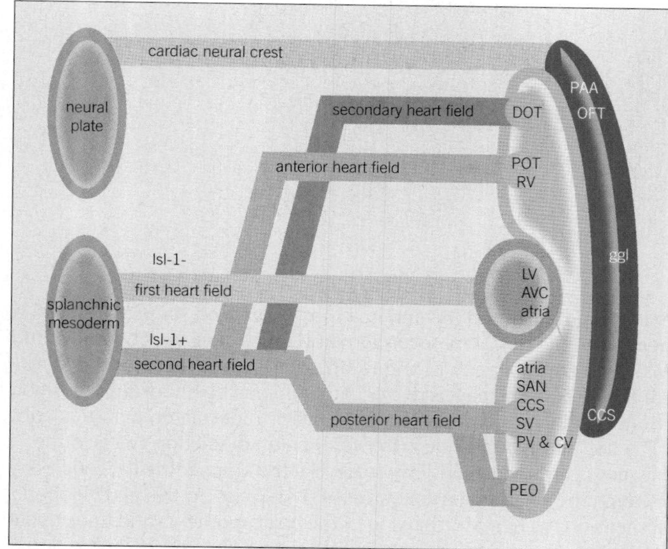

Figure 103.3 Schematic representation of the first and second heart field contribution to cardiac development. The primary heart tube is depicted in brown, and the secondary added myocardium that is derived from the second heart field is in yellow. Nomenclature is confusing, because the second heart field is divided into a *secondary heart field* (that contributes to the distal outflow tract [DOT]) and an *anterior heart field* (that contributes to the right ventricle [RV] and proximal outflow tract [POT]) at the anterior pole of the heart. At the venous pole of the heart, myocardium is added from the *posterior heart field*, which contributes to the posterior wall of the atria, the sinoatrial node (SAN), the myocardium of the sinus venosus (SV), pulmonary veins (PV), and cardinal veins (CV), including the coronary sinus, and probably part of the central conduction system (CCS). The posterior heart field also contributes to the proepicardial organ (PEO), which is the source of the epicardium and epicardium-derived cells. Cardiac neural crest cells (dark blue) migrate to the heart and enter the heart both at the arterial and venous pole. AVC, atrioventricular canal; ggl, ganglions; LV, left ventricle; OFT, outflow tract; PAA, pharyngeal arch arteries.

- The posterior and lower part of the septum secundum, forming the basis of the atrial septum, is composed of posterior heart field–derived sinus venosus myocardium (Figs. 103.4 and 103.5), extending in the wall of the coronary sinus and encompassing the pulmonary orifices in the posterior wall of the left atrium.

The above-mentioned findings have both morphogenetic and clinical implications. Morphogenetic implications arise from the recent findings that most of the smooth dorsal wall of both right and left atria as well as the atrial septal components are derived from sinus venosus myocardium. The atrial appendages develop through a ballooning process that is regulated by the balance of *Tbx* genes.[8] It is important to recognize the prominent role of tissue derived from sinus venosus for understanding the development of secundum atrial septal defects and sinus venosus defects. This becomes even more relevant if one considers that the sinus venosus myocardium forms an important basis for the formation of both the sinoatrial conduction system and possibly part of the atrioventricular conduction system. The novel finding that this posterior heart field–derived myocardium is *Nkx2.5* negative[7] sheds new light on the finding that the *Nkx2.5* gene is mutated in familial atrial septal defect and raises interesting questions as to the existence of functions of this gene other than early cardiomyocyte programming.[9]

Aortic and Tricuspid Orifice Connections and Formation of the Ventricles

On both sides of the primary ring that borders the primary interventricular foramen, the heart tube develops a ventricular segment that stands out by having a trabeculated inner myocardial wall and an outer compact layer. The left segment, which is derived from the primary heart tube and is positioned directly below the atrioventricular canal, is initially larger than its right counterpart, which derives from

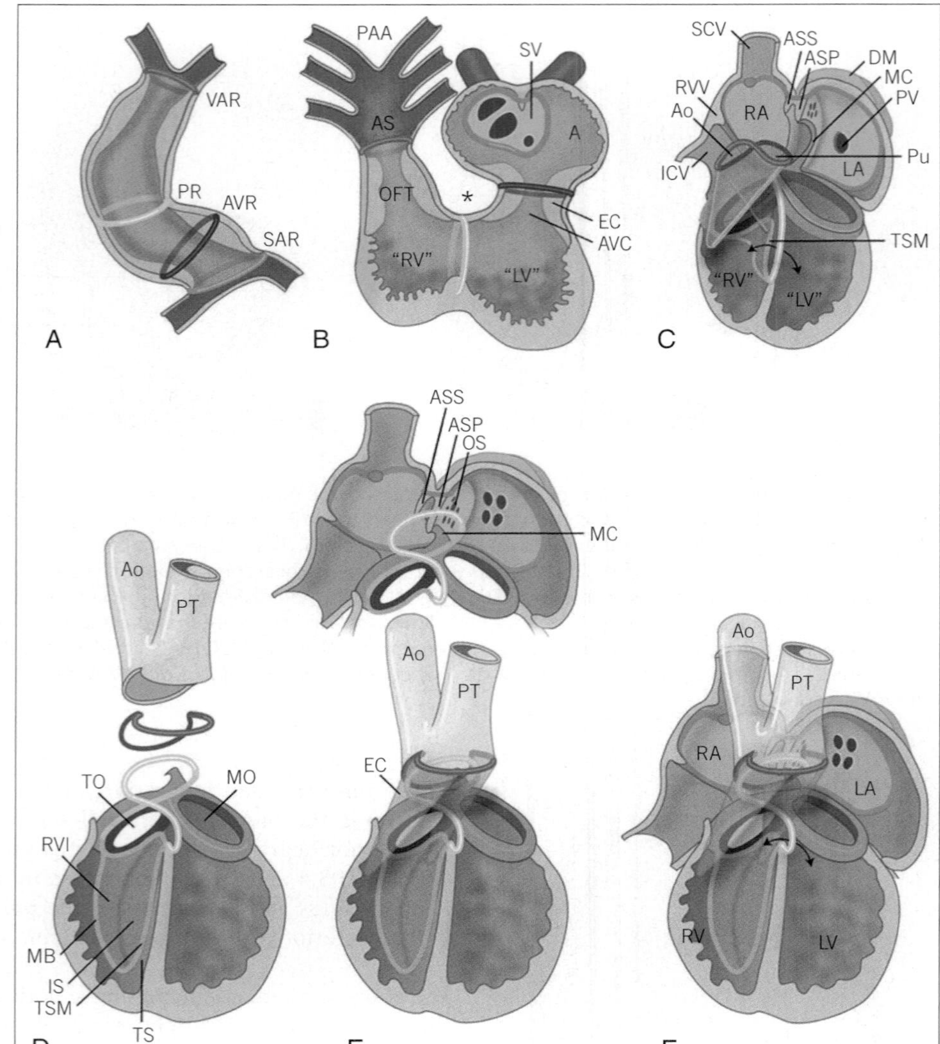

Figure 103.4 Schematic representation of the primary heart tube just after looping has started (**A**) and in a more advanced stage (**B**), showing the various segments and transitional zones. The sinus venosus (SV) is embedded in the dorsal mesocardium and receives all venous inflow into the heart. The borderline with the atrial segment (A), which is still very small, is called the sinoatrial ring (SAR), which, together with the SV, is considered to be a transitional zone. The atrioventricular ring (AVR) surrounds the atrioventricular canal (AVC) that is lined by endocardial cushion (EC) tissue. The primitive left ventricle ("LV") lined by trabeculae is already present and is separated from the smaller trabeculated primitive right ventricle ("RV") by a transitional zone referred to as the primary ring (PR). The last transitional zone is the ventriculo-arterial ring (VAR) in the ventricular outlet (OFT), with a proximal and a distal part. This zone is lined by endocardial cushion (EC) tissue, like the atrioventricular canal. The OFT connects to the mesenchymal vascular wall of the aortic sac (AS) from which the pharyngeal arch arteries (PAA) arise. In this early looped heart, all transitional zones meet in the inner curvature (*). **C,** A more three-dimensional schematic drawing of the heart segments and transitional zones after looping and initiation of atrial and ventricular septation. The SAR forms the boundary between sinus venosus and atrium. In the dorsal wall, sinus venosus tissue is continuous with the mesenchyme of the dorsal mesocardium (DM). The continuation of atrioventricular EC over the basal part of the primary atrial septum (ASP) (also visible in [**E**]), is called the mesenchymal cap (MC). In the sinus venosus part of the right atrium (RA), there is a connection with the inferior caval vein (ICV) and the superior caval vein (SCV) being bordered by the right venous valve (RVV) and the left venous valve (see Fig. 103.11). The latter has become part of the atrial septum. The coronary sinus (not shown) is also of sinus venosus origin and connects to the RA. In the left atrium (LA), the pulmonary veins (PV) are encircled by tissue from the SAR. From the atrial segment, the primitive left ventricle ("LV") is reached through the atrioventricular canal (AVC) lined by the EC tissue. The primitive left ventricle connects to the primitive right ventricle ("RV") through the PR. The saddle-shaped arterial orifice (green ring) shows the future aortic (Ao) and pulmonary (Pu) sides. During formation of the definitive RV and LV, major changes take place. **D,** Remodeling and division of the primary ring is essential for the formation of the right ventricular inlet (RVI) and positioning of the right side of the AVC above this RVI. This is the tricuspid orifice (TO); the mitral orifice (MO) remains above the LV. Formation of the TO and MO is achieved by fusion of the atrioventricular EC. The main trabeculated part of the ventricular septum, the trabeculated septum (TS), derives from the anterior part of the PR, whereas the inlet septum (IS) and the cavity of the RVI are formed by expansion of the posterior part of the PR. The borderline between RVI and trabeculated part of the right ventricle in the mature RV is still visible as the trabecula septomarginalis (TSM) and the moderator band (MB). **E** and **F**, In the OFT, the EC (pale blue) fuses to separate the left and right ventricular OFT. In this way an OFT septum is formed. In a normal heart this is recognizable as the muscular subpulmonary infundibulum. In normal septation, neural crest cells migrate into the cushions. At the ventricular level, the primary interventricular foramen (*double arrow*) is still patent but will be closed off with completion of OFT septation and connection of the aorta to the LV. At the atrial level, the primary interatrial foramen will close by fusion of the MC with the atrioventricular EC. This area is continuous with the DM and SV tissue. In the ASP, fenestrations develop that will form the ostium secundum (OS). The fusion of LVV and RVV anteriorly, and an infolding of the roof of the atrium, will form the atrial septum secundum (ASS). The free rim of the latter forms the limbus of the foramen ovale (see Fig. 103.5).

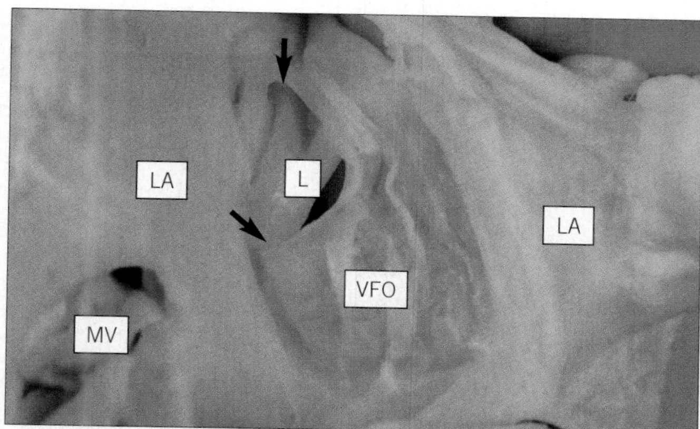

Figure 103.5 View into the left atrium (LA) depicting the attachment points (*arrows*) of the valve of the foramen ovale (VFO). The limbus fossae ovalis (L) is visible through the patent foramen. MV, mitral valve.

the second heart field (see Figs. 103.2 to 103.4). These dimensions will change even further with the late development of a right ventricular inflow tract[10] and a left ventricular outflow tract.

For correct development of the inflow and outflow tracts of the ventricles, it is essential for the aortic orifice to become connected to the left ventricle and the tricuspid orifice to the right ventricle. In this process the primary fold is remodeled (see Fig. 103.4). The aortic orifice achieves a wedged position between the tricuspid and mitral orifices and becomes connected to the left ventricle. A small part of the embryonic outflow tract is added to the primitive left ventricle to form the definitive left ventricle.[11] This process is influenced by shortening and remodeling of the inner curvature of the heart, preceded by looping. If one or both processes are disturbed, the aorta remains too far to the right and unwedged, in extreme cases resulting in a double-outlet right ventricle with an obligatory ventricular septal defect.

A similar process holds for the tricuspid orifice, which should become positioned above the right ventricular inflow tract. Initially, the trabeculated primitive right ventricle is very small. The inflow tract of the right ventricle develops secondarily by expansion of the primary fold in the posterior part of the inner curvature. Subsequently, the tricuspid orifice becomes positioned above this slit-like gully that will develop into a right ventricular inflow tract.[10,11] If this process does not proceed normally, as a result of abnormal remodeling of the inner curvature or insufficient looping, the tricuspid orifice may persist in an overriding position or even remain above the main body of the left ventricle, resulting in a double-inlet left ventricle. In that case, the expansion of the inlet of the "right ventricle" has become positioned above the left ventricle.

Septation of Ventricles

From the previous description, it becomes clear that ventricular septation is not simply the formation of a muscular septum between both ventricles, but that correct looping, wedging, and remodeling of the inner curvature are required to get the aortic and tricuspid orifices into position. The main body of the ventricular septum develops from the primary fold as the left ventricle and the right ventricular inlet expand (for mechanism, see previous section). The process of septum formation also requires compaction of the trabeculations that are part of the ventricular myocardial tube. Abnormalities in ventricular septation that lead to ventricular septal defects can be explained by the various developmental mechanisms that are involved. Insufficient progress of the compaction process can leave the myocardium in a spongy state, also referred to as noncompaction. Recent data point toward a role for epicardial derived cells in formation of the compact myocardial layer (reviewed in Lie-Venema and colleagues[12]). Other transgenic mouse models show ventricular septal defects that relate to abnormal alignment of segments and transitional zones, such as the ventricular septal defects in double-outlet and double-inlet ventricles and defects resulting from malaligned outflow tract septation.[11] In the latter category, failure of fusion of the endocardial cushions of both outflow tract and the atrioventricular canal is involved, so that the majority of such defects have boundaries that encompass a fibrous component and can therefore be designated as perimembranous defects.

The primary ring remains the boundary between inflow and outflow in each definitive ventricle. In the right ventricle, this boundary is visible as the trabecula septomarginalis, the moderator band, and the ventriculo-infundibular fold (Fig. 103.6). The remaining part of the initially muscular primary fold encircles the left outflow tract on the boundary of the aortic and mitral valves to complete the circle by ending at the left ventricular septum at the site where it connects again to the trabecula septomarginalis in the right ventricle (see Fig. 103.4). In a normal heart, the left ventricular part of the primary fold in the left ventricle cannot be distinguished as a separate structure.

Outflow Tract Septation

The myocardium of the outflow tract is derived from the second heart field (see Fig. 103.3) and is lined on the inside by proximal and distal endocardial outflow tract cushions. The outflow tract is septated by the fusion and subsequent myocardialization of the proximal part of the outflow tract ridges.[11] This results in a relatively long subpulmonary infundibulum that fuses with the remaining part of the ventricular septum in the area of the membranous septum. The lower muscle boundary of the infundibular septum forms part of the crista supraventricularis, which connects the derivatives of the primary fold: the trabecula septomarginalis and the ventriculo-infundibular fold. Because of the saddle-shaped embryonic arterial orifice level and the angle in the fully developed heart between the two arterial orifices (see Fig. 103.4), in a normal heart the posterior wall of the muscular infundibulum is not a true septum. For this reason we have chosen to refer to the outflow tract septation as a matter of separation of right (long) and left (short) ventricular outflow tracts.[11] In malalignment ventricular septal defects, the outflow tract septum can be discerned as a structure between the two arterial orifices that stands out as an actual septum between the right and left ventricular outflow tract (Fig. 103.7). The size and composition of this outflow tract septum can vary from thick and muscular to thin and fibrous. Animal experiments show that this is the result of variable myocardialization.[13] The finding that second heart field myocardium is important for outflow tract septation being linked to an essential function of *Tbx1*[14] has taken away

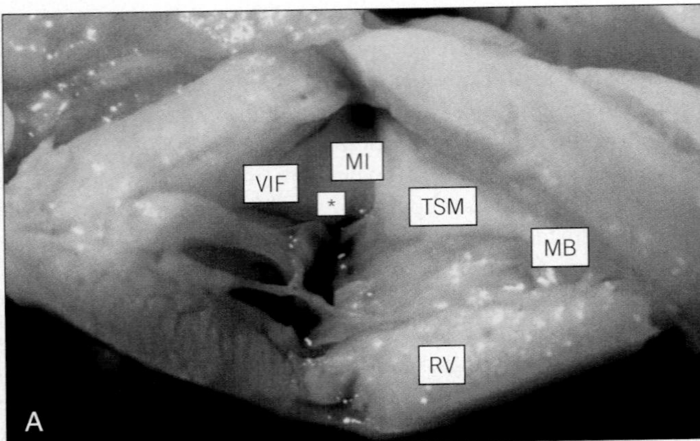

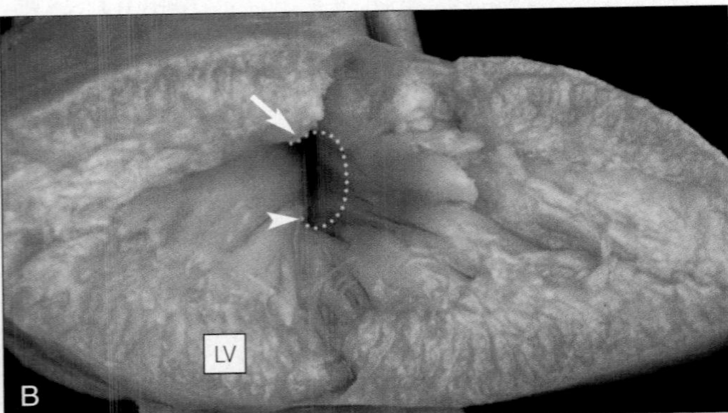

Figure 103.6 Septation of ventricles and boundaries between the inlet and outlet part of the ventricles. A, View into the normal right ventricle (RV) of a 17-week fetal human heart, where the following landmarks (see Fig. 103.3) are visible. The leaflets of the tricuspid valve are confined within the RV inlet that is bordered by the trabecula septomarginalis (TSM), the moderator band (MB), and the ventriculoinfundibular fold (VIF). The last has merged with the lower rim of the muscular subpulmonary infundibulum (MI), being the crista supraventricularis (*). **B,** View into the left ventricle (LV) of a 21-week fetal heart. The borderline of the primary foramen is indicated by a dotted line. The arrow connects to the VIF in the RV and the arrowhead to the TSM.

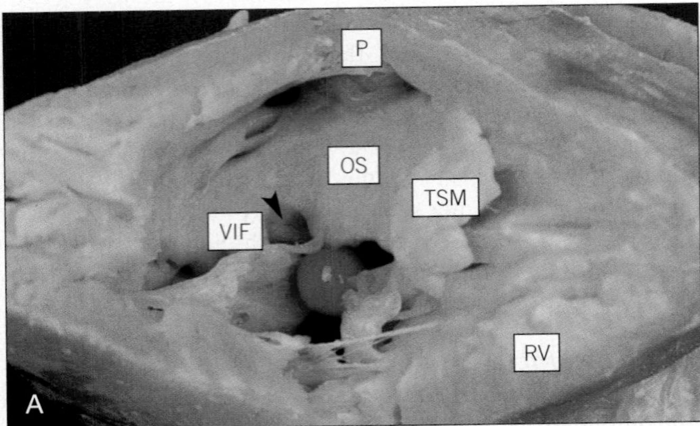

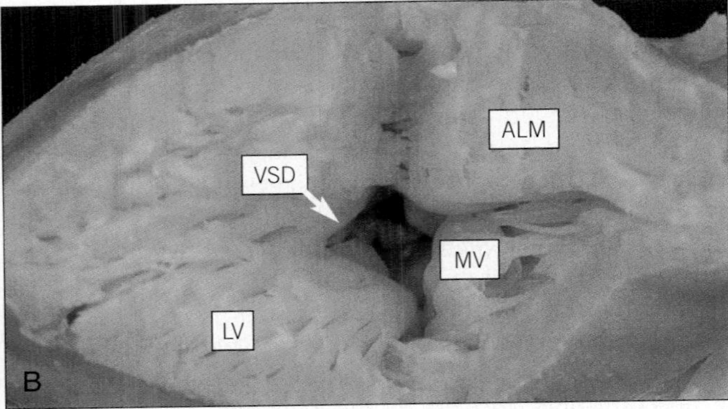

Figure 103.7 Ventricular septal defect. A, View into the right ventricle (RV) of a 28-week fetal human heart with a ventricular septal defect (VSD; site indicated by red probe). The aortic valve leaflets (*arrowhead*) are visible through the VSD. There is malalignment of the outlet septum (OS), with an anterior displacement with regard to the ventriculoinfundibular fold (VIF). The connection with the trabecula septomarginalis (TSM) is normal. This type of subaortic VSD does not lead to subpulmonary stenosis. P, pulmonary valve leaflets. **B,** View into the left ventricle (LV) of the same specimen, with a remarkably thickened anterolateral muscle (ALM) bundle being an LV part of the primary fold. MV, aortic leaflet of mitral valve.

the emphasis on the neural crest as common denominator of outflow tract malformations, as was for many years suggested for malformations linked to the 22q11 syndrome. The myocardialization process of the outflow tract endocardial cushions is most probably still linked to neural crest cells that migrate into the outflow tract cushions as mesenchymal cells.[15] These cells form the basis of the so-called condensed mesenchyme of the aortopulmonary septum, being essential for septation of the arterial orifice, and the short stretch of the aortic sac.

Formation of the ascending aorta and pulmonary trunk from the aortic sac requires very limited septation, because the distance to be bridged by the septum in the aortic sac is very small, and because the saddle shape of the arterial orifice level results in a relatively long ascending aorta and a very short pulmonary trunk that gives rise to the two small pulmonary arteries immediately above the orifice level (Fig. 103.8a). During fetal and later development, the length of the pulmonary trunk will increase. The embryonic configuration is seen in some heart malformations, for example, in the hypoplastic left heart syndrome, which features a very short pulmonary trunk. Further information on aortic arch formation is provided in a separate paragraph (see page 1401, under *Aortic Arch System*. Also see Figure 103.13). In case of complete or partial absence of outflow tract septation, a common arterial trunk results. Developmentally, this phenomenon is linked to an abnormal contribution of second heart field myocardium as well as neural crest cells to the outflow tract.[16]

ATRIOVENTRICULAR AND SEMILUNAR VALVE DEVELOPMENT

Both valve complexes and the chordae tendineae are derived from the endocardial cushions that are remodeled from thick spongy structures into thin valve leaflets. The cushions already function as valves during the peristaltic pumping stage of the heart, but this is insufficient for the increased mechanical forces that are generated in a fully beating heart. The characteristics of the tricuspid and mitral valve are the result of the left-right asymmetry of both ventricles with regard to trabecular and papillary muscle formation.

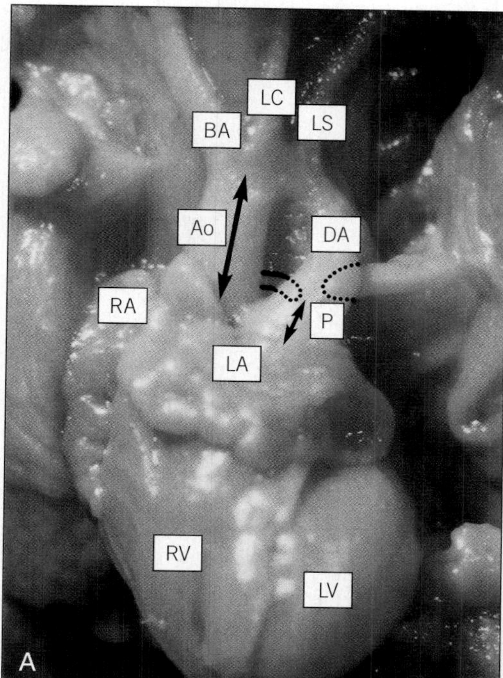

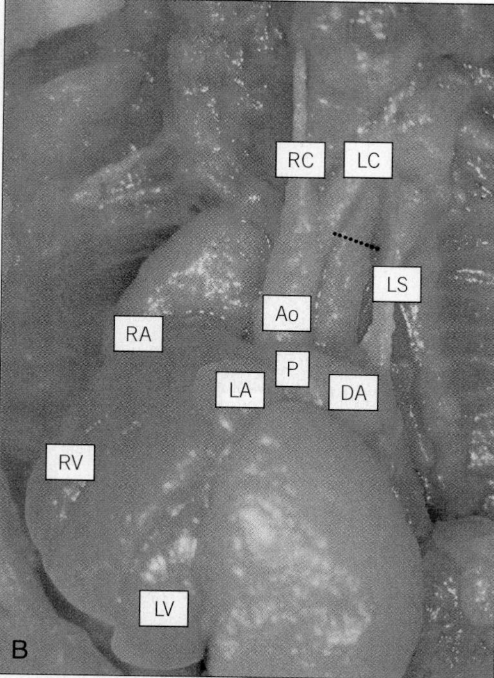

Figure 103.8 Interrupted aortic arch. A, Ventral view of an 11-week human fetal heart. There is at this stage still a marked discrepancy between the length of the ascending aorta (Ao, *long double-arrowhead line*) and the short pulmonary trunk (P, *short double-arrowhead line*). Both left and right pulmonary arteries arise very close above the P orifice level (*dotted lines*). **B,** Ventral view of a 10.5-week human fetal heart with an interruption of the B segment of the aortic arch (*dotted line*) positioned between the left carotid artery (LC) and the left subclavian artery (LS). BA, brachiocephalic artery; DA, ductus arteriosus; LA, left atrium; LV, left ventricle; RA, right atrium; RC, right carotid artery; RV, right ventricle.

Study of mouse and human embryos with immunohistochemical techniques yielded new insights into both normal and abnormal atrioventricular valve morphogenesis,[17] for example, parachute mitral valves, which should be seen as a highly asymmetric attached valve.[18] Recent investigations of our group point toward abnormalities of the atrioventricular cushions as the basis for atrioventricular septal defects and straddling valves.

The semilunar valves develop from the distal part of the endocardial outflow tract ridges. In mice and humans there are two main ridges, which are separated by the condensed mesenchyme of the aortopulmonary septum, and two smaller intercalated cushions. The ridges are remodeled into three semilunar valve leaflets in each orifice. The valve structure is comparable to that of the atrioventricular valves, but not to that of the adjoining elastic aortic or pulmonary vessel wall. Absence of outflow tract septation as seen in persistent truncus arteriosus does not hamper formation of valve leaflets. Although these valves may be abnormal in size or number, their morphogenesis and structure are essentially normal. This makes semilunar valve formation not primarily dependent on extracardiac contributions, such as neural crest cells. Current views are in favor of hemodynamic forces that might play a remodeling role.[19] Morphogenetic data derived from transgenic experiments show that certain transcription factors such as nuclear factor NFAtc are important for valve histogenesis. In the human population, absence of pulmonary valve leaflets can be encountered in neonates in combination with the 22q11 deletion syndrome[20] and mutations in the *Notch* gene have been described in case of bicuspid aortic valve.[21] The absence of an aortic semilunar valve is not compatible with late fetal life. Absence of atrioventricular valves is extremely rare in human neonates. It might be assumed that this malformation will lead to early embryonic death comparable to that seen in mouse and avian embryos.[13]

EXTRACARDIAC CELLULAR CONTRIBUTORS: NEURAL CREST CELLS AND EPICARDIAL CELLS

Cell tracing experiments have revealed the contributions of various extracardiac components to the developing heart. These cells are added to the heart tube, mostly in relation to the myocardium that is added through the second heart field. The main cell types involved are the ectomesenchymal neural crest cells originating from the neural plate, and the epicardial cells that derive from the coelomic wall and are considered by us to form a nonmyocardial population of the posterior heart field (see Fig. 103.3).

Manipulation of these cells by ablation or altered genetic information (through, for example, viral gene transfer) shows how these cells are essential in a number of already mentioned aspects of heart development.

Neural Crest Cells

Neural crest cells or ectomesenchymal cells can be traced to various parts of the embryo, including face, thymus, thoracic great vessels, and the heart. For cardiac development it is essential that these cells differentiate into the neurons of the autonomic nervous system, smooth muscle cells of

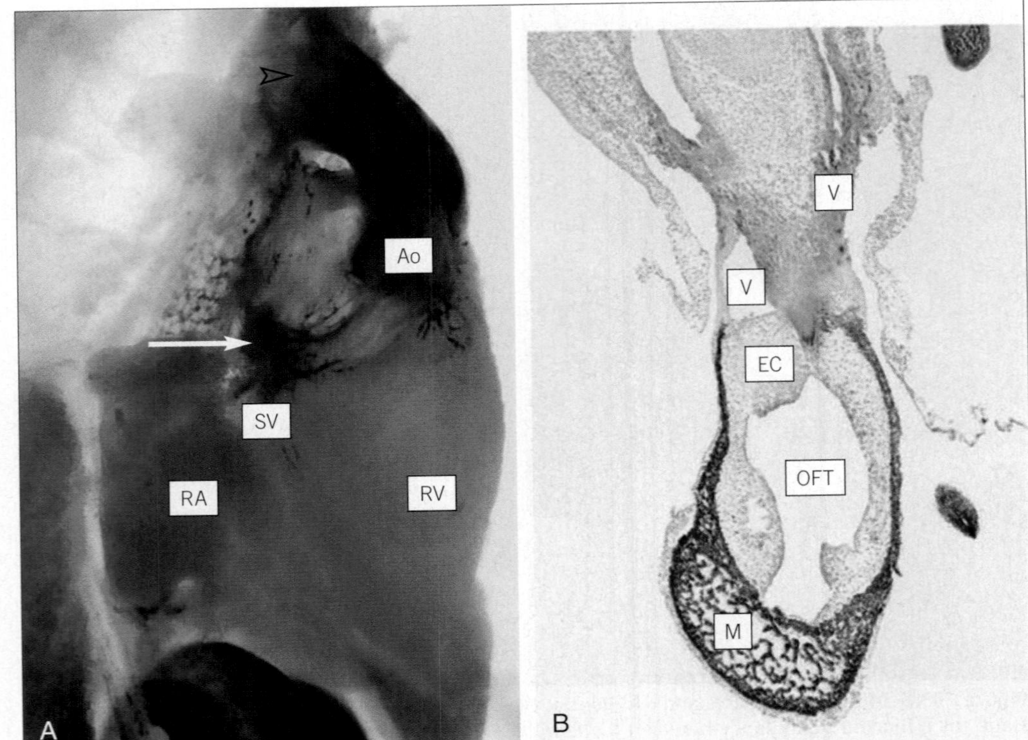

Figure 103.9 Neural crest cells. A, Right-sided view of a heart from a chicken embryo, stained using a retroviral lacZ construct to trace neural crest cells (NCC, blue). NCC can be seen at the arterial pole. The arrowhead points at the boundary between the lacZ positive and lacZ negative smooth muscle cells of the pharyngeal arch arteries and descending aorta. Neural crest cells also enter the heart at the venous pole (*arrow*). Ao, aorta; RA, right atrium; RV, right ventricle; SV, sinus venosus. (Modified from Poelmann RE, Gittenberger-de Groot AC. A subpopulation of apoptosis-prone cardiac neural crest cells targets to the venous pole: multiple functions in heart development? Dev Biol 1999;207:271-286.) **B,** Section through the outflow tract (OFT) of an HH27 heart, stained with anti–muscle actin (brown) for the myocardium (M). The blue cells derived from the NCC are present at and below orifice level in the OFT. EC, endocardial cushions; V, vessels.

many great arteries (except right and left pulmonary arteries, subclavian and distal part of the coronary arteries) and a mesenchymal population that migrates into the outflow tract and the inflow tract (Fig. 103.9).[22] It has become possible to study the contribution of neural crest cells to the heart, in so-called neural crest reporter mice. An example is the *Wnt1*-Cre reporter mouse, in which neural crest cells that once expressed this gene can be followed during their migration and differentiation in the embryo.[23] The results are highly comparable to what we have described in the chicken embryo, including an inflow tract population. The role of neuronal crest cells is still not fully appreciated especially in relation to the second heart field myocardial population with which it closely interacts. Experimental studies have revealed an influence on myocardialization of the cushion tissue that is essential for septation, differentiation of the atrioventricular conduction system, and valve histogenesis.[11] It is remarkable that most of the neural crest cells that enter the heart as mesenchymal cells go into apoptosis.

Epicardium-Derived Cells

The epicardium of the heart derives from the proepicardial organ. The epicardial cells migrate over the myocardium and thereafter go into a process of epithelial to mesenchymal transformation. The resulting epicardium-derived cells (EPDCs) also invade the myocardium. These cells differentiate into interstitial cardiac fibroblasts and into smooth muscle cells and fibroblasts of the coronary vasculature (Fig. 103.10).[24] They are important for the differentiation and formation of the compact myocardium, the atrioventricular (and possibly) the semilunar valves, the coronary arterial wall, and the Purkinje fibers of the conduction system.[12] Experiments in which outgrowth of epicardium-derived cells is inhibited show severely immature hearts with a thin compact myocardial layer, delayed looping, and absent septation. The experiments are embryolethal, because no coronary vascular system develops.[25] Because, under normal circumstances, the EPDCs provide a layer of subendocardial cells that later develop into fibroblasts, it might be speculated whether they are instrumental in the pathogenesis of endocardial fibroelastosis, which is triggered by hemodynamic stress (e.g., in some forms of the hypoplastic left heart syndrome), in addition to a genetically determined mechanism in familial forms of restrictive cardiomyopathy. There are now several indications from transgenic mouse models with defective epicardial-to-mesenchymal transformation that some forms of myocardial noncompaction might be the result of an epicardial instead of a myocardial problem.[12]

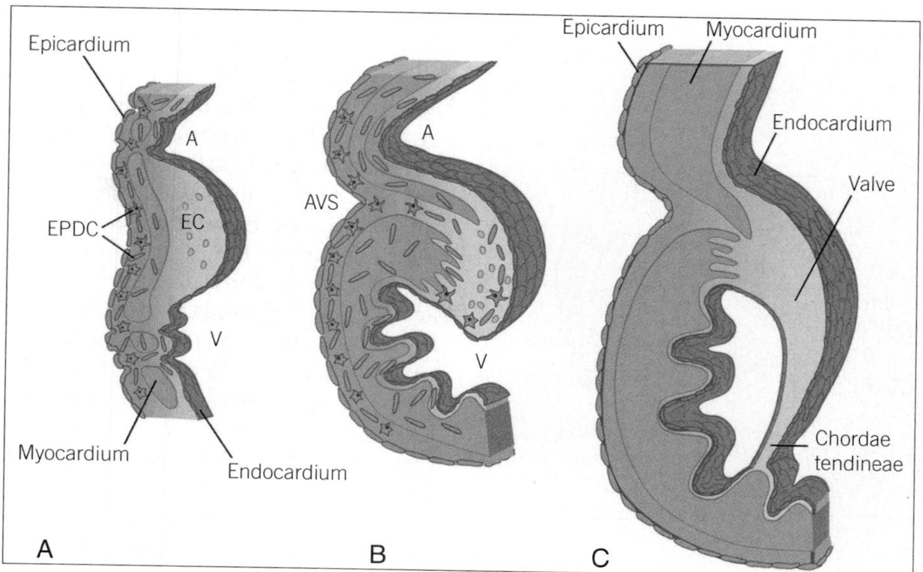

Figure 103.10 Schematic drawings of the contribution of the epicardium-derived cells (EPDCs) to myocardium and cushion tissue in early (**A**) and later (**B** and **C**) stages of development. EPDCs invade the subepicardial, myocardial, and subendocardial regions and contribute to the differentiation and architecture of the myocardium, the coronary vasculature, and the induction Purkinje fiber formation. Valve formation takes place after epithelial to mesenchymal transformation in the endocardial cushions (EC, see pink cells). EPDCs migrate into the EC and further contribute to addition of mesenchymal cells to the atrioventricular cushion tissue. The EC tissue will eventually differentiate into the fibrous valve leaflets and the chordae tendineae. A, atrium; AVS, atrioventricular sulcus; V, ventricle.

DEVELOPMENT OF THE CONDUCTION SYSTEM

The conduction system can be subdivided into a central conduction system and a peripheral Purkinje network (Fig. 103.11). Under normal circumstances, the central conduction system has sinoatrial and atrioventricular components that are connected through the atrioventricular node. Developmental data[26-28] show two main transitional zones that contribute to the formation of the central conduction system: the sinus venosus myocardium, including the sinoatrial transition; and the primary fold between the ventricular segments. The sinus venosus myocardium is initially laid down as a horseshoe-shaped Nkx2.5-negative myocardial band running along the right and left cardinal veins and encircling the pulmonary veins. It forms possibly a transient left sinoatrial node and the definitive right sinoatrial node.[7,29] The latter is connected by pathways with the right atrioventricular ring, which through developmental remodeling that includes formation of the right ventricular inflow tract, merges with part of the primary fold (see Fig. 103.4). In the sequence of their development, the following three right atrial pathways can be distinguished.

- An anterior bundle consisting of the fused right and left venous valves ends anteriorly on the right atrioventricular ring bundle behind the aortic root. This site is aligned with the position of an anterior node in some congenitally malformed hearts.
- The second pathway runs in the base of the right venous valve and is later positioned in the crista terminalis of the right atrium.
- The third pathway lies within the left venous valve and ends in the base of the sinus venosus–derived part of the atrial septum. The sinus venosus myocardium also encompasses the pulmonary veins and the coronary sinus.

The second two bundles connect to the posterior part of the right atrioventricular ring bundle, being the site of the posterior atrioventricular node, which is considered to be the regular atrioventricular node in a normal heart. This atrioventricular node connects, over the posterior part of the ventricular septum, with the common bundle or bundle of His, which splits into right and left bundle branches. Recently, a transgenic reporter mouse model was presented in which the CCS/lacZ fusion product delineates the complete cardiac conduction system.[28]

The tissue of the atrioventricular node has a dual origin, being derived from myocardium of both the sinus venosus and the primary fold.[7] It remains to be investigated whether the definitive atrioventricular node solely consists of the embryonic posterior node, or whether the anterior and the posterior anlagen fuse. This fusion is possible at the level of the sinus venosus myocardium, which runs from posterior to anterior.

These data provide an interesting insight into conduction system anomalies in which there is an anterior node or in cases with atrial automaticity with firing foci around the pulmonary veins and from other parts of the atrial embryonic pathways.

The trigger in the myocardium that is needed at the mentioned transitional zones to prompt their specialization into a functioning conduction system remains to be evaluated, but the discovery of a population of neural crest cells that enter through the venous pole into the heart provides a clue.

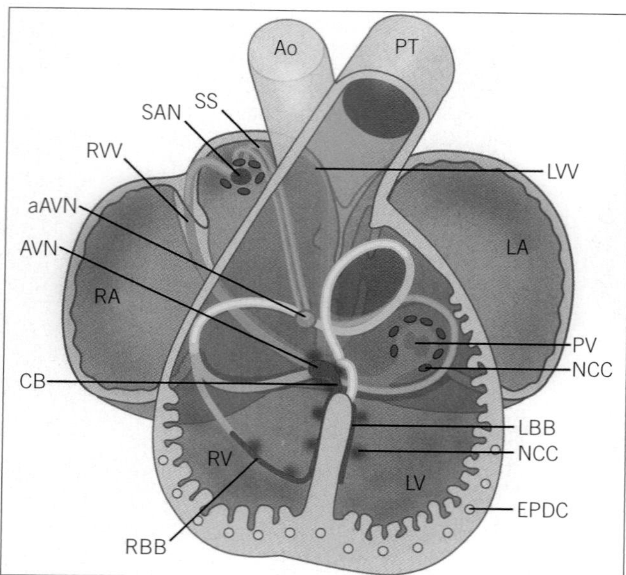

Figure 103.11 Embryonic parts of the conduction system derived from the sinus venosus and the primary fold (yellow). Additional embryonic structures, which disappear later on, are the internodal pathways (derived from the sinoatrial ring, which includes the right venous valve [RVV], the left venous valve [LVV], and the septum spurium [SS]), the myocardium around the coronary sinus and the pulmonary veins (PV), Bachman's bundle, and the right atrioventricular ring bundle that run dorsal from the aorta. The definitive conduction system consists of the sinoatrial node (SAN), the atrioventricular node (AVN), the common atrioventricular bundle (CB), the left bundle branch (LBB), and the right bundle branch (RBB), all indicated in red. It remains to be investigated whether the anterior atrioventricular node (aAVN), which is connected to the SAN by the anterior internodal pathway running in the SS, becomes part of the regular AVN or solely features as an embryonic structure in addition to persisting in some cardiac malformations. Neural crest cells (NCC) can be found in proximity to structures of the cardiac conduction system, both as precursors of the autonomic neuronal network (depicted in dark blue) and after apoptosis as possible inducing cells (depicted in shaded blue). Ao, aorta; EPDC, epicardium derived cell; LA, left atrium; LV, left ventricle; PT, pulmonary trunk; RA, right atrium; RV, right ventricle.

These neural crest cells specifically arrange themselves around the central conduction system and thereafter go into apoptosis.[22,30,31] We postulate that, as in the outflow tract, apoptosis has an active role in liberating substances that are important for myocardialization; we assume that neural crest cells might also influence the differentiation of the conduction system.

The Purkinje fiber network originates from myocardial fibers. Their differentiation seems to be dependent on induction signals from the EPDCs[12] as well as shear stress–mediated differentiation through coronary endothelium and endocardium.

CORONARY VASCULAR DEVELOPMENT

The development of the coronary vascular system is a relatively late process. It is notable that the oxygenation of the myocardium cannot sustain its function purely by diffusion from the blood flowing through the cavities. For the coronary system to develop, it is necessary to acquire a covering of the myocardial heart tube by epicardium.[24] This epicardium grows out from the proepicardial organ in the posterior heart field region (see Figs. 103.2 and 103.3). The atrioventricular groove and the inner curvature are reached first. From the inner curvature the other transitional zones are covered; the anterior part of the outflow tract is last to be encased. In the subepicardial space that is created, the endothelial cells of the coronary vasculature proliferate and form the template for the future coronary network. These endothelial cells are derived by sprouting from the sinus venosus and the liver sinusoids.[24] Initially, an endothelial network is formed that is in open connection only with the sinus venosus, resulting in a to-and-fro blood flow over the network (Fig. 103.12a). Thereafter the coronary network invaginates the aorta and the anterior part of the right atrium (Fig. 103.12b),[32] changing the direction of blood flow in the coronary system. This construction allows the blood to be pumped from the aorta, with direct shunting to the atrium. As soon as the coronary arteries connect to the aorta, a muscular media is formed. The media expands distally along the coronary arteries to the apex of the heart. During remodeling of the network, the veins and capillaries are

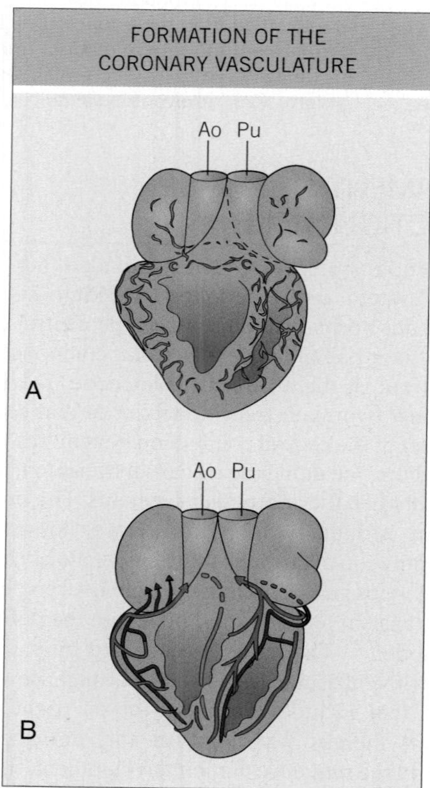

Figure 103.12 Formation of the coronary vasculature. A, An initial network of endothelial cells that line up to form a vascular network constitutes an atrioventricular and a periarterial ring. These vessels spread over the ventricles (more prominently dorsal) and grow into the myocardium. Only rarely are ventriculocoronary communications found. **B,** From the periarterial ring, the coronary network grows into the aorta and the right atrium, thus forming the main coronary artery connections and part of the coronary veins. The remaining coronary veins are in contact with the coronary sinus. The myocardial vascular network is remodeled into a system of arteries, veins, and connecting capillaries. Ao, aorta; Pu, pulmonary trunk.

formed also. Only much later, compared with the arteries, a few layers of smooth muscle cells are formed around the coronary veins. At the ostia where the coronary veins enter the atria, the veins have a myocardial sleeve, a situation that was described previously for the pulmonary veins. The origin of the smooth muscle cells and the fibroblasts is the epicardium by epithelial-mesenchymal transformation.[12]

These findings also shed new light on the origin and presence of arteriovenous collateral arteries in the adult human heart. It is clear that, during the embryonic period, the coronary network is extensive, whereas a pruning mechanism breaks it down into an arterial, venous, and an intervening capillary bed. From development it is therefore conceivable that a number of arteriovenous connections potentially persist. A similar explanation cannot be provided for the arterioluminal connections or fistulae that are present in a number of congenital heart malformations, for example, pulmonary atresia without ventricular septal defect. There is no evidence for embryonic connections as such. A possible explanation for fistula formation might be found in a very early phenomenon in which the epicardium and the endocardium are in close contact through discontinuities in the myocardium.[33] Under abnormal circumstances, these contacts might lead to fistulous connections between the ventricular lumen and the coronary arterial bed. Experimental studies in which epicardial outgrowth was inhibited and subsequently rescued showed the development of coronary vascular abnormalities, for example, single coronary artery or absence of coronary arteries. In these embryos we found ventriculocoronary communications. The parallel finding of fistulae in the human fetus with an initial pulmonary stenosis that developed into a pulmonary atresia led us to postulate that pulmonary atresia without ventricular septal defect, with and without fistulae, might developmentally be two different diseases.[34]

AORTIC ARCH SYSTEM

During development, the seemingly symmetrical aortic sac and pharyngeal arch arteries become remodeled into an asymmetrical system that forms the ascending aorta, pulmonary trunk, and their branches (Fig. 103.13).[19,35] The vascular system at the arterial pole can always be distinguished from the myocardial outflow tract on the basis of the myocardial boundary. The aortic sac is connected to the dorsal aortae by the two first pharyngeal arch arteries. This pharyngeal system expands and acquires a total of six pharyngeal arches (in mammals the fifth is missing). The development of this arch system is highly influenced by the recently discovered second heart field contribution as well as by neural crest cells migrating through that area. The neural crest cells form the core of the pharyngeal arches and provide the majority of the smooth muscle cells of the arch arteries[36] and the neuronal system surrounding the arch arteries. The second heart field provides non–neural crest-derived smooth muscle cells to the aortic sac as well as myocardium to the outflow tract.[37]

It has been shown that homeotic genes have a part in the patterning of the arches,[38] whereby the fourth arch and the sixth arch are special. The two fourth arches will remodel into a major left aortic arch in most mammals, whereas in the bird a right-sided system is formed. But a hemodynamic regulation has been postulated[19] and was recently supported in a *Pitx2* mutant model.[39] It is known, from both transgene technology and human disease, such as the 22q11 deletion syndrome, that the fourth arch can be selectively interrupted (see Fig. 103.8b). The sixth pharyngeal arch artery that persists on the left side in mammals as the ductus arteriosus is special in both histology and patterns of gene expression.[38] It is the only artery that acquires a muscular wall within an environment of elastic arteries; the reason for this pattern remains unexplained.

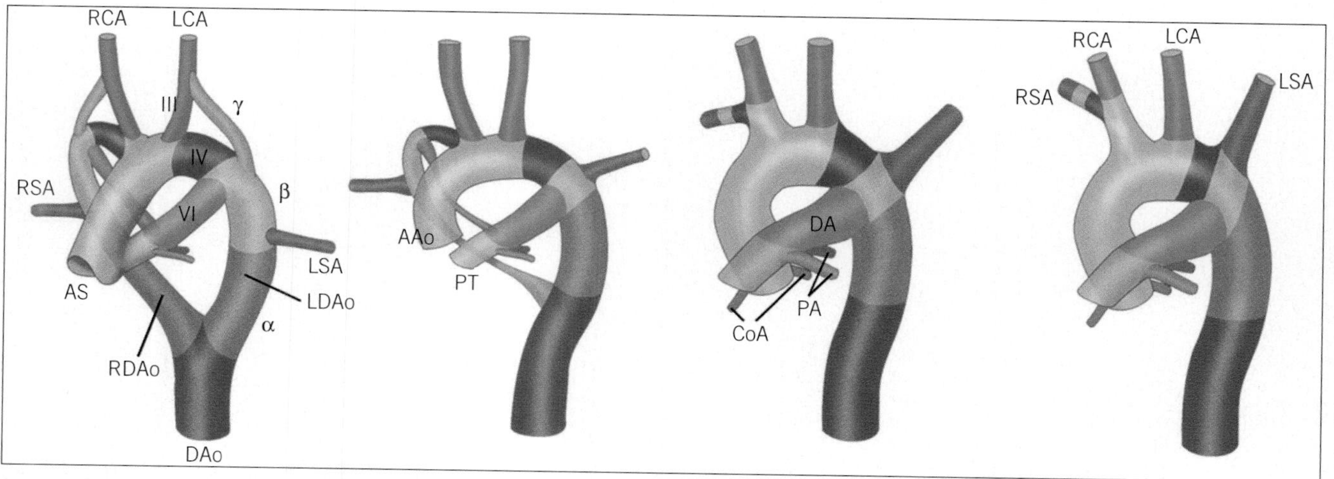

Figure 103.13 Remodeling of the pharyngeal arch arteries. From an almost symmetrical system with a slight preponderance of the left vessels, a left aortic arch develops. The right VI pharyngeal arch artery and part (the α segment) of the right dorsal aorta (RDAo) disappear in this process by apoptosis, while the right and left subclavian arteries (RSA and LSA) move cranially. The left IV pharyngeal arch artery will form part of the aortic arch, specifically the part between the left carotid artery (LCA) and the LSA, whereas the remains of the right IV pharyngeal arch artery will form the proximal part of the RSA. The III pharyngeal arch arteries will eventually form the common carotid arteries (LCA and RCA). The left VI pharyngeal arch artery forms the ductus arteriosus (DA). The aortic sac (AS) will remodel into a separate ascending aorta (AAo) and pulmonary trunk (PT). α, β, and γ, dorsal aorta segments; CoA, coronary arteries; DAo, descending aorta; LDAo, left dorsal aorta; PA, pulmonary arteries. (Modified from Molin DGM, DeRuiter MC, Wisse LJ, et al. Altered apoptosis pattern during pharyngeal arch artery remodelling is associated with aortic arch malformations in Tgf beta 2 knock-out mice. Cardiovasc Res 2002;56:312-322.)

Investigations by our group have revealed the relevance of selective apoptosis in remodeling the embryonic vascular system. In mammals, the right-sided distal aorta, the right sixth pharyngeal arch, and the ductus caroticus on both sides are the vessels that disappear. In the bird, a right-oriented system persists.[40] As mentioned previously, future research will need to concentrate on shear stress responsive genes and arch remodeling.[41]

The left-sided ductus arteriosus may remain patent after birth—a condition usually referred to as persistent ductus arteriosus. This anomaly is characterized histologically by an additional subendothelial elastic lamina.[42] The mechanism that is functional in human persistent ductus arteriosus still needs to be unraveled. DNA mapping provided evidence for a genetic background on chromosome 6.[43] Furthermore, in the rat, persistent ductus arteriosus could be linked to loci on chromosomes 8 and 9.[44]

SUMMARY

The coming years will be dominated by the hunt for genes and mutations that are responsible for disease, now that the human genome has been unraveled. However, until now most data from molecular biology studies that used transgene technology must be seen as highly simplified if attempts are made to extrapolate information on cardiac abnormalities in the mouse heart to human congenital malformations. Congenital heart malformations, and probably most of the adult myocardial and vascular diseases, are the result of highly complex cascades of gene and epigenetic interactions (including environmental factors) that necessitate fine tuning to maintain the equilibrium.

ACKNOWLEDGMENTS

Jan Lens and Ron Slagter are gratefully acknowledged for their help in preparing the figures for the manuscript.

chapter 104

Prenatal Diagnosis of Congenital Heart Disease

Yasuki Maeno

Definition

- Abnormal cardiac structure, rhythm, and function can be detected before birth by echocardiography and other modalities.

Key Features

- Congenital heart disease in the fetus can be detected by prenatal echocardiography from 13 weeks of gestation or earlier.
- Screening for fetal cardiac disease is important if a significant impact is to be made on the prenatal diagnosis of congenital heart disease.
- Intrauterine progression of anatomic and functional problems can be observed.

Clinical Implications

- Prenatal, perinatal, and postnatal management can be planned.
- Prenatal noninvasive and invasive treatment can be started.
- Ethical problems are an important issue in prenatal diagnosis.

The development of ultrasound techniques has allowed us to visualize cardiac anatomy in utero from 13 weeks of gestation by the transabdominal approach,[1-4] and from as early as 10 weeks of gestation by the transvaginal approach.[5] Because of the surrounding amniotic fluid and the fact that the fetal lung is not inflated, fetal echocardiography at 18 to 20 weeks of gestation can provide precise cardiac anatomic information—even in the pulmonary arteries and veins—some of which cannot be obtained by postnatal echocardiography. Using the technique of fetal echocardiography, it is now becoming possible to investigate the prenatal evolution of the normal and abnormal cardiac anatomy that has been seen postnatally.

Prenatal diagnosis of congenital heart disease (CHD) had been shown to improve the outcome of the affected fetuses. However, there are several issues regarding the prenatal diagnosis of cardiac disease. Skillful fetal echocardiographic technique and precise anatomic diagnosis are essential for prenatal diagnosis, but are not in themselves sufficient. Effective prenatal screening for congenital heart disease is important if prenatal echocardiography is to have a significant impact. In addition, assessment of cardiac function and hemodynamics, prediction of the development of cardiac structure during gestation, and effective perinatal management are required to improve outcomes in affected fetuses.

DESCRIPTION OF TECHNIQUE

There are two basic steps in examining the fetal heart:

- screening for the presence of abnormalities of anatomy, function, and rhythm, using three cross-sectional images, such as the four-chamber view,[1,3] the three-vessel view,[6] and the three-vessel and trachea view[7]; and
- assessment of precise cardiac and great vessel anatomy and detailed cardiac function using 2D, 3D, M-mode, and Doppler echocardiography.

Screening of the Abnormal Fetal Heart

First, the edge of the fetal heart is defined. A longitudinal section of the fetus parallel to the spine is imaged with the fetal head at the right side of the screen. Regardless of fetal position, a fetal transverse section, obtained by 90-degree clockwise rotation of the probe, should be obtained to visualize the fetus from inferior to superior, so that the side of the heart and stomach can be defined.[8]

The next step is to obtain three quite simple transverse sections of the fetal chest, the four-chamber view, the three-vessel view, and the three-vessel and trachea view, which will detect almost all major intracardiac and great vessel abnormalities. Screening using these three simple views may be completed in most cases within 3 minutes during routine obstetric ultrasonographic examination and detects up to 75% of the fetuses with heart anomaly.[9]

A four-chamber view of the fetal heart is easily obtained by a transverse section of the lower part of the fetal chest wall, because the fetal heart is positioned more horizontally, the lung is uninflated, and the diaphragm has a higher position (Fig. 104.1).[1,3] Systematic assessment of this four-chamber view can detect more than 50% of intracardiac abnormalities, such as single ventricle, atrioventricular septal defect, and Ebstein's anomaly. This view is also useful for qualitative assessment of cardiac function and rhythm.

The second transverse view of the chest, the three-vessel view (see Fig. 104.1), can be easily obtained by a simple superior sweep from the four-chamber view.[6] Systematic assessment of this three-vessel view can indirectly detect abnormal connections between the ventricles and the great arteries, such as transposition of the great arteries and tetralogy of Fallot, which are often missed by the four-chamber view alone.

The last screening view, three-vessel and trachea view (see Fig. 104.1), can be obtained by farther superior sweep from three-vessel view.[7] This three-vessel and trachea view is useful for detecting variable vascular rings, which sometimes cause marked airway problems postnatally.[10]

Three-dimensional echocardiography may have an important role for the screening of abnormal fetal heart, since these three simple transverse views for screening can be obtained from the 3D data set.[11]

Color Doppler echocardiography may provide additional information for screening. A parallel sweep from the four-chamber to the three-vessel view with color Doppler will demonstrate the cross-relation of both ventricular outflow

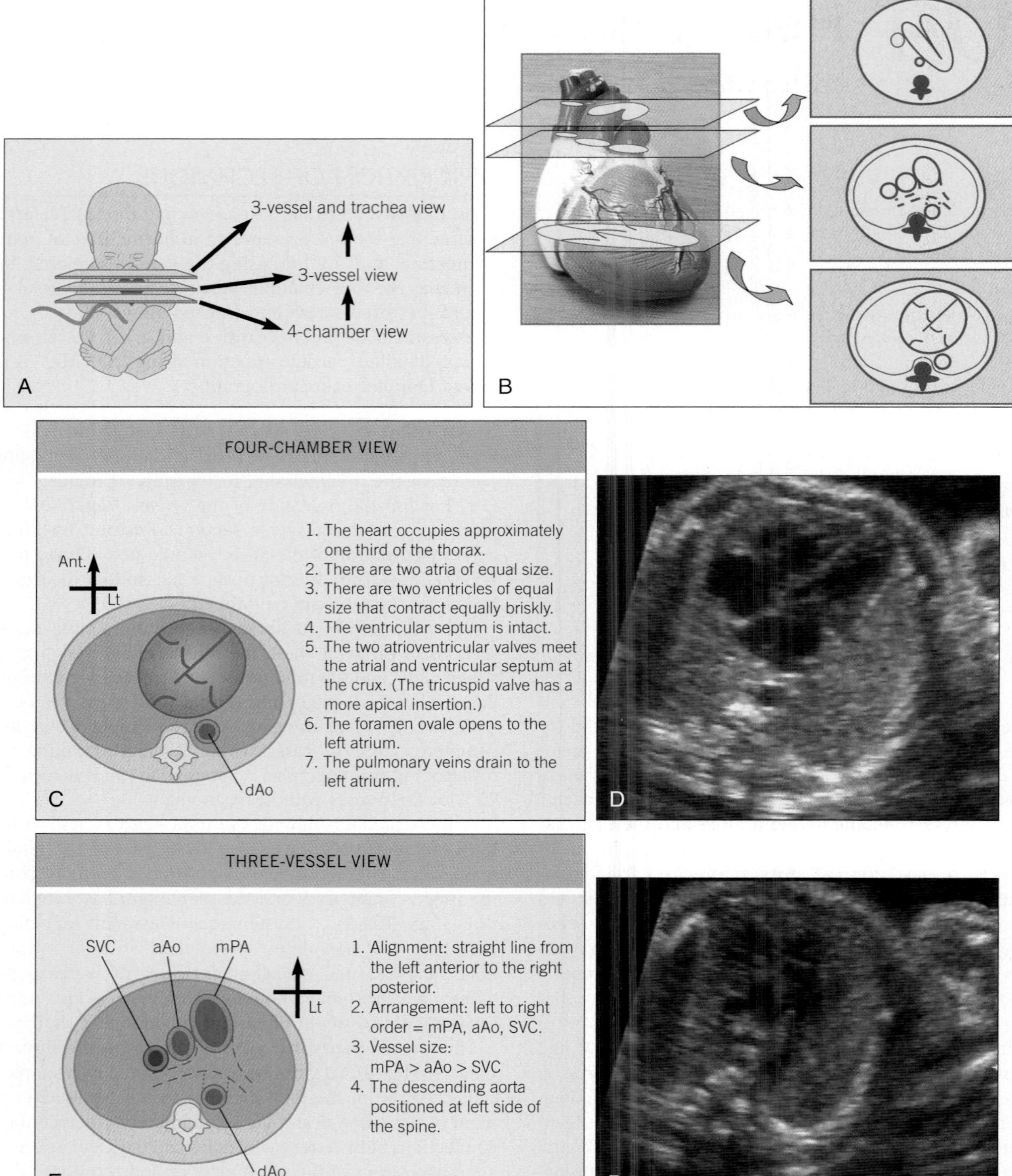

Fig. 104.1 Evaluation of four chamber, three-vessel, and three-vessel and trachea views. A, Three parallel transverse sections of the fetal chest demonstrate the four-chamber view, the three-vessel view, and three-vessel and trachea view. **B**, Relation between the cardiac structure and each view. **C**, A schema of the four-chamber view and checkpoints. **D**, An echocardiographic picture of four-chamber view. **E**, A schema of the three-vessel view and checkpoints. **F**, An echocardiographic picture of the three-vessel view. **G**, A schema of the three-vessel and trachea view and check points. **H**, An Echocardiographic picture of the three-vessel and trachea view. aAo, ascending aorta; dAo, descending aorta; mPA, main pulmonary artery; SVC, superior vena cava.

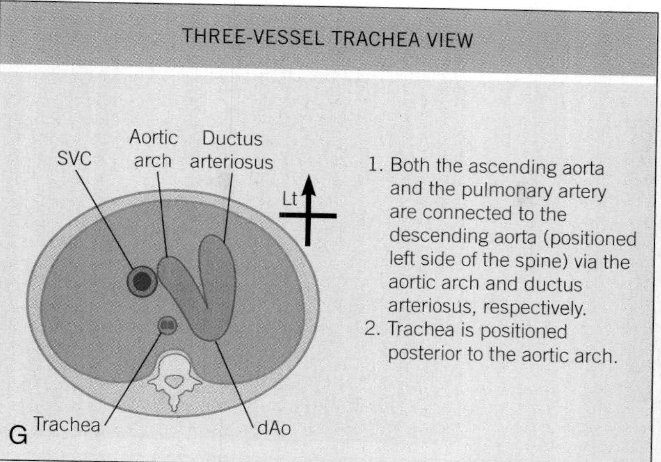

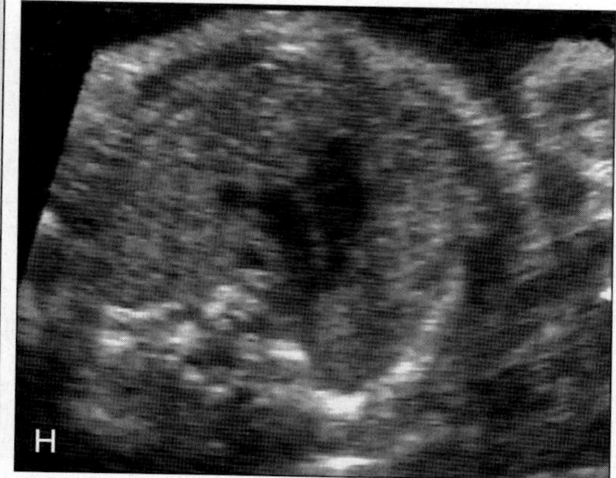

Fig. 104.1—cont'd

tracts. Location of the pulmonary venous return can be confirmed by color Doppler flow. In addition, abnormal blood flow, such as stenotic flow or regurgitant jet, can also be detected.

Recently, a new method of screening high-risk fetuses for congenital heart disease has been proposed. The presence of a thickened nuchal translucency at 10 to 14 weeks of gestation can be used to identify high-risk fetuses.[12] A clinical application for this method is now being investigated.

Evaluation of the Fetal Cardiac Anatomy

Once some abnormal finding is detected, detailed intracardiac and functional assessment is required for precise diagnosis. The cardiac anatomy is examined using a segmental approach in a similar manner to that used in postnatal echocardiography. Recent high-resolution 2D echocardiography can provide high quality images of detailed intracardiac and extracardiac anatomy as early as 14 weeks of gestation. In addition, detailed assessment of the peripheral pulmonary artery and veins, which cannot be seen by postnatal echocardiography, is possible during the fetal period because the fetal lung has not been inflated by air.

M-Mode Echocardiography

M-mode echocardiography is used to assess cardiac rhythm and function.[13,14] An M-mode trace of ventricular and atrial motion demonstrates the cardiac rhythm and rate. A simultaneous record of both ventricles and atria (Fig. 104.2) is especially useful for assessing the atrioventricular electric connection in fetuses with arrhythmias, such as complete heart block, atrial fibrillation, and ectopic beat.

An M-mode trace perpendicular to the ventricle provides qualitative information on ventricular systolic function. However, because of the variable position of the fetus, the M-mode cursor has to be carefully positioned so that it is perpendicular to the ventricular septum.

Doppler Echocardiography

Pulse and continuous-wave Doppler echocardiography are used to examine cardiac anatomy and to assess cardiac rhythm and function.[13] The interpretation of some Doppler

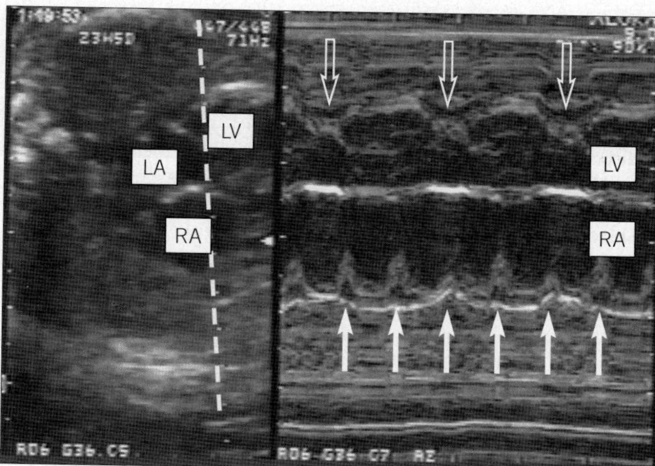

Fig. 104.2 Simultaneous M-mode recording of both ventricles and atria (dotted line). M-mode recording in a fetus with complete atrioventricular block reveals complete dissociation of atrial and ventricular contraction with a ventricular rate of 65bpm. Open arrows, ventricular contractions; closed arrows, atrial contractions. LA, left atrium. LV, left ventricle. RA, right atrium.

signals in the prenatal period require understanding of fetal hemodynamics.

The velocity of Doppler flow at the correct angle (less than 20 degrees) at either side of the inflow to[15] and outflow from the ventricles[16] and at the ductus arteriosus[17] provides the anatomic and functional information. The waveform of the pulsed Doppler is especially important to assess the cardiac function and hemodynamic condition of the fetus. Doppler waveforms obtained at the inferior vena cava,[18] pulmonary veins, foramen ovale, midcerebral artery, umbilical artery and vein, and isthmus of the aortic arch[19] change according to many fetal hemodynamic conditions, such as cardiac function and vascular resistances in various locations, including the placenta and brain.

A simultaneous record of the superior vena cava and the ascending aorta is used for assessing cardiac arrhythmias (Fig. 104.3). Beginning of reverse flow at the superior vena cava created by atrial contraction and beginning of forward flow at the ascending aorta created by ventricular

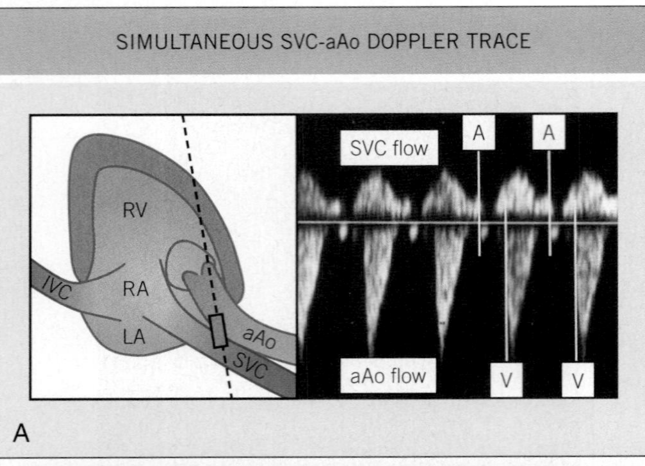

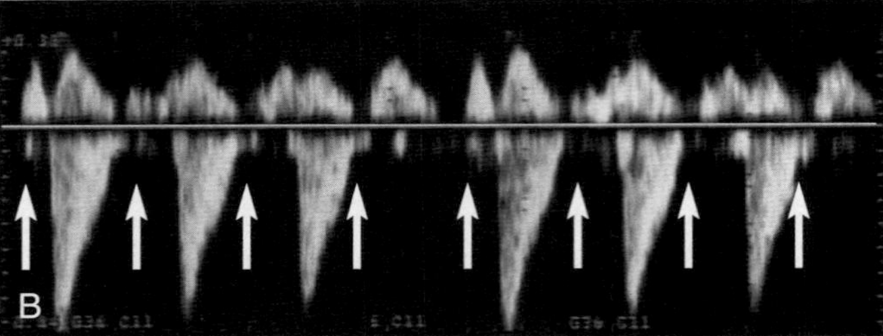

Fig. 104.3 Simultaneous Doppler trace of the ascending aorta (aAo) and the superior vena cava (SVC). A, Beginning of reverse flow at SVC (A) and forward flow at aAo (V) represent the timing of atrial and ventricular contractions, respectively. **B,** A case with a Wenckebach type of atrioventricular block revealed atrial contraction with regular rhythm *(arrows)*, atrioventricular conducting time of gradual prolongation, and block with pose of ventricular contraction.

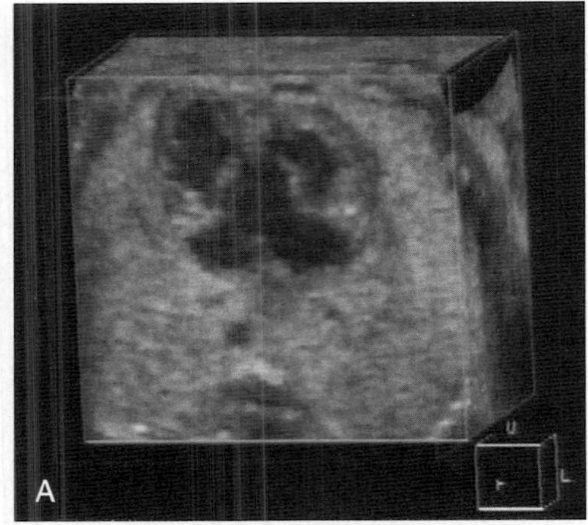

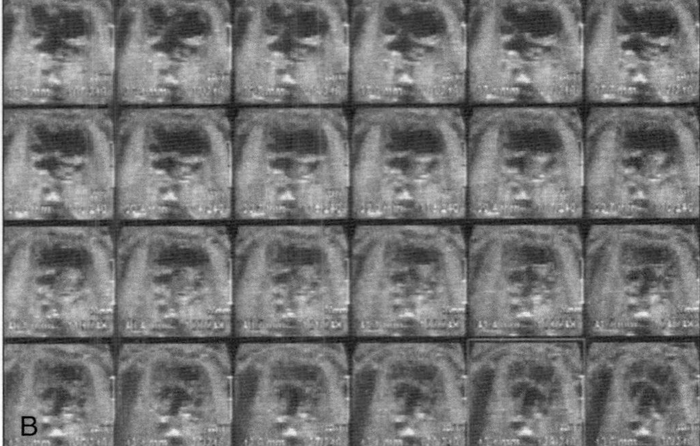

Fig. 104.4 Three-dimensional echocardiography in a case with common atrioventricular valve (asplenic syndrome). A, Optimal 2D cutting plane can be created from the 3D data set and demonstrated from optimal angle. **B,** Multiple parallel cutting planes obtained from 3D data set demonstrate the connection from the cardiac chambers to the vessels.

contraction are interpreted as the beginning of P and Q waves by electrocardiography, respectively. Hence, relation of the atrial and ventricular contraction can be assessed from this wave-form.

Color Doppler mapping is useful in the detection of abnormal blood flow. Color Doppler is examined at each valve to detect obstruction or regurgitation. Color Doppler mapping can also be used to detect abnormal vessels that are suspected in the abnormal heart, such as a coronary artery fistula[20] or, in the case of pulmonary atresia with ventricular septal defect, collateral vessels from the descending aorta to the lung.

Three-Dimensional Echocardiography

Three-dimensional echocardiography has become a powerful tool for screening and making detailed diagnosis of fetal cardiac anomalies.[11,21] For the 2D echocardiography, fetal movement and limited window caused by the fetal position often limit a detailed anatomic assessment of the fetal heart. Whereas with 3D echocardiography, any optimal 2D cutting image can be obtained without fetal movement once the 3D data set of the fetal heart is acquired and saved into the hard disk (Fig. 104.4). Especially for the spatio-temporal image correlation (STIC) method, 3D images with heartbeat can be created by automatic calculation of fetal heart rate from the acquired data set. Display of multiple parallel cutting planes is useful to assess the cardiac anatomy. Volume of the chambers and ventricular function are also accurately analyzed from this 3D data set.[21]

Interpretation of the Examination

The most important benefit of the prenatal diagnosis of CHD is making optimal plans for the perinatal management to improve the mortality and morbidity. Once the fetal cardiac problem is detected, consideration of the following issues is useful to optimize perinatal management:

- the precise anatomic and functional diagnosis, especially with respect to structures that affect the postnatal management strategy and outcome;
- anticipation of possible anatomic and functional progression of the disease during the prenatal period and planning of perinatal follow-up;
- indications for chromosome analysis;
- the plan for delivery; and
- the plan for postnatal management and estimation of the outcome.

Precise Anatomic and Functional Diagnosis

Precise anatomic assessment is essential for prenatal diagnosis. Detailed information is required about cardiac structures that affect perinatal management and postnatal outcome. Hence, possible postnatal management options are always anticipated while echocardiography is being performed. For example, when repair of a single ventricle is expected postnatally, the presence of atrioventricular valve regurgitation, cardiac function, and the size of the pulmonary arteries must be checked. The presence of subaortic stenosis is also looked for in such cases, because it presents a risk if a Damus-Kaye-Stansel (DKS) type of repair is anticipated. To give another example, when a fetus has a double-outlet right ventricle, an associated mitral valve abnormality, especially straddling of the chordae, must be excluded, because the presence of this lesion may change the surgical repair from biventricular repair to single-ventricle repair.

Doppler echocardiography provides valuable information for the investigation of detailed cardiac anatomy. Identifying the presence of valvular regurgitation or an obstructive lesion is important for an accurate diagnosis and to plan perinatal management. However, interpretation of the Doppler findings requires knowledge of fetal hemodynamics. Flow from the left atrium to the right atrium at the foramen ovale or flow from the aorta to the pulmonary artery at the ductus arteriosus, which are the complete antithesis of the normal direction of flow in the prenatal period, represents the presence of a significant congenital cardiac abnormality.[17] The pressure gradient of a stenotic aortic or pulmonary valve tends to underestimate the postnatal pressure gradient, because the main pulmonary artery and aorta, being connected by the large ductus arteriosus, have the same pressure regardless of the presence of obstructed outflow.

Functional assessment using M-mode and Doppler echocardiography is also important. The cardiac output and ventricular systolic and diastolic function are checked, and the presence of congestive heart failure should be detected before fetal hydrops develops.

Prenatal Progression

The prenatal cardiac anatomy, chamber size, and function will change during gestation, so that the appearance of the cardiac structures may be different from that usually seen postnatally. In addition, several abnormal lesions may progress during the prenatal period. The ascending aorta or the main pulmonary artery may not grow in the presence of outflow tract obstruction.[20,22] Even if the ventricle is enlarged in a fetus with severe outflow tract obstruction with intact ventricular septum, the ventricle may not grow and may become hypoplastic at birth.[22] The degree of regurgitation at the semilunar and atrioventricular valves tends to increase during gestation. Arrhythmia may develop in utero; in particular, atrioventricular block may develop in fetuses with left isomerism or discordant atrioventricular connection.[23] Restriction of the foramen ovale may appear in utero in fetuses with left-sided heart obstruction[24] or transposition of the great arteries.[25] Knowledge of all these possible developments is important when plans for follow-up and perinatal management are being made, when outcome is being predicted, and when the family is counseled.

Indication of Chromosomal Analysis

Once the presence of a congenital cardiac anomaly is diagnosed, the indication for chromosomal analysis should be considered.[26,27] In particular, when the termination of pregnancy is considered, chromosomal analysis may provide additional information to assist the family in their decision making. However, when the particular cardiac anomaly is unlikely to result from a chromosome abnormality (e.g., heterotaxy), or when the diagnosis of a chromosome abnormality will not change the management plan or the family's decision, the need for chromosome analysis should be discussed with the family, because the amniocentesis required for chromosome analysis carries some risk of premature birth.

Plan for Delivery

The delivery must take place at the tertiary care center, preferably close to the pediatric cardiac center, in all cases of major cardiac disease with some risk of deterioration at delivery. In particular, fetuses with a ductus-dependent lesion, or those in whom there is a possibility of severe hypoxemia because of a restricted foramen ovale, such as a left-heart obstructive lesion or transposition of the great arteries, must be delivered in conditions in which prostaglandin infusion and emergency balloon atrial septotomy are readily available. Prenatal echocardiographic assessment in later gestation may be able to detect some of these high-risk cases.[25]

INDICATIONS

There are two different indications for prenatal echocardiography:

- screening the fetal heart for anatomic and functional abnormality; and
- detailed prenatal echocardiography performed or assessed by a pediatric cardiologist with particular knowledge of fetal cardiology.

Screening

Effective screening of anatomic and functional abnormality of the fetal heart is essential for prenatal echocardiography. Unlike in the newborn period, the presence of severe cardiac disease in the fetus—such as heart murmur and cyanosis—cannot be detected by physical examination. Therefore fetal ultrasonographic screening of a completely healthy mother with an uneventful pregnancy is the only method of identifying the majority of cases of congenital heart disease in utero. In this regard, appropriate fetal echocardiographic assessment is indicated for all pregnant women.

The first screening ultrasound should be performed between 18 and 22 weeks of gestation if termination of pregnancy is to be considered as an option in complex cardiac problems. Screening has to be performed sufficiently early to make it possible to refer the case to a fetal cardiac center and to allow the parents to make their decision. Because some cardiac abnormalities become more obvious later in gestation, a second screening for cardiac disease should be performed at 28 to 32 weeks of gestation.

Detailed Fetal Cardiac Assessment

Detailed fetal cardiac assessment is indicated for all cases in which a structural, rhythmic, or functional cardiac abnormality is detected by screening, and those with extracardiac abnormality. The purpose of this detailed assessment is not only to make an accurate diagnosis of any cardiac disease, but also to allow an appropriate plan for perinatal management to be drawn up. From this examination, the plan for prenatal follow-up and preparation for delivery and postnatal management, such as early neonatal cardiac surgery, must be decided. Therefore the fetal echocardiography should be performed and/or reviewed by physicians with specialized skill in fetal cardiology. The indication and timing of follow-up ultrasound must be decided, in each case, on the basis of the likelihood and severity of progression of the cardiac problems.

SPECIFIC STRUCTURAL ABNORMALITIES

Atrioventricular Septal Defect

The common valve in atrioventricular septal defect can usually be easily diagnosed by the four-chamber view (Fig. 104.5a) and the short-axis view at the level of the atrioventricular valve. This anomaly is often associated with other complex cardiac anomalies. In particular, any associated right or left atrial isomerism has to be checked carefully.[2] In addition, the presence of left or right ventricular outflow obstruction, straddling of the mitral valve, and atrioventricular valve regurgitation must be checked to predict postnatal mortality and morbidity. The association of atrioventricular heart block, with or without left atrial isomerism, is also important for prognosis.[23,28]

Fetuses with this anomaly need careful follow-up during gestation, because several aspects of the fetal heart may change in utero. The size of either the ventricular or the atrial component of the septal defect may change (it may spontaneously close), and obstruction at either side of the

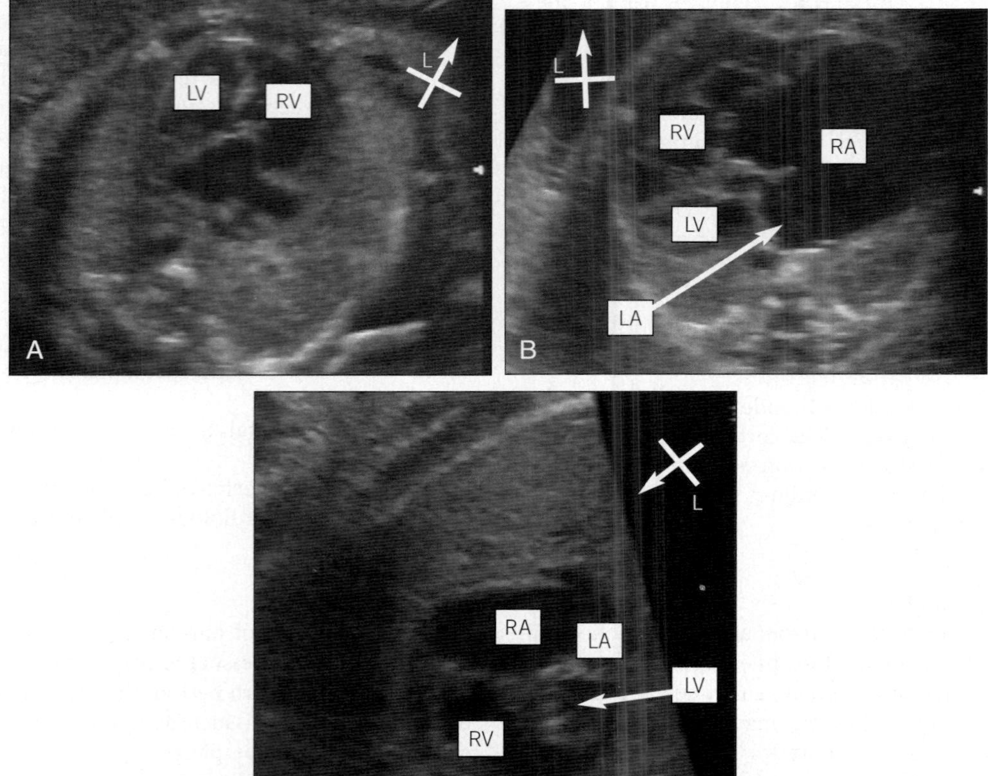

Fig. 104.5 Four-chamber view of a fetus with **(A)** atrioventricular septal defect, **(B)** tricuspid valve dysplasia, and **(C)** hypoplastic left heart syndrome. **(A)** Atrio-ventricular valve is not separated to left and right portion, and creates common atrioventricular valve. **(B)** The heart is quite enlarged and fills almost the entire chest. The right atrium (RA) is enlarged because of severe tricuspid valve regurgitation. **(C)** The left ventricle (LV) is small and endocardium of LV is high echogenic due to endocardial fibroelastosis. LA, left atrium; LV, left ventricle; RA, right atrium; RV, right ventricle.

outflow tract may appear and progress during gestation. In particular, worsening atrioventricular valve regurgitation or development of complete heart block may lead to sudden deterioration of the fetus in utero.

Complete atrioventricular septal defect, especially in the cases associated with intrauterine growth restriction, is often associated with trisomy 21. The existence of extracardiac anomalies, such as duodenal atresia and hygroma, should be carefully checked. Pleural effusion due to chylothorax and enlarged high-echogenic liver due to the transient myeloproliferative disorder are rare but important complications associated with trisomy 21.

Ebstein's Malformation/Tricuspid Valve Dysplasia

Both Ebstein's malformation and tricuspid valve dysplasia involve significant tricuspid valve regurgitation.[29,30] The severe form of these diseases produces an enlarged right atrium, which is easily detected by the four-chamber view (see Fig. 104.5b). The right atrium is sometimes considerably enlarged and fills almost the entire fetal chest. The septal leaflet of the tricuspid valve in Ebstein's malformation is displaced toward the apex of the heart. Tricuspid valve dysplasia produces a thick and nodular tricuspid valve. Both diseases show a spectrum of severity and may overlap.

Severe tricuspid valve regurgitation is often associated with functional or anatomic right ventricular outflow tract obstruction.[29,30] In the case of functional atresia, right ventricular pressure estimated from the tricuspid valve regurgitation jet is low. The presence of pulmonary valve regurgitation in the systolic phase represents penetration of the pulmonary valve.

Severe tricuspid valve regurgitation causes two serious conditions in the fetus: fetal hydrops and lung hypoplasia.[29,30] Severe regurgitation causes increased central venous pressure, in turn causing congestive heart failure and fetal hydrops. Lung hypoplasia develops secondary to the enlargement of the fetal heart, especially the right atrium, which sometimes almost fills the chest.

The fetus with these tricuspid valve abnormalities should be carefully followed during gestation to detect early signs of fetal hydrops. If fetal hydrops is already present during the middle trimester, the prognosis is extremely poor and the risk of intrauterine death is quite high.

Right Ventricular Outflow Tract (RVOT) Obstruction with Intact Ventricular Septum

Pulmonary atresia with intact ventricular septum and pulmonary valve stenosis occur in various degrees of severity.[20,31,32] Severe forms of this type of abnormality, with a severely hypoplastic right ventricle or enlarged right ventricle with severe tricuspid valve regurgitation, are easily detected by screening using the four-chamber view. However, prenatal detection of milder tricuspid regurgitation cases or those with a normal-sized right ventricle may not be possible. Critical pulmonary valve stenosis is very difficult to distinguish from pulmonary atresia.[2,20]

For fetuses in this category with associated hypoplastic right ventricle, the size of the right ventricle, the presence or absence of the outflow portion of the right ventricle, and the connections between the right ventricle and the coronary artery should be carefully assessed by prenatal echocardiography.[20] The diameter of the annulus of the tricuspid valve should be measured to assess the size of the right ventricular cavity indirectly.

The severity of pulmonary valve stenosis may progress during gestation, and, in some fetuses, valvular atresia may develop.[32] Unless the fetus develops severe tricuspid valve regurgitation, congestive heart failure may not develop and the incidence of fetal death is quite low.[2,32]

Balloon pulmonary valvuloplasty by direct puncture of the fetal heart under echocardiographic guidance has been tried in an attempt to prevent hypoplastic right ventricle at birth.[33] Although some cases of successful valvuloplasty have been reported, in others valvular atresia redeveloped.

Because the pulmonary circulation is dependent on the ductus arteriosus in all neonates with pulmonary atresia and some with pulmonary stenosis, infusion of prostaglandin should be started immediately after birth. In particular, cases of pulmonary stenosis with retrograde flow in the ductus arteriosus in the prenatal period always require a patent ductus arteriosus postnatally.

Left Ventricular Outflow Tract (LVOT) Obstruction

Left ventricular outflow tract obstruction occurs in various degrees of severity.[2,22,24,34,35] The most severe form is complete or severe obstruction of the aortic valve, associated with obstruction of the mitral valve, endocardial fibroelastosis of the left ventricle, and severe hypoplastic left ventricle (so-called hypoplastic left heart syndrome).

Most fetuses in this category have a hypoplastic or enlarged left ventricle, with or without poor cardiac function, and can be easily detected by the simple four-chamber view (see Fig. 104.5c). The enlarged, poorly contractile left ventricle may not grow during gestation and is likely to be hypoplastic at birth, especially when there is significant retrograde flow from the left to the right atrium at the foramen ovale, or a closed foramen ovale.[23] Systolic retrograde flow at the isthmus of the aortic arch represents significant obstruction at the aortic valve and probable ductus-dependent systemic circulation postnatally. In fetuses with mitral valve regurgitation, the severity of the condition may change and some of them develop fetal hydrops.

Balloon aortic valvuloplasty before 29 weeks of gestation by direct puncture of the fetal heart using echocardiographic guidance has been reported to prevent hypoplastic left ventricle at birth.[36,37] Once the left ventricle progresses to hypoplastic, Norwood-type palliative repair and single ventricular type of repair, which has much higher morbidity and mortality compared with biventricular repair, is required. Hence, prevention of the progression of hypoplastic left ventricle is very important. Successful balloon valvuloplasty and postnatal biventricular repair have been reported in recent years. To decide the indication for this procedure, accurate prediction of which fetuses develop hypoplastic left ventricle in later gestation is essential.

D-TRANSPOSITION OF THE GREAT ARTERIES

D-transposition of the great arteries cannot be detected on the four-chamber view unless there is a large ventricular septal defect, but the three-vessel view clearly demonstrates the

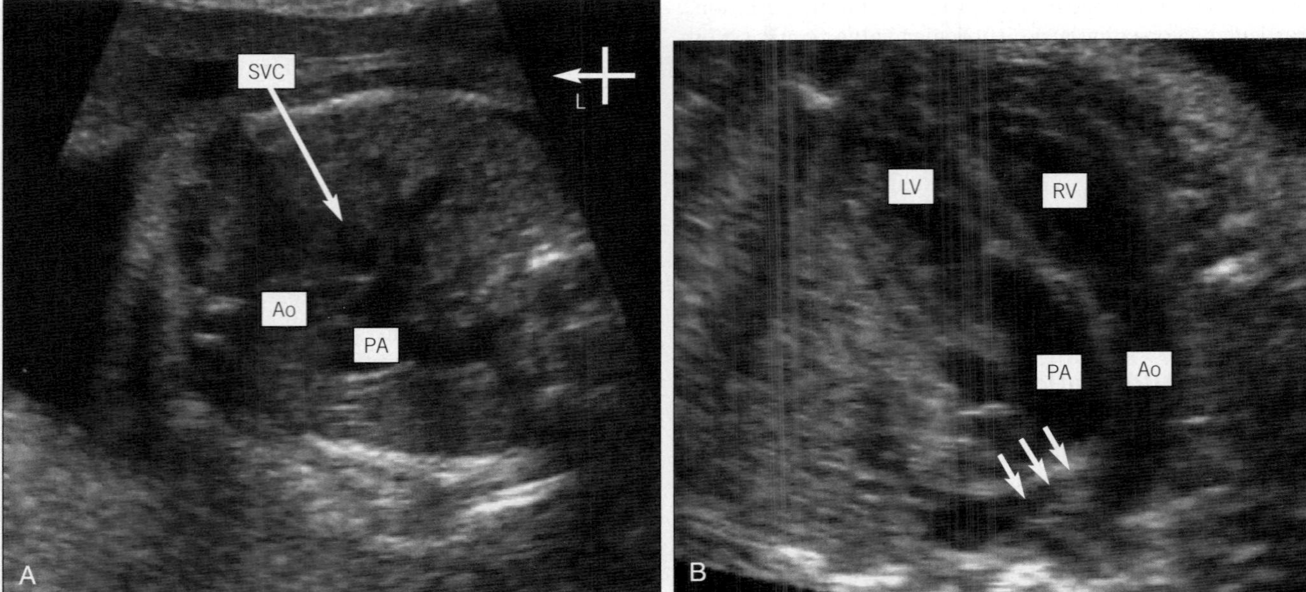

Fig. 104.6 A fetus with complete transposition of the great arteries (TGA). A, A three-vessel view reveals a right anterior ascending aorta (Ao) and left posterior main pulmonary artery (PA). **B,** A view of the outflow tract clearly demonstrates the ascending Ao arising from the right ventricle (RV) and the main PA arising from the left ventricle (LV). The great vessels lying parallel to one another can never be obtained in normal cardiac anatomy, in which the relationship between the great vessels is spiral. Of note, the ductus arteriosus (*arrows*) is narrow in many fetuses with TGA, which may lead to severe hypoxicemia immediately after birth. L, left; SVC, superior vena cava.

abnormal position of the great vessels (i.e., a right anterior ascending aorta and a left posterior main pulmonary artery) (Fig. 104.6).[6] Oblique sections visualizing the ventricular outflow tract can demonstrate the abnormal connection of the great arteries directly.[25,38] The ascending aorta and the pulmonary artery run parallel, unlike the normal heart, in which the great vessels have a spiral relation.

Once the diagnosis of transposition is made, it is very important to check for the presence of ventricular septal defect and the appearance of the foramen ovale and ductus arteriosus.[25,39] Color Doppler flow mapping is helpful in detecting the ventricular septal defect. Stenosis of the foramen ovale and the ductus arteriosus may develop during the prenatal period. High-velocity flow from the pulmonary artery to the aorta represents the presence of constricted ductus arteriosus and possible associated pulmonary hypertension. It is important to note that, even when there is a small ductus arteriosus, the Doppler velocity of the flow through the ductus may not increase if the amount of flow is reduced or pulmonary hypertension is absent. Neonates with severe constriction at either site develop severe hypoxemia soon after birth and may die within a short period. Although immediate balloon atrial septotomy in the delivery room is indicated in such cases,[25,38] exact prediction of such cases by fetal echocardiography is still difficult.[39]

Tetralogy of Fallot

The presence of tetralogy of Fallot is easily missed by the four-chamber view, but the three-vessel view demonstrates the small main pulmonary artery positioned slightly more posteriorly than usual.[6] Oblique sections to visualize both the RVOT and LVOT are the most valuable views with which to demonstrate the anteriorly deviated infundibular septum and other anatomic features.[40,41]

The patency of the pulmonary valve is sometimes difficult to ascertain in cases of severely hypoplastic RVOT obstruction. In addition, some progress in utero to pulmonary atresia.[2,40] The presence of retrograde ductal flow from the aorta to the pulmonary artery, however, indicates a postnatal ductal-dependent pulmonary circulation, regardless of the patency of the pulmonary valve. The size of both branches of the pulmonary arteries is an important factor for postnatal surgical treatment.

There is a strong relationship between tetralogy of Fallot and the microdeletion of 22q; hence, the presence of associated cleft lip or cleft palate should be checked. Associations with other chromosomal abnormalities, such as trisomy 18, or other extracardiac anomalies, have also been reported.[41] Therefore counseling of the family may require particular attention, because the prognosis of fetal tetralogy of Fallot is not always favorable.

Tetralogy of Fallot with Absent Pulmonary Valve

Tetralogy of Fallot with absent pulmonary valve complex is a relatively rare CHD, but easily detected by screening because of aneurysmally enlarged main and branch pulmonary arteries (Fig. 104.7). The ductus arteriosus is absent in most of the cases. Some of the fetuses develop to fetal hydrops and fetal death.[42,43] Postnatal mortality is high because of respiratory failure. The prediction of these worse outcomes is difficult. About 20% of the cases are associated with the microdeletion of 22q.

Univentricular Heart

Univentricular heart usually has an obviously abnormal appearance on the routine four-chamber view and is easily detected by screening. The presence of heterotaxy, such as

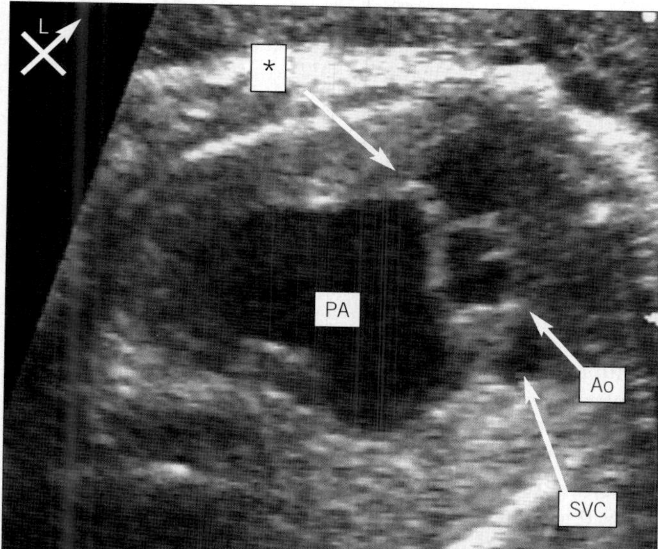

Fig. 104.7 A fetus with tetralogy of Fallot with absent pulmonary valve complex. The pulmonary valve is not well developed (*). The main and branch pulmonary arteries (PA) are aneurysmally enlarged. Ao, aorta; SVC, superior vena cava.

abdominal situs and the presence of azygos continuation, should be checked.[28,44]

The cardiac anatomy should be carefully examined to predict dependence of the postnatal circulation on the ductus arteriosus, the foramen ovale, or both. The risks of postnatal repair must also be checked during the prenatal period. This is important not only for perinatal management but also for counseling the family. In cases in which the usual type of single ventricle repair is indicated, the presence of regurgitation at the atrioventricular valves, the size of both branches of the pulmonary arteries, and ventricular function should be checked. Cases associated with subaortic or valvular aortic obstruction or arch obstruction may require a Norwood type or DKS type of arch repair during the early neonatal period and are at additional risk for postnatal morbidity and mortality.

Coarctation of the Aorta

Prenatal diagnosis of coarctation of the aorta has several limitations. When the diameter of the ascending aorta is visibly smaller than that of the main pulmonary artery, there is some possibility to develop coarctation of the aorta postnatally.[6,45-48] However, even fetuses with a relatively large isthmus may develop coarctation of the aorta if there is extension of ductal tissue into the aortic wall and ductal closure narrows the aorta, and prediction of such postnatal development is difficult.

Some fetuses with persistent left superior vena cava and enlarged coronary sinus are known to develop coarctation of the aorta.[49,50] Hence, in such cases, the diameter of the isthmus has to be carefully checked, and close follow-up is required postnatally. Although the reason for this coexistence is not clearly understood, it is speculated that enlarged coronary sinus reduces the size of the foramen ovale and mitral valve annulus and reduces the left ventricular inflow, which reduces the size of the left ventricle as well as the ascending aorta and isthmus.

Truncus Arteriosus

Although truncus arteriosus can be detected by abnormal three-vessel view during screening, differentiation from pulmonary atresia with ventricular septum is sometimes difficult.[51,52] The truncal valve is frequently stenotic, incompetent, or both. In the cases with significant regurgitation at the truncal valve, the fetus may develop fetal hydrops and may die in utero. Postnatal prognosis is also poor in such cases. About 30% to 40% of the fetuses with truncus arteriosus also have a chromosomal abnormality, such as 22q11.2, an extracardiac anomaly, or both.

Vascular Rings

There are various types of vascular rings, and the most common type is the one associated with right aortic arch, which can be detected by three-vessel and trachea view (Fig. 104.8).[7,10] Postnatally, the vascular rings may cause stenosis at the trachea, esophagus, or both. However, prediction of which cases develop stenosis after birth is not established. Nevertheless, prenatal detection is very useful because postnatal diagnosis of this vascular anomaly is often difficult and often delayed.

OTHER CARDIAC PROBLEMS

Fetal Arrhythmia

Fetal arrhythmia is found at the time of fetal heart monitoring or routine prenatal ultrasound examination. Sometimes, the mother realizes that fetal movement has decreased. Prenatal ultrasound can detect arrhythmia with or without enlarged heart and fetal hydrops. Arrhythmias are of three kinds[53,54]:

- bradycardia (heart rate <100 beats per minute);
- tachycardia (heart rate >180 beats per minute); and
- ectopic beats.

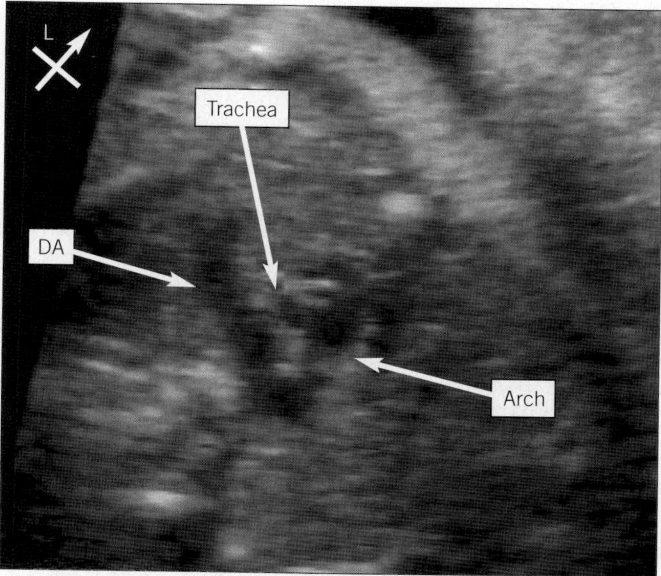

Fig. 104.8 Three-vessel and trachea view of a fetus with right aortic arch and vascular ring. The aortic arch is running on the right side of the trachea and is connected to the ductus arteriosus (DA), which is running left of and posterior to the trachea, at the right side of the spine. Of note the trachea is surrounded by the arch and the ductus arteriosus creating the vascular ring.

Detailed analysis for the type of arrhythmia in utero has become possible using M-mode (see Fig. 104.2), Doppler (see Fig. 104.3), and tissue Doppler methods.[55-57]

Bradycardia

The most common cause of fetal bradycardia is complete atrioventricular block. About 33% to 50% of cases of complete atrioventricular block are caused by associated congenital cardiac anomalies, such as left atrial isomerism, discordant connection, and septal defect, and prognosis for these fetuses is generally poor.[23,58] Most of the remaining cases of isolated atrioventricular block are caused by maternal SS-A or SS-B antibody. A heart rate of less than 55 beats per minute carries a risk for the development of fetal hydrops. It is important that transferred maternal IgG can cause pleural, pericardial, and peritoneal effusion—in addition to myocarditis and poor cardiac function—in the fetus, even if there is no hydrops.

When such atrioventricular block is detected shortly after it develops, maternal steroid treatment is reported to improve the situation.[58] Maternal steroid treatment may also improve fetal myocarditis or effusions. When this kind of atrioventricular block is discovered later in gestation, maternal administration of sympathomimetic agents appears to increase the fetal heart rate.[58,59] When the fetal heart rate progressively decreases and fetal hydrops starts to develop, early delivery and direct pacing of the ventricle may be the only option to improve congestive heart failure. Nevertheless, in cases with significant myocarditis, congestive heart failure may not improve even after pacing.

Atrial bigeminy and blocked premature atrial beats cause bradycardia and mimic 2:1 atrioventricular block. A blocked premature atrial beat has an irregular interval of atrial contraction on M-mode, whereas 2:1 atrioventricular block has a regular interval. Long QT syndrome also causes fetal bradycardia, hence a postnatal electrocardiogram to measure the QT interval is essential.

Tachycardia

Common causes of fetal tachycardia are paroxysmal supraventricular tachycardia (PSVT) and atrial flutter.[13,60] Although the tachycardia is sometimes intermittent during prenatal examination, the chance of hemodynamic complications and the development of fetal hydrops is still high.[61] Most cases of both PSVT and atrial fibrillation are successfully treated in utero by transplacental administration of antiarrhythmic drugs.

Most PSVT is caused by atrioventricular re-entry tachycardia (AVRT) caused by Wolff-Parkinson-White syndrome. A simultaneous M-mode record of atrial and ventricular contraction shows 1:1 atrioventricular conduction, with heart rates ranging from 200 to 300 beats per minute (Fig. 104.9). Measurement of the time interval from the ventricular contraction to the following atrial contraction (VA interval) is useful to distinguish AVRT (short VA interval) from the other tachycardias (long VA interval).[55] The VA interval can be measured from the simultaneous M-mode record of atrial and ventricular contraction, or from a simultaneous Doppler waveform record of the superior vena cava and the ascending aorta (Fig. 104.10).[56]

It is difficult to predict when the fetus will develop hydrops. Several Doppler echocardiographic parameters that demonstrate congestive heart failure cannot be used at this extremely high heart rate. Serial measurement of the cardiothoracic ratio may be useful for monitoring the degree of heart failure. The presence of atrioventricular valve regurgitation, especially at the mitral valve, may represent severe congestive heart failure. Usually, the fetus does not deteriorate quickly even after developing fetal hydrops. Maternal administration of digoxin, the first choice for treating AVRT, may be indicated for fetuses with early signs of heart failure or sustained tachycardia lasting more than 8 hours in a day. Sotalol, procainamide, propranolol, amiodarone, and flecainide are used as second-line drugs when digoxin fails to achieve conversion to sinus rhythm. These second-line drugs can be used from the beginning in fetuses with a long VA interval or in fetuses with severe congestive heart failure. Early delivery and administration of ATP or electrical conversion is the option when intrauterine conversion cannot be achieved.

M-mode recording of atrial and ventricular contraction for fetuses with atrial fibrillation shows a regular atrial rate of 400 to 500 beats per minute with 2:1 to 4:1 atrioventricular conduction, resulting in a ventricular rate of 200 to 300 beats

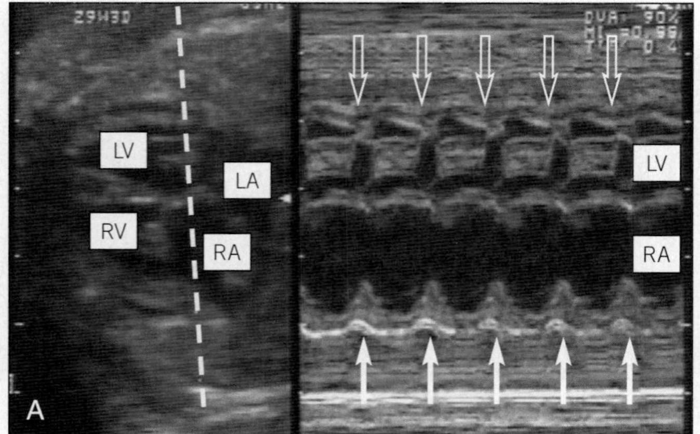

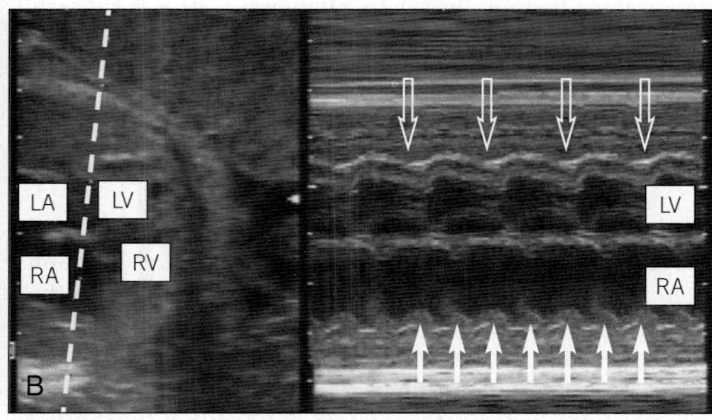

Fig. 104.9 Simultaneous M-mode recording of both ventricles and atria. A, M-mode recording in a fetus with supraventricular tachycardia reveals 1:1 relation of atrial (*solid arrow*) and ventricular contraction (*open arrow*) with a ventricular rate of 210 beats per minute. **B,** M-mode recording in a fetus with atrial flutter and 2:1 atrioventricular conduction, with an atrial (*solid arrow*) rate of 510 beats per minute and a ventricular (*open arrow*) rate of 255 beats per minute. LA, left atrium; LV, left ventricle; RA, right atrium; RV, right ventricle.

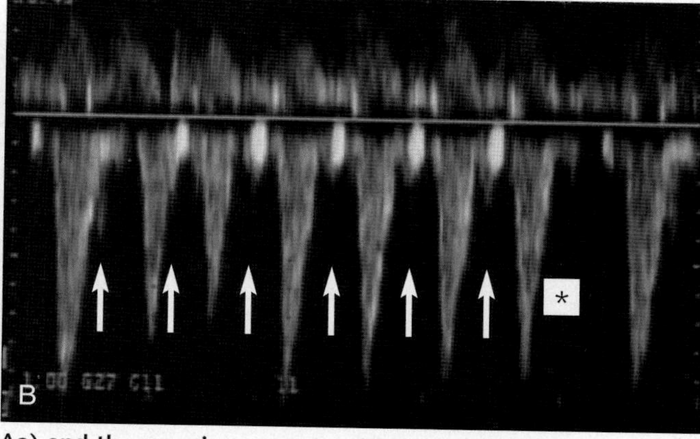

Fig. 104.10 Simultaneous Doppler trace of the ascending aorta (aAo) and the superior vena cava (SVC). A, Doppler trace of a fetus with supraventricular tachycardia with short VA interval. Although high-velocity reversal flow of SVC is almost over-rapped to the flow of Ao, the starting point of the reversal flow can be detected from the interrupted forward flow of the SVC. **B,** Doppler trace of the fetus with 1:1 atrioventricular conduction tachycardia with long VA interval. Tachycardic atrial contraction (*arrows*) disappears after the seventh ventricular contraction (*), and the tachycardia is stopped.

per minute.[62] Associated cardiac structural abnormality is more common than in PSVT. There is some tendency to develop 1:1 AV conduction and sudden deterioration; hence, all fetuses with atrial fibrillation should be treated after diagnosis. The selection of antiarrhythmic drug is similar to that for PSVT. However, the decision to start a second-line drug may be made earlier than for PSVT because of the possibility of sudden deterioration.

Fetal Cardiomyopathies

Although fetal echocardiography detects cardiac dysfunction, little is known regarding the cardiomyopathies and myocarditis in fetal life.[63] On routine fetal echocardiographic examination, the four-chamber view clearly detects the dilated, poorly contractile heart in dilated cardiomyopathy or the ventricular hypertrophy in hypertrophic cardiomyopathy. Signs of fetal hydrops are present in the case of developed heart failure. Serial assessment of systolic and diastolic cardiac function by M-mode and Doppler echocardiography is important for managing the affected fetuses.

Fetal cardiomyopathy is etiologically a heterogeneous condition, which can be the result of intrinsic pathology in addition to extrinsic factors. Noonan's syndrome, familial cardiomyopathy, α-thalassemia, and metabolic disease had been reported as intrinsic causes. Extrinsic causes include infectious disease, maternal autoantibodies,[64] and others. Although treatment for the various causes of cardiomyopathy and management of cardiac failure have been reported, the outcome of the affected fetuses is generally poor.

ACCURACY

The detection rate for congenital heart disease by screening fetal ultrasound and the accuracy of prenatal echocardiography are directly related to the quality of the examiner's technique and the reviewer's interpretation. Hence, teaching programs and sufficient experience specific to prenatal echocardiography are very important to make a significant impact on practice.

At the more advanced prenatal echocardiographic centers, quite accurate diagnosis has been reported.[2] With the new high-resolution echocardiographic machines, morphologic diagnosis has become more and more accurate. At about 18 to 28 weeks of gestation, the large volume of surrounding amniotic fluid and the less calcified fetal spine and ribs make it possible to visualize quite detailed cardiac anatomy. Even small cardiac structures with small blood flows, such as pulmonary venous return and small ventricular septal defects, can be detected by detailed prenatal echocardiographic examination combined with advanced color Doppler mapping.

COMPLICATIONS

The ultrasound technique is known to be a noninvasive imaging modality. However, there remain some concerns regarding possible adverse effects on the fetus of exposure to ultrasound, especially for Doppler echocardiography, in which the energy levels are greater. Possible adverse effects are both heat-related and non–heat-related. Although no epidemiologic report has demonstrated any adverse effects of prenatal ultrasonographic examination, particular attention should be paid to minimizing the energy level during prenatal examination. The examination time should be as short as possible, using a low power level, and use of pulse, continuous, and color Doppler should be limited to as short a time as possible.

PITFALLS AND ALTERNATIVES

Although high-resolution echocardiography provides quite accurate morphologic information, there remain some limitations, and correct knowledge of these may prevent possible misinterpretation and misdiagnosis. The limitations are divided into three categories:

- technical limitations;
- fetal hemodynamic limitations; and
- limitations resulting from prenatal and perinatal progression of disease.

The images of prenatal echocardiography are not always sufficient to provide detailed information. Movement and position of the fetus, location of the placenta, and maternal obesity are the most typical causes of inadequate images.

Less amniotic fluid and more heavily calcified bones in later gestation also limit the amount of information obtained. For fetuses in a bad position, changing the mother's position to lie on her side, having her fill her bladder by drinking water and letting her take a walk for several minutes may change the fetal position. Three-dimensional echocardiography can overcome some of these position limitations. When the position is unsuitable even after various attempts, repeat examination on a different day may be another option. When maternal obesity limits image quality, positioning the probe in the mother's navel where there is less lipid thickness may provide a better image. Despite the limitations of prenatal echocardiography, there is no alternative clinically applicable imaging modality.

The difference between fetal and postnatal hemodynamics often makes it difficult to diagnose cardiac problems in utero. Because the ductus arteriosus is widely patent, the pressures in the aorta and the pulmonary artery are the same. Hence, the presence of aortic or pulmonary stenosis may not cause a significant pressure gradient at the stenotic lesion. Functional pulmonary atresia as a result of increased pulmonary artery pressure is also difficult to distinguish from anatomic atresia. It may not be possible to diagnose patent ductus arteriosus and atrial septal defect prenatally.

Some cardiac anatomic abnormalities may progress in utero. The ventricles and the great arteries may become hypoplastic, the degree of valve stenosis and regurgitation may increase, and arrhythmia may develop. In particular, the fetus may develop atrioventricular block in left isomerism or discordant atrioventricular connection. At the present time, there is no clear method of predicting such progression. Therefore awareness of possible progression and serial prenatal examinations are important.

SUMMARY

Prenatal diagnosis of congenital heart disease has had an impact on its clinical management in several ways.[2,65] High-risk cases are delivered under cover of prostaglandin infusion and balloon atrial septostomy and are transferred to the pediatric cardiac center without deterioration. The possibility for family counseling is a clear benefit. Parents can be provided with sufficient information to make decisions and work out a strategy for perinatal management.

Prenatal pharmacologic and surgical treatment of heart disease has already begun. Fetal tachyarrhythmia has been successfully managed by pharmacologic treatment in utero.[13,58,60] Intrauterine treatment using interventional catheterization for LVOT and RVOT has also been started.[33,36,37] A number of research projects for use in future prenatal cardiac intervention and surgery, such as a very small cardiopulmonary pump for the fetus and fetoscopic surgery, have already begun.[66-69]

For the benefits of prenatal diagnosis to have a significant impact on practice, effective screening for congenital heart disease is essential.[3] The prenatal sonographic screening system for each lesion must be established. Practical methods, simple techniques, and clear interpretations within short examination times need to be taught in prenatal screening centers.

Finally, ethical problems are a very important issue in prenatal diagnosis.[70] Even before screening, the fetal ultrasonographic examination may require appropriate informed consent. Parents must be made aware that there is some chance that an anomaly in the fetus will be detected, and they may not want to know about this until the child's birth. Once the fetus is diagnosed as having congenital heart disease, the parents have to decide the management plan. The decision as to whether to continue with the pregnancy may be the most important ethical issue for prenatal diagnosis. In addition, many prenatal treatments are still experimental; hence, their efficacy and possible adverse effects on both the fetus and the healthy mother are still unknown. However, the opinion of the physician who tells the parents about fetal heart problems tends to influence the parents' decision. The support system to help parents with their decision making must be established for each lesion.

chapter 105

Diagnostic Pathways for Evaluation of Congenital Heart Disease

Tal Geva, Lisa J. Bergersen, and Jacqueline Kreutzer

Definition/Problem

- Successful treatment of congenital heart disease depends on accurate delineation of cardiovascular anatomy and physiology.

Key Features/Findings

- A variety of diagnostic techniques are currently available to pediatric cardiologists.
- To arrive at an accurate diagnosis in patients with congenital heart disease in the most timely, efficient, and cost-effective manner, cardiologists must be familiar with the strengths and limitations of all diagnostic techniques available. Whenever possible, every effort should be made to use noninvasive imaging techniques, thus reserving invasive procedures for therapeutic interventions.

Clinical Implications

- Judicious use of echocardiography, magnetic resonance imaging, x-ray angiography, computed tomography, and radionuclide perfusion studies allows clinicians to tailor treatment plans for congenital heart disease in patients of all ages.

Before the advent of cardiopulmonary bypass in the mid 1950s, little attention was given to the diagnosis of congenital heart disease (CHD), because no effective treatment was available. Progress in open heart techniques for repair of CHD required accurate and comprehensive delineation of cardiovascular anatomy and function. Physical examination, auscultation, electrocardiography, and radiography were initially the main diagnostic tools. During the 1960s and 1970s, cardiac catheterization and angiography became the principal tools used for diagnosis of CHD. Echocardiography entered the arena in the late 1970s. The diagnostic capability of M-mode echocardiography proved insufficient in patients with CHD, but the rapid evolution of two-dimensional (2D) echocardiography during the following decade transformed the field. The technological advances in transducer design, image processing and display, together with development and refinement of new imaging planes and examination technique, allowed high-quality tomographic visualization of most cardiac defects.[1] The application of Doppler ultrasound to investigate blood flow allowed comprehensive hemodynamic assessment. By the mid 1980s, much of the necessary anatomic and hemodynamic information required for patient management could be obtained noninvasively, obviating the need for a diagnostic catheterization in many patients. During the 1990s, the field of pediatric cardiac imaging experienced accelerated progress in areas such as three-dimensional (3D) echocardiography, tissue Doppler imaging, and the application of magnetic resonance imaging (MRI) to CHD. At the same time, the proportion of cardiac catheterization procedures performed solely for diagnostic purposes had drastically declined. By the end of the 1990s, the majority of catheterization procedures in pediatric cardiology were therapeutic.

ECHOCARDIOGRAPHY AND DOPPLER ULTRASOUND

Echocardiography is an ideal diagnostic tool in pediatric cardiology because of its noninvasive nature, relatively low cost, superb spatial and temporal resolutions, and ability to image cardiovascular anatomy and to evaluate physiology in real time. In addition, modern cardiac ultrasound equipment is portable and adaptable to different environments, such as the operating room, intensive care unit, the bedside, and an outpatient office setting. In today's pediatric cardiology practice, echocardiography is the primary diagnostic modality used to evaluate anatomy and physiology before, during, and after operation; during follow-up of CHD; and during the prenatal period.[1]

Description of Techniques

To obtain an echocardiographic image, a burst of ultrasound energy is generated by a transducer and travels through the soft tissue at an average speed of approximately 1540 m/second. When the propagating ultrasound wave encounters an interface between tissues with different acoustic properties, some of the energy is reflected back toward the transducer, and some of the energy is refracted and continues to travel in the medium until it encounters the next interface. The returning ultrasound energy is then converted into an electrical energy that goes through a series of electronic processes, including amplification, postprocessing, and display.

M-Mode Echocardiography

With M-mode echocardiography, a narrow beam of ultrasound energy is emitted toward the heart, and structures along the beam path reflect echoes back toward the transducer. A dot is displayed on the screen in a position corresponding to its distance from the transducer. This process is repeated rapidly to create an image. The distance from the transducer is displayed on the y-axis and time is displayed on the x-axis. This provides a unidimensional image of the heart that is characterized by excellent temporal and axial resolutions. In today's clinical pediatric echocardiography, M-mode is no longer used for anatomic imaging of the heart. 2D-directed M-mode echocardiography is used primarily for evaluation of left ventricular dimensions and functions. In selected circumstances, when superior temporal resolution is required, 2D-directed M-mode may be used to assess motion of specific structures, such as native and prosthetic valve leaflets.[2]

Two-Dimensional Imaging

An ultrasound beam is rapidly swept through an arc and multiple M-mode lines placed next to each other to construct a 2D cross-sectional image of the anatomy. This can be accomplished by rotating or rocking an ultrasonic crystal as in mechanical transducers, or by electronically sweeping the sound beam through several piezoelectric crystals (transducer elements), as in phased-array transducers. Recent advances in transducer technology and image processing permit very high frame rates (>200 Hz) and high line densities, features that greatly enhance temporal and spatial resolutions.[3]

Three- and Four-Dimensional Imaging

Accurate spatial perception of an object depends on recognition of its three dimensions—length, width, and depth. Although an experienced examiner can mentally construct a 3D image of the heart from serial 2D tomographic images obtained by sweeping the transducer across the chest, 3D echocardiography offers an enhanced perspective of cardiovascular structures and their interrelations. The addition of a fourth dimension, time, by creating dynamic 3D imaging has further enhanced comprehension of spatial features of anatomic structures and their motion throughout the cardiac cycle. Recent advances in transducer design and image processing technologies allow real-time 3D cardiac ultrasound.[4] This rapidly evolving technology is used for anatomic and hemodynamic assessments of patients with congenital heart disease.

Doppler Echocardiography

The use of Doppler ultrasound to assess normal and abnormal hemodynamics has become an integral part of the echocardiographic examination.[1] The advent of 2D-directed Doppler interrogation has greatly enhanced the clinical application of this technique by allowing evaluation of flow characteristics in specific regions within the heart and great vessels. In today's echocardiography, spectral and color-coded Doppler flow mapping are used extensively to measure velocity and direction of blood flow (Fig. 105.1). Calculations based on Doppler-derived measurements allow quantitative estimation of flow volume (such as cardiac output), pressure gradient across a stenotic region, cross-sectional flow area, and prediction of intracardiac pressures. Doppler echocardiography also provides qualitative and semiquantitative assessment of valve regurgitation, intracardiac and extracardiac shunts, and myocardial motion (tissue Doppler imaging). Detailed discussion of Doppler physics is beyond the scope of this text and can be found elsewhere.[3]

Contrast Echocardiography

As early as the late 1960s, it was noted that intravascular injection of almost any solution resulted in a contrast effect detectable by echocardiography. Initially, this technique was used to identify structures seen by M-mode echocardiography. Contrast echocardiography has been used to detect systemic[5] and pulmonary venous anomalies,[6] and to detect intracardiac shunts at the level of the great arteries.[7] In today's pediatric echocardiography, contrast studies are infrequently performed and are usually limited to detection of intracardiac shunts in patients with limited echocardiographic windows, patch or baffle leak after cardiac surgery, and pulmonary arteriovenous malformations.[1]

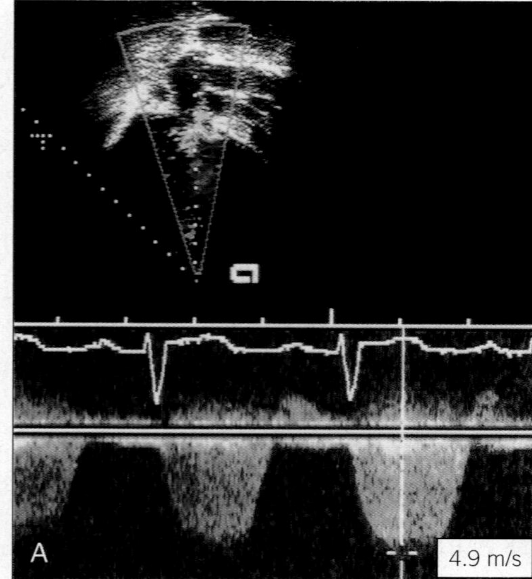

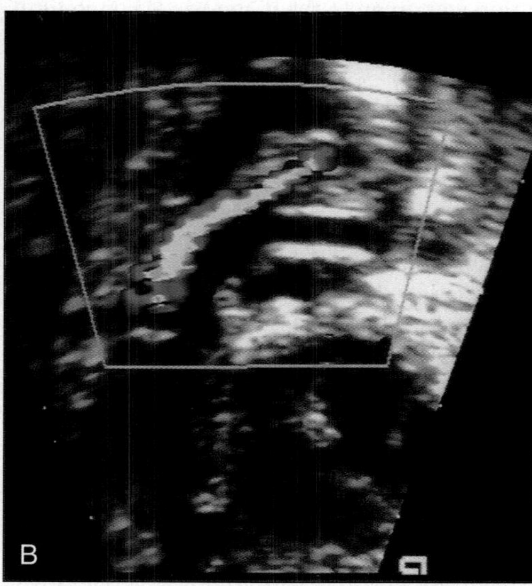

Figure 105.1 Doppler echocardiography. A, Visualization of a high-velocity jet by color Doppler aids in aligning the continuous-wave Doppler cursor in a patient with SLL (visceroatrial situs solitus [S], L-ventricular loop [L], and L-transposition [L])[1,10] transposition of the great arteries with severe subpulmonary stenosis (predicted maximal instantaneous gradient approximately 96 mm Hg). **B,** Imaging of a left-to-right flow jet through a patent ductus arteriosus by color Doppler flow mapping from the subxiphoid short-axis view.

INDICATIONS AND OBJECTIVES

The objectives of the echocardiographic examination must be tailored to the individual patient. The initial evaluation should include a comprehensive survey of all anatomic elements of the central cardiovascular system. Subsequent examinations are often targeted to answer specific clinical questions. It is important, however, to repeat complete echocardiograms during follow-up, even in patients who underwent a comprehensive initial examination, because of the dynamic nature of CHD. Examples include the late onset of discrete subaortic stenosis in patients with ventricular septal defect and/or coarctation of the aorta,[8] double-chambered right ventricle,[9] and supramitral stenosing ring.

EXAMINATION TECHNIQUE

Proper planning of the echocardiographic examination is important to ensure that all diagnostic information is obtained most efficiently. This is particularly relevant in sedated patients in whom the time available for data acquisition is limited. Ideally, a complete segmental examination of cardiovascular anatomy and function should be performed in every new patient. This includes determination of visceral situs, heart position, atrial situs, systemic and pulmonary venous connections, ventricular situs, atrioventricular and ventriculoarterial alignments and connections, and coronary and great arterial anatomy. Assessment of ventricular function, intracardiac and vessel dimensions, and flow analysis across all valves, septa, chambers, and vessels are integral parts of the examination.

In young children with suspected heart disease, the examination begins from the subxiphoid approach by determining the abdominal situs and then proceeding by scanning the heart and great vessels, using a step-by-step segmental analysis (Fig. 105.2a,b).[10] This approach is advantageous because it provides a wide-angle view of heart position and cardiovascular anatomy and function at an early stage in the examination. Subsequent 2D, 3D, and Doppler analyses from the apical, parasternal, and suprasternal notch views supplement and confirm findings from the subxiphoid window (see Fig. 105.2c-g).

The examination strategy should be tailored to the individual patient and modified according to the clinical situation as necessary. Although the standard views described previously should be obtained in almost every patient and represent the

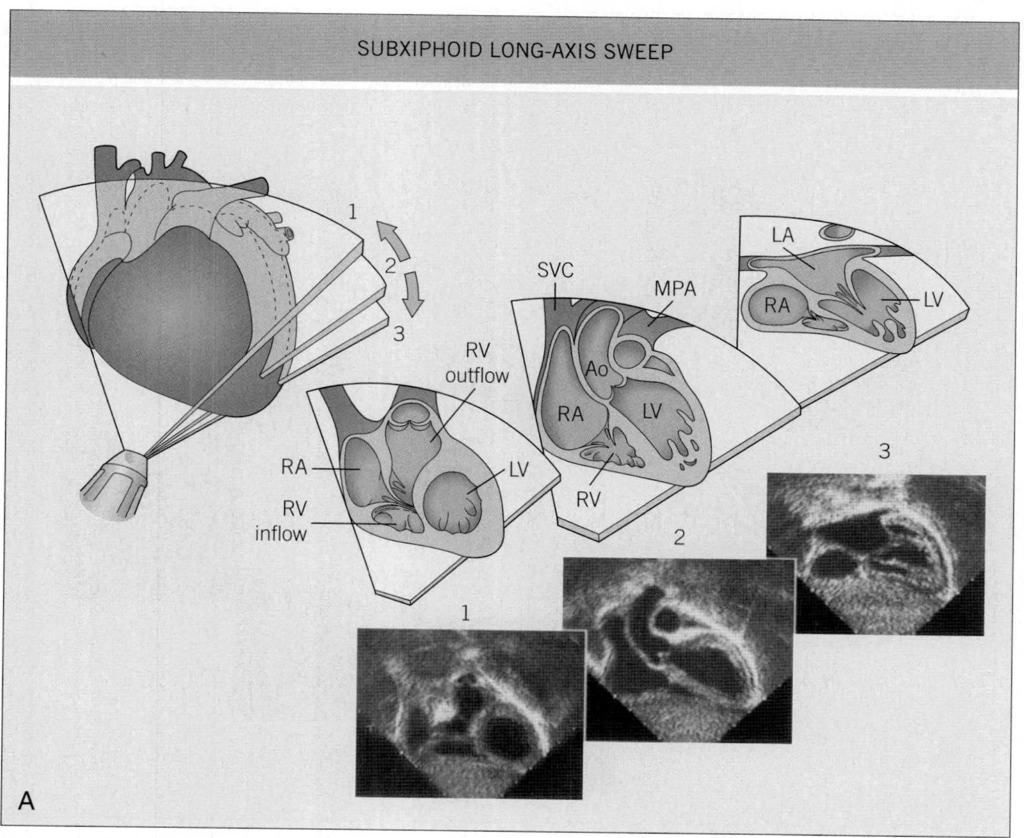

Figure 105.2 Standard two-dimensional transthoracic imaging sweeps. A, Subxiphoid long-axis sweep. Slow gradual sweep starting at the level of the upper abdomen will show the connection of the inferior vena cava to the right atrium (RA). The left atrium (LA) is seen next. The connection of the pulmonary veins and the atrial septum can be demonstrated from this view. The left ventricle (LV) is seen along its long axis. Further superior angulation of the transducer depicts the left ventricular outflow tract, aortic valve, and ascending aorta (Ao). The superior vena cava (SVC) is seen to the right of the ascending aorta and the main pulmonary artery (MPA) is seen to the left of the aorta. Further superior tilt of the transducer shows the right ventricular inflow (RV inflow) and outflow (RV outflow) and the pulmonary valve. The sweep ends with the anterior free wall of the right ventricle.

(Continued)

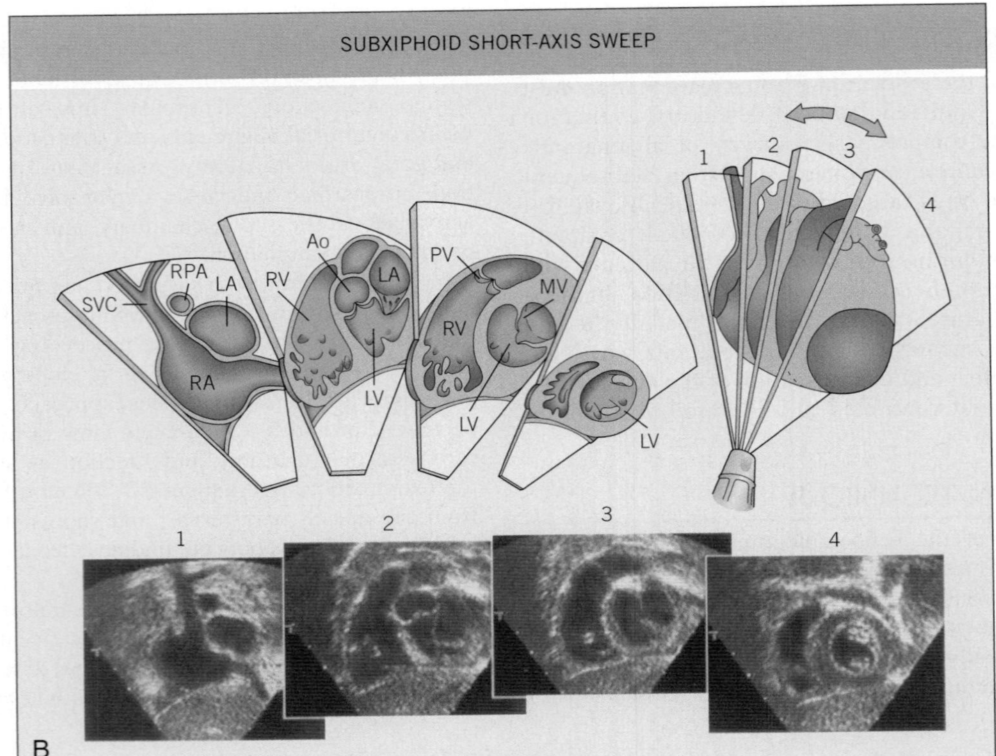

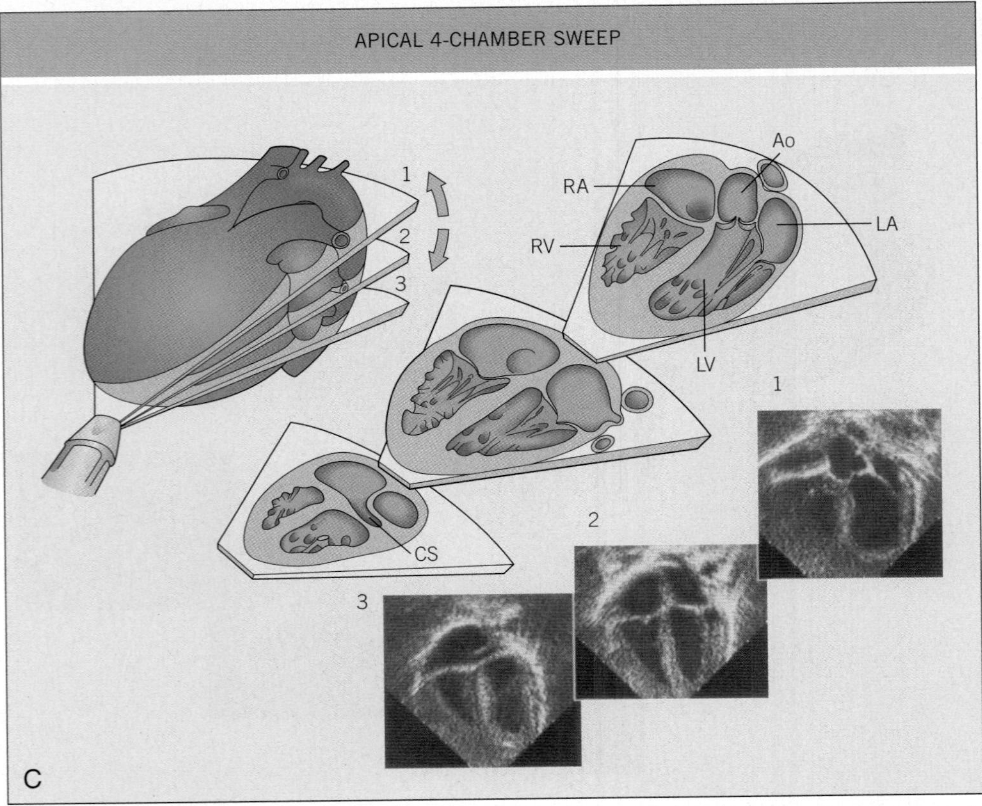

Figure 105.2—cont'd **B,** Subxiphoid short-axis sweep. From the subxiphoid long-axis view, the transducer is rotated clockwise by approximately 90 degrees. The sweep begins at the rightward-most aspect of the heart and progresses from right to left through the cardiac apex. The superior vena cava (SVC) and inferior vena cava are seen entering the right atrium (RA). The right pulmonary artery (RPA) is seen in cross section behind the SVC and above the left atrium (LA). The atrial septum is highly visible in this plane. Sweeping the transducer leftward will show the base of the left ventricle (LV) and right ventricle (RV) and the atrioventricular valves. The aortic valve is seen in cross section at this level. Further leftward tilt of the transducer depicts a cross-sectional view of the LV and mitral valve (MV), in addition to the right ventricular outflow tract and pulmonary valve (PV). The sweep ends with imaging of the mid muscular septum, the papillary muscles, and the apical portions of both ventricles. Standard two-dimensional transthoracic imaging sweeps. **C,** Apical four-chamber sweep. The transducer is positioned over the apex and angled to obtain a cross-sectional view of the atria and ventricles as shown in panel 2. The transducer is then angled posteriorly to image the posterior aspect of the heart (panel 3). In this plane, the coronary sinus (CS) can be viewed along the posterior left atrioventricular groove. Anterosuperior tilt of the transducer will show the left ventricular outflow tract and proximal ascending aorta (Ao).

PARASTERNAL LONG-AXIS SWEEP

1 2 3
RA
RV
LV
Ao
LA
RVOT
MPA
D

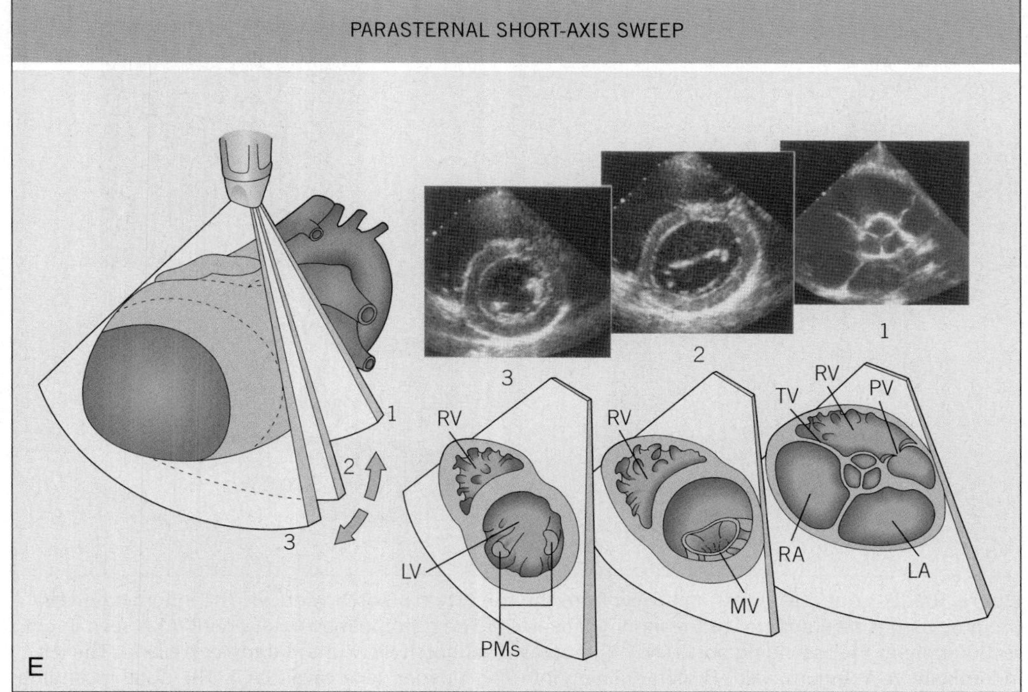

Figure 105.2—cont'd **D,** Parasternal long-axis sweep. The transducer is placed over the left precordium to the left of the sternum with the index mark toward the patient's right shoulder. A rightward and inferior tilt of the transducer toward the right hip shows the right atrium (RA), tricuspid valve, and right ventricular inflow (RV) (panel 1). The coronary sinus can be followed into the right atrium in this view. A leftward and superior tilt of the transducer toward the left shoulder depicts the right ventricular outflow tract (RVOT), pulmonary valve, and main pulmonary artery (MPA) (panel 3). Standard two-dimensional transthoracic imaging sweeps. **E,** Parasternal short-axis sweep. From the parasternal long-axis view, the transducer is rotated clockwise by approximately 90 degrees. The sweep progresses from a plane that shows right and left atria (LA and RA), the atrial septum, the tricuspid valve (TV), right ventricle (RV), pulmonary valve (PV), and main pulmonary artery (panel 1), toward the apex. Cross-sectional views of the right ventricle (RV), left ventricle (LV), ventricular septum, mitral valve (MV), and papillary muscles (PMs) are obtained.

(*Continued*)

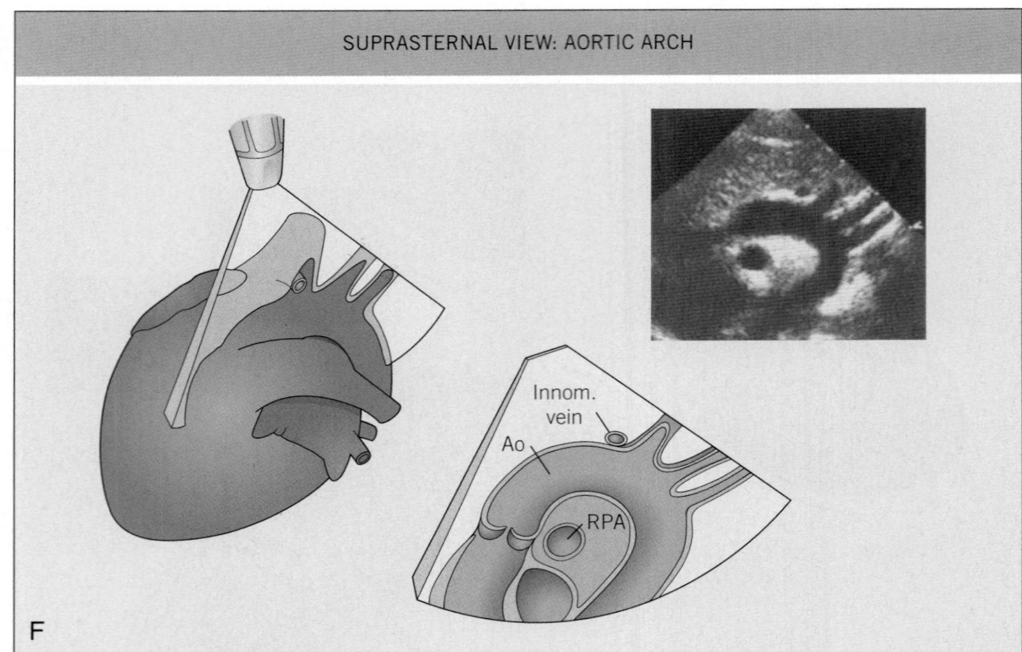

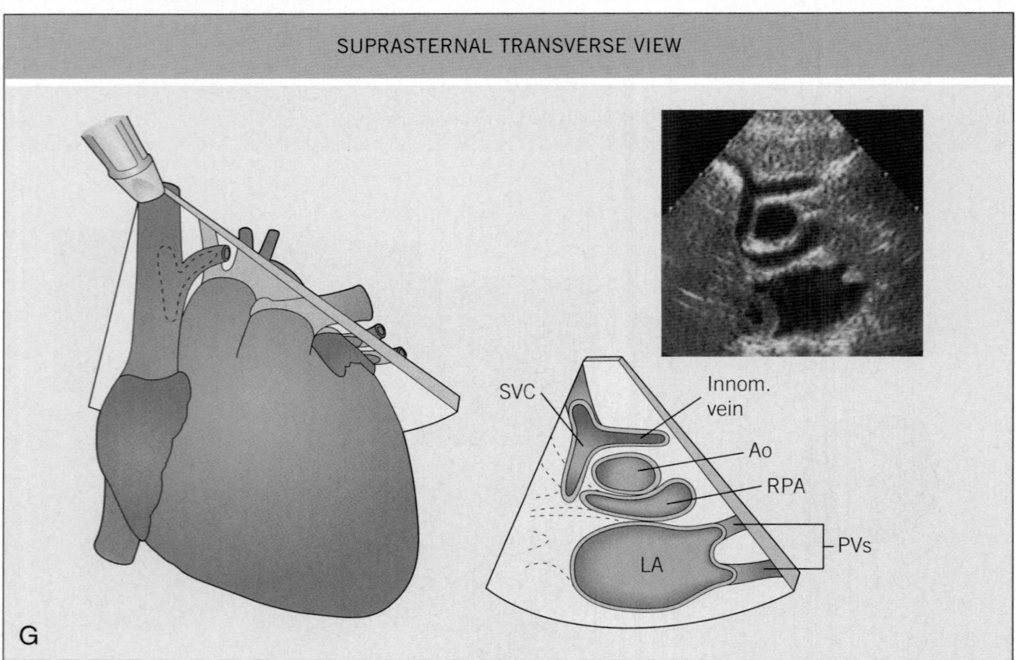

Figure 105.2—cont'd F, Aortic arch view from the suprasternal notch window. The innominate vein (Innom. vein) is seen anterior to the innominate artery. The right pulmonary artery (RPA) is seen in cross section behind the ascending aorta (Ao). **G,** Suprasternal notch view in the transverse plane. The left innominate vein (Innom. vein) is seen draining into the superior vena cava (SVC). The distal ascending aorta (Ao) is superior to the right pulmonary artery (RPA), which is visible along its length above the left atrium (LA). Note the pulmonary veins (PVs) entering the left atrium.

minimum acceptable examination, flexibility and improvisation are important to make optimal use of the full potential of echocardiography.[11]

Anatomic Analysis

When an echocardiographic examination is performed and reviewed in a patient suspected of having CHD, a stepwise segmental approach to analysis of cardiac anatomy is taken. The fundamental principle of segmental analysis of CHD is to analyze each component of the heart separately according to its unique morphologic features.[10] The heart is composed of five segments—three main segments and two connecting segments. The three main segments are the atria, the ventricles, and the great arteries. The atrioventricular canal, which includes the mitral and tricuspid valves and the atrioventricular septum, connects the atria with the ventricles. The infundibulum (or conus) connects the ventricles with the great arteries. When cardiac anatomy is analyzed, each cardiac chamber must be identified individually according to its unique anatomic-morphologic features and not according to its spatial position (right-sided or left-sided), valve of entry, or artery of exit. Throughout a systematic echocardiographic study, the examiner must go over a mental checklist of segments, their anatomic organization and position (situs), their connections and alignments with adjacent segments, and associated malformations.[10,12] Using the aforementioned principles, any potential CHD can be accurately described in specific and precise terms.

SPECIAL ECHOCARDIOGRAPHIC PROCEDURES

Transesophageal Echocardiography

Transesophageal echocardiography was first introduced in 1976 and appeared in pediatric use in 1989. The miniaturization of probes and development of multiplanar imaging has greatly increased its role as an adjunct to transthoracic imaging, during surgical repair of CHD (intraoperative transesophageal echocardiography), and to guide interventional catheterization procedures.

Indications and Objectives

A transesophageal echocardiographic examination is usually performed to answer a limited set of clinical questions. It is advisable, however, to perform a comprehensive examination of the heart and blood vessels for additional unsuspected anatomic and/or hemodynamic anomalies (Fig. 105.3). The availability of small biplane and multiplane probes designed for use in young infants weighing 3 to 3.5 kg or less has greatly enhanced the scope of transesophageal echocardiography in the pediatric age group.[13-15] Successful transesophageal echocardiographic examinations have been reported in patients weighing as little as 2.3 kg.[15] The role of transesophageal echocardiography in pediatric cardiology is continuously evolving.[16] Although the transthoracic window is adequate in most situations, transesophageal echocardiography provides many distinct advantages:

- during cardiovascular surgery[13-15];
- during video-assisted thoracoscopic procedures;
- for guidance of interventional catheter procedures;
- in the intensive care unit[13-15];
- for detection of intracardiac thrombi and vegetations;
- for assessment of prosthetic valves;
- in selected patients on mechanical assist devices and extracorporeal membrane oxygenators; and
- in selected patients with poor transthoracic windows, such as adults with CHD.

Safety and Complications

Although in expert hands transesophageal echocardiography is quite safe, complications have been reported, including oropharyngeal trauma and compression of airways and vascular structures. Transesophageal echocardiography is contraindicated in patients with an unrepaired tracheoesophageal fistula, esophageal obstruction or stricture, perforated viscus, or active gastrointestinal bleeding; in an unwilling or uncooperative patient who is inadequately sedated; or in a patient with an uncontrolled airway and respiratory or cardiac decompensation. Relative contraindications include cervical spine injury, immobility, or deformity; history of esophageal surgery; known esophageal varices or diverticulum; oropharyngeal deformities; and severe coagulopathy.[16,17]

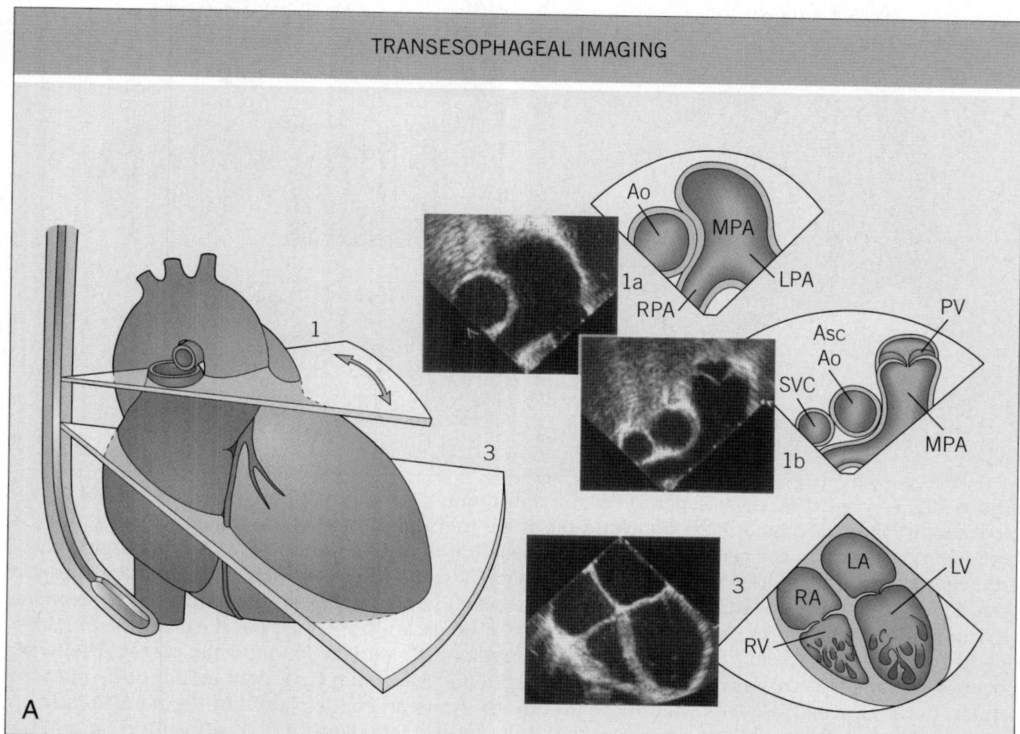

Figure 105.3 Transesophageal imaging. A, Transverse plane. Cross-sectional view at level 1a depicts the proximal ascending aorta (Ao), main pulmonary artery (MPA), and left and right pulmonary arteries (LPA and RPA, respectively). A rightward tilt of the transducer shows the RPA as it passes behind the superior vena cava (SVC) and ascending aorta (Asc Ao). To obtain a four-chamber view (level 3), the transducer is advanced in the esophagus with slight retroflexion of the scope.

(Continued)

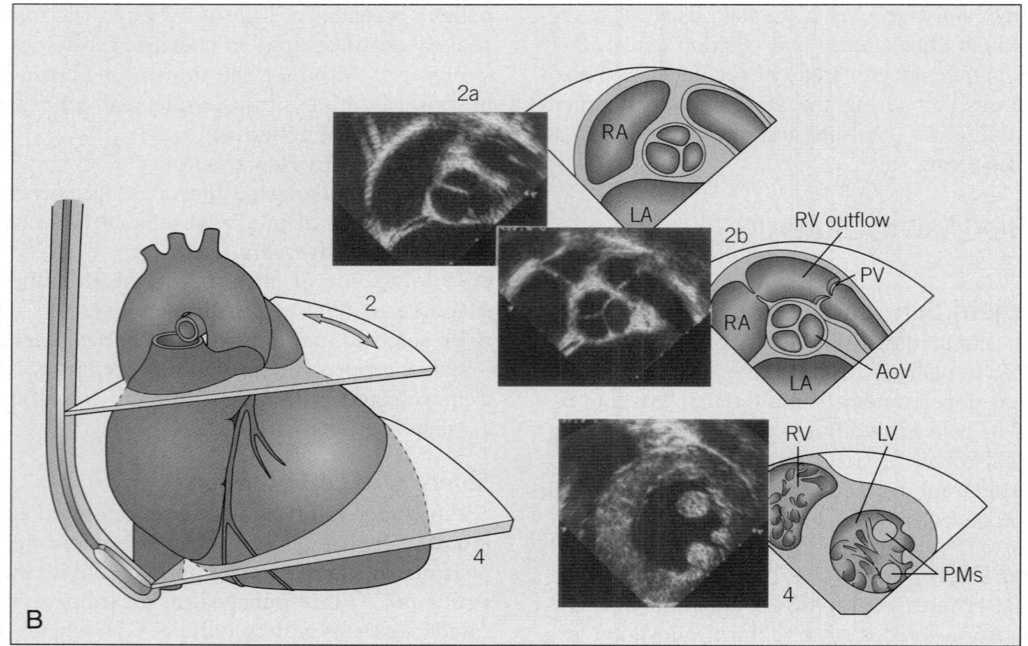

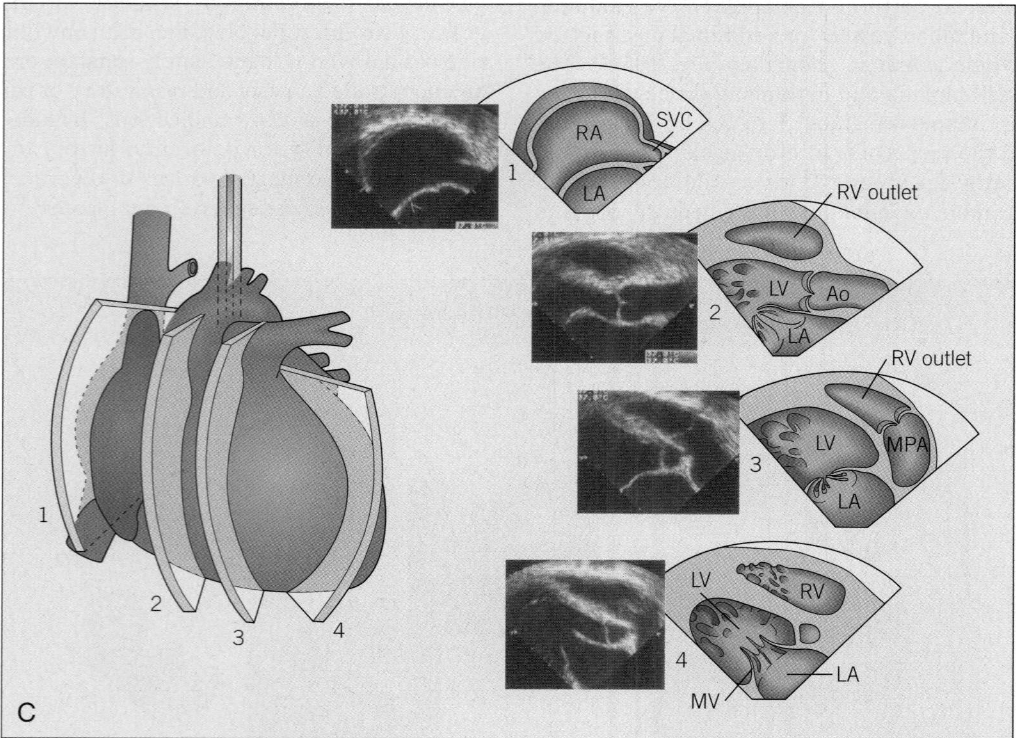

Figure 105.3—cont'd B, Level 2: parallel to the transthoracic parasternal short-axis view. In level 2a, the atrial septum is imaged by a slight rightward tilt of the transducer. In level 2b, the aortic valve (AoV) is seen in cross section in the center of the image, the left atrium (LA), right atrium (RA), tricuspid valve, right ventricular outflow (RV outflow), pulmonary valve (PV), and the proximal main pulmonary artery are seen. By advancing the transducer into the lower esophagus and anteflexing the scope, a cross-sectional view of the left ventricle (LV), mitral valve, and papillary muscles is obtained (level 4). Note that image orientation is the same as in transthoracic echocardiography. **C,** Vertical (longitudinal) planes. The sweep begins at a plane that crosses the superior vena cava (SVC), left atrium (LA), right atrium (RA), and atrial septum (level 1). Next, a leftward tilt of the transducer shows an image parallel to the transthoracic parasternal long-axis view of the left atrium (LA), mitral valve, left ventricle (LV), left ventricular outflow tract, and proximal aorta (Ao) (level 2). Further leftward tilt of the transducer (level 3) shows the right ventricular outflow tract (RV outlet), pulmonary valve, and main pulmonary artery (MPA). The sweep continues leftward to show the leftward aspects of the left atrium, mitral valve (MV), and left ventricle (level 4). Further leftward tilt depicts the left atrial appendage and the left pulmonary veins (not shown). Note that image orientation is the same as in transthoracic echocardiography.

Fetal Echocardiography

Examination of the fetal cardiovascular system in humans dates back to the late 1960s, when continuous-wave Doppler echocardiography was used to record fetal heart rate. Although Kleinman and colleagues[18] in the late 1970s had some success in detecting CHD in the fetus by M-mode echocardiography, it was not until high-resolution 2D imaging became available in the mid 1980s that accurate delineation of cardiovascular anatomy became clinically routine. Today, prenatal detection of CHD can be reliably diagnosed by 17 to 20 weeks of gestation by transabdominal imaging. Using the transvaginal window, the heart and great vessels can be imaged as early as late first trimester.[19]

Indications and Objectives

Although several studies have demonstrated a low detection rate of CHD by routine level I obstetric ultrasound,[20] cost-benefit considerations preclude universal fetal echocardiographic screening by expert pediatric echocardiographers. Alternatively, an approach based on targeting pregnancies that are at high risk for CHD is taken. Such an approach increases the yield of fetal echocardiography to approximately 30% when extracardiac anomalies are detected, to approximately 60% when level I scan detects possible CHD, and to nearly 100% when a second opinion is requested.[21] The indications for fetal echocardiography are summarized in Table 105.1. Detailed discussion of the indications for fetal echocardiography can be found elsewhere.[22]

INDICATIONS FOR FETAL ECHOCARDIOGRAPHY
Fetal risk factors
Extracardiac structural anomalies
Chromosomal abnormalities
Fetal dysrhythmias
Irregular rhythm
Tachyarrhythmia
Bradyarrhythmia
Intrauterine growth retardation
Nonimmune hydrops fetalis
Suspected cardiac anomaly on level-1 scan
Abnormal visceral situs
Maternal risk factors
Congenital heart disease
Exposure to teratogen (sample list only)
Lithium carbonate
Amphetamines
Alcohol
Anticonvulsants
Phenytoin
Trimethadione
Isotretinoin
Maternal diabetes
Phenylketonuria
Maternal infection
Rubella
Toxoplasmosis
Coxsackievirus
Cytomegalovirus
Mumps virus
Familial risk factors
Congenital heart disease
Syndromes
Down
Marfan
Noonan
Tuberous sclerosis
Velocardiofacial
Modified from Allan LD, Santos R, Pexieder T. Anatomical and echocardiographic correlates of normal cardiac morphology in the late first trimester fetus. Heart 1997;77:68-72.

Table 105.1 Indications for fetal echocardiography.

Description of Technique

Echocardiographic examination of the cardiovascular system in the fetus is based on the same principles of the segmental approach to diagnosis of CHD that is applied after birth. The main difference between examination of the fetus and the newborn is that the operator has no control over fetal position and, consequently, over the views obtained. Once fetal position is ascertained and the spatial coordinates of the fetal torso are determined, the examination then continues according to the principles outlined in the previous sections. Given optimal acoustic windows and favorable fetal position, even the most complex cardiovascular anomalies can be detected (Fig. 105.4). Defects that remain difficult to diagnose in utero include atrial septal defect, patent ductus arteriosus, small or moderate ventricular septal defect, coarctation of the aorta, anomalies of the coronary arteries, partially anomalous pulmonary venous connection, and some valve and great vessel abnormalities. It is usually not possible to distinguish between normal patency of the foramen ovale and an atrial septal defect in the fetus. Similarly, it is not possible to predict whether the normally patent ductus arteriosus will close after birth. In utero diagnosis of aortic coarctation may be difficult, because the typical isthmic narrowing may not become apparent until after ductal closure. However, the diagnosis may be suspected on the basis of abnormal morphology of the transverse aortic arch (elongation and hypoplasia) and size discrepancy between the ventricles (right ventricle larger than left ventricle).[23]

Clinical Implications

Early prenatal diagnosis of major CHD allows parents to consider the option to terminate the pregnancy. It is also common to recommend amniocentesis to detect associated genetic abnormalities. When pregnancy continues, prenatal diagnosis of CHD allows proper planning for postnatal cardiac care. When intervention is anticipated immediately or shortly after birth (e.g., ductal-dependent anomalies or balloon atrial septostomy in transposition of the great arteries), delivery in a pediatric cardiac center is arranged. From currently available data, it is not clear whether prenatal diagnosis of CHD leads to a significant reduction in mortality[24]; however, it may lead to reduced morbidity in certain lesions.[24] Other advantages, such as psychological benefits to the parents, are more difficult to measure.

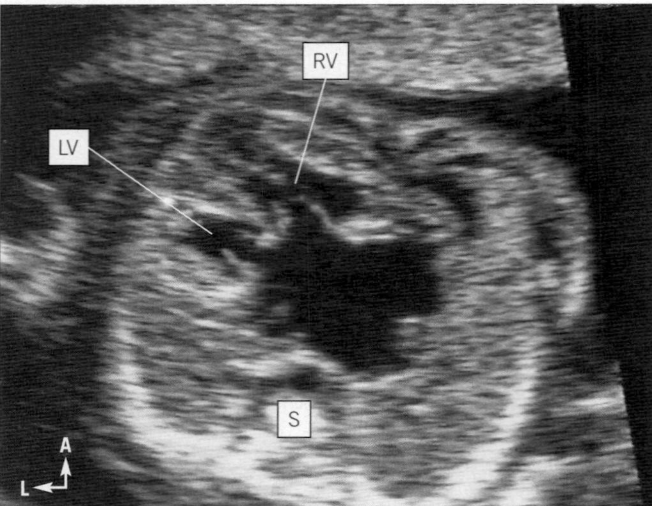

Figure 105.4 Fetal echocardiogram in a 24-week fetus with partial common AV canal as seen from a four-chamber view. The large deficiency of the atrial septum and apical displacement of the AV valve are clearly seen. LV, left ventricle; RV, right ventricle; S, spine.

Fetal Arrhythmia

One of the major reasons for referral to fetal echocardiography is arrhythmia. Most commonly, irregular fetal heart rate is caused by either conducted or blocked premature atrial contractions. These are usually benign and require follow-up only if they are frequent or associated with supraventricular tachycardia. Among the serious arrhythmias encountered in the fetus, supraventricular tachycardia and atrial flutter are the most common.[21] Premature ventricular contractions and ventricular tachycardia are rare in the fetus, but both have been reported.[21] Transplacental pharmacologic therapy is indicated in fetuses with incessant tachyarrhythmia, especially if signs of heart failure (e.g., enlargement of cardiac chambers, pericardial effusion, and hydrops fetalis) are present. Complete heart block is the most common cause of prolonged bradycardia in the fetus. The distinction between complete heart block and sinus bradycardia is important, because the latter might indicate fetal distress. In fetuses with a structurally normal heart, maternal lupus erythematosus should be suspected. The most common structural CHD associated with complete heart block are physiologically corrected SLL (S, atrial situs solitus; L, L-ventricular loop; L, L-malposition of the great arteries) transposition of the great arteries and heterotaxy syndrome with polysplenia.

Fetal arrhythmias have been traditionally diagnosed by Doppler and M-mode echocardiography.[21] Both methods rely on simultaneous recording of signals from the atria and ventricles. Fetal position, however, may not always allow optimal alignment of the M-mode cursor or the Doppler beam. A newer method, tissue Doppler imaging with a high frame rate, provides a promising alternative to standard M-mode and Doppler echocardiography (Fig. 105.5).[25]

QUANTITATIVE ANALYSIS

Modern echocardiography allows accurate measurements of cardiovascular structures.[1] These measurements are helpful in deciding whether the size of a certain structure is within normal limits and when quantifying the degree of deviation from the expected norm.

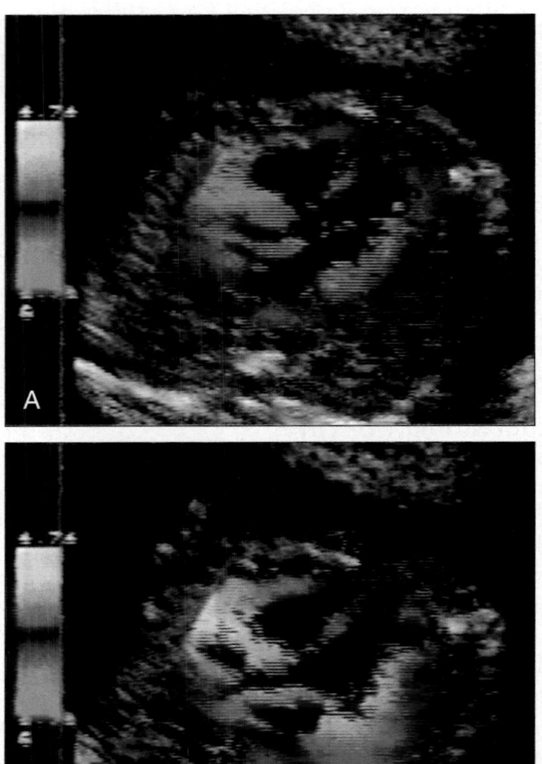

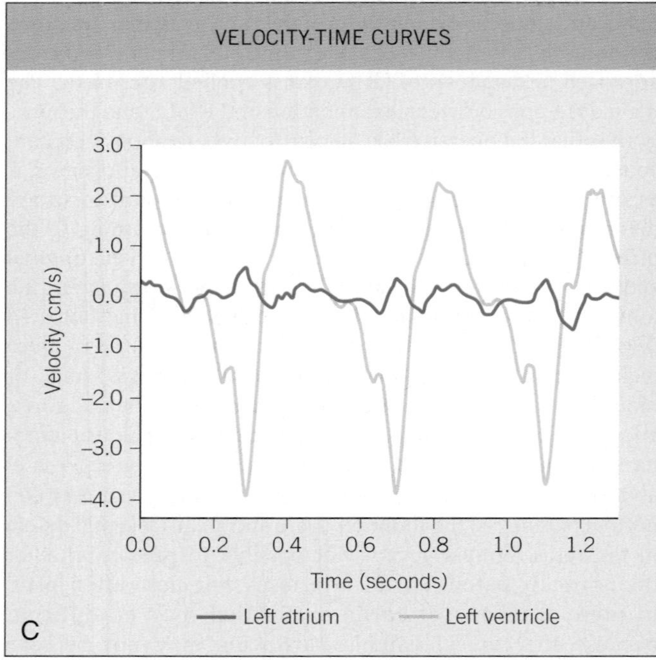

Figure 105.5 Use of tissue Doppler imaging to determine heart rhythm in the fetus. A, Diastolic frame showing left ventricular relaxation. **B,** Systolic frame showing ventricular contraction. **C,** Velocity-time curves of the left atrium (green) and left ventricle (yellow) showing the sequence of mechanical activation of the cardiac chambers in a fetus with normal AV conduction. The analysis is performed off-line using the digitally stored data.

Description of Technique

Measurements of linear dimensions (such as vessel diameter), cross-sectional areas (such as valve area), and volumetric dimensions (such as ventricular volume or mass) provide important quantitative information that can be used to assess the severity of disease process and to predict its course and prognosis. Because the pediatric age group encompasses a wide range of body sizes and because the heart and great vessels grow considerably from birth to adulthood, measured dimensions must be indexed to allow meaningful comparisons between patients of different age and body size. For example, the mean value of the aortic valve annulus diameter is 0.74 cm in a 3.6-kg newborn (body surface area [BSA] 0.24 m^2) and 1.95 cm in a 60-kg adolescent (BSA 1.66 m^2). Indexing the aortic annulus diameter to body weight yields vastly different values (0.21 cm/kg in the newborn, compared with 0.032 cm/kg in the adolescent). Indexing the aortic valve diameter to the BSA yields similarly unsatisfactory results (3.1 cm/m^2 in the newborn and 1.17 cm/m^2 in the adolescent).

Growth of cardiac structures is not necessarily a linear function of the BSA, the weight, the height, or the age.[26] These findings are to be expected because the heart and great vessels grow much faster during the first 2 to 4 years of life compared with later childhood and adolescence. It was found that linear dimensions (such as diameters of valves and great vessels) should be indexed to the square root of the BSA. Returning to the above example of the aortic valve diameter, indexing the valve diameter to the square root of the BSA yields 0.74/0.49 = 1.51 cm/$m^{0.5}$ in the 3.6-kg newborn and 1.95/1.29 = 1.51 cm/$m^{0.5}$ in the 60-kg adolescent (Fig. 105.6). Cross-sectional measurements (such as valve area) should be indexed to the BSA. Left ventricular volume should be indexed to the BSA raised to the power 1.28, and left ventricular mass should be indexed to the BSA raised to the power 1.23 (SD Colan, unpublished data).

An alternative approach to comparing measurements between individuals is the use of Z scores.[1] The Z score is a statistical expression of the position of a data point relative to the regression line of a data set. The Z score is expressed as the number of standard deviations from the expected mean. It is calculated as:

$$\text{Z value} = \frac{\text{Measured value} - \text{Mean value of normal population}}{\text{Standard deviation of normal population}}$$

Returning to the previous example of aortic valve diameter, the Z value of a 0.74-cm aortic valve diameter in a newborn with a BSA of 0.24 m^2 is 0. That means that 0.74 cm is the mean value of aortic valve diameter in infants with that body size. In the adolescent with a BSA of 1.66 m^2, the Z value of an aortic valve diameter of 1.95 cm is also 0. In other words, the same Z scores in the newborn and the adolescent indicate that both values are in the same position relative to the regression line of normal values and are comparable. An aortic valve diameter of 0.53 cm in the newborn would have a Z score of −2.0, which indicates that this value is 2 standard deviations below the expected mean. An aortic valve diameter of 0.96 cm in the same newborn would have a Z score of +2.0, which indicates that this value is 2 standard deviations above the mean. Thus, expression of measurements as Z values allows comparison between patients, regardless of differences in body size.

Estimation of left ventricular volume is an important factor in determining the adequacy of chamber size in patients with left ventricular hypoplasia and when evaluating patients with volume overload. Numerous algorithms based on several geometric models have been developed for calculation of left ventricular volume. The biplane Simpson's rule is considered among the most reliable methods for estimation of left ventricular volume. This method requires imaging of the left ventricle from two orthogonal views that share a common long axis: for example, the apical four- and two-chamber views.

Left ventricular volume (*V*) is calculated according to:

$$V = \frac{\pi}{4} \times \sum_{i=1}^{N} ai \times bi \times \frac{L}{N}$$

where a_i = slice radius in the apical two-chamber view; b_i = slice radius in the apical four-chamber view; L = left ventricular length; N = number of slices; and V = volume. Another method for estimation of left ventricular volume is the biplane area-length method, where $V = 5/6 \times \text{area} \times \text{length}$. Initial experience with assessment of left and right ventricular volumes by 3D reconstruction suggests that this technique is potentially more accurate than 2D echocardiographic techniques.[27] Left ventricular myocardial volume can be measured from the 2D echocardiogram by subtracting the endocardial volume from the epicardial volume. Left ventricular mass is calculated by multiplying the resultant myocardial volume by the density of muscle (1.055 g/mL). Because it is not influenced by acoustic windows and is independent of chamber geometry, MRI provides an excellent alternative to echocardiography in measuring chamber volume and mass, and is considered the reference standard against which other techniques are compared (see following section on MRI).

Ventricular Function

Left ventricular function can be assessed at several levels. The heart may be viewed as a pump designed to maintain adequate flow to vital organs.[28] This approach focuses on the external work performed by the heart, but it ignores the internal work and the functional state of the myocardium. The pump function of the heart can be assessed by measuring cardiac output and systemic and pulmonary venous blood pressures. It is known, however, that cardiac output and blood pressure can remain within the normal limits despite significant myocardial dysfunction.[28] Echocardiography and Doppler ultrasound allow a fairly detailed and sophisticated assessment of both pump function and myocardial performance. Understanding the techniques for assessment of ventricular function requires in-depth knowledge of cardiovascular physiology.

Doppler Evaluation of Pressure Gradients

Estimation of the pressure difference between adjacent compartments has been widely applied in clinical pediatric echocardiography (see Fig. 105.1a).[1] Among the most common uses are estimation of pressure decrease across stenotic areas and prediction of pressure in cardiac chambers. For example, the systolic pressure in the right ventricle can be predicted from the peak pressure difference between it and the right atrium, derived from the peak velocity of the tricuspid

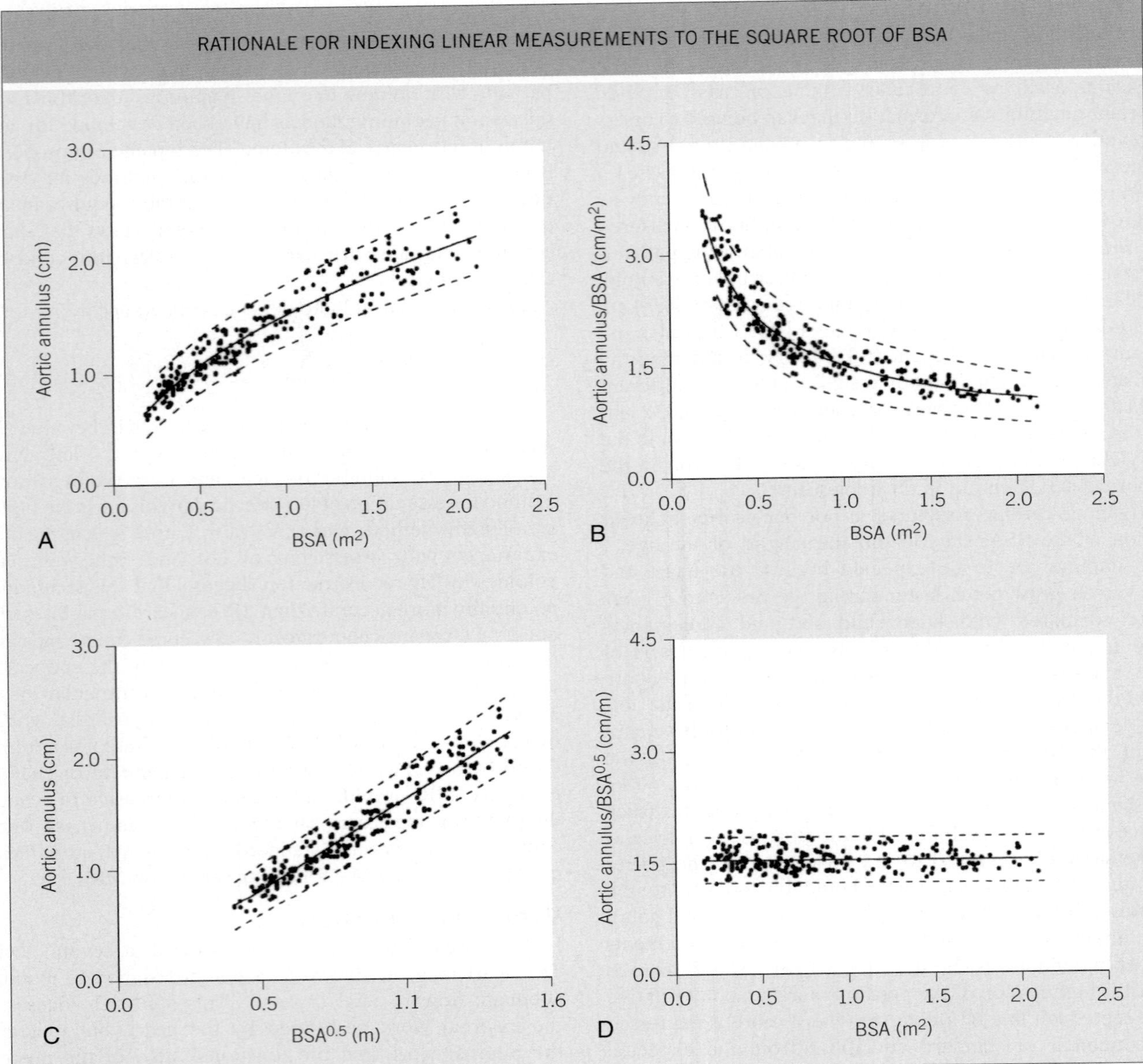

Figure 105.6 Rationale for indexing linear measurements to the square root of body surface area. A, Plot of aortic valve annulus diameter against body surface area (BSA) showing a nonlinear curve. **B,** Plot of aortic valve annulus diameter indexed to BSA against BSA shows that the indexed diameter decreases exponentially as BSA increases. **C,** Aortic valve annulus diameter plotted against the square root of BSA showing a linear relationship. **D,** Plot of aortic valve diameter indexed to the square root of BSA against BSA showing that the indexed aortic valve diameter is the same in children and adults with widely varying body size.

regurgitation jet. Right ventricular systolic pressure can also be assessed from knowledge of left ventricular pressure (by measurement of systemic blood pressure by sphygmomanometry) and the pressure decrease across a ventricular septal defect. In principle, the pressure gradient across any two compartments connected by flow can be estimated by Doppler, provided that the limitations of the technique are taken into consideration and the sources of error in the application and interpretation of the technique are eliminated.

Calculation of Pressure Gradients

The Bernoulli equation relates pressure difference (ΔP) between two points separated by a distance (s) to the velocity at the two points (V_1 and V_2, respectively), the fluid density (for blood, $\rho = 1060$ kg/L), and the velocity-dependent viscous friction according to:

$$\Delta P = \overbrace{\frac{1}{2}\rho\left(V_2^2 - V_1^2\right)}^{\text{convective acceleration}} + \overbrace{\rho \int_1^2 \frac{d\vec{V}}{dt} d\vec{s}}^{\text{flow acceleration}} + \overbrace{R\left(\vec{V}\right)}^{\text{viscous friction}}$$

For most clinical applications of the Bernoulli equation, the convective acceleration component of the formula is considered the most significant. After combining ρ for blood with conversion factors for pressure to mm Hg and velocity to m/second, the calculated coefficient is 3.98; in most clinical applications, this factor is rounded to 4.0.

The second term of the equation, flow acceleration, represents the pressure decrease generated by flow acceleration. This phenomenon, however, is important only during a very brief period at the rapid acceleration phase when there is a lag between the velocity and the pressure curves. During that time period, the pressure gradient is not considered clinically important.

The third term represents the force necessary to overcome viscous friction. When pressure decreases across a discrete orifice are considered, viscous friction becomes negligible. Hence, for most clinical applications the formula is simplified on the basis of the following assumptions:

- the velocity proximal to the obstruction (V_1) is assumed to be negligible compared with that just distal to the obstruction (V_2);
- in most clinical situations, peak flow acceleration occurs in early systole when the pressure gradient is irrelevant and can be ignored; and
- viscous friction is assumed to be trivial.

The Bernoulli equation can therefore be simplified as: $\Delta P = 4 (V_2)^2$. This formula has been shown to be valid in in vitro flow models and in a variety of clinical settings.[29] However, the assumptions that govern the use of the simplified Bernoulli equation may not always be correct. The limitations and pitfalls that can potentially lead to errors in estimation of pressure gradients have been reviewed elsewhere.[1]

Safety and Complications

Because of the widespread use of echocardiography in the diagnosis and monitoring of children with suspected heart disease, safety of the technique is of prime importance. This is particularly relevant in fetal echocardiography, where fetuses may be exposed to ultrasound energy early in gestation. To date, no reports on adverse effects from diagnostic ultrasound have been reported. Physicians involved with diagnostic ultrasound must be aware that ultrasound is a form of mechanical energy that, under certain conditions, can cause biologic damage to exposed tissue. This damage can result from conversion of mechanical energy to heat or from creation of gaseous microcavitations. To date, it appears that biologic damage has been observed only in nonclinical laboratory conditions.

MAGNETIC RESONANCE IMAGING

Cardiac MRI is a sophisticated noninvasive imaging modality that overcomes many of the limitations of echocardiography and cardiac catheterization. High resolution static and dynamic images of the heart, blood vessels, and other thoracic structures are obtained regardless of body size and acoustic barriers. Moreover, MRI provides additional unique information that is not available by other imaging techniques. As a result of the rapid technological evolution in computer sciences, electronics, and engineering over the past two decades, cardiac MRI has evolved from a technique that produced several static images in an examination that lasted 1 hour or more to a modality capable of real-time imaging,[30] succinct dynamic 3D visualization of cardiovascular anatomy,[31] and accurate quantification of blood flow[32] and myocardial function.[33] These capabilities have greatly expanded the role of MRI in pediatric cardiology.[30-33]

Description of MRI Techniques

In the course of a cardiac MRI examination, several techniques are used (Table 105.2). Each uses a different sequence of varying magnetic fields and radiofrequency pulses to create an image with specific characteristics. Three different magnetic fields are used by MRI scanners:

SUMMARY OF MAGNETIC RESONANCE IMAGING TECHNIQUES

Technique	ECG Triggering	Appearance of Blood Flow	Dynamic (cine*) vs. static**	Clinical Application
Spin echo				
Standard spin echo	Yes	Dark	Static	Anatomy, tissue characterization
Fast spin echo with inversion recovery	Yes	Dark	Static	Anatomy, tissue characterization, better blood/tissue contrast
Gradient echo				
SSFP cine MR	Yes	Bright	Dynamic	Anatomy, ventricular function, blood flow imaging
Coronary MR angiography and isotropic 3D SSFP	Yes	Bright	Static	Coronary imaging, intracardiac anatomy
Phase-velocity mapping	Yes	Bright	Dynamic	Flow quantification and characterization
Myocardial tagging	Yes	Bright	Dynamic	Analysis of myocardial mechanics and flow
Gd-enhanced 3D MR angiography	No	Bright	Static	Anatomy
MR fluoroscopy	No	Bright	Dynamic	Anatomy, function, guidance of interventional procedures
Myocardial delayed enhancement	Yes	Intermediate	Static	Myocardial viability
First-pass myocardial perfusion	Yes	Varies	Dynamic	Myocardial perfusion

*Cine: several images are obtained throughout the cardiac cycle in each anatomic location. The stacked images are then displayed on a computer screen in a cine-loop format.
**Static: a single image is obtained in each anatomic location.
Gd, gadolinium; MR, magnetic resonance; SSFP, steady-state free precession.

Table 105.2 Summary of magnetic resonance imaging techniques.

- a relatively large static magnetic field;
- much smaller but rapidly varying magnetic fields produced by magnetic field gradients; and
- radiofrequency pulses.

In general, all currently used MRI sequences are variants of just two fundamental categories: spin echo and gradient echo.[34]

To produce an image, the patient is first placed inside the scanner, which applies a static, relatively homogeneous high-strength magnetic field. Most clinical scanners use static magnetic field strengths ranging from 0.5 to 3 tesla (T) (1 tesla = 10,000 gauss [G]; the strength of earth's magnetic field at its surface is approximately 0.5 G). Higher magnetic field strengths are mostly used in research scanners, but are also used in some clinical scanners. A section of the patient's body is then excited using a radiofrequency pulse, and an echo is formed by means of a second radiofrequency pulse (spin echo), gradient pulses (gradient echo), or both. The signal from the echo is then processed by Fourier transformation, and the data are used to fill a line of matrix from which the image is generated.

Many techniques make use of additional radiofrequency and gradient pulses, either as prefixes or during the sequence, to achieve specific effects, such as suppression of a signal typical of certain tissue (e.g., fat or water suppression) or to place a "tag" on the tissue. Other techniques use various strategies to shorten the time of data acquisition, processing, and display. These techniques, designated "fast" or "turbo" by different manufacturers, are based on the acquisition of several echoes after each radiofrequency excitation. Thus several lines of matrix are filled simultaneously. This technique, also called segmented k-space, shortens the time needed for data acquisition, so that a series of images can be obtained during a period of breath-holding (12 to 30 seconds), thus improving image quality by eliminating respiratory motion.[35] Newer imaging and data processing techniques (e.g., sensitivity encoding, k-t BLAST) allow even faster image acquisition, thus shortening acquisition time. Data acquisition in the previously mentioned sequences is synchronized with the patient's electrocardiogram (ECG) using one of several triggering strategies. When the quality of the ECG signal is suboptimal, image acquisition can be triggered by a peripheral pulse sensor.

Artifacts from respiratory motion can be decreased by synchronizing data acquisition to the ventilatory cycle, either by using a flexible belt wrapped around the abdomen or by following the motion of the diaphragm using an extra pulse called navigator echo. Another technique to reduce motion artifacts and to improve signal-to-noise ratio is to acquire and average several signals. The disadvantage of this technique is increased imaging time.

When all the echoes needed to fill the matrix are acquired simultaneously from a single radiofrequency pulse, an image can be acquired in 50 to 100 ms. Such rapid image acquisition effectively "freezes" cardiac motion; thus the need for ECG or respiratory triggering is eliminated. This imaging technique, known as echo planar imaging, requires very strong and fast-acting gradients, which have become clinically available only in recent years. Echo planar imaging, however, suffers from blood flow artifacts in addition to effects of local variation in tissue magnetic susceptibility that can be severe around the heart. At present, echo planar imaging has not come into routine clinical use in cardiac MRI.

Clinical Applications of MRI in Congenital Heart Disease

Given the current capabilities of cardiac MRI and that it is used in almost all types of CHD and in patients of all ages, it is not practical to discuss its role in individual cardiac anomalies in this chapter. Instead, the discussion will focus on how the tools described in Table 105.2 are applied in the clinical arena to delineate cardiovascular anatomy and function in patients with CHD.[36]

All MRI examinations begin with localizing images that provide a "road map" and allow planning of further image acquisition. Subsequent sequences and imaging planes are then selected to address specific clinical questions. The strategy of the examination is tailored to the patient's hemodynamic and respiratory status and is influenced by whether the patient is awake or sedated. These and other factors will dictate whether breath-holding will be used.[36]

Magnetic Resonance Angiography

Gadolinium-enhanced 3D magnetic resonance angiography (MRA) is used to delineate extracardiac vascular anatomy.[36] This technique produces a 3D data set in which the signal from blood is particularly high and strongly contrasts with nonvascular structures. Intravenous administration of gadolinium (gadopentetate dimeglumine), a paramagnetic agent that shortens the T1 of blood, results in a high contrast-to-noise ratio. The 3D data set is typically acquired within a 15- to 30-second period of breath-holding, before the contrast leaves the blood vessels. We typically acquire two such sequences—the first is timed to delineate the pulmonary arterial phase, and the second shows both arteries and veins. Because of the rapid circulation time in children, it is not always possible to achieve a "pure" arterial phase. Furthermore, we have found it advantageous to image arterial and venous structures simultaneously.[36] Several techniques may be used to view the data.[31] We prefer the maximal intensity projection technique, in which the imager orients a slab within the data set.[31,36] The computer then calculates the intensity of the voxels within the slab and projects them onto a 2D plane (Fig. 105.7). The thickness and spatial orientation of the slab are defined by the imager, and production of the resultant reconstructed image is nearly instantaneous. Another useful reconstruction technique is 3D volume rendering. In contrast to cine MRI, however, 3D MRA is not time resolved.

Three-dimensional MRA is ideally suited to elucidate the anatomy of the aorta and its branches, the pulmonary arteries, pulmonary veins, and the systemic veins (see Fig. 105.7). Although this technique is mostly used for imaging of extracardiac anatomy, we have found it useful in the evaluation of intra-atrial systemic and pulmonary baffles (such as in Mustard or Senning operations and after the Fontan procedure), and for imaging of the outflow tracts (such as repaired tetralogy of Fallot and the arterial switch operation).[36] In addition to providing superb images of cardiovascular structures, 3D MRA clearly delineates the spatial relationships between vascular structures, the tracheobronchial tree, chest wall, spine, and other landmarks that may be useful for planning of interventional catheterization or surgical procedures. 3D MRA is also ideally suited for 3D surface reconstruction (Fig. 105.8).

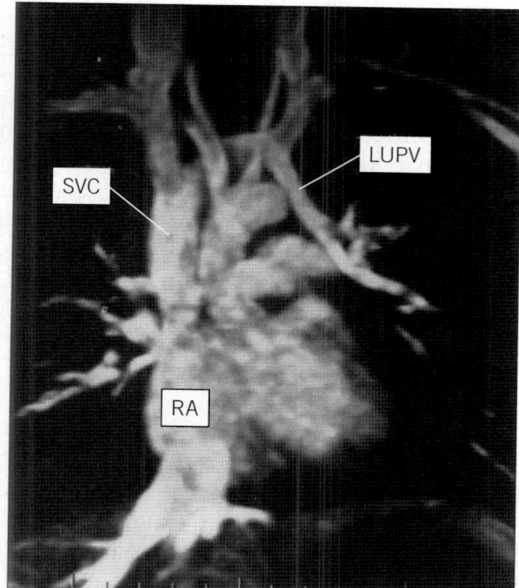

Figure 105.7 Gadolinium-enhanced 3D magnetic resonance angiography in a 9-year-old girl with partially anomalous pulmonary venous connection of the left upper pulmonary vein (LUPV) to the left innominate vein. The course of the anomalous pulmonary vein and its connection to the systemic veins, and its distance from the left atrium, are seen on this maximal intensity projection image. The 3D data set was acquired during a 21-second period of breath-holding. RA, right atrium; SVC, superior vena cava.

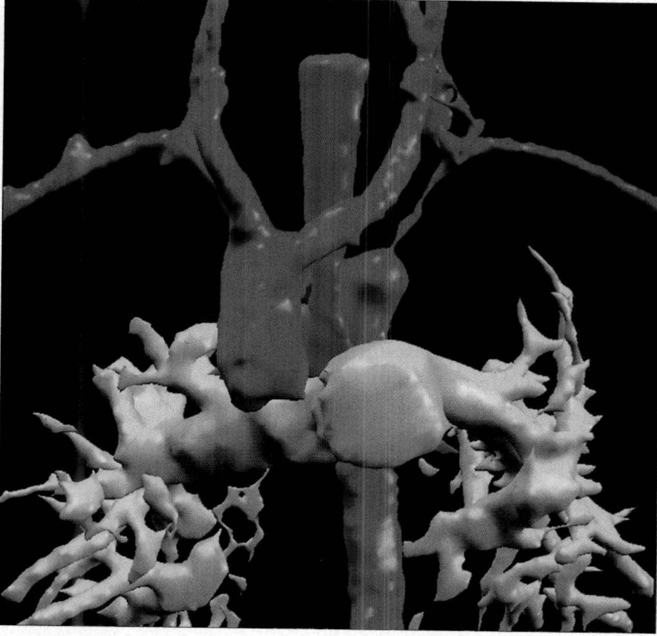

Figure 105.8 3D surface reconstruction from gadolinium-enhanced 3D magnetic resonance angiography data set in a patient with a right aortic arch and an aberrant origin of the left subclavian artery from the descending aorta. Frontal view showing the ascending aorta (red) and the aortic arch to the right of the trachea (purple). The pulmonary arteries are seen in yellow. The caliber of the left subclavian artery increases at its junction with the left vertebral artery. Phase-velocity flow mapping (not shown) demonstrated retrograde flow in the left vertebral artery, which supplies the left subclavian artery.

Cine Magnetic Resonance Imaging

Cine MRI is used to delineate cardiovascular anatomy and function. This technique uses one of several gradient echo sequences in which flowing blood produces a bright signal ("bright-blood" imaging) (Fig. 105.9b). Fast gradient echo sequences triggered by ECG produce several time-resolved images over the cardiac cycle in each anatomic location, which can then be displayed in a cine-loop format. A set of images in each anatomic location may be obtained either during 5 to 25 seconds of breath-holding or during free breathing by averaging several signals. Depending on the patient's heart rate, cine acquisition without breath-holding typically requires about 1 minute to obtain.[36] By repeating the process in several contiguous anatomic locations, it is possible to see both intracardiac and extracardiac anatomy and function with good spatial and temporal resolutions.

We currently use a steady-state free precession sequence with or without breath-holding.[36] This sequence is commonly used to evaluate the atrial and ventricular septum, intracardiac baffles and pathways (such as Fontan, Mustard,

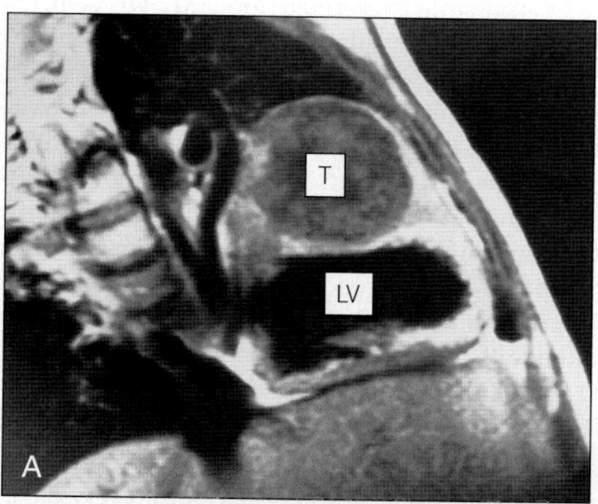

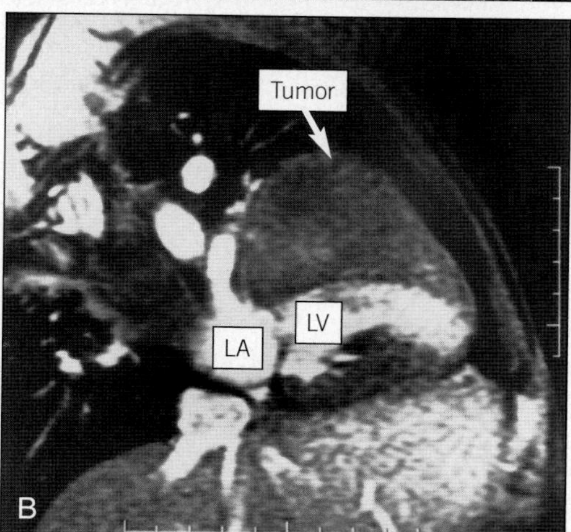

Figure 105.9 Spin echo and gradient echo MRI sequences in a 4-year-old boy with large fibroma of the left ventricle. A, Fast spin echo with double-inversion recovery showing the left ventricle (LV) and tumor (T) in the long axial oblique plane. Notice the clear definition between the dark blood pool and the myocardium, and the difference in signal intensity between the tumor and the myocardium (dark blood sequence). **B,** Diastolic frame of cine MRI obtained in the same plane as in **A**. Notice the contrast between the bright signal from the blood and the myocardium (bright blood sequence). LA, left atrium.

Senning, and Rastelli procedures), atrioventricular and semilunar valves, left and right ventricular outflow tracts and ventriculoarterial conduits, and for dynamic imaging of blood vessels. This sequence is also useful if there is a question regarding stenotic or regurgitant jets.

Ventricular Function

Steady-state free precession cine MRI is the primary sequence used in the evaluation of ventricular function. Quantitative evaluation of ventricular function is achieved by obtaining a series of contiguous cine MRI slabs that cover the ventricles.[33,35] The blood-endocardium boundary is traced and the volume of the slab is calculated as the product of its cross-sectional area and thickness (which is prescribed by the operator). Ventricular volume can then be determined by summation of the volumes of all slabs. The process can be repeated for each frame in the cardiac cycle to obtain a continuous time-volume loop, or may be performed only on a diastolic and a systolic frame to calculate diastolic and systolic volumes. From these data one can calculate left and right ventricular ejection fractions and stroke volumes. Because the patient's heart rate at the time of image acquisition is known, it is possible to calculate left and right ventricular output. Left and right ventricular mass can be calculated by tracing the epicardial borders, subtracting the endocardial volumes, and multiplying the resultant muscle volume by the specific gravity of the myocardium (1.05 g/mm^3). Because of the precise spatial and temporal registration of data, measurements of chamber volume and mass by MRI are highly accurate and reproducible and have become the accepted reference standard against which other methods are compared.[37] Table 105.3 summarizes normal MRI values of ventricular volume and mass in children, adolescents, and adults, reported by Lorenz[35] using a standard gradient echo technique.

VENTRICULAR PARAMETERS NORMALIZED TO BODY SURFACE AREA (BSA) (95% CONFIDENCE INTERVAL [1.96 STANDARD DEVIATION] IN PARENTHESES)

Parameter	All ($n = 75$)	Pediatric ($n = 8$)
LVEDV/BSA (mL/m^2)	66 ± 12 (44–89)	67 ± 9 (49–85)
RVEDV/BSA (mL/m^2)	75 ± 13 (49–101)	70 ± 11 (49–91)
LVTM/BSA (g/m^2)	87 ± 12 (64–109)	81 ± 13 (56–106)
LVFWM/BSA (g/m^2)	57 ± 8 (40–73)	53 ± 8 (38–68)
IVSM/BSA (g/m^2)	30 ± 4 (21–38)	28 ± 5 (18–38)
RVFWM/BSA (g/m^2)	26 ± 5 (17–34)	26 ± 3 (20–32)
LVSV/BSA (mL/m^2)	45 ± 8 (29–61)	44 ± 7 (31–57)
RVSV/BSA (mL/m^2)	46 ± 8 (30–62)	43 ± 7 (28–58)
CO/BSA (L/min per/m^2)	2.9 ± 0.6 (1.74–4.03)	3.2 ± 0.5 (2.17–4.28)

CO, cardiac output; IVSM, interventricular septal mass; LVEDV, left ventricular end-diastolic volume; LVFWM, left ventricular free wall mass; LVSV, left ventricular stroke volume; LVTM, left ventricular total mass; RVEDV, right ventricular end-diastolic volume; RVFWM, right ventricular free wall mass; RVSV, right ventricular stroke volume.
Modified from Lorenz CH. The range of normal values of cardiovascular structures in infants, children, and adolescents measured by MRI. Pediatr Cardiol 2000;21:37-46.

Table 105.3 Ventricular parameters normalized to body surface area (BSA) (95% confidence interval [1.96 standard deviation] in parentheses).

Cine MRI is also used to evaluate regional wall motion abnormalities and segmental wall thickening fraction.[38] Recent development of algorithms for automatic border detection has greatly facilitated the application of these techniques.[38] Another technique used in MRI evaluation of ventricular function is myocardial tagging. A saturation band ("tag") is placed on the myocardium using a preparatory radiofrequency pulse, and the motion of the myocardium throughout the cardiac cycle can then be traced and analyzed. Such analysis quantifies regional myocardial strain and stress, which are important measures of myocardial mechanics.

Flow Analysis

The most common technique used for quantification of blood flow by MRI is phase velocity contrast MRI (PVC MRI), which is a specific type of gradient echo sequence.[32] The PVC MRI technique is based on the principle that the signal from hydrogen nuclei (such as those in blood) flowing through specially designed magnetic field gradients accumulates a predictable phase shift that is proportional to flow velocity; nuclei in stationary tissue, in contrast, acquire no net phase shift. It is accomplished by briefly applying a magnetic field with a strength that varies linearly (i.e., a gradient) in the direction of blood flow. The signal emitted by protons at different locations along the gradient will develop phase differences because the rate of proton precession is proportional to the local magnetic field strength. The gradient is then reversed, so that it has equal magnitude and duration but opposite polarity. As a result, for stationary protons, the phase change induced by the first gradient is canceled and no net phase shift is accrued. Moving protons, however, will be in a new location when the second gradient is applied and will therefore be exposed to a different gradient strength. Their net phase shift accumulated during such a bipolar gradient is proportional to their velocity in the gradient-encoded direction.[32] Unintended phase shifts, however, may be induced by other factors, such as magnetic field inhomogeneity, and cause inaccuracies. Such effects are countered by acquiring a second set of phase data without velocity encoding (or with a different velocity-encoding gradient). Subtraction of the two sets of phase data from each other cancels these background phenomena and leaves only those related to motion.[32]

Flow quantification is performed by placing an imaging slab across a blood vessel or through the area at question within the heart (Fig. 105.10a). The operator then determines whether flow velocity encoding is performed only perpendicular to the imaging plane (z-axis) or in other directions also (x- and y-axes). The data are then analyzed off-line using specialized software. A region of interest (ROI) is defined by the operator around the lumen of the relevant vessel, and the instantaneous mean velocity of each voxel is calculated (Fig. 105.10b,c). Flow rate is calculated as the product of the mean velocities within the ROI and its cross-sectional area. Integration of the instantaneous flow rates over the cardiac cycle yields the stroke volume (Fig. 105.10d).

Cine phase contrast has been widely applied to measure systemic and pulmonary blood flow and their ratio, in addition to flow in individual pulmonary arteries, across the

Figure 105.10 **Flow measurements by phase velocity cine MRI. A,** The imaging plane is defined perpendicular to the vessel of interest—the ascending aorta in this example. **B, D,** The region of interest (ROI) is defined around the ascending aorta using a computer workstation and specialized software. Signal intensity of each voxel in the ROI is linearly related to velocity. **C,** By integrating the velocities of all voxels across the ROI and multiplying the mean velocity by the cross-sectional area of the ROI, the instantaneous flow rate is calculated. The process is repeated for each of the 24 frames, and a curve showing flow rate as a function of time is constructed. Stroke volume is the area under the curve.

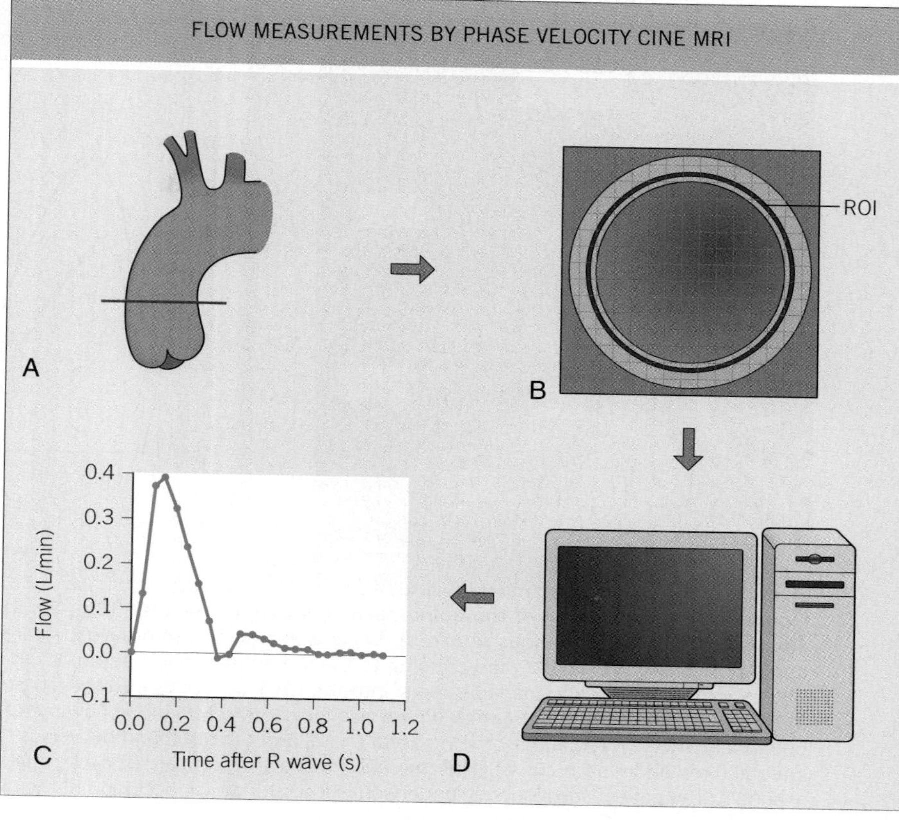

mitral and tricuspid valves, across an atrial septal defect, in systemic and pulmonary veins, and in other individual blood vessels (Fig. 105.11). This technique also allows accurate quantification of regurgitation volume and fraction across any cardiac valve. An example of an important application of this technique in pediatric cardiology is the quantification of pulmonary regurgitation in patients who have undergone repair of tetralogy of Fallot (Fig. 105.12). No other technique, including echocardiography and catheterization, provides such quantitative information. When flow encoding is performed in three spatial directions, multidimensional flow imaging and analysis can be accomplished by resolving the flow velocities and directions into flow vectors that can be viewed in cine-loop format (Fig. 105.13). This technique allows unique imaging of blood flow in five dimensions (x, y, and z spatial dimensions, velocity, and time). It also allows quantitative analysis of flow dynamics, including the ability to calculate the shear stress exerted by the flowing blood on the vessel wall.[39]

Anatomic Imaging and Tissue Characteristics

Spin echo sequences produce images in which flowing blood produces little or no signal and appears dark ("black blood" imaging) (Fig. 105.14). Other cardiac and noncardiac tissues appear in varying shades of gray. The standard spin echo sequence is triggered to the ECG. Because only one image is produced in each location, this technique provides only static anatomic information. Another disadvantage of this technique is the relatively long data acquisition time (several minutes, depending on heart rate and number of signal averages). Its advantages, however, include excellent spatial resolution, tissue characteristics, and decreased susceptibility to artifacts from certain biomedical implants (such as sternal wires, stents, and prosthetic valves). Recent development of breath-hold black-blood fast spin echo sequences allows very rapid image acquisition (10 to 15 seconds) and inversion recovery (which enhances the contrast between the blood and the myocardium) (see Fig. 105.9a).

The primary clinical use of standard T1-weighted spin echo sequences is to obtain information regarding the myocardium, epicardium, and pericardium. Examples include evaluation of the right ventricular free wall in suspected arrhythmogenic right ventricular dysplasia, evaluation of cardiac tumors, and constrictive pericardial disease. Other clinical applications include evaluation of blood vessel wall (e.g., Marfan's syndrome or to exclude dissection after balloon angioplasty) and thoracic masses. Use of T2-weighted spin echo, and the addition of preparatory pulse sequences (such as fat and water suppression) are used to evaluate specific clinical questions.[36]

Safety and Complications

Standard clinical imaging scanners present no known hazards to biologic materials. Three different magnetic fields are used by such magnets:

- the relatively large static magnetic field;
- smaller, but rapidly varying magnetic fields secondary to the magnetic field gradients; and
- radiofrequency pulses.

Guidelines set by the U.S. Food and Drug Administration keep the strength of these fields well below values that could

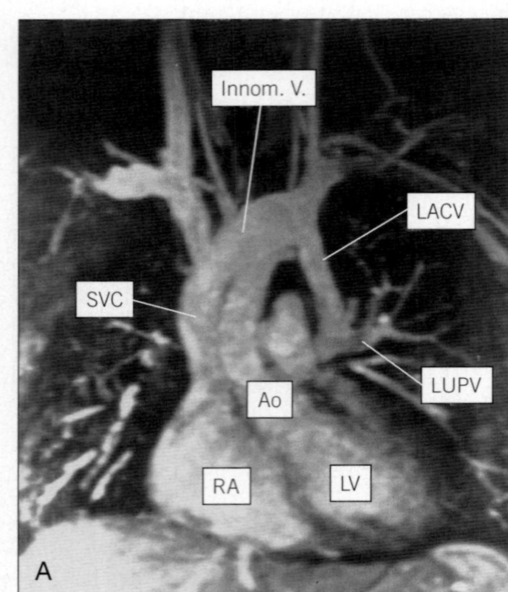

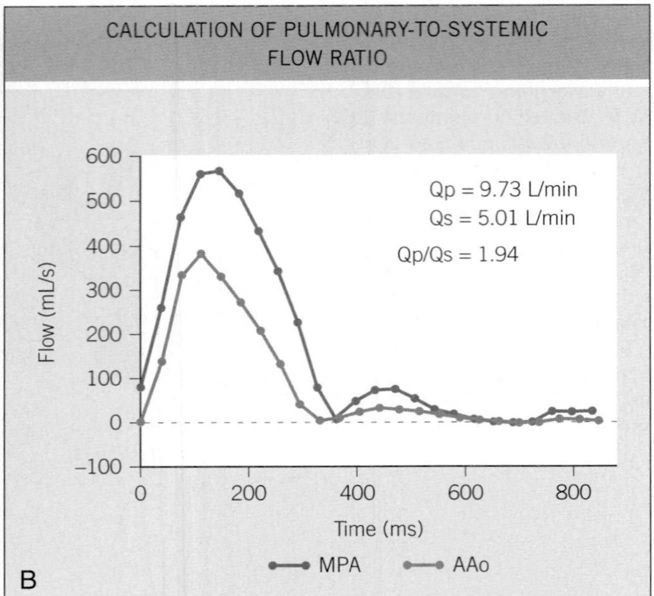

Figure 105.11 Calculation of the pulmonary-to-systemic flow ratio (Qp/Qs) in an 18-year-old man with partial anomalous pulmonary venous return. A, There is a large persistent levoatriocardinal vein (LACV) arising from the left upper pulmonary vein (LUPV) and draining to the innominate vein (Innom. V.) as shown on the gadolinium-enhanced MR angiogram. The LUPV drained directly into the LACV as well as into the left atrium. The other pulmonary veins drained normally to the left atrium. **B,** Phase velocity contrast MRI blood flow measurements were performed in the main pulmonary artery (MPA) and ascending aorta (AAo), and the resulting flow versus time curves are plotted. The flow-time integral (area under each curve) yields the net flow volume per cardiac cycle, enabling the Qp/Qs ratio to be calculated as shown. The patient subsequently underwent successful device occlusion of the distal LACV. Ao, aorta; LV, left ventricle; RA, right atrium; SVC, superior vena cava.

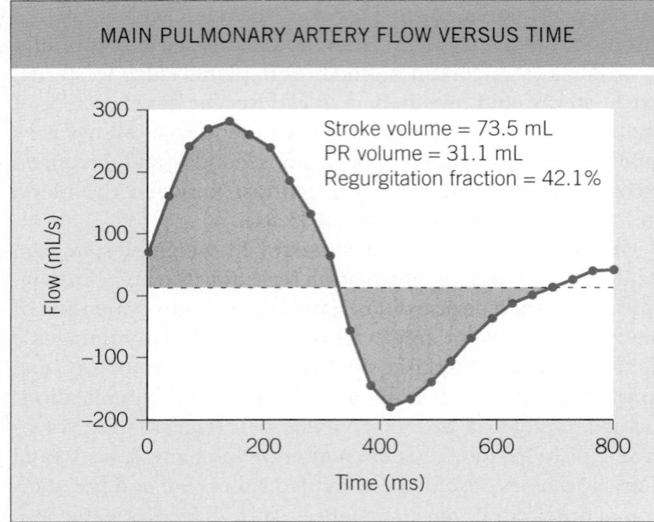

Figure 105.12 Main pulmonary artery flow versus time as measured by phase velocity contrast magnetic resonance imaging in a 26-year-old man with repaired tetralogy of Fallot and pulmonary regurgitation. Antegrade flow volume is calculated as the systolic flow-time integral above the baseline, retrograde (regurgitant) flow volume as the diastolic flow-time integral below the baseline, and regurgitant fraction as the ratio of retrograde volume to antegrade volume, expressed as a percentage. PR, pulmonary regurgitation.

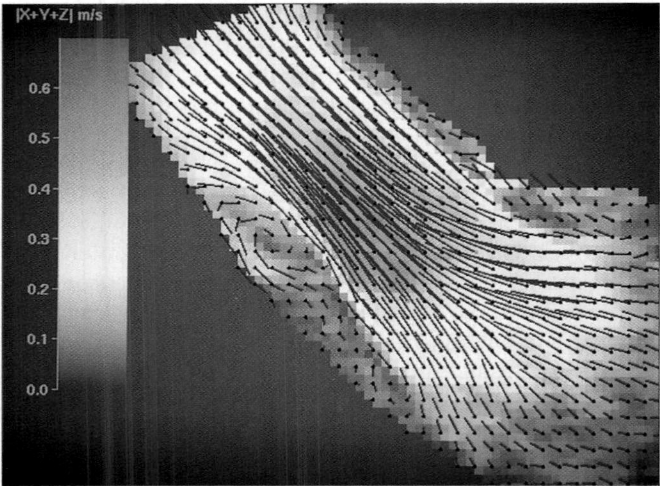

Figure 105.13 Phase velocity MRI flow vector mapping of the aortic root and ascending aorta. The origin of the flow (located in the center of the voxel) is represented by a blue dot. The length of the vector line is proportional to the instantaneous velocity and its orientation shows the direction of flow in the x-y plane. The background color map represents flow speed.

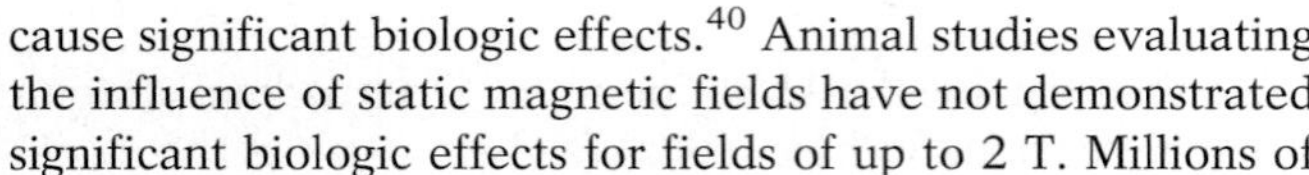
cause significant biologic effects.[40] Animal studies evaluating the influence of static magnetic fields have not demonstrated significant biologic effects for fields of up to 2 T. Millions of patients have undergone MRI studies without any noticeable immediate or long-term sequelae. Many women have undergone MRI imaging during all trimesters of pregnancy without reported ill effect on them, the fetus, or the resultant infant. When maternal and fetal health considerations require diagnostic studies, MRI imaging is preferable to methods that use x-rays, such as computed tomography or angiography.

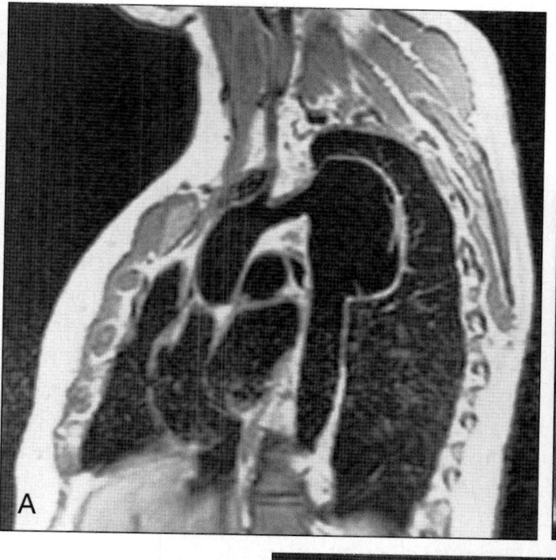

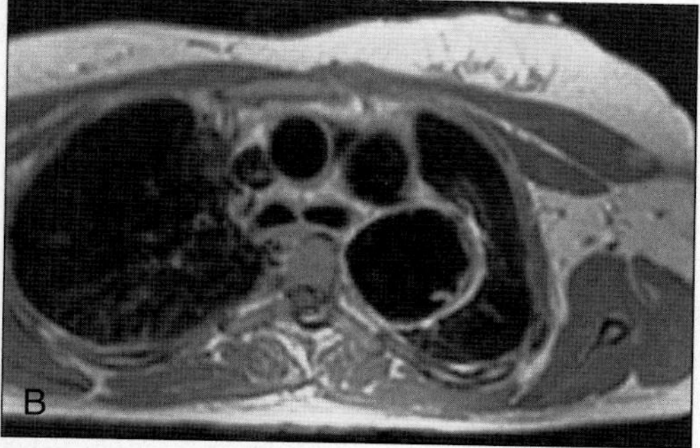

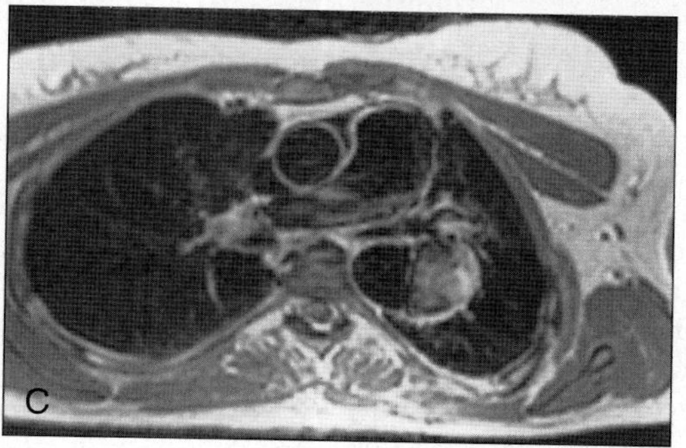

Figure 105.14 Standard T1-weighted spin echo imaging in a 27-year-old woman who underwent coarctation repair in infancy and a subsequent patch aortoplasty repair of recurrent coarctation. **A,** Oblique sagittal plane showing hypoplasia of the transverse aortic arch and a large aneurysm of the coarctation repair site. Note the dissection in the posterior wall of the aneurysm. **B,** Axial plane image through the aneurysm demonstrates dissection of the posterolateral wall. **C,** Another axial image at the base of the aneurysm demonstrates high signal intensity in the false lumen, attributable to low flow velocity (compared with the true lumen, in which there is flow void from fast-flowing blood).

Implanted metallic objects are a subject of particular concern, because they could potentially undergo undesirable torquing movements if the magnetic field were sufficiently strong and if they contained sufficient ferromagnetic material. Fortunately, surgical clips and sternotomy wires implanted in the chest and abdomen are typically only weakly ferromagnetic. Furthermore, these devices quickly become immobilized by surrounding fibrous tissue, and patients with these implants can be safely studied by MRI. The wires and clips, however, may cause image artifact. Similarly, patients with implanted intravascular coils, stents, and occluding devices can be imaged by MRI once the implants are believed to be immobile. Many centers choose to avoid exposing these patients to MRI for an arbitrarily chosen period of time after implantation (usually for several weeks), but such practice is not supported by conclusive published data. A decision to perform MRI examination shortly after cardiac surgery or implantation of a biomedical device must weigh the risk/benefit ratio for the individual patient.

A number of devices are considered either a relative or absolute contraindication to MRI. Presence of an intracranial, intraocular, or intracochlear metallic object is considered a contraindication to the procedure. Prosthetic cardiac valves are not considered a contraindication to MRI. The presence of a cardiac pacemaker is also considered a relative contraindication to MRI and some reports have suggested that it may be possible to scan patients who have modern pacemakers. A detailed listing of biomedical implants and devices considered to be relative or absolute contraindications to MRI can be found elsewhere.[41]

Because MRI scanners attract ferromagnetic objects, extreme caution should be exerted in approaching magnets with objects containing iron or other ferromagnetic materials. Only especially designed MRI-compatible physiologic monitoring equipment should be used in conjunction with MRI studies.

NUCLEAR CARDIOLOGY

Nuclear cardiology is a physiologic diagnostic modality that uses radioisotope-labeled compounds to capture and quantify blood flow, myocardial perfusion and integrity, and ventricular function. The following types of nuclear studies are available to patients with congenital heart disease.[42]

Description of Techniques

Myocardial Perfusion

The two commonly used methods are based on uptake of compounds labeled with thallium-201 (^{201}Tl) or technetium-99m (^{99m}Tc). Both ^{201}Tl and ^{99m}Tc follow potassium kinetics.

Uptake of both radioisotopes by myocardial cells depends on several factors, including coronary blood flow and isotope extraction. Underperfused myocardium will appear as a region of decreased signal intensity ("cold spot") relative to normally perfused myocardium. Exercise and pharmacologic challenges can be used to evaluate myocardial perfusion under stress. The shorter half-life of ^{99m}Tc-labeled methoxyisobutyl isonitrile (^{99m}Tc-MIBI) allows injection of a higher dose. This gives a better count rate statistic and allows potential gating of images to improve anatomic definition. Single photon emission computed tomography (SPECT), a technique similar to computed tomography, allows for expanded evaluation of regional perfusion. Myocardial perfusion studies have been reported in Kawasaki disease, after the arterial switch operation and in anomalous origin of the left coronary artery, cardiomyopathy, and atherosclerosis.

Infarct-Avid Myocardial Scintigraphy

This scan uses ^{99m}Tc-pyrophosphate to localize recent myocardial infarction.

Blood Pool Imaging

For blood pool imaging, multiple gated acquisition (MUGA) scans using ^{99m}Tc-labeled red blood cells or albumin are obtained after equilibrium of the radionuclide compound with the blood pool has been achieved. A computer with operator input to define the boundaries of the chamber's blood pool processes the data collected during the scan. Ejection fraction is determined from the end-diastolic and end-systolic counts.

This method can also be used to assess regional wall motion, cardiac output, filling and ejection times, and regurgitation fraction. Another technique, first pass radionuclide angiocardiography, allows separation of the right ventricle from the left ventricle.

Vascular Perfusion Scanning

Through the use of ^{99m}Tc-labeled macroaggregated albumin, perfusion of an organ can be investigated. This technique is commonly used in pediatric cardiology to evaluate lung perfusion. The addition of a ventilation scan using inhaled xenon-138 gives information on ventilation-perfusion mismatch. The assumption in vascular perfusion imaging is that the radionuclide tracer is trapped in the capillaries of the first vascular bed it encounters. In the absence of right-to-left shunt and pulmonary arteriovenous malformations, intravenous injection of ^{99m}Tc-labeled macroaggregated albumin will result in trapping of the tracer in the pulmonary capillary bed. Both dynamic and static tracer flow patterns can be determined. Qualitative blood flow volume is estimated from the relative count density in a defined region of interest. Potential sources of error in vascular perfusion studies include poor tagging of the albumin microaggregates with ^{99m}Tc (which will allow free ^{99m}Tc to circulate through the capillary bed and be extracted by its target organ), streaming of the injected bolus, and right-to-left shunting.

Inflammatory Disease Imaging

The technique of inflammatory disease imaging uses white blood cells labeled with gallium-67 (^{67}Ga) or indium-111 (^{111}In) to detect areas of active inflammation. This method can be used to detect myocarditis, myocardial abscess, and pericardial or mediastinal inflammation.

DIAGNOSTIC CARDIAC CATHETERIZATION AND ANGIOGRAPHY

Cardiac catheterization has developed as a diagnostic technique in pediatric cardiology over the past 50 years, becoming an essential and widely used tool for diagnosis of CHD in the 1960s and 1970s.[43] With progress in noninvasive techniques, particularly echocardiography and MRI, cardiac catheterization is currently no longer invariably necessary before surgical repair or for diagnosis of most common conditions.[44] However, it continues to play a significant part in the evaluation of complex CHD, and remains an essential diagnostic method for the hemodynamic assessment of many conditions.[45] Furthermore, all transcatheter interventions are preceded by diagnostic angiographic and hemodynamic evaluation, on the basis of which management decisions are made.

Description of Techniques

Preparation of the Patient

A thorough review of all pertinent clinical information is performed before cardiac catheterization, including previous diagnostic studies and surgical notes. A physical examination with emphasis on access sites, palpation of pulses, and search for surgical scars is performed, followed by an ECG, chest radiograms in the frontal and lateral projections, an echocardiogram, a complete blood count, and urine analysis. Informed consent is obtained both for the procedure and for possible interventions. Typed and crossmatched packed red blood cells are prepared. Specific orders regarding discontinuation of oral intake and medication schedules are given (e.g., stop digoxin the night before the procedure, or stop aspirin a week before an intervention). An intravenous cannula is inserted for administration of medications and intravenous fluids before and during the procedure. Intravenous hydration is necessary before catheterization in infants or patients with hemoglobin concentrations greater than 19 g/dL.

Patients are premedicated according to age group (chloral hydrate, meperidine hydrochloride, or diazepam). Local anesthesia with lidocaine is given at the access site. Intravenous morphine, midazolam, or ketamine is used to provide sedation, analgesia, and/or anesthesia throughout the procedure. General anesthesia is rarely necessary for diagnostic studies. However, it might be necessary in high-risk patients such as those with severe pulmonary artery hypertension or ventricular dysfunction, or in neonates receiving intravenous prostaglandin infusion.

Intravenous heparin (100 U/kg) is administered after vascular access is accomplished. Activated clotting time is monitored every hour and heparin boluses are administered to keep the activated clotting time longer than 200 seconds throughout the study.

Vascular Access

The most common sites of vascular access are the femoral artery and vein. The umbilical vessels can be used in the newborn. The most commonly used technique for vascular access is the percutaneous Seldinger technique,[46] which has become highly successful in children. As a result of this success, surgical cutdowns are no longer performed. Other access sites, such as the subclavian vein, the jugular vein, or the transhepatic approach, may be necessary when standard sites are not available. Similarly, alternative vascular access is used in patients with complex anatomy (e.g., after bidirectional Glenn shunt) or when certain interventions are planned (e.g., transhepatic access in a patient with occluded femoral vessels and need for transseptal puncture).

Catheters and Sheaths

The smallest size French (F) catheter and/or sheath that would allow adequate hemodynamic and angiographic evaluation should be selected.[47] Sheaths with backstop valves are preferred, to avoid blood loss. An arterial sheath is placed when catheter exchange is anticipated or in left-sided obstructive lesions, to allow two simultaneous arterial pressure recordings. The catheters most commonly used for hemodynamic evaluation are the 5F or 7F wedge end-hole catheter for the antegrade venous approach and a pigtail catheter for the retrograde arterial assessment. In small neonates and infants, smaller catheters such as a 4F venous and 3F arterial may be sufficient. For measurement of pressure in tortuous blood vessels, catheters with specific shapes are preferred. Examples include Berenstein, Benson, Cobra, sidewinder, and coronary catheters. Angiographic catheters most commonly used are the Berman and pigtail catheters.[47]

Hemodynamic Evaluation

Pressures and Saturations

Accurate pressure measurements are essential for hemodynamic diagnosis. Two simultaneous transducers are generally necessary and should be accurately calibrated. Normal values of pressures in the central cardiovascular system have been published and are summarized in Table 105.4.[48] The most common sequence of measurements includes:

- the superior vena cava (saturation only);
- right atrium (pressure and saturation);
- right ventricle (pressure and saturation);
- pulmonary arteries (pressure and saturation);
- bilateral wedge pressures simultaneous with left ventricular pressure
- aorta (pressure and saturation); and
- a measurement of oxygen consumption.

This sequence is sometimes followed by a second set of saturation measurements in the pulmonary artery, aorta, and superior vena cava, in addition to pullbacks from the pulmonary artery to the right atrium and from the left ventricle to the descending aorta. Exceptions to this sequence include patients with surgical caval anastomoses, transvenous pacing wires, or a history of indwelling lines, in whom a pullback with pressure tracing from the superior vena cava to the right atrium should be recorded. The sequence of measurements also varies according to the underlying condition. In patients with cyanosis, pulmonary venous saturation should be measured. Pulmonary venous wedge pressures are useful to determine distal pulmonary artery pressures in patients in whom the pulmonary arteries cannot be entered, but are only reliable at pressures less than 15 mm Hg. Double-lumen catheters or simultaneous pressure measurements are most useful to determine gradients and localize obstructions in venous pathways (e.g., Mustard or Senning pathways and Fontan circulation) and in arterial stenoses (e.g., obstructed right ventricle-to-pulmonary artery conduits, branch pulmonary artery stenosis, and supravalvar pulmonary stenosis) (Fig. 105.15). Precise localization of pressure gradients can also be achieved by a pullback recording performed using a catheter over a small guide wire with a Y adapter or long sheath over a wire. A small amount of contrast injected at the site at which the gradient is recorded allows precise localization of the obstruction.

HEMODYNAMIC VALUES IN CHILDREN WITHOUT HEART DISEASE

Site of Pressure Measurement	Average (mm Hg)	Range (mm Hg)
Right atrium, mean	3	0–8
Right ventricle (systolic/end-diastolic)	24/4	15–35/0–10
Pulmonary artery (systolic/diastolic) (mean)	21/9 (12)	11–26/2–14 (8–19)
Pulmonary capillary wedge or left atrial, mean	8	2–12
Left ventricle (systolic/end-diastolic)	96/8*	60–130/2–12*
Systemic arterial pressure (systolic/diastolic)	110/65*	Varies with age

*Variable with age normals for systemic blood pressure.
Modified from Keane JF, Lock JE. Hemodynamic evaluation of congenital heart disease. In Lock JE, Keane JF, Perry SB, eds. Diagnostic and Interventional Catheterization in Congenital Heart Disease, 2nd ed. Amsterdam, Kluwer, 2000:37-72.

Table 105.4 Hemodynamic values in children without heart disease.

Cardiac Output and Shunts

On the basis of the Fick principle, by estimating oxygen consumption ($\dot{V}O_2$) and measuring oxygen content in systemic arterial, systemic venous, pulmonary arterial, and pulmonary venous blood, it is possible to calculate cardiac output (CO or Qs), pulmonary blood flow (Qp), and shunts. Cardiac index is calculated by dividing the CO by the BSA. The oxygen saturation in the superior vena cava is considered the best representative of the mixed venous oxygen saturation in patients with shunts. Based on the Fick principle, cardiac output is calculated using the following formula:

$$\text{CO or Qs(L/min)} = \frac{\text{VO}_2(\text{mLO}_2/\text{min})}{\text{Systemic artery} - \text{mixed venous O}_2 \text{ content} \quad \text{O}_2 \text{ content} \quad (\text{mLO}_2/\text{liter blood})}$$

where oxygen (O_2) content (mL/L) = O_2 saturation × Hb (g/dL) × 1.36 mL O_2/g Hb × 10 + PO_2 × 0.03 mL O_2/L blood

where Hb is hemoglobin and PO_2 is the partial pressure of oxygen.

In patients receiving inhaled oxygen and with an arterial PO_2 more than 100 mm Hg (13.3 kPa), dissolved oxygen should be accounted for. This is particularly important for evaluation of the response of pulmonary vascular resistance to selective pulmonary vasodilators in patients with pulmonary hypertension.

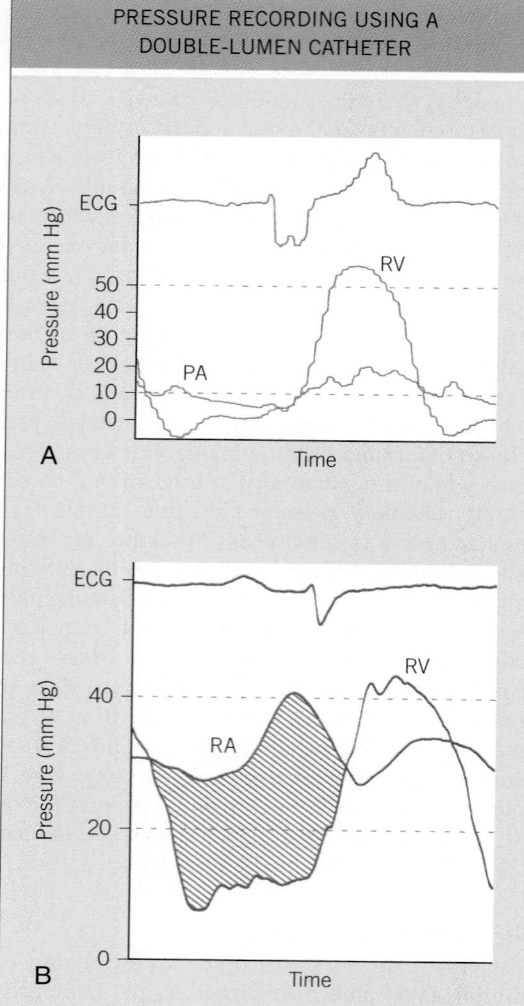

Figure 105.15 Pressure recording using a double-lumen catheter. A, Patient with right ventricle-to-pulmonary artery homograft after repair of truncus arteriosus. The distal lumen is located above the homograft valve (PA), and the proximal lumen is located in the right ventricular outflow tract (RV). A peak systolic ejection gradient of 38 mm Hg is measured, with different diastolic pressures observed for both lumens, suggesting a competent homograft valve. **B,** Patient with Bjork type of repair of tricuspid atresia using a right atrium–to–right ventricular infundibulum homograft and a classic Glenn shunt. The distal lumen is located in the right ventricle (RV), and the proximal lumen is in the right atrium (RA), indicating functional tricuspid or homograft valve stenosis (shaded area).

Based on the Fick principle, pulmonary blood flow is calculated using the following formula:

$$\text{Qp (L/min)} = \frac{VO_2(\text{ml}/O_2/\text{min})}{\text{Pulmonary artery } O_2 \text{ content} - \text{Pulmonary vein } O_2 \text{ content (ml } O_2/\text{liter blood)}}$$

The pulmonary-to-systemic flow ratio (Qp/Qs) is used to assess the clinical significance of left-to-right shunt, and is considered more useful than shunt calculations alone. The effective pulmonary blood flow (Qe) is the amount of deoxygenated blood that becomes oxygenated. Qe is calculated by the following formula:

$$Qe = \frac{VO_2 \text{ (ml } O_2/\text{min)}}{\text{Pulmonary vein } O_2 \text{ content} - \text{systemic vein } O_2 \text{ content (ml } O_2/\text{liter blood)}}$$

The absolute left-to-right shunt is the difference between Qp and Qe. Similarly, the absolute right-to-left shunt is the difference between Qs and Qe.

In patients with no source of right-to-left or left-to-right shunt, cardiac output can be accurately determined by thermodilution. This is particularly useful in patients with left-sided obstructive lesions or cardiomyopathies. Thermodilution is not accurate in patients with pulmonary regurgitation (e.g., postoperative tetralogy of Fallot), severe peripheral pulmonary artery stenosis, or tricuspid regurgitation.

Vascular Resistance

Vascular resistance is determined by the pressure difference across the vascular bed being considered (in mm Hg) divided by the flow (in L/min) across it. Vascular resistance may be expressed in mm Hg per L/min (Wood units or hybrid resistance units), converted into metric resistance units (dyn s cm^{-5}), or expressed as absolute resistance units (by multiplying the metric resistance units by 80). In children, calculated resistances are adjusted to BSA, giving a resistance index. Pulmonary vascular resistance (PVR) is calculated by the following formula:

$$\text{PVR} = \frac{\text{Mean pulmonary artery pressure} - \text{mean left atrial pressure (or pulmonary vein pressure)}}{\text{Qp (indexed to BSA)}}$$

Systemic vascular resistance is calculated by the following formula:

$$\text{SVR} = \frac{\text{Mean arterial blood pressure} - \text{mean right atrial pressure}}{\text{Qs (indexed to BSA)}}$$

Baseline calculations should be performed in room air. Depending on the patient's specific diagnosis, additional data sets are acquired under different conditions. Examples include response of pulmonary vascular resistance to inhaled oxygen or nitric oxide, test balloon occlusion of atrial septal defect in a patient with mitral stenosis or small left-sided structures, or test occlusion of a source of right-to-left shunt through an atrial septal defect or Fontan fenestration. To obtain an accurate estimate of the pulmonary vascular resistance in patients with branch pulmonary artery stenoses, it is necessary to determine the distribution of pulmonary blood flow to each lung by perfusion scintigraphy or MRI. Because the resistances are in parallel, the total resistance can then be calculated using the formula:

$$\frac{1}{\text{Total resistance}} = \frac{1}{\text{Left lung resistance}} + \frac{1}{\text{Right lung resistance}}$$

Valve Area

Calculation of valve area in pediatrics is performed the same way as in adults, using the Gorlin formula. Valve area is directly proportional to the flow across the valve considered and inversely related to the square root of the mean pressure decrease:

$$\text{Aortic or pulmonary valve area} = \frac{\text{systolic flow (ml/s)}}{44.5 \times \sqrt{\text{mean systolic gradient}}}$$

$$\text{Systolic flow (ml/s)} = \frac{\text{CO} \times \text{RR interval}}{60 \times \text{systolic ejection time}}$$

$$\text{Mitral or triscupid valve area} = \frac{\text{diastolic flow (ml/s)}}{31.5 \times \sqrt{\text{mean diastolic gradient}}}$$

$$\text{Diastolic flow (ml/s)} = \frac{\text{CO} \times \text{RR interval}}{60 \times \text{diastolic flow time}}$$

The mean pressure gradient can be accurately obtained by planimetry of the pressure tracing. It can also be estimated from the average of the gradients measured from vertical lines placed 1 mm apart throughout the area between the pressure tracings (either ventricular and arterial or atrial and ventricular).

Angiographic Evaluation

Angiography should be planned in detail before cardiac catheterization, and modified according to the hemodynamic findings. Power injections are performed using angiographic catheters (e.g., pigtail or Berman).[47] Selective injections can be performed by hand using end-hole catheters or as a power injection with a cut pigtail catheter (tail removed) over a wire with a Y adapter. This would also allow pressure measurements through the side port. Biplane angiography is preferred, and is particularly necessary in infants and in patients of any age when interventional procedures are being considered. Common angiographic views for diagnosis of congenital heart defects are summarized in Table 105.5.[47]

Contrast and Technique

Nonionic, water-soluble, iodine-based contrast agents are used for pediatric angiography.[47] The amount of contrast and flow of injection should be determined according to the chamber in question and physiologic variables. Infants, particularly those with large shunts, require larger volumes of contrast to opacify the cardiac chambers and blood vessels. If the output is low, smaller volumes may be sufficient. Generally, injection volumes of 1 mL/kg are optimal for aortic and main pulmonary artery injections in patients with normal output, and for ventriculograms in patients without significant shunts. Larger volumes (1.5 to 2 mL/kg) are necessary for large left-to-right shunts if the injection is performed in a volume-overloaded chamber. For selective right or left pulmonary artery injections or in patients with diminished pulmonary blood flow, a pulmonary arteriogram with 0.5 mL/kg should provide adequate anatomic definition.

COMMON ANGIOGRAPHIC VIEWS IN PATIENTS WITH CONGENITAL HEART DISEASE

View	AP Camera	Lateral Camera	Angiogram	Lesions
Straight AP	0°	90°	Right ventricle	Normally related great arteries, TGA, DORV, PA/IVS, postop TOF, single ventricle
			Systemic and pulmonary veins	Anomalies of the systemic and pulmonary veins
			Pulmonary arteries	Branch pulmonary artery stenosis
			Aorta/systemic arteries	Coarctation, peripheral vasculopathies, aortopulmonary collaterals, surgical shunts
Cranial frontal and straight lateral	30° cranial	90°	Right ventricle	Right ventricular outflow tract obstruction (TOF, DORV), pulmonary valve stenosis
			Pulmonary arteries	Main pulmonary artery stenosis, pulmonary bifurcation stenosis
"Laid back"	40–45° caudal ± LAO or RAO	90°	Aortogram	TOF/PA and aortopulmonary collaterals (the central pulmonary arteries have a "seagull" appearance)
			Aortogram	Coronary arteries in TGA and DORV
			Pulmonary arteries	Branch pulmonary artery stenosis at bifurcation
Long axial oblique	0° or 20–30° RAO	70°, 20–30° cranial	Left ventricle	Ventricular septal defects, left ventricular outflow tract obstruction in: VSD, TGA, DORV, TOF, truncus, hypertrophic obstructive cardiomyopathy, subvalvular and valvular aortic stenosis
Hepatoclavicular	0° or 20–30° RAO	45–50°, 40° cranial	Left ventricle	Tricuspid atresia, common atrioventricular canal

AP, anteroposterior; DORV, double outlet right ventricle; IVS, intact ventricular septum; LAO, left anterior oblique; PA, pulmonary atresia; RAO, right anterior oblique; TGA, transposition of the great arteries; TOF, tetralogy of Fallot; VSD, ventricular septal defect.

Table 105.5 Common angiographic views in patients with congenital heart disease.

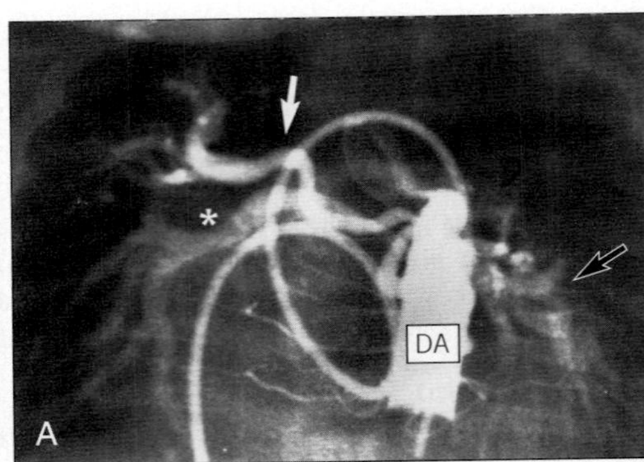

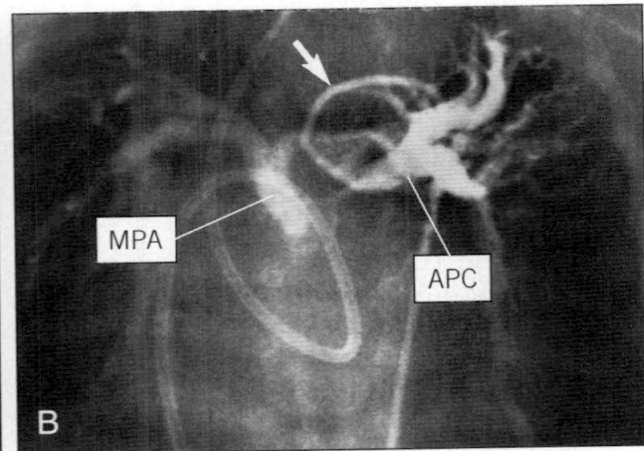

Figure 105.16 Descending aortogram in tetralogy of Fallot with pulmonary atresia. A, Balloon occlusion descending aortogram (DA) in a newborn with tetralogy of Fallot, pulmonary atresia, and multiple aortopulmonary collaterals supplying the right upper lobe (*white arrow*), the right lower and middle lobes (*), and the left lower lobe (*black arrow*). **B,** Selective angiogram (*arrow*), in the same patient, of aortopulmonary collateral to the left upper lobe (APC) demonstrating dual supply of this lung segment, connected to the central pulmonary arteries (MPA).

When anatomic definition is warranted in a ventriculogram, the injection should be as fast as possible. If ventricular function or valve regurgitation is the focus of interest, the injection rate should be slower to avoid ectopy. Angiography with balloon occlusion is used in the following conditions.

- Descending aortogram in patients with several aortopulmonary collaterals: a power injection through a Berman catheter with balloon occlusion of the descending aorta allows identification of aortopulmonary collaterals and central pulmonary arteries (Fig. 105.16).
- Ascending aortogram with a Berman catheter using an antegrade approach in patients with D-loop TGA using a "laid back" view will show the coronary origins (Fig. 105.17).
- Visualizing pulmonary venous drainage: pulmonary capillary wedge injection with end-hole wedge catheter is used; it should be performed in all lung segments in patients with suspected pulmonary vein stenosis or atresia.
- Visualizing the central pulmonary arteries: pulmonary venous wedge injection is performed when direct access is not possible (Fig. 105.18).
- Persistence of a left superior vena cava or presence of decompressing veins before a bidirectional Glenn procedure: balloon occlusion angiogram in the innominate vein is performed to determine these conditions. This angiogram can be performed either via a retrograde approach from the femoral vein using a balloon end-hole catheter or from the left subclavian vein with a Berman catheter (Fig. 105.19).
- Coronary artery fistula: a balloon occlusion coronary angiogram will determine proximal branches and define the optimal site for coil embolization.
- Documentation of test occlusion: (1) during Fontan fenestration test occlusion, a power injection through a Berman catheter allows determination of other sources

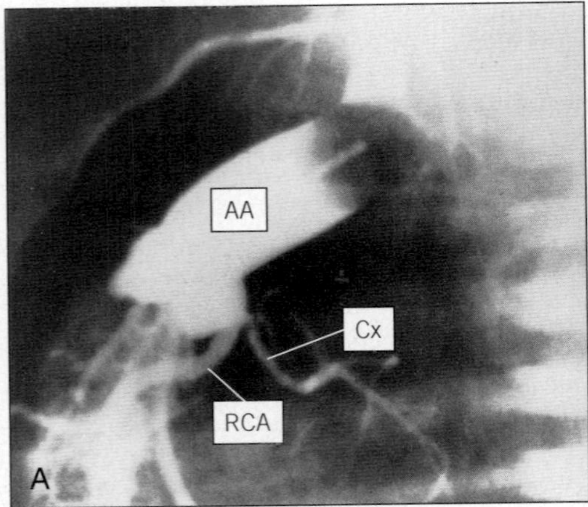

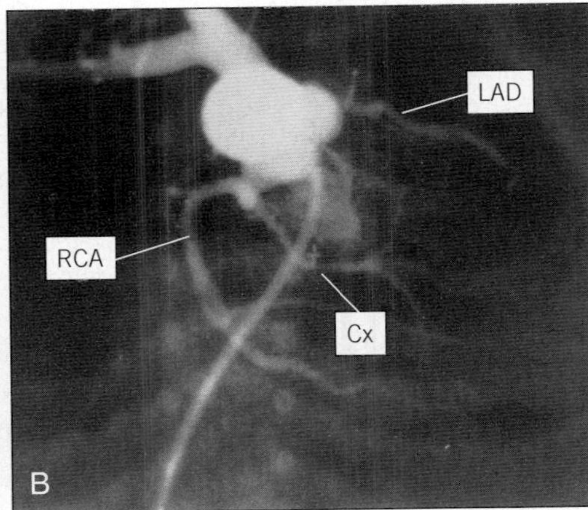

Figure 105.17 Laid-back aortogram in a patient with SDD transposition of the great arteries and circumflex coronary artery arising from the right coronary artery. A, Lateral projection. **B,** Anteroposterior projection. AA, ascending aorta; Cx, circumflex coronary artery; LAD, left anterior descending coronary artery; RCA, right coronary artery; SDD, visceroatrial situs solitus (S), D-ventricular loop (D), and D-transposition (D). (From Geva T. Echocardiography and Doppler ultrasound. In Garson A Jr, Bricker JT, Fisher DJ, Neish SR, eds. The Science and Practice of Pediatric Cardiology. Baltimore, Williams & Wilkins, 1997:789-843; Wong PC, Sanders SP, Jonas RA, et al. Pulmonary valve-moderator band distance: association with development of double-chambered right ventricle in infants with ventricular septal defect. Am J Cardiol 1991;68:1681-1686.)

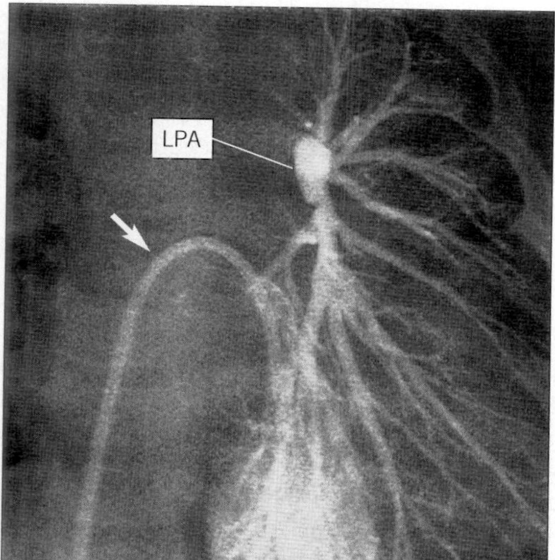

Figure 105.18 Pulmonary venous wedge injection in a patient with truncus arteriosus type A3 of Van Praagh, and absent left pulmonary artery from atretic origin of left pulmonary artery (LPA) from the descending aorta. The arrow is pointing to the catheter.

of right-to-left shunt; and (2) to test occlusion of atrial septal defect to determine additional defects.

- Anomalous pulmonary venous connection: a balloon occlusion angiogram in the pulmonary venous confluence can show the individual pulmonary veins.
- Branch pulmonary artery stenosis: a selective balloon occlusion angiogram through a Berman catheter in one branch will demonstrate stenosis in the contralateral branch.

Hand injections in selective vessels is another angiographic technique that is commonly used for coronary arteriography, pulmonary veins, small branch pulmonary arteries, small arterial or venous collaterals, and small cardiac chambers (Fig. 105.20).[49]

Indications and Objectives

Although diagnostic cardiac catheterization is generally not necessary before surgical repair of a large number of conditions, it is still essential for the preoperative evaluation of several CHDs.

Routine preoperative diagnostic cardiac catheterization is not usually required in patients with[44]

- atrial and ventricular septal defects;
- common atrioventricular canal;
- coarctation of the aorta;
- transposition of the great arteries;
- tetralogy of Fallot;
- truncus arteriosus;
- partially and totally anomalous pulmonary venous return; and
- interrupted aortic arch.

Examples of conditions in which preoperative catheterization is often useful include patients with[45]

- pulmonary atresia and intact ventricular septum;
- all forms of single ventricle before bidirectional Glenn or Fontan procedures;
- tetralogy of Fallot with pulmonary atresia associated with diminutive pulmonary arteries and aortopulmonary collaterals;
- other diagnoses associated with collaterals;
- primary or secondary pulmonary artery hypertension;
- pulmonary vein stenosis; and
- coronary artery abnormalities.

Diagnostic cardiac catheterization may also be necessary in patients with common conditions and unusual clinical presentation, and whenever symptoms cannot be explained by noninvasive testing. Hemodynamic and angiographic data will determine the need for further intervention in a large number of patients with congenital pulmonary, aortic or mitral valve stenosis, certain types of subaortic or

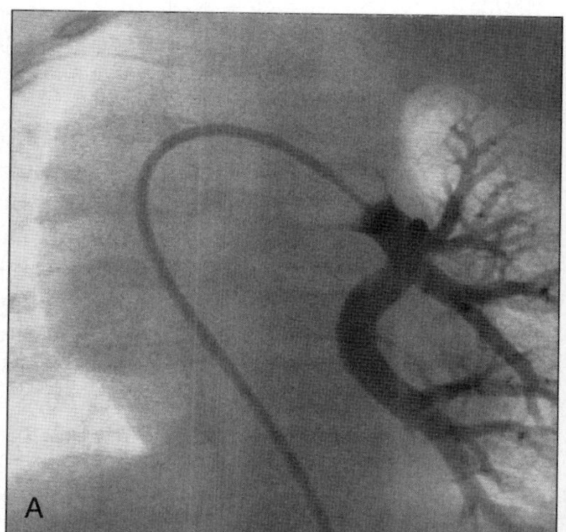

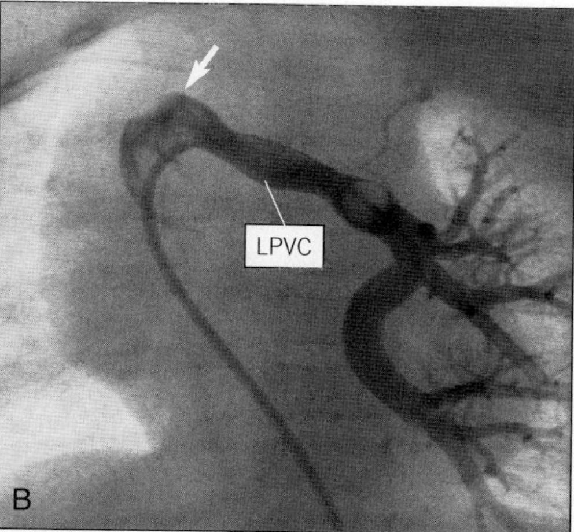

Figure 105.19 Pulmonary venous angiogram. A, Balloon occlusion angiogram in the pulmonary venous confluence in a patient with heterotaxy syndrome and complex anomalous pulmonary venous connections, showing left upper and lower pulmonary veins draining to a common confluence. **B,** As the balloon deflates, contrast fills the confluence (LPVC), draining to the high superior vena cava (*white arrow*).

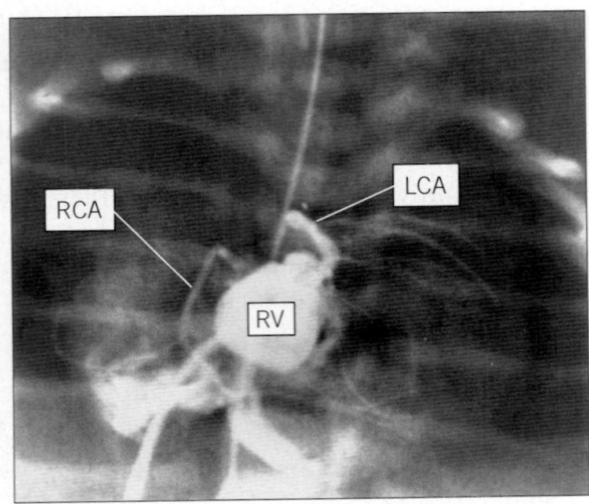

Figure 105.20 Right ventricular angiogram in a patient with pulmonary atresia and intact ventricular septum, demonstrating coronary artery anatomy. This patient has atresia of the ostia of the right coronary artery, coronary sinusoids, stenoses, and dilatations resulting in right ventricle–dependent coronary circulation. LCA, left coronary artery; RCA, right coronary artery; RV, right ventricle.

subpulmonary stenosis, and peripheral pulmonary artery stenosis. Diagnostic cardiac catheterization is complementary to noninvasive diagnostic methods to evaluate aortic arch anomalies, to determine the presence and significance of additional ventricular septal defects, and to evaluate certain anatomic features in patients with heterotaxy syndrome.

Specific diagnostic testing in the cardiac catheterization laboratory can determine candidacy for specific transcatheter or surgical interventions. For example, balloon test occlusion of an atrial septal defect can help to determine whether tricuspid stenosis is present in a patient with a borderline tricuspid valve size, atrial septal defect, and right-to-left shunting. Other examples include test occlusion of a Blalock-Taussig shunt before coil embolization, test occlusion of a patent ductus arteriosus to determine the presence of aortic coarctation or ductal-dependent hypoplastic arch, or test occlusion of a Fontan fenestration to determine candidacy for fenestration closure.

Hemodynamic testing of the effects of drugs may be indicated in certain conditions, such as pulmonary vasodilator testing in patients with pulmonary hypertension. Similarly, patients with Fontan circulation and junctional rhythm can be tested in the catheterization laboratory with atrial pacing to determine the hemodynamic benefit of pacemaker implantation.

Because diagnostic cardiac catheterization is an essential initial step in interventional studies, the indications for diagnostic catheterization are linked to the indications to intervene. These decisions are also based on data from noninvasive testing. For example, diagnostic cardiac catheterization precedes aortic balloon valvotomy in a patient with noninvasive diagnosis of severe aortic valve stenosis. In such a situation, the study would only be diagnostic if the patient did not meet criteria for intervention by hemodynamic assessment, whereas it would otherwise become interventional. Similarly, 30% to 50% of planned diagnostic cardiac catheterizations in patients with single ventricle physiology result in interventions. Examples include coil occlusion of venous or arterial collaterals, balloon dilation, and/or stent placement for venous or arterial stenoses, or device closure of baffle leaks or fenestration. Cardiac catheterization remains essential for the evaluation of a large number of postoperative conditions, including homograft or conduit stenosis, residual shunts, patients with palliated single ventricle, or unexplained abnormalities detected by noninvasive testing.

Safety and Complications

Even though diagnostic cardiac catheterizations are performed in patients with more complicated preoperative and postoperative CHD, and despite a substantial increase in the number and complexity of interventional procedures, the incidence of complications has consistently decreased over the past three decades. Depending on definitions, complication rates range from 9% to 24%, with major events occurring in 1% to 4% of cases, and mortality rates in the last decade of less than 1%. The incidence of major complications (e.g., death, cardiac arrest, cardiac perforation, complete heart block, ventricular tachycardia or fibrillation, and cardiac tamponade) is 1% to 2%. Common minor complications include nonsustained rhythm disturbances or atrial arrhythmias requiring medication during the procedure, as well as fever, hematoma, or loss of pulse in the 12 hours after the procedure. Younger age has been universally associated with a higher complication rate. Interventional cases have a higher complication rate when compared to diagnostic cases. Specific interventions such as balloon angioplasty have been associated with higher rates of both major and minor events.[50] Currently, investigators are developing risk adjustment methods to accommodate case mix complexity in congenital cardiac catheterization. With multi-institutional cooperation, these methods and the determination of benchmark rates for safety and efficacy outcomes will promote quality improvement initiatives for pediatric cardiac catheterization.

SUMMARY

Accurate diagnosis of congenital heart disease can be accomplished by the judicious use of a variety of modalities. Echocardiography has assumed a leading role as the primary diagnostic tool in pediatric cardiology, because of its noninvasive nature and its ability to provide comprehensive accurate diagnostic information in real time, in a variety of clinical settings, and at a reasonable cost. Cardiac MRI is an important diagnostic tool in pediatric cardiology because of its ability to provide anatomic and functional information that cannot be obtained by echocardiography and, in some patients, by catheterization. Diagnostic cardiac catheterization, the "gold standard" for the past 50 years, is gradually being replaced by noninvasive tools, but is still required for anatomic delineation of small blood vessels, such as the coronary arteries, for pressure measurements, and for guidance of interventional procedures.

chapter

106 Atrial Septal Defect

Ami B. Bhatt, Michael J. Landzberg, and Fred M. Wu

Definition

- An atrial septal defect (ASD) is an opening in the atrial septum allowing blood to shunt between the atria.

Key Features

- There are several types of ASD: ostium secundum, sinus venosus, coronary sinus septal, and ostium primum. Ostium secundum is the most common type of ASD.
- Atrial septal defects permit shunting of blood across the atrial septum in response to pressure gradients. The most common pattern is left-to-right, but right-to-left shunting may occur if right atrial pressures are high.
- Echocardiography is the most common test used for diagnosis of ASD in both children and adults.

Therapy

- Patients with significant ASDs should be offered elective closure upon diagnosis.
- Closure may be accomplished either surgically or with catheter-delivered closure devices.
- Atrial arrhythmias are common late complications after surgical or device closure, especially if closure is delayed until adulthood.

An atrial septal defect (ASD) is an opening in the atrial septum allowing blood to shunt between the atria, typically from the left to the right. ASDs are among the most commonly seen congenital heart defects. Their morphology and associated physiology determine the manner of presentation, and many are first diagnosed during adulthood. In this chapter, we examine the epidemiology and pathophysiology of atrial septal defects as well as the clinical presentation and role of correction in the adult. Although considered to be a normal finding, patent foramen ovale (PFO) is discussed briefly because of increasing controversy regarding its clinical significance.

Recent estimates place the prevalence of ASD at about 1 per 1000 live births.[1,2] This is higher than suggested in earlier studies,[3] but the difference may in part reflect improvements in imaging technology. The male-to-female ratio is 1:2 with similar outcomes irrespective of gender. One study suggests a slightly higher incidence in black Americans compared to whites, but the basis for this finding is not well understood.[1]

Most ASDs occur sporadically, but familial cases showing an autosomal dominant pattern of inheritance have been described. Several transcription factor mutations have been identified,[4,5] including that of the Holt-Oram syndrome, an anomaly characterized by cardiac and radial limb deformities. Other associated anomalies include the presence of a primum ASD in Down syndrome. Lutembacher syndrome is not a genetic syndrome, but refers to the combination of acquired mitral valve disease and an ASD.

ANATOMY AND PATHOLOGY

During embryonic development, the process of atrial septation involves three structures: the septum primum, the septum secundum, and the atrioventricular canal septum. A true atrial septal defect involves a deficiency of one or more components of the atrial septum. The embryology of congenital heart disease is discussed elsewhere in this text and will not be focused upon here.

Types of Atrial Septal Defects

Ostium Secundum Atrial Septal Defect

Ostium secundum atrial septal defects are the most common type of ASD (Fig. 106.1), constituting 70% of all ASDs and 6% to 10% of all congenital heart defects. The central portion of the intact atrial septum is normally occupied by the fossa ovalis, the floor of which is formed by septum primum. Contrary to its name, a secundum ASD results from an insufficiency of septum primum. As such, secundum ASDs are centrally located and are generally bounded by the superior and inferior limbic bands, which often make these defects amenable to device closure.

Patent Foramen Ovale

Although a patent foramen ovale is also located within the fossa ovalis, it is structurally and functionally distinct from secundum ASDs. During fetal life, the foramen ovale is a normal interatrial communication that is formed by the superior limb of the septum secundum on the right atrial side and the septum primum on the left atrial side. Because these two septa overlap, the higher left atrial pressure after birth forces the septum primum against the limbic septum, preventing left-to-right shunting. Conditions leading to elevated right atrial pressures can, in some instances, allow right-to-left shunting to occur.

Sinus Venosus Defect

Sinus venosus defects occur most commonly at the junction of the superior vena cava and the right atrium (the superior vena cava type). Although sometimes referred to as "sinus venosus atrial septal defects," anatomically, they are not truly defects in the interatrial septum. Rather, they

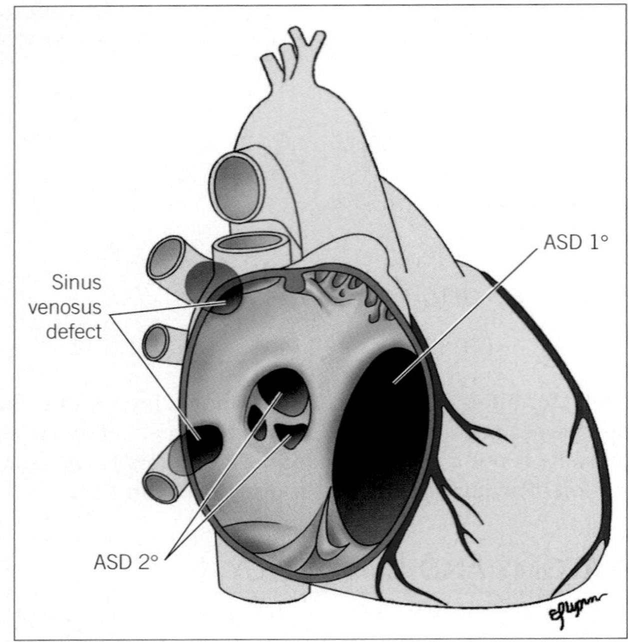

Figure 106.1 Diagram of the atrial septum showing different types of atrial septal defect. An ostium primum defect (ASD 1°) is located adjacent to the mitral and tricuspid valves. Ostium secundum defects (ASD 2°) are located centrally near the fossa ovalis. Sinus venosus defects occur in the area derived from the embryologic sinus venosus.

are thought to represent an abnormal communication between one or more right pulmonary veins and the right atrium.

In the superior vena cava type, the defect is a deficiency of the common wall between the posterolateral wall of the right superior vena cava and the anterior wall of the right upper pulmonary vein. The left atrial orifice of the right upper pulmonary vein is usually patent, thus allowing for interatrial communication. In some instances, this orifice may be atretic, creating the appearance of partially anomalous pulmonary venous connection. Rarely, a sinus venosus defect may involve the right lower and/or middle pulmonary veins and the middle or superior portion of the posterior right atrial wall. This may be referred to as the right atrial type or inferior vena cava type, although direct involvement of the inferior vena cava is extremely unusual.

Coronary Sinus Septal Defect

The coronary sinus septal defect is rare. As is the case with sinus venosus defects, coronary sinus septal defects do not result from a deficiency in the interatrial septum, but rather from a failure of development of the fold between the inferior vena cava and the sinus venosus. This results in partial or complete absence of the septum between the coronary sinus and the left atrium and permits interatrial communication through the coronary sinus ostium. The orifice is often quite large as a result of the left-to-right shunt. Coronary sinus septal defect is often associated with a persistent left superior vena cava (SVC). When the coronary sinus is completely unroofed, this left SVC enters the left atrium anterior to the orifice of the left upper pulmonary vein and posterior to the left atrial appendage.

Ostium Primum Atrial Septal Defect

Ostium primum defects fall on the continuum of atrioventricular canal defects, also referred to as endocardial cushion defects or atrioventricular septal defects (AVSDs). These defects involve the septal portions of the atrioventricular valves and the adjacent atrial and ventricular septa; cases in which there is an isolated atrial defect with little or no involvement of the ventricular septum are described as ostium primum defects. These can range from a small, hemodynamically insignificant communication to complete absence of the atrial septum. Associated abnormalities of the mitral valve including clefts and valvar regurgitation are typical. Atrioventricular canal defects are more completely addressed in a separate chapter.

Pathophysiology

The long-term effects of an atrial septal defect are the result of shunting across the atrial septum. The direction and degree of this shunting is determined by the relative compliances of the left and right ventricles. Ordinarily, the left ventricle is the thicker, more muscular chamber, a reflection of the greater workload of pumping against systemic pressures. Since the thinner right ventricle stretches more easily to accommodate blood flow during diastole, an interatrial communication initially favors a left-to-right shunt.

For this reason, conditions that cause decreased right ventricular compliance, such as pulmonary hypertension, may result in decreased shunting or, in more severe cases, shunt reversal (right-to-left shunting). Conversely, those conditions that cause decreased compliance of the left ventricle, such as systemic hypertension and aging, or those that interfere with flow across the mitral valve, such as rheumatic mitral valve disease, lead to increased left-to-right shunting. The normal decrease in left ventricular compliance associated with aging may explain in part why patients are often undiagnosed in childhood but become symptomatic as they enter their fourth or fifth decade of life.

CLINICAL PRESENTATIONS

The clinical presentation of the patient with an atrial septal defect depends on the direction and degree of shunting across the defect.

Most frequently, adult patients may be asymptomatic or report a mild reduction in functional capacity. Patients with unrepaired ASD demonstrate a reduction in peak oxygen consumption when compared with age-matched patients without ASDs. This reflects the inherent inefficiency of a left ventricle that has a continuously reduced preload and a pulmonary circulation with volume overload. After repair, exercise capacity improves within a few weeks. These functional benefits of closure extend even to mildly symptomatic adults. Importantly, this improvement has been observed regardless of age or degree of shunting.[7]

Atrial flutter and atrial fibrillation are a reflection of chronic atrial dilation and stretching of the conduction system. These seldom occur before the fifth decade of life but may be the initial presentation for some patients. Older age at the time of surgery tends to be the strongest predictor of preoperative and late postoperative atrial arrhythmias.[8]

Rarely, a patient with an ASD may present with a paradoxical embolus, even when the interatrial shunt is predominantly left-to-right. This is because transient flow reversal can often be demonstrated during the Valsalva maneuver.

Chronic pulmonary overcirculation can sometimes manifest as recurrent respiratory infections in children. In more severe cases, patients may develop heart failure or pulmonary hypertension. Pulmonary hypertension tends to be uncommon in ASD, even in the presence of large shunts. Recent studies suggest a rate of approximately 6% to 9%. When severe pulmonary hypertension does occur, the right ventricle becomes progressively hypertrophied, and compliance decreases as a result. This leads to reversal of flow across the ASD, and patients become cyanotic. This phenomenon is an example of Eisenmenger's syndrome and is outside the scope of our discussion.

Original publications on the natural history of atrial septal defects suggested that patients do well for the first two decades of life (mortality rates 0.6% and 0.7% per annum). However, the mortality rate rises in subsequent decades to 90% by 60 years of age.[9] Poor outcomes were thought to be related to pulmonary hypertension, occurring in 22% of patients, and severe pulmonary vascular disease, occurring in 14%.[10] Fortunately, with modern methods for diagnosis, monitoring, and treatment using medical optimization and percutaneous or surgical correction, atrial septal defects carry far lower mortality and morbidity in the current era.

Physical Examination

The physical examination usually reflects the size of the ASD and the relative compliance of the right and left ventricles. Small ASDs are usually silent, whereas large defects may manifest as a hyperdynamic precordium, left chest prominence in children with large shunt volumes, or a ventricular lift. Upon auscultation, the first heart sound may be accentuated or normal; the second heart sound is typically widely split and varies imperceptibly with respiration because of a fixed relative delay in pulmonic valve closure. There is often a flow murmur because of increased relative volume through the pulmonic valve, mimicking pulmonic stenosis. Rarely, with a large left-to-right shunt, a diastolic rumble may be appreciated at the lower left sternal border, resulting from turbulent flow across the tricuspid valve.

Cyanosis is an end-stage phenomenon that occurs if pulmonary vascular resistance increases to a level that reverses flow from right to left through the ASD. The typical features of pulmonary hypertension, including a right ventricular heave and a loud P_2 would accompany this finding. Patients with uncomplicated ASDs should not become cyanotic even if their saturations decrease with exercise. Exceptionally, the presence of a large eustachian valve may direct flow from the inferior vena cava directly across an ASD, but this is a rare occurrence.

Chest X-Ray

The chest x-ray may demonstrate normal cardiac size in a patient with a small or moderate-sized atrial septal defect, or a dilated right heart with greater degrees of shunting. Pulmonary vascular markings are increased, consistent with increased pulmonary flow, and the pulmonary artery is often large compared with the aorta. On the lateral view, the large right ventricle occupies a significant portion of the retrosternal space, and the upper one third of the septum may be anteriorly bowed.

Electrocardiography

The electrocardiogram (ECG) varies depending on type of interatrial communication. That of a patient with a secundum ASD typically shows sinus rhythm with a normal P wave axis. Other common rhythms are atrial fibrillation or flutter. In 50% of patients, the P waves are tall, signifying right atrial enlargement. Right ventricular forces often remain prominent in children with ASDs, and there is right axis deviation (+100 degrees) and an incomplete right bundle branch block, or rSR′ pattern, in leads V_3R and V_1 with normal T waves suggesting right ventricular volume overload. The QRS duration may be mildly prolonged because of right ventricular dilation. In adolescents and adults, right ventricular conduction delay is seen in the majority of patients.

Where there is a sinus venosus defect, the P wave axis may be abnormal. Inverted P waves in the inferior leads suggest a low atrial rhythm due to an insufficient sinus node, which occurs in superior vena cava type defects when there is involvement of the sinus node area.

The patient with an ostium primum ASD typically has a leftward or superior frontal QRS axis in addition to the findings noted previously. The ECG demonstrates sinus rhythm, often with tall, peaked P waves (usually best seen in leads II and V_2) and prolongation of the PR interval secondary to intra-atrial or bundle of His conduction delay. The presence of P mitrale signifying left atrial enlargement or left ventricular hypertrophy should alert one to the possibility of associated mitral valve regurgitation.

Echocardiography

Echocardiography has long been the standard for imaging atrial septal defects. Anatomic considerations include location and, therefore, type of defect, atrial and ventricular size, and associated defects, such as anomalous pulmonary veins, cleft mitral valve, or ventricular septal defect. Functional consequences can be determined using position of the interventricular septum on the short-axis view, which can suggest pressure (systolic flattening) or volume (diastolic flattening) overload. Estimation of shunt fractions and pulmonary artery systolic pressures are also essential and can be performed using Doppler echocardiography. Advances in transesophageal and three-dimensional echocardiography have allowed improved visualization of the atrial septum and are invaluable in planning either percutaneous or surgical ASD repair (Fig. 106.2).

Computed Tomography and Magnetic Resonance Imaging

Cardiac magnetic resonance imaging (MRI) or computed tomography (CT) can provide useful supplemental information, particularly in patients with inconclusive clinical and echocardiographic findings. Both can quantitatively assess right ventricular volume and function and confirm the size and location of the defect, its relationship to neighboring structures, and suitability for transcatheter versus surgical repair. In addition, MRI can accurately assess the

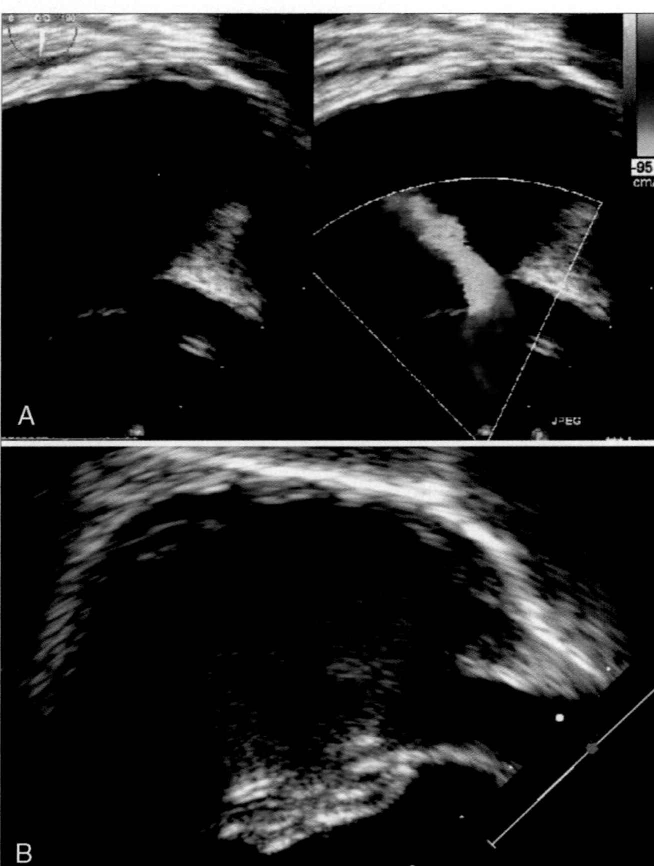

Figure 106.2 Secundum atrial septal defect. Transesophageal echocardiography. **A,** ASD preclosure. The left panel demonstrates the defect, with the right panel exhibiting simultaneous color Doppler flow from the left to right atrium. **B,** Atrial septal occluder in position across the defect as seen immediately after deployment.

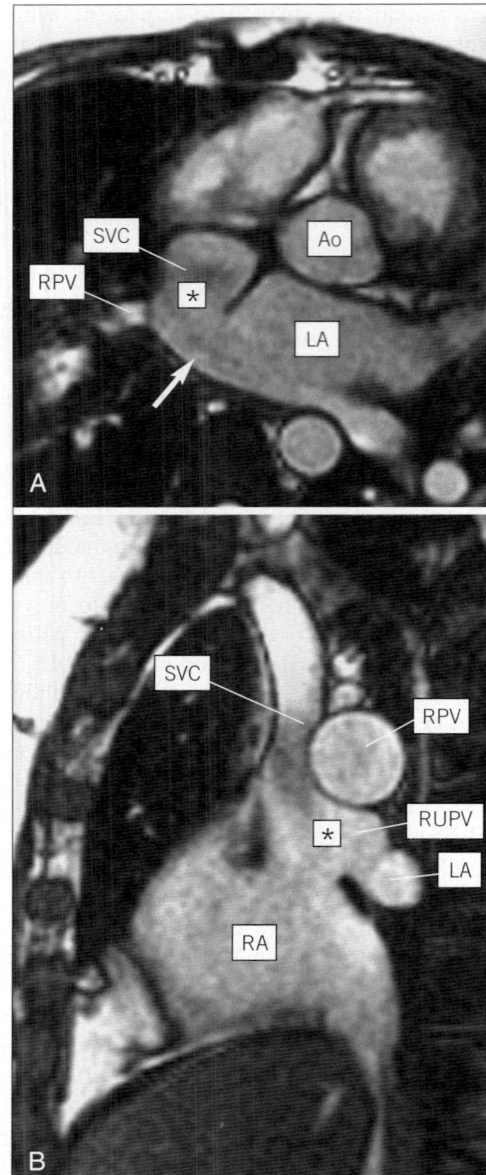

Figure 106.3 Sinus venosus defect (superior vena cava type). Steady-state free precession cine MRI. **A,** Axial plane image demonstrating the defect (*) in the wall that separates the superior vena cava (SVC) and the right upper pulmonary vein (RPV). The arrow indicates the orifice of the RPV, through which blood can flow between the right upper pulmonary vein (RUPV) and the SVC. **B,** Sagittal plane image in the same patient. RA, right atrium; RPA, right pulmonary artery.

pulmonary-to-systemic flow ratio. These imaging modalities can be particularly useful in patients with sinus venosus defects, since such lesions are often difficult to visualize by transthoracic echocardiography (Fig. 106.3).

Cardiac Catheterization

Cardiac catheterization is not necessary to diagnose an ASD, but may be indicated in those patients in whom pulmonary hypertension and vascular obstructive disease are suspected. In this situation, assessment of responsiveness to pulmonary vasodilators, such as oxygen or nitric oxide, is necessary to determine whether closure of the ASD is advisable. In addition, catheterization may be useful for confirming right heart pressures and shunt fraction and for preoperative coronary evaluation in older patients or those with coronary risk factors.

MANAGEMENT

Device Closure

There is general consensus that patients with significant ASDs should be offered elective closure upon diagnosis irrespective of age and symptomatology.

The field of transcatheter closure of atrial septal defects has advanced significantly in the past decade, and improvements and modifications of devices and techniques are continuously evolving. Indications for device closure include the presence of right ventricular volume overload from a left-to-right shunt (Qp:Qs >1.5), progressive pulmonary vascular disease (but with pulmonary vascular resistance of <8-10 indexed Wood units or pulmonary/systemic vascular resistance ratio <0.2-0.4), and development of atrial arrhythmias. There may be a role for closure in the setting of asymptomatic decreases in functional capacity as determined by exercise testing as well. In the presence of a large defect (stretched secundum ASD >36 mm); inadequate septal rims for stable device deployment; defects in proximity to atrioventricular valves, coronary sinus, or the venae cavae; or the presence of additional cardiac anomalies requiring surgical intervention, referral for surgical repair should be considered.

Percutaneous closure of ASDs is associated with improvement in right ventricular dimension, morphology, function, and exercise physiology.[7] The technique was first performed in the 1970s, and the basic device design of a dual disk structure joined by a waist has remained the cornerstone of further device development. Transesophageal and intracardiac echocardiography have proved valuable in evaluating the anatomy of the ASD, device selection, and device placement.[11] In the appropriately selected patient, device closure is well tolerated and effective, with a major complication rate (e.g., device embolization or erosion) of less than 1% in most studies.[12] Successful closure is achieved in 95% of patients, and residual shunts, if present, are usually not hemodynamically significant.[13]

Devices currently being used for ASD closure include the Amplatzer Septal Occluder (AGA Medical Corp., Plymouth, Minn), the CardioSEAL device (NMT Medical, Inc., Boston, Mass), and the HELEX Septal Occluder (W.L. Gore and Associates, Newark, Del) (Fig. 106.4). Each device carries its own advantages and disadvantages, and all have undergone repeated modifications. Outcomes range from 79% closure rates in earlier generation models to 98% successful closure in more recent models.[14] Areas of ongoing improvement include the ability to self-center, retrievability, risk of device arm fracture, rapidity of endothelialization and risk of device thrombosis, and risk of erosion or perforation. A demonstration of ASD closure is seen in Fig. 106.5.

The Amplatzer Septal Occluder allows the percutaneous closure of small to very large ASDs. The CardioSEAL/STARflex device can be used for closure of small to moderate-sized ASDs (stretch size up to 18 mm) with a 93% complete closure rate. These two devices are used most widely in clinical practice. A comparison of their use in the closure of small to moderate-sized ASDs in the late 1990s revealed that both are clinically safe and effective for ASD closure. Percutaneous closure of small to moderate-sized ASDs with the Amplatzer Septal Occluder was quicker and provided a higher rate of complete occlusion.[15] Midterm results of the relatively new HELEX Septal Occluder also reveal good efficacy with a low incidence of adverse sequelae.[16]

After device closure, there is no consensus on the recommended duration of anticoagulation and antiplatelet treatment or the recommended follow-up. Currently, patients in our practice are seen at 1 month, 6 months, 1 year, and then yearly thereafter for monitoring of device location, residual shunt, atrioventricular valve regurgitation, and intracardiac thrombosis. Aspirin alone or in combination with clopidogrel is recommended for 6 months based on device data in related fields and preliminary data on elevation of procoagulant markers after ASD device closure. Antibiotic prophylaxis is recommended for up to 12 months after device placement.

There are currently no randomized trials comparing percutaneous and surgical closure. However, a multicenter, nonrandomized study in 2000 compared the safety and efficacy of the Amplatzer Septal Occluder with surgery. Patients in the surgical group were younger (median age 4.1 years versus 9.8 years for the device group), and more patients had multiple ASDs than in the Amplatzer Septal Occluder group.

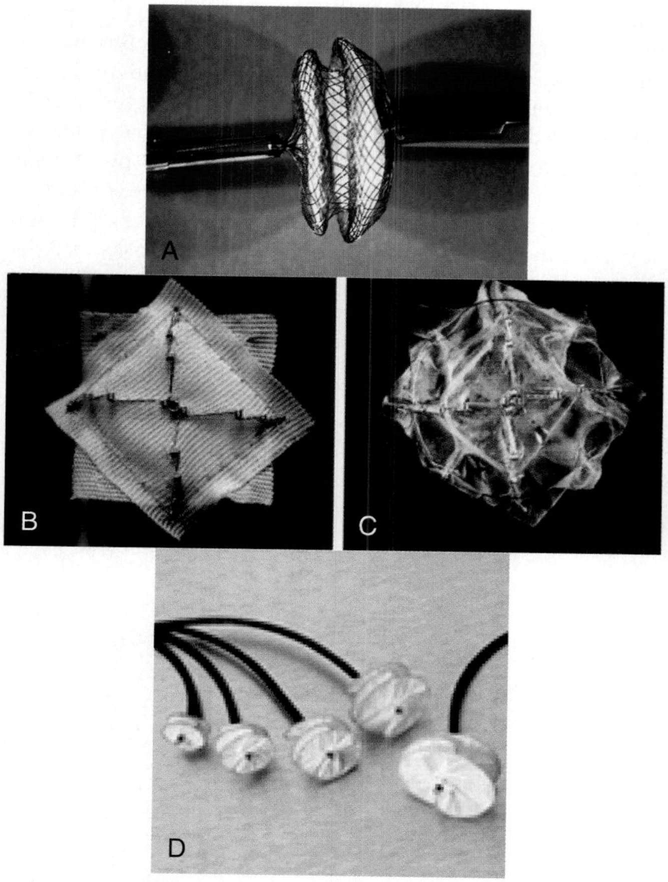

Figure 106.4 Percutaneous closure devices for atrial septal defects. **A,** The Amplatzer Septal Occluder. **B,** The CardioSEAL/STARflex device. **C,** The BioSTAR device. **D,** The HELEX Septal Occluder.

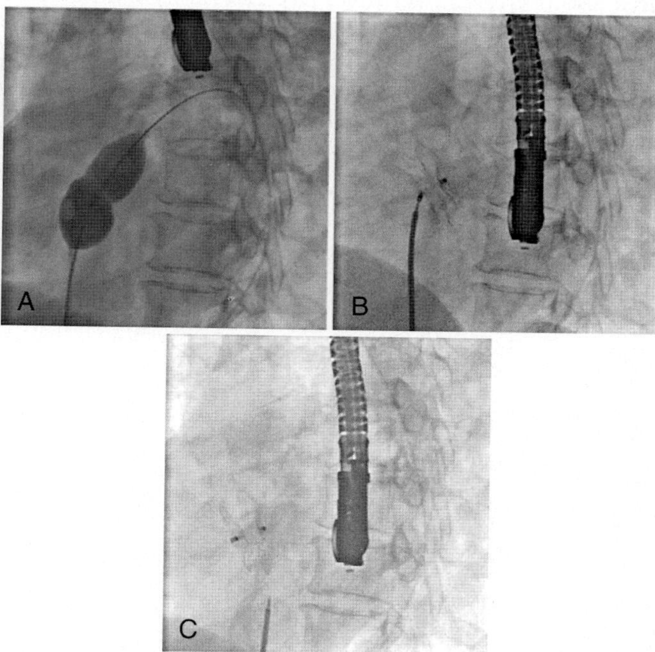

Figure 106.5 A, Balloon sizing of secundum atrial septal defect. **B,** Positioning of an Amplatzer atrial septal occluder. **C,** Release of atrial septal occluder.

The success rates were not significantly different, but the complication rate was 7.2% for the device group compared to 24.0% for the surgical group ($P < .001$), and patients in the Amplatzer Septal Occluder group had a shorter length of stay. Mortality was 0% for all subjects.[13]

Surgical Closure

When considering closure, the indications for either surgical or percutaneous closure are the same. Right ventricular volume overload (determined by cardiac imaging), a shunt fraction Qp:Qs greater than 1.5, the presence of early pulmonary vascular disease, functional limitation, or atrial arrhythmia (especially in patients under age 40 years) are all established indications for ASD closure.

In the modern era, mortality risk of surgical repair of an isolated secundum ASD at any age is less than 1%. The surgical approach generally involves a median sternotomy with either direct closure or pericardial/synthetic patch repair. However, in the appropriately selected patient with amenable anatomy and physiology, catheter-based closure techniques described previously can minimize hospital stay and procure the same hemodynamic benefits as a surgical approach.

In patients with a primum ASD or sinus venosus defect, surgical closure is almost always required. Ostium primum defects require patch closure of the ASD, may need repair of the "cleft mitral" trileaflet valve, and may have an associated ventricular septal defect. The sinus venosus repair has been modified many times, with variations on the best method of redirecting blood flow from anomalous pulmonary veins.[18-20] These repairs can be technically challenging and will not be discussed here in full detail.

As with percutaneous ASD closure, surgical closure of secundum ASDs results in decreased right atrial and right ventricular volumes at 2 years after operation. Right atrial area also decreases over time. Decrease in right atrial area is inversely proportional to age at time of ASD closure.[21] When repaired at an earlier age—before the age of 25, according to data from the Mayo Clinic—27-year survival rates are similar to those of the normal population. After the age of 25, long-term survival begins to suffer.[17] Even in patients over 40 years of age, surgical repair of ASD yields improved long-term survival and limits progression to heart failure compared with medical therapy alone. However, the incidence of new atrial arrhythmias and of cerebrovascular insults is not improved in this older population.[22] Mean pulmonary artery pressure, age at diagnosis, and cardiac index all influence the progression of disease in unrepaired ASDs.[23]

In younger patients with large ASDs or additional complicating factors or anatomy, a surgical approach may yet remain the best course of intervention. As the patient population ages, however, there may be a tendency toward percutaneous intervention. Head-to-head comparisons of the two strategies have yet to be performed.

SUMMARY

Atrial septal defects are one of the most common congenital heart defects, can be isolated or inherited, and develop from insufficiencies of the development of one or more components of the atrial septum. Presentation varies based on pathophysiology related to the size of the defect and the quantity of shunting, which is largely dependent on relative ventricular compliance. Some ASDs close spontaneously in childhood; however, for those that do not, the indications for closure include significant left-to-right shunting, right ventricular volume overload, atrial arrhythmias, paradoxical embolic events, and impaired exercise capacity. Both surgical and percutaneous closure of ASDs have good success rates with few complications. Standard physical examination, ECG and chest X-ray can all reveal classic findings for atrial septal defect, and echocardiography is the gold standard for evaluation of direction of shunt and degree of right ventricular dilation. Cardiac MRI or CT and cardiac catheterization can provide additional anatomic and physiologic information before ASD closure and, if available, should be considered to better delineate the nature of the ASD and any associated findings. As a patient ages, the risks of ASD closure increase, and prompt attention can stem the natural progression of left-to-right shunting, progressive right ventricular volume overload, atrial arrhythmias, and the risk of pulmonary vascular disease.

chapter 107 Abnormalities of the Pulmonary Veins

a. Partial Anomalous Pulmonary Venous Connections

Alexander Ellis and Gary Webb

Definition

- Abnormal connection of one or more pulmonary veins to the systemic venous circulation.

Key Features

- Partial anomalous pulmonary venous connection (PAPVC; abnormal connection of one or more of the pulmonary veins, but not all of them) results in an atrial level left-to-right shunt and increased pulmonary blood flow (a Qp:Qs > 1).

Therapy

- Medical treatment involves anticongestive therapy. Surgical correction is indicated for partial anomalous pulmonary venous connection with significantly increased pulmonary blood flow and respiratory symptomatology.

Congenital anomalies of the pulmonary venous connections are rare but heterogeneous in their presentation. There are two principal anatomic and physiologic types of anomalous pulmonary venous drainage, and the symptoms they may produce likewise range from mild exercise intolerance to severe life-threatening cyanosis. Surgical intervention is indicated for any anomaly producing symptoms, though some catheter-based therapies may also play a role after surgical repair. Noninvasive imaging techniques have allowed for quantum leaps in visualizing these anomalies, and the overall outcomes of pulmonary vein interventions have improved dramatically in recent years.

Anomalous pulmonary venous connection refers to a group of abnormalities in which one or more pulmonary veins drain to the systemic venous system. Although there are many variations, this group of anomalies can be divided into two major categories:

- partial anomalous pulmonary venous connection (PAPVC), in which one or more of the pulmonary veins, but not all of them, connect abnormally to the systemic venous circulation; and
- total anomalous pulmonary venous connection (TAPVC), in which all of the pulmonary veins connect abnormally to the systemic venous circulation. TAPVC will be discussed in the following subchapter.

A note on terminology: anomalous *connection* always denotes anomalous blood return or flow; however, anomalous *drainage* or *return* can occur without an anomalous connection. For example, in common atrium, the right pulmonary veins may connect normally to the left atrium but functionally also enter the morphologic right atrium, mixing with the systemic venous return. Likewise, with malposition of the septum, the veins may connect normally into the morphologic left atrium but malposition of the atrial septum may cause anomalous drainage of the pulmonary venous return, allowing it to mix with the systemic venous blood. Thus one cannot interchange the terms *return* or *drainage* with *connection*. For the purposes of these two subchapters, we will use anomalous "connections" to imply abnormal anatomic attachments.

ANATOMY AND PATHOLOGY

PAPVC has a reported incidence from autopsy series of 0.6% to 0.7%; however, some anomalous pulmonary venous drainage is not diagnosed during life; thus the clinical incidence is somewhat lower.[1] This anomaly was first described by Winslow in the mid 1700s, but Brody[2] more clearly summarized existing knowledge of the defect's anatomy and physiology in the mid 1900s.

The "Normal" Number of Pulmonary Veins

Normally, there are four pulmonary veins: right upper and lower, and left upper and lower pulmonary veins. Occasionally, there are deviations from this pattern that are still within the spectrum of normal. The most common variant is a single pulmonary vein on a given side, which can occur in up to 25% of individuals. There might also be three pulmonary veins on a given side (especially the right side, with the additional vein draining the right middle lobe). This can occur in about 2% of the population. There may also be a single common pulmonary vein returning to the left atrium, but this occurs typically in patients with heterotaxy and asplenia.[3]

Embryology

A brief review of the current understanding of pulmonary venous embryology is a prerequisite to appreciating the anatomic abnormalities. Different theories regarding the origin of the pulmonary veins exist and much controversy remains. However, recent work with human embryos at various stages of development has illustrated that pulmonary veins appear to be derived from the dorsal mesocardium within the posterior mediastinum. They arise as a new channel, not as an outpouching from the sinus venosus, that is forming the systemic veins that join the right atrium. This process occurs after the right atrial venous connections have been established.[4] However, some still believe the alternative concept that the pulmonary veins originate from the systemic venous sinus.[5] The veins develop in the mesenchyme of the lung then progress medially and join with the morphologic left atrium. However, perturbations in the division of the left atrium may lead to anomalous drainage patterns.

ANATOMY

As previously illustrated, numerous connections form and involute between the primitive pulmonary venous circulation and the systemic venous circulation in embryonic life. Any of these primitive connections can persist at birth as a type of PAPVC. In order of decreasing frequency, the most common anatomic variant types of PAPVC (Fig. 107A.1) are

- right pulmonary veins to right superior vena cava or azygos vein;
- right pulmonary veins to right atrium;
- right pulmonary veins to inferior vena cava (scimitar syndrome); and
- left pulmonary veins to the left innominate vein.

Anomalous connection of the right pulmonary veins is far more common than left-sided anomalous connections. However, the mechanism for this skewed ratio remains poorly understood. Partial anomalous pulmonary venous connection of the left pulmonary veins occurs infrequently and may involve the entire left lung or portions of it, mainly the upper lobe.[6,7] In this situation, the abnormal connection almost never occurs directly to the right atrium but usually through a persistent left superior vena cava that connects to the left innominate vein. Other connections, such as to the coronary sinus, do occur but they are rare.

Partial anomalous pulmonary venous connection can occur as an isolated defect or in combination with other cardiac defects. Most commonly, PAPVC is associated with an atrial septal defect (ASD), usually of the sinus venosus type, less commonly with a secundum defect. Only in approximately 20% of cases does PAPVC occur with an intact atrial septum.[8] Although sinus venosus defects do physiologically allow an atrial level of communication, they are not true ASDs in that they do not involve the atrial septum. Rather, they result from a defect in the common wall of the right upper pulmonary vein (RUPV) and the superior vena cava (SVC) or the right atrium itself. This defect produces an "unroofing," which permits drainage of pulmonary venous blood to the right side but also allows atrial level communication and shunting. PAPVC may also occur in patients with visceral heterotaxy and polysplenia.

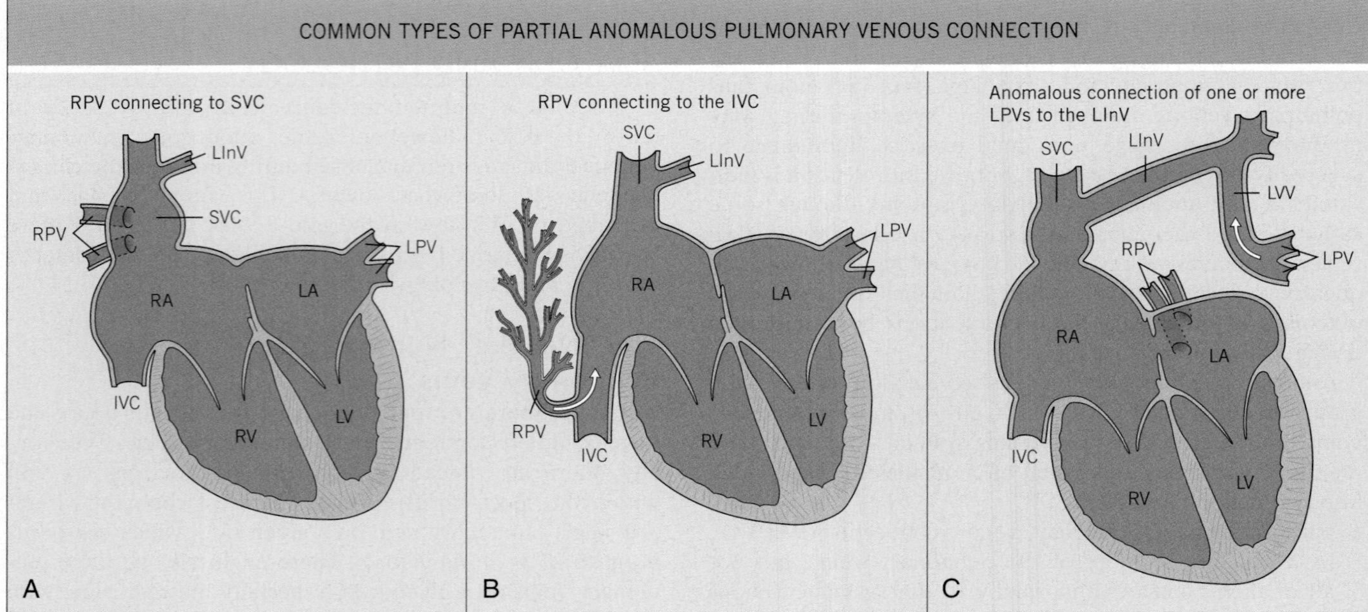

Figure 107A.1 Common types of partial anomalous pulmonary venous connection (PAPVC). A, Right pulmonary veins (RPV) connecting to superior vena cava (SVC). Usually, right upper and middle lobe veins connect separately to SVC between the azygous vein and SVC–right atrium (RA) junction. Often, a sinus venosus type of atrial septal defect is present. **B**, RPV connecting to the inferior vena cava (IVC). Usually, most or all of the RPVs form a confluence that enters the IVC as a single trunk. The trunk forms in the right hilum, passes inferiorly and to the left, and enters the IVC just above or below the diaphragm. This type of PAPVC is found in scimitar syndrome. **C**, Anomalous connection of one or more left pulmonary veins (LPVs) to the left innominate vein (LInV) by way of a left vertical vein (LVV), also called a persistent left SVC. LA, left atrium, LV, left ventricle, RV, right ventricle.

Scimitar Syndrome

Partial anomalous pulmonary venous connection of the right lung to the inferior vena cava above or below the diaphragm carries the eponym of scimitar syndrome. Other components are right lung hypoplasia and/or sequestration, diaphragmatic abnormalities, anomalous systemic arterial supply to part of the right lung, usually arising from the descending aorta, and an intact atrial septum.[9] It is named after the radiographic similarity of the vascular supply and drainage to a curved Ottoman sword (Fig. 107A.2). Other structural cardiac anomalies may be associated, including ventricular septal defects, coarctation of the aorta, and conoseptal anomalies, such as tetralogy of Fallot, and double-outlet right ventricle. Noncardiac anomalies such as horseshoe kidney and vertebral anomalies have also been recognized.

PATHOPHYSIOLOGY

In PAPVC, the principal physiologic perturbation is a left-to-right shunt causing increased pulmonary blood flow. Fully oxygenated blood from the abnormally connecting pulmonary veins recirculates back through the right atrium, right ventricle, pulmonary artery, and then lungs. This "pretricuspid" atrial level left-to-right shunt may lead to dilatation of the right heart structures and main pulmonary artery. The pulmonary to systemic blood ratio (Qp:Qs) is therefore elevated above the normal 1:1 relationship. However, the left heart chambers remain unaffected and the cardiac output is usually normal. The magnitude of the left-to-right shunt caused by PAPVC depends on

- the number of anomalously connecting pulmonary veins (as a percentage of the total pulmonary venous return);
- the degree of obstruction within the pulmonary venous system (in the anomalous or normally draining veins);
- which pulmonary segments or lobes are drained by the anomalous veins (more venous return from the middle and lower lobes when upright, more from the upper lobes when supine);
- the relative resistances of the normally and abnormally drained portions of the pulmonary vascular bed; and
- the compliance of the chamber into which the anomalous pulmonary veins connect.

As previously noted, occasionally, there is no atrial septal communication associated with PAPVC (e.g., PAPVC of the inferior vena cava [IVC] type). While the proportion of blood that enters the right heart remains influenced by the above factors, there is no possibility for right-to-left shunting. Pulmonary hypertension has not been reported with this physiology. However, pulmonary parenchymal disease or resection of the normally draining lung segments may prove fatal with this anatomy due to reduced or eliminated normal pulmonary venous return.

When PAPVC occurs with associated cardiac defects, the physiology is largely determined by the severity of the associated defect. For example, with an associated ASD, the additional left-to-right shunt increases the burden on the right heart and pulmonary circulation. It has been recognized that when one lobe connects anomalously, there is minimal right heart dilatation and an individual can expect no symptoms and a normal life span. In contrast, when more than half of the total pulmonary venous return drains anomalously, right-sided structures may become enlarged and clinical symptoms manifest. Pulmonary vascular disease has been reported with PAPVC and an atrial level shunt; however, it is unusual and, when present, occurs much later in life.

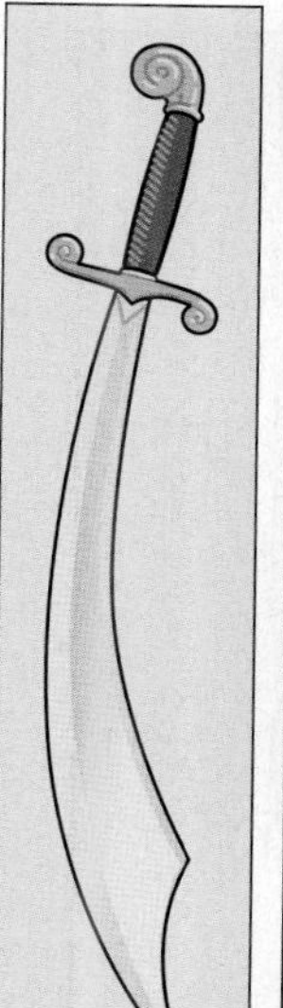

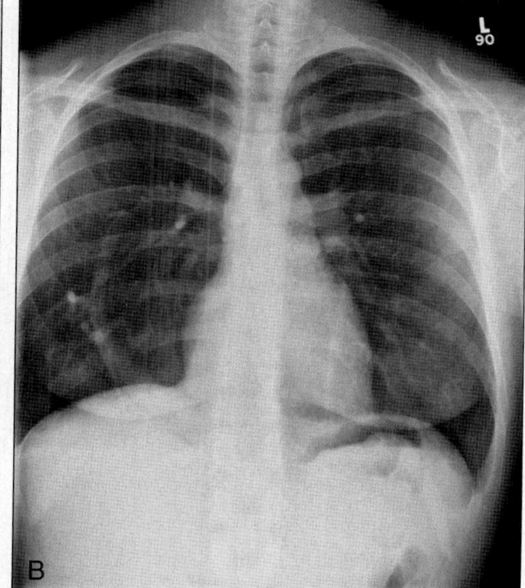

Figure 107A.2 A diagram of a scimitar or curved Turkish sword from the age of the Ottoman empire (**A**) and a chest x-ray (**B**) demonstrating a curvilinear density that represents a vessel draining the right lung. It is named scimitar syndrome after the visual similarity between the curved sword and the bowed appearance of the anomalously draining vasculature.

CLINICAL FEATURES

The majority of patients with PAPVC are asymptomatic in early life, regardless of the presence of an associated ASD. When they present, the referral may be for a cardiac murmur or an abnormal chest radiograph. When symptoms do occur at a younger age, the most common complaint is exercise intolerance. As with ASDs, symptoms usually appear in the late 20s to early 40s and consist of exertional dyspnea, recurrent respiratory infections, and palpitations.

In patients who have PAPVC of only one pulmonary vein, the physical examination is usually normal. However, a soft systolic murmur may be present. When more than one pulmonary vein drains anomalously or when there is an associated ASD, the findings on the physical examination are akin to those of an uncomplicated ASD. Specifically, there may be a

- soft systolic ejection murmur in the pulmonic area at the base of the heart;
- wide, fixed splitting of the second heart sound;
- diastolic flow rumble over the tricuspid valve area; and
- hyperactive right ventricular impulse at the lower left sternal border.

Even with an associated ASD, signs and symptoms are unusual in childhood. Though there may be some right-to-left shunting depending on the location of the PAPVC and ASD, cyanosis is rare. Dyspnea on exertion or enlarged right-sided structures may be the only clues to the presence of PAPVC in later childhood. Even in older, symptomatic patients, evidence of pulmonary artery hypertension with right-to-left atrial shunting manifested by reduced oxygen saturations or overt cyanosis is unusual. When significant hypoxemia is present, however, signs of right heart failure (hepatomegaly and jugular venous distention) are often present.

In PAPVC with only one anomalous pulmonary vein, the electrocardiogram (ECG) and chest radiograph may well be normal. In the remaining types of PAPVC, the ECG usually shows an rSR′ pattern in the right precordial leads, which is indicative of a right ventricular volume overload. A peaked P wave may be present in older patients or in those with elevated pulmonary pressures (Fig. 107A.3). The chest radiograph often shows right atrial and right ventricular enlargement with increased pulmonary vascularity. Occasionally, the chest radiograph may show findings specific for an anatomic type of PAPVC. For example, in scimitar syndrome, the shadow formed on the radiograph by the single trunk connecting the right pulmonary veins to the inferior vena cava at the level of the diaphragm resembles an Ottoman curved sword as previously shown.

DIAGNOSTIC TECHNIQUES

Echocardiography

Echocardiography is the mainstay for the initial diagnosis of abnormal pulmonary venous anatomy. However, one must thoroughly visualize the connections of all the pulmonary veins and have a very high index of suspicion that a defect is present. Special attention should be paid to ensure a connection between the left atrium and both the RUPV and left lower pulmonary vein (LLPV), because these are the most likely anomalously draining vessels. Right ventricular dilatation, flattening of the interventricular septum, or dilatation of the coronary sinus may indicate occult shunt physiology and provide indirect evidence of anomalous pulmonary venous connections. Subcostal imaging (see Fig. 107A.6) as well as the suprasternal notch view angled downward (the so-called crab view; Fig. 107A.4) typically provide the best imaging planes for visualizing all of the veins. Although identifying the veins using two-dimensional echocardiography is ideal, color flow mapping allows the rapid detection of individual pulmonary veins that are too small to visualize directly on the two-dimensional echocardiogram (Fig. 107A.5). In addition, color flow mapping provides information about the direction and velocity of flow through them, an invaluable tool in evaluating possible stenosis. Regions of aliased or disturbed flow along the pulmonary venous pathway can be quickly identified and then interrogated for further quantitative information with pulsed Doppler echocardiography.[10-14]

As previously mentioned, a very common form of PAPVC is anomalous drainage of the right upper pulmonary vein to the right side of the atrial septum or the base of the superior vena cava in patients with a sinus venosus ASD (Fig. 107A.7). As mentioned previously, however, partial anomalous pulmonary venous return can occur with any type of ASD. In 96% of patients with PAPVC, the two-dimensional echocardiogram shows evidence of dilatation of the distal structure, such as right atrial and right ventricular volume overload.[13] In rare cases (e.g., in a patient with a single anomalous pulmonary vein in the presence of a small or absent atrial shunt or in a patient with pulmonary vein stenoses), the right heart size may be normal. In older patients in whom transthoracic echocardiography windows are suboptimal, transesophageal echocardiography has been particularly useful for the detection of PAPVC.[15] It is recommended that transesophageal echocardiography be performed in any patient with right ventricular enlargement in whom the transthoracic examination is inconclusive.[16]

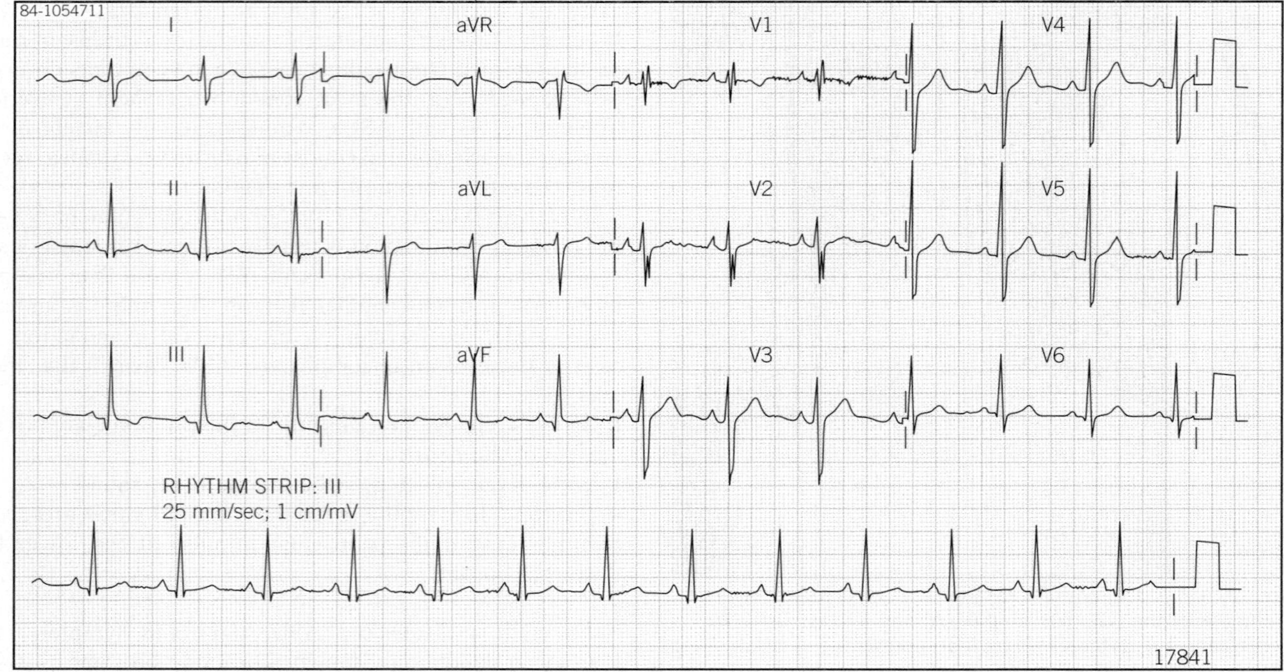

Figure 107A.3 Typical 12-lead electrocardiogram in a patient with PAPVC. There is an rSR′ pattern in lead V_1 consistent with mild right ventricular conduction delay or volume overload. The P waves are not peaked in this example. Most ECGs in PAPVC are essentially normal.

Figure 107A.4 Typical suprasternal echocardiographic view of the four pulmonary veins entering the left atrium. This view is called the crab view due to the visual similarity between the veins entering the left atrium and the legs attached to the body of a crab. It is much easier to obtain in thin patients, such as children. Although the veins are well seen in this color-compare example, pulmonary veins may be difficult to image in black and white without the aid of color Doppler. LLPV, left lower pulmonary vein; LUPV, left upper pulmonary vein; RLPV, right lower pulmonary vein; RUPV, right upper pulmonary vein.

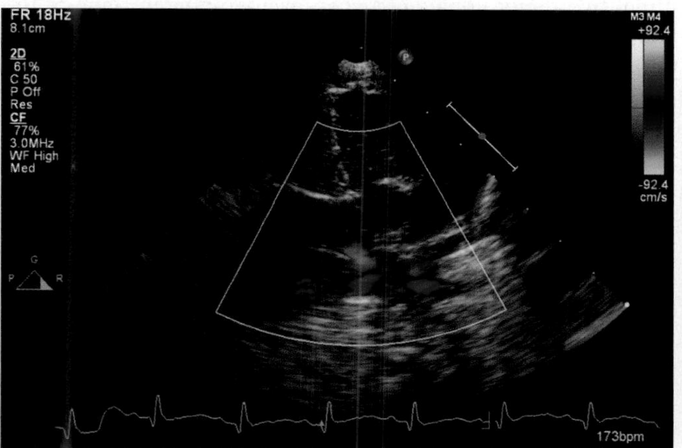

Figure 107A.5 Example of the echocardiographic evaluation of pulmonary veins from the suprasternal crab view. The veins would not be visible here without the aid of color Doppler. While hard to visualize in older or larger patients due to acoustic interference from the lungs and other soft tissues, they may be seen in younger or thinner patients from this orientation. This view allows for excellent pulsed wave Doppler interrogation of each individual vein's direction and velocity of flow.

Another type of PAPVC occurs in the scimitar syndrome, mentioned previously. In this syndrome, PAPVC or TAPVC of the right lung is usually to the inferior vena cava or azygous system.[9] The subcostal views are particularly useful for imaging the anomalous pulmonary veins in scimitar syndrome (Fig. 107A.8).

Cardiac Catheterization

As noninvasive imaging has improved, the role of cardiac catheterization has been reduced. However, there are situations in which cardiac catheterization may help elucidate the venous drainage pattern, the type of associated atrial level communication, and measure pulmonary pressures. At cardiac catheterization, the most definitive technique for

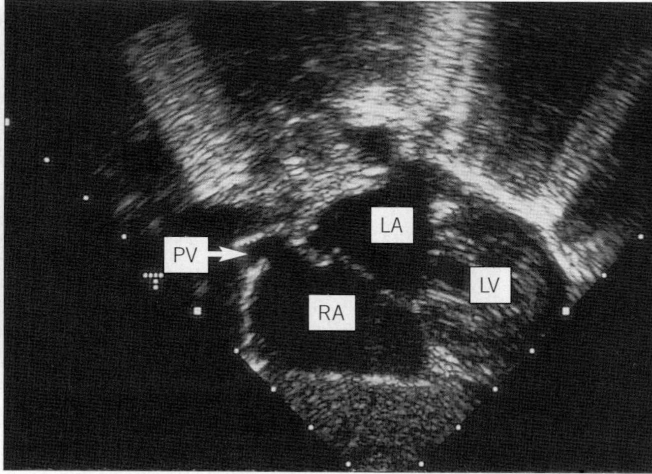

Figure 107A.6 Two-dimensional echocardiography in partial anomalous pulmonary venous connection (PAPVC). The subcostal coronal view shows PAPVC of the right upper pulmonary vein (PV) to the base of the superior vena cava. There is also a patent foramen ovale and an additional small secundum atrial septal defect. LA, left atrium; LV, left ventricle; RA, right atrium. (From Snider R, Ritter SB, Serwer GA. Echocardiography in Pediatric Heart Disease, 2nd ed. St. Louis, Mosby, 1997.)

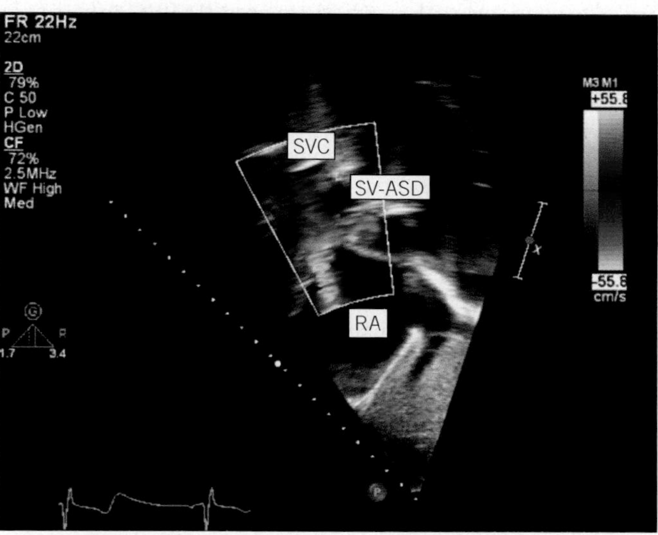

Figure 107A.7 Subcostal imaging of a sinus venosus type of atrial septal defect. Note the laminar flow of the superior vena cava (SVC) entering the right atrium. There is additional flow entering the right atrium (RA) at the junction of the SVC and the superior aspect of the atrial septum. It is here that the right upper pulmonary vein crosses to enter the left atrium, and thus pulmonary venous flow can enter into the right atrium when this type of defect is present.

diagnosing PAPVC is to enter the vein directly with the catheter and perform a selective angiogram in it. Oximetry sampling can be helpful in establishing the diagnosis; however, this depends on the site of drainage. Anomalous pulmonary venous drainage to the IVC may be missed because of the higher relative saturation level in the IVC from renal streaming. In fact, one could obtain normal results if only one pulmonary vein connects anomalously.

With regard to pressure measurements, if fewer than half of the pulmonary veins connect abnormally, intracardiac

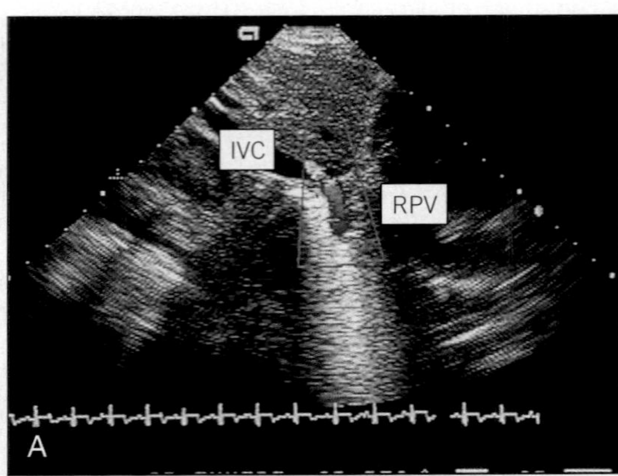

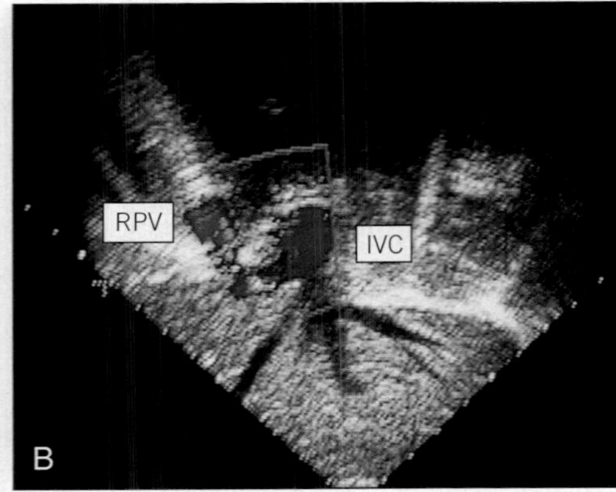

Figure 107A.8 Color Doppler examination in the scimitar syndrome. The subcostal sagittal view (**A**) and the subcostal coronal view (**B**) show partial anomalous pulmonary venous connection of the right pulmonary veins (RPV) to the inferior vena cava (IVC). At the entry of the RPV to the IVC, there is a high-velocity jet indicating pulmonary venous obstruction. In this patient, the left pulmonary veins drained normally to the left atrium. (From Snider R, Ritter SB, Serwer GA. Echocardiography in Pediatric Heart Disease, 2nd ed. St. Louis, Mosby, 1997.)

pressures are usually normal. However, the presence of long-standing increased pulmonary blood flow can lead to increased right atrial, right ventricular, and pulmonary artery pressures. Catheterization may be indicated preoperatively for older patients with newly diagnosed PAPVC to measure their pulmonary arterial pressures.

Computed Tomography

The use of computed tomographic angiography (CTA) for visualization of pulmonary venous anomalies has been burgeoning since it was first reported in the early 1990s.[17] Advantages include simultaneous visualization of the bony anatomy, lungs and airway, as well as other soft tissue and vascular structures. With the new generation of multidetector CT machines, such as the 64-slice scanner, the entire scan can be performed in a few seconds, without requiring breath-holding or multiple acquisitions. In addition, CTA, unlike magnetic resonance imaging (MRI), can be conducted by operators with little supervision or knowledge of the anatomy. In fact, as more chest CTAs are being performed for other indications, pulmonary vein anomalies are being diagnosed serendipitously. A recent retrospective series of CT scans found the prevalence of previously undiagnosed PAPVC to be 0.2% in a general adult population. However, in contrast to children, they found that the anomalous vein most commonly originated in the left upper lobe rather than the right and that it was more common in women.[18] CTA images can also be reconstructed in three dimensions, offering a clear view of the patient's thoracic anatomy. Current rendering techniques allow conversion of axial, sagittal, and coronal planes into manipulatable three-dimensional (3D) images. These can offer the surgeon the unique ability to cater their approach and technique more than ever before.

Magnetic Resonance Imaging and Magnetic Resonance Angiography

Like CTA, magnetic resonance imaging has a wide field of view and, as such, is an effective imaging modality for congenital heart defects, especially in patients with poor echocardiographic windows or for structures in multiple imaging planes. Cardiac MR (CMR) is thus ideal for pulmonary vein imaging, especially in small children or adults in whom suboptimal two-dimensional (2D) echocardiographic imaging of the veins themselves might be obtained.[19,20] Fast spin-echo CMR sequences can delineate the venous anatomy well, and new data acquisition algorithms and faster scanners permit much more rapid attainment than before, sometimes in one or two breath-holds. In addition, CMR angiography with the use of a contrast agent, such as gadolinium, may further enhance the images' diagnostic import by improving delineation of vessel borders, which may be important for surgical planning and may not be clearly visible in many patients using other modalities, such as echocardiography. Furthermore, contrast studies allow for 3D reconstruction and manipulation with appropriate software (Fig. 107A.9). As with CT, CMR allows visualization of soft-tissue structures, allowing improved understanding of thoracic spatial relationships. In addition, phase-contrast flow quantification cine sequences can be obtained within a specific pulmonary vein, helping to identify and quantify stenoses or to calculate a Qp:Qs.

CMR has been found to be a complementary modality to echocardiography or catheterization in the diagnosis of PAPVC. A recent study of adult patients with congenital defects found CMR to be 100% sensitive for PAPVC and ASDs when catheterization or echocardiography was incompletely diagnostic. Overall, CMR agreed with the catheterization or echocardiography findings in about 75% of patients and provided additional spatial relationship data with the pulmonary arteries or left atrium that was not available from other modalities.[19] CMR has become an extremely valuable modality for the diagnosis as well as the postoperative evaluation of PAPVC.

MANAGEMENT

Most children who have PAPVC are asymptomatic. However, as they progress into late adolescence or adulthood, they may experience exercise intolerance, exertional fatigue, or atrial arrhythmias. The definitive treatment of PAPVC is surgical. Surgical repair of PAPVC should be considered when

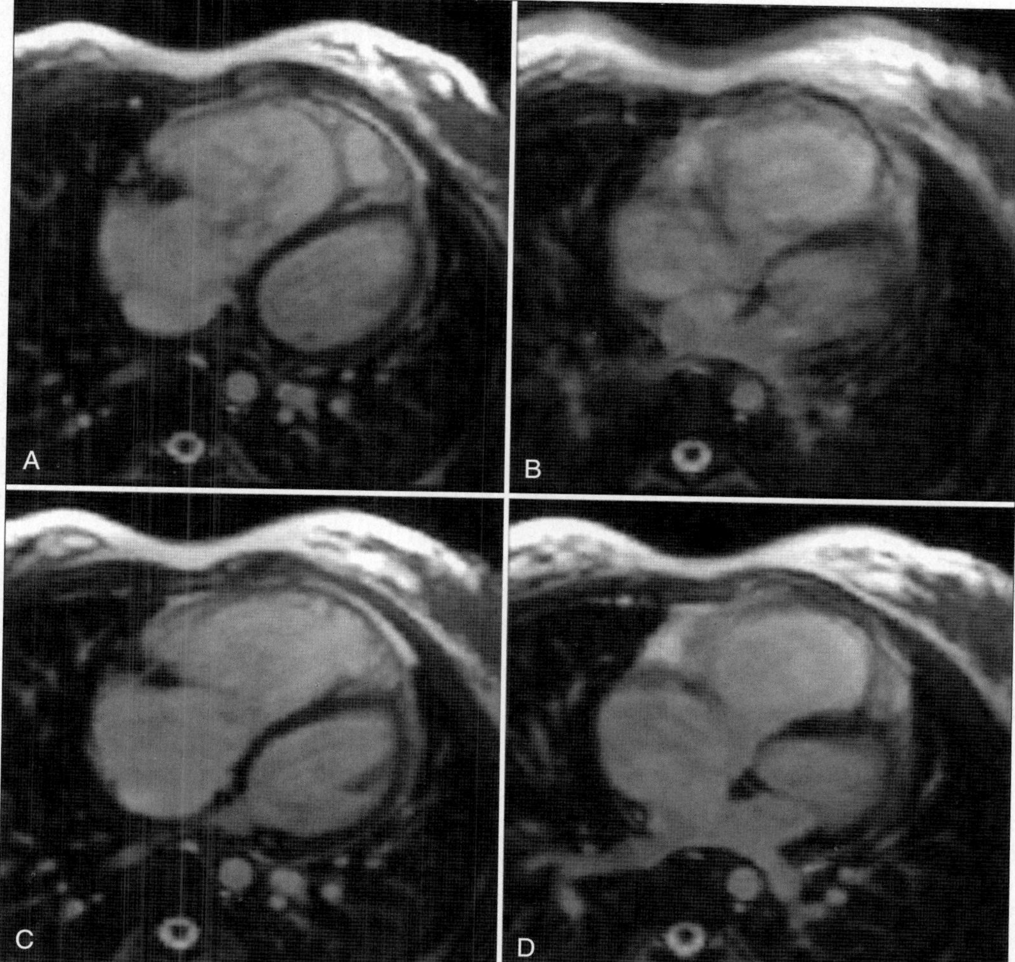

Figure 107A.9 A four-chamber cardiac MRI view in time-sequence (**A-D**) showing the posteriorly located defect that only becomes apparent in panel **C**, with the veins and defect visible in panel **D**. Note how the flow from the right upper pulmonary vein could enter the right atrium. Also notice the dilatation of the right heart structures.

- there is a hemodynamically significant left-to-right shunt leading to heart failure symptoms, atrial arrhythmias, or elevated pulmonary pressures (with a vasoreactive pulmonary bed);
- there are recurrent pulmonary infections, especially in the setting of scimitar syndrome; and
- surgical repair of other cardiac anomalies is being performed, such as an associated ASD.

The surgical approach in PAPVC should be tailored to the individual anatomy. Patients who have PAPVC with only one pulmonary vein connecting anomalously rarely require surgical intervention.[6,21]

PROGNOSIS

Partial anomalous pulmonary venous connection is usually associated with a normal or near-normal life span. Many cases of PAPVC cause no symptoms and thus are not diagnosed during life but rather are found incidentally at autopsy.[22] Of those cases that require surgical repair, operative mortality rates are low (under 3%), most patients are alive and well at long-term follow-up, and the rate of reoperation is very low. Systemic or pulmonary vein obstruction as well as sinus node dysfunction was noted, albeit rarely, in these series.[6,7] Intermittent monitoring for arrhythmias or venous obstruction may be indicated in patients who have had PAPVC repair.

b. Total Anomalous Pulmonary Venous Connections

Alexander Ellis and Gary Webb

Definition

- In patients with total anomalous pulmonary venous connection (TAPVC), all pulmonary veins have abnormal connections into the systemic venous circulation and do not directly connect to the left atrium.

Key Features

- TAPVC results in complete mixing of the pulmonary venous and systemic venous blood, causing cyanosis.
- There are four principal types of TAPVC, depending on the anatomic site of venous return.
- The size of the atrial communication and degree of pulmonary vein obstruction determine the degree of cyanosis and resultant failure symptoms.
- Obstructed pulmonary veins lead to profound cyanosis and hemodynamic instability.

Therapy

- Surgical correction is required for total anomalous pulmonary venous connection, usually in the neonatal period or early infancy. Obstructed TAPVC requires urgent surgical intervention.

We have previously reviewed partial anomalous pulmonary venous connection (PAPVC), where one or more pulmonary veins connect anomalously while the other veins return appropriately to the left atrium. These patients are typically acyanotic. In contrast, the term total anomalous pulmonary venous connection (TAPVC) implies an absence of a direct connection between the pulmonary veins and the left atrium. Instead, the pulmonary veins connect via other vessels—such as systemic veins—ultimately to the right atrium. The subsequent mixing of the deoxygenated and oxygenated blood produces cyanosis and may occur at various levels, before or at the level of the right atrium and may be circuitous and even obstructed. An atrial level communication is vital to supply left ventricular preload in this situation.

The reported incidence for TAPVC ranges from 0.4% to 2% from prior autopsy studies.[1,2] A more recent analysis from the Baltimore-Washington Infant Study, conducted from 1981 to 1987, reports an incidence of 1.5% from among all patients with congenital heart malformations. These infants were also smaller at birth, had a lower gestational age, and experienced intrauterine growth retardation. No gender preponderance was found, though other studies have found more males with infracardiac type TAPVC.[3,4] The Baltimore-Washington study also reported an association between TAPVC and maternal lead exposure.[3] While there is no known genetic inheritance pattern, there is a high incidence of associated noncardiac malformations in patients with TAPVC, such as asplenia or polysplenia heterotaxy syndrome. A brief review of our current understanding of the embryology of anomalous venous connections was provided in the prior subchapter on PAPVC.

In two thirds of patients, TAPVC is an isolated anomaly, associated only with the required interatrial communication. However, for the remaining one third of patients, significant other cardiac defects occur, including truncus arteriosus, pulmonary atresia, atrioventricular septal defect, transposition of the great arteries, single ventricle physiology, or heterotaxy syndrome (asplenia or polysplenia).

ANATOMY

As with PAPVC, TAPVC occurs in a wide spectrum of anatomic subtypes. A number of classification schemes for describing the different types of TAPVC have been proposed over time. The most widely adopted system classifies TAPVC according to the anatomic location of the anomalous connection (Fig. 107B.1).[5]

Type 1 (Supracardiac) Total Anomalous Pulmonary Venous Connection

Type 1 TAPVC is a connection that occurs at the supracardiac level and is the most common subtype of TAPVC. Connection to the left innominate vein (usually by way of a persistent left superior vena cava or vertical vein) is the most common means of a supracardiac connection, representing approximately 40% of all cases based on several series.[4,6,7] In this abnormality (Fig. 107B.1a), two pulmonary veins from each lung converge directly behind the left atrium and form a horizontal pulmonary venous confluence. Then, an anomalous vertical vein arises from the left portion of the confluence and usually passes between the left pulmonary artery and left main stem bronchus as it courses toward the left innominate vein. The left innominate vein empties normally into the right superior vena cava. Another type of supracardiac TAPVC is direct connection of the pulmonary veins to the right superior vena cava. This defect occurs less frequently and is usually associated with complex cardiac malformations.

Obstruction to pulmonary blood flow is relatively rare with supracardiac TAPVC but could occur anywhere along the anomalous connection. In addition, with this physiology, an atrial level communication (a true atrial septal defect [ASD] or a PFO) is required for survival. There will be the expected enlargement of right-sided structures found with large left-to-right shunt lesions.

Type 2 (Cardiac) Total Anomalous Pulmonary Venous Connection

Type 2 TAPVC is a connection that occurs at the "cardiac level," usually with the veins connecting to the coronary sinus or posterior midportion of the right atrium (see Fig. 107B.1b).[8] This represents the second most common form of TAPVC, accounting for 15% to 25% of all TAPVC cases.[4,6,7] The orifice of the coronary sinus may be dilated or inferiorly displaced. Obstruction is likewise unusual but could occur at several levels, including at the orifice of the coronary sinus, in the common pulmonary vein, or within the individual pulmonary veins.

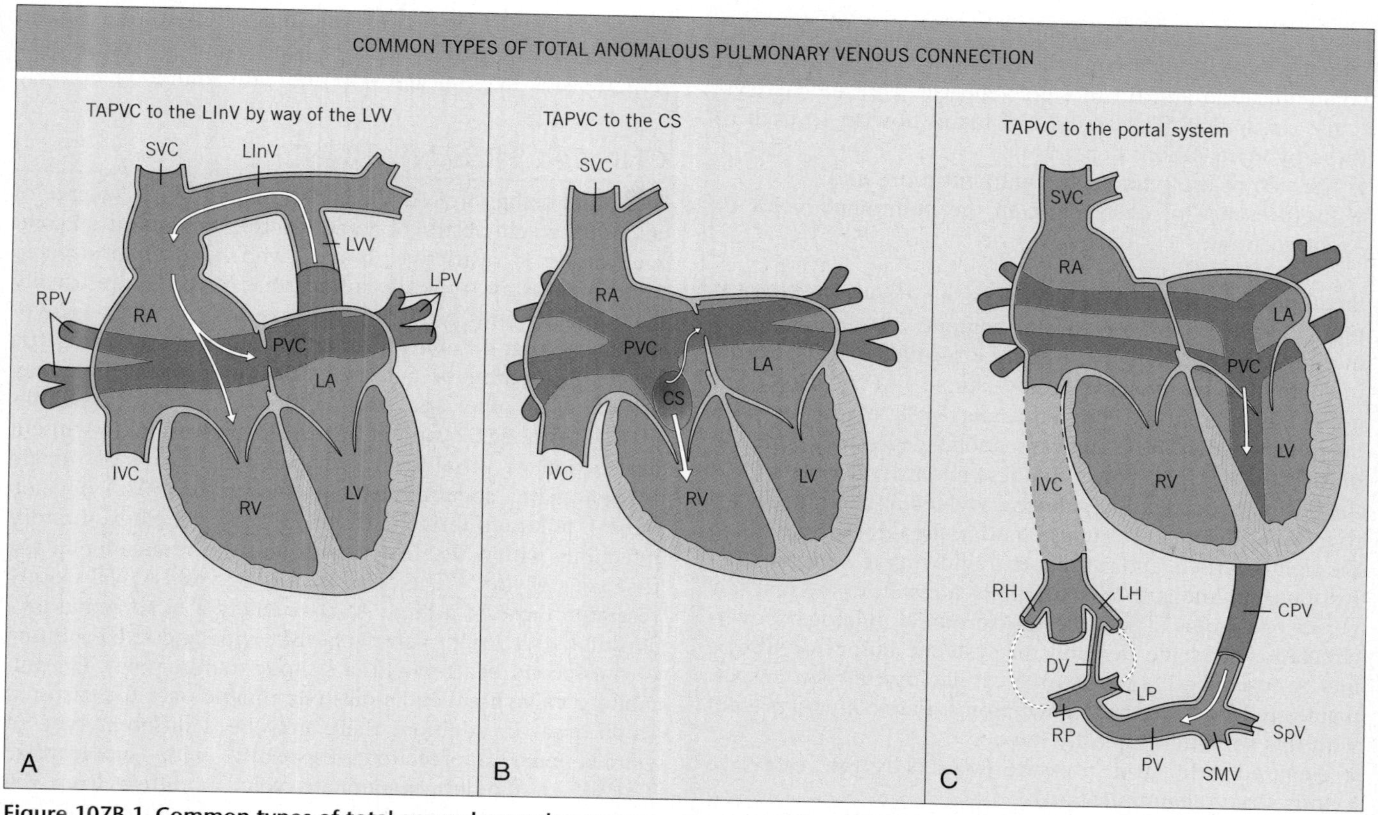

COMMON TYPES OF TOTAL ANOMALOUS PULMONARY VENOUS CONNECTION

Figure 107B.1 Common types of total anomalous pulmonary venous connection (TAPVC). A, TAPVC to the left innominate vein (LInV) by way of the left vertical vein (LVV). The right pulmonary veins (RPV) and left pulmonary veins (LPV) join to form a pulmonary venous confluence (PVC) located posterior and slightly superior to the left atrium (LA). The LVV arises from the leftward aspect of the PVC and connects to the LInV. The LInV connects to the superior vena cava (SVC), which is dilated. Flow into the systemic circulation is by way of an interatrial communication. This represents a supracardiac type of TAPVC. **B**, TAPVC to the coronary sinus (CS). The RPV and LPV join to form a PVC that connects to an enlarged CS. This represents an intracardiac or cardiac type of TAPVC. **C**, TAPVC to the portal system. The RPV and LPV course like the branches of a tree inferiorly toward the diaphragm. Here, they join to form a small PVC located posterior and slightly inferior to the LA. A common pulmonary vein (CPV) leaves the PVC, courses inferiorly through the esophageal hiatus of the diaphragm and connects to the portal vein in the abdomen. The portal vein communicates with the inferior vena cava (IVC) by way of the ductus venosus (DV) or hepatic sinusoids. This represents an infracardiac or infradiaphragmatic type of TAPVC. LH, left hepatic vein; LP, left portal vein; LV, left ventricle; RA, right atrium; RH, right hepatic vein; RP, right portal vein; RV, right ventricle; SMV, superior mesenteric vein; SpV, splenic vein.

Type 3 (Infracardiac) Total Anomalous Pulmonary Venous Connection

Unlike the prior types of TAPVC, the infracardiac type—a connection that occurs at the infradiaphragmatic level, such as into the portal venous system—is almost always associated with severe obstruction to pulmonary venous return. It represents 15% to 20% of all cases.[4,6] These patients present early in the newborn period with severe tachypnea and cyanosis. Usually, the pulmonary veins from both lungs form a confluence posterior and inferior to the left atrium (see Fig. 107B.1c). From this confluence, a common vein arises and descends through the esophageal hiatus of the diaphragm anterior to the esophagus. In the majority (70%-80%) of cases, this common pulmonary vein connects to the portal venous system, either at the splenic vein or at the confluence of the splenic and superior mesenteric veins.[5,9] It could also join the inferior vena cava (IVC) proper or the left hepatic vein. As with other types of TAPVC, obstruction can occur at several levels, including

- at the junction with the portal vein;
- at the level of the esophageal hiatus;
- at the ductus venosus after postnatal closure of this vessel; and
- at the hepatic sinusoids, in which case pulmonary venous blood entering the portal system must traverse the liver parenchyma.

Type 4 (Mixed) Total Anomalous Pulmonary Venous Connection

Type 4, or mixed connection, TAPVC involves connections at several different cardiac sites and is the rarest type, accounting for less than 5% of all cases of TAPVC.[5] The most common type of mixed connections has connection of the left pulmonary veins to a vertical vein leading to the left innominate vein along with connection of the right pulmonary veins to either the right atrium or coronary sinus. Mixed TAPVC is commonly associated with other major cardiac structural defects and can have obstruction at several levels.

PATHOPHYSIOLOGY

TAPVC is a cyanotic lesion, resulting from complete mixing of all of the pulmonary and systemic venous blood at the level of the right atrium. An atrial level shunt is necessary for survival with TAPVC. Therefore the mixed venous blood may either enter the right ventricle (RV) and the pulmonary circuit or may pass through the obligatory right-to-left atrial communication and fill the left ventricle (LV) and the systemic circulation. The amount of blood flowing to each of these two circulations depends on

- the size of the interatrial communication; and
- the presence of obstruction in the pulmonary veins or connections.

Small or restrictive atrial level shunts may severely limit LV preload and therefore cardiac output. A nonrestrictive interatrial communication, usually a secundum ASD, occurs in about 20% of infants who have simple TAPVC. However, a PFO is present in the remaining 80% of infants with uncomplicated TAPVC and causes some degree of restriction of right to left blood flow.[10] In these infants with only a PFO, the postnatal decrease in pulmonary vascular resistance leads to more of the mixed venous blood in the right atrium filling the right ventricle and subsequently flowing toward the low-resistance pulmonary circulation. As a result, in the first few weeks or months of life, there is torrential pulmonary overcirculation, and the demand for systemic output cannot be met. Consequently, progressive cardiac dysfunction ensues, manifested by heart failure symptoms. Patients who present with this condition typically have

- elevated right atrial pressure (caused by the restrictive interatrial communication);
- pulmonary blood flow that is several times higher than the systemic blood flow;
- pulmonary artery hypertension (usually moderate and caused by increased pulmonary blood flow rather than by pulmonary venous obstruction);
- decreased left atrial and left ventricular volumes;
- low cardiac output; and
- mild hypoxemia (systemic arterial oxygen saturations of 85%-90%).

With pulmonary vein obstruction, the pulmonary capillary wedge pressure increases, leading to cardiogenic pulmonary edema. In addition, as the pulmonary capillary pressure increases, so does the RV pressure, causing reduced RV compliance. Both lead to increased right atrial pressure and increased quantity of right-to-left shunting at the atrial level, aggravating systemic hypoxemia. Likewise, if the ductus arteriosus is still open, it will also shunt right-to-left, further increasing systemic cyanosis and pulmonary oligemia. This vicious cycle of worsening pulmonary oligemia, severe hypoxemia, and intractable metabolic acidosis leads to multisystem organ failure. Without relief of the pulmonary venous obstruction, death will ensue, and in this case the size of the interatrial communication has little influence on the outcome.

In the absence of pulmonary venous obstruction and the presence of a free communication between the two atria, the distribution of the mixed venous blood is determined by the relative compliances of the atria and ventricles and the relative resistances of the pulmonary and systemic circulations. In this lesion, the systemic arterial oxygen saturation depends on the amount of pulmonary blood flow. Usually, a large left-to-right shunt is present, and pulmonary artery pressures are normal or mildly elevated. The physiologic abnormalities are essentially the same as those of a patient who has a large ASD. Signs of heart failure or pulmonary hypertension may not develop until late adulthood.

CLINICAL PRESENTATION

Symptomatology in TAPVC is determined by the degree of pulmonary vein obstruction and whether the interatrial communication is restrictive. Infants who have an obstructed venous pathway (typically infracardiac TAPVC) are usually symptomatic with profound cyanosis and relentless tachypnea in the first 48 hours after birth. Other infants with little to no obstruction or a larger atrial level connection may present at an older age, many after the first several months of life. Although cyanosis is rare in these infants without obstruction or atrial-level restriction, they do not remain asymptomatic indefinitely; approximately 50% develop signs of failure to thrive, tachypnea, and frequent respiratory infections within the first month and the remainder in the first year of life.[11] The physical findings of TAPVC closely resemble those of a large ASD—namely a hyperactive precordium with a right ventricular lift, wide and fixed splitting of the second heart sound, a systolic murmur over the pulmonary valve area, and a diastolic rumble over the tricuspid valve area. In addition, there may be a different type of venous hum appreciated, especially with supracardiac TAPVC to the left innominate vein. It differs from the benign venous hum in that it is not louder in diastole nor does it extinguish with compression of the neck veins. The electrocardiogram (ECG) shows right axis deviation with right atrial and right ventricular enlargement, and the chest radiograph shows mild to moderate cardiomegaly with increased pulmonary vascular markings.

In contrast, infants with obstructed pulmonary veins or a restrictive atrial level communication manifest tachypnea, failure to thrive, and profound cyanosis at birth or shortly thereafter. In the Northern Great Plains series, nearly three quarters of infants with an obstructed pulmonary venous pathway presented shortly after birth, with the remainder in the ensuing few months.[11] Type 3 (infracardiac) TAPVC is often associated with obstructed pulmonary veins, and these infants with pulmonary venous obstruction do not manifest cardiac enlargement, either clinically or radiographically; hepatomegaly is common. Though the heart is not enlarged, there may be a prominent right ventricular impulse or heave. P_2 is often accentuated, suggesting pulmonary hypertension. Murmurs are usually absent; however, there may be a soft systolic murmur over the pulmonary outflow tract. On the ECG, most infants show a qR pattern in the right chest leads, indicating right ventricular hypertrophy, but often with no evidence of right atrial enlargement. There is often right axis deviation. The chest radiograph usually shows a variable degree of pulmonary edema, from mildly increased interstitial markings with no pulmonary venous obstruction to a "snowman in a snowstorm" appearance with obstructed type 1 (supracardiac) TAPVC (Fig. 107B.2).

Infants who have TAPVC with a restrictive atrial communication are likewise usually symptomatic at some time during the first 6 weeks of life. Unlike the obstructed veins though, their cyanosis is initially milder and their tachypnea with feeds may be less prominent initially. However, as the

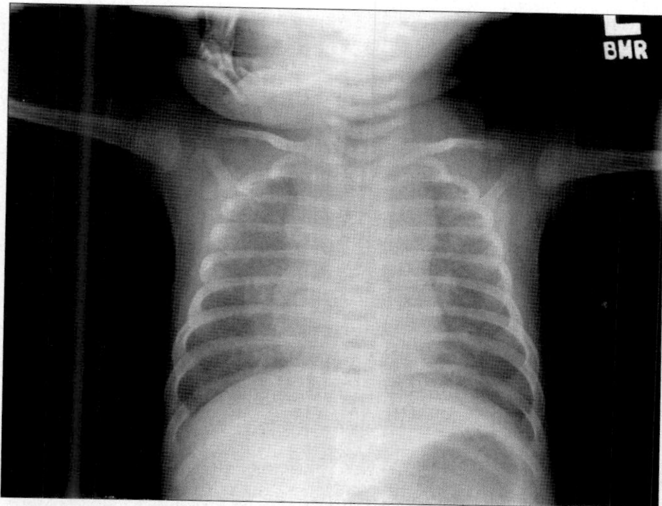

Figure 107B.2 Chest x-ray (PA view) showing diffusely hazy lung fields due to pulmonary vascular congestion characteristic of obstructed TAPVC. The pulmonary edema results from high left atrial pressure and the resultant elevated hydrostatic pressure in the lung vasculature. The lobular appearance of the heart from a vertical vein and the thymus superimposed on the hazy lung fields gives it the appearance of a "snowman in a snowstorm."

pulmonary vascular resistance drops and pulmonary blood flow increases, the interatrial communication becomes functionally more restrictive. This leads to a progressively increased work of breathing, feeding difficulties, cyanosis, and fulminant heart failure.

DIAGNOSTIC TECHNIQUES

Echocardiography

As with PAPVC, echocardiography represents the cornerstone for diagnosis and preoperative planning. Advances in ultrasound equipment and refinement of the Doppler color mapping algorithms have allowed for a diagnostic accuracy of TAPVC of 100%.[12,13] As a result, most infants who have TAPVC undergo surgical correction of their defect on the basis of the echocardiographic information and do not require invasive testing.

General Considerations

A universal finding in TAPVC is right-sided volume overload, with enlargement of the right atrium, right ventricle, and main pulmonary artery. The right ventricle is hypertrophied and there is evidence of pulmonary arterial hypertension, such as a high-velocity tricuspid regurgitation jet and an atrial septum that bows leftward. Ventricular septal motion is usually flat or frankly paradoxical. The size of the left atrium and left ventricle are normal or slightly decreased because of decreased preload.

The key to the diagnosis of TAPVC is identifying the anatomic connections of all four pulmonary veins. Echocardiography can help quantify the size of the individual veins as well as delineate abnormal flow patterns by Doppler that might indicate obstruction. An essential element is identifying the size and location of each vein and how and where they enter the heart.[14,15] This is especially important because it has been shown that the sum of the individual vein sizes is an independent risk factor for postoperative mortality. Specifically, small veins before surgery lead to higher postoperative mortality.[16]

In patients who are difficult to image with transthoracic echocardiography, transesophageal echocardiography (TEE) may provide better visualization of the pulmonary veins and their site of drainage because of their posterior location.[17]

Identification of the Pulmonary Venous Confluence

In TAPVC, there is an extracardiac antechamber or confluence of the veins that often lies posterior to the left atrium and has a separate venous egress, connecting to a systemic vein and then the heart. Echocardiography can be used to identify the confluence's size, location, and number of individual pulmonary veins that enter it. Because of its size, shape, and posterior location, the pulmonary venous confluence can sometimes be difficult to image directly, even by TEE. Moreover, because of the technical limitations associated with examining small infants with respiratory distress, it can be difficult to visualize with certainty the wall that separates the true left atrium from the common pulmonary venous chamber. Thus imaging of the pulmonary veins behind the left atrium does not prove that these veins actually drain to the left atrium. They may, in fact, be separated from the left atrium by the anterior wall of the pulmonary venous confluence. The use of high frequency transducers in conjunction with color Doppler helps visualize the wall between the left atrium and pulmonary venous confluence and is usually required for definitive information about the site of drainage of the individual pulmonary veins. Therefore in any child with TAPVC, attempts should be made using multiple two-dimensional echocardiographic views and Doppler color flow mapping to visualize the connection of all four pulmonary veins to the confluence. Whereas supracardiac TAPVC can generally best be seen from parasternal imaging, and infracardiac TAPVC is best visualized from subcostal views, some more specific echocardiographic views may be better for certain types of TAPVC.

- In cardiac TAPVC (i.e., connection to the coronary sinus or directly to the right atrium), the pulmonary venous confluence is directly posterior to the left atrium and is thus well visualized in the parasternal, apical four-chamber, and subcostal views (Fig. 107B.3). The coronary sinus itself will also be dilated; however, it can be dilated because of a persistent left superior vena cava as well. Thus, delineating the connection of the confluence into the coronary sinus is imperative.
- In supracardiac TAPVC (i.e., drainage to the superior vena cava directly or via a left vertical vein), the pulmonary venous confluence is usually superior to the left atrium and is thus best visualized in the parasternal views, especially the short-axis view. It may also be seen from the subcostal long-axis views (Fig. 107B.4).
- In infracardiac total anomalous pulmonary venous return (i.e., to the hepatic portal system or the hepatic veins), the pulmonary veins usually converge like the branches of a tree just above the diaphragm (Fig. 107B.5). Therefore the pulmonary venous confluence is often small and inferior to the left atrium or may not exist as a distinct, separate chamber. Thus the pulmonary venous confluence is usually best

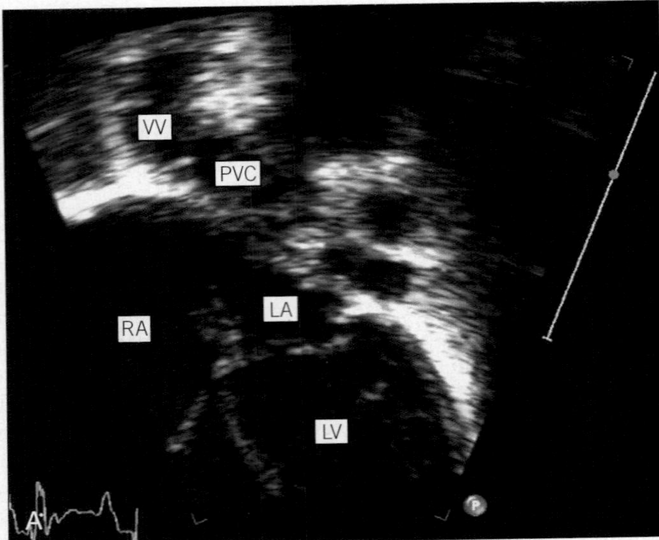

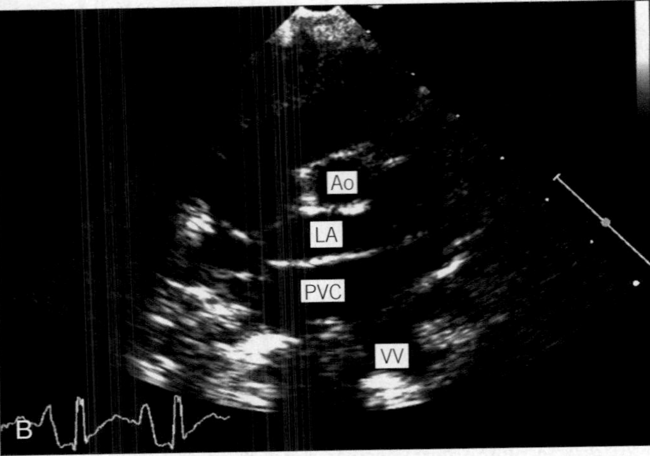

Figure 107B.3 Suprasternal (**A**) and apical (**B**) echocardiographic planes demonstrating a pulmonary venous confluence (PVC) posterior to the left atrium (LA) that is being drained by a vertical vein (VV). The apical four-chamber view (**B**) more clearly shows the VV arising from the PVC and heading cephalad. Ao, aorta; LV, left ventricle; RA, right atrium.

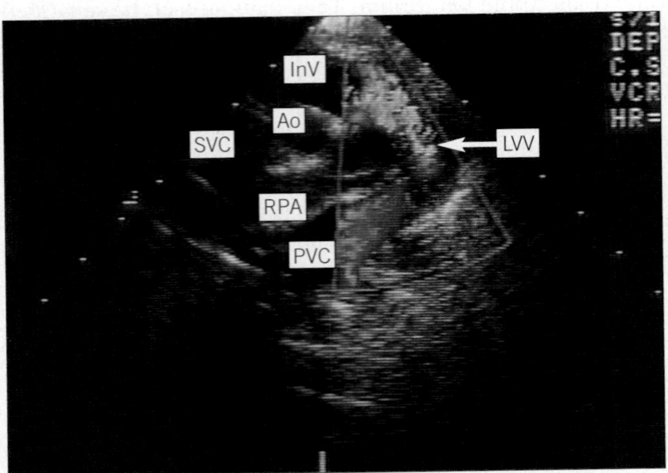

Figure 107B.4 Color Doppler examination in supracardiac total anomalous pulmonary venous connection (TAPVC). This suprasternal short-axis view shows TAPVC to the left vertical vein (LVV), to the innominate vein (InV), and to the right superior vena cava (SVC). The pulmonary veins can be seen joining inferiorly to form a pulmonary venous confluence (PVC). On the left, the LVV is seen arising from the PVC. Doppler signals from blood flow in the PVC and LVV are color-coded as red, indicating flow up the LVV toward the transducer. From the LVV, pulmonary venous return is to the InV and SVC. Beneath this abnormal vascular connection, the transverse aorta (Ao) is seen in cross section, and the right pulmonary artery (RPA) is seen in longitudinal section. (From Snider R, Ritter SB, Serwer GA. Echocardiography in Pediatric Heart Disease, 2nd ed. St. Louis, Mosby, 1997.)

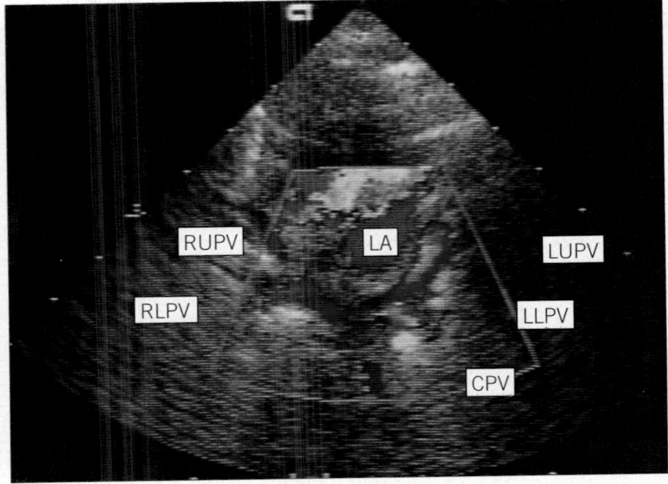

Figure 107B.5 Color Doppler examination in infracardiac total anomalous pulmonary venous connection (TAPVC). This suprasternal short-axis view shows all four pulmonary veins merging at the level of the diaphragm, like the branches of a tree. There is very little pulmonary venous confluence. The uppermost portion of the common pulmonary vein (CPV) is seen in blue, indicating flow away from the transducer. A portion of flow in the left atrium (LA) is seen above in red. LLPV, left lower pulmonary vein; LUPV, left upper pulmonary vein; RLPV, right lower pulmonary vein; RUPV, right upper pulmonary vein. (From Snider R, Ritter SB, Serwer GA. Echocardiography in Pediatric Heart Disease, 2nd ed. St. Louis, Mosby, 1997.)

visualized from subcostal short- and long-axis views, but can be seen with an apical four-chamber view as well.[14] Occasionally, with the aid of color Doppler, the four pulmonary veins, their confluence, and the upper portion of the descending common vertical vein can be imaged from the suprasternal short-axis view (see Fig. 107B.5).[12]

- In the rare mixed form of TAPVC, the pulmonary veins drain to two separate systemic venous sites. If only two pulmonary veins can be seen entering the pulmonary venous confluence despite attempted visualization in multiple imaging planes, one should suspect this mixed form of the disease. This is the most difficult form to image, because multiple views are typically required to completely define the venous drainage pattern. Special attention should be paid to the coronary sinus and the innominate vein as potential sites of drainage.

Obstruction in venous pathways is a critical element to accurately diagnose preoperatively, and echocardiography can be used to trace the egress from the confluence, including elucidating the final site of drainage into the systemic venous system. Obstruction can be recognized by turbulent flow with color Doppler echocardiography, venous flow acceleration (typically ~2 m/second), and loss of normal phasic flow patterns (Fig. 107B.6). Certain imaging views may be more helpful for certain types of TAPVC and may show the precise level of obstruction. For example, in the cardiac type of TAPVC, the pulmonary venous confluence can be seen connecting to an enlarged coronary sinus in the subcostal views, often resembling the tail of a whale (the veins representing the "fork" in the tail).[14]

In supracardiac TAPVC to the superior vena cava by way of the left vertical vein and innominate vein, the entire anomalous supracardiac connection can be seen in the suprasternal short-axis view (see Fig. 107B.4). In this view, the anomalous pulmonary venous connection resembles a large vascular collar surrounding the transverse aorta. In the parasternal long-axis view, the markedly dilated innominate vein can be seen in cross section anterior to the innominate artery. In some infants, the entire anomalous connection can be seen from the subcostal four-chamber view of the left ventricular outflow tract. Color Doppler examination of the left vertical vein shows continuous, low-velocity flow signals directed away from the heart, whereas systemic veins in the thorax would have flow directed toward the heart. In some patients, the color Doppler examination shows aliased, disturbed flow along the common pulmonary venous pathway, indicating obstruction.[18] Obstruction in this type of TAPVC would typically occur where the left vertical vein passes between the left pulmonary artery anteriorly and the left main stem bronchus posteriorly or at the junction of the innominate vein and the right superior vena cava.[19] There is often dilatation of the vein just proximal to the level of obstruction. Thus any dilated vein segment should heighten suspicion for downstream obstruction.

In infracardiac TAPVC, a common pulmonary vein leaves the pulmonary venous confluence, passes through the diaphragm (usually anterior to the aorta), and drains into a systemic vein in the abdomen. Some common sites of drainage include the hepatic portal system and the left hepatic vein. In the subcostal long-axis view in the abdomen, the common pulmonary vein is usually imaged in a plane to the left of the inferior vena cava. This vessel is usually seen anterior to the descending aorta and can be traced back through the diaphragm to its origin from the pulmonary venous confluence. Often, three large vessels (the inferior vena cava, descending aorta, and common pulmonary vein) are seen in cross section in the subcostal short-axis view.[15] Color and pulse wave Doppler examination of the common pulmonary vein shows low-velocity characteristic venous flow pattern directed away from the heart, whereas flow in systemic veins in the abdomen is continuous and directed toward the heart.

Computed Tomography and Magnetic Resonance Imaging

The advent of axial imaging techniques whose data can then be reformatted into any visual plane has greatly advanced the quantity and usefulness of data that can be obtained by noninvasive imaging for TAPVC. Just as with PAPVC, both modalities have a wide field of view and illustrate the spatial relationships between the veins and other thoracic structures, such as the airways, esophagus, and bones. Although computed tomographic angiography (CTA) may incur some radiation exposure, it is very rapid; usually does not require significant sedation for image acquisition; is not contraindicated with many implanted devices, like pacemakers and defibrillators; and is readily available at most centers. It provides superb vascular delineation as well as data on other thoracic structures during a single acquisition (Fig. 107B.7). Magnetic resonance imaging and angiography (MRI/MRA) also provides superb multiplanar imaging of these abnormal vascular

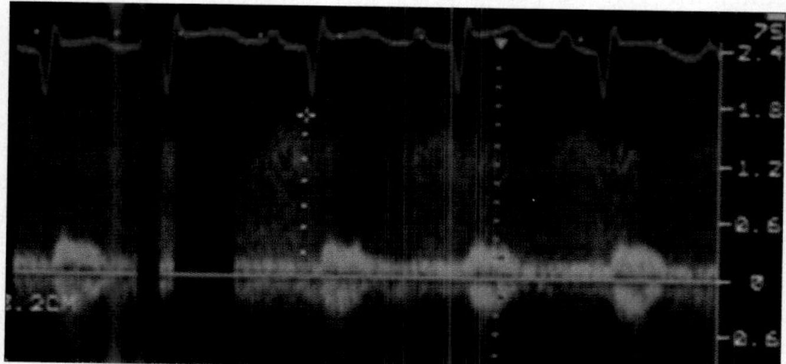

Figure 107B.6 Echocardiographic pulse wave Doppler waveform showing minimally phasic, continuous flow at high velocity (~1.8 m/sec) in a pulmonary vein. The flow pattern never returns to baseline, an obstructive pattern.

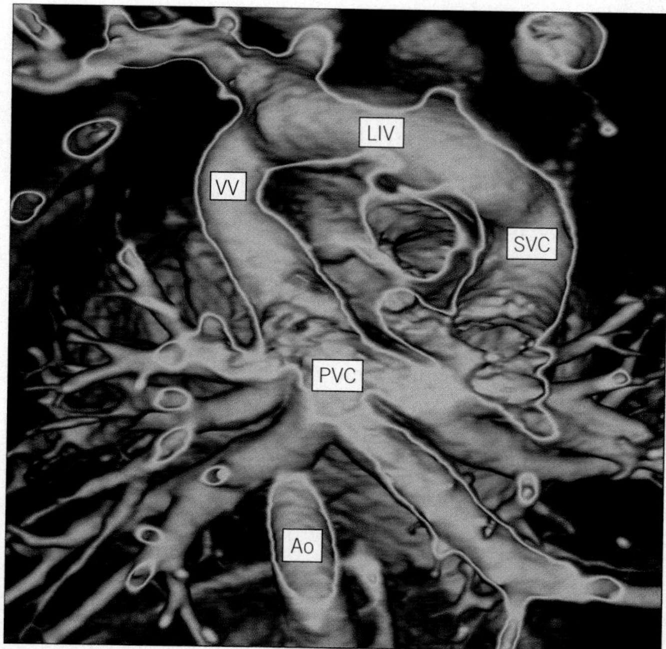

Figure 107B.7 TAPVC CTA. Three-dimensional rendering of a contrasted chest CT scan demonstrating supracardiac TAPVC. The pulmonary veins are seen returning to a pulmonary venous confluence posterior to the left atrium. Then, arising from this confluence is a vertical vein that heads cephalad and connects to the left innominate vein, which then drains into the superior vena cava. Ao, aorta; LIV, left innominate vein; PVC, pulmonary venous confluence; SVC, superior vena cava; VV, vertical vein.

structures.[20] Additional advantages include its ability to obtain functional data, such as flow velocities within individual pulmonary veins and accurate chamber volumes and function. However, though there is no radiation exposure, obtaining a study on younger patients may require sedation or anesthesia because of the longer durations required for sequence planning and acquisition. Whereas echocardiography may be sufficient for diagnosis in an infant, older children and adults may benefit from the spatial resolution in the newer modalities as well as the ability to provide comprehensive cardiac functional and anatomic analysis with MRI.

Cardiac Catheterization

Noninvasive imaging has largely eliminated the need for catheterization as a purely diagnostic modality in this disease process. In fact, caution should be employed to not further compromise these fragile patients or to delay their definitive repair by obtaining a catheterization unless there is a compelling indication. Yet, as with PAPVC, the diagnosis of TAPVC could be made by cardiac catheterization by entering the anomalous pulmonary venous channel with the catheter and performing an angiogram. Oximetry sampling is also helpful, showing a "step-up" in oxygen saturations to above 90% in the right atrium. Saturations in the right ventricle and pulmonary circulation are usually identical; however, because of streaming and incomplete mixing of blood in the right atrium, some differences do occur.[10] The right ventricular and pulmonary arterial pressures are usually suprasystemic with obstructed TAPVC, but right atrial pressures are normal or nearly so. Pulmonary artery wedge pressure is elevated, whereas left atrial pressure is low. A pullback pressure recording through the anomalous pulmonary venous channel demonstrates a discrete pressure gradient at the level of the obstruction. The size of the atrial communication is important for left heart preload and its size can be determined at catheterization using an inflated balloon catheter. An interatrial communication less than 5 mm in diameter is definitely restrictive; one that is less than 10 mm should raise suspicions of restriction.[10] Angiography may be the most diagnostic aspect of a catheterization for TAPVC. Selective pulmonary artery angiograms in the levophase may delineate the path of venous return as well as any sites of obstruction. One could also perform selective vein wedge angiograms if more detailed angiography of the veins were required. If the pulmonary venous return is seen draining to the portal system, obstruction is highly likely.

Catheter-based interventions for this disease process have generally proved ineffective and are not typically undertaken at the present time. Balloon or blade atrial septostomies were previously performed as a palliative measure, but they only delayed definitive repair. Ballooning and/or stenting individual pulmonary veins is uniformly ineffective as a management strategy despite early hemodynamic improvement. Thus interventional catheterization procedures are not currently advisable for this lesion.[21,22]

MANAGEMENT

Surgery is the only intervention with proven short- and long-term success for TAPVC. In fact, TAPVC with severe pulmonary venous obstruction requires urgent or emergent surgical intervention. In the preoperative setting, several medical treatments are useful as temporizing measures to stabilize the cardiorespiratory and metabolic systems. These include mechanical ventilation, inotropic support, treatment of acid-base disorders, treatment of pulmonary hypertension (using inhaled nitric oxide) and potentially the use of extracorporeal membrane oxygenation as the ultimate life-supporting intervention. The use of prostaglandin E1 (PGE) is often performed while transporting a cyanotic neonate with suspected congenital heart disease. Potentially, PGE could make obstructed TAPVC worse by increasing pulmonary blood flow through a PDA. However, Bullaboy et al (1984)[22a] have reported that PGE may have a beneficial effect as well, namely maintaining the patency of the ductus venosus, allowing for some decompression of obstructed infradiaphragmatic TAPVC. Furthermore, they note that there may be right-to-left shunting through the PDA which could decompress the pulmonary circulation and increase systemic blood flow. Thus, PGE may be a reasonable medication during transport or until the diagnostic evaluation has been completed.

In patients who have TAPVC without severe pulmonary venous obstruction, there is some controversy surrounding the timing of surgical repair. In some institutions, a newly diagnosed TAPVC patient is treated with balloon or blade atrial septostomy, given aggressive medical therapy and close follow-up, and then scheduled for elective surgical repair in the second year of life.[12] However, for most patients now and in most centers, surgical repair is performed as soon as the diagnosis of TAPVC is made.[23,24] As with PAPVC, the specific surgical technique used is determined by the anatomy of the defect. However, certain common principles apply. In many cases, creating an unrestrictive side-to-side anastomosis between the pulmonary venous confluence and the left atrium while resecting other means of egress from the confluence is the primary surgical approach. Similarly, in cardiac TAPVC, surgeons can unroof the coronary sinus to the left atrium and close the coronary sinus orifice with a patch.

PROGNOSIS

Without surgical repair, the majority of patients who have TAPVC do not survive past the first year of life. Since the first successful repair of TAPVC, there has been a remarkable improvement in the operative survival over the past 30 years. One study reported a significant reduction in mortality for TAPVC repair from 19% before 1995 compared with 5% in the current era.[25] Currently, operative mortality rates for surgery in the newborn period range from 0% to 5%.[23,24] Although supracardiac TAPVC is associated with a better outcome than infracardiac or mixed types,[26] the anatomic type of TAPVC is much less of a risk factor for early or late death after surgical repair of TAPVC than the size of the veins preoperatively or the presence of pulmonary vein stenoses. In one study, small individual pulmonary veins or a small pulmonary venous confluence as well as the presence of heterotaxy syndrome were all independent risk factors for mortality.[16] A separate study found that a small pulmonary venous confluence associated with diffuse pulmonary vein stenoses was an independent risk factor for early and late death as well as for the need for reoperation.[27] Morbidity and mortality have improved dramatically in concert with surgical technology. In one European series, early survivorship was 93% after TAPVC repair. However, some of these survivors will experience late pulmonary vein stenosis. In that series, pulmonary vein stenosis requiring reintervention represented 11% of the survivors and occurred an average of 41 days after surgery. Despite employing a multidisciplinary approach to relieving the stenosis (angioplasty/stenting or surgery), 56% subsequently died.[28] Likewise, unilateral pulmonary vein stenosis has a markedly improved outcome compared with bilateral disease. Thus pulmonary vein stenosis occurs with some frequency after TAPVC repair, has poor reintervention results, and remains a significant risk factor for early and late mortality.

Overall, long-term outcomes for patients after TAPVC repair appear quite good and have improved vastly since the early 1990s. A retrospective study from Philadelphia shows that most patients who had undergone isolated TAPVC repair had parentally reported excellent health (64%) or good health (27%) and exhibited above average (40%) or average (29%) school performance. Twenty-seven percent were in special education classes, but this was highly correlated with the presence of a genetic anomaly.[25] This is again attributed to the advances in diagnosis, surgical management, and postoperative care that have occurred over the past several decades.

SUMMARY

Total anomalous pulmonary venous connection is a condition in which all four pulmonary veins connect anomalously to the heart and results in the complete admixture of pulmonary venous and systemic venous blood at the atrial level. The four types of TAPVC, listed in descending order of prevalence are supracardiac, infracardiac, cardiac, and mixed. Pulmonary blood flow is increased and cyanosis is mild if there is a nonrestrictive interatrial communication and no obstruction to pulmonary venous return. Conversely, pulmonary blood flow is reduced and cyanosis may be severe with significant obstruction to pulmonary venous return, as is nearly universally found in the infracardiac type of TAPVC. Significant advances, such as noninvasive imaging, improved surgical techniques, and ICU management, have dramatically altered the outcomes of TAPVC patients. Echocardiography is the mainstay for diagnosis, making it possible to delineate all relevant anatomic features in most patients without the need for invasive diagnostic angiography. MR and CT angiography provide further anatomic detail by offering multiplanar views, clarifying the spatial relationships of the veins themselves and in relation to other thoracic structures. Although catheter-based interventions have not been shown to be effective in treating TAPVC, advances in surgical techniques and perioperative medical management have resulted in lower operative mortality and complication rates. One subgroup remains a challenge: TAPVC with pulmonary vein obstruction remains very difficult to treat and confers a grimmer prognosis. Overall, thanks to these diagnostic and management advances, most patients undergoing TAPVC surgery will have a successful, complete repair. They can expect to be largely asymptomatic and have a normal life expectancy and educational performance.

chapter

108 Ventricular Septal Defect

Mary S. Minette

Definition

- Defects of the ventricular septum can occur in any location, and they allow communication between the left ventricle and the right ventricle or right atrium.

Key Features

- Ventricular septal defects are classified according to location.
- Defects may be single or multiple and of widely varying sizes.
- Clinical features are as variable as the defects themselves and can range from no symptoms to severe congestive heart failure.
- Diagnosis is made by physical examination in conjunction with chest x-ray, electrocardiography, radiography, and echocardiography.

Therapy

- Therapy is dependent on the associated clinical features (location, size, and symptoms).
- Management strategies include observation, medical treatment, and surgical and/or transcatheter closure.

Ventricular septal defect (VSD) is the most common form of congenital heart defect in children, occurring in isolation or in association with other malformations.[1] In adults the bicuspid aortic valve is more commonly seen.[2]

Genetic factors can play a role and are divided into three categories with increasing importance: single gene disorders, chromosomal disorders, and polygenic disorders.[3] Single gene disorders are caused by deletions, missense mutations, or duplications within a gene that follow autosomal dominant, autosomal recessive, or X-linked inheritance. Chromosomal disorders are caused by absent or duplicated chromosomes. Polygenic disorders are the result of genetic and environmental factors.

ANATOMY AND PATHOLOGY

The commonly used terminology for the ventricular septum is that of Soto and coworkers.[4] The ventricular septum is divided into two morphologic components, the membranous septum and the muscular septum. The membranous septum is small and is located at the base of the heart between the inlet and outlet components of the muscular septum and below the right and noncoronary cusps of the aortic valve. Defects of the membranous septum are surrounded by fibrous tissue without extension into adjacent muscular septum. Defects that involve the membranous septum and extend into one of the three muscular components are termed perimembranous, paramembranous, or infracristal (Fig. 108.1).

The muscular septum is further divided into inlet, trabecular, and infundibular components. The inlet portion is inferioposterior to the membranous septum. It begins at the level of the atrioventricular valves and ends at their chordal attachments apically. An inlet ventricular septal defect has no muscular rim between the defect and the atrioventricular valve annulus. Defects in the inlet muscular septum are termed inlet or canal ventricular septal defects, and may be seen in association with abnormalities of the tricuspid and mitral valves.

The trabecular septum is the largest part of the ventricular septum. It extends from the membranous septum to the apex and superiorly to the infundibular septum. A defect in the trabecular septum is termed a muscular ventricular septal defect if the defect is completely rimmed by muscle. Defects in the trabecular septum are classified as anterior, midmuscular, apical, and posterior, as proposed by Kirklin and colleagues.[5] An anterior muscular defect is anterior to the septal band. A midmuscular defect is posterior to the septal band. Apical defects are inferior to the moderator band. Posterior defects are beneath the septal leaflet of the tricuspid valve.

The infundibular septum separates the right and left ventricular outflow tracts. On the right side it is bordered by the line from the membranous septum to the papillary muscle of the conus inferiorly and the semilunar valves superiorly. Defects in the infundibulum are called infundibular, outlet, supracristal, conal, conoventricular, subpulmonary, or doubly committed subarterial defects. A deficient infundibular septum may be present with corresponding degrees of malalignment.

Many defects involve more than one component of the ventricular septum. Perimembranous defects can extend into the adjacent muscular septum and have been called perimembranous inlet, perimembranous muscular, and perimembranous outlet, based on the extension.[6] Abnormalities of the tricuspid valve adjacent to these defects can be in the form of an aneurysm partially or completely occluding the defect.

Infundibular and perimembranous defects can be associated with varying degrees of malalignment of the infundibular septum with the remainder of the ventricular septum. Malalignment can be anterior, posterior, or rotational and may result in overriding of one of the semilunar valves. Although this can exist in isolation, it is most frequently associated with other defects, such as tetralogy of Fallot in the setting of anterior malalignment. Coarctation of the aorta or varying degrees of aortic hypoplasia can be seen with

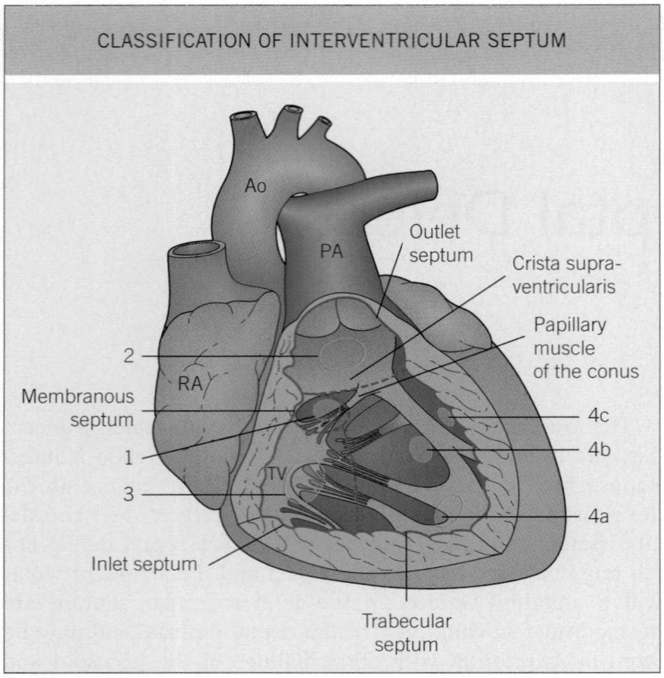

CLASSIFICATION OF INTERVENTRICULAR SEPTUM

Figure 108.1 Classification schema of the interventricular septum. Schematic representation of the anatomic classification of the ventricular septum viewed from the right ventricle. The red lines indicate the margins of the interventricular septum. Membranous septum is beneath the septal leaflet of the tricuspid valve and extends up to the aortic valve; inlet septum extends from the tricuspid valve annulus to the chordal attachments of the tricuspid valve onto the papillary muscles; trabecular septum extends from the inlet septum to the cardiac apex; and outlet septum extends from the crista supraventricularis to the pulmonary valve. Overlaid in blue on the diagram is the position of various types of ventricular septal defects: membranous (1), outlet (2), inlet (3), and muscular (apical [4a], central [4b], and marginal [4c]). Ao, aorta; PA, pulmonary artery; RA, right atrium; TV, tricuspid valve.

posterior malalignment. Straddling of the mitral valve may occur in the presence of infundibular defects.

Inlet defects can involve malalignment of the atrial and ventricular septum, resulting in annular overriding of one of the atrioventricular valves. Varying degrees of straddling of the chordal attachments of the tricuspid valve may also be present.

PATHOPHYSIOLOGY

The hemodynamic significance of ventricular septal defects is influenced by the size of the ventricular septal defect, the pressure in the right and left ventricular chambers, and the pulmonary resistance. A ventricular septal defect may not be apparent at birth because of the nearly equal pressures in the right and left ventricles and lack of shunting. With the physiologic drop in pulmonary vascular resistance in early infancy, there is an increasing pressure difference between the ventricles, and the defect may become clinically apparent.

In the absence of pulmonary hypertension or obstruction to the right ventricle, the direction of shunt is left to right. In the presence of elevated pulmonary vascular resistance, right ventricular obstruction due to muscle bundles, or pulmonary stenosis, the shunt volume is limited and may be right to left depending on the difference in pressures.

Eisenmenger's syndrome results from long-term left-to-right shunt, usually at higher shunt volumes. The elevated pulmonary artery pressure and resistance becomes irreversible and leads to a reversal in the ventricular level shunt, desaturation, cyanosis, and secondary erythrocytosis.

Muscular ventricular septal defects can undergo spontaneous closure due to muscular occlusion. Perimembranous defects can close by tricuspid valve aneurysm formation. Infundibular defects can close by prolapse of the right aortic cusp. A reduction in size of the defect by any of these mechanisms would result in changes in the hemodynamic significance of the defect.

The integrity of structures immediately adjacent to ventricular defects is a concern. For example, development of aortic valve prolapse and insufficiency in the case of infundibular defects is caused by deficiency of the aortic valve support apparatus, resulting in damage to the aortic valve leaflets.

CLINICAL PRESENTATIONS

History

Many patients are referred to a cardiologist because of the auscultatory findings associated with VSDs, usually in infancy or childhood. Patients may present with a murmur and be thriving or conversely, experiencing severe growth failure and persistent respiratory distress. As shunt volume increases, patients may present with worsening failure to thrive, increasing tachypnea, sweating, grunting, or frequent pulmonary infections. Changes in activity level or stamina may also be an indicator of increasing cardiac work and shunt volume.

Physical Examination

Vital signs performed during evaluation should include respiratory rate, heart rate, blood pressure in all extremities, and oxygen saturation. The latter two will help to exclude associated anomalies, such as coarctation of the aorta or right-to-left shunting at the VSD. Height and weight for comparison with normal percentiles and individual growth rate are valuable tools in the assessment of the clinical significance of a VSD in infants and children.

Thorough physical examination includes inspection and palpation of the precordium. A thrill would be associated with a high velocity jet. The precordium may be hyperdynamic in the setting of high cardiac output. A heave is possible with elevated right ventricular pressure. There may be evidence of left ventricular volume overload with a laterally displaced impulse. The thorax may be asymmetric in the presence of cardiac enlargement.

Accessory muscle use, intercostal retractions, nasal flaring, and abdominal muscle use may be seen with large volume of shunt into the pulmonary vasculature. Crackles or rhonchi may be heard on examination of the lung fields.

Hepatomegaly is an important and frequent sign of congestive heart failure. Unlike adults, infants and children do not typically develop extremity edema. Extremities may be cool because of increased systemic vascular resistance. Pulses may be diminished in the lower extremities if there is a coarctation in association with a posterior malalignment defect.

Murmurs associated with VSDs are typically described as holosystolic or pansystolic. The grade of murmur is dependent on the velocity of flow, and the location of murmur is dependent on the location of the defect. Smaller defects are loudest and may have a thrill. Muscular defects can be heard along the lower left sternal border and may vary in intensity, with a decrescendo as the defect size changes with muscular contraction throughout systole. Infundibular defects shunt close to the pulmonary valve and can be heard best at the left upper sternal border. Perimembranous defects may have an associated systolic click of a tricuspid valve aneurysm and can be heard at the right and left upper sternal borders.

Larger defects have murmurs of constant quality that varies little throughout the cardiac cycle and less commonly have an associated thrill. These defects will have a corresponding increase in mitral flow, resulting in a diastolic rumble at the apex. Elevated pulmonary pressure causes an increase in the intensity of the pulmonary component of the second heart sound. Large defects with little or no shunt are often without a murmur.

Defects that contribute to tricuspid regurgitation or exhibit a left ventricle to right atrial shunt will have a systolic murmur at the left lower or right lower sternal border. Defects associated with aortic insufficiency have a diastolic decrescendo murmur along the left sternal border with the patient sitting and leaning forward. A widened pulse pressure may be present.

Patients with Eisenmenger's syndrome have right-to-left shunt at the VSD. Many have cyanosis with clubbing, a right ventricular heave on palpation of the precordium, and a loud pulmonary component of the second heart sound. A ventricular septal defect murmur may not be present.

DIAGNOSTIC TECHNIQUES

Electrocardiography

The electrocardiogram is usually normal in patients with small ventricular septal defects. With increasing shunt, there may be evidence of left ventricular volume load and hypertrophy. Left atrial enlargement may be present. In cases of elevated pulmonary artery pressure, right axis deviation, right ventricular hypertrophy, and right atrial enlargement may be evident on electrocardiogram (Fig. 108.2).

Chest Radiography

Small defects have no apparent radiographic abnormality. With larger defects, chamber enlargement is present to varying degrees, depending on shunt volume. Increased

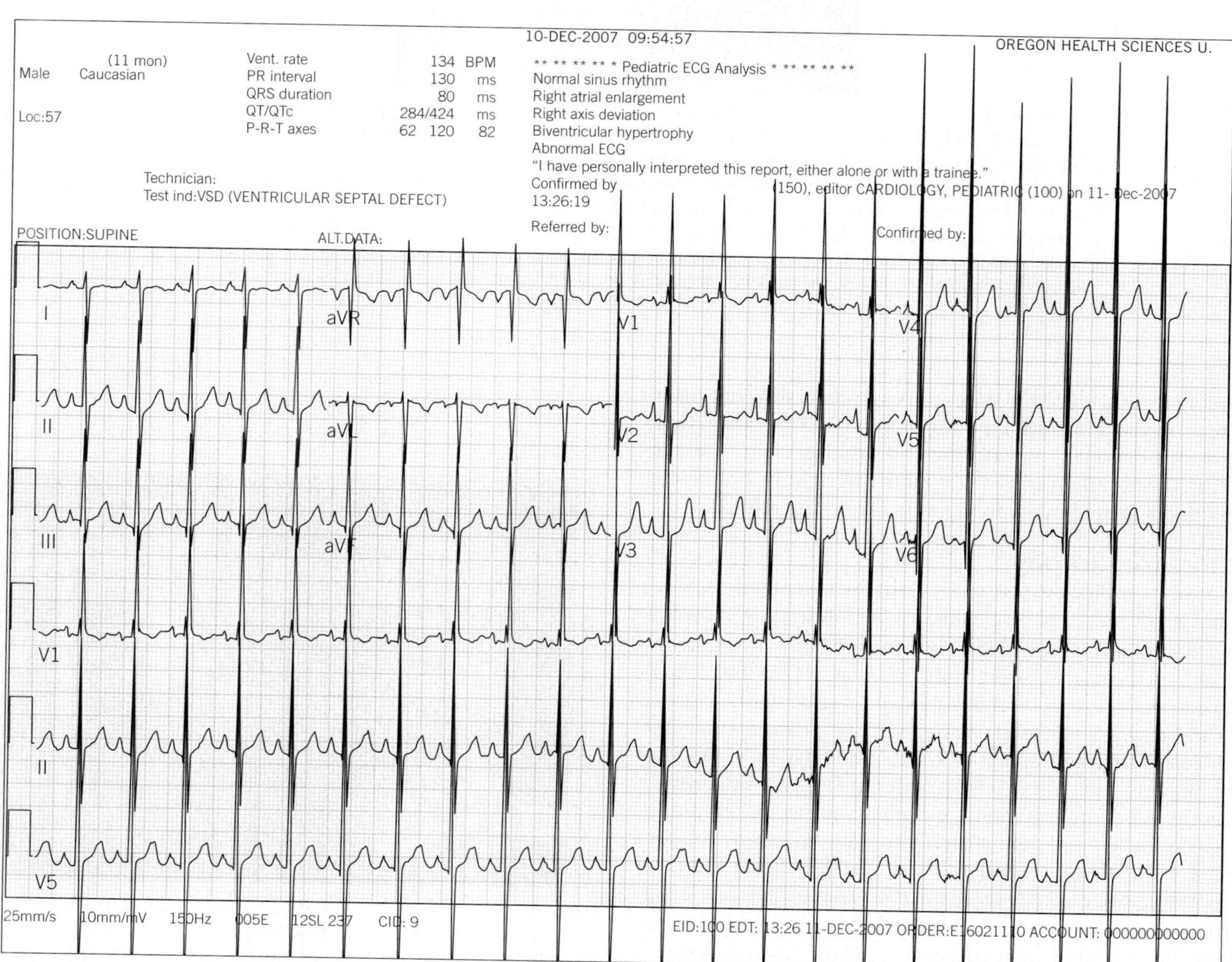

Figure 108.2 Electrocardiogram in an 11-month-old infant before surgical closure of a large ventricular septal defect. Biventricular hypertrophy, right axis deviation, and right atrial enlargement are evident.

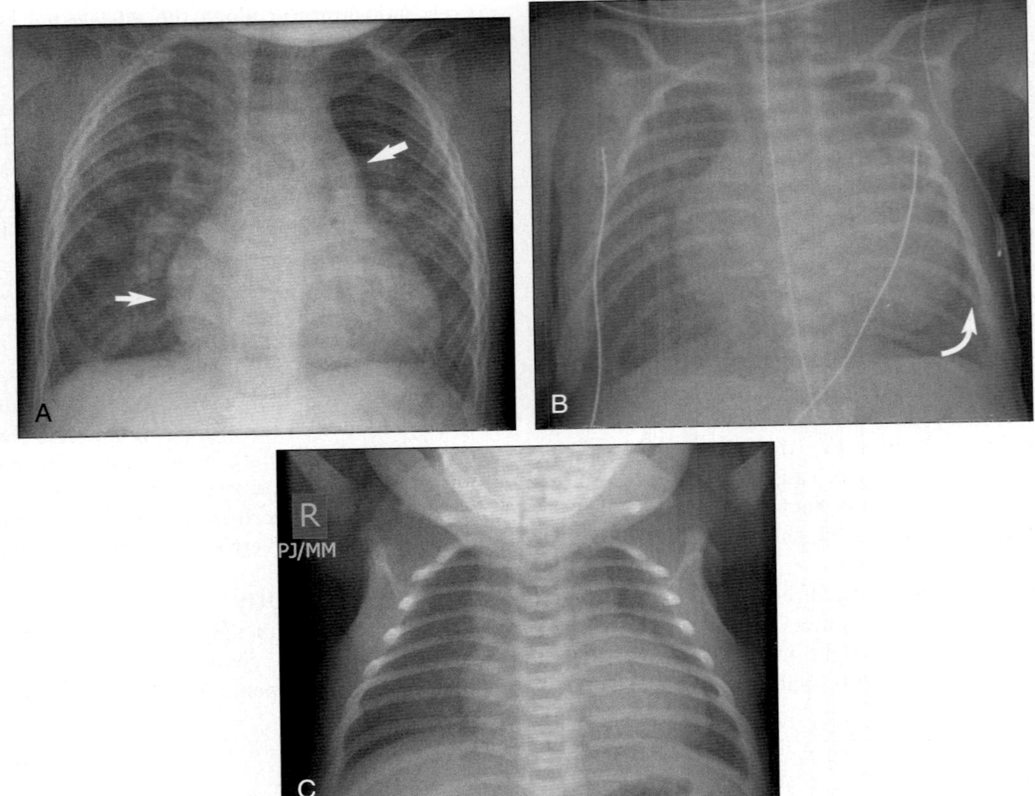

Figure 108.3 A, Chest radiography in a patient at 10 months of age with a large perimembranous ventricular septal defect before surgical closure. Cardiomegaly, increased pulmonary vascularity, right atrial dilatation (*small arrow*), and main pulmonary artery dilatation (*large arrow*) are demonstrated. This patient's ECG is seen in Fig. 108.2. **B,** Chest radiography in a 1-month-old infant with an unrestrictive inlet ventricular septal defect and a moderate secundum atrial defect. Cardiomegaly, increased pulmonary vascularity, and upward turned apex (*curved arrow*) are demonstrated. **C,** Chest radiography in a 3-month-old infant with failure to thrive and a posterior malalignment ventricular septal defect. Cardiomegaly and increased pulmonary vascularity are the predominant features demonstrated.

pulmonary vascularity is present. As patients develop Eisenmenger's syndrome or increasing pulmonary resistance, there is loss of pulmonary vascularity and pruning of the vasculature. In these patients there is evidence of right heart enlargement and a dilated main pulmonary artery (Fig. 108.3).

Echocardiography

Echocardiographic evaluation of ventricular septal defects is a noninvasive tool that is capable of demonstrating morphology, associated defects, hemodynamic characteristics, chamber enlargement, and cardiac function (Figs. 108.4 and 108.5).

Location, size, and direction of shunt can be easily assessed by careful systematic interrogation with two-dimensional (2D) and color Doppler analyses of the nonplanar ventricular septum (Figs. 108.6 and 108.7). Spectral Doppler can provide hemodynamic information, including pressure difference between the left and right chambers as determined by the simplified Bernoulli equation ($\Delta p = 4V^2$, with V being the peak Doppler velocity across the defect[7]). Spectral Doppler echocardiography can also give an estimate of right heart pressure based on tricuspid regurgitation velocity and pulmonary artery diastolic pressure based on pulmonary insufficiency velocity.

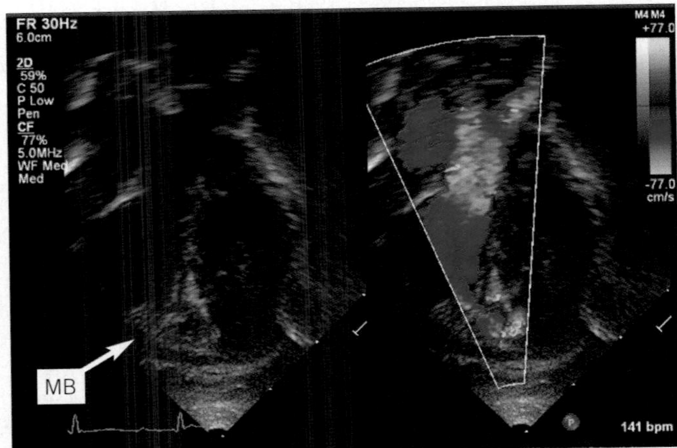

Figure 108.4 Apical four-chamber view angled anterior to the pulmonary artery. The moderator band (MB) is seen. Two muscular septal defects are present: one defect below the moderator band, termed apical muscular defect, and a second midmuscular defect above the moderator band.

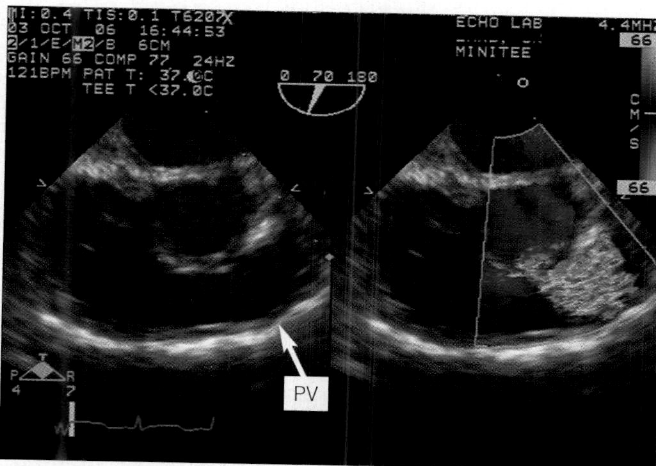

Figure 108.5 A supracristal ventricular septal defect with shunt just below the pulmonary valve (PV) is demonstrated on this transesophageal echocardiogram.

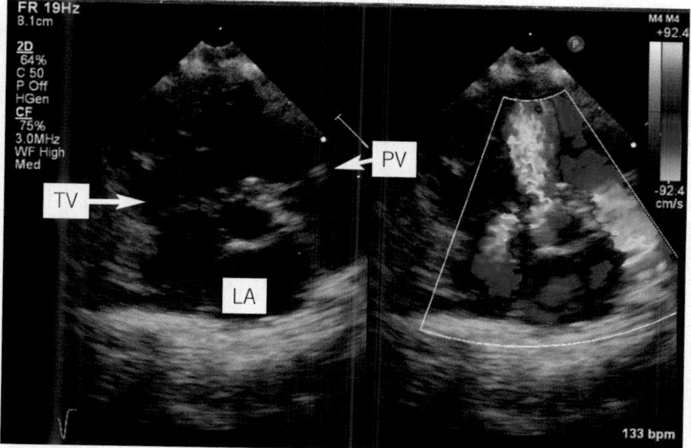

Figure 108.6 Parasternal cross-sectional view of a perimembranous defect. Tricuspid valve (TV), pulmonary valve (PV), and left atrium (LA) are seen. In contrast to Fig. 108.5, there is infundibulum separating the defect from the pulmonary valve.

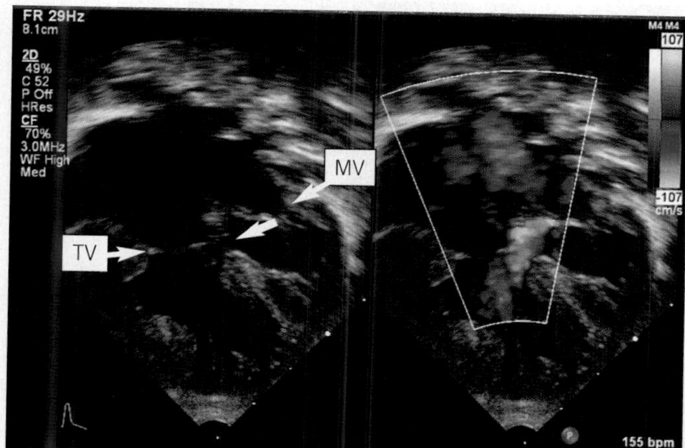

Figure 108.7 Apical four-chamber view angled posterior to the level of the mitral (MV) and tricuspid (TV) valves. An inlet defect is demonstrated (*arrow*).

Additionally, obstruction of the right ventricular outflow tract (double chamber physiology), insufficiency of the aortic valve, or distortion of the valve apparatus are all evaluated by echocardiography. When limitations in image quality of transthoracic echocardiography prevent evaluation of these aspects of the cardiovascular physiology, transesophageal imaging can be performed. Three-dimensional echocardiography has proven accurate for quantification of shunt[8] and can provide accurate visualization of defects otherwise difficult to evaluate by 2D imaging alone.[9]

Cardiac chamber size, great artery size, and annular measurements can be compared to normative data for body surface area in infants and children, which can help to guide management. Systolic function can be assessed using fractional shortening or ejection fraction methods. Combined systolic and diastolic function can be evaluated with the Tei index or myocardial performance index (MPI).[10] Tissue Doppler indices have been established in children[11] and have been shown to be normal in the setting of ventricular septal defects.[12] Echocardiography is pivotal in the diagnosis, monitoring, and management of ventricular septal defects.

Magnetic Resonance Imaging

Magnetic resonance imaging (MRI) can be used for delineation of ventricular septal defects in patients with complex associated lesions. Its use is rarely indicated for the evaluation of an isolated VSD.

Cardiac Catheterization

Though now used less commonly than in the past, catheterization can give accurate measurements of pulmonary vascular resistance, pulmonary reactivity, and volume of shunting. Response to pulmonary vasodilators can be determined and guide therapy. Angiography of the right ventricle (RV) and left ventricle (LV) and aortography can provide information on the location of a defect, number of defects, and degree of aortic insufficiency. The aortic valve can be inspected for integrity (Fig. 108.8).

MANAGEMENT

Medical Management

The small defect will likely require neither medical management nor any intervention. Each patient's condition should be followed for development of aortic insufficiency (in the case of perimembranous or supracristal defects) or tricuspid insufficiency. The medium and larger defects require varying degrees of medical management, surgical closure, or both. Congestive heart failure in the infant is treated with diuretics, digoxin, and at times, afterload reduction.[13,14]

The adult with an unrepaired ventricular septal defect in the current era would most likely have a small defect without evidence for left ventricular volume overload or alterations in the adjacent structures. Those with evidence for left ventricular volume overload or progressive aortic valve disease would be referred for closure in most institutions.

The adult who has undergone repair of ventricular septal defect needs surveillance for aortic valve dysfunction. Those adults with residual defects need continued monitoring and consideration for reoperation if there is left ventricular volume overload or progressive aortic valve dysfunction. Patients with residual defects adjacent to patch material should receive subacute bacterial endocarditis prophylaxis according to the new American Heart Association (AHA) recommendations.[15]

Patients with complex defects including Eisenmenger's syndrome need very specialized care at centers with personnel trained in the management of the myriad of potential medical problems. Arrhythmias, endocarditis, gallstones, gouty arthritis, hemoptysis, pulmonary artery thrombosis,

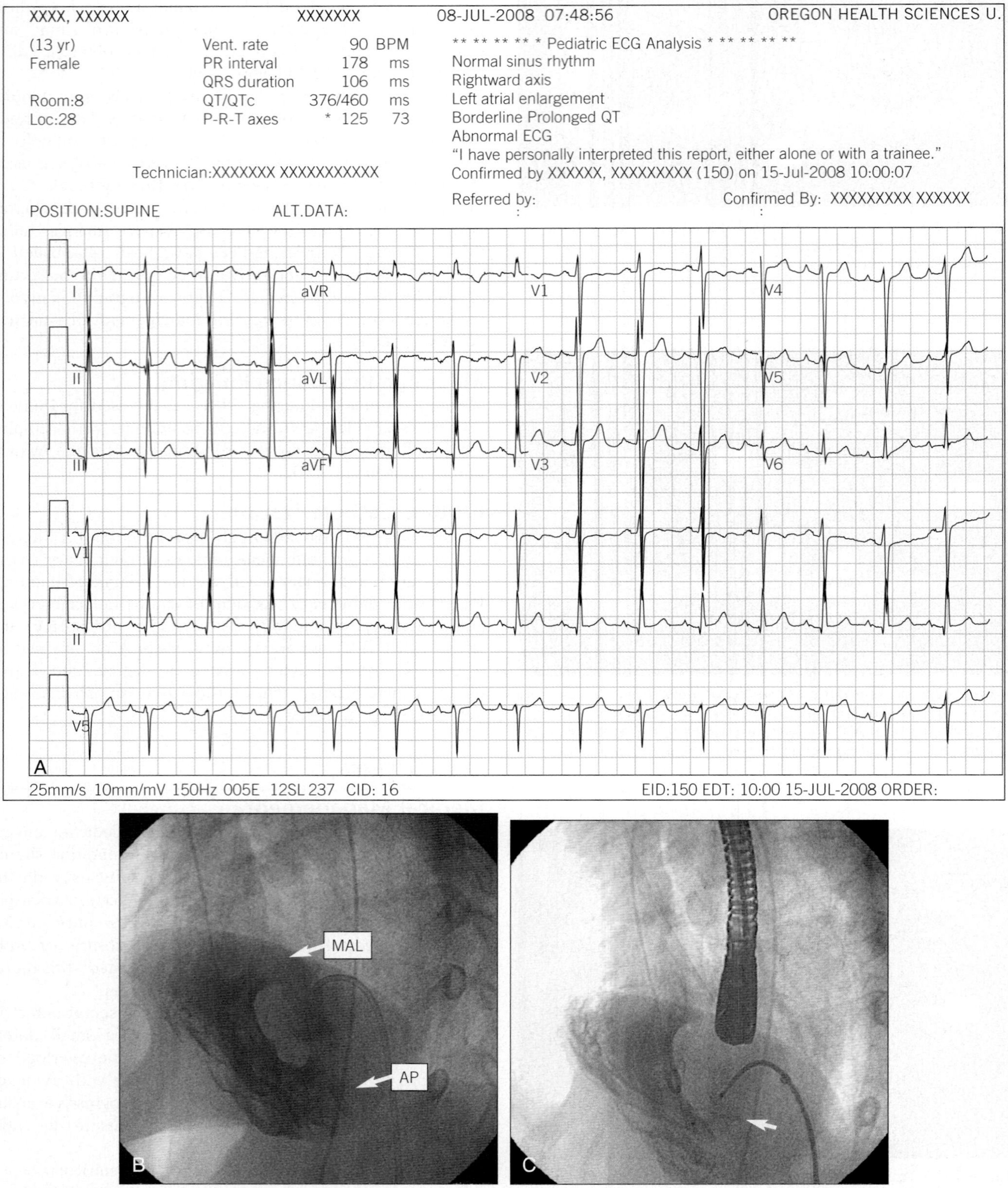

XXXX, XXXXXX XXXXXXX 08-JUL-2008 07:48:56 OREGON HEALTH SCIENCES U.
(13 yr) Female Room:8 Loc:28
Vent. rate 90 BPM
PR interval 178 ms
QRS duration 106 ms
QT/QTc 376/460 ms
P-R-T axes * 125 73
** ** ** ** * Pediatric ECG Analysis * ** ** ** **
Normal sinus rhythm
Rightward axis
Left atrial enlargement
Borderline Prolonged QT
Abnormal ECG
"I have personally interpreted this report, either alone or with a trainee."
Confirmed by XXXXXX, XXXXXXXXX (150) on 15-Jul-2008 10:00:07
Technician:XXXXXXX XXXXXXXXXXX
Referred by: : Confirmed By: XXXXXXXXX XXXXXX
POSITION:SUPINE ALT.DATA:
I aVR V1 V4 II aVL V2 V5 III aVF V3 V6 V1 II V5
A
25mm/s 10mm/mV 150Hz 005E 12SL 237 CID: 16 EID:150 EDT: 10:00 15-JUL-2008 ORDER:

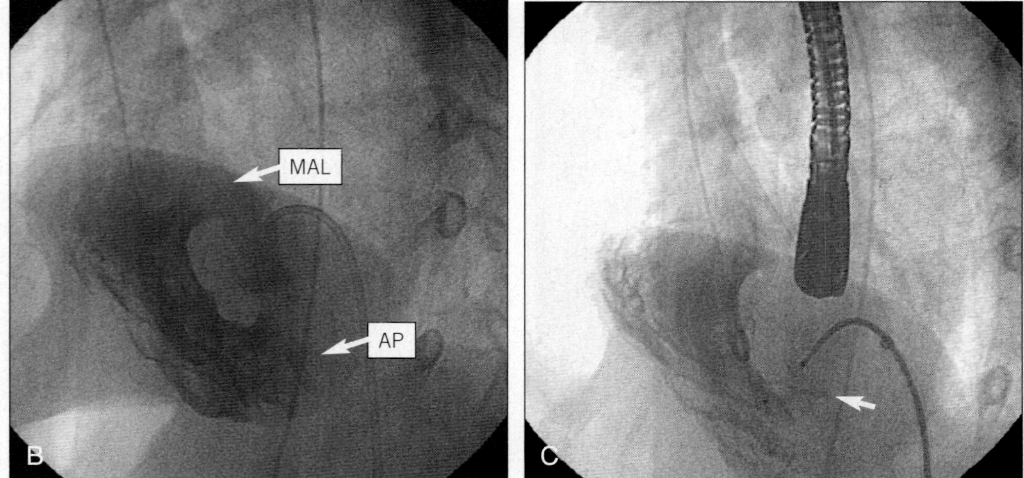

Figure 108.8 **A,** ECG in patient showing right axis deviation and left atrial enlargement. **B,** Angiography details the apical muscular defects (AP) and the large malalignment defect (MAL). **C,** The Amplatzer device is positioned within one of the apical defects (*arrow*).

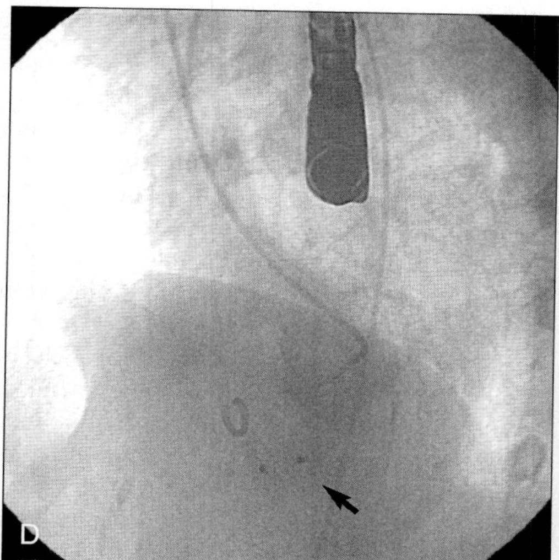

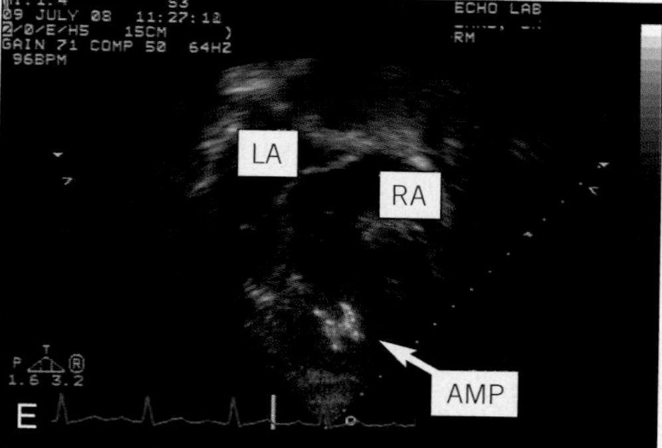

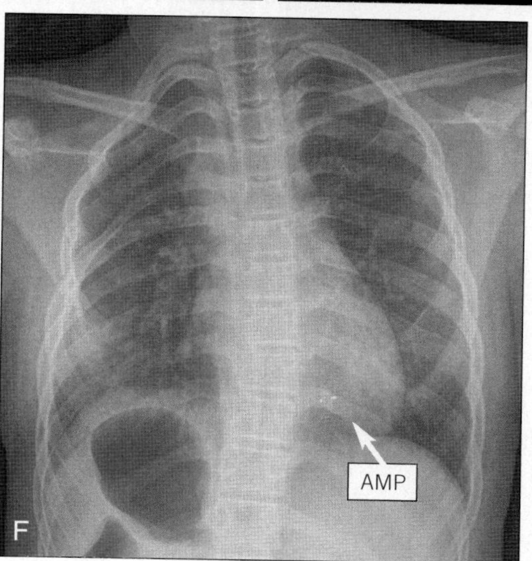

Figure 108.8—cont'd D, Postdeployment angiogram of an Amplatzer muscular ventricular septal defect occluder (*arrow*) with little residual flow seen in the apical region. **E,** Echocardiogram taken before discharge showing the Amplatzer device (AMP). RA, right atrium; LA, left atrium. **F,** Chest radiography showing visceroatrial situs inversus and the Amplatzer muscular ventricular septal defect occluder (AMP). ECG, angiography, echocardiography, and radiography in a patient with visceroatrial situs inversus, pulmonary atresia, and muscular and malalignment ventricular septal defects who underwent device closure in preparation for ventricular septation.

and symptomatic hypertrophic osteoarthropathy are frequently seen.[16] Pregnancy is poorly tolerated and many believe contraindicated in this disorder. Echocardiography and MRI are used for evaluation of right ventricular function. Cardiac catheterization is reserved for cases in which surgical or device closure is under consideration. Vasodilator therapy is an important adjunct to management and can provide functional improvement. Changes in $V{O_2}$ with exercise or Qp:Qs from MRI-derived cardiac output can be determined but are not generally used to guide therapy.

According to the new AHA guidelines, endocarditis prophylaxis is no longer recommended for ventricular septal defects. Exceptions are patients with a prior history of infective endocarditis, those patients within 6 months of surgical or device closure, or those with residual defects as mentioned previously.[15]

Surgical Closure

Indications for surgical closure vary, depending on the age of the patient and the location of the defect. In the case of infundibular defects, location has been used as an indication for surgical closure regardless of the need for medical management.[17] For all other types of defects, chamber enlargement is a measure of the degree of shunting, which may indicate the need for closure. A patient with growth failure refractory to medical therapy should be referred for closure. Catheterization can be used to help guide clinicians in some individuals by determining Qp:Qs and pulmonary artery pressure and resistance. Generally a Qp:Qs of 1.5:1 to 2:1[18] or evidence of increased pulmonary arteriolar resistance are indications for closure. In the setting of multiple muscular defects refractory to medical management, palliative pulmonary artery banding has been used rather than surgical closure.

Catheter Closure

Currently in the investigational stages are the Amplatzer ventricular septal defect occluders, of which there are muscular and perimembranous types (AGA Medical Corporation, Golden Valley, Minn). Initial experience has shown a 92% to 100% complete closure rate, with trace aortic insufficiency the primary complication seen in those series.[19] The muscular occluder has also shown similar success, with 92% to 93% complete closure rate. Device-related complications in the largest series were most common in patients weighing less than 5 kg and included cardiac perforation, embolization, complete heart block, and death.[20]

Traditionally, imaging during deployment of occluder devices has been transesophageal echocardiography (TEE). Intracardiac echocardiography (ICE) can now be used with similarly accurate measurements and safety compared to TEE.[21]

Studies using an open chest animal model and a periventricular technique for device deployment have been successful for perimembranous defects.[22] A similar technique has been used for muscular or multiple muscular defects.[23] In patients with difficult vascular access or those with contraindications to cardiopulmonary bypass, this technique provides a further reduction in the invasiveness of closure and could allow therapy for these patients in the future.

PROGNOSIS

The prognosis for small defects is very good, with most becoming smaller with time, particularly the muscular defects, which have a high rate of spontaneous closure. With medium-sized and large defects, the likelihood of spontaneous closure decreases. Advances in surgical and bypass techniques and timing of surgical repair have decreased the morbidity associated with surgical closure. The early era of repair showed an 80% closure rate in catheterized patients at long-term follow-up. In that study of 258 patients, 9 had complete heart block, 37 had transient heart block, and 168 had right bundle branch block. Endocarditis occurred in nine patients (11.4/10,000 patient-years).[24] Later studies have shown residual defects in 31% of patients, and an incidence of complete heart block of 3.1%.[25] Another study showed occurrence rates for pacemaker placement of 9.8/10,000 patient-years and occurrence rates for endocarditis of 16.3/10,000 patient-years in operated patients.[26]

SUMMARY

Ventricular septal defects are the most common congenital defect, and therapy is varied depending on the anatomic and clinical status of each patient. Morbidity and mortality with surgical therapy are clearly improving. Advances in catheter-based closure are ushering in yet another new era.

chapter 109

Tetralogy of Fallot and Common Arterial Trunk

Sonya V. Babu-Narayan, Natali A. Y. Chung, Darryl F. Shore, and Michael A. Gatzoulis

Definitions

- Tetralogy of Fallot comprises subpulmonary infundibular stenosis, right ventricle (RV) hypertrophy, rightward deviation of the aorta with biventricular origin of the aortic valve leaflets, and malalignment ventricular septal defect, all of which are explained by anterocephalad deviation of the outlet septum and hypertrophy of trabeculations on the infundibular free wall.
- Common arterial trunk is a congenital anomaly that consists of a large ventricular septal defect and a single arterial trunk (vessel) that gives rise to the coronary arteries and the pulmonary arteries. In common arterial trunk, there is no direct communication between the pulmonary arteries and the ventricular mass—not even through an atretic and miniature pulmonary trunk, as seen in some cases of tetralogy of Fallot with pulmonary atresia.

Key Features

- Tetralogy of Fallot is the most common cyanotic congenital heart disease, and the number of adults with this condition is growing since the advent of reparative surgery in the 1950s. The prognosis of repaired tetralogy of Fallot is very good, though late arrhythmia, heart failure, and sudden cardiac death remain problematic.
- Truncus arteriosus may cause congestive heart failure in early infancy and has a poor prognosis if left untreated.

Therapy

- Primary repair of tetralogy of Fallot is usual, but a Blalock-Taussig shunt may still be necessary in early infancy. Timing of reintervention, particularly for pulmonary regurgitation in adulthood, is a major clinical concern.
- Early primary cardiac repair is the treatment of choice in selected patients, but there is a high rate of reintervention.

TETRALOGY OF FALLOT

Tetralogy of Fallot accounts for up to 10% of all congenital heart diseases and is the most common cyanotic congenital heart disease. The clinical presentation is variable and depends on the degree of right ventricular (RV) outflow tract obstruction. Frequently, the diagnosis is made because of auscultation of a murmur in the neonate. But it may be made in utero with antenatal diagnosis using fetal echocardiography or in childhood when cyanosis becomes more obvious and cyanotic spells can also develop. Reparative surgery has transformed the prognosis for children born with tetralogy of Fallot and survival beyond 30 years is now greater than 90%.[1,2] There is late attrition due to arrhythmia, heart failure, and sudden death.[3,4] Clinical follow-up following repair is aimed at identifying and modifying risk factors for morbidity and mortality, throughout life's stages including pregnancy. This may involve addressing residual hemodynamic lesions or sequelae of surgical repair.

ANATOMY AND PATHOLOGY

Fallot separated the malformation to which we now ascribe his name in 1888. Although autopsy cases had been recognized previously, he was the first to show clinicopathologic correlation. The condition comprises four constants: subpulmonary infundibular stenosis, ventricular septal defect, rightward deviation of the aortic valve with biventricular origin of its leaflets, and RV hypertrophy. The unifying feature is anterocephalad deviation of the outlet septum (the muscular structure that separates the subaortic from the subpulmonary outlets), in relationship to the rest of the muscular septum, together with hypertrophy of the normally small septoparietal trabeculations, such that the outflow tract beneath the pulmonary valve becomes narrow and there is resultant RV hypertrophy, malalignment, and usually perimembranous ventricular septal defect and aortic override (Fig. 109.1). There is a spectrum of morphologic variations regarding the degree, site, and extent of RV outflow obstruction, which may extend from the subpulmonary infundibulum to involve a small (sometimes bicuspid) pulmonary valve and trunk and small branch pulmonary arteries. Tetralogy of Fallot with pulmonary atresia is discussed in Chapter 111.

Variants associated with a higher chance of having 22q11 deletion, present in 15% of cases of tetralogy of Fallot, include those with right aortic arch (25% to 30%), other aortic arch abnormalities, such as aberrant subclavian artery or double aortic arch, pulmonary atresia and major aortopulmonary collateral arteries, disconnected origin of a branch pulmonary artery (typically left), and those with absent pulmonary valve syndrome (3%). The latter is associated with aneurysmal pulmonary artery dilatation, which can be sufficiently severe to cause bronchial compression in fetal life.

Additional lesions, including secundum atrial septal defect (so called pentalogy of Fallot), patent ductus arteriosus, or patent foramen ovale, may be present, or more rarely additional muscular ventricular septal defect, and atrioventricular septal defect (<1%), particularly seen with trisomy 21. Coronary artery anomalies, including single coronary artery, are present in about 3% to 5% of patients who have tetralogy of Fallot.

Additional sources of pulmonary blood supply in severe tetralogy of Fallot include patent ductus arteriosus, coronary to pulmonary artery fistula, systemic to pulmonary collateral arteries, or aortopulmonary window.

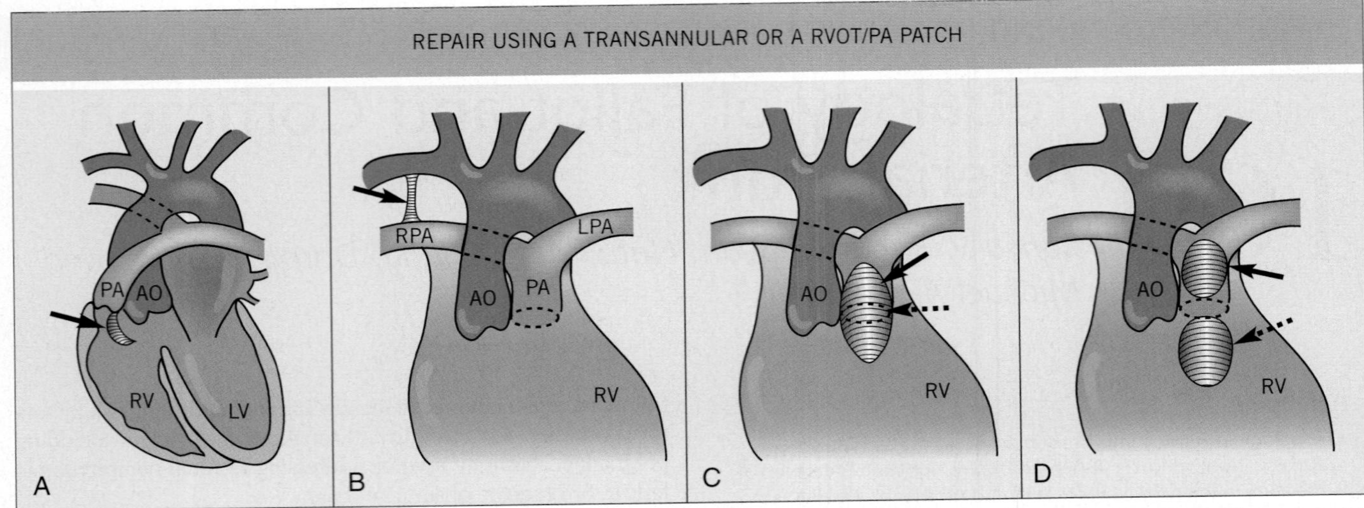

Figure 109.1 Drawings showing underlying anatomy (A), most common palliative shunt (B), repair using a transannular patch (C) and repair using a right ventricular outflow tract (RVOT) and pulmonary artery (PA) patch (D), in tetralogy of Fallot. A, The underlying anatomic substrate of tetralogy of Fallot. Anterocephalad deviation of the outlet septum (*arrow*) is the key anatomic feature leading to subpulmonary stenosis, ventricular septal defect, aortic override, and right ventricular hypertrophy. **B**, A right-sided modified Blalock-Taussig shunt (*arrow*) from the right subclavian artery to the right pulmonary artery. **C**, Use of a transannular patch (*solid arrow*) to augment the right ventricular outflow tract and main pulmonary artery (pulmonary valve annulus level, *dotted oval*; *dashed arrow*). This is associated with pulmonary regurgitation in follow-up. **D**, Use of a pulmonary artery patch (*solid arrow*) and a right ventricular outflow tract patch (*dashed arrow*), allowing augmentation of the pulmonary artery and right ventricular outflow tract while sparing the pulmonary valve (pulmonary valve annulus level marked by dotted oval). If outflow tract patching is avoidable, the patient can be spared right ventriculotomy.

CLINICAL PRESENTATIONS

Early Presentation of the Unrepaired Patient

Patients usually present in the first days of life with a murmur, which is evident from day one of life, in contrast to isolated ventricular septal defect where the murmur only becomes apparent once pulmonary vascular resistance falls. Morphologic differences explain varying degrees of cyanosis and hypoxemia and hence differing clinical presentation; for example, pulmonary stenosis may be sufficiently mild that there is so-called acyanotic or pink tetralogy. Alternatively, cyanosis may result in skin discoloration and clubbing and cyanotic spells, the pathophysiology and management of which have been previously explained.

The cardiac impulse is maximal at the lower left sternal border, indicating RV hypertrophy. On auscultation, the second heart sound, pulmonary closure, is not heard. A systolic ejection murmur is present, also at the third left sternal border. The loudness of the systolic murmur reflects pulmonary blood flow through the stenotic RV outflow tract; the loudest systolic murmur is heard in acyanotic tetralogy of Fallot, and no murmur is heard in tetralogy of Fallot with pulmonary atresia. A continuous murmur at the second left intercostal space indicates either an associated patent ductus arteriosus or a previous, patent Blalock-Taussig shunt. A continuous murmur heard at the back suggests the presence of associated major aortopulmonary collateral arteries.

Cyanosis, Hypoxemia, and Cyanotic Spells in Children

If the degree of pulmonary stenosis is very mild, the interventricular shunt remains left to right and there is no cyanosis. Occasionally, this may present with heart failure due to increased pulmonary circulation. Cyanosis may develop between 6 and 8 months as infundibular stenosis increases, producing a bidirectional or right-to-left shunt. Cyanosis may initially be apparent only when systemic venous return increases, systemic vascular resistance decreases, or pulmonary vascular resistance increases, such as during crying or bathing. Hypercyanotic attacks are consequent to dynamic outflow tract obstruction superimposed on fixed anatomic obstruction. These are caused by sudden decrease in systemic vascular resistance, which increases systemic venous return and increases pulmonary stenosis; these are classically triggered by crying, defecating, or feeding, which increase oxygen demand and are associated with increased systemic venous return. Further distress exacerbates symptoms. Because the anatomic lesion results in relatively fixed pulmonary blood flow, these events cause a decrease in aortic oxygen saturation, general hypoxia, and metabolic acidosis, which in turn stimulate the respiratory center, causing hyperventilation and increased catecholamine concentrations. Catecholamines increase dynamic infundibular stenosis, which further decreases pulmonary blood flow, further increases hyperventilation, systemic venous return increases further, and a vicious cycle occurs, causing the cyanotic spell. Decreased pulmonary blood flow results in hypercapnia, respiratory acidosis, and deeper hypoxemia. Hypoxemia causes metabolic acidosis, unconsciousness, and convulsions. Intracranial thrombosis and death may follow. Characteristically, children with symptomatic tetralogy of Fallot take a squatting position to increase systemic vascular resistance by compressing the abdominal aorta and abdominal organs and increase systemic venous return by compressing leg veins and the splanchnic venous pool. Increased venous return and increased aortic pressure open up the RV infundibulum, and these hemodynamic effects increase aortic oxygen saturation. Medical treatment involves adoption of a knee to chest position, and administration of intramuscular morphine, oxygen, and intravenous propranolol if prolonged to relieve infundibular contraction. Underlying iron deficiency anemia needs addressing, and propranolol can be prescribed prophylactically. Rarely an emergency systemic-pulmonary shunt is required.

Clinical Assessment in the Older Repaired Patient

In the absence of a clear operative history the presence of a thoracotomy will suggest previous palliative shunt, and the ipsilateral brachial pulse will be absent if there has been a classic Blalock-Taussig shunt. When assessing repaired tetralogy, a normal oxygen saturation should be expected. Signs of important pulmonary regurgitation that should be actively sought are a single second heart sound due to absent pulmonary component, a to-and-fro murmur in the pulmonary area, RV heave, a new pansystolic murmur of tricuspid regurgitation, or, in advanced cases, signs of right heart failure. The murmur of severe pulmonary regurgitation can be very short and therefore easy to underestimate. Diagnostic imaging, therefore, has an important role.

DIAGNOSTIC TECHNIQUES

Electrocardiography

Preoperatively the electrocardiogram (ECG) of tetralogy of Fallot shows dominant tall R waves in leads V_4R and V_1, and a dominant S wave in lead V_6. Sinus rhythm is expected. A right bundle branch block pattern reflecting previous ventriculotomy (Fig. 109.2) or infundibular resection/ventricular septal defect (VSD) patch sutures is very common. QRS duration and change in QRS duration should be noted from the ECG, because prolonged QRS duration, particularly above 180 msec, and increase in QRS duration with time relate to RV dilatation consequent to pulmonary regurgitation and are risk factors for sudden death.

Chest Radiography

Normal situs solitus pattern is present. A right aortic arch is present in 25% to 30% of cases. The cardiac silhouette may show a prominent RV with concavity in the main pulmonary artery area and a lifted apex sometimes referred to as a boot-shaped heart. Aneurysmal dilatation of the central pulmonary arteries or of the RV outflow tract following surgery may be evident. Calcification of an RV to pulmonary artery conduit may be present. Right heart dilatation may be apparent from retrosternal filling on a lateral chest x-ray (Fig. 109.3). The cardiothoracic ratio should be examined on the chest radiograph, because increased heart size could relate to progressive pulmonary regurgitation.

Echocardiography

Echocardiography is very useful in making a definitive diagnosis of tetralogy of Fallot and identifying additional anomalies. The diagnosis of tetralogy of Fallot can now be made antenatally with fetal echocardiography, and in general the severity of RV outflow tract obstruction can be predicted by the ratio of the main pulmonary artery to the ascending aorta in the midtrimester fetus, potentially allowing planned postnatal care in severe cases.[5] The dilated central pulmonary arteries associated with absent pulmonary valve syndrome can also be identified. In children, echocardiography includes assessment of proximal coronary arteries. An anomalous coronary artery crossing in front of the RV outflow tract will necessitate a different surgical approach (Fig. 109.4).

Echocardiography is also used to detect the presence of so-called RV restrictive physiology. This is defined as

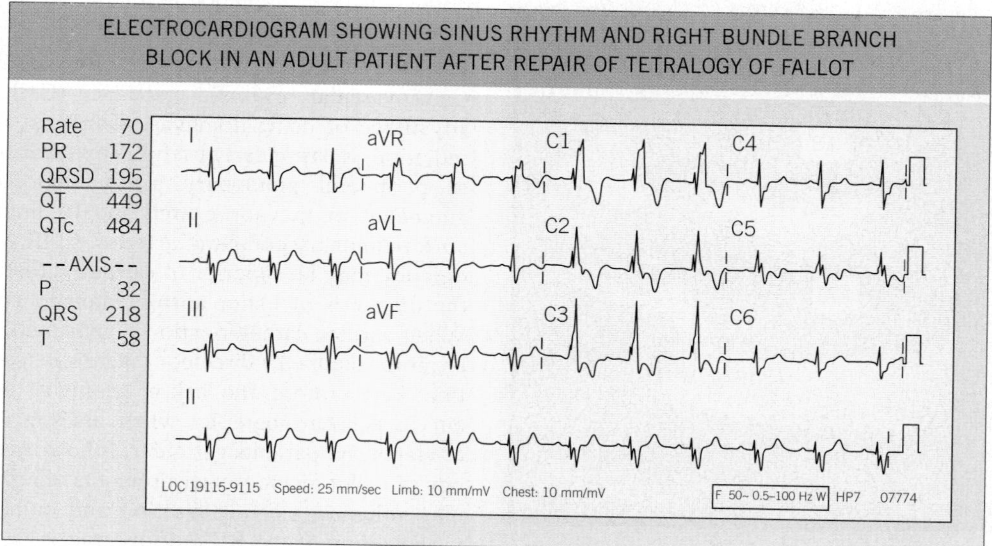

Figure 109.2 Electrocardiogram showing sinus rhythm and right bundle branch block in an adult patient after repair of tetralogy of Fallot. The patient had right bundle branch block from the time of repair due to the right ventriculotomy. The RSR pattern is typical for previous right ventriculotomy. The QRS duration is prolonged at 195 msec. This should be followed over time because increasing QRS duration may reflect increasing RV dilatation due to pulmonary regurgitation. A QRS duration above 180 msec has been shown to be a risk factor for sustained ventricular tachycardia and sudden cardiac death.

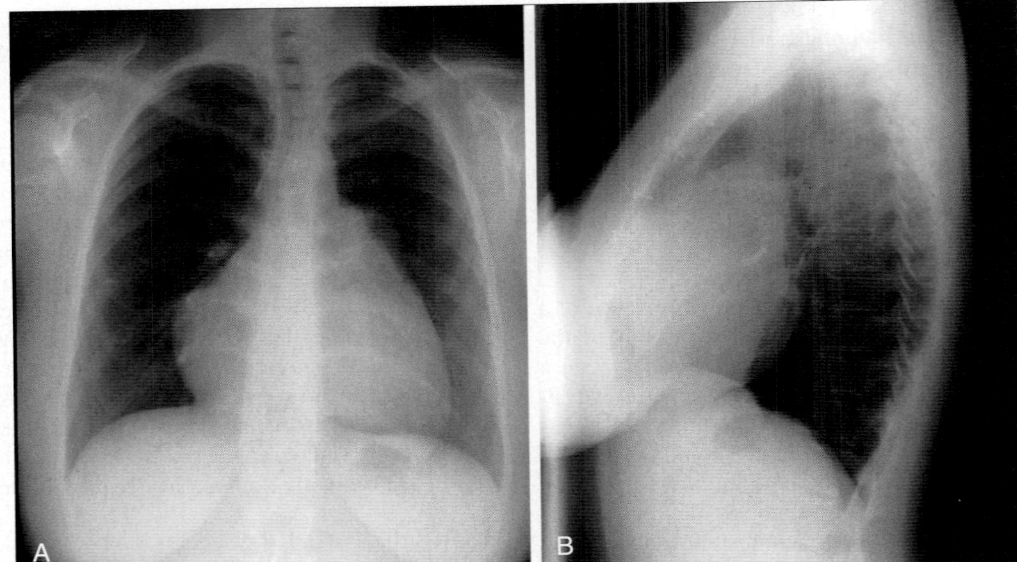

Figure 109.3 Postanterior and lateral chest x-rays. A, A posteroanterior chest x-ray after repair of tetralogy of Fallot showing sternotomy wires and evidence of left thoracotomy suggestive of previous left Blalock-Taussig shunt. There is situs solitus, levocardia, left aortic arch with small aortic knuckle relative to dilatation of right ventricular outflow tract and pulmonary artery, increased right heart border suggestive of right atrial dilatation, and cardiomegaly. The reduced pulmonary vascular markings suggest potential residual right ventricular outflow tract obstruction. **B**, A lateral chest x-ray demonstrating retrosternal filling consistent with right ventricular dilatation.

anterograde flow in the pulmonary artery in late diastole throughout the respiratory cycle on Doppler echocardiography and is discussed in the following section (Fig. 109.5).[6]

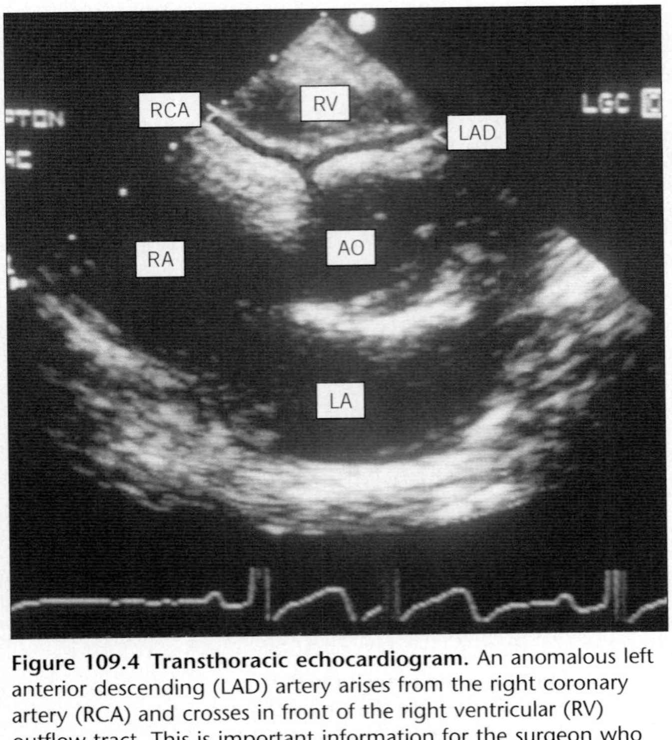

Figure 109.4 Transthoracic echocardiogram. An anomalous left anterior descending (LAD) artery arises from the right coronary artery (RCA) and crosses in front of the right ventricular (RV) outflow tract. This is important information for the surgeon who may need to insert a right ventricular to pulmonary artery conduit to avoid damage to the coronary arteries when trying to relieve native right ventricular outflow tract obstruction. AO, aorta; LA, left atrium; RA, right atrium. (Echocardiography image courtesy of Dr. Michael L. Rigby, Royal Brompton Hospital.)

Additional imaging assessment with cardiovascular magnetic resonance, computed tomography (CT) scanning, or cardiac catheterization is not usually necessary in children where echocardiographic windows are good. Additional imaging, however, may have a role in definitive diagnosis of stenosis and hypoplasia of peripheral pulmonary arteries, anomalies of the coronary arteries, anomalies of the aortic arch and its branches, and major aortopulmonary collateral arteries and in quantification of pulmonary regurgitation in follow-up after repair.

Cardiovascular Magnetic Resonance

Cardiovascular magnetic resonance (CMR), which has the advantage of being noninvasive and not requiring ionizing radiation, is particularly useful in extracardiac anatomy, such as peripheral pulmonary artery stenosis or hypoplasia, anomalies of the aortic arch and its branches, and major aortopulmonary collateral arteries. CMR with contrast angiography may be superior to cardiac catheterization alone in the diagnosis of major aortopulmonary collateral arteries.[7] When cardiac catheterization is indicated, CMR can enable a more planned, directed diagnostic study or intervention. Furthermore, the lack of geometric assumptions inherent in echocardiography when assessing RV function are obviated. As patients get older, follow-up of repaired tetralogy of Fallot includes measurements of right and left ventricular volumes, ejection fraction and myocardial mass, cine visualization of the RV outflow tract to assess presence and extent of akinetic and or aneurysmal RV outflow tract areas, measurements of left and right pulmonary arteries, measurement of any aortic root dilatation, and measurement of pulmonary regurgitant fraction by through-plane velocity mapping (Fig. 109.6). Of note, "free" pulmonary regurgitation is not usually more than 40% (diastolic reversed flow expressed as a percentage of forward flow), unless made

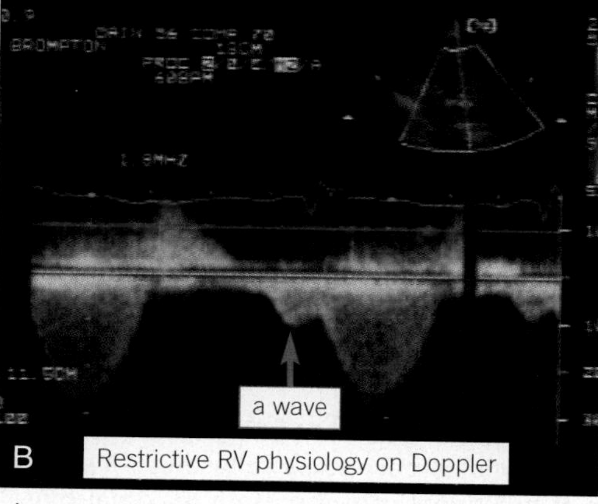

Figure 109.5 A, Four-chamber view from cardiovascular magnetic resonance imaging showing severe right ventricular dilatation with mild tricuspid regurgitation (*arrow*). **B**, Doppler echocardiography at the level of the pulmonary valve. There is pulmonary regurgitation of short duration and then anterograde flow in late diastole coinciding with atrial systole, the "a wave" (*arrow*). The latter was present throughout the respiratory cycle. This well-described phenomenon is consistent with restrictive right ventricular physiology. LV, left ventricle; RV, right ventricle. (Echocardiography image courtesy of Dr. Wei Li, Royal Brompton Hospital.)

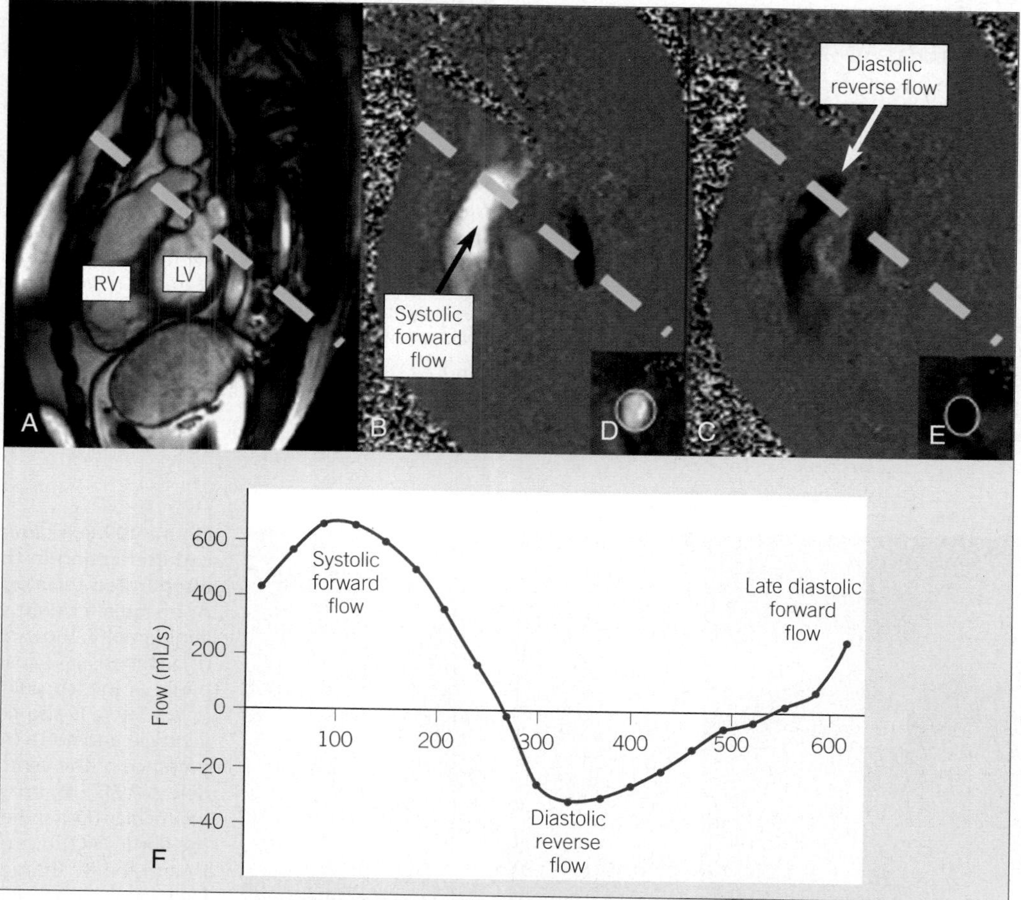

Figure 109.6 Cardiovascular magnetic resonance. A, Still frame from a steady-state free precession magnetic resonance cine image demonstrating the right ventricular (RV), RV outflow tract, and pulmonary trunk late after repair of tetralogy of Fallot. **B**, Systolic frame from a corresponding in-plane phase encoded velocity map demonstrating unobstructed forward flow into the pulmonary artery, which appears white. **C**, Diastolic frame from the same velocity map demonstrating reverse flow from the pulmonary artery into the right ventricular outflow tract, which appears black. These suggest significant pulmonary regurgitation. The in-plane velocity map and cine images can be used to pilot a through-plane velocity map through the pulmonary trunk, giving comparable systolic and diastolic images (**D** and **E**). The region of interest can be manually planimetered to derive a flow curve of pulmonary blood flow. Pulmonary regurgitant fraction can be derived from integration of areas contained by forward and reversed flow curves (**F**). Significant pulmonary regurgitation is usually above 30% and rarely above 40% in the absence of additional distal pathology, such as branch or peripheral pulmonary artery stenosis.

worse by the presence of pulmonary artery branch stenosis or other distal factors. CMR contributes to assessment of global and regional right and left ventricular function, timing of surgical pulmonary valve replacement, identification of other asymptomatic lesions that merit reintervention, and suitability for transcatheter pulmonary valve implantation. Furthermore, newly described late gadolinium enhancement imaging, which documents myocardial fibrosis, contributes to risk stratification for ventricular tachycardia and sudden cardiac death (Fig. 109.7).[8]

Cardiopulmonary Exercise Testing

Where available, cardiopulmonary exercise testing is a useful objective marker of functional capacity. Both maximal oxygen uptake and V_E/V_{CO_2} slope have prognostic value.[9-11] Interval change in these parameters provides reliable guidance on the need for and the optimal timing of reintervention and potentially can assess the benefit of interventions.

Cardiac Catheterization and Electrophysiology

Cardiac catheterization (Fig. 109.8) is generally reserved for when adequate assessment of hemodynamics cannot be obtained by noninvasive means, for transcatheter intervention, and commonly when surgical reintervention is planned in adults. Selective coronary angiography is performed when clinically indicated or as part of preoperative assessment for elective redo surgery in older patients. In selected patients, electrophysiologic study to map and treat atrial or ventricular arrhythmias and to assess the risk of sudden death may be indicated, though hemodynamic target lesions should be assessed first.[12,13] Some patients may merit secondary or primary prevention of sudden cardiac death through insertion of an internal cardiac defibrillator, which needs expert consideration given that inappropriate shocks and complications are common.[14]

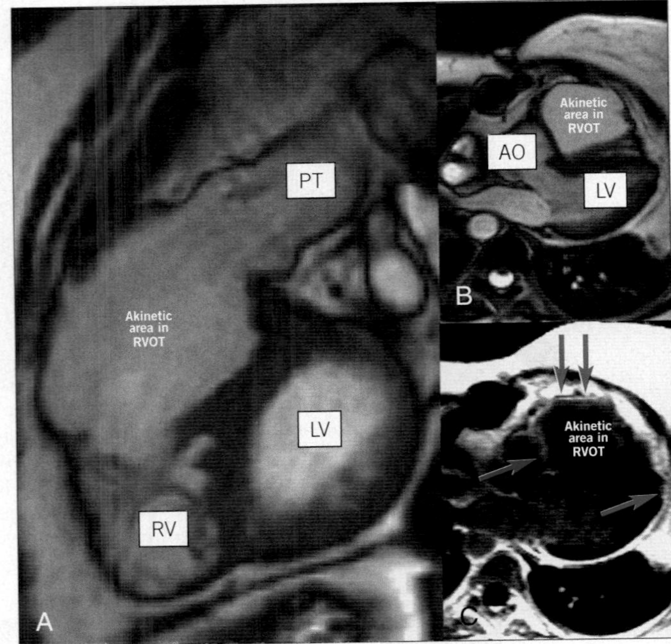

Figure 109.7 Cardiovascular magnetic resonance. A, Still frame from a steady-state free precession magnetic resonance cine image demonstrating the right ventricular outflow tract (RVOT) and pulmonary trunk (PT) late after repair of tetralogy of Fallot. Thinning of the free wall of the RVOT is seen corresponding to akinesia of this region. **B**, Still image from a left ventricular outflow tract cine image. Inversion recovery imaging after administration of gadolinium contrast in **C** shows that the akinetic region appears white compared to the normal black myocardium, suggestive of myocardial fibrosis or scarring in this region (*red arrows*). There is also scarring associated with the repair of ventricular septal defect (*blue arrow*) and use of apical vent (*green arrow*). AO, aorta; LV, left ventricle; RV, right ventricle.

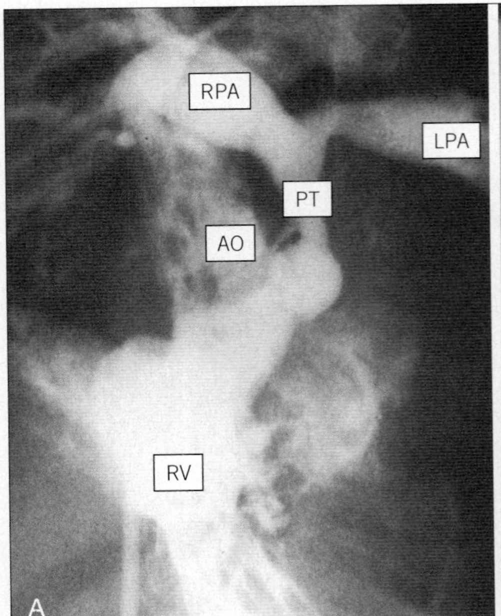

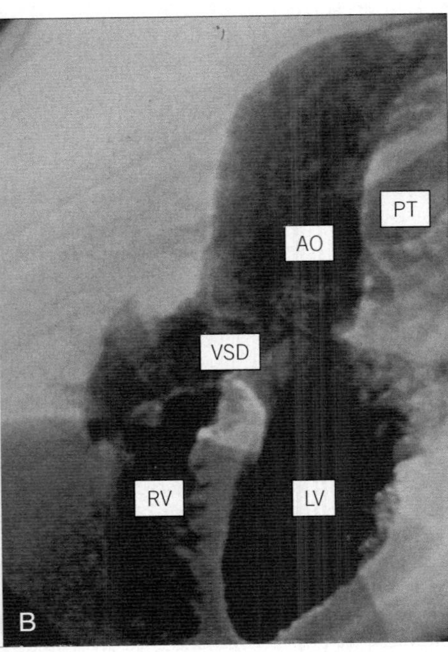

Figure 109.8 Images from cardiac catheterization in the setting of unoperated tetralogy of Fallot. A, Image after right ventricular (RV) angiography, shows pulmonary trunk (PT) stenosis and coarctation of the origin of the left pulmonary artery (LPA). There is also filling of the left ventricle and aorta (AO) due to the presence of the ventricular septal defect (VSD). **B**, Image after left ventricular (LV) angiography, shows the aortic (AO) override, filling of the LV and the RV through the VSD, and filling of the smaller pulmonary trunk (PT). RPA, right pulmonary artery. (Cardiac catheterization images courtesy of Dr. Michael L. Rigby, Royal Brompton Hospital.)

MANAGEMENT

Unrepaired Patients

Surgical Palliative Procedures

Palliative surgery includes

- the Blalock-Taussig shunt, (subclavian artery to pulmonary artery shunt; traditional is an end-to-end anastomosis and modified involves the interposition of a GORE-TEX graft);
- the Waterston shunt (ascending aorta to right pulmonary artery); and
- the Brock operation (transpulmonary infundibular resection and pulmonary valvotomy).

Most older adult patients have had one or more palliative procedures before repair, though contemporary patients frequently undergo primary repair at presentation or when symptomatic. A Blalock-Taussig shunt is still used for infants who are too small to have intracardiac repair, and for those patients in whom severe pulmonary arterial hypoplasia necessitates postponing repair to allow for pulmonary arterial growth or foregoing definitive repair.

Surgical Repair

Definitive intracardiac repair includes relief of RV outflow tract and patch closure of the ventricular septal defect. Surgical mortality in a large-volume center is less than 1%. Surgical strategies have evolved. Early cohorts were repaired via a right ventriculotomy, but currently repair is via a transatrial, transpulmonary approach where possible, to avoid the detrimental effects of ventriculotomy, including arrhythmia propensity. Transannular patching (patch augmentation that disrupts the pulmonary valve annulus) to relieve obstruction is now used sparingly if possible to preserve pulmonary valve function, and residual mild pulmonary stenosis is now seen as preferable to free pulmonary regurgitation. Younger age at repair results in better outcomes, and there appears to be no benefit in delaying elective repair of tetralogy of Fallot after the end of the first year. Neonatal repair is also advocated, but it remains unclear whether the benefits of early relief of cyanosis by primary neonatal repair versus palliative shunt and later repair outweigh neurologic concerns about cardiopulmonary bypass in neonates. It may be that the increased use of transannular patching associated with more harmful pulmonary regurgitation and increased use of finite life-span RV to pulmonary conduits will result in greater need for further bypass surgery for redo surgical intervention.

MANAGEMENT

Repaired Patients

Late Repair

The vast majority of patients with tetralogy of Fallot present in infancy. However, when the RV obstruction is not extreme, patients often have minimal cyanosis and may occasionally present in adulthood. Occasionally older patients who have had only palliative operations in childhood may also present to the adult cardiologist for follow-up. Though other comorbidity, such as acquired heart disease, must be considered, reparative surgery may still be indicated on symptomatic and prognostic grounds, albeit that late repair is associated with somewhat higher perioperative risk and more limited benefits.

Lifetime Outpatient Surveillance

Most adults with repaired tetralogy of Fallot lead unrestricted lives. Late symptoms include exertional dyspnea, palpitations, syncope, or sudden cardiac death. The latter may be the first clinical presentation of arrhythmia. Investigations are directed toward identification of late hemodynamic complications that may merit reintervention and toward preservation of biventricular function. Such investigations may vary according to the underlying anatomy, type of interventions previously performed, locally available facilities, and patient status.

Suggested regular investigations for all patients with varying interval according to their hemodynamic status are clinical examination, 12-lead ECG, posteroanterior and lateral chest x-rays, echocardiogram, cardiopulmonary exercise testing, and cardiovascular magnetic resonance imaging. Some patients may also benefit from additional investigation including Holter monitoring (when clinically indicated), quantitative lung perfusion scan (if significant branch pulmonary artery stenosis is suspected and where cardiovascular magnetic resonance is unavailable or contraindicated), multislice computed tomography, cardiac catheterization, and electrophysiologic study.

Reintervention, Arrhythmia, and Risk Stratification for Sudden Cardiac Death

A common reason for discussion of reintervention is pulmonary regurgitation and progressive RV dilatation in late follow-up, which is discussed separately in following sections. Potential indications for surgical or transcatheter reintervention dependent on severity include addressing

- pulmonary regurgitation and progressive RV dilatation;
- residual ventricular septal defect;
- RV outflow tract obstruction at subvalvar, valvar, or supravalvar levels, including branch pulmonary artery stenoses;
- patent arterial shunt causing left ventricular volume overload;
- aortic regurgitation;
- aortic root enlargement; and
- combinations of several mild lesions.

In common with other congenital heart diseases, clinical arrhythmia may need to be treated by targeting the underlying hemodynamic substrate, such as tricuspid regurgitation in the case of atrial flutter and pulmonary regurgitation in the case of ventricular tachycardia, with or without concomitant surgical cryoablation. However, in other patients electrophysiologic ablation to target arrhythmia may be indicated, particularly if there is no target hemodynamic lesion.[12] Together with a QRS duration greater than 180 msec on 12-lead ECG and left ventricular dysfunction, pulmonary regurgitation is a risk factor for sudden cardiac death.[4,15] The latter affects up to 6% of patients over the long term. Pulmonary valve implantation may lessen the risk of arrhythmia.[16] Selected patients presenting with symptomatic ventricular tachycardia, biventricular dysfunction, or inducible ventricular tachycardia on ventricular stimulation study may warrant internal cardiac defibrillator insertion.[13,14] It may be that late gadolinium cardiovascular magnetic resonance to detect burden of myocardial fibrosis has a role in risk stratification for defibrillator insertion, but this needs to be investigated.[8] Biventricular pacing has also been described. About a third of patients with repairs have evidence of asynchrony, but of note, though there is interventricular delay, a large contribution to delay is intraventricular between the RV and RV outflow tract and within the RV outflow tract itself, meaning resynchronization therapy would have to address the infundibulum.[17]

Pulmonary Regurgitation and Timing of Pulmonary Valve Implantation

Pulmonary regurgitation after repair of tetralogy of Fallot, hitherto considered relatively benign, is in fact associated with arrhythmia, late heart failure, and sudden cardiac death. If there were such a thing as a perfect pulmonary valve prosthesis, the decision regarding timing of pulmonary valve replacement would be easier. All currently available bioprostheses, however, have a finite life span and the longevity of a second homograft may be shorter than the first. Balancing the risk of late RV dysfunction, arrhythmia, and sudden cardiac death in these patients against the finite life span of a bioprosthetic valve and inherent risks of surgery leads to debate over the optimal timing of pulmonary valve replacement.[18] There is an increasingly held view that pulmonary valve replacement is happening too late for optimal benefit and that delayed intervention may risk avoidable irreversible RV damage. Our criteria for pulmonary valve implantation are one or more of the following:

- moderate/severe pulmonary regurgitation;
- RV dilatation/progressive CMR-derived end-systolic volumes;
- objective exercise intolerance (more than expected);
- progressive deterioration in exercise tolerance (objective);
- further QRS prolongation; and
- early symptoms (fatigue, mild shortness of breath, sustained arrhythmia).

Following pulmonary valve replacement, RV volume is reduced and systolic function may also improve.[19] Recently, transcatheter pulmonary valve implantation, using a stent-mounted bovine jugular venous valve in patients with pulmonary regurgitation and a degree of residual stenosis after previous surgical implantation of a valved conduit, has been introduced (Fig. 109.9).[20] This pioneering technique is not yet applicable to severe pulmonary regurgitation with a dilated RV outflow tract, but further developments will widen the group of patients for whom this technique can be used and may change the face of further interventions after surgical pulmonary valve implantation.

Restrictive Right Ventricular Physiology

Restrictive RV physiology is associated with varied clinical responses. This physiology is defined by Doppler echocardiographic studies which show anterograde diastolic flow in the pulmonary artery coinciding with atrial systole both during inspiration and expiration. In early postoperative recovery following repair, these patients can develop a low cardiac output and require considerable circulatory support and prolonged postoperative intensive care. Because the pulmonary vascular resistance is low, atrial contraction causes flow to be transmitted through a poorly compliant or "stiff" RV into the pulmonary arteries in such a way that if pulmonary incompetence is present, its duration is shortened. This leads to the view that restrictive RV physiology can also be "protective" against the effects of pulmonary regurgitation longer term and seems to restrict the extent of RV dilatation. In a study of late gadolinium CMR used to study myocardial fibrosis in adults with repaired tetralogy of Fallot, restrictive RV physiology was found to be associated with more extensive late gadolinium enhancement.[8] It is probable that increased fibrosis or scarring, whether occurring because of an early insult or late progression, is one of the underlying substrates

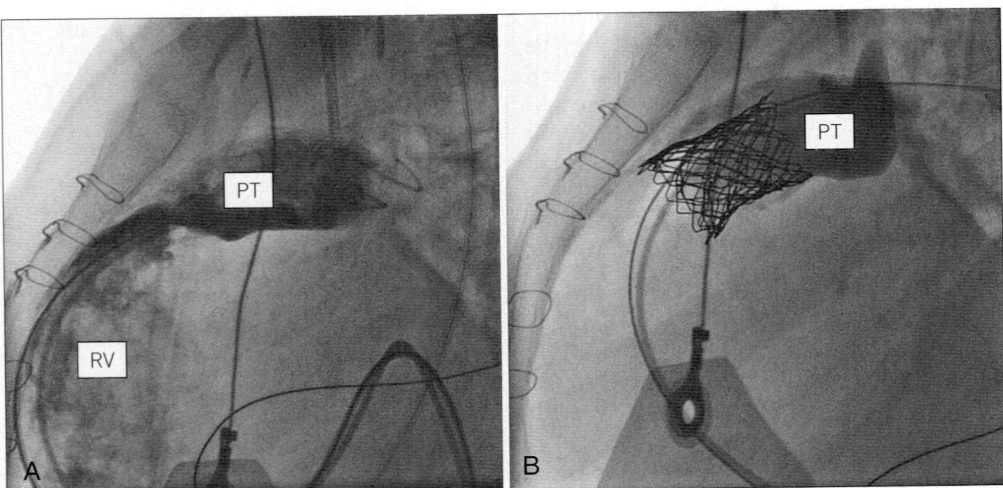

Figure 109.9 A, Severely obstructed, regurgitant right ventricular to pulmonary artery (RV-PA) conduit decades after repair of tetralogy of Fallot. Pulmonary regurgitation is clearly demonstrated outlining the RV. **B,** Relief of conduit stenosis and abolition of pulmonary regurgitation following balloon angioplasty, stent insertion and subsequent percutaneous pulmonary valve implantation. There is now no pulmonary regurgitation and thus no dye on the RV in diastole. PT, pulmonary trunk; RV, right ventricle. (Cardiac catheterization images courtesy of Dr. Michael J. Mullen, Royal Brompton Hospital.)

for restrictive RV physiology. A randomized controlled trial of ramipril 10 mg once daily for repaired tetralogy of Fallot with significant pulmonary regurgitation demonstrated improved left ventricular systolic function in the subgroup of patients with restrictive RV physiology.[21]

Biventricular Involvement

RV dysfunction is a major concern for most patients, but left heart dysfunction may also be present. The latter seems to be due to a number of factors, namely, prolonged cyanosis secondary to late repair, volume loading from palliative shunt procedures, perioperative damage, "ventricular-ventricular" interaction, and late aortic root dilatation and aortic regurgitation.[22-24] Recently, unsuspected left-sided myocardial scarring including in large territories consistent with previous infarction but not associated with obstructive epicardial coronary disease were seen in a subgroup of older patients with repaired tetralogy of Fallot.[8] Moderate to severe LV dysfunction and QRS duration greater than 180 msec have a high positive and negative predictive value respectively, for sudden cardiac death in repaired tetralogy of Fallot in a retrospective study.[15] Recent data have also shown that there are intrinsic abnormalities of the aortic medial wall in patients with tetralogy of Fallot, and cystic medial necrosis may be the mechanism for progressive aortic root dilatation seen in the late follow-up of a subgroup of patients.[25]

Endocarditis Prophylaxis

Though new guidelines may further refine practice, our institution still recommends that all patients with tetralogy of Fallot, repaired, palliated, or unoperated, have lifelong endocarditis prophylaxis, even those in whom residual intracardiac shunt has not been identified on diagnostic testing. Given these patients have prosthetic intracardiac material and that small residual patch leaks can be easily missed on routine imaging, this is currently felt to be reasonable. Patients should be advised to have regular dental checks.

Exercise

Patients with a good hemodynamic result following repair of tetralogy of Fallot, preserved biventricular function, and mild residual lesions need no exercise restrictions and can participate in athletics as well as endurance and contact sports. Patients with moderate to severe residual lesions requiring reintervention (for example, RV systolic pressure between one half and two thirds of systemic pressure, severe pulmonary regurgitation (PR), or both) may need to wait until reintervention and subsequent rehabilitation has taken place before resuming increased physical activity.

Pregnancy and Childbirth

The risk of pregnancy in repaired patients depends on hemodynamic status. It is low, approaching that of the general population, in patients with good underlying hemodynamics. In patients with significant residual RV outflow tract obstruction and severe pulmonary regurgitation with RV dysfunction, the increased volume load of pregnancy may lead to heart failure and arrhythmias, and there is mounting concern about incomplete reverse remodeling after pregnancy in the latter group.[26] If left ventricular dysfunction is present, this in turn increases the likelihood of complications during pregnancy and requires independent consideration. All patients with tetralogy of Fallot merit specialist cardiologic counseling preconception, genetic counseling, and fetal echocardiography early during the second trimester according to patient preference and follow-up during pregnancy. Genetic screening, in particular for 22q11 deletion, can be considered with the patient.

Genetics: 22q11 Deletion

Approximately 15% of patients with tetralogy of Fallot have a deletion of chromosome 22q11, which can be detected using fluorescent in situ hybridization.[27] The incidence of 22q11 deletion is suspected with certain anatomic variants as described previously; for example, it is especially high in patients with right aortic arch, pulmonary atresia, and aortic to pulmonary collaterals. 22q11 deletion is also referred to as DiGeorge syndrome and historically was summarized in the so-called CATCH 22 acronym (Cardiac defect, Abnormal facies, Thymic hypoplasia, Cleft palate, Hypocalcemia, and 22q11 deletion). Given that 22q11 deletion results in a spectrum of disease, it is therefore not always associated with cardiac abnormality, but affected subjects have a 50% risk of transmission, hence the indication for family screening and genetic counseling. Most cases seen are sporadic. Patients with 22q11 deletion may be small for dates with respect to birth weight, have nasal speech, cleft palate, learning difficulties, and a propensity to early psychiatric disorder, most commonly depression or schizophrenia in adolescence or young adulthood. In those without 22q11 deletion, there is a 3% risk of vertical transmission of congenital heart disease, which is greater for mothers with tetralogy of Fallot than for fathers.[28] Other mutations such as NKX2.5 have also been described.

Pharmacologic Therapy and Emerging Therapies

There is one randomized controlled trial of pharmacologic therapies in the setting of pulmonary regurgitation after repair of tetralogy of Fallot.[21,29] Although the potentially beneficial effects seen with ramipril therapy may in future have prognostic relevance, pulmonary valve implantation is likely to remain the mainstay of treatment. Patients with repaired tetralogy of Fallot and restrictive RV physiology have improved left heart function with ramipril and merit treatment, as potentially do patients unsuitable for pulmonary valve implantation due to comorbidity or in whom there are other indications for angiotensin converting enzyme (ACE) inhibition, such as diabetes or hypertension. The potential for medically targeting recent abnormalities demonstrated in this population group including neurohormonal activation,[30] autonomic dysfunction,[31] cystic medial necrosis in the aorta,[25] or myocardial fibrosis[8] is not yet known.

Meanwhile, therapy is generally symptom directed or empirically based on current or emerging available evidence, be it for management of arrhythmia or ventricular dysfunction.

PROGNOSIS

Unrepaired, tetralogy of Fallot has a high mortality in infancy, and about 25% of all cases with tetralogy of Fallot and severe pulmonary stenosis die by the age of 1 year and 70% by 10 years of age. Palliative surgery improves symptoms and prognosis is better, but with palliation alone most patients will have limited daily activity depending on the degree of arterial desaturation and cyanosis. Increased QRS duration greater than 180 msec, pulmonary regurgitation, and left ventricular dysfunction are associated with ventricular tachycardia and sudden death late after surgical repair. It is hoped that the rate of sudden death, described as occurring in up to 6% of patients with repaired tetralogy of Fallot at late follow-up, will further lessen because of earlier surgery, modifications in surgical technique, and improvements in medical and surgical management including reintervention, but this remains to be proved. Thirty-year survival for those operated on as children is now above 90%, and current survival of patients alive at 30 days after the operation is 98% at 20 years. Most adults with previous repair of tetralogy of Fallot lead unrestricted lives.

SUMMARY

Tetralogy of Fallot is the most common cyanotic heart disease. The prognosis for this condition has been dramatically improved by cardiac surgery. Patients with repaired tetralogy of Fallot with good hemodynamic result have an excellent prognosis. Pulmonary regurgitation is, however, an important cause of late morbidity and mortality and therefore remains of clinical concern. With increasing age, comorbidity including acquired heart disease may be contributory to late mortality. All patients should remain under lifelong follow-up and periodic review in a specialist center. Treatment is based on an overall goal of preservation of biventricular function and risk modification for arrhythmia and sudden cardiac death.

COMMON ARTERIAL TRUNK

Common arterial trunk has historically been known as truncus arteriosus, common aorticopulmonary trunk, and truncus arteriosus communis. It is an uncommon cardiovascular anomaly that accounts for 1% to 4% of congenital cardiac defects.[32] The anomaly is characterized by a common trunk arising from the ventricles that provides the aortic, pulmonary, and coronary arterial circulations. Without treatment the natural history of common arterial trunk is poor,[33] but the outlook has vastly improved over the last 30 years with surgical intervention.[34,35] Because of the nature of the repair, patients will require reintervention and thus should be under the continuing care of a congenital heart disease unit throughout later life.

ANATOMY AND PATHOLOGY

Anatomically, common arterial trunk should be distinguished from single ventricular outlet via the aorta or pulmonary trunk (with associated pulmonary atresia and aortic atresia, respectively) and single outlet via a solitary arterial trunk. The distinguishing characteristic is that the single arterial trunk gives rise to the aorta, coronary arteries, and pulmonary arteries. The truncal valve is almost always connected to both ventricles, with the orifice overriding a large ventricular septal defect. As a form of ventriculoarterial connection, truncus would be expected to coexist with all anatomic segmental connections. However, in the vast majority of cases there is usual atrial arrangement and atrioventricular concordance.[36] The anatomy of the VSD and right and left ventricular outflow tracts bear some similarity to that found in tetralogy of Fallot.

The main variation in anatomy is associated with the pattern of branching from the common trunk. Historically, two systems have been used to classify the anatomic type of common arterial trunk: the Collett and Edwards classification and the Van Praagh system.[37] A more pragmatic approach to outlining the anatomy in individual cases of truncus is to describe the position of the pulmonary arteries, associated duct or collaterals, and any abnormality of the aortic arch. This immediately provides the surgeon with the relevant anatomy and allows the description of much rarer variations. Fig. 109.10 outlines the most common patterns found, but other variations include absence of one branch pulmonary artery with arterial supply from a persistent duct or aortopulmonary collaterals. Collett and Edwards described one entity (type IV) where the pulmonary arteries are absent and the lungs are supplied by large aortopulmonary collateral arteries. This is no longer considered a form of common arterial trunk (because the pulmonary arteries are absent), but comes under the spectrum of pulmonary atresia with VSD. Other associated abnormalities are right-sided aortic arch (30%), anomalies of the coronary ostia (49%), absence of the ductus arteriosus (49%), patent foramen ovale, atrial septal defect (ASD), and peripheral pulmonary artery stenoses.

The floor of the VSD is the crest of the ventricular septum and is roofed by the leaflets of the truncal valve. The truncal valve is usually trileaflet (67%),[37] but may be bicuspid or quadricuspid. The valve leaflets tend to be in fibrous continuity with the anterior mitral valve leaflet. Valves are often dysplastic, resulting in insufficiency that contributes to early presentation with congestive heart failure. In one surgical series, preoperative data showed truncal valve insufficiency was absent or trivial in 39% of patients, mild in 47%, moderate in 8%, and severe in 6%.[38] Less commonly the valve is stenotic.

There is increasing evidence that some cases of truncus arteriosus are associated with genetic abnormalities. About 30% of patients with truncus arteriosus have DiGeorge syndrome and chromosome 22q11 deletion.[39,40] However, changes in other genes such as *sox4* and *pax3* have been implicated.[36]

PATHOPHYSIOLOGY

A more rapid fall in pulmonary vascular resistance is seen in the neonatal period in common arterial trunk compared to normal. The reason for this is unclear. The excessive pulmonary blood flow results in early presentation with congestive heart failure. Early presentation is also affected by truncal valve insufficiency or associated lesions, such as interrupted aortic arch. The increased pulmonary venous return to the left atrium results in high left atrial pressure and left ventricular volume overload, which will contribute to tachypnea and cardiac failure.

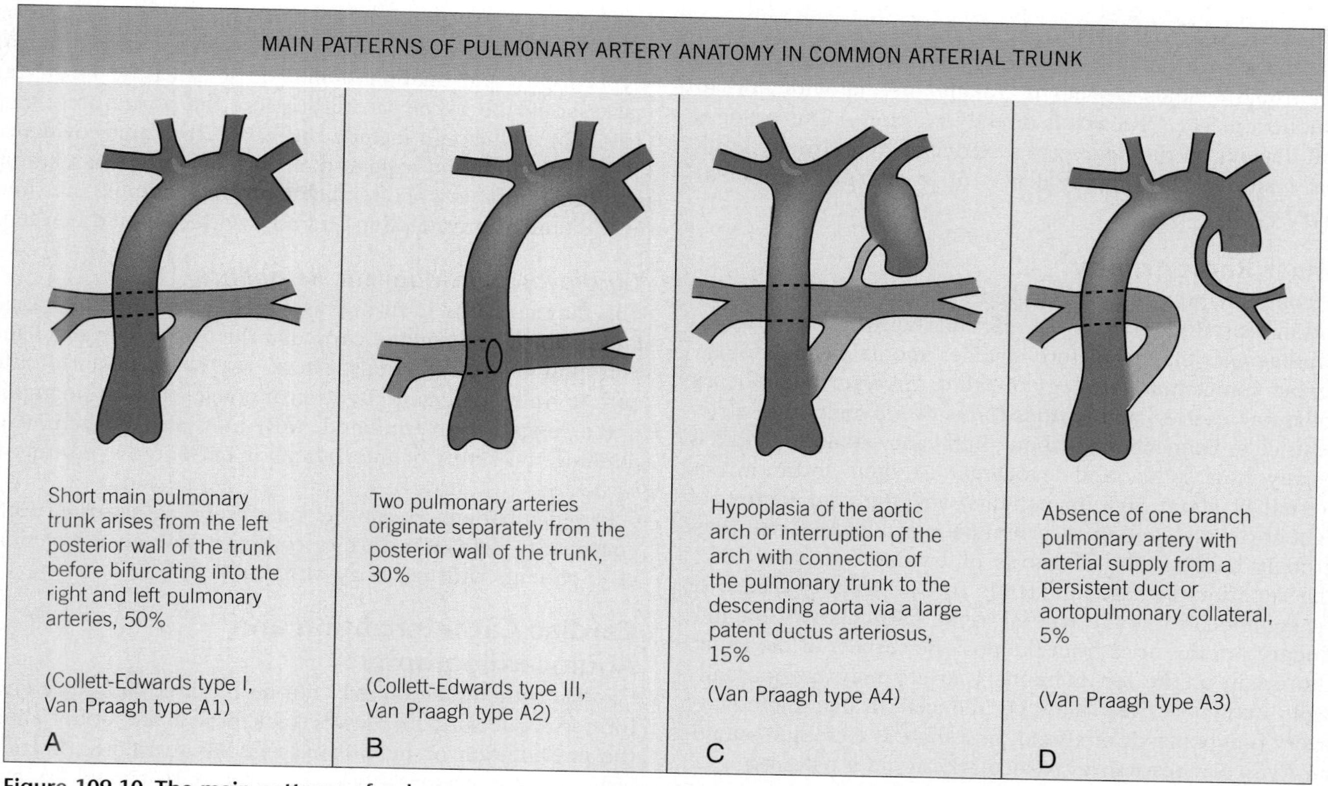

Figure 109.10 The main patterns of pulmonary artery anatomy in common arterial trunk. A, Short main pulmonary trunk arises from the left posterior wall of the trunk before bifurcating into the right and left pulmonary arteries, 50% (Collett-Edwards type I, Van Praagh type A1). **B**, Two pulmonary arteries originate separately from the posterior wall of the trunk, 30% (Collett-Edwards type III, Van Praagh type A2). **C**, Hypoplasia of the aortic arch or interruption of the arch with connection of the pulmonary trunk to the descending aorta via a large patent ductus arteriosus, 15% (Van Praagh type A4). **D**, Absence of one branch pulmonary artery with arterial supply from a persistent duct or aortopulmonary collateral, 5% (Van Praagh type A3).

Because of the nature of the defect, there will be cyanosis. However, common mixing occurs within the common trunk as well as at VSD level, and the degree of cyanosis is often mild. In some cases the fall in pulmonary vascular resistance is less marked and congestive heart failure is not seen, but the degree of cyanosis will be greater. Cyanosis will also be greater in the presence of pulmonary artery stenosis.

Right ventricular hypertrophy is usually seen in all cases because of the equalization of ventricular pressure across the VSD. Truncal valvar insufficiency will result in ventricular volume overload, and valvar stenosis results in ventricular pressure overload. Both will contribute to worsening congestive cardiac failure as well as rapidly developing ventricular hypertrophy.

CLINICAL PRESENTATION

Common arterial trunk may be found at the time of fetal echocardiography, but the majority of cases present in the neonatal period or early infancy. The two main causes of presentation are congestive cardiac failure and cyanosis.[36] As pulmonary resistance falls, the signs of heart failure, such as tachypnea, sweating, and difficulty feeding, are seen with eventual pulmonary congestion and hepatomegaly. This presentation is likely to be earlier if there is significant associated truncal valve insufficiency or an interrupted aorta with closure of the ductus arteriosus.

On examination, pulses are expected to be bouncy. Cyanosis is unlikely to be a marked feature unless there is associated pulmonary artery stenosis or raised pulmonary vascular resistance. The first heart sound is normal and the second heart sound single. However, there may be close splitting of the second heart sound due to asynchronous closure of the valvar leaflets. A loud systolic click may be heard in infants with opening of the truncal valve. A systolic murmur of varying intensity and duration is heard along the left sternal border, and occasionally a diastolic flow murmur or murmur of truncal valve insufficiency is heard.

If there is associated chromosome 22q11 deletion, there may be learning difficulties, abnormal facies, or kyphosis.

DIAGNOSTIC TECHNIQUES

The clinical differential diagnosis of common arterial trunk includes tetralogy of Fallot and pulmonary atresia, aortopulmonary septal defect, and origin of the right pulmonary artery from the ascending aorta. A combination of the investigations described in the following sections should differentiate common trunk. Moreover, in assessing common trunk it is important to accurately define each aspect of the anatomy that will affect any planned repair: origin of pulmonary arteries, evidence of pulmonary artery stenosis or raised pulmonary vascular resistance, structure of the truncal valve and insufficiency or stenosis, integrity of the aortic arch, and any other associated cardiac defect, such as an ASD or coronary artery anomaly.

Electrocardiography

There are no specific findings in patients with common arterial trunk.[35] Sinus rhythm is usually present with normal conduction. The QRS axis is directly inferiorly. The voltages will depend on the degree of ventricular hypertrophy, with the majority showing evidence of combined ventricular hypertrophy.

Chest Radiography

A common presenting radiograph is that of cardiomegaly and increased pulmonary vascular markings.[41] The differential diagnosis for this picture includes anomalous pulmonary venous connection, tetralogy of Fallot, large aortopulmonary collateral arteries, and various forms of univentricular atrioventricular connections without pulmonary stenosis. There is usually situs solitus and levocardia. A right aortic arch is present in about 30% of patients, and the combination of right aortic arch and increased pulmonary vascular markings strongly suggests the diagnosis of common arterial trunk. The superior mediastinum tends to be narrow because of the commonality of the arterial trunk, particularly if the pulmonary arteries arise from the posterior aspect of the trunk. The origin of the left pulmonary artery may be unusually high. Lung markings may be reduced if one pulmonary artery is hypoplastic or absent, or if there is increased pulmonary vascular resistance (particularly in older patients).

Echocardiography

In most cases echocardiography alone can be used to fully evaluate the anatomy in neonates and infants. The large VSD with overriding common truncal valve leaflets forming the roof of the defect is seen on the parasternal long-axis view (Fig. 109.11a). The confluent pulmonary trunk may be seen arising posteriorly in this view. The parasternal short-axis view should show the pulmonary arteries just above the level of the truncal valve. Stenosis of the origins may be seen.

The morphology of the truncal valve leaflets should be assessed. Dysplastic leaflets are more likely to be associated with significant insufficiency or stenosis. Color flow and continuous wave Doppler echocardiography should also be used to assess flow across the VSD. Evidence of ventricular hypertrophy and dilation should be seen easily. Particular care should be taken to fully assess the aortic arch (Fig. 109.11b) and should include the side of the arch, evidence of interruption, and a persistent duct or aortic coarctation. Nowadays infants will often be on prostaglandin E2 infusions at the time of presentation and a large duct should be seen.

Cardiovascular Magnetic Resonance

This may be useful in further assessing the pulmonary vasculature, aortic arch, and in particular the descending aorta and aortopulmonary collaterals. These may be particularly difficult to fully delineate by transthoracic echocardiography if the lungs are overinflated. MRI may also be helpful in defining the status of the thymus if DiGeorge syndrome is suspected.

In older patients it can be very useful in assessing right ventricle to pulmonary artery conduits and valvar function, as in patients with tetralogy of Fallot.

Cardiac Catheterization and Angiocardiography

Cardiac catheterization may not be required before referral for corrective surgery. However, if there is any doubt about the presentation or pulmonary vascular resistance, particularly in later presentations, the procedure should be performed.[35] Because of concomitant pulmonary edema and possible chest infections, pulmonary venous saturations cannot be assumed. Moreover, pulmonary artery saturations may not be the same throughout the pulmonary tree. Ideally each pulmonary artery, a systemic artery, the superior vena cava, inferior vena cava, and a pulmonary vein should be intubated. Commonly, right and left ventricular pressures are equal, there may be a small gradient across the truncal valve, and oxygen saturations are slightly higher in the systemic artery than pulmonary arteries, because of preferential streaming of blood from the right ventricle to pulmonary arteries. Pulmonary vascular resistance of less than 8 U/m^2 is necessary for surgery.

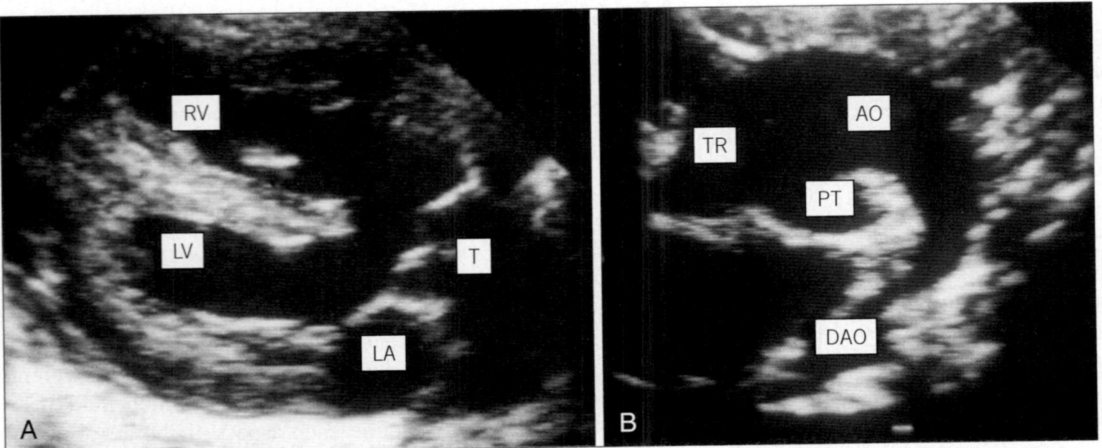

Figure 109.11 Transthoracic echocardiography. A, Parasternal long-axis view showing left atrium (LA), left ventricle (LV), right ventricle (RV), and large VSD with overriding common trunk and valve (T). **B**, Suprasternal view showing a confluent pulmonary trunk (PT) arising from the common trunk (TR), which continues as an intact aortic arch (AO) into descending aorta (DAO). (Echocardiography image courtesy of Dr. Michael L. Rigby, Royal Brompton Hospital.)

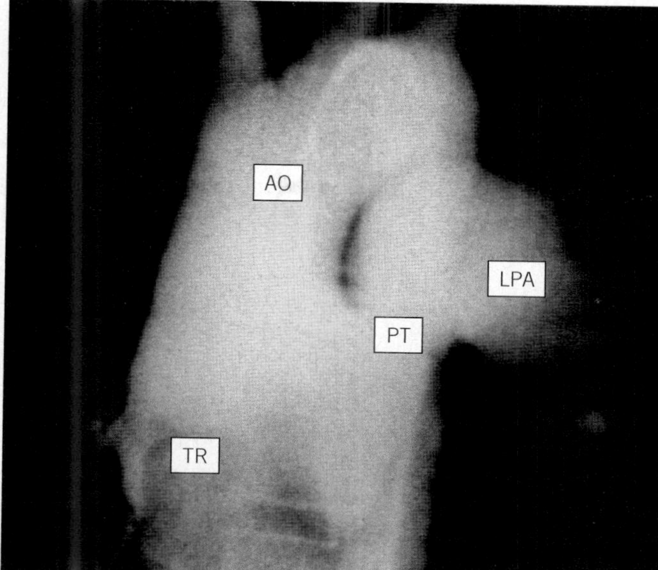

Figure 109.12 Aortogram. The common trunk (TR) giving rise to the aortic arch (AO) and common pulmonary trunk (PT). The left pulmonary artery (LPA) is seen at the pulmonary bifurcation. (Cardiac catheterization image courtesy of Dr. Michael L. Rigby, Royal Brompton Hospital.)

Angiography of the common arterial trunk reveals the anatomy of the pulmonary arteries and aortic arch, and any truncal valve regurgitation (Fig. 109.12). Rapid injections are required to avoid dilution of contrast by torrential flow in the common trunk. Further selective injections in the descending aorta may be required to further assess arterial collaterals. Angiography of the right and left ventricle shows the large VSD and overriding truncus.[41]

MANAGEMENT

The immediate medical management of the sick infant presenting with congestive cardiac failure includes the use of diuretics, intensive care support, and the use of prostaglandin E to maintain patency of the duct when appropriate.

Initial surgical intervention for a common trunk was pulmonary artery banding, either of the common pulmonary trunk when present or the individual pulmonary branches. However, although this reduces left ventricular overload and protects against increased pulmonary pressures, it exacerbates truncal valve regurgitation and cyanosis and has since been superceded by primary repair of the defects in infancy. The first successful primary repair was reported in 1968 using a valved conduit to connect the right ventricle to pulmonary arteries.[42]

The majority of cases are now repaired in the neonatal period or early infancy. An early review reported increased mortality in those with increasing pulmonary vascular resistance, greater than 8 U/m^2, or severe truncal valve insufficiency.[43] There have since been numerous reports of successful repair varying in the type of right ventricle to pulmonary artery conduit used: aortic or pulmonary allograft valved conduit, porcine or bovine valved xenografts, valveless conduits, and monocusp repair with direct attachment of the pulmonary arteries to right ventricle.[34,36,44] The VSD is usually closed from the right ventricle. Because of the problems with postoperative pulmonary regurgitation, a valved conduit should be the method of choice.

Repair of the truncal valve is indicated in the presence of significant insufficiency, which tends to be more common if the valve is quadricuspid. This may involve cusp repair, commissural plication, and leaflet suspension, or in a few cases a root replacement is required.[45,46] Successful repair of interrupted aortic arch has been reported but is still associated with significantly higher mortality rates.[47]

Because of the young age at primary repair, the majority of patients will require further surgical or catheter-based intervention. The majority of reintervention is for conduit or branch pulmonary artery stenosis at the site of anastomosis between the conduit and branch pulmonary artery. Other reasons for reintervention are truncal valve replacement (16%) and residual VSD repair (10%).[35] A significant proportion of patients will require more than one reintervention.

Continued Assessment and Management of the Adult Patient

As in those patients with tetralogy of Fallot and other areas of congenital heart disease, there is an increasing population requiring continued lifelong surveillance. There is an overlap with later symptoms, and suggested methods of regular investigations are as outlined for the patients with tetralogy of Fallot. However, the majority of those with repair of a common trunk will have stenotic rather than regurgitant lesions, at least in childhood.

Reintervention should be considered for those with

- significant right ventricle to pulmonary artery conduit stenosis or insufficiency;
- significant truncal valve (native or prosthetic) stenosis or regurgitation;
- significant branch pulmonary artery stenosis;
- significant residual VSD; and
- evidence of myocardial ischemia.

Medical treatment may be required in the presence of ventricular dysfunction, and we would suggest the empirical use of agents as for other adult patients with heart failure. A small proportion of patients who have not been repaired in early life may develop Eisenmenger's syndrome and should be assessed for advanced pulmonary arterial hypertension therapy and possible anticoagulation therapy.

All patients should be aware of the lifelong need for antibiotic prophylaxis for endocarditis.

Pregnancy and Exercise

There are very few reports of pregnancy after common arterial trunk repair. As with tetralogy of Fallot, the risk would be expected to be low in those with a good hemodynamic status at the time of pregnancy. There has been one recent report of severe and symptomatic deterioration in truncal valve regurgitation during pregnancy, with a successful outcome and recovery of valve function 2 weeks after delivery.[48] Given the high incidence of chromosome 22q11 deletion in patients with common arterial trunk (approximately one third of all patients), we would offer screening by fluoresence in situ hybridization to all women contemplating pregnancy.

Advice regarding exercise will also depend on a patient's current hemodynamic status and again reflects the advice given for those with tetralogy of Fallot. Given the high incidence of reintervention, involvement in a cardiac rehabilitation program should be encouraged.

PROGNOSIS

The prognosis in common arterial trunk is very poor without surgical repair, with congestive heart failure due to increased pulmonary blood flow, with or without truncal valve insufficiency, being the major cause of death in early infancy. In one series of 23 patients referred to the Mayo Clinic before primary repair of common arterial trunk was established, only 20% of those referred at less than 2 years of age survived beyond their second year of life.[33] Those who presented at a later age (2 to 16 years) were less likely to develop congestive cardiac failure, but average pulmonary vascular resistance was greater than 10 U/m^2. Of this group, 70% was still alive after a median follow-up period of 18 years after initial referral. All of these patients had a common pulmonary artery or both branch pulmonary arteries arising from the posterolateral aspect of the common trunk.

Recently reported early postoperative mortality following primary repair is 3.4% to 13%.[34,44,46] However, mortality rates remain high for those patients who also require repair of interrupted aortic arch. Results are better if both the common trunk and interrupted arch are repaired in one stage, but 47% of patients still die during the index admission.[47] Reintervention rates for conduit or pulmonary artery stenosis are 25% to 62% of patients followed up to a median time of 98 months postoperatively.[34,44]

SUMMARY

Common arterial trunk is an uncommon congenital heart disease. Although previous classification systems are still in use, we favor a simple descriptive approach to the anatomy of individual cases, thereby describing the origin of the pulmonary arteries in relation to the common arterial trunk along with other relevant findings, such as interrupted aortic arch and a description of the truncal valve. The natural history of the lesion is associated with high mortality, particularly in infants presenting with congestive heart failure. Primary surgical repair has significantly improved the prognosis. Even in those patients with a good outcome from initial repair, the rate of reintervention is high, often involving replacement of the right ventricle to pulmonary artery conduit.

chapter

110 Transposition of the Great Arteries

Thomas R. Kimball

Definition

- Discordant ventriculoarterial connection of the great arteries.

Key Features

- The aorta arises from the morphologic right ventricle.
- The pulmonary artery arises from the morphologic left ventricle.
- The pulmonary and systemic circulations are in parallel (deoxygenated blood is redelivered to the body; oxygenated blood is redelivered to the lungs).
- Atrial, ventricular, and/or ductal level shunts are necessary to sustain life.
- The diagnosis is established by echocardiography.

Therapy

- Acute medical: prostaglandin E_1 and balloon atrial septostomy.
- Surgical: arterial switch operation in the neonatal period.

Transposition of the great vessels accounts for 5% to 7% of congenital cardiac defects. The incidence is approximately 3 in 10,000 births,[1] with a profound male predominance (60% to 70%), and is one of the two most common cyanotic congenital heart lesions (the other being tetralogy of Fallot).[2] Before treatments were developed, almost all patients died in infancy. In 1950, the first therapeutic option—an atrial septectomy—was developed by Blalock and Hanlon.[3] Subsequently, several other treatments, such as the Senning and Mustard procedures, rapidly evolved. However, it was not until 1966, when Rashkind and Miller[1] developed the balloon atrial septostomy, that neonatal and infant survival became a reality. Today the method of surgical correction is the neonatal arterial switch operation, which is associated with 88% survival at 10 to 15 years.[4]

ANATOMY AND PATHOLOGY

The aorta and pulmonary artery are derived from the embryologic conus and truncus. The conus appears in the loop stage and constitutes the most craniad portion of the heart tube. The truncus appears in the postlooping stage and is continuous with the conus caudally and the aortic sac cranially. Initially, neither the conus nor the truncus is septated, but in the postloop stage, two conal crests of mesenchymal tissue divide the conus into anterolateral and posteromedial components (Fig. 110.1). Gradually, the conus migrates from a rightward position to an anteromedial position, so that the anterolateral conus connects to the right ventricle and the posteromedial conus connects with the left ventricle. Truncal septation is accomplished through the development of two truncal swellings and the spiral-shaped aortopulmonary septum in the aortic sac.

Two theories exist regarding the development of transposition of the great vessels:

- the straight truncal/aortopulmonary septal theory; and
- the conal growth theory.

In the former, the primary defect is blamed on a lack of spiraling of the aortopulmonary septum, leading to continuity between the anterolateral conus of the right ventricle and the aorta. However, Van Praagh and colleagues[5] have presented cases of transposition in the absence of a straight aortopulmonary septum. Van Praagh's group pointed out that the postloop stage of the developing heart resembles D-transposition, with the future aortic and tricuspid valves relatively right-sided and the pulmonary and mitral valves relatively left-sided. For ventriculoarterial concordance to occur, the pulmonary valve must migrate away from (and the aortic valve must move toward) the mitral valve and the left ventricle. This is accomplished by persistence of the subpulmonary conus lifting the pulmonary valve superiorly, rotating the pulmonary valve anteriorly and rightward, and prohibiting pulmonary–atrioventricular valve continuity. Simultaneously, the subaortic conus fails to develop, nestling the aortic valve inferiorly, posteriorly, and leftward in continuity with the atrioventricular valves. Van Praagh and coworkers[5] described three entities of transposition of the great vessels resulting from differential conal growth. The most common (92%) results from simultaneous lack of development of the subpulmonary conus (so that the pulmonary valve remains relatively leftward, in continuity with the atrioventricular valves) and persistence of the subaortic conus (so that the aortic valve rotates anteriorly). In 8% of cases, there are bilateral conuses and no semilunar–atrioventricular valve continuity (8%). Rarely (fewer than 1% of cases), there can be deficiency of both conuses and aortic–atrioventricular valve continuity. Interestingly, in these patients, the aorta is posterior and inferior to the pulmonary valve.

Transposition should be defined literally as ventriculoarterial discordance, in part because of the lack of constancy of the conal anatomy and arterial position outlined above. Indeed, hearts in which the great vessels arise from their morphologically appropriate ventricles, but are abnormally related to one another (i.e., the aorta in an anterior position) have been described (so-called anatomically corrected malposition).[6]

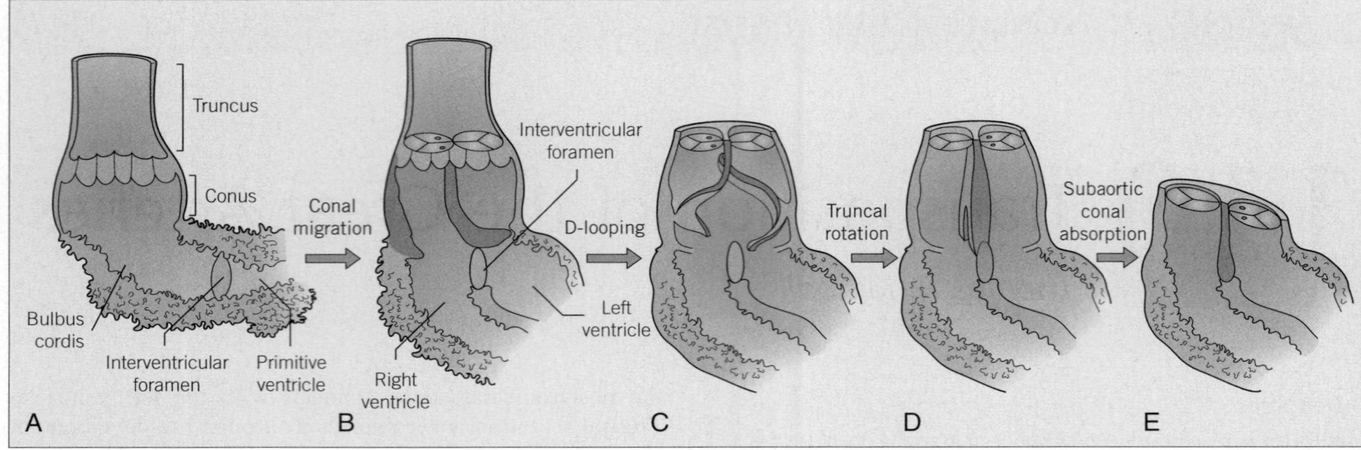

Figure 110.1 Embryologic development of the normal conotruncus. A, The truncus is continuous with the conus caudally and the aortic sac cranially. The conus overlies the bulbus cordis (the future right ventricle). **B.** Conal crests of tissue divide the conus. The conus migrates anteromedially so that a conus overlies each ventricle. **C,** D-looping of the heart tube causes rotation of the conal septum. **D,** Truncal rotation results in the transfer of the aortic truncus posterior and leftward to the pulmonary truncus and reduction of the spiral course of the conal septum. **E,** Subaortic conal absorption causes the aortic valve to drop inferiorly and allows continuity between the aortic and mitral valves.

PATHOPHYSIOLOGY

In the normal heart, the pulmonary and systemic circulations exist in series: that is, after blood courses through the pulmonary circulation, it then progresses through the systemic circulation. In this manner oxygenated blood is delivered to the body, whereas deoxygenated blood is delivered to the lungs (Fig. 110.2). Transposition of the great vessels results in the pulmonary and systemic circulations existing in parallel (a condition known as transposition physiology). Oxygenated blood is redelivered to the lungs and the deoxygenated blood is redelivered to the body. At least one communication between the two circulations is necessary for the body to receive oxygenated blood and the lungs to receive deoxygenated blood to sustain life. This is provided by a ventricular septal defect (if present), a patent foramen ovale (which can be augmented by a balloon atrial septostomy), or a patent ductus arteriosus (which can be maintained by intravenous prostaglandin administration).

Transposition physiology, with its associated shunts, leads to the creations of both anatomic and physiologic left-to-right and right-to-left shunts. The anatomic left-to-right shunt is that volume of pulmonary venous blood perfusing the pulmonary capillary bed. The anatomic right-to-left shunt is the volume of systemic venous blood perfusing the systemic capillary bed. The physiologic shunts are necessary to sustain life. They consist of a left-to-right shunt (the volume of pulmonary venous blood crossing over to perfuse the systemic capillary bed, or the effective systemic blood flow) and a right-to-left shunt (the volume of systemic venous blood crossing over to perfuse the pulmonary capillary bed, or the effective pulmonary blood flow). The degree of intercirculatory mixing is a complex phenomenon dependent on a variety of factors, including the location and number of shunts, in addition to the degree of pulmonary flow, pulmonary stenosis, and pulmonary vascular resistance.

Associated Pathology

Coronary Artery Anomalies

A variety of coronary artery distributions can exist in transposition of the great vessels (Fig. 110.3). The coronary arteries will almost always arise from the aortic sinuses facing the pulmonary valve. The most common pattern (67% of cases) is the left main coronary artery (LMCA) arising from the left facing sinus and branching into left anterior descending and circumflex arteries (Fig. 110.4a). In this instance the circumflex courses anterior to the pulmonary artery. The right coronary artery arises from the right facing sinus. The second most common distribution (16% of cases) is the left anterior descending artery arising from the left facing sinus and the right coronary artery arising from the right sinus and giving off the circumflex coronary artery (Fig. 110.4b). In this instance, the circumflex artery courses posterior to the pulmonary artery.

The proximal portion of a coronary artery may not run perpendicularly through the aortic wall, so that its epicardial exit is displaced from its ostium (intramural course) (Fig. 110.5). It is particularly important to identify this before the arterial switch operation, so that the surgeon is aware of the need to excise a wider button of aortic wall tissue when performing coronary artery transfer.

Ventricular Septal Defect

The coexistence of a ventricular septal defect (VSD) increases surgical mortality and the risk of both pulmonary vascular disease and tricuspid insufficiency. The malalignment defects are of particular surgical importance. Anterior malalignment defects are associated with override of the pulmonary artery into the right ventricle, the extreme being double-outlet right ventricle with subpulmonary VSD. Often, subaortic stenosis and associated coarctation or interruption of the aorta are present. Posterior malalignment

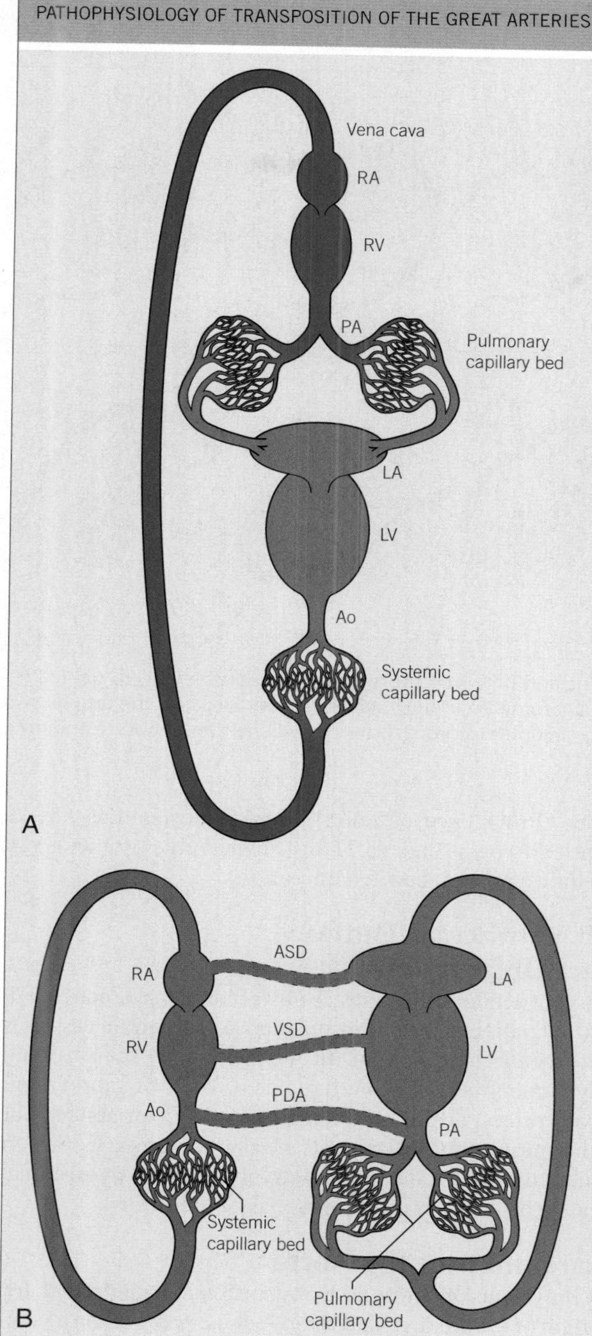

Figure 110.2 Pathophysiology of transposition of the great arteries. A, In the normal heart, the pulmonary and systemic circulations exist in series with one another, so that oxygenated blood is delivered to the tissues and deoxygenated blood is delivered to the pulmonary capillary bed. **B,** In a patient with transposition of the great arteries, the circulations exist parallel to one another, so that oxygenated blood is redelivered to the pulmonary capillary bed and deoxygenated blood is redelivered to the tissues. To sustain life, the baby must have adequate mixing of the two circulations through atrial, ventricular, and/or ductal level shunts. Ao, aorta; ASD, atrial septal defect; LA, left atrium; LV, left ventricle; PA, pulmonary artery; PDA, patent ductus arteriosus; PFO, patent foramen ovale; RA, right atrium; RV, right ventricle; VSD, ventricular septal defect.

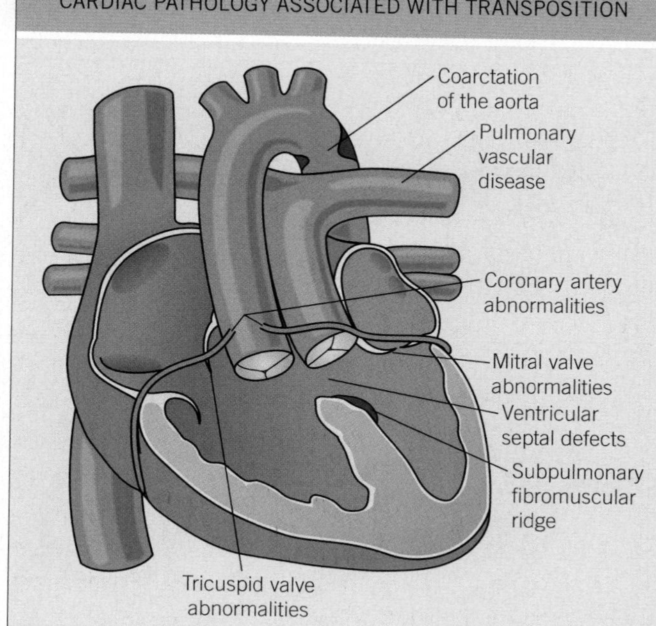

Figure 110.3 Cardiac pathology associated with transposition of the great vessels. The coronary artery origins may be abnormal, and their proximal courses may take an intramural course, complicating or prohibiting coronary artery reimplantation during arterial switch operation. Ventricular septal defects (VSD) are often of the malalignment type and will complicate surgical repair. The tricuspid and mitral valves may have abnormal morphology and/or attachments into or across a coexisting VSD. Pulmonary vascular disease may develop at an early age, particularly in the setting of a coexisting VSD. Aortic arch obstruction is relatively rare but increases in prevalence with an associated VSD and will complicate surgical repair.

defects are associated with protrusion of the infundibular septum into the left ventricular outflow tract, producing subpulmonic stenosis.

Pulmonary Vascular Disease

Usually associated with a VSD, pulmonary vascular disease can appear early and progresses rapidly. Intimal proliferation and medial thickening can occur as early as 2 months and increase markedly after 7 months. Pulmonary vascular disease may also develop even in the absence of a VSD or patent ductus arteriosus. Possible mechanisms in these cases include atrial level shunting, a shunt through the bronchial arterial circulation, and, perhaps most likely, inherent structural defects in the muscular pulmonary arteries.

Abnormalities of the Atrioventricular Valves

Tricuspid valve abnormalities are common, particularly when a VSD is present (31%). These include straddling, dysplasia, left ventricular tract obstruction, double orifice, and abnormal chordal insertions, all of which can complicate an anticipated Rastelli operation.

Mitral valve abnormalities include small annulus, restricted free margin of the anterior leaflet, attachment of the anterior leaflet to the margins of a VSD, and accessory mitral valve

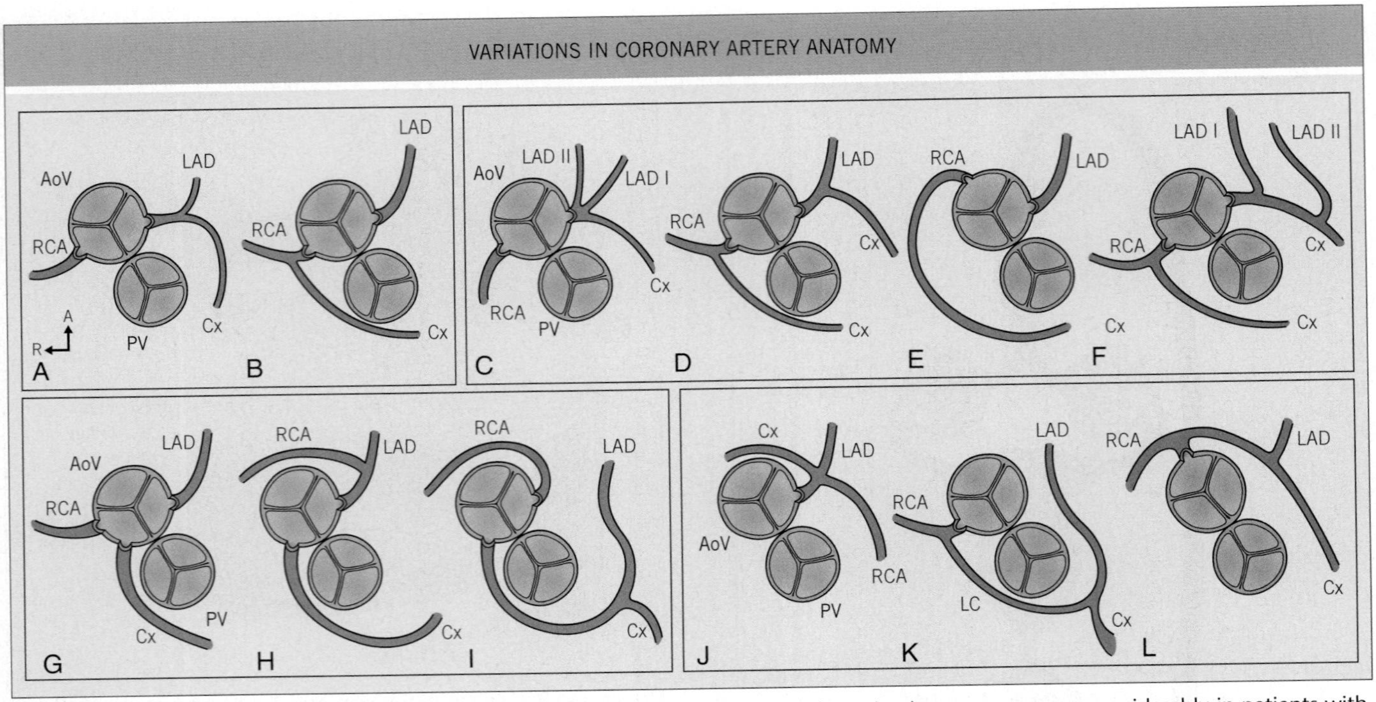

VARIATIONS IN CORONARY ARTERY ANATOMY

Figure 110.4 Variations in coronary artery anatomy. Coronary artery origins and proximal courses can vary considerably in patients with transposition of the great arteries (**A** to **I**). It is important to define coronary anatomy accurately before surgery, because the arterial switch operation involves coronary artery transfer. A, anterior; AoV, aortic valve; Cx, circumflex coronary artery; LAD, left anterior descending coronary artery; PV, pulmonary valve; R, right; RCA, right coronary artery.

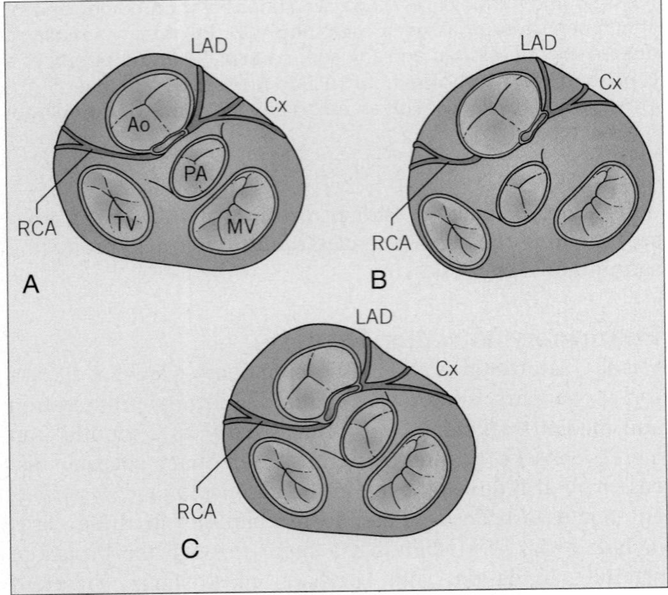

Figure 110.5 Intramural course of coronary arteries. The greatest diagnostic challenge in patients with transposition of the great vessels is determining the presence of an intramural coronary artery. An intramural coronary artery is one that is embedded in the aortic wall, so that the epicardial exit site is remote from its ostium. Preoperative diagnosis is essential so that the surgeon is prepared to excise a wider button of aortic wall that includes not only the epicardial exit but also the ostium for coronary artery transfer during the arterial switch operation. Typical associated anatomic features, perhaps more easily detected by echocardiography, include an ostium adjacent to a commissure and a coronary artery coursing between the aorta (Ao) and the pulmonary artery (PA). Cx, circumflex coronary artery; LAD, left anterior descending coronary artery; MV, mitral valve; RCA, right coronary artery; TV, tricuspid valve.

orifice. Prevalence of mitral valve abnormalities has been reported to be as high as 71%.[7] Mitral valve problems rarely preclude an arterial switch operation.

Left Ventricular Outflow Tract Obstruction

Left ventricular outflow tract obstruction can occur in 5% to 40% of patients with transposition of the great vessels and intact ventricular septum. In most patients, the obstruction is dynamic, but it may be fixed as a result of subpulmonary fibrous ridges, posterior malalignment VSD, or abnormalities of the mitral valve. Gradients measured across the left ventricular outflow tract preoperatively may be overestimated because of the increased pulmonary blood flow.

Coarctation of the Aorta

The prevalence of aortic arch obstruction in patients with transposition of the great vessels is rare but increases when a ventricular septal defect is present.[8] This combination is associated with not only particularly poor natural history but also more challenging surgical therapy. Recently it has been shown that surgical mortality with a one-stage approach consisting of both arterial switch operation and aortic arch reconstruction is 24% (all within the first month).[8] However, long-term survival (10-year survival of 76%) and residua are similar to unselected patients undergoing arterial switch operation alone.

CLINICAL PRESENTATIONS

History

Cyanosis is the most prominent symptom of transposition of the great arteries and, in the absence of a VSD, is almost always apparent within the first day of life. Murmur, cardiomegaly, and respiratory distress are inconsistent findings. Heart failure is evident only if there is an associated large VSD.

Physical Examination

Newborns are usually well-developed and without dysmorphic features. Other than cyanosis, the examination is often unremarkable. Almost 50% of neonates with transposition of the great arteries exhibit no murmur. When it is present, the murmur is believed to be a functional left ventricular outflow tract murmur resulting from increased pulmonary blood flow. In infants with transposition with VSD, the murmur from the VSD may be soft initially but gradually increases in intensity with age. In approximately 67% of newborns, the second heart sound is single. Mild tachypnea and hepatomegaly may be present.

DIAGNOSTIC TECHNIQUES

Arterial Blood Gases

Although pulmonary venous blood usually has a Po_2 as high as 110 mm Hg (14.63 kPa) and Pco_2 as low as 15 mm Hg (2 kPa) (because of hyperventilation), the systemic Po_2 is rarely greater than 35 mm Hg (4.7 kPa) and the Pco_2 is usually normal. This is because of the limited amount of intercirculatory mixing. Inspiration of 100% fractional inspired oxygen will distinguish neonates with transposition of the great vessels from those with primary pulmonary disease. In this instance, the Po_2 in babies with transposition will have only a very modest increase in Po_2 (e.g., from 30 to 35-40 mm Hg [4 to 4.7-5.3 kPa]), whereas those with primary pulmonary disease will boost the Po_2 to greater than 150 mm Hg.

Electrocardiogram

In the newborn period, the electrocardiogram (ECG) is often normal. There may be right-axis deviation and right ventricular hypertrophy.

Radiography

Like the ECG, the chest x-ray is often normal in the neonate. The heart may be slightly enlarged. The pulmonary vascular markings may be normal, diminished, or increased. The mediastinum may be narrow because of the anterior-posterior relationship of the great vessels, small thymic shadow, a more central plane of the aortic arch, or a combination of these. Because of these anatomic features, the cardiothymic silhouette may resemble an "egg-on-a-string" in approximately 33% of patients.

Approximately 50% of older (not newborn) patients will have asymmetric pulmonary blood flow with increased vascular markings in the right lung. This is due to an abnormal inclination of the main pulmonary artery into the right pulmonary artery, so that the ejection of blood from the left ventricle courses preferentially into the right pulmonary artery. This physiology may result in associated left pulmonary artery and vein hypoplasia.

Echocardiography

The transposed relationship of the great vessels is immediately evident from the parasternal window with both great vessels running parallel to one another (i.e., both coursing in their long axes in the parasternal long-axis plane or both coursing in their transverse axes in the parasternal short-axis plane). In addition, the posterior great vessel turns posteriorly almost immediately after its origin from the left ventricle, indicating that the vessel is a pulmonary artery (the aorta courses superiorly after its origin from the ventricle). Sweeping the transducer left in the parasternal long-axis plane and subsequent imaging from the parasternal short-axis plane demonstrate that the posterior great vessel bifurcates—further evidence that it is a pulmonary artery. From this latter plane, the exact relationship of the aorta to the pulmonary artery should be ascertained as right, directly anterior, or left (the D, A, or L, respectively; Van Praagh classifications). In preparation for possible arterial switch operation, the anatomy and annuli of both semilunar valves are obtained from the parasternal long and short axes. Subsequent imaging in the apical and subcostal views will demonstrate that the bifurcating great vessel (the pulmonary artery) arises posteriorly from the left ventricle (Fig. 110.6).

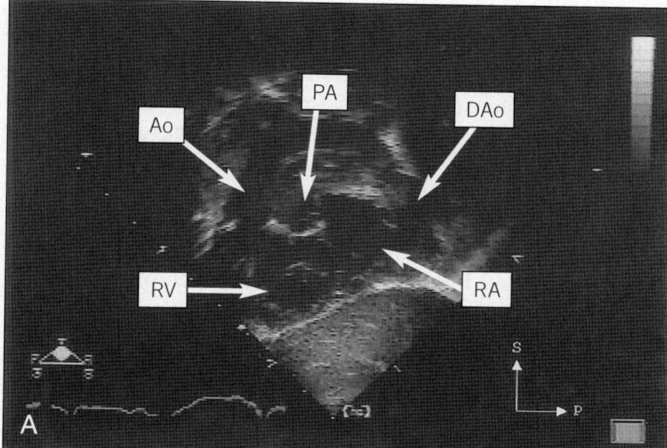

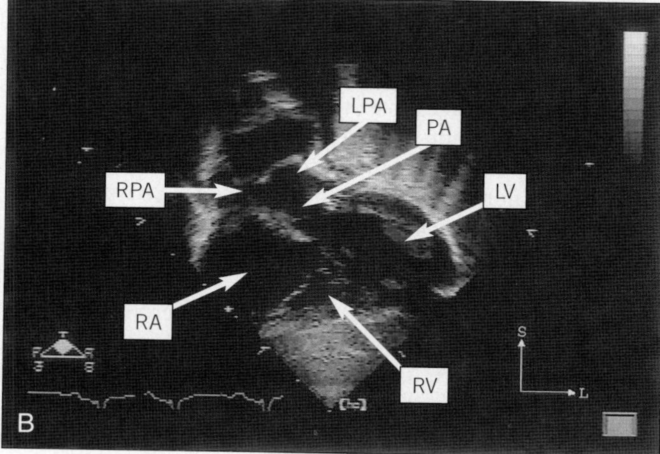

Figure 110.6 Echocardiography in transposition of the great vessels. The diagnosis of transposition of the great vessels is currently established using echocardiography. Although transposition of the great vessels is evident from the parallel alignment of the aorta and the pulmonary artery seen in the parasternal windows, the definitive views are obtained from the subcostal window. **A,** The aorta (Ao) can be seen to arise from the right ventricle (RV) in a subcostal sagittal plane. **B,** The main pulmonary artery (PA), branching into right and left pulmonary arteries (RPA, LPA), can be seen arising from the left ventricle (LV) in a subcostal coronal plane. DAo, descending aorta; L, left; P, posterior; RA, right atrium; S, superior.

The presence of life-sustaining shunts must be investigated. The presence, size, and shunting patterns of a patent ductus arteriosus and patent foramen ovale are assessed rapidly from a compilation of views. The thickness of the atrial septum should be noted before balloon atrial septostomy. Prostaglandin infusion and preparation for balloon atrial septostomy can proceed while the echocardiographic examination continues.

Associated lesions are usually easily identifiable by echocardiography. They include

- atrioventricular valve abnormalities;
- coronary artery anomalies;
- left ventricular outflow tract obstruction;
- malalignment VSDs; and
- aortic arch obstruction.

One of the greatest challenges facing the pediatric echocardiographer is evaluating the origins and proximal courses of the coronary arteries in a newborn with transposition of the great arteries, in preparation for coronary artery transfer.[9] The echocardiographer must remember that the coronary arteries will almost always arise from the sinuses facing the pulmonary artery, so that imaging should focus on these two sinuses. This is best achieved in the high parasternal short-axis view and sweeping the parasternal long-axis view. This latter view can sometimes better demonstrate the origin of the right coronary artery, so that a pericardial reflection is not mistakenly attributed to a coronary artery lumen; any suspected coronary artery lumen should be further investigated for the presence or absence of flow, using color Doppler echocardiography.

After demonstration of the main left and right coronary arteries, of particular importance is finding the origin of the left circumflex coronary artery. If it arises from a typically positioned left main coronary artery (i.e., from the left sinus), the circumflex coronary artery will run anterior to the pulmonary artery as it courses to the atrioventricular groove. If it arises from a typically positioned right coronary artery (i.e., from the right sinus), the circumflex coronary artery will run posterior to the pulmonary artery. This distinction can be made by sweeping the apical four-chamber view slowly anteriorly and ascertaining the presence or absence of a horizontally positioned coronary artery between the atrioventricular valves and the pulmonary artery (indicating a circumflex coronary artery arising from a right coronary artery).

Echocardiographic features of intramural coronary arteries include a coronary ostium arising adjacent to a commissure (rather than in the center of the sinus) and a coronary artery coursing between the aorta and the pulmonary artery.

Cardiac Catheterization

With advances in echocardiographic imaging, cardiac catheterizations are rarely needed (except for performing a balloon atrial septostomy; see following section). Occasionally, cardiac catheterization is needed to obtain better definition of the coronary arterial pattern. In this instance, simultaneous balloon occlusion of the ascending aorta and extreme caudal angulation of the anterior–posterior camera provide excellent delineation of the origins and proximal courses of the coronary arteries (see Chapter 105).

In more complex forms of transposition of the great vessels, catheterization is frequently needed to evaluate the pulmonary artery pressure and vascular resistance, the anatomy of pulmonary and subpulmonary obstruction, aortic arch problems, and relationship of VSD(s) to the great vessels.

MANAGEMENT

Medical

Prostaglandin E_1

By maintaining ductal patency, infusion of prostaglandin increases ductal flow, left atrial blood return, and mixing at the atrial level.

Other Support

Metabolic acidosis should be corrected with fluid replacement or sodium bicarbonate. If pulmonary edema develops, the patient may require mechanical ventilation. Pulmonary hypertension is quite problematic and often life-threatening, requiring pulmonary vasoactive substances, such as oxygen, nitric oxide, or both. In some of these instances, extracorporeal membrane oxygenation may be required. Even with aggressive treatment, the association of transposition of the great vessels and pulmonary hypertension carries a high mortality (up to 29% in some series).[10]

Balloon Atrial Septostomy

Because initial surgical successes in patients with transposition of the great vessels were eventually realized in atrial switch procedures that were undertaken only in later infancy (see below), palliative procedures became imperative. Early surgical experience indicated that survival through infancy could be significantly enhanced by the surgical creation or enlargement of an atrial septal defect.[3] In 1966, Rashkind and Miller[1] presented their initial experience with enlargement of an atrial septal defect by a balloon atrial septostomy using a percutaneous catheter. Now routinely performed under echocardiographic guidance, a balloon-tip catheter is introduced into the systemic venous system (usually via the femoral or umbilical vein). The tip is passed from the right atrium to the left atrium via a patent foramen ovale. The balloon is inflated while the tip is in the left atrium, care being taken to ensure that the balloon does not pass through the mitral valve or into a pulmonary vein or left atrial appendage. With the balloon fully inflated and in correct position, the catheter is withdrawn rapidly, so that the balloon passes through and tears the atrial septum. The balloon is then rapidly deflated while the tip is in the right atrium. The resulting defect is sized, and the procedure repeated if necessary. In patients with previously restrictive atrial level shunts, the balloon atrial septostomy results in a prompt increase in arterial saturation. Sometimes, volume infusion is necessary to ensure adequate mixing. Even with the advent of prostaglandin treatment, the balloon atrial septostomy remains critical. Paradoxically, newborns with restrictive atrial communications may become more cyanosed with prostaglandin therapy, because the increased left atrial blood return produces left atrial hypertension, resulting in closure of the flap of the foramen ovale and less atrial mixing, pulmonary edema, and decreased effective pulmonary blood flow. Inadequate size of the foramen ovale is an important cause of attrition before neonatal surgery, making early balloon atrial septostomy critical.[11]

Surgical

Atrial Switch Operation

Initial attempts at switching the great vessels in the 1950s were unsuccessful, because of either surgical management of the coronary arteries that included leaving one or both attached to the pulmonary artery or difficult transfer techniques. Surgeons turned their attention to more creative operative procedures with possible lower morbidity and mortality. In 1959, the Swedish surgeon Ake Senning[12] described his initial experience in four children (three of whom died) with correcting transposition "on the atrial side." The Senning operation uses native atrial wall and septal tissue to baffle pulmonary venous blood to the tricuspid valve/right ventricle and systemic venous blood to the mitral valve/left ventricle. In 1964, while at the Toronto Hospital for Sick Children, Mustard[13] reported his modification of the atrial switch procedure using pericardial tissue as the baffle material (Fig. 110.7). The use of native atrial tissue in the Senning operation has the theoretical advantage of preserving normal atrial function and growth of the venous pathways. Today, the atrial switch operations are used infrequently, but they can be useful if other lesions preclude an arterial switch, such as in transposition of the great vessels with left ventricular outflow tract hypoplasia, pulmonary valve stenosis, and a small ventricular septal defect.

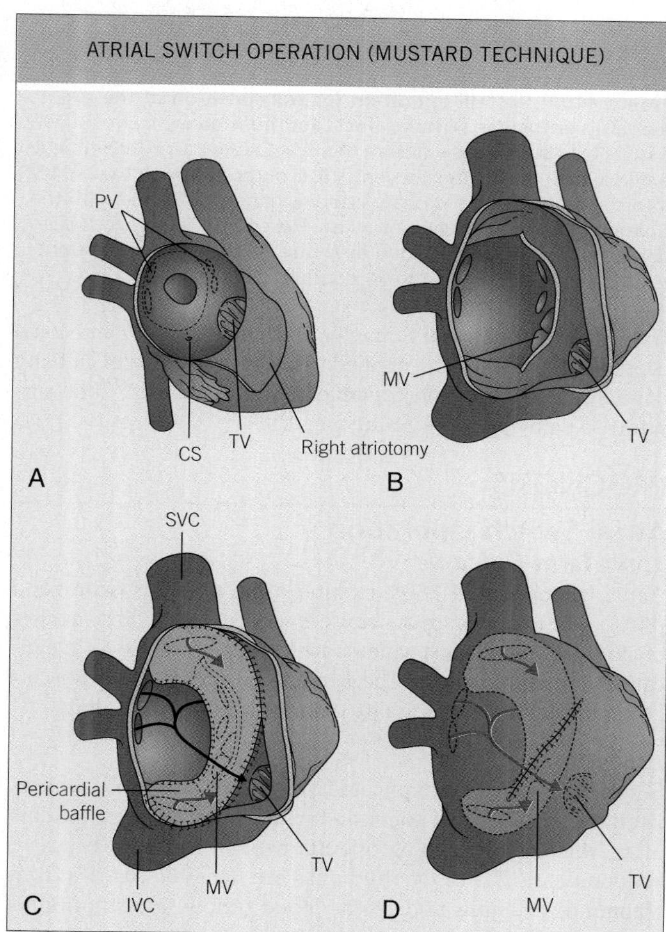

Figure 110.7 Atrial switch operation (Mustard technique) for transposition of the great vessels. An early operation for patients with transposition of the great vessels was the atrial switch operation (either a Senning or a Mustard operation pictured here). This operation consists of opening the right atrium (**A**); excising the remaining atrial septum (**B**); creating a baffle connecting the superior vena cava (SVC) and the inferior vena cava (IVC) to the mitral valve (MV), and pulmonary venous blood to the tricuspid valve (TV) (**C**); and closure of the atriotomy (**D**). CS, coronary sinus; PV, pulmonary veins.

Arterial Switch Operation

In 1976, Jatene and colleagues[14] revived interest in the arterial switch by proposing transection of the great vessels distal to the level of the pericardial reflection, and a unique coronary artery transfer technique utilizing buttons of surrounding aortic wall. This facilitated easier creation of the great vessel anastomoses, adjustment of the sizes of the great vessels, and correction of any semilunar valve leaks. It also alleviated problems with future coronary stenoses. Of note, the ascending aorta was placed in its anatomically correct position, so that the right pulmonary artery coursed posterior to it (Fig. 110.8a). This more posterior location of the right pulmonary artery often resulted in the frequent need for an interposition cylindrical prosthesis in the pulmonary outflow tract, to facilitate the lengthy anastomosis between the anterior main pulmonary artery and the posterior branch pulmonary arteries and to avoid coronary artery compression. In 1981, Lecompte and coworkers[15] placed the pulmonary arterial trunk and branch arteries in front of the aortic root, to eliminate tension in the pulmonary artery and coronary artery compression (Fig. 110.8b).

Operative mortality was approximately 11% in the early 1990s and continues to improve (7%).[4,16] Initially, abnormal coronary artery patterns and presence of a VSD were associated with increased surgical risk, but surgical experience has improved so greatly that neither is currently associated with an increased risk of death. Intramural coronary arteries, single right coronary artery, and an "inverted" coronary artery pattern (left anterior descending and circumflex from the right-facing sinus, right from the left-facing sinus) are particularly problematic.[17] However, current risk factors for death include only low birth weight and hypoplasia of the aortic arch.[18]

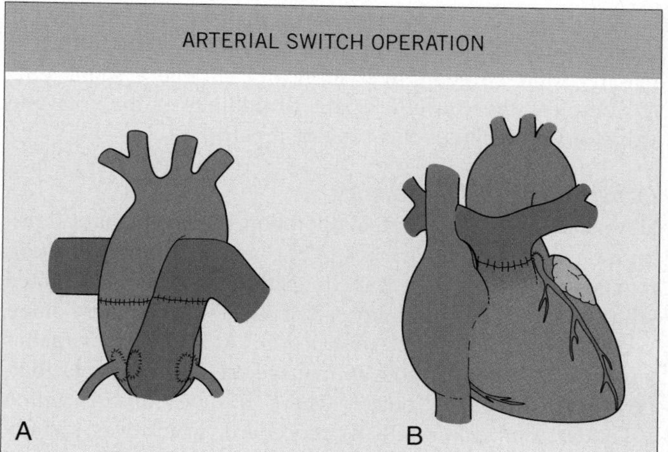

Figure 110.8 Arterial switch operation for transposition of the great vessels. A, Currently, patients undergo the arterial switch operation, which consists of transecting the great vessels and anastomosing each to the contralateral valve annulus, in addition to performing a coronary artery transfer. **B,** Because this operation stretches the right pulmonary artery, the LeCompte maneuver is usually performed as part of the arterial switch operation.

In general, the arterial switch operation should be performed within the first 2 to 3 weeks of life, while the left ventricle continues to face high pressure as a result of increased pulmonary vascular resistance, so that it can adequately function in the milieu of the relatively high systemic pressures it will face after surgery. However, some surgeons have had success with the arterial switch operation for infants presenting as late as 2 months of age.[19] Left ventricular pressure can also be maintained with associated large VSD, dynamic subpulmonary stenosis, or a large patent ductus arteriosus. However, because these patients are prone to pulmonary vascular disease, leaving (or creating) a large left-to-right shunt for even a few weeks or months may lead to irreversible pulmonary hypertension. If left ventricular pressure and therefore left ventricular mass decrease, the left ventricle must undergo preparation if an arterial switch operation is contemplated. Yacoub and colleagues[20] were the first to propose a two-stage arterial switch operation with initial placement of a pulmonary artery band to "train" an unprepared left ventricle. The duration of left ventricular training with the pulmonary artery band ranges from as long as 1 year in earlier experience to as short as 1 week more recently.[21] Using such an approach, left ventricular mass increases most rapidly in the first 2 days after band placement, with an exponential decrease in the growth rate thereafter. Recent animal studies suggest that providing a pressure overload stimulus intermittently (much like athletic training) may shorten the overall time of training.[22]

Rastelli Repair

In 1969, Rastelli and colleagues[23] described a surgical approach to repair transposition of the great vessels with VSD and pulmonary stenosis (Fig. 110.9). This operation entails closing the VSD by creating an interventricular tunnel, so that the left ventricle outflow is directed to the aorta. The right ventricular outflow is reestablished by placement of a right ventricular–pulmonary artery conduit, bypassing the pulmonary stenosis. The operation generally has excellent results.[24] For success of this operation, the VSD must be both large and free of obstruction from atrioventricular valve tissue, so that the neo–left ventricular outflow tract is patent. Some surgeons will surgically enlarge a small VSD to complete the Rastelli repair. Straddling of the tricuspid valve often precludes this type of repair.

Other Surgical Treatments

Despite the use of the Rastelli operation, management of transposition of the great arteries, VSD, and pulmonary stenosis remains a challenge. The Rastelli operation has been associated with continuing late mortality, often due to development of left ventricular outflow tract obstruction. Accordingly, surgeons have sought other methods to manage the left ventricular outflow tract from the outset. These include the *réparation à l'étage ventriculaire* (REV) procedure, which was initially described by LeCompte and associates,[25] is a modification of the Rastelli operation, emphasizing simultaneous conal resection, reconstruction of the pulmonary outflow tract without using a prosthetic conduit by wide mobilization of the pulmonary trunk to the right ventricle. The Nikaidoh[26] procedure, which consists of translocating the entire aortic root (immediately below the aortic annulus) into the left ventricular outflow

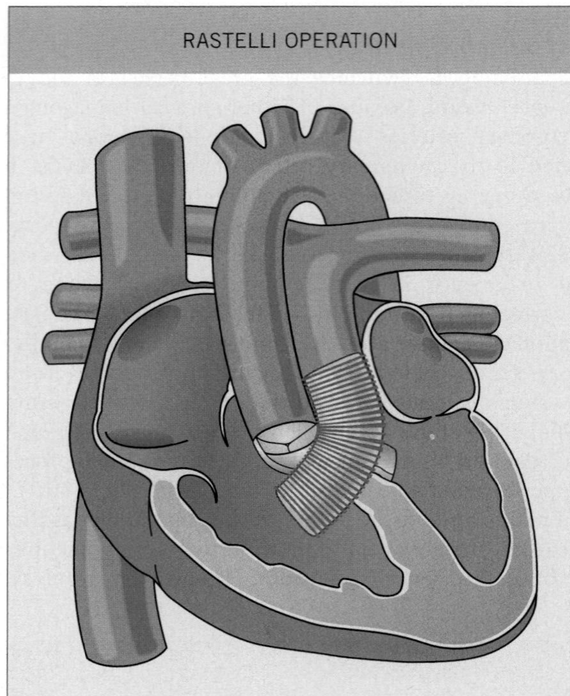

Figure 110.9 Rastelli operation for transposition of the great vessels, ventricular septal defect, and pulmonary stenosis. The Rastelli operation entails closure of the VSD using an interventricular baffle, which directs the left ventricular output through the old VSD into the aorta. The pulmonary artery is either transected with the pulmonary valve oversewn or anastomosed end-to-side to the aorta. Pulmonary artery blood flow is restored by placing a right ventricular to pulmonary artery conduit.

tract after the pulmonary annulus and subpulmonary and conal septum (if present) are divided. This procedure was initially considered to pose unacceptable technical danger[27] but currently is enjoying some resurgence.[28,29]

PROGNOSIS

Atrial Switch Operation

Long-Term Outcome

Actuarial survival at 28 years after atrial switch is quite good (80%). The major cause of demise is sudden death.[30] The quality of life is good, with most patients achieving a normal level of education and employment. The Senning procedure generally has better morbidity and mortality than the Mustard procedure.[31,32]

Arrhythmia

Sinus bradycardia complicated by recurrent atrial tachyarrhythmias is the most common management issue in patients after Mustard or Senning operations, and can be a cause of sudden death. These dysrhythmias are believed to arise from trauma to the sinus node or its blood supply, interruption of intra-atrial conduction pathways, and damage to the atrioventricular node or its blood supply from the extensive intra-atrial suture lines. Such dysrhythmias can occur in more than 50% of long-term survivors.[33]

Right Ventricular Function

The atrial switch operation places the right ventricle in the position of the systemic ventricle—a task for which it may be woefully ill-equipped. Initially, the incidence of right ventricular failure was believed to be rare (3% in the long term); however, more recent evidence indicates an incidence as high as 22%.[30,34] Possible etiologies for right ventricular dysfunction include

- the presence of a poorly contracting segment (the infundibulum);
- poor preoperative coronary perfusion;
- abnormal interventricular pressure relationships distorting right ventricular and tricuspid valve anatomy; and
- abnormal right ventricular myocardial fiber geometry and/or mismatch between right ventricular coronary blood flow and the demands of systemic ventricular work.

Even so, one study has shown that the right ventricular function may be near that of a normal subpulmonary right ventricle or even a normal subaortic left ventricle.[35] These findings have prompted investigators to study possible predictors for right ventricular failure. Early operative age (i.e., younger than 2 months) is associated with better long-term right ventricular systolic performance, whereas right ventriculotomy and VSD patch are risk factors. Because the right ventricle has unusual morphology not easily modeled by simple geometric principles, newer indices not dependent on ventricular geometry have been developed to evaluate right ventricular function and may be helpful in this population.[36] In addition, the presence of perfusion defects on single photon emission computed tomography may be a sensitive predictor (and better than exercise testing) of right ventricular dysfunction.[37]

Beta blockers may be of benefit in treating chronic right ventricular dysfunction in these patients.[38]

Intra-atrial Baffle Obstruction or Leak

Obstructions of the systemic and pulmonary venous pathways can be complications of the atrial switch operation. Pulmonary venous obstruction should be assessed in the event of pulmonary hypertension.

Arterial Switch Operation

Left Ventricular Function

The theoretical advantage of the arterial switch operation—placing the left ventricle into a systemic position—has been validated by experience in studies showing preserved ejection fraction and normal stress-velocity relationships.[39] Some studies, however, have shown that left ventricular systolic dysfunction occurs in up to 29% of patients. Symptomatic left ventricular dysfunction is rare.

Coronary Artery Perfusion

As a result of the coronary artery transfer occurring with the arterial switch operation, the coronary arteries can become stenosed, stretched, or occluded, leading to ischemia and subsequent left ventricular dysfunction and/or mitral insufficiency.[40] Sometimes, patients can succumb from myocardial infarction or sudden death—up to 10% of patients in some series.[41,42] Numerous studies have demonstrated abnormal myocardial blood flow and coronary flow reserve.[43] Although some of the investigators suggested that these abnormalities may be the result of cardiopulmonary bypass surgery, the majority of evidence indicates that these patients specifically can have decreased coronary reserve in the absence of ischemic symptoms and angiographic abnormalities. The generally global nature of perfusion abnormalities suggests altered vasoreactivity. The prognostic significance remains unknown. Stress echocardiography may be a valuable method with which to screen and follow such patients.[44] Since patients undergoing arterial switch operation seem particularly prone to abnormal coronary perfusion, they should be actively counseled to lead a healthy lifestyle including diet, exercise, hypertension screening, and avoidance of tobacco.

Neo-aorta

Up to 50% of survivors of arterial switch operations can have aortic root dilatation and associated aortic insufficiency. Potential causes include differences in pulmonary valve collagen and elastic tissue, and anatomic factors related either to transfer of the coronary ostial buttons producing enlargement of two of the sinuses or to construction of the neo-aortic root.[45] Aortic insufficiency may become sufficiently severe to require replacement of the aortic valve.[45] The incidence is greater after previous pulmonary artery banding, with older age at time of arterial switch operation, and presence of a VSD.[45,46]

Supravalvar Aortic Stenosis

Supravalvar aortic stenosis is extremely uncommon, perhaps because of the limited tension on the suture line. When it does occur, it is usually associated with preoperative pathology such as arch hypoplasia.

Supravalvar Pulmonic Stenosis

Supravalvar pulmonic stenosis can occur at the site of aorta to pulmonary artery anastomosis, or more proximally at the site where the coronary ostial buttons are removed. In some series, more than 50% of survivors have had some degree of pulmonic stenosis, with approximately 7% requiring intervention (reoperation or catheterization placement of stents). Supravalvar pulmonary stenosis may develop because of a power loss of the blood flow, resulting from the altered flow dynamics associated with the Lecompte maneuver.

Bronchial Collateral Vessels

A possible important source of intercirculatory mixing preoperatively, enlarged bronchial collateral vessels may be responsible for a significant left-to-right shunt and/or pulmonary vascular disease postoperatively. They may be present in up to 46% of patients after arterial switching. Usually clinically silent, they are often apparent only by angiography or color Doppler echocardiography. Coil embolization can be performed for significant shunts.

Rastelli Repair

Intramural Ventricular Septal Defect

The superior-rightward margin of the VSD patch must be sutured to the right ventricular free wall. Occasionally, the surgeon can mistakenly suture the patch to right ventricular trabeculations instead of the myocardial wall. Significant residual ventricular level shunts can then course through the trabeculations at the superior edge of the patch.

Left Ventricular Outflow Obstruction

If the VSD is small and has not been surgically enlarged or if atrioventricular valve tissue is associated with the defect, neo–left ventricular outflow tract obstruction may occur.

SUMMARY

Transposition of the great vessels is defined as a discordant ventriculoarterial connection and is one of the most common cyanotic heart diseases. Usually, it occurs in isolation but may be associated with ventricular septal defect, atrioventricular valve abnormalities, pulmonary vascular disease, left ventricular outflow tract obstruction, unusual coronary artery origins and courses, and aortic arch obstruction. Because the pulmonary and systemic circulations are in parallel with one another, a shunt (atrial septal defect, VSD, or patent ductus arteriosus) is necessary to sustain life. Surgery consists of switching the aorta and the pulmonary artery to the contralateral valve annulus. This surgery also necessitates transfer of the coronary arteries from the native aortic stump to the neo-aortic (native pulmonary artery) stump. Although long-term complications, such as aortic root dilatation, coronary perfusion abnormalities, and supravalvar pulmonary stenosis, can occur, survival is generally excellent.

chapter 111

Pulmonary Atresia with Ventricular Septal Defect

Malcolm J. MacDonald, Frank L. Hanley, and Daniel J. Murphy, Jr.

Definition

- Pulmonary atresia with ventricular septal defect is the most severe form of tetralogy of Fallot, with pulmonary blood flow arising solely from the systemic arterial system.

Key Features

- Spectrum of severity runs from unifocal pulmonary blood supply from a patent ductus arteriosus with confluent pulmonary arteries, to discontinuous pulmonary arteries with ductally derived pulmonary blood flow, or pulmonary flow from major aortopulmonary collateral arteries with arborization abnormalities.
- Neonatal and childhood presentation is very variable with unpredictable cyanosis or pulmonary overcirculation. Survival to adulthood is rare.

Therapy

- Prostaglandin E_1 is administered to neonates who have ductal-dependent pulmonary circulation.
- Echocardiography, computerized tomography, magnetic resonance imaging and angiography are used to define the anatomy of pulmonary arteries and major aortopulmonary collateral arteries.
- An aggressive surgical approach is recommended early in life, the aim being to unifocalize sources of pulmonary blood supply and complete intracardiac repair.

Pulmonary atresia with ventricular septal defect (VSD) generally represents the most severe end of the spectrum of tetralogy of Fallot. The variety and severity of abnormalities of pulmonary blood supply are responsible for the range of clinical presentations and the challenges encountered in surgical management. A natural history characterized by significant neonatal mortality and little chance of survival beyond the third decade is being altered by increasingly aggressive surgical management early in life, aimed at producing a septated heart with low pulmonary resistance and right ventricular pressure. The success of these management schemes depends on meticulous diagnostic studies, careful planning, and advanced surgical techniques. Whereas in the past there were few adult survivors, changes in the management of neonates who have pulmonary atresia with VSD are likely to produce dramatic changes in longevity and quality of life.

ANATOMY AND PATHOLOGY

Embryology

During early fetal development, the nutrient blood supply for the developing lungs originates from systemic segmental arteries off the dorsal aortae. In addition, by the 27th day, the pulmonary vascular plexus is also supplied by branches of the sixth aortic arches, which are destined to become the "true" pulmonary arteries. For some time, the developing lung parenchyma receives a dual blood supply, but by the 50th day of gestation the segmental arteries involute, resulting in pulmonary arterial blood flow exclusively from the right ventricle.

In pulmonary atresia with VSD, the normal connection between the right ventricular outflow tract and the central pulmonary arteries is not established or is interrupted, and blood supply to the developing lung is maintained through the ductus arteriosus or major aortopulmonary collateral arteries (MAPCAs), or both.[1] It has been proposed that MAPCAs represent aberrant bronchial vessels, though this is controversial.[2,3] MAPCAs may also represent systemic segmental arteries that do not involute in response to the pulmonary atresia.

Genetics

Microdeletions in the chromosomal region 22q11 occur in patients who have velocardiofacial syndrome, DiGeorge syndrome, and cardiac malformations that involve the ventricular outflow tracts and the aortic arch. Studies have confirmed the association between deletion of chromosome 22q11 and pulmonary atresia with VSD. Deletion of chromosome 22q11 is present in approximately 20% of patients who have tetralogy of Fallot, but the deletion is present in 40% of patients who have pulmonary atresia with VSD.[4] In patients who have pulmonary atresia with VSD, the presence of 22q11 deletion is associated with smaller central pulmonary arteries and the presence of MAPCAs.[5]

Anatomy

In most cases, the intracardiac anatomy in pulmonary atresia with VSD is similar to that in tetralogy of Fallot. The VSD is usually a large, nonrestrictive, malalignment defect with overriding of the aorta. Occasionally the VSD is restrictive, primarily because of the presence of accessory abnormal tricuspid valve tissue. Additional VSDs occur in 5% to 15% of cases.[6]

The site of pulmonary atresia is variable and may occur in the infundibulum or at the pulmonary valve, or it may extend to include the entire main pulmonary artery. When the atresia involves only the pulmonary valve, a plate-like structure may be present at valve level, with a well-developed infundibulum on one side and a main pulmonary artery on the other. The main pulmonary artery may be patent to the point of plate-like valve atresia, hypoplastic, or absent (persisting only as a fibrous cord between the right ventricular outflow tract and the central pulmonary arteries).

The aorta is dilated and overrides the VSD. Aortic valve stenosis is encountered rarely. The aortic arch is right-sided in 25% to 50% of cases. An aberrant subclavian artery is present in 18% of cases.[6]

Pulmonary Artery Anatomy

The anatomy of pulmonary blood supply distinguishes pulmonary atresia with VSD from ordinary tetralogy of Fallot, and is responsible for the variable clinical presentation and the challenges of surgical management. Blood supply to the lungs is derived entirely from the systemic arterial circulation, most commonly a patent ductus arteriosus (PDA), MAPCAs, or both.

In the simplest and most favorable form of pulmonary atresia with VSD, pulmonary blood flow is solely supplied by a PDA (unifocal pulmonary blood flow), and the central pulmonary arteries tend to be small but confluent (Fig. 111.1). The distribution of the pulmonary arteries is usually normal, with rare arborization abnormalities.[1] This arrangement occurs in 37% of cases. At the other end of the spectrum, the ductus is absent and the central pulmonary arteries are diminutive or atretic. In one large series, atretic intrapericardial pulmonary arteries were present 23% of the time.[7] All pulmonary blood flow is supplied by MAPCAs, with or without connections to the central pulmonary arteries (Fig. 111.2). Arborization abnormalities are common.

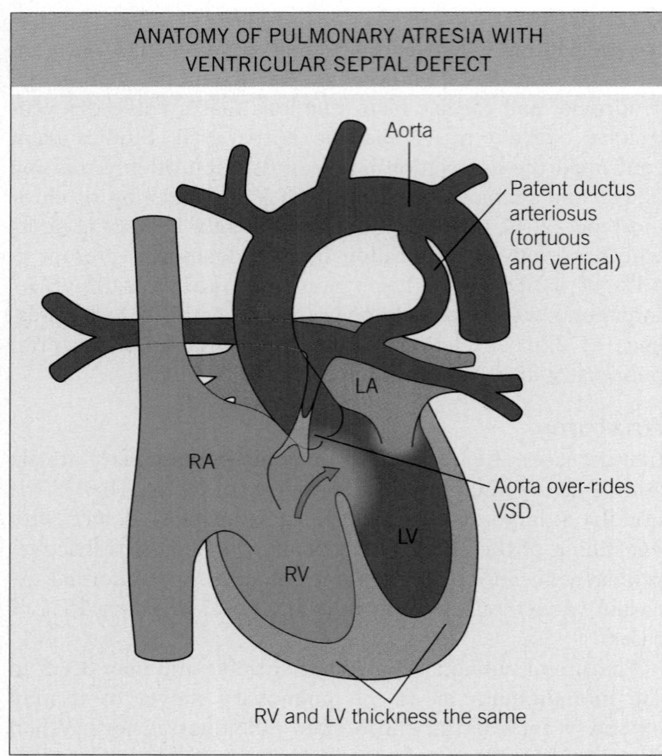

Figure 111.1 Anatomy of pulmonary atresia with ventricular septal defect (VSD). This "most favorable" type includes confluent central pulmonary arteries with a patent ductus arteriosus as the sole source of pulmonary blood flow. LA, left atrium; LV, left ventricle; RA, right atrium; RV, right ventricle.

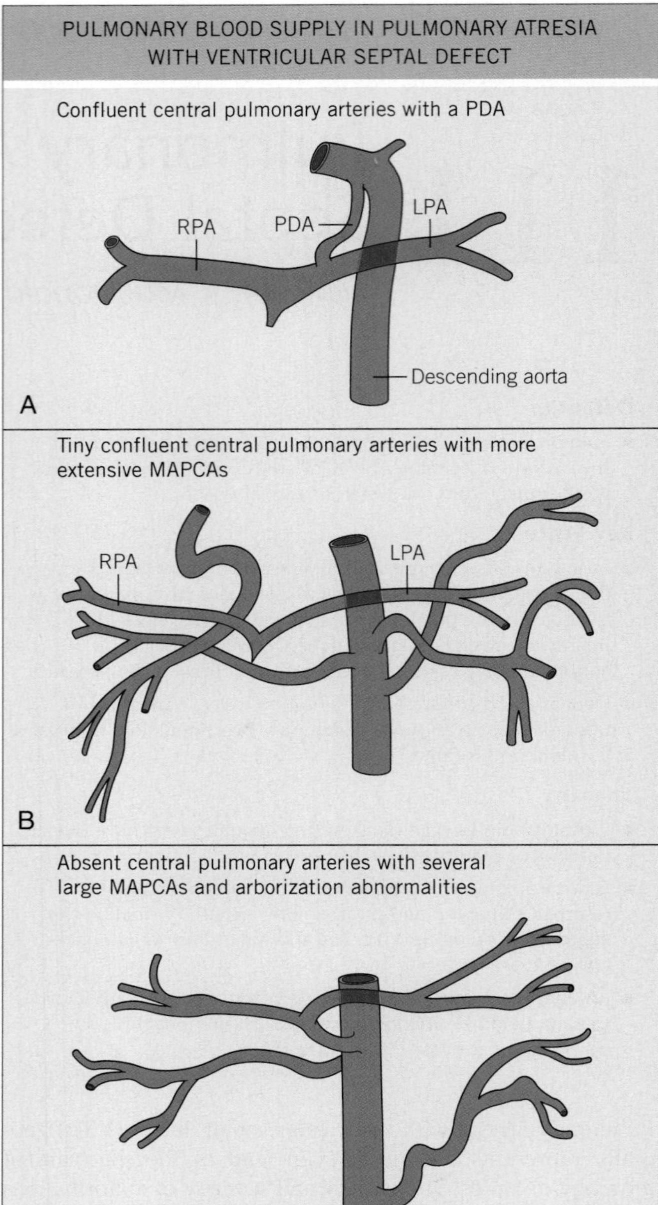

Figure 111.2 Pulmonary blood supply in pulmonary atresia with ventricular septal defect. A, Confluent pulmonary arteries with a patent ductus arteriosus (PDA). **B,** Confluent central pulmonary arteries with major aortopulmonary collateral arteries (MAPCAs) and absent PDA. There are prominent arborization abnormalities. **C,** Absent central pulmonary arteries with MAPCAs and arborization abnormalities. LPA, left pulmonary artery; RPA, right pulmonary artery.

If a patent ductus connects to confluent pulmonary arteries arborization, abnormalities are rare. If a ductus connects to one pulmonary artery (with discontinuous central pulmonary arteries PAs), that lung has normal arborization. MAPCAs to the contralateral lung may be associated with extensive arborization abnormalities.

Between 20% and 30% of patients who have pulmonary atresia with VSD have congenitally nonconfluent pulmonary arteries.[8] Confluence of the pulmonary arteries tends to be related to the presence of the ductus and the number of MAPCAs. Sixty percent of patients who have confluent pulmonary arteries have large MAPCAs, as do 100% of patients who have nonconfluent pulmonary arteries.[8] Among patients with absence of the ductus, confluent pulmonary arteries are present in 70%.

Although central pulmonary arteries are confluent in 70% to 80% of cases, they may supply only a portion of each lung, because of the presence of MAPCAs and arborization abnormalities. Arborization abnormalities occur in 50% of patients who have confluent pulmonary arteries. Such abnormalities are more severe in the presence of nonconfluent pulmonary arteries: 36% of patients who have nonconfluent pulmonary arteries have fewer than 10 pulmonary vascular segments in continuity with the central pulmonary arteries. In addition, the number of large MAPCAs correlates inversely with the incompleteness of arborization of the left and right pulmonary arteries.[8]

Stenosis of a central pulmonary artery may occur in patients who have ductal-dependent confluent pulmonary arteries, and is most likely to occur at the origin of the pulmonary artery on the side of the ductus.[9] Among patients who have ductal supply of confluent pulmonary arteries, 10% have stenosis of the origin of the right pulmonary artery and 20% have a stenosis of the left pulmonary artery caused by extension of ductal tissue into the wall of the pulmonary artery.[8]

Major Aortopulmonary Collateral Arteries

Most collateral arteries arise from the anterior surface of the descending thoracic aorta,[1,10] but MAPCAs can also originate from the coronary arteries (in approximately 10%),[9] the subclavian arteries, and, less commonly, from the cephalic arteries, the abdominal aorta, intercostal arteries, or the internal mammary artery.

Before entering the lung parenchyma, MAPCAs retain the histologic characteristics of muscular arteries. Once a MAPCA enters the lung parenchyma, the median muscular layer gradually changes to an elastic lamina that structurally resembles a true pulmonary artery.[10,11]

Major aortopulmonary collateral arteries are frequently tortuous, and up to 60% of them have areas of stenosis at the origin of the vessel or near the pulmonary artery connection.[1,10] Stenosis is caused by intimal proliferation and frequently occurs at branching points of the vessel—for example, at the junction of the MAPCA with the pulmonary artery.[10,11] The presence and severity of stenoses determine flow and pressure within the MAPCA and the pulmonary artery to which it connects. Unobstructed flow allows pulmonary vascular obstructive disease to develop in the segments of lung supplied by that MAPCA.[1]

Connections between the central pulmonary arteries and MAPCAs are observed in 40% of patients. In the other 60%, the MAPCAs enter the pulmonary hilum, travel with the bronchi as pulmonary arteries, and supply a variable number of segments. Major aortopulmonary collateral arteries may anastomose with a central pulmonary artery or its hilar or lobar branches (Fig. 111.3), usually connecting end-to-side to the central pulmonary arteries or, in the hilum, to the interlobar or intralobar pulmonary arteries. When the MAPCA does not connect to a pulmonary artery, blood flow to those lung segments is dependent upon the MAPCA, and future incorporation of those lung segments requires surgical connection to a central pulmonary artery.

The number of MAPCAs and the number of lung segments supplied is variable. In 307 consecutive patients reported by Hanley and colleagues[12] there were 3.8 ± 1.4 MAPCAs per patient. Of patients who have nonconfluent pulmonary arteries, 50% have four or more MAPCAs. All patients who have nonconfluent pulmonary arteries have at least one MAPCA; in 4% of patients, five or six MAPCAs are present.

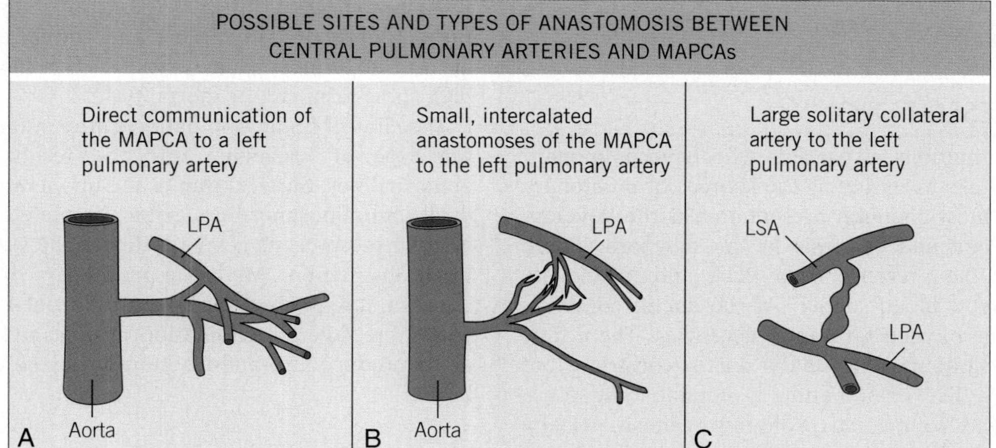

Figure 111.3 Possible sites and types of connections between central pulmonary arteries and major aortopulmonary collateral arteries (MAPCAs). A, Direct communication (with stenosis) of the MAPCA to a left pulmonary artery (LPA). This creates a dual supply to some lung segments. Other segments may be supplied entirely by other branches of that MAPCA. **B,** Small, intercalated connections of the MAPCA to the left pulmonary artery. Although blood flow from the MAPCA may enter the pulmonary arteries, the blood supply from the MAPCA is not secure. Other segments may be supplied entirely by the MAPCA. **C,** Large solitary collateral artery to the left pulmonary artery. The collateral artery may have areas of stenosis, particularly at the connection. LSA, left subclavian artery.

PATHOPHYSIOLOGY

In most cases of pulmonary atresia with ventricular septal defect the VSD is large and nonrestrictive, with equal systolic pressures in the right and left ventricles. As long as the mitral and tricuspid valves are of normal size, no atrial septal defect is required.

Because all pulmonary blood flow is derived from systemic sources, aortic and pulmonary artery oxygen saturation are identical. The eventual aortic saturation represents a mixture of pulmonary venous flow and systemic venous return. Greater pulmonary flow produces greater systemic arterial saturation. For example, a systemic arterial saturation of 85% indicates a pulmonary to systemic flow ratio of approximately 2:1. Arterial saturation of less than 80% suggests reduced pulmonary flow, and oxygen saturations greater than 85% are consistent with large amounts of pulmonary blood flow.

In the neonate, decreasing arterial saturation indicates a restrictive or closing ductus arteriosus, whereas low but stable oxygen saturation suggests collateral circulation with low pulmonary flow. High arterial oxygen saturation suggests excessive pulmonary blood flow, which can produce congestive heart failure in infants.

High flow through nonrestrictive MAPCAs may produce pulmonary vascular obstructive disease in the segments of pulmonary arteries that are supplied by those vessels. Although progressive stenosis of MAPCAs frequently occurs, stenosis may develop after irreversible vascular changes have been produced in the affected lung segments. "Perfectly balanced" MAPCAs with adequate pulmonary flow and no overcirculation are uncommon and unreliable.

Although the aortic valve is structurally normal, aortic regurgitation of some degree occurs in 77% of patients and may be moderate or severe in more than 33% of unoperated and palliated adult survivors.

Until the VSD is closed, patients who have pulmonary atresia with VSD have an intracardiac right-to-left shunt, which exposes them to the risk of brain abscess and embolic stroke, and to the effects of long-term hypoxemia.

CLINICAL PRESENTATIONS

The clinical presentations of patients who have pulmonary atresia with VSD are as varied as the sources of pulmonary blood flow. The most common presentation is the development of hypoxemia and cyanosis in the newborn infant, which occurs in the presence of a PDA and inadequate collateral pulmonary blood supply. As the ductus constricts or closes, systemic oxygen saturation decreases. There may be a transient systolic murmur as the ductus constricts, but frequently the cardiac examination is notable only for a single second heart sound and profound cyanosis, usually without respiratory distress. Such infants require treatment with prostaglandin E_1 to maintain ductal patency until a stable source of pulmonary blood supply can be created surgically. More than 50% of patients who have pulmonary atresia with VSD present with cyanosis in the neonatal period.

Infants with MAPCAs may have only mild cyanosis at birth, either because the ductus remains patent or because MAPCAs provide adequate blood supply. Such infants may appear to be "well balanced" early in life. However, pulmonary perfusion may be very heterogeneous with some segments having poor perfusion because of hypoplasia or stenoses, and other segments having severe overcirculation. Cyanosis is therefore generally progressive as the MAPCAs become stenotic or as pulmonary vascular obstructive disease develops, and lung segments are irretrievably lost.

The physical examination of infants with MAPCAs is characterized by continuous murmurs heard over the thorax on the side of the large MAPCAs. Continuous murmurs may be heard unilaterally or bilaterally, especially in the back. In the neonate, pulmonary resistance may be high enough for no continuous murmur to be produced by MAPCAs, but as pulmonary resistance decreases during the first 4 to 6 weeks of life, continuous murmurs become more apparent.

In 25% of infants with large MAPCAs, pulmonary blood flow is sufficiently increased to produce signs and symptoms of congestive heart failure (including failure to thrive, tachypnea, and hepatomegaly) once pulmonary vascular resistance has decreased from the newborn levels. Congestive heart failure in an infant who has pulmonary atresia with VSD and MAPCAs is an indication for surgical intervention, both to control the overcirculation and to prevent the development of vascular disease in the segments of lung that are supplied by large MAPCAs. Because large MAPCAs with increased flow are frequently accompanied by small central pulmonary arteries with arborization abnormalities, such infants require thorough diagnostic evaluations and a carefully coordinated surgical approach.

In a study by Bull and colleagues,[13] although 65% of patients with complex pulmonary atresia presented in infancy, 10% were first diagnosed when they were older than 10 years, demonstrating how subtle the clinical findings can be in some cases. Older patients generally present with significant cyanosis as MAPCAs become more stenotic and there is failure of very small pulmonary arteries to grow.

Unoperated adult survivors tend to be cyanotic, and none is asymptomatic. Of these patients, 50% have limitations in the activities of daily living and cardiac failure occurs in 30%. Unoperated adult survivors with heart failure face a high short-term risk of mortality.[14]

The clinical findings in patients after surgery are related to the type of procedure and the residual hemodynamic abnormalities. Surgical shunts and unoperated MAPCAs produce continuous murmurs. After complete repair, an ejection systolic murmur suggests residual right ventricular outflow tract obstruction. Moderate pulmonary regurgitation produces a low-pitched early diastolic decrescendo murmur; with more severe regurgitation, systolic and diastolic components produce a to-and-fro murmur at the upper left sternal border.

DIAGNOSTIC TECHNIQUES

Because the defect is variable and large MAPCAs are frequently accompanied by small central pulmonary arteries with arborization abnormalities, infants with pulmonary atresia and ventricular septal defect require thorough diagnostic evaluations and a carefully coordinated management approach.

Electrocardiography

The electrocardiogram in patients who have pulmonary atresia with VSD generally demonstrate right axis deviation in the frontal plane and right ventricular hypertrophy. Conduction abnormalities are unusual, but right bundle branch block is typically present after surgical repair involving a right ventriculotomy.

Chest Radiography

The classic chest radiographic finding is of a boot-shaped heart with a prominent upturned cardiac apex and a concavity in the region of the main pulmonary artery. The aortic arch is right-sided in 50% of patients, compared with 25% in patients who have tetralogy of Fallot. Pulmonary vascular markings can be quite variable, with overall increased or decreased flow and segmental differences in flow apparent on the radiograph. The presence of normal or increased pulmonary vascular markings suggests the presence of MAPCAs.

Echocardiography

Echocardiography is the definitive imaging modality for delineation of intracardiac structures. In pulmonary atresia with VSD, the typical features of tetralogy of Fallot are noted, including the large VSD and overriding aorta. The absence of a continuity between the right ventricle and the pulmonary arteries should be demonstrated and differentiated from truncus arteriosus, in which the pulmonary arteries arise from the ascending aorta. In pulmonary atresia with VSD, there is no continuity between the ascending aorta and the proximal pulmonary arteries.

The location and degree of right ventricular outflow tract obstruction are easily demonstrated from the parasternal and subcostal views. Doppler interrogation and color flow imaging confirm the absence of prograde flow from the right ventricular outflow tract into the pulmonary artery.

Left ventricular size and function are usually normal, except in the presence of significant aortic regurgitation or excessive pulmonary blood flow. Right ventricular hypertrophy is uniformly present, and right ventricular systolic function is usually normal or mildly impaired. Significant tricuspid regurgitation is uncommon.

Although echocardiography cannot be used to delineate the pulmonary arterial tree and all sources of pulmonary blood flow completely, it is a useful tool for evaluation of the proximal pulmonary arteries and identification of a PDA or MAPCAs. Careful echocardiographic examination should yield information about the size and continuity of the proximal pulmonary arteries (which can sometimes be difficult to distinguish from MAPCAs coursing from the descending thoracic aorta toward the right lung). Proximal pulmonary arteries are imaged from parasternal, subxiphoid, and suprasternal echocardiographic windows (Fig. 111.4). The right pulmonary artery can be measured in the long and short axes.[15] The origin of the left pulmonary artery is frequently seen from the high parasternal window, and the length of the left pulmonary artery is best identified from a suprasternal notch sagittal plane angled toward the patient's left. This view is particularly important in establishing continuity of the left pulmonary artery and excluding proximal coarctation of the left pulmonary artery.

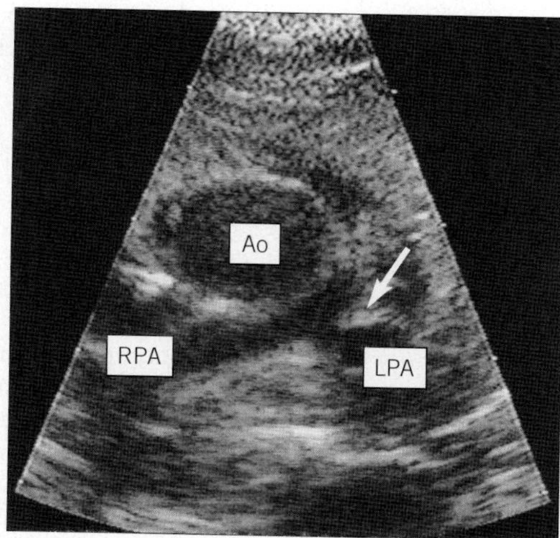

Figure 111.4 Absent connection of the main pulmonary artery to the heart with confluent central pulmonary arteries. This two-dimensional echocardiogram, from the parasternal short-axis view, also demonstrates mild proximal left pulmonary artery (LPA) stenosis (*arrow*). Ao, aorta; RPA, right pulmonary artery.

The side of the aortic arch is identified from the suprasternal notch. The initial branching pattern should be noted, and it is possible to diagnose the presence of anomalous origin of the right or left subclavian artery.[16]

The presence and location of the ductus arteriosus are demonstrated by echocardiography. The ductus is oriented vertically and is more tortuous than a normal ductus. It typically arises from the anteromedial surface of the descending thoracic aorta, but it can also arise from the innominate or subclavian arteries,[17] where it is difficult to distinguish from a MAPCA in the same location.

Echocardiography, especially with color Doppler imaging, is useful for detecting the presence of MAPCAs.[16,17] Careful color Doppler examination of the aortic arch branches and the descending thoracic aorta demonstrates continuous flow arising from collateral vessels (Fig. 111.5).

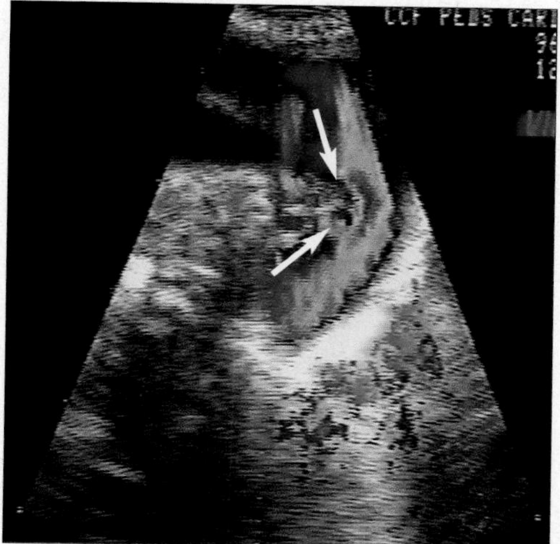

Figure 111.5 Major aortopulmonary collateral arteries (MAPCAs). This two-dimensional, color Doppler image of flow in MAPCAs reveals several MAPCAs (*arrows*) originating from the descending aorta.

However, it is not possible to define the distribution of the pulmonary arteries or MAPCAs within the lung, and distal stenoses of the pulmonary arteries are generally not visible echocardiographically.

Computed Tomography/Angiography and Magnetic Resonance Imaging/ Angiography

Recent studies[18] have demonstrated the utility of magnetic resonance imaging (MRI) in delineating pulmonary artery and MAPCA anatomy in patients with complex pulmonary blood supply. Imaging using high resolution computed tomography (CT) and CT angiography as well as MRI and magnetic resonance angiography (MRA), are increasingly used in both primary evaluation and follow-up of patients with complex pulmonary arterial anatomy. Three-dimensional reconstruction has been demonstrated to have high sensitivity and specificity in the diagnosis of pulmonary arterial stenosis and hypoplasia[19] and is frequently helpful in planning reconstructive surgical intervention (Fig. 111.6).

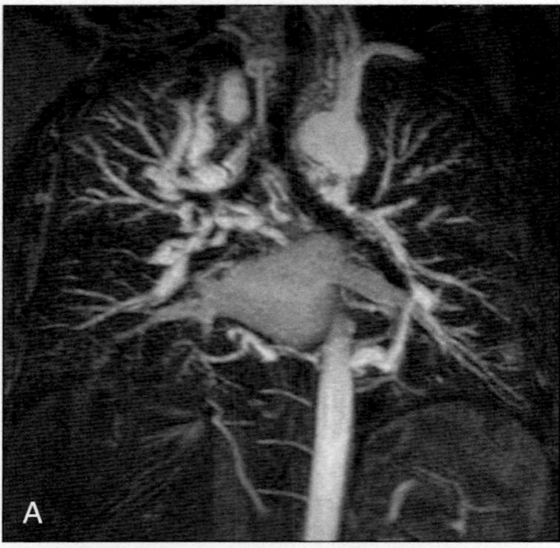

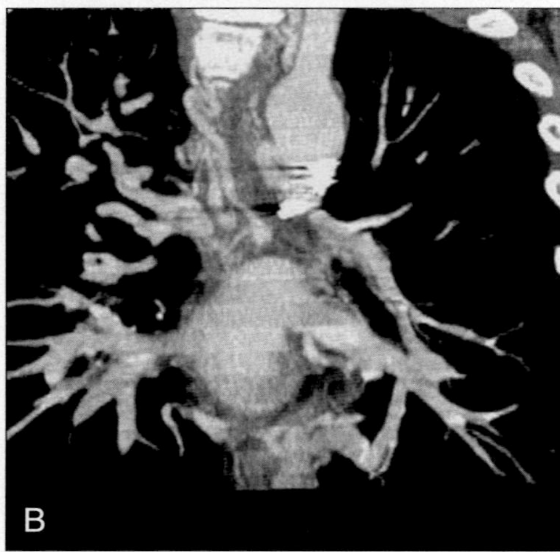

Figure 111.6 Imaging studies in a 6-year-old boy with pulmonary atresia, ventricular septal defect, and MAPCAs. Magnetic resonance imaging (**A**) and computed tomography angiography (**B**) in the same plane showing the collateral connection between a MAPCA and the left pulmonary artery.

Cardiac Catheterization and Angiography

The diagnosis of pulmonary atresia with VSD is established using echocardiography. Diagnostic cardiac catheterization is indicated after the diagnosis is established to properly define the pulmonary arterial anatomy and to plan initial surgical intervention. If a ductus arteriosus is present and the central pulmonary arteries are confluent, the newborn infant can be stabilized with prostaglandin E_1.[15] Because of the potential for progressive stenosis of MAPCAs and the development of areas of pulmonary vascular obstructive disease, even after initial surgical palliation, detailed anatomic and hemodynamic evaluations by catheterization and angiography are required early in life to provide a complete morphologic description of the sources of pulmonary blood flow, including the central pulmonary arteries, the ductus arteriosus, MAPCAs, and surgical shunts.

The central pulmonary arteries can be identified angiographically from injections in the aorta or the ductus arteriosus, or from selective injections into MAPCAs. When confluent, the hypoplastic confluent pulmonary arteries produce a characteristic Y-shaped “seagull” appearance across the mediastinum anterior to the trachea (Fig. 111.7).[20] When the pulmonary arteries are not visualized using these techniques, a pulmonary vein wedge angiogram can be useful in demonstrating the central pulmonary arteries (Fig. 111.8).[21]

Angiography should also demonstrate the origin, course, and distribution of all MAPCAs. Contrast injected into the descending thoracic aorta may help to define the number and position of MAPCAs (Fig. 111.9). Selective injections must be made into all direct and indirect MAPCAs, to obtain a complete and detailed picture of the entire pulmonary blood supply. Selective injection of MAPCAs also reveals any areas of stenosis, in addition to the points of connection between the MAPCAs and true pulmonary arteries (Fig. 111.10).[22] When there is dual supply to pulmonary segments, balloon occlusion of the MAPCA with arteriography of the true pulmonary artery can reveal the extent of central pulmonary artery distribution. In addition, balloon occlusion of the supply to the true pulmonary artery with selective injection of the MAPCA can demonstrate any additional segments supplied solely by that MAPCA.

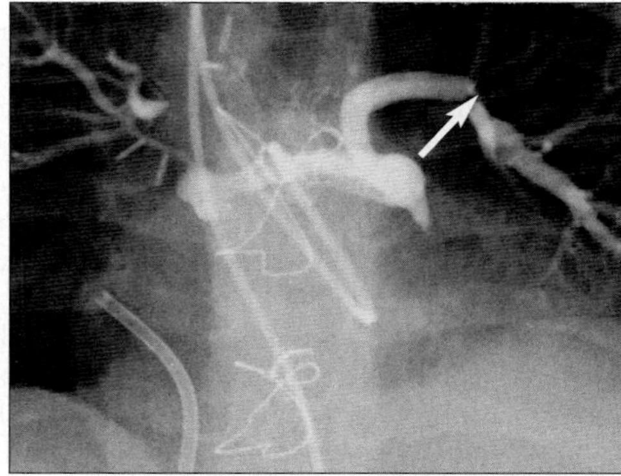

Figure 111.7 Selective injection in a central shunt. Typical “seagull” appearance of diminutive confluent pulmonary arteries. There is an area of stenosis in the left pulmonary artery (*arrow*). Arborization abnormalities are evident.

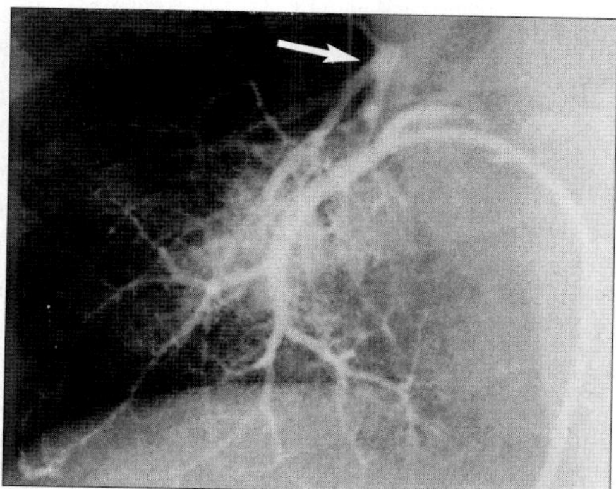

Figure 111.8 Pulmonary vein wedge angiogram in the right lower pulmonary vein. Retrograde flow fills a small right pulmonary artery (*arrow*) that is patent to the hilum, in a teenage patient with pulmonary atresia with ventricular septal defect.

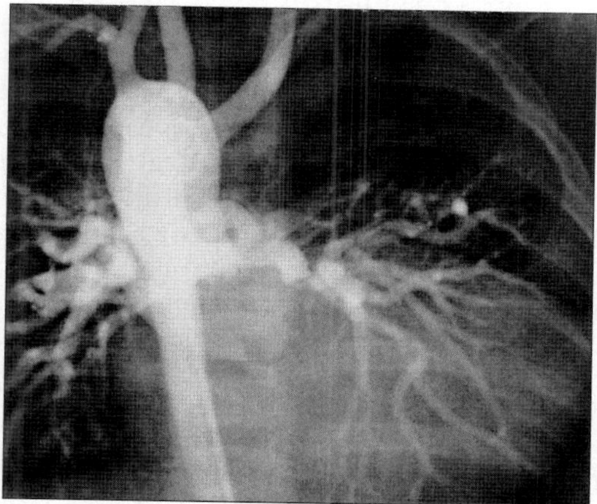

Figure 111.9 Aortogram showing major aortopulmonary collateral arteries (MAPCAs). There is a left aortic arch with normal branching. Pulmonary blood flow arises from MAPCAs, with several areas of stenosis and incomplete flow to the left upper lobe.

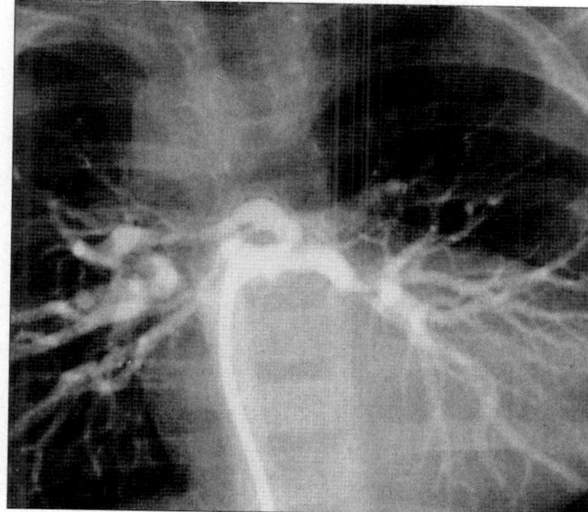

Figure 111.10 Selective injection into a large major aortopulmonary collateral artery. Bilateral flow to several lung segments is demonstrated. Several areas of stenosis are also demonstrated. This angiogram is from the same patient whose aortogram is shown in Fig. 111.9.

Data relating pulmonary artery size to eventual outcome were developed for older children and have not proved to be useful in small infants. (The Nakata index[23] is the cross-sectional area of the right and left pulmonary arteries, normalized to body surface area. The McGoon ratio[24] is the right and left pulmonary artery diameters divided by the diameter of the thoracic aorta at the level of the diaphragm. A McGoon ratio of 2 or more indicates nonrestrictive pulmonary arteries; a McGoon ratio of 0.8 indicates severely hypoplastic central pulmonary arteries). The Nakata and McGoon indices are not useful in infants partly because the maximal size of the arteries cannot be accurately measured in the presence of diminished pulmonary blood flow, and partly because the indices do not take into account the postoperative pulmonary arterial size following unifocalization. It has been shown by some authors that the outcomes of infant surgery are independent of pulmonary artery size and branching patterns.[25]

A left ventriculogram can be useful in identifying additional VSDs as well as the side and branching pattern of the aortic arch. Although a right ventriculogram confirms the diagnosis of pulmonary atresia and identifies the proximal site of obstruction, it may be precluded by the angiographic contrast limit, particularly when several sources of pulmonary blood flow dictate numerous selective injections.

MANAGEMENT

Initial Medical Management

For the subgroup of patients who have confluent pulmonary arteries and PDA, initial management consists of infusion of prostaglandin E_1 to maintain ductal patency. Such infants are usually stable until surgical palliation or repair is performed during the first few days of life.

In the small group of infants who present with excessive pulmonary blood flow and signs of congestive heart failure, attention must be paid to caloric intake, growth, and development. Anticongestive treatment includes administration of diuretics and digoxin. In some cases, administration of afterload-reducing agents, such as angiotensin-converting enzyme inhibitors, may be beneficial in reducing the pulmonary blood flow and improving systemic perfusion. Medical management should be used only to stabilize such infants until surgical palliation or correction can be carried out.

Interventional Catheterization

Interventional catheterization techniques have assumed an important role in the management of patients who have pulmonary atresia with VSD. After unifocalization or complete intracardiac repair, balloon dilatation or stenting of residual pulmonary artery stenoses improves blood flow to selected lung segments and reduces overall pulmonary vascular resistance and right ventricular pressure.[26] Stenting of stenosed aortopulmonary collaterals and shunts for palliative intervention of pulmonary atresia has been shown to be feasible and safe.[26] Stents are, however, generally best avoided because of size limitations, in-stent stenosis, and because stents tend to make future reconstructive operations considerably more difficult, particularly in infants and small children. The effects of unilateral pulmonary artery dilatation are best assessed angiographically and through the use of quantitative lung perfusion scans. After unifocalization, coil embolization may be indicated for any MAPCAs too small to be connected centrally or for MAPCAs with a demonstrated dual supply.[27]

Surgical Management

The goal of surgical therapy in patients with pulmonary atresia and ventricular septal defect is to achieve completely separated pulmonary and systemic circulations.

Infants who have ductal-dependent flow and confluent pulmonary arteries are managed surgically in the same way as patients who have critical tetralogy of Fallot with a primary neonatal repair. An initial shunt followed by a secondary repair is rarely indicated. For patients who have well-formed pulmonary arteries, outcome should be similar to that in tetralogy of Fallot.

Surgical management of patients who have pulmonary artery abnormalities, arborization defects, and MAPCAs presents a challenge. Historical management with shunt palliation or right ventricular outflow reconstruction with ligation of MAPCAs, and subsequent approaches by corrective repair without pulmonary arterial reconstruction resulted in high surgical mortality and poor survival with only approximately 50% of patients surviving to 2 years of age.[11,28] Haworth and Macartney[1] introduced the concept of preliminary unifocalization in patients with multifocal pulmonary blood supply. Unifocalization is a term used to describe incorporation of all sources of pulmonary blood flow, with eventual connection to the central pulmonary arteries.

Because the eventual pulmonary artery pressure correlates with the number of lung segments supplied by the pulmonary arterial system,[29] as many vessels as possible are incorporated into the pulmonary arterial tree. A variety of surgical techniques have been used to achieve unifocalization, including

- side-to-side anastomosis of MAPCAs to each other or to central or peripheral pulmonary arteries;
- end-to-end or end-to-side anastomoses of MAPCAs to other collaterals or to pulmonary arteries;
- anastomosis of an aortic button, giving rise to multiple collaterals to native pulmonary arteries;
- end-to-end or end-to-side anastomosis of collaterals to a central conduit;
- allograft patch plasty of stenotic distal segments of collaterals; and
- allograft patch augmentation of reconstructed central pulmonary arteries.

Emphasis is placed on early removal of all MAPCAs from the systemic circulation and achieving unifocalization by native tissue anastomoses. When necessary, stenoses within MAPCAs can be managed surgically with allograft or autograft patch augmentation. Reconstruction with circumferential nonviable conduit is rarely necessary, and should be avoided whenever possible. Major aortopulmonary collateral arteries that are the sole supply of blood flow to a segment cannot be ligated without permanent exclusion of bronchopulmonary segments, thereby reducing the effective pulmonary vascular bed. Even when a dual pulmonary vascular supply is present, unifocalization is often indicated to utilize collateral material and to optimize pulmonary vascular cross-sectional area. Important surgical concepts include aggressive mobilization, maximizing length of collaterals, creative rerouting, and flexibility regarding reconstruction. Incorporating a maximum number of pulmonary segments as well as optimally managing the pulmonary microcirculation ultimately determines the postrepair right ventricular pressure and favorable outcome. The longer the pulmonary microvasculature is exposed to systemic perfusion and the unpredictable hemodynamics of MAPCAs, the more likely it is to involute or to develop pulmonary vascular obstructive disease. The primary objective of current surgical management is thus to achieve the goal of separated circulations as early in life as possible. Management is thus based on an algorithm designed to achieve that aim (Fig. 111.11).

Unifocalization has proven to be effective for large numbers of infants and children, with a patency rate of anastomoses between 70% and 90% in older series,[30] and over 90% in more recent series.[12] Unifocalization can be performed with a low surgical mortality, providing excellent palliation in most and a preparation for complete intracardiac repair in the majority—even those who have diminutive pulmonary arteries and significant arborization defects.[7,31,32]

Several major concerns and problems accompany the unifocalization process. Progressive stenosis can develop at the site of the connection between a MAPCA and a pulmonary artery, at the surgical anastomosis, or at the edge of an augmentation patch, necessitating eventual balloon dilatation or stent placement. The use of central pericardial rolls has been associated with thrombosis in some patients and aneurysmal dilatation in others.[29] Pulmonary vascular function and structure may be altered by differential flow and pressure inhibiting growth in some segments, while at the same time causing pulmonary vascular disease in others. Completing the unifocalization procedure early in life should reduce the incidence of stenoses and localized vascular disease, allowing a majority of patients eventually to undergo successful complete repair.[25,32] Meticulous surgical technique and adherence to the techniques and principles delineated previously yields optimal results. Overall mortality and suitability for complete repair vary widely among surgical centers.

Early one-stage unifocalization and complete repair was first proposed in 1995,[25] and several groups[7,33-35] have now adopted this strategy. Although ideal age for repair of these patients is not known, if the patient is "well balanced" physiologically, repair is recommended between 3 and 6 months of age. If the patient is severely cyanotic or has severe overcirculation, earlier repair is feasible. There are significant advantages to early one-stage repair. Early normalization of cardiovascular physiology, correction of cyanosis, and protection against pulmonary hypertension are achieved; the use of nonviable materials is minimized; and the number of operations is reduced.

Timing of VSD closure is crucial. After completion of the unifocalization, the pulmonary arterial tree is assessed for suitability for closure of the VSD. Suitability for VSD closure following unifocalization is established by performing an intraoperative flow study.[35] While still on cardiopulmonary bypass, the completely unifocalized pulmonary arterial system is cannulated and perfused using a calibrated flow pump. When the flow is the equivalent of at least one cardiac

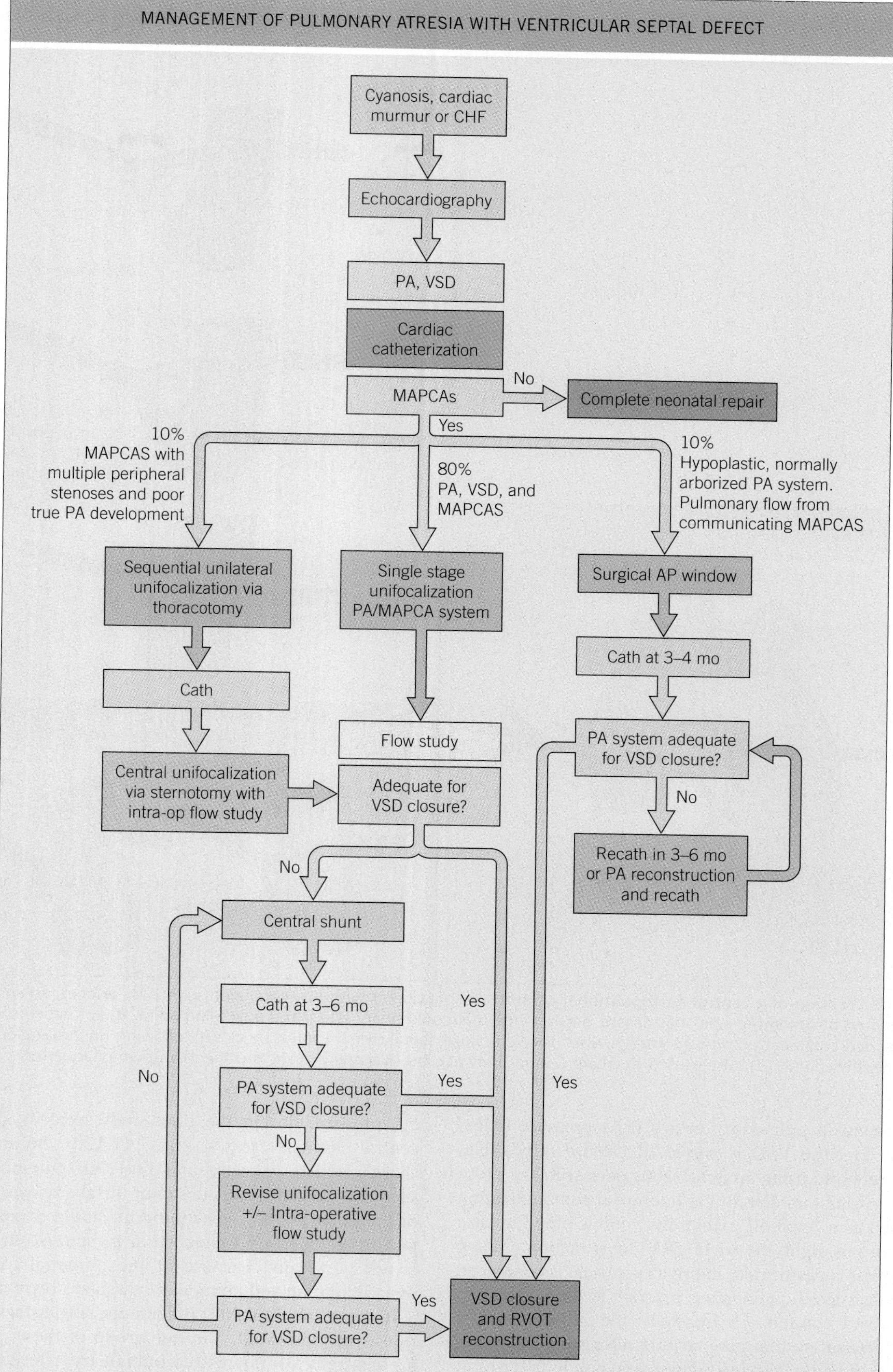

Figure 111.11 Management plan for patients born with pulmonary atresia with ventricular septal defect. Treatment is based on pulmonary blood supply as well as size and confluence of central pulmonary arteries. MAPCAs, major aortopulmonary collateral arteries.

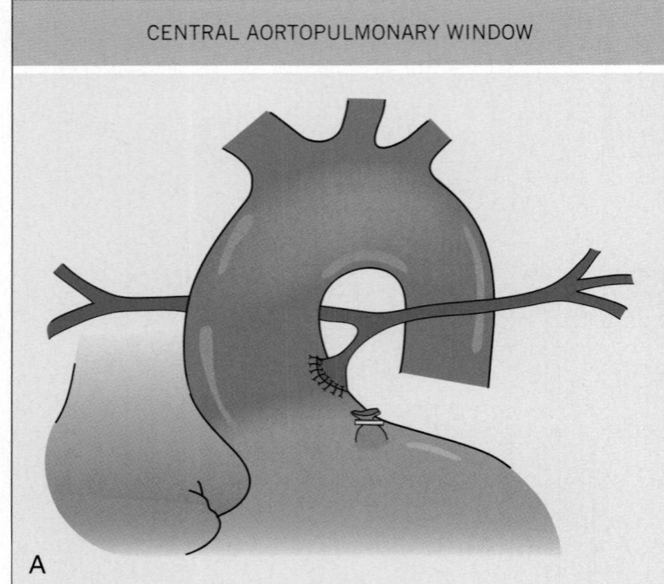

Figure 111.12 Creation of a central aortopulmonary shunt. A, For patients with tiny confluent pulmonary arteries, an aortopulmonary window is created by an end-to-side anastomosis between the main pulmonary artery and ascending aorta. **B,** For patients with intermediate-sized confluent pulmonary arteries when the ventricular septal defect cannot be closed following unifocalization, a polytetrafluoroethylene (PTFE) tube is used to create a shunt between the ascending aorta and the main pulmonary artery.

output if the mean pulmonary artery (PA) pressure is less than 25 mm Hg, the VSD is closed. If closure is possible, the VSD is repaired using an autologous pericardial or polyester patch. A small unidirectional interatrial communication is maintained as a "pop-off" valve for venous blood in case of postoperative right ventricle (RV) dysfunction. When complete repair is performed, the right ventricle is connected to the reconstructed pulmonary arterial system using an allograft valved conduit. Occasionally the intrapericardial pulmonary arterial system may require allograft reconstruction. The use of valved bovine jugular vein conduits for right ventricular outflow tract reconstruction in children as an alternative to an allograft has recently been reported with favorable early and intermediate-term results.[36] If the mean PA pressure during the flow study exceeds 25 mm Hg, a central shunt is created (Fig. 111.12b). Because a central shunt restricts pressure and flow, all pulmonary vascular segments remain protected until distal stenoses are relieved or pulmonary artery growth occurs and a complete repair is performed. RV to PA connection without closure of the VSD is not performed because of the potential for pulmonary overcirculation and pulmonary vascular obstructive disease.

In approximately 20% of patients, single stage unifocalization is not indicated.[12] In one group of these patients there are centrally confluent true pulmonary arteries with a relatively complete arborization pattern to most or all pulmonary segments, with the pulmonary blood supply from MAPCAs that share dual supply vascular distribution with the true pulmonary arteries. These patients are managed by constructing a neonatal aortopulmonary window by anastomosing the small main pulmonary artery end-to-side to the ascending aorta and ligating the MAPCAs (Fig. 111.12a). With proper patient selection the pulmonary blood flow will distribute to all lung segments, and the patients are evaluated for complete repair at 3 to 6 months of age. In the second group, true pulmonary arteries may or may not be present, and the majority of MAPCAs have stenoses at the segmental and subsegmental branches. These patients are the small minority in whom management is best achieved by sequential staged thoracotomies.

Carefully planned, surgically intensive management strategies have led to improved survival in infancy for patients who have pulmonary atresia with VSD. Short-term results are encouraging, but longer follow-up is required. Both staged unifocalization and one-stage unifocalization with repair require several operations during infancy and the possibility of interventional catheterization procedures.

Initial Postoperative Management and Follow-up Care

After surgical repair, patients with pulmonary atresia with VSD face a variety of postoperative problems. Unifocalization can result in reperfusion injury to the lungs, predominantly in segments that are severely underperfused before unifocalization. Airflow limitation is observed frequently. Reversible symptoms may be attributable to airway hyperresponsiveness, which is commonly present in up to 70% of these patients.[37] Bronchospasm may be due to extensive dissection around the tracheobronchial tree, and possibly due to disruption of lymphatic and autonomic structures. The unifocalization procedure can interrupt tracheobronchial blood supply and cause tracheobronchial necrosis, producing airway obstruction unresponsive to bronchodilators.[38] Phrenic nerve injury and resulting diaphragm paresis may occur because of the extent of necessary dissection, though with meticulous surgical technique, this is now uncommon. Splanchnic end-organ injury, particularly hepatic and intestinal dysfunction, may occur though is now infrequent. Patients with DiGeorge syndrome have metabolic abnormalities, including hypocalcemia and an increased susceptibility to infection, which complicate the postoperative course.

After unifocalization or intracardiac repair, patients who have pulmonary atresia with VSD require serial echocardiographic and clinical evaluation to assess right ventricular pressure and right ventricular outflow tract status. Echocardiographic imaging is also directed at detecting any residual septal defects, tricuspid regurgitation, or aortic regurgitation. Follow-up cardiac catheterization is recommended at 1 year after repair, particularly to assess the pulmonary anatomy. In the presence of increased right ventricular pressure, any distal stenoses should be dilated.[26] Residual MAPCAs too small to be incorporated into the pulmonary circulation should be embolized. Recent advances in computerized tomography and magnetic resonance imaging may allow these techniques to identify areas of stenosis in distal pulmonary arteries and assist in planning interventional procedures.

PROGNOSIS

The natural history of pulmonary atresia with VSD is difficult to define because of the variability of pulmonary blood supply. Before prostaglandin E_1 was available, nearly 50% of patients with ductal-dependent pulmonary atresia died during the first year of life. For patients who have confluent pulmonary arteries and MAPCAs, mortality is 50% at 5 years of age and 90% by 10 years of age without intervention. Long-term survival has been greatest in patients who have adequate but not excessive pulmonary blood flow. Initial mild cyanosis becomes progressively more severe, but may not produce symptoms until 15 to 20 years of age. Despite clinical stability in childhood, without intervention most patients in this group are dead by 30 years of age. Although shunt palliation can prolong survival into early adulthood, it does not seem to provide an adequate long-term solution. The presence of genetic syndromes, other than 22q11 deletion and trisomy 21, and the presence of pulmonary arborization defects are associated with worse outcomes after repair of tetralogy of Fallot.[39] Cardiac failure or aortic regurgitation frequently develop and are associated with a high mortality rate in adult patients, who rarely survive beyond the age of 40 years. In the University of California at Los Angeles study,[14] almost 50% of unoperated adults died during follow-up at a mean age of 33 years. For those who were alive at 20 years of age, the probability of survival to 35 years of age was 50.6%. The oldest reported surviving case is that of a 58-year-old woman.

The moderately to severely cyanotic adolescent or adult is at risk of the multiple organ system complications that are associated with cyanotic congenital heart disease, including erythrocytosis, abnormal renal function, gout, arrhythmias, and bleeding disorders. Iron stores must be maintained. All patients, whether operated or unoperated, are at risk of developing infective endocarditis.

Complete surgical repair is possible during adulthood. Early and late mortality may, however, be high. The University of California at Los Angeles group[14] reported on 10 patients, 5 of whom had previously undergone unifocalization procedures. In a follow-up ranging from 2 months to 10 years (mean 9 months) there were no reoperations and no early or late deaths. All operated patients were in New York Heart Association class I. Horer and colleagues,[40] however, recently reported corrections in 52 adult patients. There was 15% "early" mortality and an additional 12% "late" mortality during a mean follow-up period of 12 years.

The outcome after surgical repair for pulmonary atresia with VSD with ductal-dependent pulmonary flow and confluent pulmonary arteries should be identical to that for tetralogy of Fallot. The older child or young adult may benefit symptomatically from surgical palliation,[41] but he or she faces a poor long-term outcome. Selected patients in these populations may be suitable for complete repair with a relatively low surgical mortality, but delaying surgical intervention probably limits the number of patients who are suitable for complete repair.[7]

Data presented at the American Heart Association by Hanley and colleagues[12] demonstrated that in over 300 patients with pulmonary atresia, ventricular septal defect, and MAPCAs who were surgically managed according to the protocol (see Fig. 111.11) with 83% follow-up at up to 12 years there was 6.3% mortality, and Kaplan-Meier survival at 1, 5, and 10 years was 91%, 86%, and 86%, respectively. Using current surgical techniques, surgical mortality was 2%.[12] Amark and associates[42] reported on a series of 185 patients who underwent surgery and in whom repair was definitive in 75%. Overall survival from initial operation was 71% at 10 years. Risk factors for death after initial operation included younger age at repair, earlier birth cohort, fewer bronchopulmonary segments supplied by native pulmonary arteries, and initial placement of a systemic-pulmonary artery shunt. For initially palliated patients after 10 years, 68% achieved complete repair, 22% died without repair, and 10% remained alive without repair.[42]

Question remains in the opinion of some authors as to whether an aggressive surgical approach will increase the number of patients who are suitable for complete repair or improve long-term survival.[43] Current data, however, suggest that with careful management according to a rigorous protocol, many patients with MAPCAs may have long-term outcome comparable to patients with tetralogy of Fallot, and excellent long-term survival and quality of life.

Reoperation is certainly required in the majority of patients. A small percentage require closure of a residual or recurrent VSD.[28] Most reoperations are likely to be for conduit replacement. In older populations, freedom from reoperation for conduit obstruction has been found to be 99%, 95%, 59%, and 11% at 3.5 years, 5 years, 10 years, and 15 years, respectively.[44] Small conduits required in neonates and infants have a shorter reoperation interval than the larger conduits that are used in children. Whereas most studies cite statistics for reoperation for conduit obstruction, in patients who have increased distal pulmonary resistance, valve replacement is required for pulmonary regurgitation.[42] Patients who have pulmonary atresia with VSD face the same late problems and risks as those after repair of tetralogy of Fallot, including aortic regurgitation, bacterial endocarditis, right heart failure, ventricular and atrial arrhythmias, and sudden death. Progressive aortic valve regurgitation may require valve repair or replacement in an older subset of patients.[45]

SUMMARY

Pulmonary atresia with VSD is a complex congenital cardiac defect that represents the most severe end of the spectrum of tetralogy of Fallot. The clinical presentation, natural history, and surgical management of patients who have pulmonary atresia with VSD are determined by the anatomy of the pulmonary arteries and sources of pulmonary blood flow. In the most favorable form, confluent pulmonary arteries are supplied by a ductus arteriosus. After initial stabilization with prostaglandin E_1, such infants undergo complete intracardiac repair. For those who have several sources of pulmonary blood flow and arborization abnormalities, survival beyond early adulthood is unlikely unless newer surgical approaches result in improved long-term survival. Aggressive surgical management aimed at early unifocalization of sources of pulmonary blood flow has been advocated to increase the number of candidates for complete intracardiac repair and improve long-term survival and quality of life. Though the ultimate results of this surgical approach will not be evident for several decades, early and midterm outcomes strongly suggest that aggressive early management will optimize long-term outcome.

Echocardiography is used to diagnose pulmonary atresia with VSD in utero and in the newborn. Current imaging techniques, cardiac catheterization, and angiography provide detailed anatomic information about the pulmonary arteries and sources of pulmonary blood flow. The anatomic "roadmap" is then used in planning a surgical approach aimed at unifocalization of pulmonary blood supply and early complete intracardiac repair, whenever possible.

Through the availability of sophisticated diagnostic techniques and innovative surgical procedures, patients who are born with pulmonary atresia with VSD have a chance for improved survival and an enhanced quality of life. Care for these patients as infants, children, or adult survivors should be coordinated in regional centers that have sufficient experience in this rare condition to provide up-to-date diagnostic and therapeutic care.

chapter

112 Left Heart Outflow Obstructions

Gautam K. Singh and P. Syamasundar Rao

Definition

- These obstructions are congenital heart defects that cause fixed forms of hemodynamically significant left ventricular outflow tract obstruction with progressive course.

Key Features

- Obstructive lesions in the left ventricular outflow tract can be at the valvular, subvalvular, or supravalvular level.
- Neonates and young infants who have aortic valve stenosis usually develop congestive heart failure, whereas children and adolescents are mostly asymptomatic, although they carry a small but significant risk of sudden death.
- Subvalvular aortic stenosis usually appears after infancy and tends to involve aortic and mitral valves in its progressive course.
- Supravalvular aortic stenosis commonly involves coronary arteries and is often associated with stenoses of the aortic arch vessels and pulmonary artery.

Therapy

- Transcatheter or surgical intervention is indicated for symptomatic patients or those with moderate to severe left ventricular outflow tract obstruction. Many may need reintervention.

A spectrum of anatomic lesions can produce a hemodynamically significant left ventricular outflow tract (LVOT) obstruction. This chapter deals with fixed forms of obstruction to the egress of blood at three anatomic sites:

- the aortic valve (valvular aortic stenosis [VAS]);
- proximal to the aortic valve in LVOT (subvalvular aortic stenosis [SAS]); and
- distal to the aortic valve in the ascending aorta (supravalvular aortic stenosis [SVS]).

Together, these three forms account for approximately 3% to 6% of congenital heart defects and significant morbidity and mortality if untreated.[1] Each lesion is distinguished by its natural history and outcome, and each is discussed here as a separate entity.

VALVULAR AORTIC STENOSIS

INTRODUCTION

Valvular aortic stenosis, which becomes apparent in pediatric age, is almost always congenital, especially when it is isolated. It accounts for 60% to 75% of fixed LVOT obstructive lesions and occurs more frequently in males than in females by a ratio of between 3:1 and 5:1. Associated congenital heart diseases, the most common being patent ductus arteriosus, coarctation of the aorta, and ventricular septal defects, are present in 15% to 20% of patients who have VAS.

ANATOMY AND PATHOLOGY

The functional unit of a normal aortic root is built around the three aortic sinuses of Valsalva. These are formed by an expansion of the aortic wall and the semilunar attachment of its corresponding leaflet, which creates three pocket-like spaces that are separated by commissural spaces and interleaflet triangles.[2,3] The length of the free margin of a leaflet is longer than its attachment to the supporting sinus and the sum of the areas of the leaflets is greater than the cross-sectional area of the aortic root. A combination of such architecture and tissue pliability allows for a competent closure during diastole and unobstructed valve opening during systole.

Congenital VAS displays several morphologic types of abnormal valves: unicuspid, bicuspid, tricuspid, and quadricuspid.[4] The unicuspid aortic valve, most frequently seen in neonates who have critical VAS, has either an eccentric orifice with one patent commissure or a central orifice with no commissure.[2,4] The single thickened leaflet, with the length of the free edge less than that of the attachment to the sinus, has a limited flap-valve type of opening during systole, which causes marked flow obstruction and does not lend itself to balloon valvuloplasty.[3] The bicuspid aortic valve, the most common congenital heart disease with a prevalence of approximately 2% of the population,[1] has two leaflets, arranged in either[2,5]

- an anteroposterior orientation (approximately 60% of the cases); or
- a right-left orientation.

Valvular aortic stenosis results if the lengths of the free edges of the leaflets are less than those of the attachments to the sinuses, if the leaflets are dysplastic, or if commissures are fused. The majority of bicuspid aortic valves develop degenerative changes with older age, although only 1 of 50 children born with this abnormality will actually have significant obstruction or regurgitation by adolescence.

Valvular aortic stenoses in many fetuses and infants are associated with inadequate growth of left heart structure, left ventricular endocardial fibroelastosis and dysfunction, which constitute a distinct pathologic entity and management dilemma.

PATHOPHYSIOLOGY

The pathophysiology of VAS is determined by the age of the patient at onset, its severity, and any associated cardiac abnormalities.

Aortic Stenosis in the Fetus

Although organogenesis of the heart and the development of most of the congenital heart defects are complete by the first trimester, VAS may evolve throughout the gestation. Fetuses who develop severe aortic stenosis by the second trimester often demonstrate failure of growth of the aortic root and left ventricle cavity.[6] Associated hypoplasia of other left heart structures and their reduced growth rate predict the development of hypoplastic left heart syndrome.[6,7] However, in isolated VAS with unrestrictive foramen ovale and ductus arteriosus, usually the right ventricle compensates for the decreased left ventricular output, resulting in normal combined ventricular output, and gestation progresses to term.

Aortic Stenosis in Infancy

Valvular aortic stenosis in symptomatic neonates and young infants is usually critical in nature and differs in pathophysiology from the LVOT obstruction that is seen in older children. The left ventricle may be limited in its ability to match cardiac output to postnatal demand because of decreased preload, increased afterload mismatch resulting from removal of the low-resistance placental circulation after birth, and, in many cases, inadequate left heart structures and function to support the systemic circulation. With closure of the ductus arteriosus, systemic cardiac output diminishes and severe congestive heart failure develops. The timing of these developments after birth varies among neonates.

Aortic Stenosis in Children and Adolescents

The increase in LVOT obstruction in VAS in this age group is the result of a relatively unchanged effective valve orifice with growth. The increased left ventricular mass induced by increased wall stress initially overcompensates for pressure overload. The initial hemodynamics are characterized by[8]

- a subnormal wall stress;
- a normal or supranormal ejection fraction; and
- a normal cardiac output both at rest and during exercise.

Later, with progressive stenosis, cardiac output and left ventricular–aortic pressure gradient decline, and overt congestive heart failure may set in. Left ventricular hypertrophy, a key adaptive mechanism in preserving wall stress and systolic function, causes abnormalities of relaxation, increased chamber stiffness, and increased myocardial oxygen consumption. This increased oxygen consumption, when unmatched by coronary blood flow, leads to myocardial ischemia and fibrosis. These changes lead to diastolic dysfunction, with increasing reliance on atrial contribution to left ventricular filling.

CLINICAL PRESENTATIONS

Clinical findings depend upon the age of the patient at presentation, severity of the LVOT obstruction, and presence of associated cardiac lesions.

Aortic Stenosis in Fetsuses

Fetal aortic stenosis can present any time during the second or third trimester. Usually detected on fetal echocardiography as thickened and/or doming aortic valve, with or without commissural fusion or small annulus, and increased Doppler flow velocity of more than 1 m/sec, the VAS is a progressive lesion. Some fetal VAS may progress to hypoplastic left heart syndrome (HLHS) and their identification has important implications for prenatal and postnatal management. According to a study in midgestation fetuses with VAS and normal LV length, reversed flow in the transverse aortic arch and foramen ovale, monophasic mitral inflow, and LV dysfunction are predictive of progression to HLHS.[9] Additionally, reduced growth rate of the left heart structures also predicts the development of hypoplastic left heart syndrome.[6,7]

Aortic Stenosis in Infants

Most neonates who have VAS usually appear normal at birth. The neonatal and well-baby checkups perform poorly as screening test for severe VAS unless the examiner has a high index of suspicion for LVOT obstructive lesions. The majority of infants present with progressive congestive heart failure by 2 months of age. Symptomatic infants are pale, mottled, hypotensive, and dyspneic. A normal first heart sound, an ejection click, and a gallop are present in approximately 50% of those affected. An ejection systolic murmur of variable intensity is present along the mid left and right upper sternal borders, radiating to the carotid arteries. Hepatomegaly is usually mild. The presence of hypoxia (PaO_2, 30 to 40 mm Hg [4 to 5.3 kPa]) and metabolic acidosis indicates the need for immediate medical treatment and intervention.

Aortic Stenosis in Children and Adolescents

The patients in this pediatric age group are usually not symptomatic. Dyspnea, angina, or syncope, particularly on exercise, is present in 10% or fewer of older children, but because sudden death has been noted in 1% to 10% of children between the ages of 5 and 15 years who have moderate to severe VAS,[10] these symptoms in this age group deserve thorough evaluation.

The characteristic physical findings, such as arterial pulsus parvus et tardus (small amplitude and slow-rising pulse), carotid shudder, and prominent jugular venous *a* wave, which are described in adults who have VAS, are not uniformly present in children. A precordial systolic thrill over the base of the heart is present in more than 65% of patients with more than mild VAS. The first heart sound is generally normal. A narrowly split, single, or a paradoxically split second heart sound along with a fourth heart sound indicates severe VAS. An ejection click, best heard just after the first heart sound along the left lower sternal border and apex, is present in pliable and absent in immobile aortic valve. It is unaffected by respiration and absent in severe VAS. The characteristic low-pitched crescendo-decrescendo systolic murmur of VAS starts just after the ejection click and is best heard at the base of the heart, with radiation to the carotid arteries. A late-peaking and grade IV murmur indicates severe VAS. The murmur of VAS is augmented by maneuvers that increase stroke volume, such as isotonic exercise and premature ventricular contractions.

DIAGNOSTIC TECHNIQUES

Tests are usually necessary to establish the diagnosis and severity of VAS and the nature and timing of the management. To this end, the rapid and noninvasive nature of echocardiography makes it the diagnostic tool of choice in pediatric patients.

Echocardiography

Valve Morphology

An assessment of the aortic valve morphology, which in part determines the choice of intervention, is provided by the two-dimensional parasternal short-axis and long-axis views (Fig. 112.1), which demonstrate

- the anatomy of the aortic root: valve morphology and aortic root dimensions;
- the presence of commissures or raphes; and
- the position and orientation of the valve orifice.

A three-dimensional echocardiography provides a "surgeon's view" (Fig. 112.2), which can delineate the surgical anatomy and effective orifice area of the valve that may prove helpful in decision making for the type of valve surgery or intervention.

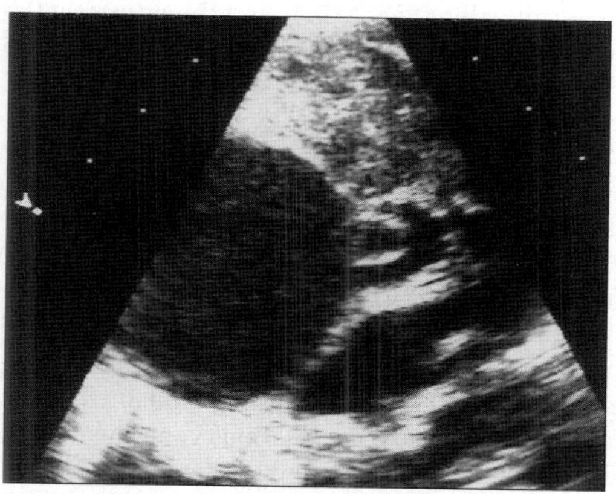

Figure 112.1 Valvular aortic stenosis with a unicuspid valve. Two-dimensional echocardiographic parasternal short-axis view of a unicuspid aortic valve in systole showing an eccentric circular orifice and a raphe.

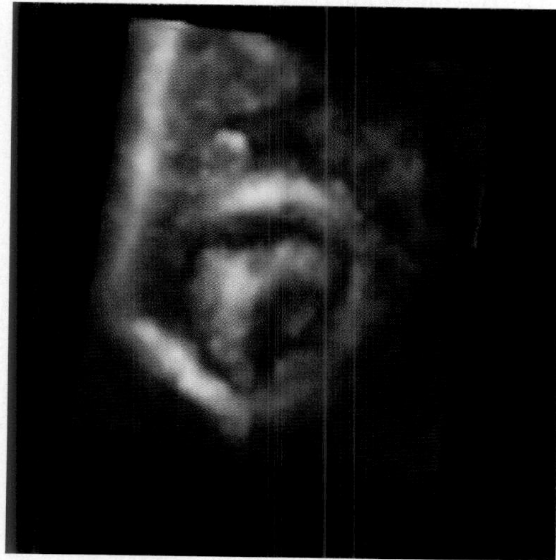

Figure 112.2 Valvular aortic stenosis with a bicuspid valve. A full volume-rendered three-dimensional echocardiographic "surgeon's view" of a bicuspid aortic valve in systole, showing fused right and noncoronary cusps with a prominent ridge, a smaller left coronary cusp (lower to the orifice), and an eccentric elliptical restricted orifice (in light blue color).

Echocardiography also provides assessment of left ventricular hypertrophy and function and aortic regurgitation.

Lesion Severity

A quantitative assessment of the severity of the valve stenosis, which determines the need for intervention, can be obtained by aortic valve pressure gradient in pediatric patients. The pressure gradient depends on the flow across the valve and downstream resistance. Because low-flow state and increased systemic vascular resistance are relatively rare in infants and children with isolated VAS, the transvalvular pressure gradient (*DP*) calculated from peak instantaneous Doppler echocardiographic velocity (*V*) using a simplified Bernoulli equation[11] is usually used to assess the severity of VAS in this age group:

$$DP = 4V^2$$

However, in clinical pediatric practice, a catheter-measured peak-to-peak LV to aortic peak pressure gradient has been traditionally used as the reference standard for the need for intervention. Because of different sites of measurements and the downstream pressure recovery phenomenon, the Doppler-derived peak pressure gradient overestimates the catheter-measured peak-to-peak pressure gradient.[12] If the recovered pressure is deducted from the Doppler peak instantaneous pressure gradient, the net pressure reliably predicts the catheter peak-to-peak gradient.[12,13] The recovered pressure can be derived by echocardiography:

$$RP = 4V^2 \times 2AVA/AOA \times [(1 - AVA)/AOA]$$

where *RP* is recovered pressure, *AVA* is aortic valve area (discussed in next section), and *AOA* is ascending aorta cross-sectional area.[12] The Doppler mean gradient has also been used as an estimate of the severity of VAS, because it is directly comparable to the catheter-measured mean pressure gradient, although a reference standard for the intervention is not yet universally established for it.

Because the pressure gradient, which is calculated from the measured velocity, may not correctly assess the severity of aortic stenosis in low-flow states, aortic valve area (*AVA*), calculated by the continuity equation, can be satisfactorily used to measure the severity of VAS, particularly in adolescents and young adults. According to the continuity equation:

$$AVA = (A_{LVOT} \times V_{LVOT})/V_{AV}$$

where A_{LVOT} is the LVOT area, V_{LVOT} is the velocity proximal to the stenotic aortic valve measured by pulsed Doppler echocardiography, and V_{AV} is the velocity across the stenotic aortic valve obtained by the continuous-wave Doppler echocardiography from multiple windows.[14] The *AVA* obtained by the continuity equation correlates closely to but often underestimates that obtained by cardiac catheterization using the Gorlin formula, which is the gold standard.[14] In clinical pediatric practice, pitfalls in calculating LVOT area makes the continuity equation a less used method to evaluate the severity of VAS. For the purpose of grading the severity, an effective valve area of less than 0.5 cm^2/m^2 of body surface area is considered as critical obstruction, whereas a valve area of more than 0.7 cm^2/m^2 indicates mild obstruction (normal is 1 to 2 cm^2/m^2).

Assessment of the Adequacy of the Left Heart Structures and Function

Because adequacy of left heart structures and function influences the outcome of intervention in infants with VAS, many echocardiographic morphometric parameters and hemodynamic variables of the left heart have been used to determine whether relieving the LVOT obstruction will achieve a two-ventricle repair or whether a staged single-ventricle repair (the Norwood procedure) or cardiac transplantation should be considered.[15,16]

The following morphometric measurements of the left heart structures favor two-ventricle repair:

- indexed aortic annulus of 3.0 cm/m^2 or more and indexed aortic root of 3.5 cm/m^2 or more;
- indexed mitral valve area of 4.75 cm^2/m^2 or more;
- a ratio of the long axis of the left ventricle to that of the heart of 0.8 or more; and
- left ventricular cross-sectional area of 2.0 cm^2 or more.

On the basis of some of the morphometric parameters, Rhodes and colleagues[15] developed a predictive equation for survival:

$$\begin{aligned}\text{Discrimination score} = {} & 14.0\ (\text{body surface area}) \\ & + 0.943\ (\text{indexed aortic root}) \\ & + 4.78\ (LAR) \\ & + 0.157\ (\text{mitral valve area}) \\ & - 12.03\end{aligned}$$

where *LAR* is the ratio of the long axis of the left ventricle to that of the heart. A discrimination score of less than −0.35 is predictive of poor outcome after two-ventricle repair. Doppler echocardiography can be used to assess hemodynamic factors. A predominant or total anterograde flow in the ascending and transverse aorta demonstrated by color Doppler echocardiography has been associated with survival after two-ventricle repair in severe VAS.[16]

Fetal Diagnosis of Valvular Aortic Stenosis

Fetuses who have VAS can be diagnosed by fetal echocardiography with high sensitivity and specificity. The progression of LVOT obstruction, left ventricle and aortic root morphometry, and flow pattern across the foramen ovale and transverse aortic arch should be assessed to aid in decision making regarding antenatal and postnatal management (see previous section on aortic stenosis in fetuses).[7,10]

Cardiac Catheterization

Cardiac catheterization for the diagnostic evaluation of VAS severity is indicated in children and adolescents with a Doppler mean gradient that is greater than 30 mm Hg or a peak gradient greater than 50 mm Hg if[17]

- they are symptomatic with angina, syncope, or dyspnea on exertion (class I);
- there is a discrepancy between clinical and noninvasive findings regarding severity of VAS (class I);
- they are asymptomatic but have developed T-wave inversion at rest over left precordium (class I);
- they are asymptomatic but are interested in athletic participation (class I); and
- there are several levels of LVOT obstruction in series that are likely to influence the therapeutic option or if interventional balloon aortic valvuloplasty is planned.

In pediatric practice, a peak-to-peak LV to aorta pressure gradient, measured by the withdrawal of an end-hole catheter from the left ventricle to the aorta, is used as the primary measure of severity:

- a gradient of 50 mm Hg or less is considered mild VAS;
- a gradient of 50 to 75 mm Hg is considered moderate VAS; and
- a gradient of more than 75 mm Hg is considered severe VAS.

The left ventricle and aortic valve are demonstrated by left axial oblique and elongated right anterior oblique views. The thickened and domed aortic valve with a thin jet of contrast displays the VAS (Fig. 112.3). The ellipsoidal orifice of bicuspid aortic valve (Fig. 112.4) and the eccentric thin jet of unicuspid valve are well visualized. The AVA can be calculated using the Gorlin formula.

Electrocardiography

Electrocardiographic (ECG) changes are neither diagnostic nor sensitive to the degree of severity of VAS in general. However, left ventricular hypertrophy with strain and ST-segment depression of 2 mm or more in the left precordial leads are relatively sensitive indicators of severe VAS. Right ventricular hypertrophy with a frontal right-axis deviation is the predominant ECG presentation in neonates.

There is a greater incidence of serious ventricular arrhythmias and sudden death in children and adolescents who have relatively long-standing moderate to severe VAS than in the normal population. A yearly ambulatory ECG monitoring is recommended in asymptomatic children and adolescents with Doppler mean gradient greater than 30 mm Hg or peak gradient greater than 50 mm Hg. Monitoring every 2 years is recommended in those with lesser gradients (class I indication).[17]

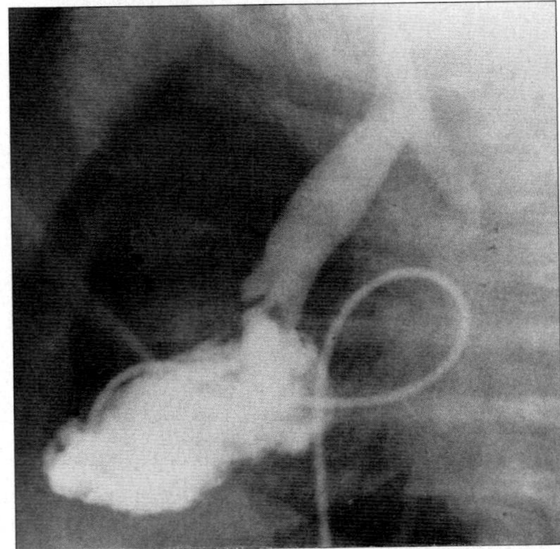

Figure 112.3 Left ventriculogram in valvular aortic stenosis. Lateral view in systole showing a thick doming aortic valve with a thin jet of contrast through the eccentric valve orifice.

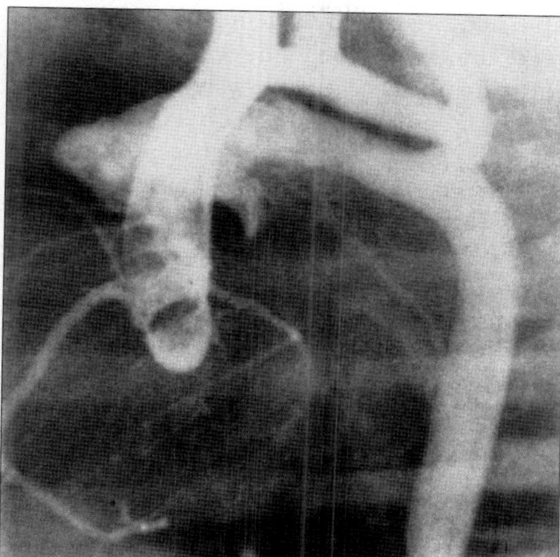

Figure 112.4 Angiographic appearance of valvular aortic stenosis. A lateral view in systole showing a bicuspid aortic valve with a fish mouth–shaped orifice, a mildly hypoplastic transverse arch, and retrogade opacification of the pulmonary artery through the patent ductus arteriosus.

Exercise Testing

Exercise testing is contraindicated in symptomatic patients. Graded exercise testing is a reasonable diagnostic evaluation in the children and adolescents with VAS who have a Doppler mean gradient greater than 30 mm Hg or a peak gradient greater than 50 mm Hg if they are interested in athletic participation (class II indication).[17] Most patients who have moderate VAS but are asymptomatic have a blunted increase in systolic blood pressure (less than 25 mm Hg) and cardiac index during exercise, which are inversely related to the transvalvular pressure gradient.[18,19] The presence of serious arrhythmias and the extent of ST-segment depression, defined as deviation from the PQ isoelectric line 60 msec after the J point, are positively related to transvalvular gradients and are indicative of myocardial ischemia. A persistent serious cardiac arrhythmia or ST-segment depression of 2 mm or more is an indication for therapeutic intervention.[18]

Chest Radiography

Cardiomegaly with rounding of the cardiac apex is the radiographic manifestation of left ventricular hypertrophy. Cardiomegaly is usually noted in children and adolescents if they have moderate or severe VAS. Cardiomegaly is present in more than 90% of symptomatic neonates with VAS who also show pulmonary venous congestion on chest radiography. Poststenotic dilatation of the aorta is not a feature in infants. Aortic valve calcification is usually not seen in pediatric patients.

NATURAL HISTORY

Congenital VAS is a progressive disorder. It carries an annual mortality rate of up to 2.1% during the first three decades and 2.4% to 4.8% beyond that in medically managed patients.[20] Fewer than 20% of cases of mild VAS are likely to remain mild after 30 years. In the Second Natural History Study, the catheter-measured peak-to-peak systolic gradient was found to be the most reliable indicator of the clinical course.[10] Beyond infancy, patients with a catheter-measured peak pressure gradient of less than 25 mm Hg have a 21% chance of requiring a valvotomy, and those with a gradient of 25 to 49 mm Hg have a 41% chance. Patients who have a gradient of 50 mm Hg or more have a 71% chance of requiring an intervention for relief of obstruction, which, if unattended, may put them at risk of serious ventricular arrhythmia, sudden death, and other morbid events at a rate of 1% to 1.5% per year.[11] A greater initial gradient predicts a greater increase in the subsequent gradient with time.

As with many congenital heart diseases, bacterial endocarditis is a potential complication of VAS. In the Second Natural History Study, the incidence of bacterial endocarditis was 27.1 per 10,000 person-years.[21] The presence of aortic regurgitation did not increase the risk of developing bacterial endocarditis.

MANAGEMENT

The management of VAS is determined by the age of the patient at presentation, the severity of the obstruction, adequacy of left heart structures, and the associated cardiac abnormalities. Depending on these factors, the current therapeutic intervention options to relieve the LVOT obstruction are percutaneous balloon aortic valvuloplasty, surgical aortic valvotomy, and valve replacement, all of which are intended for biventricular repair. The Norwood procedure is employed for single ventricular repair. The principles of therapeutic interventions are discussed here and their applications are detailed under the age-appropriate management.

Balloon Aortic Valvuloplasty

The balloon catheter is advanced retrogradely, usually via percutaneous femoral artery puncture or the umbilical artery (in the neonates), or progradely via the patent foramen ovale, and is positioned across the stenotic valve over an extra-stiff exchange length guide wire. The recommended balloon to annulus ratio is 0.8:1.0. The radial dilating force exerted by the inflation of the balloon usually tears the weakest part of the valve. In a bicuspid aortic valve, the balloon dilatation tears the fused commissures to achieve adequate relief of obstruction with some valvular insufficiency. In unicuspid valve, however, balloon dilatation tends to split the leaflet opposite the patent commissure, which results in only partial relief of obstruction and in significant valvular insufficiency.

Immediate and Intermediate Results

Immediate reduction in peak pressure gradient across the aortic valve is observed in the majority of patients after balloon aortic valvuloplasty. Among 606 patients ranging in age from 1 day to 18 years in the Valvuloplasty and Angioplasty of Congenital Anomalies Registry, the transvalvular gradients were reduced by a mean of 60%, with procedure-related mortality of 1.9%.[22] In a single-institution study of patients in the age group 1 month to 20 years, midterm results showed an 8-year actuarial survival of 95%, freedom from operation of 70%, and freedom from intervention of 50%.[23] In an intermediate-term follow-up in a series of neonatal balloon valvuloplasties, mortality was 12% and probability of survival and freedom from reintervention at 8 years were 88% and 64%, respectively.[24] Predictors of restenosis are age 3 months or less and immediate postvalvuloplasty peak gradient of 30 mm Hg or more.[22,25] Long-term follow-up data suggest that residual obstruction is low, but nearly 25% of the patients develop restenosis, requiring reintervention.[26] Aortic insufficiency at follow-up increases both in degree and frequency, some requiring reintervention.[25,26] Although the cause of progression of aortic insufficiency is not clearly understood, the severity of immediate postvalvuloplasty aortic insufficiency is predictive of late onset of aortic insufficiency.[25,26] Thus the immediate postvalvuloplasty incompetence grade and transvalvular gradient are the predictors of late reintervention.

Surgery

Surgical valvotomy is usually performed on cardiopulmonary bypass with cardioplegic and topical hypothermic myocardial protection. Through a transverse aortotomy, a commissurotomy and removal of fibrous excrescence and nodules from the aortic leaflets are performed. In patients who have an essentially uncorrectable valve, a small aortic annulus or recurrent stenosis with significant aortic regurgitation, an aortic valve replacement with a prosthetic valve or an aortic valve allograft may be performed in standard fashion. Because of its proven viability, the potential for growth, and the lack of need for anticoagulation, pulmonary autograft (the Ross procedure) is now used for valve replacement in many centers in all age groups, although it involves a previously healthy right outflow tract and predisposes it to further reoperations.

Immediate and Long-Term Results

The early mortality after surgical valvotomy in neonates with critical VAS has been more than 50% in the past.[27] With the recent approach of correctly selecting patients and treating those with associated inadequate left heart structure by staged single-ventricle repair, the surgical mortality in the neonates with isolated critical VAS has been reduced to less than 8%, and 10-year survival thereafter has improved up to 100% in some centers.[28] The surgical mortality in infants, children, and adolescents with isolated VAS has improved to 0% to 5%[28] and 10-year survival to 92% to 100%, but 10-year freedom from reoperation/reintervention and aortic valve replacement are still around 78% and 85%, respectively.[28] When mechanical valve replacements have been performed, deaths continue to occur, with 5-year and 10-year survival rates of 86% and 75%, respectively.[29] However, during the past decade, the 5- and 10-year survival rate and freedom from reoperation for autograft dysfunction after pulmonary autograft (Ross procedure) for aortic valve replacement have been 98% and 97%, respectively, and 93% and 90%, respectively, without continued attrition over that time.[30,31]

Percutaneous Transcatheter Aortic Valve Replacement

Percutaneous transcatheter aortic valve replacement (PAVR) is an emerging treatment for aortic valve disease in adults with a potential to supplant the surgical aortic valve replacement in pediatric patients. The device consists of a balloon-expandable stent xenograft valve delivered through a system consisting of lumens for the guide wire, sheath, and balloon-in-balloon system. The delivery system is available in sizes ranging from 18 to 24 mm. It has been attempted in over 100 adult symptomatic patients with severe aortic stenosis in whom the risks of conventional open heart surgery were deemed very high. Valve implantations have been successful in approximately 85% of patients, with intraprocedural mortality of 2% to 6% and 30-day mortality of 12%.[32] However, in pediatric patients with VAS, complex anatomy of the LVOT, the large sheath size of the delivery system, increased risk of dislodgement from exposure to high pressures in systole in the left heart, and therefore need for more robust mechanisms of anchoring the device in LVOT have prohibited the attempt for PAVR so far.

Management of the Fetus with Valvular Aortic Stenosis

With the purpose of improving the outcome, percutaneous echo-guided fetal balloon valvuloplasty had been attempted previously in 12 human fetuses with limited success and high mortality.[33] With improvements in fetal diagnostics, angioplasty tools and techniques, and patient selection as per criteria mentioned in the previous section on fetal aortic stenosis, a few centers have attempted balloon aortic valvuloplasty during second trimester, resulting in technically successful outcome in approximately 85% of cases. Improvement in physiology and continued growth in the left heart were noted in most cases with successful balloon dilation compared to control cases with unsuccessful or unattempted procedure. There were three deaths in the first 24 cases. A two-ventricle circulation at birth was reported in three neonates in that case series.[34,35] Although these data support the concept that fetal balloon aortic valvuloplasty is feasible and that HLHS is preventable in utero, improvements in patient identification, timing of intervention, and valvuloplasty technique are needed to make this procedure biologically successful in most fetuses with severe VAS.[34]

Currently, the conservative management consists of prenatal assessment of the dimensions, growth, and function of the left heart structure to help in decision making with regard to postnatal biventricular or single ventricle repair.[6,7] A cesarean delivery is recommended to minimize myocardial ischemia that might occur with a vaginal delivery, particularly in the case of oligohydramnios and prolonged rupture of membrane.

Management of the Infants with Critical Valvular Aortic Stenosis

Neonates and young infants who have critical VAS usually have ductus-dependent systemic circulation and present with rapidly progressive congestive heart failure as the ductus closes. They should be treated aggressively with prostaglandin E_1 infusion, inotropic support, diuretics, correction of metabolic acidosis, and mechanical ventilation to improve the systemic perfusion. To determine the therapeutic option, the Rhodes equation can be used.[15] The Congenital Heart Surgeons Society, after a large multicenter prospective study, produced a multiple linear regression equation that predicted both the magnitude and the direction of the optimum pathway for a 5-year survival benefit of Norwood (staged single-ventricle repair) compared with biventricular repair[36]:

Survival benefit = intercept + b_1 (age at entry) + b_2 (Z score of aortic valve at sinuses) + b_3 (grade of endocardial fibroelastosis) + b_4 (ascending aorta diameter) + b_5 (presence of moderate or severe tricuspid regurgitation) + b_6 (Z score of the left ventricular length).

Using their appropriate transformation factors, a positive number from the equation would favor a Norwood procedure and a negative number could favor a biventricular repair. For those selected for biventricular repair, surgical aortic valvotomy and transcatheter balloon dilatation have similar outcomes, but with greater likelihood of significant aortic regurgitation with the latter and of residual stenosis with the former.[37] Multiple centers as well as our preference is for balloon aortic valvuloplasty.[38] Among multiple routes for accomplishing the procedure, our preference is to use an anterograde, transumbilical venous route initially, followed by a retrograde, transumbilical arterial route, followed by carotid artery cut-down.[38] Most centers have found the balloon aortic valvuloplasty safe palliation for sick neonates and infants with critical aortic stenosis, with improvement in gradient and clinical status.

Management of Children and Adolescents with Valvular Aortic Stenosis

Indications for Intervention

General guidelines for therapeutic intervention are provided in Table 112.1. Because of good results comparable to those obtained surgically, good midterm palliation with little morbidity and little or no short- or intermediate-term mortality, percutaneous balloon aortic valvuloplasty is recommended in children and adolescents with catheterization peak LV–to–peak aortic gradient greater than or equal to 50 mm Hg if they are[17]

- symptomatic with angina, syncope, or dyspnea on exertion (class I);
- asymptomatic but developed ST/T-wave changes over left precordium on ECG at rest or with exercise (class I);
- asymptomatic but have a catheterization peak LV–to–peak aortic gradient greater than 60 mm Hg (class I); or
- asymptomatic but want to play competitive sports (class II).

Medical Management

Prophylaxis against infective endocarditis is no longer recommended for VAS by the guidelines from the American Heart Association (AHA) except for a prosthetic valve in the aortic position.[39] Because VAS is a progressive disorder and may be associated with exercise-induced sudden death in those who have moderate to severe obstruction, the need for careful follow-up cannot be overemphasized. For the purpose of follow-up and recommendation for participation in sports and physical exercise, the American College of Cardiology (ACC) Task Force 2 considered mild VAS with peak-to-peak catheter gradient less than 30 mm Hg (Doppler mean gradient less than 25 mm Hg and peak gradient less than 40 mm Hg), moderate VAS with peak-to-peak catheter gradient from 30 to 50 mm Hg (Doppler mean gradient from 25 to 40 mm Hg and peak gradient from 40 to 70 mm Hg), and severe VAS with peak-to-peak catheter gradient of greater than 50 mm Hg (Doppler mean gradient greater than 40 mm Hg and peak gradient greater than 70 mm Hg).[40]

Children with mild VAS should be medically managed with periodic evaluation at intervals of 1 to 2 years by two-dimensional and Doppler echocardiography. They can participate in all competitive sports if they have a normal ECG, normal exercise tolerance, and no history of exercise-related chest pain, syncope, or atrial or ventricular

INDICATORS OF SEVERE AORTIC STENOSIS AND INDICATIONS FOR INTERVENTION IN CHILDREN AND ADOLESCENTS*

Features	Description	Indication
Clinical	Presence of dyspnea on exertion, angina, or syncope	
	Arterial pulsus parvus et tardus	
	Late-peaking systolic murmur	
Echocardiographic	Transvalvular peak instantaneous pressure gradient >80 mm Hg	Class I
	Mean pressure gradient >50 mm Hg	
	Aortic valve orifice <0.5 cm^2/m^2 BSA	Class I
Catheter-measured	Peak-to-peak pressure gradient >75 mm Hg	Class I
	Peak-to-peak pressure gradient 50-75 mm Hg (+ symptoms or ECG features)	Class I
	Peak-to-peak pressure gradient <50 mm Hg (without symptoms or ECG features)	Class IIIa
	Aortic valve orifice <0.5 cm^2/m^2 BSA	Class I
ECG	Left ventricular hypertrophy with strain	
	ST-segment depression <2 mm at rest or during exercise	
Other	Plans participation in competitive sports or	Class IIa
	Pregnancy and catheter peak-to-peak gradient 50-79 mm Hg	

*A combination of clinical features and/or one of the positive test results provide indication for therapeutic intervention.
BSA, body surface area; ECG, electrocardiogram.

Table 112.1 Indicators of severe aortic stenosis and indications for intervention in children and adolescents.

tachyarrhythmia associated with symptoms. Those with moderate VAS should be evaluated at least yearly by two-dimensional and Doppler echocardiography, exercise testing, and ambulatory ECG. They can participate in low static/low-to-moderate dynamic, and moderate static/low-to-moderate dynamic competitive sports if they have mild or no LV hypertrophy by echocardiography, absence of LV strain pattern on the ECG, normal exercise test without evidence of myocardial ischemia or atrial or ventricular tachyarrhythmia and with normal exercise duration and blood pressure response, and have no symptoms as defined for mild VAS. Those with severe VAS should be followed closely and should not participate in competitive sports.[40] Delaying intervention in these patients may not be advantageous.[10]

After operation or balloon valvuloplasty, a variable degree of residual stenosis or regurgitation, or both, can be present. For these children and adolescents with residual mild, moderate, or severe stenosis the recommendations for follow-up and participation in sports are the same as those for untreated patients.[40]

PROGNOSIS

Patients with VAS have a 25-year survival rate of 85%, which is less than the 96% probability of survival for a comparable unaffected population in the United States.[10] In the Second Natural History Study,[10] 40% of medically managed patients subsequently required surgical intervention, whereas almost 40% of the operated patients required a second operation. Most patients after successful intervention or surgery remain in New York Heart Association class I, but an incidence of sudden death of approximately 5 in 1000 patient-years has been reported, mostly in those with residual lesions or endocarditis.[41]

SUMMARY

Valvular aortic stenosis is a relatively common congenital heart disease of progressive nature. Both prenatal and postnatal diagnosis and monitoring can reliably be obtained by two-dimensional and color Doppler echocardiography. There is still significant mortality in neonates who have critical VAS, and a risk of sudden death in children and adolescents who have moderate to severe VAS. These patients should be aggressively managed and closely followed. Therapeutic intervention consists of balloon valvuloplasty and surgical valvotomy or valve replacement. An overall 25-year survival rate of approximately 85%, with the majority in good functional status, can be expected. There is a significant probability of reintervention, which emphasizes the need for long-term follow-up.

SUBVALVULAR AORTIC STENOSIS

INTRODUCTION

Subvalvular aortic stenosis accounts for 10% to 20% of the fixed LVOT obstructive lesions in pediatric patients, and occurs more frequently in males than in females, by a ratio of between 2:1 and 3:1.[42] Associated congenital heart diseases are found in 25% to 60% of patients who have SAS, the most common being ventricular septal defect, followed by patent ductus arteriosus, coarctation of the aorta, bicuspid aortic valve, and persistent left superior vena cava. Although SAS is classified as a congenital heart abnormality, its absence in utero, rarity at birth and during infancy, progressive course, and high rate of postoperative recurrence suggest that it may be an acquired condition.[43]

ANATOMY AND PATHOLOGY

Subvalvular aortic stenoses have a spectrum of morphology. There are four basic anatomic variants[4,44]:

- a thin, discrete membrane that consists of endocardial fold and fibrous tissue;
- a fibromuscular ridge that consists of a thickened membrane with a muscular base at the crest of the septum;
- a fibromuscular ring or collar that is circumferentially attached to the LVOT and the base of the anterior mitral leaflet; and
- a diffuse fibromuscular tunnel-like narrowing of the LVOT.

The first two account for 70% to 80% of cases of SAS. They are located between 0.5 and 1.5 cm beneath the aortic valve and involve a variable extent of the LVOT. The distinction between the second and third types is not always clear. The tunnel-like lesion, which is unusual in patients younger than 3 years of age, accounts for 10% to 15% of cases of SAS. Histologically, the lesions consist of a composite of dense collagen fibers, short elastic fibers, and sparsely scattered fibroblasts. The LVOT obstructions that are secondary to accessory tissue, anomalous basal attachment of the anterior mitral leaflet, and anomalous chordal attachment of the mitral valve are uncommon.

PATHOGENESIS

The morphogenetic basis of the LVOT lesions that cause SAS is not fully understood. Studies have, however, suggested that certain anatomic characteristics of the LVOT are present in children who later develop SAS, including[44-46]

- a steeper (130 degrees or less) aortoventricular septal angle with an exaggerated aortic override (aortic valve dextroposition);
- an increased mitral-aortic separation; and
- a smaller left ventricular outflow tract width.

Such morphologies of the LVOT interfaced with rheologic changes from flow disturbances and shear stress may induce an abnormal endothelial proliferative response in the outflow tract. The development of aortic valve thickening and mild asymmetric poststenotic dilatation of the ascending aorta in patients with SAS are believed to be the results of repetitive trauma and vibrations from a subaortic jet. In this setting, aortic regurgitation generally develops and persists even after the removal of the SAS.

CLINICAL PRESENTATIONS

The symptoms of SAS may be masked by associated congenital heart diseases. However, in the majority of patients, it is asymptomatic and is detected by echocardiography performed either during the course of a follow-up of associated congenital heart diseases or as the evaluation of an atypical LVOT murmur. A low-pitched ejection systolic murmur is typical of an isolated SAS; it is occasionally associated with a precordial thrill and is best appreciated in the third and fourth left parasternal spaces with radiation to the suprasternal notch. An ejection click is not usually heard. A high-pitched early diastolic murmur of aortic regurgitation in the same area is present in 30% of patients. Variable cardiomegaly is seen on the chest radiograph.

DIAGNOSTIC TECHNIQUES

Echocardiography

Echocardiography is the current modality of choice to establish the diagnosis and for serial evaluation of the progress of the lesion and the result of intervention. M-mode echocardiography demonstrates early systolic closure (because of the Venturi effect of the jet formed by the SAS) and coarse flutter of the aortic valve. Two-dimensional echocardiography defines the position of the obstruction, its proximity to the aortic valve, and the extent of involvement of the LVOT in apical, parasternal, and subcostal long-axis views, respectively (Figs. 112.5 and 112.6). Biplane or multiplane transesophageal echocardiography provides superior definition of the lesion, making this an ideal tool for intraoperative evaluation of the lesion.[47] Continuous-wave Doppler interrogation provides the estimates of peak and mean pressure gradients across the LVOT that may be used as a guide to cardiac intervention, but it is not reliable in the presence of several obstructive LVOT lesions in series, ventricular septal defect with a left-to-right shunt, a tunnel-like lesion, or more than mild aortic regurgitation.

Electrocardiography

A variable degree of left ventricular hypertrophy is present in more than 50% of patients. However, occasionally, an ECG may be entirely normal, irrespective of the severity of SAS. Prominent Q waves in the left precordial leads may be present as a result of septal hypertrophy.

Cardiac Catheterization

Cardiac catheterization is indicated for discerning the contribution to LVOT obstruction by different lesions in series to help formulate the management, for preoperative hemodynamic evaluation of SAS associated with other congenital heart diseases, and for catheter intervention. A careful series of measurements of pullback pressure, using an end-hole catheter drawn from the left ventricle to aorta, usually delineates the exact site of obstruction in the LVOT. A long-axial left anterior oblique view during left ventriculography can delineate the LVOT obstructive lesion and can show aortic valve stenosis if present (Fig. 112.7).

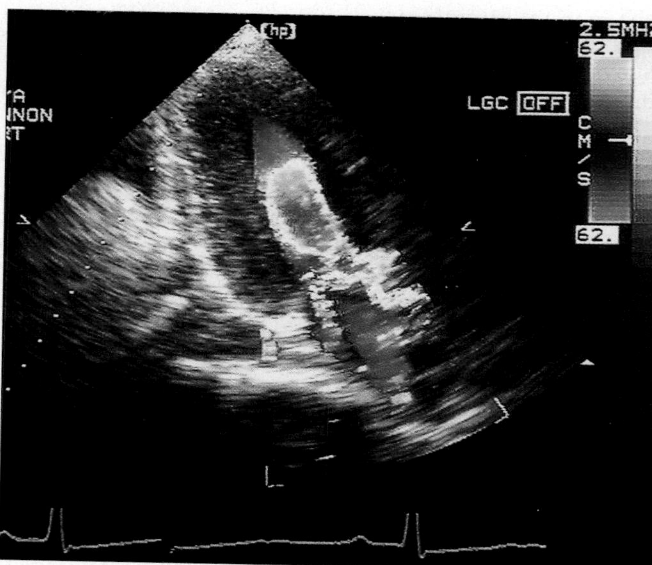

Figure 112.6 Flow turbulence caused by subvalvular aortic stenosis. Color flow mapping examination from the apical long-axis view in the same patient as in Fig. 112.5. The high-velocity jet that results from the fibrous membrane is causing a mosaic color pattern, which begins in the left ventricle well below the aortic valve. This confirms the presence of subvalvular obstruction. The mitral regurgitation jet (blue color in the left atrium) suggests anterior mitral leaflet tethering as the cause of regurgitation.

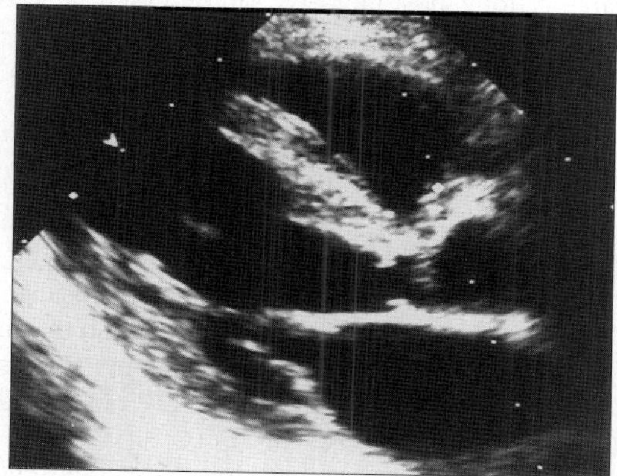

Figure 112.5 Subvalvular aortic stenosis caused by a fibrous membrane. Two-dimensional echocardiographic parasternal long-axis view showing a discrete and circumferential fibrous membrane in the left ventricular outflow tract as the cause of subaortic stenosis. The membrane is below a closed aortic valve and tethers the anterior mitral leaflet.

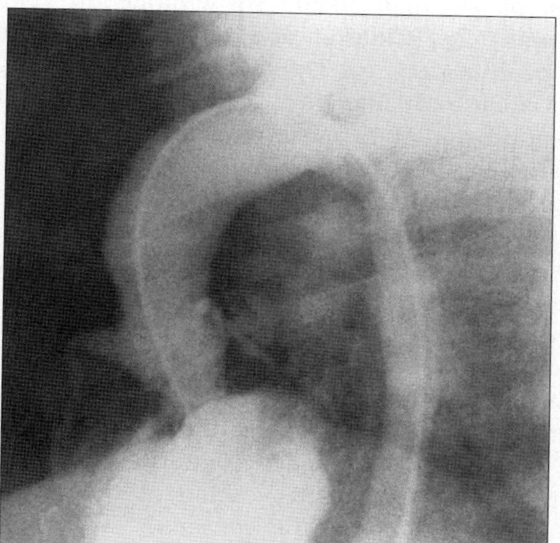

Figure 112.7 Left ventriculogram in subvalvular aortic stenosis. A left anterior oblique view in late systole in a tunnel-like subvalvular aortic stenosis caused by thick fibromuscular bands in the left ventricular outflow tract (more prominent on the ventricular septal side than on mitral valve side). The patient has mild residual coarctation of aorta after balloon angioplasty.

NATURAL HISTORY

Subvalvular aortic stenosis is a progressive lesion; however, the rate of progression is variable in the pediatric age group. Children and adolescents with an initial mild SAS (LV-to-aortic mean Doppler or catheter peak-to-peak gradient less than 30 mm Hg) may have quiescent disease and rapid progression with eventual aortic valve damage and resultant aortic regurgitation in the short and intermediate term is not "inevitable" in them, whereas those with higher initial gradient (greater than 30 mm Hg) may pursue a progressive course.[27,48,49] Besides greater initial LVOT pressure gradient, a closer proximity of the lesion to the aortic valve or its involvement of the anterior mitral leaflet, and an acute aortoventricular septal angle are also predictive of a progressive course.[46,49] Patients who have tunnel-like SAS with associated congenital heart diseases, particularly Shone's syndrome, are more likely to have progressive LVOT obstruction. Aortic regurgitation develops in up to 65% of patients, although it remains mild in the majority.

MANAGEMENT

Indication for Intervention

Because SAS is progressive in nature, intervention is required in many affected individuals during the clinical course of the disease. However, the indications and timing of intervention for discrete SAS have been controversial. Rationale for an early intervention for these types of lesions, based on the concept of inevitability of rapid progression and eventual aortic valve injury secondary to unrelieved SAS, even in its mildest form, is offset by the problem of high postoperative incidence of recurrence, late reoperation, and development of aortic regurgitation, even after successful early relief of the obstruction.[48-50] A recommended approach to the management of SAS, after risk-benefit stratification based on published data, would be nonintervention and medical follow-up for children and adolescents with stable catheter LVOT peak-to-peak (or Doppler mean) gradient of less than 30 mm Hg without left ventricular hypertrophy.[48,50] Children and adolescents with catheter LVOT peak-to-peak (or Doppler mean) gradient greater than or equal to 50 mm Hg should certainly have surgical intervention similar to those indicated for VAS.[17] Those with catheter LVOT peak-to-peak (or Doppler mean) gradient between 30 mm Hg and 50 mm Hg can be considered for surgical intervention if they are symptomatic with angina, syncope, or dyspnea on exertion (class I); asymptomatic but developed ST/T-wave changes over the left precordium on an ECG at rest or with exercise (class I); or have substrate for progressive course (mentioned in previous section on natural history), Doppler peak systolic gradient greater than 50 mm Hg, or an older age at diagnosis.[48-52] Prevention of aortic regurgitation is usually not an indication for surgical intervention in those with mild LVOT obstruction.[50] There is consensus for early surgical intervention for tunnel-like SAS.

Balloon Angioplasty

Balloon angioplasty can be used in selected patients who have a thin membranous SAS (greater than 2 mm), for immediate and short-term palliation of obstruction.[53]

Surgery

Complete resection, with or without myomectomy, is the surgery of choice for discrete SAS. Aortoventriculoplasty (the Konno-Rastan procedure) alone or in combination with "mini" aortic root replacement using aortic valve allograft or pulmonary valve autograft (Ross-Konno procedure) for tunnel-like SAS are the current surgical practices. Early postoperative complications, seen in 2% to 5% of patients, include damage to the aortic and mitral valves, variable degree of heart block, and iatrogenic ventricular septal defect. Overall surgical mortality has improved to less than 3% in recent times.[48-52,54]

PROGNOSIS

A time-related survival of 85% to 95% at 15 years postoperatively is usually seen.[55] Late mortality is mostly related to residual LVOT obstruction and reoperation. Freedom from subsequent recurrence and reoperation of 65% to 75% at 10 years have been reported in large series of follow-up.[44,48] Independent predictors of recurrence of SAS and aortic valve regurgitation are[48,51,52]

- proximity of the discrete SAS lesion to the aortic valve (less than 6 mm);
- tunnel-like lesions;
- high preoperative LVOT pressure gradient (more than Doppler mean gradient of 40 mm Hg and peak gradient of 60 mm Hg);
- intraoperative peeling of the membrane from the aortic or mitral valve at first surgery;
- greater immediate postoperative LVOT pressure gradient (more than Doppler peak gradient of 60 mm Hg); and
- longer postoperative follow-up.

The Ross-Konno procedure seems to have reduced the postoperative recurrence rate for tunnel-like SAS.

SUMMARY

Subvalvular aortic stenosis has a spectrum of anatomic variants. It has a variable progressive course, an invariable need for intervention, and a significant postintervention recurrence rate. A long postoperative time-related survival can be expected.

SUPRAVALVULAR AORTIC STENOSIS

INTRODUCTION

Supravalvular aortic stenosis can be either a localized or a diffuse narrowing of the ascending aorta beyond the superior margin of the sinuses of Valsalva. It accounts for less than 5% of all fixed forms of congenital LVOT obstruction.[56] It is equally common in both sexes.

Supravalvular aortic stenosis has three distinct presentations.

- It constitutes a feature of Williams syndrome, which is a genetic disorder caused by a deletion of the elastin gene at 7q11 (chromosome 7).[57] Other cardiovascular anomalies in Williams syndrome include multiple stenoses of peripheral pulmonary arteries; stenosis of the origins of the carotid, coronary, and subclavian arteries; and coarctation of the aorta.[56,58]

- The second presentation, a familial form of SVS caused by an autosomal dominant inheritance with variable expression, is less common. Peripheral pulmonary artery stenosis is an associated feature of this familial SVS, but features of Williams syndrome are not present.
- The third, sporadic, form of SVS is the most common presentation. Patients may have associated peripheral pulmonary artery stenosis but show no other features of Williams syndrome.

ANATOMY AND PATHOLOGY

There are three commonly recognized morphologic forms[4]:

- an external hourglass deformity with a corresponding luminal narrowing of the aorta at a level just distal to the ostia of coronary arteries, which is the most common morphologic form and is present in 50% to 75% of patients;
- a fibrous diaphragm, which is present just distal to the coronary artery ostia in approximately 25% of patients; and
- a diffuse narrowing of a variable length of ascending aorta, which is the least common form.

Similarly, three anatomic subtypes of left main coronary obstruction have been recognized and can be present in 45% of patients with SVS[59]:

- circumferential narrowing of the left main ostium;
- ostial obstruction caused by a fusion of the aortic cusp to the supravalvular ridge; and
- diffuse narrowing of the left main coronary artery.

In the absence of ostial obstruction, normal coronary arteries as well as dilated and tortuous coronary arteries have been noted. Variable degrees of thickening of intima and media are histologically evident in the wall of coronary arteries and aorta in all morphologic forms of SVS.

PATHOPHYSIOLOGY

The coronary arteries, being proximal to the site of obstruction, have the same systolic pressure as the left ventricle.[4] Consequently, in the course of time they may become dilated and tortuous and develop intimal thickening. Coronary atherosclerosis may set in prematurely. Concentric left ventricular hypertrophy as a result of SVS adds further to the problem of myocardial ischemia. In the majority of patients, the jet of blood flow from SVS demonstrates a preferential trajectory into the brachiocephalic vessels, which results in a marked increase in blood pressure in the right arm relative to the left arm (Coanda effect).[60]

CLINICAL PRESENTATIONS

Symptoms and its onset are dictated by the severity of the SVS and associated lesions. Those who have biventricular outflow obstruction present with feeding difficulties, exercise intolerance, and low cardiac output syndrome early in infancy. Most of the patients come to medical attention because of a heart murmur or the features of Williams syndrome. Dyspnea on exertion and angina develop in the course of the disease.

Discrepancies between carotid pulsations and the blood pressure in the left and right arms are the characteristic clinical findings of SVS. However, the auscultatory findings are similar to those in VAS, although an ejection click is unusual and the murmur with thrill are sited higher than in VAS. The characteristic clinical findings of additional cardiovascular abnormalities, including peripheral pulmonary artery stenosis, coarctation of aorta, and mitral insufficiency, are present in the majority of patients.

The natural history indicates that SVS is usually progressive, whereas peripheral pulmonary artery stenosis remains unchanged or lessens in severity with time.[61] The risk of sudden cardiac death, including operated patients, is 1 in 1000 patient-years and is 25 to 100 times higher than in the normal population.[62] Two anatomic abnormalities that predispose individuals with SVS and Williams syndrome to sudden death include coronary artery stenosis and severe biventricular outflow tract obstruction. The mechanisms for sudden death for both anatomic subgroups include myocardial ischemia, decreased cardiac output, and arrhythmia.[63]

DIAGNOSTIC TECHNIQUES

The clinical findings of SVS and the associated characteristic features of Williams syndrome suggest the diagnosis in approximately 50% of patients. Echocardiography can reliably make the diagnosis of SVS.

Echocardiography

In patients who have SVS with an hourglass deformity and diffuse hypoplasia, the diameter of the ascending aorta is smaller than that of the aortic root (Fig. 112.8). In the patients who have a fibrous diaphragm, an echogenic membrane is commonly seen above the sinuses of Valsalva. A turbulent color flow pattern indicates the site of hemodynamically significant obstruction (Fig. 112.9) and coronary ostial stenosis. However, Doppler peak gradient does not predict catheter-measured gradient well in patients with SVS and may not be useful in assessing its severity.[64]

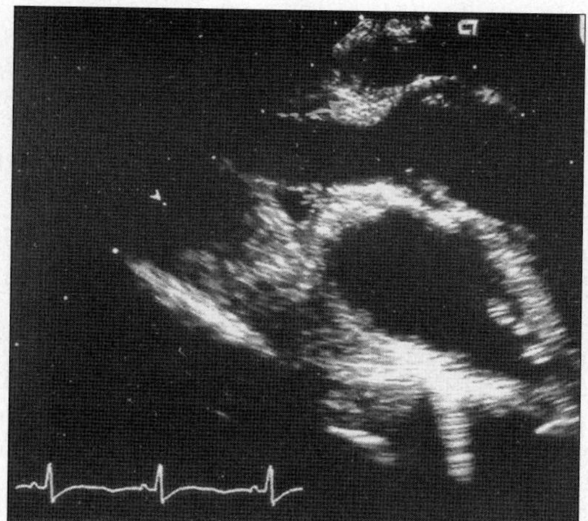

Figure 112.8 Supravalvular aortic stenosis caused by diffuse hypoplasia of ascending aorta. A multiplane transesophageal echocardiographic long-axis view in systole showing diffuse narrowing of the ascending aorta above sinutubular junction. The aortic valve, the sinuses of Valsalva, and the left ventricular outflow tract are of normal morphology.

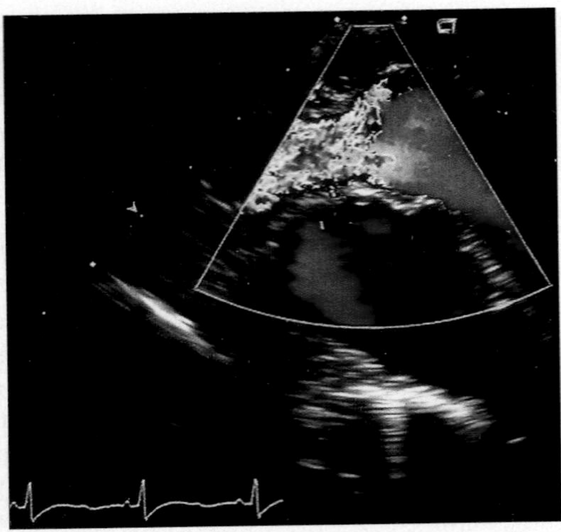

Figure 112.9 Flow turbulence caused by supravalvular aortic stenosis. Color flow mapping examination by multiplane transesophageal echocardiography in the same patient as in Fig. 112.8. The high-velocity jet resulting from the diffuse hypoplasia of the ascending aorta is causing a mosaic color pattern, which begins above the aortic valve at the level of sinutubular junction.

Cardiac Catheterization

The catheter-measured pressure gradient indicates the severity of SVS and identifies those patients who should be considered for surgery. A retrograde aortic catheterization with an end-hole catheter can localize the site of obstruction by showing the pressure gradient above the aortic valve on pullback tracing. Biplane left ventriculography and aortography can reveal the supravalvular narrowing, stenosis of the arch vessels, and abnormalities of aortic root and coronary arteries (Fig. 112.10). Right heart catheterization and right ventricular or pulmonary arterial angiography should be performed simultaneously, to discern the presence of peripheral pulmonary artery stenosis. However, cardiac catheterization carries higher risk in individuals with SVS and Williams syndrome. Two thirds of the reported cases of sudden death have been associated with anesthesia administration before or during catheterization as well as the catheterization procedure itself.[63] A risk-benefit evaluation should be considered when undertaking cardiac catheterization in individuals with SVS and Williams syndrome.

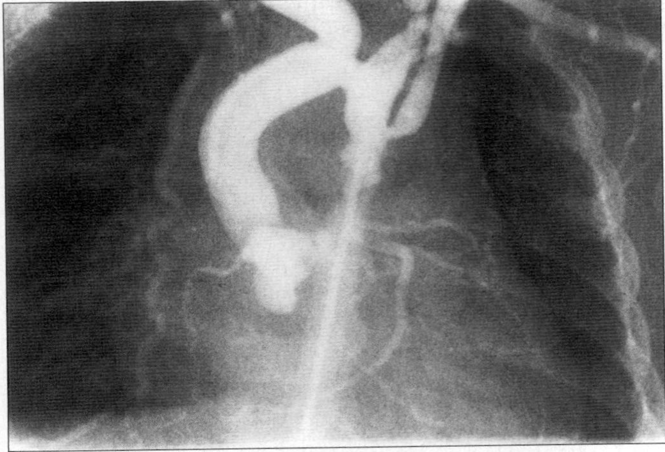

Figure 112.10 Angiographic appearance of supravalvular aortic stenosis. An anteroposterior view in early systole in supravalvular aortic stenosis showing a mild hourglass narrowing of the ascending aorta above the sinuses of Valsalva. The patient has associated stenoses in the proximal segment of the left common carotid artery and at the origin of the left subclavian artery. There is a discrete coarctation of aorta with isthmus hypoplasia. The fluorescent in situ hybridization study was negative for deletion of chromosome 7q11 (Williams syndrome).

GENETIC EVALUATION

Molecular diagnosis of Williams syndrome can now be made by fluorescent in situ hybridization using the Williams probe. Confirmation of a genetic diagnosis of Williams syndrome or a familial form of SVS is important for counseling the patient and his or her family.

MANAGEMENT

In patients who have SVS, the indications for intervention are similar to those for VAS. However, transcatheter balloon angioplasty has not been found to be an effective treatment. It is not the treatment of choice, because it carries higher risk in individuals with SVS and Williams syndrome. Surgical resection of the supravalvular obstruction and patch aortoplasty and multiple-sinus reconstructions (inverted bifurcated patch plasty and three-sinus reconstruction) are the procedures of choice for the fibrous diaphragm and hourglass deformities. In those with associated coronary artery involvement, patch aortoplasty encompassing the left main ostium for circumferential narrowing of left main ostium, excision of the fused leaflet from the aortic wall for ostial obstruction caused by a fusion of the aortic cusp to the supravalvular ridge, and bypass grafting for diffuse narrowing of the left main coronary artery are undertaken at the same sitting in addition to aortoplasty.[59] In patients who have SVS with diffuse narrowing, the ascending aorta and the arch of the aorta can be reconstructed using an aortic allograft or a pulmonary autograft. Overall early and late mortalities are 1% to 2%, respectively.[65] Surgical treatment of associated abnormalities of aortic valve and aortic arch vessels should be undertaken at the same time, to optimize the overall surgical outcome.[66]

PROGNOSIS

The actuarial survival after operative repair of SVS in one series was 98% at 10 years and 97% at both 20 and 30 years, with the majority in New York Heart Association functional class I.[60] Aortic valve insufficiency is present in approximately 25% of patients. Prognosis is influenced by the presence of genetic disorders and associated obstructive lesions of LVOT and pulmonary arteries.

SUMMARY

Supravalvular aortic stenosis constitutes a feature of Williams syndrome and other genetic disorders. It can involve coronary ostia and arch vessels. Surgical repair is the most effective treatment for long-term, recurrence-free survival.

chapter

113 Hypoplastic Left Heart Syndrome

Eric M. Graham and Girish S. Shirali

Definition

- Hypoplastic left heart syndrome (HLHS) is a spectrum of malformations characterized by underdevelopment of the left heart, including the left atrium, mitral valve, left ventricle, aortic valve, and aortic arch.

Key Features

- The right ventricle serves as a combined systemic and pulmonary pump.
- Systemic circulation depends on patency of the ductus arteriosus.
- HLHS is uniformly fatal in early infancy if not treated surgically.

Therapy

- The two options for active management are staged reconstruction (starting with the Norwood procedure or hybrid procedure [ductal stenting and pulmonary artery banding] and ending with the Fontan operation) and cardiac transplantation.
- Surgical options for HLHS are palliative and not curative.

Hypoplastic left heart syndrome (HLHS) is a spectrum of malformations characterized by underdevelopment of the left heart, including the left atrium, mitral valve, left ventricle (LV), aortic valve, and aortic arch. HLHS is a common severe congenital cardiac defect, accounting for 7% to 9% of all congenital heart disease diagnosed in the first year of life. The frequency is estimated at 0.163 to 0.184 per 1000 live births. Systemic circulation in HLHS depends on the patency of the ductus arteriosus, using the right ventricle (RV) as the combined systemic and pulmonary ventricle. With the systemic and pulmonary circulations in parallel rather than series, the cardiac output is divided with a resultant precarious balance among systemic, pulmonary, and coronary blood flows. No viable treatment choices existed before the early 1980s; as a result, death in the first month of life was the rule. In the 1980s, two radically different, innovative surgical approaches were introduced:

- Norwood and colleagues[1] devised aortic arch augmentation using the native pulmonary artery (PA); after this procedure the RV acts as the systemic ventricle; and
- Bailey and associates[2] pioneered cardiac transplantation with aortic arch reconstruction using donor aortic tissue.

Subsequent improvements in surgical technique and the evolving understanding of "single ventricle" physiology, staged reconstruction, and perioperative management have led to long-term patient survival rates of 50% to 70%, after either listing for transplantation or commencing a staged Fontan type of palliation. However, patients who complete the Fontan type of palliation exhibit a late increase in the risk of decreased functional capacity and death.[3] Similarly, cardiac transplant recipients remain at lifelong risk of allograft rejection and coronary arteriopathy. Thus both treatment pathways for HLHS are palliative rather than curative, an important distinction from most other forms of congenital heart disease.

ANATOMY AND PATHOLOGY

Cardiac position, segments, and alignments are typically normal. Systemic venous drainage is usually normal. The external appearance of the heart is remarkable for the disparity in size between the dilated right-sided cardiac chambers and the diminutive left-sided cardiac chambers (Fig. 113.1). The right atrium, tricuspid annulus, RV, pulmonary valve, and main and branch PAs are dilated. The RV is hypertrophied. The pulmonary veins usually connect to the left atrium in a normal fashion. However, if the atrial septum is intact, there may be alternative pathways of pulmonary venous drainage into the systemic veins, the coronary sinus, or the right atrium. Thus a levoatriocardinal vein may allow the left atrium to decompress into the superior vena caval system.

The left atrium may be hypoplastic and thick-walled. Left atrial endocardium may exhibit sclerosis and fibroelastosis. Possible variations of atrial septal morphology include a large secundum atrial septal defect; an intact atrial septum; an aneurysm of septum primum; malalignment of the septum primum, which may attach directly to the left atrial wall, to the left of septum secundum; and a restrictive, superiorly located foramen ovale.

The entire mitral valve apparatus is diminutive and abnormally formed. The valve itself may be stenotic, hypoplastic, or atretic. Short chordae tendineae may lead to direct attachment of the mitral valve leaflets onto the papillary muscles (arcade deformity). Interchordal spaces may be obliterated and the papillary muscles may be closely spaced or single (parachute mitral valve).

HLHS is characterized by varying degrees of global LV hypoplasia (see Fig. 113.1). The LV is almost always hypertrophied and hypoplastic, and may be a diminutive endothelium-lined slit as in the setting of mitral and aortic atresia. The ventricular septum is intact in the "classic" form of HLHS. LV endocardial fibroelastosis is commonly seen, particularly if there is prograde flow through the mitral valve in the setting of aortic atresia. Atresia of the aortic valve may be due to a diminutive and imperforate valve structure;

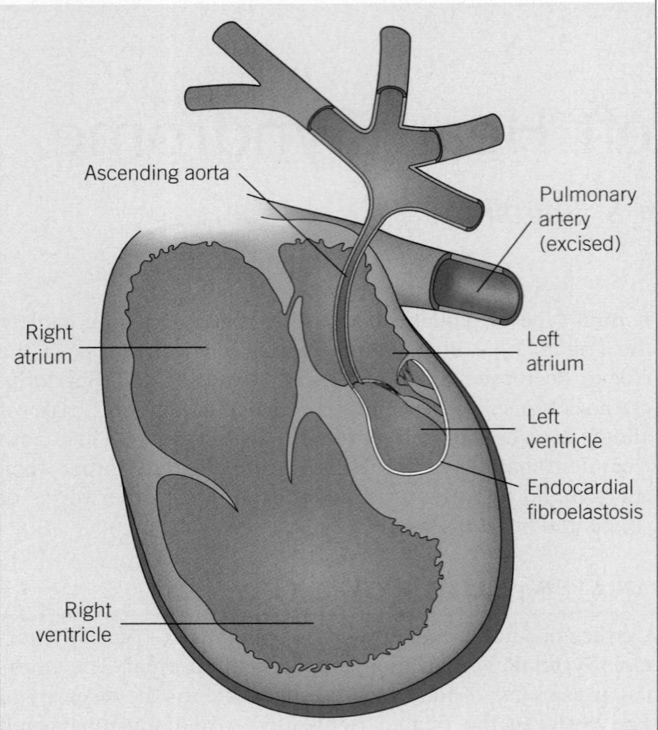

Figure 113.1 Coronal section (echocardiographic apical view) of hypoplastic left heart syndrome. The heart has been sectioned in a coronal plane, mimicking the echocardiographic apical view. The left atrium is thick-walled and hypoplastic. The mitral valve and left ventricle (LV) are diminutive. The aorta arises from the LV; the aortic valve, ascending aorta, and aortic arch are severely hypoplastic.

a membrane or a shelf may represent valve tissue. When the aortic valve is patent, the leaflets are usually thick and severely obstructed. The ascending aorta and aortic arch are hypoplastic. Typically, the ascending aorta is miniscule and serves only as a main coronary artery that fills retrograde, via the ductus arteriosus. The ductus arteriosus is normal in configuration and variable in size. Ductal tissue extension into the aorta may encircle the aortic lumen, extending proximally and distally into the aorta for variable distances. This extension of ductal tissue is believed to be the substrate for coarctation of the aorta, which is known to be present in most if not all cases of HLHS.

The coronary arteries generally originate normally from the aortic root. Although rare, anomalous origins of the right or left coronary arteries arising from the pulmonary arteries have been described. Coronary artery abnormalities in HLHS include sinusoids between the coronary arteries and the LV, tortuosity of the epicardial coronary arteries, and single (right or left) coronary artery. All of these abnormalities have been found more commonly among patients with one specific morphologic subtype of HLHS (i.e., patent [but hypoplastic] mitral valve and aortic atresia) than in those with other morphologic subtypes of HLHS (i.e., mitral and aortic atresia, or mitral and aortic hypoplasia). Coronary artery stenosis or interruption has not been reported, and dependency of the coronary circulation on the LV is probably rare. Overall, coronary artery abnormalities are less severe in HLHS than in pulmonary atresia with intact ventricular septum.

PATHOPHYSIOLOGY

Fetal hemodynamics in HLHS are similar to those encountered in a normal fetus. It is only after birth that the circulatory derangements of HLHS assume hemodynamic significance. Because the LV is essentially nonfunctional, the RV must function as a combined pump, perfusing the lungs (prograde flow into the branch PAs) and the body (systemic output via the ductus arteriosus). To allow this, both the systemic and pulmonary venous flows must return, unobstructed, to the right atrium, and thence to the RV. If the pulmonary veins drain into the left atrium, an atrial septal defect must allow unobstructed pulmonary venous flow (obligate left-to-right flow) into the right atrium. Because the RV is a combined pump, systemic output is inversely related to pulmonary output. Equilibrium between these two vascular beds is determined by the ratio of systemic to pulmonary vascular resistance. The pulmonary vascular bed is subjected to systemic perfusion pressures. Right-to-left flow across the ductus arteriosus perfuses the systemic circulation.

The first several weeks of life are notable for cardiovascular physiologic changes consisting of a gradual decline in pulmonary vascular resistance and spontaneous closure of the foramen ovale and the ductus arteriosus. Although these are usually incidental phenomena for the normal neonate, they profoundly affect the hemodynamic balance in HLHS. Thus the normal postnatal decline in pulmonary vascular resistance leads to progressively increased pulmonary blood flow, at the expense of systemic perfusion. Compromised systemic perfusion may lead to decreased coronary blood flow, and the resulting coronary insufficiency may contribute to decreased cardiac output. Pulmonary overcirculation and edema coupled with high arterial oxygen saturation, and metabolic acidosis characterize this state. Alternatively, the fetal state of elevated pulmonary vascular resistance may persist, leading to decreased pulmonary blood flow while maintaining systemic output. Low arterial oxygen saturation coupled with metabolic acidosis due to inadequate systemic oxygen delivery characterizes the latter state.

Closure of the foramen ovale, either at birth or postnatally, causes pulmonary venous obstruction, which leads to decreased prograde flow through the lungs, resulting in severe hypoxemia, metabolic acidosis, and death. Patients who are born with an intact atrial septum (so-called premature closure of the foramen ovale) have severe pulmonary venous obstruction. This may lead to pulmonary lymphangiectasis, which is associated with significant morbidity and mortality. Spontaneous closure of the ductus arteriosus leads to a decrease in systemic perfusion, metabolic acidosis, and pulmonary overcirculation, which is certainly fatal if left untreated. End-organ damage resulting from decreased systemic perfusion may manifest as hepatic necrosis and mesenteric ischemia.

Even if the atrial septum and the ductus arteriosus are nonrestrictive, the hemodynamics described previously are untenable beyond a few months of life, owing to pulmonary overcirculation and the development of irreversible pulmonary hypertension.

CLINICAL PRESENTATIONS

HLHS may be diagnosed either in utero using fetal echocardiography or in the neonatal period. There may be a family history of affected siblings or first-degree relatives with left heart obstructive lesions.[4] Pregnancy and delivery are typically uncomplicated. Neonates with HLHS are usually full-term and appropriate for gestational age, and they appear normal at birth. A male predominance has been reported. HLHS has been reported in association, although uncommonly, with several genetic syndromes, including Turner's syndrome, Noonan's syndrome, Smith-Lemli-Opitz syndrome, Holt-Oram syndrome, trisomy 13, trisomy 18, and trisomy 21. The stigmata of these syndromes may be evident. Serious extracardiac (including central nervous system) malformations have been reported in 12% to 29% of neonates with HLHS.[5] This high incidence mandates that these malformations should be sought aggressively.

Presentation within the first few hours of life is rare. When it occurs, it is clinically characterized by profound cyanosis usually due to a severely restrictive atrial septum. More typically, the neonate with HLHS usually comes to medical attention within the first 2 weeks of life, owing to a combination of pulmonary overcirculation and low systemic output. There may be a history of rapid breathing that interferes with feeding, sallow or ashen color, lethargy, and diaphoresis. Constipation and jaundice are usually due to dehydration caused by a combination of poor intake and high insensible losses resulting from tachypnea and diaphoresis. Cyanosis is variable but it is usually evident to examination and pulse oximetry. Previously undiagnosed neonates with HLHS may present in a state of circulatory collapse due to constriction of the ductus arteriosus. These neonates exhibit hypothermia, gray or ashen color, poor perfusion, cool and mottled extremities, weak or absent pulses, dyspnea, tachypnea, agonal respirations, tachycardia, cyanosis, icterus, diaphoresis, and hepatomegaly.

Cardiac examination of a neonate who has HLHS typically reveals a prominent RV impulse. The first heart sound is normal, and the second heart sound is single. A systolic click may be present owing to dilatation of the main PA. Nonspecific systolic murmurs may be present, owing to tricuspid regurgitation, a restrictive ductus arteriosus, or prograde flow across the stenotic aortic valve. A diastolic murmur due to excessive flow across the tricuspid valve may be present. Gallop rhythm, consisting of a fourth heart sound (presystolic) gallop or a third and fourth heart sound (summation) gallop may be heard.

DIAGNOSTIC TECHNIQUES

Prenatal Diagnosis

With the improvements in ultrasonography and fetal echocardiography, a significant portion of patients with HLHS are diagnosed prenatally. HLHS is an evolving process in utero, and the determinants of its evolution are not well understood. Thus the fetus may exhibit the classic echocardiographic features of HLHS as early as 16 weeks of gestation.[6] Alternatively, left heart obstruction in early gestation may be associated with a dysfunctional and either normal-sized or dilated LV. With advancing gestational age, the LV may exhibit varying degrees of growth failure, evolving into classic HLHS, critical aortic stenosis, or primary LV endocardial fibroelastosis by the time of birth. The varying patterns of left heart growth encountered in the fetus with left heart obstruction indicate the need for serial antenatal echocardiographic evaluation. Fetuses with congenital heart disease in general and HLHS in particular are at risk for aneuploidy, abnormal karyotype, and extracardiac malformations.[7] Because the presence of genetic and extracardiac malformations may profoundly influence the family's decision to intervene or not, these fetuses must undergo complete antenatal evaluation to facilitate comprehensive parental counseling before the birth of the baby.

Postnatal Diagnosis

Electrocardiography and Chest Radiography

Electrocardiogram (ECG) findings are not specific for HLHS and overlap significantly with those in the normal neonate. The most common ECG findings in HLHS include sinus tachycardia, right axis deviation, right atrial enlargement, RV hypertrophy, and paucity of LV forces.

The chest radiograph typically reveals visceroatrial situs solitus, levocardia, cardiomegaly (enlarged right atrium and RV), and indeterminate aortic arch situs. Increased pulmonary vascular markings may be encountered in the setting of low pulmonary vascular resistance or restriction to flow at either the atrial septum or the ductus arteriosus. Decreased pulmonary vascular markings may be encountered in the setting of persistent fetal circulation.

Echocardiography

Transthoracic echocardiography is the primary diagnostic modality in HLHS. Diagnostic cardiac catheterization is not necessary.

The initial echocardiogram in a patient with suspected HLHS starts with rapid evaluation of the pulsatility of the descending aortic Doppler waveform and the size and flow characteristics of the ductus arteriosus to help evaluate the need for maintaining or restoring ductal patency.

Once the patient is stable, a complete echocardiogram is performed, employing the segmental approach to cardiac diagnosis. The subcostal views of the heart are of great value. As the subcostal long-axis sweep progresses anterosuperiorly, abnormal vascular structures should be sought crossing the diaphragm. These include abnormal courses and connections of the pulmonary veins, particularly the right lower pulmonary vein to the inferior vena cava. The atrial septum may be thick or (rarely) intact. This is usually associated with the presence of a decompressing vein (the levoatriocardinal vein) from either the left atrium or the pulmonary venous confluence to the superior vena cava or its tributaries. The left atrium may be small and thick-walled. The interatrial communication may be restrictive with elevated left atrial pressure as evidenced by Doppler flow gradients. A combination of two-dimensional and color flow Doppler imaging helps to evaluate for fenestrations and multiple atrial septal defects. Septum primum may be deviated posteriorly and leftward, attaching to the left atrial free wall

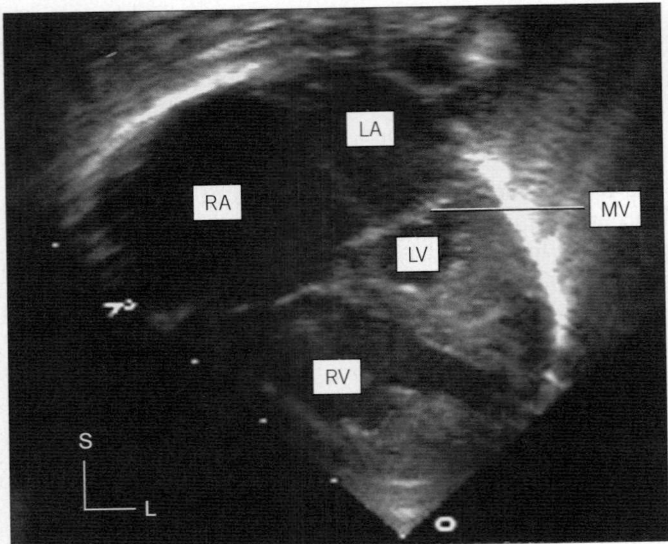

Figure 113.2 Echocardiogram in hypoplastic left heart syndrome: apical view. Dilated right heart chambers and diminutive left heart chambers (left atrium [LA] and left ventricle [LV]) are evident. The right ventricle (RV) is apex-forming. MV, mitral valve; RA, right atrium.

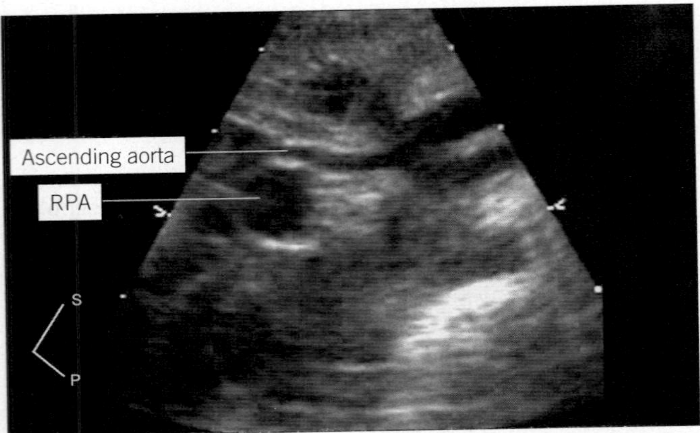

Figure 113.3 Echocardiography: hypoplastic ascending aorta in hypoplastic left heart syndrome. Suprasternal long-axis view shows a diminutive ascending aorta. The proximal and distal aortic arches are larger in caliber. The dilated right pulmonary artery (RPA) is seen in cross section.

to the left of septum secundum. This can lead to abnormal drainage of the right (and sometimes even the left) pulmonary veins to the right of the plane of the atrial septum. The subcostal views also allow estimation of the presence and severity of pulmonary regurgitation or stenosis, which is important if the Norwood procedure is being considered.

The apical four-chamber view shows obvious disparity between the dilated right heart chambers and the diminutive left heart structures (Fig. 113.2). The interatrial septum may bulge from left to right, particularly in the setting of a small or absent interatrial communication. The LV may be too small to identify, or it may be a small slit, best seen posteriorly and leftward in the left AV groove. The mitral valve annulus, supravalvar obstructive rings, and subvalvar apparatus (chordae tendineae, interchordal spaces, and papillary muscles) are best assessed from the apical view. Prograde flow across the mitral valve may be difficult to identify because of a combination of elevated LV diastolic pressure and a narrow flow jet. The LV outflow tract and the aortic valve are also well seen from the apical view. The latter is amenable to assessment for stenosis versus atresia. The RV extends to the cardiac apex. RV systolic function can be assessed qualitatively. Dilatation of the tricuspid annulus may contribute to tricuspid regurgitation.

The parasternal views demonstrate the discrepancy between the sizes of the two ventricles. The parasternal long-axis view demonstrates the diminutive aorta arising from the small LV. The LV exhibits little contractility, and may exhibit echodense areas of endocardial fibroelastosis. The mitral valve annulus and supravalvar and subvalvar levels of obstruction may be evaluated from parasternal views. These views also enable identification of a dilated coronary sinus. Drainage of a left superior vena cava to the coronary sinus is a well-known associated finding in HLHS, and is of surgical importance, given its implications for cardiopulmonary bypass cannulation.

Views from the suprasternal notch provide for clear definition of the aortic arch (Fig. 113.3). The entire aortic arch—the ascending aorta, the proximal and distal arch, and the isthmus—is amenable to echocardiographic visualization from this view. Aortic arch situs and branching pattern can be determined from this view as well. The latter allows the surgeon to plan the type of shunt or orientation of the aortopulmonary shunt as part of the Norwood procedure. The lumen of a widely patent ductus arteriosus may mask the anterior wall of coarctation of the aorta. A high index of suspicion, combined with careful scrutiny of the posterior wall of the aortic isthmus for a posterior shelf, helps avoid this diagnostic pitfall. In the presence of ductal flow, measurements of aortic arch diameters are more meaningful than Doppler gradients. Suprasternal views also help identify patterns of pulmonary venous drainage and connection. Decompressing veins that connect from the pulmonary to the systemic veins (typically the superior vena cava or its tributaries) can be identified from suprasternal views.

In HLHS, the ductus arteriosus typically exhibits systolic flow from the PA to the aorta, with diastolic flow reversal reflecting pulmonary vascular resistance lower than systemic vascular resistance. Pure right-to-left flow with absence of diastolic flow reversal in the ductus arteriosus is consistent with elevated PA diastolic pressure and implies severe elevation of pulmonary vascular resistance. This scenario is typically encountered in the setting of persistent fetal circulation, in cases with an intact atrial septum, or in infants who have been awaiting transplantation for extended periods.

HLHS is a constellation across the spectrum of severity of left heart hypoplasia. Some patients in this spectrum may be potential candidates for a biventricular approach. Echocardiographic morphometric or hemodynamic parameters may be helpful in identifying such patients.[8,9] Importantly, though, these algorithms are applicable only to specific anatomic subtypes.

Cardiac Catheterization

Interventional procedures constitute the primary indication for cardiac catheterization in HLHS. Thus balloon atrial septostomy or stent implantation in the ductus arteriosus may be indicated, typically in neonates awaiting cardiac transplantation.[10-12] Hemodynamic measurements and angiography are very rarely indicated for diagnostic purposes. Evolving hybrid procedures combining cardiac catheterization and surgery will be discussed in later sections.

MANAGEMENT

Treatment Options

The two options for active treatment of HLHS are

- staged reconstructive surgery, starting with the Norwood or hybrid procedure and culminating in a modification of the Fontan operation; or
- cardiac transplantation.

Families may also opt for nonsurgical "comfort care" (with the certainty of rapid demise).

Prenatal Management

If HLHS is diagnosed prenatally, a complete evaluation including a search for extracardiac defects and genetic syndromes is performed. In-depth counseling of the parents is essential to enable them to develop an informed plan of action. Ideally, if the family decides to proceed with either the Norwood procedure or listing for cardiac transplantation, arrangements are made to allow delivery of the neonate at the appropriate neonatal cardiac surgical center. This approach avoids the stress of neonatal transport and enables the use of expert personnel to direct the continuing care of the fetus and neonate.

Postnatal Management

Preoperative Stabilization

The success of preoperative stabilization of the neonate with HLHS determines the patient's candidacy for either transplantation or the Norwood procedure. If HLHS is suspected, an intravenous infusion of prostaglandin E_1 is begun at a dose of 0.02 to 0.1 μg/kg/minute. Evaluations for sepsis and end-organ (neurologic, hepatic, renal, and intestinal) damage are performed as appropriate for the individual patient. The preoperative management of neonates with HLHS is based predominantly on clinical experience and extrapolated data from postoperative literature and thus varies among institutions.[13] The goal of management is to achieve a balance between systemic and pulmonary flow, thus optimizing support and recovery of end-organ function.

Uncomplicated Course

Patients awaiting the Norwood procedure are usually not fed before surgery, which is generally performed within a week after birth. They usually undergo preemptive placement of umbilical arterial and venous lines to enable vascular access for perioperative management. A philosophy of watchfulness and minimal intervention has been successful in maintaining the viability of the neonate with HLHS for extended periods while awaiting cardiac transplantation.[14] Thus neonates with HLHS are not routinely intubated. The dose of prostaglandin E_1 is minimized (typically to 0.02 μg/kg/minute) to reduce untoward effects, such as apnea and pulmonary overcirculation. These patients are typically started on oral feedings as soon as possible. Tube feedings are used as necessary if the neonate is tachypneic. In order to decrease the risk of nosocomial infection, invasive monitoring is avoided. Diuretics, inotropes, and afterload-reducing agents are introduced gradually as needed, usually via the oral route. Spontaneous respiration with room air is the preferred modality of ventilation. Surveillance echocardiograms are performed periodically to evaluate the atrial septum and patency of the ductus arteriosus. Interventions such as balloon atrial septostomy and stent implantation in the ductus arteriosus are recognized as high-risk procedures, and are used only as needed for the individual patient. The successful implementation of this counter-instinctive approach requires a vigorously cooperative multidisciplinary effort.

Complicated Course

The rare neonate who presents with early and severe hypoxemia may have a restrictive atrial septum that must be addressed rapidly, usually via balloon atrial septostomy. More commonly, neonates with HLHS gradually develop pulmonary overcirculation and decreasing systemic flow, which manifests as metabolic acidosis in the face of high oxygen saturation. Pharmacologic manipulation of pulmonary vascular resistance is an effective strategy built around the concept that a low pH and an elevated carbon dioxide partial pressure will increase pulmonary vascular resistance, thus allowing improvement in systemic output. These manipulations of pulmonary and systemic blood flow using low inspired oxygen (blended with nitrogen) or high carbon dioxide arterial partial pressure ($Paco_2$) (by maintaining respiratory acidosis) may work better when the patient's lungs are mechanically ventilated and medically paralyzed to avoid spontaneous respirations.

Up to 20% of neonates awaiting transplantation may exhibit progressive restriction to flow across the atrial septum, necessitating balloon atrial septostomy.[10,11] Less commonly (in 5% of cases), patients with a restrictive ductus arteriosus may require stent implantation to ensure ductal patency.[12]

Staged Reconstruction

The aims of staged reconstruction are to completely separate the systemic and pulmonary circuits, eventually channeling all the systemic venous return to the PA without the need for a "pulmonary ventricle." When this separation is complete, only pulmonary venous blood returns to the heart. The RV pumps this blood to the systemic bed. In concept, this arrangement requires one atrium, one atrioventricular (AV) valve, one ventricle, one semilunar valve, and wide patency of the systemic and pulmonary venous inflows, PAs, and systemic outflow tract. The success of single ventricle repair is determined to a great degree by hemodynamic issues, including ventricular and valvar (AV and semilunar) function and pulmonary vascular resistance. The strategy of staged reconstruction has facilitated the physiologic transition from the native state to the eventual complete separation of pulmonary and systemic circuits.

Norwood Procedure

The goals of the Norwood procedure are to[1]

- use the RV as a combined systemic and pulmonary ventricle;
- allow unobstructed RV ejection into the systemic and the coronary circulation;

- provide pressure- and volume-controlled PA blood flow; and
- establish unrestricted mixing at the atrial level.

The components of this operation include aortic arch augmentation and the use of the pulmonary valve as the "neo-aortic" valve. The main PA is transected, thus eliminating prograde flow into the branch PAs. In the "classic" Norwood procedure, controlled PA blood flow is provided by means of an aortopulmonary shunt, typically a modified Blalock-Taussig shunt (Fig. 113.4). The ascending aorta is anastomosed to the reconstructed neo-aorta to maintain coronary perfusion. An atrial septectomy is performed to ensure free mixing at the atrial level. Meticulous surgical technique must include extended aortic arch reconstruction (to treat coarctation) without excessive arch dilatation (to avoid compression of the left PA). The aorta is aligned with the proximal PA to avoid rotation or kinking, which may obstruct coronary perfusion. An adequate interatrial communication is established. Aortopulmonary shunt size may be tailored to the individual patient.[15]

In an effort to continue to improve postoperative hemodynamics, the use of a right ventricle to pulmonary artery (RV-PA) shunt has been revisited. Larger RV-PA conduits were initially used by Dr. Norwood[1] in his original work, but were abandoned because of pulmonary overcirculation and poor outcomes. More recently smaller RV-PA shunts have gained popularity based largely on the work by Dr. Sano and colleagues[16]; this type of shunt is termed a Sano shunt at many institutions (Fig. 113.5). It has been speculated that the elimination of diastolic runoff results in an increase in coronary arterial perfusion and more stable coronary blood flow, with a resultant decrease in the incidence of interstage mortality and resilience to physiologic insults.[17,18] Nonetheless, there are some potential disadvantages of a RV-PA or Sano shunt. Concerns remain over proximal shunt obstruction, pulmonary artery distortion, or both, leading to earlier and more severe hypoxemia necessitating earlier superior cavopulmonary anastomosis. In addition the RV-PA shunt requires a small ventriculotomy and thus at least puts the patient at theoretical risk for long-term ventricular dysfunction and ventricular arrhythmias, although these concerns have not been played out in very short-term studies.[19,20] False aneurysms at the site of the ventriculotomy have been reported. Currently a multicenter prospective randomized clinical trial is underway to determine which shunt is superior; until those results are out, the "best" type of shunt really is based on the surgeon's preference.

The early postoperative period following the Norwood procedure is characterized by the potential for a labile course. With the added variability caused by shunt flow and the hemodynamic effects of cardiopulmonary bypass and circulatory arrest, the continued inverse relationship between systemic and pulmonary blood flow necessitates that a new equilibrium be established between the vascular resistances of these two circuits. Some institutions employ

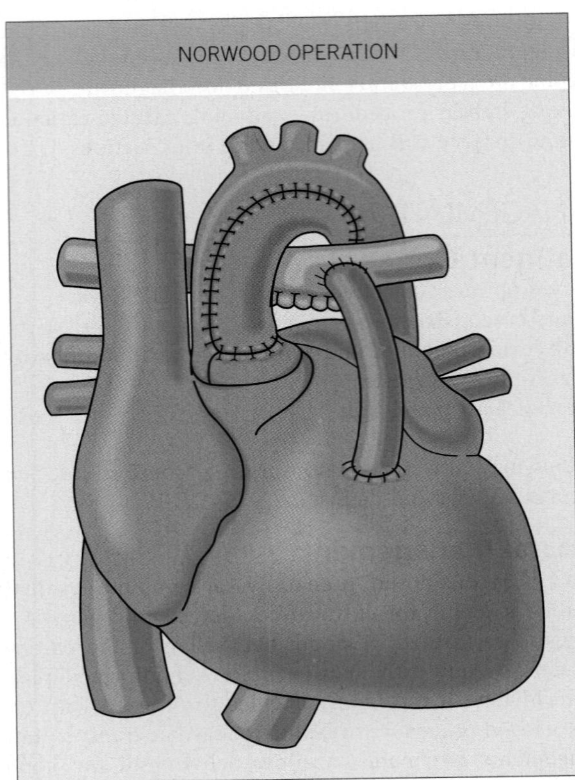

Figure 113.5 Norwood operation with the right ventricle to pulmonary artery shunt (RV-PA).

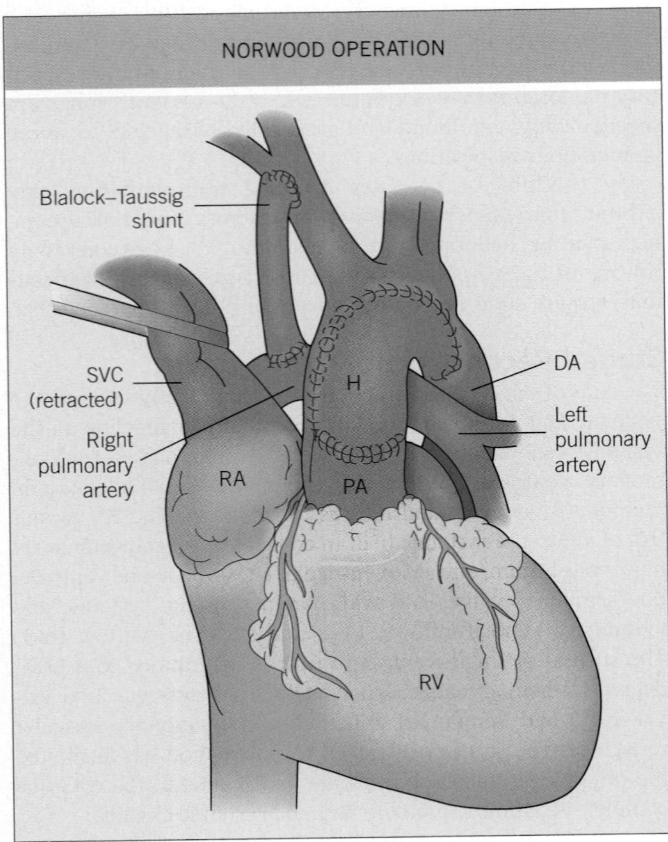

Figure 113.4 Norwood operation. The pulmonary arteries are isolated. A patch of homograft material (H) supplements the anastomosis between the proximal divided main pulmonary artery (PA) and the ascending aorta, the aortic arch and the proximal descending aorta (DA). A modified right Blalock-Taussig shunt is sutured in place. RA, right atrium; RV, right ventricle; SVC, superior vena cava.

delayed sternal closure or even routine mechanical circulatory support in the form of extracorporeal membrane oxygenation (ECMO) to facilitate successful transition.

Hybrid Procedure

Despite considerable improvements in outcomes over the last decade for the Norwood procedure, morbidity and mortality remain significant. A portion of this is thought to be related to the hemodynamic and physiologic demands of this type of circulation on an immature myocardium exposed to cardiopulmonary bypass and circulatory arrest. To eliminate the need for cardiopulmonary bypass and circulatory arrest in the neonatal period, a combined interventional and surgical approach has been developed to complete the same goals as the Norwood procedure. This hybrid procedure involves the surgical placement of bilateral branch pulmonary artery bands, stenting of the ductus arteriosus (typically by placement of the catheter sheath in the main pulmonary artery by the surgeon), and atrial balloon septostomy (Fig. 113.6).[21] Although early results appear promising, there appears to be a steep learning curve involved with this procedure and widespread acceptance awaits further studies.

Surveillance Following Norwood procedure

Potential postoperative complications following the Norwood procedure include the redevelopment of coarctation in 20% to 25% of cases, attributed to constriction of ductal tissue in the wall of the aorta.[22] The surgical shunt or the atrial septum may also become restrictive. Any of these complications may be lethal if not recognized promptly. Meticulous follow-up, including clinical evaluation, weight gain, pulse oximetry, echocardiography, and (infrequently) cardiac catheterization, is critical in the ongoing care of patients following the Norwood procedure.[23]

Echocardiographic evaluation is of particular importance. Although all of the components of the Norwood procedure may be imaged, the appearance of the post-Norwood heart is unique. The atrial septectomy should lead to a wide-open interatrial communication. Reconstruction of the aortic arch leads to disproportion between the augmented ascending aorta and the normal-sized native descending thoracic aorta. The aortopulmonary or RV-PA shunt is seen connecting to the isolated branch PAs. The anastomosis between the native ascending aorta and the neo-aorta (the so-called precoronary anastomosis) is evaluated. Pulmonary artery systolic pressure is estimated by using the peak systolic gradient across the shunt (recognizing that the length of the shunt may lead to underestimation of the gradient). Systemic (right) ventricular function and systemic AV (tricuspid) valve regurgitation are evaluated. The neo-aortic arch is evaluated for coarctation, which may occur at any location along the anastomosis. The echocardiographic diagnosis of neo-aortic arch obstruction is highly specific but may not be very sensitive. Supportive criteria, such as new AV valve regurgitation, new systemic ventricular dysfunction, and altered flow profiles in the descending aorta, have been suggested as additional indicators of arch obstruction.[22]

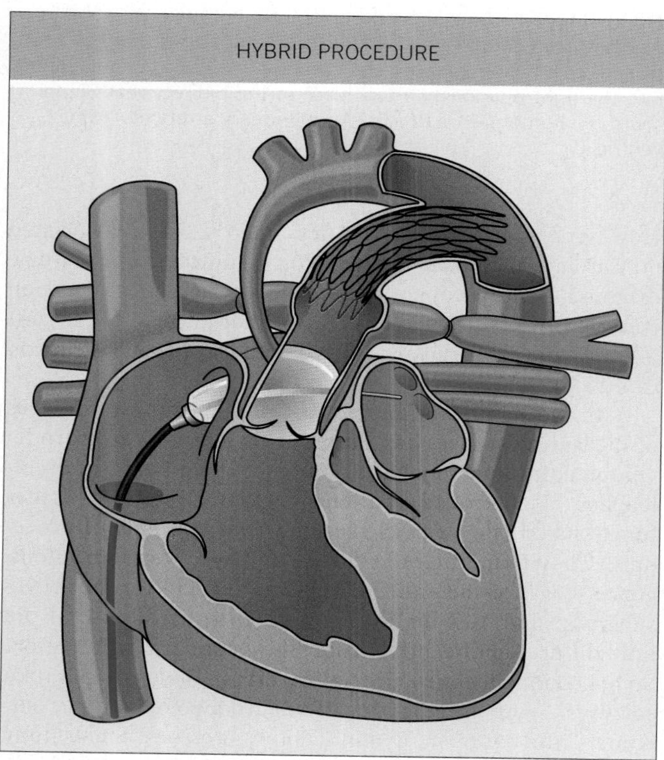

Figure 113.6 Hybrid procedure. In a combined surgical and catheterization procedure, there is placement of bilateral branch pulmonary artery bands followed by stenting of the ductus arteriosus and atrial balloon septostomy.

Subsequent Staged Surgery

Staged reconstruction following the Norwood procedure consists of two steps. The first of these is the superior cavopulmonary anastomosis (either the hemi-Fontan or the bidirectional Glenn), which is typically performed between 4 and 6 months of age. This operation consists of takedown of the previously placed aortopulmonary or RV-PA shunt and anastomosis of the superior vena cava to the right PA (Figs. 113.7 and 113.8), thus allowing superior vena caval flow to enter the PA directly. This partial separation of the systemic and pulmonary circuits achieves partial volume unloading of the RV. Potentially detrimental factors (e.g., stenotic branch PAs, tricuspid regurgitation, and obstruction to pulmonary venous return or to systemic outflow) are usually addressed at this operation.[24]

The final step in staged reconstruction is the Fontan operation (complete cavopulmonary anastomosis), which is typically performed between 18 and 36 months of age. This operation channels inferior vena caval and hepatic venous return into the PAs, thus completing the separation of the systemic and pulmonary circuits (Fig. 113.9). This results in an improvement or complete resolution of cyanosis and a decreased volume load on the single ventricle. The Fontan physiology succeeds only with very low pulmonary vascular resistance, since flow through the lungs is conducted passively without a pumping chamber.[25]

Results of the Norwood Procedure

Results of the Norwood procedure are widely variable. The best reported early survival is 92%, with the majority of institutions reporting early survival percentages in the low

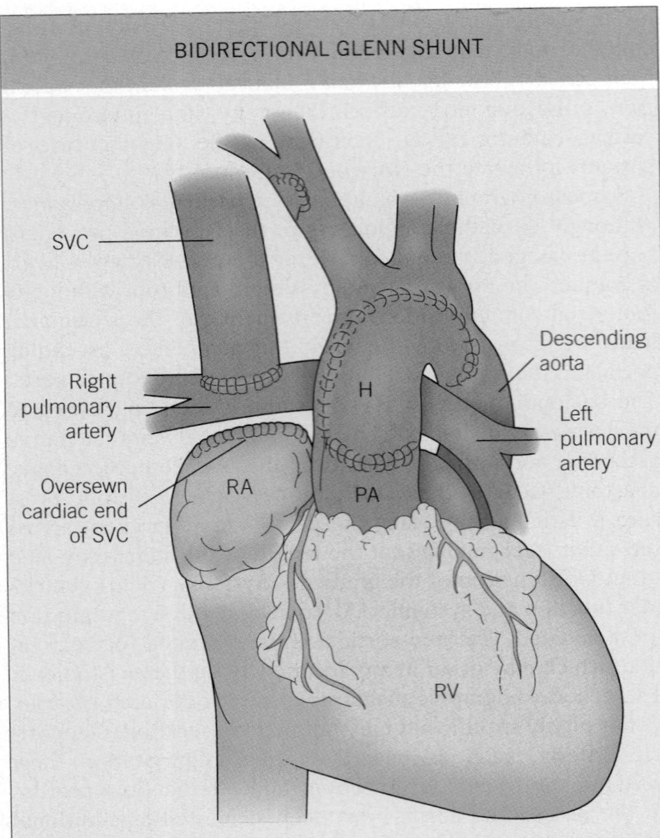

Figure 113.7 Bidirectional Glenn shunt. The previously placed Blalock-Taussig shunt is clipped. The cranial end of the divided superior vena cava (SVC) is anastomosed to the side of the right pulmonary artery. The cardiac end of the SVC is ligated. H, homograft material; PA, pulmonary artery; RA, right atrium; RV, right ventricle.

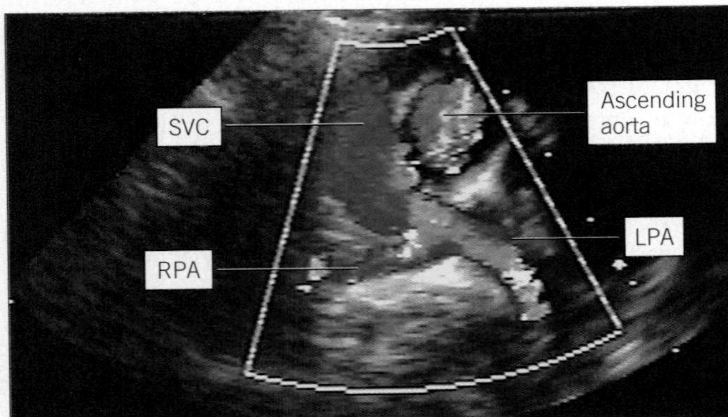

Figure 113.8 Echocardiography of bidirectional Glenn shunt. Suprasternal coronal view reveals a widely patent anastomosis between the superior vena cava (SVC) and the right pulmonary artery (RPA) with laminar flow into the pulmonary artery. LPA, left pulmonary artery.

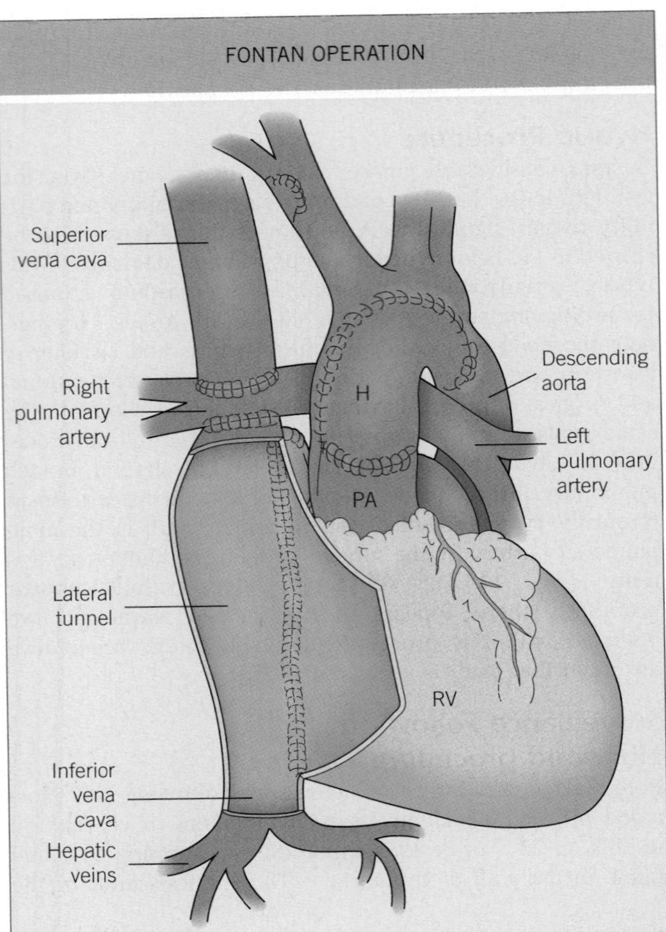

Figure 113.9 Fontan operation. A portion of the right atrial free wall has been cut away to expose the lateral tunnel that has been placed, channeling inferior vena caval (and hepatic venous) blood into the right pulmonary artery close to the bidirectional Glenn shunt. H, homograft material; PA, pulmonary artery; RV, right ventricle.

to mid 80s. Not all centers publish their results, however, and the published literature may well be representative of institutions with the best outcomes. With improvements in surgical techniques and perioperative management, many institutions have been able to overcome such risk factors as prematurity and ascending aorta diameter less than 2 mm. However, low birth weight (less than 2.5 kg), associated noncardiac anomalies (genetic or significant extracardiac diagnosis), and preoperative pulmonary venous obstruction consistently predict higher hospital mortality.[15,26] The best 5-year actuarial survival reported with staged reconstruction is 58% to 61%.[15,27]

With the significant improvement in mortality, the focus of measuring success has shifted from survival to neurodevelopmental and functional outcomes. Goldberg and colleagues[28] compared patients with HLHS to other functional single ventricle lesions after the Fontan procedure. They found that the mean Full Scale Wechsler Intelligence score for the entire group was 101 (94 for the HLHS subgroup and 107 for the non-HLHS subgroup), and did not differ significantly from the standard population. Socioeconomic status, circulatory arrest, and perioperative seizures were predictive of neurodevelopmental outcome.[28] In contrast, a multicenter, cross-sectional study compared neurodevelopmental outcomes among school-age children with HLHS; 55% had undergone Norwood palliation and 45% had undergone transplantation. They found that the mean Full Scale Wechsler Intelligence score

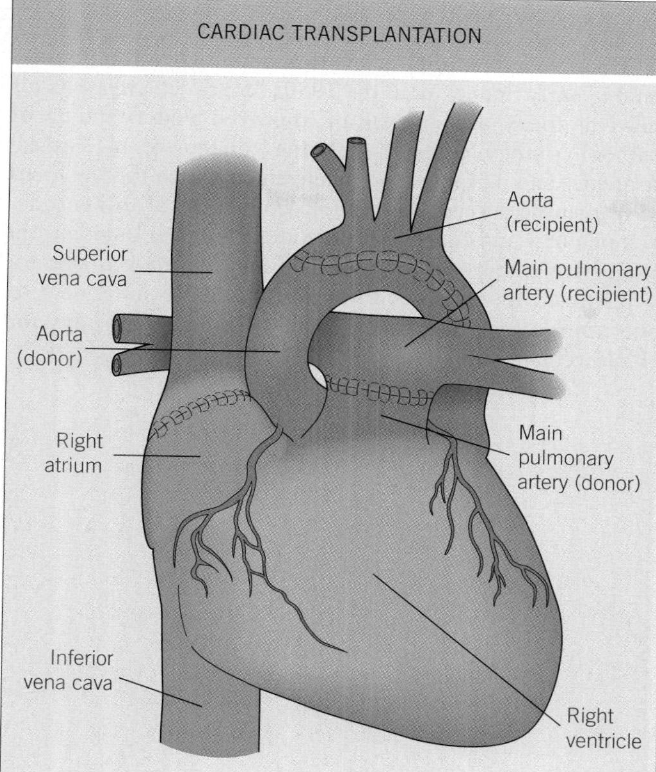

Figure 113.10 Cardiac transplantation. The donor atria are anastomosed to the posterior collar of recipient atria. An extended length of donor aorta is used to reconstruct the aortic arch well beyond the level of the ductus arteriosus.

for the entire group was 86 and did not differ between groups. They concluded that neurodevelopmental deficits were prevalent among school-age children regardless of surgical approach.[29] Despite this, most parents believe that their child's overall health, school performance, and cardiac functional status were good to excellent following Fontan palliation.[30]

Cardiac Transplantation

Transplantation offers the alternative of a single-stage operation resulting in normal biventricular physiology. In HLHS, extended reconstruction of the recipient aortic arch is performed using donor aorta (Fig. 113.10). The major drawback of transplantation is the shortage of donors. Of all infants with HLHS, 19% to 37% die while awaiting transplantation.[10,31] Maintaining the viability of the neonate with HLHS awaiting transplantation is a challenge, despite relatively short waiting times of 1.5 months.[14] This diagnosis was associated with the highest pretransplantation mortality rate among all infants listed for transplantation among the 20 member institutions composing the Pediatric Heart Transplant Study Group.[31]

The reported surgical mortality with cardiac transplantation for HLHS is widely variable. The Pediatric Heart Transplant Study Group reported post-transplant 5-year actuarial survival of 72%, with 76% of deaths occurring within 3 months of transplant. Among 1-month survivors, survival at 1 and 5 years was 92% and 85%, respectively. However, taking into account all 262 unpalliated patients with HLHS listed for transplant, survival was 68% at 3 months and 54% at 5 years.[31]

Norwood Procedure versus Cardiac Transplantation

The Norwood procedure and cardiac transplantation are based on differing philosophies, and the choice between the two approaches is far from clear. We believe that the choice between the Norwood procedure and cardiac transplantation is one best left to each family. Regardless of whether the family has chosen the Norwood procedure or transplantation, the cardiologist bears the onus for ensuring that his or her patient receives the best care. Patients with HLHS would probably be best served by the regionalization of surgery, whereby a neonate who is a candidate for a particular surgical approach would be referred to a center that has achieved the best results with that specific approach. Alsoufi and colleagues[32] have published a nice review on the various treatment strategies for HLHS.

Comfort Care

Recent improvements in survival following either surgical approach have led to questions regarding the appropriateness of a comfort care approach, which carries with it the certainty of death. However, the results of treatment are far from perfect. Current treatment choices are associated with morbidity and mortality and are not curative. The logistics of lifelong care of a child with chronic medical conditions may be unrealistic for some families and unacceptable for others. We mention the choice of nonsurgical management to the family of every child with HLHS. A family's experience with choosing comfort care is available for the interested reader.[33]

PROGNOSIS

Following staged reconstruction, long-term issues revolve around the viability of the Fontan state and the systemic RV. Patients who have completed the Fontan operation exhibit a late increase in instantaneous risk of death, which may be related to either the Fontan state, per se, or individual patient-related variables.[3] Several morphologic features place the systemic RV at a disadvantage in comparison to the LV. These features include coronary arterial supply, the conduction system, atrioventricular valve and myofiber arrangement. Whether the RV will prove functionally adequate as a lifelong systemic pump in the setting of HLHS is an unresolved issue.

Transplantation is far from being a cure. Recoarctation of the aorta occurs in 21% of infants following transplantation with aortic arch reconstruction.[34] The risk of rejection mandates lifelong immunosuppression. Heart transplant recipients may develop viral infections of the myocardium, which places them at high risk for transplant vasculopathy and graft loss.[35] Graft vasculopathy has been reported in 23% of patients transplanted for HLHS by 7 years post-transplant, and may have a rapid and malignant course.[10] There is no consensus on the management of patients with graft vasculopathy or graft failure; retransplantation may be needed.

Future developments currently being investigated to improve the outcomes of children with HLHS, focus on preventing the actual disease from developing by performing fetal cardiac interventions. This procedure involves percutaneous entry through the abdomen of the mother, through the uterus, and through the free wall of the left ventricle of the fetus. A guide wire is then passed through the stenotic aortic valve and balloon valvuloplasty is performed. Early results have been promising, although this approach is clearly not currently ready for widespread use.[36] Other areas of development include transcatheter placement of intrapulmonary flow restrictors and covered stents to reduce or eliminate the need for surgical intervention.

SUMMARY

HLHS is a complex cardiac malformation that was uniformly fatal in early infancy until the 1980s. Improved prospects for survival today are due to an improved understanding of pathophysiology coupled with the refinement of surgical strategies and perioperative management. With this the focus of measuring success has shifted from survival to neurodevelopmental and functional outcomes. Surgical outcomes in HLHS are center-specific. Survival may improve if surgery is restricted to centers with an institutional commitment to one approach or the other. Both treatment pathways for HLHS remain palliative.

chapter

114 Ebstein Malformation

Hideki Uemura and Robin Shaughnessy

Definition

- Ebstein malformation is characterized by varying degrees of downward displacement of the inferior and septal leaflets of the tricuspid valve into the right ventricle. Most cases exist as an isolated lesion but many are accompanied by an interatrial communication.

Key Features

- The physiology of the lesion varies with the degree of valvular deformity and right ventricular dysfunction. Consequently, presentation can vary from a decompensated fetus to an incidental finding at autopsy in an elderly person.
- Arrhythmias, especially supraventricular tachycardia, are not rare because of common association of Wolff-Parkinson-White syndrome or a prolongedly overloaded right atrium secondary to tricuspid regurgitation and right-sided heart failure.

Therapy

- Treatment (medical or surgical) is individualized on the basis of the age of the patient and the predominant findings.

The patient described by Wilhelm Ebstein[1] in 1866 was an emaciated 19-year-old Polish laborer with a long history of shortness of breath, palpitations, and cyanosis who died 8 days after admission to All Saints Hospital in Breslau. At autopsy, the tricuspid valve was found to be markedly abnormal. The description was accompanied by elegant illustrations drawn by Ebstein's colleague, Dr. Wyss. The septal leaflet was shown as a discoid structure lacking its posteroinferior component. The inferior mural and the anterosuperior leaflets were depicted as having annular attachments at the atrioventricular junction, while the distal edge of the inferior leaflet was illustrated as being attached to the ventricular wall and that of the anterosuperior leaflet was attached to abnormal papillary muscles. The anterosuperior leaflet was abnormally long, extending toward the apical portion of the right ventricle. A patent foramen ovale was present. In his report, Ebstein included a hypothesis of the embryology and pathophysiology. In 1927, after several reports of similar lesions had appeared in the literature, Alfred Arnstein[2] published the 14th case report and suggested that this anomaly of the tricuspid valve be known as Ebstein's disease.

Ebstein malformation is rare, occurring in approximately 5 per 100,000 live births, or 0.5% of patients with congenital heart disease.[3] There is no predilection for either sex, and although most cases occur sporadically, familial cases have been reported. The etiology remains unknown. The abnormality may be linked to mutations in the homeobox transcription factor NKX2.5.[4] Maternal ingestion of lithium carbonate, used to treat bipolar disorder, in the first trimester appears to increase the incidence in some cases. The Baltimore-Washington Infant Study Group suggested genetic, reproductive and environmental risk factors that included family history of cardiovascular malformation, white race, previous fetal loss, maternal exposure to benzodiazepine, and varnishing substances.[6] Patients with Ebstein malformation have presented as early as 18 weeks of gestation and as late as 79 years of age, making the lesion a topic of importance to pediatric and adult cardiologists alike.

ANATOMY AND PATHOLOGY

Ebstein malformation is a congenital disease in which one or two leaflets of the tricuspid valve do not attach normally to the right atrioventricular junction.[7,8] The anterior leaflet is hardly involved in terms of annular attachment of its hinge. This leaflet is usually large and redundant and has been likened to a sail. The septal leaflet and the inferior mural leaflet are plastered to the internal surface of the right ventricle to some degree. Because of this, the hinge points of these leaflets are described as being downward displaced into the right ventricle and distant from the true atrioventricular junction (Fig. 114.1). The commissure between the septal and inferior leaflets is usually the point of maximum displacement. Motion of these leaflets is limited as a consequence of the fixed leaflets and also by the abnormally structured tension apparatus for these leaflets. A part of the leaflets may not be entirely plastered onto the right ventricular mass, but often there are a certain number of very short fibrous cords present, tethering that part of the leaflets firmly. The mobile parts of two leaflets are often thickened and dysplastic.

In the normal heart, formation of the tricuspid valve leaflets and tension apparatus occurs by a process of undermining of the right ventricular wall, leading to liberation of the inner layer of ventricular muscle, continuing to the level of the atrioventricular junction.[9] Much of the apical portion of the valve tissue thus formed is normally resorbed until only papillary muscles and tendinous strands remain. In Ebstein malformation, the process of undermining is incomplete and the annulus is not reached. Resorption takes place inadequately or not at all.

The right ventricular wall can be abnormally thin for the ventricle at the region where the leaflets of the tricuspid valve are completely plastered. This finding is designated an "atrialized portion," likening the thin ventricular wall to atrial wall and to reflect the extension of the functional

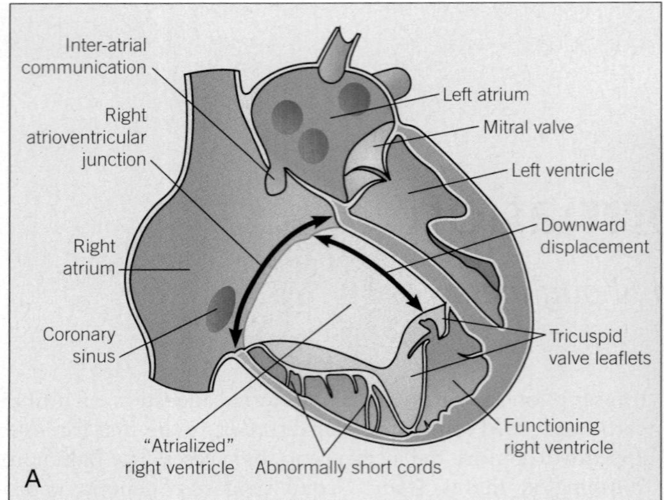

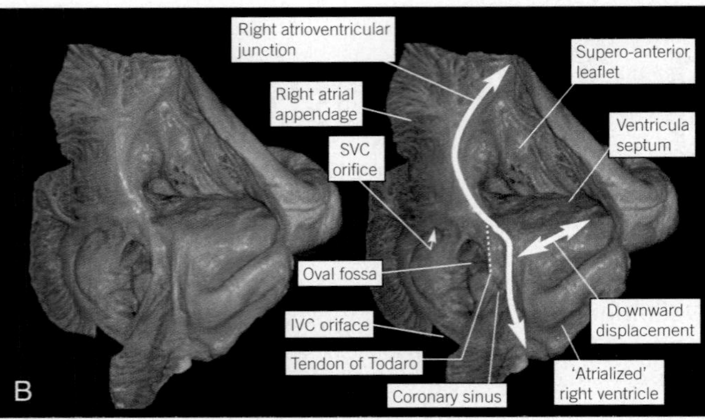

Figure 114.1 Ebstein malformation. A, Schema of Ebstein malformation of the tricuspid valve as viewed from the antero-superior aspect. Note downward displacement of the attachment of the septal and the postero-inferior leaflets produces atrialized portion of the right ventricle and makes the functional right ventricular chamber diminutive. The leaflets of the tricuspid valve have not only characteristic plastering but also short tendinous cords. **B,** Heart specimen of Ebstein malformation viewed from the antero-inferior aspect with the specimen clam-shell opened along the acute margin of the right ventricle. SVC, superior vena cava; IVC, inferior vena cava.

atrium into the right ventricle. Other parts of the right ventricle are also thinner than normal in many cases. The entire right ventricular cavity is commonly dilated. The degree of dilatation is attributed not only to the morphologically thin structure of the right ventricular wall but also to the decrease in myofibrils on a histopathologic basis.[10] There is a spectrum toward severe depletion of myocardium within the right ventricular free wall resulting in a parchment-like appearance reminiscent of Uhl's disease, although Uhl's disease does not have Ebstein malformation. In other cases, the displaced hingeline of the leaflets effectively divides the right ventricle into a thin-walled inlet part and a thick-walled trabecular-outlet part. The latter component is deemed the functional right ventricle.

The degree of downward displacement varies. In some patients with a milder morphologic form of the disease, the area of the plastered leaflets is within or around the inlet portion of the right ventricle; downward displacement is of a few centimeters in the adult. In such patients, the really functioning right ventricle possesses the trabecular apical portion as well as the outlet portion. In contrast, in other patients with a more severe morphologic form of the disease, the septal and the inferior leaflets are dysplastic and extremely displaced toward the outlet portion of the right ventricle. The apex of the right ventricle is on the nonfunctioning side, and the distorted orifice for the tricuspid valve is oriented to just guard the outlet portion of the ventricular cavity. In such a significant form, the right ventricular outflow tract tends to become larger than normal for compensation. Because of the bulging right ventricular cavity, the left ventricular outflow tract occasionally appears to be narrower than in the normally structured heart.

When the term *Ebstein malformation* is used as an entity of congenital cardiac disease, it should be less confusing to define the abnormality in a patient or a heart with normal cardiac situs, concordant atrioventricular connections (the right atrium to the right ventricle, the left atrium to the left ventricle), and concordant ventriculoarterial connections (the pulmonary trunk from the right ventricle, the aorta from the left ventricle). A possible major coexisting malformation is then interatrial communication across the oval fossa (either patent fossa ovalis or atrial septal defect), found in approximately 90%. In children, pulmonary stenosis or atresia may coexist. In a small proportion of patients, the tricuspid valve with Ebstein malformation can be imperforate.

On the other hand, when the term *Ebstein malformation* is used as a morphologic feature of the inlet valve, the phrase appears in a wider spectrum of diseases. In children, pulmonary stenosis or atresia may coexist. In these cases the right side of the heart often is markedly enlarged and produces a wall-to-wall heart on chest radiography. In the setting of congenitally corrected transposition of the great arteries (discordant atrioventricular and ventriculoarterial connections), it is well known that the left-sided atrioventricular valve (guarding the junction between the left atrium and the morphologically right ventricle that gives rise to the aorta) frequently has the morphologic feature of downward displacement.[11] The downward displacement of the valvular leaflets guarding the morphologically left ventricle is exceedingly rare. Even in the heart with a common atrioventricular valve or atrioventricular septal defect, there is evidence that the essence of the morphologic feature of Ebstein malformation can occur on the right-side component of the inlet valve.[12] In this chapter, these coexisting Ebstein phenomena in complicated cardiac malformations are excluded, and the context is focused on the entity of disease mentioned in the preceding paragraph.

The right atrium is usually enlarged. The atrioventricular junction (a normally expected annular attachment) is usually dilated and very occasionally stenotic. When a diagnosis of tricuspid stenosis is made in Ebstein malformation, the clinician needs to clarify whether the true atrioventricular junction is morphologically stenotic or the displaced valvular orifice is obstructive.

The coronary arteries in Ebstein malformation appear to be similar in distribution to that seen in the normal heart, but extensive and precise investigation has yet to be achieved. The sinus node and atrioventricular node are positioned normally. The proximal conduction axis courses also normally. The right bundle branch can be deviated. When Wolff-Parkinson-White syndrome coexists, the accessory pathway is commonly at the part of the atrioventricular junction where downward displacement is present, although rare occasions are reported.

PATHOPHYSIOLOGY

Hemodynamic features in patients with Ebstein malformation may roughly reflect the degree of morphologic abnormality, but not necessarily. Not only the degree of tricuspid regurgitation but also right ventricular function determines efficacy of the overall circulation.[13] Even after the tricuspid valve is successfully made competent by surgical repair or replacement, clinical symptoms may not improve when right ventricular performance stays at a significantly impaired level.

When an interatrial communication is present, the direction of shunt flow across the defect represents more or less the right-sided heart function. If the shunt is exclusively from right to left, the right side of the heart is not coping with the whole systemic output returning to the right atrium. In patients with the intracardiac shunt dominantly from left to right, the diseased right side of the heart is dealing with the amount of flow more than the left ventricle does. In the latter setting, closure of the interatrial communication has a theoretical benefit of volume offloading. In contrast, in the former setting, a similar change will pose more load to the right side of the heart at the expense of a noncyanotic circulation. Nonetheless, it is difficult to assess true right ventricular function and to predict potential for improvement of the right-sided heart function in Ebstein malformation.

During atrial systole, the atrialized portion of the right ventricle is in diastole and serves as a reservoir for blood. During ventricular systole, this blood is propelled back into the true right atrium rather than into the functional right ventricle. Right ventricular stroke volume is therefore decreased. Patients who are diagnosed in childhood may have significantly reduced right ventricular systolic and diastolic function compared with age-matched controls, whereas those patients who are not diagnosed until adulthood tend to have normal right ventricular systolic and diastolic function.[14]

The abnormalities of the right-sided heart structures in patients with Ebstein malformation have been shown to produce secondary effects on the shape and function of the left ventricle.[15] The atrialized portion of the interventricular septum, if any, bows toward the left ventricle during diastole, resulting in paradoxical septal motion and superior displacement of the mitral leaflets toward the left atrium. Left ventricular end-diastolic volume and ejection fraction are decreased. However, many such patients have been shown to have consistently appropriate increments in heart rate, blood pressure, and left ventricular ejection fraction with Bruce protocol exercise testing.

In patients in whom the right ventricle has little reserve capacity to drive blood into the pulmonary circulation, increase in pulmonary resistance, even of a mild degree, will burden the overall circulation. In the presence of an interatrial communication, a right-to-left shunt increases, and cyanosis becomes worse. Without a communication at the atrial level, overall cardiac output decreases because the right ventricle is unable to cope with the raised pulmonary resistance. A rise in pulmonary resistance may be induced by chest infection, a Valsalva maneuver, or exercise.

CLINICAL PRESENTATIONS

The age of presentation depends on the severity of the valvular defect, right ventricular function, and associated malformations. The displaced and highly abnormal tricuspid valve may produce functional stenosis, incompetence, or both. In the fetus, an abnormal routine prenatal ultrasound may be referred for an associated arrhythmia or a history of maternal lithium exposure.[16] The fetus may present with tricuspid valve dysfunction, cardiomegaly, congestive heart failure with or without significant right ventricular outflow obstruction. In severe cases, fetal hydrops and intrauterine death may occur. In the study by Celermajer and colleagues, the age at presentation ranged from 18 weeks' gestation to 68 years, and a median of 36 days. Routine fetal echocardiography now plays an important role in early diagnosis.

Neonates with Ebstein malformation commonly present with cyanosis, which may be intense, and signs of right heart failure. Intense cyanosis is due to elevated pulmonary vascular resistance and a right-to-left shunt through the interatrial communication. With the natural regression of the muscular layer of fetal pulmonary arterioles, pulmonary vascular resistance diminishes, resulting in improvement in tricuspid valve function, and the infant gradually becomes less cyanotic. In some cases hypoxemia and congestive heart failure may lead to an early death. In these neonates, the heart usually occupies a large proportion of the thoracic cavity and the lungs are hypoplastic. The "wall-to-wall" heart appearance on chest X-ray (where both sides of the cardiac silhouette are reaching, or nearly reaching, the thoracic cage) is recognized as a very poor prognostic sign in newborns. Infants may present with dyspnea secondary to congestive heart failure and tricuspid regurgitation, an incidental murmur, or tachyarrhythmia. Compared to older patients, children under 2 years of age are much more likely to present with hemodynamic abnormalities. Other individuals with Ebstein malformation may have no difficulty in infancy and the onset of symptoms may be delayed for several years. Children older than 2 years to adolescents are most likely to present with an incidental murmur. Often, early presentation is due to associated pulmonary stenosis or atresia. By adolescence and into adulthood, the presentation is dominated by arrhythmias, usually associated with accessory pathways and/or atrial fibrillation or flutter. Adults have also been reported to present with heart failure or an incidental murmur. Growth and development of patients who present in the older age groups are usually normal. All degrees of cyanosis and digital clubbing may be seen. Patients who have not been cyanotic previously may develop cyanosis as a result of worsening tricuspid insufficiency or deteriorating right ventricular function. Cyanosis may be seen as ruddy facial coloring, and it is usually accompanied by dyspnea. Low arterial oxygen tension contributes to dyspnea by stimulating the carotid bodies and increasing ventilation. In addition, inadequate perfusion of exercising muscles may provoke reflex ventilatory stimulation. Palpitations may be caused by single or multiple premature atrial or ventricular systoles or runs of paroxysmal tachyarrhythmias (usually supraventricular tachycardia).

Physical examination may reveal asymmetry of the chest as a result of prominence of the left or right parasternal regions secondary to right atrial enlargement. The precordium is usually normally active, and the arterial and jugular venous pulse forms are also usually normal. Patients who have an intact atrial septum are more likely to have jugular venous distention and hepatosplenomegaly.

In Ebstein malformation the auscultatory findings are usually distinctive enough to allow clinical diagnosis. The majority have a systolic murmur heard at the left sternal edge that increases with inspiration, sometimes accompanied by a thrill. Patients with severe tricuspid regurgitation have the loudest and longest murmurs. A mid-diastolic murmur of true or relative tricuspid stenosis may also be present. The first heart sound is normal or diminished in intensity and comprises two components, which are often widely split because of increased excursion of the anterosuperior leaflet and subsequent delayed closure of the abnormal tricuspid valve. The second heart sound may be normal, but it is usually widely and persistently split by the delay in pulmonary valve closure caused by right bundle branch block. The intensity of the pulmonary component may be diminished or inaudible as a result of low pulmonary pressure in the presence of a right-to-left shunt. Both atrial and ventricular filling sounds are common. Almost always present in patients with Ebstein malformation is a holosystolic murmur of tricuspid insufficiency that is heard along the left sternal border and that increases with inspiration. A mid-diastolic murmur of true or relative tricuspid stenosis may also be present. Many patients also have prominent third and fourth heart sounds, and this combination of heart sounds and murmurs contributes to the quadruple rhythm gallop or cadence that is characteristic of Ebstein malformation. The heart sounds may be difficult to analyze accurately in the newborn period.

DIAGNOSTIC TECHNIQUES

Electrocardiography

It is rare for the electrocardiogram in Ebstein malformation to be normal, so this test can be very helpful in the diagnosis. The rhythm is usually sinus. Wolff-Parkinson-White syndrome is seen in up to a quarter of patients with Ebstein malformation. Right atrial enlargement is usually seen and is characterized by tall, peaked P waves (Fig. 114.2). The PR interval is significantly prolonged (to more than 0.2 second) in many patients. Both the size of the P wave and the PR interval have been correlated with the size of the right atrium. The QRS axis in the frontal plane is usually normal, but there is right axis deviation in a significant portion of patients. The QRS complex frequently demonstrates right ventricular conduction delay in the form of right bundle branch block. The QRS complex is also usually of low voltage. Diagnostic criteria for right ventricular hypertrophy are rare, and left ventricular hypertrophy is not seen in this entity.

Arrhythmias that occur in Ebstein malformation include supraventricular tachycardia with or without Wolff-Parkinson-White syndrome. In addition, right atrial enlargement may lead to atrial flutter or atrial fibrillation; this finding is much more common in older patients. Even in young adult patients who do not have an obvious episode of arrhythmia, 24-hour Holter recording is worth arranging. Ectopic atrial beats or short and non-sustained atrial tachycardia are often present but not noticed by the patients.

Chest Radiography

The chest radiographs of patients presenting in infancy are often dramatic. Cardiomegaly dominates, leaving little of the lung fields visible (Fig. 114.3). The enlargement is primarily of the right atrium. If the lungs are visible, the pulmonary vascular markings are reduced. In older patients the cardiac size and silhouette vary considerably. The chest radiograph may appear nearly normal in the mildest cases. The right atrium may be mildly prominent, but with the most severe forms the right atrium can be so enlarged as to displace the right ventricle to the left. The right heart border shows a distinct curvature. Dilation of the right ventricular outflow tract results in displacement of the upper left cardiac border. The aortic knob commonly appears less prominent, which may be attributed to long-standing low cardiac output. The overall cardiac silhouette becomes a globular shape. Appearance on chest X-ray may change with time or with progression of decompensation of the right heart. In cyanotic patients, pulmonary vascular markings are decreased due to the right-to-left shunt.

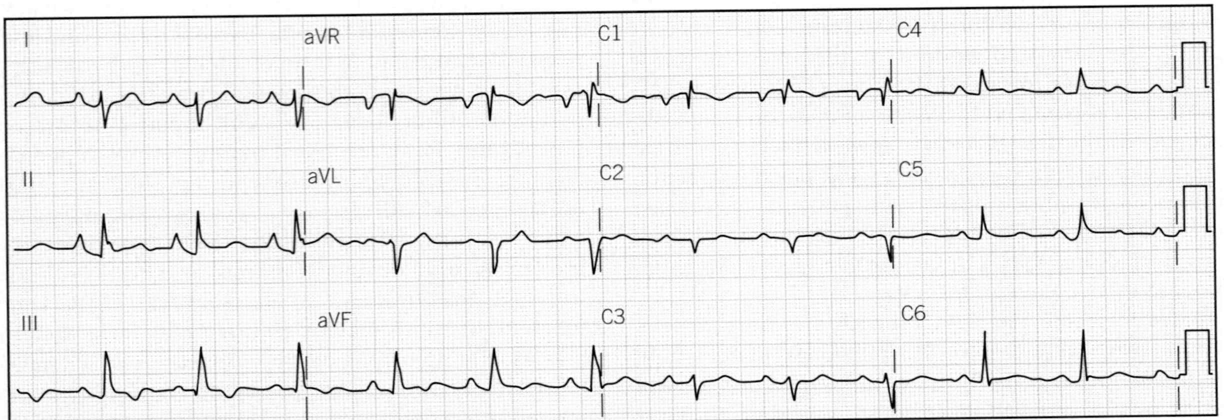

Figure 114.2 Electrocardiography. Ebstein malformation in a 19-year-old patient. Note the tall and peaked P-waves. PR interval is 240 milliseconds. QRS pattern suggests intraventricular conduction delay. QRS voltage in V leads is low.

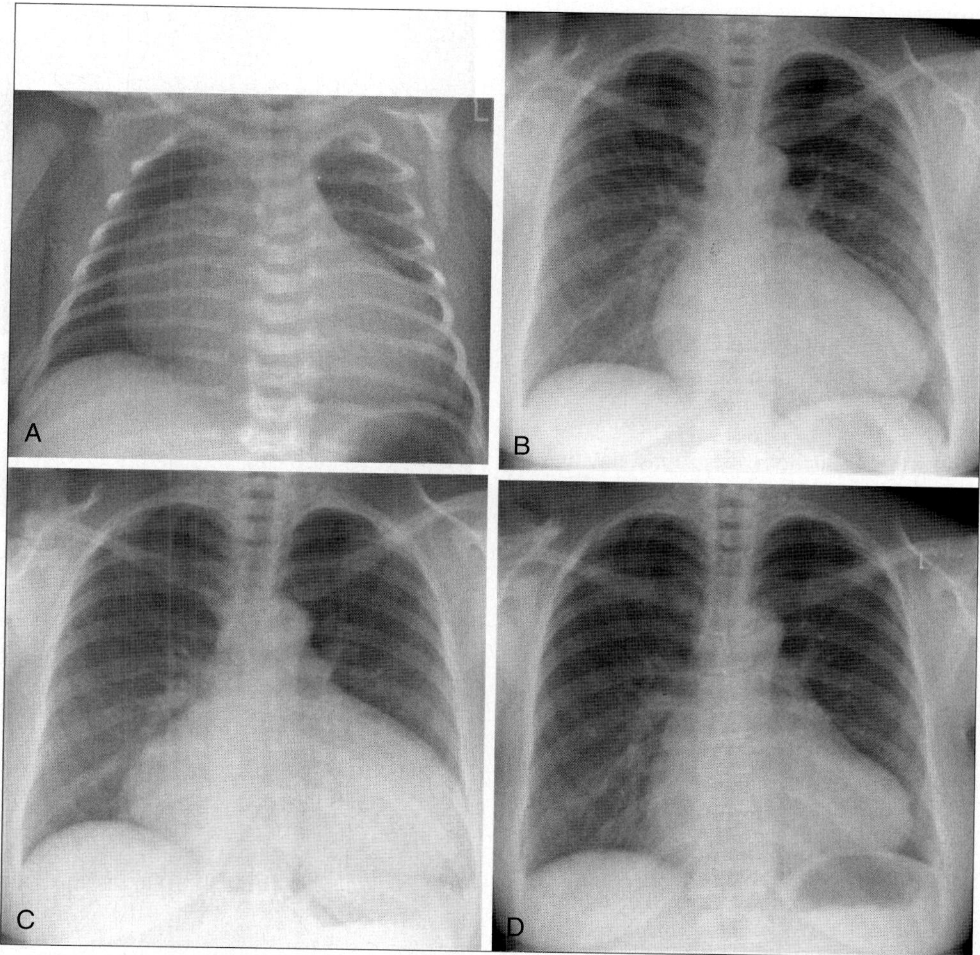

Figure 114.3 Chest radiography. A, Chest X-ray in a one-day-old newborn with severe Ebstein malformation and moderate pulmonary regurgitation. Cardiomegaly is significant (cardio-thoracic ratio 81%). This patient soon required tracheal intubation because of bradycardia. When the heart shadow reaches the thoracic cage on both sides, the radiographic appearance is called a "wall-to-wall" heart. Neonates with such a severe form of cardiomegaly usually have their lungs underdeveloped, and the impaired pulmonary condition poses difficulty in medically managing to stabilize the overall circumstance together with the circulatory impediment caused by the heart malformation. **B,** Chest X-ray of a 33-year-old patient with Ebstein malformation. The heart silhouette indicates moderate enlargement of the right heart, but not of a severe degree; cardio-thoracic ratio was 64%. Cardiomegaly due to right atrial enlargement with a narrow base is a classic radiographic appearance of this malformation. The pulmonary vasculature does not appear to be diminished in this particular patient. **C,** Six years later, the cardiac silhouette became much larger (cardio-thoracic ratio 76%) with deterioration in clinical symptoms. **D,** Chest X-ray taken 18 months after surgical repair of Ebstein malformation demonstrated vast improvement in cardiac silhouette size (cardio-thoracic ratio 61%). Repair of the tricuspid valve was carried out by Carpentier's technique. Concomitantly, the right atrium as well as the right ventricle were plicated for reduction of the enlarged right heart.

Exercise Testing

Patients with Ebstein malformation may complain of shortness of breath leading to exercise intolerance. Several factors have been suggested to account for their poor performance, including significant tricuspid regurgitation, poor right ventricular function and decreased cardiac output, right-to-left shunt and associated abnormal ventilation, cardiomegaly, and medications. Controlled testing of patients with Ebstein malformation has shown that the only major predictor of exercise tolerance in the older and unrepaired patient is the resting oxygen saturation.[17] In fact, there is a linear correlation between resting oxygen saturation and exercise tolerance as measured by maximum oxygen uptake and duration of exercise. Heart size did not prove to be predictive of exercise tolerance. Exercise tolerance does not necessarily correlate with cardiac output. Unrepaired patients who do not have an atrial septal defect may perform well and their exercise tolerance may be within the normal range. In a study among asymptomatic children with normal resting oxygen saturation, those without an atrial level right-to-left shunt perform better than those who have one.[18] Heart size is not predictive of exercise tolerance, and many patients with Ebstein malformation have been shown to have cardiac outputs in the normal range. Patients who have had surgery, either tricuspid valve repair or replacement and closure of an atrial septal defect, usually show marked improvement in their exercise tolerance. Some of them may recover to the level of normal subjects. Unrepaired patients who do not have an atrial septal defect perform similar to postoperative patients. On the other hand, those with Ebstein malformation and atrial septal defect shunting from left to right would not have much improvement in their clinical symptoms after closure of the atrial septal defect alone. This fact should be noted in the era in which catheter intervention is feasible for closure of an interatrial communication.

Echocardiography

The accuracy of cross-sectional echocardiography has markedly simplified the diagnosis of Ebstein malformation, making cardiac catheterization unnecessary in the majority of cases. The characteristic downward (apical) displacement of the septal leaflet of the tricuspid valve is seen in the apical or subcostal four-chamber views (Fig. 114.4).[19] When seen in these views the normal heart shows offsetting of the levels of annular attachments between the mitral and the tricuspid valves, with the tricuspid valve attached nearer toward the apex than the mitral valve. To distinguish normal from excessive offset, it is generally accepted that if the annular attachment of the tricuspid valve is $\geq$ 8 mm/m^2 (relative to total body surface area) below the insertion of the mitral valve, there is excessive downward displacement and the diagnosis of Ebstein malformation can be made. If this pathognomonic criterion is not met, other rare congenital or acquired diagnoses, such as tricuspid valve dysplasia or tricuspid valve prolapse must be considered. These may mimic the findings of Ebstein malformation.[20] The apical displacement of leaflet tissue also means that the tricuspid valve may be seen in the standard plane of the parasternal long-axis view and in the subcostal outlet view. Normally, tricuspid valve leaflets are not seen in these views. A comprehensive echocardiographic examination should also reveal other features of the malformation, including elongation of the anterosuperior tricuspid valve leaflet, abnormal apical attachments of the tension apparatus, leaflet tethering to underlying myocardium, absence of the septal or inferior tricuspid leaflets and enlargement of the tricuspid valve annulus. When the distal margin of the anterosuperior leaflet is fixed, normal motion is not possible and the leaflet assumes a billowing sail-like motion. The size of the functional right ventricle can be assessed from the subcostal views. The wall thickness and wall motion of the atrialized portion as well as septal motion can also be studied. With the addition of Doppler and color-flow imaging, the degree of tricuspid insufficiency or stenosis can be assessed, as well as the presence of intracardiac shunting. Serial transthoracic echocardiograms are useful in tracking the progression of disease, with or without surgical intervention.

In the fetus, echocardiography is particularly useful for making an early diagnosis when the fetus is referred for cardiomegaly or hydrops on obstetric scans (Fig. 114.5).[21] Although the inferior leaflet is difficult to visualize in the fetus, the anterior leaflet and the septal leaflet can be identified together with flow of regurgitation across the tricuspid valve. Pulmonary hypoplasia secondary to severe cardiomegaly and hydrops with pleural and pericardial effusions may progress. Arrhythmias can also be evaluated.

Intraoperative transesophageal echocardiography plays an important role in assessing the adequacy of tricuspid valve repair. The function of a prosthetic valve, if it is used, can be visualized. Color-flow imaging can determine the degree of residual tricuspid valve insufficiency after valve plication. It is also important to rule out a residual atrial septal defect before the patient leaves the operating room.

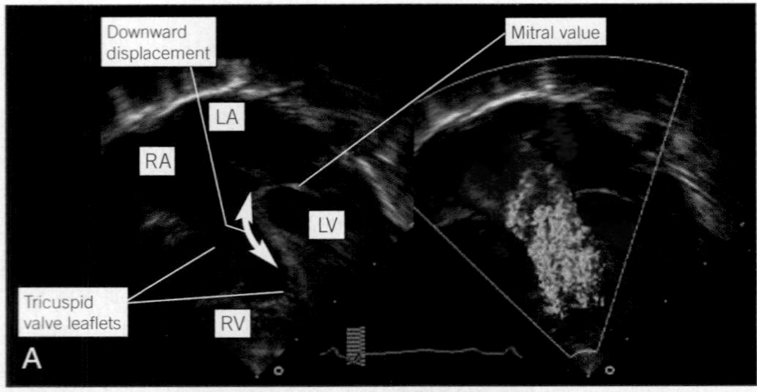

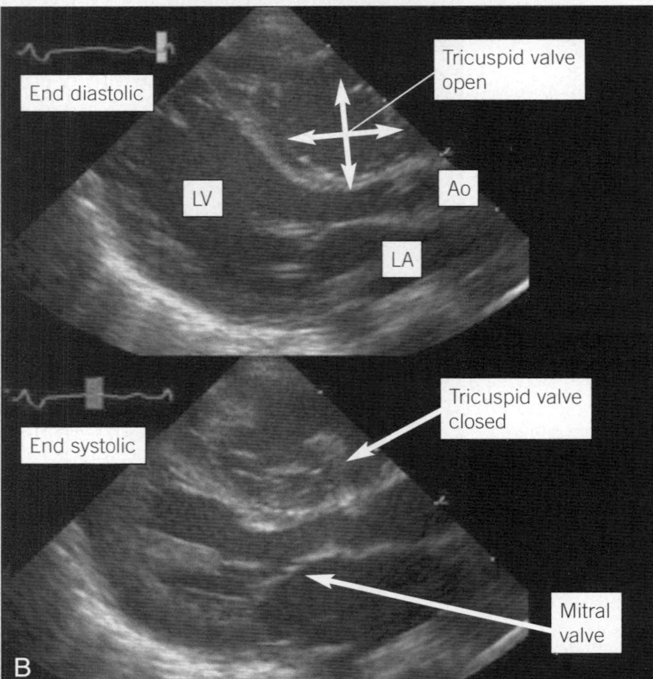

Figure 114.4 Echocardiography. A, Echocardiogram of the same newborn as in figure 114-3D. The apical four-camber view shows downward displacement of the septal leaflet of the tricuspid valve. Note that the mitral and the tricuspid valves have obviously different levels of their attachments. Color Doppler shows severe tricuspid regurgitation starting away from the right atrioventricular junction illustrated by a broad blue and least turbulent jet. **B,** In the same newborn, the left ventricular outflow tract has bulging of the ventricular septum, although no obvious obstruction is seen, related to the abnormally oriented orifice of the tricuspid valve and the atrialized portion of the right ventricle. Note that the normal tricuspid valve never appears in the long-axis view like this. LV, left ventricle; RV, right ventricle; RA, right atrium; LA, left atrium; Ao, aorta.

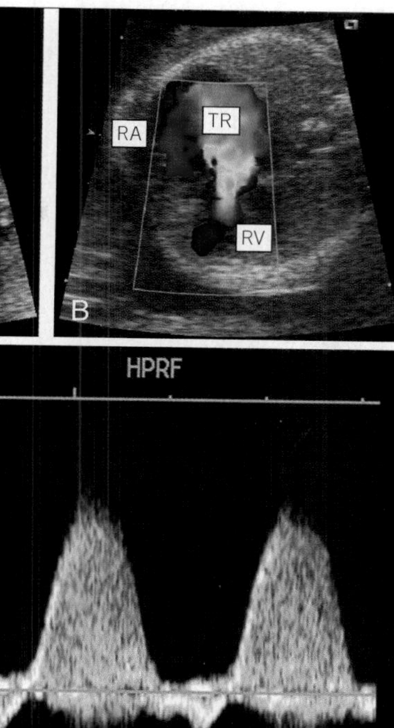

Figure 114.5 Echocardiogram in a fetus with Ebstein malformation at 27 weeks of gestation. The fetus died in utero several weeks later. **A,** Marked right atrial enlargement is seen together with tricuspid valve dysplasia and displacement. **B,** Color flow Doppler demonstrates severe tricuspid valve regurgitation shown as a broad orange jet. **C,** A pulsed-wave Doppler tracing of the tricuspid regurgitation jet illustrates pan-systolic regurgitation. LV, left ventricle; RV, right ventricle; RA, right atrium; TR, tricuspid regurgitation. (Courtesy of Dr. H. Gardiner and Dr. H. Matsui, Queen Charlotte Hospital, London, UK.)

Magnetic Resonance Imaging

Magnetic resonance imaging (Fig. 114.6), especially cine-MRI, is a useful adjunctive modality for noninvasive imaging.[22] Its three-dimensional information can equal or even surpass the quality of information gained from echocardiography. Not only morphologic features, but also functional and dynamic conditions can be evaluated through ECG-gated animation, volumetry and flow-velocity mapping. Also, orientation of the heart structures become clear in relation to the thoracic wall and the respiratory system. Current limitations of this modality remain in resolution, particularly for small structures in infants, and it cannot be performed in patients with implanted pacemakers. In small babies, anesthetic management may add another concern. Ultrafast computed tomography can also provide three-dimensional and real-time images similar to MRI, its downside being radiation.

Hemodynamics and Angiocardiography

Given the usefulness of echocardiography and MRI in the diagnosis of Ebstein malformation, cardiac catheterization now tends to be reserved for those patients who are not responding to therapy as expected or who have associated lesions in need of better definition. When it is considered that the diseased heart may not be suitable for biventricular repair, pulmonary arterial morphology and pulmonary arterial physiology (pulmonary resistance, pulmonary arterial pressure) should be investigated. In such patients, superior bidirectional cavopulmonary anastomosis may be employed to partially bypass the right heart.

In most patients with Ebstein malformation, the right atrial pressure is moderately elevated, with a dominant v wave and a steep y descent. However, if the right atrium is markedly dilated, the right atrial pressure may be normal despite severe tricuspid insufficiency. The right ventricular pressure is usually normal, but if the tricuspid valve orifice is severely displaced and stenotic, it may be very difficult to advance the catheter into the right ventricle and pulmonary artery. Patients who have severe tricuspid insufficiency may have an elevated right ventricular end-diastolic pressure. Pulmonary artery pressure is normal or decreased. Left atrial and left ventricular pressures are usually normal. In patients who have an atrial septal defect, oximetry may demonstrate systemic arterial desaturation.

An additional characteristic feature of Ebstein malformation is the demonstration of the atrialized portion of the right ventricle by use of an end-hole catheter that allows simultaneous recording of intracardiac electrocardiograms. On pullback of the catheter from the right ventricle, the intracardiac electrocardiogram demonstrates continued right ventricular electrical potentials after the pressure tracing has changed from a ventricular to an atrial contour. This technique for diagnosis of Ebstein malformation is of historic interest but is rarely used today.

The first case of Ebstein malformation reported in a living person was diagnosed with angiocardiography.[23] The right ventriculogram is usually diagnostic, demonstrating tricuspid insufficiency with a distinct notch on the anteroposterior view at the inferior cardiac border to the left of the spine. The notch represents the abnormal attachment of the displaced anterior tricuspid leaflet. A trilobed appearance may result from the enlarged right atrium, the atrialized ventricle, and the outflow portion of the functional ventricle. In the presence of moderate to severe tricuspid insufficiency, contrast material will remain in the right side of the heart through several cardiac cycles. In neonates, contrast material may fail to enter the pulmonary artery because of anatomic or functional pulmonary valve atresia. Functional pulmonary atresia is provided when pulmonary vascular resistance is elevated and the right ventricular systolic pressure cannot exceed that of the pulmonary artery. In such cases, the patent arterial duct exclusively supplies flow to the lungs.

Electrophysiology

Electrophysiologic evaluation is indicated in those patients who have Ebstein malformation and associated tachyarrhythmias. Some have recommended that all Ebstein patients who are scheduled for surgical repair undergo preoperative electrophysiologic testing to minimize the possibility of postoperative arrhythmia and sudden death.[24] One of the common dysrhythmias associated with Ebstein malformation is supraventricular tachycardia secondary to Wolff-Parkinson-White syndrome. According to the American College of Cardiology/American Heart Association Task Force report,[25] definite indications for electrophysiologic testing in patients with Wolff-Parkinson-White syndrome include consideration for nonpharmacologic

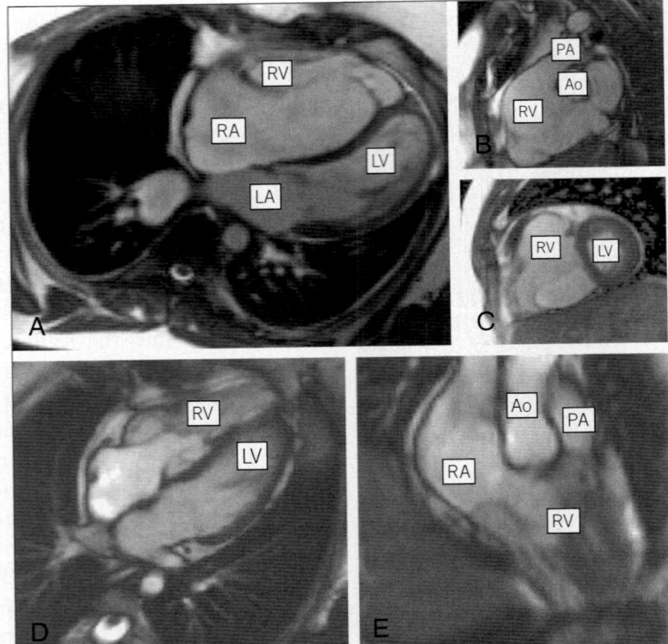

Figure 114.6 Magnetic resonance imaging. MRI is a very helpful modality for imaging of Ebstein malformation. **A,** Displaced attachment of the septal leaflet of the tricuspid valve. **B,** Right ventricular outflow tract, which has been dilated for functional compensation in this 31-year-old patient, can be seen vividly. **C,** In this patient, the ventricular septum does not possess a thin and atrialized wall despite the marked downward displacement of the septal leaflet of the tricuspid valve and moderate deformity of the left ventricular cavity. **D,** In another patient, MRI performed 18 months after surgery illustrates good repair of the tricuspid valve; the right ventricular end-diastolic volume is within a normal range. **E,** At the end-systolic phase, the tricuspid valve leaflets coapt nicely. There is only mild regurgitation as noted by flow mapping. LV, left ventricle; RV, right ventricle; RA, right atrium; LA, left atrium; PA, pulmonary trunk; Ao, ascending aorta. (Courtesy of Dr. P. Kilner, Royal Brompton Hospital, London, UK.)

treatment (ablation or antitachycardia pacing) because of life-threatening or incapacitating arrhythmias or drug intolerance. In patients with Ebstein malformation, accessory pathways are occasionally multiple and generally right-sided (either around the acute margin or near the crux of the heart). In rare occasions, they may be posteroseptal.[26] Electrophysiologic testing in Ebstein malformation can be challenging, and is therefore best performed by electrophysiologists with expertise in the evaluation of accessory pathways complicated by congenital heart disease.

In adult patients who have dilated right atrium and atrial tachyarrhythmia, electrophysiologic investigation followed by catheter ablation is one pertinent way to take. Often, one or more intra-atrial re-entry pathways are identified. Radiofrequency ablation at isthmuses is most often effective in such circumstances. Surgical ablation may be performed if a patient is already set to undergo surgery for tricuspid valve repair. Still, precise nature of atrial tachyarrhythmia should be electrophysiologically determined prior to surgery. In addition, a surgical incision to the right atrium should provide a new scar that could accommodate a re-entry circuit (the so-called incisional re-entrant). This can be minimized by prophylactic surgical ablation by creating a blocking line between the surgical right atriotomy and the wall of the inferior caval vein. When residual atrial arrhythmia is noted subsequent to surgery for tricuspid valve repair, further electrophysiologic investigation and catheter ablation should be pursued.

MANAGEMENT

Medical Management

In the presentation during the fetal period, patients should be monitored on a regular basis for the development of arrhythmias or effusions. Some fetal arrhythmias can be managed by maternal administration of antiarrhythmic agents, such as digoxin in the case of supraventricular tachycardia. Digoxin has also been administered to the mother to treat fetal hydrops.[27] Enlarging effusions and hydrops are poor prognostic signs and may be an indication for premature delivery after administration of steroids to maximize lung maturity.

For the full-term neonate who presents with cyanosis, treatment may be limited to careful observation, with improvement in the cyanosis as the pulmonary vascular resistance naturally diminishes. Prostaglandin E_1 may be indicated to maintain ductal patency to ensure adequate pulmonary blood flow until the pulmonary vascular resistance drops to a level that allows more anterograde flow from the right ventricle. Alternatively, inhaled nitric oxide therapy has been used to decrease pulmonary vascular resistance directly in the critically ill neonate, much as it is used for persistent pulmonary hypertension of the newborn.[28] If congestive heart failure is the predominant symptom, the infant may require inotropic support and diuresis.

Beyond the infantile period, in the mildest forms of Ebstein malformation, the only therapeutic intervention necessary is routine prophylaxis against bacterial endocarditis.

Arrhythmias can occur with or without the presence of Wolff-Parkinson-White syndrome, and they tend to be less well tolerated than in patients who have a structurally normal heart. Treatment is directed toward delaying conduction through the atrioventricular node or the bypass tract. However, antiarrhythmic agents can compromise cardiac output and may not be tolerated in patients who have moderate to severe Ebstein malformation. In patients whose arrhythmias cannot be managed medically or who are scheduled to undergo cardiac surgery, radiofrequency ablation should be considered. If an accessory pathway is not eliminated before or at the time of surgery, the patient runs the risk for development of supraventricular tachycardia in the immediate postoperative period, which may not be well tolerated. Atrial tachyarrhythmia unrelated to an accessory pathway is common in older patients. Prolonged hemodynamic impediments since birth make the right atrium dilated and its wall histologically damaged. Complex re-entrant circuits are likely to be formed, and atrial fibrillation, once it begins to sustain, should in turn promote histologic change of the atrial wall. On occasion, patients with Ebstein malformation will require implantation of a permanent pacemaker for atrioventricular block or sinus node dysfunction.[29]

Surgery

The surgical management of patients who have Ebstein malformation has evolved dramatically during the past 50 years. In the 1950s, pulmonary blood flow was augmented through placement of a systemic-to-pulmonary shunt, such as a Waterston or Blalock-Taussig shunt. Alternatively, pulmonary blood flow was established with creation of a superior cavopulmonary anastomosis (the Glenn shunt). The first reports of attempted tricuspid valve repair appeared in 1958, successful tricuspid valve replacement was reported in 1962, and successful valve repair was described in 1969.

Surgery is generally recommended for[30]

- patients who are in New York Heart Association (NYHA) class III or class IV;
- patients who are in NYHA class I or class II but who have a cardiothoracic ratio of 0.65 or more;
- patients who have significant cyanosis (arterial oxygen saturation of 80% or less) and polycythemia (hemoglobin concentration of 16 g/dL or more);
- patients who have experienced a paradoxical embolus; and
- patients who have supraventricular or atrial tachycardia.

If it is technically possible, repair rather than replacement of the tricuspid valve is generally preferred, with closure of the atrial septal defect under cardiopulmonary bypass. A technique conventionally used is attributed to Hardy[31] or Danielson[32] and consists of plastic reconstruction of the tricuspid valve to produce a competent monocusp valve from the large anterior leaflet. The atrialized portion of the right ventricle is horizontally plicated, and the redundant right atrial free wall may be excised. This classic technique of horizontal plication was described as the Hunter-Lillehei-Hardy method. Alternatively, Carpentier reported a technique of vertical plication of the atrialized ventricle and the tricuspid annulus together with sliding of the annular attachment of the anterior leaflet.[33] Orientation of plication is at a right angle to the conventional fashion, and reduction of the annular circumference is eminent in the plication maneuver. Some surgeons described that restoration of the shape, and therefore probably performance, of the right ventricle was better in the vertical plication. A prosthetic ring is sometimes used to remodel and to reinforce the tricuspid annulus. Artificial chordae tendineae[34] and pericardial patch augmentation of the anterior leaflet[35] have also been used to facilitate tricuspid valve repair. Any associated defects, such as an atrial septal defect or pulmonary stenosis, are addressed.

Plication of the atrialized ventricle may not be a fundamental issue. There are surgeons who focus solely on creation of a competent tricuspid valve.[36] Their opinion that preservation of the atrialized portion is preferable after reimplantation of the tricuspid leaflets onto the “true” atrioventricular junction appears to be based on the assumption that the atrialized ventricle will regain its wall thickness and strength when normal pressure load is imposed.[37] A modification proposed by Marianeschi and colleagues[38] consists of a bidirectional superior cavopulmonary anastomosis and intracardiac repair, with tricuspid valvuloplasty if indicated. Reduction of right ventricular preload alone may reduce the degree of tricuspid regurgitation and eliminate the need for tricuspid valve intervention. Additional experience with this technique has been reported by the team at Hospital Broussais.[39] When the right ventricular structure and function are too pessimistic to cope with, even half of the systemic flow, total right-sided heart bypass, the Fontan-type procedure, or total cavopulmonary connection, could be worth considering.

In approximately 20% to 35% of patients who present for surgery, the anatomy of the tricuspid valve precludes repair, and valve replacement is necessary. In such cases, the native valve tissue is usually excised. Because of frequent abnormality in subvalvular structures, preservation of the tension apparatus for better postoperative ventricular function, as employed in mitral valve replacement, is not an easy matter. The replacement valve can be either a mechanical or biologic prosthesis. Bioprostheses in the tricuspid position tend to be more durable than in other cardiac valve positions.[40] Placement of a homograft at the tricuspid position may be applicable, and there are reports supporting its use.[41] Whether the valve is repaired or replaced, the perioperative mortality is in the range of 5% to 15%. After surgery, the majority of patients experience marked improvement in their clinical status (Fig. 114.7), with approximately 90% improving to NYHA class I or class II. There remains a risk of late death, usually secondary to rhythm disturbances.[42]

In an extreme spectrum of Ebstein malformation in neonates, an alternative surgical approach was proposed by Starnes and colleagues.[43] This is the procedure that converts the complicated cardiac situation from Ebstein malformation to tricuspid atresia. Such neonates who demonstrate significant cyanosis with severe tricuspid insufficiency, massively dilated right atrium, and functional pulmonary atresia have a mortality as high as 75%. The goals of the procedure are to establish a reliable source of pulmonary blood flow, to reduce the massive cardiomegaly, and to abolish the ineffective and harmful right side of the heart, thereby creating a bridge toward a further definitive procedure or transplantation. The technique includes enlargement of an atrial septal defect, closure of the tricuspid valve, plication of the enlarged right atrium, and construction of a systemic-to-pulmonary

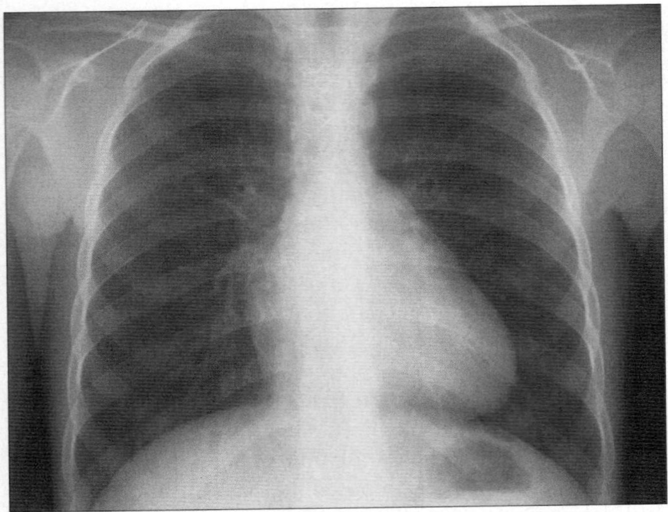

Figure 114.7 Chest radiograph after tricuspid valve repair and atrial septal defect closure. This is the same patient as shown in Figure 114.3. Note the significant reduction in heart size.

shunt. For a patient to survive the procedure, the most significant obstacle is usually very impaired pulmonary function associated with obvious hypoplasia of the lungs. Subsequently, the patients undergo the bidirectional Glenn procedure followed by the Fontan procedure or transplantation if they are not candidates for the univentricular physiology. More recently, aggressive and early biventricular repair has been advocated for the critically ill neonate with Ebstein malformation, although the number of patients addressed in this way is limited thus far.[44]

Transplantation has also been used to treat Ebstein malformation, both in infants and in older patients.[45,46] However, the number of patients with Ebstein malformation who have been treated with transplantation remains so small at this time that meaningful conclusions about its usefulness have yet to be made. Furthermore, the shortage of suitable donors may preclude its use, especially in infants. When the lungs are considerably hypoplastic, heart and lung transplantation may be needed.

Accessory conduction pathways in patients who have Ebstein malformation can also be surgically ablated, with excellent results.[47,48] Paroxysmal or chronic atrial fibrillation or flutter due to right atrial dilatation in Ebstein malformation can be surgically treated with creation of blocking lines for the right-sided atrium[49] or even with the full maze procedure, in which multiple incisions or ablations are made to the atrium to interrupt the re-entrant circuits. In addition, Chauvaud and associates[50] have demonstrated that tricuspid valve repair alone may abolish accessory pathways and reestablish sinus rhythm in a significant proportion of patients.

PROGNOSIS

The natural history of Ebstein malformation is variable, which is consistent with the varying degrees of severity of the tricuspid valve abnormalities and associated clinical findings. In general, the earlier a patient presents, the poorer the prognosis. Fetal and neonatal presentation is typically associated with a dismal outcome, but the outlook has improved. Presentation in older children and adults is usually associated with much better outcome. The oldest reported presentation was a 79-year-old man with congestive heart failure.[51] He was managed medically until his death 1 month before his 85th birthday. Regardless of the age at diagnosis, Attie and coworkers[52] found in unrepaired adults with Ebstein malformation, 25 years of age or older, an estimated cumulative overall survival of 89% at 1 year, 76% at 10 years, 53% at 15 years, and 41% at 20 years of follow-up. There was a clear correlation between severity of disease and mortality.

Celermajer and associates[53] have devised an echocardiographic grading system for the severity of Ebstein malformation that calculates the ratio of the combined area of the right atrium and atrialized right ventricle to that of the functional right ventricle, left atrium, and left ventricle in the four-chamber view at end-diastole. Grade 1 is defined as a ratio of less than 0.5, grade 2 as a ratio of 0.5 to 0.99, grade 3 as a ratio of 1.0 to 1.49, and grade 4 as a ratio of 1.5 or more. When the echocardiographic grade is treated as a continuous variable, each incremental grade is associated with a relative risk of 2.7. In their review of 46 cyanotic newborns with Ebstein malformation, Yetman and colleagues[54] found a ratio of greater than 1.0 to be 100% predictive of mortality. This index may be less useful for predicting fetal outcome.[55]

For patients with Ebstein malformation who survive to childbearing age, pregnancy (even in patients who have had surgery) is usually well tolerated, and the fetal outcome is good.[56,57] The rates of cesarean section and assisted delivery are comparable to those in the general population. However, cyanotic women have a higher incidence of premature labor and infants that are small for gestational age. The incidence of congenital heart disease in the offspring of male or female patients with Ebstein malformation has ranged from 0% to 6%. A multidisciplinary team of obstetricians, cardiologists, and obstetric anesthesiologists should monitor pregnant patients with Ebstein malformation. Care must be taken to avoid rapid fluid shifts during parturition and to monitor closely for venous thrombosis, which increases the risk of paradoxical embolism in patients who have an atrial septal defect or patent foramen ovale.

SUMMARY

Ebstein malformation describes apical displacement of the tricuspid valve but says little about the broad variability in the anatomy, clinical presentation, and management. Although patients may live long, healthy lives, the prognosis is poorest for those who are diagnosed in utero or in infancy and for those who have congestive heart failure, marked cyanosis, cardiothoracic ratio of 0.65 or more, or associated cardiac abnormalities. Mildly affected patients (those in NYHA class I or class II) can be managed medically. More severely affected patients may require surgical intervention. In the current era, two-dimensional echocardiography and magnetic resonance imaging are the diagnostic tools of choice, playing a great role in delineation of the anatomy. Patients who survive to adulthood and are asymptomatic can usually anticipate healthy pregnancies and healthy offspring.

chapter

115 Pulmonary Stenosis

Teiji Akagi

Definition

- Pulmonary stenosis can be classified as valvular, subvalvular, supravalvular, or involving the pulmonary trunk and peripheral pulmonary arterial branches. Obstruction of this right ventricular outflow at the pulmonary valve level accounts for about 10% of all cases of congenital heart disease.

Key Features

- In valvular stenosis, the pulmonary valve is thickened and has fused or absent commissures and a small orifice.
- Most patients are asymptomatic, a notable exception being infants with critical pulmonary stenosis.
- Dysplastic valves are frequently seen with Noonan's syndrome.
- Peripheral pulmonary arterial stenosis is usually associated with cardiac malformations, such as tetralogy of Fallot, and occasionally seen with Williams syndrome.

Therapy

- Balloon valvuloplasty is recommended for moderate to severe valvular pulmonary stenosis when transpulmonary peak Doppler resting gradients consistently exceed 50 mm Hg and there is corresponding right ventricular hypertrophy. Other types of right ventricular outflow obstruction with significant stenosis will require surgery.

Pulmonary stenosis can be classified as valvular, subvalvular, supravalvular, or involving the pulmonary trunk and peripheral pulmonary arterial branches. It occurs most frequently at the valvular level. These obstructive lesions of the right ventricle and pulmonary arterial tree, whether isolated or in association with other congenital heart defects, occur in 25% to 30% of all patients with congenital heart disease.[1]

Obstruction at the pulmonary valve level accounts for about 10% of all cases of congenital heart disease. There is considerable evidence that the etiology of this lesion has a genetic basis, with a number of early reports establishing recurrence rates for siblings between 2.1% and 4%.[2] Some reports have documented several families with a number of members who have pulmonary stenosis. Pulmonary stenosis is also a recognized component of several inherited syndromes, such as trisomy 18 and deletion of chromosome 22q11. In Noonan's syndrome, which may have an autosomal dominant pattern of inheritance, the pulmonary valve is frequently dysplastic.

Primary infundibular (subvalvular) stenosis with an intact ventricular septum is a rare malformation, and it may in reality represent part of the spectrum of double-chambered right ventricle. The prevalence of this entity is reported to vary from 2% to 10% of all cases of obstructive lesions to the right ventricular outflow tract.[1]

Pulmonary arterial stenosis may develop anywhere along the pulmonary arterial tree. The stenosis may be unilateral or bilateral and single or multiple. It is often associated with cardiac malformations, such as tetralogy of Fallot, transposition of the great arteries, pulmonary valve stenosis, persistent ductus arteriosus, ventricular septal defect, or other complex malformations. In Williams syndrome, characterized primarily by supravalvular aortic stenosis, multiple stenoses of the peripheral pulmonary artery are often observed. Peripheral pulmonary artery stenosis is also associated with Noonan's syndrome, Alagille syndrome, cutis laxa, and Ehlers-Danlos syndrome.

ANATOMY AND PATHOLOGY

Valvular pulmonary stenosis, the most common form of pulmonary stenosis, is almost always congenital in origin. In the classic severe form of valvular pulmonary stenosis, the pulmonary valve is conical or dome shaped and is formed by fusion of the valve leaflets. A bicuspid valve has been reported to occur in 20% of cases of pulmonary stenosis that underwent autopsy.[1] Although most patients with valvular pulmonary stenosis have some degree of valve thickening, a small portion (10% to 15%) of patients have been shown to have exceptionally thick leaflets, so-called dysplastic valves (Figs. 115.1 and 115.2).[3] The obstruction is caused by markedly thickened, immobile cusps composed of disorganized myxomatous tissue. The annulus of the valve is usually narrowed. Dysplastic pulmonary valves frequently occur in a familiar pattern and are seen in the majority of patients with Noonan's syndrome.

Secondary changes resulting from valvular pulmonary stenosis can occur in the pulmonary arteries and right ventricle. The right ventricle shows severe hypertrophy, with the chamber appearing smaller than normal. This hypertrophy is particularly noticeable in the infundibular region, producing dynamic narrowing of the outflow tract of the right ventricle. The pulmonary artery trunk almost always shows poststenotic dilatation, and the circumference of the trunk frequently exceeds that of the aorta. The only exception to this occurs in patients with dysplastic valves. The mechanism by which dilatation occurs is probably related to the high-velocity jet of blood that is ejected through the small valve orifice.

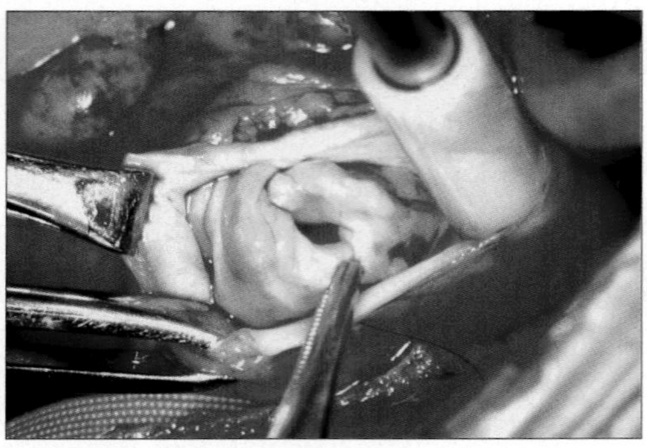

Figure 115.1 Dysplastic pulmonary valve in a patient with Noonan's syndrome. The valve is thickened and irregular.

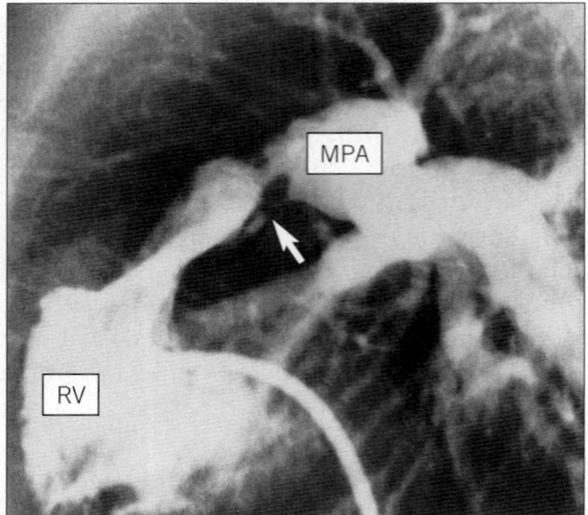

Figure 115.2 Lateral projection of right ventriculography in a patient with dysplastic pulmonary valve. The thickened pulmonary valve appears to fill the small annulus with tissue *(arrow)*. Poststenotic dilatation extends into the pulmonary distal diverticulum. Peripheral pulmonary arteries are within the normal size range. RV, right ventricle; MPA, main pulmonary artery.

Pulmonary arterial stenoses have been classified into four types[1]:

- stenoses involving the main pulmonary trunk or the right or left branches;
- stenoses involving the bifurcation of the pulmonary artery extending into both branches;
- multiple peripheral stenoses; and
- a combination of main and peripheral stenoses.

In approximately 67% of cases, the affected area is at the junction of the main and branch pulmonary arteries. When the stenosis is localized, there is usually dilatation of the vessel distal to the narrowing. On pathologic examination, there is fragmentation of media elastic tissue and intimal proliferation, with a variable degree of replacement of the media by fibrous tissue. The intimal proliferation is responsible for the reduction in the size of the lumen.

PATHOPHYSIOLOGY

The hemodynamic consequences depend on the severity of outflow obstruction.[1] This obstruction leads to an increase in right ventricular pressure, which is proportional to the degree of obstruction. Grading of the severity of the hemodynamic consequences of pulmonary stenosis, based on peak systolic pressure gradients on Doppler echocardiography, is as follows:

- trivial: less than 25 mm Hg;
- mild: 25 to 49 mm Hg;
- moderate: 50 to 79 mm Hg; and
- severe: more than 80 mm Hg.

In mild or moderate degrees of pulmonary stenosis, the hypertrophic right ventricle is able to maintain normal output with minimal or no effect on the fetal pattern of circulation. However, in severe stenosis, right ventricular output may decrease, and the pattern of circulation in the fetus may resemble that of pulmonary atresia, although the right ventricular chamber is unquestionably larger than that seen in pulmonary atresia.

During fetal life, valve stenosis stimulates right ventricular chamber hypertrophy and, in severe obstruction, results in marked reduction in the size of the right ventricular cavity. Cardiac output is maintained by an increased right ventricular pressure. In severe stenosis, the developmentally immature myocardium may not be adequate to achieve the required pressure, resulting in reduced cardiac output.[4] In some neonates, the stenosis may be of such severity as to restrict pulmonary blood flow, necessitating the continued postnatal patency of the ductus arteriosus to allow an adequate pulmonary blood flow. In this setting, central cyanosis is usually present as a result of a right-to-left shunt through the foramen ovale or an atrial septal defect. The right-to-left atrial shunting depends on the presence of a greater diastolic pressure in the right ventricle caused by the marked muscle hypertrophy and decreased compliance of the ventricle. Diminution in the size of the right ventricular cavity and in right ventricular compliance also explains the central cyanosis that is usually seen in the syndrome of pulmonary stenosis and hypoplastic right ventricle.[4]

Most patients have milder forms of obstruction and come to attention later, during the first months of life. Mild degrees of stenosis at this age tend not to worsen in severity because the valve orifice increases with age. Although right ventricular hypertrophy is present, function is not impaired, and growth and cardiac output are in the normal range. The foramen ovale may remain probe patent, but right-to-left shunting and cyanosis do not occur. In more moderate stenosis, the tendency is for increasing right ventricular pressures and hypertrophy, particularly within the first years of life, probably because of a failure of the diameter of the orifice to increase with body growth.[5] In dysplasia of the pulmonary valve, the orifice of the thickened, immobile valve rarely enlarges with body growth, and increasing obstruction is common.

In patients with infundibular (subvalvular) stenosis, the anomalous muscle bundles may not be obstructive at all, especially early in infancy, or they may cause varying degrees of obstruction within the right ventricle. During ventricular contraction, the diameter of the infundibular stenosis is markedly reduced, and sometimes the lumen of the channel adjacent to the septum may be completely obliterated. The hemodynamic consequence of the obstruction is an increased pressure within the proximal part of the right ventricle. Exercise or infusion of isoproterenol can demonstrate a markedly increased pressure gradient between the proximal and distal parts of the stenosis.

The hemodynamic features associated with peripheral pulmonary stenosis are similar to those of isolated valvular pulmonary stenosis. Depending on the degree of obstruction, there are mild to severe increases in systolic pressure in the right ventricular and pulmonary arteries (proximal to the stenosis). Because the obstruction is usually present in the central part of pulmonary arteries, the pulmonary trunk proximal to the obstruction usually has a limited volume capacity. When the obstruction is severe, right ventricular ejection is prolonged, and the pulmonary artery trunk (proximal to the stenosis) behaves like an extension of the right ventricular outflow tract.

CLINICAL PRESENTATIONS

The majority of patients who have valvular pulmonary stenosis are asymptomatic, and the condition is discovered only during a routine examination. When symptoms are present, they may vary from mild exertional dyspnea and mild cyanosis to signs and symptoms of heart failure. Most infants with typical pulmonary valve stenosis have a normal birth weight and physical appearance, a notable exception being those infants with critical pulmonary stenosis. The gestational history is usually unremarkable, and the family history is helpful only if other relations have been previously affected. In Noonan's syndrome, growth is retarded and children have typical facies and habits; however, these are difficult to identify during the neonatal period.

Auscultatory Findings

Auscultatory findings in this disease are distinctive. Diagnosis can usually be made without special laboratory techniques.

The systolic murmur of valvular pulmonary stenosis is an ejection-type systolic murmur, with maximal intensity at the upper left sternal border. The murmur is well conducted to the entire precordium, neck, and back.

The first heart sound is normal and must be distinguished from the pulmonary ejection click that occurs when the dome-shaped pulmonary valve reaches its fully open position. The intensity of the ejection click varies with ventilation, selectively decreasing during inspiration and increasing during expiration. This variation has been related to the position of the stenotic valve at the onset of ventricular contraction.

The second heart sound in pulmonary stenosis is usually split, and the degree of splitting is proportional to the degree of obstruction. The pulmonary component of the second heart sound may be normal or decreased in intensity, or it may be inaudible. With mild obstruction, splitting of the second sound is modestly increased; whereas with severe obstruction, the separation may be as great as 0.12 to 0.14 second. In severe valvular pulmonary stenosis, the split is virtually fixed because of a fixed right ventricular stroke volume. The delay in pulmonary valve closure is a useful index of the degree of obstruction, but there are shortcomings in estimating the severity of the stenosis on this basis. In addition to the splitting of the second heart sound, the intensity of the second sound is also important in estimating the severity. On occasion, in mild stenosis with marked dilatation of the pulmonary artery trunk, the pulmonary closure sound may be louder than normal. However, in the usual instance, the intensity of the pulmonary closure sound is inversely proportional to the severity of the obstruction.

A fourth heart sound is heard reasonably often at the lower left sternal border in patients who have severe pulmonary stenosis. It is associated with a large *a* wave in the right atrium and usually indicates severe stenosis. A presystolic murmur may be heard as an extension of a fourth sound; this is probably the result of some degree of tricuspid stenosis.

When a third heart sound is heard, the presence of either an associated atrial septal defect or anomalous pulmonary venous drainage should be suspected.

Early diastolic regurgitant murmurs are rare and result from distortion of the pulmonary valve ring or cusp by secondary complications, such as progressive stenotic dilatation of the pulmonary trunk, endocarditis, surgical valvotomy, or balloon valvuloplasty.

Relationship between Clinical Features and Severity of Stenosis

With mild pulmonary stenosis, the venous pressure and pulse are normal. The heart is not enlarged, the apical impulse is normal, and the right ventricle is not palpable. A relatively short pulmonary systolic ejection murmur is maximally audible over the pulmonary area. The murmur is usually preceded by a pulmonary ejection click, which is heard best at the left upper sternal border during expiration. The second heart sound is split, with a pulmonary element of normal intensity, which may be delayed.

In moderate stenosis, the venous pressure may be slightly increased, with an intrinsic *a* wave noted in the jugular pulse. A right ventricular sternal lift may be palpable. The systolic ejection murmur is prolonged later into systole, and a pulmonary ejection click may or may not be present. The second heart sound is split, with a delayed and diminished pulmonary component that may not be audible.

In severe stenosis, mild to moderate cyanosis may be noted if there is an interatrial communication. Hepatic enlargement and peripheral edema are observed in the presence of right ventricular failure. Increased venous pressure is common and is attributable to a large presystolic jugular *a* wave. The heart is moderately or greatly enlarged, and there is a conspicuous sternal and parasternal right ventricular lift that frequently extends to the midclavicular line. A loud systolic ejection murmur, frequently accompanied by a thrill, is maximally audible in the pulmonary area and may radiate widely over the entire precordium into the neck and to the back. The murmur has late systolic accentuation and frequently encompasses the aortic component of the second heart sound, but it is not preceded by an ejection sound. The pulmonary element of the second sound is usually inaudible.

In infants with critical pulmonary stenosis and heart failure, the regurgitant systolic murmur of tricuspid regurgitation is heard lower along the left sternal border. In infants, the single second sound (absence of a pulmonary closure sound), the associated cardiomegaly, and the presence of a pansystolic murmur of tricuspid regurgitation at the lower left sternal border are highly suggestive signs for the diagnosis of severe critical pulmonary stenosis.

If a dysplastic valve is present, the signs are atypical. An ejection click is uncommon, and the valve may be insufficient. Associated cardiac malformations may be present and dominate the clinical picture. Patients with Noonan's syndrome have characteristic facies with hypertelorism, an antimongoloid slant to the eyes, ptosis, maxillary hypoplasia, and webbed neck. Lymphedema is frequently seen, and both pulmonary and intestinal lymphangiectasia has been reported.

DIAGNOSTIC TECHNIQUES

Chest Radiography

The most significant feature of chest radiography in patients with pulmonary stenosis is a prominent main pulmonary artery segment caused by poststenotic dilatation of the pulmonary artery. The pulmonary trunk is sometimes aneurysmal and has been mistaken for a tumor. The greatest degree of poststenotic dilatation usually occurs with mild to moderate obstruction. In the frontal view, the pulmonary trunk is sometimes relatively inconspicuous, but this may be because of posterior projection of the dilatation. In cases of dysplastic pulmonary valve or congenital rubella syndrome with valvular or supravalvular stenosis, the pulmonary artery segment on the chest radiograph may not be prominent. In pulmonary valve stenosis, disproportionate enlargement of the left branch typically accompanies dilatation of the pulmonary trunk. Left pulmonary artery dilatation is occasionally conspicuous without evidence of enlargement of the pulmonary trunk on the plain film.

The physics of blood flow distal to the stenotic pulmonary valve sheds light on selective dilatation of the left pulmonary artery and unequal distribution of blood flow. The left pulmonary artery is a smooth continuation of the "dome" of the dilated pulmonary trunk. The jet from the stenotic valve breaks up as it strikes the dome of the left pulmonary artery. There is an accompanying increase in the pressure component of total energy and an increase in mean and peak systolic pressures in the left pulmonary artery. In about 50% of patients, a prominent right atrial segment can be seen on the chest film.

The pulmonary vasculature is usually normal, except in patients who have right ventricular failure or a right-to-left shunt at the atrial level, in whom a reduction of pulmonary vascular markings in seen as a result of reduction in pulmonary flow. In severe stenosis, the cardiothoracic ratio frequently exceeds 0.60, particularly in the presence of heart failure, tricuspid regurgitation, or atrial shunting.

Electrocardiography

In mild stenosis, the electrocardiogram is normal or characteristic of mild right ventricular hypertrophy. The only abnormality may be slight right axis deviation of the mean QRS frontal axis. Incomplete right bundle branch block is often seen in this group of patients.

In moderate pulmonary stenosis, a normal electrocardiogram is rare, occurring in less than 10% of patients. The QRS axis shows right axis deviation. Varying degrees of right ventricular hypertrophy, sometimes with a prominent spiked P wave, are seen.

In severe pulmonary stenosis, the electrocardiogram shows gross right ventricular hypertrophy, frequently accompanied by a tall, spiked P wave. The mean QRS axis may range from 110 to 160 degrees or more. A dominant R wave may be seen in lead aVR; and in the right precordial leads, a pure R, Rs, or QR pattern is usually present. In a child with severe pulmonary stenosis with hypoplasia of the right ventricle, the mean QRS axis is oriented more leftward than normal, with clear evidence of left ventricular hypertrophy. In addition, in spite of the presence of right ventricular hypertension, the anterior forces are not as prominent. Rarely, a superior axis may be present with valvular pulmonary stenosis. In these individuals, a conduction abnormality of the left bundle may be present, either in isolation or in association with Noonan's syndrome.

Echocardiography

Two-dimensional echocardiography with color-flow mapping and Doppler evaluation can provide important diagnostic information about

- the level of stenosis;
- the morphology of the valve mechanism; and
- the hemodynamic consequences of obstruction to right ventricular outflow.

The projections used to observe pulmonary valve morphology and right ventricular function are the standard and high parasternal short-axis views and the subcostal sagittal view. The thin, mobile valve becomes dome shaped during ejection, moving briskly as a single unit (Fig. 115.3). Poststenotic dilatation of the pulmonary trunk and disproportionate dilatation of the left branch can be visualized, and color-flow mapping demonstrates that the high-velocity jet is directed toward the left pulmonary artery.

In marked to severe pulmonary valve stenosis, the ventricular septum thickens together with the right ventricular free wall, and the interventricular septum appears flattened; it may move paradoxically. Color-flow mapping identifies the presence and degree of tricuspid regurgitation, and continuous-wave Doppler recording of the regurgitant jet provides an estimate of right ventricular systolic pressure. Doppler echocardiography can be also used to quantitate the pressure gradient across the stenotic pulmonary valve. For the calculation of

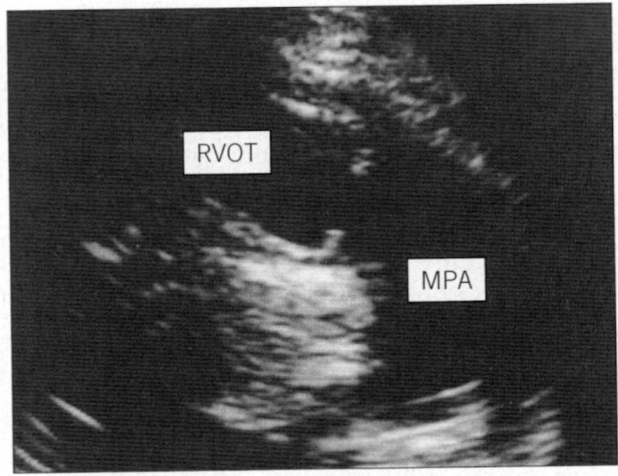

Figure 115.3 Typical appearance of valvular pulmonary stenosis on two-dimensional echocardiography. The dome-shaped valve can be seen. MPA, main pulmonary artery; RVOT, right ventricular outflow tract.

the pressure gradient, a simplified Bernoulli equation can be used:

$$P = 4V^2$$

where P is the peak instantaneous pressure gradient (in mm Hg) across the obstructed pulmonary valve and V is the peak flow velocity (in m/s) distal to the obstructive orifice.
In patients who have peripheral pulmonary arterial stenosis, hypertrophy of the right ventricular free wall can be detected by two-dimensional echocardiography and will suggest some increase in the right ventricular pressure. As the diastolic pressure in the pulmonary artery is low, the systolic time intervals of the right ventricle will be consistent with the low overall pulmonary vascular resistance. Two-dimensional echocardiography also demonstrates the main pulmonary artery and its proximal branches, in addition to the right ventricular cavity and pulmonary valves. Proximal stenosis up to the bifurcation and the origin of the left and right pulmonary artery branches may be visualized, but more distal stenoses are impossible to see. Doppler echocardiography can detect pressure gradients across stenoses in the main pulmonary trunk or its branches.

Cardiac Catheterization and Angiography

Two-dimensional echocardiography has made possible the noninvasive evaluation of a number of anatomic parameters, and with Doppler flow studies, physiologic issues can be addressed. However, in patients in whom there is a need for further definition of the right ventricular volume, level of obstruction, size of the pulmonary arteries, or possible associated lesions, angiography is required.[3] Importantly, if balloon valvuloplasty is considered for initial treatment, angiographic definition is mandatory. Pulmonary valve stenosis is best demonstrated with biplane right ventriculography, using the lateral plane with steep cranial angulation of the posteroanterior projection (Fig. 115.4). Left or right alignment of the posteroanterior projection can define the origins of the left or right pulmonary arteries.

The right ventricular cavity is usually normal in size and has prominent trabeculations. The right ventricular wall in severe stenosis is usually thickened. The thickness and size of the orifice of the pulmonary valve can be clearly seen as the jet of ejected opacified blood enters the dilated main pulmonary artery. The typical stenotic valve is slightly thickened and forms a dome shape during systole. In young children who have severe valvular pulmonary stenosis, the annulus is usually normal but moderately hypoplastic. Post-stenotic dilatation of the main pulmonary artery is usually observed; however, there is no correlation between the degree of pulmonary artery dilatation and the severity of the stenosis. In dysplastic pulmonary valve, leaflet mobility is severely restricted, and little movement is noted. Doming of the valves is not seen, and the jet of contrast medium through the valve is conspicuously absent. The annulus is frequently hypoplastic, the main pulmonary artery appears shortened, and poststenotic dilatation is not present. In patients who have Noonan's syndrome, levophase left ventriculography may outline asymmetric septal hypertrophy.

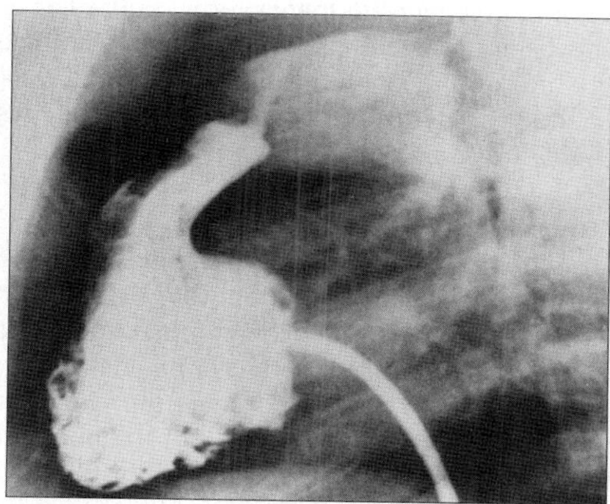

Figure 115.4 Typical appearance of valvular pulmonary stenosis on lateral projection right ventriculography. The outline of the right ventricle shows a well-formed tripartite chamber. The opacified jet can be seen leaving the hemodynamic orifice and abutting the dilated main pulmonary artery.

In patients with infundibular pulmonary stenosis, right ventriculography is the best tool for accurate diagnosis of the lesion. Biplane angiography should always be performed when evidence of a significant intraventricular pressure gradient has been found during cardiac catheterization. In the anterior projection, filling defects within the right ventricle, between the outflow and inflow areas, are observed. These filling defects are seen well below the crista supraventricularis. On the lateral projection, the right ventricular filling defects may extend from just below the crista to the anterior wall near the apex. The filling defects are constant and do not change with systole and diastole. The anterior view is the best angiographic view for the visualization of the anomalous muscle bundles.

In peripheral pulmonary stenosis, selective pulmonary angiography is the most valuable tool in the diagnosis. The exact location, extent, and distribution of the lesions can be easily visualized with this procedure. The right pulmonary artery stenosis and the multiple peripheral pulmonary artery stenoses are best seen in the anterior view, whereas stenosis involving the pulmonary trunk requires cranial angulation, and the origin of the left main branch can be well visualized in the hemiaxial oblique views. The main pulmonary trunk is usually normal or hypoplastic. In severe unilateral obstruction, a delayed filling of the respective pulmonary vein may be noted.

MANAGEMENT

Studies have revealed that individuals with mild pulmonary stenosis not requiring an operation and those who have had successful relief of moderate or severe stenosis can expect to enjoy a normal life span.[6] The chances that a child with a transpulmonary valve gradient less than 25 mm Hg will need balloon valvuloplasty (or valvotomy) are less than 5% during childhood and adolescence and virtually zero thereafter. For those with gradients of 25 to 49 mm Hg, there is an approximately 20% chance of needing some kind of procedure eventually. Most patients with gradients of 50 to 79 mm Hg will ultimately require treatment. Morbid events including ventricular arrhythmias and bacterial endocarditis rarely occur in patients with pulmonary stenosis, regardless of whether they are managed medically or surgically.

Thus, children with mild or moderate stenosis can lead a normal life, but their progress should be evaluated at regular intervals. Patients who have small transpulmonary valve gradients rarely show progression and do not need intervention, but children who have moderate stenosis are more likely to develop a more significant gradient as they grow. Worsening of obstruction may also be caused, in part, by the development of secondary subvalvular muscle and fibrous tissue hypertrophy.[1,3]

Percutaneous Balloon Valvuloplasty

Recently, experience with percutaneous balloon valvuloplasty in older infants and in children with valvular pulmonary stenosis has led to this procedure's replacing surgical intervention.[7-9] The technique of balloon valvuloplasty is relatively straightforward. The balloon catheter is advanced over an exchange guide wire that has been positioned in the left or right pulmonary artery. The balloon diameter should be at least 10% to 20% larger than the pulmonary valve annulus; if the annulus diameter is more than 20 mm, it is usually necessary to use two angioplasty balloon catheters simultaneously (Fig. 115.5). Previous studies reporting the morphologic effects of balloon valvuloplasty have described commissure splitting and tearing of the cusp. Other complications related to this procedure, such as perforation of the right ventricular outflow tract or tricuspid insufficiency, are very rare.

The immediate results of pulmonary balloon valvuloplasty have been excellent. However, in children who have a dysplastic pulmonary valve, balloon valvuloplasty has not been uniformly successful. When pulmonary stenosis is caused by a dysplastic pulmonary valve, narrowing of the valve annulus is usually present. In these patients, simple surgical valvotomy or balloon valvuloplasty does not usually relieve the pressure gradient. Removal of the thickened valve tissue and enlargement of the annulus and proximal main pulmonary artery by insertion of a patch are needed to relieve the obstruction.

The use of valvuloplasty has been extended to treatment of infants or neonates with critical pulmonary stenosis.[10-12] Infants with critical pulmonary stenosis may not tolerate the prolonged presence of a catheter across the valve because of further restriction of the functional valve area.

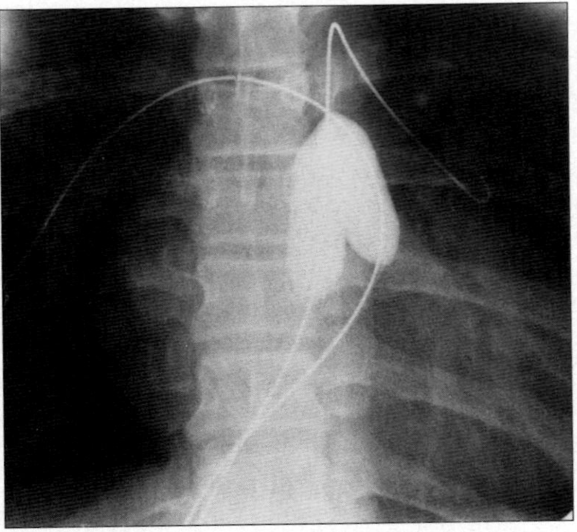

Figure 115.5 Balloon valvuloplasty of valvular pulmonary stenosis by the double-balloon technique.

In patients with systemic right ventricular pressure, the initial right ventriculography should be performed before the pulmonary valve is crossed. If the patient's condition deteriorates when the valve has been crossed, the catheter is removed without a pressure gradient measurement being made, and only the exchange wire is left in place. In these patients, a relatively small balloon is frequently used for the initial dilatation, followed by an oversized balloon for definitive dilatations (Fig. 115.6).

Two major factors make the use of balloon valvuloplasty difficult in the neonate[1]:

- the inability to position the balloon catheter across the critically narrowed pulmonary valve; and
- the frequent coexistence of pulmonary annular hypoplasia and tricuspid stenosis.

In particular, it can be difficult to cross the valve both because of the small, hypertrophied right ventricle and because of the pinhole opening in the valve. To cross the valve, a 3 or 4 French Judkins right-type catheter is usually used, rather than a balloon-tipped end-hole catheter. The catheter is manipulated to the right ventricular outflow tract. If it does not cross the valve directly, a torque-control guide wire is used to assist the technique; failure to cross the valve is then rare.

Complications after neonatal valvuloplasty have included retroperitoneal hematoma, iliofemoral venous occlusion, injury to the tricuspid valve or its chordae, rupture or perforation of the right ventricular infundibulum, and death.[13]

The long-term outcome of patients who have undergone pulmonary balloon valvuloplasty appears to be excellent,[14-20] and no serious long-term complications have been observed after this procedure. Figure 115.7 depicts the long-term follow-up measurements of the pressure gradient between right ventricle and main pulmonary artery, as evaluated by Doppler echocardiography. A significant decline in pressure gradient was observed during the first year after valvuloplasty, mainly reflecting the regression of the hypertrophied right ventricular infundibular muscle. Premature ventricular contractions are frequently observed in most patients during the procedure; however, no longer term ventricular or atrial ectopy has been reported. Pulmonary valve insufficiency is frequently present after the valvuloplasty, but long-term follow-up studies have reported that it does not cause any significant clinical problems.

Surgical Treatment

In patients who have subvalvular (infundibular) stenosis, surgical treatment is essential. When the right ventricle is opened through a transverse or longitudinal ventriculotomy, the obstructing muscle mass becomes immediately apparent and may completely or partially obscure the view of the tricuspid valve. Transection of the origin of the muscle bundle from the septum and parietal attachments of the superficial bundle is performed first. This permits reflection of the muscle mass so that injury to the anterior papillary muscle of the tricuspid valve can be avoided. A search for a ventricular septal defect should be carried out because of the frequent association of these two lesions.

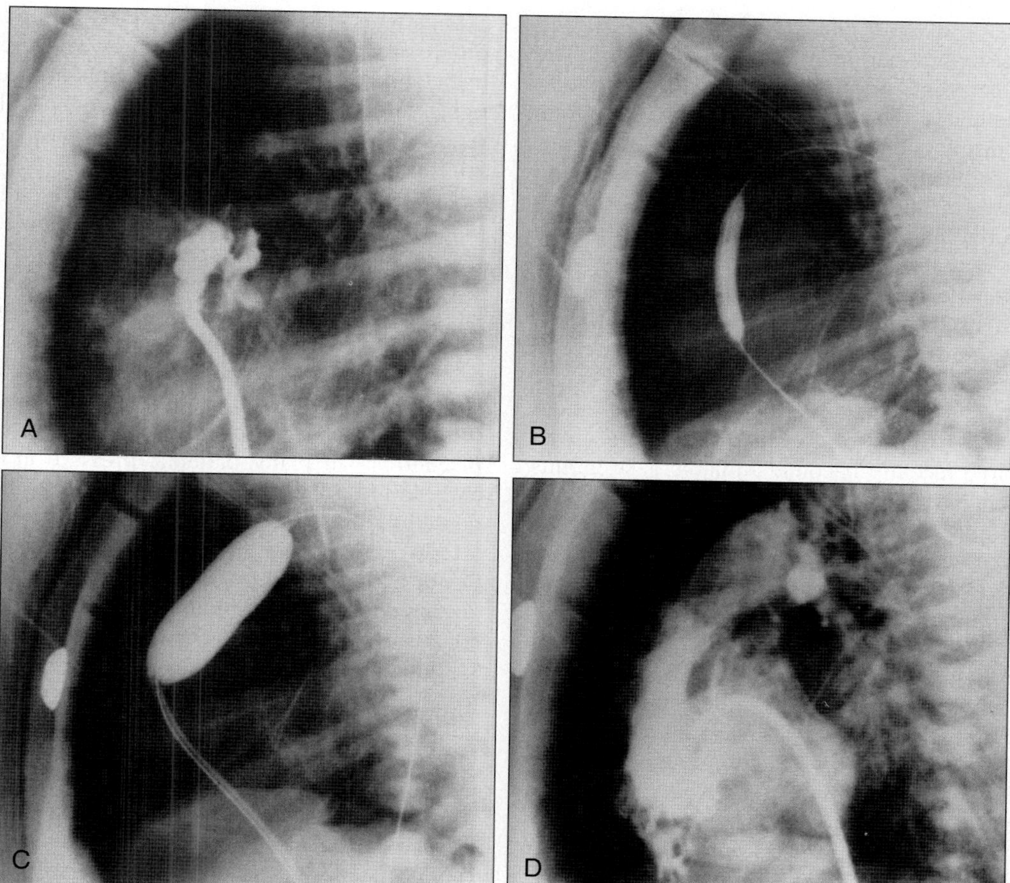

Figure 115.6 Critical pulmonary stenosis in a neonate. A, Lateral projection of right ventriculography before balloon valvuloplasty. A tiny jet of contrast material across the pinhole opening of the stenotic pulmonary valve can be seen. **B**, Initial balloon dilatation with use of a 3-mm coronary angioplasty balloon. The guide wire has crossed the ductus arteriosus and is in place in the distal descending aorta. **C**, Subsequent balloon dilatation was performed with an 8-mm balloon. **D**, Lateral projection of right ventriculography after the balloon valvuloplasty. Good anterograde blood flow from right ventricle to pulmonary artery can be observed.

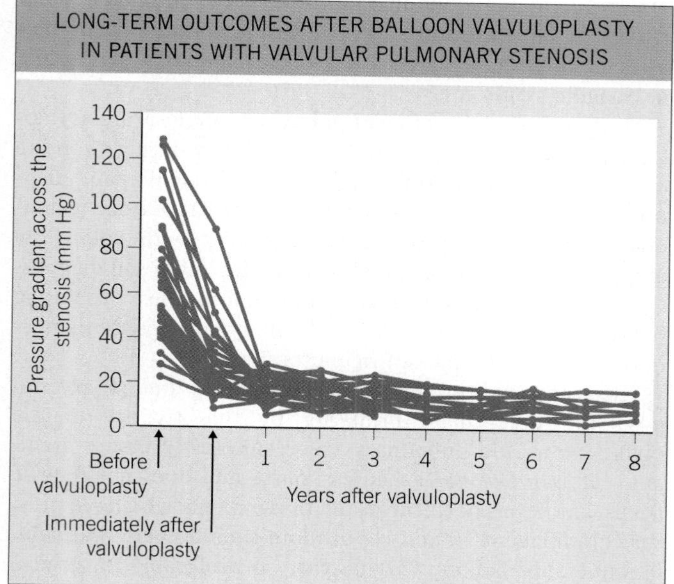

Figure 115.7 Long-term outcomes after balloon valvuloplasty in patients with valvular pulmonary stenosis. The transpulmonary pressure gradient declines significantly during the first year after the valvuloplasty, and the effect persists thereafter. (Data from the Department of Pediatrics, Kurume University, Japan.)

High-Pressure Balloon Dilatation

Because surgery produces inadequate results in patients with peripheral pulmonary stenosis, dilatation with use of a high-pressure balloon has been attempted for this lesion.[21,22] It has been reported that balloon dilatation provides significant hemodynamic relief to some patients who had peripheral pulmonary stenosis and in whom traditional operative management had usually failed.[21] The major causes of failure of dilatation include inadequate technique (e.g., balloon too small, inability to position the balloon or guide wire) and the refractory nature of the lesion itself. Nondilatable lesions appear to be more common in children older than 2 years or who have isolated pulmonary artery stenosis. Stenoses near previous systemic-to-pulmonary artery shunts and stenoses associated with the arterial-switch repair of complete transposition of the great arteries also tend to be nondilatable. Isolated lesions associated with syndromes such as Williams syndrome have been particularly resistant to balloon dilatation.

Balloon-Expandable Intravascular Stent

The efficacy of the balloon-expandable intravascular stent in the treatment of pulmonary stenosis has been investigated during the past 10 years.[23,24] The technique used for stent implantation consists of positioning a long 8 to 12 French sheath across the stenotic peripheral pulmonary artery. The balloon-expandable stent, which is mounted on a balloon angioplasty catheter, is then advanced through the long sheath into the distal pulmonary artery. After the angioplasty catheter has been positioned across the stenosis, the sheath is withdrawn off the proximal end of the angioplasty catheter and into the main pulmonary artery or right ventricle. The balloon is then inflated to a pressure of 6 to 14 atmospheres. After the stent has been positioned, the angioplasty catheter is exchanged for an angiographic catheter, and postdilatation angiography and hemodynamic assessments are performed (Fig. 115.8).

In addition to the conventional stainless steel stent (Palmaz stent), other types of stent, manufactured from new materials, have recently become available.[25] In infants or small children in particular, these new types of stent offer certain technical and therapeutic benefits because of their flexibility and relatively easy deployment.

Clinical experience with stents is increasing, and studies indicate that intravascular stenting may become the preferred treatment of individuals with refractory peripheral pulmonary stenosis.[26]

In patients in whom the angioplasty catheter or stent cannot be advanced across the stenotic lesion at the time of cardiac catheterization, intraoperative balloon angioplasty and stent implantation have been reported to be successful.[27] Restenosis of an implanted stent may develop within a few months to several years after the procedure, especially in small infants or children. The major reason for this phenomenon is intimal proliferation or external compression from related structures. It can be possible to undertake repeated dilatation of restenosis without serious complications; however, further investigation of these repeated interventions is required to clarify their true effectiveness.[28]

PROGNOSIS

The course and prognosis of patients who have valvular pulmonary stenosis are determined primarily by the severity of the obstruction. Mild pulmonary valve stenosis has a benign course and does not require treatment. However, there is still controversy about the course and prognosis of asymptomatic patients with moderate pulmonary stenosis. With the advent of pulmonary balloon valvuloplasty, most centers would now recommend valvuloplasty for all patients who have moderate or severe pulmonary stenosis, regardless of age. The Second Natural History Study of Congenital Heart Defects, which addressed the largest reported series of patients with valvular pulmonary stenosis,[29] revealed that patients in whom the transvalvular pressure gradient is less than 25 mm Hg do not experience an increase in gradient. Most patients with gradients of less than 50 mm Hg were treated medically, and those with gradients greater than 80 mm Hg were treated surgically. Less than 20% of patients treated medically during the First Natural History Study subsequently required a valvotomy (Fig. 115.9).[27] Only 4% of surgical patients required a second operation. It has been suggested that patients with gradients of 50 mm Hg or more should undergo valvotomy or valvuloplasty.

In patients who have subpulmonary (infundibular) stenosis, progressive obstruction of anomalous muscle bundles has been observed. Long-term follow-up of double-chambered right ventricle has demonstrated only mild residua and sequelae, and serious cardiac compromise has been infrequent.

The natural history of the lesions in patients who have peripheral pulmonary stenosis is not well documented.[1] The prognosis is related to the severity of the obstruction and should be more or less similar to that of valvular stenosis. However, in multiple peripheral pulmonary stenoses of severe degree, the prognosis is probably similar to that of primary pulmonary hypertension, unless angioplasty or stent placement is successful. Progressive increases in the degree of obstruction of peripheral pulmonary arteries may occur. In contrast, in many patients, pressure gradients recorded early in life disappear with growth. Poststenotic aneurysmal dilatation of the small elastic arteries may be complicated by arteritis, thrombosis, or pulmonary artery hemorrhage. Death early in infancy or later in life has been reported to occur with severe peripheral pulmonary artery stenosis; the condition is apparently very rare in late adult life.

SUMMARY

Pulmonary stenosis can be classified as valvular, subvalvular, supravalvular, or involving the pulmonary trunk and peripheral pulmonary arterial branches. Valvular pulmonary stenosis is the most common form. In the classic form of valvular stenosis, the pulmonary valve is conical or dome shaped and is formed by fusion of valve leaflets. Dysplastic pulmonary valves are frequently present in Noonan's syndrome. Primary subvalvular stenosis with an intact ventricular septum is a rare malformation and may in reality represent part of the spectrum of double-chambered right ventricle. Pulmonary arterial stenosis may develop anywhere along the pulmonary arterial tree; it may be unilateral or bilateral and single or multiple, and it is usually associated with Williams syndrome, Noonan's syndrome, or Alagille syndrome.

Most patients with valvular pulmonary stenosis are asymptomatic, and the condition is discovered only during a routine examination. Auscultatory findings are distinctive, and diagnosis can usually be made without special laboratory techniques. Two-dimensional echocardiography with color-flow mapping and Doppler evaluation provides important diagnostic information about the level of the stenosis, the morphology of the valve mechanism, and the hemodynamic consequences of obstruction to right ventricular outflow.

The course and prognosis of patients with pulmonary stenosis are determined primarily by the severity of the obstruction. Mild pulmonary valve stenosis (pressure gradient <50 mm Hg) has a benign course and does not require treatment. It has been suggested that patients who have pressure gradients of 50 mm Hg or more should have treatment. Percutaneous balloon valvuloplasty is preferable to surgical valvotomy for patients with valvular stenosis. Even in infants who have critical pulmonary stenosis, balloon valvuloplasty may be performed; if this is unsuccessful, surgery is usually needed.

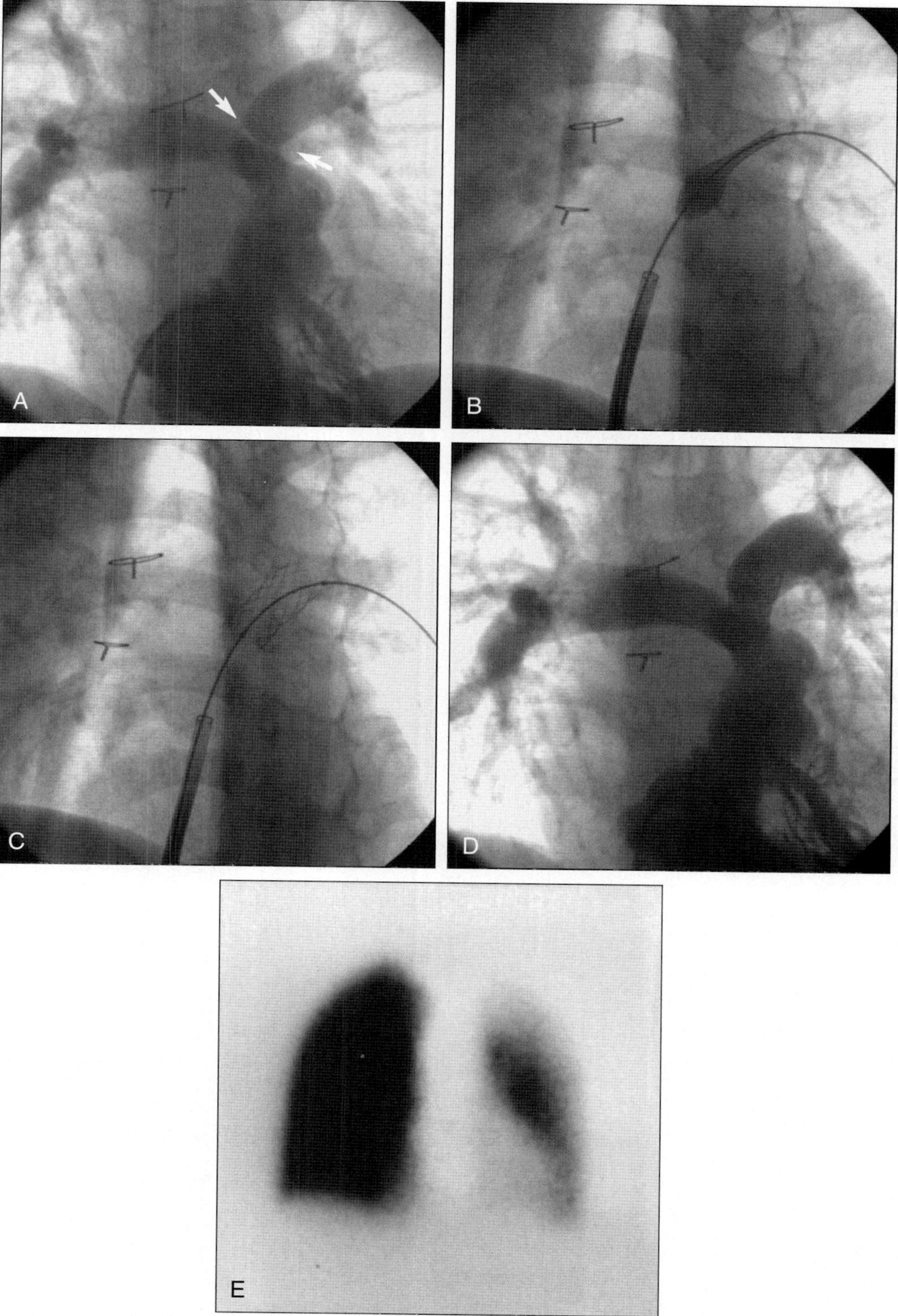

Figure 115.8 Implantation of a balloon-expandable intravascular stent. A, Cranially tilted frontal projection showing right pulmonary artery stenosis in a postoperative patient with pulmonary atresia and ventricular septal defect. **B,** The balloon-expandable intravascular stent is dilated with a high-pressure balloon. **C,** The stent fully dilated. **D,** After implantation of the stent, right ventriculography demonstrates that the pulmonary artery is dilated completely. **E,** Lung perfusion scan before implantation of the stent. After implantation of the stent, blood flow to the left lung is significantly increased.

The long-term outcome of patients who have undergone pulmonary balloon valvuloplasty appears to be excellent, and significant decline in the pressure gradient is observed during the first year after the valvuloplasty. Other types of obstruction with significant pressure gradients required surgery. If the surgical results of peripheral pulmonary stenosis are inadequate, implantation of a balloon-expandable intravascular stent by use of a high-pressure balloon should be attempted.

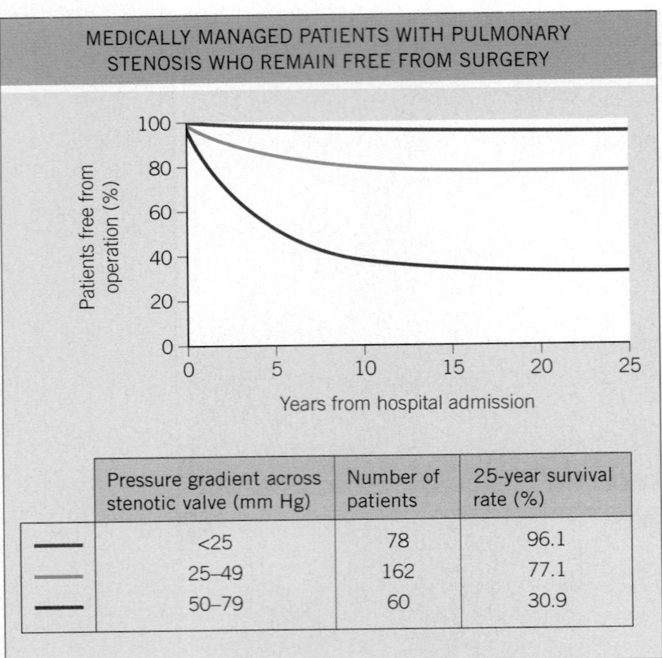

	Pressure gradient across stenotic valve (mm Hg)	Number of patients	25-year survival rate (%)
—	<25	78	96.1
—	25–49	162	77.1
—	50–79	60	30.9

Figure 115.9 Kaplan-Meier curves of percentage free from surgery for pulmonary stenosis patients who were managed medically. (With permission from Hayes CJ, Gersony WM, Driscoll DJ, et al. Second Natural History Study of Congenital Heart Defects: results of treatment of patients with pulmonary stenosis. Circulation 1993;87:I28-I37.)

chapter 116

Pulmonary Atresia with Intact Ventricular Septum

Frank Coshey Smith

Definition

- Pulmonary atresia with intact ventricular septum is a relatively rare congenital heart defect consisting of complete obstruction of right ventricular outflow in the absence of a ventricular septal defect.

Key Features

- A heterogeneous spectrum of abnormalities is defined by degrees of right ventricular hypoplasia, tricuspid valve hypoplasia, and coronary artery abnormalities.

Therapy

- Treatments vary from simple pulmonary valvotomy to cardiac transplantation, depending on the severity of the lesion.

Pulmonary atresia with intact ventricular septum (PA-IVS) is not one diagnosis but many. Its many forms require diverse treatments that result in diverse prognoses. For example, PA-IVS that involves only an imperforate pulmonary valvular membrane with a normal-sized right ventricle is, in effect, a diagnosis different from PA-IVS with extreme right ventricular hypoplasia and right ventricle–dependent coronary circulation. The former case requires only surgical or catheter-directed pulmonary valvotomy, yielding an excellent prognosis with a biventricular physiology. The latter case may require at least three surgical procedures, yielding a more guarded prognosis with a single ventricular physiology.

PA-IVS is not only heterogeneous but rare. It represents only 1% to 3% of all significant congenital heart disease,[1] and its estimated incidence is 4.5 to 4.8 per 100,000 live births.[2,3] Single-center research on its many variants is hampered by small cohort sizes. Multicenter studies are hindered by differing diagnostic and treatment approaches among the participating centers. The rarity and diversity of PA-IVS have contributed to its poor prognosis in the past relative to other cardiac defects. During the past 15 years, the prognosis has improved because investigators around the world, whose work serves as the foundation of this chapter, have raised our understanding of the heterogeneity of this lesion.

Unlike conotruncal anomalies such as pulmonary atresia *with* ventricular septal defect, PA-IVS has no particular association with chromosomal anomalies such as the 22q11 microdeletion, although 1.3% of patients in one large series had trisomy 21.[4] Rare familial cases of PA-IVS have been reported.[5]

ANATOMY AND PATHOLOGY

Although the anatomy and pathology are more complicated than its name suggests, PA-IVS primarily denotes atresia of the pulmonary valve and an intact ventricular septum. The atresia may be either membranous (an imperforate valvular membrane at the pulmonary valvular annulus) or muscular (involving severe stenosis or absence of the right ventricular infundibulum and an absent or thickened fibrous shelf at the level of the pulmonary valvular annulus).[6] PA-IVS also implies the presence of some degree of tricuspid valve inflow. Lesions with both pulmonic and tricuspid valve atresia are categorized as extreme forms of tricuspid atresia.

The heterogeneity of PA-IVS is mainly attributable to varying degrees of right ventricle and tricuspid valve hypoplasia in utero, and this can be better understood after considering the embryology of the lesion. Unlike pulmonary atresia with ventricular septal defect, the PA-IVS is presumed to occur in utero after septation of the ventricles. In early gestation, it is presumed that the pulmonary valve is severely stenotic but not atretic. The anterograde flow permitted through the right side of the heart and across the pulmonary valve encourages right-sided heart growth to some degree until complete atresia occurs later in gestation. If right ventricular outflow obstruction is relatively severe and the atresia of the pulmonary valve occurs early, then there is less prenatal anterograde flow through the right side of the heart, and the right ventricular and tricuspid valve hypoplasia is severe. If the right ventricular outflow obstruction is less severe and atresia of the pulmonary valve occurs relatively late in utero, right-sided heart structures are less hypoplastic.

Right ventricular hypoplasia to some degree is almost always associated with PA-IVS, and it involves any or all of the three parts of the morphologic right ventricle (Fig. 116.1):

- the tricuspid valve inlet;
- the body or trabecular portion; and
- the outlet or infundibulum.

By definition, the right ventricle in all cases of PA-IVS includes a tricuspid inlet of detectable size, but many cases lack one or both of the other component parts. In one large case series, the right ventricle was unipartite in 7.7%, bipartite in 33.6%, and tripartite in 58.7% of the patients.[3] The extent of the hypoplasia helps define the severity of the lesion and has been used to classify its variants (see later).

Hypoplasia of the right ventricle usually involves all of its components, including the tricuspid inlet, and it is not

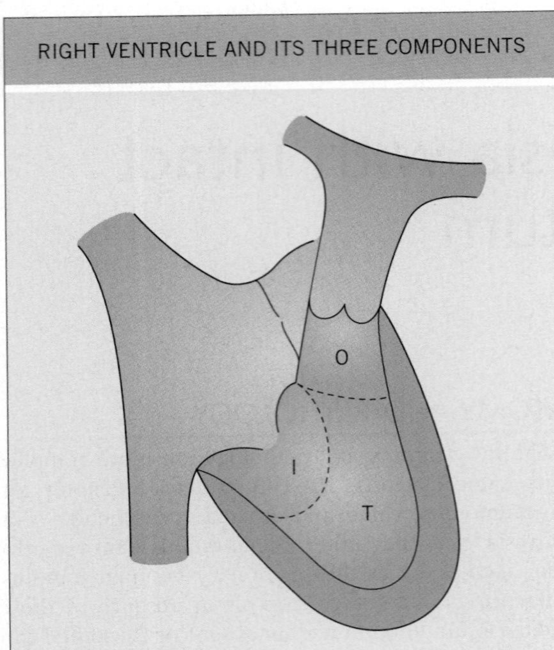

Figure 116.1 Simple diagram of the right ventricle and its three components. I, tricuspid inlet; T, body or trabecula; O, infundibulum or outlet.

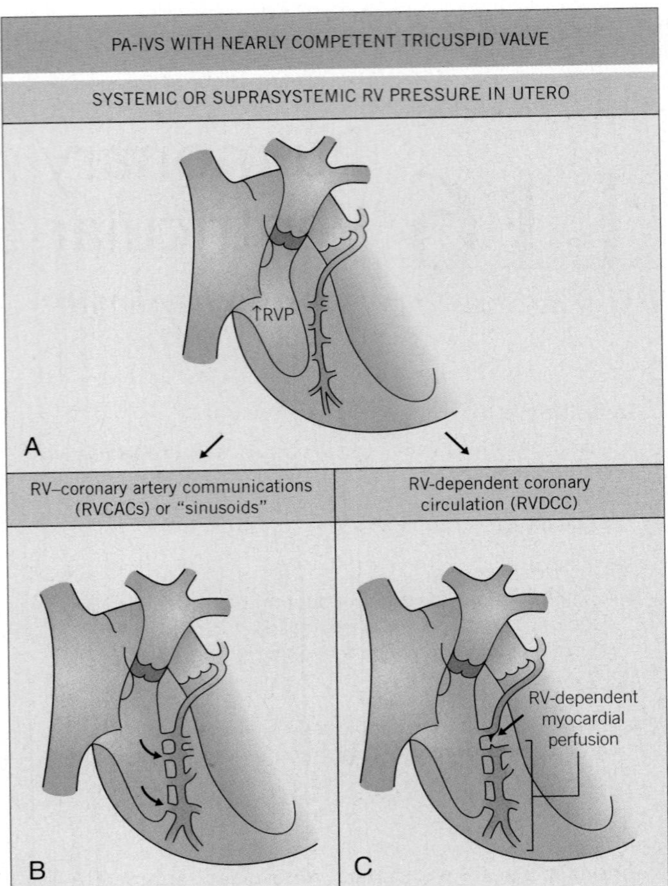

Figure 116.2 PA-IVS with nearly competent tricuspid valve. **A**, Diagrammatic representation. Right ventricular pressure (RVP) is usually systemic or suprasystemic. **B**, Right ventricular hypertension may lead to the development of coronary sinusoids that communicate with branches of the left anterior descending coronary artery (as in this diagram) or with the right coronary artery. **C**, Abnormal sinusoidal-coronary connections may lead to coronary artery stenosis or atresia *(arrow)* of the left anterior descending coronary artery (or right coronary artery). The coronary artery segment distal to the obstruction is perfused only by the right ventricle sinusoids (right ventricle–dependent coronary circulation).

surprising that tricuspid valve disease is observed in most cases of PA-IVS. There is good correlation between the degree of tricuspid valve hypoplasia and right ventricular hypoplasia.[6,7] The hypoplasia may involve the valve annulus, the valve leaflets, and their chordal attachments. In 4% to 10% of cases, the tricuspid valve is dysplastic or there is Ebstein malformation of the tricuspid valve.[3,6,8,9] These are often associated with severe tricuspid valve incompetence, right atrial enlargement, and dysplasia and thinning of the right ventricle free wall.

The pulmonary artery and its branches are relatively well developed in PA-IVS in comparison to pulmonary atresia with ventricular septal defect, presumably because antero-grade flow in the pulmonary arteries in early gestation in PA-IVS promotes growth of branch arteries.[6]

Coronary artery disease has become increasingly understood as a major complicating feature of PA-IVS, and this has led to refined surgical treatments with improved outcomes. Complete obstruction of pulmonary outflow in utero in the presence of a competent tricuspid valve leads to severe, suprasystemic right ventricular hypertension. This promotes the development of sinusoids within the right ventricular endocardium that form fistulous communications with the coronary artery branches to the right or left ventricle. Blood within the right ventricle can then decompress during systole through the coronary arterial system (Fig. 116.2). These abnormal vascular connections may be associated with coronary arterial and venous wall thickening with secondary myofiber disarray, myocardial fibrosis, and necrosis.[10] The most significant coronary artery change is stenosis or atresia of portions of the right coronary or left anterior descending coronary arteries. In these cases, the coronary artery branches that are distal to the obstruction are supplied only by the right ventricle or sinusoidal communications rather than by the proximal coronary arteries arising from the aortic root. As long as right ventricular pressure remains increased, these right ventricle–dependent coronary branches remain perfused. In contrast, surgical decompression of the right ventricle in these patients drastically reduces perfusion of the right ventricle–dependent coronary branches, leading to ventricular ischemia, hypokinesis, and death in many cases.[11]

These coronary artery abnormalities can be differentiated according to the presence of coronary artery stenosis or atresia:

- right ventricular sinusoids with fistulous communications to the coronary artery system are referred to as right ventricular fistulas or right ventricle–coronary artery connections (RVCACs) when the native coronary arteries are not stenotic or atretic.
- When coronary artery stenosis or atresia is present, those distal coronary branches that are exclusively perfused by the right ventricle are designated right ventricle–dependent coronary circulation (RVDCC).

In one series of 131 infants with PA-IVS, 54.2% had normal coronaries and 45.8% had minor or major fistula; 7.6% of all cases had RVDCC.[3] In another series, RVDCC occurred in at least 9% of the patients.[6]

Other cardiac lesions have rarely been associated with PA-IVS. These include

- primary left ventricular disease (hypertrophy, dysfunction)[12];
- mitral valve abnormalities (thickened chordal attachments)[13];
- unroofed coronary sinus;
- aortic stenosis;[8] and
- right aortic arch (3%).[3]

Major aortopulmonary collateral circulation is relatively rare in PA-IVS compared with pulmonary atresia with ventricular septal defect.[1]

Classification

PA-IVS has evaded simple classification, and this has contributed to the difficulty in analysis and comparison of treatment outcomes. PA-IVS was first classified anatomically by Greenwold and colleagues[14] in 1956 on the basis of the presence of either hypoplasia or enlargement of the right ventricle. In 1982, Bull and coworkers[7] proposed a refined classification based on the degree of right ventricular hypoplasia and, specifically, on the presence or absence of each of the three components of the right ventricle.[7] In 1993, Giglia and coworkers[11] proposed that disease severity and management be differentiated by the presence or absence of RVDCC.[11] I have attempted to combine these features into a classification in this chapter that will be useful for further discussion of management (Table 116.1).

PATHOPHYSIOLOGY

The most important pathophysiologic feature of clinical importance is complete obstruction of the pulmonary valve and absence of anterograde pulmonary flow. All newborns with PA-IVS thus depend on flow from the aorta through a patent ductus arteriosus or, in rare cases, by major aortopulmonary collaterals to portions of either lung. Because right ventricular outflow is completely obstructed, there is cyanosis as a result of obligatory right-to-left shunting across the patent foramen ovale or atrial septal defect. In most cases, the atrial communication is unrestrictive in the neonatal period. The right ventricular systolic pressure is usually systemic or suprasystemic. Right atrial pressure may be increased, depending on the degree of tricuspid incompetence. When a significant stenosis of both right and left coronary arteries is present, there may be evidence of ischemia, with left ventricular strain, hypokinesis, and increased left ventricular end-diastolic pressure.

PA-IVS with Ebstein malformation or tricuspid valve dysplasia is usually associated with severe tricuspid incompetence, right atrial enlargement, and hypertension, both prenatally and after birth. Severe cardiomegaly in utero can lead to compression of lung parenchyma, with secondary pulmonary hypoplasia and postnatal respiratory failure that severely complicates cardiac management and may render the child inoperable.

The term *functional pulmonary atresia* refers to a syndrome in which the right ventricle cannot generate sufficient pressure to open a pulmonic valve that is anatomically normal. This condition is usually associated with severe tricuspid incompetence or significantly increased pulmonary vascular resistance. In this syndrome, the pulmonary valve can be crossed by a venous catheter. Color Doppler echocardiography (or aortography through left-to-right ductal shunting) may demonstrate pulmonary valve incompetence, proving that the valve is not imperforate. Functional pulmonary atresia may resolve if pulmonary vascular resistance decreases or if tricuspid incompetence improves sufficiently to permit right ventricular outflow.

CLINICAL PRESENTATIONS

The earliest possible clinical presentation is the prenatal referral to the pediatric or fetal echocardiographer because of an abnormal four-chamber screening view on a general obstetric sonogram. Cases detected during routine obstetric imaging are more likely to have severe cardiomegaly that is often associated with tricuspid valve dysplasia or Ebstein malformation, severe tricuspid incompetence, pulmonary hypoplasia, and poor prognosis.[5,15] In one large survey in England between 1991 and 1995, there were 86 cases diagnosed prenatally, and 61% of these pregnancies were terminated.[3] In a more recent series in 2006 in the United States, fewer terminations (28%) were performed. In this study, the tricuspid valve size measured in utero was helpful in predicting tricuspid valve and right ventricle size after birth. Those fetuses with tricuspid valve sizes with a Z score lower than −3 and those with poor tricuspid valve growth during gestation required a univentricular surgical approach.[16] Prenatal diagnosis of PA-IVS may lead to a planned delivery in a tertiary center where postnatal medical and surgical management can be optimized. In selected cases, in utero balloon valve dilatation has been performed.[17]

The most common postnatal presentation of PA-IVS is severe cyanosis in the first 3 days of life. Pulmonary blood flow is duct dependent, and gradual ductal closure during the first days of life leads to restriction of pulmonary blood flow and progressive cyanosis. There is an obligatory right-to-left shunt at the atrial level. For this reason, the cyanosis is not differential (i.e., preductal and postductal oxygen saturations are the same), and it is not relieved by supplemental oxygen. As with other cyanotic congenital heart lesions, there is usually no significant history of prenatal maternal illness, premature delivery, birth asphyxia, low Apgar scores, or aspiration syndromes. The cardiac examination typically reveals a normal or a mildly increased left ventricular impulse with a single second heart sound. There may be a soft continuous or systolic murmur at the upper left sternal border, reflecting the obligatory left-to-right shunt at the ductal level, but this is not always appreciated. If tricuspid insufficiency is significant, there is a lower pitched regurgitant systolic murmur at the lower left and right sternal edges, and the precordium will be diffusely active. Hepatomegaly is usually not present unless significant tricuspid insufficiency is present. Peripheral pulses are usually normal, except when there is severe tricuspid incompetence or significant left ventricular hypokinesis related to coronary artery abnormalities.

CLASSIFICATION OF PULMONARY ATRESIA WITH INTACT VENTRICULAR SEPTUM		
Type 1	Nearly normal RV and tricuspid valve size	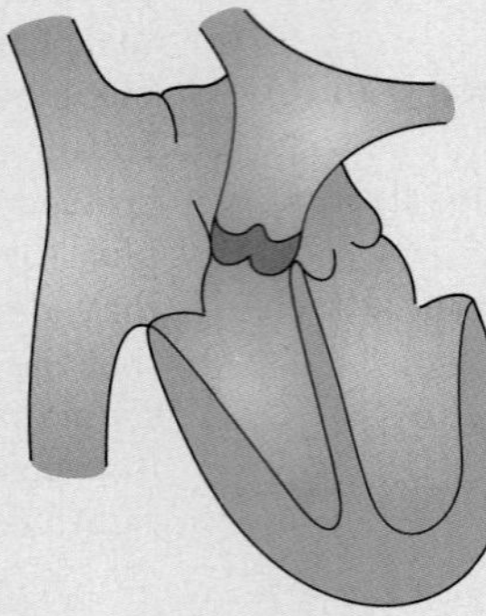
Type 2	Mild to moderate RV and tricuspid valve hypoplasia (no RVDCC)	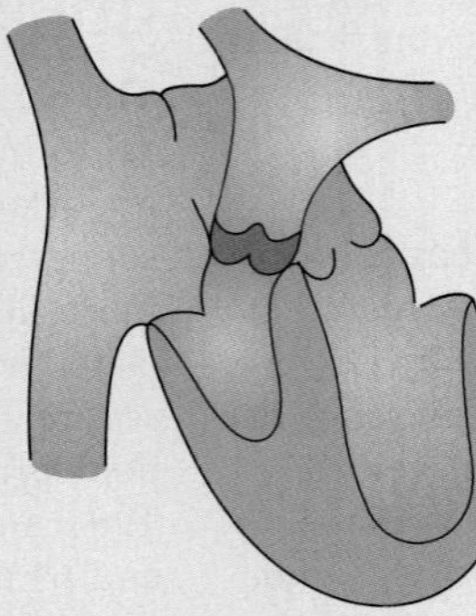
Type 3	Severe RV and tricuspid valve hypoplasia or RVDCC	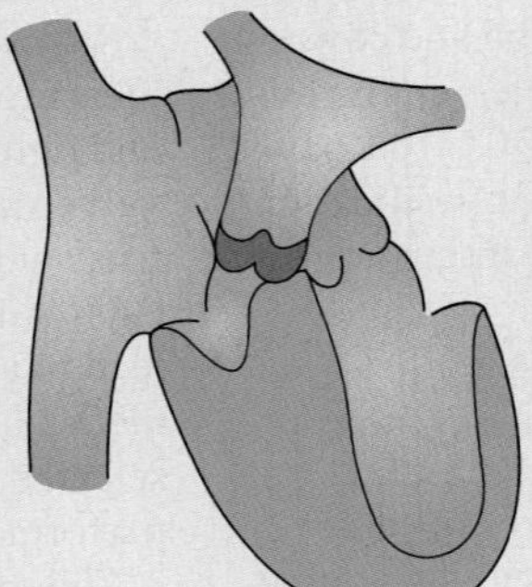 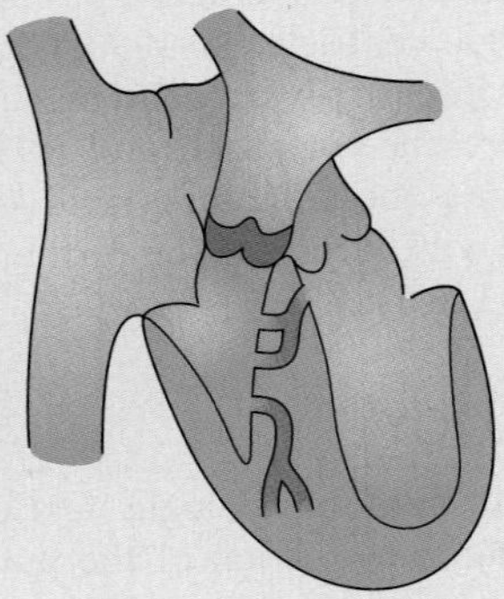
Type 4	RV enlargement and tricuspid valve dysplasia/ Ebstein malformation	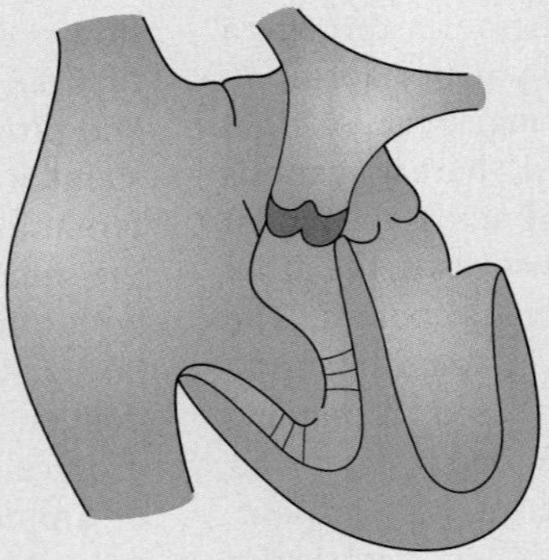
RV, right ventricle; RVDCC, right ventricle–dependent coronary circulation.		

Table 116.1 Classification of pulmonary atresia with intact ventricular septum.

DIAGNOSTIC TECHNIQUES

When congenital heart disease is suspected in a cyanotic infant, echocardiography and consultation with a pediatric cardiologist should be arranged as soon as possible. In most cases, chest radiography will be part of the initial evaluation to exclude pulmonary causes of the cyanosis and to assess the size and shape of the heart. The most characteristic radiographic finding of PA-IVS is diminished pulmonary vascular markings (Fig. 116.3). The cardiac size is usually normal.

The left upper portion of the cardiac silhouette may lack the density associated with the main pulmonary artery segment. If significant tricuspid incompetence is present, there will be cardiomegaly with an enlarged right atrial shadow (Fig. 116.4). In extreme cases, the anteroposterior projection of the heart fills the entire thorax. Other pulmonary causes of cyanosis (e.g., pneumothorax, effusion, infiltrate) should also be excluded.

The electrocardiogram may be normal, but it may provide clues as to the presence of congenital heart disease and the particular diagnosis of PA-IVS. Peaked P waves reflect right atrial enlargement (especially when severe tricuspid incompetence is present). Diminished or absent R-wave voltage in the right leads and diminished S-wave voltage in the left leads reflect severe right ventricular hypoplasia (Fig. 116.5). Left axis deviation may be present in cases of PA-IVS with extreme right ventricular hypoplasia, as with tricuspid atresia. ST-segment and T-wave changes indicating ventricular ischemia may reflect coronary artery abnormalities.

Two-dimensional color Doppler echocardiography is essential in identifying the many features of PA-IVS: the right ventricle–pulmonary artery connection, the degree of right ventricular and tricuspid valve hypoplasia, the source of pulmonary blood flow, the patent foramen ovale, and the suggestive evidence of right ventricular coronary sinusoids or RVDCC. Parasternal short-axis and long-axis views reveal either a relatively thin, atretic pulmonary valvular membrane or a thicker, more muscular ridge at the pulmonary valve annulus, with varying degrees of diffuse infundibular hypoplasia (Figs. 116.6 to 116.8). In the most severe cases, there is virtual interruption between the right ventricular infundibulum and the main pulmonary artery. In patients with a distinct pulmonary valvular membrane, the pulmonary valve annulus can be measured from modified long-axis views of the right ventricular outflow tract. This measurement is particularly helpful if catheter-directed valvotomy alone is considered. Color Doppler echocardiography fails to demonstrate a significant defect or shunt at the ventricular level. The right ventricular anatomy can be defined as tripartite, or not, and the size of the right ventricle may vary from normal to severely hypoplastic. Exact estimation of the volume of the right ventricle is difficult because of its small size and irregular shape, but an estimate can be taken by digitizing the right ventricular area from two orthogonal planes. Assessment of right ventricular size is helpful in selecting appropriate treatment. In one study, for instance, patients with a right ventricular volume of less than 6.0 mL/m^2 in addition to a tricuspid annulus diameter of less than 1.4 cm/m$^{(2/3)}$ always required shunt placement at the time of pulmonary valvotomy.[18]

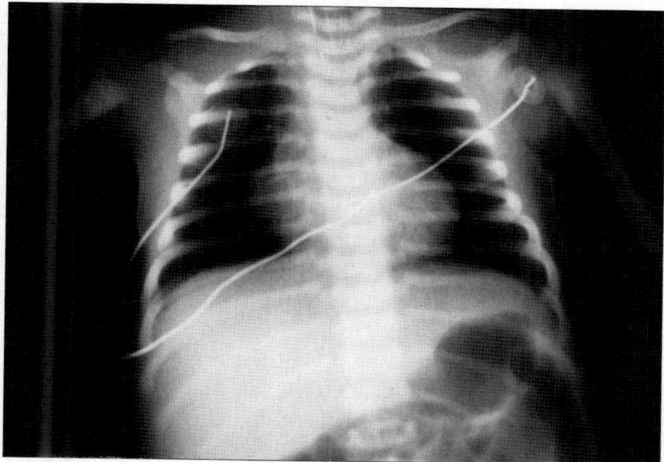

Figure 116.3 Anteroposterior chest radiograph of a newborn with PA-IVS. The heart size is normal. The pulmonary vascular markings are diminished, and there are no infiltrates.

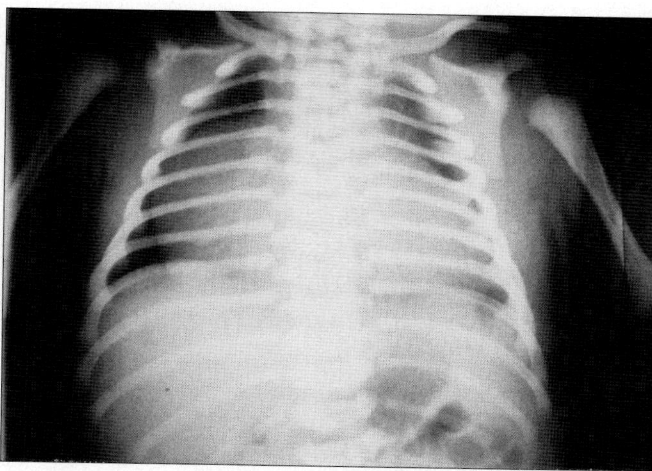

Figure 116.4 Anteroposterior chest radiograph of a newborn with PA-IVS and Ebstein malformation of the tricuspid valve. The heart is grossly enlarged, with a particularly large right border (right atrium) that extends nearly to the right lateral chest wall. Pulmonary vascular markings appear diminished, and there are no infiltrates.

Tricuspid valve hypoplasia correlates well with both right ventricular hypoplasia and the extent of right ventricular sinusoids.[19] The tricuspid valve annulus is usually measured from the apical four-chamber view, and this can be described as a Z score for the body surface area of the infant. In general, those with tricuspid valve annulus diameter Z scores of −4.0 or lower (i.e., more than 4 standard deviations below the mean for body surface area) will not tolerate a biventricular repair. Those with a tricuspid annulus Z score of −2.0 or higher will have a very good chance for eventual biventricular repair. Those with a Z score of −1.5 or higher are likely to require only valvotomy without a shunt.[18] A more recent study demonstrated the utility of indexing the tricuspid valve annulus to the mitral valve annulus (TV/MV annulus ratio); this obviates the need for estimating body surface area and the use of Z scores. All patients who eventually achieved a biventricular physiology had a TV/MV annulus ratio of 0.5 or above, and 16 of 25 patients had a ratio of 0.7 or higher.[20] The presence and degree of tricuspid incompetence should be assessed. Tricuspid valve abnormalities

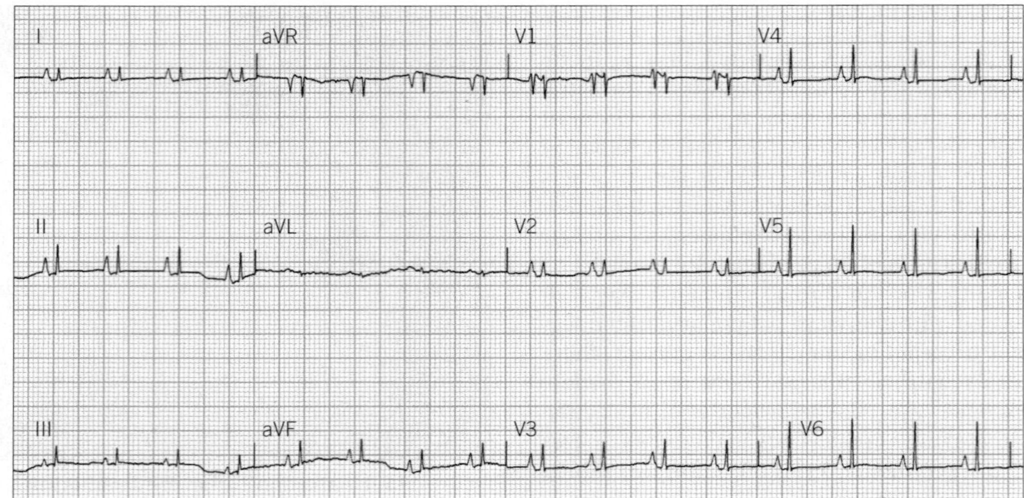

Figure 116.5 Electrocardiogram of a newborn with PA-IVS, moderate tricuspid valve and right ventricular hypoplasia, and no right ventricle–dependent coronary circulation. The P waves are peaked in leads I and II and abnormal in many other leads, consistent with atrial enlargement. There are nearly absent R waves in the right precordial leads and absent S waves in the left precordial leads, consistent with diminished right ventricular forces or left ventricular hypertrophy. There is also nonspecific T-wave flattening in most leads.

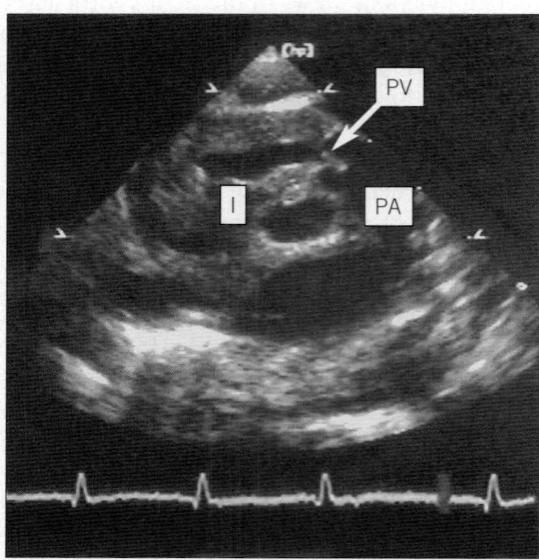

Figure 116.6 Two-dimensional echocardiogram of a newborn infant with PA-IVS and moderate right ventricular hypoplasia. This parasternal short-axis view demonstrates the atretic, thickened pulmonary valve leaflets (PV) between the pulmonary artery (PA) and the moderately hypertrophied and hypoplastic outlet or infundibulum (I).

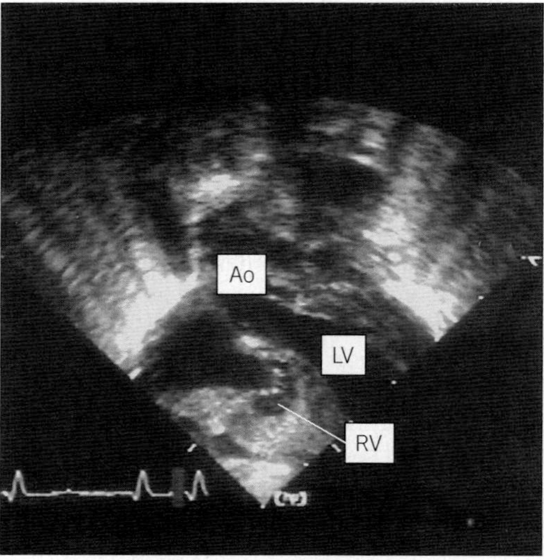

Figure 116.7 Two-dimensional echocardiogram of a newborn with PA-IVS. This subxiphoid sagittal view demonstrates the hypoplastic right ventricular inlet (RV) and tricuspid valve. Ao, aorta; LV, left ventricle.

consistent with Ebstein malformation (see Chapter 114) are best identified from apical four-chamber and right ventricle inlet views. The right ventricular systolic pressure can be estimated from the maximum gradient of the tricuspid incompetence jet, which is best obtained from the same views.

The size and shape of the patent ductus arteriosus can be assessed. The maximum ductal flow velocity is detected from high or left parasternal short-axis views to estimate pulmonary artery pressure, although the pulmonary artery pressure at birth is often increased for the first 1 or 2 days. The patent ductus arteriosus is nearly always left sided, but bilateral ductus arteriosus may occur.[21] The patent foramen ovale is identified and measured, and obligatory right-to-left shunting across the defect should be demonstrated, usually best from the subxiphoid sagittal view. Restriction of the defect is suggested if pulsed Doppler measurement of the shunt exceeds 1.5 m/s.

Color Doppler interrogation of the entire right ventricular chamber may provide clues to the presence of significant right ventricular sinusoids. The right ventricular endocardium in all patients with PA-IVS appears irregular, and there are coarse trabeculations. In many patients with right ventricular coronary sinusoids, however, color Doppler echocardiography of the right ventricular chamber will demonstrate systolic flow from the right ventricular cavity through the sinusoids into the right ventricular myocardium.[22] In some patients, systolic

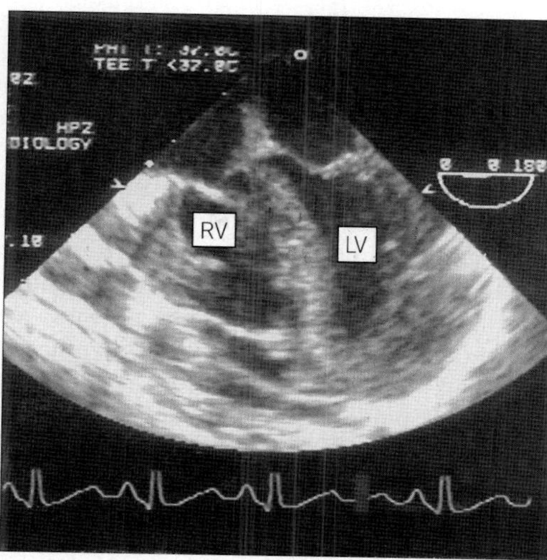

Figure 116.8 Transesophageal echocardiogram of a 3-year-old with PA-IVS undergoing bidirectional Glenn procedure. The right ventricle (RV) is moderately hypoplastic, with a length from tricuspid valve to apex that is about half the length of the left ventricle (LV).

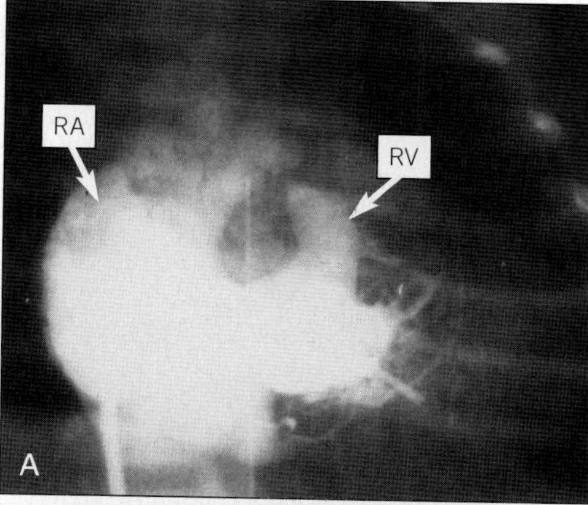

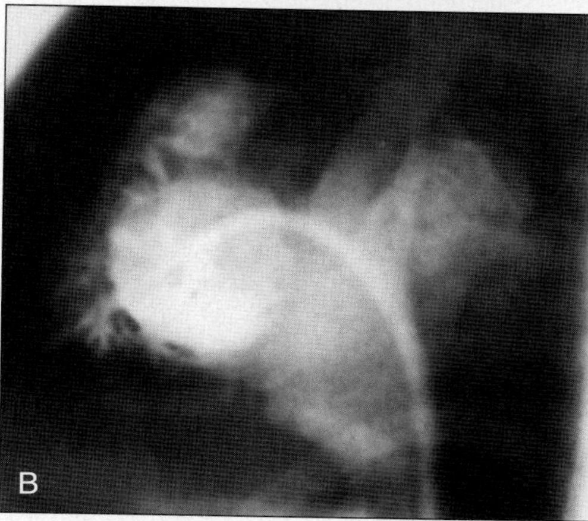

Figure 116.9 Right ventricular cine angiograms of a newborn with PA-IVS and mild right ventricular hypoplasia. A, Anteroposterior view. **B**, Lateral view. The right ventricle (RV) is tripartite with an inlet, trabecula, and outlet. There is significant catheter-induced tricuspid incompetence, with filling of an enlarged right atrium (RA). No anterograde pulmonary flow to the pulmonary artery is demonstrated. This child underwent surgical valvotomy and placement of a small modified Blalock-Taussig shunt, and the shunt was eventually ligated. He is now 15 years old. (Courtesy of Dr. Craig J. Byrum.)

retrograde flow within the proximal coronary arteries can be demonstrated. Coronary arterial and sinusoidal flow is best visualized by decreasing the color Doppler scale (Nyquist limit) to a velocity of 20 cm/s or less. The interruption of coronary artery branches is difficult to determine by color Doppler echocardiography alone, but the rarest variant of RVDCC, atresia of the origins of the right and left coronary arteries (aortocoronary atresia), may be detectable by short-axis scanning of the aortic root.[23] After right ventricle decompression in patients with non–right ventricle–dependent coronary stenoses, subtle left ventricular wall motion abnormalities may be detected by regional wall motion analysis.[24]

Ventriculography and aortography remain essential components of the diagnostic evaluation of PA-IVS in most institutions. First, the catheterization allows the potential for catheter-directed pulmonary valvotomy or balloon atrial septotomy in selected patients. For all patients, the study confirms the absence of anterograde pulmonary flow by right ventriculography and confirms the ductal source of pulmonary blood flow. In addition, the right ventricular systolic pressure can be measured. The greater the right ventricular systolic pressure, the more likely it is that coronary disease is present.[3] Right ventricular angiography provides information about the volume and shape of the right ventricle, the presence of significant tricuspid incompetence, and the size of the tricuspid annulus by demarcation of the tricuspid inflow by nonopacified right atrial blood. Left ventriculography and aortography confirm the presence of coronary anomalies and left ventricular hypokinesis (Figs. 116.9 and 116.10).

Because coronary artery disease affects postoperative survival in patients with PA-IVS, attention to coronary artery anatomy and pathology is essential.[25] Most centers define RVDCC as the presence of interruption of a portion of both right and left coronary arteries, with dependence of the distal, interrupted branches on sinusoidal communications with the right ventricle.

Right ventricular coronary sinusoidal communications to the coronary artery system are usually opacified by right ventriculography. In some patients, contrast material from the right ventricle may opacify both coronary arteries retrograde to the level of the coronary ostia. If the entire right and left coronary arteries are patent in spite of sinusoidal communications (or only one distal branch is stenotic or atretic), this does not represent RVDCC. If there is interruption of a coronary artery branch from the right coronary and the left anterior descending coronary artery with exclusively sinusoidal perfusion of the distal branches, RVDCC is present.[11] In many patients, aortography or selective coronary arteriography may be needed to exclude significant coronary arterial stenosis or atresia.[25-27]

Should a balloon atrial septotomy be performed with this lesion? If right ventricle decompression is not anticipated, balloon atrial septotomy is performed to ensure unrestricted right-to-left shunting at the atrial level, and it is usually performed in the neonatal period. In one recent series of patients undergoing a Blalock-Taussig shunt as the first procedure, one quarter of the patients who did not undergo balloon atrial septostomy before shunt placement eventually required atrial septostomy or septectomy by 8 months of age.[28] Conversely,

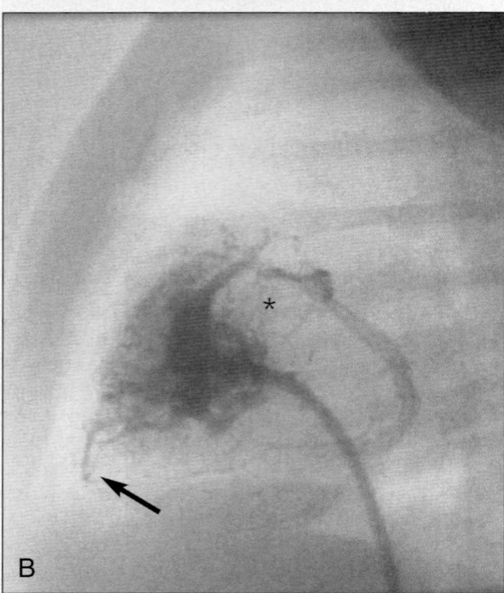

Figure 116.10 Right ventricular cine angiograms of a newborn with PA-IVS, severe right ventricular hypoplasia, and right ventricle–dependent coronary circulation. A, Anteroposterior view. **B**, Lateral view. The proximal left anterior descending coronary artery is interrupted *(asterisk)*, and several sinusoids perfuse distal segments of the coronary system *(arrow)*. (Courtesy of Dr. Daniel A. Kveselis.)

if right ventricle decompression is planned and right ventricle growth is anticipated in the future, balloon septotomy may be deferred in some centers because decompression of the right atrium across the atrial septal defect may discourage filling of the right ventricle and limit its potential for growth.[1,29]

MANAGEMENT

General Initial Therapy

Initial management of PA-IVS includes the usual assessment and treatment of airway, respiratory, circulatory, or metabolic abnormalities. After the diagnosis is confirmed by echocardiography, intravenous administration of prostaglandin E is instituted to maintain ductal patency. Prostaglandin E usually increases left-to-right ductal shunting, pulmonary blood flow, and systemic oxygen saturation. A paradoxical decrease in oxygen saturation may be observed if the infant hypoventilates as a side effect of prostaglandin E. Treatment of this may include reduction of the dose of prostaglandin E, nasal application of continuous positive airway pressure, or endotracheal intubation and mechanical ventilation of the lungs.

The management of this diverse lesion is continuing to evolve, and it varies widely, depending on the severity of the lesion. For all cases of PA-IVS without significant tricuspid incompetence, RVDCC, or the most extreme degree of right ventricular hypoplasia (types 1 and 2; see Table 116.1), the right ventricle is usually decompressed to promote filling and further growth of the right ventricle, with the hope of an eventual biventricular physiology. If the initial amount of anterograde pulmonary flow is expected to be marginal, a Blalock-Taussig shunt procedure may be performed (anastomosis of a Gore-Tex tube between a subclavian artery and the ipsilateral pulmonary artery branch). For patients with extreme right ventricular hypoplasia or RVDCC (type 3), a Blalock-Taussig shunt is placed without decompression of the right ventricle. For those patients with severe tricuspid valve disease and incompetence (type 4), varied surgical approaches have been attempted, with limited success.

The management of each patient depends on the clinical judgment of the pediatric cardiologist and cardiac surgeon and consideration of the experiences of their medical center, in addition to experiences reported by others in the literature. In one large multicenter study, among 171 neonates with PA-IVS, 30% had surgical valvotomy, 26% had transannular outflow tract patch placement, and 44% had a shunt alone as the initial procedure.[6]

Specific Therapy

Type 1: PA-IVS with Nearly Normal Right Ventricle and Tricuspid Valve Size (and usually no significant coronary artery abnormalities)

Figure 116.11 summarizes the treatment strategy for individuals with type 1 PA-IVS.

Initial Treatment

Because the right ventricle and tricuspid valve are nearly normal in size in these patients, catheter-directed or surgical pulmonary valvotomy is often all that is required (similar to the treatment of infants with severe valvular pulmonic stenosis). Several methods of catheter-directed pulmonary valvotomy for PA-IVS have been described. These include placement of the guide wire tip through the atretic valve or membrane,[30-32] radiofrequency ablation of the membrane,[31,33-35] and laser ablation of the membrane.[34] In all these studies, the patients were selected only if the right ventricle, tricuspid valve, and pulmonary valve were nearly normal in size. Several studies required that the right ventricle be tripartite also. Results of these studies in selected patients are encouraging. However, many infants required Blalock-Taussig shunt placement, balloon dilatation or stenting of the patent ductus arteriosus, or prolonged infusion of prostaglandin E (up to 49 days in one patient) to maintain oxygenation.[33]

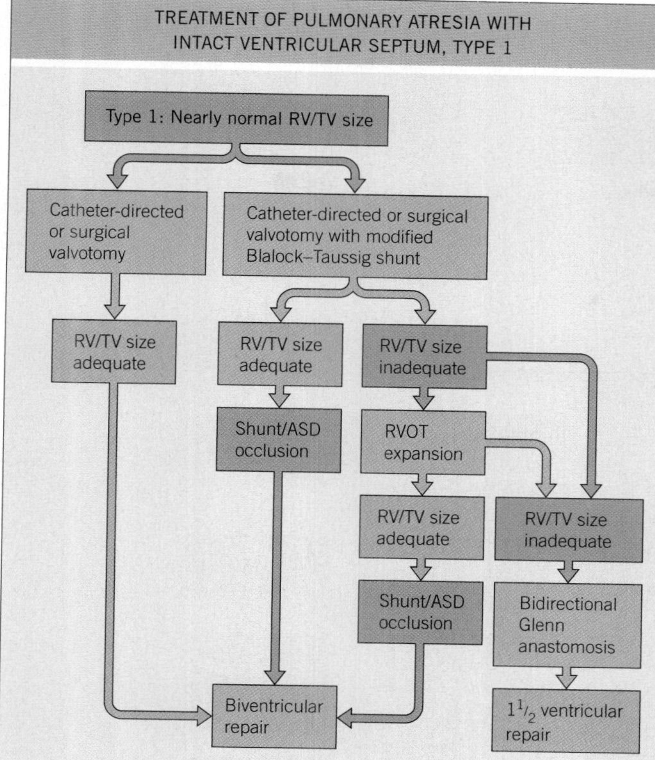

Figure 116.11 Treatment of pulmonary atresia with intact ventricular septum, type 1. ASD, atrial septal defect; RV, right ventricle; RVOT, right ventricular outflow tract; TV, tricuspid valve.

Open (rather than closed) surgical valvotomy with or without a Blalock-Taussig shunt is performed in most centers in which catheter-directed treatment of PA-IVS is not performed or is reserved only for extremely favorable cases.[4] When additional infundibular hypoplasia is present, a transannular right ventricular outflow patch placement may be needed to relieve subvalvular obstruction (similar to treatment in type 2 PA-IVS). After relief of pulmonary outflow obstruction, right ventricular volume has been shown to decrease temporarily, and it may not return to pretreatment values for more than 2 weeks. With decreased right ventricular filling and increased right-to-left shunting across the foramen ovale, significant cyanosis may persist. In these patients, some centers proceed with placement of a Blalock-Taussig shunt, whereas others continue to administer prostaglandin E for at least 14 days to allow the right ventricle to relax and remodel before shunt placement is considered.[36]

It is difficult to predict those patients with PA-IVS who will require shunt placement with valvotomy to maintain acceptable oxygenation, although preoperative echocardiographic estimates of the size of the tricuspid valve and right ventricular volume have been shown to help in predicting those who will require valvotomy alone (see earlier discussion of echocardiographic findings).

Subsequent Treatment

Infants who have had an adequate relief of pulmonary outflow obstruction demonstrate growth of the tricuspid valve and right ventricle. Some residual pulmonary outflow obstruction may be present and may require repeated catheter-directed balloon valvuloplasty or further surgery. If cyanosis is minimal, anterograde pulmonary blood flow is probably adequate. For those infants who initially underwent shunt placement, a cardiac catheterization and catheter-directed balloon occlusion of the shunt can demonstrate whether the child's oxygenation is shunt dependent. If oxygenation is acceptable during shunt occlusion, the shunt can be coil occluded during the catheterization or surgically ligated thereafter. If a significant shunt persists at the atrial level, catheter-directed device closure or surgical closure can be considered.

Ultimate Treatment

The majority of patients with type 1 PA-IVS will eventually have a biventricular physiology and an excellent prognosis. However, a study surprisingly revealed no difference in exercise capacity between those patients with PA-IVS who underwent biventricular repair and those who underwent univentricular repair, although the former group had higher peak heart rates and more efficient ventilation with exercise.[37] There may be mild residual right ventricular outflow obstruction and some degree of pulmonary incompetence related to original relief of the pulmonary outflow obstruction. Those with obligatory pulmonary incompetence related to surgical transannular patch placement may develop progressive enlargement of the right ventricle in adolescence or earlier adulthood, which could require pulmonary valve replacement.

Type 2: PA-IVS with Mild or Moderate Right Ventricular Hypoplasia (and no RVDCC)

Figure 116.12 summarizes the treatment strategy for individuals with type 2 PA-IVS.

Initial Treatment

In patients with type 2 PA-IVS, the right-sided heart hypoplasia is sufficiently significant to limit the ability of the right side of the heart to provide adequate pulmonary blood flow in the first months of life, but there is sufficient potential for eventual right-sided heart growth to justify right ventricle decompression. With more right ventricular hypoplasia, there is more right ventricle infundibular stenosis that can be effectively relieved only by transannular right ventricular outflow tract patch placement. In all patients, a modified Blalock-Taussig shunt is also performed to augment anterograde pulmonary flow in early infancy. The atrial septum is usually not enlarged because this would impede right ventricular filling and the future growth potential of the right ventricle.

Patients with RVCACs and no significant RVDCC may undergo right ventricle decompression with acceptable results.[11] The relatively rare patients with only mild or moderate right ventricular hypoplasia who have RVDCC should be considered and treated as patients of type 3 (see later).[3]

Subsequent Treatment

Patients with type 2 PA-IVS have the most unpredictable outcome and course of treatment. In some patients, right-sided heart growth will permit closure of the atrial septal defect and occlusion of the shunts, with an eventual biventricular physiology similar to that of type 1 patients.

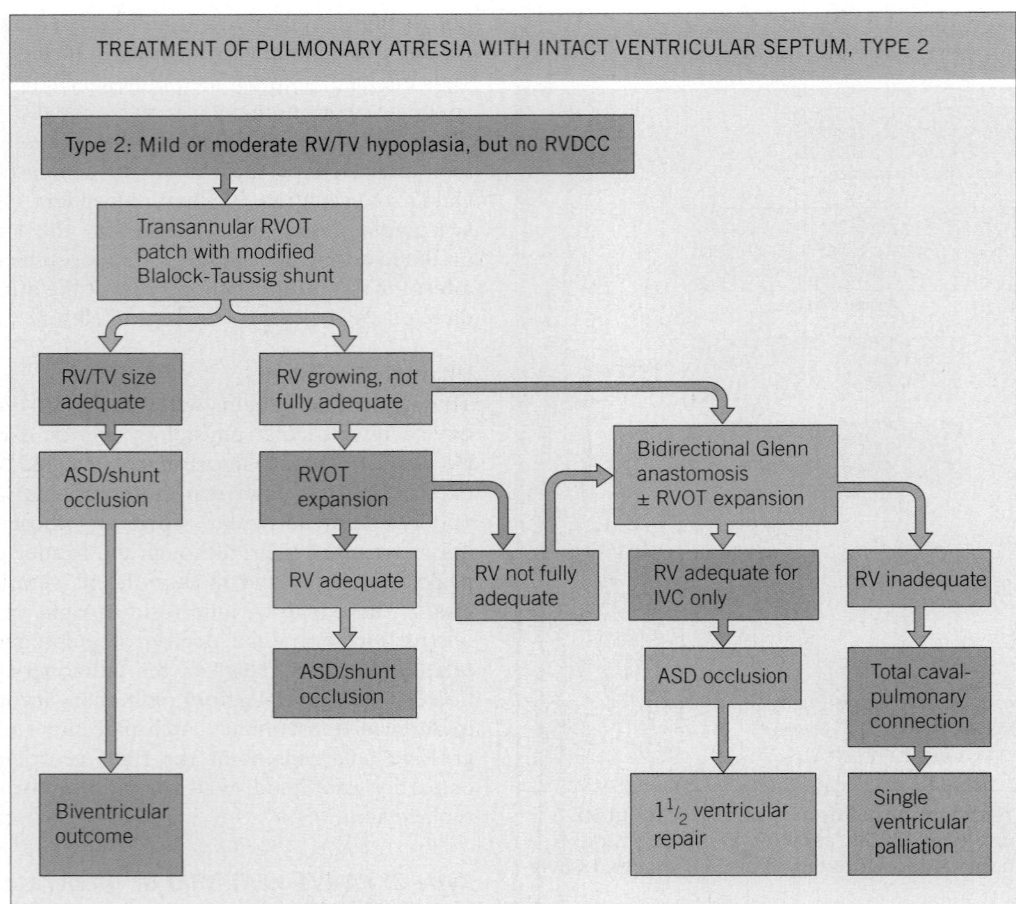

Figure 116.12 Treatment of pulmonary atresia with intact ventricular septum, type 2. ASD, atrial septal defect; IVC, inferior vena cava; RV, right ventricle; RVDCC, right ventricle–dependent coronary circulation; RVOT, right ventricular outflow tract; TV, tricuspid valve.

In patients with more severe right ventricular hypoplasia, the right ventricle may be inadequate in size to receive all the systemic venous return, yet it may still be adequate in size to receive and eject part of it (namely, inferior vena caval return). For these patients, the ultimate operation is a bidirectional Glenn anastomosis and closure of the atrial septal defect. In this situation, the superior vena caval return enters the pulmonary artery through the Glenn anastomosis. Inferior vena caval return enters the right side of the heart and is ejected anterograde by the relatively hypoplastic right ventricle. Because the right ventricle receives "half" of the systemic venous return, the result is commonly called the one-and-a-half ventricular repair. In one center, the bidirectional Glenn anastomosis was performed without disconnecting the superior vena cava from the right atrium in several cases. This afforded a 1½ ventricular repair in which each vena caval return could "choose" its entrance to the pulmonary artery (across the Glenn anastomosis to the right pulmonary artery or across the right ventricular outflow tract to the main pulmonary artery).[38,39]

In the most severe cases of type 2 PA-IVS, the right ventricle does not grow well at all, in spite of the best surgical attempts to decompress it. It is inadequate to receive any significant systemic venous return. In these patients, all systemic venous return must be connected directly to the pulmonary artery, thus bypassing the unusable hypoplastic right ventricle. Treatment first includes the bidirectional Glenn anastomosis and is followed later by the total caval-pulmonary connection, in which the inferior vena caval return is directly connected to the pulmonary artery through an intracardiac lateral tunnel within the right atrium (lateral tunnel) or through an external valveless conduit (external conduit).

Patients with type 2 PA-IVS usually have improved oxygenation after the initial right ventricular decompression and shunt placement but then become more cyanotic during later infancy. It must then be considered whether the ultimate physiology will be single ventricular, biventricular, or 1½ ventricular. Catheterization is often performed to assess the growth of the right ventricle and any significant residual right ventricular outflow obstruction. Balloon occlusion of the foramen ovale may be attempted while right atrial pressure is measured simultaneously to determine whether the tricuspid valve and right ventricle are adequate to carry total systemic venous return. If the right side of the heart is deemed adequate to receive all the systemic venous return, shunt occlusion and closure of the atrial septal defect (either surgical or catheter directed) is indicated, similar to the treatment in type 1 patients. When the right side of the heart is not completely adequate in size, further palliative surgery is necessary. Whether the ultimate outcome will be a 1½ ventricular or single ventricular physiology may be difficult to predict. Patients who have undergone the 1½ ventricular repair tend to have moderate (rather than severe) right ventricular and tricuspid valve hypoplasia. In two series of patients who underwent a 1½ ventricular repair, the preoperative tricuspid valve Z scores varied widely, from −2.5 to −6.5.[39,40] Because the bidirectional Glenn procedure is the next step in either the 1½ ventricular or single ventricular treatment pathway, it is usually performed in patients in whom the ultimate role of the right ventricle is unknown. In selected patients, further expansion of the right ventricular outflow tract may be performed at the time of the Glenn anastomosis to improve right ventricle filling and the potential for further growth.

Ultimate Treatment

As noted before, patients with type 2 PA-IVS may ultimately have a biventricular physiology (like type 1 patients), a single ventricular physiology (like type 3 patients), or the 1½ ventricular physiology.

Type 3: Pulmonary Atresia with the Most Severe Tricuspid Valve and Right Ventricular Hypoplasia, Right Ventricle–Dependent Coronary Circulation, or Both

Figure 116.13 summarizes the treatment strategy for individuals with type 3 PA-IVS.

Initial Therapy

Many clinicians question whether cases with a severely hypoplastic tricuspid valve and right ventricle have sufficient growth potential to warrant transannular right ventricular outflow tract patch placement. In those cases, only a modified Blalock-Taussig shunt is performed with balloon atrial septostomy to decompress the right atrium. In contrast, some centers have observed miraculous growth of the right ventricle and advocate right ventricle decompression as well if significant coronary disease is not present.[41] Even in those centers, however, some patients with extreme right ventricular hypoplasia are not always referred for right ventricle decompression but for a shunt alone.[42]

For patients with RVDCC, a shunt procedure alone is recommended because right ventricle decompression would lead to ischemia of myocardium perfused by the right ventricle alone. In one large series of infants with RVDCC, the authors noted that cardiopulmonary bypass was avoided during shunt placement because decompression of the right ventricle during bypass could significantly reduce perfusion to right ventricle–dependent coronary branches.[43] In two separate series of patients with RVDCC, three of three infants with RVDCC of both coronary arteries and seven of seven infants with RVDCC from atresia of the proximal portion of the left anterior descending coronary artery died after surgical decompression of the right ventricle.[8,11] Infants with aortocoronary atresia have a particularly poor prognosis. In a more recent series of patients with RVDCC, three of three infants with aortocoronary atresia died after shunt placement alone. The authors advocate cardiac transplantation as the only option for these rare cases.[43]

Some authors raise the theoretical possibility that coronary sinusoids (RVCACs) in the absence of coronary artery stenoses (RVDCC) may lead to left ventricular ischemia after shunt placement. Because right ventricular end-diastolic pressure, although increased, is still usually less than aortic diastolic pressure, the right ventricular cavity "steals" from the coronary circulation during diastole. This may be aggravated by a reduction in coronary flow as a result of reduced aortic diastolic pressure from the Blalock-Taussig shunt. Some centers have attempted to prevent diastolic steal of the coronary circulation by excluding the right ventricle and tricuspid valve from the circulation (thromboexclusion of the right ventricle).[44] Most centers advocate simple shunt placement, however, unless there is preoperative evidence of coronary steal phenomenon before surgical treatment is considered.[41]

In cases of PA-IVS with RVDCC and preoperative left ventricular hypokinesis and ischemia, the only viable option may be cardiac transplantation. One center has advocated the placement of an aortic–right ventricle conduit that maintains the right ventricular end-diastolic pressure at systemic values to decrease the coronary steal phenomenon. The results of this procedure in this rare subset of patients have been successful in some cases.[45]

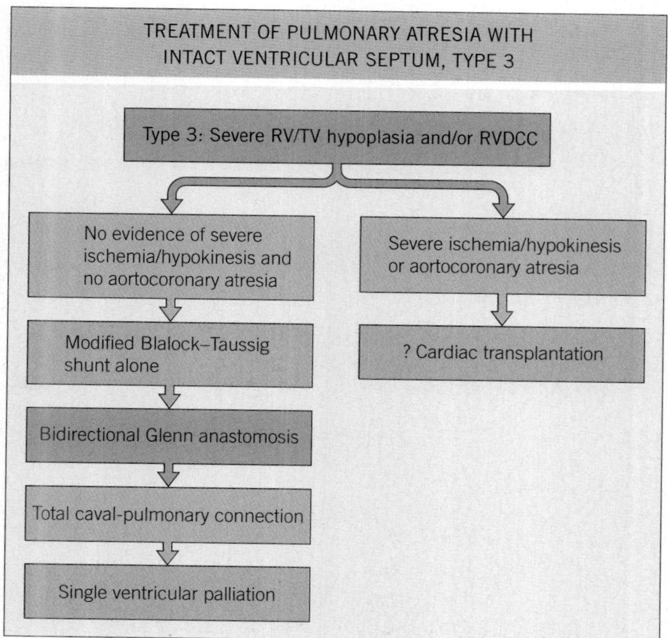

Figure 116.13 Treatment of pulmonary atresia with intact ventricular septum, type 3. RV, right ventricle; RVDCC, right ventricle–dependent coronary circulation; TV, tricuspid valve.

Subsequent Treatment

Because the ultimate surgical treatment will be a single ventricular palliation (bidirectional Glenn anastomosis followed by total caval-pulmonary connection), either an additional Blalock-Taussig shunt is placed or, more often, the bidirectional Glenn anastomosis is established as the child becomes more cyanotic during the first year of life.

Ultimate Treatment

One or more years after the bidirectional Glenn anastomosis, the total caval-pulmonary connection is performed. In patients with RVDCC, venovenous bypass has been reported to protect the RVDCC during the Glenn or total caval-pulmonary connection procedures by perfusing the right ventricle and sinusoidal-dependent coronary artery branches through the right atrium and ventricle.[46]

Type 4: PA-IVS with Ebstein Malformation or Tricuspid Valve Dysplasia and Severe Tricuspid Incompetence

Initial management is perhaps the most challenging and is arguably associated with the worst prognosis of all types. Some centers advocate simple right ventricle decompression or creation of a larger atrial septal defect (if RVDCC is not present). Other centers advocate right ventricle exclusion (patch tricuspid valvuloplasty) and placement of a modified Blalock-Taussig shunt. In one series of seven surgically treated patients, there were four deaths (57% mortality), but three have remained well at 3 to 12 years of age.[9] In another series of three patients with Ebstein malformation of the tricuspid valve, severe tricuspid incompetence, and functional pulmonary atresia, tricuspid valve patch closure and placement of a modified Blalock-Taussig shunt were performed in early infancy. All three infants survived later surgical palliation toward a single ventricular physiology.[47]

PROGNOSIS

There are no long-term studies (to adulthood) of a large, consecutive group of patients with PA-IVS. A multicenter study of consecutive patients diagnosed from 1987 to 1997 estimated survival at 1 year, 5 years, and 15 years to be 68%, 60%, and 58%. Overall 5-year survival rates for neonates enrolled in 1989, 1992, and 1997 steadily increased (49%, 63%, 79%).[48] Similar outcomes (70.8% 1-year survival and 63% 5-year survival) were observed in 183 patients born between 1991 and 1995 and entered in the U.K. and Ireland Collaborative study.[28] In both studies, approximately one third of the patients reached a biventricular or 1½ ventricular outcome. In general, survival statistics of initial surgical palliations are improving, and this may lead to steadily improving cumulative survival of all the procedures needed for each patient. For instance, although RVDCC would be expected to reduce the risk of survival of PA-IVS, there is one series in which 14 of 16 patients with RVDCC who initially underwent shunt placement eventually proceeded to bidirectional Glenn anastomosis, and one proceeded directly to a Fontan procedure.[42]

SUMMARY

Pulmonary atresia with intact ventricular septum is a heterogeneous group of diagnoses that all include total obstruction of pulmonary outflow and varying degrees of right-sided heart hypoplasia and coronary artery disease. Future studies will help clarify classification and define the management and long-term prognosis of all variants of this diagnosis. Prenatal diagnosis is increasing, and in utero intervention is currently under investigation. There is still much to be understood about the diagnosis and management of associated coronary perfusion abnormalities. In addition, many late sequelae of PA-IVS will be of research interest: the long-term right ventricular function and the effect of chronic pulmonic incompetence in patients in whom valvotomy or transannular right ventricular outflow tract patch placement has been performed, the frequency of atrial or ventricular arrhythmias, the natural history of coronary artery abnormalities, and the specific prognosis of the 1½ ventricular repair.

chapter

117 Atrioventricular Canal Defects

Craig E. Fleishman and Gerald R. Marx

Definition

- Atrioventricular (AV) canal defects represent a wide spectrum of congenital heart defects with a deficiency of the AV canal region.

Key Features

- There is a common AV valve annulus.
- One or both of the AV valves are abnormal.
- There is usually an intracardiac defect at the atrial level, the ventricular level, or both.

Therapy

- For complete AV canal defects, complete repair in early infancy is necessary.
- For partial or transitional AV canal defects, complete repair should be carried out by 2 years of age.
- Postoperative mitral regurgitation may require repeated operation.

Atrioventricular (AV) canal defects encompass a variety of congenital cardiac defects, all of which involve, to various extents, the AV septum and the AV valves. This group of congenital heart diseases has also been described as AV septal defects or endocardial cushion defects. These many combinations of anatomic defects result in multiple clinical manifestations and presentations. AV canal defects can be partial or complete. The less common partial form is characterized by an interatrial communication only, with two separate AV orifices; the complete form involves a common AV valve and large interatrial and interventricular communications.

Approximately 5% of congenital heart defects consist of some form of AV canal defect.[1,2] The incidence of AV canal defects in affected fetuses with congenital heart disease is higher, approaching 17% (based on fetal echocardiography).[3] AV canal defects are a prominent component of heterotaxy syndromes, existing in about 80% of such patients.[4,5] Almost half of all patients with Down syndrome have some form of congenital heart disease, and about 40% of these patients have an AV canal defect, usually a complete AV canal defect. Although patients with Down syndrome do not usually have heterotaxy syndrome, they can be found to have AV canal defects in combination with conotruncal anomalies such as tetralogy of Fallot and double-outlet right ventricle.[6] Molecular mapping of small regions of duplication on chromosome 21 has resulted in designation of an AV canal critical region at 21q22.1-qter.[7] This is also known as the Down syndrome critical region. The relationships of this region to the congenital heart defects seen in Down syndrome are complex.[8]

Early identification of AV canal defects, including diagnosis in utero, is important for parental education, establishment of appropriate support systems, medical interventions, and surgical decision making. Uncorrected defects can lead to congestive heart failure with pulmonary overcirculation, growth failure, pneumonia, and pulmonary vascular obstructive disease. Early surgical intervention can be undertaken to correct the various anatomic and associated cardiovascular hemodynamic alterations associated with AV canal defects.

ANATOMY AND PATHOLOGY

Embryology

Abnormal transformation of epithelial cells to mesenchymal cells during the development of the heart tube may lead to AV canal defects. The transformation of epithelial endocardial cells to mesenchymal cells in the cardiac cushions is thought to be due to signaling from protein complexes present within the cardiac jelly.[9] Endocardial cushion mesenchyme appears to differentiate into the connective tissue of the valve leaflets. Studies of the trisomy 16 mouse, a model of Down syndrome, have shown that the mesenchymal cell density is lower and that the migration of cells is slower, which results in an elongated endocardial cushion region in these mice compared with normal controls. Studies of chick embryos have established transforming growth factor β as a mediator in epithelial-mesenchymal cell transformation.[10,11] In mammals, bone morphogenetic protein 2 signaling has been shown to be essential to normal epithelial-mesenchymal cell transformation and AV canal development.[12]

In normal development, the endocardial cushions from the common canal region develop and form components of the mitral and tricuspid valves and the AV septum at this central region.[13] Specifically, during the second month of gestation, the superior and inferior endocardial cushions fuse to form separate left and right AV valve rings. Cushion tissue also extends along the ostium primum, leading to the septation of the inferior portion of the atrial septum. Failure of these cushions to fuse results in a communication at the atrial level and abnormalities of the AV valves (in particular, the anterior mitral valve leaflet is almost always affected). Lack of fusion or incomplete fusion of the superior and inferior cushions leads to a cleft in the anterior leaflet, resulting in superior and inferior components.

Complete lack of fusion between the superior and inferior cushions with a deficiency in the AV septum results in a complete AV canal defect, with a common AV valve and large

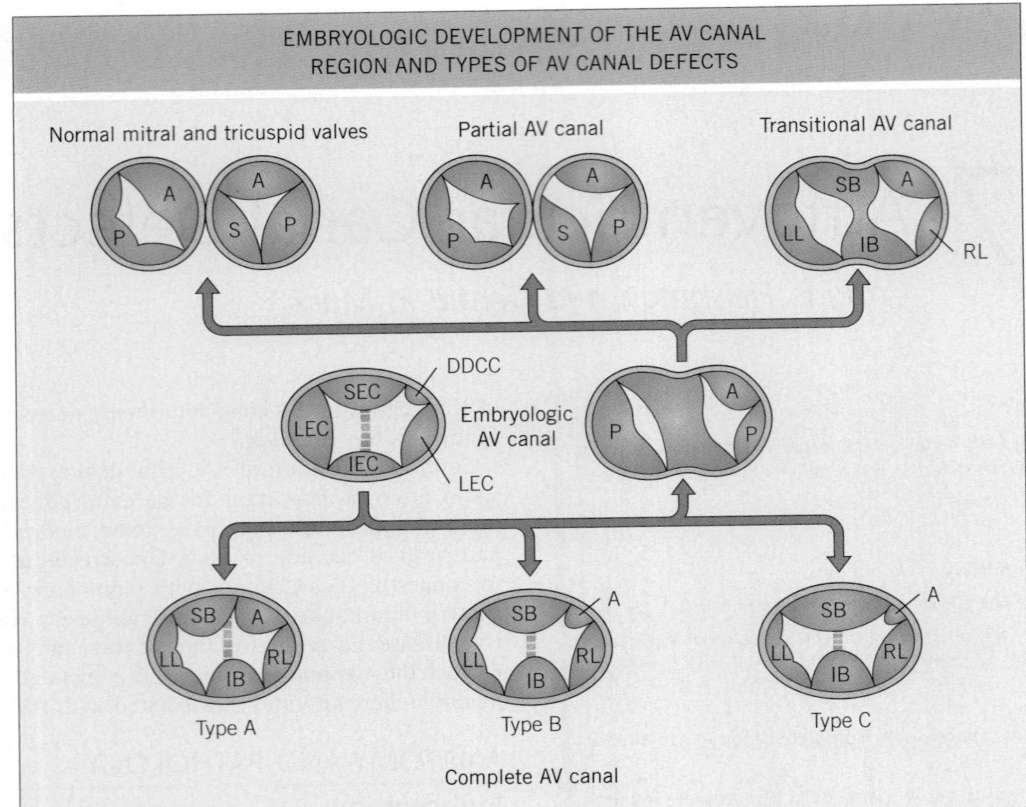

Figure 117.1 Embryologic development of the AV canal region and types of AV canal defects. Complete lack of fusion of the superior and inferior cushions results in a complete AV canal defect. Incomplete fusion results in either a partial or transitional AV canal defect. A, anterior leaflet; DDCC, dextrodorsal conus cushion; IB, inferior bridging leaflet; IEC, inferior endocardial cushion; LEC, lateral endocardial cushion; LL, left lateral leaflet; P, posterior leaflet; RL, right lateral leaflet; S, septal leaflet; SB, superior bridging leaflet; SEC, superior endocardial cushion. (Modified from Emmanouilides GC, et al, eds. Moss and Adams' Heart Disease in Infants, Children, and Adolescents: Including the Fetus and Young Adult, 5th ed. Baltimore, Williams & Wilkins, 1995:706.)

interatrial and interventricular communications (Fig. 117.1). Incomplete or partial lack of fusion between the superior and inferior cushions results in either

- a partial AV canal defect with a primum atrial septal defect, two separate AV valve orifices, and a cleft in the anterior mitral leaflet; or
- a transitional AV canal defect with a primum atrial septal defect, a common AV valve annulus, and dense chordal attachments to the ventricular septum, which results in minimal shunting at the ventricular level.

In all cases, the inlet portion of the ventricular septum appears "scooped out," resulting in a shorter distance from the crux of the heart to the apex. In addition, the aorta is no longer wedged between the tricuspid and mitral valves and becomes sprung, which increases the distance of the aorta from the apex of the heart. The combined changes of valve position and septal deficiency result in elongation of the left ventricular outflow tract. This anatomic change is visualized by echocardiography and angiography as a gooseneck deformity (Fig. 117.2). Although the left ventricular outflow tract appears narrowed, obstruction may not be present.[14] On the other hand, this anatomic substrate can be associated with left ventricular outflow tract obstruction.

Morphology

In complete AV canal defects, the common AV valve is composed of superior and inferior bridging leaflets, a left lateral leaflet, and two right (tricuspid) leaflets (anterior and lateral) (Fig. 117.3). The inferior bridging leaflet usually has dense chordal attachments to the ventricular septum. The superior bridging leaflet is more variable in its size and attachments. A nomenclature developed and revised by Rastelli and others[15,16] describes the variability of the superior bridging leaflet (Fig. 117.4). This Rastelli classification is often used because the anatomy of the superior bridging leaflet may influence the approach by the cardiovascular surgeon.

In Rastelli type A, the superior bridging leaflet is committed to the left ventricle and shares a commissure with the anterior tricuspid leaflet at the ventricular septum. Chordae attach the medial portion of the leaflet to the crest of the ventricular septum. Rastelli type A defects are frequently found in patients who have Down syndrome.

In Rastelli type B, the least common form, the superior bridging leaflet extends toward the right into the right ventricle, with a corresponding decrease in the size of the anterior tricuspid leaflet. The superior bridging leaflet has chordal attachments to papillary muscles in the right ventricle, more

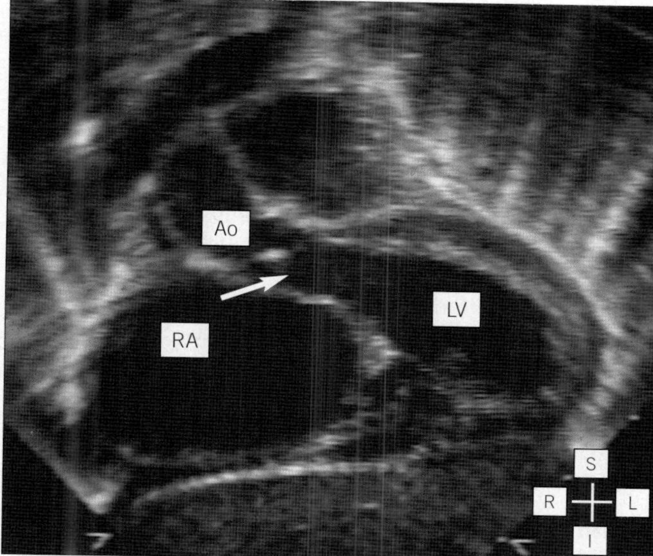

Figure 117.2 Gooseneck deformity of AV canal defect. Echocardiographic image from subcostal location demonstrating the gooseneck deformity that results from elongation and narrowing of the left ventricular outflow tract *(arrow)* in AV canal defects. The superior bridging leaflet is seen "scooping out" the subaortic region during diastole. Ao, aorta; LV, left ventricle; RA, right atrium.

inferiorly on the ventricular septum. Interventricular shunting occurs under the superior bridging leaflet.

Rastelli type C is frequently found in combination with other cardiac defects, such as tetralogy of Fallot, transposition of the great arteries, and heterotaxy syndromes.[17] The superior bridging leaflet is large, with absence of chordal attachments to the interventricular septum but attachments to papillary muscles on the right ventricular free wall. The anterior tricuspid leaflet is hypoplastic.

Quite apart from the Rastelli classification of a complete AV canal defect, the ventricles may be balanced, relatively equal in size, or unbalanced, with hypoplasia of the right or left ventricle. The relative size of the ventricles appears to be related to the alignment of the endocardial region over the corresponding ventricles. In the case of significant hypoplasia of either ventricle, complete repair may not be possible, and palliative procedures need to be employed.

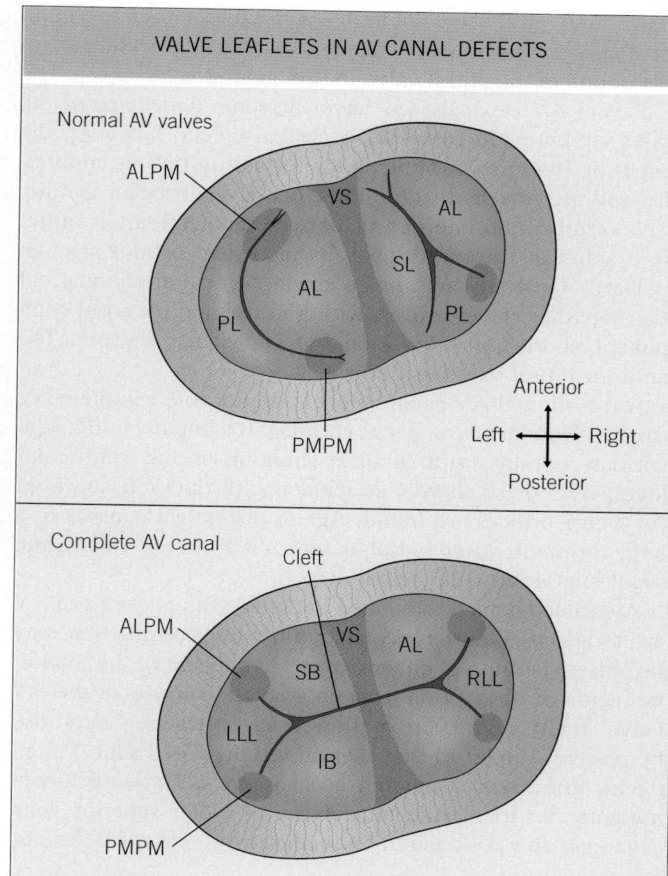

Figure 117.3 Valve leaflets in AV canal defects. Views of AV valves from above. The size and extent of the superior bridging leaflet can vary. AL, anterior leaflet; ALPM, anterolateral papillary muscle; IB, inferior bridging leaflet; LLL, left lateral leaflet; PL, posterior leaflet; PMPM, posterior medial papillary muscle; RLL, right lateral leaflet; SB, superior bridging leaflet; SL, septal leaflet; VS, ventricular septum. (Modified from Fyler DC, ed. Nadas' Pediatric Cardiology. Philadelphia, Hanley & Belfus, 1992:579.)

The papillary muscles in AV canal defects are usually abnormal in size, location, or both.[18,19] The left ventricular papillary muscles are typically shifted laterally and closer together compared with their usual location. On occasion, only one left ventricular papillary muscle may be present, resulting in

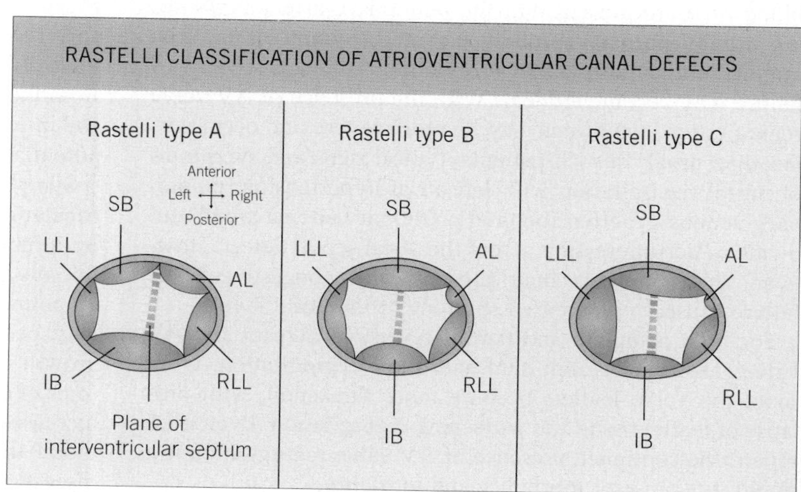

Figure 117.4 Rastelli classification of atrioventricular canal defects. In Rastelli type A, there is a superior bridging leaflet committed to the left ventricle with chordal attachments to the crest of the ventricular septum. In Rastelli type B, a superior bridging leaflet extends over the right ventricle with chordal attachments into the body of the right ventricle. In Rastelli type C, a superior bridging leaflet attaches to the free wall of right ventricle. The anterior leaflet is small. AL, anterior leaflet; IB, inferior bridging leaflet; LLL, left lateral leaflet; RLL, right lateral leaflet; SB, superior bridging leaflet.

parachute mitral valve deformity. Typical repair may result in postoperative mitral valve stenosis or may even culminate in disruption of the mitral valve tensor apparatus.[20]

Partial AV canal defects have the same deficiency of the inlet septum as in complete AV canal defect; however, the superior and inferior bridging leaflets are in fibrous continuity and are attached to the crest of the ventricular septum. This results in no interventricular communication but rather in a shunt at the atrial level (as in typical ostium primum defect). A partial canal has a single AV valve annulus but two separate valve orifices, with a mitral and tricuspid component at the same level on the ventricular septum. The anterior mitral valve leaflet is cleft.

A transitional AV canal defect is similar to a complete AV canal defect; however, dense chordal attachments to the ventricular septum result in little shunting at the ventricular level. With these chordal attachments, distinct left and right AV valve orifices are found. Again, this defect consists of a large primum atrial septal defect, cleft mitral valve, and small inlet ventricular septal defect.

Associated defects may often be found with all forms of AV canal defects. Left ventricular outflow tract obstruction may be present because of either marked hypoplasia of the subaortic region or obstruction from chordal attachments of the AV valve. Right ventricular outflow tract obstruction may also be present, similar to that seen in tetralogy of Fallot. Patent ductus arteriosus, secundum atrial septal defects, additional muscular ventricular septal defects, or a left superior vena cava may also be found in association with AV canal defects.

PATHOPHYSIOLOGY

Complete AV canal defects result in increased pulmonary blood flow secondary to left-to-right shunting at the atrial and ventricular levels. Pulmonary artery hypertension is present owing to the unrestrictive nature of the interventricular communication. Uncorrected defects will eventually lead to elevated pulmonary vascular resistance and, potentially, pulmonary vascular obstructive disease. Pulmonary vascular obstructive disease can develop as early as several months of age, especially in patients who have Down syndrome.[21]

Partial AV canal defects with an ostium primum atrial septal defect have left-to-right shunting at the level of the defect. Right ventricular dilatation and increased pulmonary blood flow are present, but the pulmonary artery pressures are usually normal or mildly elevated. Symptoms may be minimal until adulthood, when symptoms of congestive heart failure may become evident. With the presence of AV valve regurgitation, symptoms may be more severe and occur earlier than usual. In such patients, typical signs and symptoms of mitral regurgitation with left atrial hypertension, pulmonary venous hypertension, and pulmonary edema are absent owing to decompression across the atrial septal defect. However, these patients may present with congestive heart failure caused by increased shunting at the atrial level.

For both complete and partial AV canal defects, the AV valves are usually abnormal and allow regurgitation. Over time, the valve leaflets become more thickened, with prolapse of leaflet tissue and worsening regurgitation. Even after repair, the continued presence of AV valve regurgitation is a significant cause of morbidity and mortality.[22]

In complete defects, the regurgitation may be from the common valve either from left ventricle to left atrium or from right ventricle to right atrium. In partial defects, most of the regurgitation is from left ventricle to left atrium through the cleft in the anterior mitral valve leaflet. However, regurgitation can be from left ventricle to right atrium through the AV septum, resulting in the typical "left ventricle to right atrium shunt." Physiologically, this is tantamount to shunting at the atrial level and results in right atrial and right ventricular volume overload.

The manifestations of transitional AV canal defects are similar to those of partial AV canal defects. Shunting at the ventricular level is often minimal because the interventricular communication is small and restrictive. These patients may also have a left ventricle to right atrium shunt and, rarely, moderate to severe left AV valve regurgitation.

CLINICAL PRESENTATIONS

Fetal Presentations

Advances in ultrasound technology have enabled accurate diagnosis of AV canal defects as early as the first trimester. Most obstetric screening fetal ultrasound studies require accurate assessment of the four-chamber view involving the central AV septum. If abnormalities are detected, the mother should be subsequently referred by the perinatologist for specific fetal echocardiography to determine more precisely the type of AV canal defect and any associated anatomic and hemodynamic abnormalities, especially AV valve regurgitation. The presence of an AV septal defect in utero is associated with a 40% to 50% incidence of Down syndrome; therefore, fetal genetic analysis is warranted. Most often, AV canal defects are well tolerated in utero, with appropriate fetal growth and development. The exceptions to this include severe AV valve regurgitation and heart block associated with heterotaxy syndromes. The higher incidence of AV canal defects in fetuses with congenital heart disease relates to the screening evaluation necessity of a four-chamber view, which should readily diagnose most AV canal defects. Defects related to the semilunar valves or outflow tracts may be diagnosed by this technology.

Complete Atrioventricular Canal Defect

Complete AV canal defects usually present early in infancy because of congestive heart failure from increased pulmonary blood flow and biventricular volume overload. Infants typically have poor feeding, growth retardation, tachypnea, sweating, and pallor. Because of pulmonary overcirculation and interstitial pulmonary edema, microatelectasis can occur, potentially leading to respiratory tract infections.

Symptoms of heart failure may be moderated by right ventricular outflow tract obstruction from pulmonary stenosis or by infundibular stenosis associated with tetralogy of Fallot. Initially, if the degree of obstruction decreases the magnitude of pulmonary blood flow, the pulmonary-to-systemic flow may become more balanced. Such infants may have good growth and development, with absence of signs and symptoms of congestive heart failure. As the degree of obstruction increases, patients may become cyanotic as the pulmonary blood flow decreases. In rare cases of pulmonary vascular disease associated with uncorrected forms of AV canal defects, Eisenmenger's syndrome develops, with right-to-left intracardiac shunting and associated systemic cyanosis.

The patient who has a complete AV canal defect, increased pulmonary blood flow, and biventricular volume overload will have signs of congestive heart failure. The precordial impulse is increased and displaced inferiorly and laterally. The pulmonary component of the second heart sound can be increased in intensity as a result of pulmonary artery hypertension. A systolic ejection murmur is heard at the left upper sternal border because of increased blood flow across the pulmonary valve. With left AV valve regurgitation, a holosystolic murmur at the apex of the heart can be heard on auscultation, which, if it is directed toward the right atrium, radiates toward the sternum. A third heart sound or a mid-diastolic rumble can be heard at the apex secondary to increased diastolic flow across the AV valve. If pulmonary vascular disease has progressed, many of these findings will not be present owing to the decrease of pulmonary blood flow that results from increased pulmonary vascular resistance.

Partial Atrioventricular Canal Defect

The presentation of patients who have predominantly an ostium primum defect, as well as of patients who have a transitional canal defect, reflects the left-to-right shunting at the atrial level. Often, symptoms are absent until adulthood, when decreased left ventricular compliance leads to increased shunting at the atrial level. Physical examination may yield only a fixed splitting of the second heart sound and a systolic ejection murmur at the left upper sternal border due to increased blood flow across the pulmonary valve. With increased shunting, the right ventricular precordial impulse is increased, and a diastolic rumble may be present as a result of increased flow across the tricuspid valve.

Typically, some degree of left AV valve regurgitation is present. In patients who have significant mitral regurgitation, symptoms of congestive heart failure may be manifested early in life, including dyspnea, growth retardation, pallor, and recurrent respiratory tract infections. On physical examination, there is a hyperactive precordium. In association with the findings of an atrial septal defect, a high-pitched holosystolic murmur can be heard at the apex. With sufficient mitral regurgitation, a mid-diastolic rumble can be heard at the cardiac apex as a result of increased diastolic flow across the mitral valve.

Variations in Presentation

Many of these clinical presentations may be altered by the underlying pathophysiologic process. When the AV valve regurgitation is directed into the left atrium, the holosystolic murmur is typically directed toward the left side of the chest and axilla, and the diastolic rumble is heard toward the apex because of increased mitral flow. When the regurgitation is directed toward the right atrium, the murmur radiates toward the sternum, and the diastolic rumble is heard at the right lower sternal border because of increased tricuspid flow.

If the AV canal defect is unbalanced or malaligned, one ventricle receives most of the blood that flows across the AV valve. The other ventricle and, potentially, the corresponding great artery become hypoplastic. The clinical presentation depends on which ventricle is hypoplastic. In the absence of a large patent ductus arteriosus, when the left ventricle and aorta are hypoplastic, symptoms related to low cardiac output are present. When the right ventricle is hypoplastic, cyanosis may be the predominant finding.

With pulmonary vascular disease, the pulmonary outflow murmur diminishes as the flow across the pulmonary valve decreases. The murmur due to AV valve regurgitation, however, remains. The progression of pulmonary vascular disease eventually leads to systemic oxygen desaturation and cyanosis caused by right-to-left shunting.

DIAGNOSTIC TECHNIQUES

Two-dimensional Doppler echocardiography has become the main diagnostic modality for AV canal defects. However, in the preliminary evaluation, basic studies provide additional important information.

Radiography

In both complete and partial AV canal defects, cardiomegaly is secondary to the ventricular volume overload. Complete canal defects often demonstrate enlargement in all four chambers. In a large left-to-right shunt, increased pulmonary vascular markings are present. A partial AV canal defect shows enlargement of the right atrium, right ventricle, and main pulmonary artery, again with increased pulmonary blood flow. Right ventricular enlargement may be most apparent on the lateral film.

Electrocardiography

The hallmark finding of AV canal defects on electrocardiography is a superior QRS axis in the frontal plane and a counterclockwise loop (Fig. 117.5). This finding is a result of inferior displacement of the conduction system.[23] Right atrial enlargement may be present, reflecting either the shunting from left atrium to right atrium or from left ventricle to right atrium (or both) or the presence of right ventricular hypertrophy. Right ventricular volume overload, when present, is reflected by an rsR′ pattern in the right precordial leads or, less commonly, by a qR pattern. The PR interval may be prolonged. This finding is thought to be due to increased intra-atrial conduction time.[24]

Echocardiography

Echocardiography has become the major laboratory modality used to assess the anatomy and physiology of AV canal defects. Two-dimensional echocardiography, combined with Doppler echocardiography, and three-dimensional echocardiography can provide the necessary information to plan treatment strategies and timing of surgical interventions.[25,26] Many children who have AV canal defects can proceed to surgical repair after a complete echocardiographic evaluation without the need for preoperative cardiac catheterization.[27,28] Intraoperative transesophageal echocardiography has become an important adjunct during the repair of AV canal defects, especially in the assessment of AV valve regurgitation.[29,30]

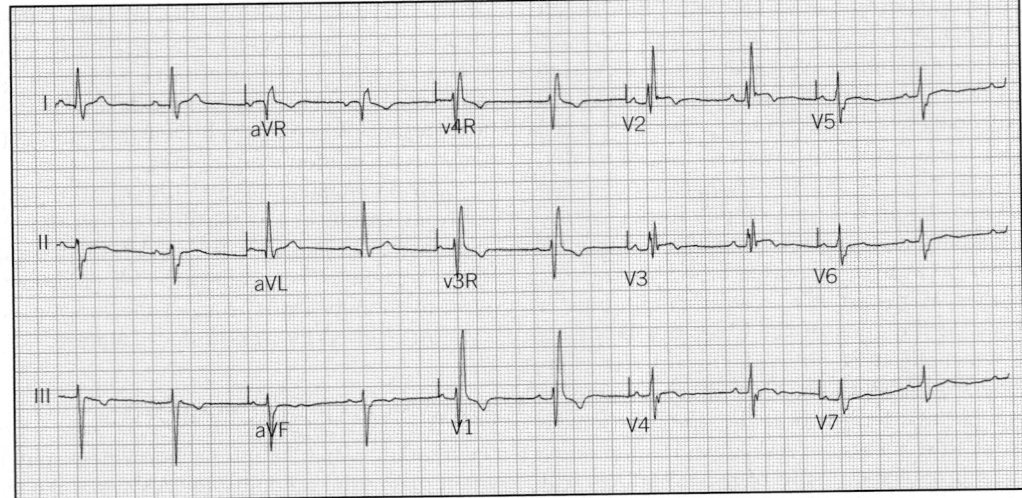

Figure 117.5 Electrocardiogram in AV canal defect. Typical electrocardiogram in an AV canal defect with a leftward and superior QRS axis.

The echocardiographic evaluation should assess for

- presence and size of atrial and ventricular level communications;
- AV valve morphology;
- orientation of the AV valve and the sizes of the right and left ventricles;
- number and location of papillary muscles;
- left ventricular outflow tract obstruction;
- right ventricular outflow tract obstruction;
- additional atrial or ventricular septal defects; and
- associated anomalies, such as abnormalities of systemic and pulmonary venous return or coarctation of the aorta.

In complete AV canal defect, a common AV valve crosses the ventricular septum, resulting in delineation of atrial and ventricular defect components (117.6). The apical or subcostal four-chamber view can readily depict an ostium primum defect (Fig. 117.7). The atrial component of the defect extends to the level of the AV valves, and the planes of both valves are seen at the same level. Although most primum atrial septal defects are reasonably large, they may occasionally be small. The size of such defects is readily diagnosed by standard two-dimensional imaging. Color-flow Doppler study documents the left-to-right shunt at the inferior border of the atrial septum. On occasion, this diagnosis can be confused with a dilated coronary sinus or an associated coronary sinus septal defect. Careful attention to ensure visualization of the floor of the left atrial cavity (or roof of the coronary sinus) and the absence of turbulent flow across the coronary sinus aid in echocardiographic determination.

From a subcostal, oblique angle, the common AV valve orifice is seen. The chordal attachment of the superior bridging leaflet can be evaluated from this view, allowing the noninvasive determination of the Rastelli classification of the valve (117.8). When the left AV valve is evaluated from a parasternal long-axis view, the valve is seen to open toward the ventricular septum, which differs from the normal appearance of opening toward the apex of the left ventricle. Two-dimensional imaging along with Doppler examination is used for assessment of the competence of the AV valve.

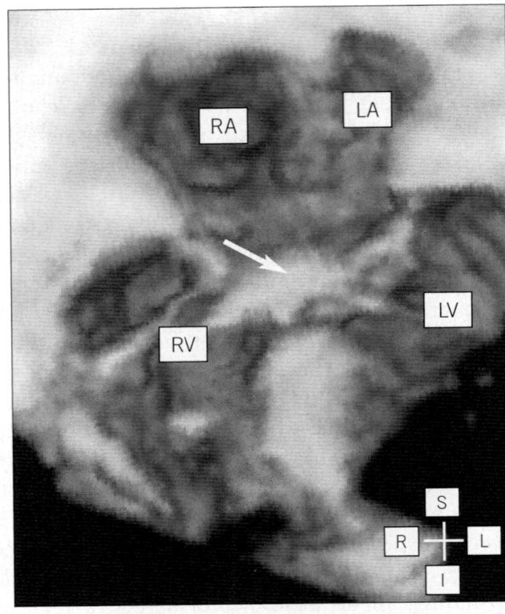

Figure 117.6 Three-dimensional echocardiogram of complete AV canal defect. Four-chamber view in systole. The common AV valve *(arrow)* crosses the canal region. LA, left atrium; LV, left ventricle; RA, right atrium; RV, right ventricle.

Color-flow Doppler study can readily depict the orientation and magnitude of AV valve regurgitation (Fig. 117.9).

The mitral valve orifice in partial AV canal defects, although separate from the tricuspid valve, is almost always abnormal and usually has a cleft (or commissure) between the superior and inferior leaflets that can be best visualized in short-axis views from the parasternal or subcostal location. A cleft in the anterior mitral valve leaflet, with appropriate visualization of the attachments of the corresponding superior and inferior components to the ventricular septum, is best appreciated in a continuous short-axis sweep from the left ventricular apex to the aortic valve. Typically, the cleft in an AV canal defect is oriented toward the ventricular septum. In non–AV canal defects, the cleft is typically oriented toward the aortic valve.[19]

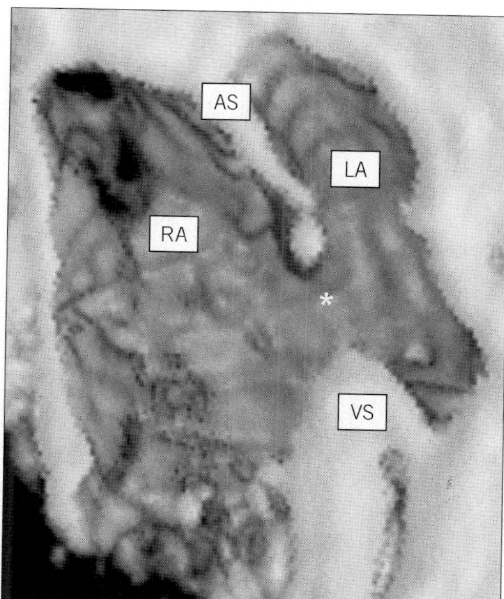

Figure 117.7 Ostium primum defect. Three-dimensional reconstruction of a four-chamber view of a partial AV canal defect. The ostium primum defect *(asterisk)* is seen above the ventricular septum. Right atrial dilatation is present. AS, atrial septum; LA, left atrium; RA, right atrium; VS, ventricular septum.

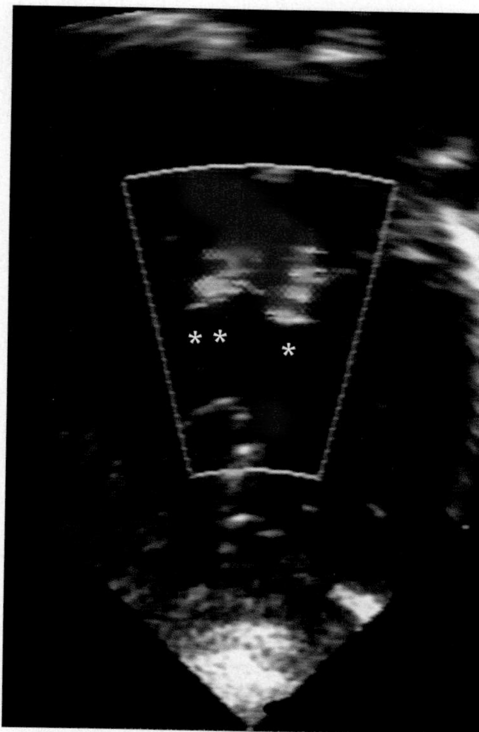

Figure 117.9 AV valve regurgitation. Two-dimensional color-flow Doppler image, four-chamber view, across common AV valve in systole. Left AV valve regurgitation *(asterisk)* and right AV valve regurgitation *(double asterisk)*.

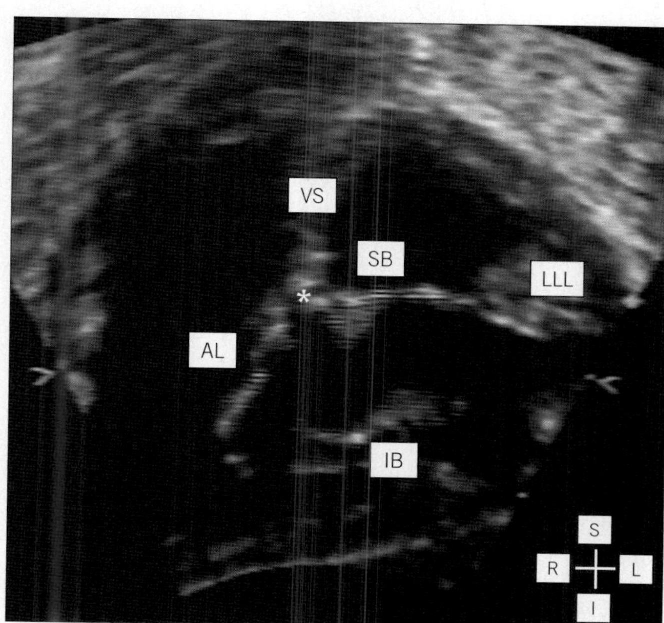

Figure 117.8 Common AV valve. Two-dimensional view of common AV valve. The superior bridging leaflet is committed to the left ventricle with attachments to the ventricular septum *(asterisk)*. AL, anterior leaflet; IB, inferior bridging leaflet; LLL, left lateral leaflet; SB, superior bridging leaflet; VS, ventricular septum.

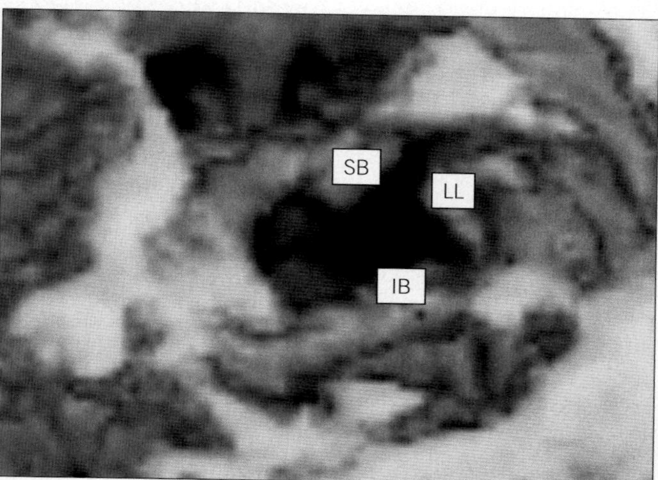

Figure 117.10 Three-dimensional echocardiographic visualization of mitral valve cleft. The reconstruction is an en face view of the mitral valve from the left ventricle in diastole. The superior and inferior bridging leaflets attach to the ventricular septum, with the cleft seen in between. IB, inferior bridging leaflet; LL, left lateral leaflet; SB, superior bridging leaflet.

Cleft mitral valves can reliably and repeatedly be rendered by three-dimensional echocardiography. En face views from the left ventricle toward the mitral valve can image the length and extent of the cleft (Fig. 117.10). En face views from above or below can detect the relative effective leaflet surface areas of the three components of the mitral valve.[31]

Two-dimensional imaging can readily diagnose the extreme forms of unbalanced AV canal defects. However, delineation of subtle forms, which would dictate a one- or two-ventricle repair, is more difficult.[32,33] A three-dimensional echocardiographic volume-based dataset can more readily depict the alignment of the endocardial region over the corresponding ventricular mass. Unique views from above the AV valve orifice, projected downward, may provide additional information as to the alignment of the endocardial region over the right or left ventricular mass.

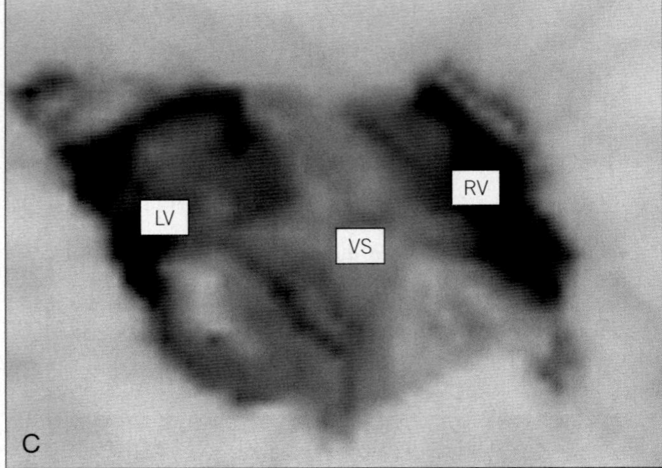

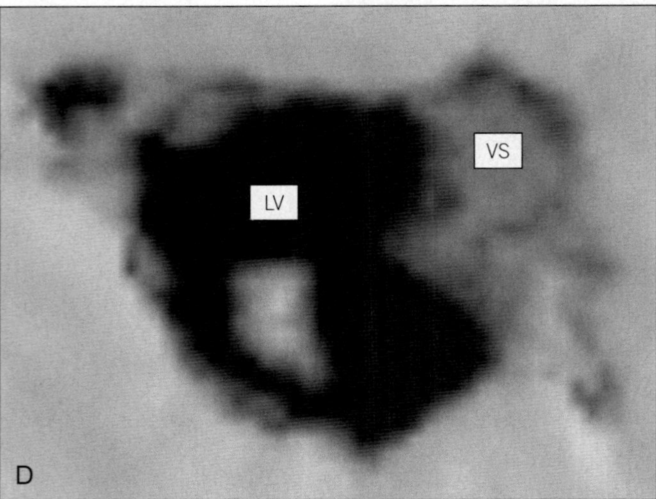

Figure 117.11 Unbalanced AV canal defect with hypoplasia of the right ventricle. A, Unbalanced ventricles and the common AV valve. A viewing plane for three-dimensional echocardiographic reconstruction is shown through the atria, oriented toward the ventricles. **B,** Viewing planes used to obtain three-dimensional reconstructions to show the commitment of the AV valve to each ventricle. **C,** Three-dimensional reconstruction oriented toward the ventricular septum, through the common AV valve orifice. **D,** Three-dimensional reconstruction oriented toward the left ventricle. Note that the size of the orifice over the left ventricle is larger than it is over the right ventricle. LV, left ventricle; RV, right ventricle; VS, ventricular septum.

We have been using three-dimensional echocardiographic reconstructions of the AV valve to evaluate the position of the common AV valve orifice relative to the corresponding ventricular mass (Fig. 117.11). When the AV canal defect is unbalanced, the common valve appears to be aligned more toward one ventricle. Extreme forms of unbalanced AV canal defects can be readily determined by echocardiographic assessment. However, delineation of adequate left or right ventricular volume can be quite difficult. The relative sizes of the ventricles can be determined from an apical view. Although three-dimensional imaging may be more appropriate for volume determination, difficulties still persist. An imaging plane must be constructed to delineate the right atrium or ventricle from the left atrium or ventricle to estimate appropriate chamber sizes.

Transitional AV canal defects are identified by the presence of an ostium primum defect and dense chordal attachments of a common AV valve to the ventricular septum, resulting in only a small degree of ventricular shunting. The degree of ventricular shunting should be assessed from parasternal, apical, and subcostal locations. Careful attention should be addressed to documenting that the ventricular septal defect is restrictive. A high left ventricle to right ventricle pressure drop confirms the restrictive nature of the ventricular septal defect. A low-velocity tricuspid regurgitant jet confirms low right ventricular systolic pressure. Caution must be exercised not to confuse the high-velocity systolic jet from a left ventricle to right atrium shunt, which usually exceeds the magnitude of the pressure drop from right ventricle to right atrium.

The papillary muscle orientation in AV canal defects can be best appreciated on short-axis imaging of the left ventricle.[34] The papillary muscles are rotated counterclockwise with decreased spacing. The presence of either a single papillary muscle or very closely opposed papillary muscles can be a harbinger for potential parachute mitral valve deformity after repair.

Subcostal imaging demonstrates the elongation of the left ventricular outflow tract that results from the deficiency of the inlet septum, the relative lengthening of the outflow tract compared with the inlet portion, and the sprung aorta due to the presence of the common AV valve. This combination of anatomic changes results in the characteristic gooseneck deformity.

On examination of the left ventricular outflow tract, potential sources of obstruction may include[35]

- accessory chordal attachments crossing the left ventricular outflow tract;
- accessory papillary muscle extending into the left ventricular outflow tract;
- discrete subaortic membrane; and
- aneurysm of membranous septum into the outflow region.

Just as the presence of an ostium primum defect confounds Doppler interrogation for mitral stenosis, the presence of a ventricular septal defect confounds the Doppler interrogation for left ventricular outflow tract obstruction. When left ventricular outflow obstruction is present, aortic arch hypoplasia with and without coarctation should be considered. Likewise, coarctation may be a harbinger for left ventricular inflow or outflow tract obstruction. In such situations, care needs to be taken to rule out left ventricular hypoplasia.

Subcostal and parasternal short-axis imaging shows the degree of infundibular narrowing in tetralogy of Fallot. Continuous-wave Doppler evaluation reliably estimates the pressure gradient across the right ventricular outflow tract. In this clinical setting, assessment of the sizes of the pulmonary arteries should also be performed.

Additional defects in the atrial septum, usually a secundum atrial septal defect, can be identified from subcostal and right parasternal views. Again, color-flow Doppler study can aid in evaluating the magnitude and direction of shunting in such defects.

A multitude of pulmonary and systemic venous abnormalities may be associated with AV canal defects as part of the heterotaxy syndrome. Partial or total anomalous pulmonary venous connection can be to the hepatic veins, superior vena cava, atria, or coronary sinus. Systemic venous anomalies may include interruption of the inferior vena cava, drainage of the hepatic veins directly to the atria, and drainage of a left superior vena cava to a coronary sinus.

A patent ductus arteriosus is a common finding associated with an AV canal defect. High parasternal imaging with color-flow Doppler evaluation is usually effective in identifying a patent ductus arteriosus with predominantly left-to-right shunting. However, in cases of severe pulmonary hypertension with elevated pulmonary vascular resistance and right-to-left shunting at the ductal level, patency of the ductus arteriosus may be difficult to discern.

Transesophageal Echocardiography

Most often, the atrial and ventricular components can be closed without undue concern. However, competence of the left AV valve after repair is often of concern to the surgeon. The degree of mitral regurgitation can be assessed by transesophageal echocardiography in the operating room immediately before and after repair. In some cases with significant residual AV valve regurgitation, further surgery on the valve may be performed before leaving the operating room; however, some controversy exists as to the relationship between immediate postoperative findings and long-term results. Changes in ventricular volume and systemic vascular resistance related to cardiopulmonary bypass will directly affect the magnitude of mitral regurgitation. Therefore, the degree of regurgitation seen in the operating room may not correspond to the degree of regurgitation seen under different hemodynamic conditions.

Cardiac Catheterization

Most patients undergo surgical repair based on two- and three-dimensional Doppler echocardiographic findings. One potential reason for catheterization is the assessment of pulmonary vascular resistance, especially in the older child. Patients with elevated pulmonary vascular resistance should have an evaluation to determine the response to oxygen and various vasodilators specific to the pulmonary artery, such as prostacyclin and inhaled nitric oxide. For patients who have upper airway obstruction, as occurs in Down syndrome, endotracheal intubation and ventilation to a normal carbon dioxide level may be necessary to determine pulmonary vascular resistance accurately.[36,37]

MANAGEMENT

Complete Atrioventricular Canal Defect

Infants who have complete AV canal defect typically develop congestive heart failure before surgical repair. Symptoms may be more severe in the presence of significant AV valve regurgitation. Medical management includes the use of digoxin and diuretics and afterload reduction (e.g., with an angiotensin-converting enzyme inhibitor). The angiotensin-converting enzyme inhibitor will decrease the left ventricular afterload, leading to a decrease in both left-to-right shunting and mitral regurgitation. Calorie supplementation is often necessary, sometimes necessitating the use of nasogastric feedings.

Because of low morbidity and nearly absent mortality and to prevent pulmonary vascular obstructive disease, elective surgical repair is recommended at approximately 3 months of age. In selected cases, surgery may be considered earlier; however, surgeons generally consider that optimal valve construction is more easily performed in patients who are older than 6 weeks.[38]

With advancements in surgical and anesthetic techniques, cardiopulmonary bypass, and postoperative management, primary complete repair in infancy has become the preferred approach, with an operative mortality now less than 3%.[39-41] Pulmonary artery banding may be used when a primary complete repair is not possible, such as with additional muscular ventricular septal defects or unbalanced AV canal defect.

Lillehei and colleagues[42] first described surgical repair of complete AV canal defect in 1955. Other associated defects, such as patent ductus arteriosus, coarctation of the aorta, left ventricular outflow tract obstruction, and right ventricular outflow tract obstruction, are approached at the same operation. Characteristics that have been found to correlate with surgical risk include the degree of AV valve regurgitation, relative hypoplasia of a ventricle, degree of congestive heart failure at operation, and presence of associated defects.[43] Over time, the increased risk associated with these characteristics has been minimized.

For complete AV canal defect, closure of the septal defect is performed with either a one- or two-patch technique or by the modified (simplified) single-patch technique. In the single-patch technique (Fig. 117.12), prosthetic patch material is placed to close the ventricular and atrial communications. The common AV valve is divided and reattached to the patch. In the two-patch technique, prosthetic patch material is used to close the ventricular septal defect, and pericardium is used to close the atrial level communication. In the modified single-patch technique, the common AV valve is directly sutured to the ventricular septum, and pericardium is used to close the atrial component of the defect. The two-patch technique and the modified single-patch technique do not require division of the common AV valve and may also result in less distortion of the valve tissue.

With any technique, the cleft in the left AV valve can be left opened or sutured closed. Closure of the cleft in the left AV valve is a controversial subject. Some investigators believe that the cleft in the left AV valve should be left open so that the repaired valve functions as a three-leaflet valve.[44] Other investigators state that the cleft should be closed, citing data that show that significant residual left AV valve regurgitation through the cleft is a frequent reason for reoperation.[45]

For patients in whom the AV canal defect is unbalanced and in whom there is significant right or left ventricular hypoplasia, a two-ventricle repair may not be possible. In such cases, the surgical goal is staging toward a single-ventricle physiology with an eventual Fontan type of palliation. The success of this approach is dependent on the competency of the AV valve and the protection of the pulmonary vascular bed. Because banding of the pulmonary artery to lower pulmonary artery pressure can lead to worsening of AV valve regurgitation, the pulmonary artery may need to be divided and pulmonary blood flow provided by a shunt from a systemic artery to pulmonary artery. With significant left ventricular outflow tract obstruction, a Damus-Kaye-Stansel type of approach may also be necessary. Subsequently, a bidirectional Glenn or hemi-Fontan procedure is performed, resulting in direct drainage of

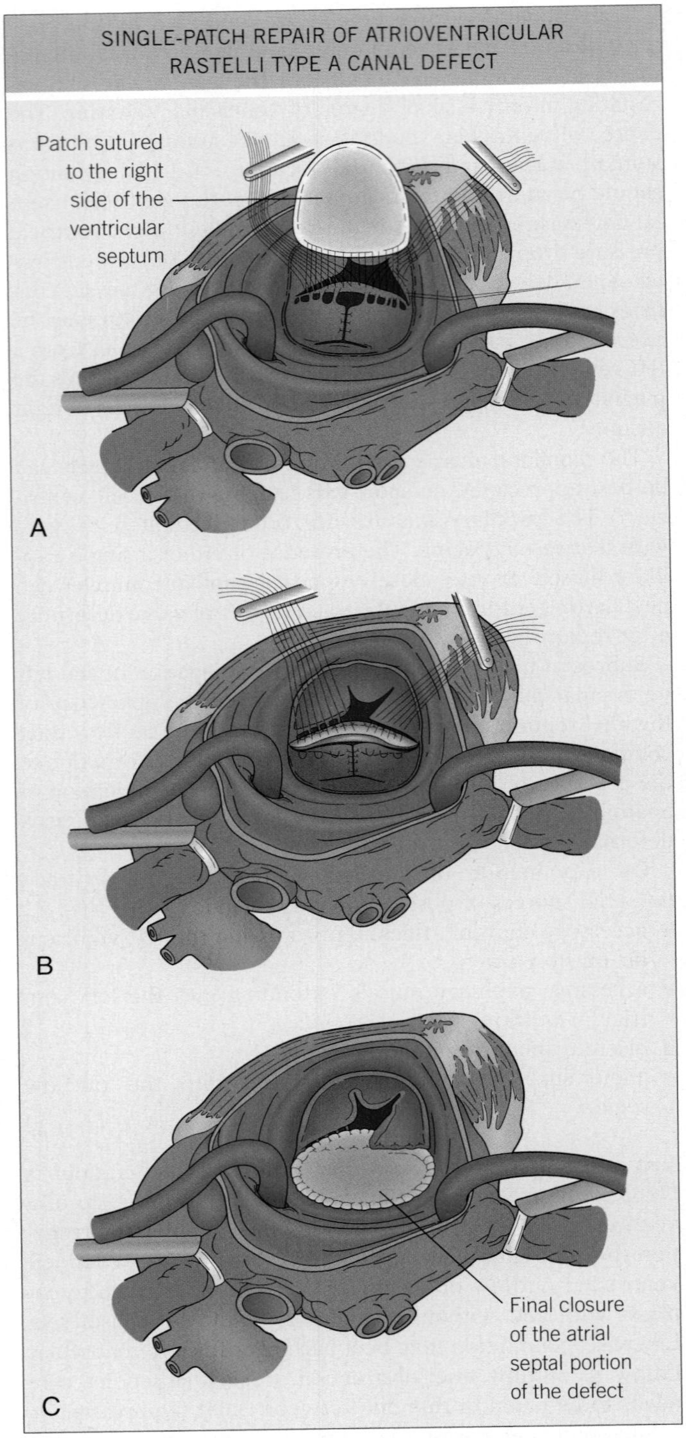

SINGLE-PATCH REPAIR OF ATRIOVENTRICULAR RASTELLI TYPE A CANAL DEFECT

Patch sutured to the right side of the ventricular septum

A

B

Final closure of the atrial septal portion of the defect

C

Figure 117.12 Single-patch repair of atrioventricular Rastelli type A canal defect. View as seen from the right atrium. **A,** The single prosthetic patch is sutured to the right side of the ventricular septum, and the mitral cleft is closed. **B,** Reconstructed septal leaflet is attached to prosthetic patch. **C,** Completion of repair with closure of atrial portion of the defect. (Modified from McMullan MH, Wallace RB, Weidman WH, McGoon DC. Surgical treatment of complete atrioventricular canal. Surgery 1972;72:905-912.)

blood from the superior vena cava to the pulmonary artery to improve systemic oxygenation and to decrease the volume load on the heart. After further growth, a modified Fontan procedure to separate the venous and arterial circulations is performed. This separation is obtained by baffling the blood return from the inferior vena cava directly to the pulmonary artery, usually with an extracardiac conduit.

Partial Atrioventricular Canal Defect

Elective surgical repair of partial AV canal defects is recommended to lessen the incidence of morbidity later in life.[46] Because of low morbidity and nearly absent mortality associated with complete repair, surgery is usually performed when the patient is 18 to 24 months of age.[47,48] On occasion, a patient requires surgery earlier in life because of severe mitral regurgitation or pulmonary artery hypertension.

Surgical repair of partial AV canal defects involves patch closure of the ostium primum defect and mitral valvuloplasty to eliminate or to minimize the mitral regurgitation. For moderate or severe mitral regurgitation, most surgeons suture the mitral valve cleft closed and perform a mitral annuloplasty when associated annular dilatation is present. Surgical closure of the cleft in the presence of mild or no mitral regurgitation is controversial.

Doppler color-flow imaging may help guide surgical management. When the regurgitation jet is medially oriented through the coaptation region of the superior and inferior components of the anterior leaflet, suturing of the cleft may suffice. Three-dimensional imaging has provided evidence that this is often related to diminished effective coaptation from the inferior leaflet. When the color-flow regurgitant jet is more laterally oriented, through the coaptation site of the anterior and posterior leaflets, this may be more amenable to an annuloplasty approach, improving the effective coaptation of the anterior and posterior leaflets. Three-dimensional imaging has shown this to be related to diminished effective coaptation from the lateral leaflet.[49] Three-dimensional imaging also provides additional information of valve morphology and function after repair.[50]

PROGNOSIS

The ultimate prognosis of an unrepaired complete AV canal defect is very poor.[21] Nearly all untreated patients go on to develop fixed pulmonary vascular resistance, as early as the second year of life.[51,52] By the second year of life, these vascular changes can reach Heath-Edwards grade 3-4, which significantly increases the operative risk.

Postoperatively, short-term morbidity and mortality for AV canal defects are related to pulmonary artery pressure, arrhythmias, residual left AV valve regurgitation, and residual left ventricular outflow tract obstruction. Postoperative pulmonary hypertension can be treated with sedation, paralysis, oxygen, fluids, and inhaled nitric oxide.[53,54]

Postoperative arrhythmias include sinus node dysfunction, junctional ectopic tachycardia, and complete heart block. Reports from large series show that the incidence of postoperative heart block varies from 0.5% to 4%.[45,55] The lowest incidence of heart block is found in patients with uncomplicated AV canal defects. Heart block in heterotaxy syndrome is progressive, regardless of surgical intervention.

Residual left AV valve regurgitation is associated with early morbidity and mortality. Long-term follow-up remains necessary to survey for recurrent mitral regurgitation that may require reoperation. Certain investigators have found postoperative mitral regurgitation to be stable in the early to intermediate postoperative period. However, worsening mitral regurgitation is the leading reason for eventual reoperation. Reoperation is necessary in 5% to 10% of cases because of significant mitral regurgitation[22,39,56] and for others because of worsening left ventricular outflow tract obstruction. Long-term follow-up is also needed to observe for the possible development of arrhythmias.[57]

SUMMARY

AV canal defects can be complete, partial, or intermediate. Variance in terminology complicates the discussion of AV valve defects; however, there is a reasonable understanding of the anatomic components and variations associated with these defects. Genetic analysis has led to the identification of an AV canal region on chromosome 21.

Echocardiography is now the primary diagnostic tool for analysis of the anatomic and physiologic characteristics of AV canal defects. Three-dimensional echocardiography can be used to assess chamber size and AV valve morphology. Cardiac catheterization is rarely needed; when it is needed, it is usually performed to determine pulmonary vascular resistance before surgical repair.

Surgical repair, usually during early infancy, is the hallmark of treatment for AV canal defects. Results of surgical repair are excellent, with little morbidity and mortality. Residual mitral regurgitation is a persistent problem that sometimes requires reoperation.

Long-term follow-up of patients should focus on residual left AV valve regurgitation. Worsening AV valve regurgitation is the leading reason for eventual reoperation.

chapter 118

Tricuspid Atresia and Single Ventricle

Luc Mertens, Donald J. Hagler, and Marc Gewillig

Definition

- Univentricular AV connections are hearts in which both atria are joined to only one ventricle. Functionally single-ventricle arrangements represent a heterogeneous group of anomalies that have in common the feature that there is only one functional chamber within the heart capable of independently supporting either the systemic or pulmonary circulation.

Key Features

- Different forms of functionally univentricular connections exist: double-inlet ventricles, with either two AV valves or a common AV valve; and single-inlet ventricles, with one (functionally or morphologically) atretic AV connection (either right or left AV valve atresia or critical stenosis).
- The morphology of the main ventricle can be right, left, or indeterminate.
- The ventricle–great artery connection can be concordant, discordant, double outlet, or single.

Therapy

- Early palliation is directed at creation of unrestricted flow to the systemic circulation and optimization of pulmonary blood flow either by reducing pulmonary flow through pulmonary artery banding or by increasing pulmonary flow through a systemic to pulmonary artery shunt.
- As an intermediate palliation, pulmonary artery flow may also be modified to be more effective by use of a bidirectional cavopulmonary shunt.
- A more definitive form of palliation is the total cavopulmonary connection (modified Fontan operation), whereby the systemic venous return is directed to the pulmonary arteries, bypassing the right ventricle.

Tricuspid atresia can be considered the prototype of the univentricular atrioventricular (AV) connection with atresia of the tricuspid valve and hypoplasia of the right ventricle. It belongs to a class of congenital malformations with a univentricular AV connection, with absent AV connection and hypoplasia of one of the ventricles.[1,2] In most patients with functionally single-ventricle hearts, there are morphologically two ventricles, one of them being too small to sustain one of the circulations.[1,2] Different terminologies have been used to describe functionally single-ventricle arrangements, causing a lot of confusion. Terms like *univentricular heart, single ventricle,* and *common ventricle* have all been used to describe the same anomalies. These terms can cause confusion because from a pathologic point of view, human hearts with a solitary ventricular chamber are extremely rare. In most cases, there is a dominant ventricle with a second hypoplastic or rudimentary chamber. From the physiologic point of view, this does not really matter, as there is only one chamber capable of sustaining systemic and pulmonary circulation.

Because the terminology used to define univentricular AV connections has been somewhat confusing, it is difficult to state the actual incidence. In different series of congenital heart disease patients, they represent about 1% to 2% of the total.[3,4] From a therapeutic point of view, patients with a functionally single-ventricle heart continue to represent a challenging group; management is often complex and needs to be adapted to the specific anatomic variability of the individual patient.

ANATOMY AND PATHOLOGY

The anatomy of complex congenital heart lesions is best approached in a systematic way. The segmental approach has generally been accepted as the standard method for analysis and categorization of congenital heart malformations.[5] This method is based on description of the four primary segments of the heart (veins, atria, ventricles, and arterial trunks) and the way they are joined together at the venoatrial, AV, and ventriculoarterial junctions. Central to the process is the use of constant "markers," which are constant morphologic characteristics of a certain segment. So, for instance, a constant feature of left atrial morphology is the left atrial appendage with the characteristic triangle shape. For each chamber, a certain number of unique "identifiers" have been established. Once the morphology of each chamber is defined, the connections can be studied. To precisely describe the type of univentricular AV connection, the atrial arrangement, the pattern of AV connection, the ventricular morphology, the ventriculoarterial connections, and the associated lesions should be accounted for.

The atrial topologic arrangement can be solitus (the usual pattern), inversus (mirror-image pattern), or ambiguus, in which there is atrial isomerism with bilateral right or left atrial morphology. Either type of AV connection can be associated with any of the four forms of atrial arrangement. The AV connection is, by definition, univentricular (Fig. 118.1), but there may be a double inlet, a common inlet, or an absent right or an absent left AV connection. In a double-inlet connection, there are two separate AV valves, and it is usually not possible to define the valves as either mitral or tricuspid valves on the basis of their morphologic characteristics. Therefore, it is better to refer to them as left and right AV valves on the basis of the anatomic position within

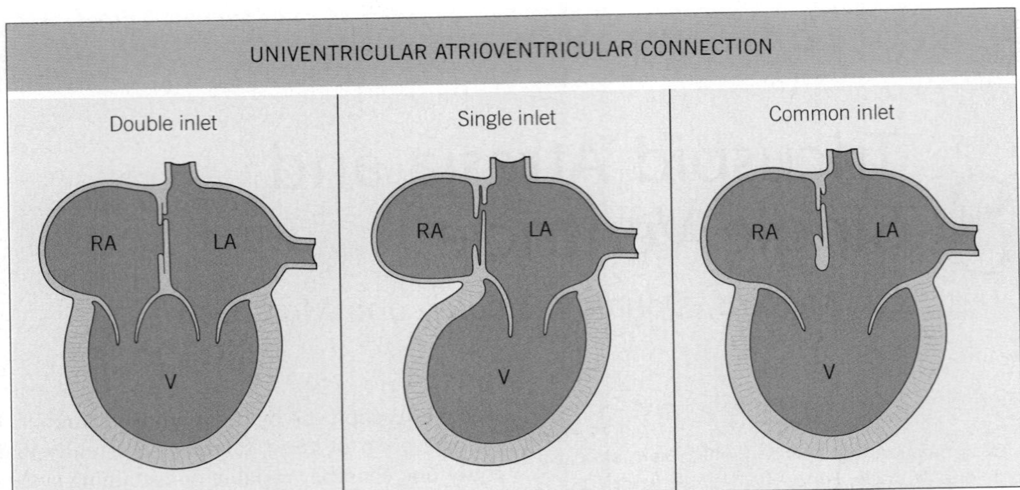

Figure 118.1 Univentricular atrioventricular connection. The three basic types of univentricular connection are shown, regardless of ventricular morphology: double inlet, single inlet, and common inlet. LA, left atrium; RA, right atrium; V, ventricle.

the chest. In case of an absent AV connection, the absent valve can be on the right side or on the left side. The remaining AV connection will usually be concordant. This describes the classic forms of "tricuspid" and "mitral" atresia. In both the double-inlet connection and the absent AV connection, the dominant ventricle can be right, left, or indeterminate. *Overriding* refers to the commitment of an AV valve annulus to the ventricular chamber and results from malalignment of the atrial and ventricular septa. The percentage of annular commitment to a ventricular chamber relative to the position of the ventricular septum determines the AV valve connection to a ventricle. In the setting of an overriding AV valve, an atrium is considered to connect to the ventricle into which more than 50% of its valve empties (Figs. 118.2 and 118.3). A univentricular AV connection requires more than 50% of both AV valves to be committed to one ventricular chamber. The remaining chamber is considered an outlet or rudimentary chamber. *Straddling* of the AV valve is a feature of the tensor apparatus (chordae and papillary muscles) and occurs if tensor insertions are present in the contralateral ventricle through a ventricular septal defect.

The identification of the ventricular myocardial morphology should be based on the most constant component of the ventricular anatomy, which is the trabecular component. A normal ventricle can be described as having an inlet, a trabecular part, and an outlet part. An abnormal ventricle can sometimes lack both inlet and outlet. In those cases, the morphology of the ventricle can still be identified on the basis of the structure of the apical trabecular component. Left ventricular myocardium typically has a relatively smooth appearance with numerous fine oblique trabeculations (Fig. 118.4), whereas right ventricular myocardium has an irregular surface with relatively few coarse trabeculations. On the basis of this, most ventricles can be recognized as being morphologically right or left. In most hearts, such left and right ventricles coexist, with the inlets and outlets being unequally shared between the apical trabecular components in those hearts with abnormal segmental connections. In rare situations, there is only one ventricular chamber in the ventricular mass, with a ventricle that has a trabecular pattern typical of neither left nor right ventricle (indeterminate or mixed ventricular morphology). Also, the *topology* (the relationship between the two ventricles in space) of the ventricle should be determined. Chirality can be used to describe ventricular topology. A ventricle is called a right-handed ventricle if the palmar surface of the right hand can be placed on the ventricular septum such that the thumb is pointing to the inlet and the fingers are pointing to the outlet, with the wrist being in the apical component. In a normal heart, the right ventricle is right-handed, reflecting the normal embryologic development with a D ventricular loop; whereas in AV and ventricular arterial discordance (also called congenitally corrected transposition), the right ventricle has left-handed topology consistent with embryologic development with an L ventricular loop (see Fig. 118.3).

As a final part of the segmental approach, the ventricle–great artery connections should be defined. This connection can be concordant, with the pulmonary artery arising from the right ventricle and the aorta from the left ventricle, or discordant, with transposed great artery relationships. Double outlet (both great arteries arising from one ventricle) and single outlet (common arterial trunk or in pulmonary or aortic atresia) may also be present.

It is also important to describe associated anomalies: outflow obstructions like associated subpulmonary, pulmonary, or suprapulmonary stenosis; subaortic or aortic valve stenosis; or associated coarctation of the aorta. Anomalies in pulmonary venous and systemic venous return commonly occur in the context of isomerism and are extremely important to identify in detail. Sidedness and branching pattern of the aorta and cranial vessels should also be recognized.

By use of the segmental approach, it is always possible to completely describe the anatomy of connections (Figs. 118.5 to 118.10).

PATHOPHYSIOLOGY

The pathophysiology of univentricular AV connection depends on the underlying anatomy and the associated lesions. In all lesions, there is a common mixing chamber in

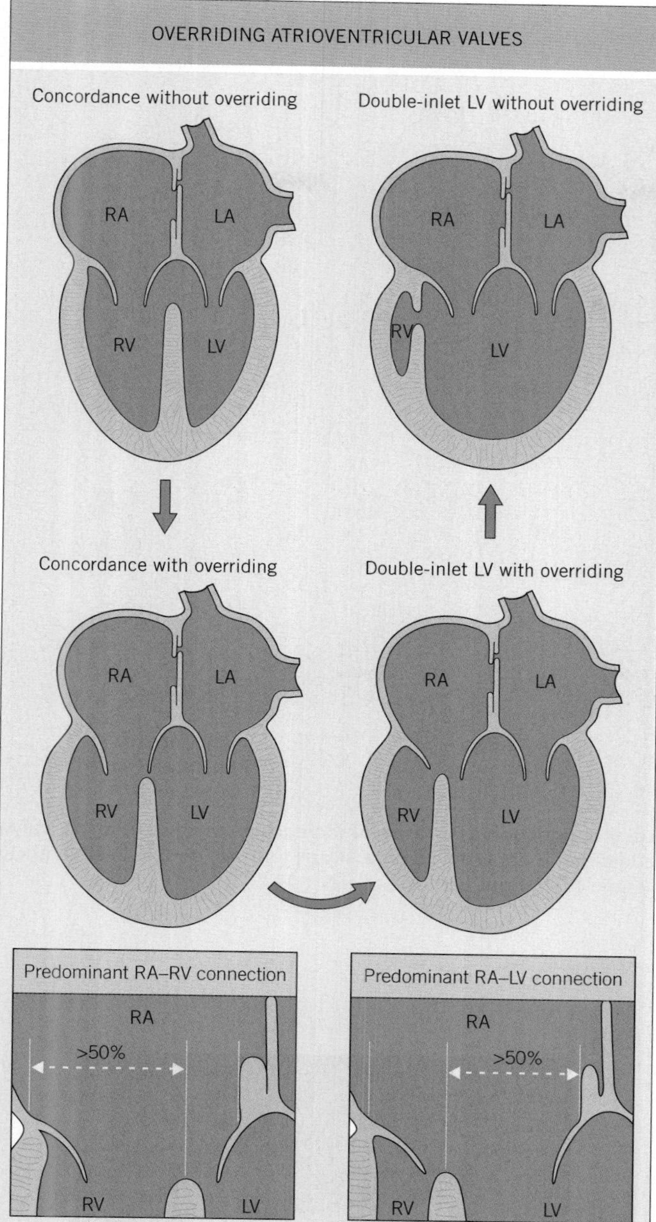

Figure 118.2 Overriding atrioventricular valves. The basic concept of univentricular AV connection necessarily includes a determination of the degree of AV connection based on the 50% rule. If 50% or more of an AV annulus overrides or is committed to a ventricle, the atrium is said to connect to that ventricle. Univentricular AV connection requires predominant connection to a single ventricular chamber. LA, left atrium; LV, left ventricle; RA, right atrium; RV, right ventricle.

which systemic venous return and pulmonary venous return come together. This results in arterial desaturation, the level of which depends on the relative amount of oxygenated and desaturated blood mixing in the single ventricle, provided there is no significant systemic obstruction (coarctation or interrupted aortic arch). Because the systemic flow index is relatively similar in different lesions (between 2 and 3 L/min • m^2), the systemic saturation will depend on the amount of blood returning from the lungs. The output from a functional single ventricle is divided between the systemic and pulmonary circulations, so the relative proportion of blood flow to both circulations depends on the relative resistances to flow in both circuits.

If there is no obstruction to pulmonary flow and the pulmonary resistance drops during the first weeks of life, the pulmonary flow will increase, reducing hypoxemia at the expense of an important volume load on the single ventricle. This will result in heart failure and pulmonary overflow. The pressures in the pulmonary artery will also be elevated, and obstructive pulmonary vascular disease is likely to develop if no surgical intervention is performed. In this case, the surgical strategy is to perform a banding of the pulmonary artery. Adequate banding is required to reduce pulmonary artery pressures and to prevent the development of pulmonary vascular disease. As discussed later, a low pulmonary vascular resistance is required for long-term palliation.

If there is obstruction to pulmonary flow caused by pulmonary stenosis or atresia or by high pulmonary vascular resistance, there will be desaturation and hypoxia. Early after birth, this may cause the pulmonary circulation to be duct dependent. In those cases, ductal patency can be prolonged with prostaglandins and afterward by ductal stenting if the arterial duct has favorable anatomy.[6] In cases in which ductal stenting is not feasible, surgical palliation is used to increase pulmonary blood flow through different types of shunting operations. This can be either a modified Blalock-Taussig shunt or a central shunt. Shunting procedures improve the arterial oxygenation often at the expense of volume loading of the single ventricle. Because of this concern for ventricular volume loading, pulmonary blood flow may be altered to be more effective by use of a bidirectional cavopulmonary shunt, which can usually be performed at 3 to 4 months of age when the pulmonary vascular resistance has become normal. This shunt is also described in Chapter 113.

In some types of single ventricle, there may be obstruction of the outflow to the systemic circulation, which may potentially compromise systemic output and cause preferential flow to the pulmonary arteries. This can result in inadequate systemic perfusion, causing metabolic acidosis and shock. In those cases, the systemic circulation is duct dependent, and prostaglandin infusion is required in the neonatal period to stabilize those infants before surgery. The pressure load caused by the obstruction can lead to ventricular hypertrophy. As discussed later, the decreased compliance associated with hypertrophy causes unfavorable ventricular mechanics for surgical palliation later in life. Many of these hemodynamic variables are similar to those encountered in hypoplastic left heart syndrome. Different surgical options are possible to relieve the obstruction. In the past, one option has been the use of surgical procedures similar to those described in the Norwood procedure (aortopulmonary window, pulmonary artery detachment, aortic arch reconstruction, and shunting with a modified central shunt). More recently, the Sano operation has been performed to provide a more direct source of pulmonary blood supply. If there is subaortic obstruction within the heart, a Damus-Kaye-Stansel procedure is used to connect both outlets to the aorta. Currently, more centers may approach this problem by a hybrid approach in the neonatal period by stenting of the arterial duct and bilateral banding of the pulmonary arteries.[7] This postpones other major surgery to later in life.

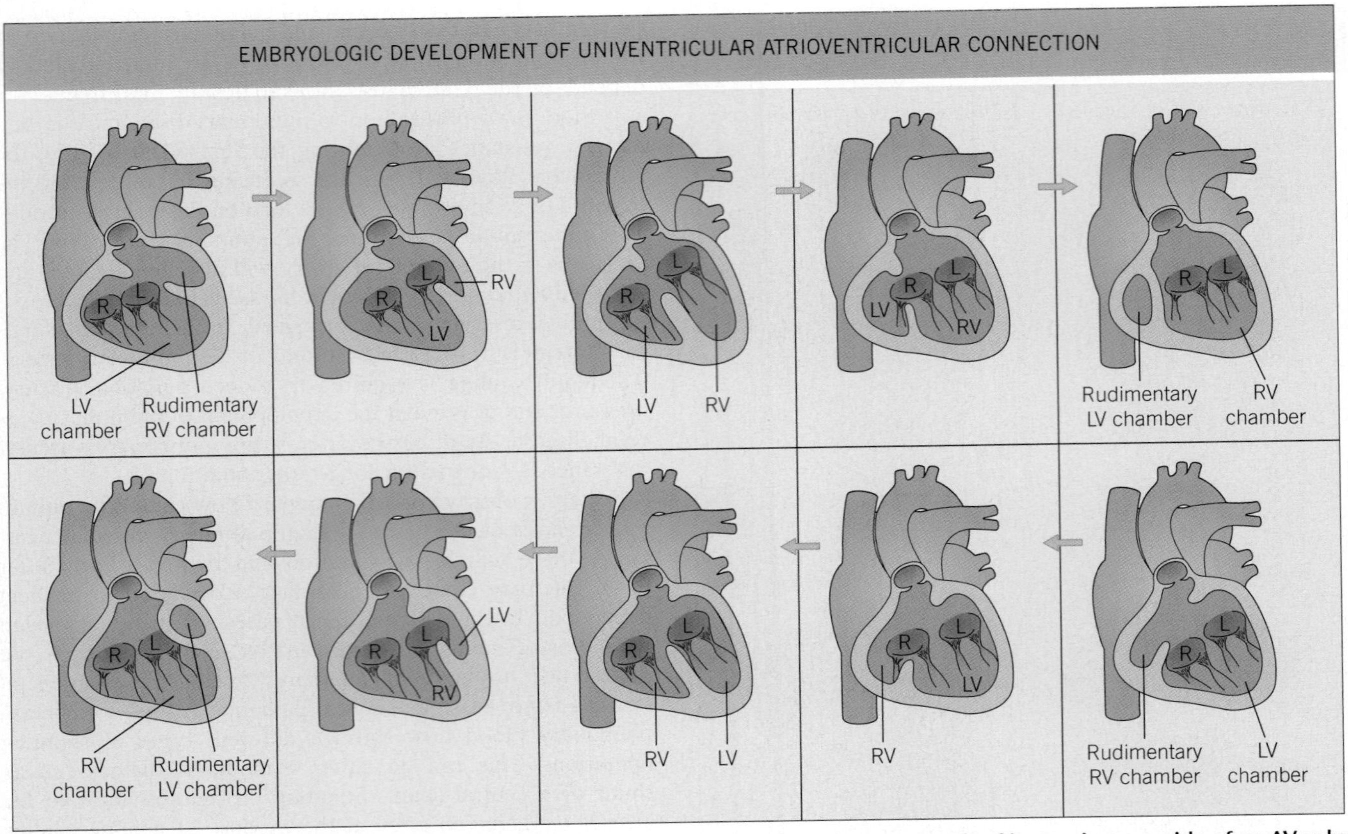

EMBRYOLOGIC DEVELOPMENT OF UNIVENTRICULAR ATRIOVENTRICULAR CONNECTION
R
L
LV chamber
Rudimentary RV chamber
R
L
RV
LV
R
L
LV
RV
LV
R
L
RV
R
L
Rudimentary LV chamber
RV chamber
R
L
RV chamber
Rudimentary LV chamber
R
L
LV
RV
R
L
RV
LV
R
L
LV
RV
R
L
Rudimentary RV chamber
LV chamber

Figure 118.3 Embryologic development of univentricular atrioventricular connection as a result of increasing override of an AV valve into the contralateral ventricle. The concept, proposed by Elliot and Gedgaudas, is applicable to virtually all forms of double-inlet ventricle whether the ventricular looping is right-handed or left-handed. LV, left ventricle; RV, right ventricle.

RV
A
LV
B

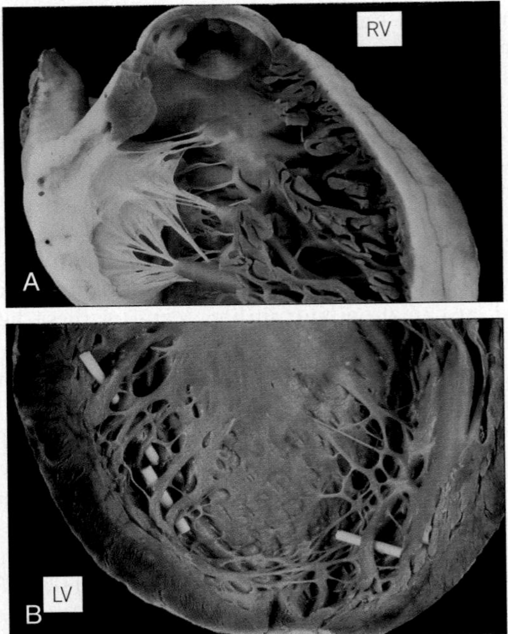

Figure 118.4 Comparative morphologic features of the right and left ventricular myocardium. Note the coarse trabeculations filling the inferior and apical portions of the right ventricle (RV) and the fine, delicate trabeculations and smooth wall of the left ventricle (LV). (Courtesy of William D. Edwards, MD.)

IVC
LA
RA
*
LV

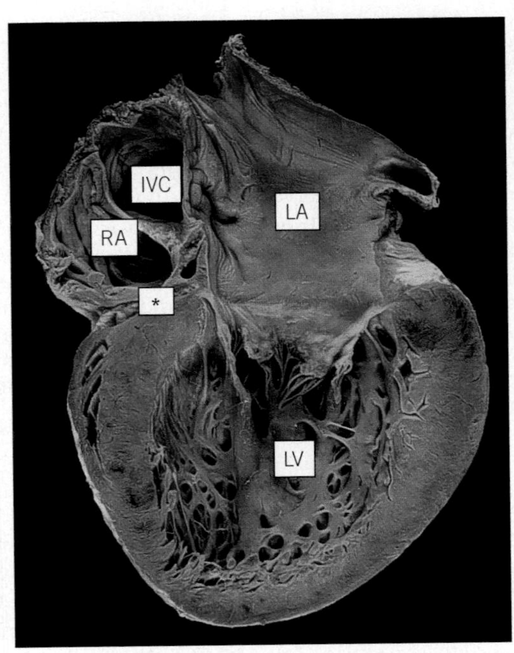

Figure 118.5 Single-inlet left ventricle with right AV valve atresia in AV concordance or classic tricuspid valve atresia. Note the atretic plate for the right AV valve *(asterisk)*. IVC, inferior vena cava; LA, left atrium; LV, left ventricle; RA, right atrium.

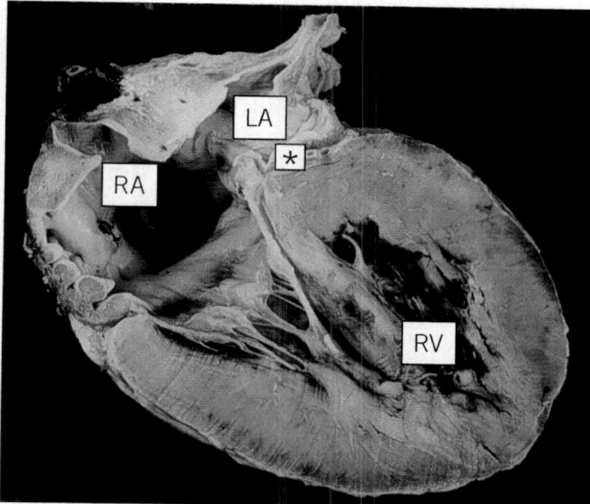

Figure 118.6 Single-inlet right ventricle with left AV valve atresia in AV concordance. Note the atretic plate of the left AV valve *(asterisk)*. LA, left atrium; RA, right atrium; RV, right ventricle.

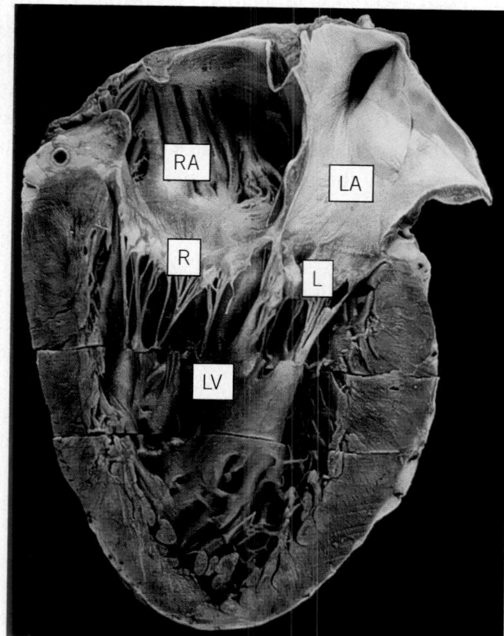

Figure 118.7 Double-inlet ventricle with left ventricular morphology (double-inlet left ventricle). L, left AV valve; LA, left atrium; LV, left ventricle; R, right AV valve; RA, right atrium.

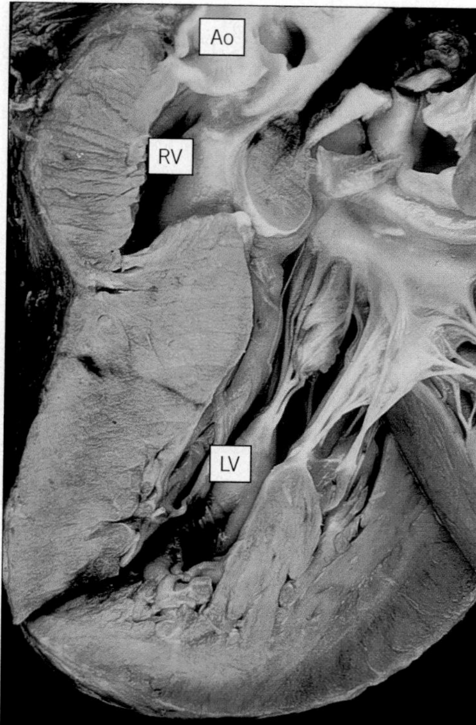

Figure 118.8 Severe subaortic obstruction at the ventricular septal defect in double-inlet left ventricle. Note the severe degree of left ventricular hypertrophy. Ao, ascending aorta; LV, left ventricle; RV, right ventricle.

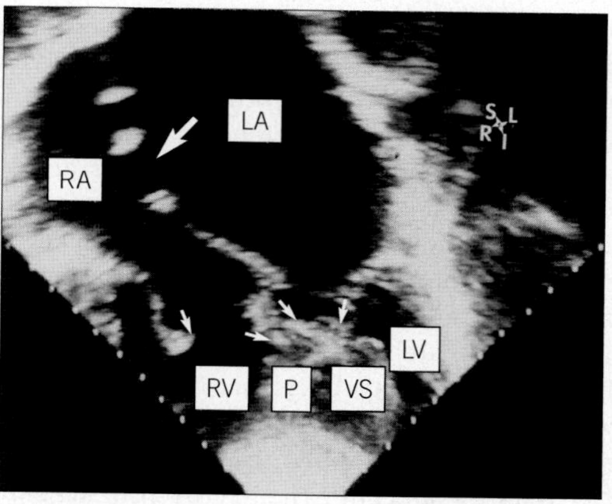

Figure 118.9 Double-inlet right ventricle with severe AV valve stenosis. LA, left atrium; LV, left ventricle; P, papillary muscle; RA, right atrium; RV, right ventricle; VS, ventricular septum.

CLINICAL PRESENTATIONS

The clinical features of univentricular AV connections are primarily determined by the presence or absence of pulmonary or systemic outflow obstruction. Patients without obstruction to the pulmonary artery blood flow present with signs and symptoms of other lesions with large left-to-right shunting (like large ventricular septal defects). The large pulmonary blood flow together with volume loading of the single ventricle causes congestive heart failure, which develops during the first 3 to 6 weeks of life, when pulmonary vascular resistance falls. The findings at that time are tachypnea, subcostal retraction, tachycardia, diaphoresis, failure to thrive, and hepatomegaly. If symptoms of congestive heart failure develop during the neonatal period, this is often secondary to associated lesions, such as AV valve abnormalities, obstruction to systemic outflow, or obstruction of pulmonary venous return (also causing more pronounced cyanosis). As pulmonary flow is high, the common mixing chamber will be associated with only mild cyanosis. A soft systolic ejection murmur secondary to flow-related relative pulmonary outflow obstruction or flow through the ventricular septal defect may often be heard. Because of the large pulmonary blood flow, a diastolic AV valve inflow murmur and a third heart sound may be present. In older patients with unobstructive pulmonary blood flow, pulmonary vascular obstructive disease may develop, resulting in progressive reduction in pulmonary blood flow and cyanosis. The second heart sound

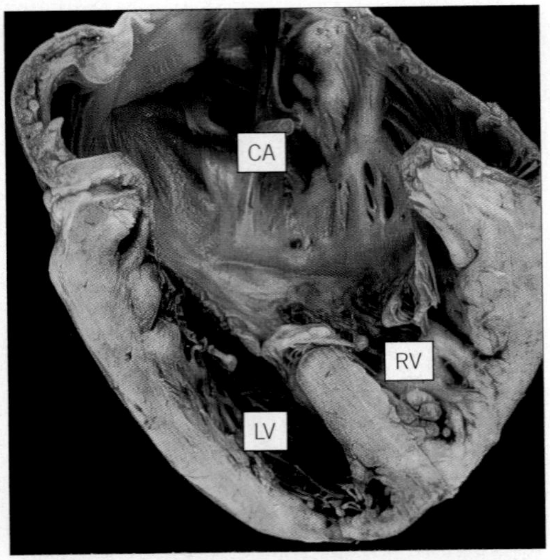

Figure 118.10 Common-inlet ventricle with ventricular inversion as observed in a left-handed ventricular loop. In this example, the two ventricles are of nearly equal size. CA, common atrium; LV, left ventricle; RV, right ventricle.

may then be loud and single. A diastolic murmur of pulmonary valve regurgitation may be present.

If pulmonary outflow obstruction or pulmonary atresia is present, hypoxemia and cyanosis are the presenting symptoms during the neonatal period. Patients with severe pulmonary stenosis or pulmonary atresia present with profound cyanosis and acidosis during the first days of life when the ductus spontaneously closes. A systolic thrill may be present with pulmonary outflow obstruction. A harsh systolic ejection murmur and single heart sound may be heard. The pulmonary valve closure sound may be audible with milder degrees of pulmonary stenosis. No murmur may be audible or there may be only a soft continuous murmur secondary to a patent ductus arteriosus or systemic-pulmonary collaterals if pulmonary atresia is present. In this case, the pulmonary circulation may be duct dependent.

If severe obstruction is present to systemic outflow (restrictive ventricular septal defect often associated with a hypoplastic aortic arch and coarctation), signs of severe organ hypoperfusion may be present during the first days of life when the ductus arteriosus spontaneously closes. This may be manifested as metabolic acidemia, oliguria, cold constricted extremities, and gut ischemia (necrotizing enterocolitis). Prompt initiation of intravenous prostaglandins is required to improve systemic cardiac output.

There may also be obstruction to the pulmonary venous return. In patients with left AV valve atresia and nearly intact interatrial septum, inadequate interatrial shunting can cause pulmonary venous hypertension because the outflow of the pulmonary venous return is severely obstructed. Symptoms may develop progressively during the first days of life as pulmonary arteriolar resistance falls and pulmonary blood flow increases. This "restrictive atrial septum" will be manifested with cyanosis and respiratory distress caused by pulmonary venous hypertension. In those cases, balloon atrial septostomy is required in the neonatal period. In rare cases, pulmonary venous hypertension may be caused by obstructed total abnormal pulmonary venous return. This is often associated with right atrial isomerism.

DIAGNOSTIC TECHNIQUES

The complete evaluation of complex congenital heart disease depends on the association of different techniques that all provide complementary information. During recent years, echocardiography has become the cornerstone in establishing the diagnosis of univentricular AV connection. It allows definition of the abnormalities in great anatomic detail and provides valuable hemodynamic information. The input of the other diagnostic modalities is discussed.

Echocardiography

Two-dimensional Doppler echocardiography has become the most important tool to establish the diagnosis of univentricular AV connections.[8-11] It allows definition of the anatomic details of the abnormal heart and the associated extracardiac abnormalities (Figs. 118.11 to 118.13). A complete description of the anatomically abnormal heart requires a careful segmental approach. First, the basic anatomy of atrial and visceral situs and location of the cardiac apex must be defined. For this purpose, subcostal views and abdominal scans are particularly useful. The same subcostal scans can be used to define the systemic and pulmonary venous connections to the atria. Abnormalities in systemic venous return, like bilateral superior caval veins or interruption of the inferior caval vein with azygos continuation, can be diagnosed echocardiographically. Abnormal pulmonary venous connections can also be identified. This is very important, especially if obstruction of pulmonary venous connection is present. Effort should be made to identify all four pulmonary veins because partial abnormal pulmonary venous connections can be present.

The diagnostic echocardiographic features of the univentricular AV connection are best viewed from an apical view delineating the crux of the heart, such as the apical four-chamber view. It can be used to describe the AV connection as being double inlet, atresia of one of the inlets, or common AV valve. In addition, parasternal and subcostal views are particularly helpful to detail the morphology of the dominant ventricle (right, left, or indeterminate), the location of the rudimentary ventricles or outlet chambers (anterior or posterior, to the left or right), the location of the papillary muscles and chordal attachments within the ventricular chambers (straddling or overriding), the status of the AV valve leaflets, and the location and commitment of the great arteries and their relationships (concordant or discordant). From the suprasternal notch, the sidedness of the aortic arch and the presence and location of a patent ductus arteriosus can be imaged. During the two-dimensional scan, it is also important to assess the size of the interatrial and interventricular communications. A restrictive interatrial communication may produce pulmonary venous obstruction, especially in left AV valve atresia. In case of tricuspid atresia, this will result in reduced cardiac output. The size of the interatrial communication should be defined by two-dimensional echocardiography, and the degree of restriction should be assessed. The size of the interventricular communication should also be evaluated. The size of the intraventricular communication between the dominant and the rudimentary ventricle can be or can become restrictive. If the aorta is originating from a small outlet right ventricle, as in double-inlet left

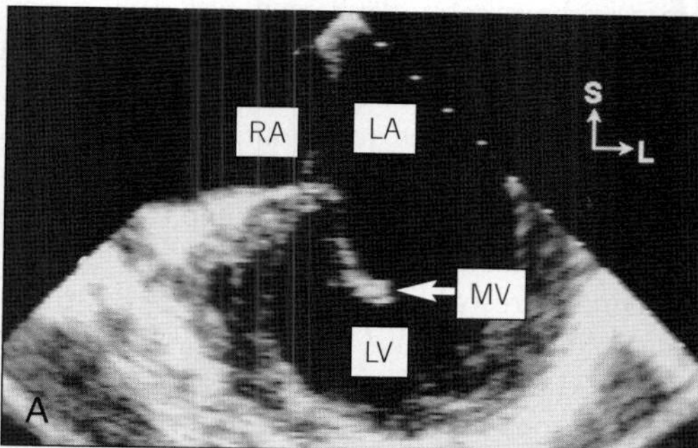

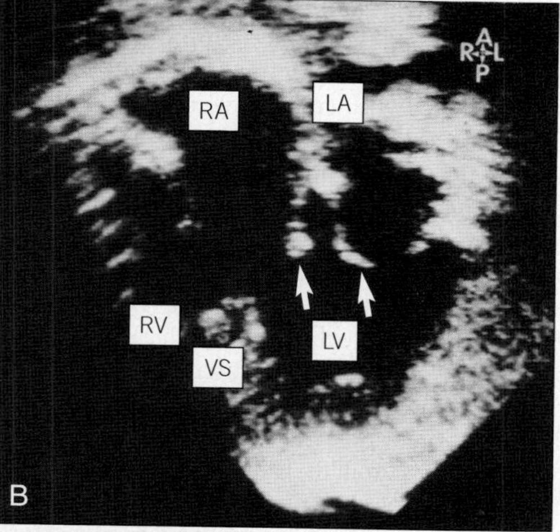

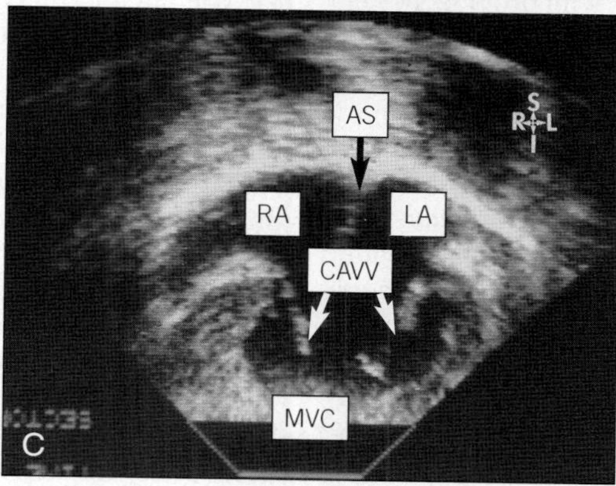

Figure 118.11 Apical four-chamber echocardiography in the diagnosis of functionally single-ventricle hearts. A, Single-inlet ventricle. **B,** Double-inlet ventricle. **C,** Common-inlet ventricle. AS, atrial septum; CAVV, common AV valve; LA, left atrium; LV, left ventricle; MV, mitral valve; MVC, main ventricular chamber; RA, right atrium; RV, right ventricle; VS, ventricular septum. The arrows point to the AV valve leaflets.

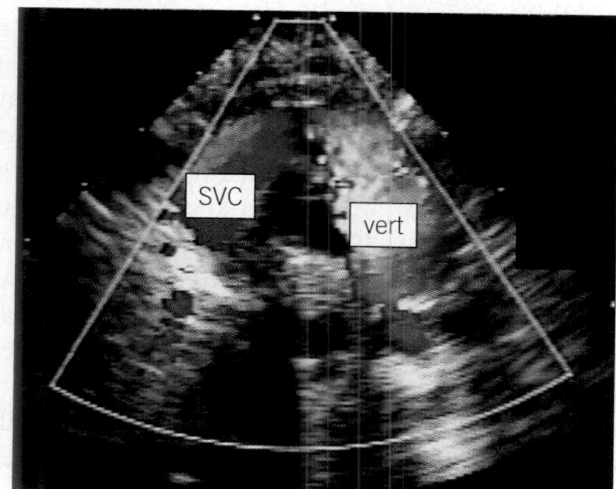

Figure 118.12 Suprasternal notch scan with color-flow imaging demonstrates total anomalous pulmonary venous connection through a vertical vein (vert) to the innominate vein in a patient with common-inlet ventricle. There is no evidence of pulmonary venous obstruction. SVC, superior vena cava.

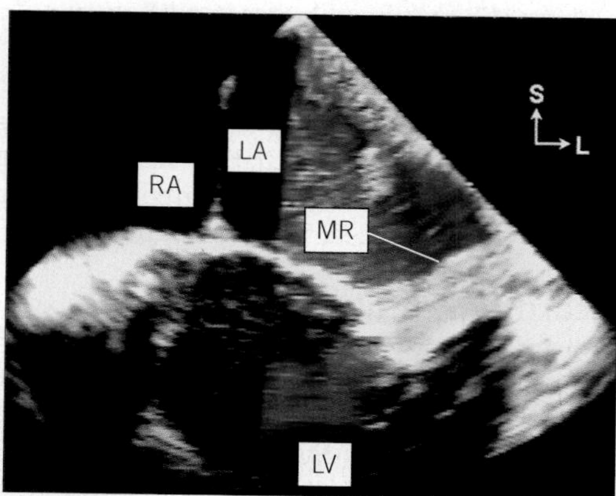

Figure 118.13 Severe left AV valve regurgitation in a patient with single-inlet ventricle and right AV valve atresia. Proximal isovelocity surface area estimates of valvular regurgitation can help in assessing the severity of regurgitation. LA, left atrium; LV, left ventricle; MR, mitral valve regurgitation; RA, right atrium.

ventricle or right AV valve atresia with transposition, a restrictive ventricular septal defect can cause severe systemic outlet obstruction. Especially the initial size of the defect is predictive of subsequent development of subaortic stenosis. Patients with an initial ventricular septal area of 2 cm^2/m^2 or less are at high risk of having associated coarctation of the aorta or even interruption of the aortic arch. They are also at risk for subsequent development of subaortic stenosis.[12]

Color-flow imaging is particularly helpful for determination of the exact location of pulmonary or systemic outflow tract obstruction. Subvalvular, valvular, or supravalvular stenosis can be defined. Ductal, interventricular, and interatrial shunting can also be evaluated by color-flow imaging.

Both the location and the degree of shunting can be viewed. Finally, color-flow imaging is extremely helpful in assessing AV valve function; stenosis and AV valve regurgitation can be recognized and evaluated with color-flow imaging. Pulsed and continuous Doppler study of the outflow tracts can be added to quantify the degree of outflow obstruction.

Two-dimensional echocardiography can also be used to assess global ventricular function. Wall motion abnormalities are common in single ventricle, limiting the usefulness of M-mode–derived measurements of shortening fraction or ejection fraction. Volumetric techniques such as biplane Simpson's volumes can provide useful estimates of ventricular volume and systolic function (ejection fraction), but these techniques are all based on geometric assumptions of a normal left ventricle. This may limit their applicability to more complex single ventricles. Possibly the further development of three-dimensional echocardiography will provide better tools to evaluate systolic function of the single ventricle, but this needs further validation.[13]

Chest Radiography

In the era of modern ultrasonography, the diagnostic value of chest radiography in patients with univentricular AV connection is probably limited. The chest film can provide information on the position of the heart within the chest (levocardia, mesocardia, or dextrocardia). The sidedness of the stomach bubble also provides information about visceral situs. Further findings on chest radiography are variable and depend on the anatomic type of single ventricle as well as on the presence or absence of pulmonary or systemic outflow obstruction. When pulmonary blood flow is unobstructed, there will be cardiomegaly with increased pulmonary vascular markings. When pulmonary flow is moderately obstructed, there may be a normal heart size and normal or slightly decreased pulmonary vascular markings. When there is severe obstruction of the pulmonary outflow or pulmonary atresia, pulmonary vascular markings are reduced or asymmetric because of systemic–pulmonary artery collaterals. If pulmonary venous obstruction is present, the lung fields may show a reticular pattern characteristic of pulmonary venous engorgement, although associated pulmonary outflow obstruction may conceal this typical picture.

Electrocardiography

An electrocardiogram will give important information about the cardiac rhythm and AV conduction.[14] In most patients, the rhythm is sinus, except in case of isomerism, when junctional or left atrial type of rhythm may be present. The PR interval is normal, although first-degree AV block has been reported in up to 30% of all cases. The frontal axis of the QRS vector is variable. Most cases with a common AV valve of the AV septal defect type have left axis deviation (−40 to 120 degrees) as commonly observed in the biventricular forms of AV septal defects. Left axis deviation, however, can also be present in other forms of single ventricle, especially right AV valve atresia (tricuspid atresia). Thus, the status of AV valves cannot be predicted from the frontal QRS axis. Depending on ventricular morphology, different patterns of right, left, and biventricular hypertrophy can be present on the electrocardiogram. The ventricular morphology (right or left) cannot be predicted on the basis of electrocardiographic characteristics.

Magnetic Resonance Imaging

In the management and preparation of patients for the different stages of palliation, magnetic resonance imaging has taken on an important role in different centers. In most infants, a detailed echocardiographic examination allows the cardiac malformation to be reliably diagnosed, and only for interventional reasons like a balloon septostomy or ductal stenting is a cardiac catheterization still required. If there is some doubt about certain connections or pulmonary blood supply, magnetic resonance imaging provides a good alternative for better description of the morphology of complex congenital heart disease before consideration and planning of a cardiac catheterization. Magnetic resonance imaging gives information not only on morphology but also on blood flow and ventricular function. Three-dimensional reconstruction techniques with use of magnetic resonance imaging have now become the "gold standard" for volume and mass assessment of unusually shaped ventricles.[15] Magnetic resonance tagging techniques also allow quantification of regional myocardial mechanics, although the clinical value of this experimental technique is still uncertain.[16] More and more, cardiac magnetic resonance imaging is replacing routine cardiac catheterization. A recent prospective randomized trial has shown that in the preoperative evaluation before a bidirectional Glenn shunt, cardiac magnetic resonance imaging can safely replace routine cardiac catheterization.[17] The same might be true in the preoperative evaluation for the total cavopulmonary connection.[18]

Cardiac Catheterization and Angiography

Because of the development of the other imaging techniques, the role of cardiac catheterization in the evaluation of univentricular AV connection has changed importantly. As the anatomy will in most cases be completely described by echocardiography or by cardiac magnetic resonance imaging, the current indications for a diagnostic cardiac catheterization are limited. Only if certain clinically relevant information cannot be reliably obtained by the echocardiographic examination or one of the other imaging modalities should a catheterization be considered. Currently, the majority of children with functionally single ventricles will undergo the first operation (like banding of the pulmonary artery, a modified Blalock-Taussig shunt, or even a Norwood-type repair) and even subsequent palliative procedures without a cardiac catheterization. If children are referred for cardiac catheterization, the indication will be interventional in most cases.

A possible indication for catheterization is the identification of systemic and pulmonary venous connections if there is any doubt on echocardiography. In addition, catheterization may be performed to determine

- adequacy of the interatrial communication;
- AV connections;
- basic ventricular morphology, ventricular volume, and systolic function;
- ventricle–great artery connections;
- pulmonary artery size, pressure, and resistance;
- systemic circulation; and
- abnormal venovenous or aorta to pulmonary collaterals.

Adequacy of the Interatrial Communication

A large interatrial communication is often present; but in some cases, the interatrial communication may be restrictive and obstructing pulmonary or systemic venous drainage.

If necessary, atrial balloon or blade septostomy or stenting of the intra-atrial septum should be performed.

AV Connections

Although echocardiography will generally provide excellent demonstration of the status of the AV connections, angiography can demonstrate AV valve commitment, determine annulus size, and assess the presence and severity of AV valve regurgitation.

Ventricular Morphology, Ventricular Volume, and Systolic Function

The basic ventricular morphology, ventricular volume, and systolic function can be evaluated by angiography. Despite the irregular shape of the ventricle, a good estimate of the ejection fraction can be obtained from ventricular volume calculations. Ventricular diastolic function can be assessed by measuring end-diastolic volume, ventricular mass, and atrial filling pressures and end-diastolic pressures.

Ventricle–Great Artery Connections

By use of angiography, the connection of the great arteries to the ventricles can be assessed. The patency of the outflow tracts can also be evaluated by careful catheter pressure measurements and angiography (Fig. 118.14).

Pulmonary Artery Size, Pressure, and Resistance

This is probably still one of the very important indications for cardiac catheterization as pulmonary artery size and distribution are critical components in planning palliative surgical procedures. Central pulmonary artery size can be measured, and distortion or stenoses of the central or distal pulmonary arteries can be excluded. A pulmonary artery index was proposed by Nakata and associates,[19] a normal value being more than 330 mm^2/m^2. Previously placed systemic-to-pulmonary or cavopulmonary shunts must be angiographically demonstrated. Preoperative assessment should also include measurement of pulmonary artery pressure and calculation of the pulmonary arteriolar resistance. Mair and colleagues[20] derived a Fontan index, which includes pulmonary arteriolar resistance (Ra_p), ventricular end-diastolic pressure (VEDP), and systemic and pulmonary flow volumes (Fontan index $= Ra_p +$ VEDP/Qs + Qp). Surgical mortality after a modified Fontan procedure was lower in patients with a Fontan index below 4. If any significant stenosis of the pulmonary arteries is present, balloon angioplasty or stent implantation can be considered.

Systemic Circulation

The aortic arch anatomy should clearly be defined by angiography. The location of the aortic arch and brachiocephalic branches, the presence of a ductus arteriosus, and systemic

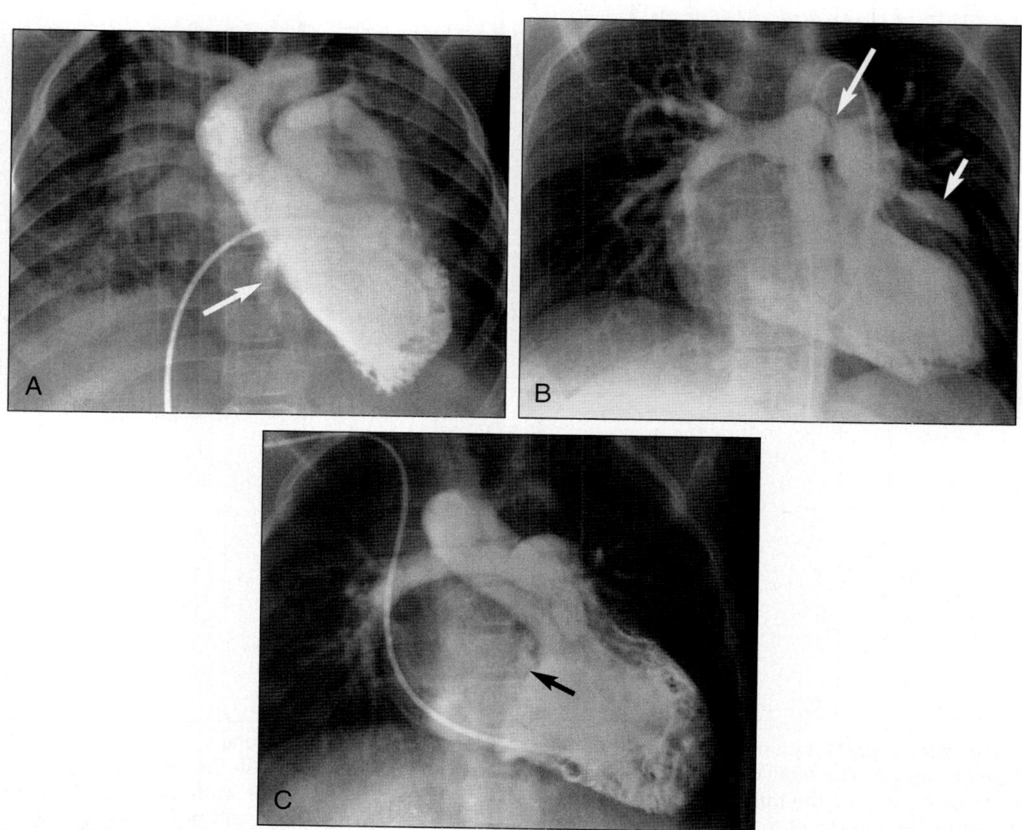

Figure 118.14 Angiographic studies in the diagnosis of functionally single-ventricle hearts. A, Typical anteroposterior and lateral angiographic features of single-inlet left ventricle with right AV valve atresia. Note the hypoplastic stenotic subpulmonary right ventricle *(arrow)*. **B,** Anteroposterior view of typical double-inlet left ventricle with a hypoplastic subaortic right ventricle *(short arrow)*. A pulmonary artery band is also evident *(long arrow)*. **C,** Anteroposterior view of common-inlet ventricle of right ventricular morphology. Note the large common AV valve orifice *(arrow)*.

to pulmonary artery collaterals should all be determined. Coarctation of the aorta should be excluded because the increased afterload would be poorly tolerated after the modified Fontan procedure.

Abnormal Venovenous or Aorta to Pulmonary Collaterals

Venovenous collaterals can be present after a bidirectional cavopulmonary anastomosis. These often originate on the innominate vein and connect to the atrium or pulmonary veins. These collaterals can be closed by coiling or use of a vascular plug. Aorta to pulmonary artery collaterals can also be present, causing additional flow to the pulmonary arteries. If significant, they need to be closed before the Fontan operation.

MANAGEMENT

A normal cardiovascular system consists of a double pulmonary and systemic circuit, connected in series, powered by two ventricular pumps—the "right" and "left" heart. A functioning single ventricle has to maintain both the systemic and pulmonary circulations, which are not connected in series but in parallel (Fig. 118.15).[21] Such a circuit has two major disadvantages: arterial desaturation, both at rest and increasing during exercise, and a chronic volume overload to the single ventricle. Chronic volume overload will in time impair ventricular function, causing from the third decade onward congestive heart failure and death. In 1971, Francis Fontan[22] reported a new approach to the surgical palliation of these malformations, separating the systemic and pulmonary circulations. In a "Fontan circulation," the systemic venous return

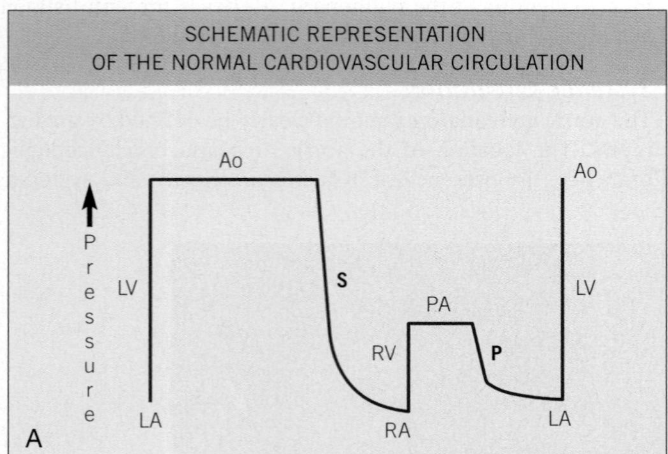

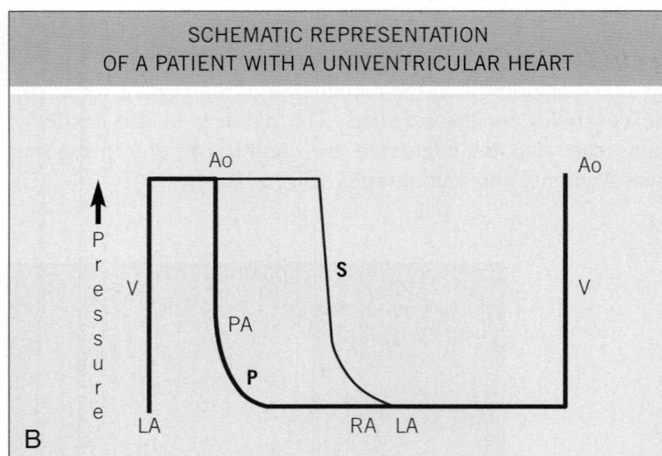

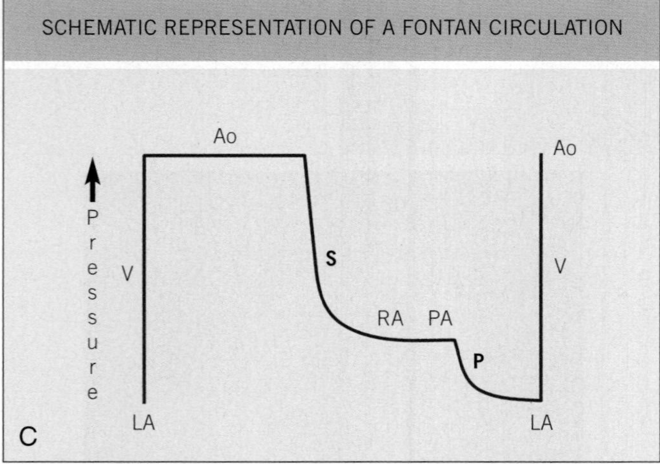

Figure 118.15 A, Schematic representation of the normal cardiovascular circulation. The pulmonary circulation (P) is connected in series with the systemic circulation (S). The right ventricle maintains the right atrial pressure lower than the left atrial pressure and provides enough energy to the blood to pass the pulmonary resistance. Ao, aorta; LA, left atrium; LV, left ventricle; PA, pulmonary artery; RV, right ventricle. **B,** Schematic representation of a patient with a univentricular heart. The systemic (S) and pulmonary (P) circuits are connected in parallel, with a considerable volume overload to the single ventricle (V). The width of the line reflects the degree of volume load. There is complete admixture of systemic and pulmonary venous blood, causing arterial oxygen desaturation. **C,** Schematic representation of a Fontan circulation. The systemic (S) and pulmonary (P) circulations are connected in series. The right atrium (RA) or systemic veins are connected to the pulmonary artery (PA). The volume overload to the single ventricle is now less than expected for body surface area. In the absence of a fenestration, there is no more admixture of systemic and pulmonary venous blood, but the systemic venous pressure is markedly elevated.

is connected directly to the pulmonary arteries without the interposition of a ventricular pump (see Fig. 118.15). Advantages of a Fontan circuit are that the arterial saturations nearly normalize and that the ventricular volume overload is relieved. This occurs at the expense of a chronic increase in systemic venous pressures and a decreased cardiac output both at rest and during exercise. The most important determinant for cardiac output in this circulation is the transpulmonary gradient, which is mainly determined by pulmonary vascular resistance and atrial pressures.

Since its original description, the Fontan circuit has known numerous modifications. Initially, surgeons used valves and created various connections between the right atrium and the pulmonary artery (anterior atriopulmonary connection, with or without inclusion of a small hypoplastic right ventricle; posterior atriopulmonary connection), with different materials (valved conduits, homografts, patches, direct anastomosis). The very high incidence of late reoperations, up to 40% in some series, did reflect the suboptimal design of the first Fontan circuits. These older circuits are no longer created and are considered obsolete; however, many patients still survive after this type of surgery. Therefore, it is important to know which type of surgery these older Fontan patients underwent before evaluating them. These initial connections were replaced by the total cavopulmonary connection. In this approach, both caval veins are connected to the pulmonary artery, bypassing not only the right ventricle but also the right atrium. The superior vena cava is connected directly to the pulmonary artery (cavopulmonary anastomosis, also referred to as bidirectional Glenn shunt). There are currently two variants to connect the inferior vena cava: the lateral tunnel and the extracardiac conduit. Introduced in the mid-1980s, the lateral tunnel is a prosthetic baffle in the atrium between the inferior vena cava and the pulmonary artery. Because of inclusion of native atrial tissue, this connection has growth potential and can therefore be created in children as young as 1 year. The disadvantage is that a minimal amount of atrial tissue remains exposed to high pressure, and there is a large suture line within the atrium that in time may be a substrate for atrial arrhythmia. Therefore, the extracardiac conduit was introduced in the 1990s; it is a tube graft between the transected inferior vena cava and the pulmonary artery. This circuit leaves the entire atrium at low pressure and avoids suture lines within the atrium. It can be performed without aortic cross-clamping or even cardiopulmonary bypass. As the extracardiac graft has no growth potential, the operation can be offered only to patients large enough to allow placement of an adult size conduit (16 to 18 mm). This influenced the current strategy to achieve the Fontan circulation and resulted in a staged approach whereby the Fontan operation is prepared through different palliative steps tailored to the patient's individual needs.

The Staged Approach to an Extracardiac Fontan Circulation

During the first 2 to 3 months of life, it is not possible to create a Fontan circulation because of the neonatal increased pulmonary vascular resistance and the small size of the vessels. During this period, there is a progressive fall in pulmonary artery resistance, making a cavopulmonary connection possible after 3 to 4 months of life. Currently, a staged approach is preferred, connecting the superior and inferior caval veins during two different steps. Such staged approach allows the cardiac condition to be better optimized for the Fontan circulation and reduces the overall operative morbidity and mortality.

Initially, in the neonatal period, management must aim to provide unrestricted flow from the heart to the aorta (if required: coarctectomy, Damus-Kaye-Stansel procedure, Norwood repair), a well-balanced limited flow to the lungs (if required: pulmonary artery band, shunt [modified Blalock-Taussig shunt, central shunt, or stent in duct]), and unrestricted return of blood to the ventricle (if required: Rashkind balloon septostomy). The infant is then allowed to grow for several months. During this time, the heart is submitted to a chronic volume overload, which is good for development of the pulmonary vasculature; but if it is excessive, negative influences are exerted on ventricular function. The infant will have mild desaturation, inversely related to mild cardiac failure. At the age of 4 to 12 months, most centers will perform a cavopulmonary connection or bidirectional Glenn shunt. This includes anastomosis of the cardiac end of the superior vena cava to the ipsilateral pulmonary artery, leaving the pulmonary arteries confluent. Through this type of shunt, the systemic venous return from the upper part of the body is directed toward the pulmonary artery, bypassing the heart. This provides pulmonary blood flow while at the same time reducing the volume load on the single ventricle if other shunts are eliminated or reduced. The creation of this type of shunt is a preparation for the later Fontan procedure, in which the inferior vena cava flow is also redirected to the pulmonary artery. The disadvantage of the bidirectional cavopulmonary anastomosis is that when the pulmonary arteries are small at the time the shunt is created, the absence of pulsatile flow might provide insufficient growth stimulus for the pulmonary arteries.[21] This can result in small pulmonary arteries at the time of Fontan completion, which can cause an unsatisfactory outcome. The bidirectional cavopulmonary shunt provides insufficient pulmonary blood flow for adequate palliation of the univentricular AV connection beyond 6 to 7 years of age. The presence of a bidirectional cavopulmonary shunt as the only source of pulmonary blood flow may also be a potent stimulus for the development of multiple systemic to pulmonary artery collateral vessels to provide more pulmonary flow. Unfortunately, these collaterals do not stimulate pulmonary artery growth and are hemodynamically unfavorable after a Fontan procedure.

Most patients will undergo Fontan completion at the age of 1 to 5 years, depending on preference of the center, growth of vascular structures, and cyanosis at rest and during exercise. The Fontan circuit is completed by connection of the inferior caval vein to the pulmonary artery, currently by putting in an extracardiac conduit or lateral tunnel. Some centers advocate the use of a residual fenestration between the conduit and the atrium as an intermediate step toward further Fontan completion. In some studies, it has been suggested that this further reduces early mortality and morbidity, especially in those patients who are considered to be at high risk for the Fontan procedure. The fenestration decompresses the systemic veins by allowing right-to-left shunting and increases preload of the single ventricle. It thus increases cardiac output at the expense of some degree of desaturation. It is possibly helpful in adapting the body to the new circulation. This fenestration can later be closed percutaneously by different devices.

In 1996, Hausdorf and colleagues[23] introduced the concept of percutaneous Fontan completion. Instead of a classic bidirectional Glenn operation, a hemi-Fontan operation is performed. In this approach, the upper part of the transected superior vena cava is connected to the right pulmonary artery; at the same time, the lower part connecting to the right atrium is connected to the pulmonary artery, but this connection is sealed off by a fenestrated patch or banding. This connection from the atrium to the pulmonary artery is used later to connect the inferior caval vein to the pulmonary artery by putting in a covered stent, opening up the restrictive communication.

The overall early mortality after Fontan-type surgery has decreased significantly during the past 10 years. Comparing early mortality in a very early cohort of patients (operation between 1973 and 1986) with that in a more recent cohort (operation between 1987 and 1992) in the Mayo Clinic, early mortality decreased from 16% to 9%.[24,25] This decline occurred despite increased anatomic complexity of patients. The very recent outcomes with the staged approach suggest a further reduction in Fontan mortality. d'Udekem and colleagues[26] reported the Melbourne experience with a hospital mortality of 6% between 1980 and 1990 and a 0% mortality of the Fontan procedure after 1990. Risk factors for early mortality include a common AV valve, elevated mean preoperative pulmonary artery resistance, and ventricular dysfunction. Early problems after surgery include low output state, prolonged pleural effusions, and atrial arrhythmias.

PROGNOSIS

Since the Fontan operation was first introduced in 1973, it is still uncertain how this type of palliation affects the long-term survival of these patients. The data are encouraging, however, as survival into adulthood and even successful outcome of pregnancy have been reported.[24,25] Current survival data show a 20-year survival of up to 84%, with a better survival for the more recent techniques (15-year survival of 94% for the lateral tunnel technique; only 81% for the atriopulmonary connection).[26] Patients report a subjective improvement in their quality of life after the Fontan operation, and exercise tolerance improves compared with their preoperative condition. Most patients are reported to be in New York Heart Association functional class I and class II. Exercise capacity continues to be subnormal in most patients, as indicated by a decreased maximal oxygen uptake and a decreased ventilatory anaerobic threshold. Exercise tolerance remains relatively stable during the range of 13 years after the Fontan operation. It seems, however, that poor functional outcome becomes more frequent with increasing duration of follow-up. Possibly, failure of the Fontan circulation related to ventricular dysfunction and the effects of chronically elevated systemic venous pressures may become a common problem beyond the third to fourth decade of life. One of the major concerns is the long-term preservation of single ventricular function. Improved management early in life aimed at maximal preservation of ventricular function by reducing volume overload and hypoxia and optimizing the pulmonary circulation by preventing pulmonary vascular disease and pulmonary hypoplasia and distortion could improve the long-term functional outcome of the Fontan operation.

Long-term problems include ventricular dysfunction, AV valve insufficiency, atrial arrhythmia, thromboembolic complications, and protein-losing enteropathy. Often, but not always, these complications appear to be secondary to excessively elevated right atrial and systemic venous pressures and chronic reduced cardiac output. This can be caused by mechanical problems in the Fontan connections, like obstruction to the atriopulmonary or cavopulmonary connections, pulmonary artery distortion or hypoplasia, pulmonary vascular disease, pulmonary venous obstruction, significant AV or semilunar valve regurgitation, and residual left-to-right shunts. Especially the occurrence of protein-losing enteropathy is a bothersome problem that often is very difficult to treat.[27] It occurs in about 1% to 5% of all Fontan patients and is associated with a very high morbidity and mortality.

The Failing Fontan Circulation

A Fontan circulation may fail, causing persistent systemic venous congestion with edema, low cardiac output, very limited exercise tolerance, tachycardia, protein-losing enteropathy, or plastic bronchitis. Immediate complete evaluation of these patients including cardiac catheterization is required. Underlying causes, such as conduit stenosis, stenosis of the pulmonary arteries, thrombosis in the conduit, extensive aorta-pulmonary collaterals, severe AV valve insufficiency, increased pulmonary vascular resistance, and ventricular dysfunction, need to be identified. Prevention of these problems is important in the preparation before the Fontan operation and also in the management afterward. Depending on the underlying cause, a treatment strategy can be developed. In some patients, no good underlying cause can be found. Classic heart failure treatment consisting of inotropes, vasodilators, and diuretics will usually show little effect. If possible, optimizing the circuit can improve the patient's condition. This can consist of dilatation or stenting of stenosis, embolization of collaterals, and conversion of older circuits to total cavopulmonary connection. For those patients in whom ventricular failure is the main problem, cardiac transplantation is often the only alternative. This can be performed with good results even for patients with complex anatomy.[28] Another important problem that might develop is a small but progressive rise in pulmonary vascular resistance by microthrombi or endothelial dysfunction in the pulmonary circulation. This often becomes obvious only after cardiac transplantation,[29] as the evaluation of pulmonary vascular resistance in this nonpulsatile lung perfusion is not evident.

SUMMARY

In patients with univentricular AV connection, the segmental approach should be used to give a complete description of the anatomy. The pathophysiology depends on the underlying anatomy and always includes common mixing physiology.

The clinical presentation can be diverse, ranging from severe cyanosis to severe congestive heart failure. Echocardiography has become the standard technique for determination of the anatomy and hemodynamics of the lesion. Cardiac catheterization often provides additional information, especially on pulmonary artery anatomy, size, and pressures. Presently, management is directed toward a modified Fontan operation. When the patient is younger than 6 months, palliative procedures, including banding of the pulmonary artery or systemic to pulmonary artery shunts, are performed if necessary. After 4 to 6 months of age, a bidirectional cavopulmonary shunt could be considered to effectively provide sufficient pulmonary blood flow while reducing ventricular volume loading. This, in conjunction with additional pulmonary flow, either through a residual systemic to pulmonary artery shunt or through anterograde pulmonary flow, may provide adequate palliation for at least the next few years of life. A more final form of palliation is a Fontan-type operation in which the entire systemic venous return is directed to the pulmonary circulation, bypassing the heart. The 20-year survival of patients with a Fontan circulation is about 90% to 95% in the current era. The life expectancy of patients with this type of palliation is still uncertain.

chapter

119 Patent Ductus Arteriosus

John Thomson and Shakeel Qureshi

The ductus arteriosus, a muscular artery present in mammalian fetuses, connects the pulmonary artery to the descending aorta. It provides an unrestrictive conduit that allows blood ejected from the right ventricle to bypass the fetal lung bed and enter the aorta.

Closure of the ductus arteriosus normally occurs in the hours after birth in response to changing arterial oxygen tension and altered concentrations of circulating prostaglandins.[1] Failure of this process leads to a persistent or patent ductus arteriosus (PDA), a cardiac defect first recognized by Galen (born AD 131). A PDA is a common lesion, representing 6% to 12% of congenital heart disease, and is particularly prevalent in premature infants as a result of immature vascular and biochemical physiology.[2,3]

After birth, an isolated PDA allows left-to-right shunting from the high-pressure aorta to the lower pressure pulmonary artery. If a large enough connection is present, clinical signs and symptoms of a significant left-to-right shunt will develop eventually.

A subgroup of infants rely on postnatal patency of the ductus arteriosus for survival in the presence of an additional important congenital heart lesion. In these infants, maintenance of the "fetal" circulation by keeping the ductus arteriosus open before definitive palliation is lifesaving.

ANATOMY AND NORMAL FUNCTION

The ductus arteriosus develops at about the sixth week of fetal life and is formed from the dorsal portion of the paired sixth aortic arch.[4] During normal development of the cardiovascular system, the common arterial trunk divides to form the aorta and the pulmonary trunk; the sixth arch remains in continuity between the newly formed pulmonary artery and the aorta to form the ductus arteriosus (Figs. 119.1 and 119.2). The normal ductus arteriosus in a fetus with a left aortic arch is a product of the left-sided dorsal sixth aortic arch after regression of the right-sided sixth dorsal arch. In the presence of a right-sided aortic arch, regression of the paired sixth aortic arches is less predictable, and the ductus arteriosus may be either left- or right-sided, connecting the aorta to either the right or left pulmonary artery. Numerous other anatomic variants are described, most of which can be explained on the basis of regression or persistence of portions of the sixth aortic arch.[5,6]

The ductus arteriosus inserts into the lesser curve of the aorta at the transition from the arch to the descending aorta (usually distal to the left subclavian artery; see Fig. 119.2). It differs histologically from both the aorta and the pulmonary artery in having both a thicker intima and a media consisting predominantly of smooth muscle cells with increased amounts of hyaluronic acid.[7]

The size of the ductus arteriosus in the fetus reflects the relative blood flow through the vessel. Before birth, right ventricular ejection is responsible for approximately two thirds of cardiac output; the proportion of cardiac output passing through the fetal lung bed is less than 10%. Therefore, the ductus arteriosus, acting as a conduit vessel from the right ventricle to the aorta, carries approximately 60% of total fetal cardiac output.

Closure of the Ductus Arteriosus

Normal closure of the ductus arteriosus occurs in two phases. The first phase of early or functional closure occurs in the first 12 hours of life in response to a number of major changes.[8] Before birth, high pulmonary vascular resistance and low arterial oxygen tension both directly favor ductal patency. In addition, the prostaglandins E_1, E_2, and prostacyclin are potent vasodilators of the ductus arteriosus and play an important role in maintaining its patency during fetal life.[1,9] Circulating prostaglandins are produced by the placenta, and during fetal life, prostaglandin metabolism in the lung tissue (where prostaglandin metabolism is most active) is almost absent as a consequence of low pulmonary blood flow.[1,10]

After birth, there is a lowering of the pulmonary vascular resistance, a rise in the arterial oxygen concentration, and a sudden and dramatic increase in pulmonary blood flow (and hence prostaglandin metabolism) along with the disconnection of an important source of circulating prostanoids (the placenta). The response of the ductus arteriosus to these changes is contraction of medial smooth muscle, leading to wall thickening, reduction in ductal length, and functional closure. This process starts at the pulmonary artery end of the ductus arteriosus and extends toward the aorta, resulting in the characteristic dome shape of the ductal ampulla at the aortic end observed even after closure (Fig. 119.3a, b).[7,11] For a time, the ductus may reopen in response to a change in homeostasis, hence the high prevalence of patent ductus in infants with low oxygen saturations, such as those with the meconium aspiration syndrome.

The second phase is anatomic closure. This occurs as a result of further shortening and thickening of the ductal wall followed by necrosis of the intimal and medial layers in response to cessation of blood flow. Proliferating muscle cells and elastic tissue infiltrate the media and intima, eventually to be replaced by collagen. By the age of 3 weeks, the process is usually irreversible, and eventually fibrosis converts the ductus arteriosus into the ligamentum arteriosum.[12-14]

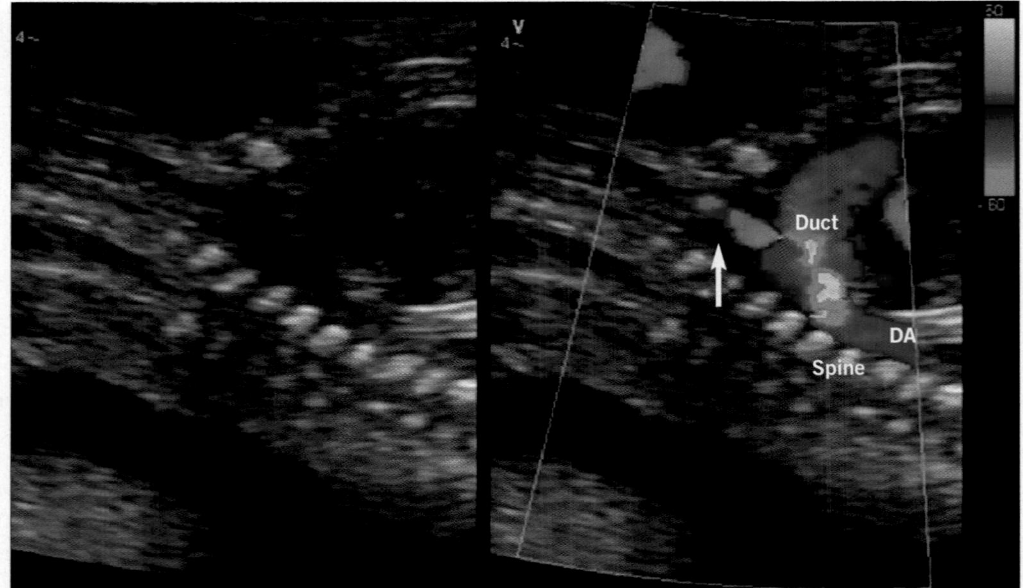

Figure 119.1 Two-dimensional and color Doppler ultrasound images of an 18-week-old fetus. Flow (blue) is across the ductus arteriosus (marked "duct") into the descending aorta (DA). Note flow away from the descending aorta in the head and neck vessels (red, *arrow*).

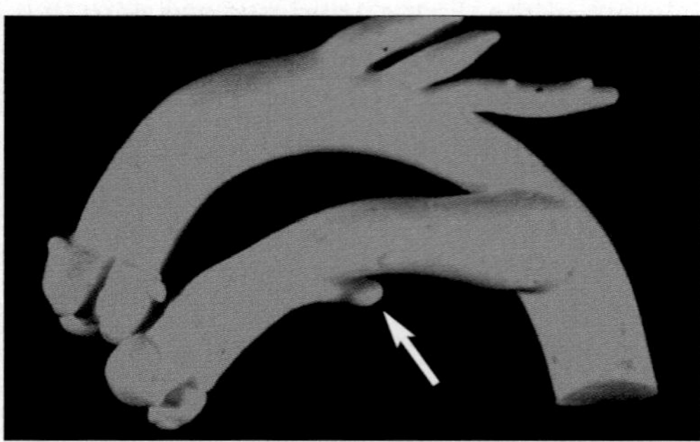

Figure 119.2 Fetal ductus arteriosus (silicon rubber cast) from week 27 of pregnancy. The right pulmonary artery branch is visible behind the ductus *(arrow);* the left pulmonary artery branch has not been prepared so that the duct can be more clearly visualized. (Courtesy of Malte Neuss, MD.)

The Persistently Patent Ductus Arteriosus

A ductus arteriosus present in a term infant of more than 3 months of age is termed persistent and is abnormal. It is a common lesion occurring in approximately 1 in 1800 live term births and represents 6% to 12% of congenital cardiac defects.[2,15] In about 15% of cases, the ductus arteriosus is associated with other congenital cardiac lesions (see later).[15,16]

A number of risk factors for persistence of the ductus arteriosus have been identified, including prematurity, maternal rubella infection (the virus interferes with the formation of normal arterial elastic tissue), and high altitude (as a consequence of lower $Pa{O_2}$). PDAs are sometimes identified in more than one member of the same family, suggesting a genetic element in some instances, an observation supported in studies of animal models.[7]

PATHOPHYSIOLOGY

The magnitude of the left-to-right shunt in a persistent ductus arteriosus is determined by the width and length of the ductus and the pulmonary vascular resistance.

Immediately after birth, the pulmonary vascular resistance remains high, so in a newborn infant, there is a small shunt regardless of the size of the PDA. As the pulmonary vascular resistance falls during the first few weeks of life, the degree of left-to-right shunting increases, and the physical characteristics of the ductus become the major determinant of the size of the shunt. A child with a large PDA, beyond the early weeks of life, will have a significant left-to-right shunt with characteristic clinical symptoms and signs. If a large ductus is left untreated for many years, the inevitable consequence of a large shunt through an unrestrictive PDA is irreversible damage to the distal pulmonary arterioles and a permanent elevation in the pulmonary vascular resistance (pulmonary vascular disease).[17] In a patient with pulmonary vascular disease as a consequence of a large PDA, the direction of flow through the ductus will eventually reverse, leading to a right-to-left shunt and central cyanosis.

CLINICAL SIGNS AND SYMPTOMS

An infant with a large PDA and a significant left-to-right shunt is usually breathless. There is a high likelihood of associated failure to thrive. The left ventricular stroke volume is increased, leading to cardiomegaly and a displaced apex beat. Aortic runoff of blood flow to the pulmonary arterial bed results in a low diastolic blood pressure, with arterial pulses of high amplitude ("collapsing"). The classic, pathognomonic auscultatory finding of a PDA is a continuous systolic-diastolic murmur (the so-called machinery murmur), which peaks around the second heart sound, is widely audible throughout the precordium, and is loudest between the first and third

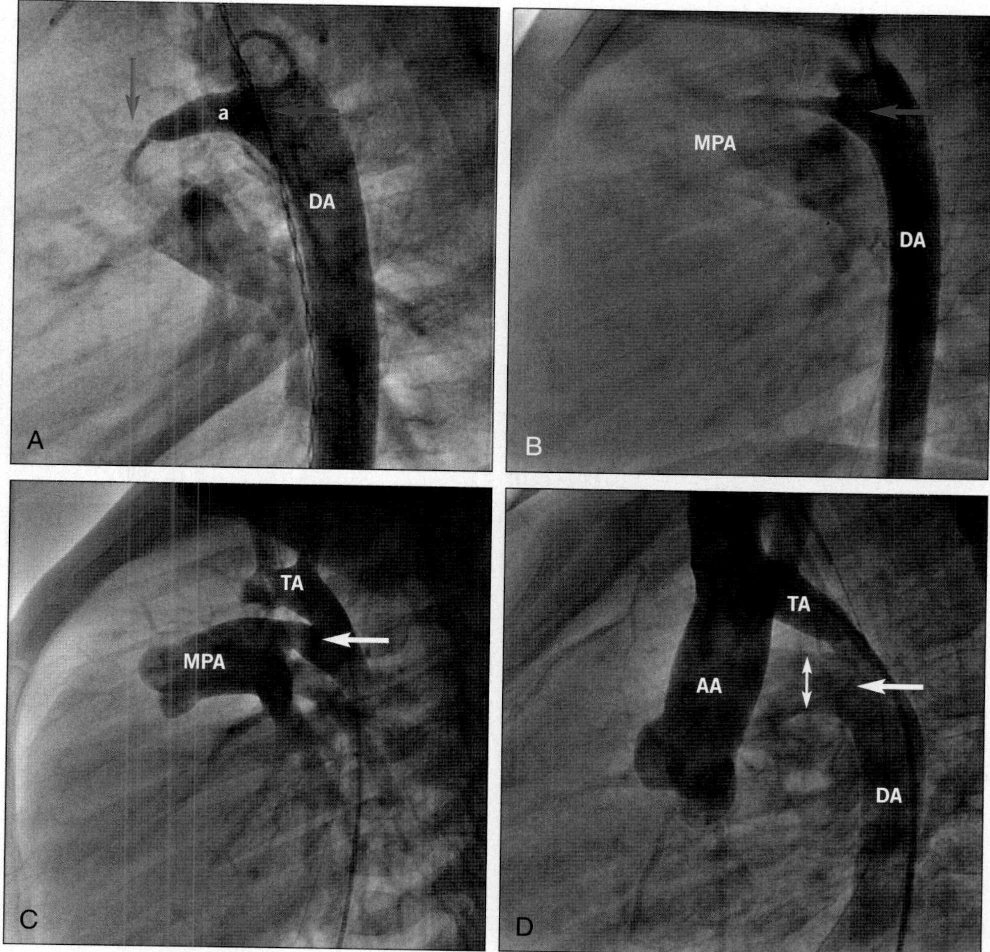

Figure 119.3 Angiograms, lateral projection. A, Small patent ductus arteriosus *(blue arrow)* with typical ampulla (a) and small connection with the main pulmonary artery *(red arrow)*. **B,** Moderate-sized patent ductus arteriosus *(blue arrow)* and connection with main pulmonary artery *(red arrow)*. **C,** Large patent ductus arteriosus *(arrow)*. **D,** Very large patent ductus arteriosus *(arrow)* with a double arrow showing the ductal width. Note this patient has pulmonary vascular disease and mild coarctation of the aorta with narrowing of the vessel proximal to the ductal insertion into the aorta. AA, ascending aorta; MPA, main pulmonary artery; DA, descending aorta; TA, transverse aortic arch.

intercostal spaces on the left side. If the ductus is large and truly unrestrictive, the aortic and pulmonary pressures may be equal during diastole, and the murmur may end just after the second heart sound.

In a patient with a small PDA, the clinical findings may be normal except for a high-pitched and continuous murmur, although sometimes the murmur is not truly holodiastolic. In the very small ductus, the murmur is often absent (the so-called silent ductus).

Pulmonary Hypertension

The clinical scenarios of pulmonary hypertension relate to either the newborn period, when the pulmonary vascular resistance may not have fallen to normal, or years later in the presence of a large PDA, when the pulmonary vascular resistance becomes elevated irreversibly.

The clinical signs are very different in the presence of raised pulmonary vascular resistance. In the newborn infant, before the pulmonary vascular resistance has fallen, the degree of left-to-right shunting is small even in the presence of a large PDA. The clinical signs are usually normal, although a difference in the arterial oxygen saturations between the upper and the lower limbs can often be detected.

In established pulmonary vascular disease as a consequence of a large PDA, there are no signs of high pulmonary blood flow, so the apex beat may be normally located, and the blood pressure and the character of the arterial pulse may be normal. The right ventricular impulse (parasternal lift) is prominent, reflecting right ventricular hypertension. Elevated pulmonary vascular resistance usually leads to a narrow split or even single second heart sound, and there is often no murmur, although a diastolic murmur typical of pulmonary regurgitation may be present. The classic sign of established pulmonary vascular disease and a right-to-left or "reversed" shunt is central desaturation (Fig. 119.4). Because desaturated blood enters the systemic arterial circuit at the level of the descending aorta, there is usually differential cyanosis between the upper and lower half of the body.

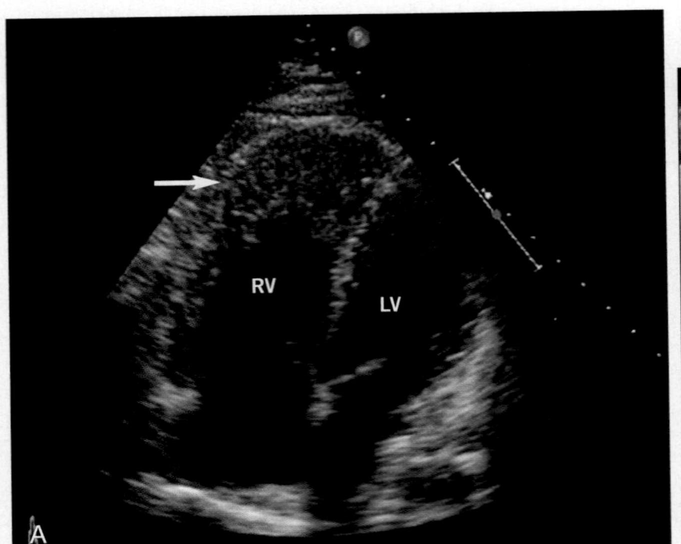

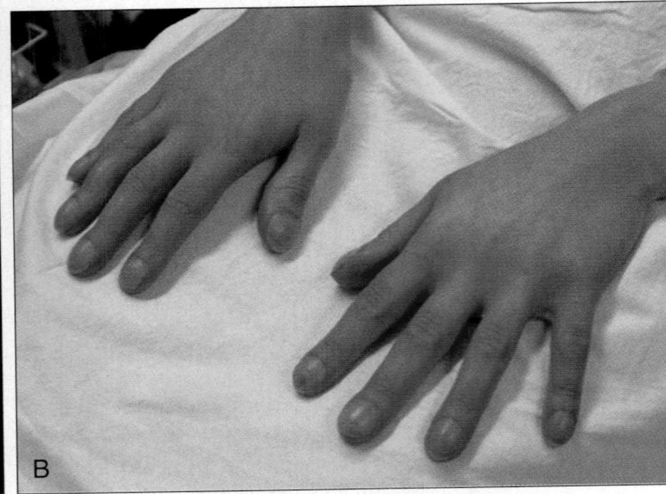

Figure 119.4 A, Significant right ventricular hypertrophy in a patient with pulmonary vascular disease as a result of a patent ductus arteriosus. LV, left ventricle; RV, right ventricle. **B,** Digital clubbing in a patient with pulmonary vascular disease.

Differential Diagnosis

A number of other conditions are manifested by either continuous murmurs or large-volume pulses.

Venous Hum

A jugular venous hum in a young child is typically continuous throughout systole and diastole. Unlike in PDA, however, the murmur varies markedly with position of the patient, particularly movement of the head.

Aortopulmonary Window

An aortopulmonary window is a rare lesion and consists of a direct connection between the ascending aorta and the pulmonary artery. There is little physiologic difference between an aortopulmonary window and a large PDA. The clinical signs are almost identical, and these conditions cannot be reliably differentiated clinically.

Truncus Arteriosus

On occasion, a harsh systolic and early diastolic murmur is audible in this condition. There are also frequently signs of high pulmonary blood flow, and prominent peripheral pulsations are often present. In contrast to a PDA, however, the second heart sound is unequivocally single, and these patients are usually mildly desaturated.

Sinus of Valsalva Aneurysm

In this condition, there is a direct connection between the aortic root and the right side of the heart, with a pressure gradient throughout systole and diastole resulting in a continuous murmur. The murmur is often louder in diastole than in a significant PDA because of the marked pressure difference between the aorta and the right atrium or ventricle. The murmur is also loudest at the lower left sternal edge, in keeping with the direction of blood flow.

Small Ventricular Septal Defect and Aortic Regurgitation

In this situation, there is a loud pansystolic murmur of a restrictive ventricular septal defect and a diastolic murmur of aortic regurgitation, which together can give the impression of a continuous murmur. With careful auscultation, separate systolic and diastolic murmurs can usually be appreciated in different positions in the precordium.

Aortopulmonary Collaterals

On occasion, an aortopulmonary collateral vessel arises from a position very similar to a PDA and may be difficult to differentiate clinically. Typically, however, aortopulmonary collaterals are multiple, and so continuous murmurs are widely heard throughout the chest and precordium. Aortopulmonary collaterals are also frequently associated with other congenital heart lesions.

NATURAL HISTORY

Surgical treatment of PDA predates the era of accurate diagnosis, and therefore the natural history of the condition is poorly described.[18,19] Deaths due to congestive cardiac failure or recurrent respiratory infections as a consequence of high pulmonary blood flow in infants with large PDAs may rarely occur.[19] Those patients with large untreated left-to-right shunts who survive beyond early childhood usually die during adult life of left ventricular decompensation.[19] Pulmonary vascular disease is another cause of death during adult life, although the prognosis in this group of patients is demonstrably better than in raised pulmonary vascular resistance as a result of other untreated congenital heart disease.

Bacterial infection of the ductus arteriosus (endarteritis) is a feared complication of the untreated PDA. Endarteritis generally occurs in older children or adults, and although deaths in older patients with PDAs without pulmonary vascular disease are rare, endarteritis may be responsible for approximately 50% of these.[19] Prevention of endarteritis is widely quoted as the clinical justification for closure of the small PDA without evidence of volume loading of the left side of the heart.

Patients with tiny PDAs but with normal clinical signs almost certainly have a normal life expectancy.

INVESTIGATIONS

Electrocardiography

The electrocardiogram may be normal in the patients with small to medium-sized PDA. In patients with large PDAs, left ventricular hypertrophy with left axis deviation will eventually develop during childhood, with deep Q and tall R waves in leads II, III, aVF, V_5, and V_6. The T waves in these leads are commonly tall and upright. Left atrial hypertrophy is uncommon. In premature infants, the electrocardiogram does not show any distinct changes, but it may show a pattern of left ventricular strain in those with congestive heart failure. In patients who have flow-related pulmonary hypertension, the electrocardiogram may show biventricular hypertrophy and peaked P waves of right atrial hypertrophy. Striking asymmetric T-wave inversion may also be present in leads V_1 to V_4.

Pulmonary vascular disease usually results in significant right ventricular hypertrophy with large R waves in lead V_1 and deep S waves in leads V_5 and V_6. Sometimes, complete right bundle branch block may be seen.

Chest Radiography

The chest radiograph is usually normal in patients with small PDAs. In those with large PDAs with significant left-to-right shunts, prominent vascular markings in addition to cardiac enlargement are often seen (Fig. 119.5). In the lateral projection, the left atrium may be enlarged. In premature infants, the chest radiograph may show increased vascular markings in the lungs along with the additional parenchymal features typical of prematurity.

In patients with pulmonary vascular disease, the peripheral pulmonary vessels are typically "pruned" and the central pulmonary arteries large and dilated. The heart size may usually be normal.

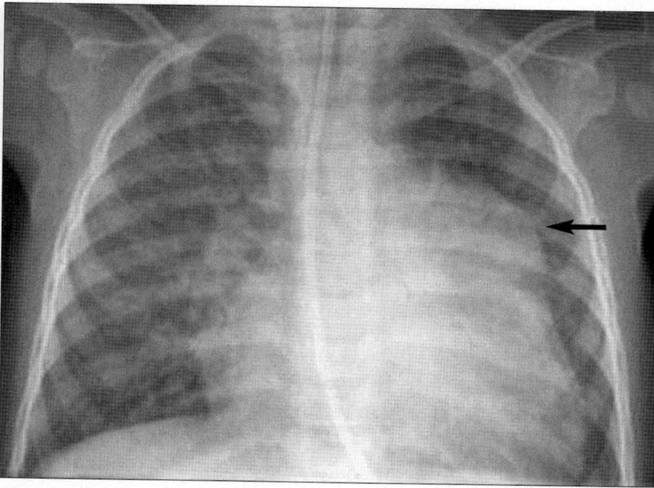

Figure 119.5 Chest radiograph of a 3-month-old child with a large patent ductus arteriosus. The heart is enlarged and the lung fields are plethoric as a result of high pulmonary blood flow. Note the prominent pulmonary artery knuckle *(arrow)*.

In the adult with a PDA, calcification of the ductus is often seen.

Echocardiography

The ductus can be reliably imaged by transthoracic echocardiography, and in the modern era, this is the primary diagnostic modality. The classic echocardiographic "window" for visualization of a PDA by both two-dimensional and color Doppler ultrasonography is the parasternal short-axis view (Fig. 119.6). Additional anatomic information can be obtained from higher parasternal and suprasternal "aortic arch" views, which show not only the flow into the pulmonary artery but also the ductal ampulla and the size of the connection between the ductus and the pulmonary artery (see Fig. 119.6). In the adult patient, poor echocardiographic

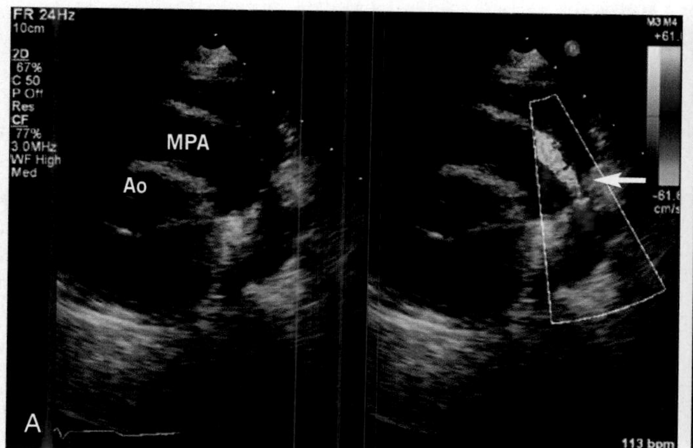

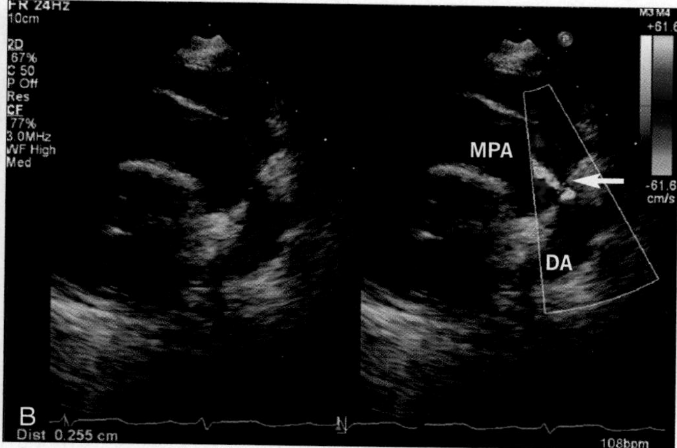

Figure 119.6 Echocardiography. A, Parasternal short-axis view, two-dimensional and color Doppler images. Typical echocardiographic appearance of a moderate patent ductus arterious *(arrow)* with high-velocity, continuous flow from the descending aorta to the main pulmonary artery. **B,** Parasternal short-axis view, two-dimensional and color Doppler images. Moderate-sized ductus measuring 2.5 mm at the connection with the pulmonary artery *(arrow)*.

(Continued)

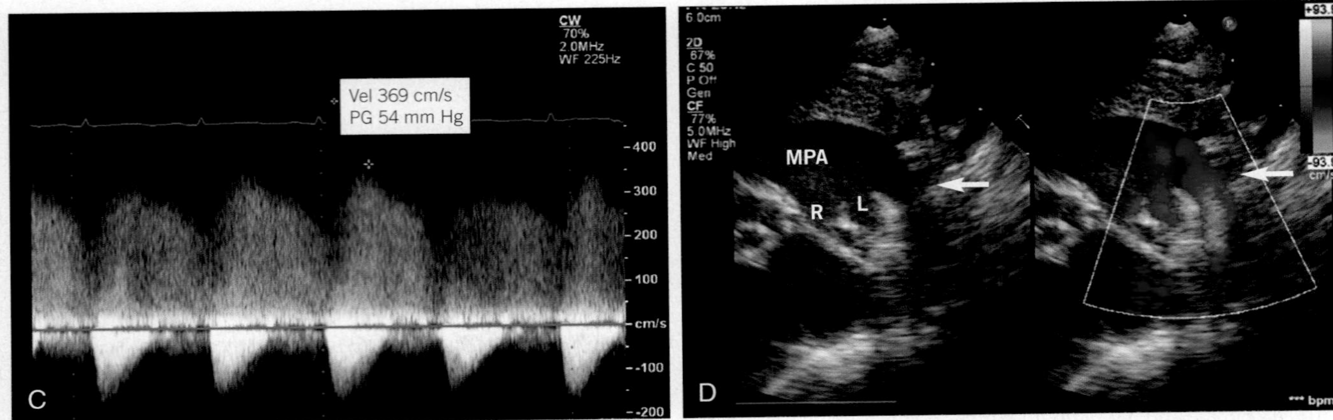

Figure 119.6—cont'd C, Continuous-wave Doppler ultrasonography. Typical pattern of continuous flow through both systole and diastole between the aorta and pulmonary artery. The peak systolic velocity *(cross)* gives an approximation of the difference between the systolic aortic and pulmonary artery pressures (in this case, 54 mm Hg). **D,** High parasternal short-axis view, two-dimensional and color Doppler images of a newborn infant with "ductus dependent" congenital heart disease. Large ductus arteriosus with bidirectional flow. Note that in this echocardiographic view, both branch pulmonary arteries are also visible (marked R and L). Ao, aorta; DA, descending aorta; MPA, main pulmonary artery.

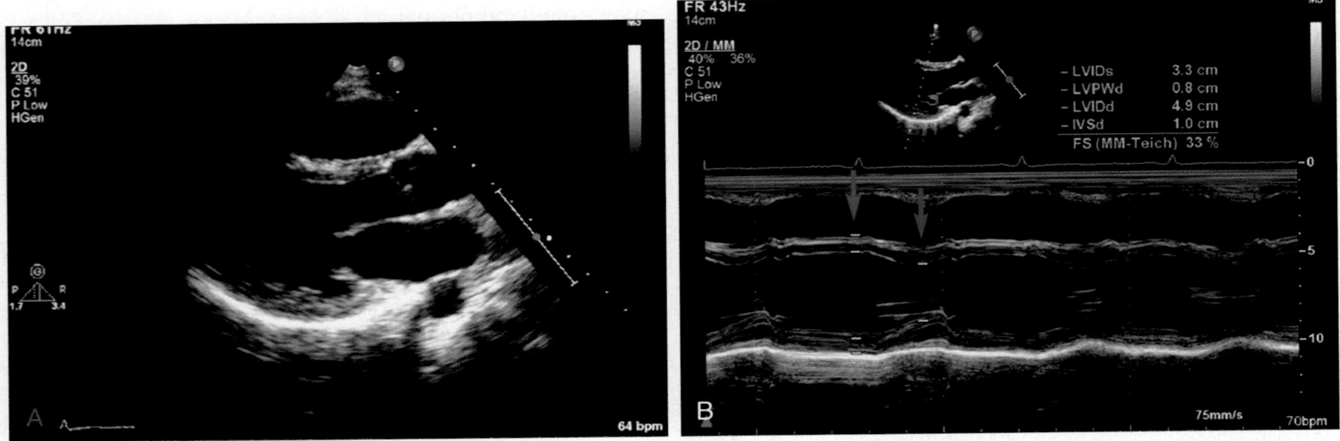

Figure 119.7 Echocardiography. A, Parasternal long-axis view. Significantly volume loaded left ventricle in a 6-year-old child with a large patent ductus arteriosus. **B,** M-mode recording. Same patient, left ventricular dimensions in systole *(blue arrow)* and diastole *(red arrow)*.

windows may limit the ability to obtain good-quality images of the PDA. Continuous-wave Doppler interrogation of the ductal flow allows the direction of flow across the ductus to be ascertained as well as an indirect assessment of the pulmonary artery pressures based on the modified Bernoulli equation (see Fig. 119.6c). Although high-velocity left-to-right flow across a ductus with a Doppler velocity of more than 4 m/s indicates low pulmonary artery systolic pressure, pressure restriction is not analogous to flow restriction, and high-velocity traces are common even in patients with significant PDAs and large left-to-right shunts.

In addition to direct imaging of the ductus arteriosus, echocardiography may give further information about the size of the shunt. In a PDA with a significant left-to-right shunt, there may be evidence of volume loading on the left side of the heart as a result of high pulmonary venous return (Fig. 119.7), with increased left ventricular end-diastolic dimension and evidence of high stroke volume. Traditionally, the ratio of the dimensions of the left atrium to the aorta on M-mode echocardiography was used as a surrogate indicator of a significant ductal shunt (>1.4), although with accurate direct measurements of ventricular dimensions, this measurement is rarely used in the current era.

Color-flow Doppler echocardiography is an extremely sensitive technique and allows the detection of the smallest of PDAs (Fig. 119.8). This has led to an "epidemic" of infants and children with normal clinical signs but with a tiny PDA on color-flow mapping (the so-called silent ductus). There is little evidence on which to guide management of this particular group of patients. However, the majority of pediatric cardiologists treat patients with unequivocally normal clinical signs as normal and do not recommend PDA closure.

Echocardiography allows the identification of additional congenital cardiac lesions. In these patients, flow patterns across the ductus will reflect the underlying cardiac problem.

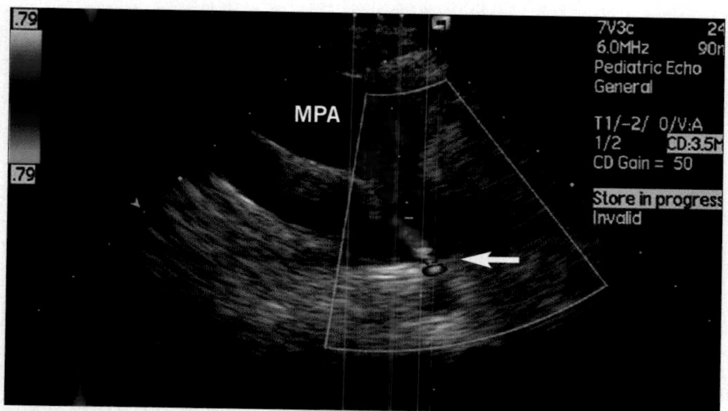

Figure 119.8 Color-flow Doppler echocardiography, parasternal long-axis view. Tiny patent ductus arteriosus with left-to-right shunt *(arrow)*. MPA, main pulmonary artery.

Cardiac Catheterization

Diagnostic cardiac catheterization is not required in a patient with an isolated PDA to confirm the diagnosis, but it is generally performed either as a prelude to transcatheter closure (discussed later) or for the assessment of pulmonary vascular resistance in older patients with large PDAs in whom pulmonary vascular disease is suspected.

Angiography in the proximal descending aorta (accessed either directly from the femoral artery or anterogradely from the right side of the heart by crossing the ductus from the pulmonary artery) in the right anterior oblique or lateral projection outlines the ductus and demonstrates the ampulla, the length of the ductus, and the size of the connection at the junction with the pulmonary artery (see Fig. 119.3). Angiography gives precise anatomic information and has shown great variation in the anatomy of the ductus from conical in shape to a direct short connection between the pulmonary artery and the aorta at the other extreme (see Fig. 119.3).

A step-up in the oxygen saturation between the right ventricle and the pulmonary artery can usually be demonstrated, but care must be taken not to overinterpret this information, particularly in quantifying the shunt and pulmonary blood flow. Preferential streaming of oxygenated blood into the pulmonary tree is common, regardless of the size of the PDA.

Pulmonary artery pressures are usually normal in smaller PDAs. Higher pulmonary artery pressures occur with larger PDAs as a result of left-to-right shunting with systemic level pulmonary artery pressures in unrestrictive connections. High systolic but low diastolic pulmonary artery pressure suggests an ongoing left-to-right shunt and potentially a degree of reversibility.

MANAGEMENT

A significant PDA in a patient with symptoms, clinical signs, and echocardiographic features of high pulmonary blood flow requires treatment. Unlike in term babies, in whom medical management is purely supportive, PDAs in premature infants will often close in response to prostaglandin inhibitors (ibuprofen or indomethacin), although these drugs are frequently associated with important side effects.[20]

Surgical ligation of an isolated PDA was first described by Gross and Hubbard[21] in 1939 in a 7-year-old girl and has subsequently been shown to be effective even in the smallest of infants.[22] The procedure requires a thoracotomy, and complications, although relatively infrequent, do occur and include chylothorax, ductal recanalization, inadvertent pulmonary artery ligation, and major blood loss. Although it is generally considered a safe procedure, the current U.K. audit data show a 30-day mortality of 8% for infants weighing less than 2.5 kg who have undergone surgical ligation of a PDA.[23] This mortality rate is likely to be a reflection of important comorbidity in sicker, often premature infants. Laparoscopic PDA ligation is a possible alternative technique, but there are few data on its safety and efficacy published in the literature.[24]

Porstmann and colleagues[25] first described a percutaneous technique for permanent closure of the ductus arteriosus in 1971. The procedure was technically complicated, unsuitable for certain types of ductal morphology, and required a large-profile sheath in the femoral artery. As such, the Porstmann PDA plug never achieved widespread clinical use but was an important landmark in transcatheter cardiovascular therapy, paving the way for the development of a large number of closure devices. The Rashkind PDA occluder was the next notable breakthrough (Fig. 119.9).[26] This device is a double-umbrella arrangement designed to occlude the ductus by trapping it between the facing disks. For many years, the Rashkind occluder was the only device available for transcatheter occlusion of the PDA and was extensively investigated and reported.[27,28] Several intrinsic problems were demonstrated, including the risk of left pulmonary artery stenosis in small infants and high late residual shunting rates (15% to 20%), which eventually rendered the device obsolete.[28,29]

Coils

Cambier and associates,[30] in 1992, first described the use of Gianturco embolization coils for the occlusion of small PDAs measuring less than 2.5 mm at the pulmonary artery end (Fig. 119.10; see also Fig. 119.9b, c). This technique has the considerable advantage, over those previously described, of allowing delivery of a device through a 4 French sheath, thus making it suitable for even the smallest of children. The procedure was further refined by the development of the Jackson or Flipper coil (William Cook Europe; see Fig. 119.9b), a device based on the Gianturco coil.[31] This coil, fully retrievable into the delivery catheter until release from a retention screw, addressed the problem of inadvertent device embolization, the main concern in the non–controlled-release variant. Numerous publications attest to the safety and efficacy of coil occlusion of the ductus arteriosus.[30-35] In 2001, Magee and colleagues[35] reported data submitted from 30 centers to a voluntary registry of 1258 patients undergoing PDA coil occlusion. These data are broadly in line with other reports showing no procedure-related mortality, the need for multiple coils in 17% of cases, and an immediate complete occlusion rate of 59% rising to 95% at 1 year. A "suboptimal" outcome, defined as hemolysis, coil embolization, residual leak needing another procedure, recanalization, and obstruction of adjacent structures, occurred in 10% of cases. The majority of these complications either settled spontaneously or were rectified with another single procedure (either additional

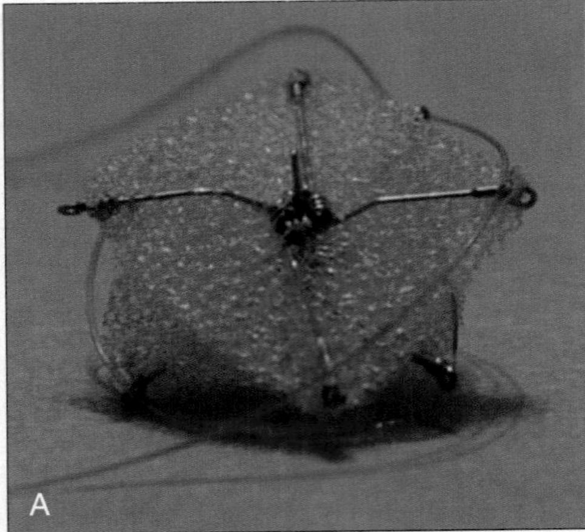

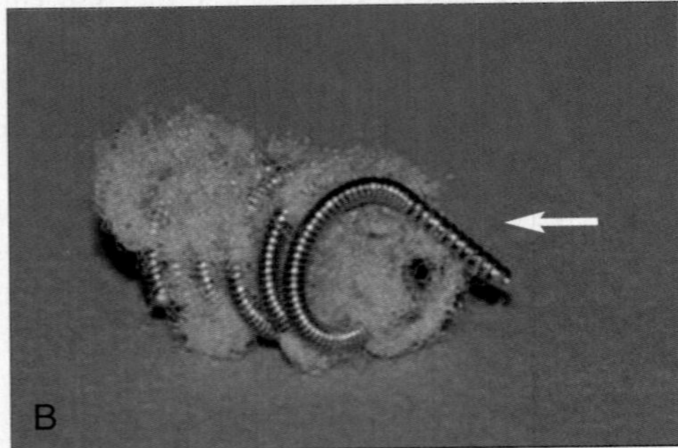

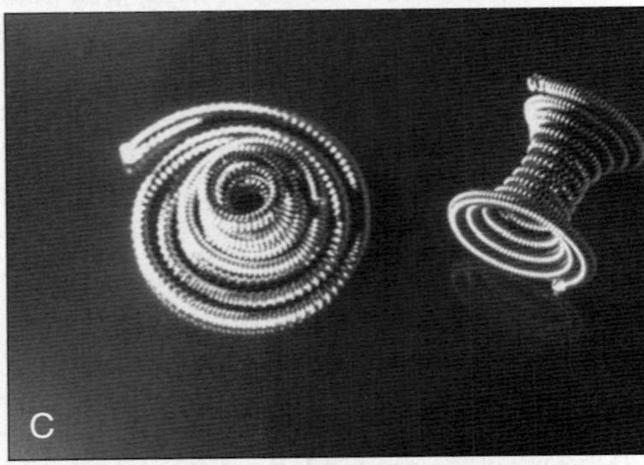

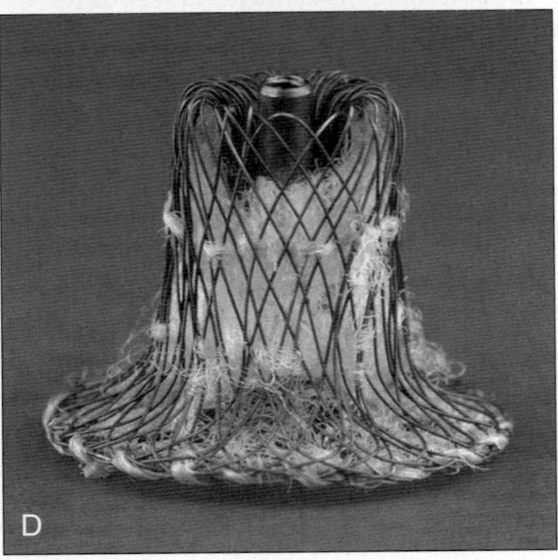

Figure 119.9 A, Rashkind device, frontal view. Double-disk occluder on a stainless steel frame. **B,** Jackson (Flipper) stainless steel controlled-release PDA coil. Note the embedded Dacron fibers to facilitate ductal occlusion and the screw mechanism *(arrow)* for attachment and release from the delivery cable. **C,** DuctOcclud embolization coil. **D,** Amplatzer duct occluder, side view. Note both the Dacron fiber filling within the metal mesh to facilitate rapid vascular occlusion and the sunken retention screw to attach the device to the delivery cable.

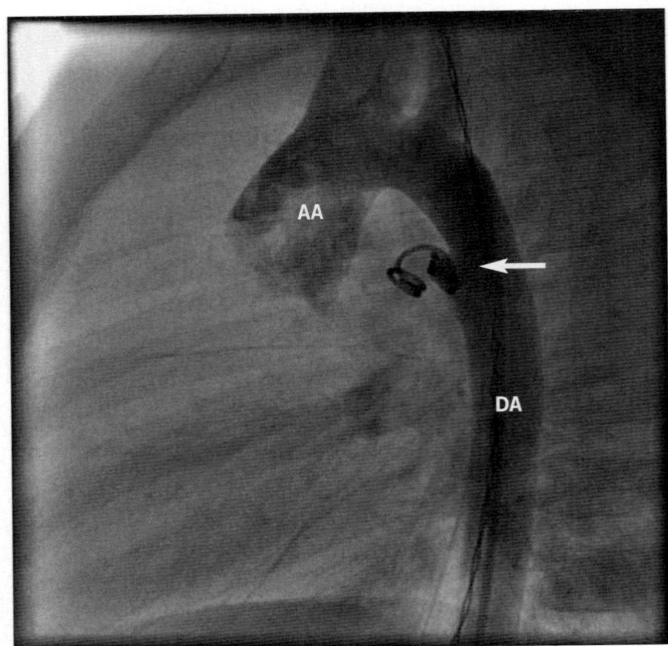

Figure 119.10 Angiogram, lateral projection. Controlled-release coils after deployment across a small duct *(arrow)*. AA, ascending aorta; DA, descending aorta.

transcatheter occlusion or surgical ductal ligation). The risk factors for a suboptimal outcome with use of coil occlusion for ductal closure in this series, as in other studies, were large ductal size (incremental risk with increasing size) and the presence of tubular ductal anatomy, compared with the more typical conical shape.

Successful PDA occlusion primarily using coils in a small group of premature infants has been reported,[36] although most operators would still consider these patients at high risk for transcatheter treatment. They are best treated surgically until devices specifically designed for the purpose are available.

In addition to the Gianturco and Flipper coils, the controlled-release DuctOcclud device (PFM, Germany) has been available for clinical use since the early 1990s.[37] This device reconfigures to a conical shape, allowing it to closely conform to the anatomy of the ductus and the ductal ampulla (see Fig. 119.9c). Like the Cook coil variants, the DuctOcclud device can be deployed through a small delivery sheath. Published data are much more limited, but clinical experience suggests a safety and efficacy profile very similar to that of other coils, with immediate residual shunts after deployment in approximately 60% of patients and eventual complete occlusion rates of approximately 95% by 12-month follow-up.[38] Given the apparent equivalence with other cheaper coils, many have questioned the need for this device.[39] However, the design of the DuctOcclud gives it the potential for safe occlusion of larger PDAs, and further design modifications may tackle the anatomically difficult PDA beyond the capability of the Cook family of coils.[40]

Large PDAs (>2.5 mm at the junction with the pulmonary artery) are a technical challenge for coil occlusion. Although multiple coils can be delivered into a large PDA, the technique is less satisfactory and the results are inferior to occlusion with the Amplatzer PDA device, described next. In particular, hemolysis as a consequence of residual shunting in a large PDA occluded with multiple coils can be troublesome to treat.

Amplatzer Duct Occluder

The Amplatzer duct occluder (Fig. 119.11; see also Fig. 119. 9d) has been available since the late 1990s and was specifically designed for occlusion of larger PDAs. The device shares many design features with other Amplatzer vascular and septal occluders. It is made from a nitinol frame, allowing it to fold into a small delivery catheter (5 to 7 French), into which it is fully retrievable before release from the delivery cable. Within the device is sewn a Dacron patch to facilitate occlusion of the shunt and to minimize the risk of hemolysis. The current-generation device is delivered from the pulmonary artery end of the ductus until the retention skirt is within the ductal ampulla, leaving the body of the device wedged into the ductus itself. A second-generation Amplatzer duct occluder with a modification to the retention skirt mechanism allowing delivery from the aortic side of the PDA through a smaller delivery sheath will soon be available.

There is now a considerable amount of safety and longer term efficacy data with regard to the first-generation Amplatzer duct occluder. Bilkis and coworkers[41] described 205 patients, median age of 1.9 years with PDAs of median size 4.5 mm, undergoing occlusion with the Amplatzer duct occluder. Successful closure was achieved in all of these patients. Immediate residual shunts were seen in 55%; but by 1 month, residual shunts were evident in just 3%, and by 12 months, all but one patient achieved complete occlusion, and this shunt had disappeared at 15-month follow-up. Device embolization to the pulmonary artery occurred in three patients (1.5%), all three of whom underwent surgical ligation with removal of the device. No obstruction to the left pulmonary artery was seen, but there was mild aortic arch obstruction in one patient. Broadly similar results were reported by Pass and colleagues[42] in the U.S. multicenter study of 439 patients undergoing ductal occlusion with the Amplatzer duct occluder. Although the median ductal diameter was slightly smaller, the age range of patients was very similar to that in the Bilkis study, and complete occlusion rates of 99.7% were achieved by 1 year of follow-up. No aortic obstruction was demonstrated in this group, but minor encroachment into the left pulmonary artery was seen in two patients (<0.5%).

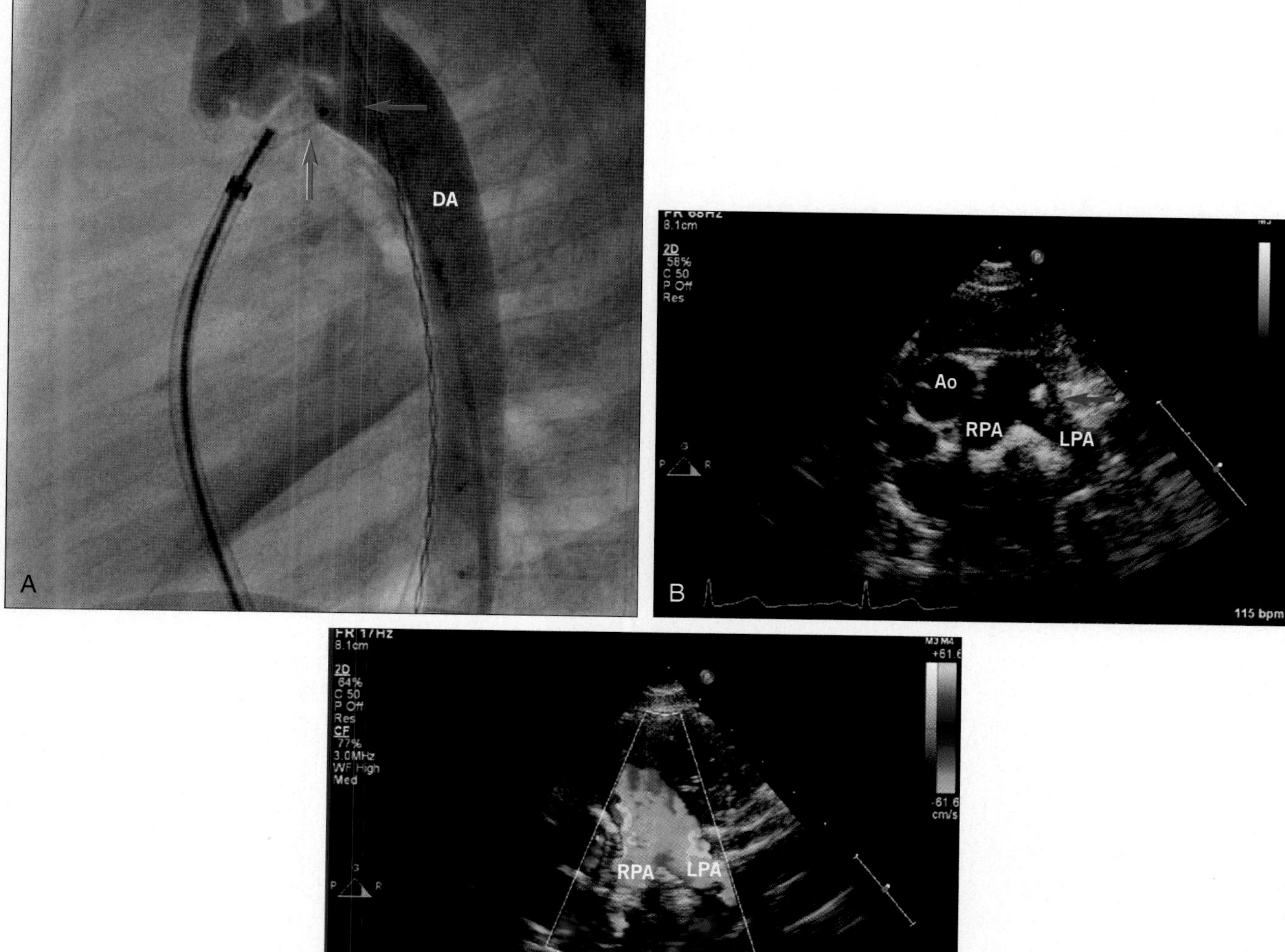

Figure 119.11 Amplatzer duct occluder. A, Aortogram, lateral projection. Amplatzer duct occluder *(red arrow)* within the ductus arteriosus *(blue arrow)* before release. **B,** Two-dimensional echocardiogram, parasternal short-axis view. Amplatzer duct occluder after release *(arrow)*. **C,** Color Doppler echocardiogram, parasternal short-axis view. Same patient as in **B,** demonstrating complete occlusion of the PDA. Ao, aortic valve; DA, descending aorta; LPA, left pulmonary artery; RPA, right pulmonary artery.

PDAs of almost any size can be occluded with the Amplatzer duct occluder, although the current design makes its use unsafe in the rare patient with a large, direct connection between the aorta and the pulmonary artery and no ampulla (see Fig. 119.3d). In these patients, procedural success has been achieved by implantation of other forms of Amplatzer occluders with two retention skirts that can be deployed in older patients without the fear of obstruction to either the aorta or left pulmonary artery. Closure of larger defects in older patients is controversial, but there are a small number of studies suggesting that it may be possible to close defects in carefully selected patients in whom pulmonary vascular disease was previously suspected.[43,44]

The Amplatzer duct occluder device is expensive relative to the Gianturco and controlled-release coils, and its use is unnecessary in small PDAs of less than 2 mm. Care must also be taken with large PDAs in very small children, as there is a risk of occlusion of other vascular structures and a higher risk of device embolization.

SUMMARY

The ductus arteriosus is a vital component of the fetal circulation. Functional ductal closure usually occurs within the first 12 hours of life. An isolated ductus present in a term infant after 3 months of age is abnormal. Our understanding of the natural history of this condition is incomplete, but occlusion of a PDA should be carried out in all patients with evidence of a large left-to-right shunt and in those with abnormal clinical signs, who may be at risk of later infection. An incidental ductus in a patient with otherwise normal clinical signs does not necessarily need treatment. Ductal occlusion can be performed surgically or by use of a transcatheter-delivered device. Occlusion of PDAs of almost any size is technically possible with modern transcatheter devices.

The PDA may be vital in bypassing an important congenital cardiac lesion in infants with "duct-dependent" congenital heart disease.

chapter

120 Coarctation of the Aorta

Barbara J. M. Mulder

Definition

- Strictly speaking, coarctation of the aorta is a localized, discrete narrowing of the thoracic aorta that occurs in connection with the embryology of patent ductus arteriosus.

Key Features

- The morphologic heterogeneity of coarctation of the aorta and associated cardiac defects may influence the presentation and prognosis of this disease.

Therapy

- Timely repair of coarctation with surgery or catheter intervention relieves symptoms and improves prognosis.

Prognosis

- Life expectancy after repair of aortic coarctation is not normal. Long-term complications are frequent; patients should be offered lifelong follow-up.

Coarctation of the aorta, a relatively common abnormality that occurs in approximately 6% to 8% of patients with congenital heart disease, has a heterogeneous anatomy and variable physiology.[1] The severity of coarctation depends not only on the degree of aortic narrowing but also on associated heart lesions. In addition, whether it is the discrete or diffuse type of narrowing, the location of coarctation of the aorta, the complexity of the associated heart defect, and the morphology of the aortic isthmus and arch may all affect clinical presentation and longer term prognosis of this malformation.

ETIOLOGY, ANATOMY, AND PATHOLOGY

Pathogenesis

The embryonic pathogenesis of aortic coarctation is not well understood, but two concepts, the ductus tissue theory and the hemodynamic theory, have been proposed.[2-4] The first theory has suggested that coarctation results from the migration of ductus smooth muscle cells into the periductal aortic wall and that the narrowing both prenatally and after ductal closure is associated with constriction of ductus tissue.[2,4] This concept is supported by the observation that coarctation often develops or is aggravated secondary to closure of patent ductus arteriosus after birth. The ductal contribution in this theory is clearly essential. It cannot explain, however, tubular isthmus hypoplasia or coarctation of the transverse arch and abdominal aorta, which may be present with a widely patent ductus arteriosus.[5] Other investigators have proposed that coarctation develops as a result of hemodynamic alterations that reduce the volume of blood flow through the fetal aortic arch and isthmus.[3] For example, if an obstructive left-sided heart lesion such as aortic stenosis or hypoplastic left heart syndrome is present, the forward flow through the ascending aorta is diminished, whereas the postductal flow to the descending aorta is increased, which may predispose to the development of coarctation—the so-called flow theory.

Anatomy

In the typical, classic form of coarctation of the aorta, the narrowing is located preductally near the thoracic end of the patent ductus arteriosus, usually just distal to the left subclavian artery, dependent on the length of the isthmus. The lesion is usually discrete and exhibits a localized indentation on external view. The external indentation corresponds internally to the ridge that eccentrically narrows the aortic lumen.[4] The distal aorta beyond the coarctation segment is usually dilated because of the jet flow after the point of narrowing, the so-called poststenotic dilatation. Coarctation of the aorta can rarely occur in the ascending intrathoracic or abdominal aorta. It may be associated with systemic diseases, such as Takayasu's aortitis, Williams syndrome, and middle aortic syndrome.

Histology

Coarctation of the aorta is a diffuse disease. Histologic examination of the coarctation site shows an intimal and medial lesion consisting of a thickened shelf that protrudes posteriorly and laterally into the aortic lumen. This shelf is continuous with the wall of the ductus and invariably contains ductal tissue, which may encircle the vessel (Fig. 120.1).[6] In longitudinal section including coarctation, ductal tissue is detected on the side of the shelf derived from the descending aorta (Fig. 120.2). These findings suggest that coarctation develops as the result of migration of ductus smooth muscle cells into the periductal aorta, with subsequent constriction and narrowing of the aortic lumen. The aortic wall is diffusely abnormal, with localized intimal hyperplasia and distortion of the medial wall architecture around the coarctation site. This appearance has been considered a potential morphologic substrate for secondary intimal proliferation, weakening of the aortic wall, aneurysm formation, or dissection.[4]

Associated Lesions

Conditions associated with coarctation of the aorta are listed in Table 120.1.

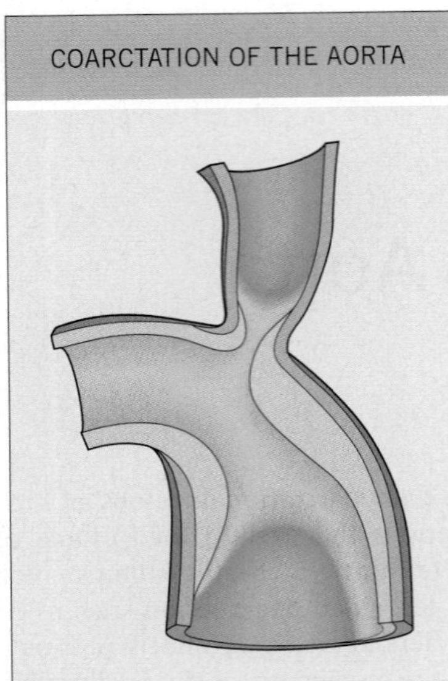

Figure 120.1 Diagram of coarctation of the aorta. The light area indicates ductal tissue.[6]

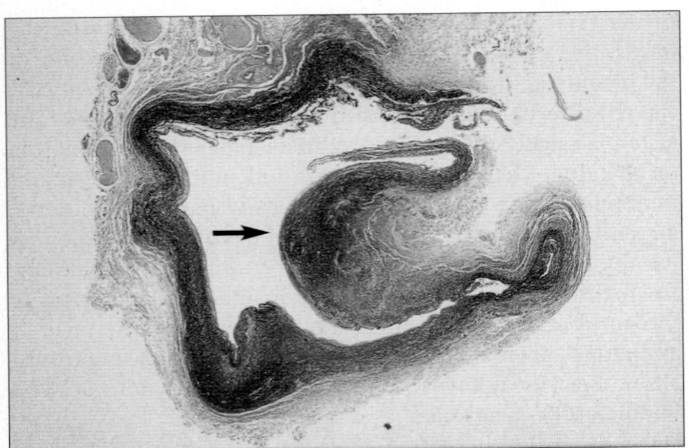

Figure 120.2 Pathologic findings of coarctation of the aorta. The arrow indicates ductal tissue at the site of the posterior shelf.

Associated Cardiac Lesions

Significant intracardiac lesions may coexist in approximately 50% of patients with coarctation of the aorta, and this is called complex coarctation.[7] In the remaining 50% of these patients, simple coarctation describes coarctation of the aorta that occurs in isolation with or without a patent ductus arteriosus. A ventricular septal defect is the most common intracardiac lesion; it is usually large, of a perimembranous type, and is often associated with posterior malalignment of the infundibular septum resulting in significant left ventricular outflow tract obstruction. Aortic valve abnormalities, such as bicuspid aortic valve, are frequently (19% to 80%) encountered. Mitral valve anomalies are also common, including supravalvular mitral ring, mitral stenosis, and single parachute papillary muscle. The association of multiple left-sided obstructive lesions with coarctation has been referred to as the Shone syndrome and constitutes a group of patients with poor prognosis who often require multiple operations.[8]

ASSOCIATED CONDITIONS WITH COARCTATION OF THE AORTA	
Lesion	**Incidence (%)**
Cardiac	
Patent ductus arteriosus	43
Ventricular septal defect	39
Atrial septal defect	20
Aortic valve abnormality	19
Hypoplastic left heart syndrome	11
Transposition of great arteries	7.7
Double-outlet right ventricle	6.7
Mitral valve abnormality	4.9
Atrioventricular septal defect	4.4
Common ventricle	3.6
Tricuspid atresia	2.4
Pulmonary stenosis	1.0
Tetralogy of Fallot	0.4
Noncardiac	
Chromosome abnormality	6.2
Prematurity	1.2
Hydrops fetalis	1.0
Tracheoesophageal fistula	0.9
DiGeorge syndrome	0.9

Table 120.1 Associated conditions with coarctation of the aorta.

Associated Noncardiac Conditions

Chromosomal abnormalities, such as Turner's syndrome, trisomy 21, trisomy 18, and prematurity are not uncommon among patients with coarctation. Moreover, extracardiac vascular anomalies, such as brachiocephalic artery anomalies, anomalous collateral circulation, and berry aneurysms of the circle of Willis, are also common.

PATHOPHYSIOLOGY

Hemodynamics

According to the site of the narrowing, coarctation of the aorta is generally classified into infantile and adult types. Infantile type is the term used for those with preductal or juxtaductal coarctation whose coarcted site is proximal to the ductus arteriosus; adult type describes those with postductal coarctation. Most coarctation in the newborn period and early infancy is of the preductal type and may migrate distally with time.

In the infantile type of coarctation, ductal patency is often critical as flow through the ductus with a right-to-left direction sustains flow into the descending aorta, including renal blood supply. After birth, with closure of the ductus arteriosus, renal blood flow and lower body perfusion decrease, and as a result, deterioration with severe metabolic acidosis develops (so-called ductal shock). In these circumstances, prostaglandin E_1 administration is mandatory to maintain ductal patency. If there is a right-to-left shunt at the ductus, the upper extremities of the infant are pink and the lower extremities are cyanotic, the so-called differential cyanosis. Oxygen administration is contraindicated in this ductus-dependent circulation, as it may promote ductal closure.

On the other hand, in the adult type of postductal coarctation, systemic blood flow to the lower half of the body is also compromised, with reduced femoral pulses and impaired renal perfusion. However, this process is a slower one, and patients develop variable degrees of collateral circulation to compensate for the restriction of flow through the coarctation. If the coarctation is severe, left ventricular dysfunction and congestive heart failure may ensue. The left ventricular dysfunction caused by afterload mismatch is so great that the mechanism of left ventricular wall hypertrophy compensating for elevated wall stress in the left ventricle does not operate. Secondary endocardial fibroelastosis may also contribute to left ventricular dysfunction in neonates and infants. Left ventricular diastolic dysfunction may also be caused by hypertrophy of the left ventricle secondary to elevated afterload.

In many patients, systemic hypertension may persist or return after successful coarctation repair, despite relief of the pressure gradient. This abnormality in vascular physiology may be caused by abnormal baroreceptor reflex function, arterial wall compliance, and abnormal structure and function of the pre-coarctation arterial conduits. Residual aortic arch gradients and a hypoplastic aortic arch may also be contributory factors.[9]

CLINICAL PRESENTATION

Clinical Symptoms

The clinical features of coarctation depend largely on the nature of the associated cardiac lesions and severity of narrowing. In isolated coarctation, most patients are asymptomatic, and clinical findings may be subtle; consequently, delayed diagnosis is common. In older children or adolescents, systolic hypertension and heart murmur are the most common presentations. On the other hand, in neonates and young infants with coarctation-associated cardiac lesions, congestive heart failure and cardiac shock often occur after closure of patent ductus arteriosus. These neonates with congestive heart failure may present with poor feeding, poor weight gain, retraction, tachypnea, and hepatomegaly. In the so-called ductal shock, after closure of the ductus, these neonates develop acute heart and renal failure with severe acidosis leading to cardiovascular collapse.

Pulse, Blood Pressure, and Oxygen Saturation

Careful evaluation of peripheral pulses and blood pressure should be made in all four limbs.

The femoral and dorsal pulses are usually diminished or absent and delayed in timing, whereas the upper limb pulses are equal and forceful. In neonates with a large ductus with right-to-left shunting, however, pulse and blood pressure in the lower extremities may sometimes be normal. In this ductus-dependent situation, the oxygen saturation in the upper extremities is normal, whereas that in the lower extremities is decreased, because of right-to-left shunting between the ductus and the post-coarctation aorta (differential cyanosis). A diminished left brachial and radial pulse suggests an anomalous origin below the coarctation or localized stenosis of left subclavian artery. A reduced right brachial and radial pulse may suggest an aberrant origin of the right subclavian artery below the coarctation.

The most consistent diagnostic sign in postductal coarctation is hypertension in the arms and hypotension in the legs. The systolic blood pressure is elevated in the arms proximal to the coarctation, and a systolic pressure gradient above 20 mm Hg between arms and legs is thought to be diagnostic of important coarctation.

Heart Murmur

Auscultatory findings vary and depend on the nature of associated cardiac lesions and hemodynamic state. A systolic ejection murmur is usually heard at the upper left sternal border, radiating to the left interscapular area posteriorly in isolated coarctation. The location of this systolic murmur identifies the site of coarctation of the thoracic aorta. A continuous murmur may be heard through the chest anteriorly and posteriorly if the collateral circulation is well developed in older children and adolescents. A ventricular septal defect may produce a pansystolic murmur at the lower left sternal border. Aortic valve stenosis will produce a systolic ejection murmur with a click heard at the apex and the right upper sternal border. A mid-diastolic rumble at the apex may be audible in patients with a large left-to-right shunt in a ventricular septal defect. The first and second heart sounds are generally normal; however, the pulmonary component of the second sound may be accelerated if pulmonary hypertension is present. Gallop rhythms may be heard in neonates and infants with congestive heart failure.

DIAGNOSTIC TECHNIQUES

Chest Radiography

In infants with coarctation of the aorta, there is almost invariably enlargement of the heart, but the outline may vary considerably. If the infant has intracardiac lesions with left-to-right shunting, there may be moderate to severe cardiomegaly with increased pulmonary vascular markings.

In older children and adolescents, the heart may be within normal limits for size or only mildly enlarged. Typically, there may be a visible indentation at the site of coarctation, especially on the posteroanterior projection, producing the so-called 3 sign. In addition, a prominent descending aorta may be visible just below the 3 sign, reflecting poststenotic dilatation. Rib notching is also evident in one third of patients with postductal coarctation, caused by erosion of the inferior surfaces of the posterior ribs by dilated and tortuous intercostal arteries (Fig. 120.3).

Electrocardiography

In general, an infant with coarctation has right axis deviation and right ventricular hypertrophy, but these may sometimes be normal for age. Although left ventricular hypertrophy with a strain pattern of ST-T segment depression is unusual in this age group, it strongly suggests the associated lesion of aortic stenosis or endocardial fibroelastosis. In older children and adolescents, left ventricular hypertrophy is usually evident because of the long-term effects of left ventricular pressure overload. If the right ventricular hypertrophy persists beyond infancy, an associated cardiac lesion, such as ventricular septal defect with pulmonary hypertension, may be present.

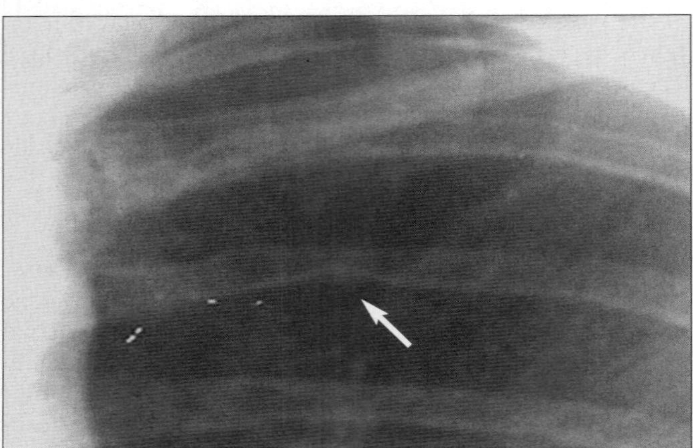

Figure 120.3 Frontal view of the chest radiograph. There are rib notchings at the inferior surface of the posterior ribs *(arrow)*.

Echocardiography

Two-dimensional echocardiography, color-flow mapping, and Doppler studies may provide noninvasive, accurate assessment of the anatomy and physiology of coarctation of the aorta, especially in children. It is important to assess not only the anatomy of coarctation but also that of associated cardiac lesions, such as type of cardiac defect, severity of left ventricular outflow obstruction, and size of aortic arch.[10]

From the suprasternal long-axis view, the aortic arch, including branching arteries, can easily be seen in most neonates and infants; however, visualization may be somewhat difficult in older patients. The localized narrowing of the thoracic aorta is usually seen just beyond the origin of the left subclavian artery (Fig. 120.4). The measurement of the ascending aorta is useful to select an option for intervention and, at older ages, to detect aortic aneurysm.

Color-flow mapping can also assist in evaluating the severity of coarctation of the aorta. A downward turbulent flow is usually detected from the site of coarctation. Its peak instantaneous flow velocity can be measured by Doppler studies. Both pulse-wave Doppler and continuous-wave Doppler studies can provide a calculation of the pressure gradient across the coarctation with use of the modified Bernoulli equation. However, aortic arch geometry (i.e., hypoplastic arch), complex flow dynamics in the aortic arch, difficulty in aligning the Doppler beam with flow, inability to measure flow velocity immediately proximal to the site of the surgical repair, segmental narrowing of the aorta, and collateral flow make Doppler gradients based on the Bernoulli equation not always reliable. Anterograde diastolic flow (diastolic runoff, i.e., "sawtooth" or diastolic "tail") in the thoracic descending aorta, as noted on spectral Doppler tracings, is considered highly specific for a hemodynamically significant recoarctation (Fig. 120.5). In neonates and young infants with cardiac failure, echocardiography is important because cardiac catheterization and angiography may be risky and can sometimes be avoided. In this setting, measurement of the aortic arch, including the isthmus, can assist in determining whether catheter intervention or surgical repair is appropriate. If there is isthmus hypoplasia, surgical repair will be preferable to balloon angioplasty.

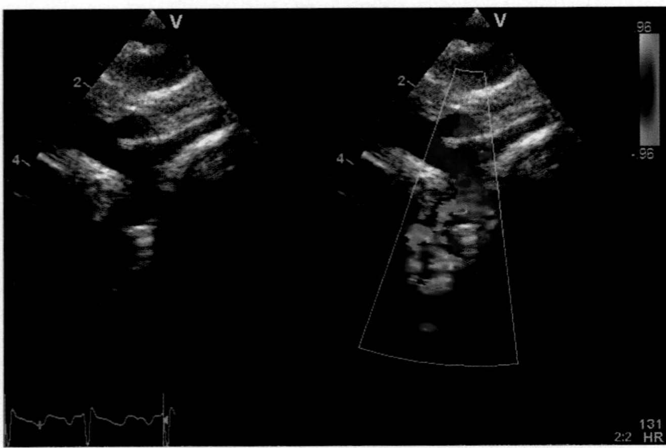

Figure 120.4 Doppler echocardiography of a discrete coarctation of the aorta *(left)*. In the suprasternal view *(right),* flow acceleration at the narrowed site is shown.

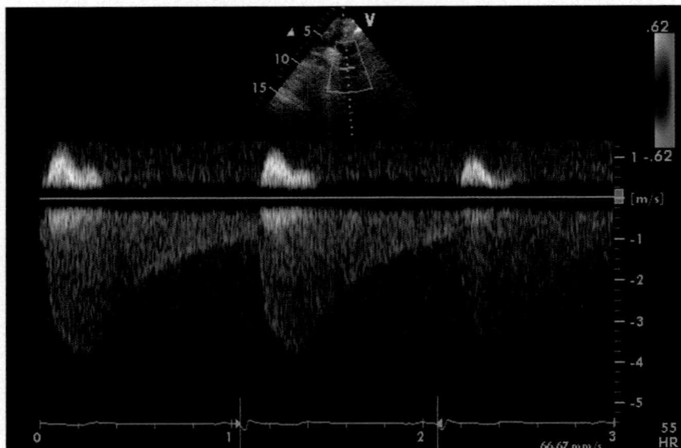

Figure 120.5 Spectral Doppler echocardiography showing anterograde diastolic flow in the descending thoracic aorta (sawtooth), highly specific for significant (residual) aortic obstruction.

Magnetic Resonance Imaging

Magnetic resonance imaging or magnetic resonance angiography in the sagittal and parasagittal projections can clearly define the location and severity of coarctation of the aorta and the anatomy of the transverse aortic arch, isthmus, and poststenotic dilatation; it may also demonstrate the presence of a patent ductus arteriosus and the extent of collateral arteries (Fig. 120.6). This examination is noninvasive, and it has largely replaced the use of diagnostic angiography in older patients. It is the "gold standard" procedure for detection of an aortic aneurysm in the ascending aorta, aortic arch, and descending aorta. After coarctation repair, magnetic resonance angiography should also be performed periodically during follow-up.[11]

Diagnostic Cardiac Catheterization and Angiography

Cardiac catheterization and angiography procedures are invasive, especially in critically ill neonates and young infants. Therefore, catheterization for diagnostic purposes

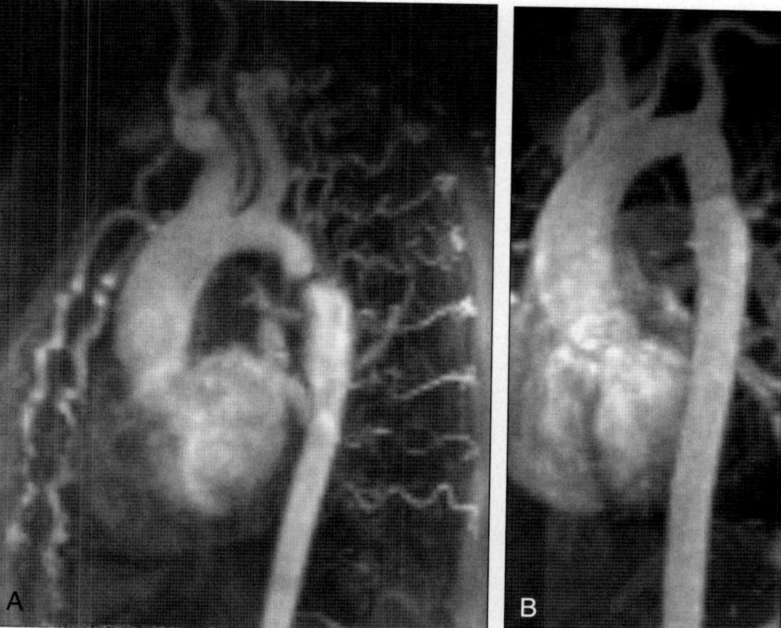

Figure 120.6 **A,** Magnetic resonance angiogram of a severe aortic coarctation and collateral arteries. **B,** Magnetic resonance angiogram of surgically corrected aortic coarctation.

only should be avoided, as clinical evaluation and noninvasive imaging delineate the anatomy and physiology in most cases. However, diagnostic catheterization should be performed if clinical questions remain about the severity of coarctation or associated cardiac lesions or when a catheter intervention is contemplated.

MANAGEMENT

Untreated aortic coarctation carries a poor prognosis. Among all infants born alive with isolated coarctation who are untreated, 10% are expected to die of heart failure within the first month. Without coarctation repair, the mean life expectancy is 35 years, whereas 90% of patients will die before reaching the age of 50 years.[12] The prognosis depends not only on the severity of coarctation but also on associated cardiac lesions.

Surgical Repair

Since surgical repair of aortic coarctation became available (in 1944), survival of these patients has dramatically improved. A variety of different operations have been used to treat coarctation, influenced largely by the age of the patient, the era at the time of repair, and the preference of the individual center. Surgical coarctectomies include resection and end-to-end anastomosis, prosthetic patch aortoplasty, subclavian flap aortoplasty, bypass graft method, and extended end-to-end anastomosis. The procedure is selected according to the extent of narrowing, and each technique has its advantages and disadvantages. Surgical coarctectomy is generally performed through a left thoracotomy incision regardless of the technique.

Resection with end-to-end anastomosis has been the classic repair for coarctation and the treatment of choice for discrete coarctation (Fig. 120.7a).[13] A disadvantage of this method is a high incidence of restenosis induced by the presence of the circumferential suture line. In prosthetic patch aortoplasty (Fig. 120.7b),[13] a longitudinal incision is made across the coarctation, and the lesion is enlarged with a patch made of Dacron or Gore-Tex. A major disadvantage of this method is the use of prosthetic material and the development of para-coarctation (para-patch) pseudoaneurysm. In the subclavian flap aortoplasty (Fig. 120.7c), the left subclavian artery is separated from the vertebral artery, ligated distally, and used to patch the isthmus and the coarcted area. The major advantage of this procedure lies in the use of an autogenous patch, with its potential for growth. The disadvantage is the potential for late growth failure of the left arm because of the sacrifice of the left subclavian artery. Moreover, as there is a ductal tissue remaining after the procedure, restenosis may occur. If the patient has a hypoplastic arch or long segmental stenosis of the aorta, an extended end-to-end anastomosis should be performed (Fig. 120.7d).[14] On occasion, an interposition tube graft is necessary in the older patient, in whom mobilization of the aorta for an end-to-end anastomosis may not be possible, whereas an extra-anatomic conduit repair may be necessary for patients with long-segment aortic arch hypoplasia or those with complex recoarctation.

The mortality rate of surgical repair for isolated coarctation of the aorta is very low in infants and older children. However, it may be higher in the presence of associated lesions. The postoperative morbidity of coarctation repair may include rebound systemic hypertension, spinal cord injury with paralysis, recurrent laryngeal nerve injury with vocal cord paralysis, phrenic nerve injury with hemidiaphragmatic paralysis, chylothorax, bleeding from suture line, and infection.

SURGICAL REPAIR FOR COARCTATION OF THE AORTA

Resection with end-to-end anastomosis

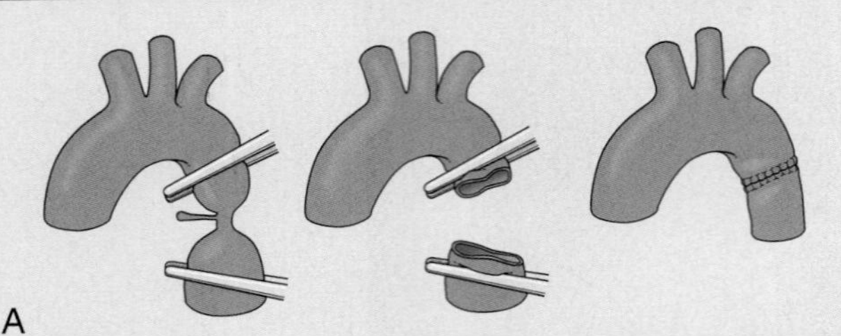

Prosthetic patch aortoplasty

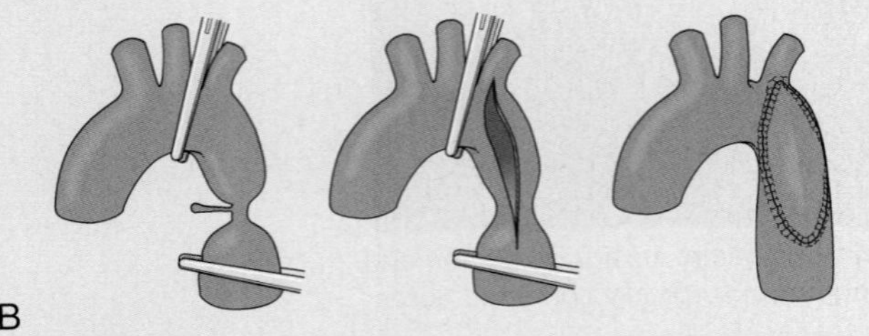

Left subclavian flap aortoplasty

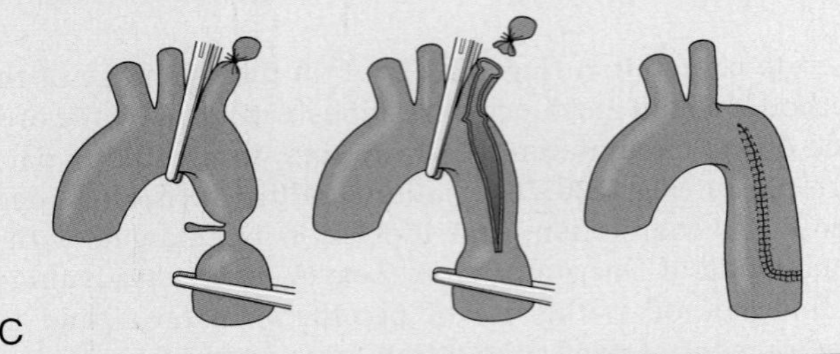

Extended end-to-end anastomosis

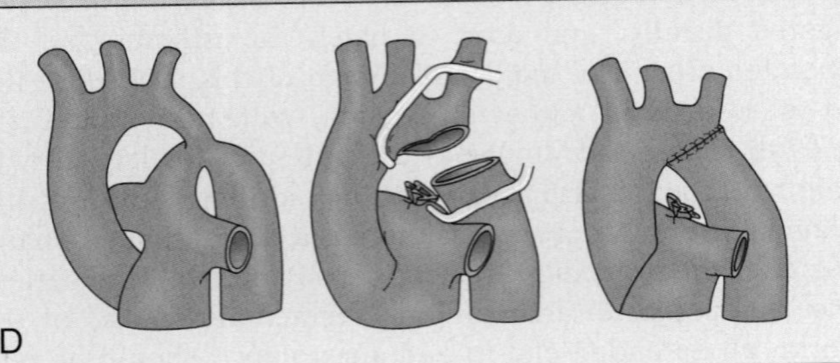

Figure 120.7 Different types of surgical repair for coarctation of the aorta.[13,14]

Catheter Intervention

Catheter intervention for treatment of coarctation has been increasingly applied as an alternative to surgical therapy. Balloon angioplasty was introduced in 1982 and was initially restricted to postoperative recoarctation. This is because the periadventitial surgical scar tissue was thought to be protective against extensive vessel damage after balloon dilatation and to limit the risk of aneurysm formation. Moreover, recurrent postoperative coarctation is difficult to repair surgically, with an increased mortality and morbidity rate, because of tissue adhesions after the previous thoracotomy. Although balloon angioplasty in recoarctation is generally accepted as a safe and effective procedure, large dissections and fatal aortic rupture have been described.

Balloon angioplasty may also be effective in patients with isolated native coarctation with discrete narrowing, with low mortality and morbidity rates similar to those of surgery (Fig. 120.8). Major complications of balloon angioplasty include aortic rupture, aneurysm, femoral artery injury, and restenosis. The incidence of aortic rupture is less than 1%, and the incidence of aortic aneurysm is less than 5%. Older age seems to be a risk factor for suboptimal outcomes, whereas restenosis is reported in approximately 20% of adult patients.[15,16]

Primary endovascular stent implantation with balloon dilatation in the fully grown pediatric or adult patient is now considered the treatment of choice for most cases, resulting in almost complete relief of the gradient in more than 95% of the patients (Fig. 120.9).[17-21] Endovascular stents can generally provide uniform vessel support and more progressive dilatation and stretch, preventing acute vessel disruption. Although some authors have applied such stenting in small children, its use is limited to older children and adults because of size limitations and the risk of stent stenosis with somatic growth. Another benefit of stent placement is the ability to address longer segment coarctations, which typically have a poorer outcome after balloon angioplasty alone. Stent implantation has also been successful in relieving long-segment lesions in Takayasu's arteritis or middle aortic syndrome. Although the short-term results for endovascular interventions are highly compelling, the long-term outcomes of this treatment are unknown at present.

LONG-TERM PROGNOSIS

Long-term outcomes after repair are consistent with those of other operations performed in congenital heart defects: they result in palliation without a cure, necessitating long-term and regular follow-up. Life expectancy is not as normal as in unaffected peers. Many studies have shown a significant late mortality in post-coarctectomy patients.[22] The age at initial repair is a critical predictor of both survival and development of hypertension. Even after early repair, before the age of 5 years, the estimated life expectancy is still reduced; of the patients operated on, 91% are alive at 20 years and 80% at 40 to 50 years after surgery.[23] The modes of death include complications related to persistent or recurrent hypertension, rupture of intracranial or other aneurysms, acute aortic dissection, acute myocardial infarction, and complications of aortic valve disease.

The frequent persistence of systemic hypertension is an important contributing factor to the increased cardiovascular risk and a major concern in post-coarctectomy patients. Despite successful repair, the prevalence of hypertension in adults 10 to 20 years after repair is 20% to 40%, and it may be even higher when patients are observed for a longer time. The most important predictor of premature death and late systemic hypertension seems to be the age at the time of initial repair. However, even after early successful repair, a prevalence of hypertension of 30% has been reported at a mean follow-up of 12 years after repair.[24] The pathogenic

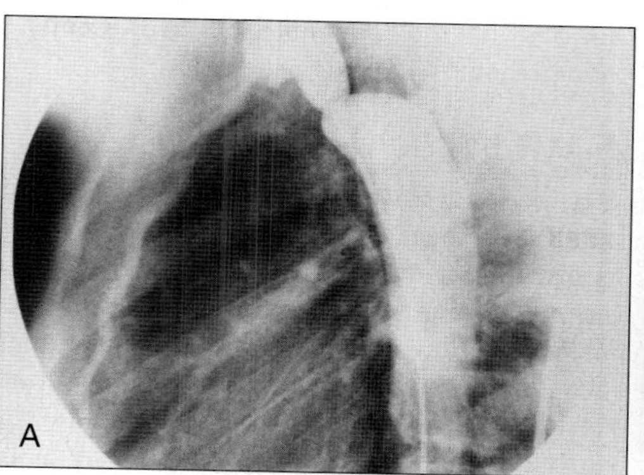

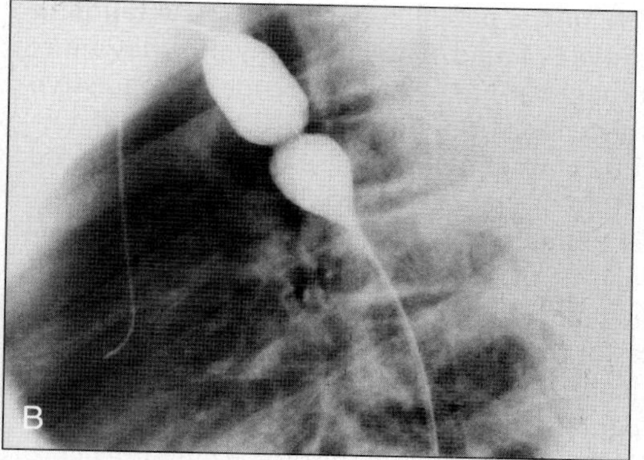

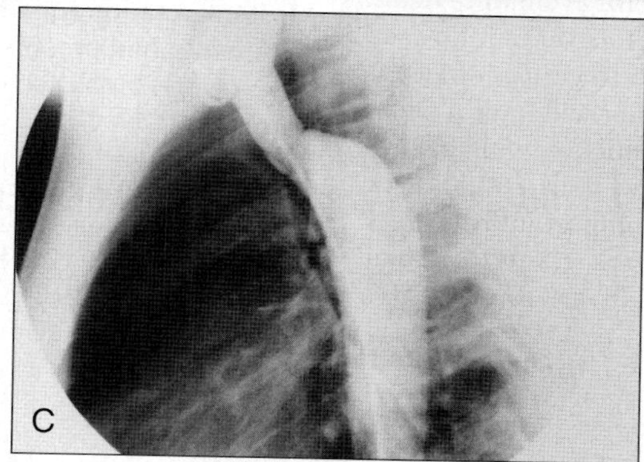

Figure 120.8 Balloon angioplasty for native coarctation of the aorta. Typical aortograms in lateral view before **(A)**, during **(B)**, and after **(C)** balloon angioplasty.

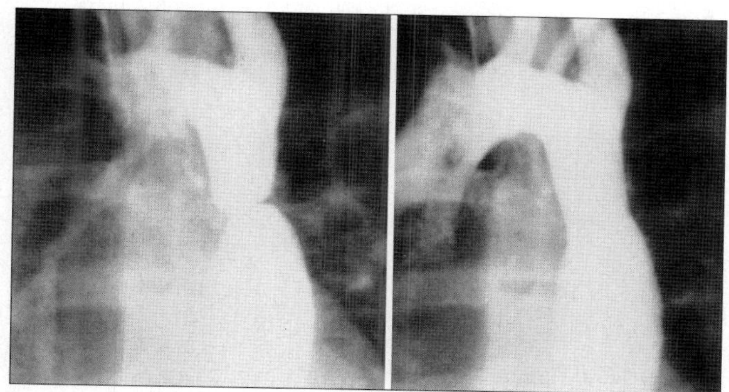

Figure 120.9 Stent implantation for a discrete-type coarctation of the aorta. Frontal view of an aortogram before *(left)* and after *(right)* stent implantation.

mechanism thought to be involved in systemic hypertension is abnormal structure and function of the pre-coarctation arterial conduits (i.e., related to ventricular load). More collagen and less smooth muscle mass are present in the aortic arch, leading to diminished arterial wall compliance and increased rigidity.[25] Untreated high blood pressure contributes to increased arterial wall stiffness, whereas arterial stiffness in turn increases systolic blood pressure. Reduced baroreceptor sensitivity and residual aortic arch gradients (recoarctation or hypoplastic arch) may also be contributing factors.

In addition to the frequently found hypertension, a considerable number of post-coarctectomy patients who are normotensive at rest show a hypertensive response to exercise. The clinical significance of exercise-induced systemic hypertension in post-coarctation repair patients and its relation to clinical outcome and organ damage are not fully elucidated. Carotid intima-media thickness was found to be significantly increased in patients with exercise-induced hypertension, probably indicating an additional risk in post-coarctectomy patients.[26]

The prevalence of recoarctation after surgery in young children ranges from 44% in neonates to 11% in older children and 9% in adult patients.[27-30] The risk is highest after end-to-end anastomosis or subclavian flap repair techniques. Recoarctation is usually defined as a peak-to-peak systolic pressure gradient above 20 mm Hg at catheterization. By use of magnetic resonance imaging, the definition of recoarctation has been variably defined as the ratio of the diameter of the aorta at the repair site to the diaphragmatic site, ranging from 0.5 to 0.9.[31,32] At Doppler echocardiography, the presence of anterograde diastolic flow (sawtooth) at the site of repair indicates hemodynamically significant narrowing. A resting arm/leg blood pressure gradient above 20 mm Hg during physical examination should prompt further investigation.

Aortic aneurysms and dissection are well-known complications after surgical or percutaneous repair of aortic coarctation. Aortic aneurysms may develop at or near the site of repair but also in the proximal aorta. The abnormal structure of the aortic wall (aortic medial disease) in combination with the frequently coexisting hypertension makes patients vulnerable to aneurysm formation or even dissection. The risk is highest after subclavian flap or patch graft repair and after balloon angioplasty. Hemodynamic and hormone-induced vascular changes may increase the risk of aortic dissection during pregnancy.

In 19% to 80% of the patients with aortic coarctation, a bicuspid aortic valve is found. The bicuspid valve may function normally throughout life, or it may develop progressive calcification with stenosis or regurgitation. The bicuspid aortic valve should be considered a disease of the entire aortic root, with accelerated degeneration of the aortic media.

Endocarditis in patients after coarctation repair may occur at the site of repair or more often at an associated abnormal aortic valve. The cumulative incidence of infective endocarditis after successful repair is 0.8% ± 0.4% at 1 year, slowly increasing to 3.5% ± 1.6% at 30 years of follow-up.[33]

It is well recognized that after successful repair of aortic coarctation, patients are at increased risk for premature death due to coronary artery disease. Although long-term follow-up of large numbers of patients with a repair in young infancy is still lacking, it seems likely that early repair will have a beneficial effect in reducing the number of patients dying of premature coronary atherosclerosis. However, residual or recurrent hypertension may still play an important role.

Another cause of premature death is a cerebrovascular accident. Aneurysms of the circle of Willis are found in 3% to 5% of the patients and are usually responsible for hemorrhage.

SUMMARY

The majority of patients with aortic coarctation now reach adulthood because of successful treatment by surgery or transcatheter intervention. Life expectancy, however, is not normal. Long-term complications are frequent and require lifelong follow-up. Magnetic resonance angiography should be performed periodically for the detection of hypoplastic aortic arch, recoarctation, and aortic aneurysms. Even after early repair, systemic hypertension may be present, exposing post-coarctation repair patients to higher cardiovascular risk. Optimal blood pressure control in these patients and elimination of other risk factors for ischemic heart disease are thus paramount.

ACKNOWLEDGEMENT

This chapter reuses part of the material originally written by Drs. Ohkubo and Ino for the previous edition of this book.

chapter 121

Vascular Compression of the Upper Airways

J. Deane Waldman

Definition

- Compression and obstruction of the upper airways by the aorta or its branches, the pulmonary arteries, or an enlarged left atrium is called vascular compression of the upper airways (VCUA).

Key Features

- VCUA is often manifested as reactive airway disease, recurrent pulmonary infections, and sometimes feeding difficulties.
- Chest radiography, echocardiography, and magnetic resonance imaging are the most useful diagnostic modalities.
- Although it is uncommon, VCUA should always be considered in children who have "obvious" intrapulmonary obstructive disease because VCUA is curable.

Therapy

- All forms of VCUA are amenable to surgical repair, which should be offered as soon as the diagnosis is made.

In children, clinical conditions that appear to be pulmonary, such as "reactive airway disease," asthma, and recurrent respiratory infections, may actually be secondary to vascular anomalies that compress and obstruct the upper airways. Such defects, called vascular compression of the upper airways (VCUA), can become manifested at any age. Presentation is not limited to the neonatal period. All such patients should have an evaluation before cardiac or pulmonary surgery. Although VCUA is not common, it should be strongly considered in the differential diagnosis of airway problems for three reasons: (1) treatment of the lung problem may partly address immediate symptoms but does not treat the root cause; (2) virtually all conditions that cause VCUA are treatable; and (3) because lung development continues until 6 to 8 years of age, the sooner normal airflow and blood flow are restored, the closer to normal the trachea, bronchi, alveoli, septa, and blood vessels (i.e., total lung function) will be. This will ultimately optimize the patient's quality of life. A differential diagnosis of the causes of VCUA is provided in Table 121.1.

COMMON PATHOPHYSIOLOGY AND PATHOANATOMY

Regardless of the anatomic basis for large airway obstruction, there are common pathophysiologic features (Fig. 121.1). The cough mechanism and ciliary function are impaired because of distortion of both laminar flow and the endothelium. Secretions and inhaled particulate matter (including microbes) are retained within the lung, causing inflammation and infection. Secondary swelling, retained secretions, and the external compressive structure all reduce the lumen of the airway and logarithmically increase the work of breathing (flow is proportional to the fourth power of the radius). There are reflex mechanisms that may induce apnea, even when hyperpnea and tachypnea would be physiologically appropriate.

In addition to the impaired function, there may be primary or secondary anatomic abnormalities of the upper airways. Primary anatomic defects include congenitally complete cartilaginous rings, congenital stenosis or hypoplasia of the airways, and anomalous or accessory bronchi. The secondary effects produce damage to the cartilaginous rings and airway narrowing.

DIAGNOSTIC MODALITIES

Until the 1970s, standard diagnostic tools for children with possible airway obstruction were history, physical examination (limited use), chest radiography (both anteroposterior and lateral), barium swallow study, and rigid tube bronchoscopy. The esophagram was used to demonstrate the indirect effect of vascular impingement, a large posterior indentation on the esophagus (Fig. 121.2a) typically caused by a right aortic arch that traverses the posterior mediastinum to become a left descending aorta in the thorax.

Echocardiography has been extensively used to evaluate the aortic arch in children. Both precordial and subxiphoid views are useful to image the relative sizes, relationships, and origins of the brachiocephalic vessel and to detect occult congenital heart disease.[1,2] Echocardiography has been reported not only externally but also within vessels and airways. Since the advent of ultrasound imaging, there has been an explosion of technologies, all aimed at increasing information about the anatomic relationships and the physiologic consequences of vascular structures impinging on neighboring airways. Furthermore, technologies such as flexible bronchoscopy and noninvasive tests seek to reduce risk, discomfort, and expense of procedures such as cardiac catheterization with angiography. Some of these new diagnostic technologies are x-ray based, such as spiral computed tomography, noninvasive controlled-ventilation computed tomography, and angiography with additional digital subtraction or balloon occlusion. Magnetic resonance imaging with three-dimensional reconstruction is becoming the definitive diagnostic modality as it provides

CONDITIONS THAT CAN PRODUCE VASCULAR COMPRESSION OF THE UPPER AIRWAYS LISTED ACCORDING TO THE ANATOMIC STRUCTURE CAUSING THE COMPRESSION	
Aortic causes	Right aortic arch with left ligament or ductus
	Left aortic arch with right ligament or ductus
	Double aortic arch
	(The first three conditions are "classic" vascular rings.)
	Right aortic arch with aberrant left subclavian artery and ligamentum arteriosum
	Innominate artery syndrome
Pulmonary artery causes	Pulmonary vascular "sling"
	Tetralogy of Fallot with absent pulmonary valve syndrome
Left atrial enlargement	Large left-to-right shunt with no atrial septal defect
	Stenosis or regurgitation of the left atrioventricular valve
	Cardiomyopathy (dilated or hypertrophic)

Table 121.1 Conditions that can produce vascular compression of the upper airways listed according to the anatomic structure causing the compression.

what is essentially a hologram of the vessels and the airways and their relationships.

Magnetic resonance imaging has become the new "gold standard."[3] In combination with three-dimensional reconstruction computational capabilities, magnetic resonance imaging is now the optimal mode of concurrent imaging of vessels and airways for evaluation of virtually any vascular cause of airway obstruction.[2]

VASCULAR RINGS

Abnormalities of the aortic arch and tributaries have been well described since Maude Abbott's *Atlas of Congenital Cardiac Disease* in 1936.[4] The pioneering work of Jesse Edwards and Maurice Lev linked the anatomic observations to the embryology that underlies vascular rings.

During cardiogenesis, all humans pass through a stage when there is a pair of ventral aortas leading to a pair of dorsal aortas; pairs of lateral aortic arches connect these aortas, one on each side of the developing trachea. Each pair of aortic arches crosses in a ventral to dorsal direction over its respective primitive bronchus. Posterior to the trachea, the two dorsal aortas fuse into a single descending aorta.[5] Researchers have identified six pairs of embryologic arches (Fig. 121.3a) that develop and partly or completely resorb sequentially. By the time that arch pair number 3 forms, at the 10-mm embryo stage, the first two pairs are no longer present. On both sides, remnants of the first two aortic arches provide substrate for the maxillary artery (arch number 1) and the hyoid and middle meningeal arteries (both arch number 2). There is no known persisting fragment of arch number 5 in the normal vascular system. Arches numbers 3, 4, and 6 form parts of the completed aortic arch and its branches (Fig. 121.3b). Maldevelopment of the aortic arches, either abnormal persistence or inappropriate resorption, can lead to vascular compression of the upper airway. Such anomalies are called vascular rings. Although there are numerous varieties of vascular rings, only the three most common ones are described here.

The first of the common types of vascular rings develops when the proximal (or ventral) fourth arch regresses when it should persist (Fig. 121.3c), eliminating the usual route to the distal right subclavian artery. The distal right dorsal aorta and the seventh intersegmental artery provide this blood

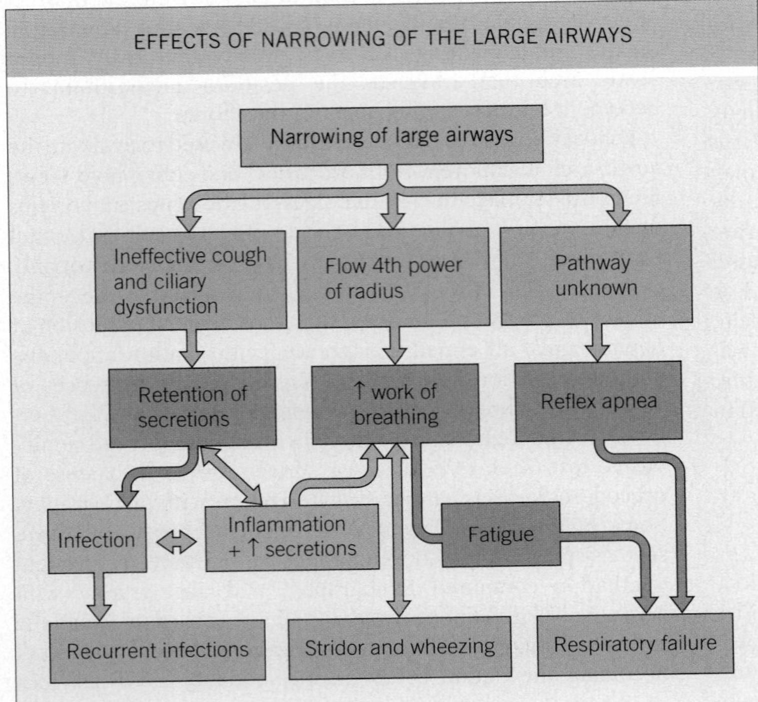

Figure 121.1 Pathophysiology of vascular compression of upper airways: effects of narrowing of the large airways. Narrowing of the upper airways can cause three clinical results: recurrent infections; stridor and wheezing; and respiratory failure. The mechanisms that lead to these outcomes are shown.

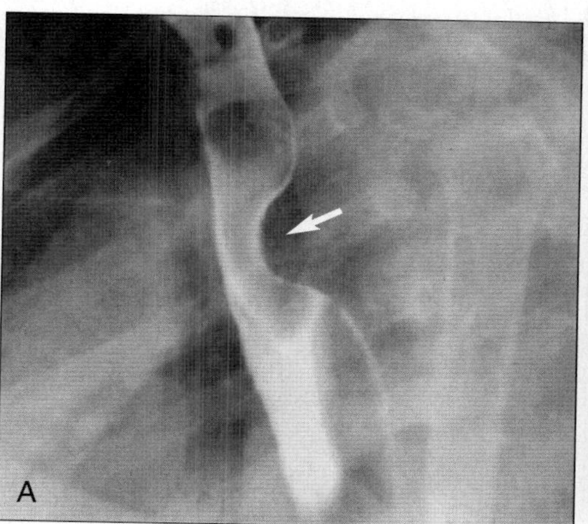

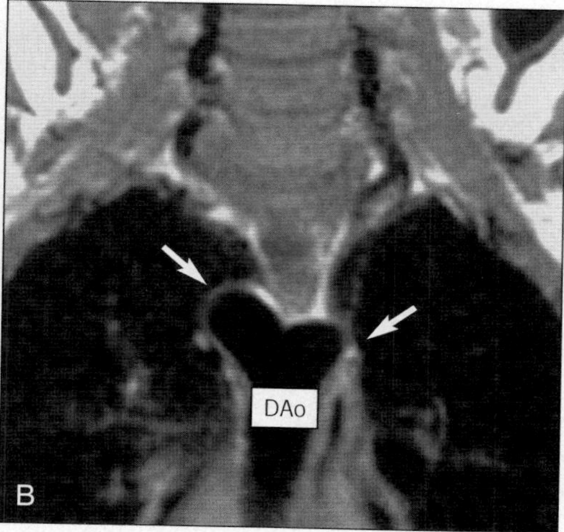

Figure 121.2 Images of vascular rings. A, Lateral view of barium swallow showing a posterior indentation *(white arrow)* made by the aorta crossing the posterior mediastinum from the right side of the patient's chest to the left as part of the vascular ring phenomenon. **B,** Frontal view of an MRI, the two limbs *(white arrows)* of the double aortic arch fuse in the posterior mediastinum to become the descending aorta (DAo).

source. As the great vessels develop, the distal right dorsal aorta is "carried" toward the head and neck vessels so that it ultimately becomes a fourth vessel arising from the proximal descending aorta. Thus, the right subclavian artery arises distal to the origin of the left subclavian artery and must traverse the posterior superior mediastinum—left to right—to supply the right arm. In its passage, this anomalously coursing right subclavian artery can compress the esophagus and trachea (Fig. 121.3d).

In the normal fetus, the distal fourth *right* arch resorbs and the distal fourth *left* arch remains. A second, relatively common type of vascular ring develops when both arches persist (Fig. 121.3e). This results in two channels connecting the ascending (ventral) aorta to the descending (dorsal) aorta. This double aortic arch encircles, compressing both the trachea and the esophagus (Fig. 121.3f).

The most commonly seen vascular ring is usually described by its shorthand name, right arch–left ligament. This type of vascular ring occurs when the left dorsal aorta resorbs abnormally, the right dorsal aorta persists abnormally and forms the only aortic arch (therefore a right aortic arch), and the ductus ligamentum arteriosum forms normally on the left (Fig. 121.3g, h).

Any vascular element that compresses the trachea can cause airway obstruction. The term *vascular ring* is usually limited to those with a complete circle of cardiovascular structures around the trachea and the esophagus. Not all of these vascular structures need be patent. For instance, the classic right arch–left ligament forms a ring of the following elements, named in a clockwise sequence: heart, ascending aorta, right arch, transverse (retroesophageal) arch, ligamentum arteriosum, pulmonary artery back to the heart, thereby completing the circle.[1,6]

There are numerous variations of great vessel anatomy that can cause vascular compression, such as the mirror image of the classic vascular ring: left arch, right descending aorta, and right ligamentum arteriosum.[7]

Typically, a child who has a vascular ring develops symptoms within the first 6 months of life. However, the obstruction may be manifested as late as adolescence, even in the adult years, when the patient may demonstrate exercise intolerance that is thought to be exercise-induced asthma. In between these two extremes are children who have recurrent pulmonary infections or reactive airway disease that is only somewhat responsive to bronchodilators. Because vascular rings can compress all structures within the circle, some of these children have feeding difficulties caused by compression of the esophagus. VCUA should be considered in children with failure to thrive, especially when the swallowing difficulty is experienced with solids more than with liquids.[8]

The treatment of all vascular rings is interruption of the ring, preferably as early as possible. For double aortic arch (Fig. 121.4), this means transection of the smaller arch, usually the left one, which courses over (i.e., runs cephalad to) the left main stem bronchus. When the child has a right arch with left ligament, the surgeon transects the ligamentum arteriosum.[9,10] The child with a double aortic arch may also have a left-sided ligamentum arteriosum, which should be transected at the same time as repair of the double arch. The usual approach is a left posterolateral thoracotomy. Repair of a vascular ring poses a risk to the recurrent laryngeal nerve during dissection around the ligamentum arteriosum.

When a vascular ring is repaired early in life, the trachea and its cartilaginous rings can remodel to achieve a normal airway. If repair is performed later (i.e., after 8 years of age), there is likely to be permanent tracheal deformity and impairment of ciliary action.

INNOMINATE ARTERY SYNDROME

Following the introduction of direct laryngoscopy in babies and infants, pulsatile compression of the trachea was noted in many children during evaluation for airway obstruction. The name given to this condition was innominate artery syndrome.[11,12] The anatomic cause of compression in innominate artery syndrome was considered to be an unusually posterior and rightward-deviated innominate artery. Extrinsic high-pressure, pulsatile impact of the anomalously coursing

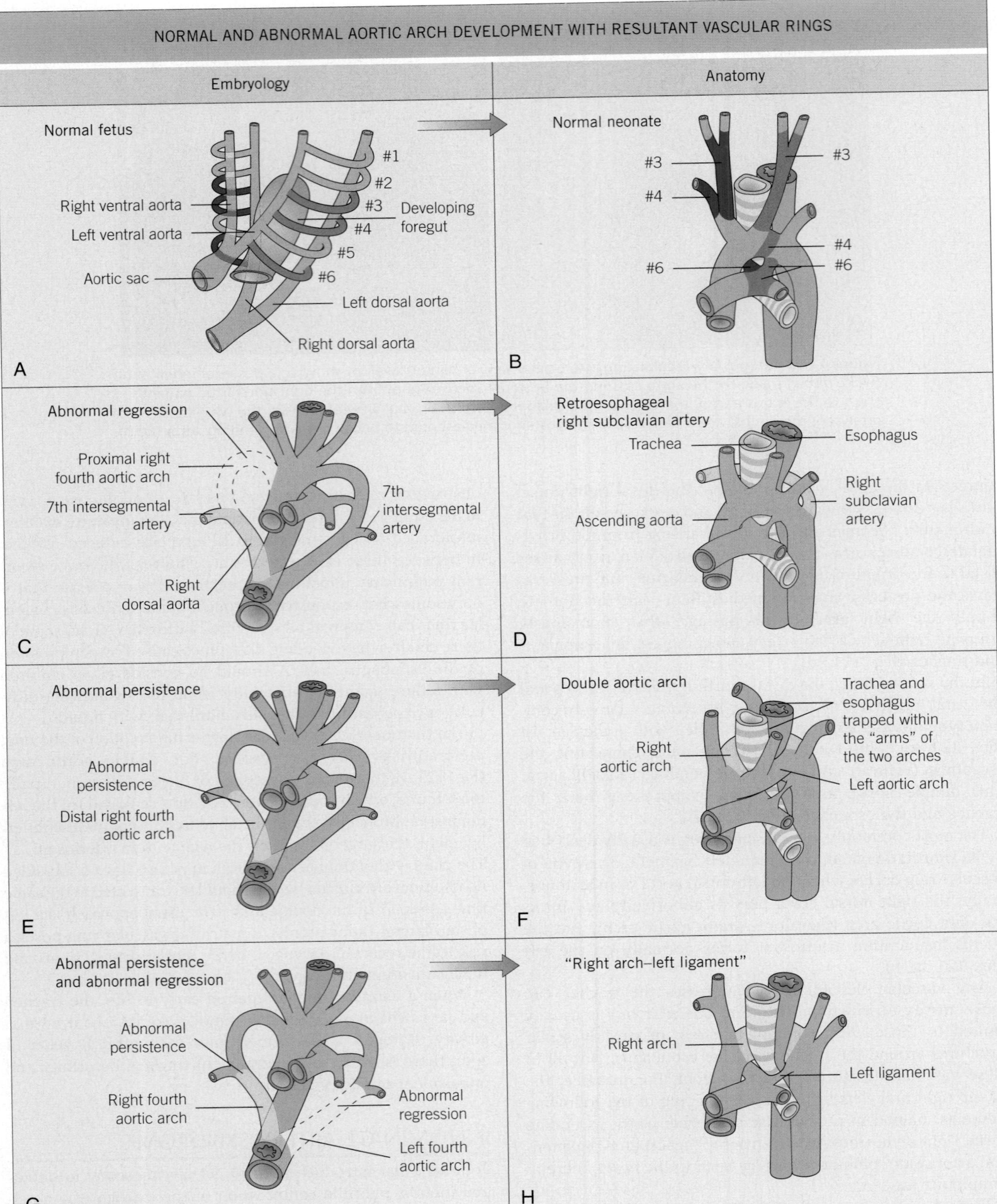

Figure 121.3 Normal and abnormal aortic arch development and the consequences. A, Cardiogenesis, with two ventral and two dorsal aortas and the lateral arch pairs connecting them. **B,** Fully developed aortic arch system, showing the parts derived from the lateral arches. **C,** Abnormal regression of proximal right fourth aortic arch (ventral view). The right dorsal aorta persists from the seventh intersegmental artery to the descending aorta. **D,** This abnormal regression results in a retroesophageal right subclavian artery, which can cause breathing or feeding difficulties. **E,** The distal fourth right arch may persist (normally it is resorbed), giving two complete fourth arches. **F,** This produces the vascular ring caused by a double aortic arch (both right and left). **G,** Regression of the fourth aortic arch may occur on the left but not on the right. **H,** The end product of the cardiovascular maldevelopment in **G** is the classic vascular ring. The yellow area behind the trachea and esophagus (i.e., the right-sided aorta) derives from the distal fourth right arch.

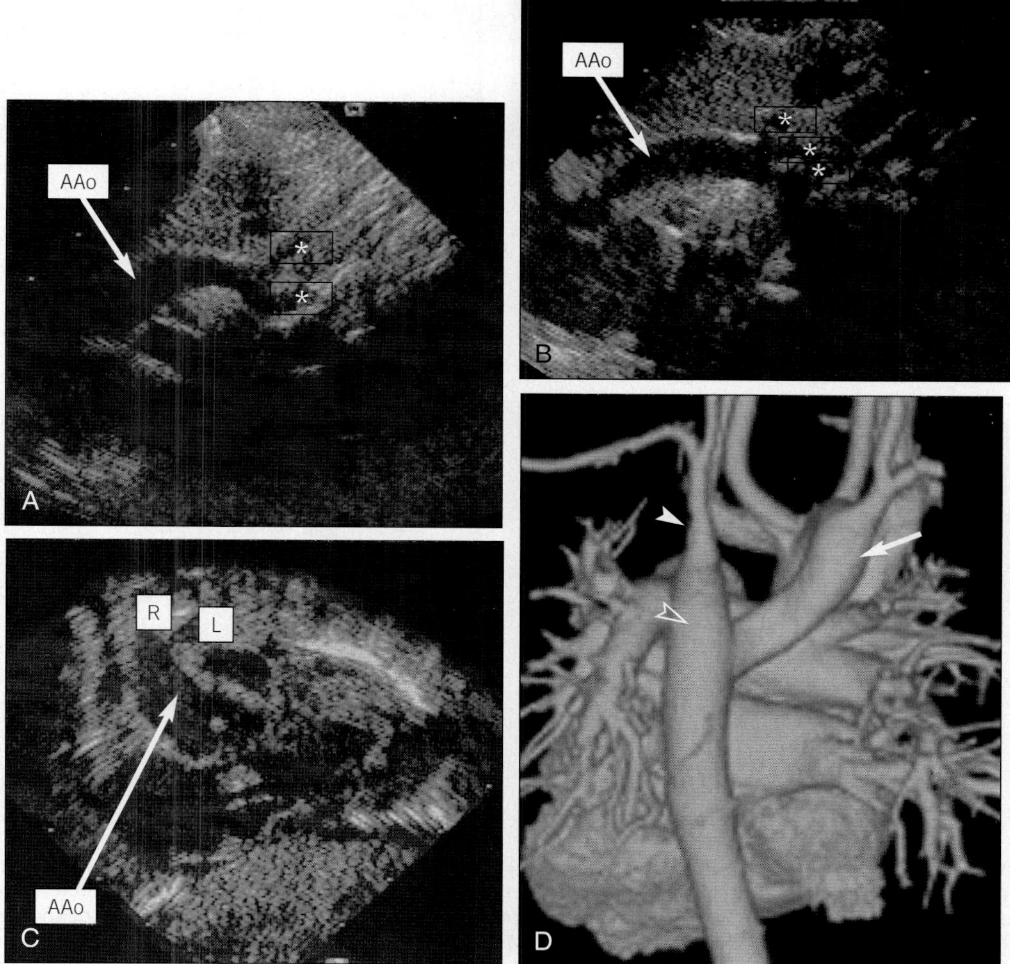

Figure 121.4 Double aortic arch images. A, Precordial echocardiography showing two brachiocephalic vessels *(asterisks)* arising from a transverse aortic arch that is in the patient's left in the chest [AAo = ascending aorta]. **B,** In the same child as in **A,** another aortic arch is shown in the patient's right chest, from which three additional brachiocephalic arteries originate *(asterisks)*. **C,** In an infant with tetraology of Fallot, a subxiphoid view shows a dilated overriding aorta from which arises a larger *right* aortic arch (R) and a smaller *left* aortic arch (L). **D,** Three-dimensional reconstruction from magnetic resonance imaging of a double aortic arch with the right arch *(closed arrowhead)* coursing directly posterior and the left arch *(solid arrow)* crossing the midline to course over the left main stem bronchus to fuse into the descending aorta *(open arrrowhead)*. (Reprinted from Yasuda K, Koyama N, Murayama H, Watabe T. Esophagel stenosis due to vascular ring. *J Pediatric* 2007;150:450).

innominate artery can cause narrowing of the tracheal lumen directly by compression and indirectly by inducing edema.

Clinical signs of wheezing and noisy breathing typically start within the first 2 to 4 months of life. Upper respiratory illnesses are more common than usual, and even when well, the child demonstrates noisy breathing. The distress and extra work associated with breathing can lead to failure to thrive (if forced to choose between eating and breathing, babies choose the latter).

Laryngoscopy was initially the standard diagnostic procedure. Routine chest radiographs are of little help, other than often showing bilateral hyperinflation with air trapping. The tracheal narrowing seen on the lateral chest radiograph, thought to be secondary to innominate artery compression, is now considered to be a common finding in normal children. Barium swallow study is of use only in that a normal study rules out vascular rings. Angiography formerly was used to provide clear delineation of the vascular-airway relationship, but the best current conventional modality is magnetic resonance imaging.[3]

Although it was suggested in 1971 that innominate artery syndrome was the most common of all vascular anomalies causing tracheal obstruction,[11] current thinking suggests that it is relatively uncommon. Whereas the condition undoubtedly exists, it is relatively rare, and other causes of airway obstruction should be aggressively sought.

Treatment of innominate artery syndrome involves either aortopexy or surgical transection and reimplantation of the innominate artery.[13] In those who truly have the innominate artery syndrome, early intervention can lead to a functionally normal trachea and should allow normal quality of life as well as normal life span.

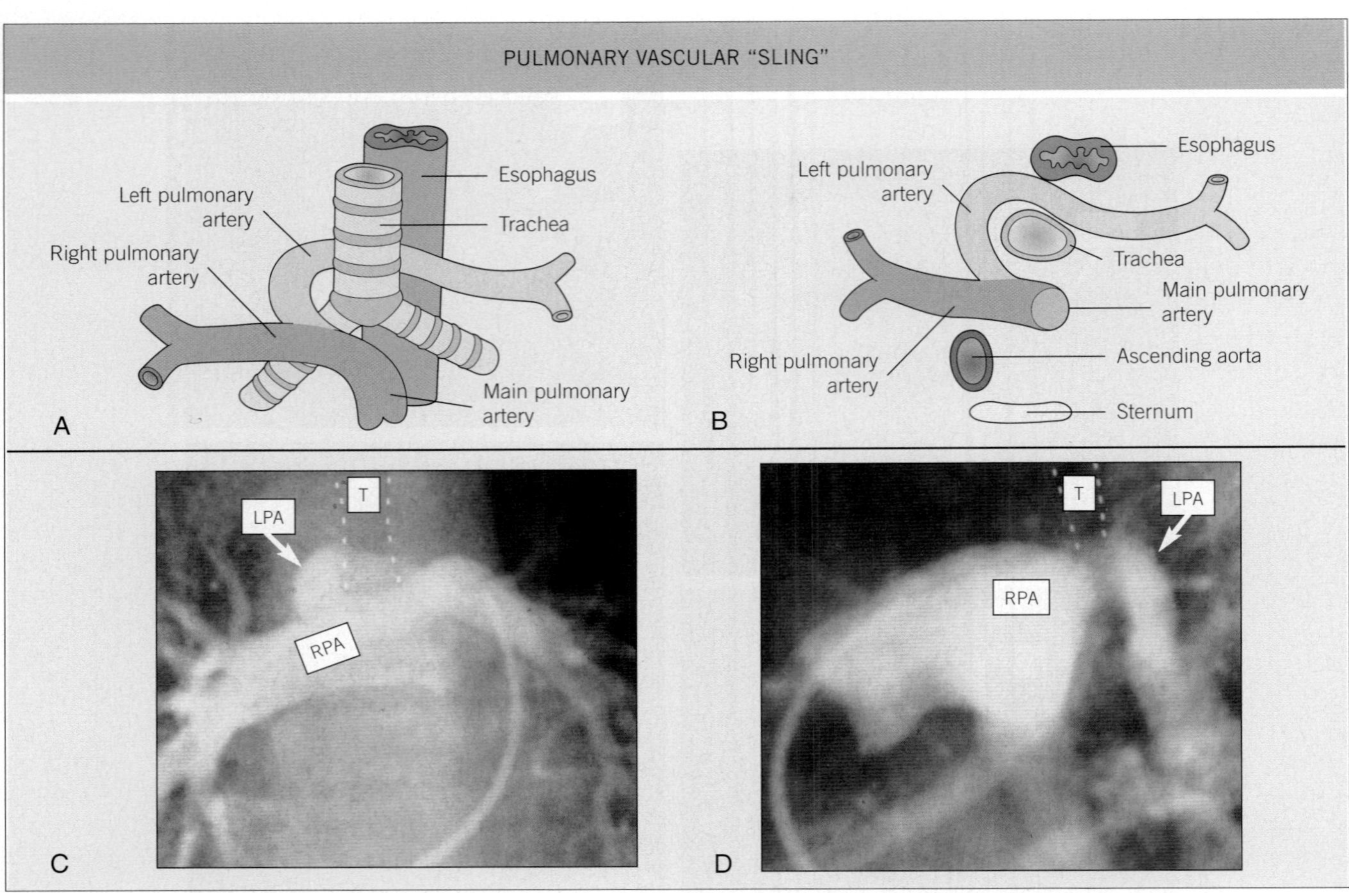

Figure 121.5 Pulmonary vascular "sling." A, Schematic drawing of a frontal view shows the left pulmonary artery arising from the right pulmonary artery and coursing between the trachea and esophagus to enter the left hilum. Both the right main bronchus and the trachea may be compressed by this vascular anomaly. **B,** Coronal view of a pulmonary artery sling. Notice that the left pulmonary artery coursing between the esophagus and trachea might be seen as a "mass" on a lateral chest radiograph. **C,** Frontal angiogram in slight coronal angulation shows a dilated right pulmonary artery (RPA) from which arises the left pulmonary artery (LPA), which turns acutely to cross the midline, seeking the left hilum. Within the hairpin turn or sling of the right pulmonary artery is the trachea and right main bronchus. Compare this angiogram to the drawing in **A**. **D,** Lateral angiogram shows the right pulmonary artery with the anomalous left pulmonary artery wrapping around the trachea (T).

ACQUIRED AORTIC ANEURYSMS

Most of the conditions that can cause VCUA are congenital. They may take years and even decades to become clinically manifested but are present "from birth." There are also acquired medical problems that can cause dilatation of the aorta or the innominate artery to produce VCUA from an acquired problem.

Some of the conditions that have been reported to produce this phenomenon include connective tissue disorders like Marfan's syndrome or Ehlers-Danlos syndrome type IV, necrotizing vasculitis, infective arteritis (such as with syphilis), Takayasu's disease, trauma, and postsurgical complications.

PULMONARY VASCULAR "SLING"

Originally described in 1897 in a postmortem description of a 7-month-old child, pulmonary vascular "sling" derives its name from the acute vascular course around the trachea taken by a left pulmonary artery aberrantly originating from the right pulmonary artery. The pathoanatomy looks as though the pulmonary arteries have wrapped the airway in a constrictive sling.

The anomalous left pulmonary artery courses over the right main bronchus, executes a hairpin turn, and crosses the midline between the trachea and esophagus to reach the hilum of the left lung (Fig. 121.5), where it ramifies normally. Blood flow to either lung is generally not a problem.[14,15] Associated cardiovascular defects are uncommon, although atrial septal defect, anomalies of systemic venous return, and even tetralogy of Fallot have been occasionally reported.[15,16] On the other hand, associated abnormalities of the tracheobronchial system are common, especially complete cartilaginous rings. These may require surgical intervention.[17]

The acutely turning left pulmonary artery compresses either the right main bronchus or the whole trachea, thereby causing obstruction either to the right lung or to both lungs. As the pulmonary vascular resistance naturally drops, flow and pulsations within the pulmonary arteries increase, which exacerbates the obstruction.

Upper airway obstruction is usually apparent within the first month of life. There is either unilateral right or bilateral hyperinflation seen on chest radiography. As there is no "ring" surrounding the esophagus, dysphagia and feeding difficulties are not usually reported.

A frontal chest radiograph often shows air trapping, and lateral views may be helpful by showing a mass in the mid-mediastinum[8]; this mass is the left pulmonary artery seen in cross section coursing between the trachea and the esophagus (see Fig. 121.5b). Bronchoscopy confirms the pulsatile extrinsic compression, and the location of the compression may suggest the diagnosis of stenosis or hypoplasia of the airway. Cardiac catheterization with pulmonary arteriography formerly was the definitive test. Echocardiography has largely supplanted catheterization because it can define the anatomy without invasive study. On ultrasound study, the right pulmonary artery is noted to be quite large (equal to or larger than the ascending aorta), and careful color mapping can identify the abnormal flow pattern of the left pulmonary artery originating from the posterocephalad aspect of the right pulmonary artery and immediately exiting from that plane. With modern rapid acquisition computer software particularly allowing three-dimensional reconstruction, magnetic resonance imaging is becoming the diagnostic procedure of choice.[2,3]

Most children who have pulmonary vascular sling demonstrate obstructive emphysema or recurrent infection that forces early intervention. Treatment is surgical repositioning of the left pulmonary artery from its right pulmonary origin to a normal position on the main pulmonary artery[18]; this usually requires cardiopulmonary bypass. Surgical resection of parts of the tracheobronchial tree has also been required.[15] When complete cartilaginous rings are present, patch tracheoplasty is performed at the same time as the left pulmonary artery reimplantation.[17]

Recent results of treatment have been excellent, with both relief of airway obstruction and preservation of good flow into the left pulmonary artery. However, it often takes months or years for the tracheobronchial tree to become normal. This should be discussed with the family and primary caregiver before surgery to ensure reasonable expectations after the operation. The best outcome for the tracheobronchial tree is achieved by early surgery, preferably within the first year of life.

TETRALOGY OF FALLOT WITH ABSENT PULMONARY VALVE SYNDROME

There has been much confusion over this condition because the term *tetralogy of Fallot* is automatically associated with central cyanosis, that is, cyanosis that is "cardiac in origin." In the more common forms of tetralogy of Fallot, cyanosis is due to abnormal blood flow within the heart. In tetralogy of Fallot with absent pulmonary valve syndrome, cyanosis is due to abnormal airflow within the lungs.

The pathologic anatomy is that of a large malalignment ventricular septal defect (as in typical tetralogy of Fallot) but without subvalvular pulmonary obstruction. There is hypoplasia of the pulmonary valve annulus, where nonfunctional nubbins of tissue are found instead of valve leaflets. Right aortic arch is common.

Pathophysiology results directly from the pathoanatomy. There is both obstruction (from the narrowed annulus) and regurgitation (from the lack of leaflets). In utero, most of these children do not have patent ductus arteriosus, and therefore they have no vent for blood that enters the main pulmonary artery. This blood must go forward toward the high-resistance (unexpanded) lungs or regurgitate backward into the right

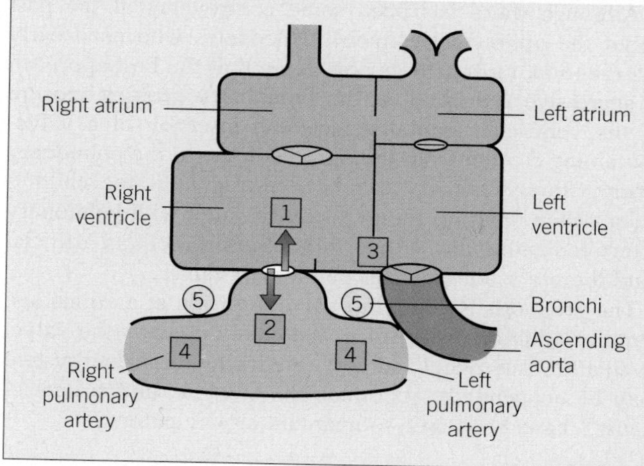

Figure 121.6 Tetralogy of Fallot with absent pulmonary valve syndrome. Because there is no functional pulmonary valve, there is severe pulmonary regurgitation (1). A stenotic pulmonary orifice creates a high-velocity jet during systole into the pulmonary artery (2). There is a large malalignment ventricular septal defect (3) allowing interventricular flow, usually left to right. There is a massive dilatation of the pulmonary arteries (4) that press on the bronchi (5), leading to upper airway obstruction and secondary cyanosis.

ventricle, from which it came. On the next contraction, the right ventricle ejects the blood that entered from the tricuspid valve as well as the blood that came back from the main pulmonary artery (Fig. 121.6).[19,20] Thus, in utero, there is progressive right ventricular enlargement and massive dilatation of the hilar pulmonary arteries. Branch pulmonary arteries in a normal term neonate measure approximately 5 to 7 mm each, but in tetralogy of Fallot with absent pulmonary valve syndrome, they often measure 25 to 40 mm. This results in compression of the bronchi and cyanosis due to airway obstruction (see Fig. 121.6).

Clinically, these patients fall into two groups: those who have severe respiratory distress as neonates and those who can tolerate the obstruction without assisted ventilation. Children in the first group require reparative surgery as neonates, with significant risk of death. Those in the second group, even though they may be tachypneic and hyperpneic, may grow well enough to enable repair to be deferred until they weigh more than 5 kg, when the operative risk is low. Tetralogy of Fallot with absent pulmonary valve syndrome can be diagnosed by physical examination; there is cyanosis of varying degree in a neonate who has respiratory distress and a loud (often grade 4 or 5) to-and-fro, not continuous, murmur. The chest radiograph shows hyperinflation and evidence of huge pulmonary arteries. The diagnosis can be confirmed by echocardiography, which shows

- the malalignment ventricular septal defect (9-o'clock to 12-o'clock position in the short-axis view);
- a small pulmonary annulus with no valve leaflets;
- the pulmonary stenosis and severe regurgitation on color mapping; and
- the massively dilated pulmonary arteries.

Cardiac catheterization is usually necessary only if there are questions about the origins and courses of the coronary arteries, given that the surgery entails a right ventriculotomy, which might pose a risk to an anomalously coursing left coronary arterial branch.

Although there has been some controversy in the past about the optimum treatment of neonates who need early intervention, most centers now agree that the best approach is aggressive reduction of the pulmonary arteries, closure of the ventricular septal defect, and insertion of a valve-containing conduit from the right ventricle to the pulmonary artery. Rarely, surgery can be deferred until the child is older, when repair of the tetralogy of Fallot with pulmonary artery reduction may suffice without insertion of an artificial (and therefore nongrowing) pulmonary valve.

The prognosis is good, but valve insertion at a young age requires additional surgery as the child outgrows the valve. Even after "successful" surgery, the tracheobronchial system may be congenitally abnormal and stenotic; endobronchial stents[21] have been used to maintain airway patency.

LEFT ATRIAL HYPERTENSION

When the left atrium is enlarged for any reason, it presses against the left main bronchus. This can cause respiratory distress, atelectasis of the left lower lobe, and pneumonia.

In virtually all circumstances in which the heart is on the left side of the chest, the left main bronchus courses directly over the left atrium and is in immediate contact with it. Any condition that raises left atrial pressure can force the roof of the left atrium to press against the inferior surface of the left main bronchus, narrowing and even obstructing it. A large interatrial communication will "vent" the left atrium. Therefore, compression of the left main bronchus secondary to left atrial hypertension occurs only in the absence of an atrial septal defect.

Conditions that can induce left atrial hypertension with secondary compression of the left main stem bronchus are

- large left-to-right shunt distal to the mitral valve, such as a large ventricular septal defect or patent ductus arteriosus;
- mitral valve disease, such as stenosis or regurgitation; and
- diastolic dysfunction of the left ventricle raising left ventricular end-diastolic pressure, such as is seen in dilated or hypertrophic cardiomyopathy.

Airway obstruction in these conditions may sometimes be missed because of the obvious signs of congestive heart failure. Coughing, rales, shortness of breath, and tachypnea may all be ascribed to the primary problem, but the chest radiograph will show atelectasis of the left lower lobe. It is not uncommon for children with dilated cardiomyopathy to present with respiratory distress and a left lower lung wedge-shaped mass as their first manifestations.

The first clue to the problem usually is the frontal chest radiograph, which shows left lower lobe collapse and a "tented-up" left main bronchus in which the air column abruptly terminates. Echocardiography delineates both the primary condition and the physiologic changes affecting the left atrium. Although bronchoscopy can "make" the diagnosis, tests other than chest radiography and echocardiography are rarely necessary.

The approach to left lower lobe atelectasis secondary to left atrial hypertension is treatment of the primary problem rather than of the secondary effect. Closure of the ventricular septal defect or repair of the regurgitant mitral valve should relieve the high pressure within the left atrium and therefore eliminate the reason for bronchial compression. Although it is preferable to re-expand a collapsed lung before an operation, this is often not possible, and therefore it may be necessary to intervene even though the probability of postoperative morbidity is higher.

Addressing the primary reason for left atrial hypertension usually solves the airway obstruction. Although damage to the left main bronchus may occur, this is usually not a long-term problem because adaptive remodeling takes place.

SUMMARY

Although VCUA is relatively uncommon, it should be considered in every child who has recurrent upper respiratory infection or reactive airway disease. The differential diagnosis involves three anatomic structures: the aorta, the pulmonary artery, and the left atrium. Virtually all children with possible VCUA should have echocardiography; additional tests, such as bronchoscopy, magnetic resonance imaging, barium swallow study, and angiography, depend on the condition under consideration. All forms of VCUA are treatable surgically with low risk. The earlier that VCUA is resolved, the greater is the chance of normal airways.

chapter

122 Kawasaki Disease

Hirohisa Kato

Definition

- Kawasaki disease is an acute systemic vasculitis syndrome in infants and young children of unknown etiology that mainly affects small and medium-sized arteries, particularly the coronary artery.

Key Features

- The clinical feature is an acute febrile illness associated with mucocutaneous involvement and lymphadenopathy. Coronary aneurysms develop in about 10% to 20% of the patients, some of which may cause myocardial infarction or develop into ischemic heart disease.

Therapy

- High-dose immune globulin and aspirin compose the essential treatment of acute Kawasaki disease.

Kawasaki disease (KD) or mucocutaneous lymph node syndrome is an acute vasculitis syndrome in infants and young children of unknown etiology that mainly affects small and medium-sized arteries, particularly the coronary artery.[1] The cardiovascular problems in KD are concerned with the coronary artery lesions, which develop aneurysm formation, thrombotic occlusion, progression to coronary artery disease, and premature atherosclerosis.[2] These may cause myocardial infarction or sudden death in the young. This disease was first described by Tomisaku Kawasaki in Japan[3]; however, it has since been recognized all over the world and is now a leading cause of acquired heart disease in children in North America and Japan.

ANATOMY AND PATHOLOGY

Pathology of Kawasaki Vasculitis

On the basis of analyses of 37 KD autopsy cases, the Japanese Kawasaki Disease Research Committee reported the following pathomorphologic findings.[4,5] KD is an acute inflammatory disease with systemic vasculitis in small or medium-sized arteries. It is distinguishable from classic periarteritis nodosa of the Kussmaul-Maier type, which is a progressive and recurrent angiitis with marked fibrinoid necrosis. KD is an acute vasculitis with rare and mild fibrinoid necrosis. Infantile polyarteritis resembles fatal KD in many pathologic aspects,[6] and it is now believed that KD and infantile polyarteritis are the same systemic arteritis.

KD is described as a systemic vasculitic syndrome with a wide spectrum of clinical symptoms and disease severity. The course of vasculitis is classified into four stages, according to the duration of illness:

- Stage 1 (1 to 2 weeks of illness): perivasculitis and vasculitis of the microvessels, small arteries, and veins; inflammation of intima, externa, and perivascular areas in the middle- and large-sized arteries; edema and inflammation with polymorphonuclear cells, rapidly followed by macrophages and lymphocytes.
- Stage 2 (2 to 4 weeks of illness): inflammatory changes of intima, media, externa, and perivascular areas in the middle-sized arteries with focal panvasculitis; aneurysms with thrombi and stenosis in the middle-sized arteries, especially in the coronary arteries; edema (exudative stage), infiltration with monocytes or necrosis (infiltrative stage), and cellular granulation with increase of capillaries.
- Stage 3 (4 to 7 weeks of illness): granulation in the middle-sized arteries.
- Stage 4 (more than 7 weeks of illness): scar formation and intimal thickening with aneurysm, thrombi, and stenosis in the middle-sized arteries (generally no acute inflammation in the vessels); these findings may persist until adult age.

Myocarditis (interstitial myocarditis with mild necrosis) involving conduction systems, pericarditis, endocarditis, cholecystitis, cholangitis, pancreatic ductitis, sialadenitis, meningitis, and lymphadenitis is frequently seen.

EPIDEMIOLOGY

Epidemiology in Japan, where KD is most prevalent, has been well documented by the Research Committee organized by the Ministry of Health and Welfare of the Japanese government.[7]

Epidemiology of KD can be summarized as follows:

- The number of patients has increased since 1968 and now totals more than 225,652 (from 1968 to 2006).
- KD affects more than 9000 children each year in Japan, and the incidence is 188.1 per 100,000 children younger than 4 years (in 2006).
- Age distribution is from 1 month of age with a peak at 1 year of age; 50% of patients are younger than 2 years; patients older than 10 years are quite rare.
- More boys than girls are affected (1.5:1).
- It is evident that this is more prevalent in Japanese (i.e., Asians) than in white individuals.

- No geographic differences in urban or rural environments, or in the south or north, have been identified, and KD is widely prevalent throughout Japan.
- Seasonal variation is not distinct; however, there are small peaks in winter-spring.
- The recurrence rate is about 3.3%, and sibling cases are 1% to 2%.
- Time-space clustering or outbreaks in the community are recognized; however, there is no evidence of person-to-person transmission. In 1979, 1982, and 1986, there were large outbreaks in Japan; but in the last 10 years, there has been no such epidemic.

The global epidemiology of KD was described by Nakamura and Yanagawa,[8] and accordingly, KD is now widely recognized all over the world. However, it is most prevalent in Japan and East Asia, and Asians are 5 to 10 times more susceptible than white people are. An estimated 3000 cases are diagnosed annually in the United States.

PATHOPHYSIOLOGY

Etiology and Pathogenesis

The etiology of KD remains unknown despite extensive investigations. On the basis of clinical features and epidemiologic data, KD is considered to be an infectious illness of unknown etiologic agent or to be an infection-triggered immune disorder with hypercytokinemia.

KD has clinical similarities to scarlet fever and toxic shock syndrome, both of which are caused by toxin-producing bacteria. These toxins have been revealed to be superantigens capable of stimulating T cell–carrying particular variable regions of the T-cell receptor β chain. A study on peripheral blood T cells in KD has shown that T cells that express T-cell receptor variable regions $V_{\beta}2$ and $V_{\beta}8$ are selectively expanded.[9] These observations suggest that KD may be caused by a toxin (superantigen)–producing microorganism. Leung and colleagues[10] suggested that the expansion of $V_{\beta}2^{+}$ T cells in most patients with KD may be caused by a new clone of toxic shock syndrome toxin-secreting *Staphylococcus aureus* by studying bacterial culture from patients with KD. However, several other studies did not support this theory.[11] Yoshioka and associates[12] reported that streptococcal pyrogenic exotoxin C (SPEC) induces activation and polyclonal expansion of $V_{\beta}2$- and $V_{\beta}6.5$-positive T cells and that SPEC-induced activation of T cells may lead to the pathogenesis of KD.

Yersinia pseudotuberculosis appears to be one of the etiologic agents of KD,[13] although this organism was implicated in only a small group of patients with KD. *Propionibacterium acnes* was isolated from the cervical lymph node of KD patients who produced the cytotoxic protein-like bacterial exotoxin,[14,15] but its etiologic role remains to be determined.

Rarely, Epstein-Barr virus may induce clinical pictures that mimic those of KD.[16] However, epidemiologic, serologic, and virologic studies do not support a causal role of Epstein-Barr virus in KD. Rowley and coworkers[17] reported that immunoglobulin A plasma cells infiltrate the vascular wall in acute KD as a monoclonal or oligoclonal response.

The acute phase of KD is associated with markedly increased production of inflammatory cytokines. Tumor necrosis factor α (TNF-α), interleukin 1β, and interferon γ induce activation antigens and adhesion molecules such as endothelial leukocyte adhesion molecule 1 and intercellular adhesion molecule 1 on endothelial cells, and TNF-α and interferon γ caused endothelial injury in in vitro studies.[18] Coronary artery endothelial cells in KD actually expressed activation antigens in a necropsy study.[19]

Many hypotheses of etiology and pathogenesis of KD have been proposed; however, no host-microbial relationship specific to KD has yet been identified. KD disperses widely in the community, has a self-limited nature, involves multiple organs, and affects infants and young children. These findings suggest that this disease may be caused in some susceptible children by ubiquitous infectious agents.

CLINICAL PRESENTATIONS

Symptoms and Diagnosis of Kawasaki Disease

The diagnosis of KD is made according to the diagnostic guidelines prepared by the Japanese Kawasaki Disease Research Committee (Table 122.1) because of the absence of a specific laboratory test. The principal diagnostic criteria of KD are persistent fever, conjunctival injection, changes in the mucosa of the oropharynx, changes in the peripheral extremities, erythematous rash, and cervical lymphadenopathy (Fig. 122.1). At least five of the six principal symptoms should be present for a diagnosis of KD to be made. However, patients with four of these symptoms can be diagnosed as having KD when coronary aneurysms are recognized by two-dimensional echocardiography or coronary angiography. Patients younger than 6 months and children older than 6 years demonstrate atypical symptoms, but coronary artery lesions may occasionally be present (see Table 122.1).

Cardiovascular Spectrum

The cardiovascular spectrum of 2180 patients with acute KD experienced during the last 31 years is shown in Table 122.2. Of all the patients, 14.9% were diagnosed as having coronary aneurysms. From 1992, we selected patients for immune globulin treatment; since then, the incidence of coronary aneurysms has declined to 8.7%. The coronary artery lesion is the most important lesion in KD; however, aneurysms in other arteries, such as in the axillary, iliac, or renal arteries, were observed in 1.0% of the patients. Valvular heart disease appeared in about 1.5% of the patients. Myocardial infarction occurred in 24 patients, 10 of whom died. Half of the fatal cases did not demonstrate any ischemic findings before the onset of myocardial infarction.

Myocardial Infarction and Death

The main cause of death in KD is acute myocardial infarction. The study of 104 fatal cases of KD in Japan suggests that 56.7% of the patients died of acute myocardial infarction and 18% died of congestive heart failure caused by ischemia. Five patients died of rupture of coronary aneurysms. In the 1970s, the fatality rate of KD was about 2%; however, in the 1990s, it declined to 0.2% in Japan. We analyzed 195 KD patients with myocardial infarction from the

DIAGNOSTIC GUIDELINES FOR KAWASAKI DISEASE
This is a disease of unknown etiology that most frequently affects infants and children younger than 5 years. The symptoms can be classified into two categories: principal symptoms and other significant symptoms or findings (Japanese Kawasaki Disease Research Committee[24]).
Principal symptoms
1. Fever persisting 5 days or more (including those cases in which the fever has subsided before the fifth day after therapy) 2. Changes of peripheral extremities: Initial stage: reddening of palms and soles, indurative edema Convalescent stage: membranous desquamation of the fingertips 3. Polymorphous exanthema 4. Bilateral conjunctival congestion 5. Changes of lips and oral cavity: reddening of lips, strawberry tongue, diffuse injection of oral and pharyngeal mucosa 6. Acute nonpurulent cervical lymphadenopathy At least five of these items should be satisfied for diagnosis of Kawasaki disease. However, patients with four of the principal symptoms can be diagnosed as having Kawasaki disease when coronary aneurysms are recognized by two-dimensional echocardiography or coronary angiography.
Other significant symptoms or findings
1. Cardiovascular: auscultation (heart murmur, gallop rhythm, distant heart sounds), electrocardiographic changes (prolonged PR or QT intervals, abnormal Q waves, low-voltage ST-T changes, arrhythmias), chest radiography (cardiomegaly), two-dimensional echocardiography (pericardial effusion, coronary aneurysms), aneurysms of peripheral arteries other than coronary (axillary, iliac), angina pectoris or myocardial infarction 2. Gastrointestinal tract: diarrhea, vomiting, abdominal pain, hydrops of gallbladder, paralytic ileus, mild jaundice, slight increase of serum transaminase 3. Blood: leukocytosis with shift to the left, thrombocytosis, increased erythrocyte sedimentation rate, positive C-reactive protein, hypoalbuminemia, increased α_2-globulin, slight decrease in erythrocyte and hemoglobin levels 4. Urine: proteinuria, increase of leukocytes in urine sediment 5. Skin: redness and crust at the site of BCG inoculation, small pustules, transverse furrows of the fingernails 6. Respiratory: cough, rhinorrhea, abnormal shadow on chest radiograph 7. Joint: pain, swelling 8. Neurologic: pleocytosis of mononuclear cells in cerebrospinal fluid, convulsion, unconsciousness, facial palsy, paralysis of the extremities
Remarks
For item 2 under principal symptoms, the convalescent stage is considered important. Nonpurulent cervical lymphadenopathy is less frequently encountered (approximately 65%) than are other principal symptoms during the acute phase. Male-to-female ratio: 1.3-1.5:1; patients younger than 5 years: 80%-85%; fatality rate: 0.1% Recurrence rate: 2%-3%; proportion of sibling cases: 1%-2% Approximately 10% of the total cases do not fulfill five of the six principal symptoms; however, if other diseases can be excluded, Kawasaki disease may be suspected. In some of these patients, coronary artery aneurysms (including so-called coronary artery ectasia) have been confirmed.

Table 122.1 Diagnostic guidelines for Kawasaki disease.

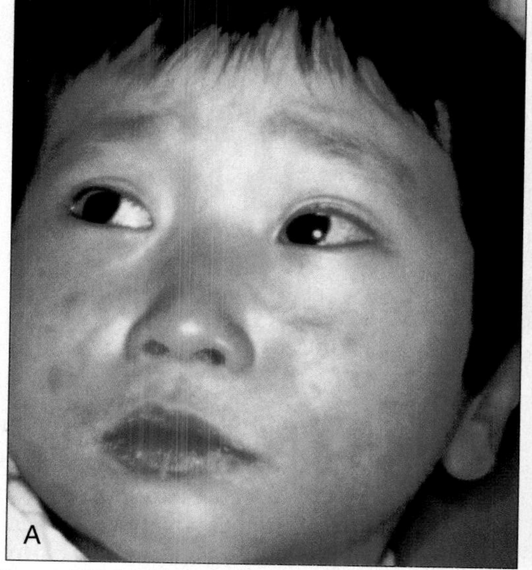

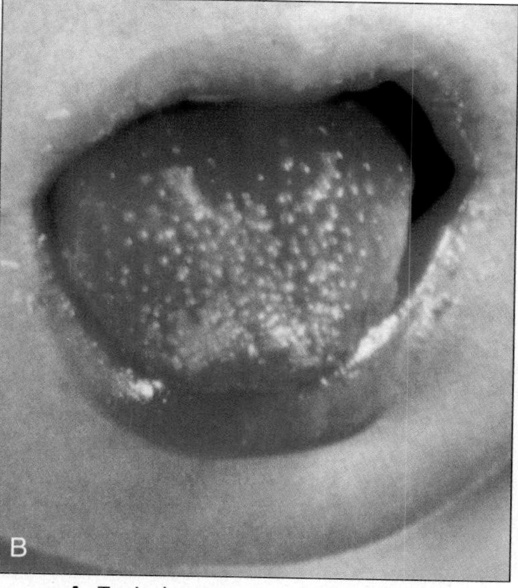

Figure 122.1 Clinical manifestations of Kawasaki disease. A, Typical appearance of face, bilateral conjunctival injection. **B**, Strawberry tongue.

(*Continued*)

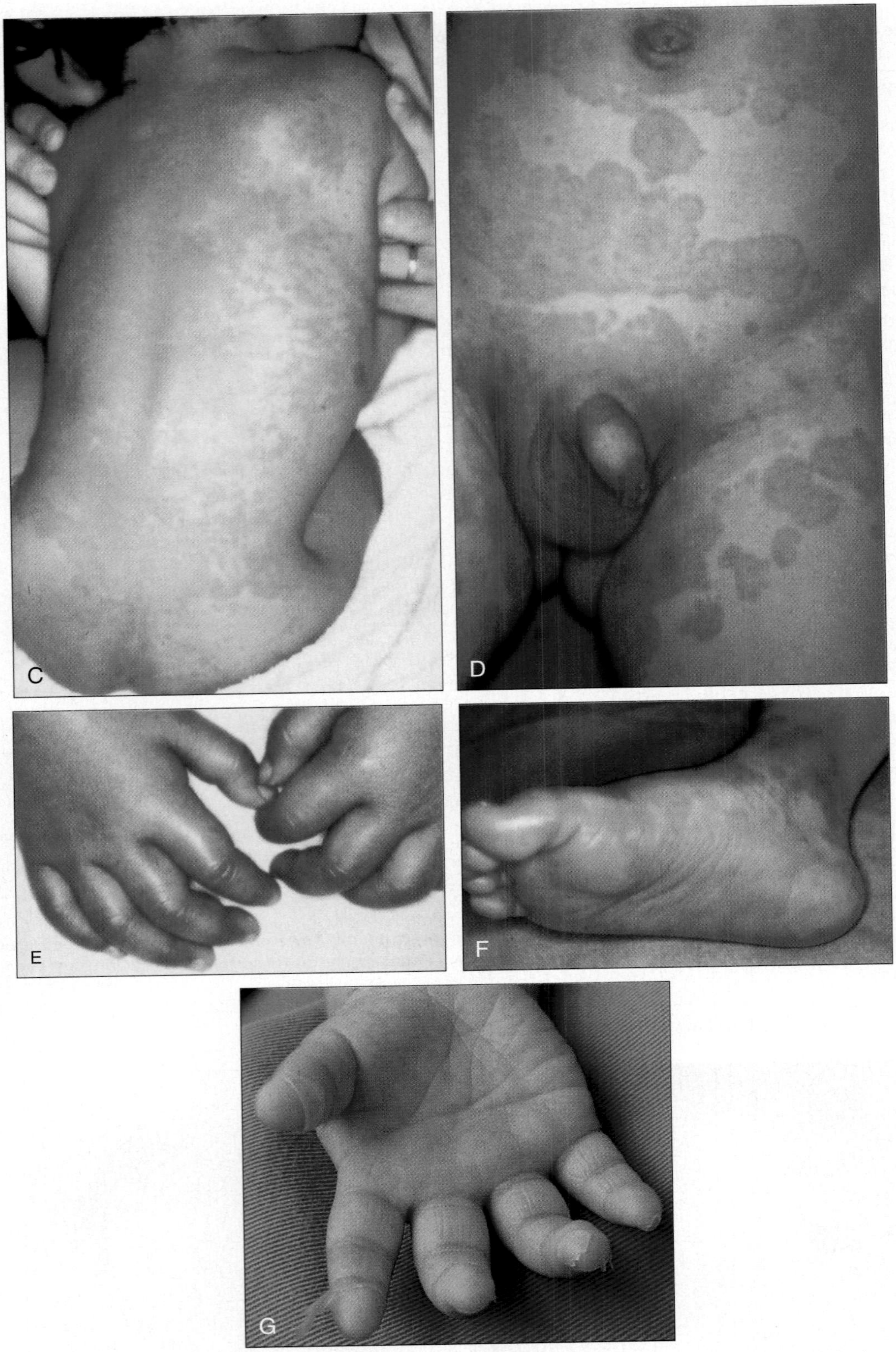

Figure 122.1—cont'd C and **D,** Polymorphous exanthema. **E,** Indurative edema of the hands. **F,** Redness and swelling of sole. **G,** Desquamation of fingers.

nationwide survey in Japan.[20] Myocardial infarction mostly occurred within 1 year of illness; however, late deaths several years after acute KD have increased relatively recently. It might occur at any time in the presence of obstructive lesions. Attacks of myocardial infarction are relatively more frequent at night, when the patient is sleeping or resting, with primary manifestations of shock symptoms, pallor, unrest, vomiting, and abdominal pain. Chest pain was more frequently recognized in the survivors of myocardial infarction and in children older than 4 years with KD.

CARDIOVASCULAR SPECTRUM IN KAWASAKI DISEASE	
Coronary artery	
Transient dilatation in acute state	282/1558 (18.1%)
Coronary aneurysm	325/2180 (14.9%)
1973-1990, aspirin treatment	253/1355 (18.6%)
1991-2001, immune globulin + aspirin	72/825 (8.7%)
Systemic artery aneurysms	
Axillary, iliac, renal, other	22/2180 (1.0%)
Mitral regurgitation	28/2180 (1.3%)
Aortic regurgitation	5/2180 (0.2%)
Pericarditis or pericardial effusion	241/1871 (12.9%)
Myocarditis	617/2180 (28.3%)
Myocardial infarction	24/2180 (1.1%)
Fatal cases	10/2180 (0.4%)
Kurume University, 1973-2003.	

Table 122.2 Cardiovascular spectrum in Kawasaki disease.

Asymptomatic myocardial infarction was seen in 37%. Twenty-two percent died at the first attack; 16% of the survivors from the first attack had a second attack. Fatality was 63% in the second attack and 83% in the third attack. From coronary angiographic studies in patients with myocardial infarction, most of the patients who died had obstructions in the left main coronary artery or in both the right main coronary artery and the anterior descending artery. In survivors, one-vessel obstruction, particularly in the right coronary artery, was frequently recognized.

Early recognition and treatment of acute myocardial infarction are critical. Recurrence of myocardial infarction is observed in about 20% of the patients who have had a previous myocardial infarction. Because the mortality of recurrent myocardial infarction is high, careful management is needed for such patients. Patients with complications after myocardial infarction, such as ventricular aneurysm, papillary muscle dysfunction, heart failure, severe arrhythmias, and postinfarction angina, are managed by medical or surgical approaches.

Systemic Artery Involvement

Coronary artery lesions are the most important lesions in KD; however, aneurysms in other arteries, such as the axillary, iliac, or renal arteries, have been observed in 1.0% of patients.[21] Although prognosis of systemic artery aneurysms is generally favorable, renovascular hypertension may develop in those with a renal artery lesion. Intrathoracic arterial lesions may cause difficulties during coronary bypass surgery. There are some reports of digital gangrenous changes.[22]

Valvular Heart Disease, Myocarditis, and Pericarditis

Valvular heart disease appears in 1% of patients. We demonstrated acute mitral regurgitation in 28 of 2180 cases (1.3%); in half of these patients, the mitral regurgitation eventually resolved after a few months to several years. The etiology of this condition may be valvulitis or papillary muscle dysfunction caused by ischemia.[23] We identified five patients with aortic regurgitation (0.2%). It is noteworthy that aortic regurgitation appeared after the acute or subacute stage of illness and developed to severe regurgitation after several years in some patients. Pericarditis or pericardial effusion appeared in 12.9% of the patients in the acute phase and was mostly subclinical and disappeared within 1 or 2 weeks. Massive pericardial effusion or cardiac tamponade was rare. There have been no reports of its progression to chronic or constrictive pericarditis. Relatively mild myocarditis was observed in about 28.3% of the patients in the acute phase, especially in the first and second weeks of illness, regardless of the presence of coronary aneurysms. Gallop rhythm, distant heart sound, ST-T segment changes, and decreased voltage of R waves on electrocardiography may suggest the presence of myocarditis. In many instances, levels of cardiac enzymes, such as creatine kinase, did not change significantly. Cardiomegaly or decreased ejection fraction of the left ventricle caused by myocarditis was noted in some patients. It generally followed an acute course to resolution, seldom developing into a chronic condition or cardiomyopathy.

DIAGNOSTIC TECHNIQUES

The evaluation of the coronary artery lesions in KD in the acute stage of illness is essential. This evaluation is usually done by two-dimensional echocardiography and coronary angiography.

Coronary Aneurysms and Evaluation

Serial two-dimensional echocardiographic studies are the most important and essential methods to evaluate coronary artery aneurysms (Fig. 122.2). The approach for two-dimensional echocardiography in KD is well described in the Japan Kawasaki Disease Research Committee's standardization of diagnostic criteria[24] and the committee report of the American Heart Association.[25] Some reports suggest that these criteria may underestimate the true incidence of coronary artery dilatation.[26,27] If a patient has abnormal findings on serial two-dimensional echocardiographic studies, coronary angiography is indicated.[28]

The method for evaluation by two-dimensional echocardiography is well described in the American Heart Association scientific statement on KD published in 2004.[29] The precordial short-axis segment is the standard approach for evaluation of the left main coronary artery, left anterior descending artery, and right main coronary artery. The posterior descending artery can be evaluated by the apical four-chamber view. The middle segment of the right coronary artery is seen by the apical four-chamber view. In our experience with two-dimensional echocardiography, it is possible to correctly diagnose left main coronary artery aneurysm with 98% sensitivity and 95% specificity compared with coronary angiography. The echocardiographic evaluation for right coronary artery lesions was less sensitive. From echocardiographic studies, it is evident that coronary artery dilatation appears at around 10 days of illness; approximately 40% of patients show coronary artery dilatation in this period. However, two thirds of these patients demonstrate a transient dilatation and regression within 3 to 5 weeks from the onset of illness (see Fig. 122.2). This means that Kawasaki arteritis may cause the various degrees of coronary artery dilatation from mild transient dilatation, to small or moderate-sized aneurysms, to giant aneurysms in

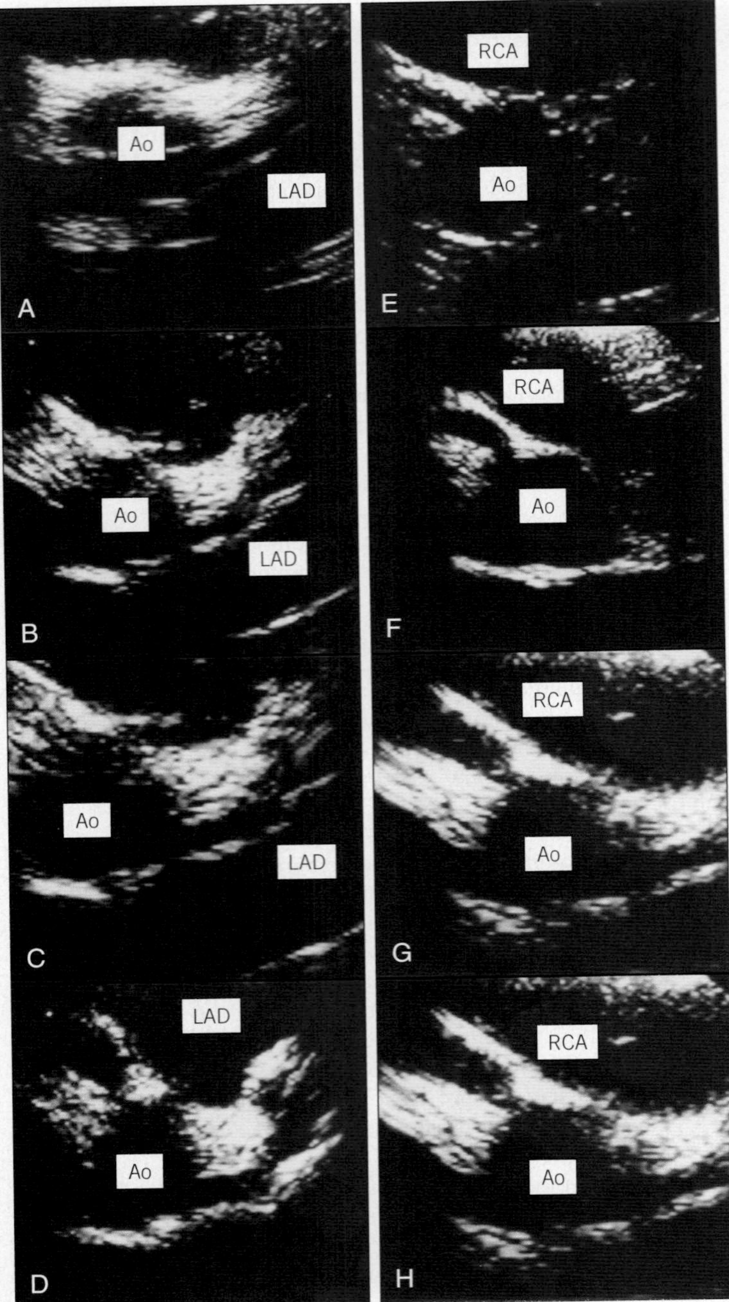

Figure 122.2 Serial two-dimensional echocardiography of the coronary artery in acute Kawasaki disease. *Left column*: left main coronary artery. At 5 days of illness, the size of the left main coronary artery was normal **(A)**. At 10 days of illness, it demonstrated mild dilatation and dense echoes in the arterial wall **(B)** and gradually dilated afterward to development of a coronary aneurysm **(C, D)**. *Right column:* right main coronary artery. At 5 days of illness, the size of the right main coronary artery looked normal **(E)**; however, the arterial wall revealed dense echoes. At 10 days of illness, it demonstrated mild dilatation **(F)** that gradually developed into an aneurysm **(G, H)**. Ao, aorta; LAD, left anterior descending artery; RCA, right coronary artery.

more than half of the patients in the acute phase of illness.[30] If the coronary artery diameter looks larger than normal without segmental dilatation, the coronary artery is considered ectatic. Follow-up echocardiography is essential to evaluate such findings to assess whether these are ectatic changes or normal variations. We performed two-dimensional echocardiography at the time of diagnosis, at 8 to 10 days after the onset of illness when coronary dilatation may appear, and at 2 and 8 weeks after the onset. The sizes of coronary artery aneurysms are classified as small (<5 mm internal diameter), medium (5 to 8 mm), and giant or large (>8 mm).

Acute coronary thrombosis is diagnosed by serial two-dimensional echocardiography. At that time, thrombolytic treatment with urokinase or tissue-type plasminogen activator is indicated. The evaluation of stenotic lesions of the coronary artery by two-dimensional echocardiography is sometimes difficult; however, by use of a high-frequency transducer and with performance of a careful examination, it may be possible. One looks for loss of uniformity or no lumen of arteries, irregular arterial walls, and dense echoes in the coronary arterial wall.

Selective coronary angiography is the most accurate method to define the presence and severity of coronary artery abnormalities in KD. The indications for coronary angiography include abnormal two-dimensional echocardiographic findings, symptoms or signs of ischemia, audible valve regurgitation during auscultation, evidence of cardiac dysfunction, and use of intracoronary thrombolytic treatment. If patients have severe coronary lesions, other systemic vascular involvement, such as axillary, iliac, renal, or intrathoracic artery aneurysms, should be looked for. Because the regression of coronary artery aneurysms or progression to stenotic lesions

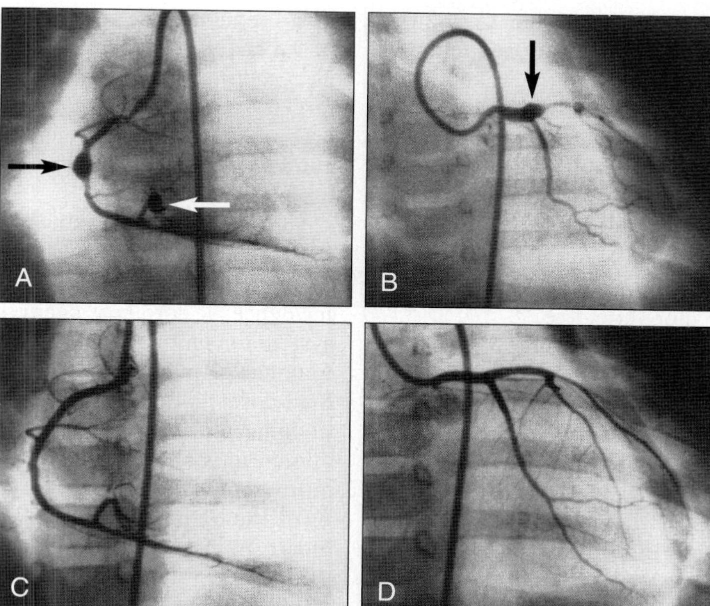

Figure 122.3 Regression of coronary aneurysms. A and **B**, Aneurysms developed in both the right and left coronary arteries of this patient with Kawasaki disease, shown at 8 months old. **C** and **D**, Two years and 2 months later, the follow-up coronary angiography demonstrated the disappearance of coronary aneurysms and normal coronary angiographic findings. There was no stenosis or irregular arterial wall in the whole coronary artery system.

mostly occurs within 2 years from the onset of illness, follow-up coronary angiography is essential, especially in patients having coronary aneurysms (Fig. 122.3). Regression of coronary aneurysms has occurred when the follow-up coronary angiography demonstrates completely normal findings in a patient who had coronary aneurysms previously. Disappearance of aneurysms and even lack of irregular arterial walls in the whole coronary artery system may be identified. Complete regression can be diagnosed by coronary angiography; however, two-dimensional echocardiography may miss some mild abnormal findings, which subsequently progress to coronary artery disease. Coronary angiography is essential for the evaluation of stenotic or obstructive lesions of the coronary artery or assessment of the collateral circulation.

The clinical feasibility of intravascular ultrasound imaging for coronary arteries has been reported in patients who had suffered from KD to assess the long-term pathologic process in vivo.[31] At the site of regressed aneurysms, it has been shown that there is marked thickening of the intima, as previously mentioned. The portion of the coronary artery with normal angiographic findings showed normal findings except in the region near to the regressed aneurysm, which showed mild intimal thickening.

The recent advances in magnetic resonance imaging and computed tomography (ultrafast computed tomography or multislice spiral computed tomography) have made it possible to evaluate the coronary artery lesions, which may decrease the performance of serial coronary angiography.[32,33]

Evaluation for Myocardial Ischemia

Because the morbidity and mortality of this disease mostly depend on the extent of associated coronary artery disease, it is particularly important to assess myocardial ischemia accurately during follow-up. However, conventional assessment methods have some limitations. Two-dimensional echocardiography can detect coronary aneurysms; however, the evaluation of stenotic lesions is not satisfactory. Similarly, the sensitivity of electrocardiography for detection of myocardial ischemia is insufficient. Coronary angiography is an accurate method to assess coronary artery involvement (Fig. 122.4), but repeated evaluation is often difficult because of the invasive nature of the technique. Although the exercise stress test can detect myocardial ischemia and this noninvasive technique is easy to repeat, the sensitivity of this method is not sufficient, even in cases complicated by significant coronary stenosis, and it is difficult to perform in young children. In this regard, myocardial single-photon emission computed tomography (SPECT) with pharmacologic stress (i.e., dipyridamole infusion) is considered the most accurate diagnostic method for identification of myocardial ischemia, especially in children in whom the exercise test cannot be performed. Because pharmacologic stress SPECT study provides a quantitative analysis, changes in the severity of myocardial ischemia can be detected on subsequent studies. The most sensitive method was dipyridamole stress SPECT (85% sensitivity); by contrast, the sensitivity of an electrocardiographic treadmill exercise test was less than 50%.[34]

MANAGEMENT

Treatment of Acute Kawasaki Disease

The combination of aspirin and high-dose immune globulin is a major therapeutic strategy in acute KD at present (Table 122.3).

In 1984, high-dose immune globulin treatment had been reported to be effective by Furusho in Japan.[35] This has been confirmed by the U.S. multicenter randomized trial.[36] These two studies indicate the use of 400 mg/kg of immune globulin for 4 or 5 days for prevention of coronary aneurysm. Immune globulin treatment is now the most effective treatment; however, the optimal dose and the indications for selection of patients for this treatment are still controversial. Some reports demonstrated a dose-dependent effect, with higher doses in a single infusion having more effect.[37] One large dose of 2 g/kg has been reported to be much more effective.[38,39] This treatment should be started at least within 10 days of illness, if possible within 7 days. It is uncertain whether early treatment within 4 days of illness is much more effective.[40]

As mentioned before, coronary aneurysms develop in only less than 20% of KD patients. If we can predict the patients who may have coronary aneurysms and select patients for immune globulin treatment, it might be more effective and can reduce the medical expenses. Harada's scoring system[41] may be useful for selection of high-risk patients for immune globulin treatment, that is, (1) white blood cell count of more than 12,000/mm^3, (2) platelet count of less than 350,000/mm^3, (3) C-reactive protein level of more than 3 mg/dL, (4) hematocrit of less than 35%, (5) serum albumin concentration of less than 3.5 mg/dL, (6) age younger than 12 months, and (7) male sex. Immune globulin treatment is indicated with more than four of the seven items.

The mechanisms of immune globulin are uncertain at present; however, possible Fc-mediated mechanisms are the down-regulation of inflammatory cytokines, the modulation of T- and B-cell functions through binding to lymphocyte Fc receptors, and the inhibition of activated complement to targets such as endothelium. As Fab-mediated mechanisms are neutralization of microbial toxins, antibodies against cytokines and anti-idiotypic reaction against autoantibodies are possible.

The problem of immune globulin treatment is that coronary artery aneurysms may develop in about 13% of immune globulin–treated patients. They may have the higher incidence of coronary aneurysms. The predictor or scoring system to identify those patients was reported.[42,43] Repeated immune globulin treatment of 2 g/kg or pulse therapy by high-dose methylprednisolone (30 mg/kg for 3 days) may be indicated.[44]

Aspirin is also an important and basic drug in KD for the antipyretic, anti-inflammatory, and antiplatelet effects; however, the optimal dose is still controversial.[45] The American Heart Association recommended high-dose aspirin (80 to 100 mg/kg, reduced to 3 to 5 mg/kg per day after the child has been afebrile for 48 to 72 hours). In Japan, middle doses of aspirin (such as 30 mg/kg per day in two doses for 2 weeks, reduced to 5 mg/kg) are generally used. If we look at the effects of aspirin on the platelet aggregation in KD, a middle dose (30 mg/kg) can successfully reduce the platelet aggregation, which usually increases in the second or third week of illness. However, a higher dose of aspirin, such as

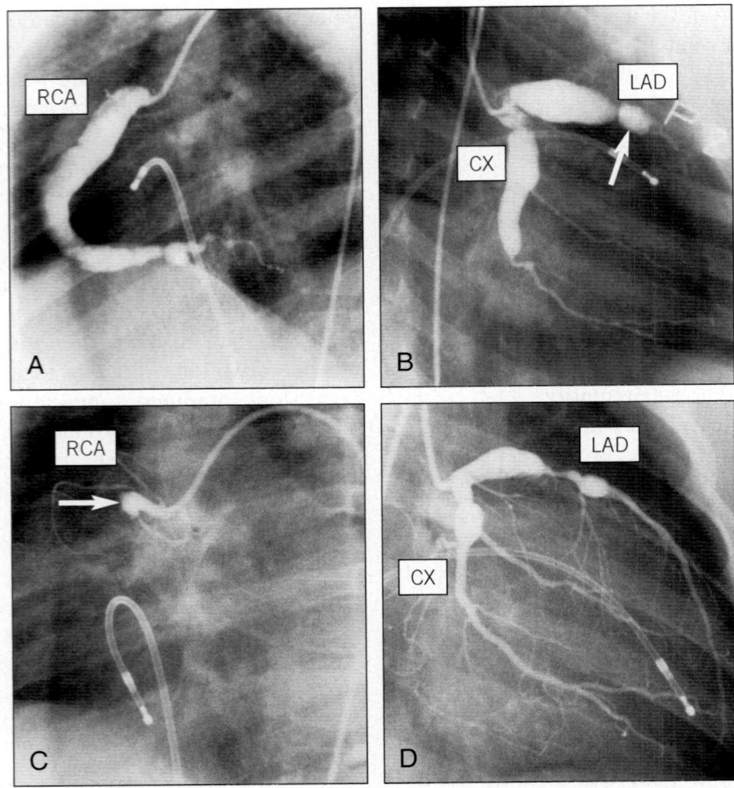

Figure 122.4 Myocardial infarction in Kawasaki disease. This 5-year-old boy with Kawasaki disease at 4 years old developed giant aneurysms in both the right and left coronary arteries **(A, B)**. Electrocardiography at that time demonstrated normal findings **(E)**. One year later, he complained of frequent chest pain, and electrocardiography **(F)** demonstrated ST elevation and deep Q waves in leads II, III, and aVF, which suggested inferior wall myocardial infarction. The follow-up coronary angiography at 6 months after myocardial infarction demonstrated complete obstruction of the right coronary artery **(C)** and persistent aneurysms in the left coronary artery with severe stenosis in the anterior descending artery **(D)**. Electrocardiography at that time revealed deep abnormal Q waves and inverted T waves in leads II, III, and aVF **(G)**. CX, circumflex artery; LAD, left anterior descending artery; RCA, right coronary artery.

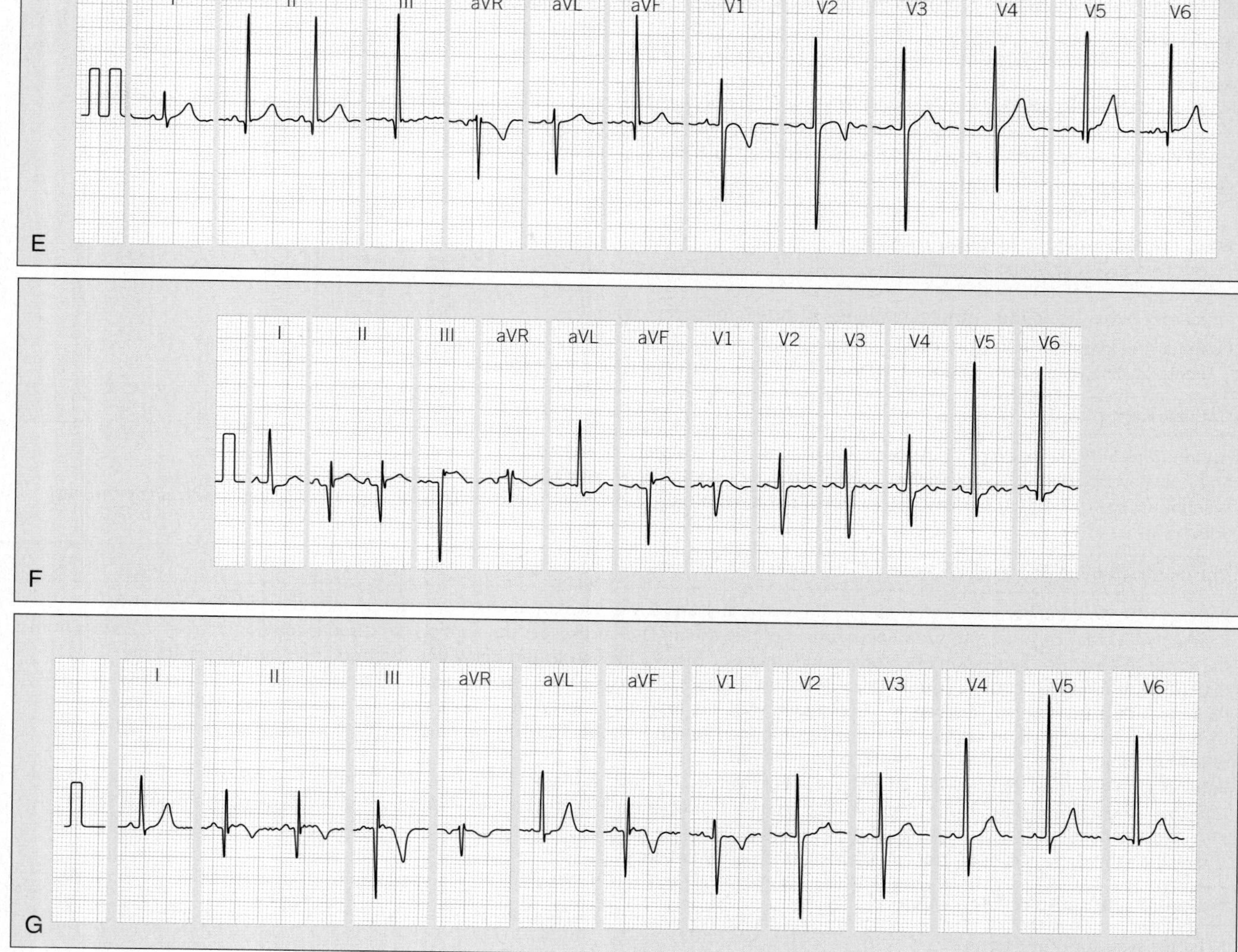

Figure 122.4—cont'd.

100 mg/kg or more, did not reveal significant effects on platelet aggregation.[46] Biosynthesis of thromboxane B_2 was completely blocked in both groups; however, the effect on platelets of plasma 6-keto prostaglandin $F_{1\alpha}$, which is a metabolite of prostacyclin, was also blocked in a certain number of cases in the high-dose group. These findings suggest that high-dose aspirin may have a disadvantage for prevention of thrombotic formation in some patients.[47] A much higher incidence of liver dysfunction was seen in the high-dose group; in such cases, we discontinued aspirin and substituted flurbiprofen. It has been reported that the absorption of aspirin in the gastrointestinal tract is impaired and that clearance may be increased in the acute stage of KD. The middle dose of aspirin may reduce aspirin intoxication, liver dysfunction, and gastrointestinal irritation and may have a lower risk for Reye's syndrome. For these reasons, we recommend 30 mg/kg in the acute stage, with reduction to 5 mg/kg in the convalescent stage. However, the optimal dose of aspirin in the acute stage is still controversial.

Is steroid therapy beneficial? In the early 1970s, steroid therapy (2 mg/kg prednisone for 2 weeks) was frequently used for KD as a treatment of vasculitis; however, I recognized a higher incidence of coronary aneurysms in patients using steroid, and also the regression of coronary aneurysms was less frequent in the steroid group. Furthermore, rupture of coronary artery aneurysms was frequently recognized in patients treated by steroid.[48] Some studies have reported that steroid pulse therapy for shorter periods with methylprednisolone resulted in a shorter fever period.[49] The steroid pulse therapy may effectively shorten the fever period and reduce the acute inflammation; however, the longer use of steroids such as prednisone for 2 weeks may have some adverse effects on vascular remodeling of coronary aneurysm and Kawasaki vasculitis. The efficacy of steroid therapy for the initial treatment of KD is still controvercial.[50,51]

The other treatments available for acute KD are pentoxifylline (specific inhibitor of TNF-α messenger RNA transcription),[52] ulinastatin (inhibiter of neutrophil elastase),[53] plasma exchange for cases refractory to intravenous immune globulin treatment,[54] infliximab (monoclonal antibody against TNF-α),[55,56] and cytotoxic agents such as cyclophosphamide and cyclosporin.[57] As an antiplatelet agent, abciximab

THERAPEUTIC RECOMMENDATIONS FOR ACUTE KAWASAKI DISEASE AND CHRONIC TREATMENT
Acute phase
Aspirin 80 to 100 mg/kg (divided into 4 doses) for 48 to 72 hours until the child is afebrile, reduced to 3 to 5 mg/kg for 6 to 8 weeks *or* 30 mg/kg (divided into 2 doses) for 2 weeks, reduced to 5 mg/kg once for 2 months Immune globulin together with aspirin 2 g/kg single-dose infusion for 12 hours Cases not responding to immune globulin Additional 2 g/kg single-dose infusion *or* Steroid pulse therapy (methylprednisolone, 30 mg/kg for 3 days IV) Optional treatment for refractory cases Pentoxifylline, ulinastatin, plasma exchange, infliximab, cyclophosphamide, cyclosporin
Convalescent phase
Aspirin: 3 to 5 mg/kg per day, single dose, for patients with coronary aneurysm Optional combination with dipyridamole, 2-5 mg/kg, or ticlopidine, 5-7 mg/kg Warfarin (0.05-0.12 mg/kg per day; international normalized ratio, 1.5-2.5) in combination with aspirin for patients with giant coronary aneurysm
Chronic treatment and management
Patients with no coronary lesion: stop aspirin; follow-up at 1 and 2 years later and at school age; no restriction of physical activity Patients with small or moderate-sized aneurysm: continue aspirin (3-5 mg/kg per day); follow-up coronary angiography at 1-2 years from the onset to check the regression of coronary aneurysms or the progression to stenotic lesion; no restriction of physical activity Patients with regressed coronary aneurysms: discontinue aspirin; follow-up every several years; no restriction of physical activity Patients with giant coronary aneurysms: aspirin with warfarin; follow-up every 3-6 months, optional coronary angiography; acute thrombosis: thrombolytic treatment by tissue plasminogen activator (bolus 1.25 mg/kg, infusion 0.1-0.5 mg/kg per hour for 6 hours), urokinase (bolus 4400 U/kg, infusion 4400 U/kg per hour) Patients with coronary stenosis with or without aneurysms: aspirin with warfarin (giant aneurysms); follow-up every 3-6 months; physical activity restricted according to stress test results; assess the indications for catheter intervention or bypass surgery; treatment of acute myocardial infarction Check the atherosclerotic risk factors at school age for every patient
Indications for catheter intervention
Ischemic symptoms or findings Localized stenosis Percutaneous transluminal coronary angioplasty is preferable in younger patients without severe calcification. Stent is indicated in children older than 10 years. Rotational ablation is indicated for patients with severe calcification.
Indications for coronary bypass surgery
Ischemic symptoms or findings of severe multivessel obstruction Obstruction in the left main trunk with stenosis in the left anterior descending artery and right main coronary artery Severe valvular disease Heart transplantation: severe ischemic cardiomyopathy (intractable)

Table 122.3 Therapeutic recommendations for acute Kawasaki disease and chronic treatment.

(platelet glycoprotein IIb/IIIa receptor inhibitor) may have efficacy for regression of coronary aneurysms.[58] All these drugs may have some efficacy for treatment of KD; however, the controlled data are lacking and reported in a small number of experiences.

Long-term Management

Long-term management of patients with KD depends on the degree of coronary arterial involvement (see Table 122.3). Low-dose aspirin (3 to 5 mg/kg per day in a single dose) is basic treatment in the convalescent phase, and it continues up to 6 to 8 weeks in patients without coronary abnormalities. If coronary arterial abnormalities are detected, low-dose aspirin should be continued until such coronary abnormalities have resolved. Coronary angiography is recommended in children in whom cardiovascular abnormalities have been found by two-dimensional echocardiography. Because the risk of progression to ischemic heart disease is high, particularly in those with giant aneurysms, these patients should be managed by pediatric cardiologists. We recommend the combination of aspirin and warfarin for patients with giant coronary aneurysms (international normalized ratio, 2.0 to 2.5). Beta blockade may be indicated for patients with ischemic symptoms.

When symptoms of acute myocardial infarction are noted, the patient should be immediately hospitalized, given oxygen, and made to rest. Vital signs and electrocardiograms must be examined and central venous pressure monitored; mechanical ventilation should be given if necessary. Because the main cause of acute myocardial infarction in KD is acute thrombotic occlusion in the stenotic coronary aneurysms, thrombolytic treatment and anticoagulation are important in the therapy for acute myocardial infarction, which includes intravenous tissue plasminogen activator, intracoronary infusion of urokinase, and heparin. Intracoronary infusion of urokinase within 6 hours after the onset of myocardial infarction is the most effective thrombolytic treatment.[59] However, tissue plasminogen activator can be administered by intravenous infusion; so when acute myocardial infarction is recognized, pediatricians should use it immediately intravenously and refer a patient to the cardiac center. Vasodilators, nitroglycerin, and diuretics are used in addition to catecholamines such as dopamine and dobutamine for cardiogenic shock and heart failure. Cardiac pacing, administration of lidocaine, and defibrillation are occasionally necessary for severe arrhythmias.

Interventional catheterization of the coronary artery in KD has been performed in limited cases, so the long-term results are still unknown. Balloon angioplasty is effective in some patients within 6 to 8 years from the onset; however, compared with the adult atherosclerotic coronary lesions, it was not so effective because of the elastic recoil and stiffness of the coronary artery.[60] We have successfully performed coronary rotational ablation in some patients for long-term severe stenosis of the coronary artery that is frequently associated with severe calcification.[61] Stent implantation may be useful in some patients. The guidelines for catheter intervention for KD have been published by the Kawasaki Disease Research Committee in Japan.[62] Catheter intervention may postpone or substitute for bypass surgery (Fig. 122.5).[63,64]

Coronary bypass surgery may be indicated for patients with serious coronary artery lesions, and the result is generally favorable.[65,66] Bypass grafting with use of an intrathoracic artery is recommended for left coronary artery bypass because the long-term patency is much more favorable (3 years, 77.1%) compared with saphenous vein grafts (3 years, 52.8%). The gastroepiploic artery is suitable for right coronary artery bypass grafting because it is usually large enough and has certain blood flow even in younger children. Surgical indications at present are three-vessel obstruction, severe occlusion in the left main coronary artery, and severe occlusion in both the left anterior descending artery and right coronary artery. Even if the patients are asymptomatic but demonstrate significant ischemic findings by exercise stress testing or by thallium myocardial scintigraphy, surgery may be indicated for such patients.[67] A native, intrathoracic arterial graft, which can

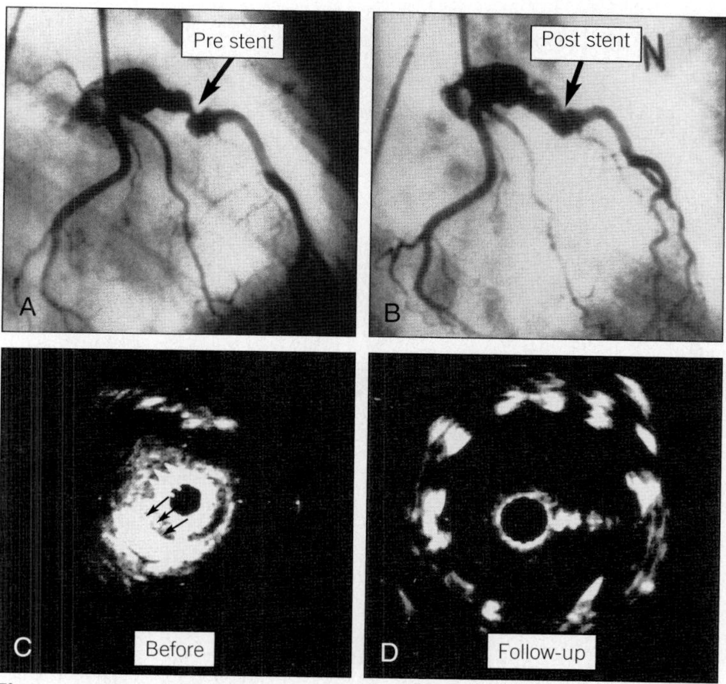

Figure 122.5 Catheter intervention by stent implantation. In this 12-year-old boy, the severe stenosis and aneurysms in the left anterior descending artery were demonstrated on coronary angiography **(A)**. After successful stent implantation with a Palmaz-Schatz stent, there was no stenosis **(B)**. Follow-up coronary angiography and intravascular ultrasound imaging demonstrated severe stenosis before intervention **(C)**. After the procedure, no restenosis was demonstrated **(D)**, and myocardial scintigraphy (not shown) demonstrated significant improvement of myocardial ischemia.

grow with age, is preferable.[68] Infants and small children younger than 3 years present technical difficulties for bypass surgery. Viability of the myocardium should be evaluated by thallium myocardial scintigraphy. Cardiac transplantation has been performed in several cases in the United States and United Kingdom.[69] It may be indicated in very rare instances of severe diffuse myocardial fibrosis due to ischemia or previous multivessel bypass surgery with difficult revascularization.

PROGNOSIS AND LONG-TERM ISSUES

Long-term Consequences of Coronary Aneurysms

The natural history or fate of coronary aneurysms is an important issue in KD (Fig. 122.6).[70] We evaluated 594 consecutive patients with acute KD between 1973 and 1983, and this cohort was followed up for 10 to 21 years.[21] In all patients, we evaluated the coronary lesions by coronary angiography just after the acute stage; 146 patients (24.6%) were diagnosed as having coronary aneurysms. A second angiographic examination was performed 1 to 2 years later in all 146 patients who previously had coronary aneurysms, which demonstrated that the aneurysm had regressed in 72 (49.3%) of these cases. This suggests that coronary aneurysm in KD shows a strong tendency toward regression. None of the patients with regression of coronary aneurysms had cardiac symptoms in the long-term follow-up periods, and electrocardiographic exercise stress test results, thallium myocardial scintigraphy, and left ventricular function were all within normal limits. In contrast, by 10 to 21 years after the onset of the illness, stenosis in the coronary aneurysms had developed in 28 cases. Myocardial infarction occurred in 11 patients, five of whom died. From this study, it is estimated that about 4% of patients with KD may develop ischemic heart disease.

When does this condition occur? We studied the time and the incidence of regression or progression to obstructive lesions from the onset of KD by the Kaplan-Meier life table method. Regression of coronary aneurysms mostly occurred within 2 years from the onset of illness, whereas the obstructive lesions developed within 2 years and gradually increased during the course of several years.

We investigated various factors that could affect the prognosis of coronary aneurysms.[71] The risk factors for coronary aneurysms to develop into ischemic heart disease are aneurysm diameter of more than 8 mm, large diffuse or saccular shape, prolonged fever for more than 21 days, and age at onset older than 2 years. In 26 patients with giant coronary aneurysms, stenotic lesions developed in 12, and no regression occurred in our follow-up study. Thus, giant coronary

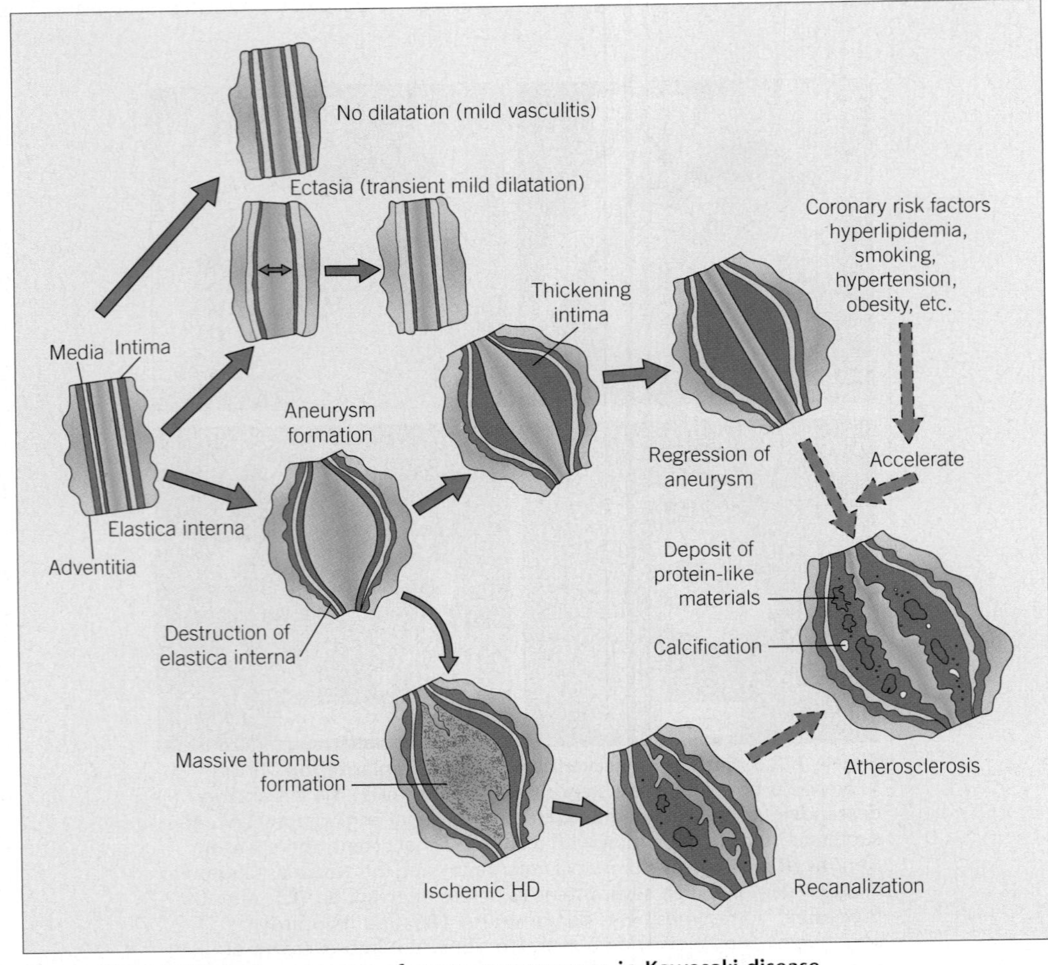

Figure 122.6 Pathologic sequence of coronary aneurysm in Kawasaki disease.

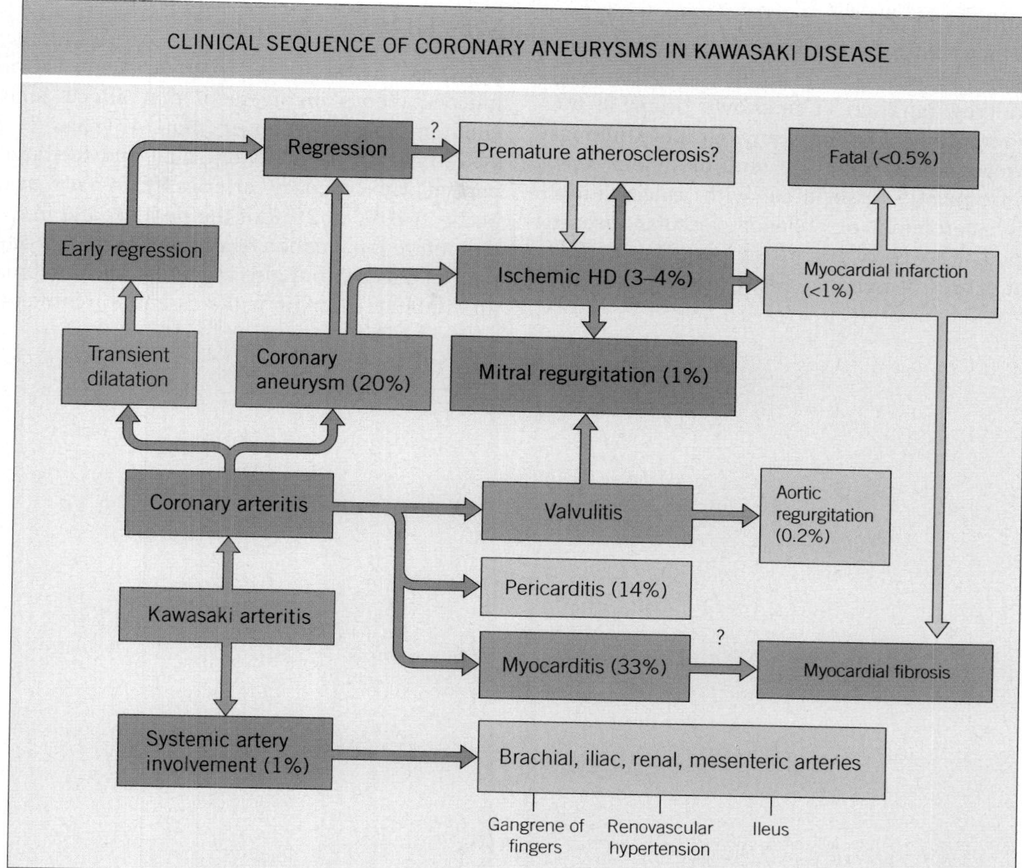

Figure 122.7 Cardiac spectrum and clinical sequence of Kawasaki disease. The incidence of coronary aneurysms and of the ischemic heart disease (HD) in this figure depends on the long-term follow-up study of the patients before immune globulin intravenous (IGIV) treatment. After IGIV is introduced, it may decline by one third to one fifth.

aneurysm is a critical problem because it has a strong potential for development into ischemic heart disease. The incidence of giant coronary aneurysms was 17.8% in the patients with coronary aneurysms and 4.4% among all KD patients in our series.

The pathologic mechanism associated with regression of aneurysms is marked proliferation of intima without massive thrombus formation, which consists of rich, smooth muscle cells and well-regenerated endothelium (Fig. 122.7).[72] Hemodynamic forces may regulate the maintenance of adequate lumens in such arteries. It is uncertain whether intimal thickening eventually develops into obstructive lesions. However, from our 10- to 21-year follow-up study, none of the patients who had regressed aneurysms developed ischemic heart disease. Our experience may indicate that stenotic lesions do not develop, at least within 1 or 2 decades, in the patients with complete regression of coronary aneurysms.

Kawasaki Vasculitis May Be an Atherosclerotic Risk Factor

The coronary artery in KD several years after onset demonstrates marked intimal proliferation and, in some patients, calcification deposits of protein-like material and hyalinized degeneration in the thickened intima. Our intravascular ultrasound study of the coronary artery after KD demonstrated the marked thickening of intima and calcification in the coronary aneurysms.[31] These findings are quite similar to arteriosclerotic lesions. Suzuki and coworkers[73] reported that the active expression of various growth factors was observed in the coronary artery in the late phase of KD, which suggests that active vascular remodeling continues even several years after onset. The endothelial function of the coronary artery in late KD was also reported to be impaired by several studies.[74-77] The important issue is whether these coronary artery lesions develop into atherosclerotic coronary artery disease in adulthood.[78]

Adult Coronary Artery Disease Due to Childhood Kawasaki Disease

It has now been more than 25 years since the first description of KD as a new clinical entity, and a certain number of the early KD children are now in adulthood. We surveyed these adults to investigate any coronary sequelae that may probably be due to their earlier KD and reported on 21 such cases and their cardiac conditions.[79] These findings suggest that some patients with coronary artery sequelae of KD may present as young adults with ischemic heart disease. The findings suggestive of this condition are as follows.

Past history in infancy or childhood is important; however, diagnosis is sometimes uncertain, and KD may have been diagnosed as other diseases during childhood. Abnormal Q waves or mitral regurgitation of unknown origin in the younger adults is important. Coronary angiographic findings are essential for recognition; these are multiple aneurysms, and stenosis is frequently associated with calcification. Familial hypercholesterolemia or collagen vascular disease should be excluded. The coronary artery sequelae of KD may be important causes of ischemic heart disease in young adults.

SUMMARY

Kawasaki disease is a common acute febrile illness with mucocutaneous involvement that affects infants and young children, mostly younger than 4 years. It is a vasculitis syndrome mostly affecting small and medium-sized arteries, particularly coronary arteries. Coronary artery aneurysms occur in 10% to 20% of the patients and may cause myocardial infarction, sudden death, and coronary artery disease not only in children but also in adults. The combination of aspirin and immune globulin is the essential treatment of acute KD.

chapter 123

Arrhythmias in Congenital Heart Disease

Victoria L. Vetter

Definition

- Patients with congenital heart disease develop a variety of arrhythmias in association with their cardiac defects.

Key Features

- Congenital cardiac defects may have anatomically abnormal conduction systems, which predispose the patient to specific arrhythmias.
- Surgical correction of congenital heart disease produces the electrophysiologic substrate that can result in atrial or ventricular arrhythmias, sinus node dysfunction, or atrioventricular block.
- Surgical correction results in hemodynamic residua, such as pulmonary regurgitation in tetralogy of Fallot and single-ventricle physiology after Fontan procedure, that predispose to specific arrhythmias.

Therapy

- The existing or potential hemodynamic and electrophysiologic effects of the arrhythmia determine treatment.
- Treatment may be pharmacologic, device (pacemaker or automatic implantable cardioverter-defibrillator), catheter ablation, or surgery.
- Alterations in surgical repairs may result in prevention of arrhythmias in patients with congenital heart disease.

In patients with congenital heart disease, arrhythmias may arise both de novo and as a result of surgical procedures used to treat the underlying condition.

Conduction system abnormalities, which result in a propensity for atrioventricular (AV) block, are seen in association with AV canal defects and L-transposition of the great arteries (L-TGA). There is an increased incidence of the Wolff-Parkinson-White anomaly in patients with L-TGA and in those with Ebstein's anomaly of the tricuspid valve. Patients with uncorrected cyanotic heart disease, atrial or ventricular pressure or volume overload and resultant myocardial ischemia, pulmonary vascular disease, or Eisenmenger's syndrome are predisposed to cardiac arrhythmias.

All patients who undergo cardiac surgery are at risk for development of cardiac arrhythmias.[1] The correction of certain defects predisposes the patient to the development of specific types of abnormal cardiac rhythms, which include supraventricular tachycardia, atrial flutter or fibrillation, ectopic atrial tachycardia, sick sinus syndrome, junctional tachycardia or junctional rhythms, AV block, ventricular tachycardia, and sudden death.

Electrophysiologic abnormalities may precede the operative repair, and postoperative arrhythmias may reflect these preexisting problems. These abnormalities may result from long-standing pressure overload and ventricular fibrosis that may be seen in patients with tetralogy of Fallot, single-ventricle complexes, and aortic stenosis, or they may result from volume overload as seen in atrial or ventricular septal defects or other lesions with left-to-right shunting. Pulmonary vascular obstructive disease may result in ventricular pressure and volume overload in addition to hypoxemia. Increases in atrial pressure with atrial dilatation may result in subsequent atrial arrhythmias, whereas abnormal hemodynamics that affect the ventricles would be more likely to result in ventricular arrhythmias. Residual hemodynamic problems, alterations in autonomic nervous system function, and intrinsic and extrinsic characteristics of the patient may also affect the development of arrhythmias.

ANATOMY AND PHYSIOLOGY

The specialized conduction system of the heart consists of the sinus node, the AV node, the bundle of His, the bundle branches, and the peripheral Purkinje fibers. The sinus node, located in the sulcus terminalis at the anterolateral margin of the junction between the superior vena cava and the right atrium, is particularly vulnerable to most surgical procedures used to correct congenital heart defects. The sinus node may sustain direct damage, or the sinus node artery, supplied by the right coronary artery in 60% and the left circumflex artery in 40% of individuals, may be damaged by the repair or during atrial cannulation. The position of the AV node, between the coronary sinus and posterior border of the membranous interventricular septum, may be somewhat variable in complex congenital heart defects; this location makes the node vulnerable to damage during ventricular septal defect (VSD) repair. The bundle of His, which is in direct continuity with the AV node, is close to the margin of many VSDs. It is beneath the aortic valve and may be vulnerable to damage in repair of VSD, in aortic or mitral valve replacement, or with myectomy for obstructive hypertrophic cardiomyopathy.

Accessory pathways are muscular connections of atrial and ventricular myocardium outside the normal area of the specialized conduction system (see Chapter 60). They occur with increased frequency in some forms of congenital heart disease.

Most arrhythmias associated with congenital heart disease result from an ectopic or automatic focus or from a re-entrant arrhythmia, involving an abnormal pathway, as in the Wolff-Parkinson-White syndrome, or an abnormal circuit from the congenital heart repair, as in atrial flutter or ventricular tachycardia.

Determination of the site of origin and the electrophysiologic mechanism of an arrhythmia allows one to select the most appropriate pharmacologic treatment or other intervention, such as ablation or surgery.

CLINICAL PRESENTATIONS

The clinical presentation will be determined by the arrhythmia and modified by the underlying hemodynamic setting, which is determined by hemodynamic sequelae of the repair of the congenital heart defect.

Sinus Node Dysfunction and Atrioventricular Block

Symptoms that occur with sinus node dysfunction and AV block include dizziness, syncope, cardiac arrest, restless sleeping patterns, nightmares, irritability, personality changes, easy or increased fatigability, and progressive exercise intolerance. Signs include low heart rate for age with failure to increase the rate with exercise, increased heart size, increased liver size, and pulmonic flow murmur secondary to the low heart rate.

Supraventricular Tachycardia and Ventricular Tachycardia

Symptoms of supraventricular tachycardia and ventricular tachycardia include palpitations or the sensation of a rapid heart rate, chest or abdominal pain, syncope, and presyncope. Signs include tachycardia (usually a heart rate of 150 to 320 beats per minute), tachypnea, hypotension, and additional findings of congestive heart failure with variable manifestations determined by the age of the patient. The symptoms and signs of ventricular tachycardia are similar to those of supraventricular tachycardia but, in the presence of poor hemodynamics, may be less well tolerated and result in progression to cardiac arrest and sudden death.

Postoperative Arrhythmias

With few exceptions, patients who undergo intracardiac surgery risk the development of postoperative arrhythmias and conduction defects. The significant abnormal postoperative arrhythmias include supraventricular tachycardia, atrial flutter, accelerated junctional rhythm or junctional ectopic tachycardia, ventricular tachycardia, sick sinus syndrome, and first-degree or second-degree AV block or complete heart block.[2] Early postoperative arrhythmias are associated with intraoperative procedural factors such as bypass time, aortic cross-clamp time, and postoperative serum concentrations of troponin as well as with inflammatory processes and other factors that affect myocardial function and electrophysiologic susceptibility.[3] Residual hemodynamic abnormalities and injury or inflammation in the electrical tissues lead to these acute arrhythmias.

Chronic Supraventricular Arrhythmias

Patients with congenital heart disease may develop atrial flutter or atrial fibrillation before or after surgical interventions. Congenital defects associated with development of atrial flutter or atrial fibrillation in the preoperative patient include those with marked right atrial enlargement or dilatation. These include lesions with a single-ventricle physiology, such as tricuspid atresia, pulmonary atresia, double-inlet single left ventricle, double-outlet right ventricle, mitral atresia, aortic atresia, and tricuspid stenosis. In addition, less complex lesions including atrial septal defects, AV canal defects, and total anomalous pulmonary venous connection result in preoperative atrial volume overload and dilatation. Supraventricular arrhythmias are more common in lesions that require extensive atrial surgery or after repairs in the presence of increased preoperative or postoperative atrial pressure. There are a number of types of congenital heart disease that require atrial surgery. These range from procedures as simple as atrial septal repair to more complex procedures, including the Mustard or Senning palliation of transposition of the great vessels and the Fontan procedure for palliation of single-ventricle physiology. The double switch repair for congenitally corrected transposition of the great arteries predisposes these patients to atrial arrhythmias similar to those experienced by the Mustard and Senning repair patients.[4] Sick sinus syndrome and atrial flutter are seen often after intra-atrial repairs such as the Mustard or Senning repair for D-transposition of the great arteries (D-TGA)[5] and the Fontan repair for complex single-ventricle lesions.[6] Late repair of atrial septal defect is associated with atrial flutter, with increasing occurrence rate according to age at repair.[7] Patients with structural heart disease often do not have the classic sawtooth electrocardiographic findings of typical atrial flutter and have variable atrial rates between 150 and 250 beats per minute. The flutter circuits in repaired or palliated congenital heart disease travel between scars created by suture lines made during surgical procedures. These patients have multiple atrial flutter circuits. The conduction may change its course in the atrium, causing the rhythm to resemble a combination of atrial flutter and atrial fibrillation. These different "flutter" characteristics have led many to refer to this as intra-atrial re-entry tachycardia rather than atrial flutter. Supraventricular arrhythmias are associated with sudden death in 2% to 8% of affected patients.[8]

Patients with L-TGA and Ebstein's anomaly are known to have a high incidence of accessory pathways that result in AV re-entrant supraventricular tachycardia. This may present as the Wolff-Parkinson-White syndrome or as concealed accessory pathways. Associated lesions resulting in AV valve regurgitation or surgical repairs can increase the likelihood of arrhythmia occurrence in these patients.

As these patients with single-ventricle physiology or systemic right ventricles age, ventricular arrhythmias are being reported more frequently. Risk factors for sudden death include tricuspid regurgitation and right ventricular dysfunction along with atrial arrhythmias.[9]

Complete or D-Transposition of the Great Arteries

The Mustard and Senning intra-atrial repairs are associated with a greater than 50% incidence of supraventricular arrhythmias, including marked sinus bradycardia, slow junctional rhythms and ectopic atrial rhythms indicating sinus node dysfunction (50% to 85%), supraventricular tachycardia, and atrial flutter (25% to 50%).[8] AV conduction disturbances, especially complete heart block and ventricular tachycardia, are seen after intra-atrial repairs. Although any of these arrhythmias may be responsible for sudden death with an incidence of 2% to 8%, recent evidence supports a significant role for atrial flutter. A 40-year follow-up found that 67% of these patients have late arrhythmias.[10,11]

It has been suggested that the etiology of the supraventricular arrhythmias after the intra-atrial repair is intraoperative damage to the sinus node or sinus node artery or interruption of intra-atrial conduction by damage to intranodal pathways. Damage to the AV node can result in AV block. The ventricular arrhythmias noted are presumed to be related to right ventricular dysfunction occurring after a period of years during which the right ventricle has functioned as the systemic ventricle.

Sinus Node Dysfunction and Atrial Flutter

More than 90% of patients who have undergone Mustard procedure will have evidence of sinus node dysfunction 10 years after their surgery, and 10% to 20% will be affected sufficiently to require implantation of a pacemaker. One study revealed that only 13.7% of patients consistently remained in sinus rhythm during a 10-year follow-up. Modifications of the intra-atrial repair made during the years have not conclusively changed the incidence of supraventricular arrhythmias.[12,13]

Late tachyarrhythmia has been reported to occur in 20% to 25% and is predominantly atrial flutter or atrial fibrillation, although ventricular arrhythmias are being seen increasingly. Late arrhythmias may be a surrogate marker for decreased ventricular function as they are correlated with decreased right ventricular ejection fraction and increased right ventricular to left ventricular end-diastolic dimensions.[13,14]

In our study of 72 patients at The Children's Hospital of Philadelphia, only 15% had normal sinus node function 5.8 ± 3.5 years after operation.[8] Ectopic atrial or junctional rhythms occurred in 53% of our patients, originating most commonly from the low right atrium. Ninety percent of these patients who were in either sinus or ectopic atrial rhythms had marked delays of intra-atrial conduction, which were most prominent in the low right atrial sites. Other abnormalities of atrial electrophysiology, including abnormal atrial refractoriness with clinical and inducible atrial flutters, have been noted in these patients.[2]

Patients with clinical episodes of atrial flutter are at high risk for the development of sudden death, with an incidence of 20% in the presence of atrial flutter, even when the rate appears to be controlled.[15] The electrocardiographic pattern of atrial flutter in these patients after atrial surgical repairs is not that of typical atrial flutter; this arrhythmia should perhaps be labeled intra-atrial re-entry. The atrial rate is slower than the expected rate, often being in the range of 180 to 260 beats per minute. AV conduction is usually excellent in these patients, often resulting in 1:1 conduction even at higher rates. The amplitude of the flutter wave is often low, and the flutter wave or atrial depolarization may be difficult to see until 2:1 AV conduction occurs (Fig. 123.1). Because most of these patients have sinus node dysfunction, a heart rate of more than 100 beats per minute after intra-atrial repair should raise the possibility of atrial flutter, and the electrocardiogram should be carefully scrutinized to exclude this arrhythmia. Although rapid AV conduction is commonly seen in these patients, the resting heart rate may be lower, at 90 to 150 beats per minute, with 2 to 3:1 AV conduction.

Sudden Death

Sudden death has been reported in 2% to 10% of patients after intra-atrial repair of D-TGA. Although initial reports suggested that sudden death was secondary to the sick sinus syndrome, it soon became apparent that many patients were dying despite normally functioning pacemakers. The recently accepted concept of sudden death implicates atrial flutter with 1:1 AV conduction, resulting in ventricular fibrillation, asystole, or electromechanical dissociation.[5,15] Underlying poor right ventricular function is a factor in this sudden death. Primary ventricular arrhythmias may be a factor, especially in those with poor ventricular function. Predictors of late death identified in a case-controlled study of 47 sudden deaths found an association with symptoms of arrhythmia including palpitations, dizziness and syncope, symptoms of ventricular dysfunction, and history of atrial flutter or fibrillation.[16] The presence of a pacemaker (approximately 15%) did not correlate with sudden death. Ventricular arrhythmias were recorded in 21 of 47 (44.7%) of these sudden death victims.

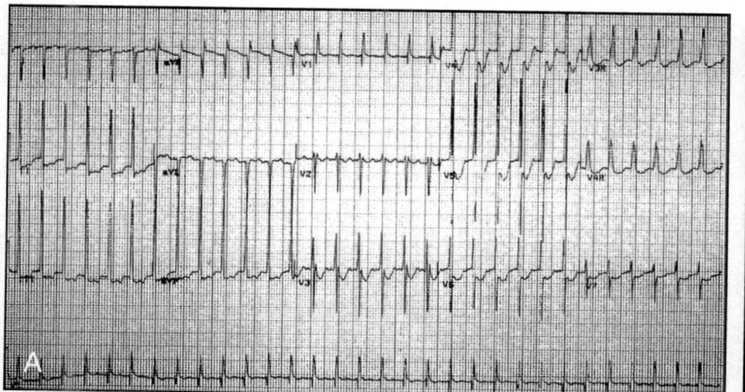

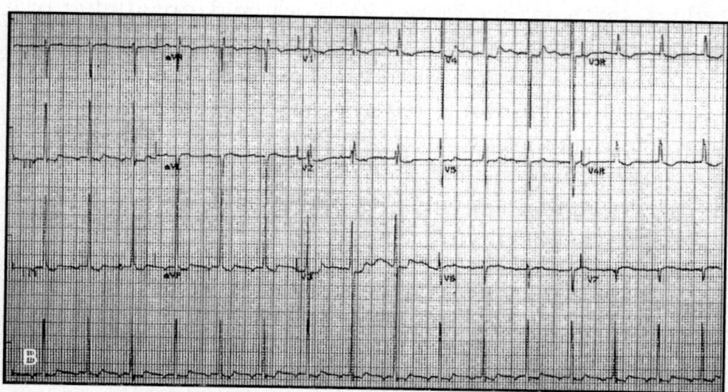

Figure 123.1 Electrocardiographic example of intra-atrial re-entrant tachycardia in a patient after intra-atrial repair of D-transposition of the great arteries. a, 1:1 AV conduction occurs with an atrial and ventricular rate of 205 beats per minute. Negative P waves are seen in leads II, III, and aVF. **b,** AV conduction is 2:1 with an atrial rate of 190 beats per minute and a ventricular rate of 95 beats per minute. The negative P waves are more easily seen in leads II, III, and aVF with the slower AV conduction.

Presence of a VSD has been correlated with increased risk of late death.[17] In a group of 61 patients who had undergone Mustard procedure and were prospectively studied electrophysiologically and observed at The Children's Hospital of Philadelphia, eight subsequently experienced sudden death. The greatest risk factors included both atrial flutter and sinus node dysfunction requiring a pacemaker. In this subset of patients, 55% experienced sudden death, compared with 4% of patients who had neither pacemakers nor atrial flutter. No patient who had a pacemaker but did not have atrial flutter experienced sudden death.[18] The predictors of sudden death in these patients include older age at repair, abnormal hemodynamics, atrial flutter and the sick sinus syndrome, and ventricular arrhythmias.

The currently preferred repair of D-TGA is the arterial switch repair (see Chapter 110). We have used the electrophysiologic study and ambulatory monitoring to evaluate these patients and have found no significant postoperative arrhythmias in early studies.[19] Some early arrhythmias, including supraventricular arrhythmias, junctional ectopic tachycardia, and ventricular arrhythmias, have been reported. This was confirmed in a large study from Japan that revealed an overall prevalence of arrhythmias of 9.6%. The presence of a VSD or older age at repair correlated with arrhythmias.[20]

Atrial Septal Defect Repairs

Preoperative atrial arrhythmias are common in adults with atrial septal defects. Atrial fibrillation occurs in approximately 25% of patients operated on after 20 years of age, compared with 5% operated on before 20 years.[21] In patients older than 35 years at the time of surgery, postoperative arrhythmias occur in more than 50%. Atrial or coronary sinus rhythms are common before operation and persist after operation. Increasing age of the patient, left-to-right shunt size, and degree of pulmonary hypertension also correlate with the incidence of atrial arrhythmias.

Early postoperative arrhythmias occur in 30% to 75% of patients after atrial septal defect repair and include sinus node dysfunction, slow junctional rhythms, AV dissociation, and ectopic atrial rhythms. These rhythms generally resolve during the first week after operation. Atrial flutter is rare in children but is relatively common in adults.

The incidence of persistent late postoperative arrhythmias varies from 2% to 9% in children and from 2% to 33% in adults.[21] These late arrhythmias consist of junctional escape rhythms, sick sinus syndrome, AV block, and atrial flutter or fibrillation. The postoperative incidence of sinus node dysfunction after sinus venosus repair has been reported to be as high as 50% but rarely requires pacemaker implantation. These abnormalities usually occur during the first year after operation but may occur up to 10 to 20 years postoperatively. Similar arrhythmias occur after repair of total anomalous pulmonary venous return.

Fontan Repair

The Fontan repair is currently the procedure of choice for congenital lesions with functional single ventricles. The postoperative arrhythmias seen in these patients are similar to those seen after the intra-atrial repair of D-TGA because of the extensive intra-atrial surgery necessary for both operations.[22]

The most common arrhythmias after Fontan repair include sinus node dysfunction (15% to 50%), supraventricular tachycardia or atrial flutter (42% to 57%), ectopic atrial rhythm (19%), junctional rhythm (8%), junctional ectopic tachycardia (48%), AV block (9.5%), ventricular arrhythmias (7.5%), and sudden death (3%).[23,24] Early postoperative arrhythmias have a reported incidence of 10% to 50%.[6,22,25]

Tachyarrhythmias during the perioperative period may be associated with hemodynamic instability and contribute to death. Atrial flutter, ectopic atrial rhythms, and junctional ectopic tachycardia occur in the early postoperative period. A prospective analysis of 33 patients at The Children's Hospital of Philadelphia revealed a 27% incidence of significant postoperative arrhythmias on the first day after operation, with a 15% incidence on day 7.[26] The most serious postoperative arrhythmia was junctional ectopic tachycardia, with rates in excess of 190 beats per minute associated with a fatal outcome. It was our experience, in contrast to that of others, that atrial flutter could be managed adequately after operation.[6] Late postoperative arrhythmias include sinus node dysfunction, ectopic atrial rhythms, atrial flutter or fibrillation, AV block, ventricular arrhythmias, and sudden death. A late risk of supraventricular tachycardia of 42% has been projected in a Mayo Clinic study. Many of the patients affected were older at the time of repair and had long-standing ventricular volume overload with ventricular hypertrophy and resultant fibrosis, providing the substrate for ventricular arrhythmias. Other studies have correlated obstruction between the right atrium and pulmonary arteries with atrial arrhythmias. Other factors associated with atrial arrhythmias include a longer follow-up period, poor preoperative functional class or preoperative atrial tachycardia, type of repair (with atriopulmonary direct connection having the greatest incidence), higher New York Heart Association functional class, and sinus node dysfunction.[23,27] As these patients are aging, postoperative atrial arrhythmias are being noted with increasing frequency. In one study, 41% had sustained atrial tachycardia or supraventricular tachycardia after the Fontan procedure. Compared with Fontan patients who did not have atrial tachycardia, those with atrial tachycardia were more likely to develop heart failure, to have an increased frequency of reoperations and of right atrial thrombus and right atrial enlargement, and to have moderate to severe systemic AV valve regurgitation.[23,24] The postoperative physiology in this group of patients necessitates a greater than normal right atrial pressure, often with associated atrial dilatation and intra-atrial scars, providing the substrate for the development of atrial arrhythmias.

A postoperative electrophysiologic study of 31 patients who had Fontan repairs at The Children's Hospital of Philadelphia revealed abnormalities of sinus node function in 57%. Abnormalities of atrial refractoriness were noted in 43% of patients and were most pronounced at faster rates. Intra-atrial conduction delays were noted in 76% of the patients. Sustained supraventricular arrhythmias were induced by programmed stimulation in 27%, with intra-atrial re-entry present in seven of eight patients. AV conduction abnormalities were noted in 10%. Repetitive ventricular responses occurred in 19%. One study showed that up to 50% developed sinus node dysfunction, but only 6.7% required pacemakers.[28]

After Fontan repair, risk factors for sudden death, which have been reported to occur with a 3% incidence, include older age at repair, ventricular dysfunction, atrial arrhythmias, and ventricular arrhythmias. Atrial arrhythmias are hypothesized to be related to atrial distention and the presence of several suture lines.

The type of repair is important; a greater incidence of atrial arrhythmias is associated with atriopulmonary connections compared with total cavopulmonary connections or right atrial to right ventricular connections.[29] Attempts to decrease the incidence of late arrhythmias have included earlier repairs and modifications of the Fontan repair by the use of lateral tunnel and extracardiac conduits.[28,30-32] In addition, conversion of atriopulmonary Fontan or right ventricle to pulmonary artery connections to a lateral tunnel type of repair has improved arrhythmia control in these patients and has improved clinical symptoms.[33]

Similarly, conversion to an extracardiac conduit has been reported to show an even lower incidence of postoperative tachyarrhythmias and sinus node dysfunction than the lateral tunnel procedure.[34-37]

Patients with heterotaxy syndrome have the highest morbidity and mortality of all patients receiving the Fontan operation, but this is improving. Up to 25% to 46% have been reported to have postoperative arrhythmias, and 22% to 27% had pacemakers.[38]

Ventricular Arrhythmias

Ventricular arrhythmias occur in association with a number of congenital heart defects, most connected by the history of preceding surgery in the ventricle, as in tetralogy of Fallot, or a previous increase in left ventricular pressure before surgery, as in aortic stenosis. Postoperative volume overload, healing of ventriculotomy scars under pressure, long-standing right ventricular hypertension, and residual left ventricular pressure overload are believed to be confounding factors. Other lesions associated with ventricular tachycardia include those with repair of VSD, AV canal defects, hypertrophic cardiomyopathy, Ebstein's anomaly, and coronary artery anomalies. In addition, 10% to 15% of patients after intra-atrial repair of complete transposition of the great arteries and the Fontan repair are now presenting with ventricular tachycardia after operation. Sudden death occurs in 5% to 10%.

Ventricular Tachycardia and Cardiomyopathies

Ventricular arrhythmias and sudden death may occur in children and young adults with both hypertrophic and dilated cardiomyopathies. These conditions are discussed in Chapter 79. Some patients with congenital heart disease develop cardiomyopathies as an end-stage manifestation of their defect. As yet, no large clinical studies of drug or device therapy have specifically addressed management of these patients.

Ventricular Tachycardia in Postoperative Aortic Stenosis

Complex ventricular arrhythmias have been known for decades to be a significant problem in patients with aortic valve disease, particularly with abnormal left ventricular function. These arrhythmias have been associated with an incidence of sudden death in postoperative patients as high as 5% to 10%.[39]

In a report of 24-hour ambulatory monitoring of patients in the Natural History Study, complex ventricular arrhythmias, including multiform premature ventricular complexes, ventricular couplets, and ventricular tachycardia, occurred in 44.8% of patients, with a 22% incidence of ventricular tachycardia noted after aortic valve surgery. The highest incidence of ventricular tachycardia occurred in patients undergoing valve replacement (13.9%). High-risk factors included increased left ventricular end-diastolic pressure and moderate to severe aortic regurgitation. The level of the transaortic gradient at the time of presentation and the presence of symptoms were also important factors. A study by Bockoven and coworkers[40] in patients who had undergone the Ross procedure revealed a 29% incidence of early postoperative ventricular tachycardia. A strong association between sudden death and ventricular systolic pressures appears to exist. It has been postulated that the high left ventricular pressure, coupled with increased left ventricular end-diastolic pressures, provides the substrate for subendocardial ischemia, leading to ventricular arrhythmias. Patients who are older at the time of the Ross procedure were found to have exercise-induced arrhythmias in 26%, which were predominantly ventricular. None of those with these arrhythmias were younger than 19 years at the time of repair.[41]

Tetralogy of Fallot

Atrial Arrhythmias

Atrial arrhythmias, a risk factor for sudden death,[42] are known to occur after repair of tetralogy of Fallot and have been noted in up to 33% of adult patients after this repair.[43] These arrhythmias are associated with right ventricular dysfunction and tricuspid regurgitation and with increased morbidity, including congestive heart failure, stroke, and death.[42] Harrison and colleagues[44] showed a prevalence of 12% of atrial arrhythmias after tetralogy of Fallot repair and found 69% with symptoms of congestive heart failure, reoperation, subsequent ventricular tachycardia, stroke, and death. A strong association of atrial arrhythmias, pulmonary regurgitation, left ventricular dysfunction, and higher mean right atrial volume was noted.

Postoperative Ventricular Tachycardia After Repair of Tetralogy of Fallot

Postoperative arrhythmias and conduction disturbances have been known to occur since the earliest total repairs of tetralogy of Fallot were performed in 1954. These arrhythmias include

- right bundle branch block (59% to 100%);
- right bundle branch block/left anterior hemiblock (7% to 25%);
- AV block (1% to 2%);
- supraventricular tachycardia or atrial fibrillation (10% to 15%);
- premature ventricular complexes (30% to 67%);
- ventricular tachycardia (10% to 15%); and
- sudden death (2% to 9%).

Early reports associated sudden death with conduction abnormalities; more recent studies have implicated the presence of ventricular arrhythmias as the most significant factor.[45] Up to 30% of patients with ventricular arrhythmias after tetralogy repair have been reported to experience sudden death.

In tetralogy of Fallot, risk factors associated with the development of ventricular tachycardia and sudden death include

- older age at repair;
- longer postoperative period;
- right ventricular systolic pressure above 60 mm Hg at rest;
- right ventricular end-diastolic pressure above 10 mm Hg at rest;
- depressed right ventricular systolic function;
- depressed left ventricular systolic function;
- moderate to severe pulmonary or tricuspid regurgitation;
- increased right ventricular end-diastolic volume; and
- history of reoperation.

The strongest correlations appear to be with moderate to severe pulmonary regurgitation with increased right ventricular end-diastolic volume and right and left ventricular dysfunction.

A number of electrocardiographic or electrophysiologic factors have been found or suggested to be of clinical significance. These include

- QRS duration of 180 ms or more;
- rate of change of QRS duration of more than 3.5 to 4 ms/year;
- QRS, QTc, or JTc dispersion;
- signal-averaged electrograms with late potentials; and
- inducible monomorphic or polymorphic ventricular tachycardia.

Some studies have suggested an association between abnormal signal-averaged electrograms with late potentials and the development of ventricular tachycardia and between abnormal signal-averaged electrograms with late potentials and the development of ventricular arrhythmia.[46,47] These findings have not been found to clearly identify those at high risk of sudden death. Others have correlated dilated right ventricles, QT dispersion, and increased QRS duration with ventricular tachycardia.[48] A wide QRS duration of 180 ms or more has been associated with ventricular tachycardia[49] and correlated with severe pulmonary insufficiency leading to right ventricular dilatation. QRS duration and degree of pulmonary regurgitation seem to be the greatest risk factors for ventricular tachycardia and sudden death.[42] Valve replacement decreases the incidence of episodes of ventricular tachycardia and atrial flutter.[50] Early studies suggested that pulmonary valve replacement does not shorten the duration of the QRS but prevented subsequent prolongation.[50] Subsequent studies have shown that QRS duration does decrease after pulmonary valve replacement, with the amount of reduction correlated to the right ventricular end-diastolic volume change.[51-53] There appears to be a steady, slow increase in QRS duration after pulmonic valve replacement.[52]

It is believed that the ventriculotomy, myocardial resection, and subsequent scarring provide the electrophysiologic substrate of slow conduction and block that predisposes the patient to development of re-entrant arrhythmias. Pathologic studies in patients with tetralogy of Fallot who have died suddenly have revealed extensive fibrosis of the right ventricular myocardium at the ventriculotomy site and the right ventricular outflow tract and septum. Electrophysiologic studies have localized the site of origin of the ventricular tachycardia to the right ventricular outflow tract and ventricular septum.

Autonomic Nervous System

Autonomic nervous system impairment may be a modulating factor in postoperative arrhythmias.

Heart rate variability is decreased in patients with arrhythmia after tetralogy of Fallot repair, who have been shown to have decreased standard deviation of all normal-to-normal intervals.[54,55]

Serious ventricular arrhythmias do occasionally occur despite good hemodynamic results, although sudden death occurs most commonly in ventricular tachycardia associated with poor hemodynamics. Patients who have undergone repair of tetralogy of Fallot earlier in life seem to have a lower incidence of ventricular tachycardia. In a mean follow-up of 28 years, sudden death occurred in 9%. In addition to age older than 12 years at the time of repair, transient complete heart block lasting more than 3 days was associated with a greater incidence of sudden death.[56] A study by Murphy and coworkers found an incidence of sudden death of 6% during a 30-year period.[56a] It was stated that there was no trend toward increased late sudden death during the follow-up period, which is in contrast to the findings of earlier studies that suggested a progressive increase in the incidence of postoperative arrhythmias with a longer postoperative interval.

Because of the high incidence of ventricular arrhythmias in postoperative patients, the precise role of premature ventricular complexes in the occurrence of sudden death is unclear. In a multicenter study of repaired tetralogy of Fallot patients undergoing programmed ventricular stimulation, both inducible monomorphic and polymorphic ventricular tachycardias were predictive of future clinical ventricular tachycardia and sudden cardiac death.[57] More sensitive and specific models are needed to risk stratify individuals who would benefit from primary prevention with implantable cardioverter-defibrillators (ICDs).

Conduction Disturbances

Right Bundle Branch Block

Postoperative right bundle branch block (RBBB) is common after repair of many cardiac anomalies, including tetralogy of Fallot, and is either central or peripheral. We found that RBBB was proximal in 50% of patients and distal in the remainder of 120 patients studied at The Children's Hospital of Philadelphia.

During the years, there has been a great deal of interest in the coexistence of left anterior hemiblock and RBBB in postoperative patients. After repair of tetralogy of Fallot, some of these patients are susceptible to the development of complete heart block.[45] As with RBBB, not all instances of RBBB with left anterior hemiblock have the same site of origin, and therefore they carry a different prognosis. Likewise, the diagnosis of trifascicular damage cannot be made from the electrocardiogram with assurance. Although the electrocardiographic pattern of RBBB and left anterior hemiblock with a prolonged PR interval has classically been associated with trifascicular damage, it may be caused by other conduction abnormalities. Conversely, trifascicular damage may be present with a normal PR interval or a normal QRS axis. The intracardiac electrophysiologic study is the only reliable method of detection of true trifascicular damage and may be predictive of late complete AV block as described in a study by Friedli and colleagues.[57a] Evaluation of HV intervals in our patients revealed a 15% incidence of HV prolongation, indicating damage in the bundle of His or the three major conduction fascicles or both.

Atrioventricular Block

Congenital Atrioventricular Block

The associated congenital heart defects in congenital complete heart block most commonly include those with L-TGA or the heterotaxy syndromes. In one study, 29% of patients with associated heart disease experienced mortality in the first year.[58]

Some infants who have congenital complete heart block will be diagnosed in utero because of low fetal heart rates. Fetal echocardiography may show fetal hydrops in 15% to 61% of cases, with survival of less than 10% unless the fetus can be delivered immediately. Although many infants with congenital complete heart block are asymptomatic at birth, others show findings typical of congestive heart failure, including cardiovascular collapse.

Sudden death has been associated with severe bradycardia, ventricular ectopy especially with exercise, prolonged pauses, increased QRS width, prolongation of the QTc interval, and junctional recovery time of more than 3 seconds.

Postoperative Atrioventricular Block

Permanent complete AV block occurs in between 0.7% and 2.0% of patients after open heart surgery. Transcatheter closure of VSDs has a reported incidence of 2-6%. The greatest risk occurs with surgery for repairs of left ventricular outflow tract obstruction, L-TGA, VSD, AV canal defects, and tetralogy of Fallot. Complete heart block occurs more commonly after repair of AV canal defects, probably because of the unusual course of the conduction system in these lesions, and may be seen in up to 7% of patients. Corrected transposition of the great arteries or L-TGA is associated with AV conduction disturbances ranging from first-degree to complete heart block in 30% to 60% of patients. These conduction disturbances may be present at birth, may develop insidiously, or may occur during or after the surgical correction of associated defects. The development of postoperative congenital heart block is increased in those with L-TGA because of the unusual course of the AV conduction system. The AV bundle and conduction system cross the pulmonary outflow tract and descend along the anterior rim of the VSD or along the right margin of the foramen between the main and outflow chambers in single ventricle with an outflow chamber. Careful attention to these facts, together with intraoperative mapping, has decreased the incidence of this form of postoperative block.

The incidence of transient complete heart block persisting for hours to weeks after operation is as high as 14%. Patients with transient complete heart block may be predisposed to the development of permanent late complete heart block, but 67% do experience recovery of AV conduction. Weindling and colleagues[59] found that recovery of AV conduction occurred by 9 days in 97% of patients who subsequently recovered. Of those who recovered, 9% did have subsequent deterioration to second-degree Möbitz II AV block. The incidence of death in patients who are not paced has been reported to be as high as 60%. Therefore, the most recent American Heart Association guidelines for pacemaker recommend implantation of a permanent pacemaker if the AV block persists at least 7 days after operation.[60] Late complete AV block can occur 10 to 15 years after repair, especially after AV canal defect repairs.[61]

Junctional Ectopic Tachycardia

An interesting postoperative arrhythmia that occurs in the acute postoperative setting is the rhythm designated accelerated junctional rhythm or junctional ectopic tachycardia. This rhythm carries a high mortality as a result of heart failure and low cardiac output if it cannot be slowed.[62] It is seen most commonly after repair of tetralogy of Fallot or AV canal defects or after the Fontan repair.

The rates often accelerate to more than 250 beats per minute and produce severe hemodynamic compromise. The electrocardiogram in junctional ectopic tachycardia shows a narrow QRS with a slower atrial than ventricular rate and AV dissociation. Pacing or cardioversion is ineffective in treating the tachycardia. Treatments used include digoxin and intravenous amiodarone, which has been quite effective. The mechanism is suspected to be one of enhanced automaticity, but little specific information is available. Decrease of inotrope dosages, treatment of fever, correction of metabolic aberrations, and supportive therapy are most important. Transient atrial pacing at rates slightly higher than the intrinsic rate can increase the cardiac output and allow time for the junctional ectopic tachycardia to resolve.

Postoperative junctional ectopic tachycardia may be fatal, but it generally subsides after 24 to 72 hours. No long-term sequelae of this arrhythmia have been identified, but no systematic studies have been reported.

DIAGNOSTIC TECHNIQUES

All requests for diagnostic studies should be made in association with periodic physical examinations by a cardiologist who is familiar with the patient's congenital heart defect and with the potential sequelae associated with the defect or its correction.

Electrocardiography, Ambulatory Monitoring, and In-Hospital Monitoring

All postoperative patients with congenital heart disease should be observed periodically with standard 12- or 15-lead electrocardiograms. Signal-averaged electrograms may be helpful in those at risk for ventricular arrhythmias, such as postoperative tetralogy of Fallot, but they have not been shown to be as useful as initially anticipated. Those in the high-risk groups, including patients undergoing intra-atrial repair of D-TGA, Fontan repairs (especially those associated with L-TGA), repair of tetralogy of Fallot, and other complex repairs, should undergo electrocardiographic follow-up yearly for an indefinite period. We perform 24-hour ambulatory monitoring in these high-risk patients once or twice yearly. Patients with intermittent symptoms may benefit from monitoring with an event recorder, which can record continuously or intermittently. Those patients with very fleeting or infrequent but serious symptoms, especially syncope, may have the arrhythmia identified by the use of an implantable event recorder.

After repair of tetralogy of Fallot, the incidence of premature ventricular contractions on routine electrocardiography has varied from 5% to 18%, with a 35% to 70% incidence on ambulatory monitoring. Similar arrhythmias are seen after other complex repairs. The Second Natural History Study reported ventricular arrhythmias on ambulatory monitoring in 36.8% of VSD repairs, 28.4% of pulmonary stenosis repairs, and more than 45% of patients after aortic valve surgery.[39] A study at The Children's Hospital of Philadelphia revealed arrhythmia in 43% of admissions to the cardiac intensive care unit.[63] Identification of these arrhythmias led to their early and appropriate management.

Exercise Stress Testing

Exercise stress testing provides significant information about the cardiovascular performance of the patient with congenital heart disease in addition to provoking significant arrhythmias. This form of testing reveals a 25% to 50% incidence of ventricular arrhythmias in patients who have had repair of tetralogy of Fallot.

We recommend exercise stress testing in patients around puberty and in those with symptoms of arrhythmias, syncope, and exercise intolerance. It may be helpful in uncovering more serious arrhythmias in patients with premature ventricular complexes on 24-hour ambulatory monitoring and in evaluating the chronotropic response to exercise in those with suspected sinus node dysfunction. Exercise stress testing is valuable in determining optimal pacemaker settings, especially with rate-responsive and dual-chamber pacemakers. It is helpful, as well, in fine-tuning ICD discriminators to avoid inappropriate shocks.

Electrophysiologic Studies in Postoperative Patients

Electrophysiologic Study of Supraventricular Tachycardia, Atrial Flutter, and Ectopic Atrial Tachycardia

Although the electrocardiogram during supraventricular tachycardia may suggest a potential mechanism, an electrophysiologic study may be needed to determine the precise mechanism of the tachycardia, if it is determined that this information is necessary. The electrophysiologic study may be used to locate the site of the accessory pathway in both Wolff-Parkinson-White anomaly and supraventricular tachycardia secondary to a concealed accessory pathway. It is also used to determine the refractory period of the accessory pathway, to induce the supraventricular tachycardia, and to determine the ventricular response to atrial fibrillation when it can be induced in patients with Wolff-Parkinson-White anomaly.

The electrophysiologic study may be used to determine the inducibility of atrial flutter or intra-atrial re-entry and to identify the location of the flutter circuit. After Fontan repair, a study found inducible intra-atrial re-entrant tachycardia in 27% of the patients.[64] The more recently developed technologies of electroanatomic mapping and noncontact mapping have enhanced the ability to locate circuits and to facilitate successful ablations.[65] Automatic or ectopic tachycardia cannot be induced by programmed stimulation, but infusion of isoproterenol during the study may initiate the tachycardia or ectopic rhythm, allowing intracardiac mapping to localize the site for possible catheter ablation.

Electrophysiologic Study of Ventricular Tachycardia

The electrophysiologic study may be used to identify the mechanism of an arrhythmia that has not been documented but is suggested by symptoms of tachycardia, presyncope, or syncope and to determine whether inducible ventricular tachycardia occurs in a patient with complex ventricular arrhythmias on ambulatory monitoring or exercise stress testing. The electrophysiologic study may be used to evaluate the propensity of postoperative patients for development of ventricular tachycardia, to evaluate specific pharmacologic treatments, to locate the site of origin of the arrhythmia in patients who are candidates for ablative therapy, and to help determine the need for implantation of an automatic ICD.

There is increasing awareness of ventricular arrhythmias postoperatively in patients with systemic right ventricles or single-ventricle physiology. After finding that 21 of 47 sudden deaths after Mustard or Senning repair for D-TGA showed evidence of a ventricular arrhythmia as the fatal event, Kammeraad and associates[16] recommended electrophysiologic study with ventricular stimulation for any of these patients who present with symptoms of arrhythmias or ventricular dysfunction.

Electrophysiologic Study After Repair of Tetralogy of Fallot and Complex Congenital Heart Disease

In a study of 120 postoperative patients with tetralogy of Fallot at The Children's Hospital of Philadelphia, 14% had had inducible ventricular tachycardia by use of an electrophysiologic procedure with single- and double-ventricular extrastimuli.[2] Only one of these patients had not had clinically documented ventricular tachycardia but had complained of palpitations and a racing heart. In our series, comparison of electrophysiologic studies in patients with and without ventricular tachycardia showed prolonged ventricular refractory periods in the right ventricular outflow tract in patients with ventricular tachycardia compared with those without ventricular tachycardia. These patients with ventricular tachycardia also had a greater dispersion of ventricular refractoriness between the right ventricular apex and right ventricular outflow tract and a propensity to development of repetitive ventricular responses to ventricular stimulation. It is possible that these parameters may be used as markers to identify those patients at high risk for the development of ventricular tachycardia.

The ventricular tachycardia in these patients can be reproducibly initiated and terminated at electrophysiologic study and has been presumed to be re-entrant.[2] Factors associated with inducibility include increased right ventricular systolic pressure or volume overload, longer period from the time of surgery, older age at electrophysiologic study, prolonged QRS duration, and complex ventricular arrhythmias. In addition to identifying ventricular tachycardia, the electrophysiologic study may be used to test the efficacy of antiarrhythmic medication in patients with inducible ventricular tachycardia. One multicenter retrospective trial did not show a correlation between sudden death and inducible ventricular tachycardia, but a variety of procedures were used.[66] A subsequent multicenter study found inducibility of monomorphic and polymorphic ventricular tachycardia predictive of clinical events of ventricular tachycardia and sudden cardiac death.[51] Determination of the usefulness of electrophysiologic study in this population awaits the appropriate controlled study.

The site of origin of the ventricular tachycardia has been localized to the right ventricular outflow tract in most instances and to the ventricular septum in others. Continuous electrical activity has been noted in the right ventricular outflow tract in these patients. Fragmented, prolonged, low-amplitude electrograms from the right ventricle have been reported and occur more commonly in patients with ventricular tachycardia (Fig. 123.2).

A QRS duration of more than 180 ms has been correlated with inducibility of ventricular tachycardia after repair of tetralogy of Fallot. Failure to induce the tachycardia is considered a favorable sign but may not predict the absence of clinical ventricular tachycardia.

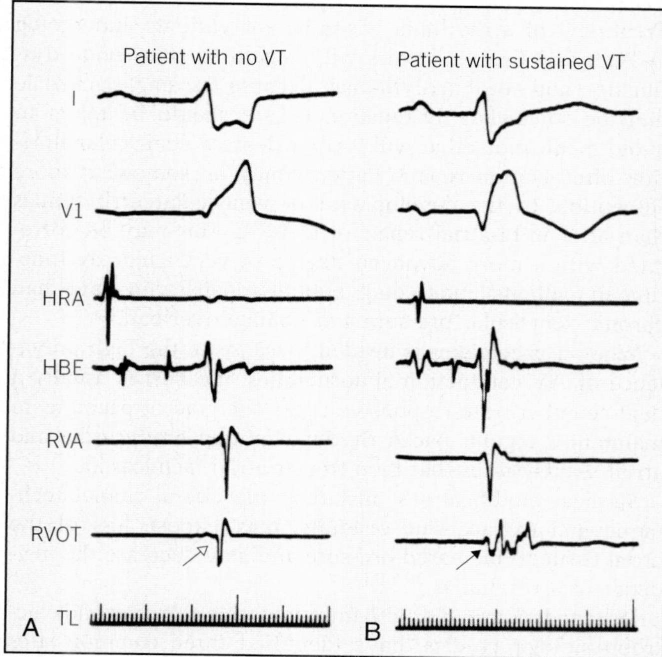

Figure 123.2 Electrograms recorded during normal sinus rhythm after repair of tetralogy of Fallot in a patient without ventricular tachycardia (VT) and in a patient with VT. In both panels, electrocardiogram leads I and V_1 are shown with electrograms recorded in the high right atrium (HRA), His bundle area (HBE), right ventricular apex (RVA), and right ventricular outflow tract (RVOT), with 10-ms time lines (TL). In **A,** recorded in a patient with no clinical evidence of VT and in whom VT could not be induced in the laboratory, note that the RVOT electrogram is relatively narrow and smooth in contour *(open arrow)*. In contrast, in **B,** the patient who had recurrent VT and in whom the tachycardia could not be induced in the clinical electrophysiology laboratory, the electrogram in the RVOT is prolonged, exceeding 100 ms in duration, and fragmented *(filled arrow)*. Such an electrogram was typical of patients in whom VT occurred after repair of tetralogy of Fallot. (Reprinted from Vetter VL, Horowitz LN. Electrophysiologic residua and sequelae of surgery for congenital heart defects. Am J Cardiol 1982;50:588-604. © 1982, with permission from Excerpta Medica Inc.)

MANAGEMENT

Treatment of Sinus Node Dysfunction

The need to treat patients with sinus node dysfunction must be determined by a combination of clinical symptoms and the results of testing. On 24-hour ambulatory monitoring, reproducible heart rates below 30 beats per minute or multiple and reproducible pauses of more than 3 seconds generally are considered to indicate a need for a pacemaker. Young patients or those with abnormal hemodynamics may require pacing for low heart rates that are more than 30 beats per minute, or with pauses shorter than 3 seconds, if they are symptomatic. The response of the heart rate to exercise stress testing is helpful in determining the need for a pacemaker. If the heart rate can accelerate to meet the patient's metabolic needs, even if it is low at rest, the patient may be observed. Close follow-up is indicated in patients who do not receive pacemakers, as postoperative sinus node dysfunction tends to be progressive. Yearly 24-hour ambulatory electrocardiographic monitoring and periodic exercise stress testing are indicated.

Treatment of Atrial Flutter

The groups of patients who most commonly require treatment for atrial flutter include those after intra-atrial repair of D-TGA and after Fontan repairs. Approximately 25% of patients will require treatment for atrial flutter after these repairs.[2] Appropriate recognition and treatment of these arrhythmias are critical to the survival of this group of patients. Simple control of heart rate is not adequate, as was shown in a large collaborative study in which there was a 20% incidence of sudden death if the patient remained in atrial flutter, even if the ventricular rate appeared to be controlled.[15] Therefore, the aim of treatment of atrial flutter should be to convert the flutter.

Pharmacologic Treatment

Digoxin is the drug of first choice and is effective in many instances in maintaining a non-flutter rhythm. It is important to monitor the underlying heart rate carefully because sinus node dysfunction may be aggravated by the treatment of the atrial flutter, resulting in low heart rates. In fact, when medications other than digoxin are needed to treat the flutter in the presence of sinus node dysfunction, pacemaker implantation is indicated in most patients. Encouraging results have been reported with use of an atrial antitachycardia pacemaker to convert episodes of atrial flutter to a slower or paced rhythm. There is a potential risk of deterioration of the atrial flutter to atrial fibrillation with more rapid ventricular response.[67] Refractory atrial flutter may require additional medications. These may include beta blockers, although consideration must be given to the effects of these medications on a dysfunctional systemic or single ventricle. Class I antiarrhythmic agents may be effective, although side effects including proarrhythmia must be carefully monitored (see Chapter 50). Class Ia agents (e.g., procainamide) have been used. These medications have potential deleterious side effects. Each has the propensity to prolong the QT interval and can be proarrhythmic, with the development of torsades de pointes. Disopyramide is a potent negative inotrope that may be detrimental to the patient with marginal ventricular function. Class Ic medications, such as flecainide and propafenone, have been used but have negative inotropic properties. Some success has been reported with these drugs. Class III medications (amiodarone and sotalol) have been used with varying degrees of success in the management of patients with chronic atrial flutter; these medications have the benefit of slowing conduction through the AV node. Amiodarone has been effective in controlling refractory atrial flutter in a number of these patients. Sotalol, with beta-blocking properties, can be a significant negative inotropic agent. It has been reported to control 60% to 90% of atrial flutter in a pediatric population,[68] but it did show a relatively high incidence of proarrhythmia, consisting predominantly of high-grade AV block.[69] As the use of any of these medications can lead to the development of significant bradycardia, patients should be monitored closely for sinus bradycardia, sinus arrest or default, or junctional escape rhythms.

Pacemakers

Antitachycardia pacing has also been used in the treatment of chronic atrial flutter in patients with congenital heart disease, with success in the termination of atrial flutter.[67] There are disadvantages to use of these devices. The currently manufactured antitachycardia pacing devices require the use of bipolar pacing, for which the patient must have two atrial epicardial wires placed on the atrium. Newer antitachycardia devices have the ability to offer backup defibrillation if there is degeneration of the rhythm to atrial or ventricular fibrillation.

In the majority of patients with complex congenital heart disease, including those who have the Fontan procedure, and in patients with right-to-left intracardiac shunts, transvenous pacing may be contraindicated because of the potential for an embolic phenomenon.

Catheter Ablation

In patients with congenital heart disease, catheter ablation can be performed on atrial and ventricular ectopic foci, atrial flutter circuits, and re-entrant circuits involving the AV node, accessory pathways, and ventricle as well as on the AV junction.[70,71]

Catheter ablation has been used in the treatment of patients with atrial flutter. An understanding of the anatomy of the lesion and of the surgical repair is essential to the success of catheter ablation in patients with congenital heart disease. Some type of three-dimensional mapping is essential in these complex cases.[72] The circuits for atrial flutter in patients with congenital heart disease are distinctly different from those seen in classic atrial flutter, often with multiple re-entrant circuits. The circuits traverse between scar lines created by the surgical procedures and natural barriers of conduction, such as the crista terminalis and the orifices of the superior vena cava and inferior vena cava. In patients with congenital heart disease, because the atrial tissue is thick, it is possible that energy delivered with conventional radiofrequency generators may not be sufficient to create a lesion that will disrupt the circuit. Irrigated ablation catheters and larger tips have helped with this problem. These unique problems lead to an overall success rate that is less than that seen with conventional atrial flutter. The acute success rate is somewhere between 80% and 90%, with recurrence rates as high as 34% to 40%.[71-74]

In right atrial re-entrant circuits, if a tricuspid valve is present, the isthmus between the valve ring and the inferior vena cava is a common element of the circuit.[75] Additional circuits are common around atriotomy sites.

All mapping for intra-atrial re-entry tachycardia should involve collection of electrograms during tachycardia from one atrium or both atria to determine the activation sequence. Entrainment mapping can be used to further define the circuit in complex cases.[76] Surgical scars and anatomic barriers can be superimposed on this model to determine the pathway of the re-entrant circuit or circuits.[77] Areas of slow conduction through a narrow isthmus can be targeted for a line of ablation with multiple contiguous lesions to produce conduction block.

Treatment of Arrhythmias After Fontan Repair

Treatment of arrhythmia is similar for patients undergoing D-TGA and Fontan repairs with regard to sinus node dysfunction and atrial arrhythmias. Because the single ventricle may be somewhat dysfunctional, care should be taken to avoid medications that will further depress ventricular function after Fontan repair. Patients may be somewhat more susceptible to the development of ventricular arrhythmias than after intra-atrial repair of D-TGA. This may be correlated with a more advanced degree of ventricular dysfunction in patients undergoing Fontan repair, who have had chronic ventricular pressure and volume overload.

When a pacemaker is needed, because of the high prevalence of AV conduction abnormalities, the best is usually a dual-chamber, rate-responsive type. The goal of pacing is to maintain a regular paced rhythm, limiting bradycardia and atrial extrasystoles that then trigger atrial tachycardia.

Surgical modifications, including the lateral tunnel technique and extracardiac conduits, may expose less of the atrial tissue to increased pressure and may decrease the incidence of arrhythmias.[33,34-37,70]

Deal and Mavroudis, with intraoperative mapping and electrophysiologic studies, have identified three common sites within the right atrium associated with re-entrant circuits, including (1) the area between the coronary sinus os and the inferior vena cava os/right-sided AV annulus, (2) the region of the atrial septal defect patch, and (3) the lateral right atrial wall.[70,78] With this information, they have used a right-sided maze. For patients with left-sided atrial re-entrant circuits or atrial fibrillation, they have added the maze–Cox III procedure, combining the right-sided atrial maze procedure with left-sided incisions and cryoablations. These procedures are combined with pacemaker placement and have shown a marked decrease in recurrence of postoperative atrial arrhythmias. In addition, those with atrial re-entrant tachycardia receive beta blockers for 3 months after surgery, and those with atrial fibrillation receive amiodarone for 3 months postoperatively. After this approach, only 12.5% of patients had recurrence of atrial tachycardia, and the majority improved their functional status significantly.[70]

The use of the extracardiac conduit has potential benefits. Some early or midterm follow-up studies suggested that the incidence of postoperative arrhythmias is decreased but without complete agreement on this issue.[79]

The majority of recent reports suggest that there is less sinus node dysfunction and pacemaker implantation after the extracardiac conduit compared with the lateral tunnel repair, although conflicting results still have been noted.[33,37,80,81] A higher occurrence of atrial tachycardia has been noted after the lateral tunnel compared with the extracardiac conduit (11% versus 38%).[79]

The consensus seems to be that those who have Fontan conversion do best if they have a total caval-pulmonary connection with an extracardiac conduit, atrial reduction, cryoablation, and postoperative pacemaker and antiarrhythmic medication.[34,36] Left atrial epicardial leads may provide better thresholds in these patients undergoing reoperation.[38] Mavroudis suggests that the result of the conversion is dependent on the underlying anatomy, type of original surgery, type of arrhythmia, and associated lesions such as AV valve regurgitation. A representation of the modified right-sided maze procedure for right atrial re-entry tachycardia and left atrial tachycardia and atrial fibrillation is shown in Figure 123.3.[36] The overall reported incidence of recurrent tachycardia after Fontan conversion is 13.5%, with a decrease in the most recent cohort of 2003-2006 to 7.8%, albeit with a shorter follow-up interval.[36]

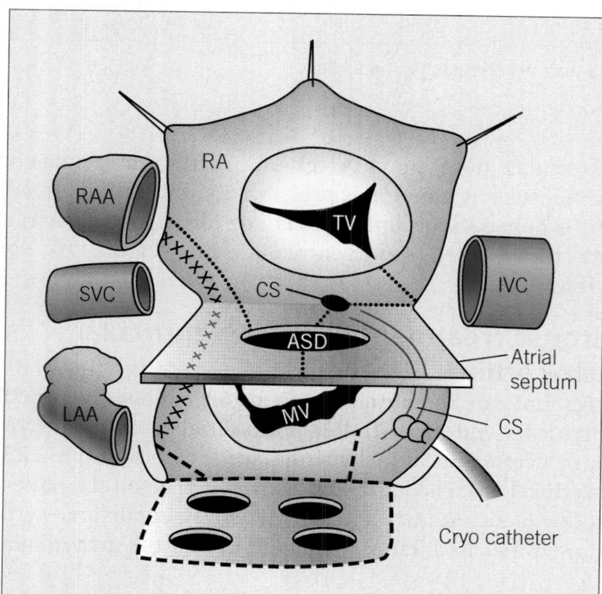

Figure 123.3 Representation of modified right-sided maze procedure for right atrial re-entry tachycardia *(dotted lines)* and the left atrial Cox-maze procedure *(dashed lines)* for atrial fibrillation and left atrial re-entry tachycardia. Significant additional cryoablation lesions are coronary sinus (CS) to atrial septal defect (ASD) for the modified right-sided maze procedure and the base of the right atrial appendage (RAA) to the base of the left atrial appendage (LAA) for the Cox-maze procedure *(x lines)*. IVC, inferior vena cava; MV, mitral valve; RA, right atrium; SVC, superior vena cava; TV, tricuspid valve. (From Mavroudis C, Deal BJ, Backer CL, et al. J. Maxwell Chamberlain Memorial Paper for congenital heart surgery. 111 Fontan conversions with arrhythmia surgery: surgical lessons and outcomes. Ann Thorac Surg 2007;84:1457-1465.)

Sites commonly seen and amenable to catheter ablation include circuits with re-entry around lateral wall atrial scars, atrial septal patches, and the area of anastomosis between the atrium and the pulmonary artery in patients having the older style Fontan operation. Circuits may be seen that are pericaval, especially in tricuspid atresia patients.[82]

Acute Treatment of Supraventricular Tachycardia in Patients with Congenital Heart Disease

Because the mechanism of supraventricular tachycardia can usually be identified, treatment can be chosen for the specific form. Treatment of any cardiac arrhythmia is determined by the clinical status of the patient. Thus, the type of treatment chosen for the patient in shock is different from that given to the patient who is asymptomatic and has only a fast heart rate (Table 123.1). In postoperative patients, atrial epicardial wires may be used with an external pacemaker to achieve rapid overdrive of the arrhythmia and to convert the patient to sinus rhythm. Adenosine may be used in acutely ill patients with AV

ACUTE TREATMENT OF SUPRAVENTRICULAR TACHYCARDIA	
Asymptomatic	Ice, vagal maneuvers
	IV adenosine
	Pharmacologic agents
	IV digoxin
	IV esmolol
	Oral propranolol
Mild congestive heart failure	Ice, vagal maneuvers
	IV adenosine
	Pharmacologic agents
	IV digoxin
	IV esmolol
	Oral propranolol
	Oral amiodarone
Moderate congestive heart failure	Ice, vagal maneuvers
	IV adenosine
	Pharmacologic agents—if IV access
	IV digoxin
	IV amiodarone
	Pacing (esophageal or intracardiac)—if no IV access or for infants
	Cardioversion synchronized
Severe congestive heart failure	Cardioversion synchronized
	IV adenosine
	Pacing, esophageal or intracardiac
	Pharmacologic agents
	IV digoxin
	IV amiodarone

IV, intravenous.
With permission from Vetter VL. Arrhythmias. In Moller JH, Hoffman JI, eds. Pediatric Cardiovascular Medicine. New York, Churchill Livingstone, 2000:833-883.

Table 123.1 Acute treatment of supraventricular tachycardia.

ACUTE PHARMACOLOGIC TREATMENT OF SUPRAVENTRICULAR TACHYCARDIA AND VENTRICULAR TACHYCARDIA		
Arrhythmia	**Agent**	**Initial Treatment (IV)**
Supraventricular tachycardia	Adenosine	50-100 μg/kg
		Increase by increments of 50 μg/kg every 2 minutes to 400 μg/kg or 12 mg maximal dose
	Digoxin	Dose is age dependent
		Give in three doses (½ TDD, ¼ TDD, ¼ TDD) at 4- to 8-hour intervals
		Give IV to ages <1 yr
		Preterm infant: 10-20 μg/kg TDD
		Term newborn to adolescent: 30-40 μg/kg TDD oral to maximal TDD of 1-1.5 mg (IV, ¾ PO)
		Oral maintenance: 10 μg/kg/day q12 h
Supraventricular tachycardia and ventricular tachycardia	Esmolol	IV load: 200-500 μg/kg/min during 2-4 minutes (maximum dose = 1000 mg/kg/min)
	Amiodarone	IV: 5 mg/kg during 10-30 minutes, followed by 2-5 mg/kg/dose IV (5-minute bolus) q6 h
	Procainamide	5 mg/kg during 5-10 minutes or 10-15 mg/kg during 30-45 minutes (maximal dose, 1 g)
		Infusion: 20-100 μg/kg/min
		Maintenance infusion: 50-200 μg/kg/min
	Propranolol	0.05-0.1 mg/kg during 5 minutes q6 h
Ventricular tachycardia	Lidocaine	1-2 mg/kg IV bolus every 5-15 minutes
		IV infusion: 20-50 μg/kg/min
	Phenytoin	3-5 mg/kg during 5 minutes, not to exceed 1 mg/kg/min
	Magnesium	0.25 mmol/kg during 1 minute; may repeat every 8-12 hours for 2-3 doses in neonates and repeat every 4-6 hours for 3-4 doses in children
		Maximum single dose: 16 mmol
		Achieve magnesium concentration of 1.5-2.5 mg/dL

IV, intravenous; PO, by mouth; TDD, total digitalizing dose.

Table 123.2 Acute pharmacologic treatment of supraventricular tachycardia and ventricular tachycardia.

re-entrant supraventricular tachycardia, but its use should not delay immediate cardioversion in severely compromised patients. For those patients who become acidotic or hypotensive, immediate synchronized DC cardioversion is advised with a dosage of 1 to 2 J/kg. The dosage may be repeatedly doubled until it is effective or until a level of 10 J/kg is reached.

Existing treatment of a patient with digoxin should not prevent the use of cardioversion when it is needed. Digoxin is one of the pharmacologic agents that may be used to treat supraventricular tachycardia. We use intravenous digoxin loading for infants 1 year of age or younger and for those in congestive heart failure (at 80% of the oral dosage). If there is evidence of digoxin toxicity, such as ventricular arrhythmia, it may be treated with intravenous lidocaine (lignocaine) (1 mg/kg), or lidocaine may be given prophylactically to prevent the occurrence of ventricular arrhythmias after cardioversion in high-risk patients. Other pharmacologic agents that may be used to treat supraventricular tachycardia include procainamide, amiodarone, esmolol, and propranolol (Table 123.2). Once the patient's rhythm has been converted and an electrocardiogram in sinus rhythm obtained, the chosen chronic treatment should be initiated immediately.

Esmolol or propranolol, which may further depress cardiac function, should be used with caution in a critically ill child or avoided in the patient with pronounced congestive heart failure. When cardiac function is not compromised, a slow intravenous dose may be given. A shorter acting beta blocker, such as esmolol, is preferable in this setting. In addition, esophageal or intracardiac overdrive pacing may be used to convert supraventricular tachycardia to sinus rhythm.

Chronic Treatment of Supraventricular Tachycardia

Drugs that can be chronically used to treat supraventricular tachycardia and atrial flutter, intra-atrial re-entry tachycardia, or ectopic atrial tachycardia are shown in Table 123.3. It is critical to consider the effect of the drug on the patient's hemodynamic status and underlying conduction system abnormalities in addition to the effects on the arrhythmia.

Catheter Ablation of Supraventricular Arrhythmias in Patients with Congenital Heart Disease

Patients with congenital heart disease and supraventricular arrhythmias may have an accessory pathway, either manifest (Wolff-Parkinson-White syndrome) or concealed, or other atrial arrhythmias, including atrial flutter or intra-atrial re-entry and ectopic or automatic atrial tachycardia. Because of the increased time required to ablate the arrhythmia surgically in combination with congenital heart surgery and a resultant increase in morbidity and mortality, catheter ablation has been recommended before surgical repair, when possible, to prevent postoperative arrhythmias.

CHRONIC ANTIARRHYTHMIC AGENTS FOR SUPRAVENTRICULAR AND VENTRICULAR TACHYCARDIA			
	Agent	**Dose (oral)**	**Concentration**
Supraventricular tachycardia	Digoxin	Dose is age dependent Give in three doses (½ TDD, ¼ TDD, ¼ TDD) at 8-hour intervals Preterm infant: 10-20 μg/kg TDD Term newborn to adolescent: 30-40 μg/kg TDD oral to maximal TDD of 1-1.5 mg (IV, ¾ PO) Oral maintenance: 10 μg/kg/day q12 h	1-2.5 ng/mL
	Verapamil	2-8 mg/kg/day q8 h	100-300 ng/mL
Supraventricular tachycardia and ventricular tachycardia	Propranolol	0.5 mg/kg/dose q6 h	50-100 μg/L
	Nadolol	0.5-1 mg/kg/dose q12 h	0.03-0.13 μg/mL
	Atenolol	0.5-1 mg/kg/day q24 h	
	Procainamide	20-100 mg/kg/day q4-6 h	PA: 4-10 mg/L, NAPA: 4-8 mg/L
	Flecainide	50-200 mg/m²/day or 3-6 mg/kg/day q12 h	0.2-1.0 mg/L
	Amiodarone	Loading dose: 10-20 mg/kg/day q12 h × 7 days Maintenance: 5-10 mg/kg/dose q24 h	RT_3 <90 ng/dL
	Sotalol	2-8 mg/kg/day q12 h or 50-210 mg/m²	
Ventricular tachycardia	Phenytoin	Loading dose: 10-20 mg/kg/day q2 h × 2 days Maintenance: 5-10 mg/kg/day q12 h	10-20 μg/mL
	Mexiletine	5-15 mg/kg/day q8 h	0.5-2.0 μg/mL

IV, intravenous; NAPA, *N*-acetylprocainamide; PA, procainamide; PO, by mouth; RT_3, reverse triiodothyronine; TDD, total digitalizing dose.
With permission from Vetter VL. Arrhythmias. In Moller JH, Hoffman JI, eds. Pediatric Cardiovascular Medicine. New York, Churchill Livingstone, 2000:833-883.

Table 123.3 Chronic antiarrhythmic agents for supraventricular and ventricular tachycardia.

In patients with a cardiac anomaly, several pathways are common and are frequently associated with the tricuspid valve.[83] The most common structural heart defects associated with accessory pathways are Ebstein's anomaly of the tricuspid valve and L-TGA or corrected transposition of the great arteries. Van Hare and colleagues[83] reported radiofrequency ablation in 15 patients with structural heart disease. Almost 50% of the patients had a second mechanism or pathway. A cure was achieved in 10 of the 15. Given the complexities of medical management in some patients with congenital defects, radiofrequency ablation is an attractive method of treatment in this group.[84] The approach to the accessory pathway may be made more difficult by the cardiac anomaly. In some lesions, such as those requiring the Fontan repair, the operation may prevent future access to the pathway.

In those patients in whom radiofrequency ablation cannot be attempted or achieved, surgical cryoablation may be used.[70]

Catheter Ablation of Supraventricular Tachycardia After Intra-atrial Repair of D-TGA

Intra-atrial re-entrant tachycardia after intra-atrial repair of D-TGA is amenable to catheter ablation. Either radiofrequency or cryothermal energy may be used. Current technology has helped to identify the location of circuits. Retrograde approaches to atrial tissue in the region of the cavotricuspid isthmus, originally right atrial but postoperatively located in the pulmonary venous atrium, may be necessary, with ablation performed in both the systemic and pulmonary venous atria.[85] These patients have also been noted to have AV nodal re-entrant supraventricular tachycardia and focal atrial tachycardias. Successful sites include near the mouth of the coronary sinus,[86] the tricuspid valve isthmus (57%), and the lateral right atrial wall (43%).[87] Linear lesions have been placed from the medial superior vena cava to the intra-atrial baffle in the systemic venous atrium, from the intra-atrial suture line to the posterior systemic venous atrium, and from the posterior and inferior pulmonary venous atrium to the tricuspid valve annulus.[88] Circuits with longer cycle lengths are more likely to be ablated successfully. Acute success has been reported in 70% to 90% of patients, with recurrence in 20% to 30%.[72,77]

Catheter Ablation of Supraventricular Tachycardia After Fontan Repair

In the Fontan repair, atrial dilatation and suture lines, including atriotomies, make intra-atrial re-entrant tachycardia more likely. After atrial repairs, a protected isthmus of conduction is often bounded by natural and surgically created barriers; split or double potentials may identify a line of block. Successful ablation consists of identifying the isthmus of slow conduction or narrow channel between barriers and creating a linear ablative lesion in this critical area. Locations of sites with acute success of 72% after Fontan repair include[87,89]

- the lateral right atrial wall (53%);
- the anterior right atrium (25%);
- the isthmus area (15%); and
- the atrial septum (7%).

Newer technologies, including noncontact mapping, electroanatomic mapping, and irrigated tip ablations, have increased success in this difficult group of patients.[72] The best outcomes occur in association with good hemodynamic results and the use of the newer technologies. Despite improvements, recurrences still develop. Given an acute success rate of 83% and a 3-year success rate of 81%, Weipert and coworkers[25] suggest catheter ablation as the first line of therapy for atrial tachycardia after Fontan operation, with surgical ablation reserved for those with conversions or failure of catheter ablation therapy.

Comparison of noncontact and electroanatomic mapping in this population showed a slight benefit of electroanatomic mapping over noncontact mapping, thought to be related to the large size of these atria.[90] An increased incidence of acquired Wolff-Parkinson-White syndrome has been reported in Fontan patients postoperatively, especially after the Fontan-Bjork procedure. This should be considered in evaluating tachycardias in these patients, as these connections are amenable to catheter ablation.[91]

Treatment of Ventricular Arrhythmias

Acute Treatment of Ventricular Tachycardia

In patients in the immediate postoperative period, arrhythmias such as ventricular tachycardia are poorly tolerated and should be treated as an emergency unless the rate is slow and the patient is clinically stable. If an extracardiac cause such as an electrolyte abnormality, hypoxia, or acidosis has been identified, the underlying abnormality should be corrected.

In patients in whom the heart function is compromised, intravenous lidocaine (1 mg/kg) should be given immediately. If the lidocaine is effective, a continuous infusion of lidocaine (10 to 50 μg/kg per minute) should be started immediately after the initial bolus dose to maintain an adequate concentration of the drug. Lidocaine concentrations should be carefully monitored to prevent toxicity. Intravenous amiodarone or procainamide may be selected for use in this setting. Synchronized cardioversion at 2 to 5 J/kg, up to 10 J/kg, should be performed if the pharmacologic treatment selected does not result in immediate conversion or if an intravenous site is not available and the patient is hemodynamically compromised.

Procainamide has been used to treat acute episodes of ventricular tachycardia. Because of its associated negative inotropic effects, the patients must be monitored very carefully during the infusion. More recently, amiodarone has been shown to be effective when it is given intravenously for ventricular tachycardia (see Table 123.2). This should be given as a slow intravenous bolus of 2.5 mg/kg per dose every 4 to 6 hours in infants and not as a continuous infusion (because of leaching of phthalate plasticizer from tubing, unless phthalate-free tubing is available).

Rapid ventricular pacing may be used to convert the rhythm to sinus if pharmacologic treatment fails or is contraindicated. Epicardial wires may be used during the immediate postoperative period.

Treatment of Chronic Ventricular Tachycardia

Once the arrhythmia has been converted, it is essential to choose an appropriate chronic regimen to maintain the stability of the patient. The drugs most commonly used are shown in Table 123.3.

If lidocaine has been successful, it may be maintained until adequate concentrations of a chronic drug have been reached or the acute causative agent is no longer present. To prevent combined toxicity of lidocaine and mexiletine when the regimen is switched from lidocaine to mexiletine, the patient should be gradually weaned from the lidocaine as the mexiletine is loaded because the side effects of these two drugs are similar.

Propranolol and other beta blockers are especially effective in patients whose arrhythmia is sensitive to sympathetic or adrenergic stimuli, but it must be used cautiously, if at all, in acute postoperative patients or in patients with decreased ventricular function. The class I agents and amiodarone are effective in more refractory arrhythmias.

Treatment of Ventricular Tachycardia After Surgery for Congenital Heart Disease

These life-threatening arrhythmias are most commonly seen in association with tetralogy of Fallot; anomalies with long-standing ventricular pressure overload, such as aortic stenosis, single ventricles, and complete transposition after intra-atrial repair; and abnormal myocardium, such as Ebstein's anomaly and hypertrophic subaortic stenosis. Sudden death occurs in up to 30% of patients with ventricular tachycardia and a congenital cardiac anomaly; therefore, these patients should be prescribed a chronic drug regimen. Studies have shown that patients with early postoperative ventricular tachycardia are likely to develop this arrhythmia during the late postoperative period, which underlies the recommendation for chronic treatment in this population as in the postoperative patient who presents months to years after surgery.

A thorough investigation is needed to exclude underlying hemodynamic abnormalities, as ventricular tachycardia is tolerated less well in this group of patients. The electrophysiologic study may be a helpful guide to medical treatment, or, in patients who are refractory to drug treatment, it may determine the site of origin of the tachycardia and direct treatment by surgical or catheter ablation. Patients with life-threatening episodes or those refractory to medical or ablative treatment may require implantation of a cardioverter-defibrillator. In patients who are having surgical repairs with use of cardiopulmonary bypass but need ICDs, we generally perform the surgery, allow the patient to recover hemodynamically, and place the ICD a week later to decrease the risk and to allow a better assessment of defibrillation thresholds.

Treatment of Ventricular Tachycardia in Tetralogy of Fallot

Although there is no absolute agreement as to the indications for treatment of ventricular tachycardia in tetralogy of Fallot, we have adopted a policy of treating patients with clinical episodes of ventricular tachycardia or with symptoms of inducible ventricular tachycardia. We generally treat patients with complex ventricular arrhythmias and abnormal hemodynamics and patients with significant symptoms and abnormal hemodynamics.

Treatment can include a combination of pharmacologic agents, catheter ablation, surgical repair, and ablation or implantation of a pacemaker or cardioverter-defibrillator. Recently, surgical or catheter ablation has been used effectively in these patients.

We use electrophysiologic study to determine the efficacy of specific drug regimens or the need for an ICD in patients in whom drug treatment is ineffective or who have hemodynamic deterioration. ICDs are used in patients who have had syncopal events or aborted sudden death or in those in whom unstable ventricular tachycardia or ventricular fibrillation is induced.

The most commonly used drug regimens include beta blockers, mexiletine, and class Ia or Ic agents. In the 1970s, phenytoin was found to be an effective drug in this population of patients, but subsequently mexiletine has been shown to be an effective drug for chronic use in patients after tetralogy of Fallot repair, as have the beta-blocker class of drugs. Class I agents and amiodarone may be effective in refractory patients.

Catheter Ablation of Ventricular Tachycardia

Postoperative ventricular tachycardia is amenable to catheter ablation, particularly in the right ventricular outflow tract, most commonly seen in tetralogy of Fallot. Scarring from the right ventriculotomy or infundibular resection allows a zone of slow conduction, producing the substrate for re-entry. Successful ablation sites include

- those with earliest activation during ventricular tachycardia;
- areas of slow conduction with low-amplitude, fractionated electrograms; and
- those sites that produce a pace map identical to the clinical or inducible ventricular tachycardia.

Critical isthmus sites have been identified and include the area between[92]

- the tricuspid annulus and the scar or patch in the anterior right ventricular outflow;
- the pulmonary annulus and the right ventricle free wall scar or patch;
- the pulmonary annulus and the septal scar or patch; and
- the septal scar or patch and the tricuspid annulus.

Newer technologies, including electroanatomic mapping and noncontact mapping, provide useful information in the mapping and ablation of complex ventricular tachycardias (see Chapters 51 and 62). These include mapping of macroreentrant circuits by sequence analysis, pace mapping, three-dimensional mapping, and entrainment techniques. Success has been noted in patients with postoperative tetralogy of Fallot; recent acute success rates approach 90%, with up to 25% recurrence.[92-94]

In patients with ventricular tachycardia after congenital heart repairs, ablation may not completely obliterate the arrhythmias but may be useful in decreasing episodes in patients receiving medication and with ICDs in place.

Treatment of Junctional Ectopic Tachycardia

Numerous treatment strategies have been developed in an attempt to treat junctional ectopic tachycardia in the postoperative patient. These have included the use of medications such as intravenous digoxin, procainamide and amiodarone, and class Ia agents.[95] We have found intravenous amiodarone to be most effective in this setting if digoxin is not effective. In using intravenous antiarrhythmics, one must be aware of the potential negative inotropic effect of these medicines. Because these drugs suppress the sinus node, transient pacing may be needed in some patients if amiodarone is used. Other treatments of junctional ectopic tachycardia include limitation of exogenous pressors, electrolyte and acid-base balance, decrease of metabolic needs by sedation or paralysis and ventilation, surface cooling, and atrial pacing at a rate slightly faster than the junctional rate if this rate is not too high and improves cardiac output.[62,96] If the heart rate can be slowed and the patient's condition stabilized for a period of 48 to 72 hours, the junctional ectopic tachycardia will resolve and normal sinus rhythm will resume, but significant morbidity and mortality can occur. Extracorporeal membrane oxygenator therapy and His bundle ablation have been reported.

Treatment of Bradycardia

Acute Management

If an increased heart rate is needed acutely, pharmacologic agents including atropine and isoproterenol may be helpful, especially if the block is in the AV node and partially mediated by vagal influences (Table 123.4). Isoproterenol may increase the heart rate by improving AV conduction or by increasing the rate of the escape pacemaker. Acutely, temporary epicardial, transthoracic, transcutaneous, or transvenous pacing may be necessary. For persistent symptomatic or high-grade AV block, permanent pacing may be needed. With postoperative heart block, temporary pacing is usually performed for 7 to 10 days. Permanent pacing should be performed if AV conduction does not return because of the high incidence of sudden death in this group of postoperative patients if they are not paced. Even the return of sinus rhythm does not ensure that heart block will not return at a later time, so close follow-up is indicated. Late complete heart block months to years after repair, especially in AV canal defect repairs, has been reported.[61]

PHARMACOLOGIC TREATMENT OF BRADYCARDIA AND ATRIOVENTRICULAR BLOCK

Drug	Dosage
Atropine	0.02-0.04 mg/kg IV (maximum, 1-2 mg)
Isoproterenol	Infusion: 0.05-2.0 μg/kg/min
Epinephrine	0.01-0.5 mg/kg (0.1 mL/kg of 1:10,000 dilution; 0.01 mL/kg of 1:1000 dilution) IV bolus
	Infusion 0.1-2.0 μg/kg/min

IV, intravenous.

Table 123.4 Pharmacologic treatment of bradycardia and atrioventricular block.

Patients with congenital complete heart block and associated congenital heart disease may present as an acute emergency. These distressed infants may require tracheal intubation and ventilation of the lungs, treatment of acidosis, and catecholamine support of heart rate and blood pressure. Temporary pacing may be performed by the transcutaneous, transthoracic, or intracardiac routes. The transcutaneous pacemaker may be effective for short-term emergency situations but should be replaced with another pacing method as soon as possible. Although infants with rates lower than 50 beats per minute or with slightly faster rates and associated congenital heart defects or cardiomyopathies may require pacing, this decision should not be made on the basis of rate alone.

Implantable Pacemakers and Implantable Cardioverter-Defibrillators

Use of permanent pacemakers was first reported in children in the early 1960s. The programmability and miniaturization of the current permanent pacemakers have significantly increased their flexibility for use in the pediatric population. The most common indications in postoperative patients are AV block and sinus node dysfunction.

Once the decision has been made to implant the pacemaker, the lead route and type of pacing system should be selected. We do not advise intracardiac leads in very small children, although it is technically possible to use them. Thrombosis or narrowing of the venous system occurs in a substantial number of these small patients.[97] Because many will require pacemakers for more than 60 to 70 years, obstruction of the venous system at an early age is undesirable and may complicate later pacing. Extraction of these leads may become necessary and can be challenging. Transvenous leads are a potential source for emboli in patients with a right-to-left shunt or sluggish circulation, as in those undergoing Fontan repairs, and we rarely use them in such patients.

The most common modes used in pediatrics are the single-chamber VVI or VVIR or AAI or AAIR and the dual-chamber DDD, DDDR, or DDIR modes (see Chapter 55 for explanation of the codes for pacemaker mode and function). The use of VDD pacing may provide AV sequential pacing with only a single lead and is especially effective in some small children. Atrial sensing may be problematic in some patients, especially as they grow. A newer mode (AAIR < = > DDDR) referred to as managed ventricular pacing is useful in patients with sinus node dysfunction to minimize ventricular pacing. The rate-responsive pacemakers allow the patient to benefit from an increased heart rate in the presence of sinus node dysfunction. Many of the newer pacemakers provide the ability to perform temporary rapid pacing or noninvasive programmed electrophysiologic testing. An implantable atrial antitachycardia pacemaker can be effective in converting atrial flutter. Electrophysiologic testing should be performed before implantation to ensure that rapid atrial pacing will not accelerate the atrial tachycardia and result in a life-threatening arrhythmia. Studies of automatic antitachycardia pacing devices in children with congenital heart disease and atrial re-entrant tachycardia indicate that 43% to 54% are successfully converted.[98] The major problem with the current antitachycardia pacemaker devices is that they cannot detect atrial tachycardia with 1:1 AV conduction, a common presentation in children.[31]

Epicardial leads are well tolerated in children and are necessary in those with single ventricles and Fontan or other repairs in which intracardiac leads cannot be placed or are not desirable.

The use of the ICD has been reported in pediatric patients. The use of transvenous nonthoracotomy leads has made implantation less invasive, but epicardial patches or other nonconventional approaches, such as subcutaneous arrays, are still necessary in smaller children because of the size of the transvenous lead system.[99] In 1993, Silka and colleagues[100] identified 177 patients younger than 20 years who had an ICD. Follow-up was obtained for 125 of these patients. The most common indications included survival of sudden cardiac death (76%), drug-refractory ventricular tachycardia (10%), and syncope with inducible ventricular tachycardia (10%). The associated cardiovascular diseases included 18% with congenital heart defects. The ICD is also efficacious for prevention of sudden death in patients with hypertrophic cardiomyopathy.[101]

Biventricular Pacing or Cardiac Resynchronization

Biventricular pacing or cardiac resynchronization has been shown to improve symptoms and cardiac function in adults with congestive cardiomyopathies. Studies in children have shown both acute postoperative and long-term benefits from biventricular or multisite pacing.[102-106] Biventricular ICD devices are available and should be used in those with life-threatening ventricular arrhythmias.

The major problem with this technique is that no large trials or small studies have been performed to aid in the selection of patients who are likely to benefit from this technology.

Pacemaker Follow-up

Pacemaker follow-up schedules recommended for adults should be altered for children. Children and adult congenital heart disease patients are more likely to show pacemaker dependence. Careful surveillance for wire fracture, impedance changes, and threshold changes requires on-site visits with the cardiology pacemaker specialist, although transtelephonic technology has reduced the number of face-to-face visits needed. At these visits, pacemaker thresholds, sensitivity, graphic analysis of rate ranges over time, and a variety of other information can be assessed to determine the best settings for the optimal function of the pacemaker. Remote monitoring of ICDs and pacemakers is now available and can be used in some instances when additional evaluation of the congenital heart lesion is not required. In addition, 24-hour ambulatory monitoring and exercise stress tests can be used to assess correct pacemaker function and to determine the most appropriate settings.

PROGNOSIS

Cardiac arrhythmias result in significant morbidity in patients with congenital heart disease, with an incidence of sudden death of 2% to 10%. The underlying hemodynamic status and electrophysiologic substrate determine the degree of symptoms and the potential for life-threatening events.

Improvements in surgical techniques and myocardial protection may prevent the late sequelae that result in ventricular dysfunction and arrhythmias. Surgical modifications or alternative procedures, such as the arterial switch repair for complete transposition or modifications of the Fontan repair, may dramatically change the arrhythmias seen in association with specific congenital heart disease lesions. Interventions such as surgical and catheter ablation provide the opportunity for improved results. Primary and secondary prevention of sudden cardiac death with defibrillators has improved the long-term prognosis of these patients.

Early repair may prevent the problems that are associated with long-standing ventricular hypertension and chronic hypoxemia, including fibrosis, subendocardial ischemia, and ventricular hypertrophy. Likewise, systematic follow-up resulting in early repair of residual defects should diminish the arrhythmogenic sequelae that are associated with altered hemodynamics. Early identification of patients at risk and appropriate treatment, including pharmacologic management, catheter ablation, surgical intervention with reoperation, and the use of ICDs and cardiac resynchronization in selected high-risk patients, may improve survival. Cardiac transplantation and heart-lung transplantation are playing an increasing role in the small population of postoperative congenital heart disease patients for whom this treatment is the recommended option.

The increasing population of adults with congenital heart disease makes understanding, identification, and successful treatment of postoperative arrhythmias even more important as long-term quality of life and survival are closely associated with freedom from arrhythmias.

SUMMARY

Cardiac arrhythmias are common in all patients with congenital heart disease; a predisposition to specific arrhythmias depends on the congenital lesion and the surgical repair. Knowledge of these potential arrhythmias and their physiologic effects, early and accurate diagnosis, and appropriate treatment should allow most of these patients to live relatively normal lives.

chapter

124 Adult Congenital Heart Disease

David S. Celermajer

Definition

- Congenital abnormalities in cardiac structure that present in subjects older than 16 years, either never having been diagnosed and treated or after palliative or corrective surgery in childhood.

Key Features

- Successful treatments for even complex congenital heart defects in childhood have resulted in increasing numbers of young adults with congenital heart disease requiring continuing surveillance and management.
- Common medical problems include hemodynamic abnormalities (shunts, pressure and volume loads), electrical sequelae (bradyarrhythmias or tachyarrhythmias), and the long-term effects of cyanosis.
- Psychosocial issues, such as employment, insurance, contraception advice, sports recommendations, and genetic counseling, are also of great importance.

Therapy

- Lesion-specific correction of hemodynamic and electrical problems.

Until the first operations for congenital heart disease were performed, more than 50 years ago,[1] outcomes of complex intracardiac lesions such as transposition of the great arteries were uniformly poor. Even relatively "simple" lesions, such as large ventricular septal defect (VSD), resulted in childhood morbidity and premature mortality. During the past half-century, however, medical and surgical advances have revolutionized outcomes in congenital heart disease, with nearly every lesion now amenable to some kind of palliation or even correction.[2] These successes have resulted in the appearance of a "new population" of young adults with congenital heart disease, now growing rapidly in both number and complexity. Indeed, by 2006, there were nearly as many adults with severe congenital heart disease as there were children.[3]

These young adults may be difficult to manage. Their medical problems can be extremely challenging, with combinations of intracardiac shunts and abnormal pressure or volume loading conditions that are the consequences of staged palliations for complex underlying anatomy (Table 124.1). Electrophysiologic abnormalities resulting from past surgery or chamber dilatation often complicate the picture further. There is often confusion as to the appropriate physician to manage these young individuals; pediatric cardiologists may not feel comfortable treating adults, and "adult" cardiologists may be inadequately trained in congenital heart medicine. Finally, the patients themselves undergo the same stresses of adolescence and young adult life as do all people and are often rebellious or reluctant to seek out regular medical follow-up. For these reasons, special multidisciplinary teams of interested cardiologists, surgeons, and allied health professionals have begun to form in major centers to provide comprehensive care facilities for young adults with congenital heart disease.[4]

The variety of complex management issues, both medical and nonmedical, may be best illustrated by considering particular problem areas that are typically present in specialty clinics of this nature. The following case problems are therefore based on actual patients to illustrate the salient diagnostic and therapeutic issues in such individuals.

SYNCOPE AFTER REPAIR OF TETRALOGY OF FALLOT

DEFINITION OF PROBLEM

In tetralogy of Fallot, cranial displacement of the infundibular part of the interventricular septum results in narrowing of the right ventricular (RV) outflow tract (and consequent RV hypertrophy), a "malalignment" VSD, and aortic override of the RV outflow. Surgical repair usually consists of VSD closure and relief of the RV outflow obstruction, which may require resection of infundibular muscle or an enlargement of the pulmonary valve annulus. When this latter is required in the repair, free pulmonary regurgitation may be created. Until recently, this surgery required a right ventriculotomy, with consequent infundibular scarring and the potential for late re-entry pathways. More recently, repair through the right atrium or pulmonary artery has been possible.[5]

Survivors of tetralogy repair also represent a large proportion of patients attending adult congenital heart disease clinics.

TYPICAL CASE

Melissa presented with a murmur at 6 weeks of age, and tetralogy of Fallot was diagnosed by echocardiography. Because of increasing cyanosis, a left modified Blalock-Taussig shunt operation was performed when she was aged 6 months. At 18 months of age, complete repair was carried out through a right ventriculotomy, requiring a transannular gusset to achieve full relief of the RV outflow obstruction. Melissa was then healthy for many years, participating in school sports. She was clinically well when she was examined by her pediatric cardiologist at the age 15 of years, with mild RV dilatation, moderate to severe pulmonary

PROBLEMS IN ADULTS WITH CONGENITAL HEART DISEASE	
Medical	**Psychosocial**
Hemodynamic	Self-esteem
Shunts	Employment
Chamber dilatation	Insurance
Ventricular dysfunction	Socialization
Valve stenosis or regurgitation	Flying or driving recommendations
Pulmonary hypertension	Sports and exercise recommendations
Electrical	Contraceptive advice
Conduction abnormalities	Genetic counseling
Re-entry circuits	
Cyanosis or hyperviscosity	
Management of pregnancy	
Endocarditis prophylaxis	

Table 124.1 Problems in adults with congenital heart disease.

regurgitation, no RV outflow obstruction, and no residual VSD on echocardiography. She was then lost to follow-up for 8 years and presented again because of palpitations followed by syncope during an aerobics class, on a background of recent gradual decline in her exercise ability. In the emergency department, 12-lead electrocardiography showed sinus rhythm with right bundle branch block (Fig. 124.1).

DIFFERENTIAL DIAGNOSIS

Late dysrhythmia, particularly tachycardia, is a well-recognized complication late after tetralogy repair.[6] In the absence of any other likely diagnosis, syncope in this setting is usually due to ventricular tachycardia. Chest radiography and echocardiography are indicated to assess the hemodynamic status of the repair. Detailed intracardiac electrophysiologic study is indicated to characterize the performance of the conducting system, to diagnose any abnormal circuits or foci for tachycardia, and potentially to treat the problem with radiofrequency ablation (Fig. 124.2).

In Melissa's case, chest radiography showed cardiomegaly and clear lung fields. Echocardiography revealed severe pulmonary regurgitation, no RV outflow obstruction or residual VSD, and severe RV dilatation with mild to moderate contractile impairment, which was markedly worse than 8 years earlier. Electrophysiologic study showed easily inducible ventricular tachycardia, causing hypotension, mapped to the RV outflow in the region of the old ventriculotomy scar. Preoperative cardiac catheterization confirmed low (normal) RV systolic pressure, absence of intracardiac shunting, and reasonable pulmonary artery anatomy.

TREATMENT OPTIONS

Although electrophysiology-guided or empiric trials of antiarrhythmic drugs might be possible in this case, the combination of progressive and probably symptomatic RV dilatation in the setting of free pulmonary regurgitation with ventricular tachycardia caused by a localized re-entry circuit suggests that operative repair would be the best strategy. Accordingly, intraoperative ventricular tachycardia mapping and radiofrequency ablation were carried out, followed by pulmonary valve replacement with a homograft. Postoperatively, Melissa remained well without cardiovascular drugs and reported a marked improvement in her aerobic exercise capacity.

SUMMARY

Late sudden death is a rare but dreaded complication after repair of tetralogy of Fallot, with an estimated incidence of approximately 0.5%.[7] Surveillance for asymptomatic, nonsustained ventricular tachyarrhythmia is not helpful as these are very common (approximately 40% of cases) and are poorly predictive of adverse events.[8] Certainly, sustained, symptomatic ventricular tachycardia requires urgent investigation and definitive treatment. In fact, all but trivial palpitations require detailed evaluation; however, supraventricular tachycardia is at least as common a cause of symptoms in this setting as is ventricular tachycardia.[6] Supraventricular tachycardia may be treated by reassurance, drugs, or (in selected cases) radiofrequency ablation. A QRS duration of more

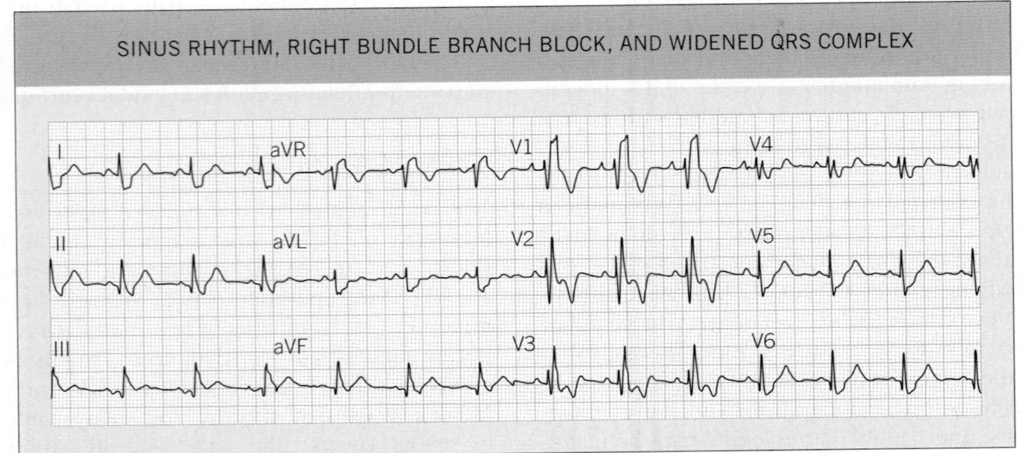

Figure 124.1 An electrocardiogram showing sinus rhythm, right bundle branch block, and widened QRS complex of more than 180 ms identifying an individual at high risk of late complications.[9]

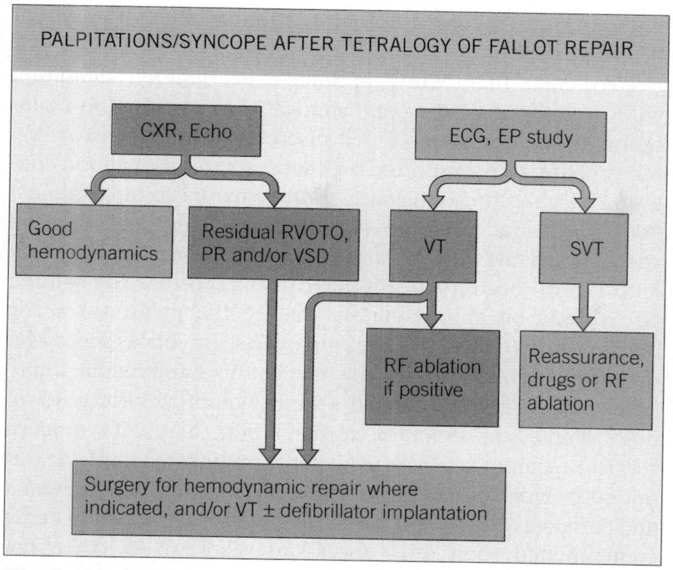

PALPITATIONS/SYNCOPE AFTER TETRALOGY OF FALLOT REPAIR

CXR, Echo

ECG, EP study

Good hemodynamics

Residual RVOTO, PR and/or VSD

VT

SVT

RF ablation if positive

Reassurance, drugs or RF ablation

Surgery for hemodynamic repair where indicated, and/or VT ± defibrillator implantation

Figure 124.2 Diagnostic work-up for arrhythmia after repair of tetralogy of Fallot. The coexistence of hemodynamic and electrical lesions may be particularly dangerous. CXR, chest radiography; ECG, electrocardiography; Echo, echocardiography; EP, electrophysiology; PR, pulmonic regurgitation; RF, radiofrequency; RVOTO, right ventricular outflow tract obstruction; SVT, supraventricular tachycardia: VSD, ventricular septal defect; VT, ventricular tachycardia.

than 180 ms on a resting electrocardiogram is an adverse prognostic feature and is useful for identification of high-risk individuals.[9] Catheter-based and surgical ablation of ventricular tachycardia may often be unsuccessful because of complex anatomy or scarring, in which case implantable defibrillator therapy may be warranted.

The timing of pulmonary valve replacement for pulmonary regurgitation with progressive RV dilatation is a difficult area. Precise measurement of RV dimensions is much less well established than the well-validated techniques for left ventricular measurement, in part related to the more complex geometry of the right ventricle. Options for assessing progressive RV dilatation on echocardiography include "eyeball" assessment, measurement of maximal end-diastolic dimensions on parasternal or apical views, and planimetry of RV area on apical views. Cardiac magnetic resonance has provided a new imaging option for the more accurate quantification of RV volumes in this setting, and recent data suggest that a cutoff value of 160 mL/m^2 most likely allows normalization of RV volumes after pulmonary valve replacement.[10]

In the setting of severe pulmonary regurgitation with progressive RV dilatation, surgical replacement of the pulmonary valve should be considered when symptoms occur or when dilatation is accompanied by progressive systolic dysfunction.[11]

RECURRENT COARCTATION OF THE AORTA

DEFINITION OF PROBLEM

In coarctation of the aorta, there is a localized aortic stenosis in the region of the arterial duct, usually just distal to the origin of the left subclavian artery. Repair can be performed by resection and end-to-end anastomosis, by use of the left subclavian artery to create a "flap" repair, or by patch aortoplasty. Late complications include hypertension with or without discrete recoarctation and localized aneurysm formation at the site of earlier repair (particularly after patch aortoplasty). Survivors of coarctation repair also represent a large proportion of adults with congenital heart disease.

TYPICAL CASE

Jane presented as a neonate with heart failure and was diagnosed by echocardiography as having a bicuspid aortic valve (with no stenosis or regurgitation) and a discrete coarctation of the aorta with a small persistent arterial duct. On day 7 of life, the duct was closed and the coarctation resected through a left thoracotomy. An end-to-end anastomosis was performed. Jane was then well for many years.

At a regular 2-yearly review at the age of 21 years, she remained asymptomatic and well. Jane had recently been married and was using a low-dose combined estrogen-progestogen contraceptive pill. She expressed a desire to become pregnant soon.

On examination, resting blood pressure was 160/100 mm Hg in the right arm, and mild radiofemoral pulse delay was noted. There was a soft systolic murmur at the base of the heart and a short early diastolic murmur. A more harsh and louder systolic murmur was heard in the back. Chest radiography and electrocardiography were within normal limits. Two-dimensional echocardiography showed borderline left ventricular hypertrophy, good left ventricular contractility, bicuspid aortic valve with mild stenosis (V_{max} = 2.5 m/s) and mild regurgitation, and a discrete area of recoarctation in the descending thoracic aorta. Doppler interrogation of the descending aorta revealed V_{max} of almost 4 m/s with continuous flow throughout diastole; the flow velocity at end-diastole was 0.5 m/s (Fig. 124.3). Magnetic resonance imaging confirmed discrete recoarctation with no aneurysm formation.

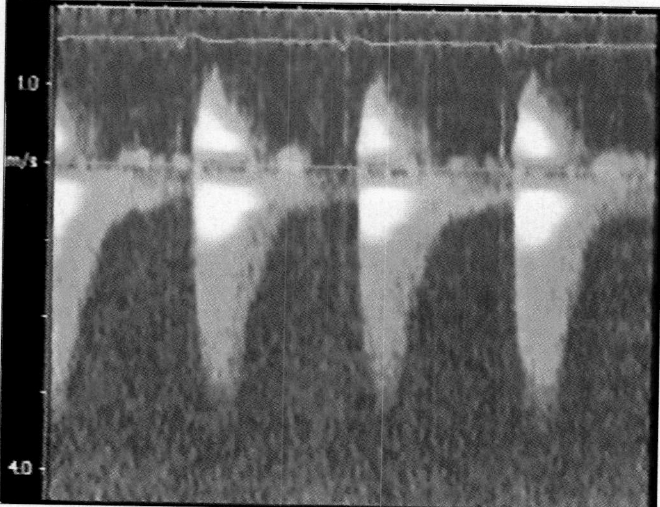

Figure 124.3 Doppler signal from the descending aorta in a case of recoarctation. The peak systolic velocity is 3.7 m/s, and the end-diastolic velocity is 0.5 m/s.

DIFFERENTIAL DIAGNOSIS

In this asymptomatic young woman, the diagnosis of hypertension with significant recoarctation is straightforward. In many survivors of "successful" early repair, however, the diagnosis is less clear. Resting blood pressure may be quite normal, with severe hypertension becoming apparent only during formal exercise testing.[12] This should be regularly checked during follow-up visits, as latent hypertension may contribute to the excess premature cardiovascular event rates in survivors of coarctation repair,[13] and abnormally increased blood pressure at rest or on exercise should be treated aggressively. This involves diagnosis and treatment of any recurrent aortic obstruction or pharmacologic antihypertensive therapy.

Diagnosis of recurrent coarctation or aneurysm formation by echocardiography may be difficult. Accelerated systolic flow (even up to 3 to 4 m/s) may be observed in the absence of discrete stenosis; the persistence of forward flow throughout diastole is much more specific for recoarctation, particularly if end-diastolic flow is greater than 0.5 m/s.[14] Late aneurysm formation is a common and occasionally fatal complication after patch aortoplasty.[15] This may not be seen well on echocardiography, and plain chest radiography is useful for screening of this complication. Magnetic resonance imaging has markedly improved the ability to diagnose recoarctation or aneurysm formation and is now the diagnostic procedure of choice in patients in whom there is clinical suspicion of complications at the site of previous repair (Fig. 124.4).

In sexually active women requiring radiologic investigations, pregnancy testing should precede the imaging studies. In Jane's case, the test result was negative.

TREATMENT OPTIONS

Relief of recoarctation is clearly indicated in this patient as there is hypertension at rest, discrete restenosis, and a desire to become pregnant (pregnancy would be poorly tolerated in the presence of aortic coarctation). The aortic valve abnormality is mild and requires expectant management only; the valve regurgitation may improve after relief of the recoarctation.

Two main therapeutic options exist: balloon dilatation with or without stenting and surgical re-repair. Balloon dilatation is mainly suitable for discrete areas of narrowing. Many centers have reported high success rates for balloon dilatation with stenting of recoarctation in such cases (up to almost 80%) with low incidence of morbidity,[16] although femoral vascular and late false aneurysm formation is a potential problem.[17] Periprocedural deaths have been reported. The balloon size should be approximately that of the measured aortic diameter just proximal to the narrowed segment. As successful dilatation involves tearing the aortic intima and media, many other centers have preferred a surgical approach for relief of both simple and complex recoarctation, and with modern surgical techniques, there is a very low incidence of serious operative morbidity in these cases (such as spinal cord ischemia and paraplegia).[18] In Jane's case, in which pregnancy was being contemplated soon after successful relief of recoarctation, a surgical approach was preferred. This proceeded without complications.

The next stage in the management of this patient was appropriate counseling for and timing of pregnancy. Four months after reoperation, Jane's resting blood pressure was 115/85 mm Hg in the right arm, increasing to 190/105 mm Hg on maximal exercise (14 METs on a Bruce treadmill test, normal for age and sex). Pregnancy was therefore considered safe.

There are few data on the incidence of preeclampsia (hypertensive disease of pregnancy) in women after coarctation repair, but clearly, appropriate blood pressure control is a major issue in this situation. Contraception in adults with congenital heart disease is also a relatively poorly studied area. The low-dose combined oral contraceptive pill is regarded as safe except in the presence of pulmonary vascular disease or systemic hypertension.[19] In these situations, progesterone-only pills are safe (although not 100% effective). Depot progesterone injections may also be considered. Intrauterine devices are usually discouraged because of the

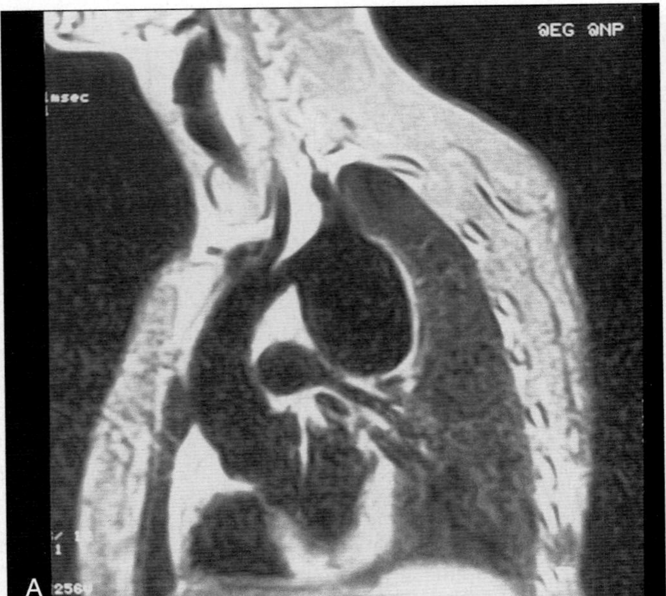

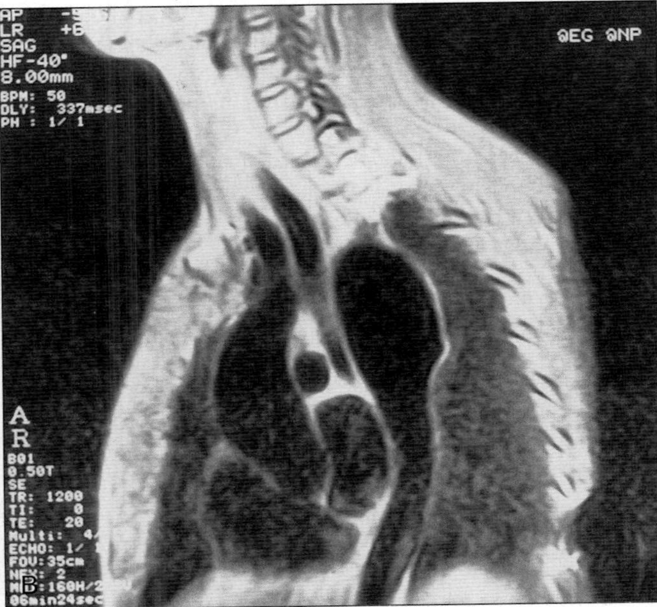

Figure 124.4 Magnetic resonance scan of the aorta showing a discrete aneurysm at the site of previous coarctation repair.

Defect in Parent	Affected Births/Live Births: Of Fathers	Affected Births/Live Births: Of Mothers	Total Risk
Tetralogy of Fallot	2/124 (1.6%)	6/132 (4.5%)	3.1%
AVSD	1/13 (7.7%)	3/38 (7.9%)	7.8%
APVC	0/10	1/17 (5.9%)	3.7%
Abnormal connections	1/22 (4.5%)	1/17 (5.8%)	5.1%
All heart defects	4/183 (2.2%)	12/210 (5.7%)	4.1%

RECURRENCE RISKS OF CONGENITAL HEART DISEASE AMONG OFFSPRING OF AFFECTED PARENTS

APVC, anomalous pulmonary venous congestion; AVSD, atrioventricular septal defect.

Modified from Burn J, Brennan P, Little J, et al. Recurrence risks in offspring of adults with major heart defects: results from first cohort of British collaborative study. Lancet 1998;351:311-316.© The Lancet Ltd., 1998.

Table 124.2 Recurrence risks of congenital heart disease among offspring of affected parents.

theoretical risk of endocarditis, and female barrier methods have high failure rates. Male barrier methods (condoms) are an effective and safe alternative if compliance can be maintained. In Eisenmenger's syndrome, in which pregnancy carries a maternal mortality of up to 50%,[20] tubal ligation should be considered.

Genetic counseling for recurrence risks of congenital heart disease should be discussed in general terms with adult survivors from the age of about 16 years and more specifically when pregnancy is being planned. The recurrence rates in offspring vary according to the index lesion and the literature consulted. Rarely, exact estimates of risk can be given when the condition is an autosomal dominant one (e.g., Holt-Oram or Noonan's syndrome). The recent recognition of a microdeletion in chromosome 22q11 as an etiologic factor in certain conotruncal defects (e.g., truncus arteriosus, tetralogy of Fallot) means that this deletion should be specifically sought in cases of clinical suspicion.[21]

In other lesions, the risk of recurrent congenital heart disease is greater if the mother rather than the father has the condition. Thus, recurrence rates appear to be approximately 2% to 5% for affected fathers and 3% to 10% for mothers (Table 124.2).[22,23] A particularly high recurrence rate has been noted for obstructive left-sided heart lesions, such as subaortic stenosis, bicuspid aortic valve, and coarctation of the aorta.[23] These issues should be discussed frankly with both prospective parents, and the role of fetal cardiac ultrasound examination at 18 to 20 weeks of gestation to screen for congenital heart disease should also be explained.

SUMMARY

Coarctation of the aorta occurs in approximately 5 in 10,000 live births and is usually treated successfully in childhood. The late risk of recoarctation is significant; after neonatal repair, it may occur in up to 30% of cases by the age 4 of years.[17] Late aneurysm formation complicates up to 25% of cases of patch aortoplasty and may even cause sudden death.[15] Hypertension is another common sequela, even in the presence of anatomically successful repair,[12] implicating residual functional abnormalities in the precoarctation vasculature.[24] As these complications are all treatable, vigilant follow-up of survivors of coarctation repair is especially important, even if these individuals are asymptomatic and well. The common concurrence of other left-sided heart obstructive lesions, especially bicuspid aortic valve (which occurs in approximately 50% to 70% of cases of coarctation), also suggests the importance of regular assessment.

Advice concerning sexuality, contraception, pregnancy, and genetic counseling is another important aspect of the management of young women and men with congenital heart disease and requires adequate time, a sensitive ear, and accurate knowledge of the correct answers. Such discussions should begin soon after puberty, as these issues often provoke anxiety in affected adolescents, even many years before they may contemplate family planning. In general, individuals with left-to-right shunts and regurgitant lesions tolerate pregnancy well, whereas those with right-to-left shunts, pulmonary vascular disease, or stenotic lesions may fare poorly.[25] Reparable conditions should be treated before pregnancy unless they are mild, and involvement of an experienced obstetrician (part of the adult congenital heart disease "team") is usually invaluable.

PALPITATIONS AFTER A FONTAN PROCEDURE

DEFINITION OF PROBLEM

The Fontan operation is a palliative one, designed for children and adults with only one effectively functioning ventricle. Initially designed for children with tricuspid atresia, it is now considered in almost all forms of "single-ventricle" hearts in which pulmonary artery size is reasonable, pulmonary resistance is low, and there is no important atrioventricular (AV) valve dysfunction but good ventricular function without outflow obstruction. The principle of the operation is connection of all the systemic venous drainage to the pulmonary arteries (usually without a subpulmonary ventricle in the circuit). The pulmonary vasculature then fills "passively," and the ventricle supplies the systemic circuit. In the original Fontan operation, the right atrium was connected directly to the pulmonary artery. Since then, a wide variety of surgical techniques have been described to allow progressively more complex congenital anomalies to be considered for this procedure.[26] Other modifications of the Fontan procedure have been designed to lessen the risk of arrhythmia and thromboembolism, two major complications of the late postoperative course.[27]

Survivors of Fontan-type operations may be well, although many complain of decreased exercise capacity or palpitations.[28] Most (but by no means all) such patients are usually managed at specialized adult congenital heart disease clinics.

TYPICAL CASE

Thomas was noted to be cyanosed on day 1 of life, after a full-term normal vaginal delivery. Early echocardiography and cardiac catheterization established the diagnosis of

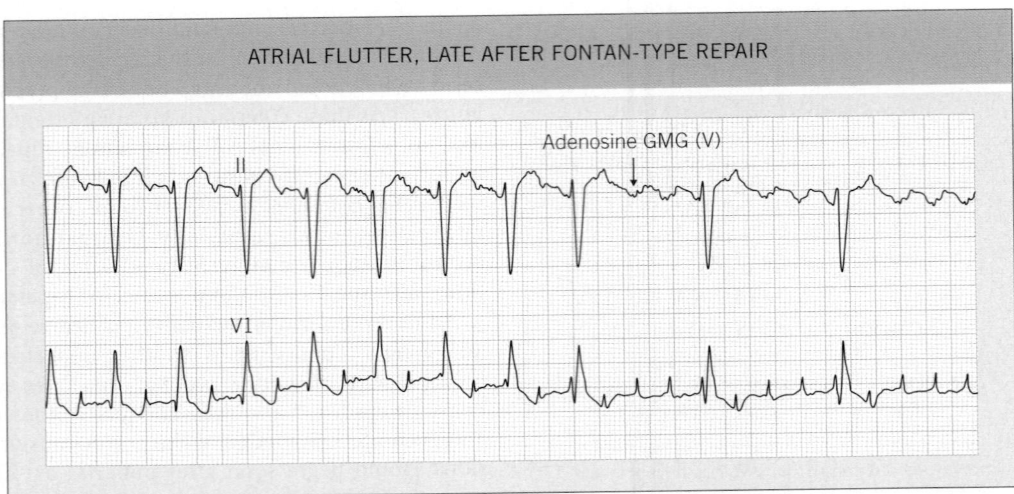

Figure 124.5 A two-lead electrocardiographic rhythm strip showing atrial flutter, late after Fontan-type repair. The ventricular rate is approximately 120 beats per minute. The flutter waves are best seen in lead V_1 on the right-hand side of the figure after the administration of adenosine to slow atrioventricular conduction temporarily.

tricuspid atresia, large atrial septal defect (ASD), large VSD, small right ventricle ("subaortic chamber"), and transposition of the great arteries. On day 3, a left Blalock-Taussig shunt operation was performed. Increasing cyanosis at the age of 2 years necessitated a right modified Blalock-Taussig shunt. At the age of 5 years, cardiac catheterization revealed upper-normal size of the pulmonary arteries, except for absent left upper lobe pulmonary artery, and low pressures and resistances in the pulmonary circuit. The left AV valve was competent, the VSD and subaortic area were nonrestrictive, and the ventricular contractility was good. Thereafter, Thomas had definitive palliation with an atriopulmonary connection (Fontan repair) with closure of the arterial shunts. Postoperatively, there was ascites, pleural effusions bilaterally, and low output for the first 10 days; however, these conditions resolved with medical management. Thomas was then well for many years and even participated in some low-intensity school sports. Serial echocardiography revealed mild ventricular contractile dysfunction, upper-normal atrial sizes, and competent left AV valve. He was maintained with low-dose aspirin and no other medical treatment. At the age of 16 years, however, Thomas started to complain of fast, regular palpitations, coming on at any time. Soon after, he presented to the emergency department at his local hospital, complaining of a prolonged palpitation that did not resolve spontaneously and some lightheadedness. His presenting electrocardiogram is shown in Figure 124.5.

DIFFERENTIAL DIAGNOSIS

The electrocardiogram clearly shows a narrow-complex tachycardia with a ventricular rate of approximately 120 beats per minute. Atrial flutter waves are also visible at a rate of approximately 240 beats per minute, suggesting the presence of 2:1 AV block.

Supraventricular arrhythmias are relatively common late after Fontan-type surgery, complicating up to 40% of cases.[29] These arrhythmias are associated with a 2.8% incidence of sudden death[30] and therefore require aggressive investigation and treatment. The underlying substrate is most commonly atrial flutter, although ectopic atrial tachycardia, junctional tachycardia, and accessory pathway–related AV re-entry are all diagnostic possibilities. Ventricular tachycardia is relatively rare in this setting and poorly tolerated when present. If flutter waves are not apparent on the surface electrocardiogram, detailed electrophysiologic study may be required to establish the diagnosis. The pathogenesis of supraventricular tachycardia after Fontan repair may relate to progressive atrial dilatation or to re-entry circuits around previous atriotomy sites. Preliminary evidence now suggests that a total cavopulmonary connection might be associated with significantly less late supraventricular tachycardia than are atriopulmonary connections because of exclusion of the atrium from the hemodynamic circuit.[31]

In general, presentation with electrophysiologic abnormalities should prompt a rigorous search for underlying hemodynamic problems in adults with repaired congenital heart disease. If residual structural lesions exist, these may require treatment to improve exercise tolerance, to minimize the abnormal loading conditions that might worsen chamber dilatation and thereby dysrhythmia, and to minimize the risk of sudden cardiac death. In this case, transthoracic and transesophageal echocardiography demonstrated good hemodynamics with upper-normal atrial sizes, no residual ASD, unobstructed atriopulmonary anastomosis, normal AV valve function, and reasonable ventricular contractility.

TREATMENT OPTIONS

As with supraventricular tachycardia in general, the therapeutic options include reassurance with a conservative approach, antiarrhythmic drugs, and consideration of specific electrical therapies such as antitachycardia pacing and radiofrequency ablation. Reassurance is appropriate only when the tachyarrhythmia is infrequent, not associated with dyspnea or dizziness and syncope, and not associated with an important underlying hemodynamic lesion. Complicating this issue in patients with atrial flutter after a Fontan procedure are the frequent findings of coexisting sinus node dysfunction in addition to several flutter pathways.[32]

Antiarrhythmic drugs are frequently ineffective in treating supraventricular tachycardia associated with repaired congenital heart disease.[32] This may be related to excessive atrial wall thickness or scarring at the re-entry sites. These agents also have the potential to depress ventricular function (which might be particularly deleterious in this setting), to exacerbate any sinus node dysfunction and thereby predispose to bradyarrhythmia, or to be proarrhythmic. Furthermore, the high prevalence of serious adverse effects with the long-term use of amiodarone[33] sometimes precludes the use of this otherwise effective agent in adolescents and young adults.

Successful catheter-based radiofrequency ablation of electrophysiologically abnormal foci or circuits may be achieved in these patients[34]; however, such procedures are not always successful. The advent of sophisticated three-dimensional mapping systems and enhanced lesion creation modalities, however, have recently improved success rates in adult congenital heart disease patients.[35]

Complicating features include distorted electrophysiologic anatomy as a result of the underlying lesion or the surgical repair technique and the frequent finding of dilated atrial chambers with or without marked hypertrophy of the chamber walls. Multiple abnormal pathways are also common.

In the case of Thomas, medical treatment with digoxin and sotalol did not reduce the frequency of episodes. At formal electrophysiologic study, three separate flutter circuits, all including the previous atriotomy site, were identified, and catheter ablation was not successful. Therefore, an antitachycardia pacing device was implanted, with marked improvement but not complete suppression of the episodes of palpitation.

SUMMARY

Palpitations are relatively common after repair of complex congenital heart disease, particularly when extensive atrial surgery has been undertaken or atrial distention is a consequence of the underlying or postsurgical anatomy.[32,36] The most common cause is supraventricular tachycardia caused by atrial flutter, although ectopic atrial tachycardia and all other forms of re-entry dysrhythmia need to be considered. Formal electrophysiologic study is often invaluable in characterizing the cardiac conduction intervals, in defining the abnormal pathways and thereby assisting with therapeutic choices, and in offering the possibility of ablative therapies. The advent of increasingly sophisticated mapping and ablating catheters, such as basket devices, may improve the success rate of ablation in this setting.

HEADACHES AND ABDOMINAL PAIN IN A CYANOSED YOUNG WOMAN WITH INOPERABLE PULMONARY ATRESIA

DEFINITION OF PROBLEM

Pulmonary atresia with VSD is the "extreme" form of tetralogy of Fallot in which the RV outflow is not connected to the pulmonary arteries (rather than just RV outflow tract narrowing). In its least severe form, only the pulmonary valve is atretic; at the other extreme, the RV infundibulum, pulmonary valve, and main or peripheral pulmonary arteries may actually be absent. In this case, the pulmonary blood supply usually originates from major aortopulmonary collateral arteries, which may be tortuous and stenosed or large and unobstructed. Management of this group of patients is particularly complex.

Cyanosis (arterial oxygen desaturation, usually <85%, with concomitant blue discoloration centrally and peripherally) is a common finding in this lesion when it is unrepaired or palliated. Erythrocytosis usually results, which in turn may be complicated by hyperviscosity symptoms. Cyanosis complicating adult congenital heart disease is becoming increasingly rare now, with improved surgical options in childhood, and is usually found complicating Eisenmenger's syndrome, systemic "mixing" of venous return (such as with palliated single-ventricle type hearts), and low pulmonary blood flow. These patients provide challenges related to both the management of the underlying condition and the cyanosis or erythrocytosis.

TYPICAL CASE

Anne presented with heart failure in 1975 as a cyanosed neonate. Early cardiac catheterization revealed pulmonary atresia, VSD, absent central pulmonary arteries, and several large, unobstructed aortopulmonary collaterals to the right and left lungs. At that stage, the condition was believed to be inoperable, and medical treatment for heart failure was prescribed. Despite some initial failure to thrive and frequent childhood respiratory infections, Anne enjoyed reasonable health in late childhood. A moderate scoliosis was noted in adolescence but not specifically treated. Cystic acne was managed by standard topical therapies. Tubal ligation was undertaken at the age of 21 years. Cardiac follow-up was initially uncomplicated; however, at the age of 28 years (after 3 years without specialist review), Anne presented with increasing tiredness, headaches, occasional dizziness, and episodic right upper quadrant abdominal discomfort. Full blood count revealed a hemoglobin concentration of 26 g/dL, a platelet count of 90,000, and a normal white blood cell count. Transcutaneous oxygen saturation was 78%.

DIFFERENTIAL DIAGNOSIS

There are several diagnostic aspects in this case: the underlying cardiac anatomy, the cause of the headaches and tiredness, and the etiology of the abdominal pain.

In pulmonary atresia with VSD and aortopulmonary collaterals, cyanosis may be caused by inadequate pulmonary flow (when the collaterals are stenosed or insufficient) or pulmonary hypertension (when the collaterals are unobstructed and cause irreversible pulmonary vascular disease). The former problem is treatable by surgical augmentation of pulmonary flow, whereas the latter is inoperable (except by heart-lung transplantation). In Anne's case, magnetic resonance imaging confirmed large, apparently unobstructed aortopulmonary collaterals bilaterally (Fig. 124.6). Magnetic resonance imaging has proved useful in delineating complex congenital heart disease anatomy, particularly of

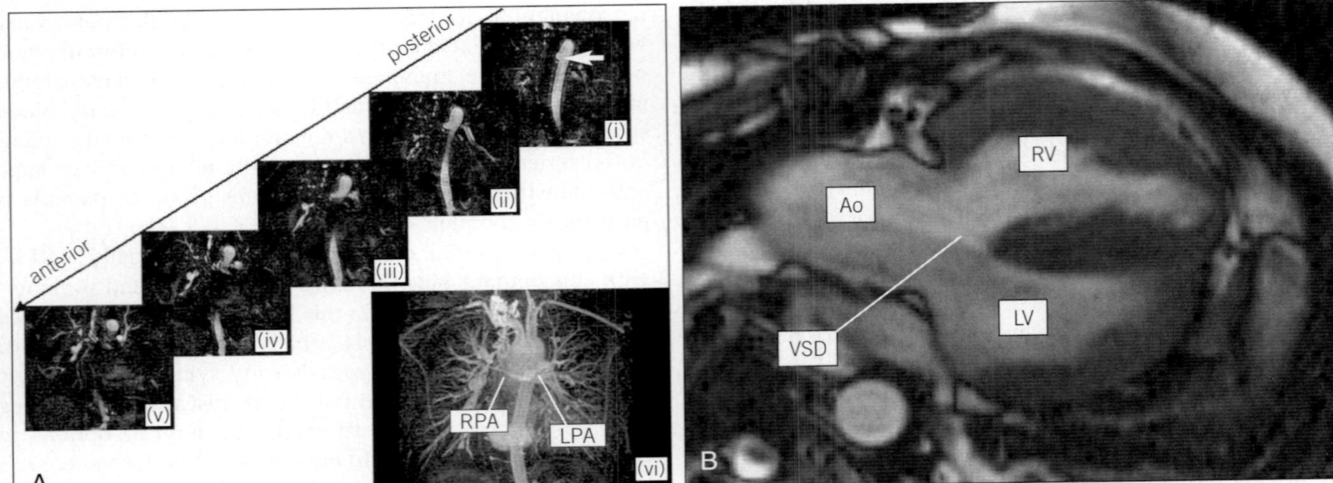

Figure 124.6 Magnetic resonance imaging in a patient with pulmonary atresia with major aortopulmonary collaterals. **A,** Contrast-enhanced magnetic resonance angiography. Selected source images in a coronal plane (i to v) and maximum intensity projection in the anteroposterior view (vi). The pulmonary trunk is atretic throughout its length. It branches into a hypoplastic right pulmonary artery (RPA) and a relatively larger left pulmonary artery (LPA) with a discrete narrowing near the origin. Note a large collateral to the right pulmonary artery arising from the anterior aspect of the descending aorta (i-v, *arrow*), numerous collaterals from the right subclavian artery to the right upper lung (vi), and a small collateral from the left subclavian artery to the left pulmonary artery. (Courtesy of Drs. Raad Mohiaddin and Jane McCrohon, Cardiovascular Magnetic Resonance Unit, Royal Brompton Hospital, London.) **B,** True fast imaging with steady-state precession (true FISP) cardiac image in a tilted transverse plane acquired in the same patient. There is an overriding aorta (Ao) and a subaortic ventricular septal defect (VSD). LV, left ventricle; RV, right ventricle. (Courtesy of Drs. Raad Mohiaddin and Jane McCrohon, Cardiovascular Magnetic Resonance Unit, Royal Brompton Hospital, London.)

extracardiac structures, for which echocardiography is often unhelpful.[37] These findings were confirmed at cardiac catheterization, with systemic pressures measured in both lungs. The most likely cause of tiredness and headache here is erythrocytosis with hyperviscosity. Other causes, particularly any psychosocial stresses, should be specifically sought and managed when possible. Dehydration must be excluded. Detailed iron studies are helpful, particularly if cyanotic patients have previously been venesected, as resulting iron deficiency with microcytosis may actually worsen hyperviscosity symptoms (as microcytic red cells are less deformable).[38] In Anne's case, the hematocrit was 69%, red cell mass and total blood volume were significantly increased, and results of iron studies were within normal limits, with no evidence of hypochromia or microcytosis.

As in other young adults, the differential diagnosis of abdominal pain is wide. Careful history and physical examination often reveal a likely cause, and in Anne's case, her pain was in the right upper quadrant and worse after fatty meals. Cholelithiasis is a common finding in cyanotic patients with high red cell turnover,[39] and abdominal ultrasound examination revealed several small gallstones. Other diagnostic possibilities include peptic ulcer disease, nonulcer dyspepsia, and pancreatitis, all of which can be investigated by standard blood test, imaging, or endoscopic means.

TREATMENT OPTIONS

Unfortunately, the underlying cardiac lesion in pulmonary atresia, VSD and absent central pulmonary vessels, complicated by pulmonary hypertension, is not operable other than by organ transplantation. Symptom relief, including treatment of complications such as hyperviscosity, cholelithiasis, gout, and bleeding, all relatively common with prolonged cyanosis, is the cornerstone of therapy. Fluid intake should be encouraged during hot months. Early assessment by a transplantation unit, particularly when dyspnea, fatigue, or hemoptysis occurs, is worthwhile in otherwise suitable candidates. Tubal ligation should be considered in women owing to the extremely high risk of pregnancy for both mother and fetus. Venesection (or phlebotomy) is actually only rarely required in adults with cyanotic congenital heart disease. Most such adults develop "compensated" erythrocytosis with stable hematocrit at about 65% and have few symptoms referable to hyperviscosity. Venesection in such individuals paradoxically often increases symptoms by creating iron deficiency in the setting of recurrent erythrocytosis.[38] We recommend venesection only in those with important hyperviscosity symptoms (fatigue, headache, dizziness, visual blurring) in whom dehydration has been excluded. In these patients, if the hematocrit is greater than 65%, judicious venesection with crystalloid volume replacement may deserve a therapeutic trial. Phlebotomy of 400 to 500 mL during 1 hour followed by isotonic saline replacement is a reasonable approach. Repeated venesections are performed for recurrent symptoms, as long as iron deficiency has been excluded or treated.

Cholelithiasis may be managed conservatively or by operation. If suitable, laparoscopic cholecystectomy may minimize risk. The major issues in noncardiac surgery for adults with congenital heart disease relate to anesthesia and endocarditis prophylaxis. In addition, cyanotic individuals usually have a mild hemostatic defect,[40] which may lead to severe surgical bleeding. Aspirin should therefore be avoided in these patients, in addition to nonsteroidal anti-inflammatory agents.

Ideally, a cardiac anesthetist should be involved, even in noncardiac surgery, for adults with cyanotic congenital heart disease. Careful volume replacement, avoidance of myocardial depressant agents, and particular attention to exclude air bubbles are especially important. When pulmonary hypertension coexists, systemic hypotension is particularly dangerous. Venesection may improve hemostasis and should be considered before surgery. Adequate blood product replacement therapy should be easily available.

SUMMARY

Some complex lesions of congenital heart disease result in persistent cyanosis in adults if lesions causing mixing, low pulmonary flow, or pulmonary hypertension with right-to-left shunting have not been repaired in childhood. This group of patients face a number of specific problems, including decreased exercise performance, hyperviscosity, and the risk of complications such as gout, acne, scoliosis, and cholelithiasis. A mild bleeding tendency is also common.

When the underlying cardiac lesion can be palliated or repaired, this is clearly the treatment of choice. When this is not possible, transplantation is a therapeutic option in some cases.[41] Aspirin and dehydration should be avoided and specific symptoms treated conventionally. Venesection should be undertaken sparingly, only in those with clear symptoms related to hyperviscosity and in whom dehydration and iron deficiency have been excluded. In general, however, the outlook for these individuals is poor, with frequent morbidity and often premature mortality.

A HEALTHY YOUNG MAN WITH LEFT ATRIOVENTRICULAR VALVE REGURGITATION AFTER PRIMUM ATRIAL SEPTAL DEFECT REPAIR

DEFINITION OF PROBLEM

Primum ASD is part of the spectrum of endocardial cushion defects or AV canal defects (see Chapter 111). There is a defect in the lowest portion of the atrial septum and a "common valve" arrangement of the normally separated tricuspid and mitral AV valves. This results in an apparent "cleft" in the medial part of the left-sided AV valve. Regurgitation of this valve is a common postoperative complication of AV canal defect repair, including closure of "simple" primum ASD.[42]

TYPICAL CASE

Mark first presented to a cardiologist at the age of 18 years, after a murmur was heard at a medical check before Army enrollment. He had been extremely well and fit at this time, excelling at football and tennis during high school. Investigations revealed sinus rhythm, a primum ASD with 3:1 left-to-right shunt, mild left AV valve regurgitation, right-sided heart volume overload, and normal pulmonary pressures. There was no VSD. ASD closure with a Dacron patch was undertaken by a specialist congenital heart surgeon, and the left AV valve was not thought to require repair during the procedure. Mild to moderate regurgitation of this valve was noted postoperatively, and recovery was uncomplicated. Mark returned to full-time manual work and was lost to follow-up for 6 years.

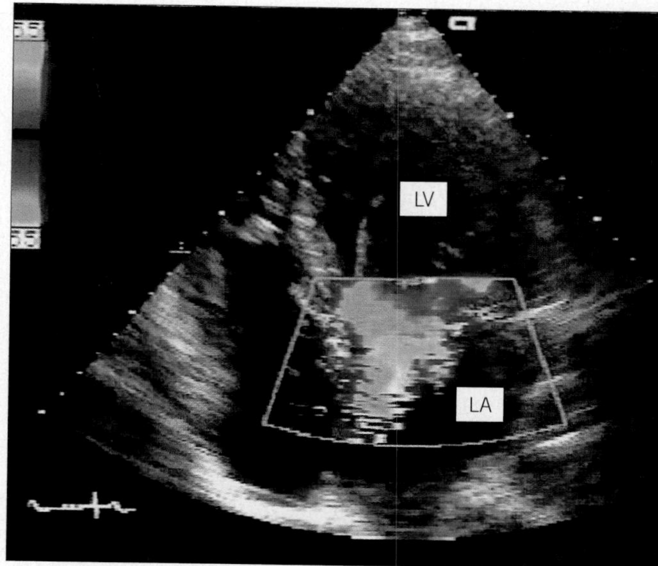

Figure 124.7 Transthoracic echocardiographic image showing severe left AV valve regurgitation after repair of primum atrial septal defect. LA, left atrium; LV, left ventricle.

At the age of 24 years, Mark presented for routine review before planned dental surgery for "wisdom" teeth. He was still feeling well and playing competitive football. Examination revealed atrial fibrillation, but a controlled ventricular rate and transthoracic echocardiography suggested at least moderate to severe left AV valve regurgitation (Fig. 124.7), severely dilated left atrium, and moderate left ventricular enlargement with good left ventricular contractile function. Transesophageal echocardiography confirmed these findings and excluded residual ASD and thrombus in the left atrial appendage.

DIFFERENTIAL DIAGNOSIS

Patients with ostium primum ASD occasionally remain asymptomatic until adult life. Coexisting abnormalities of the left AV valve are often troublesome and may require either repair or replacement of the valve if it is severely regurgitant. It is well recognized that left AV valve regurgitation may be progressive in this condition, even in the case of successful surgical closure of the ASD.[42]

In this case, the diagnosis appears straightforward. Progressive incompetence of the abnormal left AV valve may occur as part of the "natural history" and leads to atrial distention and eventually fibrillation. Endocarditis needs to be considered as another possible cause of worsening valve disease, and other contributing causes such as systemic hypertension should be excluded.

TREATMENT OPTIONS

The usual approaches to atrial fibrillation in the setting of mitral regurgitation should be considered: ventricular rate control, anticoagulation, and medical or electrical cardioversion. In Mark's case, his ventricular rate was well controlled at presentation, and 4 weeks of therapy with warfarin and sotalol was prescribed, followed by attempted electrical cardioversion, which was unsuccessful.

There are few data on the timing of left AV valve surgery in this situation. Onset of symptoms and objective evidence of progressive left ventricular dilatation are indications for operative intervention, when valve repair (with suturing of the cleft) or replacement may be necessary. This should be undertaken by an experienced congenital heart surgeon as the anatomy differs markedly from that in other cases of mitral valve disease.

In an individual who remains relatively well and in whom left ventricular dimensions are stable, expectant management may be appropriate. Angiotensin-converting enzyme inhibition should be strongly considered. Although no specific data exist in the setting of AV defects, afterload reduction would be expected to reduce the regurgitant fraction in such patients, with consequent clinical benefit.

Endocarditis prophylaxis must also be emphasized in this young man presenting before dental surgery. This issue is especially important in young adults with congenital heart disease, in whom unusual sources of bacteremia should be remembered. Ear and body piercing and tattooing, in addition to dental procedures, are potential sources of infection. Alpha streptococci and staphylococci are the two most frequent etiologic agents in adults with congenital heart disease.[43] Prevention of endocarditis relies on good daily oral hygiene, meticulous skin care (particularly in those with acne), and appropriate chemoprophylaxis. The last of these requires direct medical intervention and advice; a card to be kept in the purse or wallet of individuals at risk should be considered.

The other issue of great importance to this young man concerned recommendations about sports and exercise. In general, regurgitant valvular lesions do not limit exercise capacity to the same extent as stenotic lesions do.[44] Competitive sports are really precluded only in those with severe left-sided heart obstruction or exercise-induced arrhythmias. Recreational exercise should be actively encouraged, within the tolerance of each individual (many adults with congenital heart disease have been encouraged by family members not to participate in sports as children). Contact sports are contraindicated in those requiring anticoagulation, but in Mark's case, he was able to continue a regular exercise regimen based on cycling and swimming.

SUMMARY

Although the outlook after repair of "isolated" ostium primum ASD is usually very good,[45] surveillance for residual AV valve regurgitation is important. This case highlights several of the reasons for regular routine follow-up of even apparently well young adults with congenital heart disease: screening for residual hemodynamic lesions and intervention before complications such as atrial fibrillation arise, education and advice concerning endocarditis prophylaxis, and appropriate recommendations concerning sports and exercise.

chapter 125

Special Problems in Adult Congenital Heart Disease

a. Management of Cyanotic Heart Disease

Craig Broberg

DEFINITION OF PROBLEM

When a cyanotic individual is encountered, the reaction of many is surprise and disbelief that such a patient is still living well into adult life. Because most children today undergo palliative surgery to prevent cyanosis, one may tend to believe that cyanotic heart disease is of historical interest only. However, this is not the case. There are many surviving cyanotic individuals still carrying on decade after decade. Although they are at high risk for complications and premature death, many have adapted to their chronic cyanosis to do well and have productive lives. Therefore, the conscientious cardiologist will be wary of some of the pitfalls of cyanotic heart disease to avoid mistakes in management that can have dire consequences. There are a number of long-term considerations and complications to consider (Table 125A.1). Ideally, specialists in congenital heart disease should observe all such patients.

Cyanotic heart disease can be present in any form of heart disease wherein mixing of venous and arterial blood can occur. The degree of cyanosis depends mostly on the amount of pulmonary blood flow, which is governed by the relative resistance of flow to the pulmonary versus the systemic circulation. If there is coexistent pulmonary vascular disease, the patient has Eisenmenger's syndrome, defined as reversed or bidirectional shunting in the setting of increased pulmonary vascular resistance.

CASE

A 38-year-old man referred himself to an adult congenital heart disease clinic that he identified on the Internet. At the time of his birth, the patient was cyanotic. Early studies showed a large ventricular septal defect. He was taken to the operating room with plans for closure but was found to have a large defect that could not be repaired. Although cyanotic, the patient remained relatively asymptomatic throughout the remainder of his childhood and did not feel limited in his exertional capacity. He went to college and maintained an active career. He married and had three children.

Gradually, the patient grew more tired and fatigued. He complained of frequent headaches. His hematocrit was elevated, and so a program of regular phlebotomy had been initiated. A unit of blood was removed several times a year either because the hematocrit was above 65% or because of headache. He usually felt worse after such sessions. On one occasion, he passed out after phlebotomy and had to be fluid resuscitated because of severe hypotension.

Despite regular phlebotomy, symptoms, including dyspnea, lassitude, joint aches, right upper quadrant pain, and chest pain, worsened over time. Work-up for these various complaints included nuclear scans, computed tomographic scans, and hepatobiliary iminodiacetic acid scans, all of which were normal. Providers started him on chronic narcotics. He began to feel unable to carry on working full time. He therefore sought additional specialist treatment.

On physical examination, his blood pressure was 124/76 mm Hg; his pulse was 92 bpm. His resting oxygen saturation was 76% on room air. He was a thin, cyanotic man. His jugular venous pulse was normal. His lungs were clear in all fields. His pulse was regular, he had no murmur, and the second heart sound was loud. His peripheral pulses were all normal. His upper and lower extremities were deeply cyanotic, and there was significant clubbing of all his digits. There was no peripheral edema.

Laboratory values included a hemoglobin concentration of 16 g/dL, a hematocrit of 59%, a mean corpuscular volume of 84 fL, and a platelet count of 68×10^9/L. His serum urate concentration was mildly elevated, but his kidney and liver function test results were normal. A chest radiograph showed enlargement of the right and left pulmonary arteries without pulmonary edema (Fig. 125A.1). Magnetic resonance imaging demonstrated a double-inlet left ventricle, small hypoplastic right ventricle, and large ventricular septal defect.

DIFFERENTIAL DIAGNOSIS

The history and physical examination findings are consistent with Eisenmenger's syndrome. Specifically, he has a large shunt but no murmur, a loud second heart sound, and enlarged pulmonary arteries on chest radiography. Still, his worsening symptoms need further explanation.

LONG-TERM CONSIDERATIONS IN CYANOTIC HEART DISEASE	
Condition	**Management Strategy**
Iron deficiency	Check transferrin saturation, not just mean corpuscular volume; treat with supplemental iron until transferrin saturation is corrected
Hyperviscosity	Hydration, supplemental oxygen; exclude alternative causes of symptoms; phlebotomy discouraged and rarely necessary
Hemoptysis	Observation, bed rest, cough suppression; replace blood products if necessary; avoid bronchoscopy
Pulmonary artery thrombosis	Warfarin is justifiable but unproven; the patient should be observed closely by proper measurement of international normalized ratio with citrate-adjusted tubes
Cerebral embolism or abscess	Supportive care acutely; warfarin therapy chronically for emboli, with close follow-up and proper measurement of international normalized ratio
Arrhythmia	Supportive care acutely as needed; beta blockers can be safe but should be started with caution; cardioversion safe with minimal sedation
Thrombocytopenia	Usually no treatment needed; platelet transfusion if needed for severe bleeding
Hyperuricemia	Allopurinol in patients with gout, otherwise observation
Renal impairment	Observation, supportive care

Table 125A.1 Long-term considerations in cyanotic heart disease.

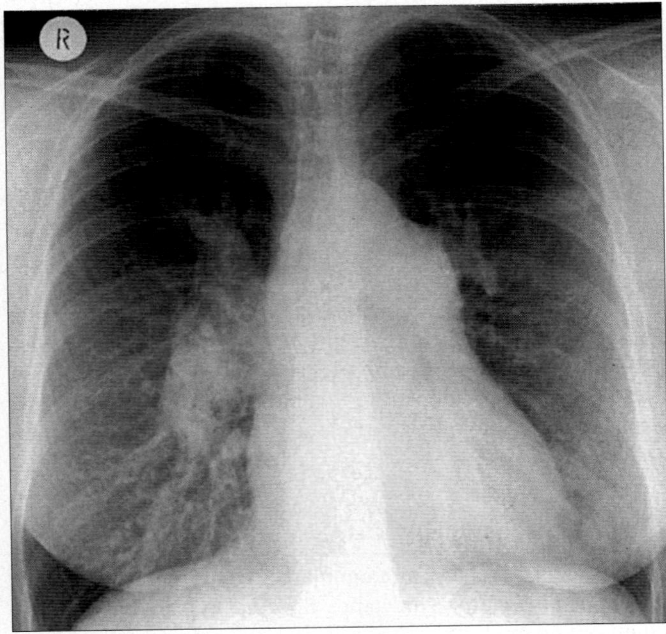

Figure 125A.1 A chest radiograph showed enlargement of the right and left pulmonary arteries without pulmonary edema.

A cyanotic patient should have an elevated hemoglobin and hematocrit. This is a necessary adaptation to maintain tissue oxygen delivery. Viewed as such, a provider will want to ensure that the hemoglobin is appropriately elevated rather than attempt to lower it to a "normal" range. In general, it is best to leave the hemoglobin alone. In this patient, however, he had been managed with increasingly frequent therapeutic phlebotomy, which may have only worsened the situation in the long term.

One of the most difficult complications to assess and to treat is hyperviscosity. Hyperviscosity symptoms can be many and include headaches, fatigue, chest pain, joint or muscle aches, paresthesias, and poor mentation. However, many of these symptoms can have other causes. Indeed, such symptoms are known to be present in cyanotic patients regardless of the measured viscosity. Although viscosity probably plays a role in symptoms, it is wrong to attribute these common symptoms to viscosity automatically without a thorough consideration of alternative causes. Early work suggests an ideal hemoglobin level may be predictable (roughly 62 minus ½ the measured oxygen saturation). Based on this, this patient's hemoglobin value of 16 g/dL is far below what one might consider ideal.

The cause of his inappropriately low hemoglobin level is most likely iron deficiency, a common finding in cyanotic heart disease. Iron deficiency is a spectrum and can be a source of symptoms even in the absence of inappropriately low hemoglobin levels. Symptoms may include fatigue, joint aches, and paresthesias. A normal mean corpuscular volume does not exclude iron deficiency, and therefore detailed iron studies should be ordered routinely.

Although many cyanotic patients will at some time complain of chest pain, atherosclerosis is rare or nonexistent. It could represent viscosity-related microperfusion abnormalities or be due to transient low myocardial oxygen delivery relative to increased demand. Nuclear perfusion studies therefore are not usually diagnostic, as this case typifies.

Even if the hemoglobin level is appropriate, Eisenmenger patients are vulnerable to slow, gradual decline. His symptoms therefore may reflect worsening pulmonary arterial hypertension and progressive cyanosis or even ventricular dysfunction.

TREATMENT OPTIONS

It is now generally accepted that routine therapeutic phlebotomy in a cyanotic patient is not appropriate, even when the hematocrit is above 65%. Unlike patients with polycythemia, in whom leukocytosis and thrombocytosis contribute to hyperviscosity, cyanotic patients have isolated erythrocytosis, and the distinction is important. Some cyanotic patients may seem "decompensated," with abrupt rise and fall of hemoglobin levels suggesting that the erythrocytotic process is unchecked. These can be difficult patients to deal with, and at times, nonjudicious use of phlebotomy can only complicate rather than clarify their management. Therefore, this practice should be stopped in this patient.

The patient needs formal assessment of his iron stores (ferritin and transferrin saturation), which are likely to be low because of his regular phlebotomy. If iron deficiency is present, most institutions advocate treatment to allow the hemoglobin to rise to a more appropriate level. This can be done with oral iron supplementation, even two or three times a day, with careful follow-up to ensure that runaway erythropoiesis does not occur.

Whenever hyperviscosity is suspected, the clinician should first ensure that the patient is adequately hydrated. Supplemental oxygen can sometimes help. Phlebotomy should be a last resort. Even in severe circumstances, such as mental status change, phlebotomy does not increase cerebral oxygen delivery, making it difficult to justify in any clinical situation. Although there may be circumstances that warrant phlebotomy, this should be the exception rather than the rule, and it should be done only with the supervision of an adult congenital heart specialist.

This patient had been treated with diuretics for shortness of breath without any evidence of hypervolemia. Although diuretics can at times be appropriate in the setting of right ventricular failure, overdiuresis can lead to hypovolemia and worsen viscosity-related symptoms.

In a patient with increased vascular resistance (Eisenmenger's syndrome), pulmonary vasodilators may be helpful. In a randomized placebo-controlled trial, one of very few such trials in congenital heart disease, bosentan was shown to have a favorable improvement in hemodynamics and 6-minute walk test distance. Nonrandomized studies of sildenafil are also promising. Most groups tend to reserve these therapies for patients with more advanced symptoms. Prostacyclin infusions are less desirable because of the need for continuous intravenous access with its risk of cerebral thromboembolism. The various merits of these drugs in patients with pulmonary arterial hypertension are discussed elsewhere in this volume.

CASE MANAGEMENT DECISIONS

The patient should probably have been referred to a specialized center years ago. Even despite multiple complications encountered, he was seen in an adult congenital heart disease center only of his own initiative. The major intervention in this patient was educating him about his condition. With informed knowledge about the nature of some of his chronic pain, he was able to wean himself from chronic narcotics, focusing instead on hydration and appropriate hemoglobin levels for control.

Phlebotomy was discontinued. Despite a normal mean corpuscular volume, his iron studies showed significant iron deficiency, and he was given oral iron supplementation. Within months, his energy level had improved. Thereafter, he was thought to be eligible for pulmonary vasodilator therapy if his symptoms declined further.

SUMMARY

The surviving adult patient with cyanosis may enjoy a productive, happy life and should be managed with this expectation in mind. The patients should receive specialized care by those familiar with their management. Survival is dependent on inherent adaptive mechanisms, namely, secondary erythrocytosis, which is best left alone. However, this adaptation leaves them vulnerable, and health issues that may be easily tolerated by another individual may be far more catastrophic for a fragile cyanotic patient. As long as mistakes are avoided, many of the complications can be successfully managed to allow the patient a prosperous future with surprising longevity.

b. Cardiopulmonary Exercise Testing in Adult Congenital Heart Disease

Konstantinos Dimopoulos

Exercise intolerance, manifested as exertional dyspnea or fatigue, is common in adults with congenital heart disease (ACHD) and can be the result of cardiac or extracardiac disorders (Table 125B.1). Cardiopulmonary exercise testing (CPET) is a powerful tool for the objective evaluation of the cardiovascular, respiratory, and muscular systems under conditions of controlled metabolic stress.[1,2] It is widely used in the assessment of patients with acquired heart failure and candidates for cardiac transplantation and in recent years has been adopted by ACHD physicians, becoming part of the routine clinical assessment of ACHD patients.

TYPICAL CASE

A 20-year-old patient with tetralogy of Fallot repaired in infancy complained of deterioration of his tolerance to strenuous efforts. CPET was performed; the patient exercised for 13 minutes, with adequate chronotropic but blunted blood pressure response. Significant exercise intolerance and marked ventilatory inefficiency were suggested by peak oxygen consumption of 24 mL/kg per minute (54% of predicted for age, sex, height, and weight), anaerobic threshold of 17 mL/kg per minute, and $\dot{V}E/\dot{V}CO_2$ slope of 39 (Fig. 125B.1a). Causes of reduced pulmonary perfusion and increased functional dead space were thus sought. Echocardiography revealed significant pulmonary regurgitation (already present in previous investigations), with good biventricular function and no residual ventricular septal defect. The left pulmonary artery was small, but no significant degree of stenosis could be detected, as echocardiographic windows were limited. Cardiac magnetic resonance imaging was thus performed, revealing significant left pulmonary artery stenosis, which was treated with balloon dilatation and stenting.

The patient reported a significant improvement in effort tolerance within a few days of the intervention. Follow-up CPET (Fig. 125B.1b) showed an objective improvement in exercise tolerance (20% increase), anaerobic threshold (30% increase), blood pressure response, and $\dot{V}E/\dot{V}CO_2$ slope (30% decrease

POSSIBLE MECHANISMS OF EXERCISE INTOLERANCE IN ADULT CONGENITAL HEART DISEASE
Cardiac
Myocardial dysfunction (systolic or diastolic, of the systemic or pulmonary ventricle)
Valve disease (stenosis, regurgitation of native or prosthetic valves)
Outflow tract obstruction (right or left)
Intracardiac shunting
Myocardial perfusion abnormalities (coronary anomalies, microvascular disease, pressure overload, significant aortic regurgitation)
Chronotropic incompetence (sinus node dysfunction, atrioventricular conduction abnormalities, medication or artificial pacing related)
Pericardial disease (absence of pericardium, constrictive pericarditis secondary to surgery)
Conduit or baffle stenosis
Great vessels
Pulmonary stenosis (valvular or peripheral)
Aortic coarctation
Lungs
Pulmonary vascular disease (pulmonary hypertension, Eisenmenger's syndrome)
Parenchymal disease
Restrictive disease (skeletal abnormalities, severe cardiomegaly)
Peripheral or other
Cyanosis
Anemia (or relative anemia in cyanotic patients)
Skeletal abnormalities
Physical deconditioning or skeletal muscle disorders
Endothelial dysfunction

Table 125B.1 Possible mechanisms of exercise intolerance in adult congenital heart disease

to 28). In this case, CPET was instrumental in detecting pulmonary stenosis as a reversible cause of the reported deterioration of exercise tolerance and in directing diagnostic and therapeutic efforts. Pulmonary stenosis resulted in significant reduction in pulmonary perfusion and contributed to the increase in physiologic dead space, leading to significant ventilatory inefficiency as well as aggravating pulmonary regurgitation. Follow-up CPET confirmed the efficacy of the intervention in improving exercise capacity and especially the ventilatory response to exercise.

DESCRIPTION OF THE TECHNIQUE AND SAFETY

CPET consists of standard exercise testing on a bicycle or treadmill with simultaneous gas exchange measurements through a mouthpiece or mask. Incremental protocols are commonly used to assess important functional and prognostic indexes, such as peak oxygen consumption (peak $\dot{V}O_2$), anaerobic threshold, ventilatory response to exercise, heart rate and blood pressure response, and oxygen saturations (Fig. 125B.2). CPET is a safe, noninvasive procedure, with a risk of death estimated well below 1/10,000 exercise tests.[2] However, appropriate training and test supervision are essential for safety of the patient. Moreover, because patients are unable to talk with the mouthpiece in place, thorough explanation of the protocol and a means of communication (hand signs) should be established beforehand.

During steady state, oxygen uptake ($\dot{V}O_2$) from the lungs reflects oxygen consumed by the cells in the periphery. Peak $\dot{V}O_2$ is the highest measured value of oxygen uptake averaged during 30 to 60 seconds and is expressed in milliliters per kilogram per minute. It approximates maximal aerobic power, that is, the upper limit of oxygen use in the body, and is a surrogate of the functional status of the cardiovascular, pulmonary, and muscular systems.[1,2] It is the most frequently reported exercise parameter because it is the simplest and most intuitive marker of exercise capacity as well as a strong prognostic marker in both acquired heart failure and ACHD.[3-5] However, peak $\dot{V}O_2$ will approximate maximal attainable $\dot{V}O_2$ only if the patient exerts himself to exhaustion.[2]

The anaerobic threshold is the level of $\dot{V}O_2$ beyond which aerobic metabolism is substantially supplemented by anaerobic processes.[1,2] Above the anaerobic threshold, lactate accumulates and is buffered by plasma bicarbonate, causing an increase in CO_2 production ($\dot{V}CO_2$). Anaerobic threshold can be identified by the V-slope method through observation of the $\dot{V}CO_2$ versus $\dot{V}O_2$ relation or by the ventilatory equivalent method through observation of the ventilation ($\dot{V}E$)/$\dot{V}O_2$ ratio over time.[1,2] Apart from its obvious pathophysiologic significance (anaerobic threshold is the point at which aerobic metabolism is unable to sustain energy requirement), the anaerobic threshold carries important prognostic information in acquired heart failure and ACHD.[3-6]

The $\dot{V}E/\dot{V}CO_2$ slope is the slope of the regression line between minute ventilation and $\dot{V}CO_2$ (see Fig. 125B.2) and is a simplification of the complex relation between ventilation and CO_2 production during exercise. In healthy subjects, the relation between ventilation and $\dot{V}CO_2$ is linear, with 23 to 25 liters of ventilation needed to eliminate 1 liter of CO_2 produced. Even though it is less intuitive than peak $\dot{V}O_2$ and anaerobic threshold, it is an important marker of exercise intolerance and reflects predominantly ventilation-perfusion ($\dot{V}/\dot{Q}$) mismatch. It is a strong independent prognostic marker in both acquired heart failure and ACHD, and unlike peak $\dot{V}O_2$, it can be calculated from submaximal testing.[7] Values of $\dot{V}E/\dot{V}CO_2$ slope exceeding 33 are considered abnormal, even though the normal cutoff depends on the convention used to measure the slope (entire exercise period versus exclusion of the period after the respiratory compensation point). The $\dot{V}E/\dot{V}CO_2$ ratio at anaerobic threshold provides information similar to the $\dot{V}E/\dot{V}CO_2$ slope.

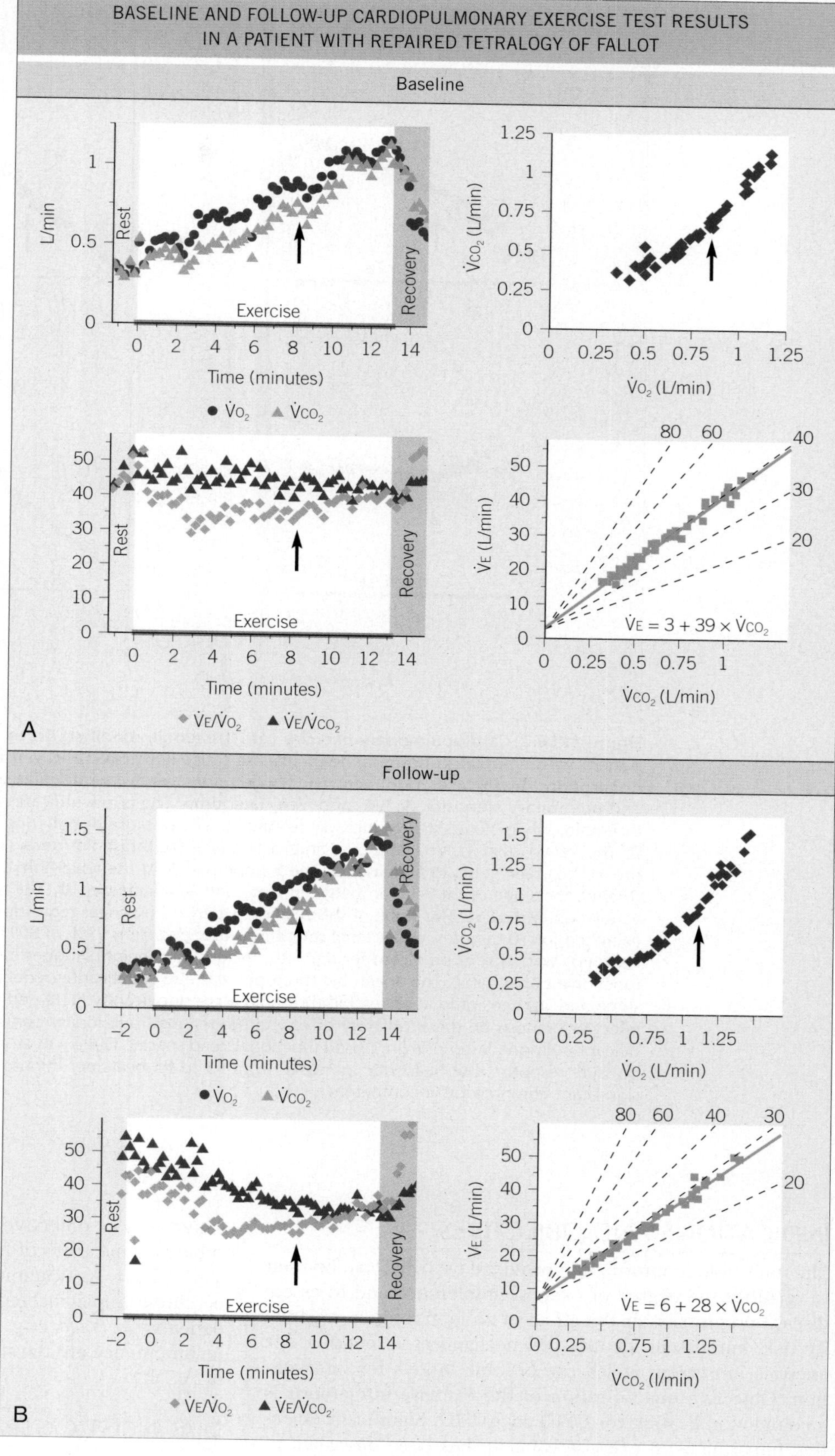

Figure 125B.1 Baseline and follow-up cardiopulmonary exercise test results in a patient with repaired tetralogy of Fallot. See text for details.

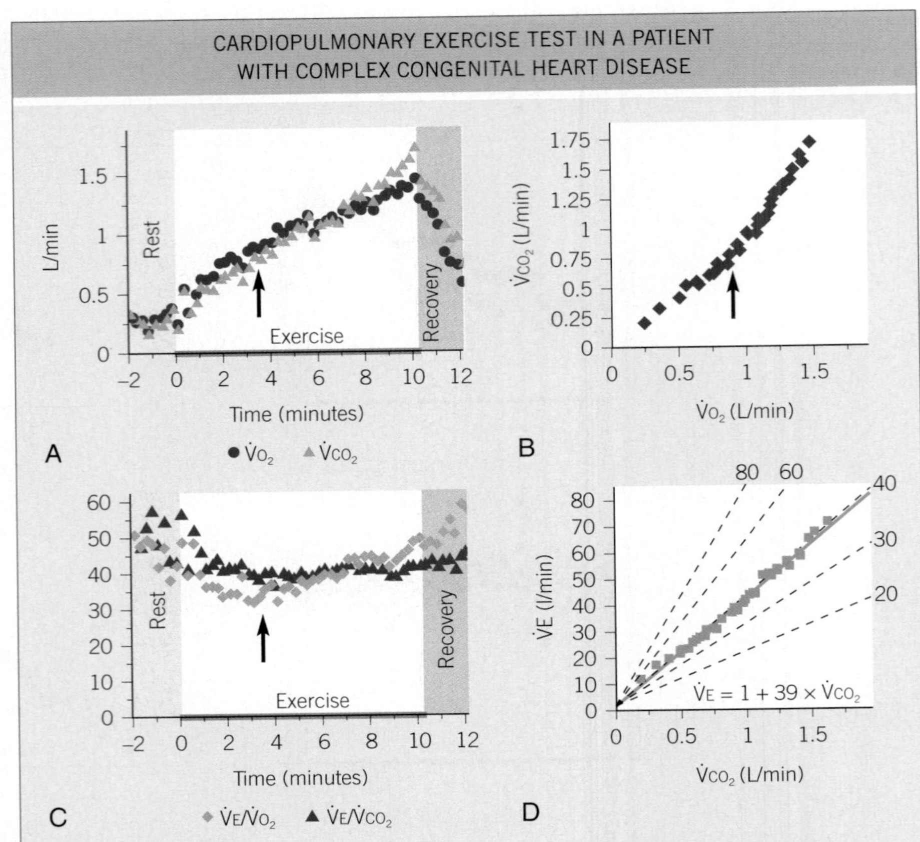

Figure 125B.2 Cardiopulmonary exercise test (treadmill, modified Bruce protocol) in a patient with complex congenital heart disease (atrioventricular and ventriculoarterial discordance, hypoplastic right ventricle, large nonrestrictive ventricular septal defect, and pulmonary stenosis). A, $\dot{V}O_2$ and $\dot{V}CO_2$ over time. The arrow indicates the anaerobic threshold, when $\dot{V}CO_2$ starts to increase relative to $\dot{V}O_2$ because of buffering of lactate. **B,** The $\dot{V}E/\dot{V}O_2$ and $\dot{V}E/\dot{V}O_2$ ratio over time. The anaerobic threshold *(arrow)* is the point when the $\dot{V}E/\dot{V}O_2$ ratio starts to increase. **C,** The V-slope panel. At the anaerobic threshold *(arrow),* the slope of the relation between $\dot{V}CO_2$ and $\dot{V}O_2$ increases. **D,** The relation between ventilation and $\dot{V}CO_2$. The slope of this relation is derived by linear regression. The patient exercised for 10 minutes, and arterial saturations dropped from 99% to 89% at peak exercise. Peak $\dot{V}O_2$ was 51% of predicted for age, sex, weight, and height, suggesting moderate functional impairment. The anaerobic threshold was also significantly reduced. The $\dot{V}E/\dot{V}CO_2$ slope and $\dot{V}E/\dot{V}CO_2$ ratio at anaerobic threshold were significantly increased because of the effect of cyanosis on the ventilatory drive and the reduced pulmonary perfusion due to significant pulmonary stenosis (increased functional dead space). There was an appropriate blood pressure response, but heart rate increased from 65 to 95 beats per minute, suggesting significant chronotropic incompetence.

INDICATIONS AND OBJECTIVES

The multitude of information provided by CPET can be used to quantify the degree of exercise intolerance and to assess disease progression or the effect of an intervention, to stratify risk, but also to identify the mechanisms responsible for exercise limitation, which can become targets for intervention. Objective quantification of the exercise intolerance is a common indication for CPET in ACHD. Significant objective impairment in exercise capacity has been described in all ACHD groups (Fig. 125B.3).[6,8-14] Interestingly, even asymptomatic ACHD patients have significantly deranged peak $\dot{V}O_2$ and $\dot{V}E/\dot{V}CO_2$ slope, further underscoring the superiority of objective assessment of exercise capacity over subjective measures of functional limitation, such as the New York Heart Association classification.[15] A high prevalence of chronotropic incompetence is also prevalent in ACHD patients. A $\dot{V}E/\dot{V}CO_2$ slope above 38 and chronotropic incompetence are the strongest prognostic exercise markers in ACHD.

DIAGNOSTIC STRATEGY

Whereas treatment of acquired chronic heart failure focuses mainly on counteraction of neurohormonal activation, in ACHD, the primary focus is identification and relief of

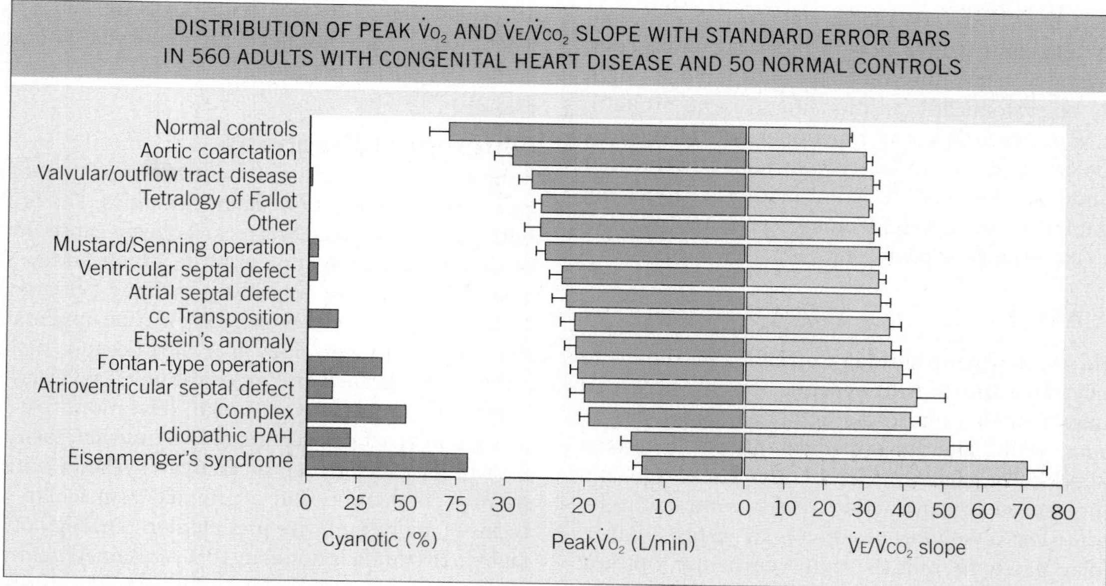

Figure 125B.3 Distribution of peak $\dot{V}O_2$ and $\dot{V}E/\dot{V}CO_2$ slope with standard error bars in 560 adults with congenital heart disease and 50 normal controls.[14] Also shown is the percentage of patients with cyanosis at rest in the various diagnostic groups. Peak $\dot{V}O_2$ is significantly lower and $\dot{V}E/\dot{V}CO_2$ slope significantly higher in ACHD patients compared with normal controls. Patients with cyanosis and pulmonary hypertension are the most impaired. cc, congenitally corrected; PAH, pulmonary arterial hypertension.

hemodynamic lesions. Combined with lung function testing, CPET can differentiate between the multitude of cardiac, pulmonary, and peripheral sources of exercise limitation in ACHD and identify targets for intervention.

SUMMARY

CPET is an essential tool for the ACHD physician and should be used routinely in assessment of all ACHD patients, independent of the degree of perceived limitation.

c. Implantable Cardioverter-Defibrillators and Cardiac Resynchronization Therapy in Congenital Heart Disease

Paul Khairy, Annie Dore, Anne Fournier and Lise-Andrée Mercier

DEFINITION OF PROBLEM

Advances in cardiac care in the young have given rise to a rapidly expanding population of patients with congenital heart disease living longer lives.[1] This remarkable achievement is, however, mitigated by the recognition that early surgical interventions were "reparative" and not "curative." After sometimes lengthy quiescent clinical courses, arrhythmias figure prominently among issues encountered in survivors with congenital heart disease.[2] Indeed, sudden cardiac death of presumable arrhythmic etiology is the most common cause of mortality in adults with congenital heart disease. In comparison to age-matched controls, an up to 100-fold increased risk of sudden death is observed, often in the third and fourth decades of life.[3,4]

As a result, implantable cardioverter-defibrillators (ICDs) are increasingly used in this population of patients. Importantly, this practice is not supported by prospective randomized clinical trials specific to congenital heart disease. However, retrospective multicenter cohort studies of ICD recipients with various forms of congenital heart disease have begun to characterize the profiles of patients most likely to benefit from this technology.[5,6] Complexities in underlying anatomy, associated extracardiac malformations, underdeveloped or obstructed vascular access, and intracardiac shunts can pose unique challenges to transvenous ICD implantation[7] and lead extraction,[8] if it is required.

Paralleling the high incidence of cardiac arrhythmias, heart failure remains a common long-term complication of congenital heart disease and is a major source of morbidity and mortality. Issues specific to this population of patients limit the generalizability of studies conducted in patients without congenital heart defects. This is true for inferences concerning pharmacologic agents[9] and cardiac resynchronization therapy (CRT). For example, in contrast to adults with heart failure and left bundle branch block, right ventricular conduction delay and right bundle branch block are more common in congenital heart disease. The morphologic right ventricle may be systemically positioned and more prone to dysfunction. Moreover, only one functional yet failing ventricle may be present, precluding biventricular pacing but not CRT by multisite pacing.[10] Current evidence supporting CRT in congenital heart disease remains sparse, yet the initial collective experience is promising.[10,11]

TYPICAL CASE 1

A 27-year-old woman with tetralogy of Fallot presented to the emergency department with syncope, briefly preceded by palpitations of sudden onset and lightheadedness, during a nonstrenuous walk. Her past medical history consisted of a right Blalock-Taussig shunt at 10 months of age and corrective surgery at 6 years with a right ventriculotomy incision, closure of a subaortic ventricular septal defect, and subannular patch to relieve right ventricular outflow tract obstruction. At 16 years of age, additional surgery was performed to alleviate residual right ventricular outflow tract obstruction. She was receiving no medical therapy and was previously asymptomatic and active (i.e., New York Heart Association [NYHA] functional class I).

On physical examination, her blood pressure was 120/60 mm Hg; heart rate, 88 beats per minute; and oxygen saturation, 98% on room air. No jugular venous distention was noted, a wide physiologically split S_2 was audible, and no third or fourth heart sounds were appreciated. A grade 2/6 systolic ejection murmur and faint diastolic decrescendo murmur were best heard over the second right intercostal space. Lungs were clear to auscultation, and no hepatosplenomegaly or peripheral edema was noted. Her 12-lead electrocardiogram is depicted in Figure 125C.1. Echocardiography revealed an 18 mm Hg gradient across the right ventricular outflow tract, mild to moderate pulmonary regurgitation, trivial tricuspid regurgitation, mild right ventricular dilatation, no residual ventricular septal defect, and normal biventricular function. A 24-hour Holter monitor 1-year prior recorded occasional single premature atrial beats, an average of 10 premature ventricular beats per hour, and a 5-beat run of asymptomatic nonsustained monomorphic ventricular tachycardia (210 beats per minute).

Differential Diagnosis

Syncope occurred in the context of normal biventricular function and otherwise stable hemodynamics. The brief prodrome with palpitations suggests a cardiogenic cause. In the absence of sinus node dysfunction or more advanced forms of conduction system disease, a bradyarrhythmic event is improbable. Notably, right bundle branch block often appears after corrective surgery for tetralogy of Fallot because of injury to the right bundle branch and myocardium,[12] whereas later broadening reflects right ventricular dilatation.[13] It is far more likely that syncope accompanied a transient tachyarrhythmia. Possibilities include atrial tachyarrhythmia with rapid ventricular conduction and a primary ventricular source. Both forms of arrhythmia are prevalent in tetralogy of Fallot; atrial tachyarrhythmia is noted in 10%, sustained ventricular tachycardia in 12%, and sudden death in 8% during a 10-year follow-up period.[14]

The patient did not have a transannular right ventricular outflow tract patch or electrocardiographic markers (e.g., QRS duration ≥180 ms) associated with ventricular tachycardia or sudden death.[14] However, several characteristics that independently predict risk for inducible sustained ventricular tachycardia were present, including age of 18 years or older, palpitations, prior palliative surgery, and nonsustained ventricular tachycardia.[15] Whereas an electrophysiologic study is not recommended to routinely screen all patients with tetralogy of Fallot, it is most helpful in those at moderate risk.[16] Inducible sustained ventricular tachycardia is associated with a nearly fivefold increased risk of clinical sustained ventricular tachycardia or sudden death, as depicted in Figure 125C.2.[15] Although imperfect, it affords predictive value above and beyond known noninvasive risk factors. An electrophysiologic study may also permit more thorough assessment of other potential arrhythmic triggers, including atrial tachyarrhythmias with rapid ventricular conduction.

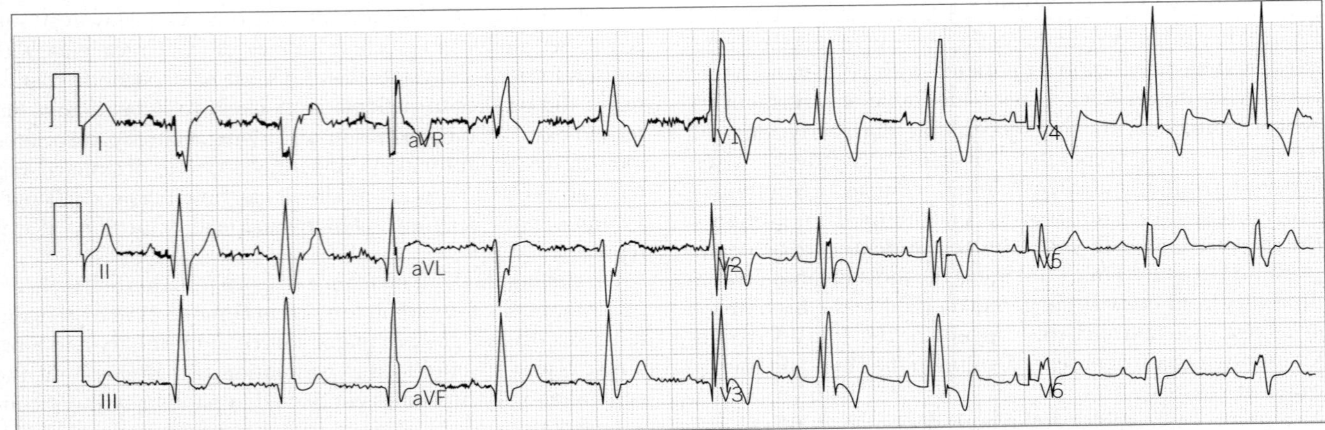

Figure 125C.1 The 12-lead electrocardiogram of a 27-year-old woman with tetralogy of Fallot and syncope. Normal sinus rhythm is present, with first-degree AV block. Note the right axis deviation, typical right bundle branch block pattern, and QRS duration of 170 ms. Right ventricular hypertrophy is suspected, with an R′ of 17 mm in V_1.

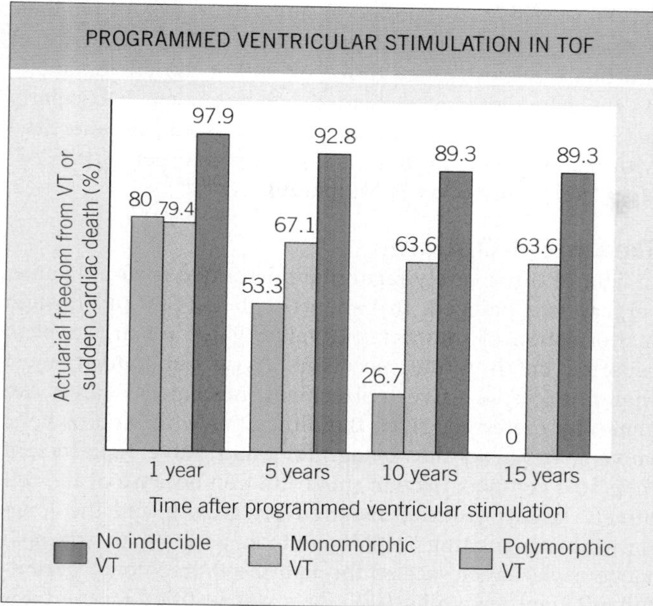

Figure 125C.2 Programmed ventricular stimulation in tetralogy of Fallot (TOF). Actuarial freedom from ventricular tachycardia and sudden cardiac death is depicted in tetralogy of Fallot patients with no inducible ventricular tachycardia (VT), inducible monomorphic VT, and inducible polymorphic VT at 1 year, 5 years, 10 years, and 15 years after programmed ventricular stimulation. (Modified with permission from Khairy P, Landzberg MJ, Gatzoulis MA, et al. Value of programmed ventricular stimulation after tetralogy of Fallot repair: a multicenter study. Circulation 2004;109:1994-2000.)

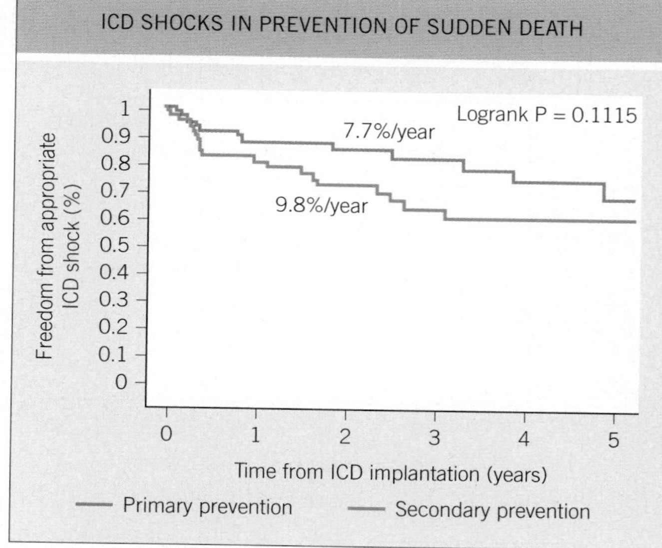

Figure 125C.3 Appropriate ICD shocks in the primary and secondary prevention of sudden death in patients with tetralogy of Fallot. Kaplan-Meier survival curves for freedom from first appropriate ICD shock are plotted and compared among patients with tetralogy of Fallot having primary versus secondary prevention indications.

Treatment Options

Programmed ventricular stimulation was performed for diagnostic assessment and risk stratification. No atrial tachyarrhythmia was inducible. However, sustained monomorphic ventricular tachycardia (220 beats per minute) with hemodynamic compromise followed two ventricular extrastimuli. Ventricular tachycardia had a left bundle branch block morphology and superior QRS axis, consistent with a right outflow tract origin. An ICD was therefore implanted for primary prevention against sudden death, and beta blockers were empirically initiated. Although catheter ablation may have been contemplated, its safety as a first-line therapy for ventricular tachycardia has yet to be demonstrated in tetralogy of Fallot.

A high rate of appropriate ICD shocks has been observed in patients with tetralogy of Fallot and primary prevention indications, as plotted in Figure 125C.3.[5] Independent risk factors for appropriate shocks include a higher left ventricular end-diastolic pressure and nonsustained ventricular tachycardia. Table 125C.1 summarizes a risk score to predict appropriate ICD shocks in tetralogy of Fallot patients with prophylactic ICDs.[5] In our patient, 8 of 12 points were tabulated, placing her in the high-risk category (i.e., 17.5% annual risk of appropriate shocks) shown in Figure 125C.4. Indeed, during follow-up, an appropriate and likely lifesaving ICD shock was delivered for rapid ventricular tachycardia that degenerated into the polymorphic form captured in Figure 125C.5.

TYPICAL CASE 2

A 12-year-old boy with congenitally corrected transposition of the great arteries (TGA), an intact ventricular septum, and Ebstein malformation of the left-sided tricuspid valve experienced increasing dyspnea and fatigue. No history of palpitations was elicited. Medical therapy consisted of an angiotensin-converting enzyme inhibitor, digoxin, and diuretics. On physical examination, S_1 was normal and S_2 single, with no third or fourth heart sound. A grade 3/6 holosystolic murmur was best heard at the apex, with transmission into the lower left part of the thorax. The electrocardiogram showed sinus rhythm with first-degree atrioventricular (AV) block (PR interval, 270 ms), left axis deviation, and intraventricular conduction delay of the left bundle branch block type with Q waves in right precordial and inferior leads, no q waves in left precordial leads, and a QRS duration of 155 ms. Echocardiography confirmed the inverted nature of the ventricles, mitral to pulmonary valve fibrous continuity, and Ebstein malformation of the tricuspid valve. Severe tricuspid regurgitation was noted, with a systemic right ventricular ejection fraction of 34%.

RISK SCORE FOR APPROPRIATE ICD SHOCKS IN PRIMARY PREVENTION

Variable	Points Attributed
Prior palliative shunt	2
Inducible sustained ventricular tachycardia	2
QRS duration ≥180 ms	1
Ventriculotomy incision	2
Nonsustained ventricular tachycardia	2
Left ventricular end-diastolic pressure ≥12 mm Hg	3
Total points	0-12

Table 125C.1 Risk score for appropriate ICD shocks in primary prevention.

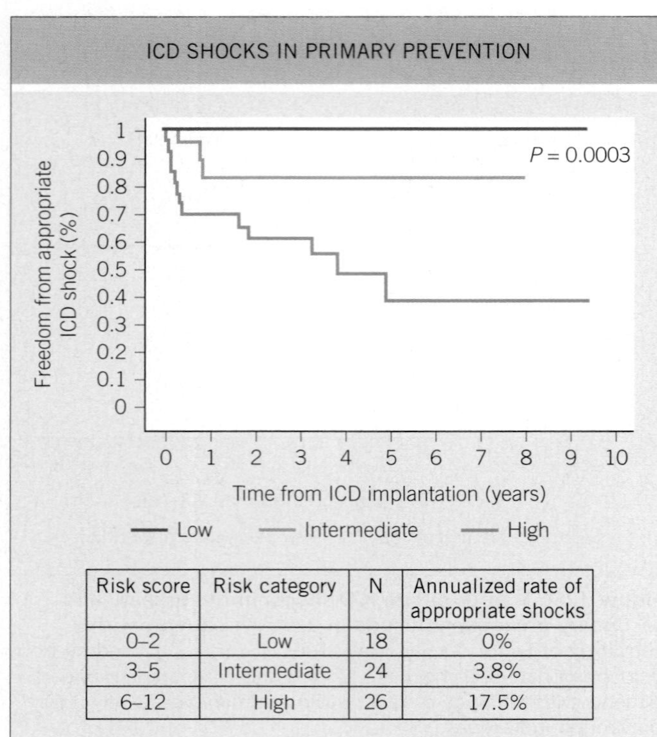

Risk score	Risk category	N	Annualized rate of appropriate shocks
0–2	Low	18	0%
3–5	Intermediate	24	3.8%
6–12	High	26	17.5%

Figure 125C.4 Freedom from appropriate ICD shocks in primary prevention patients with tetralogy of Fallot according to their risk category. In patients with primary prevention indications, Kaplan-Meier survival curves for freedom from first appropriate ICD shock are plotted and compared according to risk score classification. Risk score, corresponding risk category, number of patients, and annualized rate of appropriate shocks are summarized below.

Differential Diagnosis

In patients with complete (D) and congenitally corrected (L) TGA, the morphologic right ventricle is systemically positioned. Exposed to systolic pressures, this ventricle may fail over time, as reflected by clinical heart failure in 22% of patients with D-TGA and intra-atrial baffles in 32% with L-TGA.[17,18] The systemic ventricular ejection fraction is significantly lower in symptomatic (35% ± 16%) compared with asymptomatic (47% ± 13%) patients.[18] Moreover, at 15 years of follow-up, mortality is much higher in symptomatic patients (i.e., 47% versus 5%).[18]

In addition to systemic right ventricular dysfunction, severe tricuspid regurgitation was identified in our patient. In L-TGA, congenital tricuspid valve anomalies include a spectrum of disease that commonly involves valve leaflets and the subvalvular apparatus. Adequate valve closure may be prevented by lack of normal valve delamination from right ventricular myocardium, tethering by short chordae, or annular dilatation. As the tricuspid valve is systemic, high pressures are likely to contribute to progressive regurgitation with increasing age.

Also noteworthy is the patient's marked first-degree AV block. In L-TGA, the AV node is displaced anteriorly and laterally.[19] An elongated His bundle courses medially toward the septum, to the site of fibrous continuity between the right-sided mitral valve and pulmonary artery, and then along the anterior rim of the pulmonary valve.[19] Complete AV block has been reported in more than 20% of patients, with an estimated annual incidence of 2%.[20] The site of AV block is most often above or within the His bundle.[21] As the AV node and elongated bundle appear particularly susceptible to surgical trauma, caution should be exercised with manipulation to these areas. Complete permanent AV block commonly occurs postoperatively.[20,22]

Treatment Options

In light of the severely regurgitant deformed tricuspid valve, surgery was planned. In patients with L-TGA and Ebstein malformation of the tricuspid valve, valve repair has been reported but is rarely successful. As in our patient, most require tricuspid valve replacement. Mechanical valves are generally preferred, given the difficulties with bioprosthetic valve material in the young. Tricuspid valve replacement may be a complex issue in small children because of the relatively large prosthesis required for growth and the long-term anticoagulation requirement. In addition to tricuspid valve replacement, access through the thoracotomy permitted adjuvant epicardial CRT. This was justified on the basis of the depressed systemic ventricular ejection fraction (34%), intraventricular conduction delay (QRS, 155 ms), first-degree AV block (PR, 270 ms) with high likelihood of eventual progression to complete block (if not immediately postoperatively), difficulties with transvenous coronary sinus lead insertion in L-TGA, and epicardial access.

CRT for systemic right ventricular dysfunction was first reported in a 24-year-old man with L-TGA and complete heart block.[23] An improvement was noted in symptoms (NYHA class III to class I), ventricular dimensions, fractional area of change, and maximum oxygen uptake. Technical feasibility and hemodynamic benefits of CRT were more formally assessed in eight patients with systemic right ventricles.[24] Two had right bundle branch block and six had left ventricular pacing-induced conduction delay. Six had CRT for systemic right ventricular dysfunction despite standard medical therapy, and two received CRT as a preventive measure during thoracotomy for another indication. Three patients had concomitant surgery for tricuspid regurgitation. Encouragingly, change from baseline rhythm to CRT was accompanied by a decrease in QRS duration, reduction in interventricular mechanical delay, and immediate improvement in right ventricular filling time, Tei index, maximum right ventricular dP/dt, and aortic velocity-time integral.[24] Right ventricular ejection fraction increased by 10% on average.[24] However, no reduction in tricuspid regurgitation was noted with CRT. Concurrent tricuspid valve interventions may therefore be indicated in patients with severe regurgitation.

Our general approach to epicardial CRT in congenital heart disease is to place three bipolar epicardial leads on the right atrial surface, at the level of the basal to mid subpulmonary ventricular free wall segment, and on the systemic ventricular lateral free wall, as shown in Figure 125C.6.[10] Bipolar steroid-eluting leads are favored, with bipoles placed 1 cm apart, although ventricular screw-in leads are occasionally required to obtain acceptable thresholds in the setting of extensive fibrosis. Whereas strategies remain empiric, we systematically optimize interventricular and AV delays by tissue Doppler imaging. Cardiac index and diastolic flow patterns are

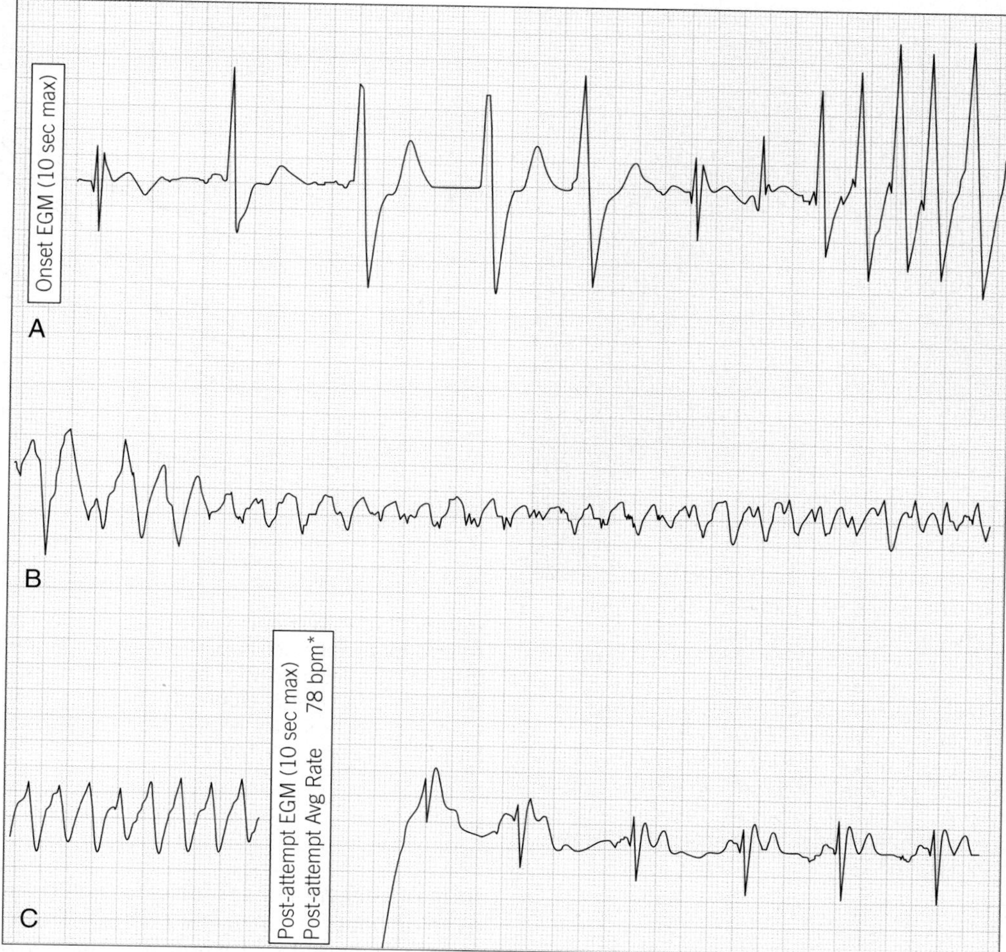

Figure 125C.5 Appropriate shock in a 27-year-old woman with tetralogy of Fallot and a prophylactic ICD. A stored ventricular electrogram is depicted with a continuous recording at 25 mm per second. Premature ventricular beats are seen in **A,** followed by onset of a rapid ventricular tachyarrhythmia. In **B,** the ventricular tachycardia degenerated into a polymorphic form. **C,** An appropriate ICD discharge is marked by the asterisk, which restored normal sinus rhythm at 78 beats per minute.

assessed over a wide range of programmable AV delays, and the systemic ventricular ejection fraction is quantified by the modified Simpson method. The optimized AV delay is defined as the value yielding the highest cardiac index and systemic AV valve flow by velocity-time integral. The interventricular conduction delay is subsequently optimized by assessing alterations of this parameter on septal to lateral wall motion delay by tissue Doppler imaging, illustrated in Figure 125C.7, and dP/dt. Delay between QRS onset and systolic wave is measured at the proximal third of the septum and lateral wall of the systemic ventricle. In this particular patient, the optimal interventricular delay consisted of right preceding left ventricular pacing by 4 ms.

In our experience with CRT in a heterogeneous group of patients with congenital heart disease, the ejection fraction significantly increased from 31.4% ± 13.5% at baseline to 50.6% ± 15.2% on follow-up, as plotted in Figure 125C.8, and dP/dt from 595 ± 178 mm Hg/s to 986 ± 162 mm Hg/s.[10] Hemodynamic improvement was similar whether or not patients had concomitant surgery, whether the systemic ventricle was right or left, and whether CRT was performed as a primary implant or as an upgrade to prior pacing.[10] At 1-year follow-up after tricuspid valve replacement and CRT, our case patient's symptoms of dyspnea and fatigue had resolved and the systemic right ventricular ejection fraction normalized to 60%.

SUMMARY

Unlike standard ICD and CRT indications based on multiple randomized clinical trials, evidence supporting this technology in patients with congenital heart disease is limited but growing. Multicenter international studies on ICDs in tetralogy of Fallot and TGA have better defined the population of patients most likely to derive benefit.[5,6] Whereas secondary prevention indications are rarely disputed, the challenge lies in identifying the subgroup of patients without clinical sustained ventricular tachyarrhythmias or resuscitated cardiac arrest at high risk for sudden death. In tetralogy of Fallot, the most common

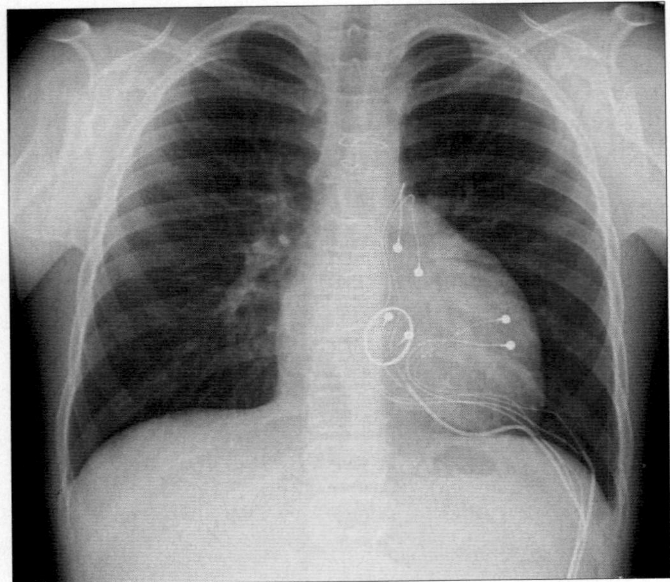

Figure 125C.6 Chest radiograph in a patient with congenital heart disease and epicardial CRT. A posteroanterior chest radiograph is shown in a patient with congenital heart disease, a mechanical mitral valve, and epicardial CRT. Note the presence and configuration of the three bipolar epicardial leads, positioned on the right atrial surface, at the level of the basal to mid right ventricular free wall segment, and on the left ventricular lateral free wall. Bipoles were placed 1 cm apart. (Reproduced with permission from Khairy P, Fournier A, Thibault B, Dubuc M, Therien J, Vobecky SJ. Cardiac resynchronization therapy in congenital heart disease. Int J Cardiol 2006;109:160-168.)

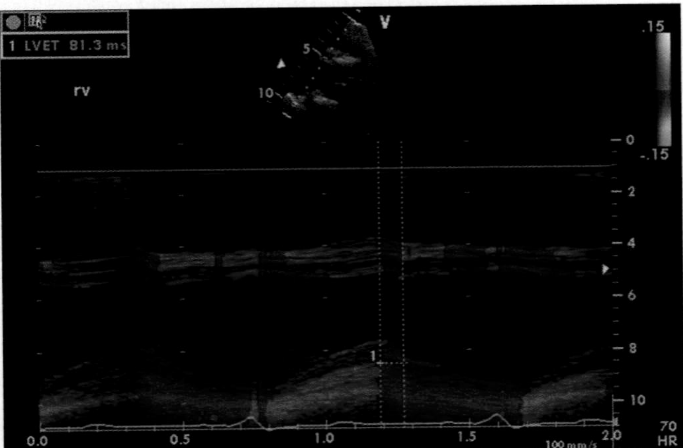

Figure 125C.7 Tissue Doppler enhanced monodimensional short-axis view. A view at the level of the papillary muscle is illustrated. The time interval between the two dotted vertical lines (labeled 1) was 80 ms, indicating delay between motion of the septum and left posterior wall, calculated as the shortest interval between the maximal posterior displacement of the septum and the maximal displacement of the left posterior wall. (Reproduced with permission from Khairy P, Fournier A, Thibault B, Dubuc M, Therien J, Vobecky SJ. Cardiac resynchronization therapy in congenital heart disease. Int J Cardiol 2006;109:160-168.)

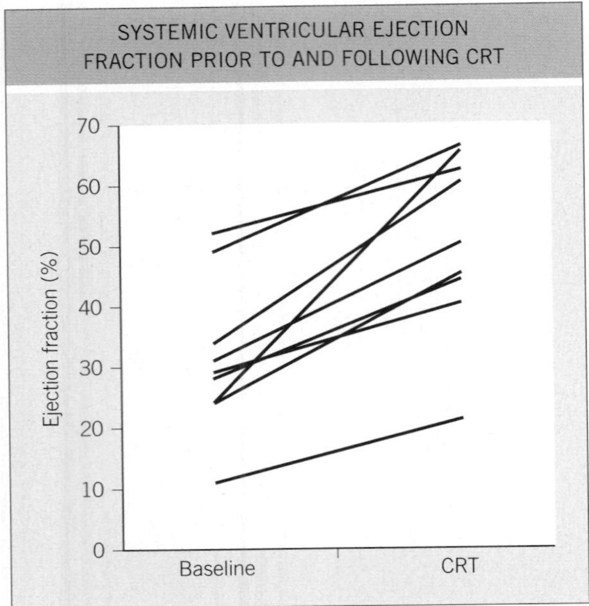

Figure 125C.8 Systemic ventricular ejection fraction prior to and following CRT in patients with congenital heart disease. (Reproduced with permission from Khairy P, Fournier A, Thibault B, Dubuc M, Therien J, Vobecky SJ. Cardiac resynchronization therapy in congenital heart disease. Int J Cardiol 2006;109:160-168.)

form of congenital heart disease in ICD recipients, risk for development of ventricular tachyarrhythmias is modulated by a combination of surgical, hemodynamic, electrocardiographic, and electrophysiologic factors.[5] Clinical characteristics are helpful in identifying candidates for further risk stratification by programmed ventricular stimulation[15,16] and, ultimately, for ICD implantation.[5]

Evidence supporting CRT in congenital heart disease has thus far been limited to case reports, case series, and small experimental acute postoperative crossover studies. The heterogeneous population of patients, technical limitations from the patient's size, vascular access issues, and unique forms of ventricular dyssynchrony encountered further obscure the selection of potential beneficiaries.[10] Nevertheless, heart failure is common in congenital heart disease, particularly in those with single or systemic right ventricles. Surgically induced intraventricular conduction delay and bundle branch block may further contribute to ventricular dyssynchrony. Studies have begun to unravel the many facets of CRT in congenital heart disease, including right bundle branch block, right (pulmonary) ventricular dysfunction, systemic right ventricular dysfunction, single-ventricle dysfunction, and acute postoperative ventricular failure. Encouragingly, experience thus far has been favorable. Although definitive evidence-based recommendations cannot be proposed at the current time, optimistic initial experience suggests that research in this field should be pursued.

d. Pregnancy and Congenital Heart Disease

Jolien Roos-Hesselink

DEFINITION OF PROBLEM

Increasing numbers of women with congenital heart disease reach childbearing age.[1,2] The majority of these women want to become pregnant, and heart disease is no bar to sexual activity; however, these women face an increased risk of cardiac and obstetric complications.[3] Heart disease is present in 0.5% to 1% of all pregnant women and accounts for about 10% to 15% of all maternal mortality.[2] There are no signs of decline of this incidence during the past decades.

During pregnancy, the peripheral vascular resistance falls, cardiac output increases by 40% to 50%, and blood volume increases by 25% (Fig. 125D.1). This adaptation process starts early in pregnancy. During labor, uterine contractions cause a further increase in cardiac output. Together with anxiety and physical effort, cardiac output may increase up to 80% of pre-pregnancy levels. During the puerperium, decompression of the inferior caval vein and the return of uterine blood into the systemic circulation (autotransfusion) result in a relatively overfilled state. After 3 to 6 months, all measurements of ventricular function and structure in the resting state are approximately at nonpregnant levels.

Other major cardiovascular adaptation mechanisms to pregnancy are the activation of the coagulation system with risk of thromboembolic events and increased distensibility and decreased stiffness of the vascular system with an increased risk of aortic dissection or rupture.

The risk of complications is strongly influenced by the kind of congenital heart defect and residual lesions. In an important study of Siu and colleagues,[4,5] predictors of adverse maternal outcome in 599 women with mainly congenital heart disease were described (Table 125D.1). However, it needs to be taken into account that some high-risk conditions, such as mechanical valve prosthesis and cyanotic lesions, might be underestimated in this risk score.[6-8] The risk factors for the fetus are depicted in Table 125D.2.

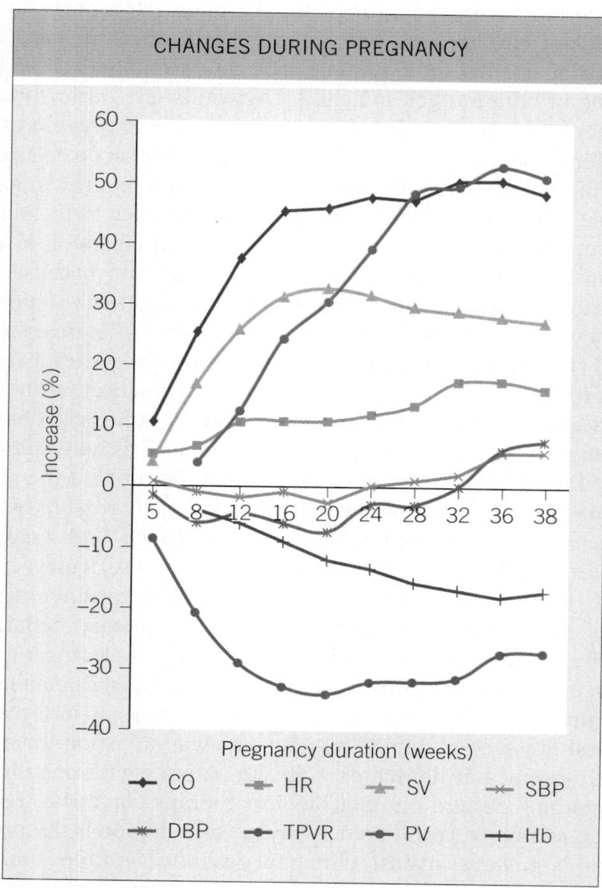

Figure 125D.1 Changes in cardiac output (CO), stroke volume (SV), plasma volume (PV), total peripheral vascular resistance (TPVR), heart rate (HR), blood pressure (SBP, systolic blood pressure; DBP, diastolic blood pressure), and hemoglobin concentration (Hb) during pregnancy.

TYPICAL CASE

A 30-year-old patient presented with shortness of breath and palpitations. She was 20 weeks pregnant and was known to have had a heart murmur in childhood, but she had not seen a physician in the last 20 years. On physical examination, we found a blood pressure of 160/80 mm Hg, a normal first heart sound, a loud systolic murmur over the second intercostal space–left sternal border, and a thrill over the precordium. The electrocardiogram showed an atrial tachycardia with a ventricular rate of 140 beats per minute. Echocardiography is the first diagnostic tool during pregnancy because it is safe and easily available. This investigation revealed

PREDICTORS OF MATERNAL COMPLICATIONS IN WOMEN WITH CONGENITAL HEART DISEASE

- History of cardiac event, such as stroke, transient ischemic attack, heart failure, or symptomatic arrhythmia
- New York Heart Association functional class >II or cyanosis (before pregnancy)
- Left-sided heart obstruction (mitral valve area <2 cm^2, aortic valve area <1.5 cm^2, or left ventricular outflow obstruction >30 mm Hg, measured with Doppler)
- Impaired systemic ventricular function (ejection fraction <40%)

Number of Risk Factors	Estimated Risk of Cardiac Events in Pregnancy
0	5%
1	27%
>1	75%

Modified from Siu SC, Sermer M, Harrison DA, et al. Risk and predictors for pregnancy-related complications in women with heart disease. Circulation 1997;96:2789-2794.

Table 125D.1 Predictors of maternal complications in women with congenital heart disease.

RISK FACTORS FOR ADVERSE FETAL OUTCOME IN WOMEN WITH CONGENITAL HEART DISEASE	
■ Maternal New York Heart Association functional class >II or cyanosis (before pregnancy) ■ Left-sided heart obstruction (mitral valve area <2 cm², aortic valve area <1.5 cm², or left ventricular outflow obstruction >30 mm Hg, measured with Doppler) ■ Smoking during pregnancy ■ Multiple gestations ■ Use of anticoagulation throughout pregnancy	
Number of Risk Factors	**Estimated Risk of Fetal or Neonatal Mortality**
0	2%
1 or more	4%
Modified from Siu SC, Sermer M, Colman JM, et al. Prospective multicenter study of pregnancy outcomes in women with heart disease. Circulation 2001;104:515-521.	

Table 125D.2 Risk factors for adverse fetal outcome in women with congenital heart disease.

a severe pulmonary stenosis at valvular level with an estimated gradient of 140 mm Hg.

Right-sided heart obstructions have been thought to be well tolerated during pregnancy. Indeed, maternal complications such as heart failure and arrhythmias are rare if the peak gradient before pregnancy is below 60 mm Hg. However, pulmonary valve stenosis is associated with an increased risk of premature labor (14%), premature delivery (15%), and intrauterine growth retardation (10%). The presence of preconceptional arrhythmias appears to be a major predictor of arrhythmias during pregnancy. This patient had not suffered from arrhythmias before. Pregnancy-related hypertensive disorders such as pregnancy-induced hypertension and preeclampsia are feared and potentially lethal conditions. The incidence of hypertensive disorders is increased in patients with aortic stenosis, pulmonary stenosis, aortic coarctation, and transposition of the great arteries.[7]

DIFFERENTIAL DIAGNOSIS

Children of mothers with heart disease are at increased risk for fetal and neonatal complications, such as preterm delivery (10% to 20%), premature delivery (with or without premature rupture of the membranes; 20%), growth retardation (8%), spontaneous abortions (12%), and respiratory distress syndrome (8%). Adverse neonatal outcome may occur in up to 30%. Overall fetal and neonatal mortality is approximately 4%, a fourfold increase in comparison with the general population.[7] In most women who are in functional class I and who experienced no complications during pregnancy, no additional peripartum actions are necessary. Epidural anesthesia has been suggested to reduce cardiovascular stress in some cases, but it must be used cautiously in patients with aortic or mitral stenosis and in patients with Eisenmenger's syndrome. The mode of delivery should be determined by obstetric reasons and the clinical status of the mother. No convincing data proclaiming either vaginal delivery or cesarean section have been reported. However, cesarean section leads to more blood loss at delivery; therefore, vaginal delivery seems preferable in most patients with heart disease, an exception being patients with Marfan's syndrome with dilatation of the ascending aorta, although this is still under debate. The puerperium is a period with further increase in volume overload and hypercoagulability. Patients at risk may develop heart failure, arrhythmias, or thrombotic events during this period. Thus, it is recommended to keep patients at risk in the hospital for 3 days post partum for clinical observation.

The overall risk of congenital heart disease in newborns with a first-degree relative with congenital heart disease is 3% and depends on the type of heart disease. In patients with a pulmonary stenosis, the risk of recurrence is about 5%; left ventricular outflow obstruction has a risk of up to 20%; and of course in the case of an autosomal dominant inherited syndrome, such as Marfan's syndrome, the recurrence rate is 50%.

TREATMENT OPTIONS

At first, treatment with bed rest and medication to reduce the ventricular rate and high blood pressure is advised. The use of cardiac medication during pregnancy is not always preventable and has a potential negative influence on fetal development. On the other hand, hemodynamic instability in the mother is also a threat for the fetus. All aspects must be taken into account, but a decision will often be made in favor of starting or continuing medication for the best well-being of both mother and child. Digoxin is safe during pregnancy; however, a higher dose is often required because of a larger plasma volume. Beta blockade also appears to be safe during pregnancy, with only mild effect on fetal growth and some effect on the fetal heart rate shortly after birth. Most experience is available with metoprolol and labetalol. Warfarin is contraindicated during the first trimester because of teratogenic effects; in addition, for the duration of pregnancy, it is associated with a higher incidence of miscarriage and stillbirth. Heparin is safe for the fetus but carries a substantial risk for the mother as a consequence of unstable anticoagulation levels. Low-molecular-weight heparins have been proved safe for various indications, such as lung emboli and thrombosis, during pregnancy; they do not pass the placenta and are safe for the fetus. However, in patients with mechanical heart valves, several case reports and smaller series of failure have been reported. During pregnancy, it is safe for the fetus to perform an electrical cardioversion. Our patient was treated with bed rest, digoxin, heparin, and a low dose of metoprolol (25 mg), and an electrical cardioversion was performed. However, although she remained in sinus rhythm (86 beats per minute) with an improved blood pressure of 140/80 mm Hg, she was still symptomatic with dyspnea at limited exercise. In patients with persistent symptoms despite optimal medical therapy, invasive treatment should be considered.[9] The use of radiation is the principal argument against percutaneous interventions during pregnancy; however, after the first trimester, the negative effect of radiation seems low. To keep the radiation dose as low as possible, echocardiographic techniques (transthoracic, transesophageal, or intracardiac echocardiography) can be used in addition to fluoroscopy.

Cardiac surgery can usually be avoided during pregnancy. Maternal mortality equals mortality in nonpregnant cardiac surgery, but fetal mortality risk is high, with an incidence of 20%. In our patient, balloon angioplasty was performed with a good result, lowering the gradient from 140 to 60 mm Hg (Fig. 125D.2). We deliberately did not choose to reach a lower gradient because during pregnancy, the risk of dissection or damage to the valve may be higher than outside pregnancy. Most interventional cardiac procedures produce a total radiation exposure to the woman of 1 to 10 mGy, with a dose to the fetus of only 1% to 2% of that total dose. Radiation risks to the fetus at a dose of less that 50 Gy have not been associated with any increase in fetal anomalies or pregnancy loss, and it would not be expected to materially increase the infant's risk of childhood cancers. However, it should be ensured that there are no other therapeutic maneuvers or imaging techniques that can be used rather than an x-ray-guided intervention, and techniques to minimize radiation exposure should be used.

After interventional treatment, our patient did well and could leave the hospital 1 day later. She was admitted again at 39 weeks of gestation and gave birth to a healthy girl through a vaginal delivery. She was observed in the hospital for 3 days and dismissed without further complications.

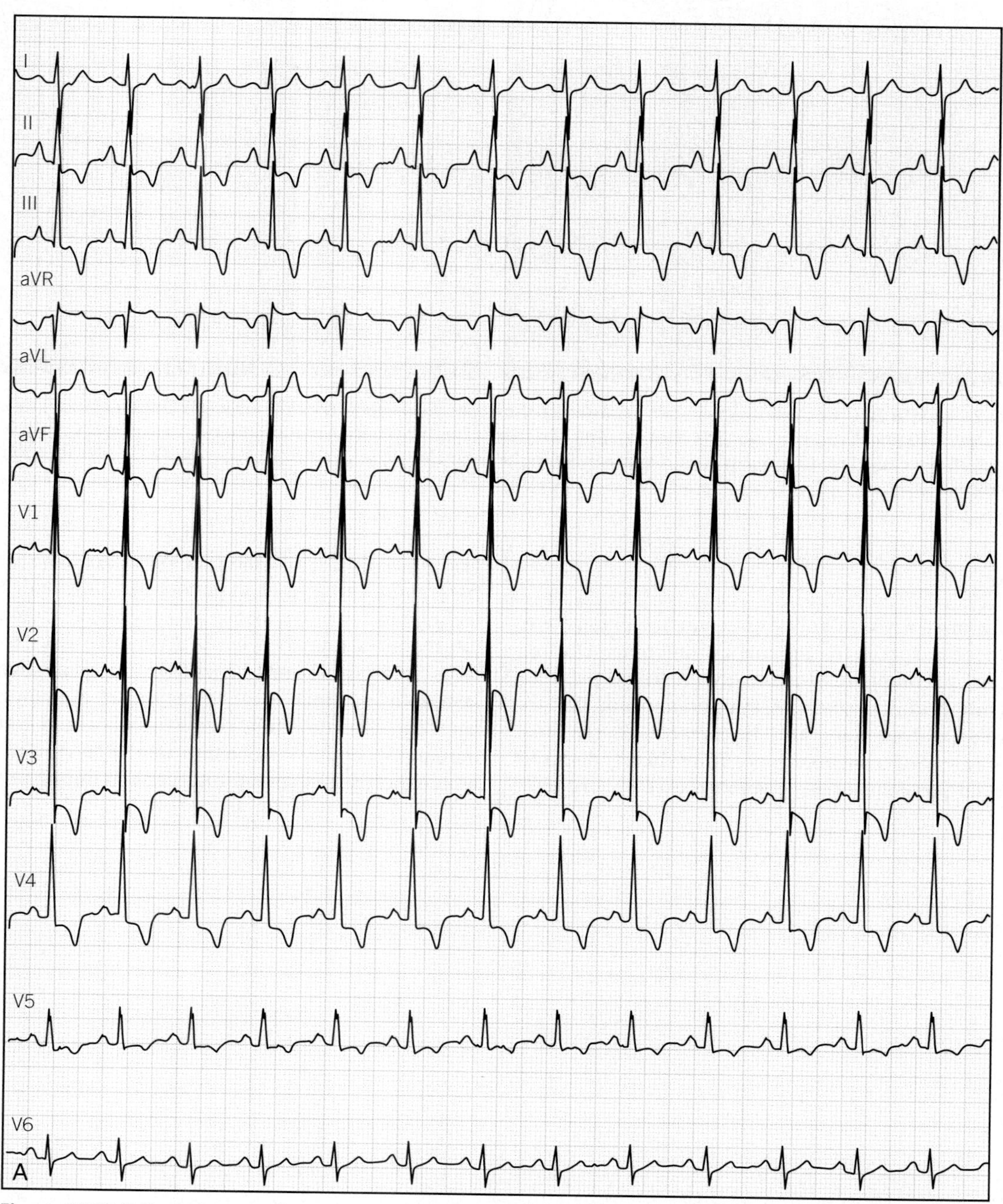

Figure 125D.2 Study images of a pregnant woman with severe pulmonic stenosis: **A,** electrocardiographic.

(*Continued*)

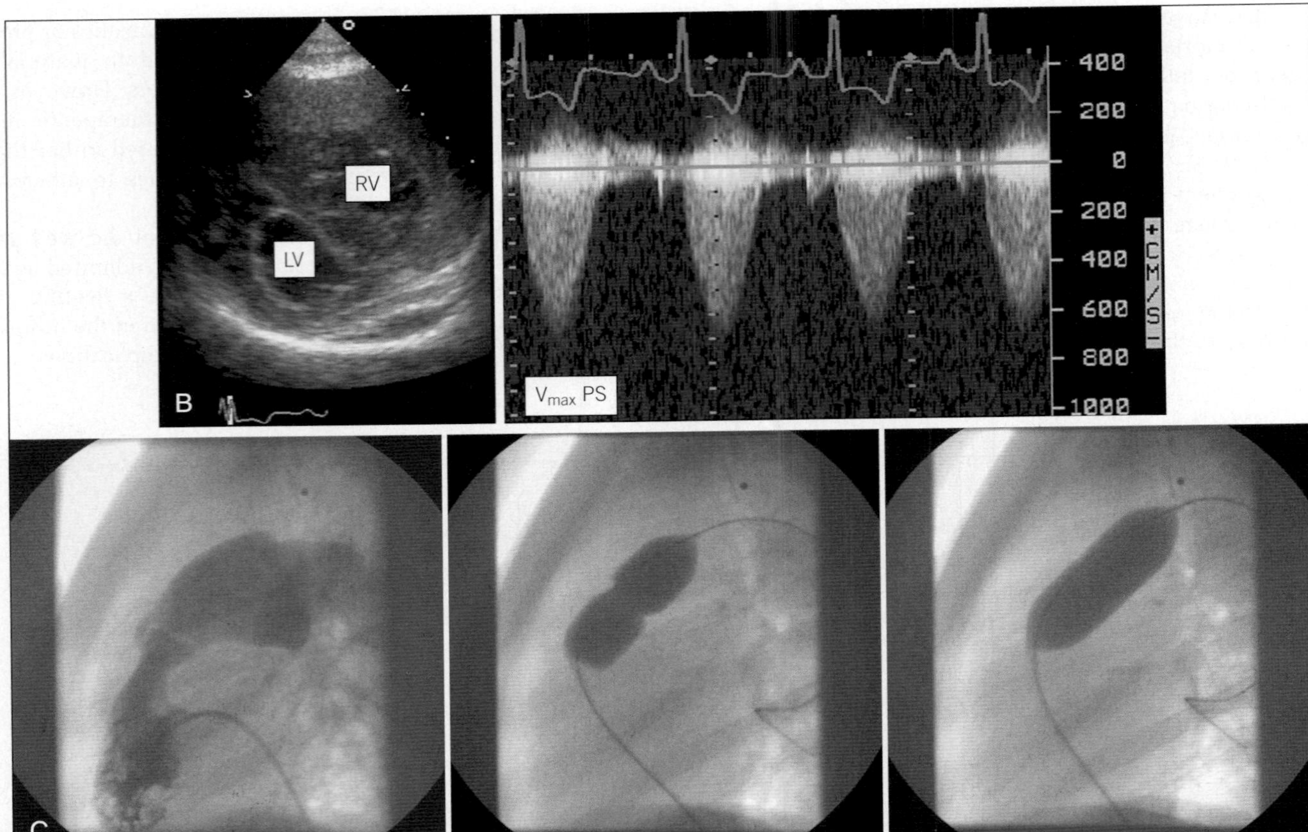

Figure 125D.2—cont'd B, echocardiographic (*left,* parasternal short-axis view; *right,* continuous-wave Doppler study); and **C,** angiographic *(left)*. The peak gradient was 144 mm Hg. She was treated with balloon dilatation during pregnancy (**C,** *middle* and *right*); the peak gradient decreased to 40 mm Hg after dilatation. RV, right ventricle; LV, left ventricle; V_{max}, maximal velocity (m/s) measured over the pulmonic valve.

SUMMARY

Optimizing a woman's health before pregnancy will improve the likelihood of a successful pregnancy outcome. During normal pregnancy, complaints such as dyspnea and palpitations may mimic cardiac disease. A systolic murmur due to the high cardiac output may also be present. It remains important to rule out congenital or other heart disease. When substantial problems occur, combined care of cardiologist, gynecologist, and anestheologist should be provided in tertiary care centers with experience in this field. Percutaneous techniques for valvular but also for coronary and arrhythmia intervention appear to carry acceptable risks to mother and fetus and significant benefit to pregnant women whose symptoms continue to be refractory to optimal medical management. The radiation risk to mother and fetus should be minimized, and the procedure should be carried out in teams with expertise in catheter intervention during pregnancy.

SECONDARY HEART DISEASE

SECTION

8

chapter

126 Chronic Kidney Disease

Dave C. Y. Chua and George L. Bakris

Summary

- Chronic kidney dysfunction is a cardiovascular disease risk equivalent.
- The two most common causes of cardiovascular disease in people with kidney disease are ischemic coronary artery disease and heart failure.
- Treatment of individuals with combined chronic kidney disease and ischemic coronary artery disease should be similar in patients with ischemic heart disease and normal kidney function.
- Therapeutic approaches in people with kidney disease are similar to those for high cardiovascular risk populations, with a focus on reducing albuminuria to allow easier fluid and edema management.
- It is very important to distinguish the primary cause of a patient presenting with symptoms of heart failure as to whether it is secondary to primary kidney disease with resultant hypoalbuminemia or primary myocardial muscle dysfunction with subsequent heart failure unrelated to kidney disease (i.e., normoalbuminemia).
- In general, the primary goal should be to lower LDL-cholesterol to values of less than 100 mg/dL and systolic blood pressure to less than 120 mm Hg. This, in addition to an aspirin a day, glucose control (hemoglobin A_{1c} <7%), and, when appropriate, angiotensin-converting enzyme inhibition, angiotensin receptor blockade, or aldosterone antagonism, could reduce the risk of a cardiovascular event by as much as 70% to 75%.

Chronic kidney disease (CKD) is traditionally defined as a glomerular filtration rate (GFR) of less than 60 mL/min/1.73 m^2 for 3 months or more irrespective of the presence or absence of kidney damage. A growing public health concern, CKD is an increasingly common, serious, and underrecognized condition, clinically manifested as an elevation in the serum creatinine level above the normal range (≥1.2 mg/dL in women or ≥1.4 mg/dL in men). This laboratory abnormality along with either a decrease in albumin (<3.5 g/L) or the presence of macroalbuminuria (>300 mg per gram creatinine) clearly indicates kidney dysfunction. Note that microalbuminuria (>30 to <300 mg per gram creatinine) is a cardiovascular risk marker and does not necessarily indicate kidney dysfunction unless it continues to increase over time to more than 300 mg per gram creatinine in a spot morning urine collection.

CKD and cardiovascular disease (CVD) are linked. Traditional cardiovascular risk factors, such as hypertension, smoking history, diabetes, dyslipidemia, and older age, are highly prevalent in individuals with CKD, and the number of cardiovascular risk factors is associated with the severity of kidney dysfunction.[1,2] Among patients with documented CVD, concurrent kidney disease correlated with a relatively worse outcome. Mild to moderate CKD independently predicted an adverse cardiovascular prognosis, even among community-based populations not originally selected for increased risk of CVD.[1,3] The risk of death, particularly from a cardiovascular cause, is much greater than the risk of eventually requiring kidney replacement therapy (dialysis).[3] About half of all deaths observed in people with end-stage renal disease (ESRD) requiring dialysis are attributable to cardiovascular causes.[4,5] The major causes that contribute to the development of heart disease in CKD patients are summarized in Figure 126.1.

CVD is frequently a preexisting condition in ESRD patients who start dialysis, and it undoubtedly contributes to the excessive morbidity and mortality observed in this population. Data from the United States Renal Data Service (USRDS) 2007 indicate that almost 50% of patients starting dialysis have structural cardiac abnormalities, ischemic heart disease, or heart failure that is predictive of future cardiovascular events.[4,6] From 2001 to 2004, death rate remains flat in the first year of hemodialysis; however, a significant decline has been noted in subsequent years.[5] Among ESRD patients 65 years and older, mortality rates are six times higher than in the general population.[5] Since 1985, mortality rates in patients who have had ESRD less than 2 years have fallen 27%, whereas rates for older patients (5 years or more) have increased 7%. Five years after a diagnosis of heart disease, the probability of survival in dialysis patients is only 18% compared with 64% in the general population.[5] In a 3-year prospective study of 1609 dialysis patients, the relative risk of myocardial infarction was 2.1 compared with age-matched controls.[7] Moreover, patients entering dialysis programs were observed to mortality from cardiovascular causes at 10.1 times that of the corresponding general population; this increased to 44 times among patients with diabetes.[8]

CKD alone is an independent risk factor for the development of CVD.[9] Furthermore, CVD can also result from the use of kidney replacement therapy because of enhanced oxidative stress and the production of proinflammatory factors.[10] Available evidence indicates that similar cardiovascular outcomes are likely with either peritoneal dialysis or hemodialysis among ESRD patients without preexisting CVD. The USRDS 2007 reported that the relative risk of

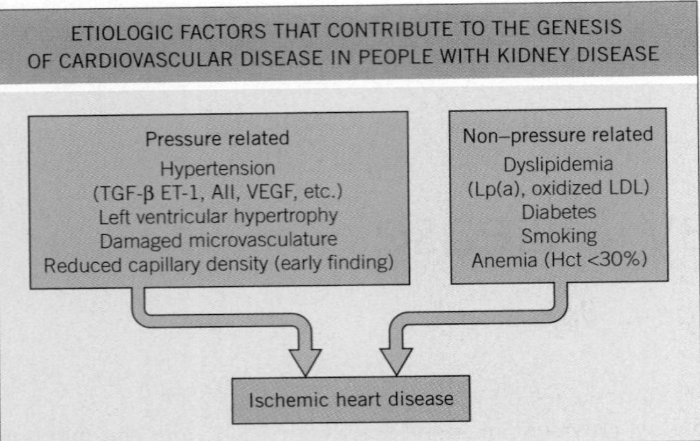

Figure 126.1 Etiologic factors that contribute to the genesis of cardiovascular disease in people with kidney disease. AII, angiotensin II; ET-1, endothelin 1; Hct, hematocrit; LDL, low-density lipoprotein; Lp(a), lipoprotein(a); TGF-β, transforming growth factor β; VEGF, vascular endothelial growth factor.

death due to coronary artery disease (CAD) in peritoneal dialysis is 1.3 compared with hemodialysis; relative risk of death from other cardiac causes is 1.08. Based on the high absolute risk of death from CVD, peritoneal dialysis patients should be considered the highest risk category (or similar to those on hemodialysis). In a Canadian study, peritoneal dialysis patients developed de novo heart failure at a lower incidence than did those on hemodialysis (16.5% peritoneal dialysis versus 28.1% hemodialysis; $P < .05$). It is notable that the hemodialysis patients had a higher prevalence of hypoalbuminemia. In the United States, CVD annual mortality was similar between these two populations (9.5%); however, peritoneal dialysis patients had 30% greater relative risk of death from myocardial infarction.[11]

CKD and CVD go hand in hand. There are two ways to view the interaction between these organ systems. The first is in the context of diseases that largely affect the heart (and to a variable degree the kidney), such as hypertension leading to heart failure. In these cases, the reduction in kidney function is due to a decline in cardiac output. Conversely, a different situation exists when primary kidney disease is present, that is, diabetes with resultant hypoalbuminemia. The kidney is unable to eliminate volume properly as a consequence of decreased oncotic pressure, whereby pulmonary edema results. Although this example may resemble the clinical presentation of heart failure, it is primarily due to kidney disease with the possible presence of diastolic dysfunction. Moreover, whereas treatment for both scenarios requires diuretics, it is not uncommon for dialysis to be required for volume removal in the latter.

ISCHEMIC HEART DISEASE

EPIDEMIOLOGY

The risk of CVD among patients with kidney dysfunction is far greater than that in the general population. The National Health and Nutrition Examination Survey reported CVD-related mortality rates of 4.1, 8.6, and 20.5 deaths per 1000 person-years among participants with estimated GFRs of more than 90, between 70 and 89, and less than 70 mL/min/1.73 m², respectively.[12] Compared with subjects with estimated GFRs of 90 mL/min/1.73 m² or higher, those with estimated GFRs below 70 mL/min/1.73 m² had significantly higher relative risks of cardiovascular deaths (1.7; 95% CI, 1.3-2.1).

In an analysis of the U.S. Medicare system, outcomes were reported for several groups, including those with CKD but no diabetes (2.2%) and those with both CKD and diabetes (1.6%).[3] At 2-year follow-up, the rates for requiring dialysis therapy were 1.6 per 100 patient-years for patients with kidney dysfunction alone and 3.4 per 100 patient-years for those with both CKD and diabetes; by comparison, the death rates were 17.7 and 19.9 per 100 patient-years, respectively. In the USRDS, after stratification by age, gender, race, and presence or absence of diabetes, cardiovascular mortality in dialysis patients is 10 to 20 times higher than in the general population.[13] More than 50% of CKD patients die within 5 years of dialysis initiation (Fig. 126.2). The most common causes of death are listed in Table 126.1.

The risk factors associated with a greater likelihood of CVD in kidney dysfunction are similar to those in non-kidney disease. Traditional cardiovascular risk factors, such as hypertension (which may be accompanied by left ventricular hypertrophy), smoking history, diabetes, dyslipidemia, and older age, are highly prevalent.[1,3,14] In addition, these patients are more likely to have the metabolic syndrome, which contributes to an increase in cardiovascular risk.[15] When Stack and Bloembergen[16] evaluated new dialysis patients in the United States, CAD was present in 38% and associated with white race, higher age, male gender, diabetes mellitus, smoking, higher residual kidney function, higher hematocrit, lower albumin levels, vascular comorbid conditions, and structural cardiac abnormalities; no association could be found with cholesterol concentration, triglyceride levels, and hypertension.

The most common cause of CKD in the Western world is diabetes. However, these individuals frequently die of cardiovascular events, even before the development of ESRD. In a study of more than 12,000 older patients with diabetes, 48% had kidney disease defined as a GFR of less than 60 mL/min/1.73 m² or proteinuria. At 3-year follow-up, mortality rates were 6%, 10%, 20%, and 30% for patients with CKD stages 2, 3, 4, and 5, respectively, compared with 5% for those with preserved kidney function at baseline. Progression to ESRD was much slower, less than 1% for stages 2 and 3 and 14% for stage 4.[17] Among enrollees in the HEMO trial, 40% had CAD that was strongly associated with diabetes, although traditional risk factors such as smoking, systolic blood pressure, and total cholesterol concentration were not.[4] Screened before kidney transplantation, as many as 30% to 50% of asymptomatic or mildly symptomatic patients with diabetes were found to have CAD.[18]

Even new-onset CKD correlates with CAD, and higher cardiovascular mortality has been reported in subjects not on dialysis (see Fig. 126.1). In a historical cohort of 281 patients with normal baseline kidney function and hypertension observed for 13 years, the 41 patients (15%) who developed CKD were significantly more likely to experience an acute myocardial infarction, angina, heart failure, stroke, or cardiovascular death compared with those with preserved

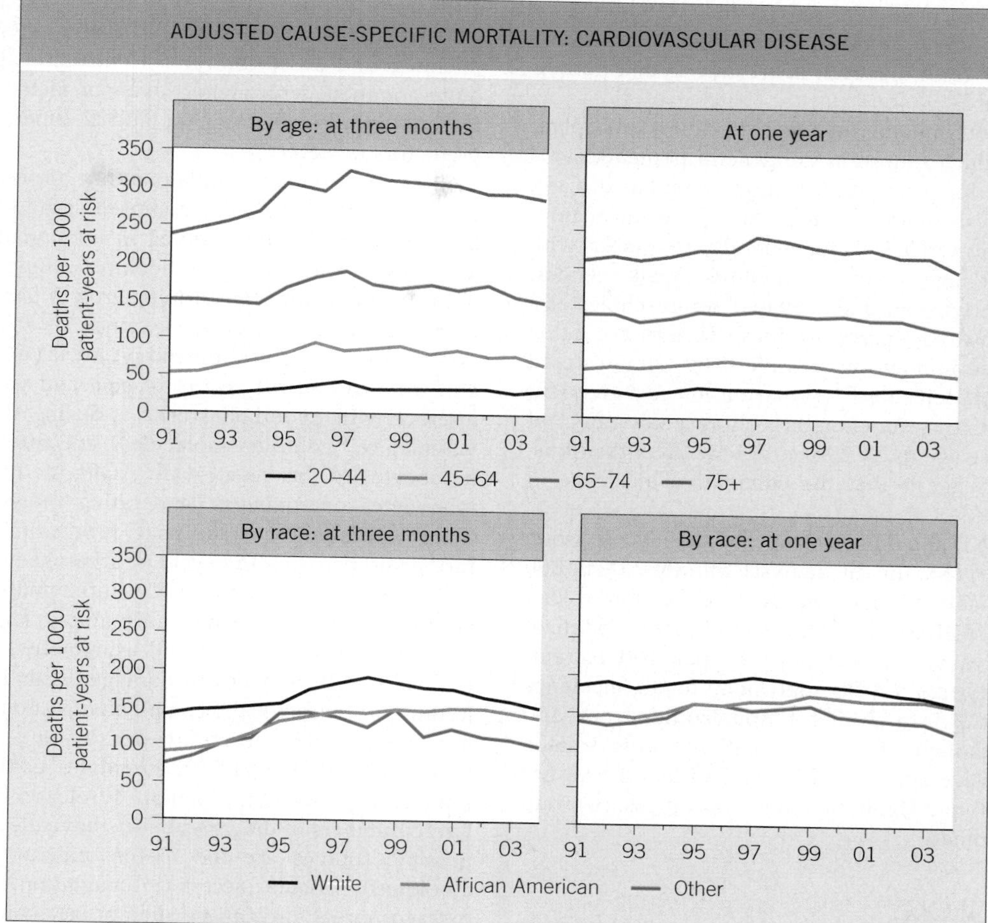

Figure 126.2 Adjusted cause-specific mortality: cardiovascular disease. Note that more than 50% of patients die within 5 years of starting dialysis. (Data from United States Renal Data Service 2007.)

MOST COMMON CAUSES OF DEATH AMONG PATIENTS WITH CHRONIC KIDNEY INSUFFICIENCY, EITHER RECEIVING OR NOT RECEIVING DIALYSIS	
Heart failure	31.2%
Myocardial infarction	15.6%
Sepsis	11.3%
Withdrawal from dialysis	5.2%
Strokes	6.4%
Malignant neoplasm	3.8%
Other	26.5%

Table 126.1 Most common causes of death among patients with chronic kidney insufficiency, either receiving or not receiving dialysis.

kidney function.[19] With multivariate analysis, the development of CKD was the most significant independent risk factor for the appearance of a cardiovascular event (hazard ratio [HR], 2.5; 95% CI, 1.3-4.8).

In a multicenter study of patients with stage 3 CKD (mean GFR, 36 mL/min) not on dialysis, the prevalence of CVD was 46%, with a 20% incidence of cardiovascular events during mean follow-up of 23 months.[20] Age and diabetes were the best predictors of events in patients without preexisting CVD. In those with preexisting CVD, predictors of progression were low diastolic blood pressure and high triglyceride levels. CVD at baseline and low diastolic blood pressure were predictors for change in New York Heart Association and Canadian Cardiovascular Society angina classification. The presence of CVD itself was found to confer a 50% increase in probability of kidney replacement therapy, but impaired kidney function had no impact on CVD.

The incidence of de novo CAD was 3.6% per year in dialysis patients,[12] whereas the risk of left ventricular hypertrophy in kidney disease was higher than in the general population and inversely proportional with the level of kidney function[21]: approximately 25% for creatinine clearance values above 50 mL/min and 50% for clearances below 25 mL/min. The USRDS estimated that in patients who recently started dialysis, 75% have left ventricular hypertrophy and 40% have CAD.[13]

Long-term survival studies of hemodialysis subjects clearly demonstrate that CVD plays a crucial role in CKD morbidity and mortality. In a study of 17 survivors receiving hemodialysis an average of 21 years, Owen and colleagues[22] compared their demographic and clinical characteristics and discovered that these patients had presented with and maintained a low cardiovascular risk profile. Family history for CVD was low (25%), about half had hypertension, and there was an absence of diabetes, heart failure, and peripheral vascular disease.

Likewise, the determinants of CVD in kidney transplant recipients are similar to those in the general population.[1,23] After accounting for pretransplantation vascular disease, multivariate analysis demonstrated that post-transplantation atherosclerotic CVD is independently associated with increasing patient age, diabetes mellitus, male gender, tobacco use, hypertension, and elevated serum cholesterol concentration. However, many of these factors are often exacerbated by the immunosuppressive drugs administered to prevent allograft rejection.[24] Hypertension is a frequent consequence of graft dysfunction as well as a side effect of immunosuppressive agents. A 15-year follow-up of the transplant population suggests that the cumulative incidence of CAD is about 23%.

Patients with CKD should be considered the highest group for cardiovascular risk. In an analysis of more than 800 people with nondiabetic CKD from the Modification of Diet in Renal Disease (MDRD) trial,[25] the rate of first hospitalizations due to all causes was 10.5 to 12 per 100 patient-years; 25% were from CVD, equivalent to an incidence of approximately 2.5 to 3 first hospitalizations per 100 patient-years. Although 91% of the patients were treated with antihypertensive agents, only 54% had blood pressure of less than 140/90 mm Hg. In fact, this lower pressure group had the best outcomes.

PATHOPHYSIOLOGY

Ischemic heart disease most commonly results from atherosclerosis of the coronary arteries. However, up to a quarter of patients with myocardial infarctions have nonatherosclerotic CAD.[26] Figure 126.1 illustrates both pressure- and non–pressure-related factors that contribute to the development of ischemic CAD in CKD; these factors are interrelated and can further accelerate the atherosclerotic process in kidney dysfunction. It is for this reason that CKD is considered a CAD risk equivalent.[1]

Both uremia and dialysis therapy markedly enhance oxidant stress through the production of proinflammatory complement fragments, cytokines, and increased adhesion molecules in endothelial cells.[10] Central to the pathobiology of atherosclerosis is alteration in vascular reactivity and endothelial dysfunction. Once endothelial injury has occurred, the ability of blood vessels to vasodilate in response to normal stimuli is lost. In extreme cases when the endothelium is partially denuded secondary to severe atherosclerosis, cytokines and other factors directly stimulate rapid vascular smooth muscle cell proliferation and hypertrophy, leading to further narrowing of the arterial luminal diameter.[27] Hence, endothelial dysfunction begets cardiac and arterial remodeling with resultant cardiovascular events.

Subjects receiving kidney replacement therapy have impaired forearm reactive (postischemic) hyperemia, and this derangement correlated significantly to markers of endothelial dysfunction (elevated levels of plasminogen activator inhibitor 1, reduced fibrinolysis, hypoalbuminemia, alteration in blood viscosity and red cell structure) as well as to markers of cardiovascular remodeling (enhancement in left ventricular mass and common carotid artery intima-media thickness and distensibility).[28] Hemostatic abnormalities are quite common, with higher levels of factor VII, fibrinogen, plasmin-antiplasmin complex, and D-dimer, all independent predictors of CAD.[29]

CKD may enhance inflammatory processes because of decreased clearance or increased production of factors directly or indirectly involved in inflammation. The serum levels of interleukin 1, interleukin 6, tumor necrosis factor α, hyaluronan, and transforming growth factor β1 have been correlated with creatinine clearance.[30,31] Also, the generation of advanced glycation end products (AGEs) is increased, and they can accrue in the plasma and vasculature. AGEs interact with endothelial cells, inducing the expression of vascular cell adhesion molecule 1 and attracting circulating monocytes to the vessel wall. AGEs then interact with the monocytes-macrophages, generating oxygen free radicals, thereby promoting additional production of AGEs and further propagating the cycle of atherogenesis.[32]

Potentially important in the inflammatory cascade and ensuing cardiovascular mortality among kidney patients are C-reactive protein (CRP) and asymmetric dimethylarginine (ADMA). CRP attaches to damaged cells in atherosclerotic lesions and activates the complement system, increases binding and aggregation of low-density and very-low-density lipoproteins (LDL, VLDL), stimulates tissue factor production, and activates interleukin 6 release from neutrophils. Large numbers of dialysis subjects have elevated CRP levels; possible sources are the uremic milieu (proinflammatory cytokines), vascular access (inflammation or infection), and extracorporeal circulation (membrane bioincompatibility or dialysate-related endotoxinemia). Elevated levels of CRP are associated with erythropoietin resistance, hypoalbuminemia, malnutrition, decreased high-density lipoprotein (HDL) concentration, raised lipoprotein(a) and fibrinogen levels, and oxidized LDL.[30,33] ADMA, a novel biochemical marker of endothelial dysfunction, is an endogenous nitric oxide synthase inhibitor. ADMA concentrations have been found to be elevated at early stages of kidney disease despite a normal-range GFR.[34] The importance of ADMA was highlighted by findings that either ADMA or CRP separately predicted intima-media thickness changes in the common carotid artery of dialysis patients, whereas their interaction was proven to be the sole independent predictor of this progression.[35]

CKD induces sympathetic nervous system hyperactivation by signals from the failing kidneys that travel through afferent kidney nerves to cardiovascular centers in the brainstem, resulting in the development of hypertension, progressive cardiovascular alterations (left ventricular hypertrophy and arterial remodeling), and atherogenesis leading to increased CVD morbidity and mortality.[36] This is particularly enhanced in the diabetic subpopulation. When Giordano and colleagues[37] examined diabetic and nondiabetic subjects receiving dialysis therapy, both groups had sympathetic hyperactivity in the predialysis period. After dialysis sessions, however, diabetic patients remained as if in the predialytic state, whereas nondiabetics were observed to have parasympathetic activation. Bilateral nephrectomy appears to normalize the increased sympathetic activity in both dialysis patients and kidney transplant recipients.[38]

Abnormalities in lipid metabolism also occur with varying degrees of CKD, with dialysis, and after kidney transplantation. Subjects with nephrotic syndrome have marked elevations in plasma cholesterol, triglyceride, and lipoprotein(a) concentrations; total HDL levels are often normal or reduced, with an obvious decline in the cardioprotective HDL2 fraction[39] due to a combination of enhanced hepatic synthesis and diminished kidney clearance. Lipoprotein(a) is an LDL-like particle with an additional protein apolipoprotein(a) that is thought to be an independent predictor of atherosclerosis.[40] For some dialysis patients, total cholesterol level may sometimes be normal or low secondary to chronic inflammation or malnutrition.[30,33] Aside from the accumulation of small, dense LDL and large chylomicron remnants, CKD decreases serum apolipoproteins A-I and A-II while increasing the circulation of complement factors C1, C2, and C3. C3 inhibits the activity of lipoprotein lipase, leading to the defective catabolism of lipoproteins, although other compound disorders have been described.[41] Furthermore, immunosuppressive therapy after kidney transplantation can also induce lipid abnormalities.[24]

In a 9-year observational study of 412 diabetic patients starting dialysis, 44% of patients died; they had considerably lower levels of apolipoprotein A-I and increased levels of fibrinogen.[42] Incidentally, type 2 diabetics had a lower mean survival time than did type 1 diabetics (34 versus 66 months; $P < .0006$). Moreover, Bommer and colleagues[43] observed that the atherosclerotic burden in 84 chronic hemodialysis subjects was comparable to that of controls who were 20 years older. Major correlates included high VLDL level, low HDL level, duration of hypertriglyceridemia, and level of VLDL-cholesterol as well as elevated parathyroid hormone (PTH) levels.

Secondary hyperparathyroidism is believed to impair energy production, transfer, and use by the myocardium, making it more susceptible to hypoxic injury. Studies in uremic animals demonstrated a reduced phosphocreatine–adenosine triphosphate ratio under hypoxic stress.[44] In addition, elevated PTH plays a key role in vascular calcification and atherogenesis through suppression of lipoprotein-regulating enzymes. In a Japanese study using electron beam computed tomography, the progressive coronary artery calcification correlated with higher triglyceride and lower HDL levels but not with other lipoprotein, calcium, or phosphate abnormalities.[45] However, in young dialysis patients, calcification was 17.5 times greater than in the general population and associated with time on dialysis, calcium × phosphate product, and use of calcium phosphate binders.[24] Postmortem examination of coronary lesions from uremic patients revealed increased media thickness and marked calcification, whereas those of patients without uremia were mostly fibroatheromatous. Although there was a trend toward higher intima thickness, no difference was found in plaque size between the groups.[46]

Another factor that contributes to CAD in subjects with kidney dysfunction is hypertension. Hypertension is the "gasoline" to the "fire" (lipid abnormalities) contributing to atherosclerosis progression. Factors that contribute to the development of hypertension include sodium and volume retention, oxidative stress, activation of the renin-angiotensin-aldosterone system (RAAS), sympathetic hyperactivity, secondary hyperparathyroidism, and erythropoietin therapy as well as the use of immunosuppressive agents after kidney transplantation. In animal models of CKD, cells are extracted and exposed to varying degrees of stretch.[47] This resulted in marked increases in growth factors that culminate in the development of left ventricular hypertrophy and further narrowing of vessel lumens because most growth factors are vasoconstrictors. The absence of nocturnal drops in blood pressure (non-dipping) is prevalent in more than 50% of dialysis patients.[48] This has been associated with left ventricular dilatation or dysfunction; it is thought to be secondary to uremic disturbances in aortic and carotid baroreflexes mediated through arterial intima-media thickness, arterial calcifications, and arterial stiffness. Studies have shown that arterial stiffness was an independent predictor of all-cause and CVD mortality; pulse pressure (related to arterial compliance and distensibility) was found to be greater in dialysis patients and correlated with cardiac mass.[49,50]

In the absence of critical CAD, ischemic symptoms may result from a reduction in coronary vasodilator reserve (atherosclerosis or left ventricular hypertrophy) or altered myocardial oxygen delivery (anemia). In general, ESRD patients display reduced exercise tolerance. This was reflected by reduced peak exercise oxygen uptake, which was significantly associated with male sex, low hemoglobin concentration, increased age, and diabetes but not with resting blood pressure, carnitine levels, or adequacy of dialysis.[51]

CLINICAL PRESENTATION

The clinical manifestations of CAD in kidney dysfunction are as varied as in the general population. Whereas many present with typical exercise-induced angina, the most common presentation is angina due to hypotension accompanying hemodialysis. Dialysis sessions stimulate cardiac work and oxygen demand with tachycardia and increased contractility but also produce hypotension, increase in hemoglobin-oxygen affinity, and reduction in blood Po_2, facilitating angina.[11] The incidence of silent ischemia is unknown, although thought to be high, particularly in diabetics.[18]

CKD patients have higher mortality rates from CAD. Forty-two percent of myocardial infarctions occur before initiation of dialysis; 29% occur within 1 year and 52% within 2 years of dialysis initiation. Among kidney transplant recipients, the incidence of myocardial infarction was 15% for the first year and 29% within 2 years after transplantation.[52] Although non–Q wave myocardial infarction was the most common presentation (80%), significantly higher in-hospital mortality was noted with transmural, anterior, and acute inferior events.

If a myocardial infarction occurs in someone during the first year of dialysis therapy, mortality is 53% compared with 25% in the non–kidney population. The mortality rate increases to 73% during the second year and 90% after 5 years.[11,53] Patients with advanced kidney failure (GFR ≤46 mL/min) had worse prognosis for in-hospital outcomes and 5-year follow-up mortality compared with those on dialysis.[54] This excess mortality correlated with arrhythmias, hemodynamic events, lower use of beta blockers, and decreased use of reperfusion therapy (angioplasty or thrombolysis). Thrombolytic therapy was associated with 33% reduction of all-cause mortality, but only 0.6% of patients received this treatment or underwent coronary revascularization.

DIAGNOSTIC TECHNIQUES

Guidelines by the National Kidney Foundation committee on cardiovascular disease in patients with kidney insufficiency have noted the following:

- The prevalence of asymptomatic CAD is 20% to 40% among people with CKD.
- Routine screening for inducible ischemia is not recommended in CKD without clinical manifestations of CVD.
- It is reasonable to use the screening guidelines recommended for the general population before noncardiac surgery in CKD patients.

Screening is recommended when the combinations of risk factors and the nature of the surgery place the patient at moderate risk for acute coronary events. The National Kidney Foundation Kidney Disease Outcomes Quality Initiative (KDOQI) also suggests that *all* patients, particularly kidney transplant candidates, undergo screening at the initiation of dialysis regardless of symptoms.[54] Many noninvasive methods are available to evaluate for the presence of CAD; Table 126.2 is a summary of the sensitivity and specificity of the most commonly used screening tests.

Comparative study of the noninvasive testing in patients receiving kidney replacement therapy found that angina pectoris had the best prognostic value for diagnosis of CAD.[55] Electrocardiographic stress testing, especially in dialysis subjects, is often of limited value, as kidney dysfunction causes resting electrocardiographic abnormalities because of the existence of left ventricular hypertrophy and electrolyte disorders. Also, many of these individuals are unable to exercise adequately because of anemia, polyneuropathy, cardiodepressant medications, and poor physical tolerance. ST depression during hemodialysis is an independent predictor of cardiac mortality.[56] During a 1-year follow-up, this finding had 46% sensitivity and 96% specificity in predicting cardiac events.

A number of studies have been performed to examine the use of noninvasive cardiac imaging and exercise stress testing either alone or in the presence of various pharmacologic stimulators of ischemia. It is noteworthy that the accuracy of the different imaging modalities may be center specific and dependent on the examiner's expertise.[18] Overall, the risk of precipitating unstable angina or myocardial infarction by stress testing appears to be fairly low.

Few data exist concerning the use of computer-aided tomography to detect coronary artery calcification in dialysis patients. The National Kidney Foundation consensus is that further study is required.

One of the most widely available methods currently used for CAD assessment is dipyridamole-thallium testing. With a 98% negative prognostic value, this test can effectively rule out significant CAD.[18,56] Unfortunately, CKD causes baseline abnormalities on thallium scintigraphy by alterations of the metabolic milieu.[57] The combination of dipyridamole infusion and exercise thallium stress imaging may provide increased accuracy. Dahan and colleagues[58] found that compared with coronary angiography, this technique had a sensitivity of 92%, a specificity of 89%, and an overall accuracy of 90% for detection of CAD in asymptomatic hemodialysis patients. Moreover, they also observed that after a median 2.8-year follow-up, 47% of the patients with an abnormal thallium uptake experienced a coronary event compared with only 9% of those who had a normal study (risk ratio of 9.2).

Serial echocardiography has prognostic value in dialysis patients for developing cardiac failure. Baseline left ventricular mass index and its change after 1 year on dialysis therapy, baseline cavity volume, and fall in fractional shortening were all associated with heart failure independent of factors like anemia and hypertension. However, neither CAD nor mortality correlated with these echocardiographic changes.[59]

Better results have been reported with dobutamine stress echocardiography. When it is used as part of a preoperative evaluation before listing for kidney transplantation, dobutamine stress echocardiography had a sensitivity of 95% (92% for one-vessel disease, 100% for disease of two or more vessels), specificity of 86%, and accuracy of 90% for the detection of CAD as well as the ability to identify a very low risk population.[60] Combined with a negative clinical cardiac evaluation, dobutamine stress echocardiography has a negative predictive value of 92%, suggesting that this tool serves as a noninvasive, low-cost screening alternative to coronary angiography in patients before kidney transplantation.[61] As such, the KDOQI guidelines have identified dobutamine stress echocardiography to be the noninvasive cardiac screening modality of choice if it is available.[54]

Coronary angiography is considered the "gold standard" for diagnosis of CAD. According to the American Society of Transplantation, angiography is not required for younger patients (younger than 50 years, without diabetes, without symptoms suggesting CAD or heart failure, and with normal

SENSITIVITY AND SPECIFICITY OF NONINVASIVE TESTS FOR CLINICAL EVALUATION OF CORONARY HEART DISEASE IN KIDNEY PATIENTS

Methods or Symptoms	Sensitivity (%)	Specificity (%)
Angina pectoris	65	66
Resting electrocardiography	67	52
In asymptomatic patients	60	61
In symptomatic patients	70	36
Exercise electrocardiography	30	100
In asymptomatic patients	100	0
In symptomatic patients	33	100
ST depression during dialysis	46	96
Echocardiography	38	92
In asymptomatic patients	100	14
In symptomatic patients	79	52
Dobutamine stress echocardiography	69-95	71-86
Dipyridamole-thallium scintigraphy	80-92	37-85

Table 126.2 Sensitivity and specificity of noninvasive tests for clinical evaluation of coronary heart disease in kidney patients.

electrocardiogram) because this method has to be reserved for high-risk patients.[18,24,62] Coronary angiography is indicated in symptomatic coronary heart disease that does not respond to medical therapy, in signs of ischemia at low exercise or low blood pressure, and in silent ischemia. If angiography is performed, the National Kidney Foundation recommends the administration of iso-osmolar radiocontrast media with a minimal amount of contrast material given and adequate hydration with intravenous half-normal saline with 2 ampules of sodium bicarbonate added before the procedure.[54]

Cardiac troponin T (cTnT) and cardiac troponin I (cTnI) are important serologic markers for the detection of myocardial injury in acute coronary syndromes. Among dialysis patients, acute events are more frequent when both troponins are increased (cTnI is suggested for diagnosis of myocardial infarction). It is notable that troponin levels, especially cTnT, are elevated in dialysis patients independent of CAD because of concentric and eccentric hypertrophy, water overload, myocardial fibrosis, decreased arterial compliance, and intima-media hypertrophy, all of them resulting in release of small amounts of intracellular proteins into the circulation. Hence, cTnT has been suggested as a long-term predictor of all-cause and cardiac mortality, alone or in combination with history of heart failure requiring hospitalization (stronger prediction). cTnI is found increased less commonly than cTnT is, possibly as a result of different modifications (in clearance rate or in relation to detection assay) during uremia. Dialysis session increases cTnT and decreases cTnI (adsorption of cTnI onto the membrane or antigenic alteration). Sensitivity and specificity values differ among studies; cTnT seems to display more ability and accuracy for the prognosis of future adverse outcomes and for exclusion (high negative predictive value) of this evaluation in dialysis patients.[63,64]

MANAGEMENT

The National Kidney Foundation, the American College of Cardiology, and the American Heart Association recommend that CKD be considered a cardiovascular risk equivalent; treatment of individuals with kidney disease and CAD should be similar to treatment of those without kidney dysfunction.[1] Data from the Choices for Healthy Outcomes in Caring for ESRD (CHOICE) study indicate that a large percentage of incident dialysis patients have the traditional risk factors for CAD, including hypertension (96%), low serum HDL-cholesterol concentration (33%), diabetes (54%), left ventricular hypertrophy by electrocardiographic criteria (22%), and increased age, with the average age of patients at the commencement of dialysis being nearly 60 years.[65]

Therapeutic interventions include risk factor reduction, antiplatelet therapy (aspirin), aggressive lipid management, blood pressure control, correction of anemia if it is present (hematocrit <30%), and possible coronary revascularization. It is notable that earlier treatment, particularly in the asymptomatic phases of CAD or before the development of irreversible structural changes, can be extremely beneficial. Moreover, a goal hematocrit between 33% and 36% is preferred—per national guidelines—because normalization of hematocrit (42%) increased mortality in patients with preexisting cardiac disease.[54,66] Perhaps the two most important factors known to reduce CAD risk in patients with kidney dysfunction are aggressive lipid-lowering therapy and tight blood pressure reduction.

Hypertension

Hypertension in kidney patients is associated with an increased cardiovascular risk; the treatment of even mild hypertension protects against *both* progressive kidney failure and CVD. For subjects of dialysis therapy, however, it is unclear when the appropriate time to measure target blood pressure is or what the preferred antihypertensive agents are to avoid the risk of intradialytic hypotension or other symptoms. Thus, until further information is available, it seems reasonable to use the predialysis blood pressure as a target blood pressure for antihypertensive therapy. One particular exception is in patients symptomatic from hypotension during the dialysis that cannot be corrected with adjustments in dialysis technique.

Hypertension is not optimally controlled in the general population and even less so in patients with CKD.[67] Moreover, this lack of aggressive blood pressure reduction has failed to alter the incidence of ESRD during the past quarter-century (Fig. 126.3). Among patients receiving kidney replacement therapy, blood pressure is better controlled on peritoneal dialysis than on hemodialysis because of factors of better volume control. Unlike in the general population, nonpharmacologic interventions are not as useful as is good

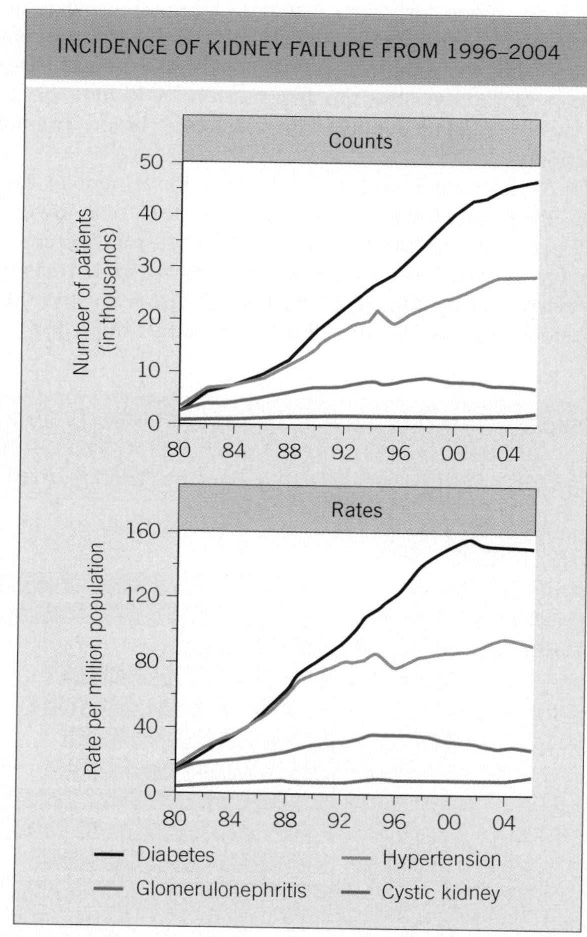

Figure 126.3 Incidence of kidney failure from 1996 to 2004. (Data from United States Renal Data Service 2007.)

antihypertensive therapy with appropriate agents. Other than sodium and volume restriction, no other significant factor has been found to alter blood pressure in a meaningful way.

The prevalence of hypertension in people with nondialysis CKD is more than 80%, depending on the target population, the cause of kidney disease, and the level of kidney function. For these individuals, the Joint National Committee Report (JNC-7) and the KDOQI Clinical Practice Guidelines recommend a blood pressure reduction to less than 130/80 mm Hg to maximize kidney and cardiovascular outcomes.[67,68] This impetus relates to data from clinical trials, the United Kingdom Prospective Diabetes Study (UKPDS) and the Hypertension Optimal Treatment (HOT) trial, in patients with kidney insufficiency for which aggressive blood pressure management reduced both the rate of kidney disease progression and cardiovascular events.[69,70]

The UKPDS trial was a 9-year follow-up of 1148 patients with type 2 diabetes. At the conclusion of the study, those randomized to "tight blood pressure control" (<150/85 mm Hg) had far less cardiovascular events than the "less tight control" (<180/105 mm Hg). Medication selection did alter the clinical outcome. Furthermore, a comparison of tight blood glucose control versus tight blood pressure control in the UKPDS trial demonstrated that tight blood pressure control provided the greatest risk reduction from cardiovascular events. Likewise, in the HOT trial of almost 19,000 people with hypertension, the subgroup of diabetics randomized to the lowest blood pressure group (<80 mm Hg, diastolic) had the most significant reduction in cardiovascular events, although this was not true for the study as a whole. Thus, one can markedly slow the progression of kidney disease and cardiovascular events with adequate blood pressure reduction.

One of the perceived limitations to achievement of these lower levels of blood pressure was the fear that lowering blood pressure too far might be harmful with an increase in coronary events, the concept of the J curve, which has not been borne out by clinical trials. The longest term study that evaluated the level of blood pressure reduction on progressive kidney disease, as assessed by change in GFR slope, is the African American Study of Kidney Disease.[71] In this trial of more than 1000 people with kidney dysfunction, the group randomized to lower blood pressure (achieved average of 127/77 mm Hg) retarded CKD progression and proteinuria without increase in the incidence of cardiovascular events or death. In addition, a meta-analysis of 1860 nondiabetic patients with kidney disease concluded that lower systolic pressures (between 110 and 129 mm Hg) may be more effective in slowing progressive kidney dysfunction and decreasing cardiac risk, although caution is advised with regard to lowering the systolic blood pressure below 110 mm Hg.[72] As such, the National Kidney Foundation KDOQI guidelines indicate that more aggressive goals may be warranted in patients with a spot urine total protein-to-creatinine ratio of 1000 mg/g or more (which represents protein excretion of more than 1000 mg/day).[72]

Achievement of these lower blood pressure levels in people with CKD will require an average of 3.5 to 4.2 different antihypertensive agents in moderate to high doses.[70,73] Figure 126.4 illustrates the need for three or more drugs per patient to appropriately lower blood pressure to the goals in various clinical trials or in kidney disease and CVD. Certain antihypertensive agents have been shown to be advantageous in reducing cardiovascular and kidney risk: angiotensin-converting enzyme (ACE) inhibitors, angiotensin receptor blockers (ARBs), nondihydropyridine calcium antagonists, diuretics, and perhaps beta blockers.[67] Although JNC-7 clearly states that there are compelling and specific indications for the use of ACE inhibitors and ARBs to lower blood pressure in individuals with diabetes or kidney disease, this report also emphasizes the fact that arterial pressure should be reduced to less than 130/80 mm Hg in such patients. It has become apparent that once a person has established nephropathy, defined as a serum creatinine concentration of more than 1.4 mg/dL (>123 mmol/L), the only factor that will slow the progression of kidney dysfunction is aggressive arterial pressure reduction.

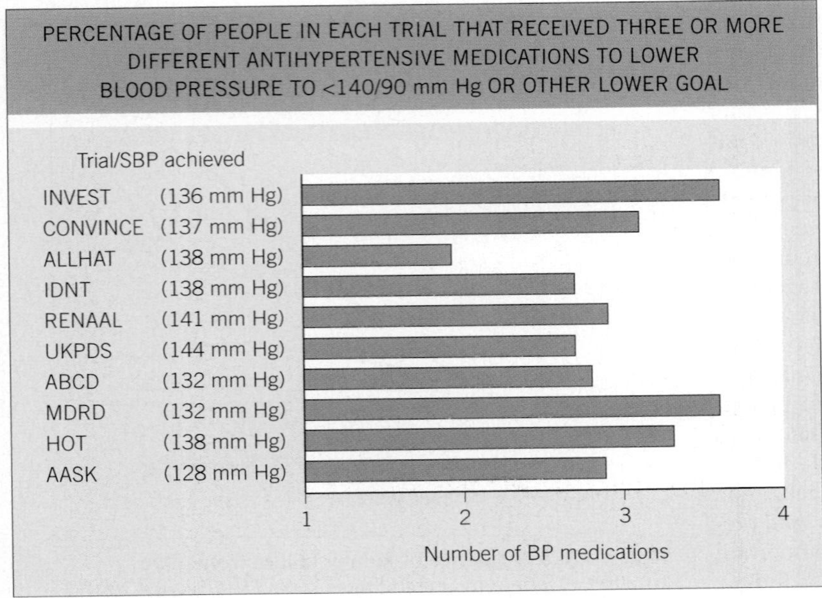

Figure 126.4 A summary of cardiovascular and kidney trials during the past decade with the percentage of people in each trial that received three or more different antihypertensive medications to lower blood pressure to below 140/90 mm Hg or other lower goal. BP, blood pressure; SBP, systolic blood pressure.

The rationale for selection of these agents to lower systemic blood pressure is based primarily on the pathophysiologic mechanism of hypertension in people with CKD. As discussed, this is attributed to sodium and extracellular volume overload, reduced kidney function, and increased vasoconstriction from activation of the RAAS system and, to a lesser extent, the sympathetic nervous system. Therefore, the concurrent use of these agents counteracts effects of these systems to restore optimum blood pressure levels and to minimize end-organ damage. Moreover, reduction in established proteinuria is also an important therapeutic target in the antihypertensive management of CKD patients.[68] This stems from epidemiologic and clinical trial data demonstrating a strong association between increased proteinuria, progressive kidney dysfunction, and higher cardiovascular mortality.[71-74] Of note, the only classes of drugs that fail to reduce proteinuria (i.e., dihydropyridine calcium antagonists, alpha blockers, hydralazine, and minoxidil) were also unsuccessful in either retarding CKD progression or decreasing cardiovascular mortality in the absence of agents that reduce proteinuria.

Data from large-scale treatment trials in people with nephropathy indicate that certain classes of antihypertensive agents should be included in the blood pressure–lowering regimen to slow CKD progression and to reduce CVD. Evidence to support the recommendation for ACE inhibitors in diabetic CKD originates from the Appropriate Blood Pressure Control in Diabetes (ABCD) trial and the Fosinopril Versus Amlodipine Cardiovascular Events Trial (FACET).[75,76] Both trials were stopped prematurely because of unacceptably high cardiovascular morbidity and mortality in the group randomized to a dihydropyridine calcium antagonist in the absence of an ACE inhibitor. It is notable that the cardiac event rate in the ABCD dihydropyridine calcium antagonist group was similar to the natural history of type 2 diabetics with untreated hypertension. Moreover, the beneficial effect of ACE inhibitors appears to extend to diabetic patients with CKD and a previous cardiovascular event or at least one other risk factor but without proteinuria, heart failure, or low ejection fraction. In the Heart Outcomes Prevention Evaluation (HOPE) and MICRO-HOPE study, ramipril lowered the risk of myocardial infarction, cardiovascular death, combined primary outcome (myocardial infarction, stroke, cardiovascular death), and total mortality.[9,77]

ARBs appear to have an antiproteinuric effect similar to that of ACE inhibitors and significantly retard the progression of CKD. The role of ARBs for management of CAD in this population was partly addressed with the Reduction of Endpoints in NIDDM with the Angiotensin II Antagonist Losartan (RENAAL) trial that evaluated 1513 patients with type 2 diabetes and nephropathy during a mean 3.4 years.[78] At the end of the study, proteinuria declined 35% with losartan ($P < .001$ compared with placebo), although the composite of cardiovascular morbidity and mortality was similar between the two groups.

Hyperlipidemia

Individuals with CKD differ from people in the general population for whom the National Cholesterol Education Program (NCEP) guidelines were intended. CKD patients have a higher frequency of lipid abnormalities that occur in the presence of normal LDL-cholesterol levels, specifically, low HDL concentration manifested concurrently with elevated triglycerides.[39,79] Even so, the prevalence of increased total cholesterol or LDL-cholesterol is highest in people with chronic kidney insufficiency and nephrotic syndrome, patients treated by peritoneal dialysis, and kidney transplant recipients. For this group, the LDL-cholesterol level can be between 45% and 85% higher than in the general population.

A paucity of studies exist to correlate dyslipidemia with CAD outcomes for persons receiving dialysis therapy. In subjects with reduced GFR, higher serum triglyceride levels and lower HDL levels were associated with a 2.5 times higher incidence of myocardial infarction than in the general population.[80] A retrospective multivariate analysis of the placebo arm of the Assessment of Lescol in Renal Transplantation (ALERT) study demonstrated that independent risk factors for myocardial infarction and cardiac and noncardiac mortality were preexisting CAD (HR, 3.69), total cholesterol level (HR, 1.55), and prior acute rejection (HR, 1.58).[81]

In the general population, the elevated total cholesterol concentration is a clear risk factor for CAD and cardiovascular death. It seems logical, therefore, that treatment decisions are directed against both hypertriglyceridemia and hypercholesterolemia in CKD. Elevated triglycerides with a low HDL level in the absence of an increased LDL-cholesterol level (i.e., >100 mg/dL) should be treated by diet and physical exercise.[68] The use of high flux dialysis and current pharmacologic therapy appear to generate a favorable improvement of lipid profiles.[79] Table 126.3 compares the recommendations for dietary intakes of the general population and CKD patients. Major differences include the slightly more liberal saturated fat intake and a lower carbohydrate intake in those with kidney disease.

RECOMMENDED INTAKE OF PROTEIN FOR ENERGY IN THE GENERAL POPULATION AND IN PATIENTS WITH KIDNEY DISEASE COMPARED WITH THAT OF THE NATIONAL CHOLESTEROL EDUCATION PROGRAM AND THE AMERICAN DIABETES ASSOCIATION

	Protein (g/kg per day)
General population	0.80
Hemodialysis	1-1.2
Peritoneal dialysis	1.2-1.5
Low-protein diet, CKD stages late 3 and 4	0.55-0.60
NCEP Step III	1.2
American Diabetes Association and National Kidney Foundation (diabetes)	0.6-0.8

Note that the recommended amount of fat is less than 30% of the diets.
CKD, chronic kidney disease; NCEP, National Cholesterol Education Program.

Table 126.3 Recommended intake of protein for energy in the general population and in patients with kidney disease compared with that of the National Cholesterol Education Program and the American Diabetes Association.

The KDOQI guidelines recommend a goal LDL-cholesterol level of less than 100 mg/dL in patients with CKD, although the NCEP revision suggests the LDL-cholesterol goal of less than 70 mg/dL in high-risk individuals.[68,82] Statins are the first line of therapy on the basis of post hoc analyses of large clinical trials. Among mildly hyperlipidemic subjects with a history of myocardial infarction and creatinine clearance calculated to be less than 75 mL/min in the Cholesterol And Recurrent Events (CARE) trial, pravastatin was associated with decreased major coronary events and coronary revascularization but not total mortality.[83] Only one randomized trial, the 4D trial, has evaluated the efficacy of lipid lowering in ESRD; 1255 hemodialysis patients with type 2 diabetes and elevated serum LDL concentration were randomly assigned to placebo or atorvastatin (20 mg/day). At a median follow-up of 4 years, there was a reduction in the rate of myocardial events in the atorvastatin group, although this was balanced by an increase in the rate of fatal stroke.[84]

Because lipid abnormalities in people with CKD are far more severe in those with greater degrees of proteinuria, it is important to tailor therapy. Virtually all patients with proteinuria of 3 g/day or more will have abnormal lipid profiles. Hyperlipidemia is most often characterized by increased total cholesterol and LDL levels, whereas triglycerides may not be as elevated. The best pharmacologic intervention in this situation is to reduce cholesterol synthesis from the liver, with medications such as statins, and to reduce leakage of protein through the kidney, with agents such as ACE inhibitors, ARBs, and nondihydropyridine calcium antagonists. Data from small observation studies suggest that combination therapy with ACE inhibitors and nondihydropyridine calcium antagonists can actually reduce total cholesterol concentration by as much as 32%, simply by decreasing proteinuria in nephrotic patients.[85]

Hyperhomocysteinemia

Elevated homocysteine levels are a predictor for CAD and CVD in the general population. Because homocysteine is cleared by the kidney, serum concentrations are often increased in CKD and inversely related to kidney dysfunction. In studies of dialysis patients and kidney transplant recipients, hyperhomocysteinemia was associated with a greater risk for atherosclerotic disease (2.1-fold) or mortality (2.44 times) than in patients with normal levels.[86,87]

Whereas the most common mechanism for hyperhomocysteinemia appears to be alterations in kidney metabolism, absolute or relative deficiency of vitamin B_6, vitamin B_{12}, and folate has been implicated. The combination of high-dose folic acid (usually 4 to 5 mg/day), vitamin B_{12}, and vitamin B_6 lowers homocysteine by 25% and may restore normal levels in patients with CKD or after kidney transplantation but not for those on hemodialysis or peritoneal dialysis. Vitamin B_6 is a major player in homocysteine metabolism. Because of vitamin B_6 deficiency, subjects on dialysis or with lesser degrees of CKD have low concentrations of the vitamin B_6 metabolites pyridoxal 5-phosphate and pyridoxal in plasma and red blood cells. Both groups have elevated levels of the metabolic end-product pyridoxic acid and homocysteine, fasting or post–methionine load (PML). In patients with CKD, vitamin B_6 did not change fasting levels of homocysteine but prevented PML increase; folic acid coadministration had no additional effect. Among dialysis patients, fasting levels were reduced by only vitamin B_6 and PML by the simultaneous use of folic acid.[88]

Coronary Revascularization in Patients with Kidney Insufficiency

Other than appropriate kidney dosing, the management of CAD is the same in patients with and without kidney disease. Many of the pharmacologic agents and invasive techniques available for management of individuals with an acute coronary event can be used regardless of kidney function.[89] Hence, if there are no contraindications, aspirin, beta blockers, ACE inhibitors, statins, or nitroglycerin should be given as indicated in the CKD and dialysis patient. In contrast, the optimal use of thrombolytic agents, heparin, and platelet glycoprotein IIb/IIIa inhibitors is less clear, as many of the large trials evaluating the efficacy of these drugs included patients with only mild kidney dysfunction.[89,90] In any case, KDOQI guidelines specify that control of extracellular fluid volume and partial correction of anemia, with erythropoietin for a target hematocrit between 33% and 36%, are critical for reducing cardiovascular risk in dialysis patients.[54]

Revascularization appears to be superior to medical therapy in uremic patients. When it is indicated, patients can be revascularized by either percutaneous coronary intervention or coronary artery bypass grafting. Whereas indications for these procedures are similar to those in nonuremic subjects, percutaneous coronary intervention is the preferred modality as recommended by the National Kidney Foundation.[54] Survival after myocardial infarction in relation to treatment modality was 45% in medically treated patients, 54% in patients treated with percutaneous transluminal coronary angioplasty, and 69% in patients treated by bypass surgery. In these numbers, a selection bias may have an influence. Restenosis is common after percutaneous transluminal coronary angioplasty in CKD patients, and stents are preferred to straightforward angioplasty. Whether the generalized use of drug-eluting stents will improve these statistics is unknown at present. Coronary artery bypass grafting is associated with a three times higher perioperative mortality. Although improvements in surgical technique have increased 5-year survival from 26.5% to 65% during the last decade, this is still far lower than in those without uremia (90%).[18]

HEART FAILURE

EPIDEMIOLOGY

Heart failure is more common among individuals with chronic kidney dysfunction than in the general population. About 40% of people starting dialysis therapy have a history of heart failure symptoms, which is a risk factor for significant morbidity and mortality in this group.[8,13] For those without heart failure symptoms at the commencement of dialysis, 25% will develop it within 3½ years (7% per year).[91] Approximately 75% of kidney transplant recipients have hypertrophic cardiomyopathy, whereas more than 50% have systolic dysfunction or dilated cardiomyopathy.[11,24] In a similar vein, mild to moderate CKD in patients with left ventricular systolic dysfunction and heart failure conferred an increase in all-cause mortality, pump failure death, and heart failure hospitalization as seen in the Studies of Left Ventricular Dysfunction (SOLVD) trial and the Candesartan in Heart Failure: Assessment of Reduction in Mortality and Morbidity (CHARM) program.[92,93]

Both concentric and eccentric left ventricular hypertrophy can be observed in hemodialysis patients. As in the general population, concentric left ventricular hypertrophy is associated with pressure overload; eccentric left ventricular hypertrophy (also known as left ventricular dilatation) is associated with volume overload. Moreover, the relationship of left ventricular hypertrophy to subsequent outcomes is similar to that in the general population. The risks of heart failure and death, however, are significantly higher in CKD patients with left ventricular hypertrophy compared with those without.

In a Canadian study of subjects starting dialysis, 41% had concentric left ventricular hypertrophy, 28% had left ventricular dilatation, and 16% had systolic dysfunction, whereas 16% had a normal echocardiogram. For patients with either hypertrophy or dilatation, heart failure developed within 38 months in comparison to 19 months for those with systolic dysfunction; mean survival was 48 months for dialysis patients with left ventricular hypertrophy, 56 months with left ventricular dilatation, and only 38 months with systolic dysfunction. Regardless, the presence of concentric left ventricular hypertrophy, cardiac dilatation, or systolic dysfunction correlated with a threefold increase in the risk for subsequent heart failure, which when present during dialysis initiation amplified the risk of death by 93% and preceded two thirds of all deaths.[11,66] The incidence of de novo heart failure was 7.6% per year, and this increased the risk of death fivefold compared with dialysis patients without heart failure.

In the U.S. experience, heart failure was recorded in 36% of dialysis patients. Age (risk increased by 30% for every 10 years), female sex, hypertension, diabetes (doubling likelihood), conditions of atherosclerosis (CAD, cerebrovascular or peripheral vascular disease), pericarditis, and structural cardiac abnormalities (left ventricular hypertrophy, clinical cardiomegaly) were all associated with heart failure. Elevated serum phosphate ($\geq$6.8 mg/dL) and calcium ($\geq$8.0 mg/dL) concentrations as well as low serum cholesterol and low albumin concentrations (as a consequence of malnutrition because of heart failure or as a cause of myofibrillar atrophy–cardiac fibrosis) were also significantly associated. Patients with heart failure had greater residual kidney function (because of earlier initiation of dialysis) and infrequent visits to a nephrologist or dietitian.[94]

The prevalence of heart failure in CKD is shown in Figure 126.5a. The survival of ESRD patients with systolic dysfunction is far less than that of those with a transplant (Fig. 126.5b). The 18-month survival probabilities among incident hemodialysis, peritoneal dialysis, and CKD patients are comparable after the onset of heart failure, at approximately 53% annually versus 87% for renal transplant recipients. In the prevalent population, the probability of 2-year survival after a diagnosis of congestive heart failure is 49% for hemodialysis patients and 69% for renal transplant recipients.[5] A prospective analysis that included the careful characterization of patients' baseline cardiac status by echocardiography observed that the median time to onset of heart failure was 24 months in those with ischemic heart disease at dialysis initiation compared with 55 months in those without. This effect was independent of age, diabetes, and underlying cardiomyopathy.[95] For CKD patients with ischemic disease, the median survival was 44 months, whereas for those without ischemia, it was 56 months. This adverse relationship was independent of age and diabetes mellitus, but when heart failure was considered, ischemic heart disease was no longer an independent predictor of survival.

PATHOPHYSIOLOGY

CAD and hypertension occur with increasing frequency in CKD patients and are important causes of heart failure in this population. Furthermore, accelerated atherosclerosis, vascular calcification, anemia, sodium and water retention, alterations in neurohumoral regulation (sympathetic nervous system, RAAS system, and natriuretic peptides), and hemodialysis vascular access shunting can contribute to hemodynamic overload as well as to the development of concentric and eccentric left ventricular hypertrophy. Both systolic and diastolic function may be impaired with associated reductions in overall cardiac reserve. Table 126.4 summarizes the neurohumoral changes that occur in heart failure.

The etiology of systolic and diastolic dysfunction in dialysis subjects has been attributed to abnormalities in the uremic milieu. Experimental studies demonstrate inhibition of the Na^+,K^+-ATPase activity in cardiac myocytes, resulting in increased force of contraction as well as impaired relaxation and recovery of calcium concentration. This was mediated by increases of cytosolic sodium or sodium changes limited to specific compartments or modification of signal transduction pathways resulting in Na^+-Ca^{2+} exchange impairment with subsequent increase of cytosolic calcium concentration.[96]

Anemia is an important, independent risk factor for left ventricular hypertrophy and heart failure as well as for cardiovascular mortality in this population. Anemia contributes to left ventricular hypertrophy by reduced oxygen delivery to the myocardium (thus, myocyte necrosis and apoptosis), increased cardiac output, enhanced oxidative stress, and stimulation of the sympathetic nervous system.[11,53] Patients with CKD have lower mean hemoglobin concentration; hemoglobin levels of 8 g/dL or lower correlated with a twofold increase in the odds of death. Partial correction with erythropoietin regressed left ventricular hypertrophy, although there was no benefit for hemoglobin levels above 11 g/dL[66]; complete correction of anemia can prevent left ventricular dilatation only in patients with normal ventricular volume. As heart failure progresses, worsening anemia ensues, perpetuating a vicious circle. In a cohort study of patients with pre–end-stage kidney failure, the prevalence of left ventricular hypertrophy increased with decreasing hemoglobin level, increasing creatinine concentration, and systolic blood pressure; anemia was a predictor of hospitalization.[53,66]

Secondary hyperparathyroidism may also be involved in the pathogenesis of left ventricular hypertrophy and heart failure in kidney dysfunction. As discussed before, elevated PTH levels impair myocardial energy production, transfer,

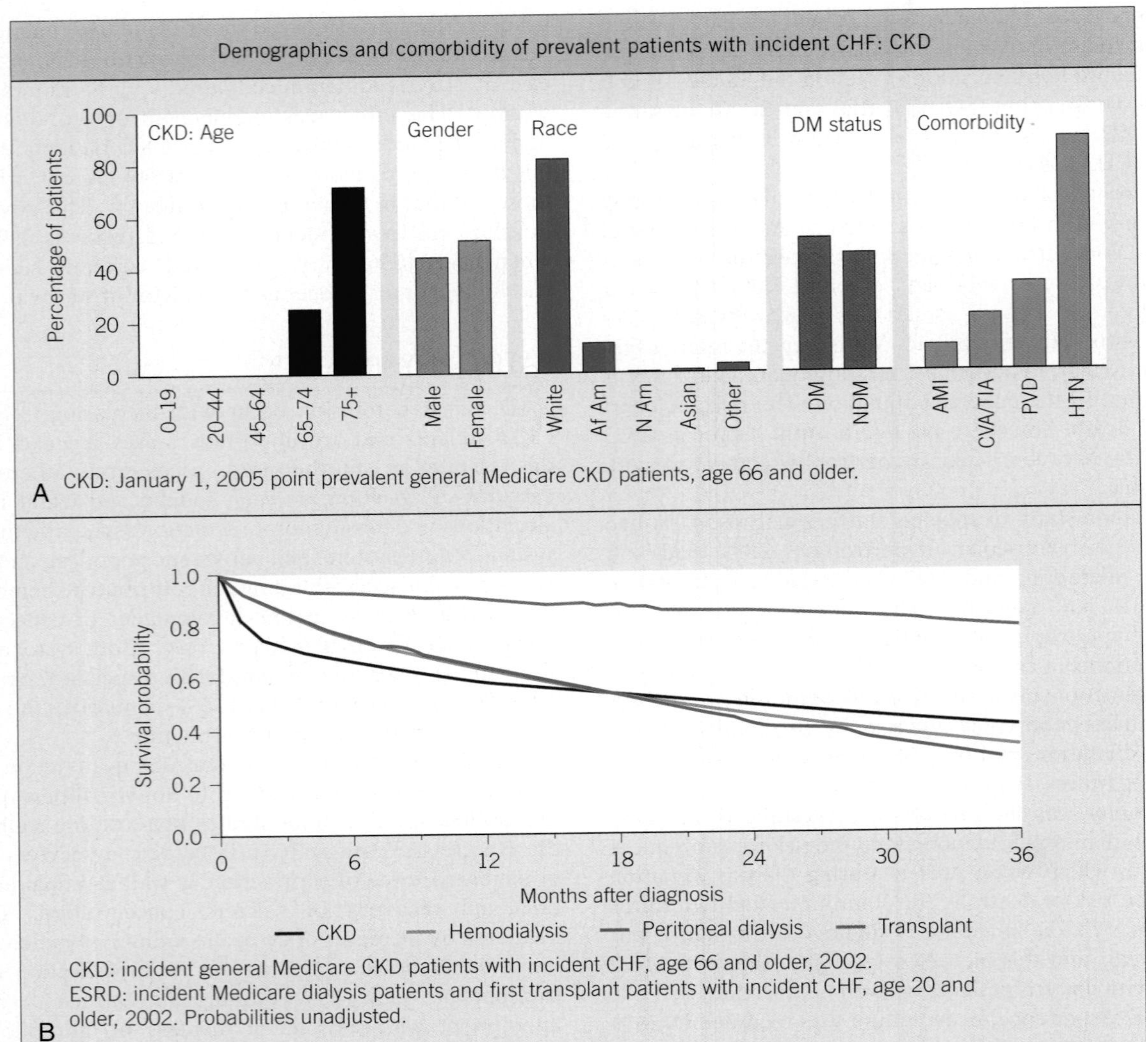

Figure 126.5 **A,** Demographics and comorbidity of prevalent patients with incident heart failure who have CKD. AMI, acute myocardial infarction; CVA/TIA, cerebrovascular accident/transient ischemic attack; DM, diabetics; HTN, hypertension; NDM, nondiabetics; PVD, peripheral vascular disease. **B,** Survival in people starting dialysis with systolic dysfunction and left ventricular hypertrophy. (From United States Renal Data Service 2007.)

and use.[44] PTH is strongly correlated with changes in cardiac mass and angiotensin II. Intravenous calcitriol partially corrects secondary hyperparathyroidism with associated decline in left ventricular hypertrophy as well as a decrease in renin, angiotensin II, and atrial natriuretic peptide levels. This beneficial effect of calcitriol is attributed to direct action on cardiac myocytes through vitamin D receptors as well as to reductions in angiotensin II.[97] Furthermore, elevated PTH, in conjunction with comorbidities frequently found in CKD patients, predisposes to myriad valvular heart abnormalities (regurgitant or stenotic) and their concomitant sequelae on cardiac mass and function.[98] Newer specific vitamin D receptor agonists have also been shown to have this effect with no increase in vascular calcifications.[99]

Hyperphosphatemia in kidney dysfunction has been linked with higher risks for sudden cardiac death and cardiovascular mortality. For sudden cardiac death, there was significant correlation to higher calcium × phosphate product and PTH levels.[100] Moreover, there is higher diastolic and mean blood pressure, hyperkinetic circulation, increased cardiac work, and high arterial tensile stress, factors independent of interdialytic weight gain or PTH concentrations.[101]

Reduced heart rate variability has been suggested to be an independent risk factor for sudden cardiac death in dialysis patients. This value was independent of conditions such as ejection fraction of less than 0.45, multivessel coronary stenosis, and ventricular tachycardia on 24-hour electrocardiography. This is attributed to CAD or congestive heart failure and has been associated with anemia and longer period of dialysis therapy. Its presence reflects autonomic dysregulation (depressed vagal activity or sympathetic hyperactivity), which can be involved in the pathogenesis of ventricular tachycardia and sudden death.[102]

The RAAS is an essential regulatory system that maintains sodium balance, fluid volume, and vascular tone. Because CKD essentially induces a state of kidney hypoperfusion, the juxtaglomerular cells of the kidney stimulate RAAS, with the resultant adverse cardiovascular consequences of sympathetic

EFFECTS OF ACTIVATED NEUROHUMORAL SYSTEMS AND THEIR BLOCKADE ON KIDNEY HEMODYNAMICS IN HEART FAILURE

	Sympathetic Nerves	ANG II	Aldosterone	ANP	AVP	Diuretics*	Alpha Blockers	ACEI	ARBs	Aldosterone Receptor Blockade	V_2 Antagonist
Kidney blood flow	↓	↓		↑		↑	↑	↑	↑		
Efferent arteriole constriction	↑	↑			↑			↓	↓		
Proximal sodium reabsorption	↑	↑		↓				↓	↓		
Distal sodium absorption			↑	↓	↑	↓		↓	↓	↓	
Water absorption					↑	↓		↓	↓		↓
Renin release	↑	↓		↓		↑		↑	↑	↑	
Aldosterone release		↑		↓		↑		↓		↑	

*This section refers only to loop diuretics. Moreover, if volume depletion occurs with diuretics, kidney blood flow is reduced with these agents and an indirect increase in efferent arteriolar tone is observed.

ACEI, angiotensin-converting enzyme inhibitors; ANG II, angiotensin II; ANP, atrial natriuretic peptide; ARBs, angiotensin receptor blockers; AVP, arginine vasopressin.

Table 126.4 Effects of activated neurohumoral systems and their blockade on kidney hemodynamics in heart failure.

hyperactivation, endothelial dysfunction, progressive atherosclerosis, and fibrinolytic system inhibition.[103] Furthermore, components of the RAAS system (angiotensin II and aldosterone) add insult to injury with direct profibrotic effects on the heart and kidney, culminating in worsening hypertension, CKD, left ventricular hypertrophy, and heart failure.

Atrial natriuretic peptide (ANP) is released by atria myocytes in response to stretch from increased atrial pressure and by ventricular myocytes in left ventricular hypertrophy. Brain natriuretic peptide (BNP) is produced from ventricular myocytes, being more slowly regulated by alterations of its gene expression by pressure overload. Both peptide levels have been found to be elevated in dialysis patients, particularly in those with CAD. In this subgroup, BNP levels correlated with reduced left ventricular (LV) ejection fraction, increased LV end-systolic and LV end-diastolic volume indexes; while in those without CAD, an association to LV mass and systolic BP was found. Furthermore, ANP and BNP are associated with the risk of overall and cardiovascular mortality. The correlation was stronger for BNP, which, after adjustments, remained an independent predictor of mortality. Both of them could be used for exclusion of left ventricular dysfunction (high negative predictive value of 97% and 96% for ANP and BNP, respectively) and for identification of left ventricular hypertrophy (high positive predictive value of 92% and 87%, BNP having more sensitivity than ANP: 88% versus 51%).[104-106]

CLINICAL PRESENTATION

Heart failure is an independent predictor of death in individuals with CKD, particularly for those receiving kidney replacement therapy. As discussed previously, myriad factors contribute to heart failure development in this population. In practice, it can be quite challenging to differentiate the clinical picture of left ventricular dysfunction and extracellular fluid overload because these conditions can present singularly or in tandem. The typical symptoms of dyspnea on exertion can be exacerbated by predialysis extracellular fluid overload, which may be managed with ultrafiltration. Clinical suspicion should be raised for left ventricular dysfunction in dialysis subjects with particularly low blood pressure or intradialytic hypotension in the absence of extracellular volume overload. Furthermore, ESRD patients are likely to have ventricular and atrial arrhythmias as their primary clinical presentation of myocardial dysfunction and heart failure.[107]

MANAGEMENT

Given the marked incidence of heart failure and poor overall cardiovascular prognosis in dialysis patients, they should be evaluated for systolic and diastolic dysfunction. The KDOQI guidelines recommend that at the initiation of dialysis, all patients should undergo baseline echocardiography and electrocardiography.[54] Echocardiography should be performed after dry weight is attained (which usually occurs after 1 to 3 months) and should be repeated routinely at 3-year intervals. For patients who clinically present with heart failure, it is crucial that they be evaluated for CAD, because traditional cardiovascular risk factors, such as hypertension, smoking history, diabetes, dyslipidemia, and older age, are rampant in people with CKD. Moreover, additional risk is incurred with the hemodynamic and metabolic onslaughts of proteinuria, increased extracellular fluid volume, electrolyte imbalance, anemia, and higher levels of thrombogenic factors. Thus, approaches toward risk factor reduction are key in this setting.

The evaluation and treatment of heart failure in CKD should be based on the pathophysiology of the disease. Figure 126.6 outlines a management strategy in people already receiving or about to start kidney replacement therapy. Optimal volume control is a significant factor in the management; the KDOQI guidelines indicate that consistent maintenance of euvolemia is a major component of effective therapy.[54] As in nonuremic subjects, pharmacologic approaches to heart failure management can significantly reduce morbidity and mortality. Table 126.4 summarizes the neurohumoral changes that occur

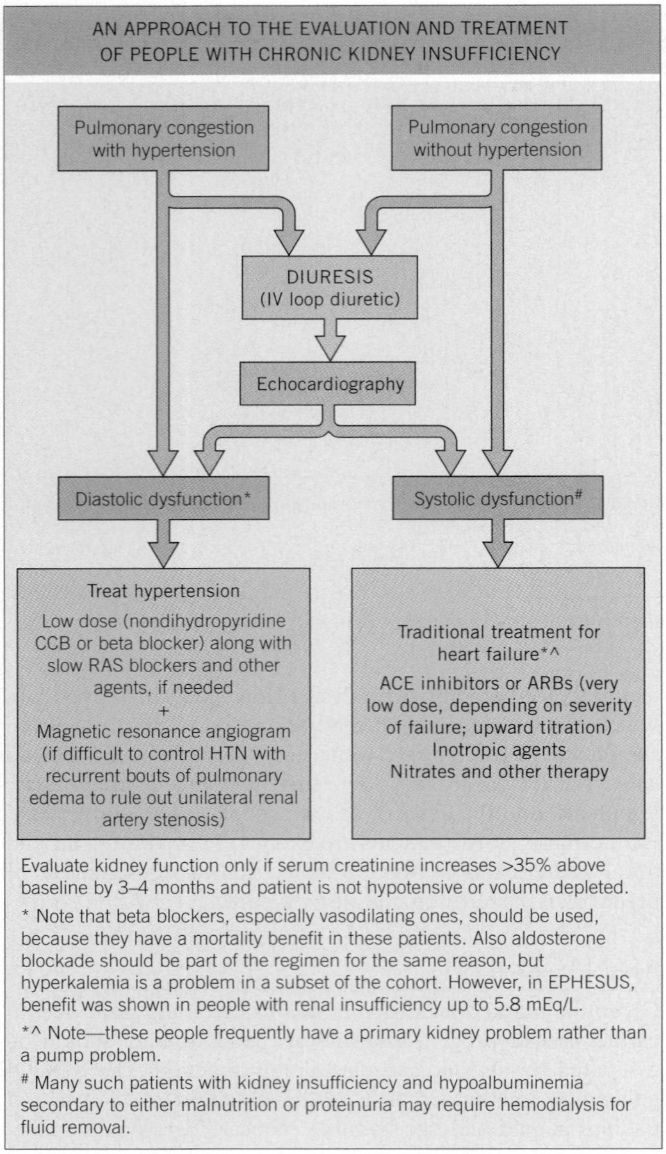

AN APPROACH TO THE EVALUATION AND TREATMENT OF PEOPLE WITH CHRONIC KIDNEY INSUFFICIENCY

Pulmonary congestion with hypertension

Pulmonary congestion without hypertension

DIURESIS
(IV loop diuretic)

Echocardiography

Diastolic dysfunction*

Systolic dysfunction#

Treat hypertension
Low dose (nondihydropyridine CCB or beta blocker) along with slow RAS blockers and other agents, if needed
+
Magnetic resonance angiogram (if difficult to control HTN with recurrent bouts of pulmonary edema to rule out unilateral renal artery stenosis)

Traditional treatment for heart failure*^
ACE inhibitors or ARBs (very low dose, depending on severity of failure; upward titration)
Inotropic agents
Nitrates and other therapy

Evaluate kidney function only if serum creatinine increases >35% above baseline by 3–4 months and patient is not hypotensive or volume depleted.

* Note that beta blockers, especially vasodilating ones, should be used, because they have a mortality benefit in these patients. Also aldosterone blockade should be part of the regimen for the same reason, but hyperkalemia is a problem in a subset of the cohort. However, in EPHESUS, benefit was shown in people with renal insufficiency up to 5.8 mEq/L.

*^ Note—these people frequently have a primary kidney problem rather than a pump problem.

\# Many such patients with kidney insufficiency and hypoalbuminemia secondary to either malnutrition or proteinuria may require hemodialysis for fluid removal.

Figure 126.6 An approach to the evaluation and treatment of people with chronic kidney insufficiency (creatinine clearance <60 mL/min). ACE inhibitors, angiotensin-converting enzyme inhibitors; ARBs, angiotensin receptor blockers; CCB, calcium channel blockers; HTN, hypertension; RAS, renin-angiotensin system.

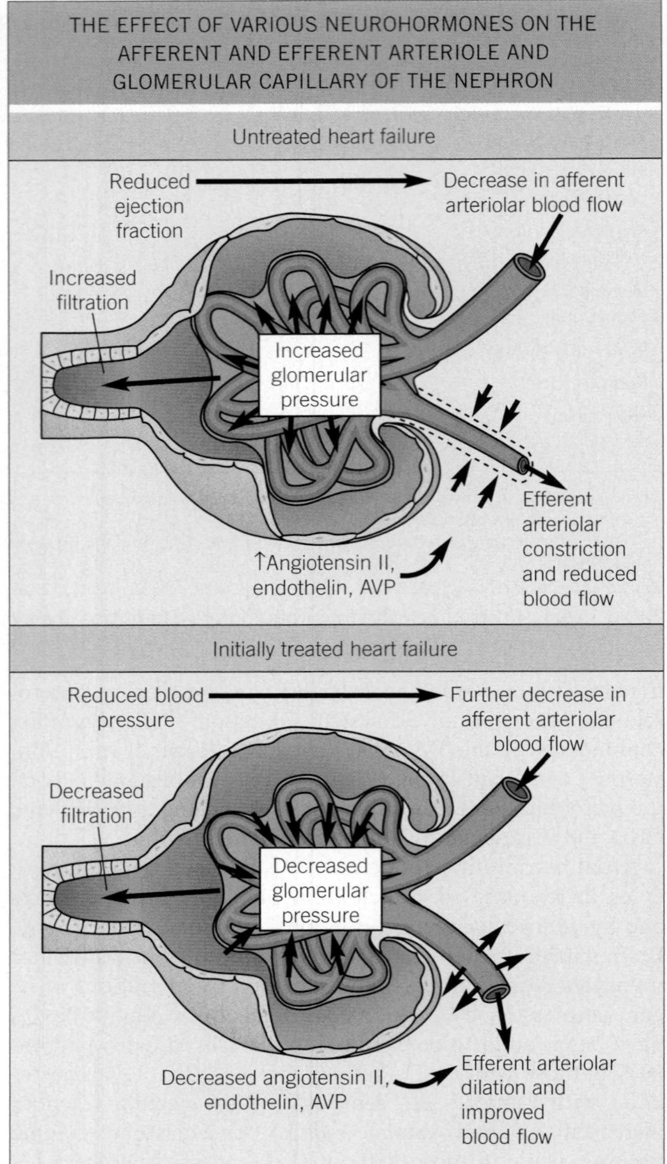

Figure 126.7 The effect of various neurohormones that help maintain glomerular filtration on the afferent and efferent arteriole and glomerular capillary of the nephron and the impact of various therapies used in heart failure. Note: These are the initial changes seen when blockade of the renin-angiotensin system is applied. Over time, with improvement of cardiac function, kidney function also improves because of reduced neurohumoral influence and improved perfusion. AVP, arginine vasopressin.

in heart failure and the effects of their blockade. This is further illustrated in Figure 126.7. The 2007 National Kidney Foundation guidelines for the management of CKD are summarized in Table 126.5.

Kidney Aspects of Heart Failure Pharmacotherapy

Angiotensin-Converting Enzyme Inhibitors and Angiotensin Receptor Blockers

Inhibition of the RAAS system with either an ACE inhibitor or an ARB provides both cardiovascular and kidney protection, which is most significant for reducing heart failure morbidity and mortality in CKD patients. This benefit applies not only to individuals with kidney disease alone, as shown in the RENAAL trial, but also to CKD and underlying heart failure, as shown in the Randomized Evaluation of Strategies for Left Ventricular Dysfunction (RESOLVD) pilot study and the CHARM trial, as well as to CKD and left ventricular dysfunction after an acute coronary event, as demonstrated in the Valsartan in Acute Myocardial Infarction Trial (VALIANT) and the Survival And Ventricular Enlargement (SAVE) trial.[78,93,108-110] Thus, the National Kidney Foundation guidelines recommend ACE inhibitors and ARBs in the management of heart failure in patients with kidney dysfunction.[54]

A rise in serum creatinine concentration occurs in about 10% to 11% of patients with significant heart failure (ejection fraction <20%) treated with ACE inhibitors or ARBs.

KDOQI CLINICAL PRACTICE GUIDELINES FOR MANAGEMENT OF CHRONIC KIDNEY DISEASE		
Parameters	**Goals**	**Treatment**
Blood pressure	<130/80 mm Hg	Reduction in dietary salt
CKD stages 1-5		ACEI or ARB (diuretics), CCB in transplant recipients
		Reduction in dietary salt and fluid intake; ultrafiltration in dialysis patients
		Any medication, except diuretics
Lipid management		Diet (daily, ≤30% fat, <7% saturated fat, <200 mg cholesterol)
LDL (primary)	<100 mg/dL	Agents: statin, niacin, fibrate
HDL (secondary)	>35 mg/dL	
Triglycerides (secondary)	<200 mg/dL	
Weight management	Especially with hypertension and elevated glucose or triglyceride levels. Low protein (0.6 g/kg per day) if GFR <30 mL/min/1.73 m^2	

Other recommendations: cessation of smoking; physical activity (at least 30 minutes of moderate-intensity activity three or four times a week); aspirin, 75 to 150 mg/day. Other agents individualizing benefit: angiotensin-converting enzyme inhibitors, angiotensin receptor blockers, or beta blockers (post–myocardial infarction), estrogens (postmenopausal women); hemoglobin A_{1c} <7%, preferably <6.5%.

Separately, in diabetic patients, an angiotensin-converting enzyme inhibitor and an angiotensin receptor blocker, alone or together, are very important if albuminuria is above 300 mg per gram creatinine on maximal dose of either alone, with other agents added for strict blood pressure control.

ACEI, angiotensin-converting enzyme inhibitor; ARB, angiotensin receptor blocker; CCB, calcium channel blocker; CKD, chronic kidney disease; GFR, glomerular filtration rate.

From the Kidney Disease Outcome Quality Initiative (KDOQI) Clinical Practice Guidelines for Chronic Kidney Disease and Diabetes. Am J Kidney Dis 2007;49 (Suppl 2):S12–S154.

Table 126.5 KDOQI clinical practice Guidelines for management of chronic kidney disease.

Mechanisms for this rise in creatinine (reflecting a fall in GFR) include (1) loss of angiotensin II effect on the efferent arteriole, leading to a fall of filtration pressure within the glomerulus; and (2) severe reduction of blood pressure associated with intravascular volume depletion, leading to a fall in kidney perfusion (see Fig. 126.7). In the SOLVD trial, patients assigned to enalapril had a 33% greater likelihood of decreased kidney function than controls did. Multivariate analysis revealed that older age, diuretic therapy, and diabetes correlated with reduced kidney function, whereas beta-blocker therapy and higher ejection fraction were renoprotective.[111] The magnitude of kidney dysfunction seen with ACE inhibitor or ARB therapy is directly proportional to the degree of heart failure. Therefore, the lower the ejection fraction, the greater the initial increase in serum creatinine concentration; but as cardiac function improves, serum creatinine concentration will start to fall.

Of note, ACE inhibitors may cause hyperkalemia in some heart failure patients, particularly in those with baseline GFRs below 50% before initiation of ACE therapy. Hyperkalemia may be due to reduction in GFR and hence the amount of sodium presented to the distal nephron where potassium excretion typically occurs, or to blockade of aldosterone production and release, or to a combination of both of these processes. ARBs may be an alternative in this setting because they cause smaller rises in potassium compared with ACE inhibitors.[112]

Aldosterone Antagonists

Competitive binding of the mineralocorticoid receptor reduces the avidity of the distal nephron for sodium and volume reabsorption, thereby providing another avenue for the inhibition of RAAS. Aldosterone antagonists such as spironolactone and eplerenone have been demonstrated to significantly abrogate morbidity and mortality in CKD patients with advanced heart failure alone, as in the Randomized Aldactone Evaluation Study (RALES), or in conjunction with an acute myocardial infarction, as in the Eplerenone Post–Acute Myocardial Infarction Heart Failure Efficacy and Survival Study (EPHESUS). Aldosterone inhibition substantially reduces the likelihood of hypokalemia from diuretic therapy, but at the same time, it increases the risk of hyperkalemia.[113,114] The use of these agents is extremely controversial in dialysis patients, particularly when they are administered concurrently with ACE inhibitors or ARBs. Moreover, aldosterone antagonists may decrease potassium excretion in the colon as well as the translocation of potassium into tissues, thereby exacerbating the issue. The risk of hyperkalemia exists even for anuric dialysis patients.

SUMMARY

Chronic kidney disease is a cardiovascular risk equivalent similar to diabetes alone. The two most common presentations of cardiovascular disease in individuals with kidney dysfunction are ischemic coronary artery disease and heart failure. Therapeutic approaches in these patients are similar to the guidelines recommended for the general population, with the exception that more aggressive goals should be sought. It is particularly important to distinguish whether a patient presenting with symptoms of heart failure has a primary kidney cause or truly has heart failure. Patients with occult bilateral renal artery stenosis and hypertension can frequently present with "flash pulmonary edema." In this case, a work-up of the kidney, *not* the heart, should ensue. In general, the recommendations for high-risk patients with cardiovascular and kidney disease should be the same as for high-risk, non-kidney patients. The goal should be to lower both LDL-cholesterol level and mean arterial pressure in addition to an aspirin a day and reduction of homocysteine levels, which would reduce risk by as much as 60% to 70%.

chapter

127 Obesity

Scott M. Grundy and Nicola Abate

Definition

- Overweight is defined as a body mass index (BMI) of 25 to 29.9 kg/m^2. Obesity is defined as a BMI greater than 30 kg/m^2. In this chapter, the term *obesity,* unless otherwise indicated, encompasses both overweight and categoric obesity.

Key Features

- Obesity, particularly truncal obesity, increases the risk for various forms of cardiovascular disease (CVD); it usually presents as coronary heart disease but can manifest as arrhythmia, heart failure, or stroke. Weight loss in obese patients is accompanied by improved CVD outcomes.

Therapy

- Gradual weight loss, brought about by combined use of a low-calorie diet, behavioral modification, and drug therapy, reduces the risk for CVD. Surgical therapy occasionally may be indicated for severely obese patients.

Approximately 97 million adults in the United States are overweight or obese.[1,2] The increasing prevalence of these conditions, which have reached epidemic proportions in the United States and throughout the Western world, constitutes a significant obstacle to the favorable outcome of current public health strategies for reducing cardiovascular disease (CVD). A wealth of epidemiologic data shows a close relationship between excessive accumulation of body fat and premature cardiovascular morbidity and mortality.[3] Obesity increases the risk for coronary heart disease (CHD) and also predisposes to ventricular hypertrophy, heart failure, and arrhythmia. Obesity seemingly increases the risk for CVD both directly and indirectly by engendering comorbid conditions that, in turn, predispose to CVD.

ANATOMY AND PATHOLOGY

Obesity is characterized by the accumulation of excessive fat in adipose tissue. Fat deposition may be generalized or may occur preferentially in different adipose tissue compartments. Two major variants of obesity are distinguished for their different impact on CVD morbidity and mortality. Truncal obesity (also referred to as *abdominal obesity, upper body obesity* and *android obesity*) is characterized by a predominant accumulation of fat in the truncal area, which includes subcutaneous and visceral adipose tissue compartments. This form of obesity is more frequently found in men and is associated with a high risk for CVD independent of generalized adiposity. Peripheral obesity (also referred to as *lower body obesity* and *gynoid obesity*) is characterized by a predominant accumulation of fat in the gluteofemoral area. This form of obesity is more frequently found in premenopausal women and apparently is not associated with an increased risk for CVD. In fact, peripheral fat distribution is often associated with a decreased prevalence of traditional cardiovascular risk factors among obese patients.

Autopsy and echocardiographic studies in obese patients have revealed various anatomic changes in the heart; these include fatty infiltration of the heart's conduction system, left ventricular hypertrophy (LVH) (mainly with eccentric geometry), right ventricular hypertrophy, and left atrium enlargement. Concentric LVH in obesity has been traditionally attributed to coexisting hypertension; however, recent magnetic resonance imaging (MRI) studies raise the possibility that concentric LVH is a result of obesity per se, independent of hypertension.

PATHOPHYSIOLOGY

Obesity affects CVD morbidity and mortality, mainly by promoting the occurrence of CVD risk factors or comorbidities, such as insulin resistance, type 2 diabetes, dyslipidemia, hypertension, cardiac hypertrophy, cardiac electric abnormalities, low-grade systemic inflammation, and a prothrombotic state. These clinical and subclinical conditions related to obesity often coexist in what is now identified as the metabolic syndrome, a condition that creates an enhanced risk for cardiovascular disease. The following is a discussion of the proposed pathophysiologies of the comorbidities of obesity that frequently cluster in the metabolic syndrome.

Obesity and Insulin Resistance

Insulin resistance (Fig. 127.1) is a predisposing risk factor for CVD and may constitute the main pathophysiologic mechanism that underlies most of the comorbidities that accompany obesity. The mechanisms by which obesity, particularly abdominal obesity, leads to insulin resistance are still incompletely understood. Recent advances in the understanding of the molecular pathophysiology of adipose tissue have revealed that adipose tissue may affect insulin signaling in other cells through the release of nonesterified free fatty acids or through secretion of various proteins, peptides, and cytokines that may affect insulin signaling. For example, adipocytes have been shown to produce tumor necrosis factor α (TNF-α), a cytokine secreted at higher levels with obesity that may affect insulin-mediated glucose disposal signaling in the skeletal muscle surrounding adipocytes through a paracrine effect.

Leptin is another important product of adipocytes; it not only controls appetite, but also regulates intracellular metabolism by mediating fatty acid utilization for energy production. Obesity

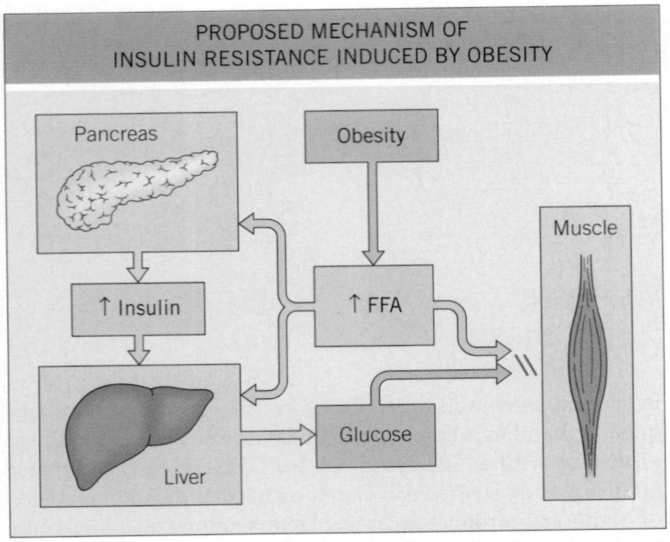

Figure 127.1 Proposed mechanism of insulin resistance induced by obesity. Excessive release of free fatty acids (FFAs) from excessive adipose tissue may decrease insulin-mediated glucose disposal in the skeletal muscle and induce hypersecretion of insulin by the beta cells of the pancreas.

is associated with increased production of leptin, but also with leptin resistance, which results in an increase in intracellular accumulation of triglycerides in various cell types. Leptin resistance promotes triglyceride accumulation in adipocytes, hepatocytes, pancreatic beta cells, and skeletal and myocardial myocytes, thus predisposing to multiple tissue and organ dysfunctions; these dysfunctions, in turn, lead to the clustering of health complications of obesity, such as steatohepatitis, heart failure, insulin resistance, and type 2 diabetes.

More recently, adiponectin has been identified as an important product of adipocytes that affects insulin sensitivity. Reduced adiponectin production in patients with obesity has been associated with insulin resistance. Less clear is the role of resistin, another adipose tissue product that has been linked to insulin resistance in animals.

Another important product of adipocytes is nonesterified free fatty acids (NEFAs). Excessive release of free fatty acids (FFAs) from an excess of adipose tissue may play a major role in insulin resistance. Indeed, the excessive availability of plasma fatty acids to muscle and other tissues dictates the preferential use of fatty acids for energy production. This abundance of fatty acids in tissues appears to inhibit the oxidation of glucose.

Insulin resistance, defined as decreased insulin-mediated glucose disposal, contributes to compensatory hyperinsulinemia. Because insulin resistance frequently accompanies truncal obesity, the question of which compartment of truncal adipose tissue (subcutaneous or visceral) contributes more to insulin resistance has evoked considerable interest. Several investigators propose that visceral ("portal") adipose tissue is mainly responsible for the insulin resistance of obesity. Portal adipocytes have been shown to have a greater sensitivity to lipolytic stimulation in vitro. According to this theory, excessive FFAs that reach the liver through the portal circulation stimulate higher hepatic glucose output and decrease hepatic insulin clearance, thus predisposing to insulin resistance. Recent studies, however, have challenged this hypothesis and have suggested that subcutaneous adipose tissue in the truncal area contributes more to peripheral insulin resistance than does visceral adipose tissue.

Although most investigators believe that truncal obesity precedes the development of insulin resistance, it is possible that truncal obesity could be the result of insulin resistance. Support for this possibility comes from two diseases: Cushing's disease and polycystic ovary syndrome (PCOS). Both conditions appear to have a primary insulin resistance, and the truncal fat distribution appears to be a secondary phenomenon. It has further been proposed that a mild form of hypercorticoidism underlies both truncal obesity and insulin resistance. Recent studies in our laboratory suggest that insulin resistance is not entirely due either to generalized or to regional obesity, but rather is determined by genetic predisposition.[4]

Obesity and Type 2 Diabetes

Obesity is a major risk factor for type 2 diabetes (Fig. 127.2).[5] Furthermore, truncal obesity is a better predictor for type 2 diabetes than is overall obesity. The insulin resistance that accompanies obesity promotes the development of hyperglycemia by increasing hepatic glucose output and impairing the uptake of glucose by skeletal muscle. However, abnormalities in the ability of pancreatic beta cells to secrete insulin must also be present for the development of categoric hyperglycemia. Insulin resistance typically precedes the development of type 2 diabetes by several years. Initially, insulin resistance results in normoglycemic hyperinsulinemia. However, once relative beta-cell decompensation ensues, overt hyperglycemia develops. The mechanisms that lead to beta-cell decompensation are not completely understood. Inherited abnormalities in beta-cell function may accelerate the decline in insulin secretion that typically occurs with advancing age. Beta-cell accumulation of amylin, which is produced along with insulin, has been observed in some patients with diabetes. Recently, accumulation of triglycerides in beta cells (lipotoxicity) has been implicated in the decline of insulin secretion.

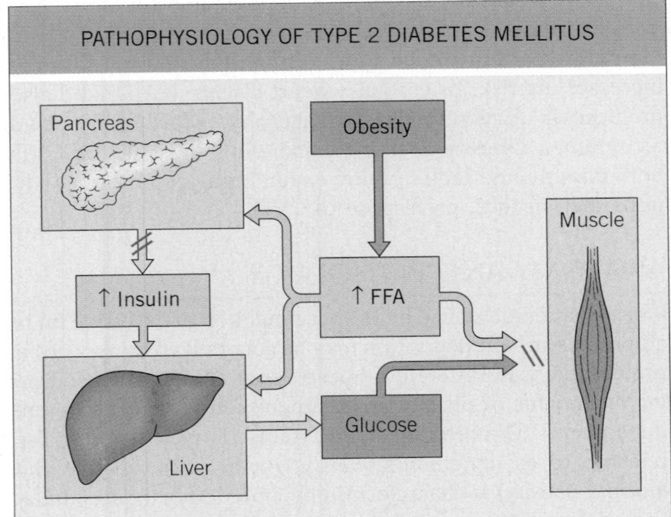

Figure 127.2 Pathophysiology of type 2 diabetes mellitus. Excessive release of free fatty acids (FFAs) from excessive adipose tissue may worsen the insulin resistance of patients predisposed to diabetes. Coexisting beta-cell dysfunction reduces the hyperinsulinemic response to circulating FFAs and favors the onset of hyperglycemia.

Obesity and Dyslipidemia

Several cross-sectional and prospective studies have shown that obesity, particularly truncal obesity, gives rise to various lipoprotein abnormalities (Fig. 127.3).[6] Although elevated plasma levels of triglycerides, low plasma levels of high-density lipoprotein (HDL) cholesterol, and qualitative changes in low-density lipoprotein (LDL) particles (defined as small, dense LDL) are often found in obese subjects, significant elevation of LDL-cholesterol levels has not been uniformly described. Kinetic studies have shown that the production rate of very-low-density lipoprotein (VLDL) is increased in obese patients.[7] The increased VLDL production may be related to the increased FFA levels in obese persons, because FFAs accumulate in the liver and enhance the formation of triglyceride-enriched VLDL. In some obese subjects, the response to greater VLDL production is an increase in the lipolysis of VLDL triglycerides; other patients develop hypertriglyceridemia. High circulating levels of VLDL lead to an increased exchange of VLDL-triglycerides for cholesterol esters in HDL and LDL. This bidirectional exchange reduces HDL-cholesterol levels, engenders cholesterol-depleted LDL (small, dense LDL), and increases the cholesterol content of VLDL. For these reasons, although LDL-cholesterol may not be overtly elevated in patients with obesity, qualitative abnormalities in LDL particles probably contribute to the increased risk for CHD. If an obese patient has coexisting reductions in LDL-receptor activity, which impair LDL removal, frank elevation in LDL-cholesterol may occur.

Obese patients also have greater hepatic triglyceride lipase activity; this mechanism contributes to the lowering of HDL-cholesterol levels that is observed in obese patients.

Obesity and Blood Pressure

Blood pressure often is high in obese subjects (Fig. 127.4). Population studies have shown a correlation between body weight and blood pressure in both normotensive and hypertensive persons.[5] Despite the recognition that obesity and hypertension are associated, the mechanisms by which obesity raises blood pressure are still not completely understood. Obese patients have been reported to retain sodium and water. When volume retention is accompanied by arteriolar vasoconstriction, blood pressure increases. Hyperinsulinemia/insulin resistance, which is commonly found in obesity, may affect blood pressure by

- reducing the physiologic peripheral vasodilatory action of insulin, thus promoting vasoconstriction;
- stimulating kidney resorption of sodium; and
- stimulating sympathetic nervous system activity.

Long-standing hyperinsulinemia may also induce thickening of the arterioles. Activation of the renin-angiotensin system may be a cause of increased tubular reabsorption of sodium, which raises blood pressure in obese patients. Even small increases in the levels of angiotensin II can elevate blood pressure, especially when accompanied by volume expansion. Tuck and coworkers[8] reported that both plasma renin activity and aldosterone levels are elevated in obese patients. Moreover, weight reduction lowers plasma renin activity and aldosterone concentrations in obese subjects.

Recently, Hall and Louis[9] proposed an alternative mechanism for increased volume retention in obesity. From experiments in dogs, they found that large increases in interstitial fluid hydrostatic pressure were observed in the presence of obesity. This condition could cause increased resistance to

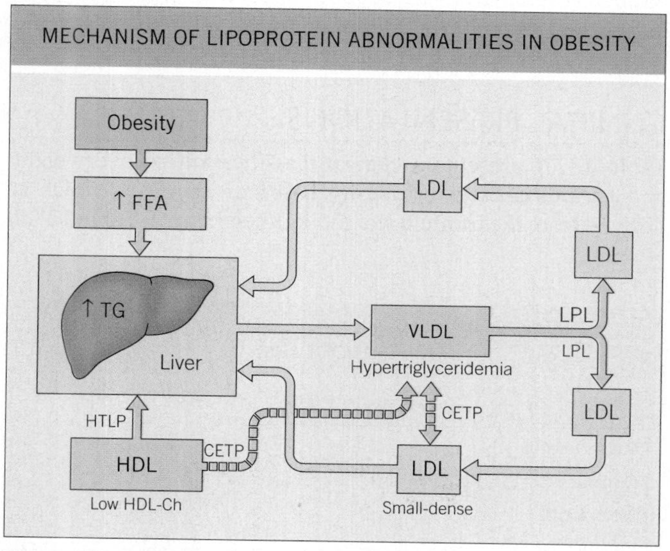

Figure 127.3 Mechanism of lipoprotein abnormalities in obesity. Excessive release of free fatty acids (FFAs) from excessive adipose tissue induces excessive production and secretion of triglyceride-enriched very-low-density lipoprotein (VLDL) in the liver. Hypertriglyceridemia induces changes in the physicochemical composition of low-density lipoprotein (LDL) and high-density lipoprotein (HDL). CETP, cholesterol ester transfer protein; HDL-Ch, HDL-cholesterol; LPL, lipoprotein lipase; TG, triglycerides; HTLP, hepatic lipoprotein lipase.

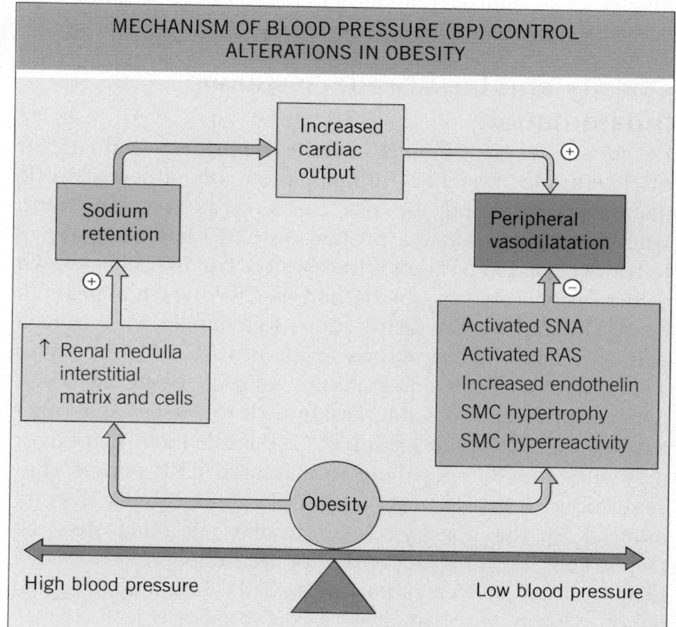

Figure 127.4 Mechanism of blood pressure (BP) control alterations in obesity. Volume retention, accompanied by impaired peripheral vasodilatation, often accompanies obesity. SNA, sympathetic nervous system activity; RAS, renin-angiotensin system; SMC, smooth muscle cell.

flow through the loop of Henle and, consequently, a reduction in the tubular flow rate and increased sodium reabsorption.

Obesity and Cardiac Hypertrophy

Left ventricular mass has been reported to be increased in obesity, independent of hypertension.[10] Several studies in obese adults reported increased left ventricular mass, left ventricular wall thickness, and left ventricular cavity size compared with lean subjects. Obesity could increase left ventricular mass by various mechanisms. One likely mechanism is an increased circulatory blood volume secondary to sodium and water retention. As a consequence, cardiac output rises because of a high stroke volume. The increases in circulating blood volume and cardiac output produce an increase in the cavity size of the left ventricle, which puts stress on the left ventricular wall, in accordance with Laplace's law. The resulting greater afterload predisposes to eccentric LVH, which in turn engenders diastolic dysfunction. However, concentric LVH has also been described in obesity, even in the absence of hypertension.[11] More recently, evidence in animal models of obesity is accumulating for intramyocardial accumulation of triglyceride, which likely contributes to the anatomic and functional abnormalities of the heart observed in obese patients.[12]

Obesity and Cardiac Electric Abnormalities

Obesity increases the risk of sudden death.[13] This could result from cardiac electrical abnormalities secondary to ventricular changes. The main electrical abnormality described in obese patients is a prolongation of the QT interval. In addition, autopsy and echocardiographic studies in obese patients have revealed fatty infiltration of the conduction system of the heart, as well as enlargement of the left ventricle and atrium. Finally, sleep apnea, frequently found in obese patients, may contribute to sudden arrhythmias.

Obesity and Low-Grade Systemic Inflammation

Recent studies have emphasized the importance of the effect of low-grade systemic inflammation on atherosclerotic plaque stability and the risk for a cardiovascular event. High-sensitive C-reactive protein (hs-CRP) has been shown to be increased in patients with obesity. The IRAS has shown a correlation between obesity and hs-CRP, which appears to be modulated by fat distribution. Individuals with truncal adiposity have higher plasma levels of hs-CRP. Adipocytes and macrophages residing in the adipose tissue of obese patients produce more interleukin 6 (IL-6), which may play a major role in the production of CRP in the liver. Fatty liver may also directly contribute to increased CRP plasma concentrations. It is also possible that plaque instability directly induced by the obesity-related insulin resistance may be responsible for the propensity of obese patients to have higher plasma concentrations of hs-CRP. This may independently contribute to enhanced cardiovascular risk.[14]

Obesity and Fatty Liver

Increased plasma concentrations of fatty acids, leptin resistance, and insulin resistance[15,16] have been identified as major pathogenetic factors in the development of the fatty liver and nonalcoholic steatohepatitis observed in obesity. The increased availability of free fatty acids in plasma promotes storage in the hepatocytes. Leptin resistance decreases fatty acid oxidation, and hyperinsulinemia stimulates fatty acid synthesis in hepatocytes. Increased fatty acid flux from adipocytes also contributes to triglyceride accumulation in hepatocytes (fatty liver) and may trigger tissue inflammation (nonalcoholic steatohepatitis).

A strong association between BMI and fat content in the hepatocytes has been described in a typical U.S. population.[17] The prevalence of this condition is high among obese patients undergoing bariatric surgery, ranging from 84% to 96%. In these patients, 25% to 55% have nonalcoholic steatohepatitis, 34% to 47% have fibrosis, and 2% to 12% have bridging fibrosis or cirrhosis.[18]

Obesity and a Prothrombotic State

Elevated plasma concentrations of plasminogen activator inhibitor 1 (PAI-1) and fibrinogen levels have been described in the obese patient.[19] These abnormalities may accelerate atherogenesis and, in the presence of coronary plaque rupture, increase the size of the resulting coronary thrombosis Recent studies indicate that PAI-1 is secreted by adipose tissue, and this secretion may be increased in obese subjects.

Obesity and the Metabolic Syndrome

Obesity, particularly truncal obesity, which typically presents with a waist circumference exceeding 40 inches (100 cm) in men and 35 inches (87.5 cm) in women, is frequently associated with the metabolic abnormalities discussed previously. The clustering of these metabolic abnormalities seemingly has its roots in obesity-related insulin resistance and poses a significantly increased risk for CVD. The metabolic syndrome has been estimated to affect about one fourth of the U.S. population and recently was identified by the ATP III as a specific target of therapy for CVD prevention.

CLINICAL PRESENTATIONS

Table 127.1 presents a clinical classification of overweight and various degrees of obesity based on the BMI, which is derived from the formula weight (kg)/height (m^2). Table 127.2

CLASSIFICATION OF OVERWEIGHT AND OBESITY BY BODY MASS INDEX (BMI)

	Obesity Class	BMI (kg/m2)
Underweight		<18.5
Normal		18.5-24.9
Overweight		25.0-29.9
Obesity	I	30.0-34.9
	II	35.0-39.9
Extreme obesity	III	>40.0

Data from the National Heart, Lung, and Blood Institute.[20] North American Association for the Study of Obesity.

Table 127.1 Classification of overweight and obesity by body mass index (BMI).

CLASSIFICATION OF OVERWEIGHT AND OBESITY BY BODY MASS INDEX (BMI), WAIST CIRCUMFERENCE, AND ASSOCIATED DISEASE RISK				
			Disease Risk Relative to Normal BMI and Waist	
	BMI (kg/m²)	Obesity Class	Men <102 cm Women <88 cm	>102 cm >88 cm
Underweight	<18.5			
Normal	18.5-24.9			
Overweight	25.0-29.9		Increased	High
Obesity	30.0-34.9	I	High	Very high
	35.0-39.9	II	Very high	Very high
Extreme obesity	≥40.0	III	Extremely high	Extremely high

Data from the National Heart, Lung, and Blood Institute.[14] North American Association for the Study of Obesity.

Table 127.2 Classification of overweight and obesity by body mass index (BMI), waist circumference, and associated disease risk. Obesity is characterized by the accumulation of excessive fat in adipose tissue. Fat deposition may be generalized or may occur preferentially in different adipose tissue compartments. Two major variants of obesity are distinguished.

includes the waist circumference in the estimation of the relative risk for CVD in each category of BMI.

Heart disease in obese patients often presents as CHD. However, LVH, heart failure, and arrhythmia are other frequent clinical manifestations of obesity-related heart disease.

DIAGNOSTIC TECHNIQUES

A number of accurate methods are available to assess body fat; these include underwater weighing, total body water, total body potassium, bioelectrical impedance, and dual-energy x-ray absorptiometry. Because the equipment frequently is not readily available and measuring body fat by these techniques often is expensive, a more practical approach in the clinical setting is measurement of the BMI. Epidemiologic and observational studies have shown that the BMI provides an acceptable approximation of total body fat for most patients.

Computed tomography (CT) and MRI scans are the most accurate methods for evaluating fat distribution, particularly the degree of fat accumulation in internal adipose tissue compartments (e.g., intra-abdominal adipose tissue). However, these techniques are also laborious and expensive. For clinical and epidemiologic purposes, a more acceptable approach is the use of anthropometric measurements, such as the waist circumference, waist-to-hip circumference ratio, and skinfold thickness; these measurements are taken with calipers. The waist circumference is an acceptable indicator of the presence of truncal obesity, and skinfold thickness provides an acceptable measure of total body fat in most patients. Moreover, the sum of truncal skinfold thickness measurements provides an alternate measure of truncal fat, and studies in our laboratory have shown that this sum correlates strongly with whole body insulin sensitivity.

MANAGEMENT

The management of obese patients should be influenced by the degree of obesity and by the overall risk status for CVD.[20] Management includes both reducing excess body weight and instituting other measures to control accompanying risk factors. Obesity should be assessed in terms of the BMI, waist circumference, and the patient's motivation to lose weight. Table 127.1 summarizes the classification of overweight and obesity by BMI. The presence of preferential accumulation of fat in the abdomen is an independent predictor of the risk for CVD. Waist circumference is positively correlated with abdominal fat content, including both subcutaneous and visceral fat. It provides a clinically acceptable measurement for assessing a patient's abdominal fat content (Table 127.2).

Assessment of a patient's absolute risk status requires examination for the presence of comorbidities, such as

- dyslipidemia: LDL-cholesterol = 160 mg/dL (4.1 mmol/L), HDL-cholesterol <35 mg/dL (0.9 mmol/L), and triglycerides >200 mg/dL (2.3 mmol/L);
- type 2 diabetes: fasting plasma glucose >126 mg/dL (6.1 to 7.0 mmol/L);
- hypertension;
- LVH; and
- sleep apnea.

A fasting glucose of 100 to 126 mg/dL (7.0 mmol/L) (impaired fasting glucose) is also common in obese patients and is a risk factor both for CHD and for type 2 diabetes.

Other CVD risk factors unrelated to obesity, such as age (men >45 years, women >55 years or postmenopausal); family history (definite myocardial infarction or sudden death at or before age 55 years in father or first-degree relative, or at or before age 65 years in mother or other female first-degree relative); and smoking status, should be evaluated. Management of coexisting risk factors in obese patients is just as important as weight reduction for reducing the risk for future development of CVD.

The initial goal of weight loss therapy is to reduce the body weight to approximately 10% below the baseline. If this goal is achieved, additional weight loss can be attempted, if indicated. For patients who are unable to achieve significant weight loss, prevention of further weight gain is an important goal; these patients may also need to participate in a weight management program.

STRATEGIES FOR WEIGHT LOSS AND WEIGHT MAINTENANCE

Dietary Therapy

A diet should create a deficit of 500 to 1000 kcal/day. Depending on the patient's risk status, the low-calorie diet should be consistent with the therapeutic lifestyle changes defined by the National Cholesterol Education Program.[20a] Apart from reducing saturated fat, total fat should be 30% or less of total calories. Saturated fat should not exceed 7%. Reducing the percentage of fat alone does not produce weight loss; the total number of calories also must be decreased. Fiber intake should be encouraged.

Physical Activity

An increase in physical activity is an important component of weight loss therapy, although physical activity alone does not usually produce significant weight loss in obese patients. Most weight loss occurs because of a decreased caloric intake. Nonetheless, sustained physical activity is helpful for maintaining a lower weight. In addition, regular exercise reduces cardiovascular and diabetes risks beyond the effect of weight reduction alone.

Behavior Therapy

Strategies based on learning principles, such as reinforcement, help the patient overcome barriers to compliance with dietary therapy and/or increased physical activity. Specific strategies include self-monitoring of both eating habits and physical activity, stress management, stimulus control, problem solving, cognitive restructuring, and social support.

A combined intervention of behavioral therapy, low-calorie diet, and increased physical activity offers the most effective therapy for achieving weight loss and weight maintenance. This type of intervention should be maintained for at least 6 months before pharmacotherapy is considered.

Pharmacologic Therapy

In carefully selected patients, weight loss drugs can augment weight loss from a low-calorie diet, increased physical activity, and behavior therapy. Weight loss drugs that have been approved by the U.S. Food and Drug Administration (FDA) for long-term use may be useful for some patients with a BMI greater than 30 kg/m^2 with no concomitant risk factors or diseases. The risk factors (or comorbidities) that warrant consideration of weight loss drugs at a BMI of 27 to 29.9 kg/m^2 are hypertension, dyslipidemia, type 2 diabetes, sleep apnea, and clinical cardiovascular disease.

One approved weight loss drug is sibutramine. It can induce moderate weight loss and can help facilitate maintenance of a lower weight. Monitoring is required for side effects, particularly increases in blood pressure and heart rate. Sibutramine should not be used in patients with CHD, heart failure, arrhythmias, or a history of stroke; the presence of hypertension is a relative contraindication.

Another weight loss drug that has been approved for the treatment of obesity in the United States is orlistat. Orlistat is a pancreatic lipase inhibitor that blocks digestion and absorption of dietary fat. It causes increased fecal fat loss in patients who eat diets that are more than 30% fat. It can induce moderate weight loss and can facilitate weight maintenance. Orlistat has frequent gastrointestinal side effects.

Surgical Therapy

Weight loss surgery is one option for weight reduction in a limited number of patients with clinically severe obesity (i.e., BMI = 40 kg/m^2 [men] or 35 kg/m^2 [women]) with comorbid conditions. Weight loss surgery should be reserved for patients for whom efforts at medical therapy have failed and who are suffering from the complications of extreme obesity. Gastrointestinal surgery for weight loss is an intervention for motivated subjects with acceptable operative risks. It includes gastric restriction procedures (vertical or horizontal banded gastroplasty, vertical ring gastroplasty), adjustable silicone gastric banding, gastric bypass, and biliopancreatic bypass.

The vertically banded gastroplasty and Roux-en-Y gastric bypass have become the standard procedures used in most obese patients. Although the operative mortality appears to be low, these procedures are associated with a variety of side effects and complications. Intraoperative or postoperative complications, such as anastomotic leakage and infection, are more common with the Roux-en-Y procedure. This procedure also may cause vitamin B_{12} deficiency, anemia, and neuropathy.

Rapid weight loss generally follows any of these surgical procedures and often results in an increased incidence of gallstones. A need for revision also is a frequent complication of weight loss surgery.

PROGNOSIS

Epidemiologic studies reveal that risk factors and comorbidities begin to increase with a BMI above 25 kg/m^2. The increase in total mortality generally tends to be modest until a BMI of 30 kg/m^2 is reached. For patients with a BMI above 30 kg/m^2, mortality rates are increased by 50% to 100% above those of patients with a BMI in the range 20 to 25 kg/m^2.

Several factors affect the relationship between BMI and mortality. The correlation between cardiovascular risk factors and type 2 diabetes has already been discussed in detail. Other factors that affect the prognosis include the age of onset and duration of obesity, degree of weight gain, weight cycling, ethnicity, and cardiovascular fitness.

Overweight children and adolescents are at increased risk for premature morbidity and mortality, independent of adult BMI.[21] A recent study by Gunnell and colleagues[22] on a cohort of 2990 subjects followed for 57 years revealed that a childhood BMI above the 75th centile was associated with a twofold increase in the risk for CHD compared with those with a BMI between the 25th and 49th centiles. The risk of CVD with increasing BMI is higher in young adults and seems to attenuate with aging.[23] The impact of weight gain on the CVD risk of an increasing BMI was recently emphasized in an analysis of the Nurse Health Study cohort; this study showed that the relative risk for CVD morbidity and mortality rises with increasing BMI, beginning at age 18 years.[24] In addition, the study showed that each kilogram of weight gain from age 18 years was associated with a 3.1% higher relative risk for CVD.

Obesity affects CVD morbidity and mortality differently in different ethnic groups. Although most studies are available in populations of European descent, various epidemiologic studies conducted in different ethnic groups have given inconsistent results. For example, African American women and men have high mortality rates from CVD,[25] but only a weak association between obesity and CVD was found in some studies. Studies in Native Americans[26] have revealed that obesity is related to CVD in this population, but the risk rises only at much higher degrees of obesity than in Caucasians.

Few data are available on Mexican Americans on the relation between BMI and morbidity and mortality. An increased prevalence of obesity and truncal obesity in Mexican Americans has not been reported to be associated with increased mortality; for this reason, the impact of obesity on CVD in this population has been questioned.[27] Interestingly, a 10-year prospective study by Hodge and associates[28] revealed that an increased BMI in Micronesian Nauruans (an ethnic group from the central Pacific Ocean with a rapidly increasing prevalence of obesity) and Melanesian and Indian Fijians does not confer increased risk for cardiovascular mortality. Finally, the excessive CVD morbidity and mortality in Asian Indians is not associated with an increased prevalence of obesity.[29]

Although the strength of the association between obesity and the risk of CVD may vary in different ethnic groups, secular trends in many populations have demonstrated that long-standing overweight and obesity eventually lead to the emergence of chronic diseases. Therefore, obesity cannot be ignored, even when associated health problems have not reached the levels that would be expected on the basis of data for the Caucasian population.

Weight cycling is frequently found in obese patients. Although it remains unknown whether weight cycling is causally linked with increased mortality or whether it is an indirect health marker of subclinical disease, several studies have indicated that weight variability is associated with an increased risk of death.

A high level of physical fitness has been reported to reduce CVD morbidity and mortality, independent of obesity.[30] Sedentary, lean men with a BMI of 25 kg/m^2 or lower are at greater risk of developing heart disease than fit, overweight men with a BMI of 27 kg/m^2 or higher who exercise regularly. Because overweight and obese subjects tend to have a more sedentary lifestyle, their lower levels of physical activity may independently account for their increased risk of CVD morbidity and mortality.

These obesity-related factors may account for the variability in strength of the association between obesity and morbidity and mortality from CVD observed in different population studies. The interaction of these different factors may also account for the U- or J-shaped relationship between BMI and mortality. The higher mortality with very low body weight observed in population studies is probably the result of concomitant chronic diseases and involuntary weight loss. Voluntary weight loss has been associated with an improved prognosis in prospective studies.

SUMMARY

Obesity, particularly truncal obesity, is associated with increased morbidity and mortality from CVD. Obesity seemingly increases the risk for CVD both directly and indirectly by promoting the onset of comorbid conditions that predispose to CVD. More commonly, obesity-related heart disease presents as CHD. However, LVH, heart failure and arrhythmia are other common clinical manifestations. Voluntary weight loss may prevent or even reverse CVD in obese patients. Therapeutic intervention for weight loss and coordinated management of obesity-related comorbidities are essential for adequate prevention and treatment of CVD in obesity.

chapter 128

Central Nervous System: The Neurogenic Heart

Alexander Kopelnik and Jonathan Zaroff

Definition

- Neurocardiogenic injury is a syndrome of cardiac abnormalities and dysfunction that occurs in the setting of diverse central nervous system diseases. This syndrome may present with any of the following: electrocardiographic (ECG) changes, cardiac arrhythmias, abnormal cardiac biomarkers, ventricular dysfunction, and sudden death.

Key Features

- Neurocardiogenic injury is often associated with lesions in the autonomic centers of the cortex (right insula), the diencephalon (hypothalamus), the medulla, and the stellate ganglia. Experimental and clinical data indicate that excessive release of catecholamines from sympathetic nerve terminals into the myocardium is the central mechanism of this syndrome.

Therapy

- Close cardiac monitoring is recommended, including screening for elevated cardiac biomarker levels and echocardiographic abnormalities in high-risk patients.
- Treatment priority should be given to the underlying neurologic condition, even in the setting of cardiac dysfunction, for which cardiac care is mostly supportive in nature.

Cardiac function is highly dynamic, and the heart can adjust its output based on systemic metabolic demands. Because these demands may change rapidly, the heart is regulated by specific centers in the central nervous system (CNS) and not solely by circulating catecholamines. Considerable experimental evidence and a moderate degree of clinical evidence indicate that acute brain injury is associated with autonomic activity imbalance, with subsequent myocardial injury, arrhythmias, and sudden death.

The interconnection of the central nervous system and the heart was first described by Cushing at the turn of the twentieth century. Cardiac abnormalities were described thereafter, associated with various CNS diseases, including trauma, ischemic stroke, and intracerebral hemorrhage (ICH). Neurocardiogenic injury is particularly common in patients with subarachnoid hemorrhage (SAH). Less common etiologies include tumors, electroconvulsive therapy, and CNS infections, such as meningitis. In 2003, more than 157,000 Americans died of stroke,[1] and a cardiac cause could be implicated in up to 6% to 19% of these deaths.[2,3]

Because they are frequently consulted in the care of neurologic patients who develop signs of neurocardiogenic injury, cardiologists must have a knowledge of clinical detection and the monitoring and treatment of high-risk patients.

In previous editions, the anatomy and neurophysiology of cardiac control were emphasized. In this third edition, we focus more on the cardiac aspects of neurocardiogenic injury and on updated clinical observations and management recommendations.

NEUROANATOMY AND NEUROPHYSIOLOGY OF CARDIAC CONTROL

CNS regulation of cardiovascular function involves different levels of the nervous system and is very complex. Several nuclei in the diencephalon and brainstem regions act as centers of autonomic cardiovascular regulation. Recent investigations have localized cortical areas within the insular cortex that play an important role in the regulation of central autonomic processes. Afferent impulses from receptors are sent to the petrosal and nodose ganglion and from there to the nucleus tractus solitarius. The impulses then are processed at medullary limbs, with regulatory input from the hypothalamus. Efferent sympathetic response starts at the cortical levels in the right insular cortex and hypothalamus; preganglionic fibers are sent to the intermediolateral cell column, where they synapse with sympathetic nerves, sending postganglionic fibers through the upper thoracic roots, then via the stellate and superior cervical ganglion to effector sites in the heart.

PATHOPHYSIOLOGY

Experimental models indicate that the direct release of catecholamines from myocardial sympathetic nerve terminals is a central factor in brain injury–associated cardiac dysfunction. After acute brain injury, a marked increase in myocardial interstitial catecholamine levels, without a significant increase in plasma levels, has been observed. Furthermore, the cardiovascular effects of experimental brain injury can be prevented by both C2 spinal section and stellate ganglionectomy. High sympathetic tone is known to occur after SAH, and circulating levels of catecholamines remain elevated for at least 10 days after the event. Plasma levels of catecholamines correlate with the severity of neurologic injury and neurologic outcome.

The systemic release of catecholamines may cause cardiac injury by increasing myocardial oxygen demand (tachycardia, increased inotropy, and systolic blood pressure) or by causing coronary vasospasm. Excessive release of norepinephrine from the myocardial sympathetic nerves has been hypothesized to cause cardiac injury and dysfunction by means of persistent activation of the β_1-adrenergic receptors, resulting (through G-protein activation) in persistent opening of cardiomyocyte calcium channels. It also is possible that excessive interstitial levels of catecholamines result in the formation of free radicals, which cause membrane perforations, allowing cellular calcium influx. The excessive influx of calcium may result in myocardial contraction band necrosis, which is histologically distinct from the coagulative necrosis seen in myocardial infarction secondary to coronary thrombosis. The lesions are characterized by their multiplicity, seemingly random locations, and loss of sarcoplasm and striations of the affected myocytes (Fig. 128.1). Under the electron microscope, these lesions are found near the intracardiac nerves.

Certain single nucleotide polymorphisms (SNP) of the β- and α-adrenergic receptors, which modulate the catecholamine sensitivity of the adrenoceptors, are associated with an increased risk of cardiac injury and dysfunction after SAH; this supports the hypothesis that cardiac injury after SAH is neurogenic and catecholamine mediated.[4] Specific combinations of adrenoceptor SNP genotypes result in a 10-fold to 15-fold increase in the odds of myocardial necrosis and left ventricular contractile dysfunction developing after SAH.

A significant proportion of cardiac arrhythmias occur in patients with normal cardiac function, suggesting neurogenic mechanisms. The type and location of the stroke may determine the type of arrhythmia, with each cerebral hemisphere having a different influence on cardiac function.[5] Animal studies show that the sinoatrial node is under right-sided autonomic control and that stimulation or inhibition of the right medulla, hypothalamus, and cerebral hemisphere exerts a greater influence on heart rate than do comparable manipulations on the left. Bradycardia and vasodepressor effects are more common with injury to the right insula, whereas tachycardia and hypertension are more common with injury of the left insular region. Supraventricular arrhythmias are more common after stimulation of the right hemisphere. Because supraventricular tachycardia can be activated by an increase in sympathetic tone, it is hypothesized that the impaired parasympathetic tone caused by right hemispheric injury is responsible for the excess in arrhythmias. QT prolongation also is more common after right middle cerebral artery occlusion, which explains the higher incidence of fatal arrhythmias and sudden death after right hemispheric strokes.

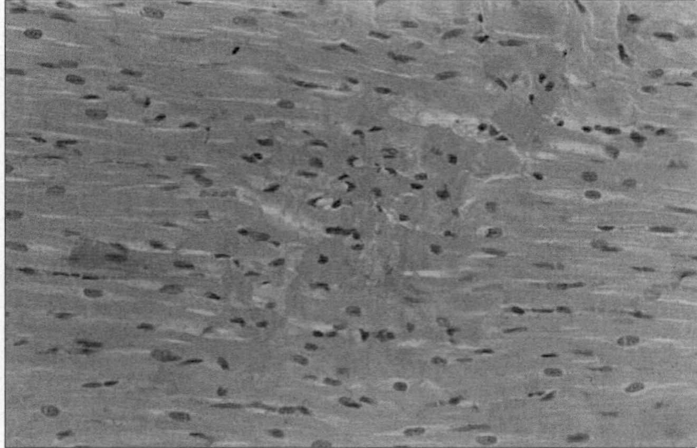

Figure 128.1 Example of contraction band necrosis from an experimental canine model of subarachnoid hemorrhage (SAH). The characteristic pattern of myofibrillar degeneration is noted. This lesion is histologically distinct from coagulative necrosis, which is typical for myocardial infarction. (From Zaroff JG, Rordorf GA, Titus JS, et al. Regional myocardial perfusion after experimental subarachnoid hemorrhage. Stroke 2000;31:1136-1143.)

CLINICAL PRESENTATIONS

Neurocardiogenic injury typically occurs in patients with clinically obvious neurologic disorders. The neurocardiogenic injury itself, however, is clinically silent in many cases, either because no symptoms are evident or the patient is neurologically impaired and unable to communicate about cardiac symptoms. For this reason, most cases are detected by electrocardiographic changes, elevation of cardiac biomarkers, pulmonary edema on chest radiograph, or echocardiographic abnormalities. A minority of the patients develop cardiac arrhythmias or overt signs of cardiac impairment with pulmonary edema or hemodynamic instability. In some patients, sudden, unexpected death, presumably from arrhythmia, is the presenting feature.[6,7]

Electrocardiographic Abnormalities

In 1947, Byer and colleagues described several cases, including at least two patients with SAH whose ECGs showed marked QT prolongation with large T and U waves.[7a] Subsequently, in 1954, Burch and colleagues described an ECG pattern, most pronounced in the septal leads, that consisted of large, inverted T waves, prolonged QT intervals, and large U waves; this pattern has since been considered distinctive of cerebrovascular accidents.[8] ECG abnormalities are common in the setting of stroke. Their incidence ranges from 49% to 100% in different series. ECG changes are seen more commonly in patients with ICH (60% to 70%) or SAH (40% to 70%) than among those with ischemic stroke (15% to 40%).[9]

The most common stroke-related ECG abnormality is QT prolongation, found in 45% to 71% of patients with SAH, 64% of patients with intraparenchymal hemorrhage, and 38% of patients with ischemic stroke.[10-12] In patients with SAH, ventricular tachyarrhythmias, including sudden death and torsades de pointes, often are preceded by QT prolongation.[12] ST-segment changes (including ST elevations) occur in 22% to 35% of patients with ischemic stroke. New T-wave abnormalities appear in approximately 15% of patients with acute stroke, even in the absence of electrolyte disturbances or primary ischemic heart disease. New Q waves have been identified in about 10% of patients with acute ischemic or hemorrhagic stroke. U waves unrelated to any electrolyte abnormality are common after stroke and may occur in isolation or with T waves and QT abnormalities. Studies found new U waves in 13% to 15% of patients with acute ischemic stroke and SAH.[12] One study showed that standard ECG criteria for left ventricular hypertrophy (LVH) were met in 14% of patients with SAH, none of whom had a history of coronary artery disease (CAD), and 43% had no history of hypertension.[13] The data on the prognostic significance of ECG changes in SAH are inconsistent, at least partly because the available studies were retrospective and had limited power to adjust for comorbid factors.

Cardiac Arrhythmias

Arrhythmias are seen in 20% to 40% of patients with ischemic stroke or ICH and in virtually all patients with SAH.[14] In a retrospective study of 150 patients with acute stroke, Goldstein[15] found a 25% incidence of new arrhythmias, compared with 3% in the control group. Atrial fibrillation was the most common, occurring in 14% of patients; ventricular arrhythmias occurred in about 5% of patients. Sinus bradycardia and supraventricular tachycardias were seen more commonly with traumatic frontal lobe hemorrhage (33%), whereas atrial and ventricular ectopy was seen more frequently with temporal-parietal bleeding episodes. In one prospective study of ischemic stroke patients, ventricular extrasystoles were the most common cardiac arrhythmia, followed by atrial extrasystoles, supraventricular tachycardia, and atrial fibrillation.[16]

The importance of continuous ECG monitoring, especially early in the course of a subarachnoid hemorrhage, was underscored by Di Pasquale and coworkers,[11] who found that the frequency and severity of arrhythmias were significantly higher in patients studied within 48 hours of the onset of SAH. In patients with SAH, sinus bradycardia was noted in 23%, multifocal ventricular ectopy in 54%, asystolic intervals in 27%, and atrial fibrillation in 4%.[17] In one study of monitored patients, rhythm disturbances occurred in 35%, most commonly sinus tachycardia or bradycardia. Ventricular arrhythmias, such as asystole and fibrillation, were also recorded, and 5% of these patients suffered a life-threatening event.[18] A polymorphic ventricular tachyarrhythmia (torsades de pointes) could be detected in about 4% of SAH patients; it has been shown to correlate with prolongation of the QT interval on the ECG.[12]

Myocardial Injury and Dysfunction

Cardiac Biomarkers

Cardiac biomarker elevations are common in ischemic stroke and hemorrhagic stroke and provide evidence that myocardial necrosis may occur. Elevations of the creatine kinase (CK) or CK-MB isoenzyme level are seen in 10% to 45% of stroke patients, and good correlation is seen between elevation in the CK-MB level and stroke-induced ECG changes or cardiac arrhythmias.[9] In contrast to acute myocardial infarction, a stroke-induced increase in serum CK-MB levels occurs more slowly and peaks at a much lower value, on average approximately 4 days after stroke. Cardiac troponin I elevations have been described in 20% to 25% of patients with SAH. The degree of neurologic injury and female gender are strong predictors of myocardial necrosis after SAH.[19] The severity of the initial neurologic injury (Hunt-Hess grade) is a strong independent predictor of myocardial necrosis and suggests a neurally mediated form of cardiac injury that occurs early in the course of SAH. Elevated B-type natriuretic peptide (BNP) levels early after SAH have been associated with myocardial necrosis, pulmonary edema, and both systolic and diastolic dysfunction of the left ventricle.[20]

The clinical implications of neurocardiogenic injury extend beyond the observed cardiac morbidity and mortality. Several studies have demonstrated an association between myocardial injury and adverse neurologic outcomes, especially in patients with SAH. Evidence indicates that troponin elevation after SAH is associated with an increased risk of cardiopulmonary complications, delayed cerebral ischemia, and death or poor functional outcome at discharge.[21] Elevated BNP levels are also independently associated with adverse neurologic outcomes and predict mortality after SAH (Fig. 128.2).[22,23]

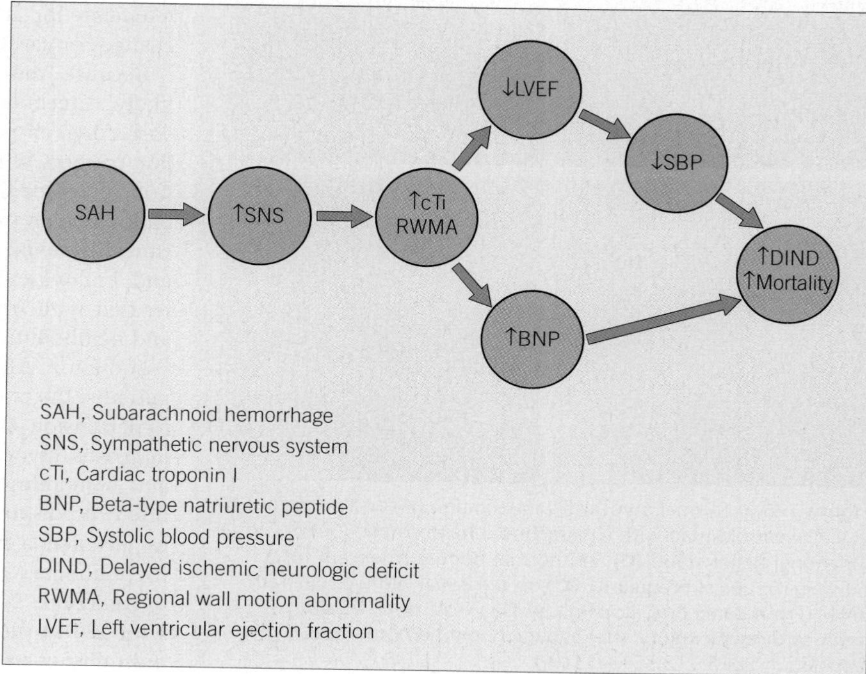

Figure 128.2 Paradigm for the association between cardiac dysfunction and death after subarachnoid hemorrhage (SAH). The figure proposes a mechanistic pathway to explain the effects of cardiovascular abnormalities on the risk of delayed ischemic neurologic deficits and mortality. (From Yarlagadda S, Rajendran P, Miss JC, et al. Cardiovascular predictors of in-patient mortality after subarachnoid hemorrhage. Neurocrit Care 2006;5:102-107.)

Left Ventricular Dysfunction

Global or regional left ventricular (LV) systolic dysfunction has been described after SAH, with an approximate incidence of 10% to 28%, and up to 15% of patients develop a depressed LV ejection fraction.[12] Diastolic dysfunction is quite common after SAH (up to 71% of patients). It is associated with the severity of neurologic injury and may be the cause of pulmonary edema in many patients with SAH.[24]

Despite recent advances in diagnostic techniques for cardiac disease, the pathophysiology remains unclear. Proposed hypotheses, such as myocardial ischemia or infarction from CAD, vasospasm, and supply-demand mismatch, have not been proven. A neurogenic catecholamine-mediated mechanism of injury, or the "catecholamine hypothesis," has been demonstrated in experimental and clinical studies. A study by Banki and colleagues[25] found an association between regions of contractile dysfunction and abnormalities in myocardial sympathetic innervation while demonstrating normal perfusion. This study used a combination of echocardiography with a scintigraphic evaluation of myocardial innervation and perfusion in patients with SAH. Patients with functional sympathetic denervation had worse regional wall motion scores and more troponin release than patients without evidence of denervation. All study subjects had normal perfusion imaging, which suggests a neurogenic mechanism of cardiac injury (Fig. 128.3).[25]

The patterns of regional wall motion abnormalities observed in SAH patients differ from the typical patterns seen in coronary artery disease. SAH patients show a well-demonstrated, apical-sparing pattern. The most frequently affected segments are the basal and midventricular portions of the anteroseptal and anterior walls.[12] Younger age and an anterior position of the aneurysm were independent predictors of this pattern.[26] This apical-sparing pattern of LV dysfunction argues against an obstruction or vasospasm of coronary arteries and provides indirect evidence of a neurally mediated mechanism of injury.

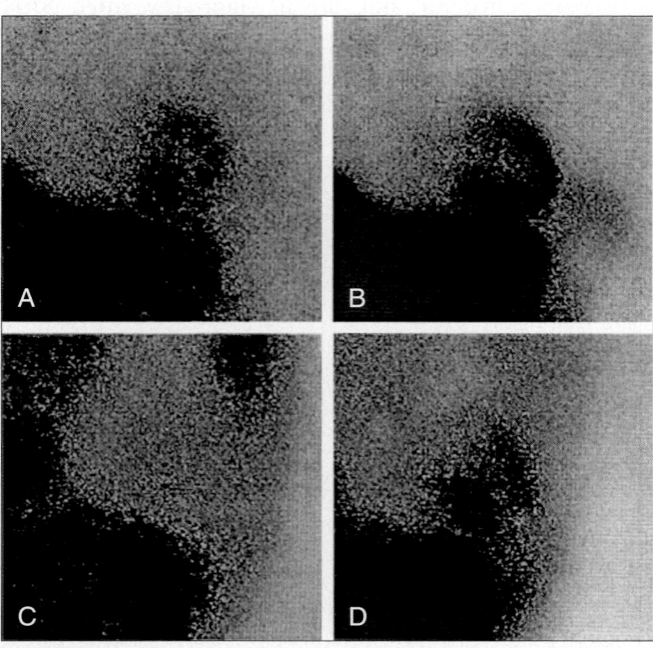

Figure 128.3 Normal myocardial innervation (**A**) and perfusion (**B**) in a 71-year-old man with subarachnoid hemorrhage (SAH). Global functional denervation (**C**) and normal perfusion, except for a nonspecific apical irregularity (**D**), in a 41-year-old woman with SAH. (From Banki NM, Kopelnik A, Dae MW, et al. Acute neurocardiogenic injury after subarachnoid hemorrhage. Circulation 2005;112:3314-3319.)

Ischemic Stroke and Coronary Artery Disease

Unlike SAH patients, patients who have an ischemic stroke are more likely to have concomitant coronary artery disease.[27] Angina, myocardial infarction (MI), and cardiac ischemia complicate about 6% of acute strokes and constitute serious or life-threatening medical events in 1%.[28] A number of clinical studies have established a strong association between cerebrovascular disease and CAD. In the longitudinal Framingham study, patients with carotid bruits had a higher incidence of transient ischemic attack (TIA), stroke, MI, and vascular death than patients without bruits. In patients with TIA, the risks for MI and sudden death (21%) and stroke (23%) were similar, although cardiac events are more likely to be fatal (63%) than stroke (16%).[29] A significant incidence of CAD (35% severe, 28% surgically correctable) was found by coronary angiography among 506 consecutive patients evaluated for possible carotid endarterectomy in one study.[30] Thallium stress imaging also has demonstrated significant CAD in 45% to 60% of patients with TIA or stroke.[31]

MANAGEMENT

All patients with intracranial pathology should have a 12-lead ECG and probably cardiac biomarker measurements on admission. Our knowledge of the role of the right insula (right middle cerebral artery territory stroke) and hypothalamus (hypertensive diencephalic or subarachnoid hemorrhages or intracranial hypertension) in the generation of arrhythmias suggests that patients with lesions at these sites should have telemetry for at least 72 hours, as should patients with ECG changes or cardiac enzyme elevation on admission.

Because the mechanism of neurocardiogenic injury is likely catecholamine mediated, treatment should focus on correcting or palliating the underlying neurologic process. For patients with SAH, current treatments include prevention of rebleeding with early aneurysm-clipping surgery or endovascular treatment. Evidence indicates that no significant difference in cardiac morbidity exists between surgical and endovascular therapies. Cerebral vasospasm may be treated with triple-H therapy (hypertension, hypervolemia, and hemodilution) and nimodipine, a potent cerebrovascular vasodilator. Although these therapies are tolerated by most patients, the potential for cardiac toxicities exists. Permissive hypertension may improve cerebral blood flow, but it also increases myocardial wall stress and oxygen consumption, and hemodilution reduces oxygen delivery to the myocardium, predisposing to further injury. In addition, iatrogenic hypervolemia may cause increased filling pressures, leading to pulmonary edema, especially in patients with diastolic dysfunction. Nevertheless, these therapies should not be withheld in most cases, given the increased morbidity and mortality of untreated vasospasm.

In patients with SAH, cardiac abnormalities during the clinical window of cerebral vasospasm are poor prognostic indicators. From a therapeutic standpoint, the data suggest that treatment for cerebral vasospasm with high-dose phenylephrine (a current vasopressor agent of choice) is relatively ineffective in patients with a reduced left ventricular ejection fraction (LVEF). Treatment with milrinone or dobutamine may be more effective in this setting.[32]

Electrocardiographic changes usually do not require specific treatment. Apart from intensive cardiovascular monitoring, appropriate investigations should be arranged to identify other causes or contributors that may require specific treatment, such as electrolyte abnormalities, toxic effects of medications, or myocardial ischemia or infarction. Cardiac arrhythmias should be managed in accordance with current guidelines.

Given the role of excessive local catecholamine levels as the likely cause of cardiac injury after SAH, beta blockers may play a part in providing cardioprotection if administered early in the hospital course. However, only a few small studies have investigated this therapy, and these suggest resolution of abnormal ECG changes associated with SAH after administration of a beta blocker. A randomized, double-blind, placebo-controlled trial of 12 patients compared 80 mg of propranolol and 20 mg of phentolamine with placebo given within the first 48 hours.[33] Although no mortality benefit was seen in the treatment group, necrotic myocardial lesions were present in all six patients who died in the placebo group; in contrast, no myocardial lesions were seen in the six patients who died in the treatment group. This small study suggests that beta blockade may protect myocytes from the hostile environment caused by massive levels of catecholamines released from cardiac sympathetic nerve terminals after SAH. Although beta blockers may provide cardioprotection from the hyperadrenergic milieu around myocytes, to date they have no proven mortality benefit. Larger studies would be helpful for determining the role of early administration of beta blockers in patients with LV dysfunction after SAH.

Coronary plaque rupture is an uncommon occurrence in SAH patients with LV systolic dysfunction; therefore, cardiac catheterization usually is not indicated. The current focus of treatment should be on the underlying neurologic injury. In most cases, treatment of the cardiac injury should be supportive. In the uncommon event that an SAH patient shows evidence of cardiogenic shock, a more aggressive diagnostic evaluation is recommended, including echocardiography, cardiac catheterization, and placement of a pulmonary artery catheter in conjunction with intra-aortic balloon counterpulsation, if necessary, to maintain adequate cerebral perfusion pressure.

Given the high prevalence of CAD in ischemic stroke patients, if clinical suspicion arises, several diagnostic modalities can be used to detect significant coronary disease. Based on the patient's risk level and functional status, these include an echocardiogram, an exercise or pharmacologic stress test (nuclear or echocardiographic), or a coronary angiogram. Once clinically evident CAD has been detected, it should be managed in accordance with current guidelines.

PROGNOSIS

After an ischemic stroke, the 30-day risk of cardiac death or nonfatal MI is estimated to be 0.6%, the 1-year risk is 3.3%, and the 5-year risk is 8.7%.[34] Not surprisingly, this risk increases significantly with age and the presence of CAD. Interestingly, left insular stroke is associated with an increased risk of adverse cardiac outcome compared with stroke in other locations and TIA. This difference is particularly marked in patients without CAD.[35]

Cardiac dysfunction that occurs after SAH may normalize over time. The onset of LV dysfunction occurs early in the course of SAH. In the largest study to date, a regional wall motion abnormality was most likely to be present within the first 2 days.[12] The prevalence then declined during days 3 to 8. Complete or partial resolution of LV dysfunction is seen in most patients during the acute hospitalization. No important difference in cardiac outcomes is seen between surgical aneurysm clipping and percutaneous aneurysm coiling. Risks associated with neurocardiogenic injury after hospitalization are unclear; however, it seems that although sympathetic denervation may persist, LV systolic dysfunction appears reversible over 6 months in most cases.

Similar to victims of head trauma and anoxic brain injury, SAH patients may experience brain death and become potential heart donors. Many of these hearts are declined because of LV dysfunction observed on the preliminary transplant workup. Because LV dysfunction after SAH likely is reversible and not related to CAD, an initial cardiac evaluation, which often is obtained under suboptimal conditions, may not be an accurate reflection of long-term LV contractile function. Optimization of volume status and inotropic support, with careful echocardiographic evaluation and possibly left heart catheterization, may allow the use of some donor hearts that otherwise would be rejected.

SUMMARY

Cardiac disturbances are diverse and frequent in the setting of stroke and are associated with adverse cardiac and neurologic outcomes. The pathophysiology of neurocardiogenic injury is likely related to intracardiac catecholamine excess and cardiotoxicity. Close cardiac monitoring of stroke patients is recommended, including screening for elevated cardiac biomarker levels and echocardiographic abnormalities in high-risk patients. Treatment priority should be given to the underlying neurologic condition, even in the setting of cardiac dysfunction. Cardiac injury that occurs after SAH seems to be reversible. In contrast to SAH patients, patients with ischemic stroke are more likely to have concomitant coronary artery disease. In cases of brain death, cardiac evaluation under optimal conditions may help increase the organ donor pool.

chapter

129 Endocrinology and the Heart

Alice Y. Y. Cheng

Definition

- Disorders of the endocrine glands often lead to increases or decreases in hormone levels, which can have detrimental effects on the cardiovascular system.

Key Features

- Diabetes—premature atherosclerotic disease, autonomic dysfunction
- Hyperthyroidism—atrial fibrillation
- Hypothyroidism—bradycardia
- Pheochromocytoma—hypertension
- Adrenal insufficiency—hypotension
- Cushing's syndrome—hypertension, premature atherosclerotic disease
- Hyperaldosteronism—hypertension
- Acromegaly—hypertension, biventricular hypertrophy
- Carcinoid—valvular disease

Therapy

- The general principle of therapy is to normalize hormone levels by means of drugs or surgery.

DIABETES MELLITUS

ANATOMY AND PATHOLOGY

The incidence of atherosclerotic heart disease in people with diabetes is approximately three times that of a person without diabetes, and coronary heart disease (CHD) is the leading cause of death.[1] In addition, CHD develops prematurely; is generally more diffuse, with involvement of small vessels; and is more often fatal, particularly for women[1] It has been shown that diabetes places one at a similar risk of myocardial infarction as someone who has had a previous myocardial infarction.[2] Similar results have been shown with stroke.[3] Because of this increased risk, a number of practice guidelines around the world have designated diabetes a CHD risk equivalent and have recommended aggressive risk factor modification.[4,5] Two types of vascular disease are seen: macrovascular disease, which causes stroke, myocardial infarction, and heart failure; and microvascular disease, which causes retinopathy, nephropathy, neuropathy, and possibly small artery occlusion in the heart.

PATHOPHYSIOLOGY

Type 1 diabetes is characterized by autoimmune destruction of the pancreatic islet cells, resulting in insulin deficiency and hyperglycemia. Type 2 diabetes differs in that it is characterized by insulin resistance and relative islet cell dysfunction, again resulting in hyperglycemia. Associated with the insulin resistance, or perhaps partially because of it, several other metabolic derangements coexist, which all contribute to the increased risk of vascular disease. These include increased flux of free fatty acids, atherogenic dyslipidemia, hypertension, obesity, microalbuminuria, and a procoagulant state characterized by increases in fibrinogen, plasminogen activator inhibitor 1 (PAI-1), and platelet aggregation. Chronic hyperglycemia results in the nonenzymatic glycosylation of arterial proteins, or advanced glycation endproducts (AGEs). These cause the increased basement membrane permeability that is characteristic of diabetic vasculopathy. Increased permeability to low-density lipoprotein (LDL) cholesterol causes inflammation of the arterial wall by inducing chemotaxis of mononuclear leukocytes, as well as secretion of platelet-derived growth factor (PDGF) and various cytokines, such as tumor necrosis factor (TNF), interleukin 1, and insulin-like growth factors (IGF-I and IGF-II). Glycation also modifies the apoB-100 found on LDL-cholesterol, making it more susceptible to oxidation and to uptake by macrophages in the arterial wall, initiating the process of the fatty streak.

The function of high-density lipoprotein (HDL) cholesterol in reverse cholesterol transport also is deranged by diabetes. Hyperglycemia, therefore, appears to be a major contributor to the premature atheroslcerotic disease; however, other significant players include blood pressure, dyslipidemia, and a procoagulant state. Consequently, treatment must be multifactorial to reduce the risk of macrovascular disease.

CLINICAL PRESENTATIONS

Coronary Artery Disease

Angina and myocardial infarction often are manifested by atypical symptoms. Among patients with diabetes, only 4% of those with ischemia also have painful angina; in patients without diabetes, 30% to 40% of those with ischemia also have painful angina.[6] Painless infarction is common in up to one third of people with diabetes, and many present with symptoms of congestive heart failure (CHF) rather than ischemia. Epidemiologic studies suggest that the presence of diabetes ameliorates the protective cardiovascular effects of female gender.[7]

Congestive Heart Failure

Men with diabetes have a 2.4-fold increase in heart failure, but women with diabetes have a particularly high incidence—5.1 times that of those without diabetes. CHF most often is due to macrovascular disease of the coronary arteries, which causes an ischemic cardiomyopathy. It also may result from hypertension, which causes left ventricular hypertrophy. Diabetic cardiomyopathy can occur in the absence of epicardial vessel disease and hypertension; some maintain that it is caused by a preponderance of small-vessel disease and metabolic alterations in the diabetic myocardium.[8] The cardiomyopathy, which occurs particularly in women, is characterized by myocardial hypertrophy, fibrosis, increased interstitial connective tissue, and microangiopathy with microaneurysms, and it can result in both systolic and diastolic dysfunction (see Chapter 71).[9]

Autonomic Dysfunction

Autonomic neuropathy is common and results in sympathetic denervation, which is manifested by a fixed tachycardia. Subsequent parasympathetic damage results in a lowering of the heart rate. Complete autonomic cardiac denervation occurs, resulting in a heart rate that is no longer responsive to physiologic stimuli, such as standing. A patient can be considered to have autonomic neuropathy if two or more of the following are present[10]:

- increased resting heart rate (above 100 beats per minute [bpm] after supine position for 15 minutes);
- decreased beat-to-beat heart rate variation (below 10 bpm during inspiration and expiration);
- abnormal ratio of R-R interval (less than 1.1 after and during the Valsalva maneuver);
- abnormal ratio of R-R interval (less than 1.0 at 30th beat/15th beat in response to standing); and
- excessive fall in blood pressure with standing (above 30 mm Hg at 1 minute).

DIAGNOSTIC TECHNIQUES

The diagnosis of diabetes mellitus is established when the fasting glucose measurement is found to be greater than or equal to 7.0 mmol/L on two occasions or when the random glucose value is greater than 11.0 mmol/L with hyperglycemic symptoms. Noninvasive cardiac risk assessment is not recommended routinely for all patients with diabetes.[11] However, clinical suspicion should be high, because patients with diabetes are considered in the high-risk category, and clinical judgment should mandate the use of noninvasive testing for management decisions. Many patients with diabetes have neuropathy, foot ulcers, amputations, and peripheral arterial disease, and these patients need pharmacologic stress testing with Persantine or dobutamine for adequate evaluation. Patients with multiple risk factors or unstable coronary disease and those in whom medical therapy has failed should undergo coronary angiography to determine the extent of their disease, because the incidence of multivessel disease is high. Echocardiographic studies have shown abnormal systolic function in 70% to 90% of patients with diabetes, and diastolic dysfunction occurs in 10% to 30%. Impaired diastolic filling may be one of the earliest manifestations of diabetic cardiomyopathy.

MANAGEMENT

Hyperglycemia

Comprehensive, multifactorial management of the patient with diabetes is critical for reducing the risk of cardiovascular disease and mortality.[12] Meticulous attention should be paid to achieving blood pressure and lipid targets, smoking cessation, lifestyle modifications, and correction of hyperglycemia. Evidence exists that good glycemic control improves macrovascular outcomes, but it is not as strong as for blood pressure and lipid control.[13,14] However, reduction of microvascular complications, including neuropathy, has been well proven. Diet, exercise, oral antihyperglycemic agents, and insulin remain the mainstays of therapy. At the present time, the glycemic target for all patients with diabetes should be an A1c below 7%.[4,5]

Hypertension

Control of blood pressure is an important factor in the reduction of the macrovascular burden of diabetes. Early, vigorous antihypertensive and lipid-lowering therapy is recommended. Angiotensin-converting enzyme (ACE) inhibitors or angiotensin receptor blockers (ARBs) are preferred for control of hypertension. The goal is a blood pressure below 130/80 mm Hg, as suggested by the American Diabetes Association and the Canadian Diabetes Association.[4,5] Combination therapy with beta blockers, calcium channel blockers, and diuretics often is necessary, and most patients with diabetes require at least three antihypertensive agents to reach this goal. Although thiazides and beta blockers can aggravate dyslipidemia slightly, they are effective antihypertensive agents and should be used. Beta blockers are indicated in patients with recent myocardial infarction.

Dyslipidemia

Treatment of dyslipidemia should be directed at lowering LDL-cholesterol to below 100 mg/dL.[15] β-Hydroxy-β-methylglutaryl coenzyme A (HMG-CoA) reductase inhibitors (statins) are the initial drugs of choice for lowering LDL-cholesterol. With patients considered to be at very high risk, the clinician may opt to reduce the LDL-cholesterol further, to below 70 mg/dL. In addition, triglycerides often are found to be elevated with a low HDL-cholesterol. No specific targets have been established for triglycerides or HDL-cholesterol. However, in cases of severe hypertriglyceridemia (triglyceride level >1000 mg/dL), fibrates generally are indicated. Unfortunately, few agents are available that raise HDL-cholesterol, and it remains a frustrating lipid parameter to improve.

Cardiovascular Disease

The management of cardiovascular disease in patients with and without diabetes is generally the same. However, a few notable differences exist. In acute coronary syndrome, aggressive glycemic control appears to reduce cardiovascular morbidity and mortality and should be an important consideration in the management of these patients. In addition, in patients with diabetes and coronary disease, surgical revascularization, when possible, is preferred over angioplasty because of the higher restenosis rates among those with diabetes.

PROGNOSIS

Patients with diabetes have a higher mortality from, and frequent recurrence of myocardial infarction. They also have a poor long-term prognosis, with a higher incidence of CHF and ventricular rupture compared to patients without diabetes. However, early, aggressive, multifactorial treatment of diabetes with blood pressure and lipid control, glucose control, smoking cessation, lifestyle changes, antiplatelet therapy, and ACE-inhibitor therapy can significantly reduce cardiovascular morbidity and mortality among patients with diabetes.[12]

THYROID DISEASE AND THE HEART

THYROTOXICOSIS (HYPERTHYROIDISM)

Anatomy and Pathology

The thyroid gland is a bilobed, butterfly-shaped gland in the anterior neck, below the thyroid cartilage and anterior to the trachea. Its primary responsibility is the synthesis, secretion, and storage of the thyroid hormones, thyroxine (T_4) and triiodothyronine (T_3). T_3 is the biologically active form. Thyroid hormone production is under the control of a feedback system in which the pituitary secretes thyroid-stimulating hormone (TSH), which stimulates synthesis and secretion of T_4 and T_3. Circulating thyroid hormone levels act as feedback to the pituitary to increase or decrease TSH levels. Disruption of this feedback system results in the clinical syndromes of excess (thyrotoxicosis) or deficient (hypothyroidism) thyroid hormone.

The term *thyrotoxicosis* refers to the symptom complex of excess thyroid hormone; the term *hyperthyroidism* applies only to causes of thyrotoxicosis that originate from the thyroid. These terms often are confused and used interchangeably in everyday practice.

The potential causes of thyrotoxicosis include Graves' disease, thyroiditis, toxic adenoma, toxic multinodular goiter, exogenous thyroid hormone ingestion, or other rare causes. Graves' disease and thyroiditis account for the vast majority of diagnoses. Both causes are autoimmune. In Graves' disease, an autoantibody stimulates the thyroid directly and increases production of thyroid hormone, under no feedback. This differs from thyroiditis, in which autoantibodies cause inflammation of the thyroid gland and release of stored thyroid hormone, without any increase in production. Irrespective of the cause of thyrotoxicosis, the effects on the cardiovascular system are the same, because the high levels of thyroid hormone, specifically T_3, result in the cardiovascular changes outlined in the following discussion.

Pathophysiology

Thyroid hormone, specifically T_3, has multiple effects throughout the body and influences changes in virtually every organ system. Thyrotoxicosis, therefore, results in a host of clinical manifestations. T_3 has direct and indirect effects on cardiac muscle, the peripheral vascular system, and the sympathetic nervous system. In thyrotoxicosis, the cardiovascular system is placed into a hyperdynamic state.[16,17] The heart rate, cardiac contractility, cardiac output, diastolic relaxation, and myocardial oxygen consumption are increased. Systemic vascular resistance and diastolic pressure are decreased. These effects are brought on by the direct effects of T_3 binding to nuclear receptors and altering gene expression within cardiac myocytes. Enhanced contractility in humans is due predominantly to the fact that thyroid hormone increases calcium ATPase in the sarcoplasmic reticulum and decreases its inhibitor, phopholamban, thereby regulating the intracellular calcium concentration and increasing inotropy.[18]

In general, the hyperdynamic cardiovascular system is similar to the effect of other conditions in which the sympathetic nervous system is activated with the release of catecholamines. Although systolic contraction and diastolic relaxation are augmented, the heart functions near its maximal capacity, with little cardiac reserve. Surprisingly, catecholamine levels are low or normal in hyperthyroidism, and the catecholamine-like effects are believed to be due to the direct effects of T_3 on contractile elements and sinoatrial node automaticity that are not mediated through the autonomic nervous system (Table 129.1).[19,20]

EFFECTS OF THYROID HORMONE ON THE CARDIOVASCULAR SYSTEM

Direct Thyroid Hormone Effects	Catecholamine-Like Effects
Tachycardia	Tachycardia
Palpitations	Palpitations
Atrial fibrillation	Exertional dyspnea
Increased oxygen consumption	Increased pulse pressure
Weight loss	Hyperdynamic precordium
Muscle weakness	Resting tremor
Increased bone tumover	Heat intolerance
Increased bowel movements	Stare, lid lag
Oligomenorrhea	Anxiety

Table 129.1 Effects of thyroid hormone on the cardiovascular system.

Clinical Presentations

Cardiovascular Symptoms and Signs

The clinical manifestations of the hyperdynamic cardiovascular system are presented in Table 129.2. These symptoms are very common in thyrotoxicosis and may dominate the presentation in some patients. Signs and symptoms can include

CARDIOVASCULAR MANIFESTATIONS OF HYPERTHYROIDISM

- Atrial arrhythmias
- Tachycardia
- Systolic hypertension
- Cardiomegaly
- Congestive heart failure

Table 129.2 Cardiovascular manifestations of hyperthyroidism.

tachycardia, palpitations, exertional dyspnea, atypical chest pain, and systolic hypertension with widened pulse pressure. Resting sinus tachycardia is the most common cardiovascular sign of thyrotoxicosis. Cardiac arrhythmias are also common, especially atrial fibrillation, atrial flutter, and atrial premature contractions. Atrial fibrillation appears to be the most common arrhythmia, occurring in 5% to 10% of patients with thyrotoxicosis.[21] In the elderly, atrial fibrillation may be the only manifestation of a condition known as apathetic hyperthyroidism. The increased risk of atrial fibrillation is present even in subclinical hyperthyroidism, in which patients have a low TSH level but normal thyroid hormone levels.

Despite the increased contractile function seen in thyrotoxicosis, exercise intolerance and dyspnea on exertion can occur. The exertional dyspnea usually is due to respiratory or skeletal muscle weakness rather than heart failure. However, heart failure also can develop as a complication of atrial fibrillation. Most of these patients have underlying cardiac disease.[17] Those who do not have underlying cardiac disease are believed to have a rate-related cardiomyopathy that results from prolonged, marked sinus tachycardia with no clear histopathologic correlate.

In patients with preexisting coronary disease, hyperthyroidism can precipitate more angina because of the increased demands placed on the heart by the thyrotoxic state. The angina improves once the thyrotoxicosis has been treated.

Systemic Signs and Symptoms

In addition to the cardiovascular system, virtually every other organ system in the body can be affected by thyrotoxicosis. Patients often complain of fatigue and weight loss despite an increased appetite, which helps distinguish this condition from other wasting conditions. Occasionally, the appetite may be so great as to result in weight gain. Patients may also complain of nervousness, anxiety, insomnia, mood swings, irritability, and heat intolerance. Proximal muscle weakness with brisk reflexes may be present. The patient may have an increased number of bowel movements (hyperdefecation), which is caused by decreased intestinal transit time. Women may exhibit disturbances of the menstrual cycle (lighter menses or oligomenorrhea). With Graves' disease, Graves' ophthalmopathy can develop as a direct effect of the autoantibody interaction with the extraocular muscles, resulting in diplopia or other visual abnormalities.

Physical Examination

On observation, the patient may appear agitated or nervous. Often a fine resting tremor of the hand is present. Examination of the eyes reveals a stare, lid retraction, and lid lag because of the sympathetic effects. Exophthalmos, proptosis, and diplopia may be seen only in Graves' disease as a result of hypertrophy of the extraocular muscles. In most cases, examination of the neck reveals a goiter. The skin has an unusually soft, velvety texture and often is sweaty. Proximal muscle weakness with brisk deep tendon reflexes is present. Dermopathy or localized myxedema may be present on the shins in Graves' disease. Acropachy (subperiosteal resorption of the distal digits) can look like clubbing of the fingers.

The cardiovascular examination reveals a hyperdynamic precordium with a loud first heart sound and an accentuated pulmonic component of the second, reflecting accelerated flow. These physical signs, especially when accompanied by atrial fibrillation, often can be mistaken for mitral stenosis. Systolic ejection murmurs may be heard, reflecting increased flow across the aortic and pulmonic valves. The pulse is rapid and bounding even at rest and during sleep, and the precordial impulse may be visible. Peripheral vasodilatation is accompanied by systolic hypertension with a wide pulse pressure.

Diagnostic Techniques

Laboratory Findings

The diagnosis of thyrotoxicosis is made by measurement of a low TSH and elevated free T_4 and free T_3. Other blood tests that may be helpful include antithyroid peroxidase antibody or antithyroglobulin antibody levels, which are elevated in thyroiditis. Alternatively, TSH receptor antibodies are elevated in patients with Graves' disease. Although antibody levels may be helpful, they are not reliably elevated in all patients with thyroiditis or Graves' disease; therefore, radioactive iodine uptake testing is more useful for differentiating between thyroiditis and Graves' disease, because it is a test of thyroid function. Uptake would be expected to be high in Graves' disease because of increased production of thyroid hormone, and it would be expected to be low in thyroiditis because production is not increased, merely the release of stored hormone. Thyroid scans are useful only in the context of a structurally abnormal thyroid gland (i.e., nodule), for which they can determine whether the nodule or nodules are functioning.

Electrocardiography and Echocardiography

Sinus tachycardia usually is present, although any supraventricular tachycardia can be seen. Atrial fibrillation is present in 5% to 10% of patients. On echocardiography, a hypercontractile state is seen, with rapid filling of a highly compliant ventricle.[22] Increased left ventricular mass and left ventricular hypertrophy can be seen.[23] Asymptomatic reversible pulmonary hypertension can also be seen, with elevated pulmonary artery systolic pressure.[24]

Management

Treatment of thyrotoxicosis is directed at rapidly improving symptoms and reducing demands on the heart (Table 129.3). Symptomatic relief is achieved with beta blockers. Initial treatment of patients with cardiac-related symptoms is with beta blockers, which target the tachycardia-mediated component of ventricular dysfunction without adversely affecting the inotropic effects of thyroid hormone.[25] Tremor and tachycardia improve almost immediately with beta-blocker therapy. Of the oral beta blockers, propranolol is preferred, because it also prevents the peripheral conversion of T_4 to T_3. The dose should be titrated to the patient's pulse; it usually is 20 to 80 mg given two to four times daily. Occasionally, high doses of propranolol (80 to 320 mg given four times daily) are required in thyroid storm.

Beta-blocker therapy provides only symptomatic relief; it does not treat the underlying thyroid problem. In thyroiditis, no additional therapy is required, because the underlying thyroid problem is self-limited. Once the inflammation has resulted in the release of all the stored hormone, the patient

AGENTS USED IN THE TREATMENT OF THYROTOXICOSIS			
Agents		**Dose**	**Mechanism of Action**
Thionamides	Propylthiouracil	50-300 mg orally q8h	Inhibits thyroid hormone synthesis Inhibits T_4 conversion to T_3
	Methimazole	10-30 mg orally qday	Inhibits thyroid hormone synthesis
Beta blockers	Propranolol	10-80 mg orally q6h	Decreases β adrenergic activity
	Atenolol	50-100 mg/day orally q12h	Decreases β adrenergic activity
	Nadolol	80-160 mg/day orally q12h	Decreases β adrenergic activity
	Metoprolol	100-200 mg/day orally q12h	Decreases β adrenergic activity
Iodides	SSKI	1-5 drops orally q6-8h	Prevents thyroid hormone release
	Lugol's solution	2-5 drops orally q6-8h	Prevents thyroid hormone release
	Ipodate	3 g orally every 2-3 days or 0.5 g/day	Prevents thyroid hormone release
	131	Dose calculated	Destroys overfunctioning thyroid
Other agents	Lithium	Monitor blood levels	Prevents thyroid hormone release
	Hydrocortisone	50-100 mg IV q6-8h	Decreases conversion of T_4 to T_3 Prevents thyroid hormone release

Table 129.3 Agents used in the treatment of thyrotoxicosis. SSKI, supersaturated potassium iodide; T_3, tri-iodothyronine; T_4, thyroxine.

actually may become hypothyroid. However, Graves' disease behaves differently, and more definitive therapy is required. This is achieved with antithyroid drugs, radioactive iodine thyroid ablation, or, rarely, surgery. Thionamides (antithyroid drugs) are used to prevent thyroid hormone synthesis and release by blocking iodine oxidation, organification, and iodotyrosine coupling. Propylthiouracil and methimazole are the thionamides available for use in North America. Potential side effects of thionamides include nausea, rash, elevated liver enzymes, and, rarely, agranulocytosis. Because of these potential side effects, thionamides are not used long term in North America. Generally, if remission is not achieved after 12 to 18 months of therapy with a thionamide, radioactive iodine thyroid ablation is performed. Other drugs, including lithium, iodides, and steroids, usually are reserved for the prevention of life-threatening conditions, such as thyroid storm.

Radioactive iodine is the definitive treatment for thyrotoxicosis in patients with a high percentage of radioactive iodine uptake (typically Graves' disease). Because thyroid tissue is the only tissue that requires iodine (for thyroid hormone synthesis), radioactive iodine is used for thyroid gland destruction. Advantages of radioactive iodine include the fact that customarily only a single treatment is needed and that it is relatively safe and inexpensive. Because treatment usually requires 3 to 6 months before the hyperthyroidism resolves, most patients need interim therapy with thionamides. Ultimately, the patient usually is rendered hypothyroid and is treated with long-term thyroid hormone replacement.

Patients with toxic adenoma or toxic multinodular goiters require surgery for definitive treatment of these problems. Pregnant patients must not receive ^{131}I and therefore should be treated with small doses of propylthiouracil, with or without beta blockers, or with subtotal thyroidectomy in the second trimester.

Treatment of CHF, angina, and atrial fibrillation is essentially the same as for a euthyroid individual. However, the physician should be aware that treatment of atrial fibrillation is limited to control of the ventricular rate, because cardioversion will not be successful as long as the thyrotoxicosis is present.[26] Attempted cardioversion should be postponed until 3 to 4 months of euthyroidism have been attained, because spontaneous conversion often occurs during this period.[26] In addition, patients may be relatively resistant to digoxin because of the increased volume of distribution and a decrease in the atrioventricular node refractory period, normally prolonged by the glycosides. Anticoagulation should be considered until the patient is euthyroid and in sinus rhythm.

Prognosis

The prognosis generally is excellent for most thyrotoxic conditions. Once the patient is rendered euthyroid, the hyperdynamic cardiovascular manifestations disappear. Atrial fibrillation should convert to normal sinus rhythm in more than 60% of patients. Angina should improve because of decreased demand on the heart. In the absence of preexisting underlying cardiac disease, treatment of thyrotoxicosis should result in a return to normal cardiac function. However, some population-based studies have suggested that patients with hyperthyroidism have a slightly higher mortality from circulatory diseases compared with the general population.[27]

HYPOTHYROIDISM

Anatomy and Pathology

The most common cause of hypothyroidism in industrialized countries is Hashimoto's thyroiditis, a consequence of autoimmune destruction of the thyroid gland. It occurs most often in women between the ages of 30 and 60 years. Hypothyroidism also can be caused by ablation of the thyroid gland with radioactive iodine, thyroidectomy, or drugs (e.g., amiodarone or lithium). Iodine deficiency, although once a common cause of hypothyroidism, is rare now because of widespread iodine supplementation in salt and bread.

Pathophysiology

The cardiovascular findings in hypothyroidism are the opposite of those of hyperthyroidism.[17] Cardiac contractility and the heart rate are reduced, and peripheral vascular resistance is increased. Cardiac output is reduced. Ventricular diastolic relaxation is impaired, leading to reduced compliance and diastolic filling. Myocardial oxygen consumption appears to be decreased below levels expected by the reduced workload.[16] Systemic vascular resistance is increased, and blood volume is reduced, causing prolongation of circulation time and a decrease in blood flow to the periphery. In most tissues, this decrease in tissue perfusion is accompanied by decreased oxygen consumption; therefore, the mixed arteriovenous oxygen difference remains normal. The hemodynamic alterations resemble those of CHF, except that pulmonary congestion does not occur, and the pulmonary artery and right ventricular pressures often are normal.[17] In addition, hypothyroidism may be associated with atherosclerosis. Proposed explanations include the dyslipidemia of hypothyroidism (high LDL-cholesterol), diastolic hypertension, elevated C-reactive protein, and endothelial dysfunction.

Clinical Presentations

Cardiovascular Symptoms and Signs

Unlike in hyperthyroidism, the cardiovascular manifestations of hypothyroidism (Table 129.4) are not commonly present. Marked hypothyroidism must be present for several months before cardiovascular manifestations occur. These may include exertional dyspnea, decreased exercise tolerance, and easy fatigability. In addition, bradycardia may be present. Hypertension also has been described, despite the reduction in cardiac output. The increase in systemic vascular resistance is thought to explain the predominantly diastolic hypertension that is seen.[28,29] As the hypothyroidism worsens, increased capillary permeability can result in pleural or pericardial effusions.[17] The pericardial effusions are rarely hemodynamically significant and typically resolve slowly after treatment of the hypothyroidism. Hypothyroidism rarely causes heart failure; therefore, most hypothyroid patients with heart failure have some intrinsic cardiac disease that is exacerbated by the hypothyroid state, resulting in a reduction of myocardial contractility. Despite an increased incidence of coronary artery disease, angina is uncommon, and the incidence of myocardial infarction is not increased.[16] This likely is due to the decreased metabolic demands placed on the heart in the hypothyroid state.

Myxomatous valve abnormalities also have been described in patients with autoimmune thyroid disease (Hashimoto's thyroiditis or Graves' disease). These lesions typically affect the mitral and aortic valves and, less commonly, the tricuspid valves. They occur as a consequence of deposition of glycosaminoglycans and have been linked with thyroid autoimmunity. They are rarely clinical significant, but the presence of a murmur may justify an echocardiogram.[16]

CARDIOVASCULAR MANIFESTATIONS OF HYPOTHYROIDISM
■ Bradycardia
■ Exertional dyspnea
■ Diastolic hypertension
■ Pericardial effusion
■ Combined dyslipidemia

Table 129.4 Cardiovascular manifestations of hypothyroidism.

Systemic Signs and Symptoms

Hypothyroidism is an insidious disease and may be subtle in its progression and presentation. As mentioned, cardiovascular manifestations occur infrequently and rarely are the initial presenting symptoms. Patients typically complain of weight gain, weakness, lethargy, fatigue, depression, muscle cramps, constipation, cold intolerance, dry skin, and coarse hair. Women often have menstrual disorders (menorrhagia), whereas men may have decreased libido or erectile dysfunction, or both.

Physical Examination

On observation, the patient may appear pale with periorbital edema, facial puffiness, or coarsened features. The voice may also have deepened. The hair and skin are usually coarse and dry. Goiter is present in patients with Hashimoto's thyroiditis, congenital enzyme deficiencies, iodine deficiency, and thyroid hormone resistance. Reflexes characteristically are delayed in the return phase. In severe hypothyroidism, neurologic findings are prominent and may progress to "myxedema coma."

On cardiovascular examination, bradycardia with weak arterial pulses and mild hypertension, particularly diastolic hypertension, are characteristic vital signs. Pericardial examination may reveal an enlarged heart and distant heart sounds, especially if pericardial effusion is present. Percussion of the chest may reveal pleural effusions that result from increased capillary permeability and leakage of proteins into the interstitial space.

Diagnostic Techniques

Laboratory Findings

In primary hypothyroidism, TSH is elevated, and free T_4 and free T_3 levels are reduced. Antithyroid antibodies (antithyroglobulin and thyroid peroxidase antibodies) are elevated in Hashimoto's thyroiditis. Creatine kinase isoenzymes are increased in hypothyroidism and can confuse the evaluation of the hypothyroid patient with chest pain, although the isoenzyme pattern is usually MM and not MB. Dyslipidemia also is commonly found in patients with hypothyroidism. Approximately 56% of hypothyroid patients have elevated cholesterol (LDL-cholesterol), 34% have both elevated LDL-cholesterol and triglycerides, and 1.5% have high triglycerides alone. Only 8.5% have a normal lipid profile.

Electrocardiographic and Echocardiographic Findings

Electrocardiographic changes include sinus bradycardia, a prolonged PR and QT interval, low voltage complexes, and flattened or inverted T waves (Fig. 129.1). Atrial, ventricular, and intraventricular conduction delays are three times as likely in patients with myxedema as in the general population. Pericardial effusion probably is partly responsible for these ECG changes. Echocardiography shows that pericardial effusions occur in as many as 30% of all hypothyroid patients. Cardiac tamponade is unusual because of the slow accumulation of fluid, which does not increase pericardial pressure excessively.[30] Other findings on echocardiography may include mitral, aortic, or tricuspid valve abnormalities.

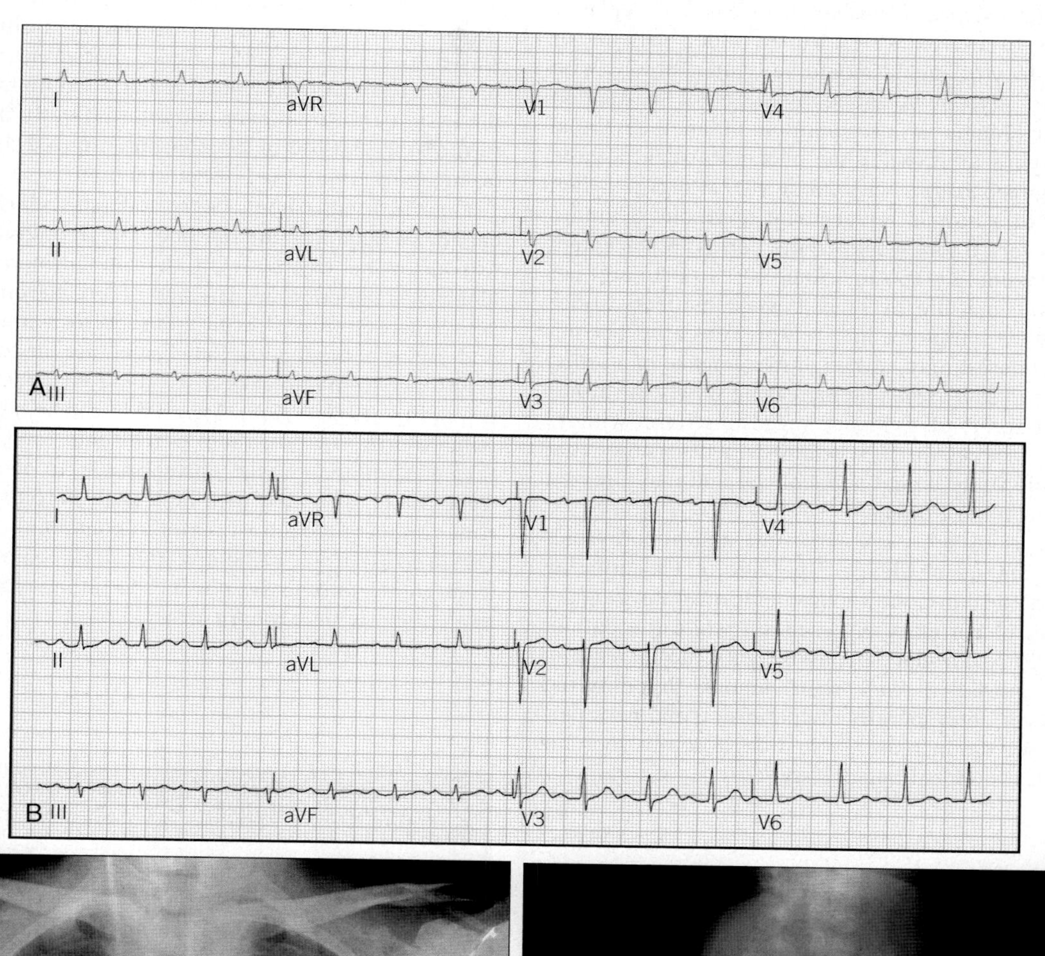

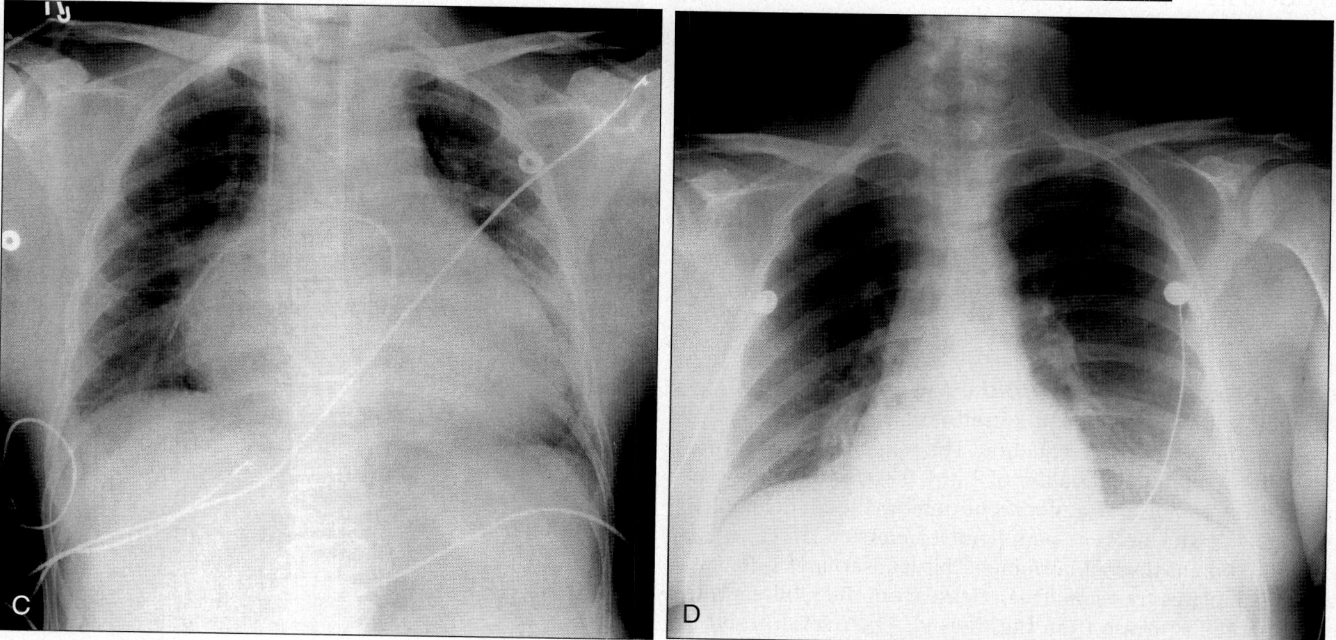

Figure 129.1 Hypothyroidism. **A**, Twelve-lead electrocardiogram (ECG) of a profoundly hypothyroid patient in heart failure. Note the low voltage, widened QRS, and flattened T waves. **B**, Twelve-lead ECG from the same patient 5 months later, after thyroid hormone replacement. The ECG is now normal except for first-degree atrioventricular block. **C**, Chest radiograph on admission for a patient in heart failure with a pericardial effusion. **D**, Chest radiograph before discharge 3 weeks later, showing a normal cardiac silhouette.

Management

All the cardiovascular signs and symptoms of hypothyroidism are reversed with thyroid hormone therapy.[16,17] The most important consideration with thyroid hormone replacement is the speed of rendering the patient euthyroid. Young patients without evidence of cardiac disease can be replaced with full doses of thyroxine. However, older patients or those with a history of angina should be treated slowly, with judicious use of thyroid hormone replacement to prevent exacerbation of angina or precipitation of an arrhythmia due to underlying atherosclerotic or myocardial disease. The typical regimen begins with 25 μg (0.025 mg) per day, or one quarter of a normal replacement dose, and is gradually increased every 6 to 8 weeks to the normal replacement dosage of approximately 100 to 150 μg (0.1 to 0.15 mg) per day. Because the half-life of T_4 is 1 week, patients notice alleviation of their symptoms in 1 to 2 months after becoming euthyroid. Interestingly, although the practice of starting with a low dose of thyroxine and increasing slowly in cardiac patients is well accepted, evidence suggesting harm with T_4 replacement is lacking. In fact, some evidence shows that adequate thyroid replacement is beneficial and may prevent progression of coronary disease.[31]

Patients with acute coronary syndrome and hypothyroidism present a unique challenge. The risk of exacerbating angina with thyroid hormone replacement must be weighed against the risk of coronary intervention while the patient is hypothyroid. For coronary bypass surgery, no increase in perioperative mortality was seen among hypothyroid patients; however, intraoperative hypotension and perioperative heart failure did increase.[32] No difference was seen for percutaneous transluminal angioplasty.[33]

Prognosis

In the absence of coexisting heart disease, treatment with thyroid hormone and restoration of euthyroid status correct the hemodynamic, electrocardiographic, and serum enzyme alterations and restore heart size to normal. Therapy is lifelong, and relapses occur if the patient is noncompliant or taken off therapy for any reason. The long-term cardiovascular outcomes of patients treated for hypothyroidism are not entirely clear. One population-based study suggested an increase in cardiovascular morbidity from arrhythmias and nonfatal ischemic heart and cerebrovascular disease but no increase in all-cause mortality.[34]

Amiodarone and the Thyroid

Normally, the thyroid gland secretes approximately 20% of the T_3 in the peripheral circulation. The remaining 80% is produced from monodeiodination of T_4 by the enzyme 5′ deiodinase. Propranolol and amiodarone inhibit the 5′ deiodinase enzyme[35,36] and prevent peripheral conversion of T_4 to T_3, the more potent thyroid hormone. This leads to low T_3 levels, which stimulates transient TSH release from the pituitary and consequent T_4 release from the thyroid. The overall result is a slightly elevated T_4 with a low-normal T_3 and a transiently elevated TSH.[35,36] Typically, the patient remains clinically euthyroid in the face of the elevated T_4 level.

Iodine is a major component of amiodarone and results in a massively expanded iodine pool. Normally, the thyroid gland adjusts to increased iodine substrate; however, in individuals with an underlying predisposition to thyroid disease, amiodarone-induced thyrotoxicosis (AIT) from iodine excess or destructive thyroiditis, as well as hypothyroidism, may occur. The overall incidence of thyroid dysfunction is estimated to be 2% to 24%. Serial measurements of thyroid function tests should be obtained at 2-month intervals during the first year of treatment and intermittently thereafter. Due to the long half-life of amiodarone, thyroid dysfunction can occur up to 1 year post discontinuation.

Thyroid disease should be treated, particularly if the patient cannot be taken off amiodarone. The hypothyroid individual can easily be treated with thyroid hormone replacement along with amiodarone. Therapy of amiodarone-induced thyrotoxicosis often is difficult and requires a knowledge of the underlying pathogenesis; that is, whether the condition is type 1 AIT due to iodine excess or type 2 AIT due to destructive thyroiditis (Table 129.5). Type 1 AIT can be treated with thionamide drugs or potassium perchlorate (or both) and even thyroidectomy in cases unresponsive to medical therapy. Type 2 AIT is treated with high-dose steroids. Like amiodarone, radiologic contrast material containing iodine, such as that used in cardiac catheterization, has the potential to cause transient thyrotoxicosis, possibly resulting in decompensation in a patient with coronary artery disease.

CHARACTERISTICS AND MANAGEMENT OF AMIODARONE-INDUCED THYROTOXICOSIS (AIT)

Type 1 AIT	Type 2 AIT
Pathogenesis: excess thyroid hormone synthesis from large iodine load released as a result of iodine-induced destructive thyroiditis	Pathogenesis: excess thyroid hormone
Exam: multinodular or diffuse goiter	Exam: occasional goiter, small, diffuse, often present and may be tender
Labs: thyroid peroxidase Ab often absent; markedly elevated IL-6; elevated ESR; elevated thyroglobulin	Labs: thyroid peroxidase Ab often present; normal or elevated IL-6
RAIU: low or normal	RAIU: very low
Therapy: thionamides (PTU or methimazole); potassium perchlorate may be necessary; thyroidectomy may be necessary, d/c amiodarone if possible	Therapy: high-dose steroids (40 mg prednisone), d/c amiodarone if possible

Ab, antibody; IL-6, interleukin-6; RAIU, radioactive iodine uptake; PTU, propylthiouracil; ESR, erythrocyte sedimentation rate; d/c, discontinue.

Table 129.5 Characteristics and management of amiodarone-induced thyrotoxicosis (AIT).

PARATHYROID DISEASE AND THE HEART

HYPERPARATHYROIDISM

Anatomy and Pathology

The parathyroid glands are located behind the thyroid gland and secrete parathyroid hormone (PTH), which is responsible for the maintenance and regulation of serum calcium levels within a fairly narrow physiologic range. Primary sources of calcium are the diet and bone. The secretion of PTH stimulates the release of calcium from bone. It also stimulates the conversion of 25-hydroxy-vitamin D to the active 1,25-dihydroxy-vitamin D by the kidney. The increase in active vitamin D stimulates intestinal absorption of dietary calcium. In addition, PTH has direct effects on the kidneys to increase calcium reabsorption. All these effects result in an increase in serum calcium. Hyperparathyroidism occurs when an excess of parathyroid hormone is present. Causes of hyperparathyroidism are divided into primary, secondary, and tertiary causes. In primary hyperparathyroidism, the predominant abnormality is at the level of the parathyroid; excess PTH, under no feedback, results in high serum calcium levels. In secondary hyperparathyroidism, the abnormality does not lie within the parathyroid glands. In fact, the parathyroid glands respond normally to a secondary stimulus, such as hypocalcemia or vitamin D deficiency, and increase secretion of PTH. In tertiary hyperparathyroidism, the parathyroid glands have been exposed to a secondary stimulus for such a long time that they become abnormal and the secretion becomes autonomous. With respect to cardiovascular effects, the limited data available focus on primary hyperparathyroidism, which is the focus of the remainder of this section.

Pathophysiology

Approximately 85% of cases of primary hyperparathyroidism are due to one or more adenomas that are autonomously producing PTH. Most of the remaining cases are due to diffuse hyperplasia.[37] In primary hyperparathyroidism, hypercalcemia is present, which can manifest in many ways clinically. However, nowadays, many primary hyperparathyroid cases are detected on routine blood tests at an early, asymptomatic phase of hypercalcemia. It is difficult to determine whether the cardiovascular manifestations of primary hyperparathyroidism are due to the PTH, the hypercalcemia, or both. PTH has effects beyond the bone and kidney. It has been found to stimulate vascular smooth muscle by binding to the PTH/PTH-related peptide (PTHrP) receptor, thereby increasing intracellular cAMP levels and reducing influx of calcium.[37]

Interestingly, studies have produced contradictory results on the effect of PTH on endothelial function. Some studies have shown significantly impaired endothelium-dependent vasodilatation, whereas others have not. Results also are contradictory on whether structural alterations in the vascular wall occur with primary hyperparathyroidism; some studies suggest an increased intima media thickness in the carotid artery wall, whereas others do not.

Beyond the vascular wall and endothelium, PTH appears to have an effect on cardiac hypertrophy. An association has been seen between left ventricular hypertrophy and primary hyperparathyroidism. This finding has several potential explanations. PTH can directly affect the cardiomyocyte because it shares receptors with PTHrP. Binding to the PTH/PTHrP receptor on the cardiomyocyte results in a rise in intracellular calcium and activation of the protein kinase C cascade, which leads to activation of hypertrophic processes within the cell. An effect on the chronotropic pacemaker cells in vitro also is seen. It is important to remember that differentiating the effects of PTH from those of simultaneous hypercalcemia is very difficult in these patients.

Clinical Presentations

Cardiovascular Signs and Symptoms

Primary hyperparathyroidism does not typically present with prominent cardiovascular features, particularly in this day and age, when most patients are diagnosed at an early, asymptomatic phase. However, some potential effects are noteworthy. Patients with symptomatic primary hyperparathyroidism have a higher mortality rate, and the prevalent cause of death appears to be cardiovascular (myocardial infarction). No particular parameter has been demonstrated to be an effective predictor of death (i.e., PTH level, calcium level). Whether parathyroidectomy corrects the risk increase is unclear, although if a benefit truly exists, it becomes apparent years after surgery. Whether asymptomatic primary hyperparathyroidism is associated with any increase in mortality remains unknown. Other cardiovascular signs or symptoms include left ventricular hypertrophy, with correction several years after parathyroidectomy. Systolic function usually is not affected; however, diastolic function can be impaired. Hypertension also can be found in conjunction with hyperparathyroidism, but establishing a cause-and-effect relationship is difficult. Some reports have demonstrated more valvular and myocardial calcification of unknown significance.

Systemic Signs and Symptoms

The vast majority of signs and symptoms occur outside the cardiovascular system. The classic symptoms of hypercalcemia include fatigue, weakness, polyuria, polydipsia, nausea, vomiting, constipation, confusion, nephrolithiasis, and bony pain. Bone density is reduced, and the patient is at risk of low-trauma fractures. Recognition of these signs and symptoms is important; however, fortunately, most people with primary hyperparathyroidism are diagnosed early, in an asymptomatic state.

Diagnostic Techniques

Laboratory Findings

The main diagnostic laboratory findings are an elevated serum calcium and a simultaneously high PTH level; these findings are in keeping with a primary cause (not a secondary or tertiary cause). The presence of renal insufficiency relates to the duration and severity of the hyperparathyroidism, Phosphate levels may be low or low normal. Bone radiographs may demonstrate classic changes of osteitis fibrosa cystica, which now is rare. Subperiosteal bone resorption is seen on the radial aspect of the middle phalanges. Once the biochemical diagnosis of primary hyperparathyroidism has been established, imaging can be arranged, which may include a parathyroid radionuclide scan to try to identify the culprit lesion, with or without a neck ultrasound scan to help localize the lesion or lesions.

Management

The definitive management of primary hyperparathyroidism is surgical removal of the parathyroid adenoma or, in the case of parathyroid hyperplasia, removal of 3.5 parathyroid glands. Before surgical intervention, the hypercalcemia can be addressed conservatively with adequate fluid maintenance. Rarely, a patient with untreated primary hyperparathyroidism may present with a parathyroid crisis with marked hypercalcemia, often accompanied by an intercurrent illness. These patients require rapid correction of the marked hypercalcemia through fluid resuscitation, and once the patient is euvolemic, furosemide could be added. In addition, intravenous bisphosphonate (pamidronate or zolendronic acid) could be used in severe cases. However, the definite treatment remains surgical removal of the adenoma or hyperplastic tissue.

Prognosis

As previously mentioned, mortality, particularly cardiovascular mortality, is increased among patients with symptomatic primary hyperparathyroidism. However, this increase remains unproven in the asymptomatic primary hyperparathyroid population. The mortality risk might be expected to return to baseline once "cure" is provided through a parathyroidectomy; however, this remains controversial. Some studies have shown a marked reduction in mortality risk, whereas others have shown only a slight reduction or no reduction in certain subgroups. With respect to left ventricular (LV) mass, parathyroidectomy appears to reduce the LV mass, but this effect can take years to manifest. Whether the high PTH levels or the hypercalcemia, or a combination of two, causes the cardiovascular manifestations remains unknown; it is reasonable to think that the earlier detection and correction of all of these parameters is helpful, but this hypothesis has not been proven. Clearly, further research is needed in this area to provide a better understanding of the interrelationship of PTH, calcium, and the heart.

HYPOPARATHYROIDISM

Neck or thyroid surgery is the most common cause of hypoparathyroidism, which develops postoperatively. Less commonly, hypoparathyroidism can have a primary autoimmune cause, often linked with other endocrinopathies. A functional hypoparathyroidism can occur in patients with magnesium deficiency, because magnesium is a cofactor for PTH. Patients usually complain of tingling around the mouth and in the hands and feet. Cardiovascular manifestations are insignificant. The physical examination reveals positive Chvostek's and Trousseau's signs. Laboratory evaluation reveals a low serum or free calcium with a low or inappropriately low-normal PTH level. Hypoparathyroidism is associated with a prolonged QT interval on an electrocardiogram because of ST-segment lengthening; the T wave usually is normal (Fig. 129.2). Occasionally, impaired left ventricular dysfunction is detected.[38,39] Restoration of eucalcemia may improve cardiac function.

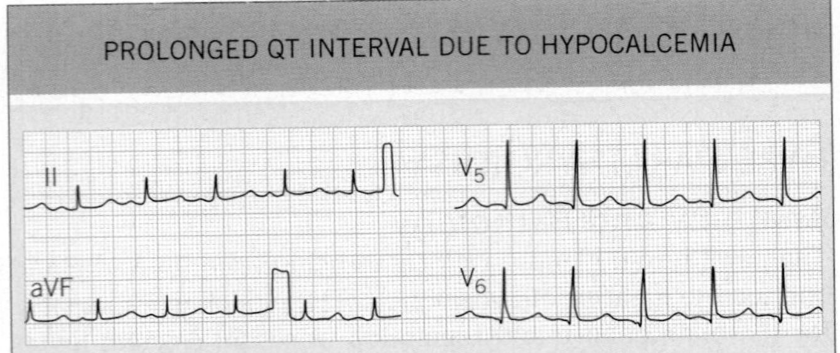

Figure 129.2 Prolonged QT interval due to hypocalcemia. Four ECG leads showing a prolonged QT interval caused by hypocalcemia.

ADRENAL DISEASE AND THE HEART

PHEOCHROMOCYTOMA

Anatomy and Pathology

Pheochromocytomas are catecholamine-producing tumors of the chromaffin cells. Eighty percent of these cells are located in the adrenal medulla. Of these, 20% occur along the sympathetic chain (paragangliomas), anywhere from the base of the brain to the testicle but most commonly in the abdomen. Pheochromocytomas can be life-threatening and cause hypertension, arrhythmia, and hyperglycemia. Most tumors are benign, but malignancy can occur. Although a main manifestation is hypertension, pheochromocytoma accounts for less than 0.1% of the causes of hypertension in the general population.

Pathophysiology

Most pheochromocytomas occur sporadically, but germ-line mutations are seen in up to 24% of cases.[40] These germline mutations include von Hippel-Lindau (VHL) syndrome, multiple endocrine neoplasia (MEN) IIa and IIb, succinate dehydrogenase subunit B or D, and neurofibromatosis type 1. In VHL disease, associated problems include cerebelloretinal hemangioblastomas, pancreatic cysts, renal cell cysts and carcinoma, and epididymal cystadenoma. In MEN IIa, other problems include medullary thyroid cancer and hyperparathyroidism. In MEN IIb, other problems include medullary thyroid cancer, mucosal neuroma, and marfinoid habitus. In patients with familial syndromes, all members of the family should be screened, particularly because certain syndromes are more highly associated with malignant pheochromocytoma. Pheochromocytomas secrete catecholamines (norepinephrine or epinephrine, or both). A small subset may secrete dopamine only or cosecrete other active hormones, such as vasoactive intestinal peptide (VIP) or PTHrP. Most pheochromocytomas (80%) are unilateral.

Clinical Presentations

Cardiovascular Signs and Symptoms

Some 85% of patients have hypertension, which may be either sustained or paroxysmal. The effects of catecholamines on the heart are mediated by β_1 receptors and include an increased heart rate, enhanced contractility, and augmented conduction velocity, all of which contribute to an increase in cardiac output. Patients without hypertension most probably secrete dopamine, which can be vasodilating. Orthostatic hypotension may be noted, although not as often as was previously thought. The combination of severe hypertension and orthostasis should suggest the possibility of pheochromocytoma. Light-headedness and syncope occur rarely.

Both dilated and hypertrophic cardiomyopathies and myocarditis have been described with pheochromocytoma. Exposure to high levels of catecholamines can cause contraction band necrosis and fibrosis. The cardiomyopathy is reversible if the excessive catecholamine stimulus is removed early, before extensive replacement fibrosis occurs. Chest pain, angina, and acute myocardial infarction may occur in the absence of coronary artery occlusive disease and are frequently diagnosed in these patients. Catecholamine-induced increases in myocardial oxygen consumption, myocarditis, and coronary artery spasm probably contribute to the infarction.[41]

Cardiac arrhythmias occur, such as atrial and ventricular fibrillation, especially in the setting of surgical resection of the tumor. Sudden death is a not uncommon presentation for patients with pheochromocytoma. Pulmonary edema and shock may also be presentations, especially with epinephrine-secreting tumors. Shock may be associated with myocarditis or infarction or may occur after hypertensive crisis. Cerebral infarction also can occur because of catecholamine effects on vasospasm and coagulation.

Systemic Signs and Symptoms

The release of catecholamines from the tumor is unpredictable and usually causes explosive attacks of headache, palpitations, and sweating.[41] The absence of this triad is very helpful in excluding the diagnosis of pheochromocytoma. Patients may also complain of increased nervousness, irritability, and a sense of impending doom. Mild abdominal pain and constipation are relatively common. Pallor, hypertension, orthostatic drop, and hyperventilation may be noted on examination. A pheochromocytoma should be suspected in any patient who develops a sudden elevation in blood pressure during anesthesia induction or a paradoxic response to beta-blocker therapy, as well as in a patient with wildly fluctuating blood pressures.

Certain prescription medications may precipitate hypertensive crisis. Beta blockade, when not given after alpha blockade, can cause unopposed alpha vasoconstriction. Desipramine, metoclopramide, and naloxone all have been reported to precipitate attacks.

Diagnostic Techniques

Laboratory Findings

Elevations in catecholamines or their metabolites are necessary for the diagnosis, along with localization/imaging studies. Indications for diagnostic testing include symptoms of pheochromocytoma; hypertension resistant to triple-drug therapy; accelerated or malignant hypertension; paradoxical blood pressure response to a beta blocker; family history of MEN II or von Hippel-Lindau syndrome; and hypertensive paroxysm with anesthesia induction or parturition. The most useful tests are 24-hour collections of urinary catecholamines and metanephrines, particularly while elevated blood pressure is present. Most clinicians favor this as the initial investigation, because the sensitivity is 98% to 99%. If the urinary results are equivocal, plasma free metanephrines (where available) should be measured. Plasma catecholamines can also be measured, but this can be affected by a number of other environmental parameters, such as emotional stress. Having the patient avoid drugs, foods, and conditions that may affect the tests should minimize false-positive results.

Imaging

Computed tomography (CT) scanning is the most widely used method of preoperative localization. It can identify adrenal masses larger than 1 cm and abdominal masses larger than 2 cm. T2-weighted magnetic resonance imaging (MRI) is superior to CT in detecting extra-adrenal tumors and is the procedure of choice in pregnant women. ^{123}I-metaiodobenzylguanidine scanning can help detect small tumors in unusual locations, but the results will be falsely negative if tricyclic antidepressants and labetalol are also administered.

Electrocardiographic and Echocardiographic Findings

Electrocardiographic changes are common; NSST-T wave changes, including inverted T waves and prominent U waves, may be seen. Sinus tachycardia, sinus bradycardia, and atrial and ventricular tachyarrhythmias all have been noted. Conduction disturbances sometimes occur, including right and left bundle branch block and ventricular strain patterns. Clinically significant cardiomyopathy and increased left ventricular mass have been noted on echocardiography, as have systolic anterior motion of the anterior mitral leaflet, paradoxic septal motion, and proximal excursion of the posterior wall during hypertensive crisis.

Management

Treatment involves surgical removal of the tumor and prevention of cardiovascular complications, such as myocardial infarction, heart failure, hypertensive crisis and stroke, arrhythmias, and sudden death. Resection of the tumor is associated with multiple perioperative complications caused by excessive release of catecholamines during handling of the tumor and a decrease in catecholamine levels postoperatively. Recent advances in laparoscopic adrenalectomy, along with proper medical preparation before surgery, have reduced the morbidity and mortality significantly.[42]

Alpha and beta blockade are used preoperatively to reverse the effects of excessive catecholamines and to prevent hypertensive crisis. Because most pheochromocytomas secrete norepinephrine, alpha blockade should be given before beta blockade to prevent aggravation of hypertension and precipitation of coronary spasm or pulmonary edema from unopposed alpha-receptor stimulation. The most frequently used alpha blockers are phenoxybenzamine, started at 20 mg/day and increased to 80 to 120 mg/day as tolerated; prazosin, 2 to 5 mg given two to four times daily; terazosin, 1 to 20 mg/day; and doxazosin, 1 to 16 mg/day, typically started 1 week before surgery. Beta blockade with propranolol or labetalol to control hypertension and arrhythmias can be started several days before surgery. Adequate volume repletion is also critical.

Phenoxybenzamine causes orthostasis and should be titrated according to the severity of the orthostasis before the beta blocker is added. Blood pressure control should be attempted for 2 weeks before surgery. Metyrosine is a drug that inhibits the rate-limiting step in catecholamine synthesis by 40% to 80% and is associated with a number of side effects. It can be used in inoperable patients with pheochromocytoma or can be used preoperatively if the hypertension is difficult to control. The dose is 250 mg four times daily, increased by increments of 250 to 500 mg to a maximum of 4 g/day. Resection can be done laparoscopically if the tumor localizes to the adrenal gland and is less than 5 cm in size.

Intraoperative treatment of hypertension during manipulation of the tumor can be done with nitroprusside and phentolamine. Cardiac arrhythmias are best managed by esmolol or lidocaine. Postoperative hypotension can be avoided by adequate volume expansion both before and during surgery. The use of morphine or phenothiazines also should be avoided, because they can cause both hypotensive and hypertensive crisis.

One to 2 weeks after surgery, a 24-hour urine collection for catecholamines should be obtained; if the result is normal, a cure is likely. If the level is abnormally elevated, incomplete resection, a second lesion, or metastases should be suspected. In patients with an inoperable lesion, chronic alpha and beta blockade, coupled with radiation therapy, is helpful.

Prognosis

Surgical removal of the pheochromocytoma usually corrects hypertension. For patients with benign tumors, the prognosis is excellent. The 5-year survival rate is 96% with benign pheochromocytomas and 44% with malignant tumors.[41] About 10% of patients have recurrences; therefore, yearly checks of catecholamines for the first 5 years after resection are recommended. Hypertension may persist in up to 25% of patients because of irreversible vascular and/or renal damage, but this usually is well controlled with standard antihypertensive therapy. If surgical cure is achieved before irreparable damage to the cardiovascular system has been sustained, cardiovascular health will be restored completely.

ADRENAL INSUFFICIENCY

ANATOMY AND PATHOLOGY

The adrenal glands are situated above the kidneys and are divided into two main sections, the adrenal cortex and the adrenal medulla. The adrenal medulla was discussed previously in the section on pheochromocytoma. The adrenal cortex is divided further into three sections, which produce glucocorticoids, mineralocorticoids, or sex hormones. The term *adrenal insufficiency* refers to an insufficiency of the adrenal cortex that results in deficient production of glucocorticoids, with or without a deficiency of mineralocorticoids. Both glucocorticoids and mineralocorticoids can have potent effects on volume homeostasis, maintenance of blood pressure, and electrolytes; therefore, deficiencies of these hormones can significantly affect the cardiovascular system.

PATHOPHYSIOLOGY

Adrenal insufficiency is classified into two types: primary adrenal insufficiency, in which the abnormality originates at the level of the adrenals; and secondary adrenal insufficiency, in which the abnormality originates at the level of the pituitary. In the developed countries, the most common cause of primary adrenal insufficiency is autoimmune destruction of the adrenal cortex (also known as Addison's disease). Worldwide, the most common cause of primary adrenal insufficiency is tuberculosis. Other causes include adrenal hemorrhage, other granulomatous diseases (e.g., histoplasmosis), metastasis, and acquired immunodeficiency syndrome (AIDS).[43]

The most common cause of secondary adrenal insufficiency is sudden withdrawal of exogenous steroids that had suppressed the hypothalamic-pituitary-adrenal axis. Sudden withdrawal of the exogenous steroids results in a glucocorticoid deficiency, because the suppressed axis is unable to compensate so quickly. Other secondary causes include hypopituitarism as a result of surgery, other tumors, autoimmune and infiltrative diseases, and hemorrhage.

Because the abnormality in primary adrenal insufficiency lies with the adrenal cortex, both glucocorticoids and mineralocorticoids are reduced. In contrast, the abnormality in secondary adrenal insufficiency lies with the pituitary; consequently, there is a deficiency of adrenocorticotrophic hormone (ACTH), which is primarily responsible for stimulating the secretion of glucocorticoids. For this reason, mineralocorticoids often are not affected in secondary adrenal insufficiency.

CLINICAL PRESENTATION

The clinical presentation of adrenal insufficiency differs, depending on the level of acuity. In acute adrenal insufficiency, the presentation can be very dramatic and life-threatening. Chronic adrenal insufficiency presents more insidiously, and the diagnosis often can be missed until the patient develops an acute illness and presents with an acute adrenal crisis.

Cardiovascular Signs and Symptoms

The major cardiovascular finding is hypotension. Mineralocorticoid or aldosterone deficiency causes renal sodium and bicarbonate wasting, resulting in profound volume depletion, hyponatremia, hyperkalemia, and acidosis. Acute adrenal insufficiency, or adrenal crisis, occurs when the patient is exposed to the stress of infection, trauma, or surgery and cannot compensate adequately with augmented steroid release. Hypotension, often orthostatic, is present in 90% of patients and may cause syncope. In an acute adrenal crisis, the patient may present in hypovolemic shock.

Systemic Signs and Symptoms

In chronic adrenal insufficiency, the patient often presents with a long history of progressive fatigue, malaise, anorexia, nausea, vomiting, weight loss, abdominal pain, and hypotension with orthostasis. The physical examination in primary insufficiency can demonstrate hyperpigmentation of the skin due to compensatory high levels of ACTH, which shares a promolecule with melanocyte-stimulating hormone. In acute situations, patients can present with hypotension, depressed mentation, nausea, vomiting, abdominal pain, hypoglycemia, and fever.

DIAGNOSTIC TECHNIQUES

Laboratory Findings

Hyponatremia, hyperkalemia, hypercalcemia, hypoglycemia, elevated creatinine, and acidosis can be seen in primary adrenal insufficiency. Patients with secondary adrenal insufficiency do not have hyperkalemia, because the renin-angiotensin system is able to stimulate aldosterone production. The diagnostic test of choice is the ACTH stimulation test. The baseline cortisol level is measured, and synthetic ACTH then is administered; the cortisol level is measured again 60 minutes later. Failure to increase cortisol indicates adrenal insufficiency. The ACTH level also is helpful for distinguishing between primary (high ACTH), and secondary (low ACTH) causes. Once the biochemical diagnosis has been made, the appropriate imaging studies can be ordered. Electrocardiographic evidence of conduction defects, most often first-degree heart block, can occur in as many as 20% of patients. Echocardiography reveals small cardiac chambers with normal function.

MANAGEMENT AND PROGNOSIS

The treatment of adrenal crisis is lifesaving. If the patient is in serious shock, delaying treatment to make the diagnosis of adrenal crisis is unwise and dangerous. Immediate volume resuscitation is critical and often sufficient to temporize for the hour until the ACTH stimulation test can be completed. Then stress doses of steroids (e.g.,100 mg of hydrocortisone given intravenously every 6 to 8 hours) should be administered immediately. If an ACTH stimulation test cannot be done in a timely fashion, blood should be drawn for measurement of the cortisol level and the stress dose of steroids then should be administered. In this situation, a very low cortisol level in the face of acute illness, shock, and hypotension is diagnostic.

The treatment of chronic adrenal insufficiency involves both glucocorticoid and mineralocorticoid replacement. Glucocorticoid replacement can be given in the form of hydrocortisone, cortisone acetate, or prednisone (prednisolone). Hydrocortisone routinely is started at 20 mg in the morning and 10 mg in the evening to mimic the body's circadian secretion of cortisol. The lowest doses possible that render the patient asymptomatic with normal electrolyte levels are preferred, to prevent the long-term effects of glucocorticoid excess. Mineralocorticoid is given in the form of oral fludrocortisone, 0.05 to 0.1 mg per day, in patients with Addison's disease. The prognosis for both primary and secondary adrenal insufficiency is excellent with appropriate steroid replacement.

CUSHING'S SYNDROME

ANATOMY AND PATHOPHYSIOLOGY

Cushing's syndrome is a clinical syndrome of excess cortisol, which results in a number of adverse systemic effects, particularly on the cardiovascular system.[44] The syndrome has many possible causes. Primary causes originate from the adrenals themselves. The usual primary cause is an adrenocortical tumor that is hypersecreting cortisol. Secondary causes originate from the pituitary and usually are due to an ACTH-secreting tumor of the pituitary (Cushing's disease). Alternatively, the source of ACTH could be ectopic and originate from other tissue, usually a malignancy. The most common cause of Cushing's syndrome is exogenous intake of glucocorticoids.

CLINICAL PRESENTATIONS

Cardiovascular Signs and Symptoms

Systemic Signs and Symptoms

Other symptoms of Cushing's syndrome include fatigue, proximal muscle weakness, thinning of the skin, hirsutism, irregular menses, blurry vision, and confusion. The physical examination demonstrates hypertension and central adiposity with thin arms and legs. Often a dorsal fat pad, supraclavicular fat pad, and moon facies with plethora are present. The patient also may have premature cataracts, central bruising, and abdominal striae. Severe cases of Cushing's syndrome have all of the physical features outlined above. Diabetes and hyperglycemia can also manifest in Cushing's syndrome, along with decreased bone density and an increased risk of fractures.

DIAGNOSTIC TECHNIQUES

Laboratory Findings

The diagnosis of Cushing's syndrome can be fairly challenging. The initial screening test is a 24-hour urine collection to measure free cortisol or a dexamethasone suppression test. In this test, 1 mg of dexamethasone is given overnight; in a healthy individual, the morning cortisol level is suppressed. If the screening test produces a positive result, measurement of the ACTH level sometimes can be helpful for distinguishing between primary and secondary causes. In addition, an 8-mg overnight dexamethasone suppression test can be helpful for distinguishing between pituitary disease and other diseases. In pituitary disease, a small degree of feedback to the pituitary tumor still is expected with high-dose dexamethasone, resulting in suppression of the cortisol level. Failure to suppress the cortisol level indicates an ectopic or adrenal source. Once the biochemical diagnosis has been made, imaging can be helpful for further identifying the area of abnormality. In addition to identifying the source of the problem, the physician must always identify and treat associated cardiometabolic risk factors (i.e., assess blood pressure and the lipid profile and measure the glucose level).

MANAGEMENT

Once the etiology of Cushing's syndrome has been identified, the usual treatment is surgical removal of the offending adrenal or pituitary tumor. Ketoconazole can be given temporarily to reduce the production of cortisol to better prepare the patient for surgery. As mentioned previously, it is important to treat associated cardiometabolic risk factors both before and after surgical management. If left untreated, Cushing's syndrome often is fatal because of cardiovascular, thromboembolic, hypertensive, and infectious complications.

PRIMARY HYPERALDOSTERONISM

ANATOMY AND PATHOPHYSIOLOGY

Increased and autonomous production of aldosterone by the adrenal gland is known as primary hyperaldosteronism. Hyperaldosteronism is believed to account for up to 20% of all patients with systemic hypertension, and it is the most common form of secondary hypertension. Consequences of excessive aldosterone production by the adrenal gland include sodium retention with plasma volume expansion and hypertension; renal loss of potassium and bicarbonate, resulting in hypokalemia and alkalosis; and suppression of renin and angiotensin. The hallmarks of primary hyperaldosteronism, therefore, are hypertension and hypokalemia.[45]

Thus far, six subtypes of primary hyperaldosteronism have been described.[45] Aldosterone-producing adenoma (APA) and idiopathic hyperaldosteronism (IHA) are the two most common types; primary adrenal hyperplasia and renin-responsive APA are uncommon. The two familial forms are glucocorticoid-remediable aldosteronism and familial occurrence of APA, IHA, or both.

The elevation in aldosterone results in volume expansion, which increases systemic vascular resistance and exacerbates hypertension. In addition, direct potassium-secreting actions on the kidney contribute to the resulting hypokalemia. From a cardiovascular perspective, beyond hypertension, patients with primary hyperaldosteronism have an increased cardiovascular risk. This partly may be explained by direct effects on the mineralocorticoid receptors of the heart and vasculature that can impair endothelial function.

CLINICAL PRESENTATION

Cardiovascular Signs and Symptoms

Patients usually come to medical attention because of hypertension and hypokalemia. The hypertension may be severe, requiring several antihypertensives, but malignant hypertension is rare. The heart usually is only modestly enlarged, and heart failure is rarely seen. Interestingly, patients with primary hyperaldosteronism appear to have an increased risk of stroke, myocardial infarction, and atrial fibrillation, even when the blood pressure is controlled. However, this was demonstrated in a retrospective analysis and requires further clarification.[45a]

Systemic Signs and Symptoms

Hypokalemia can be associated with muscle weakness, cramping, headaches, palpitations, polydipsia, and polyuria. Although diuretics are the most common culprit responsible for hypokalemia in hypertensive patients, marked hypokalemia in a patient taking diuretics should precipitate a search for hyperaldosteronism.[45] Despite sodium retention, edema is not a feature of hyperaldosteronism; the kidney presumably can compensate for the excess sodium retention.

DIAGNOSTIC TECHNIQUES

Laboratory Findings

Hypokalemia in a patient with hypertension should trigger investigations for primary hyperaldosteronism. However, not all patients have hypokalemia, particularly if the patient routinely eats a low-sodium diet. Other suggestive laboratory results include mild metabolic alkalosis and relative hypernatremia. A random sample can be drawn for measurement of the plasma renin activity and aldosterone level for screening in an ambulatory patient. The basal plasma renin activity should be suppressed with an elevated aldosterone level (i.e., above 20 ng/dL). A ratio of aldosterone to renin greater than 20 is a positive screening test result. If the screening result is positive, confirmation entails demonstrating failure of the elevated aldosterone to suppress normally with a sodium load. Subtype differentiation involves imaging of the adrenal glands with CT and adrenal vein sampling for aldosterone; these tests should be performed at centers familiar with subtype differentiation. Electrocardiography typically demonstrates mild left ventricular hypertrophy and signs of hypokalemia.

MANAGEMENT

The cause of the primary hyperaldosteronism determines the treatment. Treatment of an aldosterone-producing adenoma involves surgical resection, currently through a laparoscopic approach. Patients with unresectable tumors and those with other subtypes are treated medically with the aldosterone antagonist spironolactone (100 to 200 mg/day), amiloride (10 to 40 mg/day), calcium channel blockers, and ACE inhibitors. Spironolactone has the troubling side effect of gynecomastia in men, particularly when dosages higher than 200 mg/day are used. Dexamethasone at a dosage of 2 mg/day is used for glucocorticoid-remediable aldosteronism; this returns the potassium level, blood pressure, and aldosterone level to normal within 3 weeks. Hypertension and hypokalemia are cured in as many as 70% of patients who undergo resection of an aldosterone-producing adenoma. However, return of the blood pressure to normal may require several months.

OTHER ENDOCRINE DISEASES AND THE HEART

ACROMEGALY

Anatomy and Pathophysiology

Acromegaly is a rare condition caused by excessive secretion of growth hormone (GH), typically from a pituitary adenoma.[46] GH stimulates the liver to produce insulin-like growth factor I (IGF-I), which mediates GH action on peripheral tissues. In children and adolescents, GH and IGF-I play critical roles in longitudinal bone growth and other aspects of development. In adults, the hormones continue to play important roles in body composition, bone density, and lipid and glucose metabolism. Cardiovascular morbidity and mortality are increased in acromegaly. The proposed mechanisms through which GH and IGF-I may exert their cardiovascular effects are outlined in the following discussion.

Both GH and IGF-I appear to have direct effects on cardiac myocytes to stimulate hypertrophy and enhancement of contractile performance. In addition, high levels of GH and IGF-I induce hypertension by means of expansion of plasma volume through renal sodium retention and an inhibitory effect on atrial natriuretic peptide. GH and IGF-I excess leads to abnormalities of glucose metabolism, with the prevalence of diabetes mellitus ranging from 19% to 56%, depending on the series. Lipid abnormalities are also increased, marked by elevated triglycerides and lipoprotein (a) and low HDL-cholesterol. Both the glucose and lipid abnormalities certainly can contribute to the atherosclerotic process. Furthermore, GH and IGF-I are vascular growth factors and may play a direct role in the development of atherosclerosis through stimulation of collagen deposition.

Clinical Presentation

Cardiovascular Signs and Symptoms

The cardiovascular effects of acromegaly occur in stages.[46] The first stage is characterized by a hyperkinetic left ventricle with increased contractility and cardiac output. The second stage is marked by biventricular hypertrophy, diastolic filling abnormalities, and impaired cardiac performance with exercise. The final stage is characterized by valvular disease (atrial regurgitation, mitral regurgitation) and systolic and diastolic dysfunction with congestive heart failure. Some patients with acromegaly have CHF that is particularly resistant to conventional treatments. In general, this resistance correlates with the duration of uncontrolled GH secretion.

Hypertension, diabetes, and dyslipidemia coexist with acromegaly, worsening the cardiovascular problem. The hypertension usually is mild and easily treated with antihypertensives, especially diuretics.

Cardiac arrhythmias may also be present, particularly ectopic beats, paroxysmal atrial fibrillation, paroxysmal supraventricular tachycardia, sick sinus syndrome, ventricular tachycardia, and bundle branch blocks. Rarely, acromegaly can present as part of Carney's syndrome, which also can include atrial or cutaneous myxoma, Sertoli cell tumors, cutaneous hyperpigmentation, and pigmented nodular adrenocortical disease. Family members of these patients should be screened for myxomas.

Systemic Signs and Symptoms

Excessive growth hormone causes disfiguration, which is characterized by coarsened facial features with frontal bossing and a prominent jaw, malocclusion, excessive growth of the hands and feet, a large tongue, and skin tags. Patients may complain of symptoms related to local expansion of the tumor, such as headache and bitemporal hemianopsia. Other symptoms include excessive sweating, hoarseness, central sleep apnea, and carpal tunnel syndrome. Because of the role of GH as a counter-regulatory hormone for hypoglycemia, most patients with acromegaly have either glucose intolerance or frank diabetes, which further contributes to the increased incidence of premature coronary artery disease. Sleep apnea, evident in nearly half of patients with acromegaly, may also contribute to cardiovascular mortality.

Diagnostic Techniques

The diagnosis of acromegaly is based on clinical findings and elevated IGF-I or somatomedin C levels, as well as demonstration of nonsuppressibility of serum growth hormone levels after glucose infusion.[47] Dynamic MRI of the pituitary should confirm the presence of an adenoma. On echocardiography, both symmetric and asymmetric cardiac hypertrophy out of proportion to the hypertrophy of other organs in this condition have been seen. Electrocardiographic abnormalities include ST depression and nonspecific T-wave changes, left ventricular hypertrophy, and intraventricular conduction defects. Cardiac arrhythmias often occur, and ventricular ectopies and atrial fibrillation or flutter are the most frequent types.

Management

Successful treatment of acromegaly, which suppresses GH and IGF-I, improves most of the clinical signs and symptoms. First-line therapy of acromegaly involves surgical removal of the pituitary adenoma. Medical therapy also is available, involving somatostatin analogues, growth hormone receptor antagonist, or dopamine agonists (less effective). Surgical therapy is preferred over medical therapy in the vast majority of cases. However, medical therapy can be a helpful preoperative tool for reducing some of the signs and symptoms of acromegaly that may render the surgery more difficult (e.g., oropharyngeal soft tissue swelling). Medical therapy certainly is used postoperatively in many cases to maintain the GH and IGF-I levels in the normal range. Rarely, radiation therapy can be considered in cases of surgical or medical failure. The goal of all therapies is to normalize IGF-I levels and GH response to an oral glucose tolerance test.

Prognosis

The mortality rate for individuals with untreated acromegaly is significantly greater than that of the general population. However, with treatment that successfully lowers the GH and IGF-I levels to the normal range, survival can be improved to that of the age-matched population.[48]

CARCINOID AND THE HEART

ANATOMY AND PATHOLOGY

Carcinoid neoplasms are uncommon neuroendocrine tumors that contain vasoactive secretagogues, which most commonly secrete serotonin or its metabolites, or both. The incidence of these neoplasms is low, or approximately 1.2 to 2.1 cases per 100,000 per year.[49] They can arise anywhere in the body and are derived from the tissues of the foregut, midgut, or hindgut.

Depending on the location of the primary tumor, symptoms and complications may differ. The most common locations are the midgut (gastrointestinal tract) or the foregut (bronchus). Some patients may present with bowel obstruction if the bowel is involved. However, 20% to 30% of patients present with symptoms caused by the hormones secreted (carcinoid syndrome).[50] These symptoms include flushing, diarrhea, and others.

Serotonin is one of the major hormones that cause the symptoms of carcinoid syndrome. However, it is metabolized in the liver. Therefore, patients do not develop symptoms of carcinoid syndrome until liver metastases are present such that the vasoactive substances are released directly into the systemic circulation. Ovarian or bronchial carcinoids also may release directly into the circulation. Carcinoid heart disease eventually develops in 60% of those with carcinoid syndrome.[51] The main manifestation of carcinoid heart disease is right-sided valvular disease. Because of the pulmonary degradation of serotonin, carcinoid heart disease affects the right side of the heart and not the left side unless a right-to-left shunt or bronchial or pulmonary metastasis is present.

PATHOPHYSIOLOGY

Serotonin is thought to be the direct cause of the valvular abnormalities seen. In fact, higher serotonin levels are associated with more severe carcinoid heart disease. Similar cardiac problems are seen with the use of ergot-alkaloid derivatives or the anorectic drugs fenfluramine and dexfenfluramine, which also increase serotonin levels. However, the exact mechanism by which serotonin causes these abnormalities is unclear. The valvular disease is characterized by distinctive deposits of fibrotic plaques, with absence of elastic fibers that adhere to the endocardium of the tricuspid and pulmonic valves, atria, and ventricles.[51] The carcinoid plaques are composed of smooth muscle cells, myofibroblasts, and an overlying endothelial layer. The morphology of the valve leaflet is not disrupted; rather, retraction and fixation of the tricuspid or pulmonic leaflets (or both) result in reduced motion, poor closure, and typically regurgitation but occasionally stenosis. Rarely, carcinoid tumors can metastasize to the heart.

CLINICAL PRESENTATIONS

Cardiovascular Signs and Symptoms

In early carcinoid heart disease, the symptoms are subtle. When the tricuspid or pulmonic regurgitation becomes more severe, failure of the right side of the heart can develop, and at that point, symptoms may arise. These may include fatigue, dyspnea on exertion and when severe, peripheral edema, ascites, and hepatomegaly. If left untreated, right-sided heart failure is a frequent cause of death. The physical examination may show a palpable right ventricular impulse and murmurs of tricuspid or pulmonic regurgitation. Murmurs of stenosis are less frequently heard. As the valve disease progresses, the physical features of right-sided heart failure become more apparent.

Systemic Signs and Symptoms

The presentation of the patient depends on the location or site of the carcinoid. Based on the location, different hormones may be secreted, with accompanying symptomatology. The more common form of carcinoid arises from the midgut and occurs in the gastrointestinal tract. Serotonin is one of the major substances secreted by these carcinoid tumors, and symptoms include diarrhea, facial flushing, low blood pressure, and wheezing. Carcinoid crisis can occur with alarming symptoms of profound hypotension, which is particularly aggravated by anesthetics.

DIAGNOSTIC TECHNIQUES

Laboratory Findings

The diagnosis of carcinoid is made by documentation of high levels of urinary 5-hydroxyindoleacetic acid (5-HIAA) in a 24-hour urine collection. Testing must be done while the patient is on a diet free of serotonin-rich foods for several days. Localization should be attempted with bowel series, abdominal CT, a liver-spleen scan, or octreotide isotope scanning.

The diagnosis of carcinoid heart disease can be established by noninvasive means. All patients with carcinoid syndrome should have echocardiography to check for heart involvement. Most commonly, both the tricuspid and pulmonic valves have carcinoid plaques that cause thickening and retraction of the tricuspid valve leaflets, resulting in regurgitation and immobility of the pulmonic valves. Tricuspid regurgitation is found in virtually all patients with carcinoid heart disease. Pulmonic stenosis is present in 53%, and pulmonic regurgitation in 81%.[52] Left-sided heart disease is uncommon and present only in patients with a right-to-left shunt or a carcinoid tumor involving the lung. It should be remembered that carcinoid is the only condition in which both right-sided valves are involved, potentially causing devastating right-sided failure. An electrocardiogram demonstrates a low-voltage QRS.

MANAGEMENT

Treatment of carcinoid is surgical removal if the tumor has not metastasized. However, most patients develop symptoms only after metastasis to the liver has occurred; therefore, removal of the primary tumor may not be beneficial in these cases. Debulking of the liver metastases and hepatic artery embolization are undergoing evaluation.

The mainstay of symptom control remains medical therapy with a somatostatin analogue. In fact, because use of an anesthetic may precipitate a carcinoid crisis, it is imperative that medical treatment be instituted before any attempt is made at a surgical remedy.

From a cardiac perspective, the valvular lesions do not regress with treatment of the carcinoid. Most patients will require cardiac surgery with valve replacement. In fact, liver surgery for debulking can be done only after cardiac surgical intervention, even in patients with less severe right-sided heart failure, because the high right-sided pressures pose a high risk of hepatic hemorrhage.

PROGNOSIS

Patients with carcinoid heart disease have a reduced 3-year survival compared with those without echocardiographic evidence of cardiac involvement (31% versus 68%).[52] However, with treatment, the prognosis improves slightly. In a Mayo Clinic analysis of 200 patients that covered 20 years, comparisons of survival were made between groups diagnosed at different times. Among those diagnosed most recently (1995 to 2000), the median survival was significantly better at 4.4 years. Among those who underwent valve replacement in that era, the postoperative mortality was only 9%, compared with 25% in the group diagnosed from 1981 to 1989.[53] Therefore, earlier screening for asymptomatic heart involvement, as soon as the diagnosis is made, and earlier intervention, before right-sided heart failure develops, are thought to improve survival in carcinoid heart disease.

chapter

130 Rheumatologic Diseases

Carlos A. Roldan

Definition

- System lupus erythematosus, rheumatoid arthritis, scleroderma, ankylosing spondylitis, polymyositis and dermatomyositis, and mixed connective tissue disease are immune-mediated inflammatory diseases primarily of the musculoskeletal system; however, they frequently involve the cardiovascular system.

Key Features

- The pericardium, myocardium, valve leaflets, conduction system, and great vessels are affected with variable frequency and degrees of severity.
- Heart disease in patients with immune-mediated inflammatory disease contributes significantly to their morbidity and mortality; however, a large discrepancy exists between infrequent clinical recognition of the heart disease and its universally present effects as seen postmortem.

Therapy

- In addition to standard therapy, corticosteroids, cytotoxics, and tumor necrosis factor inhibitors may be useful for treating cardiac inflammation.

SYSTEMIC LUPUS ERYTHEMATOSUS

VALVULAR DISEASE

Clinically, valvular disease is the most important and frequent type of heart disease associated with systemic lupus erythematosus (SLE). It is categorized as Libman-Sacks vegetations, valvular thickening, regurgitation or, rarely, stenosis.[1,2] Recent series have demonstrated that valvular disease, especially valvular vegetations, are highly associated with and are independent predictors of stroke or transient ischemic attacks (TIAs), nonfocal neurologic dysfunction (cognitive dysfunction, acute confusional state, seizures, and psychosis), and focal brain injury (cerebral infarcts and white matter abnormalities) on magnetic resonance imaging (MRI).[3-5]

Anatomy and Pathology

The incidence of valvular disease in postmortem studies ranges from 13% to 100%. Libman-Sacks vegetations are cauliflower-like or flat, red, multiple spreading masses, 2 to 4 mm in diameter, that are found on leaflet closure lines. Active vegetations have central fibrinoid degeneration with variable degrees of fibroblastic proliferation and fibrosis, surrounded by mononuclear and polymorphonuclear cellular infiltration, small hemorrhages, and peripherally by platelet or fibrin thrombus. Healed masses have central fibrosis and minimal or no inflammatory cell deposition. Thrombus often is absent or minimal; if present, it is hyalinized and endothelialized. Active, healed, and mixed masses can be seen in the same valve. Most valve masses have associated and usually diffuse leaflet fibrosis.

Pathophysiology

Current data suggest that subendothelial deposition of immunoglobulins and complement leads to increased expression of $\alpha3\beta1$ integrin on the endothelial cells; an increased amount of collagen IV, laminin, and fibronectin; proliferation of blood vessels; inflammation; thrombus formation; and fibrosis. Antiphospholipid antibodies (aPLs) are believed to cause valvular injury by the following mechanisms:

- they activate endothelial cells and up-regulate the expression of adhesion molecules and the secretion of cytokines and also induce abnormal function of prostacyclins;
- they increase the uptake of oxidized low-density lipoprotein (LDL) cholesterol by macrophages, leading to macrophage activation and damage to endothelial cells;
- they interfere with the regulatory functions of prothrombin and reduce the production of prostacyclin and endothelial-relaxing factor, protein C, protein S, and tissue factor; and
- they cause a heparin-like induced thrombocytopenia.[6]

Clinical Presentations

More than 50% of patients with SLE have valvular disease; however, because it usually is mild, it is clinically evident only in about 20% of patients. The physical examination is inaccurate in patients who have mild regurgitation, valve masses, or thickening without regurgitation. Moreover, valvular regurgitation may be mistaken for functional murmurs caused by anemia, hypertension, or volume overload, which are frequently present in these patients. If moderate to severe valvular dysfunction is present, the physical examination usually detects regurgitant or stenotic murmurs. Severe valvular regurgitation results from recurrent or acute valvulitis; leaflet perforation, including bioprosthetic leaflets; noninfective mitral valve chordal rupture; and infective endocarditis. Chronic severe regurgitation results from progressive leaflet thickening and retraction or recurrent subclinical valvulitis.

Patients with SLE have a greater than 15% incidence of stroke and TIA, which are associated with significant morbidity and mortality. Recent series report that valvular disease,

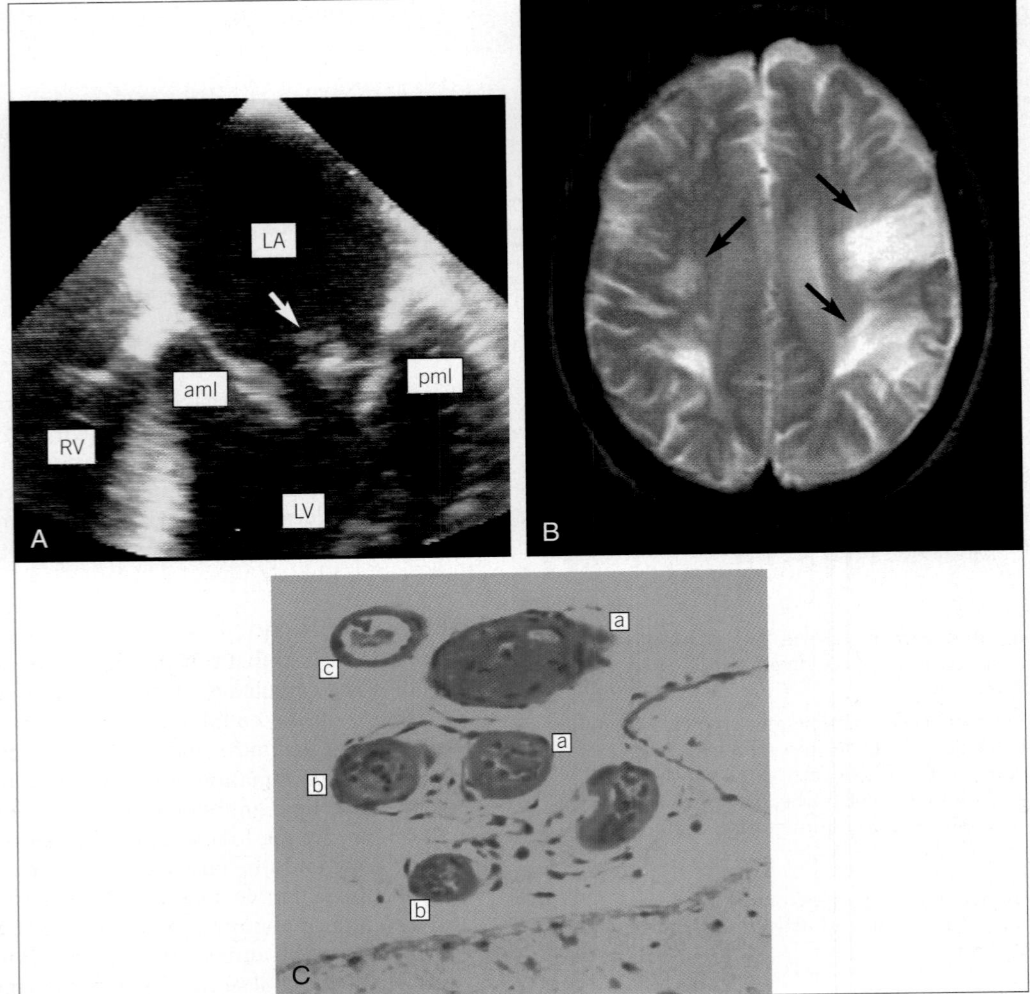

Figure 130.1 Mitral valve Libman-Sacks vegetation, the cause of a recurrent and fatal stroke in a 47-year-old woman with systemic lupus erythematosus (SLE). **A**, A transesophageal echocardiographic view demonstrating severe thickening of the midportion and tip of the anterior (aml) and posterior (pml) mitral leaflets, with a large Libman-Sacks vegetation on the midportion and atrial side of the posterior leaflet *(arrow)*. **B**, In this patient, a T2-weighted magnetic resonance imaging (MRI) brain scan demonstrates multiple areas of old cerebral infarcts, characterized by loss of both gray and white matter (large areas of hyperintensity, *arrows*) in a cortical and subcortical pattern; multiple areas of deep white matter abnormality consistent with widespread ischemic cerebrovascular disease; and generalized cortical atrophy. **C**, Histopathologic examination of the brain demonstrated (a) occlusion of cerebral vessels by fibrin thrombi; (b) intimal hyperplasia, vessel wall thickening, and platelet thrombi; and (c) an occasional patent blood vessel. LA, left atrium; LV, left ventricle; RV, right ventricle. (Modified from Roldan CA. Echocardiography Findings in Systemic Diseases Characterized by Immune-mediated Injury. In Otto C, ed. The Practice of Clinical Echocardiography. 3rd ed. Philadelphia, WB Saunders, 2007:877-901.)

especially mitral vegetations and valve thickening, is two to four times more common in patients with SLE who have a stroke or TIA than in those who do not; in those with nonfocal neuropsychiatric manifestations of cognitive dysfunction, acute confusional state, seizures, or psychosis; and in those with focal ischemic brain injury on MRI studies (Figs. 130.1 and 130.2).[3-5] In these series, valvular vegetations and valve thickening were strong independent predictors of focal or nonfocal neurologic dysfunction and brain injury on MRI. These data suggest that in patients with SLE, valvular disease frequently associated with hypercoagulability is a source of fibrin or platelet macroembolism or microembolism to the brain (Fig. 130.1).

Infective endocarditis can mimic, accompany, or trigger a flare of SLE. It also may be the initial presentation of SLE valvular disease, and it may lead to severe valvular dysfunction, heart failure, and septic death. Flares of SLE that require treatment with high-dose corticosteroids and cytotoxic agents frequently precede or accompany an infection. Antibody-mediated granulocyte dysfunction, leukopenia, hypocomplementemia, abnormal immunoglobulin synthesis, and functional asplenia are predisposing factors.

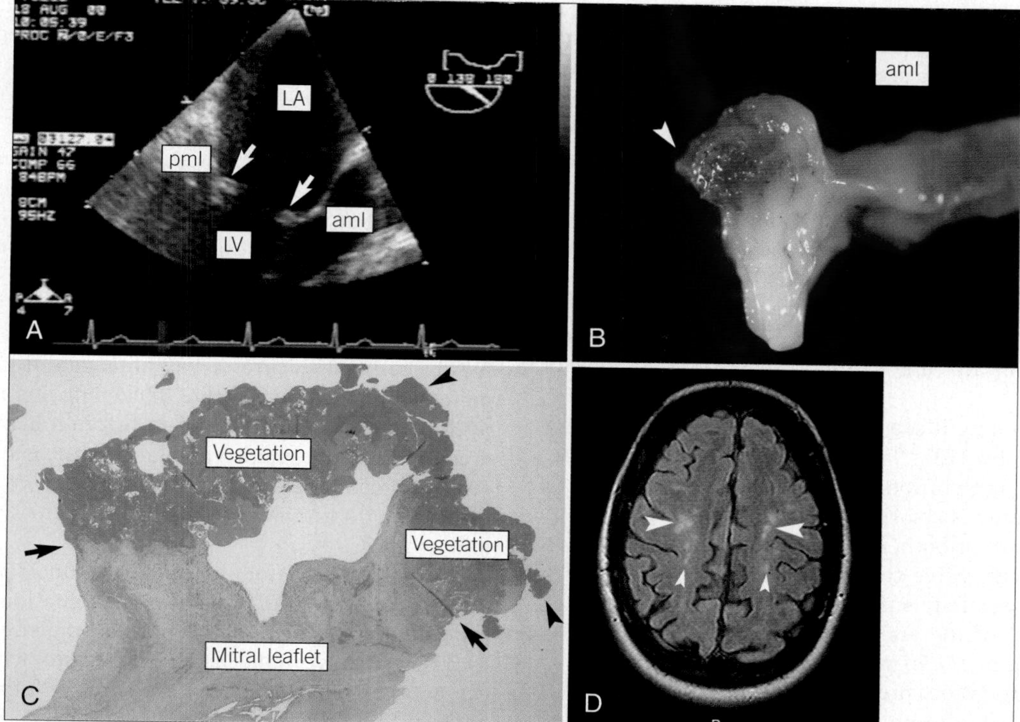

Figure 130.2 Mitral valve Libman-Sacks vegetations, which caused cerebral infarcts, acute confusional state, and cognitive dysfunction in a 28-year-old woman with systemic lupus erythematosus (SLE). **A**, A transesophageal echocardiographic view demonstrates small vegetations *(arrows)* on the atrial side and tip portions of the anterior (aml) and posterior (pml) mitral leaflets associated with thickening and decreased mobility of the leaflets. Because of associated symptomatic severe mitral regurgitation, the patient underwent mitral valve replacement. **B**, Libman-Sacks vegetation on the atrial side and tip portion of the anterior leaflet *(arrowhead)* associated with diffuse thickening of the leaflet. **C**, Libman-Sacks vegetation attached to the leaflets *(arrows)* demonstrates amorphous, eosinophilic, fibrinous to granular deposits admixed with histiocytes, inflammatory cells, and superficial microthrombi *(arrowheads)*. The mitral leaflet demonstrated focal areas of myxoid degeneration and fibrinoid necrosis but no inflammation. **D**, A FLAIR image shows multifocal hyperintensities in the subcortical white matter typical of small cerebral infarcts *(arrowheads)*. LA, left atrium; LV, left ventricle; FLAIR, fluid-attenuated inversion recovery. (Modified from Roldan CA. Echocardiography Findings in Systemic Diseases Characterized by Immune-mediated Injury. In Otto C, ed. The Practice of Clinical Echocardiography. 3rd ed. Philadelphia, WB Saunders, 2007:877-901.)

Pseudoinfective endocarditis is a syndrome of active SLE that mimics infective endocarditis.[7] It is characterized by

- fever;
- cardiac murmurs;
- splinter hemorrhages;
- valvular vegetations on echocardiography;
- high DNA antibody titers;
- low complement;
- moderately to highly positive antiphospholipid antibodies; and
- negative results on blood cultures.

A low leukocyte count, moderately elevated antiphospholipid antibodies, and a negative or low-positive C-reactive protein (CRP) value indicate active SLE.

Acute rheumatic endocarditis may mimic SLE endocarditis. Both diseases occur in young or middle-aged women, and their clinical and serologic markers are similar except that antistreptolysin antibodies are elevated in rheumatic carditis.

Diagnostic Techniques

Transthoracic echocardiography (TTE) shows a greater than 40% prevalence of valvular disease, compared with 60% to 70% by transesophageal echocardiography (TEE).[1,2,5] The prevalence of Libman-Sacks vegetations is less than 10% by TTE and up to 40% by TEE. In a recent series, 81 patients with SLE (73 women and 8 men) and 75 healthy volunteers (40 women and 35 men) underwent paired TTE and TEE studies to detect valvular vegetations; thickening; or regurgitation. Libman-Sacks endocarditis was significantly more commonly detected by TEE than by TTE ($P \leq .05$); TTE and TEE demonstrated poor agreement rates (κ = 0.02-0.54); and when TEE was considered the standard, TTE demonstrated a low sensitivity (63% overall, 11% for valvular vegetations), low specificity (58%), low negative predictive value (40%), and a moderate positive predictive value (78%) for detection of Libman-Sacks endocarditis.[8] Therefore, TEE should be considered as a complement to a nondiagnostic TTE or as the initial test in patients with SLE suspected of having cardioembolism, acute or subacute

Libman-Sacks endocarditis with moderate or worse valve dysfunction, or superimposed infective endocarditis.

Valvular vegetations are seen mostly on the mitral and aortic valves and rarely on the valves on the right side of the heart. They usually are less than 1 cm^2 in size and have irregular borders, heterogeneous echoreflectance, and no independent motion. They can be located on any leaflet portion, on the atrial side in the case of the mitral valve and on the vessel or ventricular side in the case of the aortic valve, and they mostly have associated valve thickening or regurgitation (see Figs. 130.1 and 130.2). By serial TEE, Libman-Sacks vegetations resolve, appear de novo, or change morphology over time, independent of SLE activity, severity, duration, or therapy.[2]

Valvular thickening is seen in 30% to 50% of patients by TTE and in 70% by TEE.[5,8] It generally is diffuse but is predominant on the midportion and tip of the mitral and aortic valves. It commonly is associated with valvular regurgitation or valvular masses, or both, and it may cause reduced leaflet mobility. However, valve stenosis occurs in fewer than 3% of patients. Associated leaflet calcification is uncommon, and involvement of the annular and subvalvular apparatus is rare, occurring in 1% of patients.

Valvular regurgitation, predominantly of the mitral valve, is common (occurring in up to 79% of patients) but usually mild. However, moderate regurgitation is not uncommon (15% to 30% of patients) and usually is associated with valvular thickening.

In contrast to Libman-Sacks vegetations, infective vegetations usually are located at the line of closure of the leaflet and show a homogeneous echoreflectance and independent vibratory motion. However, these echocardiographic characteristics overlap with those of Libman-Sacks vegetations, and the two types can coexist.

In rheumatic valvular disease, in contrast to SLE valvular disease, leaflet tip thickening and marked chordal thickening, fusion, tethered motion, and calcification are characteristic. Valvular masses, which are uncommon in chronic rheumatic disease, usually are located near the tip of the leaflet and frequently are calcified. In acute rheumatic endocarditis, as in SLE, mild mitral and aortic regurgitation are predominant, but moderate to severe lesions are not uncommon. Valvular masses are seen predominantly on the mitral valve (more than 80% of patients). As in SLE, rheumatic valvular regurgitation and masses frequently resolve over time. However, when these masses are in the chronic state, their echocardiographic characteristics may be similar to those of SLE valvular disease.

Management

Current data have not established whether corticosteroid or cytotoxic therapy has an effect on the presence or evolution of SLE valvular disease. Prospective, longitudinal, and controlled data are not available. In patients with SLE with focal or nonfocal central nervous system disease, a TEE and, uncommonly, a TTE that demonstrates valvular vegetations establishes a likely embolic cause of cerebral dysfunction and supports the use of anticoagulant therapy. In addition, in patients who have recurrent systemic embolism, surgical excision of noninfective valvular masses may not prevent recurrent events. Valve replacement or repair has been performed successfully in patients with severe valvular disease.[9]

Infective endocarditis should be excluded in a febrile patient with active SLE and clinically suspected or known valvular disease.

Prognosis

A unique feature of SLE is that valvular abnormalities frequently resolve (24% of patients), appear de novo (12%), or persist but change over time (40%).[2] Intermittent or recurrent valvulitis, the formation and spontaneous resolution of thrombotic vegetations as a result of underlying hypercoagulability, and embolization of valvular vegetations may explain these changes.

As a result of recurrent valvulitis or thrombosis, or both, patients with SLE with valve thickening and moderate valve dysfunction have a threefold to fourfold higher rate of progression to symptomatic valvular disease, need for valve surgery, and death over a 2- to 8-year follow-up compared with those who do not have valvular disease or who have only a mild form.[7]

During a 5-year follow-up, a 21% incidence of symptomatic acute or chronic severe regurgitation and the need for valve replacement was reported. In addition, the mortality rate for valve replacement in patients with SLE patients can go as high as 25%, compared with 3% to 5% in patients without SLE.[9] Other causes of death include refractory heart failure caused by severe valvular dysfunction and coronary artery disease, infective endocarditis, a complicated postoperative course, and cerebrovascular events.

PERICARDITIS, MYOCARDITIS, AND ARRHYTHMIAS OR CONDUCTION DISTURBANCES

Pericarditis, with or without effusion or pericardial thickening, is seen in about two thirds of patients with SLE in postmortem series; however, a clinical diagnosis is made in only one fourth of these patients.

Myocardial disease in SLE has three etiologies:

- primary acute, chronic, or recurrent myocarditis, the most common cause;
- myocardial ischemia or infarction caused by coronary atherosclerosis, coronary thrombosis, coronary embolism, or rarely by coronary arteritis; or
- myocardial dysfunction secondary to valvular regurgitation.

The prevalence of myocarditis in autopsy series ranges from 10% to 70% of patients with SLE, but fewer than 15% of cases are detected clinically. Myocarditis is associated with the antinuclear antibody to the ribonucleoprotein Ro (SSA), but its primary pathogenic role has not been defined.

The prevalence of arrhythmias or conduction disturbances in patients with SLE is unknown, but they are commonly associated with myocarditis.

Clinical Presentations

Pericarditis

Because acute pericarditis frequently is symptomatic, it is the SLE heart disease most often detected clinically, usually during SLE flares, but it generally is uncomplicated.[10]

Symptomatic pericardial disease occurs in patients with active or flares of SLE and is manifested by clinical pericarditis with or without pericardial effusion on echocardiography or, uncommonly, by cardiac tamponade. Constrictive pericarditis rarely complicates acute pericarditis (fewer than 2% of cases). Acute pericarditis or, rarely, cardiac tamponade, or both, can be the initial manifestation of SLE. Complicating infectious pericarditis can occur, most often caused by *Staphylococcus aureus*. Pericardial effusions in patients with SLE may be secondary to severe uremia or nephrotic syndrome.

Myocarditis

Acute myocarditis manifests with fever, tachycardia, or chest pain and in rare cases with heart failure, arrhythmias, or conduction disturbances. Rarely, it can be associated with peripheral myositis. The myocarditis generally is mild and usually does not cause myocardial systolic dysfunction; however, severe dilated cardiomyopathy is well described.[11] Myocardial dysfunction secondary to coronary arteritis, small-vessel vasculitis, coronary atherosclerosis, microvascular coronary artery disease caused by endothelial dysfunction, severe valvular disease, and chloroquine sulfate–induced dilated or restrictive cardiomyopathy is uncommon, occurring in fewer than 6% of patients. Acute coronary thrombosis without underlying atherosclerosis and coronary embolism from aortic or mitral valve noninfective vegetations are rare.

Arrhythmias and Conduction Disturbances

Atrial and ventricular tachyarrhythmias or conduction disturbances can occur during acute myopericarditis or myocarditis and are due to inflammation and fibrosis of the conduction system.

Diagnostic Techniques

The electrocardiographic manifestations of SLE-associated pericardial and myocardial diseases are similar to those seen with other inflammatory etiologies.

Echocardiography demonstrates small pericardial effusions in about 50% of patients with clinical pericarditis. Laboratory analysis of an usually exudative pericardial fluid demonstrates the presence of antinuclear antibodies and immune complexes and low complement levels.

In acute myocarditis, echocardiography generally shows no abnormalities. When the myocarditis is severe, diffuse or regional wall motion abnormalities with chamber enlargement and biventricular dysfunction may be present. In young patients with active SLE and no pericardial or valvular disease, diastolic dysfunction has been reported in 15% to 35% by Doppler echocardiography.[12] Also in young patients with active SLE and normal coronary arteries, a high prevalence of reversible, fixed, and mixed myocardial perfusion defects has been demonstrated. These findings suggest subclinical SLE myocardial or small-vessel coronary artery disease.

Mild elevation of troponin I can occur and is more common than elevation of creatine phosphokinase (CPK).

Endomyocardial biopsy is indicated to diagnose myocarditis, because the degree of inflammation determines the need for high-dose corticosteroids, azathioprine, or cyclophosphamide.

Management

For symptomatic pericarditis, most rheumatologists recommend low-dose prednisone (10 to 20 mg/day for 7 to 14 days). Use of oral nonsteroidal anti-inflammatory drugs (NSAIDs) in patients with SLE frequently is limited by associated renal disease, thrombocytopenia, or anticoagulation. Chronically recurrent pericarditis is treated with hydroxychloroquine or immunosuppressives. High-dose oral prednisone (1 mg/kg/day) is recommended for a complicating large pericardial effusion without tamponade and for early cardiac tamponade that is seen by echocardiography but is not clinically evident. Pericardiocentesis is performed when large effusions are unresponsive to corticosteroids or when cardiac tamponade is present clinically. Pericardiectomy has been performed for chronic constrictive pericarditis.

Acute myocarditis is treated with high-dose oral prednisone in out-patients and with intravenous methylprednisolone in in-patients (1 to 2 mg/kg/day). A course of 7 to 14 days generally is recommended, but the dose and duration are titrated based on the clinical response.

THROMBOTIC DISEASES AND CORONARY ARTERY DISEASE

A high proportion of patients with SLE have anticardiolipin antibodies, lupus anticoagulant antibodies, or antiendothelial cell antibodies, which may relate to the high prevalence of arterial or venous thrombotic events and pulmonary hypertension in patients with this disease.

The improved longevity of patients with SLE has resulted in a higher incidence of coronary artery disease (CAD), which has become one of the leading causes of death in SLE. After controlling for traditional risk factors for CAD, the risk of functional (abnormal vasodilatation or microvascular disease) or, less often, atherosclerotic epicardial CAD in patients with SLE is four to eight times higher than in matched controls.[13] Coronary artery disease, including myocardial infarction, affects women with SLE in the third and fourth decade more commonly than in age-matched women without SLE.

Risk factors for the development of coronary artery disease include a longer mean duration of SLE, a longer mean duration of corticosteroid therapy, a high disease damage score, and a high Framingham risk score. Patients with inactive SLE have high levels of very-low-density lipoprotein (VLDL) cholesterol, low-density lipoprotein (LDL) cholesterol, and triglycerides, as well as low levels of high-density lipoprotein (HDL) cholesterol. These abnormalities are worse in patients with active SLE. Antiphospholipid antibodies also have been associated with coronary artery disease. Coronary arteritis and coronary obstruction from embolism of a Libman-Sacks vegetation or an in situ thrombosis rarely occur.

Anatomy and Pathology

Postmortem studies in patients with SLE have demonstrated up to a 25% prevalence of epicardial atherosclerotic coronary artery disease, but functional or small-vessel coronary artery disease is more common. Medium-sized or smaller arteries usually are affected and show focal or diffuse obstruction by hyaline deposits and intimal proliferation. In coronary arteritis, accumulation of polymorphonuclear cells and edema of all vessel wall layers lead to arterial obstruction.

Pathophysiology

The pathogenesis of thrombosis described for the formation of Libman-Sacks vegetations also applies to the generalized thrombogenesis in patients with SLE (see page 1719).

Coronary artery disease has four pathogenic mechanisms.

1. Activation of cellular and humoral immunity (including aPLs), along with activation of macrophages, CD4+CD28− T cells, and dendritic cells. These cells, which are cytotoxic to the endothelium, cause decreased production of prostacyclin and prostaglandin I and, ultimately, vasoconstriction and thrombosis through release of platelet-derived growth factor and thromboxane A_2. Cytotoxic cells also produce interferon γ, which destabilizes atherosclerotic plaques by 1) suppressing synthesis of collagen, 2) increase proliferation of smooth muscle cells, and 3) activation of macrophages to release free radicals and matrix metalloproteinases.
2. Increased production of inflammatory cytokines and chemokines, such as heat shock proteins, CRP, rheumatoid factor, tumor necrosis factor α, and interleukins. These cytokines, which are expressed on the endothelium of coronary arteries, recruit inflammatory cells, promote abnormal vascular smooth cell proliferation, and induce oxidative stress, endothelial apoptosis, and further up-regulation of adhesion molecules and chemokines.
3. Increased oxidation of LDL-cholesterol and exacerbation of dyslipidemia (high levels of VLDL-cholesterol and triglycerides and low levels of HDL-cholesterol), homocystinemia, and insulin resistance.
4. Uncommon pathogenic factors include coronary arteritis, in situ coronary thrombosis, and embolization from a Libman-Sacks vegetation.

Clinical Presentations and Diagnosis

Pleuritic chest pain, which often is related to pericarditis or pleuritis, should also prompt suspicion of pulmonary emboli. Focal transient or permanent neurologic deficits are more commonly related to cardioembolism than to vasculitis or cerebritis.[1,3-5,14] Therefore, in patients with focal neurologic deficits or peripheral arterial thrombosis, TEE is indicated to exclude cardioembolism. The manifestations of coronary artery disease in patients with SLE are similar to those in the general population. Coronary arteritis should be suspected in a young patient with an acute ischemic syndrome with active SLE and evidence of vasculitis affecting other organs. Coronary embolism or in situ thrombosis warrants consideration when a myocardial infarction occurs in association with a cardioembolic substrate (valvular vegetations) or a procoagulant state (moderate to high levels of aPLs). Although multiple stenotic lesions or aneurysms suggest coronary arteritis, angiography cannot reliably differentiate arteritis from coronary atherosclerosis.

The diagnostic value of electrocardiography, exercise testing with or without perfusion scanning, echocardiography, and coronary angiography for the detection of coronary artery disease in patients with SLE is similar to that in the general population. Electron beam computed tomography (CT) has demonstrated a high prevalence (up to 40%) of coronary calcification in selected asymptomatic patients with SLE.[15] However, none of these techniques can reliably differentiate functional coronary artery disease or coronary arteritis from coronary atherosclerosis. Therefore, in patients suspected of having acute coronary syndrome, coronary angiography may be warranted because of the confounding clinical, echocardiographic, and myocardial perfusion features of functional or small-vessel CAD and lupus myocarditis.

Management

The role of corticosteroids and immunosuppressive agents in patients who have antiphospholipid antibodies and thrombosis is undefined. Anticoagulants have demonstrated efficacy in preventing recurring events in patients with previous venous or arterial thrombosis or thromboembolism.

The treatment of epicardial coronary artery disease in patients with SLE is no different from that for the general population. Both percutaneous coronary intervention (PCI) and bypass surgery have been performed successfully in patients with SLE, but morbidity and mortality during these procedures are higher for these patients.

Because functional and small-vessel coronary artery disease results from an active inflammatory process or a microvascular thrombotic process, or both, therapeutic interventions should be directed toward suppression of these pathogenic factors.

If coronary arteritis is suspected, intravenous high-dose corticosteroids (1 to 2 mg/kg/day) are used initially, followed by intravenous cyclophosphamide or oral mycophenylate. The duration of therapy is based on the clinical response. Corticosteroids may increase the incidence of myocardial rupture after an acute transmural myocardial infarction.

ANKYLOSING SPONDYLITIS

AORTIC ROOT AND VALVULAR DISEASE AND CONDUCTION DISTURBANCES

Aortic root and valvular disease and conduction disturbances are the most common and clinically important cardiovascular manifestations of ankylosing spondylitis (AKS).[16] They generally follow the arthritic syndrome by 10 to 20 years, but they sometimes precede it. Although cardiovascular disease in AKS has important clinical and prognostic implications, clinical recognition has been lower than that of postmortem series.

Anatomy and Pathology

The prevalence of aortic root and valvular disease associated with AKS has ranged from 24% to 100% in postmortem series. The disease has been categorized as

- proximal aortitis that leads to aortic root thickening and dilatation;
- thickening of the aortomitral junction, or a “subaortic bump”;
- aortic valvulitis that results in cusp thickening and retraction; and
- aortic and mitral regurgitation.

Pathophysiology

The pathophysiology of the selective involvement of the left side of the heart skeleton and proximal aortic root is unknown. Animal data suggest an HLA-B27–mediated mononuclear cellular inflammatory process. Moreover, increases in platelet-aggregating activity and platelet-derived growth factors probably are linked to the proliferative endarteritis of aortic root and valvular disease. The aortic root inflammation results in a fibroblastic response and a vascularized fibrous tissue thickening that extends to the aortic annulus and cusps; to the aortomitral junction, where it results in a subvalvular fibrous ridge, or subaortic bump; and to the proximal septum and atrioventicular (AV) node. Aortic root thickening, dilatation, and stiffness in association with valvular thickening lead to aortic regurgitation. A subaortic bump reduces anterior mitral leaflet mobility and causes leaflet retraction and an asymmetric or incomplete leaflet coaptation, leading to mitral regurgitation. Rarely, aortic or mitral regurgitation is caused by acute valvulitis.

Conduction disturbances result from the subaortic fibrotic process that extends to the basal septum and AV node, leading to destruction or dysfunction of the AV node, the proximal bundle of His, and the bundle branches or the fascicles.

Clinical Presentations

The clinical prevalence of aortic root and valvular disease probably is under 10%. Aortitis, valvulitis, and valvular regurgitation generally are mild and clinically silent. Rarely, severe aortic or mitral regurgitation occurs as a result of acute valvulitis or infective endocarditis. Clinically silent aortic root and valvular disease is present in one third of patients before AKS itself is clinically apparent. Severe aortic regurgitation rarely presents with mild or no articular disease.

The prevalence of conduction disturbances varies greatly but is probably about 20%. Sinus node dysfunction and bundle branch or fascicular blocks follow AV blocks; they generally are asymptomatic. High-degree blocks occasionally are transient or in rare cases may precede the diagnosis of AKS.

The importance of traditional clinical, radiologic, and serologic parameters of skeletal inflammation as predictors of cardiovascular disease is still uncertain.[16,17]

Diagnostic Techniques

Transesophageal echocardiography in ARS patients younger than 60 years of age has demonstrated aortic root and valvular disease in 82%, compared with 27% in age- and gender-matched controls.[16] Aortic root thickening, predominantly of the posterior wall, which is seen in 60% of patients, and aortic root dilatation, which is seen in 25% of patients, are associated with aortic root stiffness. Aortic thickening and mitral valve thickening are seen in 41% and 34% of patients, respectively.

Thickening of the aortic valve consists predominantly of small nodularities that can be located on any cusp portion. Thickening of the mitral valve is almost always localized to the basal anterior leaflet and forms the subaortic bump. The subaortic bump is associated with aortic root thickening (Figs. 130.3 and 130.4). The fixed basal anterior mitral leaflet combined with the normal diastolic mobility of the midportion and distal portion give the leaflet the appearance of an elbow (the "elbow sign") (see Fig. 130.3). Aortic regurgitation and mitral regurgitation are seen in 16% and 32% of patients, respectively, and up to 40% of these lesions are moderate

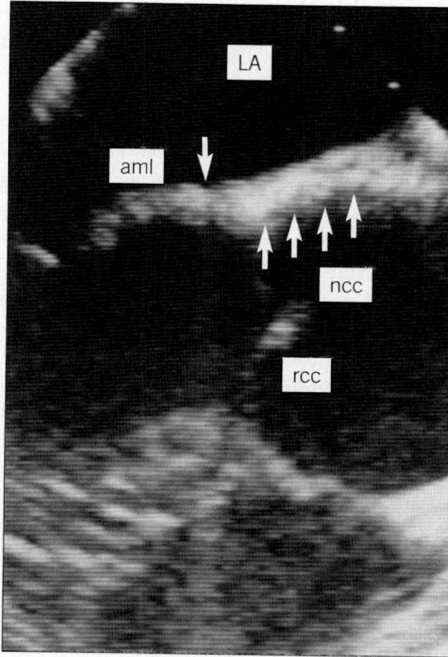

Figure 130.3 Aortic root disease and valvular disease in a 31-year-old man with ankylosing spondylitis. This transesophageal echocardiographic view shows marked thickening, predominantly of the posterior aortic root wall *(arrows)*, that extends to the base and midportions of the anterior mitral leaflet (aml) and forms a subaortic bump *(single arrow)*. Mild nodular thickening of the right coronary cusp (rcc) tip and mild aortic root dilatation should be noted, as should the immobility of the basal and midportions of the anterior mitral leaflet, in contrast with the tip ("elbow sign"). LA, left atrium; ncc, noncoronary cusp.

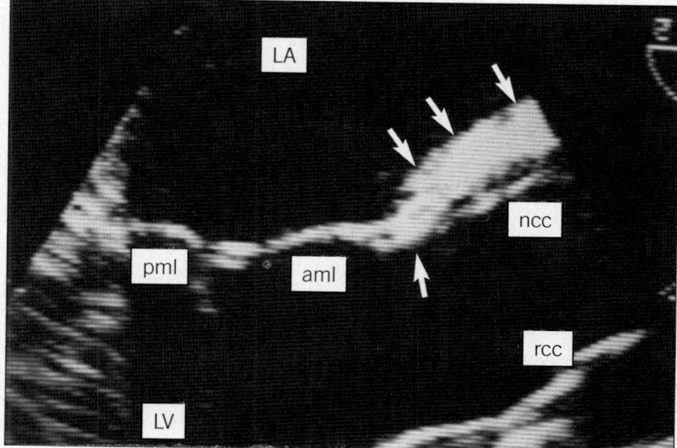

Figure 130.4 Aortic root disease and valvular disease in a 43-year-old man with ankylosing spondylitis. This transesophageal echocardiographic view demonstrates sclerosis of the aortic root, predominantly of the posterior wall *(arrows)*, that extends to the base of the anterior mitral leaflet (aml) and forms a subaortic bump *(single arrow)*. The aortic valve cusps appear normal, and no aortic regurgitation was detected. LA, left atrium; LV, left ventricle; pml, posterior mitral leaflet; ncc, noncoronary cusp; rcc, right coronary cusp.

to severe. Conduction abnormalities are also associated with aortic root thickening and the subaortic bump.

Management

The role of corticosteroids in the treatment of the aortic root, valvular, and conduction system disease associated with AKS is uncertain. Use of tumor necrosis factor α inhibitors results in a significant, sustained, clinical and serologic improvement in AKS. The anti-inflammatory effect of these drugs on the associated aortic root and valvular disease of AKS is unknown.[18] Aortic and mitral valve replacement has been performed successfully in patients with severe valvular dysfunction.

Mild to moderate valvular abnormalities can progress without being recognized, and clinically unrecognized mild valvular regurgitation and thickening can be complicated by infective endocarditis. The prevalence of subclinical aortic root and valvular disease is higher in patients older than 45 years of age who have had AKS for longer than 10 years; therefore, echocardiography may be required in these patients.[19]

Prognosis

The cardiovascular disease seen in AKS demonstrates similar rates of progression (12%), resolution (20%), and de novo appearance (24%) as in SLE or rheumatic endocarditis. Current data suggest that patients with AKS who are younger than 60 years of age and who have cardiovascular and cerebrovascular disease have a higher mortality than patients without these conditions. Because of the absence of multiorgan disease and the infrequent use of corticosteroids or cytotoxic agents in AKS, the mortality of patients undergoing valve replacement is no higher than in those who do not have AKS.

MYOCARDITIS AND PERICARDITIS

Clinically apparent primary myocarditis is rare in AKS, and its pathogenesis is unknown. It is characterized by a diffuse increase in myocardial interstitial connective tissue and reticulum fibers. It is manifested more commonly (in up to 40% of cases) as left ventricular diastolic dysfunction and may be related to age and the duration or activity of the disease.[19] Left ventricular systolic dysfunction and dilatation occur in fewer than 20% of patients. Secondary myocardial dysfunction relates to chronic valvular regurgitation.

Similarly, the prevalence and pathogenesis of pericardial disease is unknown, but it is rare (occurring in fewer than 1% of patients) and generally asymptomatic and uncomplicated. In contrast to systolic dysfunction, left ventricular diastolic dysfunction generally is asymptomatic. Clinical pericarditis is uncommon, and small pericardial effusions or pericardial thickening usually is detected incidentally on echocardiography. No specific therapy for primary myocardial or pericardial disease associated with AKS has been defined, and the prognostic implications are not known.

RHEUMATOID ARTHRITIS

VALVULAR DISEASE

In previous series, predictors of cardiovascular disease, including valvular disease in patients with rheumatoid arthritis (RA), included male gender; advanced age at the onset of the disease; hypertension; corticosteroid therapy early in the disease; long-standing disease; active extra-articular, erosive polyarticular and nodular disease; systemic vasculitis; high serum titers of rheumatoid factor; high levels of haptoglobin, von Willebrand factor, and plasminogen activator inhibitor; and an erythrocyte sedimentation rate greater than 55 mm Hg.[17,20,21] These findings suggest an inflammatory and prothrombotic pathogenesis. However, in a recent prospective series using TEE, no correlation was found between valvular disease and the duration, activity, severity, pattern of onset and course, extra-articular disease, serology, or therapy of rheumatoid arthritis.[22] Therefore, a clinical or laboratory predictor or marker for rheumatoid valvular disease remains undefined.

Rheumatoid valvular heart disease is more commonly subclinical and can manifest in four forms:

- healed valvulitis with residual leaflet fibrosis and regurgitation and, rarely, stenosis;
- valvular nodules;
- acute or chronic valvulitis with variable degrees of regurgitation and with Libman-Sacks–like vegetations[23]; and, rarely,
- aortitis with aortic root dilatation and aortic regurgitation.

Acute and chronic valvulitis, with resulting leaflet thickening and fibrosis, is indistinguishable from that seen in SLE. In contrast, valvular nodules appear to be unique to rheumatoid arthritis.

Pathophysiology and Pathology

Rheumatoid valvular heart disease is caused by a nonspecific, acute, chronic, or recurrent immune complex inflammatory process, vasculitis, or deposition of granulomas on the valve leaflets.[21] The pathogenesis of the granulomas is unknown.

Histologically, valvulitis consists of infiltration with plasma cells, histiocytes, lymphocytes, and eosinophils, which leads to leaflet thickening and retraction. The valvular granulomas resemble rheumatoid nodules and consist of central fibrinoid necrosis and variable fibrosis surrounded by mononuclear cells, histiocytes, Langhans' cells, and giant cells. They appear as yellow, firm, smooth, and focal or coalescent lesions. They generally are multiple, located within the leaflets, and surrounded by a thin border of fibrous tissue. These granulomas most commonly are seen on the base of the leaflets and the valve rings; they are less commonly seen on the papillary muscle tips and the atrial or ventricular endocardium, and they are rarely seen on the aortic root wall.

Diagnosis and Management

Valvular disease is evident clinically in fewer than one third of patients with RA, but prospective data are limited. Rarely, acute or chronic mitral or aortic valvulitis, valvulitis with leaflet prolapse, coalescent valve granulomas, rupture of a granuloma, aortitis, or infective endocarditis can cause severe valvular regurgitation. Cardio embolism may be a primary manifestation of RA valvular disease.[23]

Transthoracic echocardiography has reported up to a 30% prevalence of nonspecific valvular thickening. In a recent series using TEE in 34 patients with RA, 20 patients (59%) had mainly left-sided valvular disease (valve nodules in 11

[32%], valve thickening in 18 [53%], at least moderate mitral or mild aortic regurgitation in 7 [21%], and valve stenosis in 1 [3%]).[22,24] Valve nodules generally were single and small (4 to 12 mm); had homogeneous echoreflectance and an oval shape with regular borders; typically were located at the leaflets' basal portion or midportion; and equally affected the aortic and mitral valves (Fig. 130.5). In one patient, mitral and aortic valve thickening was associated with mitral valve Libman-Sacks–like vegetations (Fig. 130.6). Valve thickening was equally diffuse or localized; when localized affected any leaflet portion; was usually mild; involved similarly the mitral and aortic valves; and rarely involved the annulus and subvalvular apparatus.

No specific anti-inflammatory or antithrombotic therapy for RA valvular disease has been established. However, treatment with corticosteroids or cytotoxic agents in a few cases of severe valvulitis and with anticoagulation in those with associated Libman-Sacks–like vegetations has resulted in significant improvement.[23] Treatment of RA with tumor

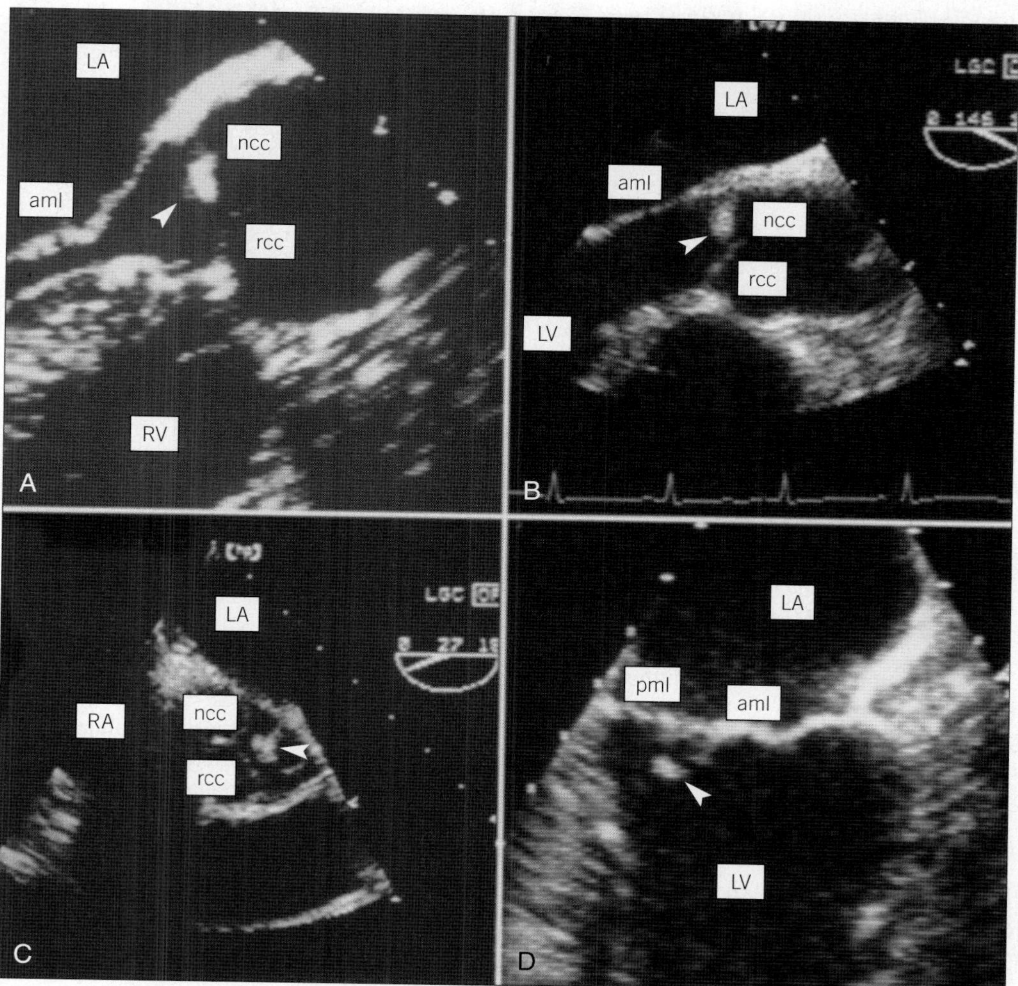

Figure 130.5 Asymptomatic patients with rheumatoid valve nodules. **A**, A transesophageal echocardiographic view in a 43-year-old man demonstrates an oval nodule with well-defined borders and homogeneously increased echocardiographic reflectance within the midportion of the aortic noncoronary cusp (ncc) *(arrowhead)*, with otherwise normal-appearing cusps. No aortic regurgitation was detected. **B**, A transesophageal echocardiographic longitudinal view in a 48-year-old woman demonstrates an oval nodule with soft tissue echocardiographic reflectance within almost the entire length of the aortic noncoronary cusp *(arrowhead)*. The appearance of the right coronary cusp (rcc) is normal. Aortic valve regurgitation was not demonstrated. **C**, This transesophageal echocardiographic view of the aortic valve in a 44-year-old man demonstrates a well-defined nodule with homogeneously increased echocardiographic reflectance within the tip and midportion of the left coronary cusp *(arrowhead)*. Note the normal appearance of the noncoronary cusp (ncc) and the right coronary cusp (rcc). Mild aortic valve regurgitation was detected. **D**, This transesophageal echocardiographic view demonstrates an oval nodule at the tip and chordal junction of the posterior mitral leaflet (pml) that has characteristics similar to those of the aortic valve. Associated mild mitral regurgitation was noted. LA, left atrium; aml, anterior mitral valve leaflet; RV, right ventricle; LV, left ventricle; RA, right atrium. (Modified from Roldan CA, Delong C, Qualls CR, Crawford MH. Characterization of valvular heart disease in rheumatoid arthritis by transesophageal echocardiography and clinical correlates. Am J Cardiol 2007;100:496-502.)

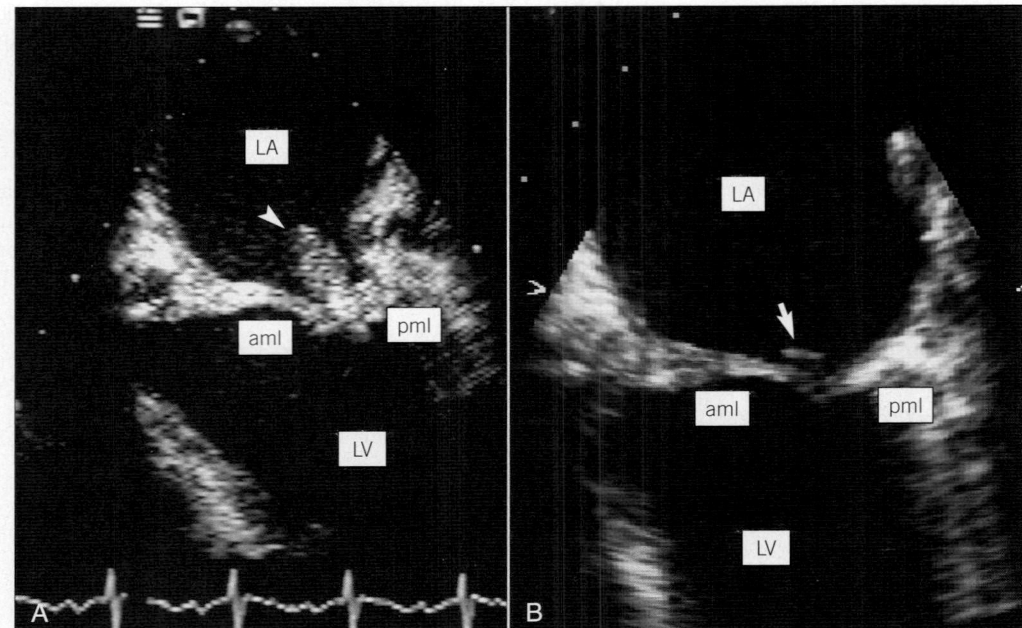

Figure 130.6 Severe mitral valvulitis with Libman-Sacks-Like vegetations as a cause of recurrent transient ischemic attacks in a 52-year-old female with severe rheumatoid arthritis. **A**, A transesophageal echocardiographic (TEE) view demonstrates severe thickening with soft tissue echocardiographic reflectance of the anterior (aml) and posterior mitral leaflets (pml). A large, elongated, oval mass is seen on the atrial side and at the coaptation point of the anterior and posterior mitral leaflets *(arrowhead)*. The valve mass has regular borders and soft tissue echocardiographic reflectance. **B**, A close-up, four-chamber TEE view after 6 months of therapy with warfarin and tumor necrosis factor α blockers demonstrates significant improvement in the thickening of the mitral leaflets and a residual small mass on the tip and atrial side of the posterior mitral leaflet *(arrow)*. LA, left atrium; LV, left ventricle. (Modified from Roldan CA, Delong C, Qualls CR, Crawford MH. Characterization of valvular heart disease in rheumatoid arthritis by transesophageal echocardiography and clinical correlates. Am J Cardiol 2007;100:496-502.)

necrosis factor α inhibitors may also result in improvement of associated valvulitis.

The morbidity and mortality rates of patients with RA who undergo valve replacement are higher than in patients without RA, but uncomplicated valvular disease may not affect the prognosis.

PERICARDITIS, MYOCARDITIS, AND CONDUCTION DISTURBANCES

Rheumatoid pericarditis, myocarditis, and conduction disturbances occur by four mechanisms: a nonspecific immune complex inflammatory process; vasculitis; uncommonly granulomatous or nodular deposition; and, rarely, amyloid infiltration.[21] Recently, a dilated or restrictive cardiomyopathy resulting from chloroquine therapy has been reported. The clinical prevalence of pericarditis and myocarditis associated with RA is probably less than 10%, compared with 30% to 40% in postmortem series. The prevalence of conduction disturbances in patients with RA may be higher than in age-matched controls without RA.

In acute pericarditis, mononuclear cellular infiltration and edema of the pericardium are seen. Fibrinous changes, fibrous adhesions, and granulomas can be seen. In myocarditis, focal or generalized mononuclear cell infiltration is the most common pathologic condition, followed by granulomas and, rarely, amyloid deposition. Rheumatoid granulomas differentiate RA pericarditis and myocarditis from that arising from other etiologies.

Pericarditis generally is uncomplicated and is evidenced by pleuritic chest pain and pericardial rub in two thirds of patients. Cardiac tamponade or constrictive pericarditis is rare (occurring in 1% of patients).[25]

Myocarditis is commonly mild and asymptomatic and usually clinically unrecognized. Pleuritic chest pain suggests the presence of myopericarditis. Rarely, severe acute myocarditis leads to left ventricular systolic dysfunction, heart failure, or symptomatic atrial or ventricular arrhythmias.

Patients with conduction disturbances generally are older than 60 years of age and have severe RA with nodular disease that requires corticosteroid or other immunosuppressive therapy. Conduction disturbances generally are mild and diagnosed incidentally. They sometimes are transient and may be reversed with corticosteroids.

Electrocardiography shows classic signs of pericarditis in fewer than 20% of patients. Echocardiography demonstrates pericardial effusions in most patients with clinical pericarditis.

In patients with myocarditis, left ventricular diastolic dysfunction may be present.[26] Radionuclide myocardial scanning shows focal patchy or diffuse myocardial uptake, which is indicative of myocardial inflammation or necrosis, or both.

Laboratory analysis of serosanguineous, exudative pericardial fluid is positive for rheumatoid factor and reveals low glucose and complement levels and generally a leukocyte count greater than 2000/dL, predominantly neutrophils. Pericardial immunofluorescence shows granular deposits of IgG, IgM, C3, and C1q in the interstitium and blood vessel walls. In severe myocarditis, troponin I, CPK, and the CPK-MB isoenzyme levels are elevated.

Management of pericarditis or myocarditis in RA is similar to that in SLE. High-dose oral prednisone (1 to 2 mg/kg/day) frequently is beneficial in unresponsive or severe cases. Echocardiographically guided pericardiocentesis can be performed safely in patients with hemodynamically significant pericardial effusions.[25] The use of intrapericardial corticosteroids is controversial, and the value of cytotoxic agents is unknown.

Treatment of high-degree AV or intraventricular block associated with acute RA myocarditis consists of temporary pacing and high-dose corticosteroids. Patients who are unresponsive should receive a permanent pacemaker.

The prognosis for patients with RA who have pericarditis is unaltered when the pericarditis is mild. Cardiac tamponade or constrictive pericarditis, however, increases morbidity and mortality. The natural history and prognostic implications of myocarditis and conduction disturbances are unknown.

CORONARY ARTERY DISEASE

Patients with rheumatoid arthritis have two to three times more common epicardial and small-vessel CAD than matched controls after controlling for traditional atherogenic risk factors.[27] With the exception of antiphospholipid antibodies, the pathogenic factors for CAD in patients with RA are similar to those described for patients with SLE. Obstructive epicardial CAD probably is as common as abnormal coronary artery vasodilatation or microvascular disease. Patients older than 50 years of age are more prone to epicardial atherosclerotic CAD. About two thirds of asymptomatic patients with a long duration of rheumatoid arthritis have coronary artery calcification on electron beam CT, compared with 40% of those with a recent onset of the disease. Patients with chronically active inflammation have reduced elasticity in the small and large arteries and a twofold independent risk for myocardial infarction, heart failure, stroke, and cardiovascular mortality compared with matched controls. Also, patients RA who have acute coronary syndromes have a two times higher recurrence rate of events and mortality than matched controls.[28,29] Coronary arteritis is rare, affects the small or medium-sized intramyocardial arteries, and spares the epicardial vessels.

Most patients with coronary artery disease are either asymptomatic or have angina pectoris that is overshadowed by arthritic symptoms. Symptomatic disease presents as stable or unstable angina or myocardial infarction. Coronary arteritis more commonly presents as acute ischemic syndromes.

Amelioration of systemic inflammation with low-dose corticosteroids, tumor necrosis factor α blockers, or statins may reduce vascular inflammation and endothelial dysfunction and, consequently, native coronary events and stent or graft stenosis or thrombosis. In addition, in patients with suspected or known CAD, cyclooxygenase-2 selective inhibitors and, to a lesser extent, NSAIDs, which inhibit prostaglandin I_2 (an inhibitor of platelet aggregation and a vasodilator) increase the risk of acute coronary syndromes; therefore, their use should be avoided or minimized. Coronary arteritis initially can be treated with high doses of corticosteroids and intravenous cyclophosphamide or oral mycophenylate in conjunction with heparin, aspirin, nitrates, and beta blockers. Limited data are available about coronary angioplasty or stenting in coronary arteritis. The morbidity and mortality of patients with RA during surgical coronary revascularization is higher than expected, due to the risk of infection and abnormal wound healing induced by corticosteroid or cytotoxic therapy.[29]

SCLERODERMA

CORONARY ARTERY DISEASE, MYOCARDITIS, AND CONDUCTION DISTURBANCES OR ARRHYTHMIAS

Heart disease in scleroderma manifests more commonly as coronary artery disease, myocarditis, and pulmonary hypertension with or without cor pulmonale.[30] Pericarditis, conduction disturbances, and arrhythmias are less common. However, overt heart disease is reported in fewer than one fourth of patients; in contrast, the percentage is as high as 80% in autopsy series. Intramural coronary artery disease leading to myocardial dysfunction is the most common and clinically important heart disease associated with scleroderma.[31,32] Ischemic heart disease, heart failure, and sudden death are the major causes of cardiac death in these patients. Conduction defects occur in up to 20% of patients and are more common in those who have myocarditis.

Anatomy and Pathology

The epicardial coronary arteries usually are normal. The intramural coronary arteries and arterioles frequently show endothelial proliferation, intimal hypertrophy, fibrinoid necrosis, fibrosis, and vessel narrowing. The high frequency of focal and diffuse myocardial fibrosis and contraction band necrosis suggests recurrent intramyocardial coronary vasospasm, or "intramyocardial Raynaud's phenomenon." These pathologic findings differ from those of atherosclerotic coronary disease in that there is a lack of relation to epicardial coronary arteries and frequent involvement of the right ventricle and subendocardium. Fibrous replacement of the sinus and AV nodes, bundle branches, and surrounding myocardium causes conduction disturbances.

Pathophysiology

Endothelial responses to thrombosis, inflammation, and vasodilatation are impaired by

- immune-mediated endothelial cell injury;
- increased production of platelet-derived growth factor;
- stimulation of fibroblasts;
- collagen deposition; and
- mast cell degranulation of histamine, prostaglandin D_2, and leukotrienes C_4 and D_4.

Clinical Presentations

Angina and myocardial infarction are uncommon, even in patients who have resting or stress-induced myocardial perfusion defects or wall motion abnormalities. The most common manifestations are those of myocardial dysfunction or heart failure. Although intramyocardial coronary vasospasm is the rule, severe vasospasm of the epicardial coronary arteries, leading to myocardial infarction, has been reported. Almost all patients who have intramyocardial coronary artery disease have peripheral Raynaud's phenomenon.

Clinically apparent myocarditis is rare, and the most common form is due to recurrent but asymptomatic intramyocardial ischemia, leading to focal patchy necrosis and fibrosis. A second uncommon form, of unknown pathogenesis, is an acute inflammatory myocarditis. Myocarditis is more common in patients with diffuse cutaneous involvement, anti-Scl70 antibodies, peripheral myopathy, and those older than 60 years of age. Patients with scleroderma who have active peripheral myopathy have up to a 21% prevalence of myocarditis, compared with a 10% prevalence in those without active peripheral myopathy. Focal or diffuse myocardial fibrosis may result in significant left ventricular diastolic or systolic dysfunction and heart failure. Acute clinical heart failure and sudden death rarely occur.

Atrial or ventricular premature contractions, supraventricular tachycardias, and nonsustained ventricular tachycardias are common in patients with active myocarditis or myocardial perfusion defects. Syncope caused by high-degree AV block or ventricular arrhythmias occasionally is the primary manifestation of scleroderma.

Diagnostic Techniques and Management

Most patients have a normal electrocardiogram (ECG), which is highly predictive of normal left ventricular (LV) function. The presence of a left or right bundle branch block or bifascicular block generally correlates with resting or exercise-induced LV systolic dysfunction. Also, complex atrial and ventricular arrhythmias or conduction abnormalities on an ECG are common and correlate with LV dysfunction or myocardial perfusion defects. Electrocardiography may show a septal or anteroseptal pseudoinfarction pattern that correlates with septal and anteroseptal perfusion abnormalities. A bundle branch or bifascicular block and ventricular arrhythmias on an ambulatory ECG correlate with resting or exercise-induced LV systolic dysfunction. Electrophysiologic studies show a high prevalence of abnormal function of the sinus and AV nodes and His-Purkinje system.

In most patients, echocardiography shows preserved LV systolic function. Echocardiographic findings typical of transmural myocardial infarction are uncommon because of the predominant involvement of the intramyocardial coronary arteries. In patients without clinical evidence of ischemic heart disease, contrast-enhanced pulse-wave Doppler echocardiography demonstrates a reduction in coronary flow reserve ($\leq$2.5) in the left anterior descending coronary artery during adenosine infusion in 52% of patients, compared with 4% of matched controls.[32] Reduction in coronary flow reserve is more common in the diffuse form of scleroderma and is related to the duration and severity of the disease. As a result of functional or obliterative microvascular disease, LV diastolic dysfunction is common.[33,34] Occasionally, a transmural myocardial infarction caused by epicardial coronary vasospasm can occur. The cold pressor test during echocardiography demonstrates transient wall motion abnormalities in patients with angiographically normal or mild epicardial CAD. LV diastolic dysfunction correlates with high levels of soluble vascular cell adhesion molecule 1 and ESR as well as the duration and severity of Raynaud's phenomenon. Similarly, a high prevalence (40%) of right ventricular (RV) diastolic dysfunction independent of pulmonary hypertension has been reported and is due to myocardial interstitial collagen deposition and fibrosis.[35,36]

Exercise testing has limited sensitivity because of the low prevalence of epicardial coronary artery disease. Resting or exercise-induced reversible, fixed, or mixed myocardial perfusion abnormalities on radionuclide studies are common (Fig. 130.7). Moreover, cold-induced reversible or partially reversible perfusion defects or transient wall motion abnormalities suggest coronary vasospasm. In fewer than 20% of patients, radionuclide ventriculography shows an abnormal resting ejection fraction, but almost 50% of patients have an abnormal ventricular function response to exercise.

Coronary angiography usually shows normal epicardial coronary arteries and slow dye flow, indicative of increased intramyocardial coronary resistance. Endomyocardial biopsy to diagnose myocarditis is nonspecific and of limited sensitivity, owing to the heterogeneity of myocardial involvement.

Nifedipine and nicardipine have demonstrated short-term improvement in the number and severity of perfusion defects, but their long-term benefit is unknown. Captopril has shown similar beneficial effects. Also, RV dysfunction in patients with

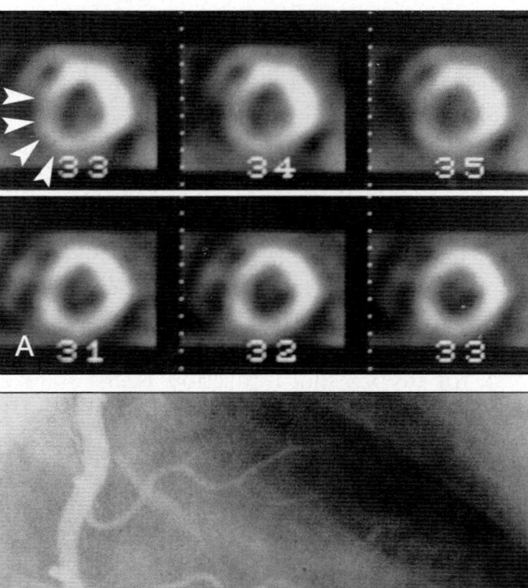

Figure 130.7 Intramyocardial coronary artery disease and dilated cardiomyopathy in a 52-year-old patient with scleroderma. **A**, A short-axis myocardial perfusion scan shows marked left ventricular dilatation and a decrease in radioisotope uptake in the inferior septum and inferior walls during exercise *(arrows)*, which partially improved at rest *(bottom)*.These findings suggested right coronary artery disease. **B**, Cardiac catheterization demonstrated a normal epicardial right coronary artery. Therefore, the patient was thought to have intramyocardial coronary artery disease.

normal pulmonary artery pressure improves with nicardipine therapy. These data support functional microvascular CAD as the cause of RV diastolic dysfunction. The use of intravenous methylprednisolone in acute inflammatory myocarditis is controversial. Otherwise, symptomatic LV systolic or diastolic dysfunction is treated with the current standard therapy. A pacemaker is indicated for symptomatic high-grade conduction disturbances, and antiarrhythmic or implantable defibrillator therapy is appropriate for symptomatic arrhythmias.

Prognosis

Pulmonary, renal, and then heart diseases are the major causes of mortality. The major causes of cardiac death are ischemic heart disease, followed by refractory heart failure, sudden death, and pericarditis. The presence on an ambulatory ECG of frequent ventricular and supraventricular arrhythmias predicts a mortality risk two to six times higher than that of patients without arrhythmias and predicts up to a 50% mortality at 6 years. Because arrhythmias are strong independent predictors of sudden cardiac death, 24-hour ambulatory ECG monitoring should be considered in patients with scleroderma to identify those at high risk of sudden cardiac death. Cardiac conduction defects on the resting ECG also indicate a poor prognosis, with a mortality rate of 50% by 6 years after diagnosis.

Left ventricular systolic dysfunction and heart failure increase the risk of death by five times, and these patients have a 100% mortality at 7 years; however, the highest mortality (80%) occurs during the first year after diagnosis.

PERICARDITIS, VALVULAR DISEASE, AND PULMONARY HYPERTENSION

Pericarditis is more common in patients who have limited cutaneous scleroderma and is clinically recognized in about 10% of patients.[30] Pulmonary hypertension is the most important cause of secondary heart disease in patients with scleroderma. It occurs more commonly in the limited cutaneous type of scleroderma (in which it is seen in 11% of patients) than in the diffuse cutaneous type (fewer than 1% of patients) or the overlap syndrome (2% of patients), but its true prevalence is unknown. It can lead to cor pulmonale in up to 44% of patients. Pulmonary fibrosis is the most common cause of pulmonary hypertension; inflammatory vasculopathy or pulmonary vasospasm are less common causes.

Pericarditis in postmortem series is seen with a frequency of up to 70%. Postmortem series report a prevalence of up to 18% of nonspecific left-sided valvular thickening and mild valvular regurgitation. Mitral valve masses, similar to those of SLE, have been reported.

Pericardial disease usually is asymptomatic. Cardiac tamponade and chronic constrictive pericarditis are rare. Valvular disease is rarely recognized clinically. However, aortitis and aortic valvulitis with cusp perforation and severe aortic regurgitation have been reported as a complication of infective endocarditis, and cardioembolism also has been reported.

Echocardiography commonly shows asymptomatic pericardial effusions and thickening. Chronic loculated pericardial effusions are rare. Nonspecific thickening of the mitral or aortic valves without significant regurgitation and an unexplained high prevalence (up to 67%) of mitral valve prolapse has been described. Laboratory analysis of exudative or transudative pericardial fluid does not demonstrate immune complexes or complement activation. Abnormal pulmonary function tests, abnormal lung uptake of gallium and technetium 99m sestamibi, and radiographic abnormalities often precede cor pulmonale on echocardiography.

Patients with a moderate or large pericardial effusion have a cumulative survival of only 25% after 6 to 7 years, but mortality is higher during the first year after diagnosis. This association probably is related to accompanying progressive renal failure in patients with chronic effusions or to sudden cardiac death in patients with acute myopericarditis. Pulmonary hypertension is associated with a 50% mortality at 8 years.

POLYMYOSITIS AND DERMATOMYOSITIS

Myocarditis and pericarditis are the most common heart diseases of polymyositis and dermatomyositis.[37] They are detected clinically in about 25% of patients with postmortem evidence of disease. Coronary artery disease, conduction disturbances, valvular disease, and pulmonary hypertension are uncommon and may be secondary because of the advanced age of the patients and their high frequency of risk factors for heart disease.

Clinically overt heart disease associated with polymyositis and dermatomyositis is uncommon. It occurs more commonly in polymyositis and overlap syndrome than in dermatomyositis or in malignant and childhood polymyositis or dermatomyositis. Heart disease is similar among men and women, but whether it correlates with the activity, severity, or duration of polymyositis or dermatomyositis is uncertain.

Acute myocarditis has been reported to mimic acute myocardial infarction. Acute myocarditis can also manifest with fatal cardiac arrhythmia, heart failure, and dilated cardiomyopathy. Restrictive cardiomyopathy is rare.[38] A high association is seen between active myositis and pericarditis. Acute pericarditis occurs more commonly in children with dermatomyositis and in patients with overlap syndrome. Uncomplicated pericarditis with small or moderate pericardial effusions has been described in more than 20% of adults, but cardiac tamponade and chronic constrictive pericarditis are rare. Rarely, pericarditis may be the initial clinical manifestation of polymyositis or dermatomyositis.

Atrial and ventricular ectopy are common. Supraventricular and ventricular arrhythmias and sudden cardiac death are rare. Bundle branch, fascicular, and AV blocks are uncommon and rarely progress to severe forms or require permanent pacing. Arrhythmias and conduction disturbances are related to active myocarditis or residual myocardial fibrosis of the sinus and AV nodes and bundle branches.

Except for an unexplained high prevalence of mitral valve prolapse, no other specific valvular disease has been reported. Pulmonary hypertension and cor pulmonale secondary to interstitial lung disease and primary pulmonary vasculopathy have been reported. Coronary arteritis is rare.

The ECG infrequently shows abnormal Q waves in those with myocarditis. About half of patients with peripheral myositis (as indicated by uptake of technetium 99m pyrophosphate) also have myocardial uptake. Approximately 10% to 20% of them have dilated cardiomyopathy.

Laboratory analysis in patients with active myositis frequently shows high levels of CPK and CPK-MB isoenzymes. In contrast to patients with myocardial infarction, these patients have persistently high levels for days to weeks. Active myositis leads to regeneration of skeletal muscle cells to a more primitive or embryonic form with a high content of CPK-MB, which explains this finding. A negative troponin I or T confirms the diagnosis of polymyositis.

Corticosteroids may be beneficial for patients who have myocarditis, pericarditis, or conduction disturbances.[39] Patients with polymyositis or dermatomyositis have a cumulative mortality of 25% to 50% after 6 to 8 years as a result of malignancy, sepsis, and cardiovascular disease. Poor prognostic indicators include age over 45 years, cardiopulmonary disease, and cutaneous necrotic lesions. However, the natural history, effects of therapy, and prognosis of heart disease in these patients are still uncertain.

MIXED CONNECTIVE TISSUE DISEASE

Pericarditis is the most common heart disease associated with mixed connective tissue disease (MCTD). It manifests with small pericardial effusions or pericardial thickening, or both.[37] Pericarditis is more common in children and is rarely the initial presentation of the disease.[40]

Mitral valve prolapse has been reported with an unexplained high prevalence of 32% in these patients. Moreover, verrucous thickening of the mitral valve and mitral regurgitation that are indistinguishable from those seen in SLE have been described. Supraventricular arrhythmias and conduction disturbances are uncommon.

Despite the intimal hyperplasia of coronary arteries and the perivascular and myocardial leukocytic infiltration described in postmortem examinations, clinical coronary arteritis or myocarditis is rare.[41] One case of fatal myocarditis complicated by congestive heart failure has been reported.

Because of the high frequency of pulmonary disease in these patients (up to 80%), pulmonary hypertension associated with proliferative pulmonary vasculopathy can occur, more commonly in patients with features of scleroderma.

Treatment of MCTD heart disease is similar to that for heart disease in SLE, RA, and scleroderma. The overall mortality of patients with MCTD is 13% at 6 to 12 years, but the prognostic implications of its associated heart disease are unknown.

SUMMARY

The rheumatologic diseases are immune-mediated inflammatory diseases that manifest predominantly with signs and symptoms of musculoskeletal and mucocutaneous inflammation. However, they frequently affect the heart valves, pericardium, myocardium, coronary arteries, and conduction system (Table 130.1). It is important to note that heart disease is associated with substantial morbidity and is the third leading cause of mortality in these patients. The poorest prognosis of heart disease in these patients is related to the chronicity and debilitating nature of the illness, the high prevalence of multisystem disease, and immunosuppression. These factors underscore the importance of early recognition, prevention of complications, and proper clinical or echocardiographic follow-up. However, the prevalence rates of clinically detected heart disease are low compared with postmortem findings and echocardiographic series. This discrepancy is related to lack of awareness, overshadowing of cardiovascular manifestations by the predominant musculoskeletal inflammatory symptoms and signs, and lack of a systematic application of the cardiovascular history and physical examination or echocardiography for detecting subclinical abnormalities.

RELATIVE CLINICAL PREVALENCE OF HEART DISEASE IN RHEUMATOLOGIC DISEASES

Type of Heart Disease	Systemic Lupus Erythematosus	Ankylosing Spondylitis	Rheumatoid Arthritis	Scleroderma	Polymyositis and Dermatomyositis	Mixed Connective Tissue Disease
Valvular disease	++++	++++	++++	++	++	+
Pericarditis	+++	++	+++	+	++	++
Myocarditis	++	+	++	++	++	+
Arrhythmias	++	++	++	++	+	+
Conduction disturbances	++	+++	++	++	++	++
Coronary artery disease (including intramyocardial coronary artery disease, coronary arteritis, and coronary atherosclerosis)	++	+	++	+++	++	+
Arterial or venous thrombosis	+++	+	+	+	+	+

\+ Rare
++ Uncommon
+++ Common
++++ Frequent

Table 130-1 Relative Clinical Prevalence of Heart Disease in Rheumatologic Diseases.

RELATIVE PREVALENCE OF ECHOCARDIOGRAPHIC ABNORMALITIES IN RHEUMATOLOGIC DISEASES

Abnormality	Systemic Lupus Erythematosus	Ankylosing Spondylitis	Rheumatoid Arthritis	Scleroderma	Polymyositis and Dermatomyositis	Mixed Connective Tissue Disease
Valvular masses or nodules	+++	+	+++	+	+	+
Valvular thickening	++++	+++	++++	++	++	+
Valvular regurgitation	++++	+++	+++	++	++	++
Valvular stenosis	+	–	+	–	–	–
Pericardial effusion or thickening	+++	++	+++	++	++	++
Cardiac tamponade or constriction	++	+	++	+	+	+
Left ventricular diastolic dysfunction	+++	+++	+++	+++	++	++
Left ventricular systolic dysfunction	++	++	++	++	++	++
Aortic root dilatation or thickening	+	++++	++	+	+	+
Subaortic bump	–	+++	–	–	–	–

– Absent or not reported
\+ Rare
++ Uncommon
+++ Common
++++ Frequent

Table 130.2 Relative Prevalence of Echocardiographic Abnormalities in Rheumatologic Diseases.

Several cardiac abnormalities, especially on echocardiography, are predominantly seen in or are unique to a specific rheumatologic disease (Table 130.2). Libman-Sacks vegetations, valvular nodules, and a subaortic bump are characteristic of SLE, RA, and AKS, respectively. Intramyocardial coronary disease, predominantly vasospastic, is typical of scleroderma.

In general, the treatment of heart disease associated with rheumatologic disorders is similar to that for heart disease of other etiologies. Anti-inflammatory therapy may have a beneficial effect on the acute cardiac manifestations of the rheumatologic diseases, but prospective, controlled, cross-sectional, and longitudinal data are limited.

chapter 131

Human Immunodeficiency Virus Infection

Priscilla Hsue and Henry Masur

Definition

- Before the introduction of highly active antiretroviral therapy (HAART), the most frequently observed cardiac abnormalities in patients infected with the human immunodeficiency virus (HIV) were dilated cardiomyopathy, myocarditis, and pericardial disease. Since the introduction of antiretroviral therapy, premature atherosclerosis has become increasingly common.

Key Features

- The widespread use of combination antiretroviral therapy, especially protease inhibitors, has been associated with the development of metabolic abnormalities, including hyperlipidemia and hyperglycemia, which represent significant atherosclerotic risk factors in patients infected with HIV.
- A growing number of studies suggests that accelerated atherosclerosis may be a consequence of traditional risk factors and of the use of protease inhibitors in patients with HIV.
- Many drug interactions between protease inhibitors and benzodiazepines, narcotics, warfarin, and other antimicrobial agents can cause substantial adverse effects if not anticipated and if dosages or regimens are not modified.
- In the pre-HAART era, HIV-related cardiac disease occurred primarily in patients with substantial immunosuppression; however, premature atherosclerosis occurs in patients across the entire spectrum of immunosuppression.
- Current hypotheses concerning the pathogenesis of HIV-associated cardiomyopathy include infection of myocardial cells with HIV, coinfection with other cardiotropic viruses, or an autoimmune process. How HIV accelerates atherosclerosis over and above the effects of traditional risk factors is not clear.
- Other factors that may contribute to cardiac disease in patients with HIV include malnutrition, depletion of trace elements, and use of nontherapeutic drugs, such as ethanol and cocaine.

Therapy

- Recognition and treatment of antiretroviral-induced hyperlipidemia and hyperglycemia and modification of traditional cardiovascular risks to reduce the risk of atherosclerosis are necessary.
- Conventional therapy to treat pericarditis and cardiomyopathy also must be instituted.

Before the introduction of highly active antiretroviral therapy (HAART) in 1995, the most frequently observed cardiac abnormalities in patients infected with the human immunodeficiency virus (HIV) were pericardial disease, dilated cardiomyopathy, and myocarditis.[1,2] In that era, clinically significant cardiac disease was not common in patients infected with HIV and usually was detected only at autopsy. In the pre-HAART era, several autopsy series of patients infected with HIV revealed evidence of endothelial pathology; that is, inflammation of the endothelium with lymphocytes and mononuclear giant cells, which had led both to fragmentation of elastin fibers and intimal fibrosis, resulting in luminal narrowing.[3,4] The interest of most investigators focused on possible infectious and immunologically mediated causes of these conditions.[5]

During the past 15 years, the mean age of patients infected with HIV has risen for two major reasons: patients are living longer as a result of HAART, and older patients in relatively good general health are sexually active and thus become infected with HIV.[6] Atherosclerosis, therefore, has become an increasingly important issue because of traditional risk factors (notably tobacco use, which is consistently overrepresented in HIV-infected cohorts compared with matched HIV-uninfected groups) and antiretroviral-related risk factors. The actual mechanism by which HIV infection may increase cardiovascular risk remains unclear; traditional risk factors, adverse effects of HAART, altered immunity, and inflammation all may contribute to increased atherogenesis in patients with HIV. In particular, health care providers have come to recognize that protease inhibitors, and perhaps other antiretroviral agents, are associated with insulin resistance, hyperglycemia, and hyperlipidemia.[7] These biochemical abnormalities are associated with disorders of fat distribution. Furthermore, an increasing number of reports suggest that accelerated atherosclerosis may be related to exposure to antiretroviral agents, especially protease inhibitors.

Clinicians should be vigilant in addressing known risk factors for coronary disease in their patients with HIV, and they also should be aware of the clinical importance of cardiovascular and cerebrovascular events in this population.

This chapter reviews the pathophysiology, diagnosis, and management of the cardiac complications most commonly encountered in patients infected with HIV.

ACCELERATED ATHEROSCLEROSIS

Initial reports of myocardial infarction in young patients with HIV who were receiving protease inhibitors focused on the role antiretroviral therapies play in increasing the cardiovascular risk. Retrospective data and previous studies have produced differing results. In the future, controlled prospective data are needed to establish the interrelationship of HIV infection, treatment, and atherosclerosis.

Several cohort studies have reported an increased incidence of myocardial infarction after the introduction of HAART.[8] In one cohort of nearly 5000 patients, the incidence of myocardial infarction per 1000 patient-years increased from 0.59 in 1991 to 1994 to 3.41 in 1995 to 1998. Reporting bias and changing risk factor profiles had an impact on the results.[8] Other retrospective studies have found up to a fivefold increased risk of myocardial infarction in patients treated with protease inhibitors compared with those who were not. The role of protease inhibitors has been controversial, however, because other series have suggested that traditional risk factors are responsible for most of the observed coronary artery disease.[9]

In a small French study, patients treated with protease inhibitors had an almost threefold increase in the risk of myocardial infarction (MI) compared with untreated patients with HIV, which suggests that rapidly forming, drug-induced plaques are unstable and prone to rupture.[10] Data from a large managed care database in northern California showed that the rates of hospitalization from coronary heart disease were higher in patients with HIV than in controls (6.5 versus. 3.8, $P = .003$) and that patients with HIV had a higher rate of MI (4.3 versus 2.9, $P = .07$).[11] No association with protease inhibitors or other antiretroviral therapy was found.

A retrospective analysis of two large cohorts of patients with HIV during an 8-year period showed that MI rates in patients receiving protease inhibitors were five times greater than those not receiving this therapy.[12] However, a larger retrospective study reported no relationship between cardiovascular events and the use of protease inhibitors or other retroviral therapy.[13] This study evaluated records of more than 36,000 patients with HIV in the U.S. Veterans Administration database. It found a decrease in hospital admission for cardiovascular events after the dates by which combination antiretroviral therapy began to be used widely. This study's findings are in contrast to the DAD study, a prospective study of 23,000 patients with HIV. During the study period, 126 patients had a myocardial infarction. During the first 4 to 6 years of combination therapy, a 26% relative increase was seen in the rate of MI per year of exposure to antiretroviral medication. There was not sufficient power to permit comparisons among patients receiving different types of antiretroviral regimens.[14] In a follow-up study from this same group, the incidence of myocardial infarction was found to be increased to 6.01 per 1000 person-years in patients exposed to protease inhibitors (PIs) for longer than 6 years, compared with an incidence of 1.53 per 1000 person-years in patients who were not exposed to protease inhibitors. Even after adjustment for other cardiovascular risk factors, including serum lipid levels, the effect of exposure to protease inhibitors was reduced to 1.10 (95% CI, 1.04-1.18)[15] Of note, the magnitude of increased cardiovascular risk due to protease inhibitors was less than the relative risk due to each traditional factor, such as age, male gender, cigarette smoking, or a history of cardiovascular disease.

Data from a large health care database in Boston showed that the acute myocardial infarction rate was 11.13 per 1000 person-years in patients with HIV (95% CI, 9.58-12.68), compared with 6.98 in patients without HIV (95% CI, 6.89-7.06). Even after adjustment for age, gender, race, hypertension, diabetes, and dyslipidemia, patients with HIV had a higher relative risk of acute myocardial infarction than patients without the virus.[16] Of note, data on cigarette smoking were available for only 22% of patients in this study.

At San Francisco General Hospital, we have performed a retrospective study of patients with HIV discharged with the ICD-9 diagnosis of myocardial infarction or unstable angina and have compared these patients to a control group without the virus. The patients with HIV were more than a decade younger than the controls and were more likely to be cigarette smokers and to have a lower high-density lipoprotein (HDL) cholesterol level. Patients with HIV had lower scores for risk assessment for the prediction of cardiac disease (thrombolysis in myocardial infarction, TIMI) and were more likely to have single-vessel disease. Interestingly, patients with HIV who had undergone coronary angioplasty had a significantly higher rate of restenosis than their HIV-negative counterparts.[17] The role of drug-eluting stents has not been investigated in patients with HIV.

Whether protease inhibitors, independent of their metabolic effects, contribute directly to endothelial dysfunction remains unclear. Noninvasive studies have shown the use of protease inhibitors to be associated with endothelial dysfunction and with atherogenic lipoprotein abnormalities.[18] Likewise, in six healthy volunteers, short-term treatment (4 weeks) with the protease inhibitor indinavir was shown to induce endothelial dysfunction, possibly suggesting a direct toxicity from the drug.[19] However, in contrast, a study of lopinavir-ritonavir in healthy volunteers without HIV showed no adverse effects on endothelial cell function.[20]

Inflammation and the immune response are likely to play an important role in the pathogenesis of premature atherosclerosis among patients with HIV. The SMART Study revealed some provocative data: intermittent HAART was associated with more cardiovascular events than continuous HAART.[21] Therefore, intermittent therapy, although potentially sparing cost and certain adverse effects, was associated with an increase in several clinically important endpoints. Continuous therapy has definite advantages in terms of cardiovascular risk. Data from the AIDS Clinical Trials Group A 5152s showed that antiretroviral-naïve patients assigned to three different drug regimens (PI sparing, nucleoside reverse transcriptase inhibitor [NRTI] sparing, and non-nucleoside reverse transcriptase inhibitor [NNRTI] sparing) all displayed significant improvement in endothelial function as early as 4 weeks after treatment.[22]

ANTIRETROVIRAL-INDUCED HYPERGLYCEMIA, HYPERLIPIDEMIA, AND LIPODYSTROPHY

Patients receiving HAART have an increased risk of hyperglycemia (insulin resistance), hyperlipidemia, and body fat abnormalities compared with patients with HIV who are not receiving HAART. These laboratory abnormalities have been seen both in patients experiencing a positive virologic response to antiretroviral drugs and in those in whom virologic failure was seen. The effect of these drug-induced metabolic complications on the life expectancy of patients with HIV remains to be seen; it has yet to be determined whether these abnormalities create a risk for cardiovascular disease in patients with HIV that is equivalent to the risk they would produce in patients without HIV.

HYPERGLYCEMIA (INSULIN RESISTANCE)

About 2% to 10% of patients receiving any of the protease inhibitors (e.g., saquinavir, ritonavir, nelfinavir, indinavir, amprenavir and lopinavir) experience new or worsening hyperglycemia or insulin resistance.[7] In patients with HIV with evidence of fat loss or fat accumulation, 7% of individuals have diabetes mellitus compared with 0.5% of uninfected controls.[23] In a 3-year follow-up, men with HIV who were treated with antiretroviral therapy were more than three times as likely to develop diabetes mellitus as uninfected individuals.[24]

Some have proposed that, although glucose metabolism is deranged in a large proportion of patients treated with protease inhibitors, only those with a predisposition to diabetes will manifest clinically evident, sustained fasting hyperglycemia. Several plausible explanations can be given for this. First, antiretroviral therapy is associated with changes in glucose homeostasis, including decreases in peroxisome proliferator-activated receptor γ (PPAR-γ) expression in adipocytes,[25] accumulation of intramyocellular lipids,[26] changes in adipokine levels,[27] and changes in free fatty acids.[28] The lack of ketones and the response to sulfonylureas suggest a pathogenesis similar to that of type 2 diabetes mellitus, with insulin resistance playing a key role. In addition, increases in fasting plasma insulin and C peptide suggest that a resistance to the peripheral effect of insulin could be partially responsible.[7] Several protease inhibitors have been associated with insulin resistance in vitro[29] and with alterations in insulin sensitivity.[30,31]

HYPERLIPIDEMIA

In the absence of antiretroviral drug therapy, HIV causes hypertriglyceridemia, low HDL-cholesterol, and increased numbers of small, dense, low-density lipoprotein (LDL) cholesterol particles.[7] With the use of highly active antiretroviral agents, notably the protease inhibitors, a new pattern of lipoprotein abnormalities has been seen in 30% to 70% of patients.[7] Some investigators report only hypertriglyceridemia, which in itself is a risk for pancreatitis and possible heart disease; others describe significant increases in both cholesterol and triglycerides.[32] The predominant changes that have been noted are increased LDL-cholesterol and very-low-density lipoprotein (VLDL) cholesterol associated with decreased HDL-cholesterol; this is a profile known to be a risk factor for accelerated atherosclerotic disease.

Hyperlipidemia is linked to lipodystrophy, a syndrome characterized by the accumulation of fat in some areas but peripheral fat wasting in others. Hyperlipidemia and insulin resistance can occur independently of body changes or hyperglycemia.[33]

The largest collection of data has come from the Data Collection of Adverse Events of Anti-HIV Drugs (DAD) Study Group, a co-ordination of 11 large cohorts (from Europe, North America, and Australia). In more than 20,000 patients stratified by class of antiretroviral exposure, this group found that the odds ratio for having an increased total cholesterol was 1.9 for those on a regimen based on non-nucleoside reverse transcriptase inhibitors, 2.48 for those on a regimen based on protease inhibitors, and 5.8 for those on regimens involving both classes of drugs.[14] Data from the recent DAD study suggest that the increased risk of myocardial infarction associated with protease inhibitors is only partially explained by dyslipidemia.[15] The protease inhibitor ritonavir has been associated with increased triglyceride levels,[34] whereas another PI, atazanavir, is not associated with hypertriglyceridemia.[35]

No consensus has been reached on the mechanism by which protease inhibitors cause hyperlipidemia. One plausible explanation is that these agents have a high affinity for the catalytic site of proteases; some homologous human proteins that are involved in lipid metabolism are bound as well as sites on the virus. The binding of the protease inhibitors to these homologous human regions interferes with chylomicron clearance and the cytochrome P450 3A system. This results in reduced storage of triglycerides and promotes the release of lipid into the circulation.[36] Other proposed mechanisms include the formation of atherosclerosis by up-regulation of CD36 and the accumulation of sterol in macrophages.[37]

LIPODYSTROPHY

Between 15% and 30% of patients with HIV who are treated with protease inhibitors experience body changes as a result of alterations in fat distribution. The data are difficult to interpret, because a universally accepted definition of HIV-related lipodystrophy is lacking. Some studies are based on self-reporting by patients, whereas other investigations rely on more objective measures, such as dual-energy x-ray absorptiometry scans and computed tomography, to demonstrate the redistribution of fat.[7,38] Several terms had been used to describe these unusual body changes: visceral fat accumulation ("protease paunch," "crix belly"), buffalo humps, and peripheral lipodystrophy. Women with HIV treated with PIs have reported breast enlargement and increased abdominal girth, along with a reduction in fat mass in the calves, thighs, and glutei. Such fat accumulations can be detected after 6 to 12 months of therapy.

Some investigators have termed the constellation of fat, glucose, and lipid changes "lipodystrophy"; this includes increased triglycerides and cholesterol, hyperglycemia, and body fat redistribution comprising loss of limb fat, truncal obesity, buffalo humps, and loss of facial fat.[7] The physical and metabolic characteristics of these patients are markedly similar to the metabolic syndrome ("syndrome X"), which is a recognized risk for heart disease in patients without HIV. It is biologically plausible that the changes in body habitus, perhaps caused by protease inhibitors and other drugs, can contribute to the development of the metabolic abnormalities. However, some think that these findings could represent overlapping, unconnected syndromes; that is, some of those affected may experience redistribution of fat in some areas of the body without associated evidence of metabolic abnormalities.

Many of the metabolic and body habitus changes linked to HAART have some similarities to the changes seen in Cushing's disease. However, these Cushing-like findings have not been associated with hypercortisolism.[39]

Hadigan and colleagues[40] described metabolic abnormalities and cardiovascular risk parameters in men and women with lipodystrophy by comparing their clinical characteristics with those of healthy participants in a population-based observational study of cardiovascular disease risk factors (the Framingham study). The risk of cardiovascular disease in the patients with HIV with lipodystrophy was greater than the expected risk in healthy individuals of similar age and weight. In particular, the risk factors of hypertriglyceridemia, hypercholesterolemia, and low HDL-cholesterol were significantly more common among the patients with HIV with lipodystrophy. Risk prediction equations for patients with HIV that incorporate protease inhibitor exposure and traditional risk factors have been proposed[41,42] and appear to work well in men and women, as well as in smokers and non-smokers.[41] Although the Framingham model works well for many patients with HIV, it underestimates coronary heart disease (CHD) events in patients with HIV who also smoke.[41]

Diagnosis

The diagnosis of coronary artery disease in patients with HIV is no different from diagnosis in individuals without HIV; it includes exercise treadmill testing, pharmacologic stress testing, stress echocardiography, or cardiac catheterization.

Noninvasive tests have been evaluated as surrogate markers in the assessment of subclinical cardiovascular disease in patients with HIV. In cross-sectional studies of carotid intimal thickening (cIMT) as assessed by carotid ultrasound scans, older age, male gender, smoking, and an increased body mass index (BMI) were associated with an increased cIMT.[43-51] One AIDS Clinical Trial Group (ACTG) study was uniquely designed, with triads of patients enrolled simultaneously: patients with HIV with a history of PI use; patients with HIV with no PI exposure; and controls without HIV who were age, gender, ethnicity, smoking history, blood pressure, and menopausal status matched.[47,52] No correlation was found between PI use or HIV infection and cIMT, but traditional risk factors of age, HDL-cholesterol, and BMI were associated with a higher rate of subclinical atherosclerosis. The sample size was small in all of these studies, and follow-up was limited in duration. In one longitudinal study, 148 patients with HIV and 68 controls without HIV were studied for 1 year.[53] Increasing age, an elevated LDL-cholesterol level, a history of smoking, Latino ethnicity, hypertension, and HIV infection were associated with an increased cIMT.[53] The 1-year progression of cIMT in patients with HIV was more accelerated than in controls without HIV (0.074 pack-years of cigarette smoking versus 0.006 mm/year). Age, race, and CD4 nadir all were associated with progression of cIMT. Each of these studies used different methodologies to evaluate the cIMT and studied different patient populations.

The coronary calcium score (CCS) has been assessed in seven cross-sectional studies in individuals with HIV. In one study, 17 individuals with HIV were compared to controls without HIV; the CCS appeared to be higher in the individuals with HIV.[54] Other studies have demonstrated that higher scores were associated with the PI nelfinavir alone or with PI use in general.[55-57] Another study, however, showed no association with HIV infection or with PI use when individuals with HIV were compared to individuals without the virus. In univariate analysis of a cohort of 327 individuals with HIV, an abnormal CCS was predicted by age, triglycerides (TG), and remnant lipoprotein C in both men and women.[50] The duration of HIV infection tended to be associated with an increased risk for an abnormal CCS in both men and women. In studies that reported the CCS in cocaine users, cocaine was associated with an increased CCS.[55,56] The sample size in all these studies was small (17 to 98 participants), and populations were biased (entirely African American or cocaine users, or both).

Management

Aggressive modification of traditional risk factors is recommended for patients with HIV for primary prevention of coronary artery disease. Management of hyperlipidemia in patients with HIV involving lipid-reducing agents should follow the same guidelines established for uninfected individuals by the National Cholesterol Education Program (see Chapter 7). Measurements of fasting lipids and glucose should be performed before initiation of protease inhibitor therapy and at regular intervals of 2 to 3 months after a change in antiretroviral therapy. Cessation of tobacco use, dietary management of fat and carbohydrate consumption, regular physical exercise, and counseling regarding recreational drug use, including alcohol, are appropriate. The importance of smoking cessation should be emphasized, because smoking is a common risk factor in patients with HIV.

Prophylactic aspirin therapy also should be considered for patients with HIV; the criteria for starting this treatment should be addressed by the primary care provider.

Lipid-lowering agents may cause serious and even life-threatening drug interactions in patients undergoing certain HAART regimens. Both hydroxymethyl-glutaryl-coenzyme A reductase inhibitors and protease inhibitors are metabolized by the hepatic cytochrome P450 (CYP3A4) system.[58] Rhabdomyolysis and death[59] have been reported; because of an increased area under the curve for simvastatin and lovastatin with PIs, these drugs should not be used concurrently.[60] Pravastatin and fluvastatin are the least likely to cause a drug interaction with a protease inhibitor, because they are not CYP3A4 substrates; they therefore are generally safe to use with PIs. However, high levels of pravastatin were reported when the drug was used in combination with darunavir/ritonavir.[61] The Adults AIDS Clinical Trial Group has published recommendations for managing dyslipidemia.[60] These guidelines are similar to the National Cholesterol Education Program Adult Treatment Panel III (NCEP ATPIII) guidelines.

Fibrates produce better effects on triglycerides than do statins. Fibrates are not metabolized by CYP450 and thus are potentially safe when used with protease inhibitors. More large, controlled studies are needed to evaluate the effects of lipid-lowering agents in patients with HIV.

A new class of antiretroviral medications, the integrase inhibitors (raltegravir), has not been associated with lipid abnormalities.[62]

Prognosis

Evidence continues to emerge that drug-induced metabolic abnormalities translate into enhanced cardiovascular risk. Long-term cohort studies currently in progress may take years to establish the rate of diseases. Based on current data, aggressive management of traditional cardiovascular risk factors, with strict attention to preventing adverse drug interactions, is appropriate for patients with HIV.

PERICARDIAL DISEASE

Clinically significant pericardial disease is uncommon in patients with HIV in the United States. However, the pericardium is the most common site of cardiovascular involvement; as many as 25% of patients with severe immunosuppression have echocardiographic or autopsy evidence of effusions, but most of these effusions are small and clinically insignificant.[63] Occasionally, pericarditis may be the initial presentation of acquired immunodeficiency syndrome (AIDS).[1,2,63]

Pathophysiology

Most cases of pericardial effusion in patients with HIV are idiopathic and presumably related to HIV itself. However, many specific etiologic agents can cause pericarditis, such as

- bacterial, fungal, or mycobacterial infections; and
- neoplasms, such as lymphoma or Kaposi's sarcoma.[64]

HIV has been detected in macrophages in the pericardium, which suggests that the virus may play a part in the pathogenesis of pericardial effusion.

Clinical Presentations

The clinical presentation of pericarditis is similar in patients with or without HIV:

- chest pain;
- a pericardial friction rub on the physical examination; and
- an enlarged cardiac silhouette on chest radiograph.

In contrast to patients with HIV who have idiopathic pericarditis, those with purulent pericarditis arising from bacterial causes, particularly infection with *Staphylococcus aureus*, usually are severely ill and have fever and chest pain. Without early intervention (i.e., drainage and antibiotic therapy), these patients usually die as a result of tamponade and sepsis.

Diagnostic Techniques

When pericardial disease is clinically significant, fluid and tissue tests are necessary to determine whether the disease has an identifiable and treatable cause. Culture for routine bacteria, mycobacteria, and fungi are indicated: antigen tests and molecular diagnostics are useful and should be chosen in consultation with infectious disease specialists. Cytology also is useful for detecting lymphoma, primary effusion cell lymphomas, or solid tumors. Pericardial involvement from Kaposi's sarcoma is asymptomatic unless a concomitant bacterial infection is present; however, malignant pericardial effusions may cause recurrent pericardial effusion or tamponade.[65]

In patients unlikely to have pericarditis caused by conventional bacteria, clinicians should consider the possibility of malignancy or granulomatous disease. In immigrants from developing countries, tuberculosis should be a major consideration, regardless of whether evidence of the disease is present in other organs. *Mycobacterium tuberculosis* involving patients with HIV may represent primary infection or primary reinfection rather than reactivation, and extrapulmonary infection is common.[66] Pericardial disease in patients with HIV is largely caused by *M. tuberculosis*. A large percentage of those affected are symptomatic and progress to tamponade. Other species of mycobacteria, including *M. kansasii* and *M. avium complex*, have also been recovered from pericardial fluid.

Management

Management of pericardial disease in patients with HIV is no different from management of pericardial disease in other patient populations.[67-69] An asymptomatic patient with a small to moderate pericardial effusion (generally exudates) can be observed without undergoing pericardial drainage.[67] These effusions may be benign and may resolve spontaneously,[67] but the possibility of infectious or neoplastic processes should be considered. In symptomatic patients with respiratory complaints caused by a large effusion or tamponade, pericardiocentesis or pericardotomy with window placement is indicated to relieve the hemodynamic effects of tamponade.

Prognosis

The presence of pericardial effusion creates a poor prognosis for patients with HIV.[63] CD4 cell counts usually are lower in these patients. The 6-month survival is reduced compared with survival in those without effusion (60% compared with 93%).[63]

MYOCARDIAL DISEASE

Myocardial disease in patients with HIV includes myocarditis and dilated cardiomyopathy. The findings of autopsy studies suggest that myocarditis may be present in 33% of patients with AIDS,[2,70] although the frequency with which it occurs during the course of HIV infection probably is much lower. Clinical congestive heart failure in patients with AIDS has been uncommon, although autopsy reports suggest dilated cardiomyopathy is responsible for approximately 33% of all deaths from AIDS.[1]

Pathophysiology

Myocarditis and infection with the human immunodeficiency virus type 1 (HIV-1) are the most studied causes of dilated cardiomyopathy (DCM) in HIV disease.[71] In the era before antiretroviral drugs were available, global left ventricular dysfunction was detected by echocardiography in 15% of patients with HIV in one study.[72] In almost all cases, myocardial biopsy revealed myocarditis with cardiotropic viral infection.[73] No treatable causes of cardiomyopathy were seen other than HIV infection. In autopsy studies of patients with HIV, myocarditis was identified in more than half of the 71 patients evaluated, and biventricular dilatation was present in 10% of cases.[74] In children with HIV, increased left ventricular wall thickness and depressed left ventricular function were common compared with uninfected cohorts and were independent predictors of mortality.[75]

Zidovudine (AZT, ZDV) causes mitochondrial myopathy in skeletal muscles, providing a possible link to involvement of myocardial muscle.[76] Studies performed on transgenic mice suggest that AZT is associated with diffuse destruction of cardiac mitochondrial ultrastructures and with inhibition of cardiac mitochondrial DNA replication.[77] In one study of six patients, cardiac dysfunction was associated clinically with AZT and dideoxyinosine (didanosine) therapy.[78] Three patients improved after AZT was discontinued. However, another study found that patients taking AZT did not have worse left ventricular function or more frequent evidence of diastolic dysfunction than those not taking the drug.[80] These findings are consistent with those of a previous study by the same authors, which showed that AZT does not affect left ventricular function during short-term use.[81]

The origin of myocarditis has been the subject of much debate; however, a particularly intriguing issue has been the hypothesis that myocarditis caused by the effects of HIV may play a part in the pathogenesis of dilated cardiomyopathy and ventricular dysfunction.[2,65,70,73,81] Infectious causes, including opportunistic agents and viral pathogens, have been implicated, but they are rarely recovered from myocardial tissue.

A nonspecific lymphocytic myocarditis, attributed to a specific pathologic effect of HIV on myocardial tissue, accounts for most AIDS-associated myocarditis. Histopathologically, three patterns can been seen in AIDS-associated myocarditis:

- nonspecific focal inflammatory infiltrates without myocyte necrosis;
- myocyte damage without cellular inflammatory infiltrates; and
- lymphocytic infiltration with necrosis of the myocyte.[2,80]

Diffuse fibrosis may cause the myocardium to undergo a compensatory hypertrophy and dilatation, eventually leading to dilated cardiomyopathy.[82]

Several investigators have used in situ hybridization, polymerase chain reaction, and culture techniques at autopsy and biopsy in patients with congestive cardiomyopathy and have demonstrated HIV-1 genomic material within cardiac myocytes.[70,83] Whether this represents a direct effect of HIV, an autoimmune process, or the effects of other cardiotropic viruses is unclear.[5,73,83,84] The mechanism of viral entry into CD4 receptor–negative cells, such as myocytes, remains elusive, although injured myocytes may allow entry of HIV virions into the cell. In one study, a primary culture of human fetal cardiac myocytes did not become infected with wild-type HIV-1, which suggests that direct infection of myocytes is not the primary means of pathogenesis of HIV-1 cardiomyopathy.[85] However, the same study demonstrated that HIV-based vectors may be promising for ex vivo cardiovascular gene therapy, because cardiac myocytes support the HIV-1 life cycle. The presence of viral hybridization and the increased myocardial expression of major histocompatibility complex class I molecules strongly suggest the presence of an active immune process within the myocardium.[73,81] Cardiac autoantibodies also have been detected in patients with AIDS who have DCM.[86]

OTHER CAUSES OF DILATED CARDIOMYOPATHY

Other factors may contribute to dilated cardiomyopathy in patients with AIDS. Malnutrition and wasting are important independent predictors of cardiac-related morbidity and mortality and of overall mortality in children with HIV.[87] The mechanism by which malnutrition contributes to dilated cardiomyopathy is unknown. The virulence of the coxsackie virus with respect to cardiac tissue has been reported to be increased in the presence of concomitant selenium deficiency.[5] Selenium repletion in selenium-deficient patients with HIV who have symptomatic ventricular dysfunction has improved cardiac function. L-Carnitine deficiency has also been noted in HIV-infected adults.

Patients with HIV produce excessive amounts of cytokines (including tumor necrosis factor, interferon α, and interleukins 1 and 2). It remains to be determined whether these are present in quantities sufficient to reduce myocardial function.[88] Cardiotoxicity from nontherapeutic drugs such as ethanol, cocaine, and heroin must also be considered as possible causes of dilated cardiomyopathy.

Clinical Presentations

The clinical presentation of AIDS-related cardiomyopathy is similar to that of dilated cardiomyopathy of any cause. Symptoms such as dyspnea are nonspecific and frequently are attributed to pulmonary disease. More specific findings of cardiac dysfunction may be present, including an S_3 gallop, pulmonary edema, pathologic murmurs, and pericardial friction rub. In patients with clinical findings of heart failure, an increased cardiac silhouette on chest radiograph and an echocardiogram with ventricular dilatation may be seen.[89]

Diagnostic Techniques

A thorough cardiovascular history and baseline routine cardiac physical examination are essential in the diagnosis of cardiac disease in patients with HIV. The frequency and type of cardiac evaluation should be determined by the patient's symptomatology. Impairment of systolic and diastolic function may be detected by echocardiogram in asymptomatic patients with HIV.[90] The degree of left ventricular dysfunction correlates with the extent of immune dysfunction at baseline but not in the long term; this suggests that the CD4 cell count may not be a useful surrogate marker of HIV-associated left ventricular function.[91]

Endomyocardial biopsy is useful as a research tool; clinically, biopsy does not alter therapy. Immunosuppressive therapy with prednisone and azathioprine has not affected the course of myocarditis in patients not infected with HIV (see Chapter 77). However, the use of monthly intravenous immunoglobulin recently has been reported to have promising effects on left ventricular structure and function in pediatric patients with HIV; this warrants further investigation.[92]

Management

Cardiac function in patients with HIV can improve significantly with medical therapy. In patients with asymptomatic left ventricular dysfunction, the primary treatment goal is prevention of further deterioration of left ventricular performance; in patients with chronic heart failure, the goals should be symptomatic relief, improvement of quality of life, and prevention of progression of left ventricular dysfunction.[90]

The mainstays of treatment for dilated cardiomyopathy continue to be diuretics, digoxin, afterload reduction with angiotensin-converting enzyme (ACE) inhibitors, beta-blocker therapy, and referral for an automatic implantable cardioverter defibrillator (AICD) or biventricular pacemaker as indicated clinically. The introduction of potent antiretroviral therapy (ART) regimens seems to influence the course of HIV-associated dilated cardiomyopathy, with a lower rate of mortality for congestive heart failure.

The incidence and prevalence of dilated cardiomyopathy in patients with HIV in the HAART era remains unknown.

In a study performed in 1999 in the Netherlands involving 105 ambulatory patients with HIV, the prevalence of myocardial systolic dysfunction was low (3%), and none of the patients developed end-stage DCM.[93] The authors suggested a myocardial protective effect of antiretroviral therapy to explain this low prevalence of cardiac dysfunction compared with previous studies. A decrease in the prevalence of global cardiac involvement has been shown in a retrospective study conducted in Italy among patients with HIV treated with ART, compared with those treated with nucleoside reverse transcriptase inhibitors.[94]

The epidemiology of HIV-associated dilated cardiomyopathy in the antiretroviral era and the role of HIV medication in improvement of left ventricular dysfunction remain unknown. The HIV-HEART study, a long-term cohort study of more than 800 patients, will help to assess the prevalence of myocardial dysfunction in a contemporary group of patients with HIV.[95]

Prognosis

Dilated cardiomyopathy usually occurs late in the course of HIV infection.[96,97] It has been associated with reduced survival; the mean survival in those affected was 101 days, compared with 472 days in patients with normal hearts but a similar stage of disease.[97] Interestingly, the presence of HIV encephalopathy is one of the strongest predictors of cardiac involvement in patients with HIV.[91]

OTHER PATHOLOGIC CONDITIONS ASSOCIATED WITH ACQUIRED IMMUNODEFICIENCY SYNDROME

Pulmonary Hypertension

Severe pulmonary disease occurs frequently in patients with advanced HIV disease and cardiac abnormalities; right ventricular dilatation and failure are not unusual. At San Francisco General Hospital in the 1980s, six patients with advanced HIV disease were found to have pulmonary hypertension (proven by catheterization) and right ventricular hypertrophy.[98] Other authors since have reported similar patients with pulmonary hypertension.[99-101] Pulmonary hypertension has been reported in patients with HIV who have no history of thromboembolic disease, intravenous drug use, or pulmonary infection.[102]

Primary pulmonary hypertension has been described in a disproportionate number of individuals with HIV, and in the 1980s, it was estimated to occur in 0.5% of hospitalized patient with AIDS.[98] One review of the literature concluded that only one third of patients with HIV who had pulmonary hypertension had AIDS and that the development of pulmonary hypertension did not require the presence of AIDS, pulmonary infection, a low CD4 cell count, or hypoxemia.[100] Before the advent of antiretroviral therapy, HIV-associated pulmonary hypertension warranted a poor prognosis; in a review of 131 cases, half of the patients died during a median follow-up period of 8 months, with a median time interval between diagnosis of pulmonary hypertension and death of only 6 months.[103]

The prevalence of pulmonary hypertension in treated patients with HIV remains poorly described. In several preliminary studies, a high pulmonary artery systolic pressure (PASP) was detected on echocardiography in 4.7% of patients with HIV[104]; in another study, the prevalence of pulmonary artery hypertension (PAH) was 0.21%.[105] In a study from San Francisco, an elevated PASP was detected in 6% of patients; HIV infection was independently associated with an elevated PASP.[106] The effect of antiretroviral therapy on pulmonary hypertension is not known; in a retrospective report from the Swiss Cohort Study, pulmonary artery pressure increased in untreated patients but decreased in patients treated with HAART.[107] The oral endothelin receptor antagonist bosentan improved exercise tolerance and hemodynamic measurements in a small study of patients with HIV.[108]

Neoplasms

The two neoplasms known to involve the heart in patients with AIDS are Kaposi's sarcoma (KS) and non-Hodgkin's lymphoma. Cardiac involvement with KS usually is seen in widely disseminated disease. The tumor usually involves the epicardium and pericardium and causes pericardial effusion.[1] The incidence of KS involving the heart in autopsy series of patients with AIDS has ranged from 20% to 30%. KS most often involves the visceral and parietal pericardium, although involvement of the myocardium, coronary artery adventitia, great vessels, epicardium, and epicardial fat also has been described.[109] Cardiac KS is not usually associated with obstruction or with clinical cardiac dysfunction, morbidity, or mortality. Therefore, cardiac KS remains occult and is rarely diagnosed during life. Pericardial involvement usually does not affect underlying myocardial function, but in rare cases, it may cause tamponade or constriction.

Primary cardiac lymphoma has been reported, but non-Hodgkin's lymphoma of the heart in patients with AIDS usually occurs as a result of widely metastatic disease. The malignancy is characterized most commonly by diffuse myocardial infiltration. Although many patients are asymptomatic, this diffuse infiltration can result in congestive heart failure, atrial and ventricular dysrhythmia, and heart block. The tumor also can extend into the cardiac chambers and across valves, causing mechanical obstruction of blood flow. Surgical resection may be appropriate in patients with tumors that are significantly obstructing blood flow. Pericardial involvement can result in pericardial effusion and tamponade. Responses to chemotherapy and radiotherapy are variable and usually short lived.[110] The introduction of potent ART led to a reduction in the overall incidence of cardiac involvement by KS and non-Hodgkin's lymphoma. This change may be attributed to patients' improved immunologic state and to prevention of the pathogens (human herpes virus type 8 and Epstein-Barr virus) known to play an etiologic role in these neoplasms.[111]

Valvular Heart Disease

Infective endocarditis in patients with AIDS most often occurs in intravenous drug users the condition otherwise is rare.[112] It also may occur in patients with intravascular catheters. In such patients, the predominant organism is *Staphylococcus aureus*, and a growing fraction of these staphylococci are resistant to methicillin (MRSA).[112] Infection with HIV should not preclude cardiac surgery.[113] Case reports describe both nonbacterial thrombotic endocarditis[114] and infective endocarditis in patients with HI, with infections at times caused by unusual organisms such as

Candida or *Aspergillus*. Among patients infected with HIV, infective endocarditis is seen almost exclusively in intravenous drug users, in whom the prevalence varies from 6.3% to 34%; the condition otherwise is rare.[113] Right-sided valves are affected predominantly, and the most frequent pathogens are *S. aureus* (>75% of cases), *Streptococcus pneumoniae, Haemophilus influenzae, Candida albicans, Aspergillus fumigatus*, and *Cryptococcus neoformans*.[116]

The presentation of infective endocarditis and survival rates for the condition generally are similar in patients with and without HIV. The survival rate is 85% in patients with HIV and 93% in patients without HIV.[117] However, patients with late-stage HIV infection have a 30% higher mortality with endocarditis than asymptomatic patients with HIV; this may be related to the degree of immunodeficiency.[117]

Before the advent of antiretroviral therapy, marantic endocarditis was reported with a prevalence of 4% to 10% among autopsied patients with HIV. Currently, it is much less commonly encountered, which suggests that its prevalence was overestimated in the past. The disorder is seen mostly in patients with HIV wasting syndrome. It is characterized by friable endocardial vegetations that affect predominantly the left-sided valves and consist of platelets and inflammatory cells within a fibrin mesh. Systemic embolization from marantic endocarditis is a rare cause of death in patients with HIV who are treated with ART.

CARDIAC SURGERY AND HUMAN IMMUNODEFICIENCY VIRUS INFECTION

A small retrospective study of 37 patients from 1994 to 2000 showed that after 3 years of follow-up, 81% of patients were free of repeat revascularization, myocardial infarction, and angina; no patients died; and no patients progressed to AIDS during the study period.[118] Another retrospective study showed that cardiac surgery in patients with HIV did not blunt the CD4 response from antiretroviral therapy.[119] Patients with HIV who had thoracic surgery at a large managed health care system in northern California had fewer complications than patients who did not have the virus.[120]

Two case reports of heart transplantation in patients with HIV are reported in the literature.[121,122] The optimal timing of surgery with respect to HIV infection remains unclear, and future studies are needed to further elucidate the clinical outcomes of patients with HIV after cardiac surgery.

Occasionally concern is expressed about the risk to the surgical team posed by patients with HIV. However, HIV infection has never been convincingly transmitted in the operating room or by needle injury with solid needles. Meticulous observation of universal precautions and careful attention to prevention of sharps injuries should be sufficient to provide the surgical team with a high degree of protection from HIV transmission.

SUMMARY

Patients infected with HIV who have access to medical care and who can adhere to antiretroviral regimens have an excellent long-term prognosis for avoiding the opportunistic complications of HIV. In doing so, these patients will live to age ranges in which they will be subject to the same morbidities as people who are not infected with HIV, and they will need to be treated for these morbidities. In addition, as patients infected with HIV are treated for more years, unique metabolic complications are occurring that appear to accelerate the development of atherosclerotic disease. Understanding the basis for this accelerated disease will allow better management of these patients and insight into the pathogenesis of atherosclerosis. Whether new morbidities, such as pulmonary hypertension, will emerge as major challenges to survival remains to be seen.

In addition to patients receiving antiretroviral therapies, there will continue to be a population without access to care. These individuals will develop opportunistic processes that involve the myocardium. A subset of these patients who abuse intravenous drugs also will develop cardiovascular complications, such as endocarditis. More than 600,000 people in the United States have HIV, and 40,000 to 70,000 new cases are seen each year; most cardiologists, therefore, will be confronted with management of these patients.

A careful cardiac examination should be done at the time of diagnosis of HIV infection, and the patient should be monitored throughout the course of the disease. The mechanism underlying the increased risk of atherosclerosis in individuals with HIV infection remains unknown, as do the methods of diagnosis of cardiovascular disease and optimal treatment for individuals with HIV infection. The epidemiology and natural history of many cardiovascular complications of HIV infection await additional studies in the antiretroviral era. Clinicians must be vigilant in considering the possibility of cardiovascular disease in their patients with HIV and must also try to address aggressively all traditional risk factors.

Further investigation should focus on epidemiologic and clinicopathologic studies to gain a better understanding of cardiovascular disease in patients infected with HIV who are receiving highly active antiretroviral therapy.

chapter

132 Cardiac Tumors

Colette Guiraudon

Definition

- Primary cardiac tumors arise from the three layers of the heart (pericardium, myocardium, and endocardium) and from the nonspecialized connective tissue within the heart. Some entities in this group are not true neoplasms (hamartomas, heterotopias) or have a controversial histogenesis.
- Secondary cardiac tumors are metastases from an extracardiac tumor disseminated via blood vessels or lymphatics, or both. Direct propagation from a nearby tumor, most often a mediastinal lesion, also is seen.
- Carcinomas are the main source of cardiac metastases, followed by secondary hematologic malignancies (see Chapter 133).

Key Features

- Primary tumors are rare, particularly in individuals under age 16 years. Tumors are different in adults and children.
- Eighty percent of tumors are histologically benign, but they may have disabling or lethal complications.
- The clinical presentation is protean and often misleading. Sudden cardiac death is possible in all cases.
- Modern diagnostic tests have made earlier diagnosis easier; they also aid treatment planning.
- Secondary tumors are much more common than primary tumors.
- Secondary tumors may involve the three layers of the heart, but they are rare in the endocardium.
- Cardiac metastases often are discovered only at autopsy.
- The most common metastatic tumors seen at autopsy are carcinomas of the lung and breast.
- In at least 10% of cases, death is directly related to the cardiac involvement.

Therapy

- Surgery is the treatment of choice for benign tumors. Because of the tumor's size and location, complex reconstructive procedures may be required.
- Malignant primary tumors cannot be resected completely. Chemotherapy and radiotherapy may slow the evolution in some cases.
- In metastases, treatment is only palliative and symptomatic. Survival generally is very short.

The incidence of primary cardiac tumors in autopsies ranges from 0.002% in general hospitals up to 0.1% in tertiary hospitals. Multiple case series have been published and show different proportions of each tumor type, depending on whether the study was based on autopsies, surgical experience, or reference center material and whether it was based on a pediatric or general population.[1,2] Approximately 80% of primary cardiac tumors are benign.

The types of tumors predominantly seen in adults (older than 16 years) (Fig. 132.1) are very different from the types predominantly seen in children (younger than 16 years) (Fig. 132.2); 85% of benign tumors in adults are myxomas, lipomatous tumors, and papillary fibroelastomas, whereas 82% of benign tumors in children are rhabdomyomas, teratomas, and fibromas. The four more common malignant tumors in adults are angiosarcomas, rhabdomyosarcomas, mesotheliomas, and fibrosarcomas; in children they are rhabdomyosarcomas, fibrosarcomas, malignant teratomas, and neurogenic sarcomas.

Because of the rarity of primary cardiac tumors and the diversity of their clinical presentation, they often are mistaken for more common cardiac or systemic diseases. This partly explains the morbidity and mortality associated with benign tumors. When symptoms point to the heart, echography often provides the first clue to the diagnosis. In the absence of cardiac symptoms, the diagnosis may be mistaken for some time. Modern noninvasive diagnostic techniques allow for preoperative tumor diagnosis. Surgery is indicated in most cases of benign tumors and should be performed as an emergency to prevent unpredictable complications. With malignant tumors, metastases already are present in 80% of cases, and complete resection generally is impossible.

No good classification scheme has yet been devised for primary cardiac tumors (Table 132.1). The most common benign tumors have an uncertain histogenesis or are hamartomas or heterotopias. Most of malignant tumors are sarcomas and are classified by their tissue of origin.

PRIMARY CARDIAC TUMORS

ANATOMY AND PATHOLOGY

Benign Primary Tumors

Myxomas

Myxomas account for more than half of the benign tumors resected in adults. A myxoma is an intracavitary mass measuring 4 to 8 cm in diameter (Fig. 132.3). In 85% of cases, it originates on the septal surface of the left atrium over the foramen ovale. More rarely, it is found in the right atrium or in the ventricles. Multiple myxomas (synchronous, successive, or recurrent) are a fixture of the myxoma syndromes (which occur in 7% of cases). Multiple myxomas

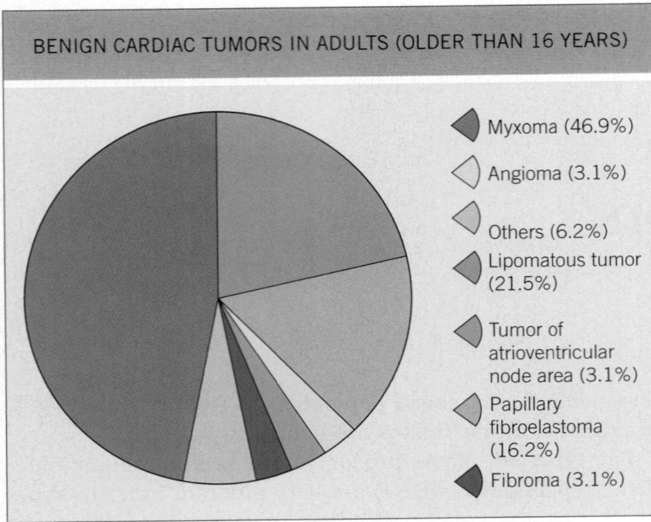

Figure 132.1 Benign Cardiac Tumors in Adults (Older than 16 Years) The three most common tumors (myxomas, lipomatous tumors, and papillary fibroelastomas) account for 85% of benign cardiac tumors in this age group.

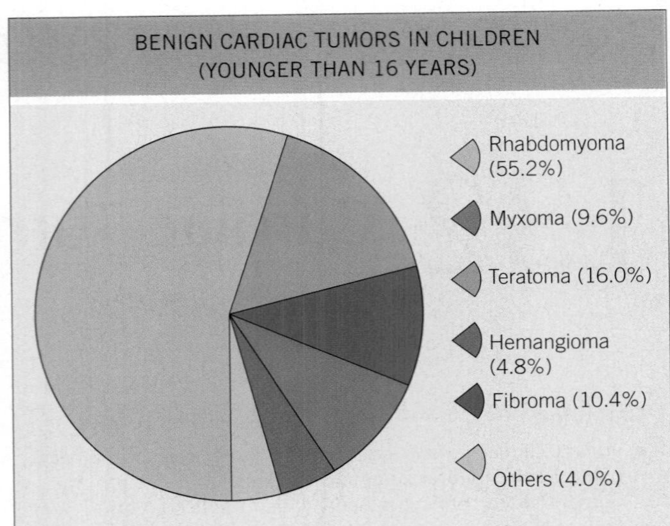

Figure 132.2 Benign Cardiac Tumors in Children (Younger than 16 Years) The three most common tumors (rhabdomyomas, teratomas, and fibromas) account for 82% of benign cardiac tumors in this age group.

CLASSIFICATION OF PRIMARY CARDIAC TUMORS

	Benign Tumors		
Histogenesis	**True Neoplasms?**	**Hamartomas, Ectopias, Pseudotumors**	**Malignant Tumors**
Unknown	Myxoma Papillary fibroelastoma		Unclassified sarcoma
Cardiomyocytes		Rhabdomyoma Histiocytoid cardiomyopathy	Rhabdomyosarcoma
Endothelial cells	Hemangioma Lymphangioma	Varix Congenital valvular blood cysts	Angiosarcoma
Fibrocytes	Fibroma	Inflammatory pseudotumor	Fibrosarcoma Malignant fibrous histiofibrome
Adipose cells	Lipoma	Lipomatous hypertrophy of atrial septum	Liposarcoma
Mesothelial cells		Cysts	Malignant mesothelioma
Miscellaneous		Tumor of atrioventricular node area teratoma	Leiomyosarcoma malignant teratoma

Table 132.1 Classification of primary cardiac tumors. Only the most common primary tumors in adults and children have been included.

often are familial and tend to start at a younger age than single myxomas; familial multiple myxomas are associated with diverse endocrinologic and skin tumors (Table 132.2). Familial cases have an autosomal dominant transmission.[3]

Myxomas may be sessile or pedunculated, spheric or polypoid. They have a smooth, glistening surface with areas of hemorrhage or thrombosis. The typical "lepidic" cells may be single with a stellate appearance, or they may form cords and rings around vessels; they float in a myxoid matrix with thin-walled vessels (Fig. 132.4). Chronic inflammatory cells, hemosiderin, fibrosis, calcium, bone, and even bone marrow are commonly seen. Because of these changes, some considered a myxoma to be an organized thrombus; however, modern pathologic and molecular techniques favor a neoplastic origin.

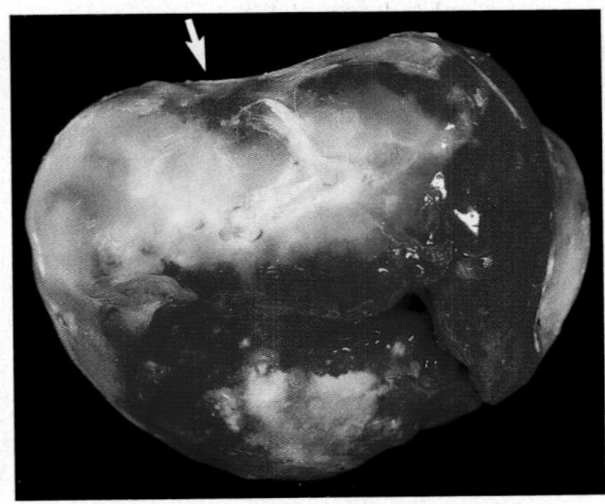

Figure 132.3 Large, spheric left atrial myxoma. The tumor has a smooth, shiny surface with thrombosed, red areas. A broad attachment base can be seen *(arrow)*.

"LAMB"	"NAME"	Other associations
Lentiginosis	Nevi	Breast fibroadenoma
Atrial myxoma	Atrial myxoma	Pituitary adenoma
Mucocutaneous myxomas	Mucocutaneous myxomas	Cortical adenoma
Blue nevi	Ephelides	Sertoli cell tumor
		Melanotic schwannoma

Table 132.2 Myxoma syndromes. Several skin and glandular tumors can be associated with cardiac myxoma in familial myxomas.

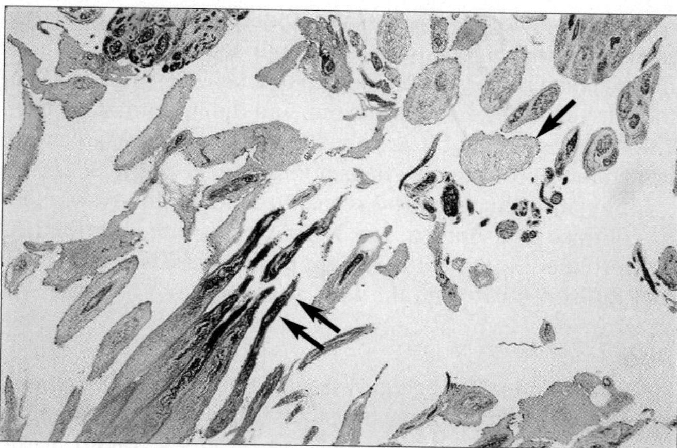

Figure 132.5 Papillary fibroelastoma. The tumor is made up of slender fronds with a flat endothelial cell lining *(single arrow)*, a myxoid matrix, and focal accumulation of elastic tissue *(double arrow)*. Movat's pentachrome stain.

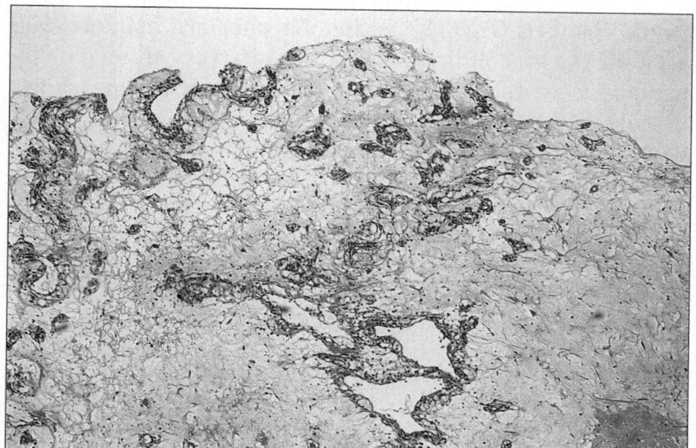

Figure 132.4 Myxoma. Most of the lepidic cells are arranged around thin-walled blood vessels. Others are dispersed within the myxoid matrix. Hematoxylin and eosin stain.

Papillary Fibroelastomas

Papillary fibroelastomas, another type of benign intracavitary tumor, account for 15% of resected tumors in adults. These are papillary tumors made up of slender fronds (Fig. 132.5) that grow on any one of the cardiac valves or on the surrounding endocardium. Multiple tumors sometimes are seen. The fronds are lined with endothelial cells and have a core of connective tissue with a myxoid matrix, a variable amount of collagen, and elastic tissue. A neoplastic origin for these tumors is not unanimously accepted; some favor a reactive process.

Rhabdomyomas

Rhabdomyomas are the most common benign tumors in children, accounting for 55% of childhood cases. Most cases are diagnosed in utero or before 1 year of age. Rhabdomyomas are hamartomas, and they originate from cardiac myocytes.[4] They may be sporadic and isolated, but in 50% of cases, they are associated with tuberous sclerosis.

Rhabdomyomas are found in the ventricular walls more often than in the atrial walls, and they generally are multiple. They are firm, light tan, lobular masses that range in size from a few millimeters to a few centimeters, and they can protrude into the cavities of the heart. Rhabdomyomas are composed of clear, glycogen-rich cells with a central nucleus. Some of the cells, known as spider cells, have thin filaments that radiate from the nucleus to the periphery.

The cardiomyocyte origin of these tumors is proven by positive tests for myoglobin and desmin and by electron microscopy, which shows abundant glycogen, myofibrils with Z bands, primitive T tubules, and poorly formed, intercalated disks.

Histiocytoid Cardiomyopathy

Histiocytoid cardiomyopathy, a much rarer hamartoma of children, accounts for 3% of benign cardiac tumors in children. Histiocytoid cardiomyopathies originate from Purkinje cells and are associated with other cardiac or systemic malformations in 25% of patients.[5,6] They consist of small, yellow, multicentric nodules that measure a few millimeters in diameter. They generally are located in the left ventricle and rarely in the right ventricle or atria. The cells are found in small clusters; they appear pale, foamy, and poor in glycogen. They stain weakly positive for myoglobin and desmin. On electron microscopy, they have abundant mitochondria, few if any fibrils, and no T tubules.

Fibromas

Fibromas are the third most common tumor in children, accounting for 10% of cases. Fibromas are solitary tumors that grow in the ventricular myocardium and that have a predilection for the septum and the left anterior ventricular wall.[7] They are whitish, have a whorled appearance, and are well circumscribed but not encapsulated. They measure a few centimeters in diameter. They are made up of fibroblasts within a variable amount of collagen and elastic fibers. They may be calcified or cystic. Occasionally fibromas are associated with multiple basal cell carcinomas and skeletal abnormalities in Gorlin's syndrome.

Lipomas and Lipomatous Hypertrophy of the Interatrial Septum

Lipomas and lipomatous hypertrophy of the interatrial septum are two different conditions. Lipomas are true neoplasms, whereas lipomatous hypertrophy of the interatrial septum is the accumulation of adipose tissue in the interatrial septum.

Lipomas generally are sessile or polypoid and sit on either surface of the myocardium, although some are intramural. Lipomas can be large, weighing up to 2 kg. They mostly affect the left ventricle, the right atrium, and the interatrial septum. They are made up of mature adipose tissue and may contain brown fat, fibrous tissue, and smooth muscle cells.[8]

Lipomatous hypertrophy is seen in obese, elderly women. In contrast to a lipoma, the lesion is not circumscribed or encapsulated; rather, it is made up of mature adipose tissue that infiltrates between the cardiac myocytes.[9]

Angiomas

Angiomas and other benign vascular tumors are uncommon, accounting for 5% of benign lesions. They are less than 5 cm in diameter. Angiomas are found in the myocardium of the right atrium and rarely in the right ventricle. They are subendocardial, but they protrude into the cavity. As elsewhere in the body, cavernous and capillary hemangiomas are differentiated from arteriovenous (AV) malformations. Angiomas are further classified on the basis of their cytologic characteristics and the vessel of origin (blood vessels or lymphatics). Many of these lesions probably are not true neoplasms, but rather are malformations or hamartomas. This is the case with varices (cystic lesions of the right atrium that are lined by endothelium and contain blood) and congenital valvular blood cysts.

Cystic Atrioventricular Nodal Tumors

Cystic atrioventricular (AV) nodal tumors make up 3% of the benign tumors, and they have the same incidence in adults and children. They are thought to be heterotopia or metaplasia. These tumors are tiny lesions, only 10 to 15 mm across, and are found in the area of the AV node. Histologically, they are small cysts lined by flat or cuboid cells in a fibrous background. The cysts may be distended with eosinophilic material. The cells are epithelial (they test positive for cytokeratin and epithelial membrane antigen) and also endodermal (they test positive for carcinoembryonic antigen [CEA]). Electron microscopy shows glandular spaces suggestive of an endodermal origin.[10]

Teratomas

Teratomas are neoplasms that contain endodermal, mesodermal, and ectodermal tissue (bronchogenic cysts may be mistaken for teratomas, but they have no ectodermal layer). Teratomas account for 16% of pediatric benign tumors, but they are rare in adults. Teratomas are found in the pericardium, the right atrium and ventricle, or the interventricular septum. Histologically, they show a variety of benign tissues from the three germinal layers.

Ectopic Tissue

Ectopic tissues and their tumoral counterparts have been found in the heart. Paragangliomas arising in the left epicardium, the interventricular septum, or from ectopic cells have been described. Likewise, benign thyroid tumors and thymomas may develop in the heart.

Pericardial Cysts

Pericardial cysts may be unilocular or multilocular and are covered by a single layer of mesothelial cells.

Malignant Primary Tumors

Malignant primary tumors consist of primary cardiac sarcomas, the most common cardiac tumors after myxomas (15% to 35% of all cardiac tumors); malignant mesothelioma of the pericardium; and malignant germ cell tumors. Hematologic malignancies are presented in Chapter 133.

Angiosarcomas

Angiosarcomas represent 35% of malignant sarcomas. They occur in adults, most often men in the third or fourth decade. Angiosarcomas originate in the atria, into which they protrude and form a polypoid, hemorrhagic mass that may extend into the afferent veins and the AV valves (Fig. 132.6). They invade the pericardium rapidly.[11] They are hypercellular, have necrotic foci, and are made up of pleomorphic cells. They may be arranged in bundles of spindle cells or in solid or papillary areas, or they may form vague channels (Fig. 132.7). Immunochemical markers (factor VIII, CD34) confirm the endothelial origin, although they may be only focally positive. Electron microscopy shows vascular channels lined with large pleomorphic cells mixed with single cells that have basal lamina and, occasionally, intracellular lumina (Fig. 132.8). Weibel-Palade bodies are

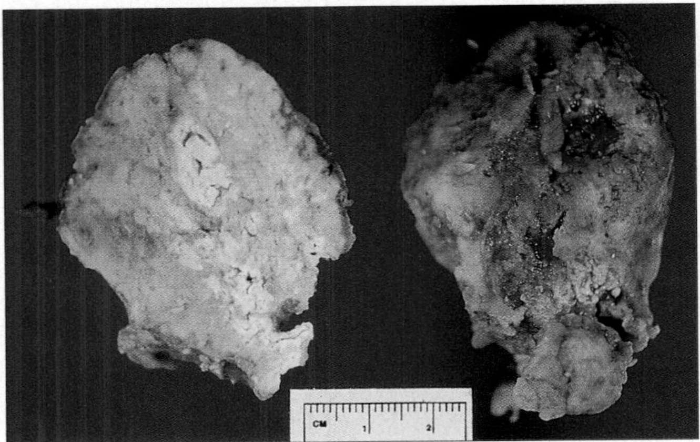

Figure 132.6 Right atrial angiosarcoma. This large, necrotic, thrombosed tumor was filling the atrium and had largely invaded the pericardium and the posterior mediastinum.

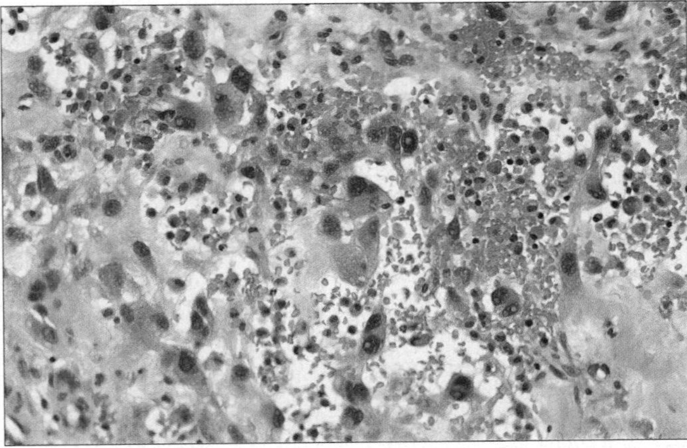

Figure 132.7 Right atrial angiosarcoma. Large, pleomorphic cells with multilobular nuclei are loosely arranged around vascular spaces. Hematoxylin and eosin stain.

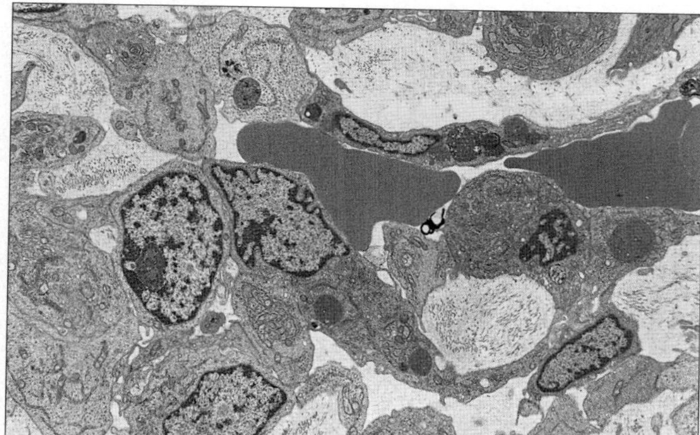

Figure 132.8 Left atrial angiosarcoma. This electron micrograph shows pleomorphic endothelial cells with large nuclei lining small vascular spaces filled with erythrocytes.

inconspicuous. Kaposi's sarcoma, found in 5% of patients with AIDS at autopsy and in sporadic cases, is a variant of angiosarcoma.

Unclassified Sarcomas

The incidence of unclassified sarcomas is difficult to evaluate. It ranges from 0 to 24%, depending on the reporting institution.[12] Most of these tumors occur in the left side of the heart. They have several histologic patterns (small, round cells; spindle cells; and epithelioid or pleomorphic cells). However, no histologic, immunologic, or electron microscopic indicator has been found that allows them to be assigned to a specific type of sarcoma or to suggest that they are a metastasis of an extracardiac tumor.

Rhabdomyosarcomas

Rhabdomyosarcomas, which account for 5% of cardiac sarcomas, are derived from striated muscle.[12] They are large and grow in the myocardium. They can involve the atria or ventricles, where they form polypoid masses that protrude into the cavities. They often are gelatinous. The embryonal pattern or, less often, the pleomorphic pattern is found in the heart. The cells are rhabdomyoblasts, which have abundant glycogen and, occasionally, cross-striations. The cells test positive for desmin and myoglobin, and electron microscopy shows filaments, Z bands, glycogen, and numerous mitochondria.

Malignant Fibrohistiocytomas

Malignant fibrohistiocytomas represent 15% to 20% of the cardiac sarcomas. They arise from the posterior or septal wall of the left atrium. They are large, soft, polypoid, sessile or pedunculated, and often multiple. They show a myxoid or storiform-pleomorphic pattern. The cells are spindly or pleomorphic and test positive for vimentin; some test positive for KP1. Electron microscopy shows fibroblasts and histiocytoid cells but, more important, helps to rule out more characteristic sarcomas.

Fibrosarcomas

Fibrosarcomas account for 5% of cardiac sarcomas. They are soft, polypoid tumors, with areas of necrosis and hemorrhage, that infiltrate the myocardium and fill the cavities (often the left atrium). They also may originate in the pericardium. They are composed of spindle cells with a herringbone pattern in a stroma that contains a variable proportion of collagen and myxoid tissue. They stain for vimentin and sometimes for actin, but they test negative for all other markers. Electron microscopy shows fibroblasts.

Other Sarcomas

Myxosarcomas, osteosarcomas, leiomyosarcomas, liposarcomas, synoviosarcomas, and malignant nerve sheath tumors are rare. They have the same histologic, immunologic, and ultramicroscopic characteristics as their extracardiac counterparts.

Malignant Mesotheliomas

Malignant mesotheliomas are rare tumors of the pericardial mesothelial cells.[13] Exposure to asbestos is rarely documented. Nodules of firm, white tissue with necrotic areas fill the cavity and may compress the large arteries and the venae cavae. They are formed of epithelioid or spindle (sarcomatoid) cells, or a mixture of the two. All the epithelioid cells and a large portion of the sarcomatoid cells test positive for high-molecular-weight keratin; the test result for vimentin may be positive, mainly in the sarcomatoid cells. The cells test negative for CEA and Leu-M1. Electron microscopy shows long microvilli.

Malignant Teratomas

A malignant teratoma is a rare tumor found in children. These tumors generally are located in the pericardium and show early extracardiac invasion and metastases.

PATHOPHYSIOLOGY

The location of the tumor is the main pathophysiologic factor, followed in importance by size and type (benign or malignant).

Intracavitary tumors are prone to embolize and occlude valves and vessels. Left-sided tumors embolize in the systemic circulation and may also cause mitral or aortic stenosis, with their respective hemodynamic consequences. Right-sided tumors embolize in the pulmonary circulation and can obstruct the tricuspid and pulmonary valves, causing right cardiac failure, pulmonary hypertension, and occlusion of the venae cavae.

Intramyocardial tumors cause cardiac failure and arrhythmias. Pericardial tumors cause effusions, which sometimes are hemorrhagic, and result in tamponade, constrictive pericarditis syndrome, or constriction of the large vessels. Intracavitary or intramyocardial malignant tumors also may invade the pericardium and provoke the same complications.

Sudden death is possible with all cardiac tumors. Several mechanisms can account for this, including:

- arrhythmias;
- coronary artery or distal emboli;
- tamponade;
- cardiac rupture;
- valvular obstruction; and
- cardiac failure.

Some tumors (myxomas, sarcomas, endocrine tumors) cause general symptoms. These are due to the release of tumor products, such as interleukin 6, tumor necrosis factor, and neuroendocrine factors.[14]

CLINICAL PRESENTATIONS

The clinical presentations are protean and may suggest any type of cardiac, extracardiac, or systemic disease. Given the extreme rarity of cardiac tumors, congestive heart failure, chest pain, valvular symptoms, arrhythmias, thromboembolic events, fatigue, and fever are more suggestive of other etiologies.

Cardiac Symptoms

Cardiac symptoms vary with the location of the tumor. Sudden death may be the first manifestation of most cardiac tumors.

Myocardial tumors may expand to a large volume before becoming symptomatic. Arrhythmias of all types are common, and their nature may suggest their location. Bundle branch blocks, ventricular tachycardia, and fibrillation are found in infiltrating tumors of the ventricular walls. Cystic tumors of the AV node or angiomas can cause complete heart block. Infiltration of the ventricular walls may result in congestive heart failure or may simulate restrictive or hypertrophic cardiomyopathy. Myocardial rupture with tamponade is possible.

Intra-atrial masses mimic valvular diseases. In the left atrium, tumors (most of them myxomas) that prolapse across the mitral valve suggest mitral disease and cause chest pain, dyspnea, cough, pulmonary edema, and hemoptysis. Fever and fatigue are present and may suggest an endocarditis. Symptoms may be present only when the patient adopts a certain position. Right intra-atrial and intraventricular tumors provoke right-sided cardiac failure with hepatomegaly, peripheral edema and ascites, and tricuspid valve regurgitation or stenosis, revealed by de novo murmurs. With malignant tumors, vena caval syndrome, pulmonary hypertension, and tamponade secondary to pericardial invasion are possible.

Pericardial tumors are revealed by chest pain, dyspnea, signs of constrictive pericarditis, or tamponade.

Thromboembolic Events

Thromboembolic events are the revealing factors in up to 60% of intracavitary masses. Systemic emboli originate from left-sided tumors. Cerebral emboli are common, and seizures or strokes often are the earliest symptoms. Emboli also are seen in the renal, femoral, and coronary arteries. Multifocal systemic emboli or vascular aneurysms, occasionally associated with general symptoms, may suggest bacterial endocarditis or polyarteritis nodosa. The discovery of neoplastic material consistent with a cardiac origin in biopsy samples or excised thrombi occasionally is the first clue to the diagnosis of a cardiac tumor. Right-sided tumors embolize in the lungs, producing the possibility of infarction, pulmonary hypertension, and cor pulmonale.

General Findings

General findings are common with myxomas but also may be seen with other tumors, particularly malignant tumors. Fever, fatigue, arthralgias associated with anemia, hyperglobulinemia, leukocytosis, and an elevated erythrocyte sedimentation rate orient more toward a systemic disease than a cardiac tumor. In some cases, metastases are the first indication of malignant tumors.

Clinical Examination

The clinical examination is poorly specific in cardiac tumors. However, cardiac signs in a patient who has had no previous cardiac problems, in association with general symptoms and embolic events, should initiate cardiac investigations.

Auscultation anomalies often are found with intracavitary tumors. Tumors of the left atrium, most of them myxomas, can produce a loud first heart sound and a holosystolic and diastolic murmur, which suggests mitral valve disease. However, a loud first heart sound with a normal PR interval and no diastolic murmur should suggest a tumor, especially if an early diastolic sound (tumor "plop") is detected. In the right atrium, a protodiastolic tumor plop has been described both with and without a holosystolic murmur and an early diastolic murmur. These de novo murmurs should raise the possibility of a tumor, because tricuspid valve disease is uncommon. In the right ventricle, signs of tricuspid valve dysfunction may be found in addition to a third heart sound and a delayed pulmonary component of the second heart sound. In the left ventricle, a systolic murmur can reveal aortic valve stenosis. All these abnormalities may be present only in some positions.

DIAGNOSTIC TECHNIQUES

Modern diagnostic techniques allow preoperative diagnosis of cardiac tumors, differentiation between benign and malignant tumors in some cases, and the design of an operative strategy.

Noninvasive Techniques

Electrocardiography and chest radiography are poorly specific, although a large pericardial effusion, irregular cardiac contours, or calcifications may be suggestive. Calcification is seen with several cardiac tumors and is particularly significant in children.

Echocardiography (Fig. 132.9) has completely transformed the way cardiac tumors are explored, and it often is the only test needed to diagnose most types of tumors (except for

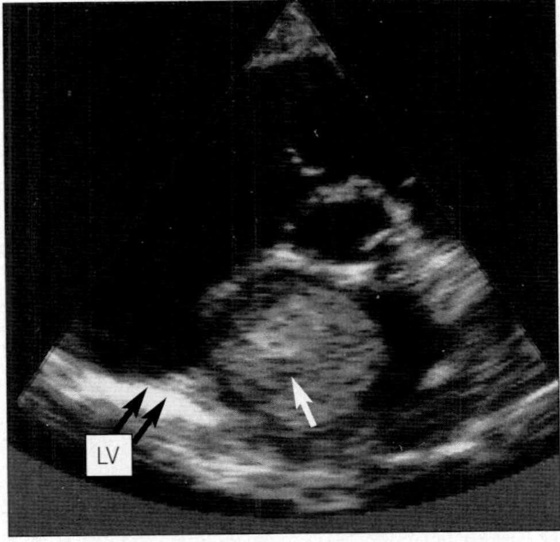

Figure 132.9 Large left atrial myxoma. A two-dimensional echocardiogram (short-axis view) shows a large left atrial myxoma *(arrow)* prolapsing into the left ventricle (LV; *double arrow*) during diastole. (Courtesy Dr. J. G. Pickering.)

pericardial masses). In the presence of many cardiac symptoms, echocardiography makes it possible to visualize the tumor and to rule out the more common differential diagnoses. M-mode echography was the first modality to provide a good image of left atrial intracavitary tumors; however, it was not very reliable for ventricular masses. Transthoracic two-dimensional echocardiography and now transesophageal echocardiography[15,16] can detect even small tumors; determine their size, location, and mode of attachment; and allow assessment of their mobility. These modalities can detect cardiac tumors in utero and can differentiate between tumors and thrombi. Doppler ultrasound can evaluate changes in valvular hemodynamics.

The transesophageal approach is superior to the transthoracic approach for the diagnosis of right atrial tumors and the study of their attachment. It also provides good visualization of the great vessels; however, it is not adequate for intramural and even intracavitary ventricular lesions. Spiral computed tomography (CT) scanning allows multiplanar and three-dimensional reconstructions that can clarify the tumor's anatomic relationships.[17]

Radionuclide imaging is less sensitive than echography and contrast injection angiography for the diagnosis of small intracavitary masses, but it may be useful for ventricular and intramural tumors.

CT is excellent for evaluating intramural and pericardial involvement and for studying the surrounding structures to detect extracardiac invasion. Increased resolution is obtained with electrocardiogram (ECG)-gated CT. Ultrafast CT reduces the number of motion artifacts.[18,19]

Magnetic resonance imaging (MRI), especially if ECG gated, gives the best resolution in three dimensions, allows exact localization of the tumor in the three cardiac layers and beyond, and may differentiate fat from a thrombus or tumor. It is particularly valuable for intramyocardial and malignant tumors (Fig. 132.10). Contrast imaging enhances the results. Dynamic study of the myocardium is possible.

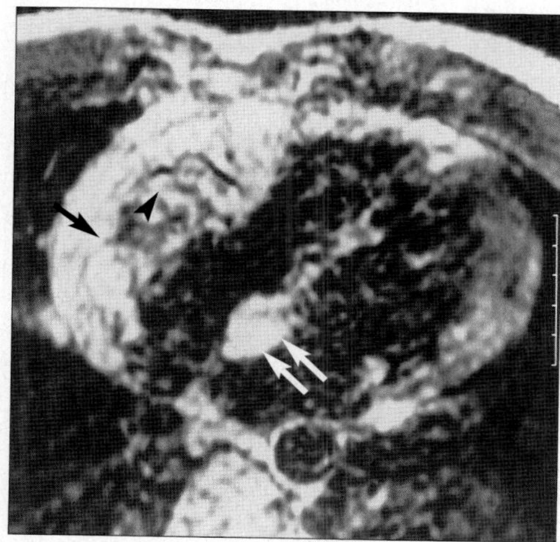

Figure 132.10 Angiosarcoma of the right atrium. Axial T1-weighted magnetic resonance imaging scan (four-chamber view) after gadolinium-DTPA enhancement. An infiltrative component can be seen in the free wall *(arrow)*, a nodular mass in the septum *(double arrow)*, and a thrombus in the atrium *(arrowhead)*. The thrombus was found to be a necrotic tumor. (Courtesy Dr. L. Thain.)

Although echography often is sufficient to make the diagnosis and assist in designing the surgery, MRI certainly is the best tool to use when echographic results are suboptimal.[19,20]

Invasive Techniques

Cardiac catheterization and selective angiography, once the best methods for diagnosing and characterizing cardiac tumors, have been replaced by echography, CT, and MRI. Only a few indications remain for the use of these techniques, such as poor visualization of the mass and its attachment, incomplete evaluation of all four chambers, and suspicion of malignancy or other cardiac disease. Invasive techniques pose a risk of embolization of tumor material, particularly in the trans-septal approach to the left atrium, and echography should be performed before catheterization if a tumor is suspected. Digital subtraction angiography, with injection of the contrast material far away from the tumor, reduces the risk of embolic events and allows this technique to be used safely if noninvasive techniques are unsatisfactory.

Endomyocardial biopsy has been performed to diagnose cardiac tumors. It is easily done in the right side of the heart, where sarcomas are more common. Complications (e.g., emboli, perforation) are uncommon.

Cytologic aspiration and transcutaneous biopsy play major roles in the diagnosis of pericardial tumors. Ancillary techniques (immunochemistry, electron microscopy) can help clinicians reach a definitive diagnosis.

MANAGEMENT AND PROGNOSIS

Benign Tumors

Complete surgical excision is the ideal treatment for benign tumors and should be performed without delay.[21] Unfortunately, severe complications (emboli, arrhythmias) and even sudden death may occur before the diagnosis of a cardiac tumor is made. With the exception of pericardial tumors, open heart surgery with extracorporeal circulation is necessary to allow adequate visualization of the mass and its attachment, as well as exploration of all the cavities. Minimal invasive surgery has been used lately for small, accessible tumors.[22] The perioperative mortality is close to 8% overall but is only approximately 1% for myxomas.

Myxomas

Myxomas by far are the most frequently resected tumors. Excision of a small rim of atrium around the stalk is mandatory and prevents recurrence in more than 95% of cases. Other measures have been used to prevent recurrence, including laser coagulation around the base of the tumor[23] and complete excision of the fossa ovalis area, followed by repair (generally with a pericardial patch).[24,25] In fewer than 5% of cases, the myxoma recurs or growth of a second myxoma is seen.[26] In familial cases, the risk of recurrence reaches 20%. Familial screening is warranted in familial cases.

Rhabdomyomas

Rhabdomyomas may regress spontaneously, especially in patients younger than 4 years of age. For this reason, and because removal of multiple intramural tumors is difficult, surgery generally is reserved for children with hemodynamic problems or arrhythmias. In particular, tumors close to cardiac valves that are obstructing the ventricular outflow tract and intractable arrhythmias should be excised. However, only the troublesome lesions should be removed, and partial excision is acceptable if the symptomatic area is removed.[27] Repeat procedures may be necessary, and careful follow-up is advised.

Other Benign Tumors

The other benign tumors also can be resected, with excellent results. However, large or critically located intramyocardial tumors may require complex surgical measures (e.g., ventricular or atrial patches, valvular replacement, valvular repair, or pacemaker implantation). Autotransplantation has been performed in some technically difficult cases, and orthotopic transplantation has been done when reparative surgery was impossible.

Malignant Tumors

Malignant tumors carry a dire prognosis, and the treatment is palliative. The large size of the tumor, associated with early extracardiac invasion and metastases, makes complete excision almost impossible. Even so, most patients undergo surgery, either because the diagnosis of malignancy is not determined before surgery or for debulking of the tumor. Iterative excisions have been done occasionally. The operative mortality is approximately 17% for cardiac sarcomas. Chemotherapy, radiotherapy, or a combination of the two may prolong life, but survival for longer than 3 years is rare.

SUMMARY

Primary tumors of the heart are rare. About 70% are histologically benign; however, they have a relatively high morbidity and mortality. The diagnosis of cardiac tumor often is delayed, because the clinical presentation can mimic that of many cardiac or systemic diseases. Emboli in the systemic or pulmonary circulation are common and are a cause of delay in diagnosis, as well as morbidity and mortality. The now extensive use of transthoracic or transesophageal echocardiography in many cardiac diseases allows earlier, noninvasive diagnosis of cardiac tumors and aids the planning of surgical treatment. Echography generally is the only imaging test needed. Other investigative methods (e.g., CT scans, MRI, and angiography) may be used in selected cases, particularly for intramyocardial and malignant tumors. Differentiation of benign and malignant tumors is not always possible preoperatively.

The most common cardiac tumor in adults is the myxoma. Surgical resection cures the patient in more than 95% of cases. Recurrences are few and occur in sporadic cases. Most other benign tumors can be cured surgically, although some cases require complex reparative surgery. In rhabdomyomas, surgery is recommended only if life-threatening symptoms develop.

Malignant tumors also have a protean clinical presentation. Malignancy may be obvious in advanced cases and with the help of modern imaging techniques, but some cases are diagnosed only at surgery. Complete eradication is impossible, despite attempts through surgery, chemotherapy, and radiotherapy.

SECONDARY CARDIAC TUMORS

Secondary cardiac tumors are found at autopsy in 10% to 15% of patients with generalized cancer and in 1% to 3% in the general population. Based on autopsy studies, secondary tumors occur 1000 times more frequently than primary tumors.[28]

Most malignant tumors can metastasize to the heart. The most common are carcinomas from the lung and breast because of these tumors' frequency, near vicinity, and metastatic propensity (Fig. 132.11). Melanomas, malignant germ cell tumors, and sarcomas have a high metastatic rate, including in the heart. Cardiac manifestations often are overlooked or misinterpreted among all the other problems of terminal cancer. This is the reason the diagnosis often is made at autopsy.

Fifty-two percent of metastases are located mostly in the pericardium, 42% in the myocardium, and 6% in the endocardium.[29] Carcinomas metastasize mostly to the pericardium; the lung, breast, stomach, and esophagus are the most common sources of metastases to this location. As do all carcinomas, they invade by lymphatic propagation, mostly retrograde, following obstruction of the regional lymph nodes. Direct extension also is possible because of the anatomic proximity of the heart to the primary tumor.

Melanomas; sarcomas; and renal, adrenal, liver, and uterine tumors metastasize by hematogenous propagation; they mostly involve the myocardium and less often the endocardium. Intracavitary tumors may have propagated by direct extension through the inferior vena cava from the kidney or through the pulmonary veins from the lung.

The microscopic characteristics of the metastases are identical to those of the primary tumor. When metastases are diagnosed but no primary tumor has been identified, pinpointing the organ of origin may be difficult, especially in the case of adenocarcinoma, because specific stains are not available for each organ.

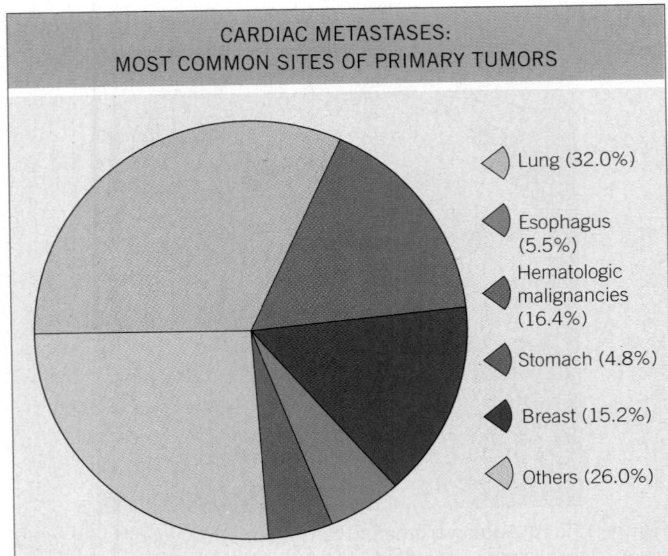

Figure 132.11 Cardiac Metastases: Most Common Sites of Primary Tumors. The three most common metastatic tumors to the heart are lung and breast carcinomas and hematologic malignancies (lymphomas and leukemias).

CLINICAL PRESENTATIONS

Pericardial metastases can provoke cardiac constriction and tamponade. Stricture of the vessels can cause caval syndrome and constriction of the coronary arteries and pulmonary vessels. Invasion of the sinus node can provoke arrhythmias.

Myocardial metastases are responsible for cardiac failure and arrhythmias, the type of which depends on the location of the metastases. Cardiac rupture also has been documented.

Intracavitary metastases are rare. They can impinge on valves, causing them to become stenotic or regurgitant, or both. They also can embolize in the pulmonary circulation or the systemic circulation, causing infarction and giving rise to new metastases.

The most common symptoms are dyspnea and cough, which can be related to cardiac failure, pleural effusion, and valvular obstruction. Chest pain may be related to pleural or pericardial effusion or to coronary obstruction. Right-sided heart failure with ascites, peripheral edema, and tender hepatomegaly suggests pericardial effusion or obstruction of the right-sided heart vasculature, with possible vena caval syndrome. Systemic emboli are revealed by myocardial infarction, cerebrovascular manifestations, renal pain and hematuria, and acute limb ischemia.

All types of arrhythmias are possible. Death may be due to an acute cardiac event such as tamponade, cardiac rupture, myocardial infarction, or arrhythmias.

DIAGNOSTIC TECHNIQUES

The same diagnostic techniques used for primary tumors are used for metastases. However, the indications are different. In patients with secondary cardiac tumors, the diagnosis of malignancy generally is known, and the problem is to confirm that the cardiac symptoms are secondary to metastases and not to the treatment or to previous cardiac disease. Histologic confirmation is the most useful test.

Low voltage on an ECG suggests pericardial effusion.

The chest radiograph may show widening of the cardiac silhouette consistent with pericarditis, pleural effusions and, in some cases, a primary carcinoma of the lung; or, it may show pulmonary and skeletal metastases and hilar and mediastinal node involvement.

Two-dimensional echography is the technique of choice in the imaging of metastases. Although it gives better results in intracavitary tumors, which are uncommon in metastases, it also can detect pericardial effusions and intramyocardial lesions.[30]

MRI, gallium, and CT scans are also useful. They can detect small lesions and are excellent for showing intramyocardial lesions and pericardial involvement. Because they are more difficult to obtain and more expensive, they are used mainly when active surgical treatment is considered or when the diagnosis of secondary tumor is uncertain.

Pericardiocentesis and pericardial biopsy (surgical, endoscopic, or transcutaneous) are performed routinely to diagnose pericardial effusions. They provide a tissue diagnosis, which is useful for establishing the treatment. Right endomyocardial biopsy is useful for intramyocardial tumors.

MANAGEMENT AND PROGNOSIS

With malignant tumors, treatment nearly always is only palliative and symptomatic, because cardiac involvement often is only one location of a generalized cancer. Pericardial involvement is the most common problem in cardiac metastases. Creating a pericardial window is more efficient than performing repeated pericardiocentesis.

Several agents have been used to dry up the effusion, including tetracycline, local chemotherapy, isotopes, and radiotherapy. Emergency treatment is needed if tamponade occurs.

Surgery is indicated only in a few cases of myocardial metastases. A variety of metastatic tumors has been excised, at least partially, under bypass surgery. The optimal indications are a single, well-circumscribed metastasis, no obvious spread elsewhere, and no intractable arrhythmias or obstruction of blood flow. Renal and hepatic neoplasms and, less often, adrenal and stromal uterine tumors can extend up to the right side of the heart through the inferior vena cava and occasionally are removed.

Bold surgical procedures may prolong the life of some patients. However, survival for patients with intramyocardial invasion generally is limited to a few months at most. Survival is longer for intracavitary tumors. Occasional patients have survived several years.

Chemotherapy and radiotherapy also are used, but the cardiotoxicity of these techniques must be weighed against their expected efficiency. Many patients are being treated or already have been treated with either or both of these modalities. Radiotherapy has been responsible for worsening cardiac failure and is used only as a last resort.

Too often, only compassionate care with symptomatic treatment of cardiac failure or arrhythmias is possible.

SUMMARY

Secondary cardiac tumors are more common than primary tumors, and they carry a dismal prognosis. Many are discovered only at autopsy. Those discovered premortem often are found in cases of generalized cancer, and even patients with only cardiac metastases have a short survival. The two most common secondary neoplasms are from the lung and the breast; however, other, less common tumors, such as melanomas, sarcomas, and germ cell tumors, are also seen because of their high metastatic potential.

Pericardial metastases are common and cause persistent pericardial effusions, which often are hemorrhagic; they also pose the risk of tamponade. Aspiration or biopsy can provide a histologic diagnosis in many cases. Pericardial window and fibrosing agents lessen the need for repeated aspiration. Intramyocardial metastases are secondary to hematogenous dissemination and therefore occur frequently with melanomas and sarcomas. Clinical symptoms include heart failure and arrhythmias. New imaging techniques are necessary to demonstrate them.

Palliative symptomatic treatment most often is the only resource. Chemotherapy can be used, with monitoring of the cardiotoxicity. Radiotherapy is used only as a last resort because of the risks of acute cardiac failure. Surgical excision is rarely indicated and does not improve survival significantly.

chapter

133 Hematologic Diseases

Stuart J. Hutchison

Definition

- Hematologic diseases comprise a diverse array of disorders: anemias and polycythemia; hypercoagulable states and bleeding diathesis; cellular and molecular elements; hereditary and acquired disorders; self-limited disease; and those that result from radiotherapy and chemotherapy.

Key Features

- Hematologic diseases have diverse effects on the cardiovascular system.
- In patients with a hematologic disorder, cardiovascular disease may precipitate symptoms of ischemia or heart failure, or both.

Therapy

- Determination of the optimal course of therapy requires collaboration between the cardiologist and the hematologist.

The diverse hematologic disorders—anemias and polycythemias, hypercoagulable states and bleeding diatheses, blood cellular elements and molecular elements, self-limited diseases and malignancies, hereditary and acquired disorders—can affect the cardiovascular system in similarly diverse ways, as can the treatment of these disorders. Hematologic disease and its treatment may cause heart disease, and heart disease may have hematologic complications. The optimal course of treatment for an individual patient often is best arrived at through close collaboration of the treating cardiologist and the hematologist, so that the risks to each system of the possible therapeutic options can be weighed.

ANEMIA

EFFECTS ON THE CARDIOVASCULAR SYSTEM

Pathophysiology

Mild and moderate degrees of anemia have no perceivable effect on a normal cardiovascular system. More severe degrees of anemia result in the expected structural changes of a high-output state. As hemoglobin concentrations decrease to less than 9 gm/dL, cardiac output increases in the resting state. Cardiac output increases progressively with further decreases in hemoglobin as a result of lower blood viscosity and lower systemic arterial resistance, which reduce afterload; increased venous return, which increases preload; and eccentric hypertrophic remodeling of the heart, which increases stroke volume.[1] Severe anemia may be associated with increased markers of sympathetic nervous system activation, such as plasma catecholamines.

Clinical Presentation

The first symptoms of anemia are dyspnea and exertional limitation from fatigue and dyspnea. These generally are seen at a hemoglobin concentration of approximately 7 gm/dL. As the hemoglobin concentration decreases further, symptoms become more severe and increasingly occur at rest. When erythrocyte transfusion is considered because of symptoms of severe anemia, careful attention should be paid to volume to avoid precipitating congestive heart failure.

Marked anemia results in congestive heart failure even in a normal circulatory system. This generally is seen at hemoglobin concentrations around 4 gm/dL. In this setting of hypervolemia, transfusion should be undertaken with concurrent diuresis.

Symptoms of chest pain generally are not attributable to anemia. The normal coronary circulation and myocardium are able to tolerate marked anemia without myocardial ischemia because of both structural and functional adaptations; increases in capillary density, collateral formation, and a shift of the oxygen dissociation curve maintain the delivery of oxygen despite marked anemia.

Diagnostic Techniques

On examination, vital signs may be normal or consistent with a hyperdynamic state, with an increased heart rate and increased pulse pressure. The precordium is dynamic. Systolic flow murmurs are common, and in severe anemia, anterograde diastolic flow rumbles may be present, as may an S_3 gallop rhythm. Cardiomegaly is evident radiographically. Echocardiography shows increased cardiac chamber end-diastolic dimensions, which are responsible for the cardiomegaly. Electrocardiography often is unremarkable but may show nonspecific repolarization abnormalities.

The cardiovascular changes of anemia reflect both the severity of the anemia and the rate at which it develops. Correction of the anemia eliminates symptoms and normalizes cardiovascular findings; therefore, the prognosis is heavily influenced by the natural history of the anemia.

EFFECTS OF ANEMIA ON THE CARDIOVASCULAR SYSTEM IN THE PRESENCE OF CARDIOVASCULAR DISEASE

Aggravation of Cardiovascular Symptoms

With underlying cardiovascular disease, symptoms become evident at lesser degrees of anemia. However, mild anemia is very unlikely to cause symptoms.[2] Moderate anemia also is generally fairly well tolerated, although with some aggravation of symptoms. Adults with renal failure or who are undergoing dialysis exemplify how commonly a moderate degree of anemia is tolerable despite mild to moderate coronary disease and hypertensive heart disease. Hemoglobin concentrations of less than 8 gm/dL may precipitate symptoms in patients with coronary artery disease or valvular or myopathic disease. The more severe the cardiovascular abnormality, the less severe the degree of anemia that will worsen the symptoms (Fig. 133.1).

Anemia as a Marker of Excess Risk

A considerable body of data has emerged indicating that the presence and severity of anemia is associated with a higher risk of adverse events across a broad range of cardiovascular diseases.

Coronary artery bypass surgery involves dilution of the patient's blood volume with volume used to prime the bypass pump and its circuit, unless red blood cell volume is used. Preoperative anemia is associated with an increase in renal and cerebral adverse events after coronary artery bypass surgery[3] and with increased mortality.[4,5] Although the level of preoperative anemia does not accurately predict the degree of intraoperative or postoperative anemia, the nadir of the intraoperative hemoglobin concentration predicts the degree of renal insufficiency associated with coronary artery bypass surgery.[6] Unfortunately, transfusion support in the context of coronary artery bypass surgery is itself associated with an increased risk of morbidity, cost in-hospital, and long-term mortality.[7-10] The free hemoglobin inadvertently delivered in red cell transfusions diminishes the availability of vascular nitric oxide. Whether anemia is the cause of adverse outcomes or a marker/risk factor, or both, is unclear, as is its optimal management.[11]

Similarly, the presence of anemia is associated with adverse outcomes in congestive heart failure. The presence and severity of anemia with congestive heart failure are associated with worse symptoms,[12] an increased risk of death,[12,13] longer hospital stays, and readmission.[14,15] Studies are underway on the risk/benefit ratio of chronic erythropoietin use and intravenous iron in patients with heart failure.[16]

With coronary artery disease, the presence and severity of anemia are associated with a greater risk of myocardial infarction and death in stable[17] and unstable coronary syndromes.[18] Anemia probably is the most common secondary cause of unstable angina. The combination of reduced oxygen-carrying capacity of the blood, flow-limiting stenoses, and increased myocardial oxygen demand reduces the threshold for ischemia, resulting in a worsening intensity of ischemic pains and a decreasing threshold for angina. Rest pains are less common and likely indicate primary unstable angina in a patient with anemia.

SICKLE CELL ANEMIA

Sickle cell anemia represents a specific cardiovascular disease state because of the combined effects of this hemolytic anemia and the vaso-occlusive effects of intravascular sickling.

Pathophysiology

Sickle cell anemia is caused by one of several inherited hemoglobinopathies, usually homozygous sickle cell disease, but also S-C and S-α thalassemia hemoglobinopathies.

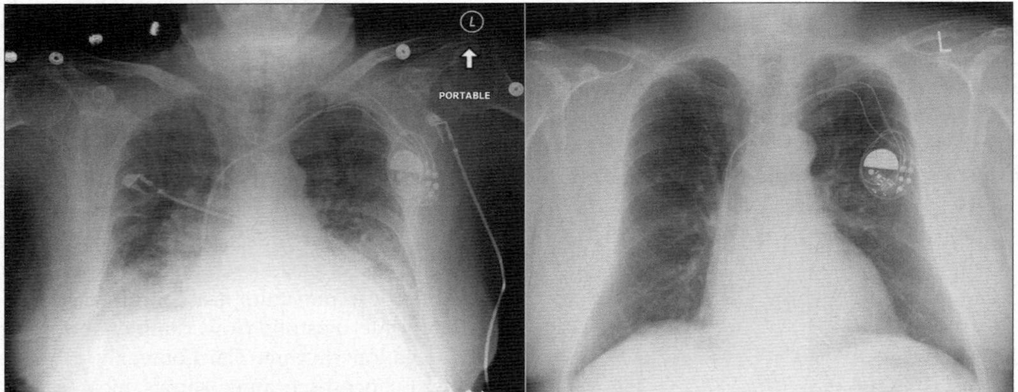

Figure 133.1 Anemia and heart failure. A 65-year-old man presented with class IV dyspnea, orthopnea, paroxysmal nocturnal dyspnea (PND), and gross edema. Three years before, he had undergone aortic valve replacement for aortic stenosis. At that time, other than moderate left ventricular hypertrophy, the left ventricle was normal. When he presented with heart failure, the valve and ventricular systolic function both were normal. His hemoglobin (Hgb) level was 51 gm/L. Chronic lower gastrointestinal bleeding was identified and treated endoscopically. With recovery of the Hgb level to 75 gm/L, the patient's resting heart failure symptoms subsided; at an Hgb of 110 gm/L, his functional class normalized. The heart failure had occurred as a result of high-output demands on a hypertrophied heart that had had aortic stenosis and consequently had limited compliance. *Left image*: At presentation with heart failure (Hgb 51 gm/L). *Right image*: Improvement is seen, and the patient had limited symptoms of heart failure (Hgb 75 gm/L).

Heterozygous sickle cell state, or "trait," usually is asymptomatic and associated with only a mild anemia. Deoxygenated sickle hemoglobin polymerizes in hypoxic conditions, elongating the erythrocyte and rendering it less flexible. Consequently, microvascular and macrovascular occlusive phenomena occur. Hypoxic areas of the body are the usual sites of infarction. Erythrocyte longevity is shortened. The degree and duration of hypoxia influence the frequency and severity of occlusive phenomena. In sickle cell trait, sickle hemoglobin generally is insufficient to cause sickling. In sickle cell disease, moderate to severe anemia results from markedly decreased erythrocyte survival.

Clinical Presentations

Infarction in numerous locations may occur in sickle cell disease. Bone, splenic, cerebral, pulmonary, and myocardial infarction may occur. Bone infarction is common and usually is very painful. Splenic infarction is common to the point of being invariable and renders most patients with sickle cell anemia asplenic. Pulmonary infarction also is common. Myocardial infarction in sickle cell disease is only rarely the result of epicardial coronary artery thrombosis. It is mainly subendocardial and typically affects the papillary muscles, presumably because papillary muscles are supplied by end-arteries and are the most hypoxic locality of the heart.[19,20] Whether myocardial ischemia occurs during sickle cell crises is the subject of controversy.[21]

Pulmonary hypertension may be caused by thromboembolism or by in situ thrombosis. Right-sided heart failure may occur, as may pulmonary infarction.

Congestive heart failure may occur in sickle cell anemia. The major factors responsible for this are the high-output demands of marked anemia and myocardial depression caused by iron overload from transfusion support. Whether an intrinsic myocardial depression occurs in sickle cell disease is the subject of debate. Diastolic dysfunction and pulmonary hypertension are independent risk factors for death.[22] Myocardial responses to exercise often are subnormal in sickle cell anemia,[23] despite factors favoring enhanced myocardial performance, such as increased preload and reduced afterload.

Whether mitral valve prolapse is more common in sickle cell disease is unclear and a matter of debate.[24]

The physical examination commonly demonstrates flow murmurs and findings typical of anemia. As mentioned previously, the findings may be consistent with congestive heart failure, isolated right-sided heart failure, pulmonary hypertension, or mitral insufficiency. Echocardiography generally reveals eccentric hypertrophy but may show impaired systolic function in patients with iron overload.[25] Diastolic inflow parameters frequently are abnormal. The electrocardiogram usually is normal but may show left ventricular hypertrophy, first-degree atrioventricular block, or nonspecific repolarization abnormalities.[26]

Management

Avoidance of hypoxic conditions as well as hydration and analgesia during sickle cell vaso-occlusive crises form the cornerstones of treatment. Transfusion and exchange transfusion may be necessary to maintain adequate hemoglobin concentrations and a low proportion of cells prone to sickling. Specific complications are treated accordingly.

THALASSEMIA

The term thalassemia refers to several inherited hemoglobinopathies caused by impaired production of hemoglobin chains.

Pathophysiology

The human body has four hemoglobin chains, two alpha and two beta. The most important thalassemic disorder of adults is thalassemia major, or Cooley's disease. This disorder is caused by defective production of both β-hemoglobin chains and, consequently, results in severe anemia. This anemia is largely unresponsive to substrate supplementation and requires continuing transfusions.

Clinical Presentations

Cardiovascular complications are the most common cause of death in patients with thalassemia major. Untreated or insufficiently treated anemia is severe and is responsible for the expected full range of cardiovascular alterations in response to severe anemia, including heart failure. In addition (and a point that is very important), repeated transfusions to correct anemia frequently lead to iron overload, cardiac hemosiderosis, and consequent heart failure. Pericardial disease is common among patients with thalassemia, including typical acute pericarditis with fever, leukocytosis, a pericardial rub, and electrographic changes. Asymptomatic pericardial effusions also are seen. Conduction disease of the atrioventricular node is common.

HEMOCHROMATOSIS

Iron metabolism normally is carefully regulated in the body, because both iron deficiency and iron overload result in life-shortening disease. Iron deficiency leads to hypochromic microcytic anemia and is the most common cause of anemia.

Pathophysiology

Iron absorption is carefully regulated at the intestinal level. Iron overload is caused either by inappropriate excessive absorption of iron (primary iron overload) or by repeated erythrocyte transfusions (secondary iron overload). Iron absorption is inappropriately increased in the inherited disorder of hemochromatosis. Iron overload results in the deposition of ferritin in tissues, with the resultant release of lysosomal acid hydrolases and tissue fibrosis. Alcohol enhances iron absorption generally and in hemochromatosis.

Clinical Presentations

Extracardiac manifestations of hemochromatosis include endocrine pancreatic failure with diabetes, hepatic cirrhosis and liver failure, hepatoma arising from cirrhosis, pituitary failure, and "bronzing" of the skin. Cardiac disease is responsible for death in approximately 33% of patients with hemochromatosis (Fig. 133.2).[27] Cardiac involvement includes conduction disturbances,[28] arrhythmias, and heart failure and is seen in advanced iron deposition.[29] Conduction system disturbances are common, as are both atrial and ventricular arrhythmias. Myocardial fibrosis and hypertrophy with a picture of dilated or restrictive cardiomyopathy are common. Cardiac disease can be

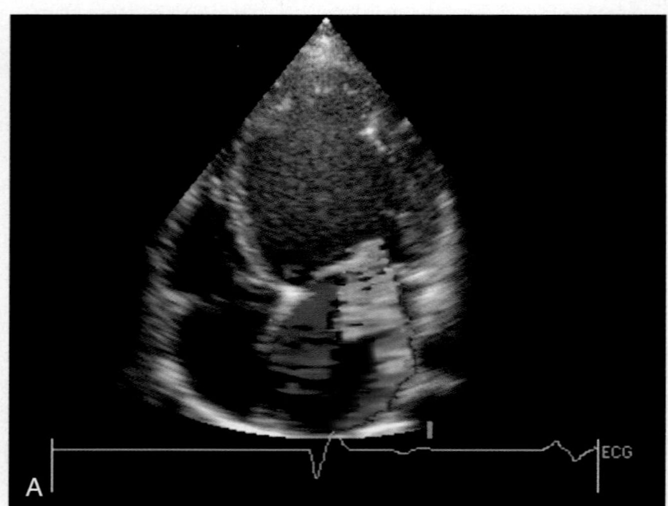

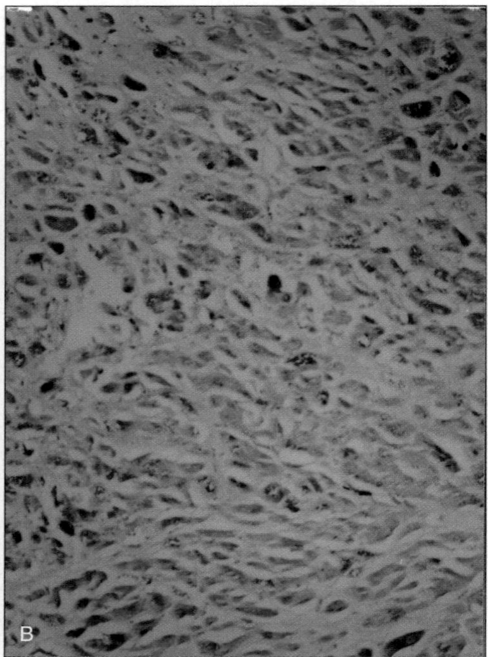

Figure 133.2 Cardiac hemochromatosis. A 20-year-old man presented with episodes of syncope and palpitations and symptoms of congestive heart failure (New York Heart Association class III). The examination demonstrated increased venous pressure, a dilated apex, and S_3 gallop. No murmurs were detected. The chest radiograph demonstrated cardiomegaly. Echocardiography revealed enlargement of all four cardiac chambers **(A)**, with biventricular severe systolic dysfunction. The electrocardiogram (ECG) showed sinus rhythm with a first-degree atrioventricular block, posterior hemiblock, and right bundle branch block. Frequent episodes of monomorphic ventricular tachycardia were demonstrated. The patient died of a ventricular fibrillation arrest. Autopsy demonstrated markedly positive Prussian blue staining for iron throughout the myocardium **(B)**, consistent with advanced hemochromatosis leading to dilated cardiomyopathy and recurrent ventricular arrhythmias.

prevented with a high degree of success by regular phlebotomy, particularly when tissue concentrations of iron are not markedly increased.

Repeated transfusion support (in the absence of chelation therapy) for chronic, symptomatic, severe anemia results in iron overload. Fifty to 100 erythrocyte transfusions result in severe iron overload and the likelihood that myocardial dysfunction will develop. In addition, iron overload from transfusion therapy for thalassemia is compounded by increased intestinal absorption of iron.

Management

Phlebotomy is effective in improving myocardial function in more advanced cases, although the success per case is variable. Cases have been described of recovery from class IV heart failure to class I. Phlebotomy is a highly efficient means of removing iron (200 to 250 mg of iron per treatment). Because phlebotomy cannot be used to remove iron in cases of anemia, iron chelation therapy with agents such as desferrioxamine is needed to prevent tissue iron overload. Iron chelation therapy is considerably less effective at removing iron than is phlebotomy, and it is important to institute such treatment before iron overload is advanced and established organ dysfunction is present. Aggressive iron chelation therapy concurrent with transfusion therapy has been demonstrated to retard myocardial dysfunction and reduce mortality. In occasional cases of advanced disease, improvement of myocardial function has been demonstrated with desferrioxamine treatment.[30]

INTRAVASCULAR HEMOLYSIS

The list of causes of hemolytic anemia (a shortened erythrocyte life span; 110 days is the norm) is considerable, but of note to cardiologists and internists is intravascular hemolysis caused by intracardiac flow disturbances. Such disturbances are characterized by high-velocity jets that increase shear forces; these, in turn, disrupt erythrocyte membranes and result in hemolysis. Intravascular hemolysis may occur with hemolysis-prone erythrocytes (those with enzyme or hemoglobin abnormalities) or, if shear forces are great enough, with normal erythrocytes.

The most common cardiovascular cause of intravascular hemolysis is paravalvular insufficiency around a prosthetic valve; intravascular hemolysis in a patient with a mechanical prosthesis should prompt a search for a paravalvular leak. Hemolysis is evidenced by abnormal erythrocyte morphology on a blood smear (schizocytes, indicating cellular disruption), an increased serum hemoglobin, a reduced serum haptoglobin, and urinary hemosiderin. If the rate of hemolysis exceeds the marrow reserve, anemia develops. The resultant anemia worsens the hemodynamic burden of valvular insufficiency, and congestive heart failure is common in these circumstances (Fig. 133.3). Moderate anemia may be tolerable, but severe anemia as a result of paravalvular insufficiency may require reoperation to eliminate the insufficiency. Hemolytic anemia is seen more often with older models of valve prostheses, such as ball-cage and single disk–occluder types, than with current bileaflet-occluder

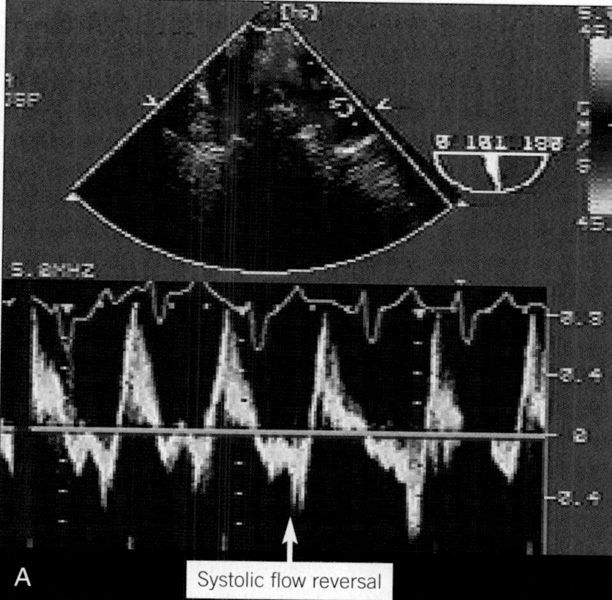

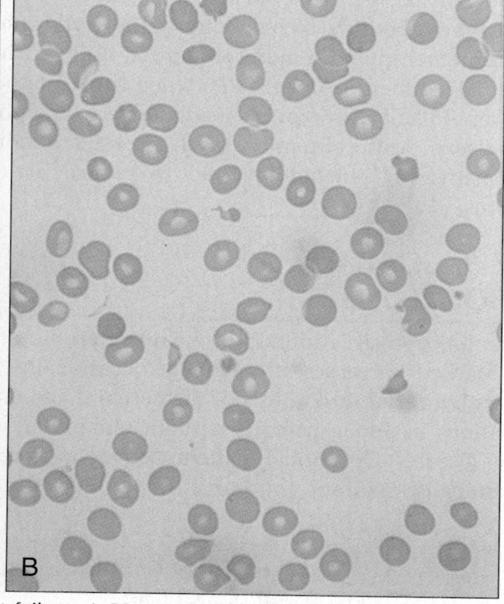

Figure 133.3 Paravalvular leak with hemolytic anemia and heart failure. A 58-year-old woman with a mechanical mitral prosthesis presented with marked ankle edema and shortness of breath that had worsened for 6 months. The mitral prosthesis had been inserted 9 months earlier for rheumatic mitral valve disease. The patient was in biventricular heart failure, with a murmur of mitral insufficiency and findings of pulmonary hypertension. Transesophageal echocardiography demonstrated a large jet of mitral regurgitation and flow reversal on the pulmonary veins **(A)** consistent with a severe paravalvular regurgitation. The hemoglobin concentration was 68 gm/dL. Schistocytes were seen on the blood smear **(B)**, and hemosiderin was recovered in the urinary sediment. The patient underwent successful surgical closure of the paravalvular leak. The markers of hemolysis subsided postoperatively, and the hemoglobin level rose to and stayed within the normal range.

mechanical prosthesis.[31] Bioprostheses and mitral repairs may also cause hemolysis. Hemolysis is not uncommonly seen after cardiac surgery; it may reflect trauma to erythrocytes from extracorporeal bypass, transfusion incompatibility, or drug-related hemolysis.

Other intracardiac flow disturbances, such as native valve insufficiency or stenosis; hypertrophic obstructive cardiomyopathy; and congenital lesions with a high gradient, occasionally may be responsible for intravascular hemolysis.

MYELOPROLIFERATIVE SYNDROMES

CARDIOVASCULAR DISTURBANCES CAUSED BY POLYCYTHEMIA

An increased hematocrit increases blood viscosity and predisposes to stasis and thrombosis. Blood viscosity increases exponentially with increasing hematocrit; consequently, oxygen transport decreases hematocrit greater than 45%. The optimal hematocrit, therefore, is approximately 40%. Symptoms of hyperviscosity are common when the hematocrit is greater than 60% and are indicative of low tissue flow. Arterial hypertension and pulmonary hypertension also are common and are caused by increased resistance from thrombosis in both the venous and arterial vasculature.[32,33]

Clinical Presentations

Polycythemia (an increased hematocrit and hemoglobin) may occur for a wide range of reasons and therefore is considered in these categories:

- Relative polycythemia;
- Secondary polycythemia; and
- Primary polycythemia, or polycythemia rubra vera.

Polycythemia may be relative or "spurious"; rather than an increased red cell mass (absolute polycythemia), it may reflect plasma depletion that increases the hematocrit. The hematocrit seldom is greater than 60%. The treatment is expansion of plasma volume.

Secondary Polycythemia

Causes of secondary polycythemia are classified as those causing an appropriate increase in erythropoietin secretion and those causing inappropriate secretion. An appropriate increase in erythropoietin is seen in chronic hypoxic conditions such as chronic lung disease and cyanotic congenital heart disease and at high altitudes. Inappropriate causes include paraneoplastic phenomena of renal cell carcinomas, hepatomas, and lung carcinomas. Treatment consists of phlebotomy and is undertaken when the hematocrit is greater than 45% and disturbances attributable to the polycythemia are seen.

Primary Polycythemia

Primary polycythemia, also known as polycythemia rubra vera, is a myelodysplastic syndrome in which malignant proliferation of bone marrow progenitor cells results in increases in erythrocytes, platelets, and neutrophils. The symptoms are attributable to hyperviscosity and thrombosis. Despite increased platelet concentrations, patients with polycythemia rubra vera are predisposed to bleeding. Occasional patients have nonspecific valve thickening or marantic endocarditis. Treatment consists of phlebotomy (or erythropheresis) and chemotherapy with antiproliferative drugs such as hydroxyurea. Treatment is undertaken when the hematocrit is greater than 45% if disturbances attributable to the polycythemia are seen. Antiproliferative drugs are used to reduce the requirements for phlebotomy and to reduce platelet concentrations.

PRIMARY (ESSENTIAL) THROMBOCYTOSIS

Essential thrombocytosis is another of the myeloproliferative disorders. Marked increases in platelets occasionally are associated with arterial thrombosis of the cerebral and coronary circulations in young patients without underlying atherosclerotic disease. Occasional patients have nonspecific valve thickening or marantic endocarditis.

HEMATOLOGIC MALIGNANCY AND THE CARDIOVASCULAR SYSTEM

MALIGNANT LYMPHOMA

Cardiac involvement by malignant lymphoma is relatively common and may occur by extension to cardiac structures, either by direct contiguous invasion from adjacent lymph nodes in the chest or by hematogenous seeding.[34] Cases of primary cardiac lymphoma are extremely rare and questionable.

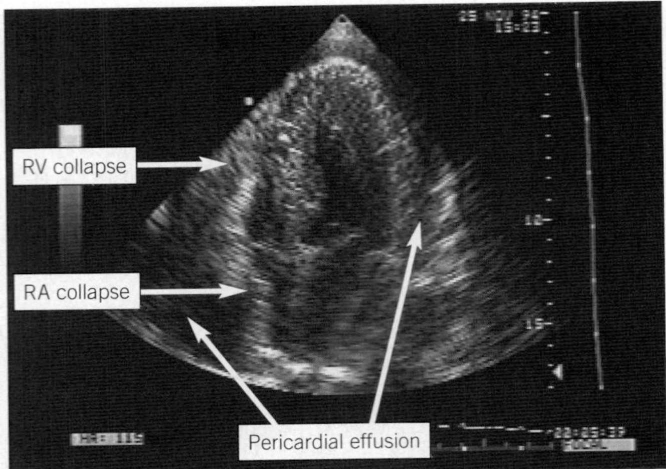

Figure 133.4 Cardiac tamponade with lymphomatous involvement of the pericardium. A 17-year-old man with a well-functioning renal transplant of 5 years presented with shortness of breath, jugular venous distention, ankle edema, hypotension, and a pulsus paradoxus of 45 mm Hg. Cardiomegaly was noted on radiographs. The electrocardiogram (ECG) showed sinus tachycardia and low voltages in the standard limb leads. Echocardiography confirmed tamponade with the findings of a large pericardial effusion with diastolic collapse of the cavities in the right side of the heart. Pericardiocentesis resulted in normalization of the heart rate and blood pressure. Cytology yielded a diagnosis of large cell non-Hodgkin's lymphoma. After chemotherapy, the patient remained in remission 2 years later. RA, right atrium; RV, right ventricle.

Clinical Presentations

Pericardial Disease

Although an almost unlimited number of types of cardiac involvement have been described in cases of malignant lymphoma, the most common involvement remains direct extension of the malignancy into the pericardial space, with accumulation of intrapericardial fluid. Pericardial effusions and tamponade, therefore, are the clinical complications of malignant lymphoma most commonly recognized (Fig. 133.4). Tumor encasement of the heart may occur with a large bulk of intrathoracic disease and may result in a compressive, pericardial constriction–like syndrome.

Treatment of lymphoma may also result in pericardial disease, such as pericarditis from irradiation, hemorrhagic pericarditis from high-dose cyclophosphamide, and constrictive pericarditis from previous irradiation.

Cardiac Masses

Myocardial involvement is far less common than pericardial involvement. Intramyocardial masses have been reported in all areas of the heart. Most masses are seen within the cardiac cavities or within the pericardial cavity. Occasionally, an obstructive effect occurs either when a bulky mass lesion obstructs an intracardiac cavity or when a bulky paracardiac mass compresses a cardiac structure or vascular structure, such as the pulmonary artery or veins or superior vena cava.[35]

Myocardial Involvement

Most myocardial involvement in malignant lymphoma relates to preexisting myopathic disease, disease resulting from chemotherapy with anthracyclines or cyclophosphamide or, rarely, from studding of the myocardium with lymphoma masses. Congestive heart failure in a patient with lymphoma likely is the result of preexisting myopathic or valvular disease, but it may occur because of myocardial depression caused by chemotherapy. Occasionally, in a patient with lymphoma, a hyperviscous state caused by a paraproteinemia contributes to congestive heart failure.

Coronary Disease

Coronary disease in a patient with lymphoma is more likely a comorbid condition than attributable to the lymphoma. Worsening of ischemia often reflects an anemia caused by marrow suppression from chemotherapy or radiotherapy, or both, in a patient with coexisting coronary artery disease. Occasionally, coronary artery disease may be caused by previous irradiation to the heart, especially if higher doses of radiation and lesser shielding were used.

Other Signs

Occasional patients with malignant lymphoma may have nonspecific valve thickening or marantic endocarditis.

MULTIPLE MYELOMA

Multiple myeloma, a malignant proliferation of B-lymphocyte tissue with a propensity to produce high serum concentrations of antibody components, may involve the heart through amyloidosis, mass involvement, hyperviscosity syndrome, or high-output states. Some patients have more than one cardiovascular manifestation.

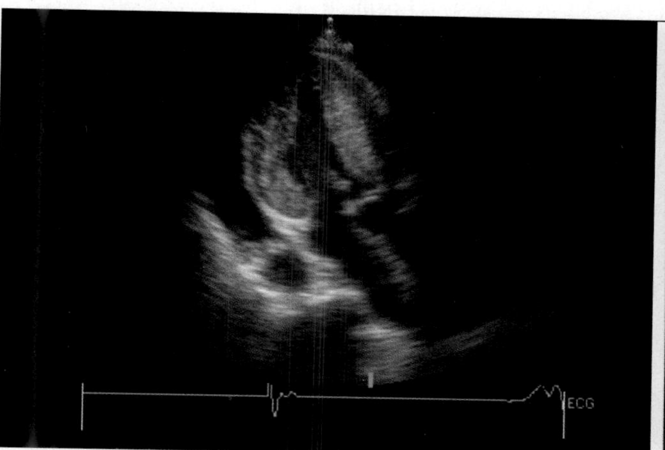

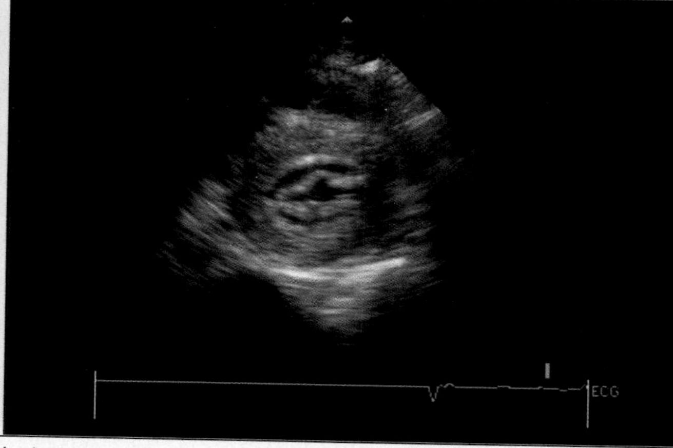

Figure 133.5 Cardiac amyloidosis. A 51-year-old man presented with signs and symptoms of biventricular heart failure (New York Heart Association class III). He had no history of hypertension or coronary artery disease. He also had macroglossia and findings of peripheral neuropathy. The electrocardiogram (ECG) revealed sinus rhythm with right bundle branch block, left anterior fascicular block, and a pseudoinfarction pattern. Echocardiography demonstrated marked thickening of the left ventricular wall (27 mm) and the right ventricular wall (9 mm), with small cavities, moderate systolic dysfunction, and biatrial enlargement. The myocardial appearance was bright and unusually echoreflective, consistent with restrictive cardiomyopathy caused by cardiac amyloidosis. The valves were mildly and nonspecifically thickened and mildly to moderately insufficient. In addition, a small pericardial effusion was seen. Mitral inflow demonstrated the impaired relaxation pattern of diastolic dysfunction. Rectal biopsy confirmed systemic amyloidosis.

Cardiac amyloidosis, or infiltration of the heart with amyloid fibrils, may occur in multiple myeloma (in addition to other plasma cell dyscrasias), resulting in a picture of restrictive cardiomyopathy. Symptoms of heart failure in a patient with myeloma are most likely to result from cardiac amyloidosis (Fig. 133.5). Mass involvement (plasmacytomas) is rare but has been described. Involvement of the myocardium usually is clinically bland. Involvement of the pericardium may lead to effusions and tamponade. Hyperviscosity syndromes may occur as a result of production of antibody fragments by the myeloma that render the serum unusually viscous. Syndromes that may result include arterial and venous thrombosis and congestive heart failure. High-output states may occur because of the increased flow to plasmacytomas in the bone marrow.[36] Occasionally, this is responsible for congestive heart failure.

LEUKEMIA

Cardiac involvement in acute leukemia is common at autopsy, but clinically identified involvement is rare. Tamponade may occur.[37] Autopsy series reflecting the most severe cases of leukemia commonly describe microscopic involvement of the heart with leukemic infiltrates. With chronic leukemias, anemias (which reflect failure of the marrow as a result of leukemic infiltration or chemotherapy, or both) may precipitate myocardial ischemia in individuals with underlying coronary artery disease, as well as congestive heart failure in individuals with underlying myopathic or valvular disease. Patients with plasma cell leukemia may have symptomatic hyperviscosity.

HYPERCOAGULABLE STATES

Hypercoagulable states may be caused by molecular coagulation deficiencies, antiphospholipid antibodies, and predisposing states. An underlying hypercoagulable state is sought when recurrent thrombotic episodes have occurred with a frequency beyond that expected by chance alone.

Predisposing states include a range of clinical circumstances associated with thromboembolism, such as the use of certain drugs, recent surgery, hormonal states, and immobilization. Predisposing states are responsible for most recurrent cases of venous thromboembolism.

MOLECULAR COAGULATION DEFICIENCIES

Several molecular deficiencies are associated with hypercoagulable states and predispose to arterial and venous thrombosis. Antithrombin III deficiency, protein S deficiency, and protein C deficiency all are associated with arterial and venous thrombosis,[38] including myocardial infarction.[39] The list of recognized molecular bases that predispose to thrombosis is continually lengthening, as are the recognized associations (Fig. 133.6).[40] For example, diagnosticians increasingly test for the common prothrombin mutation. Many of the assays required for detection of the deficiencies are not widely available.

ANTIPHOSPHOLIPID ANTIBODIES

Antiphospholipid antibodies may be present in association with connective tissue diseases (lupus anticoagulant) or may represent an isolated disease state. The cardiovascular associations of antiphospholipid antibodies are principally arterial and venous thrombosis.[41] Marantic endocarditis (involving the mitral valve more than the aortic valves) is not uncommon; however, significant valvular dysfunction (usually insufficiency) is uncommon, as is embolism of a vegetation. However, some patients require valve replacement. Pulmonary hypertension may occur because of thromboembolism or in situ pulmonary artery thrombosis (Fig. 133.7).[42] Antiphospholipid antibodies have been associated with simultaneous arterial and venous thrombosis, microvascular and macrovascular thrombosis, and myocardial infarction (Fig. 133.8).[43]

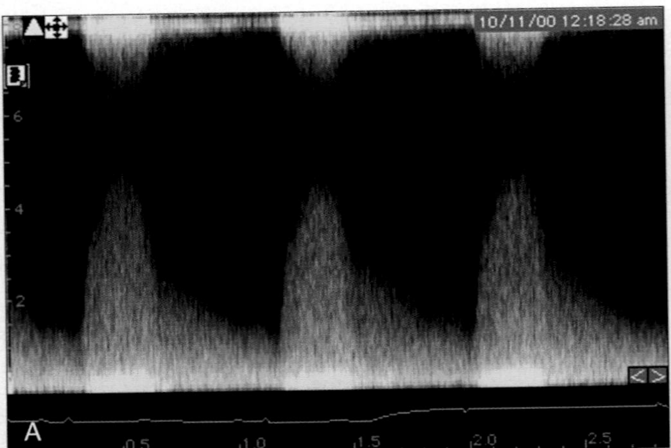

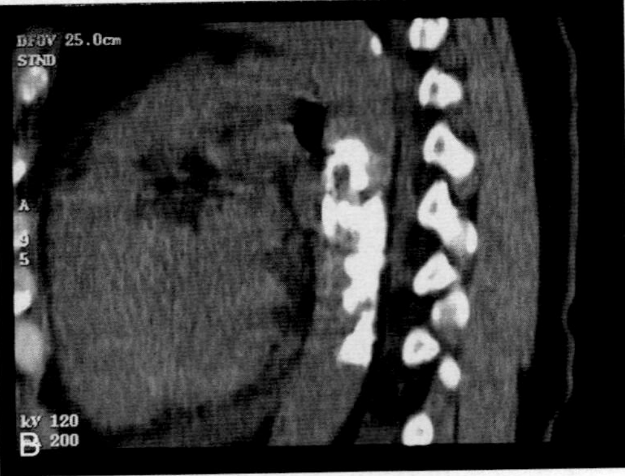

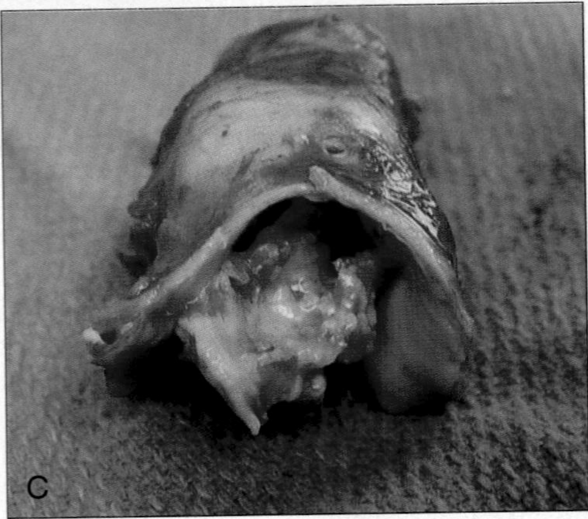

Figure 133.6 Aortic obstruction caused by a calcified thrombus associated with the common prothrombin mutation. A 49-year-old woman, who had had 8 years of recognized hypertension for which no secondary cause could be found, developed lower back pain. Magnetic resonance imaging suggested an aortic intramural hematoma; however, a transesophageal echocardiogram demonstrated a large mass in the lumen of the thoracic aorta that was obstructing flow (gradient >100 mm Hg **[A]**). Collaterals also were present, consistent with chronicity of the obstruction. **B**, Computed tomography scanning showed that the mass was calcific and was not outside the aorta. **C**, Surgical removal was successful and alleviated the hypertension. Pathologically, the mass was a calcified thrombus, and the patient was found to have the common prothrombin mutation.

PREDISPOSING STATES

States such as immobilization, stroke with limb paralysis, and congestive heart failure lead to low flow and predisposition to venous thrombosis. Pregnancy and the postpartum state are associated with an excess of thromboembolism, such that pulmonary embolus is one of the major maternal risks at delivery. Older formulations of oral contraceptives and hormone replacement therapy clearly were associated with an excess of venous thrombosis and probably of arterial thrombosis, because they contained a considerably greater (several-fold greater) estrogen content than do currently used preparations. Current preparations of oral contraceptives are not associated with an increased risk of thromboembolism; however, current regimens of hormone replacement therapy may be. Other medications, such as tamoxifen, which is a mixed estrogen antagonist/agonist, and other forms of chemotherapy are associated with thromboembolism. Use of heparin may lead to heparin-induced thrombocytopenia and venous or arterial thrombosis (Fig. 133.9). Cancer itself is a risk factor for thromboembolism. Indwelling catheters commonly are associated with thrombosis, which may obstruct the catheter, occlude the vessel into which the catheter is inserted, or generate embolism.

CARDIOVASCULAR COMPLICATIONS OF CHEMOTHERAPY AND RADIOTHERAPY

CHEMOTHERAPY

The major cardiac complication of chemotherapy is myocardial depression from the use of anthracyclines (described elsewhere in this text). However, other chemotherapeutic and antiproliferative drugs also may cause notable cardiac complications. High-dose cyclophosphamide (>1 gm/m^2) may cause hemorrhagic myopericarditis, resulting in concurrent myocardial depression and hemorrhagic pericarditis.[44] Tamponade is not uncommon, and interventions such as

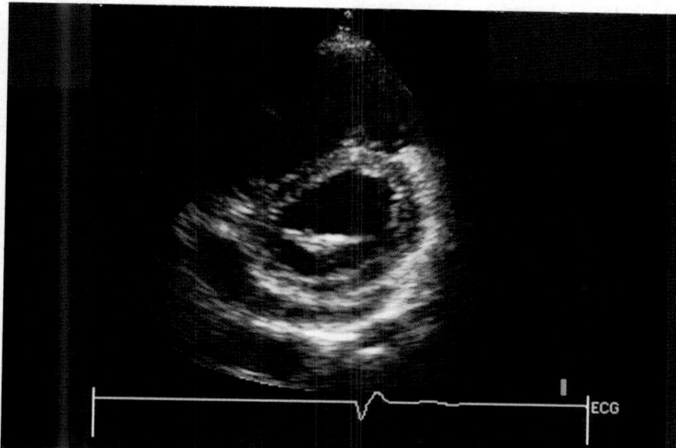

Figure 133.7 Antiphospholipid antibody and pulmonary hypertension. A 51-year-old woman presented with progressive exertional dyspnea. Eight months previously, she had developed a deep venous thrombosis in her right leg. While undergoing anticoagulation with warfarin, and with an international normalized ratio (INR) that averaged 2.5, she developed a deep venous thrombosis of the left leg. She was treated with higher doses of warfarin (INR 4 to 5). Progressive symptoms of dyspnea developed. Examination revealed an elevated venous pressure, a left parasternal lift, and an accentuated P2, with the murmur of tricuspid insufficiency. Chest radiographs demonstrated cardiomegaly, with prominence of the central pulmonary arteries and right side of the heart. Echocardiography demonstrated marked dilatation of the right side of heart and a right ventricular pressure overload pattern of septal motion (O shape in diastole and D shape in systole). Severe tricuspid insufficiency was detected, which yielded a resting ventricular systolic pressure of 115 mm Hg. An antiphospholipid antibody was strongly positive; this was believed to be responsible for the recurrent thrombosis. The patient refused further treatment.

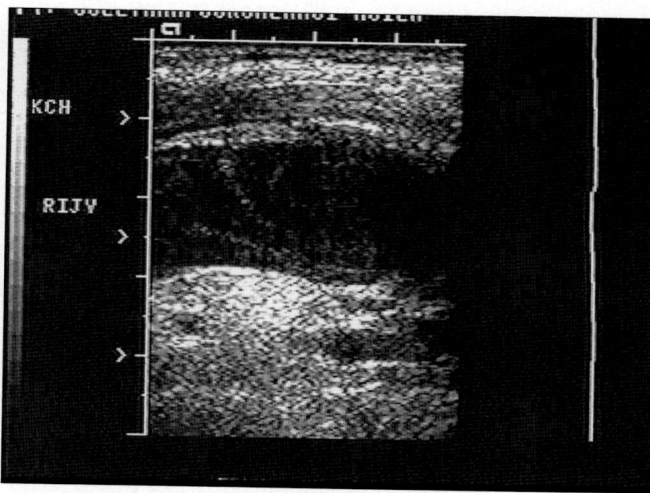

Figure 133.9 Heparin-associated thrombocytopenia and venous thrombosis. A 79-year-old woman was admitted to the hospital with respiratory failure secondary to pneumonia and congestive heart failure from atrial fibrillation and mitral stenosis. A right-side heart catheter was inserted via the right internal jugular vein for hemodynamic monitoring of therapy during the first 3 days. After 5 days of gradual improvement in response to antibiotics, rate-controlling medications, and heparin, the patient developed rapid swelling of the right arm and the right side of the face. The platelet count decreased to 50,000/mm. A heparin-induced thrombocytopenia assay was strongly positive. Venous duplex scanning of the right internal jugular and right subclavian vein demonstrated thrombosis of both vessels. Heparin-induced thrombocytopenia was believed to be responsible for the venous thrombosis, with the central line also possibly predisposing to thrombosis.

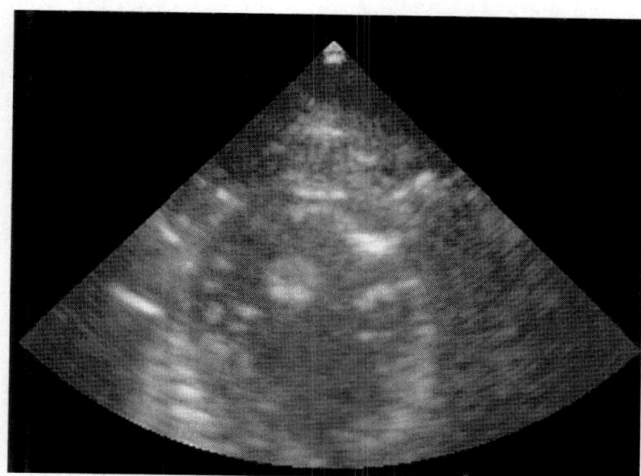

Figure 133.8 Myocardial infarction and apical thrombosis in a patient with an antiphospholipid antibody. A 28-year-old woman presented with a large anterior wall infarction. She was obese and mildly dyslipidemic. Cardiac catheterization demonstrated angiographically normal coronary arteries. The patient suffered a deep venous thrombosis of the calf while in the hospital. She recovered from the initial heart failure and was discharged, free of angina and heart failure. She received anticoagulation treatment for 6 months because of an apical aneurysm. Ten days after the warfarin was discontinued, an apical thrombus was seen on echocardiography that had not been present the week before cessation of anticoagulation therapy. A strongly positive antiphospholipid antibody was identified. This was believed to be responsible for the coronary, venous, and left ventricular thromboses. The patient subsequently remained well on warfarin.

pericardiocentesis may be lifesaving. Platelet transfusion frequently is necessary, because the thrombocytopenia that results from treatment with high-dose cyclophosphamide often is the precipitating cause of intrapericardial hemorrhage. 5-Fluorouracil and vincristine may cause myocardial infarction.

RADIOTHERAPY

Radiotherapy of the mediastinum for treatment of Hodgkin's lymphoma, testicular carcinoma, or breast or lung carcinoma with superior vena caval compression may result in acute or chronic cardiac damage. Acute damage is the inflammatory type; chronic damage is the fibrotic sequela of early inflammation. Similarly, total body irradiation, given as an ablative treatment before bone marrow transplantation, may result in cardiac damage.[45]

Pericardium and Myocardium

Acutely, pericarditis, effusions, and tamponade may occur. Subacutely, effusoconstrictive pericarditis has been described. Chronic constrictive pericarditis may be seen among longer term survivors.[46] Complicating the assessment of constrictive pericarditis secondary to previous radiotherapy is the possibility of concurrent radiation-induced myocardial fibrosis that results in restrictive cardiomyopathy. If restrictive cardiomyopathy dominates the hemodynamic disturbances, pericardiectomy may confer incomplete hemodynamic improvement.

Coronary Arteries

Irradiation, particularly with inadequate cardiac shielding, may lead to precocious coronary artery disease as a result of accelerated atherosclerosis or fibrointimal hyperplasia. Such complications were more common when less shielding was used, but they still may be encountered. Characteristic lesions are notably proximal in the coronary arterial tree and are seen in the absence of lesions or even irregularities elsewhere.[46,47]

Conduction System

Conduction system disturbances are seen with increased frequency in patients who have undergone mediastinal irradiation. The basis likely is patchy fibrosis that involves components of the atrioventricular node, bundles, or fascicles.[46]

Valves

Valvular dysfunction caused by fibrosis has been reported after mediastinal irradiation, concurrent with extensive fibrosis elsewhere in the heart.[48]

chapter 134 Neuromuscular Disease

Alison Knauth Meadows

The relationship between the cardiovascular and neuromuscular systems is complex and often difficult to elucidate. In addition, the neuromuscular disorders are a diverse group of diseases that have different and often variable degrees of cardiac involvement. Regardless, cardiac disease, including both cardiomyopathy and arrhythmias, is a major cause of morbidity and mortality in patients with neuromuscular diseases. This chapter explores the neuromuscular diseases with which dilated cardiomyopathy or arrhythmias, or both, are more commonly associated. The discussion is divided into disorders that affect the muscular system and those that affect the neuromuscular system. The epidemiology and genetics, pathophysiology, clinical presentations, diagnostic testing and monitoring, therapy, and prognosis are discussed for each disorder.

DISORDERS OF MUSCLE

DUCHENNE'S MUSCULAR DYSTROPHY

Epidemiology and Genetics

Duchenne's muscular dystrophy is the most common form of muscular dystrophy, with an incidence of 30 per 100,000 live births. Duchenne's muscular dystrophy also is the most severe form of progressive muscular dystrophy, presenting early and progressing rapidly. Duchenne's muscular dystrophy is transmitted by means of an X-linked recessive pattern. Two thirds of affected individuals are found to have mothers who are carriers; the remaining one third are found to have new, spontaneous mutations.[1] The genetic locus is an abnormality in the dystrophin gene on chromosome Xp21; in Duchenne's muscular dystrophy, dystrophin is absent or nearly absent.

Cardiac involvement is common in Duchenne's muscular dystrophy and can manifest in various forms, including cardiomyopathy or arrhythmias, or both. At least 10% of female carriers of the dystrophin gene defect are likely to develop a progressive cardiomyopathy.[2,3]

Pathophysiology

Dystrophin is expressed primarily in skeletal, cardiac, and smooth muscle, although small amounts can be found in the brain. Dystrophin and dystrophin-associated glycoproteins provide a structural connection between the myocyte cytoskeleton and the extracellular matrix functioning to link contractile proteins to the cell membrane. Absence of dystrophin in the cell membrane results in an inadequate or fragile membrane that is more easily damaged during muscular contraction. With increased membrane breakdown, an influx of calcium occurs, leading to enhanced proteolysis and cell death. This leads to muscle inflammation and necrosis and, ultimately, replacement by fibrous tissue.[4]

The typical histology in Duchenne's muscular dystrophy demonstrates widespread degeneration and regeneration of individual muscle fibers with extensive connective tissue proliferation. This connective tissue proliferation, called endomysial fibrosis, is thought to inhibit muscle fiber regeneration. As a result, the number of muscle fibers progressively decreases, and connective tissue content progressively increases.

The incidence of cardiomyopathy associated with Duchenne's muscular dystrophy increases with age and is progressive. The cardiomyopathy is characterized by extensive myocardial fibrosis and thinning. Interestingly, disproportionately more scarring occurs in the posterobasal left ventricular wall. Patients with Duchenne's muscular dystrophy usually have mild to moderate left ventricular dilatation and dysfunction, which remain only slowly progressive for a long period before entering a phase of rapid progression. Some hypothesize that as left ventricular dilatation progresses, wall tension rises to a critical level. Once this critical point is reached, the rate of muscle fiber degeneration increases, wall tension rises more rapidly, and cell loss accelerates. This cycle rapidly leads to congestive heart failure and death.[5]

Mitral valve prolapse and mitral regurgitation can be seen in patients with Duchenne's muscular dystrophy. The ultrastructure of the papillary muscles shows multifocal and confluent areas of loss of myofibrils, creating a moth-eaten appearance (Fig. 134.1); this suggests that dystrophic changes in the papillary muscles are responsible for this burden. Postmortem examination of valve leaflets, chordae tendineae, and annuli fail to show any morphologic abnormalities, which makes valvular pathology a less likely etiology.[6]

Regional myocardial perfusion defects, as seen on nuclear and positron emission tomography (PET) imaging, have been described in patients with Duchenne's muscular dystrophy. Autopsy findings have demonstrated the small, intramural coronary arteries to be thick walled and to have luminal narrowing, which may be responsible for the perfusion defects.

Coronary vascular reserve also has been studied in patients with Duchenne's muscular dystrophy. Although patients with Duchenne's muscular dystrophy seem to have a normal resting myocardial blood flow (when adjusted for a higher heart rate),[7] they appear to have a significant reduction in coronary vasodilator reserve.[8]

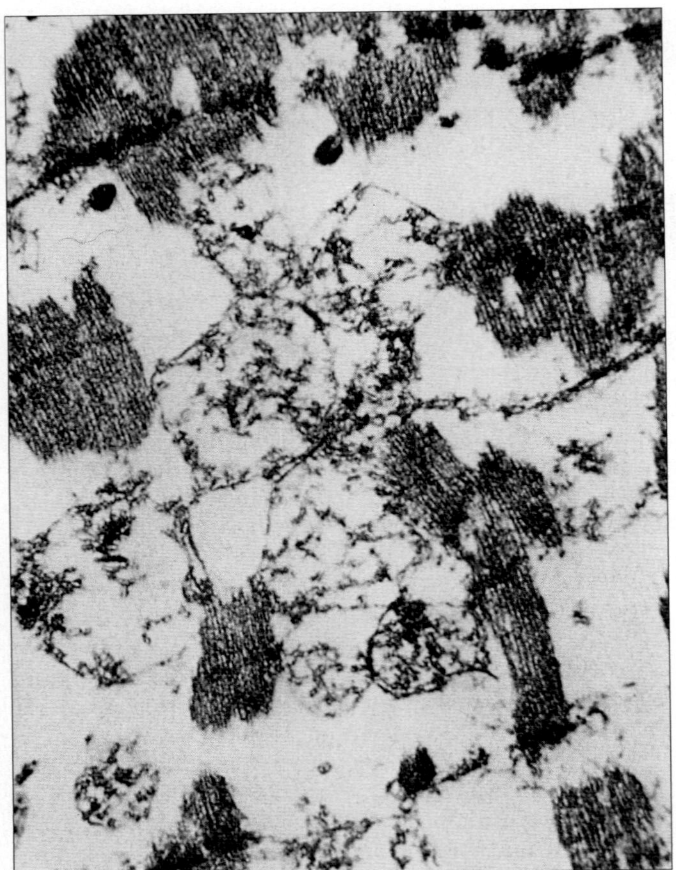

Figure 134.1 The moth-eaten appearance of a posterior papillary muscle in a patient with Duchenne's muscular dystrophy is indicative of myofibrillar lysis with loss of thick and thin myofilaments.

The cardiac conduction system frequently is affected in patients with Duchenne's muscular dystrophy. Dystrophin appears to be an important component of the membrane in the Purkinje conduction fibers. Bundle branch block and atrioventricular (AV) node block are common. Interestingly, sinus tachycardia is quite common. This sinus tachycardia often begins in the early stages of disease, before significant systolic dysfunction develops, and it does not appear to correlate with the degree of dysfunction. It may be related to enhanced sympathetic drive secondary to diminished ventricular function, but the etiology has not been entirely elucidated.[8]

Arrhythmias, particularly ventricular arrhythmias, can occur. They are thought to be related to the patchy myocardial fibrosis typically seen in Duchenne's muscular dystrophy. Sudden death is most common in patients with severe ventricular dysfunction and those with documented ventricular arrhythmias. QT dispersion has been shown to define the level of risk for sudden death.[9] Atrial flutter and fibrillation also are quite common toward the end stages of cardiomyopathy.

Clinical Presentation

Although the genetic abnormalities are present at birth, and elevated sarcoplasmic enzymes can be found early on, the first signs of weakness usually become obvious in the second year of life. These signs begin with the classic waddling gate and progress rapidly to an inability to walk before the child reaches young adolescence. Other neuromuscular manifestations follow, including lumbar lordosis, pseudohypertrophy of calf muscles, and shortening of the Achilles tendon. Contractures progress in the later stages of the disease process. Dystrophy of skeletal muscles of the chest wall leads to respiratory difficulties and pulmonary complications. Cognitive delay is quite common; 35% of these patients have a Full-scale Intelligence Quotient (FIQ) of less than 70,[10] and the mean IQ is shifted about one standard deviation below the normal population mean.[11]

The development of cardiomyopathy is invariable. Left ventricular dilatation and dysfunction usually are noted by 10 years of age and are universal by the late teens. Symptoms of systolic dysfunction often are masked by the profound skeletal myopathy. In addition, if respiratory muscle weakness is present and goes untreated, the patient may develop pulmonary arterial hypertension and cor pulmonale.[12] Although both the skeletal weakness and the cardiac muscle weakness are progressive, they do not always progress at the same rate. For this reason, they must be assessed separately.

Death usually occurs before 20 years of age, and few of these patients reach their thirties. The cause of death is estimated to be a respiratory disruption in 75% of cases and congestive heart failure or sudden cardiac death in 25%. It is important to note that patient's with Duchenne's muscular dystrophy are surviving longer as a result of more aggressive ventilatory support and improved supportive care.[13] However, with this increased survival comes increased cardiac complications.

Diagnostic Testing and Monitoring

The physical examination is an important and inexpensive diagnostic tool. Lung disease can be evaluated. Signs of poor systolic function can manifest as a boggy impulse and poor perfusion. Diastolic dysfunction can be suggested by pulmonary edema and crackles (left sided) and by jugular venous distension, ascites, and peripheral edema (right sided). Auscultation can be performed to check for a click of mitral valve prolapse and a murmur of mitral regurgitation. If pulmonary hypertension is present, a prominent pulmonary component of the second heart sound often can be heard.

Most patients with Duchenne's muscular dystrophy manifest characteristic electrocardiographic (ECG) abnormalities, including tall R waves in the anterior precordial leads and deep, narrow Q waves in the lateral precordial leads. These findings give the appearance of a posterolateral infarct and may be secondary to the disproportionate fibrosis in the posterobasal left ventricular wall. Inappropriate sinus tachycardia, premature ventricular contractions, and varying degrees of AV block also are common ECG findings. A typical ECG in a patient with Duchenne's muscular dystrophy is shown in Fig. 134.2.

Electrocardiography is essential in patients with Duchenne's muscular dystrophy; it is a simple, noninvasive test that can detect early myocardial involvement. Serial Holter monitoring also is helpful in looking for asymptomatic rhythm disturbances. However, ECG and rhythm investigation alone may underestimate the degree of a developing cardiomyopathy. Echocardiography is useful for diagnosing and following the progression of cardiomyopathy. The echocardiographic appearance is that of an "atrophic heart."[14]

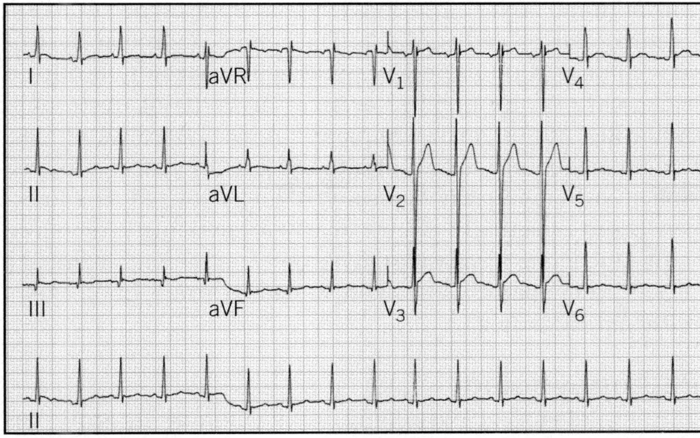

Figure 134.2 The typical electrocardiogram of a patient with Duchenne's muscular dystrophy. Note the tall precordial R waves and the deep, narrow S waves in leads V_1 to V_3.

The left ventricular posterior wall thickness is less and the cavity dimensions are smaller than in controls, and the left ventricular wall thickness and short-axis dimensions decrease inappropriately with age. Echocardiography also can demonstrate regional wall motion abnormalities, mitral valve prolapse and regurgitation, and pulmonary hypertension by Doppler assessment of the tricuspid valve.

Many patients with Duchenne's muscular dystrophy ultimately develop poor echocardiographic windows secondary to progressive chest wall deformity and lung disease. For this reason, serial magnetic resonance imaging (MRI) has become an important tool for monitoring the progression of ventricular dysfunction. MRI can quantify the biventricular chamber size and function, discern regional wall motion abnormalities, and evaluate mitral valve prolapse and regurgitation. Special MRI techniques, namely, delayed enhancement with gadolinium contrast, can be used to look for myocardial fibrosis and scarring.[15] In addition, newer MRI techniques allow assessment of myocardial wall strain,[16] as well as coronary perfusion and coronary flow reserve if these are in question.[17]

Perfusion defects may be evident by single photon emission computed tomography (SPECT) imaging using thallium 201. Reduced uptake of radiotracers, such as 13N-ammonia, also confirms reduced perfusion. PET imaging can show simultaneous perfusion and metabolic mismatches (Fig. 134.3).[18]

Investigators have proposed the use of neuroendocrine screening to identify early or incipient cardiomyopathy. More specifically, levels of atrial and brain natriuretic peptide have been shown to be elevated in a small group of patients with Duchenne's muscular dystrophy and may serve as a noninvasive monitoring tool.[19]

Current recommendations suggest that, at a minimum, patients with Duchenne's muscular dystrophy should have a cardiac evaluation, including a physical examination, ECG, Holter monitor, and echocardiography, at the time of diagnosis. They should have a repeat cardiac evaluation every 2 years until age 10 years and annually thereafter. Patients with Duchenne's muscular dystrophy also should have a cardiac evaluation before any major surgical intervention. Because respiratory failure is common in Duchenne's muscular dystrophy, assessment and treatment of respiratory function should be performed in parallel with the cardiac evaluation.[20]

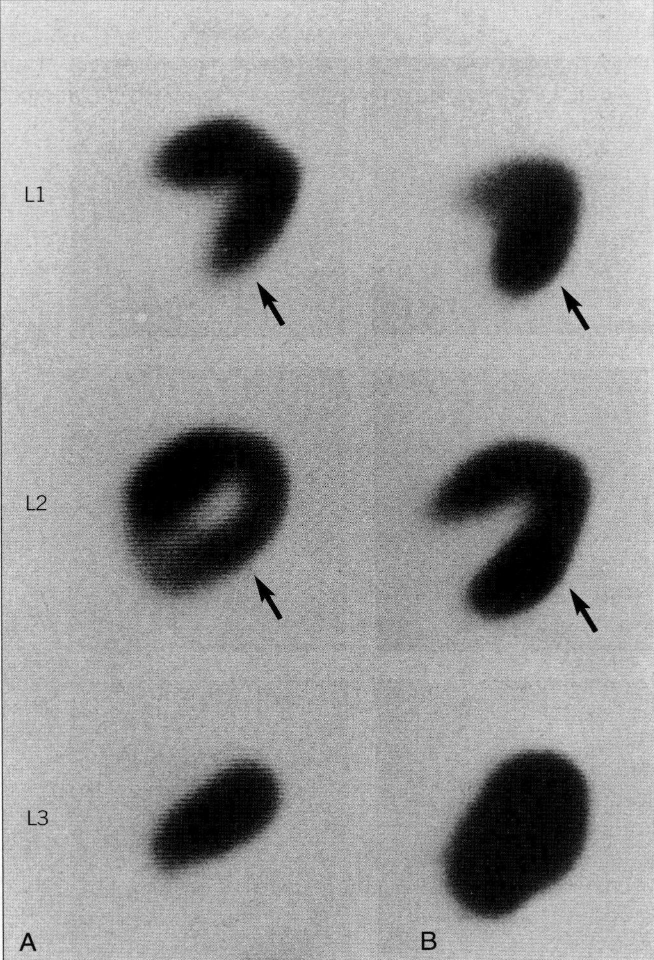

Figure 134.3 Reduced uptake of radiotracers and positron emission tomography (PET) show perfusion and metabolic mismatches in Duchenne's muscular dystrophy. Regional myocardial 13NH3 (**A**) and fluorine-18 deoxyglucose (FDG) (**B**) uptake is seen in three contiguous positron CT images of the left ventricle in a patient with Duchenne's muscular dystrophy. A segmental decrease in activity in the posterolateral wall *(arrows)* is seen, with a discordant increase in FDG in the same segment.

Therapy

The current era of heart failure management has brought new options for treating patients with Duchenne's muscular dystrophy and cardiomyopathy. Angiotensin-converting enzyme (ACE) inhibitors and beta blockers have been shown to improve outcomes and prolong survival in patients with ischemic and nonischemic forms of dilated cardiomyopathy.[19,21] Diuretics are a well-established standard of care for patients with symptoms of volume overload. Such conventional therapies are effective for the management of cardiomyopathy in patients with Duchenne's muscular dystrophy.

Recent evidence suggests that treatment of patients with Duchenne's muscular dystrophy with ACE inhibitors before any impairment of ventricular function is detectable by echocardiography may delay the onset and progression of cardiomyopathy and may improve survival.[22,23] Concerns about the impact of ACE inhibition on left ventricular development in young children limit the treatment in the very young to the context of formal clinical trials.

Fatal arrhythmias are not uncommon in patients with Duchenne's muscular dystrophy. Antiarrhythmic medications can and should be used. Based on data from adult patients with cardiomyopathy, placement of an implantable cardioverter-defibrillator in patients with documented ventricular arrhythmias or a severely reduced ejection fraction should be considered.[24] This option should be discussed in the context of the patient's prognosis and the patient's and family's desire for aggressive strategies.

Corticosteroids are the mainstay of therapy for patients with Duchenne's muscular dystrophy. In a double-blind, randomized, controlled trial, they were found to stabilize muscle strength.[25] Patients with Duchenne's muscular dystrophy who are treated with long-term steroids develop respiratory insufficiency later and have fewer cardiac symptoms. The mechanism by which steroids slow the dystrophic process is not fully understood and currently is under investigation.[26]

A number of gene-specific approaches are being explored to restore dystrophin expression in Duchenne's muscular dystrophy. Oligonucleotide-induced exon skipping has been shown in a murine model of dystrophin deficiency to induce dystrophin expression in skeletal muscle, but it has not been shown to be efficacious for the heart.[27,28]

A second approach, stop codon–based therapy, is undergoing investigation. Approximately 15% to 30% of patients with Duchenne's muscular dystrophy have disease based on a small mutation that creates a premature stop codon.[29] The aminoglycoside antibiotic gentamicin can induce a read-through of normal stop codons, particularly those that are premature and mutation produced.[30,31] Although gentamicin has been demonstrated to be effective in a mouse model,[32] such positive results were absent in human trials. This disappointing result was partly secondary to the drug's ototoxicity and nephrotoxicity.[33] Novel agents with fewer side effects currently are being tested in patients with Duchenne's muscular dystrophy.

Gene replacement strategies for Duchenne's muscular dystrophy have been explored using adenoviruses and adeno-associated viruses.[34,35] This approach has been limited primarily by the fact that such viruses are unable to carry as large a molecule as dystrophin. Truncated molecules have been used but likely are insufficient.

Other approaches to strengthening the weakened cell membrane in dystrophin deficiency are currently being explored but are far from widespread use.[36]

Unfortunately, the multiple other complications that patients with Duchenne's muscular dystrophy experience, including scoliosis, progressive muscular deterioration, and respiratory failure, make them poor candidates for cardiac transplantation.

Prognosis

Despite the aforementioned therapies for Duchenne's muscular dystrophy, the prognosis for these patients is grim. Death usually occurs by the third decade of life as a result of respiratory complications, congestive heart failure, or arrhythmia.

BECKER'S MUSCULAR DYSTROPHY

Epidemiology and Genetics

Similar to Duchenne's muscular dystrophy, Becker's muscular dystrophy is an X-linked recessive form of muscular dystrophy caused by abnormalities in the dystrophin gene on chromosome Xp21. The incidence is 3 cases per 100,000 live male births. In contrast to Duchenne's muscular dystrophy, the mutation in Becker's muscular dystrophy results in a decrease in the number or size (or both) of dystrophin molecules, rather than complete absence. Because of this, the clinical course is that of later onset and slower progression. Cardiomyopathy typically is first detected in adolescence and eventually affects nearly all patients. Compared with Duchenne's muscular dystrophy, a similar incidence of cardiomyopathy is seen in female carriers of Becker's muscular dystrophy.[3]

Pathophysiology

The importance of dystrophin for membrane integrity has been discussed for Duchenne's muscular dystrophy. The decreased amount or size (or both) of the dystrophin gene in Becker's muscular dystrophy similarly leads to membrane fragility, muscle fiber degeneration, and replacement with fibrosis. Pathologic examination of the heart shows extensive areas of fatty infiltration and fibrosis in the subepicardial and middle regions of the myocardium, with a predilection for the lateral wall.[37]

Becker's muscular dystrophy does not spare the right side of the heart. Patients develop progressive dilatation of all four cardiac chambers. In fact, symptomatic right ventricular failure may be the first presenting sign of cardiomyopathy. In comparison with Duchenne's muscular dystrophy, the left ventricular dimensions of patients with Becker's muscular dystrophy are larger. By the time patients with Becker's muscular dystrophy develop symptoms associated with cardiomyopathy, indices of advanced and persistently elevated myocardial workload are present, including increases in the ventricular chamber dimensions, the mitral annular size, and the ratio of the pre-ejection period to the ejection time (PEP/ET).[37] Mitral regurgitation is due to failure of coaptation of the leaflets rather than insufficiency of the posterior papillary muscle as is observed in Duchenne's muscular dystrophy. The syndrome of heart failure that develops may be due to inherent ventricular dysfunction coupled with sustained mitral regurgitation. Figure 134.4 shows an echocardiogram for a 35-year-old man with a history of Becker's muscular dystrophy who presented with increasing fatigue on exertion. The echographic findings support the presence of a severe cardiomyopathy.

Interestingly, in patients with Becker's muscular dystrophy, in contrast to those with Duchenne's muscular dystrophy, coronary lesions have not been described, and coronary vascular reserve has been reported to be normal.[7]

As in Duchenne's muscular dystrophy, the cardiac conduction system is affected in patients with Becker's muscular dystrophy. Bundle branch block and AV node block are common. Atrial and ventricular arrhythmias have been reported and appear to correlate with the severity of ventricular dysfunction.

Clinical Presentation

Cardiomyopathy in Becker's muscular dystrophy often is first detected in adolescence. It usually is present by the third decade and eventually affects nearly all patients. A striking lack of correlation exists between the degree of skeletal muscle weakness and the severity of the cardiomyopathy. In fact,

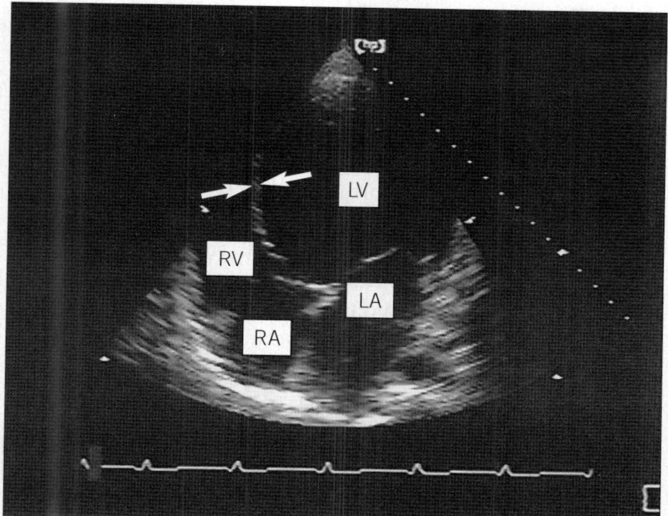

Figure 134.4 Echocardiogram of a 35-year-old man who had been diagnosed with Becker's muscular dystrophy. The patient's main symptom was extreme fatigue in daily living activities. Symptoms were difficult to differentiate with the muscular disease. Note the thinning of the ventricular walls and the marked ventricular dilatation. The left atrium (LA) and the right atrium (RA) also are dilated. LV, left ventricle; RV, right ventricle.

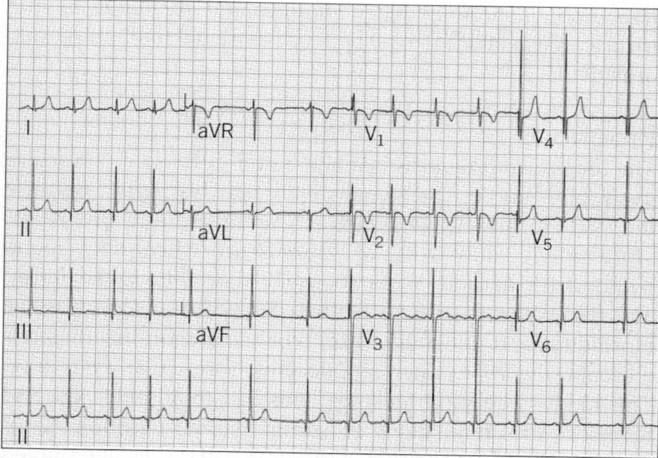

Figure 134.5 Electrocardiographic features of Becker's muscular dystrophy. This ECG, from the same patient as in Figure 134.4, shows the tall R waves in V_2 to V_5, with generalized flattening of T waves in III and aVF and T-wave inversion in V_1 and V_2.

some patients can have severe myocardial dysfunction before manifesting any skeletal muscle weakness, and it is not uncommon for young patients with Becker's muscular dystrophy to be functionally most limited by their cardiomyopathy.[12,37] Because the skeletal muscle weakness is less severe, only 10% of patients are wheelchair bound by the fifth decade. Even so, early mortality is the norm, and few patients survive beyond 50 years of age. Cardiac morbidity and mortality are common.

Diagnostic Testing and Monitoring

The physical examination is useful for monitoring the signs of cardiomyopathy. Signs of poor systolic function can manifest as a boggy impulse and poor perfusion. Diastolic dysfunction can be suggested by pulmonary edema and crackles (left sided) and by jugular venous distention, ascites, and peripheral edema (right sided). A murmur of mitral regurgitation can be heard. If pulmonary hypertension is present, a prominent pulmonary component of the second heart sound can be heard.

ECG abnormalities are present in more than 75% of patients with Becker's muscular dystrophy. These abnormalities can be nonspecific or can include evidence of right or left ventricular hypertrophy; prominent R waves in the precordial leads V_1 to V_4; incomplete right bundle branch block, which may be related to early involvement of the right ventricle; left bundle branch block in patients with congestive heart failure; and pathologic Q waves in the anterolateral leads, suggesting lateral wall damage. Conduction disturbances can include fascicular block or complete heart block. Figure 134.5, which shows an ECG from the same patient as in Figure 134.4, demonstrates a prominent R wave in leads V_2 and V_3.

ECG is essential as a first tool for detecting early cardiac involvement, but it is rarely sufficient. Holter monitoring is useful for finding asymptomatic arrhythmias that may portend a poor outcome, but it, too, is rarely sufficient. Most clinicians rely on echocardiography to diagnose and monitor the severity and progression of the cardiomyopathy and mitral valve disease.

Echocardiographic windows typically are not as poor in patients with Becker's muscular dystrophy as in those with Duchenne's muscular dystrophy. Regardless, serial MRI can be an important tool for monitoring the progression of ventricular dysfunction. MRI can quantify the biventricular chamber size and function, discern regional wall motion abnormalities, quantify and characterize mitral valve regurgitation, and detect areas of myocardial fibrosis and scarring.

The current recommendations for evaluating cardiac involvement in patients with Becker's muscular dystrophy include a full cardiac evaluation, consisting of a history, physical examination, ECG, Holter monitoring, and echocardiogram, at the time of diagnosis and then every 5 years at minimum. If cardiomyopathy is found or if symptoms develop, more frequent follow-up is recommended.

Therapy

Conventional therapies for heart failure, such as ACE inhibitors, beta blockers, and diuretics, are effective and recommended for the management of cardiomyopathy, ventricular dysfunction, and symptomatic congestion in patients with Becker's muscular dystrophy. Unfortunately, no prospective data have shown that corticosteroids ameliorate the progression of skeletal muscle disease.[38]

Prophylactic afterload reduction, gene-specific approaches, and therapies to strengthen the cell membrane are being studied (see the section on therapy in Duchenne's muscular dystrophy). To date, none have found widespread clinical use, but some are showing promise.

Because patients with Becker's muscular dystrophy are older at presentation, in contrast to those with Duchenne's muscular dystrophy, other treatable causes of heart failure, such as coronary artery disease, should not be overlooked. In addition, because patients with Becker's muscular dystrophy have lesser neuromuscular limitations and greater longevity, cardiac transplantation may be a viable treatment in this group of patients.[38-40]

Prognosis

The long-term prognosis is much better in Becker's muscular dystrophy than in Duchenne's muscular dystrophy. Because the skeletal muscle weakness is less severe and progresses more slowly, only 10% of patients are wheelchair bound by the fifth decade. Even so, early mortality is the norm, and few patients survive beyond 50 years of age. Cardiac morbidity and mortality are more common in Becker's muscular dystrophy than in Duchenne's muscular dystrophy. This likely is because these patients live to an older age and therefore are more likely to suffer the complications associated with a progressive cardiomyopathy. As mentioned previously, these patients may benefit from cardiac transplantation. Multiple studies have shown this to be a useful therapeutic option for patients with severe cardiomyopathy or dangerous arrhythmias.

MYOTONIC DYSTROPHY (STEINERT'S DISEASE)

Epidemiology and Genetics

Myotonic dystrophy is an autosomal dominant, systemic disorder associated with myotonia, frontal balding, gonadal dysfunction, cataracts, cardiac conduction abnormalities and, more rarely, cardiomyopathy. It is quite common, with an incidence of 1 in 8000 live births. The genetic defect is a variably increased number of cytosine-thymine-guanine (CTG) trinucleotide repeats in the 3′ untranslated portion of the myotonic dystrophy protein kinase gene located on chromosome 19q13.[41,42] A known association exists between a greater number of repeats and both earlier age at onset of symptoms and more severe disease. In addition, the clinical severity is greater when the mother is the transmitting parent.

Pathophysiology

In skeletal muscle, the myotonia of myotonic dystrophy manifests as impaired relaxation. In fact, this is the most common presenting symptom. Cardiac disease is common and progressive. It usually presents after the onset of skeletal muscle symptoms. Cardiac manifestations usually are in the form of conduction abnormalities and arrhythmias. Myocardial involvement is less common but when present takes the form of diastolic dysfunction; not surprising, given that the pathophysiology of the skeletal muscle dysfunction is impaired relaxation. The molecular etiology of myotonic dystrophy recently has been elucidated. It has been shown that the transcribed CTG repeat is toxic and leads to abnormal ribonucleic acid (RNA) splicing.[43] The messenger ribonucleic acids (mRNAs) encoding a chloride channel and cardiac troponin T have been identified as having abnormal splice forms in myotonic dystrophy patients; chloride channels are implicated in myotonia, and defects in troponin splicing are thought to contribute to cardiomyopathy.[44,45]

Myocardial histology in myotonic dystrophy demonstrates fibrosis and fatty infiltration of the sinoatrial (SA) and AV nodes, conduction system, and ventricular myocardium. Fatty infiltration can range from focal to diffuse. Mitral valve prolapse also is described frequently and likely occurs secondary to dystrophy of the papillary muscle rather than because of valve pathology.

Conduction abnormalities are the most common cardiac manifestation of myotonic dystrophy, occurring in more than 90% of cases. These abnormalities include first-degree AV block in as many as two thirds of patients, and intraventricular conduction delays, in the form of right bundle branch block or left anterior hemiblock, in one third. Left bundle branch block is less common. The range of arrhythmias seen in myotonic dystrophy is broad and includes sinus bradycardia, atrial ectopy, sustained atrial arrhythmias (atrial flutter and fibrillation), and ventricular arrhythmias. The rate of progression of the conduction system involvement parallels the progression of systemic disease. Sudden death can result from complete heart block or ventricular arrhythmias.

Generalized cardiomyopathy is less common. Symptomatic cardiac involvement usually is absent, and systolic function usually is preserved; however, diastolic dysfunction has been reported. Diastolic dysfunction is manifested in early diastole, suggesting impaired relaxation.[46,47] The etiology of diastolic dysfunction is not entirely clear. It may be secondary to the same mechanisms causing impaired skeletal muscle relaxation. Alternatively, or additionally, diastolic impairment may be secondary to the aforementioned conduction defects. Sudden death occurs and is more commonly related to AV node block than to ventricular tachycardia. Of course, diastolic dysfunction is associated with depressed preload reserve, and thus intolerance of bradycardia, which may explain this observation.

Clinical Presentation

The onset of symptoms in myotonic dystrophy is variable and ranges from 10 to 60 years of age. Weakness of the flexor muscles of the neck give the face a sagging appearance (Fig. 134.6). Myotonia affects other muscles as well, particularly those of the hands, forearms, tongue, and jaw.

Conduction abnormalities typically present after the onset of skeletal muscle symptoms. In an attempt to identify the likelihood of rhythm abnormalities, Antonini and colleagues[48] studied 50 patients from 36 families. They found that major rhythm disturbances developed in 38% of the patients: major conduction abnormalities in 48%; major arrhythmias in 26%; and all in 26%. Placement of a cardiac pacemaker was required in 8% of the patients. Myocardial involvement is relatively well tolerated, and symptomatic heart failure is rare (fewer than 7% of patients).

Less commonly, infantile (congenital) cases occur.[49] The infantile form is associated with symptoms from birth, including hypotonia of skeletal muscles that leads to respiratory compromise, feeding difficulties, and contractures. These children also suffer cognitive delay. Neonatal mortality nears 25%. In the children who survive, cardiac symptoms usually present in adolescence.

Diagnostic Testing and Monitoring

In patients with known myotonic dystrophy, an annual cardiac evaluation should be performed, including a thorough history and ECG. ECG findings do not reliably predict progression and risk of sudden death, although one study

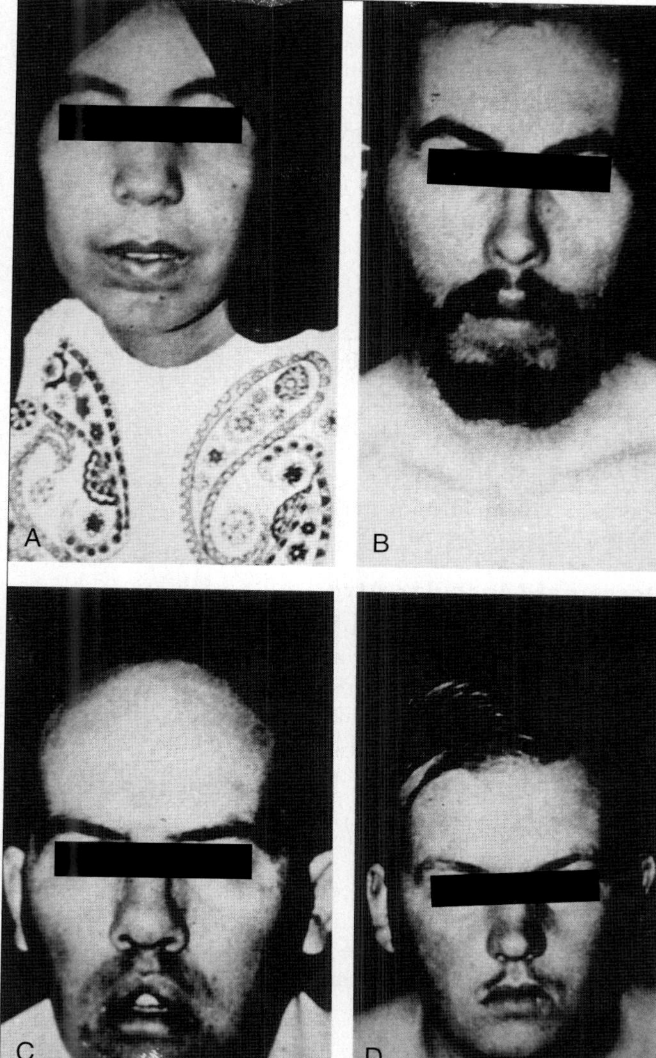

Figure 134.6 Myotonic dystrophy facies. Note the sagging appearance, the weakness of the flexor muscles of the neck, and the premature balding.

suggested that a PR interval greater than 240 msec was a significant risk factor for atrial fibrillation, syncope, and sudden death in patients older than 40 years of age.[50]

If the history provides suspicion of arrhythmias, a 24-hour Holter recording or an event monitor is recommended. A Holter monitor also is recommended if the annual ECG demonstrates an increasing PR interval or other risk factors for bradycardia.

Because ventricular tachyarrhythmias are suspected to be an etiology of sudden death in patients with myotonic dystrophy, any wide complex arrhythmia or symptoms suggestive of a tachyarrhythmia should be investigated further with electrophysiologic testing.[51] Surface ECG may be normal despite the presence of an important intra-hisian conduction delay on electrophysiologic testing. In fact, invasive electrophysiology testing, when performed in patients with abnormal ECGs, typically detects more widespread conduction abnormalities than are suggested by the surface recording and may have prognostic value.[41] Regardless, the role of electrophysiologic testing in patients with normal ECGs is not well established.

MRI has been used as a method of identifying right ventricle abnormalities, such as right ventricular wall thinning or fatty replacement. Such imaging abnormalities have been strongly correlated to inducibility of ventricular arrhythmias.[52]

Therapy

Atrial tachyarrhythmias are common and, if symptomatic, may justify antiarrhythmic therapy. Caution should be used, however, because antiarrhythmic drugs may aggravate any preexisting tendency to bradycardia or ventricular tachyarrhythmias. Catheter ablation of atrial tachyarrhythmias also is an option. Treatment with a pacemaker is indicated when a progressive bradyarrhythmia is detected, even before symptoms arise. If malignant ventricular arrhythmias are identified, implantable defibrillators or catheter ablation should be considered, although no large series has been reported.[51] Despite reports of ventricular tachyarrhythmias, the incidence is not sufficiently high to justify implantable defibrillator therapy routinely when permanent pacing is indicated.

The management of diastolic or systolic dysfunction should follow standard clinical care guidelines.

Prognosis

In one representative study of 367 patients with myotonic dystrophy, 75 died over a 10-year follow-up at a mean age of 53 years, with the youngest death at 24 years.[53] Sudden death can occur even at an early stage of disease. Although cardiac involvement generally is well tolerated, approximately 7% of patients have clinical heart failure.

X-LINKED HUMEROPERONEAL DYSTROPHY (EMERY-DREIFUSS MUSCULAR DYSTROPHY)

Epidemiology and Genetics

X-linked humeroperoneal dystrophy, or Emery-Dreifuss muscular dystrophy, is characterized by early contractures, slowly progressive muscle wasting and weakness with a distinctive humeroperoneal distribution and later limb-girdle involvement, and cardiac involvement (conduction abnormalities and cardiomyopathy). The disease has two main modes of inheritance; X-linked and autosomal dominant. Rare autosomal recessive inheritance has been described. Emery-Dreifuss muscular dystrophy is relatively rare, with a disease frequency estimated at 1 in 100,000 for the X-linked form (the frequency of the autosomal dominant form is unknown).[54]

The X-linked form of Emery-Dreifuss muscular dystrophy is caused by mutations of the STA gene at Xq28, which encodes the nuclear membrane protein emerin.[54-56] Emerin is an inner nuclear membrane protein anchored to the inner nuclear membrane in skeletal, cardiac, and smooth muscle. The primary role of the emerin nuclear protein complex is to stabilize the nuclear membrane against the mechanical stresses generated in muscle cells during contraction.[57]

The autosomal dominant form, although clinically similar to the X-linked form, is caused by mutations of the LMNA gene at 1q11-q23. This gene encodes the lamins A and C.[54,56,58] The autosomal-recessive form is likely also due to mutations of the LMNA gene. Lamins A and C are components of the nuclear envelope that interact with chromatin, other proteins of the inner nuclear membrane, and emerin. These proteins have many roles, including mechanical stabilization of the nucleus.[54]

Pathophysiology

Conduction abnormalities and arrhythmias are the most commonly described cardiac complications. Cardiomyopathy is rare. Regardless, myocardial histopathology can demonstrate myocyte hypertrophy, interstitial fibrosis, and nuclear hyperchromaticity, which suggests myocardial involvement. The interstitial fibrosis and hypertrophy can result in end-stage cardiomyopathy similar to that described for other dystrophic diseases.

Conduction system abnormalities include reduced atrial contraction, permanent atrial paralysis, atrial fibrillation and flutter, and complete heart block. Sudden death has been attributed to complete heart block, although terminal ventricular arrhythmias also can be observed, particularly with a background cardiomyopathy.

Clinical Presentation

The onset of Emery-Dreifuss muscular dystrophy typically occurs in early childhood, with subsequent slow progression of disease. The first manifestations of Emery-Dreifuss muscular dystrophy are early contractures of the elbows, Achilles tendons, and post cervical neck muscles, even before muscle weakness is manifest. After this stage, a slow progression of muscle wasting and weakness occurs, in a humeroperoneal distribution early (proximal in the upper limbs and distal in the lower limbs), then with extension to the limb-girdle muscles later. Muscle weakness rarely is severe, and loss of ambulation is uncommon.

Cardiac involvement is the most serious complication in Emery-Dreifuss muscular dystrophy. It usually becomes evident as muscle weakness progresses but may be present before any significant skeletal muscle symptoms are manifest; the first symptoms of Emery-Dreifuss muscular dystrophy can be sudden cardiac death. Nearly all patients with Emery-Dreifuss muscular dystrophy have cardiac involvement by age 30.

Diagnostic Testing and Monitoring

A surface ECG should be obtained at diagnosis and annually thereafter. Holter monitoring for tachy- or bradyarrhythmias is recommended annually as well. Echocardiography to evaluate ventricular function can be performed on a less regular basis, the frequency dictated by a history of myocardial involvement and symptoms. In the presence of SA or AV nodal conduction abnormalities on surface ECG, the role of electrophysiology is unclear. Invasive electrophysiology testing probably adds little to the decision to implant a permanent pacemaker.

As with Duchenne's muscular dystrophy and Becker's muscular dystrophy, some female carriers of this X-linked disease may manifest cardiac disease. Published cases of manifesting carriers may have been diluted by cases of autosomal dominant disease. Carrier status should be established in females at risk. These women should be offered periodic ECG surveillance to detect SA or AV nodal conduction disease.

Therapy

Permanent pacemaker implantation is justified, even in asymptomatic patients, when the surface ECG begins to show abnormalities of SA or AV node disease. Nocturnal AV-Wenckebach may be a normal finding in young people, and pacemaker implantation in this setting may be deferred.

The management of heart failure should follow standard clinical care. Cases of cardiac transplantation in patients with severe cardiomyopathy have been reported.[59]

Prognosis

The prognosis for these patients is directly related to the severity of cardiac involvement.

LESS COMMON DISORDERS OF MUSCLE

The less common muscular disorders are presented in Table 134.1.

Peroneal Muscular Atrophy (Charcot-Marie-Tooth Syndrome)

Peroneal muscular atrophy, also known as Charcot-Marie-Tooth syndrome, is an autosomal dominant disorder characterized by distal muscle weakness along the distribution of the peroneal nerves. The muscle groups involved most commonly include the everters and occasionally the intrinsic muscle groups of the hands. The onset of muscle weakness typically occurs in the second or third decade of life, and the weakness is progressive.

Cardiac manifestations associated with peroneal muscular atrophy are unusual. Conduction abnormalities, such as right bundle branch block, complete heart block, atrial tachyarrhythmias, and dilated cardiomyopathy, have been reported.[60,61]

CARDIAC MANIFESTATIONS OF LESS COMMON MUSCULAR DISORDERS	
Charcot-Marie-Tooth syndrome	■ Right bundle branch block ■ Complete heart block ■ Atrial fibrillation and flutter ■ Dilated cardiomyopathy
Facioscapulohumeral dystrophy	■ Atrial paralysis ■ Atrial fibrillation and flutter ■ Cardiomyopathy
Limb-girdle dystrophy	■ Bradycardia ■ First-degree atrioventricular block ■ Left bundle branch block ■ QRS prolongation ■ Complete heart block
Kearns-Sayre syndrome	■ Atrioventricular nodal delay ■ Infranodal conduction delay ■ Complete heart block
Periodic paralysis	■ Hyperkalemic or hypokalemic changes on electrocardiogram ■ First-degree atrioventricular block ■ Bidirectional ventricular tachycardia

Table 134.1 Cardiac manifestations of less common muscular disorders.

Facioscapulohumeral Muscular Dystrophy (Landouzy-Dejerine Dystrophy)

Facioscapulohumeral muscular dystrophy, also known as Landouzy-Dejerine dystrophy, is an autosomal dominant disorder characterized by facial muscle weakness followed by progressive upper and proximal lower extremity weakness. It is a rare disorder, with an incidence of 3 to 10 cases per 1 million. The onset of weakness typically occurs in the first or second decade of life.

Cardiac abnormalities associated with facioscapulohumeral muscular dystrophy include atrial paralysis with loss of P waves and absence of atrial response to direct stimulation.[62] Other conduction abnormalities and cardiomyopathy also have been described.

Limb-Girdle Dystrophy (Erb's Spastic Paraplegia)

Limb-girdle dystrophy is an autosomal recessive disorder characterized by progressive muscle weakness beginning in the lower extremities and progressing to the upper extremities. The age of onset of symptoms is variable, ranging from the first to the fourth decades of life. Regardless, patients ultimately are wheelchair bound. At least 15 genetically unique types have been described.[56]

Cardiac involvement in limb-girdle dystrophy is uncommon. When present, conduction abnormalities are most common, including bradyarrhythmias and tachyarrhythmias, first-degree AV block, infranodal conduction abnormalities with left bundle branch block, QRS prolongation, and complete heart block. Even less often is the myocardium involved. Case reports have described left ventricular apical hypertrophy with biopsy-proven histologic changes resembling those of skeletal muscle, namely, muscle fiber atrophy and hypertrophy and mild interstitial fibrosis.[63] Cases of associated dilated cardiomyopathy have been reported as well.[64,65]

Kearns-Sayre Syndrome

Kearns-Sayre syndrome is a mitochondrial disease characterized by the pathologic triad of progressive external ophthalmoplegia, pigmentary retinopathy, and heart block. All patients with Kearns-Sayre syndrome have a deletion of nucleotide positions 8483 to 13483 of mitochondrial DNA.[66] The histology of skeletal muscle demonstrates the classic "ragged red fibers."

Cardiac involvement in Kearns-Sayre syndrome has been reported in as many as 50% of patients.[67] Cardiac manifestations consist primarily of slowly progressive infranodal and AV nodal conduction delay. Although the rate of progression is variable, fascicular block is likely to progress to high-grade AV block. The risk of sudden death is significant (up to 20%) and has been attributed to heart block and a prolonged QT interval. To obviate this risk, some advocate pacemaker implantation when a prolonged HV interval or block below the His bundle is elicited with atrial pacing.[68] Myocardial manifestations include asymmetric septal hypertrophy.

Periodic Paralysis

Periodic paralysis is an autosomal dominant disorder of skeletal muscle characterized by recurrent episodes of paralysis associated with either hyperkalemia or hypokalemia. As a rule, the onset of weakness occurs in the lower extremities, with progression of weakness to the upper extremities. Surface ECG abnormalities are consistent with either hyperkalemia (peaked T waves, widened QRS complex, and increased PR interval) or hypokalemia (flattened T waves, U waves, and sinus bradycardia). In addition, arrhythmias such as bidirectional ventricular tachycardia or fusion beats have been described. Arrhythmias can occur independently of the paralysis episodes. A mild form of cardiomyopathy has been reported in elderly patients with periodic paralysis, but the etiology is unclear.[69]

DISORDERS OF NERVES

FRIEDREICH'S ATAXIA

Epidemiology and Genetics

Friedreich's ataxia is an autosomal recessive disease characterized by progressive spinocerebellar degeneration. Although the degeneration typically occurs in the spinocerebellar tracts, the dorsal columns, pyramidal tracts, cerebellum, and medulla also can be affected to a variable degree. Friedreich's ataxia is characterized by ataxia, areflexia, and muscle weakness in all extremities. The genetic defect responsible for this disease is a mutation and unstable triplet expansion of GAA repeats in the first intron of the gene encoding fataxin on chromosome 9q13.[70] Up to 90% of patients with Friedreich's ataxia may demonstrate various cardiac abnormalities, the most common being cardiac hypertrophy.

Pathophysiology

Two types of cardiac involvement appear to occur in Friedreich's ataxia: a hypertrophic form (the most common) and a segmental dystrophic form. The hypertrophic form is described either as an asymmetric septal hypertrophy or as a concentric left ventricular hypertrophy with normal cavity size and function. Histologic findings include extensive fibrosis and foci of necrosis intermingled with hypertrophied myocardial cells. Typically, no evidence is seen of the cellular disarray associated with hypertrophic cardiomyopathy. Intimal proliferation of intramural coronary arteries occurs. The dystrophic form is also known as minimally dilated cardiomyopathy. This form likely represents a late stage of involvement and is associated with segmental dystrophy but global hypokinesis.

Whether the cardiac anomalies in Friedreich's ataxia are directly related to the genetic defect in fataxin or indirectly related to the spinocerebellar degeneration has not been clearly established. Some hypothesize that the etiology is the elevated levels of catecholamines in patients with Friedreich's ataxia. Support for this hypothesis is seen in the fact that many patients with Friedreich's ataxia have inappropriate sinus tachycardia. In one series of 23 patients, 15 had evidence of catecholamine elevation, primarily in the form of norepinephrine. Interestingly, 12 patients with both left ventricular hypertrophy and catechol elevation had more severe neuromuscular disease.[70a] Parasympathetic activity also has been implicated, in the form of a nighttime decrease in heart rate variability.[71] Arrhythmias and heart failure are late occurrences and are associated with progressive neuromuscular disease.[72]

Clinical Presentation

The onset of cardiac abnormalities in Friedreich's ataxia is variable and can occur before or up to 20 years after the onset of neurologic symptoms. The earlier the onset of neurologic symptoms, the more frequent is the occurrence of left ventricular hypertrophy.

Dyspnea and palpitations are the most common symptoms of cardiac involvement. The physical examination can include a harsh systolic murmur of left ventricular outflow tract obstruction, as well as pathologic heart sounds.

Heart failure is rare and manifests late in the course of the disease. Similarly, although arrhythmias are uncommon, persistent arrhythmias may manifest late in the disease course. In the absence of ECG abnormalities, cardiac signs and symptoms are rare.

A subset of patients may develop a dilated cardiomyopathy, which tends to have a worse prognosis. Arrhythmias and overt cardiac failure tend to be more common with this group.

Diagnostic Testing and Monitoring

ECG abnormalities are found in more than 90% of patients with Friedreich's ataxia. In one study of 75 patients, 79% had ST-T wave changes, 40% had right-axis deviation, 24% had a short PR interval, 20% had an abnormal R wave in V_1, 14% had abnormal inferolateral Q waves, and 16% had evidence of left ventricular hypertrophy.[73]

Echocardiography has been instrumental in defining the functional abnormalities of the heart associated with Friedreich's ataxia. Diastolic function may be abnormal and manifested by a prolonged isovolumic relaxation period with an E/A ratio that is decreased compared with normal controls. In addition, the left ventricular mass index often is greater than it is in controls.[74] The left ventricular cavity dimensions usually are normal or small, and septal motion usually is normal. In contrast to the muscular dystrophies described previously, perfusion defects detected by thallium 201 imaging are rare, which suggests that ischemia does not play a pivotal role.[75]

Therapy

Symptomatic atrial and ventricular arrhythmias in Friedreich's ataxia should be managed as in any other arrhythmic disorder. In patients who develop the dilated form of cardiomyopathy, pharmacologic therapy for heart failure should be initiated. Antioxidants, such as coenzyme Q_{10}, vitamin E, and idebenone, have been used to attempt to reverse left ventricular hypertrophy in patients with cardiomyopathy with promising results.[76,77]

Prognosis

Friedreich's ataxia is an unremitting, progressive neurologic disorder that leads to limb weakness and ataxic gait. The concentric hypertrophy associated with Friedreich's ataxia has a more benign course than hypertrophic cardiomyopathy. Patients who develop the alternate form of dilated cardiomyopathy can have progressive and terminal heart failure. Because the neurologic component of Friedreich's ataxia is relentless, these patients ordinarily are not considered for cardiac transplantation.

LESS COMMON NEUROLOGIC OR NEUROMUSCULAR DISORDERS

Cardiac features of the less common neurologic or neuromuscular disorders, Guillain-Barré syndrome and myasthenia gravis, are presented in Table 134.2.

Guillain-Barré Syndrome

Guillain-Barré syndrome is an autoimmune polyneuropathy that presents as an acute onset of nerve demyelination. Guillain-Barré syndrome typically occurs days to weeks after an acute respiratory or gastrointestinal viral illness. Ascending muscle weakness with paresthesias is the hallmark of this syndrome. Ultimately, progressive weakness of the respiratory muscles leads to the need for mechanical ventilation. Although this disorder is potentially reversible, mortality remains as high as 20%.[78] Mortality typically is secondary to respiratory failure but may also be secondary to autonomic dysfunction.

Cardiac arrhythmias are common in Guillain-Barré syndrome, particularly in patients with severe neurologic involvement. Surface ECG abnormalities tend to be limited to nonspecific repolarization abnormalities. Sinus tachycardia is common. Other tachyarrhythmias also have been described, such as atrial fibrillation, atrial flutter, and ventricular tachycardia. Bradyarrhythmias secondary to vagal hypersensitivity, such as sinus bradycardia and sinus arrest, can occur and may account for sudden cardiac death in some patients. Tracheal tube manipulation and suction have been associated with the development of asystole. Atropine may help overcome this intense vagal stimulation. Most authors advocate the use of pacemakers when bradycardia is present.

Other manifestations of autonomic neuropathy that frequently accompany Guillain-Barré syndrome include refractory orthostatic hypotension, hypertension, excessive sweating, and wide fluctuations in heart rate and blood pressure. The relationship between the severity of paralysis and the degree of autonomic neuropathy is unclear.

CARDIAC INVOLVEMENT IN LESS COMMON NEUROLOGIC DISORDERS

Disorder	Cardiac Manifestations
Guillain-Barré syndrome	■ Nonspecific repolarization abnormalities ■ Sinus bradycardia ■ Asystole ■ Atrial flutter and fibrillation ■ Ventricular tachycardia ■ Sudden cardiac death ■ Myocarditis
Myasthenia gravis	■ QT prolongation ■ Nonspecific repolarization abnormalities ■ Ventricular tachycardia ■ Sudden cardiac death ■ Myocarditis

Table 134.2 Cardiac Involvement in less common neurologic disorders.

Myasthenia Gravis

Myasthenia gravis occurs secondary to the formation of autoantibodies to acetylcholine receptors at the neuromuscular junction. Generalized weakness and fatigue, which worsen with repetitive movements and improve with rest, are the classic symptoms associated with this disorder. Myasthenia gravis affects women more often than men. Antibodies against β_1- and β_2-adrenergic receptors have been implicated in patients with myasthenia gravis who have cardiac involvement.[79] The result on histology is a myocarditis. Surface ECG abnormalities include QT prolongation and nonspecific repolarization abnormalities. Cardiac arrhythmias, including ventricular tachycardia, are common and pose a significant risk of sudden death.

ACKNOWLEDGEMENT

This chapter reuses part of the material originally written by Drs. Piña and Sanchez for the previous edition of this book.

chapter

135 Aging and Geriatric Heart Disease

J. M. Stolker and M. W. Rich

Definition

- The prevalence of cardiovascular disease increases progressively with age, and heart disease is the leading cause of death in both men and women older than age 65.

Key Features

- The effects of aging on cardiovascular structure and function, prolonged exposure to cardiac risk factors, and advances in therapy for common medical problems all contribute to the high prevalence of cardiovascular disease in older individuals.
- Cardiovascular disease in the elderly is characterized by atypical symptoms, delayed presentation, multiple comorbid illnesses, and a worse prognosis.

Therapy

- Management of the older patient with cardiovascular disease must be individualized, with due consideration given to coexisting illnesses, the risks and benefits of therapeutic interventions, and personal preferences regarding quality versus quantity of life.

The prevalence of cardiovascular disease increases progressively with age, and more than three fourths of Americans 75 years of age or older have clinically recognized cardiovascular disease (Fig. 135.1).[1] Nearly two thirds of all cardiovascular hospitalizations occur in individuals age 65 or older, and 83% of cardiovascular deaths occur in this age group. With the projected doubling in size of the geriatric population between 2010 and 2030,[2] older patients with cardiovascular disease will consume an increasing proportion of clinicians' time and national health care resources. It therefore is essential that practitioners have an understanding of the effects of aging on cardiovascular structure and function, and the implications of these changes for the care of the older cardiac patient.

Despite the high prevalence of cardiovascular disease in the geriatric population, most clinical trials either have excluded elderly individuals or have enrolled small numbers of relatively healthy older patients. Consequently, recommendations for the management of elderly patients often are derived from findings in younger, healthier populations, and such findings may not apply to elderly patients with more advanced disease, multiple coexisting medical illnesses, and a shorter life expectancy.

Care is further hampered by atypical clinical features, delayed presentations, polypharmacy, alterations in drug distribution and metabolism, cognitive impairment, behavioral changes, and social and financial issues. Furthermore, older patients exhibit considerable variability in personal preferences regarding the relative importance of quality versus quantity of life, a factor that has important implications for therapeutic decision making.

For all of these reasons, optimal management of the elderly cardiac patient requires an individualized approach that involves careful assessment of the risks and benefits of each therapeutic intervention in the context of the patient's overall health status, prognosis, and desire for an aggressive or conservative treatment strategy.

ANATOMY AND PATHOLOGY

Aging is associated with extensive alterations in cardiovascular anatomy and biochemistry that predispose to the development of cardiovascular disease (Table 135.1).[3] Left ventricular (LV) wall thickness and left atrial size increase with age, and progressive fibrosis and sclerosis occur in the aortic and mitral valves, cardiac exoskeleton, and conduction system.[4] Increased collagen deposition and cross-linking are noted throughout the heart and vasculature; this, in conjunction with degeneration of elastin fibers, leads to increased myocardial and vascular stiffness. Focal myocyte apoptosis and hypertrophy of residual myocytes are accompanied by a decrease in the number of mitochondria and in the nucleus to myofibril size ratio.

Biochemical changes include numerous alterations in enzyme content and activity that affect most metabolic pathways. The synthesis of catecholamines and acetylcholine declines with age, as does the activity of nitric oxide synthase.[5] The number of functioning sinus node pacemaker cells declines by about 90% by age 75, and degeneration and fibrosis of sinus node transition cells occur.[6] The number of conduction cells in the atrioventricular (AV) node and His-Purkinje system also declines with age.

With increasing age, the aorta and large muscular arteries become dilated, elongated, and tortuous, and wall thickness increases as a result of increased connective tissue and calcification. Vascular endothelial function becomes impaired, and the distensibility of the large and medium-sized arteries is reduced. The responsiveness of the heart and blood vessels to β-adrenergic and cholinergic stimulation is attenuated, and responses to baroreceptor stimulation and the Valsalva maneuver decline with age. Although circulating catecholamine levels increase with age, tissue catecholamine levels are diminished.

PATHOPHYSIOLOGY

The anatomic and biochemical changes described previously result in clinically significant alterations in physiology and function with increasing age.

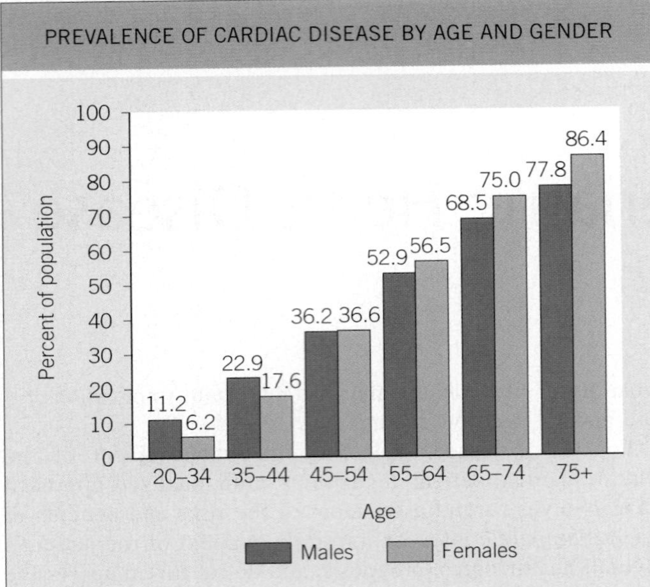

Figure 135.1 Prevalence of cardiac disease by age and gender. Prevalence of cardiovascular diseases (including coronary heart disease, heart failure, stroke, and hypertension) by age and gender in the United States, 1999 to 2002. (From Rosamond W, Flegal K, Friday G, et al: Heart disease and stroke statistics: 2007 update. Circulation 2007;115:e69-e171.)

Age-Related Cardiovascular Changes

Increased arterial stiffness contributes to the progressive rise in systolic blood pressure and pulse pressure observed with increasing age.[7,8] Arterial stiffening also results in increased impedance to LV ejection (i.e., afterload), thereby increasing myocardial work and oxygen requirements. The concurrent rise in arterial pulse wave velocity with age results in earlier reflection of the pulse wave back to the heart, which further increases impedance to ejection in late systole.

Increased myocardial stiffness in conjunction with impaired myocardial relaxation results in diminished LV filling during early diastole and a compensatory increase in the proportion of filling that occurs during atrial contraction (i.e., increased reliance on the "atrial kick" to preserve LV end-diastolic volume, or preload). Taken together, these changes contribute to an age-related increase in left atrial size, predisposing to the development of atrial fibrillation (AF) and to the progressive rise in prevalence of diastolic heart failure (HF) with increasing age.[9-11]

Impaired responsiveness to β_1-adrenergic stimulation results in a progressive decline in the maximum attainable sinus heart rate (HR) with increasing age, exemplified by the formula

$$\text{Maximum HR} = 220 - \text{Age}$$

Because cardiac output (CO) varies directly with HR and stroke volume (SV)

$$\text{CO} = \text{SV} \times \text{HR}$$

it follows that peak CO declines progressively with age. The stress-induced increase in contractility mediated by β_1-adrenergic stimulation also is attenuated with age, which further limits peak CO. Impaired responsiveness to β_2-adrenergic stimulation limits bronchodilatory capacity and peripheral arteriolar vasodilatation, an important mechanism for increasing blood flow to exercising muscles and to the skin (the latter function plays a key role in thermoregulation).

EFFECTS OF AGING ON THE CARDIOVASCULAR SYSTEM	
Gross anatomy	↑ Left ventricular wall thickness
	↓ Left ventricular cavity size
	Endocardial thickening and sclerosis
	↑ Left atrial size
	Valvular fibrosis and sclerosis
	↑ Epicardial fat
Histology	↑ Lipid and amyloid deposition
	↑ Collagen degeneration and fibrosis
	Calcification of fibrous skeleton, valve rings, and coronary arteries
	Shrinkage of myocardial fibers with focal hypertrophy
	↓ Mitochondria, altered mitochondrial membranes
	↓ Nucleus/myofibril size ratio
Biochemical changes	↓ Protein elasticity
	Numerous changes in enzyme content and activity affecting most metabolic pathways, but no change in myosin ATPase activity
	↓ Catecholamine synthesis, especially norepinephrine
	↓ Acetylcholine synthesis
	↓ Activity of nitric oxide synthase
Conduction system	Degeneration of sinus node pacemaker and transition cells
	↓ Number of conducting cells in the AV node and His-Purkinje system
	↑ Connective tissue, fat, and amyloid
	↑ Calcification around the conduction system
Vasculature	↓ Distensibility of large and medium-sized arteries
	Impaired endothelial function
	Aorta and muscular arteries become dilated, elongated, and tortuous
	↑ Wall thickness
	↑ Connective tissue and calcification
Autonomic nervous system	↓ Responsiveness to β-adrenergic stimulation
	↑ Circulating catecholamines, decreased tissue catecholamines
	↓ α-Adrenergic receptors in the left ventricle
	↓ Cholinergic responsiveness
	Diminished response to Valsalva and baroreceptor stimulation
	↓ Heart rate variability

Modified from Stolker JM, Rich MW. Diagnosis and management of heart disease in the elderly. In Arenson C, Reichel W, eds. Reichel's Care of the Elderly. 6th ed. Lippincott Williams & Wilkins, 2009.

Table 135.1 Effects of aging on the cardiovascular system.

The decline in functioning sinus node pacemaker cells and associated diffuse changes throughout the cardiac conduction system predispose older adults to the development of bradyarrhythmias, conduction disturbances, and supraventricular and ventricular tachyarrhythmias. Sick sinus syndrome, which is associated with both inappropriate bradycardia and supraventricular tachyarrhythmias, is a hallmark of cardiovascular aging and the leading indication for permanent pacemaker implantation in older adults.[3]

Endothelium-mediated vasodilatation also declines with age, primarily as a result of diminished production of nitric oxide due to reduced activity of nitric oxide synthase.[5] Because coronary blood flow is regulated by nitric oxide and other endogenous vasodilators, impaired endothelium-mediated vasodilatation limits peak coronary blood flow. As a result, the myocardium may become ischemic even in the absence of significant obstructive coronary artery disease (CAD). Hypertension, dyslipidemia, diabetes, and tobacco use accentuate age-related endothelial dysfunction, further predisposing to myocardial ischemia. Endothelial dysfunction also is an important mechanism contributing to the pathogenesis and progression of CAD, and it likely contributes to the widespread prevalence and increased severity of CAD in older adults.

Altered baroreceptor responsiveness results in an impaired ability to adapt rapidly to positional changes and other stimuli to maintain blood pressure and cerebral perfusion. Consequently, older individuals are at increased risk for orthostatic hypotension, falls, and syncope, particularly with coexisting cardiovascular disease and use of a wide range of common medications.[12]

Taken together, these changes greatly increase the risk for the development of cardiovascular disease in older individuals and simultaneously reduce cardiovascular reserve and the ability of the older patient to respond to stress, whether physiologic (e.g., exercise) or pathologic (e.g., myocardial ischemia, pneumonia). In particular, aging is associated with alterations in all four of the principal determinants of CO: preload, afterload, HR, and contractility. As a result, maximum cardiopulmonary performance declines progressively with advancing age (Fig. 135.2).[13] The marked decline in cardiovascular reserve, in turn, plays a crucial role in the exponential increase in the incidence of HF with increasing age and in the striking increase in mortality associated with cardiovascular disease in older adults.

Age-Related Changes in Other Organ Systems

In parallel with cardiovascular aging, increasing age is associated with substantive changes in other organ systems that affect both cardiovascular function and the clinical features and management of cardiovascular disorders in older adults (Table 135.2).[3] Renal function declines progressively with age, and the glomerular filtration rate decreases gradually, averaging about 8 cc/min/decade. Impaired fluid and electrolyte homeostasis contributes to the propensity of older patients to develop HF and increases the risk of diuretic-induced electrolyte disturbances. Ventilatory capacity declines with age, and ventilation-perfusion mismatching is increased; as a result, older patients are more susceptible to exertional dyspnea and hypoxemia, especially in the context of superimposed cardiovascular disease.

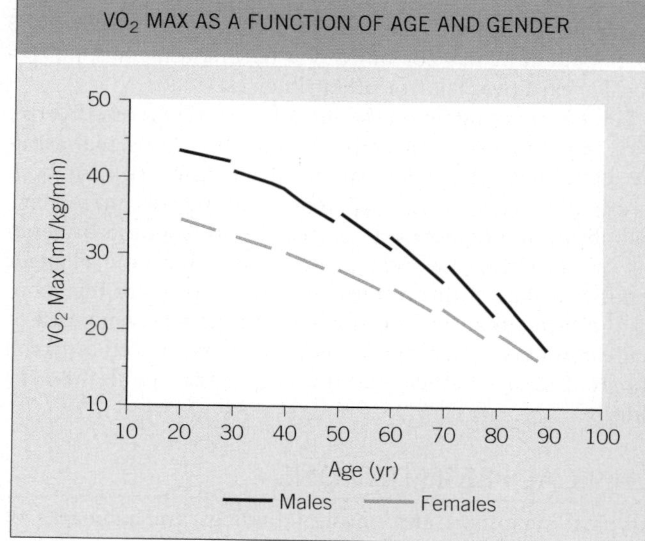

Figure 135.2 VO_2 max as a function of age and gender. Peak treadmill oxygen consumption (VO_2 max) as a function of age and gender in healthy subjects. (From Fleg JL, Morrell CH, Bos AG, et al: Accelerated longitudinal decline of aerobic capacity in healthy older adults. Circulation 2005;112:674-682.)

EFFECTS OF AGING ON OTHER ORGAN SYSTEMS	
Kidneys	Gradual ↓ in glomerular filtration rate (~8 cc/min/decade)
	Impaired fluid and electrolyte homeostasis
Lungs	↓ Ventilatory capacity
	↑ Ventilation/perfusion mismatching
Neurohumoral system	↓ Cerebral perfusion autoregulatory capacity
	Diminished reflex responsiveness
	Impaired thirst mechanism
Hemostatic system	↑ Levels of coagulation factors
	↑ Platelet activity and aggregability
	↑ Inflammatory cytokines and C-reactive protein
	↑ Inhibitors of fibrinolysis and angiogenesis
Musculoskeletal system	↓ Muscle mass (sarcopenia)
	↓ Bone mass (osteopenia), especially In women

Modified from Stolker JM, Rich MW. Diagnosis and management of heart disease in the elderly. In Arenson C, Reichel W, eds. Reichel's Care of the Elderly. 6th ed. Lippincott Williams & Wilkins, 2009.

Table 135.2 Effects of aging on other organ systems.

The ability of the central nervous system's autoregulatory capacity to maintain cerebral perfusion declines with age. As a result, older patients are at risk for alterations in cognitive function with modest reductions in blood pressure, as well as falls or syncope with more pronounced changes in systemic arterial pressure. The thirst mechanism (mediated in the hypothalamus) also declines with age, predisposing older individuals to dehydration (e.g., in response to diuretic therapy). Important changes in the musculoskeletal system include sarcopenia and osteopenia, both of which contribute to impaired functional capacity in older adults and place the older patient at risk for functional decline after hospitalization for cardiovascular or other illnesses.

The effects of aging on the hemostatic system are diverse, with impairments in thrombosis and fibrinolysis that paradoxically place the older patient at increased risk for both thrombotic events (e.g., deep venous thrombosis, pulmonary embolism) and hemorrhage (especially in response to heparin or warfarin). Overall, age-related hemostatic changes result in a shift of this intrinsic balance in favor of thrombosis,[14] a factor that likely contributes to the increasing risk of acute coronary syndromes in older patients, as well as to the apparent reduced efficacy of fibrinolytic therapy in the very elderly.

CLINICAL PRESENTATIONS

Atypical symptoms and physical findings are hallmarks of clinical aging and often lead to delays in presentation while posing diagnostic and therapeutic challenges. Plausible mechanisms for these changes include altered pain sensitivity, cognitive and memory impairment, and medical comorbidities that confound symptom analysis. In conjunction with more advanced disease at the time of presentation, these issues contribute to worsened clinical outcomes for most cardiovascular conditions as age increases.

Atherosclerotic Coronary Disease

Of the approximately 2 million Americans hospitalized each year with CAD as the primary diagnosis, almost two thirds are age 65 or older.[15] Nearly 83% of people who die as a result of atherosclerotic CAD belong to this age group, and more than 60% of deaths from CAD occur in the 6% of the population 75 years of age or older. The incidence of acute myocardial infarction (MI) also increases progressively with age (Fig. 135.3).[16] Of note, in the geriatric population, the number of men and women with CAD is nearly equal, and by age 90 or older, more than two thirds of patients presenting with acute coronary syndromes are women.[17] Nonoctagenarians with CAD are less likely to have traditional CAD risk factors, such as diabetes (20% versus 34% for ages 75 to 89), hyperlipidemia (25% versus 45%), family history (15% versus 25%), recent tobacco use (2.5% versus 8.8%), or obesity (8% versus 19%).

Elderly patients with CAD frequently present without substernal chest discomfort, and the proportion of patients with acute MI who present with chest pain decreases with age.[3] Common presentations of acute coronary syndrome in older individuals include dyspnea or HF, nausea or gastrointestinal distress, presyncope or syncope, generalized malaise, fatigue, diaphoresis, or altered mental status (Fig. 135.4).[18] In patients with chronic CAD, diagnosis may be delayed because a sedentary lifestyle or limitations in functional capacity reduce the likelihood of exertional symptoms. Silent ischemia and clinically unrecognized MIs also become increasingly more common with advancing age.[19]

Although the diagnostic utility of the physical examination is limited in patients with acute coronary syndromes, older patients are more likely than younger ones to present with signs of HF or shock, and AF also is more common in the elderly. Approximately 4% to 5% of older patients have a systolic blood pressure below 90 mm Hg; 25% to 30% have tachycardia; and more than 33% have signs of HF at

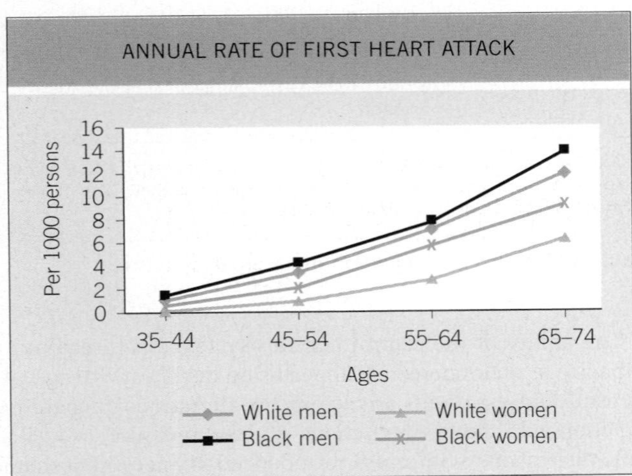

Figure 135.3 Annual rate of first heart attack. Annual rate of first heart attack by age, gender, and race in the Atherosclerosis Risk in Communities (ARIC) study, 1987 to 2000. (Data from NHLBI's ARIC surveillance study, 1987-2000.)

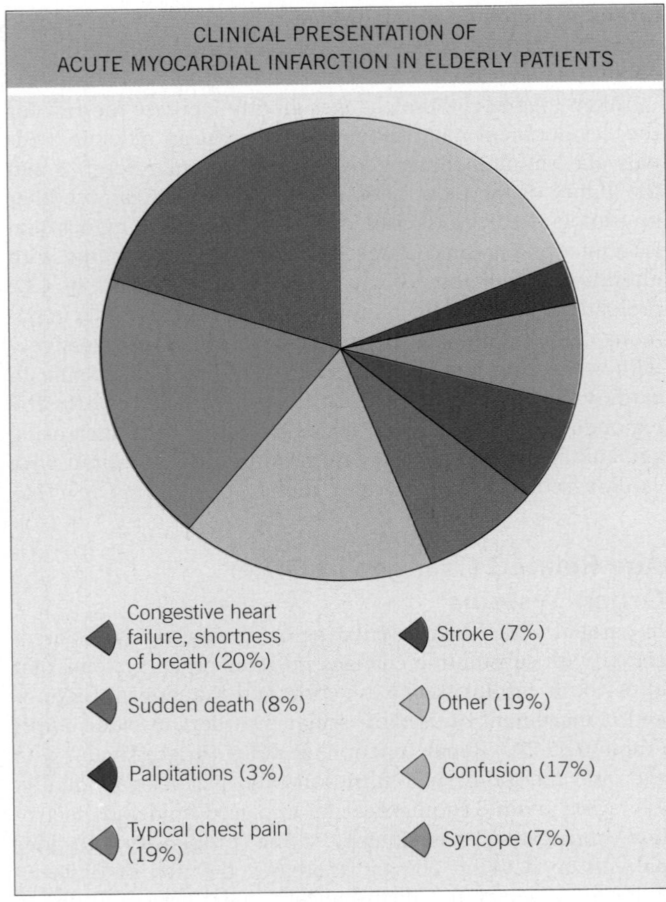

Figure 135.4 Clinical presentation of acute myocardial infarction in elderly patients. Clinical presentation of acute myocardial infarction in patients age 85 or older. (Modified from Keller NM, Feit F: Coronary artery disease in the geriatric population. Prog Cardiovasc Dis 1996;38:407-418.)

presentation (a proportion that increases to 45% in patients age 90 or older).[17] Other signs may include pallor, confusion, diaphoresis, tachycardia or bradycardia (especially with heart block), or low-grade fever.

Heart Failure

The incidence and prevalence of HF increase with age, and nearly 80% of hospitalizations for HF occur in patients age 65 or older; more than 50% occur in patients older than age 75.[15,20] In addition, HF is the most costly Medicare diagnosis-related group (DRG) in the United States by a factor of almost two. Exertional shortness of breath, orthopnea, and edema remain the most common symptoms in older patients with HF, but elderly patients often present with nonspecific complaints, such as generalized fatigue, lethargy, anorexia, bloating, gastrointestinal disturbances, or altered mental status.[21] Because older individuals tend to be more sedentary, exertional symptoms may play a less prominent role and HF may be more advanced at the time of presentation.

The physical examination findings of HF, such as an S_3 gallop, elevated jugular venous pressure, hepatojugular reflux, and bilateral pitting edema of the lower extremities, all occur less commonly in older patients with HF. Resting tachycardia also occurs less frequently because of impaired β-adrenergic responsiveness, sinus node dysfunction, and medication use (especially beta blockers). Pulmonary rales, if present, may be due to chronic lung disease or atelectasis. Peripheral edema may be due to chronic venous insufficiency, medication use (especially calcium channel blockers), poor nutrition with hypoalbuminemia, or hepatic or renal disease.

Arrhythmias and Conduction Abnormalities

Arrhythmias and conduction system disturbances increase with increasing age, and more than 85% of cardiac pacemakers and two thirds of implantable defibrillators in the United States are placed in patients age 65 or older.[3] The clinical presentation of heart rhythm disorders generally is similar in older and younger patients, except that older patients may be less tolerant of acute changes in rhythm because of their diminished cardiac reserve. More problematic is the fact that common symptoms associated with rhythm disturbances (i.e., fatigue, diminished exercise tolerance, weakness, dizziness, palpitations, and syncope) are common in older patients, and correlating symptoms with specific arrhythmias may prove challenging. Nonetheless, such correlation often is critical to the implementation of effective therapy.

Bradycardia may occur abruptly, such as during an acute inferior MI or as a result of high-degree AV block, but the clinical presentation often is gradual when related to sick sinus syndrome or hypothyroidism. Symptoms may range from life-threatening syncope to nonspecific complaints such as fatigue or decreased exercise tolerance. Tachyarrhythmias may be asymptomatic or associated with abrupt paroxysms of dizziness, palpitations, syncope, or HF; occasionally, sudden death is the initial presentation. Geriatric patients may become symptomatic upon termination of a tachyarrhythmia as a result of a prolonged pause before resumption of the baseline heart rate and rhythm (i.e., "tachy-brady syndrome").[3] Other symptoms may be related to frequent atrial or ventricular premature beats, some of which may initiate sustained arrhythmias.

AF is the most common arrhythmia in the geriatric population; the prevalence increases from fewer than 1% before age 40 to around 10% after age 80 (Fig. 135.5).[22] Patients with paroxysmal AF often are more symptomatic than those with chronic AF. They typically develop symptoms at the onset or termination of the arrhythmia that range from palpitations to chest pain, shortness of breath, or acute pulmonary edema. Older patients with paroxysmal AF are particularly prone to acute HF because of the loss of the atrial contribution to LV end-diastolic volume; this, in conjunction with a shortened diastolic filling period during tachycardia, results in an abrupt fall in cardiac output and a marked increase in left atrial pressure. Conversely, older patients with chronic AF often are less symptomatic than younger patients because of their slower ventricular response rates (as a result of slower conduction through the AV node) and decreased activity levels.

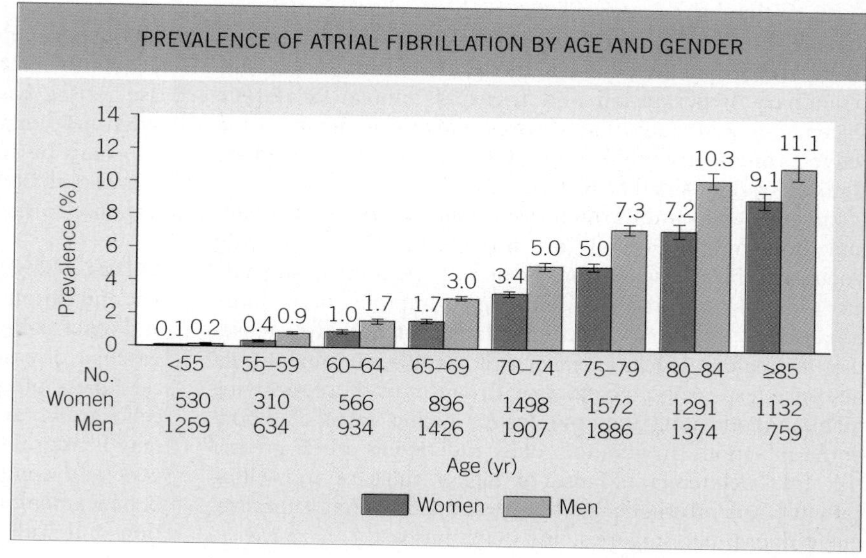

Figure 135.5 Prevalence of atrial fibrillation by age and gender. Prevalence of atrial fibrillation by age and gender in a large health maintenance organization, 1996 to 1997. (From Go AS, Hylek EM, Phillips KA, et al: Prevalence of diagnosed atrial fibrillation in adults: national implications for rhythm management and stroke prevention: the Anticoagulation and Risk Factors in Atrial Fibrillation (ATRIA) study. JAMA 2001;285:2370-2375.)

Syncope

Dizziness, falls, near-syncope, and syncope represent a spectrum of symptoms that are potentially attributable to a transient reduction in cerebral perfusion and that occur with increasing frequency at older age. Up to 30% of people age 65 or older experience an unexplained fall or syncopal episode each year[23]; the incidence rates are even higher in the very elderly and among residents in nursing homes. Older patients may be unable to provide a detailed history after a fall or syncopal event because of cognitive impairment or retrograde amnesia; therefore, establishing the etiology may be difficult. Common causes of syncope in older patients include arrhythmias, acute MI, aortic stenosis, carotid hypersensitivity, orthostatic hypotension, and vasovagal reactions. In addition, many syncopal events occur as a result of medication side effects, dehydration, postprandial hypotension, or neurologic disorders (e.g., Parkinson's disease). Notably, whereas younger patients frequently experience neurocardiogenic syncope, older individuals more commonly lose consciousness or fall as a result of structural heart disease, arrhythmias, or acute medical conditions such as pulmonary embolus.[12]

Valvular and Pericardial Diseases

Apart from differences in etiology, the clinical presentation of valvular heart disease generally is similar in older and younger patients. Aortic stenosis is the most common valvular abnormality that requires surgery in older adults.[24] As with CAD and HF, the clinical presentation may be delayed because of physical inactivity and medical comorbidities in patients with increasing age, and many cases are diagnosed in the setting of other medical illnesses or at the time of noncardiac surgery. Calcific aortic stenosis in geriatric patients often is associated with significant CAD, conduction system abnormalities, LV dysfunction, or arrhythmias.

Other valvular conditions also increase in prevalence with age. Aortic insufficiency may occur as a result of long-standing arterial hypertension, myxomatous leaflet degeneration, aortic aneurysm and dilatation, or calcific aortic valve disease.[3] Mitral annular calcification may involve the valve leaflets, but unlike with rheumatic stenosis in younger patients, calcific narrowing of the mitral orifice rarely causes severe symptoms. Mitral regurgitation may occur as a result of myxomatous degeneration or annular dilatation, but ischemic etiologies also are common in the geriatric population. Tricuspid regurgitation in elderly individuals commonly arises from progressive pulmonary hypertension and tricuspid annular dilatation. Pacemaker and defibrillator wires traversing the tricuspid valve promote tricuspid regurgitation and may exacerbate findings of right-sided heart failure.

Infective endocarditis often is subacute in older individuals, and the symptoms usually are nonspecific. Compared with younger subjects, significant fever and peripheral stigmata are less common, whereas neurologic symptoms occur more frequently.[25] Age-associated valvular degeneration increases the risk for the development of endocarditis, and immunosenescence (especially in patients with cancer or those receiving immune-modulating therapy) fosters higher rates of blood-borne infections. In addition, older individuals are at greater risk for bacteremia because of higher rates of indwelling catheters and prosthetic heart valves or pacemakers, more frequent noncardiac surgeries, and dental disease.

Diseases of the pericardium are common in older people because of the rising prevalence of predisposing conditions such as hypothyroidism, recent MI, uremia, chest malignancy or surgery, and radiation therapy. As a late complication of infectious or inflammatory pericarditis, pericardial constriction may occur in elderly patients who previously underwent heart surgery or chest irradiation.

DIAGNOSTIC TECHNIQUES

Image acquisition and interpretation of diagnostic studies in older individuals often are confounded by preexisting conditions (e.g., a previous MI) or other comorbidities (e.g., chronic lung disease). In addition, invasive studies carry a greater risk in older patients than in younger ones.

Electrocardiogram

In a large study of ambulatory geriatric patients, abnormalities of the electrocardiogram increased with age.[26] In particular, major conduction abnormalities, AV block, pathologic Q waves, LV hypertrophy, ST-segment or T-wave changes, or AF were identified in 12.4% of subjects age 65 to 69 without CAD or hypertension, versus 40.4% of similar subjects age 85 or older. The prevalence also increased with age in the cohort with known CAD or hypertension, from 30.6% at age 65 to 69 to 48.2% at age 85 or older.

Among patients with acute chest symptoms subsequently attributed to MI, 1% to 6% have a normal electrocardiogram at presentation.[27] In contrast, in a study of patients age 85 or older diagnosed with acute MI, approximately 25% had no definite acute or chronic ischemic changes on the initial electrocardiogram.[28] Despite its limitations, the electrocardiogram remains a vital component of the initial assessment of elderly patients suspected of having cardiac disease, particularly given the high prevalence of CAD and the increased frequency of atypical presentations in this population.

Stress Testing

Baseline abnormalities may confound analysis of both the electrocardiogram and the imaging portion of stress tests in geriatric patients. Diseases of the chest may prevent adequate imaging with stress echocardiography, particularly during stress-induced tachycardia. Functional capacity is lower than in younger subjects,[13] and orthopedic or pulmonary disorders frequently limit exercise tolerance. Despite these issues, exercise testing has similar diagnostic and prognostic utility in older and younger populations.[29,30] Nonischemic conditions also may be revealed, such as chronotropic incompetence, exercise-induced arrhythmias, or an abnormal blood pressure response to exercise.[31]

Echocardiography

The indications for echocardiography are similar in younger and older patients,[32] although the high prevalence of cardiovascular disease and the subacute or atypical nature of clinical illness often result in a lower threshold for performing echocardiograms in older individuals. Image acquisition may be more difficult in the elderly, but advances in transducers and computer analysis, in conjunction with contrast enhancement, have improved assessment of LV systolic function and wall motion abnormalities.[33] Optimal imaging of the heart valves (e.g., to evaluate for vegetations or severe mitral regurgitation), atrial structures, and the proximal aorta and great vessels may necessitate a transesophageal study, and selected patients with AF may require a transesophageal echocardiogram to rule out intracardiac thrombus before cardioversion.[34]

Advances in echocardiography in the past decade have greatly improved the assessment of LV diastolic function. Tissue Doppler imaging complements mitral inflow patterns for quantifying diastolic function and estimating LV filling pressures.[35,36] However, Doppler measures of LV diastolic filling change with age, independent of volume status or level of cardiovascular conditioning (Fig. 135.6).[37] Echocardiography therefore must be used in conjunction with clinical assessment in the evaluation of older patients with symptoms potentially attributable to HF.

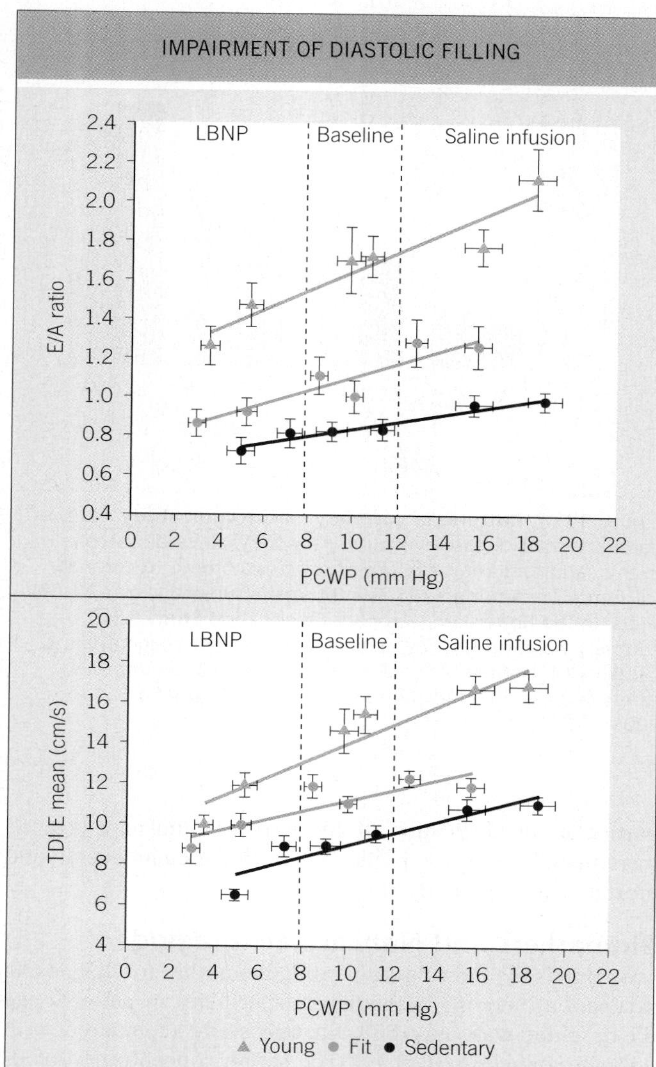

Figure 135.6 Impairment of diastolic filling. Impairment of diastolic filling across various loading conditions in young (mean age, 32) versus geriatric subjects, regardless of whether cardiovascular conditioning is present ("fit" seniors, mean age 70) or absent ("sedentary" seniors, mean age 68). E/A ratio, early to late transmitral Doppler velocity ratio; LBNP, lower body negative pressure; PCWP, pulmonary capillary wedge pressure; TDI E mean, mean early mitral annular velocity by tissue Doppler imaging. (From Prasad A, Popovic ZB, Arbab-Zadeh A, et al: The effects of aging and physical activity on Doppler measures of diastolic function. Am J Cardiol 2007;99:1629-1636.)

Ambulatory Monitoring

Recommendations for ambulatory electrocardiographic monitoring are similar in older and younger patients.[38] However, because more than two thirds of geriatric patients experience supraventricular and ventricular arrhythmias, interpretation of the ambulatory recording may be difficult, and correlation of symptoms with a specific arrhythmia may be challenging. Event-driven ambulatory monitoring may assist in the diagnosis and management of AF, including the assessment of rate control and determination of the frequency of recurrences, because asymptomatic AF is common in elderly individuals.[34]

An implantable monitor may be required to evaluate infrequent events, such as falls or syncope, if arrhythmia is suspected but not documented by external monitors.[23] In one study, an implantable monitor was diagnostic in 52% of patients with unexplained syncope, compared with a 20% yield in patients undergoing conventional testing.[39] Ambulatory blood pressure monitoring may be useful for assessing blood pressure control and in the diagnosis of dizziness and syncope.

Cardiac Catheterization

Since the late 1990s, more than 1.2 million cardiac catheterizations have been performed annually in the United States; it is the most frequently performed procedure in the Medicare population.[40,41] Most of these procedures are performed in patients 65 to 75 years of age, partly because increasing age "is generally considered to be a significant factor related to cardiovascular mortality after coronary angiography."[41] Older individuals are more likely to have tortuous or calcified arteries, which contribute to the higher rates of vascular access and embolic complications seen in elderly patients. Compared with younger patients, the risk of significant hemorrhage is threefold higher in patients age 75 or older who undergo an early invasive approach to acute coronary syndrome.[42] In addition, reduced creatinine clearance with age increases the risk for contrast nephropathy.[43,44] As a result, increasing age is associated with a marked reduction in the use of catheterization during hospitalization for an acute coronary syndrome (Table 135.3).[45] Despite these concerns, clinical trials and observational studies indicate that most older patients with acute coronary syndromes derive significant benefit from an early invasive assessment of the coronary anatomy.[42]

Electrophysiology and Tilt Table Testing

Most electrophysiologic studies are performed in patients with palpitations and potentially ablatable atrial arrhythmias or when unexplained syncope occurs in the presence of structural heart disease with a high clinical suspicion for ventricular tachycardia.[12] Complication rates rise with increasing age (3.3% in geriatric patients versus 2% in younger ones),[46] but procedural success was not affected by age in one multicenter trial of radiofrequency ablation for ventricular tachycardia.[47]

EARLY UTILIZATION OF THERAPY DURING ACUTE CORONARY SYNDROMES				
	<65 yr (%)	65-74 yr (%)	75-84 yr (%)	≥85 yr (%)
Medications				
Aspirin	93.1	90.6	89.6	88.5
Beta blocker	79.7	78.1	76.1	75.8
Any form of heparin	84.8	83.7	80.4	72.8
Clopidogrel	45.2	40.8	35.0	29.9
GP IIb/IIIa inhibitors	44.6	35.9	25.8	12.8
Procedures				
Catheterization	83.1	77.8	64.0	32.2
Cath <48 h	62.8	53.5	40.4	18.0
PCI	50.4	42.2	33.4	18.8
PCI <48 h	38.7	29.6	21.0	10.1
Bypass surgery	14.5	16.8	12.1	3.1

From Alexander KP, Roe MT, Chen AY, et al: Evolution in cardiovascular care for elderly patients with non-ST-segment elevation acute coronary syndromes: results from the CRUSADE national quality improvement initiative. J Am Coll Cardiol 2005;46:1479-1487.
GP, glycoprotein; PCI, percutaneous coronary intervention.

Table 135.3 Early medication and procedural utilization after acute coronary syndromes (among patients with no contraindications to each therapy) in the CRUSADE National Quality Improvement Initiative when stratified by age groups.

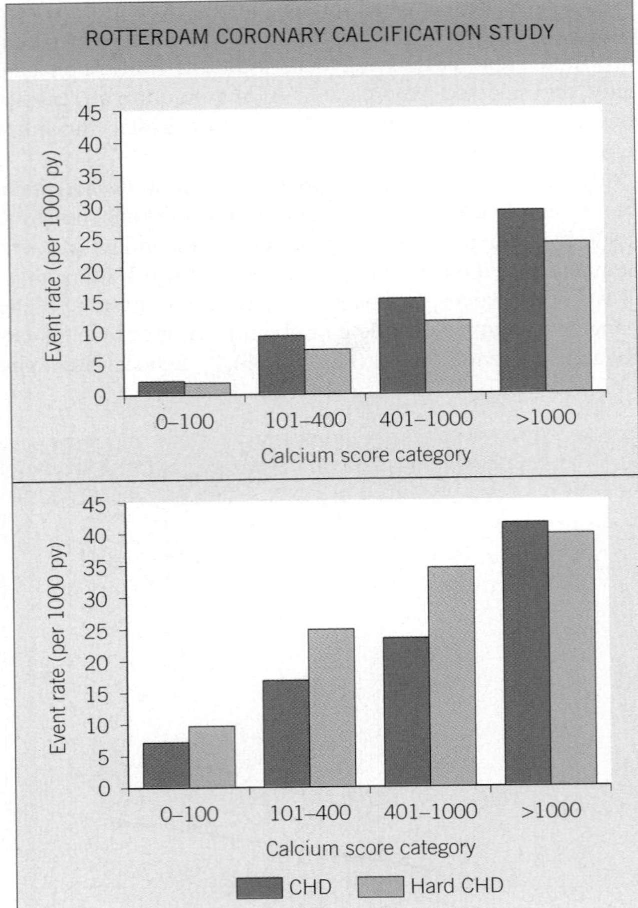

Figure 135.7 Rotterdam coronary calcification study. Rates of coronary heart disease events *(upper panel)*, all cardiovascular events, and total mortality *(lower panel)* according to coronary calcium score among 1795 asymptomatic subjects, age 62 to 85 years, in the Rotterdam Coronary Calcification Study. CHD, coronary heart disease; py, patient-years. (From Vliegenthart R, Oudkerk M, Hofman A, et al: Coronary calcification improves cardiovascular risk prediction in the elderly. Circulation 2005;112:572-577.)

Tilt table testing may be performed to diagnose neurocardiogenic syncope or to quantify orthostatic hypotension. However, national guidelines have questioned the sensitivity, specificity, diagnostic yield, and reproducibility of tilt table findings in clinical practice.[12] In one study, carefully screened elderly subjects without a previous episode of syncope or presyncope had relatively high rates of abnormal responses to head-up tilt (28%) or carotid sinus massage (13%).[48] These tests, therefore, should be used only for select elderly patients with unexplained syncope.

Other Noninvasive Cardiac Imaging Procedures

Recent advances in magnetic resonance imaging and computed tomography have allowed improved imaging of the heart and blood vessels, including the coronary arteries. However, the rapid evolution of noninvasive technology generally has outstripped clinical outcomes data in all populations, including the elderly. Published guidelines mention few, if any, age-related factors as affecting the acquisition and interpretation of these studies.[49,50] More diffuse and severe coronary calcification with increasing age may confound evaluation for luminal stenosis,[50] and other technical factors, such as breath-holding or heart rate irregularities, may adversely affect imaging in older patients. Nevertheless, these technologies may be helpful in selected geriatric patients (e.g., individuals at intermediate risk for CAD). In particular, quantification of coronary calcium may provide incremental value for predicting cardiovascular events and mortality in the elderly (Fig 135.7).[51]

Biomarkers and Noncardiac Imaging

Troponin is the most discriminating biomarker for diagnosing myocardial necrosis, although its specificity in patients age 65 or older was only 83% in one study (compared with 94% in younger patients).[52] The serum concentration of B-type natriuretic peptide increases with age, especially in women,[53,54] but retains its diagnostic utility in patients with acute dyspnea.[55] C-reactive protein provides additional risk stratification in selected patients (usually intermediate risk), including elderly individuals.[56,57] The utility of the ankle-brachial index also has been well documented in the geriatric population.[58] Other methods of risk stratification (e.g., carotid intima media thickness, brachial artery reactivity, and novel cardiac biomarkers, such as hemoglobin A_{1c}) remain inadequately studied in older patients.

MANAGEMENT

The management of geriatric patients with cardiovascular disease must be undertaken in the context of altered disease presentation and prognosis, prevalent coexisting cardiac and noncardiac conditions, and individual patient preferences. In general, medications should be started at lower dosages and titrated more gradually, and the clinician must take into consideration the potential effects of diminished renal and hepatic function and the likelihood of drug interactions with concomitant medications. The higher risks associated with invasive procedures and interventions, including cardiac catheterization and surgery, must be acknowledged, especially in frail patients older than age 80 to 85, and appropriate measures should be implemented to minimize risk whenever possible. Physicians also must keep in mind that most "standard" cardiac therapies have not been well studied in the very elderly or in patients with multiple comorbidities, therefore the indications for these treatments often are less clear-cut in these populations. As a result, a high degree of clinical judgment is essential for designing an appropriate therapeutic strategy. With these caveats in mind, indications for treatment of most cardiac conditions generally are similar in older and younger patients.

Atherosclerotic Coronary Disease

Despite the high prevalence of CAD in the geriatric population, more than half of the major clinical trials excluded older subjects, and few trials included patients older than 80 years of age.[18] In the absence of robust evidence from clinical trials, current guidelines recommend the use of "therapeutic interventions in a similar manner as younger patients," with management decisions also taking into consideration an elderly individual's "general health, functional and cognitive status, comorbidities, life expectancy, and patient preferences and goals."[27] In clinical practice, the use of all pharmacologic and mechanical interventions for CAD declines with advancing age (see Table 135.3), even though adherence to guidelines is associated with improved clinical outcomes, including in patients older than age 90.[17,45]

Antiplatelet Therapy

The absolute 35-day mortality benefit of aspirin in acute MI increases with age, from 1% in patients younger than age 60 to 4.7% for those age 70 or older.[59] The addition of clopidogrel to aspirin improves cardiovascular outcomes in patients with non-ST-elevation acute coronary syndromes who are older than 65 years of age, but the risk of bleeding complications is higher, and the value of clopidogrel in patients older than 75 years of age is unproven.[60] Few studies of glycoprotein IIb/IIIa inhibitors have enrolled subjects older than age 75, but both clinical trials and observational studies suggest higher bleeding risks with fewer benefits in elderly patients[61,62]; these agents, therefore, should be used judiciously in the geriatric population.

Antithrombotic Therapy

The risk of bleeding with heparin therapy increases with age,[63] which in part may reflect excessive dosing in the elderly.[64] In one study of Medicare beneficiaries with acute MI, patients receiving heparin derived no mortality benefit but had more bleeding complications and required more transfusions than patients who did not receive heparin.[65] Older patients also are at increased risk for bleeding with low-molecular-weight heparins (LMWHs) partly because of age-related decline in renal function. In addition, the effects of LMWHs on cardiovascular endpoints in elderly patients have been mixed, with some studies showing benefit relative to unfractionated heparin, whereas other studies show no benefit.[66]

Beta Blockers

The value of intravenous beta-blocker therapy in acute MI recently has been questioned, because higher rates of cardiogenic shock have been demonstrated during the first 24 hours of treatment,[67] and patients older than age 70 are significantly more likely to experience adverse outcomes than younger patients. Conversely, a meta-analysis of intravenous beta-blocker trials restricted to patients at low risk for cardiogenic shock found significant benefits from early treatment.[68] Therefore, intravenous beta blockers remain an important component of therapy in carefully selected patients with acute MI, including the elderly.

In the absence of contraindications, long-term treatment with a beta blocker is recommended for all patients after acute MI. An observational analysis of Medicare patients demonstrated relative risk reductions with administration of a beta blocker in patients age 65 to 74 (16% reduction), 75 to 84 (21%), and 85 or older (13%).[68] In a pooled analysis, chronic beta-blocker therapy was associated with 6 lives saved per 100 older patients treated, versus only 2.1 lives saved per 100 younger patients.[3] Therefore, advanced age is not a contraindication to beta-blocker therapy, although close attention to dosing is required to minimize the risk of side effects.

Angiotensin and Aldosterone Inhibitors

Intravenous angiotensin-converting enzyme (ACE) inhibitor therapy has been associated with increased hypotension in patients with acute MI,[69] and routine treatment with an oral ACE inhibitor within 24 hours of MI presentation did not reduce mortality in patients age 70 or older enrolled in two large trials.[68] Nonetheless, lisinopril had a beneficial effect on the 6-month composite outcome of death or severe LV dysfunction in one of these studies.[70] Treatment with an oral ACE inhibitor, beginning 2 to 16 days after acute MI, in patients with clinical HF or decreased LV systolic function (ejection fraction $\leq$40%) reduces mortality during long-term follow-up, and the benefits are at least as great in patients older than age 65.[68] Although few subjects age 75 or older were enrolled in these trials, a retrospective analysis of more than 14,000 Medicare patients with MI found that prescription of an ACE inhibitor at hospital discharge was associated with improved survival in patients 65 to 80 years of age, as well as in those age 80 or older.[71]

Angiotensin receptor blockers (ARBs) are acceptable alternatives for patients intolerant to ACE inhibitors because of cough; the risks of hyperkalemia and worsening renal function are similar for the two classes of drugs and higher in the elderly. Combination therapy with an ACE inhibitor and an ARB after acute MI is associated with an increased risk of side effects without improvement in outcomes and therefore is not recommended in older patients. The selective aldosterone antagonist eplerenone has been associated with improved outcomes after acute MI in patients with a decreased LV ejection fraction and concomitant HF or diabetes, but benefits are limited to patients younger than 65 years of age. Because the risk of hyperkalemia with this agent is significantly higher in older patients, use of eplerenone after acute MI is not recommended.[68]

Statins

An observational study of Medicare beneficiaries with acute MI demonstrated that statin therapy at hospital discharge improved outcomes in patients age 65 to 79 but not in those older than age 80.[72] However, in a randomized, controlled trial involving subjects age 70 to 82 with known vascular disease or significant risk factors for CAD, statin therapy was associated with a 15% reduction in MI, stroke, or cardiovascular mortality.[73] Other studies also support the use of statins in elderly subjects with CAD, including individuals with a low-density lipoprotein (LDL) cholesterol equal to or less than 125 mg/dL.[68,74] As are other medications, statins are associated with higher rates of side effects in older patients.

Other Medications

Nitrates have not been shown to reduce mortality after an acute MI, but in one trial, the subgroup of patients age 70 or older experienced a reduction in the combined endpoint of death, HF, or severe LV dysfunction with transdermal nitroglycerin.[70] Calcium channel blockers may be used as adjunctive therapy to treat persistent ischemia, hypertension, or AF in patients with acute MI, but side effects such as hypotension and bradycardia are more common in the elderly.

Reperfusion in ST-Elevation Myocardial Infarction

The role of fibrinolytic therapy in the treatment of ST-elevation MI in the very elderly remains controversial. A meta-analysis of clinical trials found that the absolute mortality benefit of fibrinolytic therapy relative to placebo for an individual older than 75 years of age was three times higher than for a patient younger than age 55.[68] Conversely, the risk of intracranial hemorrhage in patients undergoing fibrinolysis increases progressively with age, with an absolute risk of 1% to 2% in patients older than age 75.[3] In addition, several observational studies have questioned the benefits of fibrinolytic therapy in the very elderly. In one large registry, fibrinolysis was associated with decreased mortality in patients age 65 to 75 but with increased mortality in those older than age 75.[75] Based on these findings, careful selection of very elderly patients is of paramount importance. The risk/benefit ratio is most favorable when treatment is initiated within 6 hours of the onset of ischemia and the risk of major hemorrhage is low. Lower doses of anticoagulants should be used, and glycoprotein IIb/IIIa inhibitors should be avoided in elderly patients receiving fibrinolytic therapy.[68]

When initiated in a timely fashion (i.e., a "door to balloon" time of less than 90 to 120 minutes), percutaneous coronary intervention (PCI) is superior to fibrinolysis for ST-elevation MI in the geriatric population, although very limited data are available in patients older than age 85. In the largest trial to date comparing primary PCI with fibrinolysis in older patients, PCI was associated with a significant reduction in the combination of death, stroke, or reinfarction relative to fibrinolytic therapy (11.6% versus 18%).[76] The risk of hemorrhagic stroke is substantially lower with PCI than with fibrinolysis,[68] although the overall risk of bleeding is higher with PCI because of hemorrhagic complications at the arteriotomy site. Older patients also are at increased risk for worsening renal function from contrast nephropathy, and efforts should be made to minimize this risk whenever possible. Overall, pooled analyses indicate that the number of older patients who need to be treated with PCI relative to fibrinolytic therapy to save one life is about eight, compared with 23 patients younger than age 60.[68]

In patients with MI complicated by cardiogenic shock, routine early revascularization did not improve outcomes in subjects age 75 or older in a small subgroup ($n = 56$) of a clinical trial.[77] However, survival rates were significantly higher in elderly patients enrolled in the registry component of the trial who underwent early PCI.[78] These data suggest that carefully selected elderly individuals with cardiogenic shock may benefit from early revascularization, but use of an invasive therapeutic approach must be individualized.

Reperfusion for Non-ST-Elevation Acute Coronary Syndromes

Several large trials have compared PCI with medical management in non-ST-elevation acute coronary syndromes, but most of these were conducted before the advent of intracoronary stents and intensive antiplatelet regimens (i.e., clopidogrel, glycoprotein IIb/IIIa inhibitors). In addition, enrollment of elderly subjects in these trials was limited. Nonetheless, the available evidence suggests that an early invasive approach is associated with improved clinical outcomes in older patients.[66] In the trial with the largest number of older individuals, a strong interaction with age was seen, such that the combination of death or recurrent MI was reduced more significantly with early PCI in older than in younger patients (Fig. 135.8).[79] The number needed to treat with PCI to prevent one death or MI was 250 for patients younger than age 65, 21 for patients age 65 or older, and 9 for patients age 75 or older. Therefore, although complications from invasive therapy are higher in the elderly, early PCI appears to be beneficial in appropriately selected geriatric patients with non-ST-elevation acute coronary syndromes.

Chronic Coronary Artery Disease and Secondary Prevention

Management of geriatric patients with chronic CAD generally follows the recommendations for younger individuals, including aggressive control of blood pressure, lipids, and diabetes in conjunction with lifestyle modifications appropriate for secondary prevention of ischemic events (i.e., smoking cessation, regular exercise, weight loss if indicated).[80] Aspirin, statins, beta blockers, and ACE inhibitors should be prescribed in the absence of contraindications. Clopidogrel is recommended for at least 3 to 6 months after PCI and for 1 year after an acute coronary syndrome or placement of a drug-eluting stent. Cardiac rehabilitation reduces mortality and improves exercise capacity and quality of life

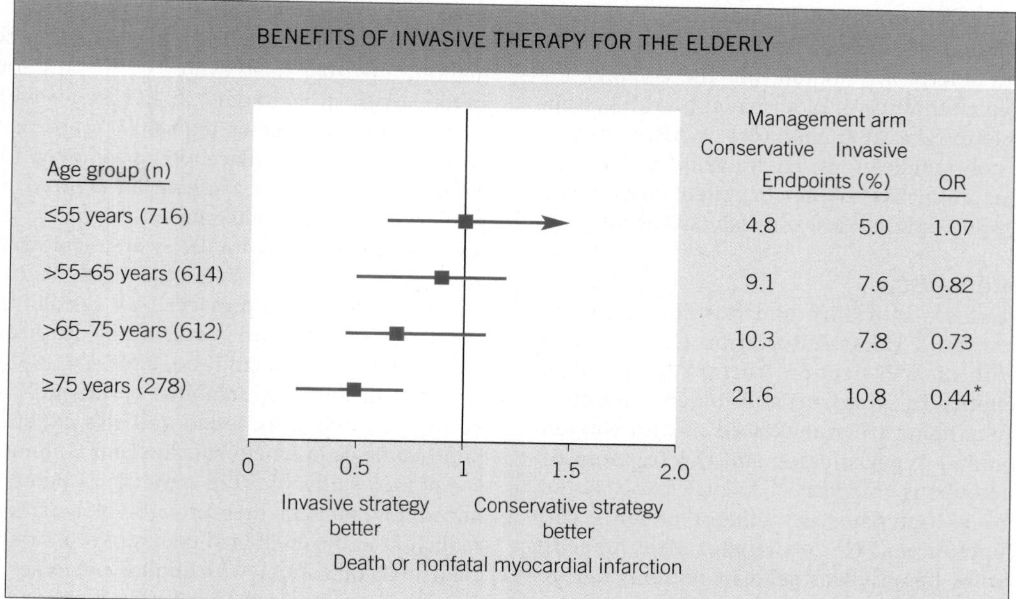

Figure 135.8 Benefits of invasive therapy for the elderly. Benefits of invasive therapy for elderly subjects with non-ST-elevation acute coronary syndromes enrolled in the TACTICS-TIMI 18 trial. (From Bach RG, Cannon CP, Weintraub WS, et al: The effect of routine, early invasive management on outcome for elderly patients with non-ST-segment elevation acute coronary syndromes. Ann Intern Med 2004;141:186-195.)

in elderly patients after an MI or bypass surgery,[81] yet referral rates for cardiac rehabilitation decline markedly with age.[82] Annual influenza vaccination is recommended for all geriatric individuals, and pneumonia vaccination also is indicated.

Beta blockers, calcium channel blockers, and nitrates are standard therapy for the treatment of chronic angina pectoris in younger and older patients. Ranolazine reduces the frequency and severity of angina when added to conventional therapy, although side effects such as syncope and dizziness are more common in elderly subjects receiving higher doses.[83] Enhanced external counterpulsation (EECP) may be an option for refractory angina in select individuals.[84]

Coronary revascularization using PCI or bypass surgery reduces symptoms and improves quality of life in geriatric patients, although the effect on mortality is unclear.[85,86] Complication rates generally are higher in the elderly; in-hospital mortality rates for octogenarians undergoing elective PCI or isolated bypass surgery are approximately 3% to 4% and 7% to 10%, respectively.[3] Despite these risks, clinical outcomes after PCI and bypass surgery are quite favorable in geriatric individuals, even those older than age 80.[87]

Heart Failure

HF is the prototypical disorder of cardiovascular aging, reflecting the convergence of age-related changes in cardiovascular structure and function with the rising prevalence of age-associated diseases that predispose to the development of HF (e.g., hypertension and CAD). Once a diagnosis of HF has been established, the primary goals of treatment are to alleviate symptoms, maximize functional capacity and quality of life, reduce the risk of acute exacerbations, and improve survival. In contrast to younger patients, HF in the elderly often is multifactorial. Optimal management involves treatment of underlying disease processes, as well as identification of other factors contributing to exacerbations, such as nonadherence to medications, excess sodium or fluid consumption, or concomitant illness (e.g., ischemia, pneumonia, AF). Concurrently, a therapeutic regimen should be implemented to improve the prognosis by restoring hemodynamic stability and euvolemia, reducing the progression of HF symptoms, and stabilizing or reversing cardiac or valvular dysfunction.

Beta Blockers

Beta blockers reduce hospitalizations and improve survival in elderly patients with systolic HF, including patients older than age 80.[88,89] Older patients are more susceptible to hypotension, bradycardia, and orthostasis; dose titration, therefore, must be gradual, and side effects may limit dose escalation.

Angiotensin-Converting Enzyme Inhibitors and Angiotensin Receptor Blockers

ACE inhibitors reduce hospitalizations and mortality by 25% to 30% in patients with systolic HF. They have similar effects in younger and older patients, but the benefits are attenuated in patients older than age 75.[90] Adverse drug effects, such as cough, hypotension, renal insufficiency, and hyperkalemia, may limit use in the geriatric population, but individuals treated with ACE inhibitors at doses studied in clinical trials experience improved clinical outcomes.[20] As in younger patients, ARBs are acceptable substitutes in elderly individuals who are allergic or intolerant to ACE inhibitors.

Other Oral Vasodilators

The combination of hydralazine and nitrates improves survival in systolic HF but to a lesser degree than ACE inhibitors. This combination also has been associated with improved outcomes when added to standard therapy (including ACE inhibitors) in middle-aged African Americans with systolic HF.[20] Data in the elderly are limited, but the combination offers a reasonable alternative in older patients with systolic HF who are unable to take ACE inhibitors or ARBs because of side effects or contraindications. Hydralazine and nitrates also may be used as adjunctive therapy in patients with persistent symptoms despite optimal doses of standard agents.

Aldosterone Antagonists

Spironolactone reduces mortality and hospitalizations in patients with New York Heart Association class III or IV HF and those with an LV ejection fraction below 30%, with similar benefits in younger and older patients.[91] However, elderly patients are at increased risk for worsening renal function and hyperkalemia, and careful monitoring of these parameters is essential.[92] As previously noted, eplerenone improves outcomes in younger patients with LV systolic dysfunction and HF or diabetes after an acute MI, but no apparent benefit was seen in patients age 65 or older.[68]

Diuretics

Diuretics are the most effective agents for restoring and maintaining euvolemia in patients with acute decompensated or chronic HF, although loop diuretics have not been shown to improve survival. In addition, older patients are at increased risk for diuretic-induced dehydration, worsening renal function, and electrolyte disturbances such as hyponatremia and hypokalemia.[3] Therefore, diuretics should be used judiciously and at the lowest effective dose in older patients to minimize the risk of adverse effects.[20] Patients resistant to standard doses of loop diuretics may require the addition of metolazone to enhance diuresis, but electrolytes should be monitored very closely when this combination is used in elderly individuals.

Digoxin

Digoxin has no effect on total mortality but reduces HF mortality and hospitalizations, with similar effects in younger and older patients.[93] Recent retrospective analyses suggest that total mortality may be reduced when serum digoxin levels are less than 1.0 ng/mL,[94] although these findings have not yet been confirmed in prospective studies. Low-dose digoxin, therefore, is a reasonable option for elderly HF patients with persistent symptoms, but careful monitoring is warranted because polypharmacy and renal dysfunction increase the risk of adverse drug effects.

Intravenous Infusions

Inotropic agents, such as dobutamine, dopamine, and milrinone, are associated with higher mortality rates and are recommended only for short-term treatment of patients with severe decompensated HF.[3,20] Nesiritide (recombinant B-type natriuretic peptide) reduces filling pressures more effectively than intravenous nitroglycerin in patients with acute decompensated HF, but the clinical outcomes for the two agents are similar. Nesiritide may precipitate hypotension or worsening renal function, especially in patients with preexisting renal impairment; therefore this drug should be used with caution in elderly patients.[95]

Diastolic Heart Failure

Despite the high prevalence of diastolic HF in the geriatric population, few trials have evaluated therapy for these patients. In the largest study to date, 3023 patients with HF and an LV ejection fraction greater than 40% were randomized to the ARB candesartan or placebo and followed for an average of 37 months. Although candesartan showed no effect on the primary composite outcome of mortality or hospitalization for HF, readmissions for HF were significantly reduced, by approximately 18%.[96] In another study involving 850 elderly patients with HF and preserved LV systolic function, a strong trend was seen toward reduction of death or hospitalization for HF at 1 year (hazard ratio, 0.69; $P = .055$) in patients randomized to the ACE inhibitor perindopril versus placebo.[97] Patients treated with perindopril also experienced significant improvements in functional class and 6-minute walk distance.

Another study of 2128 geriatric patients with HF randomized to the beta blocker nebivolol demonstrated a 14% reduction in the combined endpoint of mortality or cardiovascular hospitalization, with similar outcomes in subjects with preserved or impaired LV systolic function.[98] In the Digitalis Investigation Group (DIG) ancillary study, among 988 patients with HF and an LV ejection fraction equal to or greater than 45%, digoxin therapy for a mean of 37 months was associated with reduced hospitalizations for HF, but a commensurate increase in hospitalizations for unstable angina was seen, along with no effect on total mortality.[99]

In summary, several HF therapies appear to reduce hospitalizations for HF in elderly patients with diastolic heart failure, but no trials to date have demonstrated a reduction in mortality. Consequently, optimal management of patients with diastolic HF remains undefined. Current recommendations for the management of diastolic HF include aggressive treatment of underlying etiologies, such as hypertension and ischemia.[20] Diuretics should be administered to maintain euvolemia, but overdiuresis should be avoided to prevent prerenal azotemia and worsening renal function. A beta blocker should be prescribed for patients with CAD, and an ACE inhibitor or ARB is indicated for patients with atherosclerotic disease, renal dysfunction, or diabetes. The role of other agents in the management of diastolic HF awaits the results of future studies.

Nonpharmacologic Therapies

Management of HF in the elderly frequently is complicated by the presence of multiple comorbid conditions, cognitive dysfunction, impaired mobility, sensory deficits, and limited finances. Multidisciplinary management programs for HF disease that provide comprehensive care and close follow-up have been shown to reduce hospitalizations and improve quality of life in older patients with HF; in some settings, mortality and the cost of care also may be reduced.[20]

Dietary counseling is indicated for all patients with HF, emphasizing sodium restriction and avoidance of excess fluid intake. Regular exercise is recommended but should be tailored to each individual's functional capacity and limitations (e.g., caused by arthritis or neurologic conditions).

The patient should be provided with a complete list of medications to be taken, along with explicit instructions about when to take each medication and the importance of adhering to the medication regimen and dietary restrictions.

Biventricular pacing improves symptoms and exercise tolerance in patients with New York Heart Association class III to IV HF, an LV ejection fraction less than 30% to 35%, and wide QRS morphology (especially left bundle branch block). Benefits are similar in younger and older patients, and meta-analysis data suggest that this therapy is associated with improved survival.[100] Based on these findings, biventricular pacing is a suitable option in appropriately selected elderly patients with refractory HF symptoms despite intensive medical therapy.

Implantable cardioverter-defibrillators (ICDs) reduce mortality caused by ventricular tachyarrhythmias in patients with New York Heart Association class II to III HF and an LV ejection fraction less than 30% to 35%,[101,102] and the mortality benefit is similar in older and younger patients. However, the role of ICDs for primary prevention of sudden cardiac death in the very elderly remains controversial, partly because no mortality benefit is seen within the first 12 to 18 months after ICD implantation, and the overall effect on survival is modest. In addition, ICD shocks adversely affect quality of life, an important consideration for many elderly patients with HF. Therefore, although advanced age is not a contraindication to ICD therapy, patient selection is of paramount importance, because elderly patients with limited life expectancy are unlikely to benefit from this treatment. Disabling of the device to prevent recurrent, painful ICD shocks during the last days or weeks of life also should be discussed.

Ventricular-assist devices and heart transplantation are not usually recommended for elderly patients with HF. However, newer devices that are implanted percutaneously or with minimally invasive procedures may expand the role of device therapy in selected older patients with advanced HF.

Arrhythmias and Conduction Disorders

Management of symptomatic bradycardia begins with a careful evaluation for treatable causes, such as medications, ischemia, hypothyroidism, or electrolyte abnormalities. Dose reduction or discontinuation of beta blockers, non-dihydropyridine calcium channel blockers, digoxin, and antiarrhythmic drugs may be required. Pacemaker implantation is recommended in symptomatic patients without a reversible etiology and in patients requiring bradycardia-inducing therapy for other conditions (e.g., beta blockers for angina or HF).[103] In one trial, dual-chamber pacing for sick sinus syndrome was associated with a lower risk for the development of AF or requiring hospitalization, compared with single-chamber pacing, although mortality was not affected, and subjects older than age 75 derived less benefit.[104]

The treatment of supraventricular and ventricular tachyarrhythmias is similar for older and younger patients, although elderly patients are more likely to experience symptomatic bradycardia from pharmacologic therapies (i.e., tachy-brady syndrome). Metabolic and electrolyte abnormalities should be corrected, and underlying cardiac and noncardiac conditions should be treated appropriately. Mechanical interventions, including ablation procedures and implantable devices, should be considered in accordance with current guidelines.

In elderly patients with paroxysmal or chronic AF who are asymptomatic or mildly symptomatic, rate control in combination with warfarin is associated with equivalent or better outcomes than a strategy aimed at maintaining normal sinus rhythm with antiarrhythmic drugs.[34] Effective rate control may be complicated by symptomatic bradycardia requiring pacemaker implantation in some patients. Moderate or severe symptoms that fail to respond to medical therapy alone may require catheter-based ablation or the surgical "maze" procedure. AV node ablation with permanent pacemaker implantation often is effective in reducing symptoms and improving quality of life in elderly patients with AF unresponsive to AV nodal–blocking agents; however, the procedure does not obviate the need for lifelong antithrombotic therapy. Although pulmonary vein isolation is effective in selected younger patients with paroxysmal AF, limited data are available on the safety and efficacy of this procedure in elderly patients.

Advanced age is a major risk factor for stroke in patients with AF,[105] and the proportion of strokes attributable to AF increases with age. For example, in the Framingham Heart Study, AF accounted for 1.5% of strokes among subjects in their 50s, compared with 23.5% for subjects in their 80s.[34] In addition, older patients often have concomitant risk factors for stroke, such as a previous stroke, structural or valvular heart disease, hypertension, diabetes, or HF. Clinical trials of anticoagulation for stroke prevention demonstrate significant benefit with warfarin therapy for patients age 65 or older, but few subjects older than age 85 have been studied. Although the risk of bleeding also increases with age, the beneficial effect of warfarin in preventing strokes consistently outweighs the potential risk of bleeding. Therefore, warfarin is recommended for stroke prophylaxis in older patients with AF or atrial flutter. For patients with major contraindications to warfarin, aspirin is a reasonable but less effective alternative.

Postoperative AF occurs in nearly one third of older individuals undergoing major cardiac surgery, resulting in a longer hospital stay and higher costs. Increasing age is the strongest predictor of postoperative AF (Table 135.4),[106] such that patients older than age 70 should be considered at high risk for AF after coronary bypass or other cardiac operations. Perioperative beta-blocker therapy reduces the risk, and clinical trials have shown lower rates of AF with perioperative administration of sotalol, amiodarone, non-dihydropyridine calcium channel blockers, and magnesium sulfate and biatrial pacing.[107] Prevention of AF is associated with shorter intensive care and in-patient hospitalization requirements, but a reduction in mortality has not been demonstrated.

Syncope

Compared with younger patients, syncope in older patients is more likely to be cardiac in origin and carries a worse prognosis. In addition, syncope remains unexplained in approximately 40% of cases even after an appropriate diagnostic evaluation.[12] When a reversible etiology is not identified, supportive care with compression stockings and maintenance of hydration may reduce symptoms and falls. Some elderly individuals require sodium supplementation or fludrocortisone to maintain intravascular volume, and midodrine may be effective in patients with chronic orthostatic hypotension. Indications for pacemakers and other devices are similar in older and younger patients presenting with syncope.

PREDICTORS OF ATRIAL FIBRILLATION AFTER BYPASS SURGERY			
Predictor	**Incidence (%)**	**Odds Ratio**	**Risk Score***
Age <30 yr	0	1.75†	6
30-39	5.6		12
40-49	8.3		18
50-59	20.1		24
60-69	33.0		30
70-79	46.1		36
≥80	58.8		42
Previous atrial fibrillation	53.0	2.11	7
Chronic obstructive lung disease	42.8	1.43	4
Concurrent valve surgery	53.9	1.74	6
Withdrawal of beta blockers	50.5	1.91	6
Withdrawal of ACE-I	46.2	1.69	5
Preoperative and postoperative beta blocker Rx	17.7	0.49	−7
Preoperative and postoperative ACE-I Rx	20.1	0.62	−5
Postoperative beta blocker Rx	17.7	0.32	−11
Potassium supplementation Rx	28.8	0.53	−5
NSAID Rx	18.5	0.49	−7

*The risk of postoperative atrial fibrillation is calculated from the summation of risk scores for an individual patient; a combined score <14 indicates a 10% to 13% risk; a score of 14-31 indicates a 28% to 32% risk; and a score >31 indicates a 60% to 65% risk.

†Odds ratio for each 10-year increment of age.

Modified from Mathew JP, Fontes ML, Tudor IC, et al: A multicenter risk index for atrial fibrillation after cardiac surgery. JAMA 2004;291:1720-1729.

ACE-I, angiotensin-converting enzyme inhibitor; NSAID, nonsteroidal anti-inflammatory drug.

Table 135.4 Multivariable predictors of postoperative atrial fibrillation, odds ratios, and calculated risk scores in a multinational registry of patients undergoing coronary bypass surgery.

Valvular Heart Disease

Because older patients have a reduced activity level, symptoms from valvular abnormalities often are atypical or occur later in the course of disease. Associated medical comorbidities frequently increase the perioperative risk, and many complications arise in geriatric patients during the recovery phase rather than at the time of surgery (e.g., ileus, infectious colitis, prolonged deconditioning). Coronary angiography generally is recommended before valve surgery in older individuals, and concurrent coronary bypass procedures increase complication rates relative to isolated bypass or valve surgery.[24] Despite these risks, elderly individuals who undergo elective valve surgery generally have a good prognosis. Quality of life is improved after aortic valve replacement for severe aortic stenosis, and long-term survival is excellent, even for patients older than age 80.[3] Bioprosthetic valves are preferred in the geriatric population, because the long-term durability of these valves is very good and lifelong anticoagulation is unnecessary. Percutaneous aortic valve replacement currently is under investigation and may provide a suitable option for selected elderly patients in the near future.

The management of acute or chronic aortic insufficiency is similar in younger and older patients, and therapy should be implemented in accordance with current guidelines.[24] The operative mortality for aortic valve replacement in older patients with aortic insufficiency is approximately 5%, with improved long-term outcomes demonstrated in observational studies. Vasodilator therapy is indicated for elderly subjects with symptomatic aortic insufficiency, although treatment may be limited by hypotension or organ hypoperfusion.

The use of diuretics in elderly patients with mitral stenosis may be limited by renal insufficiency or hypotension.[24] In addition, elderly patients often are unsuitable candidates for mitral valvuloplasty because of heavy annular calcification, leaflet thickening, or concomitant mitral regurgitation. As a result, most geriatric patients with severe, symptomatic mitral stenosis are best served with surgical valve repair or replacement. The operative mortality after mitral valve replacement in older patients ranges from 5% to 15%, and postoperative AF is a common complication.[107]

Management of mitral regurgitation is similar in older and younger patients. Medical therapy has not been shown to reduce the progression of symptoms or to improve the prognosis.[24] Although most mitral valve surgeries in the United States are performed in the Medicare population, the operative mortality increases after age 75 and exceeds 14% with mitral valve replacement in this age group; the decision to undertake mitral valve replacement, therefore, must be considered carefully in elderly individuals. Mitral valve repair is associated with more favorable outcomes and is preferred when feasible.

Infective endocarditis in older patients often presents at a more advanced stage with more atypical symptoms, especially HF. Although the indications for surgery in younger and older patients with endocarditis are similar, surgery in the elderly is associated with higher complication rates and lower success rates. Hospitalization is significantly longer for geriatric individuals with endocarditis, and the mortality rate is close to 30%, approximately twice the rate in younger patients.[25]

PROGNOSIS

The prognosis for nearly every cardiac condition worsens with increasing age because of a combination of diminished cardiovascular reserve, more advanced disease, increased comorbidity, and higher complication rates. Mortality rates for atherosclerotic CAD, acute MI, and HF increase exponentially with age (Table 135.5).[108,109] Similarly, mortality rates after PCI, bypass surgery, and valve surgery all increase progressively with age, especially after age 80. In addition, complication rates after these procedures are substantially higher in elderly patients.

Age (yr)	CHD*	MI*	HF†
MORTALITY RATES FOR CHD, MI, AND HF IN THE UNITED STATES			
65-74	487.2	237.7	32.2
75-84	1252.2	554.6	130.8
≥85	3743.9	1382.4	633.5

From Centers for Disease Control and Prevention: Changes in mortality from heart failure: United States, 1980-1995. Available at http://www.cdc.gov/MMWR/preview/mmwrhtml/00054249.htm. Accessed 3/15/2009; and Centers for Disease Control and Prevention: Mortality from coronary heart disease and acute myocardial infarction: United States, 1998. Available at http://www.cdc.gov/MMWR/preview/mmwrhtml/mm5006a2.htm. Accessed 3/15/2009.

*1998.

†1995.

CHD, coronary heart disease, MI, acute myocardial infarction; HF, heart failure.

Table 135.5 Age-specific mortality rates per 100,000 population for coronary heart disease, acute myocardial infarction, and heart failure among age subgroups in the U.S. geriatric population.

In addition to age, other factors associated with a worse prognosis in older patients include the number and severity of comorbid illnesses. Chronic kidney disease, pulmonary disease, diabetes, peripheral arterial disease, cerebrovascular disease, and cognitive impairment consistently have been shown to be associated with a poor prognosis in elderly patients with cardiovascular disease. Frailty, depression, and poor social support also have been associated with adverse outcomes in elderly patients, whereas anemia has been associated with worse outcomes in some but not all studies.

Women tend to have a worse prognosis than men after acute MI, PCI, or bypass surgery, but a somewhat more favorable prognosis with chronic HF (partly because HF in older women is more likely to be nonischemic and associated with preserved LV systolic function). Nonetheless, 5-year survival rates in elderly men and women with HF are only 20% to 25%, compared with up to 50% in younger patients.[110]

SUMMARY

Normal aging is associated with diffuse structural and functional changes throughout the heart and vascular tree, and these changes contribute to a progressive rise in the incidence and prevalence of cardiovascular disease with increasing age. As a result, cardiovascular disease is a major cause of morbidity and mortality in the geriatric population, and the prognosis is less favorable compared with younger patients. In addition, older patients often present with atypical features and more advanced disease at the time of diagnosis. Diagnostic and therapeutic options are less well studied in older individuals, and medical comorbidities and other factors (e.g., polypharmacy, hearing or vision loss, and memory changes) may influence both the choice and effectiveness of therapy. Care, therefore, must be individualized based on a patient's unique set of medical problems, psychosocial milieu, degree of frailty, functional status, and personal preferences. In light of the progressive aging of our population, considerable research is needed to develop more effective strategies for the prevention and treatment of cardiovascular disease in older people.

chapter 136

Pregnancy in the Heart Disease Patient

Laura J. Collins and Pamela S. Douglas

Definition

- Approximately 1% of pregnancies per year in the United States are complicated by preexisting cardiovascular disease.

Key Features

- The hemodynamic changes associated with pregnancy are well tolerated by women with a normal cardiovascular system.
- Pregnancy poses the highest maternal and fetal morbidity and mortality for patients with significant obstructive valvular lesions, pulmonary hypertension, significant pathology of the thoracic aorta (dilatation or uncorrected coarctation), New York Heart Association class III or IV heart failure, or uncontrolled hypertension.

Therapy

- As a rule, a spontaneous vaginal delivery is preferable for most patients with cardiac disease.
- Venous thromboembolic disease remains the leading cause of maternal mortality, but no consensus has been reached as to which patients benefit from prophylaxis.
- Pregnancy-induced hypertension and pre-eclampsia complicate 8% to 10% of all pregnancies. Early parturition and medical control of severe hypertension remain the treatments of choice.

Preexisting maternal heart disease or hypertension is estimated to complicate up to 10% of pregnancies. To put this in better perspective, that is approximately 400,000 pregnancies in the United States each year (based on an annual birth rate of just over 4 million).[1] Pregnancy in patients with congenital heart disease will be encountered more frequently in the future, owing to the increased survival of children with these conditions into the reproductive years (85% now live to adulthood).[2] Although many patients with known heart disease or hypertension already are under the care of a cardiologist or other physician before their pregnancy, many experience the initial presentation during pregnancy and may require a more rapid diagnostic assessment and treatment plan. The obstetrician or family practitioner must remain vigilant and must suspect heart disease early in pregnancy in such patients, because in many cases, the lives of both the mother and the fetus depend on prompt diagnosis and early prenatal care.

PATHOPHYSIOLOGY

Effects of Pregnancy on the Normal Cardiovascular System

Pregnancy in a woman with a normal cardiovascular system imposes hemodynamic changes that generally are well tolerated. Blood volume increases by an average of 50%, with most of the increase occurring within the first trimester of pregnancy. This volume overload induces a mild dilatation of all the cardiac chambers; it resembles the physiologic process that occurs in the athletic heart, which helps to meet increased demand. Concurrently, cardiac output increases by 30% to 50%, mostly because of an increase in stroke volume, with a smaller contribution from an increase in the heart rate (by 10 beats per minute [bpm]) (Fig. 136.1). Although red cell volume also increases, the rise in plasma volume is greater, resulting in the physiologic anemia of pregnancy.

Pregnancy also alters components of the fibrinolytic system, resulting in a relative decrease in protein S activity, stasis, and venous hypertension, which predispose to a hypercoagulable state. Higher concentrations of circulating estrogen can inhibit collagen deposition within the media of muscular arteries and, in conjunction with a higher level of circulating collagenases, predispose to arterial dissection even in patients without connective tissue disease.

CLINICAL PRESENTATIONS

Because of all the changes previously described, pregnant women with a normal heart not uncommonly present with complaints of shortness of breath, exercise intolerance, or fatigue. It is imperative to identify patients who will benefit from a more extensive cardiovascular diagnostic work-up. The clinician can best accomplish this by taking a thorough history, including pertinent information about the patient's prepregnant state, and by focusing on exercise tolerance and symptoms of shortness of breath. A careful physical examination should be performed, focusing on

- the presence of cardiac murmurs and gallops of pathologic significance;
- the quality of heart sounds (especially the pulmonic second sound);
- an assessment of heart size;
- auscultation and percussion of the lungs to assess for signs of pulmonary congestion; and
- assessment of the central venous pressure and for peripheral edema and cyanosis.

A third heart sound and a low-grade systolic ejection murmur are common in normal pregnancy, owing to the increased cardiac output. A history of cardiovascular symptoms in the prepregnant state should alert the practitioner that further diagnostic work-up is warranted (i.e., an electrocardiogram [ECG] and an echocardiogram). However, it should be remembered that pregnancy often uncovers

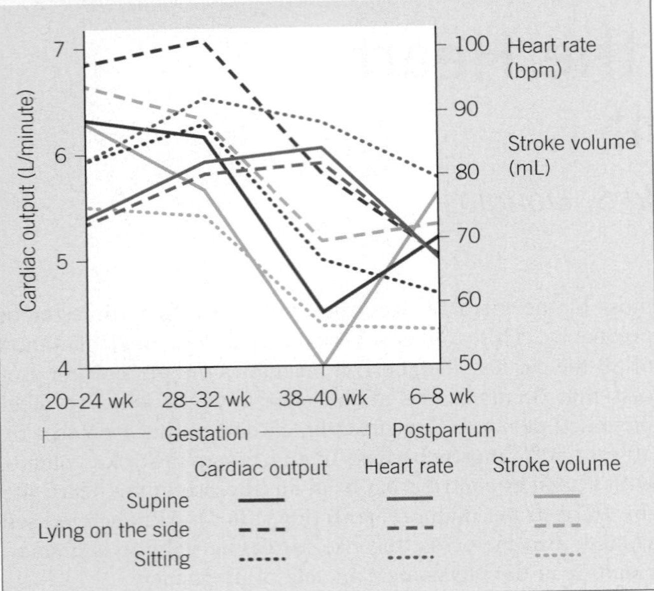

Figure 136.1 Cardiovascular hemodynamic effects of pregnancy as a function of maternal position. bpm, beats per minute. (Modified from Metcalfe J, Ueland K. Maternal cardiovascular adjustments to pregnancy. Progr Cardiovasc Dis 1974;16:363-374.)

previously silent valvular or other cardiovascular disease. With significant valvular or left ventricular systolic dysfunction, the normally well-tolerated changes in cardiac output and blood volume can pose difficulties during the gestational and peripartum periods, causing hemodynamic compromise with worsening or precipitation of congestive heart failure.

MANAGEMENT

Planning of Pregnancy in Women with Heart Disease

When counseling a woman with heart disease who wants to become pregnant, the clinician should discuss the following issues. An accurate diagnosis and prognosis in the pregnant and the nonpregnant state for the woman with heart disease and her fetus must be established. This should take into account how the hemodynamic and coagulation changes associated with pregnancy are likely to affect the underlying heart disease during the gestational and peripartum periods, as well as the longer term sequelae. Two recent prospective studies have found a 13% to 19.4% incidence of primary cardiac events in pregnant women with heart disease, the most common being arrhythmias, heart failure, and pulmonary edema.[3,4] Predictors of these events included a history of a previous cardiovascular event (congestive heart failure [CHF], transient ischemic attack [TIA], or stroke), arrhythmia, poor functional class (New York Heart Association [NYHA] class higher than 2), cyanosis, significant left heart obstruction (a mitral valve area <2 cm^2 or an aortic valve area <1.5 cm^2; or a peak left ventricular outflow tract gradient >30 mm Hg), and a left ventricular ejection fraction of less than 40%.[5] These same authors found an incremental increase in adverse neonatal outcomes when pregnant women with heart disease also had obstetric risk factors (smoking, multiple gestation, older age, or anticoagulation). Accordingly, women with heart disease should be strongly encouraged to discontinue smoking and should be followed at a regional high-risk center if they have any of the previously mentioned obstetric risk factors.

Next, the effects of maternal drugs and the mother's underlying cardiac disorder must be considered with regard to fetal development. A woman with congenital heart disease also should be counseled that her child would have an approximately 7% chance of having congenital heart disease,[4] which is tenfold higher than the overall population. In many cases, referral to a qualified genetic counselor is advised for the woman and her partner so that they will fully understand the risks of congenital cardiovascular disease in the child. Once pregnancy has occurred, fetal echocardiography may help to exclude this possibility or, if the condition is present, may help the couple plan for abortion or for delivery in the appropriate setting.

Management of Labor and Delivery

Choice of Vaginal or Cesarean Delivery

In most circumstances, spontaneous vaginal delivery is the preferred mode of delivery in patients with congenital or ischemic heart disease, including those with pulmonary hypertension. Vaginal delivery often is assisted with vacuum extraction or forceps to avoid the hemodynamic stress associated with pushing. Contrary to popular belief, cesarean delivery is associated with more hemodynamic changes than is a spontaneous vaginal delivery, and it may be less well tolerated in a woman with heart disease. Major abdominal surgery (which characterizes a cesarean delivery) is associated with the hemodynamic effects of blood loss, anesthesia and analgesia, intubation, and rapid fluid shifts, which can contribute to a more rapid increase in preload in the postpartum period than is seen with a vaginal delivery.

The need for cesarean delivery should be individualized on the basis of the status of the fetus and the hemodynamic stability of the mother; in general, it is reserved for obstetric indications. Exceptions to this are patients with Marfan's syndrome who have a dilated aortic root (>4.0 cm) or uncorrected severe aortic coarctation with poorly controlled hypertension. Patients with these aortic pathologies should not be allowed to labor and should be delivered by elective cesarean section so that blood pressure can be better controlled and a potential aortic rupture prevented. Hypertension and pre-eclampsia may necessitate the induction of labor or, if severe, cesarean section.

Anesthetic Choices

Patients with pulmonary hypertension are at greatest risk of complications from anesthesia during pregnancy. Agents that cause myocardial depression and hypoxemia should be avoided. Narcotics should be used with caution. If general anesthesia is required, an agent such as isoflurane (an inhalant anesthetic that has the fewest myocardial depressant effects) should be considered.

Although use of invasive hemodynamic monitoring with a pulmonary artery catheter during labor and delivery has become a standard of care in patients with severe pulmonary hypertension, the clinical utility of this procedure is uncertain, and it poses a significant risk of pulmonary artery rupture. Epidural anesthesia has been used safely in patients with severe valvular disease (e.g., severe aortic stenosis). However, care must be taken to avoid significant hypotension; this is done through slow induction of anesthesia. Spinal anesthesia is not a safe mode of anesthesia for cardiac patients because of its unpredictable effect of hypotension.

Cardiac Effects of Tocolytic Agents

Although terbutaline has been widely used for more than 20 years for tocolysis, the U.S. Food and Drug Administration (FDA) has not yet approved its use in the United States for this indication. In the United Kingdom, terbutaline has been approved by the Medicine Control Agency for the management of uncomplicated preterm labor. Terbutaline has no known teratogenic effects, but several adverse maternal effects have been reported, including tachycardia, hyperglycemia, hypokalemia, and pulmonary edema.

Ritodrine, another β-receptor agonist, was approved by the FDA for the prevention of preterm labor; however, the manufacturer voluntarily withdrew this drug from the U.S. market in 1998 because of marketing and regulatory pressures. Ritodrine is contraindicated in patients with pulmonary hypertension or any cardiac disease. Cardiovascular effects, such as arrhythmias (including ventricular tachycardia), increased contractility, and chest pain with or without ECG changes, have been reported in 1% to 2% of patients. Maternal pulmonary edema and even death also have been reported.

Cardiac arrest caused by hypermagnesemia has been reported in pre-eclamptic patients receiving magnesium sulfate for seizure prevention.

Cardiovascular Drugs and Pregnancy

Currently, the only cardiovascular drugs that have been clearly proven to be teratogenic are angiotensin-converting enzyme (ACE) inhibitors and warfarin. Other cardiovascular drugs have fetal side effects that make their use during pregnancy less than optimal (Table 136.1).

Anticoagulants

The various indications for anticoagulation therapy during pregnancy are the same as in the nonpregnant state (see Chapter 145). They include

- previous thromboembolic disease with a history of deep venous thrombosis or pulmonary embolism;
- left atrial thrombus or atrial fibrillation in a patient with valvular heart disease or mechanical prosthetic valves; and
- rheumatic mitral stenosis.

Pregnancy confers a hypercoagulable state, which complicates the administration and monitoring of typically utilized anticoagulants. Unfractionated heparin (UFH) long has been the anticoagulant of choice in pregnant patients because it does not cross the placenta. However, UFH is best administered intravenously, has a narrow therapeutic index, and requires frequent monitoring. The use of adjusted-dose UFH administered subcutaneously requires high doses and aggressive monitoring. Long-term use of heparin can cause osteopenia and platelet deficiency.

Warfarin crosses the placenta and has been associated with an embryopathy with skeletal abnormalities and central nervous system defects when used in the first trimester. The risk of warfarin embryopathy results primarily from the use of warfarin between 6 and 12 weeks of gestation. The reported incidence of warfarin embryopathy has varied widely in the literature, ranging from less than 5% to 67%[6,7]; however, the true estimated incidence of embryopathy generally is accepted to be 4% to 10%.[8] The use of warfarin during pregnancy also increases the risk of fetal intracerebral bleeding, because the immature fetal liver produces inadequate vitamin K–dependent clotting factors, and maternal procoagulant factors do not cross the placenta. Both heparin and warfarin have been associated with an increased risk of fetal loss.[9]

Low-molecular-weight heparin (LMWH) has several advantages over unfractionated heparin. It has increased bioavailability and a longer half-life, which permits once-daily dosing. It also has a more reliable pharmacokinetic profile; therefore, dosing is more standardized, and monitoring (by phlebotomy) is not required. Long-term use of LMWH also has a reduced risk of causing the thrombocytopenia sometimes seen with unfractionated heparin. In addition, despite the smaller size of LMWH drugs, they do not cross the placenta.[10] Most experience with the use of LMWH drugs during pregnancy has been for the prophylaxis of venous thromboembolic disease. The results of a small, nonrandomized trial of 61 patients suggested that a daily subcutaneous dose of 40 mg of enoxaparin is adequate for prophylaxis of venous thromboembolism in pregnant women at high risk of venous thromboembolic disease.[11] The role of these agents is not well established for patients with prosthetic valves, arterial thrombi, or intracardiac thrombi. Labeling approved by the FDA in 2004 states that the use of LMWH for anticoagulation in pregnant women with mechanical prosthetic heart valves has not been adequately studied. Fetal death has been reported in a few cases in patients taking enoxaparin (i.e., early and midtrimester miscarriages in women with antiphospholipid syndrome). However, none of these deaths has been definitively associated with the use of the drug.[11]

The American College of Chest Physicians Conference on Antithrombotic and Thrombolytic Therapy[12] has recommended one of three approaches to anticoagulation for pregnant patients with mechanical heart valves: (1) Use of LMWH or UFH during weeks 6 through 12 of gestation and close to term, with warfarin used at other times; (2) aggressive use of dose-adjusted UFH throughout pregnancy; or (3) aggressive use of dose-adjusted LMWH throughout pregnancy.

European experts recommend the use of warfarin throughout pregnancy because of poor maternal outcomes with heparin, and because some think that the risk of warfarin embryopathy (particularly at low doses, ≤5 mg/day) may have been overstated.[13] They additionally recommend that warfarin dosing should be adjusted to an international normalized ratio (INR) of 3.0 (range, 2.5 to 3.5), and subcutaneous UFH should be initiated at high doses (17,500 to 20,000 units every 12 hours) and adjusted to an activated partial

USE OF SELECTED CARDIOVASCULAR DRUGS IN PREGNANCY				
	Drug	**FDA Pregnancy Category***	**Indications**	**Adverse Effects**
Drugs that are safe to use in pregnancy	Beta blockers	C	Hypertension, arrhythmias, hypertrophic cardiomyopathy, fetal bradycardia, hyperthyroidism	Intrauterine growth retardation, uterine contractions
	Acebutolol	B		
	Labetalol	C		
	Metoprolol	C		
	Propranolol	C		
	Atenolol	D		
	Quinidine	C	Atrial or ventricular arrhythmias	Rare fetal thrombocytopenia
	Methyldopa	B	Hypertension	Rare maternal hepatotoxicity
	Hydralazine	C	Hypertension, congestive heart failure	Rare neonatal thrombocytopenia
	Digoxin	C	Congestive heart failure, atrial fibrillation	Low birth weight
	Adenosine	C	Supraventricular tachycardia	None known
Drugs that should be used with caution because of possible safety concerns	Diuretics	C (furosemide)	Congestive heart failure, hypertension	Intrauterine growth retardation, hypotension
		B (thiazides)	Congestive heart failure, hypertension	Electrolyte imbalance
	Heparin	C	Anticoagulation	Prematurity, thrombocytopenia, osteopenia
	Sodium nitroprusside	C	Hypertension, congestive heart failure	Thiocyanate toxicity
Drugs for which safe use in pregnancy cannot be fully established	Calcium channel blockers (all classes)	C	Hypertension, arrhythmia, angina	Hypotension, neonatal congestive heart failure
	Procainamide	C	Atrial or ventricular arrhythmias	None known
	Low-molecular-weight heparin	B	Prophylaxis of venous thromboembolism	None known
	Nitrates	C	Angina, congestive heart failure	None known
Drugs that are unsafe to use in pregnancy or are teratogenic	Angiotensin-converting enzyme inhibitors	D (all trimesters)	None	Teratogenesis, fetal loss, neonatal renal failure
	Warfarin	C	Anticoagulation	Embryopathy, fetal skeletal abnormalities, hemorrhage
	Amiodarone	C	Ventricular arrhythmias	Intrauterine growth retardation, hypothyroidism, congenital goiter, hyperthyroidism, transient bradycardia, prolonged QT in the newborn, prematurity, fetal hypothyroidism

*The U.S. Food and Drug Administration (FDA) pregnancy categories are defined as follows:

Category B: Animal studies do not indicate a risk to the fetus, and there are no controlled human studies; *or,* animal studies show an adverse effect on the fetus, but well-controlled studies in pregnant women have failed to demonstrate a risk to the fetus.

Category C: Studies have shown that the drug exerts teratogenicity or embryocidal effects in animals, but there are no controlled studies in women; *or,* no studies are available in either animals or women.

Category D: Positive evidence of human fetal risk exists, but benefits in certain situations (e.g., life-threatening conditions or serious diseases for which safer drugs cannot be used or are ineffective) may make use of the drug acceptable despite its risks.

Table 136.1 Use of selected cardiovascular drugs in pregnancy.

thromboplastin time [aPTT], drawn 6 hours after injection of at least twice control. These guidelines suggest that further information is necessary on the dosing of LMWH in pregnant patients, but they recommend that if used, the drug should be administered twice daily to achieve anti-Xa levels of 0.7 to 1.2 units/mL (4 to 6 hours after injection). The European guidelines also state that low-dose aspirin (75 to 100 mg) can be considered in addition to therapy with Coumadin or heparin to reduce the risk of thrombosis, but with the recognition of an increased risk of bleeding. Patients need to be counseled that even when warfarin, the anticoagulant that affords the greatest maternal protection, is used throughout pregnancy (with a target INR of 2.0 to 3.0), a 5.7% risk of maternal death or thromboembolism still exists.[14]

Antiarrhythmic Agents

Type Ia Agents

Quinidine and Procainamide

Both quinidine and procainamide have been safely used to treat maternal and fetal supraventricular arrhythmias, although experience is more limited with procainamide. Although no teratogenic effects have been reported with therapeutic dosages of these drugs, toxic doses of quinidine have been associated with premature labor, spontaneous abortion, and damage to the fetal eighth cranial nerve. Clinically insignificant amounts of these drugs are present in breast milk, which makes them good options for nursing women. Disopyramide has not been associated with any teratogenic effects, but information on its safety profile is limited. It therefore should probably not be used during pregnancy unless use of other type Ia agents fails or the patient is unable to tolerate the other type Ia agents (see Chapter 50).

Lidocaine

Lidocaine (lignocaine) is also safe to use during pregnancy as long as levels are carefully monitored.[15] Elevated levels have been associated with fetal central nervous system depressant effects, including apnea. Fetal seizures and bradycardia also have been reported.

Mexiletine and Flecainide

Based on limited information, mexiletine and flecainide have been safely used during pregnancy to treat tachyarrhythmias without evidence of teratogenic or long-term effects on the fetus.[16,17]

Propafenone

Although teratogenic studies in animals have been negative,[15] limited safety data are available on the teratogenic effects of propafenone in humans. Therefore, at this time, use of this agent during pregnancy cannot be recommended.

Sotalol

Sotalol, a class III antiarrhythmic, has been associated with embryonic deaths in animal studies.[18]

Amiodarone

Because of a 9% incidence of fetal hypothyroidism and a 21% incidence of infants born small for gestational age among those exposed to amiodarone in utero, this agent cannot be routinely recommended during pregnancy and should be reserved for patients with refractory arrhythmias. Nursing mothers should not use this drug, because it is secreted into breast milk and its long-term effects on the infant are unknown.

Beta Blockers

No teratogenic effects have been observed with beta blockers.[15] Rare adverse fetal and neonatal effects, which appear to occur more frequently when beta blockers are used in the first or second trimester, include intrauterine growth retardation, low birth weight, hypoglycemia, bradycardia, hyperbilirubinemia, and respiratory depression. Beta blockers readily cross the placenta, and some experts have suggested discontinuing their use just before birth to prevent possible depressive effects on the neonatal respiratory or nervous system.

Although breast-fed infants appear to tolerate beta blockers at the levels present in breast milk, close observation is warranted, because the immature neonatal liver may be unable to clear the drug optimally. Some experts have advocated the use of β_1-selective blockers because of the presence of uterine β_2-receptors; a nonselective antagonist may precipitate uterine contraction.

Calcium Channel Blockers

Verapamil is safe to use for maternal or fetal supraventricular arrhythmias,[19] and it can be safely used by nursing mothers. Multiple studies also have confirmed the safety of nifedipine during pregnancy, as it has become more widely used to treat pre-eclampsia, hypertension, and tocolysis.[20] A myocardial infarction was reported in a patient who had been treated with both nifedipine and ritodrine, a tocolytic agent.[21] Experience with the other calcium channel blockers is limited, and their safety profile, therefore, is unknown.

Angiotensin-Converting Enzyme Inhibitors

The use of ACE inhibitors during pregnancy, including the first trimester, is contraindicated, owing to the risk of several teratogenic effects, including renal tubular dysplasia with resulting neonatal renal failure, hypocalvaria, intrauterine growth retardation, patent ductus arteriosus, oligohydramnios, premature delivery, and even fetal demise.[22,23] A recent report confirmed the teratogenic effects of ACE inhibitors after first-trimester exposure; consequently, it is extremely important that physicians counsel any woman who is not pregnant before initiating this therapy and that they strongly consider alternative treatments.[23]

Diuretics

Continuation of diuretic therapy in pregnancy for the treatment of hypertension or heart failure does not appear to be harmful to the mother or fetus. However, initiation of diuretic therapy during pregnancy is not recommended, owing to a reduction in effective blood volume and placental perfusion.

Digoxin

Digoxin has been used safely to treat maternal and fetal supraventricular arrhythmias and congestive heart failure. Although no evidence of teratogenesis has been seen, low birth weight has been reported, and whether this results from more premature births or from intrauterine growth retardation is a matter of controversy. Lactating women may also be treated safely with digoxin, because the calculated dose ingested by the infant is 1% of the recommended pediatric dose.

Preferred Antihypertensive Agents

Labetalol and methyldopa are the preferred antihypertensive agents during the gestational period, and many years of clinical experience support their use. Other agents include beta blockers, such as metoprolol or propranolol (atenolol should be avoided, because it has been associated with a higher incidence of intrauterine growth retardation); hydralazine; nifedipine; and prazosin.[24,25]

SPECIFIC DISEASES

CONGENITAL HEART DISEASE

Acyanotic Congenital Heart Disease

Atrial Septal Defects

Atrial septal defects (ASDs) rarely present any significant problems during pregnancy, owing to the rare incidence of pulmonary hypertension and atrial arrhythmias until the fifth decade of life (see Chapter 106). Despite how well this defect is tolerated during pregnancy, it is recommended that ASDs be closed before conception when possible.[26] Two unusual but potentially serious problems that may result in pregnant patients with an atrial septal defect are a paradoxic embolism and hemodynamic collapse caused by a sudden loss in volume (e.g., significant hemorrhage), prompting a marked increase in left-to-right shunting with a subsequent decline in forward cardiac output. If necessary, closure of a secundum ASD can be performed during pregnancy with a catheter closure device. Prophylaxis for subacute bacterial endocarditis is not required for any type of delivery (Table 136.2).

CONDITIONS ASSOCIATED WITH THE HIGHEST RISK OF ENDOCARDITIS

- Prosthetic cardiac valve
- Previous infective endocarditis (IE)
- Unrepaired cyanotic congenital heart defect (CHD), including palliative shunts and conduits
- Congenital heart defect completely repaired with prosthetic material or a device, whether placed by surgery or by catheter intervention, during the first 6 months after the procedure†
- Repaired CHD with residual defects at the site or adjacent to the site of a prosthetic patch or prosthetic device (which inhibit endothelialization)
- Cardiac transplantation recipient who develops cardiac valvulopathy

†Although routine antibiotic prophylaxis no longer is recommended for vaginal delivery (or GI/GU procedures), the presence of these conditions or an active infection may prompt the use of prophylaxis. Recommended antibiotic guidelines can be found in Wilson et al.[47]

Table 136.2 Conditions associated with the highest risk of endocarditis.

HIGH-RISK CONDITIONS IN PREGNANCY

- Pulmonary hypertension (pulmonary artery systolic pressure >70 mm Hg)
- Symptomatic left-sided obstructive lesions
- Marfan's syndrome with dilated aorta
- Dilated cardiomyopathy with heart failure

In patients who have these conditions, pregnancy should be avoided or terminated because of the high risk of maternal and fetal morbidity and mortality.

Table 136.3 High-risk conditions in pregnancy.

Ventricular Septal Defects and Patent Ductus Arteriosus

If the ventricular septal defects or patent ductus arteriosus are small and the pulmonary artery systolic pressure is normal, no hemodynamic problems are anticipated during pregnancy. Prophylaxis for infective endocarditis is recommended during a surgical delivery but not for a vaginal delivery (see Table 136.2). Patients who have undergone previous repair of these lesions should be assessed for symptoms of dyspnea before pregnancy. If right ventricular function is at least moderately impaired or if significant pulmonary artery hypertension is noted on echocardiography, the woman should be advised against pregnancy (Table 136.3; see also Chapters 108 and 119).

Complex and Cyanotic Congenital Heart Disease

Owing to anatomic variability and the resultant diverse palliative procedures, each case of complex congenital heart disease should be considered individually in the assessment of maternal and fetal risks of pregnancy. The maternal and fetal risks depend on the adequacy of the repair and the nature of residua of specific conditions. For example, for a well-repaired tetralogy of Fallot without significant residua or sequelae, the overall risk of pregnancy[27] is low, compared with the risk for patients with right or left ventricular dysfunction, severe pulmonary hypertension, or severe pulmonary regurgitation, all of whom have a higher incidence of adverse maternal events.[4,27] Cyanosis poses a significantly increased risk of pregnancy for the mother and fetus. In patients with right-to-left shunts, air bubble filters should be used to prevent paradoxic embolus. In general, the degree of risk is proportional to the systolic pulmonary artery pressure.

VALVULAR HEART DISEASE

Pulmonary Stenosis

Mild and moderate degrees of pulmonary stenosis do not usually present any difficulty during pregnancy. A recent small study showed that unlike left-sided obstructive valvular lesions, pulmonary valve stenosis, regardless of severity, has no significant impact on maternal or fetal outcomes.[28] This finding needs to be confirmed in a larger group of patients to allow definitive management recommendations in patients with severe pulmonary valve stenosis (a peak right ventricular outflow tract gradient of >50 mm Hg at rest). Patients with severe pulmonary valve stenosis should be considered for balloon valvuloplasty before pregnancy.[29] Case reports have shown valvuloplasty to be a safe, effective procedure during pregnancy if deemed necessary (see Chapter 97).[30,31]

Aortic Stenosis

Patients with mild or moderate degrees of obstruction usually tolerate the hemodynamic changes of pregnancy without sequelae; however, patients with severe fixed stenosis, including those with significant subvalvular obstructions (i.e., membranes) or supravalvular obstructions, are at high risk of morbidity and mortality during pregnancy.[32,33] A recent retrospective analysis by Hameed and coworkers[34] found unfavorable maternal and fetal outcomes in patients with moderate to severe aortic or mitral stenosis. Pregnancies in these patients were complicated by a 38% incidence of maternal congestive heart failure, a 15% incidence of maternal arrhythmias, and significantly higher rates of hospitalization during pregnancy. In addition, a higher incidence of intrauterine growth retardation, preterm deliveries, and lower birth weights were noted in patients with severe left-sided valve stenoses.[34] If the patient has moderate or severe aortic stenosis, an exercise treadmill test before pregnancy may offer further prognostic information. Both failure of the blood pressure to rise, indicating a fixed stroke volume, and ST depression consistent with subendocardial ischemia are poor prognostic markers, and valve replacement should be considered before conception (Fig. 136.2).

If a patient with severe aortic stenosis presents in the pregnant state and refuses abortion, careful monitoring with serial ECGs and echocardiograms should be done. Hospital admission should be considered if the velocity across the aortic valve (as measured by Doppler echocardiography) decreases during pregnancy or if the patient becomes symptomatic with angina, congestive heart failure, or syncope. If left ventricular function is normal, careful treatment with a beta blocker and nitrates to reduce venous return is indicated. Aortic valvuloplasty[35,36] can be considered in an emergency situation and may be preferred over valve replacement, because cardiothoracic surgery during pregnancy is associated with high fetal loss. The development of severe aortic regurgitation is a possible consequence of this procedure. Valvuloplasty in such patients is clearly a temporary solution and only delays anticipated valve replacement (see Chapter 93).

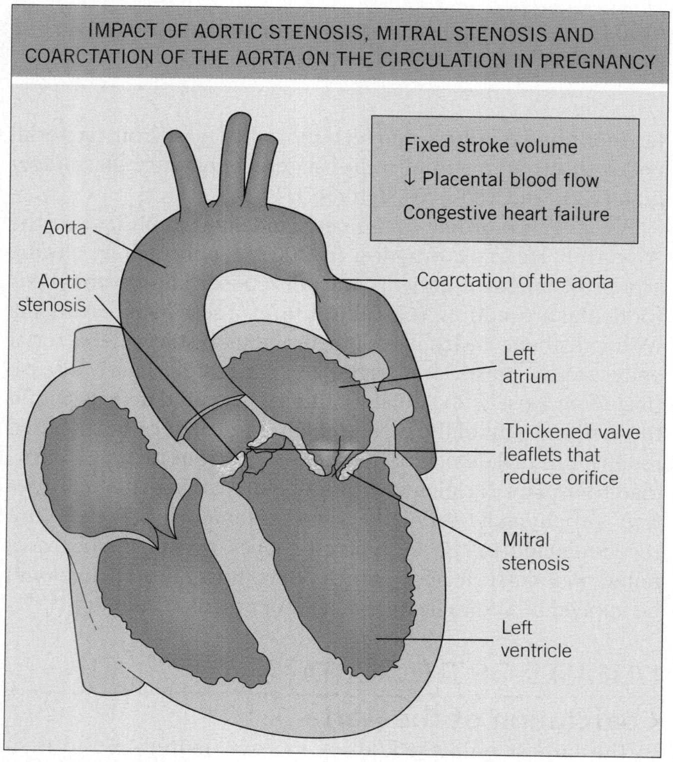

IMPACT OF AORTIC STENOSIS, MITRAL STENOSIS AND COARCTATION OF THE AORTA ON THE CIRCULATION IN PREGNANCY

Figure 136.2 Impact of aortic stenosis, mitral stenosis, and coarctation of the aorta on the circulation in pregnancy.

Mitral Stenosis

Mitral stenosis is the most common valvular lesion in women of childbearing years (see Chapter 89), and in many cases symptoms may not become apparent until after the patient is pregnant and has the typical hemodynamic changes. The classic murmur of mitral stenosis can be difficult to detect. If a patient presents with symptoms of unexplained dyspnea or congestive heart failure, echocardiography is indicated to rule out the possibility of occult mitral stenosis.

Because of the stenosis, stroke volume cannot be increased, which results in a worsening of tachycardia to preserve or augment cardiac output, decreased left ventricular filling, a rise in left atrial pressures, and acute pulmonary edema. For those with mild to moderate mitral stenosis, careful treatment with small doses of a diuretic and a beta blocker (metoprolol should be chosen over atenolol, which has been associated with a higher incidence of fetal growth retardation) to reduce the heart rate and improve diastolic left ventricular filling are indicated. Mortality among pregnant patients with mild to moderate mitral stenosis typically is less than 1%.[37] In contrast, those with severe symptomatic mitral stenosis have a maternal mortality of 3.5% and a neonatal mortality of 7.5%.[38] Accordingly, if medical management fails, the patient should be evaluated for a percutaneous balloon mitral valvuloplasty; this can be done by performing a transesophageal echocardiogram to evaluate the suitability of the valve and to exclude the presence of a left atrial or appendage thrombus. Percutaneous balloon mitral valvuloplasty has proved to be safe and successful in pregnant patients.[39,40] This procedure preferably should be delayed until the second trimester because of the risk of radiation exposure of the fetus, and transesophageal echocardiographic guidance may be helpful in reducing radiation. Although cardiac surgery usually can be performed on pregnant patients with low maternal morbidity and mortality, fetal mortality remains high (20% to 38%) because of reduced placental blood flow and hypothermia.[41,42]

Regurgitant Valve Disease

Regurgitant valve disease usually is well tolerated in pregnancy, owing to the associated hemodynamic changes. Systemic vasodilatation actually reduces the regurgitant volume and murmur. Mitral valve prolapse is the most common cause of mitral regurgitation in pregnancy and generally is well tolerated. Tachycardia is well tolerated when left ventricular filling is unimpeded, and diuretic therapy is indicated only in the setting of pulmonary congestion. Pharmacologic vasodilatation usually is not required, unless associated hypertension is present. Because ACE inhibitors are contraindicated, hydralazine is the agent of choice. The etiology of the regurgitant disease is important in assessing the patient's suitability for pregnancy. Aortic regurgitation secondary to aortic root dilatation from Marfan's syndrome or other causes of cystic medial necrosis carries a higher risk of aortic rupture or dissection than aortic regurgitation secondary to a congenitally abnormal valve (see Marfan's syndrome; also see Chapters 12 and 95).[43]

Prosthetic Heart Valves

A woman may want to become pregnant after the placement of a prosthetic valve (see Chapter 101b). The best course is to discuss the issue of pregnancy and its risks with every woman of childbearing potential before placement of a prosthesis. Bioprosthetic valves have the advantage of not requiring anticoagulation; however, accelerated deterioration has been reported during pregnancy. In addition, owing to the limited life span of these valves, placement of such a valve in a young woman almost invariably necessitates a second operation. Mechanical valves often are the optimal choice for young patients. Homograft placement or a Ross procedure might be the best option for a young woman who needs aortic valve replacement and is planning pregnancy in the future.

For patients with a preexisting valve prosthesis, it is important that the integrity of the valve and the patient's functional status be assessed before pregnancy. Patients with NYHA class I or class II symptoms and a normally functioning prosthetic valve probably will tolerate pregnancy without difficulty. However, owing to the hypercoagulable state of pregnancy and the difficulty in achieving a stable pattern of anticoagulation with subcutaneous heparin, these patients are at higher risk of valve thrombosis, thromboembolic events, and even death.

Patients with older, single-disk prosthetic valves (e.g., Björk-Shiley valves) and those with mitral prostheses appear to have a higher risk of thromboembolic events.[9] If a patient is at relatively low risk of valve thrombosis (i.e., status post valve replacement with a mechanical bileaflet valve, such as a St. Jude valve, in the aortic position), anticoagulation with subcutaneous heparin may suffice throughout pregnancy. Patients at high risk of valvular thrombosis should be considered for an approach that involves intravenous heparin at the onset and end of pregnancy (which requires hospitalization) and oral anticoagulation in the middle (Fig. 136.3). The role of LMWH in anticoagulation in either group of patients is uncertain, but it may provide a more efficacious and safe approach (see previous discussion of LMWH).

Infective Endocarditis

Before publication of the American Heart Association's current guidelines for the prevention of infective endocarditis, antibiotic prophylaxis was not recommended for patients with valvular disease undergoing uncomplicated vaginal delivery or cesarean section unless infection was suspected, and prophylaxis was considered optional for high-risk patients. In clinical practice, antibiotic prophylaxis was used liberally, with many citing several studies that showed a significant incidence of bacteremia (5% to 19%) in patients immediately after labor with organisms capable of causing bacterial endocarditis.[44,45]

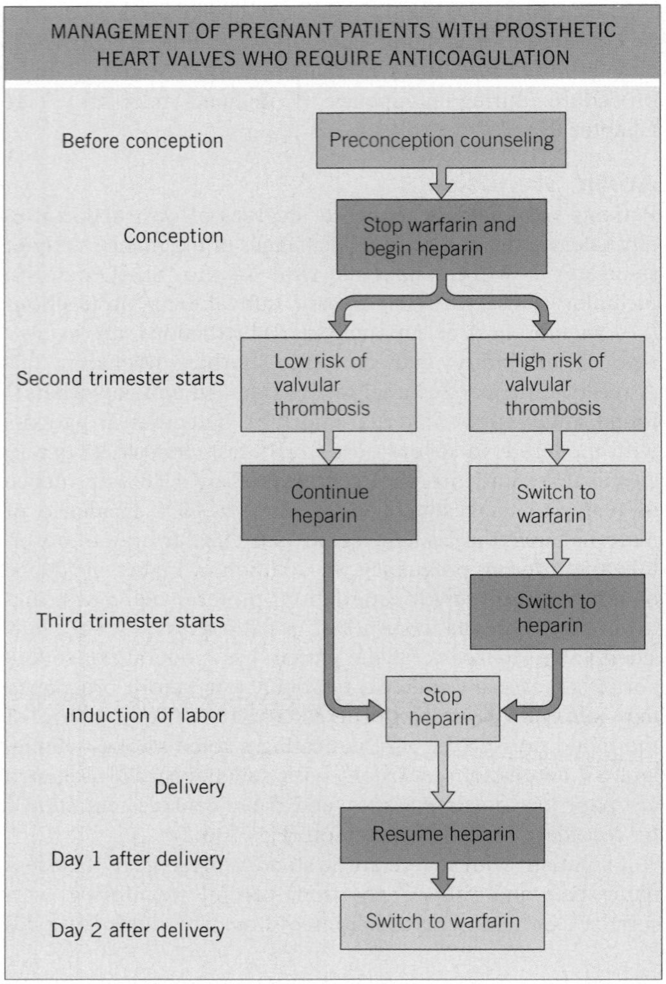

MANAGEMENT OF PREGNANT PATIENTS WITH PROSTHETIC HEART VALVES WHO REQUIRE ANTICOAGULATION

Before conception
Preconception counseling
Conception
Stop warfarin and begin heparin
Second trimester starts
Low risk of valvular thrombosis
Continue heparin
High risk of valvular thrombosis
Switch to warfarin
Third trimester starts
Switch to heparin
Induction of labor
Stop heparin
Delivery
Day 1 after delivery
Resume heparin
Day 2 after delivery
Switch to warfarin

Figure 136.3 Management of pregnant patients with prosthetic heart valves who require anticoagulation.

Furthermore, maternal and fetal mortality rates from bacterial endocarditis as a complication of pregnancy are alarmingly high (22% and 15%, respectively).[46]

However, according to the new guidelines published by the American Heart Association in 2007,[47] only a few specific groups of pregnant patients warrant endocarditis prophylaxis for dental procedures (see Table 136.2). These include patients with prosthetic heart valves, a previous history of bacterial endocarditis, unrepaired cyanotic congenital heart disease (including those with palliative shunts), repaired defects within the first 6 months of the repair (either surgical or catheter-based repair), residual defects at the site of a previous repair, and cardiac transplant recipients with a valvulopathy. Although routine prophylaxis for labor and vaginal delivery is not recommended in the current guidelines except in the cases noted previously, it is too early to know how the guidelines will be applied in a complicated vaginal or cesarean delivery.

DISEASES OF THE AORTA

Coarctation of the Aorta

In the largest published series to date, maternal and neonatal outcomes were retrospectively assessed for 50 women with coarctation.[48] The incidence of miscarriages and pre-eclampsia in women with coarctation did not seem to differ from that in the general population. The greatest morbidity in this group of patients appears to be maternal hypertension, which was found to occur more frequently in patients with a hemodynamically significant coarctation (gradient ≥20 mm Hg). In this series only one maternal death occurred, in a woman with Turner's syndrome who died in week 36 of pregnancy from a type A aortic dissection. This woman had undergone repair of the coarctation as a child and had a normal-sized ascending aorta. Given the morbidity and mortality from maternal hypertension, these findings suggest that surgical correction of any coarctation with a gradient equal to or greater than 20 mm Hg should be performed before pregnancy. Surgical or percutaneous correction should be considered in the gestational period in cases of uncontrollable maternal hypertension or left ventricular failure. Cesarean section probably is the preferred mode of delivery in women with a coarctation and a significant gradient, an enlarged aorta, or uncontrolled hypertension. The role of percutaneous correction of coarctation of the aorta during pregnancy to prevent an aortic catastrophe is undefined (see Chapter 120).

Marfan's Syndrome

Patients with Marfan's syndrome, especially those with aortic root dilatation, are at increased risk of aortic dissection or further dilatation of the aorta during pregnancy (see Chapter 12). The absence of aortic root dilatation appears to reduce but does not eliminate the risk of aortic dissection.[49] Recently, a prospective study found no significant difference in the growth of the aortic root during 6.4 years of follow-up in pregnant patients with Marfan's syndrome, compared with a matched childless group. A subgroup of patients with aortic roots equal to or greater than 40 mm showed a small but significant increase in growth of the aortic root. The only dissection in this study was a type B in a patient with a previous type A dissection. This study therefore suggests that pregnancy may be relatively safe in patients with Marfan's syndrome who have had no previous aortic dissection and whose aortic root measures less than 45 mm.[50] Data are lacking on the safety of pregnancy in a patient with Marfan's syndrome whose aortic root is larger than 45 mm and on the long-term effects of pregnancy on the cardiac status of patients with Marfan's syndrome.

Currently, both the Canadian[29] and European[51] guidelines discourage pregnancy in patients with an aortic root greater than 45 mm or 40 mm, respectively. In contrast, the guidelines established by the American College of Cardiology and the American Heart Association (ACC/AHA) advise against pregnancy in all women with Marfan's syndrome because of an increased risk of aortic rupture or dissection during pregnancy, even in patients with a normal or minimally dilated aortic root.[13]

All patients with Marfan's syndrome need to be counseled about the risk of pregnancy, and the patient should be advised against pregnancy if she has even mild preexisting aortic root dilatation or a personal history of previous aortic dissection. Further genetic counseling should be offered to inform parents about the 50% risk of transmission of this syndrome to their children.

Pregnant patients with Marfan's syndrome should be followed closely with periodic echocardiograms, regardless of aortic size, and surgery should be considered if aortic root dilatation progresses or if the aortic root reaches 5.5 cm.[49] Physical activity should be minimized, and beta-blocker therapy should be used throughout pregnancy to reduce the risk of aortic root dilatation and dissection.

If dissection is suspected, diagnostic assessment of the aortic root and arch is most safely performed during pregnancy by transesophageal echocardiography or magnetic resonance imaging (MRI) to avoid exposure to ionizing radiation. Currently, elective cesarean delivery is advised in patients with significant aortic root dilatation or dissection to decrease the risk of increased shear stress on the aorta from labor. Patients without cardiovascular involvement generally tolerate a vaginal delivery.

CARDIAC ARRHYTHMIAS DURING PREGNANCY

Palpitations are a common complaint of pregnant women. During normal pregnancy, the heart rate increases 10 bpm above baseline. Greater degrees of sinus tachycardia, supraventricular tachycardia, or even nonsustained ventricular tachycardia (including a new onset) are not uncommon during pregnancy. Some investigators have reported up to a fivefold increase in the onset of paroxysmal supraventricular tachycardia during pregnancy,[52] indicating the possibility of an independent gestational (hormonal) arrhythmogenic effect. A study by Rosano and colleagues[53] showed that the incidence of supraventricular tachycardia correlated with hormonal fluctuations during the menstrual cycle. They concluded that the incidence of supraventricular tachycardia showed a positive correlation with the progesterone level but an inverse relationship with the estrogen level.

An increase in the frequency of arrhythmias in patients with mitral valve prolapse or preexcitation syndromes also is seen.[54] In the absence of underlying structural or organic heart disease, most of these arrhythmias resolve in the postpartum period. However, a symptomatic arrhythmia may be the first clue to the presence of significant structural heart disease. Any suspected or documented sustained arrhythmia should prompt an evaluation by a cardiologist and a screening echocardiogram to rule out obstructive valvular lesions, intracardiac shunts, or cardiomyopathy. Prompt and appropriate management of the maternal cardiovascular condition may prove crucial in preventing fetal hemodynamic compromise.

Analysis of data from the International LQTS (long QT syndrome) Registry by Seth and colleagues[55] found a reduced risk of cardiac events for women with long QT syndrome during pregnancy. Interestingly, they found an increased risk (2.7-fold for any cardiac event, 4.1-fold for fatal events) during the first 9 months postpartum; the risk returned to the baseline prepregnancy level after this period of transient increase. In confirmation of a previous report,[56] women with the LQT2 genotype were at considerably higher overall risk for cardiac events, compared with those with the LQT1 or LQT3 genotypes. The authors suggested that several physiologic changes that occur abruptly in the postpartum state (i.e., fluid shifts that affect preload, a decline in cardiac output compared with the pregnant state, an increase in afterload, and a marked decline in estrogen levels) all may contribute to the increased risk of arrhythmias during this period. The Registry analysis[55]

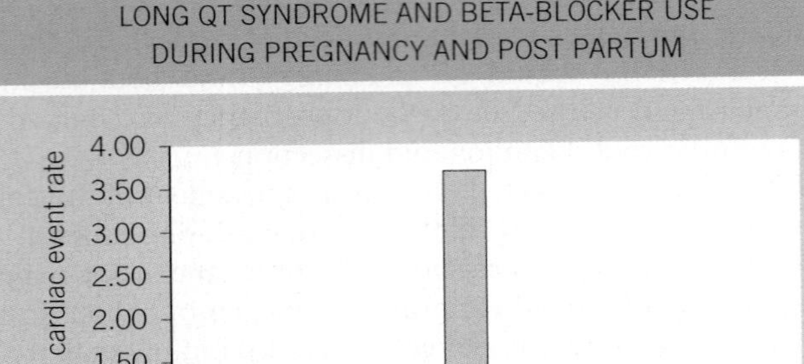

Figure 136.4 Long QT syndrome and beta-blocker use during pregnancy and the postpartum period. In women with long QT syndrome, beta-blocker use in the 9-month postpartum period is associated with a greater than fourfold reduction ($P = .01$) in the cardiac event rate. No significant effect of beta-blocker therapy was noted during pregnancy or during the post-postpartum period (>9 months after parturition).[55]

also found that women who took beta blockers had a significant reduction ($P = .01$) in cardiac events during the postpartum period (Fig. 136.4). This finding is consistent with previous hypotheses,[57,58] which suggested that increased adrenergic activity in the postpartum period may cause an increase in postpartum cardiac events. It currently is recommended that all women, even those breast-feeding, who have long QT syndrome be prescribed beta blockers post partum.[55]

For women with implantable cardiac defibrillators (ICDs), a recent study revealed that pregnancy does not result in an increased number of discharges or complications related to the ICD.[59] This finding suggests that, in the absence of significant underlying structural heart disease, women with an ICD should not be discouraged from pregnancy.

CARDIAC ARREST

Cardiac arrest is a rare complication during pregnancy, occurring only once in every 30,000 deliveries. The significant hemodynamic changes that take place during the gravid period, including compression of abdominal vessels, which results in decreased venous return and reduced cardiac output, must be taken into consideration during an arrest. In addition to resuscitation, identification of the etiology of the cardiac arrest is mandatory. Causes may include amniotic fluid embolism, pulmonary embolism, cardiac arrhythmia, hemorrhage, aortic dissection, congestive cardiomyopathy, or drug toxicity (particularly with magnesium sulfate). To prevent an impending arrest or during an arrest, the patient should be placed in the left lateral decubitus position, or the uterus should be manually positioned to relieve aortocaval compression, and a fluid bolus and 100% oxygen should be administered. Basic life support procedures and advanced life support procedures should be followed routinely, and an emergency cesarean section should be considered within 5 minutes of the arrest to preserve fetal viability.[60]

ISCHEMIC HEART DISEASE

Acute Myocardial Infarction during Pregnancy

Myocardial infarction (see Chapter 27) during pregnancy is rare, with an overall incidence of 6.2 cases per 100,000 live births.[61] This incidence is a threefold to fourfold increase over that of nonpregnant women of reproductive age.[61] Significant risk factors for pregnancy-related myocardial infarction include age older than 30 years, hypertension, thrombophilia, diabetes mellitus, smoking, transfusion, and postpartum infection.[61] Of note, smoking during pregnancy is associated with an eightfold increase in the risk of myocardial infarction, compared with a twofold increase in nonpregnant smokers.[61] The highest incidence of myocardial infarction occurs in the third trimester (commonly during labor and delivery) in women older than 33 years.[62] A recent study found a lower maternal mortality rate (5.1%)[61] compared with previous reports, which reported a high maternal death rate (21%), with most deaths occurring at the time of the infarction or within the first 2 weeks after it.[62] This difference may be attributed to improvements in care, earlier recognition, possible underreporting of less severe cases in the past, and changes in the definition of acute myocardial infarction. A review of 125 cases found the most common etiology of the infarct to be atherosclerotic disease, with or without associated thrombus (43%). A fair number of cases (21%) were due to coronary thrombosis without atherosclerotic disease, which suggests a hypercoagulable state. Coronary dissection was evident in 16% of the cases, and up to one third of the patients were found to have normal coronary arteries, which suggests transient thrombus formation or spasm as the etiology.[62]

The amount of experience with systemic thrombolysis in pregnancy is not considerable, and the potential risk of fetal or placental bleeding, or both, would favor primary percutaneous coronary intervention (if available) as the preferred treatment.

CARDIOMYOPATHIES

Hypertrophic Obstructive Cardiomyopathy

Patients with hypertrophic obstructive cardiomyopathy (see Chapter 79) should be counseled in the prenatal period, because a 50% risk exists that a child will be affected as a result of autosomal dominant inheritance. Most patients who have hypertrophic obstructive cardiomyopathy do well during pregnancy, because increases in blood volume also increase left ventricular size, relieving outflow obstruction, and significant diastolic dysfunction rarely is present in young patients. Left ventricular volume typically is able to increase to meet the hemodynamic demands of pregnancy, and the gradient and the typical systolic murmur may even be reduced (see Fig. 136.4). Sudden death has been reported infrequently, and no evidence exists that it is increased during pregnancy. Treatment with pharmacologic agents is warranted only for symptomatic relief of dyspnea or angina and is best accomplished with a beta blocker.

No agreement has been reached on the anesthetic choice in pregnant patients with significant left ventricular outflow obstruction. Some advocate general anesthesia with pulmonary artery catheter placement,[63] whereas others[64,65] have safely used regional anesthesia (epidural or spinal) during both labor and cesarean delivery, despite concerns of vasodilatation. In general, most believe that cesarean section typically should be performed only for obstetric indications or cardiac instability. Clearly, more investigation is warranted to define the safest mode of delivery and the anesthetic choice in this group of patients.

Sustained supraventricular or ventricular arrhythmias are uncommon in this young age group. During delivery and in the early postpartum period, it is important to prevent significant blood loss and to maintain an adequate blood pressure and heart rate to ensure adequate left ventricular volume, cardiac output, and placental perfusion.

Peripartum Cardiomyopathy

Peripartum cardiomyopathy is defined as the development of a dilated cardiomyopathy (of unexplained etiology) that results in congestive heart failure, which is temporally related to the gestational period. Heart failure most often occurs from 1 month before to 6 months after childbirth. It is a rare condition, with an estimated incidence of 1 in 4000 live births.[66] A large, population-based study in southern California highlighted significant racial differences, finding much higher incidences in African Americans (1:1421) and Asians (1:2675).[66] A higher incidence also is found in twin gestations, in women over age 30, and in multiparous women.[67,68] The observed mortality rate now is believed to be lower than previously thought, ranging from 2.1% to 3.3%.[66,68]

The etiology of this illness is not fully understood, and several causes have been suggested, including myocarditis of viral or immune origin, nutritional deficiency, small-vessel coronary artery abnormalities, hormonal effects, and toxemia. The incidence of biopsy-proven myocarditis is unclear; although an infrequent finding in most series, some have indicated a higher incidence.[67] The diagnosis is one of exclusion, and the spectrum of the illness is broad, ranging from mild to severe. The disorder is manifested by the typical presenting signs and symptoms of congestive heart failure. Other potential causes of pulmonary edema or compromise must be excluded.

The more fulminant cases tend to occur within days of childbirth. A transthoracic echocardiogram should be obtained immediately to assess cardiac chamber sizes, right and left ventricular function, and valve function. The diagnosis of acute myocardial infarction must be entertained and can be difficult to make in this group of patients, because ECG changes consistent with myocardial infarction, segmental wall motion abnormalities on echocardiogram, and elevated creatine kinase-MB or troponin biomarkers can be seen in patients with peripartum cardiomyopathy. For these reasons, prompt cardiac catheterization may be warranted in some patients to rule out epicardial coronary disease or other pathology, such as dissection. The mother also should be questioned about the use of cocaine as a possible etiology of myocardial infarction. Treatment with ergonovine or bromocriptine, which are used to prevent uterine hemorrhage and lactation, also has been implicated (rarely) as an iatrogenic cause of myocardial infarction by causing coronary spasm.[69] Other causes of pulmonary edema need to be excluded in a postpartum patient who presents in respiratory distress, including the use of β_2-agonists (e.g., ritodrine or terbutaline) for premature labor, venous thromboembolism, or amniotic fluid embolism. Hemodynamic decompensation from a preexisting, undiagnosed dilated cardiomyopathy may be difficult to distinguish from a true peripartum cardiomyopathy.

Immediate supportive care should be initiated with oxygen, an ACE inhibitor (or hydralazine if the patient is still pregnant), digoxin, and diuresis. If fulminant congestive heart failure is present, respiratory support and inotropic support with a β_1-agonist or even an intra-aortic balloon pump or a left ventricular assist device should be considered. Anticoagulation should be considered, especially with a left ventricular thrombus or severe left ventricular dysfunction. Immunosuppressive therapy with corticosteroids or azathioprine rarely is used unless biopsy evidence of myocarditis is seen. A biopsy result consistent with active myocarditis would defer the decision for potential cardiac transplantation.

More than half of patients have complete or nearly complete recovery of left ventricular systolic function within 6 months. Patients who have had a fulminant course or who have residual left ventricular dysfunction should be discouraged from future pregnancies because of the risk of relapse. Some think that the left ventricles of patients who apparently have made a complete recovery have decreased contractile reserve, which may impair their ability to respond to hemodynamic stress.[70] Unfortunately, even patients who fully recover left ventricular function have an increased risk of a recurrent cardiomyopathy and even death with subsequent pregnancies.[71-73] Further work is needed to define better the group of patients at increased risk of recurrent peripartum cardiomyopathy despite seemingly full recovery of cardiac function. All patients should be counseled that future pregnancies are not without risk.

PREGNANCY IN THE HEART TRANSPLANT PATIENT

Limited information is available about maternal and fetal morbidity and mortality after transplantation. Most patients are able to tolerate the hemodynamic changes of pregnancy, and no episodes of rejection during pregnancy have been reported. High incidences of maternal hypertension, preeclampsia, and maternal infections (e.g., *Cytomegalovirus* infection) have been observed.[73,74] No fetal deaths have been reported; however, many of the births (up to 40%) are preterm with fetal growth retardation.[74,75]

Frequent monitoring of cyclosporin levels is necessary because of unpredictable fluctuations. No direct teratogenic effects of immunosuppressive therapy have been detected. Breast-feeding is discouraged because of the presence of cyclosporin A and Imuran in breast milk. Excess late mortality may be an issue, because at least three maternal deaths have been reported within 30 months of gestation.[76] Given the current experience, patients with a heart transplant can safely tolerate pregnancy without an excessively adverse outcome. However, they must be informed of the possible maternal and fetal morbidity associated with pregnancy and lactation and of the possible limitation of life expectancy, given the reports of late deaths.

PULMONARY HYPERTENSION

Pregnancy is contraindicated in patients with pulmonary hypertension, regardless of the etiology, because of high maternal and fetal morbidity and mortality. The peripartum maternal mortality rate in primary pulmonary hypertension has been reported to be as high as 30% to 40%,[77,78]; a high incidence of fetal loss (at least 10%) and prematurity also are seen.[78] Close postpartum monitoring is warranted, because maternal death has been reported to occur as late as 1 week after delivery.[78] A recent review shows that patients with secondary pulmonary hypertension caused by vasculitis, illicit drug or appetite suppressant use, or chronic venous thromboembolic disease have an even greater maternal mortality (>50%) than patients with idiopathic pulmonary hypertension (30%) or pulmonary hypertension resulting from Eisenmenger's syndrome (36%).[78]

The maternal prognosis appears to depend on early diagnosis and early hospital admission.[78] Patients should be encouraged to undergo an elective abortion early in gestation. If the patient insists on continuing the pregnancy, physical activity should be limited, and the patient should be closely monitored for evidence of hypoxemia. The use of anticoagulant therapy is controversial, and adverse outcomes have been reported both with and without its use. Symptoms of right ventricular failure, syncope, and chest pain typically occur in the second trimester, and hospitalization with careful monitoring should be instituted immediately. A spontaneous vaginal delivery with close hemodynamic monitoring is preferable; however, if anesthesia is necessary for a cesarean section, negative inotropic agents should be avoided because of preexisting right ventricular failure. Likely mechanisms responsible for death include right ventricular failure, pulmonary embolism, and arrhythmia (see Chapter 83).

HYPERTENSION DURING PREGNANCY

In the United States, hypertension complicates 8% to 10% of all pregnancies and is an important cause of maternal and fetal morbidity and mortality. Hypertension during pregnancy is defined as an increase in the systolic blood pressure of 30 mm Hg or more or an increase in the diastolic blood pressure of 15 mm Hg or more. The Working Group on High Blood Pressure in Pregnancy has classified hypertension into four categories[79]:

- chronic hypertension;
- pre-eclampsia or eclampsia;
- pre-eclampsia or eclampsia superimposed on chronic hypertension; and
- gestational or transient hypertension.

Chronic hypertension is defined as a systolic blood pressure (BP) greater than 140 mm Hg or a diastolic blood pressure greater than 90 mm Hg (or both) diagnosed before pregnancy or before 20 weeks' gestation or that persists longer than 6 weeks postpartum. Patients with chronic hypertension have a 15% maternal and fetal complication rate. The value of bed rest for any type of hypertension during pregnancy is controversial and without evidence from large randomized trials.[80] Nevertheless, some degree of bed rest is recommended for the theoretical benefit of improving uteroplacental flow when the mother is in the left lateral decubital position. Benefits of strict bed rest must be weighed against the potential increased risk of venous thromboembolic disease. Currently it is recommended that, for women with uncomplicated (no end-organ damage), mild hypertension (a systolic BP of 140 to 159 mm Hg or a diastolic BP of 90 to 99 mm Hg), antihypertensive therapy should be tapered off during pregnancy and the maternal blood pressure should be monitored closely.[79] These women not uncommonly continue to have acceptable blood pressure readings in the absence of their usual therapy because of the normal physiologic decrease in blood pressure during the second trimester.

Controlled studies have not demonstrated that pharmacotherapy for mild hypertension lowers the risk of pre-eclampsia or convincingly improves fetal or maternal outcomes. Some evidence indicates that antihypertensive agents in these patients may reduce the incidence of severe hypertension; however, many think that this potential benefit is outweighed by the potential for intrauterine growth retardation in neonates exposed to these agents.[81] Drug therapy is recommended for any patient with a systolic blood pressure greater than 150 to 160 mm Hg or a diastolic blood pressure greater than 100 to 110 mm Hg or for evidence of end-organ damage (left ventricular hypertrophy or renal insufficiency).[79] In women without end-organ damage, the blood pressure goal is a systolic pressure of 140 to 150 mm Hg and a diastolic pressure of 90 to 100 mm Hg.[82]

Subgroups of patients with mild hypertension who may benefit from institution of antihypertensive therapy outside of the previously discussed guidelines include women with secondary hypertension (i.e., concomitant renal disease, collagen vascular disease, or coarctation of the aorta), end-organ damage, dyslipidemia, maternal age older than 40, microvascular disease, a history of stroke, diabetes, and previous perinatal loss.[82] Methyldopa is the treatment of choice because of its proven safety and efficacy. It also is the treatment with the longest follow-up (longer than 8 years) with regard to long-term effects on children whose mothers were treated with it (see Chapters 45 and 46). Intravenous labetalol is recommended for acute therapy.[83]

Pre-eclampsia or eclampsia is defined as the development of hypertension (as stated previously) in a previously normotensive woman after more than 20 weeks' gestation that is accompanied by new proteinuria (>0.3 g/24 hours) or edema, or both. If the fetus is mature enough, the best treatment for the hypertension is parturition. If the fetus is too immature for delivery, the mother needs to be treated medically, with the goal of reducing the diastolic blood pressure to at least 85 to 100 mm Hg. In general, the guidelines for initiation of antihypertensive therapy would be followed; however, more intensive control could be considered, depending on the severity of the pre-eclampsia and any associated symptoms. If the blood pressure cannot be controlled or if clinical findings are predictive of an adverse fetal or maternal outcome (Table 136.4), labor should be induced regardless of fetal maturity.

Pre-eclampsia or eclampsia superimposed on chronic hypertension is defined as a further increase in blood pressure compared with the prepregnant state (as outlined previously) and the development of pre-eclampsia or eclampsia. Patients with preexisting chronic hypertension, especially

PREDICTORS FOR HIGH MATERNAL AND FETAL RISK IN WOMEN WITH PRE-ECLAMPSIA
▪ Systolic blood pressure ≥60 mm Hg or diastolic blood pressure ≥110 mm Hg ▪ New proteinuria ≥2.0 g/24 hr (2+ or 3+ on qualitative examination) or a decrease in urine volume ▪ New increased serum creatinine level (>2.0 mg/dL) ▪ Platelet count <100,000/L or evidence of microangiopathic hemolytic anemia (e.g., schistocytes or increased levels of lactic acid dehydrogenase and direct bilirubin) ▪ Elevated hepatic enzymes (aspartate aminotransferase or alanine aminotransferase) ▪ Upper abdominal pain (especially epigastric and right upper quadrant) ▪ Headache and other cerebral or visual disturbances ▪ Cardiac decompensation (e.g., pulmonary edema) ▪ Retinal hemorrhages, exudates, or papilledema ▪ Intrauterine growth retardation
Modified from Lindheimer MD. Hypertension in pregnancy. Hypertension 1993;22:127-137.

Table 136.4 Predictors for high maternal and fetal risk in women with pre-eclampsia.

those with chronic renal disease, are three to seven times more likely to develop pregnancy-induced hypertension and pre-eclampsia than normal women.[84]

Gestational or transient hypertension is defined as hypertension that develops after 20 weeks' gestation or within 24 hours postpartum but that is not associated with other manifestations of pre-eclampsia. Patients with this condition need to be treated according to the guidelines stated previously and followed carefully, because some will develop proteinuria and thus be considered pre-eclamptic. Hypertension in this group of patients tends to predict the development of hypertension in the future (unrelated to pregnancy), as well as atherosclerotic disease. The etiology of pre-eclampsia and pregnancy-induced hypertension is not fully understood, but it most likely involves endothelial dysfunction. Trials examining prophylaxis with low-dose aspirin[85-87] or calcium[88] have not shown any benefit.

VENOUS THROMBOEMBOLIC DISEASE

Pulmonary embolism (see Chapter 85) remains the leading cause of maternal death in developed countries.[89] The incidence of lower extremity deep venous thrombosis during pregnancy is estimated to be 0.1% as diagnosed by ultrasound,[90] whereas the incidence of pregnancy-related pulmonary embolism has been found to be 0.01% to 0.03%.[91] The coagulopathy associated with pregnancy and venous stasis caused by uterine compression increase the incidence of deep venous thrombosis and subsequent pulmonary embolism during pregnancy.

Patients with a previous history of gestational or "estrogen associated" venous thromboembolism should be treated with prophylactic anticoagulation during subsequent pregnancies. Owing to the lack of adequately controlled trials, the optimal management of pregnant women at risk of thromboembolic disease (i.e., those with a past history of venous thromboembolism unassociated with pregnancy or estrogen use) is controversial. However, because of the high incidence of pulmonary embolism (24%) and high mortality (15%) in patients with untreated deep venous thrombosis and the increased incidence of venous thromboembolic events during pregnancy, many recommend anticoagulation.[92,93] The American College of Obstetrics and Gynecology, in a comprehensive review, recommended treatment or prophylaxis of all pregnant women with a previous history of venous thromboembolism, except in cases associated with trauma.[93]

To prevent fetal radiation exposure, Doppler ultrasound of the lower extremities is strongly preferred to venography for diagnosis of deep venous thrombosis, and a ventilation-perfusion scan is preferred to pulmonary angiography for diagnosis of pulmonary embolism. Because of the high morbidity and mortality associated with pregnancy-associated venous thromboembolic disease, the clinician should proceed to the invasive procedures for a more definitive diagnosis if clinical suspicion remains high and the results of the noninvasive studies are negative or uncertain.

A diagnosis of venous thromboembolism during pregnancy requires anticoagulation throughout the remainder of the pregnancy or at least for 6 months. Treatment and thromboprophylaxis should be done with unfractionated heparin; the role of LMWH for these indications is evolving (see Chapter 145). Caval filters have been placed successfully and have been found effective in a limited number of patients. In the event of a large pulmonary embolism that causes hemodynamic compromise, consideration must be given to systemic thrombolysis or emergency thrombectomy. One case report showed successful thrombolysis using urokinase during pregnancy, without apparent harm to the fetus.[94]

SUMMARY

During the coming decades, the population of women giving birth will be increasingly complex. Mothers will be older and will be more likely to have cardiovascular disease (whether congenital or acquired) and cardiovascular complications during pregnancy. In addition, more multiple births will occur, and an increased number of children will have congenital heart defects. A recent task force recommended that, to ensure optimal medical care for these mothers and infants, pregnant women with heart disease who are at intermediate or high risk for cardiovascular complications be managed at a high-risk perinatal unit by a multidisciplinary team composed of an obstetrician, a cardiologist, an anesthesiologist, and a pediatrician. Although much remains to be learned in important areas, a knowledge of the physiologic changes associated with pregnancy and their impact on the heart's ability to compensate for chronic and acute diseases will facilitate the care of pregnant women with heart disease.

chapter 137

Athlete's Heart and Causes of Sudden Death in Athletes

Barry J. Maron

We chaired you through the market-place;
Man and boy stood cheering by,
And home we brought you shoulder high.
Today, the road all runners come,
Shoulder-high we bring you home,
And set you at your threshold down,
Townsman of a stiller town.
"To an Athlete Dying Young"
ALFRED EDWARD HOUSMAN, 1896

"Death should stay away from young men's games. Death belongs in musty hospital rooms, sickbeds. It should not impinge its terrible presence on the celebrations of youth, reap its frightful harvest in fields where cheers ring and bands play and banners wave."

JIM MURRAY
LOS ANGELES TIMES

Sudden deaths of competitive athletes are personal tragedies that have a great impact on the lay and medical communities.[1,2] These deaths are caused by a variety of usually unsuspected cardiovascular diseases,[1-19] as well as by low-energy blows to the chest.[20,21] Such events often assume a high public profile because of the widely held perception that young, trained athletes constitute the healthiest segment of our society, and the occasional but highly visible death of a well-known elite athlete exaggerates this visibility.[1,9,21] These athletic field catastrophes also have substantially increased impact on the role and efficacy of preparticipation screening for the detection of cardiovascular disease.[20-26]

For these reasons, the present comprehensive discussion related to young competitive athletes includes an analysis of the epidemiology and cardiovascular causes responsible for sudden death; the differential diagnosis of physiologic athlete's heart and structural cardiovascular disease; the strengths and limitations of preparticipation screening for early detection of these cardiovascular abnormalities, as well as their cost-efficiency, feasibility, and medical-legal implications[20-26]; and consensus recommendations and guidelines for sports eligibility or disqualification when cardiac abnormalities are identified.[27-29] Given the large number of competitive athletes in the United States and many other countries, as well as the recent public health initiatives on physical activity and exercise, these issues have become particularly timely.

PATHOPHYSIOLOGY

Definitions and General Considerations

The present considerations focus on the competitive athlete, defined as one who participates in an organized team or individual sport requiring systematic training and regular competition against others and places a high premium on athletic excellence and achievement.[30] The purpose of cardiovascular screening, as described here, is to provide medical clearance for participation in competitive sports through routine and systematic evaluations intended to identify clinically relevant and preexisting abnormalities and thereby reduce the risks associated with organized sports. It should be underscored, however, that raising the suspicion of a cardiovascular abnormality on a standard screening examination is only the first tier of recognition, after which referral to a specialist for further diagnostic investigation likely will be required. When a definitive cardiovascular diagnosis is made, expert consensus panel guidelines (e.g., those of the Thirty-Sixth Bethesda Conference, sponsored by the American College of Cardiology)[27] and a similar document from the European Society of Cardiology[29] may be used to formulate recommendations for continued participation or disqualification from competitive sports.

Guidelines established by the American Heart Association[24] focus on the process of mass screening for high school and college student-athletes. These recommendations may be extrapolated to athletes in youth, middle school, masters, or professional sports and in some instances to participants in intense recreational sporting activities. It also should be emphasized that the overall preparticipation screening process extends well beyond the cardiovascular considerations discussed here, potentially involving many other organ systems and medical issues.

Eligibility and disqualification guidelines and screening programs are predicated on the assumption that intense athletic training is likely to increase the risk for sudden cardiac death (or disease progression) in susceptible trained athletes with clinically important and underlying structural cardiovascular disease; however, currently it is not possible to quantify that risk with precision. Indeed, the vast majority of young athletes who die suddenly do so during or just after physical exertion while engaged in athletic training or competition.[1,3,5,10,16,19] These observations support the proposition that intense exercise can be an important trigger for sudden death, and in fact a risk factor, given the presence of certain underlying (but unsuspected) cardiovascular diseases.

Early detection of clinically significant cardiovascular disease through preparticipation screening may well permit timely therapeutic interventions that prolong life either by withdrawal from physical conditioning,[20-26] or with an implantable cardioverter-defibrillator (ICD)[31-33] in certain high-risk individuals with genetic cardiovascular diseases such as hypertrophic cardiomyopathy (HCM), ion channelopathies, or arrhythmogenic right ventricular dysplasia.

Causes of Sudden Death in Athletes

A variety of cardiovascular abnormalities represent the most common causes of sudden death in young competitive athletes.[1-19] Based on a large autopsy-based registry of more than 1800 sudden deaths in competitive athletes younger than 40 years of age, which was assembled over 27 years, the vast majority of events are due to a variety of largely congenital cardiac malformations (Figs. 137.1 to 137.3).[13] Virtually any disease capable of causing sudden death in young people potentially may do so in young competitive athletes. It should be emphasized that although these cardiovascular diseases may be relatively common among athletes who die suddenly, all are uncommon within the general population. Also, diseases responsible for sudden death do not occur with the same frequency, and most are responsible for only 5% or fewer of all such deaths (see Fig. 137.1). Most of these events occur in team sports, such as basketball and football, which require intense physical exertion but also are associated with high levels of participation.

Hypertrophic Cardiomyopathy

The single most common cardiovascular cause of sudden death in young athletes is hypertrophic cardiomyopathy, usually without obstruction, to left ventricular (LV) outflow.[1,2,5,6,9,10,13,19,34-36] This type of HCM accounts for about one third of such athletic field deaths (see Figs. 137.2 and 137.3).[3,10,13] HCM is a genetic cardiac disease with a heterogeneous clinical and phenotypic expression, complex pathophysiology, and diverse clinical course. It is caused by mutations in 11 genes encoding proteins of the cardiac sarcomere, and >500 disease-causing mutations have been reported,[34,37] including β-myosin heavy chain, cardiac myosin–binding protein C, cardiac troponin T and I, α tropomyosin, essential and regulatory light chains of myosin, α actin, α-myosin heavy chain, titin, and muscle limb protein (MLP). In the general population, HCM is the most common genetic disease, occurring in about 1 in 500 individuals.[38]

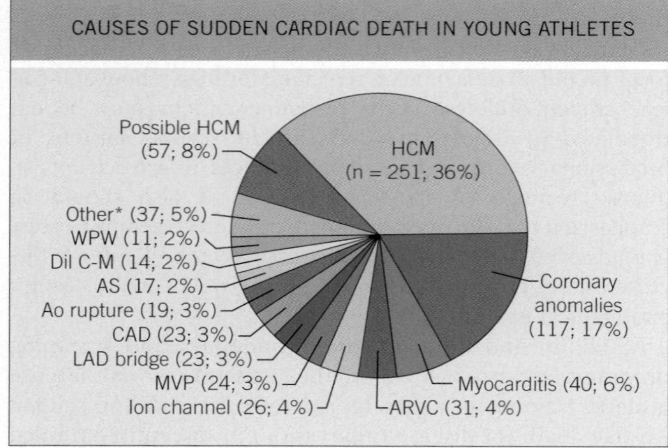

Figure 137.1 Causes of sudden cardiac death in young competitive athletes based on systematic tracking of deaths in the United States over 27 years, 1980 to 2006. HCM, hypertrophic cardiomyopathy; WPW, Wolff-Parkinson-White syndrome; Dil C-M, dilated cardiomyopathy; AS, aortic stenosis; Ao, aortic; CAD, coronary artery disease; LAD, left anterior descending; MVP, mitral valve prolapse; ARVC, arrhythmogenic right ventricular cardiomyopathy. (From Maron BJ, Doerer JJ, Haas TS, et al: Sudden death in young competitive atheletes: Analysis of 1,866 deaths in the United States 1980-2006. Circulation 2009;119:1085-1092.)

Not uncommonly, HCM is responsible for sudden cardiac death in young and asymptomatic individuals, frequently occurring in association with moderate or severe exertion.[34] The stress of intense training and competition (and associated alterations in blood volume, hydration, and electrolytes) undoubtedly increases the risk to some degree in certain susceptible athletes. With HCM, particularly strenuous physical activity during sports may act as a trigger mechanism (Fig. 137.4), generating potentially lethal ventricular tachyarrhythmias, given the underlying electrophysiologically unstable myocardial substrate composed of replacement fibrosis (probably the consequence of small-vessel disease–mediated ischemia) and disorganized myocardial architecture (see Fig. 137.2).

Disease variables that appear to identify individuals with HCM at greatly increased risk include a previous aborted cardiac arrest or spontaneous and sustained ventricular tachycardia; a family history of sudden or other premature HCM-related death; multiple-repetitive, nonsustained ventricular tachycardia on 24-hour ambulatory Holter electrocardiographic (ECG) recordings; unexplained syncope, particularly in the young; massive LV hypertrophy (wall thickness ≥ 30 mm); and a hypotensive blood pressure response to exercise.[31,39-41] Patients with HCM who are judged to be at high risk for sudden death based on one or more of these markers and are considered for primary prevention of sudden death with a prophylactic ICD.[31] In a cohort of high-risk patients with HCM, the annual appropriate ICD discharge rate is 5.5% overall and about 4% for primary prevention.[31]

Although HCM may be suspected during preparticipation sports evaluations by the previous occurrence of syncope, a family history of HCM or premature cardiac death, or detection of a systolic heart murmur, these features are relatively uncommon among all individuals affected by the disease.[24,26,34] In particular, a loud heart murmur rarely is encountered in screening for HCM, because a substantial proportion of affected individuals have the nonobstructive form of the disease under resting conditions (which is associated with no or only a soft systolic murmur).[24] Consequently, screening procedures for high school and college-aged competitive athletes, limited to a history and physical examination (as is customary in the United States), cannot be expected to consistently identify HCM.

Hypertrophic Cardiomyopathy and Athlete's Heart

In young athletes with mild segmental ventricular septal thickening (13 to 15 mm), it may be difficult to distinguish the physiologic and benign form of LV hypertrophy, which represents an adaptation to athletic training (i.e., "athlete's

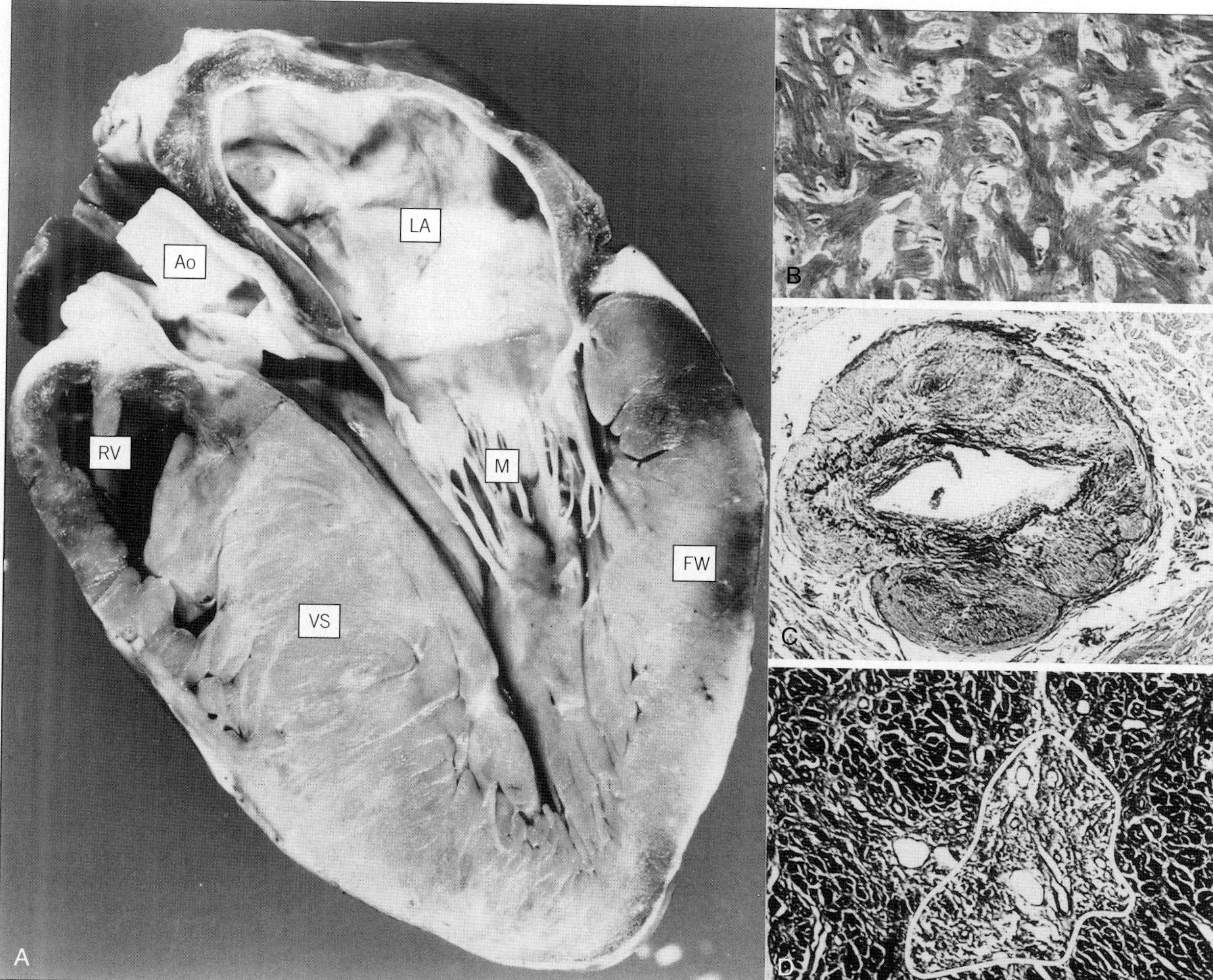

Figure 137.2 Morphologic components of the disease process in hypertrophic cardiomyopathy (HCM), the most common cause of sudden death in young competitive athletes. **A,** A gross heart specimen sectioned in a cross-sectional plane similar to that of the echocardiographic (parasternal) long axis. Left ventricular wall thickening shows an asymmetric pattern and is confined primarily to the ventricular septum (VS), which bulges prominently into the left ventricular outflow tract. The left ventricular cavity appears reduced in size. **B** to **D** show histologic features characteristic of left ventricular myocardium in HCM. **B,** Markedly disordered architecture with adjacent hypertrophied cardiac muscle cells arranged at perpendicular and oblique angles. **C,** An intramural coronary artery with a thickened wall, primarily from medial hypertrophy, and an apparently narrowed lumen. **D,** Replacement fibrosis in an area of ventricular myocardium adjacent to an abnormal intramural coronary artery. Ao, aorta; FW, left ventricular free wall; FW, left atrium; RV, right ventricle. (From Maron BJ, Shirani J, Poliac LC, et al: Sudden death in young competitive athletes: clinical, demographic and pathological profiles. JAMA 1996;276:199-204.)

heart") from a pathologic condition such as HCM (albeit with a mild morphologic expression), which conveys a risk for sudden death.[42] Athletes in this ambiguous morphologic "gray zone"[2,42,43] represent an important and not uncommon clinical dilemma, for which the differential diagnosis between HCM and athlete's heart often can be resolved by noninvasive testing (Fig. 137.5).[42] This distinction may have particularly important implications, given that young athletes with an unequivocal diagnosis of HCM are discouraged from participation in intense competitive sports to reduce arrhythmic risk, with the possible exception of low-intensity activities (e.g., golf and bowling).[36] On the other hand, improper diagnosis of cardiac disease in an athlete may lead to an unnecessary withdrawal from athletics, thereby depriving that individual of the varied benefits of participation in sports.

Congenital Coronary Anomalies

The second most frequent cause of sudden death in young athletes is a variety of congenital coronary anomalies of wrong aortic sinus origin, which account for about 15% to 20% of these deaths.[3,28,31] The most common of these lesions appears to be anomalous origin of the left main coronary artery from the right (anterior) sinus of Valsalva[44-46] or, less commonly, anomalous right coronary artery from the left aortic sinus (the mirror image malformation).[45] Such malformations are exceedingly difficult to recognize during life, including with customary preparticipation history and

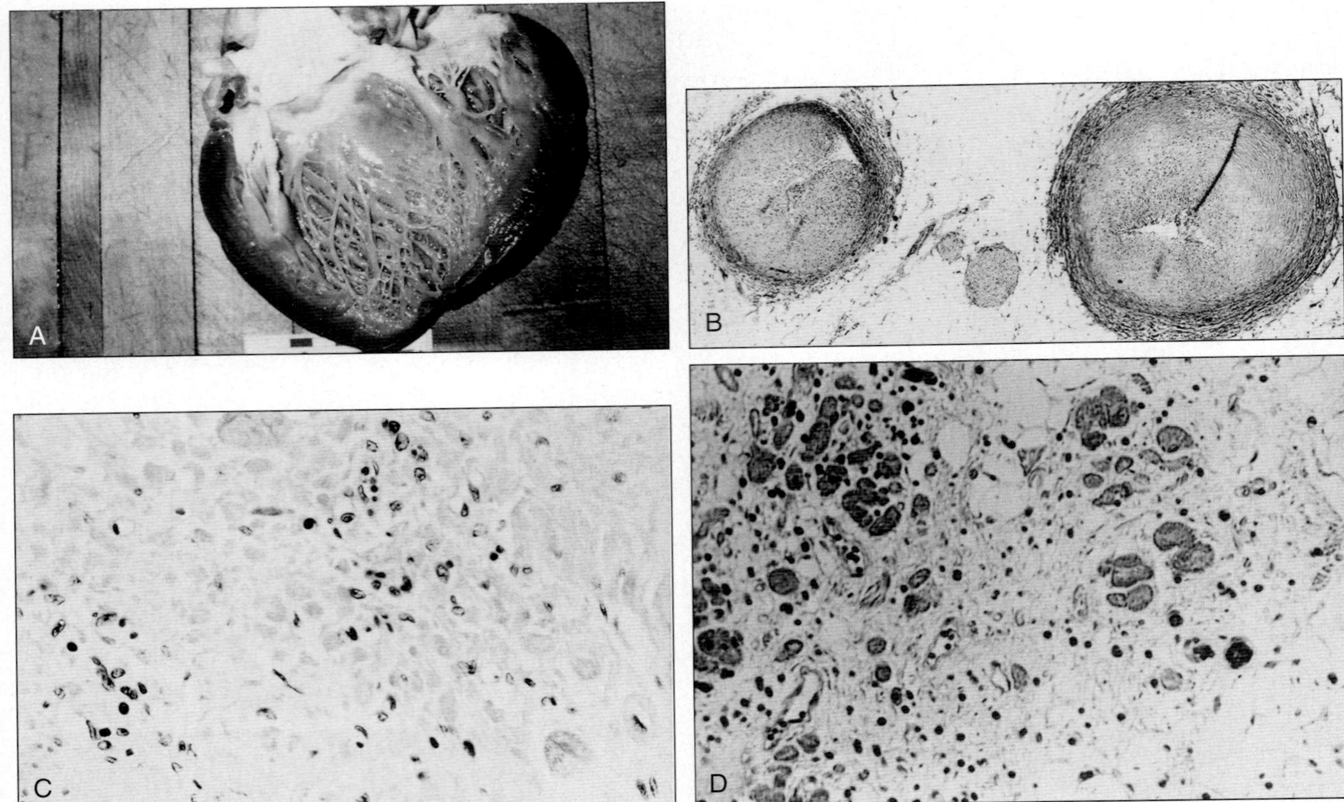

Figure 137.3 Cardiac morphologic findings at autopsy in four competitive athletes who died suddenly of causes other than HCM. **A,** Gross specimen from an athlete with greatly enlarged ventricular cavities, consistent with dilated cardiomyopathy. **B,** Histologic section of the left anterior descending coronary artery *(left)* and a diagonal branch *(right)* showing severe (>95%) cross-sectional luminal narrowing by atherosclerotic plaque. **C,** Foci inflammatory cell infiltrate consistent with myocarditis. **D,** Histologic section of the right ventricular wall showing islands of myocytes within a matrix of fatty and fibrous replacement, characteristic of arrhythmogenic right ventricular dysplasia. (Modified from Maron BJ, Shirani J, Poliac LC, et al: Sudden death in young competitive athletes: clinical, demographic and pathological profiles. JAMA 1996;276:199-204.)

physical examination screening, given an uncommon association with symptoms (such as exertional syncope or chest pain) or alterations in the scalar 12-lead or exercise ECG.[44] Therefore, clinical diagnosis requires a high index of suspicion, utilizing imaging with coronary arteriography, cardiac magnetic resonance, two-dimensional echocardiography, or computed tomography angiography.[46] When identified, coronary anomalies of wrong sinus origin are amenable to surgical correction.[44]

Myocardial ischemia in young people (and athletes) with congenital coronary artery anomalies probably occurs in infrequent bursts, cumulative with time and ultimately resulting in patchy myocardial necrosis and repair in the form of replacement fibrosis. This scarring can predispose to lethal ventricular tachyarrhythmias by creating an electrically unstable myocardial substrate.

Potential mechanisms proposed for myocardial ischemia resulting from coronary anomalies of wrong sinus origin, particularly during exercise and in the presence of aortic expansion, include (1) acute angled takeoff and kinking or flap-like closure at the origin of the coronary artery; and (2) compression of the anomalous artery between the aorta and pulmonary trunk during exercise, particularly when the coronary artery is intramural (i.e., within the aortic tunica media). Other coronary anomalies rarely reported to cause sudden death in athletes include hypoplasia of the right coronary and left circumflex arteries, left anterior descending or right coronary artery from the pulmonary trunk, virtual absence of the left coronary artery, and spontaneous coronary arterial intersusception and dissection.[45]

Atherosclerotic Coronary Artery Disease

Atherosclerotic coronary artery disease may be responsible for sudden death during physical exertion in youthful athletes,[3-7,10,47,48] often associated with acute plaque rupture.[49] Corrado and coworkers[47] emphasized the occurrence of premature atherosclerotic coronary disease as a prominent cause of sudden death in young people (including competitive athletes) in the Veneto region of northeastern Italy. In that report, coronary artery disease usually was confined to the left anterior descending coronary artery and resulted from obstructive fibrous and smooth muscle cell plaques in the absence of an acute thrombus.

Myocarditis

Myocarditis is an acknowledged cause of sudden death in young athletes, even in the absence of previous symptoms. Definitive diagnosis may be difficult clinically (or even at autopsy, particularly in the healed phase).[1,3,6,9,50] The

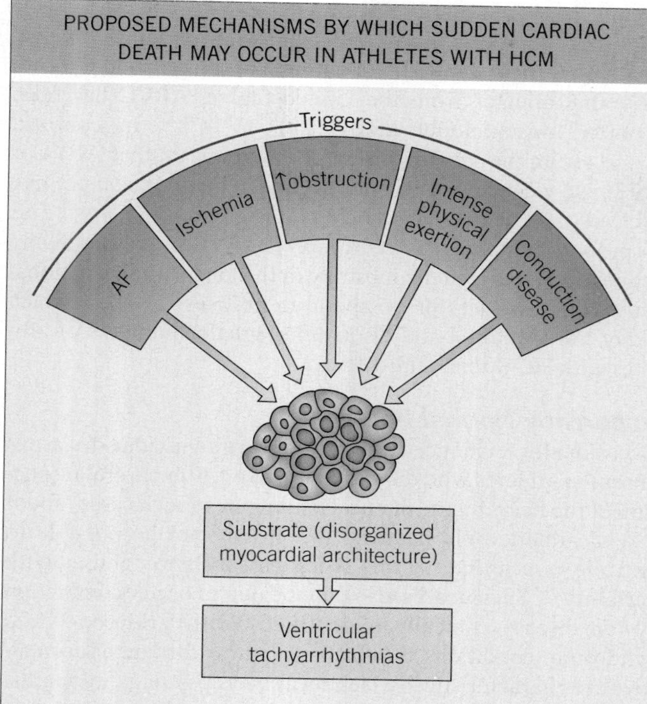

Figure 137.4 Proposed mechanisms by which sudden cardiac death may occur in athletes with hypertrophic cardiomyopathy (HCM). AF, atrial fibrillation.

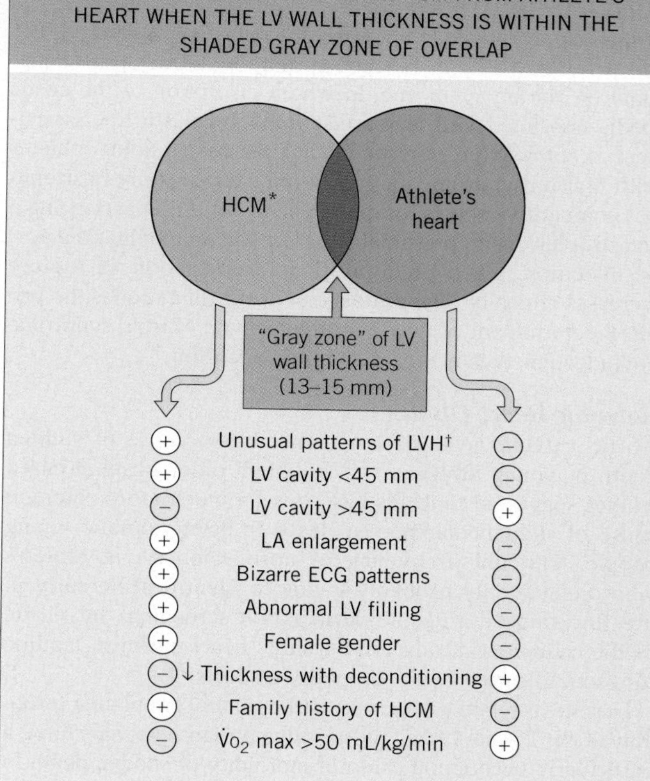

Figure 137.5 Criteria used to distinguish hypertrophic cardiomyopathy (HCM) from athlete's heart when the left ventricular (LV) wall thickness is within the shaded gray zone of overlap, consistent with both diagnoses. *Assumed to be the nonobstructive form of HCM in this discussion, because the presence of substantial mitral valve systolic anterior motion would confirm, per se, the diagnosis of HCM in an athlete. †May involve a variety of abnormalities, including heterogeneous distribution of left ventricular hypertrophy (LVH) in which asymmetry is prominent and adjacent regions may be of greatly different thicknesses, with sharp transitions evident between segments; also, patterns in which the anterior ventricular septum is spared from the hypertrophic process and the region of predominant thickening may be in the posterior portion of the septum; anterolateral or posterior free wall or LVapex. ↓, decreased; ECG, electrocardiogram; LA, left atrial; $\dot{V}O_2$max, maximum oxygen consumption. (From Maron BJ, Pelliccia A, Spirito P: Cardiac disease in young trained athletes: insights into methods for distinguishing athlete's heart from structural heart disease with particular emphasis on hypertrophic cardiomyopathy. Circulation 1995;91:1596-1601.)

importance of myocarditis as an etiology for sudden death in the young may have been previously exaggerated as a result of overinterpretation of histologic findings, as well as a lack of standardized morphologic criteria.[50] In a large autopsy-based registry of competitive athletes, only about 5% showed areas of myocardium with inflammatory and necrotic changes diagnostic of acute myocarditis or idiopathic myocardial scarring consistent with healed myocarditis.[13] The inflammatory process of myocarditis (see Fig. 137.3) can be triggered by a number of viral agents, most often enterovirus but also adenovirus[51]; however, it also can be associated with chronic cocaine use.[52] Although myocarditis can be overlooked at routine autopsy examination, the diagnosis can be verified by direct analysis of the viral genome.[49]

A diagnosis of myocarditis does not necessarily require permanent withdrawal from competitive athletics.[36] The guidelines of the Thirty-Sixth Bethesda Conference permit athletes to undergo a prudent convalescent period of about 6 months after the onset of clinical manifestations; they can return to competition if ventricular function and cardiac dimensions normalize and clinically relevant arrhythmias are absent on ambulatory monitoring and stress testing.[36]

Coronary Arterial Bridging

An unresolved question is whether short "bridged" segments of the left anterior descending coronary artery (usually 1 to 3 cm) completely surrounded by LV myocardium per se constitute a potentially lethal anatomic variant responsible for sudden death in otherwise healthy young individuals during physical exertion.[53-55] Some observers regard such muscle bridges as harboring the potential to produce critical systolic arterial narrowing (and residual diastolic compression) responsible for myocardial ischemia and, in one report associated with, an increased risk for cardiac arrest in young patients with HCM.[53] Short-acting beta blockers have been reported to alleviate anginal symptoms and ischemia by increasing the luminal diameter of tunneled coronary segments and normalizing flow velocities.[54] Nevertheless, coronary blood flow occurs predominantly during diastole, and necropsy studies frequently have documented tunneled coronary arteries to be a common incidental finding in patients who died of chronic noncardiac diseases. The finding that 3% to 5% of young athletes who die suddenly have no other pathologic finding is at least circumstantial evidence favoring tunneled coronary arteries as the cause of death in that population.[1,3,13]

Aortic Dissection/Rupture (and Marfan Syndrome)

Uncommonly, young athletes die suddenly as a result of rupture of the aorta,[1,3,5,6,9,10,13] including some with the physical stigmata of Marfan syndrome, in whom disruption of the aortic media associated with decreased numbers of elastic fibers is evident at autopsy (i.e., "cystic medial necrosis"). Some athletes with Marfan syndrome may participate successfully in strenuous competitive sports for many years without experiencing a catastrophic event, presumably before the time of marked aortic dilatation, when predisposition for dissection or rupture increases critically. The presence of aortic dilatation is the primary determinant of whether athletes with Marfan syndrome are judged medically ineligible for competition.[36]

Valvular Heart Disease

Aortic valvular stenosis is an uncommon cause of sudden death in young athletes,[3,5,13] although older hospital-based studies suggested that this lesion was a much more common cause of sudden unexpected death in asymptomatic young people. The low frequency of aortic stenosis in athletes who die suddenly probably is due to identification early in life (including during preparticipation screening) by virtue of the characteristically loud systolic heart murmur, leading to disqualification from competitive sports.[24]

Despite its relative frequency in the general population (probably about 2% to 4%),[56] mitral valve prolapse appears to be a particularly uncommon cause of morbidity or sudden death in young competitive athletes.[24,36] In most cases, this diagnosis does not lead to disqualification from competitive sports.[36] Reliable stratification of risk level in the mitral valve prolapse population has proved to be particularly challenging.[57]

Cardiac Conduction System Abnormalities

Congenital or acquired abnormalities confined to the cardiac conduction system (in the absence of other structural cardiac abnormalities) have been regarded as occasional causes of sudden death in competitive athletes and other young people, presumably by producing heart block and bradyarrhythmias.[3,5,6,9,10] These include malformations of the atrioventricular conduction tissue (e.g., accessory atrioventricular pathways) and morphologically abnormal small intramural arteries (serving the sinoatrial or atrioventricular nodes) with thickened walls and narrowed lumen. Such vascular abnormalities have been incriminated as determinants of myocardial ischemia and sudden death by virtue of the observed tissue degeneration, scarring, and hemorrhage in the surrounding conducting tissue.

Arrhythmogenic Right Ventricular Cardiomyopathy

Arrhythmogenic right ventricular cardiomyopathy (ARVC) is a familial condition caused by mutations in seven disease genes (desmoplakin, cardiac ryanodine receptor, plakophilin-2; transforming growth factor, desmoglein 2, plakoglobin, and desmocollin 2), which are responsible for cell-to-cell adhesion or calcium homeostatis.[7,8,58,59] ARVC may be associated with important ventricular or supraventricular arrhythmias and has been cited as a cause of sudden cardiac death in young people, including athletes.[1,3,15,16] ARVC is characterized morphologically by myocyte death in the right ventricular wall with replacement by fibrous or adipose tissue as part of a repair process, often associated with myocarditis (see Fig. 137.3). ARVC may be segmental or may diffusely involve the right ventricle. In autopsy studies of sudden death in young athletes from the United States, ARVC has been reported uncommonly (i.e., <5%).[1,3-6,9,10,13] In contrast, reports from the Veneto region of Italy indicate that ARVC is the single most common cause of sudden death in competitive athletes (and, conversely, HCM is uncommon).[7,8,15,22,25] This disproportionately high occurrence of ARVC in Italy probably is due to a unique genetic substrate or the long-standing national screening program for competitive athletes,[15,22,23,25] which likely has identified and disqualified greater numbers of athletes with HCM than with ARVC.[22]

Apparently Normal Hearts

Occasionally, evidence of structural cardiovascular disease is absent in athletes who die suddenly, even after careful inspection of the heart by the medical examiner. In such cases (about 2% of athletic field deaths)[3,10,13] it may not be possible to exclude noncardiac factors, such as substance abuse, with certainty.[60] Such deaths also may be due to occult conduction system disease, clinically unidentified Wolff-Parkinson-White syndrome, conditions in which structural cardiac abnormalities are characteristically lacking at necropsy (e.g., idiopathic ventricular fibrillation or right ventricular outflow tract tachycardia), ion channel disorders (e.g., long QT and Brugada syndromes), unrecognized segmental forms of ARVC, and HCM in the prehypertrophic phase.

Older Athletes

Older athletes (those more than 35 years of age) also may harbor occult cardiac disease and die suddenly and unexpectedly while participating in intense athletic activities (Fig. 137.6). Unlike in youthful athletes, the cause of death in older conditioned athletes usually is atherosclerotic coronary artery disease.[3,4,9] The remaining small proportion of deaths in older athletes is due to nonatherosclerotic diseases, such as HCM or valvular heart disease.

Trained athletes who died suddenly of coronary heart disease, as reported in several necropsy-based investigations, comprise a heterogeneous athletic population that includes runners training for competitive long-distance road racing and recreational joggers, as well as participants in sports such as rugby, squash, and golf.[9,61-63] These deaths usually occur during or just after periods of physical activity. Most older athletes who die of coronary heart disease have known risk factors, cardiovascular symptoms, or a previous myocardial infarction associated with obstructive atherosclerotic coronary artery disease (stenosis of two or three major extramural coronary arteries) and myocardial scarring (see Fig. 137.6).

CLINICAL PRESENTATION

Epidemiology

Prevalence and Significance

Sudden unexpected death during competitive sports as a result of cardiovascular disease is rare in high school students participating in organized interscholastic sports (i.e., about 1 in 200,000 participants per year or 1 in 60,000 participants over a 3-year high school period)[17,18]; somewhat lower estimates for the risk of sudden death have been reported for

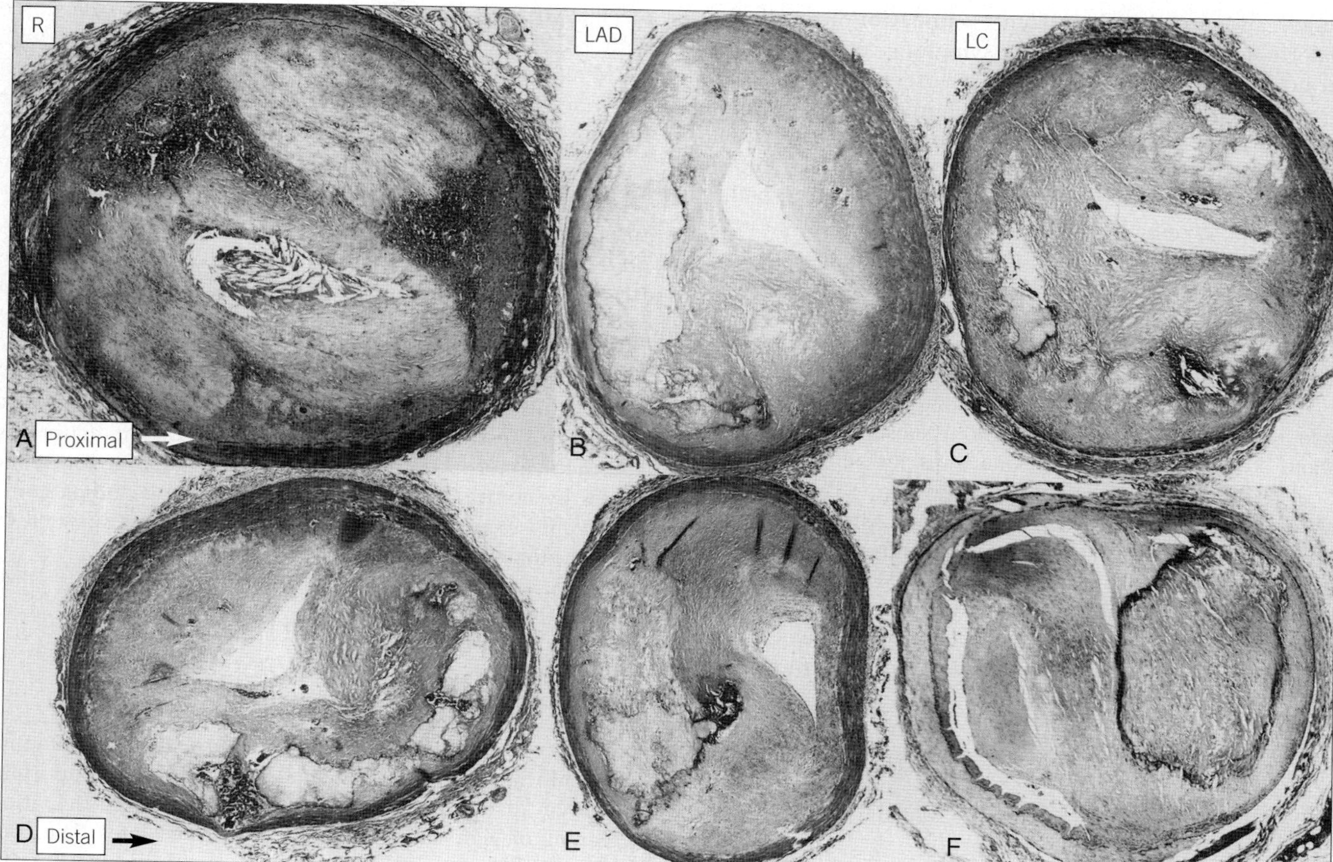

Figure 137.6 Atherosclerotic coronary artery disease. Sections of coronary arteries from a 49-year-old man who ran an average of about 170 km a week and successfully completed six marathons and seven 10-km races, but who died suddenly of coronary heart disease. The right (R), left anterior descending (LAD), and left circumflex (LC) coronary arteries are shown at the sites of maximal narrowing by atherosclerosis, both in the proximal *(upper panels)* and distal *(lower panels)* portions of the respective arteries. (From Maron BJ, Epstein SE, Roberts WC: Causes of sudden death in competitive athletes. J Am Coll Cardiol 1986;7:204-214.)

adult joggers and marathon and other road racers.[11,12,61] Automated external defibrillators have proven effective in reducing sudden death on the race course during a marathon.[12] Preliminary data from a 27-year national registry of sudden death in young athletes showed that such events in U.S. competitive athletes number about 120 each year, from all causes about fivefold more common than previously estimated, but nevertheless a relatively small number, considering the overall at-risk population.[13] Extrapolation of these data suggests that one young athlete dies suddenly in the United States every 3 days, and that one such athlete with HCM dies every 2 weeks.

Independent of incidence, the emotional and social impact of athletic field deaths remains high. The competitive athlete symbolizes the healthiest segment of our society, and the unexpected collapse of such young people is a powerful event that inevitably strikes to the core sensibilities of both the lay public and the physician community.[1,2,17,19] For these reasons, sudden death in young athletes will continue to represent an important medical issue and public health problem. It is the responsibility of the medical community to create a fully informed public and to pursue early detection of the cardiovascular and other causes of catastrophic events in young athletes when prudent and practical. On the other hand, because such events are particularly uncommon with respect to the vast number of athletes participating safely in sports, it also is important that such information about athletic field deaths should not create undo and unnecessary anxiety among young athletes and their families.

Demographics

Based primarily on data assembled from broad-based U.S. populations, a profile of young competitive athletes who die suddenly has emerged.[1-6,9,10,13,17-19] Such athletes participate in a large number and variety of sports, the most common being basketball and football (about 60%), which probably reflects the high participation level in these popular team sports as well as the intensity of physical activity required. In Europe, sudden death in athletes most frequently is associated with soccer.[1]

The vast majority of athletic field deaths occur in men (about 90%). The relative infrequency of these events in women probably reflects lower participation rates, sometimes less intense levels of training, and the fact that women do not engage in some sports with an implicitly higher risk (e.g., football). Most athletes are involved in high school sports at the time of death (about 75%), and less commonly in college or professional competition.

Most athletes who die suddenly with HCM or some other underlying disease are free of symptoms or suspicion of cardiovascular disease. Sudden collapse usually occurs in association with physical exertion, predominantly in the late afternoon and early evening hours, which correspond to peak periods of competition and training, particularly in organized team sports such as football and basketball.[1,3] In addition, genetic heart diseases are more likely to cause sudden unexpected death in trained athletes than in their sedentary counterparts.[16] These observations substantiate the belief that (in the presence of cardiovascular disease), physical activity represents a trigger and an important precipitating factor for sudden death in young athletes.

Although most sudden deaths in competitive athletes have been reported in Caucasian males, a substantial proportion (about 30%) occur in African Americans, including the majority of HCM-related athletic field deaths (Fig. 137.7).[10,13] The number of these sudden deaths in young African American male athletes contrasts sharply with the infrequent identification of African American patients with HCM in hospital-based populations.[10] These observations probably reflect the disproportionate access to subspecialty medical care of young African Americans compared with Caucasians, which in turn makes it less likely that young African American men will be diagnosed with HCM. Consequently, African American athletes with HCM also are less likely to be disqualified from competition to reduce their risk for sudden death, in accordance with the recommendations of the Thirty-Sixth Bethesda Conference.[27]

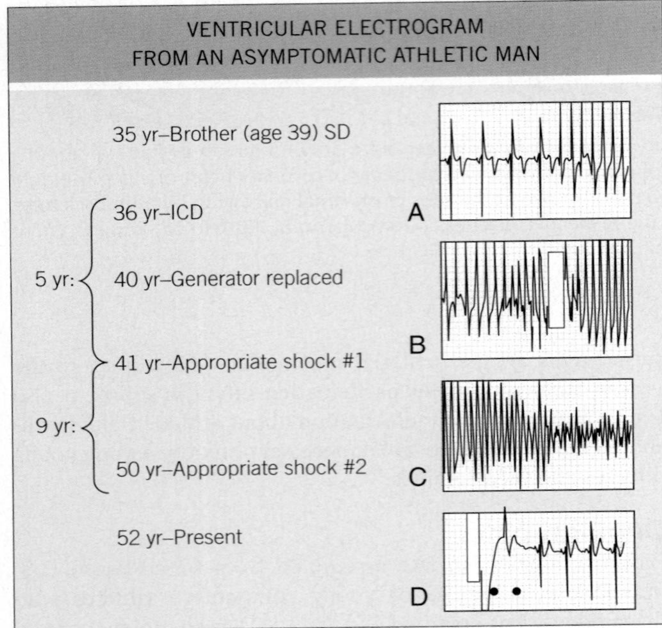

Figure 137.7 Stored ventricular electrogram from an asymptomatic athletic man. The man received a defibrillator prophylactically because of a family history of sudden death related to hypertrophic cardiomyopathy and marked ventricular septal thickness (31 mm). The electrogram was obtained 4 years and 8 months after implantation of the defibrillator. The data were recorded at 1:20 AM, while the patient was asleep. A continuous recording, at 25 mm/s, is shown in four panels, with the tracing recorded from left to right in each. **A,** After four beats of sinus rhythm, ventricular tachycardia begins abruptly, at a rate of 200 beats per minute. **B,** The defibrillator senses ventricular tachycardia and charges. **C,** Ventricular tachycardia deteriorates into ventricular fibrillation. **D,** The defibrillator discharges appropriately (a 20-J shock is denoted by the bar) during ventricular fibrillation and restores sinus rhythm. SD, sudden death; ICD, implantable cardioverter-defibrillator.

Mechanisms and Resuscitation

In most athletes with HCM and other cardiac diseases, cardiac arrest results from electrical instability and primary ventricular tachyarrhythmias (see Fig. 137.7). The major exception is Marfan syndrome, in which death usually results from aortic dissection or rupture. However, regardless of the mechanism, only a small proportion of athletes with cardiovascular disease who collapse on the athletic field are resuscitated successfully. More widespread dissemination of automatic external defibrillators that are available for public access by nontraditional responders in schools and at sporting events would be expected to result in the survival of greater numbers of athletes.[64]

SCREENING AND PREPARTICIPATION DETECTION OF CARDIOVASCULAR ABNORMALITIES

Detection of cardiovascular abnormalities with the potential for significant morbidity or sudden death is the important objective of the widespread practice of preparticipation screening of high school and college-aged athletes. The consensus is that in a benevolent society, physicians have a responsibility to initiate prudent efforts to identify life-threatening diseases in athletes to minimize the cardiovascular risks associated with sports participation.[15,22,24-26] Identification of high risk patients with genetic diseases such as HCM, ARVC, and the ion channelopathies (long QT and Brugada syndromes) has taken on much greater significance with the application of ICDs for primary prevention of sudden death.[31-33] However, a consensus also exists that the return of athletes to competition with potentially lethal cardiovascular disease, based explicitly on the presence of an ICD, is not advisable.[27,29,65]

Major obstacles to any preparticipation screening program are the large reservoirs of young competitive athletes eligible for evaluation (about 10 million to 15 million in the United States) and the uncommon occurrence of cardiovascular disease–related sudden death in a young athlete population.[24,26] Customary cardiovascular screening practice for U.S. high school and college athletes is confined to a history and physical examination,[24,66-69] a strategy that likely lacks sufficient power to identify certain important cardiovascular abnormalities on a consistent basis.[24,66] For example, although the nonobstructive form of HCM (at rest) is the single most common disease entity to be targeted in a mass screening effort, clinical recognition probably occurs relatively infrequently, given that potential diagnostic markers (e.g., a loud heart murmur, syncope, or a family history of sudden death) often are absent. In one retrospective study, only 3% of trained athletes who died suddenly of HCM or other heart disease were suspected by preparticipation screening to have had those cardiovascular abnormalities, and none were disqualified from competition.[3]

The quality of the cardiovascular screening process for U.S. high school and college athletes has come under critical scrutiny (Figs. 137.8 and 137.9).[66-69] However, the design of approved history and physical examination questionnaires for high school preparticipation screening has improved during the past decade in many states (see Fig. 137.8).[67] This is likely to translate into identification of greater numbers of student-athletes with cardiovascular disease, although this judgment will be difficult to document with any precision. Furthermore, legislation in several states continues to allow screening by health care workers with vastly different levels of training and expertise (including chiropractors and naturopathic clinicians), and who often perform preparticipation sports examinations under suboptimal conditions (see Fig. 137.9).[67] National standardization of high school and college preparticipation medical examinations, incorporating American Heart Association (AHA) recommendations,[24] would provide the most practical and effective strategy for achieving the goal of detecting athletes who unknowingly harbor clinically relevant cardiovascular abnormalities.

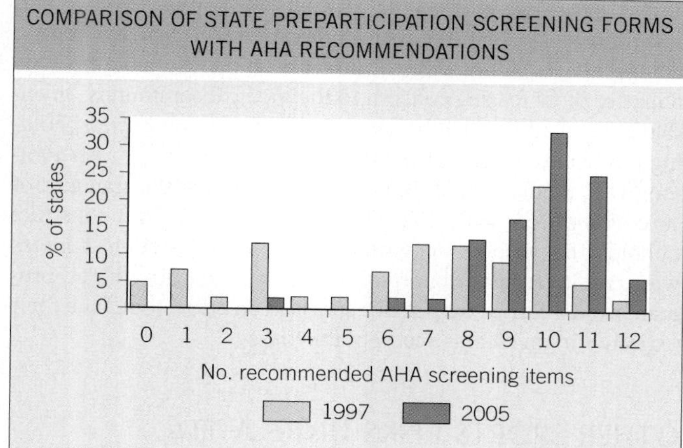

Figure 137.8 Comparison of state preparticipation screening questionnaires (1997 versus 2005) analyzed with respect to the American Heart Association (AHA) recommendations. Screening forms were available in 43 states in 1997 and for 48 states in 2005. (From Glover DW, Glover DW, Maron BJ: Evolution in the process of screening United States high school student-athletes for cardiovascular disease. Am J Cardiol 2007;100:1709-1712.)

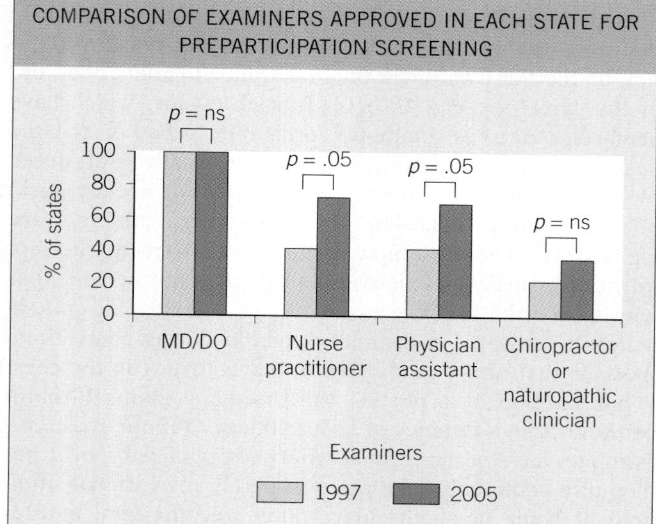

Figure 137.9 Comparison of examiners approved in each state for preparticipation screening (1997 versus 2005). MD, doctor of medicine; DO, doctor of osteopathy.

A unique circumstance has existed in Italy for the past 25 years. Federal government legislation (Medical Protection of Athletic Activities Act) has mandated national preparticipation screening and medical clearance for all young athletes engaged in organized sports programs.[15,23] Annual sports medicine evaluations in Italy routinely include a history and physical examination, as well as a 12-lead ECG. Because the ECG can be abnormal in up to 95% of patients with HCM,[70,71] this test ultimately permits identification of many athletes previously undiagnosed with this disease.[22]

Italian investigators have also attributed a decline in the sudden cardiac death rate associated with competitive sports in the northeastern Veneto region to the long-standing systematic preparticipation screening program in that country, particularly the routine inclusion of a 12-lead ECG.[15,22-24] Specifically, they report a 90% decline in the annual incidence of sudden cardiovascular death in competitive athletes (due largely to a reduced mortality from cardiomyopathy). The Veneto experience has been used to promote the concept of ECG screening to athletic populations in other countries.[15]

Obstacles to implementation of obligatory, government-sponsored national screening in the United States with ECG or echocardiography (or both) are outlined in detail in the 2007 AHA consensus statement on preparticipation screening.[24] These factors include the particularly large "at risk" athlete population to be screened, major cost-benefit considerations, and recognition that achieving a zero risk circumstance in competitive sports is not realistic. Other obstacles include the absence of a federal law in the United States (as currently exists in Italy) to govern eligibility and disqualification decisions and, most importantly, the lack of existing resources in the form of dedicated medical personnel (including physicians) available to perform the examinations and interpret ECGs.[24] Large population preparticipation screening with noninvasive testing also is limited by the expected large number of false-positive (i.e., borderline) examinations.[72,73] Furthermore, the possibility of false-negative tests in which subtle but important lesions go undetected exists, such as when echocardiography is performed in the prehypertrophic phase of HCM (individuals younger than 14 years of age)[74] or when coronary anomalies cannot be reliably identified.[44] Preparticipation screening using ECG, conducted in research settings in relatively small athlete cohorts, produced a particularly low yield of cardiovascular abnormalities.[72-75]

CRITERIA FOR SPORTS ELIGIBILITY AND DISQUALIFICATION

When a cardiovascular abnormality is identified in a competitive athlete, several considerations arise: (1) the level of risk for sudden death if participation in organized sports continues; (2) the likelihood that risk would be reduced if systematic training and competition were terminated; and (3) the criteria to formulate appropriate eligibility or disqualification decisions. Unfortunately, on occasion the medical disqualification decision-making process can become polarized, given the personal aspirations of the athlete versus the mandate of the physician to protect patients from circumstances associated with unacceptable risks.[1,2]

It should be underscored that the risk associated with intense physical exertion for sports participants with cardiovascular abnormalities is difficult to quantify with any precision, given the extreme and unpredictable physiologic circumstances to which individual athletes may be exposed. Only some HCM-related sudden deaths are associated with intense physical activity,[34] and not all trained athletes with this disease die suddenly during the competitive phase or even while diretly engaged in sporting activities.[3,13]

In this regard, the American College of Cardiology (ACC) Thirty-Sixth Bethesda Conference[27] and the European Society of Cardiology (ESC) consensus panel[29] offer expert recommendations and clear benchmarks for clinical practice. Panel guidelines for athletic eligibility or qualification start with the premise that intense sports training and competition increase sudden death risk in susceptible athletes with most forms of heart disease and that the risk is likely to be reduced or minimized by temporary or permanent withdrawal from sports participation. The unique pressures of organized athletics do not allow participants to exert strict control over their level of exertion or reliably discern when cardiac symptoms make it prudent to withdraw from the physical activity. The U.S. appellate court decision in *Knapp v. Northwestern*[28] upholds the use of national association medical guidelines (e.g., those of the Bethesda Conference) in making disqualification decisions for athletes. Therefore, team physicians would be wise to rely on the guidelines established by the Thirty-Sixth Bethesda Conference[27] in making difficult eligibility versus disqualification recommendations, because this document likely will play an important role as precedent in resolving future medical-legal disputes.

Under these guidelines, young athletes with the unequivocal diagnosis of HCM are discouraged from competitive athletic participation, except for low-intensity sports (e.g., golf and bowling).[27] Some acquired diseases that are potentially reversible (e.g., myocarditis) can justify temporary withdrawal from competition, followed by resumption of organized sports activity after reversal and resolution of the disease state. The ESC consensus report[29] is modeled largely after the recommendations of the Bethesda Conference.[27] Although the two sets of guidelines are very similar, the European recommendations are more restrictive in selected instances.

Decisions to withdraw athletes from sports because of heart disease may be confounded by complex societal considerations and can prove difficult to implement and enforce, particularly when elite sports careers and substantial economic gain are involved.[2] Many such athletes are highly motivated to remain in the competitive arena, may not fully appreciate the implications of the relevant medical information, or are willing to accept the risks while resisting prudent recommendations to withdraw.[2] National medical standards for disqualification are linked to law in Italy,[23] but such mandatory processes generally are not part of the U.S. health care system.

Improper overdiagnosis of cardiac disease may lead to unnecessary disqualification from athletics, depriving some individuals of the psychological and economic benefits of competitive sports. In the United States, the physician's judgment in making medical eligibility and disqualification decisions can be impaired insidiously by extrinsic pressures imposed by relatives, fans, alumni, coaching staff and administrators, particularly when athletes participate in "shopping" for multiple medical opinions until one is secured that supports continued sports participation.[1,2,24] Such situations often become particularly complex, attributable to the societal attitudes that often attach exaggerated importance and materialism to organized sports.[1]

In the United States, the relationship between sports medicine and the law is complex and involves tenuous relationships between physicians, athlete-patients, teams, and institutions.[76,77] Liability issues relevant to the management of competitive athletes with cardiovascular disease have become a matter of increasing concern to the medical community, given that several athlete deaths have triggered disputes in court holding physicians accountable for alleged grievances.[76,77] An evolving U.S. medical-legal framework is clarifying the standard of care associated with this clinical practice.[76] This construct upholds the wisdom of withholding selected student-athletes with cardiovascular abnormalities from access to athletic programs and intense competitive sports in an effort to reduce their exposure to medically unacceptable risks.[27]

OTHER SPORTS RISKS UNRELATED TO CARDIOVASCULAR DISEASE

Commotio Cordis

Although sudden death in young athletes as a result of unsuspected cardiovascular disease has achieved considerable visibility, other risks of organized (or recreational) sports activity that lead to cardiac arrest have emerged more recently.[1,20,21,78] For example, virtually instantaneous cardiac arrest may result from a relatively modest, nonpenetrating precordial blow (Figs. 137.10 and 137.11) in the absence of underlying cardiovascular disease or structural injury to the chest wall or heart itself. This impact may leave a contusion on the chest wall over the precordium in about one third of the cases (see Fig. 137.10). In such events, which have been referred to as commotio cordis ("disturbed or agitated heart motion"), blunt precordial impact usually is produced by a projectile (most commonly a baseball or hockey puck) or by bodily collision with another athlete (see Fig. 137.11). The chest blow usually is of low energy (except for hockey pucks and lacrosse balls) and is not perceived as unusual for the sporting event nor of sufficient magnitude to result in death. A common scenario during competitive sports is that of a young baseball player struck in the chest (while batting) by a pitched ball thrown at about 40 miles per hour from a distance of about 40 feet. Of note, these catastrophes have occurred in a variety of organized sports, but they also commonly take place in purely recreational situations at home or on the playground, and the fatal injuries often are caused by friends or relatives (see Fig. 137.11).

An experimental model in juvenile swine closely simulated the clinical profile of commotio cordis and provided important

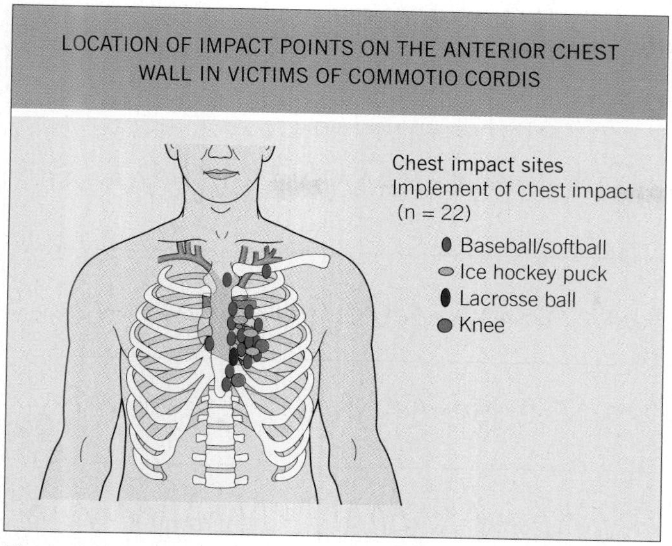

LOCATION OF IMPACT POINTS ON THE ANTERIOR CHEST WALL IN VICTIMS OF COMMOTIO CORDIS

Chest impact sites
Implement of chest impact
(n = 22)
Baseball/softball
Ice hockey puck
Lacrosse ball
Knee

Figure 137.10 Location of impact points on the anterior chest wall judged to be produced by projectiles such as baseballs, softballs, ice hockey pucks, lacrosse balls, or blunt bodily contact that were identified in victims of commotio cordis. The estimated contour of the heart is demarcated by the solid line. The lesions are oval or circular contusions, abrasions, or bruises located in the midprecordial area, usually to the left of the sternum, extending laterally to the nipple line and vertically from the angle of Louis to the xiphoid process.

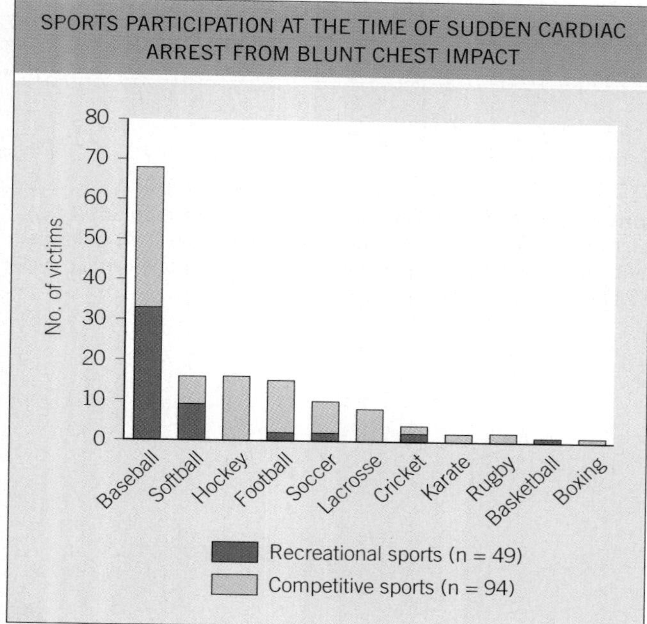

Figure 137.11 Sports participation at the time of sudden cardiac arrest induced by blunt chest impact (commotio cordis), shown separately for competitive and recreational athletic activities.

insights into the mechanisms responsible for these events.[79-81] This model demonstrated that a precordial blow can create devastating electrophysiologic consequences, largely by virtue of its precise timing and location over the heart. Low-energy chest impact during a very narrow window of 15 to 30 ms before the peak of the T wave (representing only about 1% of the overall cardiac cycle) reproducibly resulted in ventricular fibrillation (Fig. 137.12).[79] Conversely, when the precordium was struck during depolarization (on the QRS complex), transient complete heart block usually occurred.

Recognition of commotio cordis as a risk of athletic participation raises consideration for possible preventive strategies.[82] While softer than normal safety baseballs reduced the risk for ventricular fibrillation in the swine model,[79] such projectiles have not proven to be absolutely protective against sudden cardiac death on the athletic field.[20] Commotio cordis events are not uniformly fatal, and approximately 15% of reported victims are known to have survived, usually when afforded prompt cardiopulmonary resuscitation and defibrillation.[20,21] With enhanced public awareness of this syndrome, emergency measures, including the use of automated external defibrillators, are more likely to be implemented on the athletic field in a timely fashion, possibly preventing many future deaths.

Although undoubtedly uncommon, the precise frequency with which commotio cordis occurs is unknown. Nevertheless, among all causes of sudden death in young athletes, commotio cordis ranks second in occurrence, behind only hypertrophic cardiomyopathy.[1] Cardiac arrest induced by blunt chest impact has been so poorly understood in the lay community that some events have been regarded as criminal acts rather than physiologically based catastrophic accidents.[83]

Neck Blows

Virtually instantaneous death has been reported during ice hockey competition when high-velocity blows to the neck by the puck triggered arterial rupture and subarachnoid hemorrhage[78] (Fig. 137.13). Reflex hyperextension of the head, causing vertebral artery dissection at its fixed anchor point in the foramina transversaria, was the likely mechanism for these deaths. Such events underscore the broad spectrum of causes and mechanisms that may be responsible for sudden death in young athletes while engaged in competitive sports.

SUMMARY

Athletic training commonly results in benign cardiac remodeling, but it also incurs a very low risk for sudden death, usually as a result of a variety of unsuspected congenital cardiovascular diseases; or less commonly, due to nonpenetrating chest blows (commotio cordis). Sudden death in young athletes usually occurs during physical exertion, with hypertrophic cardiomyopathy and congenital coronary artery anomalies of wrong sinus origin most commonly the cause of these tragic events. In adults (over age 35) participating in sports, atherosclerotic coronary artery disease is the predominant cause of sudden death. Preparticipation screening of athletes can raise the suspicion or diagnosis of cardiovascular abnormalities, permitting timely therapeutic intervention to reduce risk, including disqualification from intense competitive sports.

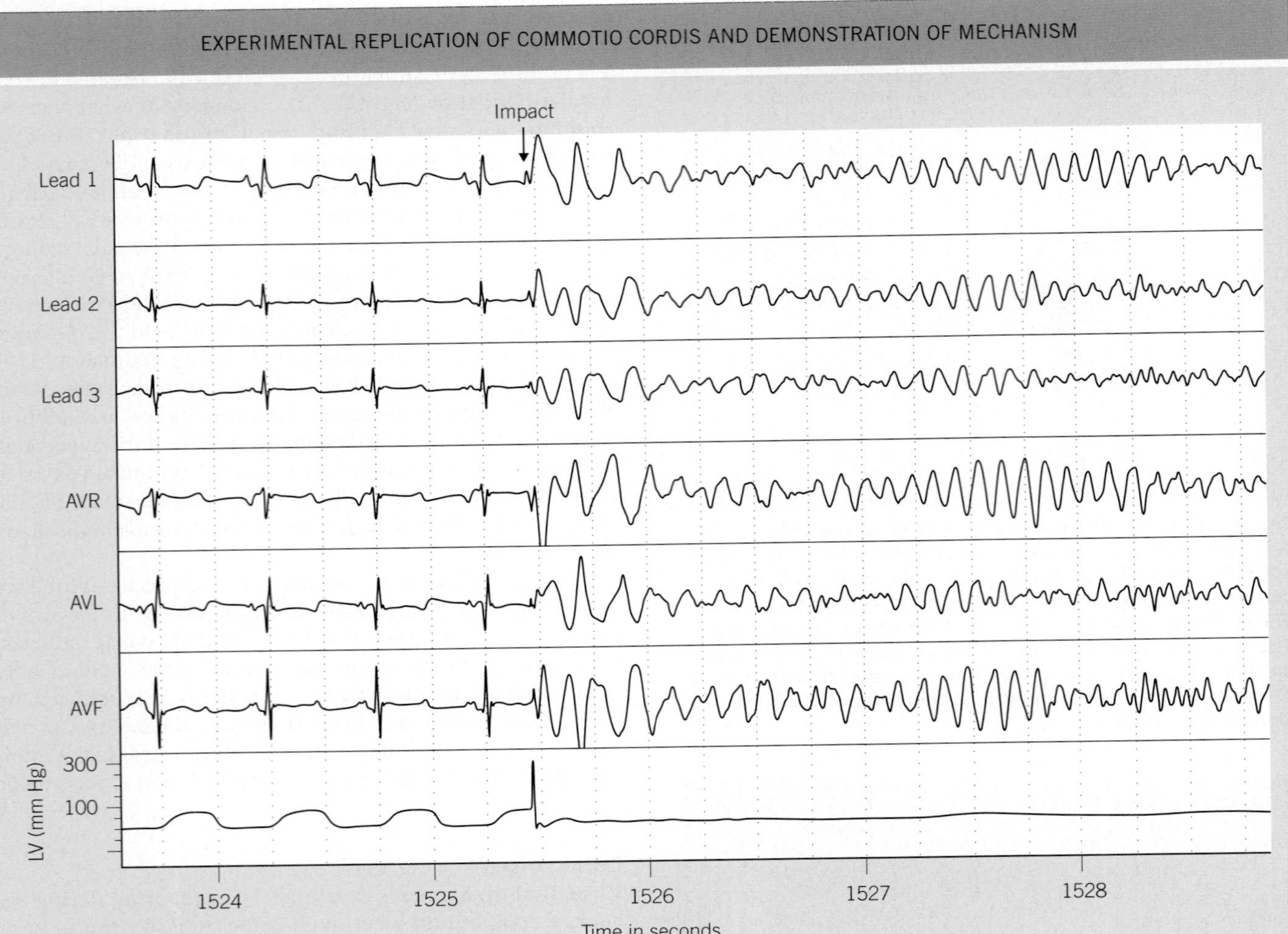

Figure 137.12 Experimental replication of commotio cordis and demonstration of mechanism. A six-lead electrocardiogram (ECG) shows the electrophysiologic and hemodynamic consequences of an impact to the chest from a wooden object traveling at 30 miles per hour, timed to occur 15 ms before the peak of the T wave in a 9-kg pig. Ventricular fibrillation began immediately (within one cardiac cycle) after the chest impact, which was associated with instantaneous loss of effective left ventricular (LV) pressure.

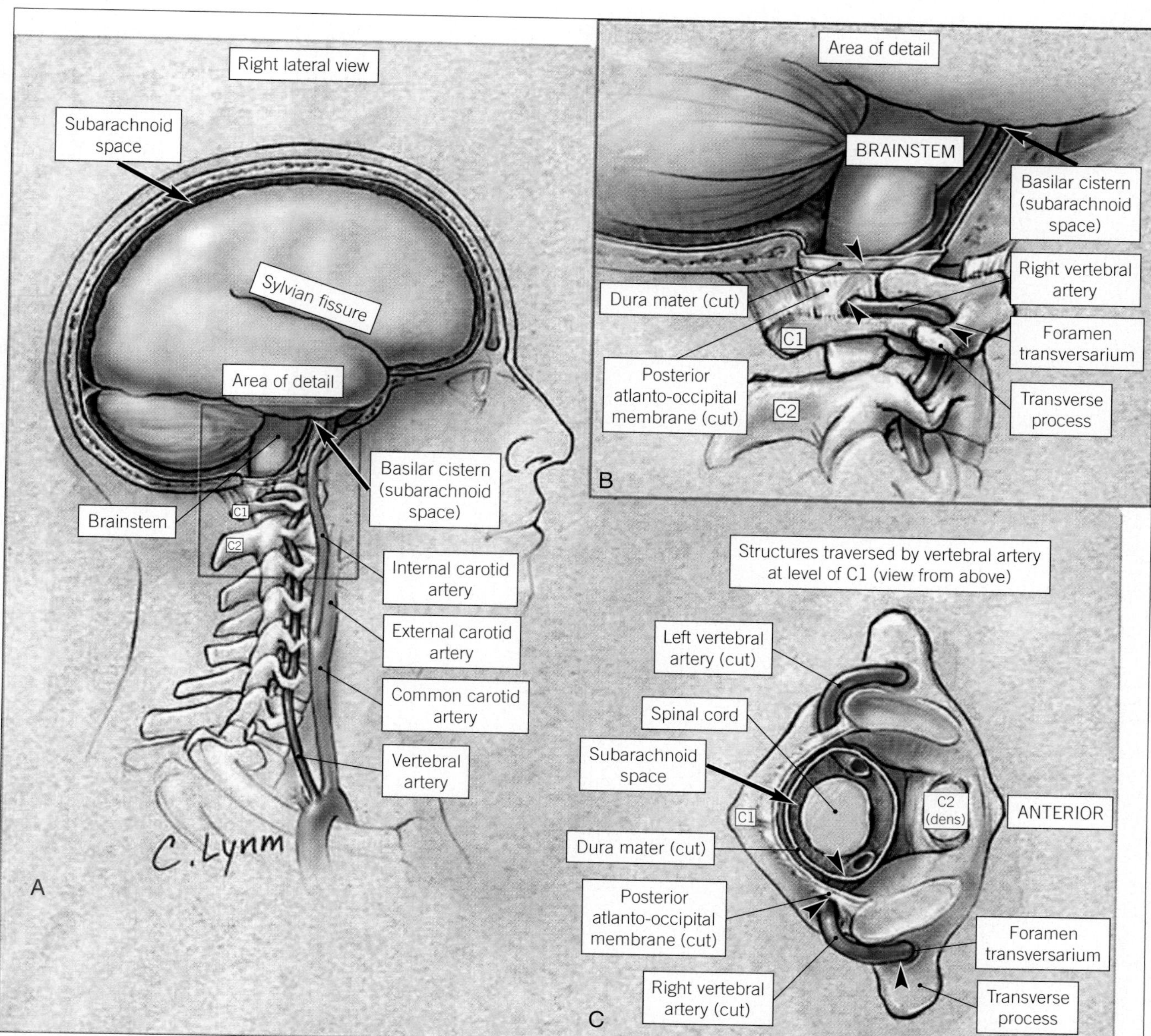

Figure 137.13 A blow to an unprotected area of the upper neck by a hockey puck (accompanied by abrupt reflex hyperextension) can result in sudden death *(upper panel).* The mechanism involves arterial dissection and rupture at the anatomic point where the vertebral artery courses through the bony canal of the foramen transversarium and penetrates the posterior atlanto-occipital membrane or dura mater *(lower panel).* The vertebral artery is rigidly anchored at this point (as it enters the transverse process of the first cervical vertebra) and becomes the point of rupture, leading to massive hemorrhage into the subarachnoid space and, consequently, instantaneous death. (From Maron BJ, Poliac LC, Ashare AB, et al: Sudden death due to neck blows among amateur hockey players. JAMA 2003;290:599-601.)

chapter 138 Psychosocial Influences on the Heart

Kristina Orth-Gomér, Gerdi Weidner, David E. Anderson, and Margaret A. Chesney

Definition

- Psychosocial influences are independent risk factors for cardiac disease that work by directly affecting physiologic parameters and by affecting behaviors that are associated with increased risk.

Key Features

- Stressful social environments: low socioeconomic status, stressful work and family situations, social strain.
- Individual characteristics: emotional response styles, lifestyle behaviors, inhibited breathing patterns.

Therapy

- Improve coping skills for managing stressful social environments, including increasing social support.
- Reduce emotional reactions to environmental stress, particularly anger and depression.
- Intervene to modify lifestyle behaviors associated with stress, including smoking, physical inactivity, and unhealthy eating habits.
- Consider stress management techniques, including those emphasizing breathing, that have been shown both to reduce stress and improve respiration.

Research in industrialized countries has shown that psychosocial factors contribute to the risk of cardiovascular disease (CVD) over and above the standard risk factors of hypertension, dyslipidemia, and smoking.[1-3] Psychosocial risk factors for CVD arise in a context of the dynamic interactions between people and their social environments and lead to physiologic adaptations that increase cardiac risk. Recent evidence suggests that psychosocial factors also increase the risk of CVD in the developing world. In the INTERHEART Study,[4] a case-control investigation of acute myocardial infarction (MI) in 52 countries representing every continent, a considerable percentage of the attributable risk was due to psychosocial stress (25.3% in men; 40% in women) at work or at home, from financial status, life events, and depression.

The multivariate nature of psychosocial factors, including environmental components (e.g., work stress) and individual components (e.g., pathogenic emotional, behavioral, and physiologic responses), presents a challenge to the development of a systematic approach for incorporation into cardiology. In this chapter, we propose a conceptual framework that organizes these factors into a system of interacting pathways by which psychosocial factors can influence the heart. As shown in Fig. 138.1, environmental factors, such as stressful working conditions or low socioeconomic status, create conditions that increase cardiac risk through three interacting pathways. The first consists of emotional response styles or adaptations to stressful environments, such as trait anger or depression. The second consists of lifestyle behaviors, such as sedentary behavior and smoking, each of which has been shown to be sensitive to environmental stress. Recent research suggests a third pathway, which involves stress-induced changes in breathing habits that alter the set point for blood gases and plasma volume. By understanding these different factors as separate but interacting routes to common cardiovascular outcomes, the empiric evidence for psychosocial influences on the heart may contribute to more effective clinical practice.

INFLUENCE OF STRESSFUL SOCIAL ENVIRONMENTS

Low Socioeconomic Status

Much of the research during the past decades on the influence of stressful social environments on CVD in developed countries has focused on low socioeconomic status (SES). SES is assessed by low education, income, or occupational status (or all three). Specifically, men and women of low SES have an increased all-cause, as well as CVD, mortality risk, which is reflected in an increased risk of acute MI and other acute coronary syndromes. A similar SES gradient is found in most of the risk factors for CVD, including behavioral, psychological, and biologic risk factors. Several attempts have been made to "explain" the SES gradients in CVD in developed countries, with evidence focused on individuals' responses to challenges associated with lower SES and lack of coping resources.[5]

In the classic Whitehall studies of British civil servants, Marmot and colleagues[6] showed that the risk of ischemic heart disease was four times higher in men in the lowest occupational categories than in administrative personnel in top positions. However, the standard risk factors (cholesterol, blood pressure, smoking) also were more prevalent in lower occupational levels. Controlling for these factors reduced the gradient but did not eliminate it. More recently, the extent of atherosclerosis found in carotid arteries also was shown to be inversely related to SES.[7] The social gradient of carotid atherosclerosis reflected a similar gradient in coronary disease in a preclinical cohort of middle-aged Finnish men.

It should be noted that women were under-represented in early SES studies.[8] One exception was the Stockholm Female

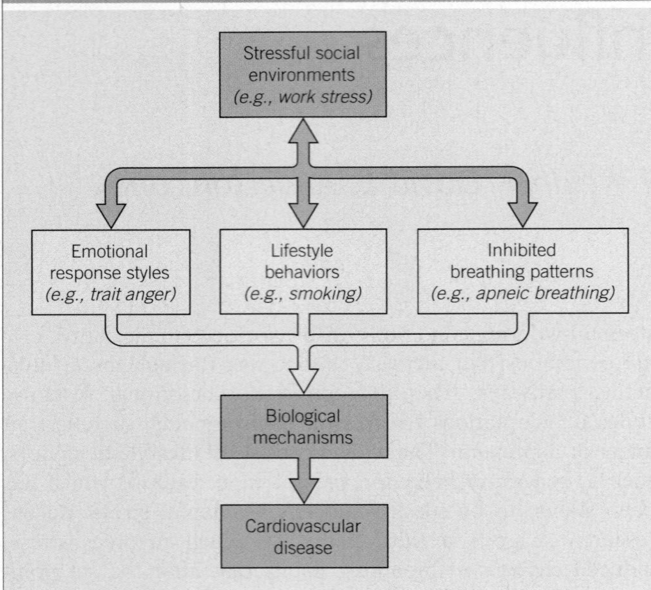

Figure 138.1 Conceptual framework: pathways by which stressful social environments contribute to cardiovascular disease.

Coronary Risk Factor Study, a population-based study of Swedish middle-aged women with acute coronary syndromes; this study provided the first comprehensive information on the influence of low SES on the risk of MI in women.[9,10] Women with low educational status had twice the risk of MI, and women with low-status manual work had four times the risk, of women working in higher status academic settings. The most pronounced SES gradients were associated with other specific environmental stress factors; work environments characterized by lack of control, influence, and decision latitude; and social environments low in social support and social integration.

Consistent with the model proposed in this chapter, the Stockholm Female Coronary Risk Factor Study[9,10] showed that more than half of the association with the risk of MI was explained by poor lifestyle behaviors and emotional adaptations to stress, which were more common in low-SES women. Specifically, low-SES women were more likely than higher-SES women to smoke, to be less physically active, and to have poor dietary habits, with a higher intake of total fat and a lower intake of fiber. Consequently, obesity was more prevalent in low-SES women, particularly central obesity with abdominal fat distribution. Low-SES women also showed more emotional reactions to stress, marked by decreased personal capacity to cope with stressors, more depressed mood, and greater hostility. Consistent with the model, the SES gradient also was associated with increased physiologic risk factors, including higher systolic and diastolic blood pressure, higher low-density lipoprotein (LDL) cholesterol, and lower high-density lipoprotein (HDL) cholesterol, all of which are also influenced by intervening factors, such as physical inactivity, diet, and consequential obesity.

Stress in Work and Home Settings

Stressful working conditions and lack of control at work are factors that become more salient as the demands and strains of working life increase globally.[4] These sources of lifestyle stress were among the first to be tested in empiric investigations, which provided information for models that linked environmental stress to biomedical outcome variables. The leading stressful work environment model, the demand-control model, originally proposed by Karasek and Theorell[11] includes two characteristics of the work environment that, when combined, may lead to work strain. The first is high demand in terms of workload, time pressure, or consequences of making errors; the second is low control or decision latitude. When these two conditions coexist, the work strain is greater than for either alone. Illustrating the dynamic interplay between various environmental stressors, high work strain is found in many low-SES jobs. In addition, many relatively high-SES jobs are becoming high-strain jobs according to this model. For example, being dependent on computer technology without being able to influence and control the computer systems may be associated with increased work strain.

Several studies have tested the demand-control model in various settings and study groups. Alfredsson, Theorell, and others[12] have shown prospectively in large population samples that high demand and low control at work doubles the risk of acute MI. Furthermore, once an acute MI has occurred, the risk of recurrence increases dramatically if the patient returns to the same work situation.

Subsequent models of work stress also have considered worker characteristics. Eriksen and Ursin[13] argue that whether the worker expects to cope with the situation is as important as the extent of control. In the effort-reward paradigm of Siegrist,[14] strain from high demand and low control is combined with the extent to which the worker feels that reward is appropriate. If reward is insufficient, the worker becomes frustrated, overwhelmed, and "submerged" by the demands of the working conditions. Reaching a state of submersion constitutes a strong risk of impending CVD. A recent test of the combined strain and reward models resulted in an augmented risk of CVD in both men and women.[15]

Cardiovascular research long has reported that life stress not only exists in the workplace, but also arises with migration, war, natural disasters, and strain in the home. The dramatic health decline in Central and Eastern Europe over the past four decades, more than half of which has been due to an increase in CVD mortality, has been attributed to the stresses of social change, marked by economic hardship, social disruption, and a poor outlook for the future.[8] Regarding stress in the home, several authors have cautioned against generalizing results from men's to women's work situations and other stressors.[16] In women, the issue of total workload from both paid and unpaid work is more germane than in men. Frankenhaeuser and associates[17] have shown that women in industrialized countries with small children had a total workload of several hours more per week than men in the same situation.

Social Strain

Research on social networks indicates that a lack of social ties, characterized by social isolation and poor social relations, increases overall mortality. At least five large-scale,

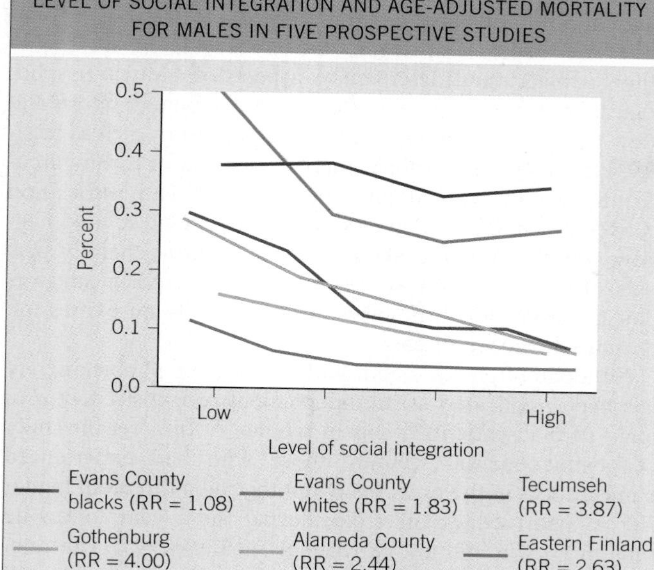

Figure 138.2 Level of social integration and age-adjusted mortality for males in five prospective studies. The relative risk (RR) ratios of mortality at the lowest versus highest level of social integration are shown. (Modified from House JS, Landis KR, Umberson D. Social relationships and health. 1988;241:540-545.)

population-based studies from three different countries have shown that poor social networks increase CVD mortality (Fig. 138.2). In their classic review, House and colleagues[18] summarized the evidence, "This effect of poor social networks and the patterns of prospective association between social integration (i.e., the number and frequency of social relationships and contacts) and mortality are remarkably similar with some variation by race, sex, and geographic locale."

Consistent with the model proposed here, people who are low in social support are more likely to be depressed. The absence of social support may potentiate the health hazards of stressful life events and multiply the health risks of such events several times. In population-based studies of older men born in Gothenburg, those who both experienced stressful events and had poor emotional support had five times the mortality risk of men with more social support.[19] Good emotional support, therefore, was protective against the adverse health effects of a life crisis, such as loss of a friend or a job or economic difficulties.

A primary source of social support for many is the spousal relationship. Problematic spousal relationships both contribute to the development of CVD and worsen the prognosis of patients with CVD. In Swedish women, for example, the chronic experience of a stressful spousal relationship was found to increase the risk of a recurrent cardiac event by a factor of three, even after adjustment for clinical markers of poor prognosis. Most of those women were employed outside the home, but stress at work alone did not carry the same risk.[20] Women may also receive less emotional support from their spouses than men. In a large, population-based survey, men were more than twice as likely to name their spouse as their primary provider of social support, whereas women were more likely to name another female relative. Furthermore, being single was not a risk factor for CVD in those women, as it is in men. Contrary to the common finding in men, being married or a cohabitant did not improve the cardiovascular health risk in the women.[20]

Management of Stressful Social Environments

Intervening at the environmental level to reduce or eliminate stress, such as improving social equity to address the adverse effects of low SES, certainly is feasible and advisable, although not within the domain of traditional cardiology. Several interventions attempt to increase the ability of individuals to cope with stress and its effects on their lives. An example of such an intervention is coping effectiveness training (CET), which trains individuals to distinguish between stressors over which they have potential control and those over which they do not and then apply different coping strategies for each of these contingencies. Specifically, people are taught to apply a wide range of problem-solving approaches to increase effectiveness in the social environment, including negotiation and communication skills. For situations beyond individual control, persons are taught skills, such as meditation, or cognitive approaches to reduce depression and enhance positive moods.[21,22] In addition, CET teaches specific skills for identification of the type of social support needed and for matching the characteristics of the support to the skills and resources of the provider. Thus CET is similar to a number of other programs that emphasize empowerment and enhance a person's potential to gain control and take self-determined actions.[5] The recent program, "Tackling Inequalities in Health" reported that participants who were actively engaged in the project's planning and implementation personally experienced an increase in social integration.[23]

Trials of group interventions for cardiac patients often teach skills for coping with environmental stress as part of a comprehensive, psychological approach to reducing emotional reactions to stress and providing social support. A recent meta-analysis of 43 randomized trials containing psychological treatments concluded that psychological treatment reduced mortality by 27% for follow-up of 2 years or less and reduced event recurrence by 43% at follow-up longer than 2 years.[24] Other, more comprehensive projects that include management of environmental stress and increasing social support in multi–risk factor intervention programs have demonstrated improvements, including the Lifestyle Heart Trial, which documented a reversal of coronary artery disease progression and a reduction in clinical events.[25] Underscoring the importance of adherence to the intervention, the extent to which patients practiced stress management (yoga and meditation) was related to the reduction in percent diameter stenosis at both the 1-year and 5-year follow-ups.[26] Similarly, among 440 patients with coronary artery disease participating in the Multisite Cardiac Lifestyle Intervention Program, the frequency of support group attendance over 1 year was associated with improvements in blood pressure, health behaviors, and quality of life.[27] In the earlier Recurrent Coronary Prevention Project,[28] the intervention group had a substantially lower risk of relapse during the following 2 years. Although this trial aimed at reducing hostility and stress-related behaviors, one of the important effects was an increase in social support.[28]

PATHWAYS FOR REDUCING RISK ASSOCIATED WITH ENVIRONMENTAL STRESS

Stressful social environments exert their effects through three major pathways. Each pathway is characterized by dynamic interplay between individuals and their social situations, consisting of their socioeconomic status, work, and family milieus. In this section, we discuss each of these pathways, documenting how they can lead either to increased risk or, when disrupted, to risk reduction (see Fig. 138.1).

Pathway 1: Emotional Response Styles

The concept that emotional reactions, such as anger or depression, exert a powerful influence on the heart has a long history but a short scientific past. More than a century ago, the noted physician Sir William Osler stated that, "Mental worry, severe grief, or sudden shock may precede directly the onset of the attack of anginal chest pain." Not until the second half of the 20th century, however, did large epidemiologic studies identify emotional reaction to stress or psychological characteristics such as anger and depression as independent risk factors for coronary heart disease (CHD).[2,3]

Anger, or its underlying predisposition, hostility, is viewed here as an emotional adaptation to environmental stress. In some individuals, the pattern becomes chronic, characterized by mistrust and cynicism, and can lead to antagonistic or aggressive behavior. Interest in anger or hostility evolved from early research on the type A behavior pattern,[29] as characterized by a sense of time urgency, loud and explosive speech, impatience, hostility/anger, and competitiveness. Early studies documented the association between overall type A behavior and the development of CHD. More recent studies have indicated that the anger/hostility component of the original type A construct accounted for the increased risk for the development of CHD.[2,3,30,31]

Research on potential mechanisms that link anger to increased CVD risk increased the focus on both physiologic and behavioral pathways.[32] Laboratory and field studies indicate that individuals with high levels of anger or hostility spend more time than their less angry counterparts in states of heightened autonomic arousal. Studies indicate that they are more likely to perceive their social environments as a challenge, often accompanied by feelings of anger and hostility. Chronically elevated sympathetic nervous system activity has been implicated in the development of atherosclerosis and coronary heart disease. Expressions of anger have been shown to trigger MI, and recall of anger-provoking situations can also produce an acute impairment of ventricular function in patients with CHD.[31,32]

Illustrating the interactions among the three pathways linking stressful social environments to cardiovascular disease, individuals with high levels of anger or hostility also tend to engage in unhealthy behavior, including smoking, physical inactivity, and consumption of foods high in cholesterol and saturated fat. Another illustration of the interactions of these pathways is the fact that individuals with high anger levels also are less likely to receive social support, which increases their risk.

Depression, like anger or hostility, is another emotional adaptation that has been extensively investigated in relation to CVD. Depression, anger, and anxiety often are highly intercorrelated and described as aspects of a single psychological construct, negative affect. The evidence supports the view that depression and related characteristics such as anxiety, like anger and hostility, increase the risk of cardiovascular disease in women and men.[3,31,33-35] The association between increases in depressive symptoms (and related negative emotions) and cardiovascular mortality generally persists after control for severity of disease, which suggests that the psychological factors are not merely an expression of more advanced disease.

Although often coexistent with depression, phobic anxiety has been implicated as an independent prognostic factor in male cardiac patients[36] and in women.[37] In a recent study of postmenopausal women, those who had experienced panic attacks in the previous 6 months had a threefold higher risk of heart attack or stroke during the 5-year follow-up than those who did not experience such attacks.[34] The relationship between panic disorders and cardiovascular disease is complex. On the one hand, many patients who present with panic attacks (anxiety, palpitations, dizziness, dyspnea, and other somatic manifestations) have no clinical signs or symptoms of CHD. However, an increased cardiovascular mortality risk, in particular sudden cardiac death, has been confirmed in these patients.

Research investigating potential mechanisms linking depression to increased CVD risk has focused on elevations in neurotransmitters, such as catecholamines and serotonin, which are central to dysregulation theories of affective disorders and have been shown to increase platelet aggregation and facilitate thrombogenic events. Although the release of epinephrine in the face of real physical threat can be adaptive, frequent release in response to stressful social environments is thought to be associated with an elevated risk of CVD. Like anger, depression has been linked to life-threatening arrhythmias and resulting mortality in humans.[32] In addition, new evidence indicates that individuals with high levels of depression show inflammatory processes and lower levels of omega-3 polyunsaturated fatty acids, both of which have been implicated in an elevated CHD risk.[38] As with anger and hostility, people with a high level of depression tend to engage in unhealthy behaviors, such as smoking, physical inactivity, delay in seeking treatment, and nonadherence to medical regimens.[38]

Management of Emotional Reactions to Environmental Stress

Recognizing the increased risk associated with anger and depression, cardiac rehabilitation facilities have incorporated programs to reduce this risk. Consistent with the framework presented here, most of these programs are described as involving "stress management" and focus on training individuals to modify cognitive, behavioral, and physiologic responses to stressful social environments. In general, these programs help patients to recognize their reactions to stress, particularly anger and depression, and to examine the sources of these feelings and their likely consequences. Patients are encouraged to consider alternatives to these responses and taught specific skills to reinforce more socially effective strategies, thus improving coping and social competence.

The previously mentioned Recurrent Coronary Prevention Project successfully reduced hostility and other stress-related behaviors and reported a significantly lower recurrence rate in the treatment group compared with control participants.[28] Significant long-term reductions in hostility, in addition to improvements in the cardiac risk profile, clinical events, and coronary stenosis, were observed in the aforementioned Lifestyle Heart Trial.[35] These findings were replicated in the previously cited Multisite Cardiac Lifestyle Intervention Program.[39]

In the previously mentioned recent meta-analysis of psychological treatments of cardiac patients, the effects of such treatment were isolated from those of exercise, diet, and smoking cessation.[24] The results indicated that psychological treatments that focused primarily on reducing depression and distress reduced mortality and the recurrence of cardiovascular events. The effects were confined to trials that initiated treatment at least 2 months after the cardiac event and were most pronounced among male patients. Studies that initiated psychological treatment less than 2 months after a cardiac event showed little benefit compared with usual care controls. The authors speculated that early recruitment may capture patients who have sufficient psychological resources to recover without professional help. Indeed, this may be one explanation for the failure of the ENRICHD trial conducted in the United States, which found no benefit of treatment to reduce depression and increase social support, compared with a standard care group.[40] Secondary gender specific analyses, however, suggested a decreased CVD mortality in caucasian men, whereas in women, CVD prognosis did not change significantly. In contrast, in a recent long term follow-up of Swedish women with CVD, survival improved dramatically in those women, who received a psychosocial intervention program specifically adapted for women's needs. This group-based program focused on skills to cope with both family and work-related stress.[41]

Pathway 2: Lifestyle Behaviors

Lifestyle behaviors, such as smoking, physical inactivity, and unhealthy eating habits, are more prevalent among people who live in stressful social environments, such as those characterized by low SES.[41a] Indeed, unhealthy lifestyles explain approximately 25% of the variance in health outcomes associated with low SES.[41] Similarly, people who live in environments characterized by high levels of work or family stress have been shown to engage in unhealthy behavior, such as smoking or physical inactivity. As noted in the previous section, a potential for synergism in the adverse effects is seen in the fact that people who respond to environmental stress with anger and depression are also more likely to smoke or to be less physically active, or both.

Management of Lifestyle Behaviors

Cardiac rehabilitation programs routinely place considerable attention on improving lifestyle behaviors, particularly increased exercise and smoking cessation. Effective management strategies are discussed in other chapters in this volume. Of relevance here is the importance of the social environment in the extent to which it potentiates or deters positive lifestyle changes. For example, low-SES environments have been shown to limit physical activity and access to healthier food while providing more ready access to tobacco and alcohol products.[5,42] Similarly, it has been shown that after MI, women in problematic spousal relationships had a higher rate of recurrence.[43] Therefore, establishment of healthier lifestyles is facilitated by consideration of the social environment, social norms, and resources available to patients. Moreover, it is important to take into account the patient's emotional response styles, such as anger and depression, which can undermine lifestyle changes. It is well known, for example, that increased anger mediates relapse to smoking after attempts to stop, and depression is associated with nonadherence to medical instructions concerning lifestyle changes.

The coexistence of negative emotional adaptations and unhealthy lifestyles indicates a need for interdisciplinary programs that address those behaviors in a comprehensive manner (see the Guidelines of the Third and Fourth Joint Task Forces of the European and Other Societies on Cardiovascular Disease Prevention).[44,45] Interventions incorporating such approaches include the Multisite Cardiac Lifestyle Intervention Program,[39] which emphasizes a group format, thus creating a social environment likely to reinforce positive health practices and reduce CVD risk.

Pathway 3: Inhibited Breathing Patterns

Another link between environmental stress and CVD is suggested in studies that investigate conditions under which apneic breathing can be observed. It is well known that sleep apnea is an established risk factor for chronic hypertension,[46] but intermittent breath-holding also has been observed in hypertensive patients during the daytime.[47] Disordered breathing is characteristic of chronic heart failure[48,49] and is a marker for increased cardiovascular mortality in these patients.[50] Other research with normotensive individuals has documented that inhibited breathing can be the result of environmental stress. Specifically, in the Baltimore Longitudinal Study on Aging, normotensive women with high chronic perceived stress were found to breathe more slowly (but not more deeply) at rest than those who reported less chronic stress.[51] In addition, a slow breathing pattern at rest recently was found to be a risk factor for blood pressure responsiveness to changes in dietary sodium intake in older women.[52] By contrast, faster breathers showed no changes in blood pressure in response to changes in dietary sodium intake. Associated studies have indicated that breathing inhibition could affect blood pressure regulation through effects on renal regulation of sodium, plasma volume, and natriuretic factors involved in the regulation of vascular tone.[53]

Management of Respiratory Stress Responses

The observation that stress can be associated with inhibited breathing and increased blood pressure responsiveness to dietary sodium intake suggests that breathing exercises might have therapeutic value in the treatment of hypertension and other cardiovascular disorders. Clinical studies have reported that meditation, yoga, and other stress-reducing interventions that focus on deep breathing can have salutary effects on blood pressure.[54] It is noteworthy that some of these interventions, such as meditation and yoga, also have been shown to reduce stress and hostility, as discussed previously. Other studies in which guided breathing procedures slowed rates below resting values also have been reported to reduce blood pressure.[55] The physiologic mechanisms by which such changes in breathing habits are effective have yet to be clarified but could include improved ventilation and homeostatic blood gas levels (e.g., carbon dioxide).[48] Therefore, research into the role that inhibited breathing plays in the development of and interventions for various cardiovascular disorders merits increased attention, as does the potential beneficial effects of breathing exercises on this risk.

SUMMARY

Traditional risk factors alone cannot explain the incidence of CVD, and efforts to modify heart disease by focusing on traditional risk factors alone have not been successful. Interventions focusing on traditional risk factors conferred no added benefits in the Multiple Risk Factor Intervention Trial, the Gothenburg Primary Prevention Trial, or the World Health Organization European Factory Study. In contrast, psychosocial interventions show promising effects on CVD outcomes,[24] which suggests that more work should focus on investigation of these effects and exploration of ways they can be integrated into cardiology practice.

This chapter discussed the dynamic interactions that occur between people and aspects of their social environment, such as low SES and stressful work and family situations. These interactions can set up at least three pathways that can affect the individual's risk of CVD. Specifically, stressful social environments create conditions that engender negative emotional response styles, unhealthy lifestyles, and respiratory maladaptations that alter circulatory function. These three adaptations to social stress are associated with physiologic patterns that have been shown to have deleterious effects on the cardiovascular system. Future investigations can benefit from interdisciplinary, multifactorial approaches that integrate psychosocial strategies with standard risk factor reduction. Efforts to help patients reduce their risk of CVD will be more successful if, along with addressing standard risk factors, psychosocial risk factors are taken into account.

chapter

139 Trauma

M. L. Myers and L. Ray Guo

Definition

- Cardiac trauma is conventionally classified as a penetrating and blunt or a nonpenetrating injury.

Key Features

- Penetrating injuries or blunt injuries that cause myocardial rupture generally present with manifestations of pericardial tamponade or hemorrhagic shock, or both.
- Most myocardial contusions present with nonspecific chest pain and electrocardiographic (ECG) changes; they rarely result in significant long-term sequelae.

Therapy

- Most patients with potential myocardial contusions require limited diagnostic testing (electrocardiogram, cardiac troponin I, and/or echocardiogram) or therapeutic intervention.
- Although penetrating injuries, particularly gunshot wounds, have a high fatality rate, survival has improved with rapid transport systems and a systematic, coordinated team approach to evaluation and management.

Trauma is the leading cause of death in individuals younger than 45 years. It also results in huge direct and indirect costs to health care systems and societies throughout the world.

The management of patients with cardiac trauma has become a relatively common practice in many level I trauma centers. During the past two decades, urban centers in the United States have seen a significant increase in the relative frequency of gunshot wounds, compared with knife wounds, and an increasing proportion of these injuries are caused by high-velocity weapons.[1] In other health care facilities, blunt cardiac trauma, most commonly secondary to motor vehicle accidents, is a more predominant cause of injury.

In the past, most victims of penetrating cardiac trauma died at the scene. However, the potential for survival with such injuries has improved with the development of coordinated rapid transport systems and facilities with specialized teams for emergency care.

Traumatic myocardial injury can occur by itself or with other significant injuries. A consistent, systematic approach to the initial evaluation and management is imperative. The advanced trauma life support course of the American College of Surgeons[2] provides an excellent reference source for the management of patients with obvious or suspected cardiac trauma. Successful management of these patients also requires appropriate triage to hospitals equipped and prepared to deal with the suspected or identified injuries. In addition, aggressive and complete early resuscitation is necessary to normalize arterial perfusion pressure, maintain adequate tissue oxygen delivery, and prevent subsequent development of multiple organ dysfunction syndrome. This may present a particular challenge in the hypotensive patient with cardiac trauma, in whom the need to restore arterial pressure is accompanied by an urgent requirement to identify and control the precipitating cause.

PENETRATING INJURY

The penetrating cardiac injuries seen in civilian practice are caused mainly by gunshots, knives, and ice picks. Nail gun injuries to the heart and other organs also are increasingly seen.[3] On rare occasions, inward displacement of sternal and rib fragments may cause penetrating injury.

Penetrating cardiac injuries most commonly are seen with precordial wounds, but they also may occur with wounds elsewhere in the chest, neck, back, or upper abdomen. Cardiac injuries originating from sites other than the precordium typically are more complex and are predictive of a high mortality rate.

Single cardiac chambers are involved most frequently, but penetrating trauma also can result in injury to the cardiac valvular structures, the aorta, pulmonary artery, the atrial or ventricular septa, the coronary arteries, or the superior or inferior vena cava. Because of its anterior location, the right ventricle most commonly is injured. In a review of 109 patients with penetrating cardiac injuries, Attar and coworkers[4] found that the right ventricle was involved in 63 cases, the left ventricle in 35 cases, the right atrium in 15 cases, the left atrium in six cases, and the superior vena cava in three cases. Multiple-chamber injury was found in 13 cases.

CLINICAL PRESENTATIONS

Penetrating cardiac trauma results in pericardial tamponade or hemorrhagic shock, or both. The predominant clinical manifestations depend on the extent of both the cardiac and pericardial wounds, as well as the completeness of resuscitation, because tamponade may not become apparent until a patient with significant concomitant blood loss receives adequate fluid resuscitation. Pericardial tamponade is the most frequent presentation in patients with stab injuries. With a limited pericardial wound, thrombus formation may effectively seal the pericardial defect. With ongoing intrapericardial bleeding, however, tamponade occurs, with Beck's triad of hypotension, increased central venous pressure, and distant heart sounds. These patients also generally have a sinus tachycardia and acute respiratory distress. Pulsus paradoxus, the decrease in systolic blood pressure seen during inspiration, may exceed the normal physiologic limit of 10 mm Hg. Kussmaul's sign, an increase in venous pressure with inspiration, also may be noted with tamponade. However, if blood loss beyond the pericardium is significant, central venous distention may be absent.

Patients with gunshot wounds most often present with hemorrhage that may prove rapidly fatal, although approximately 20% present with tamponade.

Penetrating cardiac injuries frequently are accompanied by wounds that involve the lung and pleural space, the internal thoracic and intercostal vessels and, occasionally, the liver and other abdominal viscera.

MANAGEMENT

A rapid but systematic approach must be taken to the assessment and management of patients with penetrating cardiac injuries. An airway must be secured if the patient has respiratory distress, hypoventilation secondary to a depressed level of consciousness, or a need for airway protection. Persistent ventilatory impairment raises the question of hemopneumothorax, for which chest tubes should be inserted. Large-bore catheters should be inserted for rapid volume infusion in patients found to be in shock.

In addition to the initial assessment and institution of resuscitative measures, the patient must be evaluated for evidence of other injuries and exit wounds. After the airway is secured, patients are rapidly stratified into five categories: lifeless, critically unstable, cardiac tamponade, thoracoabdominal injury, or benign presentation (Fig. 139.1).[5] Emergency room thoracotomy (ERT) is not indicated for lifeless patients if vital signs have been absent for longer than 5 minutes before arrival in the emergency department if not intubated, or 10 minutes if intubated. In reviewing a 20-year experience involving 228 patients with penetrating cardiac injuries, Ivatury and colleagues[6] found that 45 of 89 patients who arrived in extremis and underwent ERT were resuscitated to the extent that they could be transported to the operating room for more definitive repair. Of these patients, 29% ultimately survived to be discharged from the hospital.

Critically unstable patients show signs of life but are profoundly hypotensive, and cardiac arrest appears imminent. These patients should be intubated immediately and resuscitated with fluid. In the absence of rapid improvement, ERT should be performed without delay. Patients who show clinical improvement, as well as patients with cardiac tamponade, should be transferred immediately to the operating room for sternotomy. If ERT is not appropriate, a subxiphoid pericardiocentesis may result in a level of hemodynamic improvement that allows transfer to the operating room for definitive treatment.

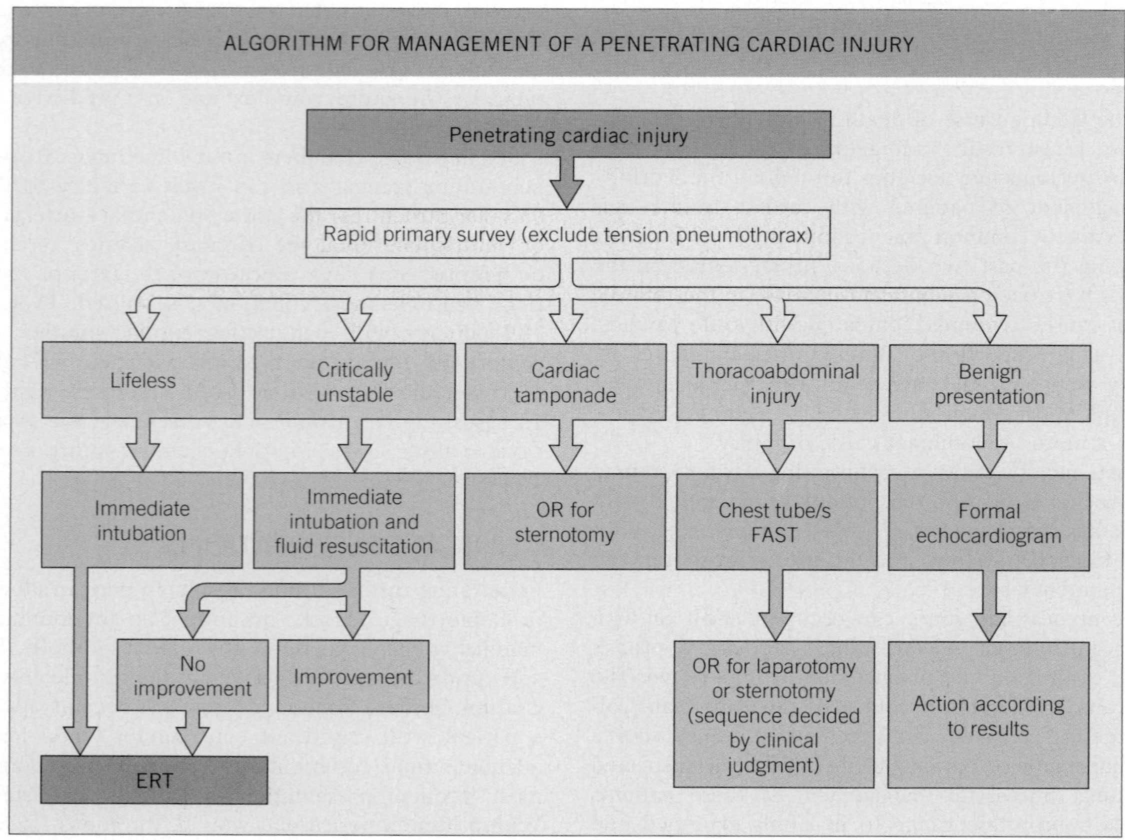

Figure 139.1 Algorithm for management of a penetrating cardiac injury. ERT, emergency room thoracotomy; OR, operating room. (Modified from Degiannis E, Loogna P, Doll D, et al. Penetrating cardiac injuries: recent experience in South Africa. World J Surg 2006;30:1258-1264.)

Pericardiocentesis also should be performed expeditiously in patients with vital signs present who remain in shock after initial resuscitative measures. The pericardial sac is a fixed, fibrous structure, and aspiration of as little as 20 to 40 mL of blood may result in significant improvement in hemodynamic status, thereby increasing the potential for successful surgical intervention.

Patients with thoracoabdominal injury may have sustained a single penetrating injury that damaged both sides of the diaphragm or multiple, separate thoracic and abdominal injuries. An accurate preoperative diagnosis may be very difficult, and evidence of cardiac tamponade, chest tube drainage, or abdominal distention should provide clues to the site of the most life-threatening pathology. Cardiac tamponade may be masked by hemorrhage within the peritoneal cavity.

Penetrating cardiac injury may present without symptoms or clinical signs of tamponade, and small myocardial wounds may stop bleeding after initial resuscitation. Focused abdominal sonogram for trauma (FAST) ultrasound can be used to rapidly diagnose the presence of pericardial blood with high levels of accuracy.[7] However, FAST ultrasound also may be falsely negative, and a high index of suspicion is required. Formal echocardiography may be needed to assess the situation more definitively, and accurate views and reliable interpretation depend on well-trained personnel. An initial negative study should not be considered definitive and should be followed by a second study in 8 to 10 hours.

A subxiphoid pericardial window (Fig. 139.2) occasionally can be used in unusual circumstances, although false-positive results can occur. Brewster and associates[8] reported on 108 patients with no obvious signs of cardiac injury but with penetrating wounds potentially involving the heart who were managed with subxiphoid windows. Of 30 patients with a positive result (i.e., blood in the pericardial sac), two were false positives, and seven of the 28 injuries were not sufficiently significant to require suture repair.

ERT generally is performed through a left anterolateral approach, most commonly through the fourth intercostal space. After insertion of a large thoracotomy retractor, the lung is retracted laterally, and the pericardium is opened vertically, anterior to the phrenic nerve. Thrombus is quickly evacuated and blood aspirated with a sterile suction device. Digital pressure is used to control the site of bleeding. If necessary, the thoracotomy may be extended across the sternum to control right atrial or caval injuries. In most cases, the patient then is transported to the operating room for more definitive repair, further exploration, and wound closure.

Ventricular repair generally is carried out with interrupted mattress sutures of 3-0 or 4-0 polypropylene using Teflon or pericardial pledgets. Care must be taken to insert the sutures in normal-appearing tissue approximately 1 cm from the wound edges and to avoid tissue strangulation. Atrial and caval defects generally are repaired with continuous 4-0 or 5-0 polypropylene sutures. Wounds close to coronary arteries are repaired by placing sutures beneath the artery (Fig. 139.3).

Most cardiac injuries can be repaired without the use of cardiopulmonary bypass. Although injuries that involve distal arterial segments or smaller branches can simply be ligated, injury to the proximal or midportions of major vessels (usually the left anterior descending or right coronary artery) generally should be managed with bypass grafting; cardiopulmonary bypass may also be required for missiles embedded in the heart or free within a cardiac chamber. The latter should be removed because of the potential for embolization; also, foreign bodies embedded in the myocardium generally should be removed, particularly if they are large or have jagged edges. However, studies have shown that embedded missiles do not necessarily result in erosion, infection, or embolization, and some may best be left alone, particularly if extraction likely would cause significant damage.[9]

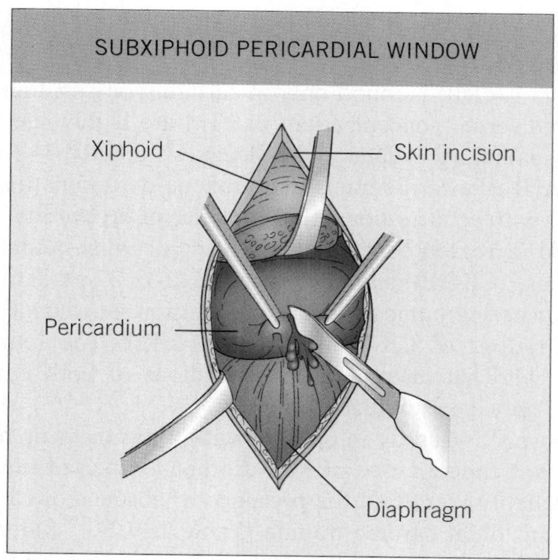

Figure 139.2 Subxiphoid pericardial window. A short vertical incision is made, centered over the xiphoid process. The tip of the xiphoid is elevated, and blunt dissection is used to expose the junction of the pericardium and diaphragm. A small vertical incision is made in the distal aspect of the pericardium.

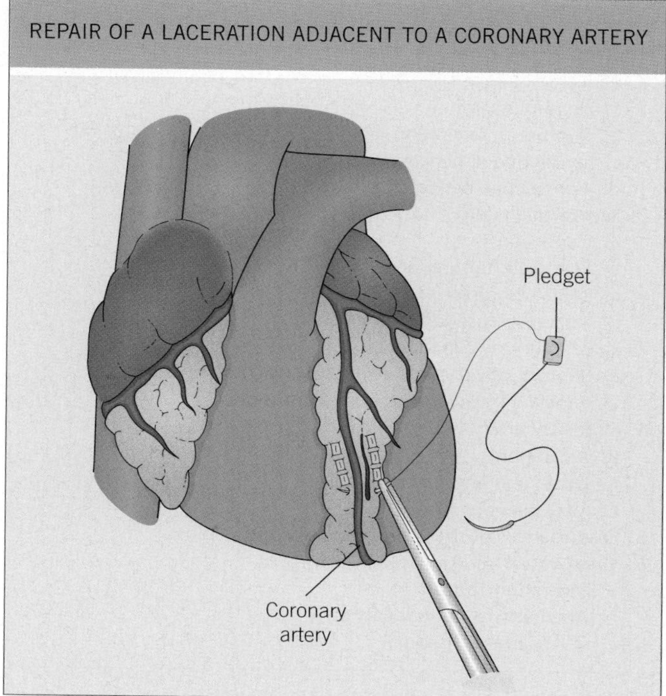

Figure 139.3 Repair of a laceration adjacent to a coronary artery. A laceration adjacent to the left anterior descending artery is repaired with pledgeted horizontal mattress sutures placed beneath the artery.

BLUNT INJURY

Blunt cardiac trauma occurs most commonly in association with motor vehicle accidents; however, it may occur secondary to other mechanisms, such as falls, crush injuries, explosions, or direct blows to the chest. Because of differing diagnostic criteria, the reported incidence of cardiac injury varies significantly; it appears to be about 15% of patients with a history of blunt chest trauma.[10] Cardiac injury from motor vehicle accidents is declining overall because of the increasing use of passive and active restraining devices in contemporary vehicles.

The mechanism of injury may be direct compression between the sternum and vertebral column, or the injury may occur secondary to sudden deceleration or rapid increases in intrathoracic or intra-abdominal pressure. The anterior position of the right ventricle makes it a more vulnerable target, but a wide variety of injuries have been described (Table 139.1). Sudden death in association with a blow to the chest (so-called commotio cordis) has been described in a variety of settings and appears to be the result of ventricular fibrillation.[11]

MYOCARDIAL CONTUSION

Clinical Presentations

The reported incidence of myocardial contusion varies greatly, as does the physiologic significance of these injuries. They comprise a broad spectrum of pathology, ranging from mild epicardial ecchymosis to frank myocardial necrosis. The diagnosis of myocardial contusion should be considered in any individual who suffers significant blunt chest trauma. A careful history with respect to the etiology of the injury, from the victim or witnesses, is valuable in determining the mechanism or significance (or both) of the injury.

Characterization of chest pain may be problematic with multiple injuries, but a description of angina-type pain that is unrelieved by nitrates may be suggestive. Patients may have evidence of external trauma, such as rib fractures or the impression of a steering wheel on the anterior chest wall. Dyspnea and hypotension may be present in moderate to severe contusion injuries, although severe signs and symptoms of cardiac failure should raise the question of additional major pathology, such as hemopericardium with cardiac tamponade or rupture of a cardiac valve. The diagnosis of myocardial contusion also should be entertained in any patient who shows an inadequate hemodynamic response to appropriate resuscitative measures.

CLASSIFICATION OF BLUNT CARDIAC INJURY
1. Pericardial injury
a. Hemopericardium
b. Rupture or laceration
c. Serofibrinous pericarditis
d. Constrictive pericarditis
2. Myocardial injury
a. Contusion
b. Free wall rupture/laceration
c. Septal rupture
d. Aneurysm/pseudoaneurysm
3. Valve injury/dysfunction
a. Rupture of valve leaflets, cusps, or chordae tendineae
b. Papillary muscle/ventricular contusion
4. Coronary artery injury
a. Laceration
b. Dissection and/or thrombosis
c. Arteriovenous fistula
5. Disturbances of rhythm or conduction
6. Great-vessel injury
a. Laceration/rupture
b. Aneurysm/pseudoaneurysm
c. Aortocameral fistula
Modified from Symbas PN. Traumatic Heart Disease: the Heart. 8th ed. New York, McGraw-Hill, 1994:2033.

Table 139.1 Classification of blunt cardiac injury.

Diagnostic Techniques

No uniformly accepted diagnostic criteria have been established for myocardial contusion; therefore, to some extent, the incidence of the diagnosis is in direct proportion to the aggression with which it is sought.[12]

Electrocardiogram

Electrocardiographic abnormalities, most commonly nonspecific repolarization changes, are consistently present with contusion, although the overall specificity is somewhat limited. Diagnostic specificity may be reduced by other factors, including hypoxia, acid-base or electrolyte abnormities, alcohol or drug use, and head trauma or preexisting cardiac disease. Right bundle branch block, ST elevation, heart block, and dysrhythmias, such as atrial fibrillation or flutter and atrial or ventricular premature beats, may be more indicative of acute injury.[13] It has been recommended that a patient with blunt chest trauma and no additional significant injuries who has a completely normal ECG and is hemodynamically stable requires no additional testing to rule out blunt cardiac injury.[14]

Cardiac Markers

Troponin I (cTnI) is found only in cardiomyocytes; therefore, increased serum concentrations of cTnI are highly specific to myocardial injury. Adams and colleagues[15] studied 44 patients with serial echocardiograms and enzyme determinations. Six patients with echocardiographic evidence of myocardial injury also had increased concentrations of myocardial-bound creatine kinase (CK-MB) and cTnI, whereas 26 of 37 patients without echocardiographic evidence of contusion showed increased concentrations of CK-MB but not of cTnI. The remaining patient who had increased concentrations of both enzymes showed only a pericardial effusion.

A prospective study in patients with blunt thoracic trauma found that concordance of ECG findings and cTnI measurement reliably identified the presence or absence of clinically significant blunt cardiac trauma (Table 139.2).[16] Individuals with both an abnormal ECG and cTnI need close monitoring for at least 24 hours. Conversely, those with a normal admission ECG and cTnI can be safely discharged in the absence of other injuries.

DIAGNOSTIC VALUE OF ECG, SERUM cTnI, AND THEIR COMBINATION IN DETECTING CLINICALLY SIGNIFICANT BLUNT CARDIAC TRAUMA			
	ECG (%)	cTnI (%)	ECG + cTnI (%)
Sensitivity	84	68	100
Specificity	56	85	88
Positive predictive value	28	48	62
Negative predictive value	95	93	100

Modified from Salim A, Velmahos GC, Jindal A, et al. Clinically significant blunt cardiac trauma: role of serum troponin levels combined with electrocardiographic findings. J Trauma 2001;50:237-243.
ECG, electrocardiogram; cTnI, cardiac troponin I.

Table 139.2 Diagnostic value of ECG, serum cTnI, and their combination in detecting clinically significant blunt cardiac trauma.

Echocardiography

Echocardiography is a very useful tool in the evaluation of possible cardiac contusion. The main diagnostic findings include wall motion abnormalities in up to 25% of cases, increased echo brightness, and increased end-diastolic wall thickness of the contused segment.[17] Transthoracic echocardiography (TTE) also is useful in detecting pericardial effusion and intracardiac shunts. Its main limitation is the difficulty of image acquisition in cases of chest wall and lung injuries and in intubated patients.[18,19]

Transesophageal echocardiography (TEE) now is recognized as an excellent technique for the evaluation of cardiac injuries after trauma.[18] It provides high-quality images of the right and the left ventricles and the proximal ascending and descending thoracic aorta. The introduction of biplane and multiplane TEE has allowed for better image acquisition and improved diagnostic capabilities. In a multicenter prospective study of 134 patients, TEE was found to be superior to ECG and cardiac enzymes for the diagnosis of cardiac contusion.[17] TEE may be problematic in patients with associated head and neck trauma and requires experienced personnel for accurate interpretation.

Management

The initial assessment should include an ECG and cTnI measurement, which generally should be repeated in 6 to 8 hours. In patients with a significant contusion injury, the major therapeutic concern is cardiac arrhythmia, although most arrhythmias in this setting tend to be benign and self-limited. No unique approach has been devised to the treatment of arrhythmias in such patients, and no serious outcomes specifically related to these arrhythmias have been seen. As in other situations, appropriate measures should be instituted to treat hypoxia and hypothermia, in addition to normalizing pH and the potassium and magnesium concentrations.

Treatment with pharmacologic agents that have been shown to be effective in suppressing ventricular arrhythmias in acute myocardial ischemia occasionally may be warranted, and supraventricular arrhythmias with a rapid ventricular response should be treated pharmacologically for rate control.

As recommended by Fildes and coworkers,[20] patients presenting with blunt chest trauma who are younger than 55 years of age, have no history of cardiac disease, and are hemodynamically stable, with no requirement for surgery or neurologic observation, do not require admission to the hospital for monitoring if they have a completely normal ECG. Individuals with an abnormal ECG should be admitted to hospital for a brief period of monitoring and observation. Additional cardiac imaging studies (usually TTE) should be done if a specific clinical concern exists based on the patient's signs and symptoms or if the individual requires urgent operative intervention for other injuries.

Invasive monitoring with arterial and pulmonary artery catheters may be indicated in patients with suspected blunt cardiac injury who have hemodynamic instability, preexisting cardiac disease, and/or severe multisystem trauma, and particularly in those who require a general anesthetic. The right ventricular stroke work index is maintained in patients with a right ventricular contusion by means of an increase in the right ventricular end-diastolic volume. Therefore, appropriate fluid resuscitation is an important consideration in optimizing hemodynamic function. Individuals with severe dysfunction and hemodynamic compromise may require inotropic and, very rarely, intra-aortic balloon pump support. It is important to exclude traumatic injury of the aorta before a balloon pump is inserted.

VALVULAR INJURY

Valvular rupture is a relatively rare but well-recognized complication of blunt cardiac trauma. Sudden increases in intravascular or intraventricular pressure, or both, may lead to valvular injury or rupture, with a range of clinical decompensation, depending on the extent of the injury. Acute bioprosthetic valve dysfunction also has been reported after blunt chest trauma.[21]

Clinical Presentations

The aortic valve has been most commonly reported to be injured.[22] The underlying anatomic derangement may be leaflet laceration or avulsion, or commissural avulsion or dissection may occur secondary to localized aortic injury. The signs and symptoms of aortic insufficiency may develop immediately after injury but more commonly evolve over several weeks, depending on the severity of the injury. A variable systolic murmur secondary to turbulent flow around the disrupted valve may be present in addition to the diastolic murmur of aortic insufficiency. The timing of intervention depends on the patient's hemodynamic and clinical status. Valve replacement most often is required, but occasionally, repair of a torn leaflet or resuspension of a disrupted commissure may be possible.

The most common mitral valve injury is papillary muscle rupture, followed by ruptured chordae tendineae and, rarely, isolated leaflet tear. As with aortic valve injuries, symptoms secondary to mitral injury may occur immediately or may be somewhat delayed in onset, depending on the underlying pathology. Papillary muscle avulsion results in severe acute mitral insufficiency with acute pulmonary edema, and it generally requires urgent or emergency surgical intervention. As with acute mitral insufficiency that complicates myocardial infarction, insertion of an intra-aortic balloon pump may provide significant benefit in the face of rapid hemodynamic deterioration. More limited chordal rupture or partial leaflet tears may result in a more subacute presentation, with progression of symptoms over weeks to months. Papillary muscle rupture generally requires valve replacement, but other types of injury may be amenable to repair, with excellent long-term results.

Although traumatic tricuspid valve injury may present with acute decompensation, most reports document progressive chronic symptoms. The classic constellation of findings includes a history of trauma, isolated right heart failure, a systolic murmur, right bundle branch block, and echocardiographic evidence of severe tricuspid insufficiency. Although some patients may do well for many years with medical management, others derive benefit from surgical intervention, as documented in a report from the Mayo Clinic.[23] This study outlined the cases of 13 patients who had surgery for traumatic tricuspid insufficiency. The specific pathology included chordal rupture in nine, rupture of the anterior papillary muscle in three, anterior leaflet tear in one, and septal leaflet fibrosis and retraction in one. Valve repair was carried out in five patients, and valve replacement was required in eight. Although the patients did well during follow-up, it was suggested that earlier surgery might increase the possibility of repair and attenuate the sequelae of long-standing right heart dysfunction, including the development of chronic atrial fibrillation.

MYOCARDIAL RUPTURE

Clinical Presentations

Most patients with rupture of a cardiac chamber or the great vessels (aortic or pulmonary arteries) die at the scene of the accident, although a review of autopsy series suggests that 10% to 20% of patients potentially could survive long enough to undergo surgical intervention if expeditious transport and resuscitation could be carried out.[2] Sudden compressive forces transmitted to the atria at the end of ventricular systole or to the ventricle at end-diastole appear to be the mechanism of rupture, whereas sudden severe torsion probably is the mechanism responsible for tears at the atrial-caval junction. Autopsy reports most commonly document rupture of the ventricles; the right atrium appears to be most commonly involved in patients who survive with rupture of a cardiac chamber. Isolated pericardial rupture may result in herniation of the heart, with catastrophic sequelae.

As with penetrating injuries, the clinical presentation is one of tamponade or hemorrhagic shock (or both), depending on whether concomitant rupture of the pericardium is a factor. Additional injuries may confuse the initial clinical evaluation. In many instances, the diagnosis is made after emergency thoracotomy or sternotomy in the face of severe shock or a rapidly deteriorating hemodynamic picture. Such an injury should be suspected in any patient with a history of severe chest trauma who has persistent hypotension that is unresponsive to fluid administration or disproportionate to the estimated blood loss. In patients whose condition is stable, echocardiography may demonstrate pericardial accumulation of fluid or evidence of myocardial disruption or dyskinesia. Repair of cardiac lacerations follows the same general principles as outlined for the management of penetrating injuries.

TRAUMATIC VENTRICULAR SEPTAL DEFECT

Isolated traumatic ventricular septal defect (VSD) is a rare occurrence in the setting of blunt trauma. Autopsy data suggest an incidence of about 1% for isolated VSD and 5% for VSD associated with other cardiac injuries.[24] The most common site for the rupture is near the apex.[24] Septal rupture is believed to occur as a result of cardiac compression between the spine and the sternum, although a sudden increase in intrathoracic pressure during deceleration may also be contributory. As with free wall rupture, the greatest vulnerability of the septum is during late diastole and early systole, when the ventricles are full and the valves are closed.[25] In cases of delayed traumatic VSD, initial damage to the nutrient vessels of the septum is thought to result in infarction, which progresses to subsequent rupture. VSD also can result from penetrating cardiac injury involving any part of the septum.

Individuals with traumatic VSD initially may be asymptomatic or may present with signs and symptoms of acute pulmonary edema. VSD associated with a free wall rupture typically presents with acute cardiac tamponade and shock. Echocardiography generally should be diagnostic. Right-heart catheterization can detect a step-up in oxygen saturation between the right atrium and ventricle and permit calculation of the pulmonary to systemic flow ratio.

The decision to proceed with surgical repair must be individualized and based on a number of factors, including the ability to improve hemodynamic status with inotropic or intra-aortic balloon pump support (or both), the potential contribution of myocardial contusion to the clinical findings, and the presence of other noncardiac injuries. As with acute postinfarction VSD repair, surgical closure requires cardiopulmonary bypass support with ventriculotomy and patch closure and/or exclusion and may be associated with a very significant mortality.

CORONARY ARTERY INJURY

Autopsy results suggest an incidence of coronary artery involvement in blunt cardiac injury of 1% to 2%.[26] Because of its anterior location, the left anterior descending artery most commonly is injured, resulting in an acute anteroseptal myocardial infarction with a high subsequent incidence of aneurysm formation. Postulated mechanisms of coronary occlusion include intimal injury and thrombosis, rupture of preexisting atherosclerotic plaque, and acute dissection. Coronary spasm superimposed on preexisting coronary disease probably plays a significant role in trauma-associated myocardial infarction in older individuals. Penetrating cardiac trauma involves the coronary arteries in 4% of cases and can result in acute tamponade, infarction, or intrathoracic bleeding, or all of these. The involved artery can fistulize to a major vein or cardiac chamber, or an aneurysm may develop in the infarction territory.

Echocardiography can identify a regional wall motion abnormality, pericardial fluid collection, and evidence of

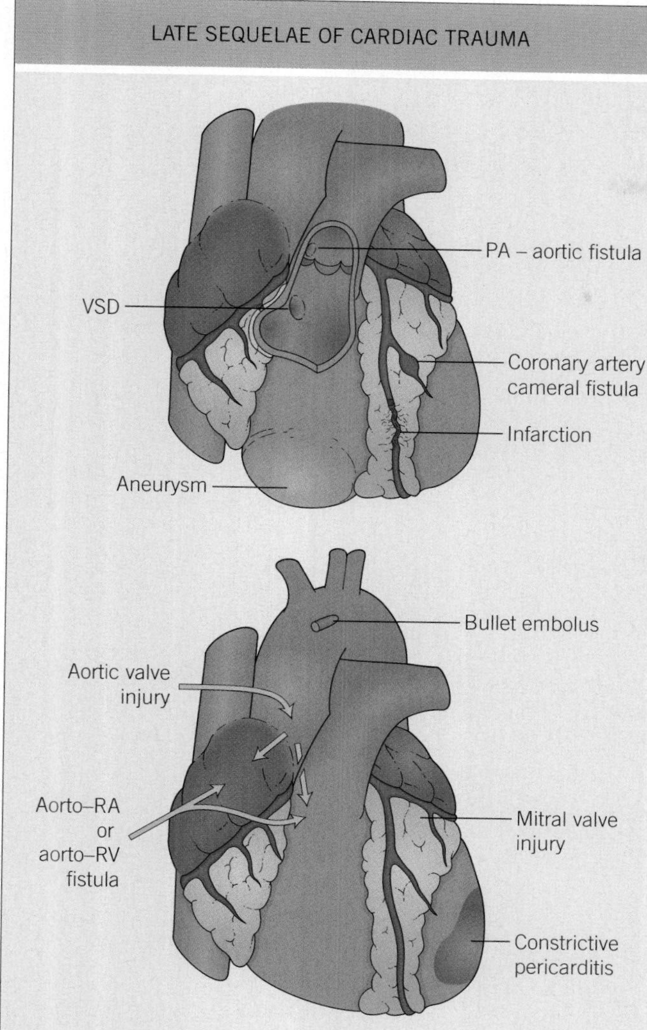

Figure 139.4 Late sequelae of cardiac trauma. Signs of heart failure or the presence of murmurs in a patient who has suffered cardiac trauma requires investigation for residual defects. PA, pulmonary artery; RA, right atrial; RV, right ventricular; VSD, ventral septal defect.

tamponade. Under unusual circumstances, coronary angiography may be indicated to delineate the nature of the injury. Proximal coronary injuries often require bypass with either an internal thoracic artery or saphenous vein graft. Injury to distal arterial segments generally can be treated with ligation without the use of cardiopulmonary bypass.

PROGNOSIS

A variety of abnormalities have been reported as delayed findings after blunt and penetrating trauma (Fig. 139.4). Good evidence indicates that myocardial contusion rarely results in permanent sequelae. A review of more than 2500 patients treated for blunt chest trauma during a 15-year period at the Maryland Institute for Emergency Medicine failed to identify a single individual with a significant sustained abnormality.[27] Similar findings have been reported by others,[28] with normalization of ventricular function within days to weeks after injury. Other abnormalities, such as ventricular aneurysms and pseudoaneurysms, atrial and ventricular septal defects, constrictive pericarditis, valvular insufficiency, and sinus of Valsalva to atrial fistulas, may be detected in follow-up. The decision to intervene surgically generally is based on the same clinical and hemodynamic parameters used when such abnormalities present with another etiologic basis.

SUMMARY

Cardiac injury is an important cause of trauma deaths. Many of these patients die after reaching the hospital. Prompt diagnosis with initial assessment, resuscitation, and treatment are essential. Cardiac tamponade most commonly results from penetrating injuries. Pericardiocentesis is indicated early for patients who do not respond to the usual methods of resuscitation for hemorrhagic shock and who have the potential for cardiac tamponade. Myocardial contusion, although difficult to diagnose, is relatively common after blunt chest trauma. Rupture of the heart or great vessels most often is fatal at the scene of the accident. Rarely, patients with cardiac trauma may develop delayed findings requiring elective surgical intervention.

chapter

140 Radiation-Induced Heart Disease

M. Jacob Adams, Louis S. Constine, and Steven E. Lipshultz

Definitions

- Radiation-associated heart disease consists of a broad spectrum of clinical and subclinical damage caused by exposure of various tissues of the heart to radiation.
- Units of radiation: gray (1 gray [Gy] = 100 centigray [cGy] = 100 rads).

Key Features

- The increased risk of cardiac damage from radiation is lifelong and probably increases with time.
- Patients at highest risk include survivors of Hodgkin's disease and left-sided breast cancer treated with chest radiotherapy.
- Screening of patients at risk for radiation-induced heart disease is necessary, but the optimal methods and frequency remain unclear.
- Mediastinal radiation increases the likelihood that anthracyclines will have a negative effect on the heart.

Therapy

- Appropriate therapy may include no intervention, medical therapy, or surgery, possibly including heart transplantation.

As late as the 1960s, the association between radiation therapy and cardiac damage remained controversial. By 1975, reports of cardiac damage in patients treated with thoracic radiation for Hodgkin's disease (HD) firmly established the existence of radiation-associated heart disease. Heart disease is the leading cause of noncancer death among survivors of HD, whose risk of fatal cardiovascular disease appears to be about three times greater than that of the general population.[1]

In addition, accumulating evidence during the past two decades has shown that the risk of mortality from cardiovascular disease is elevated in survivors of left-sided breast cancer who received adjuvant radiotherapy that included the inner mammary lymph nodes (IMNs) in the treatment field.[2] Historically, the IMNs were included in the radiation treatment after mastectomy but generally not after breast-conserving surgery. However, current practice is to avoid irradiating the IMNs unless absolutely necessary. Various techniques have reduced the radiation dose and the volume of the heart exposed to radiation, reducing cardiac damage, but whether the most serious effects are simply delayed remains unclear.

Therapeutic chest irradiation, essentially as used to treat cancer, has created a large population at risk for long-term cardiac sequelae. Several variables confound the determination of risk, however, including the technique used, dosage, patient's age, time since irradiation, other cancer therapies received, and other traditional cardiovascular disease risk factors.

The spectrum of radiation-induced cardiac injury is broad and includes direct and indirect cardiovascular effects. This chapter concentrates on direct effects. However, the clinician should keep in mind the broad range of indirect effects when evaluating and treating patients exposed to therapeutic doses of radiation.

ANATOMIC PATHOLOGY

All cardiac structures are at risk for radiation-induced injury. The following discussion focuses on those that undergo clearly visible morphologic changes.

In the pericardium, dense collagen and fibrin replaces the normal adipose tissue of the outer layer of the heart. Fibrosis occurs in the stroma and on the mesothelial surfaces. Small blood vessels proliferate throughout. The parietal surface is more severely affected than the epicardium.

Nonspecific, diffuse interstitial fibrotic lesions may occur in the myocardium. These lesions measure from a few millimeters to several centimeters in diameter but usually do not involve the entire myocardium. The severity of fibrosis from one region to another can be markedly different. Collagen not only increases as a whole, but type I collagen also increases in proportion to type III. Both changes are thought to affect the compliance of the myocardium. This change may contribute to the marked diastolic dysfunction seen in patients who have undergone irradiation.[3] Myocardial cells involved with conduction also are sensitive to radiation-induced fibrosis.

The cusp or leaflets (or both) of valves may undergo fibrotic change with or without calcification. Changes to valves on the left side of the heart are more common and severe than on the right side, regardless of the dose distribution. This asymmetry suggests that the higher pressures of the systemic circulation are involved in pathogenesis, and valvular disease, therefore, probably is progressive. However, stenosis of the entire pulmonary outflow tract has been reported in five cases after chest radiotherapy at doses above 40 Gy.[4]

The coronary arteries show disease in locations relative to the dose distribution of radiation. The left anterior descending and right coronary arteries most often are affected after anterior-weighted mantle radiotherapy (Fig. 140.1). After such treatment, left main coronary artery disease occurs more often in irradiated patients than in the general population.[5] However, with modern radiotherapy techniques, the distribution of disease sites is similar to that in the general

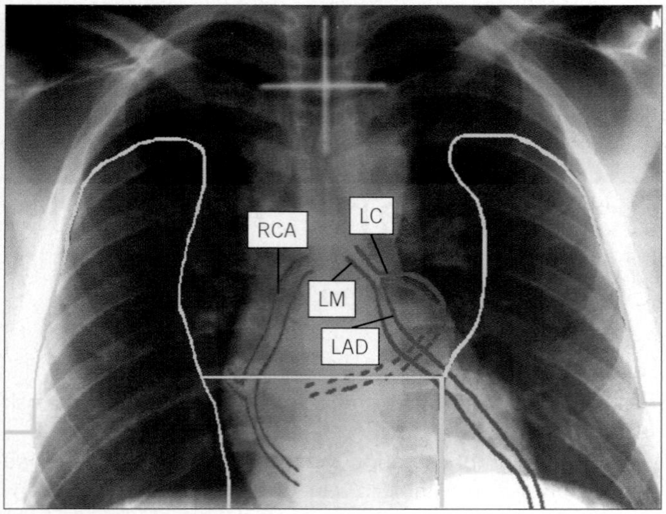

Figure 140.1 Location of the coronary vessels on a standard mantle field. LAD, left anterior descending; LC, left circumflex; LM, left main; RCA, right coronary artery. (From King V, Constine LS, Clark D, et al: Symptomatic coronary artery disease after mantle irradiation for Hodgkin's disease. Int J Radiat Oncol Biol Phys 1996;36:881-889.)

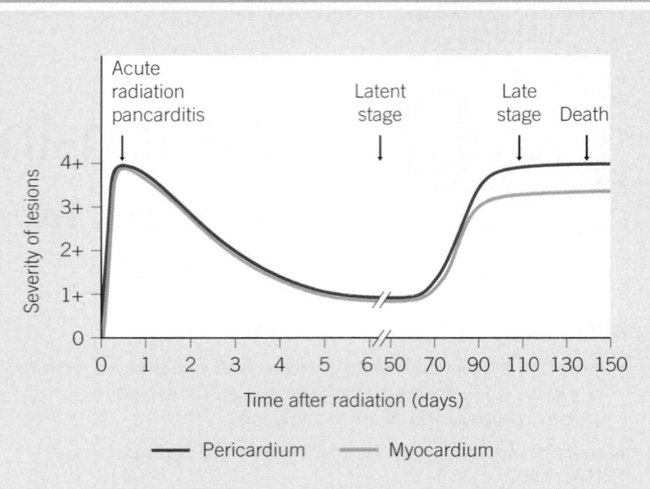

Figure 140.2 Development of radiation heart disease in white rabbits as observed by light microscopy after a single dose of 20 Gy. The curve indicates the severity of the lesions at different times. See text for variation in the nature of the lesions. (From Fajardo LF, Stewart JR. Experimental radiation-induced heart disease. 1. Light microscopic studies. Am J Pathol 1970;59(2):299-316.)

population.[6] The artery generally narrows proximally and often involves the coronary ostia. Smooth muscle in the media tends to be greatly decreased. The media and adventitia are densely thickened with fibrous tissue compared with the generic coronary lesion. Yet intimal plaques may be both lipid laden and fibrotic.[5,7,8] Consequently, histologic discrimination of radiation damage from typical atherosclerosis may be difficult. Nevertheless, fibrosis in any portion of the heart is the characteristic pathology caused by radiation, although such changes are nonspecific.

PATHOPHYSIOLOGY

Landmark experimental work on white rabbits exposed to a single or fractionated lethal dose or doses of radiation revealed three phases of microscopic cardiac injury (Fig. 140.2).[9] Few lesions, if any, were seen immediately. The early or transient phase began 6 hours after exposure. A neutrophilic infiltrate involving all layers of the heart appeared, with small and medium-sized arteries showing acute inflammation. The latent phase began as the acute exudate resolved, about 2 days after exposure. This phase was notable for remarkably healthy-appearing pericardium and myocardium on light microscopy, which showed only a slight increase in fibrosis. However, serial electron microscopy of the myocardial capillary endothelial cells revealed progressive damage that obstructed the lumen with thrombi of fibrin and platelets. Although the healthy endothelial cells responded by replicating to provide unobstructed capillaries, replication was inadequate. This reduction in capillaries caused ischemia, leading to myocardial cell death and fibrosis. The animals began to die at the start of the late phase, around day 70. The hallmark of this stage was the previously described extensive fibrosis.

The alterations seen in white rabbits during the latent and late stages under gross and light microscopy are identical to those described in humans, although the timing is different, which suggests that the pathogenesis probably is the same in humans.

Radiation probably injures coronary artery endothelial cells in a similar way. It causes fibrointimal hyperplasia, which leads to thrombus formation and possibly lipid deposition, similar to the typical mechanism of coronary artery disease. However, the effect of lipid deposition on radiation-induced coronary artery disease is unclear. Pathologic studies differ greatly in the amount of lipid deposits and foam cells seen in lesions. Coronary artery spasm also may be important in some cases of sudden cardiac death.[10]

The pericardial microvasculature also is injured, causing increased permeability. Fibrosis of the venous and lymphatic channels of the heart and mediastinum reduces the ability of extracellular fluid to drain, leading to the accumulation of a protein-rich effusion. Vascular damage also causes ischemia and eventual fibrosis. Fibrin accumulation may be expedited by the disruption of fibrinolysis. Fibrinolysis depends on plasminogen activator, which is deficient in the lungs of irradiated dogs and humans. This deficiency interferes with the resorption of fibrin; therefore, the fibrin is more likely to become organized by the invasion of fibroblasts and the subsequent production of collagen. This process also may occur in pericardial fibrosis.

CLINICAL PRESENTATIONS

The range of radiation-associated cardiovascular disease and its indirect effects is broad (Tables 140.1 and 140.2), and the severity and types of manifestations depend on several risk factors (Table 140.3). After anterior-weighted therapy, the rate of hemodynamically important cardiac complications has been estimated to be 15% to 30% within 5 to 10 years of follow-up.[11] The prevalence of asymptomatic abnormalities is even higher. Similar follow-up data are not available for

SPECTRUM OF RADIATION-INDUCED CARDIOVASCULAR DISEASE		
Manifestation	**Comments**	**References**
Pericarditis	1. During therapy: associated with mediastinal tumor and some chemotherapeutic agents, such as cyclophosphamide.	9
	2. Post therapy: acute effusion, chronic effusion, pericarditis, constrictive pericarditis.	9
Myocarditis	1. Fibrosis secondary to microvasculature changes.	9
	2. Frequently with normal left ventricular dimensions, ejection fraction, and fractional shortening as measured by radionuclide scan or echocardiogram.	49
	3. Can have progressive, restrictive cardiomyopathy with fibrosis; can cause pulmonary vascular disease and pulmonary hypertension.	49
	4. Diastolic dysfunction often occurs alone, as well as with systolic dysfunction.	49
Coronary artery disease	1. Premature fibrosis and also probably accelerates atherosclerosis.	7, 50
	2. Distribution of arteries affected tends to be anterior with anterior-weighted therapy.	9
	3. Lesions tend to be proximal and even ostial.	7, 50
	4. ↑ Rates of silent ischemia, acute myocardial infarction, and possibly the proportion of clinically unsuspected infarctions (see autonomic effects).	17
Valvular disease	1. Left-sided valve damage predominates.	16, 17
	2. ↑ Regurgitation and stenosis with ↑ time since therapy.	16
	3. May progress to significant disease 10 to 20 years later, even in those with normal valves at the completion of therapy.	2
Conduction system/ arrhythmia	1. High rate of complete or incomplete right bundle branch block is suggestive of right bundle branch fibrosis.	34
	2. Can progress to complete heart block and cause congestive heart failure, requiring a pacemaker.	34
	3. Complete heart block rarely occurs without other radiation-induced abnormalities to the heart.	34
	4. ↑ Left ventricular fibrosis associated with ↑ high-grade ventricular ectopic activity.	34
	5. ↑ Right atrial pressure associated with ↑ risk of atrial arrhythmia.	34
Autonomic dysfunction	1. Frequent cardiac dysfunction with tachycardia, loss of circadian rhythm, and respiratory phasic heart rate variability.	17
	2. This is similar to a denervated heart, suggesting autonomic nervous system damage.	17
	3. ↓ Perception of anginal pain.	17
Vascular changes	1. May cause significant pulmonary artery stenosis and hypoplasia, especially in those treated in early childhood.	49

Table 140.1 Spectrum of radiation-induced cardiovascular disease.

INDIRECT EFFECTS OF MEDIASTINAL RADIATION ON THE CARDIOVASCULAR SYSTEM		
Manifestation	**Comments**	**References**
Mediastinal fibrosis	↓ Success of cardiovascular surgery	44, 45
Lung fibrosis	Chronic, restrictive, and can be progressive	51
Scoliosis and ↓ skeletal muscle	↓ Cardiovascular and lung function	51
Thyroid	Usually hypothyroid; affects cardiovascular function and lipid profile	37

Table 140.2 Indirect effects of mediastinal radiation on the cardiovascular system.

current radiotherapy techniques. Although survivors of mediastinal radiotherapy are at increased risk for coronary artery disease and functional abnormalities, the risk from radiotherapy in left-sided breast cancer survivors has been clearly documented only for coronary heart disease, although isolated changes in the myocardium may be visible with perfusion imaging techniques, which suggests that damage can occur to the heart muscle directly.[12] Moreover, treatment with chemotherapy, especially anthracyclines, and biologics (e.g., trastuzumab) put these women at risk for functional abnormalities.

Pericarditis

Historically, 20% to 30% of patients who had radiotherapy to the entire pericardium for HD developed pericarditis. However, at one center, restricting the total dose to 30 Gy, weighting anterior and posterior fields equally, using subcarinal blocking, and reducing the daily fraction size to 2.0 Gy or less reduced the incidence from 20% to 2.5%.[13] Pericarditis can remain clinically silent, or it can present with the sudden onset of typical signs and symptoms: pleuritic chest pain, dyspnea, fever, friction rub, ST-segment and T-wave changes, and decreased QRS voltage. Early, acute-onset pericarditis is defined as occurring during radiotherapy and usually is associated with a large tumor contiguous to the heart. It is thought to be a reaction to necrosis of the tumor and

RISK FACTORS FOR THE DIFFERENT MANIFESTATIONS OF RADIATION-INDUCED HEART DISEASES							
Risk factor	Pericarditis	CM	CAD	Arrhythmia	Valvular Disease	All Causes of CD	Reference
Total dose (>30-35 Gy)	+	+	+	+	+	+	9, 16, 24
Fractionated dose (≥2.0 Gy/day)	+	+	+	Likely	Likely	+	9
Volume of heart exposed	+	+	+	Likely	Likely	+	9
Relative weighting of radiation portals and thus the amount of radiation delivered to different parts of the heart without subcarinal blocking	+	+	+	Likely	Likely	+	9, 21
Presence of tumor next to the heart	+	–	–	–	–	–	9
Younger age at exposure	–	+	+	Likely	Likely	+	9, 22, 45
Increased time since exposure	–	+	+	+	+	+	21, 31, 34, 52
Type of radiation source	+	+	+	Likely	Likely	+	9
Use of adjuvant cardiotoxic chemotherapy	–	+	–	+	+	+	9
Presence of other known risk factors in each individual (e.g., current age, weight, lipid profile, and habits, such as smoking)	–	–	+	–	–	+	9, 28

–, no known association; likely, unknown but likely association; +, association of specific risk factors with specific presentation. CAD, coronary artery disease; CD, cardiac death; CM, cardiomyopathy; Gy, gray.

Table 140.3 Risk factors for the different manifestations of radiation-induced heart diseases.

does not have long-term consequences. Radiotherapy generally is continued.

If it occurs, delayed pericarditis develops 4 months to several years after radiotherapy, although most cases occur within the first year. Both delayed acute pericarditis and delayed chronic pericardial effusion may occur. The former presents as described previously, and it may be recurrent. Of patients with delayed acute pericarditis, about half develop some degree of tamponade, presenting with paradoxic pulse or Kussmaul's sign. Delayed chronic pericardial effusion often is discovered on routine chest radiography, which reveals an enlarged cardiac silhouette; a minority of patients present with tamponade. Most effusions clear spontaneously, but clearance may take up to 2 years.

About 20% of patients with delayed pericarditis experience chronic or constrictive pericarditis 5 to 10 years after therapy. The risk for development of chronic pericarditis is substantially greater if pericardial effusion was present previously.[14] Chronic pericarditis also can develop without antecedent acute pericarditis.

Pancarditis, or severe inflammation throughout all layers of the myocardium, often occurs with pericarditis. Although it is rare and probably requires at least 60 Gy of mediastinal irradiation, most patients with pancarditis have severe, often intractable congestive heart failure.

Cardiomyopathy

Cardiac dysfunction, as evidenced by congestive heart failure or asymptomatic cardiomyopathy, may result from mediastinal radiotherapy. However, cardiac dysfunction caused by radiotherapy differs from that caused by anthracyclines. Radiation causes myocardial fibrosis, which leads to a restrictive cardiomyopathy characterized by diastolic dysfunction. In contrast, systolic dysfunction usually is the primary abnormality in survivors treated with anthracyclines without irradiation. Nevertheless, given high enough doses and time, mediastinal radiotherapy has been shown to lead to systolic dysfunction.[2]

Recent studies have documented this greater impact on diastolic dysfunction than on systolic dysfunction after mediastinal radiotherapy.[15-18] The frequency of diastolic dysfunction ranges from 12% to 83% when measured at a mean 15 to 17 years after diagnosis, whereas the prevalence of systolic dysfunction is lower, ranging from 9% to 36%. In a study by Heidenreich and colleagues[15] of 294 HD survivors treated with at least 35 Gy of mediastinal irradiation at any age, a substantial percentage of survivors with diastolic dysfunction experienced ischemia with exercise. Adams and associates[17] noted that in 48 HD survivors treated with mediastinal radiotherapy between 15 and 25 years of age, 14 had an abnormally low peak oxygen consumption with exercise.[17] These two studies established, respectively, that HD survivors with diastolic dysfunction have substantially worse cardiac event–free survival and worse quality of life than those without diastolic dysfunction.[15,17] The prevalence of dysfunction increases with higher radiation dose-volumes, higher anthracycline dose, and longer follow-up. Prevalence also depends on the screening modality.

Radiation also increases the cardiotoxicity of anthracyclines, which directly damage myocardiocytes and can cause dilated cardiomyopathy. In long-term survivors of childhood cancer, left ventricular function has been shown to be lower in survivors who received anthracyclines and chest irradiation than in those who received chest irradiation alone and than in a group that received anthracyclines alone at a substantially higher mean total dose.[19] In a Dutch cohort of 1474 survivors of HD treated before age 41 (between 1965 and 1995), anthracyclines greatly added to the elevated risks of congestive heart failure and valvular disorders from mediastinal radiotherapy alone, which was already increased twofold to sevenfold for myocardial infarction, angina, congestive heart failure, and valvular disorders.[20] The 25-year cumulative incidence of congestive heart failure was 10.7% after combined radiation and anthracycline therapy but just 7.5% after radiotherapy alone.

Coronary Artery Disease and Overall Cardiac Mortality

High-dose mediastinal radiation (>30 to 35 Gy), especially during childhood, increases the risk of coronary artery disease. Coronary artery disease may be silent or may cause anginal pain or sudden death. Silent myocardial infarction appears to occur more often in survivors of mediastinal radiotherapy than in the general population.

A retrospective review of 635 patients treated before age 21 years for HD at Stanford University between 1961 and 1991 reported a relative risk for fatal myocardial infarction of 41.5 over that of the age-matched general population.[21] Death occurred 3 to 22 years after therapy, but only among those exposed to 42 Gy or more of mediastinal radiation. Although few children today are treated with more than 30 Gy, survivors of childhood malignancy who received higher doses are still alive.

The Stanford group also retrospectively evaluated 2232 patients of all ages treated for HD between 1960 and 1991. The relative risk for cardiac death from all causes increased when total mediastinal radiation was greater than 30 Gy, and the risk rose with increasing dose. These studies included patients treated with both older and current techniques, in terms of portal weighting, use of blocks, and daily fraction size.[22]

Data relating to coronary artery disease and overall mortality from cardiac causes in HD survivors who have received mediastinal radiotherapy with modern techniques are encouraging but not as conclusive. A multicenter study of 4655 adults and children treated for HD from 1940 to 1966 and from 1967 to 1985 found no significant increase in myocardial infarction mortality after an average follow-up of 7 years in those treated with mediastinal radiotherapy, compared with those who did not receive irradiation.[23] Although the relative risk for fatal myocardial infarction was 6.33 for those treated during the early period, the risk fell to 1.97 for the later period, and the confidence interval for the estimate crossed 1.00 and therefore was not significant.

The study by the Stanford group of 2232 patients found that the relative risk of non–myocardial infarction cardiac deaths, compared with that in the general population, declined from 5.3 to 1.4 with subcarinal blocking, but the relative risk for fatal myocardial infarction did not change significantly (3.7 versus 3.4).[22] These apparently contradictory findings can be explained. Some preventive maneuvers, such as subcarinal blocking, do not protect the proximal part of the coronary arteries but do protect other parts of the heart. Therefore, the incidence of coronary artery disease would not be expected to change as much as disease caused by radiation damage to other structures of the heart. Other confounding factors include a shorter follow-up time in those treated with newer forms of therapy and lack of control for other cardiac risk factors in both studies.

One retrospective study of 352 HD patients treated with modern mediastinal radiotherapy, except that total doses exceeded 40 Gy in some cases, found a significantly higher than expected incidence of fatal myocardial infarctions or sudden death at a mean follow-up of 11.2 years.[24] The risk of fatal or nonfatal cardiac events in patients without other known cardiac risk factors, however, was not significantly different from that predicted for the age-matched population. This finding underscores the fact that radiotherapy is one of several risk factors for cardiac disease.

Breast cancer survivors treated with adjuvant radiotherapy for a left-sided malignancy also appear to be at 1.5 to two times the risk of coronary heart disease, depending on the dose-volume of exposure. Evidence comes from follow-up studies comparing cardiac mortality in patients treated with or without irradiation,[25] studies comparing cardiac mortality and morbidity in left- versus right-sided survivors treated with irradiation,[26] and similar but smaller studies comparing myocardial perfusion defects using stress testing with radionuclide imaging techniques.[12,27]

Treatment of the IMNs with older techniques exposed the heart to larger dose-volumes of radiation, and multiple studies have reported that such exposure increases the risk of ischemic heart disease.[26,28] Although some follow-up studies have not found a significantly increased risk of myocardial infarction with radiotherapies used since the mid-1990s, these studies obviously have relatively shorter follow-up periods (median, 10 years) than those that have found an increased risk.[27] Furthermore, studies that have looked at time since radiation as a risk factor have noticed an increased risk only after 10 to 15 years.[28-30] Taken together, these studies suggest that the increased risk of ischemic heart disease depends on the heart's dose-volume of exposure, the length of time since irradiation, and the presence of traditional coronary heart disease risk factors, such as smoking.

Valvular Disease

Although autopsy studies reported a prevalence of valvular fibrosis of 70% to 80% after radiation doses in excess of 35 Gy,[50,51] as late as the early 1990s, clinically important valvular disease was believed to be uncommon after mediastinal radiotherapy.[31]

Recent studies have found that valvular disease is quite common and that the need for cardiac valve surgery is elevated in HD survivors. In their studies of HD survivors, both Adams and associates[17] and Heidenreich and colleagues[16] reported that the rate of valve disease for which endocarditis prophylaxis should be considered was significantly greater than that expected in historical age- and gender-matched controls. In both studies, valvular insufficiency was more common, particularly aortic regurgitation (19% and 26%, respectively, in the two studies), but aortic stenosis was also quite common (6% and 4%). Heidenreich also found that the rate of left-sided valvular insufficiency increased with age and time since therapy, which suggests that radiation-associated valvular disease is progressive.

A study of 415 HD survivors treated between 1962 and 1998 revealed the impact of radiation-associated valvular disease by finding that the observed-to-expected ratio for valve surgery was 8.42 (95% confidence interval, 3.20 to 13.65).[32] Signs and symptoms of valvular abnormalities are no different from those seen for regurgitation and stenosis arising from other causes, although these patients may be less symptomatic.

In general, the radiotherapy techniques used to treat breast cancer have not been associated with abnormal cardiac function, but they do worsen the effects of cardiotoxic chemotherapy agents. However, the largest study to date of breast cancer survivors treated with adjuvant radiotherapy suggests that those whose IMNs were exposed to radiation had an increased risk of valvular defects and congestive heart failure and that this risk did not decrease significantly with more modern techniques, in contrast to the reduced risk of myocardial infarction.[28] However, this IMN-treated cohort was more likely to be exposed to cardiotoxic chemotherapy because they had a less favorable prognosis, and whether the analysis was adjusted for this likelihood is unclear.

Arrhythmias and Conduction Disturbances

Life-threatening arrhythmias and conduction disturbances may occur years after radiation exposure and are quite distinct from the common asymptomatic, nonspecific, and transient repolarization abnormalities that occur soon after irradiation. Serious abnormalities reported after radiotherapy range from bradycardia (including atrioventricular nodal bradycardia), to prolonged QTc intervals, and all levels of heart block (including complete heart block and sick sinus syndrome).

Cardiac dysfunction often is seen with persistent, monotonal tachycardia and loss of circadian and respiratory phasic heart rhythms.[17] This picture is similar to a denervated heart, which suggests autonomic nervous system dysfunction. Patients who have received radiation to the heart also may have a decreased perception of anginal chest pain.

Radiation may increase the risk of potentially serious ventricular arrhythmia in children receiving anthracyclines. With outdated, anterior-weighted mediastinal radiotherapy techniques, the prevalence of conduction abnormalities in childhood cancer survivors has been observed to be as high as 12.5% for prolonged QTc interval and 11% for complete or incomplete heart block; however, the length of follow-up and cumulative radiation doses were not provided.[33] Given that other cardiac late effects seem to increase with time, arrhythmias and conduction defects also may be progressive.

In general, symptoms associated with dysrhythmias are uncommon but can range from palpitations to syncope to sudden death. These conditions may not occur until years after exposure; therefore establishing causation is difficult. Irradiation of implanted pacemakers can cause them to malfunction or fail entirely.

Criteria have been proposed for associating atrioventricular heart block with radiation therapy, based on a review of 19 cases (Table 140.4).[34] Radiation also causes infranodal blocks more commonly than nodal blocks. Symptomatic conduction delays rarely occur in isolation and may worsen. The presence of a bundle branch or bifascicular block suggests imminent life-threatening problems.

PROPOSED CRITERIA FOR ASSOCIATING CARDIAC CONDUCTION ABNORMALITIES WITH RADIATION THERAPY

- Radiation dose to the heart >40 Gy
- Appearance 10 years or more after therapy
- Abnormal interval on electrocardiogram (ECG), such as bundle branch block
- Previous pericardial involvement, not necessarily requiring clinical intervention
- Cardiac conduction abnormalities that occur with other cardiac or mediastinal abnormalities or in patients who have had such abnormalities

From Slama MS, Le Guludec D, Sebag C, et al: Complete atrioventricular block following mediastinal irradiation: a report of six cases. PACE 1991;14:1112-1118.

Table 140.4 Proposed criteria for associating cardiac conduction abnormalities with radiation therapy.

Indirect Effects on the Heart

Radiation may damage other structures in the neck and chest that the heart depends on to function properly (see Table 140.2).[35] Fibrosis in the lung and its vessels may greatly affect cardiopulmonary function. Stenosis and fibrosis may occur to the major arteries, including but not limited to the carotid arteries, the aorta, and the branch pulmonary arteries. Clinical presentations have included transient ischemic attacks, stroke, carotid bruits, vertebrobasilar insufficiency, and arterial insufficiency in the extremities. The lymphatic system also may be disrupted by radiation-induced fibrosis, which leads to chylous pleural effusions.[36]

Thyroid dysfunction after mantle irradiation is common and occurs from 6 months to longer than 10 years after therapy. Hypothyroidism may cause decreased ventricular contractility, ventricular diastolic dysfunction, arrhythmias, abnormalities of peripheral vessels, congestive heart failure, dyslipidemias, and coronary artery disease.[37] Myxedema may cause a chronic effusion that may lead to symptoms and, rarely, tamponade. Prevention is the key element, because cardiovascular dysfunction may not resolve when the patient is treated and becomes euthyroid.

Other neuroendocrine functions, such as those of the hypothalamus-pituitary axis, may be affected by radiation exposure or chemotherapy, and their effects on the heart and coronary heart disease risk factors need to be considered as well (see Chapter 129). In particular, growth hormone deficiency is a common problem in children who received cranial irradiation of 20 Gy or greater, and growth hormone deficiency has been associated with metabolic syndrome abnormalities.[38,39] Furthermore, growth hormone deficiency may prevent optimal recovery from cardiac injury; growth hormone replacement therapy has been shown to be beneficial in increasing wall thickness in childhood acute lymphocytic leukemia survivors who had been treated with anthracyclines and were growth hormone deficient.[40]

DIAGNOSTIC TECHNIQUES

The large number of possible radiation-associated abnormalities may require screening with multiple diagnostic modalities (Table 140.5). Nevertheless, the cardiac evaluation of a person previously exposed to radiation still begins with a thorough history and physical examination. The evaluation should begin by assessing the medical record for at least

EVALUATION OF PATIENTS AT RISK FOR LATE EFFECTS OF MEDIASTINAL RADIATION

Late Effects	Treatment*	Signs and Symptoms	Screening and Diagnostic Tests	Management and Intervention
Pericarditis	>35 Gy	Fatigue, dyspnea on exertion, chest pain, cyanosis, ascites, peripheral edema, hypotension, friction rub, muffled heart sounds, venous distention, pulsus paradoxus, Kussmaul's sign	ECG Chest radiograph Echocardiogram	Pericardiocentesis Pericardiectomy
Cardiomyopathy (myocardial)	>35 Gy or >25 Gy and anthracycline	Fatigue, cough, dyspnea on exertion, peripheral edema, hypertension, tachypnea, rales, tachycardia, murmur, extra heart sounds, hepatomegaly, syncope, palpitations	ECG ECG and/or radionuclide angiography (evaluate diastolic and systolic function) Pulmonary function testing and NT-proBNP with symptoms of congestive heart failure	Education regarding risks of alcohol, isometric exercise, smoking and other drug use, pregnancy, and anesthesia Afterload reducers, antiarrhythmics, diuretics, digoxin Cardiac transplantation
Coronary artery disease	>30 Gy	Chest pain, dyspnea, diaphoresis, hypotension, pallor, nausea, arrhythmia	Lipids and hsCRP Exercise stress test with or without radionuclide angiography, or dobutamine stress echocardiography (frequency depends on risk factor profile and symptoms) Consider thin slice CT for coronary artery calcium scoring Troponin and cardiac enzymes with chest pain	Risk factor modifications, including diet and conditioning regimens Cardiac medications and lipid-lowering agents Coronary artery bypass graft or angioplasty
Valvular disease	>40 Gy	Cough, weakness, dyspnea on exertion, new murmur, rales, peripheral edema or any other sign of congestive heart failure	Echocardiogram Cardiac catheterization	American Heart Association antibiotic recommendations for endocarditis prophylaxis Valve replacement
Arrhythmia	>35 Gy	Palpitations, light-headedness, syncope	ECG and 24-hour ECG Evaluation for other abnormalities	Pacemaker

Modified from Constine LS: Late effects of cancer treatment. In Halperin EC, Constine LS, Tarbell NJ, et al, eds. Pediatric Radiation Oncology. 3rd ed. New York, Lippincott, Williams & Wilkins, 1999:457-537.

*Total cumulative radiation exposure of the chest at this level or higher clearly indicates increased risk for the specific complication and thus the need to screen for it; however, the complication may occur at lower doses as well.

CT, computed tomography; ECG, electrocardiogram; Gy, gray; hsCRP, highly sensitive C-reactive protein; NT-proBNP, serum N-terminal pro-BNP brain natriuretic peptide.

Table 140.5 Evaluation of patients at risk for late effects of mediastinal radiation.

the 10 risk factors listed in Table 140.3. Habits related to coronary artery disease risk factors should be discussed, as should any family history of cardiac disease.

Cardiomegaly apparent on chest radiography may represent a pericardial effusion and can be definitively diagnosed by echocardiography. However, asymptomatic pericarditis generally does not require treatment; therefore screening for it makes little sense. On the other hand, because electrical conduction abnormalities may remain silent until fatal, electrocardiographic (ECG) screening for these abnormalities is quite important. Screening tests for indirect effects also should be performed, particularly for pulmonary function and thyroid function, as well as routine screening for other coronary artery disease risk factors (e.g., lipid profile and highly sensitive C-reactive protein [hsCRP]).

Myocardial function can be assessed by echocardiography and radionuclide angiography. Both are reliable, noninvasive methods of measuring left ventricular systolic performance. Echocardiography has the added advantage of allowing visualization of particular portions of the heart, such as the pericardium, valves, aorta, and branch pulmonary arteries. Diastolic function can (and should) be measured indirectly by echocardiography.

Unfortunately, echocardiograms are of poor quality in some adults because of body habitus and bone density. Radionuclide imaging, therefore, may be preferable for repeated quantitative analysis of systolic function in certain patients. Such imaging also may be adapted to look at myocardial perfusion, and it is a strong predictor of future ischemic heart events. However, diastolic function is difficult to measure with the radionuclide technology available in most hospitals.

Other modalities also may be useful for assessing myocardial function. Cardiac magnetic resonance imaging appears to be a powerful modality for evaluating both cardiac function and perfusion, but its limited availability and expense make it unrealistic to use for regular screening. Continued research to determine whether it provides significant advantages in irradiated patients with possible cardiac damage should be encouraged (see relevant chapters on cardiac imaging modalities). Serum N-terminal pro-BNP brain natriuretic peptide (NT-proBNP) appears to be a very useful tool for evaluating whether dyspnea is caused by heart failure, but its usefulness for serial screening for asymptomatic cardiomyopathy is less clear.[41]

In summary, myocardial function should clearly be assessed with echocardiography, with or without radionuclide studies, depending on the quality of each in a particular patient, while other modalities are reserved for answering specific questions.

The increased risk of fatal coronary artery disease may occur as soon as 5 years after therapy. Investigating other risk factors for coronary artery disease is extremely important in all survivors of high-dose irradiation, regardless of age. Exercise stress testing is a noninvasive method to assess ischemia. Radionuclide myocardial perfusion scanning during exercise has a sensitivity and specificity for detecting ischemic heart disease of about 90% in the general population. Heidenreich and colleagues[42] reported the usefulness of such screening in their series of 294 HD survivors treated with more than 35 Gy of mediastinal radiotherapy who had no history or symptoms of cardiovascular disease.[42] Of these patients, 21.4% had abnormal ventricular images at rest, suggesting myocardial injury, and 42 patients (14%) experienced perfusion defects with exercise. Of the 44 patients who proceeded to have angiography, half had 50% or greater stenosis in one coronary artery, and seven went on to have coronary bypass graft surgery. Furthermore, 23 of the 294 patients experienced coronary events during a median of 6.5 years of follow-up, and 10 had acute myocardial infarctions.

Maximal myocardial oxygen consumption during exercise provides additional information about myocardial health and has had prognostic value in patients with cardiomyopathy. We found myocardial oxygen consumption to be surprisingly low in some patients with a history of mediastinal irradiation who did not have marked symptoms.[17] Hypotension, syncope, and rate-related conduction changes or rhythm abnormalities also were found unexpectedly in some of these same patients during exercise testing.

Coronary calcium scoring using magnetic resonance imaging (MRI) or thin slice computed tomography (CT) scanning also may be useful for assessing the risk of ischemic heart disease, but research specific to this population has not been performed. Angiography and cardiac catheterization are appropriate to evaluate symptoms of angina and heart failure. Some experts argue that these procedures should be done if any other clinically important cardiac lesions are found, because coronary artery disease often occurs with other abnormalities in survivors exposed to greater than 35 Gy of radiation, and it often is asymptomatic.[43] Cardiac biopsy may be helpful in evaluating a patient in congestive heart failure.

Although data do not exist to support definitive recommendations on test frequency, we recommend annual evaluations of survivors of childhood malignancy exposed to radiation. The course of cardiac disease progression is unknown and may vary considerably among patients. In addition, cardiac complications can be life-threatening but in some cases may be easily identified with routine testing. Children may be at higher risk because maturation of the irradiated heart may not keep pace with the growing body. Echocardiograms should be obtained annually to assess systolic and diastolic function, valvular and pericardial abnormalities, and coronary flow. Annual ECG, Holter monitoring, and exercise stress testing is performed to detect high-grade ectopy, conduction defects, ischemia, and abnormal hemodynamic response to exercise. Lipid profiles and thyroid and pulmonary function tests are also performed regularly. Radionuclide imaging is not performed regularly, but others have proposed that it should be done at least every 5 years because of the risk of silent ischemia.[24]

MANAGEMENT

Prevention is the best way to "treat" radiation-induced cardiotoxicity. Although modern radiation techniques seem to reduce the risk of most types of cardiac disease, they do not appear to eliminate it, nor is it clear whether they substantially reduce the most serious risk, that of fatal myocardial infarction in HD survivors. Modern techniques include the use of a linear accelerator as a radiation source, a daily fraction size less than 2 Gy, equally weighted anterior-posterior portals each treated daily, a subcarinal block implemented before a cumulative dose of 30 Gy is reached, and shrinking field technique to minimize the dose-volume of exposure to the heart.

Although permanent complications tend to occur less frequently at total doses less than 40 Gy, systematically limiting therapy to this dose is not a good idea, because such a dose may not control the cancer. Steroids should not be used prophylactically to prevent fibrosis. They have little clinical effect and have an unacceptably high incidence of side effects with long-term administration. Dexrazoxane, an agent that binds iron and, when delivered before each dose of anthracycline, reduces the amount of free radical myocardial injury from the formation of iron-anthracycline complexes, may also hold promise as a cardioprotectant against radiation damage.

Acute pericarditis rarely requires extensive treatment. More than half of patients require no treatment, and another 40% respond to bed rest, nonsteroidal anti-inflammatory medications, and mild diuretics. Asymptomatic effusions may be followed while awaiting spontaneous resolution, which may take 2 years. Chronic effusions that cause symptoms or hemodynamic abnormalities of cardiac compression should be treated with a subtotal parietal pericardiectomy. In one series, pericardiocentesis alone was completely unsuccessful in treating radiation-induced chronic effusions that required intervention.[44]

Pericardiectomy may reduce the propensity of radiation-related effusions to evolve into constrictive pericarditis, and it is more easily carried out if an effusion is present. Waiting until constriction occurs is associated with a higher mortality from acute dilatation and heart failure. However, if tamponade is present, pericardiocentesis should be performed using a local anesthetic just before pericardiectomy because of the higher risk of general anesthesia in such conditions. This operation usually is successful unless myocardial fibrosis or constrictive pericarditis is present, in which case the prognosis is poor. Before surgery, however, hypothyroidism should be ruled out, because it is common after mantle irradiation and may cause chronic effusion. Also, the pericardial fluid and the pericardium should be analyzed to rule out tumor invasion and infectious agents.

Coronary artery bypass surgery may be preferable for relieving acute coronary blockage in these patients, even in those whose lesions are treatable with percutaneous transluminal coronary angioplasty. Complications during angioplasty may require placement of an emergency coronary artery bypass graft. However, under emergency conditions, coronary bypass can be especially difficult because of extensive fibrosis in the mediastinum. In addition, left main coronary artery and ostial lesions are quite common in these patients and have been reported not to be amenable to angioplasty. Several studies report good long-term results with nonemergency bypass surgery in these patients.[5,45,46]

Hicks[45] described his experience in operating on 14 patients who had received greater than 35 Gy of chest radiotherapy. Standard operative technique (moderate hypothermia and cold blood cardioplegia) was used in all patients, with good results. He recommends that anterior pericardiectomy be routine, with the initial operation on the heart, regardless of whether the pericardium is thickened, because this seemed to reduce complications. Postoperative complications depended largely on the extent of radiation injury to the lungs and right ventricle and on the maintenance of normal sinus rhythm. Many patients had moderate to severe right ventricular fibrosis with an elevated right atrial pressure and failure of the right ventricle to empty on cardiopulmonary bypass. Therefore, the right ventricle must be protected by maintaining higher filling pressures and by restoring normal sinus rhythm with its coordinated atrial contraction after bypass. Although the internal mammary artery is preferable to the saphenous vein for the bypass graft, the internal mammary artery was too damaged for use in 11 of the 14 patients. Therefore, shielding the mammary arteries from radiation is a good idea if it does not minimize therapy.

A recent single institution review of 230 cancer survivors treated with chest radiotherapy who subsequently underwent surgery showed that HD survivors had significantly more complications and worse surgical outcomes, whereas women treated with tangential radiotherapy for breast cancer had similar outcomes to the general population.[47] These researchers recommended that for the highest risk survivors, the techniques chosen should minimize the length of time pulmonary function is compromised in recovery and the time during the surgery that the heart is kept ischemic. They noted that, at a minimum, operations must be carefully planned and executed and that definitive repairs must be performed to minimize the risk of future surgeries.

Heart block or valve disease requiring surgery often occurs with other manifestations of radiation-induced heart disease, such as chronic pericarditis or coronary artery disease. These other manifestations may explain why a 1991 retrospective review found the mortality rate among 35 patients with valvular disease undergoing surgical repair to be 66%.[31] More recent reports suggest that patients do well even when valve repair is performed concurrently with coronary artery bypass.[48] Appropriate endocarditis prophylaxis should be given as well, regardless of surgical intervention. Atrioventricular sequential pacing is important for patients with complete heart block, because they tend to have stiff ventricles. In some cases, the appropriate treatment for survivors with severe radiation-induced heart disease in whom other therapies have failed is heart or heart-lung transplantation. Such patients should not be denied this option solely because of their history of cancer, and they deserve an appropriate and careful transplant evaluation.

In summary, manifestations of radiation-induced heart disease are treated in the same way as these problems would be treated in the general public. However, extra precautions and a special appreciation of the changes irradiation causes in the heart and other structures in the chest should be kept in mind in the treatment of affected patients.

PROGNOSIS

Although most people who receive therapeutic mediastinal irradiation remain asymptomatic from a cardiac perspective, virtually all patients with HD who are treated with radiation using older techniques have subclinical dysfunction 5 to 10 years after therapy. Clinically important dysfunction can occur during therapy or many years later. Subclinical dysfunction may be progressive and eventually may cause complications and death. Although refined therapeutic radiation techniques generally have reduced the percentage of patients with subclinical abnormalities and clinically meaningful problems,[49] follow-up has been shorter with these newer techniques. In addition, the absolute risk of cardiac mortality for a given dose also appears to increase with longer follow-up. This suggests that the higher risk of cardiac complications associated with chest irradiation is lifelong. Continued evaluations for longer periods are needed to determine whether newer radiation techniques have eliminated the increased risk of cardiovascular disease or simply delayed the appearance of its manifestations.

SUMMARY

Radiation-induced heart disease has been a major cause of complications and death among patients treated with mediastinal radiation. The spectrum of disease is broad, in terms of both manifestation and severity. Radiotherapy for left-sided breast cancer causes a lesser degree but still seriously increased risk of ischemic heart disease. Damage is caused primarily by microvascular injury. The resulting symptoms may not occur until decades later, although subclinical abnormalities commonly occur much earlier. Radiation should be considered one of many cardiac risk factors, which emphasizes the need to reduce other risk factors as much as possible. Unfortunately, radiation is not widely recognized as a risk factor for cardiac disease, even among cardiologists; therefore, it is incumbent on those of us who recognize this fact to inform our colleagues. More important, we must also teach this awareness to those who routinely care for these patients (primary care providers) and those who might care for these patients in a crisis (emergency department doctors). Longitudinal monitoring of patients exposed to radiation is needed not only to provide the best care for individual patients, but also to identify the best treatment options for those exposed to therapeutic irradiation as a group.[49]

chapter

141 High Altitude Medicine

Stuart J. Hutchison

Definition

- The progressive hypoxia of exposure to high altitude may result in a number of cardiovascular events ranging from subtle to increasing morbidity (acute mountain sickness with progression to high altitude pulmonary edema or high altitude cerebral edema) and death.

Key Features

- Acute mountain sickness, the most common altitude-related medical disorder, is not itself life-threatening; however, it is a marker of poor acclimatization and indicates a risk of complicated forms of altitude illness (high altitude pulmonary edema and high altitude cerebral edema), which may prove fatal.
- Acute mountain sickness, in all its forms, is likely to occur at higher altitudes, after a more rapid ascent, and when greater levels of exertion are performed on attaining altitude.

Therapy

- The primary strategy is prevention—a progressive ascent to altitude.
- Several pharmacologic means (the vasodilators nifedipine, sildenafil/tadalafil, and salbutamol and dexamethasone) have been shown in small trials to prevent forms of high altitude illness. Bosentan has been shown to reduce pulmonary pressures but has not been established as preventive or therapeutic for pulmonary edema.
- Once symptoms have developed, prompt descent of more than 1000 vertical meters, together with supplemental oxygen, is effective.
- Pulmonary and cerebral edema are medical emergencies.

Exposure to high altitude may initiate life-threatening medical illness and may also aggravate preexisting medical disorders. Exposure of a few hours to moderate altitude is seldom a risk to individuals with or without recognized cardiovascular disease, but longer stays may incite altitude-related illness. The most common altitude-related medical disorder is acute mountain sickness (AMS). Although not life-threatening, this nonspecific disorder is a marker of poor acclimatization and of susceptibility to the life-threatening forms of altitude-related illness. The life-threatening forms of altitude-related illness are high altitude pulmonary edema (HAPE) and high altitude cerebral edema (HACE). HAPE is a noncardiogenic pulmonary edema of unpredictable nature. It typically affects healthy and fit individuals who ascend rapidly to high altitude and promptly engage in strenuous exertion. Similarly, HACE is of unknown medical basis and affects individuals who ascend rapidly to high altitude; it can be viewed as a terminal and fulminant state of AMS. Although debate persists concerning the optimal treatment of all forms of altitude-related disorders, there is no debate that prevention should be the primary strategy, and that once significant symptoms have developed, no further altitude gain should be attempted—and risk incurred.

Exposure to high altitude occurs principally in the great mountain ranges of the world, which are visited by tourists and recreational adventurers such as skiers, trekkers, and climbers. Across America, more than 1 million individuals ski at or over moderately high altitudes of 3050 m (10,000 feet) each year. More than 1500 individuals attempt to climb Mount McKinley (Denali) in Alaska each year, and approximately 50% reach the 6198-m (20,320 feet) summit each year. Roads enable vehicular ascent to the summit of the Rocky Mountains, including the summit of Pike's Peak (4300 m [14,100 feet]), to which hundreds of thousands of individuals drive yearly. Similarly, more than 300,000 individuals a year drive from sea level to two thirds of the way up Japan's Mount Fuji (i.e., to 2440 m [8000 feet]), and many thousands continue the ascent to the summit (3776 m [12,380 feet]). Increasing numbers of individuals trek and climb to very high and extreme altitude in the Himalayas; the numbers have dipped only in 2002.

An individual must be exposed to altitude for 6 to 24 hours for AMS, HAPE, or HACE to ensue. The fact that most individuals who ascend rapidly do so in one "tourist" mode or another and spend only a few hours at altitude likely accounts for the relatively low incidence of altitude-related health problems. Individuals who engage in recreational or other pursuits for longer intervals and those who venture into higher and more remote regions assume a greater risk, both of contracting an altitude-related disorder and of adverse outcomes to the disorder.

Fatalities have occurred at altitudes as low as 2135 m (7000 feet), but altitude-related symptoms generally are very mild between 1525 m (5000 feet) and 2440 m (8000 feet) above sea level. Altitude-related disorders start at approximately 2440 m (8000 feet), and most cases occur between 3050 m (10,000 feet) and 4575 m (15,000 feet). The threshold effect of 2440 m (8000 feet) on altitude illness is best seen at alpine ski resorts:

- those such as Tahoe, at 2135 m (7000 feet), have very few cases of altitude illness;
- those such as Vail, at 2440 m (8000 feet), have occasional cases; and
- those such as Mammoth, at 2745 m (9000 feet), have more cases.

Interestingly, the elevation at which the individual sleeps is a greater influence on the development of altitude-related illness than is the altitude attained during the day—the elevation of the ski resort matters at least as much as the height of the ski hill—hence the climber's dictum, "carry high, sleep low."

Above 4575 m (15,000 feet), the incidence of altitude-related illness increases. Therefore, most cases of altitude-related disorders are suffered by tourists, mainly at moderately high altitude and generally in areas with better facilities and access to treatment. The absolute number of cases in those who proceed to greater heights is smaller, but the incidence is greater, as is the mortality. Few definitive medical treatments are available for high altitude pulmonary and cerebral edema; the principal "treatment" is prevention.

PHYSIOLOGIC EFFECTS OF ALTITUDE AND ACCLIMATIZATION

The goal of acclimatization is to minimize intracellular hypoxia. Acclimatization to high altitude occurs principally at the pulmonary level but also at the peripheral cellular level. Acclimatization to extreme altitude represents a complex and notable physiologic feat. The scientific community initially held that survival, let alone exertion, at the summit of Mount Everest (8854 m [29,028 feet]) was impossible. However, early British climbs in the 1920s established that, with and without supplemental oxygen, strenuous exertion could be performed at extreme altitude. In 1978, the summit of Mount Everest was reached for the first time without supplemental oxygen by Reinhold Messner; he subsequently repeated his feat, to be followed over many years by many others.[1]

Exposure to the hypobaric hypoxia of altitude results in an immediate decrease in the resting (and exertional) partial pressure of oxygen (Pao_2) and in oxygen (O_2) saturation. The extent of the decrease in Pao_2 and O_2 saturation is altitude dependent. At 2135 m (7000 feet), the Pao_2 is 8.0 kPa (60 mm Hg) and O_2 saturation is still high (92%). However, above 2440 m (8000 feet), the decrease in O_2 saturation accelerates as the decline in the O_2 saturation curve accelerates. Concentrations of 2,3-diphosphoglycerate in the red blood cells increase.

Decreases in O_2 saturation stimulate carotid body chemoreceptors, which in turn stimulate an increase in ventilation by means of a greater increase in tidal volume than in rate of ventilation. This hyperventilation persists throughout the stay at altitude. As a result of the hyperventilation, the partial pressure of carbon dioxide ($Paco_2$) decreases, and respiratory alkalosis develops. Over 3 to 4 days, renal adaptation occurs and blood pH is normalized, although the $Paco_2$ remains low. With further hypoxia, further hyperventilation occurs. Alkalosis shifts the O_2 dissociation curve to retain greater saturation for any degree of hypoxia. The extent of hyperventilation is considerable, and at the summit of Mount Everest, an end-alveolar $Paco_2$ concentration as low as 1.0 kPa (7.5 mm Hg) has been measured.[1] With an extremely low $Paco_2$, a greater Pao_2 can be achieved, but the extreme hypoxic ventilatory response is believed to contribute to the cerebral artery vasoconstriction and neurologic sequelae of climbing to extreme altitude.[2]

Exposure to altitude-related hypoxia, as with exposure to any form of hypoxia, stimulates complex changes in sympathetic output. Field and laboratory studies have yielded widely divergent observations on indices of sympathetic activity at altitude. A predominance of data affirms that sympathetic output increases promptly and decreases to normal or even subnormal levels after several days, and thus potentially may be viewed as a marker of acclimatization.[3] For several days after altitude is attained, the heart rate and blood pressure are increased, resting cardiac output increases (mainly as a result of the increase in heart rate), venoconstriction occurs, and basal metabolic indices are increased. An increased heart rate is consistent with a nonacclimatized state, and tachycardia suggests HAPE.

For the first several days at altitude, total blood volume decreases as a result of a reduction in serum plasma volume; often, within hours of altitude being attained, plasma volume has decreased by 10% to 15%. This is caused partly by a shift of fluid out of the intravascular compartment; the proportion of shift into the interstitial compartment compared with that into the intracellular compartment is unclear.

The basis of the fluid shift is not understood, but vascular integrity and permeability are a factor in most altitude-related diseases. In addition, fluid intake often does not match fluid shifts and insensible loss, and degrees of intravascular hypovolemia are common. Therefore, edema is not unusual after exposure to altitude, before acclimatization has occurred, and intravascular depletion may occur concurrently.

Because of loss of plasma volume, the hematocrit increases acutely. Also, the circulating erythrocyte mass increases slightly as a result of reduced splenic sequestration of erythrocytes. The total erythrocyte mass does not increase significantly unless exposure to altitude and hypoxia are of sufficient duration that erythrogenesis, with its 10-day intramedullary phase, has occurred. Most individuals acclimatize to altitudes such as 3050 m (10,000 feet) within 3 to 4 days and clearly do so without relying on erythrogenesis and an increase in the hematocrit. Notably, the llama, an animal that performs the most efficiently and powerfully at altitude, has a hemoglobin concentration of less than 100 g/dL. Rather than being essential to acclimatization, polycythemia is only a late and minor contributor to acclimatization, and it is strongly suspected of contributing to some cases of altitude-related ischemic events.

Initially, the cardiac response to altitude exposure consists of a decrease in cardiac chamber cavitary size (as a result of plasma volume contraction) and stroke volume, but proportionally a greater increase in heart rate, such that resting cardiac output increases. The resting heart rate tends to normalize with acclimatization; however, the maximum heart rate is very significantly reduced—130 beats per minute (bpm) at 6100 m (20,000 feet)[4] —throughout the time at altitude.

The most striking aspect of arriving at altitude is the profound decrease in exercise capacity. Several factors contribute, and the dominant cause is unknown. A lower maximum cardiac output occurs at the cardiac level because of the lower maximum heart rate and also at the pulmonary vascular level because of hypoxic-induced vasoconstriction. Decreased O_2 saturation and a greater decrease in saturation with exertion impair exercise capacity by reducing intracellular O_2 tension.

Peripheral cellular responses are important in adaptation to altitude. The intracellular machinery of respiration (i.e., oxidative enzymes, myoglobin, mitochondrial numbers, and capillary density) all increase with hypoxic exposure at altitude. This has been well demonstrated in hypobaric chamber experiments with quadriceps muscle biopsy sampling.

In summary, the principal adaptation to altitude occurs at the pulmonary level and is achieved through hyperventilation; the secondary response occurs through peripheral cellular respiratory changes. Consequently, any pulmonary disease acquired at altitude, such as HAPE, is potentially life-threatening. Respiratory alkalosis has the important effect of increasing the saturation at any Pa_{O_2}. This confers only a very small and clinically insignificant benefit at elevations of 3050 m (10,000 feet) or so; however, above 6100 m (20,000 feet), it confers a very important advantage in terms of maintaining O_2 saturation (Fig. 141.1).

PATHOPHYSIOLOGY

Acute Altitude Exposure

As with loss of pressurization in an aircraft, acute exposure to altitude may compromise an individual through both acute hypoxia and acute hypobaria. The severity of the symptoms relates to the severity of the hypoxia. Increasing hypoxia causes initially mild sensory impairment, then mild cognitive impairment, then worsening cognitive impairment, then lethargy, loss of consciousness, coma, and death. In the 20th century, several early French balloonists ascended to remarkable heights, greater than 15,250 m (50,000 feet), in hot air paper balloons and then returned to earth as fatalities of hypoxia. Acute decompression syndromes (the formation of nitrogen bubbles within the joints, organs, and bloodstream) also can occur with abrupt loss of pressurization, similar to the acute decompression syndromes related to

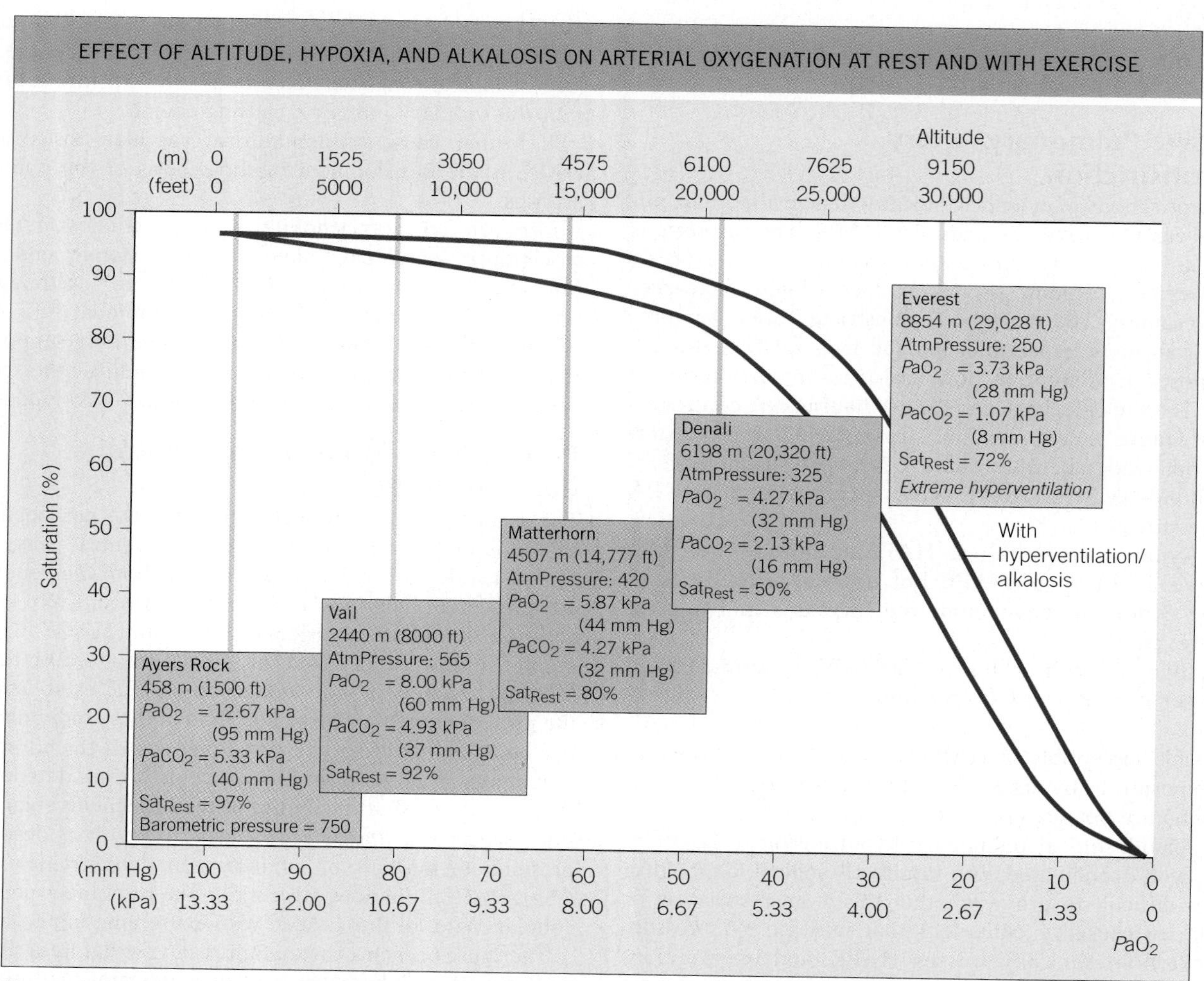

Figure 141.1 Effect of altitude, hypoxia, and alkalosis on arterial oxygenation at rest and with exercise. Above 2440 m (8000 feet), arterial saturation (Sat) begins to decline. Hyperventilation and alkalosis confer increasing benefit at higher elevations. Exertion leads to increasing desaturation with increasing altitude. Atm, atmospheric; Pa_{CO_2}, partial pressure of carbon dioxide; Pa_{O_2}, partial pressure of oxygen.

scuba diving. Climbers who are poorly acclimatized and who ascend using inadequate supplies of supplemental oxygen that become depleted may experience acute hypoxic symptoms as described previously.

High Altitude Pulmonary Edema

Few pathologic studies have been done on individuals who succumb to HAPE. Dickinson and colleagues[5] described the autopsy findings in seven trekkers who died of altitude-related illness. All had wet lungs, edematous with exudative, protein-rich fluid; many had alveolar hemorrhage; and some had hyaline membranes. In 50% of these individuals, thrombosis was observed in pulmonary arteries, which suggests that in situ thrombosis of the pulmonary arteries may complicate the course of HAPE. The right ventricles were dilated, consistent with pressure strain on the right side of the heart.

The pathophysiology of HAPE is incompletely understood, despite decades of observational studies, and is the subject of a high degree of debate. Four schools of thought attempt to explain the development of the disorder:

- an abnormal pulmonary vascular response underlies HAPE;
- permeability alone is the central cause of the disorder;
- increased pulmonary capillary pressure causes HAPE; and
- impaired sodium-driven clearance of alveolar fluid may underlie susceptibility to HAPE.

Excessive Pulmonary Artery Vasoconstriction

A substantial body of evidence indicates that an abnormal pulmonary vascular response underlies HAPE. The response is abnormal in two ways: an excessive pulmonary artery (PA) vasoconstrictor response occurs, as does a highly heterogeneous response. The patchy vasoconstricted areas are protected from local hyperemia, but the less constricted areas are exposed to disruptive flow and pressure that result in edema. The site of leakage and the mechanisms are controversial, but failure of hemodynamic stress of capillaries or arterioles is believed to be responsible. It has been shown that[6,7]:

- individuals with HAPE have severely increased PA pressures;
- individuals susceptible to HAPE at altitude (i.e., who have a history of HAPE but do not currently have the condition) have moderate increases in PA pressure; and
- individuals with no history of HAPE at altitude have lesser increases in PA pressure.

Individuals susceptible to HAPE have greater PA pressures after exposure to hypoxia and with exercise than do individuals who are not susceptible to the condition.[8]

The relationship of pulmonary hypertension to HAPE is strong, well documented, and intuitively logical, although it remains difficult to prove whether this is an association or a matter of causality. Situations that increase PA pressure (e.g., exertion) clinically worsen HAPE, and interventions that reduce PA pressure (e.g., supplemental O_2, descent from altitude, nifedipine, and nitric oxide) improve HAPE.

The mechanism of the excessive and patchy pulmonary vasoconstriction is not well understood, but a number of studies support the concept that endothelial injury or activation underlies HAPE. Concentrations of endothelin 1 increase twofold at 4575 m (15,000 feet), and correlate with PA pressure. Bosentan, a mixed Eta/Etb endothelin receptor antagonist, has been shown to attenuate altitude-induced increases in pulmonary artery pressure.[9] Nitric oxide markers may be reduced in individuals with HAPE,[10] and nitric oxide supplementation does improve HAPE.[6] Concentrations of E-selectin, which is produced only by endothelial cells, increase at altitude, which supports the suggestion that endothelial injury participates in HAPE.[11]

Specific endothelial nitric oxide gene polymorphisms have not yet been associated with HAPE.

A magnetic resonance imaging (MRI) study using a spin labeling technique demonstrated that the relative dispersion of pulmonary blood flow was no different in normoxic conditions between HAPE-susceptible, HAPE-resistant, and unselected patients; however, when under hypoxic stress, HAPE-susceptible individuals showed greater pulmonary blood flow heterogeneity, whereas HAPE-resistant and unselected individuals did not show heterogeneity.[12] The theory that regional heterogeneity of pulmonary vasoconstriction incites high altitude pulmonary edema proposes that lung regions that develop greater arteriolar vasoconstriction protect their capillary beds from excess hydrostatic forces, but regions with lesser constriction do not adequately protect the capillary beds, exposing them to excess physical forces that disrupt the capillary integrity, causing edema.

A further cause of nonuniform vascular obstruction in HAPE is the development of thrombosis of the pulmonary arteries.

Intra-arterial acetylcholine infusion studies in HAPE-susceptible individuals have shown systemic endothelial function to be impaired by hypoxic stress.[13] Although this observation pertains solely to the endothelial nitric oxide pathway, the study indirectly and considerably supports the theory that endothelial dysfunction, including other components of pulmonary endothelial function, is involved.

Permeability Alone as the Central Cause of HAPE

The second school of thought regarding the pathogenesis of HAPE is that permeability alone is the central cause of the disorder. Edema is common at altitude, both the generalized edema seen in individuals who have nonspecifically failed to acclimatize and the disorders of HAPE and HACE. Bronchoscopic studies carried out at 4422.5 m (14,500 feet) on Mount McKinley, in individuals with HAPE, established that the protein content of bronchial fluid in these individuals was the same as that of serum, providing one of the cornerstone arguments of the permeability concept.[14] More detailed studies have shown that the nature of the bronchoalveolar lavage fluid suggests a “large pore” leak[15] and that, despite the presence of markers of inflammation (leukotrienes B4 and C5a), HAPE fluid does not contain the prominent neutrophil cellular material that is seen with acute lung injury states.[15]

The cause of such an acute failure of vascular integrity is not well understood, but some evidence indicates that inflammation participates in the process.[16] The 12- to 24-hour interval between exposure to altitude and the development of HAPE is intriguing and indirectly may suggest a number of cellular transcriptional mechanisms that result in uncontrolled permeability. Inflammation has been proposed as a central mediator of permeability in HAPE[16] but has been refuted as such by others.[17]

Increased Pulmonary Capillary Pressure

The third school of thought holds that HAPE is caused by increased pulmonary capillary pressure. Although increased pulmonary capillary pressure customarily is equated with cardiogenic pulmonary edema, hypoxic pulmonary venoconstriction[18] (which may account for 20% of the increase in pulmonary resistance in pulmonary edema[19]) direct PA-capillary connections increase capillary pressure.[20] A recent study demonstrated increased pulmonary capillary wedge pressure (PCWP) in individuals with early HAPE:

Early HAPE cases	PCWP: 22 mm Hg
HAPE-susceptible individuals	PCWP: 16 mm Hg
Controls	PCWP: 12 mm Hg

In addition, increased pulmonary permeability (as measured by the transport of gallium 67–labeled transferrin protein) has been reported to occur when the capillary pressure was greater than 19 mm Hg.[21]

Experimental work in dogs has shown that lung weight increases when the capillary pressure exceeds 17 to 24 mm Hg.[22] However, older studies demonstrated low-normal capillary pressures (4 mm Hg), mildly reduced cardiac indices (3l/min/m^2), and greatly increased pulmonary vascular resistance (19 Woods units) and pulmonary arterial hypertension.[23-26]

Therefore, no evidence indicates that HAPE is a cardiogenic pulmonary edema, but increased capillary pressure may participate through complex mechanisms of small-vessel vasoreactivity. Left ventricular diastolic dysfunction, documented in healthy mountaineers ascending to altitude, is believed to be imparted by secondary changes in left-sided heart filling caused by acute right ventricular hypertension. The occurrence of overt diastolic heart failure has not been established.[27]

Impaired Sodium-Driven Clearance of Alveolar Fluid

The most recent school of thought proposes that impaired sodium-driven clearance of alveolar fluid may underlie susceptibility to HAPE.[28] HAPE-susceptible individuals are approximately four times as likely to have a patent foramen ovale, intracardiac shunting as a result of it, and worse hypoxemia as HAPE-resistant individuals.[29] Although the patent foramen ovale has been proposed to worsen hypoxemia and thereby aggravate pulmonary vasoconstriction, its significance in HAPE is unclear.

High Altitude Cerebral Edema

Most patients who develop HACE have previously had AMS, and a prior history of HACE is common. Brain edema occurs in all cases, and petechial hemorrhages are common, as is spongiosis. In affected individuals who die, focal necrosis and brain herniation have been observed.[5]

The pathophysiology of HACE is poorly understood. Initially, volume overload was thought to be the cause; however, even moderate to severe volume overload does not cause cerebral edema.

The current theory is that HACE is vasogenic in origin; that is, it is the result of a local failure of maintenance of fluid compartment partitioning of the intracranial vasculature. Recent MRI data have characterized the pattern of edema in HACE[25] as reversible white matter edema; however, a vasogenic basis for the disorder has not been conclusively established.[30]

CLINICAL PRESENTATIONS

Acute Mountain Sickness

As mentioned, AMS is a nonspecific disorder that is not life-threatening but that serves as a marker of poor acclimatization to date and therefore of the risk of development of more severe altitude illness. It is far more common than HAPE or HACE, and generally takes 6 to 24 hours at altitude to develop.

The principal symptom of AMS is headache. It typically is worse in the morning, which suggests that sleep-impaired hyperventilation may contribute. The headache typically is bifrontal and throbbing. The mountains beside the 4819 m (15,800 feet) Kilik Pass in Afghanistan are known as the Great Headache and Little Headache Mountains. In addition to headache, nonspecific complaints are common, such as fatigue, lethargy, irritability, anoxia, nausea, vomiting, light-headedness, personality changes, and insomnia. No physical findings are specific to the diagnosis of AMS. Edema is common but is not specific for AMS. Nocturnal periodic breathing also is not specific for AMS. Overt neurologic findings (especially ataxia) are strongly suggestive of HACE, severe hypoxia from HAPE, or other lung disease.

Susceptibility to AMS is highly variable. Some individuals show no AMS symptoms, whereas others are incapacitated. Prediction on the basis of patient-related parameters remains elusive. Physical conditioning does not reduce the incidence of AMS. Older individuals are not more likely to develop AMS, but children are. Rapid ascent (e.g., traveling from sea level to a ski resort at 2440 m [8000 feet] in a day), exertion (e.g., skiing), and male gender typify most patients with AMS. Individuals who spend 2 days at an intermediary elevation (e.g., Denver on the way to Vail) have few symptoms of AMS. The irresistible accessibility of mountain resorts and recreational areas contributes to most cases of AMS, as does neglecting the process of acclimatization.

High Altitude Pulmonary Edema

High altitude pulmonary edema is a life-threatening disorder. Its basis is incompletely understood, and no fully reliable treatment, other than descent and supplemental oxygen, is available. HAPE accounts for most deaths from high altitude medical illness and for an important proportion of all deaths at altitude (Fig. 141.2).

The first death likely from HAPE was recorded in AD 403, involving a Chinese monk who died foaming at the mouth while traveling at high altitude in Afghanistan. The first recorded impression that HAPE was an acute edema was made nearly a century ago, by a physician on an expedition to climb the Abruzzi Ridge of K2. The physician recorded that a young member died of "fluid on the lungs." For many decades, HAPE was not understood, and cases invariably

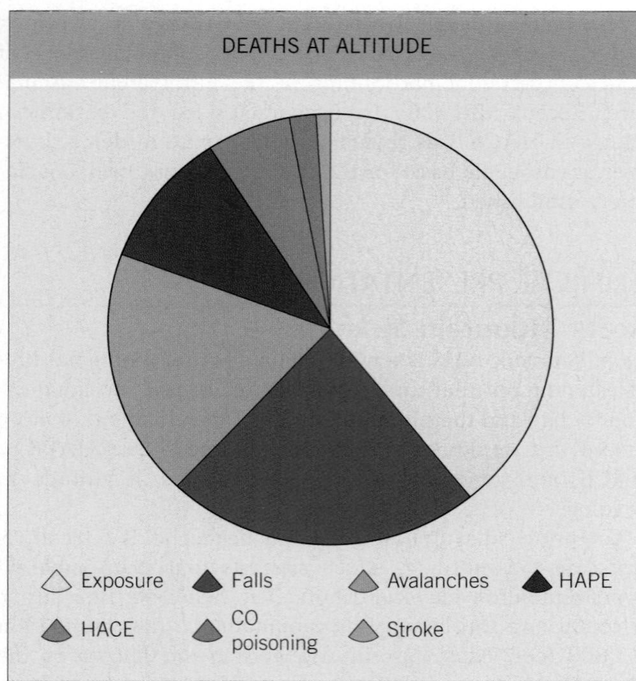

Figure 141.2 Deaths at altitude. Deaths observed on 10 Alaskan climbs and four Himalayan climbs. Exposure (death from cold) and falls are the most common causes of death. High altitude pulmonary edema (HAPE) and high altitude cerebral edema (HACE) are the next most common causes of death. CO, carbon monoxide.

were regarded as pneumonia. HAPE was first documented and described in the modern era in 1965.[31]

The incidence of HAPE is influenced both by the altitude to which the individual is exposed and the rate of ascent to that altitude. It is

- much less than 1 in 1000 for skiers at resorts at 2135 m (7000 feet);
- approximately 1 in 1000 for those at resorts at 2440 m (8000 feet);
- 1 in 100 for those who ascend rapidly to higher than 3050 m (10,000 feet); and
- approximately 5 in 100 at altitudes approaching 4575 m (15,000 feet).

Cases have occurred at altitudes higher than 8500 m (27,869 feet) on Mount Everest. Some individuals appear to harbor a susceptibility to HAPE and repeatedly develop HAPE at the same elevation. Children appear to be particularly predisposed to HAPE.[32]

The third factor that influences the incidence of HAPE is exertion performed at altitude: exertion increases cardiac output and pulmonary artery pressures. The individuals who incur the greatest risk are fit and strong individuals who ascend rapidly to above 3050 m (10,000 feet) and engage in strenuous exertion upon arriving at altitude and before having acclimatized.

An unusual form of high altitude pulmonary edema is seen among individuals who live at high altitude and who return to altitude after several days or weeks at low altitude (i.e., "re-entry" or "reascension" pulmonary edema).[33]

Unusual basic grounds of HAPE include backgrounds such as congenital absence of a pulmonary artery[34] or previous pneumonectomy.[35]

The natural history of HAPE is variable and unpredictable. In addition to the pulmonary features, cerebral symptoms frequently are observed as a result either of concurrent disorders (50% of those with HAPE have AMS, and 15% have HACE[36]) or of severe hypoxia. Many cases stabilize, and some improve even without therapeutic intervention, but some progress to a fatal outcome. Loss of consciousness portends death within the day. One of the most distinctive features is nocturnal progression. The reasons for this are unclear, but many deaths occur at night. Nocturnal hypoventilation may contribute to this nocturnal deterioration. Mortality rates are increased by unavailability of treatment, unavailability of descent or evacuation, and higher altitude at which HAPE occurred. In the author's experience, three of 21 cases (14%) died.

High Altitude Cerebral Edema

High altitude cerebral edema is a potentially life-threatening altitude-related disorder. As with HAPE, it is much less common than nonspecific AMS and can be viewed as the end-stage and worst form of AMS. The reported incidence is about 25% that of HAPE. HACE may be present in an individual who also has HAPE.

The principal symptom is headache. Nausea, vomiting, visual disturbances, lethargy, and personality changes may occur. Loss of consciousness precedes death. Seizures are uncommon but may occur. Lack of coordination, ataxia, mental status changes, abnormal reflex responses, and retinal hemorrhages and papilledema are common.

DIAGNOSTIC TECHNIQUES

Acute Mountain Sickness

No serologic or radiologic tests are available to assist with the diagnosis of AMS. It therefore remains a clinical diagnosis consisting of:

- a context of recent altitude gain;
- headache; and
- nonspecific symptoms.

For most individuals, as long as no progressive altitude gain has occurred, AMS is a time-limited disorder and symptoms will subside within several days. A small subset of patients never acclimatizes.

High Altitude Pulmonary Edema

The diagnosis of HAPE is made clinically based on the following factors:

1. A susceptible individual (one who has ascended rapidly to altitude)
2. An individual who develops respiratory distress after a short latent period
3. The presence of at least two of the following symptoms:
   - Dyspnea at rest
   - Cough
   - Exertional intolerance
   - Chest pressure
   - Undue weakness

4. The presence of at least two of the following physical findings:
   - Rales
   - Wheezing
   - Tachycardia
   - Tachypnea at rest
   - Central cyanosis
5. An individual in whom no other cause of pulmonary disease is likely.

The most compelling and elegant description of the symptoms of HAPE was provided in a personal account by a prominent physician, James Wilkerson III: fatigue, possible mild AMS symptoms a few days before, shortness of breath on exertion, a sensation of breathing deeper when at rest, but not of frank shortness of breath at rest, and no orthopnea.[37]

The principal findings are respiratory. Patients with HAPE appear agitated and distressed from hypoxia and increased ventilatory effort. The ventilatory rate and effort typically are greatly increased. Tachycardia is a valuable sign. Crepitations inevitably are heard throughout the lung fields, and wheezing is common. Cyanosis is present in all severe cases. A few patients have overtly frothing pink bubbly secretions. Somnolence suggests respiratory fatigue and an increased mortality as a result either of the terminal state of pulmonary edema or concurrent cerebral edema. Jugular venous pressures are rarely described in the literature. In the author's experience, despite the increased right ventricular and systolic pressures, jugular pressures tend to be low, usually as a result of concurrent volume depletion because of the high insensible water losses in the low-humidity environment of high altitude. Abnormalities on cardiac auscultation are seldom detected. Low-grade fever is quite common for the first several days among patients with substantially increased respiratory work.

Differential Diagnosis

It is important to recall the differential diagnosis of respiratory distress at altitude. Bronchial and tracheal irritation from the dry if not desiccating air at high altitude is clearly the most common reason for cough at altitude. The "Himalayan hack" or "Karakoram cough" is nearly ubiquitous among expedition members to very high altitude peaks. Up to 10% of individuals taking part in high attitude expeditions have fractured ribs as a result of intractable dry cough. This cough is not associated with airflow obstruction.

Some individuals develop an exacerbation of bronchial asthma as a result of the cold air or exercise (or both) at altitude. Bronchitis and bronchopneumonia are encountered among Western climbers who go to altitude and in local porters and Sherpas.

Some fulminant cases of HAPE, with an abrupt onset, low-grade fever, and red, frothy secretions may be misinterpreted as pneumococcal pneumonia. Pulmonary embolism has been described among expedition members who ascend to high altitude, particularly those immobilized for a period of days, typically waiting out storms in small tents. An inadequate fluid intake and immobility are the presumed precipitants of venous thrombosis and subsequent embolization.

Radiographic Findings

The typical radiographic findings of HAPE differ from those of cardiogenic edema and other noncardiogenic edemas.[38] The radiographic features of HAPE (interstitial, central, with peribronchial cuffing, ill-defined vessels, and patchy air space consolidation) have been elegantly summarized by Gluecker and associates.[38] Typically, the size of the heart in individuals with HAPE is normal, and the pattern of HAPE, in contradistinction to that of cardiogenic pulmonary edema, is typically supradiaphragmatic sparing (Fig. 141.3a). With descent and/or supplemental oxygen, complete resolution within 24 to 48 hours is common (Fig. 141.3b).

Patients who develop HAPE in remote settings generally never undergo chest radiography because of a lack of immediate availability and because the survivors, once evacuated down to developed areas, have clinically recovered. Given the lag phase of clearance of pulmonary edema, infiltrates often persist at least 48 hours after clinical resolution.

Echocardiographic Findings

The typical echocardiographic findings, described in research studies of HAPE, are an increase in the right ventricular systolic pressure. The degree of increase is greater among individuals susceptible to HAPE than it is among those who are not susceptible (i.e., have no previous history of pulmonary edema): 58±10 mm Hg, compared with 37 mm Hg (P =.0001) at 4575 m (15,000 feet).[7] In cases of HAPE that

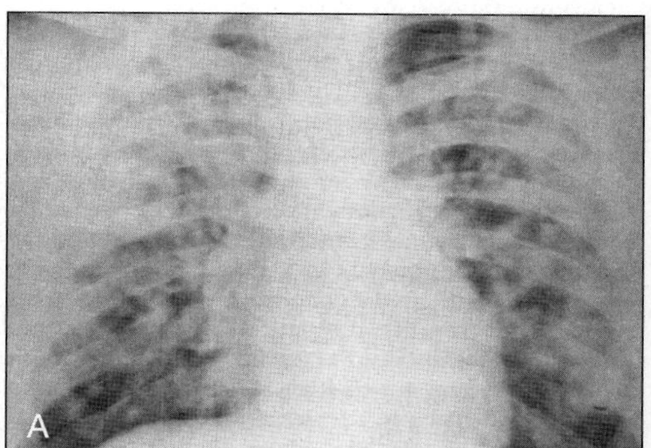

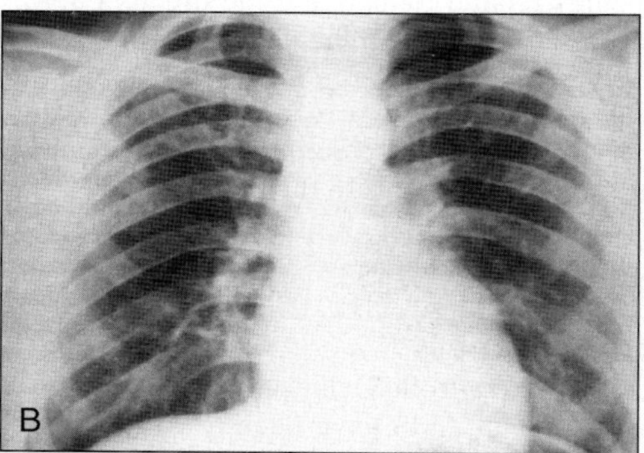

Figure 141.3 Chest radiographs of a young man with high altitude pulmonary edema (HAPE). **A,** The patchy supradiaphragmatic distribution, normal-sized heart, and prominent pulmonary arteries are typical. **B,** Near-complete resolution after 48 hours of supplemental oxygen is typical.

occurred in research studies, right ventricular systolic pressures greater than 100 mm Hg have been described.[39] Patent foramen ovale with right-to-left shunting is observed more frequently in HAPE-susceptible individuals than in those who are HAPE resistant.

Predictive Testing

No laboratory tests are available that predict with sufficient clinical accuracy those who will develop HAPE. Standard pulmonary function testing that assesses lung volumes and flow rates has no clinical value in this regard. Hypoxic-induced ventilation testing has been proposed as predictive, but clinical data are lacking. For individuals who have previously been to high altitude and remained healthy, the risk of development of HAPE is low. Conversely, in individuals who have previously developed pulmonary edema, the likelihood of developing pulmonary edema again is considerable; specifically, there is a 60% recurrence rate in individuals who ascend to the same altitude.

Stress echocardiography appears to offer some ability to differentiate HAPE-susceptible individuals; they appear to be those individuals who develop a right ventricular systolic pressure greater than 45 mm Hg during supine bicycle exercise in normoxic conditions.[8]

Most cases of HAPE develop in a milieu of unrestrained rapid ascent followed promptly by heavy exertion on achieving altitude. The disorder, therefore, can be considered preventable, other than in a small number of individuals who are unusually susceptible to it.

High Altitude Cerebral Edema

The diagnosis of HACE is a clinical one and is based on the following factors:

- the context of recent altitude gain (within 1 week);
- development of a change in mental status or of ataxia in an individual with previous AMS; or
- development of a change in mental status and ataxia in an individual without AMS.

Truncal ataxia is a useful finding, because it is seldom observed in individuals with HAPE.

Other neurologic disorders that may manifest at altitude should be recalled when the diagnosis of HACE is considered. Stroke and transient ischemic attack have been described at altitude. They may be caused by a number of mechanisms, including sympathetic activation and relative polycythemia. Seizures related to high altitude (hypoxic seizures) have been described in individuals both with and without a previously recognized seizure disorder. Subarachnoid hemorrhage at altitude has occurred and may have an increased incidence at high altitude. Some individuals with HACE have focal findings that confuse the diagnosis.

MANAGEMENT

Acute Mountain Sickness

Appropriately sized and controlled clinical studies on the prevention and treatment of AMS have been few. The best prevention is graded, or progressive, ascent to altitude,[40] with a rate on average of less than 305 m (1000 feet) per day above 2440 m (8000 feet). Staged intervals of rest, maintaining the same approximate overall rate of ascent, may be helpful and often is more practical.

For individuals who are mildly or moderately symptomatic, descent of 500 to 1000 m (1640 to 3280 feet) or supplemental oxygen, if available, is the treatment of choice. Most of these individuals experience complete improvement. Further ascent can be entertained after improvement, but with caution. Severely symptomatic individuals improve with supplemental oxygen, if available, and with descent of 1000 m (3280 feet).

Both acetazolamide and dexamethasone are used to prevent symptoms of AMS. However, the clinical evidence for use of these drugs is scant; there is no proven basis that either prevents the development of life-threatening forms of altitude-related disease. Acetazolamide, 250 mg given every 12 hours by mouth, reduces symptoms of AMS when given prophylactically or for established AMS.[31] Unwanted side effects include diuretic effects, tingling of the fingers or toes, myopia (dose dependent), and hypersensitivity. A dose of 125 mg given every 12 hours by mouth is less likely to produce finger and toe tingling and probably is as effective.

Dexamethasone, 4 mg given orally every 6 hours, has been shown to reduce the symptoms of AMS both prophylactically[41] and for established symptoms.[42] The prophylactic effect appears greater. However, the use of dexamethasone is controversial. Clinical evidence of its efficacy is scant, whereas evidence exists that it is simply an antinausea and mood-enhancing drug. Dexamethasone is not recommended for routine use to prevent or treat AMS because of its side effects. In fact, its use is discouraged.

Dexamethasone and acetazolamide may reduce the symptoms of AMS but in so doing may potentially mask failure to acclimatize and continuing susceptibility to more serious forms of altitude illness. Furthermore, the actual benefit of these medications is widely overestimated by both physicians and patients. Neither medication should be used as a substitute for graded or staged acclimatization. Too commonly, and out of convenience, the drugs are taken in lieu of a graded acclimatization.

High Altitude Pulmonary Edema

It must be emphasized that prevention is the principal desired strategy for HAPE. Most individuals do very well, particularly when the disease occurs in developed areas; however, cases that occur in remote settings, particularly those in remote settings at high or extreme altitude, may easily be fatal. It also is important to recall that fulminant and fatal cases of HAPE have occurred at altitudes below 3050 m (10,000 feet).

All patients should be treated with rest if they are not in descent, because exertion increases cardiac output and thus pulmonary artery pressures.

The definitive treatment for HAPE, whether mild or severe, is prompt descent of more than 1000 vertical meters (3280 feet); this is effective in terminating the disorder in most individuals. Supplemental oxygen is useful to increase O_2 saturation, and leads to symptomatic and objective improvement; it is the definitive treatment in most cases of mild to moderate HAPE.[43] It can reduce pulmonary artery pressures by up to 50%.

A review of 166 cases of HAPE demonstrated the clinical impact of descent and supplemental oxygen: when descent was impossible and oxygen unavailable, the mortality of HAPE was 44%; with descent and supplemental oxygen, the overall mortality was 11%.[44] Patients who do not improve with descent likely are suffering from complicated forms of

HAPE, such as pulmonary arterial thrombosis, or have a concurrent or alternative diagnosis, such as pneumonia.

Portable hyperbaric chambers (Gamov bags) are widely available and have the advantage over oxygen cylinders of being more portable, renewable, and safer to airdrop. The additional 13.8 kPa (2 psi) of pressure confers equivalence to a descent of 1500 m (4918 feet) if applied at 4575 m (15,000 feet), and a greater equivalence of descent at higher altitudes (2000 m [6557 feet]) when applied at 6100 m (20,000 feet). It is important to note that supplemental oxygen cannot be administered to an individual on the inside of a Gamov bag because of the fear that static electricity may initiate a spark.

Sartori and coworkers[28] recently demonstrated that prophylactic administration of salmeterol reduced the incidence of HAPE by more than 50% in susceptible individuals and improved arterial saturation, the AMS score, and the radiographic score. Given the acceptable safety profile of salmeterol, its use to prevent HAPE in susceptible individuals should be considered. Corroborative studies of this therapy are eagerly awaited.

Acetazolamide, regularly used to ward off the morning headaches of uncomplicated AMS, has not been shown to reduce the incidence of HAPE. The use of diuretics is controversial and even illogical, because elevated filling pressure on the left side of the heart is not the dominant cause of the edema, and no proven evidence supports the benefit of diuretics. Indeed, many cases of HAPE are associated with moderate or severe hypotension as a result of volume depletion; such hypotensive cases of HAPE should not be treated with diuretics. Similarly, the use of morphine sulfate to reduce preload is illogical, and its use in remote settings is justly controversial because narcotic-induced hypoventilation or apnea may ensue without the availability of resuscitative equipment.

Nifedipine, and similarly tadalafil, have been shown in small trials to reduce the incidence of HAPE in susceptible individuals (those with a history of HAPE).[45] The benefit observed in these small trials of select individuals supports the concept of pulmonary vasoconstriction as a participant in the development of HAPE. A single study has shown that dexamethasone reduces the incidence of HAPE,[45] potentially by stabilizing endothelial function against inflammation.

Nifedipine, inhaled nitric oxide, and tadalafil have been shown to afford acute improvement in the clinical profile of HAPE. Nifedipine has been reported to reduce pulmonary artery pressures by 25% to 55%, improve arterial saturation, reduce the alveolar-arterial pressure gradient, improve the radiographic score, and improve symptoms.[39] Similar findings have been observed with tadalafil, another pulmonary vasodilator.[45] Inhaled nitric oxide reduces the pulmonary artery pressure and improves O_2 saturation in individuals with HAPE. Nitric oxide (40 ppm) has been shown to reduce pulmonary artery pressure by an average of 25 mm Hg.[6] However, the combination of supplemental oxygen and nitric oxide is more effective than either alone in reducing pulmonary artery resistance. Compared with the values in ambient air, pulmonary resistance decreased by 23% with supplemental oxygen, by 36% with nitric oxide (15 ppm), and by 54% with nitric oxide plus oxygen (1:1). Similarly, the combination of supplemental oxygen and nitric oxide was superior in reducing the alveolar to arterial oxygen difference and increasing saturation.

Bosentan (a nonselective endothelin receptor antagonist) has been shown in healthy individuals to reduce the increase in pulmonary artery pressures incurred with altitude ascent, but it has not yet been studied in a preventive or therapeutic role for HAPE. Bosentan was associated with reduced urinary volume and free water clearance.[9]

Most patients who survive experience complete recovery.

High Altitude Cerebral Edema

As with HAPE, the principal treatment for HACE should be prevention of the disorder. Individuals who develop HACE may be difficult to evacuate because of the neurologic compromise. No definitive medical interventions are available for HACE. Acetazolamide, dexamethasone, and nifedipine have not been shown to prevent HACE. Diuretics (acetazolamide and furosemide), nifedipine, mannitol, and dexamethasone have been found to improve cases of HACE.

Administration of supplemental oxygen, if available, and descent of more than 1000 m (3280 feet), if possible, are the best therapeutic options. As with HAPE, most cases improve, if not normalize, with this strategy.

Like supplemental oxygen, the portable hyperbaric chamber (Gamov bag) may improve temporarily the symptomatology and findings of HACE, but it is not considered definitive treatment for the disorder. Its contribution may be to stabilize the patient while evacuation is planned.

Other Clinical Manifestations

Edema

Peripheral edema is common in individuals who have ascended rapidly to altitude. The edema generally is mild, but approximately 10% of individuals gain 4.54 kg (10 pounds) of edema. Edema occurs during the preacclimatized period and is generalized to the legs, hands, and face. Upon acclimatization, the edematous state subsides, often with conspicuous diuresis. The pathophysiologic basis is incompletely understood but may involve atrial natriuretic peptides. Edema of the hands but not of the legs is a spurious finding and is not attributable to a lack of acclimatization or to a cardiovascular abnormality; rather, it generally is the result of backpack straps that are too tight and compress the subclavian veins. Few individuals who develop edema go on to develop a life-threatening form of altitude-related disease, such as pulmonary edema or cerebral edema.

Coronary Artery Disease

Until a decade or so ago, only a few individuals with recognized coronary artery disease (CAD) ascended to altitude. The great explosion in the number of people who ascend to altitude means that many individuals with coronary disease, both recognized and unrecognized, now make such ascents. In addition, up to 60% of individuals who ascend to altitude are older than 60 years.

The augmented sympathetic output engendered by altitude-related hypoxia increases both the heart rate and blood pressure in patients with CAD, thereby increasing the incidence of angina, particularly during the first several days at altitude but lasting for a week.

Twenty veterans of the U.S. 10th Mountain Division (mean age, 68 years), most of whom had known CAD or were at high risk of CAD, underwent cardiopulmonary testing at low altitude (Dallas, Texas) and at an altitude of 2440 m (8000 feet) (Vail, Colorado).[46] Predictably, the threshold to ischemia in the presence of the ambient hypoxia of moderate altitude was lower, and plasma catecholamines were increased at altitude.

Pulmonary artery pressure increased by more than 40%, and maximal oxygen consumption ($\dot{V}O_2max$) decreased by 12% acutely but normalized after 5 days of acclimatization. Unpredictably, a patient who had a stable anginal syndrome at low altitude experienced a myocardial infarction on exertion during the study at moderate altitude. Although these findings constitute a small body of data, they underscore the unpredictability of coronary disease in the ambient milieu of hypobaric hypoxia and an increased sympathetic activation at altitude. Ascent to altitude by those with a low threshold to ischemia at low altitude appears unwise.

Altitude-related myocardial infarction has been described in an individual without apparent atherosclerosis. A notable case occurred in a 28-year-old elite athlete who experienced a prodrome of angina on effort at high altitude[47] and then an acute ST-segment-elevation inferior wall infarction. Subsequent coronary angiography was normal, and thus the mechanism of altitude-related infarction remains unclear. In susceptible younger individuals, it may involve hyperventilation-induced spasm of the coronary arteries, whereas in older individuals with CAD, the mechanism may be sympathetic activation–mediated infarction.

For individuals with recognized CAD who intend to ascend to altitude, several general recommendations can be made[48]:

- a moderate or better functional capacity;
- a more gradual and graded ascent than usual;
- tight control of blood pressure;
- avoidance of exertion while at altitude, especially for the first several days;
- availability of or access to medical facilities (i.e., supplemental oxygen); and
- ability of the patient to check the blood pressure and heart rate.

Such considerations may reduce the incidence of ischemia but may not alter the incidence of infarction. For individuals with recognized CAD who recently have experienced unstable coronary syndromes or who have a low threshold to ischemia, ascent to or beyond moderate altitude is relatively contraindicated.

Roach and colleagues[49] observed that an older group of patients (59 to 83 years), most of whom had a history of CAD or hypertension, acclimatized generally well to an altitude of 2440 m (8000 feet) over 5 days, with a lower incidence of AMS than in younger individuals and without significant problems. However, the complex considerations that may surround older patients with respiratory distress at altitude were highlighted by Basnyat and associates,[50] who reported a case of myocardial infarction in a previously well, 60-year-old man who developed pulmonary edema caused by myocardial infarction and not by HAPE.

Hypertension

Many individuals experience an increase in blood pressure when ascending to altitude. The mechanism for this is not well understood, but it generally is held to pertain to the sympathetic activation that occurs with exposure to hypoxic conditions. Many individuals with hypertension expose themselves to altitude during recreational pursuits such as skiing and hiking. Such individuals, even those receiving antihypertensive treatment, are more likely to have uncontrolled hypertension on exposure to altitude. Because it generally is held that hypertension is recognized in only 50% of individuals who have it and only 50% of those with recognized hypertension have it well controlled, it is not surprising that many cases of hypertension are recognized for the first time or are exacerbated at altitude. It seems prudent to ensure that the blood pressure is well controlled before an individual ascends to altitude and to advise individuals with uncontrolled hypertension not to attempt such ascents.

Permanent Tissue Damage from Altitude and Frostbite

Most altitude-related illness is acute and without residua in survivors. However, some evidence indicates that lasting tissue damage occurs. "Everest nails"[51] (Fig. 141.4) and lingering subtle and pervasive neurologic deficits afflict those who travel to extreme altitude.[2]

Previous frostbite injury is a strong risk factor for repeat frostbite. Previously affected extremities are often bothersomely cold. Vascular function in previously frostbitten territory is abnormal, which may underlie the greatly impaired resistance to repeat injury.

Subacute and Chronic Altitude Illness

Principally seen in the Andes, chronic altitude illness is a rare form of altitude illness that arises in a few individuals who live in the sparse permanent settlements at altitudes above 3050 m (10,000 feet). Bolivia has the largest number of extremely high permanent settlements, and these are among the best studied populations with true chronic (versus subacute) high altitude disorders.[52] Cyanosis and right-sided heart failure as a result of pulmonary hypertension and polycythemia cause fatigue and dyspnea. The findings and complaints resolve with descent. The maximum altitude at which pregnancy can reliably be carried to term determines the maximum elevation of permanent habitation, and the stress of altitude-related hypoxia has been well characterized in infants (dyspnea, cyanosis, and edema).[53] Indian soldiers, rotated through outposts at moderate to high altitudes, have been observed to develop dyspnea, cough, and peripheral edema, consistent with right-sided heart failure incited by hypoxic altitude stress.[54] The bovine disorder "brisket disease," an altitude-dependent edema in cows caused by right ventricular dysfunction, behaves similarly.[55]

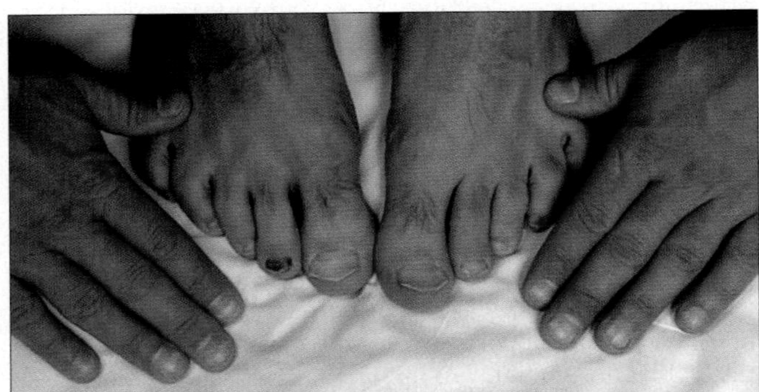

Figure 141.4 "Everest nails" in a 40-year-old man who climbed Cho Oyu (8254 m [27,063 feet]) in the Everest region. White bands are seen on all nail beds; the bands' width and distance from the base plate are proportional to the time spent at high altitude and to the time since exposure to high altitude.

chapter 142

Alternative Cardiovascular Medical Therapies

William J. Kostuk

Definition

- Alternative medicine for cardiovascular disease is in high demand by health consumers.
- Popular forms of therapy are chelation therapy, antioxidant vitamin supplementation, and herbal therapies.

Key Features

- The major concern is the lack of any scientific evidence for clinical benefit.
- Randomized trials have shown no beneficial effect of vitamin E in preventing cardiovascular disease.
- A large, randomized trial to assess chelation therapy will complete enrollment in 2009.

Clinical implications

- Currently, these alternative therapies cannot be recommended either to prevent or to treat atherosclerotic disease.

Complementary or alternative medicine is in demand by health consumers throughout the developed world. These therapies, which can be defined as "medical interventions that are not taught widely in Western medical schools or generally available at major hospitals,"[1] have an impact on all medical specialties, including cardiovascular medicine.

The major difference between alternative medicine and conventional medicine is the lack of scientific evaluation. Moreover, the proponents of alternative medicine do not see any need for such evaluation and rely instead on the testimonials and anecdotes of patients. These therapies are widely available to the general public through all means of communication, including the Internet, which is becoming a popular and primary source of information for many people. Given that people in the United States spend approximately $21 billion on these therapies each year, there must be reasons patients seek out and use such remedies, either in addition to or instead of conventional medicine.

Chelation therapy, high-dose vitamins, and herbal therapies are among the myriad alternative measures that are being popularized for the treatment of cardiovascular disorders.[2]

REASONS PATIENTS SEEK ALTERNATIVE THERAPIES

During the past decade, a general shift has occurred toward nonconventional or alternative approaches to health care in many disease processes. Some think that these alternative approaches are safer and better than so-called Western medicine. However, despite the great popularity of various supplements, general agreement on their benefits is lacking. Myths and false information abound both in print and on the Internet.

In the United States, more visits are made to alternative practitioners than to primary care physicians.[1] In Europe and Australia, up to 50% of the population uses alternative therapies.[3,4] Most patients do not tell their physicians that they are consulting alternative medical practitioners. If the scientific message is, "Alternative therapies do not work," why do so many people, physicians included, use them? The diverse reasons patients seek alternative therapies are summarized in Table 142.1.[5]

CHELATION THERAPY

The term *chelate,* coined by the analytic chemist G. T. Morgan in 1920, has its origin in the Greek *chele* (meaning claw), which refers to the claw-like chemical structure of the compound. In chelation, a metallic ion is firmly bound into a ring within the chelating molecule.

The use of natural chelators has a long history in medicine. In 1917, sodium tartrate was used in the treatment of antimony poisoning; in 1938, fruit juices were prescribed for nickel-induced eczema, primarily because of the citrate and tartrate in the fruit juices.

Synthetic chelators are abundant and serve as analytic and research tools in chemistry. Chelation therapy was applied to humans during the World War II, when the chelating agent dimercaprol (also known as British antilewisite or BAL) was developed and used to treat arsenic poisoning caused by the war gas lewisite. In 1938, ethylenediamine tetraacetic acid (EDTA) was developed and used by chemists. EDTA is a water-soluble chemical that forms soluble complexes with bivalent and trivalent cations such as calcium, magnesium, iron, mercury, copper, aluminum, copper and nickel, cobalt, zinc, cadmium, and magnesium. In the late 1940s, EDTA was used to treat industrial workers with lead poisoning. When injected into the blood, EDTA binds the heavy metal, which subsequently is excreted in the urine; this has remained the treatment of choice for lead poisoning.[6] EDTA also was investigated for use in the treatment of hypercalcemia and radiation poisoning caused by plutonium. In the 1960s, it was used in the treatment of digitalis toxicity, until it was supplanted by digitalis-specific antibodies.

REASONS PATIENTS EXPLORE ALTERNATIVE THERAPIES
■ The patient wants to promote good health and prevent disease.
■ Conventional therapies have been exhausted.
■ Conventional therapy is ineffective or risky.
■ No conventional therapy is available.
■ Conventional therapy is perceived to be emotionally or spiritually without benefit.

Table 142.1 Reasons patients explore alternative therapies.

Rationale for Use in Cardiovascular Disease

After EDTA was found to be effective in chelating and removing toxic metals from the blood, some investigators in the early 1950s postulated that atherosclerotic vessels could be "softened" if the calcium in the walls was removed.[7] During the past four decades, numerous theoretical mechanisms have evolved to justify the use of EDTA chelation in patients with atherosclerotic disease. These include[8]

- the simple removal of calcium from the atherosclerotic lesions;
- an effect on endothelial enzymatic function, such that the availability of calcium or some other metallic ion is altered;
- an anticoagulant effect, resulting from a decrease in platelet stickiness;
- improved arterial elasticity, resulting from a reduction in metallic cross-linkages in arterial walls;
- vasodilatory effects, resulting from calcium channel blocker–like activity; and
- prevention of free radical production and thus lipid peroxidation.

None of these proposed mechanisms has been validated.

Procedure for Chelation Therapy

The American College of Advancement in Medicine (ACAM) was founded in 1973 for the study of complementary and alternative medical therapies. A major focus of ACAM is the promotion of chelation therapy.

ACAM's procedure for chelation therapy calls for intravenous infusion of approximately 500 mL of a solution that contains the ingredients listed in Table 142.2.[9] The solution is infused slowly over 3 to 4 hours one to three times a week. Renal function is checked before each infusion. In addition to the infusions, patients are prescribed supplemental nutrients (vitamins and minerals) and lifestyle modification, including stress reduction, avoidance of caffeine, limitation of alcohol intake, cessation of smoking, exercise, and nutritional counseling. The number of treatments required for patients with symptomatic disease ranges from 20 to 50 separate infusions, depending on the patient's health status; the average number required for "optimal benefit" is 30 treatments. Some patients eventually receive more than 100 chelation infusions over several years. The protocol states that "full benefit does not normally occur for up to 3 months after a series is completed" and that "follow-up treatments may be given once or twice monthly for long-term maintenance, to sustain improvement, and to prevent recurrence of symptoms." The cost is $80 to $125 per treatment.

CHELATION INFUSION MIXTURE	
■ Sterile water	440 mL
■ EDTA (150 mg/mL)	50 mg/kg lean body weight
■ Sodium bicarbonate	(50 mmol per 50 mL)
■ Vitamin C	3.0 g
■ Magnesium sulfate	500 mg/mL
■ Heparin	2500 U
■ Folic acid	2.5 mg
■ Pyridoxine (vitamin B_6)	100 mg
■ Hydroxycobalamin (vitamin B_{12})	1000 U
■ B-complex-100	1 mg
■ Lidocaine (2%)	200 mg

EDTA, ethylenediamine tetra-acetic acid.

Table 142.2 Chelation infusion mixture.

Purported Indications

Chelation therapy is promoted and practiced throughout the world as an alternative form of medical therapy for the treatment of atherosclerotic disease. Unfortunately, the claims for the efficacy of chelation therapy for atherosclerotic vascular disease have been based on uncontrolled studies. These studies have involved small numbers of participants, the diagnostic and evaluation criteria were largely subjective, and controls were not used. The effects of other medications were not given, and follow-up periods were short. Most of these reports have been confined to the holistic literature. The proponents of chelation therapy state that "more than 75% of chelation patients have improved dramatically."[10] However, this statement is based on personal testimonials and not on scientific evidence. Until recently, no randomized, placebo-controlled, double-blind trials of chelation therapy had been conducted that might provide any support for this statement.

The possibility that EDTA could be used as a treatment for atherosclerotic disease was suggested by Clarke and colleagues[7] in 1955. These investigators studied the effect of EDTA on serum calcium in patients. A patient with bilateral nephrocalcinosis showed radiographic improvement in kidney stones, which implied direct evidence of removal of metastatic calcium. The authors speculated on the possible inter-relationship of calcium and atherosclerotic plaque.[7] They subsequently reported that anginal symptoms improved in 19 of 20 patients with coronary and peripheral arterial disease.[11]

Kitchell and colleagues[12] initially reported subjective improvement of anginal symptoms in nine of 10 patients. A subsequent follow-up study of 28 patients who received EDTA for treatment of angina showed that after 18 months, seven (25%) were dead; the condition of two (7%) was worse; the condition of six (21%) was unchanged; and the condition of the remaining 13 (46%) had improved. The authors concluded that "chelation as used in this study did not benefit patients more than commonly used therapeutic methods. It is not a useful clinical tool in the treatment of coronary artery disease at the present time."[12]

No reports appeared in the medical literature of EDTA chelation therapy regarding cardiovascular disease until 2002, when Knudtson and others[13] reported a double-blind, randomized, placebo-controlled study conducted from January 1996 to January 2000. In this study, 84 individuals with documented disease (coronary angiography and/or a myocardial infarction with stable angina and evidence of ischemia on treadmill testing) received an infusion of weight-adjusted (40 mg/kg) EDTA (n = 41) or a placebo (n = 43). Infusions were given over 3 hours twice weekly for 15 weeks and then monthly for an additional 3 months, a total of 33 treatments. Patients in both groups took multivitamins in accordance with the ACAM protocol. The primary endpoint in this study was the change in time to ischemia (1 mm of ST-segment depression) at the 27-week evaluation. Thirty-nine patients in each group completed the procedure; one patient in the EDTA group was withdrawn because of an increase in serum creatinine. At 27 weeks, exercise time to ischemia improved significantly in both groups (by 54 and 63 seconds in the placebo and EDTA groups, respectively), but no significant difference was seen between the times to ischemia in the two groups. Exercise capacity and quality of life scores improved in a similar fashion in both groups. The improvement is related not only to the placebo and training effects commonly seen in studies of patients with angina, but also to the optimal risk reduction therapy in both groups. The authors concluded that "the use of chelation therapy to increase ischemic threshold and improve quality of life cannot be supported for patients with ischemic heart disease." They also stated that larger trials with a broader range of patients would be required to assess the impact of EDTA therapy.

The National Institutes of Health currently is supporting a large, randomized trial of chelation therapy to assess clinical outcomes in individuals with coronary artery disease. This study, Trial to Assess Chelation Therapy (TACT), is supported jointly by the National Center for Complementary and Alternative Medicine and the National Heart, Lung and Blood Institute. TACT commenced enrollment in September 2003, and completion is expected by July 2009. The planned enrollment is 1950 patients age 50 years or older who had had a heart attack at least 6 weeks earlier. Centers across the United States and Canada are involved. This study is large enough to determine whether chelation therapy has any benefit (Table 142.3) More information about the study is available at *www.clinicaltrials.gov/ct/show/NCT00044213or*.

TRIAL TO ASSESS CHELATION THERAPY (TACT)

1. To enroll 1950 patients (nonsmokers > 3 months) > 50 years with previous myocardial infarction > 6 weeks
2. Randomized (factorial 2 × 2) to:
   - Chelation therapy or placebo
   - High-dose vitamin supplements or placebo
3. Infusions:
   - Weekly × 30
   - Bimonthly × 10
4. Average follow-up 3.5 years
5. Primary endpoint composite of:
   - Major vascular events:
     - Myocardial infarction
     - Stroke
     - Admission to hospital for angina
     - Coronary revascularization
   - Death

Table 142.3 Trial to Assess Chelation Therapy (TACT).

The evidence from randomized, placebo-controlled, double-blind trials for EDTA treatment for patients with peripheral vascular disease has been reviewed.[14] Studies were identified using computerized literature searches (MEDLINE 1966-1996; CISCOM 1996, a database specializing in complementary/alternative medicine; bibliographies of relevant papers) and suggestions from six leading experts and national societies. Studies were selected if they were randomized, placebo-controlled, double-blind trials of intravenous chelation therapy for peripheral arterial occlusive disease. Outcomes included walking distances, ankle and arm blood pressures, transcutaneous oxygen tension, and the results of angiography. Four papers reported on three trials that involved patients with intermittent claudication. None of the studies found between-group differences for patients receiving chelation therapy and those receiving placebo.

A small trial of 10 men reported no between-group differences in walking distance or ankle and arm blood pressures for patients who received 10 intravenous injections of EDTA (totaling 1.5 g), compared with patients who received placebo. Nevertheless, the authors concluded that "EDTA had a significant impact in causing the improvements seen in the patient's clinical status."[15]

A trial of 153 patients allocated to 20 treatments of either disodium EDTA (3 g) or isotonic saline over 5 to 9 weeks found no between-group differences in the outcome parameters (walking distance, ankle/brachial index, or subjective evaluation) at the end of treatment or after 6 months.[16] A subgroup of 30 patients from this trial underwent digital angiography before and after treatment. Most of the angiograms were unchanged; only two were improved, one in the placebo group and one in the treatment group.[17]

A study of 32 patients allocated to 20 infusions of EDTA (n = 15) or saline (n = 17) over 10 weeks likewise found no difference for walking distances or ankle and arm blood pressures at the 3-month follow-up. The proportion of patients who improved was similar in each group (60% for the EDTA group versus 59% for the saline group).[18]

Compared with this paucity of controlled clinical trials for chelation therapy, case report series are abundant. A retrospective review of 2870 patients treated with EDTA showed "marked improvement" in 76.9%; "good improvement" occurred in 17% of treated patients with ischemic heart disease. In treated patients with peripheral vascular disease and intermittent claudication, marked improvement occurred in 91% and good improvement in 8%.[19] There was no comparison group.

The claims of improvement for chelation therapy are not limited to the treatment or prevention of atherosclerosis. Proponents claim that chelation is effective against arthritis, multiple sclerosis, psoriasis, Alzheimer's disease, and problems with vision, hearing, smell, and sexual potency.[10] None of these claimed benefits has ever been demonstrated.

Because no evidence showing that treatment has modified the disease process is available, the "benefits" described clearly are the result of other factors. These include not only a placebo effect, but also the compassionate care given to the patient's problems and the encouragement given to them to cope with their symptoms and to changes in lifestyle. These lifestyle and diet changes (i.e., smoking cessation, regular exercise, proper diet, and weight loss) are extremely valuable for improving the quality of life and the patient's sense of well-being.

Complications

EDTA is not a benign drug, and it has been associated with serious adverse effects. These are most likely to occur if EDTA is infused either too rapidly or in too large a dose. In such instances, profound hypocalcemia and nephrotoxicity with renal failure have occurred. Other adverse effects are minor discomfort at the injection site, vasculitis, hypotension, hypoglycemia, and prolongation of the prothrombin time.

Perhaps the most serious adverse effect, and the one of greatest concern, is that chelation therapy, which is unproven, may prevent patients from receiving the benefits of effective methods of treatment, or at least delay them. Also, the repeated and prolonged course of chelation therapy leads to needless expense.

Conclusions

Without scientific evidence to support either the efficacy or safety of chelation therapy in treating atherosclerosis, its use is discouraged. Absolutely no proof indicates that this therapy either relieves symptoms or alters the atherosclerotic process. Important toxicity may include hypocalcemia, renal injury, and thrombophlebitis. At worst, there is a significant risk to patients in believing chelation therapy to be an accepted treatment for vascular disease and thus perhaps depriving themselves of the well-established benefits of recognized modes of therapy, including lifestyle modification, medications, and surgical procedures.

In 1998, ACAM agreed to settle charges by the U.S. Federal Trade Commission (FTC) that it made unsubstantiated and false advertising claims that chelation therapy is effective in treating atherosclerosis or any other circulatory disorder.

ANTIOXIDANT VITAMINS

The link between increased total cholesterol and atherosclerosis is well established. The oxidation of low-density lipoprotein (LDL) cholesterol, particularly by macrophages, is thought to play a significant role in the formation of atherosclerotic plaques. Oxidized LDL-cholesterol also is thought to play a part in the precipitation of clinical events such as plaque rupture and thrombosis. This has stimulated interest in the role of antioxidants that may prevent or retard the process. The major lipid-soluble antioxidant vitamins are vitamin E (alpha-tocopherol) and beta-carotene, a precursor of vitamin A. The major water-soluble antioxidant vitamin is vitamin C.

Indications

Evidence for the antioxidant vitamin–cardiovascular disease hypothesis has accumulated from several lines of research. Laboratory research has identified biochemical properties of the antioxidant vitamins that could explain their possible role in inhibiting and delaying coronary atherosclerosis.[20] Supplemental concentrations of vitamin E inhibit platelet function.[21] In addition, endothelial-dependent vasodilatation, although improved with cholesterol reduction, is further enhanced when antioxidant therapy (probucol) is added to an agent that lowers LDL-cholesterol.[22] Also, antioxidants may modify smooth muscle proliferation.[23]

Observational Studies

Epidemiologic studies have provided support for the antioxidant vitamin–cardiovascular disease hypothesis by showing that individuals who consume large amounts of antioxidant vitamins through diet or supplements, or those with high concentrations of these nutrients in their blood, have reduced morbidity and mortality from coronary artery disease.

Descriptive studies that examine the characteristics of a population and its associated disease rates have shown an inverse relationship between consumption of fresh fruit and vegetables and rates of cardiovascular disease.[24] Case-control studies support an association between lower plasma concentrations of vitamin E in individuals with angina compared with controls,[25] which suggests that this antioxidant might reduce the risk of cardiovascular disease.

In the past decade, large prospective cohort studies, such as the Nurses Health Study[26] and the Health Professionals Study,[27] showed a 31% to 40% risk reduction for nonfatal myocardial infarction and death from cardiovascular disease among individuals whose vitamin E intake was in the upper quintile during follow-up for 4 to 8 years. This benefit was greatest in those who took vitamin E supplements (more than 100 IU/day) for at least 2 years. In these same studies, a high intake of vitamin C or beta-carotene was not associated with a lower risk of coronary artery disease. A smaller prospective cohort study in Finland, which involved a follow-up for a mean of 14 years, showed a significant reduction in cardiovascular death only in women who were in the highest tertile of vitamin E intake (Table 142.4).[28]

Muntwyler and coworkers[29] obtained data on the use of vitamin E, vitamin C, and multivitamin supplements by means of a self-administered questionnaire given to the 83,693 male physicians participating in the Physicians Health Study in the United States. They found that 29% of the men (24,270) were current users of one or more of these supplements, most commonly a multivitamin (in 24.6% of the cohort). During a mean follow-up of 5.5 years (and after adjusting for several cardiovascular risk factors, including hypertension, hypercholesterolemia, current and past smoking, alcohol intake, physical activity, and body mass index), Muntwyler's researchers found that the use of supplements was not associated with any decrease in total cardiovascular or coronary heart disease mortality.[29]

In a study of 34,486 postmenopausal women with no cardiovascular disease who were followed for 7 years, Kushi and colleagues[30] observed that vitamin E supplementation did not provide any benefit in reducing death from coronary disease. However, they did observe an inverse association of vitamin E intake from food and coronary deaths. The women in the highest quintile of vitamin E intake from food had less than half the risk of women in the lowest quintile (relative risk [RR], 0.42 versus 1.0). The reason for the lack of association with supplementation is not clear.[30] It is important

CARDIOVASCULAR ENDPOINTS AND VITAMIN E TREATMENT

Study	n	Risk Reduction	95% CI
Observation Studies			
Nurses Health Study[26]	87,245	0.66	0.50-0.87
Health Professionals[27]	39,910	0.63	0.47-0.84
Finland men[28]	2748	0.42	0.66-1.11
Finland women[28]	2348	0.14	0.35-0.88
Postmenopausal women[30]	34,486	0.96	0.82-1.51
Randomized Trials			
ATBC[31]	29,133	0.96	0.9-1.03
CHAOS[33]	2002	0.60	0.40-0.89
GISSI[39]	11,324	0.98	0.87-1.10
HOPE[38]	9541	1.04	0.94-1.15
HPS[40,41]	20,536	1.00	0.94-1.06
Su.Vi.Max[37]	13,017	0.97	0.77-1.20
WACS[42]	8171	0.94	0.85-1.04

CI, confidence interval; ATBC, alpha-tocopherol, beta-carotene.

Table 142.4 Cardiovascular endpoints and vitamin E treatment.

to emphasize that observational studies do not prove cause and effect; that is, they are unable to exclude the possibility that individuals who consume antioxidant-rich diets or who take vitamin supplements also share important lifestyle or dietary practices that actually account for their lower disease rates. Because of these uncertainties, the only definitive way to determine whether antioxidants have any part to play in reducing cardiovascular risk is through large-scale, randomized clinical trials.

Randomized Trials

The large-scale, randomized trials of antioxidants have shown mixed results in terms of reduction in cardiovascular events (see Table 142.4). Several of these trials were designed specifically to address outcome from cancer and not from cardiovascular disease. In the Alpha-Tocopherol, Beta-Carotene Cancer Prevention Study (ATBC), middle-aged Finnish smokers were treated daily with beta-carotene, vitamin E, both, or neither for 5 to 8 years. Neither vitamin E nor beta-carotene provided any benefit for mortality from cardiovascular disease. However, in this trial, the dose of vitamin E (50 mg) was below the protective range suggested by the epidemiologic studies.[31] Also in this study, no beneficial effect was seen from supplemental vitamin E or beta-carotene in the male smokers who had had a previous myocardial infarction upon entry. In fact, more deaths occurred in the beta-carotene and vitamin E groups.[32] Among 22,000 physicians, no difference was seen in cardiovascular death rates between those who took beta-carotene and those who did not.[33]

In the Cambridge Heart Antioxidants Study (CHAOS), patients with angiographically documented coronary artery disease were randomly allocated to groups to receive daily treatment with vitamin E (400 to 800 IU) or placebo. During the median follow-up of 510 days, a 77% reduction in nonfatal myocardial infarction (14% compared with 41%) was seen in the group receiving vitamin E. However, a nonsignificant, slight excess of cardiovascular deaths was noted in the vitamin E group (27 compared with 23 in the placebo group).[34]

In a double-blind, primary prevention trial, smokers, former smokers, and workers exposed to asbestos were randomly allocated to receive daily beta-carotene (30 mg) and vitamin A (25,000 IU) or placebo. After an average of 4 years of supplementation, the combination of beta-carotene and vitamin A showed no protective benefit and may have had an adverse effect on the incidence of lung cancer and cardiovascular death; this led to premature termination of the study.[35]

The results of a small, randomized, double-blind, placebo-controlled trial of probucol, beta-carotene, and vitamins C and E are of interest. Probucol, a lipid-soluble, cholesterol-lowering drug with potent antioxidant properties, was administered alone or together with the vitamins in patients undergoing coronary angioplasty. Therapy was commenced 4 weeks before angioplasty and continued for 6 months after it. Follow-up angiograms showed a smaller reduction in luminal diameter in the patients who had received probucol; no significant difference was seen in those who did or did not receive vitamins. Moreover, the rates of repeat angioplasty were lowest (at 11%) in the probucol group, compared with 16% in the combined treatment group, 24% in the multivitamin group, and 27% in the placebo group.[23]

Several large-scale, randomized trials are in progress or have recently been completed. The Women's Health Study (WHS), which examines primary prevention of coronary artery disease, involves more than 40,000 healthy postmenopausal nurses.[36] In this randomized, double-blind, placebo-controlled trial using a 2 × 2 factorial design, women age 45 or older received vitamin E (600 IU every other day), or placebo and aspirin (100 mg every other day), or placebo. Randomization, which began in February 1993 and ended in January 1996, was stratified on 5-year age groups. The primary endpoint is the reduction of vascular events and a decrease in the incidence of total malignant neoplasms of epithelial cell origin. The study has been extended through March 2009. Additional observational follow-up is available at *http://clinicaltrials.gov/ct/show/NCT00000479.*

The Supplementation en Vitamines et Mineraux Antioxydants study, which commenced in 1994, involved 13,017 men and women age 35 to 60. The participants were randomly allocated to a single capsule of a combination of vitamin C, vitamin E, beta-carotene, and minerals (selenium and zinc) or a placebo. After a median follow-up of 7.5 years, no difference was seen between the groups for incidence of ischemic heart disease (2.1% versus 2.1%), cancer (4.1% versus 4.5%), or all-cause mortality (1.2% versus 1.5%). However, the total cancer incidence and all-cause mortality were lower in the men.[37]

The Heart Outcomes Prevention Evaluation (HOPE) enrolled 9541 women and men age 55 or older who were at high risk for cardiovascular events because of cardiovascular disease or diabetes and one other risk factor. In this simple, double-blind, 2 × 2 factorial design trial, patients were randomly assigned to groups to receive the angiotensin-converting enzyme (ACE) inhibitor ramipril (up to

10 mg/day), or vitamin E (400 IU/day), or placebo.[38] The primary endpoint was the combination of cardiovascular death, myocardial infarction, or stroke. The trial (ramipril/placebo arm) was stopped early after 4.5 years by the independent data and safety monitor board when it was determined that individual endpoints clearly were reduced by ramipril (by 13.9%, compared with 17.5% for placebo). In contrast to the excellent results achieved with ramipril, the results from the vitamin E arm of the HOPE study were disappointing. Active vitamin E treatment showed a neutral effect across the range of cardiovascular outcomes (16% for vitamin E compared with 15.4% for placebo) (Fig. 142.1).

In the randomized, open-label Gruppo Italiano per lo Studio della Sopravuivenza nell' Infarto Miocardico Prevenzione study (GISSI) involving 11,324 patients who had recently suffered myocardial infarction, the investigators compared the effects of an n-3 polyunsaturated fatty acid (PUFA; 1 g/day), vitamin E (300 mg/day), both supplements, and no supplements, on the combined primary endpoints of death, nonfatal myocardial infarction, and stroke over 3.5 years. Intention-to-treat analyses were completed by factorial design (two way) and treatment group (four way). Treatment with an n-3 PUFA, but not with vitamin E, significantly reduced the relative risk of the primary endpoint by two-way and four-way analysis (10% and 15%, respectively). By four-way analysis, benefit was attributed to relative decreases in overall mortality and cardiovascular mortality (20% and 30%, respectively). This study, therefore, demonstrated a modest benefit from n-3 PUFAs, but no benefit from vitamin E, for the secondary prevention of cardiovascular events after myocardial infarction.[39]

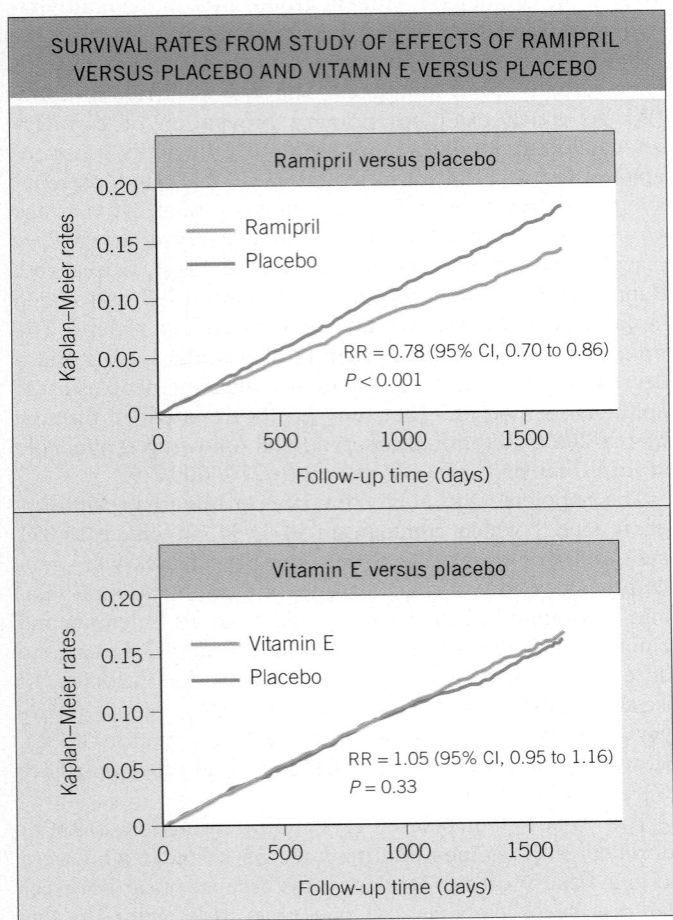

Figure 142.1 Survival rates from study of effects of ramipril versus placebo and vitamin E versus placebo. RR, relative risk; CI, confidence interval.

The landmark Heart Protection Study (HPS) assessed the long-term effects of treatment with statins (hydroxymethyl glutaryl [HMG]-CoA reductase inhibitors) and antioxidant vitamin supplementation in 20,536 individuals age 40 to 80[40,41] who had coronary artery disease (previous myocardial infarction or angina), other occlusive vascular disease, or diabetes, and in men older than age 65 who had hypertension that was being treated. In a factorial 2×2 design, patients were randomly allocated to groups to receive simvastatin (40 mg daily), combination vitamins (600 mg of vitamin E, 250 mg of vitamin C, and 20 mg of beta-carotene), both, or neither. After an average of 5.5 years of follow-up, vitamin supplementation did not reduce the risk of death, myocardial infarction, strokes, or cancer. Participants assigned to simvastatin had significantly lower mortality (12.9%) than those given placebo (14.7%). The coronary death rate was 18% lower with simvastatin (5.7% compared with 6.9%). After the first year, statin treatment provided significant protection against major vascular events (i.e., nonfatal infarctions, stroke, and coronary or noncoronary revascularization), which were 24% lower with simvastatin (19.8% compared with 25.2%) (Fig. 142.2).

The Women's Antioxidant Cardiovascular Study (WACS) assessed the effects of ascorbic acid (500 mg/day), vitamin E (600 IU every other day), and beta carotene (50 mg every other day) on the prevention of cardiovascular events. The study involved 8171 female health professionals age 40 or older who had a history of cardiovascular disease (CVD) or three or more risk factors. Follow-up, for a mean of 9.4 years, lasted from 1995-1996 to 2005. In the study, 1450 women experienced one or more CVD outcomes, but no overall effects of ascorbic acid, vitamin E, or beta carotene were seen on cardiovascular events among women at high risk for CVD.[42]

The Women's Antioxidant and Folic Acid Cardiovascular Study (WAFACS), a randomized trial of the roles of folic acid and B vitamins in the prevention of cardiovascular (CV) events, involved 5442 women age 40 or older who had either preexisting heart disease or at least three major risk factors. This trial was a subset of the larger WACS trial. The participants received folic acid (2.5 mg/day), vitamin B_6 (50 mg/day), vitamin B_{12} (1 mg/day), or placebo. Over the 7.3 years of follow-up, 796 women (14.6%) experienced a CV event; no significant difference was seen between the groups. Furthermore, supplementation was ineffective at preventing CV events in the women with CV disease (AHA Scientific Sessions Nov 2006).

These studies further underscore the importance of randomized controlled trials to test hypotheses generated by experimental and observational data.

A recent study adds further interest to the issue of vitamins and heart disease. In a study of 1739 children of the Framingham Heart Study participants (average age, 59), researchers observed that those with low blood levels of

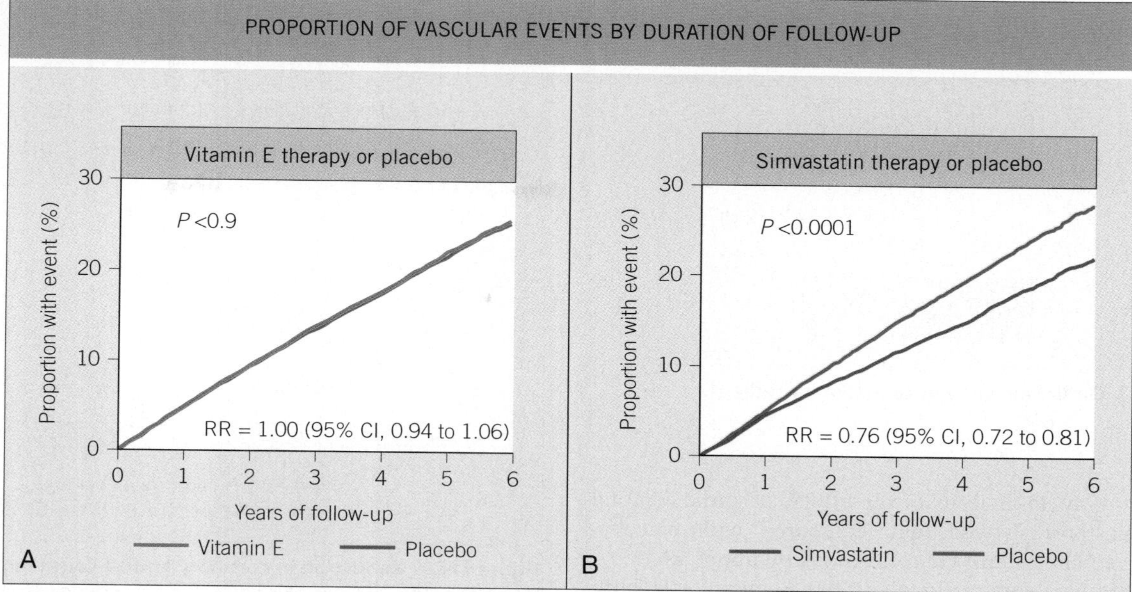

Figure 142.2 Proportion of vascular events by duration of follow-up. A, Individuals allocated to vitamin E therapy or placebo. **B,** Individuals allocated to simvastatin therapy or placebo. RR, relative risk; CI, confidence interval. (Data from Heart Protection Study Collaborative Group. MRC/BHF heart protection study of cholesterol lowering with simvastatin in 20,536 high-risk individuals: a randomized placebo-controlled trial. Lancet 2002;360:7-22; and Heart Protection Study Collaborative Group. MRC/BHF heart protection study of antioxidant vitamin supplementation in 20,536 high-risk individuals: a randomized placebo-controlled trial. Lancet 2002;360:23-33.)

vitamin D (<15 ng/mL) had twice the risk of a cardiovascular event (myocardial infarct, heart failure, or stroke) in the next 5 years as those with higher levels of vitamin D. This risk remained when adjusted for traditional cardiovascular risk factors; a 62% higher risk was seen in those with low vitamin levels. The highest rate of events, a twofold increase, was seen in those with both hypertension and vitamin D deficiency.[43]

This observational study is exactly that: observational. Whether vitamin D deficiency actually causes an increased risk of cardiovascular disease would require a large randomized trial to show that correcting the vitamin D deficiency resulted in a reduction in cardiovascular risk (Table 142.5).

Complications

Vitamins have been associated with few major side effects, and epidemiologic studies and previous trials suggest that supplementation with antioxidant vitamins is safe. The observation of a greater number of deaths from cardiovascular disease and lung cancer with beta-carotene supplementation needs to be carefully addressed in future trials. Also, further studies are needed to determine whether a link exists between vitamin D deficiency and cardiovascular risk.

VITAMIN E AND CARDIOVASCULAR DISEASE
■ Observational studies suggest benefit. ■ Randomized trials have shown no benefit. ■ Long-term use of vitamin E is safe. ■ A balanced diet and lifestyle modification, rather than supplemental vitamin E, are the best strategies for prevention of cardiovascular events.

Table 142.5 Vitamin E and cardiovascular disease.

Conclusions

Large, randomized clinical trials with vitamin E supplementation have shown no benefit in reducing fatal or nonfatal cardiovascular events. Likewise, no evidence indicates that beta-carotene or vitamin C supplementation provides any benefit with respect to cardiovascular disease. In fact, supplemental beta-carotene may be harmful. Although vitamins are safe, no evidence supports the routine use of antioxidant vitamins to prevent cardiovascular events.[44] The American Heart Association states, "Vitamin supplementation should not be encouraged until they are proven beneficial." Vitamin supplements are not a substitute for a healthy diet (rich in vegetables, whole grain foods, and fruit) or lifestyle. They cannot compensate for the risk associated with smoking, obesity, or inactivity.

HEART HERBS

Herbs are plants that have some of the qualities of food and some of the properties of drugs. A perfect example is garlic. Allicin is considered the most important biologically active compound. Allicin is a derived product, formed by enzymatic action from alliin, a crystalline amino acid that occurs in garlic oil. When the garlic bulb is crushed, alliinase converts alliin to allicin. Cooking and acid destroy the activity of the enzyme; the benefits of garlic, therefore, are obtained when it is ingested raw. Unfortunately, the daily dose of raw garlic required for therapeutic efficacy results in halitosis (Fig. 142.3).

Indications

During the past two decades, a number of human studies have demonstrated the lipid-lowering effects of garlic. Most of these studies used a garlic powder tablet standardized to

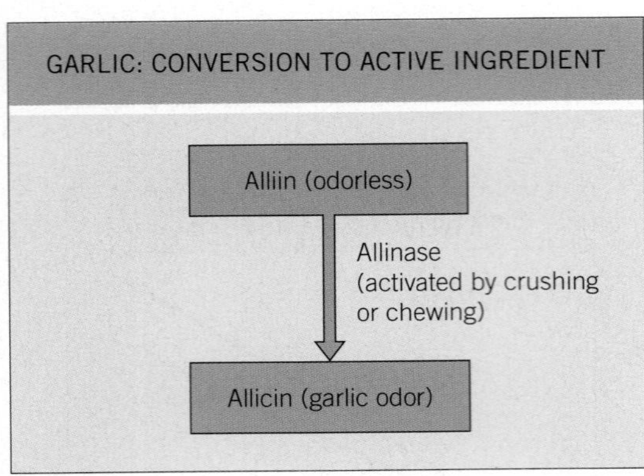

Figure 142.3 Garlic: conversion to active ingredient.

1.3% alliin. A meta-analysis of the effects of garlic on total serum cholesterol showed that, compared with placebo, garlic reduced cholesterol concentrations by about 9%.[45]

A recent review commissioned by the Agency for Healthcare Research and Quality (AHRQ) evaluated 37 randomized trials evaluating the effect of garlic preparations on blood cholesterol. Although statistically significant reductions in total cholesterol were seen at 1 and 3 months, this effect was not sustained at 6 months. Changes in LDL-cholesterol levels and triglycerides mirrored total cholesterol results; no significant changes were seen in high-density lipoprotein (HDL) cholesterol levels. The review concluded that garlic does not appear to have any benefits that endure beyond 6 months and does not offer long-term protection against cardiovascular disease.[46]

Complications

Daily consumption of moderate amounts of garlic (either natural, powder tablet, or capsules) should not pose any health risks. The larger doses required for any potential therapeutic effect may cause heart burn, garlic aftertaste, or body odor.

Conclusions

Garlic supplementation can produce a significant reduction in the concentrations of both total cholesterol and LDL-cholesterol. However, the reductions are not sustained and therefore of no benefit. Individuals with hypercholesterolemia that requires treatment are best served by taking an HMG-CoA reductase inhibitor (statin). Several large clinical trials (primary and secondary prevention) have demonstrated not only a favorable effect of statins on the lipid profile, but also, most important, a reduction in cardiovascular events and mortality (Fig. 142.4).

COENZYME Q_{10}

Coenzyme Q_{10} is a fat-soluble quinone present in the mitochondria of the heart, liver, and kidneys, where it is involved in electron and proton transfer during oxidative phosphorylation. Coenzyme Q_{10} was isolated from beef heart mitochondria in 1957. It is an antioxidant and free radical scavenger. It inhibits the oxidation of LDL-cholesterol. In animal models, coenzyme Q_{10} has been found to protect left ventricular function from ischemic reperfusion injury.

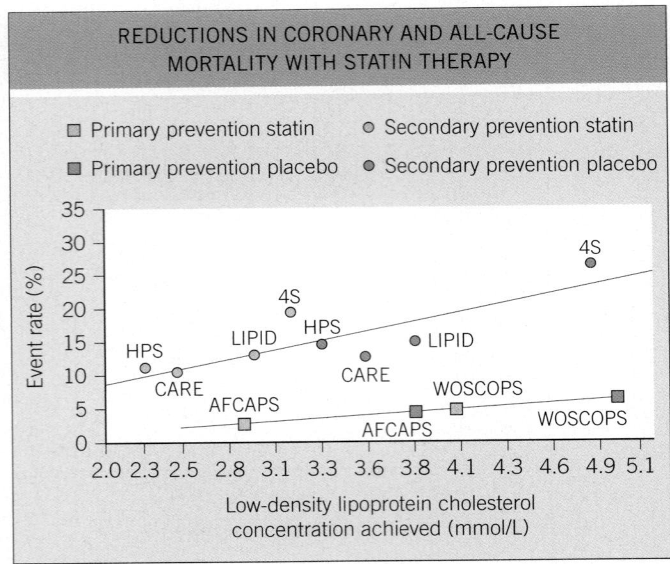

Figure 142.4 Reduction in coronary and all-cause mortality with statin therapy. AFCAPS, Air Force Texas Coronary Atherosclerosis Prevention Study; CARE, Cholesterol and Recurrent Events study; HPS, Heart Protection Study; LIPID, Long-term Intervention with Pravastatin in Ischemic Disease; 4S, Scandinavian Simvastatin Survival Study; WOSCOPS, West of Scotland Coronary Prevention Study.

In patients with heart failure, the myocardial tissue concentration of coenzyme Q_{10} has been shown to be low. Some have postulated that this low concentration may contribute to the heart failure. Moreover, some suggest that coenzyme Q_{10} may be useful for treating not only cardiac failure, but also other cardiac disorders, such as angina and diastolic dysfunction. Currently, coenzyme Q_{10} is a popular supplement among those who use alternative medicines.

During the past decade, numerous studies have claimed an improvement in symptoms, quality of life, left ventricular ejection fraction, and prognosis in patients with heart failure after oral treatment with coenzyme Q_{10}. However, these studies have lacked adequate randomization, placebo controls, and blinding.

A randomized, double-blind, cross-over study in Australia enrolled 30 patients with ischemic or idiopathic dilated cardiomyopathy who were in chronic heart failure (mean 41 months, with a mean ejection fraction of 26%).[47] The patients were clinically stable with traditional medications, including maximal doses of ACE inhibitors. The patients received coenzyme Q_{10} (33 mg every 8 hours) and placebo for 12 weeks each, separated by a 1-week washout period. Cardiac function was measured with transthoracic echocardiography and right-sided heart catheterization at baseline and after each treatment period. Quality of life was measured by means of a questionnaire. Compared with placebo, coenzyme Q_{10} had no effect on echocardiographic or hemodynamic data and no effect on well-being or functional capacity (Table 142.6). These results occurred despite an increase in plasma coenzyme Q_{10} concentrations during active therapy to more than twice the basal value.

Conclusions

Currently, although coenzyme Q_{10} is a popular dietary supplement and is touted as useful for patients with left

Parameter	Baseline	Coenzyme Q_{10}	Placebo
Left ventricular diastolic volume (mL)	220 ± 72	209 ± 75	220 ± 68
Left ventricular systolic volume (mL)	167 ± 54	149 ± 61	155 ± 58
Ejection fraction (%)	26 ± 6	31 ± 9	31 ± 9
Cardiac index	2.7 ± 0.7	2.9 ± 0.7	2.9 ± 0.7
Pulmonary wedge pressure (mm Hg)	16 ± 6	16 ± 7	16 ± 7
Systemic vascular resistance (U)	16 ± 4	15 ± 4	15 ± 5

ECHOCARDIOGRAPHIC AND HEMODYNAMIC DATA ON COMPARISON EFFECTS OF COENZYME Q_{10} AND PLACEBO

Table 142.6 Echocardiographic and hemodynamic data on comparison effects of coenzyme Q_{10} and placebo.

ventricular dysfunction, clinical data are insufficient to recommend its use as a cardiovascular agent.

SUMMARY

Medicine is a process in constant evolution. The science of today may be the disaster of tomorrow, and therapies about which medical practitioners are skeptical today may prove to be useful. The medical community must continue to establish evidence-based and outcome-based standards for all therapeutic measures. Because a therapy is labeled "alternative" does mean that the need for scientific scrutiny can be overlooked. Testimonials from patients are not adequate evidence. Only a systematic evaluation—that is, a randomized, double-blind, placebo-controlled clinical trial—can determine whether an alternative therapy has positive or negative results. If efficacy is demonstrated, the medical community should be willing to accept such therapies and make them available to their patients.

chapter 143

Perioperative Evaluation and Management of the Cardiac Patient

Michael H. Crawford

Definitions

- Cardiac events account for 40% of perioperative mortality in noncardiac surgery. One third of patients who undergo noncardiac surgery have cardiovascular disease, but the overall cardiac event rate is less than 1%. Can a cost-effective approach to reducing this risk be devised?

Key Features

- A high-risk subset of patients can be identified by clinical evaluation, the type of surgery, and selected testing.

Therapy

- In high-risk patients, the risk may be lowered by appropriate therapy, such as beta blockers.

Cardiac complications in patients undergoing noncardiac surgery account for 40% of perioperative mortality. This figure corresponds to the frequency of complications caused by sepsis. By contrast, the overall rate of major cardiac events (death, cardiac arrest, and myocardial infarction) is 1.4%, which is low considering that about one third of patients who undergo noncardiac surgery have cardiovascular disease if hypertension is included. The prevalence of cardiovascular disease in patients undergoing surgery is explained by the fact that patients age 45 or older are most likely to have surgery, and the incidence of cardiac disease increases with advancing age.

The most important cardiac complications of surgery are cardiac death, myocardial ischemia or infarction, cardiac arrest, and pulmonary edema. Considerable effort, therefore, is devoted to trying to predict these complications and to prevent them.

Major surgery has many features that can provoke unsuspected cardiovascular disease–related complications.[1] General anesthesia results in increased activation of the sympathetic nervous system and increased catecholamine excretion, especially during phase II of induction. Studies of surgical patients have shown that phase II is the most vulnerable time for precipitating cardiac events such as arrhythmias and myocardial infarction. Postoperative patients may have anemia, hypoxia, infection, and reduced or excess blood volume, all of which can stimulate the sympathetic nervous system. These complications frequently cause tachycardia and hypertension postoperatively, which can increase myocardial oxygen demand and precipitate unstable angina, myocardial infarction, or arrhythmias in the presence of ischemic heart disease. In addition, increased catecholamine excretion can increase the coagulable state; this, when coupled with arrhythmias such as atrial fibrillation, can predispose the patient to systemic emboli and stroke. Cardiac complications are more common when other complications of surgery, such as anemia, occur.

Major surgery, therefore, is associated with a greater risk of cardiac complications than is minor surgery. In addition, the likelihood of underlying ischemic heart disease influences this risk. Patients undergoing vascular surgery often have multiple risk factors for coronary disease, including atherosclerotic vascular disease. Consequently, patients undergoing vascular surgery usually are a high-risk group.[2]

Despite the fact that cardiovascular disease is common, cardiac morbidity and mortality from surgery is low. However, patients undergoing major surgery or vascular surgery are at higher risk, and surgeons are particularly concerned with preventing cardiac complications in these individuals. The issue is whether physicians and surgeons can identify from among these higher risk patients a very high risk group, whose members either should avoid nonessential surgery, or for whom interventions could be planned to reduce the risk of a cardiac complication with surgery.

The problem of identifying high-risk patients has received considerable attention. Cardiac consultants have a battery of tests that could fairly accurately define the risk in such patients; however, this would involve a tremendous increase in the cost of health care. When surgery is essential or emergency surgery is necessary to save a life, the risks must be balanced against the potential benefits, and a clinical decision must be made based on the information available and the testing that is feasible in that situation.

The incidence of cardiovascular events during the perioperative period increases with advancing age of the patient, the urgency and type of surgery, and the likelihood and severity of coronary artery disease (CAD). Therefore, the first goal of risk assessment is to estimate the likelihood that the patient has CAD. The next step is to determine the prognosis of the patient with cardiovascular disease independent of noncardiac surgery. Patients with high-risk cardiovascular disease may benefit from treatment alterations based on this fact alone. Next, the consultant should consider the effect of the cardiovascular disease on the risk of surgery and whether this risk can be reduced by specific therapy of the heart disease, prophylactic treatments, or other special considerations. Then, the risk of cardiac events with the planned surgical procedure is estimated. This figure is given to the surgical team, and they decide whether the risk to benefit ratio is acceptable. The consultant does not "clear" the patient for surgery; this is the surgeon's decision, based on the information provided.

One factor that influences the surgeon's decision is whether a specific management strategy or treatment of the cardiovascular disease will reduce the risk of surgery. Examples of specific management strategies include diuresis before surgery in fluid-overloaded patients, insertion of a Swan-Ganz catheter during surgery to monitor the patient's fluid status, and careful selection of anesthetic agents. Examples of prophylactic therapy include administration of beta blockers before and during surgery and revascularization before surgery. Invasive coronary interventions, which carry their own risks, rarely are necessary to lower the risk of surgery. An invasive approach is justified in only a small percentage of high-risk patients. Usually these are patients who would greatly benefit from the intervention anyway, regardless of the noncardiac surgery.

ASSESSING PATIENT RISK

The most challenging cardiovascular disease to assess is CAD, because many patients either are asymptomatic or have minimal, nonspecific symptoms. Although cardiac catheterization with coronary angiography can detect CAD readily, the cost and risks of the procedure prohibit its widespread use. Clinical information has great value and has proven useful for risk stratification of preoperative patients. In the 1970s, several clinical risk prediction models were promulgated by cardiologists, internists, and anesthesiologists. In the 1980s, noninvasive stress testing became popular and dominated the risk assessment approaches recommended. By the 1990s, the cost-effectiveness of the more expensive testing protocols was questioned, and algorithms that involved more selective testing were advocated. This more selective approach is preferred, because although CAD is prevalent in the general surgical population, perioperative cardiac events rates are low.

More recently, Lee and colleagues[3] developed a prospectively validated preoperative risk stratification tool for patients age 50 or older who are undergoing elective, major, noncardiac procedures. These researchers found six independent predictors of major cardiac complications (Table 143.1). Major cardiac complications occurred in 2% of more than 4000 patients studied. Giving each of the six variables a score of 1 resulted in a total score of 0 to 6, which corresponded to the incidence of major complications (Table 143.2). High-risk surgery is defined as an intraperitoneal, intrathoracic, or a suprainguinal vascular procedure. Ischemic heart disease was noted if the patient had a history of myocardial infarction, a positive result on a stress test, angina pectoris, used nitrates, or had pathologic Q waves on an electrocardiogram (ECG). Congestive heart failure was present if the patient had a history of it, pulmonary edema, or paroxysmal nocturnal dyspnea; bibasilar rates or a third heart sound; or a chest radiograph showing pulmonary vascular redistribution. Cerebral vascular disease was described as a history of stroke or transient ischemic attacks. As can be seen in Table 143.2, as soon as a patient has two risk factors, perioperative events jump to high levels. However, in this study, only about 12% of patients were taking beta blockers, and many think that event rates are lower when the patient is taking these drugs, even in high-risk patients.

THE SIX INDEPENDENT RISK FACTORS FOR PREDICTING MAJOR CARDIAC EVENTS

1. High-risk surgery
2. Ischemic heart disease
3. History of congestive heart failure
4. History of cerebrovascular disease
5. Insulin therapy for diabetes
6. Preoperative serum creatinine >2.0 mg/dL

Table 143.1 The six independent risk factors for predicting major cardiac events.

CARDIAC RISK INDEX AND THE OCCURRENCE OF MAJOR CARDIAC COMPLICATIONS

Score	Event Rate (%)
0	0.4
1	0.9
2	6.6
≥3	11.0

Table 143.2 Cardiac risk index and the occurrence of major cardiac complications.

It is important that the consultant be involved during the entire perioperative period. Intraoperative myocardial ischemia is common; however, in 18% of surgical patients, cardiac events are more common on days 2 to 5 postoperatively. Many patients go home during this period; therefore, the management strategy and prophylactic treatment to prevent cardiac events must extend to the outpatient arena. Cardiac problems are more likely to occur after the patient is out of the recovery room or intensive care unit and on the hospital floor. Physicians need to pay particular attention to the patient during this time and shortly after discharge, because further evaluation or treatment may be needed during this vulnerable period.

Systematic Approach

The first consideration is the type of surgery the patient requires. Data from the CASS registry in patients who underwent noncardiac surgery defined high-risk surgery as procedures with mortality or myocardial infarction rates higher than 4%.[2] These included abdominal, vascular, thoracic, and major head and neck surgery. All others were low risk because the mortality and myocardial infarction rates were less than 1%. However, more recent data from the BARI study suggests that only vascular and thoracic surgery have a mortality or myocardial infarction rate greater than 4%.[4] Abdominal and major head and neck procedures, therefore, are intermediate-risk surgery. Low-risk surgeries had event rates less than 1% in the CASS registry and less than 2% in the BARI study (Table 143.3). Consequently, extensive evaluation of patients undergoing low-risk surgery is not warranted, because treatment is unlikely to affect these low event rates.[5]

The second consideration is the likelihood the patient has CAD (Table 143.4). Age correlates with the incidence of CAD and is almost always a prognostic factor in patients undergoing higher risk surgeries.[6] However, no particular age triggers a more extensive evaluation. Self-reported poor

RISK OF MAJOR PERIOPERATIVE CARDIOVASCULAR EVENTS BY TYPE OF SURGERY
High Risk—Death or Myocardial Infarction (>4%) ■ Thoracic ■ Vascular
Intermediate Risk (2% to 4%) ■ Abdominal ■ Head and neck
Low Risk (≤1%) ■ Breast ■ Eye ■ Gynecologic ■ Skin ■ Urologic

Table 143.3 Risk of major perioperative cardiovascular events by type of surgery.

CLINICAL RISK STRATIFICATION OF MEN UNDERGOING NONCARDIAC SURGERY AND THE RISK OF PERIOPERATIVE MYOCARDIAL INFARCTION

Risk Class	Criteria	Risk of MI (%)
High	CAD almost certain: myocardial infarction by history/ECG; typical angina; previous angiography or revascularization	4.1
Intermediate	Peripheral vascular disease; previous stroke/transient ischemic attack (cerebral); atypical chest pain but no evidence of CAD	0.8
Low	Risk factors for CAD but no obvious disease; age >75 years; ECG abnormal	0.0
Negligible	None of the above	0.0

CAD, coronary artery disease; ECG, electrocardiogram; MI, myocardial infarction.

Table 143.4 Clinical risk stratification of men undergoing noncardiac surgery and the risk of perioperative myocardial infarction.

exercise tolerance predicts increased events and may be related to the presence of cardiovascular disease.[7] More specifically, the presence of risk factors for CAD are important (i.e., diabetes, hypertension, hypercholesterolemia, cigarette smoking, and a family history of CAD). Symptoms suggestive of CAD also are powerful predictors (i.e., angina, dyspnea, edema, syncope, palpitations, and a history of heart failure). A history of definite CAD is the most useful information (i.e., prior myocardial infarction, catheterization, percutaneous coronary intervention, coronary bypass surgery, or positive findings on stress tests).

In patients with a greater likelihood of CAD or with known CAD, determining the severity of the disease is the next step. Certain clinical conditions are useful in this regard, such as unstable angina, overt heart failure, acute myocardial infarction (MI), or hypotension. Such high-risk clinical conditions deserve attention regardless of impending surgery and would preclude all but the most urgent life-saving surgery until the condition had been stabilized. Historical information may be of value, such as previous cardiac catheterization results; percutaneous interventions or bypass surgery; stress test results; or echocardiographic findings. All these considerations usually are sufficient in patients with a high likelihood of or known CAD to characterize the disease as mild, moderate, or severe. If uncertainty still exists, then further testing may be necessary.

Systemic Testing

When ischemic heart disease is suspected, a resting ECG is appropriate to detect silent myocardial infarction, evidence of ischemia, and conduction abnormalities.[8] Evidence of left ventricular hypertrophy, which carries a poor prognosis, also may be seen. Left atrial enlargement frequently is seen in patients with hypertensive heart disease, valvular disease, and CAD and may be a harbinger of atrial fibrillation, which can complicate surgery. Conduction abnormalities are important, because prophylactic pacing may have to be considered in some individuals. However, prophylactic pacing is rarely indicated unless pacing is required for other reasons.[9]

Occasionally the ECG reveals a rhythm disturbance, such as atrial fibrillation or premature ventricular or atrial contractions. Atrial fibrillation is important because of the issue of anticoagulation management and rate control during the perioperative period. Premature ventricular contractions may be a result of ongoing myocardial ischemia and may increase the risk of ventricular arrhythmias in the perioperative period. Premature atrial contractions increase the incidence of atrial fibrillation. Therefore, the resting ECG alone often provides sufficient information, along with the clinical information, to enable risk stratification of the patient before surgery. Most of the clinical approaches to risk assessment include an assessment of the ECG.

If ischemic heart disease is likely or if it is known but its severity is unclear, a stress test often is useful. Stress tests may be exercise based or pharmacologically based. Exercise testing is preferred, because it has a high diagnostic yield and provides considerable additional information, such as functional status and inducibility of arrhythmias. Exercise testing can be accomplished with a treadmill or with upright or supine bicycle exercise. Treadmill exercise usually provides the highest level of myocardial oxygen demand and therefore is preferred to bicycle exercise. Pharmacologic stress testing is reserved for those who cannot exercise adequately. The two types of pharmacologic stressors are exercise mimics, such as dobutamine, and vasodilators, such as dipyridamole or adenosine. Dipyridamole is a precursor to adenosine; therefore, the results with the two drugs are very similar. Adenosine causes more intense side effects but has a much shorter duration of action.

The other component of stress testing is an ischemia detection system. Electrocardiography frequently is used to detect ST-wave transients indicative of ischemia. Exercise ECG testing can be up to 85% accurate, depending on the patient population, the adequacy of exercise, and the characteristics of the resting ECG. Good exercise performance with a normal ECG, no signs or symptoms of heart disease during exercise, and a normal blood pressure response indicate a good prognosis even if CAD is missed. As mentioned, pharmacologic stress usually is selected for patients who cannot exercise.

Imaging also can function as an ischemia detection method. It usually is accomplished by echocardiography or nuclear perfusion scintigraphy. Because dobutamine is an exercise mimic, echocardiography usually is used to detect wall motion abnormality. Myocardial perfusion imaging usually reveals differences in perfusion more reliably with vasodilator drugs. However, both vasodilators and dobutamine have been used with echocardiography and perfusion imaging with relatively good results. The current practice in the United States is to use dobutamine echocardiography and either dipyridamole or adenosine nuclear perfusion imaging.

Indications for Testing

Because cardiac catheterization and revascularization are not usually performed just to improve surgical risk, stress testing usually is done only if the patient has an active cardiac problem that requires therapy or if such testing will change the management strategy.[10,11] Either surgical or percutaneous revascularization delays noncardiac surgery; the former for healing and the latter because of the need for aggressive antiplatelet therapy. Although surgery can be accomplished while the patient is taking aspirin and clopidogrel, the risk of bleeding is increased such that surgeons delay all but life-saving surgery.

Occasionally the diagnosis of CAD or defining its severity changes the management strategy. For example, when the decision about noncardiac organ transplantation is borderline, knowledge of the presence of severe CAD could tip the decision. The use of prophylactic beta blockers also might be affected, but in borderline cases this therapy usually is used, because the risk of adverse events from beta blockers is low.

Assessment of left ventricular function can be valuable in selected patients and usually is accomplished with echocardiography. The discovery of wall motion abnormalities may help clarify the significance of nonspecific ECG findings. Also, patients with unexplained dyspnea or a change in status of chronic heart failure may benefit from knowledge of left ventricular function. However, routine assessment of left ventricular function has not been shown to be useful.

STRATEGY

The complexity of preoperative evaluation of the cardiac patient for noncardiac surgery has occasioned the publication of several algorithms to aid the process. Most were derived retrospectively, and some have been prospectively tested. The American College of Cardiology and the American Heart Association produced a guideline and algorithm on this topic by committee.[12] It relies heavily on clinical predictors, an assessment of the patient's ability to exercise, and test results. It also considers the urgency and type of surgery. Although comprehensive, the algorithm is very complex, which limits its usefulness.

Despite the attractiveness of some of these algorithms, they do not cover all patients and all situations. Highly skilled anesthesia care also can help to get high-risk patients through surgery without complications. In addition, the cost of risk-stratifying strategies must be considered in relation to benefit. If a patient with known coronary disease and recent revascularization is asymptomatic and exercises every day, little will improve the individual's risk for surgery.[13]

PREOPERATIVE RISK REDUCTION

Once risk stratification is accomplished, the consultant advises the surgeon and anesthesiologist of the risk of cardiac events. The surgeon then assesses the risk to benefit ratio of surgery, and a decision is made to cancel surgery, to go ahead with the operation, or to try to modify the risk. Risk modification can be as simple as controlling blood pressure, heart failure, or angina by adjusting the patient's medical regimen. On the other hand, it can be as aggressive as coronary artery bypass surgery before noncardiac surgery. If surgery is performed, the consultant's role continues in the management of the patient to reduce the risk of perioperative morbidity and mortality. This may include the choice of anesthesia, the surgical approach, specific monitoring, perioperative prophylactic therapy, and postoperative rehabilitation.

Ischemic Heart Disease

Considerable information exists concerning the use of prophylactic beta blockers for higher risk patients undergoing major noncardiac surgery. Although early studies showed significant reductions in perioperative events, several recent randomized trials have shown no benefit.[14,15] Examination of these data suggest that these drugs are beneficial in high-risk patients, especially those with ischemic heart disease, undergoing high-risk noncardiac surgery.[16,17] In lower risk patients or those undergoing low-risk surgery, the risks of beta blockers probably outweigh any potential benefits. If beta blockers are given, data suggest that long-acting agents are better than short-acting ones and that titration of dose to a resting heart rate less than 70 beats per minute (bpm) is important. Also, beta blockers should be continued for at least 1 week postoperatively and longer in selected cases when recovery takes longer. In addition, patients already taking a beta blocker for clear indications should be kept on it for surgery.

The use of other drugs prophylactically in the perioperative period is less well established. α_2-Agonists, such as clonidine, have been shown in several trials to reduce the incidence of myocardial infarction and death.[18] These drugs may be most useful when the preoperative patient has hypertension. Intravenous nitrates have not been shown to influence outcomes favorably. Calcium channel blockers have been shown to reduce perioperative ischemia and supraventricular arrhythmias but not death or infarction.[19] Statins may be beneficial, based on observational studies and one small, randomized trial, but they cannot be routinely recommended at this time.[20-22]

Despite the attractiveness of angioplasty, especially for patients with one- or two-vessel disease, no prospective, randomized trials have supported the efficacy of this approach for reducing preoperative risk in patients undergoing noncardiac surgery. However, retrospective observational studies do suggest a benefit.[13] Currently, the indications for angioplasty are similar to the indications if surgery were not being considered. Whether stents would improve the results obtained is unknown.

The major issue with stents is the timing of surgery after stent placement because of the need for intensive antiplatelet therapy for weeks to months after placement of the stent.

Patients who have undergone percutaneous coronary procedures before surgery present special challenges.[23] Balloon angioplasty causes endothelial injury at the site that takes 2 to 4 weeks to heal, and aspirin therapy is important during this time. The peak incidence of restenosis after balloon angioplasty is 8 to 12 weeks. Therefore, the ideal timing of noncardiac surgery would be 1 month after angioplasty. If bare metal stents are placed, the peak incidence of in-stent thrombosis is during the first 2 weeks, and 4 to 6 weeks are required for complete endothelialization. Restenosis is rare before 12 weeks. Also, a thienopyridine usually is administered for the first 4 weeks after placement of a bare metal stent. Therefore, the ideal time for noncardiac surgery after bare metal stent replacement is 6 to 12 weeks after stenting. The thienopyridine can be stopped after 4 weeks, which allows time for it to clear the system before surgery.

Because drug-eluting stents require longer to endothelialize, patients need to take thienopyridines for a longer period. Premature cessation of aspirin and thienopyridines may result in acute stent thrombosis if endothelialization is not complete. Also, each brand of drug-eluting stent is different; therefore, the manufacturer's information should be consulted. However, after 1 year with any drug-eluting stent, stopping thienopyridine therapy and proceeding with noncardiac surgery is relatively safe.

Valvular Heart Disease

Of the valvular lesions, stenosis carries a higher risk than regurgitant lesions. Because mitral stenosis is unusual in developed countries, where more surgery is done, aortic stenosis is the most common lesion of concern. In a recent study, more than 5000 patients with aortic stenosis were compared with more than 10,000 controls matched for age and type of surgery.[24] The rate of acute myocardial infarction was 2% in the control group versus 4% in the aortic stenosis patients. After correcting for heart failure and coronary artery disease, which frequently are associated with aortic stenosis, aortic stenosis was associated with a 55% higher incidence of perioperative myocardial infarction even in low-risk surgeries. However, death rates were not significantly different. The data were not stratified by severity of aortic stenosis, and other outcomes, such as heart failure, were not reported. Nevertheless, aortic stenosis modestly increases the rate of perioperative myocardial infarction.[25,26] Whether prophylactic pharmacologic therapy would reduce this risk is not known, but many prophylactic drugs for the perioperative period lower blood pressure, which could be dangerous in patients with severe aortic stenosis.

Very few data are available on the advisability of performing valvular surgery to improve preoperative risk. If the criteria are met for valvular surgery and the noncardiac surgery can be delayed, it would make sense to do the valvular surgery first. Hemodynamic derangements during surgery that reduce blood pressure or fluid levels can cause a cardiac arrest, and significant aortic stenosis makes resuscitation extremely difficult. Therefore, patients with severe aortic stenosis should avoid noncardiac surgery, or the stenosis should be addressed before noncardiac surgery, if possible.

Those who refuse valvular surgery or are not candidates for aortic valve replacement can undergo noncardiac surgery, but the perioperative major cardiac event rate is 10% or higher in these patients. Also, percutaneous aortic balloon valvuloplasty can be considered as a bridge to noncardiac surgery when comorbidities that prevent valvular surgery may be corrected by the noncardiac surgery. Balloon valvuloplasty is an even better option for patients with severe mitral stenosis who need major noncardiac surgery because, unlike aortic valvuloplasty, it may have lasting benefit.

Regurgitant lesions are better tolerated than stenosis even if they are severe. Reduced left ventricular filling pressure is almost never an issue, even with bleeding and reduced intravascular fluid, because the regurgitation provides adequate filling for the left ventricle. Valve regurgitation patients are at higher risk of increases in blood pressure during surgery, which can increase the amount of regurgitation and result in congestive heart failure. However, elevated blood pressure is readily controlled during surgery. Patients with heart failure caused by valvular disease usually have aggressive treatment that reduces or controls the heart failure and makes surgery more feasible.

Patients who require chronic anticoagulation for cardiovascular disease present special problems in management. If surgery can be safely accomplished with the patient taking anticoagulants or with a reduced international normalized ratio (INR; 1.8 to 2.5), there is no major issue; however, if anticoagulation therapy has to be stopped, management depends on the risk of thrombosis. In patients with mechanical prosthetic valves, the risk of valve thrombosis increases rapidly after 48 hours off anticoagulation. These patients must have a heparin bridge until surgery, then 48 hours off heparin, and then resumption of heparin, followed by warfarin when safe. Patients with a history of deep venous thrombosis, atrial fibrillation, or left ventricular aneurysm probably can tolerate being off anticoagulation for 7 to 10 days with a low risk of thrombotic events, but the more conditions the patient has, the greater the risk.

Heart Failure

A history of congestive heart failure is important in most preoperative risk algorithms for predicting major cardiac events. However, in patients with clinically stable heart failure who are undergoing elective surgery, the risk may not be as high as previously reported. The 1-month mortality is higher than in non–heart failure populations, but the absolute risk is 1% to 2%.[27] These patients need more care postoperatively; therefore, the length of stay is about 1 day longer on average, and 1-month readmission rates are twice that of non–heart failure patients. There are several reasons for these more encouraging recent experiences. Many patients today have heart failure caused by diastolic dysfunction rather than systolic dysfunction, and the former have a lower risk of perioperative mortality. Also, elective surgery allows time for optimizing the patient's clinical status. Furthermore, advances in anesthesia care and less invasive and traumatic surgery put less stress on the dysfunctional heart. For these reasons, a history of heart failure should not automatically exclude a patient from needed surgery.

Arrhythmias and Electrophysiology Devices

For patients with supraventricular arrhythmias, consideration should be given to ablation, cardioversion, or rate control, as appropriate for the type of arrhythmia. In patients with intermittent atrial arrhythmias, no indication exists for prophylactic digitalization as a preventive measure, and most supraventricular arrhythmias can be dealt with effectively in the perioperative setting.

Patients in chronic atrial fibrillation who are taking anticoagulants present a special problem. Although few data exist on how to manage noncardiac surgery in such patients, it would seem prudent to switch them to heparin preoperatively and then to reverse the heparin for the surgery and the immediate postsurgical period, when bleeding is most likely to occur. The risk of stroke is less than 5% a year in such patients who are not taking anticoagulation drugs, and the advisability of switching patients preoperatively to heparin for stroke prevention is problematic, especially if surgery can be accomplished with the patient taking warfarin or during a brief period of lower INR values.

Ventricular arrhythmias usually are not a problem unless they induce a hemodynamic abnormality in the patient. Prophylactic therapy usually is not indicated, because ventricular arrhythmias during surgery can be readily treated with intravenous lidocaine (lignocaine) or procainamide.

The indications for temporary pacing for patients undergoing noncardiac surgery are similar to the indications for permanent pacing; namely, advanced atrioventricular block and severe bradycardia.[9] Therefore, most patients should have permanent pacers placed before surgery. In addition, the availability of transthoracic pacing has made the use of prophylactic temporary pacing much less important. Intraventricular conduction defects and bifascicular block, with or without first-degree atrioventricular block, should not be taken as indications for temporary pacing if the patient has no symptoms of syncope or documented episodes of advanced block.

Patients with implanted electrophysiologic devices may experience device malfunction during electrocautery. If the patient is pacemaker dependent, the pacemaker should be reprogrammed to an asynchronous mode, or a magnet should be placed over it during surgery. Patients with implantable defibrillators may experience unwanted shocks if the electrocautery discharges are interpreted as tachycardias. Therefore, the tachycardia treatment function should be shut off just before surgery and a defibrillator should be available in the operating room. If defibrillation is necessary, the paddles should be placed anteroposteriorly away from the device. After surgery, full functionality of the device should be restored.

PERIOPERATIVE MYOCARDIAL INFARCTION

Troponin elevation is now considered the cornerstone of myocardial infarction diagnosis; however, it must be accompanied by two of the following: typical chest pain, ECG changes, or imaging evidence of infarction. Because anesthesia and postoperative pain medications may blunt or abrogate chest pain, ECG changes or cardiac imaging become much more important in the diagnosis of myocardial infarctions. If troponins are measured in all postoperative patients, numerous false-positive myocardial infarctions will be chased in patients who do not have ECG or imaging abnormalities consistent with infarction. Therefore, troponin should be measured only if hemodynamic abnormalities are present or infarction is suspected for other reasons, such as ventricular arrhythmias. If troponin measurement is done, an ECG also should be done. If the troponin result is positive and the ECG is nonspecific, imaging is necessary. If the ECG shows ST elevation, an echocardiogram should be done immediately to confirm an evolving infarction.

Generally, two types of myocardial injury occur perioperatively: supply-demand mismatch ischemic events and plaque rupture coronary artery thrombosis events. The latter usually show ECG ST-segment elevation or significant new wall motion abnormalities and should be treated as any ST-elevation myocardial infarction. Preference should be given to invasive management, because thrombolysis may be problematic in a postoperative patient. The supply-demand events, or "demand MIs," frequently are associated with small elevations of troponin; minor, nonspecific ECG changes; and normal wall motion on echocardiography. These patients can be observed for hemodynamic or arrhythmic events and not treated prophylactically. If all goes well, the prudent course is to perform an outpatient stress test after the patient has recovered from surgery, because many of these patients have underlying ischemic heart disease.

SUMMARY

Cardiac events are a significant cause of morbidity and mortality during major noncardiac surgery. Therefore, risk stratification of preoperative patients is important to identify those at high risk of such an event. These high-risk patients should not have surgery, or the surgery should be delayed until the risk can be reduced, providing it is not emergency life-saving surgery. Clinical indices of risk and algorithms have been developed, but they are complex and not easily remembered. Simple, more intuitive approaches are preferable, but they require considerable experience and judgment.

One such approach recently was described by Goldman (Table 143.5). Patients with no history of heart disease, who do not have any symptoms, and who are fully active, need no further evaluation, not even an ECG. Patients with stable, known CAD or who have a high likelihood of coronary disease based on risk factors (e.g., a vascular surgery patient) and who are functional class I need a resting ECG and careful perioperative management. High-risk patients, such as those with a very recent myocardial infarction, overt heart failure, or advanced arrhythmias, who are functional class III or IV, need a full cardiac evaluation and appropriate therapy. This could include cardiac catheterization and coronary revascularization in some cases, because this therapy is necessary for optimal management of the heart disease.

Invasive procedures solely for the purpose of lessening the risk of surgery are rarely justified.

The situation becomes more difficult in patients with known CAD or diabetes; those older than 75 years; and those undergoing vascular surgery whose functional class is II or III or unknown. Noninvasive testing probably can stratify these patients into a lower risk group (the majority) or a high-risk group (few); however, even in these patients, the risk of perioperative myocardial infarction is 1% to 2%, and mortality is less frequent. Nevertheless, the risk of perioperative myocardial infarction probably can be reduced to less than 1% in these patients by appropriate interventions, such as beta blockers. For these reasons, this selective testing and intervention approach has become the accepted method for the management of the perioperative cardiac patient.

SIMPLIFIED APPROACH TO PREOPERATIVE CARDIAC EVALUATION AND MANAGEMENT				
Clinical Assessment	**Recommended Tests**		**Cardiac Event Risk* (%)**	**Therapy**
No history or symptoms of CAD Fully active	None		<1	None
High likelihood of CAD Known CAD, stable Functional class I	ECG		1-2	None
High likelihood of CAD Known CAD, stable Functional class II or unknown	Stress test	Negative Positive	1-2 2-4	None Beta blockers
Known CAD, unstable Functional class III or IV	Cardiac catheterization		2-4	Revascularization

*Cardiac events include cardiac arrest, death, myocardial infarction, and pulmonary edema.
CAD, coronary artery disease; ECG, electrocardiogram.

Table 143.5 Simplified approach to preoperative cardiac evaluation and management.

chapter

144 Employment and Insurability

William Dafoe, Laura Cupper, and Bill Williams

Issues/Problems

- For best results, the return to work process requires active involvement by the treating cardiologist.
- To ensure maintenance of work, patients need ongoing assessment of their medical and psychosocial health and the job conditions so that the risk of job strain can be evaluated.
- Assessment for licensing to drive or to fly a plane requires the establishment of an acceptable level of risk for the individual and society.

Key Findings

- At least 20% of cardiac patients do not return to work after a cardiac event; this results in considerable economic and social costs.
- Return to work rates are similar across various procedural and diagnostic groups (e.g., percutaneous transluminal coronary angioplasty, coronary artery bypass grafts, myocardial infarction).
- Factors that influence return to work reflect individual, societal, and employment issues and vary with the patient's career stage.
- Most of the predictive information comes from demographic and socioeconomic factors, then from physical and emotional measures, and finally from clinical variables.
- The assessment for return to work should include physical requirements, environmental factors, and employer issues.
- Work capacity can be determined by stress testing and in some cases by simulating work demands.
- Jobs characterized by chronic job strain (high psychological demands and low decision latitude) may pose an increased risk of repeat cardiovascular events for patients returning to work.
- Between 1% and 5% of sudden cardiac deaths occur while the individual is driving; fewer than 2% of these incidents result in injury or death in bystanders.

In general, vocational issues are assuming greater importance, with the expectation that cardiac patients can be gainfully employed. This is related to the cost of cardiac procedures, such as heart transplantation surgery or coronary artery bypass graft (CABG) surgery, and the economic costs incurred when cardiac patients fail to return to work. Moreover, for many cardiac patients, returning to work is an important objective. Work is considered psychologically therapeutic for the recovering cardiac patient, and the economic survival of many patients and their families depends on gainful employment. In addition, returning to work can signify the transition from a "sick" to an "active" role.

MEANING OF WORK

Work is considered central to well-being. The two hallmarks of adult functioning, as identified by Freud, are the ability to love and the ability to work.[1] Work can have an intrinsic or extrinsic value; if a person works for intrinsic reasons, it is expected that the work is interesting, meaningful, and even self-actualizing.

RELATIONSHIP OF WORK TO HEALTH

Jin and others[2] reviewed the evidence for an association, and possibly a causative association, between unemployment and adverse health outcomes. They found a positive association between unemployment and all-cause mortality, cardiovascular mortality, suicide, higher rates of traffic accidents, and use of health care resources. Studies of mortality attributable to cardiovascular disease showed an increase in relative risk from 1.3 to 1.8. They concluded that unemployment is strongly associated with a greater risk of morbidity and mortality.

The effect of unemployment on cardiac risk factors is complex and depends on many factors. For example, the financial loss may be an economic incentive to stop smoking; or, conversely, the resultant stress of unemployment may make it "impossible" for the patient to consider stopping smoking.

Unemployed people may demonstrate a mild to moderate depressive affect and in some cases a clinical depression. Work offers opportunities for interpersonal contact, improved finances, valued social position, and a purpose and structure to life.[3] Boudrez and De Backer[4] have shown that 1 year after returning to work, individuals have fewer somatic and cognitive complaints and a more positive affect.

ECONOMIC COSTS OF CARDIOVASCULAR DISEASE AND WORK-RELATED ISSUES

Despite major advances in medical and surgical management of heart disease, little or no improvement has been seen in return to work rates after cardiac events. Studies have reported rates that vary from 47% to 93%, depending on the population, treatment modality, duration of follow-up, and outcome criteria. Estimates are that about 20% of previously employed people do not return to work after a myocardial infarction or CABG surgery. It generally is accepted that good health makes people more productive and reduces expenditures of societal resources; the converse is also true: bad health adversely affects productivity and increases expenditures of resources. Therefore, the failure of those with cardiovascular disease to return to work has an enormous economic impact.

Even an unnecessary delay in resuming work can result in significant societal economic loss. A prospective study assessed the cost associated with absence from work for 53 patients who underwent percutaneous transluminal coronary angioplasty. The study found the direct costs to be $5,160 per patient, and the indirect costs to be $2,848 per patient.[5]

From a Canadian perspective, the most recent statistics show that the total cost of cardiovascular disease in 2000 to 2001 was $20.5 billion, with a direct cost of $7.1 billion and an indirect cost of $13.4 billion (Table 144.1).[6]

The direct and indirect costs of cardiovascular disease (CVD) in the United States for 2007 have been estimated at $431.8 billion.[7] In Europe, on average, cardiovascular disease represents 49% of all-cause mortality, with significant national variability.

The average time for returning to work in patients with ischemic heart disease has declined, from 4 months in 1970 to approximately 15 to 70 days in more recent studies.[8-10] In a study comparing return to work rates of patients undergoing percutaneous transluminal coronary angioplasty and CABG surgery, Hlatky and colleagues[11] found that patients in the angioplasty group returned to work significantly earlier than those in the CABG group (6 weeks compared with 11 weeks); however, after their return, the number of hours spent working did not differ significantly between the groups. Similar results were reported by Pocock and coworkers,[12] who found that the CABG group returned to work more slowly, with only 9% back in employment after 2 months. However, by 5 months after the procedure, the angioplasty and CABG groups were very similar, with return to work rates of 52% and 50%, respectively. Froelicher and associates[13] reported that 21% of patients who had had a myocardial infarction returned to work by 3 weeks, 62% between 4 and 12 weeks, and 11% between 12 and 24 weeks; 6% did not return at all. Kovoor and associates[10] demonstrated that low-risk patients who had had a myocardial infarction (MI) could return to normal activities, including work, at 2 weeks. At a 2-week return, this group showed no differences in reinfarction or revascularization rates compared with the group that returned at 6 weeks. However, the 6-week group was able to participate in a cardiac rehabilitation program and showed greater exercise capacity than the group that returned to work earlier. In addition, no quality of life indicators were assessed. Therefore, selected low-risk patients who need to return to work at an early stage can do so without apparent harm.

ECONOMIC COST OF CARDIOVASCULAR DISEASE*			
	Total Cost	Direct Cost	Indirect Cost
Canada	20.5	7.1	13.4
United States	431.8	283.2	148.6

*Cost is given in billions of dollars.

Table 144.1 Economic cost of cardiovascular disease.

Dennis and coworkers[9] demonstrated that a work evaluation intervention designed to promote timely return to work reduced the period of convalescence by 32% and resulted in savings of $2,102 per patient (based on earned income). If these savings are extrapolated to include patients in general who have suffered acute myocardial infarction, the findings of this study suggest that early counseling about returning to work could lead to significant savings in disability compensation.

FACTORS THAT INFLUENCE THE RETURN TO WORK

A complex amalgam of individual factors, societal issues, and employment aspects influence the process of return to work. These factors vary with age and with the patient's career stage. Table 144.2 presents these various factors, along with possible interventions.

Individual Factors

One of the most important factors in the return to work is the individual's "self-efficacy," which may reflect a summary gestalt of the other predictive factors. Self-efficacy has been defined as "an evaluation of the ability to execute a specific action with confidence"[14]; from a vocational perspective, it refers to the confidence in returning to work. A less severe "perception of illness" is seen in patients who anticipate minimal problems with returning to work and subsequently have a greater rate of return to work.[15,16] Petrie and others[17] outlined a schema of five cognitive components that patients use to interpret their symptoms and health risk and to determine subsequent actions after discharge:

- Identity—the label used to describe the illness and to understand the symptoms
- Cause—personal ideas about the cause of the illness
- Time line—how long the illness will last
- Consequences—anticipated effects and outcome of the illness
- Cure or control—how the patient recovers or controls the illness

The perceptions that correlated with return to work in 6 weeks were that the illness would last a short time and have less serious consequences. While the patient is in the hospital, the treating cardiologist should ascertain the individual's "self-efficacy" of returning to work and should clarify any false perceptions about the disease. It is important that the patient understand the physician's viewpoint.

The patient's clinical status is one of the basic determinants of returning to work. Obviously, patients with unstable medical conditions, severe left ventricular dysfunction, or life-threatening arrhythmias cannot return to work.

Years of education is a significant predictor of returning to work and may be associated with favorable socioeconomic and job-related factors.

Depression, as assessed in the hospital using the Hospital Anxiety and Depression Scales–depression subscale (HADS-D), predicted failure to return to work with an odds ratio of .4. Interestingly, the Beck Depression Inventory–Fast Scale was nonpredictive.[18]

FACTORS THAT INFLUENCE RETURN TO WORK AND POSSIBLE INTERVENTIONS				
Factor		**More Likely to Return to Work**	**Less Likely to Return to Work**	**Possible Interventions**
Individual factors	Self-perception of return to work and of illness	Strong self-efficacy	Poor self-efficacy	Assess self-efficacy at early stage to clarify patient's perceptions of illness
	Perception of the view of the treating physician	Favors return to work	Does not approve of return to work	Ensure patient and family understand treating physician's view
	Age	≤55 yr	>55 yr	
	Education	Postgraduate degree	Less education	
	Clinical status	None or mild	Significant	Clarification of medical status
	Left ventricular impairment			
	Number of cardiac events	One	Numerous	Clarification of medical status
Social issues	Family attitudes	Supportive	Not supportive, overprotective, or believes that work caused the event	Early family involvement in discussions about returning to work
		Involved in rehabilitation	May sabotage efforts regarding return to work	Family awareness of patient's improvement in rehabilitation
	Labor market	Previous job still available or other jobs available	Job market poor	Early vocational intervention (community agency)
Employment aspects	Career stage	Advancement or maintenance	Retirement stage	
	Job satisfaction	High	Low	Clarification of job-interest mismatch
	Work stress	Manageable	High; believed that "stress caused cardiovascular problems"	Stress management strategies
	Type of work	White collar, self-employed	"Blue collar"	
	Time off work	Working at time of event	Off work before the event; has not worked for 6 months	Early vocational intervention
	Financial situation	Needs work for income	Sufficient alternative funds	
	Employer aspects	Job modification possible; contact maintained with employees	No job modification possible; no contact while off work	Trial of altered job requirements
	Coworkers' attitudes	Supportive, encouraging, and help to reduce work stressors	Minimal assistance; resentful	Advocacy for worker in discussions with employer and coworkers

Table 144.2 Factors that influence return to work and possible interventions.

Societal Issues

Societal issues are important in determining return to work.[19,20] For most patients, the family can provide a positive or negative influence with respect to returning to work. If the family believes that the "stress" of the job caused the cardiac event or that the job places the patient at risk, efforts to delay returning to work may ensue. Women generally have less social support, which may inhibit return to work.[21] Obviously, the local labor market helps to dictate job availability.

Employment Aspects

The influence of employment-related factors in determining return to work is well recognized.[22,23] Work or unemployment becomes an integral part of a person's life, and the patient's pre-event working status, therefore, is an important determinant of return to work. The individual's career stage also helps determine return to work options, both for the patient and for the employer. The career stages are career advancement (workers consider career a top priority), maintenance/stabilization, and retirement. More recently, the concept of retirement is changing as the baby boomer generation rewrites the expectations of the various stages of life. Bolles and Nelson[24] state that "retirement implies a kind of parole from a thing called *work,* which is assumed to be onerous and tedious. It implies 'disengagement' from both work and life, as one patiently, or impatiently, waits to die." Thus, a certain percentage of workers may continue to work at their full job or at modified jobs, or they may engage in a new career. "White collar" or self-employed patients who had a high level of job satisfaction and manageable levels of stress are likely to return to work. Conversely, those with "blue collar" jobs who perceive their jobs to have high degrees of stress and low job satisfaction are unlikely to return to work. Financial incentives or disincentives for returning to work are related to the availability of sick leave, disability, or pension plans. The characteristics of the job and the attitude of the employer, coworkers and, in some instances, the union can influence the possibility of job availability and the ease of returning to work.

Multivariate Analyses

Smith and O'Rourke[25] assessed 151 patients after myocardial infarction and found that 72% returned to work. Univariate analyses showed that education, the energy demands of employment, the severity of the myocardial infarction, the patient's perception of his health status, financial incentives, socioeconomic status, social status, locus of control, satisfaction with work, and early entry into the job force all were associated with returning to work. A multivariate analysis indicated that the most important predictor for return to work was a higher level of education, followed by decreased energy demands of the job, less severe myocardial infarction, and a favorable general health rating index.

Mark and colleagues[26] correlated various factors at angiography with work status 1 year later. Functional capacity, as reported subjectively by the Duke Activity Survey, was the most important predictor, followed by older age, black race, presence of congestive heart failure, lower education level, presence of extracardiac vascular disease, poorer psychological status, and lower job classification.

Mittag and associates[27] evaluated 132 male patients participating in a cardiac rehabilitation program. The predictive variables for work return at 1 year were derived from the perspectives of both patient and physician. The physicians derived their prognosis from medical variables (cardiac status and comorbidity), whereas the patient's perspective concerned his or her overall health status, the former job status, job satisfaction, and negative incentives for return for work. A multivariate analysis found three variables that predicted return to work in 85% of cases: age, the patient's perception of the degree of disability from cardiac problems, and the physician's views of the extent of disability derived from the overall medical situation. As with other studies, the cardiac status had little relevance with regard to the return to work status.

Samkange-Zeeb and coworkers[28] reported that return to work rates in Germany varied from 43% to 67%. A risk tool was developed in hopes of identifying individuals at risk of not returning to work. The screening instrument had a positive predictive value (PPV) of 33%. In other words, it predicted the non–return to work (non-RTW) of 33% of the participants starting the rehabilitation program. It had a negative predictive value (NPV) of 93%; that is, it had excellent discriminating properties for identifying individuals not at risk of early retirement; therefore, intervention programs were not required. The significant factors in the multiple regression analysis included greater age, profession, positive expectations concerning return to work, and level of depression.

These four prospective studies have slightly different indicators in terms of predictors of return to work. In general, they corroborate categories of predictive information recognized by Mark and colleagues,[26] which indicate that demographic and socioeconomic characteristics provide 45% of the total, followed by physical and emotional measures (27%), and clinical variables (20%).

MULTIVARIATE ANALYSIS OF PREDICTORS OF RETURN TO WORK

Study	Predictive Factors (from multivariate analysis)	Possible Related Factors
Smith and O'Rourke[25]	Years of education	Socioeconomic class, "white collar" job
	Physical requirements of job	"Blue collar" job, high job stress
	Severity of myocardial infarction	
	General health rating index	
Mark and colleagues[26]	Functional capacity	Self-efficacy
	Age	Career stage, financial disincentives
	Black race	Socioeconomic status
	Congestive heart failure	Self-efficacy, job requirements
Mittag and coworkers[27]	Age	May reflect situation in the labor market, employer attitudes
	Patient's perception of cardiac disability	Self-efficacy
	Physician's perception of vocational disability by overall medical condition	Self-efficacy
Samkange-Zeeb and others[28]	Age	Career stage
	Profession	
	Positive expectations concerning return to work	Self-efficacy
	Level of depression	
Mark and colleagues[26]	Predictive factor	Predictive value (%)
	Demographic and socioeconomic factors	45
	Physical and emotional measures	27
	Clinical variables	20

Table 144.3 Multivariate analysis of predictors of return to work.

WORK PERFORMANCE

Although consideration of strategies for work return and identification of predictive variables are important, equal attention is required for the quality of work return and work retention. Ellis and associates[29] defined work performance as "the physical, psychological and social functioning of an individual while at work." In a cross-sectional study, these researchers used a mail survey to evaluate 490 patients previously diagnosed with an acute coronary syndrome. They were evaluated over a 3-year period after the index event. More than 84% of the patients had worked longer than 1 year since the most recent cardiac event.

Perceived work performance was evaluated using the Work Performance Scale (WPS) of the Functional Status Questionnaire.[30] This particular cohort was primarily Caucasian, well educated, and had a higher socioeconomic status. About half the group rated their heart disease severity to be moderate to very severe. Findings showed that 84% of patients had a perceived high level of work performance. Symptom burden, perceived disease severity, age, time since the event, and physical function were most associated with work performance. Symptoms and physical parameters seem to have a stronger effect on perceived work performance than on predictors for work return.

Similar findings by Drory and associates[31] showed that early resumption of employment after an acute myocardial infarction is primarily a function of the sociodemographic and vocational characteristics of the person, as opposed to the specific medical condition. Long-term maintenance of work mainly is related to the medical condition.

Assessment for Licensing to Drive or Fly

Heart disease always has been associated with an unpredictable aspect, and this has challenged the authorities responsible for the public safety of roads and airways. Concern about sudden incapacitation haunts cardiac patients and their families and physicians, in addition to transportation policy workers. About 33% of myocardial infarctions are fatal, and 50% of patients who suffer a myocardial infarction die suddenly before reaching the hospital. The challenge is to identify these patients before they can put others in harm's way by operating a moving vehicle on the ground or in the air.

Case Presentation

Lee Wulff was a great guru of Atlantic salmon fishing. In fact, a famous salmon fly bears his name: the Royal Wulff. In his 80s, he still enjoyed flying around the Adirondack countryside in his Piper Super Cub, which he had owned for 30 years. However, one day Wulff did not return home. He was found crumpled up with his Piper Cub in his beloved Adirondack woods.

Should he have still been flying? Did he pose a risk to anyone but himself? How good is the mandatory annual medical examination in detecting heart disease? How accurate are existing techniques for assessing cardiac risk? What are the health and safety implications of a rapidly aging pilot population? These are questions that pertain to Lee Wulff and to anyone with a heart condition who assumes responsibility for heavy equipment that is set in motion in the public domain.

Other Cardiac Conditions: Implications for Licensing to Drive or Fly

Although problems relating to ischemia are most likely to evoke concern for commercial drivers and pilots, other conditions such as cardiomyopathy, hypertension, arrhythmias, and valvular and congenital heart disease raise issues that demand evaluation.

Treatment of hypertension with medications free of adverse side effects, such as hypotension, excessive somnolence, or untoward bradycardia, must be documented. A combination of potassium-sparing thiazide diuretics, beta blockers, long-acting calcium channel blockers, and angiotensin-converting enzyme inhibitors or angiotensin receptor blockers often suffices.

CARDIAC ARRHYTHMIAS AND FITNESS TO FLY	
Arrhythmia	**Response**
Premature atrial contractions or premature ventricular contractions	Report if symptomatic
Paroxysmal tachycardias	Report
Atrial flutter or atrial fibrillation	Report
Sinus node dysfunction	Report
Heart block and bundle branch block	Report if block is second or third degree
Pacemakers	Report
Cardioverter defibrillator	Unfit

Table 144.4 Cardiac arrhythmias and fitness to fly.

Cardiac arrhythmias cover a wide spectrum of risk, from the chronically benign to the capriciously malignant. The presence of structural heart disease and the likelihood of loss of consciousness dictate the degree of operator restriction (Table 144.4).

Valvular and congenital heart disease must be assessed individually. Recipients of prosthetic valves require periodic review because of the risk of thromboembolism, valve failure, and anticoagulant-induced bleeding. Congenital heart disease usually is assessed at the time of the initial application for licensing, but it may present with symptoms that mandate a report. Patients with cardiomyopathy must meet minimal left ventricular functional criteria, usually an ejection fraction greater than 50%. They also must demonstrate that they do not have potentially incapacitating ventricular arrhythmia.

Managing Risk: Identifying and Responding to Cardiac Patients

Licensing restrictions generally are predicated on the cardiac patient's perceived risk for sudden incapacitation and the consequences such incapacitation would have for the patient and others. The physician must balance the dual roles of advocate for the patient's individual human rights and protector of the public from potential harm. The most common tasks are assessing risk and determining the appropriateness of commercial drivers and pilots returning to work after myocardial infarction. Bus drivers and pilots face the greatest hurdle.[32] However, recent initiatives to abort evolving myocardial infarctions by prompt revascularization using thrombolytic agents or primary angioplasty have improved outcomes, with better ventricular function and less recurrent ischemia, leading to a more favorable prognosis.

Generally, the more severe the functional class of cardiac impairment, the greater the restriction. For example, patients with a New York Heart Association class IV impairment are prohibited from all driving. Those who have stable angina or New York Heart Association class II or III functional impairment are restricted to driving a private vehicle. Asymptomatic patients who have good exercise tolerance may drive any type of vehicle.[33] Patients with unstable angina or non-ST-elevation myocardial infarction (NSTEMI) may resume private driving as soon as 48 hours after successful coronary angioplasty; the requirement is 7 days for commercial drivers and 6 months for pilots in the absence of provocable ischemia by stress test.

Details about specific guidelines for assessing fitness to drive must be obtained from publications such as Determining Medical Fitness to Operate Motor Vehicles.[34] Guidelines for assessing cardiac patients with rhythm disturbances, valvular heart disease, or congenital heart disease are itemized in publications dedicated to this purpose.

Establishing the Acceptable Level of Risk

Regulations that govern the operation of a vehicle or aircraft tend to reflect the concern of society for tolerating risk to an innocent third party. This often defies logic. Risk-adverse citizens concerned about the perils of fluorinated water and nuclear power generation are more sanguine about the inevitable health hazards of smoking and alcohol consumption. With respect to cardiac patients on the road, it has been suggested that the accepted level of risk from a sudden incident amounts to 1 in 20,000 fatalities or injuries per driver-year. This extremely low risk is achieved when the probability of sudden cardiac incapacitation at any time during the year is 1% or less for commercial drivers and 20% or less for private drivers.[33]

A mathematical function attempts to estimate the risk of harm that results from a cardiac patient being granted a driver's license:

$$\text{Risk of harm} = T_o \times V \times SCI \times Ac$$

where T_o is the fraction of the day spent driving, V is the type of vehicle driven, SCI is the risk of a sudden cardiac incapacitation, and Ac is the probability that such an event will result in injury or fatality for a third party.

Using this type of model, it has been estimated that fewer than 0.2% of all road accidents are caused by sudden driver illness. Although 5% of sudden cardiac deaths occur while the individual is driving, the risk to a third party is very small, with fewer than 2% of these incidents resulting in injury or death for bystanders.[35]

Generally accepted guidelines permit a driver of a heavy vehicle to return to work 3 months after an acute myocardial infarction, provided that New York Heart Association functional class I activity has been achieved, with a negative stress test at 7 metabolic equivalent of task units (METs), and no disqualifying arrhythmias. Using the previous formula for calculating the risk of harm, such a driver would be associated with a risk of causing death or injury to others of approximately 1 in 20,000 over 1 year. This generally is acceptable. Interestingly, the expenditure to achieve public safety per quality-adjusted life-year saved far exceeds that deemed acceptable for more conventional medical treatment such as dialysis.

Fitness to Fly: the Pilot's Position

Greater rigor is brought to bear in assessing a pilot's fitness to fly because of the dependence of passengers on the welfare of the pilot. A high degree of international coordination of fitness criteria has been achieved under the aegis of the International Civil Aviation Organization and its affiliates. The pilot is responsible for grounding himself or herself, and the physician is responsible for reporting to an aviation medical adviser any medical condition that may compromise flight safety.

Heart problems are the second most common cause of incapacitation in flight. Commercial airline travel remains exceedingly safe, with less than 1 fatality per 1 million passengers each year[35]; this amounts to fewer than 25% of the traffic fatalities in the United Kingdom alone. An inverse relationship exists between the size of an aircraft and the accident rate. Private pilots have fatal accidents 10 to 20 times more often than professional airline transport pilots.

The likelihood of a serious accident resulting from sudden pilot incapacitation in the modern, highly automated, multicrew cockpit is virtually negligible. In more than 300 million flying hours, no fatalities to passengers in multicrew aircraft have occurred as a result of a pilot having a cardiovascular event.

In most jurisdictions, a pilot's license is not legal without an appropriate medical validation certificate. The frequency and standard of the aviation medical examination are determined by the type of license and the pilot's age.

The most consistent risk factor contributing to cardiac disqualification for medical validation to fly is advancing age. The cardiovascular mortality rate of a 65-year-old man is about 1% annually. This approximates to a rate of 1 event in 1 million flying hours. This 1% rule can be extrapolated to a medical-cause accident rate in multicrew operations of 1 incident in 100 million to 1 billion flying hours.[35] However, in the single-crew commercial environment, the 1% per year risk is considered too high, necessitating a license restricted to flying with a copilot.

Ironically, the benefits of medical screening are lost by middle age, as accumulating flying experience more than compensates for the increasing age-related medical hazard. This evokes an aphorism well known to all pilots: "There are old pilots and there are bold pilots, but there are no old, bold pilots."

Assessing and Controlling Cardiovascular Risk in the Pilot

In addition to the clinical history, physical examination, and compilation of cardiac risk factors, a routine resting electrocardiogram (ECG) is a required item of the pilot medical examination. Minor ST-segment and T-wave changes occur in 2% to 3% of pilots. Of these, fewer than 20% have an abnormal exercise ECG, and of these, only 33% have significant coronary disease at angiography.[36] Consequently, in keeping with Bayesian theory, the pretest likelihood of coronary disease in an apparently healthy aircrew is so low that an exercise ECG is likely to yield a false-positive and misleading result. Stress testing remains useful when special scrutiny is required, such as among those with suspected angina, multiple risk factors, or known coronary disease after a myocardial infarction or revascularization. However, an exercise ECG is not part of the routine examination for aircrews.

Establishing the level of risk and fitness to fly for those who have valvular or congenital heart disease, cardiomyopathy, dysrhythmias, or vascular disorders requires reference to a detailed manual of guidelines for assessing cardiovascular fitness to fly.

PREREQUISITES FOR PILOT RECERTIFICATION AFTER A CORONARY EVENT
■ Symptom: limited exercise electrocardiogram (ECG) to Bruce stage IV without ischemia; scintigraphy may be required to show absence of reversible ischemia
■ Left ventricular ejection fraction ≥50%
■ No significant arrhythmia by ambulatory monitoring
■ No stenosis >30% in a vessel that is remote from the infarct-related artery
■ Annual cardiologic follow-up with physiologic testing

Table 144.5 Prerequisites for pilot recertification after a coronary event.

Pilot Recertification after a Coronary Event

Unstable angina and acute myocardial infarction need not be the death knell for a pilot's flying career. Timely thrombolytic treatment or primary angioplasty quickly performed during a myocardial infarction can preserve substantial myocardium, resulting in a better ejection fraction and an improved prognosis. Revascularization by CABG surgery or coronary angioplasty and stenting can eliminate residual ischemia in many cases. A well-preserved left ventricle with an ejection fraction of at least 50% and an absence of ischemia on physiologic testing are two compelling recommendations that support unrestricted recertification after a suitable hiatus, usually 6 months.[37]

The interpretation of tests and written reports in support of pilot recertification (Table 144.5) requires deft judgment by the physician, who must find a balance between being the pilot's advocate and being a protector of public safety. Licensing issues for driving a vehicle or flying a plane should leave an important element of discretion with respect to the way the plethora of transportation rules and regulations that govern operator fitness are applied.

INSURABILITY OF THE CARDIAC PATIENT

In 2009, 1.2 million Americans will have a coronary attack; of these, more than one third will die. Heart attack, therefore, ranks as the United States' single leading cause of death.[7] Better prediction of outcome has enabled insurance companies to devise a more accurate risk assessment of applicants. This results in more equitable and less costly premiums for policy holders. Identification and control of risk factors such as hypertension, diabetes mellitus, hyperlipidemia, and smoking have improved access to insurance at more reasonable rates. The mortality rate from coronary heart disease has reduced by 50% between 1980 and 2000, and half of this decline has been attributed to better control of major risk factors.[38]

Risk can be usefully characterized by the mortality ratio, which is defined as the number of observed deaths over the number of expected deaths in a cohort of a certain age and gender within a defined period. A mortality ratio of 100% is standard, whereas 150% implies 50% more deaths than expected. Generally, companies do not insure anyone with a mortality ratio greater than 40% than expected. Actuarial tables relate mortality ratios to the number of expected deaths over an interval (e.g., 10 years) to determine the additional premium to be charged.

Insurance underwriters rely on standard prognostic indicators when assessing an applicant's insurability and calculating the premium. For example, poor left ventricular function or evidence of residual ischemia after a myocardial infarction signal a poor prognosis, and most insurance companies decline the risk in these cases. However, successful revascularization may improve the insurance rating, as may compliance with risk factor control and adherence to a prescribed rehabilitation program.

In summary, insurance companies demand access to all relevant clinical and laboratory information about an applicant with heart disease. They then apply a risk stratification strategy to determine the cardiac prognosis and the implications for insurability. The Orwellian prospect of genetic profiling to estimate the risk of coronary heart disease is on the horizon. The ethical implications of this technology for the insurability of susceptible individuals will be the topic of a vigorous public policy debate in the years to come.

ASSESSMENT FOR RETURN TO WORK

General Concepts

The physician plays a major role in determining whether a patient can return to work. The focus of an occupational work evaluation is to determine whether the cardiovascular demands produced by physical, psychological, and environmental stressors exceed the threshold for a safe working capacity. Three factors must be considered: the capability of the patient to perform the job; the risk involved in performing the job; and the risk to society if the patient performs the job.

Some patients should not return to work for medical or psychological reasons. Or, as Lewin[39] eloquently states, "Return to work is not necessarily the optimal outcome and is a rather naïve audit point; a contented pensioner may represent a better outcome than a frightened and unwilling company man." If, however, returning to work appears feasible, a proactive approach is required to reduce the risk factors for nonreturn. Patients who have not returned to work within 6 months of a myocardial infarction or coronary bypass surgery are unlikely to do so.[40] Conversely, if return to work is prescribed too early, before the patient is capable of managing the work demands, problems may occur (e.g., fatigue) that lead the patient to quit.

Assessment of the Job

Physical Requirements

The physician must have accurate information about the demands of the patient's job. Job titles generally provide little insight into the requirements of a position and may be misleading. The tasks that are performed on the job can be categorized in terms of metabolic cost as METs and found in tables that describe occupational activities in METs. This allows the work tasks to be compared with the individual's peak or symptom-limited functional capacity, as determined by a recent stress test. The current recommendation is that tasks performed regularly in an 8-hour working day should fall within the range of 25% to 40% of the maximum METs achieved on the stress test, and peak tasks performed occasionally should be no greater than the maximum METs.

The patient may be unable to provide all the information that pertains to the job. Therefore, a visit to the individual's work site facilitates a thorough assessment of the work environment, work culture, labor relations, and technologic processes.[41] This assessment may be performed in some settings by the cardiac rehabilitation staff.

Environmental Factors

Working conditions can include shift work, fumes, extremes of temperature, and low job control (Table 144.6). Shift work has been postulated to increase the risk of coronary heart disease[42] and can add to energy demands, particularly if the shifts are irregular. Workplace fumes should be considered; for example, exposure to carbon monoxide can result in the formation of carboxyhemoglobin, which reduces the oxygen-carrying capacity of the blood. Patients may experience angina with less effort when working in cold temperatures.[15] Hard work with an isometric component performed in a cold environment increases the risk of cardiovascular complications.[43,44] Working in hot conditions causes the heart rate and myocardial oxygen consumption to increase disproportionately to keep up with increasing metabolic demands.[45]

If low job control or an imbalance between personal efforts and rewards (or both) is a factor, the risk of coronary heart disease is increased.[46] Earlier literature suggested that high job demands were damaging; however, recent findings indicate that low job control is a requisite cofactor. Aboa-Eboulé and coworkers[47] demonstrated that the risk of a recurrent coronary event after a first MI was greater if the individual experienced chronic job strain. Job strain was defined as high psychological demands and low decision latitude.

Employer Issues

Employers must be reassured that a patient who has cardiovascular disease can resume work with a manageable risk of adverse sequelae. Froom and colleagues[48] showed that individuals attempting to resume employment had a 1.2% risk of having an ischemic event at work. Employers usually resist modifying jobs; however, medical persuasion might allow a graduated return to full duties and hours of work. Continuing contact between the employer and employee can facilitate the patient's return to work; failure of an employer to contact an employee is demoralizing and can inhibit return to work.[49] Social support from supervisors tends to reduce the risk of early retirement caused by disability.[50]

Assessment of the Patient

Exercise Capacity

It is axiomatic that vocational tasks should not exceed the functional capacity of the patient or provoke untoward cardiovascular symptomatology (e.g., ischemia or arrhythmias). A patient's current exercise capacity can be estimated by functional scales, such as the Duke Activity Scale.[51] However, such functional scales may be misleading, because they do not ascertain peak capacity, blood pressure response, or signs or symptoms of ischemia. Some patients are evaluated while they are at work, undergoing Holter monitoring to

EFFECTS OF CHEMICAL AND PHYSICAL AGENTS ON THE CARDIOVASCULAR SYSTEM		
Agent	**Mechanism**	**Effects**
Carbon monoxide	Carboxyhemoglobin	Reduced tolerance to exercise Earlier-onset angina Increased vulnerability to cardiac arrhythmias
Metal and metalloids		
Cobalt	Nephrosclerosis	Dilated cardiomyopathy
Mercury	Arteriolar vasoconstriction	Hypertension
Cadmium		Renal hypertension
Lead		Hypertension
Nitrates	Absorption through respiratory system and skin Excessive nitrate absorption Withdrawal	Vasodilatation, orthostatic hypotension Coronary vasospasm Sensitization to epinephrine (adrenaline)
Organic solvents		
Freon Chlorinated hydrocarbons	Cardiac sensitization to epinephrine, decreased inotropism, suppressed sinus and atrioventricular (AV) nodes	Arrhythmias Arrhythmias
Heat	Shunting of blood from core to periphery	At >75° F (24° C), increased heart rate response of 1 beat per minute (bpm) per degree (C) increase in temperature; with exercise, a heart rate response of 2-4 bpm per degree (C) increase in temperature
	Loss of electrolytes (through sweating)	Possible arrhythmia
Cold	Reflex vasoconstriction of the coronary arteries	Lowered ischemic threshold Decreased workload
Noise	Activation of the autonomic nervous system	Increased heart rate and blood pressure at all workloads

Table 144.6 Effects of chemical and physical agents on the cardiovascular system.

record the heart rate response to various tasks. The implicit assumption is that the heart rate response seen on the Holter recordings serves as proxy for the workload and that any untoward effects (e.g., ischemia) will be detected. It is important to note that the chronotropic response may increase as a result of demands that are unrelated to exercise-related demands (e.g., stress).

Most cardiac patients have a stress test as part of their evaluation. The exercise capacity, in terms of oxygen uptake, may be estimated from the time on the treadmill (Table 144.7). The functional capacity is the oxygen uptake achieved before any signs of ischemia or arrhythmias. The Bruce protocol is ideal for unmasking ischemic changes; however, the estimated oxygen uptake may be in error by as much as 1 MET (1 MET is equivalent to 3.5 mL/kg/min). Exercise protocols with smaller increments (e.g., the Balke protocol) more closely approximate measured oxygen uptakes. The gold standard is the cardiopulmonary test using a metabolic cart. This test can assess whether a maximal effort has been performed, detect any respiratory abnormalities, and determine the workload equivalent to the anaerobic threshold (i.e., the threshold above which prolonged work cannot be maintained).

Other Medical Conditions

Other medical problems may have an adverse effect on a successful return to work. Some conditions that predated the cardiac event may have changed. For example, a patient with chronic lung disease and mild shortness of breath may become more dyspneic, with superimposed left ventricular dysfunction. A number of musculoskeletal, neurologic, or psychological problems may result from CABG surgery.

Work Simulation

The myocardial oxygen requirements for any task may be increased by factors unique to the job, such as superimposed mental stressors, environmental conditions, or mechanical factors. The estimated work capacity from the stress test (using the leg musculature) may not easily translate to arm work, which provokes greater myocardial oxygen demands. If necessary, simulated tasks can approximate actual working conditions and can include lifting, stacking, and carrying (Table 144.8). During the simulation, the myocardial oxygen demands can be estimated from the heart rate and blood pressure response, and any untoward aspects can be recorded.

Work simulation may be appropriate for individuals with a reduced functional capacity (<7 METs) with left ventricle dysfunction who perform work with regular isometric demands.

CASE STUDY

A 50-year-old man complained of shortness of breath and fatigue during work. He was employed as a framing carpenter, a job that required arm work above his head for extended periods (Fig. 144.1). These particular vocational activities provoked most of the symptoms. An echocardiogram at rest showed the presence of mild aortic valve disease that was presumed to be attributable to a congenital bicuspid valve. The maximum gradient was 34 mm Hg, with a mean gradient of 21 mm Hg. He was able to perform 9 minutes on the Bruce protocol with no symptoms, ischemia, or arrhythmias, and nuclear images showed normal ventricular functioning and no perfusion defects.

As the patient's medical condition deteriorated, a work simulation was performed using arm weights to replicate his duties in the work setting. After 2 minutes, he developed dyspnea, and the peak gradient at that time was greater than 90 mm Hg. He subsequently had aortic valve replacement and now is asymptomatic.

Thus a work simulation was able to expose the underlying pathophysiology.

TREATMENT STRATEGIES FOR THE INDIVIDUAL PATIENT

Table 144.9 summarizes strategies that can be used to optimize the likelihood that a patient will return to work.

Increased Exercise Capacity

One of the most efficacious modalities of improving vocational capacity is exercise training. Exercise training includes aerobic training, strength training, and flexibility improvement. Improvement in peak exercise capacity, as determined by peak oxygen consumption, depends on many variables, but it generally can improve from 11% to 56% (mean, 26%)[52] with an exercise program that lasts at least 3 months.

An effective training regimen increases the efficiency with which external work can be performed. Therefore, any particular task can be performed with a reduced heart rate and blood pressure response (and hence a reduced myocardial oxygen demand). This can improve exercise-related myocardial ischemia and allow the patient to accomplish greater external workloads before exceeding the ischemic threshold. Reductions in the ischemic burden by 34% to 54%[53] have been determined by thallium perfusion scans. A strengthening program has been shown to reduce the mean blood pressure response by 17% and the mean heart rate response by 15% in men lifting the same absolute weight.[54] Mittleman and associates[55] have shown that regular exercise, with an intensity of at least 6 METs, is protective against myocardial infarction that may be precipitated by intense physical activity or anger.

Specificity of training in exercise physiology relates to the selective training effect of the exercising musculature, with the lack of effect in the untrained portion. Thus, a cardiac patient whose only aerobic activity is walking derives little benefit for arm activities. In a similar way, vocational counselors can arrange for a work-hardening program, such that the actual job elements are performed either in a rehabilitation setting or in a reduced capacity at work. As the patient acclimates to the job requirements, work hours or job tasks can be added until it is appropriate to resume the complete job.

Most cardiac patients benefit by pursuing an exercise training program within a formalized cardiac rehabilitation program.[56] Such programs provide advice, training, and support for individuals, many of whom are deconditioned and possibly fearful of pursuing an exercise program. Participation in a 12-month cardiac rehabilitation program has demonstrated an earlier return to work and an improved vocational status at 5-year follow-up.[57] Mital and others[58] showed that

METS CORRELATED WITH TIME IN THE BRUCE PROTOCOL						
				METs Requirement		
Stage	MPH	Grade	Min	Men	Women	
I	1.7	10%	1	3.2	3.1	3.6
			2	4.0	3.9	4.3
			3	4.9	4.7	4.9
II	2.5	12%	4	5.7	5.4	5.6
			5	6.6	6.2	6.2
			6	7.4	7.0	7.0
III	3.4	14%	7	8.3	8.0	7.6
			8	9.1	8.6	8.3
			9	10.0	9.4	9.0
IV	4.2	16%	10	10.7	10.1	9.7
			11	11.6	10.9	10.4
			12	12.5	11.7	11.0
V	5.0	18%	13	13.3	12.5	11.7
			14	14.1	13.2	12.3
			15	15.0	14.1	13.0

METs, metabolic equivalent of task units.

Table 144.7 METs correlated with time in the Bruce protocol. (Data from ACSM. Guidelines for exercise testing and prescription. 4th edition. Lea and Febiger, 1991:60.)

individuals who participate in a cardiac rehabilitation exercise program that contained real elements of their work had an increased likelihood of returning to the same job they held before the myocardial infarction.

DESIGNING A WEIGHT-LIFTING AND WEIGHT-CARRYING WORK SIMULATION TEST

The following information should be obtained from the patient or observed at the work site.

- The type of weight lifting performed in the workplace
- Is the object lifted and stacked?
- Is the object lifted and carried?
- Is the object lifted and held?
- The differing amounts of weight that are lifted
- How the object is lifted and carried
- Is the object carried with one arm?
- Is the object lifted and carried on one shoulder?
- Is the object held against the body?
- The amount of time for each lifting episode and the rest period between lifting episodes
- The position of the object before it is lifted and after it has been put down
- Is the object at floor level?
- Is the object at waist height?
- Is the object above the shoulders?

In addition, the following should be done:

1. Blood pressure should be taken in the nonexercising arm immediately before the weight is lifted and just before it is released.
2. Continuous electrocardiographic (ECG) monitoring should be performed.
3. The patient should lift weights with no warm-up and at a rate that would be followed in the workplace (i.e., self-determined).

Table 144.8 Designing a weight-lifting and weight-carrying work simulation test.

Decreased Risk

All patients with ischemic cardiac disease require aggressive risk factor modification for optimal secondary prevention. The control of risk factors improves the prognosis, but it also presumably stabilizes the fibrous plaque, preventing acute rupture. Increased cholesterol concentrations predispose patients to rupture of vulnerable plaques, and cigarette

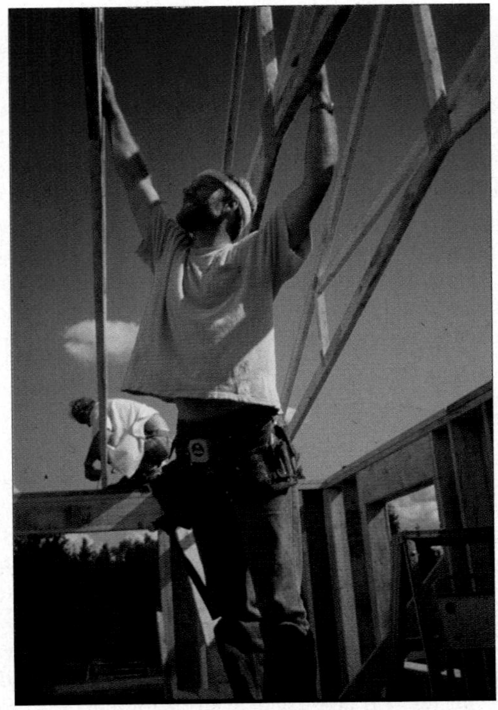

Figure 144.1 The patient at work as a framing carpenter.

INDIVIDUAL STRATEGIES FOR IMPROVING RETURN TO WORK		
Strategy	**Modality**	**Anticipated Outcome**
Increase exercise capacity	Aerobic training Strength training Flexibility Task-specific training ("work hardening")	Enhanced external workloads Decreased myocardial demands for similar external workload Higher workloads accomplished before onset of ischemia
Optimal risk factor control	Exercise, diet, smoking cessation, hypertension control, lipid management	Decreased risk of work-related adverse cardiac outcome
Stress management	One-on-one or group	May reduce cardiovascular risk on returning to work
	Specific modification of work-related stressors	Enhanced likelihood of returning to work
Family issues	Involvement in all aspects of the return to work process	Enhanced likelihood of returning to work and compliance for other strategies

Table 144.9 Individual strategies for improving return to work.

smoking predisposes them to an acute thrombosis.[59] A post-mortem study of men with hypercholesterolemia who had died suddenly during physical exertion suggested the cause to be rupture of vulnerable plaques.[60] Left ventricular hypertrophy in hypertensive patients is associated with plaque rupture that may result in sudden cardiac death.[61] Aggressive lipid lowering can result in a marked decrease in ischemia, as detected by ambulatory Holter monitoring.[62,63]

Self-Perception and Stress Management

A patient's self-efficacy or belief system is a key determinant of return to work. It is important to ascertain these perceptions so that any misperceptions can be corrected. Petrie and colleagues[64] used such a therapeutic approach for MI patients seen in the hospital to alter the patients' inaccurate perceptions. The interventional group was assessed by the Illness Perception Questionnaire. They then took part in specific sessions at which the pathophysiology of an MI, the distinction of cardiac and noncardiac symptoms, plans for minimizing future risk, and an action plan for recovery were explained. The control group received the usual in-patient education. Compared with the controls, the intervention group developed significant positive views for coping with the MI, reported less angina and, an important factor, had an earlier return to work.

Patients often consider the perceived stress of a job as either a causative factor in their cardiac disease or a factor that prevents them from returning to work. Stress can be described as "excessive environmental demands combined with inadequate coping resources, yielding the presence of emotional distress or characteristic patterns of maladaptive behaviors, or both."[65] Recent studies have indicated that low work control, not high work demands, put workers at greater relative risk of cardiovascular mortality,[66] with a 43% increase in the chance of death if the individuals has worked in low-control jobs throughout his or her working life.[67] Stress management programs, through either individual counseling or group efforts, are beneficial.

Treatment of Depression

Depression requires treatment, because it is known to increase the chances of further cardiovascular events and negatively affect the likelihood of an individual returning to work. Brisson and colleagues[68] showed that psychological distress was more prevalent in individuals who had returned to work than in the general working population, particularly among women. Wang and coworkers[69] and others have found that effective treatment can improve workplace outcomes. They showed that overall work functioning improved by 2.6 hours per week through a combination of greater job retention and more hours worked.

Family Issues

The individual's return to work affects the entire family, and the family ideally should be involved in the decision making. Overprotection can inhibit return to work; however, too much support seems preferable to not enough support.[20]

SUMMARY

Work can be one of the most important factors for the cardiac patient. For some, unemployment leads to adverse health; for others, the resumption of work may be equally deleterious. The economic burden of unemployment and disability accounts for a significant portion of the health care costs attributable to cardiovascular disease. Return to work rates are remarkably similar across various diagnostic groups and have changed little over the past decade.

The factors that influence return to work are predominantly demographic and socioeconomic, followed by physical and emotional measures, and then by clinical variables. Multivariate analyses appear to indicate that years of education, functional status, perception of health, and the severity of the medical condition are the most powerful predictors.

The treating physician plays a key role in the process of return to work. While the patient is in the hospital, his or her self-perceptions with regard to return to work can be determined. Categorizing the probability of return to work, as follows, may be helpful:

- No return to work: Return is contraindicated because of impaired medical status, or the individual elects to retire and has adequate finances.

- Possible return to work: The medical risk is acceptable, but significant barriers to return to work exist.
- Probable return to work: The medical risk is acceptable, but some barriers may prevent or delay a return to work.
- Definite return to work: Work poses an acceptable medical risk. The patient has high self-efficacy, derives considerable satisfaction from the job, or must return to work for financial reasons.

The assessment for returning to work should include the patient's capability to perform the job mentally and physically and the risk of an untoward event either for the patient or for society after the return to work. Risk determination is particularly important if the patient is to resume driving or flying. The physician must balance carefully the patient's human rights against the public's right to protection from harm.

The assessment for returning to work should include an assessment of the physical requirements of the job, any superimposed environmental factors that may augment work demands, and any employer issues that need to be addressed. The individual's physical capacity can be ascertained with a stress test or a work simulation to mimic job requirements. Patients should reach their optimal physical capacity by exercise training, both aerobic and strength training, and ideally this can be accomplished through a cardiac rehabilitation program. Vocational stressors should be addressed, either through one-on-one counseling or through a stress management program. Optimal risk factor control can both minimize ischemia and reduce the risk of untoward events. The family should be involved in all aspects of the process. A vocational counselor or cardiac rehabilitation team, or both, can help with all these factors.

chapter 145

Anticoagulation in Heart Disease

Rangadham Nagarakanti, Binu Malhotra, Abhay J. Dhond, Pavlo I. Netrebko, and Michael D. Ezekowitz

Anticoagulation is indicated in several common cardiac conditions. The number of patients requiring anticoagulation therapy is rising steadily in an aging population with an increased prevalence of atrial fibrillation (AF), congestive heart failure (CHF), and survivors of acute myocardial infarction (MI).

This chapter describes emerging and commonly used drugs for anticoagulation, their mechanisms of action, clinical indications, and side effects. The uses of anticoagulant therapy are described, consistent with current guidelines established by the American College of Chest Physicians (Tables 145.1 to 145.5).

UNFRACTIONATED HEPARIN

Unfractionated heparin (UFH) consists of a heterogeneous group of negatively charged, highly sulfated glycosaminoglycan molecules of different sizes and structures. The overall molecular weight ranges from 5 to 30 kDa (mean, 15 kDa).[1]

Mechanism of Action

Unfractionated heparin mediates its anticoagulant effect through a unique pentasaccharide sequence that binds to and catalyzes antithrombin III (AT-III). Thrombin (factor II) and factor Xa are the most sensitive to inactivation by the antithrombin-heparin complex. Heparin increases vessel wall permeability and inhibits platelet function, independent of its anticoagulant activity, by inhibiting thrombin generation on the platelet surface through inhibition of factor Va. UFH shows very high nonspecific protein binding, which explains its low bioavailability, nonlinear anticoagulation effect, and the need for a loading dose and monitoring of therapy.[2]

Heparin must be administered by intravenous or subcutaneous injection. Intramuscular injection is contraindicated because of the danger of producing large hematomas by accidental puncture of an intramuscular blood vessel. Heparin therapy is monitored by the activated partial thromboplastin time (aPTT). Maintaining the aPTT ratio above 1.5 is associated with protection against thrombosis. The intravenous route is preferred when rapid anticoagulation is indicated.[3] Weight-based dosing nomograms are recommended, because they have been shown to reduce recurrent thromboembolism and bleeding complications. An example of a weight-based nomogram for intravenous treatment of venous thromboembolism is presented in Table 145.6. When the subcutaneous route is used for therapeutic anticoagulation, an initial heparin dosage of 17,500 U given every 12 hours is suggested.

Increased procoagulant activity in pregnancy, malignancy, acute thrombosis, and major surgery may be associated with heparin resistance (i.e., a need for heparin doses greater than 35,000 U every 24 hours to maintain the therapeutic aPTT).

Indications

Heparin is indicated for prophylaxis and treatment of venous thromboembolism (VTE), including pulmonary embolism (PE); as well as treatment of unstable angina (UA), acute MI (with or without thrombolytic therapy); and during cardiac procedures (coronary angioplasty, stent placement, and cardiopulmonary bypass). In addition, heparin may be used to initiate chronic anticoagulation therapy until warfarin reaches the desired therapeutic level. Heparin also is the preferred agent for anticoagulation during all trimesters of pregnancy.[2]

Heparin reduces mortality and reinfarction rates in acute coronary syndrome.[4] Treatment with heparin and aspirin during the acute phase of unstable angina reduces death and infarction rates better than aspirin alone.

In ST-elevation myocardial infarction (STEMI), careful, weight-adjusted dosing of unfractionated heparin in conjunction with thrombolytics confers a mortality benefit.[5] The most recent studies compared low-molecular-weight heparin (LMWH) and UFH to determine the equivalent efficacy of the two agents, and some practical advantages were seen with the use of LMWH.[6]

During coronary angioplasty and stenting, intravenous heparin in higher doses is used. If percutaneous coronary intervention (PCI) is attempted with anti-Gp IIb/IIIa coverage, the dose of heparin must be reduced. Details on the treatment of acute coronary conditions are presented in Chapter 28 and 29.

In cases of heparin resistance, when dosages greater than 35,000 U every 24 hours are required, anti-Xa levels, rather than the aPTT, should be used for dosage correction. Maintenance of the anti-Xa level at 0.35 to 0.7 IU/mL provides adequate anticoagulation and leads to a significantly lower heparin dose.[7]

Complications

Bleeding

Heparin may induce bleeding by inhibiting blood coagulation, by impairing platelet function, and by increasing capillary permeability. Variables that influence bleeding include the dose of heparin, the mode of heparin administration, and patient factors, such as concurrent illness, concurrent medications (e.g., aspirin), age, gender, renal failure, poor blood pressure control (with an increased risk for

RECOMMENDATIONS FOR ANTICOAGULATION IN CHRONIC STABLE CORONARY ARTERY DISEASE*
1. For all patients with chronic stable coronary artery disease (CAD), aspirin, 75 to 160 mg PO daily, is recommended. It should be continued indefinitely. 2. If the risk profile of the chronic coronary disease indicates a high likelihood of acute myocardial infarction (MI), long-term therapy with clopidogrel in addition to aspirin is recommended. 3. Chronic CAD without a previous MI is *not* an indication for anticoagulation.
From Harrington RA, Becker RC, Ezekowitz M, et al. Antithrombotic agents in coronary artery disease. Chest 2004;126:513S-548S. *From American College of Chest Physicians (CCP) guidelines on anticoagulation in CAD.

Table 145.1A Recommendations for anticoagulation in chronic stable coronary artery disease.

RECOMMENDATIONS FOR PRIMARY PREVENTION OF CORONARY ARTERY DISEASE*
1. Patients with at least a moderate risk for a coronary event (based on age and risk factor profile with a 10-year risk of a cardiac event >10%) should take aspirin, 75 to 162 mg PO daily, over no antithrombotic therapy or a vitamin K antagonist (grade 2A). 2. Patients at a particularly high risk of a coronary event, in whom the international normalized ratio (INR) can be monitored without difficulty, should be given a low dose of a vitamin K antagonist, with a target INR of 1.5 (grade 2A).
From Harrington RA, Becker RC, Ezekowitz M, et al. Antithrombotic agents in coronary artery disease. Chest 2004;126:513S-548S. *American College of Chest Physicians (ACCP) guidelines for primary prevention of CAD.

Table 145.1B Recommendations for primary prevention of coronary artery disease.

intracerebral bleeding), and chronic alcohol abuse. Aspirin increases operative and postoperative bleeding in patients who receive the very high doses of heparin that are required during open heart surgery. However, the benefits of the combination of aspirin and heparin outweigh the risk in treatment of acute coronary syndromes.[8]

Hemorrhagic complications during intravenous heparin infusion are managed by stopping the infusion. The half-life of the intravenous therapeutic dose of heparin is approximately 30 to 60 minutes. With cessation of therapy, the anticoagulant effect is rapidly lost. In the case of a heparin overdose or life-threatening bleeding, the heparin effect may need to be reversed more rapidly with protamine sulfate. The dose of protamine sulfate is determined by the concentration of circulating heparin, which in turn depends on the dose of heparin administered and the time elapsed since the last heparin dose. The full neutralizing dose is 1 mg of protamine sulfate for every 100 U of heparin; the dose must be reduced to one half at 1 hour and to one quarter at 2 hours after stopping the heparin. The maximum dose should not exceed 50 mg. Caution must be exercised, because an overdose of protamine sulfate induces bleeding and paradoxically increases the activated clotting time (ACT). Also, the benefits of protamine use should be carefully weighed against

RECOMMENDATIONS FOR ANTITHROMBOTIC THERAPY IN PATIENTS WITH NON-ST-ELEVATION MYOCARDIAL INFARCTION AND ACUTE CORONARY SYNDROME*
1. Aspirin in initial dose of 160 to 325 mg, then 75 to 162 mg orally daily indefinitely (grade 1A). 2. Patients with aspirin-induced bleeding should receive lower doses of aspirin: <100 mg orally daily (grade 1C+). 3. Patients intolerant to aspirin should receive clopidogrel: 300-mg bolus, followed by 75 mg orally daily indefinitely (grade 1A). 4. In patients in whom diagnostic catheterization will be delayed or coronary artery bypass grafting (CABG) is not planned for at least 5 days: clopidogrel bolus, 300 mg, followed by 75 mg orally daily, in addition to aspirin for 9 to 12 months. 5. In patients with non-ST-elevation myocardial infarction (NSTEMI) in whom angiography is planned within 24 hours: clopidogrel should be given only after the coronary anatomy has been determined. 6. In patients with NSTEMI: low-molecular-weight heparin (LMWH) administered subcutaneously is recommended over unfractionated heparin (UFH) administered intravenously for acute management (grade 1B), and heparin is recommended over no heparin. 7. In patients at moderate to high risk with non-ST-elevation acute coronary syndrome: glycoprotein (Gp) IIb/IIIa inhibitors (eptifibatide, tirofiban) administered intravenously are recommended in addition to aspirin and heparin (grade 1 A). This therapy also is used in high-risk patients who also are receiving clopidogrel. 8. Abciximab administered intravenously is used as an initial treatment only when the coronary anatomy is known and percutaneous coronary intervention (PCI) is planned within the next 24 hours.
From Harrington RA, Becker RC, Ezekowitz M, et al. Antithrombotic agents in coronary artery disease. Chest 2004;126:513S-548S. *American College of Chest Physicians (ACCP) guidelines for use of antithrombotics in non-ST-elevation myocardial infarction.

Table 145.2 Recommendations for antithrombotic therapy in patients with non-ST-elevation myocardial infarction and acute coronary syndrome.

potential complications, which include hemodynamic "protamine reactions" (systemic hypotension and pulmonary hypertension), noncardiogenic pulmonary edema, and allergic and anaphylactoid reactions. Protamine should be infused over 10 minutes to prevent hypotension. Administration may need to be repeated because of its rapid clearance. Smaller repeated doses of protamine are required to reverse therapeutic doses of subcutaneous heparin.[2,8]

Heparin-Induced Thrombocytopenia

Heparin-induced thrombocytopenia (HIT) is caused by an IgG–heparin–platelet factor 4 immune complex. The incidence of HIT is approximately 3% to 5% but may vary widely with the type of preparation, dose, duration, and route of therapy. HIT is a diagnosis based on clinical and serologic features. It should be suspected in the event of an unexplained fall in the platelet count greater than 50%, skin lesions at injection sites, or venous thromboses. HIT is less common in patients treated with LMWHs than in those treated with UFH.

Arterial thrombosis may occur as a complication of HIT in up to 30% of affected patients. Thrombocytopenia usually begins 3 to 10 days after the start of heparin therapy; however,

RECOMMENDATIONS FOR ANTIPLATELET AND ANTICOAGULATION THERAPY IN ST-ELEVATION MYOCARDIAL INFARCTION WITH THROMBOLYSIS*
1. Patients with acute ST-elevation myocardial infarction (STEMI), irrespective of fibrinolytic therapy, should receive aspirin, 160 to 325 mg PO, followed by indefinite therapy with 75 to 162 mg PO orally daily. 2. Patients allergic to aspirin should receive clopidogrel at a loading dose of 75 mg and then a maintenance dose of 75 mg daily (grade 2C). 3. Intravenous heparin bolus, followed by a drip to target a partial thromboplastin time (PTT) of 50 to 75 sec (grade 2A). 4. Patients with normal renal function younger than age 75: low-molecular-weight heparin (LMWH) is administered subcutaneously with tenecteplase intravenously for 7 days (grade 2B). 5. Glycoprotien (Gp) IIb/IIIa inhibitors are not recommended with thrombolysis. 6. Direct thrombin inhibitors are not recommended with thrombolysis.
From Menon V, Harrington R, Hochman J, et al. Thrombolysis and adjunctive therapy in acute myocardial infarction. Chest 2004;126:549S-575S. *American College of Chest Physicians (ACCP) guidelines for treatment of ST-elevation myocardial infarction with thrombolysis.

Table 145.3 Recommendations for antiplatelet and anticoagulation therapy in ST-elevation myocardial infarction with thrombolysis.

in patients previously exposed to the drug, it has been reported within hours of the start of heparin therapy. If arterial thrombosis develops, heparin should be stopped and treatment with alternative antithrombotic agents, such as danaparoid, lepirudin (recombinant hirudin), or argatroban, should be started if continued anticoagulation is needed or if HIT-associated thrombosis develops.[8-10] The platelet count usually returns to baseline levels within 4 days of stopping heparin. Warfarin should not be used alone while HIT-induced thrombosis is treated because of the risk of warfarin-associated venous thrombosis and limb gangrene. Although LMWHs are contraindicated in the treatment of HIT because of cross-reactivity, danaparoid has been used successfully for this indication.[9,10] (NOTE: Danaparoid is not available in the United States.)

Other Side Effects

Heparin-induced osteoporosis is seen in patients who receive moderately high doses of heparin (>20,000 U every 24 hour) for longer than 1 to 3 months. Adverse cutaneous reactions to heparin include three distinct types of skin lesions: urticarial lesions, erythematous papules and plaques, and skin necrosis. Urticarial lesions occur at the site of subcutaneous injection and may be caused by a contaminant in the heparin preparation. Changing to a different salt or heparin of a different animal origin may be beneficial.

Skin necrosis is the most serious complication of heparin. A less severe form presents as erythematous papules and plaques. Skin necrosis usually occurs as a complication of subcutaneous heparin, but it also has been observed in association with the intravenous route of administration. These lesions usually develop after 5 days or more of therapy. Skin necrosis seems to be unrelated to the source of the heparin; therefore, treatment with alternative antithrombotic agents, such as danaparoid, r-hirudin, or argatroban, is indicated. Other reported complications include generalized hypersensitivity

RECOMMENDATIONS FOR ANTICOAGULATION WITH PROSTHETIC HEART VALVES*
Mechanical Heart Valves 1. Patients with mechanical valves must receive a vitamin K antagonist for anticoagulation. Unfractionated heparin (UFH) should be used concomitantly until the international normalized ratio (INR) is therapeutic for 2 consecutive days. ■ St. Jude valve in the aortic position: target INR = 2.5. ■ Tilting disk valve and bileaflet mechanical valves in the mitral position: target INR = 3 (range, 2.5-3.5). ■ Cage-disk or ball-cage valves: target INR = 3, in combination with 75 to 100 mg of aspirin daily. ■ Carbomedics bileaflet valve or Medtronic Hall tilting disk mechanical valves in the aortic position, normal left atrial (LA) size and sinus rhythm: target INR = 2.5. ■ Mechanical valves and additional risk factors (e.g., atrial fibrillation, myocardial infarction, LA enlargement, low ejection fraction): target INR = 3, in combination with low-dose aspirin. 2. If a patient with mechanical heart valves suffers systemic embolism despite a therapeutic INR, a combination of low-dose aspirin and an INR of 3 is recommended. **Bioprosthetic Heart Valves** *First 3 Months* 1. Bioprosthetic valves in the mitral position: vitamin K antagonist, with target INR of 2.5, for the first 3 months. 2. Bioprosthetic valves in the aortic position: vitamin K antagonist, with a target INR of 2.5, or aspirin for the first 3 months. 3. Bioprosthetic valves and a history of systemic embolism: vitamin K antagonist for 3 to 12 months. 4. Bioprosthetic valves and left atrial thrombus at surgery: vitamin K antagonist life long or until thrombus disappears. *Long-Term Treatment* 1. Bioprosthetic valves and atrial fibrillation: long-term anticoagulation with a vitamin K antagonist. 2. Bioprosthetic valves, patient in sinus rhythm: may be maintained on long-term aspirin.
From Salem DN, Stein PD, Ahmad AA, et al. Antithrombotic therapy in patients with valvular heart disease: native and prosthetic. Chest 2004;126:457S-482S. *American College of Chest Physicians (ACCP) guidelines for anticoagulation in patients with prosthetic heart valves.

Table 145.4 Recommendations for anticoagulation with prosthetic heart valves.

GUIDELINES FOR ANTICOAGULATION IN PATIENTS WITH ATRIAL FIBRILLATION*		
Age (yr)	**Risk Factors†**	**Recommendations**
>75	Present/absent	Warfarin (target INR, 2-3)
65-75	Absent	Either aspirin or warfarin (target INR, 2-3)
	Present	Warfarin (target INR, 2-3)
<65	Absent	Aspirin 325 mg/day
	Present	Warfarin (target INR, 2-3)

From Singer DE, Albers G, Dalen J, Go S, Halperin J, Manning W. Antithrombotic therapy in atrial fibrillation. Chest 2004;126:429S-456S.
*American College of Chest Physicians (ACCP) 2004 guidelines.
†Risk factors include age older than 75 years, hypertension, diabetes, congestive heart failure or left ventricular systolic dysfunction, and a history of a previous transient ischemic attack or stroke.

Table 145.5 Guidelines for anticoagulation in patients with atrial fibrillation.

INTRAVENOUS HEPARIN PROTOCO				
aPTT (seconds)	**Repeat Bolus (U/kg)**	**Stop Infusion (min)**	**Change Infusion (U/kg/h)**	**Next aPTT (h)**
<35 (<1.2 × control)	80	0	Increase by 4	6
35-45 (1.2-1.5 × control)	40	0	Increase by 2	6
46-70 (1.5-2.3 × control)	0	0	0	Next AM
71-90 (2.3-3.0 × control)	0	0	Decrease by 2	6
>90 (>3 × control)	0	60	Decrease by 3	6

Modified from Raschke RA, Reilly BM, Guidry JR, et al. The weight-based heparin dosing nomogram compared with a "standard care" nomogram. A randomized controlled trial. Ann Intern Med 1993;119(a):874-881.

Table 145.6 Intravenous heparin protocol. Initial intravenous (IV) heparin bolus, 80 U/kg body weight; maintenance IV heparin infusion at 18 U/kg/h; activated partial thromboplastin time (aPTT) after 6 hours of initial bolus and adjust IV heparin as shown.

reactions, anaphylactic shock, heparin-induced hypoaldosteronism, priapism, and bilateral adrenal hemorrhagic necrosis.[2]

LOW-MOLECULAR-WEIGHT HEPARINS

LMWHs are smaller heparin molecules derived from unfractionated heparin by chemical or enzymatic depolymerization. They have a mean molecular weight of 4 to 6 kDa (range, 1 to 10 kDa). LMWHs produce their anticoagulant effect by binding to AT-III through the same unique pentasaccharide sequence as UFH. However, because of the smaller molecular size of the LMWHs, the resulting complex has reduced binding to thrombin and a higher anti-Xa to anti-IIa activity ratio. Low nonspecific binding results in better bioavailability and a more predictable anticoagulant response. Low nonspecific binding and predominant clearance through nonsaturable renal mechanisms provide a longer half-life. A half-life of 4 to 5 hours allows for once or twice a day subcutaneous dosing.

Routine monitoring of LMWH therapy is not required because monitoring does not offer any clinical benefits over weight-adjusted dosing,[11] a significant advantage over UFH. Monitoring is recommended in cases of renal insufficiency, morbid obesity, and prolonged therapy (months) and in newborns.[12] Because of the LMWHs' weak effect on thrombin, aPTT values are not an accurate measure of their anticoagulation efficacy; instead, the peak anti-Xa activity should be measured at 4 hours after subcutaneous injection.

The therapeutic range is 0.6 to 1.0 IU/mL (international anti-Xa units) for twice a day dosing and 1.0 to 2.0 IU/mL for once a day dosing.

The side effect profile of LMWHs has several advantages over UFH. The decreased affinity for platelets leads to a lower incidence of HIT. However, LMWHs cross-react with HIT antibodies and are contraindicated in patients with a previous history of HIT. LMWHs are associated with a lower incidence of osteoporosis than is seen with UFH.

LMWHs tend to produce fewer hemorrhagic complications than UFH when used in patients with deep venous thrombosis (DVT), pulmonary embolism, and acute coronary syndromes and, most recently, in conjunction with thrombolysis in patients with STEMI.[2,13] Unfortunately, in case of bleeding, LMWH-induced anticoagulation is not readily reversible. The longer half-life of the LMWHs results in significant anticoagulation activity up to 12 to 14 hours after the last subcutaneous dose. Protamine sulfate is only a partial antidote, and definitive clinical confirmation of its effectiveness is lacking. Protamine neutralizes anti-IIa activity and normalizes the aPTT, but it is only minimally effective in neutralizing anti-Xa activity. The recommended dosage is 1 mg of protamine per 100 anti-Xa U of LMWH if used within 8 hours of the last subcutaneous dose. If bleeding continues or the aPTT is prolonged 2 to 4 hours after the first protamine injection, an additional dose of 0.5 mg per 100 anti-Xa U is given.

All the LMWHs[14] have been shown to be equally or more effective than standard heparin in the prevention and treatment of venous thromboembolism in orthopedic, general surgical, and high-risk medical patients, including for anticoagulation during pregnancy. As with standard heparin, LMWHs do not cross the placental barrier and are not excreted in breast milk; studies suggest that they are safe in pregnancy.[14a]

The efficacy of LMWHs and UFH in the treatment of unstable angina and non-ST-elevation MI (NSTEMI) has been compared in randomized trials. LMWH with concurrent aspirin therapy was found to be equally or more effective than heparin in the treatment of UA and NSTEMI, and sustained benefit was seen at 1 year from use of enoxaparin in this setting.[15,16] The role of LMWH in conjunction with thrombolysis in patients with STEMI recently was evaluated in clinical trials, but the findings are not reflected in any of the current guidelines thus far.

In summary, LMWHs offer equal or superior anticoagulation compared with standard heparin; convenient once or twice a day dosing; no need for laboratory monitoring; a lower incidence of side effects, such as thrombocytopenia, bleeding, and osteoporosis; lower costs; and the possibility of outpatient therapy. Growing experience with LMWHs predicts their use as a standard of care. The LMWHs approved for use in the United States are enoxaparin, dalteparin, and tinzaparin. These drugs have minor differences in their chemical composition, pharmacokinetics, and clinical uses (Table 145.7). The results of clinical trials with one agent cannot be generalized to others, because studies involving head-to-head comparisons among them are lacking.

Heparinoids

Danaparoid sodium is a combination of different low-molecular-weight sulfated glycosaminoglycans derived from animal tissues. It contains heparan sulfate (83%), dermatan sulfate (12%), and chondroitin sulfate (5%). Danaparoid exerts its antithrombotic effect primarily through factor Xa inhibition; it has minimal anti-IIa activity and no influence on platelets. Danaparoid has almost 100% bioavailability and a half-life of 8 hours after subcutaneous injection. Elimination of danaparoid is kidney dependent; therefore, the half-life is prolonged in kidney failure. Danaparoid has little effect on the aPTT and the international normalized ratio (INR), and it is monitored using an appropriately calibrated anti-Xa assay. However, when the drug is used at approved prophylactic doses, no laboratory monitoring is required. Periodic complete blood counts, including a platelet count, and stool occult blood tests are recommended during treatment with danaparoid sodium.[17]

Side effects of danaparoid sodium include hemorrhage, anemia, thrombocytopenia, and generalized hypersensitivity reactions. The long half-life and the inability of protamine sulfate to neutralize the drug are disadvantages.

In contrast to the LMWHs, danaparoid sodium is essentially heparin free and has virtually no in vivo cross-reactivity with heparin. It has been used successfully in patients with HIT.[18] Compared with lepirudin, which also is used in HIT treatment, danaparoid appears to have fewer hemorrhagic complications.[19] One study found danaparoid to be effective in the treatment of patients with large artery atherosclerotic stroke.[20] However, the drug has not been approved by the U.S. Food and Drug Administration (FDA); it is not available in the United States but is available and used in other countries, such as Canada.

FACTOR Xa INHIBITORS

Fondaparinux (Pentasaccharide)

Fondaparinux is a synthetic pentasaccharide identical to the active pentasaccharide sequence of heparin. It is a selective anti-Xa agent that requires AT-III for its action. Fondaparinux does not affect thrombin activity, platelet function, or fibrinolytic activity. It is eliminated unchanged by the kidneys, and the elimination half-life is approximately 15 to 20 hours. Fondaparinux is administered once a day by subcutaneous injection. Caution should be used in patients with mild to moderate renal impairment. Fondaparinux is contraindicated in patients with severe renal failure and those who weigh less than 50 kg.

With prophylactic doses, no anticoagulation monitoring is usually required; however, renal function, thrombocyte counts, and clinical symptoms of bleeding should be evaluated. Fondaparinux does not affect bleeding time or conventional anticoagulation tests. When required, anticoagulation intensity may be assessed with a pentasaccharide-calibrated anti-Xa test. Bleeding is the major side effect. Because of the drug's long half-life, anticoagulant effects may persist for up to 2 to 4 days. No antidote is available. Rarely, severe

COMPARISON OF DIFFERENT LOW-MOLECULAR-WEIGHT HEPARINS IN PHARMACOKINETIC PROFILE AND INDICATIONS FOR USE

	Enoxaparin	Dalteparin	Tinzaparin
Bioavailability	~ 100%	~ 90%	87%
Peak anti-Xa effect	3-5 hours	4 hours	4-5 hours
Metabolism	Hepatic	Renal	Desulfation, depolymerization
Excretion	40% in urine	20% in urine	Urine
Indications	NSTEMI, DVT Rx, STEMI	NSTEMI, DVT Rx	Rx for DVT and PE
	DVT prophylaxis in surgical patients	DVT prophylaxis in surgical patients	Not established for use in NSTEMI, STEMI

DVT, deep venous thrombosis; NSTEMI, non-ST-elevation myocardial infarction; PE, pulmonary embolism; STEMI, ST-elevation myocardial infarction.

Table 145.7 Comparison of different low-molecular-weight heparins in pharmacokinetic profile and indications for use.

thrombocytopenia may occur. Besides VTE prophylaxis, fondaparinux shows promise in the management of unstable angina/NSTEMI and in thrombolysis in STEMI.[21]

Recent data from the OASIS-5 and OASIS-6 studies show noninferiority of fondaparinux to enoxaparin when the former is used as an anticoagulant in patients with acute coronary syndrome ACS). Current guidelines from the American College of Cardiology (ACC) support the use of fondaparinux in patients with ACS/NSTEMI with a class I recommendation, and its use is preferred over UFH in patients with an increased risk of bleeding (Ic) and those managed conservatively (IIa).[22,23]

The FDA has approved fondaparinux for VTE prophylaxis only in patients undergoing surgery for hip fracture, hip replacement, or knee replacement.

Idraparinux

As does fondaparinux, idraparinux selectively inhibits activated factor X. However, it has a much longer half-life of 80 hours, which allows it to be administered subcutaneously once a week. A phase II trial by the PERSIST investigators suggested that a fixed-dose subcutaneous injection given once a week is effective and safe. This recently was tested by the van Gogh investigators in the phase III trials; they found noninferiority of idraparinux compared with a combination of heparin and vitamin K antagonist in patients with DVT. However, idraparinux was less efficacious than standard therapy in patients with pulmonary embolism.[24]

An open label phase III atrial fibrillation trial of monitored, adjusted-dose vitamin K antagonist, comparing the efficacy and safety with unadjusted SanOrg 34006/idraparinux (AMADEUS) study was intended to compare subcutaneous idraparinux with dose-adjusted warfarin (target INR, 2.5; range, 2.0 to 3.0) in about 7000 patients with AF and at least one additional risk factor for stroke. However, the trial was terminated early because of safety concerns about bleeding. Another phase III trial in AF is ongoing.

DIRECT THROMBIN INHIBITORS

The direct thrombin inhibitors directly bind and inhibit free and clot-bound thrombin; they do not require AT-III for action. Members of this class currently approved by the FDA include the polypeptides r-hirudin and bivalirudin and the low-molecular-weight inhibitor argatroban. The orally administered direct thrombin inhibitors, ximelagatran and dabigatran, do not require routine laboratory monitoring.

Hirudin

Hirudin (lepirudin) is a recombinant DNA product originally isolated from the salivary glands of the medicinal leech *Hirudo medicinalis.* r-Hirudin is a potent and specific inhibitor that binds both to the catalytic site and to the fibrinogen-binding exosite of thrombin and forms a slowly reversible complex with thrombin. r-Hirudin is predominantly cleared by the kidneys; therefore, dose adjustment is necessary in renal failure.[25] The drug usually is administered intravenously, and it has a plasma half-life of 40 to 60 minutes. For DVT prophylaxis, it also could be given by subcutaneous injection every 12 hours. The intensity of anticoagulation is monitored by the aPTT level, with a target range of 1.5 to 2.5 times the control.

r-Hirudin does not have an antidote. Desmopressin, prothrombin complex, hemofiltration, and plasma exchange have been reported to reverse r-hirudin anticoagulation.[26] However, the short half-life provides for rapid reversal upon discontinuation of infusion. The formation of antihirudin antibodies was observed in about 40% of patients with HIT who were treated with hirudin. This may increase the anticoagulant effect of r-hirudin, possibly as a result of delayed renal elimination of active hirudin-antihirudin complexes. Consequently, strict monitoring of the aPTT is necessary during prolonged therapy.

r-Hirudin has no interaction with platelets and no cross-reactivity with heparin and may safely be administered to patients who have developed HIT. It also has been shown to be effective and safe for thromboprophylaxis in patients undergoing elective hip arthroplasty, and these are the only two indications for which it has been approved for use by the FDA.[27] In patients with acute coronary syndromes, r-hirudin appears to lower the death and MI rates compared with heparin, but at a price of higher bleeding rates. Although r-hirudin increased the risk of major bleeding, no increase was seen in life-threatening bleeding.[28]

Bivalirudin

Bivalirudin is a hirudin-related bivalent synthetic thrombin inhibitor. Unlike hirudin, it produces only transient inhibition of the active site of thrombin. Bivalirudin has a half-life of 25 minutes. Only 20% of bivalirudin is eliminated through the kidneys. It is relatively safe for patients with mild to moderate renal failure.[29] It is administered by intravenous infusion and produces an immediate anticoagulation response, prolonging the aPTT, prothrombin time (PT), thrombin time (TT), and ACT in a dose-dependent manner.

ACT monitoring is recommended in patients with renal impairment. The mechanism of action and shorter half-life of bivalirudin may render it safer than hirudin. Coagulation parameters return to normal 1 hour after bivalirudin infusion is stopped. Bivalirudin holds special value for interventional cardiology because of its high efficacy, favorable safety profile, and easy reversibility of anticoagulation.[30] In a large, randomized, urgent coronary intervention trial in patients with ACS (ACUITY), bivalirudin alone, with provisional use of Gp IIb/IIIa inhibitors (on an as-needed basis in 9% of the patients), was comparable in efficacy to the combination of heparin and Gp IIb/IIIa inhibitors and conferred a lower risk of bleeding.[31-33] Bivalirudin was found to reduce both ischemic endpoints and bleeding complications, compared with heparin, in patients with unstable angina undergoing balloon angioplasty.[34] Bivalirudin also was found to be effective in the management of acute MI in combination with fibrinolysis.[30] Bivalirudin is approved in North America as an alternative to heparin in patients undergoing coronary angioplasty.

Argatroban

Argatroban is a small-molecule carboxylic acid derivative. It binds noncovalently to the active site of thrombin. Argatroban undergoes hepatic metabolism; therefore, it could be used in patients with renal failure.[35] Argatroban is administered by intravenous infusion and has a half-life of approximately 40 minutes. Anticoagulation is well correlated with the aPTT. With an initial infusion rate of 2 mcg/kg/min, the aPTT is checked at 2 to 4 hours and the dose is adjusted to maintain the value above

1.5 the control. No specific antidote is available for argatroban; however, anticoagulation parameters return to baseline 2 to 4 hours after the infusion is discontinued. Argatroban is a weak antithrombotic agent, compared with UFH, and is not indicated for use in ACS.[36] A major indication for argatroban is the treatment of HIT, and the FDA has approved it for this use.[37]

Ximelagatran

Ximelagatran is the first oral direct thrombin inhibitor tested in clinical trials. It is a prodrug that is well absorbed from the gastrointestinal tract. It undergoes rapid biotransformation into the active compound melagatran, a small-molecule direct thrombin inhibitor. The drug produces a predictable anticoagulant response after oral administration and reduces the need for laboratory monitoring. Phase III studies comparing ximelagatran with warfarin for the prevention of cardioembolic events in patients with atrial fibrillation and for VTE prophylaxis in orthopedic surgery showed noninferiority of ximelagatran with respect to warfarin.[36,38,39] However, ximelagatran failed to receive FDA approval because of safety concerns regarding elevated liver transaminases and some cases of fulminant hepatic failure.

Dabigatran

Dabigatran is a novel oral anticoagulant. It is a potent, competitive, and reversible direct inhibitor of thrombin. Like ximelagatran, dabigatran produces a predictable anticoagulant response with no known drug or food interactions, which reduces the need for laboratory monitoring. The half-life of dabigatran is about 8 hours after single-dose administration and up to 14 to 17 hours after multiple doses. It usually is given twice daily. The efficacy and safety of dabigatran in preventing venous thrombosis have been demonstrated.[40] Compared with enoxaparin, VTE was significantly lower in patients receiving 150 mg twice daily (17.4% versus 24%, odds ratio [OR], 0.65; 95% confidence interval [CI], 0.43 to 0.98; $P = .04$), 300 mg once daily (OR, 0.61; 95% CI, 0.40 to 0.92; $P = .02$), and 225 mg twice daily (OR, 0.47; 95% CI, 0.30 to 0.73; $P = .0007$).

The first evaluation of dabigatran in patients with atrial fibrillation in a phase II trial has been completed.[41] Major bleeding events were limited to patients treated with dabigatran (300 mg) plus aspirin, and thromboembolic episodes were limited to the groups receiving 50 mg of dabigatran. The two highest doses of dabigatran (150 mg and 300 mg) suppressed D-dimer concentrations to a degree similar to warfarin, suggesting adequate anticoagulation. Two doses of dabigatran (110 mg and 150 mg given twice daily) currently are undergoing testing in comparison with warfarin (INR, 2 to 3) in a very large, phase III, noninferiority, randomized, controlled trial, the Randomized Evaluation of Long-Term Anticoagulant Therapy (RELY).

ORAL FACTOR XA INHIBITORS

Rivaroxaban

Rivaroxaban is an orally active, specific, competitive direct factor Xa inhibitor. It has high bioavailability (60% to 80%) and a rapid onset of action, and it is excreted by renal (two thirds) and fecal (one third) routes. It has a half-life of 6 to 9 hours. Rivaroxaban has completed extensive phase II studies in two indications (DVT prevention and treatment) and has entered large-scale phase III studies in three indications (VTE prevention, VTE treatment, and stroke prevention in patients with AF).

Apixaban

Apixaban is an orally active factor Xa inhibitor that does not require antithrombin for its action. This drug is a follow-up to razaxaban, which was discontinued because of concerns about increased bleeding.

Apixaban has shown positive results after knee replacement surgery compared with enoxaparin and warfarin. It currently is under study in a phase II trial for use in patients with unstable angina and MI. It also is being studied in a phase II pilot study for prevention of VTE in patients with metastatic carcinomas.

WARFARIN

Warfarin is the most commonly used oral anticoagulant. This coumarin derivative exists in two optically active isomers (the R and S forms), which are present in the drug in approximately equal amounts. S-warfarin is more important clinically because this isomer is five times more potent as a vitamin K antagonist than the R form.

Mechanism of Action

Warfarin produces its anticoagulant effect by inhibiting the enzymatic reduction of vitamin K epoxide in the liver microsomes. This interferes with the production of vitamin K–dependent procoagulant factors II, VII, IX, and X and of two natural inhibitor proteins, C and S. Warfarin is rapidly absorbed from the gastrointestinal tract into the blood. It binds to plasma proteins and then accumulates in the liver, where it is metabolized.[42] It has a half-life of 36 to 42 hours. The dose-response relationship of warfarin is affected by several factors: the general health of the patient, concomitant drug use, diet, and certain disease states. The variations in dose-response in individual patients require close monitoring. The prudent course is to take special care when any new drug is added to the regimen of patients taking warfarin. Some of the common food and drug interactions are listed in Table 145.8.[43]

The prothrombin time is used to monitor oral anticoagulant therapy. The PT is responsive to depressions of three of the four vitamin K–dependent clotting factors (factors II, VII, and X). Thromboplastins used in this test vary in potency, depending on their tissue origin, phospholipid content, and method of preparation. Recognition of this variation in thromboplastin responsiveness led to the development of the international normalized ratio in 1982. The International Sensitivity Index (ISI) is a measure of the responsiveness of a given thromboplastin. The lower the ISI, the more responsive the reagent. The calibration used to standardize the reporting of the PT by converting the PT ratio observed with the local thromboplastin into an INR is expressed by the following equation[42]:

FOOD AND DRUG INTERACTIONS WITH WARFARIN		
Potentiation	**Inhibition**	**No Effect**
Phenylbutazone, amiodarone, alcohol (with liver disease), cimetidine, sulfinpyrazone, anabolic steroids, clofibrate, cotrimoxazole, isoniazid, erythromycin, omeprazole, propranolol, propafenone, metronidazole, fluconazole, miconazole, acetaminophen, chloral hydrate, ciprofloxacin, disulfiram, dextropropoxyphene, itraconazole, phenytoin, tamoxifen, tetracycline, flu vaccine, aspirin, disopyramide, flourouracil, ifosfamide, ketoprofen, lovastatin, metolazone, moracizine, nalidixic acid, norfloxacin, ofloxacin, propoxyphene, sulindac, tolmetin, topical salicylates, cefamandole, cefazolin, gemfibrozil, heparin, indomethacin, sulfisoxazole	Griseofulvin, barbiturates, carbamazepine, chlordiazepoxide, cholestyramine, nafcillin, rifampin, sucralfate, avocado, dicloxacillin, azathioprine, cyclosporine, etretinate, trazodone, high vitamin K content, foods/enteral feeds	Alcohol, antaclds, atenolol, bumetadine, enoxacin, famotidine, fluoxetine, ketorolac, metoprolol, naproxen, nizatidine, psyllium, ranitidine, ibuprofen, ketoconazole, diltiazem, tobacco, vancomycin

Table 145.8 Food and drug interactions with warfarin.

$$\text{INR} = (\text{Patient PT}/\text{Mean normal PT})^{\text{ISI}}$$

or

$$\log \text{INR} = \text{ISI} \times \log(\text{Patient PT}/\text{Mean normal PT})$$

After administration of warfarin, an observable anticoagulant effect is delayed until the circulating clotting factors are metabolized and removed from the circulation. Depending on the dose administered, the delay may range from 2 to 7 days.

Pharmacogenomics

Warfarin inhibits the regeneration of vitamin K–dependent clotting factors by inhibiting vitamin K epoxide reductase (VKOR), a multiprotein enzyme complex. Warfarin is metabolized to 7-hydroxywarfarin by the liver cytochrome CYP2C9, a polymorphic enzyme. Studies have shown that variations in the expression of genes for these enzyme complexes (VKOR and CYP2C9) are responsible for the variations in dose-response and outcomes in patients treated with warfarin.[44] Clinical trials studying the pharmacogenomics of warfarin are ongoing.

Clinical Indications

Warfarin is indicated in the prevention and treatment of venous and arterial thrombosis, unstable angina, myocardial infarction, atrial fibrillation, and coronary artery disease (CAD) and for patients with prosthetic heart valves. The current guidelines established by the American Association of Chest Physicians (AACP) recommend an INR of 2.0 to 3.0 as the optimum range of anticoagulation for most indications. This includes patients with bileaflet mechanical valves in the aortic position and all bioprosthetic valves. Higher intensity anticoagulation, with an INR range of 2.5 to 3.5, is recommended for all other mechanical valves and for the prevention of recurrent MI, for patients with antiphospholipid syndrome, and when the moderate-intensity regimen fails.[42]

If rapid anticoagulation is indicated, heparin (UFH or LMWH) is started in combination with warfarin. Heparin is discontinued when the INR has been in the therapeutic range for at least 2 days.

Warfarin alone can be given if rapid anticoagulation is not required (e.g., chronic stable atrial fibrillation). For initiation of anticoagulation, a dose of 5 or 10 mg can be used. Starting therapy at a dosage of 5 mg/day is recommended for patients older than age 70 and for those at high risk of bleeding. This achieves a steady-state anticoagulant effect in 5 to 7 days. The INR usually is monitored daily, starting on day 3, until the therapeutic range is reached and held for at least 2 consecutive days. Monitoring then is done weekly for 1 to 2 weeks, and then less often, depending on the stability of the INR results. If the INR response remains stable, the frequency of testing can be reduced to intervals of approximately 4 weeks. If dose adjustments are required, the cycle of more frequent monitoring is repeated until a stable dose-response is again achieved. Dose adjustment of a 1-mg increment or decrement at a time is advised.

Some patients undergoing long-term warfarin therapy are difficult to manage because they have unexpected fluctuations in dose-response. The fluctuations could be due to changes in diet, inaccuracy in PT testing, undisclosed drug use, poor patient compliance, surreptitious self-medication, or intermittent alcohol consumption. Keeping tight control of the anticoagulation level is very important, because hemorrhagic or thromboembolic complications occur predominantly when the INR is outside the target range. An INR below 2.0 increases the incidence of thromboembolism, and an INR above 3.5 increases the risk of bleeding.

Although randomized trials are lacking, overall evidence suggests that better control may be achieved in patients referred to anticoagulation clinics.[45] Selected groups of patients may benefit from implementation of self-monitoring. Point of care (POC) coagulation monitors approved by the FDA for home use provide estimated INR levels from a finger-stick capillary blood sample. Further studies are required to define their role in standard management of warfarin anticoagulation.

In patients taking warfarin who have a low risk of thrombosis and who require surgery, the risk of bleeding can be reduced by stopping warfarin 4 to 5 days before surgery and, if the INR remains elevated, giving a dose of vitamin K_1 24 to 48 hours before surgery. Prophylactic low-dose heparin or LMWHs should be started during the preoperative or postoperative period. However, in patients with a high risk of thrombosis (e.g., those with prosthetic heart valves), full-dose intravenous heparin therapy should be started after the warfarin is stopped when the INR becomes subtherapeutic; the heparin then is withheld for 5 to 6 hours before surgery. A simpler regimen of subcutaneous LMWH, started when the INR is subtherapeutic and withheld 12 to 18 hours before surgery, also is widely used, except in patients with mechanical valves. Another approach is to continue warfarin at a lower dose and to perform the surgery when the INR is in the range of 1.3 to 1.5.[42]

Anticoagulation does not need to be reversed for the usual dental procedures. If the patient has an increased risk of bleeding, tranexamic acid or epsilon-aminocaproic acid mouth washes can be used.

Complications

Bleeding

Bleeding is the main complication of oral anticoagulant therapy. The reported incidence is anywhere from 4% to 6% in patients with an INR range of 2.0 to 3.0, but it is much higher for an INR above 3.5. The risk of bleeding is influenced by the patient's age, the intensity of anticoagulant therapy, the patient's underlying clinical disorder, and concomitant use of aspirin or other antiplatelet drugs. The risk of major bleeding has been reported to be increased if the patient is older than age 65, has a history of stroke or gastrointestinal bleeding, AF, and serious comorbid conditions, such as renal insufficiency or anemia. Important preventable causes of bleeding are uncontrolled hypertension and poor anticoagulation control.[42,46] Guidelines for the management of patients with a high INR are presented in Table 145.9. The management of patients who bleed during warfarin therapy is a challenge. In such patients, every effort should be made to treat and reverse the primary cause of bleeding.

Skin Necrosis

Skin necrosis, although uncommon, is the most serious nonhemorrhagic complication of warfarin therapy. This complication is caused by extensive thrombosis of the venules and capillaries in the subcutaneous fat, and it usually is seen on the third to eighth day of therapy.[47] Warfarin-induced skin necrosis is known to occur in patients with protein C or protein S deficiency; however, this complication also has been reported in nondeficient individuals. Continuing warfarin is relatively contraindicated, and long-term heparin is inconvenient and associated with osteoporosis. In these patients, therapeutic anticoagulation first should be achieved with heparin, and warfarin then should be restarted at a low dose (e.g., 2 mg/day). The dose of warfarin is increased slowly over several weeks. This regimen prevents an abrupt fall in

RECOMMENDATIONS FOR MANAGEMENT OF PATIENTS WITH A HIGH INTERNATIONAL NORMALIZED RATIO (INR)
1. If the INR is above the therapeutic range but below 5.0, the patient is not bleeding, and rapid reversal is not indicated for reasons of surgical intervention, the dose can be lowered or one dose can be omitted and warfarin therapy can be resumed at a lower dose when the INR approaches the therapeutic range. 2. If the INR is above 5.0 but below 9.0 and the patient is not bleeding, the next one or two doses of warfarin can be omitted. Alternatively, one dose of warfarin may be omitted and vitamin K_1 can be given orally at a dose of 1.0 to 2.5 mg. Warfarin therapy can be resumed at a lower dose when the INR approaches the therapeutic range. When rapid reversal is desired because the patient requires elective surgery, vitamin K_1 at a dose of 2 to 4 mg can be given orally. If the INR remains high at 24 hours, an additional dose of 1 to 2 mg of vitamin K_1 can be given. 3. If the INR is above 9.0 and the patient is not bleeding, a higher dose of vitamin K_1 (3 to 5 mg) should be given orally with the expectation that the INR will be reduced substantially by 24 to 48 hours. The INR should be monitored closely, and vitamin K_1 can be repeated, if necessary. 4. If a very rapid reversal of an anticoagulant effect is required because of serious bleeding or major warfarin overdose (e.g., INR > 20.0), vitamin K_1 in a dose of 10 mg should be given by slow intravenous (IV) infusion (e.g., over 20 to 30 min) and the INR checked every 6 hours. It may be necessary to repeat vitamin K_1 every 12 hours and supplement with plasma transfusion or prothrombin complex concentrate, depending on the urgency of the situation. 5. In case of life-threatening bleeding or serious warfarin overdose, replacement with prothrombin complex concentrate is indicated, supplemented with IV vitamin K_1 (10 mg), which should be repeated as necessary, depending on the INR. 6. If continued warfarin therapy is indicated after administration of high doses of vitamin K_1, heparin can be given until the effects of vitamin K_1 have been reversed and the patient becomes responsive to warfarin.
Modified from Ansell J, Hirsh J, Poller L, Bussey H, Jacobson A, Hylek E. Pharmacology and management of vitamin K antagonists. Chest 2004;126:204S-233S.

Table 145.9 Recommendations for management of patients with a high international normalized ratio (INR).

the protein C level before the reduction in the levels of factors II, IX, and X, and it has been shown to be free of the recurrence of skin necrosis.[48]

Embryopathy

Warfarin is contraindicated in the first trimester of pregnancy. If possible, it should be avoided throughout pregnancy. Warfarin can cross the placenta. When given during pregnancy, it has been known to produce a characteristic embryopathy, central nervous system abnormalities, or fetal bleeding.[49] Warfarin inhibits the action of vitamin K on osteoblasts and interferes with the carboxylation of Gla proteins (osteocalcin) synthesized in bone. This could lead to bone abnormalities in neonates of women treated with warfarin during pregnancy (see Chapter 136). Heparin and LMWHs are the preferred anticoagulants in pregnancy. However, in patients at very high risk of thrombosis or in certain cases in which heparin is contraindicated, warfarin use during pregnancy may be justified. Convincing evidence indicates that warfarin therapy in a nursing mother does not induce an anticoagulant effect in the breast-fed infant; therefore, breast-feeding is not contraindicated.[50]

ORAL ANTICOAGULATION IN SELECTED CARDIAC CONDITIONS

Chronic Stable Coronary Artery Disease

Aspirin is the drug of choice for primary prevention of CAD. In patients at high risk who are intolerant to aspirin, clopidogrel may be used. Warfarin also is effective in some subgroups of patients, as was shown in one trial.[51]

In patients with chronic stable CAD, aspirin is the drug of choice for secondary prevention. Coumadin is not recommended except in very high risk patients whose INR can be followed closely. Warfarin remains a viable option in patients intolerant to aspirin.

A hypercoagulable state and risk of thrombosis persist for up to 6 months after MI, with the highest risk of reinfarction and death within 1 month. Aspirin consistently has reduced the risk of MI, death, and stroke and is a standard of care for secondary prophylaxis of CAD. Analysis of pooled data compared the efficacy of oral anticoagulation of different intensity versus aspirin or placebo or a combination of warfarin and aspirin. Warfarin alone or a combination therapy of low-intensity INR (<2.0) and aspirin is inferior to aspirin. In a smaller trial of moderate intensity, an INR of 2.0 to 3.0 in combination with aspirin was superior to aspirin alone in reducing endpoints and had similar safety.[52] The positive results of these studies were closely correlated with high-quality anticoagulation management. The recommendations for anticoagulant therapy in CAD are given in Tables 145.1 to 145.3.[53] The details of treatment of acute coronary conditions are presented in Chapter 28 and 29.

Chronic Heart Failure and Dilated Cardiomyopathy

The rates of thromboembolism in heart failure vary from 1.5% to 3.5% per year in unselected patients with chronic heart failure (CHF) and a New York Heart Association (NYHA) classification of class II or III. The risk increases to 20% in patients hospitalized with dilated cardiomyopathy.[54] The risk is greatest for patients with heart failure with severe left ventricular dysfunction (and increases steadily as the ejection fraction [EF] drops below 35%), a past history of thromboembolism, atrial dysrhythmias, and echocardiographic evidence of cardiac thrombus.[55]

Several observational studies in the past suggested efficacy of anticoagulation in preventing embolism in patients with heart failure and dilated cardiomyopathy, and one trial even found an additional decrease in mortality from the reduced number of cardiac events in the warfarin arm.[56] However, these studies did not take into account the INR achieved or other confounding factors, such as the prevalence of AF and left ventricular (LV) thrombus. Many randomized, controlled trials, such as the WATCH trial, a prospective study with more than 3000 participants, compared the efficacy of warfarin and aspirin in patients with heart failure in sinus rhythm; these studies have not shown any benefit in the use of antithrombotics. Therefore, without clear indications, such as AF, LV thrombus, or previous thromboembolic events, the use of anticoagulants in CHF is not encouraged. Recent ACC guidelines also do not endorse the routine use of anticoagulation in CHF; rather, they recommend evaluation of the risks and benefits for each patient.[56] The use of aspirin may have some benefit in patients with CHF who have an underlying coronary artery disease, given the benefit of aspirin in coronary artery disease.[57,58]

In nonischemic cardiomyopathy, however, aspirin should be avoided because of concern over its interaction with angiotensin-converting enzyme (ACE) inhibitors and interference with renal perfusion (7th consensus conference on antithrombotic therapy).[70] AF warrants long-term anticoagulation (see discussion later in the chapter). The current recommendation for the intensity of long-term anticoagulation with warfarin for AF is a target INR of 2.5 (range, 2.0 to 3.0) (see Chapter 72).[42]

Prosthetic Heart Valves

Heart valves can be classified into two broad categories: bioprosthetic heart valves and mechanical prosthetic heart valves; the latter require a higher degree of anticoagulation (see Chapter 100).

Mechanical valves require lifelong anticoagulation to prevent valve thrombosis and systemic embolism. In patients with bioprosthetic valves who are in sinus rhythm, anticoagulation usually is stopped after the initial 3 months and long-term aspirin therapy is substituted, provided the patient has no other indication for prolonged anticoagulation.

Warfarin has never been compared with a placebo in patients with prosthetic heart valves, for obvious ethical reasons. However, warfarin has been compared with a combination of antiplatelet drugs (aspirin-dipyridamole and aspirin-pentoxifylline) in a randomized trial. The patients receiving warfarin were found to have a significantly lower rate of thromboembolism than the other two groups, with a relative risk reduction of 60% to 79%.[59]

Studies of minimum effective intensity of anticoagulant therapy demonstrated that moderate-intensity warfarin treatment was as effective and was safer than a high-dose regimen. In patients with bioprosthetic heart valves, a less intense regimen (INR, 2.0 to 2.25) was as effective as the more intense regimen (INR, 2.5 to 4.0) and produced less bleeding. Also, patients with aortic mechanical valves do just as well with a moderate degree of anticoagulation (INR, 2 to 3) as they do with the conventional regimen (INR, 3.0 to 4.5).[60,61] Another randomized trial has shown that the addition of low-dose aspirin (100 mg/day) to high-intensity warfarin anticoagulation (INR, 2.5 to 3.5) results in a significant reduction in mortality and stroke without a significant increase in major bleeding or in cerebral hemorrhage.[62,63] A retrospective study of 16,081 patients showed that the incidence of thromboembolic events rose sharply when the INR fell below 2.5, and the incidence of bleeding increased sharply when the INR rose above 5.0.[64] The current recommendations for anticoagulation for patients with prosthetic heart valves are given in Table 145.4.[65]

Atrial Fibrillation

The most feared complication of atrial fibrillation is thromboembolic stroke. AF is an important independent risk factor for stroke, with an event rate of approximately 5% per year. The risk of stroke in AF is age related; it increases from 1.5% in those age 50 to 59, to greater than 10% in those age 80 to 89. Prospectively validated independent predictors of a higher risk of thromboembolism in atrial fibrillation are age older than 75, a history of hypertension, a history of diabetes mellitus, a previous transient ischemic attack (TIA) or stroke, and impaired left ventricular function (heart failure or an EF below 35%) (see Chapter 58).

The approach to anticoagulation in the patient with AF depends on the clinical presentation. In unstable patients, heparinization is desirable both before and (an important factor) after cardioversion. In stable patients, warfarin anticoagulation is indicated for at least 3 to 4 weeks before and after chemical or electrical cardioversion because of the stunning phenomenon; in this development, mechanical function of the left atrium does not recover for up to 4 weeks after restoration of sinus rhythm, and the risk of thromboembolism persists. Long-term anticoagulation with warfarin is indicated for patients with chronic AF.

Five primary prevention trials have shown a decisive benefit in reducing thromboembolic complications of AF with anticoagulant therapy. The pooled risk reduction was 68% (the stroke rate was reduced from 4.5% to 1.4% per year), and this proved the superiority of warfarin over both aspirin and placebo. The European Atrial Fibrillation Study, a secondary prevention trial, evaluated the efficacy of warfarin, aspirin, or placebo for patients with nonrheumatic AF who had had a recent TIA or minor ischemic stroke. Anticoagulant therapy was associated with a 66% risk reduction (the stroke rate was reduced from 12% to 4% per year). Also, no statistically significant increase in major bleeding events was seen in anticoagulated patients in these randomized trials. The SPAF III trial revealed that full-dose warfarin therapy (target INR, 2 to 3) was more effective than a combination of aspirin and fixed low-dose warfarin therapy (stroke rates of 2.6% and 7.8%, respectively).[42,66,67] The Birmingham AF Treatment of the Aged (BAFTA) study of high-risk patients reported annual stroke rates of 3.8% and 1.8% in patients assigned to aspirin and warfarin, respectively.[68] Perhaps the most striking demonstration of the superiority of vitamin K antagonist anticoagulation over an antiplatelet regimen comes from ACTIVE-W trial, which showed that oral anticoagulation with warfarin (INR, 2 to 3) was superior to a combination of aspirin and clopidogrel for the prevention of stroke (annual stroke rates of 3.9% and 5.6%, respectively).[69]

Therefore, conclusive evidence indicates the beneficial effects of anticoagulation in reducing the risk of stroke and morbidity associated with AF. Current recommendations for long-term oral anticoagulation in AF are summarized in Table 145.5.[70]

The recommended treatment for patients with AF and valvular heart disease is long-term anticoagulation with warfarin (target INR, 2.5; range, 2 to 3). If systemic embolism occurs despite warfarin therapy, the addition of aspirin (80 to 100 mg/day), dipyridamole (400 mg/day), or clopidogrel (75 mg/day) to the anticoagulation regimen is recommended. However, if these patients develop infective endocarditis, anticoagulation is not recommended if a native or bioprosthetic valve is present. In the case of a mechanical prosthetic valve, warfarin therapy may be continued; however, it should be noted that the risk of intracranial hemorrhage is very high.[65]

SUMMARY

Anticoagulation in heart disease is indicated in a variety of clinical situations, both acute and chronic. Emergency and acute coronary syndromes generally are managed with parenteral anticoagulants (heparin, LMWHs, direct thrombin inhibitors). Antiplatelet drugs (aspirin, thienopyridines, Gp IIb/IIIa receptor antagonists) often are used as adjuncts to anticoagulation in these situations. Chronic cardiac conditions require long-term anticoagulation, which is achieved with warfarin, which can be used orally. However, in special clinical situations (e.g., pregnancy), heparin or LMWHs may be used for long-term anticoagulation. Bleeding continues to be a major side effect of anticoagulation; however, in most situations, the benefits of anticoagulant therapy far outweigh the risks.

chapter

146 Special Problems for the Cardiology Consultant

a. Radiotherapy

Stuart J. Hutchison

A 55-year-old woman had undergone aortic valve replacement and coronary bypass surgery after two episodes of acute pulmonary edema. Six years earlier, she had first become symptomatic with mild (class 2) dyspnea. She had no symptoms of angina, presyncope, or syncope. She was a lifelong nonsmoker, nonhypertensive, and nondiabetic and had no family history of coronary disease.

Thirty-five years previously, she had undergone chest radiotherapy treatment for a stage II Hodgkin's lymphoma. No details were obtainable concerning the dose or field details of radiotherapy. Nine years previously, she had undergone bilateral mastectomy, chemotherapy, and radiation therapy for breast carcinoma. No details were directly available concerning treatment for this malignancy either.

Cardiology consultation was requested 7 days after surgery because of a persistent low output state despite elevated filling pressures.

Review of preoperative consultations revealed that the cause of the acute pulmonary edema episodes was frustratingly unclear. The first episode occurred when the patient was walking with her husband, the second occurred 5 months later when she was at rest. Neither episode occurred with hypertension documented at the time. Radiographic evidence was unequivocal in one case and borderline in the other case. Murmurs were detected, which resulted in echocardiograms that described low aortic valve areas, in the context of left ventricular (LV) dysfunction and low transvalvular gradients.

Preoperative and postoperative 12-lead electrocardiograms demonstrated an incomplete left bundle branch block pattern with secondary repolarization abnormalities (Fig. 146A.1).

Posteroanterior and lateral chest radiographs revealed no cardiomegaly or heart failure. Mitral valve and mitral annular calcification was evident on the lateral film (Fig. 146A.2).

The patient had undergone two coronary angiograms and an intravascular ultrasound. The first coronary angiogram revealed an occluded right coronary artery, a "normal" left coronary artery, and "no" gradient on LV to aortic pullback. After the second episode of acute pulmonary edema, reconsultation was done, and a second angiogram and catheterization were performed. A second coronary angiogram confirmed the right coronary occlusion and revealed a 40% to 50% left main stem lesion (Fig. 146A.3). Intracardiac hemodynamics revealed a right atrial pressure of 12, a right ventricular pressure of 47/10, a pulmonary artery pressure of 45/21, a pulmonary capillary wedge pressure of 29 with a prominent V wave, a LV end-diastolic pressure of 20, and a mean aortic valve gradient of 16 mm Hg. The cardiac index was 2.1 L/min/m^2. The Gorlin calculation of aortic valve area was 0.6 cm^2. Ventriculography demonstrated moderate to severe LV systolic dysfunction.

Echocardiography had revealed extensive valvular abnormalities. The aortic and mitral valves were diffusely and irregularly thickened with an unusual appearance, as were the aortic and mitral annuli (Fig. 146A.4). The echocardiographic calculations of the aortic valve area also were low (0.8 to 0.9 cm^2); however, notably, the left ventricular outflow tract (VTI) also was low (14 cm), which was consistent with LV systolic dysfunction and "low flow." The mean aortic valve gradients were low (12 and 15 mm Hg) and not commensurate with the calculations of aortic valve area severity (Fig. 146A.5). Mild to moderate insufficiency of the mitral valve was noted, and color Doppler evidence of flow convergence across it was seen, but the mean gradient was only 4 mm Hg (Fig. 146A.6). The pulmonic valve also was thickened and moderately to severely insufficient (Fig. 146A.7). Determinations of LV systolic function essentially were irreconcilable with three different echocardiograms that found normal, mild, and severe dysfunction without regional wall motion abnormalities. One echocardiogram described concentric left ventricular hypertrophy (LVH), and another did not. Two different contrast ventriculograms deemed LV systolic dysfunction moderate and also severe, and one included a comment on an anterior wall motion abnormality. A gated blood pool scan calculated normal systolic function. Tissue Doppler assessment recorded severely abnormal indices (Fig. 146A.8).

No investigations described right heart function.

The patient had undergone a third preoperative coronary assessment with intravascular ultrasound of the left main coronary artery stenosis to refute a significant lesion. The left main stem lesion was assessed to be borderline significant and, driven by the clinical history, the patient was referred for coronary bypass surgery. With a primary indication for bypass surgery resolved by the referring physicians, a

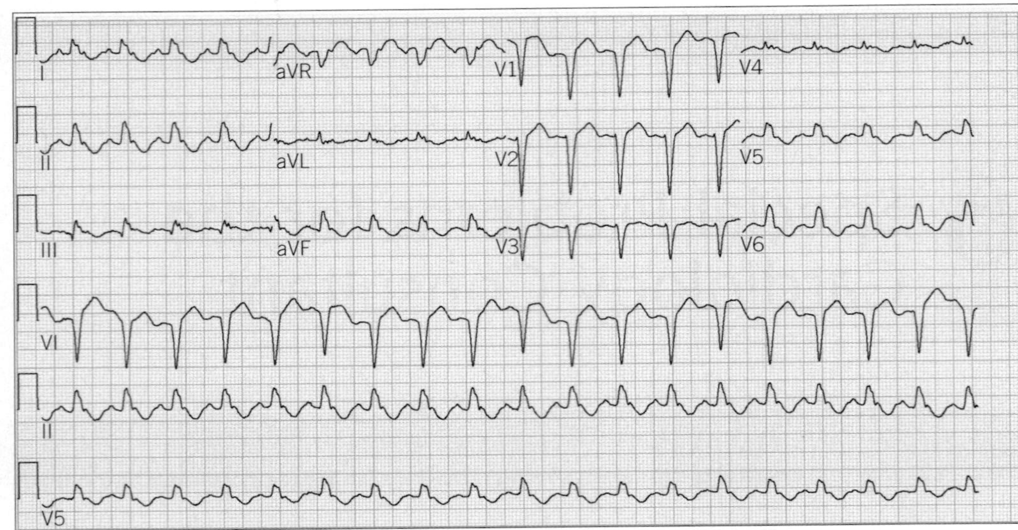

Figure 146A.1 Twelve-lead electrocardiogram (ECG) indicating incomplete left bundle branch block.

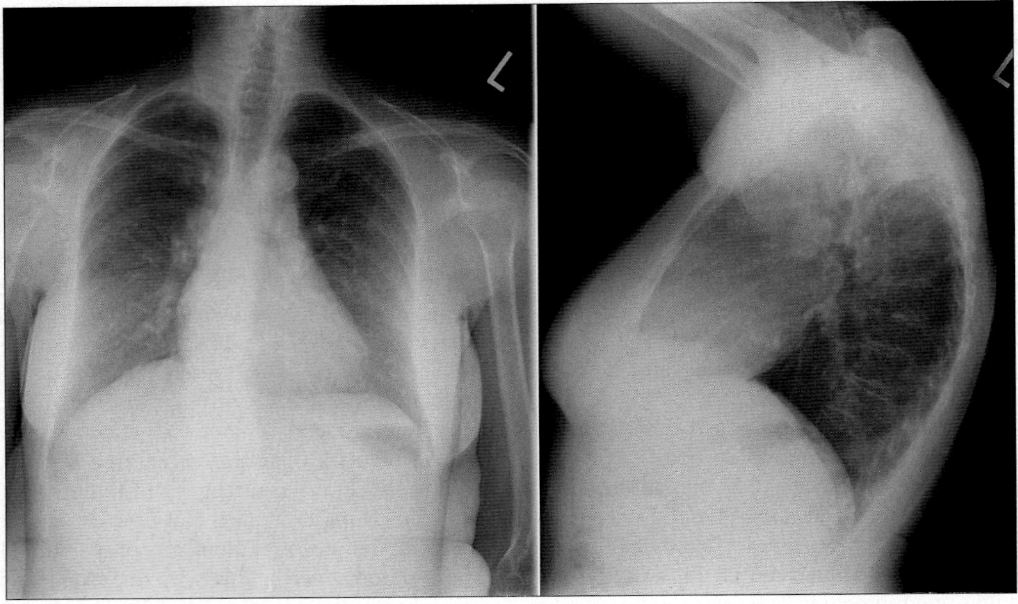

Figure 146A.2 Posteroanterior *(left)* and lateral *(right)* radiographs. No cardiomegaly or sign of left-sided heart failure is present. Calcification of the mitral apparatus is apparent on the lateral radiograph.

secondary indication for aortic valve replacement had been accepted because of calculations of moderate aortic stenosis and low aortic valve area both by echocardiography and by the second cardiac catheterization.

Electrocardiographic (ECG) gated cardiac computed tomography (CT) demonstrated extensive calcification of the proximal left and right coronary arteries, mild calcification of the aortic valve and annulus, and extensive calcification of the mitral valve leaflets and annulus. Some regions of pericardial thickening were noted. Streak artifact from the valve calcification was extensive. The internal mammary arteries were both patent despite previous chest irradiation, the concern that prompted the CT scan (Fig. 146A.9). Lung scarring also was apparent on CT scanning (Fig. 146A.10).

Intraoperative findings were notable. Intraoperative transesophageal echocardiography (TEE) demonstrated only mild thickening of the aortic valve, mild aortic insufficiency, low V1 flow (VTI, 14 cm), and a low gradient of only 12 mm Hg (Fig. 146A.11). Intraoperative TEE revealed that the mitral valve was morphologically severely calcified through its leaflets and exuberant calcification of the annulus was present, but with only moderate insufficiency and a small gradient of 4 mm Hg. Exophytic extensions of annular calcification into the left atrium were seen (Fig. 146A.12). Moderate biventricular systolic dysfunction was seen.

The patient underwent coronary bypass surgery with an internal mammary artery graft to the left anterior descending coronary artery and a saphenous vein bypass graft to the obtuse

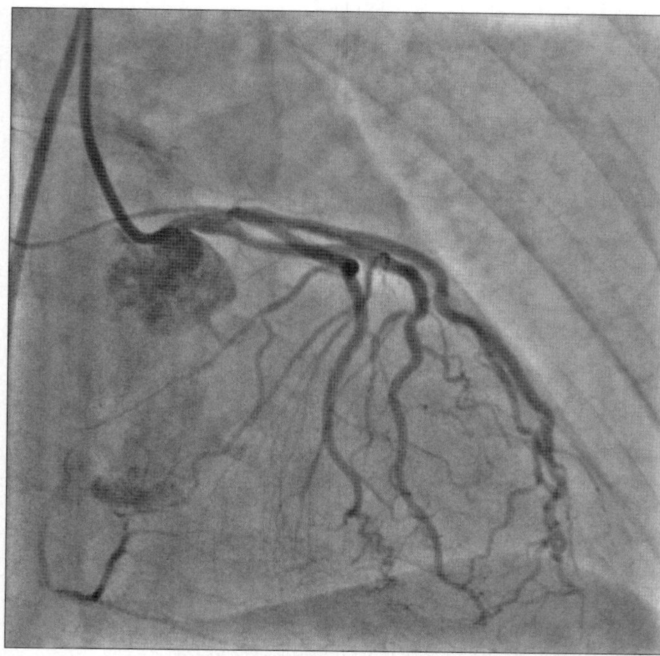

Figure 146A.3 Left coronary injection, right anterior oblique (RAO) projection. A borderline ostial left main stem stenosis is present, as is extensive collateralization to the (proximally occluded) distal right coronary artery.

marginal system, as well as mechanical aortic valve replacement. The calcific protrusions from the mitral valve were removed. The posterior pericardium was noted to be firmly fibrosed to the underlying heart chambers. Restarting the heart

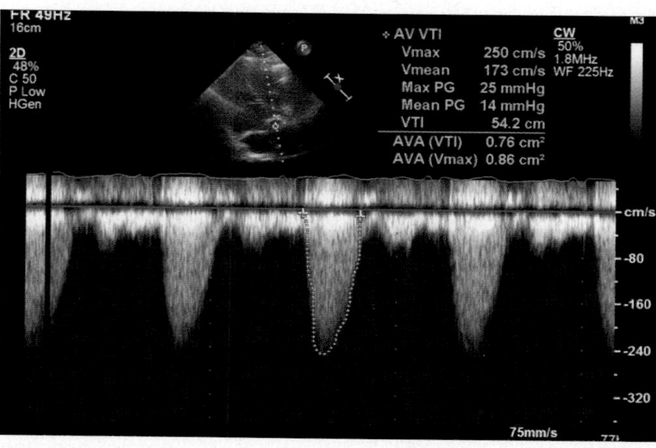

Figure 146A.5 The continuous-wave Doppler sampling of the aortic valve gradient demonstrates a mean gradient of only 14 mm Hg. The low subvalvular velocity generates the calculation of a low aortic valve area.

was slow and difficult, and a critical low output state was present. Right ventricular systolic function was poor; high doses of inotropes and intra-aortic balloon counterpulsation were required. The night after surgery, excessive blood return through mediastinal and pericardial chest tubes necessitated opening of the chest and identification and elimination of several bleeding sources. In the intensive care unit (ICU), the patient languished in a critically low output state. A central venous pressure (CVP) of 20 mm Hg was the minimum required to maintain output, but the elevated venous pressures

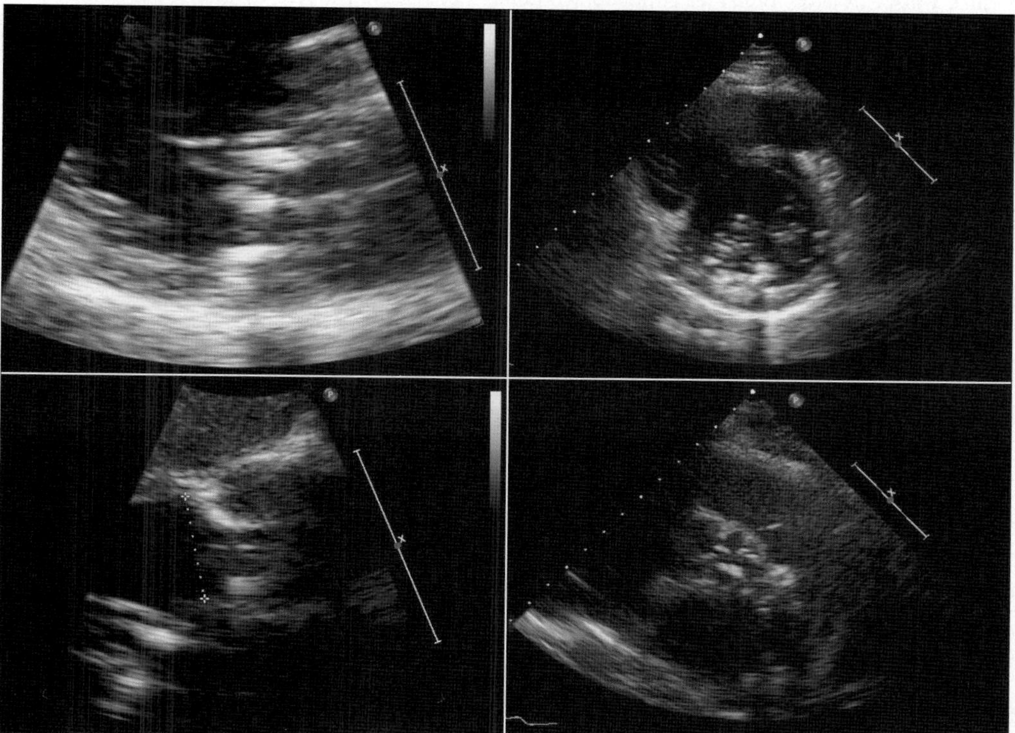

Figure 146A.4 Transthoracic images. *Upper images:* Mitral valve. *Lower images:* aortic valve. The mitral valve is extensively and irregularly thickened and appears calcified, as does the medial portion of the mitral annulus. The aortic valve also is eccentrically thickened.

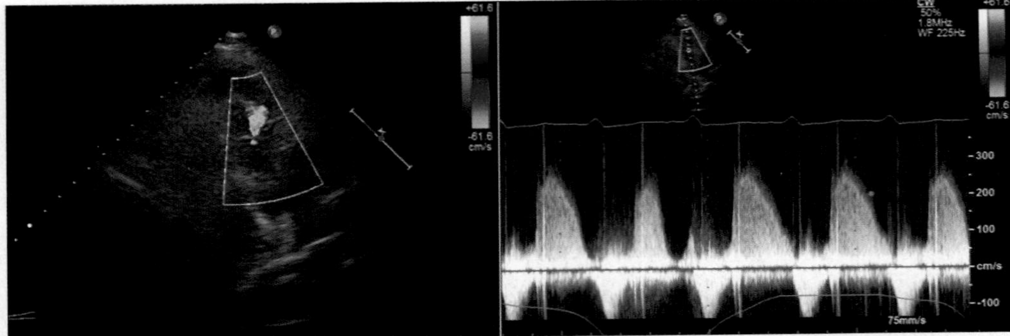

Figure 146A.6 The mitral valve is thickened, and its annulus appears calcified. Color Doppler interrogation depicts diastolic flow convergence at the valve and a broad diastolic jet. Spectral display of pulsed Doppler sampling reveals increased velocity of the transmitral flow but no significant stenosis. Color Doppler flow mapping also revealed mild to moderate mitral regurgitation but no evident pulmonary venous systolic flow reversal. The color Doppler flow mapping and pulsed-wave pulmonary venous sampling were of lower than average quality, possibly because of attenuation by the thickened mitral valve tissue.

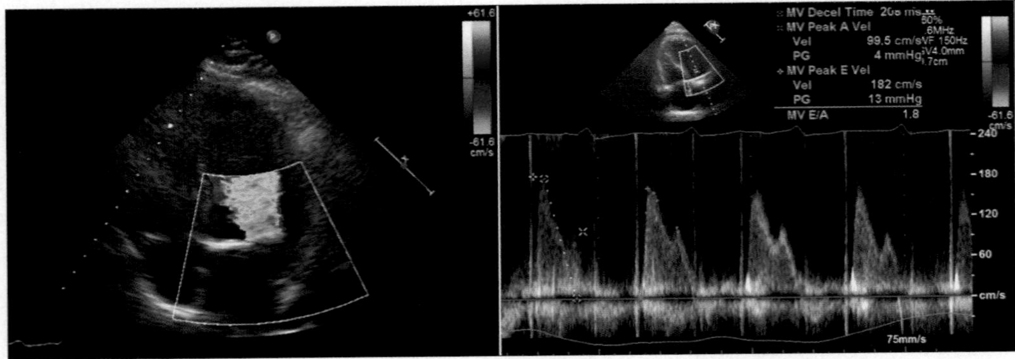

Figure 146A.7 A large, broad jet of pulmonic insufficiency is demonstrated by color Doppler flow mapping, and the spectral display demonstrates a steep velocity decay consistent with severe pulmonic insufficiency.

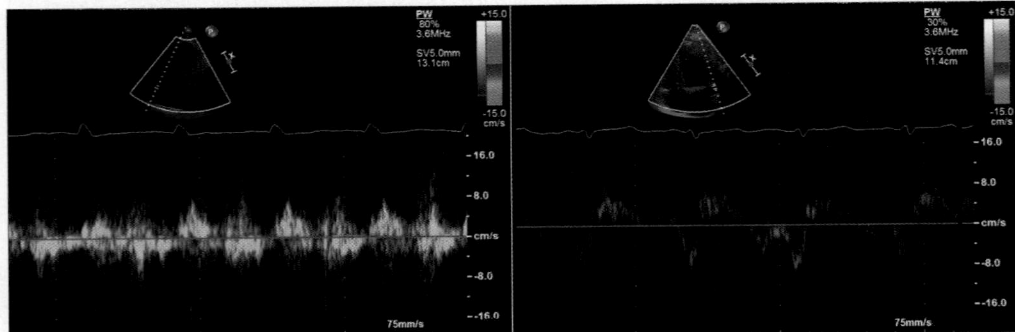

Figure 146A.8 Tissue Doppler sampling of the septal *(left)* and lateral *(right)* mitral annulus demonstrates subnormal early (E′) velocities consistent with diastolic dysfunction.

resulted in the development of large pleural effusions and hindered ventilation. Some ventricular interdependence signs were present, which were worrying for the presence of residual constrictive physiology worsened by right heart failure (Fig. 146A.13). Over 3 weeks, higher cardiac output and renal function returned. Six weeks later, the patient was discharged from the ICU. Nine weeks later, she was discharged to a rehabilitation facility.

Sixteen weeks later, the patient was discharged home with New York Heart Association class III dyspnea and no angina.

DISCUSSION

This case was complex and frustrating because the immediate postoperative hemodynamic state, with the aortic stenosis alleviated, was worse than the preoperative state with aortic stenosis. Also, consultation was challenging because the preoperative data were internally inconsistent, and most of them were unavailable for direct review. The preoperative assessment, despite the extent of it, was incomplete with regard to aortic valve disease severity and possible radiation-induced myopathy.

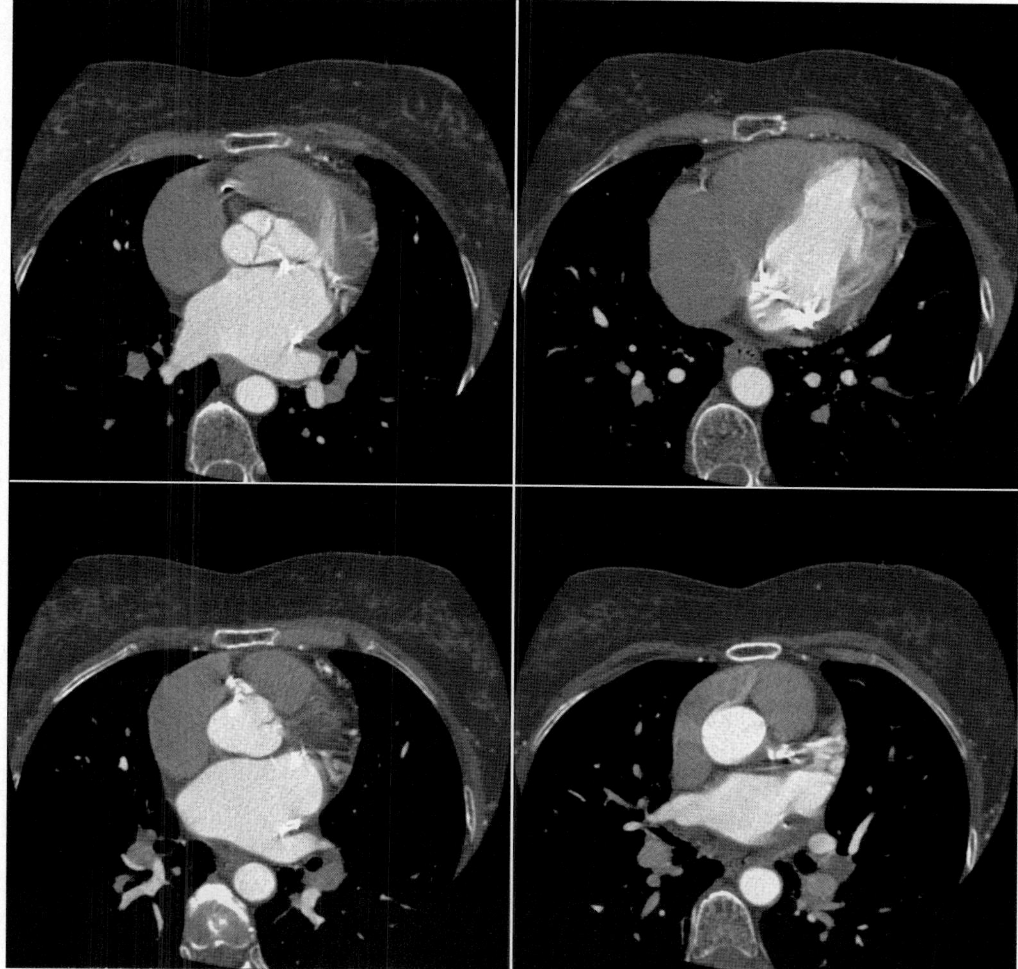

Figure 146A.9 Electrocardiograph (ECG) gated cardiac computed tomography (CT) scanning demonstrates mild thickening of the aortic valve and some calcification. The mitral valve is severely calcified. The proximal right coronary artery and left coronary arteries are severely calcified.

Numerous pathophysiologies likely were contributing to the low output state that dominated the postoperative period.

Postoperatively, right heart failure was prominent. Inadequate myocardial protection may have contributed to postoperative right ventricular dysfunction. However, in this case, the usual procedures had been observed, and the bypass and pump run times were less than average for coronary bypass, aortic valve replacement, and mitral valve repair. There was a prominent requirement for high right-sided heart filling pressures to maintain cardiac output, and that fact, as well as the absence of significant pulmonary hypertension postoperatively, augured that intrinsic right heart dysfunction was primary. The intolerance to cardioplegia and the early and dominant right-sided heart failure were consistent with radiation-induced myopathic dysfunction.

Frustratingly, little preoperative characterization of right-sided heart function or pathology had been done. The right-sided heart catheterization provided the only documentation of right-sided heart dysfunction (moderately elevated right atrial and right ventricular diastolic pressures). The usefulness of intraoperative TEE to comprehensively review cardiac findings that were not fully evaluated preoperatively is evident in this case.

The postoperative course was complicated by heart failure caused by radiation-induced myopathy. A preoperative endomyocardial biopsy in pursuit of the cause of the systolic dysfunction or an intraoperative biopsy would have clarified the nature of the heart failure.

The fibrocalcific changes in the aortic valve were consistent with radiation damage.[1] The underlying valve morphology was trileaflet, not bicuspid. Other pathologies that result in fibrotic degeneration of the aortic valve, such as rheumatic disease, seemed improbable because the mitral valve leaflets were not thickened along the commissures, nor were the chordae thickened. The peculiar and exuberant calcification arising off the mitral valve was unusual for any common pathology. The severity of the aortic stenosis was unclear. A low output state clearly existed, and the aortic valve area calculations were more severe than were the gradient determinations. Both Gorlin and continuity equations are less accurate at low flow states, where notably, the Gorlin equation "constant" is not constant.

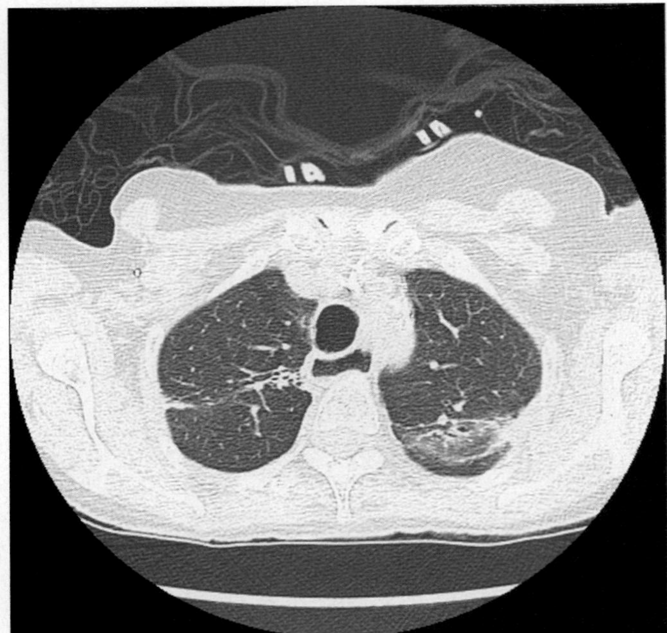

Figure 146A.10 Chest computed tomography (CT) scan: lung windows. Apical scarring of the lung parenchyma is especially pronounced on the left side.

Reliance on the valve area calculation appeared to have influenced the perception of aortic valve severity more than gradient determination.

The thickening of the pericardium both anteriorly and especially posteriorly, where it also was severely adherent to the heart, likely also was due to widespread radiation damage throughout the heart structures. A constrictive component to the hemodynamics is probable, given the posterior pericardial thickening and fusion to the posterior chambers.

The proximal pattern of the coronary disease also is consistent with radiation damage.[2] The discordance of the findings of the initial and the repeat angiograms can be explained by either of two circumstances: (1) the catheter on the first angiogram was inserted too deeply into the left main stem to recognize a short and moderate ostial stenosis; or (2) catheter-induced damage to the left main stem by the first angiogram resulted in a stenosis that was detected on the second angiogram.

Specific radiation damage to the heart may have predominated, but ultimately, global damage was likely to have occurred.[3] Cardiac surgery is fraught with risk when one aspect of the cardiac anatomy or physiology compromised by previous radiation repair prompts surgical repair, as damage of that degree to one component of cardiac anatomy is inevitably accompanied by damage to other cardiac structures and by some degree of dysfunction.

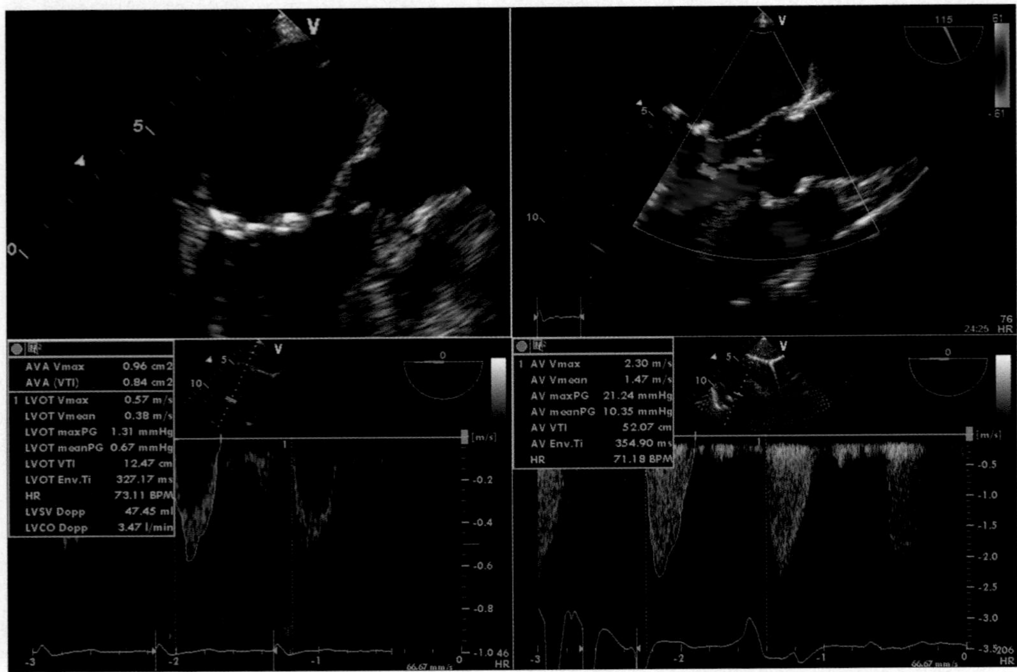

Figure 146A.11 Intraoperative transesophageal echocardiographic (TEE) images of the aortic valve. The valve is thickened but not as much as the mitral valve, and it also is much less calcified. Doppler sampling reveals low subvalvular flow velocity (VTI 13 cm) and a mean gradient of only 11 mm Hg.

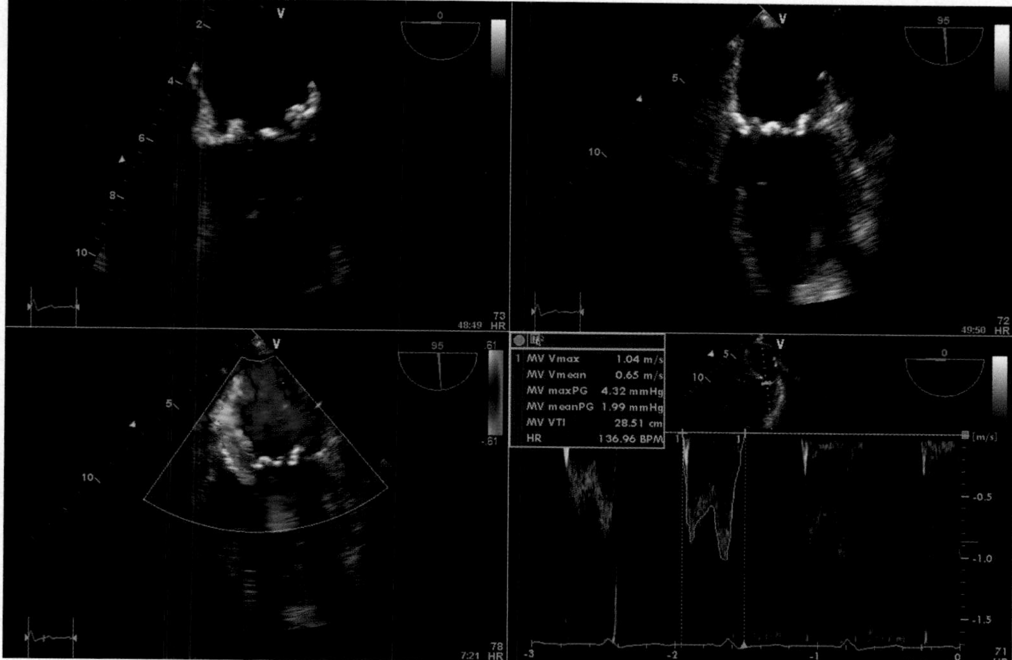

Figure 146A.12 Intraoperative transesophageal echocardiographic (TEE) images of the mitral valve. Severe and exuberant mitral valve calcification of the valve leaflets and annulus is present, as is mild to moderate mitral insufficiency. Despite the calcification and thickening of the mitral valve, there is no significant gradient.

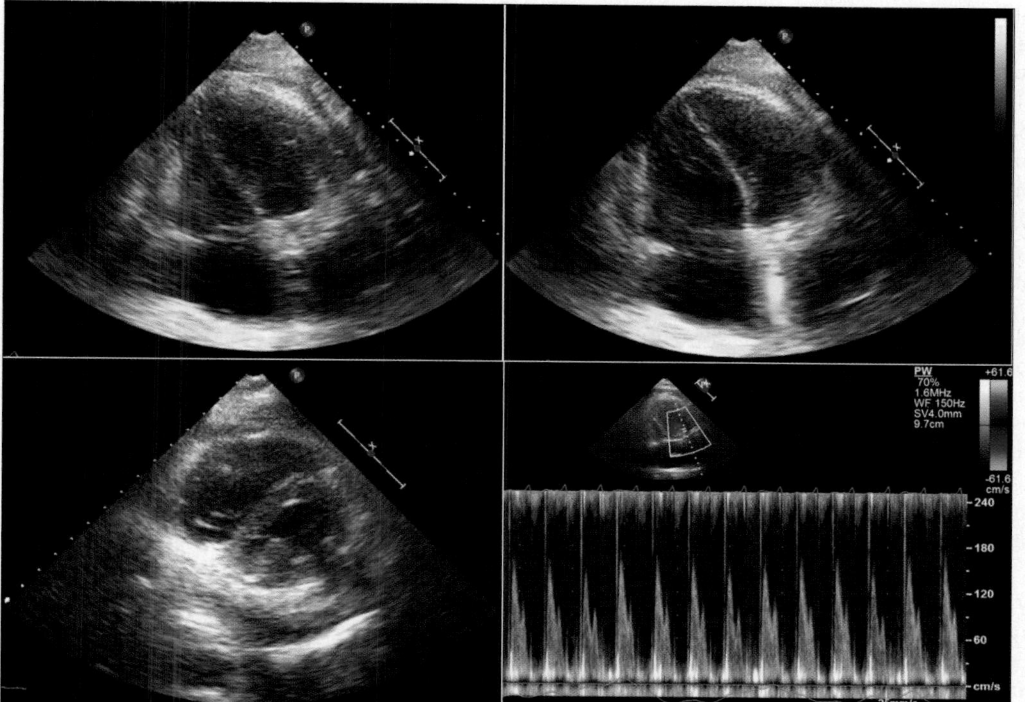

Figure 146A.13 Postoperative transthoracic images. *Upper images:* Apical four-chamber views at expiration *(left upper image)* and at inspiration *(right upper image)*. With inspiration a prominent septal shift to the left side occurs, a finding consistent with constrictive compressive physiology and also with acute right-sided heart failure. *Left lower image:* Parasternal short-axis image showing the leftward septal shift in inspiration. *Right lower images:* Mitral inflow does not show a greater than 25% fall in early inflow velocity as is usually seen with constriction.

b. Bariatric/Gastric Bypass

Stuart J. Hutchison

A 46-year-old man was scheduled to undergo laparoscopic gastric bypass for weight loss (bariatric) surgery. He weighed 565 pounds, and his body mass index (BMI) was 63 kg/m^2. His preoperative evaluation was negative for symptoms other than increased dyspnea over the preceding several months. He had no orthopnea or paroxysmal nocturnal dyspnea (PND). His ankles had been swollen for years, ever since his weight exceeded 350 pounds. He was physically almost completely inactive and could not recall not being short of breath on exertion. He had no history of chest pains. He was a lifelong nonsmoker. He had been recognized as hypertensive for 8 years and was poorly compliant with his antihypertensive medications. The glycosylated hemoglobin A_{1c} was 9%. His family history was unknown to him. He lived alone. Simply by virtue of his weight, he was assumed to have sleep apnea, but he had not participated in investigations or treatments.

Preoperatively, his blood pressure was 145/90 mm Hg, and his heart rate was 90 beats per minutes. The fit of the blood pressure cuff on his large arm was uncertain, and therefore so was the accuracy of the recording. The respiratory rate was 15 per minute at rest but rose to 30 per minute with slight exertion. The heart sounds were distant. No gallops or murmurs were audible. The apex was too distant to palpate. No adventitious breathing sounds were noted. Edema of the forelegs was seen, with chronic venous stasis dermatitis.

Preoperative laboratory investigations were limited to a chest radiograph, which was interpreted as unremarkable for his body size, and a 12-lead electrocardiogram (ECG) that also was unremarkable, with no criteria of left ventricular hypertrophy (LVH) or ST deviations.

Surgery was performed uneventfully, and the patient was under general anesthesia for 2 hours. Recovery was slower than expected. The early recovery period was characterized by significant sleep apneas and airway obstruction and the need for higher oxygen supplementation than expected. The patient spent 2 days in the intensive care unit (ICU) and another 14 days in the hospital before discharge.

Over the next 6 months, the patient lost weight at an average rate of 12 to 15 pounds a month. His dyspnea, however, worsened despite the weight loss of more than 100 pounds. By 8 months after surgery, then weighing 470 pounds, he was markedly dyspneic at rest and clearly experienced arterial desaturation with slight exertion or when lying supine. He complained of a chronic but variable and at times episodic chest pressure. He was admitted to the hospital. Other than tachypnea and respiratory distress, the physical examination findings were similar to those at the time of surgery. He was afebrile. The 12-lead ECG was unchanged and did not vary with chest pain episodes. The chest radiograph was unchanged (Fig. 146B.1).

The cause of the respiratory distress and chest pains was unclear. The means to investigate were limited by the patient's marginal respiratory state. Left-sided heart failure was considered, given the possible interstitial prominence on the chest radiograph, as was pulmonary embolism. The image quality of bedside echocardiography was poor. Left ventricular systolic function was grossly normal; poor endocardial definition precluded regional wall motion assessment. No left-sided valvular lesions were seen. Left ventricular inflow and tissue Doppler findings were consistent with the impaired relaxation pattern of diastolic dysfunction. The E/E′ ratio was 10, neither definitive for a normal pulmonary venous pressure nor indicative of a significantly elevated one. The right side of the heart was not obviously dilated, but the cavity was not well defined. Tricuspid insufficiency was inadequate to establish the right ventricular systolic pressure (RVSP). There was 3 cm of lucency around the cardiac chambers, which initially was thought to be pericardial fluid; however, the coarse specular pattern was believed to be more consistent with copious epicardial and pericardial fat. Computed tomography (CT) scanning was not feasible, given the orthopnea, and transesophageal echocardiography (TEE) was not feasible at the time, given the respiratory distress. D-dimers were elevated at 550 mg/L. Venous Duplex scanning was negative for proximal deep venous thrombosis. The serum brain natriuretic peptide (BNP) was mildly elevated at 247 pg/mL. Troponin I was normal. The serum albumin level was low at 13 g/L, and ketones were elevated, consistent with caloric deprivation.

Empiric diuresis was performed to the point of volume contraction, and a 20% rise in serum creatinine incurred, with a mild and transient improvement in respiratory effort. However, during the next 5 days, the patient's condition progressively worsened, necessitating mechanical ventilation. Intubation was notable for considerable difficulty maintaining saturation with manually "bagging" and for moments of severe desaturation. Hemodynamically, the patient remained stable throughout. Once he was intubated, TEE was performed, which demonstrated LVH with normal or borderline reduced systolic function and no flow disturbances. Right ventricular hypertrophy (RVH) was seen, but right-sided heart function was normal. Again, no tricuspid insufficiency or Doppler evidence of a patent foramen ovale (PFO) or right-to-left shunting was detected. No thrombus was seen with TEE at the main pulmonary artery bifurcation, in the proximal left main pulmonary artery, or in the right main pulmonary artery.

CT scanning of the chest was obtained with difficulty. The image quality was very suboptimal. Pulmonary venous size was equivocally increased. The appearance of the heart was normal. No evidence of pulmonary embolism was seen in the central or lobar arteries. A possible thrombus may have been present in the right lower lobe segmental arteries. The image quality was not adequate to evaluate the subsegmental pulmonary arteries. The right pleural effusion was seen, and the patient was started on intravenous heparin.

Ventilation was prolonged, and with no improvement apparent after 2 weeks, other causes of respiratory failure were considered. The elevated BNP and equivocal chest radiographic findings generated the concern of unrecognized left-sided heart failure. To exclude this, a pulmonary artery

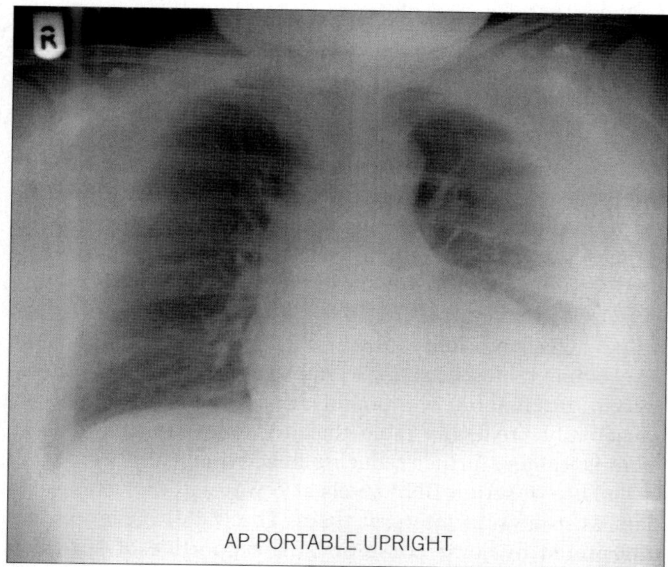

Figure 146B.1 Anteroposterior chest radiograph. The cardiopericardial silhouette is unremarkable. The overlying fat accentuates lung and vascular markings and also blurs them.

catheter was inserted via the right internal jugular vein. Access was difficult (through 14 cm of soft tissue), and the carotid artery was punctured inadvertently. Compression through the soft tissue was difficult, and a significant hematoma developed. A repeat attempt 2 days later was successful. On 10 mm Hg of positive end-expiratory pressure (PEEP), the right atrial pressure was 10 mm Hg, the pulmonary artery pressures were 78/20 mm Hg, the pulmonary capillary wedge pressure was 16 mm Hg, and the cardiac index was 2.0 L/min/m^2. Left-sided heart failure finally was excluded. The mild elevation of the pulmonary capillary wedge pressure was attributed to long-standing LVH. The pulmonary hypertension was attributed to the thromboembolic disease process and presumed sleep apnea and hypoventilation.

An attempt to aspirate pleural fluid yielded fluid of a transudative quality, normal glucose, and negative stains, cultures, and cytology. However, the aspiration resulted in a pneumothorax that required a chest tube because of ongoing air leakage. Consideration of a lung biopsy was deferred until the respiratory status stabilized. The patient developed a fever and gram-positive sepsis.

With the sepsis treated and a further 3 weeks in the ICU, the patient finally improved enough to be extubated. Ward recovery also was slow, but eventually the patient was discharged.

The cause of the respiratory failure was held to be pulmonary thromboembolic disease, some of which may have been chronic and started postoperatively.

DISCUSSION

This case was notable for the frustrations of imprecise cardiac assessment in a morbidly obese individual and the pursuit of a diagnosis of left-sided heart failure that was difficult, procedurally complicated, and ultimately fruitless. The development of chest pains concurrent with the worsening dyspnea established a pretest probability of cardiac (coronary) disease that subsequently was disproved.

Most deaths after bariatric weight loss surgery are reported to be due to technical complications, such as anastomotic leaks, abscesses, sepsis, hemorrhage, and bowel obstruction.[1,2] Death as a result of pulmonary embolism has been repeatedly described with bariatric surgery.[1,2] Fatal thromboembolism is described despite prophylaxis for deep venous thrombosis. One series described an 80% incidence of microscopic evidence for pulmonary embolism, clearly beneath the resolution of imaging in normal-weight patients, let alone in those who are morbidly obese. One pathology series described half of deaths as cardiac (arrhythmia).[1] The younger age of patients undergoing bariatric surgery is a significant reason for the low cardiac event rate. In an autopsy series of 10 patients who died after bariatric gastric bypass surgery, the average age was 40 years (range, 30 to 49 years), and the mean BMI was 60 kg/m^2. In this series, microscopic evidence of coronary disease was seen in 60% of cases, LVH in 80%, and RVH in 30%.[1] If or when larger numbers of older patients begin to undergo bariatric surgery, cardiac events likely will become more common.

The physical examination was low yield and consistently without confidence about the presence or absence of gallops, softer murmurs, or abnormal heart sounds. No physical diagnosis findings consistent with the moderate to severe pulmonary hypertension were detected. Jugular venous pressure and contour assessments were clinically impossible, and until pulmonary artery catheterization was performed, volume status could only be inferred by the creatinine response to diuresis.

The heart of an individual who is morbidly obese will be hypertrophic. LVH results as adaptation to hypertension associated with the obesity and the increase in blood volume. RVH develops in response to sleep apnea and pulmonary hypertension.[3] Surface ECGs in morbidly obese patients reveal a higher incidence of low QRS voltage, leftward shift of the P, QRS, and T axes, and LVH criteria.[4]

Although RVH is common, as is leg swelling, right-sided heart failure/cor pulmonale is not. Leg swelling usually is due to venous insufficiency, inactivity, and the effect of large groin fat folds on the femoral veins. Significant right-sided heart dysfunction or failure would render laparoscopic surgery, the preferred means to achieve gastric bypass, hemodynamically riskier, because the right side of the heart would tend to be deprived of preload during abdominal insufflation. Compared with nonobese patients undergoing laparoscopy, morbidly obese patients have significantly greater increases in systemic blood pressure during pneumoperitoneum.[5] In patients undergoing open gastric bypass procedures, normally, no change occurs in right ventricular systolic function when the abdomen is opened.[3] Bedside and objective evaluation of the right side of the heart in morbidly obese individuals is at least as difficult as evaluation of the left side of the heart.

Chest radiography of patients with morbid obesity is invariably of lesser quality than usual. Epicardial fat and pericardial fat layers increase the dimensions of the heart. The superimposition of attenuation from soft tissue of the chest wall onto that of the lung tissues generates blended findings. Some enhancement of interstitial markings is common. In this case, opinion initially was divided as to whether the finding was significant.

Transthoracic echocardiographic image quality suffered from the supine position of the patient and the unusually distant location of the heart with respect to the chest wall. Normally, parasternal and apical windows afford 2 to 3 cm of subcutaneous, intercostal, pericardial, and epicardial soft tissue between the transducer and the heart. In this case, more than 12 cm of soft tissue was interposed between the transducer and the transthoracic windows, and more than 30 cm between the transducer and the subcostal window. Endocardial definition was extremely poor, beneath clinical confidence. Doppler interrogation was better, because it often is despite poor two-dimensional images, but it was inconclusive. Echocardiographic Doppler findings were variably interpreted toward the consideration of left-sided heart failure. The abnormal left ventricular inflow pattern was viewed by most consultants as an early sign of diastolic dysfunction, inevitable given the history of hypertension and the finding of LVH on that basis, and unlikely to be associated with diastolic heart failure. Others interpreted it as significantly pathologic and supportive of left-sided heart failure. The use of the E/E′ ratio to ascertain left ventricular filling pressures was undertaken with the knowledge of its lack of validation in the clinical context of morbid obesity. However, it eventually proved correct in excluding left-sided heart failure.

Available bedside noninvasive testing was inconclusive in establishing or refuting a diagnosis of heart failure. More sophisticated imaging testing was more difficult to arrange and obtain.

Angiography databases demonstrate that ischemic testing is less sensitive (75%) and specific (40%) in morbidly obese patients. In such series, the obese patients have a lower prevalence of coronary artery disease than nonobese patients and their referral for angiography is generated by the higher prevalence of false-positive noninvasive tests. Use of radial access is more common in morbidly obese patients.[6] Dobutamine stress-TEE has been performed successfully in a small series of patients to evaluate coronary risk in bariatric patients.[7]

CT scanning also was of less adequate image quality than usual because of noise generated by the body size. The ability to exclude pulmonary embolism is imperfect, even with 64-slice scanners and normal body habitus. The negative predictive value of CT–pulmonary angiography in usual patient populations is approximately 90% in published series. The value in the morbidly obese is unknown but surely less. The sliding table of the CT scanner has a maximum bearable weight, often about 650 pounds. Excess weight is less likely to actually break the table than to deflect the table away from isocenter, further reducing image quality.

The use of serum BNP levels also was without established data as to how to interpret them. The (mild) elevation was interpreted by some consultants as supportive of left-sided heart failure; others did not view the elevation as sufficient to be commensurate with the clinical picture. The elevated right-sided heart diastolic pressures were the likely etiology.

The optimal prophylactic and therapeutic coagulation regimen for morbidly obese patients has not been established and essentially borrows from algorithms used far more commonly in nonobese individuals. Systemic thrombolytic therapy (intravenous urokinase) has been used successfully to treat massive pulmonary embolism in a morbidly obese patient.[8]

In this case, typical of the tribulations of cardiac assessment of the morbidly obese, noninvasive assessment was not conclusive. Ischemic testing in obese patients typically is confounded by greater false-negative findings and lesser feasibility. Invasive procedures also were difficult and resulted in more complications than usual.

c. Amphetamine Acute Aortic Dissection

Stuart J. Hutchison

A 38-year-old male was transferred from a rural town with a confirmed diagnosis of acute aortic dissection. He was confused and agitated but did not have a specific motor deficit. Six hours earlier, he had developed chest pain and dysarthria, both of which were resolving. Details were reluctantly afforded by a companion. The patient had abused multiple drugs over a 72-hour period: a small amount of cocaine, a large amount of methamphetamine, and (probably) a small amount of morphine, as well as 3 L of whiskey. After the last ingestion of methamphetamine, he developed chest pain of an intense, searing, and sharp quality, as best he could recall and express.

Upon presentation to a rural community hospital, he was treated with naloxone, to no effect, and referred for computed tomography (CT) scanning. The description of his verbal state varied from dysarthric to inebriated/slurred. CT scanning identified dissection of the aortic arch, the basis of his referral.

Upon transfer, his blood pressure was 165/85 mm Hg and the heart rate was 110 beats per minute. No pulse deficits, pulsus paradoxus, murmur of aortic insufficiency, venous distention, or pericardial rub was seen. He was mildly confused but could follow commands. His speech was slurred but not dysarthric.

Toxicology was positive for numerous agents, principally methamphetamine but also morphine, codeine, cocaine, and a high level of alcohol (3.1 g/L).

Review of the CT scan confirmed the presence of an aortic dissection involving the aortic arch, without complications (Fig. 146C.1). Transthoracic echocardiography confirmed the lack of an intimal flap in the proximal ascending aorta, aortic valve insufficiency, and pericardial and pleural effusion.

The patient was managed medically with intravenous labetalol to normalize blood pressure and reduce the heart rate (and dP/dt). The speech difficulty was due only to intoxication. Labetalol was given only for 18 to 24 hours; beyond that, the patient was intolerant of labetalol because of marked hypotension and bradycardia. His usual blood

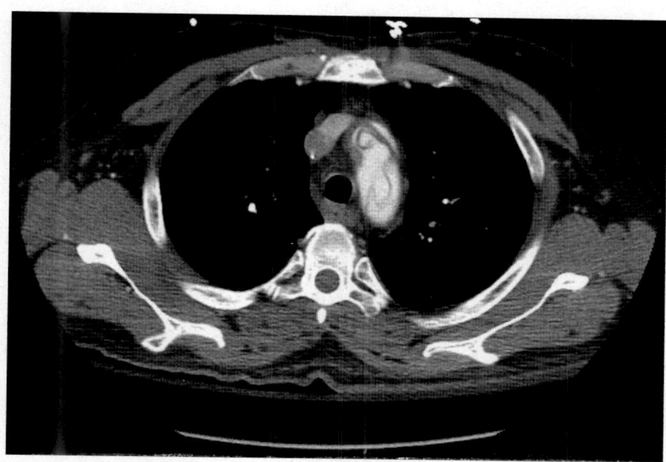

Figure 146C.1 Contrast-enhanced computed tomography (CT) scan demonstrating an intimal flap within the aorta only at the arch level. The initially described dysarthria may have been produced by transient malperfusion of the left common carotid artery.

pressure was low normal, and his usual resting heart rate was bradycardia. He was discharged on a low dose of a beta blocker. Medication compliance was improbable. He did not maintain follow-up.

DISCUSSION

Acute aortic dissection in younger individual (younger than 40 years of age) is due to heritable disorders such as Marfan's syndrome, bicuspid aortic valve–associated aortopathy, and other diverse causes, including pregnancy, aortic instrumentation, surgery, and trauma. Sympathomimetic substance abuse also may result in aortic dissection or aortic rupture, or both, typically in younger and middle-aged patients. The profile of drugs of abuse associated with acute aortic dissection varies according to local "recreational" drug use patterns and availability.

Cocaine is second only to cannabis in illegal recreational drug abuse. It is produced in different salt and base forms, allowing abuse by several means (i.e., injection, inhalation, snorting, and ingestion). Crack cocaine, named after the sound that occurs when the water-based form splits when heated, is held to be the most hemodynamically potent and variable form of cocaine. Several aortic complications with cocaine abuse have been reported, including severe vasoconstriction, dissection and redissection, intramural hematoma, rupture, malperfusion, and thrombosis.[1-5] Cocaine-related aortic dissection, unlike usual acute aortic dissection, appears more frequently to involve the descending aorta. Its true incidence is unknown, and although a plausible (by virtue of associated hypertension) distinct entity, it is poorly characterized and understood.[6,7]

Abuse of methamphetamine (methylamphetamine or desoxyephedrine), a powerful psychostimulant and sympathomimetic vasoconstrictor, has increased steadily across urban and rural North America. Although worldwide cocaine production and abuse exceeds that of methamphetamine severalfold, local abuse of methamphetamine, including in rural North America, may equal or exceed that of cocaine. Methamphetamine also may be abused concurrently with cocaine and even may be used to "cut" cocaine. The methylization ("meth") of amphetamine increases lipid solubility and reduces monoamine oxidase (MAO) breakdown. Methamphetamine reverses the direction of noradrenaline, dopamine, and serotonin transporters, increasing stimulation of postsynaptic receptors. Withdrawal is more intense than with cocaine, and addiction is intense, As with cocaine, reported complications with the abuse of methamphetamine include severe hypertension and aortic dissection.[8] In an autopsy series of 85 cases of aortic dissection, 35 were positive for drugs of abuse, of which seven were positive for methamphetamine.[9]

Many issues confound the association and understanding of aortic dissection in substance abusers, including paucity of data, unreliable and under-reporting, polydrug and substance abuse, and presumption of mechanism. This patient tested positive both for methamphetamine and for cocaine, and by history had abused far more methamphetamine over the preceding 3 years.

Index

Note: Page numbers followed by *f* indicate figures; page numbers followed by *t* indicate tables.

A

B

C

D

E

G

H

I

M

N

Q

R

T

U

V

W

X

Y

Z